MICHIGAN STATE UNIVERSITY
LIBRARY
JUL 31 2025
WITHDRAWN

Veterinary Pharmacology and Therapeutics

8th Edition

8th Edition

Veterinary Pharmacology and Therapeutics

EDITED BY H. RICHARD ADAMS

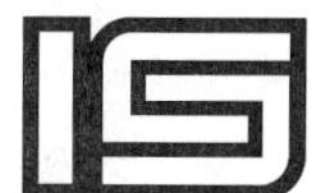

IOWA STATE UNIVERSITY PRESS / AMES

H. RICHARD ADAMS has specialized in veterinary pharmacology and pathophysiology, with emphasis in cardiovascular and autonomic drugs and research in circulatory shock. He has taught pharmacology to veterinary medical students and medical students for 30 years. He was on the faculty in the Department of Pharmacology at the University of Pittsburgh and in the Department of Pharmacology of Southwestern Medical School at the University of Texas Health Science Center at Dallas. He served as Professor in the Department of Pharmacology in the School of Medicine, Professor and Chairman of the Department of Veterinary Biomedical Sciences, and Dean of the College of Veterinary Medicine at the University of Missouri, Columbia. He holds Professor Emeritus and Dean Emeritus titles from the University of Missouri and is an Honorary Diplomate of the American College of Veterinary Emergency and Critical Care. Dr. Adams currently is Dean of the College of Veterinary Medicine at Texas A&M University, College Station. He is a member of the American Academy of Veterinary Pharmacology and Therapeutics, the American Society of Pharmacology and Experimental Therapeutics, the American Physiological Society, and the Shock Society (serving as its 1994–1995 president). He received B.S. and D.V.M. degrees from Texas A&M University and a Ph.D. degree in pharmacology from the University of Pittsburgh.

© 1954, 1957, 1965, 1977, 1982, 1988, 1995, 2001 Iowa State University Press, Ames, Iowa 50014-8300
All rights reserved

Copyright is not claimed for Chapter 56, which is in the public domain.

Portions of Chapter 17, "Drugs Affecting Animal Behavior," are from Dawn Merton Boothe, *Small Animal Clinical Pharmacology and Therapeutics,* Philadelphia: WB Saunders Company; copyright © 2000 Mosby, Inc., a Harcourt Health Series Company. All rights reserved.

Portions of Chapters 16, 22, 29, 51, and 54 also appear in Dawn Merton Boothe, *Small Animal Clinical Pharmacology and Therapeutics,* Philadelphia: WB Saunders Company, 2000.

Authorization to photocopy items for internal or personal use, or the internal or personal use of specific clients, is granted by Iowa State University Press, provided that the base fee of $.10 per copy is paid directly to the Copyright Clearance Center, 222 Rosewood Drive, Danvers, MA 01923. For those organizations that have been granted a photocopy license by CCC, a separate system of payments has been arranged. The fee code for users of the Transactional Reporting Service is 0-8138-1743-9/2001 $.10.

∞ Printed on acid-free paper in the United States of America

First, second, and third editions 1954, 1957, and 1965 edited by L. Meyer Jones; fourth edition 1977 edited by L. Meyer Jones, Nicholas H. Booth, and Leslie E. McDonald; fifth and sixth editions 1982 and 1988 edited by Nicholas H. Booth and Leslie E. McDonald; seventh edition 1995 edited by H. Richard Adams. Copyright © Iowa State University Press.

Eighth edition, 2001

Iowa State University Press
2121 South State Avenue, Ames, Iowa 50014-8300

Orders: 1-800-862-6657
Office: 1-515-292-0140
Fax: 1-515-292-3348
Web site: www.isupress.com

Library of Congress Cataloging-in-Publication Data

Veterinary pharmacology and therapeutics—8th ed. / edited by H. Richard Adams
p. cm.
Includes bibliographical references and index.
ISBN 0-8138-1743-9 (alk. paper)
I. Veterinary pharmacology. I. Adams, H. Richard.

SF915.V49 2001
636.089′57—dc21 00-053953

Last digit is the print number: 9 8 7 6 5 4 3 2 1

05 98956

CONTENTS

Contributors ... vii
Preface ... ix

Section 1. Principles of Pharmacology ... 3

1. Veterinary Pharmacology: An Introduction to the Discipline *Scott Anthony Brown and Lloyd E. Davis* ... 3
2. Pharmacodynamics: Mechanisms of Drug Action *Mark J. Novotny* ... 9
3. Pharmacokinetics: Disposition and Fate of Drugs in the Body *Scott Anthony Brown* 15
4. Clinical Pharmacology: Principles of Therapeutics *Mark J. Novotny* ... 57

Section 2. Drugs Acting on the Autonomic and Somatic Nervous Systems ... 69

5. Introduction to Neurohumoral Transmission and the Autonomic Nervous System *H. Richard Adams* ... 69
6. Adrenergic Agonists and Antagonists *H. Richard Adams* ... 91
7. Cholinergic Pharmacology: Autonomic Drugs *H. Richard Adams* ... 117
8. Neuromuscular Blocking Agents *H. Richard Adams* ... 137

Section 3. Drugs Acting on the Central Nervous System ... 153

9. Introduction to Drugs Acting on the Central Nervous System and Principles of Anesthesiology *Eugene P. Steffey* ... 153
10. Therapeutic Gases: Oxygen, Carbon Dioxide, Water Vapor, and Nitric Oxide *Eugene P. Steffey* ... 172
11. Inhalation Anesthetics *Eugene P. Steffey* ... 184
12. Injectable Anesthetics *Keith R. Branson* ... 213
13. Opioid Agonists and Antagonists *Keith R. Branson and Marjorie E. Gross* ... 268
14. Tranquilizers, α_2-Adrenergic Agonists, and Related Agents *Marjorie E. Gross* ... 299
15. Local Anesthetics *Khursheed R. Mama and Eugene P. Steffey* ... 343
16. Anticonvulsant Drugs and Analeptic Agents *Dawn M. Boothe* ... 360
17. Drugs Affecting Animal Behavior *Dawn M. Boothe* ... 383
18. Euthanizing Agents *Eugene P. Steffey* ... 397

Section 4. Autacoids and Anti-inflammatory Drugs ... 403

19. Histamine, Serotonin, and Their Antagonists *H. Richard Adams* ... 403
20. Peptides: Angiotensin and Kinins *H. Richard Adams* ... 413
21. Prostaglandins, Related Factors, and Cytokines *H. Richard Adams* ... 420
22. The Analgesic, Antipyretic, Anti-inflammatory Drugs *Dawn M. Boothe* ... 433

Section 5. Drugs Acting on the Cardiovascular System ... 453

23. Digitalis and Vasodilator Drugs *H. Richard Adams* ... 453
24. Antiarrhythmic Agents *H. Richard Adams* ... 482

Section 6. Drugs Affecting Renal Function and Fluid-Electrolyte Balance ... 501

25. Principles of Acid-Base Balance: Fluid and Electrolyte Therapy *Deborah T. Kochevar* ... 501
26. Diuretics *Deborah T. Kochevar* ... 534

Section 7. Drugs Acting on Blood and Blood Elements **553**

27. Antianemic Agents *Martin J. Fettman and H. Richard Adams* 553
28. Hemostatic and Anticoagulant Drugs *H. Richard Adams* 571
29. Blood and Blood Components *Dawn M. Boothe* 586

Section 8. Endocrine Pharmacology **593**

30. Hypothalamic and Pituitary Hormones *Duncan C. Ferguson and Margarethe Hoenig* 593
31. Hormones Affecting Reproduction *Frederick N. Thompson* 612
32. Thyroid Hormones and Antithyroid Drugs *Duncan C. Ferguson* 626
33. Glucocorticoids, Mineralocorticoids, and Steroid Synthesis Inhibitors *Duncan C. Ferguson and Margarethe Hoenig* 649
34. Drugs Influencing Glucose Metabolism *Margarethe Hoenig* 672

Section 9. Nutritional Pharmacology **683**

35. Fat-Soluble Vitamins *Martin J. Fettman* 683
36. Water-Soluble Vitamins *Martin J. Fettman* 702
37. Calcium, Phosphorus, and Other Macroelements *Martin J. Fettman* 722
38. Trace Elements and Miscellaneous Nutrients *Martin J. Fettman* 744

Section 10. Chemotherapy of Microbial Diseases **783**

39. Antiseptics and Disinfectants *Mark C. Heit and Jim E. Riviere* 783
40. Sulfonamides *Jerry W. Spoo and Jim E. Riviere* 796
41. Penicillins and Related β-Lactam Antibiotics *Shelly L. Vaden and Jim E. Riviere* 818
42. Tetracycline Antibiotics *Jim E. Riviere and Jerry W. Spoo* 828
43. Aminoglycoside Antibiotics *Jim E. Riviere and Jerry W. Spoo* 841
44. Chloramphenicol and Derivatives, Macrolides, Lincosamides, and Miscellaneous Antimicrobials *Mark G. Papich and Jim E. Riviere* 868
45. Fluoroquinolone Antimicrobial Drugs *Mark G. Papich and Jim E. Riviere* 898
46. Antifungal and Antiviral Drugs *Mark G. Papich, Mark C. Heit, and Jim E. Riviere* 918

Section 11. Chemotherapy of Parasitic Diseases **947**

47. Antinematodal Drugs *Craig R. Reinemeyer and Charles H. Courtney* 947
48. Anticestodal and Antitrematodal Drugs *Craig R. Reinemeyer and Charles H. Courtney* 980
49. Antiprotozoan Drugs *David S. Lindsay and Byron L. Blagburn* 992
50. Ectoparasiticides *Byron L. Blagburn and David S. Lindsay* 1017

Section 12. Specialty Areas of Pharmacology **1041**

51. Drugs Affecting Gastrointestinal Function *Dawn M. Boothe* 1041
52. Chemotherapy of Neoplastic Diseases *Kenita S. Rogers and Gordon L. Coppoc* 1064
53. Dermatopharmacology: Drugs Acting Locally on the Skin *Jim E. Riviere and Jerry W. Spoo* 1084
54. Drugs Affecting the Respiratory System *Dawn M. Boothe* 1105
55. Ophthalmic Pharmacology *Cecil P. Moore* 1120

Section 13. Regulatory Considerations **1149**

56. Legal Control of Veterinary Drugs *Stephen F. Sundlof* 1149
57. Dosage Forms, Drug Prescription Orders, and Veterinary Feed Directives *Scott Anthony Brown* 1157
58. Chemical Residues in Tissues of Food Animals *Jim E. Riviere and Stephen F. Sundlof* 1166

Index 1175

CONTRIBUTORS

H. Richard Adams, DVM, PhD
Dean
Professor of Veterinary Physiology and Pharmacology
College of Veterinary Medicine
Texas A&M University
College Station, TX 77843-4461

Byron L. Blagburn, PhD
Distinguished University Professor
Department of Pathobiology
College of Veterinary Medicine
Auburn University
Auburn, AL 36849-5519

Dawn M. Boothe, DVM, PhD
Associate Professor
Department of Veterinary Physiology and Pharmacology
College of Veterinary Medicine
Texas A&M University
College Station, TX 77843-4466

Keith R. Branson, DVM, MS
Clinical Assistant Professor of Veterinary Anesthesiology
College of Veterinary Medicine
University of Missouri-Columbia
Columbia, MO 65211

Scott Anthony Brown, DVM, PhD
Director, Animal Health Drug Metabolism
Pharmacia & Upjohn Animal Health
7926-190-45
7000 Portage Road
Kalamazoo, MI 49001

Gordon L. Coppoc, DVM, PhD
Professor and Head
Department of Basic Medical Sciences
School of Veterinary Medicine
Purdue University
West Lafayette, IN 47907-1246

Charles H. Courtney, DVM, PhD
Professor and Associate Dean
College of Veterinary Medicine
Box 100125
University of Florida
Gainesville, FL 32611-0633

Lloyd E. Davis, DVM, PhD
Professor, retired
Department of Veterinary Clinical Medicine
College of Veterinary Medicine
University of Illinois
Urbana, IL 61801

Duncan C. Ferguson, VMD, PhD
Professor
Department of Veterinary Physiology and Pharmacology
College of Veterinary Medicine
University of Georgia
Athens, GA 30602

Martin J. Fettman, DVM, PhD
Mark L. Morris Professor of Clinical Nutrition
Department of Pathology
College of Veterinary Medicine and Biomedical Sciences
Colorado State University
Fort Collins, Colorado 80523-1671

Marjorie E. Gross, DVM, MS
Clinical Assistant Professor of Veterinary Anesthesiology
College of Veterinary Medicine
University of Missouri-Columbia
Columbia, MO 65211

Mark C. Heit, DVM, PhD
Associate Director, Animal Health
ICON Clinical Research
212 Church Road
North Wales, PA 19454

Margarethe Hoenig, Dr.med.vet., PhD
Professor of Physiolology and Small Animal Medicine
Department of Physiology and Pharmacology
College of Veterinary Medicine
University of Georgia
Athens, Ga 30602

Deborah T. Kochevar, DVM, PhD
Associate Professor
Department of Veterinary Physiology and Pharmacology
College of Veterinary Medicine
Texas A&M University
College Station, TX 77843-4466

David S. Lindsay, PhD
Associate Professor
Center for Molecular Medicine and Infectious Diseases
Department of Biomedical Sciences and Pathobiology
Virginia-Maryland Regional College of Veterinary Medicine
Virginia Tech University
1410 Prices Fork Road
Blacksburg, Virginia 24061-0342

Khursheed R. Mama, DVM
Assistant Professor of Anesthesiology
Department of Clinical Sciences
College of Veterinary Medicine and Biomedical Sciences
Colorado State University
Fort Collins, CO 80523

Cecil P. Moore, DVM, MS
Professor of Veterinary Ophthalmology
Chairman, Department of Veterinary Medicine and Surgery
Director, Veterinary Medical Teaching Hospital
College of Veterinary Medicine
University of Missouri
Columbia, MO 65211

Mark J. Novotny, DVM, MS, PhD
Principal Clinical Research Investigator
Animal Health Clinical Affairs
Pfizer Global Research and Development
Groton, CT 06340

Mark G. Papich, DVM, MS
Associate Professor of Clinical Pharmacology
Department of Anatomy, Physiological Sciences, and Radiology
College of Veterinary Medicine
North Carolina State University
Raleigh, NC 27606

Craig R. Reinemeyer, DVM, PhD
President, East Tennessee Clinical Research, Inc.
4315 Papermill Drive
Knoxville, TN 37909
Adjunct Associate Professor
Department of Comparative Medicine
College of Veterinary Medicine
University of Tennessee
Knoxville, TN 37901-1071

Jim E. Riviere, DVM, PhD
Burroughs Wellcome Fund Distinguished Professor
Director, Center for Cutaneous Toxicology and Residue Pharmacology
College of Veterinary Medicine
North Carolina State University
Raleigh, N.C. 27606

Kenita S. Rogers, DVM, MS
Associate Professor
Department of Small Animal Medicine and Surgery
Staff Oncologist and Chief of Medicine
College of Veterinary Medicine
Texas A&M University
College Station, TX 77843-4474

Jerry W. Spoo, DVM
Research Toxicologist
Center for Life Sciences and Toxicology
Manager, Toxicology and Health Assessment Program
Research Triangle Institute
Research Triangle Park, NC 27709-2194

Eugene P. Steffey, VMD, PhD
Professor
Department of Surgical and Radiological Sciences
School of Veterinary Medicine
University of California
Davis, CA 95616

Stephen F. Sundlof, DVM, PhD
Director, Center for Veterinary Medicine
U.S. Food and Drug Administration
Rockville, MD 20855

Frederick N. Thompson, DVM, PhD
Professor
Department of Veterinary Physiology and Pharmacology
College of Veterinary Medicine
University of Georgia
Athens, GA 30602

Shelly L. Vaden, DVM, PhD
Associate Professor
Department of Clinical Sciences
College of Veterinary Medicine
North Carolina State University
Raleigh, NC 27606

PREFACE

Welcome to the 21st century and the eighth edition of *Veterinary Pharmacology and Therapeutics*. The first edition of this textbook was authored almost 50 years ago by a pioneer in veterinary pharmacology, Dr. L. Meyer Jones. He dedicated the first edition primarily to professional students learning pharmacology as part of their quest to become doctors of veterinary medicine. Now, almost one-half century and seven revisions later, the eighth edition of *Veterinary Pharmacology and Therapeutics* is likewise dedicated to veterinary medical students enrolled in professional colleges and schools of veterinary medicine.

The authors and editor of this text have compiled in one book a comprehensive resource for students to learn basic and applied principles of veterinary pharmacology and therapeutics. Although this textbook is directed to the professional veterinary student, expanded coverage of pharmacology has broadened its audience to also include graduate students in the biomedical sciences, residents and interns in medicine and surgery, laboratory animal specialists, and research investigators who utilize animals, to name just a few. Furthermore, because practicing veterinarians who already have earned their DVM or VMD are lifetime students of veterinary medicine, this text is also intended as a desktop reference for veterinary practitioners to review details about drugs, drug mechanisms, and their clinical applications. The authors and editor sincerely seek critical feedback from students, practitioners, academic colleagues, and others as to whether the book is meeting its goals and how future editions can be improved.

Veterinary pharmacology has changed dramatically in many complex ways since the first edition of this textbook was published. This evolving complexity is reflected in the changing faces of the different editions of this book. A single veterinary pharmacologist, Dr. Jones, was able to author the entire textbook in excellent fashion by himself in 1954. By the third edition in 1965, several more contributors had joined Dr. Jones, and by the seventh edition in 1995, more than two dozen authors were necessary to adequately cover the breadth of veterinary pharmacology necessary for the "fountainhead" textbook in this field. Pharmacology and its sister disciplines, veterinary pharmacology and veterinary clinical pharmacology, have simply become too complex to be adequately covered by only a few authors. We are fortunate that the eighth edition includes chapters authored by 27 contemporary pharmacologists, each one a recognized and well-published expert in some aspect of veterinary pharmacology and veterinary clinical pharmacology.

The 1990s witnessed an explosion of new drugs and increased understanding of the cellular and molecular mechanisms responsible for the pharmacodynamic actions of both new and older pharmacologic agents. However, the full clinical relevance of such exciting discoveries is adequately understood only in a few cases. This textbook focuses on those aspects of pharmacology that have clinical applications in veterinary medicine and surgery. Attempts were not made to address every available drug or to continue to discuss older drugs that are infrequently used. Rather, the authors focused on basic mechanisms of representative drugs from the most important classes of therapeutic agents. An understanding of basic drug mechanisms and their pharmacotherapeutic applications in the presence of disease provides the basis for problem solving in clinical medicine. We believe this approach provides the most effective way to learn pharmacology and therapeutics, rather than rote memorization of pyramiding facts.

This edition includes considerable revision of existing materials, again reflecting the changing contents of veterinary pharmacology. A new chapter, "Drugs Affecting Animal Behavior," was added to reflect the expanding importance of animal behavior and its therapeutic modulation. Continuing its success from the seventh edition, a section on specialty areas of pharmacology was included to cover those important aspects of pharmacology that overlap multiple facets of pharmacotherapeutics which do not readily fit into single traditional drug groups.

As the editor of this textbook, I have the pleasure of expressing appreciation to the many people who made the eighth edition of *Veterinary Pharmacology and Therapeutics* a reality. Sherry Adams provided special contributions as my staff assistant, and Dr. Gheorghe Constantinescu of the University of Missouri College of Veterinary Medicine provided several original illustrations. We are all indebted to Dr. L. Meyer Jones for his pioneering contributions as a veterinary pharmacologist and educator and for establishing this textbook. Special acknowledgment also goes to former editors Dr. Nicholas H. Booth and Dr. Leslie E. McDonald for leading this textbook through earlier revisions necessary for its transition into the modern era of veterinary pharmacology. Special recognition and appreciation also are extended to Dr. Lloyd Davis, a retired former author and major contributor to veterinary pharmacology for many decades. Dr. Davis helped secure disciplinary stature for veterinary pharmacology and was central to formation of the American Academy of Veterinary Pharmacology and Therapeutics and the American College of Clinical Veterinary Pharmacology.

It is especially important to acknowledge and thank all the authors: the authors of previous editions, who composed the foundation upon which we now stand, and the new authors for assuming the responsibility to prepare new chapters and to update previous ones. Our common goal is to help carry forth the tradition of excellence set by previous editions of *Veterinary Pharmacology and Therapeutics* and to provide the seminal resource for veterinary pharmacology and therapeutics that will help the veterinary profession successfully enter the 21st century.

H. Richard Adams

Veterinary Pharmacology and Therapeutics

8th Edition

SECTION 1
Principles of Pharmacology

1 VETERINARY PHARMACOLOGY: AN INTRODUCTION TO THE DISCIPLINE

SCOTT ANTHONY BROWN AND LLOYD E. DAVIS

Scope of Pharmacology
Role of Pharmacology in the Veterinary Medical Curriculum

Throughout recorded history, humans have employed drugs for treating disease as well as for social and religious purposes. Sir William Osler (1849–1919), a prominent medical educator of the latter 19th century, stated, "A desire to take medicine is, perhaps, the great feature which distinguishes people from other animals."

The discovery of drugs was undoubtedly through the process of trial and error as people tried various plant, animal, and mineral substances in their environment as potential sources of food. Through such activity it soon became apparent that ingestion of certain plants would produce diarrhea or vomiting and that chewing the bark of trees would cause constipation. It was then probably recognized that if one were suffering from diarrhea, ingestion of tannins in bark would relieve symptoms. Such accumulated knowledge gave rise to oral traditions within tribes, and a folklore on drugs developed.

Primitive tribal folklore evolved into attempts to organize knowledge of drug substances. The earliest written compilation of drugs is the Chinese herbal formulary *Pen Tsao,* which is attributed to Emperor Shen Nung, who lived in about 2700 BC. Veterinary and human medicine were well developed in Asia Minor during antiquity. Ancient Hindu records mention eating chaulmoogra fruit to treat leprosy. The Code of Hammurabi (about 2200 BC) described penalties for malpractice by practitioners. The oldest record of Egyptian drug codification is the Kahun papyrus, which was written about 2000 BC. It deals with veterinary medicine and uterine disease of women and contains a number of prescriptions. The Ebers papyrus (1550 BC) is a compilation of a number of disease conditions and 829 prescriptions for medicaments employed in Egyptian medicine. Medicine also was highly developed in Sumeria during the millennium preceding the Christian era. Evidence for this is provided by a library of clay tablets assembled by Ashurbanipal (626–568 BC) and discovered at Nineveh during the 19th century.

The codified drug lore of Egypt was transmitted to Greek civilization. Foremost among early Greek physicians was Hippocrates (460–375 BC), a great teacher of medicine. There formed about him a group of physicians known as the Hippocratic school. They were astute diagnosticians and brilliant surgeons who maintained high ethical standards. They had little use for drugs, as they recognized that sick people usually tended to get well regardless of treatment. This concept of the healing power of nature became known as the *Vis medicatrix naturae.* A precept from the Hippocratic school, which still provides an ethical basis for the practice of therapeutics, is "Above all, do no harm." Both these concepts had to be relearned again and again throughout subsequent history. Hippocratic physicians adapted the notion of a humoral basis for disease from philosophers in Asia Minor. The four elements of natural philosophy were water, fire, air, and earth. Combinations of these elements gave rise to four humors of the body related to a scale of life from most alive to death. They were blood (sanguine temperament), phlegm (phlegmatic), yellow bile or urine (bilious), and black bile (melancholic). Treatment consisted of attempting to balance these humors by replenishment of deficiencies or removing excesses. Thus arose the practices of bleeding, purging (including vomiting), and sweating that continued well into the 19th century. Hippocrates also promoted the use of inorganic salts as medicine.

Works of Galen (131–201) dealing with physiology and materia medica became authoritative and were used widely for the next 1400 years. Galenic medicine consists of preparations of plants by soaking (infusion) or boiling (decoction). Galenic medicine has rebounded today as more people embrace herbal remedies. A scientific basis for medicine was begun by Aristotle (384–322 BC), who made and recorded numerous observations on animals. His pupil Theophrastus (380–287 BC) systematically classified medicinal plants on the basis of their individual characteristics rather than their recommended use in treatment. This work was improved upon by Dioscorides, a surgeon with the armies of Nero, who compiled the first *Materia Medica.* This treatise consisted of six volumes describing about 600 plants. Drugs were discussed from the standpoint of name, source, identification, tests for adulteration, preparation of the dosage form, what it would do, and for what conditions it would be used. This contribution was important because it established the framework for later pharmacopeias (officially recognized books of drug preparations). With the decline of the Roman Empire, scholarship transferred to Byzantium, where during the 5th century Publius Vegetius compiled a veterinary treatise that included prescriptions for farm animals.

Following the fall of Rome, Europe entered the Dark Ages, during which time there was little advancement in intellectual development. Custodians of knowledge and developers of medical thought during this period were found in Muslim culture. They developed the practice of pharmacy to a high level and were the first to distill wines and beers to obtain ethanol for preparing tinctures. Also they were the first to regulate the practice of pharmacy to standardize the preparation of prescriptions. An influential Persian writer during this period was Geber Ibn Hajar (702–765). He classified drugs and poisons of his time and recognized that the difference between a drug and a poison was a matter of dosage. Any drug can be toxic if given in large enough amounts.

The spirit of inquiry was reestablished in Europe during the Renaissance and was given impetus by the development of printing. The first pharmacopeia was compiled by the German Valerius Cordus (1514–1544). He carefully described techniques to be employed in preparation of drugs, in marked contrast to the secrecy prevailing prior to his time. The most influential person during this period was the Swiss physician Theophrastus Bombastus von Hohenheim (1493–1541), who called himself Philippus Aureolus Paracelsus. He introduced the clinical use of laudanum (opium) and a number of tinctures of various plants, the active principles of which are used to this day. He advocated using drugs in a directed or rational manner as opposed to the following of recipes.

The 17th and 18th centuries were an era of nationalism and flowering of individual genius. Drug trade flourished and medical experimentation began. Drugs such as cinchona (quinine), coffee, tea, and cocoa (methylxanthines), curare, digitalis, and a variety of alkaloids were discovered. The energetic and brilliant English physician John Hunter (1728–1793) influenced a group of physicians to conduct controlled clinical experimentation. The most notable contribution to therapy was William Withering's (1741–1799) *An Account of the Foxglove and Some of Its Medical Uses,* published in 1785. His observations on the use of digitalis in the treatment of dropsy (ascites due to congestive heart failure) are still pertinent. Edward Jenner (1749–1823) discovered and established the principle of prophylactic immunization against smallpox and was the first to describe anaphylaxis. Thus he set the stage for later development of preventive medicine and immunologic therapy. William Harvey (1578–1657) discovered the circulation of blood and indicated that drugs were distributed to various parts of the body by this means. The great English architect Christopher Wren (1632–1723) made the first intravenous injection of drugs into a dog, but it was not until 1853 that the hypodermic needle and syringe were devised by Alexander Wood (1817–1884). This was to have a major influence on later pharmacologic experimentation. During this period scientific societies developed as scientific information was disseminated. Pharmacopeias were well developed at this time and were the principal sources of information concerning drugs. Prescriptions were carefully devised by the practitioner for treatment of the individual patient.

The 19th century marked the development of chemistry, which paved the way for detailed characterization and experimental study of active pharmacologic principles derived from natural sources. Friedrich Sertürner (1783–1841), a German pharmacist, isolated the specific narcotic substance from opium and named it morphine after Morpheus, the Roman god of sleep. There followed in rapid succession isolation of active alkaloids from a variety of medicinal plants through the work of Joseph Caventou (1795–1877), Pierre Pelletier (1788–1842), Philipp Geiger (1785–1836), Georg Merck (1825–1873), and Albert Neimann (1840–1921).

The association between Pelletier and François Magendie (1783–1855) led Magendie to develop organized experiments to elucidate physiologic processes and action of drugs in the body. Magendie and his illustrious pupils Claude Bernard (1813–1878) and James Blake (1814–1893) established the foundations for modern pharmacology and outlined its unique scientific problems: dose-response relationships, drug disposition in the body, mechanism of action of drugs, site of action of drugs, and structure-activity relationships. The first laboratory devoted exclusively to the study of pharmacology was established by Rudolph Buchheim (1820–1879) at the University of Dorpat in Estonia. Extensive research was performed there to elucidate actions of drugs within the body. This stimulated development of pharmacology as a distinct scientific discipline. One of Buchheim's students, Oswald Schmiedeberg (1838–1921), was an excellent teacher who attracted students from around the world to the pharmacology institute of the University of Strasbourg. He led in establishing pharmacology as an independent scientific discipline based upon experimental methodology. Many of his students became leaders in the development of pharmacology throughout the world. These included Hans Meyer (1853–1939) at Vienna and John J. Abel (1857–1938), who is regarded as the "father of pharmacology" in the USA. Abel established departments of pharmacology at the University of Michigan and later at Johns Hopkins University. He trained many young scientists who became prominent pharmacologists. He founded the *Journal of Biological Chemistry* and *Journal of Pharmacology and Experimental Therapeutics* and was instrumental in the formation of the American Society of Pharmacology and Experimental Therapeutics (Abel 1926).

During the 20th century the science of pharmacology flourished in the medical and pharmacy schools, and the focus of leadership shifted from Europe to the USA. This was due in part to the occurrence of two world wars and the emergence of the USA as an industrial power. The almost exponential growth of knowledge and development of new drugs during this century were the result of the development of organic chemistry and the existence of an abundance of well-trained scientific investigators. The ability of chemists in the pharmaceutical industry to synthesize new chemical substances removed our dependence on natural products as a source of drugs. All aspects of the science progressed rapidly during this century, with appreciable gains in effective treatment and control of diseases. Most notable has been development of drugs effective in the treatment of infectious diseases. For a more detailed and scholarly review of the historical development of pharmacology, the reader is referred to Leake 1975 and Burger 1986.

The development of veterinary pharmacology is the same as that for humans. Throughout much of medical history little distinction was made between human and animal medicine, and both professions share common roots. Early European schools of veterinary medicine were established in conjunction with schools of human medicine. Near the beginning of the 20th century the two professions and their schools separated and developed more or less independently. Since that time a cultural lag has existed between human and veterinary medicine due to differences in size and economic factors. The teaching of materia medica as a didactic course persisted in veterinary schools until the early 1950s. Little was known or taught about pharmacology of drugs in domesticated animals.

L. Meyer Jones was instrumental in shifting emphasis in the veterinary curriculum from materia medica to the science of veterinary pharmacology. The decisive event in this transition was publication of the first edition of this textbook by Jones in 1954. As with most aspects of veterinary medicine, veterinary pharmacology has lagged behind its human counterpart by several years. Today, however, veterinary pharmacology is a vital part of veterinary medical education and research. Several professional organizations are dedicated to the furtherance of veterinary pharmacology as a research and clinical discipline, including the American Academy of Veterinary Pharmacology and Therapeutics, the European Association of Veterinary Pharmacology and Toxicology, the European College of Veterinary Pharmacology and Toxicology, and the American College of Veterinary Clinical Pharmacology.

SCOPE OF PHARMACOLOGY. *Pharmacology* is an experimental science dealing with the properties of drugs and their effects on living systems. It has included study of sources of drugs (pharmacognosy), action and fate of drugs in the body (pharmacodynamics), use of drugs in the treatment of disease (therapeutics), and poisonous effects of drugs or xenobiotics (toxicology). The word *drug* is derived from the Old French *drogue,* which meant herb. Drugs have been defined officially by the US Food, Drug, and Cosmetic Act to include all articles recognized in the *United States Pharmacopeia* (USP) and the *National Formulary* (NF); articles intended to be used in the diagnosis, mitigation, treatment, or prevention of disease in humans or other animals; and articles other than food intended to affect the structure or function of the body.*Pharmacodynamics* refers to study of the response of an organism to the action of drugs in the absence of disease. *Pharmacotherapy* refers to the use of drugs in the treatment of disease, whereas *therapeutics* is a term describing treatment of disease in general and includes use of drugs, surgery, radiation, behavioral modification, and other modalities. *Pharmacokinetics* is defined as the mathematical description of temporal changes in concentration of drugs and/or their metabolites within the body (Baggot 1977). Such studies provide the experimental basis for drug dosage regimens in various animal species.

Clinical pharmacology is considered in human medicine to be synonymous with human pharmacology (Smith 1978). In its broader sense, *clinical* means "pertaining to or founded on actual observation and treatment of patients, as distinguished from theoretical or basic sciences" (Anderson 1994). The discipline forms a foundation for the application of pharmacologic principles in the development of drug therapy for animal patients (Brumbaugh and Davis 1987). Controlled evaluation of the efficacy and safety of drug therapy in animal patients is a major concern of veterinary clinical pharmacology.

Chemotherapy is a branch of pharmacology dealing with drugs that selectively inhibit or destroy specific agents of disease such as bacteria, viruses, fungi, and other parasites. Use of this term has been extended to the use of drugs in treatment of neoplastic diseases. The notion of selective toxicity is central to chemotherapy. Drugs that are useful as chemotherapeutic agents affect the pathogen or abnormal cell more adversely than normal cells of the host.

Toxicology classically has been defined as the study of poisons. The subject is concerned with the adverse effects of xenobiotics. Its scope classically includes not only drugs used in therapy but also the many other chemicals that may be responsible for household, environmental, or industrial intoxication through food additives, industrial wastes, radioactive substances, pesticides, and ingestion of natural substances (Benet 1996). Others have defined toxicology as the science that defines the limits of safety of chemical agents for human and animal populations (Casarett 1996).

Posology is the study of medicine dosage, which varies with the species of animal, the intended effect of the drug, and individual tolerance or susceptibility. In general, the effective dose of a drug is that amount necessary to elicit the desired therapeutic response in the patient. The student should differentiate between the terms *dose* and *dosage.* A dose is the quantity of medication to be administered at one time, whereas dosage refers to determination and regulation of doses.

Metrology is the study of weights and measures as applied to preparation and administration of drugs. The reader is referred to Chapter 57 for a more complete discussion.

Pharmacy is a separate and complementary health care profession concerned with collection, preparation, standardization, and dispensing of drugs. By training, the pharmacist is well-equipped to advise the veterinarian on matters relevant to dosage forms, incompatibilities, drug interactions, and medicinal chemistry as well as to fulfill the traditional role of compounding and dispensing appropriate dosage forms of drugs.

Materia medica is an obsolete didactic subject that was concerned with pharmacy, posology, pharmacognosy, and indications for therapeutic use of drugs. This subject was purely descriptive in nature and has been replaced in the modern veterinary medical curriculum by the science of comparative pharmacology.

Nutraceuticals are nutritional products which allegedly have some therapeutic value in addition to their scientifically recognized nutritional content. These are not regulated as drugs by the US Food and Drug Administration and as such do not have the supporting data regarding their safety or efficacy for the alleged (or implied) claim.

ROLE OF PHARMACOLOGY IN THE VETERINARY MEDICAL CURRICULUM. The purpose of an education is to assist the individual in becoming an independent person who can think. Veterinary medical curricula are designed to facilitate the acquisition of factual material, skills, and an understanding of concepts to enable the student to practice the profession of veterinary medicine. Practice is the application of knowledge, skills, and thought for purposes of maintaining the health of animals, relieving suffering, and serving the best interests of the clients. Thus the student must endeavor to understand the concepts and facts of the veterinary medical sciences to be able to make decisions regarding diagnosis, treatment, and management of animal patients.

Pharmacology, like pathology, is a bridging medical science in that its study is dependent on an understanding of anatomy, physiology, microbiology, biologic and organic chemistry, and mathematics. Conversely, thorough understanding of pharmacology, toxicology, and pathology is requisite to studies of internal medicine, surgery, and other clinical subjects.

The number of products—from approved drug products to nutraceuticals and homeopathic remedies—that can be acquired worldwide and used legally by the practicing veterinarian is staggering. Literally hundreds of new products become available every year, although only a very few are new compounds, and even fewer are approved new animal drugs. While this growth in available therapeutic products has provided an unprecedented armamentarium of potent pharmacotherapeutic agents, it has also greatly increased the incidence of therapy-related disorders (iatrogenic diseases). No one can have an intimate knowledge of all drugs available, and even if it were possible, it would be unnecessary to the optimal medical care of animal patients. Efforts are being made by educators in veterinary pharmacology to define the 50–100 drugs essential to the practice of veterinary medicine for detailed discussion in veterinary pharmacology courses and emphasis in clinics. Monographs describing several of these veterinary drugs appear in the *United States Pharmacopeia Dispensing Information.*

The veterinarian must keep in mind that there is no completely "safe" drug unless the compound is pharmacologically inert. Thus the art of rational therapeutics requires consideration of potential risks as well as possible benefits of drugs to the patient's well-being

(Nierenberg and Melmon 1992) and consideration of the public health implications of such intervention. Considerable risk might be tolerated in treatment of a life-threatening disease, whereas even a small risk might be unacceptable in management of a self-limiting disease. The veterinarian must, therefore, understand the actions of the drug on the body, how it is absorbed and eliminated, its toxic effects, its clinical indications and contraindications, and its dosage in the species of animal to be treated. The student should attempt to incorporate this specific information into an intellectual framework of pharmacologic principles. Subsequent chapters of this book will develop the ideas underlying veterinary pharmacology and provide specific information concerning a number of drugs.

A convenient guide for the student to organize a course of study has been developed (Coppoc and Stuckey 1977). The purpose of the Minimal Essential Drug Information Checklist (MEDIC) is to encourage a problem-solving approach to learning pharmacology, i.e., to ensure that the student possesses an adequate knowledge base to make rational decisions regarding use of a particular drug in a given patient. This checklist is given below with permission from the authors and publisher (Coppoc and Stuckey 1977):

DRUG

1. What is your therapeutic goal? What specific pathologic process do you wish to alter by using a drug from this class and this drug in particular? Is it absolutely necessary that you use this or any drug?

2. By what routes can the drug be given for the indication in question and which are you going to use? On what basis did you make this decision? What are, e.g., the relative advantages or disadvantages of intravenous vs. oral administration in this case?

3. What dosage form are you going to use?

4. What dose in units/kg or mg/kg is generally recommended and how much are you using in this particular animal? How did you arrive at this dose? Are there items considered under "precautions" that should modify the dose in this animal?

5. What is the dosage interval? Is this going to be frequent enough to prevent the drug from dropping below effective concentrations? Will it be too frequent and precipitate cumulation and toxicity?

6. What is the probable duration of therapy?

7. For food animals? Is the drug approved for use in this food-producing species? What is the withdrawal time?

8. How much does the drug cost per treatment and per expected duration of therapy? (This should include administration expenses such as syringes, technician time, and special dispensers as in a water supply.) Does the cost of treatment exceed the value of the animal or the desire of the owner to pay? Is the cost appropriate to the seriousness of the disease?

9. What special precautions must be observed to enhance its effectiveness or safety? Examples: What if the drug is eliminated by the kidney and renal function is compromised? Will the drug interact with other drugs in the regimen?

10. What are contraindications to the use of this drug; i.e., under what conditions should it not be used?

11. What adverse reactions might one reasonably expect to see? How would you monitor the animal to detect potentially serious reactions before they are permanent or endanger the animal's life?

12. What course of action will you take if you elicit one of the drug reactions outlined above? Do you have the requisite drugs and/or equipment on hand?

13. What plans do you have for evaluating the results of your therapy? By what parameter(s) will you judge whether the animal is responding to treatment? When can you reasonably expect to see the first response? How will you judge whether you have cured the animal? What follow-up procedures should be instituted?

Veterinary pharmacology is not an easy subject to master because of the multiplicity of species concerned and plethora of available drugs that can be legally obtained. The veterinarian is asked to care for the health of the entire animal kingdom with the exception of humans. In studying this text, the student should constantly be alert to the fact that various species of animals may respond differently to certain drugs. These species differences, and the fact that many of the animals we treat enter the human food supply, distinguish veterinary pharmacology from medical pharmacology.

Diligent study of comparative pharmacology is an essential part of becoming an effective veterinarian who is capable of applying or prescribing rational drug therapy without harming the patient. This has been a central problem of medicine since antiquity and continues to the present time.

As Aristotle (384–322 BC) said in *Nichomachean Ethics,* book 9, "Even in medicine, though it is easy to know what honey, wine and hellebore, cautery and surgery are, to know how and to whom and when to apply them so as to effect a cure is no less an undertaking than to be a physician [veterinarian]."

REFERENCES

Abel, J. J. 1926. J Pharmacol Exp Ther 27:266.
American Medical Association (AMA). 1971. Drug Evaluations.
Anderson, D. M. 1994. Dorland's Illustrated Medical Dictionary, 28th ed., p. 341. Philadelphia: W. B. Saunders.
Aviado, D. M. 1972. Pharmacologic Principles of Medical Practice, 8th ed., p. 9. Baltimore: Williams & Wilkins.
Baggot, J. D. 1977. Principles of Drug Disposition in Domestic Animals, p. 144. Philadelphia: W. B. Saunders.
Benet, L. Z. 1996. In J. G. Hardman, L. E. Limbird, P. B. Moninoff, R. W. Ruddon, and A. G. Gilman, eds., Goodman and Gilman's The Pharmacological Basis for Therapeutics, 9th ed., p. 2. New York: McGraw-Hill.
Brown, E. A. 1955. J Am Med Assoc 157:814.
Brumbaugh, G. W., and Davis, L. E. 1987. Equine Practice: Clinical Pharmacology, p. ix. Veterinary Clinics of North America. Philadelphia: W. B. Saunders.
Burger, A. 1986. Drugs and People: Medicines, Their History and Origins, and the Way They Act. Charlottesville: Univ. Press of Virginia.

Casarett, L. J. 1996. In L. J. Casarett, C. D. Klaasen, M. O. Amam, and J. Doull, eds., Toxicology: The Basic Science of Poisons, 5th ed. New York: McGraw-Hill.

Coppoc, G. L., and Stuckey, W. J. 1977. J Vet Med Educ 4:171.

Davis, L. E. 1977. Fed Proc 36:119.

———. 1979. In J. D. Powers and T. E. Powers, eds., Proceedings of the 2nd Equine Pharmacology Symposium, p. 9. Golden, Colo.: American Association of Equine Practitioners.

Leake, C. D. 1975. An Historical Account of Pharmacology to the Twentieth Century. Springfield, Ill.: Charles C. Thomas.

Nierenberg, D. W., and Melmon K. L. 1992. In K. L. Melmon, H. F. Morelli, B. F. Nierenberg, and D. W. Nierenberg, eds., Clinical Pharmacology: Basic Principles in Therapeutics, 3rd ed. New York: McGraw-Hill.

Smith, W. M. 1992. In K. L. Melmon, H. F. Morelli, B. F. Nierenberg, and D. W. Nierenberg, eds., Clinical Pharmacology: Basic Principles in Therapeutics, 3rd ed. New York: McGraw-Hill.

Tumbleson, M. 1975. Am Soc Vet Physiol Pharmacol (Bus Meet).

2 PHARMACODYNAMICS: MECHANISMS OF DRUG ACTION

MARK J. NOVOTNY

Pharmacodynamic Terms
Receptor
Agonists, Affinity, Efficacy, and Potency
Antagonism
Selectivity and Specificity
Quantitative Responses in the Patient
Quantitative Aspects of Drug-Receptor Interaction
Dose Titration Studies

Pharmacodynamics is the study of physiologic and biochemical effects of drugs and how these effects relate to a drug's mechanism of action. Pharmacodynamics focuses on the action and effects of drugs within the body. For example, a drug may interact with a receptor on the surface of a myocardial cell to initiate a series of reactions that cause the myocardial cell to contract more forcefully (a positive inotropic effect); the result is an increase in cardiac output and peripheral tissue perfusion, culminating in an increase in exercise tolerance of a patient with congestive heart failure. The study of the effects of a drug can span from basic biochemical and molecular mechanisms to cellular responses, to effects on organs or systems, to the whole animal, or even to populations of animals. Thus, pharmacodynamics is relevant to all aspects of pharmacology: from basic pharmacologic research in the laboratory to applied therapeutics in the clinical patient. In general, pharmacodynamics characterizes what a drug does to the patient. In contrast, the study of pharmacokinetics (Chapter 3) addresses what the patient's body does to a drug. The patient absorbs the drug into the systemic circulation, distributes the drug to tissues in the body, metabolizes the drug, and eliminates the drug from the body. Effective use of a drug requires knowledge of the drug's pharmacokinetic and pharmacodynamic properties.

PHARMACODYNAMIC TERMS

Important to the discussion of pharmacodynamics is an introduction to the terms used to define the pharmacodynamic properties of a drug.

Receptor. A *drug receptor* is the macromolecular component of body tissue with which a drug interacts to initiate its pharmacologic effects. Only the initial consequence of a drug-receptor interaction is correctly termed the "action" of the drug. The succeeding effects are more properly called drug "effects." Receptors can be proteins, enzymes, nucleic acids, or other cellular constituents. Protein receptors are often well characterized. Examples include the muscarinic receptors on cells of the heart, smooth muscle, or exocrine glands and nicotinic receptors on cells at neuromuscular junctions or preganglionic synapses. The endogenous neurotransmitter acetylcholine (ACh) activates both muscarinic and nicotinic receptors. The widely used drug atropine competes with ACh for muscarinic receptors as its mechanism of drug action.

Enzymes associated with key regulatory or metabolic processes are particularly useful receptors. As an example, the neurotransmitter ACh is metabolized by acetylcholine esterase (AChE), an endogenous enzyme that terminates the action of ACh. The drug pyridostigmine inhibits AChE, prolonging the action of endogenous ACh, and is therefore useful for treating myasthenia gravis, a disease characterized by a reduction in functional nicotinic receptors at neuromuscular junctions. In the presence of pyridostigmine, ACh is available longer to activate the remaining functional nicotinic receptors. As another example, the synergistic antimicrobial effect of the trimethoprim-sulfonamide combination results from actions on sequential steps in the enzymatic pathway by which microorganisms synthesize folic acid from precursor molecules.

Other cellular constituents can serve as receptors. Examples include nucleic acids, ion channels, and intracellular proteins such as tubulin, the respective sites of action of cancer chemotherapeutic agents, calcium channel blockers, and the antifungal agent griseofulvin. For certain drugs a therapeutic effect occurs in the absence of clearly defined, macromolecular tissue receptors. Examples include the osmotic diuretic mannitol (Chapter 26) and analogs of purine and pyrimidine bases (Chapter 52) that serve as suicide substrates for DNA or RNA synthesis.

Maximal tissue response to a drug may occur when only a fraction of the total number of receptors are occupied by the drug. This situation can come about, e.g., when a step subsequent to occupancy of the receptor by the drug is limiting the expression of the drug-receptor response. The term *spare receptor* applies to the situation when maximal response is elicited by occupancy of a fraction of the tissue receptors.

Agonists, Affinity, Efficacy, and Potency. An *agonist* is a drug that possesses affinity for a particular receptor and causes a change in the receptor that results in an observable effect. Agonists are further characterized as *full agonists,* producing a maximal response by occupying all or a fraction of receptors, or *partial agonists,* producing less than a maximal response even when the drug occupies all of the receptors. *Affinity* describes the tendency of a drug to combine with a particular kind of receptor, whereas *efficacy* or *intrinsic activity* of a drug refers to the maximal effect the drug can produce. A partial agonist has less intrinsic activity than a full agonist. *Potency* is a term that is frequently misunderstood when comparing two or more drugs that give rise to the same observable effect. Potency of a drug refers to the dose that must be administered to produce a particular effect of given intensity. Potency is influenced by the affinity of a drug for its receptor sites and by pharmacokinetic processes that determine drug concentration in the immediate vicinity of its site of action (biophase). Potency of a drug varies inversely with dose; the lower the dose required to produce a stated response, the more potent the drug. Potency is a relative, rather than an absolute, expression of drug activity. For potency determinations a standard must be defined, and potency comparisons are valid only for drugs that produce the stated response by the same mechanism of action. Potency of a drug is not necessarily correlated with its efficacy or safety, and the most potent drug within a series is not necessarily clinically superior. Low potency is a disadvantage only if the effective dose is so large that it is too costly to produce or too cumbersome to administer.

Antagonism. An *antagonist* is a drug that blocks the response produced by an agonist. Antagonists interact with the receptor or other component of the effector mechanism, but antagonists are devoid of intrinsic activity. Antagonists can be further characterized as *competitive antagonists* or *noncompetitive antagonists.* Competitive antagonism is completely reversible; an increase in the concentration of the agonist in the immediate vicinity of its site of action or biophase will overcome the effect of the antagonist. Although lacking intrinsic activity, the "efficacy" of an antagonist is measured in terms of reversing or blocking the effects of the receptor's agonist. Therapeutic agents acting by competitive antagonism include atropine (antimuscarinic agent), diphenhydramine (antihistamine or H_1-receptor blocker), propranolol (β-adrenergic blocking drug), and spironolactone (aldosterone antagonist).

A *noncompetitive antagonist* conceptually removes the receptor or response potential from the system. Addition of more agonist to the biophase of the inhibited receptor will not overcome the antagonism achieved by a noncompetitive antagonist. Thus the essential feature of noncompetitive antagonism is that the agonist has no influence upon the degree of antagonism or its reversibility. The maximal effect achievable by the agonist is reduced accordingly by a noncompetitive antagonist. Examples of noncompetitive antagonists include the α-adrenergic blocking drug phenoxybenzamine and the platelet-inhibiting action of aspirin. The thromboxane synthase enzyme of platelets is irreversibly inhibited by aspirin, a process that is reversed only by production of new platelets (Chapter 22).

Selectivity and Specificity. A drug is usually described by its most prominent effect or by the action thought to be the basis of that effect. However, rarely does a drug produce only a single effect; most drugs produce multiple effects. *Selectivity* of a drug depends on its capacity to preferentially produce a particular effect. The characteristic effect of the drug is produced at lower doses than those required to elicit other responses. For example, the sympathomimetic amine clenbuterol has a high degree of selectivity for β_2 receptors in airways and is useful in the treatment of respiratory disease in horses with bronchospasm. At high doses manifestation of activity on cardiac β_1 receptors may be apparent. A truly selective drug produces only a single effect. The anticoagulant heparin is an example of a drug that has selective action. For therapeutic applications, selectivity of a drug is one of its more important characteristics. The route of administration (e.g., topical administration) or the pattern of drug distribution to sites of action (e.g., restricted from the central nervous system) may confer selectivity of action on certain drugs that are ordinarily nonselective.

When all the effects produced by a drug are due to a single mechanism of action, the drug is said to be *specific.* A specific drug acts at only one type of receptor but may produce multiple pharmacologic effects because of location of receptors in various organs. Atropine is a specific drug in that its varied effects can be attributed to its antimuscarinic action. Effects of a nonspecific drug result from several mechanisms of action. The potential effects of phenothiazine tranquilizers (e.g., acepromazine) include sedation (increase the rate of dopamine turnover in the brain), an antiemetic action (depress activation of the chemoreceptor trigger zone), hypotension (α-adrenergic receptor blockade), an antispasmodic effect on the gastrointestinal smooth muscle (anticholinergic action), and hypothermia (interference with hypothalamic control of temperature regulation).

QUANTITATIVE RESPONSES IN THE PATIENT.

The purpose of administering a drug to an animal is to produce a particular response of desired intensity. This response will usually be produced by establishing and maintaining for a certain time an effective concentration of the drug in the immediate vicinity of its site of action. A fundamental principle of pharmacology is that the intensity of response elicited by a drug is a function of the dose administered. The response of a patient to different doses of a drug, or the dose-response relationship, conforms to the principles discussed below for drug-receptor interactions. The patient response can be represented graphically in at least two ways, as shown in Fig. 2.1. In Fig. 2.1A the relationship is depicted between the drug dose and the response. More commonly, the concentration of the drug is expressed on a logarithmic scale as shown in Fig. 2.1B. The slope of the log dose-response indicates the range of dosage over which the drug acts, from minimally detectable to maximally effective. The variability in the response can be related to physiologic, pathologic, or drug-induced variation in the patient or to variation in a population of patients. Thus, variability in effectiveness of a drug given to the same patient at different times or to different patients within the same species can be due to circadian changes, age, the state of the patient's health, genetic variation, or environmental effects, or it may be drug induced, as for instance by receptor down-regulation (see Chapter 4).

The relationship between dose and response may be interpreted in one of two ways: (1) as the dose of a drug is increased, the intensity of the response is increased (graded dose-response); or (2) as the dose is increased, the number or proportion of animals exhibiting a particular, stated response is greater (quantal dose-response). A graded dose-response relationship can be measured on a continuous scale, whereas a quantal response is an all-or-none response. Thus, for an individual patient, the dose-response may be graded or quantal depending on which criterion of response has been adopted. For example, if the response criterion for dogs with atrial fibrillation is reduction in the rate of contraction of the ventricles in response to increasing doses of the cardiac glycoside digoxin, then the ventricular rate can be measured on a continuous scale with an electrocardiograph. Therefore, the dose-response relationship is graded. However, if the response criterion is reduction of the ventricular rate to ≤140 beats per minute (bpm) for a population of dogs with atrial fibrillation, then the response of each dog to a given dose of digoxin will be all-or-none; the ventricular rate either did or did not decrease to ≤140 bpm for each animal. The more-sensitive dogs in the population may experience a decline in ventricular rate to ≤140 bpm at a relatively low dose of digoxin; more-resistant cases of atrial fibrillation will require higher doses. Thus, the effect of a drug and its variability can be monitored in a population, not necessarily by measuring the graded response in individuals in the population to a range of different doses, but by measuring the dose required to produce a measured effect among the individuals.

In practice, an end point to a response or an effect is defined, and the dose of drug required to achieve that end point is determined in a group of individuals from the population. Fig. 2.2 shows the result of such a procedure. A frequency distribution curve is obtained with

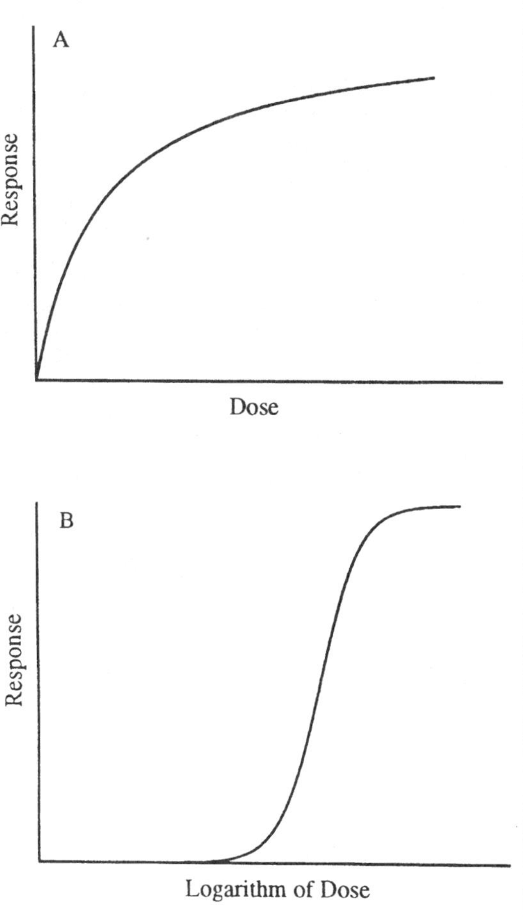

FIG. 2.1

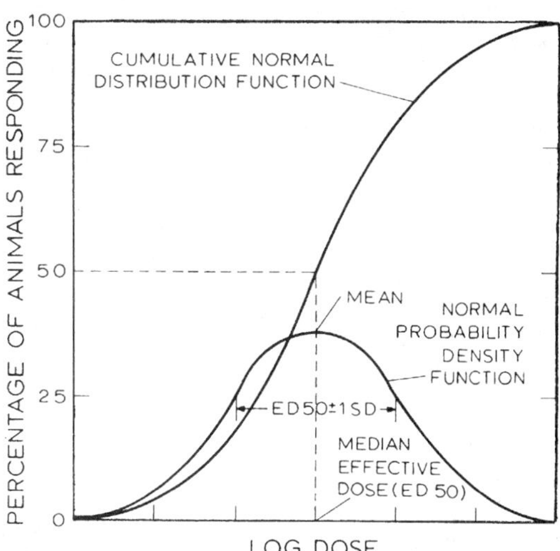

FIG. 2.2—Graphic presentation of the quantal dose-response relationship. Both normal and cumulative forms of the frequency distribution curve are shown.

the most-sensitive members of the population responding and reaching the end point at the lowest dose of the drug and with the most-resistant members of the population requiring the highest doses. As Fig. 2.2 illustrates, the sensitivity of a drug is distributed normally with respect to the logarithm of the dose. In this population, the dose required to produce the effect in 50% of the individuals is known as the *median effective dose* and is abbreviated ED_{50}. When the frequency distribution curve is plotted as a cumulative frequency distribution curve, the familiar logarithmic dose-response curve is obtained (Fig. 2.1B). This is the form of the curve commonly used for ease of understanding some of the principles of drug dosage.

At any given dose, the cumulative (quantal log dose-response) curve gives the percentage of animals responding to that dose and to all lower doses. Although both the graded and quantal dose-response curves are sigmoidal in shape, they represent different interpretations of the dose-response relationship. The graded curve relates the intensity of response to the size of dose (see below), whereas the quantal curve expresses individual variation in the dose needed to produce a specified (predetermined) response.

A useful measure of variability of the normal distribution curve is the standard deviation (SD). The area under the curve enclosed by 1 SD on either side of the median represents about 68% of the total area enclosed by the entire distribution curve (Fig. 2.2). That is, approximately two-thirds of the total number of animals tested would respond to a dose lying within 1 SD of the ED_{50}.

As noted previously, for the individual dose-response curve, the slope of the curve gives an indication of the range over which a drug elicits its effects. In a population, the slope is similarly important in indicating the range over which a population is affected. If one considers only the desirable effect of a particular drug, then the importance of the slope lies in its ability to predict the dose of the drug which will produce the desired effect in all or any fraction of the population. The steeper the slope, the narrower the range of doses which encompasses the majority of the population. In the unlikely and "ideal" case where a drug has no undesirable side effects, the ED_{99} (the dose sufficient to be effective in almost all individuals in the population) can be used effectively in virtually all patients. However, for most drugs, as the dose increases, undesirable or side effects become increasingly common. Because at high doses these may include severe toxicity and even death, the safety margin between an effective dose and a toxic or lethal dose is of extreme importance. Therefore, the greater the gap between the effective dose and the dose that causes toxicity or death, the safer the drug. The positioning and slope of the cumulative frequency distribution curves for the desired effect, side effects, toxic effects, and lethal effect are important indicators of the safety of the drug and our ability to use the drug successfully.

The ratio of the drug dose which produces an undesired effect and the dose which causes the desired effects is a *therapeutic index* and indicates the selectivity of the drug and consequently its usability. A single drug can have many therapeutic indices, one for each of its undesirable effects relative to a desired drug action, and one for each of its desired effects if the drug has more than one action. Consequently, a single therapeutic index derived from the ratio of the ED_{50} and the median lethal dose (LD_{50}) values is only a gross assessment of the safety margin. Also, this is likely to be misleading if the dose-response curves from which the values are derived are shallow.

Fig. 2.3 shows two cumulative frequency distribution curves, one for the effective doses of a particular drug and one for the lethal doses. In this hypothetical and extreme case, the effective dose in only 50% of the population (ED_{50}) will cause death in the most-sensitive individual in the population. The dose of the drug sufficient to be effective in almost all the individuals in the population (the ED_{99}) is also the LD_{50} and therefore sufficient to kill half of the population. The margin of safety for this drug is unacceptable.

Fig. 2.4 demonstrates that the slope of the cumulative frequency distribution curve is important in the separation of desirable from undesirable effects. Shown in the figure are the dose-response curves for two drugs (A and B) that have identical ED_{50}'s and identical LD_{50}'s but different slopes to the dose-response curves. To understand the importance of the slope, compare the doses of the two drugs required to produce the desired effect in all members of the population with the range of doses causing death. Drug A, with the steeper dose-response slope, can be used effectively on the whole population without causing death, while drug B, with the shallower curves, cannot be used in this way. The dose of drug B that yields a therapeutic effect in the majority of the patient population will also be lethal to a significant number of patients. Rather than death as the end point for comparing therapeutic cumulative frequency distribution curves, a more clinically meaningful comparison is

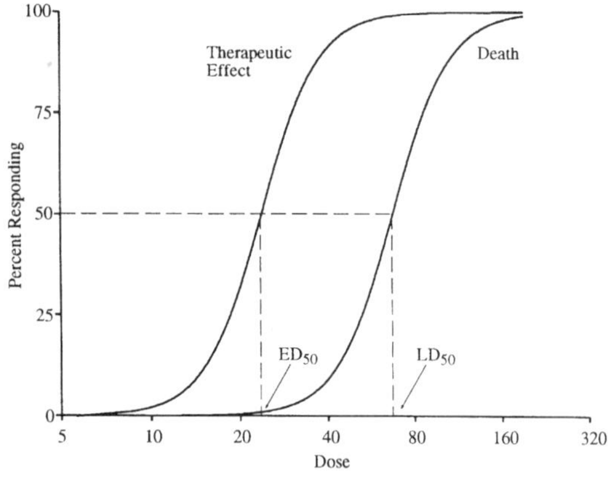

FIG. 2.3

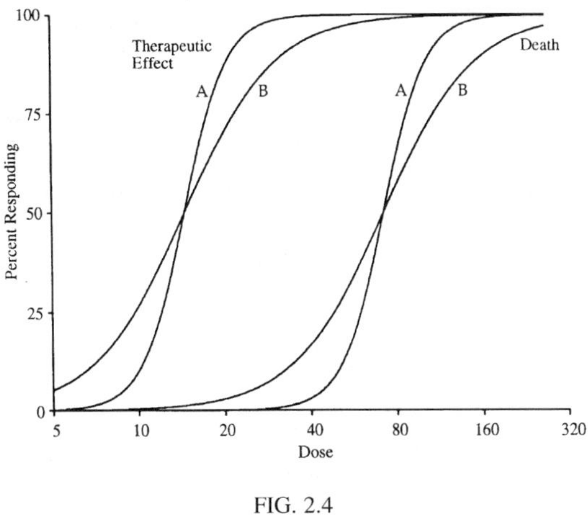

FIG. 2.4

with distribution curves for the relationship between dose and the onset of the manifestations of a drug's toxic principle (e.g., the onset of vomiting, anorexia, or bradycardia for the cardiac glycoside digoxin).

Thus, the use of a drug cannot be predicted on the basis of a therapeutic index derived from the ED_{50}'s and LD_{50}'s alone. A wider knowledge of a drug's properties is required. With respect to effective doses, lethal doses, or doses associated with the onset of toxic drug effects, the important factor is the safety margin and a clear gap between the maximum dose required to produce the therapeutic effect and the minimum dose that will initiate a toxic drug effect or cause death.

QUANTITATIVE ASPECTS OF DRUG-RECEPTOR INTERACTION. The drug concentration in the biophase depends on the amount of drug (dose) administered, route of administration, factors that influence distribution of the drug to the biophase, and the rate of elimination of drug from the biophase and patient. Presence of the drug in the biophase leads to interaction between drug molecules and receptors and thus to a change at the receptor level. The magnitude of this change depends on the concentration of the drug in the biophase, the affinity of the drug for the receptors, and the drug's intrinsic activity. The result of the drug-receptor interaction is the formation of a *stimulus*. The stimulus has a linear relationship to the number of occupied receptors. Action of the stimulus on the effector system results in the quantifiable pharmacologic effect.

Thus, a pharmacologic response is considered to be the result of a reversible interaction of a drug with its receptors. The intensity of response elicited by a drug is a function of the dose administered. In certain instances a drug-receptor response may be characterized as quantal in nature; however, the preponderance of dose-response relationships at the receptor level are better described in terms of a graded response. The drug-receptor-response relationship is summarized in the following equation:

drug + receptor ↔ drug-receptor complex → response

The magnitude of response is assumed to be proportional to the number of receptors occupied by the drug, with a maximal response corresponding to occupancy of all receptors. Alternatively, maximal tissue response to a drug may occur when only a fraction of the total number of receptors are occupied by the drug, as previously discussed for the situation when a step subsequent to occupancy of the receptor by the drug is limiting the expression of the drug-receptor response.

Two important assumptions are inherent in the dose-response relationship: (1) the drug response is directly proportional to the percentage of the total number of receptors occupied by the drug and (2) a negligible fraction of the total amount of drug in the body combines with its receptors. The reacting substances are the drug and the unoccupied (free) receptors for the drug:

$$\underset{(C_x)}{\text{drug}} + \underset{(100 - Y)}{\text{free receptors}} \underset{k_2}{\overset{k_1}{\leftrightarrow}} \underset{(Y)}{\text{drug-receptor complex}}$$

where C_x is the concentration of the drug in the biophase and Y is the percentage (concentration) of receptors occupied by the drug. Peculiar to this situation is that neither of the reacting substances can be accurately measured, yet conclusions may be deduced from the interaction. At equilibrium,

$$k_1 \cdot C_x(100 - Y) = k_2 \cdot Y$$

Rearranging, $Y/[C_x(100 - Y)] = k_1/k_2 = K_x$, where K_x is the affinity constant of the reaction. The affinity constant is an association constant that relates to the equilibrium attained in the formation of the drug-receptor complex.

Since effective concentration of the drug remains essentially unchanged during the reaction, the ratio of concentration of occupied receptors to that of unoccupied receptors is proportional to the dose administered. That is, the dose that will occupy half of the receptors in the drug-receptor complex gives a 50% response. This will correspond to a situation in which $Y/(100 - Y) = 1$ and $1/ED_{50} = K_x$ so that the median effective dose (ED_{50}) is the reciprocal of the affinity constant of the tissue receptor for the particular drug.

Graphic representation of a graded response with increase in dose has the form of the hyperbola seen previously for quantal dose-response relationships. The response is the dependent variable and the dose is the independent variable. On a semilogarithmic graph, the hyperbola is converted to the familiar sigmoid curve, again analogous to the quantal log dose-response curve. Drugs that produce a particular effect by the same mechanism of action but differ in potency yield a series of parallel log dose-response curves.

DOSE TITRATION STUDIES. An application of the dose-response relationship is in the regulatory approval process for new animal drugs. Traditionally, the dose-response relationship of a new animal drug can be characterized in a manner described above. A clearly defined end point (or end points) of drug efficacy that is related to the proposed clinical indication is evaluated in a population of animals across a range of doses. The critical aspects of the dose-response relationship for the dose or dose range of the drug under study include the lower plateau of the curve at which the dose is ineffective, the slope of the curve, and the upper plateau at which effectiveness is not improved by increasing the dose. When a drug is proposed as being effective over a dose range, efficacy should be demonstrated in such a way that one can determine from the dose-response data that the drug will be effective at all doses within the range. Thus, the lower limit of a dose range may be based, e.g., upon the cumulative frequency distribution curve for the therapeutic effect, whereas the upper limit of a dose range may be based upon some other practical aspect such as safety to the target animal, the potential for drug residues in food products from treated animals, length of withdrawal times for food animals, injection site volume, or development costs pertaining to synthesizing and presenting the drug in its final formulation for the market.

REFERENCES

Angehrn, P., and Then, R. 1973. Investigations on the mode of action of the combination sulfamethoxaole-trimethoprim. Chemotherapy 19:1–10.

Ariëns, E. J. 1954. Affinity and intrinsic activity in the theory of competitive inhibition. Part I. Problems and theory. Arch Int Pharmacodyn Ther 99:32–49.

Baggot, J. D. 1988. Mechanisms of drug action. In N. H. Booth and L. E. McDonald, eds., Veterinary Pharmacology and Therapeutics, 6th ed., pp. 25–37. Ames: Iowa State Univ Press.

Barlow, R. B. 1964. Introduction to Chemical Pharmacology, 2nd ed., p. 27. London: Methuen.

Paton, W. D. M. 1961. A theory of drug action based on the rate of drug-receptor combination. Proc R Soc Lond (Biol) 154:21–69.

Schultz, W. B. 1997. Substantial evidence of effectiveness of new animal drugs. Fed Reg 62:59830–59840.

Sharp, G. W. G., and Oswald, R. E. 1995. Pharmacodynamics: Mechanisms of drug action. In H. R. Adams, ed., Veterinary Pharmacology and Therapeutics, 7th ed., pp. 9–17. Ames: Iowa State Univ Press.

Stephenson, R. P. 1956. A modification of receptor theory. Br J Pharmacol 11:379–393.

3 PHARMACOKINETICS: DISPOSITION AND FATE OF DRUGS IN THE BODY

SCOTT ANTHONY BROWN

Passage of Drugs across Biologic Membranes
- **Nature of Biologic Membranes**
- **Drug Passage across Membranes**
- **The pH Partition Hypothesis**
- **Carrier-Mediated Transport**

Drug Administration
- **Parenteral Administration**
- **IV Injection**
- **Extravascular Administration**
- **Percutaneous Absorption**
- **Pulmonary Absorption**
- **Drug Administration by the Oral Route**
- **Comparative Aspects of Drug Absorption**
- **Quantitating Drug Absorption**
- **Species Variations in Bioavailability**
- **Bioequivalence**

Distribution of Drugs
- **Plasma Protein Binding**
- **Quantitating Drug Distribution**

Mechanisms of Drug Elimination
- **Drug Metabolism (Biotransformation)**
- **Excretion of Drugs**
- **Quantitating Drug Elimination**

Pharmacokinetic Analysis
- **Compartmental Analysis**
- **Noncompartmental Analysis**

Some Aspects of Drug Dosage
- **Drug Administration**
- **Therapeutic Plasma Concentrations**
- **Application of Pharmacokinetics to Dosage**
- **Dosage Regimen**
- **Steady-State Concentration**

Interspecies Scaling
- **Body Weight**
- **Body Surface Area**
- **Allometry**

Glossary of Pharmacokinetic Terms
- **Primary Pharmacokinetic Terms**
- **Volume and Clearance Terms**
- **Terms Associated with Dosage**

Pharmacokinetics is concerned with study and characterization of the time course of drug absorption, distribution, metabolism, and excretion. Specifically, it is defined as the mathematical description of drug concentration changes in the body. Additionally, it is concerned with the relationship of these processes to intensity and duration of characteristic effects of drugs. An understanding of the dose-effect relationship can generally be obtained by linking pharmacokinetic behavior with information on pharmacodynamic activity (Holford and Sheiner 1981).

The usual reason for administering a drug to an animal is to produce a certain pharmacologic response. This objective may sometimes be achieved, at least in part, by giving a recommended dose of the drug without appreciation of the basis of the recommendation. The most effective use of drugs, based on an understanding of pharmacodynamics and pharmacokinetic principles in the clinical patient, together with some knowledge of product formulations, is the essence of clinical pharmacology. This enlightened approach provides an insight to mechanisms of drug interactions and potential usefulness (or otherwise) of combination preparations.

To produce its characteristic effect(s), a drug must attain effective concentrations at its site of action. In veterinary medicine, this requirement is complicated by the variety of animal species to which therapeutic agents and anesthetics are administered. Wide variations in intensity and duration of pharmacologic effect are commonly observed among species of domestic animals when a drug is given at the same dose level (mg/kg). These variations in response can be attributed to species differences either in the availability of the drug at the site of action or in the inherent sensitivity of tissue receptor sites. Clinical pharmacologic studies suggest that, for the majority of therapeutic agents, the species variations in response are largely due to differences in disposition kinetics of the drugs. This implies that a drug has the same range of therapeutic plasma concentrations, once defined, in the different species. When a drug is administered by the oral route, the rate and extent of its absorption from the gastrointestinal (GI) tract are likely to vary, in particular between monogastric and ruminant animals. Consequently, by influencing the plasma concentrations attained, drug absorption can contribute to species variations in the response to a given dose.

PASSAGE OF DRUGS ACROSS BIOLOGIC MEMBRANES. Absorption and distribution of a

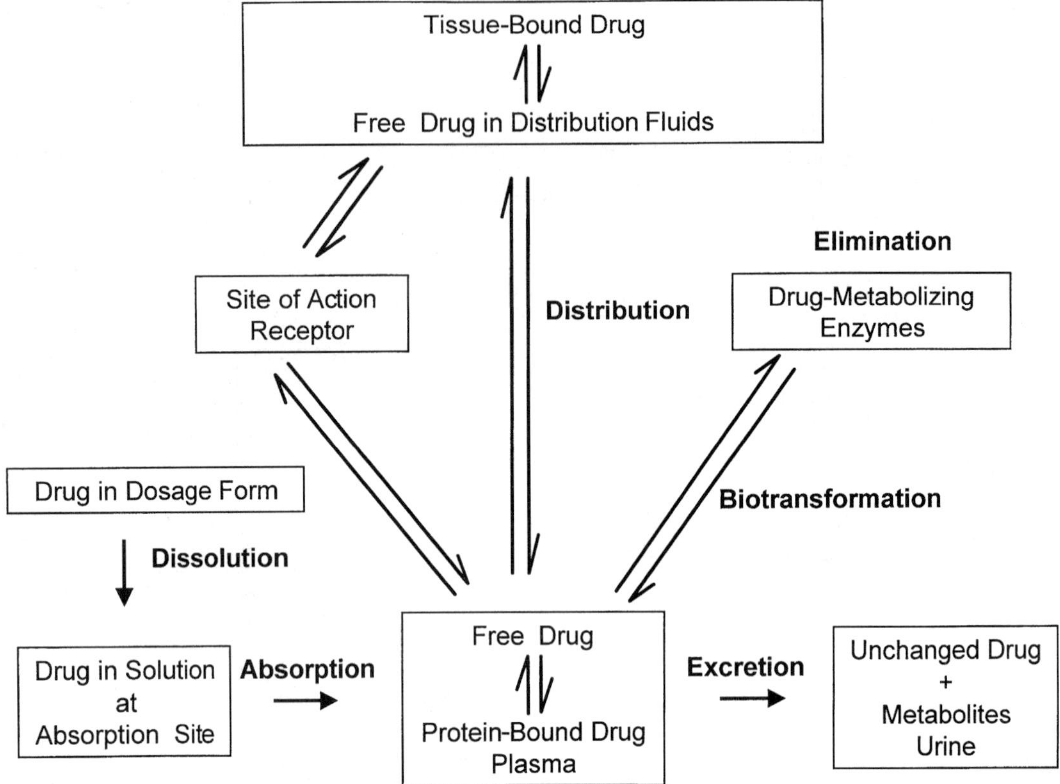

FIG. 3.1—Schematic representation of various processes that determine duration of drug action.

drug influence the concentration attained in the immediate vicinity of its receptor sites, while biotransformation (metabolism) and excretion are responsible for terminating action of the drug. The interrelationship of the various processes that determine duration of drug action is shown in Fig. 3.1. Either directly or indirectly, all these processes involve passage of drugs across membranes. It is important, therefore, to consider briefly the general nature of the biologic membrane and mechanisms by which drugs traverse this cellular barrier.

Nature of Biologic Membranes. Biologic membranes may be viewed as fluid mosaics of functional units composed of lipoprotein complexes (Dowben 1969). The characteristic feature of cell membranes is a bilayer of amphipathic phospholipid molecules, oriented perpendicular to the plane of the membrane, with polar head groups aligned at both surfaces and long hydrocarbon chains extending inward, forming a continuous hydrophobic phase (Benet et al. 1996). Individual lipids can move laterally, endowing the membrane with fluidity, flexibility, imperviousness to polar molecules, and high electrical resistance. The lipid molecules can even flip from one bilayer of the membrane to the other. In this model, proteins integral to the membrane are a heterogeneous set of globular molecules, each arranged in an amphipathic structure, i.e., with their ionic and highly polar groups located largely on membrane surfaces in contact with the extra- and intra-cellular aqueous media and with their nonpolar residues sequestered from contact with water in the membrane interior. These proteins are partially embedded in a discontinuous, fluid bilayer of phospholipids that forms the matrix of the mosaic. Aqueous channels appear to be present in the core of the globular intrinsic (integral) proteins and may be gated (i.e., channels may open and close) by conformational changes in the proteins. Extrinsic proteins are bound to exposed surfaces of the intrinsic proteins by electrostatic or hydrophobic interactions, but they are not involved in lipid-protein interactions critical to the membrane structure and its functions. Cell membranes are approximately 8 nm thick.

Drug Passage across Membranes. Drug molecules move across membranes either by passive transfer or by active participation of the membrane (Benet et al. 1996). In passive transfer, the membrane behaves as an inert lipoid-pore boundary, and drug molecules traverse this barrier either by diffusing through the lipid region or, if of sufficiently small size, by filtering through the postulated aqueous pores (channels). Both nonpolar lipid-soluble compounds and polar water-soluble substances that possess sufficient lipid solubility can cross the predominantly lipoid plasma membrane by passive diffusion. Rate of translocation (diffusion) is directly proportional to concentration gradient across the membrane and lipid-to-water partition coefficient of the drug. Passive diffusion, characterized by movement of drug molecules down a concentration gradient without the cellular expenditure of energy, is by far the most important mechanism for passage of drugs across membranes.

Filtration is a common mechanism for transfer of many small, water-soluble, polar, and nonpolar substances. The apparent diameter of membrane channels differs among various body membranes. Channels in the capillary endothelial membrane are large (4–8 nm depending on capillary location), while those in the intestinal epithelium and most cell membranes are only about 0.4 nm in diameter. Drug permeation through aqueous channels is important in renal excretion (glomerular filtration), removal of drugs from the cerebrospinal fluid (CSF) (arachnoid villi), and passage of drugs across the hepatic sinusoidal membrane.

In terms of drug distribution, penetration into extracellular fluid of the brain and CSF is similar to diffusion into intracellular fluid elsewhere in the body. Capillaries of the brain are unlike the fenestrated (porous) capillaries in muscle and most other tissues; their endothelial cells are joined one to another by continuous tight intercellular junctions. Passage of a drug from cerebral circulation into brain extracellular fluid can take place only by diffusion through capillary endothelial cells (blood-brain barrier). In the choroid plexus, capillary endothelial cells have open intercellular junctions, but choroidal epithelial cells are in close apposition to one another. For a drug to enter CSF from the systemic circulation, it must diffuse through the choroidal epithelial cells (blood-CSF barrier). Likewise, the penetration of drugs into aqueous humor of the eye involves diffusion through the blood-aqueous barrier. The capacity of drugs to penetrate these barriers may be increased in the presence of fever and certain inflammatory conditions.

The pH Partition Hypothesis. Most drugs are weak organic acids or bases and exist in solution as both nonionized and ionized forms. The nonionized form is usually more lipid-soluble and can more readily diffuse across the cell membrane to achieve the same equilibrium concentration on either side. In contrast, the ionized moiety is often virtually excluded from transmembrane diffusion because of its low lipid solubility.

The degree of ionization of an organic electrolyte depends on its pK_a value and the pH of the environment. For an acid this is

$$\%\ \text{ionized} = \frac{100}{1 + \text{antilog}\ (pK_a - pH)} \qquad (3.1)$$

and for a base,

$$\%\ \text{ionized} = \frac{100}{1 + \text{antilog}\ (pH - pK_a)} \qquad (3.2)$$

The pK_a value, the negative logarithm of the acidic ionization (or dissociation) constant, is a constant for an acid or a base. The majority of therapeutic agents have pK_a values between 3 and 11 and exist accordingly as both nonionized and ionized forms within the range of physiologic pH. The ratio of nonionized to ionized drug at a given pH can be calculated from the Henderson-Hasselbalch equation. For an acid this is

$$pH - pK_a = \log \frac{(\text{conc. ionized})}{(\text{conc. nonionized})} \qquad (3.3)$$

and for a base,

$$pH - pK_a = \log \frac{(\text{conc. nonionized})}{(\text{conc. ionized})} \qquad (3.4)$$

From Eqs. 3.3 and 3.4 it is apparent that when pH and pK_a values are equal, 50% of the drug exists in either form. When the pH is one unit below the pK_a, an acid is 9% ionized and a base, 91%. In the case of an acid (vice versa for a base), each one pH unit change to the acid side of the pK_a results in a tenfold increase in nonionized form relative to ionized form; the converse occurs when shifts to the alkaline side of the pK_a are made. Because of the relationship between pH and degree of ionization, a relatively small pH change will produce a large change in the proportion of drug present in nonionized form, particularly when the pH of the solution is numerically close to the pK_a of the weak organic electrolyte.

Distribution of a weak electrolyte is usually determined by its pK_a value and pH gradient across the membrane. The nonionized moiety diffuses across the membrane at a rate determined by its lipid solubility. Because of the pH difference on either side of the membrane, the degree of ionization will differ. At equilibrium, there will be a higher total (nonionized plus ionized) concentration of drug on the side of the membrane where the degree of ionization is greater. This phenomenon is known as the ion-trapping mechanism. To illustrate the effect of pH on distribution of drugs, partitioning of a weak organic acid (pK_a 4.4) between plasma (pH 7.4) and gastric juice (pH 1.4) is depicted in Fig. 3.2. It is assumed that the gastric mucosal membrane behaves as a simple lipoidal barrier permeable only to the lipid-soluble, nonionized form of the acid. At equilibrium, the total drug concentration ratio between plasma and gastric juice would be approximately 1000:1. Accordingly, weak organic acids such as aspirin (pK_a 3.5), phenylbutazone (pK_a 4.4), sulfadiazine (pK_a 6.4), and phenobarbital (pK_a 7.4) are well absorbed from the GI tract of dogs and cats. Likewise, the acidic urinary reaction of the carnivorous species promotes passive reabsorption of acidic drugs (pK_a values between 3.0 and 7.2) from the distal portion of the nephron. Conversely, urinary alkalinization will

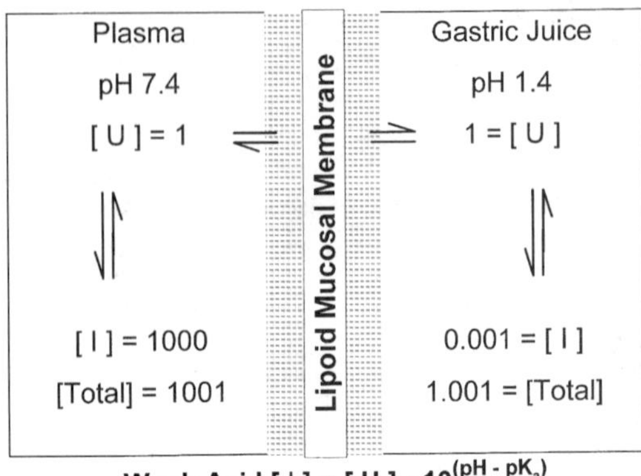

FIG. 3.2—Effect of pH gradient on distribution of a weak organic acid (pK_a 4.4) between blood plasma (pH 7.4) and gastric juice (pH 1.4). In this figure, [I] and [U] represent the concentrations of the ionized and nonionized fractions of the drug, respectively. A dynamic equilibrium exists between ionized and nonionized drug.

promote their excretion by favoring ionization of organic acids. Although the excretion rate of several drugs may be altered by changing urinary pH, this technique will have little clinical application in management of overdosage unless a significant fraction of the dose is excreted unchanged (unmetabolized) as the parent drug in the urine. It may be significant that weak organic bases (alkaloidal substances), tetracyclines, and macrolide antibiotics, administered parenterally, diffuse passively into the rumen of cattle and sheep and into the colon of horses as part of their usual distribution pattern. At these important sites of microbial digestion, those drugs may interfere with functioning of microorganisms or be inactivated by them. Basic drugs (narcotic analgesics, phenothiazine tranquilizers, ketamine, xylazine, diazepam, antiarrhythmic agents) tend to concentrate in fluids that are acidic relative to plasma, such as intracellular fluid (pH 7.0).

The theoretical equilibrium concentration ratio ($R_{x/y}$) of a drug on opposite sides of a biologic membrane may be calculated according to the following equations (Jacobs 1940). For an acid this is

$$R_{x/y} = \frac{1 + 10^{(pH_x - pK_a)}}{1 + 10^{(pH_y - pK_a)}} \quad (3.5)$$

i.e.,

$$R_{x/y} = \frac{1 + \text{antilog}\,(pH_x - pK_a)}{1 + \text{antilog}\,(pH_y - pK_a)} \quad (3.6)$$

and for a base,

$$R_{x/y} = \frac{1 + 10^{(pK_a - pH_x)}}{1 + 10^{(pK_a - pH_y)}} \quad (3.7)$$

The validity of these equations for predicting passage of antimicrobial agents from the systemic circulation into the milk of lactating animals is well documented (Table 3.1). It has been shown that only the lipid-soluble nonionized moiety of an organic electrolyte in the water phase of blood plasma diffuses into milk (Rasmussen 1966). This indicates that the mammary gland epithelium behaves as a lipoidal membrane that separates blood of pH 7.4 from milk, which has a somewhat lower pH value (normal range is 6.5–6.8). In normal lactating cows, weak acids give milk ultrafiltrate to plasma ultrafiltrate concentration ratios less than or equal to unity; organic bases, excluding aminoglycoside antibiotics (which are polar in nature), attain concentration ratios greater than one. In mastitis, the milk pH reaction may be increased up to 0.7 of a pH unit, so higher concentration ratios than those in normal animals will be obtained for the organic acids (Ziv et al. 1983). Choice of antimicrobial agent for systemic therapy of mastitis should be based upon susceptibility of the infecting microorganism to the drug and upon the active drug concentration that can be attained in the milk with usual dosage. The former can be determined in vitro, and the latter may be predicted by Eq. 3.5 or 3.7.

Carrier-Mediated Transport. Carrier-mediated transport across membranes implies a rapidly reversible interaction between components of the membrane and the transported substance. This kind of transport shows relative selectivity toward the chemical nature of the substance moved across the membrane. Since a carrier (membrane component) is involved in transport, the process is saturable, and substances of a similar chemical nature may compete for the carrier. Competitive inhibition is a characteristic of carrier-mediated transport.

Active transport and facilitated diffusion are both carrier-mediated processes but differ in that the former requires direct expenditure of energy. The rapid transfer into urine and bile of drugs that are strongly acidic or basic as well as most drug metabolites takes place by active transport. It is also responsible for removal of certain drugs (e.g., penicillins) from the central nervous system (CNS) at the choroid plexus. This is now believed to be accomplished through reverse transport from the CSF back into the bloodstream by the *p*-glycoprotein pump (Miyama et al. 1998). Generation of the pH gradient across a biologic membrane is an active process.

Facilitated diffusion is neither an energy-dependent process nor does it move substances against a concentration gradient. Transport is facilitated, however, by attachment to a carrier and is more rapid than simple diffusion. Entry of glucose into most cells takes place by facilitated diffusion (enhanced by insulin), but its passage across the GI mucosa and excretion by proximal renal tubular cells are active processes.

Most inorganic ions are sufficiently small to penetrate membranes pores, but their concentration gradient across the cell membrane is generally determined by the transmembrane potential (e.g., chloride ion) or by active transport (e.g., sodium and potassium ions). The

TABLE 3.1—Passage of antimicrobial agents from the systemic circulation into milk

Drug	pK_a	Milk pH	Concentration ratio (milk ultrafiltrate:plasma ultrafiltrate)		Reference
			Theoretical	Experimental	
Organic acids					
Benzyl penicillin (G)	2.7	6.8	0.25	0.13-0.26	Ziv et al. 1973
Cloxacillin	2.7	6.8	0.25	0.25-0.30	Ziv et al.1973
Ampicillin	2.7, 7.2	6.8	0.26	0.24-0.30	Ziv et al 1973
Cephaloridine	3.4	6.8	0.25	0.24-0.28	Ziv et al. 1973
Sulfadimethoxine	6.1	6.6	0.20	0.23	Stowe and Sisodia 1963
Sulfamethazine	7.4	6.6	0.58	0.59	Rasmussen 1958
Organic bases					
Tylosin	7.1	6.8	2.0	3.5	Ziv and Sulman 1973a
Lincomycin	7.6	6.8	2.83	2.50–3.60	Ziv and Sulman 1973b
Trimethoprim	7.6	6.5–6.8	2.8–5.3	2.90–4.90	Rasmussen 1970
Erythromycin	8.8	6.8	3.9	8.7	Rasmussen 1959
Kanamycin	(7.8)	6.8	3.1	0.60–0.80	Ziv and Sulman 1974a
Amphotericin					
Oxytetracycline		6.5–6.8		0.75	Ziv and Sulman 1974b

Note: Individual references should be consulted for the design of each experiment. It is important to know the method of drug administration, since equilibrium will not be established after a single IV injection.

potassium-sustaining diuretic agents appear to inhibit sodium-potassium exchange mechanisms in the distal nephron (specifically, the cortical collecting tubules) either by competitively antagonizing tubular action of aldosterone (e.g., spironolactone) or by interfering directly with tubular transport of these cations (triamterene, amiloride).

DRUG ADMINISTRATION. For a drug to act and produce its characteristic systemic effects, it must first be absorbed and then attain an effective concentration at its site of action. Drug absorption is generally defined as passage of the drug from its site of administration into the bloodstream. Drugs are administered in prepared dosage forms called drug products rather than as raw drug substances. The drug product contains a certain amount of the pharmacologically active drug substance(s) incorporated into a dosage form. The dosage form and route of administration can influence the selectivity of a drug product and thereby its clinical indications. The absorption process is governed by solubility of the dosage form, route of administration, and certain physicochemical properties of the drug substance. A balance is needed between water solubility (necessary for the drug to dissolve in the intestinal fluid and for distribution in the extracellular fluids of the body) and the lipid solubility required to enhance membrane transit across the GI tract as well as other membranes in the body.

A drug can be given either orally (by mouth) or by a parenteral route when systemic effects are desired. Parenteral administration indicates that the GI tract is bypassed and the drug is given by injection or inhalation (as in the case of inhalant anesthetics). Topical application and intramammary and intrauterine infusions are employed when local effects are sought. A variable degree of drug absorption takes place from these sites of administration, the extent of which depends largely on the formulation of the preparation administered and also on the drug itself.

Parenteral Administration. The major routes of parenteral administration are intravenous (IV), intramuscular (IM), and subcutaneous (SC). Other parenteral routes include tissue infiltration and intra-articular, subconjunctival, and epidural injections, which are used when localized action is sought. Parenteral injection necessitates that strict asepsis be maintained to avoid infection.

IV Injection. Injection of a drug solution directly into the bloodstream gives a more predictable concentration of the drug in plasma and produces immediate plasma concentrations which can produce a pharmacologic response. This is true because the entire dose of the drug is administered directly into the systemic bloodstream rather than being administered extravascularly and requiring the drug to be absorbed from the injection site into the systemic circulation. Another advantage of the intravascular route is that, by controlling the infusion rate, the veterinarian can control the rate of introduction of a drug into systemic circulation, and hence the effects may be immediately titrated (i.e., administering a drug to effect). IV injection should be performed slowly, except in special circumstances. Induction of anesthesia by rapid introduction into the bloodstream of a small dose of thiopental (thiobarbiturate) as an IV bolus is a special application of IV drug administration. Rapid penetration of the blood-brain and blood-CSF barriers by this lipophilic thiobarbiturate allows an almost immediate onset of anesthesia.

The duration of anesthetic effect is related mainly to redistribution of the drug from highly perfused CNS and visceral organs to the less well perfused muscle and other tissues. In some instances, as in induction of surgical anesthesia with pentobarbital in dogs and small ruminant species, the exact dose is not predetermined but the amount of drug administered is determined by the response of the animal. Certain irritating and hypertonic solutions can be given only by the IV route. One must ensure that the tip of the needle is in the lumen of the vein, so that the drug solution can be injected freely without causing either intimal or perivascular damage. Drugs in an oily vehicle or drug suspensions should not be given by the IV route.

Continuous IV infusion is an effective technique for achieving and maintaining steady-state concentration of a drug. A particular infusion rate is determined simply by fixing the rate of flow and concentration of drug in the infusion solution. While the rate of infusion determines the steady-state concentration achieved, time taken to reach the steady state is determined solely by the value of the overall elimination half-life of the drug (see the section below on quantitating drug elimination). The more rapidly a drug is eliminated (i.e., the shorter the half-life of the drug), the shorter the time required to achieve a steady state. To immediately establish the desired concentration, the classic procedure is to administer a loading dose as an IV bolus and at the same time start infusing the drug at a constant rate.

Although the IV route has many advantages, it is potentially the most dangerous route of drug administration. Great care must be exercised in computing the total dose to be administered (this applies to all parenteral routes) and rate of injection. Furthermore, rapid IV injection will result in transiently high concentrations in the bloodstream, and hence other tissues, enhancing the likelihood of acute toxicities (among the most important of which are CNS toxicities).

Extravascular Administration. Absorption of most drugs from IM and SC injection sites is rapid when given as aqueous solutions; the peak concentration in plasma is usually attained within 30 minutes. The rate of drug absorption is determined mainly by the vascularity of the injection site. However, other factors that affect the rate of drug absorption include the drug concentration in parenteral solution, the degree of ionization and lipid solubility of the nonionized form, and area of the absorbing surface to which the drug is exposed. Differences in drug absorption may exist not only between IM and SC injection sites but also between various IM locations. As an example, absorption of atropine, scopolamine, and glycopyrrolate was more rapid when administered IM to humans in the deltoid muscle compared with the gluteal region (Ali-Melkkila et al. 1993). A drug may influence its own rate of absorption and uptake of another drug administered simultaneously if it alters the blood supply or capillary permeability at the injection site. Addition of epinephrine, usually to give a final concentration of 1:100,000, to solutions of local anesthetics (procaine, lidocaine) is a good example. By causing local vasoconstriction (α-adrenoceptor activation), it delays absorption of the local anesthetic and thereby prolongs duration of analgesia, decreases the amount of anesthetic required, and lessens the danger of systemic toxicity.

The assumption that drugs are completely available systemically from all parenteral products injected intramuscularly is invalid, as shown for diazepam (Gamble et al. 1973), digoxin (Greenblatt et al. 1973), and florfenicol (Lobell et al. 1994; Soback et al. 1995). Incomplete availability may be attributed to low solubility of a drug at the pH of the tissue or to a damaging effect caused by the preparation at the injection site. Certain parenteral preparations (droperidol-fentanyl, ketamine) cause pain when injected intramuscularly, which can only be attributed to their formulation.

Sustained-release preparations, mostly of antimicrobial agents, are designed to give long duration of therapeutically effective plasma drug concentrations, e.g., procaine penicillin G (buffered aqueous suspension or in oil containing aluminum monostearate), amoxicillin trihydrate (aqueous suspension), oxytetracycline base in 2-pyrrolidone, and tilmicosin phosphate. The prolonged action provided by these preparations is due to their limited rate of absorption, which may be attributed to slow dissolution and/or absorption of the drugs. Formulation of sustained-release preparations must be such that their IM injection will not cause significant tissue damage with residual levels persisting at the site of administration at the time the food-producing animals go to slaughter (Nouws et al. 1990). The main disadvantages are loss of flexibility in dosage, but this is often offset by the tremendous added convenience of these products for the practicing food-animal veterinarian and by the reduction in animal stress associated with repeated capture and restraint.

Extremely slow absorption can be achieved by incorporating an insoluble drug into a compressed pellet or polymer suitable for SC implantation. Several steroid hormones (desoxycorticosterone acetate, trenbolone acetate, testosterone) are effectively administered in this manner. This is the basis for hormonal implants placed in the ear of feedlot cattle to improve feed efficiency and promote weight gain.

Percutaneous Absorption. The ability of a drug, applied topically as a dermatologic preparation, to be absorbed through the skin depends on three consecutive events. It must first dissolve and be released from the vehicle, then penetrate the keratin layer (stratum corneum) and cells of the epidermis, and finally be taken up by the capillary blood supply. Since absorption takes place by passive diffusion, lipid solubility is the most important physicochemical property of the drug. Concentration of a drug in its formulation is an obvious factor influencing its absorption. In terms of the vehicle, drug absorption is enhanced from an oil in water emulsion base, e.g., aqueous cream, which contains the anionic surface-active agent sodium lauryl sulfate. Surfactants increase skin penetration of water-soluble substances, possibly by increasing the permeability of the skin to water. Dimethyl sulfoxide, a skin irritant in humans, is a sorption promoter that passes rapidly through the stratum corneum (Ponec et al. 1990; Sodicoff et al. 1990) and has been found to accelerate penetration through the skin of water, fluocinolone acetonide, salicylic acid, and other substances. The percutaneous absorption of corticosteroids is also increased by so-called occlusive dressings (e.g., polyethylene). Since the stratum corneum is the barrier to skin penetration, presence of a de-epithelialized surface permits absorption of substances that are poorly absorbed through intact skin. Toxic effects may sometimes follow percutaneous absorption of lipid-soluble substances such as pesticides in an organic solvent.

When a skin infection is located in the deeper layers of the epidermis or in the dermis, systemic therapy with an antibacterial or antifungal agent is often more effective than topical application. Based on culture and sensitivity alone amoxicillin is often the antibiotic considered first for such infections, but it is worth considering other agents with good tissue-penetrating capacity (clindamycin, erythromycin, lincomycin, trimethoprim/sulfadiazine) for treatment of deep-seated or persistent dermatoses. Mycotic disease of the skin, hair, claws, and nails caused specifically by *Microsporum*, *Epidermophyton*, or *Trichophyton* species responds well to oral dosage with griseofulvin (using micronized preparations), provided the drug is given for an adequate time.

Agents that are primarily used topically for their local action are discussed elsewhere in this text.

Pulmonary Absorption. Gaseous and volatile liquid anesthetic agents, given by inhalation, are rapidly absorbed into the systemic circulation by diffusing across the pulmonary alveolar epithelium. Inhalant anesthetics are highly soluble in lipids but differ widely in their blood solubility (blood/gas partition coefficient) and blood/brain partitioning. These properties determine the rate of induction, ease with which level or depth of anesthesia can be changed, and speed of recovery. With agents of high blood solubility (halothane, methoxyflurane) these processes, like the equilibration in body water, take place slowly. The converse situation holds true for an agent of very low blood solubility (nitrous oxide). Blood solubility of an inhalant anesthetic also determines the extent to which the physiologic parameters of pulmonary ventilation (high-solubility agents) and cardiac output (low-solubility agents) influence rates of induction and recovery in clinical anesthesia. Both physiologic parameters influence the induction of and recovery from halothane anesthesia, which has an intermediate blood solubility.

Drug Administration by the Oral Route. Although some oral solutions, either aqueous or elixirs, and suspensions are available commercially, most oral dosage forms are solids and include the tablet, bolus for large animals, pellet, capsule, and a variety of specialized sustained-release products for ruminants.

Before entering the systemic circulation, a drug administered as a solid dosage form must undergo three events: release from the dosage form, diffusion and/or transport across the GI mucosal barrier into the portal circulation, and passage through the liver (Fig. 3.3). Each of these events has the potential to decrease the amount of drug reaching the systemic circulation intact (unchanged); the net effect is reflected in the bioavailability profile.

Dissolution is the rate-limiting step that determines release of drug from a solid dosage form, and it frequently controls the rate of drug absorption. The dissolution process can be enhanced by administering the drug in salt form (phenytoin sodium, propranolol hydrochloride) or by decreasing the particle size, oftentimes using a technique called micronization (griseofulvin, spironolactone). Following its dissolution, the drug in solution must be stable in the environment within the stomach (reticulorumen) and small intestine and must be sufficiently lipid-soluble to diffuse through the mucosal barrier to enter the hepatic portal venous blood. A drug that is stable (neither chemically nor enzymatically inactivated) in GI fluids, with a sufficient degree of both water solubility and lipid-solubility, would be expected to be well absorbed. Penicillin V potassium, which is the potassium salt of the phenoxymethyl analog of penicillin G, is more stable in an acidic medium than the latter; therefore, a greater fraction of the dose should be available for absorption. In small animals, amoxicillin has far greater systemic availability (60–70%) than ampicillin (20–40%). To increase the systemic availability of ampicillin, the prodrug hetacillin (which is rapidly hydrolyzed to ampicillin in the bloodstream) was developed. Cephalexin is an acid-stable cephalosporin that, in contrast to cefazolin and cephalothin (parenteral cephalosporins), is well absorbed from the GI tract. This antibiotic is available as the monohydrate in several oral dosage forms. Erythromycin, administered as the acid-resistant estolate ester, is well absorbed from the small intestine. Oral preparations of all the tetracyclines are available, mostly as the hydrochloride salts. These antibiotics are adequately although incompletely absorbed and, because of their tendency to cause GI disturbances, should not be given to a fasting animal. Milk or milk products and antacids, however, impair absorption of tetracyclines. This interaction may be attributed to chelation or an increase in gastric pH. Systemic sulfonamides (sulfamethazine; sulfadiazine sulfamethoxazole and sulfadoxine, which are combined with trimethoprim) are well absorbed, whereas the enteric sulfonamide succinylsulfathiazole is poorly absorbed. The aminoglycoside antibiotics (neomycin, streptomycin, kanamycin, gentamicin), because of their low solubility in lipid, are poorly absorbed from the GI tract. As a consequence, administration of these polar antibiotics by the oral route should not even be considered in

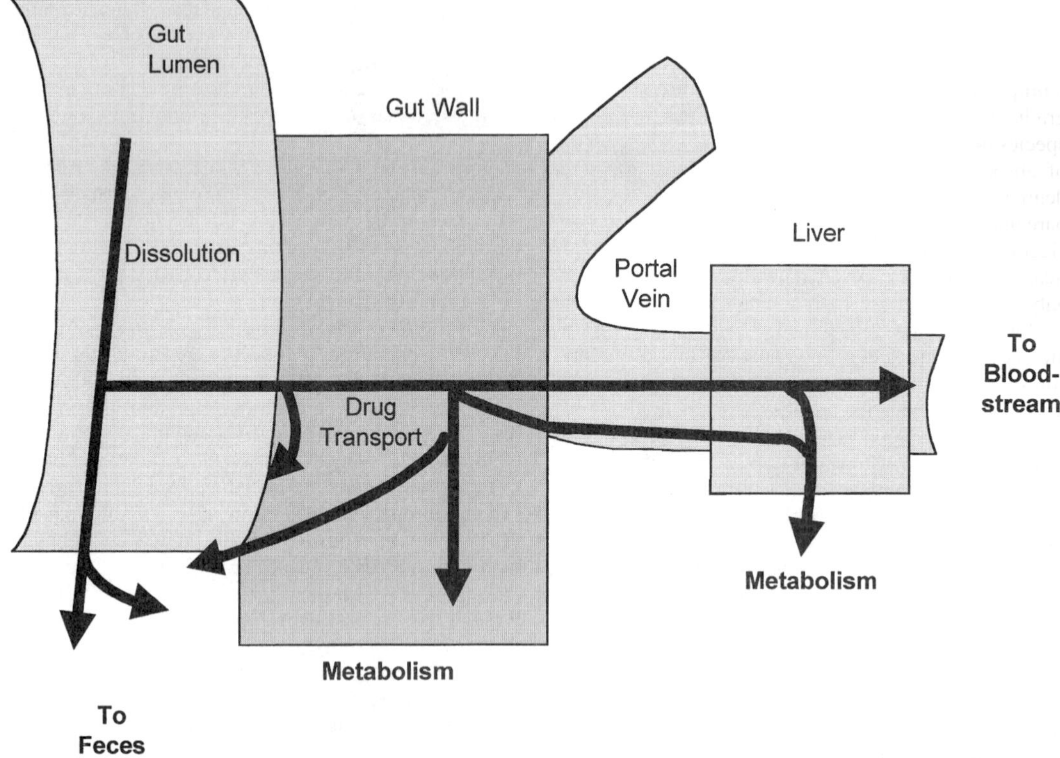

FIG. 3.3—A drug, given as a solid, encounters several barriers and sites of loss in its sequential movement during gastrointestinal absorption. Dissolution, a prerequisite to movement across the gut wall, is the first step. Incomplete dissolution or metabolism in the gut lumen or by enzymes in the gut wall is a cause of poor bioavailability. Removal of drug as it first passes through the liver further reduces bioavailability.

treatment of systemic and urinary tract infections. They are completely available systemically from parenteral preparations injected intramuscularly or subcutaneously.

Because of the extensive surface area and rich blood supply of its mucosal surface, the small intestine is the principal site of absorption for all drugs given orally, regardless of whether they are weak acids, weak bases, or neutral compounds. The rate of gastric emptying is therefore an important determinant of drug absorption. Gastric emptying depends on various physiologic factors such as autonomic and hormonal activity as well as the volume and composition of gastric contents. A change in gastric emptying or intestinal motility is of most importance with poorly soluble drugs and enteric-coated or slow-release formulations.

An effective pH of 5.3 in the microenvironment at the mucosal surface of the intestinal epithelial barrier, rather than the pH of intestinal contents (pH 6.6), is consistent with observations on the absorption of organic electrolytes. It has been shown that in the normal intestine, weak acids with pK_a values above 3 and bases with pK_a less than 7.8 are very well absorbed (Hogben et al. 1959). Changes in the intestinal blood flow will alter the rate of absorption of lipid-soluble drugs (Ther and Winne 1971; Rowland et al. 1973). Absorption of quaternary ammonium compounds such as the antimuscarinic agents propantheline and methscopolamine is slow and incomplete, which may explain their relatively selective antispasmodic effect. Absorption of loperamide is also minimal, relegating its opiate receptor actions to its local effects on intestinal motility.

Recent observations of relatively low oral absorption for compounds with physicochemical properties lending themselves to absorption across biological membranes (e.g., cyclosporine) have led to the discovery of a tandem system of a reverse transport system and metabolizing enzymes in the intestinal mucosa that significantly reduce oral absorption of such compounds. The substrate specificity for the *p*-glycoprotein pump (also known as the multiple drug resistance protein), oriented to pump drugs from the mucosa into the intestinal lumen, and that for the cytochrome P-450 isoenzyme found in the intestinal mucosa work in unison to significantly impair absorption of several therapeutic compounds (Zhang et al. 1998). The significance of this system is only now being elucidated.

Comparative Aspects of Drug Absorption. The pH gradients between plasma and GI fluids of various species play an important role in determining the extent of absorption of orally given drug products and the degree of distribution or excretion into the GI tract of parenterally administered drugs that are weak organic electrolytes. These gradients differ in different domesticated species and are largely dependent on dietary habits.

Domestic animals may be divided on the basis of dietary habit into herbivorous (horse, cow, sheep, goat, chicken, turkey), omnivorous (pig), and carnivorous (dog, cat) species. The physiology of digestion and drug absorption is, in general, similar in the pig, dog, and cat and not unlike that in humans. The rate of gastric emptying is probably the most important physiologic factor controlling drug absorption rate, since the small intestine is the principal site of absorption. Precise information on the physiologic factors that control absorption of drugs in horses is lacking. The horse is a continuous feeder and its stomach, which has a relatively small capacity, is seldom empty. The mean pH of gastric contents is usually higher in the horse (pH 5.5) than in the dog and pig (usual pH range is 3–4). However, unlike most species, neither the dog nor the cat are basal acid secretors; rather, their gastric pH varies from 1 to 6 based on the temporal relationship to feeding stimuli (Gupta and Robinson 1988). For this reason, dissolution of some types of formulations (i.e., those dependent upon an acidic environment for dissolution) may be drastically different in fasted dogs and cats compared with those administered the drug postprandially. Absorption of some drugs (e.g., phenylbutazone) administered orally to horses after feeding takes place mainly in the large intestine. The microbial digestion of polysaccharides, which takes place in the colon, is an essential digestive process in the horse. Disturbance of the microorganisms indigenous to this region of the digestive tract, resulting from either disease or antimicrobial therapy, can have serious consequences.

The principal feature of digestive physiology in the ruminant animal is that microbial fermentation takes place continuously in the reticulorumen. The forestomach contents vary from fluid to semisolid consistency, and the pH reaction is normally maintained within a relatively narrow range (pH 5.5–6.5) in spite of the high concentrations of volatile fatty acid produced. This is accomplished by buffers secreted in alkaline saliva (pH 8.0–8.4) and, it appears, directly by the forestomach epithelium. Despite the stratified squamous nature of its epithelial lining, the rumen has been shown to have considerable absorptive capacity (Phillipson and McAnally 1942; Masson and Phillipson 1951). After comminution by both microbial digestion and rechewing, the liquid portion of reticuloruminal contents, in which small particles of feed are suspended, is pumped by the omasum into the abomasum. Based on average values of salivary flow and volume of the rumen liquid pool (60 L in cattle, 4.5 L in sheep), the turnover rate for reticuloruminal fluid is estimated to be 2.0/day for cattle and 1.1–2.2/day for sheep (Hungate 1966). Reaction of abomasal contents does not vary much and is usually about pH 3 (Masson and Phillipson 1952).

Due to the large volume of ruminal fluid, a drug can attain only a relatively low concentration in this organ, whether it is given in solution or as a solid dosage form. This diluting effect may deter rate but not necessarily extent of absorption. The nonionized, lipid-soluble form of weak organic acids in particular should normally be well absorbed from the rumen. Indigenous microflora may inactivate certain drugs by metabolic transformations of a hydrolytic or reductive nature. Chronic oral dosage with an antimicrobial agent can suppress microflora activity and thereby disturb carbohydrate digestion, which is an essential function of the forestomach. Lipid-soluble, parenterally administered organic bases diffuse from the systemic circulation into ruminal fluid, in which they may become trapped by ionization, depending on their pK_a values. At pH reactions below the pK_a, acids exist mainly in the nonionized form, whereas bases are predominantly ionized. The concentration of a weak organic electrolyte in ruminal fluid is influenced by the dose administered, route of administration, lipid solubility and pK_a of the drug, relative rates of uptake from and passage into the ruminal fluid (both of which take place by nonionic diffusion), rate of salivary flow (for organic acids), extent of drug binding to plasma proteins, and efficiency of elimination (biotransformation and excretion) processes.

Quantitating Drug Absorption. The processes of absorption, distribution, metabolism, and excretion are often quantitated retrospectively so that dosage regimens that target therapeutic concentrations can be prospectively predicted. Quantitation of drug absorption includes both a rate component and an extent component.

One of the fundamental approaches is to quantitatively describe the plasma drug concentrations observed over time after one or more administered doses of a formulation. Mathematical or empirical curves can be fitted to the plasma concentrations over time. From those graphical representations of drug disposition over time, several useful parameters can be calculated. One of the most fundamental parameters is the area under the plasma concentration versus time curve (AUC), which is proportional to the systemic exposure to a drug. Graphically, plasma concentration is plotted on the Y-axis, and time is plotted on the X-axis (Fig. 3.4). The AUC may be calculated by the trapezoidal rule, with extrapolation to infinite time (Baggot 1977). By itself, the AUC has little relevance. However, the AUC can be used in the calculation of several more physiologically meaningful pharmacokinetic terms.

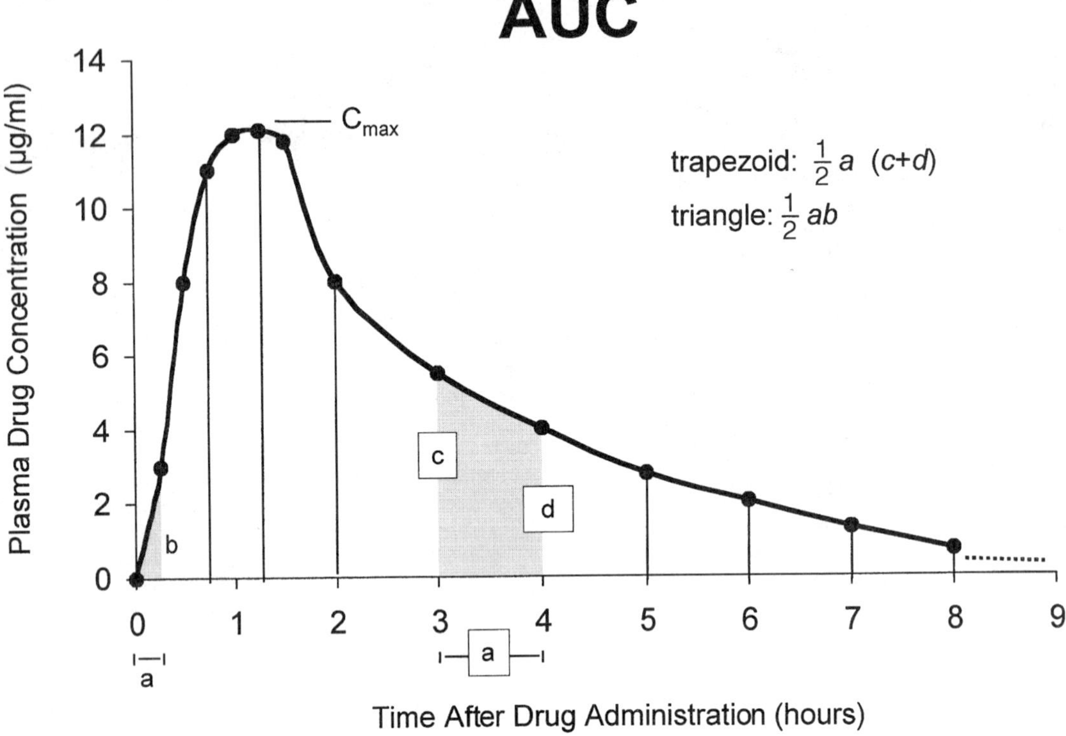

FIG. 3.4—The area under the concentration–time curve (AUC)is estimated by the sum of all the trapezoids and triangles bounded by the curve and is mathematically calculated as the integral of the curve.

A related term necessary for further calculations is the area under the first statistical moment curve (AUMC). This is defined as the area under the (plasma drug concentration · time) versus time curve. The Y-axis in this case is the product of the observed plasma concentration and the time after dosing that the plasma concentration was observed, whereas the X-axis is simply time after drug administration (Fig. 3.5).

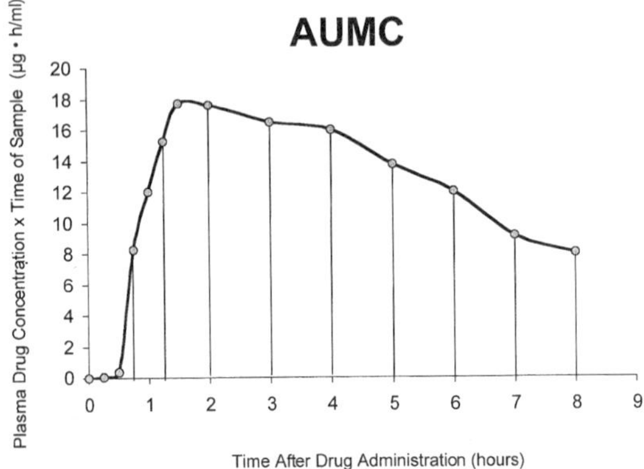

FIG. 3.5—The area under the moment curve is the integral of the curve plotting the product of concentration and time by the time the concentration was observed.

RATE OF ABSORPTION. An estimate of absorption rate of a drug from a particular dosage form is given by the time at which the peak is reached on the plasma concentration versus time curve. Remember, however, that absorption continues after peak concentration has been reached. Alternatively, rate of absorption can be characterized by the half-life of absorption, which is the time it takes for half of the drug waiting to be absorbed reaches the systemic circulation.

EXTENT OF ABSORPTION. Bioavailability is defined as the extent to which a drug administered as a particular dosage form enters the systemic circulation intact. This pharmacokinetic parameter is but the first of many factors determining the relationship between drug dosage and intensity of action. The usual technique for estimating the systemic availability (F) or extent of absorption of the drug employs the method of corresponding areas, which entails comparison of the total AUC obtained after administration via the oral or other nonvascular route with the AUC observed after IV administration of equal doses of

TABLE 3.2—Systemic availability of some drugs given orally to dogs

Drug (dosage form)	Dose	Systemic availability	Contributing factor(s)	Reference
	(mg/kg)	*(%)*		
Digoxin (tablet)	1 mg (total)	80	Dissolution	De Rick et al. 1979
Propranolol (tablet)	80 mg (total)	2–7	Hepatic metabolism	Kates et al. 1979
Lidocaine (solution)	10	15	Hepatic metabolism	Gugler et al. 1975
Salicylamide (solution)	30	22	Metabolism (intestinal wall and the liver)	Gugler et al. 1975
Levodopa (solid in gelatin capsules)	25	44	Metabolism (gastrointestinal lumen and/or intestinal wall)	Cotler et al. 1976
Sulfadimethoxine (suspension)	55	50	(Dissolution and hepatic metabolism?)	Baggot et al. 1976; Sams and Baggot 1977

the drug (in appropriate dosage forms) to the same animals:

$$F = AUC_{oral}/AUC_{IV} \quad (3.8)$$

By definition, IV injection of a drug substance represents complete systemic availability. If an IV preparation of the drug is not available, a reference formulation and route of administration (usually a well-established aqueous solution or elixir) may be used for comparison, in which case the relative bioavailability rather than absolute bioavailability is measured.

When the systemic availability of a drug is incomplete, the ratio of the areas (Eq. 3.8) at equal doses is less than 1.0 (or 100%). This situation could arise for a variety of reasons that may be physicochemical and/or physiologic in nature. They include poor dissolution of the drug product (solid dosage form) in GI fluids, instability or inactivation of the drug substance in luminal contents, poor passage through the mucosal (epithelial) barrier, and metabolism in either the intestinal mucosa or liver preceding entry of the drug into the systemic circulation (first-pass effect). Incomplete systemic availability of a drug due to first-pass effect could be misinterpreted as defective absorption. The systemic availability of some drugs from oral preparations administered to dogs is shown in Table 3.2.

High clearance by the liver is a characteristic of drugs that show a significant first-pass effect (lidocaine, propranolol, diazepam). Phenytoin has a short half-life and is poorly available systemically in dogs (Sanders and Yeary 1978). Wide variation in the bioavailability profile occurs among individual dogs given a single dose (30 mg/kg) of phenytoin in capsules. Time taken to reach the peak serum phenytoin concentration varies from 2 to 12 hours, and the peak concentration ranges from 2.66 to 7.90 g/mL. Appearance in the serum of a metabolite in large amounts indicates that the liver may be largely responsible for reducing systemic availability of phenytoin.

Species Variations in Bioavailability. Considerable variations in bioavailability of drugs from oral dosage forms are likely to exist, particularly between monogastric and ruminant species. When chloramphenicol is given orally (capsules) at the same dose (22 mg/kg) to ponies, goats, pigs, dogs, and cats, areas under the plasma concentration-time curves vary widely (Fig. 3.6). Based on the relative areas, the extent of chloramphenicol absorption is greatest in cats and decreases in the following order: cats, dogs and swine (approximately similar areas), ponies, goats. In goats, the antibiotic is rapidly inactivated by reduction of the aromatic nitro group to an arylamine by rumen microflora (Theodorides et al. 1968; De Corte-Baeten and Debackere 1978); consequently, chloramphenicol is not even available for absorption.

Interspecies variation became evident in a comparative study of salicylate (pK_a 3.0) absorption in which sodium salicylate contained in gelatin capsules was administered orally at three dose levels (18.5, 50, and 133 mg/kg) to dogs, swine, ponies, and goats (Davis and Westfall 1972). Inspection of the plasma salicylate concentration-time curves (Fig. 3.7) shows that a considerably larger amount of salicylate is available systemically in dogs and swine than in ponies and goats.

Critical comparison of dosage regimens for aspirin (pK_a 3.5) is most informative (Table 3.3). Although the dose (10 mg/kg) that will produce analgesia is the same for dogs and cats, the interval between successive doses to maintain analgesia is much longer for cats (Davis 1979). This can be attributed mainly to the slow rate of hepatic biotransformation of salicylate in the cat, since this species has a relative deficiency in microsomal glucuronyl transferase activity. A direct consequence of the difference in rate of salicylate metabolism is that the half-life ($t_{1/2}$) of the drug is four to five times longer in cats than in dogs. To maintain an effective plasma concentration of salicylate in cows, the dose (100 mg/kg) is far higher than in monogastric species and might be attributed to the diluting effect of ruminal fluid. The dosage interval, 12 hours, is based on the rate of salicylate absorption ($t_{1/2,a}$ [absorption half-life] = 2.9 hours) rather than on the elimination half-life ($t_{1/2}$ = 0.54 hour) of the drug.

Bioequivalence. Bioequivalence assessment relies on the concept that pharmaceutically equivalent drug

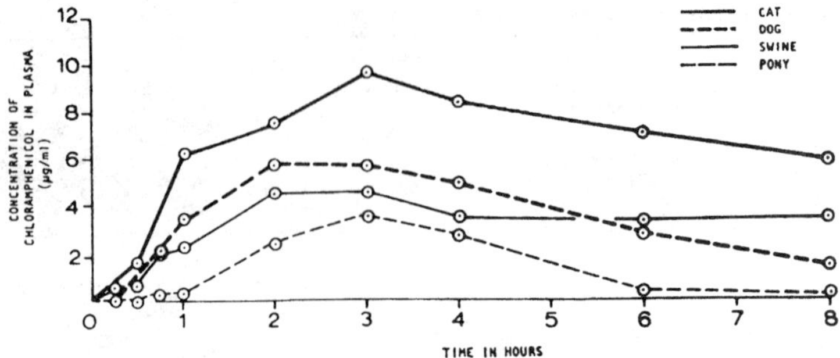

FIG. 3.6—The time course of chloramphenicol concentrations in plasma of domestic animals after oral administration of chloramphenicol (22 mg/kg) in capsules. The drug was undetectable in plasma of goats. Each point represents the mean drug concentration determined in 4 cats or dogs and 8 swine, ponies, and goats (Davis et al. 1972).

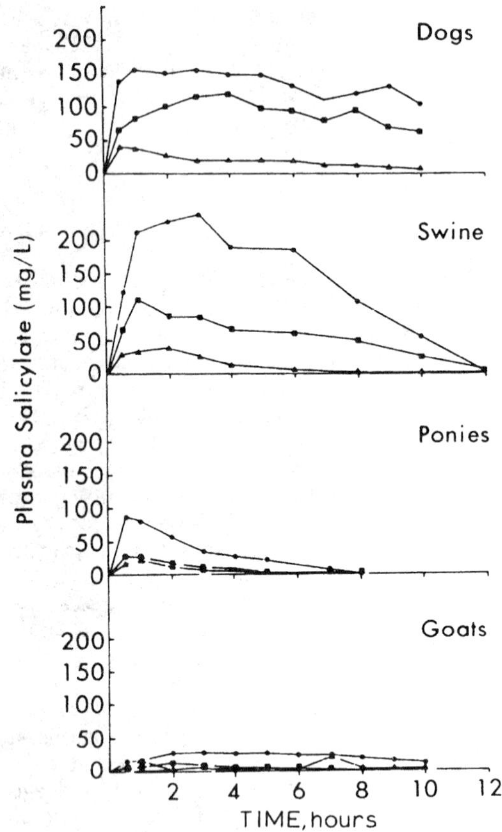

FIG. 3.7—Species differences in absorption of sodium salicylate after oral administration of the drug contained in gelatin capsules. Three dose levels (18.5, 50, and 133 mg/kg) were studied. Data points represent means from at least 4 animals (Davis and Westfall 1972).

products which provide essentially equivalent plasma concentration profiles, in terms of rate and extent of absorption, will produce the same pharmacologic response (therapeutic effect). Two drug products are considered to be bioequivalent when the rates and extents of absorption of the active ingredient in the two products are statistically equivalent to each other according to predetermined criteria under controlled test conditions. The intended analysis should dictate the design of a bioequivalence study, since design constrains the analysis that can be performed. Comparison of the test product (often generic) with a reference product (often pioneer) is based on an estimate of relative bioavailability together with a measure of the uncertainty (variance) of the estimate. Certain parameters obtained from plasma concentration-time curves provide the best estimate of relative bioavailability. These parameters include AUC, observed peak plasma concentration (C_{max}), and time of the observed peak (t_{max}). The AUC, often estimated by the trapezoidal rule, measures extent of absorption. The C_{max} and t_{max} provide an indication of the rate of absorption. When designing bioequivalence studies, blood-sampling times should be selected to characterize C_{max} and t_{max} well, and sample collection should extend for a period that will enable complete description of the plasma concentration profile (from time of drug administration to limit of quantification of the drug). The latter ($AUC_{0\text{-}LOQ}$) should capture 90% of the total AUC extrapolated to infinite time.

Statistical evaluation of bioequivalence studies should be based on confidence interval estimation rather than hypothesis testing (Westlake 1988). The confidence interval approach, using $1 - 2\alpha$ or 90%, is applied to the difference of individual parameters (AUC, C_{max}, and t_{max}). The entire 90% confidence interval should lie within the limits of –0.2 to +0.2 multiplied by the mean of that parameter for the reference product. The values of –0.2 and +0.2 are historical limits which may be constrained or expanded based on the characteristics of the drug (i.e., the safety margin or

TABLE 3.3—Dosage regimens for aspirin in different species

Species	Dose	Dosage interval	Steady-state plasma salicylate concentration	Reference
	(mg/kg)	*(hr)*	*(μg/mL)*	
Dog	10	12	—	Davis 1979
Cat	10	48	—	Davis 1979
Cow	100	12	40–60	Gingerich et al. 1975

TABLE 3.4—Body composition of various species (% liveweight)

Organ /tissue	Horse	Dog	Goat	Ox	Human
Blood	8.6		4.7	7.8	
Brain	0.21	0.51	0.29	0.06	2.0
Heart	0.66	0.82	0.48	0.37	0.47
Lung	0.89	0.89	0.88	0.71	1.4
Liver	1.30	2.32	.95	1.22	2.6
Spleen	1.11	0.26	0.25	0.16	0.26
Kidney	0.36	0.61	0.35	0.24	0.44
GI tract	5.8	3.9	6.4	3.8	1.7
GI contents	12.3	0.72	13.9	18.4	1.4
Skin	7.45	9.3	9.2	8.3	3.7
Muscle	40.1	54.5	45.5	38.5	40.0
Bone	14.6	8.7	6.3	12.7	14.0
Tendon	1.71	—	—	—	2.0
Adipose	5.1	—	—	18.9	18.1
Total weight, kg	308	16	39	620	70
Reference	Webb and Weaver 1979	Neff-Davis et al. 1975		Matthews et al. 1975	Int. Comm. Radiol. Prot. 1975

therapeutic window for the compound). Ratios of the parameters can also be used instead of differences, with the corresponding limits being 0.8 to 1.25.

DISTRIBUTION OF DRUGS. Drugs are conveyed throughout the body in the circulating blood and reach tissues of each organ in an amount determined by blood flow and blood concentration to the organ. Concentrations attained in the tissues depend upon the ability of the drug to penetrate capillary endothelium (influenced mainly by binding to plasma proteins) and diffuse across cell membranes.

The pattern of distribution describes the relative amount or concentration of drug that enters each organ and tissue. This can be found only by measuring drug concentrations in each part of the body (including the GI contents) at an appropriate time after its administration. Differences in body composition (Table 3.4), notably in the contribution of the GI tract with its contents and the skeletal muscle to the percentage of body weight, may largely account for species variations in drug distribution. In general, the kinetics of drug distribution in blood, organs, and tissues depend on dose and route of administration, lipid solubility of the drug, extent of binding to plasma proteins and extravascular tissue constituents, and blood flow rates through organs and tissues. Certain drugs such as thiopental undergo redistribution into poorly perfused tissues (e.g., fat and muscle) after initially attaining high concentrations in well-perfused tissues, such as brain, liver, and kidney. The biphasic distribution pattern of this drug can be attributed to differences in blood supply to various tissues.

An outline of the distribution pattern of a drug can be obtained by use of whole-body autoradiography. Uneven distribution of a drug within an organ such as the kidney (Whelton et al. 1971) can affect the success of therapy. Since critical areas for bacterial infection in the kidney are medullary and papillary tissues, knowledge of the intrarenal distribution pattern of antibiotics would greatly assist with selection of an antibacterial agent for treatment of pyelonephritis.

Plasma Protein Binding. Binding of a drug to plasma proteins restricts its distribution, thereby limiting its receptor availability, and can influence elimination of the drug from the body. Protein binding is a reversible interaction, which implies that the drug-protein complex serves as a circulating reservoir of potentially active drug. As an example, the principal active metabolite of ceftiofur, desfuroylceftiofur, is extensively protein bound, which serves to increase the half-life from the typical 1 hour observed with most cephalosporins to approximately 10 hours in cattle (Brown et al. 1991). Microbiological activity after ceftiofur has a similar prolonged half-life (Clarke et al. 1996). Among factors that can affect equilibrium between the free and bound drug are the protein concentration, drug affinity for the binding sites, presence of disease states that alter concentration of certain

TABLE 3.5—Plasma protein binding of drugs in dogs at therapeutic concentrations

Drug	Concentration	Extent of binding
	(μg/mL)	*(%)*
Sulfadimethoxine	100	81
Sulfisoxazole	100	68
Sulfadiazine	100	17
Chloramphenicol	20	39
Thiopental	10	75
Morphine	1	12
Propranolol	0.15–0.18	97
Chlorpromazine	0.1	94
Amphetamine	0.1	27
Digitoxin	0.05	89
Digoxin	0.01*	27

*This concentration exceeds therapeutic range for digoxin (cf. Table 3.19).

endogenous compounds (free fatty acids) in the plasma, and presence of other drugs or their metabolites. The plasma protein to which the majority of drugs bind is albumin. Each drug binds to a characteristic extent, usually expressed as a percentage of the total concentration of the drug in plasma (Table 3.5). Binding of different drugs in the same chemical class (sulfonamides, penicillins) can vary widely. The influence that an alteration of molecular structure can have on the percent of drug binding is clearly shown by comparing the binding of digitoxin (89%) and digoxin (27%) in dogs, since these complex molecules differ only in the presence of a hydroxyl group.

The binding capacity of plasma proteins for a drug (moles/g protein) and the dissociation constant of the drug-protein complex (moles/L) quantitatively describe the interaction. Values of these parameters characterizing the binding of some drugs in horse plasma are given in Table 3.6.

The extent of protein binding can be measured by in vitro techniques (equilibrium dialysis, ultrafiltration), which can be compared with the value obtained by measuring equilibrium concentrations of the drug in plasma and transcellular fluid collected simultaneously. Only the lipid-soluble, nonionized moiety of an organic electrolyte that is free (unbound) in the plasma can penetrate cell membranes, diffuse into transcellular fluids (cerebrospinal, synovial, ocular), and enter the milk. At equilibrium the concentration of drug in transcellular fluid will approximate free drug concentration in plasma, which may be only a fraction of total concentration in plasma. This relationship has been shown in vivo for penetration of amphetamine (Baggot et al. 1972) and diazepam (Kanto et al. 1975) into CSF and passage of cloxacillin and ampicillin (Howell et al. 1972) into synovial fluid. The same principle can be applied to the passage of weakly acidic (pK_a >9) and basic (pK_a <5) drugs as well as neutral molecules (chloramphenicol, digoxin) into milk and saliva. For most organic electrolytes the degree of ionization in milk (pH 6.5–6.8) and saliva (pH varies with species) will influence the final concentration attained.

Extensive (>80%) protein binding of a drug restricts its extravascular distribution and may either hinder or facilitate elimination, depending on the mechanism of the process. In terms of renal handling of drugs, protein binding decreases availability of a drug for glomerular filtration (a passive process) but does not interfere with carrier-mediated tubular excretion. Certain disease conditions, such as hypoalbuminemia (nephrotic syndrome) or the uremic state (chronic renal failure), and competition between drugs for albumin-binding sites (drug displacement effect, e.g., warfarin by phenylbutazone) can cause an increase in the percentage of free drug in plasma. Consequently, more is available for distribution to the site of action (as well as other tissues) and an enhanced pharmacologic response can result. Decrease in protein binding is likely to assume clinical importance only for drugs that are extensively bound (Table 3.7). Protein binding can be seen in perspective by considering the fraction in plasma compared with overall distribution of the drug in the body.

Conversely, conditions that increase the amount of protein in the extracellular fluid or that allow increased plasma protein leakage extravascularly (e.g., infection) can enhance total drug concentrations locally in the protein-rich fluid. Clarke et al. (1996) showed this for ceftiofur in infected tissue chambers.

Even though variation among species in protein binding of a number of drugs is statistically significant, classification of drug binding as extensive (>80%), moderate (50–80%), and low (<50%) generally negates interspecies variation; however, this is adequate for clinical purposes. Species variation in binding does not relate to total protein concentration in plasma (apart from avian species versus mammals) due to the excess amount of protein molecules to which drug molecules can bind, but may be attributed at least tentatively to

TABLE 3.6—Parameters describing quantitative aspect of drug-protein binding in horse plasma

Drug	Binding capacity	Dissociation constant	Reference
	(moles/g)	*(molar)*	
Penicillin G	39.0×10^{-6}	2.13×10^{-3}	Dürr 1976
Ampicillin	46.5×10^{-6}	22.70×10^{-3}	Dürr 1976
Oxytetracycline	3.9×10^{-6}	2.25×10^{-4}	Pilloud 1973a
Chloramphenicol	9.12×10^{-6}	5.07×10^{-4}	Pilloud 1973b
Sulfamethazine	12.99×10^{-6}	4.29×10^{-4}	Tschudi 1972
Sulfadimethoxine	9.77×10^{-6}	3.61×10^{-5}	Tschudi 1972

TABLE 3.7—Drugs that are extensively (>80%) bound to plasma proteins

Drug	Principal pharmacologic effect
Phenylbutazone*	Antiinflammatory
Warfarin*	Anticoagulant
Furosemide*	Diuretic
Digitoxin	Positive inotropic effect, heart rhythm stabilizer
Ceftiofur	Antimicrobial agent
Propranolol	β-adrenergic receptor blockade, antiarrhythmic
Quinidine	Antiarrhythmic, myocardial depressant
Phenytoin*	Anticonvulsant, antiarrhythmic
Diazepam*	Sedative, anticonvulsant
Valproate	Anticonvulsant

*Decreased binding in plasma of uremic patients causes an increase in the percentage of free (unbound) drug.

TABLE 3.8—Range of drug binding to plasma proteins in a variety of mammalian species

Drug	Range of binding (%)
Propranolol	88–99
Digitoxin	83–93
Phenytoin	73–85
Sulfisoxazole	65–86
Amphetamine	20–40
Digoxin	18–36
Morphine	12–34

Note: Total protein concentration in plasma of all mammalian species is within the range 6.0–8.5 g/mL.

differences in composition and conformation of plasma albumin. The range of plasma protein binding of some drugs at therapeutically relevant concentrations is given in Table 3.8 for various species. Species represented include the human, monkey, horse, cow or goat, dog, cat, and rabbit.

Quantitating Drug Distribution. Just as with drug absorption, the distribution of drugs in the animal can be quantified in terms of rate and extent of distribution by evaluation of plasma concentrations over time. However, such evaluation cannot determine the rates and extents of distribution to specific tissues without actually acquiring data over time in those tissues. Rather, the rate and extent of systemic distribution is defined as a weighted average of the rates and extents of distribution to specific tissues within the body.

RATE OF DISTRIBUTION. Plasma concentrations decline very rapidly shortly after administration of an IV dose. The rate of that decline is dependent upon the ability of the drug to distribute from the bloodstream into extracellular fluids and tissues. The rate of distribution can be described as a half-life of distribution, interpreted as the time it takes for 50% of the drug in the plasma to distribute outside of the bloodstream.

EXTENT OF DISTRIBUTION. The extent of distribution is described in terms of volumes of hypothetical fluid compartments, with larger volumes of distribution reflecting more extensive distribution from plasma into tissues. Recall that no relationship exists between distribution volumes for drugs and physiologic spaces. Rather, the value of Vd serves as a proportionality constant relating plasma concentration of a drug to total amount of drug in the body at any time after pseudodistribution equilibrium has been attained:

$$\text{Vd} = \frac{A_{B(t)}}{C} \tag{3.9}$$

where C_p and $A_B(t)$ are plasma concentration and amount of drug in the body respectively at time t. This pharmacokinetic term can be defined as the volume of fluid that would be required to contain the amount of drug in the body if it were uniformly distributed at a concentration equal to that in the plasma. While the volume of distribution provides an estimate of the extent of distribution of a drug, it does not distinguish between widespread distribution and high affinity (selective) binding with restricted distribution. The pattern of distribution must be related to both value of Vd and physicochemical properties of the drug (lipid solubility, ionic character of functional groups) that govern diffusion across biologic membranes and binding to tissues. One cannot tell in which tissue the drug concentrates by looking at the volume of distribution, but one can determine the fraction of drug that is outside the plasma (f_o):

$$f_o = A_{B(t)} - (C \cdot \text{V}_p) \tag{3.10}$$

where V_p is the plasma volume in the animal.

An estimate of the extent of distribution of a drug is given by the pharmacokinetic term, apparent volume of distribution (Vd, mL/kg), which can be calculated according to

$$\text{Vd}_{\text{area}} = \frac{D \cdot F}{\text{AUC} \cdot \beta} \tag{3.11}$$

where AUC represents the total area under the plasma drug concentration versus time curve from $t = 0$ to ∞, F is the bioavailability of the dose administered by that route of administration, D is the administered dose, and β represents the slope of the terminal disappearance portion of the plasma concentration-time profile when plotted as the natural logarithm of concentration (Y-axis) versus time (X-axis).

A more straightforward but less accurate method for calculating volume of distribution entails extrapolating the linear terminal phase of the drug disposition curve to its intercept on the ordinate (plasma drug concentration axis) and substituting this value (B, mg/L) in the expression

$$\text{Vd}_B = \frac{D \cdot F}{B} \tag{3.12}$$

Since the extrapolation method neglects the distribution phase of drug disposition, it is valid only for drugs that behave according to a one-compartment model (distribute almost instantaneously). Otherwise, this method gives an overestimate of the Vd value.

The volume of distribution at steady-state (Vd_{ss}) provides an estimate of drug distribution which is independent of elimination processes, and which is most useful for predicting plasma concentrations upon multiple dosing to a steady-state, or pseudo-equilibrium (Martinez 1998a). The Vd_{ss} is proportional to the amount of drug in the body versus the plasma drug concentration at steady-state. The following equation defines Vd_{ss}:

$$Vd_{ss} = \frac{D \cdot F \cdot \text{AUMC}}{\text{AUC}^2} \qquad (3.13)$$

All of the various volumes of distribution may be calculated from a plasma concentration-time profile. In general, Vd_B overestimates the true volume of distribution, and Vd_{area} is generally an overestimate relative to Vd_{ss}.

Species differences in volume of distribution, notably between monogastric (dogs, cats) and ruminant (cattle, sheep, goats) animals, have been found, particularly with lipid-soluble organic bases. Following parenteral administration, these drugs diffuse into ruminal liquor (in which they may become trapped by ionization) as part of their normal pattern of distribution. The colon of the horse, by acting similarly as a reservoir, can contribute to a value of Vd (in L/kg) intermediate between those found in small animals and ruminant species.

Knowledge of volume of distribution is required for calculating the dose that must be administered to provide a certain (therapeutic) concentration of drug in plasma (C_{ther}):

$$\underset{(\text{mg/kg})}{D} = \underset{(\text{mg/L})}{C_{ther}} \cdot \underset{(\text{L/kg})}{Vd_{area}/F} \qquad (3.14)$$

When the drug is administered by other than the IV route, its bioavailability (F) may be less than 1.0 and must be taken into account.

MECHANISMS OF DRUG ELIMINATION.

Mechanisms of drug elimination are biotransformation (metabolism) and excretion. Although it is usual for one mechanism to predominate, both hepatic metabolism and renal excretion are involved in elimination of most drugs. The fate of a drug is largely determined by certain of its physicochemical properties, specifically lipid solubility and degree of ionization. Lipid solubility appears to be a prerequisite for biotransformation of drugs by the hepatic microsomal enzyme system. Polar drugs and many drug metabolites are excreted by the kidneys. Widespread extravascular distribution, which is a feature of lipophilic organic bases, and selective tissue binding, such as localization of thiopental in body fat, reduce the rate of elimination of a drug by limiting its accessibility to eliminating organs (drug concentration in the blood flowing to the organs of elimination is very low). Influence of extensive plasma protein binding on elimination of a drug appears to be determined by renal and hepatic mechanisms involved in this process. Apart from the liver, metabolism of drugs takes place in blood plasma and lumen of the gut, where hydrolytic and reductive reactions may occur, as well as in other tissues (intestinal mucosa, kidney, lung). Plasma pseudocholinesterase, which varies in activity according to species, hydrolyzes drugs of widely different pharmacologic classes. An ester linkage is a feature of drugs that undergo hydrolysis. These include acetylcholine, succinylcholine, atropine, procaine, meperidine, aspirin to salicylate, ceftiofur to desfuroylceftiofur, and hetacillin to ampicillin. The selective toxicity of malathion (an organophosphate) for insects rests on the difference in metabolism of the drug between insects and mammals. Insects preferentially convert malathion to malaoxon, which is the effective pesticide, whereas mammals rapidly deesterify the compound to an inactive metabolite. Halogenated volatile anesthetics (halothane, methoxyflurane) are eliminated predominantly unchanged by the lungs (pulmonary excretion) but undergo some degree (5–20%) of metabolism in the liver. Although metabolism is the minor mechanism of their elimination, accumulation of metabolites, which can occur in patients with impaired renal function, can give rise to toxicity.

Drug Metabolism (Biotransformation). Drugs undergo metabolic changes in the body that are directed primarily toward formation of metabolites that have physicochemical properties favorable to their excretion. Products of biotransformation are generally less lipid-soluble and more polar in nature. The latter feature renders metabolites suitable for carrier-mediated excretion processes as well as more likely to be partitioned into the aqueous fluids of the body such as the bloodstream, rendering higher concentrations being presented to the organs of excretion (e.g., kidneys).

Elimination of drug by metabolic alteration can be either limited by the rate of presentation to the organs of biotransformation, or limited by the capacity of the enzymatic system involved in the biotransformation. For drugs that are presentation-limited, alterations in blood flow to the liver (or other organs responsible for metabolism) can dramatically alter the rate of alteration. Changes in the rate of metabolism of coumarin, a flow-rate limited xenobiotic, are predictive of liver blood flow in beagle dogs (Ritschel and Vachharajani 1993).

Drug metabolism has been generally divided into two types of reactions, termed phase I and phase II reactions (Fig. 3.8). The initial phase consists of reactions that can be classified as oxidative, reductive, and

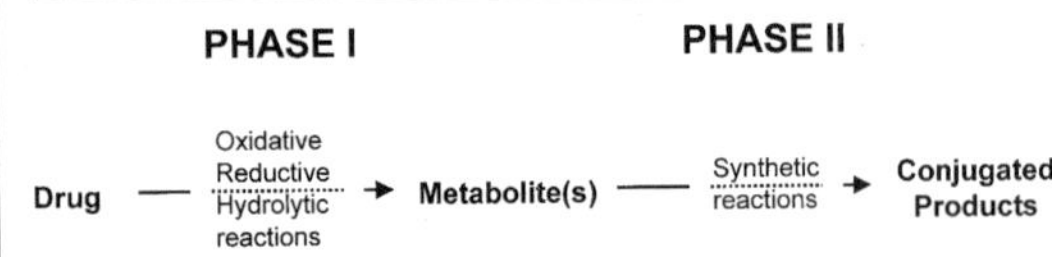

FIG. 3.8—The general pattern of drug metabolism. (Adapted from Williams 1967)

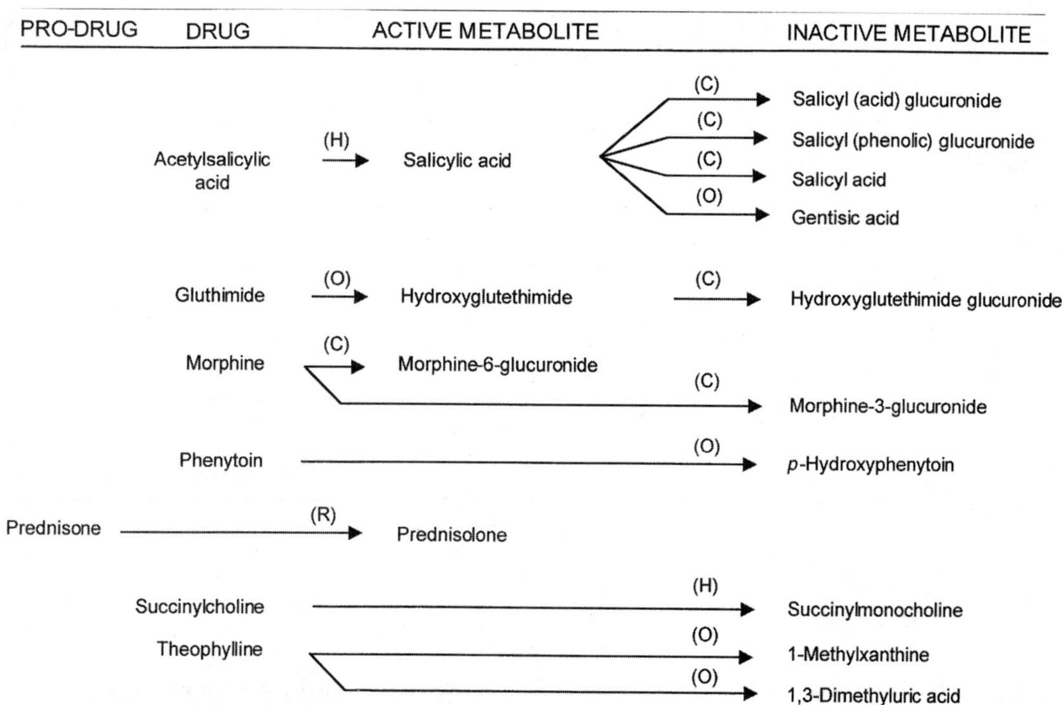

FIG. 3.9—Patterns of biotransformation of representative drugs. Only representative metabolic pathways are shown for some drugs. Inactive concentrations obtained following the therapeutic administration of the parent drug. (O) = oxidation; (R) = reduction; (H) = hydrolysis; (C) = conjugation.

hydrolytic, while the second phase includes the synthetic reactions (conjugations). Phase I transformations usually unmask or introduce into the drug molecule polar groups such as —OH, —SH, —COOH, and —NH_2. These functional groups enable the compound to undergo conjugation with endogenous substances such as glucuronic acid, acetate (acetylation), sulfate (sulfuric acid ester formation), and various amino acids (primarily glutathione, cysteine, and glycine). The drug conjugates formed are water soluble and almost invariably inactive pharmacologically (Fig. 3.9). The most likely metabolic pathway can be qualitatively predicted on the basis of the functional group in a compound (Table 3.9) and the predominant metabolizing reactions found in each species. The results of in vitro studies of drug metabolic pathways for various model compounds show that species differences in metabolic activity are principally quantitative (Table 3.10). It should be noted, however, that it is virtually impossible to quantitatively predict the relative concentrations of metabolites that will be produced after administration of a drug in any given species.

TABLE 3.9—Probable biotransformation pathways for drugs

Functional group	Biotransformation pathways
Aromatic ring	Hydroxylation
Hydroxyl	
Aliphatic	Chain oxidation, glucuronic acid conjugation, sulfate conjugation (to lesser extent)
Aromatic	Ring hydroxylation, glucuronic acid conjugation, sulfate conjugation, methylation
Carboxyl	
Aliphatic	Glucuronic acid conjugation
Aromatic	Ring hydroxylation, glucuronic acid conjugation, glycine conjugation
Primary amines	
Aliphatic	Deamination
Aromatic	Ring hydroxylation, acetylation, glucuronic acid conjugation, methylation, sulfate conjugation
Sulfhydryl	Glucuronic acid conjugation, methylation, oxidation
Ester linkage/ amide bond	Hydrolysis

PHASE I REACTIONS. Although phase I metabolic reactions usually yield products with decreased activity, some may give rise to products with similar or even greater activity (Table 3.11). Divergence between

TABLE 3.10—Comparative cytochrome P450 levels, oxidative drug metabolism (phase I), and conjugation (phase II) activities for various substrates in rats, rabbits, and ruminant species in vitro

	Rat	Rabbit	Goat	Sheep	Cattle
P450[a]	0.6–0.8	0.6	0.6	0.4–0.6	0.5–0.6
Oxidation[b]					
Benzo(a)pyrene	0.8	0.7	ND	0.2	0.1–0.3
Ethoxycoumarin	0.3	ND	0.5–1.0	0.6–0.7	0.6–0.8
Benzphetamine	2.7–3.8	1.7	2.3	1.5–3.4	1.3–4.7
Aniline	0.2–0.4	0.1–0.6	0.2–1.1	0.2–0.7	0.3
p-nitroanisole	13.9	23.6	30.9	24.4	10.3
Ethylmorphine	5.1–12.0	4.0	ND	2.0–3.6	1.2–8.9
Glucuronidation[b]					
1-naphtol	6.4	ND	ND	3.6–17.3	2.9–3.0
p-nitrophenol	2.6–4.5	6.4	14.3	6.3–11.3	4.2–4.8
Sulphation[b]					
2-naphtol	0.8–4.1	4.8	5.2	2.1–4.3	3–9
Acetylation[c]					
Sulfadimidine	9–26	304	0.3	0.8–4.2	2.5–5.4

Source: van't Klooster 1992.
ND = not determined.
[a]nmol/mg microsomal protein.
[b]nmol/mg protein · min.
[c]pmol/mg protein · min.

TABLE 3.11—Effect of phase I metabolic reactions on pharmacologic activity of some drugs

Drug	Metabolite
Conversion of active drug to inactive metabolite (drug inactivation)	
Pentobarbital	Pentobarbital alcohol
Phenobarbital	*p*-hydroxyphenobarbital
Phenytoin	*p*-hydroxyphenyl derivative
Amphetamine	*p*-hydroxyamphetamine, phenylacetone
Phenothiazine	Phenothiazine sulfoxide
Procaine	*p*-aminobenzoic acid
Conversion of active drug to active metabolite	
Phenylbutazone	Oxyphenbutazone
Aspirin	Salicylic acid
Propranolol	4-Hydroxypropranolol
Diazepam	N-desmethyldiazepam
Ceftiofur	Desfuroylceftiofur
Primidone	Phenobarbital, phenylethymalonamide
Spironolactone	Canrenone
Conversion of inactive drug (pro-drug) to active drug	
Prontosil	Sulfanilamide
Hetacillin	Ampicillin
Parathion	Paraoxon

decline in plasma concentrations and effects of a drug suggests that one or more of its metabolites may have pharmacologic activity. The only way to determine the activity of a metabolite is to administer the metabolite and study its pharmacokinetic/pharmacodynamic relationship. Many compounds are metabolized to active metabolites, either with therapeutic implications (e.g., ceftiofur to desfuroylceftiofur, procainamide to *N*-acetylprocainamide, ramipril to ramiprilat) or toxicologic implications. Metabolic conversion of parathion (nontoxic per se) to paraoxon (a powerful inhibitor of cholinesterase) and the formation of fluorocitrate (a specific inhibitor of the enzyme aconitase) from fluoroacetic acid and fluoroacetamide are examples of lethal synthesis.

Oxidation is the most prominent reaction in the metabolism of most compounds, including lipid-soluble drugs and steroid hormones. Specifically, many of these enzymes that are located predominantly in parenchymal cells of metabolizing organs (liver, kid-

$$NADPH + A + H^+ \rightarrow AH_2 + NADP^+$$

$$AH_2 + O_2 \rightarrow \text{"active oxygen complex"}$$

$$\text{"active oxygen complex"} + \text{drug} \rightarrow \text{oxidized drug} + A + H_2O$$

FIG. 3.10—Hepatic microsomal drug-oxidizing system. The oxidative mechanism requires that equivalent amounts of NADPH, oxygen, and drug substrate be utilized in the reaction. A represents the oxidized form, and AH_2 is the reduced form of cytochrome P450.

TABLE 3.12—Oxidative reactions mediated by the liver microsomal enzyme system

Oxidative reaction	Drug	Metabolite
Aromatic hydroxylation	Phenylbutazone*, phenobarbital*	Oxyphenbutazone*, *p*-hydroxyphenobarbital
Aliphatic oxidation	Pentobarbital*	Pentobarbital alcohol
O-dealkylation	Phenacetin*	Acetaminophen*
N-dealkylation	Diazepam*	*N*-desmethyldiazepam*
Oxidative deamination	Amphetamine*	Phenylacetone
Desulfuration	Parathion	Paraoxon*
Sulfoxidation	Phenothiazine tranquilizers*	Corresponding sulfoxide

*Pharmacologically active compound

ney, intestinal epithelium), where they are associated with the smooth-surfaced endoplasmic reticulum. When many tissues including liver are homogenized, endoplasmic reticulum is broken down to form small vesicles known as microsomes. These enzymes, which have a specific requirement for reduced nicotinamide adenine dinucleotide phosphate (NADPH) and molecular oxygen, have been classified as mixed-function oxidases and are termed *microsomal enzymes* because of their association with, and continued activity within, microsomes.

Ability of the microsomal drug-metabolizing enzymes to mediate a wide variety of oxidative reactions may be ascribed to a common mechanism, hydroxylation (Brodie et al. 1958; Gillette 1963, 1966). The mixed-function oxidase mechanism requires that NADPH reduce cytochrome P-450, which is the oxidizing enzyme found in microsomes. Reduced cytochrome P-450 reacts with molecular oxygen to form an active oxygen intermediate. Interaction between this complex and a lipid-soluble drug or steroid substrate yields a hydroxylated substrate, oxidized P-450, and an equivalent molar fraction of water (Fig. 3.10). There are several isoenzymes of cytochrome P-450, each of which has certain substrates it most efficiently metabolizes (Benet et al. 1996). This results in a wide variety of oxidative reactions known to occur in microsomes and include aromatic hydroxylation, aliphatic oxidation, *O*- and *N*-dealkylation, oxidative deamination, replacement of S by O (desulfurization), and sulfoxide formation. In Table 3.12, examples are given of drugs that are metabolized predominantly by hepatic microsomal oxidation. It is common for a drug to be metabolized along two or more pathways simultaneously, in which case, amounts of the metabolites formed depend on the relative activities of different metabolizing enzyme systems. The prevalence of these various isoenzymes is different from organ to organ within an species, by species for a specific organ (Witcamp et al. 1991), and by age within a species and organ type (Kawalec and El Said 1990, 1994). As an example, amphetamine is metabolized along two oxidation pathways (aromatic hydroxylation and oxidative deamination), and the metabolites in turn undergo conjugation reactions (Fig. 3.11). The extent to which these metabolic reactions take place appears to vary with the species (Dring et al. 1970; Baggot and Davis 1973). Acetaminophen, an analgesic and antipyretic agent, has a free hydroxyl group that makes this molecule suitable for conjugation reactions (Fig. 3.12). The glucuronide and sulfate ester formed are highly polar and pharmacologically inactive compounds that are rapidly excreted in urine. Cats are particularly susceptible to acetaminophen toxicity due, in part, to defective conjugation of the drug and conversion to a reactive electrophilic metabolite. Phenacetin and acetanilid, which are precursors of the more polar acetaminophen, are transformed to the latter by the microsomal oxidative reactions of *O*-dealkylation and aromatic hydroxylation respectively (Brodie and Axelrod 1948; Brodie and Axelrod 1949). Biotransformation of phenylbutazone involves aromatic hydroxylation to oxyphenbutazone (an anti-inflammatory agent and drug

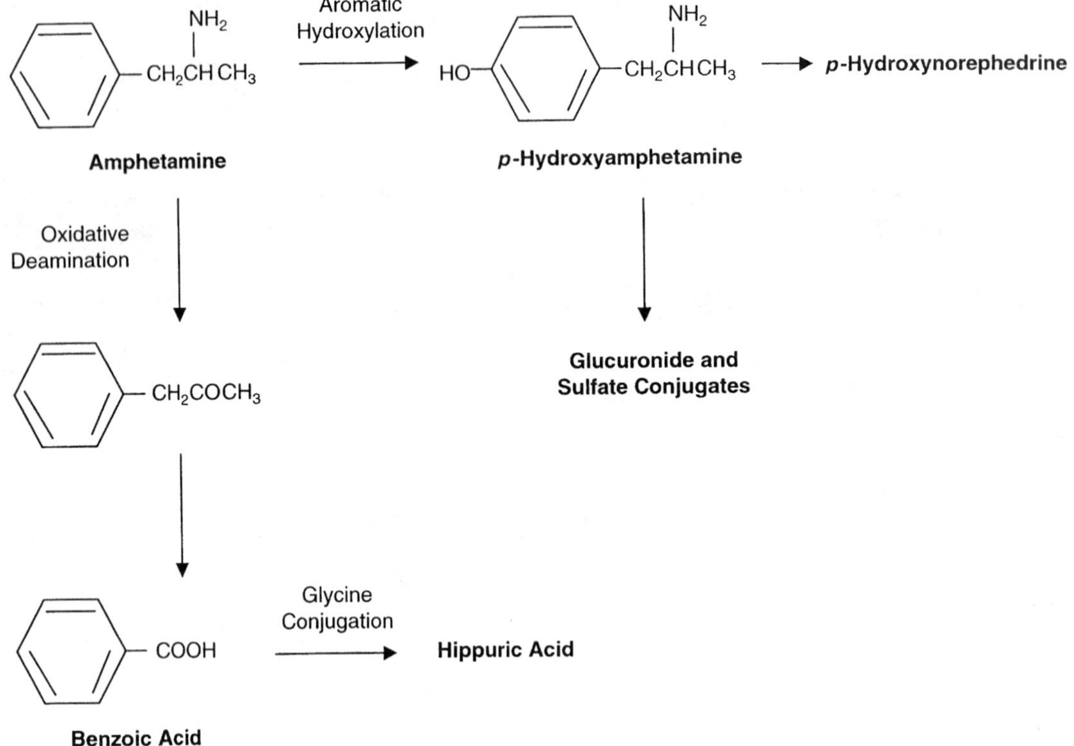

FIG. 3.11—Pathways of amphetamine metabolism in a variety of species.

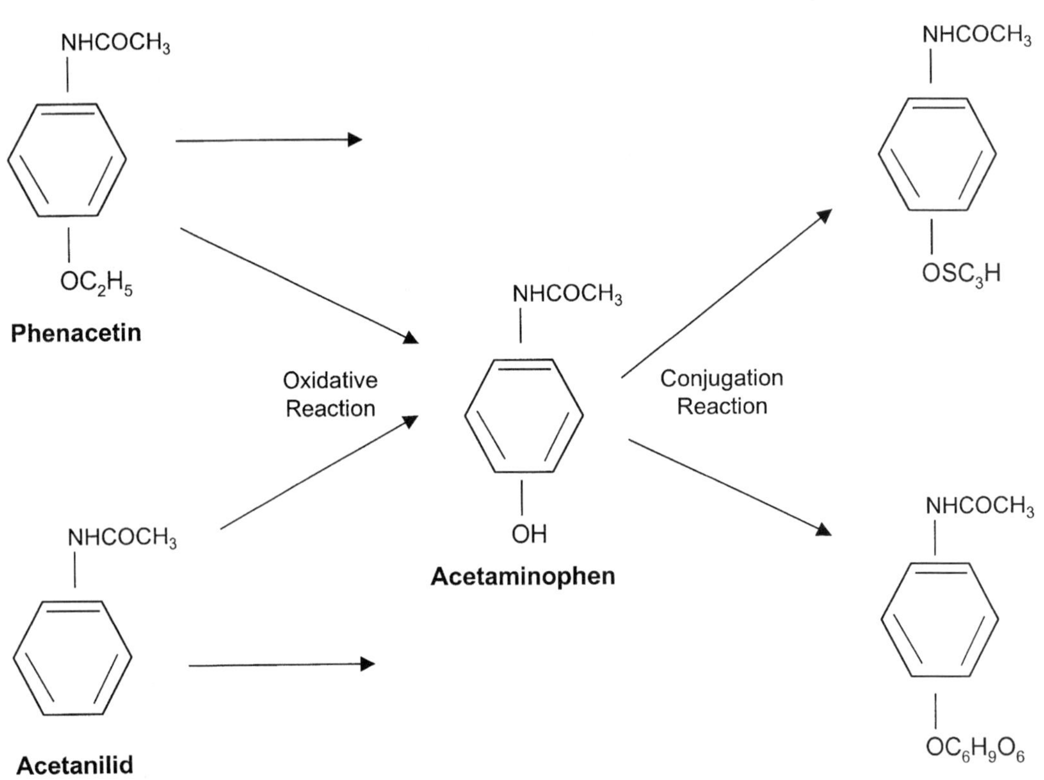

FIG. 3.12—Metabolism of acetaminophen and its precursors, phenacetin and acetanilid.

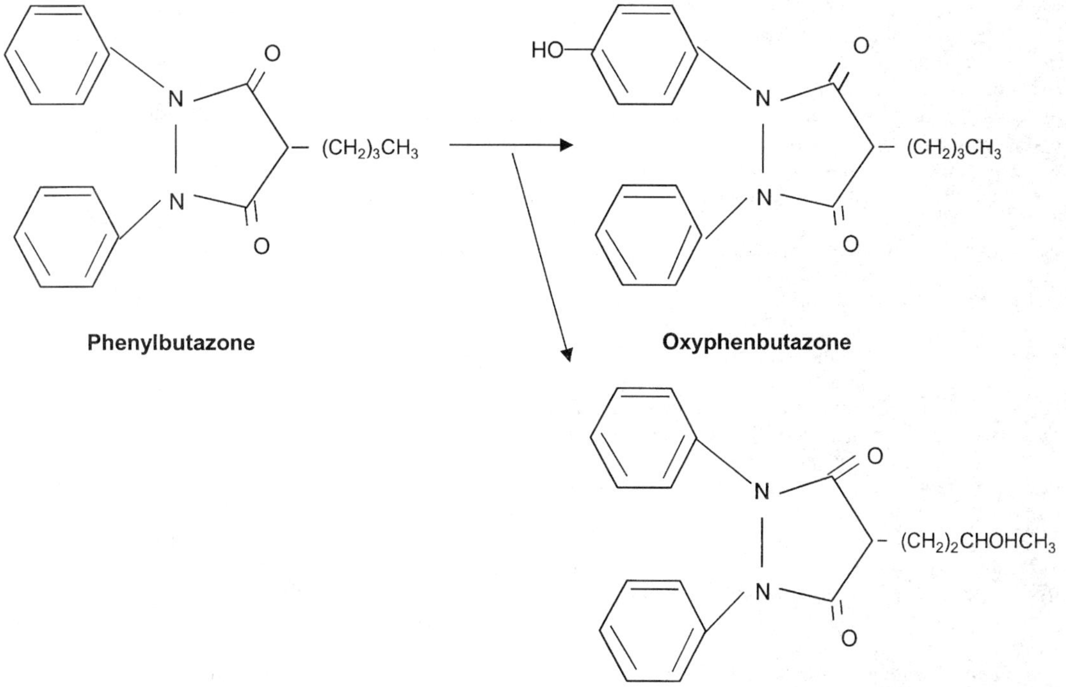

Phenylbutazone

Oxyphenbutazone

FIG. 3.13—Oxidative metabolic transformations of phenylbutazone.

in its own right) and oxidation of the side chain to a metabolite with only uricosuric action (Fig. 3.13). Oxyphenbutazone in turn forms a glucuronide and sulfate ester. Extensive plasma protein binding of phenylbutazone and its metabolites prior to conjugation limits their availability for glomerular filtration. While long-chain fatty acids undergo microsomal ω oxidation, side-chain alkyl substituents in otherwise lipophilic molecules are characteristically metabolized in the subterminal (ω-1) position, e.g., as in pentobarbital, meprobamate, and ethosuximide. This seems to be a metabolic reaction to avoid formation (by ω oxidation) of a lipophilic carboxylic acid that, like the long-chain fatty acids themselves, would inhibit cytochrome P-450 by detergent action on the lipophilic membrane to which it is attached and on which it is dependent (Stenlake 1979).

Species variations in duration of action of a lipid-soluble drug can often be attributed to differences in the rate of its biotransformation (Dalvi et al. 1987). Reduction of cytochrome P-450 may be rate-limiting in hepatic microsomal oxidative reactions; species differences in P-450 reductase activity have been shown to parallel differences in rates of drug oxidation (Davies et al. 1969). Comparison of half-lives of some drugs that are eliminated to a large degree by hepatic microsomal oxidative reactions shows that the activity of this system is far lower in humans than in domestic and laboratory animal species.

In addition to catalyzing various oxidative reactions, hepatic microsomes can reduce azo and nitro compounds to corresponding amines. Both reductive reactions involve anaerobic conditions, require NADPH, and are almost certainly mediated by enzymes that contain flavine adenine dinucleotide (Mueller and Miller 1950). Azo compounds undergo reductive cleavage to primary aromatic amines. Prontosil, an azo dye, is reduced to sulfanilamide, which has antibacterial activity. The nitroreductase system is partly responsible for inactivation of chloramphenicol. Ruminal microflora and intestinal bacteria can very effectively carry out these reductive reactions. Reductive dehalogenation of volatile anesthetics (halothane, methoxyflurane) is almost certainly mediated by hepatic microsomal enzymes.

Foreign compounds (xenobiotics) can be metabolized by other than the microsomal enzyme system. Nonmicrosomal metabolic reactions include oxidation of alcohols and aldehydes, reduction of ketones, deamination by monoamine oxidase (MAO), and most types of synthetic (i.e., phase II) reactions. Hydrolysis of esters and amides is readily catalyzed by a variety of hydrolytic enzymes present in blood plasma and other tissues, including liver and kidney. Ruminal microorganisms and gut bacteria mediate hydrolytic and reductive reactions (Williams 1972).

Alcohol dehydrogenase and aldehyde dehydrogenase are rather nonspecific enzymes found in the soluble fraction of liver that catalyze important oxidative transformations. Substrates include endogenous compounds (vitamin A, retinine) as well as some drugs (ethanol, propranolol, chloral hydrate). The major metabolic pathway for the hypnotic drug chloral hydrate is reduction to trichloroethanol, which is pharmacologically active. In catalyzing this reaction, alcohol dehydrogenase functions as a reductase (Friedman and Cooper 1960). Chloral hydrate has an apparent half-life of 3 minutes in the dog; the drug is rapidly and quantitatively converted to trichloroethanol (Garrett and Lambert 1973). This metabolite undergoes conjugation with glucuronic acid, and the conjugate is excreted in urine and bile. Likewise, metabolism of ethylene glycol (the primary component in antifreeze) is converted to toxic metabolites including oxalic acid by alcohol dehydrogenase. For this reason, an historic treatment for antifreeze intoxication was administration of ethanol, which competitively inhibits the formation of the toxic metabolite.

MAO, a flavoprotein located in the outer membrane of the mitochondria, is widely distributed in a variety of tissues (liver, kidney, intestinal mucosa, lung, blood vessels and plasma, heart muscle, brain, neurons). Tissue distribution of this enzyme is such that it is readily available to deaminate the biogenic amines. Following release of norepinephrine from adrenergic nerve terminals, it interacts with certain adrenergic receptors on effector cells. Excess is removed from the extracellular region largely by reuptake into the nerve terminal by active transport and to some extent by diffusion away from the site and subsequent enzymatic inactivation by extraneuronal catechol-*O*-methyl-transferase. Within the nerve terminal, norepinephrine is partitioned between a cytoplasmic mobile pool and intragranular pools. That portion present in the former is susceptible to oxidative deamination by MAO. Drugs that inhibit MAO (isocarboxazid, phenelzine, tranylcypromine) can cause an increase in the level of norepinephrine in the brain and other tissues and is accompanied by a variety of pharmacologic effects.

Hydrolysis is an important metabolic pathway for compounds with an ester linkage (—COO—) or an amide bond (—CONH—). Most amides are hydrolyzed more slowly than the corresponding esters. Use of procainamide as an antiarrhythmic is based on its slow rate of hydrolysis compared with that for procaine. Elimination mechanisms for procainamide include hepatic biotransformation (hydrolytic reaction) and renal excretion (Galeazzi et al. 1976). In dogs, over 50% of the dose is excreted unchanged in urine. Formation of the active metabolite *N*-acetylprocainamide is a major metabolic pathway of procainamide in humans and rhesus monkeys (Dreyfuss et al. 1971; Giardina et al. 1976). Since dogs are less able to acetylate primary aromatic amines, they would not form this metabolite as effectively (Papich et al. 1986). Lidocaine undergoes extensive hepatic biotransformation, which varies in pattern among species (Keenaghan and Boyes 1972). The principal metabolic pathways are microsomal oxidation (aromatic hydroxylation, *N*-dealkylation) and hydrolysis of the amide bond, catalyzed by amidases in the soluble fraction of the liver. Phase I metabolites are excreted in urine as such and in the form of conjugates (presumably glucuronides).

PHASE II (SYNTHETIC) REACTIONS. Synthetic (conjugation) reactions may take place when a drug or phase I metabolite contains a chemical group such as hydroxyl (—OH), carboxyl (—COOH), amino (—NH_2), or sulfhydryl (—SH) and is suitable for combining with a natural compound provided by the body to form readily excreted water-soluble polar metabolites (Williams 1971). Conjugating agents include glucuronic acid, glutathione, glycine, cysteine, methionine (for methylation), sulfate (for ethereal sulfate formation), and acetate (for acetylation). These conjugating agents do not, however, react directly with the drug or its phase I metabolite but do so either in an activated form or with an activated form of the drug (as an example, acetyl-coenzyme A rather than acetate). These activated forms are usually nucleotides, and the reaction between the nucleotide and drug or conjugating agent is catalyzed by an enzyme. A conjugation reaction requires a conjugating agent, a nucleotide containing either the conjugating agent or the foreign compound, and a transferring enzyme. Species variations in conjugation reactions can thus depend on occurrence of the conjugating agent, ability of the body to form the necessary nucleotide, or amount of transferring enzyme. In contrast to phase I metabolic reactions, which appear to be ubiquitous throughout mammalian species (at least qualitatively), certain synthetic reactions are either defective or absent in particular species (Table 3.13). The cat synthesizes glucuronide conjugates at a slow rate, as this species is deficient in the transferring enzyme glucuronyl transferase (Dutton 1966). The dog and fox are unable to acetylate aromatic amino groups. Unlike the enhanced potential for drug toxicity imposed on cats by defective glucuronide synthesis, lack of ability to acetylate a particular type of amino group does not appear to hinder elimination of drugs in dogs.

Glucuronide synthesis is a most important phase II metabolic pathway for drugs and certain endogenous compounds (steroid hormones, thyroxine, bilirubin). The activated form of glucuronic acid is the nucleotide uridine diphosphate glucuronic acid (UDPGA), formation of which is catalyzed by enzymes in the soluble fraction of the liver. Synthesis of the glucuronide involves transfer of the conjugating agent from the nucleotide to an acceptor molecule; transfer is mediated by the microsomal enzyme glucuronyl transferase (Isselbacher et al. 1962). This conjugation reaction is unique in that the transferring enzyme is associated with the microsomes, mainly in the liver but also in other tissues.

Some drugs that are excreted largely as glucuronides include morphine, salicylates, acetaminophen, chloramphenicol, iopanoic acid, sulfadimethoxine

TABLE 3.13—Domestic animals with defect in certain conjugation reactions

Species	Conjugation reaction	Major target groups	State of synthetic reaction
Cat	Glucuronide synthesis	–OH, –COOH, –NH_2, –SH, >NH,	Present but slow rate
Dog	Acetylation	Ar–NH_2	Absent
Pig	Sulfate conjugation	Ar–OH, Ar–NH_2	Present but low extent

(humans), and the phase I metabolites of diazepam (oxazepam), phenylbutazone (oxyphenbutazone), phenobarbital, and phenytoin. Glucuronide conjugates may be extensively excreted into the bile, the degree of which appears to be determined largely by its molecular weight. This route of excretion may predominate for compounds with molecular weights above 500 and is relatively more common in rats, dogs, and chickens than in other species. Glucuronides that are excreted in bile may undergo hydrolysis (mediated by β glucuronidase) in the intestine. The hydrolytic reaction liberates the drug or the phase I metabolite, which may then be reabsorbed, and an enterohepatic cycle may be established. Not all glucuronides are hydrolyzed by β glucuronidase in the gut (the ester glucuronide of iopanoic acid). Certain breeds of fish do not synthesize glucuronides, which is apparently due to deficiency of the nucleotide UDPGA. Defective synthesis of glucuronides in cats is related to the low level of the transferring enzyme glucuronyl transferase rather than a deficiency of UDPGA. In insects, glucuronide formation is replaced by β-glucoside conjugation (Parke 1968).

Sulfate conjugation is an important alternative metabolic pathway to glucuronidation in metabolism of phenols and, to a much lesser extent, aliphatic alcohols. Some drugs that form ethereal sulfates include phenol, acetaminophen, morphine, isoproterenol, and ascorbic acid. Various endogenous compounds such as chondroitin, heparin, and certain steroids form sulfate esters. Enzymes that catalyze formation of the nucleotide and transfer of the conjugating agent to the acceptor molecule are found in the soluble fraction of the liver (Robbins and Lipmann 1957; Nose and Lipmann 1958). Capacity for sulfate conjugation in the pig is limited and hence can become saturated, yielding a change from a constant fraction of drug metabolized (first order) to a constant amount of drug metabolized (zero order). It appears that the total pool of sulfate in the body can be readily exhausted. For this reason, conjugation with glucuronic acid usually predominates over sulfate formation.

Acetylation of all types of amino groups takes place in humans and several species of animals except the dog and fox, which do not acetylate the aromatic amino group (Williams 1967). The dog appears to have a specific deficiency in arylamine acetyltransferase, although some evidence has been presented that dog liver contains a natural specific inhibitor of this enzyme (Leibman and Anaclerio 1962). Acetylation is the principal metabolic pathway for sulfonamide compounds in humans, rabbits, and rats but is accompanied by aromatic hydroxylation in ruminant species. Sulfanilamide, e.g., undergoes acetylation at both the aromatic and sulfonamido NH_2 groups in a variety of species except the canine, which suggests that transacetylases may be specific for the type of amino group (Fig. 3.14). The acetylation reaction takes place in two stages; the first step involves formation of acetyl coenzyme A and is followed by a nucleophilic attack by the amino-containing compound on the acetylated enzyme. This reaction takes place in the reticuloendothelial rather than parenchymal cells of liver, spleen, lungs, and intestinal mucosa (Govier 1965).

Acetylation decreases water solubility as well as lipid solubility (which is usual for conjugates) of sulfonamide compounds. Sulfapyrimidine and probably sulfadoxine and sulfadimethoxine are exceptions in that their acetyl derivatives are more water-soluble. Increased aqueous solubility decreases the potential for crystalluria. Urinary alkalinization increases the solubility of sulfonamides in urine and the fraction of dose excreted unchanged by the kidney.

Sulfhydryl-containing drugs and/or phase I metabolites are subject to conjugation with other molecules containing free —SH groups. These may be either endogenous compounds or xenobiotics. Many of these compounds, including glutathione (G—SH)and cysteine (C—SH), are critical in the maintenance of the proper redox potential within the body and may exist as either the reduced monomer (G—SH or C—SH) or the oxidized dimer (G—SS–G or C—SS–C, namely cystine). Likewise, conjugation of xenobiotics containing free —SH groups with these endogenous redox modulating compounds are subject to interconversion between the reduced form (e.g., desfuroylceftiofur) and the oxidized conjugate (e.g., desfuroylceftiofur glutathione, desfuroylceftiofur cysteine) (Olson et al. 1998). This is one of the few covalently bound conjugations that is readily reversible, depending upon the redox potential of the local environment.

METABOLIC TRANSFORMATIONS MEDIATED BY GI MICROORGANISMS. GI microflora are capable of mediating a wide variety of metabolic transformations, the most prominent of which are hydrolytic and reductive reactions (Scheline 1968, 1973). Microbial metabolism may occur after oral administration of a drug product or following passive diffusion of the nonionized form of a drug from the systemic circulation

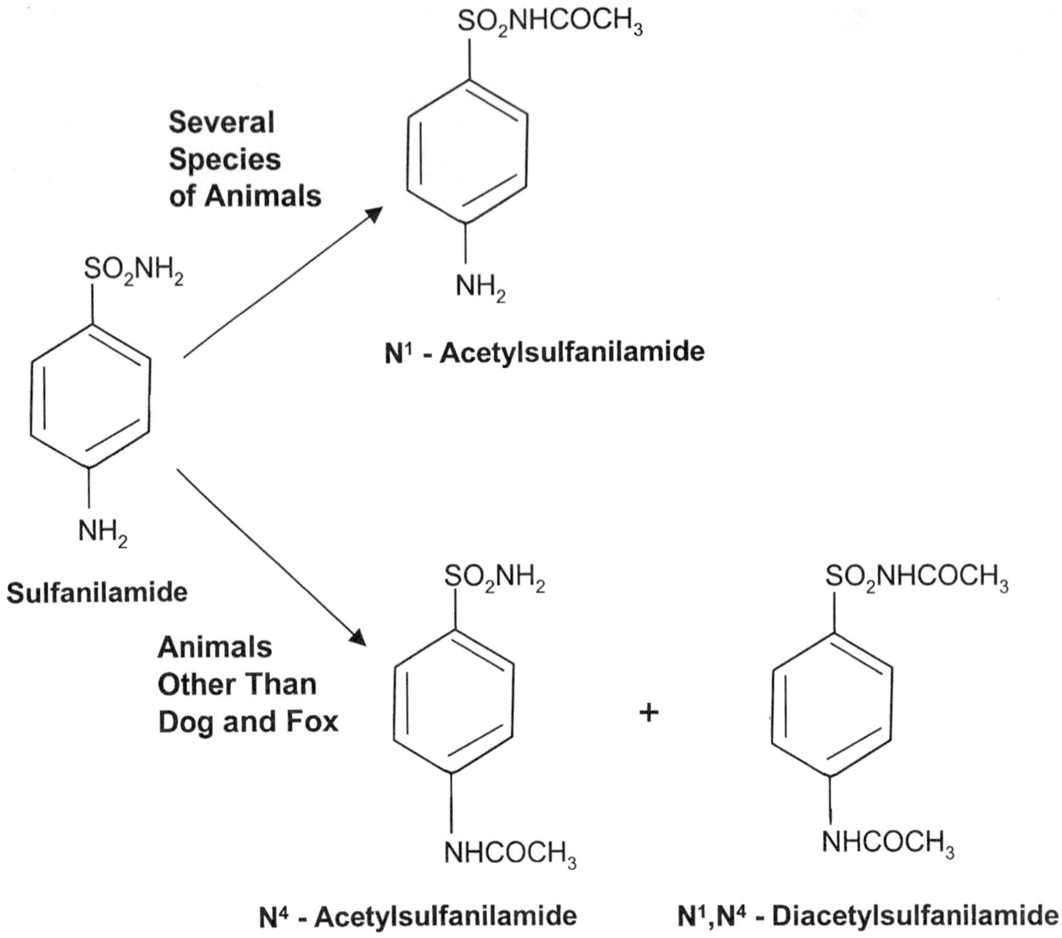

SO_2NH_2

NH_2

Sulfanilamide

Several Species of Animals

$SO_2NHCOCH_3$

NH_2

N^1 - Acetylsulfanilamide

Animals Other Than Dog and Fox

SO_2NH_2

$NHCOCH_3$

N^4 - Acetylsulfanilamide

+

$SO_2NHCOCH_3$

$NHCOCH_3$

N^1,N^4 - Diacetylsulfanilamide

FIG. 3.14—Acetylation reactions of sulfanilamide in several species of animals. The dog and fox do not form the N^4-acetyl derivative; i.e., these animals are unable to acetylate the aromatic amino group.

into the lumen of the GI tract. Enteric sulfonamides (phthalylsulfathiazole, succinylsulfathiazole) depend on release of sulfathiazole for their antibacterial action. Hydrolysis, mediated by bacterial enzymes in the large intestine, is also responsible for activation of the anthraquinone glycosides (cascara sagrada, senna). Hydrolysis of glucuronide conjugates that are excreted in bile underlies the phenomenon of enterohepatic circulation, since only the drug itself is lipid-soluble and can be reabsorbed. The enzyme responsible for this hydrolytic reaction, β glucuronidase, is found principally in bacteria (*Escherichia coli*) of the large intestine. Microbial glucuronide hydrolysis is necessary for release of bile acids from their conjugates in the intestine, enabling them to play their essential role in fat absorption. Both azo- and nitro-reductase activity are also associated with gut bacteria.

Ruminal microflora catalyze hydrolytic and reductive reactions; e.g., cardiac glycosides are hydrolyzed in the rumen, and chloramphenicol is inactivated by reduction of the nitro (—NO_2) group. Parathion, which is the precursor of the active pesticide paraoxon, may undergo nitroreduction in the rumen. This metabolic reaction reduces both the activity and toxicity of the irreversible anticholinesterase agent.

While GI microorganisms can mediate certain metabolic transformations of drugs, chronic administration of antimicrobial agents can adversely affect activity of these bacteria. Since they are located mainly in the large intestine and rumen, microflora may be exposed to action of an antimicrobial agent irrespective of the route of administration. The extent of bacterial exposure to a drug depends on the extent of absorption from the small intestine and, following parenteral administration, the amount of drug that is excreted into the large intestine and rumen. These translocation processes are determined by the lipid solubility and degree of ionization of the drug.

DRUG BIOTRANSFORMATION IN THE DEVELOPING ANIMAL. Hepatic drug metabolism generally increases from birth, to reach a maximum when the animal is a young adult. As animals age thereafter, metabolism gradually diminishes, with the rate of decrease in biotransformation efficiency increasing as the animal approaches geriatric age. These generalities are fraught with exceptions, and specific situations must be addressed.

In dogs, most mixed function oxidases mature by the fifth to eighth week after birth, with slight decreases after weaning (Kawalek and El Said 1990). Sulfation reactions mature early in dogs, but glucuronidation matures more slowly. This impacts on the metabolism and disposition of acetaminophen, phenobarbital, and phenytoin in dogs (Ecobichon et al. 1988).

In ruminants, clear changes in metabolism result when preruminant animals become ruminants. Cytochrome P-450 and NADPH-dependent reductases increase by 50%; analine hydroxylase increases by threefold; and ethoxycoumarin *O*-deethylase, UDP glucuronic acid glucuronyl transferase, and glutathione *S*-transferase all are increased subsequent to the development of a functional rumen (Kawalek and El Said 1994). Such maturational changes, likely because of the increased complexity of the nutrients being exposed to the liver as a result of the dietary change, is consistent with the quantum increase in the rate of elimination of ceftiofur and desfuroylceftiofur-related metabolites in ruminant cattle compared with preruminant cattle (Brown et al. 1996).

DRUG-INDUCED CHANGES IN RATE OF METABOLISM. Metabolism of a drug generally facilitates its removal from the body. Therefore, an alteration of the rate of metabolism will affect duration of drug action. Among factors that can alter rate of metabolism are certain lipophilic drugs and environmental chemical substances (pesticides, carcinogens) and a reduction in the hepatic blood flow. Decreased binding of extensively bound drugs can increase their availability for metabolism. A number of drugs are capable of stimulating (inducing) the hepatic microsomal enzyme system (phenobarbital, diazepam, phenytoin, phenylbutazone). Enhanced metabolizing capacity represents an increase in concentration of enzyme protein (increased synthesis) rather than increased activity and is referred to as enzyme induction (Conney and Burns 1972). Any drug that is lipid-soluble at physiologic pH is potentially capable of inducing microsomal enzymes when administered on a chronic basis. This phenomenon also has physiologic implications, since the steroid hormones, thyroxine, and bilirubin are substrates for microsomal enzymes.

Drug interactions are manifested as the sequelae attending concurrent use of two or more drugs. A drug such as phenylbutazone, which is extensively bound to plasma albumin and capable of inducing microsomal enzymes, can considerably increase the metabolism of other (particularly acidic) drugs. The influence of induction on pharmacologic action of a drug depends on relative activity of the parent drug and its oxidized product (phase I metabolite).

The rate of drug metabolism can be decreased by inhibition of the process. In addition to microsomal enzymes, others such as plasma pseudocholinesterase and monoamine oxidase are subject to inhibition. Delayed elimination is a direct consequence of inhibited metabolism, and the effect of this on pharmacologic action depends largely on the fraction of the dose normally eliminated by the inhibited metabolic reaction. When a major metabolic pathway is inhibited, the metabolite of a minor pathway may assume greater importance, particularly if this product has toxic potential.

Drugs that inhibit microsomal enzyme activity include cimetidine, chloramphenicol, quinidine, organophosphorus insecticides, and ketaconazole. Chloramphenicol increases duration of pentobarbital anesthesia in dogs and decreases body clearance of both phenobarbital and phenytoin, commonly used anticonvulsant drugs. The ability of some drugs to stimulate or depress the microsomal drug-metabolizing system requires that this possibility be kept in mind when considering multiple drug therapy. Alterations in the half-life of drugs in patients with thyroid dysfunction appear to result mainly from accelerated hepatic microsomal metabolism in hyperthyroidism and retarded biotransformation in hypothyroid patients (Vesell et al. 1975).

Irreversible inhibition of plasma pseudocholinesterase by organophosphorus compounds may in itself cause toxicity or, when inhibition is partial, can provide the circumstance for a drug that is metabolized by this enzyme (succinylcholine) to produce an adverse effect.

Excretion of Drugs. Most drugs are eliminated by a combination of biotransformation and excretion processes. Biotransformation generally enhances the water solubility of drugs, so their metabolites are readily excreted. Polar drugs and compounds with low lipid solubility are eliminated mainly by excretion. Although the kidney is by far the most important organ of excretion, certain compounds are excreted mainly in bile. The liver; salivary, sweat, and mammary glands; and lungs constitute nonrenal routes of excretion. Pulmonary excretion involves diffusion of volatile substances from systemic circulation into pulmonary alveolar spaces, from which they are removed by exhalation.

Drug excretion is a first-order process except in the situation when plasma concentration of a substance exceeds the capacity of a carrier-mediated transport mechanism, in which case excretion obeys zero-order kinetics. When the drug concentration declines to the level at which the system is no longer saturated, the excretion process becomes first order.

RENAL EXCRETION. Renal excretion is the principal process of elimination for drugs that are predominantly ionized at physiologic pH and for compounds with limited lipid solubility. Drugs excreted unchanged (not altered by a metabolic reaction) mainly in urine include many antibiotics (most penicillins, cephalosporins, aminoglycosides, and oxytetracycline), most diuretics (with the notable exception of ethacrynic acid), the competitive neuromuscular blocking agents (*d*-tubocurarine, gallamine), and possibly the cardiac glycoside digoxin.

Renal handling of drugs and drug metabolites is complex and, depending on the physicochemical properties of the substance, the following mechanisms may be involved: glomerular filtration of molecules that are free (unbound) in the plasma; carrier-mediated excretion of certain polar organic compounds by the proximal tubular cells; and pH-dependent passive reabsorption, by nonionic diffusion, of lipid-soluble substances (weak organic electrolytes) in the distal portion of the nephron. In general, compounds that have low lipid solubility and those that are predominantly ionized in blood plasma are rapidly excreted by the kidney, whereas weak organic electrolytes, which are partly nonionized and lipid-soluble, are excreted more slowly.

Extensive (>80%) protein binding hinders a drug's passage through the porous glomerular capillary membrane. The amount of drug that enters the glomerular filtrate is determined by its concentration in plasma water and the rate of glomerular filtration (GFR). Any pharmacologically active substance that lowers arterial blood pressure or constricts renal arterioles will reduce the GFR. The extent of this effect on renal excretion of the drug, however, might be lower than expected if the substance is transported into tubular fluid by a carrier-mediated process.

Carrier-mediated transport of certain drugs and drug metabolites into tubular fluid takes place in the proximal tubule. This process requires an energy source and intracellular carrier substances. The carriers are relatively nonspecific in that they transport either organic acids or organic bases, but their capacity is limited. Above a certain concentration of drug in plasma, the carrier-mediated system becomes saturated and transport proceeds at a constant rate (obeys zero-order kinetics). Some substances excreted by this process are listed in Table 3.14. Extensive protein binding does not hinder tubular excretion of drugs, presumably because the drug-albumin complex dissociates upon removal of free drug from the plasma. Cloxacillin and ampicillin, which are excreted by the same renal mechanisms, have the same half-life (1.2 hours in cows), even though cloxacillin is 80% bound to plasma albumin and ampicillin is only 20% bound.

Concurrent administration of two drugs (either acids or bases) that are substrates for the same carrier-mediated excretion process will cause delayed excretion of the less readily transported substance, e.g., probenecid decreases the rate of elimination of penicillin G and ceftiofur by reducing tubular excretion of the antibiotic (Kampmann et al. 1972; Whittem et al. 1995). Substrate inhibition provides conclusive evidence that a transport process is carrier-mediated.

TABLE 3.14—Drugs excreted by carrier-mediated process in the proximal renal tubule

Acids	Bases
Penicillin G	Procainamide
Ampicillin	Dopamine
Ceftiofur	Neostigmine
Sulfisoxazole	*N*-methylnicotinamide
Phenylbutazone	Trimethoprim
Furosemide	
Probenecid	
p-aminohippurate	
Glucuronic acid conjugates	
Ethereal sulfates	

While a drug may enter tubular fluid by glomerular filtration and proximal tubular excretion, its renal clearance may nonetheless be low. This situation can be explained by substantial reabsorption taking place in the distal nephron. Renal handling of salicylate (an organic acid, pK_a 3.0) in dogs and cats exemplifies this point. Since tubular reabsorption takes place by passive diffusion, only the lipid-soluble nonionized form of a weak organic electrolyte can be reabsorbed. The extent of reabsorption depends on concentration of the drug and its degree of ionization in distal tubular fluid; e.g., weak organic acids are more highly ionized, and thus less well absorbed, in an alkaline than an acidic environment. This concept forms the basis of urinary alkalinization and, perhaps even more effective, the induction of alkaline diuresis to promote excretion of organic acids in cases of overdosage. An underlying requirement for this therapeutic procedure to be effective is that a substantial fraction of the amount of drug in the body be excreted unchanged in urine; i.e., renal excretion constitutes a significant mechanism of elimination for the drug. In humans and probably in dogs, urinary alkalinization increases the excretion rate of salicylate (pK_a 3.0), sulfisoxazole (pK_a 5.0), and phenobarbital (pK_a 7.4), whereas acidification of urine hastens removal of amphetamine (organic base, pK_a 9.9).

The usual urinary pH of carnivorous animals such as dogs and cats is acidic (5.5–7.0), while that of herbivorous species (horses, cattle, sheep) is alkaline (7.0–9.0). In any species, however, urinary pH is dependent mainly on dietary habit. In humans, the urinary reaction is generally acidic but can vary over a wide range of pH (5.0–8.5). Suckling and milk-fed herbivores generally excrete an acid urine; however, following maturity they characteristically excrete an alkaline urine.

BILIARY EXCRETION. Although the kidney is the principal organ of excretion for drugs that are eliminated unchanged and for most drug metabolites, some compounds are excreted mainly by the liver into bile. Properties of a compound that appear to facilitate its biliary excretion include a molecular weight greater than 300–500 and presence of polar groups. Conjugation with glucuronic acid, which takes place in the hepatocytes, may be the determining factor for excretion of a drug or phase I metabolites and certain endogenous substances in bile. Biliary excretion is an important elimination mechanism for organic anions and cations that are too polar to be reabsorbed from the intestine.

Some drugs (nafcillin, erythromycin, digitoxin), iopanoic acid (contrast agent used in cholecystography), certain endogenous substances (steroid hormones), and glucuronide conjugates of a variety of compounds (chloramphenicol, morphine, bilirubin) are excreted to a substantial extent in bile. The relative importance of the biliary excretion route depends mainly on the particular substance and to some extent on species, which may be grouped together as good (rats, dogs, chickens), moderate (cats, sheep), and poor (guinea pigs, rabbits, rhesus monkeys, probably humans) biliary excretors (Williams 1971). This grouping of species is based on the minimum molecular weight for extensive biliary excretion of polar compounds. Species variation in the extent of biliary excretion of drugs is likely to occur with compounds of molecular weight between 300 and 500. When molecular weight of a polar compound exceeds 500, which may be a glucuronide, it will be excreted predominantly in bile of all species. The rate of bile flow has been shown to affect excretion of a number of substances, including bromsulfophthalein and bilirubin (Roberts et al. 1967).

Compounds excreted in bile enter the small intestine. Depending on their lipid solubility, some drugs (e.g., tetracyclines) are reabsorbed. Glucuronide conjugates may be hydrolyzed by β glucuronidase, which is present in the intestinal microorganisms, and the liberated compound may then be reabsorbed. This cycle, consisting of biliary excretion followed by reabsorption from the intestine, is known as the enterohepatic circulation of a drug (Fig. 3.15). When a significant fraction of the dose undergoes enterohepatic circulation, this process delays elimination of the drug. It is usual for the drug and its metabolites to be gradually removed from the body by renal excretion. Enterohepatic circulation increases the half-life of drugs that are eliminated by renal excretion.

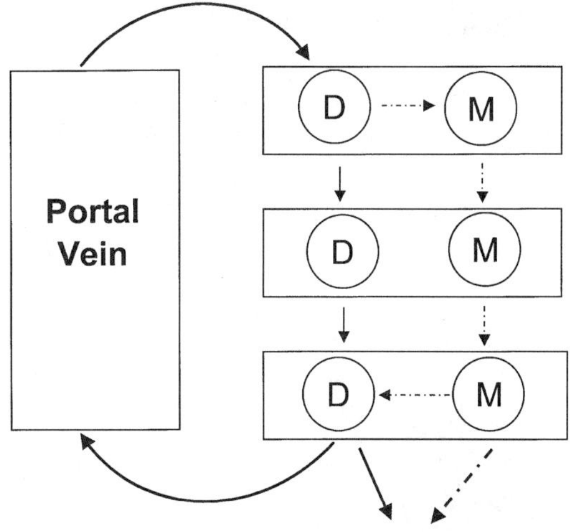

FIG. 3.15—When a drug (D) is absorbed from the intestine, excreted in bile, and reabsorbed from the intestine, it has undergone enterohepatic cycling (solid arrows), a component of distribution. Similarly, when a drug is converted to a metabolite (M) that is secreted in bile, converted back to drug in the intestine, and drug is reabsorbed (dashed arrows), the drug has also undergone enterohepatic cycling, in this case indirectly through a metabolite.

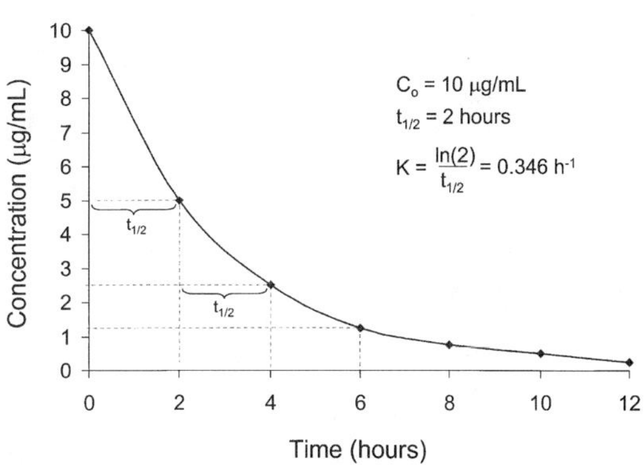

FIG. 3.16—Normal Cartesian graph showing first-order (exponential) decline in plasma concentration of a drug with time. The solid line represents the elimination (linear terminal) phase of the disposition curve.

Quantitating Drug Elimination. The rate of elimination of a drug is determined mainly by the mechanism(s) of the process. It may be influenced by extensive (>80%) binding to plasma proteins, degree of perfusion of the eliminating organ(s), activity of drug-metabolizing enzymes, and efficiency of renal excretion. Plasma drug concentrations typically decline according to a first-order rate process, meaning that a constant *fraction* of drug is eliminated for each unit of time. In contrast, elimination by a zero-order rate process would indicate that a constant *amount* of drug is eliminated for each unit of time. Graphically, using the same data elimination by a first-order rate process appears curvilinear when plotted as concentration versus time (Fig. 3.16), but appears as a straight line when plotted as the logarithm of concentration versus time (Fig. 3.17).

HALF-LIFE. The elimination half-life of a drug, defined as the time required for the body to eliminate one-half of the remaining drug, is given by the expression:

$$t_{1/2} = 0.693/\beta \quad (3.15)$$

where β (sometimes defined as K), the overall elimination rate constant, is the negative value of the slope of

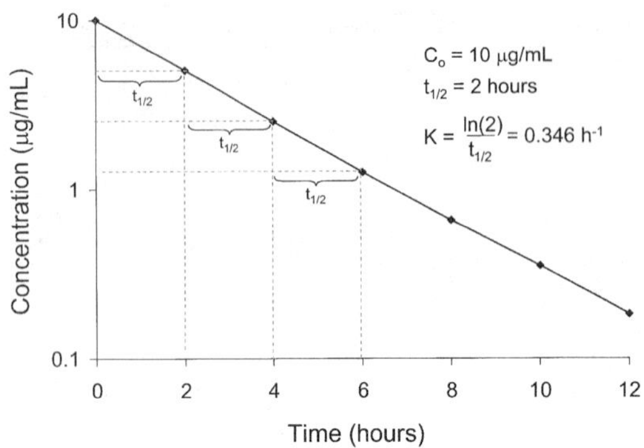

FIG. 3.17—Semilogarithmic graph showing first-order (exponential) decline in plasma concentration of a drug with time. The solid line represents the elimination (linear terminal) phase of the disposition curve.

the elimination (linear terminal) phase of the plot of the logarithm of concentration versus time. A large value of β (or K), corresponding to a short half-life, indicates rapid elimination. The half-life is found simply by measuring the time required for any given plasma concentration of the drug to decline by 50% during the linear phase of the drug concentration-time profile (this can be determined graphically; see Figs. 3.16 and 3.17).

Half-life values of the majority of therapeutic agents are independent of the dose administered, since their overall elimination obeys first-order kinetics. When drug absorption from the GI tract or an injection site is rapid, the half-life is independent of the route of administration. IV injection of a single dose is, however, the only foolproof procedure on which to base the calculation of the true elimination half-life. To ascertain whether a drug has linear pharmacokinetic characteristics, the disposition kinetics should be studied at two or more dose levels.

When drug elimination obeys zero-order (constant-rate) kinetics, the "half-life" becomes progressively longer as the dose is increased, and the drug is said to have nonlinear (or dose-dependent) pharmacokinetics, implying that concentrations at any time after administration are not proportional to the dose administered. The usual cause of dose-dependent elimination is the limited capacity of certain drug-metabolizing enzyme systems (e.g., microsomal glucuronyl transferase activity in cats). Mathematical treatment of nonlinear kinetics is invariably complex (Wagner 1973). The half-life of salicylate is dose-dependent in cats (Yeary and Swanson 1973), phenylbutazone elimination follows zero-order kinetics in dogs (Dayton et al. 1967) and horses (Piperno et al. 1968), and phenytoin half-life is dose-dependent in humans (Houghton and Richens 1974).

The rate of elimination of a drug is usually an important determinant of duration of pharmacologic effect. In this context, half-life is used, along with the range of

TABLE 3.15—Application of half-life to estimate fraction of the dose remaining in the body, assuming first-order elimination

Time after dosing (multiples of $t_{1/2}$)	Fraction of dose in the body
1	1/2
2	1/4
3	1/8
4	1/16
5	1/32
6	1/64

therapeutic plasma concentrations, to estimate the dosage interval for a drug that is given repeatedly to maintain a particular effect, e.g., digoxin (in treatment of congestive heart failure), phenytoin (as an anticonvulsant), aspirin or acetaminophen (for relief of mild to moderate pain), and theophylline oral dosage forms (bronchodilating effect). When absorption is rapid and complete, the amount of drug remaining in the body at fixed times after administration of a single dose can be estimated from knowledge of the half-life (Table 3.15).

FACTORS INFLUENCING HALF-LIFE. Any physiologic state or disease condition that alters either access of a drug to the organs of elimination or activity of the eliminating mechanism is likely to cause change in the usual half-life of the drug. For drugs that behave pharmacokinetically according to a two- or three-compartment model (described later), the half-life is a function not only of elimination but also of distribution.

In neonatal animals the biotransformation pathways associated with the microsomal drug-metabolizing enzyme system (oxidation and reduction reactions and glucuronic acid conjugation) are deficient. Their development appears to be biphasic, consisting of a rapid and nearly linear increase in activity during the first 3–4 weeks, followed by slower development up to the 10th week postpartum (Short and Davis 1970). Renal function (both rate of glomerular filtration and, even more so, carrier-mediated proximal tubular excretion processes) is inefficient in neonatal animals of most species, excluding the bovine (Dalton 1968a,b,c). It follows that the half-life of drugs eliminated by microsomal metabolic reactions or by renal excretion will be prolonged in neonatal animals.

Various types of interaction between drugs that are administered concomitantly can affect the half-life. Interference with carrier-mediated transport mechanisms (probenecid decreases proximal tubular excretion of penicillins), displacement from binding sites on plasma proteins (phenylbutazone displaces warfarin from plasma albumin), and stimulation of the hepatic microsomal drug-metabolizing enzyme system (by chronic administration of phenobarbital) or its depression (by chloramphenicol) are interactions that may have clinical significance. Drugs that alter activity of hepatic microsomal enzymes affect the metabolism of endogenous steroids.

TABLE 3.16—Half-life (hours) of some drugs in domestic animals

Drug	Cattle	Horse	Pig	Dog	Cat
Hepatic metabolism					
Salicylate	0.8	1.0	5.9	8.6	37.6[a]
Pentobarbital	0.8	1.5	—	4.5	4.9
Amphetamine	0.6	1.4	1.1	4.5[b]	6.5[b]
Chloramphenicol	4.2	0.9	1.3	4.2	5.1[c]
Ivermectin	60–72	50–90	35	44	—
Hepatic metabolism and renal excretion					
Sulfadimethoxine	12.5	11.3	15.5	13.2	10.2
Sulfadoxine	11.7	14.0	8.2	—	—
Trimethoprim	1.5	3.2	2.3[d]	4.6[cd]	—
Ceftiofur	10	3–4	6	3–4	—
Renal excretion					
Penicillin G	0.7	0.9	—	0.5	—
Ampicillin	1.2	1.55	—	0.8	—
Kanamycin	1.9	1.45	—	1.0	—
Oxytetracycline	9.1	10.5	—	6.0	—

[a]Dose dependent.
[b]Eliminated by hepatic metabolism and renal excretion (30-35%); half-life influenced by urinary pH.
[c]Eliminated by hepatic metabolism and renal excretion (20%).
[d]Influenced by urinary pH reaction.

Urinary pH can influence the half-life of a drug for which tubular reabsorption, a passive nonionic diffusion process, is a feature of its handling by the kidney. The extent of this effect depends on the concentration and degree of ionization of the drug in tubular fluid. An alteration of urinary pH from acidic to alkaline reaction can reduce considerably the reabsorption of weak organic acids with pK_a values within the range 3.0–7.2 and thereby decrease their half-life. The converse will apply to the excretion rate of weak organic bases.

Increase in the half-life of drugs, which are eliminated in healthy animals mainly by renal excretion, is a direct and important consequence of impaired renal function. The relationship between the half-life and body clearance of a drug is given by

$$t_{1/2} = 0.693 \cdot Vd_{area}/Cl_B \tag{3.16}$$

where Vd_{area} is apparent volume of distribution of the drug and Cl_B is body clearance. When renal clearance represents a substantial fraction of body clearance of a drug, the half-life can be estimated from Eq. 3.11. In patients with reduced renal function, increase in dosage interval, based on the longer half-life, will offset excessive accumulation and toxic effects that might otherwise ensue. Likewise, in patients that have an altered volume of distribution, the half-life will be affected because the concentration of drug being presented to the organs of elimination will be altered. For example, the volume of distribution of gentamicin in neonatal animals is larger due to a larger extracellular fluid volume in neonatal animals compared with adults (Clarke et al. 1985). The resultant apparent elimination half-life of gentamicin is longer in neonates than in adults.

Superimposed on numerous factors influencing the half-life of a drug in an individual animal are intra- and interspecies variations. Considerable variation exists among the species of domestic animals in the half-lives of several drugs (Table 3.16). Although it is not feasible to rank species according to the rate at which they eliminate drugs (expressed as half-life), herbivorous species (in particular, ruminant animals) appear to eliminate drugs that undergo extensive hepatic metabolism (biotransformation) more rapidly than carnivorous species. Most impressive is the rapid elimination of salicylate in ruminant animals and horses compared with the long and dose-dependent half-life of this drug in cats (Davis and Westfall 1972). Clinical application of this wide variation in salicylate elimination is manifest in the dosage interval for sodium salicylate in horses (35 mg/kg, IV at 6-hour intervals) and aspirin in dogs (10 mg/kg, orally at 12-hour intervals) and cats (10 mg/kg, orally at 48-hour intervals) (Davis 1979).

Trimethoprim is generally used in conjunction with a sulfonamide, the choice of which does not appear to be critical in terms of antibacterial action but is supposedly related to their relative rates of elimination in different species. For use in humans trimethoprim is combined with sulfamethoxazole. Since both drugs have approximately the same half-life (10.6 hours), any appropriate dosage interval will take advantage of their synergistic action. Veterinary preparations contain trimethoprim combined with sulfadoxine or sulfadiazine for use in large or small animals respectively. These preparations have been found very effective, even though half-lives of the trimethoprim and sulfonamide do not coincide. Presumably, the dose rates recommended aim at maintaining therapeutic concentrations of sulfonamide with intermittent synergistic action of the combination. Trimethoprim undergoes extensive hepatic biotransformation in domestic animals compared with humans (Table 3.17).

The half-lives of drugs eliminated by renal excretion, in particular by filtration alone, may be shorter in dogs than herbivorous species. This observation is consistent with the higher rate of glomerular filtration in dogs. Apart from these general trends, the only

TABLE 3.17—Half-life and urinary excretion of trimethoprim

Species	Average half-life	% dose excreted unchanged in 24-hour urine	References
	(hr)		
Human	10.6	47	Schwartz et al. 1970
Pony	3.8	10	Alexander and Collett 1974
Dog	3.0	20	Kaplan et al. 1970
Pig	2.25	15	Nielsen and Rasmussen 1975
Cow	1.0	3	Nielsen and Rasmussen 1975
Goat	0.65	2	Nielsen and Rasmussen 1975

TABLE 3.18—Overall pharmacokinetics of antimicrobial agents in dogs

Drug	$t_{1/2}$	V_d	Cl_B	Process(es) of elimination
	(min)	*(mL/kg)*	*(mL/min)/kg*	
Penicillin G	30	156	3.6	E(r)
Ampicillin	48	270	3.9	E(r)
Tylosin	54	1700	21.8	E(b + r) + M
Kanamycin	58	255	3.05	E(r)
Gentamicin	75	335	3.10	E(r)
Trimethoprim	278*	1849	4.77	M + E(r)
Chloramphenicol	252	1770	4.87	M
Sulfisoxazole	270*	300	0.77	E(r) + M
Sulfadiazine	338*	422	0.92	M + E(r)
Enrofloxacin	201	2454	8.56	E(r) + M
Oxytetracycline	360	2096	4.03	E(r)
Sulfadimethoxine	792*	410	0.36	M + E(r)

E(r) = excess renal excretion.
M = metabolism.
E(b) = biliary excretion.
*Half-life influenced by urinary pH reaction.

conclusion that can be drawn is that half-life should not be extrapolated from one species to another.

BODY CLEARANCE. Body clearance, which represents total clearance, is considered to be a better index of efficiency of drug elimination than the commonly used half-life. It is based on the concept of the body as a whole acting as a drug-eliminating system and represents the sum of clearances of the drug by eliminating organs (liver, kidneys). Accordingly, body clearance may be defined as the volume of plasma cleared of the drug by various elimination processes per unit time and is expressed in terms of (mL/min)/kg. The value of this parameter can be calculated by dividing the systemically available dose of drug by the total area under the plasma concentration-time curve:

$$\mathrm{Cl}_B = F \cdot \mathrm{dose/AUC} \qquad (3.17)$$

which is equivalent to the expression

$$\mathrm{Cl}_B = 0.693 \cdot \mathrm{Vd}_{\mathrm{area}}/t_{1/2} \qquad (3.18)$$

when the drug is completely available systemically (i.e., $F = 1.0$ when the drug is administered IV).

Body clearance differs from half-life in that it allows expression of the rate of elimination of a drug in a manner that is independent of disposition kinetics of the drug (i.e., distribution). The terms body clearance and half-life, which is a hybrid parameter, can be distinguished by comparing the pharmacokinetics of ampicillin and digoxin in dogs. These two drugs have the same body clearance (3.9 mL/min)/kg); the half-life of ampicillin is 48 minutes compared with 1680 minutes for digoxin and is influenced by the apparent volumes of distribution, which are 0.27 L/kg and 9.46 L/kg, respectively. It can be concluded that for drugs with a given clearance value, the smaller the apparent volume of distribution, the shorter the half-life. Values of the major pharmacokinetic parameters describing the disposition kinetics of some antimicrobial agents in dogs are given in Table 3.18.

Since body clearance is the sum of the individual clearance processes, it can be viewed simply as

$$\mathrm{Cl}_B = \mathrm{Cl}_r + \mathrm{Cl}_{nr} \qquad (3.19)$$

where Cl_r is renal clearance and Cl_{nr} is nonrenal clearance of the drug. In the case of a drug that undergoes extensive hepatic biotransformation, the nonrenal clearance represents hepatic (metabolic) clearance and may well approximate body clearance. For a drug that is excreted unchanged in the urine, its renal clearance is principally the sole or at least predominant component of body clearance. Contribution of an eliminating organ to body clearance of a drug can be determined if the fraction of IV dose cleared by the particular organ is known. For the kidney,

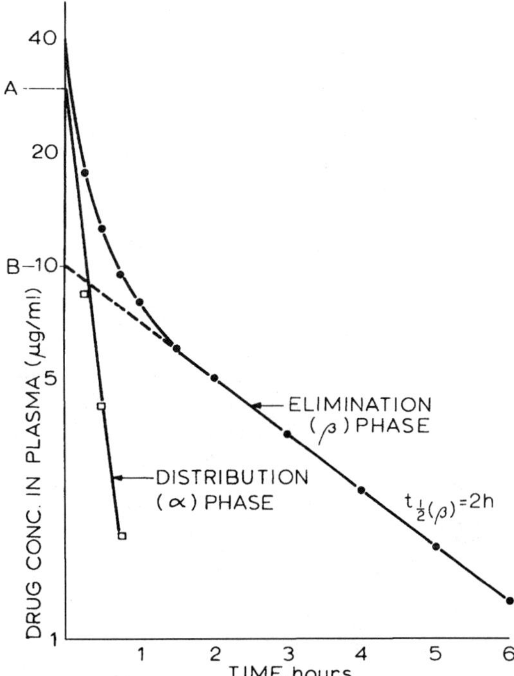

FIG. 3.18—Semilogarithmic graph depicting time course of drug in plasma after IV administration of a single dose. Data points represent experimental (•) and residual (□) plasma drug concentrations. Zero-time intercepts of the distribution and elimination phases of the biphasic disposition curve are *A* and *B*, respectively.

$$Cl_r = f_{ex} \cdot Cl_B \qquad (3.20)$$

where Cl_r is renal clearance of the drug and f_{ex} is the fraction of dose excreted unchanged in the urine. Based on this concept, the Cl_B of insulin and *p*-aminohippurate, which are handled by known renal mechanisms and excreted unchanged (i.e., have f_{ex} approximating 1.0), are used to measure the glomerular filtration rate and effective renal plasma flow, respectively.

PHARMACOKINETIC ANALYSIS. Mathematical expression of the relationship between plasma concentrations and time following administration of a drug allows not only for the description of the former, but also estimation of drug plasma profiles following different dosage regimens, disease conditions, and physiologic states. From these estimations, the efficacy and/or toxicity of a drug under these conditions may be more effectively predicted. What follows is only an introduction into this field. Other textbooks provide substantially more detail (Gibaldi and Perrier 1982; Rowland and Tozer 1995).

Compartmental Analysis. Compartmental analysis, in which the body is conceived as consisting of distribution compartments interconnected by first-order rate constants defining drug transfer (i.e., constant fraction of drug transfered per unit of time), is used to describe the pharmacokinetic behavior of drugs. Usually these compartments, which are mathematical entities, have no physiologic counterpart.

Following an IV injection of a single dose of drug, the decline in plasma concentration of the drug is expressed graphically by the disposition curve. For most drugs this curve, plotted in a semilogarithmic manner (i.e., as the logarithm of concentrations over time), is biphasic (Fig. 3.18). The initial steep decline in the plasma drug concentration can be attributed mainly to the combined effect of intravascular mixing and distribution (by passive diffusion) of the drug into tissues and organs of the body. Elimination contributes to a lesser extent to this phase of drug disposition. Once distribution pseudoequilibrium has been established, the rate of decline in plasma concentration decreases and is determined by elimination of the drug from the body. Elimination refers to biotransformation and excretion, i.e., the processes responsible for removal of the drug per se from the body.

It is assumed that a drug introduced directly into the systemic circulation equilibrates very rapidly in the fluids and tissues that compose the central compartment. For many drugs, the central compartment consists of the blood and tissues of highly perfused organs such as lungs, liver, and kidneys. Distribution throughout the remainder of the body space available to the particular drug (peripheral compartment) takes place more slowly. The peripheral (tissue) compartment may be considered to consist of less well perfused tissues such as muscle, skin, and the rumen of cattle and sheep or the colon of horses. The apparent volumes of central and peripheral compartments for a drug depend upon the characteristics of blood flow to their component tissues, partitioning of the drug between blood and tissues (determined by lipid solubility and degree of ionization), and extent of binding to plasma proteins and tissue constituents. An assumption associated with compartmental models is that drug elimination takes place exclusively from the central compartment. Furthermore, distribution and elimination processes associated with the model are assumed to obey first-order kinetics. Accordingly, the rate at which a drug is removed from a compartment is proportional to concentration of the drug in the compartment.

It is usual for drug concentrations in plasma and those organs and tissues that contain a significant fraction of the total amount of drug in the body to decline in a parallel fashion. The linear terminal portion of the disposition curve is appropriately called the elimination phase, and from its slope ($-\beta/2.303$) is derived the half-life of the drug. The extrapolated zero-time intercept of the elimination phase is denoted by the letter *B* and is expressed in units of concentration. Resolving the biexponential disposition curve into its components by the method of residuals (feathering technique) yields a second linear segment called the distribution phase (Rowland and Tozer 1995). The distribution phase has a slope of $-\alpha/2.303$ and a zero-time intercept designated *A*. If the ordinate of the semilogarithmic graph were in natural logarithms (base *e*), the slopes of the two exponential phases of the disposition curve would be simply $-\alpha$ and $-\beta$.

The disposition curve is described mathematically by the biexponential equation

$$C = Ae^{-\alpha t} + Be^{-\beta t} \tag{3.21}$$

where *C* is the concentration of drug in the plasma at time *t* (in minutes); *A* and *B* are intercept terms with dimensions of concentration (g/mL); α and β are the overall distribution and elimination rate constants, respectively, which are expressed in units of reciprocal time (e.g., min^{-1}); and *e* represents the base of the natural logarithm. In drug disposition studies the coefficients (*A, B*) and the rate constants (α, β) are calculated from the experimental data by nonlinear least-squares regression analysis. The sum of *A* and *B* gives the initial concentration of drug in the plasma (C_0).

The two-compartment open model (Fig. 3.19) adequately describes the disposition kinetics of most therapeutic agents in humans and animals. Values of the actual pharmacokinetic rate constants (k_{12}, k_{21}, k_{el}) can be calculated from the derived hybrid constants (*A, B,* α, β) by means of appropriate equations (Riegelman et al. 1968; Baggot 1977). The absorption rate constant after extravascular administration, K_a, can be estimated from the data after determining the hybrid rate constants. Determination of the microconstants permits assessment of the relative contribution of distribution and elimination processes (either or both of which may be altered in disease states or, possibly, by concurrent administration of more than one drug) to disposition of a drug.

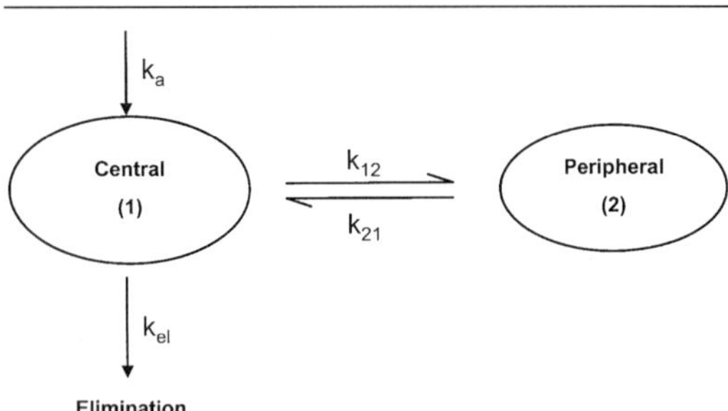

FIG. 3.19—Schematic diagram of the two-compartment open model. The drug is introduced into the central compartment, where it equilibrates almost instantaneously. Distribution between the central and peripheral compartments takes place more slowly; k_{12} and k_{21} are first-order rate constants for drug transfer between the two compartments. Elimination is assumed to take place exclusively from the central compartment; k_a is the absorption rate constant from the extravascular site of administration and k_{el} is the first-order rate constant for drug elimination from the central compartment.

While a biexponential expression describes the plasma concentration-time course of most drugs given by IV injection, the disposition curve for some drugs can be approximated mathematically by the monoexponential equation:

$$C = Be^{-\beta t} \tag{3.22}$$

where *B* is the zero-time intercept of the extrapolated first-order decline in the plasma drug concentration with time, and β is the apparent overall elimination rate constant of the drug. The value of *B* is an estimate of initial concentration of the drug in plasma, based on the premise that pseudodistribution equilibrium is instantly or at least very rapidly attained. Eq. 3.22 can also be applied to describe decline in plasma drug concentration during the postabsorption phase following IM, SC, or oral administration of the drug. When the rate of absorption is slower than the rate of elimination, the decrease in plasma concentrations is governed by the absorption rate, a phenomenon termed *flip-flop* pharmacokinetics.

The pharmacokinetic behavior of drugs that have a high affinity for a particular tissue (perhaps through selective binding) or undergo redistribution is best interpreted according to a three-compartment open model. The following mathematical expression describes the triexponential disposition curve:

$$C = Ae^{-\alpha t} + Be^{-\beta t} + Ce^{-\gamma t} \tag{3.23}$$

Although the experimental constants (*A, B, C,* α, β, γ) may be calculated by iterative least-squares linear regression in conjunction with the method of residuals for determining distribution and redistribution phases (termed *curve-stripping*), the best method for determining these constants is to fit the disposition curve by nonlinear least-squares regression analysis. There are indications that the three-compartment open model may be necessary to completely characterize the pharmacokinetic profile of digoxin (Kramer et al. 1974), pentazocine (Vaughan and Beckett 1974), and diazepam (Kaplan et al. 1973) in humans; oxytetracycline in dogs (Baggot et al. 1977); sulfadoxine in horses (Rasmussen et al. 1979); sulfadimethoxine in cattle (Boxenbaum et al. 1977); and gentamicin in various species (Brown and Riviere 1991).

Noncompartmental Analysis. Because artificial, mathematical compartments that have no direct relationship to physiologic spaces within the animal are confusing at times, a method of quantitating the same pharmacokinetic terms that do have physiologic relevance (Vd, Cl, $t_{1/2}$) has been derived. In this approach, called noncompartmental analysis (Martinez 1998), the plasma concentration-time profile or curve is described in terms of slopes, heights, areas, and moments (SHAM). The previous pharmacokinetic equations (Eqs. 3.21, 3.22, 3.23) can be generalized as follows:

$$C = \sum_{i=1}^{n} C_i e^{-\lambda_i t} \tag{3.24}$$

where the C_i and λ_i represent the heights and slopes of the n different linear terms that sum together (denoted by the Σ) to describe the plasma concentrations over time t. If one or more of the linear terms describe the appearance (e.g., absorption) of drug in the plasma, the height term is negative (e.g., $-C_i$). The AUC and AUMC are then described as follows:

$$\text{AUC} = \sum_{i=1}^{n} \frac{C_i}{\lambda i} \quad (3.25)$$

$$\text{AUMC} = \sum_{i=1}^{n} \frac{C_i}{\lambda_i^2} \quad (3.26)$$

From these SHAM values, any of the respective half-lives and Vd_{area} can be calculated:

$$\text{Vd}_{\text{area}} = F \cdot \frac{D}{\text{AUC} \cdot \lambda_i} \quad (3.27)$$

Clearance, Vd_{ss}, and bioavailability can be calculated as previously described (Eqs. 3.8, 3.13, and 3.17).

Thus, the vital pharmacokinetic values that can be related to physiologic states or pathologic conditions can be obtained using either compartmental or non-compartmental analysis. The biggest limitation to non-compartmental analysis is that no inference regarding drug localization in the body can be made, whereas compartmental analysis provides understanding of whether drug resides primarily within or outside the plasma and whether more tightly bound drug exists outside the bloodstream in peripheral tissues.

SOME ASPECTS OF DRUG DOSAGE. The term *dose* (D) is simply the amount of drug administered to an animal at any particular time. The term *optimum dose* is a historical term used to estimate the amount of drug that, when administered by a particular route to a certain species, is most likely to produce a certain intensity of response. The desired response is almost invariably a therapeutic effect. Clearly, there is no one optimum dose for every animal, due to the biological variation associated with the pharmacokinetics and pharmacodynamics of the drug from animal to animal. Information obtained from clinical studies lends support to the hypothesis that the intensity of effect produced by a drug is more closely correlated with plasma concentrations of the drug than with dose administered. Simply described, this is because observation of the plasma concentrations has already taken into account much of the variation associated with the pharmacokinetics of the drug. This reflects the situation that exists after pseudodistribution has been attained, in that the tissue drug concentrations and plasma concentrations, although not equal, decline in parallel for most therapeutic agents. The validity of pharmacokinetic predictions based solely on plasma drug concentrations is critically dependent on the assumption that this ratio is relatively constant in any given species.

Knowledge of body clearance of a drug is essential for determining the dosing rate (dose per unit time) that would be required to produce a given average steady-state concentration of the drug (C_{ss}):

$$FD/\tau = C_{ss}\text{Cl}_B \quad (3.28)$$

where F is the fraction of the dose absorbed, D, that enters the systemic circulation intact, and τ is the dosage interval. When the mode of administration is by continuous IV infusion, the right-hand side of Eq. 3.28 gives the infusion rate that will gradually achieve a desired C_{ss} of the drug. Following a period of infusion equal to 3.3 times the half-life of the drug, the plasma concentration will have reached 90% of the eventual steady-state (plateau) concentration.

Drug Administration. Medication may entail administration of a single dose (atropine or morphine when used for preanesthetic medication, thiopental given as an IV bolus dose for induction of anesthesia) or multiple doses at fixed time intervals (chronic dosage of phenytoin and/or phenobarbital for prevention of convulsive seizures, use of digoxin in treatment of congestive heart failure, phenylbutazone therapy for management of lameness in horses, treatment of bacterial infections with antimicrobial agents). The dosing rate of a drug refers to the dose per unit time (dose/dosage interval, or D/τ). When the drug is administered extravascularly, the systemic availability (F) of drug from the dosage form (preparation) administered must be taken into account in calculating a dosing rate.

The most reliable method of drug dosage involves titration by the therapeutic response of the patient, which requires that the intensity of the pharmacologic effect be quantifiable clinically. The continuous IV infusion technique is the best mode of drug administration for allowing adjustment of dose according to response. In antimicrobial therapy, recovery from bacterial infection is the best indicator of effectiveness of treatment. A satisfactory response would indicate that the antimicrobial agent had been given at an appropriate dosing rate and for an adequate duration.

Therapeutic Plasma Concentrations. Major factors that determine concentration of a drug in plasma include the size of the dose and the dosage regimen, formulation of the drug preparation, route of administration, systemic availability of the drug substance and its rate of absorption, extent of distribution and plasma protein binding, and rate of elimination. In addition to these factors, drug accessibility, which usually involves tissue penetration, to the site of action influences concentration attained at the receptor, which along with the affinity and intrinsic activity of the drug for the receptor determines the intensity of response elicited. With an appreciation of factors inherent in quantitatively relating pharmacologic response to plasma concentrations, the value of the plasma drug concentration range for a therapeutic agent (or even for an antimicrobial drug) can be seen in perspective.

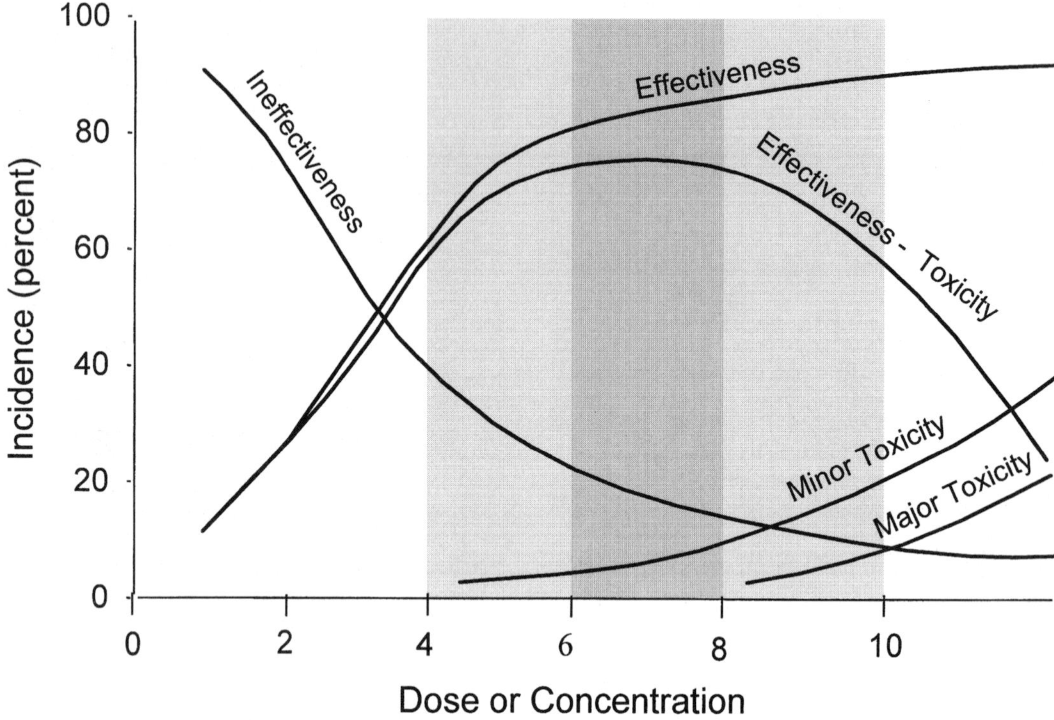

FIG. 3.20—Schematic representation of the incidence (%) of ineffective therapy, effective therapy, minor side effects, serious toxicity, and "therapeutic effectiveness" by dose on plasma concentration. (Adapted from Okita and Archeson 1973.)

TABLE 3.19—Tentative range of therapeutic plasma concentrations and principal pharmacologic effect

Drug	Therapeutic plasma concentrations	Principal pharmacologic effect
	(μg/mL)	
Salicylate	25–100	Analgesia
	200–350	Antiarthritic
Acetaminophen	10–30	Analgesia
Pentazocine	0.04–0.16	Analgesia (central)
Phenytoin	10–20	Anticonvulsant, antiarrhythmic
Procainamide	4–10	Antiarrhythmic
Procainamide + *N*-acetyl procainamide	20–30	Antiarrhythmic
Propranolol	0.02–0.08	β-adrenergic blockade, antiarrhythmic
Digoxin	0.6–2.5 (ng/mL)	Positive inotropic, rhythm stabilizer

The therapeutic (safe and effective) range of plasma concentrations for a drug is defined by careful clinical evaluation (which often entails precise physiologic and biochemical measurements) of the response in a sufficient number of appropriately selected individuals. Definition of the therapeutic plasma drug concentration range relies on elucidation of the concentration-effect relationship as well as the concentration-toxicity relationship (Fig. 3.20). As can be seen from the figure, there is a transition from therapeutic concentrations to nontherapeutic concentrations, rather than a clear demarcation between the two. The tentatively accepted range and the principal pharmacologic effect of a variety of drugs are given in Table 3.19. The effective range of concentrations may differ with the therapeutic indication, as with salicylate. The effective concentrations and width of the therapeutic range might be considered to reflect inherent activity and relative safety of a drug respectively. This statement must be interpreted with caution, because chronic administration of some drugs allows tolerance to develop or a side effect to assume prominence. The principles associated with application of the therapeutic concentration range as the basis for establishing the usual dosage regimen are the same for all pharmacological classes of drugs.

Application of Pharmacokinetics to Dosage. Drug disposition studies provide the data necessary for calculating the size of dose that will produce a therapeutic effect for a certain time. The dose (or dose level) in mg/kg represents the product of desired plasma concentration and the apparent specific volume of distribution of the drug (Eq. 3.14). The margin of safety (therapeutic index) and rate of elimination (half-life) of a drug are factors limiting the dose size and duration of action respectively.

Assuming that elimination is first-order and the metabolites are pharmacologically inactive, duration of a therapeutic concentration of a drug, tC_{ther}, is given by

$$tC_{ther} = [\ln(A_0/A_{min})] \cdot t_{1/2} \qquad (3.29)$$

in which A_0 is the dose administered, A_{min} is the minimally effective dose, and $t_{1/2}$ is the apparent elimination half-life of the drug. It follows from Eq. 3.29 that geometric increases in dose (minimum effective dose times 2, 4, 8) produce only linear increases in duration of therapeutic plasma concentrations (half-life times 1, 2, 3, respectively). The longer the half-life of a drug, the longer the duration of drug action for a given dose ratio. The tolerable limit of geometric increases in drug dosage is determined by the dose-related toxicity of a particular drug.

Since effective use of antimicrobial drugs relates to their action on pathogenic microorganisms, both the microbiologic (quantitative susceptibility) and pharmacokinetic properties of these drugs must be considered in calculating dosage (Prescott and Baggot 1993). The potential of an antimicrobial drug to produce adverse effects may vary with the animal species. The success of antimicrobial therapy depends on the attainment of effective drug concentrations at the site of infection. This requires that dosage be appropriate for the drug preparation (pharmaceutical dosage form) selected. Except in severe infections when intravenous administration is required, it is usual to administer antimicrobial drugs by other routes. The route selected (oral, IM or SC injection) depends on the species of animal to be treated and the dosage forms available.

Dosage Regimen. In treating diseased animals, it is usual to administer multiple doses of the therapeutic agent at intervals appropriate for the drug preparation selected. The variables (size of dose and interval between successive doses) are described by the dosage regimen, the objective being to maintain plasma concentrations of the drug within the therapeutic range for the duration of treatment. Such is the case with many kinds of drugs that affect mammalian physiology (e.g., drugs affecting the central and peripheral nervous systems) and some kinds of antimicrobials (compounds such as β-lactam antibiotics which kill bacteria based upon the time that active drug concentrations remain above the minimum inhibitory concentration, or MIC). The C_{max} in the serum or plasma determines the rate of penetration and concentration attained at the active site (Bergan 1978) and can be a critical predictor of efficacy for antibacterial agents that kill bacteria in a concentration-dependent fashion (e.g., aminoglycosides).

In management of disease conditions other than bacterial infections, the first decision is whether to administer a drug. When making this decision, one must recognize that drugs are potentially toxic substances that are likely to produce a therapeutic effect only after correct diagnosis and when administered in proper dosage. Effectiveness of therapy with a drug can be greatly influenced by formulation of the drug preparation (pharmaceutical dosage form). The range of therapeutic plasma concentrations is the only feature of dosage estimation that can be assumed to be constant in different species. Size of the dose depends on apparent volume of distribution, while dosage interval is related to the half-life of the drug. Regardless of the drug dosage form and route of administration, body clearance is the pharmacokinetic parameter that dictates the dosing rate. Since clearance, volume of distribution, and half-life vary among species, it is reasonable to conclude that dosage regimens for most drugs can be expected to vary. The marked differences in dietary habit and digestive system of domestic animals will contribute to variations in bioavailability of drugs from oral preparations.

Steady-State Concentration. Steady state is defined as the time during which concentrations remain stable or consistent from dose to dose. For continuous infusion, steady state is the time during which concentrations plateau; for intermittent dosing, the plasma concentration at steady state fluctuates over time within a dosing interval, but the concentration-time curve is superimposable from interval to interval. True steady state is asymptotically approached as dosing is continued at the same rate, with 90% of steady state achieved after 3.3 apparent elimination half-lives, 95% within 5 apparent elimination half-lives, and 99% within 7 apparent elimination half-lives. As an example, the terminal half-life of desfuroylceftiofur, the active metabolite of ceftiofur, is approximately 10 hours in cattle (Brown et al. 1991). Therefore, concentrations are at approximately 90% of steady state after 33 hours of any particular dosage regimen and are virtually at steady state after the first 3 days of dosing.

The steady-state concentration of a drug can be achieved by various methods of administration. One way is to administer a loading (priming) dose, usually parenterally, and continue with a series of maintenance doses at regular intervals (Fig. 3.21). The loading dose provides an amount of drug in the body that produces an immediate effect, in essence immediately producing steady-state concentrations that are maintained by the maintenance dose. The decision as to whether a course of therapy should be initiated with a loading dose depends on the urgency of treatment and half-life of the drug. For drugs that have a long half-life (digoxin) and for antimicrobial agents that exert a bacteriostatic action (sulfonamides, tetracyclines, chloramphenicol), the loading approach to dosage is desirable. In the case

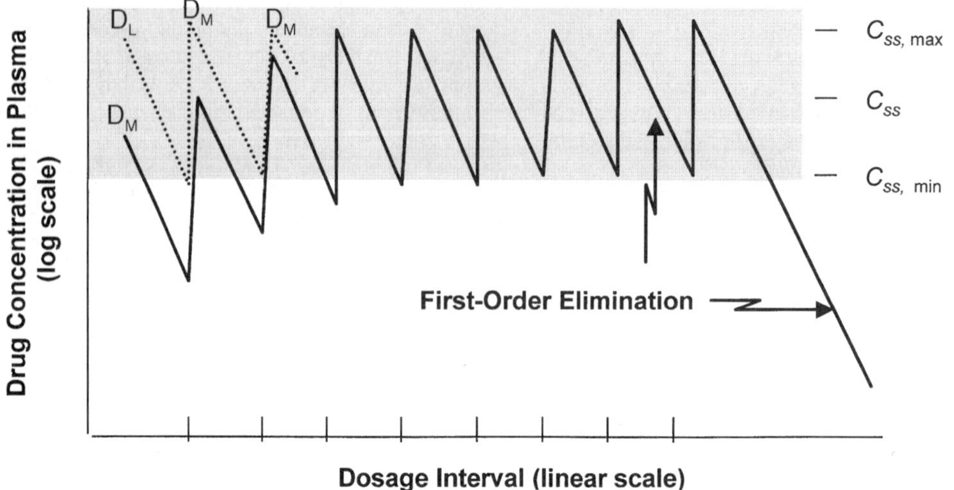

FIG. 3.21—Fluctuation in steady-state plasma concentrations of a drug given at constant intervals. The therapeutic range of plasma drug concentrations is between $C_{ss,min}$ and $C_{ss,max}$. Drug concentrations within the therapeutic range can be achieved either rapidly by giving a loading dose (D_L) or gradually by accumulation through repeated administration of the maintenance dose (D_M). Both methods will yield the same steady-state levels. Upon cessation of dosage, the drug will be eliminated exponentially at the same rate as after administration of a single dose.

of digoxin, which has a narrow margin of safety, the loading dose is given in fractions at short intervals rather than as a single dose. The loading dose (D_L) can be calculated by the following:

$$D_L = (\mathrm{Vd}/F) \cdot C_{ss,\max} \tag{3.30}$$

where D_L is the loading dose and $C_{ss,max}$ is the maximum therapeutic concentration desired at steady state. Typically, a loading dose is not needed unless the interval between doses is much longer than the $t_{1/2}$ and rapid initiation of effective concentrations is required. Pitfalls of a loading dose all relate to rapid achievement of high concentrations and include increased probability of acute toxicities (especially CNS toxicities), inconvenient dosage sizes (volume of injection or number of tablets or capsules), and preclusion of adaptation on the part of the animal to any altered behavioral or cognitive function.

The same steady-state concentration can be achieved gradually by accumulation, without a loading dose (Wagner et al. 1965). This method simply entails administration of a fixed dose repeatedly at constant intervals (the maintenance dose, or D_M). The D_M required to maintain concentrations within the target therapeutic range (i.e., between $C_{ss,max}$ and $C_{ss,min}$) is calculated by the following:

$$D_M = (\mathrm{Vd}/F) \cdot (C_{ss,\max} - C_{ss,\min}) \tag{3.31}$$

The interval between D_M required to maintain concentrations within the therapeutic range (T_M) is calculated as

$$T_M = \ln(C_{\max}/C_{\min}) \cdot t_{1/2} \tag{3.32}$$

Based on this concept, the average (mean) steady-state plasma concentration of drug, C_{ss}, can be predicted:

$$C_{ss} = (F \cdot D)/(\mathrm{Cl}_B \cdot \tau) \tag{3.33}$$

where F is the fraction of the dose, D, that enters the systemic circulation intact; Cl_B is body clearance of the drug; and τ is dosage interval. This relationship holds true for any route of administration and pharmacokinetic model, provided absorption, distribution, and elimination of the drug can be described by a set of linear differential equations. By administering fixed doses repeatedly at intervals, each corresponding to the half-life of the drug, a steady-state concentration should be achieved after six doses. To foster owner compliance with drug administration, a dosage interval of 4, 6, 8, 12, or 24 hours, depending on duration of action of the drug, is normally recommended.

A third method of attaining steady-state concentrations of a drug is by continuous IV infusion at a constant rate (zero-order input). The infusion rate, R_0, that will gradually achieve the desired plateau (steady-state) concentration of the drug in plasma is given by

$$R_0 = C_{ss} \cdot \beta \cdot \mathrm{Vd}_{ss} \tag{3.34}$$

where C_{ss} and Vd_{ss} are the plateau plasma drug concentration and the steady-state volume of distribution, respectively, and β is the overall elimination rate constant of the drug (as defined in Eq. 3.11). The alternate techniques for establishing a plateau concentration are described in the section on drug administration (IV injection). It is sufficient here to say that the plateau can be achieved either rapidly (by simultaneously administering an IV priming dose and starting the infusion) or gradually (by infusing the drug at a constant rate). The magnitude of the plateau plasma concentration depends upon the infusion rate, value of β, and volume of distribution. Since pharmacokinetic terms are constant for a given drug, the rate of infusion determines the plateau concentration. Doubling the infusion rate leads to doubling in magnitude of plateau concentration but does not influence the rate at which plateau concentration is attained. Continuous IV infusion of a drug attains a steady-state at a rate that depends only upon the elimination rate constant (β) or the half-life (0.693/β) of the drug. After infusing the drug for a period corresponding to four times the half-life, the plasma concentration will be within 90% of the eventual steady-state value. Continuous infusion of a drug that has a narrow margin of safety and short half-life value offers the distinct advantage of control over the steady-state concentration, which remains constant when attained. Upon terminating the infusion, the drug is eliminated by first-order kinetics and at the same rate as that following an IV bolus dose; i.e., the half-life is the same.

Administration of single doses of a drug at specified dosage intervals gives fluctuations in the steady-state concentrations around the average value (Fig. 3.21). The extent of fluctuation may be considered to represent the fraction of the amount of drug in the body that is eliminated during the dosage interval. The value of this term, f_{el}, is given by

$$f_{el} = 1 - e^{-\beta\tau} \qquad (3.35)$$

where β is the overall elimination rate constant of the drug and τ is the dosage interval. When the interval between successive doses corresponds to the half-life of the drug, the extent of fluctuation in steady-state concentrations is 50%. A dosage interval of twice the half-life would cause a 75% fluctuation in steady-state plasma concentrations. The wider the fluctuation that is acceptable for a drug, the longer the time (in terms of half-life) that may elapse between successive doses (Baggot 1977). In clinical practice, choice of dosage interval usually represents a compromise between the need for minimizing the extent of fluctuation in steady-state concentrations (based on the therapeutic concentration range of the drug) and the inconvenience of frequent dosing. In veterinary medicine a dosage interval of twice the half-life might be considered suitable for most antimicrobial agents, analgesics, and anticonvulsant drugs. Digoxin, which has a narrow margin of safety, is given to dogs at 24-hour intervals. The half-life of digoxin in normal dogs (mean ± SD, $n = 7$) is 28 ± 4 hours. In azotemic animals the (total) body clearance of the drug is reduced significantly (Gierke et al. 1978). The range of therapeutic serum concentrations is narrow (0.6–2.5 ng/mL), with evidence of toxicity at concentrations exceeding the therapeutic range. Because systemic availability of the drug can vary widely among different oral preparations, the same digoxin product should be used continuously in an animal on maintenance therapy.

Size of the maintenance dose, which replaces the amount of drug eliminated during the preceding interval, depends on the extent of fluctuation and can be calculated in the following manner as well as from Eq. 3.31:

$$D_M = D_L \cdot f_{el} \qquad (3.36)$$

When the route of administration is other than IV, an appropriate correction must be made for systemic availability of the drug from the particular dosage form.

INTERSPECIES SCALING. Several approaches exist to adjust drug administration from one animal to another, even from one species to another. These approaches range from adjusting the dose administered by body weight to adjustments based upon detailed information regarding physiologic differences between the animals.

Body Weight. The simplest approach to adjusting drug doses from one animal to another is simply to dose on a body weight basis. This approach will tend to underdose smaller animals and overdose larger animals, due to the more rapid metabolic rate in the former on a body weight basis. However, for most therapeutic agents, the therapeutic margin (range between effective dose and toxic dose) is sufficiently large that such discrepancies are clinically irrelevant.

Body Surface Area. Dosing based on body surface area is a more precise method of scaling drug administration from one animal to another. In general, body surface area increases more gradually than body weight (proportional to volume), a fundamental principle of geometry of 3-dimensional objects (e.g., a 1 cm cube has 1 cm^3 volume and 6 cm^2 surface area, whereas a 2 cm cube, 2 × 2 × 2, has 8 cm^3 volume and 24 cm^2 surface area; volume increases eightfold, whereas surface increases fourfold). Many cancer chemotherapeutics and other drugs with a narrow therapeutic range can be effectively scaled across different body weight individuals within the same species based on body surface area nomograms. Pragmatically, few veterinarians have body surface area nomograms for their patients, and body surface area nomograms are unavailable for many species.

Allometry. For allometric pharmacokinetic scaling across species, pharmacokinetic profiles are described for several different species across a broad range of normal body weights, using a similar type of pharmacokinetic model. Then, the pharmacokinetic parameters of the model are scaled by the following equation:

$$Y = aW^b \qquad (3.37)$$

where Y is the pharmacokinetic parameter of interest, W is body weight (usually expressed in kg), and log(a) and b are the intercept and slope, respectively, obtained from the plot of log(Y) versus log(W). This equation describes a power function.

Allometric scaling is scientifically rooted in the paradigm that metabolism, as well as many other physiologic functions, is normally higher in small mammalian species than in larger mammals (Mordenti 1986). Organ weights, blood flows to organs, heart rate, and cardiac output are larger (when normalized by body weight) in smaller species than in larger species. Since physiologic processes such as these govern drug disposition and elimination, it is entirely rational that drugs highly dependent on organ weight and blood flows can be scaled accordingly. As an example, when evaluated on a time basis, ceftizoxime half-life ranged from less than 15 minutes in the mouse and approximately 20 minutes in the rat to nearly 90 minutes in humans. When the differences in basal metabolic rate were factored in by describing ceftizoxime half-life in heartbeats, all of the species evaluated (mouse, rat, monkey, dog, and human) had 50% of the drug eliminated in approximately 7300 heartbeats (Mordenti 1986) (Fig. 3.22). Jezequel (1994) evaluated fluconazole pharmacokinetics across several species (mouse, rat, guinea pig, rabbit, cat, dog, and human) and reported very strong allometric relationships for $Cl_{B,}$ $Cl_{R,}$ and elimination half-life (Fig. 3.23). He noted that volume of distribution corrected for body weight was relatively constant across the species, consistent with the notion that time-related pharmacokinetic properties ($t_{1/2}$, Cl_B), rather than time-static pharmacokinetic parameters (volumes), are most altered across species and cannot be simply corrected by normalizing for body weight. Amphotericin B has a similar interspecies scaling profile (Hutchaleelaha et al. 1996).

Using the Food Animal Residue Avoidance Databank, Riviere et al. (1997) evaluated the half-life of 44 veterinary drugs by this allometric method. Eleven of the drugs had half-lives that significantly correlated with interspecies body size. These drugs were mostly antibiotics, and were drugs with primarily renal excretion, drugs in which their metabolism is dependent upon hepatic blood flow rather than enzyme capacity, and low plasma protein binding. Fourteen of the drugs clearly did not have a significant correlation across species, owing to either capacity-limited metabolism and/or high plasma protein binding. The remaining 19 drugs may have had insufficient data to determine a significant relationship, or may not be good candidates for allometric scaling. The general conclusion is that drugs which have low protein binding and are eliminated either by renal mechanisms or by flow-limited metabolism are likely to be scalable across species with the allometric approach.

The physiologic approach to interspecies scaling uses organ weights and organ blood flows to describe a complex hydraulic system which can be tailored to each species. This approach is tremendously useful when concentrations presented to specific organs are important, as is the case with many cancer chemotherapeutic agents. This is a very data-intense approach and does not lend itself to prediction of a pharmacokinetic profile for a new species without substantial organ weight and blood flow data for that new species.

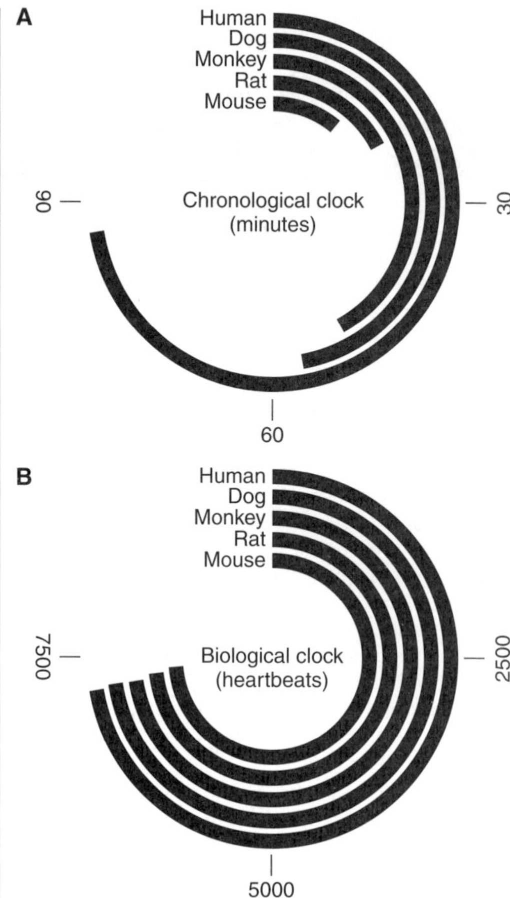

FIG. 3.22—Ceftizoxime half-life in various mammals using *(A)* chronological time (minutes) and *(B)* physiological time (heartbeats). (Copyright © 1986, from Mordenti 1986; Reprinted by permission of Wiley–Liss, Inc., a subsidiary of John Wiley & Sons, Inc.)

GLOSSARY OF PHARMACOKINETIC TERMS

Primary Pharmacokinetic Terms:

C_p = concentration of drug in the plasma at time t.

$A_B(t)$ = amount of drug in the body at time t.

A, B, C = intercept terms, which represent plasma drug concentrations at time 0, based on the distribution, apparent elimination, and deep tissue elimination phases, respectively, of the disposition curve.

α, β, γ = hybrid rate constants associated with a polyexponential expression that mathematically describes the disposition curve. Values of α, β, and γ are related to slopes of the distribution, apparent elimination, and deep tissue elimination phases, respectively, of the disposition curve; β, the overall elimina-

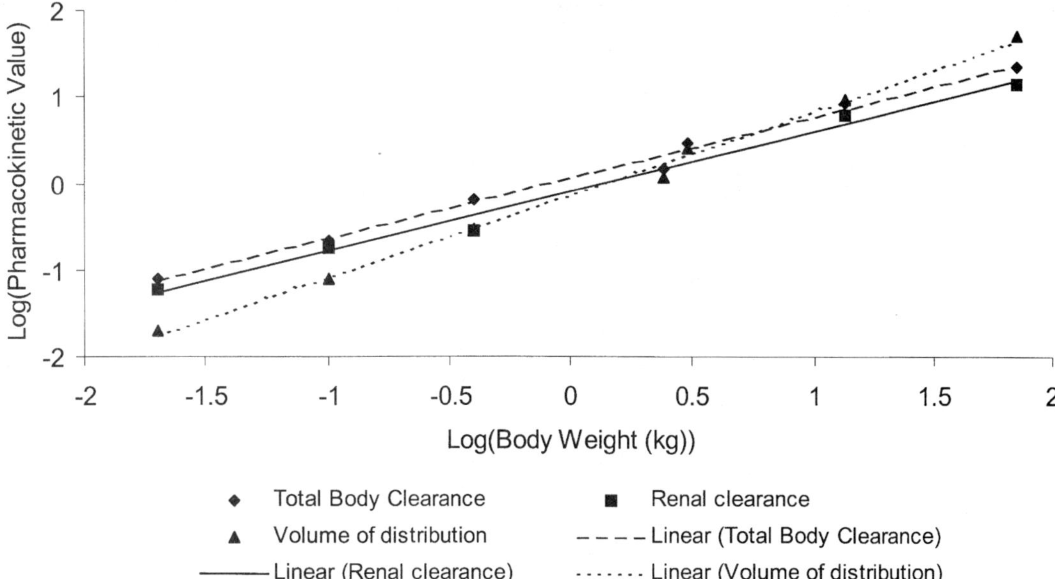

FIG. 3.23—Allometric scaling of volume of distribution (L), total body clearance (mL/min), and renal clearance (mL/min) by body weight (kg). Plotting the logarithm of the pharmacokinetic parameter by the logarithm of body weight linearizes the relationship, the basis of allometric scaling.

tion rate constant, is the negative value of the slope of the linear terminal phase of the plot in C versus time.

C_0 = initial concentration of drug in the plasma following IV injection of a single dose ($C_0 = A + B + C$).

λ_i = general first-order rate constant for the i different exponential phases in a polyexponential predictive mathematical equation that describes the disposition curve.

C_i = general coefficients for the i different exponential phases in a polyexponential predictive mathematical equation that describes the disposition curve.

k_{12}, k_{21} = first-order transfer rate constants for drug distribution between central and peripheral compartments of the two-compartment open model.

k_{el} = first-order rate constant for elimination of a drug from the central compartment.

$t_{1/2}$ = the half-life of a drug (0.693/β), based on first-order (exponential) elimination.

e = base of natural logarithm (ln).

Volume and Clearance Terms:

V_c = apparent volume of central compartment.

Vd = apparent volume of drug distribution; proportionality constant relating plasma concentration of a drug to total amount of drug in the body at any time after pseudodistribution equilibrium has been attained.

Vd_B = apparent volume of distribution obtained by neglecting the α (distribution) phase of drug disposition (extrapolation method).

Vd_{area} = apparent volume of distribution based on total area under the plasma drug concentration versus time curve (area method).

Vd_{ss} = steady-state volume of distribution of a drug.

AUC = total area under the plasma drug concentration versus time curve from $t = 0$ to $t = \infty$ after administration of a single dose.

AUMC = total area under the plasma drug concentration multiplied by time versus time curve from $t = 0$ to $t = \infty$ after administration of a single dose.

Cl_B = body clearance of a drug. This term, which represents total clearance, is the sum of individual clearance processes for the drug. Clearance is expressed as (mL/min)/kg.

Cl_r = renal clearance. This term represents volume of blood cleared of a drug by the kidneys per unit time.

Cl_{nr} = nonrenal clearance. This term represents volume of blood cleared of a drug by other than renal (mainly metabolic) processes per unit time.

f_{ex} = fraction of dose excreted unchanged in the urine.

Terms Associated with Dosage:

D = administered dose.

D_L = loading (or priming) dose.

D_M = maintenance dose.

D/τ = maintenance dose (dosing) rate, i.e., dose per unit time.

τ = dosage interval.

F = systemic availability of a drug, i.e., fraction of the dose that enters systemic circulation intact (unchanged).

f_{el} = fraction of the amount of drug in the body that is eliminated during a dosage interval. This term represents the extent of fluctuation in steady-state concentrations of a drug that takes place during the interval between successive doses.

C_{ther} = therapeutic range of plasma (or serum) drug concentrations.

C_{ss} = plateau (steady-state) concentration of a drug achieved by continuous IV infusion; or average steady-state concentration of a drug in the plasma achieved by a dosage regimen.

C_{max} (or $C_{ss,max}$) = maximum plasma or serum concentration achieved either by a single dose or at steady state.

C_{min} (or $C_{ss,min}$) = minimum plasma or serum concentration achieved prior to a subsequent dose, either prior to or at steady state.

T_M = interval required between maintenance doses to maintain concentrations in the therapeutic range.

R_0 = IV infusion rate.

Terms Associated with Allometry:

Y = pharmacokinetic parameter of interest.

W = body weight (usually in kg).

a,b = antilog of the intercept *(a),* and the slope *(b)* obtained from the plot of log *(Y)* versus log *(W);* also known as the power function.

REFERENCES

Alexander, F., and Collett, R. A. 1974. Br J Pharmacol 52:142.

Ali-Melkkila, T., Kanto, J., and Iisalo, E. 1993. Acta Anaesthesiol Scand 37:633.

Baggot, J. D. 1977. Principles of Drug Disposition in Domestic Animals: The Basis of Veterinary Clinical Pharmacology. Philadelphia: W. B. Saunders.

Baggot, J. D., and Davis, L. E. 1973. Res Vet Sci 14:207.

Baggot, J. D., Davis, L. E., and Neff, C. A. 1972. Biochem Pharmacol 21:1813.

Baggot, J. D., Ludden, T. M., and Powers, T. E. 1976. Can J Comp Med 40:310.

Baggot, J. D., Powers, T. E., Powers, J. D., et al. 1977. Res Vet Sci 24:77.

Benet, L. Z., Kroetz, D. L., and Sheiner, L. B. 1996. In J. G. Hardman, L. E. Limbird, P. B. Molinoff, R. W. Ruddon, and A. G. Goodman, eds., Goodman and Gilman's The Pharmacological Basis of Therapeutics, 9th ed., p. 3. New York: McGraw-Hill.

Bergan, T. 1978. Scand J Infect Dis (Suppl) 14:36.

Boxenbaum, H. G., Fellig, J., Hanson, L. J., et al. 1977. Res Vet Sci 23:24.

Boyce, J. R., Wright, F. J., Cervenko, F. W., et al. 1976. Anesthesiology 45:629.

Brodie, B. B., and Axelrod, J. 1948. J Pharmacol Exp Ther 94:29.

———. 1949. J Pharmacol Exp Ther 97:58.

Brodie, B. B., Gillette, J. R., and LaDu, B. N. 1958. Annu Rev Biochem 27:427.

Brown, S. A., Jaglan, P. S., and Banting, A. 1991. Acta Vet Scand (Suppl):97.

Brown, S. A., and Riviere, J. E. 1991. J Vet Pharmacol Ther 14:1.

Brown, S. A., Chester, S. T., and Robb, E. J. 1996. J Vet Pharmacol Ther 19:32.

Cabana, B. E. 1976. Arzneim Forsch 26:151.

Clarke, C. R., Brown, S. A., Streeter, R. N., Clarke, J. M., Hamlow, P. J., Callahan, J. K., Hubbard, V. L., Speedy, A. K., and Burrows, G. E. 1996. J Vet Pharmacol Therap 19:376.

Clarke, C. R., Short, C. R., Hsu, R.-C., and Baggot, J. D. 1985. Am J Vet Res 46:2461.

Conney, A. H., and Burns, J. J. 1972. Science 178:576.

Cotler, S., Holazo, A., Boxenbaum, H. G., et al. 1976. J Pharm Sci 65:822.

Dalton, R. G. 1968a. Br Vet J 124:371.

———. 1968b. Br Vet J 124:451.

———. 1968c. Br Vet J 124:498.

Dalvi, R. R., Nunn, V. A., and Juskevich, J. 1987. J Vet Pharmacol Therap 10:164.

Davies, D. S., Gigon, P. L., and Gillette, J. R. 1969. Life Sci 8:85.

Davis, L. E. 1979. J Am Vet Med Assoc 175:1210.

Davis, L. E., and Westfall, B. A. 1972. Am J Vet Res 33:1253.

Davis, L. E., Neff, C. A., Baggot, J. D., et al. 1972. Am J Vet Res 33:2259.

Davson, H., and Danielli, J. F. 1952. The Permeability of Natural Membranes, 2nd ed., p. 57. London: Cambridge Univ Press.

Dayton, P. G., Cucinell, S. A., Weiss, M., et al. 1967. J Pharmacol Exp Ther 158:305.

De Corte-Baeten, K., and Debackere, M. 1978. J Vet Pharmacol Ther 1:129.

De Rick, A., Chakrabarti, S., Belpaire, F., et al. 1979. J Vet Pharmacol Ther 2:27.

Dowben, R. M. 1969. In R. M. Dowben, ed., Biological Membranes, p. 1. Boston: Little, Brown.

Dreyfuss, J., Ross, J. J., and Schreiber, E. C. 1971. Arzneim Forsch 21:948.

Dring, L. G., Smith, R. L., and Williams, R. T. 1970. Biochem J 116:425.

Dürr, A. 1976. Res Vet Sci 20:24.

Dutton, G. J., ed. 1966. Glucuronic Acid: Free and Combined Chemistry, Biochemistry, Pharmacology, and Medicine, p. 185. New York: Academic Press.

Ecobichon, D. J., D'Ver, A. S., and Ehrhart, W. 1988. Fund Appl Toxicol 11:29.

Fouts, J. R. 1961. Biochem Biophys Res Commun 6:373.

Friedman, P. J., and Cooper, J. R. 1960. J Pharmacol Exp Ther 129:373.

Galeazzi, R. L., Sheiner, L. B., Lockwood, T., et al. 1976. Clin Pharmacol Ther 19:55.

Gamble, J. A. S., Mackay, J. S., and Dundee, J. W. 1973. Br J Anaesth 45:926.

Garrett, E. R., and Lambert, H. J. 1973. J Pharm Sci 62:550.

Giardina, E.-G. V., Dreyfuss, J., Bigger, J. T., Jr., et al. 1976. Clin Pharmacol Ther 19:339.

Gibaldi, M., and Perrier, D. 1982. Pharmacokinetics, 2nd ed. New York: Marcel Dekker.

Gibaldi, M., Nagashima, R., and Levy, G. 1969. J Pharm Sci 58:193.

Gierke, K. D., Perrier, D., Mayersohn, M., et al. 1978. J Pharmacol Exp Ther 205:459.

Gillette, J. R. 1963. Recent Prog Drug Res 6:13.

———. 1966. Adv Pharmacol 4:219.

Gingerich, D. A., Baggot, J. D., and Yeary, R. A. 1975. J Am Vet Med Assoc 167:945.

Govier, W. C. 1965. J Pharmacol Exp Ther 150:305.

Greenblatt, D. J., Duhme, D. W., Koch-Weser, J., et al. 1973. N Engl J Med 289:651.

Gugler, R., Lain, P., and Azarnoff, D. L. 1975. J Pharmacol Exp Ther 195:416.

Gupta, P. K., and Robinson, J. R. 1988. Int J Pharmaceut 43:45.

Hogben, C. A. M., Tocco, D. J., Brodie, B. B., et al. 1959. J Pharmacol Exp Ther 125:275.

Holford, N. H. G., and Sheiner, L. B. 1981. Clin Pharmacokinet 6:429.

Houghton, G. W., and Richens, A. 1974. Br J Clin Pharmacol 1:155.

Howell, A., Sutherland, R., and Robinson, G. N. 1972. Clin Pharmacol Ther 13:724.

Hungate, R. E. 1966. The Rumen and Its Microbes, p. 218. New York: Academic Press.
Hutchaleelaha, A., Chow, H.-H., and Mayersohn, M. 1997. J Pharm Pharmacol 49:178.
International Commission on Radiological Protection. 1975. Report of the Task Group on Reference Man, 1st ed. Oxford, England: Pergamon.
Isselbacher, K. J., Chrabas, M. F., and Quinn, R. C. 1962. J Biol Chem 237:3033.
Jacobs, M. H. 1940. Cold Spring Harbor Symp Quant Biol 8:30.
Jezequel, S. G. 1994. J Pharm Pharmacol 46:196.
Kampmann, J., Molholm Hansen, J., Siersboek-Nielsen, K., et al. 1972. Clin Pharmacol Ther 13:516.
Kanto, J., Kangas, L., and Siirtola, T. 1975. Acta Pharmacol Toxicol (Kbh) 36:328.
Kaplan, S. A., Weinfeld, R. E., Cotler, S., et al. 1970. J Pharm Sci 59:358.
Kaplan, S. A., Jack, M. L., Alexander, K., et al. 1973. J Pharm Sci 62:1789.
Kates, R. E., Keene, B. W., and Hamlin, R. L. 1979. J Vet Pharmacol Ther 2:21.
Kawalek, J. C., and El Said, K. R. 1990. Am J Vet Res 51:1742.
———. 1994. Am J Vet Res 55:1579.
Keenaghan, J. B., and Boyes, R. N. 1972. J Pharmacol Exp Ther 180:454.
Kramer, W. G., Lewis, R. P., Cobb, T. C., et al. 1974. J Pharmacokinet Biopharm 2:299.
Leibman, K. C., and Anaclerio, A. M. 1962. In B. B. Brodie and E. G. Erdös, eds., Metabolic Factors Controlling Duration of Drug Action, Proceedings of the First International Pharmacological Meeting, vol. 6, p. 91. Oxford, England: Pergamon.
Lobell, R. D., Varma, K. J., Johnson, J. C., Sams, R. A., Gerken, D. F., Ashcraft, S. M. 1994. J Vet Pharmacol Therap 17:253.
Martinez, M. N. 1998a. J Am Vet Med Assoc 213:974.
———. 1998b. J Am Vet Med Assoc 213:1122.
Mason, H. S. 1957. Science 125:1185.
Masson, M. J., and Phillipson, A. T. 1951. J Physiol (Lond) 113:189.
———. 1952. J Physiol (Lond) 116:98.
Matthews, C. A., Swett, W. W., and McDowell, R. E. 1975. J Dairy Sci 58:1453.
Miyama, T., Takanaga, H., Matsuo, H., Yamano, K., Yamamoto, K., Iga, T., Naito, M., Tsuroio, T., Ishisuka, Hl, Kawahara, Y., Sawada, Y. 1998. Antimicrob Agents Chemother 42:1738.
Mordenti, J. 1986. J Pharm Sci 75:1028.
———. 1986. Antimicrob Agents Chemother 27:887.
Mueller, G. C., and Miller, J. A. 1950. J Biol Chem 185:145.
Neff-Davis, C., Davis, L. E., and Powers, T. E. 1975. Am J Vet Res 36:309.
Nielsen, P., and Rasmussen, F. 1975. Acta Pharmacol Toxicol (Kbh) 36:123.
Nose, Y., and Lipmann, F. 1958. J Biol Chem 233:1348.
Nouws, J. F., Smulders, A., and Rappalini, M. 1990. Vet Q 12:129.
Olson, S. C., Beconi-Barker, M. G., Smith, E. B., Martin, R. A., Vidmar, T. J., and Adams, L. D. 1998. J Vet Pharmacol Therap 21:112.
Papich, M. G., Davis, L. E., Davis, C. E., McKiernan, B. C., and Brown, S. A. 1986. Am J Vet Res 47:2351.
Parke, D. V. 1968. The Biochemistry of Foreign Compounds, p. 127. Oxford, England: Pergamon.
Phillipson, A. T., and McAnally, R. A. 1942. J Exp Biol 19:199.
Pilloud, M. 1973a. Res Vet Sci 15:224.
———. 1973b. Res Vet Sci 15:231.
Piperno, E., Ellis, D. J., Getty, S. M., et al. 1968. J Am Vet Med Assoc 153:195.
Ponec, M., Haverkort, M., Soei, Y. L., Kempenaar, J., and Bodde, H. 1990. J Pharm Sci 79:312.
Prescott, J. F., and Baggot, J. D. 1993. Antimicrobial Therapy in Veterinary Medicine, 2nd ed. Ames: Iowa State Univ Press.
Rasmussen, F. 1958. Acta Pharmacol Toxicol (Kbh) 15:139.
———. 1959. Acta Pharmacol Toxicol (Kbh) 16:194.
———. 1966. Studies on the Mammary Excretion and Absorption of Drugs. Copenhagen: Carl Fr. Mortensen.
———. 1970. Vet Rec 87:14.
Rasmussen, F., and Høgh, P. 1971. Nord Vet Med 23:593.
Rasmussen, F., and Ladefoged, O. 1974. Acta Vet Scand 15:636.
Rasmussen, F., and Svendsen, O. 1976. Res Vet Sci 20:55.
Rasmussen, F., Gelsä, H., and Nielsen, P. 1979. J Vet Pharmacol Ther 2:245.
Riegelman, S., and Rowland, M. 1975. In T. Teorell, R. L. Dedrick, and P. G. Condliffe, eds., Pharmacology and Pharmacokinetics, p. 87. New York: Plenum.
Riegelman, S., Loo, J. C. K., and Rowland, M. 1968. J Pharm Sci 57:117.
Ritschel, W. A., and Vachharajani, N. N. 1993. Arzneim-Forsch 43:963.
Riviere, J. E., Martin-Jimenez, T., Sundlof, S. F., and Craigmill, A. L. 1997. J Vet Pharmacol Therap 20:453.
Robbins, P. W., and Lipmann, F. 1957. J Biol Chem 229:837.
Roberts, R. J., Klaassen, C. D., and Plaa, G. L. 1967. Proc Soc Exp Biol Med 125:313.
Rowland, M., Benet, L. Z., and Graham, G. G. 1973. J Pharmacokinet Biopharm 1:123.
Rowland, M., and Tozer, T. N. 1995. Clinical Pharmacokinetics. Concepts and Applications, 3rd ed. Baltimore: Williams & Wilkins.
Sams, R. A., and Baggot, J. D. 1977. Can J Comp Med 41:479.
Sanders, J. E., and Yeary, R. A. 1978. J Am Vet Med Assoc 172:153.
Schanker, L. S. 1964. In N. J. Harper and A. B. Simmonds, eds., Advances in Drug Research, vol. 1, p. 71. New York: Academic Press.
Scheline, R. R. 1968. J Pharm Sci 57:2021.
———. 1973. Pharmacol Rev 25:451.
Schwartz, D. E., Vetter, W., and Englert, G. 1970. Arzneim Forsch 20:1867.
Shoaf, S. E., Schwark, W. S., and Guard, C. L. 1989. Am J Vet Res 50:396.
Short, C. R., and Davis, L. E. 1970. J Pharmacol Exp Ther 174:185.
Singer, S. J., and Nicolson, G. L. 1972. Science 175:720.
Soback, S., Paape, M. J., Filep, R., and Varma, K. J. 1995. J Vet Pharmacol Therap 18:413.
Sodicoff, M., Lamperti, A., and Ziskin, M. C. 1990. Radiat Res 121:212.
Stenlake, J. B. 1979. Foundations of Molecular Pharmacology, vol. 2, p. 232. London: Athlone.
Stowe, C. M., and Sisodia, C. S. 1963. Am J Vet Res 24:525.
Theodorides, V. J., Di Cuollo, C. J., Guarini, J. R., et al. 1968. Am J Vet Res 29:643.
Ther, L., and Winne, D. 1971. Annu Rev Pharmacol 11:57.
Tschudi, P. 1972. Zentralbl Veterinaermed (A) 19:851.
Ullberg, S. 1954. Acta Radiol (Suppl) (Stockh) 118:1.
———. 1961. In O. H. Lowry and P. Lindgren, eds., Methods for the Study of Pharmacological Effects at Cellular and Subcellular Levels, Proceedings of the First International Pharmacological Meeting, vol. 5, p. 29. Oxford, England: Pergamon.
van't Klooster, G. 1992. Drug metabolism in ruminants: an in vitro approach. PhD thesis, Utrecht Univ.

Vaughan, D. P., and Beckett, A. H. 1974. J Pharm Pharmacol 26:789.
Vesell, E. S., Shapiro, J. R., Passananti, G. T., et al. 1975. Clin Pharmacol Ther 17:48.
Waddell, W. J., and Brinkhous, W. K. 1967. J Biol Photogr Assoc 35:147.
Wagner, J. G. 1973. J Pharmacokinet Biopharm 1:363.
———. 1974. Clin Pharmacol Ther 16:691.
Webb, A. I., and Weaver, B. M. Q. 1979. Equine Vet J 11:39.
Westlake, W. J. 1988. In K. E. Peace, ed., Biopharmaceutical Statistics for Drug Development, p. 329. New York: Marcel Dekker.
Whelton, A., Sapir, D. G., Carter, G. G., et al. 1971. J Pharmacol Exp Ther 179:419.
Whittem, T., Freeman, D. A., Hanlon, D., and Parton, K. 1995. J Vet Pharmacol Therap 18:61.
Williams, R. T. 1967. Fed Proc 26:1029.
———. 1971. In B. N. LaDu, H. G. Mandel, and E. L. Way, eds., Fundamentals of Drug Metabolism and Drug Disposition, p. 187. Baltimore: Williams & Wilkins.
———. 1972. Toxicol Appl Pharmacol 23:769.
Witkamp, R. F., Lohuis, J. A. C. M., Nijmeijer, S. M., Kolker, H. J., Noorhoek, J., and van Miert, A. S. J. P. A. M. 1991. Xenobiotica 21:1483.
Yeary, R. A., and Swanson, W. 1973. J Am Vet Med Assoc 163:1177.
Zhang, Y., Guo, X., Lin, E. T., and Benet., L. Z. 1998. Drug Metab Disposit 26:360.
Ziv, G., and Sulman, F. G. 1973a. Am J Vet Res 34:329.
———. 1973b. Br Vet J 129:83.
———. 1974b. Am J Vet Res 35:1197.
Ziv, G., Shani, J., and Sulman, F. G. 1973. Am J Vet Res 34:1561.
Ziv, G., Soback, S., and Bor, A. 1983. J Vet Pharmacol Therap 6:41.

4 CLINICAL PHARMACOLOGY: PRINCIPLES OF THERAPEUTICS

MARK J. NOVOTNY

Rational Drug Therapy
Therapeutic Decision Making
Drug Formulation
Dosage Regimen
Margin of Drug Safety
Contraindications
Adverse Drug Experiences
Drug Interactions
Drug Therapy in Special Patient Populations
Drug Therapy during Pregnancy
Drug Therapy in Neonatal and Pediatric Patients
Drug Therapy in Geriatric Patients
Drug Therapy in Patients with Liver Failure
Drug Therapy in Patients with Renal Failure
Monitoring Response to Therapy
Therapeutic Drug Monitoring

Veterinary clinical pharmacology is a clinical science that integrates disease pathophysiology with fundamental concepts of pharmacology to provide a rational basis for drug therapy in animal patients (Davis 1978). In a review of the discipline Brown (1997) stated that the goal of veterinary clinical pharmacology is to apply the principles of pharmacology to more successfully treat patients and to more rationally use medications in veterinary medical practice. In selecting and understanding pharmacologic approaches to the management of diseases, veterinarians must consider the benefits and risks of drug therapy, methods of monitoring responses to therapy, the financial and safety impact of therapeutic decisions, and the impact of the disease process on pharmacokinetics and pharmacodynamics (Coppoc and Stuckey 1977; Novotny 1993a; Wilcke 1986). These concepts shape the principle of rational drug therapy.

RATIONAL DRUG THERAPY. Rational drug therapy is the development and execution of a plan of therapy centered on the pharmacologic and clinical rationale for the selection of drugs to target distinct pathophysiologic processes. Rational drug therapy consists of the selection of the proper drug and dosage regimen appropriate for the species and the disease state in order to normalize bodily functions or to eliminate a pathogen. The decision-making process should be conducted with regard for benefit, risk, and economic considerations and with knowledge of the divergent opinions or controversies frequently associated with approaches to managing certain diseases. The reality of controversy, principally due to insufficient knowledge in drug selection and use for certain diseases, needs to be recognized when striving to optimize therapeutic decisions for individual patients (Ingenito et al. 1992).

A prerequisite to the rational use of any drug is an accurate diagnosis. Diagnoses should be in pathophysiologic terms. For example, one would diagnose streptococcal pneumonia rather than simply pneumonia, nocardial mastitis rather than mastitis, or ascariasis rather than intestinal parasites. Specific pathophysiologic diagnoses lead to specific therapeutic goals. These goals should be established prior to the institution of therapy, and therapy should be monitored against these goals while recognizing and minimizing the undesired effects of drugs (Ingenito et al. 1992).

Rational drug therapy requires a knowledge of the pharmacodynamics and pharmacokinetics of drugs in the species to be treated. Consideration should be given to the relationship between the pathophysiology of the disease and the potential impact of the disease process on pharmacodynamics so that drug effects can be anticipated. For example, sulfonamide antimicrobials competitively inhibit para-aminobenzoic acid (PABA) incorporation into folic acid in bacterial cells, a drug action that may be reversed by an excess of PABA in tissue exudate, necrotic tissue, or purulent wounds (Prescott and Baggot 1993). Similarly, the disease process may alter the drug's pharmacokinetics such that drug absorption, distribution, metabolism, or elimination changes in a predictable or unpredictable manner. Failure to adjust the regimen for the aminoglycoside antibiotic gentamicin in a patient with diminished glomerular filtration could result in drug accumulation and toxicity. Patients should be observed for drug efficacy and toxicity. These observations are needed to determine if therapeutic objectives are attained and will enable a course to be set for continued therapy.

THERAPEUTIC DECISION MAKING. Therapeutic goals are a logical extension of disease pathophysiology. Once established, clear therapeutic goals or end points should guide therapeutic decision making and monitoring therapeutic outcome. The first question to be considered is the need for drug therapy to achieve the therapeutic goals. Once the decision is made that drug therapy is needed, there are several practical considerations surrounding drug selection and the drug of first choice. Detailed below is a problem-solving approach to therapeutic decision making that includes practical considerations of the drug or drugs of choice and a benefit-risk assessment process.

Drug Formulation. When selecting the drug of first choice, available formulations must be considered. Choices may include proprietary formulations, generic products, use of approved veterinary products in an extra-label fashion, human products, or compounding a drug formulation. Often the veterinarian must select from several different formulations or brand name products of the same generic drug product. In other cases no veterinary-approved formulation exists and a human product must be used. Consideration should be given to the approval status when several formulations, including human preparations, are at the veterinarian's disposal. Approved products generally have met regulatory requirements for efficacy and safety in the target animal species for the approved indication and dosage regimen. Such products are produced to high manufacturing standards.

Generic versions of an approved off-patent (pioneer) product are often available to practitioners. Generic drugs are less expensive and may allow practitioners to use certain drugs on a routine basis that otherwise would be very expensive. Generic formulations can differ from a pioneer product in many ways, including the concentration of the active drug and the nature and amount of inactive ingredients (Koritz 1980). A pharmaceutical equivalent is a generic formulation that contains the same amount of active drug but not necessarily the same inactive ingredients as the pioneer reference product. A pharmaceutical alternative is a generic formulation that contains the same active drug but not necessarily the same amount or in combination with the same inactive ingredients as the pioneer reference product. The ultimate test of equivalence of two drug formulations is therapeutic equivalence, or the demonstration of the same pharmacologic effect in the same individual. A more practical comparison is biological equivalence, in which bioequivalence, the rate and extent of drug absorption, is evaluated. Two products are considered bioequivalent when they are equal in the rate and extent to which the active ingredient is absorbed and becomes available at the site of drug action. Regulatory guidelines exist for the design, conduct, statistical analysis, and interpretation of in vivo bioequivalence studies. Typically, key pharmacokinetic variables such as area under the concentration-time curve, maximum plasma drug concentration, and time-to-maximum concentration are compared between the generic and pioneer formulations using a confidence interval statistical analysis. Bioequivalent drugs are generally statistically indistinguishable based on these concentration-time end points (Riviere 1994).

Extra-label use of drugs (ELUD) is any use of a drug product other than in accordance with the directions for use that appear on the label, with the exception that the concurrent use of two approved drugs is not considered an extra-label use unless such concurrent administration is contraindicated by the labeling (Mitchell 1988). The specific ways in which a drug can be used in an extra-label manner include route of administration, dose, duration of therapy, species, indicated disease, or failure to follow the withdrawal period. In the USA, the Animal Drug Use Clarification Act of 1994 provides veterinarians with greater flexibility in extra-label prescribing of certain approved animal drugs and approved human drugs. However, major concerns about ELUD exist, and veterinarians must be selective about using drugs in an extra-label fashion. The chief concern is the potential for drug residues in food products from animals that received drugs in an extra-label manner (Mercer 1990; Sundlof et al. 1986). In general, residue depletion data are not available for the multitude of potential extra-label uses of a drug product. Extra-label use of drugs must occur within the context of a veterinarian-client-patient relationship, and such usage must not result in violative residues in food products from these animals.

A second major concern of ELUD relates to the well-being of the patient and the standards of veterinary practice. For example, penicillin G procaine is an effective antibiotic agent for the treatment of several bacterial diseases but not at the label dose of 6600 units/kg once daily. Rather, doses ranging from 3 to 10 times the label dose are frequently recommended (Plumb 1999). To use 6600 units/kg simply because this is the label dose may result in therapeutic failure.

The US Food and Drug Administration—Center for Veterinary Medicine (US FDA—CVM) restricts extra-label use in certain circumstances, such as when usage practices pose a risk to public health. In 1997, the US FDA—CVM prohibited the extra-label use of fluoroquinolone (e.g., enrofloxacin and sarafloxacin) and glycopeptide (e.g., vancomycin) antimicrobial agents, citing the increasing resistance of zoonotic pathogens in treated animals. Other drugs prohibited from use in food-producing animals are listed in Table 4.1.

Human-labeled drugs are widely used in veterinary medicine, a practice that likely will not change in the future. Many diseases of companion and nonfood animals cannot be treated without the use of human-labeled drugs because appropriate veterinary-labeled drug products often do not exist. Veterinarians have administered cephalexin, diazepam, insulin, lidocaine, morphine, phenobarbital, and antineoplastic agents for many years to companion animals, yet none of these drugs have ever been approved for veterinary use (Reid 1988). As with extra-label use of veterinary-approved drugs, the use of human-labeled drugs in animals raises efficacy and safety concerns, since studies that demonstrate efficacy and safety in domestic animals are lack-

TABLE 4.1—Drugs prohibited by the US FDA—Center for Veterinary Medicine for use in food-producing animals

Chloramphenicol	Other Nitroimidazoles
Clenbuterol	Furazolidone (except for approved topical use)
Diethystilbestrol	Nitrofurazone (except for approved topical use)
Dimetridazole	Sulfonamide drugs in lactating dairy cattle (except approved use of sulfadimethoxine, sulfabromomethazine, and sulfaethoxypyridazine)
Ipronidazole	

ing. Potentially harmful and illegal residues following administration of human products to food animals and adverse drug experiences in animals are major safety concerns. Thus, if an appropriate and effective veterinary-labeled product is available, the practitioner should use the approved veterinary product according to label directions. In the absence of a veterinary-labeled product, the veterinarian may consider use of human-labeled drugs, realizing the greater responsibility assumed for the effective and safe use of such products. The human-labeled product should be used only if a veterinarian-client-patient relationship has been established. The practitioner should be reasonably confident that the human product will be safe and effective when administered at the selected dose, route, and duration and for the specific disease. Administration should be consistent with current usage practices and with existing evidence in the veterinary literature on efficacy and safety. Finally, if the use of a human-label product is unavoidable in a food animal species, then adequate measures must be taken to avoid illegal residues in edible products. The veterinarian should be aware of the best available toxicologic, tissue distribution, and tissue depletion data for the drug in the animal species. The veterinarian should provide for an extra-long drug withdrawal period prior to marketing of the animal or animal product for human consumption.

In certain specific instances drug formulations may need to be compounded. Compounding is any manipulation to produce a dosage form of a drug other than manipulations described in the directions for use on the labeling of the drug product. The veterinarian must be aware of efficacy, safety, and legal issues associated with compounding. Safety concerns can range from lack of efficacy, leaving the disease process essentially untreated, to adverse or toxic drug reactions. The mixing of two different drug formulations in the same syringe prior to administration is a form of compounding that could inactivate one or both of the active drug components because of physical or chemical incompatibilities. Drugs in common use that should not be mixed with other drugs in the same syringe or solution include penicillins, cephalosporins, aminoglycosides, tetracyclines, antineoplastic agents, diazepam, and barbiturates (Griffiths 1988). The safety of excipients and vehicles used in compounded formulations may be unknown or they may pose risks if safe usage regimens have not been established in certain domestic animal species. For example, following intravenous administration, propylene glycol, a common vehicle for many drugs, may cause profound adverse cardiovascular reactions, characterized by cardiac asystole, systemic hypotension, and decreased pulmonary and renal arterial blood flow (Gross et al. 1979). The pharmacokinetics and drug depletion for compounded formulations are frequently not known, creating the potential for harmful residues if administered to a food animal species. As a vehicle for compounded drug formulations, dimethyl sulfoxide may contribute to the occurrence of violative drug residues in food products from the treated animals (Mercer 1990).

Dosage Regimen. Once the drug and formulation have been selected, a dosage regimen must be determined. "Dosage" is defined as the determination and regulation of the size, frequency, and number of doses. A "dose" is a quantity to be administered at one time. "Regimen" refers to a systematic course or strictly regulated scheme of treatment. Thus, a "dosage regimen" describes several practical features of therapy, including the dose to be administered, the route of administration, the frequency of administration, and the duration of therapy. Determining a dosage regimen may range from an empirical process to a well-defined process needed to achieve regulatory approval of the drug and regimen. Regulatory approval typically requires adequate and well-controlled studies to characterize the dose-response relationship in the target animal species. The selected dose is then confirmed in laboratory models and in patients during controlled, blinded clinical trials. The randomized, controlled, and blinded clinical trial is recognized as a valuable research method for evaluating new therapies in veterinary patients (Lund et al. 1998). Recently the US FDA—CVM has eliminated the requirement for dose titration studies to identify and select an optimal dosage, but it continues to require pharmaceutical sponsors to demonstrate substantial evidence that a new animal drug is effective and safe for each indication at the proposed dose or dose range (Sundlof 1998). Prudent therapeutic decisions generally include use of approved doses.

The route of drug administration may be limited simply by the available formulation; e.g., tablets, capsules, boluses, and elixirs are designed for oral administration. Suspensions designed for subcutaneous or intramuscular injection generally are not recommended for intravenous administration. The disease process may preclude administration of drugs by certain routes. Vomiting generally precludes oral administration. Severe dehydration may delay absorption of drugs administered subcutaneously. Administration of lidocaine by other than the intravenous route may not effectively control ventricular arrhythmias. When considering administration by a route other than the approved route, one again must consider the efficacy, safety, and legal issues of such extra-label use practices. For example, tilmicosin phosphate (Micotil®) is an effective antimicrobial agent for treating bovine respiratory disease associated with *Pasteurella haemolytica* when administered at the approved dose by the subcutaneous route in cattle. Intravenous injection is fatal (Arrioja-Dechert 1999).

The frequency of dosing is determined by a drug's pharmacokinetics, pharmacodynamics, and demonstrated duration of efficacy. Drugs with brief half-lives, such as lidocaine and dobutamine, may require frequent administration or administration by continuous, intravenous infusion in order to sustain effective drug concentrations at the site of drug action. In contrast, drugs with long half-lives, sustained drug-receptor action, or sustained therapeutic effects require less frequent administration. Aspirin is administered to cats once every 48–72 hours because of the long half-life in this species. The duration of effect of phenoxybenzamine, an irreversible α-receptor blocker used to reduce urethral resistance in cats (Barsanti et al. 1992), is related to the drug's pharmacokinetic properties and the rate of synthesis of new α receptors on the target cell (Hoffman and Lefkowitz 1990). Dexamethasone has a longer anti-inflammatory effect than hydrocortisone, allowing less frequent administration of dexamethasone.

The next step in therapeutic decision making is setting the probable duration of therapy. Many diseases are amenable to a single dose or short-term therapy, while other diseases require days, weeks, or months of therapy, reinforcing the need to understand pathophysiologic processes. With certain drugs the duration of therapy is influenced by the development of tachyphylaxis or receptor down-regulation. With other drugs induction or inhibition of drug metabolic and/or elimination processes accompanies intermediate or prolonged therapy. Prolonged antimicrobial therapy ostensibly contributes to the development of antimicrobial resistance through selection of resistant populations of bacteria (Prescott and Baggot 1993). As with selection of formulation, dose, route, and frequency, the duration of therapy should be determined with careful consideration of the benefits and risks of short-, intermediate-, or long-term therapy.

Well-designed therapeutic regimens (formulation, dose, route, frequency, and duration) may be meaningless should the client fail to comply with prescribed treatment for the patient. In humans certain diseases are associated with compliance failures (Gibaldi 1996). These include illnesses that lack symptoms, such as hypertension; drugs having delayed benefits, such as lipid-lowering treatments; or prophylactic therapy. Veterinary patients that are intractable and cannot be medicated also pose compliance challenges. Types of diseases that encourage compliance are those associated with noticeable and rapid repression of symptoms. Thus compliance improves with therapy of short duration involving simple regimens for which the frequency of dosing is convenient, efficacy is evident, and the drug is associated with a low incidence of adverse drug experiences.

Margin of Drug Safety. The benefit-risk assessment continues with consideration of the relative safety of the drug. For an approved drug, the margin of safety is established during the drug development process with characterization of the toxic features of the drug through evaluation of multiples of the predicted dose using the predicted formulation, frequency, and route in the target species. For other drugs, relative safety may be discerned from usage patterns described in the veterinary pharmacology literature, including reports of adverse drug experiences in animals, or from human applications. Gauging safety through these latter approaches is not a substitute for well-designed target animal safety studies; assumptions regarding cross-species safety may be false. For some drugs the relative safety is low, perhaps with adverse experiences likely even with the use dose in some patients. This does not preclude use of the drug, depending on the severity of the disease and the potential benefit of treatment with the drug. For other, quite safe drugs the precise margin of safety may not be established because assessing a multiple of the use dose may require such high doses to demonstrate an adverse experience that it is impractical and unnecessary. The veterinarian may use these drugs with confidence that adverse experiences are unlikely. Frequently the safety of a drug is refined following regulatory approval and use of the drug in a larger number of patients in the target species.

Contraindications. The next component of risk assessment is consideration of the contraindications for use of the drug and determination of whether any of the contraindications exist in the patient. Contraindications can be characterized as absolute or relative. The severity of the disease and the potential benefit of drug therapy in a specific patient may warrant using a drug when a relative contraindication is present.

Adverse Drug Experiences. Consideration should be given to the likelihood of adverse drug experiences (ADEs) in the patient. An ADE is an unintended or noxious response to a drug that occurs within a reasonable time frame following drug administration (Aronson and Riviere 1989; Davis 1995; Novotny 1993b). Some ADEs are predictable and possibly avoidable; many others are unpredictable. Although any drug potentially can cause an adverse experience, certain drug usage patterns are associated with a higher incidence of ADEs. These include (1) use of human-label drugs in animal patients for which drug safety and efficacy data may be lacking; (2) use of drugs with low therapeutic indices; (3) inappropriate or "trivial" drug use; (4) failure to set therapeutic goals or end points; (5) use of multiple drugs simultaneously in a patient or fixed-dose drug combinations; and (6) failure to weigh the benefits versus the risks of drug therapy. Adverse drug experiences are more likely to occur in younger

TABLE 4.2—Categories of adverse drug experiences

Lack of efficacy
Pharmacologic or side effect
Allergic drug reaction
Adverse drug experience resembling allergic reaction
Toxic drug reaction
Idiosyncratic reaction

(pediatric) and older (geriatric) patients, in animals that are obese or emaciated, in pregnant animals, and in animals with diseases of the principal organs of drug metabolism and elimination (liver and kidneys). Modifications in drug disposition patterns in young, old, obese, emaciated, and pregnant patients and during hepatic and renal failure may allow drug accumulation or predisposition to ADEs.

Adverse drug experiences can be classified into six categories (Table 4.2). The first type is lack of efficacy when an appropriate drug is administered at the proper dose, route, interval, and duration to treat a disease for which efficacy previously had been established (based on approved indications or previous clinical experience).

The second category of ADEs is pharmacologic or side effects. These reactions are extensions of the usual pharmacodynamic properties of the drug and, therefore, relate to the mechanism of drug action. For example, α_1-receptor blockers, such as phenothiazine tranquilizers, may cause hypotension as a potential side effect. A gastrointestinal disturbance resulting from overgrowth of nonsusceptible bacteria in patients receiving antimicrobial therapy is a side effect due to suppression of susceptible, normal bacterial flora of the GI tract. Nonsteroidal anti-inflammatory drugs inhibit the enzyme cyclooxygenase and reduce synthesis of prostaglandins that mediate inflammation. As side effects, prostaglandin E_2 and I_2 synthesis by the gastric mucosa and thromboxane A_2 synthesis by platelets are also reduced, resulting in gastric ulcers and decreased platelet aggregation and adhesiveness, respectively. Because pharmacologic or side effects are extensions of the usual pharmacologic response and are often dose related, this form of ADEs frequently can be anticipated and possibly avoided.

The third category of ADEs is allergic drug reactions. Unlike side effects, a first occurrence of this type of ADE cannot be anticipated in a patient. Further, allergic drug reactions are not dose related. Clinical manifestations of allergic drug reactions follow known allergic patterns and range from mild skin reactions to anaphylaxis. Other types of drug allergy include skin eruptions, serum sickness–like (type III) reactions, hemolytic anemia, thrombocytopenia, allergic gastroenteritis, and systemic lupus erythematosis (SLE). The usual mechanism of allergic drug reactions consists of the drug or a drug metabolite forming a covalent bond with an endogenous substance, resulting in an allergen. Because some drugs have common structures or metabolites, cross-reactivity between different drugs can occur. For example, patients allergic to one penicillin may be allergic to most penicillins. Cephalosporins share the β-lactam structure with penicillins, and although the incidence in animals is not known, as many as 20% of humans allergic to penicillins demonstrate cross-reactivity to cephalosporins (Mandell and Petri 1996). However, a much smaller percentage of these people will manifest clinical signs of an allergic reaction to cephalosporins.

The fourth type of ADEs includes reactions that resemble allergic reactions but do not have an immunological basis. These reactions might consist of cardiovascular or pulmonary effects such as those manifested following rapid intravenous administration of certain drugs dissolved in a polyethylene glycol vehicle (Gross et al. 1979). Hematologic reactions that resemble autoimmune hemolytic anemia but lack an immunological basis may occur following intravenous administration of dimethyl sulfoxide if the concentration is greater than 20% (Jenkins 1985). Drug fever, or hyperpyrexia, also is included in this category. Hyperpyrexia induced by acetylsalicylic acid (aspirin) is believed to stem from uncoupling of oxidative phosphorylation at the cellular level by salicylate (Riviere 1985).

Toxic drug reactions represent the fifth category of ADEs. Direct organ damage occurs through complex mechanisms that, in general, are not related to the pharmacologic effects of the drug. For example, the nephrotoxic effects of aminoglycoside and outdated tetracycline antimicrobial agents have no relationship to the binding of these drugs to bacterial ribosomal subunits and the decreasing bacterial protein synthesis that results in an antimicrobial effect. Similarly, the hepatotoxic effects of acetaminophen are mediated through reactive drug intermediates that have no bearing on the antipyrexic and analgesic properties of the drug.

The final category of ADEs comprises the idiosyncratic or unexpected reactions in an individual animal that cannot be classified in the previous five categories. The term applies to unusual effects of a drug that occur in a small percentage of the patient population and, like allergic drug reactions, are unrelated to drug dose. Often idiosyncratic reactions have a genetic basis.

Recognition of ADEs can be challenging, especially when the manifestations of an ADE resemble the disease the drug is being used to manage. For example, aspirin may be used to manage pain, inflammation, and pyrexia, yet the drug has the potential to induce fever. If most of the other disease symptoms of a patient receiving aspirin are ameliorated, yet pyrexia presents, drug fever should be suspected. With most ADEs, a definable temporal relationship exists between drug administration and manifestation of the adverse experience. However, this may be seconds, minutes, hours, days, or even weeks, as is possible with hemolytic anemia or SLE-like reactions. An ADE usually improves with discontinued drug administration. When reoccurrence is expected with repeated administration, the risk of reinstituting therapy with the offending drug must be weighed against the benefits of therapy with the drug.

An ADE initially manifested as a minor skin rash may, upon subsequent use, result in more severe reactions.

Managing ADEs can be equally challenging (Davis 1995, 1989). General principles of managing ADEs include (1) providing life support where appropriate (e.g., for anaphylactic reactions); (2) ceasing therapy with or modifying dosage of the offending drug; (3) selecting an alternative drug should therapy continue to be required; (4) enhancing drug elimination; (5) where available and appropriate, administering specific antagonists or antidotes; and (6) managing organ (e.g., liver, kidney) toxicity using strategies similar to those used to treat such toxicity from other causes. Mild, acute hypersensitivity reactions may be managed by allowing time for clearance of the offending drug. In other cases, such as hemolytic anemia or SLE-like reactions, immunomodulation may be required. Epinephrine is the drug of choice for treating anaphylaxis, owing to the effects of epinephrine on vascular α_1 receptors (causing vasoconstriction and supporting blood pressure), cardiac β_1 receptors (causing positive inotropic and chronotropic effects and supporting cardiac output), and respiratory β_2 receptors (causing bronchodilation and supporting ventilation). Corticosteroids and antihistamines are of lesser clinical value in anaphylaxis but may be useful in managing less severe allergic drug reactions.

Preventing ADEs is also a challenge. Allergic and idiosyncratic reactions are unpredictable. Once a reaction is observed in a patient, the reaction should be recorded and efforts undertaken to guard against repeated administration of the offending drug to the patient. Additional measures to prevent ADEs include (1) cautious use of human-label drugs until safety and efficacy of specific products become established in veterinary patients; (2) avoidance of polypharmacy (refer to section on drug interactions) and fixed-dose drug combination products; (3) setting of clear therapeutic goals and end points; and (4) assessing the benefit-risk aspects of drug therapy. Potential ADEs frequently are detected during drug development. However, in many instances ADEs are not noted until postapproval use in the larger target animal population. Adverse experiences may be general to a class of drugs or specific to a member of a drug class. Adverse experiences also may be specific to a domestic animal species or even to subpopulations within a species. When ADEs are suspected, an attempt should be made to determine the probable association between the drug and the ADE and to characterize the ADE. Suspected ADEs may be reported to the drug sponsor or the drug regulatory authorities (e.g., US FDA—CVM). Suspected ADEs are listed in product monographs at the time of drug approval, and those reported to the US FDA—CVM are published annually (Grassie 1997).

Drug Interactions. Frequently, concurrent administration of more than one drug is needed to achieve therapeutic goals. In these circumstances the potential for drug interactions becomes part of risk assessment. A drug interaction is the change in magnitude of the pharmacologic effect of a drug due to some other factor (Griffiths 1988). The other factor may be another drug, the focus of this discussion. However, drug vehicles, food, nutrients, plastic components of syringes or intravenous infusion sets, and environmental chemicals are among the factors that potentially impact the pharmacologic effect of drug. Drug interactions may occur in vitro when incompatible drugs are mixed in the same syringe or vial or when drugs are mixed in incompatible solvents. For example, solutions of the following drug pairs are incompatible: epinephrine and sodium bicarbonate, gentamicin and carbenicillin, ketamine and barbiturates, and methylprednisolone sodium succinate and calcium gluconate (Trepanier 1994). Types of in vitro reactions that can occur from mixing these drugs include hydrolysis, oxidation, reduction, complexation, acid-base reactions (incompatible pH), and precipitation (Paul 1987). In vivo drug interactions may result in diminished or enhanced drug effects, expression of a new or different effect, or perhaps no obvious pharmacodynamic change but altered pharmacokinetics that may not be clinically apparent. Some drug interactions are advantageous and are exploited in therapy. Many others are potentially deleterious. A documented or potential drug interaction is rarely an absolute contraindication for concurrent administration and hence becomes a component of risk assessment in therapeutic decision making.

Most drug interactions of clinical significance result in changes in pharmacokinetics. These include changes in absorption, distribution, metabolism, or excretion of a drug as a result of concurrent administration of a second drug. Cimetidine or other H_2-receptor antagonists alter gastric pH and may affect absorption of other drugs across the gastric mucosa. Drugs such as metoclopramide, anticholinergic agents, and sympathomimetics alter gastric emptying and delivery of other drugs to the small intestine, which is the site of adsorption of most orally administered drugs. Hence the rate of absorption of other drugs may be altered by agents that alter gastric emptying. Competition between drugs for binding to plasma proteins may alter drug distribution and transiently increase free plasma drug concentrations. Clearance of the drug also is likely to change; however, an adverse drug experience may occur should one or both of the interacting drugs have a low therapeutic index. Changes in hepatic drug metabolism can occur with certain drugs, leading to enzyme induction or inhibition. A drug that induces hepatic enzyme activity may increase clearance of itself and other drugs administered concurrently, thus reducing drug efficacy. Enzyme induction takes time to occur but may persist for several days, weeks, or months after withdrawal of the inducing agent. Hepatic enzyme inhibition generally develops quickly after administering the inhibiting drug and similarly reverses quickly upon withdrawal of the drug. A drug that inhibits hepatic enzyme activity may decrease clearance of other drugs administered concurrently, thus increasing the potential for adverse or toxic drug experiences. Drugs that alter hepatic blood flow (e.g., propranolol) may also limit clearance of a second drug should the later drug normally be efficiently extracted from plasma by the liver.

While there are few examples of specific drug interactions stemming from altered glomerular filtration, any drug that may alter hemodynamics and renal blood flow may interact with the elimination of a second drug that is chiefly dependent on glomerular filtration for elimination. Tubular secretion may be inhibited competitively by drugs that compete for the same transport mechanism. Tubular reabsorption of a drug may be altered by a second drug that changes urine pH or urine flow rate.

Changes that occur in pharmacodynamics stemming from concurrent administration of two drugs might be predicted from the mechanisms of drug action. Two drugs may have additive or antagonistic effects on the same drug receptor. Alternatively, physiologic additive or antagonistic actions may occur through independent effects on receptors associated with antagonistic arms of physiologic processes, as might occur through simultaneous effects of one drug on the parasympathetic nervous system and of a second drug on the sympathetic nervous system. Synergism occurs when the pharmacologic effect of the interaction exceeds additive effects that might be predicted from concurrent administration. Synergism is frequently leveraged in the treatment of bacterial infections through combination antimicrobial therapy with a penicillin and an aminoglycoside or use of a potentiated sulfonamide (Stowe 1984).

While there are many potential adverse drug interactions, drugs with narrow therapeutic indices are more likely to be associated with interactions that result in diminished, enhanced, or toxic drug effects. Under such circumstances adjustments in the dosage regimens may be appropriate.

DRUG THERAPY IN SPECIAL PATIENT POPULATIONS

Drug Therapy during Pregnancy. Pregnancy poses a number of challenges for designing rational therapeutic strategies because the potential benefits of therapy to the dam must be balanced against the potential risks to the embryo or fetus (Murray and Seger 1994). Relatively few drugs are specifically approved for or have demonstrated safety in pregnant animals. Changes in physiology from the nonpregnant state include increased gastric pH, decreased GI motility, decreased plasma protein binding of drugs, increased cardiac output, and progesterone-mediated induction of hepatic biotransformation. These differences in physiology potentially affect absorption, distribution, metabolism, and elimination of drugs administered to pregnant animals. When treating pregnant animals, one must prevent teratogenic or other possible adverse effects on the developing embryo or fetus. The factors that most affect placental transfer of drug, and thus exposure of the fetus to drugs administered to the dam, are the dose of the drug, frequency of drug administration, volume of distribution, extent of plasma protein binding, clearance in the dam, blood flow to the placenta, drug metabolism by the placenta, and the rate of drug diffusion across the placenta. Of these, the drug diffusion rate is the most important factor and is dependent upon the concentration difference between maternal and fetal plasma, the surface area for diffusion, and the drug's lipid solubility. Because maternal fluids are slightly more alkaline than fetal fluids, basic drugs, such as atropine, epinephrine, propranolol, quinidine, erythromycin, and trimethoprim, have a tendency to concentrate in fetal plasma. Acidic drugs, such as penicillin, aspirin, furosemide, and phenobarbital, diffuse slowly across the placenta.

In addition to teratogenic effects, other potential adverse effects include prevention of implantation and early termination of pregnancy, mutagenesis, and fetal growth retardation. Later in pregnancy, drug effects in the fetus may be manifestations of the pharmacodynamics of the drug. Predicting the fetal toxicant nature of a particular drug in the absence of data supporting safety during all stages of pregnancy is difficult. When selecting drugs for use in pregnant animals, consideration should be given first to drugs specifically approved for use and with demonstrated safety in pregnant animals of the species. For other drugs a conservative and prudent approach is to regard such drugs as potential development toxicants. Papich and Davis (1986) and Murray and Seger (1994) reviewed relative risks in pregnancy of a large number of drugs in common use in veterinary and human medicine, respectively. These reviews are useful when considering options for treating pregnant animals with drugs that have not been evaluated specifically for safety during pregnancy in the target species.

Drug Therapy in Neonatal and Pediatric Patients. As with treating pregnant animals, drug therapy in neonatal and pediatric patients poses unique challenges. Few drugs are specifically approved for young animals, and physiologic differences from adults of the species lead to important differences in drug disposition. Following topical administration, the rate and extent of drug absorption are enhanced due to an immature barrier to percutaneous absorption (Besunder et al. 1988). Absorption from the GI tract may be affected by variable gastric emptying rates, irregular peristalsis, and increased permeability of the intestinal mucosa during the neonatal period (Papich and Davis 1986; Besunder et al. 1988). The volume of distribution of most drugs is greater in neonates due to proportionally greater body water content, particularly extracellular fluid volume, and decreased plasma protein binding due, in part, to lower plasma albumin concentrations in neonates. Further, full development of the blood-brain barrier may not be complete during the first few days postpartum, facilitating distribution of drugs to the central nervous system that otherwise would be restricted from it (Short 1984). The proportionally lower amount of adipose tissue in neonates limits drug sequestering in or redistribution to adipose, a process important in terminating the effects of short-acting thiobarbiturate anesthetic agents (Branson and Booth 1995).

Although species differences exist, hepatic biotransformation mechanisms are relatively immature in neonates. Biotransformation processes mature within a few days postpartum in foals but may take 3–6 weeks in other domestic animal species (Papich and Davis 1986; Short 1984). Glomerular filtration by the kidneys appears limiting only during the first few days postpartum. However, tubular secretion, important for elimination of many acidic or basic drugs, may take 3–4 weeks to fully develop (Short 1984). Applying dosage regimens designed for mature animals to neonatal and pediatric patients may result in drug accumulation due to differences in drug disposition and adverse or toxic drug reactions. In other situations, drugs safe in mature animals are inherently unsafe or potentially toxic in young animals. Examples of the latter drugs include the antimicrobial agents tetracyclines, sulfonamides, and fluoroquinolones. Based on known differences in drug disposition patterns in young animals, it may be possible to adjust adult dosage regimens to minimize the risk of adverse experiences in young animals. For example, aminoglycoside antibiotics may be safe and effective in neonates if the dose and dosing interval are both increased to account for the larger volume of distribution (Wilcke 1991) and reduced renal clearance.

Drug Therapy in Geriatric Patients. As with pediatric patients, tailoring drug therapy to the individual takes on great importance in geriatric patients. Among animals within a species the aging process can proceed at different rates, as is seen among different breeds of dogs. Older animals are more likely than younger animals to receive multiple drugs to manage diseases of a more chronic nature. Aging results in physiologic changes that potentially alter drug disposition and may lead to enhanced or toxic drug effects. Although information on specific age-related changes in drug disposition in domestic animals is scarce, qualitative predictions of effects of aging on drug absorption, distribution, metabolism, and elimination can be based on general knowledge of age-related physiologic changes.

With age, gastric pH is increased, gastric emptying is prolonged, and GI motility is weakened (Ritschel 1987). The consequences of these physiologic changes may include a delay in disintegration of tablets and capsules, alteration of the degree of drug ionization, and decreased mixing of GI contents, causing slower dissolution of orally administered drugs. Prolonged gastric emptying may delay transit of drugs from the stomach to the small intestine, the site of absorption of most orally administered drugs. The surface for absorption from the GI tract also decreases with age as macrovilli and microvilli atrophy. The sum effect of these physiologic changes may be a decrease in the rate of drug absorption with lesser or no effect on the extent of absorption.

With age lean body mass decreases as the proportion of adipose tissue increases and total body water decreases. The volume of distribution of lipid-soluble drugs may increase, thus prolonging half-life. It is likely that drug distribution into body fat does not correspond to distribution to the desired site of action for most drugs. Thus efficacy could be diminished (Aucoin 1989). In contrast, water-soluble drugs will exhibit a smaller volume of distribution (Ritschel 1987). Also potentially affecting volume of distribution is a reduction in plasma albumin concentration and a decrease in the amount of drug bound to plasma protein. For drugs highly bound to albumin, the proportion of free drug may increase, leading to more drug available for interacting with receptors and augmenting the intensity of drug action or leading to adverse or toxic effects.

Drug metabolism consists of biotransformation of drugs to more polar compounds. Metabolism generally occurs in the liver; however, biotransformation can occur in the kidneys, other tissues, and plasma. The effects of aging on drug metabolism appear minimal. Reduction in hepatic blood flow, which occurs with aging, decreases biotransformation of drugs whose hepatic metabolic rate is blood flow dependent, as discussed in the next section (Ritschel 1987; Aucoin 1989).

The greatest difference in drug disposition between older and younger patients is the rate of drug elimination (Reidenberg 1987). Functional renal mass and the number of functional nephrons decrease with age. This leads to a reduction in effective renal plasma flow and glomerular filtration rate (Ritschel 1987). These aging changes in renal function, analogous to changes observed in patients with chronic renal failure, lead to a decrease in the rate of elimination of drugs and drug metabolites normally excreted by the kidneys (see below).

Drug Therapy in Patients with Liver Failure. With reduction in hepatic blood flow, drugs with blood-flow-limited hepatic metabolism may accumulate. Although the content and activity of both phase I and phase II liver enzymes decrease, hepatic metabolism of drugs is probably not overwhelmed until an extreme loss (greater than 80%) of liver function has occurred. No adequate routine biochemical test exists that correlates with hepatic drug metabolism, and thus close patient monitoring is needed for evidence of drug toxicity. Many drugs in common use are well tolerated in patients with hepatic dysfunction. In general, β-lactam antimicrobial agents are safe, whereas lincosamides, macrolides, sulfonamides, and chloramphenicol are best avoided in hepatic-failure patients (Bunch 1995; Tams 1984). The glucocorticoids prednisone and cortisone require reduction of the keto group at C-11 by hepatic enzymes before these drugs are biologically active (Chastain and Ganjam 1986) and are best avoided in advanced hepatic insufficiency. Prednisolone and hydrocortisone are suitable alternatives, whereas long-acting glucocorticoids are generally avoided unless potential benefits outweigh the risks of prolonged half-lives.

Drug Therapy in Patients with Renal Failure. In relation to drug therapy, the most profound changes in drug disposition accompany renal failure. With age, functioning nephron mass diminishes, as does tubular secretion and the ability to concentrate and acidify urine. Chronic renal failure is common in aging animals. Drug disposition changes associated with chronic renal failure include diminished clearance of drug excreted by the kidneys and alterations in drug distribution patterns. With uremia, protein binding and hepatic biotransformation of some drugs are decreased. Hence drugs that normally are excreted by the kidneys may accumulate, increasing the risk of ADEs. Drugs such as aminoglycosides that are nephrotoxic and undergo renal elimination have enhanced nephrotoxic potential. Thus, nephrotoxic drugs should be avoided in patients with chronic renal failure. Further, drugs requiring renal excretion should be avoided unless accumulation is relatively innocuous. Alternatively, to compensate for decreased clearance, formulas for adjusting the drug dose, dosing interval, or both may be applied to drugs that may accumulate in renal failure (Papich 1995; Polzin et al. 2000). These formulas are based on the reduction of glomerular filtration rate, generally estimated from a reduction in creatinine clearance in chronic renal failure. For some drugs plasma concentrations may be measured readily in the clinical setting through therapeutic drug-monitoring programs, with dosage adjustments based on established safe and effective plasma drug concentrations (see below).

MONITORING RESPONSE TO THERAPY. A final and important consideration in designing drug therapy is establishing a priori what end points, and changes in those end points, will be monitored to assess response to therapy (Coppoc and Stuckey 1977; Novotny 1993a). Plans should be established to evaluate the results of theory. Variables should be monitored to determine whether the animal is responding to treatment. Criteria should be established for what constitutes a "cure" or for concluding there is a lack of a therapeutic response. The clinician should determine when an initial response to therapy might occur. Consideration should be given also to follow-up procedures and alternative therapeutic strategies.

For many diseases the end points for monitoring therapeutic response may be simple clinical observations. For other diseases monitoring may include responses seen in clinical pathology variables or radiographic findings. Monitoring end points in chronic diseases of older patients is particularly important and challenging, as follow-up care may be forgotten, prescriptions may not be filled, enthusiasm, compliance, and vigilance may wane, and economic factors may limit what the client is willing and able to provide for the animal (Kay 1994).

Therapeutic Drug Monitoring. Therapeutic drug monitoring (TDM) can provide the practitioner with information useful in tailoring drug therapy to the individual patient. A clinical need for TDM may arise from a lack of therapeutic response, suspected drug toxicity, or the desire to confirm a therapeutic approach. Therapeutic drug monitoring of plasma (or serum) is the quantification of either the free or the total plasma concentration of drug to assess whether a particular patient has attained subtherapeutic, therapeutic, or toxic plasma concentrations (Neff-Davis 1988). Generally, drugs have a characteristic plasma concentration–response relationship, and clinical response correlates better with plasma concentrations than with the administered dosage (Jernigan 1991). Much of the variability in pharmacokinetics (drug absorption, distribution, metabolism, and elimination) between animals is reflected in plasma drug concentrations for any given dose administered. Insight into the effect of a disease process on pharmacokinetics may be gleaned from knowledge of the plasma concentration profile of the drug.

Limitations of TDM in veterinary medicine restrict its practical application to only a few drugs at present (Papich 1991). Therapeutically effective plasma concentrations must be defined. Similarly, plasma concentrations that are subtherapeutic or toxic need to be established. A cost-effective, clinically applicable method for analyzing the plasma (or serum) concentration of the drug must be available, and for some drugs, the results of the analysis should be available prior to administering the next dose to a patient so that dosage adjustments may be made. For drugs applied topically or that have transient effects, there is no value in measuring plasma concentrations. For drugs with minimum interpatient variability in drug absorption, distribution, metabolism, and elimination, it is less likely that the optimum dosage regimen differs much between patients.

Thus, TDM is of value when a drug assay is available in the clinical setting, therapeutic and toxic drug concentrations are known, the pharmacologic effect is proportional to the plasma drug concentration, and pharmacokinetic properties in the species are well characterized, with significant interpatient variability in pharmacokinetics (Papich 1991). Drugs that have been monitored in veterinary medicine include the cardiac glycoside digoxin, the anticonvulsant phenobarbital, methylxanthines (e.g., aminophylline, theophylline), cardiac antiarrhythmic agents such as lidocaine and procainamide, and antimicrobial agents. Of the latter, TDM is particularly useful for monitoring plasma concentrations of aminoglycoside antibiotics (e.g., gentamicin, amikacin), as these drugs have a low therapeutic index, and pharmacokinetics can be quite variable between patients. For drugs with small therapeutic indices, TDM can aid in optimizing dosage regimens to maximize benefits and minimize risk. While TDM is a valuable tool that increases the likelihood of therapeutic success, TDM will not replace the clinician's good judgment or good observational skills in monitoring response to therapy (Jernigan 1991).

REFERENCES

Aronson, A. L., and Riviere, J. E. 1989. Adverse drug reactions. In R. W. Kirk, ed., Current Veterinary Therapy IX: Small Animal Practice, pp. 169–176. Philadelphia: W. B. Saunders.

Arrioja-Dechert , A. 1999. Compendium of Veterinary Products, 5th ed., p. 1663. Port Huron: North American Compendiums.

Aucoin, D. P. 1989. Drug therapy in the geriatric animal: the effect of aging on drug disposition. Vet Clin North Am: Small Anim Prac 19:41–47.

Barsanti, J. A., Finco, D. R., and Brown, S. A. 1992. Feline urethral obstruction: medical management. In R. W. Kirk and J. D. Bonagura, eds., Current Veterinary Therapy XI: Small Animal Practice, pp. 883–885. Philadelphia: W. B. Saunders.

Besunder, J. B., Reed, M. D., and Blumer, J. L. 1988. Principles of drug biodistribution in the neonate: a critical evaluation of the pharmacokinetic-pharmacodynamic interface. Clin Pharmacokinetics 14:189–216.

Branson, K. R., and Booth, N. H. 1995. Injectable anesthetics. In H. R. Adams, ed., Veterinary Pharmacology and Therapeutics, 7th ed., pp. 209–273. Ames: Iowa State Univ Press.

Brown, S. A. 1997. Perspectives in clinical veterinary pharmacology. J Vet Pharmacol Ther 20 (Suppl 1):121–126.

Bunch, S. E. 1995. Specific and symptomatic medical management of diseases of the liver. In S. J. Ettinger and E. C. Feldman, eds., Textbook of Veterinary Internal Medicine, 4th ed., pp. 1358–1371. Philadelphia: W. B. Saunders.

Center for Veterinary Medicine, US Food and Drug Administration. 1992. Human-Labeled Drugs Distributed and Used in Animal Medicine. Compliance Policy Guide. Rockville, MD.

———. 1996a. Bioequivalence Guidance (Final). Docket no. 94D-0401. Rockville, MD.

———. 1996b. FDA Publishes Final Rule on Extralabel Drug Use in Animals. Rockville, MD.

———.1996c. Compounding of Drugs for Use in Animals. Compliance Policy Guide. Rockville, MD.

———. 1997. Docket no. 97N-0172. Extralabel Animal Drug Use; Fluoroquinolones and Glycopeptides; Order of Prohibition. Rockville, MD.

Chastain, C. B., and Ganjam, V. K. 1986. Glucorticoid therapeutics, iatrogenic secondary hypoadrenocorticism, and iatrogenic hyperadrenocorticism. In Clinical Endocrinology of Companion Animals, pp. 409–430. Philadelphia: Lea & Febiger.

Coppoc, G. L., and Stuckey, W. J. 1977. MEDIC: an approach to student responsibility in drug usage. J Vet Med Educ 4:171–173.

Davis, L. E. 1978. Role of clinical pharmacology in veterinary medicine. In C. R. Short, ed., Proc First Symp Vet Pharmacol Ther, p. 147. Baton Rouge: Louisiana State Univ.

———. 1989. Clinical management of adverse drug reactions. In R. W. Kirk, ed., Current Veterinary Therapy IX: Small Animal Practice, pp. 176–183. Philadelphia: W. B. Saunders.

———. 1995. Adverse drug reactions. In S. J. Ettinger and E. C. Feldman, eds., Textbook of Veterinary Internal Medicine, 4th ed., pp. 326–335. Philadelphia: W. B. Saunders.

Dorland's Illustrated Medical Dictionary. 1974. 25th ed., pp. 472 and 1340. Philadelphia: W. B. Saunders.

Gibaldi, M. 1996. Failure to comply: a therapeutic dilemma and the bane of clinical trials. J Clin Pharmacol 36:674–682.

Grassie, L. A. 1997. CVM—annual report of adverse drug experiences—1996. FDA Vet 12:I1–I28.

Griffiths, J. P. 1988. Drug interactions. Vet Clin North Am 6:1243–1265.

Gross, D. R., Kitzman, J. V., and Adams, H. R. 1979. Cardiovascular effects of intravenous administration of propylene glycol and of oxytetracycline in propylene glycol in calves. Am J Vet Res 40:783–791.

Hoffman, B. B., and Lefkowitz, R. J. 1990. Adrenergic receptor anatagonists. In A. G. Gilman, T. W. Rall, A. S. Nies, and P. Taylor, eds., The Pharmacological Basis of Therapeutics, 8th ed., pp. 221–243. New York: Pergamon Press.

Ingenito, A. J., Noble, B. G., and Wooles, W. R. 1992. The case conference approach to teaching clinical pharmacology. J Clin Pharmacol 32:502–510.

Jenkins, W. L. 1985. Pharmacologic control of inflammation. In L. E. Davis, ed., Handbook of Small Animal Therapeutics, pp. 127–148. New York: Churchill Livingstone.

Jernigan, A. D. 1991. Therapeutic drug monitoring: benefits to the clinical case. Vet Med Report 3:164.

Kay, N. D. 1994. Rational methods to monitor chronic disease therapy. In Proc. 12th ACVIM Forum, pp. 436–440. San Francisco.

Koritz, G. D. 1980. Bioequivalence of drug products. J Am Vet Med Assoc 177:279–281.

Lund, E. M., James, K. M., and Neaton, J. D. 1998. Veterinary randomized clinical trial reporting: a review of the small animal literature. J Vet Intern Med 12:57–60.

Mandell, G. L., and Petri, W. A. 1996. Penicillins, cephalosporins, and other β-lactam antibiotics. In J. G. Hardman, L. E. Limbird, P. B. Molinoff, and R. W. Ruddon, eds., Goodman and Gilman's The Pharmacological Basis of Therapeutics, 9th ed., pp. 1073–1101. New York: McGraw-Hill.

Mercer, H. D. 1990. How to avoid the drug residue problem in cattle. Compen Contin Educ Pract Vet 12:124–126.

Mitchell, G. A. 1988. The veterinary practitioner's right to prescribe. Can Vet J 29:689–692.

Murray, L., and Seger, D. 1994. Drug therapy during pregnancy and lactation. Emerg Med Clin North Am 12:129–149.

Neff-Davis, C. A. 1988. Therapeutic drug monitoring in veterinary medicine. Vet Clin North Am: Small Anim Prac 18:1287–1307.

Novotny, M. J. 1993a. A case-based approach to veterinary clinical pharmacology. J Vet Med Educ 20:50–52.

———. 1993b. Perspectives in veterinary clinical pharmacology: adverse drug reactions. New Brunswick Veterinary Medical Assoc Newsl, December, pp. 16–21.

Papich, M. G. 1991. Therapeutic drug monitoring: a realistic assessment. Vet Med Report 3:165.

———. 1995. Pharmacologic principles. In S. J. Ettinger and E. C. Feldman, eds., Textbook of Veterinary Internal Medicine, 4th ed., pp. 264–272. Philadelphia: W. B. Saunders.

Papich, M. G., and Davis, L. E. 1986. Drug therapy during pregnancy and in the neonate. Vet Clin North Am: Small Anim Prac 16:525–539.

Paul, J. W. 1987. Drug interactions and incompatibilities. Vet Clin North Am: Equine Prac 3:145–151.

Plumb, D. C. 1999. Veterinary Drug Handbook, 3rd ed., pp.489–493. Ames: Iowa State Univ Press.
Polzin, D. J., Osborne, C. A., Jacob, F., and Ross, S. 2000. In S. J. Ettinger and E. C. Feldman, eds., Textbook of Veterinary Internal Medicine, 5th ed., pp.1634–1662. Philadelphia: W. B. Saunders.
Prescott, J. F., and Baggot, J. D. 1993. Antimicrobial Therapy in Veterinary Medicine, pp. 21, 230. Ames: Iowa State Univ Press.
Reid, J. S. 1988. Use of human-label drugs in veterinary medicine. J Am Vet Med Assoc 192:247–249.
Reidenberg, M. M. 1987. Drug therapy in the elderly: the problem from the point of view of a clinical pharmacologist. Clin Pharmacol Ther 42:677–680.
Ritschel, W. A. 1987. Pharmacokinetic changes in the elderly. Meth and Find Exptl Clin Pharmacol 9:161–166.
Riviere, J. E. 1985. Clinical management of toxicosis and adverse drug reactions. In L. E. Davis, ed., Handbook of Small Animal Therapeutics, pp. 657–683. New York: Churchill Livingstone.
———. 1994. Unique problems associated with the determination of veterinary drug product bioequivalence. J Vet Pharmacol Therap 17:86–88.
Short, C. R. 1984. Drug disposition in neonatal animals. J Am Vet Med Assoc 184:1161–1162.
Stowe, C. M. 1984. Antimicrobial drug interactions. J Am Vet Med Assoc 185:1137–1141.
Sundlof, S. F. 1998. Legal and responsible drug use in the cattle industry: the Animal Drug Availability Act. Vet Med 93:681–684.
Sundlof, S. F., Craigmill, A. C., and Riviere, J. E. 1986. Food Animal Residue Avoidance Databank (FARAD): a pharmacokinetic-based information resource. J Vet Pharmacol Therap 9:237–245.
Tams, T. R. 1984. Management of liver disease in dogs and cats. Mod Vet Prac 65:107–114.
Trepanier, L. A. 1994. Avoiding adverse drug reactions: a review of clinically relevant drug interactions. In Proc. 12th ACVIM Forum, pp. 267–269. San Francisco.
Wilcke, J. R. 1986. Development of clinical pharmacology over the next decade. In H. R. Adams, ed., Proc 5th Symp Vet Pharmacol Ther, p. 229. Lake Ozark, MO.
———. 1991. Clinical pharmacology of antimicrobial drugs for the treatment of septic neonatal calves. Vet Clin North Am: Food Anim Prac 7:695–711.

SECTION 2

Drugs Acting on the Autonomic and Somatic Nervous Systems

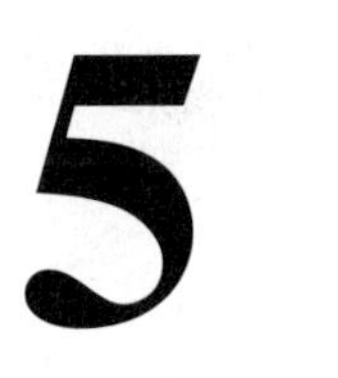

INTRODUCTION TO NEUROHUMORAL TRANSMISSION AND THE AUTONOMIC NERVOUS SYSTEM

H. RICHARD ADAMS

Organization of the Autonomic Nervous System
Sympathetic Nervous System
Parasympathetic Nervous System
General Concepts of Autonomic Function
Autonomic Interrelationships
Organ Responses to Autonomic Discharge
Information Transmission
Central Integration of Autonomic Activity
Neurohumoral Transmission
General Concepts
Physiologic Events
Adrenergic Neurohumoral Transmission
Catecholamines
Adrenergic Receptors
Receptor Subtypes
Cholinergic Neurotransmission
Synthesis, Storage, Release, and Catabolism of ACh
Cholinergic Receptors
Pharmacologic Considerations
Autonomic Receptor Sites on Nerve Terminals
Putative Neurohumoral Substances
Nitric Oxide
Nitric Oxide Biosynthesis
Pharmacologic Modulation of Nitric Oxide Synthesis and Action
Physiologic Roles Proposed for Nitric Oxide
G Proteins and Cyclic Nucleotides
Autonomic Drugs

Primary diseases of the autonomic nervous system are infrequently encountered in domestic animals, and yet drugs that alter autonomic activity are used daily in the clinical practice of veterinary medicine. Physiologic functions of diseased organs often are still responsive to their nervous supply and may favorably respond to drugs that induce autonomic effects. Also, autonomic blocking drugs are often used prior to anesthesia to prevent inadvertent stimulation of autonomic influences on visceral tissues and, furthermore, certain autonomic drugs are life-saving antidotes to particular types of chemical intoxicants.

It is obvious, therefore, that a thorough comprehension of autonomic pharmacology is required for a rational approach to therapeutic management of a wide variety of clinical disorders in animals.

ORGANIZATION OF THE AUTONOMIC NERVOUS SYSTEM. The autonomic nervous system is a peripheral complex of nerves, plexuses, and ganglia that are organized to modulate the involuntary activity of secretory glands, smooth muscles, and visceral organs. This system functions to sustain homeostatic conditions during periods of reduced physical and emotional activity and, equally important, to assist in internal bodily reactions to stressful circumstances. The autonomic nervous system also has been termed the visceral, involuntary, or vegetative nervous system.

In relation to clinical pharmacology, the most important components of the autonomic nervous system are the outflow (efferent) nerve tracts. Efferent autonomic tracts supply motor innervation to visceral structures. The efferent segment of the autonomic nervous system is divided into two principal components: the sympathetic nervous system and the parasympathetic nervous system. Sympathetic and parasympathetic outflow tracts comprise preganglionic neurons and postganglionic neurons. The cell body of a preganglionic neuron is located within the central nervous system (CNS). The synapse (junction) of a preganglionic axon with a ganglionic neuronal body occurs outside the CNS within an autonomic ganglion. An axon of a ganglionic cell passes peripherally and innervates its effector organ or organ substructure. The junction of a postganglionic axonal terminal with its effector cell is termed a neuroeffector junction.

Sympathetic Nervous System. The sympathetic nervous system is often synonymously referred to as the thoracolumbar outflow because of its anatomic origin (Fig. 5.1). Sympathetic preganglionic fibers (axons) originate from cell bodies localized within the intermediolateral columns of the thoracic and lumbar regions of the spinal cord. These fibers are myelinated; they exit the spinal cord with the ventral (anterior) nerve roots and then form bundles (white rami communicantes) before entry into the paravertebral chain of sympathetic ganglia. Gray rami communicantes are composed of nonmyelinated postganglionic fibers that exit the sympathetic chain and reenter spinal nerve roots to be distributed to target structures (sweat glands, blood vessels, hair follicles) within the limbs and body trunk.

Paravertebral (or vertebral) ganglia are located bilaterally to the ventral aspects of the vertebral column. Ganglia on each side are interconnected by nerve fibers to form sympathetic ganglionic chains that extend into the cervical and sacral regions; however, ganglia in these areas receive fibers only from the thoracolumbar spinal cord.

Upon entering the sympathetic ganglionic chain, a preganglionic fiber may terminate in one of several manners. It may synapse with a neuronal body located within the immediately adjacent ganglion, it may ascend or descend the sympathetic chain and synapse with a neuron of a distant ganglion, or it may pass through the chain and synapse in a prevertebral ganglion rather than in the vertebral chain. Prevertebral ganglia are located more peripherally than the vertebral chain and include the celiac, cranial (anterior) mesenteric, and caudal (posterior) mesenteric ganglia. They supply fibers to abdominal and pelvic viscera. Sympathetic control to the head and neck arises from cranial (anterior, or superior), middle, and caudal (posterior, or inferior) cervical ganglia. Fibers from the cervical ganglia and the anterior thoracic ganglia innervate the thoracic organs.

Sympathetic postganglionic fibers are usually relatively long since most sympathetic ganglia are located in close proximity to the spinal cord (Fig. 5.1). Sympathetic preganglionic fibers may ramify, form plexuses, and subsequently synapse with numerous different postganglionic cell bodies. Furthermore, one sympathetic ganglionic neuron may be innervated by preganglionic fibers originating from several different nerve bodies. Sympathetic discharge may, therefore, affect several different target organs and organ substructures.

The adrenal medulla is an extremely important component of the sympathetic nervous system. It is embryologically and functionally homologous to a sympathetic ganglion but does not contain postsynaptic neuronal cells. Instead, secretory chromaffin cells are present. They are innervated by typical preganglionic fibers that issue from the midthoracic spinal cord. Adrenal chromaffin cells contain epinephrine and norepinephrine; these hormonal substances are released from the adrenal gland into the circulatory system.

Parasympathetic Nervous System. Parasympathetic outflow tracts originate from the midbrain, medulla oblongata, and sacral spinal cord (Fig. 5.2). The parasympathetic component of the autonomic nervous system is referred to anatomically as the craniosacral outflow.

The vagus nerve (the 10th cranial nerve) is the most important parasympathetic nerve trunk. It arises from the medulla oblongata and sends efferent fibers to all thoracic and abdominal viscera from the caudal pharyngeal region to the cranial portions of the large colon. Fibers from the spinal accessory nerve (11th cranial nerve) may also join the vagus trunk. The facial (7th cranial nerve) and glossopharyngeal (9th cranial nerve) nerves arise from the medulla oblongata and carry parasympathetic fibers to various glands and smooth muscles within the head. The oculomotor nerve (3rd cranial nerve) carries preganglionic efferent fibers from the Edinger-Westphal nucleus of the midbrain to the ciliary ganglion that then supplies postganglionic autonomic motor fibers to ocular structures.

The sacral portion of the parasympathetic system comprises nerve fibers arising from the sacral spinal cord. These fibers form the pelvic nerves; they terminate in ganglion cells located in the colon, bladder, and sex organs.

Parasympathetic ganglia are localized more peripherally than sympathetic ganglia and usually are close to innervated structures. In many cases, parasympathetic

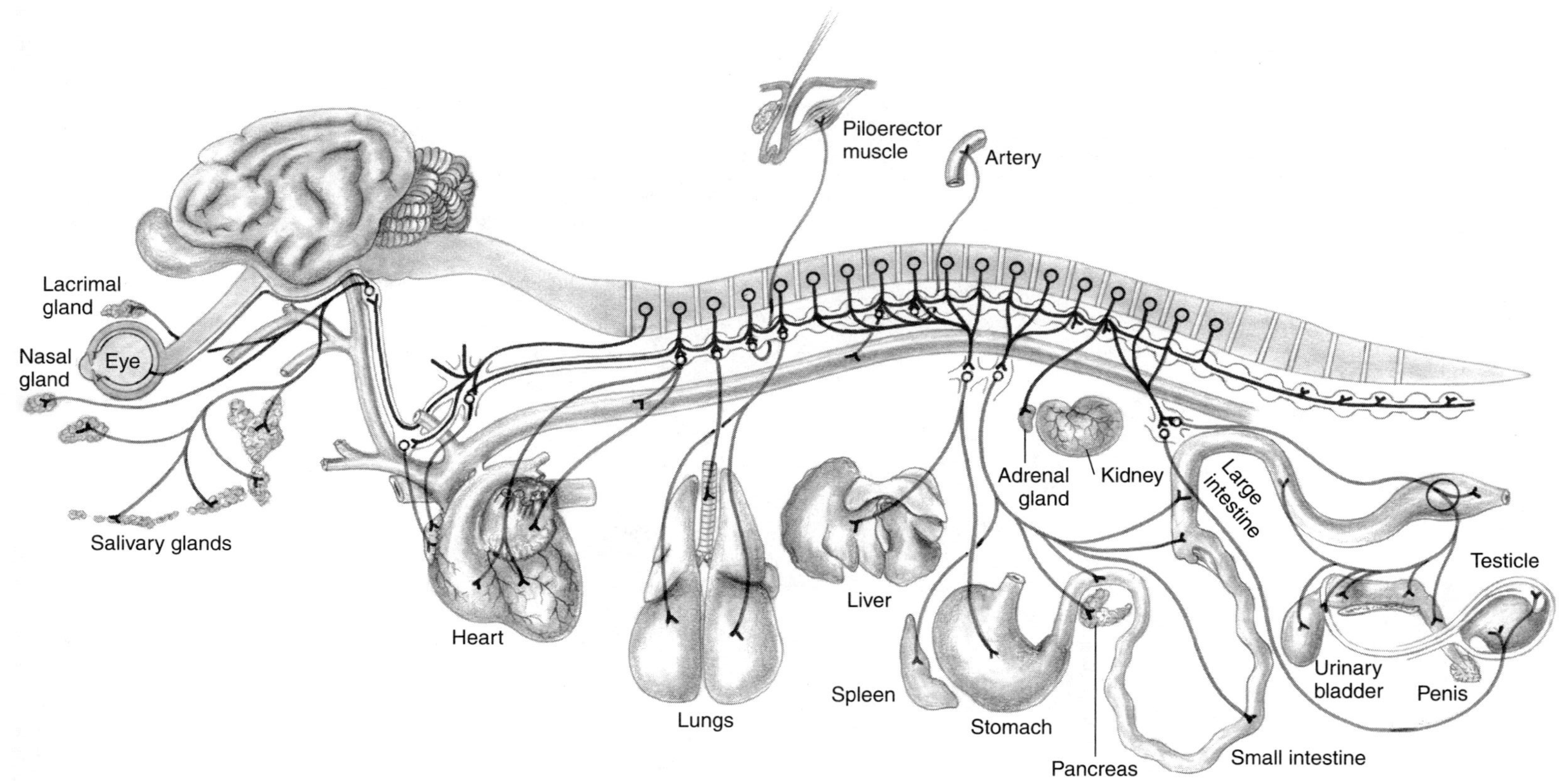

FIG. 5.1.—Anatomical representation of motor innervation from the sympathetic nervous system to various body organs and tissues. Preganglionic sympathetic neuron bodies within the thoracolumbar region of the spinal cord send axons peripherally to synapse with ganglionic neuron bodies comprising the sympathetic ganglionic chains located along each side of the vertebral column. Postganglionic axons exit the sympathetic ganglionic chains and pass peripherally to innervate those cells regulated by the sympathetic (thoracolumbar) division of the autonomic nervous system. Preganglionic fibers are red; postganglionic fibers are blue. Drawn by Dr. Gheorghe M. Constantinescu, University of Missouri. (*See also color plates following p. 118.*)

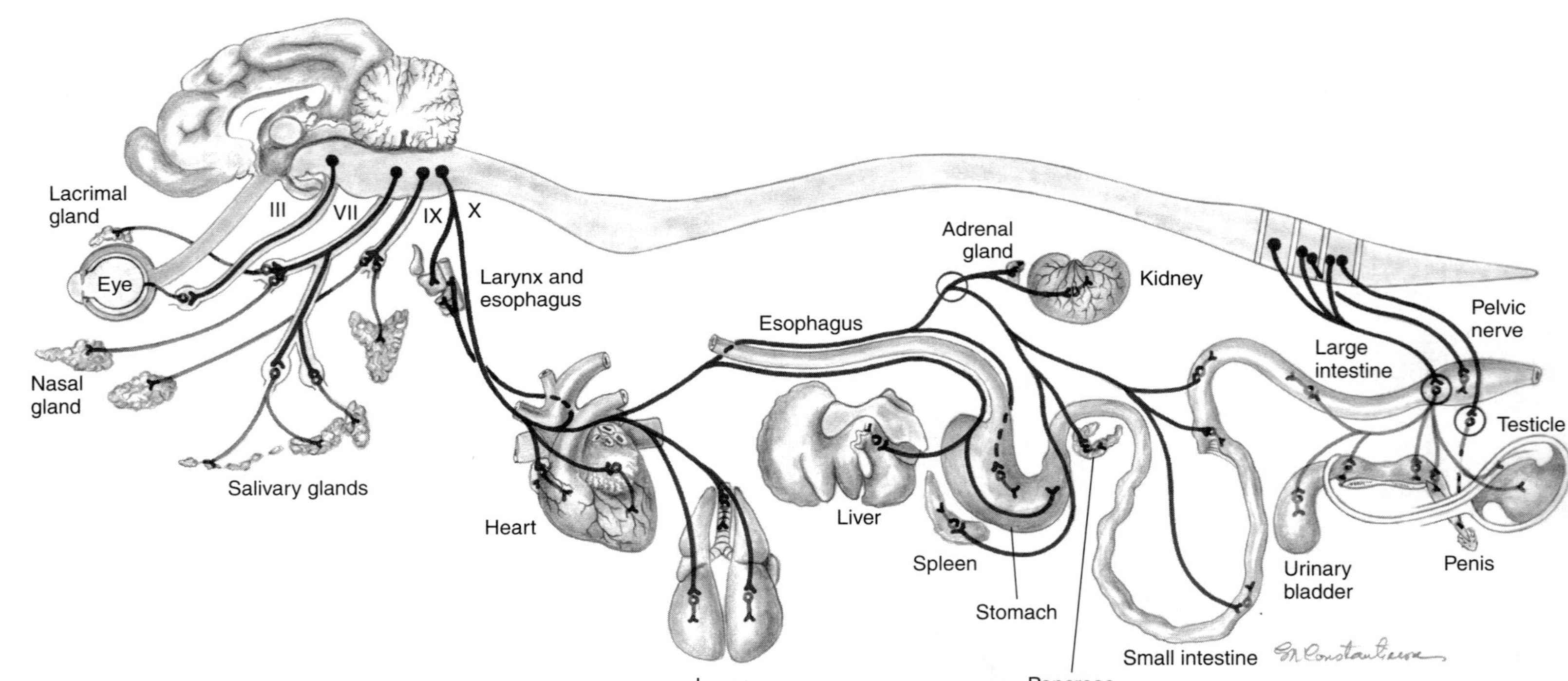

FIG. 5.2.—Anatomical representation of motor innervation from the parasympathetic nervous system to various body organs and tissues. Preganglionic parasympathetic neuron bodies within cranial and sacral zones of the central nervous system send axons peripherally to synapse with ganglionic neuron bodies localized within or adjacent to visceral tissues. Postganglionic axons exit parasympathetic ganglia and innervate those cells regulated by the parasympathetic (craniosacral) division of the autonomic nervous system. Roman numerals depict cranial nerves carrying parasympathetic neurons. Preganglionic fibers are red; postganglionic fibers are blue. Drawn by Dr. Gheorghe M. Constantinescu, University of Missouri. (*See also color plates following p. 118.*)

TABLE 5.1—Typical responses of effector tissues to sympathetic and parasympathetic nerve impulses

Effector tissues	Sympathetic-mediated responses[1]	Parasympathetic-mediated responses[2]
Heart	General excitation	General inhibition
Sinoatrial (SA) node	β_1—increase heart rate	Decrease heart rate
Atria	β_1—increase contractile force, conduction velocity	Decrease contractile force
Atrioventricular (AV) node	β_1—increase automaticity, conduction velocity	Decrease conduction velocity; AV block
His-Purkinje system	β_1—increase automaticity, conduction velocity	. . .
Ventricles	β_1—increase contractile force, conduction velocity, irritability[3]	Decrease contractile force[4]
Blood vessels		
Coronary	α_1—constriction; β_2—dilation[5]	Dilation[6]; constriction[6]
Cutaneous, mucosal	α_1—constriction	Dilation[7]
Cerebral	α_1—constriction; β—dilation	Dilation[7]
Skeletal muscle	α_1—constriction; β_2—dilation[8]	Dilation[7]
Splanchnic	α_1—constriction; β_2—dilation[9]	Dilation[7]
Renal	α_1—constriction; β_2—dilation[9]	Dilation[7]
Genital	α_1—constriction	Dilation[10]
Veins	α_1—constriction	
Endothelium	α_2—dilation	
GI tract	General inhibition	General excitation
Smooth muscle	β_1—relaxation; α—relaxation[11]	Increase motility and tone
Sphincters	α—contraction	Relaxation
Secretions	Decrease (usually)	Increase
Gallbladder and ducts	Relaxation	Contraction
Bronchioles		
Smooth muscle	β_2—relaxation	Contraction
Glands	Inhibition (?)	Stimulation
Eye		
Radial muscle, iris	α_1—contraction (mydriasis)	. . .
Sphincter muscle, iris	. . .	Contraction (miosis)
Ciliary muscle	β—relaxation; far vision	Contraction; near vision
Urinary bladder	Urinary retention	Urination
Fundus	β_1—relaxation	Contraction
Trigone, sphincter	α—contraction	Relaxation

continued

ganglia are within innervated organs. Accordingly, postganglionic parasympathetic fibers are usually quite short. Parasympathetic discharge usually is discrete and affects specific effector systems individually.

GENERAL CONCEPTS OF AUTONOMIC FUNCTION

Autonomic Interrelationships. Most visceral organs are innervated by both parasympathetic and sympathetic divisions (Figs. 5.1 and 5.2), often producing contrasting effects on the same structure. For example, parasympathetic fibers of the vagus nerve elicit a decrease in heart rate, whereas sympathetic cardiac nerves accelerate heart rate. Such reciprocating relationships allow varying degrees of qualitative, as well as quantitative, changes in organ function, depending upon the relative needs of the organism (Stuesse et al. 1979; Low 1993). Principal organ responses mediated by sympathetic and parasympathetic discharge are summarized in Table 5.1.

Another important aspect involves the unmasking of parasympathetic or sympathetic activity when the opposing system is blocked. For example, gastrointestinal (GI) functions are normally under parasympathetic dominance. Enhanced activity of this division elicits a pronounced increase in GI secretion and smooth muscle motility. However, sympathetic nerve traffic causes an inhibition of smooth muscle activity and secretory processes in the GI tract. Abolishment of parasympathetic control produces a quiescent, hypoactive GI tract characterized by sympathetic dominance. Blockage of sympathetic control to the GI tract accentuates parasympathetic activity. Such relationships are important to clinical pharmacology and explain why the response of an individual to a specific autonomic drug may present as a complex change in sympathetic and parasympathetic activity (Freeman and Miyawaki 1993).

Organ Responses to Autonomic Discharge. The sympathetic outflow tract and closely associated adrenal medulla are often referred to as the sympathoadrenal (or sympathoadrenomedullary) axis. This axis is extremely reactive. Activity varies discretely on a moment-to-moment basis consistent with the needs of the organism. Thus small changes required for homeostasis are readily accomplished. The sympathoadrenal axis can also discharge in a mass action affecting virtually all sympathetically innervated structures. Such a

TABLE 5.1—*continued*

Effector tissues	Sympathetic-mediated responses[1]	Parasympathetic-mediated responses[2]
Splenic capsule	α—contraction, β_2—relaxation	. . .
Sweat glands	Secretion (cholinergic);[12] β_2—secretion (horse)	
Salivary glands	α_1—scant, viscous secretion	Profuse, watery secretion
Piloerector muscles	α—contraction	. . .
Kidney renin release	α_2—decrease; β_1—increase	. . .
Uterus[13]	α_1—contraction; β—relaxation (nonpregnant > pregnant)	Contraction[14]
Genitalia		
Male	α—ejaculation	Erection[15]
Female	. . .	Erection[15]
Adrenal medulla	Secretion of epinephrine > norepinephrine (cholinergic)	. . .
Autonomic ganglia	Ganglionic discharge (cholinergic)	Ganglionic discharge[16]
Liver	β_2—glycogenolysis and gluconeogenesis (α in some species)	. . .
Pancreas		
Islet cells	α_2—decrease secretion; β_2—increase secretion	. . .
Acini	α—decrease secretion	Increase secretions
Fat cells	β_1—lipolysis	. . .
Adrenergic nerve terminals	α_2—decrease release of norepinephrine β_2—increase release of norepinephrine	± Release of norepinephrine[17]
Platelets	α_2—aggregation	. . .

Note: Superscript numbers are defined as follows: (1) α and β designate the principal adrenoceptor type subserving a tissue response. α_1, α_2, β_1, and β_2 designate the receptor subtype. The usual receptor types are presented; considerable interspecies variation exists, particularly with reference to subtypes. (2) Except when otherwise designated (e.g., ganglia), parasympathetic responses are subserved by muscarinic receptors. (3) Catecholamine-induced irritability of the myocardium may be associated with β_1 and α receptors; systemic pressor response may contribute. (4) Muscarinic receptors subserving decreased contractility are demonstrable in ventricular muscle, but the significance is not definitely known. (5) In small coronary arteries, β receptors are more numerous, more sensitive, and/or more responsive than α receptors. In large coronary arteries α receptors can be demonstrated. β_1 and β_2 subtypes differ depending upon species. (6) Depending upon experimental conditions, cholinergic effects on coronary blood vessels have been reported as both constriction and dilation (Kalsner 1989). (7) Arterial smooth muscle generally is not innervated by the parasympathetic nervous system (exceptions include blood vessels of genitalia). Thus cholinergic receptors in most arterial beds are not associated with parasympathetic nerves. In certain regions (e.g., arteries of skeletal muscles) sympathetic cholinergic vasodilator fibers are present, but their physiologic importance is poorly understood. (8) In skeletal muscle arteries β receptors are more sensitive than α receptors. (9) β receptors of visceral blood vessels seem less important than α receptors. (10) Parasympathetic-induced dilation of genital blood vessels (which contributes to erection) is not mediated by ACh; the neurotransmitter is believed to be nitric oxide; see (15) below. (11) β-inhibitory receptors may be localized on smooth muscle cells, whereas α-inhibitory receptors may be localized on parasympathetic cholinergic (excitatory) ganglionic cells of Auerbach's plexus. (12) In humans, sweat glands are innervated by postganglionic sympathetic axons that release ACh (i.e., cholinergic) rather than norepinephrine (i.e., adrenergic). In domestic animals, however, sweat glands are regulated by adrenergic (e.g., horse) or cholinergic mechanisms, depending upon species and type of gland (Robertshaw 1980). (13) Uterine responses vary depending on species and stage of estrus, pregnancy, and menstrual cycle (when present). (14) Contractile responses dominate; cholinergic drugs can induce severe myometrial contractions and abortion. (15) Smooth muscle erectile tissue is relaxed by parasympathetic impulses, thereby leading to vascular space engorgement and erection. The neurotransmitter at these sites is not ACh but is believed to be nitric oxide. (16) Ganglionic transmission is subserved predominantly by nicotinic receptors. (17) See Chap. 6 for distribution of α_1 and α_2 receptor subtypes in arteries. In many blood vessels endothelial α_2 receptors mediate vasodilation through the release of endothelium-derived nitric oxide. In contrast, α_2 receptors of vascular smooth muscle subserve vasoconstriction.

unitary sympathoadrenal discharge occurs in response to severe rage or fear and readies the organism for "fight or flight." Accordingly, cardiovascular activity is accelerated; an increase in heart rate, myocardial contractile strength, cardiac output, and blood pressure is observed. Blood is redistributed from splanchnic and cutaneous beds to voluntary skeletal muscles; bronchioles dilate and respiration increases; pupils enlarge; and blood glucose concentration increases. The organism is now better prepared to effectively react to the stimulus that instigated the sympathetically mediated fight-or-flight reaction.

Conversely, the parasympathetic nervous system functions mainly to regulate localized organ changes and is not organized for mass action. Whereas sympathetic activation results in expenditure of energy, the parasympathetic system reacts to generate and maintain biologic energy. Parasympathetic activity therefore has been referred to as a "live-and-let-live" type of response (Adams 1977). Digestive breakdown of nutrients, e.g., is enhanced by increased parasympathetic activity to the GI system. Myocardial oxygen consumption and energy utilization are decreased by vagal-mediated decreases in heart rate and contractile strength of the heart.

How an individual organ will respond to sympathetic or parasympathetic impulse traffic can be predicted by considering whether a particular physiologic activity would benefit the fight-or-flight response (sympathetic) or the live-and-let-live response (parasympathetic). This physiologic concept is important to the pharmacology student, because an understanding of how tissues respond to autonomic nervous activity often can be extrapolated to understanding how tissues will respond to autonomic drugs. This can save much memorization work; e.g., it is logical that an increase in heart rate, myocardial contractile strength, and cardiac output would be beneficial to an effective fight-or-flight reaction to rage or fear. Conversely, cardiac rest would be consistent with the sedentary condition of the live-and-let-live state. Thus activation of the heart would be a result of sympathetic discharge, whereas diminished cardiac activity would be a result of parasympathetic discharge. Accordingly, a sympathomimetic drug would increase cardiac function, and a parasympathomimetic drug would reduce cardiac function.

Digestion of food obviously would not be required for an immediate sympathetic reaction to stressful environmental changes. Thus sympathetic nervous system activity inhibits GI function, whereas parasympathetic (live-and-let-live) discharge increases GI function. Accordingly, a sympathomimetic drug reduces GI activity, and a parasympathomimetic drug enhances GI activity.

One apparently contradictory aspect of sympathetic-parasympathetic control is quite familiar to veterinarians. Occasionally, some animals (especially dogs and nonhuman primates) that experience profound fright will exhibit signs of increased intestinal and urinary bladder activity (i.e., defecation and micturition). However, it should be appreciated that in severe incidences of fear it is likely that parasympathetic centers in the brain will be activated by overspill of central sympathetic impulses that originate from emotional centers. Thus sympathetic inhibition of intestinal and urinary bladder activity may momentarily be overridden by parasympathetic discharge.

Information Transmission. Information is communicated from nerve to nerve and from nerve to effector organ by a process termed "neurohumoral transmission." This process involves release from a nerve terminal of a chemical neurotransmitter that reacts with specialized receptor areas on the innervated cell. Activation of the receptor instigates characteristic physiologic responses in the effector cell.

The neurotransmitter at all ganglia (both parasympathetic and sympathetic) and at most parasympathetic neuroeffector junctions is acetylcholine (ACh). In a few regions (e.g., erectile tissue of genitalia) the neurotransmitter at parasympathetic neuroeffector junctions is not ACh (Klinge and Sjöstrand 1974; Klinge et al. 1978). Norepinephrine (noradrenalin) is the transmitter released at the majority of sympathetic neuroeffector junctions and is considered to be "the" sympathetic neurotransmitter. At a few sympathetic neuroeffector junctions (e.g., sweat glands in humans) ACh is the transmitter.

Nerves that release ACh are classified chemically as cholinergic nerves. Nerves that release norepinephrine are classified chemically as adrenergic or noradrenergic nerves. A third type of nerve is classified as nonadrenergic-noncholinergic (NANC) since these neurons release neither norepinephrine nor ACh. Instead, these NANC neurons release nitric oxide as their neurotransmitter substance (Lowenstein et al. 1994). It now seems clear, e.g., that nitric oxide is the NANC neurotransmitter responsible for penile erection (see the section on nitric oxide later in this chapter).

Preganglionic and postganglionic relationships of sympathetic and parasympathetic efferent fibers are shown schematically in Fig. 5.3, which should be studied thoroughly. Often, difficulty is encountered in correlating classifications of sympathetic and parasympathetic nerves with chemical classifications of adrenergic and cholinergic nerves. An adrenergic nerve releases norepinephrine and is a sympathetic postganglionic nerve. A cholinergic nerve releases ACh but can be a parasympathetic preganglionic nerve; a parasympathetic postganglionic nerve; a sympathetic preganglionic nerve; and, in a few regions, a sympathetic postganglionic nerve. The proposed relationships for NANC nerves, which release nitric oxide, are also included in Fig. 5.3 (Änggard 1994; Adams 1996).

Central Integration of Autonomic Activity. Attention is usually directed toward the efferent adrenergic and cholinergic pathways of the autonomic nervous system. However, afferent fibers and brain nuclei that influence peripheral motor function are equally important when physiologic interactions of the autonomic nervous system are considered. Afferent fibers transmit information concerning visceral pain, cardiovascular activity, respiration, and numerous other organ functions from peripheral receptive areas to the CNS (Lang and Szilagyi 1991).

Afferent fibers are usually nonmyelinated and pass into the CNS along autonomic nerve trunks such as the vagus, pelvic, and splanchnic nerves. Sensory fibers often make up a considerable portion of autonomic nerve trunks. Nerve bodies of sensory afferent fibers are believed to be located in the dorsal root ganglia of spinal nerves and in specialized sensory ganglia of autonomic nerve trunks.

An autonomic reflex arch involves passage of information along an afferent pathway, reaction of CNS sites to the received impulse, and resulting change in efferent discharge. Well-known examples involve the baroreceptor (pressure- or stretch-sensitive) areas localized in the aortic arch and carotid sinus and the chemoreceptive cells localized in the aortic arch and carotid bodies. Information concerning blood pressure, blood O_2 and CO_2, and respiration is relayed from these sites via afferent fibers to CNS areas.

The hypothalamus is the principal supraspinal site involved in modulation of both sympathetic and

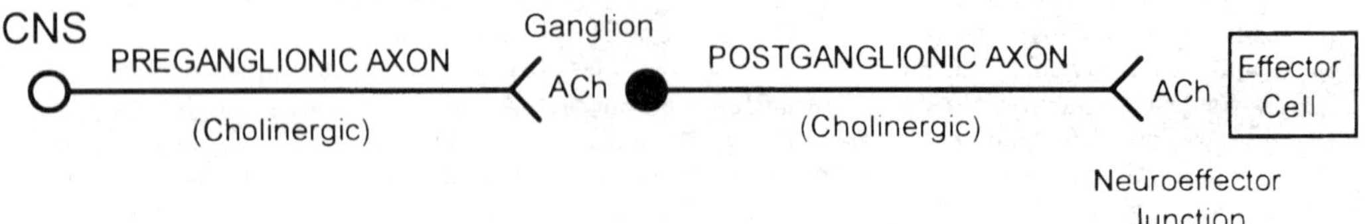

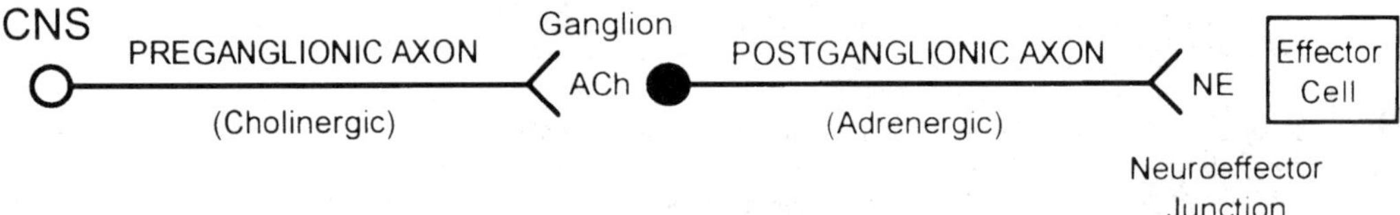

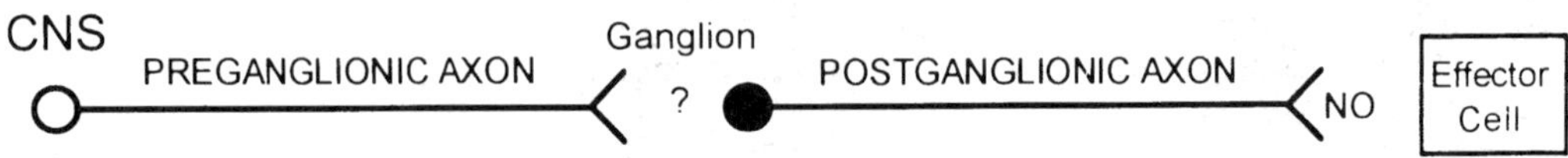

FIG. 5.3—Schematic representation of the preganglionic and postganglionic relationships of sympathetic and parasympathetic outflow tracts. ❍ = CNS preganglionic nerve bodies; ● = ganglionic cell bodies. ACh is the neurotransmitter released at sympathetic and parasympathetic ganglia and at most parasympathetic neuroeffector junctions. Norepinephrine (NE) is the neurotransmitter released at adrenergic sympathetic neuroeffector junctions. (See text for exceptions.) Cholinergic fibers release ACh. Adrenergic fibers release NE. Some autonomic nerves are classified as nonadrenergic-noncholinergic (NANC) neurons; they release nitric oxide (NO), which diffuses into effector cells without the necessity of cell surface receptors. Pre- and postganglionic relationships for NANC nerves are putative. ? = the ganglionic transmitter serving NANC neurons is believed to be ACh.

parasympathetic outflow traffic. Autonomic participation in regulation of blood pressure, body temperature, carbohydrate metabolism, water-electrolyte balance, sexual responses, emotions, and sleep is mediated through hypothalamic pathways. The medulla oblongata contains nuclei that integrate blood pressure and respiration, often interacting with hypothalamic regions.

Cerebral cortical foci may also influence autonomic activity. The Pavlovian experiments are classic examples of conscious and emotional brain centers affecting peripheral autonomic activity. In these experiments, a dog was repeatedly fed only after the ringing of a bell. Eventually, ringing a bell would evoke an increase in secretory activity of the GI tract in anticipation of a meal. Such basic experiments led numerous research workers to subsequently propose that certain disorders of body viscera may actually represent psychic influence on central autonomic sites rather than organic disease.

The pharmacologic activity of certain drugs is characterized by dominant CNS effects rather than peripheral-mediated responses. Amphetamine, e.g., affects peripheral adrenergic neuroeffector junctions; however, the overall response to amphetamine in an intact animal is characterized by CNS stimulation. Conversely, some drugs used for their CNS effects (tranquilizers) may also have profound peripheral autonomic actions. The phenothiazine tranquilizers, e.g., may depress blood pressure rather markedly by blocking the interaction of norepinephrine with adrenergic receptor sites in blood vessels (Popovic et al. 1972). Such peripheral and central interactions should always be kept in mind when the total pharmacologic profile of a drug is evaluated prior to its clinical use.

NEUROHUMORAL TRANSMISSION. Most autonomic drugs used clinically exert primary pharmacologic activities by altering some essential step in the neurohumoral transmission process. In the remaining portions of this chapter, the physiologic steps involved in neurohumoral transmission will be summarized. In subsequent chapters, autonomic drugs that affect the neurohumoral transmission process in the parasympathetic and sympathetic nervous systems will be examined.

General Concepts. Discovery and subsequent characterization of events involved in communication of information from nerve to nerve and from nerve to effector organ represent major scientific achievements. Although numerous investigators have provided various relevant information, the first definitive evidence of chemical neurotransmission seems to have been obtained by Loewi (1921) and coworkers. In these simple but scientifically elegant experiments, Loewi electrically stimulated the vagus nerve of an isolated perfused frog heart. The perfusate leaving this preparation was perfused through another frog heart. Upon stimulation of the vagus nerve to the first heart, Loewi observed that this heart was immediately depressed. Within a few seconds, the second heart was also depressed. Certainly, the most logical explanation for this finding was that stimulation of the vagus nerve liberated a chemical "myocardial inhibitory" substance that was carried in the perfusate to the second heart. This substance, referred to as *Vagusstoff* (vagus substance), was later identified as ACh.

The basic techniques proved by Loewi have been modified and utilized by numerous investigators to map other adrenergic and cholinergic pathways. ACh was found to be the chemical released from all (parasympathetic and sympathetic) autonomic preganglionic fibers and most postganglionic parasympathetic fibers. Norepinephrine is the neurotransmitter released at the majority of sympathetic neuroeffector junctions (Fig. 5.3). Nitric oxide is the neurotransmitter discharged by certain NANC neurons innervating regions of the GI tract, the vasculature, and the external genitalia (Änggard 1994; Lowenstein et al. 1994).

Several criteria should be met before a chemical can be accepted as a neurotransmitter: (1) stimulation of a nerve should markedly increase the concentration of the active substance in the effluent, (2) the proposed mediator should be chemically and pharmacologically identified and characterized, (3) exogenous administration of the chemical should identically simulate nerve stimulation, (4) other drugs should have basically similar effects on responses to nerve stimulation and the proposed transmitter substance, and (5) cellular mechanisms capable of manufacturing, storing in an inactive form, and inactivating the neurotransmitter should be demonstrable (Lefkowitz et al. 1990).

Physiologic Events. Events involved in neurohumoral transmission at neuroeffector junctions can be subdivided into axonal conduction, synthesis and release of the neurotransmitter, receptor events, and catabolism of the neurotransmitter.

AXONAL CONDUCTION. Axonal conduction refers to the passage of an impulse along a nerve fiber. It is dependent upon selective changes in the permeability of the axonal membrane to electrolytes. At rest, membrane potential within mammalian axons is approximately −85 mV. This negative intracellular potential is maintained at rest basically because the axonal membrane is relatively more permeable to K^+ than to Na^+. Na^+ ions are in higher concentration in extracellular than in intracellular fluid, whereas K^+ ions are in greater concentration in intracellular than in extracellular fluid. The relatively small amounts of K^+ that leak into the interstitial space in conjunction with the large number of organic anions that are intracellular result in a net negative charge within the axon.

An action potential reflects a reversal of the polarization state present at rest and is the result of permeability changes that occur at the axonal surface as an impulse is propagated along a nerve fiber. A suprathreshold stimulus initiates a localized change in the permeability of the axonal membrane. Suddenly, permeability of the fiber to Na^+ is greatly increased in relation to K^+; Na^+ moves inward in the direction of its large electrochemical gradient. This movement is detected by an instantaneous change in the membrane potential in a positive direction. The positively charged Na^+ increases in concentration within the axon; the membrane potential moves from −85 mV toward zero and then overshoots to the extent that momentarily the inside of the fiber is positive in relation to the exterior of the cell.

Repolarization of the membrane occurs rapidly as the selective permeability characteristics of the axonal membrane are quickly reestablished. The axon once again becomes relatively impermeable to Na^+ and relatively more permeable to K^+, and the negativity of the interior of the cell is quickly reestablished. A schematic representation of axonal conductance and resulting neurohumoral transmission events is presented in Fig. 5.4.

Although the localized permeability changes associated with an action potential are extremely short-lived, they elicit similar alterations in membrane function in immediately adjacent quiescent areas of the axon. Thus the action potential is self-propagating, and in this manner an action potential is conducted along an axonal fiber. Over long periods the absolute concentration gradients of electrolytes are maintained by energy-utilizing transport systems such as the sodium pump. The axonal membrane is refractory for a brief interval after the passage of an action potential, thereby preventing antidromic and excess impulse traffic.

Axonal conduction is insensitive to most drugs. Even local anesthetics must be used in high concentrations in immediate contact with the nerve before excitability is blocked. However, subsequent events in neurohumoral transmission are quite susceptible to drug actions.

NEUROTRANSMITTER RELEASE. Release of neurotransmitter substance is triggered by arrival of the axonal action potential at the nerve terminal (Fig. 5.4) (Klein 1973; Winkler and Hörtnagl 1973). Ca^{++} acts to link or couple the excitation of the membrane (action potential) with discharge of neurotransmitter from the axon terminal. The action potential initiates an inward movement of Ca^{++} into the nerve terminal from the interstitial space and/or superficial membrane binding sites at the axon terminal. Inward movement of Ca^{++}

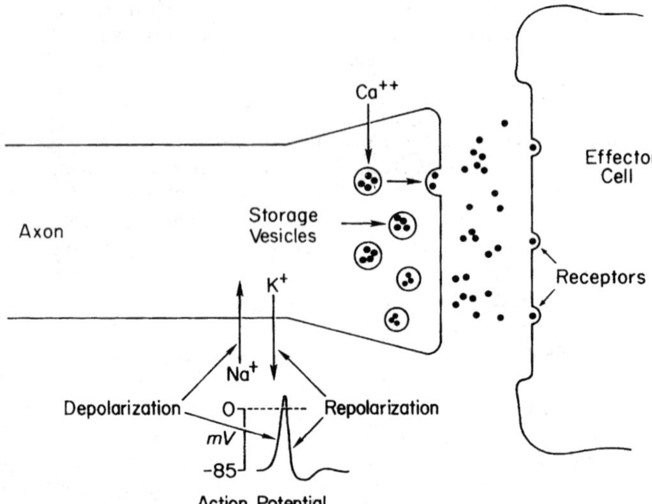

FIG. 5.4—Schematic representation of neurohumoral transmission. The axonal action potential represents a self-propagating depolarization-repolarization of the axon that is characterized by an influx of Na^+ and an efflux of K^+. As the action potential arrives at the nerve terminal, it facilitates an inward movement of Ca^{++}, which triggers the discharge of neurotransmitter (●) from storage vesicles into the junctional cleft. Neurotransmitter reacts with specialized receptor areas on the postjunctional membrane and initiates a physiologic response in the effector cell.

triggers exocytotic discharge of neurotransmitter from the vesicles into the junctional cleft (Rubin 1982). Nitric oxide is not stored in synaptic vesicles. Instead, the increase in cytosolic Ca^{++} activates a Ca^{++}-dependent enzyme: nitric oxide synthase. The activated form of this enzyme utilizes molecular oxygen and a nitrogen moiety from the amino acid L–arginine to yield nitric oxide. The latter is highly lipophilic and it rapidly diffuses to effector cells (Adams 1996).

RECEPTOR EVENTS. After rapid migration of neurotransmitter across the cleft, the mediator substance bonds with receptive areas on the postsynaptic membrane. Cell surface receptors are specialized macromolecular structures of the cell that a neurotransmitter interacts with to elicit a response (Abramson and Molinoff 1984). Many types and subtypes of receptors have now been isolated and cloned. The clinical utility of all such discoveries remains to be defined.

Receptor events caused by interaction of neurotransmitter substance with the receptor may be of two general types: excitatory or inhibitory. If the neurotransmitter initiates an excitatory response in the cell, receptor activation triggers a general increase in permeability of the postsynaptic membrane to all ions. Thus, in a manner analogous to the axonal action potential, there is a sudden depolarization-repolarization of the postsynaptic membrane characterized by a net inward movement of Na^+ and an efflux of K^+ along their respective concentration gradients. Electrically, these changes are characterized as an excitatory postsynaptic potential, which then propagates localized permeability changes in adjacent portions of the cell membrane, and an action potential is conducted along the remainder of the innervated cell.

An inhibitory postsynaptic potential occurs when the neurotransmitter initiates a selective increase in permeability of the postsynaptic membrane to only smaller ions (e.g., K^+, Cl^-). Thus outward movement of K^+ and inward movement of Cl^- along their respective concentration gradients increase the net negative charge within the cell and actually hyperpolarize the postsynaptic membrane. The resulting hyperpolarization of the membrane increases the threshold to stimuli and, in effect, elicits an inhibitory response in the cell.

CATABOLISM OF NEUROTRANSMITTER. Termination of the duration of action of released neurotransmitter substances involves different mechanisms. The adrenergic neurotransmitter norepinephrine is metabolized by both intraneuronal and extraneuronal enzymes. However, the uptake of norepinephrine back into the adrenergic nerve terminal and diffusion of norepinephrine away from receptor sites are probably more important pathways for termination of norepinephrine activity. Extraneuronal ACh is rapidly hydrolyzed by acetylcholinesterase (AChE), a quite specific enzyme localized in close proximity to the synaptic cleft. Nitric oxide is a highly reactive free radical, and it undergoes oxidation to nitrites and nitrates within seconds.

ADRENERGIC NEUROHUMORAL TRANSMISSION. For critical examination of adrenergic mecha-

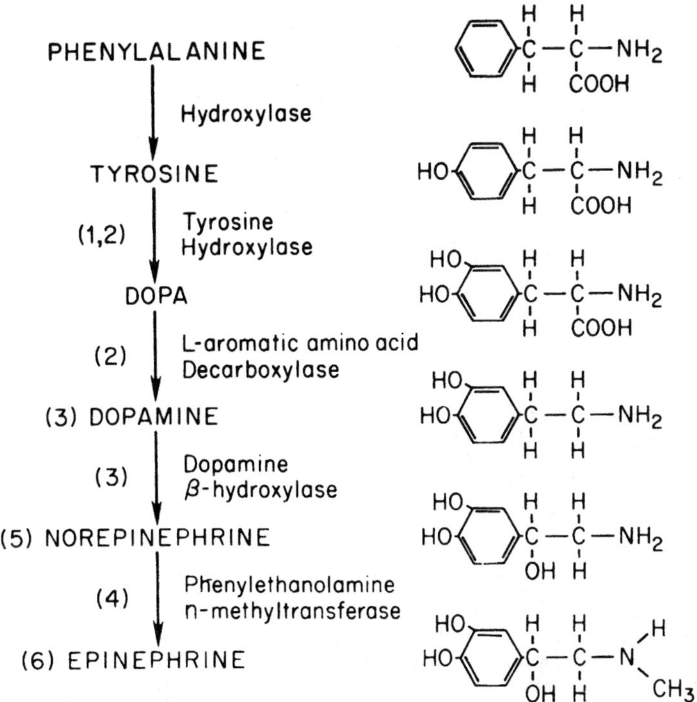

FIG. 5.5—The biosynthetic pathway of norepinephrine and epinephrine. (1) = the rate-limiting step, (2) = occurs within axoplasm, (3) = occurs within amine storage granule, (4) = occurs primarily within cytoplasm of adrenal medullary chromaffin cells, (5) = stored primarily within amine storage granule of adrenergic neurons, (6) = stored within amine storage granule of chromaffin cells.

nisms, the interested reader is referred to the detailed bibliography accumulated by Lefkowitz et al. (1990).

Catecholamines. Norepinephrine, epinephrine, and dopamine are endogenous catecholamines; they are the sympathetic neural and humoral transmitter substances in most mammalian species. Norepinephrine and dopamine are believed to transmit impulse information in specific areas within the CNS; norepinephrine is also the neurotransmitter at most peripheral sympathetic neuroeffector junctions. Epinephrine is the major hormone released from the adrenal medulla. Catecholamines are stored in an inactive form within granular structures in nerve terminals and chromaffin cells (Hokfelt 1973).

SYNTHESIS. Norepinephrine is synthesized from the amino acid phenylalanine in a stepwise process summarized in Fig. 5.5. The aromatic ring of phenylalanine is hydroxylated by action of an enzyme, phenylalanine hydroxylase. This reaction yields tyrosine, which is converted to dihydroxyphenylalanine (dopa) by the enzyme tyrosine hydroxylase. This reaction involves additional hydroxylation of the benzene ring, and it is believed to represent the rate-limiting step in catecholamine synthesis (Vulliet et al. 1980).

Dopa is decarboxylated by the enzyme L–aromatic amino acid decarboxylase (dopa decarboxylase) to dihydroxyphenylethylamine (dopamine). Conversion of tyrosine to dopa to dopamine is believed to occur within the cytoplasm. Dopamine is taken up into the storage granule. In some central anatomic sites (e.g., mammalian extrapyramidal system), dopamine seems to act as the primary neurotransmitter rather than its metabolites, norepinephrine and epinephrine (Aghajanian and Bunney 1973; Bartholini et al. 1973).

In peripheral adrenergic neurons and adrenal medullary chromaffin cells, intragranular dopamine is hydroxylated in the β position of the aliphatic side chain by dopamine-β-hydroxylase to form norepinephrine. In the adrenal medulla, norepinephrine is released from the granules of chromaffin cells and is *N*-methylated within the cytoplasm by phenylethanolamine *N*-methyltransferase to form epinephrine. Epinephrine is subsequently localized in what seems to be another type of intracellular storage granule prior to its release from the adrenal medulla.

STORAGE, RELEASE, REUPTAKE, AND METABOLISM. Physiologic events involved in adrenergic neurotransmission and susceptibility of these events to pharmacologic agents are outlined schematically in Fig. 5.6.

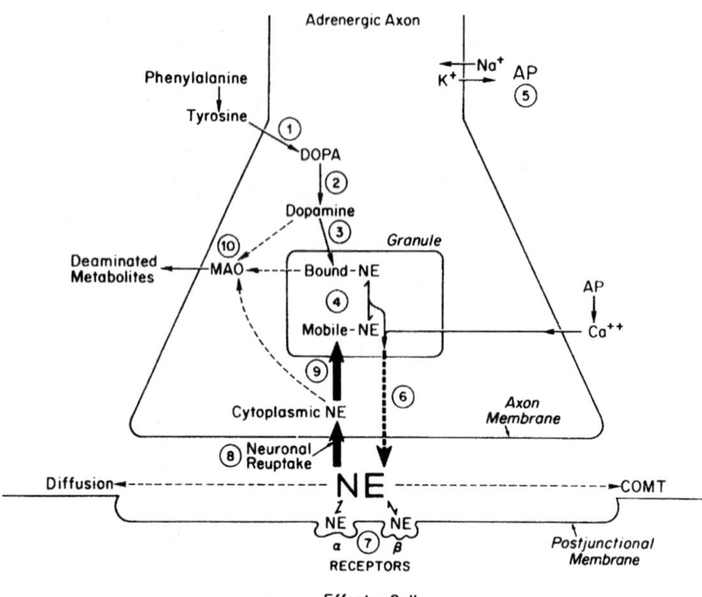

FIG. 5.6—Neurohumoral transmission at the adrenergic neuroeffector junction: proposed physiologic pathways and sites of action susceptible to modification by pharmacologic agents. (1) Tyrosine is hydroxylated to dopa. This reaction, considered to be the rate-limiting step in catecholamine synthesis, is inhibited by α-methyl-*p*-tyrosine. (2) Dopa is decarboxylated to dopamine. Dopa decarboxylase inhibitors (e.g., α-methyldopa) inhibit this step. (3) Dopamine is taken up into the storage granules and oxidized to norepinephrine (NE). α-Methyldopamine inhibits conversion of dopamine to NE and is converted to α-methylnorepinephrine. α-Methyl NE is then stored in the granule and upon nerve stimulation may be released as a "false neurotransmitter." (4) NE is stored in the granule in a bound and free (mobile) form. Tyramine-like drugs release NE from adrenergic neurons. (5) The axonal action potential is a self-propagating depolarization process that upon reaching the nerve terminal increases influx of Ca^{++}, which then triggers the discharge of NE from the nerve terminal. Bretylium inhibits NE release. (6) NE is released from the neuron via exocytotic emptying of the contents of storage granules into the junctional cleft. Newly synthesized NE may be preferentially released. (7) Released NE reacts with receptor sites on the postjunctional membrane of the effector cell. This step is blocked by adrenergic blocking agents (e.g., α-phentolamine, β-propranolol). Receptive areas (that modify NE release) may also be located on the prejunctional membrane of the nerve terminal (see Fig. 5.7). (8) Extraneuronal NE can be taken back up into the nerve terminal by an active Na^+-dependent uptake process. This step is inhibited by cocaine and imipramine-like drugs. Extraneuronal NE may also diffuse from the junction or be catabolized by catechol-O-methyltransferase. (9) Cytoplasmic NE may be taken up into the granule by a Mg^{++}-ATP-dependent uptake process. Reserpine-like drugs inhibit this step. (10) Monoamine oxidase (MAO) can deaminate cytoplasmic NE and dopamine. MAO inhibitors (e.g., pargyline) suppress this step. The bold dashed line = release of NE from the granular pool into the junctional cleft. Small dashed lines = catabolic pathways. Bold solid lines = uptake processes. Double-headed arrows = reversible pathways.

Catecholamines are taken up from the cytoplasm into granules by an active transport system that is adenosine triphosphate (ATP) and Mg^{++} dependent. Storage within the granular vesicles is accomplished by complexation of the catecholamines with ATP and a specific protein, chromogranin. This complexation renders the amines inactive until their release (Shore 1972). The intragranular pool of norepinephrine is the principal source of neurotransmitter released upon nerve stimulation. The cytoplasmic amine pool is taken up by the granules for storage or inactivated by a deaminating enzyme, monoamine oxidase (MAO), that is located in the neuronal mitochondria.

Excitation-secretion coupling and release of norepinephrine from adrenergic nerve terminals are dependent upon an inward movement of Ca^{++}. Released norepinephrine migrates across the synaptic cleft and interacts with specific adrenergic receptor sites on the postjunctional membrane.

A very active amine uptake system is present in the axonal membrane of postganglionic sympathetic nerve terminals. This transport system is Na^+ and energy dependent, and it functions to recapture or reuptake catecholamines that have been released from the nerve. Exogenously administered norepinephrine and epinephrine are taken up into sympathetic nerve endings by this uptake process (Iverson 1973). Conservation of catecholamine neurotransmitters by reuptake is one of the first examples of recycling used products.

The adrenergic neuronal uptake mechanism is referred to as $Uptake_1$. $Uptake_2$ signifies the extraneuronal uptake of catecholamines into surrounding tissue.

The duration of action of norepinephrine can be terminated by active reuptake via $Uptake_1$ into the nerve across the axoplasmic membrane (the amine reuptake pump), diffusion from the cleft via extracellular fluid, or metabolic breakdown by an extraneuronal enzyme, catechol-*O*-methyltransferase (COMT). Activity of COMT involves methylation of one of the ring hydroxyl groups (3-OH).

Norepinephrine that has been taken back into the nerve may be restored in granules or deaminated by MAO. Deamination of norepinephrine or epinephrine by MAO initially yields the corresponding aldehyde, which in turn is further oxidized to 3,4-dihydroxymandelic acid. Alternatively, the 3-hydroxyl group of norepinephrine and epinephrine can first be methylated by COMT to yield normetanephrine and metanephrine respectively. The *O*-methylated or deaminated metabolites can then be acted upon by the other enzyme to yield 3-methoxy-4-hydroxymandelic acid. The deaminated *O*-methylated metabolites can then be conjugated with sulfate or glucuronide prior to excretion by the kidneys.

PHARMACOLOGIC CONSIDERATIONS. Many drugs exert their pharmacologic activity by altering the synthesis, storage, and release mechanisms of catecholamines. Most of these agents are used in humans to control hypertension or affect central autonomic centers (e.g., tranquilization, antidepression, antiparkinsonism). Few of these drugs are commonly employed in clinical veterinary medicine. Some of these drugs are briefly mentioned, however, because they are often used as model drugs in research to characterize the mechanism of action of new drugs intended for clinical veterinary use.

Certain drugs act as false substrates for the catecholamine-synthesizing enzymes; e.g., α-methylparatyrosine inhibits tyrosine hydroxylase, the rate-limiting step in norepinephrine formation. Thus norepinephrine stores are not replenished by newly synthesized norepinephrine. Alpha-methyldopa may be converted to α-methyldopamine to α-methylnorepinephrine by dopa decarboxylase and dopamine-β-hydroxylase respectively. The α-methylnorepinephrine is active at CNS α_2 receptors, which reduce sympathetic efferent nerve traffic to the cardiovascular system.

Reserpine-like drugs block the granular uptake process (Shore 1972). Catecholamine stores are depleted and adrenergic functions are markedly altered by prolonged treatment with even small doses of reserpine (Adams et al. 1971, 1972). Guanethidine can slowly deplete norepinephrine and interfere with its release. Bretylium blocks the neuronal release of neurotransmitter. The experimental drug 6-hydroxydopamine produces a functional peripheral sympathectomy by destroying adrenergic nerve terminals (Gauthier et al. 1974).

Other drugs (e.g., cocaine, imipramine) inhibit the neuronal reuptake process so that released norepinephrine is available for a longer period for reaction with receptor sites. Inhibition of MAO by drugs can result in accumulation of catecholamines. Drugs like tyramine and amphetamine release intraneuronal stores of catecholamines.

Most adrenergic drugs important to clinical veterinary medicine act primarily by activating or blocking postjunctional adrenergic receptors in peripheral tissues or the CNS.

Adrenergic Receptors. The interaction of neurohormone with an adrenergic receptor (i.e., adrenoceptor) may elicit either an excitatory or an inhibitory response. Following isolation and identification of norepinephrine as the adrenergic neurotransmitter, attention was directed to differences in postjunctional events that might explain such contrasting results. In his classic paper, Ahlquist (1948) proposed that there were two basic types of adrenergic receptors: α and β. Epinephrine is the most potent α-receptor stimulant, norepinephrine is intermediate, and isoproterenol is the least active. On the other hand, isoproterenol is the most potent β-receptor agonist, epinephrine is intermediate, and norepinephrine is least active. Epinephrine is therefore classified as a mixed α-β agonist, whereas isoproterenol is virtually a pure β agonist with few, if any, α-receptor effects. Norepinephrine is primarily an α agonist; however, it does activate the excitatory β receptors in the heart.

Receptor Subtypes. The concept of dissimilar adrenoceptors has been strongly supported by observations that certain adrenergic antagonists block only α or β receptors (Moran 1973). Furthermore, studies with selective antagonists and agonists have demonstrated that β receptors can be divided into two subtypes: β_1 and β_2 (Lands et al. 1967). Beta receptors in the heart are β_1; they are associated with excitatory responses. Isoproterenol, epinephrine, and norepinephrine activate β_1 adrenoceptors. $Beta_2$ receptors are localized in vascular smooth muscle and bronchiolar smooth muscle; they instigate inhibitory (relaxant) effects. Norepinephrine has little effect on β_2 receptors, whereas epinephrine and isoproterenol are very active at β_2-receptor sites.

Alpha receptors located at adrenergic nerve terminals show a somewhat different responsiveness to drugs when compared to the classic α receptors of effector cells, leading to their designation as α_2 (Starke et al. 1977; Langer 1980). Other studies have supported the existence of different α-receptor populations but indicate that α_1 and α_2 subtypes are not necessarily restricted to postjunctional and prejunctional localizations respectively (U'Prichard and Snyder 1979).

Designation of adrenoceptors as either α_1, α_2, β_1, or β_2 is now well accepted. A summary of the different adrenergic receptor types in various sympathetically innervated tissues is given in Table 5.1. Numerous studies have now established that classification of receptor types and subtypes is far more complex than Ahlquist (1948) envisioned. Indeed, there may be many

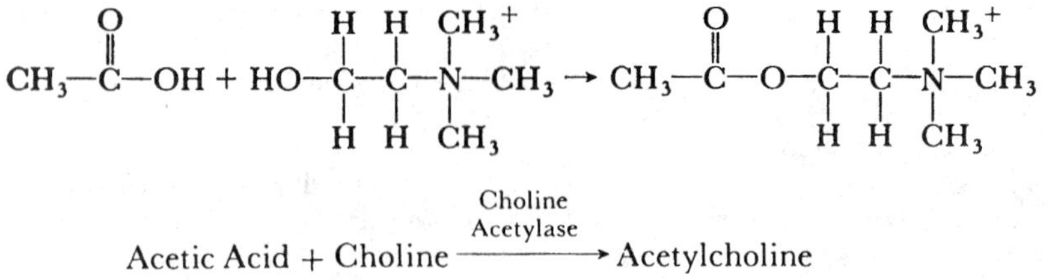

$$CH_3{-}\overset{O}{\overset{\|}{C}}{-}OH + HO{-}\underset{H}{\overset{H}{C}}{-}\underset{H}{\overset{H}{C}}{-}\underset{CH_3}{\overset{CH_3^+}{N}}{-}CH_3 \rightarrow CH_3{-}\overset{O}{\overset{\|}{C}}{-}O{-}\underset{H}{\overset{H}{C}}{-}\underset{H}{\overset{H}{C}}{-}\underset{CH_3}{\overset{CH_3^+}{N}}{-}CH_3$$

$$\text{Acetic Acid} + \text{Choline} \xrightarrow{\text{Choline Acetylase}} \text{Acetylcholine}$$

FIG. 5.7—Formation of ACh involving choline acetylase, choline, and acetic acid. Source of the acetic acid moiety is acetyl coenzyme A.

types of α receptors, β receptors, muscarinic receptors, nicotinic receptors, and others (Alberts 1993). Because the clinical importance of such complexities remains to be established, this textbook will consider clinically relevant receptor nomenclatures.

CHOLINERGIC NEUROTRANSMISSION. ACh is the neurotransmitter substance at most parasympathetic neuroeffector junctions, autonomic ganglia, the adrenal medulla, somatic myoneural junctions, and certain CNS regions (Brimblecombe 1974; Waser 1975; Goldberg and Hanin 1976). Neurohumoral transmission processes seem to be basically similar at all cholinergic junctions. Autonomic ganglionic and somatic myoneural transmission will be discussed in greater detail in subsequent chapters.

Synthesis, Storage, Release, and Catabolism of ACh. ACh is synthesized within cholinergic nerves by the enzymatic transfer of an acetyl group from acetyl coenzyme A to choline. This reaction is catalyzed by the enzyme choline acetylase (also referred to as choline acetyltransferase) and is summarized in Fig. 5.7. The acetyl coenzyme A is formed by the action of an enzyme, acetyl kinase, which mediates the transfer of an acetyl group from adenylacetate (formed from acetate and ATP) to the coenzyme A molecule. Choline is transported from the extracellular fluid into the cholinergic nerve by an energy-requiring axoplasmic uptake process. ACh is stored within axonal vesicular structures in a concentrated solution or bound to membranes or both.

ACh is released from the nerve terminal upon arrival of an axonal action potential. ACh within the junctional space is rapidly inactivated by hydrolysis by a specific enzyme, AChE. AChE is present in cholinergic nerves, autonomic ganglia, and neuromuscular and neuroeffector junctions. A somewhat similar enzyme, pseudocholinesterase (butyrocholinesterase), is present in serum and other body tissues.

Cholinergic Receptors. There are two basic types of cholinergic receptors within the peripheral efferent autonomic nerve tracts: nicotinic and muscarinic. Early studies demonstrated that small doses of nicotine mimicked certain actions of ACh, and large doses inhibited the same ACh responses. The nicotinic responsive sites were found to be present in autonomic ganglia, adrenal medullary chromaffin cells, and also the neuromuscular junction of the somatic nervous system. Accordingly, these sites have been referred to as nicotinic cholinergic receptors.

Nicotine does not, however, simulate or block the action of ACh at the parasympathetic neuroeffector junctions in heart muscle, smooth muscle, or secretory glands. The plant alkaloid muscarine was found to simulate the activity of ACh at these sites but not at the previously described nicotinic receptors. Muscarinic receptors therefore designate the type of receptor present at cholinergic neuroeffector junctions in muscle and glands.

A nicotinic response usually denotes an excitatory response, whereas muscarinic receptor activation may elicit an excitatory or inhibitory response, depending on the tissue. This seems to be related to either a general increase in permeability to all ions (depolarization-excitatory) or a selective increase in permeability to small ions like K^+ (hyperpolarization-inhibitory) respectively. Nicotinic and muscarinic cholinergic receptors have been placed into different subtypes (Birdsall et al. 1983; Chassaing et al. 1984), but the relevance of these subclassifications to clinical veterinary medicine is unclear at this time.

Pharmacologic Considerations. A wide variety of chemical and biologic agents affect cholinergic neurotransmission. The synthesis of ACh is inhibited by hemicholinium, which blocks the entrance of choline into the cholinergic nerve. Botulinum toxin interferes with the release of ACh. The plant alkaloids nicotine and muscarine have been mentioned in preceding paragraphs. Atropine and related alkaloids block muscarinic receptors, whereas curare blocks nicotinic receptor sites. The activity of endogenous and exogenous ACh is markedly augmented by many chemicals that act as cholinesterase inhibitors (anticholinesterase agents). The therapeutic importance of cholinergic and anticholinergic agents will be discussed in Chap. 7.

AUTONOMIC RECEPTOR SITES ON NERVE TERMINALS. Release of autonomic transmitters from nerve terminals can be influenced by other transmitters interacting with specific receptor sites present on the nerve terminal (for reviews, see Adams 1983, 1984).

Muscarinic cholinergic receptors at adrenergic nerve endings mediate an inhibition of the neuronal release of norepinephrine (Muscholl 1973). Such receptors may well explain the reduced cardiac responses to sympathetic nerve activity when vagal influence is increased (Stuesse et al. 1979). Several unrelated autacoids (e.g., histamine, prostaglandins) also inhibit norepinephrine release from adrenergic nerves, evidence for inhibitory presynaptic receptors specific for certain autacoids (Horton 1973; Langer 1980).

There also is evidence for α_2- and β_2- adrenoceptive sites on adrenergic nerve terminals (Starke et al. 1977; Langer 1980). Prejunctional α_2 receptors mediate a decrease in the amount of norepinephrine released upon nerve stimulation. The function of these α_2 sites has been envisioned as a local feedback control mechanism through which norepinephrine can inhibit its own release once a threshold concentration has been obtained in the junctional space. Conversely, the prejunctional β_2 receptors subserve increased release of norepinephrine (Adams 1984).

It is tempting to speculate on the physiologic significance and implications of such local inhibitory-facilitatory feedback mechanisms. However, although these extremely complex interrelationships most likely exist, neither the complete physiologic nor the complete pharmacologic significance of all presynaptic receptors has been definitely established at this time. The clinical relevance of the α_1- and α_2-receptor subtypes and β_1- and β_2-receptor subtypes is considered in Chap. 6.

PUTATIVE NEUROHUMORAL SUBSTANCES. Biologic substances other than ACh and the catecholamines have been proposed as probable (putative) neurotransmitter substances. Histamine, e.g., has been suggested as a potential neurotransmitter at certain peripheral and CNS sites, as have different neuropeptide substances. There is even evidence now that certain peptides coexist in the same neuron as primary neurotransmitters (Iverson et al. 1983). It remains unclear whether these peptides serve as primary neurotransmitters themselves or, more likely, modulate either the axon or the effector cell process in the neurohumoral communication event.

Considerable evidence has revealed that serotonin (5-hydroxytryptamine) acts as a neurotransmitter in specific brain centers and some peripheral nerves. The functional consequences of tryptaminergic transmission have not been completely defined, but it is likely that 5-hydroxytryptamine participates in thermoregulation, sleep cycles, and extrapyramidal influences on motor control of skeletal muscles. Gamma-aminobutyric acid has been shown to be an inhibitory neurotransmitter at certain CNS sites.

Although several putative neurotransmitter substances are involved in information transfer in the central and peripheral nervous systems, the pharmacologic activity of most autonomic drugs and numerous centrally acting agents can best be explained by actions on cholinergic or adrenergic pathways.

NITRIC OXIDE. Nitric oxide is an unlikely candidate for an endogenously synthesized messenger for physiologic and pathophysiologic communications in living organisms (Lowenstein et al. 1994; Adams 1996). Compared to classical neurotransmitters and polypeptides, nitric oxide is an exceptionally small and simple molecule comprising a single atom each of nitrogen and oxygen and existing under atmospheric conditions as a gas. With an unpaired electron in its outer orbit, nitric oxide is a radical species with a biological half-life of only a few seconds; it reacts rapidly with oxygen or with iron moieties of heme-containing proteins. Nitric oxide also is a combustion product generated in cigarette smoke, smog, and jet engine exhaust.

Despite considerable interest in nitric oxide as an environmental pollutant, it gathered little notice from biomedical scientists until the recent discovery that this compound is actively synthesized by different cell types, where it serves as a key regulator of a wealth of different bodily functions. These include immunomodulation, antimicrobial defenses, tumoricidal activity, neurotransmission in both the central and peripheral nervous systems, respiration, intestinal peristalsis, penile erection, and cardiovascular dynamics. The idea that a small molecule of gas can be synthesized by mammalian cells and then serve as a key controller of physiologic functions truly represents a new frontier in medicine (Adams 1996).

The surge of biomedical interest in nitric oxide can be traced directly to several lines of investigation involving the biochemistry of carcinogenesis, immunomodulatory and antimicrobial characteristics of activated macrophages, and control of hemodynamics (Änggard 1994; Langrehr et al. 1993). Relative to vascular effects, the discovery of endothelium-derived relaxing factor (EDRF) by Furchgott and Zawadzki (1980) unquestionably was a pivotal step in the recognition that mammalian cells can synthesize nitric oxide. These investigators observed that ACh produced vasodilation in isolated blood vessels only when the vascular endothelium was intact. This classical observation prompted an explosion of interest in vascular endothelium as a necessary intermediary in the vascular smooth muscle relaxation induced not only by ACh but also by many other vasodilators, including bradykinin, thrombin, oxytocin, adenosine diphosphate, and substance P. It became clear that when such agents interacted with vascular endothelium, the latter released an endogenous factor responsible for vasorelaxant responses to the former—hence, the discovery of EDRF (Furchgott and Zawadzki 1980). Depending on species and vascular bed, some vasodilator agents exert both endothelium-dependent and endothelium-independent actions as part of their pharmacodynamic profiles (Cogswell et al. 1995).

Following studies with exogenous nitrovasodilators that release nitric oxide (such as nitroglycerin and nitroprusside) and endothelium-dependent vasodilators (such as ACh and bradykinin), different investigators concluded that the pharmacodynamic and pharmacokinetic characteristics of EDRF closely mimicked those of nitric oxide. It is now widely accepted that EDRF is in fact either authentic nitric oxide, a closely related nitrosothiol that releases nitric oxide to target cells, or both. Nitric oxide migrates from the endothelium and activates the cytosolic form of guanylyl cyclase in adjacent vascular smooth muscle cells. This activation accelerates conversion of guanosine triphosphate (GTP) to cyclic guanosine monophosphate (cGMP), with the latter leading in turn to relaxation of vascular smooth muscle and its accompanying vasodilation.

Endothelium-derived nitric oxide was not simply an experimental curiosity of isolated blood vessels. Indeed, pharmacologic inhibition of nitric oxide biosynthesis in intact animals elicits a pronounced systemic hypertensive response owing to a substantial increase in peripheral vascular resistance. Because this peripheral vasoconstriction is expressed under basal conditions, it became clear that EDRF is an important modulator of normal vasodilator tone regulated by a dynamic release of endothelium-derived nitric oxide on a moment-to-moment basis. These remarkable findings revolutionized long-held concepts about control of peripheral vasomotion, prompting robust searches for different agents that would selectively modulate the biosynthesis of nitric oxide.

Nitric Oxide Biosynthesis. Details of the complex biochemical and electron-transfer steps culminating in the formation of nitric oxide have been reviewed (Ånggard 1994; Langrehr et al. 1993; Lowenstein et al. 1994; Schulz and Triggle 1994). In brief, nitric oxide is synthesized from an N^G-guanidino nitrogen of the amino acid L–arginine. The D–enantiomer of arginine is inactive. The enzyme family responsible for nitric oxide biosynthesis is nitric oxide synthase (NOS). Because this enzyme family utilizes molecular oxygen, NOS is classified as a dioxygenase. Cofactors required for nitric oxide formation include flavin adenine dinucleotide, flavin mononucleotide, nicotinamide adenine dinucleotide phosphate (NADPH), heme, and tetrahydrobiopterin. In addition to nitric oxide, the amino acid citrulline is a coproduct in a 1:1 stoichiometric relationship with nitric oxide. The production of tritiated citrulline from tritiated L–arginine is commonly used as an indirect assay for NOS activity and nitric oxide synthesis.

Several different isoforms of NOS have been characterized, and the identifying nomenclatures are still undergoing modification as new molecular and cofactor requirements are discovered. The two original isoforms described were the constitutive NOS (cNOS) and the inducible NOS (iNOS).

The NOS prototypically present in endothelium and neurons is cNOS; this enzyme is constitutively present under basal conditions, and its activation is dependent upon calmodulin and Ca^{++}. Nitric oxide synthesis from cNOS is activated within seconds to minutes after intracellular Ca^{++} is increased in response to classical cell surface receptors and affiliated signal-transduction mechanisms that culminate in elevated cytosolic Ca^{++}. The cNOS synthesizes nitric oxide in relatively small amounts; synthesis dynamically ceases as cellular Ca^{++} falls to basal concentrations. The biosynthesis of endothelium-derived nitric oxide and its subsequent role as an activator of guanylyl cyclase in vascular smooth muscle are schematized in Fig. 5.8.

The iNOS is prototypically induced in macrophages and hepatocytes, but it is not present in these or other cell types under basal conditions. When macrophages are exposed to LPS and/or certain cytokines such as tumor necrosis factor-α or interleukin-1, de novo synthesis of nascent iNOS is initiated by transcriptional regulation. Several hours are required for maximal expression of iNOS, which produces amounts of nitric oxide large enough to destroy pathogenic microorganisms. Although calmodulin is an integral subunit component of iNOS, its regulatory role is unknown in that Ca^{++} does not seem to be required for iNOS activity.

Recent experiments have provided evidence that iNOS is not restricted to macrophages and hepatocytes; it can also be induced in a rather impressive spectrum of different cell types including vascular smooth muscle, endothelium, Kupffer cells, neutrophils, and possibly cardiac myocytes (Schulz and Triggle 1994).

Nitric oxide is a nonpolar gas and it readily crosses cellular membranes, providing access to intracellular structures in nearby cells. Unlike classical neurotransmitters and hormones, nitric oxide does not seem to require a specific macromolecular protein for its receptor site. Nitric oxide is oxidized rapidly upon contact with oxygen, yielding the much less active nitrites and nitrates. Alternatively, nitric oxide can interact with the heme constituent of iron-containing enzymes, leading to configurational modifications that adjust catalytic activity of the affected enzyme.

Activation of cytosolic guanylyl cyclase through nitrosation of its heme moiety is considered a cardinal mechanism of action of nitric oxide in platelets and smooth muscles. The resulting increase in cGMP is the intracellular messenger subserving the physiologic response to nitric oxide (Fig. 5.8). Smooth muscle relaxation and anti-platelet-aggregating actions of nitric oxide are mimicked by cell-permanent forms of cGMP and are potentiated by inhibitors of the cGMP phosphodiesterase enzyme. Activation of quanylyl cyclase by nitric oxide not only is responsible for dilation of blood vessels and inhibition of thrombogenesis but is involved in neuronal signaling and cytotoxicity responses to nitric oxide as well.

Because of amino acid heterogenicity in the structural motif of the different isoforms of NOS, the following nomenclature modification has been proposed: the neuronal cNOS has been referred to as NOS-I, the macrophage iNOS as NOS-II, and the endothelial cNOS as NOS-III. This nomenclature will no doubt continue to evolve as new discoveries are made.

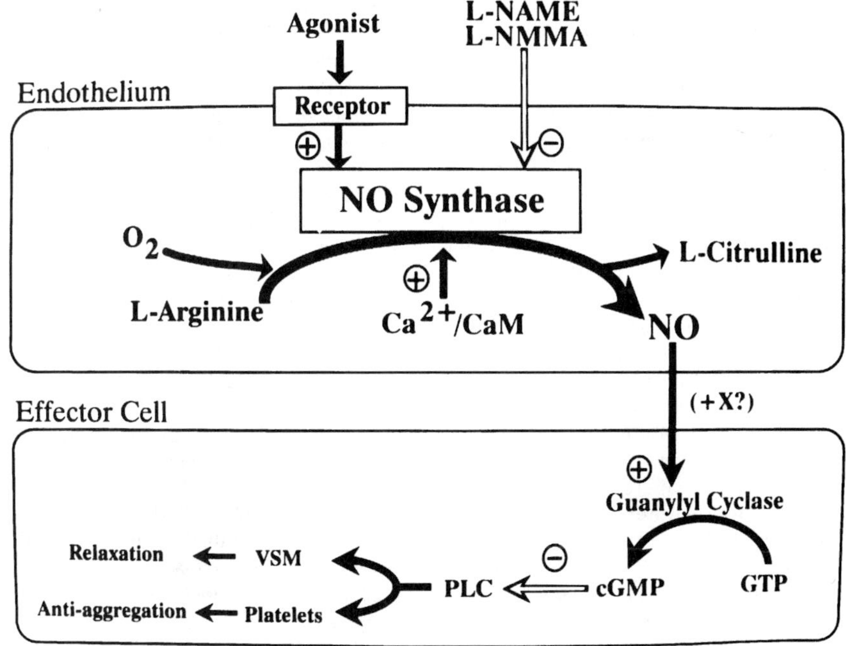

FIG. 5.8—The biosynthetic pathway for nitric oxide (NO) in vascular endothelial cells. Increased intracellular Ca^{++} activates the Ca^{++}-calmodulin (CaM)-dependent enzyme NO synthase, which utilizes O_2 and L-arginine to form NO. NO activates guanylyl cyclase in nearby platelets and vascular smooth muscle (VSM), leading to increased formation of cyclic guanosine monophosphate (cGMP). The latter inhibits phospholipase C (PLC) and exerts other effects that lead to changes in cellular functions, e.g., vasodilation and antiaggregation of platelets. L-arginine analogs such as L-nitroarginine methylester (L-NAME) and L-nitromonomethyl arginine (L-NMMA) inhibit NO synthase. (+X?) = possible biological carrier of NO. ⊖ = activates; ⊕ = inhibits.

Pharmacologic Modulation of Nitric Oxide Synthesis and Action. Organic compounds containing nitrate or nitroso moieties such as nitroglycerine, nitroprusside, *S*-nitroso-*N*-acetylpenicillamine, $NaNO_3$, and sydnonimines undergo tissue-catalyzed metabolism or spontaneous breakdown to yield exogenous-source nitric oxide. These and related compounds serve as nitric oxide donors, and their pharmacodynamic actions mimic in many respects the physiologic effects of endogenously synthesized nitric oxide.

There are several different types of NOS inhibitors, including congeners of the substrate L–arginine. The N^G-substituted L-arginine analogs include *N*-nitro-L–arginine methylester (L–NAME), *N*-nitro-L–arginine, and *N*-methyl-L–arginine (L–NMA). These inhibitors generally are competitive when administered concomitantly with L–arginine, and studies are under way to identify arginine analogs that are more selective for either iNOS or cNOS. Arginine analogs are routinely described as "specific" inhibitors of NOS, and yet few studies have systematically tested whether these agents also possess pharmacologic actions unrelated to NOS inhibition. In this regard, for instance, recent studies have indicated that L–NAME is a muscarinic receptor antagonist and may therefore inhibit effects of ACh by muscarinic receptor blockade. As another example, apparently L–NMMA) can be metabolized to L–arginine and actually accelerate NOS activity under some circumstances. Such pharmacologic limitations should be considered when drugs are assumed to be "specific" inhibitors of NOS.

Other inhibitors of NOS include calmodulin antagonists for cNOS, flavoprotein binders for iNOS and cNOS, heme binders such as carbon monoxide for iNOS and cNOS, and inhibitors of iNOS induction. Inhibitors of iNOS induction include corticosteroids and certain cytokines such as transforming growth factor-α and interleukins-4 and -10. Although tumor necrosis factor-α is a strong inducer of iNOS, recent experiments indicate this cytokine may inhibit synthesis or accelerate breakdown of cNOS.

Physiologic Roles Proposed for Nitric Oxide. Proposed physiologic roles for nitric oxide undergo dynamic revision almost weekly, and many areas overlap. The following points are quite selective but provide a brief glimpse of the wealth of bodily functions that may be modulated by nitric oxide.

CIRCULATION. The discovery of EDRF initially focused interest on endothelial cell cNOS as a source of vasodilatory nitric oxide. Indeed, as mentioned previously, basal release of EDRF is a primary determinant of vasodilation and blood flow through vascular networks, including coronary, cerebral, renal, and skeletal muscle arteries. Release of nitric oxide from endothelial cNOS is stimulated not only by certain receptor agonists but also by shear stresses exerted over the intimal surface by flowing blood. Nitric oxide from endothelial cNOS participates in vascular autoregulatory control mechanisms, e.g., in hypoxia-induced vasodilation and metabolic demand–induced vasodilation associated with ischemia-reperfusion.

Recent studies have shown that immunomodulatory-inflammatory stimuli can induce an iNOS in both endothelium and vascular smooth muscle. Thus, nitric oxide derived from both the intimal layer and the blood vessel wall may play important pathophysiologic roles in the local circulatory response to infection and inflammation (Parker and Adams 1993).

Nitric oxide exerts antiaggregating actions in platelets, thereby eliciting thrombolytic or antithrombogenic effects. Inhibition of aggregation is not restricted to platelets; nitric oxide also slows leukocyte adhesion and aggregation onto the vascular intimal surface. Inhibition of platelet aggregation and adhesion by nitric oxide is believed to be an important constituent of the antithrombogenic characteristic of the intimal surface of the blood vessel lumen. Impaired synthesis of nitric oxide has been implicated in the formation of atherosclerosis and the affiliated loss of vasodilator function.

NEUROTRANSMITTER. Nitric oxide is believed to act as a neuronal messenger in both the central and peripheral components of the nervous system. In the brain, nitric oxide participates in experience-driven synaptic plasticity that may control learning and memory retention. Nitric oxide may well be the mediator of neuronal responses to certain excitatory amino acids. And because of its ability as a gas to be "broadcast" and diffuse from a single neuron to large numbers of nearby cells, nitric oxide may be an important controller of neuronal development and spatial orientation of neuronal centers. This exciting theory is quite distinct from the classical concept of one neuron releasing a signal molecule that interacts with specific receptor sites only on one adjacent neuron.

Peripheral neuronal control of intestinal peristalsis and synchronous opening-closing of GI sphincters has been ascribed historically to NANC nerves because the responsible neurotransmitter was unknown. It now seems that certain NANC nerves may be reclassified as nitric oxide neurons because this gas may be a NANC neurotransmitter in the alimentary tract, external genitalia, and the respiratory tract.

RESPIRATORY TRACT. There is increasing evidence that NANC nerves innervating bronchiolar smooth muscle release nitric oxide, which serves as a mediator of neurogenic bronchodilator tone. End-stage chronic obstructive pulmonary disease has been associated with decreased nitric oxide production, and it has been proposed that oxidation of nitric oxide may be accelerated in inflamed airways, leading to loss of bronchodilator reserves. Hypoxia-induced pulmonary vasoconstriction is an important compensatory reaction diverting or shunting blood flow away from nonperfused pulmonary zones and toward selective perfusion of oxygenated alveoli. Loss of this reflex may be an important component of acute respiratory distress syndrome (ARDS) and may also occur during prolonged periods of general anesthesia. Because of its conjoint bronchodilator and vasodilator activities, nitric oxide has not escaped the attention of pulmonary care centers. Inhalation of exogenous nitric oxide is undergoing evaluation as a selective vasodilator in oxygenated alveoli since inhaled gas would be delivered only to ventilated regions of the lung; this would selectively enhance perfusion only of oxygenated alveoli, thereby improving ventilation-perfusion matching.

PENILE ERECTION. Neurogenic control of penile erection is issued through the sacral division of the parasympathetic nervous system, and yet drugs that block receptors for the classical parasympathetic neurotransmitter ACh fail to prevent erection. This decades-old perplexity may have been resolved by the discovery of NANC neurons containing NOS in pelvic nerve plexuses. Immunohistochemical evidence exists that these nitric oxide neurons extend into the cavernous nerve and affect processes in the corpus cavernosum and its affiliated penile blood vessels. Functionally, pharmacologic inhibitors of NOS forestall electrically stimulated erection in animals and inhibit relaxation of corpus cavernosum smooth muscle. It has therefore been proposed that nitric oxide is the final chemical mediator controlling relaxation of corpus cavernosum smooth muscle and its supplying blood vessels, leading to vascular tumescence necessary for erection. Future studies no doubt will focus on the putative role of NOS and nitric oxide in impotence and priapism.

GASTROINTESTINAL FUNCTION. Peristalsis of the alimentary tract and synchrony of GI sphincter functions are believed to be regulated by nitric oxide released from neurons. Nitric oxide production and NOS have been localized to the enteric nerve plexuses formerly classified as intestinal NANC neurons. Nitrate concentration is elevated in diarrhea, and colonic production of nitric oxide is increased in patients with ulcerative colitis. Abnormalities of nitric oxide production have been implicated in esophageal motility disorders associated with esophageal achalasia and pyloric motility dysfunction in infantile hypertrophic pyloric stenosis. These interrelations between nitric oxide and GI function suggest more than an incidental role for nitric oxide in regulation of intestinal smooth muscle function.

G PROTEINS AND CYCLIC NUCLEOTIDES. Cyclic adenosine 3′,5′-monophosphate (cAMP), a cyclic nucleotide, acts as a "second messenger" to link

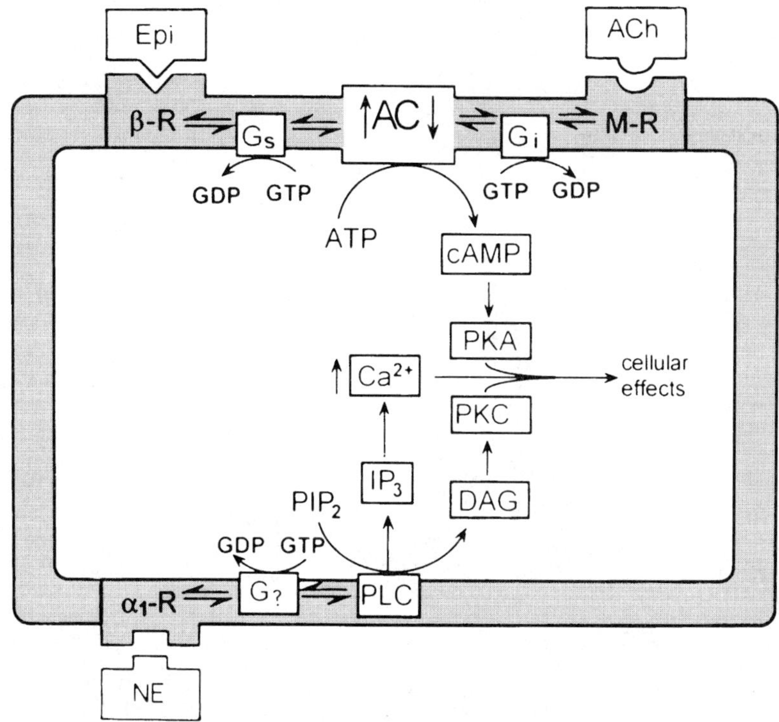

FIG. 5.9—Signal transduction pathways involving cell surface receptors (R), guanine nucleotide-binding regulatory proteins (G), and intracellular Ca^{++}. Activation of β-R by epinephrine (Epi) involves a stimulatory G (G_s), which serves as a GTPase (converting GTP to GDP) and activates the enzyme adenylyl cyclase (AC). The latter converts ATP to cyclic adenosine 3′,5′monophosphate (cAMP), which activates protein kinase A (PKA). Acetylcholine (ACh) binds with a muscarinic-R (M-R) linked to an inhibitory G (G_i), which reduces catalytic activity of AC and hence PKA. Activation of α_1-R by norepinephrine (NE) activates another G ($G_?$), which in turn activates phospholipase C (PLC). PLC hydrolyzes a membrane phospholipid phosphatidylinositol-4,5-bisphosphate (PIP_2), releasing inositol-1, 4,5-trisphosphate (IP_3) and diacylglycerol (DAG), which release endoplasmic reticulum Ca^{++} and activate protein kinase C (PKC), respectively. PKA and PKC phosphorylate various cellular constituents that, in concert with elevated cytosolic Ca^{++}, elicit characteristic changes in cellular functions. (Modeled after Lefkowitz et al. 1990; Lambert 1993; Schwinn 1993; and Levitzki et al. 1993.)

certain agonist-receptor interactions with cellular responses (Sutherland and Rall 1960; Robison et al. 1967; Robison 1971; Rall 1972). Cyclic AMP is formed from ATP by the catalytic action of the enzyme adenylyl cyclase. It is broken down to 5′-adenosinemonophosphate by another enzyme, phosphodiesterase. Adenylyl cyclase is believed to be localized in the cell membrane in mammalian cells that contain the cAMP system (Gilman 1984). Adenylyl cyclase is closely linked to numerous hormonal receptor sites, and changes in intracellular concentration of cAMP explain the pharmacologic activity of certain autonomic drugs and hormones.

It is known, e.g., that the adrenergic drugs norepinephrine, epinephrine, and isoproterenol increase the concentration of cAMP in the liver. This effect is mediated through acceleration of the activity of adenylyl cyclase. Isoproterenol, primarily a β agonist, has the greatest effect, whereas norepinephrine, primarily an α agonist, has the least potent action. These relationships correspond closely with catecholamine-mediated glycogenolysis in the hepatocytes, which has now been attributed to cAMP-mediated increase in phosphorylase activity.

Alteration of adenylyl cyclase and resultant change in cAMP by various adrenergic drugs have been demonstrated in numerous other mammalian tissues, including spleen; kidney; brain; adipose cells; and cardiac, skeletal, and smooth muscles. An increase in the tissue concentration of cAMP is generally associated with β-receptor activation, whereas a decrease in cAMP seems to be mediated in some tissues by α_2 receptors. Numerous endocrine hormones may also act via alteration of tissue levels of cAMP. In contrast, the inositol triphosphate pathway is the intracellular mechanism linked to α_1-receptor activation. The cellular pathways linking hormone receptors to guanine nucleotide-binding regulatory proteins (i.e., G proteins), cyclic nucleotides, and associated enzymes are schematized in Fig. 5.9 (also see Lambert 1993; Schwinn 1993; Levitzki et al. 1993).

The interrelationship of β adrenoceptors and cAMP has been intensely studied in heart muscle.

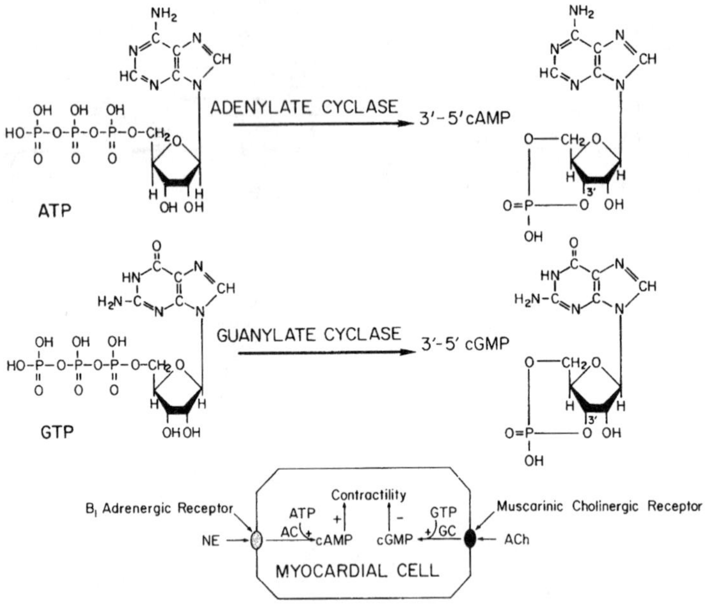

FIG. 5.10—Structures and biosynthetic pathways of cyclic AMP (cAMP) and cyclic GMP (cGMP) and a schematic of their potential roles as intracellular messengers for autonomic neurotransmitters. Activation of β-adrenergic receptors by NE increases activity of adenylate cyclase (AC), an enzyme that catalyzes (+) the conversion of ATP to cAMP. Increased intracellular cAMP leads to increased (+) contractility (via several mechanisms) of the myocardial cell. ACh activates muscarinic receptors, which leads to activation of guanylate cyclase (GC), an enzyme that catalyzes (+) the conversion of guanosine triphosphate to cGMP. Increased intracellular concentration of cGMP leads (via several mechanisms?) to decreased myocardial contractility.

Catecholamines increase the concentration of cAMP in the myocardium by activating adenylyl cyclase secondary to their agonist effects at the cardiac β_1 adrenoceptors. Increases in cAMP correspond with an increase in heart rate and contractile strength, and effects of catecholamines in the heart are mediated by the formation of cAMP.

Several groups of drugs have been known to elicit autonomic-like activity in various tissues, but attempts to associate these effects with change in neurohumoral transmission have failed. It now seems that certain of these drugs bypass receptor sites and act on the same cAMP system as the catecholamines. The methylxanthines (caffeine, theobromine, theophylline), e.g., elicit changes in heart function reminiscent of β-receptor activation in that they elicit positive inotropic and chronotropic responses. However, β blockers do not prevent the cardiac actions of the methylxanthines. These drugs are phosphodiesterase inhibitors. By inhibiting the phosphodiesterase enzyme, the catabolism of cAMP is impaired and the cellular concentration of this nucleotide increases. Furthermore, the methylxanthines potentiate the effect of catecholamines and other drugs that activate adenylyl cyclase (Samir Amer and Kreighbaum 1975).

Another related nucleotide, cyclic guanosine 3′,5′-monophosphate (cGMP), is also important as an intracellular messenger in some cell types (Robison 1971). Specifically, cGMP is the second messenger for the effects of ACh mediated through activation of the muscarinic receptor. The structures and biosynthetic pathways of cAMP and cGMP are presented in Fig. 5.10 along with a model of their potential antagonistic actions on myocardial contractility (George et al. 1975; Nawrath 1976).

AUTONOMIC DRUGS. Drugs that exert pharmacologic effects simulating activation, intensification, or inhibition of either the sympathetic or the parasympathetic nervous system have been historically referred to as autonomic drugs. As a rule, autonomic drugs are classified according to the physiologic activity they mimic. Table 5.2 summarizes the classification of the basic types of autonomic drugs that will be discussed in subsequent chapters.

TABLE 5.2—Classification of autonomic drugs

Classification	Other terms	Pharmacologic effects	Mechanisms and examples
Sympathomimetic	Andrenergic* Adrenomimetic*	Resemble effects caused by stimulation of adrenergic neurons Simulate effects of epinephrine and norepinephrine	Direct acting—α,β-adrenergic receptor agonists (α-phenylephrine; β-isoproterenol; α,β-epinephrine) Indirect acting—release endogenous stores of catecholamines (tyramine, amphetamine) Increase sympathetic discharge (nicotinic cholinergic agonists)†
Sympatholytic			
Receptor blocking effects	Adrenergic blocking drugs	Inhibit effects of sympathomimetic drugs; inhibit responses caused by stimulation of adrenergic neurons	Block α or β receptors (α blocker—phentolamine; β blocker—propranolol)
Neuronal blocking effects	Adrenolytic	Inhibit responses caused by stimulation of adrenergic neurons	Deplete endogenous catecholamines (reserpine) Inhibit release of morepinephrine from nerve terminals (bretylium)
Parasympathomimetic	Cholinergic§ Cholinomimetic§	Resemble effects caused by stimulation of postganglionic parasympathetic neurons Simulate effects of ACh	Direct acting—cholinergic receptor agonists (ACh, carbachol) Indirect acting—cholinesterase inhibitors (neostigmine, organophosphates)
Parasympatholytic			
Receptor blocking effects	Cholinergic§ blocking drugs	Inhibit effects of ACh; inhibit responses caused by stimulation of postganglionic parasympathetic neurons	Block nicotinic§ or muscarinic receptors (muscarinic blocker—atropine; nicotinic blocker—hexamethoruum)
Neuronal blocking effects	Anticholinergic§	Inhibit responses caused by stimulation of postganglionic parasympathetic neurons	Inhibit release of ACh from nerve terminals (botulinum toxin)

*These terms refer specifically to activities at adrenergic synapses, adrenergic neuroeffector junctions, and adrenergic receptors.

†Sympathomimetic effects may be produced by nicotinic cholinergic agents by their excitatory action on sympathetic ganglia, the adrenal medulla, and adrenergic nerve terminals, causing sympathetic discharge and release of epinephrine and norepinephrine. However, these activities should be considered as secondary when broad-based classifications of autonomic drugs are considered.

§These terms also refer to nonautonomic sites (e.g., somatic neuromuscular junction, CNS). Thus the terms parasympathomimetic and parasympatholytic are reserved to describe activities at the parasympathetic neuroeffector junction (i.e., in relation to muscarinic receptors; see text).

REFERENCES

Abramson, S. N., and Molinoff, P. B. 1984. In vitro interactions of agonists and antagonists with beta-adrenergic receptors. Biochem Pharmacol 33(6):869–875.

Adams, H. R. 1977. In L. M. Jones, N. H. Booth, and L. E. McDonald, eds., Veterinary Pharmacology and Therapeutics, 4th ed., p. 86. Ames: Iowa State Univ Press.

———. 1983. Pharmacologic problems in circulation research: alpha adrenergic blocking drugs. Circ Shock 10(3):215–223.

———. 1984. New perspectives in cardiopulmonary therapeutics: receptor-selective adrenergic drugs. J Am Vet Med Assoc 185(9):966–974.

———. 1996. Physiologic, pathophysiologic, and therapeutic implications for endogenous nitric oxide. J Am Vet Med Assoc 209:1297–1302.

Adams, H. R., Smookler, H. H, Clarke, D. E., Jandhyala, B. S., Dixit, B. N., Ertel, R. J., and Buckley, J. P. 1971. Clinicopathologic effects of chronic reserpine administration in mongrel dogs. J Pharm Sci 60(8):1134–1138.

Adams, H. R., Dixit, B. N., Smookler, H. H., Buckley, J. P. 1972. Clinical and biochemical effects of chronic reserpine administration in mongrel dogs. Am J Vet Res 33(4):699–707.

Aghajanian, G. K., and Bunney, B. S. 1973. In E. Usdin and S. Snyder, eds., Frontiers in Catecholamine Research, p. 643. Elmsford, NY: Pergamon.

Ahlquist, R. P. 1948. A study of the adrenotropic receptors. Am J Physiol 153:586–600.

Alberts, P. 1993. Subtype classification of presynaptic α_2-adrenoceptors. Gen Pharmac 24:1–8.

Änggard, E. 1994. Nitric oxide: mediator, murderer, and medicine. Lancet 343:1199–1206.

Bartholini, G., Stadler, H., and Lloyd, K. G. 1973. In E. Usdin and S. Snyder, eds., Frontiers in Catecholamine Research, p. 471. Elmsford, NY: Pergamon.

Birdsall, N. J., Hulme, E. C., and Stockton, J. M. 1983. Muscarinic receptor subclasses: allosteric interactions. Cold Spring Harbor Symp Quant Biol 48, pt. 1:53–56.

Brimblecombe, R. W. 1974. Drug Actions on Cholinergic Systems. Baltimore: University Park Press.

Campbell, W. B. 1990. Lipid-derived autacoids: eicosanoids and platelet-activating factor. In A. G. Gilman, T. W. Rall, A. S. Nies, and P. Taylor, eds., Pharmacological Basis of Therapeutics, 8th ed. New York: Pergamon.

Chassaing, C., Dureng, G., Baissat, J., and Duchene-Marullaz, P. 1984. Pharmacological evidence for cardiac muscarinic receptor subtypes. Life Sci 35(17):1739–1745.

Cogswell, A. M., Johnson, P. J., and Adams, H. R. 1995. Evidence for endothelium-derived relaxing factor/nitric oxide in equine digital arteries. Am J Vet Res 56:1637–1641.

Freeman, R., and Miyawaki, E. 1993. The treatment of autonomic dysfunction. J Clin Neurophysiol 10:61–82.

Furchgott, R. F., and Zawadzki, J. V. 1980. The obligatory role of endothelial cells in the relaxation of arterial smooth muscle by acetylcholine. Nature 288:373–376.

Gauthier, P., Nadeau, R. A., and de Champlain, J. 1974. Cardiovascular reactivity in the dog after chemical sympathectomy with 6-hydroxydopamine. Can J Physiol Pharmacol 52(3):590–601.

George, W. J., Busuttil, R. W., Paddock, R. J., White, L. A., and Ignarro, L. J. 1975. Opposing regulatory influences of cyclic guanosine monophosphate and cyclic adenosine monophosphate in the control of cardiac muscle contraction. Rec Adv Stud Cardiol Struc Metab 8:243–250.

Gilman, A. G. 1984. Guanine nucleotide-binding regulatory proteins and dual control of adenylate cyclase. J Clin Invest 73(1):1–4.

Goldberg, A. M., and Hanin, I., eds. 1976. Biology of Cholinergic Function. New York: Raven.

Hokfelt, T. 1973. In E. Usdin and S. Snyder, eds., Frontiers in Catecholamine Research, p. 439. Elmsford, NY: Pergamon.

Horton, E. W. 1973. Prostaglandins at adrenergic nerve-endings. Br Med Bull 29(2):148–151.

Iverson, L. L. 1973. In E. Usdin and S. Snyder, eds., Frontiers in Catecholamine Research, p. 403. Elmsford, NY: Pergamon.

Iverson, L. L., Iverson, S. D., and Snyder, S. H. 1983. Handbook of Psychopharmacology, vol. 16, pp. 519–556. New York: Plenum.

Kalsner, S. 1989. Cholinergic constriction in the general circulation and its role in coronary artery spasm. Circ Res 65:237–257.

Klein, R. L. 1973. In E. Usdin and S. Snyder, eds., Frontiers in Catecholamine Research, p. 423. Elmsford, NY: Pergamon.

Klinge, E., Fränkö, O., and Sjöstrand, N. O. 1978. Cholinergic and adrenergic innervation of the penis artery of the bull: transmitter concentrations and synaptic vesicles. Experientia 34(12):1624–1626.

Klinge, E., and Sjöstrand, N. O. 1974. Contraction and relaxation of the retractor penis muscle and the penile artery of the bull. Acta Physiol Scand Suppl 420:1–88.

Lambert, D. G. 1993. Signal transduction: G proteins and second messengers. Br J Anaesthesia 71:86–95.

Lands, A. M., Arnold, A., McAuliff, J. P., Luduena, F. P., and Brown, T. G., Jr. 1967. Differentiation of receptor systems activated by sympathomimetic amines. Nature 214(88):597–598.

Lang, E., and Szilagyi, N. 1991. Significance and assessment of autonomic indices in cardiovascular reactions. Acta Physiol Hung 78:241–260.

Langer, S. Z. 1980. Presynaptic regulation of the release of catecholamines. Pharm Rev 32(4):337–362.

Langrehr, J. M., Hoffman, R. A., Lancaster, J. R., and Simmons, R. L. 1993. Nitric oxide—a new endogenous immunomodulator. Transplantation Overview 55:1205–1212.

Lefkowitz, R. J., Hoffman, B. B., and Taylor, P. 1990. Neurohumoral transmission: the autonomic and somatic nervous systems. In A. G. Gilman, T. W. Rall, A. S. Nies, and P. Taylor, eds., The Pharmacological Basis of Therapeutics, 8th ed., p. 109. New York: Pergamon.

Levitzki, A., Marbach, I., and Bar-Sinai, A. 1993. The signal transduction between β-receptors and adenylyl cyclase. Life Sci 52:2093–2100.

Loewi, O. 1921. Pfluegers Arch Ges Physiol 189:239.

Low, P. A. 1993. Autonomic nervous system function. J Clin Neurophysiol 10:14–27.

Lowenstein, C. J., Dinerman, J. L., and Snyder, S. H. 1994. Nitric oxide: a physiologic messenger. Ann Intern Med 120:227–237.

Moran, N. C. 1973. In E. Usdin and S. Snyder, eds., Frontiers in Catecholamine Research, p. 291. Elmsford, NY: Pergamon.

Muscholl, E. 1973. In E. Usdin and S. Snyder, eds., Frontiers in Catecholamine Research, p. 537. Elmsford, NY: Pergamon.

Nawrath, H. 1976. Cyclic AMP and cyclic GMP may play opposing roles in influencing force of contraction in mammalian myocardium. Nature 262(5568):509–511.

Parker, J. L., and Adams, H. R. 1993. Selective inhibition of endothelium-dependent vasodilator capacity by *E. coli* endotoxemia. Circ Res 72:539–551.

Popovic, N. A., Mullane, J. F., and Yhap, E. O. 1972. Effects of acetylpromazine maleate on certain cardiorespiratory responses in dogs. Am J Vet Res 33(9):1819–1824.

Rall, T. W. 1972. Role of adenosine 3′,5′-monophosphate (cyclic AMP) in actions of catecholamines. Pharm Rev 24(2):399–409.

Robertshaw, D. 1980. Handb Exp Pharmacol 53:345.

Robison, G. A. 1971. Cyclic AMP. New York: Academic Press.

Robison, G. A., Butcher, R. W., and Sutherland, E. W. 1967. Adenyl cyclase as an adrenergic receptor. Ann NY Acad Sci 139(3):703–723.

Rubin, R. P. 1982. Calcium and Cellular Secretion. New York: Plenum.

Samir Amer, M., and Kreighbaum, W. E. 1975. Cyclic nucleotide phosphodiesterases: properties, activators, inhibitors, structure-activity relationships, and possible role in drug development. J Pharm Sci 64(1):1–37.

Schulz, R., and Triggle, C. R. 1994. Role of NO in vascular smooth muscle and cardiac muscle function. TIPS—July 15:255–259.

Schwinn, D. A. 1993. Adrenoceptors as models for G protein–coupled receptors: structure, function and regulation. Br J Anaesthesia 71:77–85.

Shields, R. W., Jr. 1993. Functional anatomy of the autonomic nervous system. J Clin Neurophysiol 10:2–13.

Shore, P. A. 1972. Transport and storage of biogenic amines. Ann Rev Pharm 12:209–226.

Starke, K., Taube H. D., and Browski, E. 1977. Presynaptic receptor systems in catecholaminergic transmission. Biochem Pharm 26(4):259–268.

Stuesse, S. L., Wallick, D. W., and Levy, M. N. 1979. Autonomic control of right atrial contractile strength in the dog. Am J Physiol 236(6):H860–865.

Sutherland, E. W., and Rall, T. W. 1960. In J. R. Vane, F. E. W. Wolstenholme, and M. O'Conner, eds., Adrenergic Mechanisms, p. 295. Boston: Little, Brown.

Taylor, P. 1990. Cholinergic agonists. In A. G. Gilman, T. W. Rall, A. S. Nies, and P. Taylor, eds., Pharmacological Basis of Therapeutics, 8th ed., pp. 600–617. New York: Pergamon.

U'Prichard, D. C., and Snyder, S. H. 1979. Distinct alpha-noradrenergic receptors differentiated by binding and physiological relationships. Life Sci 24(1):79–88.

Vulliet, P. R., Langan, T. A., and Weiner, N. 1980. Tyrosine hydroxylase: a substrate of cyclic AMP–dependent protein kinase. Proc Natl Acad Sci USA 77(1):92–96.

Waser, P. G., ed. 1975. Cholinergic Mechanisms. New York: Raven.

Winkler, H., and Hörtnagl, H. 1973. In E. Usdin and S. Snyder, eds., Frontiers in Catecholamine Research, p. 415. Elmsford, NY: Pergamon.

6

ADRENERGIC AGONISTS AND ANTAGONISTS

H. RICHARD ADAMS

Adrenergic (Sympathomimetic) Drugs
Adrenergic Receptors
Structure-Activity Relationships
Adrenergic Receptor Subtypes: Pharmacologic Applications
Catecholamines
Epinephrine, Norepinephrine, and Isoproterenol
Dopamine
Dobutamine
Noncatecholamines
Ephedrine
Amphetamine
Phenylephrine
Methoxamine and Metaraminol
α_2-Selective Agonists
β_2-Selective Bronchodilators
Antiadrenergic Drugs
Adrenergic Antagonists
Pharmacologic Considerations
Adrenergic Neuron-Blocking Drugs and Catecholamine-Depleting Agents
Miscellaneous Agents

Amine substances that cause physiologic responses similar to those evoked by the endogenous adrenergic mediators epinephrine and norepinephrine are known as adrenergic drugs. They are referred to as sympathomimetic agents because their pharmacologic effects mimic sympathetic nervous system activity. Sympathetic neurons and affiliated receptors of innervated cells are depicted in Fig. 6.1. Most clinically relevant adrenergic agonists exert their principal pharmacodynamic actions through receptor activation. Just the opposite, adrenergic receptor antagonists prevent receptor activation and thereby reduce sympathetic activity. "Sympatholytic," "adrenolytic," and "adrenergic blocking" are terms used to describe pharmacologic effects that, in general, simulate a decrease in adrenergic nerve activity. These terms are not synonymous, and they have been used to describe different types of antiadrenergic actions, as will be discussed later in this chapter.

ADRENERGIC (SYMPATHOMIMETIC) DRUGS. Pharmacologic effects of sympathomimetic amines are mediated by activation of adrenergic receptors of effector cells innervated by the sympathetic nervous system (Fig. 6.1). Noninnervated adrenoceptors also are present in some cell types. In general, therefore, pharmacologic effects of adrenergic agonists can be equated to physiologic effects resulting from increased sympathoadrenal discharge. A thorough understanding of basic adrenoceptor concepts is important to the future practitioner because this information has direct application to the clinical use of all adrenergic agonists and antagonists (Adams 1984).

Adrenergic Receptors. Adrenergic receptors (i.e., adrenoceptors) are macromolecular structures localized on or within the surface membrane of cells innervated by adrenergic neurons (and certain noninnervated cells). The basic physiologic function of the adrenergic receptor is to recognize and interact with the endogenous adrenergic mediators norepinephrine and epinephrine. This interaction triggers a series of complex intracellular events that yield a characteristic change in effector cell activity.

A classic simplification of the complex field of adrenergic receptors was formulated by Ahlquist in 1948; he proposed the existence of two basic types of adrenergic receptors, which he designated as alpha (α) and beta (β). This classification system is based on the relative potencies of several adrenergic agonists to elicit excitatory and inhibitory effects in different tissues.

Structure-Activity Relationships. Several factors have complicated determination of optimal structural requirements for adrenergic drugs. Most adrenergic drugs affect both α and β receptors, and the ratio of α and β activity varies tremendously between drugs and species. Some adrenergic agents cause indirect effects mediated by release of endogenous norepinephrine. Despite these various and often conflicting interrelationships, some general and some rather specific aspects of the structure-activity relationship of sympathomimetic amines have been determined.

The basis for sympathetic-like activity of various drugs depends upon the similarity of their chemical

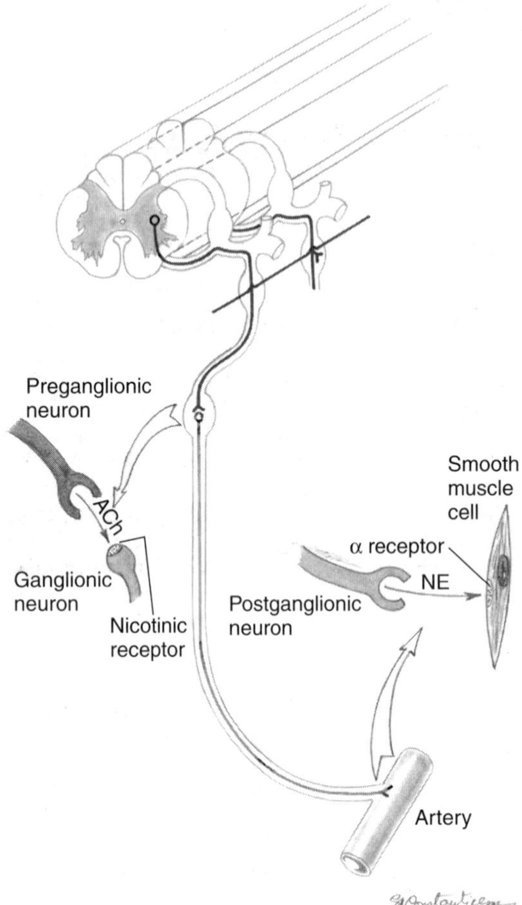

FIG. 6.1.—Anatomical relationships of sympathetic neuronal outflow tracts and affiliated receptors of innervated cells. Sympathetic preganglionic axons exit the thoracolumbar region of the spinal cord and synapse with ganglionic neurons in an adjacent ganglion, or pass through the latter to synapse with a neuron within a distant ganglion (shown). The preganglionic axon terminal releases the neurotransmitter acetylcholine (ACh), which activates nicotinic cholinergic receptors on the ganglionic neuron body. The resulting stimulation of the ganglionic neuron promotes release of the neurotransmitter norepinephrine (NE) from the axon terminal at the postganglionic sympathetic neuroeffector junction at blood vessels (shown) or other tissues innervated by sympathetic neurons. NE activates α- (shown) or β-adrenergic receptors present on cells innervated by the sympathetic division of the autonomic nervous system. Preganglionic fibers are red; postganglionic fibers are blue. Drawn by Dr. Gheorghe M. Constantinescu, University of Missouri. (*See also color plates following p. 118.*)

structure to that of the endogenous adrenergic mediators norepinephrine and epinephrine. The nucleus of this chemical structure, β-phenylethylamine, is a benzene ring and an ethylamine side chain. Substitution may be made on the aromatic ring, on the α and β carbons of the side chain, and on the amine moiety. (The α and β nomenclature of the carbon atoms represents organic chemical terminology and has no relationship to the α- and β-receptor classification.)

The chemical structures and related pharmacologic characteristics of several adrenergic drugs are summarized in Table 6.1. Epinephrine, norepinephrine, dopamine, and isoproterenol have a hydroxyl group on both the 3 and 4 positions of the benzene ring. Because 3,4-dihydroxybenzene is also known as catechol, sympathomimetic amines containing this nucleus are termed catecholamines. In general, the catechol nucleus is required for maximum α and β potencies. Removal of one or both hydroxyl groups from the aromatic ring especially reduces β activity; e.g., phenylephrine is identical in structure to epinephrine except for the lack of one hydroxyl group on the ring (Table 6.1). Phenylephrine is almost exclusively an α agonist, whereas epinephrine is a mixed α-β agonist. Substitution of a ring hydroxyl group similarly reduces potency and may actually yield an antagonist (i.e., an adrenergic blocking drug such as the β blocker dichloroisoproterenol).

Substitution on the β-carbon atom of the side chain results in less active central actions in relation to peripheral effects. Substitution on the α-carbon atom yields a compound that is not susceptible to oxidation by monoamine oxidase (MAO).

Alkyl substitutions on the amino moiety affect the ratio of α- and β-agonistic properties. Within limits, increasing the size of the aliphatic substitution increases β activity. Epinephrine (*N*-methylnorepinephrine) is a more potent β agonist than norepinephrine. Isoproterenol (*N*-isopropylnorepinephrine) is a more potent β agonist than epinephrine or norepinephrine. Naturally occurring norepinephrine and epinephrine are in the levo configuration at the β-carbon atom. Dextrorotatory substitution on the β carbon yields the many times less potent *d*-isomers.

Adrenergic Receptor Subtypes: Pharmacologic Applications. Historically, the principal events responsible for information transmission across noradrenergic neuroeffector junctions were believed to include only the following: biosynthesis and storage of norepinephrine in the neuron terminal; exocytotic discharge of norepinephrine from the neuron; activation of effector cell α- or β-adrenergic receptors by released norepinephrine; and active "reuptake" of a portion of the free norepinephrine back into the axon terminal, thereby decreasing transmitter availability at the postjunctional receptors. We now know, however, that α- and β-adrenergic receptors of effector cells exist as subclasses and, furthermore, that several types of receptor-linked mechanisms operate within the adrenergic nerve endings themselves (Langer 1980; Adams 1984).

PREJUNCTIONAL α Receptors. The α-adrenergic receptors on the sympathetic neuron are believed to be important physiologically and pharmacologically; they

TABLE 6.1—Chemical structures and related pharmacologic activities of some commonly used sympathomimetic amines

Drug	Ring (5 6 / 4 1 / 3 2)	β CH	α CH	NH	Activity	Clinical use
β-phenylethylamine	. . .	H	H	H	. . .	. . .
β-phenylethanolamine	. . .	OH	H	H	. . .	. . .
Catecholamines						
Dopamine	3-OH, 4-OH	H	H	H	α, $β_1$, D	P, C, K
Norepinephrine	3-OH, 4-OH	OH	H	H	α,$β_1$	P, C
Epinephrine	3-OH, 4-OH	OH	H	CH_3	α, β	P, C, A, B
Isoproterenol	3-OH,4-OH	OH	H	$CH(CH_3)_2$	β	C, B
Noncatecholamines						
Metaraminol	3-OH	OH	CH_3	H	α	P
Phenylephrine	3-OH	OH	H	CH_3	α	P, Rb
Tyramine	4-OH	H	H	H	I	. . .
Hydroxyamphetamine	4-OH	H	CH_3	H	I	CNS
Amphetamine	. . .	H	CH_3	H	I	CNS
Methamphetamine	. . .	H	CH_3	CH_3	I	CNS
Ephedrine	. . .	OH	CH_3	CH_3	I, α, β	P, C, CNS

Note: α = α receptor; β = β receptor; A = allergic reactions; B = bronchodilator ($β_2$ receptor); C = cardiac stimulation ($β_1$ receptor); CNS = central nervous system excitation; D = dopamine may interact with α, $β_1$, and dopaminergic receptors; I = indirect-acting, causes release of endogenous norepinephrine that acts on α and β receptors; K = renal vasodilation (dopaminergic receptors); P = pressor activity; Rb = reflex bradycardia from pressor activation of baroreceptor-vagal reflex.

subserve an autoinhibitory regulation of norepinephrine release mechanisms. The physiologic role of α-receptor prejunctional events is envisioned as a local servomechanism through which norepinephrine can govern its own release once a threshold concentration of transmitter has been exceeded within the junction (Saeed et al. 1982).

PREJUNCTIONAL β Receptors. Epinephrine also can activate the prejunctional autoinhibitory α receptors, with potency about equal to that of norepinephrine. Interestingly, however, low concentrations of epinephrine actually accelerate norepinephrine release. This facilitatory action is shared by the β agonist isoproterenol and prevented by β-blocking drugs. These findings indicate that noradrenergic nerve endings possess β receptors that subserve a stimulatory effect on transmitter release mechanisms, an action opposite to that of the prejunctional α receptor.

Norepinephrine itself seems to have little influence on the prejunctional β-autostimulatory receptors, perhaps because this receptor population is more representative of $β_2$ rather than $β_1$ subtype. Thus the α-controlled autoinhibitory cycle probably dominates during usual communication between neuron and effector cell. A model of noradrenergic neurohumoral transmission incorporating prejunctional α and β receptors is presented in Fig. 6.2, along with representative effector cells, their prototypical receptor classes, and associated physiologic responses (Adams 1984).

ADRENERGIC RECEPTOR CLASSIFICATION. The original differentiation of adrenergic receptors into the two main classes, α and β, was based mainly on the relative potencies of the agonists norepinephrine, epinephrine, and isoproterenol in eliciting excitatory or inhibitory effects in a series of tissues (e.g., heart, vasculature, lungs) (Ahlquist 1948). Excitatory responses were generally designated as α-receptor events, and, for the most part, inhibitory responses were designated as β-receptor events. The excitatory β receptors of the heart represented an important exception to this rule and pointed toward different types of β receptors.

$β_1$-$β_2$ ADRENERGIC RECEPTOR SUBTYPES. Partly because of the potent β-stimulatory properties of norepinephrine in some tissue (e.g., the heart), but not others (e.g., the lungs), it was suggested that β receptors actually comprised a heterogeneous population of two distinct subtypes: $β_1$ and $β_2$ (Lands et al. 1967). Many tissues contain both $β_1$ and $β_2$ receptors in various ratios, depending on species and other variables. One subtype usually dominates and provides the tissue and organ with their functional classification as being under either $β_1$ or $β_2$-receptor control. A compilation of the predominant β-receptor subtype in several tissues is included in Table 5.1.

CARDIAC $β_1$ RECEPTORS. The functionally prevalent β receptor in the myocardium of most if not all mammalian species is the $β_1$ subtype. These receptors are activated in the following order of potency: isoproterenol > epinephrine ≥ norepinephrine. Activation of cardiac $β_1$ receptors leads to the characteristic sympathomimetic response of the heart as schematized in Fig. 6.3. In brief, this entails positive inotropic effects

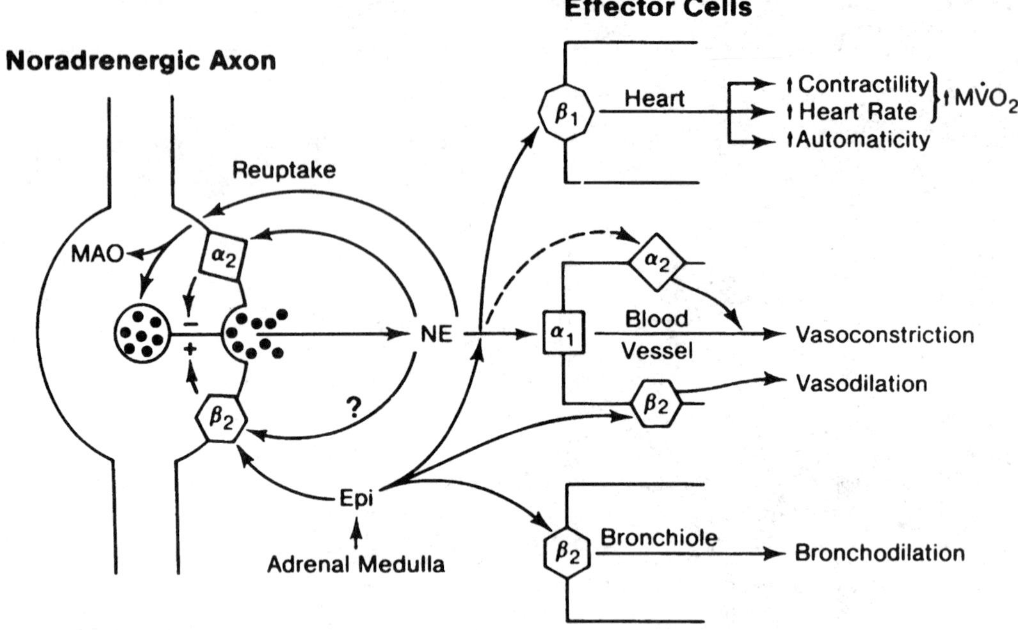

FIG. 6.2—Schematic diagram of peripheral noradrenergic neuroeffector junctions with a model axon terminal varicosity on the left and typical effector cells on the right. The predominant adrenoceptor subtypes and associated physiologic responses of the heart, blood vessel, and bronchiole are depicted. Norepinephrine (NE) released from the neuron can interact postjunctionally with innervated α_1 or β_1 receptors of effector cells and perhaps overflow (dashed line) to other nearby postjunctional receptors. NE also can activate prejunctional α receptors (α_2 subtype) to inhibit further release of NE. NE is removed from the junctional cleft by diffusion, extraneuronal uptake, and active uptake (reuptake) into the neuron, where it is metabolized by monoamine oxidase (MAO) or reincorporated into storage vesicles. Prejunctional β receptors (β_2 subtype) subserve a facilitatory effect on NE release, but it is questionable (?) whether NE itself activates this β_2-autostimulatory feedback loop. NE also has little β_2-agonist activity in blood vessels or bronchioles, whereas epinephrine (Epi) can activate all types of α and β adrenoceptors. $\dot{M}VO_2$ = myocardial oxygen demand (Adams 1984).

(increased contractility), positive chronotropic effects (increased heart rate), positive dromotropic effects (accelerated conduction of the cardiac impulse), and emergence of latent pacemaker activity. Increased heart rate and contractility lead in turn to increased myocardial oxygen demand and metabolic coronary vasodilation.

PULMONARY AND VASCULAR SMOOTH MUSCLE β_2 RECEPTORS. The β-adrenergic receptors of the pulmonary airways and peripheral vascular beds are mainly the β_2 subtype (Fig. 6.2). These receptors are activated potently by isoproterenol and epinephrine but quite poorly by norepinephrine. The β_2-pulmonary receptors subserve relaxation of bronchiolar smooth muscle and its accompanying bronchodilation, leading to an improvement in airway conductance. Vascular smooth muscle β_2 receptors are present in various tissues, where they mediate vasodilation and reduced vascular resistance. Although there is some uncertainty, most β_2-vascular receptors are probably noninnervated and, as with the pulmonary β_2 receptors, depend mainly on circulating epinephrine for activation and basal adrenergic tone (Fig. 6.2).

α_1-α_2 RECEPTOR SUBTYPES. Alpha receptors also can be divided into two distinct subpopulations: α_1 and α_2. This nomenclature began with the realization that the prejunctional α-receptor population responded to drugs somewhat differently than did the usual α receptors of effector cells. This led to classification of the typical effector cell α receptor as α_1 subtype, while the nerve terminal receptor was designated as α_2 (Fig. 6.2).

Alpha$_2$ receptors are not restricted anatomically to neuronal elements. They also are located on some noninnervated cell types, e.g., thrombocytes. Moreover, α_2 receptors also share certain tissue and functions with the α_1 subgroup. Pressor responses mediated by norepinephrine and epinephrine, e.g., involve activation of α_1- and α_2-receptor types in vascular smooth muscle. The α_1 receptor represents the innervated vascular receptors, whereas the α_2 type in this tissue is believed to localize predominantly in extrasynaptic regions of vascular smooth muscle cells. Endothelial cells of blood vessels also have α_2 receptors, which subserve release of endothelium-derived relaxing factor (EDRF) leading to vasodilation. EDRF has been identified as nitric oxide or a closely related compound that releases

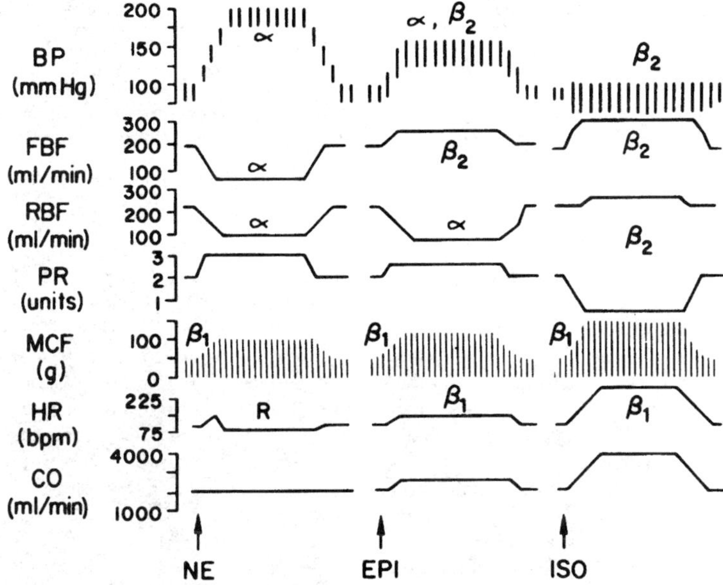

FIG. 6.3—Cardiovascular effects of intravenously administered norepinephrine (NE), epinephrine (Epi), and isoproterenol (ISO) in a dog. Schematic representations of effects of equivalent doses of these amines on blood pressure (BP), femoral blood flow (FBF), renal blood flow (RBF), peripheral vascular resistance (PR), myocardial contractile force (MCF), heart rate (HR), and cardiac output (CO). α = response mediated primarily by α-adrenergic receptor; β = response mediated primarily by β-adrenergic receptor (β_1 or β_2 subtype); R = reflex mediated. Characteristics of cardiovascular excitation evoked by these agents are due to differences in their α-β agonistic properties (Table 6.2). See text for explanation of each response.

nitric oxide (see Chap. 5; Lowenstein et al. 1994; Änggard 1994).

Based on the foregoing summary of α_1-α_2 and β_1-β_2 receptor subtypes and respective tissue responses, it should be apparent that all adrenergic drugs do not necessarily produce identical effects. Their pharmacologic profiles vary depending upon their basic chemical structure and resulting activities as α, β, or mixed α-β agonists. Nevertheless, sympathomimetic amines exhibit many similar pharmacodynamic properties. Therefore, only representative adrenergic drugs will be examined in detail; other agents will be compared in relation to differences they may exhibit in agonistic properties (i.e., activity at α or β receptors) and in mechanisms of action (i.e., direct- or indirect-acting sympathomimetic activity).

It also is important to realize that the α_1-α_2 and β_1-β_2 classification of receptors is an oversimplification of receptor subtypes. There are multiple subtype divisions of α_1, α_2, β_1, and β_2 receptors (Alberts 1993; Feldman 1993; Barnes 1993). However, the clinical relevance of adrenergic receptor classifications beyond α_1-α_2 and β_1-β_2 remains to be clarified.

CATECHOLAMINES. Catecholamines are direct-acting sympathomimetic amines. They activate receptors of effector cells; therefore, adrenergic nerves are not required for their effects.

Epinephrine, Norepinephrine, and Isoproterenol. Epinephrine (adrenaline) and norepinephrine (noradrenaline, levarterenol, arterenol) are endogenous biogenic amines; isoproterenol (isopropylarterenol) is not found in the body but is chemically synthesized. Subtle differences in the pharmacologic effects of structurally related adrenergic drugs can be demonstrated by comparing cardiovascular effects of these three agents, as shown schematically in Fig. 6.3.

Different cardiovascular responses seen with epinephrine, norepinephrine, and isoproterenol in Fig. 6.3 are due to differences in the ratios of their α- and β-agonistic properties. Classification of adrenergic receptors in the heart and blood vessels, related effects, and the order of potency of epinephrine, norepinephrine, and isoproterenol are shown in Table 6.2.

Norepinephrine, because of its α-agonist properties, activates the α-vascular receptors, resulting in intense vasoconstriction; peripheral resistance increases and femoral and renal blood flows decrease (Fig. 6.3).

Although epinephrine is a potent α stimulant, it also is very active at β receptors. Beta$_2$ receptors in blood vessels subserve vasodilation. In response to epinephrine, vasoconstriction occurs in vascular beds that have predominantly α receptors (e.g., abdominal viscera); however, vasodilation can occur in beds that contain β_2 receptors (e.g., skeletal muscle). Blood flow increases in areas in response to regional vasodilation (e.g.,

TABLE 6.2—Adrenergic receptor activation by catecholamines

Receptor type	Tissue	Response	Potency of agonists
α	Blood vessels	Vasconstriction	Epinephrine > norepinephrine >>> isoproterenol
β_1	Heart	Positive inotropic and chronotropic effects	Isoproterenol > epinephrine ≧ norepinephrine
β_2	Blood vessels	Vasodilation	Isoproterenol > epinephrine >>> norepinephrine

Note: > = greater than; ≧ = greater than or equal; >>> = many times greater.

femoral flow) but decreases if vasoconstriction dominates (e.g., renal flow) (Fig. 6.3).

Because isoproterenol is a selective β agonist, it causes vasodilation, fall in diastolic blood pressure, decrease in peripheral resistance, and increase in blood flow to areas containing β receptors (e.g., femoral blood flow). The renal vasculature has few β receptors and is therefore little affected by isoproterenol (Fig. 6.3).

The heart is activated by epinephrine, norepinephrine, and isoproterenol (Fig. 6.3). Isoproterenol is the most potent of the three and causes a relatively greater increase in myocardial contractile force, heart rate, and cardiac output than the similarly acting epinephrine. Norepinephrine also increases myocardial contractile force, but bradycardia occurs at the peak pressor effect of this amine. This is due to an increase in vagal tone reflexly instigated by the pronounced norepinephrine-induced increase in mean blood pressure. Norepinephrine-mediated peripheral vasoconstriction may decrease venous return so cardiac output does not increase, although the heart is activated.

These examples demonstrate differences in selective cardiovascular effects of these closely related catecholamines. Nevertheless, it should be apparent that all three agents elicit the same basic result, a net increase in cardiovascular activity.

Pharmacologic Effects

BLOOD PRESSURE. Norepinephrine administered intravenously either by slow infusion or bolus injection causes a dose-related increase in systolic and diastolic blood pressures due to bodywide vasoconstriction. Mean blood pressure increases accordingly; little change is seen in pulse pressure.

Slow intravenous (IV) infusion of small amounts of epinephrine usually causes a fall in diastolic blood pressure that may or may not be accompanied by a slight increase in systolic pressure. This response is due to regional vasodilation (β_2-receptor-mediated), which causes a decrease in peripheral resistance. However, a bolus IV injection of a large amount of epinephrine (e.g., 1-3 μg/kg) causes a pronounced increase in blood pressure that is as remarkable as that produced by norepinephrine. It should be appreciated that epinephrine is an extremely potent pressor agent. This pressor response depends upon vasoconstriction, myocardial stimulation, and tachycardia. Bradycardia can occur at the peak pressor response as a result of reflex vagal activity. A depressor effect may be observed after the pressor response to a large dose of epinephrine. This secondary response is related to residual activation of β_2 receptors in blood vessels.

Following a single bolus injection of norepinephrine or epinephrine, the pressor response lasts for several minutes, then gradually decreases and returns to normal within 5-10 minutes. Isoproterenol increases pulse pressure predominantly by lowering diastolic pressure. This effect is due to β_2-receptor-mediated vasodilation.

VASCULAR SMOOTH MUSCLE. This type of tissue can contain both α_1- and α_2-receptor subtypes (which subserve vasoconstriction) and β_2 receptors (which subserve vasodilation). Epinephrine and norepinephrine are very potent constrictors of cutaneous and mucosal blood vessels in mammalian species. Adrenergic receptors in these vessels are almost exclusively α. Intense vasoconstriction, increased vascular resistance, and decreased blood flow occur in these regions in response to norepinephrine and epinephrine. This is often seen as a blanching type response in skin or mucosal membranes.

Since epinephrine is a more potent α agonist than norepinephrine, it is 2-10 times more active than norepinephrine in constricting cutaneous and mucosal vessels. Smaller arterioles and precapillary sphincters are particularly responsive to the vasoconstrictor catecholamines. They are active regardless of whether they are applied topically to blood vessels, sprayed upon mucosal surfaces, injected perivascularly, or administered systemically. Isoproterenol has little if any effect on cutaneous and mucosal vessels, because of the relative lack of β receptors in these tissues.

The renal vasculature has predominantly α receptors. Epinephrine and norepinephrine cause vasoconstriction in the kidney and a generalized increase in vascular resistance in this organ. Renal blood flow is decreased even in the presence of an elevated systemic blood pressure (Fig. 6.3). Large doses of α-agonistic catecholamines may actually induce a functional renal shutdown caused by decreased perfusion of the kidney. During this period, urinary output is substantially decreased from lowered glomerular filtration rate.

Isoproterenol has little effect on renal arteries because of the small number of β receptors in kidney vasculature. However, direct injection of the drug into the renal artery increases renal blood flow. In addition, there are β_1 receptors in the kidney, which upon activation cause a release of renin into the circulation for angiotensin formation.

Mesenteric arteries are constricted by norepinephrine and epinephrine as a result of activation of α receptors. Mesenteric arterial resistance is markedly increased and splanchnic blood flow decreases proportionately. In some circumstances, i.e., with small doses, epinephrine may cause slight vasodilation of splanchnic arteries because of the presence of β_2 receptors.

Skeletal muscle blood vessels have both α and β receptors. Vasoconstriction or vasodilation can be induced, depending upon the α- and β-agonistic profiles of a vasostimulatory amine. Norepinephrine, because of its relative lack of effect on β-vascular receptors, elicits vasoconstriction in skeletal muscles caused by activation of α receptors. Vascular resistance increases and blood flow decreases proportionately.

Beta receptors in skeletal muscle blood vessels are more sensitive to epinephrine than are the α receptors. Therefore, small amounts of epinephrine actually cause a decrease in vascular resistance and an increase in blood flow to voluntary muscles through vasodilation. However, large doses of epinephrine cause vasoconstriction in skeletal muscles from the α-receptor-mediated contraction overriding β-mediated relaxation. If α receptors are blocked, the response to epinephrine is converted to vasodilation from unmasking of the β effect. If a β blocker is used, the α-mediated constrictor effects of epinephrine are accentuated.

Isoproterenol causes relaxation of skeletal muscle blood vessels, increased blood flow to voluntary muscle masses, and decreased vascular resistance in these structures caused by activation of the vascular β receptors. Since isoproterenol has little effect on α receptors, β blockade abolishes the vasodilator effect of isoproterenol but does not convert the response to vasoconstriction.

Coronary arteries dilate in response to catecholamines (isoproterenol > epinephrine ≥ norepinephrine). The major portions of this vasodilator response are secondary to increased myocardial contractility and heart rate and resulting metabolic demands of the heart. Alpha receptors that subserve vasoconstriction can be demonstrated in the coronary vasculature; however, they are more prevalent in larger vessels than in smaller nutrient arteries. Beta receptors dominate, causing vasodilation and increased coronary blood flow in response to catecholamines. Studies with isolated vessels suggest that coronary receptors are of the β_1 subtype (Cornish and Miller 1975), while in vivo studies indicate the β_2 subtype (Moreland and Bohr 1984). This is different from most other vasodilator β receptors that have generally been characterized as β_2, irrespective of in vivo or in vitro setting.

Cerebral arteries are less responsive to adrenergic agonists than most other vascular beds. This is compatible with the concept that cerebral blood flow, like coronary blood flow, is controlled principally by local metabolic needs rather than by the nervous system. Nevertheless, both α-vasoconstrictor and β-vasodilator receptors can be demonstrated in cerebral blood vessels.

VASCULAR MECHANISMS. Mechanical function of a vascular smooth muscle cell depends upon the availability of free intracellular Ca^{++} in the vicinity of contractile proteins. Norepinephrine and epinephrine produce vascular contraction by initially causing release of an intracellular (sequestered) source of Ca^{++} to the contractile proteins in response to activation of α_1 receptors. The signal-transduction mechanism linking α_1 receptors to vasoconstriction involves the G protein, phospholipase C, and inositol triphosphate pathway (Brodde and Michel 1992).

Cyclic adenosine 3′,5′-monophosphate (cAMP) is increased in response to β_2-receptor activation; this mechanism utilizes the stimulatory G protein (G_s) and adenylyl cyclase pathway (Feldman 1993; Schwinn 1993; Levitzki et al. 1993) (Fig. 5.9).

MYOCARDIAL EFFECTS. Isoproterenol, epinephrine, and norepinephrine are potent myocardial stimulants. They increase the strength of myocardial contractile force and accelerate heart rate. These changes represent direct effects that are not dependent upon changes in venous return (preload), afterload, or other hemodynamic variables. Contractile and rate effects of catecholamines are mediated via direct activation of β receptors of the myocardial and pacemaker cells. Myocardial β receptors are subtyped predominantly as β_1. Isoproterenol is 10-20 times more active in the heart than epinephrine; norepinephrine is somewhat less potent than epinephrine.

The increase in myocardial contractility (positive inotropic effect) seen with each of the three agents is produced in both atrial and ventricular muscles. The positive inotropism in the whole heart is characterized by more rapid and forcible systolic ejection. The rate of pressure changes in the ventricular chambers is increased. The systolic interval is shortened and diastolic relaxation takes place more quickly. Oxygen consumption is accelerated to a relatively greater extent than the heart work is increased. Therefore, cardiac efficiency is sacrificed at the expense of absolute increase in myocardial contractility produced by catecholamines.

Acceleration of heart rate (positive chronotropism) induced by catecholamines is due to changes in the automaticity of pacemaker cells. The spontaneous depolarization process in the sinoatrial node cells is accelerated; velocity of the action potential is enhanced in these and other conduction system cells. Purkinje fibers are similarly affected by epinephrine and norepinephrine. Latent or normally inactive pacemaker cells are activated by these agents; they become more excitable and fire more easily or even spontaneously.

Norepinephrine, epinephrine, and isoproterenol increase myocardial irritability, resulting in serious tachyarrhythmias, especially in sensitized animals or with large doses. This can be partially blocked by an α blocker (Benfry 1993). However, pure α agonists such as phenylephrine and methoxamine are weak arrhythmogenic agents. Also, a β blocker such as propranolol

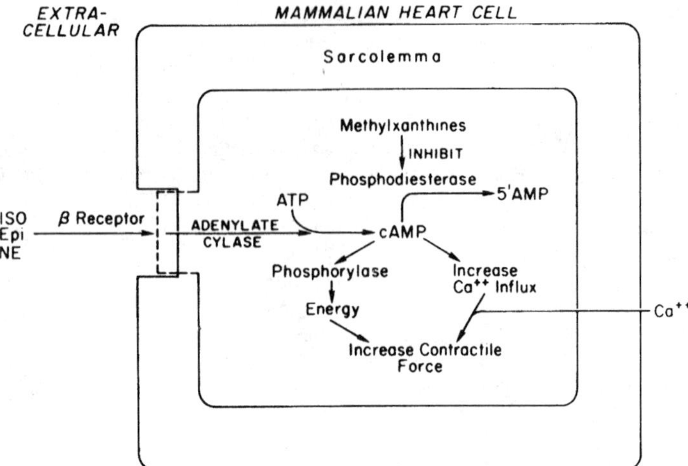

FIG. 6.4—Representation of proposed involvement of cyclic adenosine monophosphate (cAMP) in the myocardial effects of catecholamines. ISO = isoproterenol; Epi = epinephrine; NE = norepinephrine; ATP = adenosine triphosphate; 5′AMP = 5-adenosine monophosphate. The intracellular receptor for cAMP is protein kinase A, which phosphorylates different cellular substrates, resulting in changes in cell function (Feldman 1993). The stimulatory G protein (G_s) links the β-receptor recognition site to the catalytic component of adenylyl (adenylate) cyclase (Levitzki et al. 1993); see Fig. 5.9. Phosphorylase represents this and other biochemical reactions influenced by cAMP (see text).

is more active than an α blocker in decreasing the arrhythmias evoked by epinephrine and norepinephrine. Certain halogenated anesthetics (halothane, chloroform) increase the sensitivity of the heart to cardiac rhythm irregularities induced by catecholamines.

Bradycardia often occurs during the peak pressor response seen after administration of epinephrine or norepinephrine to intact animals. This can be blocked by vagotomy or atropine; it is dependent upon the hypertensive response causing an increase in vagal discharge via the baroreceptor reflex mechanisms. It is usually more pronounced with norepinephrine than with epinephrine because of the relatively greater increase in mean blood pressure seen with the former. Tachycardia is invariably produced by isoproterenol.

MYOCARDIAL MECHANISMS. In a heart muscle cell, contractile Ca^{++} is believed to originate in part from superficial sarcolemmal sites. Calcium bound at these sites is in rapid equilibrium with Ca^{++} within the extracellular space (Langer 1974; Parker and Adams 1977). Ca^{++} influx from superficial sites links membrane excitation (i.e., the cardiac action potential) to contraction of the myofibers. Catecholamines enhance the influx of Ca^{++} into the myocardial cell, due to increased intracellular concentrations of cAMP.

Activation of the cardiac β_1 receptor by epinephrine, norepinephrine, and isoproterenol increases the activity of a G_s-protein-linked adenylyl cyclase (Brodde and Michel 1992; Feldman 1993). This enzyme catalyzes the conversion of adenosine triphosphate (ATP) to cAMP. Cyclic AMP causes an increased Ca^{++} influx through the slow Ca^{++} channels of the sarcolemma, resulting in increased availability of Ca^{++} at the contractile proteins (Watanabe and Besch 1974). Cyclic cAMP activates protein kinase A, which phosphorylates various substrates, culminating in changes in cellular functions responsible for positive inotropic and chronotropic responses to β_1-receptor activation.

Several drugs alter the cAMP system in complementary ways; e.g., the methylxanthines inhibit the enzyme (phosphodiesterase) that inactivates cAMP (Fig. 6.4). These drugs, termed phosphodiesterase inhibitors, cause increase in cAMP concentrations and a positive inotropic effect in heart muscle. They potentiate inotropic activity of the catecholamines.

RESPIRATORY EFFECTS. Epinephrine is a potent bronchodilator as a result of relaxation of bronchial smooth muscle. This effect is particularly pronounced if bronchial muscle is contracted by other drugs (e.g., acetylcholine, histamine) or by anaphylactoid or asthmatic conditions. Adrenergic receptors in bronchiolar muscle are of the β_2 type. Isoproterenol is therefore a potent bronchiolar dilator, whereas exogenous norepinephrine has relatively less effect. Epinephrine and isoproterenol have been used clinically to dilate bronchiolar passageways during episodes of allergic reactions. As bronchodilators, however, selective β_2 agonists such as terbutaline and salbutamol have advantages over conventional catecholamines. The former drugs relax bronchiolar smooth muscle (β_2) with less cardiac excitatory effects (β_1) than seen with epinephrine (α-β_1-β_2 agonist) or isoproterenol (β_1-β_2 agonist), as discussed later in this chapter.

GASTROINTESTINAL SYSTEM. Adrenergic drugs inhibit gastrointestinal (GI) activity in a manner similar to that seen upon stimulation of the sympathetic nerves. The frequency and amplitude of peristaltic contractions in the gut are decreased as a result of relaxation of the intestinal smooth muscle. These effects are from activation of β-adrenergic receptors of the smooth muscle cells. Adrenergic drugs also inhibit the function of excitatory parasympathetic nerves via α_2 effects. This action contributes further to GI quiescence. Isoproterenol, as a result of β effects, exerts a rather potent inhibitory effect on GI smooth muscle. GI sphincters are generally contracted by α-sympathomimetic agents. This is in basic agreement with the overall slowing down of GI activity produced by sympathetic nerve stimulation.

Secretion of digestive juices is also decreased by α-sympathetic agents. Although salivary glands are activated in response to sympathetic activity, the saliva produced is scant and viscous, in contrast to the profuse and watery salivation seen with parasympathetic activity.

Catecholamines can exert both an inhibitory and a stimulatory effect on secretion of insulin by β cells of the pancreatic islets. The facilitatory effect is mediated via β-receptor activation, the inhibitory effect via α-receptor activation. The α-inhibitory effect is strongly predominant in vivo in most species. Since insulin is antagonistic to many of the metabolic actions of adrenergic mediators (e.g., gluconeogenesis, hyperglycemia), inhibition of insulin release by the catecholamines reinforces their metabolic effects.

Adrenergic drugs have no application as GI inhibitory agents in clinical situations. Cardiovascular effects are usually concurrently produced by dosages required to inhibit GI function. Also, parasympathetic activity in the GI system can quickly override the depressant effects exhibited by most sympathomimetic drugs.

UTERINE MUSCLE. Both α and β receptors are present in the uterus. Responses of uterine smooth muscle to catecholamines are quite variable, depending on species and stage of the estrous and gestational cycles; e.g., in the cat, epinephrine relaxes the nongravid uterus but contracts the uterus during late pregnancy. In the rabbit, epinephrine contracts the gravid and nongravid uterus. In humans, epinephrine contracts the pregnant or nonpregnant uterus when examined in vitro. In situ, however, responses vary; epinephrine may cause relaxation of the uterus during late pregnancy. Isoproterenol usually exerts relaxant effects in uterine muscle even in the presence of epinephrine-induced contraction. The presence of circulating hormones such as estrogen and progesterone modify responses of the uterus to other agents. There is presently little clinical application of catecholamines as effectors of uterine motility. However, selective β_2 agonists (e.g., salbutamol, ritodrine) have been used in human obstetrics to relax the uterus and delay premature labor.

SPLEEN. Smooth muscle of the splenic capsule is contracted by epinephrine and norepinephrine via α effects. The size of the spleen decreases and blood is discharged into the circulation. This response is probably functional in physiologic states such as acute hypoxia, severe fear or rage, hemorrhage, or other conditions that elicit a generalized activation of the sympathoadrenal axis.

The splenic effects of catecholamines are easily and decisively demonstrable in dogs anesthetized with pentobarbital. Under these circumstances, the spleen is enlarged and engorged with blood. Injection of small amounts of norepinephrine or epinephrine into the splenic artery causes a pronounced contraction of the spleen and a remarkable diminution of its size. Injection of these agents directly under the splenic capsule causes intense localized contraction of the capsule. These effects are associated with α receptors. Relaxation of the splenic capsule via β receptors also has been demonstrated.

PILOMOTOR EFFECTS. Norepinephrine and epinephrine cause contraction of piloerector muscles; hairs become erect. This effect is mediated by α receptors; it is often seen in animals during severe reaction to fear or rage.

OCULAR EFFECTS. Mydriasis occurs in response to stimulation of the sympathetic innervation to the eye. IV administration or topical application of epinephrine or norepinephrine causes pupillary dilation via α effects. Parasympathetic activity easily overrides adrenergic activity in the eye, however, and responses to adrenergic drugs may vary considerably. The nictitating membrane, or third eyelid, is contracted by norepinephrine and epinephrine; conjunctival and scleral blood vessels are constricted. Intraocular pressure may decrease slightly upon local instillation of epinephrine; this effect is sometimes useful in treating wide angle glaucoma.

CENTRAL NERVOUS SYSTEM EFFECTS. Catecholamines do not readily cross the blood-brain barrier. Therefore, epinephrine and norepinephrine have little effect on the central nervous system (CNS). Certain noncatecholamine adrenergic agents, like amphetamine, readily cross the blood-brain barrier and elicit pronounced stimulation of the CNS.

METABOLIC EFFECTS. Catecholamines exert several rather striking effects on anabolic and catabolic activities in different organs and tissues. In mammals, there is an overall calorogenic effect (increase in general metabolism) associated with a 20-30% increase in oxygen consumption. Glycogenolysis occurs in the liver and skeletal and cardiac muscles following exposure to epinephrine, norepinephrine, or isoproterenol. There is also an acceleration of fatty acid mobilization and lactic acid formation. Accordingly, concentrations in the blood of glucose, free fatty acids, and lactic acid are increased. The order of potency of catecholamines in eliciting these metabolic changes varies in different tissues and species. In general, the glycogenolysis effect in muscles and liver follows the potency order of that associated with β receptors.

The metabolic activities of catecholamines have been associated with alterations of tissue concentration of cAMP. In hepatic and muscle tissue, e.g., adenylyl cyclase activity is increased by catecholamines, resulting in an accelerated conversion of ATP to cAMP, which in turn activates protein kinase A; the latter accelerates conversion of the inactive phosphorylase enzyme (phosphorylase b) to an active form (phosphorylase a) that then catalyzes the catabolism of glycogen to glucose. Similarly, the catecholamines have been associated with changes in the relative activities of other protein kinases, lipases, and phosphofructokinases by increases in cAMP formation.

ABSORPTION AND BIOTRANSFORMATION. Epinephrine and norepinephrine are not absorbed to any appreciable extent following oral administration because of destruction within the GI tract. The liver rapidly inactivates by oxidative deamination and conjugation any norepinephrine or epinephrine that is absorbed into the portal system. Isoproterenol is absorbed following oral or sublingual administration but often in such an erratic manner as to be therapeutically nonuseful. Catecholamines are readily absorbed from aerosolized sprays or after parenteral administration. Subcutaneous (SC) dosages are more slowly absorbed than intramuscular (IM) injections.

Injected norepinephrine and epinephrine are metabolized by MAO and COMT (catechol-*O*-methyltransferase) enzymes; the inactive metabolites are excreted in urine. A portion of the *O*-methylated and deaminated metabolites are conjugated prior to excretion. MAO and COMT are present in many tissues; breakdown of catecholamines does not depend entirely upon the liver or kidney. Uptake of norepinephrine and epinephrine into adrenergic neurons away from their active receptor sites is an important pathway for termination of their pharmacologic activities (see Chap. 5). This is demonstrated by injecting a drug that blocks the amine uptake pump, e.g., cocaine, which potentiates the pressor response to norepinephrine and epinephrine. Inhibition of MAO and COMT has little effect on responses to single injections of catecholamines.

PREPARATIONS. *Epinephrine,* USP, the free base, is obtained from adrenal medullary extracts of domestic farm animals or is chemically synthesized. It is a white or light brown crystalline powder that is relatively insoluble in water but readily forms the water-soluble salt epinephrine hydrochloride upon addition to dilute hydrochloric acid. Solutions are unstable in alkaline mediums or upon exposure to light or heat and discolor to pink and eventually brown. Discoloration indicates oxidation of epinephrine to an inactive form; such solutions should be discarded.

Epinephrine Injection, USP, and *Epinephrine Solution,* USP, are aqueous solutions of epinephrine hydrochloride (adrenaline hydrochloride) prepared in a 1:1000 (1 mg/mL; 0.1%) solution; they are probably the most commonly used preparations of epinephrine. The former solution is sterile. Addition of small amounts of sodium bisulfite retards oxidative breakdown of epinephrine.

Sterile Epinephrine Suspension, USP, is a sterile suspension of epinephrine, usually 2 mg/mL, in sesame or peanut oil for IM injection only. This product is used when prolonged activity is desired.

Epinephrine Bitartrate, USP, is available in aerosol and ophthalmic solutions.

Norepinephrine (levarterenol) Bitartrate, USP (*l*-norepinephrine bitartrate), is a white crystalline powder (monohydrate salt) that readily dissolves in water. Solutions turn pink upon exposure to light, heat, or air and should be discarded if discoloration occurs.

Norepinephrine (levarterenol) Bitartrate Injection, USP, is a sterile aqueous solution usually containing 0.2% (2 mg/mL) of the salt (equivalent to 0.1% or 1 mg/mL of norepinephrine base). Bisulfite is included to delay oxidation.

Isoproterenol Hydrochloride, USP (Isuprel hydrochloride), is the water-soluble hydrochloride salt. Solutions of this compound also oxidize when exposed to light or air.

Isoproterenol Hydrochloride Injection, USP, is a sterile aqueous solution of isoproterenol hydrochloride for parenteral injection. Available preparations usually contain 0.2 mg/mL (0.02%).

Isoproterenol Hydrochloride Tablets, USP, are available in 10 mg and 15 mg sizes.

CLINICAL USE

WITH LOCAL ANESTHETICS. Epinephrine is commonly used in concentrations of 1:100,000 to 1:20,000 in local anesthetic solutions. It causes pronounced local vasoconstriction and thereby localizes the action and delays the absorption of the infilterable anesthetic. Since norepinephrine is a less potent α agonist than epinephrine, it is infrequently used in local anesthetic solutions.

LOCAL HEMOSTATIC. Vasoconstrictor effects of epinephrine (1:100,000 to 1:20,000 solution) may be used to control superficial bleeding of mucosal and SC surfaces by application of moistened gauze sponges or by aerosol sprayed directly onto the damaged region. Epinephrine solutions have been used topically during ophthalmic surgery to control hemorrhage. Epistaxis and dental extractions are other indications. Epinephrine is effective only against hemorrhage from capillaries and arterioles and should not be used in attempts to control bleeding from larger vessels. Although smooth muscle of large vessels contracts in response to amines, this effect is by no means sufficient to occlude the lumen. During surgery, topical application of epinephrine should be considered only as a temporary aid for controlling bleeding to assist in visualization of the operative field. Serious bleeding may well recur subsequent to termination of activity of this catecholamine if routine ligation of blood vessels is disregarded.

HYPOTENSION. Pressor amines are often used to maintain blood pressure during spinal surgery, and epinephrine is quite effective in treating hypotension associated with anaphylactic shock. The peripheral vasoconstrictor effects of norepinephrine, epinephrine, and other adrenergic drugs have also been used in attempts to treat and prevent hypotension occurring during other shock syndromes. However, blood pressure elevation due to peripheral vasoconstriction is not an adequate substitution for correcting serious underlying problems such as hypovolemia, undetected hemorrhage, and electrolyte and fluid imbalances. Some shock states are characterized by peripheral vasoconstriction secondary to a generalized sympathoadrenal discharge. Under such circumstances, administration of epinephrine or norepinephrine may serve to compound the problem by causing further intensification of vasoconstriction in vital areas (e.g., splanchnic and renal vascular beds) (Adams and Parker 1979). In some cases, the exact opposite effect (blockade of α-adrenergic receptors) has been proposed as a treatment in shock. These factors should always be considered when use of sympathomimetic amines during shock therapy is considered.

In shock cases characterized by loss of vascular tone, use of pressor amines has been suggested. Also, reestablishment of normal blood volume in some shock patients does not seem to correct the vascular complications, and blood pressure remains seriously depressed. Pressor agents may be of some use. Norepinephrine has been used under these circumstances. Usually, a 4 mL vial of 0.2% norepinephrine bitartrate (0.1% of free norepinephrine base; 1 mg/mL) is added to 1 L of sterile isotonic saline solution or 5% dextrose solution, which gives a final concentration of norepinephrine base of 4 μg/mL of solution. This solution is slowly infused intravenously until blood pressure is maintained somewhat lower than normal. Usually, an infusion rate of 0.1-0.2 μg/kg/min proves effective; however, administration should be to effect. The pressor response to norepinephrine can be readily controlled since it disappears within 1 or 2 minutes after stopping the infusion. Blood pressure should be closely monitored during the infusion process. An attempt should always be made to closely monitor cardiovascular function during treatment with any of the catecholamines. Isoproterenol has been used in some low cardiac output stages of shock. Soma et al. (1974) recommend a slow IV infusion of a 0.1-0.2 μg/mL solution of isoproterenol.

CARDIAC EFFECTS. Catecholamines are indicated in treatment of certain cardiac disorders: cardiac arrest, partial or complete atrioventricular (AV) block, and Stokes-Adams syndrome (Adams 1981). With cardiac arrest, an attempt is first made to restore heartbeat by mechanical means such as a precordial blow, electrical shock, or external cardiac massage. If the heart starts contracting, isoproterenol or epinephrine can be given by slow IV drip to maintain heart rate and cardiac output after circulation is restored. Care should be taken with IV infusion, since epinephrine may precipitate ventricular fibrillation if prefibrillatory rhythm is presented.

If asystole persists, norepinephrine, epinephrine (0.5-1.0 mL of a 1:10,000 solution; i.e., 50-100 μg), or isoproterenol (20-40 μg) may be administered directly into the left ventricular chamber in an attempt to restore contraction. Larger doses may be required in some instances. The heart should then be massaged to ensure circulation of the catecholamine through the coronary vasculature. Peripheral circulation should be maintained by cardiac massage until myocardial contraction is restored.

Isoproterenol is used for treating heart block. Complete AV heart block in a dog was treated with 0.05 mg (approximately 3.5 μg/kg) of isoproterenol administered intravenously; the heart rate increased almost immediately from 44 beats/minute to 68 beats/minute (Buchanan et al. 1968). Because of its potency, isoproterenol should be administered by slow IV infusion rather than rapid bolus injection. Slow IV drip of a diluate solution can be instituted until the heart rate is maintained at 80-100 beats/minute. Thereafter, IM injections of 0.1-0.2 mg isoproterenol every 4 hours may prove effective. Isoproterenol tablets (15-30 mg) have been given every 4 hours; however, patients should be closely monitored because absorption after oral administration is erratic. Buchanan et al. (1968) found that orally administered isoproterenol (30 mg twice daily) was ineffective in treating complete AV block in a dog. Ettinger (1969) infused isoproterenol (5 μg/mL in dextrose and water) intravenously at a rate (usually 1 mL/minute) sufficient to maintain the ventricular rate at 80/minute. Isoproterenol was then administered subcutaneously every 6 hours at the dose of 0.2 mg. Oral administration of an isoproterenol tablet (30 mg) every 6 hours was prescribed for several weeks. Catecholamines should not be used in the presence of acute or chronic heart failure. These agents decrease efficiency of myocardial contraction by increasing oxygen demands of the heart muscle and compound the heart failure syndrome.

ANAPHYLACTIC AND ALLERGIC REACTIONS. Epinephrine is extremely effective and often lifesaving in treatment of acute anaphylactic shock. It quickly reverses the precipitous fall in blood pressure and cardiac irregularities associated with this type of syndrome. Histamine-like constriction of bronchiolar smooth muscles occurs during anaphylaxis; these effects are rapidly antagonized by epinephrine. Bronchiolar passageways are dilated by epinephrine as a result of relaxation of the smooth muscle, and dyspnea is quickly counteracted. Care should be taken that allergic signs do not recur after epinephrine activity has terminated.

BRONCHIAL ASTHMA. Isoproterenol and epinephrine have been useful for providing immediate relief from bronchial asthma. These agents activate the β_2 receptors of the bronchial smooth muscle cells, causing relaxation and prompt relief by dilating the airways. Norepinephrine is ineffective in dilating passageways even though it may transiently decrease mucosal congestion by constricting mucosal blood vessels. For systemic relief from allergic and anaphylactoid reactions, epinephrine can be administered subcutaneously or intramuscularly, because with these routes effective blood levels are quickly achieved. However, if a patient is presented in late stages of anaphylactic shock or other similar life-threatening situations, IV administration may be required.

In large domestic animals (cattle, horses) 4-8 mg epinephrine can be given intramuscularly or subcutaneously by injection of 4-8 mL of a 1:1000 dilution of epinephrine solution. Sheep and swine may be administered 1-3 mL of the 1:1000 dilution. Dogs and cats are usually given 1-5 mL of a 1:10,000 (0.1 mg/mL) dilution. Based on a body weight range of approximately 5-25 kg, this represents a dosage schedule of approximately 20 μg/kg. A dose this large should be administered only by IM or SC injection. Response of animals to adrenergic drugs may vary considerably; therefore, repeat injections or somewhat larger doses may be required in some cases. If IV administration is necessary, one should proceed cautiously and give no more than 0.25-0.5 μg/kg. In experimental animals, 1-2 μg/kg epinephrine or norepinephrine administered by IV bolus injection causes a pronounced increase in cardiovascular activity, and even slightly larger doses may well lead to serious arrhythmias. Selective β_2 agonists (e.g., terbutaline, metaproteronol) may supplant epinephrine and isoproterenol as bronchodilators (see β_2-selective bronchodilators).

TOXICITY. As implied in the preceding discussion, toxicity of the catecholamines is usually characterized by untoward cardiovascular responses. In particular, cardiac dysrhythmias such as tachycardia and even fatal ventricular fibrillation may occur following inadvertent overdosage. Hyperthyroid conditions, thyroid therapy, digitalis therapy, halogenated hydrocarbon anesthetics, and thiobarbiturates predispose a patient to the myocardial toxicity of catecholamines. The influence of anesthetics on the arrhythmogenicity of catecholamines is believed to be due to sensitization of the heart muscle. Myocardial sensitization to catecholamines is evoked by trichlorethylene, ethyl chloride, cyclopropane, halothane, chloroform, methoxyflurane, and fluroxene (listed in order of decreasing effect) (Katz and Katz 1966). Thiobarbiturates increase the incidence of epinephrine- and norepinephrine-induced arrhythmias in chloroform-anesthetized dogs (Claborn and Szabuniewicz 1973; Wiersig et al. 1974).

Hypertensive crises occur from norepinephrine or epinephrine overdosage; cerebral vascular accidents and ruptured aneurysms may result. The latter represents a potential problem in horses because of a fairly common incidence of undiagnosed verminous aneurysms. Large or repeated dosages of epinephrine and isoproterenol have been associated with myocardial ischemia and necrosis; these effects are prevented by β-blocking agents. Local necrosis and sloughing of tissue may occur at injection sites because of intensive vasoconstriction and resulting ischemia.

In short, the catecholamines are extremely potent agents; under no circumstances should they be considered innocuous. Therapeutic use of these drugs should always be carefully monitored by a trained individual familiar with their indications, limitations, and toxicities.

Dopamine. Dopamine (3,4-dihydroxyphenylethylamine) was thought to be important only as the immediate precursor to norepinephrine. Dopamine itself is now known to have important physiologic functions in mammalian species and is receiving attention in certain clinical circumstances in humans (Caccavelli et al. 1992). Parkinson's disease, e.g., has been related to decreased concentrations of dopamine in the basal ganglia, and treatment with *l*-dopa has proved effective in controlling motor disorders in some Parkinsonism patients. *l*-Dopa crosses the blood-brain barrier (dopamine does not in significant quantities) and is decarboxylated to dopamine.

Experimental hemodynamic studies indicate that dopamine also has use as a selective cardiovascular agent. In anesthetized dogs, IV injection of 1-9 μg/kg dopamine induces a slight depressor response associated with a decrease in total peripheral resistance, a decrease in renal vascular resistance, an increase in renal blood flow, and an increase in cardiac output. Large amounts, 9-81 μg/kg, produce pressor responses and a more pronounced increase in myocardial contractile force (Setler et al. 1975). Cardiovascular effects of dopamine depend on activation of different types of catecholaminergic receptors. The pressor response is blocked by an α blocker (e.g., phenoxybenzamine), and the cardiac stimulatory effects are blocked by a β blocker (e.g., propranolol). Part of the myocardial effects of dopamine are thought to be indirect and mediated by release of norepinephrine from cardiac sympathetic nerves (Fig. 6.5).

The depressor effects of dopamine are not blocked by a β blocker but are blocked by haloperidol. Because the latter drug is a dopamine antagonist in the brain, it has been proposed that there are specific dopamine receptors in certain vascular beds (Goldberg and Rajfer 1985). The dopamine-responsive or dopaminergic receptors of vascular beds can be considered a fifth adrenergic receptor subtype. Although the physiologic purpose of the vascular dopamine receptors is unknown, this receptor type is important to clinical pharmacology because it subserves vasodilatory responses in the renal, visceral, coronary, and cerebral

DOPAMINE

A. Releases Endogenous NE
Activates B_1 Receptors
NE
HEART
Increased Contractility
:Blocked by Propranolol

B. Activates Alpha Adrenoceptors (>10 μg/kg)

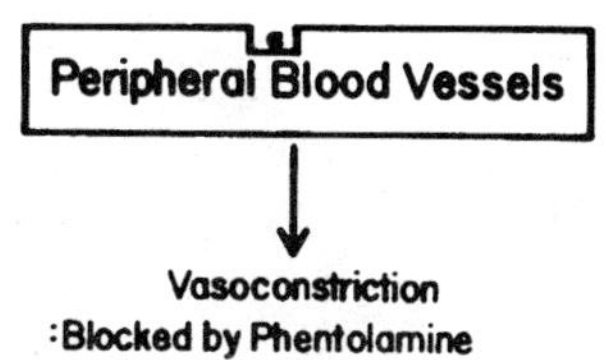

C. Activates Dopaminergic Vascular Receptors (<10 μg/kg)

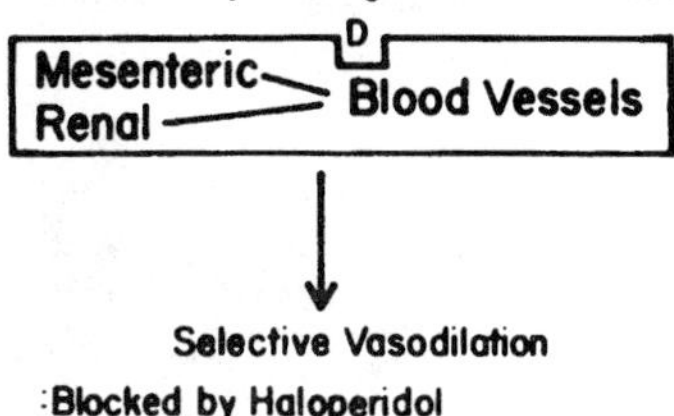

FIG. 6.5—Cardiovascular activities of dopamine. (A) Dopamine increases heart rate and myocardial contractility by directly activating β_1 adrenoceptors and releasing neuronal stores of endogenous norepinephrine (NE); these activities are blocked by the β-blocking agent propranolol. (B) Dopamine in large doses activates α adrenoceptors of blood vessels, resulting in vasoconstriction and a pressor response. This is blocked by the α-blocking agent phentolamine. (C) Dopamine in low doses can selectively dilate mesenteric and renal arterial beds (and perhaps cerebral and coronary arterial beds) by activation of dopamine-response (dopaminergic) receptors. It is not blocked by an α- or β-blocking agent but is blocked by the CNS dopamine antagonist haloperidol (Adams and Parker 1979).

beds. Dopamine activates these receptors rather selectively, whereas other catecholamines have unimportant agonist activity at these sites.

Dopamine causes decreased vascular resistance and increased blood flow to the kidneys and mesenteric circulation concurrent with myocardial stimulation. This particular aspect may be an advantage over conventional catecholamines in treatment of shock, because norepinephrine and epinephrine markedly constrict renal and mesenteric arteries as a result of α-receptor effects, and because isoproterenol has little effect on resistance in these regions owing to a relative lack of β-vascular receptors in these tissues (Adams and Parker 1979).

Selective vasodilation of renal and splanchnic beds by dopamine has prompted use of this agent in clinical cases of cardiovascular dysfunction. The optimal dose range of dopamine for selective vasodilation and cardiac stimulation in dogs is about 1-10 μg/kg/min administered by IV infusion; higher doses run the risk of α-vasoconstrictor effects owing to loss of dose-dependent dopamine receptor selectivity (Fig. 6.5). One study indicated that dopamine (about 5 μg/kg/min) was effective in terminating advanced AV heart block in 4 ill foals that were refractory to atropine (Whilton and Trim 1985).

Dopamine receptors of vascular smooth muscle are categorized as dopamine_1 (DA_1), and the inhibitory dopamine receptors of peripheral sympathetic neurons are DA_2 subtype (Goldberg and Rajfer 1985). The relevance of this nomenclature to cardiovascular therapeutics in veterinary medicine remains to be established.

Dobutamine. Dobutamine hydrochloride (Dobutrex) is a synthetic catecholamine that evokes a positive inotropic response in the heart. Importantly, dobutamine elicits this activity via an activation of β_1 receptors subserving increased myocardial contractility, with less activity at β_1 receptors subserving chronotropic effects and β_2 receptors subserving peripheral vasodilation. This compound was formulated and synthesized by Tuttle and Mills (1975) in a search for agents that would selectively increase cardiac contractility without affecting heart rate, cardiac rhythmicity, or blood pressure. The net cardiovascular response to dobutamine actually comprises different effects of its sterioisomers as well as important reflex adjustments (Swanson et al. 1985).

Potential advantages of dobutamine over conventional catecholamines relates to the relative multiplicity of actions of the latter agents. Isoproterenol, for instance, is the most powerful inotropic catecholamine presently available; however, it usually produces this effect accompanied by excessive tachycardia, which substantially increases myocardial oxygen demands. The positive inotropic activity of norepinephrine is limited by peripheral vasoconstriction and, hence, increased afterload and cardiac workload. Also, the tachyarrhythmogenic potential for isoproterenol, norepinephrine, epinephrine, and even dopamine is an important consideration. Dobutamine, because of its relative inotropic cardioselectivity, may therefore have advantages over other adrenergic amines in the therapy of low-output cardiac failure.

The hemodynamics of dobutamine were studied in dogs by Hinds and Hawthorne (1975) and Willerson et al. (1976). Dobutamine produces a dose-related increase in myocardial contractility, velocity of myocardial fiber shortening, ejection fraction, and stroke work. Importantly, these increments in cardiac contractility occur without changes in ventricular preload or heart rate when dobutamine is infused in doses of 5-20 μg/kg/min; cardiac output increases and total peripheral resistance is slightly decreased. After

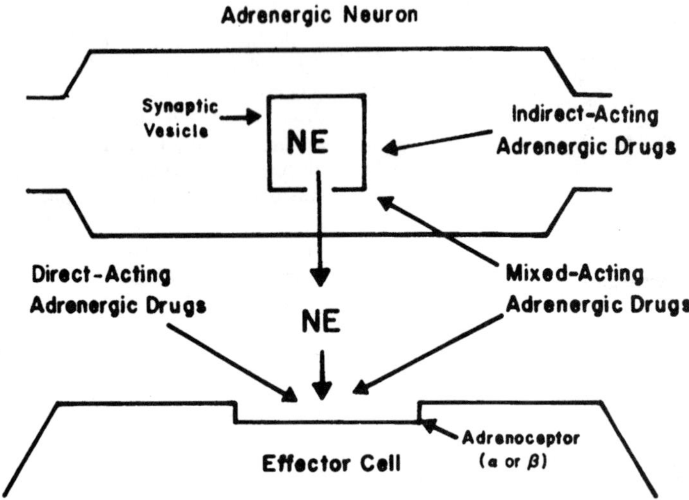

FIG. 6.6—Pathways of adrenoceptor activation by adrenergic drugs. Norepinephrine (NE) is stored in neuronal vesicles. Direct-acting adrenergic drugs activate the receptors of the effector cell; indirect-acting agents evoke release of endogenous NE. Arrows point to sites of action (Adams and Parker 1979).

cardiopulmonary bypass in dogs, mortality rate and cardiovascular function were improved by dobutamine infusion (5 μg/kg/min); an increase in automaticity or arrhythmia was not detected (Eyster et al. 1975).

In dogs anesthetized with pentobarbital, Willerson et al. (1976) found increased ST-segment elevation during infusion of dobutamine after coronary artery ligation; heart rate also increased under these conditions. Tachycardia, arrhythmia, and blood pressure changes are likely if optimal dosage levels are exceeded. More information is needed about the cardiac and hemodynamic actions of dobutamine, particularly in different species and under clinical conditions. However, dobutamine is an important adrenergic agent because of its relative inotropic cardioselectivity when the desired goal of therapy is to improve ventricular function by direct inotropic stimulation (Loeb et al. 1977).

NONCATECHOLAMINES. Although the 3,4-dihydroxybenzene structure yields maximum potency, many drugs lacking the catechol nucleus have proved to be clinically useful. As with the catecholamines, the end effects of these drugs are mediated by the adrenergic receptors of effector cells. However, the mechanism of obtaining receptor activation varies considerably from one drug to another. Surgical sympathetic denervation abolishes or markedly reduces the effects of some agents (e.g., tyramine, an experimental sympathomimetic amine) but does not reduce effects of epinephrine. Reserpine causes a functional sympathectomy by depleting adrenergic neurons of their stores of norepinephrine. Pretreatment with reserpine markedly decreases the response to tyramine but does not decrease effects of epinephrine. An α-blocking agent, however, prevents effects of tyramine, epinephrine, and norepinephrine. These findings indicate that tyramine acts presynaptically to cause a release of endogenous norepinephrine from the nerve, which in turn acts on postjunctional receptors. Based on these types of findings, adrenergic drugs can be classified into three groups: direct-acting (effects not decreased by denervation), mixed-action (effects partially reduced by denervation), and indirect-acting (effects markedly reduced by denervation) (Fig. 6.6).

Despite these complex interrelationships, the peripheral effects of adrenergic drugs can be explained by activation, whether direct or indirect, of the α and/or β receptors. Therefore, effects of these drugs can be compared with the previously discussed pharmacologic effects of the direct-acting agents norepinephrine, epinephrine, and isoproterenol.

Ephedrine. *Ephedrine,* USP, was originally isolated from the Chinese shrub *Ma huang (Ephedra)* but is now chemically synthesized. The natural product has been used in oriental medicine for centuries and was introduced into modern therapeutics during the 1920s (Chen and Schmidt 1930). The structure of ephedrine and related pharmacologic effects are shown in Table 6.1. The levo isomer is the most active form of this component. Ephedrine exerts its sympathomimetic effects by direct activation of adrenergic receptors and release of endogenous norepinephrine.

PHARMACOLOGIC EFFECTS

CARDIOVASCULAR. IV administration of ephedrine produces hemodynamic changes similar to those caused by bolus injection of epinephrine. Systolic and diastolic blood pressures increase, myocardial contractile force increases, heart rate increases if vagal reflexes are blocked, and cardiac output increases if venous return is adequate. Vasoconstriction occurs in kidney, mesenteric, and cutaneous circulations; blood flow to these regions decreases. Blood flow may increase, however, through coronary, cerebral, and skeletal muscle vascular beds. Ephedrine is many times less potent a pressor agent than epinephrine, but its effects last 7-10 times longer. Cardiovascular effects are obtained after oral administration of ephedrine, whereas epinephrine is inactive if given by mouth.

In contrast to epinephrine and norepinephrine, repeated injections of ephedrine evoke progressively smaller pressor responses in intact animals. This condition, tachyphylaxis, is probably dependent upon different factors. First, because ephedrine causes a release of endogenous amines, stores of norepinephrine may eventually be depleted, so less and less is available for release. The long duration of action of ephedrine may also contribute to development of tachyphylaxis. During long courses of cardiovascular stimulation, reflex mechanisms attempt to return hemodynamic function toward normal. Blood pressure may return to somewhat normal values, although ephedrine, because of its delayed elimination, is still present at receptor sites. Repeated injections therefore prove less effective if occupation of the receptors by prior administration of ephedrine still exists.

CENTRAL NERVOUS SYSTEM. Ephedrine is a CNS stimulant. It stimulates corticomedullary regions and, in large doses, causes excitement, apparent anxiety, and muscular tremors. Respiratory centers of the medulla oblongata are activated by appropriate doses of ephedrine. This effect has been used clinically to reverse respiratory depression, particularly if respiratory problems are associated with barbiturate overdosage. Ephedrine is infrequently used for this purpose now, since other central stimulants have proved more effective or more reliable. Other adrenergic drugs such as amphetamine stimulate the CNS to a greater extent than ephedrine.

OCULAR. Mydriasis occurs after local or systemic administration of ephedrine as a result of active stimulation of the radial muscle of the iris. A 10% solution has been used to enlarge the pupillary space to facilitate ophthalmic examination.

BRONCHIAL SMOOTH MUSCLE. Ephedrine is effective in causing relaxation of bronchial smooth muscle and increasing the diameter of bronchiolar passageways; these effects are believed to be due to direct activation of β receptors.

CLINICAL USE. *Ephedrine Hydrochloride,* USP, is used rarely in veterinary medicine. It offers no particular advantage over epinephrine except that its duration of action is longer and it is effective when given orally. Indications for use of an adrenergic drug in veterinary medicine usually require an immediate response, which can often best be obtained with injection of epinephrine.

The prolonged duration of the pressor effect of ephedrine may be of some benefit in maintaining blood pressure without having to resort to repeated injection or constant perfusion with a catecholamine. Use of 10-20 mg ephedrine administered by IV or IM injection has been advocated for pressor effects in dogs (Soma et al. 1974).

Ephedrine solution, 1-1.5%, can be applied topically onto congested mucosal membranes to evoke vasoconstriction and decongestion. Ephedrine is effective in reducing allergic responses, but the onset of action is slower than with epinephrine. Ephedrine is sometimes included in cough suppressant preparations for relief from bronchiolar congestion and vascular constriction.

Amphetamine. *Amphetamine Sulfate,* USP, or β-phenylisopropylamine, induces pronounced stimulation of the CNS as well as causing marked peripheral α and β effects. A considerable portion of the pharmacologic effects of amphetamine is due to release of endogenous norepinephrine. Cardiovascular effects of amphetamine are somewhat similar to those produced by ephedrine. An increase of systolic and diastolic blood pressures is observed. Heart rate is reflexly slowed and cardiac output is not affected to any appreciable extent. Cardiovascular effects are observed after the drug is given by the oral route. The *l*-isomer is a somewhat more active pressor agent than the *d*-isomer. The chemical structure of amphetamine is shown in Table 6.1.

Amphetamine is active if given by mouth; CNS effects persist for several hours. The entire CNS is affected, but effects on the cerebrum are most evident in humans: increased alertness, loss of fatigue, euphoria, and a sense of exhilaration. The performance of athletes is improved; this is attributed to improvement of activities requiring mental and physical coordination. After effects of amphetamine have dissipated, pronounced depression may occur. In humans amphetamine is most often used in treatment of neuropsychiatric disorders such as mild but chronic depression, narcolepsy, alcoholism, and in some cases of hyperkinesis in children.

Amphetamine is no longer available for use in veterinary medicine in the USA and is subject to strict control under the 1970 Controlled Substances Act. Prior to the strict control of amphetamine it was used in veterinary therapeutics for its stimulatory effects on the respiratory centers in the medulla oblongata. The entire cerebrospinal axis is affected, but particularly the brain stem and cortex. The *d*-isomer, dextro-amphetamine, is the most centrally active. Its analeptic potency is similar to that of pentamethylenetetrazol. Amphetamine increases both the rate and depth of inspiration in anesthetized animals. It was used intravenously (4-4.5

mg/kg) in the dog to overcome respiratory depressant effects of barbiturate overdose.

Phenylephrine. *Phenylephrine Hydrochloride,* USP (Neo-Synephrine), is similar in structure to epinephrine except that it lacks the 4-OH group on the benzene ring; the chemical structure and pharmacologic characteristics of phenylephrine are shown in Table 6.1. Phenylephrine is a direct-acting sympathomimetic amine at α_1 receptors and does not depend upon release of endogenous norepinephrine for its effects. Similar to norepinephrine, phenylephrine causes peripheral vasoconstriction by direct activation of α_1 receptors of blood vessels. However, dissimilar to norepinephrine, it has very little effect at cardiac β receptors. Systolic and diastolic blood pressures are increased by phenylephrine; reflex bradycardia usually occurs. The predictable reflex-mediated slowing of the heart rate by phenylephrine has led to use of this agent in human patients to control episodes of paroxysmal atrial tachycardia.

Phenylephrine is a less potent pressor agent than norepinephrine but has a longer duration of action. The IV dose for dogs is 0.088 mg/kg; approximately twice this amount should be given if administered by the SC or IM route.

Methoxamine and Metaraminol. The chemical structure of *Methoxamine Hydrochloride,* USP (Vasoxyl), is β-hydroxy-β-(2,5-dimethoxyphenyl)-isopropylamine. The chemical structure and related pharmacologic effects of *Metaraminol Bitartrate,* USP (Aramine), are included in Table 6.1. Like phenylephrine, these drugs act almost exclusively as direct-acting sympathomimetic amines at peripheral α receptors. They have minimal detectable myocardial stimulatory properties. Their pressor effects on systolic and diastolic blood pressures can be explained by peripheral vasoconstriction and increased peripheral resistance. Reflex bradycardia usually results. These drugs are used as pressor agents. After IV injection, the pressor response to methoxamine occurs rapidly and may persist for 1 hour. With IM administration, 15 minutes is usually required for the pressor response to take effect and it usually lasts 1-1.5 hours.

α_2-SELECTIVE AGONISTS. The CNS contains α_2 receptors on neurons involved in control of blood pressure and heart rate. CNS α_2 receptors also modulate CNS perception of pain as well as levels of sedation. Activation of CNS α_2 receptors by α_2 agonists can lower systemic blood pressure, explaining their role as antihypertensive agents in human medicine. In veterinary medicine, α_2 agonists are used for their sedative and analgesic properties, thereby gaining chemical restraint and relief from pain.

β_2-SELECTIVE BRONCHODILATORS. The β_2-agonist effects of isoproterenol have been used successfully to improve airway diameter and conductance in obstructive pulmonary disorders such as bronchitis, emphysema, and asthmatic-like syndromes. Because of equipotent β_1 activity, however, cardiac excitation and tachydysrhythmias represent limiting side effects of isoproterenol when only β_2-bronchodilator action is sought. Similar limitations apply to epinephrine, although it is still the drug of choice for treating acute anaphylaxis when a combination of β_2 bronchodilation, β_1-cardiac stimulation, and α vasoconstriction is needed. Cardiac side effects with epinephrine or isoproterenol can develop after any route of administration but are more pronounced after parenteral injection than with aerosol inhalation. For these reasons, considerable effort has been expended in the development of drugs with more selective β_2 activity and therefore less propensity for β_1-cardiac excitation.

Metaproterenol, isoetharine, terbutaline, salbutamol, pirbuterol, and clenbuterol are new drugs that meet the requirements for high β_2- and relatively less β_1-agonist activity. Indeed, these drugs are generally classified as β_2-selective bronchodilators. Most of these compounds are absorbed after oral administration and have prolonged duration of bronchodilator action, other distinct advantages over the short-lived response to isoproterenol and epinephrine.

Clenbuterol was shown to improve airway conductance in horses for several hours after a single IV injection at a dose of 0.8 μg/kg; heart rate increased dramatically but for less than 2 minutes (Shapland et al. 1981). The brief tachycardia may have been reflexly mediated due to transient β_2 vasodilation and hypotension. Unanticipated blood pressure responses may therefore represent a concern after systemic administration of β_2 bronchodilators. Blood pressure changes should be less pronounced after aerosol inhalation. However, untoward side effects, including β_1-cardiac stimulation, can be expected with any route of administration if optimal dosage ranges of the β_2 bronchodilators are exceeded.

Patients often become refractory to bronchodilator effects of adrenergic agonists during long-term therapy, and this is believed to reflect "down-regulation" or agonist-induced loss of the β_2-pulmonary receptor population. An alternative approach involves concomitant administration of a methylxanthine, such as aminophylline, along with the β_2 agonist. Methylxanthines inhibit the intracellular enzyme known as phosphodiesterase. This enzyme is responsible for the metabolism of cAMP, which is the intracellular messenger for β-receptor activation and mediates the resulting cellular reactions that culminate in bronchodilation. Because the results of β-receptor stimulation are mediated through an increase in cAMP synthesis and because methylxanthines inhibit the breakdown of cAMP and prolong its intracellular sojourn, combined therapy with a β_2 agonist and aminophylline can result in accentuated bronchodilator effects.

ANTIADRENERGIC DRUGS. Numerous agents have been discovered that prevent either the pharmacologic effects of sympathomimetic drugs, the physiologic responses evoked by stimulation of adrenergic nerves, or both. The terms adrenolytic and sympatholytic have been used to describe such activities; however, more precise terminology is presently in use. Adrenergic antagonists interact with adrenergic receptors and by occupying these sites do not allow an adrenergic agonist access to the receptor. Adrenergic neuron blocking drugs do not block receptors; instead, they act presynaptically at the nerve terminal to cause a decreased release of the endogenous neurotransmitter norepinephrine.

Adrenergic Antagonists. In 1906 Dale reported that pretreatment of cats with ergot alkaloids prevented some of the hemodynamic effects of epinephrine. These studies presented the first evidence of the drug action now commonly referred to as adrenergic blockade. Adrenergic blocking drugs exert their pharmacologic effects by interlocking with and occupying adrenergic receptors. In this manner, adrenergic agonists are prevented from affixing to the receptor site; effects of the agonist are abolished or markedly decreased.

The adrenergic blocking effects of ergot alkaloids (and some drugs like phentolamine that were subsequently synthesized) were identified as being present only at those adrenergic receptors designated by Ahlquist (1948) as α. In fact, for over 50 years the only adrenergic blocking agents identified inhibited α-receptor-mediated effects. This problem delayed full acceptance of Ahlquist's (1948) differentiation of α- and β-receptor sites. However, Powell and Slater (1958) and Moran and Perkins (1958) demonstrated that the 3,4-dichlorophenyl analog of isoproterenol selectively inhibited those responses ascribed by Ahlquist (1948) to be mediated by β receptors. This drug, dichloroisoproterenol, blocked the vasodilation, cardiac stimulation, and bronchial smooth muscle relaxing effects of catecholamines but had no effect on α-mediated effects. *Propranolol Hydrochloride,* USP (Inderal), was subsequently identified as a β-blocking agent, and it serves as the prototype for this drug group.

Pharmacologic Considerations

RECEPTOR BLOCKADE. The α- or β-inhibitory effects of representative adrenergic blocking drugs (e.g., α blockade with phentolamine and β blockade with propranolol) on the blood pressure and myocardial effects of sympathomimetic drugs are shown in Fig. 6.7. Alpha blockade abolishes the pressor response to norepinephrine. Epinephrine is a mixed α-β agonist; α blockade by phentolamine not only prevents the pressor response to epinephrine, it actually converts it to a depressor response. This is called epinephrine reversal. Since the α receptors are occupied by phentolamine, only the vasodilator β_2 receptors are available for interaction with epinephrine. Thus epinephrine causes a fall in blood pressure. Alpha blockade does not affect the β_2-receptor-mediated depressor effect of isoproterenol nor does it affect the cardiac stimulant effects of the catecholamines.

Propranolol, a nonselective β_1-β_2 blocker, inhibits the β_1-cardiac stimulant effects of isoproterenol, epinephrine, and norepinephrine (Fig. 6.7). It also blocks the β_2-depressor response to isoproterenol but does not prevent the α-receptor-mediated pressor response to norepinephrine. The secondary depressor effect of epinephrine seen in the control situation is due to residual β_2-receptor-mediated vasodilation; this too is inhibited by propranolol.

PHARMACOLOGIC EFFECTS. The degree of autonomic nervous system activity at any one time plays an important role in determining the extent of pharmacologic effects that will be produced by an adrenergic blocking agent. For example, administration of a β-blocking drug to a trained quiescent patient does not cause profound cardiovascular effects because at rest the heart is not under pronounced sympathetic influence. Upon physical exertion, however, an increase in heart rate and cardiac output is produced as a result of increased sympathetic nervous system activity. If the patient is required to exercise during treatment with propranolol, these characteristic cardiac responses are not obtained since the β-adrenergic receptors of the heart are blocked by this drug.

Effects of an α-blocking agent are similarly influenced by the existing state of autonomic nervous system activity. If the cardiovascular system is under pronounced sympathetic dominance (e.g., during fright or severe hypovolemia), an α-blocking drug will cause a decrease in blood pressure. This occurs because the α receptors of blood vessels are occupied by the α-blocking agent and are no longer available to norepinephrine or to circulating epinephrine.

Pharmacologic effects of adrenergic blocking agents can be reliably predicted by considering the distribution of α and β receptors in the body and the respective physiologic functions they subserve. Distribution of α and β receptors in various organs and tissues and their pharmacologic characteristics are summarized in Tables 5.1 and 6.3.

α-ADRENERGIC BLOCKING AGENTS

ERGOT ALKALOIDS. Ergot alkaloids are not used clinically in humans or lower animals for α-blocking effects. They affect a variety of organs at concentrations less than those required for α blockade. Therefore, they are not truly prototypical α blockers; however, they were the first adrenergic blocking agents identified (Dale 1906).

Ergot is a fungus *(Claviceps purpurea)* that parasitizes rye and other grains. Ingestion of contaminated grain products has caused outbreaks of ergotism in humans and domestic animals throughout the world. Ergot is a mixture of different types of alkaloids that

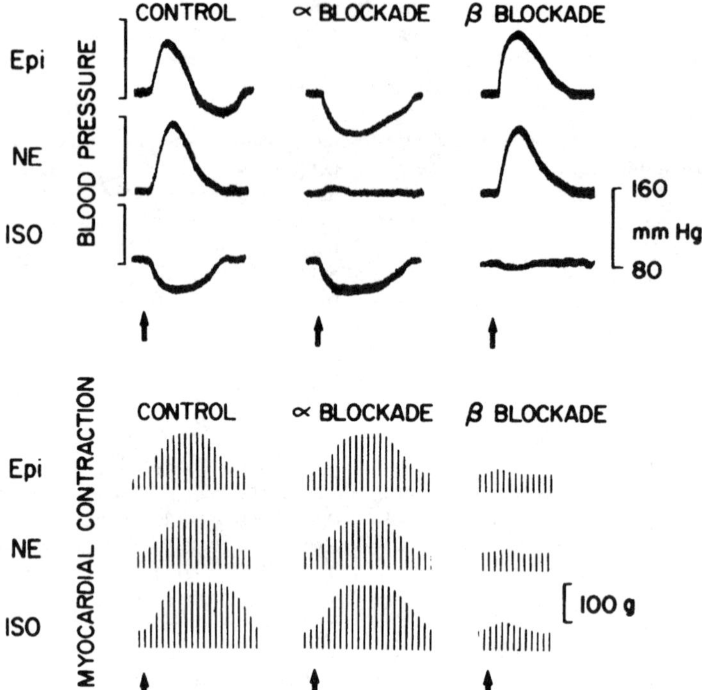

FIG. 6.7—Effects of α- and β-adrenergic blockade on the blood pressure and myocardial effects of epinephrine (Epi), norepinephrine (NE), and isoproterenol (ISO) in a dog. Control = effects of amines in the absence of an adrenergic blocking drug. α blockade = effects of amines after administration of an α blocker (e.g., phentolamine); β blockade = effects of amines after administration of a β blocker (e.g., propranolol). Epi, NE, or ISO was injected intravenously at arrow. α blockade inhibits the pressor response to NE, does not affect the depressor effect of ISO, converts the pressor effect of Epi to a depressor effect (Epi reversal), and does not affect the cardiac stimulant effects of the amines. β blockade does not affect pressor responses to NE, inhibits depressor effect of ISO, inhibits the secondary depressor effect of Epi, and inhibits myocardial stimulant effects of all three amines (see text for details).

TABLE 6.3—Classification and characteristics of catecholaminergic receptors

	Receptor types			
Characteristics	α	β_1	β_2	Dopamine
Potency of agonists	E > NE > D > I	I > E ≥ NE > D	I > E > NE > D	D > E, NE, I
Antagonists				
α blockers (PHEN)	Block	No	No	No
β blockers				
General (PROP)	No	Block	Block	No
β_1 (PRACT)	No	Block	Weak block	No
β_1 (BUT)	No	Weak block	Block	No
Dopamine antagonist (HAL)	No	No	No	Block

Note: E = epinephrine; NE = norepinephrine; D = dopamine; I = isoproterenol; PHEN = phentolamine; No = no blocking effect; PROP = propranolol; PRACT = practolol; BUT = butoxamine; HAL = haloperidol. See Table 6.4 for further breakdown of α receptors into $\alpha_1 - \alpha_2$ subtypes.

have biologic effects. The ergonovine group lacks a polypeptide side chain; it does not cause adrenergic blockade but has potent oxytocic activity. The ergotamine group causes adrenergic blockade but has little effect on nonvascular smooth muscle.

The predominant vascular effect of ergot is not α blockade but is related to intense peripheral vasoconstriction. These compounds cause a direct stimulation of smooth muscle, including that of peripheral blood vessels. Because of peripheral vasoconstriction, ergot initially causes a pressor response that may persist for a fairly long time. Larger doses eventually block the α-adrenergic receptors; α-receptor-mediated effects of norepinephrine, epinephrine, and

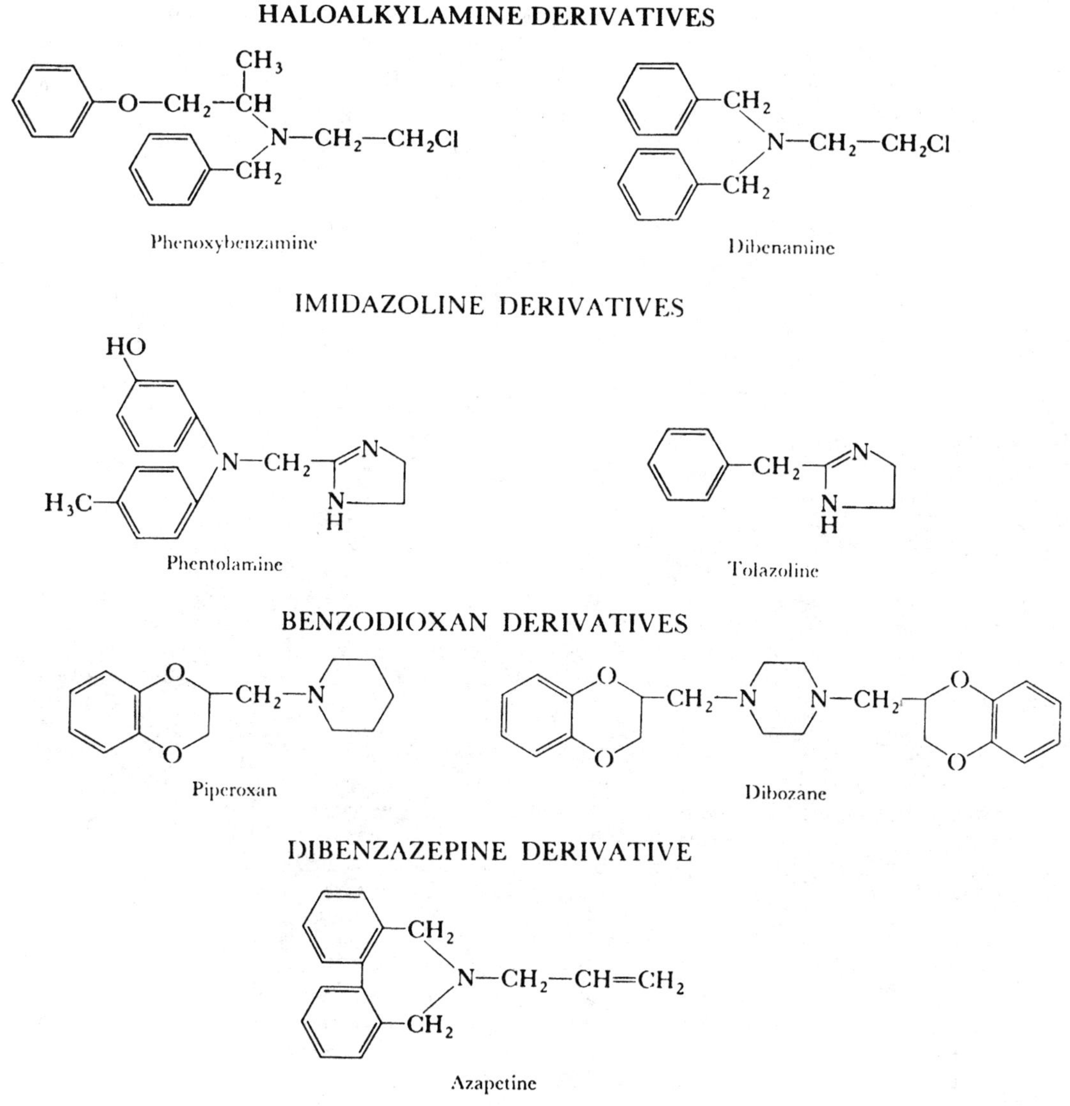

HALOALKYLAMINE DERIVATIVES

Phenoxybenzamine

Dibenamine

IMIDAZOLINE DERIVATIVES

Phentolamine

Tolazoline

BENZODIOXAN DERIVATIVES

Piperoxan

Dibozane

DIBENZAZEPINE DERIVATIVE

Azapetine

FIG. 6.8—Chemical structures of some α-adrenergic blocking drugs.

other agonists are inhibited. Beta receptors are not affected.

Because of α-blocking effects, ergot produces epinephrine reversal as previously described (Fig. 6.7). In ergot-treated animals, vasodilation and hypotension occur after administration of epinephrine (or other mixed α-β agonists) resulting from β-receptor dominance in the presence of α blockade. Although this is not the most prominent effect of ergot, it is the most interesting, since it led to identification of other, more selective α blockers. Large doses of ergot cause serious circulatory disturbances because of intense and persistent vasoconstriction of peripheral vessels. This is characterized by stasis of blood in the capillaries and arterioles, thrombosis, and eventually obliterative endarteritis, leading to gangrene of the extremities. Sloughing of portions of the feet, hooves, tails, ears, and tongues have occurred in ergot-poisoned animals.

SYNTHETIC α-BLOCKING AGENTS. The synthetic α blockers fall into several classes of structurally unrelated chemical compounds; structure-activity relationships have not been clarified. There are several groups of α blockers such as the haloalkylamine derivatives (phenoxybenzamine, dibenamine), the imidazoline derivatives (phentolamine, tolazoline), the benzodioxans (piperoxan, dibozane), and the dibenzazepine derivatives (azapetine); see Fig. 6.8 for chemical structures.

Members of the phenothiazine derivative tranquilizers also have α-adrenergic blocking properties. These drugs are discussed in detail in relation to their CNS effects in a later chapter; their peripheral vascular actions are also of interest. Chlorpromazine and several other related compounds can cause blockade of α receptors. These agents alter pressor effects of catecholamines (they can cause epinephrine reversal) but it seems likely that the total cardiovascular effects are from a variety of factors such as concomitant antihistaminic, antiserotonergic, and anticholinergic effects.

Inhibition of pressor responses to catecholamines by the other synthetic α blockers, however, can be ascribed almost entirely to α-receptor blockade. Phentolamine and phenoxybenzamine are older α-blocking drugs. Their site of action is the α receptor; β responses are not blocked. *Phenoxybenzamine Hydrochloride,* USP (Dibenzyline), and other related haloalkylamines such as dibenamine produce a noncompetitive block; increasing the dosage of an α agonist will not overcome the α blockade produced by phenoxybenzamine. This characteristic seems to be due to the drug binding in a very stable manner to the receptor or nearby structures. *Phentolamine Hydrochloride,* USP (Regitine hydrochloride), and *Tolazoline Hydrochloride,* USP (Priscoline hydrochloride), however, cause a competitive blockade of α receptors that can usually be antagonized by increasing the availability of agonist.

Cardiovascular Effects. Slow IV infusion of phenoxybenzamine or phentolamine to a normal patient usually does not cause a remarkable change in blood pressure. Usually, a slight to moderate fall in pressure occurs; however, these drugs will cause a marked hypotensive response if a patient's cardiovascular system is under pronounced sympathetic tone. This is particularly evident during hypovolemia, since in this state sympathetic discharge increases to maintain adequate blood pressure in the presence of low circulating blood volume.

If phenoxybenzamine or other potent α blockers are given by rapid IV injection, severe hypotension and other adverse cardiovascular effects are seen; however, these effects probably involve factors other than α blockade.

In humans, α blockade evokes little change in blood pressure if the patient is supine, but pronounced hypotension occurs when the patient stands. This response is called postural or orthostatic hypotension. It is due to blockade of the vascular α receptors that are normally active in the efferent limb of reflex blood pressure pathways.

Other reflex changes are also altered. Reflex hypertension caused by anoxia is prevented by α blockade, as is the pressor response to occlusion of the carotid arteries (the bilateral carotid artery occlusion reflex depends upon increased sympathetic vasoconstrictor tone and increased release of epinephrine from the adrenal gland). Because of their occupation of α receptors, α-blocking agents prevent transmission of the nerve impulse to the α receptors of blood vessel cells and also block interaction of circulating epinephrine with α receptors. In this manner, reflex pressor responses are inhibited. Alpha-blocking agents increase blood flow through capillaries and arterioles as a result of α-receptor blockade and perhaps some direct relaxing effect on vascular smooth muscle.

Positive inotropic and chronotropic effects of catecholamines in heart muscle are not prevented by phentolamine or phenoxybenzamine. However, studies have shown that drugs having α-blocking effects decrease arrhythmias caused by catecholamines (Claborn and Szabuniewicz 1973; Wiersig et al. 1974; Benfry 1993). This has been demonstrated in nonanesthetized subjects and after sensitization of the myocardium by halogenated hydrocarbon anesthetics. It is not known if this is mediated entirely by α blockade. The haloalkylamines have a slight direct depressant effect on the heart that may be involved. Also, inhibition of the pressor effects of catecholamines (known to contribute to sensitization of the myocardium to arrhythmias) may also contribute (Katz and Katz 1966).

Under certain conditions, α-blocking agents partially decrease the inotropic effects of catecholamines in isolated heart muscle. This response varies from species to species, and in some cases it is demonstrable only during abnormally low temperatures. Although heart muscle contains α_1 receptors that increase myocardial contractility, the positive inotropic and chronotropic effects of catecholamines are predominately β-receptor-mediated events.

Other Effects. Phentolamine and phenoxybenzamine cause relaxation of the nictitating membrane (3rd eyelid); contractile responses caused by stimulation of sympathetic nerves or administration of an α agonist are blocked in this structure. The ocular effects of epinephrine and norepinephrine are inhibited by α blockers, as are pilomotor effects. The GI tract is variably influenced by α blockers, caused in part by the presence of β receptors in this system that also subserve relaxation.

Pharmacokinetics. The haloalkylamines and the imidazolines are effective whether administrated by mouth or injection. However, the former group is absorbed inefficiently after oral administration; only 20-30% of the drug is absorbed in active form from the GI tract. The onset of action of phenoxybenzamine and dibenamine is prolonged even after IV administration. These drugs may be converted to active intermediates, which then exert α-blocking effects. Their local irritating properties restrict their clinical use to oral or IV administration. Effective blood levels of tolazoline may not be obtained after oral administration, since it is slowly absorbed from the GI tract and is rapidly excreted by the kidneys. Phentolamine is less than 30% as active when given by mouth as when injected. Biotransformation pathways of the α-adrenergic blocking agents have not been clarified. Several of these drugs may localize in body adipose tissue because of their relatively high fat solubility.

Clinical Use. The α-receptor blocking drugs have been used with varying degrees of success in attempts to reduce vasoconstriction in the treatment of peripheral vasospasm, hypertension, pheochromocytoma, and visceral ischemia during circulatory shock syndromes. Early members of the α-antagonist group have not achieved appreciable cardiovascular application in veterinary practice and they have proved only slightly more useful in human medicine.

Certain types or stages of shock syndromes have been reported to respond favorably to an α-blocking agent. This is believed to be due to antagonism of catecholamine-induced peripheral vasoconstriction in vital visceral regions (e.g., renal and splanchnic circulation). Phenoxybenzamine (0.44-2.2 mg/kg diluted in 500 mL isotonic saline or glucose) administered by slow IV infusion has been suggested as a treatment procedure for preventing ischemia of the microcirculation during shock in animals. If hypotension occurs upon administration of an α-blocking agent during shock, adequate fluid replacement has not been achieved. It is essential that additional administration of blood or plasma expanders be instituted prior to continuing the infusion of the α-blocking agent. Currently, α-blocking agents are used infrequently, if at all, during the management of circulatory shock.

NONSELECTIVE α_1-α_2 BLOCKERS. An important limitation to therapy with the older α blockers such as phentolamine and phenoxybenzamine is their paradoxic sympathomimetic activity, especially in the heart. Administration of α blockers can result in cardiac excitation and increased plasma concentrations of epinephrine and norepinephrine (Saeed et al. 1982). Historically, these effects were attributed to a triphasic adjustment in autonomic nerve activity instigated reflexly by the hypotensive response to inhibition of α-vasoconstrictor tone. These three phases are increased sympathetic efferent traffic over the cardioaccelerator nerves, decreased vagal impulses to the sinoatrial pacemaker, and increased sympathetic firing to the adrenal medulla. Study indicates, however, that the cardiac response to α-blocking agents is even more complex than originally surmised and involves yet a fourth pathway that incorporates the α_2-adrenergic neuronal receptors.

It is now known that phenoxybenzamine and especially phentolamine can block both α_1-and α_2-receptor subtypes (Table 6.4). Thus these drugs not only inhibit the α receptors of the vascular smooth muscle cell but can likewise block the α_2 receptors of the noradrenergic nerve endings (Fig. 6.2). Since the prejunctional α_2-receptor subtype controls the previously discussed feedback inhibition of norepinephrine and epinephrine release mechanisms, α_2 blockade would thereby free the noradrenergic neuron and adrenal chromaffin cell from a resident suppressor system (Saeed et al. 1982).

TABLE 6.4—Relative order of selectivity of several α antagonists for α_1- and α_2-adrenergic receptor subtypes

Prazosin	α_1
Trimazosin	
Corynathine	
WB 4101	
Phenoxybenzamine	
Clozapine	
Phentolamine	
Piperoxan	
Tolazoline	
Yohimbine	
Rauwolscine	α_2

Source: Adams 1984.

Note: α_1-blocking activity diminishes and α_2-blocking activity increases as the list is traversed from top to bottom. Drugs in the middle are nonselective blockers of both receptor subtypes.

An important consequence of such action would be an augmentation of the net quantity of catecholamines mobilized and released by reflex mechanisms. This sequence would not be manifested at either α_1- or α_2-vasoconstrictor receptors, owing to the original nonselective α-receptor blocking action of the drug. In the heart, however, the increased availability of catecholamines can explain the β_1-receptor stimulation and accentuated cardiac responses that can be associated with use of nonselective α antagonists.

SELECTIVE α_1 BLOCKERS. Prazosin is an α antagonist with selectivity for the α_1-receptor subtype (Table 6.4). Since it leaves the prejunctional α_2 receptors operational, prazosin should exert less reflex sympathomimetic response than would a nonselective α_1-α_2 antagonist. Confirming this theory is a study that compares the hemodynamic effects of prazosin and phentolamine in conscious dogs (Saeed et al. 1982). Both drugs induced equivalent reductions in peripheral vascular resistance and blood pressure. Phentolamine also evoked significant increases in heart rate, cardiac output, oxygen consumption, and plasma concentrations of norepinephrine and epinephrine. Prazosin did not elicit these sympathomimetic side effects despite equivalent reduction in systemic blood pressure. The differences between prazosin and phentolamine can be explained by the α_1-receptor selectivity of the former, leaving intact the α_2-autoinhibitory mechanisms for catecholamine release (Fig. 6.2).

In addition, since extrasynaptic α_2 receptors of vascular smooth muscle also remain unblocked during therapy with prazosin, these vasoconstrictor receptors are available to help maintain vasomotor tone in the resistance and capacitance beds. Thus orthostatic hypotension seems to be less of a problem with α_1-selective blockers such as prazosin than with nonselective α_1-α_2 blockers such as phentolamine.

Because of reduced frequency of reflex cardiac excitation and orthostatic hypotension, prazosin and other

α_1-selective antagonists have established an important niche in antihypertensive therapy in humans. These agents may also prove useful as peripheral vasodilators for reducing cardiac workload without reflex tachycardia in heart failure syndromes. Indeed, a study indicated that peripheral vasodilation with prazosin was effective in 4 dogs with congestive heart failure that were refractory to digoxin (Atwell 1979). However, digoxin was continued at reduced dosage in 3 of the dogs. It is unclear whether the beneficial responses in these patients were attributable to unloading of the heart by prazosin, to improvement in digoxin dosage management, or to both.

SELECTIVE α_2 BLOCKERS. Yohimbine and rauwolscine are experimental drugs that have prominent blocking actions at α_2 receptors with little or no activity at α_1 receptors. These drugs are used commonly to investigate α_2-receptor-dependent mechanisms in different tissues. Also, there is considerable interest in yohimbine as an antidote to CNS depressant drugs that have α_2-receptor agonist activity in the brain. Table 6.4 ranks the order of selectivity of several α blockers relative to their antagonistic activity at α_1- and α_2-receptor subtypes.

β-ADRENERGIC BLOCKING AGENTS. Dichloroisoproterenol was the first drug demonstrated to cause a specific blockade of β-adrenergic receptors. Because it also caused an initial stimulation of the same receptors, subsequent studies were directed to identification of other β-blocking agents that lacked agonistic properties. Propranolol is structurally related to its precursors; it is many times more potent than pronethalol and has very minimal agonistic effects. Propranolol and related β antagonists are somewhat similar in structure to the β agonist isoproterenol, as seen in Fig. 6.9. These compounds have an isopropyl-substituted secondary amine on the carbon side chain; this moiety appears to be important for effective interaction with the β receptor. The levoconfiguration of the asymmetric carbon atom on the side chain of propranolol yields the many times more potent β-blocking isomer than does the *d*-configuration.

CARDIOVASCULAR PHARMACOLOGIC EFFECTS. Propranolol causes minimal depression of heart rate, myocardial contractile force, and cardiac output during normal conditions, because at rest the heart is not under pronounced sympathetic tone. However, if the heart is functioning under sympathetic nervous system dominance (e.g., during exercise), a relative bradycardia and a rather pronounced decrease in myocardial contraction and cardiac output will be produced. This drug prevents the positive inotropic and chronotropic effects of catecholamines in the heart as a result of β_1-receptor blockade and antagonizes the arrhythmogenic actions of the catecholamines.

Under most physiologic conditions, β_2-vascular receptors participate only in a limited manner to homeostatic regulation. Thus β-blocking agents affect blood pressure primarily through their effects on cardiac output rather than by peripheral vascular effects. Vasodilation produced by isoproterenol or epinephrine is blocked by propranolol, however, and the vasoconstrictor response to epinephrine (α response) may be somewhat accentuated. The vasoconstrictor effects of norepinephrine or other α agonists are not blocked by propranolol.

Bronchiolar airways are under sympathetic dominance, resulting in an active state of relaxation of the bronchiolar smooth muscle. By blocking β_2 receptors, propranolol inhibits sympathetic bronchodilator activity and causes bronchiolar constriction. This effect is especially prominent during episodes of allergic reactions and bronchiolar asthma; nonselective β_1-β_2-blocking drugs are contraindicated in these and related conditions.

PHARMACOKINETICS. Effective blood concentrations of propranolol are obtained after oral administration,

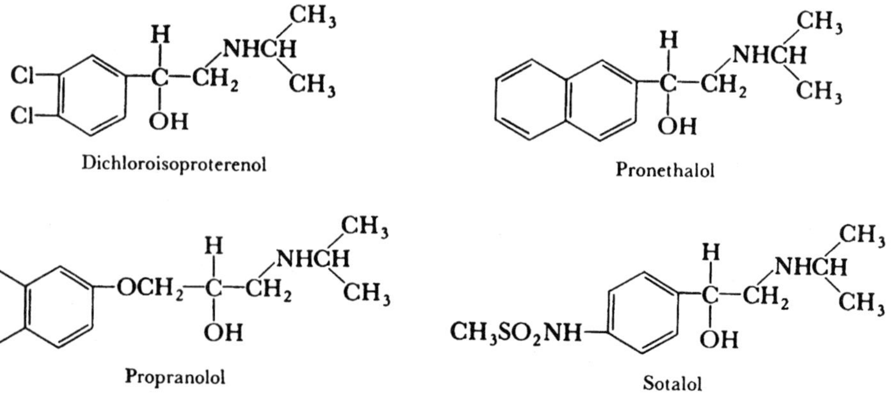

Dichloroisoproterenol

Pronethalol

Propranolol

Sotalol

FIG. 6.9—Chemical structures of some β-adrenergic blocking drugs.

but a large dose is required when given by this route. Biotransformation takes place primarily within the liver, and several active metabolites have been identified. In some species, 4-hydroxypropranolol is as active a β-adrenergic blocking agent as the parent compound. Propranolol causes a competitive blockade of β receptors. Therefore, large doses of β agonists can overcome the β-blocking effects of this drug. Pharmacokinetic features of propranolol and other β blockers were reviewed by Muir and Sams (1984).

CLINICAL USE. In human medicine, the β-receptor antagonists are used rather extensively to help manage several important medical problems, including hypertension, angina, cardiac dysrhythmias, hypertrophic obstructive cardiomyopathies, hyperthyroidism, anxiety-related muscle tremors, glaucoma, and myocardial reinfarction. The β blockers are utilized considerably less in veterinary practice but have application for controlling cardiac dysrhythmias provoked by overactivity of the sympathetic nervous system. Controlled clinical trials are generally lacking; however, β blockers also have potential benefit in domestic animals for reducing cardiac work effort in obstructive cardiomyopathies and perhaps for lowering myocardial oxygen demand in chronic heart failure syndrome. By blocking the β_1 receptors of the heart, the drugs decrease the inotropic, chronotropic, and arrhythmogenic effects of the endogenous catecholamines and other β-adrenergic agonists.

Wiersig et al. (1974) reported that 1 mg/kg racemic propranolol administered intravenously to dogs markedly decreased the incidence of ventricular fibrillation induced by epinephrine and norepinephrine during halothane and thiobarbiturate anesthesia. In this respect, propranolol was more effective than chlorpromazine or acepromazine. Adrenergic antagonists should be infused very slowly when given by the IV route, since cardiovascular depression may occur if they are administered by bolus IV injection.

Beta-blocking drugs are frequently effective in decreasing AV conduction and thereby controlling ventricular rate in patients with atrial fibrillation or flutter. Propranolol has been shown to be effective in controlling atrial and ventricular arrhythmias induced by digitalis excess and in treating paroxysmal arrhythmias that prove resistant to digitalis and quinidine. In dogs, slow IV infusion of propranolol (1-3 mg) has been proposed for treatment of digitalis-induced supraventricular tachycardia, idiopathic sinus tachycardia, and supraventricular tachycardia. The oral dose is 10-40 mg every 8 hours.

β_1-SELECTIVE ANTAGONISTS. The preceding clinical uses of β antagonists depend on their block of the β_1-receptor subtype. Thus a drug with selective β_1-blocking action would have therapeutic capabilities equivalent to propranolol or other nonselective β_1-β_2 antagonists, but with reduced risk for loss of important β_2-receptor events as unwanted side effects. Propranolol and other β_1-β_2 blockers, e.g., are potentially harmful in certain patient populations owing to β_2-receptor inhibition in lung airways, leading to bronchoconstriction; in vascular smooth muscle, leading to changes in blood pressure and distribution of cardiac output; and in hepatocytes, leading to disruption of glucose metabolism. The latter condition is especially important in insulin-dependent diabetics, while loss of bronchodilator tone obviously is critical in patients with reduced respiratory reserve.

Some of the newly discovered β antagonists were found to be relatively more selective for the β_1- than for the β_2-receptor subtype. Metoprolol is protypical for this group. These drugs are commonly referred to as cardioselective β blockers because the mainstay of their clinical uses pertains to antagonism of the cardiac β_1 receptors. Some β blockers and associated affinities for receptor subtypes are included in Table 6.5, along with approximate biologic half-life values. Some of these compounds are lipophilic and undergo rather rapid biotransformation by liver enzymes, while others are lipophobic and depend upon renal excretory mechanisms for a longer half-life (Muir and Sams 1984).

β BLOCKERS AND REDUCED CARDIAC RESERVES. It should be remembered that β-blocking drugs, whether of the β_1-selective or β_1-β_2-nonselective group, should be administered cautiously in patients with preexisting heart disease. Under such conditions, cardiac performance may well depend on increased dominance of sympathetic activity as part of the compensatory attempt to maintain hemodynamics. Blockade of sympathetic input to the β_1 receptors of the heart, especially if sudden, can precipitate cardiac decompensation and failure. As a good example, Kittleson and Hamlin (1981) reported that propranolol caused cardiac decompensation in a dog with congestive heart failure that had been responding favorably to a vasodilator (hydralazine). If β blockade is attempted in the setting of reduced myocardial contractile reserves, it should be implemented cautiously with strict scrutiny of the patient's hemodynamic status.

INTRINSIC SYMPATHOMIMETIC ACTIVITY. An interesting facet of the pharmacodynamic profile of certain β blockers is their intrinsic sympathomimetic activity (ISA) (Table 6.5). This means that these agents exert partial agonist effects; hence, they maintain a slight basal stimulation of the β receptors while also preventing further receptor activation through their primary antagonistic action. An advantage of ISA might be that basal tone to the cardiac β_1 receptors and pulmonary β_2 receptors may forestall cardiac depression and bronchoconstriction respectively. Another advantage of low-grade β-receptor stimulation might be a reduced tendency for the up-regulation of β-receptor numbers that can follow long-term therapy with β antagonists. Administration of any of the β blockers should be discontinued gradually after chronic treatment to prevent supersensitivity to agonists secondary to the receptor

TABLE 6.5—Pharmacodynamic characteristics and empiric dosage schedules for several β-adrenergic-blocking drugs

Drug	β_1-Receptor block	β_2-Receptor block	ISA*	Half-life† (hr)	Oral dose (mg, TID)	IV dose‡ (mg)
Propranolol	Yes	Yes	No	1–2	5–40	1–5
Timolol	Yes	Yes	No	1–2	0.5–1	0.4–1
Nadolol	Yes	Yes	No	3–8	5–40	. . .
Oxprenolol	Yes	Yes	Yes	≈2	5–40	1–12
Alprenolol	Yes	Yes	Yes	≈2	20–80	5–10
Pindolol	Yes	Yes	Yes	2–4	1–4	0.4–2
Metoprolol	Yes	No§	No	1–2	5–40	. . .
Atenolol	Yes	No§	No	3–6	20–80	. . .
Practolol	Yes	No§	Yes	No longer used	. . .	. . .

Sources: Adams 1984; Muir and Sams 1984.

Note: The biologic half-life values and dosage ranges for all β-blocking drugs have not been determined for domestic animals under clinical conditions. This table represents an empiric extrapolation based on data from either experimental studies in dogs or clinical studies in humans. Dosage schedules should be considered only as fundamental guidelines, and actual therapy should be implemented with lower dosages while patient response is closely monitored.

*ISA = intrinsic sympathomimetic activity.

†Biologic half-life values vary considerably, and variations among patients regarding therapeutically effective plasma concentrations reach 4- to 20-fold.

‡Intravenous therapy with β blockers to control cardiac dysrhythmias should be done slowly and cautiously with dilute solutions while the electrocardiogram is monitored.

§β_1 selectivity is lost with higher dosages.

"up-regulation" or antagonist-induced receptor sensitivity phenomenon.

In human medicine, many questions remain about the clinical relevance of ISA, receptor up-regulation, and even cardioselective blocking profiles with the β-receptor antagonists. Even less is known about the practical relevance of these aspects in veterinary medicine. Until more data are available, metoprolol or other β_1-selective antagonists should be considered when β-blocking effects are deemed necessary in patients with preexisting pulmonary disease or diabetic-related disorders.

Adrenergic Neuron-Blocking Drugs and Catecholamine-Depleting Agents. These drugs act presynaptically at the adrenergic nerve terminal and prevent release of norepinephrine; they do not block the postsynaptic adrenergic receptor. Therefore, responses to direct-acting sympathomimetic amines are not prevented. However, effects of indirect-acting sympathomimetic amines (agents that cause release of endogenous norepinephrine) are attenuated by neuron-blocking and amine-depleting drugs, since the latter agents affect neuronal mechanisms that are active in the norepinephrine release process. For example, reserpine is a catecholamine-depleting agent that causes a severe reduction of the neuronal stores of norepinephrine. Therefore, less is available for release by an indirect-acting amine such as tyramine. Pressor effects of tyramine are thereby attenuated. Adrenergic neuron-blocking and amine-depleting drugs have not been used in clinical veterinary medicine to any appreciable extent.

Reserpine has been used for treating hypertension and psychic disorders in humans and is extensively used in research as a pharmacologic tool to deplete endogenous catecholamines from peripheral and CNS adrenergic pathways. Chronic daily treatment of dogs with reserpine (approximately 26 μg/kg, administered orally) induces a marked decrease in the concentration of norepinephrine in the hypothalamus, pons-medulla oblongata, and heart (Adams et al. 1971, 1972). Pronounced disturbances in peripheral and central sympathetic functions occur, and myocardial damage has been suspected. The mechanism of action of reserpine is related to an impairment of the Mg^{++}- and ATP-dependent capacity of intraneuronal vesicles to accumulate and store catecholamines. After treatment with reserpine, amines are released from granular storage sites into the neuronal cytoplasm, where they are metabolized by MAO (Shore 1972).

Guanethidine is another agent that depletes catecholamines from adrenergic nerves. However, responses to adrenergic nerve stimulation are inhibited by guanethidine before detectable amine depletion occurs. A local anesthetic-like effect at the adrenergic nerve terminal is thought to be involved. Guanethidine does not effectively pass the blood-brain barrier and has relatively less effect on central adrenergic pathways than reserpine. Guanethidine is used in antihypertensive therapy in humans; propranolol is sometimes given concurrently to block the reflex tachycardia resulting from guanethidine-induced hypotension.

Bretylium is an adrenergic neuron-blocking drug originally used in attempts to control hypertension. Side effects such as postural hypotension precluded the extensive use of this drug in clinical situations. Bretylium is often used in research to prevent the release of norepinephrine from adrenergic nerves. This drug does not deplete adrenergic neurons of their catecholamine stores; in this respect, it is dissimilar to reserpine and guanethidine. Bretylium seems to exert a local anesthetic-like effect at the adrenergic nerve terminal and, by this mechanism, decreases the amount of norepinephrine discharged from the nerve. Interestingly, because of its direct prolonging effect on refractoriness of ventricular tissue, bretylium has been approved for control of certain types of cardiac arrhythmias.

Miscellaneous Agents. A chemical sympathectomy is produced by 6-hydroxydopamine. This compound is taken up into adrenergic nerves and causes anatomic destruction of the nerve terminal. Several weeks are required for regeneration of these structures after treatment with 6-hydroxydopamine.

α-Methyldopa is taken up into the adrenergic nerves, where it is biotransformed by the catecholamine-synthesizing enzymes into α-methylnorepinephrine, which is then stored in the amine granules. The α-methyl group protects this compound from oxidation by MAO. Therefore, endogenous norepinephrine may be displaced from the granule, metabolized by MAO, and replaced by α-methylnorepinephrine. The α-methylnorepinephrine is a potent α_2 agonist, thereby decreasing sympathetic efferent outflow from the CNS.

α-Methyl-para-tyrosine inhibits tyrosine hydroxylase, the rate-limiting enzyme in the synthesis of norepinephrine. Norepinephrine stores are not replenished, and depletion of this amine occurs after cessation of synthesis.

MAO inhibitors are used in humans as mood elevators or antidepressants. These drugs interfere with the oxidative deamination of catecholamines; these amines accumulate in the neuron after treatment with a MAO inhibitor. Responses to peripheral nerve stimulation do not seem to be markedly augmented by MAO inhibitors; however, effects of indirect-acting sympathomimetic amines are markedly potentiated by pretreatment with them. This is due partly to the increased concentration of amine that is available for release by the indirect-acting agent. Hypertensive crises and cerebral vascular accidents have occurred in human patients who ingested tyramine-containing foods (e.g., cheese, wine) while they were taking MAO inhibitors.

Cocaine inhibits the neuronal amine uptake pump of adrenergic nerves. This pump functions to take norepinephrine back up into the nerve. Other amines (e.g., tyramine) gain access into the neuron by this uptake mechanism. Thus cocaine potentiates the effect of norepinephrine but blocks the effect of tyramine. Imipramine and desmethylimipramine are tricyclic antidepressants; they, too, block the neuronal amine uptake mechanism.

REFERENCES

Adams, H. R. 1981. Cardiovascular emergencies: drugs and resuscitative principles. Vet Clin North Am 11:77-102.

———. 1984. New perspectives in cardiopulmonary therapeutics: Receptor-selective adrenergic drugs. J Am Vet Med Assoc 185(9):966-74.

Adams, H. R., Dixit, B. N., Smookler, H. H., Buckley, J. P. 1972. Clinical and biochemical effects of chronic reserpine administration in mongrel dogs. Am J Vet Res 33(4):699-707.

Adams, H. R., Parker, J. L. 1979. Pharmacologic management of circulatory shock: cardiovascular drugs and corticosteroids. J Am Vet Med Assoc 175:86-92.

Adams, H. R., Smookler, H. H., Clarke, D. E., Jandhyala, B. S., Dixit, B. N., Ertel, R. J., Buckley, J. P. 1971. Clinicopathologic effects of chronic reserpine administration in mongrel dogs. J Pharm Sci 60(8):1134-38.

Ahlquist, R. P. 1948. A study of the adrenotropic receptors. Am J Physiol 153:586-600.

Alberts, P. 1993. Subtype classification of presynaptic α_2-adrenoceptors. Gen Pharmac 24:1-8.

Änggard, E. 1994. Nitric oxide: mediator, murderer, and medicine. The Lancet, 343:1199-1206.

Atwell, R. B. 1979. The use of alpha blockade in the treatment of congestive heart failure associated with dirofilariasis and mitral valvular incompetence. Vet Rec 104:114-16.

Barnes, P. J. 1993. β-Adrenoceptors on smooth muscle, nerves and inflammatory cells. Life Sci 52:2101-9.

Benfry, B. G. 1993. Antifibrillatory effects of α_1-adrenoceptor blocking drugs in experimental coronary artery occlusion and reperfusion. Can J Physiol Pharmacol 71:103-11.

Brodde, O. E., Michel, M. C. 1992. Adrenergic receptors and their signal transduction mechanisms in hypertension. J Hypertens 10(Suppl 7):S133-S145.

Buchanan, J. W., Dear, M. G., Pyle, R. L., et al. 1968. Medical and pacemaker therapy of complete heart block and congestive heart failure in a dog. J Am Vet Med Assoc 152:1099-109.

Caccavelli, L., Cussac, D., Pellegrini, I., Audinot, V., Jaquet, P., Enjalbert, A. 1992. D_2 dopaminergic receptors: normal and abnormal transduction mechanisms. Horm Res 38:78-83.

Chen, K. K., Schmidt, C. F. 1930. Ephedrine and related substances. Medicine 9:1-117.

Claborn, L. D., Szabuniewicz, M. 1973. Prevention of chloroform and thiobarbiturate cardiac sensitization to catecholamines in dogs. Am J Vet Res 34:801-4.

Cornish, E. J., Miller, R. C. 1975. Comparison of the beta-adrenoceptors in the myocardium and coronary vasculature of the kitten heart. J Pharm Pharmacol 27:23-30.

Dale, H. H. 1906. On some physiological actions of ergot. J Physiol (Lond) 34:163-206.

Ettinger, S. 1969. Isoproterenol treatment of atrioventricular block in the dog. J Am Vet Med Assoc 154:398-405.

Eyster, G. E., Anderson, L. K., Bender, G., et al. 1975. Effect of dobutamine in postperfusion cardiac failure in the dog. Am J Vet Res 13:1285-89.

Feldman, A. M. 1993. Modulation of adrenergic receptors and G-transduction proteins in failing human ventricular myocardium. Circulation 87(Suppl IV):IV27-IV34.

Goldberg, L. I., Rajfer, S. I. 1985. Dopamine receptors: Applications in clinical cardiology. Circulation 72:245-48.

Hinds, J. E., Hawthorne, E. W. 1975. Comparative cardiac dynamic effects of dobutamine and isoproterenol in conscious instrumented dogs. Am J Cardiol 36:894-901.

Katz, R. L., Katz, G. J. 1966. Surgical infiltration of pressor drugs and their interaction with volatile anaesthetics. Br J Anaesth 38:712-18.

Kittleson, M. D., Hamlin, R. L. 1981. Hydralazine therapy for severe mitral regurgitation in a dog. J Am Vet Med Assoc 179:903-4.

Lands, A. M., Arnold, A., McAuliff, J. P., Luduena, F. P., Brown, T. G., Jr. 1967. Differentiation of receptor systems activated by sympathomimetic amines. Nature 214(88):597-98.

Langer, G. A. 1974. Calcium in mammalian myocardium: localization, control, and the effects of digitalis. Circ Res 35(Suppl 3):91-98.

Langer, S. Z. 1980. Presynaptic regulation of the release of catecholamines. Pharm Rev 32(4):337-62.

Levitzki, A., Marbach, I., Bar-Sani, A. 1993. The signal transduction between β-receptors and adenylyl cyclase. Life Sci 52:2093-2100.

Loeb, H. S., Bredakis, J., Gunner, R. M. 1977. Superiority of dobutamine over dopamine for augmentation of cardiac output in patients with chronic low output cardiac failure. Circulation 55:375-78.

Lowenstein, C. J., Dinerman, J. L., Snyder, S. H. 1994. Nitric oxide: a physiologic messenger. Ann Intern Med 120:227-37.

Moran, N. C., Perkins, M. E. 1958. Adrenergic blockade of the mammalian heart by a dichloro analogue of isoproterenol. J Pharmacol Exp Ther 124:223-37.

Moreland, R. S., Bohr, D. F. 1984. Adrenergic control of coronary arteries. Fed Proc 43:2857-61.

Muir, W. W., Sams, R. S. 1984. Clinical pharmacodynamics and pharmacokinetics of beta-adrenoceptor blocking drugs in veterinary medicine. Comp Cont Ed Prac Vet 6:156-67.

Parker, J. L., Adams, H. R. 1977. Drugs and the heart muscle. J Am Vet Med Assoc 171:78-84.

Powell, C. E., Slater, I. H. 1958. Blocking of inhibitory adrenergic receptors by a dichloro analog of isoproterenol. J Pharmacol Exp Ther 122:480-88.

Saeed, M., Sommer, O., Holtz, J., et al. 1982. Alpha-adrenoceptor blockade by phentolamine causes beta-adrenergic vasodilation by increased catecholamine release due to pre-synaptic alpha-blockade. J Cardiovasc Pharmacol 4:44-52.

Schwinn, D. A. 1993. Adrenoceptors as models for G protein-coupled receptors: structure, function and regulation. Br J Anaesthesia 71:77-85.

Setler, P. E., Pendleton, R. G., Finlay, E. 1975. The cardiovascular actions of dopamine and the effects of central and peripheral catecholaminergic receptor blocking drugs. J Pharmacol Exp Ther 192:702-12.

Shapland, J. E., Garner, H. E., Hatfield, D. G. 1981. Cardiopulmonary effects of clenbuterol in the horse. J Vet Pharmacol Ther 4:43-50.

Shore, P. A. 1972. Transport and storage of biogenic amines. Annu Rev Pharmacol 12:209-26.

Soma, L. R., Burrows, C. F., Marshall, B. E. 1974. In R. W. Kirk, ed., Current Veterinary Therapy, V: Small Animal Practice, p. 26. Philadelphia: W. B. Saunders.

Swanson, C. R., Muir, W. W., Bednarski, R. M., et al. 1985. Hemodynamic responses in halothane-anesthetized horses given infusions of dopamine or dobutamine. Am J Vet Res 46:365-70.

Tuttle, R. R., Mills, J. 1975. Dobutamine: development of a new catecholamine to selectively increase cardiac contractility. Circ Res 36:185-96.

Watanabe, A. M., Besch, H. R., Jr. 1974. Cyclic adenosine monophosphate modulation of slow calcium influx channels in guinea pig hearts. Circ Res 35:316-24.

Whilton, D. L., Trim, C. M. 1985. Use of dopamine hydrochloride during general anesthesia in the treatment of advanced atrioventricular heart block in four foals. J Am Vet Med Assoc 187:1357-61.

Wiersig, D. O., Davis, R. H., Jr., Szabuniewicz, M. 1974. Prevention of induced ventricular fibrillation in dogs anesthetized with ultrashort acting barbiturates and halothane. J Am Vet Med Assoc 165:341-45.

Willerson, J. T., Hutton, I., Watson, J. T., et al. 1976. Influence of dobutamine on regional myocardial blood flow and ventricular performance during acute and chronic myocardial ischemia in dogs. Circulation 53:828-33.

7 CHOLINERGIC PHARMACOLOGY: AUTONOMIC DRUGS

H. RICHARD ADAMS

Parasympathomimetic Agents
Direct-Acting Parasympathomimetic Agents
  Choline Esters
  Naturally Occurring Cholinomimetic Alkaloids
Cholinesterase Inhibitors
  Pharmacologic Considerations
  Reversible Inhibitors
  Organophosphorus Compounds
Parasympatholytic Agents
  Atropine and Scopolamine
  Synthetic Muscarinic Blocking Agents
Autonomic Ganglionic Blocking Drugs
  Mechanisms
  Nicotine
  Synthetic Ganglionic Blocking Agents

Acetylcholine (ACh) acts as the messenger between nerve endings and innervated cells of autonomic ganglia, parasympathetic neuroeffector junctions, some sympathetic neuroeffector junctions, somatic neuromuscular junctions, the adrenal medulla, and certain regions of the central nervous system (CNS). It has been recognized for many years that considerable therapeutic benefit could be derived from drugs that would selectively mimic the action of ACh only at certain of these sites or, alternatively, that could selectively prevent only unwanted effects of this biogenic substance. Although ideal drugs have yet to be identified, some agents have been found to be relatively more active at certain cholinergic sites than at others. In this chapter, drugs that influence postganglionic parasympathetic neuroeffector junctions and autonomic ganglia by ACh-like or ACh blocking effects will be examined. Parasympathetic neurons and affiliated receptors of innervated cells are depicted in Fig. 7.1.

PARASYMPATHOMIMETIC AGENTS. "Cholinergic" is used to describe an ACh-like effect without distinction as to anatomic site of action. "Parasympathomimetic" is used specifically to describe an ACh-like effect on effector cells innervated by postganglionic neurons of the parasympathetic nervous system (Fig. 7.1). Most of the cholinergic drugs considered here are used clinically for their parasympathomimetic activities. However, the scope of pharmacologic activity of several of these compounds is not restricted to parasympathomimetic effects but includes cholinergic actions throughout the body.

Based on mechanism of action, drugs that cause parasympathomimetic effects can be divided into two major groups: direct-acting agents, which like ACh activate cholinergic receptors of the effector cells, and cholinesterase inhibitors, which allow endogenous ACh to accumulate and thereby intensify and prolong its action.

DIRECT-ACTING PARASYMPATHOMIMETIC AGENTS. Direct-acting parasympathomimetic agents consist of esters of choline and naturally occurring cholinomimetic alkaloids.

Choline Esters. Choline, a member of the B vitamin group, possesses the characteristic depressor action of a cholinergic drug when injected intravenously in large unphysiologic amounts; however, its potency is multiplied thousands of times when it is esterified with acetic acid to yield ACh.

ACh, although essential for maintenance of body homeostasis, is not used therapeutically for two important reasons. First, it acts simultaneously at various tissue sites and no selective therapeutic response can be achieved. Second, its duration of action is quite brief because it is rapidly inactivated by the cholinesterases. Several derivatives of ACh are more resistant to hydrolysis by cholinesterase and have a somewhat greater selectivity in their sites of action. Of several hundred choline derivatives that have been synthesized, carbachol, bethanechol, and methacholine have proved effective for certain clinical uses and will be discussed here.

MECHANISM OF ACTION. Pharmacologic effects of ACh and related choline esters are mediated by activation of specific ACh-responsive sites (i.e., cholinergic receptors or cholinoceptors) located on cells innervated by cholinergic nerves and, in some cases, on cells that lack cholinergic innervation. Choline esters act directly on postsynaptic receptors and do not depend upon endogenous ACh for their effects. Based on differential responsiveness to cholinergic agonists and antagonists, two basic types of cholinoceptors have been identified

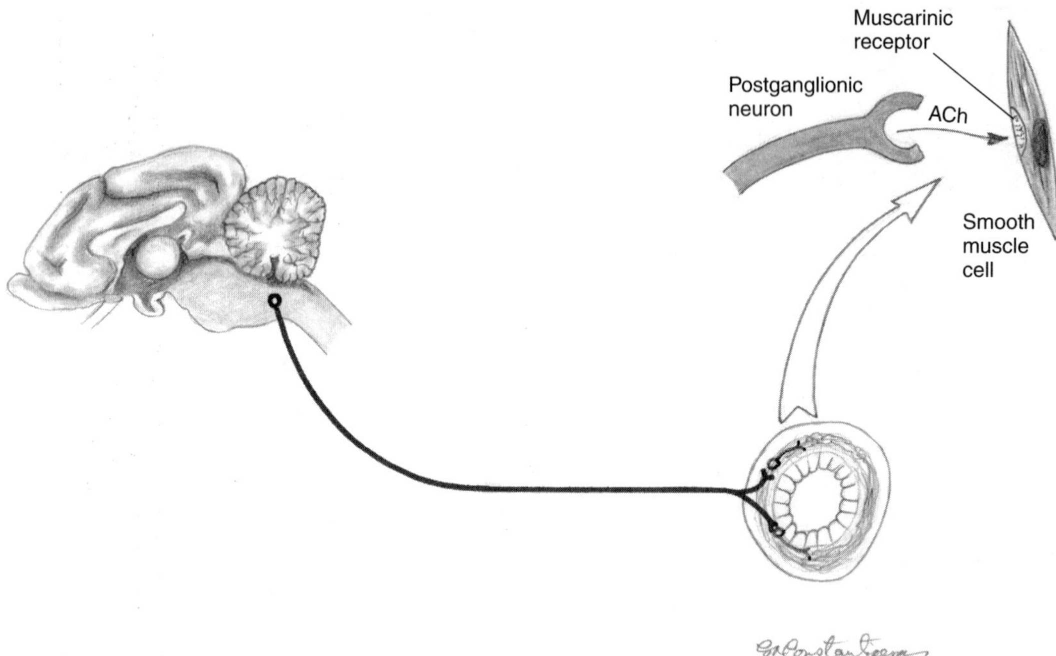

FIG. 7.1.—Anatomical relationships of parasympathetic neuronal outflow tracts and affiliated receptors of innervated cells. Parasympathetic preganglionic axons exit cranial (shown) or sacral zones and pass peripherally to synapse with a neuron body located within (shown) or adjacent to innervated tissue. The preganglionic neuron releases the neurotransmitter acetylcholine (ACh), which activates nicotinic cholinergic receptors on the ganglionic neuron body. The resulting stimulation of the ganglionic neuron promotes release of ACh from the axon terminal at postganglionic parasympathetic neuroeffector junctions within the intestinal tract (shown) or other tissues innervated by parasympathetic neurons. ACh activates muscarinic cholinergic receptors present on cells innervated by the parasympathetic division of the autonomic nervous system. Preganglionic fibers are red; postganglionic fibers are blue. Drawn by Dr. Gheorghe M. Constantinescu, University of Missouri. (*See also color plates following p. 118.*)

within the peripheral efferent pathways of the mammalian autonomic nervous system (Fig. 7.1).

NICOTINIC RECEPTORS. Beginning with the early studies by Dale (1914), it was known that nicotine in small doses mimics certain actions of ACh and in larger doses blocks these same cholinergic effects. As summarized in Chap. 5, nicotinic responsive sites are present in autonomic ganglia, adrenal medullary chromaffin cells, and neuromuscular junctions of the somatic nervous system. Accordingly, receptors at these sites are called nicotinic cholinergic receptors, and effects of cholinergic drugs at these sites are described as nicotinic effects. Nicotinic receptors at ganglia are different subtypes from those localized to voluntary skeletal muscle.

MUSCARINIC RECEPTORS. Nicotine does not mimic ACh at postganglionic parasympathetic neuroeffector junctions, i.e., parasympathetic innervation to heart muscle, smooth muscle, and exocrine glands. The mushroom alkaloid muscarine was found to selectively mimic activity of ACh at these sites, but not at the previously mentioned nicotinic receptors. Muscarinic receptors, therefore, designate the type of cholinoceptors present at postganglionic parasympathetic neuroeffector junctions (Fig. 7.1). Muscarinic receptors are also present in some blood vessels that lack cholinergic innervation and at neuroeffector junctions of the sympathetic nervous system that are cholinergic (see Chap. 5). The parasympathomimetic, or muscarinic, effects produced by drugs examined in this chapter are equivalent to the physiologic changes evoked by postganglionic parasympathetic nerve impulses, as listed in Table 5.1.

Atropine is a cholinergic blocking agent that selectively blocks muscarine receptors without blocking nicotinic sites; whereas hexamethonium, *d*-tubocurarine, and large doses of nicotine block nicotinic but not muscarinic receptors.

ACh evokes an excitatory response in some tissues, e.g., smooth muscle of the gastrointestinal (GI) tract, but causes inhibitory responses in other tissues, e.g., myocardium. In general, excitatory effects of ACh are due to depolarization of the postsynaptic membrane characterized by an increase in permeability of the membrane to both Na^+ and K^+ ions. Inhibitory effects have been associated with an inhibitory G protein (i.e.,

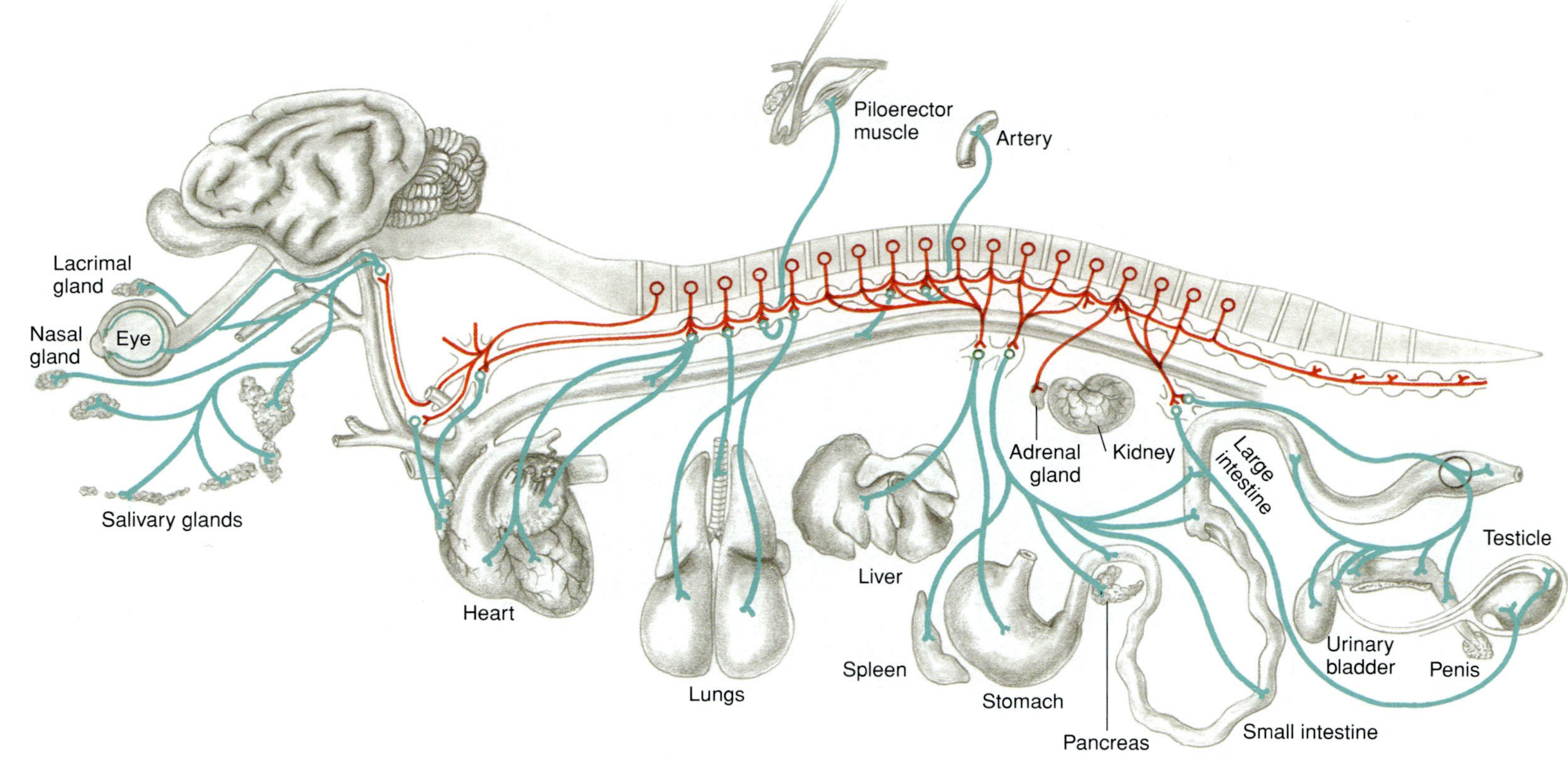

FIG. 5.1.—Anatomical representation of motor innervation from the sympathetic nervous system to various body organs and tissues. Preganglionic sympathetic neuron bodies within the thoracolumbar region of the spinal cord send axons peripherally to synapse with ganglionic neuron bodies comprising the sympathetic ganglionic chains located along each side of the vertebral column. Postganglionic axons exit the sympathetic ganglionic chains and pass peripherally to innervate those cells regulated by the sympathetic (thoracolumbar) division of the autonomic nervous system. Preganglionic fibers are red; postganglionic fibers are blue. Drawn by Dr. Gheorghe M. Constantinescu, University of Missouri.

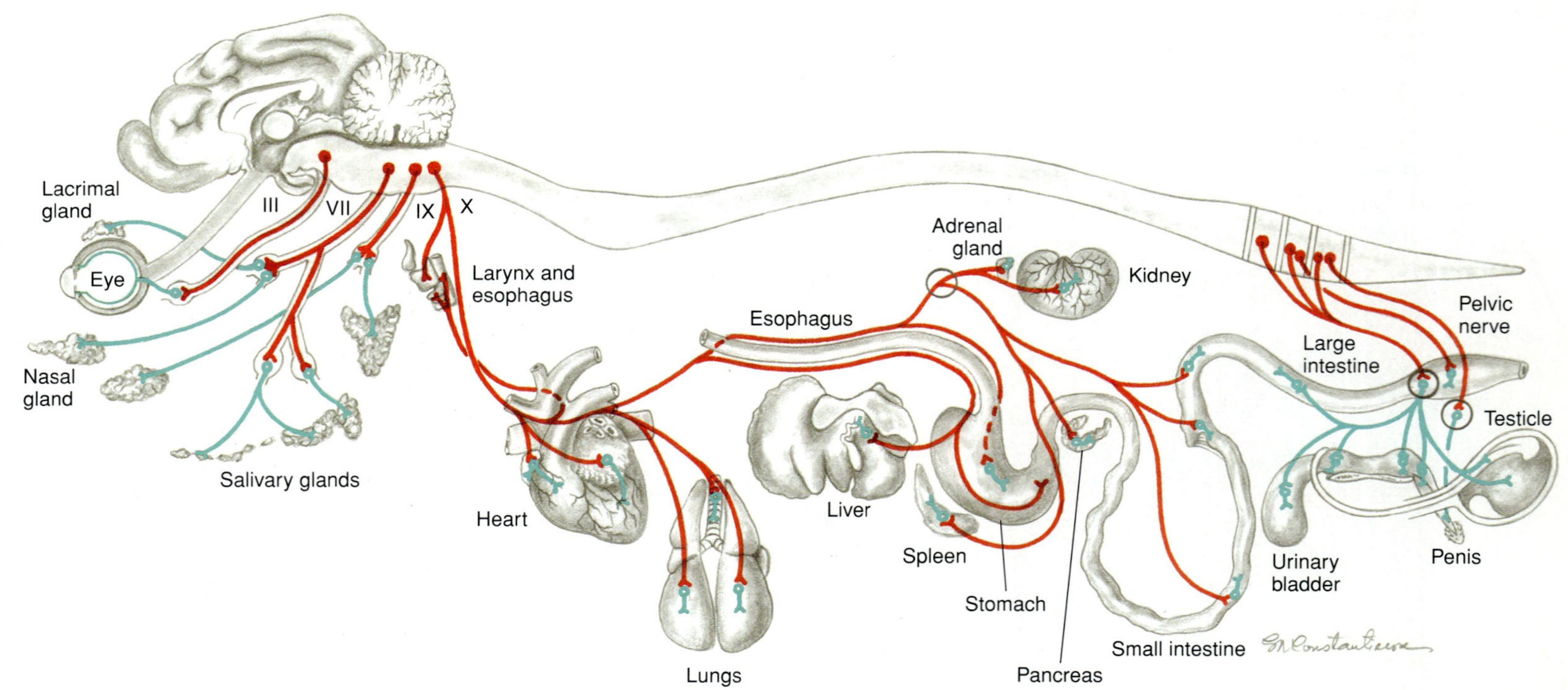

FIG. 5.2.—Anatomical representation of motor innervation from the parasympathetic nervous system to various body organs and tissues. Preganglionic parasympathetic neuron bodies within cranial and sacral zones of the central nervous system send axons peripherally to synapse with ganglionic neuron bodies localized within or adjacent to visceral tissues. Postganglionic axons exit parasympathetic ganglia and innervate those cells regulated by the parasympathetic (craniosacral) division of the autonomic nervous system. Roman numerals depict cranial nerves carrying parasympathetic neurons. Preganglionic fibers are red; postganglionic fibers are blue. Drawn by Dr. Gheorghe M. Constantinescu, University of Missouri.

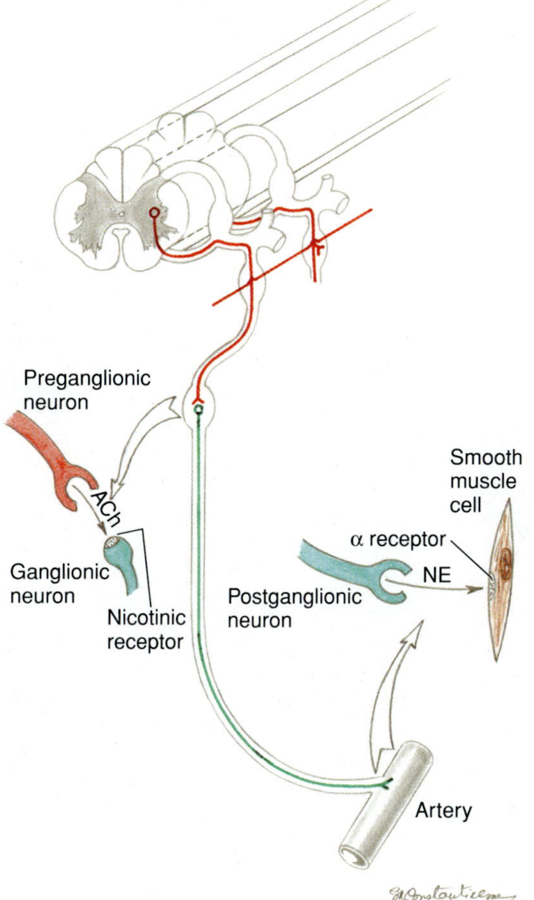

FIG. 6.1.—Anatomical relationships of sympathetic neuronal outflow tracts and affiliated receptors of innervated cells. Sympathetic preganglionic axons exit the thoracolumbar region of the spinal cord and synapse with ganglionic neurons in an adjacent ganglion, or pass through the latter to synapse with a neuron within a distant ganglion (shown). The preganglionic axon terminal releases the neurotransmitter acetylcholine (ACh), which activates nicotinic cholinergic receptors on the ganglionic neuron body. The resulting stimulation of the ganglionic neuron promotes release of the neurotransmitter norepinephrine (NE) from the axon terminal at the postganglionic sympathetic neuroeffector junction at blood vessels (shown) or other tissues innervated by sympathetic neurons. NE activates α- (shown) or β-adrenergic receptors present on cells innervated by the sympathetic division of the autonomic nervous system. Preganglionic fibers are red; postganglionic fibers are blue. Drawn by Dr. Gheorghe M. Constantinescu, University of Missouri.

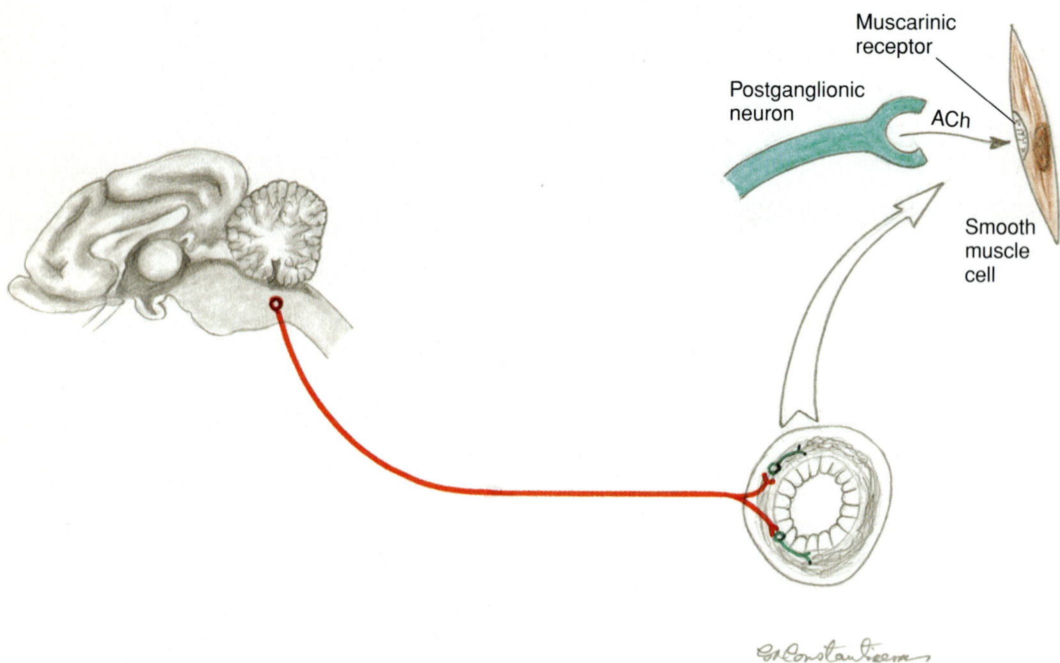

FIG. 7.1.—Anatomical relationships of parasympathetic neuronal outflow tracts and affiliated receptors of innervated cells. Parasympathetic preganglionic axons exit cranial (shown) or sacral zones and pass peripherally to synapse with a neuron body located within (shown) or adjacent to innervated tissue. The preganglionic neuron releases the neurotransmitter acetylcholine (ACh), which activates nicotinic cholinergic receptors on the ganglionic neuron body. The resulting stimulation of the ganglionic neuron promotes release of ACh from the axon terminal at postganglionic parasympathetic neuroeffector junctions within the intestinal tract (shown) or other tissues innervated by parasympathetic neurons. ACh activates muscarinic cholinergic receptors present on cells innervated by the parasympathetic division of the autonomic nervous system. Preganglionic fibers are red; postganglionic fibers are blue. Drawn by Dr. Gheorghe M. Constantinescu, University of Missouri.

G_i) linked to diminution of adenylyl cyclase and resulting decreased formation of cAMP and protein kinase A (Lambert 1993). In some tissues, muscarinic receptors are linked to activation of guanylyl cyclase with increased formation of cGMP (Lefkowitz et al. 1990; Lambert 1993).

STRUCTURE-ACTIVITY RELATIONSHIPS. Direct-acting cholinergic agonists contain structural groupings that allow interaction of the agent with cholinergic receptors and result in similar changes in membrane configuration and thus ion permeability as caused by ACh (Rand and Stafford 1967). Choline esters contain a quaternary nitrogen atom to which three methyl groups are attached. Except for some naturally occurring cholinomimetic alkaloids, a quaternary nitrogen moiety is usually required for a direct potent action on cholinergic receptors. Like its counterpart the ammonium ion, the quaternary nitrogen group carries a positive charge; this cationic group electrostatically binds with a negatively charged (anionic) site of the cholinergic receptor. The anionic site is believed to be the main determinant of receptor events, and interaction of the cationic head of ACh with the anionic site is the primary instigator of conformational changes that lead to alterations in membrane permeability.

Receptive macromolecules (i.e., cholinergic receptors and cholinesterases) that recognize and bind ACh have, in addition to the anionic site, a region that combines with the ester component of ACh (Fig. 7.2) (Hucho et al. 1991). In cholinesterase, this region is called the esteratic site and its combination with the carboxyl group results in hydrolysis of the ester (see discussion later in this chapter). Hydrolysis of ACh does not occur upon its interaction with a receptor, however, and the ester-attracting region of the receptor is called the esterophilic site (Inestrosa and Perelman 1990; Taylor 1990a, 1991; Massoulie et al. 1993).

ACh is ideally arranged structurally so that it combines with the esterophilic and anionic sites of both nicotinic and muscarinic receptors and acetylcholinesterases (Hucho et al. 1991). When both components of the ester moiety of ACh (i.e., the carbonyl group and the ether oxygen) are replaced by methylene molecules, agonistic properties at both muscarinic and nicotinic sites are reduced. If only the ether oxygen of ACh is substituted by a methylene group, the muscarinic potency is markedly decreased but nicotinic properties are little affected. Introduction of a methyl group on the β-carbon atom of the choline segment considerably reduces nicotinic properties but does not reduce muscarinic activities. These findings indicate that the esterophilic sites are arranged somewhat differently in muscarinic than in nicotinic receptors and therefore influence specificity of agonistic and antagonistic properties of different drugs. The esterophilic region may contain subunits that individually attract either the ether oxygen or the carbonyl oxygen by hydrogen bonding and dipole-dipole interaction respectively (Fig. 7.2B) (Khromov-Borisov and Michelson 1966).

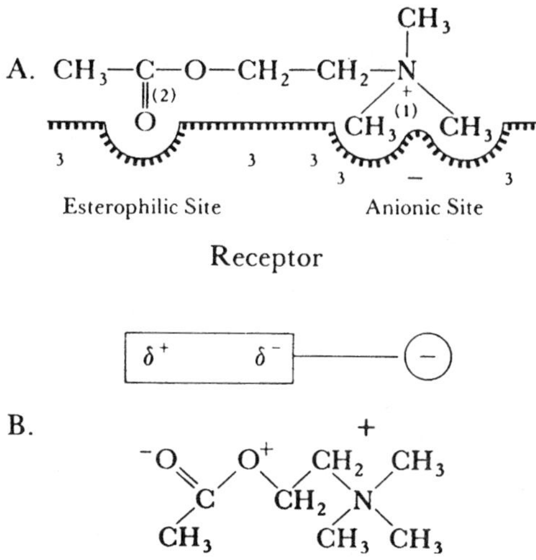

FIG. 7.2—Interaction of ACh and its receptor. **A.** (1) = electrostatic bond between cationic (quaternary N^+) group of ACh and the anionic site of the receptor. (2) = dipolar binding of ester of ACh with the esterophilic site of the receptor [note: in ACh-cholinesterase interaction, (2) = covalent bonding of carboxyl carbon to a protonated acidic group of the esteratic site of the enzyme]. (3) = probable existence of hydrophobic bonds between the various methyl groups and adjacent proteins of the receptor surface. Based on the postulated interaction of ACh and cholinesterase (modified from Eldefrawi 1974). **B** Electrical charge distribution of ACh and its receptor (Khromov-Borisov and Michelson 1966).

ACh is the prototypical cholinergic agent; it acts at all cholinoceptor sites and therefore evokes both nicotinic and muscarinic effects. Acetyl-β-methylcholine (methacholine) is identical in structure to ACh except for the substitution of a methyl group on the β-carbon atom of the choline group. This structural change yields a compound that is primarily a muscarinic receptor agonist lacking significant nicotinic effects when given in usual dosages. Further, it is more active on the cardiovascular system than on the GI tract. Duration of action of methacholine is considerably longer than that of ACh because the former drug is hydrolyzed by acetylcholinesterase (AChE) at a much slower rate than is ACh and methacholine is almost totally resistant to breakdown by pseudocholinesterase.

Carbachol and bethanechol each have a carbamyl (NH_2COO-) group substituted for the acetic moiety of ACh, and bethanechol also has a β-methyl group. Both of these agents are almost completely resistant to inactivation by the cholinesterases. Their duration of action is therefore considerably longer than that of ACh. Carbachol is active at both muscarinic and nicotinic receptor sites (therefore it is cholinomimetic and not just parasympathomimetic), whereas bethanechol is primarily a muscarinic agonist. Unlike methacholine, both these drugs are somewhat more active on smooth muscles of the GI tract and urinary bladder than on

TABLE 7.1—Chemical structures (A) and scope of cholinergic receptor activating properties (B) of some choline esters

A.	Compound	Structure
	Choline	$(CH_3)_3N^+ \cdot CH_2 \cdot CH_2 \cdot OH$
	Acetylcholine	$(CH_3)_3N^+ \cdot CH_2 \cdot CH_2 \cdot O \cdot COCH_3$
	Methacholine	$(CH_3)_3N^+ \cdot CH_2 \cdot CH_2 \cdot O \cdot COCH_3$
	Carbachol	$(CH_3)_3N^+ \cdot CH_2 \cdot CH_2 \cdot O \cdot CONH_2$
	Bethanechol	$(CH_3)_3N^+ \cdot CH_2 \cdot CH(CH_3) \cdot O \cdot CONH_2$

	Susceptibility to cholinesterase		Agonistic properties				
			Muscarinic receptors				
B.	True	Pseudo	CV	GI	UB	E	Nicotinic receptors
Choline							
Acetylcholine	+ + +	+ + +	+ + +	+ + +	+ +	+	+++
Methacholine	+	–	+ + +	+ +	+ +	+	±
Carbachol	–	–	+	+ + +	+ + +	+ +	+ + +
Bethanechol	–	–	±	+++	+ + +	+ +	–

Note: CV = cardiovascular; GI = gastrointestinal; UB = urinary bladder; E = eye.

cardiovascular function. Chemical structures of these choline esters and their related pharmacologic characteristics are shown in Table 7.1.

ACETYLCHOLINE. Although ACh is not used clinically, it is the prototypical cholinergic agonist, and an understanding of its activity is imperative for a comprehension of the pharmacologic effects of other cholinomimetic drugs. The biosynthesis, neuronal release, cellular activities, and inactivation of endogenous ACh are examined in Chap. 5 and should be reviewed in conjunction with this chapter.

Since ACh is a mixed nicotinic-muscarinic agonist, different effects can be produced by administration of this agent, depending upon the relative dominance of muscarinic (parasympathomimetic) or nicotinic actions. These effects can be differentiated by use of small and large doses of ACh and by using selective cholinergic blocking drugs. In general, parasympathomimetic effects dominate with small doses, whereas with large doses cholinergic effects at other tissue sites are also produced. Therefore, muscarinic receptors seem to be more susceptible than nicotinic receptors to ACh. Use of cholinergic blocking drugs and small and large doses of ACh to differentiate muscarinic and nicotinic effects of ACh is shown in Fig. 7.3. This figure is discussed in greater detail in the following sections.

PHARMACOLOGIC EFFECTS

Cardiovascular Effects of Small Doses of ACh. Intravenous (IV) administration of small amounts of ACh (5-10 µg/kg) produces a brief but rapid fall in systolic and diastolic blood pressures. This is due to a decrease in peripheral resistance resulting from dilation of blood vessels. Most blood vessels receive little or no parasympathetic innervation (see Chap. 5). Therefore, most vascular smooth muscle is different from other smooth muscle in that its muscarinic receptors are noninnervated.

Interestingly, muscarinic receptors subserving dilation of blood vessels are located on the endothelium rather than on the smooth muscle itself. Activation of endothelial muscarinic receptors by ACh causes the endothelial cells to release endothelium-derived relaxing factor (EDRF) (Furchgott and Zawadzki 1980), identified as nitric oxide (Lowenstein et al. 1994). Nitric oxide transfers to the vascular smooth muscle cells and therein activates cytosolic guanylyl cyclase; the resulting increase in cGMP provokes vascular smooth muscle relaxation and vasodilation, as summarized in Fig. 5.8 (Adams 1996).

Somewhat larger doses of ACh (10-30 µg/kg) produce pronounced muscarinic effects; therefore, a pronounced decrease in peripheral resistance and blood pressure is produced. In addition to the hypotension response, a slowing of the heart rate occurs after administration of ACh (a transient tachycardia may initially occur from the hypotensive response affecting baroreceptor reflex activity). Atrial myocardial cells contain muscarinic receptors associated with vagal fibers that mediate negative chronotropic and inotropic effects. The chronotropic effects predominate; they are due to a decreased slope of phase 4 (spontaneous depolarization) of the pacemaker action potential of the sinoatrial (SA) node.

ACh, in addition to its pronounced slowing effect on heart rate, exerts important effects on impulse conduction. In the atria, cholinergic activation slows conduction velocity but shortens action potential duration and the effective refractory period. These actions reinforce atrial dysrhythmias and lead to atrial flutter and fibrillation. In the atrioventricular (AV) node, however, ACh slows conduction velocity but prolongs the refractory period. Thus, although cholinergic drugs can exacerbate atrial tachyarrhythmias, the number of aberrant impulses that effectively traverse the AV junction into the ventricular cells can be decreased concomitantly by the same agent. The net effect is a slowing of ventricu-

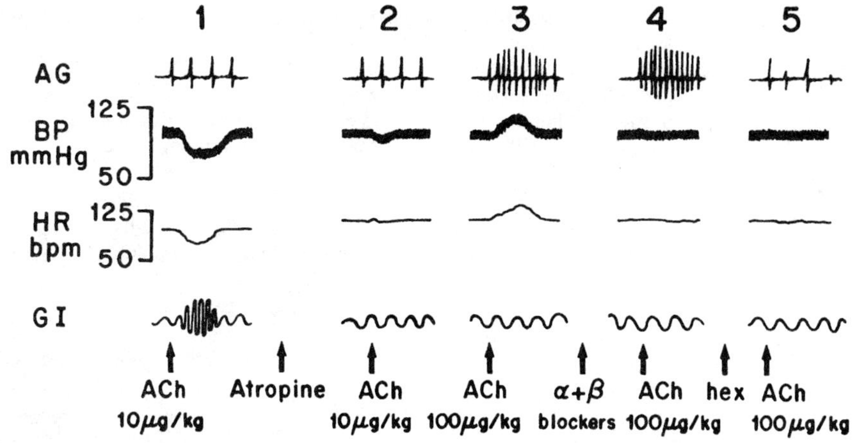

FIG. 7.3—Muscarinic and nicotinic effects of ACh on blood pressure, heart rate, intestinal motility, and autonomic ganglionic action potentials in an anesthetized dog. Schematic reproductions: 1. A small dose of ACh (10 µg/kg) administered intravenously causes hypotension, bradycardia, and intestinal contractions caused by direct stimulation of muscarinic receptors of blood vessels, heart, and intestinal smooth muscle respectively. These effects are brief because of rapid destruction of ACh by cholinesterase. 2. Atropine blocks the muscarinic receptors and thereby prevents the effects seen in (1). 3. Large doses of ACh (100 µg/kg) stimulate, in addition to muscarinic receptors, nicotinic receptors of parasympathetic and sympathetic ganglionic neurons, causing an increase in frequency and amplitude of ganglionic action potentials. Although all autonomic ganglia are activated, impulses arising from parasympathetic ganglia do not reach their effector cells because of blockade of parasympathetic postganglionic neuroeffector junctions by atropine. Sympathomimetic responses (pressor effect and tachycardia) result. 4. Impulses arising from sympathetic ganglia are prevented from reaching their effector cells by adrenergic blocking drugs; however, ganglionic nicotinic receptors are still activated by ACh. 5. Hexamethonium (hex) blocks nicotinic receptors of ganglia and thereby inhibits the nicotinic ganglionic stimulating effect of ACh and reduces ganglionic action potentials. AG = action potentials of autonomic ganglionic neuron; BP = systemic blood pressure; HR = heart rate; GI = intestinal peristaltic waves.

lar rate; this mechanism has pharmacologic importance, because the beneficial slowing effects of digitalis on ventricular rate in patients with atrial fibrillation or flutter is mediated in part by increased vagal tone.

Different arrhythmias that can result from use of cholinergic drugs include sinus arrest, severe bradycardia, incomplete and complete heart block, notching and decreased amplitude of the P wave, momentary ventricular asystole, and atrial fibrillation and flutter.

Smooth Muscle. GI motility and secretions are enhanced by ACh in a manner identical to that seen upon stimulation of the parasympathetic innervation to the alimentary tract. These effects may be difficult to detect with small doses because duration of action of ACh is brief owing to rapid destruction by cholinesterase. Larger doses markedly increase secretions and peristaltic movements of the GI tract.

ACh stimulates smooth muscle of the urinary bladder and uterus to contract. Bronchiolar smooth muscle is also contracted by ACh, resulting in decreased diameter of airways. The smooth muscle effects of ACh are blocked by atropine and therefore are due to muscarinic receptor activation.

Central Nervous System. Because of its highly charged quaternary nitrogen group, ACh is lipophobic and poorly penetrates cell membranes and the blood-brain barrier. Thus CNS effects are not observed when usual dosages are administered. However, intra-arterial injection into cerebral arteries of large amounts of ACh or its direct application into the CNS produces increased electrical activity, excitation, and possibly convulsions. Both muscarinic and nicotinic receptors are present in the CNS.

Muscarinic and Nicotinic Effects of Large Doses of ACh. With high doses (50-100 µg/kg), muscarinic effects of ACh on postganglionic effector cells are accentuated. Profound hypotension is caused by extensive peripheral vasodilation. Duration of this effect is prolonged. Heart rate slows dramatically and momentary asystole can occur. The GI tract and other visceral smooth muscles are markedly activated; defecation, urination, and vomiting may result.

Large doses of ACh produce, in addition to the muscarinic (i.e., parasympathomimetic) effects described above, stimulation of the nicotine receptors of autonomic ganglia (both parasympathetic and sympathetic) and the adrenal medulla. These effects are particularly evident when the muscarinic receptors of the parasympathetic neuroeffector junctions are blocked by atropine. Under these circumstances large doses of ACh stimulate nicotinic receptors of both sympathetic and parasympathetic ganglia. However, because the muscarinic receptors of the parasympathetic neuroeffector junctions are blocked by atropine, impulses originating from parasympathetic ganglia will not reach their effector cells. Only impulses originating from sympathetic ganglia will do so; therefore, only sympathomimetic responses will be evident. These are characterized by an increase in blood pressure, tachycardia, and other typical sympathetic-mediated effects, which can be blocked by use of appropriate adrenergic blocking drugs (see Chap. 6) or by use of a ganglionic blocking agent (Fig. 7.3).

Adrenal Medulla. The adrenal medulla is functionally analogous to autonomic ganglia, and nicotinic receptors of adrenal medullary chromaffin cells are innervated by typical preganglionic cholinergic fibers. These receptors are stimulated by ACh to cause release of epinephrine and norepinephrine from chromaffin cells into the circulation. This effect contributes to the overall nicotinic-mediated sympathomimetic effect evoked by large doses of ACh in the presence of muscarinic blockade.

Skeletal Muscle. Intra-arterial injection of significant quantities of ACh will produce skeletal muscle fasciculations caused by penetration of some of the agent to motor end-plates and resulting activation of nicotinic receptors of skeletal muscle cells. Continued exposure to excessive amounts of ACh causes severe fasciculations and asynchronous contractions and terminates in a depolarizing paralysis. Also, if an atropine-like drug has not been given, an increase in blood flow to the injected muscle occurs as a result of vasodilation from stimulation of the muscarinic receptors of blood vessel endothelial cells and the resulting release of EDRF.

METHACHOLINE, CARBACHOL, AND BETHANECOL. The pharmacologic effects of these choline esters are equivalent to the previously outlined parasympathomimetic effects of ACh and thus are similar to the physiologic changes evoked by stimulation of postganglionic parasympathetic nerves as listed in Table 5.1. Carbachol also has marked nicotinic agonistic characteristics; however, differences between the parasympathomimetic actions of these choline esters are primarily quantitative and vary principally in relative selectivity for one organ system or another (Table 7.1).

Methacholine (acetyl-β-methylcholine) is a synthetic choline ester used occasionally in human therapeutics but infrequently employed in veterinary medicine. Methacholine causes muscarinic effects on cardiovascular function similar to those produced by ACh, but it is considerably less active on the GI system and has few agonist properties at nicotinic receptors.

Carbachol (Lentin, carbamylcholine chloride, Doryl) is an extremely potent choline ester that is active at both muscarinic and nicotinic receptors and therefore causes pharmacologic effects similar to changes evoked by ACh. These are particularly prominent on the nicotinic receptors of autonomic ganglia; however, this drug is also very potent at muscarinic sites. For example, IV injection of doses as small as 2 μg/kg causes a transient slowing of heart rate and hypotension owing to muscarinic effects.

Bethanecol (Urecholine, carbamylmethylcholine) is somewhat similar to methacholine and carbachol in scope of pharmacologic activity. Unlike carbachol, however, it is primarily a muscarinic agonist and has little stimulant effects on nicotinic receptors.

PHARMACOLOGIC EFFECTS

Cardiovascular Effects. Methacholine is more active on the cardiovascular system than on the GI or urinary tracts. The opposite selectivity is seen with carbachol and bethanechol. IV administration of methacholine, like ACh, produces a depressor response and slowing of heart rate caused by activation of muscarinic receptors of blood vessels and the heart respectively. Cardiac rhythm is altered by methacholine, and the AV node is particularly sensitive to this agent. Conduction velocity through the AV node is decreased. Various degrees of heart block, including complete AV disassociation, can occur with large doses. IV administration of methacholine to normal nonanesthetized animals can produce atrial fibrillation, as can ACh. These effects are blocked by atropine. Carbachol evokes blood pressure changes similar to those seen with methacholine except relatively less pronounced, whereas bethanechol is considerably less active on cardiovascular function.

GI Tract. Carbachol and bethanecol are relatively more active on the GI and urinary tracts than on the cardiovascular system. Methacholine is also active on the alimentary canal but only in large doses. Carbachol is a potent GI stimulant. It evokes profuse salivation and an increase in peristaltic movements of the gut resulting in increased fluidity of feces and defecation. These responses are due to activation of muscarinic receptors. GI stimulant effects of choline esters are relatively well defined in simple-stomached animals, but responsiveness of ruminants may vary. Effects of carbachol and various other autonomic drugs on the GI tract of ruminants are summarized in previous editions of this text.

Other Smooth Muscle. Uterine musculature, in in vitro strips and the intact animal, is contracted by carbachol. This response is more evident during the latter stages of gestation. Carbachol should not be used during pregnancy, because abortion or uterine rupture might result. After parturition, carbachol may be useful in expelling uterine contents.

Similar to ACh, carbachol causes contraction of bronchiolar smooth muscle, resulting in a decreased airway. The urinary bladder is contracted by carbachol and bethanechol, and frequent urination results. Effects of carbachol and bethanechol on these as on other smooth muscles are muscarinic and blocked by atropine.

Skeletal Muscle. Carbachol does not discernibly affect skeletal muscle when usual dosages are employed. If a high dose is inadvertently given, muscle fasciculations and even paralysis may occur. This is a nicotinic effect due to carbachol causing a persistent depolarization block of the postjunctional membrane of the neuromuscular junction. Because of relative lack of agonistic effects at nicotinic sites, bethanechol and methacholine have little effect on voluntary muscles.

Sweating. Profuse sweating in the horse is evoked by carbachol. It is not known if this is due to a direct effect on sweat glands, a ganglionic stimulating effect, an increase in circulating catecholamines (as a result of adrenal medullary stimulation), or local release of catecholamines from adrenergic neurons. Because sweat gland mechanisms in the horse seem to be β_2 adrenergic (Bijman and Quinton 1984), either of the latter two mechanisms could be involved.

Other Effects. Carbachol, like ACh, is a mixed nicotinic-muscarinic agonist. It therefore has a potent stimulating effect on autonomic ganglia and the chromaffin cells of the adrenal medulla. Such an effect on the adrenal medulla would cause an increased discharge of epinephrine and norepinephrine into the bloodstream, which in turn could produce diffuse sympathomimetic effects. This relationship may explain why adrenergic-like effects have occasionally been encountered during the use of carbachol. Nicotinic effects of carbachol on autonomic ganglia can be demonstrated by the hypertensive response obtained with large doses after the postganglionic muscarinic receptors have been blocked with atropine (Fig. 7.3).

CLINICAL USES. Methacholine and bethanechol are not used frequently in clinical veterinary medicine. Methacholine has been used in humans and animals to produce peripheral vasodilation in treating different vascular disorders such as Raynaud's disease and ergot poisoning respectively. It has been used in human medicine to control tachycardia of supraventricular origin. Ventricular tachycardia and nodal paroxysmal tachycardia (in which the origin is in the AV node) are not amenable to methacholine therapy. Bethanechol, 1 mg administered subcutaneously twice daily, has been used to treat urinary bladder atony in cats after incidences of urolithiasis; however, care should be taken to ensure that the urethra is completely patent.

Carbachol is a potent drug, and care should be taken to avoid overstimulation of the GI tract and uterus during its clinical use. It has been used for treatment of colic and impactions of the intestinal tract; however, its use in such cases should be closely monitored. If excessive peristaltic movements are induced in a patient suffering from intestinal obstruction, rupture or intussusception may occur. Before resorting to a potent cholinomimetic compound such as carbachol, consideration should first be given to more conservative approaches to GI therapy such as the use of mineral oil, saline cathartics, water, or other stool softeners. If these measures are not successful, carbachol may be cautiously added to the therapeutic regimen. Repeated small subcutaneous (SC) doses of 1-2 mg carbachol at 30- to 60-minute intervals have been used in treating colic in mature horses after treatment with oils and saline cathartics had been instituted. Dosages should be decreased to 0.25-0.5 mg in foals.

When administered during the middle of farrowing, carbachol (2 mg subcutaneously) has been reported to decrease the incidence of stillbirths in litters from sows and gilts by increasing uterine contractions (Sprecher et al.. 1975). However, severe salivation, vomiting, diarrhea, and frequent urination were adverse side effects.

Carbachol has been used in treatment of rumen atony and impaction in cattle. After conservative treatment with stool softeners, repeated doses of 1-2 mg have proved effective in stimulating rumen motility. However, single doses greater than 4 mg may be ineffective and in some cases may actually inhibit ruminoreticular activity. Carbachol should not be given by IV or, probably, intramuscular (IM) injection because of its potency. It is given by the SC route; however, the dosage is still critical. Fatalities have occurred in human patients after IM injection of carbachol.

Naturally Occurring Cholinomimetic Alkaloids. Pilocarpine, muscarine, and arecoline are plant alkaloids that exert parasympathomimetic effects with minimal activity at nicotinic sites. Although all three agents are used in research, only pilocarpine has been used to any appreciable extent in clinical medicine.

Pilocarpine nitrate is the water-soluble salt of the alkaloid pilocarpine, obtained from leaves of the Brazilian shrubs *Pilocarpus jaborandi* and *P. microphyllus.* Arecoline is an alkaloid found in the betel nut, the seed of the betel palm *(Areca catechu).* Muscarine is found in the poisonous mushrooms *Amanita muscaria.* The chemical structures of these three compounds are given in Fig. 7.4.

PHARMACOLOGIC MECHANISMS AND EFFECTS. Pilocarpine, arecoline, and muscarine are rather selective parasympathomimetic agents; i.e., their cholinomimetic activity is exerted primarily at muscarinic sites with minimal nicotinic effects. Even the slight ganglionic-stimulating effects of pilocarpine and arecoline are believed to be from activation of the secondary muscarinic pathway involved in ganglionic transmission (see latter part of this chapter). These cholinomimetic alkaloids evoke their parasympathomimetic effects by direct stimulation of the muscarinic receptors of cells innervated by postganglionic cholinergic nerves. They do not inhibit cholinesterase. Also, because their effects are produced in chronically denervated tissue, they are not dependent upon release of endogenous ACh.

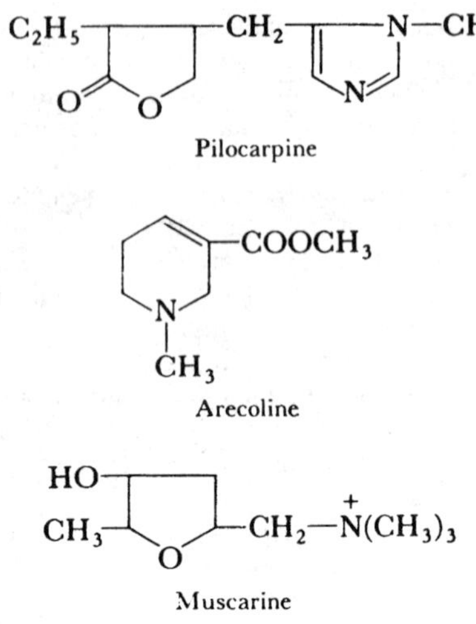

Pilocarpine

Arecoline

Muscarine

FIG. 7.4

Pilocarpine is particularly effective in stimulating flow of secretions from exocrine glands, including salivary, mucous, gastric, and digestive pancreatic secretions. As with ACh it causes contraction of GI smooth muscle, thereby increasing smooth muscle tone and peristaltic activity. Of considerable importance, pilocarpine has a potent constrictor effect on the pupil.

Arecoline activates muscarinic receptors of cholinergically innervated effector cells of glands, smooth muscles, and myocardium and therefore produces the usual parasympathomimetic effects. It is similar to pilocarpine in scope of activity but is considerably more potent. Arecoline depresses heart rate and blood pressure and may produce dyspnea by constricting the bronchioles. Dyspnea generally is not marked except in cases where the dose is toxic or the animal has previously been affected with a respiratory ailment such as acute pulmonary emphysema. Arecoline stimulates secretion of the glands of the digestive tract and increases peristaltic movements of the gut. Increased flow of saliva, occurring within 5 minutes following a SC injection and lasting for an hour, is particularly noticeable. Arecoline contracts the urinary bladder.

Muscarine has been employed experimentally for many years because it has a selective excitatory effect on the effector cells of tissues innervated by postganglionic cholinergic nerves. It does not stimulate the nicotinic receptors of autonomic ganglia or skeletal muscle as does ACh.

CLINICAL USES. Pupillary constriction (miosis) occurs when pilocarpine is administered systemically or applied topically to the eye. Clinically, solutions of 0.5-2% are used for instillation into the conjunctival sac for treatment of glaucoma. Pilocarpine stimulates the sphincter muscle of the iris and the ciliary muscle of the lens, causing pupillary constriction and spasm of accommodation. Intraocular pressure momentarily increases, followed by a persistent decrease. Fixation of the lens for near vision lasts only 1-2 hours; however, miosis, which develops within about 15 minutes after instillation, persists 12-24 hours. Pilocarpine is also used alternately with mydriatics to prevent synechiation, but it is contraindicated in patients with iridocyclitis.

TOXICOLOGY. Toxic doses of the cholinomimetic alkaloids evoke severe colic and diarrhea and exocrine gland secretions. The pupil is markedly constricted. Dyspnea occurs because of constriction of the bronchioles and accumulation of mucus in the airways. Hypotension and extreme cardiac slowing, complicated by excessive bronchoconstriction and bronchial secretions, lead to death. Arecoline or systemic exposure to pilocarpine is contraindicated in animals with heart failure, depression or disease of the respiratory tract, and spasmodic colic and during gestation. Atropine is a specific antidote to toxic doses of arecoline, pilocarpine, and muscarine. Toxic action of the poisonous mushroom in humans results from the parasympathomimetic action of muscarine.

CHOLINESTERASE INHIBITORS. The function of AChE in terminating the transmitter action of endogenous ACh at cholinergic synapses and neuroeffector junctions is discussed in Chap. 5. Cholinesterase inhibitors (anticholinesterase agents) inactivate or inhibit AChE and pseudocholinesterase and thereby intensify activity of endogenous ACh. In addition, the activity of drugs that are biotransformed by cholinesterase (e.g., succinylcholine) is also prolonged by cholinesterase inhibitors. Because these drugs magnify the actions of endogenous ACh at all cholinergic receptors, their scope of activity is not limited to parasympathomimetic effects but includes cholinomimetic actions throughout the body.

Physostigmine, neostigmine, and edrophonium are examples of the type of anticholinesterase agent that produces a reversible inhibition of cholinesterase, whereas organophosphate compounds such as diisopropyl fluorophosphate (DFP) produce an irreversible inhibition. Although there is considerable distinction between these two groups of anticholinesterases, their pharmacologic effects are similar because of a common basic mechanism of action.

Pharmacologic Considerations

MECHANISM OF ACTION. The pharmacologic effects of cholinesterase inhibitors can be explained almost entirely by their characteristic inhibitory action on AChE. This results in decreased hydrolysis of neuronally released ACh and intensification of its action at cholinergic receptors. This is particularly true with the irreversible organophosphate compounds and can be demonstrated by lack of miotic effect of topically

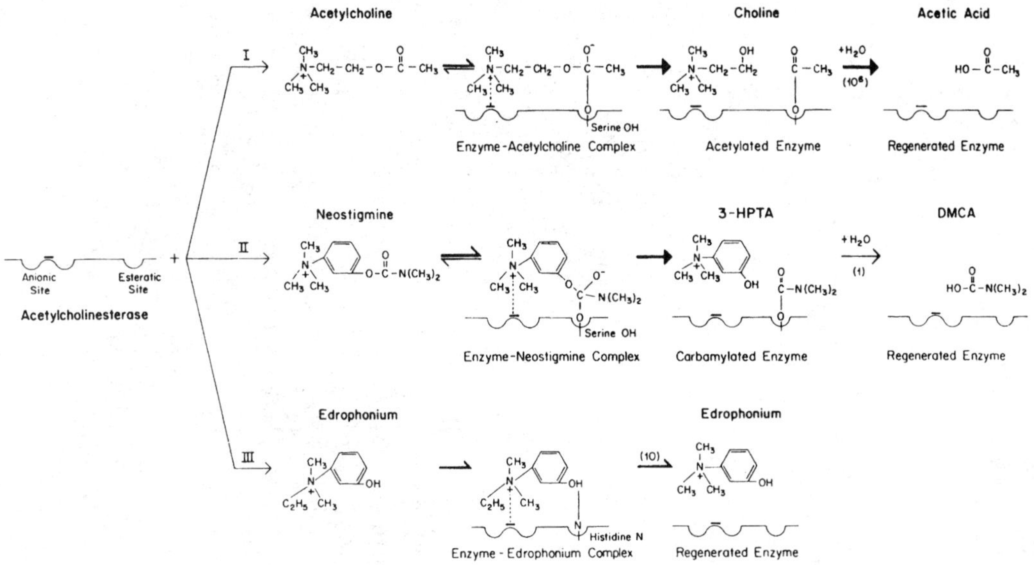

FIG. 7.5—Interaction of ACh, neostigmine, and edrophonium with AChE. I. ACh complexes with AChE via electrostatic binding of the quaternary (cationic) N^+ of the choline group with the anionic site of the enzyme and by interaction of the carbonyl group with a serine hydroxyl group of the esteratic site. Choline is split off, yielding the acetylated enzyme, which interacts with H_2O to yield acetic acid and the reactivated enzyme. II. Neostigmine complexes with AChE to yield 3-hydroxyphenyltrimethylammonium (3-HPTA) and carbamylated enzyme, which then react with H_2O to give *N,N*–dimethylcarbamic acid (DMCA) and the reactivated enzyme; this reaction is $\simeq 10^{-6}$ slower than the comparable reaction involving ACh and AChE. III. Edrophonium complexes with AChE via electrostatic interaction at the anionic site and by H bonding to the imidazole N atom of histidine at the esteratic site; this complex is reversible, yielding reactivated AChE and edrophonium. The numbers in parentheses refer to relative rates of reaction (Taylor 1990a; Inestrosa and Perelman 1990; Massoulie et al. 1993).

applied DFP in a chronically denervated eye, where there is no source of ACh. Neostigmine and other quaternary nitrogen anticholinesterase agents exert some direct effects (either agonistic or antagonistic) on cholinergic receptors in addition to inhibition of cholinesterase. At the somatic neuromuscular junction, e.g., muscle twitch stimulant effects of neostigmine are attributed to direct receptor activation as well as to cholinesterase inhibition. The direct effect is not uniform throughout the body. Neostigmine, like DFP, is miotically inactive in the denervated eye. Effects of physostigmine, a tertiary amine, can be explained almost entirely by its anticholinesterase activity.

MOLECULAR. The enzymatic interactions of AChE, ACh, and cholinesterase inhibitors are shown schematically in Fig. 7.5 and can be summarized as follows (Taylor 1990a, 1991; Inestrosa and Perelman 1990; Massoulie et al. 1993). AChE contains two active sites that recognize specific parts of the ACh molecule: an anionic (negatively charged) region where electrostatic binding occurs with the cationic nitrogen of the choline moiety, and an esteratic site where the carboxyl portion of the acetyl ester binds to it by covalent bonding. After ACh-AChE interaction occurs, the choline portion is split off, leaving the acetylated esteratic site. Acetic acid is rapidly formed as water reacts with the acetyl group, and the enzyme is thereby reactivated (Wilson 1954).

Neostigmine, physostigmine, and other carbamate derivatives interact with the anionic and esteratic sites of the enzyme, thereby preventing ACh from affixing to the enzyme. Neostigmine and physostigmine are believed to be hydrolyzed in a manner similar to but much slower than that of ACh (Wilson et al. 1960); i.e., the alcoholic portion of the anticholinesterase compound is split off, leaving a carbamylated esteratic site. A carbamic acid is then formed upon reaction with water, and the enzyme is regenerated (Fig. 7.5). Although the rate of combination of inhibitor with AChE is only a few times slower than the analogous combination of ACh with the enzyme, the rate of hydrolysis is probably over 10^6 times faster for ACh. Therefore, neostigmine and related drugs are reversible cholinesterase inhibitors as a result of their acting as competitive substrates hydrolyzed at a much slower rate than the endogenous substrate ACh (Taylor 1990a, 1991; Massoulie et al. 1993).

Edrophonium and tetraethylammonium ions are complex and simple quaternary nitrogen compounds respectively that interact with the anionic site of cholinesterase. Therefore, they are not hydrolyzed but act as simple competitive reversible inhibitors. Accordingly, the duration of action of edrophonium is much shorter than that of neostigmine or physostigmine.

Organophosphate compounds interact with AChE at the esteratic site and form an extremely stable enzyme-inhibitor complex that does not undergo significant spontaneous disassociation. The esteratic site is persistently phosphorylated, and recovery of cholinesterase activity is dependent upon *de novo* synthesis of new enzyme. Some organophosphates (e.g., echothiophate) may interact with both the anionic and esteratic sites. Because cholinesterase synthesis requires days, organophosphates cause an irreversible inhibition. As discussed below, however, certain oxime compounds exhibit such high affinity for the organophosphate that they can actually cause detachment of the inhibitor from the esteratic site, resulting in cholinesterase reactivation (see Fig. 7.8).

PHARMACOLOGIC EFFECTS. Effects of cholinesterase inhibitors can be reliably predicted by considering the anatomic location of cholinergic nerves and the respective physiologic processes they modulate in their innervated cells. Parasympathomimetic (muscarinic) effects of these agents are equivalent to the effects associated with postganglionic parasympathomimetic nerve impulses. Cholinesterase inhibitors also cause intensification of ACh activity at nicotinic sites. Therefore, these drugs can cause the following effects: stimulation of postganglionic muscarinic receptors of effector cells, resulting in typical parasympathomimetic activity; stimulation of adrenal chromaffin cells to discharge catecholamines into the circulation; initial stimulation and subsequent depolarization block of nicotinic receptors of autonomic ganglia and skeletal muscle fibers; and marked CNS cholinergic effects.

Although all these activities can be seen with excessive doses, therapeutic doses usually result in more selective actions; e.g., neostigmine and other quaternary nitrogen compounds do not easily penetrate the blood-brain barrier and therefore exert little CNS activity. These compounds are relatively more active at nicotinic receptors of the skeletal neuromuscular junction than at muscarinic sites of autonomic effector cells. Tertiary amines and organophosphates are less lipophobic and can cross the blood-brain barrier and evoke CNS effects. These compounds are relatively more active with low doses at autonomic receptor sites than on voluntary muscles.

Reversible Inhibitors. *Physostigmine,* USP (Eserine), is an alkaloid extracted from the dried ripe seed of a vine, *Physostigma venenosum,* which grows in tropical West Africa. This seed, also called the Calabar or "ordeal" bean, was used by tribal Africans in witchcraft ordeals. A person accused of a crime was forced to eat the bean. If vomiting occurred, the accused did not die and was considered innocent. If there was no vomiting, however, death resulted and the suspect was declared guilty.

Neostigmine Bromide, USP (Prostigmine), is the salt of a synthetically produced substance discovered in a research investigation of compounds structurally related to physostigmine. Physostigmine also can be synthesized. *Edrophonium Chloride,* USP (Tensilon), is a synthetically derived agent that produces pharmacologic effects similar to neostigmine except that its duration of action is considerably shorter. It is used primarily as an anticurare agent. *Pyridostigmine Bromide,* USP (Mestinon, Regonol), and *Ambenonium Chloride,* USP (Mytelase, Mysuran), are moderately long acting, chemically synthesized cholinesterase inhibitors used primarily in management of myasthenia gravis and curare overdosage. The chemical structures of physostigmine, neostigmine, and edrophonium are shown in Fig. 7.6.

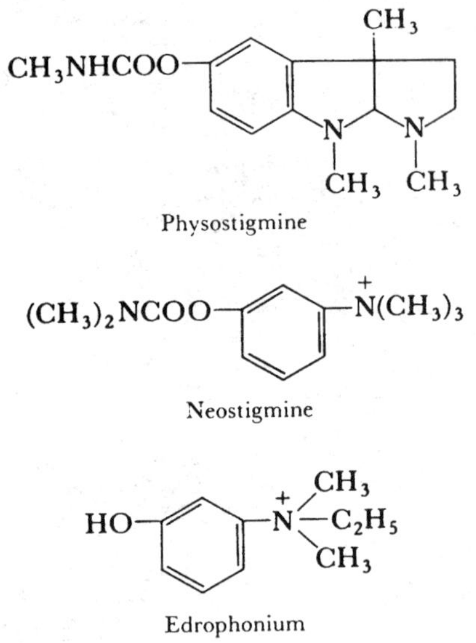

Physostigmine

Neostigmine

Edrophonium

FIG. 7.6

MECHANISM OF ACTION. These agents produce their effects by combining with cholinesterase and thereby preventing the enzyme from hydrolyzing ACh. ACh released during normal cholinergic nerve impulses has a prolonged and uninterrupted action upon cholinergic receptors. The interaction with cholinesterase is reversible, so as the inhibitor-enzyme complex breaks down, the enzyme is reactivated and it will now hydrolyze ACh and terminate its activity. At certain sites, neostigmine may act directly on receptors and evoke release of ACh from nerve endings; however, these are considered to be secondary actions.

PHARMACOLOGIC EFFECTS

DIGESTIVE TRACT. Physostigmine and neostigmine cause contraction of smooth muscle, thereby increasing motility and peristaltic movements of the gut. Frequency and strength of peristaltic waves are increased, and movement of intestinal contents is accelerated. Physostigmine has been used in animals for initiating peristaltic movements and evacuating the digestive tract. Excessive peristalsis leading to intestinal spasm and colic complicates use for this purpose. Physostigmine is given by SC or IM injection; its action after oral administration is unreliable. Neostigmine is not absorbed effectively after oral administration because of its quaternary nitrogen structure.

OCULAR EFFECTS. Physostigmine causes pupillary constriction and spasm of accommodation when applied locally to the eye or when injected for systemic effect. Intraocular pressure decreases, and physostigmine has been used in treating glaucoma to relieve elevated intraocular pressure.

SKELETAL MUSCLE. Besides its major action of inactivating AChE at the somatic myoneural junction, neostigmine is believed to directly stimulate nicotinic receptors of skeletal muscle fibers. Physostigmine is not active in denervated muscle. The skeletal muscle effects of neostigmine are relatively more pronounced at low doses than the smooth muscle effects of this agent. Twitching of skeletal muscles may be observed when a large dose of physostigmine or neostigmine is injected.

Physostigmine, neostigmine, pyridostigmine, and edrophonium are anticurare agents; they are antagonists to *d*-tubocurarine and other nondepolarizing (competitive) neuromuscular blocking agents at the somatic myoneural junction. These drugs can be used clinically to counteract an excessive dose of true curarimimetic agents but should not be used in attempts to antagonize the depolarizing neuromuscular blocking agents (e.g., succinylcholine), since synergism may actually occur (see Chap. 8).

OTHER EFFECTS. A therapeutic dose of physostigmine or neostigmine does not produce pronounced effects on cardiovascular function. Effects of higher doses are complicated by concurrent ganglionic stimulation and muscarinic effects on the heart and blood vessels. Usually, hypotension and a bradycardia leading to arrhythmias are produced. Smooth muscle of the bladder is cholinergically innervated and therefore is contracted by cholinesterase inhibitors. Bronchiolar smooth muscle is also contracted by these agents.

CLINICAL USES. *Physostigmine Salicylate,* USP (Isopto Eserine), or *Physostigmine Sulfate,* USP, can be used to produce miosis of the pupil and reduce intraocular pressure in the treatment of glaucoma. A solution of 0.5-1% physostigmine salicylate can be applied topically three times a day. The maximum miotic effect is obtained within an hour and may persist 12-24 hours, depending upon the dosage. Physostigmine may also be used alternately with atropine to prevent or break down synechia formed between lens and iris, such as occurs with periodic ophthalmia in horses.

Physostigmine has been used in a SC dose of 30-45 mg in cattle to stimulate ruminal activity in treatment of simple impaction or nonobstructive atony. Physostigmine, neostigmine, pyridostigmine, and edrophonium can be used to overcome the effects of true curare-like drugs in voluntary muscles, but the latter two agents are used more commonly for this purpose (Chap. 8).

Neostigmine has been used extensively in treating myasthenia gravis in humans. In myasthenia-like syndromes in dogs, neostigmine has also proved beneficial (Hall and Walker 1962). Marlow (1977) reported problems in controlling signs of myasthenia gravis in a dog treated with 60 mg neostigmine administered orally twice daily; difficulty was encountered in differentiating myasthenia crisis from cholinergic crisis. The former indicates an exacerbation of muscle weakness disease, whereas the latter refers to overdosage of the cholinesterase inhibitor with its attendant muscle weakness caused by excessive accumulation of ACh at the neuromuscular junction. Edrophonium, because of its brief duration of action, has been used to differentiate cholinergic and myasthenic crises in humans. If IV injection of this agent improves muscle function, myasthenia crisis is indicated and the dose of cholinesterase inhibitor used in maintenance therapy should be increased. However, if muscle weakness is accentuated by edrophonium, a cholinergic crisis is indicated and the dose of the cholinesterase inhibitor used in maintenance therapy should be reduced accordingly.

Impaction or other obstructions of the alimentary tract constitute a contraindication to the systemic use of cholinesterase inhibitors. Violent peristalsis produced by these drugs can cause rupture or intussusception of the gut. These drugs should not be used during pregnancy, particularly late in term, because of the danger of producing abortion.

TOXICOLOGY. Large doses of physostigmine first stimulate and then depress the CNS; small to moderate doses have little effect, whereas massive doses can produce convulsions. Neostigmine does not cross the blood-brain barrier to an appreciable extent. Toxic doses of these agents produce marked skeletal muscle weakness, nausea, vomiting, colic, and diarrhea. The pupil is markedly constricted and fixed. Dyspnea is characteristically seen from constriction of the bronchiolar musculature. Bradycardia and lowered blood pressure are also characteristic signs. Respiratory paralysis caused by depolarization block of the neuromuscular junction and compounded by excess bronchiolar secretions is the usual cause of death. Atropine is the most effective pharmacologic antagonist for physostigmine or neostigmine toxicity.

Organophosphorus Compounds. Diisopropyl fluorophosphate (diisopropyl phosphorofluoridate, DFP) is the prototypical organophosphate anticholinesterase agent. Related compounds include the alkyl pyrophosphates such as hexaethyltetraphosphate, tetraethylpyrophosphate (TEPP), and octamethyl pyrophosphortetramide (Taylor 1991). Organophosphates were

TABLE 7.2—Structural formulas of several organophosphate anticholinesterase agents

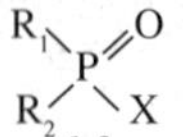

R_1, R_2, X attached to P=O

General formula

R_1	R_2	X	Agent
Isopropyl	Isopropyl	Fluoride	DFP
Pinacolyl	Methyl	Fluoride	Soman
Dimethylamino	Ethoxyl	Cyanide	Tabun
Isopropylamino	Isopropylamino	Fluoride	Mipafox
Ethoxyl	Ethoxyl	*S*-(2-Trimethylaminoethyl)	Echothiophate

Source: Modified from Volle 1971, p. 602.

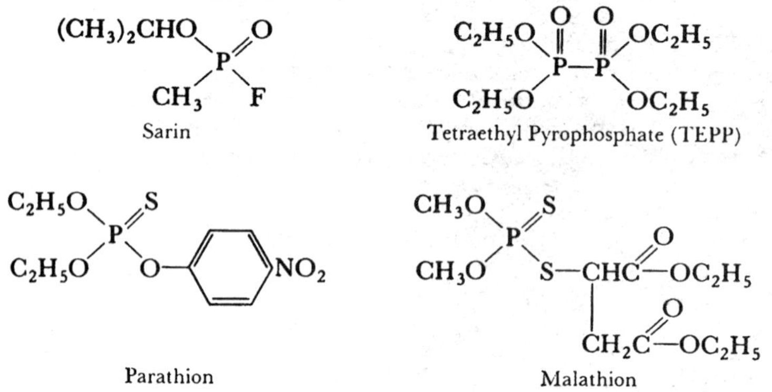

$(CH_3)_2CHO$, CH_3, F, P=O

Sarin

C_2H_5O, C_2H_5O, O, O, OC_2H_5, OC_2H_5, P—P

Tetraethyl Pyrophosphate (TEPP)

C_2H_5O, C_2H_5O, S, P, O, NO_2

Parathion

CH_3O, CH_3O, S, P, S—CHC(=O)—OC_2H_5, CH_2C(=O)—OC_2H_5

Malathion

FIG. 7.7—Representative structural formulas for organophosphate compounds.

originally introduced as pesticides by German scientists prior to and during World War II; however, there was considerable speculation by many scientists as to the potential use of these highly toxic substances as antipersonnel devices in chemical warfare. Subsequently, a wide variety of organophosphorus compounds have been synthesized and extensively investigated. Some of the more important of these used as pesticides are parathion [Thiophos, diethyl *O*–(4-nitrophenyl) phosphorothioate]; malathion [*O,O*–dimethyl *S*–(1,2-dicarbethoxyethyl) phosphorodithioate]; ronnel [*O,O*–dimethyl *O*–(2,4,5-trichlorophenyl) phosphorothioate]; and Co-ral. Soman, tabun, and sarin are extremely potent synthetic compounds that have been referred to as nerve gases. Dichlorvos (*O,O*–dimethyl-2,2-dichlorovinyl phosphate or 2,2-dichlorovinyl dimethyl phosphate) has been used as an oral anthelmintic in veterinary medicine and impregnated in flea collars as a pesticide.

Although the chemical structures of organophosphate compounds vary considerably, the basic moiety is a phosphate with various organic groups attached to it, as described in Table 7.2. Representative structural formulas are shown in Fig. 7.7.

MECHANISM OF ACTION, EFFECTS, AND TOXICITY. Organophosphates act as irreversible inhibitors of the cholinesterases in mammals. These compounds irreversibly phosphorylate the esteratic site of both AChE and the nonspecific or pseudocholinesterase throughout the body (Fig. 7.8). Endogenous ACh is not inactivated, and the resulting effects are due to the excessive preservation and accumulation of endogenous ACh (Taylor 1990a, 1991; Gutman and Besser 1990). Organophosphate poisoning produces diffuse cholinomimetic effects: profuse salivation, vomiting, defecation, hypermotility of the GI tract, urination, bradycardia, hypotension, severe bronchoconstriction, and excess bronchial secretions. These signs reflect excess activation of muscarinic receptors of postganglionic parasympathetic neuroeffector junctions with typical parasympathomimetic actions.

In addition to the muscarinic effects, skeletal muscle fasciculations, twitching, and, subsequently, muscle paralysis occur. These effects are due to persistent excessive stimulation of the nicotinic receptors of skeletal neuromuscular junctions, resulting in the depolarizing type of striated muscle paralysis (Gutman and Besser 1990). Convulsions and frequently death are seen in organophosphate poisoning, caused by penetration of the agent into the CNS and subsequent intensification of the activity of ACh at CNS sites (Gutman and Besser 1990).

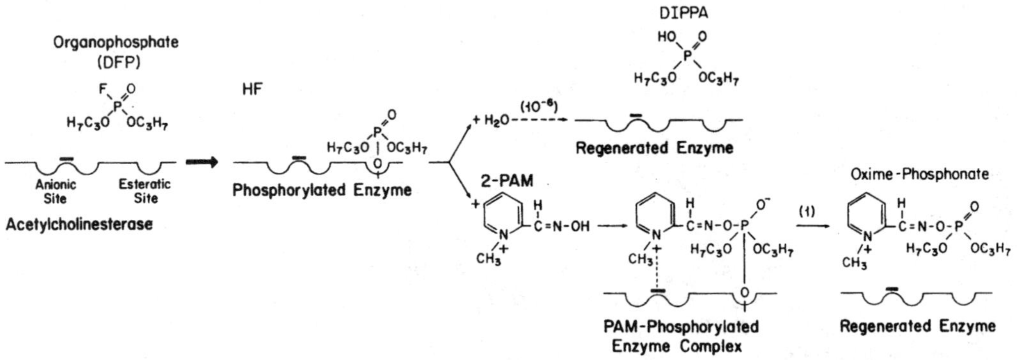

FIG. 7.8—Interaction of organophosphate diisopropyl fluorophosphate (DFP) with AChE and reversal by pralidoxime (2-PAM). DFP interacts irreversibly with the esteratic site of AChE to yield a phosphorylated enzyme complex with virtually no spontaneous release of diisopropylphosphoric acid (DIPPA) and regeneration of active enzyme. However, 2-PAM and other oximes can interact with the phosphorylated enzyme complex via electrostatic binding at the anionic site of AChE and binding at the P atom; the oxime-phosphonate is split off, yielding a regenerated enzyme. The numbers in parentheses refer to relative rates of reactions (Taylor 1990a; Inestrosa and Perelman 1990; Massoulie et al. 1993).

Antagonists and Antidotes

ATROPINE. Because atropine blocks muscarinic receptors, it not only lessens severity of the parasympathomimetic effects but also increases the quantity of organophosphate required to produce death; e.g., the ratio of the median lethal dose (LD_{50}) of sarin in atropine-treated dogs to the LD_{50} in nonatropinized dogs may be 150:1 (DeCandole and McPhail 1957). These ratios vary with the animal species and organophosphate, but atropine is almost invariably beneficial. In addition, because atropine is a competitive antagonist to ACh, large doses are effective even if administered after exposure to an organophosphate.

CHOLINESTERASE REACTIVATORS. Although phosphorylation of the esteratic site of cholinesterase by organophosphates yields a normally irreversible complex, certain compounds cause a disassociation of the enzyme bondage. Pralidoxime (pyridine-2-aldoxime-methiodide, 2-PAM) was synthesized based on structural requirements postulated by Wilson (1958) to be necessary for a selective antidote to organophosphate-cholinesterase interaction. This compound causes an effective removal of the phosphate group from the enzyme, so the enzyme is reactivated (Fig. 7.8). This and related oxime compounds are undoubtedly the most valuable adjunct to atropine therapy in treating organophosphate poisoning; e.g., pretreatment of animals with 2-PAM increases by several times the LD_{50} of various organophosphates. If atropine is given in conjunction with 2-PAM, the lethal dose is increased many more times.

Similarly, animals previously exposed to toxic doses of organophosphates experience considerable improvement after treatment with 2-PAM. In dogs, 10-20 mg/kg 2-PAM administered by slow IV injection is usually effective; this dose may have to be repeated. In horses and cattle, 20 mg/kg and 10-40 mg/kg respectively are used. Since 2-PAM significantly reverses the combination of organophosphate with cholinesterase, the reactivated enzyme can then perform its normal function. The phosphorylated enzyme complex tends to age with time and to become resistant to reactivation by oximes. Thus treatment with 2-PAM should not be delayed once organophosphate intoxication is diagnosed. Although treatment with 2-PAM alone has been used successfully in human incidences of organophosphate poisoning, atropine should always be used first to block muscarinic receptor sites.

Various other reactivator oximes such as pyridine-2-aldoxime dodecaiodide (designed for CNS effects), monoisonitrosoacetone, and diacetylmonoxime have also been investigated. Oxime reactivators are probably ineffective in antagonizing the carbamate cholinesterase inhibitors and in some cases apparently can act synergistically.

CLINICAL USES OF ORGANOPHOSPHATES. Organophosphorus compounds have achieved widespread use as anthelmintics and pesticides because they are highly toxic to a wide variety of internal and external parasites. Their introduction in the late 1940s and 1950s had considerable impact on pest control. Concurrent with their widespread use, however, is the potential for immediate and/or delayed damage to humans, domestic animals, and wildlife. The ecologic impact of organophosphate pesticides has received considerable attention from various conservation organizations, and there is some evidence that certain of the compounds may be tumorigenic when given in large doses to experimental animals. Dichlorvos-impregnated collars can occasionally cause hypersensitivity skin reactions on the animal's neck and, less frequently, on pet owners.

Organophosphates such as DFP and TEPP have been used locally to constrict the pupil in human patients for treatment of glaucoma; DFP (0.1% in peanut oil) and echothiophate (phospholine iodide, 0.03-0.25% solutions) are sometimes used for this purpose in dogs. Effects of these compounds are relatively long lasting and the dosage must be carefully controlled.

PRECAUTIONARY NOTE ABOUT CLINICAL USES OF CHOLINESTERASE INHIBITORS. As repeatedly emphasized, cholinesterase inhibitors are highly reactive molecules capable of influencing functions of cholinergic nerves throughout the body. This is particularly true with the organophosphates. At no time should their clinical use be considered as an innocuous procedure. Care should always be taken by the clinician to insure that the patient is not exposed either to drugs that are metabolized by cholinesterase (e.g., succinylcholine) or to other cholinesterase inhibitors (e.g., pesticide dips or sprays) for several days before and after administering either a reversible or irreversible anticholinesterase agent. If not, serious and even fatal synergistic interactions can occur (Hines et al. 1967). Other types of drugs (e.g., phenothiazine tranquilizers) may decrease cholinesterase activity as a potential side effect; their concurrent use with anticholinesterase drugs should be avoided or closely monitored.

Severely ill, debilitated animals should not be exposed to a cholinesterase inhibitor except in emergency situations. If hepatic disease is presented, synthesis of cholinesterase may be markedly reduced and effects of cholinesterase inhibitors can be intensified and/or prolonged. Respiratory illness may be exacerbated by excessive bronchiolar constriction and secretion. Abortion may occur, particularly during the latter gestational periods. Because of the potency of cholinesterase inhibitors, especially organophosphate compounds, care should always be taken to closely follow the manufacturer's individual dosage recommendations and procedural directions.

PARASYMPATHOLYTIC AGENTS. Parasympatholytic drugs prevent ACh from producing its characteristic effects in structures innervated by postganglionic parasympathetic nerves. They also inhibit effects of ACh on smooth muscle cells that respond to ACh but lack cholinergic innervation; i.e., these drugs inhibit the muscarinic actions of ACh and related cholinergic agonists. In fact, "muscarinic blocking" or "antimuscarinic" is actually more completely descriptive of the effects of this group of drugs than is "parasympatholytic," because muscarinic receptors are blocked irrespective of whether they are innervated by a parasympathetic nerve. Clinically, however, these drugs are used almost exclusively for their parasympatholytic activities. This group of drugs includes atropine and related alkaloids and numerous synthetically derived compounds.

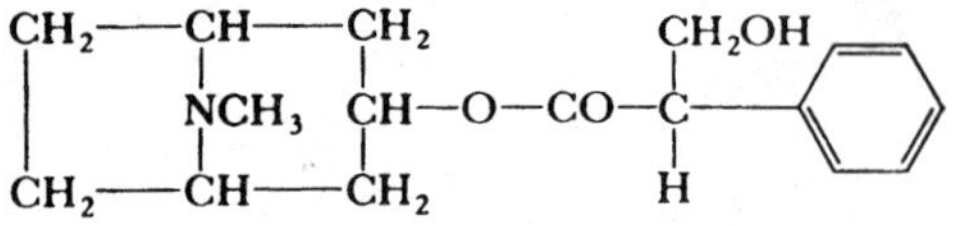

Atropine

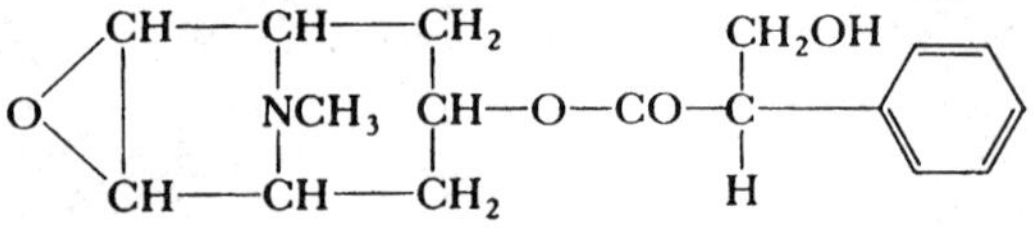

Scopolamine

FIG. 7.9

Atropine and Scopolamine. Atropine, the prototypical muscarinic blocking agent, is an alkaloid extracted from the belladonna plants that belong to the Solanaceae (potato family) and include *Atropa belladonna* (deadly nightshade), *Datura stramonium* (jimsonweed), and *Hyoscyamus niger* (henbane). Alkaloids obtained from *Atropa belladonna* are atropine (which is a racemic mixture of *d*-hyoscyamine and *l*-hyoscyamine, racemization occurring during the extraction procedure), scopolamine (*l*-hyoscine), and others of lesser significance. Because atropine is actually an equal mixture of *d*- and *l*-hyoscyamine and the dextro form of hyoscyamine is biologically inactive, a given quantity of atropine is about one-half as potent as the same quantity of *l*-hyoscyamine. Despite the inactive dextrorotatory component, atropine is nevertheless effective in very small doses. Chemically, the atropine molecule consists of two components joined through an ester linkage: tropine, which is an organic base, and tropic acid. Other related alkaloids also contain the aromatic tropic acid moiety combined by ester linkage to either tropine or another organic base, scopine. The chemical structures of atropine and scopolamine are given in Fig. 7.9.

MECHANISM OF ACTION. *Atropine Sulfate,* USP, *Scopolamine Hydrobromide,* USP (Hyoscine), and other related alkaloids interact with muscarinic receptors of effector cells and by occupying these sites prevent ACh from affixing to the receptor area. Physiologic responses to parasympathetic nerve impulses are thereby attenuated. Pharmacologic effects of exogenously administered ACh and other muscarinic agonists are similarly blocked by atropine and scopolamine. Although muscarinic receptors have been divided into M_1, M_2, M_3 and perhaps other subtypes (Chassaing et al. 1984; Brown 1990), the utility of this nomenclature to clinical veterinary medicine is unclear at this time.

Blockade of muscarinic receptors of smooth muscle, cardiac muscle, and glands by atropine-like drugs involves a competitive antagonism. Therefore, large doses of ACh or other cholinomimetic drugs (e.g., carbachol, cholinesterase inhibitors) can overcome or surmount inhibitory effects of atropine at these sites.

Although atropine and related compounds act immediately distal to all postganglionic cholinergic nerve endings, this block is not equally effective throughout the body. Salivary and cholinergic sweat glands are quite susceptible to small doses of atropine, whereas somewhat larger doses are required for a vagolytic effect upon the heart. GI and urinary tract smooth muscles are less sensitive to atropine, and even larger dosages are required to inhibit gastric secretion. Except for effects on salivation and cholinergic sweating, it is difficult to achieve a selective action on targeted structures without concurrently inducing side effects on other, more susceptible sites. Net pharmacologic effects of atropinic drugs in a particular organ are influenced by the relative dominance of parasympathetic or sympathetic tone in that structure. After cholinergic impulses are blocked, adrenergic nerves become dominant and sympathomimetic-like effects may contribute to the final effect.

Pharmacologic Effects

CARDIOVASCULAR SYSTEM. The usual therapeutic doses of atropine do not markedly affect blood pressure; however, pulse rate is altered. Tachycardia is the dominant effect, and large doses of atropine invariably produce an increased heart rate. Small doses may initially produce a slight slowing of heart rate, but this effect is believed to be due to transient stimulation of vagal nuclei of the medulla oblongata and perhaps to transient stimulation of peripheral receptors prior to their block (Averill and Lamb 1959; Ashford et al. 1962). The ease with which atropine produces tachycardia is dependent in part upon the degree of vagal tone of the individual patient. Because atropine blocks transmission of vagal impulses to the heart, animals with a preexisting high vagal tone would show a relatively greater tachycardia than those with low vagal tone.

Cardiac output tends to increase with atropine primarily because of increase in heart rate. Arterial blood pressure either remains unchanged or increases slightly in a normal animal. In animals exposed to exogenous ACh or other cholinomimetics (e.g., cholinesterase inhibitors), atropine can cause a relative increase in blood pressure, because muscarinic effects of the agonists will be blocked. Also, atropine unmasks the hypertensive response to high experimental doses of cholinergic agonists resulting from their nicotinic effects (see Fig. 7.3).

Because atropine blocks the cardiac vagus, it markedly reduces or abolishes cardiac inhibitory effects of drugs acting through a vagal mechanism and will attenuate vagal-mediated reflex responses. Accordingly, the pressor effects of epinephrine and norepinephrine are accentuated in atropinized animals by blockade of the cardiac limb of vagal-baroreceptor reflexes. Large doses of atropine are directly depressant to the myocardium and also cause cutaneous dilation as a result of a direct vascular smooth muscle effect.

GI SYSTEM. Atropine causes relaxation of GI smooth muscle by inhibiting contractile effects of cholinergic nerve impulses. Thus, atropine and related drugs can be helpful in treatment of intestinal spasm and hypermotility. Inhibition of smooth muscle motility extends from stomach to colon, although the degree of blockade may not be uniform. Insofar as rumen motility is concerned, adequate doses are consistently inhibitory, and atropine is one of the few agents that can be relied upon to produce cessation of rumen motility.

Secretions of the GI tract are also blocked by atropine. Salivation is reduced quite markedly. Similarly, secretions of intestinal mucosa are inhibited; however, gastric secretions are reduced only with exceedingly high doses that also block virtually all other muscarinic sites.

BRONCHIOLES. Cholinergic innervation to the bronchioles modulates secretion of mucus and contraction of bronchiolar smooth muscle. Atropine and other drugs of the belladonna group block effects of cholinergic impulses and thereby decrease secretions and increase luminal diameter of the bronchioles. The dilator action of atropine is valuable in counteracting constriction of bronchioles following overdosage of a parasympathomimetic drug.

Atropine often will give temporary symptomatic relief from the dyspnea of "heaves" in horses, and it has been used by unscrupulous individuals for this purpose. A SC dose of atropine (30 mg) may produce immediate relief in the horse lasting 1-3 hours; however, dyspnea worsens after effect of the drug has terminated. A crude form of the drug, such as belladonna leaves, administered orally produces its effect within 30 minutes, with a duration of about 24 hours. When atropine medication is suspected, the following signs should be detectable: dry oral mucosa, dilated and relatively fixed pupils, and tachycardia.

OCULAR EFFECTS. Atropine blocks the cholinergically innervated sphincter muscle of the iris and the ciliary muscle of the lens, resulting in mydriasis and cycloplegia after topical or systemic administration. Because atropine blocks cholinergic effects, adrenergic nerve impulses dominate and the pupil actively dilates. Atropine is contraindicated in the presence of increased intraocular pressure from acute angle glaucoma because the drainage system of the anterior chamber of the eye is impeded during mydriasis.

URINARY TRACT. Atropine relaxes smooth muscle of the urinary tract. The spasmolytic effect on the ureters may be of some benefit in treatment of renal colic. Atropine tends to cause urine retention because it inhibits smooth muscle tone. This effect may be of some use in reducing frequency of micturition that accompanies cystitis; however, the deleterious effects of only partially emptying the bladder should be considered.

SWEAT GLANDS. Atropine has a definite anhydrotic action in species such as humans, who have a cholinergic mechanism in control of sweat secretion, and a large dose may cause a hyperpyrexic response. Atropine does not directly affect sweating in species that have adrenergic mechanisms in control of sweating (e.g., equines) and has minimal effect in species that do not use cholinergic sweating as an important component of thermoregulation.

CENTRAL NERVOUS SYSTEM. Therapeutic doses of atropine produce minimal effects on the CNS. Excessive doses may cause hallucinations and disorientation in humans and mania and excitement in domestic animals. Excessive motor activity followed by depression and coma is the usual sequence of events. Scopolamine has a slight sedative effect; when combined with morphine it produces analgesia and amnesia (referred to as "twilight sleep") in human patients. These effects of scopolamine usually are not detectable in domestic animals. While small doses may be depressant in dogs and cats, larger doses produce delirium and excitement in these species and also in horses.

TOXICOLOGY. There is considerable interspecies variation in the toxicity of belladonna and atropine; the route of administration is also important. Herbivora are usually more resistant than Carnivora. Certain strains of rabbits are quite resistant to a diet of belladonna leaves, because an esterase (atropinase) of the liver hydrolyzes and thus inactivates atropine. However, rabbits fed on such a diet may prove toxic if eaten by dogs, cats, or humans because of the large amount of alkaloid present in muscle tissues. Horses, cattle, and goats are relatively resistant to belladonna when it is administered orally; however, these species are quite susceptible to atropine when it is injected parenterally. Swine are not resistant to belladonna ingested from eating the deadly nightshade plant.

Signs of atropine poisoning are similar in all mammalian species. Dry mouth, thirst, dysphagia, constipation, mydriasis, tachycardia, hyperpnea, restlessness, delirium, ataxia, and muscle trembling may be observed; convulsions, respiratory depression, and respiratory failure lead to death. A drop of urine obtained from a patient suspected of atropine toxicosis causes mydriasis when placed in the eye of a cat. Also, the tested pupil will not constrict when exposed to light, while the untreated eye will. This simple procedure may prove helpful in the differential diagnosis of belladonna intoxication.

CLINICAL USES. Parasympatholytic drugs are used to control smooth muscle spasm as antispasmodics or spasmolytics. Antispasmodics can be used to decrease or abolish GI hypermotility and depress hypertonicity of the uterus, urinary bladder, ureter, bile duct, and bronchioles. Parasympatholytics are not as effective as epinephrine or other adrenergic amines in dilating the bronchioles, but atropine is effective in antagonizing excessive cholinergic stimulation at these sites.

Atropine is used routinely as an adjunct to general anesthesia, particularly with inhalant anesthetics, to decrease salivary and airway secretions. Also, atropine is frequently given in conjunction with morphine to reduce salivary secretions that may be produced by the latter drug. When used prior to anesthesia, the dose of atropine in dogs is 0.045 mg/kg, administered subcutaneously.

The newer inhalant anesthetics produce minimal respiratory irritation, and bronchiolar secretions are considerably less pronounced than with older agents like ether. Thus the routine preoperative use of atropine in all patients has been questioned, especially because this drug may increase the potential for certain cardiac arrhythmias. Moreover, use of atropine in cattle often results in several days of inappetence concomitant with postoperative rumen stasis (Garner et al. 1975). In the horse, use of atropine is sometimes questioned because of the possibility of reducing intestinal motility to the degree that colic develops (Klavano 1975). However, some clinicians cautiously use IV atropine (0.01 mg/kg) to prevent the second degree heart block induced by xylazine in horses. Because of the incidence or potential for anesthesia-associated tachyarrhythmias with atropine, glycopyrrolate (see below) has been advocated as an alternative to atropine for muscarinic blockade in routine preanesthetic medication.

Atropine is used routinely to facilitate ophthalmoscopic examination of internal ocular structures and functions and also for treatment of various ocular disorders. Homatropine hydrobromide, because of its shorter duration of action, has largely replaced atropine for ophthalmoscopic purposes in human patients. Application of a few drops of 1-2% solution of atropine into the conjunctival sac causes mydriasis within 15-20 minutes. Maximum pupillary dilation occurs in about 2 hours and may be detectable for several days. The time course of the cycloplegic action of atropine is similar to that of mydriatic action. Mydriatics like atropine are helpful in preventing or breaking down adhesions between the iris and the lens when used alternately with miotics.

Atropine is an essential antidote to anticholinesterase overdosage or poisoning.

Synthetic Muscarinic Blocking Agents. Synthetic muscarinic blocking agents were chemically synthesized in attempts to find atropine substitutes that would act selectively at certain muscarinic sites and therefore would have fewer undesirable side effects than the alkaloids.

GLYCOPYRROLATE. *Glycopyrrolate,* NF, is a quaternary nitrogen anticholinergic agent that has received attention for preanesthetic use in veterinary medicine.

It exerts potent antimuscarinic activity but reportedly has some benefits when compared to atropine. The tachycardia response associated with muscarinic block at the SA node, e.g., seems to be somewhat less of a problem with glycopyrrolate. In dogs this compound effectively diminishes the volume and acidity of gastric secretions and reduces intestinal motility; it also reduces and controls excessive secretions of the respiratory tract. Similar control of respiratory secretions by glycopyrrolate has been reported in cats, and its duration of action exceeds that of atropine. Also, because of its more polar nitrogen moiety, glycopyrrolate penetrates the blood-brain barrier less effectively than atropine, with less propensity for unwanted CNS side effects. The muscarinic blocking action of glycopyrrolate is evident within minutes after IV injection. After SC or IM administration, maximal effects generally develop within 30-45 minutes, and vagal blocking action can be demonstrated for 2-3 hours, while the antisialagogue response is evident for up to 7 hours. The glycopyrrolate dose is approximately 10 μg/kg by SC, IM, or IV routes, administered 15 minutes or so prior to anesthetic induction (Short et al. 1974; Short and Miller 1978).

HOMATROPINE. *Homatropine Hydrobromide,* USP, is similar in structure to atropine except that it is an ester of mandelic acid rather than of tropic acid. Homatropine closely resembles atropine in most of its pharmacologic actions, particularly the ocular effects. Mydriasis and cycloplegia are produced in the eye by topical application of a 2-5% solution of homatropine, but these effects last for a shorter duration than those resulting from atropine. Homatropine produces fewer side effects on cardiovascular and GI functions than atropine and is considerably less toxic than the parent drug.

METHANTHELINE, PROPANTHELINE, AND METHYLATROPINE. *Methantheline Bromide,* USP, *Propantheline Bromide,* USP, and *Methylatropine Nitrate,* INN, are quaternary amines used primarily as smooth muscle relaxants. Because of the charged quaternary group, these compounds do not cross the blood-brain barrier to an appreciable extent. Accordingly, they are considerably less effective than atropine as antagonists to organophosphates, since the CNS effects of the latter agents would not be blocked. In addition to muscarinic blocking effects, these drugs act as autonomic ganglionic blockers, which most likely contributes to their antispasmodic effect on GI smooth muscle.

AUTONOMIC GANGLIONIC BLOCKING DRUGS

Mechanisms. Following Langley's investigations in 1889, it has been known that small doses of nicotine stimulate autonomic ganglion cells, and larger doses block the transmitter function of ACh at these same sites. Therefore, the cholinergic receptors of ganglion neurons have been classified as nicotinic. Considerable evidence is now available indicating that impulse transmission within autonomic ganglia is much more complicated than originally believed. Studies have demonstrated a secondary excitatory cholinergic pathway in autonomic ganglia that is apparently muscarinic, and an inhibitory catecholaminergic mechanism has also been recorded (Eccles and Libet 1961; Libet 1970; Akasu 1992). The different putative pathways involved in synaptic transmission in sympathetic autonomic ganglia are shown schematically in Fig. 7.10.

The physiologic purposes of these different ganglionic pathways are poorly understood. Evidence for participation of different types of receptors has been gained primarily from studies of sympathetic ganglia. Parasympathetic ganglia are studied less frequently because of their poor accessibility. The nicotinic receptor represents the primary ganglionic transmission pathway present in all autonomic ganglia. The muscarinic receptors on the postganglionic neuron may facilitate impulse transmission events that are normally dominated by the nicotinic mechanisms. The adrenergic component may act as a modulator to prevent excessive impulse traffic.

Nicotine. Nicotine is an alkaloid obtained from leaves of the tobacco plant. Nicotine sulfate, the most commonly produced salt, is available commercially in an aqueous solution that contains 40% alkaloidal nicotine. This solution long has been designated by the proprietary name of Blackleaf 40. Nicotine was the original autonomic ganglionic blocking agent; however, it is not used clinically for this purpose. Nicotine first stimulates and then in higher doses blocks nicotinic receptors by producing a persistent depolarization of the receptor area.

PHARMACOLOGIC EFFECTS

CENTRAL NERVOUS SYSTEM. Alkaloidal nicotine is an extremely toxic substance that transiently stimulates and then severely depresses the CNS. Death is from respiratory paralysis of the diaphragm and chest muscles resulting from descending paralysis and depolarization block of the nerve-muscle junction of skeletal muscle. Nicotine is absorbed through the chitinous shell of insects after a direct spraying or after contacting a sprayed surface and kills by paralysis of the CNS.

CARDIOVASCULAR SYSTEM. Both cardioaccelerator and cardioinhibitor nerves are activated by small amounts of nicotine, which cause stimulation of all autonomic ganglia. Since the cardioinhibitor nerve (vagus) is predominant, the response to a small dose, or the initial response to a large dose, of nicotine is a decreased pulse rate. Because of paralysis of all autonomic ganglia, the heart rate returns toward normal after a large dose has taken full effect, and a relative

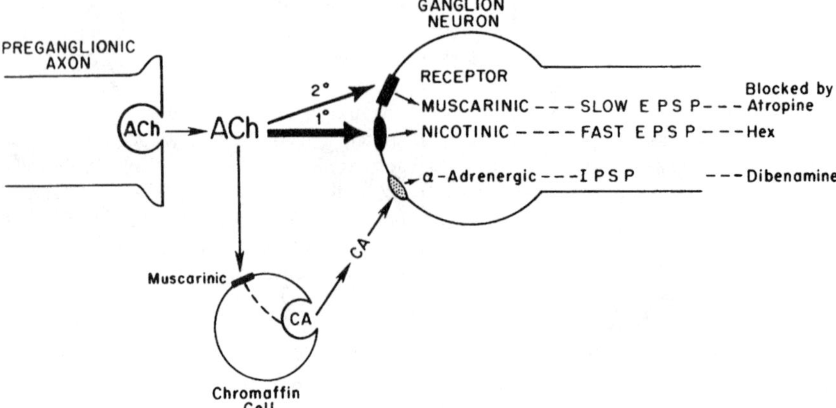

FIG. 7.10—Impulse transmission in sympathetic autonomic ganglia. ACh is discharged from the preganglionic nerve terminal and interacts with a nicotinic receptor on the ganglionic neuron to cause a rapid depolarization measured electrically as a fast excitatory postsynaptic potential (EPSP). ACh also interacts with a muscarinic receptor on the ganglionic neuron to cause a delayed depolarization measured electrically as a slow EPSP. In addition, ACh activates nearby chromaffin cells through a muscarinic receptor, which results in a release of catecholamine (CA: dopamine or epinephrine). CA interacts with an α receptor on the ganglionic neuron to cause an inhibitory (hyperpolarization) response measured electrically as an inhibitory postsynaptic potential (IPSP). 1° and 2° indicate primary (nicotinic) and secondary (muscarinic) pathways of excitatory ganglionic impulses respectively; hex = hexamethonium (Eccles and Libet 1961; Libet 1970; Nishi 1974; Akasu 1992).

tachycardia may result. Similarly, small doses of nicotine can cause a pressor response, by stimulation of the predominating sympathetic ganglia that furnish postganglionic vasoconstrictor fibers to arterioles. However, peripheral vasodilation results from ganglionic block after large doses.

GASTROINTESTINAL. Nicotine activates the smooth muscles and secretory glands of the digestive tract with the following clinical signs: excessive salivation, increased gastric secretion, vomiting, increased peristalsis, and defecation.

SKELETAL MUSCLE. Nicotine initially stimulates nicotinic receptors of the motor end-plate and in large doses produces a depolarizing muscle paralysis. This effect has been used in attempts to immobilize wild animals for capture.

ACUTE NICOTINE POISONING. Accidental ingestion of the 40% solution of nicotine sulfate results in acute toxicosis characterized by excitement, hyperpnea, salivation, pulse rate irregularities, diarrhea, and emesis in species that vomit. After this transient stimulatory phase, a depressed state occurs and is characterized by incoordination, tachycardia, dyspnea, coma, and death from respiratory paralysis.

Synthetic Ganglionic Blocking Agents. Nicotine is not used clinically in animals or humans as a ganglion blocker, since it activates nicotinic sites before blockage occurs and affects functions of various tissues throughout the body. However, several drugs have been discovered that preferentially block autonomic ganglia by a nondepolarizing (competitive) mechanism. These drugs are bis-quaternary compounds, i.e.,

$$(CH3)_3\overset{+}{N}(CH_2)_n\overset{+}{N}(CH_3)_3$$

In cases where the methonium groups are separated by 5 or 6 methylene groups (i.e., n = 5 or 6), a selective site of action at autonomic ganglia is obtained. These compounds interact with nicotinic receptors of the ganglion cells and thereby block impulse transmission across the ganglionic synapse. Dissimilar to nicotine, they do not cause initial depolarization. Members of this group of ganglionic blocking agents include hexamethonium (n = 6; *C*-6), pentamethonium (n = 5; *C*-5), chlorisondamine, pentolinium, trimethidinium, and azamethonium. In addition, there are several other ganglionic blocking drugs that are not bis-quaternary compounds, such as tetraethylammonium ions, mecamylamine, and pempidine.

PHARMACOLOGIC EFFECTS AND USES. Because of the blockade of impulse transmission at the ganglia, effects of ganglionic blocking agents are manifested on effector organs innervated by the postganglionic fibers of the sympathetic or parasympathetic nervous system. The overall effects of these agents on various functions are dependent upon the predominance of sympathetic or parasympathetic tone in a particular structure, as indicated in Table 7.3 (Taylor 1990b). Because the GI system functions predominantly under parasympathetic tone, ganglionic blockade will result in a relative parasympatholytic effect; decreased motility and secre-

TABLE 7.3—Usual predominance of sympathetic or parasympathetic tone in various tissues and consequent effects of autonomic ganglionic blockade

Structures	Predominant tone	Effects of ganglionic blockade
Cardiovascular		Overall depression; block reflexogenic changes
Arterioles	Sympathetic	Vasodilation: increased peripheral blood flow; hypotension
Veins	Sympathetic	Vasodilation: pooling of blood; decreased venous return
Heart	Parasympathetic	Tachycardia
Gastrointestinal	Parasympathetic	Decreased tone and motility; constipation
Eye		
Iris	Parasympathetic	Mydriasis
Ciliary muscle	Parasympathetic	Cycloplegia
Urinary bladder	Parasympathetic	Urinary retention
Salivary glands	Parasympathetic	Dry mouth
Sweat glands	Sympathetic	Annidrosis

Source: Taylor 1990b.

tions and constipation result. Similarly, because heart rate is under dominant vagal tone, a relative tachycardia may result. However, because tone of peripheral blood vessels is dominated by sympathetic impulses, vasodilation and hypotension occur after ganglionic block. Similarly, the output of catecholamines by the adrenal medulla is also reduced. Severe postural hypotension and even syncope may result. The hypotensive effect has occasionally been utilized in surgery to decrease the chance of hemorrhage in highly vascular areas; however, ganglionic blocking agents have achieved no significant purpose in clinical veterinary medicine.

REFERENCES

Adams, H. R. 1996. Physiologic, pathophysiologic, and therapeutic implications of endogenous nitric oxide. J Am Vet Med Assoc 209:1297-1302.

Akasu, T. 1992. Synaptic transmission and modulation in parasympathetic ganglia. Japan J Physiol 42:839-64.

Ashford, A., Penn, G. B., Ross, J. W. 1962. Cholinergic activity of atropine. Nature 193:1082-83.

Averill, K. H., Lamb, L. E. 1959. Less commonly recognized actions of atropine on cardiac rhythm. Am J Med Sci 237:304-18.

Bijman, J., Quinton, P. M. 1984. Predominantly beta-adrenergic control of equine sweating. Am J Physiol 15:R349-R353.

Brown, J. H. 1990. Atropine, scopolamine, and related antimuscarinic drugs. In A. G. Gilman, T. W. Rall, A. S. Nies, P. Taylor, eds., The Pharmacologic Basis of Therapeutics, 8th ed., pp. 150-65. New York: Pergamon.

Chassaing, C., Dureng, G., Baissat, J., Duchene-Marullaz, P. 1984. Pharmacological evidence for cardiac muscarinic receptor subtypes. Life Sci 35(17):1739-45.

Dale, H. H. 1914. The action of certain esters and ethers of choline, and their relation to muscarine. J Pharmacol Exp Ther 6:147-90.

De Candole, C. A., McPhail, M. K. 1957. Sarin and paraoxon antagonism in different species. Can J Biochem Physiol 35:1071-83.

Eccles, R. M., Libet, B. 1961. Origin and blockade of the synaptic responses of curarized sympathetic ganglia. J Physiol (Lond) 157:484-503.

Eldefrawi, M. E. 1974. In J. I. Hubbard, ed., The Peripheral Nervous System, p. 181. New York: Plenum.

Furchgott, R. F., Zawadzki, J. V. 1980. The obligatory role of endothelial cells in the relaxation of arterial smooth muscle by acetylcholine. Nature 288:373-76.

Garner, H. E., Mather, E. C., Hoover, T. R., et al. 1975. Anesthesia of bulls undergoing surgical manipulation of the vas deferentia. Can J Comp Med 39:250-55.

Gutmann, L., Besser, R. 1990. Organophosphate intoxication: pharmacologic, neurophysiologic, clinical, and therapeutic considerations. Sem Neurology 10:46-51.

Hall, L. W., Walker, R. G. 1962. Suspected myasthenia gravis in a dog. Vet Rec 74:501-3.

Hines, J. A., Edds, G. T., Kirkham, W. W., et al. 1967. Potentiation of succinylcholine by organophosphate compounds in horses. J Am Vet Med Assoc 151:54-59.

Hucho, F., Jarv, J., Weise, C. 1991. Substrate-binding sites in acetylcholinesterase. Trends Pharmacol Sci 12:422-26.

Inestrosa, N. C., Perelman, A. 1990. Association of acetylcholinesterase with the cell surface. J Membr Biol 118:1-9.

Khromov-Borisov, N. V., Michelson, M. J. 1966. The mutual disposition of choline receptors of locomotor muscles, and the changes in their disposition in the course of evolution. Pharmacol Rev 18:1051-90.

Klavano, P. A. 1975. Proc Am Assoc Equine Pract, p. 149.

Lambert, D. G. 1993. Signal transduction: G proteins and second messengers. Br J Anaesth 71:86-95.

Lefkowitz, R. J., Hoffman, B. B., Taylor, P. 1990. Neurohumoral transmission: the autonomic and somatic nervous systems. In A. G. Gilman, T. W. Rall, A. S. Nies, P. Taylor, eds., The Pharmacological Basis of Therapeutics, 8th ed., p. 109. New York: Pergamon.

Libet, B. 1970. Generation of slow inhibitory and excitatory postsynaptic potentials. Fed Proc 29:1945-56.

Lowenstein, C. J., Dinerman, J. L., Snyder, S. H. 1994. Nitric oxide: a physiologic messenger. Ann Intern Med 120:227-37.

Marlow, C. A. 1977. Myasthenia gravis in a dog [letter]. Vet Rec 101:123.

Martyn, J. A. J., White, D. A., Gronert, G. A., Jaffe, R. S., Ward, J. M. 1992. Up-and-down regulation of skeletal muscle acetylcholine receptors. Anesthesiology 76:822-43.

Massoulie, J., Pezzementi, L., Bon, S., Krejci, E., Vallette, F. M. 1993. Molecular and cellular biology of cholinesterases. Prog Neurobiol 41:31-91.

Nishi, S. 1974. In J. I. Hubbard, ed., The Peripheral Nervous System, p. 225. New York: Plenum.

Rand, M. J., Stafford, A. 1967. In W. S. Root and F. G. Hofman, eds., Physiological Pharmacology. Vol. 3, The Nervous System. Parc C, Autonomic Nervous System Drugs, p. 1. New York: Academic Press.

Short, C. E., Miller, R. L. 1978. Comparative evaluation of the anticholinergic agent glycopyrrolate as a preanesthetic agent. Vet Med Small Anim Clin 73(10):1269-73.

Short, C. E., Paddleford, R. R., Cloyd, G. D. 1974. Glycopyrrolate for prevention of pulmonary complications during anesthesia. Mod Vet Pract 55:194-96.

Sprecher, D. J., Leman, A. D., Carlisle, S. 1975. Effects of parasympathomimetics on porcine stillbirth. Am J Vet Res 36:1331-33.

Taylor, P. 1990a. Anticholinesterase agents. In A. G. Gilman, T. W. Rall, A. S. Nies, P. Taylor, eds., The Pharmacological Basis of Therapeutics, 8th ed., pp. 131-49. New York: Pergamon.

———. 1990b. Agents acting at the neuromuscular junction and autonomic ganglia. In A. G. Gilman, T. W. Rall, A. S. Nies, P. Taylor, eds., The Pharmacological Basis of Therapeutics, 8th ed., pp. 166-86. New York: Pergamon.

———. 1991. The cholinesterases. J Biol Chem 266:4025-28.

Volle, R. L. 1971. In J. R. DiPalma, ed., Drill's Pharmacology in Medicine, 4th ed., p. 584. New York: McGraw-Hill.

Wilson, I. B. 1954. In W. D. McElroy and B. Glass, eds., Symposium on the Mechanism of Enzyme Action, p. 642. Baltimore: Greenwood.

———. 1958. A specific antidote for nerve gas and insecticide (alkylphosphate) intoxication. Neurology 8:41-43.

Wilson, I. B., Hatch, M. A., Ginsburg, S. 1960. Carbamylation of acetylcholinesterase. J Biol Chem 235:2312-15.

8 NEUROMUSCULAR BLOCKING AGENTS

H. RICHARD ADAMS

Development
The Nicotinic Receptor and Structure-Activity Relationships
Impulse Transmission at the Somatic Neuromuscular Junction
Physiologic and Anatomic Considerations
Pharmacologic Considerations
Postjunctional Mechanisms of Neuromuscular Blockade
Competitive (Nondepolarizing) Agents
Depolarizing Agents
Pharmacologic Effects of Neuromuscular Blocking Agents
Skeletal Muscle
Autonomic Effects
Histamine Release
Central Nervous System
Cardiovascular Effects
Ocular Effects
Serum Potassium
Pharmacokinetics
Interactions
Clinical Use
Margin of Safety of Neuromuscular Transmission
Clinical Reversal of Neuromuscular Paralysis

Numerous drugs have been identified that inhibit transmission of nerve impulses at the somatic neuromuscular junction. Neuromuscular blocking agents used clinically act by interfering with the effectiveness of the endogenous neurotransmitter acetylcholine (ACh) to activate nicotinic cholinergic receptors of skeletal muscle cells. The end results of this action are skeletal muscle paralysis and muscular relaxation. Neuromuscular blocking agents are most often used as adjuvants to anesthesia to facilitate tracheal intubation, abdominal muscle relaxation, and orthopedic manipulations, and as part of balanced anesthesia procedures to reduce the amount of general anesthetic required.

DEVELOPMENT. Development of neuromuscular blocking drugs originated with the discovery of curare, a tarlike mixture of plant material used as a poison by South American Indians. The actual ingredients of the poison for arrows, blowgun darts, and spears were known only to the local "pharmacist," who was often the tribal medicine man or witch doctor. Thus the botanical preparations obtained by explorers could not be identified as to content; they were simply classified according to the containers in which they were packaged. Tubo-, para-, or bamboo-curare was contained in cutoff bamboo tubes; this mixture was usually obtained from southern Amazon tribes. The plant origin of tubecurare preparations was primarily Menispermaceae (*Chondodendron tomentosum*). Calabash-curare was packaged in hollow gourds or calabashes; it was the most active preparation. Pot-curare came in small earthenware pottery from the central part of the Amazon basin; this concoction often contained plants other than Menispermaceae. The most important constituent isolated from curare is *d*-tubocurarine. Complete discussions of the colorful and interesting history of curare have been presented by McIntyre (1972) and Waser (1972).

Original studies in the nineteenth century by Claude Bernard (1856) demonstrated that curare prevented the muscle contraction elicited by stimulation of the motor nerve. It did not, however, affect the central nervous system (CNS), prevent response to direct stimulation of the muscle, or depress axonal conductance. It was proposed that curare acted at the nerve-muscle junction. Reports since then have substantiated, clarified, and extended observations concerning the neuromuscular blocking properties of curare alkaloids. Early results stimulated active research into the chemical structural requirements of curare-like compounds, leading to the discovery of other types of neuromuscular blocking agents.

THE NICOTINIC RECEPTOR AND STRUCTURE-ACTIVITY RELATIONSHIPS. Neuromuscular blocking agents possess chemical structural groups that allow interaction of the agent with the nicotinic cholinergic receptor. However, these drugs cause distinctly different effects from the endogenous mediator ACh. One group of neuromuscular blocking drugs, competitive agents, occupies the receptor so that ACh cannot act. The other group, depolarizing agents, acts in a more complicated manner and initially causes depolarization before blockage occurs.

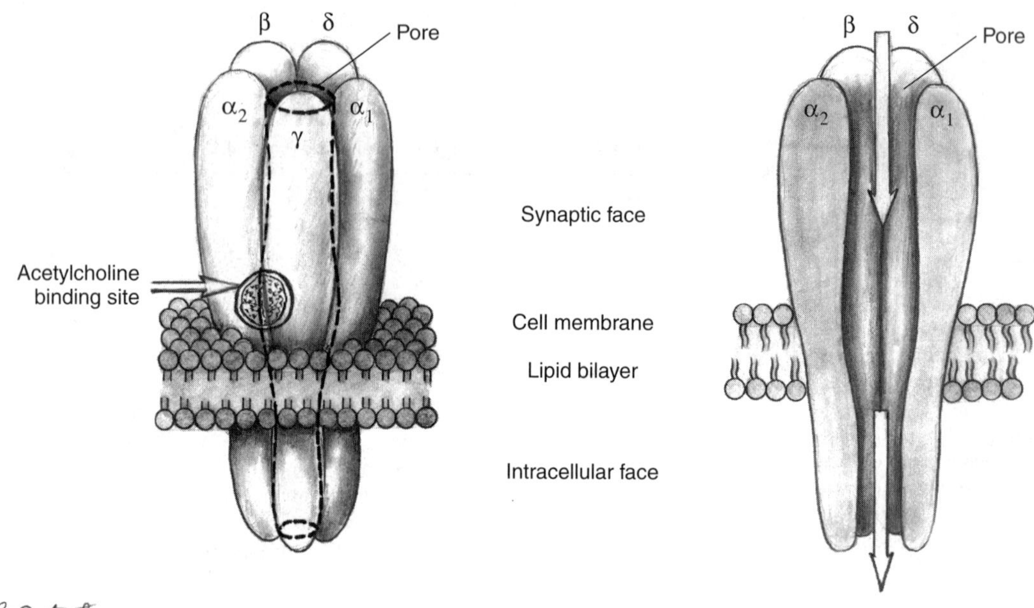

FIG. 8.1—Schematic representation of the nicotinic cholinergic receptor. The receptor is embedded across the cell membrane lipid bylayer, presenting a synaptic face to the neuroeffector junction between the neuron and innervated cell, and an intracellular face within the cytoplasm. The receptor comprises a pentameric configuration of four separate subunits with a stoichiometric ratio of $\alpha_2\beta\gamma\delta$; in adult muscle $\alpha_2\beta\varepsilon\delta$. The α subunits contain the primary ligand binding sites for recognition of acetylcholine and related agents. Subunit arrangement forms an internal pore that allows passage of select ions upon receptor activation and resulting membrane depolarization (see text). Redrawn from Unwin et al. (1988) by Dr. Gheorghe M. Constantinescu, University of Missouri.

Based on general chemical structural characteristics, Bovet (1951) placed neuromuscular blocking agents into two large categories. One group is characterized by large, bulky, and nonflexible molecules; members of this group include *d*-tubocurarine, dimethyl (or trimethyl) tubocurarine, gallamine, and pancuronium, all of which produce a competitive (nondepolarizing) block. The other group is characterized by long, slender, flexible molecules that allow free bond rotation. Decamethonium and succinylcholine are in this group; these agents cause a depolarizing block. The dichotomy in basic structural arrangement of competitive and depolarizing agents has been offered as a partial explanation for dissimilar effects evoked by interaction of these agents with the nicotinic cholinergic receptor.

The proposed charge distribution of the cholinergic receptor was shown in Chap. 7, and a schematic of the nicotinic cholinergic receptor is illustrated in Fig. 8.1. Among other requirements, receptors contain anionic (negatively charged) binding sites separated by set distances. These negative sites are essential for electrostatic bonding of the cationic (positively charged) nitrogen moiety of ACh (and exogenous chemicals) to the receptors.

Occupation of negative binding sites by ACh activates influx of Na^+ and efflux of K^+ along their respective concentration gradients, resulting in membrane excitation. Occupation of these sites by the molecularly rigid competitive agents stabilizes the receptors so that the membrane pores are not easily affected. Depolarizing agents initially act similarly to ACh. Because of their flexible structure, they allow initial channel activation but for some reason cause a persistent short-circuiting of the receptor so that additional changes in electrical potential are not achieved.

Different investigative groups have now isolated the nicotinic cholinergic receptor from the electric eel and electric ray (Taylor 1990a,b; Unwin et al. 1988) and also from mammalian skeletal muscle (Dolly and Barnard 1977). The cobra neurotoxin, α-bungarotoxin, binds irreversibly and with high specificity to ligand recognition sites of the nicotinic receptor. This toxin, when radiolabeled, has allowed remarkable achievements in isolating and characterizing the nicotinic receptor (Kistler et al. 1982).

The nicotinic cholinoceptor is a pentameric asymmetric molecule (8 × 14 nm) of about 250 kilodaltons that spans the bilayer of the postjunctional membrane (Fig. 8.1). The receptor comprises five individual subunits in a stoichiometric ratio of $\alpha_2\beta\gamma\delta$; the γ-subunit is replaced by an ε-subunit in muscle from adult animals. Each subunit has an extracellular and intracellular

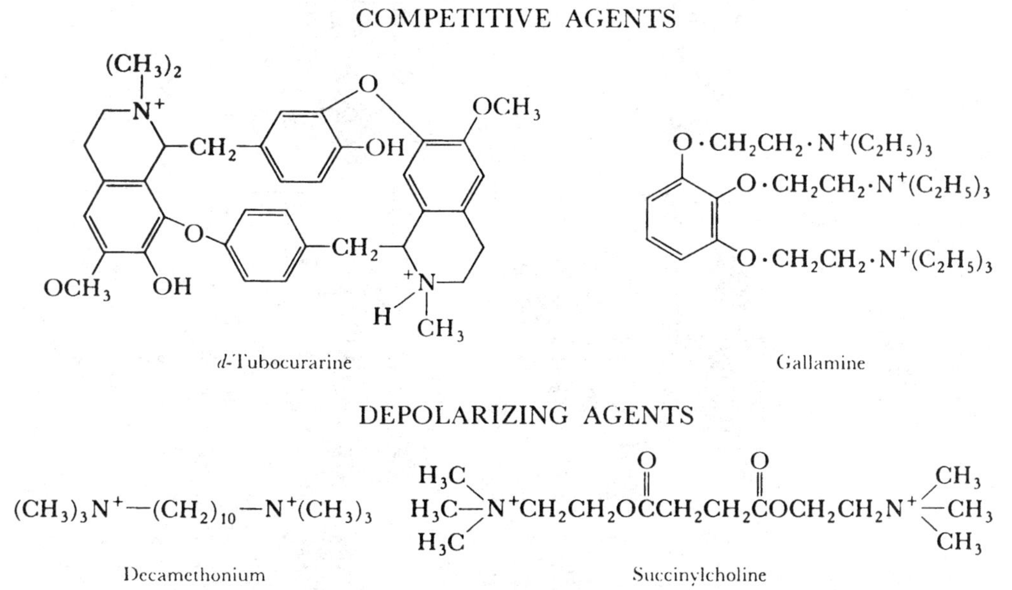

COMPETITIVE AGENTS

d-Tubocurarine

Gallamine

DEPOLARIZING AGENTS

$(CH_3)_3N^+—(CH_2)_{10}—N^+(CH_3)_3$

Decamethonium

$(H_3C)_3N^+CH_2CH_2OCOCH_2CH_2COOCH_2CH_2N^+(CH_3)_3$

Succinylcholine

FIG. 8.2—Chemical structures of some commonly used neuromuscular blocking agents.

exposure and also contains sequences of hydrophobic amino acids that are the likely regions embedded within the membrane bilayer (Taylor 1990b). In vivo, the pentamerous receptor complex occurs as a dimer or couplet, with two adjacent receptors connected via a disulfide bond between two δ-subunits. The five subunits of each monomere receptor complex are elongated perpendicular to the postjunctional membrane and are arranged circumferentially to form a rosette around a central lumen (Fig. 8.1). This central transmembrane channel of the receptor complex represents the previously discussed membrane pore for ion fluxes instigated by agonist activation of the receptor. Agonist and antagonist binding sites are believed to be restricted to the α-subunits (Kistler et al. 1982). Whereas acetylcholine evokes receptor activation upon binding to the α-subunits, occupation of these same sites by antagonists prevents effective receptor activation. The muscle becomes paralyzed, whether in response to a competitive blocking agent or to transient activation by a depolarizing blocking agent.

Chemical structures of several commonly used neuromuscular blocking agents are shown in Fig. 8.2 to demonstrate structural differences of the competitive and depolarizing types.

IMPULSE TRANSMISSION AT THE SOMATIC NEUROMUSCULAR JUNCTION. Prior to discussing neuromuscular blocking agents, impulse transmission at the somatic neuromuscular junction will be reviewed in relation to sites of action of different drugs. General concepts of cholinergic transmission were mentioned in Chap. 5.

Physiologic and Anatomic Considerations. The majority of investigations aimed at identifying cholinergic transmission mechanisms have utilized the somatic myoneural junction because of its accessibility in relation to other cholinergic synapses. Although the term synapse was originally proposed to describe a nerve-nerve junction, it is commonly used in reference to neuroeffector junctions. A representation of a somatic neuromuscular junction (synapse) and proposed sites of drug actions are shown in Fig. 8.3.

Terminal branches of a motor axon lose their myelin sheath and embed within invaginations of the cell membrane of the skeletal muscle cell; these invaginations are termed synaptic gutters. A synaptic gutter, in turn, has many microinvaginations or infoldings called either junctional folds or subneural folds. The space within the synaptic gutter between the nerve ending and the muscle cell is called the synaptic cleft. "Presynaptic" refers to axonal elements, whereas "postsynaptic" refers to constituents of the muscle cell.

Vesicular structures localized within cholinergic nerve terminals represent storage sites for ACh (see Chap. 5). As an axonal action potential arrives at the nerve terminal, it increases the release of ACh from the storage vesicles into the synaptic cleft. This step (excitation-secretion coupling) is dependent upon mobilization into the neuron of extracellular Ca^{++} and/or Ca^{++} bound to superficial membrane areas of the nerve terminal. Released ACh reacts with the specialized

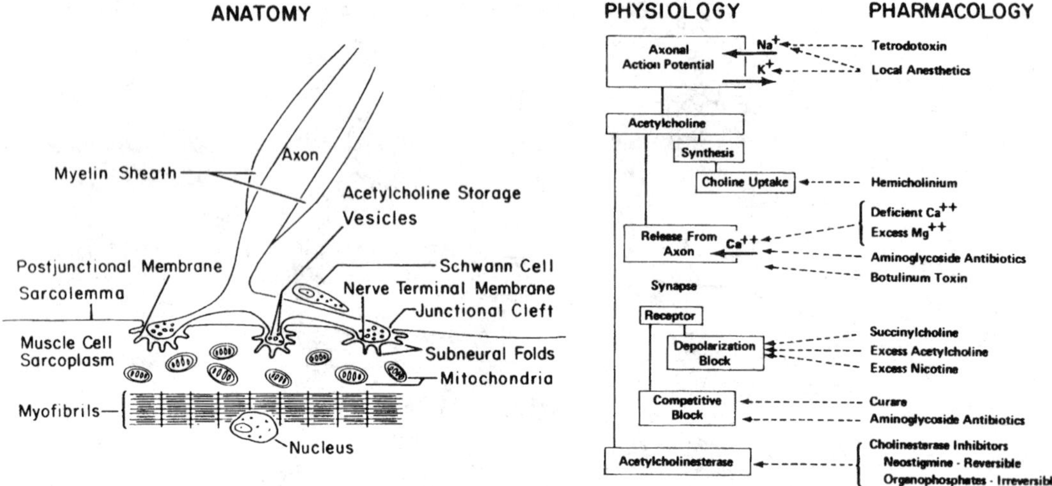

FIG. 8.3—Schematic representation of a somatic neuromuscular junction (synapse), related physiologic pathways, and proposed sites of action of various pharmacologic agents. An axonal action potential (AP) is characterized by an influx of Na^+ and an efflux of K^+. Tetrodotoxin and saxitoxin inactivate Na^+ pathways. Local anesthetics block Na^+ and K^+ pathways. Choline uptake into the neuron is blocked by hemicholinium; synthesis of ACh is prevented. As the AP arrives at the nerve terminal, it instigates inward movement of Ca^{++}; this triggers discharge of ACh into the junctional cleft. A lack of Ca^{++} or an excess of Mg^{++} decreases release of ACh. Aminoglycoside antibiotics also interfere with Ca^{++}-dependent release of ACh. Botulinum toxin inhibits ACh release. Decamethonium and succinylcholine (depolarizing neuromuscular blocking agents) cause persistent depolarization block of the motor end-plate region, as do excess ACh and nicotine. Curare, gallamine, and pancuronium (competitive neuromuscular blocking agents) compete with ACh for postjunctional receptors but do not cause depolarization. Aminoglycoside antibiotics decrease sensitivity of the postjunctional membrane to ACh. Catabolism of ACh by acetylcholinesterase is inhibited by reversible and irreversible anticholinesterase agents; ACh accumulates. (Modified from Taylor 1990b; Couteaux 1972.)

receptor sites of the subsynaptic membrane and causes depolarization of this structure. Cholinergic receptors of somatic myoneural junctions are classified as nicotinic; they are located on the outer membrane of the muscle cell and are almost exclusively confined to the postsynaptic membrane. After denervation, sensitivity to ACh spreads over the entire muscle cell.

Extraneuronal ACh is rapidly metabolized by acetylcholinesterase (AChE) enzyme, which is localized in the end-plate region. Although it may be bound in part to presynaptic elements, it is concentrated at the postsynaptic membrane (Inestrosa and Perelman 1990; Hucho et al 1991).

ACh-induced depolarization of the subsynaptic membrane can be measured as a change in the electric potential of the motor end-plate region, i.e., the end-plate potential. If the end-plate potential is above a threshold level, it instigates a muscle action potential, leading to depolarization of immediately adjacent areas of the postsynaptic membrane. Subsequently, the muscle action potential is propagated along the remainder of the muscle cell membrane. Contraction of skeletal muscle is initiated by the muscle action potential causing a release of Ca^{++} into the cytoplasm from the intracellularly located sarcoplasmic reticulum. The increased free intracellular Ca^{++} binds with troponin, a protein constituent of tropomyosin that acts to inhibit sliding of the actin and myosin filaments during the resting state. Ca^{++}-bound troponin loses this function; cross-linkages are formed between actin and myosin, and sliding of these filaments occurs. The muscle contracts. Miniature end-plate potentials represent subthreshold depolarizations of the motor end-plate region that are due to spontaneous neuronal release of small amounts of ACh; they do not instigate muscle contraction.

Pharmacologic Considerations. The neuromuscular junction is quite susceptible to alteration by selective pharmacologic agents. Various drugs, toxins, electrolytes, and other agents alter in different manners the synthesis, storage, release, receptor interactions, and catabolism of ACh. Several important factors affecting cholinergic transmission are outlined in Fig. 8.3.

Hemicholinium and triethylcholine compete with choline for choline uptake into cholinergic neurons; ACh synthesis is prevented by lack of choline. Existing vesicular stores of ACh are exhausted upon nerve stimulation, and a gradual weakening and eventual paralysis result.

Nerve conduction is affected by only a few substances. The local anesthetics, when in high concentration and immediate contact with the axon, act to stabilize the nerve by inactivating both Na^+ and K^+ channels so that axonal action potential propagation is halted. The pufferfish poison tetrodotoxin and the shellfish poison saxitoxin decrease the permeability of excitable membranes to Na^+ (but not K^+); thus axonal action potentials are not generated, and paralysis results. These toxins do not cause an initial depolarization of nerves; they act noncompetitively, are approximately 100,000 times more potent than cocaine or procaine, and are frequently used in research. Clinical cases of fatal food poisoning have been attributed to ingestion of these substances.

Botulinum toxin is an extremely potent substance (lethal dose for a mouse is 4×10^7 molecules) produced by *Clostridium botulinum.* It is ingested occasionally by humans and lower animals and often is fatal. It decreases the amount of ACh released from cholinergic nerves.

Magnesium ions (Mg^{++}) interfere with release of ACh from the nerve terminal by competing for the transport mechanisms responsible for mobilization of Ca^{++} into the nerve. Mg^{++} uncouples the excitation-secretion coupling process. An insufficient concentration of Ca^{++} produces similar effects. Mg^{++} also acts postsynaptically to decrease the effectiveness of ACh to activate receptors.

Aminoglycoside antibiotics (i.e., neomycin-streptomycin group) inhibit release of ACh from motor nerves by decreasing availability of Ca^{++} at superficial membrane binding sites of the axonal terminal, thereby inhibiting the excitation-secretion coupling process. These antibiotics also reduce sensitivity of the postsynaptic membrane to ACh (Adams 1984).

Cholinesterase inhibitors (see Chap. 7) decrease the hydrolytic activity of AChE and pseudocholinesterase (Taylor 1990a, 1991). ACh rapidly accumulates at receptor sites. Muscle fasciculations, spasms, convulsions, and eventually apnea occur after overdosage with cholinesterase inhibitors.

POSTJUNCTIONAL MECHANISMS OF NEUROMUSCULAR BLOCKADE. The preceding examples illustrate the complexity of neuromuscular transmission and the numerous sites susceptible to many agents and toxins. However, the pharmacologic effects of clinically useful neuromuscular blocking drugs can best be explained by a direct alteration of the effectiveness of ACh to activate postjunctional (postsynaptic) receptors. According to the mechanisms of postjunctional action, neuromuscular blocking agents are classified as either a competitive (nondepolarizing) or a depolarizing agent.

Competitive (Nondepolarizing) Agents. These drugs compete with ACh for available cholinergic receptors at the postsynaptic membrane and, by occupying these receptors, prevent the transmitter function of ACh. A prototype of this group of drugs is *d*-tubocurarine (*Tubocurarine Chloride,* USP, Tubarine). Other similarly acting agents include *Metocurine Iodide,* USP (Metubine) (previously referred to as dimethyl tubocurarine iodide), gallamine (*Gallamine Triethiodide,* USP, Flaxedil), and pancuronium (*Pancuronium Bromide,* Pavulon). Newer competitive agents include fazadinium, a rapidly acting drug that undergoes hepatic biotransformation; alcuronium; atracurium, a synthetic compound that undergoes spontaneous and enzymatic degradation to inactive metabolites; and vecuronium, a derivative of pancuronium (Taylor 1990b; Agoston et al. 1992). Pharmacologic characteristics of several neuromuscular blocking agents are summarized in Table 8.1.

Ultrarefined experimental techniques (e.g., measurement of single-cell electrical activity and microionophoretic application of drugs) have verified the primary site of action of competitive blocking agents as the subsynaptic membrane (Bowen 1972; Hubbard and Quastel 1973). At this region, *d*-tubocurarine is believed to have the same or similar affinity as ACh for cholinergic receptors; i.e., *d*-tubocurarine can interact with these sites as well as ACh. However, *d*-tubocurarine does not exhibit agonistic properties, whereas ACh is extremely active. Although *d*-tubocurarine binds to or in some way interlocks with the cholinoceptors, it has no depolarizing activity and therefore does not cause an end-plate potential. Moreover, the *d*-tubocurarine-receptor interaction renders affected receptors unavailable for interaction with ACh. ACh-induced end-plate potentials are reduced to subthreshold levels or abolished in curarized muscles. In the absence of induced end-plate potentials and subsequent muscle action potentials, the muscle relaxes and is, in fact, paralyzed.

The competitive mechanism of nondepolarizing agents is readily demonstrable. In essence, *d*-tubocurarine blockade of receptors increases the threshold of the end-plate region to ACh. Increasing the concentration of ACh will overcome the blockade produced by *d*-tubocurarine and restore neuromuscular transmission. Correspondingly, reincreasing the concentration of *d*-tubocurarine will again decrease the effectiveness of ACh.

Based on competitive interaction between nondepolarizing agents and ACh, cholinesterase inhibitors were found to be effective in antagonizing effects of these blocking agents. Cholinesterase inhibitors prevent the enzymatic catabolism of ACh. More ACh is available for interaction with cholinoceptors and thereby decreases effectiveness of competitive blocking agents. This relationship has been exploited clinically in successful efforts to terminate effects of nondepolarizing agents. However, cholinesterase inhibitors do not antagonize effects of the other class of neuromuscular blockers, the depolarizing drugs.

Depolarizing Agents. *Succinylcholine Chloride,* USP (Quelcin, Anectine, Sucostrin, Suxamethonium), and *Decamethonium Bromide,* USP (Syncurine, C-10), are members of this group of agents. These drugs exert their skeletal muscle paralyzing effects by interfering with ACh-mediated depolarization of the postsynaptic

Table 8.1—Characteristics of neuromuscular blocking agents

Generic name	Trade name	Chemical class	Duration properties	Onset (min)	Duration (min)	Biotransformation
Depolarizing Agents						
Succinylcholine	Anectine	Choline ester	Ultrashort	<2	6-8	Hydrolysis by plasma cholinesterases
Nondepolarizing (Competitive) Agents						
d-Tubocurarine		Natural alkaloid (cyclic benzylisoquinoline)	Long	4-6	80-120	Renal elimination; liver clearance
Atracurium	Tracrium	Benzylisoquinoline	Intermediate	2-4	30-40	Spontaneous degradation; hydrolysis by plasma cholinesterases
Doxacurium	Nuromax	Benzylisoquinoline	Long	4-6	90-120	Renal elimination; liver metabolism and clearance
Mivacurium	Mivacron	Benzylisoquinoline	Short	2-4	12-18	Hydrolysis by plasma cholinesterases
Pancuronium	Pavulon	Ammonio steroid	Long	4-6	120-180	Renal elimination; liver metabolism and clearance
Pipecuronium	Arduan	Ammonio steroid	Long	2-4	80-100	Renal elimination; liver metabolism and clearance
Rocuronium	Zemuron	Ammonio steroid	Intermediate	1-2	30-40	Liver metabolism; renal elimination
Vecuronium	Norcuron	Ammonio steroid	Intermediate	2-4	30-40	Liver metabolism and clearance; renal elimination

Source: Modified from Taylor 1996.

membrane. In contrast to the well-defined mechanism of the competitive agents, certain aspects of the mechanism(s) of depolarizing neuromuscular blockers are continually debated.

Succinylcholine and related drugs interact with postsynaptic cholinergic receptors but cause distinctly different effects than curare-like drugs. Initially, an end-plate potential and a corresponding muscle action potential are elicited upon exposure to succinylcholine. These depolarization changes in membrane potential are similar to those produced by the endogenous mediator ACh. However, ACh is immediately hydrolyzed by cholinesterase; the postsynaptic membrane repolarizes and is prepared for subsequent activation by additional quanta of ACh. Succinylcholine elicits a prolonged depolarization of the end-plate region that does not allow the subsynaptic membrane to completely repolarize and renders the motor end-plate nonresponsive to the normal action of ACh.

Because of the initial depolarizing action, transient contraction of muscle cells occurs after administration of succinylcholine and related agents. This is characterized in vivo as momentary asynchronous muscle twitches and fasciculations. Because of the persistent depolarization of the postsynaptic membrane, however, subsequent impulse transmissions are blocked and a flaccid type of paralysis ensues. The molecular mechanism(s) of depolarizing neuromuscular blocking agents is not completely understood but may be biphasic.

PHASE I BLOCK. Depolarization of the motor end-plate region by ACh is characterized by increased permeability of the subsynaptic membrane to Na^+ and K^+. As ACh is catabolized by AChE the selective permeability characteristics of the postsynaptic membrane are rapidly reestablished. Repolarization occurs. Succinylcholine, however, causes a persistent increase in permeability of the postsynaptic membrane to Na^+ and K^+. ACh cannot act as a transmitter, and impulse transmission fails. It should be remembered that ACh, when in excess, also causes persistent depolarization block of cholinergic synaptic junctions.

PHASE II BLOCK. Phase II block occurs in some instances after prolonged exposure to a depolarizing agent and is characterized by a change from the depolarizing block to one that in some ways resembles that caused by curare. The actual mechanisms involved are poorly understood and opinion is contradictory as to this transition. Zaimis (1959) believes, e.g., that confusion has occurred because in some species some blocking agents have a "dual mechanism"; i.e., they cause some effects that resemble depolarization block and cause other effects that resemble competitive blockade.

After exposure of isolated nerve-muscle preparations to succinylcholine, the initial peak level of depolarization subsides. Subsequently, the end-plate becomes transiently sensitive to depolarizing agents. Gradually, a competitive-like blockade results and

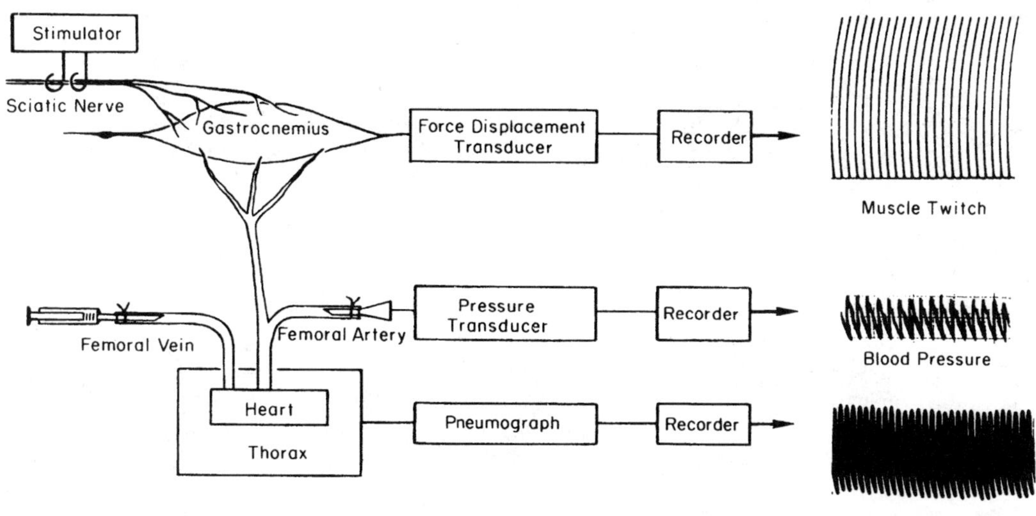

FIG. 8.4—Schematic representation of a sciatic nerve-gastrocnemius muscle preparation in an anesthetized cat. Stimulation of the isolated and decentralized sciatic nerve evokes contraction (muscle twitch) of the gastrocnemius muscle. Femoral arterial blood pressure and respiratory movements can be measured concurrently. Neuromuscular blocking drugs can be administered intravenously and changes in muscle twitch height observed.

seems to be at least partially susceptible to reversal by cholinesterase inhibitors. Tachyphylaxis to depolarizing agents quickly develops and the receptors now appear to be insensitive to ACh. However, the importance of Phase II has not been clearly defined for each depolarizing neuromuscular blocking agent.

As a group the depolarizing neuromuscular blocking agents cause depolarization of receptor areas of muscle fibers sometime during their course of action. Increasing availability of ACh by administration of a cholinesterase inhibitor has no effect or in some cases may actually intensify the neuromuscular block of a depolarizing agent. Just the opposite, cholinesterase inhibitors can be quite effective in antagonizing the competitive block produced by nondepolarizing curaremimetic agents.

PHARMACOLOGIC EFFECTS OF NEUROMUSCULAR BLOCKING AGENTS

Skeletal Muscle

COMPETITIVE NEUROMUSCULAR BLOCKING AGENTS. Nondepolarizing curare-like drugs paralyze skeletal muscle by neuromuscular blockade. These agents interact with nicotinic cholinergic receptors of skeletal muscle cells and render them inaccessible to the transmitter function of ACh. Flaccid paralysis occurs. Neither axonal conductance nor response to direct stimulation of muscle is blocked by curare agents.

A schematic representation of an in vivo nerve-muscle preparation is shown in Fig. 8.4. This sciatic nerve-gastrocnemius muscle preparation of anesthetized cats is often used to examine actions and interactions of neuromuscular blocking agents. In this preparation, stimulation of the sciatic nerve causes contraction (kg of isometric tension) of the gastrocnemius muscle.

Fig. 8.5 demonstrates the neuromuscular blocking effect of *d*-tubocurarine on indirectly stimulated muscle twitch of the sciatic nerve-gastrocnemius muscle preparation of a cat, as described in Fig. 8.4. In this example, muscle twitch quickly decreases after intravenous (IV) injection of *d*-tubocurarine, reaches peak depression within a few minutes, and then gradually returns to normal in approximately 15 minutes. Tubocurarine does not evoke an initial increase in muscle twitch; this lack of facilitation is a consistent finding with nondepolarizing agents. Gallamine, metocurine, and pancuronium produce similar characteristics of neuromuscular paralysis. Metocurine is 3-10 times more active than *d*-tubocurarine, pancuronium is 5-7 times more potent than *d*-tubocurarine, and gallamine is somewhat less active.

Antagonism of the neuromuscular blocking effects of *d*-tubocurarine by administration of a cholinesterase inhibitor, neostigmine, is shown in Fig. 8.5. By comparing the two tracings in this figure, it is readily apparent that neostigmine markedly hastens recovery from the muscle twitch depression caused by *d*-tubocurarine. This antagonistic interaction is primarily attributed to the anticholinesterase activity of neostigmine. Inhibition of cholinesterase delays the catabolic breakdown of ACh and allows its accumulation at receptor

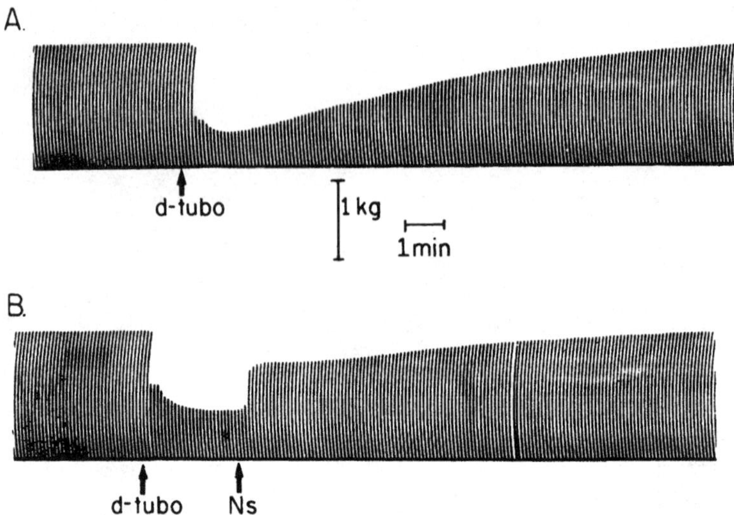

FIG. 8.5—Neuromuscular blocking effect of *d*-tubocurarine (*d*-tubo) and reversal of the *d*-tubo by neostigmine in a sciatic nerve-gastrocnemius muscle preparation of a cat. The cat was anesthetized with pentobarbital; muscle twitch was monitored as described in Fig. 8.4. (A) Typical depression of muscle twitch by *d*-tubo (0.2 mg/kg) administered intravenously at designated arrow. (B) Antagonism of *d*-tubo (0.2 mg/kg) induced depression of muscle twitch by neostigmine (Ns; 0.1 mg/kg). Agents were administered intravenously at arrow. Notice rapid antagonism of the neuromuscular blocking effect of *d*-tubo by Ns. Compare this with the lack of antagonism by Ns of the muscle twitch depressant effect of succinylcholine in Fig. 8.6.

sites. Newly available ACh, now in increased concentration at the post-synaptic membrane, effectively competes with *d*-tubocurarine for the cholinoceptors. ACh-mediated depolarization of the end-plate, muscle action potentials, and muscle contraction are restored; muscle twitch quickly returns to normal.

DEPOLARIZING NEUROMUSCULAR BLOCKING AGENTS. Succinylcholine and decamethonium elicit transient muscle fasciculations prior to causing neuromuscular paralysis. This is due to initial depolarization of the motor end-plate and is characterized in the intact animal by asynchronous muscular contractions of the head, body trunk, and limbs. Fasciculation does not always occur in anesthetized animals.

The in vivo neuromuscular blocking effect of a small dose of succinylcholine in a cat nerve-muscle preparation is shown in Fig. 8.6. Initially, there is a slight and transient facilitory effect of succinylcholine on neuromuscular transmission; muscle twitch height momentarily increases by a small increment as a result of the initial depolarizing effect of the drug. Subsequently, however, muscle twitch rapidly decreases and within 1-2 minutes maximum depressant effect is obtained. Shortly thereafter, the neuromuscular effects of succinylcholine subside and muscle twitch returns to normal within an additional 5-8 minutes. The magnitude and duration of neuromuscular paralysis is dependent upon the dosage of succinylcholine. The relatively short duration of succinylcholine activity is from rapid biotransformation of this drug by plasma pseudocholinesterase. Decamethonium causes similar characteristics of neuromuscular blockade, but the duration of action of this drug is considerably longer than that seen with succinylcholine.

The effects of a cholinesterase inhibitor, neostigmine, on the neuromuscular paralysis produced by succinylcholine are demonstrated in Fig. 8.6. By comparing the two tracings in this figure, it is apparent that neostigmine potentiated the muscle twitch depression evoked by succinylcholine and prolonged recovery from the effects of this agent. This synergistic interaction is primarily attributed to the anticholinesterase activity of neostigmine, resulting in decreased biotransformation of both succinylcholine and endogenous ACh. Thus succinylcholine and ACh are available at receptor sites for longer periods and the duration of depolarizing neuromuscular paralysis is prolonged.

The potency of neuromuscular effects of succinylcholine varies in different species (Hansson 1958), as shown schematically in Fig. 8.7. Bovine and canine species are quite sensitive to succinylcholine, whereas horses and pigs are considerably less responsive. This difference is probably dependent upon species differences in the activity of pseudocholinesterase, the enzyme that biotransforms succinylcholine (Radeleff and Woodard 1956; Palmer et al. 1965). Cattle and sheep, e.g., have considerably less detectable pseudocholinesterase activity than horses and pigs. Administration of purified pseudocholinesterase preparation to dogs increases resistance to succinylcholine (Hall et al. 1953).

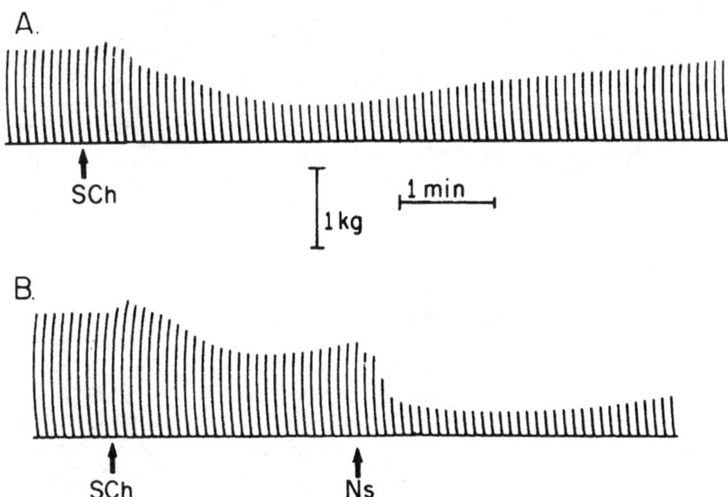

FIG. 8.6—Neuromuscular blocking effect of succinylcholine (SCh) and augmentation of its effect by neostigmine (Ns) in a sciatic nerve-gastrocnemius muscle preparation of a cat. The cat was anesthetized with pentobarbital; muscle twitch was monitored as described in Fig. 8.4. (A) Typical depression of muscle twitch by SCh (0.04 mg/kg) administered intravenously at designated arrow. (B) Augmentation of the muscle twitch depressant effect of SCh (0.04 mg/kg) by Ns (0.1 mg/kg). Agents were administered intravenously at designated arrows. Notice augmentation of the degree and duration of effect of SCh by Ns. Compare this with the antagonism by Ns of the neuromuscular blocking effect of *d*-tubo in Fig. 8.5.

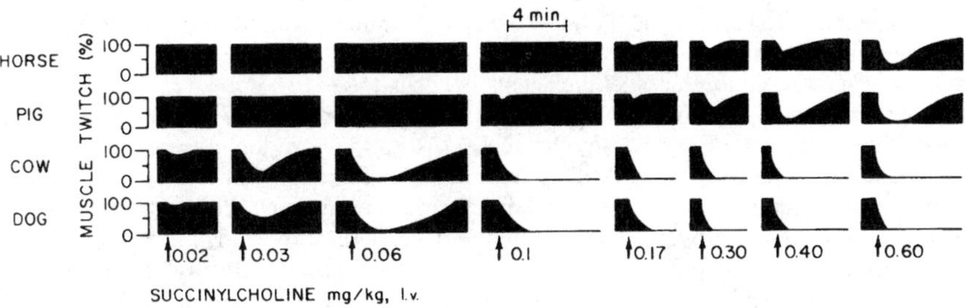

FIG. 8.7—Schematic representations of the neuromuscular blocking effect of succinylcholine iodide in nerve-muscle preparations of different species during barbiturate anesthesia. Notice interspecies differences in degree and duration of paralysis caused by succinylcholine. (Modified from Hansson 1956, after Lumb and Jones 1973.)

Autonomic Effects. Synaptic transmission at autonomic ganglia involves activation by ACh of nicotinic receptors of the postganglionic nerve body (see Chap. 7). It is not surprising, therefore, that neuromuscular blocking agents (which act at somatic nicotinic sites) may also alter ganglionic transmission.

Tubocurarine is an excellent example of a drug selected for site of action at nicotinic receptors of the somatic myoneural junction that as a side effect also acts at ganglionic nicotinic receptors. Tubocurarine interacts with ganglionic receptors, renders them inaccessible to ACh, and thereby increases the threshold of the postganglionic nerve to ACh. However, as a general rule, autonomic ganglia are less sensitive to curare than are the myoneural junctions. Ganglionic impulse transmission involves, at least partially, a muscarinic pathway (see Chap. 7); *d*-tubocurarine has little blocking effect on muscarinic receptors. Thus in most cases it would be anticipated that ganglionic transmission is functional during treatment with curare-like drugs. Nevertheless, hypotension believed to be partly dependent upon ganglionic blockade can occur after administration of *d*-tubocurarine.

Other neuromuscular blocking drugs, both competitive and depolarizing types, have been shown experimentally to alter ganglionic transmission, but in clinically insignificant amounts. Succinylcholine induces transient ganglionic stimulation prior to blockade evoked by larger doses. The former effect may partially explain hypertension that has occurred subsequent to succinylcholine administration.

Parasympathetic effects of neuromuscular blocking agents are usually minimal. Pancuronium has anticholinesterase activity. Succinylcholine and decamethonium are approximately 1000 times and 100 times less potent respectively than ACh in eliciting contraction of guinea pig ileum. In dogs, large doses of succinylcholine induce salivation; this is antagonized by pretreatment with atropine (Hansson 1956).

Histamine Release. Tubocurarine causes release of histamine. The magnitude of this response varies, depending on species, dosage, and rate and route of administration. Intra-arterial infusion of *d*-tubocurarine evokes histamine release in the perfused hind-limb preparation of dogs, and histamine-like wheals can be produced by subdermal and intra-arterial administration of *d*-tubocurarine. In vivo, increased respiratory tract secretions and bronchospasm seen after administration of *d*-tubocurarine have been attributed to histamine release, as has the hypotensive effect of *d*-tubocurarine. Pretreatment with antihistamine drugs antagonizes these side effects; they are not inhibited by atropine or neostigmine.

Metocurine, succinylcholine, decamethonium, and gallamine are very weak histamine-releasing agents.

Central Nervous System. Although synaptic transmission in the brain is altered by direct application of neuromuscular blocking drugs into the brain, CNS effects are nondetectable when these drugs are administered by other routes. Neuromuscular blocking agents do not gain entry into the CNS to any appreciable extent because of the presence of the highly charged quaternary ammonium moieties. Therefore, neither CNS depression nor tranquilization is produced by neuromuscular blocking agents. Nonambulation results only from peripheral myoneural paralysis. This was decisively confirmed when Smith (Smith et al. 1947) allowed himself to be paralyzed with *d*-tubocurarine. At no time during the experiment did he experience hypnosis, tranquilization, amnesia, anesthesia, or analgesia. He simply could not voluntarily breathe or move, an experience described as quite frightful.

Cardiovascular Effects. As outlined above, *d*-tubocurarine often induces hypotension, particularly if rapidly administered to dogs. Slight increases in heart rate and cardiac output have been observed after administration of gallamine, apparently from a vagolytic effect on the heart (Longnecker et al. 1973). Others have reported no significant cardiovascular changes after IV administration of gallamine to anesthetized dogs (Evans et al. 1977). In cats, mild atropine-like effects on the heart were observed after injection of gallamine, pancuronium, and alcuronium chloride (Alloferin) (Hughes and Chapple 1976).

Studies with pancuronium in humans and dogs indicated that this agent evokes slight increases in heart rate, blood pressure, and cardiac output during thiobarbiturate anesthesia (Coleman et al. 1972; Reitan and Warpinski 1975). Cardiovascular effects of this agent were absent if patients were pretreated with atropine. Others have reported no significant cardiovascular changes with pancuronium (Brown et al. 1973). Similarly, studies have indicated that neither pancuronium nor gallamine significantly altered heart rate or blood pressure in anesthetized horses (Klein et al. 1983). Atracurium (up to 0.6 mg/kg) and vecuronium (up to 0.2 mg/kg) were reported to have negligible effects on arterial blood pressure in dogs (Jones 1985).

Succinylcholine usually evokes minimal cardiovascular changes in horses or dogs if administered during general anesthesia; blood pressure remains fairly constant if artificial breathing is provided (Evans et al. 1977; Benson et al. 1979).

Subparalytic doses of succinylcholine increase the arrhythmogenicity of epinephrine during light halothane anesthesia in dogs (Tucker and Munson 1975). In dogs not treated with succinylcholine, an average dose of 4.15 μg/kg epinephrine was required to evoke premature ventricular contractions, whereas an average dose of 1.6 μg/kg epinephrine was the arrhythmogenic dose in dogs pretreated with 0.25 mg/kg succinylcholine. However, *d*-tubocurarine provides a slight protection against epinephrine-induced arrhythmias. Mechanisms involved in these drug interactions have not been clarified. If deemed essential, catecholamines should be used cautiously in patients treated with depolarizing neuromuscular blocking agents.

Also, succinylcholine has been reported to increase susceptibility to the myocardial irritant effects of digitalis preparations, and it has been suggested that succinylcholine may be contraindicated in digitalized patients (Dowdy et al. 1965).

Pronounced cardiovascular side effects have been reported in horses after administration of succinylcholine (Larson et al. 1959; Hofmeyer 1960; Lees and Tavernor 1969). In general, these effects seem to be more pronounced in unanesthetized and nontranquilized animals than during general anesthesia. Severe hypertension, initial bradycardia followed by tachycardia, atrioventricular conduction disturbances, and extrasystoles have been reported, and myocardial damage has been suspected. Early institution of artificial respiration has been reported to block the blood pressure effect. The hypertensive response seems to be at least partially mediated by the succinylcholine-induced dyspnea and the accompanying blood PO_2-PCO_2 disturbances, causing a reflexogenic increase in blood pressure. Direct activation of autonomic ganglia by succinylcholine may also be involved.

It should be remembered that neuromuscular blocking agents do not depress the brain unless or until apnea-induced hypoxia actually causes syncope. Prior to hypoxic states, skeletal muscle paralysis affords no depression whatsoever of conscious centers of the brain of nonanesthetized animals. It seems likely, then, that the novel sensations experienced by conscious animals as they are being paralyzed evoke profound fright. This can cause activation of autonomic centers within the brain. Autonomic discharge may be altered markedly resulting in cardiovascular side effects. Autonomic blocking agents (ganglionic block with hexamethonium, β-adrenergic block with propranolol) substantially decrease the cardiovascular side effects of succinylcholine.

Ocular Effects. Clinically important ocular effects depend upon the pronounced contracture of ocular muscles that occurs after treatment with depolarizing neuromuscular blockers. These agents are contraindicated in glaucoma, since intraocular pressure may be increased.

Serum Potassium. Depolarizing neuromuscular blocking agents cause a release of K^+ from skeletal muscle. Elevation of serum K^+ may result, particularly if repeated injections are given.

Pharmacokinetics. Neuromuscular blocking agents with quaternary nitrogen groups are ionized at all levels of physiologic pH. Therefore, they are highly charged, lipophobic compounds and cross lipoprotein membrane barriers poorly. Little if any absorption occurs after oral administration of these drugs. South American Indians were well aware of this, since they ingested flesh of curare-poisoned animals without concern. Inefficient absorption after oral administration has little importance to modern medicine, however, because these agents should be given by the IV route so that muscle relaxation can be quickly evaluated. Whereas South American Indians were concerned only with one end point, death, and were worried only about underdosage, practitioners are concerned with facilitating muscle relaxation and are extremely concerned with overdosage. Administration of neuromuscular blocking agents should be closely monitored and correlated at all times, with effects observed in the patient.

Intramuscular (IM) injection of neuromuscular blocking agents is occasionally used to immobilize nondomestic animals. Absorption occurs rapidly after IM injection, and effective blood concentrations are obtained shortly thereafter.

Tubocurarine is distributed primarily in the extracellular space throughout body tissues, but it concentrates at myoneural junctional regions (Waser 1967). It penetrates cells poorly because of the charged state of the molecule. The liver and kidney participate in the biologic fate of *d*-tubocurarine; however, duration of action of this agent normally does not depend upon biotransformation. Rather, redistribution of *d*-tubocurarine away from the neuromuscular junction and into nonspecific body compartments is believed to account for the short duration of action of a single dose of this drug. Repeated treatment or excessive amounts of *d*-tubocurarine tends to saturate nonspecific sites. Under these circumstances, renal excretion becomes important as a mechanism for termination of activity of *d*-tubocurarine. If injection must be repeated, less drug is needed to evoke muscle relaxation. Cumulative neuromuscular blockade occurs when injections are repeated, since *d*-tubocurarine is excreted rather slowly by the kidneys.

Gallamine and metocurine are probably handled similarly to *d*-tubocurarine. Gallamine is excreted virtually unchanged in the urine, as are decamethonium and pancuronium. These agents are thought to bind only minimally to tissues. Renal failure markedly prolongs their duration of action.

Atracurium is one of a series of new competitive agents that was developed to overcome pharmacokinetic disadvantages of the older drugs. Atracurium is rapidly inactivated by plasma esterases and also, importantly, by a spontaneous chemical degradation instigated at physiologic pH and body temperature (Table 8.1). Atracurium is therefore noncumulative, and the duration of action of the same dose does not increase with repetitive injections (Agoston et al. 1980). In dogs, Jones (1985) recommended that atracurium be administered initially at 0.5 mg/kg, followed by increments of 0.2 mg/kg. The duration of neuromuscular blocking action of vecuronium, another new agent, is similar to that of atracurium and is about one-third to one-half that of pancuronium. Vecuronium undergoes hepatic biotransformation and is excreted predominantly in the bile; it is somewhat cumulative, and this characteristic can be expected to be more pronounced in the presence of hepatic disease (Jones 1985). Because of its short duration of action and affiliated ease of control, atracurium has become a frequently used neuromuscular blocking agent in veterinary anesthesiology.

Succinylcholine is rapidly disposed of by the body, since it is a suitable substrate for plasma pseudocholinesterase. This enzyme quickly hydrolyzes succinylcholine to the considerably less active metabolite succinylmonocholine. This metabolite is more slowly broken down by pseudocholinesterase to succinic acid and choline, natural body constituents. The interspecies potency of succinylcholine varies considerably. This has been attributed to species differences in activity of pseudocholinesterase.

INTERACTIONS. Various drugs influence the pharmacologic effects of muscle relaxants. Neuromuscular blocking agents themselves alter activity of other neuromuscular agents. As would be expected, competitive agents summate with each other. Similarly, depolarizing agents also interact synergistically with one another. However, tubocurarine decreases the muscle twitch depressant effects of succinylcholine and decamethonium. This is related to persistent occupation of a certain portion of receptors by tubocurarine, although muscle twitch may have recovered (see margin of safety of neuromuscular transmission below). Depolarization of the end-plate by succinylcholine or decamethonium is partially impeded by the stabilizing effects of tubocurarine. Succinylcholine antagonizes the effects of curare as a result of the partial agonistic characteristics of the former agent. These complex antagonistic interactions, however, have no clinical application, since they depend upon complicated treatment and time and dosage schedules. During clinical situations, neuromuscular blocking agents should not be used in attempts to reverse the effects of other types of neuromuscular blocking agents, since potentiation may occur despite experimental results to the contrary.

The interaction of cholinesterase inhibitors with neuromuscular blocking agents has been discussed above. Cholinesterase inhibitors decrease responsiveness to the competitive agents, while they tend to increase intensity and duration of action of depolarizing agents (Sunew and Hicks 1978). Organophosphate pesticides and anthelmintics, carbamates, and any other cholinesterase inhibitor may cause interactions. The phenothiazine family of tranquilizers has some anticholinesterase activity. Use of succinylcholine in a patient exposed to an organophosphate may be particularly hazardous if a phenothiazine tranquilizer has also been administered.

Many general anesthetics, in addition to depressing the CNS, depress impulse transmission at somatic myoneural junctions. Halothane acts synergistically with curare-like drugs but to a lesser extent than ether. Methoxyflurane and pentobarbital also have depressant effects on myoneural transmission events.

Aminoglycoside antibiotics (neomycin, streptomycin, dihydrostreptomycin, kanamycin, gentamicin) decrease the release of ACh from the nerve and also the sensitivity of the end-plate to ACh (Pittinger and Adamson 1972; Adams et al. 1976a). They do not cause depolarization. Their effects in many ways resemble those of low Ca^{++} or excess Mg^{++}. The presynaptic effect of antibiotics is believed to be due to interruption of Ca^{++}-dependent events at the axonal membrane (Adams 1984). Cholinesterase inhibitors such as neostigmine antagonize the post-synaptic depressant effect of these antibiotics. Ca^{++} antagonizes the presynaptic action and is usually more effective than neostigmine in reversing the neuromuscular paralyzing effects of aminoglycoside antibiotics. These antibiotics interact synergistically at the myoneural junction with neuromuscular blocking agents, anesthetics, and other antibiotics. The clinical significance of neuromuscular interactions of antibiotics and other drugs has been well established in humans and has been suggested in lower animals (Adams and Bingham 1971). These subjects have been reviewed (Pittinger et al. 1970; Adams et al. 1976b; Keller et al. 1992).

Different disease states influence pharmacologic effects of neuromuscular blocking agents. Hepatic synthesis of pseudocholinesterase is decreased in the presence of liver disease. The duration of succinylcholine activity will be prolonged if the liver is seriously affected. Administration of purified pseudocholinesterase preparation hastens recovery from effects of succinylcholine (Scholler et al. 1977).

Renal problems delay excretion of *d*-tubocurarine, gallamine, pancuronium, and decamethonium. Anand et al. (1972) successfully reversed persistent gallamine-induced neuromuscular paralysis in a renally incompetent human patient by use of artificial diuresis.

CLINICAL USE. Muscle paralysis proceeds at different rates in different body regions after administration of a neuromuscular blocking agent. Usually, head and neck muscles are affected first, often within 0.25-1 minute after injection. This characteristic is employed in a biologic assay (i.e., head-drop test in rabbits) for determining potency of an unknown concentration of curare. The tail is usually affected with the head and neck. Subsequently, muscles of the limbs are paralyzed, then the deglutition and laryngeal muscles. Abdominal muscles, intercostal muscles, and the diaphragm are then paralyzed in this order. Recovery usually proceeds in the reverse of this sequence (Hall 1971).

Attempts have been made in clinical practice to use the sequential development of muscle paralysis by administering doses of neuromuscular blocking agents adequate to paralyze ambulatory muscle but insufficient to affect the diaphragm. This has not always proved effective, because respiratory insufficiency may still occur, although the diaphragm is seemingly spared. Therefore, it is imperative that apparatus for administering artificial respiration be available when neuromuscular blocking agents are used clinically. To circumvent the need for immediate establishment of an adequate airway and other emergency procedures, it would seem wise to routinely perform tracheal intubation and institute artificial respiration whenever a neuromuscular blocking agent is used.

Muscle relaxants have been used in clinical practice for several purposes: to facilitate tracheal intubation; to paralyze respiratory muscle so that artificial respiration can be easily controlled; to increase muscle relaxation to facilitate surgical access to difficult anatomic regions; to evoke muscle relaxation to facilitate orthopedic manipulations and, particularly, fracture reduction; and as part of balanced anesthesia procedures to reduce the amount of general anesthetic required.

Tracheal intubation may be performed in a nonanesthetized animal immediately after a paralyzing dose of neuromuscular blocking agent has taken effect. Prior administration of a sedative or tranquilizer is advisable for humane reasons and to circumvent potential side effects that may be precipitated by fear reaction to paralysis.

A wide range of dosages of neuromuscular blocking agents has been reported for use of these drugs during anesthesia (Hansson 1956; Tavernor 1971; Lumb and Jones 1973). Often this variance reflects differences in investigative procedures of the original studies, e.g., the use of different anesthetics and sedatives, different salts of the neuromuscular blocking agent, different nerve-muscle preparations, and in some cases the use of nonanesthetized subjects. Neuromuscular blocking agents should be given to effect rather than by bolus administration of a set precalculated dose. It is advisable for these drugs to be administered by titration during anesthesia and to be continuously correlated with muscle relaxation much in the way that barbiturates are administered for induction of general anesthesia.

In dogs, 0.4-0.5 mg/kg *d*-tubocurarine administered intravenously will cause generalized skeletal muscle relaxation, but hypotension frequently occurs as a side effect in this species. In pigs, 0.2-0.3 mg/kg *d*-tubocurarine will usually afford acceptable muscular relaxation; blood pressure effects are less in this species than in the dog. Tubocurarine is somewhat more potent in ruminants; doses of 0.05-0.06 mg/kg have been suggested for use in young lambs and goats.

Approximately 1 mg/kg gallamine causes complete muscle paralysis in both dogs and cats within 1-2 minutes after IV injection and lasts 15-20 minutes. A hypotensive response may be induced in cats with gallamine but is infrequently observed in dogs. In young ruminants (lambs and calves), 0.4 mg/kg gallamine is effective, whereas the dose in horses is 0.5-1 mg/kg.

Solutions of succinylcholine should always be refrigerated and kept on ice in the field, since this agent undergoes spontaneous hydrolysis. Hansson (1956) reported that the IV ED_{50} (dose that reduced muscle twitch by 50%) of succinylcholine in the sciatic nerve-gastrocnemius muscle preparation of anesthetized dogs was 0.045-0.060 mg/kg. This dose did not effectively paralyze the respiratory muscles, however, and 0.085 mg/kg was required to induce transient apnea, whereas 0.11 mg/kg and 0.22 mg/kg were needed to cause apnea for 18-21 minutes and 23-27 minutes respectively. In unanesthetized dogs, IM administration of 0.12 mg/kg succinylcholine caused ataxia in 5 minutes and forced abdominal respiration in 7 minutes; recovery was apparently complete in 30 minutes. In clinical situations, 0.3 mg/kg succinylcholine administered intravenously will usually afford good muscle relaxation in dogs, whereas in the cat, 1 mg/kg may be required. In dogs, Hansson (1956) reported that 0.15 mg/kg succinylcholine was effective in paralyzing the diaphragm during thoracotomy procedures. However, Eyster and Evans (1974) suggested the use of 0.5 mg/kg succinylcholine for muscle relaxation in dogs during thoracotomy for open-heart surgery. This dose was also reported to control muscle twitches evoked by inadvertent stimulation of nerves during use of electrocautery. Duration of paralysis varies and should be closely monitored.

In rhesus monkeys, 1-2 mg/kg succinylcholine administered intravenously has been used for restraint for tuberculosis testing and endotracheal intubation (Lindquist and Lau 1973). In pigs, approximately 2 mg/kg succinylcholine is effective. Much smaller amounts (0.01-0.02 mg/kg) are required in cattle and sheep. Hansson (1956) reported that 0.13-0.18 mg/kg succinylcholine is required to immobilize nonanesthetized horses. However, the generally accepted dose of succinylcholine in horses, when used alone, is 0.088 mg/kg (Lumb and Jones 1973).

Succinylcholine has been used without anesthesia in horses for casting and restraint during brief surgical procedures such as castration. This practice should not be condoned, because no anesthesia is afforded for painful procedures, severe fright is seemingly evoked, and pronounced cardiovascular disturbances and even myocardial damage may result. Succinylcholine should not be used as a sole restraining agent during surgical procedures but only in conjunction with a general or local anesthetic.

Moreover, care should always be taken during the use of neuromuscular blocking agents to ensure that the patient does not simply remain paralyzed after recovery from the anesthetic. This has occurred in human patients and has led to successful lawsuits by patients and receipt of monetary compensation. Although lower animals cannot complain, it behooves us as veterinarians to ensure that our patients are not inadvertently subjected to such excruciatingly painful incidents.

Margin of Safety of Neuromuscular Transmission. The concept of a margin of safety of neuromuscular transmission bears discussion in relation to clinical use of these drugs. It has been estimated that a relatively large percentage of the cholinergic receptors must be occupied by a curare agent before muscle twitch fails. In the cat diaphragm, e.g., muscle twitch is not affected until about 80% of the receptors are blocked by *d*-tubocurarine, and twitch is not completely abolished until about 90% of the receptors are occupied (Waud and Waud 1972). A somewhat greater margin of safety was found in dogs. Accordingly, for recovery of the diaphragm from the effects of a previous injection of *d*-tubocurarine, only a small percentage (5% in dogs, 18% in cats) of the receptors need to be free. Therefore, and most important, although to all outward signs recovery seems complete, over 80% of the receptors can still be blocked.

Recognition of this aspect becomes clinically important in the postoperative recovery room and should be considered in patients that have been exposed to neuromuscular blocking drugs and/or other myoneural depressants such as anesthetics. As a patient regains some control of voluntary muscles, spontaneous respiration returns and may seem completely normal. However, it must be remembered that at this time an extremely small margin of safety of neuromuscular transmission exists. That is, only a small percentage of the postsynaptic receptors are available for interaction with ACh; this small fraction of receptors is now responsible for maintaining muscle contraction. Therefore, if the patient is then exposed to another drug that as a side effect depresses neuromuscular function (even though it may be minimal or even nondetectable normally), disastrous complications may result. Anesthetic mortality has occurred in humans that can be attributed to such interactions. For example, Pridgen (1956) reported the anesthetic deaths of two children who were given neomycin intraperitoneally immediately after completion of successful laparotomies under ether anesthesia. Initially, respiration was adequate, but within a short time after administration of the antibiotic, persistent apnea occurred. Death followed several hours later. It seems likely that the margin of safety of neuromuscular transmission was reduced in these infants by ether, resulting in marked augmentation of the neuromuscular blocking properties of neomycin. Pittinger et al. (1970) estimated a 9% death rate in human patients experiencing antibiotic-induced respiratory problems in conjunction with anesthetics and neuromuscular blocking agents. Apnea and eventual death in a traumatized dog were attributed to antibiotic (dihydrostreptomycin)-induced neuromuscular paralysis (Adams and Bingham 1971).

These examples illustrate potential problems that may be inadvertently introduced in a patient that seemingly is recovering quite well from anesthesia and surgery. The margin of safety of neuromuscular transmission should be considered any time that anesthetics, neuromuscular blocking agents, or any other drug that depresses myoneural function are used in multiple drug regimens.

Clinical Reversal of Neuromuscular Paralysis. Treatment of persistent neuromuscular paralysis and/or treatment of inadvertent overdosage of neuromuscular blocking agents should be approached conservatively (Bevan et al. 1992). The initial step should be immediate artificial respiration and withdrawal of administration of the involved agent. Often, artificial respiration will allow adequate time for the drug to be disposed of by the patient's system. Exposure to other drugs that may synergistically interact with neuromuscular blocking agents should be avoided. If a competitive neuromuscular blocking agent was used, paralysis can usually be effectively antagonized by administration of a cholinesterase inhibitor such as neostigmine or edrophonium (Hildebrand and Howitt 1984). Neostigmine can be administered to small and large animals by slow IV injection at the dose of 0.022 mg/kg. It should be remembered that cholinesterase inhibitors will cause intensification of ACh activity at both muscarinic and nicotinic receptors. Atropine (0.04 mg/kg) should be administered prior to or in conjunction with neostigmine to circumvent the muscarinic effects of the latter drug (Klein et al., 1983; Jones 1985). Care should be taken to ensure that paralysis does not recur after antagonism by neostigmine; additional injection of neostigmine may be required.

Because cardiovascular complications occasionally occur after treatment with atropine and neostigmine, new ideas have evolved in management of persistent paralysis in patients treated with nondepolarizing neuromuscular blocking drugs. These include substitution of quaternary ammonium muscarinic antagonists in place of atropine (to avoid potential CNS effects of atropine) and substitution of pyridostigmine and edrophonium for neostigmine. Pyridostigmine in combination with propantheline or glycopyrrolate, e.g., produced less abrupt changes in heart rate than combined therapy of either atropine-neostigmine or atropine-pyridostigmine. Pyridostigmine (0.05-0.08 mg/kg), a moderately long-acting drug, and edrophonium (0.2-0.4 mg/kg), a short-acting agent, when combined with either propantheline (0.03-0.06 mg/kg) or glycopyrrolate (0.004-0.006 mg/kg), were reported to produce a rapid and effective reversal of pancuronium-induced neuromuscular block in humans, with minimal changes in heart rate and almost no incidence of arrhythmias (Gyermek 1977). The clinical effectiveness of the above regimen in reversing neuromuscular paralysis produced by competitive agents other than pancuronium or in other species should be examined.

A new drug, 4-aminopyridine, was found to antagonize curare-induced neuromuscular block; however, this agent is not a cholinesterase inhibitor. Instead, it evokes release of ACh from the somatic nerve terminal. Advantages of 4-aminopyridine over cholinesterase inhibitors include longer duration of action without muscarinic side effects. Thus concurrent therapy with atropine-like drugs is unnecessary. The CNS excitatory effects of 4-aminopyridine limit its use in doses adequate to completely antagonize curare block. However, this agent markedly potentiates the anticurare activity of cholinesterase inhibitors. This combined therapy of low doses of 4-aminopyridine and a cholinesterase inhibitor has considerable potential application to clinical reversal of the nondepolarizing type of neuromuscular blocking agents (Miller 1979).

Neostigmine or other cholinesterase inhibitors should not be used in attempts to reverse the effects of a depolarizing agent (Sunew and Hicks 1978). Reliable chemical antidotes are not available for this group of agents. Artificial respiration may be required for a prolonged period. Injection of purified pseudocholinesterase preparation has been shown to hasten recovery from the effects of succinylcholine (Scholler et al. 1977).

Because of the small therapeutic index of neuromuscular blocking agents, their clinical use should always be supervised by qualified experienced personnel who are thoroughly familiar with the indications, limitations, hazards, and methods of administration of these highly active drugs.

REFERENCES

Adams, H. R. 1984. Pharmacodynamic actions of antimicrobial agents in host cell membranes. J Am Vet Med Assoc 185:1127-30.

Adams, H. R., Bingham, G. A. 1971. Respiratory arrest associated with dihydrostreptomycin. J Am Vet Med Assoc 159:179-80.

Adams, H. R., Mathew, B. P., Teske, R. H., et al. 1976a. Neuromuscular blocking effects of aminoglycoside antibiotics on fast- and slow-contracting muscles of the cat. Anesth Analg (Cleve) 55:500-507.

Adams, H. R., Teske, R. H., Mercer, H. D. 1976b. Anesthetic-antibiotic interrelationships. J Am Vet Med Assoc 168:409-12.

Agoston, S., Salt, P., Newton, D., et al. 1980. The neuromuscular blocking action of ORG NC 45, a new pancuronium derivative, in anaesthetized patients: a pilot study. Br J Anaesth 52:53S-59S.

Agoston, S., Vandenbrom, R. H. G., Wierda, J. M. K. H. 1992. Clinical pharmacokinetics of neuromuscular blocking drugs. Clin Pharmacokinet 22:94-115.

Anand, J. S., Mehta, R. K., Munshi, C. A., et al. 1972. Reversal of neuromuscular blockade by artificial diuresis: case report. Can Anaesth Soc J 19:651-53.

Benson, G. J., Hartsfield, S. M., Smetzer, D. L., et al. 1979. Physiologic effects of succinylcholine chloride in mechanically ventilated horses anesthetized with halothane in oxygen. Am J Vet Res 40:1411-16.

Bernard, C. 1856. C R Acad Sci (Paris) 43:825.

Bevan, D. R., Donati, F., Kopman, A. F. 1992. Reversal of neuromuscular blockade. Anesthesiology 77:785-805.

Bovet, D. 1951. Some aspects of relationship between chemical constitution and curare-like activity. Ann NY Acad Sci 54:407-37.

Bowen, J. M. 1972. Estimation of the dissociation constant of d-tubocurarine and the receptor for endogenous acetylcholine. J Pharmacol Exp Ther 183:333-40.

Brown, E. M., Smiler, B. G., Plaza, J. A. 1973. Cardiovascular effects of pancuronium. Anesthesiology 38:597-99.

Coleman, A. J., Downing, J. W., Leary, W. P., et al. 1972. The immediate cardiovascular effects of pancuronium, alcuronium and tubocurarine in man. Anaesthesia 27:415-22.

Couteaux, R. 1972. In J. Cheymol, ed., Neuromuscular Blocking and Stimulating Agents, vol. 1 , p. 7. Elmsford, NY: Pergamon.

Dolly, J. O., Barnard, E. A. 1977. Purification and characterization of an acetylcholine receptor from mammalian skeletal muscle. Biochemistry 16:5053-60.

Dowdy, E. G., Duggar, P. N., Fabian, L. W. 1965. Effect of neuromuscular blocking agents on isolated digitalized mammalian hearts. Anesth Analg (Cleve) 44:608-17.

Evans, A. T., Anderson, L. K., Eyster, G. E., et al. 1977. Cardiovascular effects of gallamine triethiodide and succinylcholine chloride during halothane anesthesia in the dog. Am J Vet Res 38:329-31.

Eyster, G. E., Evans, A. T. 1974. In R. W. Kirk, ed., Current Veterinary Therapy, V: Small Animal Practice, p. 255. Philadelphia: W. B. Saunders.

Gyermek, L. 1977. Clinical pharmacology of the reversal of neuromuscular block. Int J Clin Pharmacol 15:456-62.

Hall, L. W., ed. 1971. Wright's Veterinary Anaesthesia and Analgesia, 7th ed., p. 1. Baltimore: Williams & Wilkins.

Hall, L. W., Lehman, H., Silk, E. 1953. Response in dogs to relaxants derived from succinic acid and choline. Br Med J 1:134-36.

Hansson, C. H. 1956. Succinylcholine iodide as a muscle relaxant in veterinary surgery. J Am Vet Med Assoc 128:287-91.

———. 1958. Studies on the effect of succinylcholine in domestic animals. Nord Vet Med 10:201-16.

Hildebrand, S. V., Howitt, G. A. 1984. Antagonism of pancuronium neuromuscular blockade in halothane-anesthetized ponies using neostigmine and edrophonium. Am J Vet Res 45:2276-80.

Hofmeyer, C. F. B. 1960. Some observations on the use of succinylcholine chloride (suxamethonium) in horses with particular reference to the effect on the heart. J S Afr Vet Med Assoc 31:251-59.

Hubbard, J. I., Quastel, D. M. 1973. Micropharmacology of vertebrate neuromuscular transmission. Annu Rev Pharmacol 13:199-216.

Hucho, F., Jarv, J., Weise, C. 1991. Substrate-binding sites in acetylcholinesterase. Trends Pharmacol Sci 12:422-26.

Hughes, R., Chapple, D. J. 1976. Effects of non-depolarizing neuromuscular blocking agents on peripheral autonomic mechanisms in cats. Br J Anaesth 48:59-68.

Inestrosa, N. C., Perelman, A. 1990. Association of acetylcholinesterase with the cell surface. J Membr Biol 118:1-9.

Jones, R. S. 1985. New skeletal muscle relaxants in dogs and cats. J Am Vet Med Assoc 187:281-82.

Keller, R. S., Parker, J. L., Adams, H. R. 1992. Cardiovascular toxicity of antibacterial antibiotics. In D. Acosta, ed., Cardiovascular Toxicology, 2d ed. New York: Raven Press.

Kistler, J., Stroud, R. M., et al. 1982. Structure and function of an acetylcholine receptor. Biophys J 37:371-83.

Klein, L., Hopkins, J., Beck, E., et al. 1983. Cumulative dose responses to gallamine, pancuronium, and neostigmine in halothane-anesthetized horses: neuromuscular and cardiovascular effects. Am J Vet Res 44:786-92.

Larsen, L. H., Loomis, L. N., Steel, J. D. 1959. Muscle relaxants and cardio-vascular damage: with special reference to succinyl-choline chloride. Aust Vet J 35:269-75.

Lees, P., Tavernor, W. D. 1969. The influence of suxamethonium on cardiovascular and respiratory function in the anaesthetized horse. Br J Pharmacol 36:116-31.

Lindquist, P. A., Lau, D. T. 1973. The use of succinylcholine in the handling and restraint of rhesus monkeys (*Macaca mulatta*). Lab Anim Sci 23:562-64.

Longnecker, D. E., Stoetling, R. K., Morrow, A. G. 1973. Cardiac and peripheral vascular effects of gallamine in man. Anesth Analg (Cleve) 52:931-35.

Lumb, W. V., Jones, E. W. 1973. Veterinary Anesthesia, p. 343. Philadelphia: Lea & Febiger.

Martyn, J. A. J., White, D. A., Gronert, G. A., Jaffe, R. S., Ward, J. M. 1992. Up-and-down regulation of skeletal muscle acetylcholine receptors. Anesthesiology 76:822-43.

Massoulie, J., Pezzementi, L., Bon, S., Krejci, E., Vallette, F. M. 1993. Molecular and cellular biology of cholinesterases. Prog Neurobiol 41:31-91.

McIntyre, A. R. 1972. In J. Cheymol, ed., Neuromuscular Blocking and Stimulating Agents, vol. 1, p. 187, Elmsford, NY: Pergamon.

Miller, R. D. 1979. Recent developments with muscles relaxants and their antagonists. Can Anesth Soc J 26:83-93.

Palmer, J. S., Jackson, J. B., Younger, R. L., et al. 1965. Normal cholinesterase activity of the whole blood of the horse and angora goat. Vet Med 58:885-86.

Pittinger, C., Adamson, R. 1972. Antibiotic blockade of neuromuscular function. Annu Rev Pharmacol 12:169-84.

Pittinger, C. B., Eryasa, Y., Adamson, R. 1970. Antibiotic-induced paralysis. Anesth Analg (Cleve) 49:487-501.

Pridgen, J. E. 1956. Respiratory arrest thought to be due to intraperitoneal neomycin. Surgery 40:571-74.

Radeleff, R. D., Woodard, C. T. 1956. Vet Med 51:512.

Reitan, J. A., Warpinski, M. A. 1975. Cardiovascular effects of pancuronium bromide in mongrel dogs. Am J Vet Res 36:1309-11.

Scholler, K. L., Goedde, H. W., Benkmann, H. 1977. The use of serum cholinesterase in succinylcholine apnoea. Can Anaesth Soc J 24:396-400.

Smith, S. M., Brown, H. O., Toman, J. E. P., et al. 1947. Lack of cerebral effects of *d*-tubocurarine. Anesthesiology 8:1-14.

Sunew, K. Y., Hicks, R. G. 1978. Effects of neostigmine and pyridostigmine on duration of succinylcholine action and pseudocholinesterase activity. Anesthesiology 49:188-91.

Tavernor, W. D. 1971. In L. Soma, ed., Textbook of Veterinary Anesthesia, p. 111. Baltimore: Williams & Wilkins.

Taylor, P. 1990a. Anticholinesterase agents. In A. G. Gilman, T. W. Rall, A. S. Nies, P. Taylor, eds., The Pharmacological

Basis of Therapeutics, 8th ed., pp. 131-49. New York: Pergamon Press.
———. 1990b. Agents acting at the neuromuscular junction and autonomic ganglia. In A. G. Gilman, T. W. Rall, A. S. Nies, P. Taylor, eds., The Pharmacological Basis of Therapeutics, 8th ed., pp. 166-86. New York: Pergamon.
———. 1991. The cholinesterases. J Biol Chem 266:4025-28.
———. 1996. Agents acting at the neuromuscular junction and autonomic ganglia. In J. G. Hardman and L. E. Limbird, eds. The Pharmacological Basis of Therapeutics, 9th ed., p. 182. New York: McGraw-Hill.
Tucker, W. K., Munson, E. S. 1975. Effects of succinylcholine and d-tubocurarine on epinephrine-induced arrhythmias during halothane anesthesia in dogs. Anesthesiology 42:41-44.
Unwin, N., Toyoshima, C., Kublaek, E. 1988. Arrangement of the acetylcholine receptor subunits in the resting and desensitized states determined by cryvelectromicroscopy of crystalized Torpedo postsynaptic membranes. J Cell Biol 107:1123-38.
Waser, P. G. 1967. Receptor localization by autoradiographic techniques. Ann NY Acad Sci 144:737-55.
———. 1972. In J. Cheymol, ed., Neuromuscular Blocking and Stimulating Agents, vol. 1, p. 205. Elmsford, NY: Pergamon.
Waud, B. E., Waud, D. R. 1972. The margin of safety of neuromuscular transmission in the muscle of the diaphragm. Anesthesiology 37:417-22.
Whittaker, V. P. 1990. The contribution of drugs and toxins to understanding of cholinergic function. TIPS 11:8-13.
Zaimis, E. J. 1959. In D. Bovet, F. Bovet-Nitti, G. B. Marini-Mettolo, eds., International Symposium on Curare and Curare-like Agents, p. 191. Amsterdam: Elsevier.

SECTION 3

Drugs Acting on the Central Nervous System

9 INTRODUCTION TO DRUGS ACTING ON THE CENTRAL NERVOUS SYSTEM AND PRINCIPLES OF ANESTHESIOLOGY

EUGENE P. STEFFEY

Introduction to CNS Drugs
Neuroanatomy and Neurophysiology
Action of Drugs in the CNS
Principles of Anesthesiology
Anesthetic Use
Anesthesia Classified
Basics of Clinical Anesthesia
Evaluation of the Response to Anesthesia

Drugs that act in the central nervous system (CNS) are of fundamental importance to health care delivery. Some agents are administered to animals to directly improve their well-being. For example, without general anesthesia, modern surgery would not be possible. Some drugs alter behavior and improve animal-human interaction. They may induce sleep or arousal or prevent seizures. Drugs that act in the CNS are sometimes administered in an attempt to understand the cellular and molecular basis for CNS actions (i.e., physiology and pathophysiology) and/or identify the sites and mechanisms of action of other drugs. Finally, CNS actions of some drugs come as unwanted "side effects" when those drugs are used to treat conditions elsewhere in the body. For example, seizures may result from the injection of too much local anesthetic.

The purpose of this chapter is to, first, review principles of organization and function of the CNS. The intent is to lay a foundation from which later discussion on principles and applied aspects of CNS pharmacology can meaningfully follow. Behavior-altering drugs and anesthetics are routinely administered to animals by veterinarians and allied personnel. Appropriate use of these drugs is an important application of our knowledge of CNS pharmacology. Therefore, this chapter will conclude with a review of the principles of contemporary veterinary anesthesiology.

INTRODUCTION TO CNS DRUGS

NEUROANATOMY AND NEUROPHYSIOLOGY. The CNS consists of the brain and spinal cord. As opposed to the peripheral nervous system, which is mainly concerned with relaying sensory information to the brain and conveying signals to the effector organs, the CNS is involved with control and coordination of movement and higher functions such as consciousness and memory. A detailed discussion of neuroanatomy and physiology is beyond the scope of this chapter and is available elsewhere, but a brief review is in order. A great deal of the information to follow has been synthesized from more extensive reviews (Bradley 1989; Guyton and Hall 1996; Nicoll 1998; Bloom 1996; Cooper et al. 1996; Sihra and Nichols 1993; Unwin 1993).

The basic functional unit of the nervous system is the nerve cell, or neuron. The neuron has three parts: a cell body, a dendritic tree, and an axon. The CNS comprises billions of neurons, many of which are linked and form diffuse networks. Because of the complex arrangements of these transmission lines, an impulse may be (1) blocked in its transmission from one neuron to another, (2) changed from a single impulse into repetitive impulses, or (3) integrated with impulses from other neurons to result in highly intricate patterns of impulses in subsequent neurons (Guyton and Hall 1996).

Nerve impulses are transmitted from one neuron to the next via specialized structures called synapses. Synapses determine the path of spread of signals within the nervous system. For example, some synapses easily transmit signals from one neuron to another; others do it with more difficulty. Other areas of the nervous system can alter function, sometimes facilitating synaptic transmission by "opening" synapses for transmission and at other times "closing" them. Thus, synapses are junction points and as such are sites of focus for control of signal transmission. There are two types of synapses: the chemically mediated and the electrical synapses. The electrical synapse is characterized by channels that conduct impulses directly from one cell to the next. However, the vast majority of signal transmission in the CNS is via chemically mediated synapses. An important characteristic of chemically mediated synapses is that unlike the electrical synapse they always transmit signals in one direction. Transmission is initiated when the first neuron (i.e., the presynaptic neuron) releases a chemical substance known as a neurotransmitter, which impinges on the surface of the other cell (the postsynaptic neuron) (Fig. 9.1). Usually the cell body or dendritic region is the receiving end of the neuron, and the axon terminals are the transmitting end of the cell. However, other synaptic arrangements, such as axoaxonic and dendrodendritic, also exist.

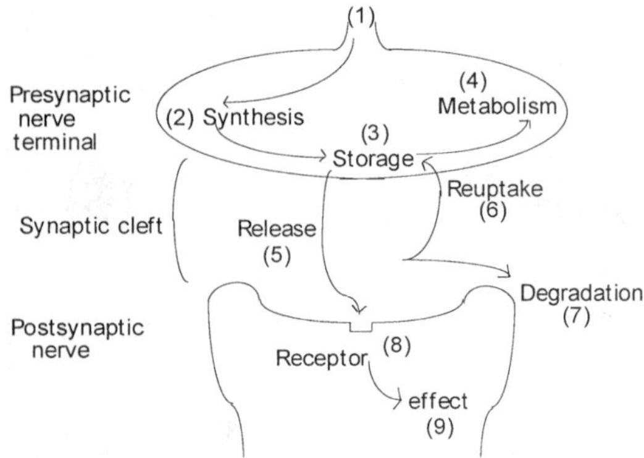

FIG. 9.1—Simplified schematic of steps in interneuron transmission of a nerve impulse. (1) Action potential propagated in the presynaptic nerve, (2) transmitter synthesis, (3) transmitter storage, (4) interneuron transmitter breakdown or inactivation, (5) transmitter release into the synaptic cleft, (6) transmitter reuptake into presynaptic terminal, (7) transmitter synaptic degradation, (8) transmitter attachment to postsynaptic receptor, and (9) receptor-induced increase or decrease in ionic conductance or altered cellular process.

Figure 9.2 shows the basic physiologic anatomy of the synapse. The presynaptic terminal is separated from the postsynaptic neural stroma by a synaptic cleft. Transmitter vesicles are located in the presynaptic terminal. These vesicles contain transmitter chemicals that when released either excite or inhibit postsynaptic neuronal functions by way of receptor proteins on the postsynaptic neuron.

The events involved in the release of transmitter from the presynaptic terminal are initiated by an impulse (action potential) that is propagated in the presynaptic fiber and travels to the synaptic terminal (Fig. 9.2). There are a large number of voltage-gated calcium channels at this location, and the action potential activates these channels (Sihra and Nichols 1993). Calcium ions then flow into the terminal. The rapid increase in intraterminal calcium concentration promotes the fusion of transmitter-containing synaptic vesicles with the presynaptic membrane. The transmitter is then released from the vesicles into the synaptic cleft and diffuses to receptors on the postsynaptic membrane. The amount of transmitter released is directly related to the number of calcium ions that enter the terminal.

Receptor proteins on the membrane of the postsynaptic neuron have two important components: a binding component (binds with the neurotransmitter) and an inophore component. The inophore component passes through the membrane to the interior of the postsynaptic neuron. There are two types of inophore components. One type is an ion channel. Membrane ion channels can be pictured as water-filled tunnels through the cell membrane and provide an aqueous route for specific types of ions to traverse the hydrophobic membrane interior. Cationic channels most often allow passage of sodium ions but sometimes potassium or calcium and serve to excite the postsynaptic membrane (i.e., excitatory transmitters open these channels). Anionic channels allow mainly chloride to pass through and are opened by inhibitory transmitters; open chloride channels inhibit neuronal function. Ion channels provide for rapid activation or inhibition of neuronal function. The other type of inophore component is a "second-messenger" activator; i.e., the component protrudes into the cell cytoplasm and activates substances within the neuron that

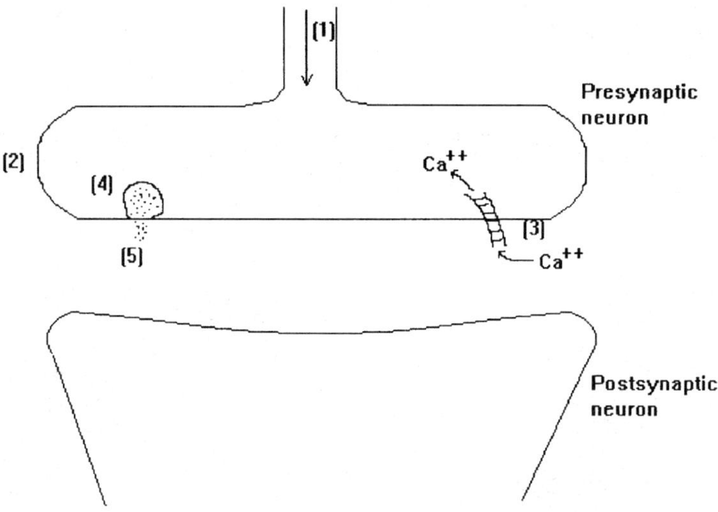

FIG. 9.2—Release of neurotransmitter at the synapse. The action potential (1) arrives at the nerve terminal (2) and stops here. It causes the opening of calcium channels (3) (voltage gated), allowing Ca^{++} to enter the presynaptic terminal. The Ca^{++} within the terminal catalyzes a reaction leading to liberation of transmitter (4) from the terminal's vesicles into the synaptic cleft (5).

TABLE 9.1—Summary of small-molecule neurotransmitters located in the CNS

Transmitter	Anatomic location in CNS	Receptor subtypes	Predominant postsynaptic action
Actetylcholine	Cell bodies at all levels	Yes	Excitatory (and inhibitory)
Monoamines			
Norepinephrine	Cell bodies in pons and brain stem	Yes	Excitatory (and inhibitory)
Dopamine	Cell bodies at all levels	Yes	Inhibitory
5-hydroxytryptamine (serotonin)	Cell bodies in brain stem and pons	Yes	Inhibitory (and excitatory)
Amino acids			
Gamma-aminobutyric acid (GABA)	Supraspinal interneurons involved in presynaptic inhibition	Yes	Inhibitory
Glycine	Spinal and brain stem interneurons	—	Inhibitory
Glutamate and aspartate	Relay neurons at all levels	—	Excitatory

Sources: Guyton and Hall 1996; Nicoll 1998; Bloom 1996; Cooper et al. 1996; Bradley 1989.

in turn serve as "second messengers" to alter cell functions. Unlike the results of ion channel activation by neuronal changes, the neuronal changes activated by a second-messenger system cause prolonged (i.e., seconds to months) neuronal effects. One of the most common types of second-messenger systems in neurons uses a protein complex known as G proteins.

Over 40 different neurotransmitter substances have been identified. They are usually classified into two major groups: small-molecule, rapidly acting transmitters (Table 9.1) and slowly acting, neuropeptide transmitters (Table 9.2) (Guyton and Hall 1996). Many of these transmitters are operational in the CNS. An alternative transmitter classification scheme has been proposed (Strange 1988) and is favored by some authors (Cooper et al. 1996). Further evidence may require that the more traditional classification presented here be modified.

TABLE 9.2—Examples of neuropeptide neurotransmitters located in the CNS

β Endorphin	Substance P
Vasopressin	Somatostatin
Oxytocin	Cholecystokinin
Growth hormone	Angiotensin II
Enkephalin	Neurotensin

Neurotransmitters in the CNS. The small-molecule, rapidly acting transmitters are the ones of most concern to us in this discussion (Table 9.1). They are synthesized in the cytosol of the presynaptic terminal and cause most of the responses in the CNS. Their actions on receptors usually occur within a millisecond or less after release. Afterward they either are destroyed (degraded) locally by enzymes, diffuse out of the cleft, or are absorbed by active transport back into

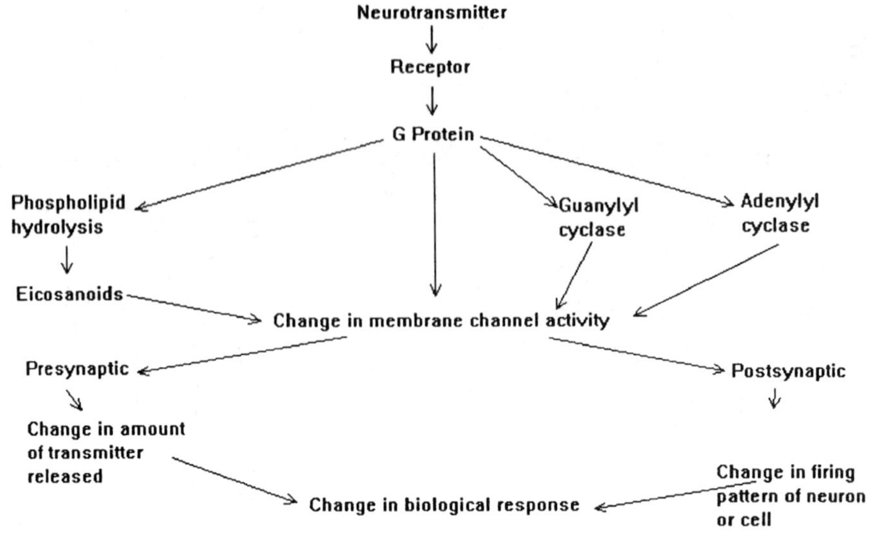

FIG. 9.3—Synaptic transmission pathway. (From Cooper et al. 1996.)

transmitter vesicles (i.e., reuptake) (Fig. 9.1). The larger group of neurotransmitters comprises the neuropeptides (Table 9.2), which are very potent, slower to act, and present in much smaller quantities than the small-molecule transmitters. They are synthesized by ribosomes in the neuronal cell body. Some, such as the endorphins, will be discussed later in this and other chapters.

As noted above, the effect of the transmitters on the postsynaptic neuronal membrane is usually to increase or decrease conductance through ion channels; e.g., increased sodium conductance from outside the cell to inside causes excitation, and increased potassium (from inside to outside) or chloride (from outside to inside) conductance causes inhibition (Unwin 1993). At other times the transmitters stimulate receptor-activated enzymes that in turn change the intracellular metabolic processes. Many neuropeptides and biogenic amines act via this latter method. That is, the neurotransmitter (the "first messenger") links with receptor proteins of the postsynaptic membrane. The resultant conformational change occurring in the receptor protein enables the receptor to interact with a second element in the system, the G protein. The G protein in turn transduces the signal to an amplifying enzyme (a third component). This activity activates a "second messenger." The second messenger then interacts with various cellular processes to invoke the ultimate action (Fig. 9.3). Currently, three major biochemical cascades have been described as second messengers in the CNS. They are the adenylyl cyclase (cyclic AMP), guanylyl cyclase, and phospholipid hydrolysis (eicosanoid) systems (Cooper et al. 1996). The amines (Table 9.1) are an example of neurotransmitters acting (via cyclic AMP) in this general way.

Knowledge of the CNS sites at which given neurotransmitters operate and the degree of specificity by which such sites are affected is rapidly mounting, but in many cases a clear picture is not yet formed.

Characteristics of Some of the More Important Small-Molecule, Rapidly Acting Type of Neurotransmitters

ACETYLCHOLINE. Acetylcholine is widely distributed throughout the CNS. The mechanisms by which acetylcholine functions as a synaptic transmitter in the CNS are similar to those operant in the periphery (e.g., the neuromuscular junction). The transmitter is released from vesicles at the presynaptic terminal and diffuses across the synaptic cleft to act upon postsynaptic receptors. It is then inactivated via hydrolysis (acetylcholinesterase). As in the periphery, cholinergic receptors are of two classes: muscarinic and nicotinic. To date, five muscarinic receptors (M_1-M_5) are known (Caulfield and Birdsall 1998), and M_1 is abundant in the brain. They are coupled to G proteins and either act directly on ion channels or are linked to a variety of second-messenger systems (Cooper et al. 1996). Their effect is primarily to close K^+, Ca^{++}, or Cl^- channels depending on cell type, leading to either depolarization or hyperpolarization. In most regions of the CNS the effects of acetylcholine seem to be the result of an interaction with a mixture of nicotinic and muscarinic receptors (Bloom 1996). While most actions are believed to be related to postsynaptic receptors, it is known that presynaptic receptors for acetylcholine exist at many nerve terminals in the CNS. The function of these presynaptic terminals is to modulate release of neurotransmitter (Bradley 1989). Only relatively recently have nicotinic cholinergic receptors been identified in the CNS. Multiple subtypes are known (Kerlavage et al. 1987). There is as yet only limited evidence for a physiological role for nicotinic receptors in synaptic function in the mammalian brain (Role and Berg 1996). Recent review on muscarinic receptors are summarized in Caulfield and Birdsall 1998.

NOREPINEPHRINE. Like acetylcholine, the mechanisms by which norepinephrine functions in synaptic transmission in the CNS are very similar, if not identical, to those in the periphery. However, unlike acetylcholine, norepinephrine has an uneven distribution in the CNS, although the distribution is similar among most mammals. Two regions of the CNS that are most important in this regard are the locus ceruleus (caudal central gray matter of the brain stem) and the lateral and ventral trigeminal regions of the medulla (reticular formation). From neurons arising in these locations, axons innervate target cells in cortical, subcortical, and spino-medullary fields.

Norepinephrine mechanisms are considered important in the control of sleep and wakefulness, mood and emotional behavior, and temperature, among other functions. In most but not all of these areas norepinephrine probably activates excitatory receptors.

Both α and β adrenoreceptors are present in the CNS, and as in the periphery their actions are further differentiated into α_1 and α_2 and β families, each with their own further subtypes. Both pre- and postsynaptic receptors are present. Norepinephrine is secreted by most of the postganglionic neurons of the sympathetic nervous system. The α_2 family is of particular investigative interest at present, and our knowledge in this area is rapidly increasing. More on this subject is presented later in this volume (see also Ruffolo et al. 1993; Limbird 1988).

EPINEPHRINE. The direct influence of epinephrine in CNS synaptic transmission was recognized only relatively recently. Epinephrine-containing neurons are found in the reticular formation of the medulla. The physiological properties of CNS neurons using epinephrine as a neurotransmitter are poorly understood.

DOPAMINE. In the CNS dopamine is a major neurotransmitter in addition to its role as a precursor in the synthesis of norepinephrine. It is distributed heterogeneously throughout the CNS. The largest concentration of dopamine in the brain is in the basal ganglia and the limbic system. Dopamine in the CNS is linked to fine control of movement, to disturbances of behavior, and to the hypothalamic-pituitary endocrine system. Dopamine has primarily an inhibitory function.

Before 1992 two classes of dopamine receptors were recognized as distinct molecular entities, utilizing different messenger systems and having different distributions in the brain. Dopamine-1 (D_1) receptors are located postsynaptically and activate adenylyl cyclase as a second messenger and increase levels of cyclic AMP. Dopamine-2 (D_2) receptors are located both pre- and postsynaptically and inhibit or have no effect on the synthesis of cyclic AMP. Molecular biological approaches have identified additional forms of the dopamine receptor. Results indicate that the D_1 and D_2 subtypes represent families of dopamine receptors. For example, subtypes D_3 and D_4 receptors are similar in action to D_2 and are prototypic of G-protein-coupled receptors that inhibit adenylyl cyclase. The D_5 receptor is similar to D_1; it couples to the G protein and activates adenylyl cyclase. The D_3 receptor is of particular interest because of its hypothesized role as a therapeutic target for treatment of schizophrenia and drug abuse in humans (Levant 1997; Missale et al. 1998).

5-HYDROXYTRYPTAMINE. This neurotransmitter is also known as 5-HT or serotonin and has strong inhibitory actions. It inhibits pain pathways in the spinal cord and is believed to help control behavioral mood. Inhibition results from membrane hyperpolarization caused by an increase in K^+ conductance.

The neurotransmitter 5-HT is present in highest concentration in blood platelets and the gastrointestinal tract. Most of the 5-HT-associated neuronal pathways originate from the pons and upper brain stem regions and project to many brain and spinal cord areas. Multiple distinct 5-HT receptors and subtypes have been identified in the brain (14 according to Bloom 1996). Proposed CNS regulatory functions of 5-HT-containing neurons include sleep and wakefulness, mood and emotion, temperature, and appetite and neuroendocrine control. Presynaptic autoreceptors on 5-HT terminals have been found in the brain. Stimulation of these receptors inhibits the release of more transmitter. Presynaptic 5-HT receptors have also been found on nerve terminals that release other neurotransmitters, e.g., dopamine (Bradley 1989).

HISTAMINE. Only recently has evidence been accumulated to support the hypothesis that histamine functions as a neurotransmitter in the brain (Schwartz et al. 1991). Most of these neurons are located in the posterior hypothalamus. Three subtypes of histamine receptors have been described (H_1, H_2, and H_3), and all are found in peripheral tissues and brain (Bloom 1996; Hill et al. 1997). The function of this system in the brain is uncertain but it is thought to be involved in the regulation of arousal, temperature, and vascular dynamics.

AMINO ACIDS. High concentrations of certain amino acids are contained in the CNS. From a quantitative standpoint they are likely the major transmitters in the mammalian CNS. They fall into two categories: (1) the predominantly inhibitory, neutral acids, γ-aminobutyric acid (GABA) and glycine, and (2) the predominantly excitatory, acidic acids, glutamate and aspartate. They are all extremely potent modifiers of neuronal excitability.

GABA. In 1954, γ-aminobutyric acid (GABA) was first proposed as an inhibitory neurotransmitter in the mammalian CNS. It is distributed widely in the CNS; however, its concentration varies in different regions, with the greatest concentrations found in the basal ganglia, hippocampus, cerebellum, and hypothalamus in the brain and in the substantia gelatinosa of the dorsal horn of the spinal cord. Large concentrations are also found in the retina. In both the brain and the spinal cord, many of the GABA-containing neurons are short interneurons. GABA has a major functional role in the control of spinal and cerebellar reflexes. GABA is involved in the induction of convulsions and may also be important in anxiety states. It is considered the major inhibitory transmitter receptor in the CNS. Stimulation causes a shift in postsynaptic membrane permeability to inorganic ions, primarily chloride. This results in hyperpolarization of the receptive neuron in the case of postsynaptic inhibition or depolarization with presynaptic inhibition.

There are two major types (families) of GABA receptors (Barnard et al. 1998): $GABA_A$ (Bowery 1989) and $GABA_B$ (Olsen and Tobin 1990; Bowery 1993). The types are pharmacologically separate and have different second-messenger mechanisms and different locations within the CNS. Both receptor families have pre- and postsynaptic locations.

$GABA_A$ is the most prevalent family. The $GABA_A$ receptor is a ligand-gated Cl^- ion channel that opens after release of GABA from presynaptic neurons. Classes of subunits are described as α, β, γ, δ, ε, π, and ρ. Many neuroactive substances (e.g., alcohol, barbiturates and benzodiazepines) facilitate the effects of $GABA_A$ on Cl^- conductance. Further information is given in Sieghart 1995 and Barnard et al. 1998.

The $GABA_B$ receptor acts via G protein to increase conductance in K^+ channels. The functional role of $GABA_B$ receptors in the CNS is poorly understood.

GLYCINE. Glycine appears to serve as the inhibiting transmitter between spinal interneurons and motor neurons. Like GABA it acts by increasing conductance of Cl^-. Its actions are poorly understood but seem restricted to the spinal cord, lower brain stem, and retina. Glycine subtypes have been described but their functional significance is not known.

GLUTAMATE AND ASPARTATE. Glutamate and aspartate occur in uniquely high concentrations in the brain. Glutamate is considered the primary excitatory transmitter in the brain and spinal cord; it is estimated to be responsible for 75% of the excitatory transmission in the brain. Aspartate is also likely a principal excitatory transmitter throughout the CNS but its function has been less well studied.

Glutamate receptors are classified as two types: metabotropic (G-protein-coupled) receptors and ionotropic (ligand-gated ion channel) receptors. The ion-gated receptors resemble $GABA_A$ receptors and are further divided into three types named for the cogeners of glutamate to which they respond. These are the kainate receptors, the α-amino-3-hydroxy-5-methyl-4-isoxazole propionic acid (AMPA) receptors, and the *N*-methyl-D-aspartate (NMDA) receptors. The kainate and AMPA receptors are simple ion channels that permit Na^+ influx and K^+ efflux, while the NMDA receptor permits passage of Ca^{++} (Kaczmarek et al. 1997).

In recent years the NMDA receptor has become a major focus of attention because it may be involved in a wide range of both neurophysiological and pathological processes. For example, actions of these receptors are very selectively blocked by the dissociative anesthetics ketamine and phencyclidine, which enter and block the open ion channel. There are considerable potential therapeutic benefits from this action, e.g., inhibition of epilepsy and the neurotoxic effects of brain ischemia.

NITRIC OXIDE. Nitric oxide (NO) occurs in regions of the brain that are responsible for long-term behavior and memory. It differs from other small-molecule transmitters in that it is not preformed and stored in vesicles in the presynaptic terminal but instead is synthesized nearly instantly as needed and then rapidly diffuses out of the terminal. It also usually does not alter membrane potential but acts by changing intracellular functions that in turn modify neuronal excitability.

NEUROPEPTIDES. The peptides differ in many ways from the neurotransmitters thus far reviewed. They are greater in number of known substances, present in smaller quantities, and far more potent. Their synthesis is directed by messenger RNA and is much more complicated than that of the classic neurotransmitter, taking place in ribosomes. The prohormone so produced is larger than the ultimate transmitter and biologically inactive. It is packaged into vesicles in the smooth endoplasmic reticulum and transported to the nerve terminal for later release by a calcium-dependent (like the classic transmitter) process. After release, the peptides are probably not recycled but inactivated by enzymatic breakdown.

The neuropeptides are thought to act on specific receptors; however, few have actually been identified or characterized. Like other neurotransmitters, some of the postsynaptic effects are probably mediated by direct alteration of ion channel conductance or indirect regulation of ion channels via second-messenger systems (Cooper et al. 1996). Current thought also includes the possibility that they act in concert with the small-molecule neurotransmitters discussed above. That is, in many cases the neuropeptides are present in the same terminals as the small-molecule neurotransmitters and are released together with them. Investigators thus speculate that the action of neuropeptides may be to simply expand the armamentarium of the messenger molecules to enable transmission of an enriched message that requires more than one type of transmitter for its full effect; that is, the peptide embellishes what the primary transmitter "seeks" to accomplish.

For example, the action of the peptide might be to strengthen or prolong the primary transmitter actions (Cooper et al. 1991).

Many peptide families acting as neurotransmitters have been characterized to date (Table 9.2), with more surely to come. Only two of these will be briefly introduced here as examples.

SUBSTANCE P. Substance P has been known for more than six decades, being initially identified in the brain and intestine. The primary effect of substance P release in the brain is an excitatory action on dopaminergic neurons (Bradley 1989). Prolonged duration of action is a prominent finding associated with substance P. It is commonly accepted that it is the neurotransmitter released by primary afferent nerve fibers in the dorsal horn of the spinal cord and mediates sensation of noxious stimuli.

OPIOID PEPTIDES. These peptides have agonist activity at opiate receptors. An opiate is a substance derived from the opium poppy that has analgesic properties, e.g., morphine. An endorphin is any chemical substance naturally formed in the living animal (i.e., endogenous) that exhibits pharmacological properties of morphine. The endorphins are transmitters at a number of synapses in the pain-modularity mechanism, such as those related to the periaqueductal and periventricular gray matter of the CNS. The term *endorphin* actually encompasses what has become a family of opioid peptides currently viewed as comprising three branches: the pro-opiomelanocortin-derived peptides (e.g., β endorphin, the most potent of the natural opioids), the proenkephalin-derived peptides (e.g., Met-enkephalin and Leu-enkephalin), and the prodynorphin-derived peptides (e.g., dynorphin). The peptides derived from proenkephalin and prodynorphin are widely distributed throughout the CNS and often found in the same area, whereas those derived from the pro-opiomelanocortin branch have more restricted distribution, e.g., anterior and intermediate lobes of the pituitary gland. Current thought is that likely the shorter-acting enkephalins are neurotransmitters, and the longer-acting peptides like β endorphin have more of a modulating (hormonal) effect on the CNS. The enkephalins and β endorphins are involved in mediating analgesia. Subtypes of opiate receptors are generally recognized and include mu (μ), delta (δ), and kappa (κ). It is presently unclear whether or not a fourth type, the sigma (σ) receptor, is actually a true opiate receptor. There are also some data to indicate that μ (Pasternak and Wood 1986), δ (Wild et al. 1991; Negri et al. 1991), and κ (Rothman et al. 1990; Unterwald et al. 1991) receptors consist of multiple subtypes.

The μ receptor is thought to be the site at which analgesia is mediated in the brain. Morphine and β endorphin are potent agonists (enkephalins less so) of receptor activity, and naloxone is a potent antagonist of receptor activity. Stimulation of this receptor is also associated with respiratory depression, dependence, miosis, and decreased gastrointestinal propulsive motility. The δ receptor is strongly influenced by Leu-enkephalin, followed in order by Met-enkephalin, β endorphin, and morphine. In addition to analgesia these receptors are thought to mediate behavioral and sedative actions. The κ receptor is stimulated by dynorphin and mediates spinal analgesia but also causes dysphoria.

ACTION OF DRUGS IN THE CNS

Sites of Drug Action. Drug action in the CNS may be specific or nonspecific. Many drugs produce their effects by specifically modifying some step or mechanism in the chemical synaptic transmission of nerve impulses that was reviewed above (Fig. 9.1). For example, nerve impulse conduction can be prevented by applying local anesthetic to the nerve fiber, as occurs with epidural anesthesia. Synaptic transmission can be blocked or depressed at the presynaptic site by halting transmitter synthesis or storage. For example, reserpine interferes with the intracellular storage of monoamines and thereby limits their availability for release from the presynaptic cell terminal. Other drugs increase the release of transmitter (e.g., amphetamine), thereby causing a heightened (in this example, stimulant) response. Drugs may affect the reuptake (e.g., cocaine) or degradation (e.g., physostigmine) of drugs once they are released into the synaptic cleft. On the postsynaptic membrane drugs may act like the neurotransmitter on the receptor (e.g., opioids) or block receptor function at the level of the receptor or affect further transduction of the signal from the receptor (i.e., ion channels, enzyme systems, etc.).

On the other hand, some drugs are nonspecific in nature; i.e., a drug may affect many different target cells by diverse or poorly understood mechanisms. The inhaled anesthetics represent one such class of CNS drugs.

Blood-Brain Barrier. The boundary between the blood and tissues of the CNS is less permeable to large, water-soluble, and/or ionic molecules than that between blood and other tissues. The barrier that limits the penetration into the brain of hydrophilic substances like dissociated acids, bases, and proteins is known as the blood-brain barrier and has important pharmacological characteristics. The barrier exists both in the brain tissue capillaries and in the choroid plexus (i.e., the blood-cerebrospinal fluid barrier) and is created by the uniquely tight junctions between the brain's capillary endothelial cells or the epithelial cells of the choroid plexus and by the close association to capillary walls of glial cells. The barrier, however, is not absolute. Water, carbon dioxide, oxygen, and most lipid-soluble substances like anesthetics freely pass through cell membranes and gain entrance to the brain. However, the blood-brain barrier makes it very difficult to achieve effective concentrations of non-lipid-soluble drugs in the cerebrospinal fluid or parenchyma of the brain.

A selective active-transport mechanism is available for some substances. Recent evidence indicates that both the choroid plexus and the brain parenchymal capillaries have separate, specific, carrier-mediated transport mechanisms to transfer micronutrients (e.g., vitamins), macronutrients (e.g., glucose, amino acids), ions, and certain other substances between the blood and the extracellular space of the brain and cerebrospinal fluid (Spector 1990). Several types of carrier-mediated transport systems exist in plasma membranes and other parts of the cell. Water-soluble and ionic substances must use carrier mechanisms on each side of the cell to penetrate the brain parenchyma. These systems are broadly classified into three groups: (1) active transport, (2) facilitated diffusion, and (3) endosomal transport, in which substances are taken up by an energy-requiring system into endosomal sacs and transported into or out of the cell via these sacs.

PRINCIPLES OF ANESTHESIOLOGY

Anesthesiology is defined as the art and science of administration of anesthesia. The term also describes a clinical specialty of medicine (including veterinary medicine) that emerged during the early 1900s when a few physicians began devoting full time to the clinical administration of anesthetics. Anesthesiology was officially recognized as an organized specialty in medicine with the establishment in 1938 of a peer-certifying body of physicians, the American Board of Anesthesiologists (ABA). The ABA was an affiliate board of the American Board of Surgery and in 1941 became an independent board. In addition, in 1940 a section of anesthesiology was formed within the American Medical Association. In 1975 the American College of Veterinary Anesthesiologists was officially recognized by the American Veterinary Medical Association as the body to certify veterinarians as specialists in veterinary anesthesia. Broader summaries of the development of anesthesiology are available elsewhere (Smithcors 1971; Vandam 1994). The central role of the anesthetist is (1) to apply methods to minimize or eliminate pain, relax muscles, and facilitate patient restraint during surgical, obstetrical, and other medical, diagnostic, and therapeutic procedures and (2) to monitor and support life functions in patients during the operative period as well as in critically ill, injured, or otherwise seriously ill patients. The skills and knowledge that have developed in the field have extended the clinical practice of anesthesiology into intensive care, cardiac and pulmonary resuscitation, and the control of pain problems unrelated to surgery. The word anesthesia is derived from the Greek for "insensible" or "without feeling." The word does not necessarily imply loss of consciousness. In the realm of veterinary anesthesiology, anesthesia and anesthetics are used for a variety of reasons (Table 9.3).

TABLE 9.3—Use of anesthetics in animals

Elimination of sensibility to noxious stimuli
Humane restraint (e.g., protect animal, facilitate diagnostic or surgical procedure)
Technical efficiency (e.g., protect personnel, facilitate diagnostic or surgical procedure)
Specific biomedical research tool (e.g., sleep time)
Control of convulsions
Euthanasia

ANESTHETIC USE

Perception of Noxious Stimuli (Pain). Prevention of the perception of a noxious stimulus during surgery is the primary justification for anesthesia. A noxious stimulus is defined as a stimulus that is potentially damaging to body tissue. Nociception has no emotional or perceptional connotation. The stimulus triggers a reaction in an animal, including the feeling of pain in humans (Bonica 1990). Pain is an unpleasant sensory and emotional experience; it is a perception, not a physical entity. The perception of pain depends on a functioning cerebral cortex. The concept of pain includes several interdependent dimensions: the sensory/discriminative and motivational/affective.

It is not the intent to sidetrack here into semantic issues or to belabor what are to some fine points, but it is necessary for completeness to stress that contemporary reasoning holds that pain is a subjective response in conscious human beings. When considering "pain" in animals, it is important to recognize that our knowledge of pain in animals is largely inferential. We approach the subject with "the tacit assumption . . . that stimuli are noxious and strong enough to give rise to the perception of pain in animals if the stimuli are detected as pain by human beings, if they at least approach or exceed tissue damaging proportion and if they produce escape behavior in animals" (Kitchell and Erickson 1983).

Classical Approach to Mechanisms of Pain. Before further discussion of methods by which insensitivity is produced, it is helpful to briefly review the mechanisms whereby an individual becomes aware of and reacts to a noxious stimulus (Fig. 9.4). This inclusion here is justified on the basis that knowledge of these mechanisms offers the clinician targets for single or multiple attacks in an attempt to abolish or minimize pain.

Acute pain that is provoked by disease or injury (planned or unplanned) is the net effect of many interacting and complex anatomic paths and physiological mechanisms. The stimulus excites a specialized receptor organ, the nociceptor. Nociceptors are distributed throughout the body but are frequently grouped as somatic (cutaneous, muscle, bone, joint, fascia) or visceral. Nociceptors are located at the termination of free nerve endings of small poorly myelinated or nonmyelinated A-delta and C afferent nerves. The nociceptors transduce the stimuli into nociceptive impulses that are

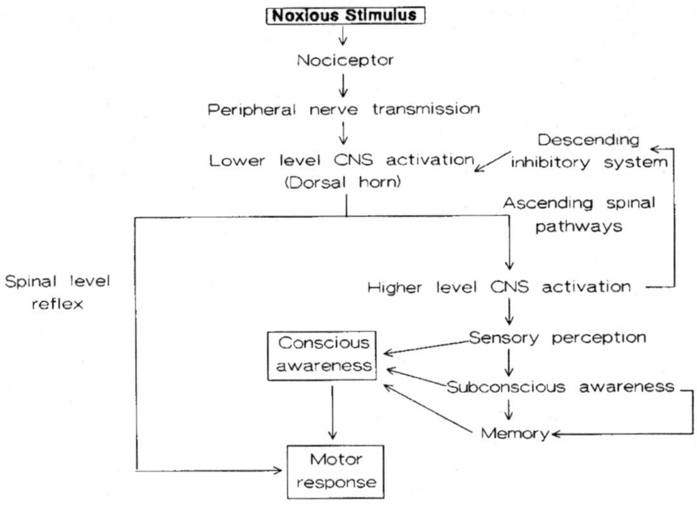

FIG. 9.4—Events in the reaction to a noxious stimulus.

transmitted to the CNS. Impulses that originate from areas below the head are transmitted via fibers that synapse with interneurons or second-order neurons in the dorsal horn of the spinal cord. Impulses from the head travel via fibers within the cranial nerves to the medulla, where they synapse with neurons in the trigeminal nuclei (medullary dorsal horn). In the spinal cord, the signal is subjected to a variety of potential modulating influences in the dorsal horn. For a long time the dorsal horn was considered to perform simply as a relay station. More recent evidence indicates it contains an incredibly complex circuitry and rich biochemistry that permits not only reception and transmission of nociceptive impulses but also a large degree of signal processing. After being subjected to these modulating influences, some of the impulses may then stimulate somatomotor and preganglionic sympathetic neurons and provoke nocifensive reflex responses. Nociceptive impulses also activate other neurons making up the ascending systems that pass to the brain stem and brain. Supraspinal systems that are probably involved in processing nociceptive information to progressively higher levels of awareness include the reticular formation, limbic system, hypothalamus, thalamus, and cortex.

Activation of the reticular formation results in abrupt awakening, diffuse alertness, and initiation of protective homeostatic responses. In turn, affective (emotional) alertness is obtained through cortical arousal. The animal is now fully knowledgeable regarding the cause and strength of the noxious stimulus and its relationship to the environment. The animal in turn reacts with a coordinated response.

For more detailed information the reader is referred to Bonica 1990, from which much of this summary has come, Willis 1985, and Wall and Melzack 1994.

Immobility. Although the primary reason for anesthetic delivery is to render the animal insensible to pain, restraint and technical efficiency are also long-recognized important considerations. Although viewed as an extreme in approach today, Alexandre Liautord, a Frenchman, noted in his 1892 *Manual of Operative Veterinary Surgery:* "In veterinary surgery, the indication for anesthesia has not, to the same extent as in human, the avoidance of pain in the patient for its object, and though the duties of the veterinarian include that of avoiding the infliction of *unnecessary* pain as much as possible, the administration of anesthetic compounds aims principally to facilitate the performance of the operation for its own sake, by depriving the patient of the power of obstructing, and perhaps even frustrating its execution, to his own detriment, by the violence of his struggles, and the persistency of his resistance. To prevent these, with their disastrous consequences, is the prime motive in the induction of the anesthetic state" (quoted in Smithcors 1971). More in keeping with contemporary thought are the words of George H. Dadd written in 1854 in *The Modern Horse Doctor:* "We recommend that, in all operations of this kind, the subject be etherized, not only in view of preventing pain, but that we may, in the absence of all struggling on the part of our patient, perform the operation satisfactorily, and in much less time after etherization has taken place than otherwise. So soon as the patient is under the influence of that valuable agent, we have nothing to fear from his struggles, provided we have the assistance of one experienced to administer it" (quoted in Smithcors 1971). Many of these same clinical principles can and should also be applied directly to the research environment.

TABLE 9.4—Routes by which anesthetic or anesthetic adjuvant drugs are administered to animals

1. Topical
   a. Cutaneous
   b. Mucous membrane
2. Injection
   a. Intravenous
   b. Subcutaneous
   c. Intramuscular
   d. Intraperitoneal
   e. Intraosseous
3. Gastrointestinal tract
   a. Oral
   b. Rectal
4. Respiratory system (e.g., inhalation)

TABLE 9.5—Techniques of anesthesia based on extent of loss of sensation

1. Local/regional: drugs placed in close proximity to nerve membranes, causing conduction block
   a. Topical or surface
   b. Area infiltration
      i. Subdermal
      ii. Intravenous regional
   c. Perineural (i.e., nerve trunk)
   d. Peridural (i.e., epidural or caudal)
   e. Subarachnoid (i.e., spinal)
2. General anesthesia: state of controlled, reversible CNS depression (including unconsciousness) produced by one or multiple drugs
   a. Injectable
   b. Inhalation
   c. Balanced

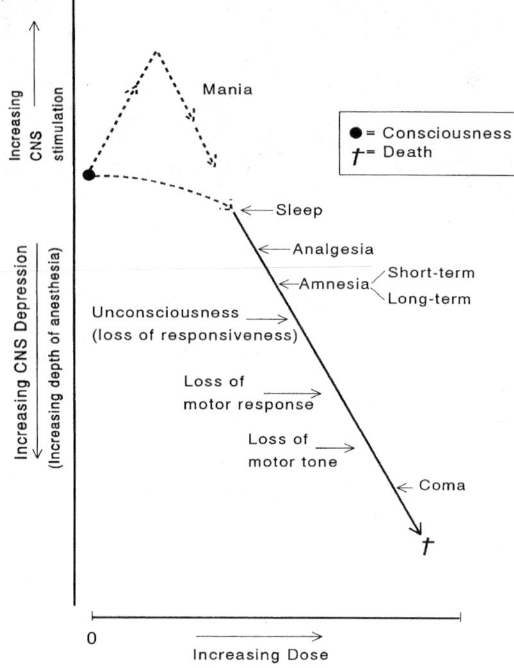

FIG. 9.5—The anesthetic continuum as viewed clinically in a healthy subject.

ANESTHESIA CLASSIFIED. Anesthesia is produced by both chemical (i.e., drugs) and physical (e.g., sensory nerve destruction) means. Anesthetic drugs are frequently classified according to their route of administration (Table 9.4). Some drugs are only suited for common delivery via one route, e.g., the inhalation anesthetics, while many of the injectable agents may be administered in a variety of different manners depending on the drug and the desired end point of effect.

Local and Regional Anesthesia. Anesthetics are also classified according to the region of the body influenced (Table 9.5). For example, a local anesthetic is administered, usually to conscious or mildly sedated animals, to desensitize a localized or regional area of the body. It is deposited in close proximity to a nerve membrane, causing nerve conduction blockade.

General Anesthesia. General anesthesia is a condition induced by pharmacological or other means that results in controlled, reversible CNS depression. It is true that some drugs in the process of producing anesthesia cause excessive stimulation and activity in the brain, but all anesthetic agents ultimately reduce and stop electrical activity in the brain and decrease brain oxygen consumption. On this basis it is proper to characterize anesthetic agents as CNS depressants.

Basic elements of general anesthesia in humans in addition to reversibility include loss of awareness (unconsciousness), no recall of events at the conscious level (amnesia), conscious insensitivity to pain (analgesia), and muscle relaxation and diminished motor response to noxious stimulation. In recent years the importance of minimal autonomic nervous system response to noxious stimulation has been also emphasized in clinical applications.

General anesthesia has traditionally been considered a dose-related continuum of a series of events passing into each other (Fig. 9.5), from alert wakefulness through lethargy and drowsiness (sedation), unconsciousness (with and without somatic and visceral response to external stimuli), coma, and death. The wakefulness to coma series implies progressive loss of higher CNS (cortical) function followed by depression of brain stem functions. While portions of this scheme have been challenged (Winters et al. 1967; Winters et al. 1972), its use is generally acceptable and offers a convenient method to set the stage for further discussion of principles of general anesthesia.

TECHNIQUES OF GENERAL ANESTHESIA. General anesthesia is pharmacologically induced and maintained in animals via one of two general methods. The oldest approach, which is still widely used in certain animal applications, is the single-agent technique. With this technique, an agent such as pentobarbital, thiopental, or ketamine (or perhaps two agents such as xylazine and ketamine given simultaneously or in close time proximity) is administered at sufficient dose to provide the complete spectrum of characteristics of general anesthesia. This method is simple but may be more life threatening, especially under adverse circumstances, including animal ill health. Because *all* anesthetic agents have some undesirable effects when used alone, modern anesthetic practice increasingly involves the use of combinations of drugs. This technique is known as *balanced anesthesia.* With this technique, multiple drugs in low dosage are used, each drug for a specific purpose. The ultimate intent is to take advantage of the desirable features of selected drugs while minimizing their potential for harmful depression of homeostatic mechanisms. This technique is especially advantageous when used with physiologically compromised individuals. An example of such an approach is the combined use of a low dose of a hypnotic-sedative drug for unconsciousness and amnesia, an opioid for profound analgesia with little cardiovascular insult, a neuromuscular blocking drug for muscle relaxation, and intermittent positive pressure ventilation with oxygen to facilitate respiratory gas exchange in the face of total skeletal muscle paralysis. Unfortunately, the balanced technique is complex, and inexperienced or careless use of a drug combination may aggravate undesirable drug actions and/or other common difficulties encountered by the anesthetist.

MECHANISM OF ACTION CAUSING GENERAL ANESTHESIA. There have been many attempts to explain the mechanism of general anesthesia at a molecular level. Three simple observations limit possible explanations. The rate at which anesthesia can be induced and wakefulness resumed effectively rules out long-term biochemical events and focuses attention on drug-induced alterations of short-term biochemical events. In addition, the diverse chemical structures of anesthetic agents also pose a problem in arriving at a common theory of action. For example, anesthetic drugs range from inert gases such as xenon, relatively simple inorganic (nitrous oxide) and organic (chloral hydrate and chloroform) compounds, to progressively more complex molecules such as pentobarbital, ketamine, and alphaxalone (Fig. 9.6). The absence of a common chemical structure reduces the possibility of a specific-receptor-mediated action. Finally, explanation of their anesthetic action must in some way be linked with their ability to cause superimposed selective and specific anesthetic "side effects," such as reductions in myocardial contractility.

An important neurophysiological action common to most general anesthetics is to depress both spontaneous and evoked neuronal activity in many regions of the brain. Actions exerted on synaptic transmission seem most sensitive, whereas nerve conduction is little influenced. Anesthetics may reduce synaptic transmission by interfering with neurotransmitter release from presynaptic nerve terminals, by altering reuptake of neurotransmitter after release, by altering binding of neurotransmitter to postsynaptic receptor sites, or by influencing ionic conduction following activation of postsynaptic receptors. At this point in time, ionic mechanisms thought to be involved are varied and the focus of extensive study. For example, barbiturates are known to act on the GABA-receptor-mediated chloride channel, and at least some of the inhaled anesthetics are reported to cause hyperpolarization of neurons via activation of potassium currents. In both examples there is a decreased ability to initiate action potentials; i.e., the cellular threshold for firing is increased (Bradley 1989; Halsey 1989; Koblin 1994).

A striking physiochemical characteristic of inhalation anesthetic drugs is their lipid solubility—a physical property shown to correlate best with anesthetic potency. This correlation is commonly referred to as the *Meyer-Overton rule* after the two individuals who independently (1899 and 1901, respectively) noted that the potency of anesthetics increased directly in proportion to their partition coefficient between olive oil and water (i.e., the concentration ratio of the agent in oil and water at equilibrium). Because inhalation anesthetic molecules are hydrophobic and therefore distribute to sites in which they are removed from aqueous environments, and because of the close correlation between potency and lipophilicity, it is theorized that these anesthetics act in the cell membrane lipid layer. It is thought that their presence distorts the membrane structure, which in turn causes occlusion of the pores through which ions pass, e.g., the sodium channel (this is the so-called membrane expansion theory) (Halsey 1989; Koblin 1994).

Although there is no pharmacologic antagonist to inhalation anesthesia, very high ambient pressure (e.g., 50–100 atmospheres of pressure) causes reversal of the anesthetic state. This observation is another important clue to the mechanism of anesthesia. Because pressure acts by reducing volume, the reversal of anesthesia with pressure suggests that an increase in lipid volume (i.e., less-orderly arrangement of the membrane lipid molecules and thereby a small volume expansion) is somehow involved in the process.

Unfortunately, the membrane expansion theory is not without its faults, and a unitary theory of narcosis (i.e., the thought that all anesthetics have a common mode of action on a specific molecular site) may not be achievable. However, popular dogma has been challenged with observations that suggest anesthetic drugs do act at specific sites (Firestone 1988). During the past 10–15 years there has been increasing evidence that specific neuronal membrane proteins that permit translocation of ions during membrane excitation are the primary targets for anesthetic action. Debate is ongoing whether at least inhalation anesthetics disrupt ion flow through membrane channels by an indirect action on surrounding lipids or via a second messenger

a. Xe
Xenon

b. O / \ N=N
Nitrous oxide

c. Cl–C(Cl)(Cl)–H
Chloroform

d. Cl–C(Cl)(Cl)–C(OH)(OH)–H
Chloral hydrate

e. Pentobarbital

f.

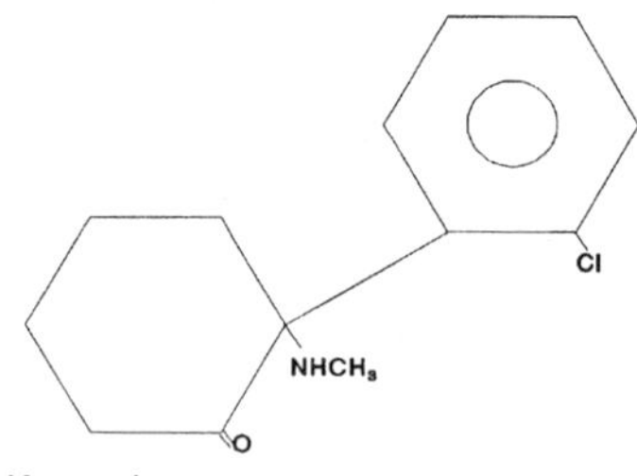

Ketamine

g. Alphaxalone

FIG. 9.6—Chemical structures of examples of drugs causing general anesthesia.

or alternatively whether they link directly to membrane channel proteins. Regardless, the molecular mechanism of action of general anesthetic drugs is still far from clear, and there is still much to learn regarding this phenomenon. Readers are referred elsewhere for more in-depth analysis of this topic (Halsey 1989; Firestone 1988; Albrecht and Miletich 1988; Franks and Lieb 1987; and especially Koblin 1994).

BASICS OF CLINICAL ANESTHESIA. A favorable anesthetic course begins with a good plan—a plan based on sound pharmacological and physiological principles. There is no rigid format. *No anesthetic technique is unequivocally the best for all animals under all circumstances.* Each plan is adapted to prevailing circumstances. Accordingly, appropriate anesthetic management requires a broad understanding of the physiology of bodily life support systems (e.g., respiratory, circulatory, central and autonomic nervous systems), the pathology and pathophysiology of the condition(s) necessitating anesthesia and surgery, the pharmacology and principles and techniques of administration of anesthetic and adjuvant drugs, and monitoring and support of vital organ function. The rationale that underlies the selection of an appropriate anesthetic protocol is outlined in Table 9.6.

Drug selection for anesthetic management is accomplished by considering the pharmacological requirements for the individual case, reviewing and selecting major drug classes that are appropriate for the specific needs, and then reviewing characteristics and selecting the specific drug(s) within the desired drug class(es). Frequently, the best drug and technique are those with which the clinician is most experienced; i.e., there is an art to the clinical administration of potent, life-threatening drugs such as those used in anesthetic management.

Drugs used in anesthetic management can be conveniently classified according to time frame of use: the preanesthetic, perianesthetic, and immediate postanesthetic periods.

TABLE 9.6—Considerations in the selection of appropriate anesthetic protocol and drugs

1. Animal characteristics (e.g., species, age, physical status)
2. Capabilities and confidence of anesthetist
3. Capabilities of surgeon and surgical requirements
4. Available drugs, facilities, and ancillary personnel
5. Wishes of client

TABLE 9.7—Goals for preanesthetic medication

1. Alleviate or minimize pain
2. Allay apprehension
3. Facilitate handling
4. Minimize undesirable reflex autonomic nervous system activity
   a. Parasympathetic
      i. Vagal nerve
      ii. Secretions: salivary, bronchial
   b. Sympathetic
      i. Arrhythmic
      ii. Arterial blood pressure alterations
5. Supplement general anesthesia
   a. Add to level of analgesia, sedation
   b. Reduce anesthetic requirement
6. Minimize undesirable postanesthetic recovery complications
7. Prevent infection
8. Continue treatment of intercurrent disease

Preanesthetic Period. Drugs are usually administered to animals (usually 15–45 minutes) before induction of general anesthesia. The primary aims of preanesthetic medication are to calm the animal, facilitate handling, and relieve preoperative pain. These along with secondary goals are listed in Table 9.7. Unfortunately, preanesthetic medication is not without its complications, which also must be considered in formulating the anesthetic management plan (Table 9.8). The concurrent use of two or three drugs is usually required to accomplish the desired preanesthetic conditions in the patient. These are selected from a variety of major drug classes (Table 9.9). The extent of drug combinations advocated by individuals attests to the variety of circumstances commonly encountered clinically and to the lack of agreement on optimal drug effects.

TRANQUILIZER-SEDATIVES. Tranquilizers (ataractics or neuroleptics) are frequently administered to animals to produce a calming effect, i.e., tractability or "chemical restraint." This group of drugs includes the phenothiazine, the butyrophenone, and the benzodiazepine subclasses. They are frequently used in combination with other preanesthetic drugs (e.g., opioids), because lower doses can be used than would be the case if each drug were used alone and the degree of sedation accomplished by the drug combination is often potentiated without causing further severe circulatory and respiratory depression.

TABLE 9.8—Complications of preanesthetic medication

1. Depressed vital organ function
   a. Direct effects
   b. Interaction with anesthetic and other adjuvant drugs
2. Anti-analgesia
3. Prolonged sedation influencing recovery from anesthesia
   a. Prolonged recumbency
   b. Ataxia

TABLE 9.9—Major classes of drugs (and specific drug examples) commonly considered for preanesthetic medication

1. Tranquilizer-sedative
   a. Acepromazine
   b. Diazepam
   c. Midazolam
   d. Droperidol
   e. Azaperone
2. Hypnotic-sedative
   a. Pentobarbital
   b. Chloral hydrate
3. Opioid
   a. Agonist
      i. Morphine
      ii. Meperidine
   b. Agonist-antagonist
      i. Butorphanol
4. α_2-adrenergic agonist
   a. Xylazine
   b. Detomidine
   c. Medetomidine
5. Dissociative
   a. Ketamine
6. Commercially prepared combinations of sedating drugs
   a. Telazol (tiletamine + zolazepam)
   b. Innovar-neuroleptanalgesia (fentanyl + droperidol)
7. Parasympatholytic
   a. Atropine
   b. Glycopyrrolate

The phenothiazines have received widespread use for many years. Their potency facilitates easy administration, and favorable tranquilization is usually realized. They have antiarrhythmic, antihistaminic, and antiemetic effects that may be particularly desirable. The α_1-adrenergic blocking action of the phenothiazines is likely to be of special concern in some patients because it results in usually unwanted arterial hypotension.

The butyrophenones also have α_1-adrenergic blocking activity, but better cardiovascular stability accompanies their use compared to the phenothiazines. Largely on the basis of cost and the lack of broad-based, clear advantages, the butyrophenones are less frequently used for anesthetic management of veterinary patients than other drugs in the tranquilizer grouping.

Although representatives of the benzodiazepines are increasingly used with other drugs to induce and maintain general anesthesia, especially in some animals their use in the preanesthetic period is, like the butyrophenones, very limited. Pain and occasional erratic absorption after intramuscular injection are characteristic of some benzodiazepines (e.g., diazepam). Also, sedative actions in otherwise healthy animals are quite variable across animal species commonly encountered in veterinary practice. Sedation caused by benzodiazepines can be reliably reversed by a specific antagonist at least in some species.

HYPNOTIC-SEDATIVES. Drugs of this class, including the barbiturates and chloral hydrate, cause a dose-dependent spectrum of CNS depression, sedation, sleep, anesthesia, coma, and death. They produce minimal ventilatory and circulatory depression in sedative doses. Disadvantages of their use include a lack of analgesia and the absence of a specific antagonist. Use of drugs from this class have largely been replaced in the preanesthetic period by the α_2-adrenergic agonist drugs.

α_2-ADRENERGIC DRUGS. Drugs such as xylazine cause dose-related sedation and analgesia. They are widely used across species lines singly and in combination with, especially, opioids and dissociative agents. Bradycardia, mild arterial hypertension followed by more prolonged hypotension, hyperglycemia, and increased urine volume are commonly attendant effects. Direct antagonists of varying purity and effectiveness are now available.

OPIOIDS. Potent analgesia, sedation, and the absence of direct myocardial depression are important advantages of the use of opioids in the preanesthetic period. Patients with preexisting preoperative pain or who will require painful diagnostic or therapeutic procedures before anesthetic induction are likely candidates for opioid preanesthetic medication. Opioid premedication is also appropriate prior to anesthetic management techniques that use opioids as a predominant component (i.e., a balanced technique, see above). Predominant adverse effects of opioids when used prior to anesthesia include depression of medullary ventilatory control centers resulting in decreased responsiveness to carbon dioxide and in turn hypoventilation. Opioids commonly induce a vagotonic affect so heart rate may also be decreased to variable degrees depending on agent, dose, and animal species. In some species (e.g., the dog) opioids commonly cause CNS sedation, while in others (e.g., the horse) excitement or CNS arousal are predominant concerns. Opioid-induced vomition in some species (e.g., dog) may be wanted (e.g., a newly presented patient with a full stomach requiring anesthesia for a diagnostic or minor surgical procedure) or unwanted (e.g., risk of pulmonary aspiration of vomitus in elderly or depressed patients). They also decrease intestinal propulsive and ruminal activity.

DISSOCIATIVE DRUGS. Drugs such as ketamine reliably cause a state of somatic analgesia and sedation in some species (e.g., cat) and may be of benefit in special clinical situations (e.g., highly fractious animals under conditions of limited management choices). Its relatively wide margin of safety in otherwise healthy animals is of special benefit under conditions of limited patient control or knowledge base.

The most prominent disadvantage of its use is that, depending on dosage, this class of drugs may cause CNS arousal in some species (e.g., horse) leading to animal excitement or frank convulsions.

DRUG COMBINATIONS. Sometimes drug combinations are marketed to provide ready access to clinical benefits of two drugs while attempting to minimize their individual disadvantages. For example, Telazol® is a combination of tiletamine, a dissociative agent, and zolazepam, a benzodiazepine tranquilizer-sedative. The combination improves the reliability of the sedative properties of either drug used alone without adding extensively to further vital organ depression (e.g., cardiopulmonary depression). However, as a consequence of the fixed combination, a prolonged duration of effect may be an unwanted result.

Innovar® is a combination of a short-acting opioid (fentanyl) and a longer-acting butyrophenone tranquilizer (droperidol). Its commercial availability to the North American veterinary community has varied greatly in recent years. Its use in, especially, dogs and swine provides reliable sedation and potent analgesia, again with limited vital organ depression. Bradycardia is commonly an unwanted side effect but can be countered by the administration of an anticholinergic drug such as atropine. The different duration of actions of the two component drugs is an important aspect of redosing considerations.

PARASYMPATHOLYTIC (ANTICHOLINERGIC) DRUGS. The most common reason for administering drugs such as atropine or the more potent, longer-acting glycopyrrolate before induction of general anesthesia is to reduce upper-airway and salivary secretions (antisialagogue effect) and counteract reflex bradycardia occurring with, e.g., concurrent opioid use or certain surgical manipulations (e.g., ocular).

In years past it was routine to use anticholinergics as part of the premedication scheme. However, this is no longer so. Contemporary anesthetic drugs are much less irritating to the respiratory tract, minimizing the likelihood of excessive respiratory tract secretions, and in the absence of potent vagotonic preanesthetic drugs it is thought that heightened vagal tone is best treated just prior to its anticipated occurrence or at first sign of its presence. Sparing use of anticholinergic drugs reduces the risk of other unwanted effects such as tachycardia or reduced gastrointestinal motility. Avoidance of gastrointestinal stasis is of special importance in herbivorous animals, for whom preanesthetic gastrointestinal emptying is almost never desired or

TABLE 9.10—Major classes of CNS drugs (and examples) commonly considered for general anesthesia

1. Hypnotic-sedatives a. Ultrashort acting i. Thiopental b. Short acting i. Pentobarbital 2. Dissociatives a. Ketamine 3. Opioid a. Morphine b. Oxymorphine c. Fentanyl d. Alfentanil	4. Drug combinations a. Innovar b. Telazol 5. Others a. Guaifenesin b. Propofol c. Etomidate d. Saffan 6. Tranquilizer-sedatives* a. Benzodiazepines

*Never used alone.

accomplished. Mydriasis is another effect (e.g., of atropine) that is often undesirable because it confounds interpretation of some clinical signs of anesthesia and/or exposes the patient to potential retinal damage in some uncontrolled postanesthetic circumstances.

Anesthetic Period. The administration of anesthesia requires a combination of knowledge, skill, and ingenuity. The anesthetic drugs selected and their dose and method of delivery will largely depend on the animal, the facilities available, and the skill of the individual who will administer them.

General anesthetics are usually given by inhalation or injection; on rare occasions anesthetic drugs may be given orally or per rectum. More specific information on anesthetic delivery is given later in this volume and in Short 1987, Hall and Clarke 1991, and Andrews 1990.

Drugs of several classes of injectable agents (Table 9.10) are commonly used for general anesthesia. These are preferably given intravenously (IV); however, because of the varied circumstances associated with clinical conditions in veterinary medicine, the intramuscular (IM) route is also widely used. The IV route is the preferred means of inducing general anesthesia because anesthetic induction with the loss or reduction of many of the patient's life-protecting reflexes is consistently the most crucial maneuver in managing general anesthesia. The IV administration permits incremental dosing and thus titration of the level of anesthetic to a desired end point. This technique is often desired especially in critically ill patients or in unfamiliar circumstances because of the likelihood of unpredictable animal responses to a "routine" dose of drug. Drugs of a single class are used alone or in combination with other drugs listed in Table 9.10 (e.g., inhalation anesthetics and neuromuscular blocking drugs) to achieve suitable anesthetic conditions. Many of the drugs from the classes listed in Table 9.10 are also used at lower dosage for preanesthetic medication (Table 9.9).

The barbiturates likely continue as overall the most popular intravenous anesthetic for animals. They have universal (or at least nearly so) geographic and species application. Accurate information is not readily available but likely the dissociative class of drugs has become a close second choice in popularity to the barbiturates. For example, ketamine may be used alone in some species or combined with other drugs to produce a state that enables restraint and surgery and can be administered via a variety of routes, a decided advantage for fractious animals and/or treatment outside the controlled hospital environment.

Opioids in large doses are the basis for balanced anesthetic techniques for human patients—especially those patients with circulatory system instability or those undergoing cardiac surgery. This method is also applicable to some veterinary patients (e.g., dogs) and is presently used to varying degrees. An important point to keep in mind is that opioids, even in large doses, do not predictably produce unconsciousness, so other drugs are used concurrently to accomplish the individualized goals of general anesthesia. Also, some animal species (e.g., horses) are excited by even moderate (by comparison to other species, e.g., dogs) opioid doses.

Immediate Postanesthetic Period. The immediate postanesthetic period is also known as the anesthetic recovery period. It begins with the discontinuation of the administration of anesthetic drugs. Recovery of healthy animals from routine anesthetic techniques is usually, but not always, uneventful and routine. Circumstances such as compromised physical status and unfamiliar anesthetic techniques heighten the likelihood of recovery problems. The immediate goal of this period is the rapid return of the patient's independent, uncompromised ability to maintain normal respiratory and circulatory systems function and to return sensory and motor abilities to preanesthetic levels as soon as possible. Despite this overriding philosophy, when the needs of different species and circumstances are considered, the actual broad plan is less clear. For example, most of the contemporary inhalation anesthetics do not have potent or persistent analgesic properties at alveolar concentrations associated with awakening. The sooner a patient recovers following surgery, the sooner there is potential for pain and an uncomfortable situation for the patient. Consequently, the question arises, is it better for a patient to awaken quickly following surgery and then receive, as needed, analgesic drugs, or is it more desirable and beneficial for the patient to receive analgesic drugs toward the end of the anesthetic period and as a result have a slower recovery from general anesthesia and transition to sensation? The same therapeutic dilemma applies to the patient who may emerge from anesthesia excited and risk a particularly "stormy" recovery with attendant physical injury. The various combinations of drugs used in anesthetic management coupled with unique species characteristics make it impossible to describe here all of the patterns

TABLE 9.11—Hazards of the immediate postanesthetic period

1. Circulatory system complications
   a. Arterial hypotension
   b. Arterial hypertension
   c. Cardiac dysrhythmias
2. Respiratory system complications
   a. Hypoxemia
   b. Hypoventilation
3. Pain
4. Emergence excitement (physical trauma)
5. Hyperthermia/hypothermia
6. Vomiting
7. Delayed awakening

of recovery that occur and appropriate therapeutic schemes. In the end, individualized therapy is the most desirable plan.

Hazards of the recovery period that may require therapeutic intervention are listed in Table 9.11.

EVALUATION OF THE RESPONSE TO ANESTHESIA. Since very early in the history of general anesthesia attempts have been made to correlate observations of the effects of anesthetics with "depth" of anesthesia. To be able to define the depth of anesthesia is important for a number of reasons. For example, too little or too much anesthesia is a threat to life. Consequently, if one can determine the magnitude of anesthesia with reasonable accuracy, patient safety is improved and optimal operating conditions are facilitated for the health care providers. Furthermore, specific guidelines help the novice anesthetist provide appropriate anesthetic conditions. Finally, in investigative circumstances an accurate means for describing and comparing anesthetic levels within or between studies is essential so that we may account for the effects of the anesthetic in our overall understanding versus other variables that may be operant and of interest at the time of study. It would be very helpful to be able to precisely define the depth of anesthesia in every animal from moment to moment regardless of the anesthetic technique. Unfortunately, this is presently not possible, so we rely on estimates.

More than 50 years ago Guedel (Guedel 1920, 1927) published his classic description of the four stages of anesthesia (Table 9.12). The traditional classification is based on a progressive depression of a continuum of CNS function. Guedel extended the descriptions of earlier workers such as Plomley (1847) and Snow (1847) to divide the state of anesthesia into distinct "packages," each correlating with a particular set of physiological responses or reflexes, i.e., clinical signs. The organizational scheme (Table 9.12) includes four stages of anesthesia and subdivides the third stage into four strata (i.e., planes). Guedel's system has been

TABLE 9.12—A summary of the classical description of the four stages of general anesthesia

1. Stage I
   a. Stage either of analgesia, induction, and voluntary excitement or of analgesia and amnesia
   b. Period from beginning of induction to loss of consciousness
   c. Voluntary resistance to restraint and to anesthetic vapors
   d. In humans: loss or obtundation of pain sensation; mental facilities controllable throughout this stage but progressively depressed until unconsciousness
2. Stage II
   a. Stage of delirium, involuntary excitement, or uninhibited action
   b. Period from loss of consciousness to onset of automatic respiration
   c. In humans: dream stage
3. Stage III
   a. Surgical stage
   b. Period from onset of automatic respiration to respiratory arrest
   c. Subdivided into four planes of anesthesia:
      i. Plane I: light surgical
      ii. Plane II: moderate surgical
      iii. Plane III: deep surgical
      iv. Plane IV: excessive surgical
4. Stage IV
   a. Stage of respiratory paralysis or overdose
   b. Interval between respiratory and cardiac arrest

Source: Modified from Steffey 1983.

prominent in pharmacology texts (including earlier editions of this text) and anesthesia texts for more than five decades. The concept is included here in abbreviated form because its importance in the discussion of fundamental principles of anesthesia is becoming more limited.

The classic signs and stages are partly recognizable with many general anesthetics (e.g., the barbiturates), but they are incomplete or are obscured when using modern anesthetics (e.g., ketamine) and/or techniques. It is important to remember that Guedel's description was based on his observation of the actions of diethyl ether administered to otherwise unmedicated human patients who were breathing spontaneously. This is a situation far different from contemporary practice, in which controlled mechanical ventilation is common and newer and multiple anesthetic and adjuvant drugs are an important part of the anesthetic plan. There are unique differences in the way different species react to conditions of general anesthesia that also must be taken into consideration. Because of diethyl ether's characteristics and the methods of delivery, the onset and "deepening" of anesthesia were slow. This situation facilitated a slow (relative to today's standards) unfolding. In addition, numerous physiological responses to anesthetics that are widely monitored today (Table 9.13) are not included in the classic description.

With the emergence of anesthetics such as ketamine and enflurane the concept that all anesthetics are depressants required reconsideration. Winters et al.

TABLE 9.13—Useful signs in clinical assessment of anesthetic depth

1. Cardiovascular system
   a. Heart rate and rhythm[a]
   b. Arterial blood pressure[b]
   c. Mucous membrane color
   d. Capillary refill time
2. Respiratory system
   a. Breathing frequency[a]
   b. Ventilatory volumes (tidal and minute ventilation)[a]
   c. Character of breathing[a]
   d. Arterial or end-tidal CO_2 partial pressure[b]
3. Eye
   a. Position and/or movement of eyeball[b]
   b. Pupil size[a]
   c. Pupil response to light
   d. Palpebral reflex
   e. Corneal reflex
   f. Lacrimation
4. Muscle
   a. Jaw or limb tone[a]
   b. Presence or absence of gross movement[a]
   c. Shivering or trembling[a]
5. Miscellaneous
   a. Body temperature
   b. Laryngeal reflex[a]
   c. Swallowing[a]
   d. Coughing[a]
   e. Vocalizing[a]
   f. Salivating
   g. Sweating
   h. Urine flow

Source: From Steffey 1983.
[a]Moderate or [b]High specificity in assessment of anesthetic depth for various animal species and anesthetic agents.

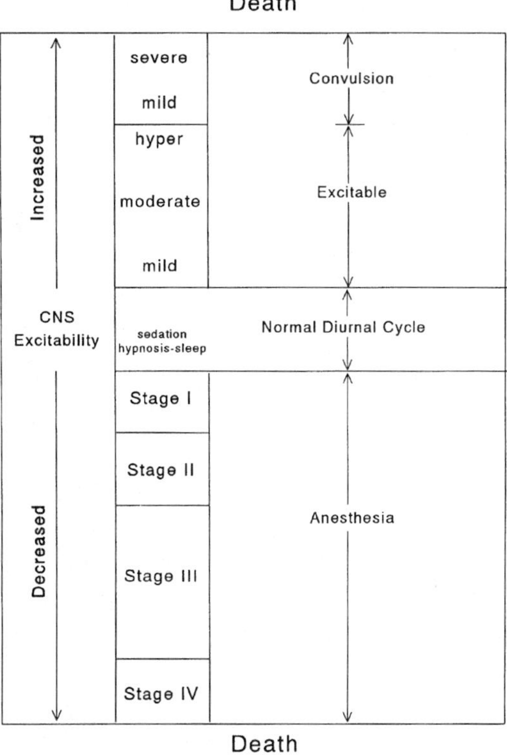

FIG. 9.7—The classic unidimensional schema of CNS excitation and depression. (Modified from Winters 1976.)

(1967) proposed replacement of the classic, unidirectional schema (Fig. 9.7) of CNS excitation and depression with a new schema that included a description of progressive states of both CNS depression and excitation (Fig. 9.8). The new schema recognized bidirectional influences of drugs acting on the CNS and was based on results of electrophysiological studies of anesthetic, excitatory, hallucinogenic, and convulsive agents in cats (Winters et al. 1967; Winters et al. 1972; Winters 1976).

Guedel's scheme also does not take into consideration the modifying influences of such things as duration of anesthesia (Dunlop et al. 1987; Steffey et al. 1987a; Steffey et al. 1987b) or varying magnitudes of surgical stimulus intensity on the signs of anesthesia (Eger et al. 1972; Steffey 1983). In modern clinical anesthetic practice it is recognized that no single observation is always reliable as a sign indicating a specific magnitude of anesthesia. Accordingly, anesthetists are encouraged to develop a basic background knowledge of both the individual to be anesthetized and the selected drugs. Current advice for anesthetic management under clinical conditions is to use an initial anesthetic loading dose just necessary to suppress purposeful movement and to observe all signs possible in each patient (Table. 9.13) and then to manipulate further anesthetic dose in relation to continual stimulus-patient response assessment. If the level of anesthesia is in doubt err on the side of an animal that is too lightly anesthetized.

Stimulus assessment is of special importance since the intensity of stimulus applied to an anesthetized animal may rapidly and markedly alter the observed signs (Eger et al. 1972; Steffey 1983). A quiet animal with reasonable vital signs may quickly show evidence of light to moderate anesthesia in the presence of intense visceral stimulation despite no change in anesthetic delivery. Common responses to anesthetic dose-stimulus interaction are given in Table 9.14.

More precise quantitative measures of anesthetic depth are of obvious interest for the clinician and essential in research. Measurement of end-expired (alveolar) concentration of inhaled anesthetics is a more precise indication of anesthetic level than clinical signs when this type of anesthetic agent is used. In addition, there is continued interest in using electrophysiological approaches to measure depth of anesthesia in both the laboratory and the operating room. For a more complete review of this focused area, see Stanski 1990.

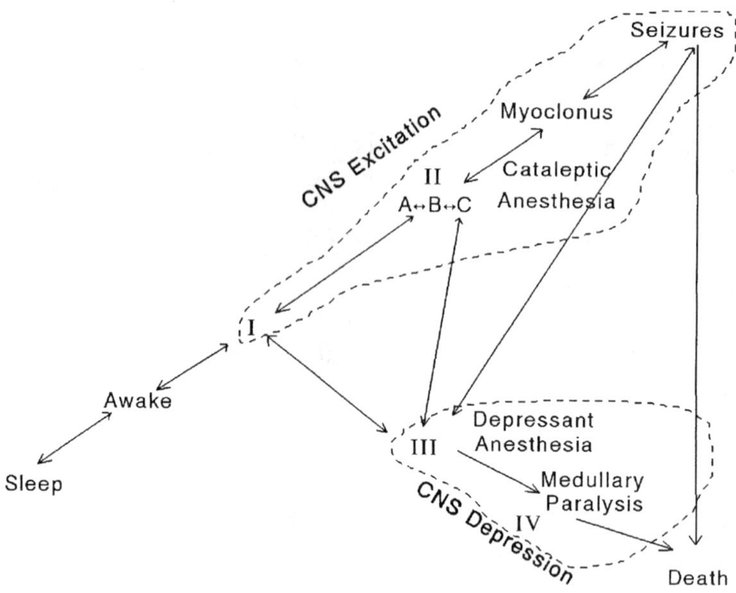

FIG. 9.8—Schematic representation of the stages of anesthesia according to Winters et al. 1972 and Winters 1976. The schematic has been modified slightly from its original description. I-IV refer to the classic stages of anesthesia.

TABLE 9.14—Common responses to anesthetic dose stimulus interaction

1. Signs of presurgical anesthesia
   a. Bradycardia, tachycardia, arrhythmia
   b. Arterial hypertension
   c. Pupillary dilation, lacrimation, globe rotation
   d. Tachypnea or breath holding
   e. Deep breathing
   f. Reduced alveolar/arterial PCO_2
   g. Limb/body movement
   h. Salivating, vomiting
   i. Swallowing
   j. Laryngeal spasm
   k. Phonating
2. Signs of deep surgical anesthesia
   a. Bradycardia, tachycardia, arrhythmia, cardiac arrest
   b. Arterial hypotension
   c. Pupillary dilation, dry cornea, centrally fixed eye
   d. Shallow breathing, respiratory arrest (*not* breath holding)
   e. Elevated alveolar/arterial PCO_2
   f. Muscle flaccidity

Source: Steffey 1983.
Note: Importance of a given sign in a specific species and/or individual varies.

REFERENCES

Albrecht, R. F., and Miletich, D. J. 1988. Speculations on the molecular nature of anesthesia. Gen Pharmac 19:339–46.

Andrews, J. J. 1990. Inhaled anesthetic delivery systems. In R. D. Miller, ed., Anesthesia, 3rd ed., pp. 171–223. New York: Churchill Livingstone.

Barnard, E. A. Skolnick, P., Olsen, R. W., Mohler, H., Sieghart, W., Biggio, G., Braestrup, C., Bateson, A. N., and Langer, S. Z. 1998. International union of pharmacology XV. Subtypes of γ-aminobutyric acid$_A$ receptors: classification on the basis of subunit structure and receptor function. Pharmacol Rev 50:291–313.

Bloom, F. E. 1996. Drugs acting on the central nervous system. In J. G. Hardman, L. E. Limbird, P. B. Molinoff, R. W. Ruddon, and A. G. Gilman, eds., Goodman and Gilman's The Pharmacological Basis of Therapeutics, 9th ed., pp. 267–293. New York: McGraw-Hill.

Bonica, J. J. 1990. The Management of Pain, 2nd ed. Philadelphia: Lea & Febiger.

Bowery, N. 1989. GABA-b receptors and their significance in mammalian pharmacology. Trends Pharmacol Sci 10:402–407.

———. 1993. GABA(b) receptor pharmacology. Annu Rev Pharmacol Toxicol 33:109–147.

Bradley, P. B. 1989. Introduction to Neuropharmacology. Boston: Wright/Butterworth.

Caulfield, M. P., and Birdsall, N. J. M. 1998. International union of pharmacology XVII. Classification of muscarinic acetylcholine receptors. Pharmacol Rev 50:279–290.

Cooper, J. R., Bloom, F. E., and Roth, R. H. 1996. The Biochemical Basis of Neuropharmacology, 7th ed. New York: Oxford Univ Press.

Dunlop, C. I., Steffey, E. P., Miller, M. F., and Woliner, M. J. 1987. Temporal effects of halothane and isoflurane in laterally recumbent ventilated male horses. Am J Vet Res 48:1250–1255.

Eger, E. I., II, Dolan, W. M., Stevens, W. C., Miller, R. D., and Way, W. L. 1972. Surgical stimulation antagonizes the respiratory depression produced by Forane. Anesthesiology 36:544–549.

Firestone, L. L. 1988. General anesthetics. Int Anesthesiol Clin 26:248–256.

Franks, N. P., and Lieb, W. R. 1987. What is the molecular nature of general anaesthetic target sites? Trends Pharmacol Sci 8:169–174.

Gasic, G. P., and Hollmann, M. 1993. Molecular neurobiology of glutamate receptors. Annu Rev Physiol 54:507–536.

Guedel, A. E. 1920. Third stage ether anesthesia: a sub-classification regarding the significance of the position and movements of the eyeball. Am J Surg 24 (Suppl):53–57.

———. 1927. Stages of anesthesia and reclassification of the signs of anesthesia. Anesth Analg 6:157–162.

Guyton, A. C., and Hall, J. E. 1996. Textbook of Medical Physiology, 9th ed. Philadelphia: W. B. Saunders.

Hall, L. W., and Clarke, K. W. 1991. Veterinary Anaesthesia, 9th ed. London: Bailliere Tindall.

Halsey, M. J. 1989. Molecular mechanisms of anaesthesia. In J. F. Nunn, J. E. Utting, and B. R. Brown, eds., General Anaesthesia, 5th ed., pp. 19–29. Boston: Butterworths.

Hill, S. J., Ganellin, C. R., Timmerman, H., Schwartz, J. C., Shankley, N. P., Young, J. M., Schunark, W., Levi, R., and Haas, H. L. 1997. International union of pharmacology XIII. Classification of histamine receptors. Pharmacol Rev 49:253–278.

Kaczmarek, L., Kossut, M., and Skangiel-Kramska, J. 1997. Glutamate receptors in cortical plasticity: molecular and cellular biology. Physiol Rev 77:217–255.

Kerlavage, A. R., Fraser, C. M., and Venter, J. C. 1987. Muscarinic cholinergic receptor structure: molecular biological support for subtypes. Trends Pharmacol Sci 8:426–431.

Kitchell, R. L., and Erickson, H. H. 1983. Introduction: what is pain? In R. L. Kitchell and H. H. Erickson, eds., Animal Pain: Perception and Alleviation, pp. vii–viii. Bethesda: American Physiological Society.

Koblin, D. D. 1994. Mechanisms of action. In R. D. Miller, ed., Anesthesia, 4th ed., pp. 67–99. New York: Churchill Livingstone.

Levant, B. 1997. The D_3 dopamine receptor: neurobiology and potential clinical relevance. Pharmacol Rev 49:231–252.

Limbird, L. E., ed. 1988. The Alpha-2 Adrenergic Receptors. Clifton: Humana Press.

Missale, C., Nash, S. R., Robinson, S. W., Jaber, M., and Caron, M. G. 1998. Dopamine receptors: from structure to function. Physiol Rev 78:189–225.

Negri, L., Potenza, R. L., Corsi, R., and Melchiorri, P. 1991. Evidence for two subtypes of delta opioid receptors in rat brain. Eur J Pharmacol 196:335–336.

Nicoll, R. A. 1998. Introduction to the pharmacology of CNS drugs. In B. G. Katzung, ed., Basic and Clinical Pharmacology, 7th ed., pp. 343–353. Stamford: Appleton & Lange.

Olsen, R. W., and Tobin, A. J. 1990. Molecular biology of GABA-a receptors. FASEB J 4:1469–1480.

Pasternak, G. W., and Wood, P. L. 1986. Multiple mu opiate receptors. Life Sci 38:135.

Plomley, F. 1847. Stages of anaesthesia. Lancet 1:134.

Role, L. W., and Berg, D. K. 1996. Nicotinic receptors in the development and modulation of CNS synapses. Neuron 16:1077–1085.

Rothman, R. B., Bykov, V., De Costa, B. R., Jacobson, A. E., Rice, K. C., and Brady, L. S. 1990. Interaction of endogenous opioid peptides and other drugs with four kappa opioid binding sites in guinea pig brain. Peptides 11:311–331.

Ruffolo, R. R., Jr., Nichols, A. J., Stadel, J. M., and Hieble, J. P. 1993. Pharmacologic and therapeutic applications of α_2-adrenoceptor subtypes. Annu Rev Pharmacol Toxicol 32:243–279.

Schwartz, J.-C., Arrang, J.-M., Garbarg, M., Pollard, H., and Ruat, M. 1991. Histaminergic transmission in the mammalian brain. Physiol Rev 71:1–51.

Short, C. E., ed. 1987. Principles and Practice of Veterinary Anesthesia. Baltimore: Williams & Wilkins.

Sieghart, W. 1995. Structure and pharmacology of gamma-aminobutyric $acid_A$ receptor subtypes. Pharmacol Rev 47:181–234.

Sihra, S. T., and Nichols, R. A. 1993. Mechanisms in the regulation of neurotransmitter release from brain nerve terminals: current hypotheses. Neurochem Res 18:47–58.

Smithcors, J. F. 1971. History of veterinary anesthesia. In L. R. Soma, ed., Textbook of Veterinary Anesthesia, pp. 1–23. Baltimore: Williams & Wilkins.

Snow, J. 1847. On the Inhalation of the Vapour of Ether in Surgical Operations: Containing a Description of the Various Stages of Etherization, and a Statement of the Results of Nearly Eighty Operations in which Ether has been Employed in St. George and University College Hospitals. London: Churchill.

Spector, R. 1990. Drug transport in the central nervous system: role of carriers. Pharmacology 40:1–7.

Stanski, D. R. 1990. Monitoring depth of anesthesia. In R. D. Miller, ed., Anesthesia, 3d ed., pp. 1001–1029. New York: Churchill Livingstone.

Steffey, E. P. 1983. Concepts of general anesthesia and assessment of adequacy of anesthesia for animal surgery. In R. L. Kitchell and H. H. Erickson, eds., Animal Pain: Perception and Alleviation, pp. 133–150. Bethesda: American Physiological Society.

Steffey, E. P., Farver, T. B., and Woliner, M. J. 1987a. Cardiopulmonary function during 7 h of constant-dose halothane and methoxyflurane. J Appl Physiol 63:1351–1359.

Steffey, E. P., Kelly, A. B., and Woliner, M. J. 1987b. Time-related responses of spontaneously breathing, laterally recumbent horses to prolonged anesthesia with halothane. Am J Vet Res 48:952–957.

Strange, P. G. 1988. The structure and mechanism of neurotransmitter receptors. Biochem J 249:309–318.

Unterwald, E. M., Knapp, C., and Zukin, R. S. 1991. Neuroanatomical localization of K 1 and K 2 opioid receptors in rat and guinea pig brain. Brain Res 562:57–65.

Unwin, N. 1993. Neurotransmitter action: opening of ligand-gated ion channels. Cell 72(Suppl):31–41.

Vandam, L. D. 1994. History of anesthetic practice. In R. D. Miller, ed., Anesthesia, 4th ed., pp. 9–19. New York: Churchill Livingstone.

Wall, P. D., and Melzack, R. E. 1994. Textbook of Pain, 3rd ed. New York: Churchill Livingstone.

Wild, K. D., Vanderah, T., Mosberg, H. I., and Porreca, F. 1991. Opioid delta receptor subtypes are associated with different potassium channels. Eur J Pharmacol 193:135–136.

Willis, W. D. 1985. The Pain System: The Neural Basis of Nociceptive Transmission in the Mammalian Nervous System. Basel: Karger.

Winters, W. D. 1976. Effects of drugs on the electrical activity of the brain: anesthetics. Ann Rev Pharmacol Toxicol 16:413–426.

Winters, W. D., Mori, K., Spooner, C. E., and Bauer, R. O. 1967. The neurophysiology of anesthesia. Anesthesiology 28:65–80.

Winters, W. D., Ferrar-Allado, T., Guzman-Flores, C., and Alcaraz, M. 1972. The cataleptic state induced by ketamine: a review of the neuropharmacology of anesthesia. Neuropharmacology 11:303–315.

10 THERAPEUTIC GASES: OXYGEN, CARBON DIOXIDE, WATER VAPOR, AND NITRIC OXIDE

EUGENE P. STEFFEY

Physical Principles
- **Compressed Gases**
- **Behavior of Gases**

Oxygen
- **Oxygen Lack**
- **Oxygen Excess**
- **Therapeutic Uses of Oxygen**
- **Administration of Oxygen**

Carbon Dioxide
- **Hypercapnia**
- **Hypocapnia**

Water Vapor
- **Therapeutic Uses of Water Vapor**
- **Administration of Water Vapor**

Nitric Oxide
- **Therapeutic Use of Inhaled NO**
- **Administration of NO**

This review of therapeutic gases centers on oxygen (O_2) and carbon dioxide (CO_2). Because of the increased interest in and effectiveness of respiratory therapy in veterinary patients and the need to administer water in the inspired breath, water vapor is also briefly discussed. Although the therapeutic value of these three gases is not uniquely associated with the central nervous system, they are discussed in this section because they have a prominent role in the management of general anesthesia. Information on nitric oxide (NO) has been briefly added to this chapter (and supplements information in Chap. 5) because it is now recognized as a major endogenous mediator of multiple physiologic processes, and as a result it offers promise as an inhaled drug for use in the clinical practice of anesthetic management and critical patient care.

PHYSICAL PRINCIPLES

Compressed Gases. Gases are normally commercially available compressed and stored in cylinders. Cylinder sizes are designated by letters, beginning at A. For medical applications, the E and H cylinder sizes are most commonly used (Table 10.1). These cylinders are normally attached directly to anesthetic or respiratory care delivery equipment, and gas inflow is regulated by calibrated gas flow meters. Users of large volumes of O_2 often have a bank of cylinders attached to a manifold supplying a hospital-wide piping system. Users of very large volumes of O_2 may also consider supply in the form of liquid O_2 (Dorsch and Dorsch 1984).

TABLE 10.1—Physical properties of gases

	Carbon dioxide	Oxygen
Chemical formula	CO_2	O_2
Molecular weight	44.01	32.00
Density (g/L at 1 atm, 15°C)	1.867	1.352
Specific gravity (air = 1 at 21°C,* 1 atm)	1.52	1.11
Boiling point (°C)	—	–183
Cylinder fillings		
Physical state in cylinder	liquid	gas
Cylinder pressure (psi at 21°C, 1 atm)	750	2200
Cylinder gas volume (L)		
Style E	1590	622
Style H	—	6900
Cylinder color code (U.S.)	gray	green

*21.1°C = 70.0°F.

Behavior of Gases. The behavior of gases in entering, leaving, and moving within the body is an important consideration in anesthesia and respiratory system therapy. Gases are composed of molecules that move about at random. The gas expands or contracts to fill the space available to it. The random movement and collision of gas molecules with the surface of the surrounding vessel exert a pressure that can be measured. The more molecules per unit volume, the greater the pressure. Temperature is important because, e.g., when a gas is heated, the activity of the molecules increases, and either the volume of the gas increases (no limit to the gas container) or the pressure of the gas increases (i.e., the volume is fixed and the number of molecular collisions therefore increases).

A mixture of gases contained within a space also imparts a pressure. In this case the total pressure of the mixture is the sum of the pressure of each gas in the mixture. That is, each gas exerts a certain fraction (F) of the total pressure. This is known as the gas's partial pressure. The usual notation for partial pressure is P_X, where the subscript X denotes the source. The unit of expression is usually mm Hg. Thus $P_{gas} = P_{total} \times F_{gas}$. The fraction is the percentage of gas in the whole/100 and is without units.

TABLE 10.2—Partial pressure (*P*) of respiratory gases during air and 100% oxygen breathing

	Inspired gas (dry)		Alveolar gas		Arterial blood	
	Air	O_2	Air	O_2	Air	O_2
PO_2 (mm Hg)	159	760	104	673	100	640
PCO_2 (mm Hg)	0.3	0	40	40	40	40
PH_2O (mm Hg)	0	0	47	47	47	47
O_2 saturation (%)	—	—	—	—	97	100
O_2 content (mL/100 mL)	—	—	—	—	019.80	22.02

Note: These values generally apply to terrestrial mammals at sea level (760 mm Hg).

Gases enter the pulmonary capillary blood from the lung alveoli (e.g., O_2) or leave the blood (e.g., CO_2) en route to the external environment via the alveoli. Blood of course acts as a medium of transport for gases and vapors between the lungs and the tissues. Gases are carried in blood simply in solution or they are reversibly combined with some constituents in the blood. Chemical combination enables more gas to be carried than would be the case with the gas simply dissolved in the liquid. The gas molecules move passively by the process of diffusion, from a place where there is a higher partial pressure of the gas to one of a lower pressure. When there is no difference in pressure of the gas molecules between the two locations, there is no net movement or transfer of molecules. The greater the difference (i.e., the steeper the partial pressure gradient), the more easily the gas exchange occurs. While the inward movement of gases from the air to alveoli is aided by mechanical means (i.e., ventilation), the passage of gas to and from tissues is solely dependent upon diffusion. In addition to the pressure gradient, the rate of gas diffusion is influenced by the distance for diffusion, the cross-sectional area of the membrane across which diffusion may occur, and the molecular weight of the gas. When gases are exposed to a gas-free liquid, an additional factor requires consideration: that of solubility. The gas molecules diffuse into the liquid until the partial pressure of the gas in the liquid equals the partial pressure in the gas phase. The number of gas molecules that enter the liquid before equilibrium is reached (i.e., equal partial pressure of the gas in the two media) is determined by the solubility of the gas. This fact is known as Henry's law (Nunn 1993). Therefore, at the same partial pressure there will be more molecules of a gas of high solubility in a liquid compared to a gas of low solubility. Henry's law applies only to gas in solution and not to a gas in chemical combination with the liquid or its constituents (e.g., O_2 with hemoglobin). Temperature also plays a role in the amount of gas dissolved in a solvent. The higher the temperature, the less the amount of gas that goes into solution.

While these principles are likely most easily understood in the context of the respiratory gases O_2 and CO_2, they also apply to absorption and elimination of other gases that pass into and out of the tissues, e.g., nitrogen and anesthetic gases. Normal values for the partial pressure of respiratory gases in terrestrial mammals breathing air at sea level (760 mm Hg) are given in Table 10.2.

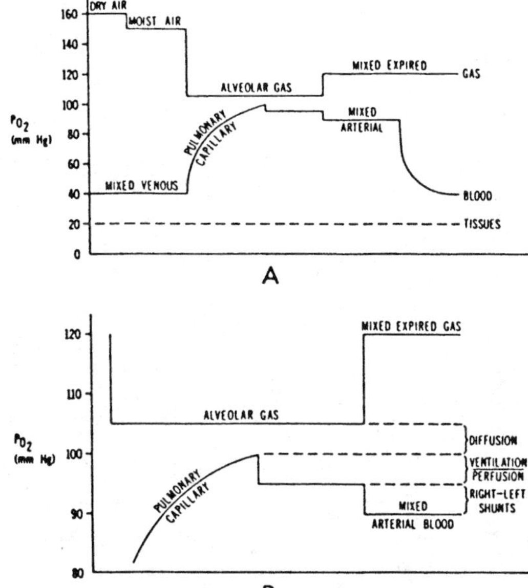

FIG. 10.1.—Oxygen tensions in blood and gas phases. Graph A shows the oxygen partial pressure (PO_2, mm Hg) in blood and gas phases of the respiratory system. Graph B shows blood and gas PO_2 within the lung and factors involved in the alveolar-arterial PO_2 difference. (From Steffey and Robinson 1983, with permission.)

OXYGEN Most of the energy used in the mammalian body is derived from biochemical pathways that consume O_2 and are located in the mitochondria. Anaerobic pathways also exist for energy production, but they are less efficient.

About one-fifth (20.9%) of the air inhaled in each breath consists of O_2. Thus the partial pressure of O_2 (P_aO_2) of dry air at sea level is 159 mm Hg. Oxygen moves down a partial pressure gradient from ambient air through the respiratory tract. Moisture is added in the upper airway, and it mixes with alveolar gas so the PO_2 in the alveoli is reduced from 159 mm Hg (Table 10.2). Further reductions in partial pressure occur in the arterial blood, the tissue, the capillaries, and the cell, and the partial pressure ultimately reaches its lowest level within the mitochondria (Fig. 10.1). These steps in the decrease of the PO_2 are commonly referred

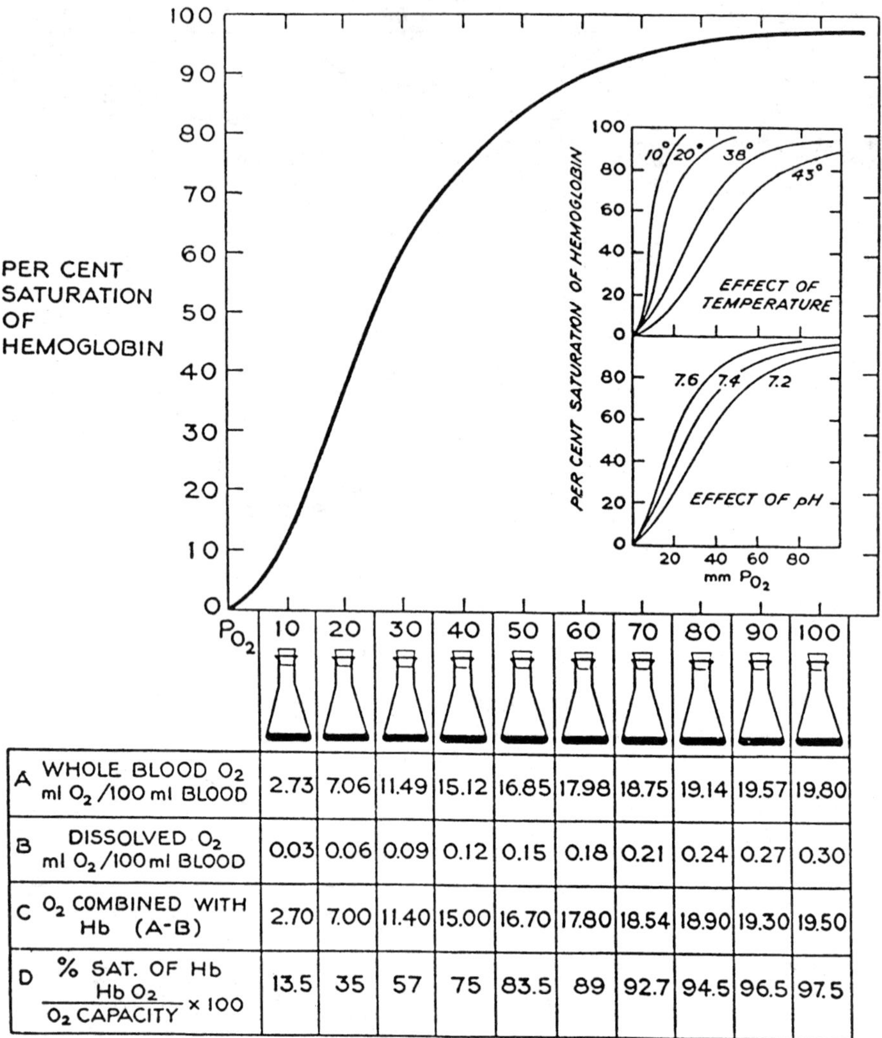

P_{O_2}	10	20	30	40	50	60	70	80	90	100
A WHOLE BLOOD O_2 ml O_2/100 ml BLOOD	2.73	7.06	11.49	15.12	16.85	17.98	18.75	19.14	19.57	19.80
B DISSOLVED O_2 ml O_2/100 ml BLOOD	0.03	0.06	0.09	0.12	0.15	0.18	0.21	0.24	0.27	0.30
C O_2 COMBINED WITH Hb (A-B)	2.70	7.00	11.40	15.00	16.70	17.80	18.54	18.90	19.30	19.50
D % SAT. OF Hb $\frac{\text{Hb O}_2}{\text{O}_2\text{ CAPACITY}} \times 100$	13.5	35	57	75	83.5	89	92.7	94.5	96.5	97.5

FIG. 10.2.—Oxygen dissociation curves. The large graph shows a single dissociation curve for human blood when pH of the blood is 7.40 and temperature is 38°C. Effects on the curve of changes in temperature and pH are shown on the smaller graphs. The positioning of the curve is also influenced slightly according to species (not shown). (From Comroe 1965, with permission.)

to as the O_2 cascade and are more thoroughly reviewed elsewhere (Comroe 1965; Guyton and Hall 1996; Nunn 1993; Steffey and Robinson 1983; West 1992).

Oxygen is carried in the blood in two forms. About 75% is transported to the tissue in loose chemical combination with hemoglobin (Fig. 10.2). Each gram of hemoglobin can combine with about 1.34 mL of O_2. A normal value for hemoglobin concentration that broadly reflects species of importance in veterinary medicine is 15 g/dL of whole blood. Thus in the presence of normal hemoglobin concentration, arterial blood will carry about 20 mL of O_2 when the hemoglobin is fully saturated (1.34 × 15).

Hemoglobin saturation is defined as the actual O_2 content of a sample and is expressed as a percentage of the possible total carrying capacity of the sample. The saturation of hemoglobin with O_2 at different partial pressures of O_2 in blood is described by the S-shaped hemoglobin dissociation curve (Fig. 10.2).

Only about 0.03 mL of O_2 is in physical solution (dissolved in plasma) in 100 mL of blood when the PO_2 is 100 mm Hg. Although this quantity is not large, O_2 solubility has importance since it is via this pathway that O_2 passes to and from hemoglobin and the tissues. Furthermore, although the amount of O_2 carried by hemoglobin cannot increase beyond that quantity at

TABLE 10.3—Etiology of hypoxia

I. Prepulmonary cause
  A. Deficiency of O_2 in the inspired breath
    1. Low inspired O_2 concentration at normal ambient pressure (e.g., improper O_2/N_2O mixture during anesthesia)
    2. Normal O_2 concentration at low ambient pressure (e.g., high altitude)
  B. Reduced ventilation
    1. Anatomic obstruction to gas flow (e.g., airway obstruction)
    2. Mechanical deficit (e.g., neuromuscular block)
    3. System control deficit (e.g., drug- or disease-induced CNS depression)
II. Pulmonary cause
  A. Impaired diffusion at alveolar-capillary membrane (e.g., pulmonary edema)
  B. Increased right to left (i.e., venous to arterial) pulmonary vascular shunt (e.g., congenital cardiac disease)
  C. Mismatching of ventilation to perfusion
III. Postpulmonary cause
  A. Inadequate circulatory system transport of O_2
    1. Reduced hemoglobin concentration (e.g., anemia)
    2. General dicrulatory deficiency (e.g., decreased cardiac output)
    3. Localized circulatory deficiency (e.g., decreased regional blood flow)
  B. Inadequate tissue oxygenation
    1. Inadequate unloading of O_2 from hemoglobin (e.g., defiency in 2, 3-DPG)
    2. Tissue diffusion impairment (e.g., edema)
    3. Abnormally high tissue O_2 demand (e.g., local hyperthermia)
    4. Cellular enzyme system malformation (e.g., cyanide poisoning)

which hemoglobin is fully saturated, the total amount in solution increases directly with an increase in P_aO_2.

The O_2 content of blood is the sum of the volume of O_2 carried in solution and that transported via hemoglobin per unit volume of blood (again by convention, 1 unit volume is usually considered 100 mL). Changes in the amount of hemoglobin per 100 mL of blood will alter O_2 content but not the percent saturation of hemoglobin or P_aO_2.

A number of factors influence the amount of O_2 transported by hemoglobin and so shift the oxygen-hemoglobin dissociation curve to the left or to the right. Acidosis, increased body temperature, and increased concentrations of 2,3-diphosphoglycerate (2,3-DPG, a product of erythrocyte metabolism) all shift the curve to the right (i.e., decrease the affinity of hemoglobin for O_2 and facilitate unloading of O_2); and increased blood pH, decreased body temperature, and decreased concentration of 2,3-DPG all have an opposite effect (Fig. 10.2).

When the O_2 content of arterial blood is very low, unpigmented mucous membrane color may change from pink to blue. This is known as cyanosis and is due to the darker color of deoxyhemoglobin. Cyanosis appears when about 5 g/dL of deoxyhemoglobin are present in arterial blood.

Oxygen Lack. The lack of O_2 represents a serious threat to the vitality of the organism and is variously described. *Hypoxia* is a general term that signifies a decrease in O_2 below normal levels in inspired gas, alveolar air, blood, or tissues (Comroe 1965). In recent times it has been most commonly used to designate insufficient oxygenation of tissues. *Hypoxemia* signifies a decrease in arterial hemoglobin O_2 saturation below normal or a below-normal P_aO_2 or both.

The causes of hypoxia can be conveniently classified according to prepulmonary, pulmonary, and postpulmonary sites (Table 10.3). Hypoxemia is not surprisingly associated with prepulmonary and pulmonary etiologies. Indeed, multiple etiologies frequently occur simultaneously under clinical conditions.

Physiological responses to hypoxia may be considered direct or indirect. The direct responses relate largely to the cardiovascular and respiratory systems, and the indirect effects are those secondary effects due to hypoxia-associated failure of vital organs such as the heart, brain, kidney, and liver. When O_2 delivery to the tissues falls below a critical level, vigorous compensatory mechanisms come into play to attempt to minimize harm to the individual.

The direct responses are usually robust and tend to over ride conflicting mechanisms. Some compensatory mechanisms may be impaired by concurrent drug therapy (e.g., anesthetics) or vary in extent depending on species (Comroe 1965; Guyton and Hall 1996; Nunn 1993).

Cardiac output and regional blood flow to vital organs increase largely as a result of an increase in heart rate and a decrease in peripheral vascular resistance. Tachypnea and hyperventilation are the prominent respiratory system responses due to stimulation of the peripheral chemoreceptors. Pulmonary arterioles constrict, and pulmonary artery blood pressure increases, presumably in an attempt to better balance pulmonary blood flow with regional lung ventilation.

Lack of O_2 impairs tissue function and if prolonged causes cellular death and necrosis. Cellular survival times depend on many factors but are largely influenced by inherent tissue characteristics of O_2 consumption and local O_2 stores. Survival conditions can be improved by, e.g., decreasing cellular metabolism (e.g., hypothermia). Hyperbaric oxygenation improves O_2 stores.

The cerebral cortex is especially vulnerable to hypoxia, and change in cerebral function is a very sensitive indication of O_2 lack. In humans, a change in mood is an early sign of hypoxia, and with continued insult or an increased magnitude of hypoxic conditions, mental performance gradually deteriorates and consciousness may ultimately be lost. In anesthetized animals anesthetic requirement is decreased (Cullen and Eger 1974). Skeletal muscle, on the other hand, is much less sensitive to an insult of similar magnitude. Heart and hepatic cells are intermediary in their vulnerability to hypoxic conditions, and hepatic centrilobular necrosis is a consequence of some mishaps.

OXYGEN-DERIVED FREE RADICALS AND CELL INJURY. Organ survival after a period of hypoxia depends also on factors that influence O_2 transport during the recovery phase. Restored tissue perfusion and oxygenation before hypoxic cell death can sometimes paradoxically result in an accelerated form of cell injury (ischemia-reperfusion injury). Events associated with reperfusion following ischemia produce further tissue injury via the generation of O_2 free radicals. The resulting injury is distinct from that occurring as a result of the preceding ischemic period.

A free radical is a molecule containing an odd number of electrons. This state is chemically very reactive. Of the radicals formed in biological systems, most attention is focused on superoxide, a species formed when O_2 is reduced by a single electron (Bhagavan 1992; McCord 1985, 1987; Pryor 1986). Superoxide anion is also produced by O_2-reducing enzymes of phagocytes (neutrophils, mononuclear phagocytes), which defend the host against invading organisms. Current thinking regarding the etiology of ischemia-reperfusion injury is that the initial hypoxic stress results in the production of hypoxanthine and O_2-radical-producing xanthine oxidase. During reperfusion, molecular O_2 is reintroduced into the tissues, where it supports the burst production of more superoxide anion and hydrogen peroxide, which in turn yields highly reactive cytotoxic components. Granulocytes are attracted to this area, are activated, and adhere to microvascular endothelium. These granulocytes then in turn cause further endothelial cell damage via release of superoxide and various proteases (Granger 1988; McCord 1987; Welbourn et al. 1991).

Dysfunction induced by free radicals is likely a major component of ischemic diseases of the heart, bowel, liver, kidney, brain, and skeletal muscle (McCord 1985; Granger et al. 1981; Perry and Fantini 1987; Karmazyn 1991). In addition, reperfusion of ischemic tissue may lead to an inflammatory reaction that is not just confined to the region of injury (Welbourn et al. 1991; McCord 1987).

Reperfused tissues are protected in a variety of laboratory models by scavengers of superoxide radicals (superoxide dismutase) and hydroxyl radicals (dimethyl sulfoxide) or by inhibitors of xanthine oxidase (allopurinol) (Welbourn et al. 1991; McCord 1985).

CHRONIC OXYGEN LACK. A gradual decline in O_2 tension occurs as the vertical distance from sea level increases. The decrease in PO_2 is a direct result of the decrease in barometric pressure with increasing altitude since O_2 concentration in the earth's atmosphere remains at slightly less than 21% of the total barometric pressure. For example, the PO_2 of ambient air at sea level is 159 mm Hg (0.21 × 760 mm Hg; Table 10.2) but 110 mm Hg (0.21 × 523 mm Hg) at 10,000 feet and only 47 mm Hg (0.21 × 226 mm Hg) at 30,000 feet.

Adaptations to high altitude and the associated lowered inspired PO_2 depends to a certain degree on whether the individual has resided at high altitude since birth or has only recently (within weeks) traveled there. However, in general, the adaptation process includes an increase in alveolar ventilation, hemoglobin and 2,3-DPG production, respiratory gas-diffusing capacity in the lungs, and vascularity of tissues. There is also an improved ability of the cells to use a more limited PO_2. Occasionally, adjustments fail to occur in individuals, and their health and well-being are affected (Guyton and Hall 1996; Nunn 1993; West 1992).

Oxygen Excess. *Hyperoxia* refers to an increase in P_aO_2 above normal for animals breathing air at sea level and can be produced in two ways. First, an elevation in P_aO_2 at sea level can result from increasing the inspired O_2 fraction (concentration). Common clinical examples of O_2 enrichment of the inspired breath include the practice of using O_2 as an anesthetic carrier gas or to supplement the inspired breath of a critically ill, hypoxemic patient. Alternatively, hyperoxia may be produced by elevation of the ambient pressure with or without a change in the oxygen concentration, i.e., hyperbaric oxygenation.

Hyperoxia can be detrimental in a number of ways, including depression or cessation of ventilation (apnea), retrolental fibroplasia, fire, and O_2 toxicity. Retrolental fibroplasia is a condition that frequently develops in prematurely born infants who in the treatment of prematurity are exposed to high concentrations of O_2 (Ashton 1979; Patz 1965). The condition may cause permanent blindness as a result of O_2-associated retinal damage. The crucial determinant appears to be the magnitude of P_aO_2. The incidence of this problem has been reduced via monitoring P_aO_2 and controlling the inspired O_2 concentration to facilitate a P_aO_2 of 60–70 mm Hg in the infant.

All tissues of the body can be directly injured by sufficiently high PO_2, but because the lung is exposed to the highest partial pressure, it is very vulnerable. Normobaric O_2 toxicity of the lung is related to the magnitude of inspired O_2 concentration and the duration of exposure. Except for tracheitis, which develops early in the exposure, normal humans can likely tolerate an elevated inspired O_2 concentration at sea level for at least 24 hours without any serious lung tissue injury. Longer exposure times and/or underlying disease or other physiological factors that reduce the subjects' tolerance (e.g., age, nutrition status, previous exposure to O_2 or other oxidants) will result in parenchymal injury.

Hyperbaric O_2 accelerates the effects of O_2 toxicity and rapidly induces convulsions, suggesting the cells of the central nervous system are also very sensitive to hyperoxia (Deneke and Fanburg 1982).

The pathology of O_2 toxicity based on studies of animals and human beings is nonspecific and includes atelectasis, pulmonary edema, inflammation, and alveolar membrane thickening. The endothelial cells of the lung seem to be affected earliest, resulting in altered cell permeability and ultimately noncardiogenic edema. Damage to the alveolar type 1 epithelial cells contributes to loss of alveolar stability and later local fibrosis. Although the pathogenesis of hyperoxic O_2 toxicity is not fully established, the formation of excess O_2 free radicals and associated cytotoxic species is currently viewed as the probable mechanism. Thus xanthine oxidase and neutrophil-induced O_2-metabolite-mediated injury seem to participate in both pulmonary O_2 toxicity and ischemia-reperfusion injury. Readers will find reviews by Deneke and Fanburg (1982), Crapo et al. (1983), Repine and Tate (1983), Jackson (1985), and Nunn (1987) helpful for further information on this subject.

Therapeutic Uses of Oxygen. There are two primary clinical uses of O_2 in veterinary patients: correction of hypoxemia and hypoxia and as a diluent or carrier gas for inhalation anesthetics. The absolute O_2 concentration used as therapy for hypoxemia varies with clinical circumstances and the physical status of the patient. Because of its potential for harm, especially with prolonged respiratory care and O_2 use, the inspired O_2 concentration used for treatment of hypoxemia needs to be closely monitored and controlled. Usually an inspired O_2 concentration less than 50% is desirable if prolonged (12 hours or more) administration is anticipated. The adequacy of oxygenation is monitored via serial determination of sampling of arterial blood and measurement of P_aO_2. On the other hand, because of the relatively short duration of exposure and the added complexities of multiple gas delivery, an inspired O_2 concentration greater than 90% is the common, if not usual, circumstance associated with the management of inhalation anesthesia of veterinary patients.

A third clinical use of supplemental O_2 administration is to facilitate the absorption of inert gas(es) from gas pockets within the body. Gas spaces exist in the body under usual and sometimes under abnormal circumstances. Sites within the body include the gastrointestinal tract, peritoneal and pleural cavities, alveoli whose gas entrance/exit paths are not in free communication with airways, and subcutaneous locations. The gas contained within these pockets (largely nitrogen) will be absorbed into the blood and lost from the body more rapidly if O_2 is inhaled because of the individual gas partial pressure differences between the gas space and the blood.

Finally, O_2 can be administered at more than one atmosphere (hyperbaric conditions) if the patient is placed in a rigid container. The clinical application of hyperbaric O_2 delivery to veterinary patients is a rare event. Its use with animals is more commonly associated with investigative activities. It has application to human patients with specific clinical conditions such as gas gangrene caused by clostridial organisms, decompression sickness, or air embolism (the therapeutic goal is for an increased hydrostatic pressure and the establishment of a gradient for outward diffusion of inert gas) or those patients who require a P_aO_2 in excess of that at normobaric circumstances (e.g., P_aO_2 in these patients is normal but blood flow to a region is reduced) (Eckenhoff and Longnecker 1990; Guyton and Hall 1996; Nunn 1993).

Administration of Oxygen. Oxygen is usually administered by inhalation using a variety of available equipment (Dorsch and Dorsch 1984; Shapiro et al. 1975; Short 1987; Hall and Clarke 1991; Haskins 1986). An exception occurs in circumstances in which extracorporeal blood circulation is used (e.g., open heart surgery), in which case O_2 is made to come in direct contact with blood. Terminal devices used to supplement O_2 in the inspired breath of awake or lightly sedated/depressed animals include masks, nasal cannulas, and specially designed gas delivery cages. To facilitate maintenance of the airway during O_2 delivery in anesthetized or markedly depressed critically ill patients, endotracheal intubation is used. The endotracheal tube provides direct access to the airway and seals off the walls of the airway to minimize any possibility of lung aspiration of foreign material. The tube also allows better control of inspired gases and facilitates use of mechanical ventilation in patients with compromised ventilatory function (Short 1987; Hall and Clarke 1991; Haskins 1986).

CARBON DIOXIDE. Carbon dioxide (CO_2) is present in the atmosphere in minute proportions (0.03%). It is stored in cylinders and available commercially for medical use. Carbon dioxide is a waste product of tissue metabolism and is carried in blood primarily in three forms: physical solution, combined with proteins as carbamino-compounds in the red blood cell (about 85% of the total) and plasma, and as bicarbonate in plasma (CO_2 readily combines with water to form carbonic acid, which then dissociates to bicarbonate and hydrogen ions). The CO_2 dissociation curve relates P_aCO_2 to the CO_2 content of blood. Unlike the oxyhemoglobin dissociation curve, this curve has no plateau, so that as P_aCO_2 increases, blood CO_2 also increases (Comroe 1965; Guyton and Hall 1996; Nunn 1993). The CO_2 produced in the body is lost primarily via the lungs. The alveolar PCO_2 is inversely related to the magnitude of alveolar ventilation. Since there is virtually no diffusion impediment to pulmonary capillary-alveolar diffusion of CO_2, P_aCO_2 mirrors the P_ACO_2. Thus P_aCO_2 and alveolar ventilation are also inversely related.

The normal range for the P_aCO_2 in terrestrial mammals is 35–45 mm Hg. Each species usually exhibits a narrower range within this broader range. Clinically, hypoventilation is present when P_aCO_2 exceeds normal (i.e., hypercapnia), and hyperventilation is indicated by a lower than normal P_aCO_2 (i.e., hypocapnia). When alveolar ventilation is decreased (or CO_2 is inhaled), the P_aCO_2 increases and blood pH decreases. This change in pH_a is referred to as respiratory acidosis. Conversely, when alveolar hyperventilation occurs (e.g., overzealous mechanical ventilation), P_aCO_2 decreases and pH_a increases, resulting in respiratory alkalosis. Since CO_2 is freely diffusible, rapid intracellular pH changes also occur.

Changes in the magnitude of P_aCO_2 have important pharmacological effects. However, as pointed out by Nunn (1987), a number of issues relevant to our understanding of the etiology of these effects must be appreciated. First, species differences, especially in the magnitude of response to alterations in P_aCO_2, sometimes make interpretation of findings in the target species difficult. Second, the pharmacological effects of CO_2 may occur because of its direct effect on tissues or via its ability to alter intracellular and extracellular pH. Finally, because of its universal nature and ability to rapidly equilibrate throughout the body, its effects are rapidly produced at different sites so that there may be additive, synergistic, or antagonistic influences on a resultant effect. For example, a direct effect of CO_2 is to depress muscle function, which in the heart results in a decreased myocardial contractility. This in turn will cause a decreased cardiac output. At the same time it causes an endogenous release of catecholamines, which in turn results in an overriding increase in cardiac output in the healthy, sympathetically intact subject. The influence of changes in P_aCO_2 will be briefly reviewed below keeping in mind these difficulties. Also, since the effects of hypocapnia are less well defined than those of hypercapnia, discussion emphasis will be on effects of increased P_aCO_2. The review will emphasize effects related to general anesthesia and the unconscious, critically ill patient.

Hypercapnia. Hypercapnia has important effects on the cardiovascular system, the central and autonomic nervous systems, and the respiratory system. General influences on other organs (e.g., kidneys) are largely related to more direct effects on control of organ function via the nervous system or blood flow.

CARDIOVASCULAR SYSTEM. The observed response represents a balance between the direct effect of CO_2 on the target tissues and excitatory effects mediated via the nervous system (Cullen and Eger 1974; Guyton and Hall 1996; Nunn 1993).

Carbon dioxide causes a direct depression of myocardial contractility (as determined from isolated heart muscle preparations) as well as a depressant effect on myogenic activity in the blood vessels. Consequently, direct unopposed actions of CO_2 foster a decrease in cardiac output and a reduction in peripheral vascular resistance.

In the subject with intact autonomic control of cardiovascular function, the direct effect of CO_2 is overcome by the stimulant effect of the sympathetic nervous system. Consequently, with hypercapnia cardiac output is increased (increased stroke volume), and if there is a change in arterial blood pressure, an increase is the predominant change (Cullen and Eger 1974; Cullen et al. 1990). At superhigh levels of P_aCO_2, cardiac output may decrease (Nunn 1993).

The incidence of cardiac arrhythmias increases with an elevation in P_aCO_2. The impact of this change is related to other factors (e.g., anesthetic agent, anesthetic dose, species, and the animal's physical status).

Regional blood flow is also heavily influenced by an increase in P_aCO_2. For example, cerebral vessels are dilated by hypercapnia. The loss of autoregulation and the increase in cardiac output accompanying hypercapnia result in an increase in intracranial (an enclosed space) pressure, which may be further influenced by some anesthetic agents and techniques (Cullen et al. 1990). These actions are usually not good for the patient's well-being, especially in the presence of any underlying cerebral pathology.

CENTRAL NERVOUS SYSTEM. Three basic consequences of an increase in P_aCO_2 on the central nervous system are relevant to this discussion: (1) effects on cerebral blood vessels and the secondary effects on cerebrospinal fluid and intracranial pressure, (2) the effect on breathing, and (3) the effect on general neuronal activity (Nunn 1993).

Intracranial pressure tends to increase with hypercapnia largely as a result of cerebral vascular vasodilation, as discussed above.

In spontaneously breathing individuals, the addition of CO_2 to the inspired breath causes an increase in P_aCO_2 that in turn causes ventilation to increase. The CO_2 acts primarily by changing the H^+ concentration at the central chemoreceptor area which is located close to the ventrolateral surface of the medulla (Guyton and Hall 1996; Nunn 1993; West 1992). Concurrent hypoxia adds to the response to hypercapnia via peripheral chemoreceptor stimulation, and anesthetics depress the response, usually in a dose-dependent manner (Nunn 1993; Weiskopf et al. 1974; Hickey et al. 1971).

Hypercapnia depresses general neuronal function and if sufficiently high causes general anesthesia (Clowes et al. 1955; Eisele et al. 1967; Klemm 1964; Mattsson et al. 1972). In dogs a P_aCO_2 above 95 mm Hg has been shown to be progressively narcotic and reduces the amount of concurrently administered halothane required to maintain a constant depth of anesthesia. Anesthesia was achieved with CO_2 alone at a P_aCO_2 above 245 mm Hg (Eisele et al. 1967). It is advocated as a sedative for small laboratory animals prior to euthanasia (Urbanski and Kelley 1991; Blackshaw et al. 1988; Danneman et al. 1997). Use of CO_2 as an anesthetic for minor surgery in human beings has also been reported (Leake and Waters 1928). At concentrations below those causing general anesthesia, CO_2 may cause sedation or convulsions in some otherwise-unmedicated individuals. Indeed, review of available literature suggests that especially in susceptible individuals like human beings there is a progressive depression of central nervous system activity as the P_aCO_2 is increased up to about 150 mm Hg; above this a stage of central nervous system excitation and convulsions occurs. With a continued increase in P_aCO_2 (beyond 35%, inspired) this second stage is followed by progressive depression of cerebral electrical activity and general anesthesia (Clowes et al. 1955).

AUTONOMIC NERVOUS AND ENDOCRINE SYSTEMS. Increased sympathetic adrenergic activity is widely recognized as the cause for many of the actions or modification of actions of hypercapnia. Effects originate both centrally and peripherally (Nunn 1993). Hypercapnia results in an increase in plasma concentrations of both epinephrine and norepinephrine (Millar 1960).

EFFECTS OF CO_2 ON OXYGENATION. A major consequence of hypercapnia is a decrease in alveolar O_2 concentration. The O_2 reduction is of particular concern if the inspired gas mixture also includes nitrogen and/or nitrous oxide. Additional CO_2 molecules occupy space in the lung previously available for O_2. This situation thereby reduces the alveolar PO_2, and hypoxemia may result.

Hypercapnia can ultimately influence arterial and tissue oxygenation in other ways. For example, hypercapnia can induce improvements in ventilation and cardiac output in spontaneously breathing animals. An increase in P_aCO_2 also causes hemoglobin to have a reduced affinity for O_2. Both of these effects oppose the alveolar-O_2-diluting effect and maintain or enhance O_2 delivery. However, further discussion on this is beyond the scope of this review; interested readers are referred to appropriate sections in textbooks of respiratory physiology for additional information (Comroe 1965; Guyton and Hall 1996; Nunn 1993).

EFFECTS ON DRUG ACTIONS. Hypercapnia may affect concurrently administered drugs a number of ways. Altered regional blood flow caused by an increase in P_aCO_2 may change drug distribution. In addition, an increase in P_aCO_2 decreases blood pH (respiratory acidosis), thereby influencing the degree of ionization of drugs. Either or both of these consequences may be substantial enough to alter the drug's pharmacokinetic characteristics to a point of investigative or clinical concern.

CLINICAL USE OF CO_2. The main therapeutic indication for the administration of CO_2 is to stimulate ventilation. There is evidence to show that at least mild hypercapnia improves cardiac output and arterial blood pressure, especially in anesthetized patients. Carbon dioxide is used to rapidly render unconscious and euthanize small laboratory animals.

Hypocapnia. As previously noted, pharmacological effects of hypocapnia are less well defined than those of hypercapnia. The effects manifested during conditions of lower than normal P_aCO_2 are also dependent on whether conditions relate to active pulmonary hyperventilation as might occur in states of anxiety or in spontaneously breathing patients in light planes of anesthesia or alternatively in anesthetized or critically ill patients whose ventilation is mechanically controlled to cause hypocapnia. The presence or absence of mechanical effects of altered intrathoracic pressure swings on blood circulation modifies any pharmacological effects of CO_2 or accompanying pH changes.

In the anesthetized subject the prominent effects of hypocapnia include a general reduction in cardiovascular performance (e.g., decrease in cardiac output and arterial blood pressure) that may be considerable in magnitude. For example, cerebral blood flow is decreased as P_aCO_2 is decreased from 40 to 20 mm Hg. Hypocapnia also causes decreased activity of respiratory control centers and an accompanying decrease in alveolar ventilation.

There is a clinical impression that lowering P_aCO_2 during the anesthetic management of patients contributes to the anesthetic effect (Geddes and Gray 1959). However, studies of dogs (Cullen and Eger 1971; Eger et al. 1965) and humans (Bridges and Eger 1966) could not demonstrate a reduction in halothane anesthetic requirement.

CLINICAL USES. Decreasing P_aCO_2 via hyperventilation during anesthesia is a common tactic to facilitate controlled mechanical ventilation in the absence of neuromuscular blockade or excessive anesthetic depth. It is also used to attempt to minimize or prevent neurological complications that might arise from increased intracranial pressure in patients with central nervous system pathology and/or to shrink brain size (via reduced blood flow) and facilitate surgery within the cranial cavity.

WATER VAPOR. Humidity is water in its vapor state: invisible moisture. It is not technically a gas, because the critical temperature of water has not been reached (Scanlan et al. 1990). When air is inspired, it is normally warmed and humidified to saturation at body temperature. This process is largely complete by the time the gas reaches the larynx. In clinical circumstances in which the nasal cavity, mouth, and pharynx are bypassed, as with tracheostomy or endotracheal intubation, the process of hydrating inspired air is accomplished less efficiently by the mucosa and the mucous blanket of the trachea and more distal airways. Normal individuals can withstand this shift in site of air hydration without apparent clinical consequence, but patients with airway injury often cannot.

Humidity can be described in a number of ways. For example, the absolute humidity is the actual water content of a gas and is recorded in terms of weight per

TABLE 10.4—Water vapor pressures and content (saturated) at selected temperatures

Temperature	Vapor pressure	Water vapor content*
(°C)	*(mm Hg)*	*(mg/L)*
20	17.5	17.3
21	18.7	18.4
22	19.8	19.4
23	21.1	20.6
24	22.4	21.8
25	23.8	23.1
26	25.2	24.4
27	26.7	25.8
28	28.3	27.2
29	30.0	28.8
30	31.8	30.4
31	33.7	32.1
32	35.7	33.8
33	37.7	35.6
34	39.9	37.6
35	42.2	40.0
36	44.6	41.7
37	47.1	43.9
38	49.7	46.2
39	52.4	48.6
40	55.3	51.2

Source: From Dean 1985, pp. 10–26 and 10–81.
*Absolute humidity.

volume, e.g., mg/L (Table 10.4). Relative humidity is the relationship of the actual water vapor content of a gas and its capacity to carry water at a given temperature and is expressed as a percentage (of that capacity). Capacity increases with an increase in temperature.

Water as a vapor acts like a gas. The molecules of a liquid, like those of a gas, are in constant motion. Some of the molecules at the air-liquid interface escape from the liquid and enter the gaseous space above. At equilibrium the number of molecules leaving the surface of the liquid equals the number returning from the gas space above. The greater the temperature, the greater the liquid molecules' kinetic energy and therefore their tendency to leave and enter the gas phase. Water molecules in the vapor state exert a pressure, and as the temperature increases, the partial pressure of water vapor also increases. Therefore, we can describe water vapor in terms of its vapor pressure: the pressure (commonly in mm Hg) that water can exert at a given temperature. This is true regardless of the ambient pressure. When the atmosphere is completely saturated with water vapor at a given temperature, the relative humidity is 100%. This temperature-pressure relationship is well known (Table 10.4) and is an important concept in our therapeutic application of respiratory and anesthetic vapors. For example, as noted in Table 10.4, the vapor pressure of water at a body temperature of 38° C (100.4° F) is 50 mm Hg. We know that as air is inhaled, it is humidified to saturation. Recall that the total pressure exerted by the atmosphere is the sum of the pressures exerted by its component gases (i.e., the partial pressure of each of the component gases of the gas mixture; Dalton's law) (Scanlan et al. 1990; Comroe 1965; West 1992). The water vapor added to inspired gas (remember this is temperature dependent) thus reduces the partial pressure of O_2 in the inspired gas. That is, the PO_2 of moist inspired gas in the trachea of an animal with a body temperature of 38° C is 20.9% of 760 – 50 mm Hg (149 mm Hg), not 20.9% of 760 (159 mm Hg) as in dry air (the atmospheric or total gas pressure at sea level is taken as 760 mm Hg). This can be stated in general form as partial pressure of humidified sample = fractional concentration of dry gas × (barometric pressure – saturated vapor pressure).

Therapeutic Uses of Water Vapor. The humidification of inspired air normally helps maintain the hydration of the mucous blanket of the airways. A decrease or loss of this action promotes crusting of the respiratory mucosa, thick airway secretions, and reduced efficiency of mucociliary transport. Some clinical examples in which administration of water vapor is indicated include a patient whose upper airways are bypassed for a prolonged period via tracheostomy or oro-endotracheal intubation. Another may be the long-term delivery of inspired gases derived in part or totally from cylinders. The gas delivered from these sources is dry and can have a rapid drying effect on respiratory system mucosa.

Administration of Water Vapor. Water vapor may be delivered as a vapor (humidity) or as a suspension of very fine particles of liquid (water droplets) in a gas (aerosol) (Scanlan et al. 1990; Shapiro et al. 1975; Haskins 1986). Water may also be directly instilled into the tracheobronchial tree. Water can be given alone or with various medically active constituents, including electrolytes (e.g., saline). Humidifiers can deliver water vapor at room temperature to make the gas more comfortable to breathe or at body temperature to increase the amount of water that is delivered in a breath (Table 10.4). Water volume over that limited by temperature can be accomplished with aerosol generators. In addition, particle size of aerosols can be varied and determines the site of water deposition within the respiratory tract. Therefore, if the clinician knows the preferred level of aerosol deposition in the airway, the device best suited for the therapeutic effect can be selected.

Likely the greatest problem related to this mode of therapy is infecting a patient via contaminated respiratory therapy equipment. Other potential problems include thermal injury to the respiratory mucosa, fluid overload via water absorption, and airway obstruction, especially in very young or small patients.

NITRIC OXIDE. In 1987 Palmer et al. and Ignarro et al. (1987) separately proposed that the biological actions of endothelium-derived relaxing factor (Furchgott and Zawadski 1980) are due to the endogenous release of nitric oxide (NO). Nitric oxide is formed from the amino acid L-arginine by a family of enzymes, the NO synthases, and is recognized as a major endogenous mediator of a variety of diverse physiological processes (see Chap. 2), including smooth muscle relaxation, platelet inhibition, central and autonomic neurotransmission, tumor cell lysis, bacteria killing, and stimulation of hormonal release. Its formation in vascular endothelial cells in response to chemical and physical stimuli helps to maintain a vasodilator tone that is essential for regulation of local blood flow and pressure (Moncada et al. 1989; Vanhoutte 1989; Furchgott 1990). Following its formation in the endothelium, NO diffuses into adjacent vascular smooth muscle and activates soluble guanylate cyclase; the subsequent increased synthesis of the second-messenger cyclic guanylate 3′,5′-monophosphate produces smooth muscle relaxation and vessel dilation (Ignarro 1989).

Therapeutic Use of Inhaled NO. Nitric oxide is not effective when administered directly into the bloodstream because it is extremely rapidly inactivated (in 3–5 seconds) by hemoglobin (Gibson and Roughton 1957).

The potential beneficial role of nitro-compounds in problems of the lung has been appreciated for many years. In the past five years there has been an explosion of knowledge related to the therapeutic applications of NO in the lung. It is now widely appreciated that alterations of NO metabolism or the therapeutic and diagnostic use of NO or its derivatives may play an important role in pulmonary hypertension (including hypoxic pulmonary vasoconstriction, or HPV) and some other reversible lung diseases. With pulmonary hypertension the vasodilatory action specific to the pulmonary versus the systemic vasculature is of critical importance.

Frostell et al. (1991) reported that inhalation of 5–80 ppm NO caused pulmonary vasodilation during pulmonary vasoconstriction (e.g., caused by severe hypoxia; HPV). Exogenous inhaled NO diffuses from the alveoli to the pulmonary vascular smooth muscle and produces pulmonary vasodilation. The action is selective since any NO that diffuses into the blood is rapidly inactivated before it can produce any systemic effects (Frostell et al. 1993). In addition, inhaled NO is known to cause bronchodilation in the guinea pig (Dupuy et al. 1991). Thus, as a result, the use of inhaled NO is being widely and intensely investigated as a therapeutic possibility in pulmonary medicine.

Although published reports of its use in clinical practice (e.g., Frostell et al. 1993; Rossaint et al. 1993; Wysocki et al. 1994) are increasing in number, its use is still considered experimental. The many unresolved issues include the potential pulmonary toxicity of inhaled NO. Toxicity may be due to either NO itself or its reactive metabolite NO_2 (nitrogen dioxide) (Stavert and Lehnert 1990; Hugod 1979); both have been the subject of study for many years (Morrow 1984). Nitric oxide is a common air pollutant, and acute lung injury can occur at levels over 50–100 ppm. In addition, NO binds to hemoglobin to form nitrosylhemoglobin, which is rapidly converted to methemoglobin (Gibson and Roughton 1957).

In the presence of O_2, NO is converted to NO_2. The rate of NO_2 production in simulated and actual clinical conditions has been reported (Foubert et al. 1992; Bouchet et al. 1993; Lindberg and Rydgren 1998). Nitrogen dioxide has long been recognized as responsible for Silo Fillers Disease (a syndrome of pulmonary edema, hemorrhage, and bronchiolitis; NO_2 is a product of grain fermentation) and other related lung injury syndromes (Williams et al. 1971). Occupational safety and health guidelines recommend 5 ppm as the upper limit of exposure to NO_2 (Centers for Disease Control 1988), and recent guidelines for NO_2 exposure during therapeutic use of inhaled NO recommend less than 1 ppm (Zapol et al. 1994).

Administration of NO. Nitric oxide is a gas at room temperature (and down to −152° C) and is usually supplied in a cylinder as an inert mixture with nitrogen (NO-N_2). These preparations may, if not carefully prepared, contain higher oxides of nitrogen, including NO_2. Nitric oxide has a density relative to air of 1.227 and a water/gas solubility of 4.6 (20° C).

Guidelines for appropriate administration of NO have been published (Tibballs et al. 1993; Zapol et al. 1994; Nishimura et al. 1995; Lindberg et al. 1997; Body et al. 1995). The mode of delivery of inhaled NO must allow for precise, rapid control of NO concentration. Waste and excess gases should be scavenged to reduce potential dangers associated with occupational exposure to NO or NO_2.

Both NO and NO_2 concentrations in the inspired limb of the breathing circuit and in the immediate environment should be continuously monitored by chemiluminescence or electrochemical analyzers. The "gold standard" method is chemiluminescence (Body et al. 1995; Kavanagh and Pearl 1995), but other more economical and "user-friendly" monitors are becoming commercially available.

Dose recommendations for inhaled NO are variable and circumstance dependent, but most suggestions lie in the region of 0.1–40 ppm, with recent emphasis on the lower concentrations (Rossaint et al. 1993; Puybasset et al. 1994; Kavanagh and Pearl 1995). Inhaled NO effectiveness may be enhanced if NO is combined with adjunctive agents such as almitrine bismesylate (Wysocki et al. 1994; Lu et al. 1995).

In summary, at present NO inhalation is a promising therapy for some patients with reversible lung disease. However, its present use with human and veterinary patients continues to be considered in the experimental phase.

REFERENCES

Ashton, N. 1979. The pathogenesis of retrolental fibroplasia. Ophthalmology (Rochester) 86:1695–99.

Bhagavan, N. V. 1992. Medical Biochemistry. Boston: Jones & Bartlett Publishers.

Blackshaw, J. K., Fenwick, D. C., Beattie, A. W., and Allan, D. J. 1988. The behaviour of chickens, mice and rats during euthanasia with chloroform, carbon dioxide and ether. Lab Anim 22:67–75.

Body, S. C., Hartigan, P. M., Shernan, S. K., Formanek, M., and Hurford, W. E. 1995. Nitric oxide: delivery, measurement and clinical application. J Cardiothorac Vasc Anesth 9:748–763.

Bouchet, M., Renauden, M.-G., Raveau, C., Mercier, J.-C., Dehan, M., and Zupan, V. 1993. Safety requirements for use of inhaled nitric oxide in neonates. (Letter.) Lancet 341:968–969.

Bridges, B. E. J., and Eger, E. I. 1966. The effect of hypocapnia on the level of halothane anesthesia in man. Anesthesiology 27:634–637.

Centers for Disease Control. 1988. Recommendations for occupational safety and health standards. MMWR 37:21.

Clowes, G. H. A., Jr., Hopkins, A. L., and Simeone, F. A. 1955. A comparison of the physiological effects of hypercapnia and hypoxia in the production of cardiac arrest. Ann Surg 142:446–459.

Comroe, J. H., Jr. 1965. Physiology of Respiration: An Introductory Text. Chicago: Year Book Medical Publishers.

Crapo, J. D., Freeman, B. A., Barry, B. E., Turrens, J. F., and Young, S. L. 1983. Mechanisms of hyperoxic injury to the pulmonary microcirculation. Physiologist 26:170–176.

Cullen, D. J., and Eger, E. I. 1971. The effect of extreme hypocapnia on the anaesthetic requirement (MAC) of dogs. Br J Anaesth 43:339–343.

———. 1974. Cardiovascular effects of carbon dioxide in man. Anesthesiology 41:345–349.

Cullen, L. K., Steffey, E. P., Bailey, C. S., Kortz, G., da Silva Curiel, J., Bellhorn, R. W., Woliner, M. J., Elliott, A. R., and Jarvis, K. A. 1990. Effect of high P_aCO_2 and time on cerebrospinal fluid and intraocular pressure in halothane-anesthetized horses. Am J Vet Res 51:300–304.

Danneman, P. J., Stein, S., and Walshaw, S. O. 1997. Humane and practical implications of using carbon dioxide mixed with oxygen for anesthesia or euthanasia of rats. Lab Anim Sci 47:376–385.

Dean, J. A., ed. 1985. Lange's Handbook of Chemistry. 13th ed. New York: McGraw-Hill.

Deneke, S. M., and Fanburg, B. L. 1982. Oxygen toxicity of the lung: an update. Br J Anaesth 54:737–749.

Dorsch, J. A., and Dorsch, S. E. 1984. Understanding Anesthesia Equipment: Construction, Care, and Complications. 2nd ed. Baltimore: Williams & Wilkins.

Dupuy, P. M., Shore, S. A., Drazen, J. M., Frostell, C., Hill, W. A., and Zapol, W. W. 1991. Bronchodilator action of inhaled nitric oxide in guinea pigs. J Clin Invest 90:421–428.

Eckenhoff, R. G., and Longnecker, D. E. 1990. The therapeutic gases: oxygen, carbon dioxide, helium, and water vapor. In A. G. Gilman, T. R. Rall, A. S. Nies, et al., eds., The Pharmacological Basis of Therapeutics, 8th ed., pp. 332–344. New York: Pergamon Press.

Eger, E. I., Saidman, L. J., and Brandstater, B. 1965. Minimum alveolar anesthetic concentration: a standard of anesthetic potency. Anesthesiology 26:756–763.

Eisele, J. H., Eger, E. I., and Muallem, M. 1967. Narcotic properties of carbon dioxide in the dog. Anesthesiology 28:856–865.

Foubert, L., Fleming, B., Latimer, R., Jonas, M., and Oduro, A. 1992. Safety guidelines for use of nitric oxide. (Letter.) Lancet 339:1615–1616.

Frostell, C. G., Fratacci, M. D., Wain, J. C., and Zapol, W. M. 1991. Inhaled nitric oxide: a selective pulmonary vasodilator reversing hypoxic pulmonary vasoconstriction. Circulation 83:2038–2047.

Frostell, C. G., Blomquist, H., Hedenstierna, G., Lundberg, J., and Zapol, W. M. 1993. Inhaled nitric oxide selectively reverses human hypoxic pulmonary vasoconstriction without causing systemic vasodilation. Anesthesiology 78:427–435.

Furchgott, R. F. 1990. Studies on endothelium-dependent vasodilation and the endothelium-derived relaxing factor. Acta Physiol Scand 139:257–270.

Furchgott, R. F., and Zawadski, J. V. 1980. The obligatory role of endothelial cells in the relaxation of arterial smooth muscle by acetylcholine. Nature 288:373–376.

Geddes, I. C., and Gray, T. C. 1959. Hyperventilation for the maintenance of anaesthesia. Lancet 2:4–6.

Gibson, Q. H., and Roughton, F. J. W. 1957. The kinetics of equilibria of the reactions of nitric oxide with sheep hemoglobin. J Physiol (London) 136:507–526.

Granger, D. N. 1988. Role of xanthine oxidase and granulocytes in ischemia-reperfusion injury. Am J Physiol 255:H1296–H1275.

Granger, D. N., Rutili, G., and McCord, J. M. 1981. Superoxide radicals in feline intestinal ischemia. Gastroenterology 81:22–29.

Guyton, A. C., and Hall, H. E. 1996. Textbook of Medical Physiology. 9th ed. Philadelphia: W. B. Saunders.

Hall, L. W., and Clarke, K. W. 1991. Veterinary Anaesthesia. 9th ed. London: Bailliere Tindall.

Haskins, S. C. 1986. Physical therapeutics for respiratory disease. Seminars in Vet Med Surg (Sm Anim) 1:276–288.

Hickey, R. F., Fourcade, H. E., Eger, E. I., Larson, C. P. J, Bahlman, S. H., Stevens, W. C., Gregory, G. A., and Smith, N. T. 1971. The effects of ether, halothane, and Forane on apneic thresholds in man. Anesthesiology 35:32–37.

Hugod, C. 1979. Effect of exposure to 43 ppm nitric oxide and 3.6 ppm nitrogen dioxide on rabbit lung. Int Arch Occup Environ Health 42:159–167.

Ignarro, L. J. 1989. Biological actions and properties of endothelium-derived nitric oxide formed and released from artery and vein. Circ Res 65:1–21.

Ignarro, J. L., Bugo, G. M., Wood, K. S., Byrns, R. E., and Chaudhuri, G. 1987. Endothelium derived relaxing factor produced and released from artery and vein is nitric oxide. Proc Natl Acad Sci USA 84:9265–9269.

Jackson, R. M. 1985. Pulmonary Oxygen Toxicity. Chest 88:900–906.

Karmazyn, M. 1991. Ischemic and reperfusion injury in the heart: cellular mechanisms and pharmacological interventions. Can J Physiol Pharmacol 69:719–730.

Kavanagh, B. P., and Pearl, R. G. 1995. Inhaled nitric oxide in anesthesia and critical care medicine. Intern Anesth Clinics 33:181–210.

Klemm, W. R. 1964. Carbon dioxide anesthesia in cats. Am J Vet Res 25:1201–1205.

Leake, C. D., and Waters, R. M. 1928. The anesthetic properties of carbon dioxide. J Pharmacol Exp Therap 33:280–281.

Lindberg, L., and Rydgren, G. 1998. Production of nitrogen dioxide in a delivery system for inhalation of nitric oxide: a new equation for calculation. Br J Anaesth 80:213–217.

Lindberg, L., Rydgren, G., Larsson, A., Olsso, S., and Nordstrom, L. 1997. A delivery system for inhalation of nitric oxide evaluated with chemiluminescence, electrochemical fuel cell and capnography. Crit Care Med 25:190–196.

Lu, Q., Mourgeon, E., Law-Kowne, J. D., Roche, S., Vezinet, C., Abdennour, L., Vicant, E., Puybasset, L., Diaby, M., Coriat, P., and Rouby, J.-J. 1995. Dose response curves of inhaled nitric oxide with and without intravenous almitrine in nitric oxide–responding patients with acute

respiratory distress syndrome. Anesthesiology 83:929–943.
Mattsson, J. L., Stinson, J. M., and Clark, C. S. 1972. Electroencephalographic power-spectral changes coincident with onset of carbon dioxide narcosis in rhesus monkey. Am J Vet Res 33:2043–2049.
McCord, J. M. 1985. Oxygen-derived free radicals in postischemic tissue injury. N Engl J Med 312:159–163.
———. 1987. Oxygen-derived radicals: a link between reperfusion injury and inflammation. Fed Proc 46:2402–2406.
Millar, R. A. 1960. Plasma adrenaline and noradrenaline during diffusion respiration. J Physiol 150:79–90.
Miller, R. D., ed. 1990. Anesthesia. New York: Churchill Livingstone.
Moncada, S., Palmer, R. M. J., and Higgs, E. A. 1989. Biosynthases of nitric acid from L-arginine: a pathway for the regulation of cell function and communication. Biochem Pharmacol 38:1709–1715.
Morrow, P. E. 1984. Toxicological data on NO_x: an overview. J Toxical Environ Health 13:205–207.
Nishimura, M., Gess, D., Dacmarek, R. M., Ritz, R., and Hurford, W. E. 1995. Nitrogen dioxide production during mechanical ventilation with nitric oxide in adults: effect of ventilator internal volume, air versus nitrogen dilution, minute ventilation and inspired oxygen fraction. Anesthesiology 82:1246–1254.
Nunn, J. F. 1993. Applied Respiratory Physiology. 4th ed. Boston: Butterworths.
Palmer, R. M. J., Buga, G. M., Wood, K. S., Byrns, R. E., and Chaudhuri, G. 1987. Nitric oxide release accounts for the biological activity of endothelium-derived relaxing factor. Nature 327:524–526.
Patz, A. 1965. The effect of oxygen on immature retinal vessels. Invest Ophthalmol 4:988–999.
Perry, M. O., and Fantini, G. 1987. Ischemia-profile of an enemy-reperfusion injury of skeletal muscle. J Vasc Surg 6:231–235.
Pryor, W. A. 1986. Oxy-radicals and related species: their formation, lifetimes, and reactions. Ann Rev Physiol 48:657–667.
Puybasset, L., Rouby, J. J., Mourgeon, E., Stewart, T. E., Cluzel, P., Arthand, M., Poete, P., Bodin, L., Korinek, A. M., and Viars, P. 1994. Inhaled nitric oxide in acute respiratory failure: dose-response curves. Intens Care Med 20:319–327.
Repine, J. E., and Tate, R. M. 1983. Oxygen radicals and lung edema. Physiologist 26:177–181.
Rossaint, R., Falke, K. J., Lopez, F., Slama, K., Pison, U., and Zapol, W. M. 1993. Inhaled nitric oxide for the adult respiratory distress syndrome. N Engl J Med 328:399–405.
Scanlan, C. L., Spearman, C. B., and Sheldon, R. L., eds. 1990. Egan's Fundamentals of Respiratory Care. 5th ed. St. Louis: C. V. Mosby.
Shapiro, B. A., Harrison, R. A., and Trout, C. A. 1975. Clinical Application of Respiratory Care. Chicago: Year Book Medical Publishers.
Short, C. E., ed. 1987. Principles and Practice of Veterinary Anesthesia. Baltimore: Williams & Wilkins.
Stavert, E. M., and Lehnert, B. E. 1990. Nitric oxide and nitrogen dioxide as inducers of acute pulmonary injury when inhaled at relatively high concentrations for brief periods. Inhalation Toxicol 2:53–67.
Steffey, E. P., and Robinson, N. E. 1983. Respiratory system physiology and pathophysiology. In S. J. Ettinger, ed., Textbook of Veterinary Internal Medicine: Diseases of the Dog and Cat, 2nd ed., pp. 673–691. Philadelphia: W. B. Saunders.
Tibballs, J., Hochmann, M., Carter, B., and Osborne, A. 1993. An appraisal of techniques for administration of gaseous nitric oxide. Anaesth Intens Care 21:844–847.
Urbanski, H. F., and Kelley, S. T. 1991. Sedation by exposure to a gaseous carbon dioxide-oxygen mixture: application to studies involving small laboratory animal species. Lab Anim Sci 41:80–82.
Vanhoutte, P. M. 1989. Endotheluim and control of vascular function. Hypertension 13:658–667.
Weiskopf, R., Raymond, L. W., and Severinghaus, J. W. 1974. Effects of halothane on canine respiratory responses to hypoxia with and without hypercapnia. Anesthesiology 41:350–359.
Welbourn, C. R. B., Goldman, G., Valeri, C. R., et al. 1991. Pathophysiology of ischaemia reperfusion injury: central role of the neutrophil. Br J Surg 78:651–655.
West, J. B. 1992. Respiratory Physiology: The Essentials. 4th ed. Baltimore: Williams & Wilkins.
Williams, R. A., Rhodes, P. A., and Adams, W. S. 1971. The response of lung tissue and surfactant to nitrogen dioxide exposure. Arch Intern Med 128:101–108.
Wysocki, M., Dalclaux, C., Roupie, E., Langeron, O., Liu, N., Herman, B., Lemaire, F., and Brochard, L. 1994. Additive effect of gas exchange of inhaled nitric oxide and intravenous almitrine bismesylate in the adult respiratory distress syndrome. Inten Care Med 20:254–259.
Zapol, W. M., Rimar, S., Gillis, N., Marletta, M., and Basken, C. H. 1994. Nitric oxide and the lung. Am J Resp Crit Care Med 149:1375–1380.

11

INHALATION ANESTHETICS

EUGENE P. STEFFEY

Physiochemical Characteristics
- **Chemical Characteristics**
- **Physical Characteristics**

Properties Determining Methods of Administration
- **Gas versus Vapor**
- **Methods of Description**
- **Vapor Pressure**
- **Boiling Point**

Properties Influencing Drug Kinetics: Solubility
- **Blood/Gas Partition Coefficient**
- **Oil/Gas Partition Coefficient**
- **Other Partition Coefficients**

Pharmacokinetics: Uptake and Elimination of Inhalation Anesthetics
- **Delivery to the Alveoli**
- **Removal from the Alveoli: Uptake by Blood**
- **Anesthetic Recovery**
- **Biotransformation**
- **Anesthetic Dose: The Minimum Alveolar Concentration**

Pharmacodynamics: Actions and Toxicity of the Inhalation Anesthetics
- **Central Nervous System**
- **Respiratory System**
- **Cardiovascular System**
- **Liver**
- **Kidneys**
- **Skeletal Muscle**
- **Actions by Agent**

Trace Concentrations of Inhalation Anesthetics: Occupational Exposure

Inhalation anesthetics are unique among the anesthetic drugs because they are administered, and in large part removed from the body, via the lungs. They are used widely for the anesthetic management of animals in part because their pharmacokinetic characteristics favor predictable and rapid adjustment of anesthetic depth. In addition, a special apparatus is usually used to deliver the inhaled agents. This helps minimize patient morbidity or mortality because it facilitates accurate and controlled anesthetic delivery, lung ventilation, and improved arterial oxygenation.

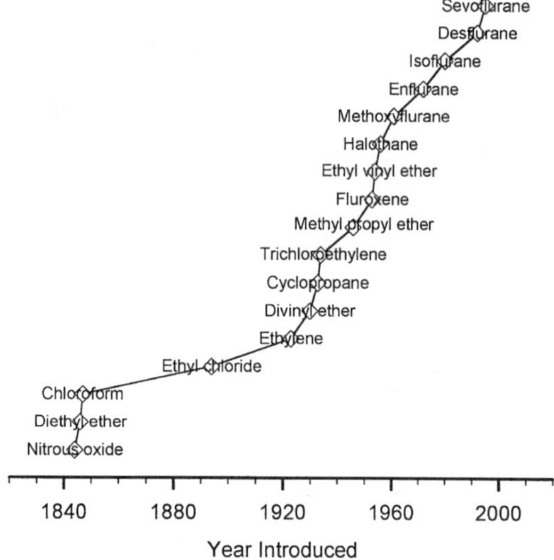

FIG. 11.1—Inhalation anesthetics introduced for widespread clinical use. (Adapted from Eger 1985a; reprinted with permission from Steffey 1995.)

The search for anesthetic agents with ever greater safety and fewer side effects is ongoing. Over the 150 years that inhalation anesthesia has been used in clinical practice, fewer than 20 agents have actually been introduced and approved for general use with patients (Fig. 11.1). Fewer than 10 of these have had any history of widespread clinical use in veterinary medicine, and only 5 are of current clinical importance in North America. This chapter will focus on this last group of anesthetics (Table 11.1). The group includes halothane and isoflurane, which together are the most widely used inhaled anesthetics. In addition, nitrous oxide (N_2O), methoxyflurane, and enflurane enjoy varying, but lesser, degrees of popularity. Unfortunately, none of these is the ideal inhalation anesthetic. An ideal agent would have characteristics that include a stable shelf life without preservatives and compatibility with existing delivery equipment. It would be inexpensive to purchase, nonflammable, and easily vaporized under

Parts of this chapter have appeared in a chapter by E. P. Steffey in J. C. Thurmon, W. Tranquilli, and G. J. Benson, eds., *Veterinary Anesthesia* (Baltimore: Lea & Febiger, 1996). Reprinted with permission.

TABLE 11.1—Inhalation anesthetic agents

Group 1: Agents in current clinical use for animals
Major use
Halothane
Isoflurane
Minor use
Enflurane
Methoxyflurane
Nitrous oxide
Diethyl ether
Group 2: New agents
Desflurane
Sevoflurane
Group 3: Agents of historical interest
Chloroform
Cyclopropane
Fluroxene
Trichloroethylene

ambient conditions. Such an agent would have a low blood solubility to foster rapid changes in anesthetic depth and permit rapid, controlled recovery from anesthesia. The ideal agent would be very potent, thereby allowing anesthesia at low inspired concentrations and maximizing flexibility of adjustments of inspired oxygen concentration. There would be no cardiopulmonary depression; the agent would not be irritating to airways and would be compatible with catecholamines and other vasoactive drugs. Finally, it would produce good skeletal muscle relaxation, resist degradation in the body, and be nontoxic to kidneys, liver, and gut.

Since the search for the ideal agent continues, new anesthetics are found. A few years ago desflurane and sevoflurane were released in the U.S. for general clinical use with human patients. Although at this time these agents have only very limited direct impact on the anesthetic management of animals, a review of the characteristics of these agents here is important.

A third group is comprised of agents that once enjoyed variable popularity for veterinary application (Table 11.1). These agents are no longer broadly used in clinical circumstances so they will not be discussed beyond brief mention of examples here. Data of typical contemporary interest regarding their action in species of clinical importance to veterinary medicine are generally lacking, but readers interested in further information on agents in this group are referred to early editions of pharmacology (Booth and McDonald 1988) and veterinary anesthesia textbooks (Soma 1971; Hall 1971; Lumb and Jones 1973; Short 1987). This third group of anesthetics includes agents like chloroform and cyclopropane. These agents have long been discarded for general use in human and veterinary medical practice because they cause liver failure (chloroform) or are explosive (cyclopropane). Diethyl ether, on the other hand, was widely used for clinical anesthetic management of human patients and a variety of animals up to about 20 years ago but then was largely replaced by newer agents because it is flammable (Duncalf 1982). This characteristic negates its use in the environment of the modern operating room, which

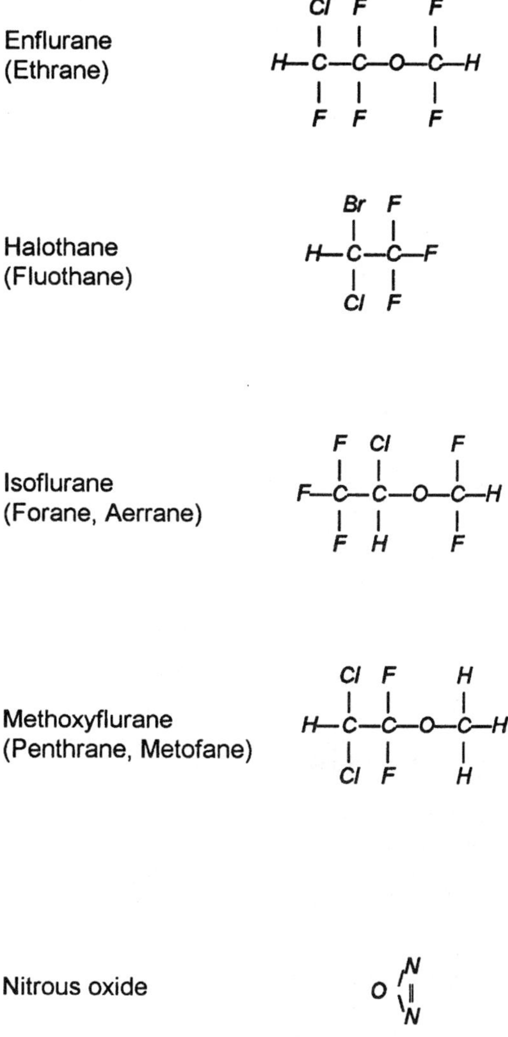

FIG. 11.2—Chemical structure of inhalation anesthetics in current use for animals. Trade names are given in parentheses.

ordinarily includes a variety of electrical surgical support (e.g., electrocautery), anesthetic delivery, and patient monitoring and ventilating devices. However, it is still used in some laboratory situations and in selected clinical circumstances, especially outside North America. Accordingly, there is continued justification to provide a brief overview of its pharmacology.

PHYSIOCHEMICAL CHARACTERISTICS. The their physical properties are important determinants of their actions and safety of administration. Consequently, brief discussion of aspects of Figs. 11.2 and 11.3 and Tables 11.2 and 11.3 is appropriate because

Desflurane (Suprane, I653)

```
     F  H     F
     |  |     |
  F—C—C—O—C—H
     |  |     |
     F  F     F
```

Sevoflurane (Ultane)

```
              F
              |
      H   F—C—F
      |       |
   F—C—O—C—H
      |       |
      H   F—C—F
              |
              F
```

FIG. 11.3—Chemical structure of two new inhalation anesthetics. Trade name is given in parentheses.

physiochemical characteristics determine and/or influence practical considerations such as how the agents are supplied by the manufacturer (e.g., as a gas or as a liquid), the stability of the anesthetic molecule to degradation by physical factors (e.g., heat, light) and by substances it contacts during use (e.g., metal, soda lime). The equipment necessary to safely deliver the agent to the patient (e.g., vaporizer, breathing apparatus) is influenced by some of these properties as are the agent's uptake by the patient and its distribution within and elimination (including potential for metabolic breakdown) from the patient.

Chemical Characteristics. All contemporary inhalation anesthetics are organic compounds except nitrous oxide (N_2O) (Table 11.1). Agents of current interest are further classified as either aliphatic (i.e., straight or branch chained) hydrocarbons or ethers (i.e., two organic radicals [R] attached to an atom of oxygen; the general structure is R–O–R).

In the continued search for a less reactive, more potent, nonflammable inhalation anesthetic, focus on halogenation (i.e., addition of fluorine, chlorine, or bromine; iodine is least useful) of these compounds has predominated. Chlorine and bromine especially convert many compounds of low anesthetic potency to more potent drugs. Historically, interest in fluorinated derivatives was delayed until the 1940s because of difficulties in synthesis, and thus quantities available for study were limited. Methods of synthesis, although difficult, have improved considerably and have facilitated discovery of new agents (Fig. 11.1). Interestingly, organic fluorinated compounds are a group of extreme contrasts: some are toxic, others are not; some are extremely inert, others are highly reactive. In some anesthetics fluorine is substituted for chlorine or bromine to improve stability but at the expense of reduced anesthetic potency and solubility.

TABLE 11.3—Properties of two new inhalation anesthetics

Property	Desflurane	Sevoflurane
Molecular weight	168[a]	200[a]
Liquid specific gravity at 20°C (g/mL)	1.47[b]	1.52[b]
Boiling point (°C)	23.5[a]	59[d]
Vapor pressure (mm Hg) at		
20° C (68°F)	664[c]	160[d]
24° C (75°F)	798[e]	188
Milliliters of vapor/milliliters of liquid at 20°C	209.7	182.7
Preservative	None	None
Stability in soda lime	Yes	No

[a]Jones 1990.
[b]Laster et al. 1994.
[c]Miller and Greene 1990.
[d]Wallin et al. 1975.
[e]Eger 1993.

TABLE 11.2—Some physiochemical properties of inhalation anesthetics in current clinical use for animals

Property	Enflurane	Halothane	Isoflurane	Methoxyflurane	Nitrous oxide
Molecular weight	185	197	185	165	44
Liquid specific gravity (20° C) (g/mL)	1.52	1.86	1.49	1.42	—
Boiling point (° C)	57	50	49	105	–89
Vapor pressure (mm Hg)					
20° C (68° F)	172	244	240	23	—
24° C (75° F)	207	288	286	28	—
Milliliters of vapor/milliliters of liquid at 20° C	197.5	227	194.7	206.9	—
Preservative	None	Required	None	Required	None
Stability in					
Soda lime	Stable	Decomposes	Stable	Decomposes	Stable
UV light	Stable	Decomposes	Stable	Decomposes	Stable

Sources: Lowe and Ernst 1981; Eger 1982.

Halothane (Fig. 11.2) is a halogenated aliphatic saturated hydrocarbon (ethane). Predictions that halogenated structure would provide nonflammability and molecular stability encouraged the development of halothane in the early 1950s. However, soon after clinical introduction it was observed that the concurrent presence of halothane and catecholamines increased the incidence of life-threatening cardiac arrhythmias, especially in human patients. An ether linkage in the molecule favors a reduced incidence of cardiac arrhythmias. Consequently, this chemical structure is a predominant characteristic of all agents developed or proposed for clinical use since the introduction of halothane (Figs. 11.2 and 11.3).

Despite many favorable characteristics and improvements over earlier anesthetics, including improved chemical stability, halothane is susceptible to decomposition. Accordingly, halothane is stored in dark bottles, and a very small amount of a preservative, thymol, is added to it to retard breakdown. Thymol is much less volatile than halothane and over time collects within the devices used to control delivery of the volatile anesthetic (i.e., vaporizers) and causes them to malfunction. To achieve greater molecular stability, fluorine is substituted for chlorine or bromine in the anesthetic molecule. This chemical manipulation adds shelf life to the substance and negates the need for additives such as thymol. Unfortunately, the fluorine ion is also toxic to some tissues (e.g., kidneys), which is of substantial concern if the parent compound (e.g., methoxyflurane, enflurane, sevoflurane; Figs. 11.2, 11.3) is not resistant to metabolism.

Physical Characteristics. In simplest form the administration of inhalation anesthetics requires a carrier gas that must include oxygen, a source of anesthetic, and a patient breathing circuit. For very small animals (e.g., laboratory rodents or small birds) this may mean nothing more than placing the animal in a closed air-filled chamber that contains a cotton pledget saturated with liquid anesthetic (e.g., methoxyflurane). With larger animals and/or to provide more controlled delivery of anesthetic and O_2 it is more appropriate to use specialized equipment. Such equipment, though more complex, greatly improves the safety of the anesthetic technique. It includes what is commonly referred to as an anesthetic machine, one or more vaporizers, and a patient breathing circuit. The anesthetic machine with two vaporizers attached is shown in schematic form in Fig. 11.4. Extensive reviews of anesthetic equipment are available (Short 1987; Dorsch and Dorsch 1984; Andrews 1990 Thurmon et al. 1996).

The chain of events whereby anesthetic is transferred under control from a container to sites of action in the central nervous system (CNS) involves many physical characteristics that can be quantitatively described (Tables 11.2–11.5). The practical clinical applications of these quantitative descriptions will be briefly reviewed here. More in-depth background information is available elsewhere (Lowe and Ernst 1981; Hill 1980; Eger 1990; Butterworth and Strichartz 1990).

The physical characteristics of importance to this review are divided into two general categories; those that determine the means by which the agents are administered and those that help determine their kinetics in the body. This information is applied in the clinical manipulation of anesthetic induction and recovery and in facilitating changes in anesthetic levels in timely fashion.

PROPERTIES DETERMINING METHODS OF ADMINISTRATION. A variety of physical properties determine the means by which inhalation anesthetics are administered. These include molecular weight, boiling-point, liquid density (specific gravity), and vapor pressure.

Gas versus Vapor. Inhalation anesthetics are either gases or vapors. In relation to inhalation anesthetics the term "gas" refers to an agent, like N_2O (or cyclopropane), that exists in its gaseous form at room temperature and sea-level pressure. The term "vapor" indicates the gaseous state of a substance that at ambient temperature and pressure is a liquid. With the exception of N_2O, all the contemporary and new anesthetics fall into this category. Desflurane (Table 11.3), one of the new volatile liquids, comes close to the transition stage and has some unique (among the inhalation anesthetics) properties, to be discussed later in this chapter.

Regardless whether inhalation agents are supplied as a gas or volatile liquid under ambient conditions, the same physical principles apply to each agent when in the gaseous state.

Methods of Description. Quantities of inhalation anesthetic agent are usually characterized by one of three methods: pressure (e.g., in mm Hg), concentration (in volumes %), or mass (in mg or g). The form most familiar to clinicians is that of concentration (e.g., *X*% of agent A in relation to the whole gas mixture). Modern monitoring equipment samples inspired and expired gases and provides concentration readings for inhalation anesthetics. Precision vaporizers used to control delivery of inhalation anesthetics are calibrated in percentage of agent, and effective doses are almost always reported in percentages. Pressure is also an important way of describing inhalation anesthetics and will be discussed next. Finally, the molecular weight and agent density are used in many calculations to convert from liquid to vapor volumes and mass (Hill 1980).

Vapor Pressure. The vapor pressure of an anesthetic is a measure of its ability to evaporate; i.e., it is a measure of the tendency for molecules in the liquid state to enter the gaseous (vapor) form. The vapor pressure of a volatile anesthetic drug must at least be sufficient to provide enough molecules of anesthetic in the vapor state to produce anesthesia at ambient conditions. The *saturated vapor pressure* represents a maximum concentration of molecules in the vapor state that can

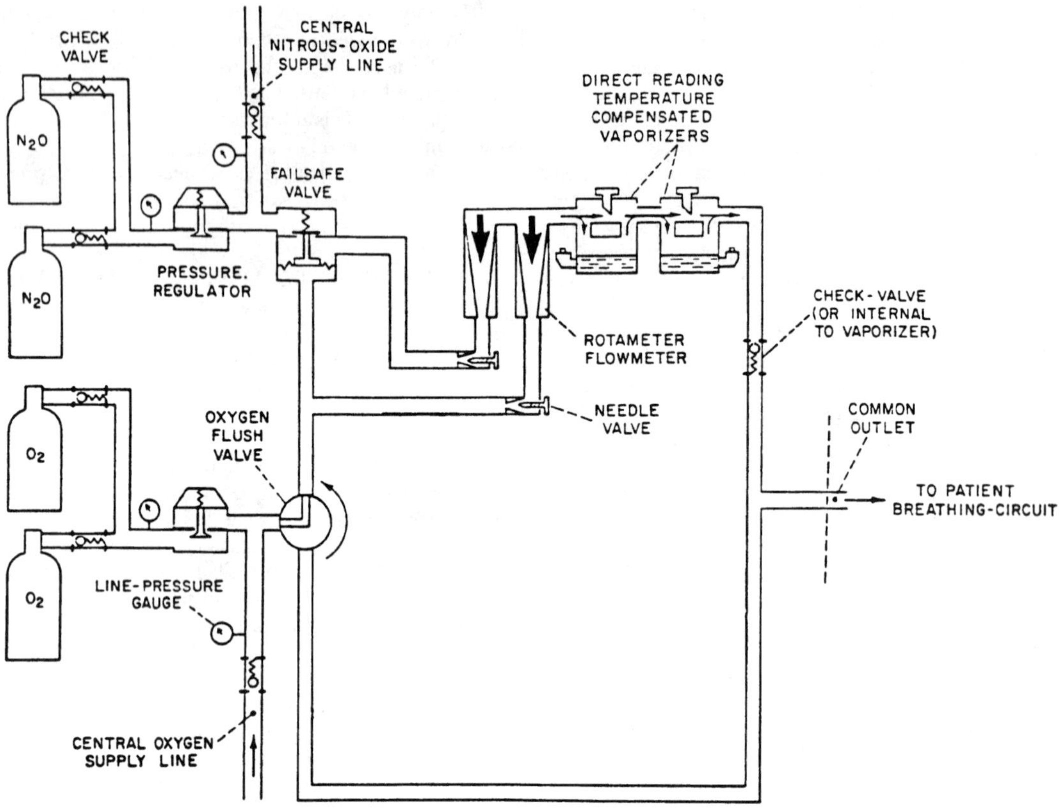

FIG. 11.4—Schematic diagram of the internal circuitry of a generic anesthetic machine. The common outlet directs the fresh gas flow to the patient via a breathing circuit (not shown). Reprinted with permission of the publisher (Stoelting and Miller 1989).

TABLE 11.4—Partition coefficients at 37°C

Agent	Blood/ gas	Oil[a]/ gas	Brain/ blood	Lung/ blood	Kidney/ blood	Muscle/ blood	Fat/ blood
Desflurane	0.42	18.7	1.3	1.4	1	2	27
Nitrous oxide	0.47	1.4	1.1	0.8	—	1.2	2.3
Sevoflurane	0.69	47	1.7	1.8	1.2	3.1	48
Isoflurane	1.4	91	1.6	1.8	1.2	2.9	45
Enflurane	1.8	98	1.4	2.1	—	1.7	36
Halothane	2.5	224	1.9	2.1	1.2	3.4	51
Diethyl ether	12	65	2	1.9	0.9	1.3	5
Methoxyflurane	15	970	1.4	2	0.9	1.6	38

Note: Values are for human tissue, from Eger (Butterworth and Strichartz 1990).

[a]Data for olive oil from Eger 1974, 1985a, 1987, 1992; and Strum and Eger 1987.

TABLE 11.5—Rubber or plastic/gas partition coefficients at room temperature

Solvent	Desflurane	Enflurane	Halothane	Isoflurane	Methoxyflurane	Nitrous oxide	Sevoflurane
Rubber	19	74	120	62	630	1.2	29
Polyvinyl chloride	35	120	190	110	—	—	68
Polyethylene	16	~2	26	~2	118	—	31

Sources: Eger 1985a, 1992.

exist for a given liquid at each temperature. The saturated vapor concentration can be easily determined by relating the vapor pressure to the ambient pressure. Using halothane and associated information from Table 11.2 as an example, we see that a maximal concentration of 32% halothane is possible under usual operating-room conditions; that is, 244/760 × 100 = 32%, where 244 mm Hg is the vapor pressure at 20° C and 760 mm Hg is the barometric pressure at sea level. Thus, other variables considered constant, the greater the vapor pressure, the greater the concentration of the drug deliverable to the patient. Therefore, again from Table 11.2, halothane, for example, is more volatile than methoxyflurane under similar conditions.

Boiling Point. The boiling point of a liquid is defined as the temperature at which the vapor pressure of the liquid is equal to the atmosphere pressure. Customarily, the boiling temperature is stated for the standard pressure of 760 mm Hg. The boiling point decreases with increasing altitude since the vapor pressure does not change but the barometric pressure decreases.

The boiling point of N_2O is –89° C (Table 11.2) at 1 atmosphere pressure, sea level. It is thus a gas under operating-room conditions. Because of this it is distributed for clinical purposes in steel tanks compressed to the liquid state at about 750 psi (pounds per square inch; 750 psi/14.9 psi [1 atmosphere] = 50 atmospheres). As the N_2O gas is drawn from the tank, liquid N_2O is vaporized, and the overriding gas pressure remains constant until no further liquid remains in the tank. At that point only N_2O gas remains, and the gas pressure decreases from this point as remaining gas is vented from the tank. Consequently, the weight of the N_2O plus tank rather than the gas pressure within the tank is a more accurate guide to the remaining contents of the tank (Haskins and Sansome 1979).

Desflurane, the newest clinically available volatile anesthetic, poses an interesting problem since its boiling point (Table 11.3) is near room temperature. This characteristic accounted for an interesting engineering challenge in developing an administration device (i.e., vaporizer) for routine use in the relatively constant environment of the operating room and limits its use to a narrow range of circumstances commonly encountered in veterinary medical applications. For example, because of its low boiling point, even evaporative cooling has large influences on the vapor pressure and thus on the vapor concentration of gas mixtures delivered to the patient.

PROPERTIES INFLUENCING DRUG KINETICS: SOLUBILITY. Anesthetic gases and vapors dissolve in liquids and solids. The solubility of an anesthetic is a major characteristic of the agent and has important clinical ramifications. For example, anesthetic solubility in blood and body tissues is a primary factor in the rate of uptake and distribution within the body. It is therefore a primary determinant of the speed of anesthetic induction and recovery. Solubility in lipids bears a strong relationship to anesthetic potency, and the tendency to dissolve in anesthetic delivery components such as rubber influences equipment selection and other aspects of anesthetic management.

The extent to which a gas will dissolve in a given solvent is usually expressed in terms of its *solubility coefficient* (Table 11.4). With inhalation anesthetics solubility is most commonly expressed as a partition coefficient (PC). Other expressions of solubility include the Bunson and Ostwald solubility coefficients (Hill 1980; Eger 1974).

The PC is the concentration ratio of an anesthetic in two solvent phases, for example, blood and gas. It thus describes the affinity or capacity of an anesthetic for one solvent phase relative to another, that is, how the anesthetic will *partition* itself between two phases after equilibrium has been reached. Anesthetic gas movement occurs because of a partial pressure difference in the two phases so that when there is no longer any anesthetic partial pressure difference between the two phases, there is no longer any net movement of anesthetic in either phase direction, and equilibrium has been achieved. Solvent/gas PCs are summarized in Table 11.4. Values noted in this table are for human tissues since they are the most widely valued and thus the data are available in the anesthesia literature. Rubber/gas and plastic/gas PCs are given in Table 11.5. It is important to emphasize that many factors besides species can alter anesthetic agent solubility (Eger 1974; Mapleson et al. 1972; Eger and Eger 1985; Lerman et al. 1986). Perhaps most notable after the nature of the solvent is that of temperature.

Of all the PCs that have been described or are of possible interest, two are of particular importance in the practical understanding of anesthetic management. They are the blood/gas and the oil/gas solubilities.

Blood/Gas Partition Coefficient. The blood/gas solubility (Table 11.4) is a measure of the speed of anesthetic induction, recovery, and change of anesthetic levels. For example, other factors considered constant, the lower the blood/gas PC, the more rapid the anesthetic induction or rate of change of anesthetic level in response to a stepwise change in anesthetic delivery. Further information regarding the influence of anesthetic blood solubility on practical aspects of anesthetic management is presented in the section on pharmacokinetics.

Oil/Gas Partition Coefficient. The oil/gas PC is another solubility characteristic of clinical importance (Table 11.4). This PC describes the ratio of concentration of an anesthetic in oil (in this case olive oil is the generally agreed upon standard) and gas phases at equilibrium. The oil/gas PC correlates directly with anesthetic potency (see section in this chapter titled Anesthetic Dose: The Minimum Alveolar Concentration) and describes the capacity of lipids for anesthetic.

Other Partition Coefficients. Solubility characteristics for tissues (Table 11.4) and other media like rubber and plastic (components of anesthetic delivery equipment; Table 11.5) are also important. For example, tissue solubility determines in part the quantity of anesthetic removed from the blood to which it is exposed. The higher the tissue solubility, the longer it will take to saturate the tissue with anesthetic agent. Thus, other things considered equal, agents very soluble in tissues will require a longer period for induction and recovery. If the rubber goods are of substantial amount in the apparatus used to deliver the anesthetic to the patient and anesthetic agent solubility in rubber is large, the amount of uptake of anesthetic agent by the rubber may be of clinical significance.

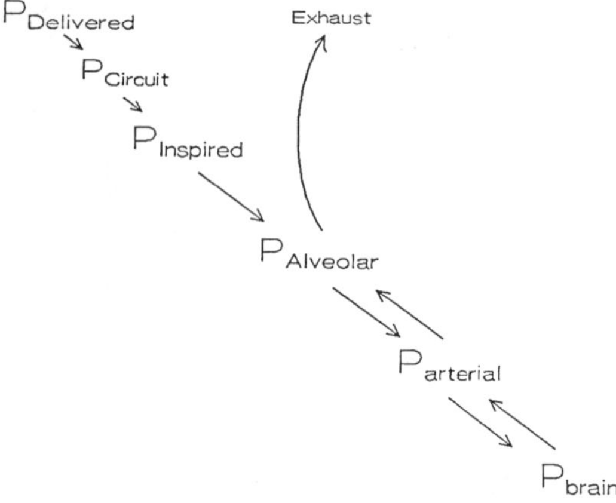

FIG. 11.5—The flow pattern of inhaled anesthetic agents during anesthetic induction and recovery. Inhalation anesthesia may be viewed as the development of a series of partial pressure (tension) gradients. During induction there is a high anesthetic tension in the vaporizer that decreases progressively as the flow of anesthetic gas moves from its source to the brain. Some of these gradients are easily manipulated by the anesthetist; others are not or are done so with difficulty. (From Steffey 1994, with permission of the publishers.)

PHARMACOKINETICS: UPTAKE AND ELIMINATION OF INHALATION ANESTHETICS. The aim in administering an inhalation anesthetic to a patient is to achieve an adequate partial pressure, or tension, of anesthetic (P_{anes}) in the brain to cause a desired level of anesthesia. Anesthetic depth varies directly with P_{anes} in brain tissue. The rate of change of anesthetic depth is of obvious clinical importance and is directly dependent upon the rate of change in anesthetic tensions in the various media in which it is contained before reaching the brain. This section will not provide an extensive review of these principles. If more information is desired, readers are directed to reviews by Eger (1974, 1990), Butterworth and Strichartz (1990), Mapleson (1989), and Steffey (1994, 1991, 1995).

Movement of molecules of inhalation anesthetics, like O_2 and CO_2, occurs down partial pressure gradients (Fig. 11.5). Gases move from regions of higher tension to those of lower tension until equilibrium (i.e., equal pressure in the two media) is established. Thus, during anesthetic induction, the P_{anes} at its source, say in the vaporizer, is high (which, in turn as we recall, is dictated by the vapor pressure) and is progressively less as anesthetic travels from vaporizer to patient breathing circuit, from circuit to lungs, from lungs to arterial blood, and, finally, from arterial blood to body tissues (e.g., brain; Fig. 11.5). Of these, the alveolar partial pressure (P_A) of anesthetic is most crucial to our further understanding. The reasoning for this is as follows. The brain is very rich in blood supply, and the anesthetic in arterial blood (P_aAnes) rapidly equilibrates with brain (P_{brain}Anes). Usually gas exchange at the alveolar level is sufficiently efficient when the P_aAnes is close to P_AAnes. Thus, the P_{brain}Anes closely follows P_AAnes, and controlling the P_AAnes is a reliable indirect way for controlling P_{brain}Anes and anesthetic depth.

At this point it may also be helpful to recall that although the partial pressure of anesthetic is of primary importance, we frequently define clinical dose of an inhaled anesthetic in terms of concentration (*C;* i.e., volumes %). As previously noted, this is because it is common practice for the clinician to regulate and/or measure respiratory and anesthetic gases in volumes %. In addition, in the gaseous phase the relationship between the P_{anes} and the C_{anes} is a simple one:

$$P_{anes} = \text{fractional anesthetic concentration} \times \text{total ambient pressure}$$

The fractional anesthetic concentration is of course $C_{anes}/100$. However, as we reviewed in the section above, in the blood or tissue phases, for example, the actual quantity of anesthetic vapor contained in this solvent phase depends on both the P_{anes} and the anesthetic solubility (or PC) in the solvent phase. Consequently, at equilibrium, the partial pressure in all phases will be equal, but the concentration will vary.

The P_A of anesthetic is a balance between anesthetic input (i.e., delivery to the alveoli) and loss (uptake by blood and body tissues) from the lungs (Fig. 11.5). A rapid rise in P_A of anesthetic is associated with a rapid anesthetic induction or change in anesthetic depth. Factors that contribute to a rapid change in P_A of anesthetic are summarized in Fig. 11.6.

Delivery to the Alveoli. Delivery of anesthetic to the alveoli and therefore the rate of rise of the alveolar concentration or fraction (F_A) toward the inspired concentration or fraction (F_I) depend on the inspired anesthetic concentration itself and the magnitude of alveolar ventilation. Increasing either one of these or both increases the rate of rise of the P_A of anesthetic; that is, other things considered equal, there is an increase in speed of anesthetic induction or change in anesthetic level.

- A. Increased alveolar delivery of anesthetic
  - 1. Increased inspired anesthetic concentration
    - a. Increased vaporization of agent
    - b. Increased vaporizer dial setting
    - c. Increased anesthetic laden fresh gas inflow to the patient breathing circuit
    - d. Decreased gas volume of patient breathing circuit
    - e. Vaporizer positioned in a patient rebreathing circuit
  - 2. Increased alveolar ventilation
    - a. Increased minute ventilation
    - b. Decreased ventilation of respiratory system dead space
- B. Decreased removal of anesthetic from the alveoli
  - 1. Decreased blood solubility of anesthetic
  - 2. Decreased cardiac output
  - 3. Decreased alveolar-venous anesthetic gradient

FIG. 11.6—Factors related to a rapid change in alveolar anesthetic tension (Lockhart et al. 1991a; modified from Steffey 1994).

INSPIRED CONCENTRATION. The inspired concentration has a number of variables controlling it. First of all, the upper limit of inspired concentration is dictated by the agent vapor pressure, which in turn is dependent on temperature. This may be especially important considering the breadth of veterinary medical application of inhaled anesthesia and methods of vaporizing volatile anesthetics under widely diverse conditions (e.g., some environmental conditions are quite hostile).

Characteristics of the patient breathing system in use can also be a major factor in generating a suitable inspired concentration under usual operating-room conditions. Characteristics of special importance include the volume of the system, the amount of rubber or plastic in the system, the position of the vaporizer relative to the breathing circuit (i.e., within or outside the circuit), and the fresh gas inflow to the patient breathing circuit.

The solubility of especially some anesthetics (e.g., methoxyflurane; Table 11.5) in rubber and plastic will also delay development of an appropriate inspired anesthetic concentration. The loss of anesthetic to these equipment "sinks" serves to increase the apparent volume of the anesthetic circuitry and may, in some cases, be clinically important (e.g., use of rubber hoses and a large rubber rebreathing bag on circuits designed for anesthetic management of horses).

ALVEOLAR VENTILATION. An increase in alveolar ventilation increases the rate of delivery of inhalation anesthetic to the alveoli. If unopposed, alveolar ventilation would rapidly increase the alveolar concentration of anesthetic so that within minutes the alveolar concentration would equal the inspired concentration. However, in reality the input created by alveolar ventilation is countered by absorption of anesthetic into blood. Predictably, hypoventilation reduces the rate at which the alveolar concentration increases over time compared to the inspired concentration; that is, anesthetic induction is slowed. Alveolar ventilation is altered by changes in anesthetic depth (increased depth usually means decreased ventilation), mechanical ventilation (usually increased ventilation), or changes in dead-space ventilation (i.e., for constant minute ventilation, a decrease in dead-space ventilation results in an increase in alveolar ventilation).

Removal from the Alveoli: Uptake by Blood. As noted by Eger (1990) anesthetic uptake is the product of three factors: solubility (*S;* the blood/gas solubility, Table 11.4), cardiac output (CO), and the difference in the anesthetic partial pressure between the alveoli and venous blood returning to the lungs ($P_A - P_v$; expressed in mm Hg); that is,

$$\text{Uptake} = S \cdot \text{CO} \cdot [(P_A - P_v)/P_{\text{bar}})],$$

where P_{bar} = barometric pressure in mm Hg. Note that if any of these three factors equals zero, there is no further uptake of anesthetic by blood.

SOLUBILITY. The solubility of an inhalation anesthetic in blood and tissues is characterized by its partition coefficient (PC; Table 11.4).

Compared to an anesthetic agent with high blood solubility (PC), an agent with low blood solubility should be associated with a more rapid equilibration between tissue phases because a large amount of the highly soluble anesthetic must be dissolved in the blood before equilibrium is reached with the gas phase. In the case of the agent with a high blood/gas PC, the blood acts like a large "sink" into which the anesthetic is poured, and accordingly blood is "reluctant" to give up agent to other tissues (like the brain). For purposes of the present discussion, the blood only serves as a conduit for drug delivery to brain and as such can be visualized as a large or small pharmacologically inactive reservoir that is interposed between the lungs and the agent's site of desired pharmacological activity (i.e., brain). Therefore, an anesthetic agent with a low blood/gas PC is usually more desirable than a soluble

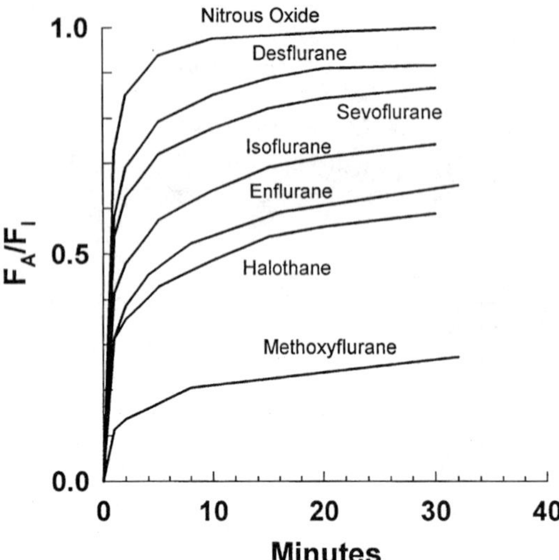

FIG. 11.7—The rise in the alveolar (F_A) anesthetic concentration toward the inspired (F_I) concentration. Note the rise is most rapid with the least soluble anesthetic, N_2O, and slowest with the most soluble anesthetic, methoxyflurane. All data are from studies of humans. The curves are redrawn from Eger 1985a, 1992.

agent, because it is associated with (1) a more rapid anesthetic induction (i.e., more rapid rate of rise in alveolar concentration during induction; Fig. 11.7); (2) more precise control of anesthetic depth (i.e., alveolar concentration during the anesthetic maintenance phase of anesthesia); and (3) a more rapid elimination of anesthetic and recovery from anesthesia (i.e., a rapid decrease in alveolar concentration during the anesthetic recovery phase).

CARDIAC OUTPUT. The amount of blood flowing through the lungs and on to body tissues (cardiac output, or CO) also influences anesthetic uptake from the lungs. The greater the CO, the more blood passing through the lungs carrying away anesthetic from the alveoli. Thus, a large CO, like increased anesthetic agent blood solubility, delays the alveolar rise of P_{anes}. Patient excitement is an example in which a relatively large CO is anticipated. Conversely, a reduced CO should be anticipated with a patient in shock. Such a situation is associated with a relative increase in the rate of rise of the P_A of anesthetic and makes anesthetic induction more risky.

ALVEOLAR TO VENOUS ANESTHETIC PARTIAL PRESSURE DIFFERENCE. The magnitude of difference in anesthetic partial pressure between the alveoli and venous blood is related to the amount of uptake of anesthetic agent by tissues. Not surprisingly, the largest gradient occurs during induction. Once the tissues no longer absorb anesthetic (i.e., equilibrium between the two phases is reached), there is no longer any uptake of anesthetic agent from the lungs (i.e., the venous blood returning to the lungs contains as much agent as when it left the lungs). The changes in gradient in between these extremes result from the relative distribution of CO. In this regard it is important to recognize that roughly 70–80% of the CO is normally directed to only a small volume of body tissues in a lean individual (Webb 1985; Staddon et al. 1979). That is, tissues such as brain, heart, hepatoportal system, and kidneys represent only about 10% of the body mass but normally receive about 75% of the total blood flow each minute. As a result these highly perfused tissues equilibrate with arterial anesthetic tension fairly rapidly (actual timing is influenced by agent solubility). Since the venous anesthetic tension equals that in the tissue within 10–15 minutes, about 75% of the blood returning to the lungs is the same as the alveolar tension. This presumes there has been no change in the mean time in arterial tension. Thus uptake is reduced. Skin and muscle compose the major bulk of the body (about 50% in humans) but at rest receive only about 15–20% of the CO, so saturation of this tissue group takes up to a few hours to accomplish. Fat is a variable component of body bulk and receives only a small proportion of blood flow. Consequently, anesthetic saturation of this tissue group is very slow, especially given that all anesthetics are considerably more soluble in fat than in other tissue groups (Table 11.4).

Other factors can further influence the magnitude of the alveolar-to-arterial anesthetic partial pressure gradient. They include abnormalities of lung ventilation/perfusion (Eger and Severinghaus 1964), loss of anesthetic via the skin (Stoelting et al. 1969; Fassoulaki et al. 1991; Lockhart et al. 1991b) and into closed gas spaces (Eger 1974, 1990, 1985b), and metabolism (Eger 1974, 1990).

Anesthetic Recovery. Recovery from inhalation anesthesia results from the elimination of anesthetic from the brain. This requires a decrease in alveolar anesthetic partial pressure (concentration), which in turn fosters a decrease in arterial and then brain anesthetic partial pressure (Fig. 11.5). Prominent factors accounting for recovery are the same as those for anesthetic induction. Therefore, factors such as alveolar ventilation, CO, and especially agent solubility play prominent roles in recovery from inhalation anesthesia. Indeed, the graphic curves representing the wash out of anesthetic from the alveoli versus time (Fig. 11.8) are essentially inverse of the wash-in curves seen earlier (Fig. 11.7). That is, the wash out of the less soluble anesthetics is high at first, then rapidly declines to a lower output level that continues to decrease but at a slower rate.

The output with the more soluble agent is also high at first, but the magnitude of decrease in alveolar anesthetic concentration is less and only more gradually decreases with time (Fig. 11.8). Thus recovery from the two newest agents, desflurane and sevoflurane, is faster than with isoflurane and even more so than the older agents (Eger and Johnson 1987; Frink et al. 1992).

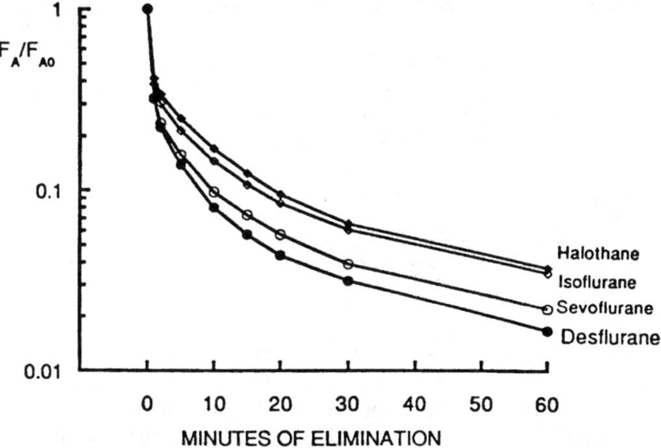

FIG. 11.8—The fall in alveolar (F_A) concentration relative to the alveolar concentration at the end of anesthesia (F_{AO}). Note that the newest, most insoluble volatile anesthetic, desflurane, is eliminated in humans more rapidly than the other contemporary potent anesthetics. Not shown is information for methoxyflurane—if present, the curve for methoxyflurane would appear above that for halothane. (From Eger 1992; reprinted with permission.)

A factor that is important in the rate of recovery but not during the induction period is the duration of anesthesia. Because there is a greater reserve in the body of a highly soluble agent like methoxyflurane after a prolonged administration, its alveolar concentration will be slow to fall in comparison to a less soluble agent like isoflurane.

Other factors that are important to varying but smaller degrees to inhalation anesthetic elimination from the body include percutaneous loss (Stoelting and Eger 1969; Lockhart et al. 1991b; Fassoulaki et al. 1991; Cullen and Eger 1972) and intertissue diffusion of agents (Carpenter et al. 1987, 1986a). Metabolism may also play a small role with some inhalation anesthetic agents (e.g., methoxyflurane and perhaps even halothane; Baden and Rice 1994; Carpenter et al. 1986b, 1987; Cahalan et al. 1981), especially in cases of clinically unusual, prolonged anesthesia. No appreciable effect on recovery by metabolism is expected for isoflurane, desflurane and sevoflurane.

Biotransformation. Inhalation anesthetics are not chemically inert (Van Dyke et al. 1964). They undergo varying degrees of metabolism (Table 11.6), primarily in the liver but also to lesser degrees in the lung, kidney, and intestinal tract (Stier et al. 1964; Rehder et al. 1967; Holaday et al. 1970; Baden et al. 1994; Mazze et al. 1989). The importance of this is twofold. First, in a very limited way with older anesthetics, metabolism may facilitate anesthetic recovery (supra vide). Second and more important is the potential for acute and chronic toxicities by intermediary or end metabolites of inhalation agents on, especially, kidneys, liver, and reproductive organs (Baden and Rice 1994; Mazze and Fujinaga 1989).

TABLE 11.6—Biotransformation of inhalation anesthetics in humans

Anesthetic	Anesthetic recovered as metabolites (%)	Reference
Methoxyflurane	50	Holaday et al. 1970
Halothane	20-25	Cascorbi et al. 1970; Rehder et al. 1967
Sevoflurane	3	Eger 1994
Enflurane	2.4	Chase et al. 1971
Isoflurane	0.17	Holaday et al. 1975
Desflurane	0.02	Eger 1994
Nitrous oxide	0.004	Hong et al. 1980a

For further information on the biotransformation of inhalation anesthetics and for details regarding individual anesthetic agents, see reviews by Baden and Rice (1994) and Mazze and Fujinaga (1989).

Anesthetic Dose: The Minimum Alveolar Concentration. In 1963 Merkel and Eger described what has become the standard index of anesthetic potency for inhalation anesthetics: MAC (Merkel and Eger 1963). MAC is the minimum alveolar concentration of an anesthetic that prevents gross purposeful movement in 50% of subjects exposed to a supramaximal noxious stimulus. Thus, MAC corresponds to the effective dose-50, or ED_{50}; half of the subjects are anesthetized and half are not. The dose that corresponds to the ED_{95} (95% of the individuals are anesthetized), at least in humans, is 20–40% greater than MAC (De Jong and Eger 1975); and 2.0 times the MAC (i.e., 2 MAC) represents a deep level of anesthesia, in some cases even

TABLE 11.7—The minimum alveolar concentration (MAC) of inhalation anesthetics

Anesthetic	Bird	Cat	Dog	Horse	Human
Methoxyflurane	—	0.23	0.29	0.28	0.16
Halothane	1.04 (duck)	1.04	0.87	0.88	0.74
Isoflurane	1.30 (duck)	1.63	1.30	1.31	1.15
Enflurane	—	2.37	2.06	2.12	1.68
Sevoflurane	—	2.58	2.36	2.31	2.05
Desflurane	—	9.79	7.20	—	7.25
Nitrous oxide	220 (pigeon)	255	222	205	104

Note: Values are expressed in volumes % and selected from a review by Steffey (1995).

an anesthetic overdose. MAC values for contemporary inhalation anesthetics for a variety of animals commonly encountered in clinical veterinary medicine and humans are summarized in Table 11.7.

The anesthetic potency of an inhaled anesthetic is inversely related to MAC (i.e., potency = 1/MAC). From information presented above it also follows that MAC is inversely related to the oil/gas PC. Thus, a very potent anesthetic (e.g., methoxyflurane) has a low MAC value and a high oil/gas PC; an agent of low anesthetic potency (e.g., N_2O) has a high MAC and a low oil/gas PC.

A number of characteristics of MAC deserve emphasis (Eger 1974). MAC is defined in terms of a percentage of 1 atmosphere and therefore represents an anesthetic partial pressure at the anesthetic site of action (i.e., remember $P_x = C/100 \cdot P_{bar}$, where P_x stands for the partial pressure of the anesthetic in the gas mixture, C is the anesthetic concentration in volumes %, and P_{bar} is the barometric, or total, pressure of the gas mixture). Thus, although the concentration at MAC for a given agent may vary depending on ambient pressure conditions (e.g., sea-level vs. high-altitude locations), the anesthetic partial pressure at MAC would be the same.

Second, the A in MAC represents *a*lveolar concentration, not the inspired or delivered (as, e.g., from a vaporizer) concentration. This is important because as we reviewed above, after sufficient time for equilibration (i.e., minutes), alveolar partial pressure represents arterial and brain anesthetic partial pressures. In addition, the alveolar concentration is easily monitored with contemporary technology.

Finally, MAC is normally determined in healthy animals under controlled laboratory conditions in the *absence* of other drugs and other circumstances common to clinical use that may modify the requirements for anesthesia. Many factors can influence MAC (anesthetic requirement); some increase and some decrease MAC. (See reviews by Eger [1997] and Quasha et al. [1980]).

PHARMACODYNAMICS: ACTIONS AND TOXICITY OF THE INHALATION ANESTHETICS. Inhalation anesthetic agents influence vital organ function. Some actions are associated with the use of all agents while other actions are a special or prominent feature of one or a number of the agents. The differences in actions, and in particular undesirable actions, of specific anesthetic agents are major considerations when selecting one agent over another for clinical use. Undesirable actions also provide important impetus for development of new agents and/or anesthetic techniques.

The following review of the actions and toxicity of inhaled anesthetics draws from results of studies of many different species, including humans (in some cases humans are the most completely studied species). Species- or agent-specific reviews include those by Eger (1985a,b, 1993), Haskins and Klide (1992), and Steffey (1991, 1994, 1995).

It is important to stress that many variables commonly accompany anesthetic management of animals in both clinical and laboratory settings. These variables influence drug pharmacodynamics and may cause individuals to respond differently from test subjects that were studied under standardized conditions. Examples of such confounding variables include species, duration of anesthesia, noxious (surgical) stimulation, mechanical ventilation, coexisting disease, concurrent medications, and extremes of age.

Central Nervous System. Inhalation anesthetics produce a reversible generalized CNS depression for which the degree of depression is often described as depth of anesthesia. The mechanism of action of inhalation anesthetics is still poorly understood. (See Chap. 9.)

Several anesthetic agents in contemporary use have epileptogenic potential. Enflurane is most prominent in this regard among the potent inhalation anesthetics.

The fragile relationship between cerebral blood flow, intracranial pressure, and cerebral metabolic rate for oxygen is an especially important consideration in some types of patients. For example, an increase in intracranial pressure can reduce cerebral perfusion pressure to the extent that cerebral blood flow is reduced. This situation may in turn result in a reduction of oxygen delivery below that of metabolic oxygen demands required for brain vitality.

Inhalation anesthetics are potent vasodilators and tend to increase cerebral blood flow. Anesthetic-induced cerebral vasodilation and associated increases in cerebral blood flow increase intracranial pressure usually to a trivial extent in normal individuals but perhaps to a life-threatening extent in patients with preexisting reduced intracranial compliance (e.g., tumor, hemorrhage). In such cases isoflurane with hyperventilation (changes in arterial carbon dioxide tension, P_aCO_2, result in corresponding directional changes in cerebral blood flow; Drummond and Shapiro 1994) is preferred over a similar anesthetic management plan incorporating halothane.

Respiratory System. All contemporary inhalation anesthetics depress alveolar ventilation. As a consequence, the P_aCO_2 is increased in direct relation to anesthetic dose (MAC multiple; Fig. 11.9). The magnitude of P_aCO_2 is also species related (Fig. 11.10). In addition, the normal stimulation to ventilation caused by an increased P_aCO_2 and/or a low arterial oxygen tension (P_aO_2) is reduced (Pavlin and Su 1994; Knill and Gelb 1978).

Bronchospasm is associated with some diseases and other patient conditions and contributes to increased airway resistance. Among the volatile anesthetics, halothane appears to be the most effective bronchodilator (Coon and Kampine 1975; Klide and Aviado 1967).

Volatile inhalation anesthetics may affect reflex hypoxic pulmonary vasoconstriction and thereby contribute to a maldistribution of ventilation to perfusion and an increase in the alveolar-to-arterial partial pressure of oxygen and decrease in P_aO_2 (Pavlin and Su 1994; Marshall et al. 1984).

Cardiovascular System. All of the volatile inhalation anesthetics cause dose-dependent and drug-specific changes in cardiovascular performance. The mechanisms of cardiovascular effects are diverse but often include direct myocardial depression by the inhaled anesthetic and a directly or indirectly induced decrease in sympathoadrenal activity.

All of the volatile anesthetics decrease cardiac output, usually via a decrease in myocardial contractility (Pagel et al. 1991a, 1993; Eger 1985a; Warltier and Pagel 1992; Boban et al. 1992; Eisele 1985) and, in turn, stroke volume. The magnitude of change is dose related and dependent on agent (Eger 1985a; Steffey and Howland 1978b, 1980; Klide 1976; Steffey et al.

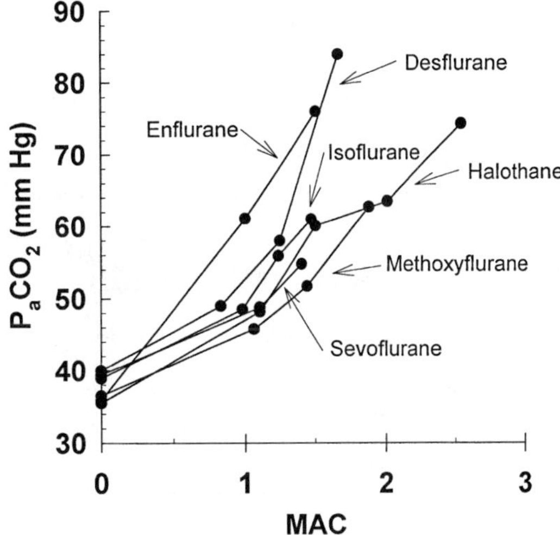

FIG. 11.9—A summary of the effects of contemporary volatile anesthetics on P_aCO_2 in humans, the species for which data are most complete. (Data from Lockhart et al. 1991a; Munson et al. 1966; Larson et al. 1969; Doi and Ikeda 1987; Calverley et al. 1978a; Fourcade et al. 1971.)

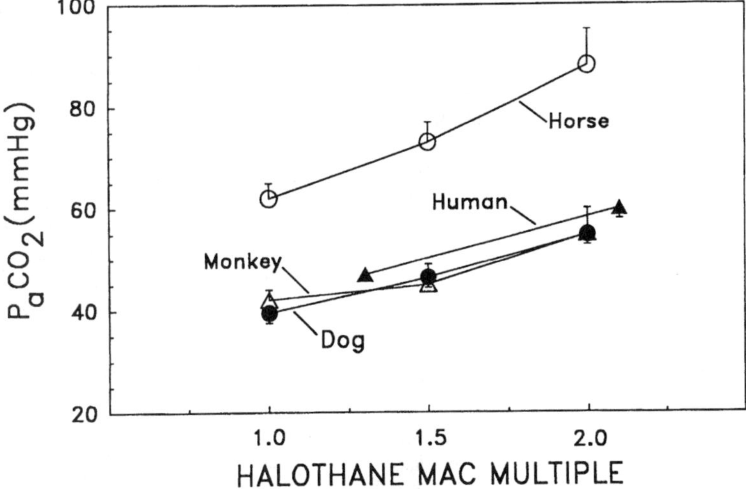

FIG. 11.10—The P_aCO_2 (mean ±1 SE; mm Hg) in spontaneously breathing, healthy dogs, horses, humans, and monkeys during halothane-oxygen anesthesia. The anesthetic dose is expressed as a multiple of the minimum alveolar concentration (MAC) for each species. (Reproduced from Steffey 1991, by permission.)

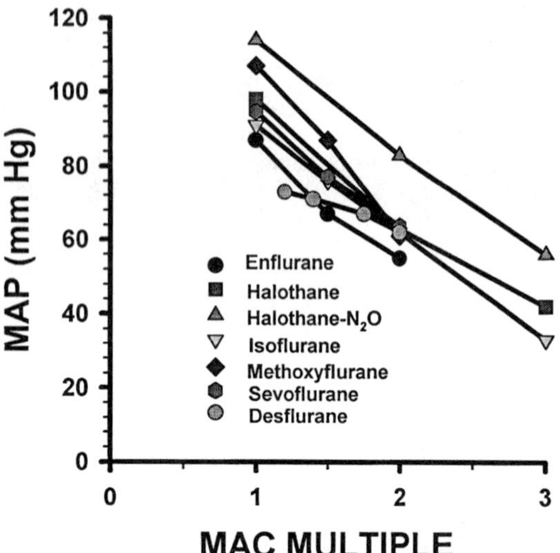

FIG. 11.11—Inhalation anesthetics cause a dose-dependent (expressed as multiples of MAC) decrease in mean arterial blood pressure (MAP) in dogs whose ventilation is mechanically controlled to produce eucapnia. (Data from Steffey et al. 1984; Steffey and Howland 1978b; Steffey et al. 1974b; Frink et al. 1992b; Merin et al. 1991.)

1984; Sommer 1987; Eger 1994; Merin et al. 1991; Weiskopf et al. 1988; Pagel et al. 1991b; Warltier and Pagel 1992). Arterial blood pressure is also decreased in a dose-related manner (Steffey et al. 1974b, 1974c, 1984; Steffey and Howland 1977, 1978b; Frink et al. 1992b; Merin et al. 1991) (Fig. 11.11). The decrease in arterial blood pressure is usually related to a decrease in cardiac output, but in some cases (agent or species related) a decrease in peripheral vascular resistance may also play an important but lesser role.

Inhalation anesthetics affect the cellular mechanisms of myocardial contraction at multiple steps. They decrease free calcium concentration (1) by interfering with Ca^{++} movement through the sarcolemma and by decreasing the availability and release of Ca^{++} from the sarcoplasmic reticulum and (2) by altering the sensitivity of regulatory and contractile proteins to available Ca^{++}. Halothane and enflurane are the most potent of the contemporary agents in this regard. These cellular effects are consistent with the rank order of agent-induced myocardial depression seen in the intact animal (Pavlin and Su 1994).

The distribution of blood flow to organs is altered during inhalation anesthesia (Eger 1985a; Warren and Webb 1986; Bernard et al. 1991; Haskins and Sansome 1979). For example, volatile anesthetics cause a dose-dependent increase in cerebral blood flow (supra vide) and decreases in blood flow to liver and kidneys (infra vide).

CARDIAC RHYTHM AND CATECHOLAMINES. Inhalation anesthetics may increase the automaticity of the myocardium (Price 1966). This effect is exaggerated by adrenergic agonists (Katz and Epstein 1968). Inhalation anesthetics, especially halothane, also may sensitize the heart to arrhythmogenic effects of catecholamines (Raventos 1956; Eger 1985a, 1994; Moore et al. 1993; Munson and Tucker 1975; Navarro et al. 1994; Joas and Stevens 1971; Weiskopf et al. 1989a; Johnston et al. 1976). Temporal changes in cardiovascular function have also been reported in a variety of animals during inhalation anesthesia (Steffey et al. 1987b,c,d, 1993a; Dunlop et al. 1987).

Liver. Hepatocellular injury may result as a general consequence of a reduction in hepatic blood flow or by direct anesthetic agent toxicity. Of the contemporary volatile agents, halothane is most often associated with direct hepatotoxicity.

Kidneys. All of the volatile anesthetics reduce renal blood flow and glomerular filtration rate in a dose-related manner. As a consequence, during anesthesia even healthy animals produce small volumes of concentrated urine. This response is a common finding regardless of the species studied. A transient increase in serum urea nitrogen, creatinine, and inorganic phosphate also may accompany inhalation anesthesia, especially if prolonged (Eger 1985a; Steffey et al. 1979, 1980; Stover et al. 1988; Pohl et al. 1988). In most cases the effects of inhalation anesthesia on renal function are rapidly reversed after anesthesia. Beyond these general responses, methoxyflurane is notable with regard to its potential for causing nephrotoxicity (see below).

Skeletal Muscle. The volatile anesthetics are associated with some small amount of skeletal muscle relaxation, likely a direct result of their CNS depression. They also enhance the muscle relaxation induced by the nondepolarizing neuromuscular blocking drugs that are sometimes used as adjuvants in the anesthetic management of patients.

Malignant hyperthermia, a life-threatening pharmacogenetic myopathy, is most commonly associated with halothane anesthesia. It is further discussed below.

Actions by Agent. Actions by agent will be discussed in this section; the volatile agents presented first, followed by the gaseous agent, N_2O. The agents can be divided into three groups based on broad use in veterinary medicine. Emphasis here is on the properties of halothane, isoflurane, and, later on, N_2O because they are currently the most widely used, and specific data derived from laboratory and clinical investigations are readily available. The second group includes methoxyflurane, enflurane, and diethyl ether. Methoxyflurane never was widely used for anesthetic management of large animals but is still (although increasingly less) selectively used for the management of small animals. Enflurane was never used a great deal for animals, especially in the clinical environment, and its current use overall is at best infrequent. Diethyl ether continues to have value in nonclinical aspects of animal anesthesia and locations outside North America. The remaining group of agents is composed of desflurane and sevoflurane. They are the newest agents; both now are approved for general use in humans in North America and elsewhere. Because chloroform is now used principally as a toxicological tool (to cause reproducible liver damage) and as an industrial solvent, its actions will not be covered.

HALOTHANE. *Halothane,* USP (Fluothane), a multihalogenated ethane, is a clear, volatile liquid. Introduction of halothane into clinical practice in 1957 represented a significant advance in anesthesia pharmacology, since the drug possesses characteristics of rapid induction and recovery, potency, and nonflammability, with minimal side effects (Brown and Sipes 1977). By 1960 halothane was the most popular potent anesthetic agent used in humans in the Western world. Human patients accept the anesthetic without difficulty because of its minimal unpleasant side effects. The most frequently used potent inhalation agent now used in humans is isoflurane.

BIOTRANSFORMATION. About 60–80% of administered halothane is eliminated unchanged in the exhaled breath. The remainder is eliminated via other routes either unchanged or as metabolites. Biotransformation of halothane occurs primarily in the liver; most as a result of the cytochrome P-450 system in the endoplasmic reticulum of the hepatocytes. It has been well established that a major metabolite of halothane metabolism in humans and animals is trifluoroacetic acid (Van Dyke and Wood 1975; Baden and Rice 1994). Other metabolites resulting from oxidative metabolism via the cytochrome P-450 pathway are inorganic chloride (Cl^-) and to a lesser extent bromine (Br^-). Since the bond for fluorine (F^-) is much stronger than for Cl^- or Br^-, little F^- is released. In humans, Br^- from halothane breakdown will induce headache, ataxia, lethargy, and EEG alterations (Tinker et al. 1976). In the dog (Pedersoli 1980) and horse (Rice and Steffey 1985b), serum bromide concentrations increase significantly during and following a period of halothane anesthesia.

An alternative route of halothane metabolism is via a reductive pathway requiring anaerobic conditions and the presence of an electron donor. Both Br^- and F^- are metabolites of this pathway (Baden and Rice 1994). An increase in halothane metabolism occurs in experimental animals when inducing agents such as phenobarbital and isoniazid are given prior to halothane (deGroot et al. 1982; Rice et al. 1987). Prolonged administration of low-dose halothane can also result in increased drug metabolism (Linde and Berman 1971; Ross and Cardell 1978). Such circumstances may have clinical consequences.

CENTRAL NERVOUS SYSTEM. Halothane depresses CNS function in a dose-related fashion until respiratory and cardiovascular collapse and death. The MAC for halothane in the dog is 0.9%; values for other species are given in Table 11.7.

Cerebral blood flow usually increases during halothane anesthesia and may result in an accompanying increase in cerebrospinal fluid pressure (Drummond and Shapiro 1994). Halothane is the most potent of the contemporary volatile anesthetics in this regard, making it a less desirable anesthetic for animals with preexisting space-occupying intracranial lesions and/or increased cerebrospinal fluid pressure. The cerebral metabolic oxygen consumption is reduced in dose-related fashion.

Shivering during recovery from halothane is common. Its cause is related to heat loss associated with general anesthesia and other ill-defined mechanisms (Sessler et al. 1988). Some drowsiness remains evident for several hours after halothane anesthesia even in ambulatory animals.

CARDIOVASCULAR SYSTEM. Halothane depresses circulatory system function. Studies of a variety of mammals, including humans, indicate that cardiac output, stroke volume, and arterial blood pressure are less during halothane anesthesia compared to the awake, unmedicated individual. Further decreases in cardiovascular function accompany increasing alveolar doses of halothane (Pavlin and Su 1994; Bergman 1976; Steffey et al. 1974b,c, 1977; Steffey and Howland, 1978a, 1980; Eger et al. 1970; Ingwersen et al. 1988; Grandy et al. 1989). For example, as halothane dose is increased, mean arterial blood pressure decreases because cardiac output decreases. Total peripheral vascular resistance changes very little; thus, generalized peripheral vasodilation is not the primary cause of hypotension. The reduction in cardiac output is caused by a decrease in stroke volume as a result of a direct drug-induced depression in myocardial muscle contractility.

Effects on heart rate vary widely depending on species and associated conditions. Often there is little change in heart rate over a range of clinical anesthetic doses. The rhythm of the heart beat may vary during halothane anesthesia. Especially at light levels of anesthesia spontaneous arrhythmias may appear. There is some evidence that deeper levels of halothane anesthesia decrease this incidence (Purchase 1966; Muir et al. 1959).

Halothane is especially well noted for its likelihood to predispose the heart to premature ventricular extrasystoles in the presence of catecholamines (Purchase 1966). It is the most potent of the contemporary volatile anesthetics in this regard. Increased endogenous release of catecholamines may occur as a result of surgical stimulation and insufficient anesthesia or from an elevation in P_aCO_2 secondary to hypoventilation. Catecholamines (e.g., epinephrine) and other sympathomimetic amines are sometimes injected during anesthesia and surgery to facilitate patient management or reduce localized bleeding. Thus, anesthetic influence on heart beat rhythm is not a trivial matter. Some anesthetic adjuvant drugs may increase (e.g., xylazine, thiopental, and thiamylal; Tranquilli et al. 1986; Bednarski et al. 1985), and others may decrease (e.g., acepromazine, lidocaine; Muir et al. 1975; Horrigan et al. 1978), the arrhythmogenic dose of epinephrine during halothane anesthesia.

The baroreceptor reflex is a short-term central mechanism to aid in arterial blood pressure homeostasis. Halothane depresses the sensitivity of the baroreceptor reflex (Pavlin and Su 1994).

The cardiovascular effects of halothane change with duration of anesthesia. A time-related increase in arterial blood pressure, stroke volume, and cardiac output has been a common finding in studies of dogs (Steffey et al. 1987b), horses (Dunlop et al. 1987; Steffey et al. 1990a,b, 1993a, 1987d), and humans (Price et al. 1970; Bahlman et al. 1972).

RESPIRATORY SYSTEM. Halothane depresses respiration in a dose-related manner. As a result, the P_aCO_2 increases and there is less efficiency in oxygenating arterial blood and perhaps hypoxemia (Steffey et al. 1977, 1975, 1974c; Steffey and Howland 1978a, 1979a; Grandy et al. 1989). The volume of expired minute ventilation decreases initially as a result of a decrease in tidal volume; respiratory frequency also tends to decrease from awake conditions but the extent is species and condition variable. As anesthetic depth is increased, breathing rate also decreases. In otherwise unmedicated healthy dogs and horses the alveolar halothane concentration that is associated with complete respiratory arrest is 2.9 MAC (Regan and Eger 1967) and 2.6 MAC (Steffey et al. 1977) respectively.

Because halothane has bronchodilator action (Klide and Aviado 1967; Colgan 1965), it has been long considered the anesthetic agent of choice for patients with either a history of asthma or upon anticipated or real bronchospasm during induction or maintenance of anesthesia (Pavlin and Su 1994).

LIVER. Hepatic blood flow is decreased during halothane anesthesia, mostly as a passive consequence of reduced cardiac output and decreased liver perfusion pressure. The reduced blood flow per se, unless extreme, is not usually of a magnitude to result in clinical consequences.

Hepatic dysfunction that sometimes occurs following inhalation anesthesia is most often associated with halothane. The etiology is unknown but the syndrome is likely actually multiple entities (Baden and Rice 1994; Pohl and Gillette 1982). One entity is a mild transient form of hepatic dysfunction that is associated with all of the inhaled (or other) anesthetics and may result from hepatocyte hypoxia (perhaps as a result of reduced tissue oxygen delivery) (Harper et al. 1982a,b; Shingu et al. 1982a,b; Ross and Daggy 1981). Another entity, "halothane hepatitis," is rarer but far more severe and often fatal. The most frequently invoked theories regarding its etiology include the metabolism of halothane to a (hepatic) reactive metabolite (Plummer et al. 1982) and the occurrence of an immune-mediated hypersensitivity (allergic) reaction, a process that is more directly hepatocellularly damaging. The immunological basis for halothane hepatitis has been extensively reviewed (Pohl et al. 1988, 1989; Hubbard et al. 1988).

Laboratory and clinical studies of some clinically important veterinary species (e.g., horses and ponies) indicate there are alterations in hepatic function and cellular integrity associated with halothane anesthesia (Engelking et al. 1984; Gopinath and Ford 1976; Gopinath et al. 1970; Joyce et al. 1983; Steffey et al. 1993c).

KIDNEY. Halothane is not known to have a direct nephrotoxic effect. However, diminution of renal function may occur secondary to an anesthetic reduction in renal blood flow and glomerular filtration rate. The effects reverse rapidly after anesthesia is discontinued (Steffey et al. 1980, 1991, 1993c; Stover et al. 1988).

SKELETAL MUSCLE. Halothane causes some relaxation of skeletal muscle via its action on the CNS. It also increases the magnitude and duration of muscle relaxation induced by nondepolarizing neuromuscular blocking drugs (e.g., pancuronium).

Rarely, induction of anesthesia triggers a rapidly developing hypermetabolic reaction in the skeletal muscle of susceptible individuals. The syndrome was originally described as associated with halothane, but other inhaled anesthetics have also since been implicated. The resultant syndrome of malignant hyperthermia is characterized by muscle rigidity, a rapid rise in body temperature, large consumption of oxygen, and consequent production of CO_2. Death rapidly ensues in most cases unless very aggressive therapy is instituted. Dantrolene is currently the drug of choice for specific therapy.

It is most commonly reported in susceptible swine (Landrace, Pietrain, and Poland China) and human patients and is caused by an acute loss of intracellular control of calcium. The subject has been reviewed by Gronert and Antognini (1994).

Undoubtedly malignant hyperthermia has been wrongfully diagnosed in the past as a cause for hyperthermia in veterinary patients when a more detailed investigation would have revealed other causes.

ISOFLURANE. *Isoflurane,* USP (Forane, Aerrane), is a halogenated methyl ethyl ether. Isoflurane and enflurane are structural isomers. Both compounds contain the same number of atoms of fluorine, chlorine, carbon, hydrogen, and oxygen.

Isoflurane was first synthesized in 1965, and its widespread clinical use for human patients began in 1981. At least in North America, it is now the most widely used volatile anesthetic agent for human patients. Isoflurane is also in widespread clinical use in veterinary patients. It is probably the most commonly used inhaled agent for dogs, cats, horses, and birds.

BIOTRANSFORMATION. In humans and animals isoflurane resists biodegradation. In humans less than 0.2% of the isoflurane taken up by the body is metabolized (Holaday et al. 1975); this rate of metabolism is far less than for halothane, methoxyflurane, and enflurane (Table 11.6). Both inorganic fluoride and trifluoroacetic acid have been identified as end products of isoflurane metabolism (Baden and Rice 1994). The resistance of isoflurane to metabolism accounts for the very small increase in serum fluoride concentration even after prolonged isoflurane administration (Cousins et al. 1973; Dobkin et al. 1973; Mazze et al. 1974a).

Isoflurane is defluorinated by cow, dog, lamb, and rat hepatic microsomes (Rice and Steffey 1985a). In contrast to adult horses, it is not significantly metabolized by neonatal horses (Rice and Steffey 1985b).

The small quantities of degradation products account for the lack of direct renal or hepatic toxicity. Isoflurane also does not appear to be a mutagen, teratogen, or carcinogen (Eger et al. 1978; Eger 1985a).

CENTRAL NERVOUS SYSTEM. Isoflurane, unlike its isomer enflurane, does not produce seizure activity. Cats given isoflurane display "sharp waves" (isolated spiking) on the EEG. This activity is also seen in cats with halothane, enflurane, and methoxyflurane and may be a species peculiarity (Julien and Kavan 1974; Kavan and Julien 1974; Hodgson et al. 1985a).

Isoflurane has become the agent of choice for critically ill animal patients and birds. The MAC for isoflurane is in the range 1.2–1.7% depending upon the species of focus (Table 11.7).

Isoflurane has anticonvulsant effects (Koblin et al. 1981). Electrical silence is seen on the EEG at 2 MAC (Clark and Rosner 1973).

Most studies in animals have shown that isoflurane causes less cerebral vasodilation than halothane (Drummond et al. 1986; Eger 1985a). Cerebral circulation autoregulation is maintained with isoflurane but is impaired by halothane (Todd and Drummond 1984; Miletich et al. 1976). For these reasons isoflurane is usually preferred over halothane for neurosurgery.

CARDIOVASCULAR SYSTEM. Isoflurane depresses cardiovascular function in a dose-related fashion (Steffey and Howland 1977; Steffey et al. 1977, 1987a; Corbally and Brennan 1990; Berl 1990; Eger 1985a; Ludders et al. 1989). The magnitude of its effect on arterial blood pressure is similar to halothane, although with isoflurane the cause is more related to a decrease in the calculated systemic vascular resistance. Also like halothane it decreases cardiac contractility and stroke volume, resulting in a decrease in cardiac output. However, results of studies in a number of species indicate that isoflurane, especially at light and moderate levels, affects cardiac output less than halothane does. Isoflurane thus affords a wider margin of patient safety.

Heart rate tends to be better maintained during isoflurane and may be increased from awake conditions. It remains relatively constant over a range of alveolar isoflurane doses. Heart rhythm is usually little affected by isoflurane, and the incidence of dysrhythmias after injection of vasoactive substances (including catecholamines) is substantially reduced in comparison to halothane (Bednarski and Majors 1986; Eger 1985a; Joas and Stevens 1971; Johnston et al. 1976; Tucker et al. 1974).

As with halothane, duration of isoflurane anesthesia influences the magnitude of cardiovascular function, at least in some species (Dunlop et al. 1987; Steffey et al. 1987c).

RESPIRATORY SYSTEM. Isoflurane, like halothane, depresses respiration and increases P_aCO_2 (Steffey et al. 1977; Steffey and Howland 1977, 1980; Pavlin and Su 1994; Eger 1985a). The magnitude of depression is dose and time related and is at least equal to or greater than that caused by halothane under similar conditions (Steffey et al. 1977, 1985, 1987c; Pavlin and Su 1994; Eger 1985a; Hodgson et al. 1985a; Fourcade et al. 1971; Cromwell et al. 1971).

In some species, like the horse, during light and moderate levels of anesthesia respiration is characterized by large tidal volume and low breathing rate (Hodgson et al. 1985a,b; Steffey et al. 1977). Respiratory depression accompanying isoflurane anesthesia may be increased in magnitude by concurrent administration of opioids (Ossipou and Gebhart 1984; Steffey et al. 1993b), a common practice in clinical circumstances.

The alveolar concentration that causes apnea is 2.5 MAC for the dog (Steffey and Howland 1977) and 2.3 MAC for the horse (Steffey et al. 1977).

The work of Hirshman in dogs sensitized to ascaris antigen suggests that isoflurane (and enflurane) is as effective in decreasing the constrictive ability of airway smooth muscle as halothane (Hirshman et al. 1982). Thus, isoflurane may serve as an acceptable alternative to halothane in animals with elevated airway resistance (Hirshman et al. 1982; Englesson 1974).

LIVER. Blood flow to the liver is altered less by isoflurane than halothane, so isoflurane might be preferable to halothane in patients at risk for hepatic injury (Gelman et al. 1984a,b; Seyde and Longnecker 1984; Gelman 1987; Yasuda et al. 1991). Results of tests of hepatic function and cellular integrity show only minimal changes following isoflurane anesthesia, and the changes are only transient in nature (Daunt et al. 1992; Steffey et al. 1979; Eger 1985a). Transient hepatic insult has been reported with hypoxemia and halothane but not isoflurane anesthesia (Whitehair et al. 1996).

KIDNEY. As with halothane, renal blood flow and urine volume are depressed with isoflurane. Changes in blood components related to renal function and/or injury are not seen or are small in magnitude and are rapidly reversed following anesthesia (Eger 1985a; Daunt et al. 1992; Steffey et al. 1979).

Isoflurane resists metabolism and the release of F^- is small, so direct renal toxicity by this drug is unlikely.

SKELETAL MUSCLE. Isoflurane is more potent than halothane in its ability to enhance the neuromuscular blocking effect of nondepolarizing neuromuscular blocking drugs (Miller et al. 1972; Eger 1985a).

Isoflurane is among the anesthetic drugs reportedly able to trigger malignant hyperthermia (Gronert and Antognini 1994).

Muscle blood flow was better maintained in rats, dogs, and humans anesthetized with isoflurane than with halothane (Seyde and Longnecker 1984; Gelman et al. 1984b; Eger 1985a).

METHOXYFLURANE. *Methoxyflurane,* USP (Metofane, Penthrane), was first synthesized in 1958 and was introduced clinically a few years later. It was a popular inhalation anesthetic for anesthetic management of small companion and laboratory animals throughout most of the 1970s and 1980s. Its use for human patients rapidly declined following discovery of its ability to cause vasopressin-resistant polyuria renal failure (Crandell et al. 1966). Over the past 5–10 years its use in clinical veterinary medicine has also been declining as newer anesthetic agents and anesthetic techniques have appeared. Reliable statistics regarding the frequency of its use in clinical practice are not available, but it is judged by this author to be used less than halothane and isoflurane. Because of its extreme blood solubility, imposing costly delays in manipulating anesthetic dose, it was never widely advocated for use with large domestic species. Its use for avian anesthesia has been replaced by isoflurane. Because less objective information is available for methoxyflurane compared to newer volatile anesthetics and because of its perceived decline in use, information on this drug will be more limited in this edition. See earlier editions of this text for additional information.

BIOTRANSFORMATION. Methoxyflurane undergoes substantial biotransformation; in humans about 50% of the absorbed dose can be recovered as metabolites (Table 11.6) (Holaday et al. 1970). It is the most extensively metabolized of the inhaled anesthetics. The major metabolites are F^-, dichloroacetic acid, and oxalic acid. Both cytochrome P-450-dependent and noncytochrome mechanisms can be involved in its breakdown. The metabolism is increased following administration of enzyme-inducing drugs such as phenobarbital and diazepam (Baden and Rice 1994; Mazze et al. 1974b; Biermann et al. 1986).

CENTRAL NERVOUS SYSTEM. Methoxyflurane is the most potent of the inhalation anesthetics. The MAC for methoxyflurane for the dog is 0.2–0.3% (Eger et al. 1965; Steffey et al. 1984). Values for some other species are given in Table 11.7.

CARDIOVASCULAR SYSTEM. Arterial blood pressure and cardiac output decrease in a dose-related manner (Steffey et al. 1984; Walker et al. 1962). The magnitude of effect in dogs is at least equal to that found with halothane (Steffey et al. 1984; Dobkin and Fedoruk 1961; Bagwell and Woods 1962). As with halothane, the decrease in cardiac output is a result of a decrease in myocardial contractility (Brown and Crout 1971; Merin and Borgstedt 1971). Heart rate changes little over a range of doses, and as is true with all of the anesthetic ethers, cardiac arrhythmias are rare.

RESPIRATORY SYSTEM. Methoxyflurane is a potent respiratory depressant. The increase in P_aCO_2, as with the other volatile anesthetics, is dose related (Steffey et al. 1984). The dose of methoxyflurane resulting in at least 60 seconds of apnea is 3.4 MAC (Regan and Eger 1967).

LIVER. Methoxyflurane along with other inhalation anesthetics reversibly depresses hepatic performance. Though objective data are limited (Pedersoli 1977a), years of uncomplicated use (in relatively healthy dogs) in veterinary practice support the notion that incidence of damage is not great. However, the possibility of liver injury is apparently present in at least some circumstances (Giesecke et al. 1966).

KIDNEY. Renal blood flow, glomerular filtration rate, and urine volume are reduced, as they are with other volatile anesthetics. In especially humans and certain strains of rats (Fischer 344) (Mazze et al. 1972) resultant products (notably F^-) from the metabolism of methoxyflurane reliably result in nephrotoxicity that is characterized by an inability to concentrate urine (Crandell et al. 1966; Baden and Rice 1994). In addition to rats and humans, the cow, dog, lamb, and probably horse are able to biodegrade methoxyflurane and release F^- (Rice and Steffey 1985a,b). Thus, high serum F^- is attainable in species other than man and rat following exposure to methoxyflurane. An increase in serum F^- following methoxyflurane anesthesia in dogs has been reported (Pedersoli 1977b; Pedersoli 1977a; Fleming and Pedersoli 1980) but under conditions of study clinical signs of renal failure were not obvious. However, anesthetic adjuvant drugs may increase the likelihood of toxicity to methoxyflurane (Matthews et al. 1990).

ENFLURANE. *Enflurane,* USP (Ethrane), was synthesized in 1963, introduced for clinical trial in human patients in 1963, and released for general clinical human use in 1972. Its introduction was encouraged because of the clinical need for an alternative inhalation anesthetic to halothane for human patients. It was investigated for use with small companion animals and horses but received at best only brief clinical exposure.

It is a chemical isomer of isoflurane (Fig. 11.2).

BIOTRANSFORMATION. About 2–10% (Table 11.6) of the enflurane that is administered to humans is biodegraded in the liver (Chase et al. 1971; Carpenter et al.

1986b), with F^- as one of its metabolites. Treatment with drugs that induce hepatic enzymes (e.g., phenobarbital) enhances enflurane metabolism (Baden and Rice 1994). The degree of biotransformation occurring with enflurane is substantially less than that found with methoxyflurane and halothane but more than with isoflurane and the two newest inhalation anesthetics.

CENTRAL NERVOUS SYSTEM. The MAC for enflurane in a variety of animal species averages about 2.2% (Table 11.7).

The occurrence of motor hyperactivity such as twitching of the muscles of the face and extremities at moderate levels of anesthesia was noted early in the use of enflurane in both humans and animals. These signs were accompanied by EEG evidence of seizure patterns (Neigh et al. 1971; Clark and Rosner 1973; Joas et al. 1971; Julien and Kavan 1972; Bassell et al. 1982; Steffey and Howland 1978b; Steffey et al. 1977; Steffey 1978; Klide 1976). Enflurane's epileptogenic nature is unique among the commonly used inhaled anesthetics. Hypocapnia seems to potentiate seizurelike activity during enflurane anesthesia (Neigh et al. 1971). Consequently, hyperventilation is usually avoided in the clinical management of patients.

Other effects by enflurane on the CNS are similar to those for halothane and include cerebrovascular dilation, increased cerebral blood flow, and increased intracranial pressure (Michenfelder and Cucchiara 1974; Drummond and Shapiro 1994).

CARDIOVASCULAR SYSTEM. Enflurane causes dose-related depression in cardiovascular function (Calverley et al. 1978a,b; Skovsted and Price 1972; Steffey and Howland 1978b; Steffey et al. 1977; Klide 1976), and overall its effects are considered more profound than those of halothane and isoflurane (Pavlin and Su 1994). Arterial blood pressure is progressively decreased as dose of enflurane is increased. The magnitude of reduction in blood pressure is at least equal to that caused by halothane. Cardiac output also is decreased in a dose-related manner due to a profound depression in myocardial contractility and in turn a decrease in stroke volume. The magnitude of depression in contractility is at least as severe or more so than that produced by halothane (Iwatsuki et al. 1970; Brown and Crout 1971; Merin et al. 1976).

Heart rate may be increased with enflurane. It is intermediate between halothane and isoflurane in its arrhythmogenic potential in the presence of catecholamines (Johnston et al. 1976).

RESPIRATORY SYSTEM. Enflurane is a potent respiratory depressant. The increase in P_aCO_2 is directly related to anesthetic dose (Klide 1976; Steffey and Howland 1978b; Steffey et al. 1977; Calverley et al. 1978a). Enflurane is about equally effective as halothane in decreasing lung airway resistance (Hirshman and Bergman 1978).

LIVER. As with other volatile anesthetics, liver blood flow is reduced in proportion to anesthetic dose and to changes in cardiac output. Hepatic necrosis has been only rarely reported in human patients following enflurane anesthesia (Lewis et al. 1983; Ona et al. 1980; Van der Reis et al. 1974). The influence of accompanying severe hypoxic conditions may have played a prominent role in at least some of these cases (Baden and Rice 1994; Eger et al. 1986). As with halothane, enflurane should probably be avoided in patients suspected of hepatic dysfunction.

KIDNEY. Enflurane, like halothane, depresses renal function. It causes reductions in renal blood flow, glomerular filtration rate, and urine volume that are equivalent in magnitude to those seen with halothane.

The metabolism of enflurane by the liver to F^- is much less than that for methoxyflurane. The amount of F^- produced is usually below the toxic threshold level (Cousins et al. 1976), so it is unlikely to cause clinically significant renal dysfunction except in unusual circumstances like prolonged anesthetic conditions (Barr et al. 1974; Mazze et al. 1977).

SKELETAL MUSCLE. Skeletal muscle relaxation occurs with enflurane, and nondepolarizing neuromuscular blocking drugs are more potent in the presence of enflurane (Fogdall and Miller 1975; Lebowitz et al. 1970). Malignant hyperthermia is induced in susceptible individuals by enflurane (Caropreso et al. 1975; Gronert and Antognini 1994).

DESFLURANE. *Desflurane,* USP (Suprane), is the newest inhalation anesthetic released for general clinical use in human patients in North America, United Kingdom, and other parts of Europe. Its actions have been investigated in humans and in a variety of animal species, including dogs, horses, and pigs. Reviews of its actions are in Eger 1993 and 1994.

Desflurane, formally known as I-653, was first synthesized in the 1960s along with similar agents such as enflurane and isoflurane. It was not actively investigated at that time because it was difficult to produce and its greater anesthetic potency compared to other prospects was considered undesirable (Eger 1993).

Desflurane has a high vapor pressure (Table 11.3) and required a newly designed, temperature-controlled, pressurized vaporizer for predictable delivery (Andrews and Johnston 1993). It has a very low solubility (Eger 1987) in blood (Table 11.4), contributing to greater precision of control over the maintenance of anesthesia and a very rapid emergence from anesthesia (Eger 1992).

BIOTRANSFORMATION. Desflurane resists degradation by the body to a greater degree than any of the other volatile anesthetics (Koblin 1992; Koblin et al. 1988); actual amounts of degradation are too small to measure accurately. Results to date do not indicate any toxicity associated with its use in a variety of species. Although the magnitude of breakdown is different, desflurane is expected to be metabolized in a manner similar (parallel) to that for isoflurane (Baden and Rice 1994). Resulting products are free fluoride ions, trifluoroacetic acid, and CO_2 and water (Eger 1993).

CENTRAL NERVOUS SYSTEM. Desflurane is less potent than other contemporary volatile agents (Table 11.7). For example, the MAC for the dog is 7.2%.

Desflurane causes dose-related depression of EEG activity comparable to effects seen with an equipotent dose of isoflurane (Rampil et al. 1988, 1991). Epileptiform EEG activity is not reported.

Desflurane causes dose-dependent decreases in cerebrovascular resistance (vasodilation) and cerebral metabolic rate of oxygen consumption similar to actions by halothane and isoflurane (Lutz et al. 1990). As is the case with isoflurane, desflurane may also result in an increase in brain volume and associated intracranial pressure increase (Young 1992). Although these effects are trivial in animals without intracranial pathology (Lutz et al. 1990, 1991), the agent must be used carefully in patients with decreased intracranial compliance. Desflurane is similar to isoflurane in that cerebrovascular responsiveness to carbon dioxide is maintained (Lutz et al. 1991).

CARDIOVASCULAR SYSTEM. The cardiovascular actions of desflurane are similar to those of isoflurane (Weiskopf et al. 1988, 1989b, 1991; McMurphy and Hodgson 1994; Warltier and Pagel 1992). Like isoflurane and halothane, desflurane decreases mean arterial blood pressure and stroke volume in dose-related fashion. But cardiac output during desflurane, as with isoflurane, is better maintained compared to conditions during halothane anesthesia. Heart rate is usually higher and peripheral vascular resistance less with desflurane compared to the other volatile agents (Pagel et al. 1991b). Myocardial contractility is depressed (Pagel et al. 1991a; Boban et al. 1992). Desflurane does not predispose the heart to ventricular arrhythmias, nor does it sensitize it to arrhythmogenic effects of epinephrine (Moore et al. 1993; Weiskopf et al. 1989a).

RESPIRATORY SYSTEM. Desflurane, like other contemporary volatile anesthetics, causes a dose-related respiratory depression (Lockhart et al. 1991a). Its effects in this regard in humans are most comparable to those of enflurane (i.e., more depressing than isoflurane). Apnea occurs in pigs at alveolar desflurane concentrations between 1.2 and 1.6 MAC, while the apneic threshold in dogs is 2.38 MAC (Warltier and Pagel 1992).

LIVER. Desflurane depresses hepatic blood flow only minimally. In a study of dogs, total hepatic blood flow (portal plus hepatic arterial) was significantly decreased by desflurane only at the two highest anesthetic concentrations (1.75 and 2.0 MAC) (Merin et al. 1991). These actions were not significantly different from isoflurane.

Desflurane is not associated with hepatic toxicity in humans (Jones et al. 1990; Weiskopf et al. 1992), swine (Holmes et al. 1990), or rats (Eger et al. 1987).

KIDNEY. Renal blood flow is not substantially altered by desflurane (Merin et al. 1991). Because desflurane is extremely resistant to degradation, it is not expected to possess, and has not to date shown, nephrotoxic potential (Baden and Rice 1994; Jones et al. 1990; Weiskopf et al. 1992).

SKELETAL MUSCLE. Desflurane, like isoflurane and enflurane, causes muscle relaxation and enhances the action of neuromuscular blocking drugs (Caldwell et al. 1991). Desflurane is also a trigger of malignant hyperthermia in susceptible swine (Wedel et al. 1991).

SEVOFLURANE. *Sevoflurane* (Ultane) was synthesized in the early 1970s, and its characteristics were first described in 1975 (Wallin et al. 1975). It has been approved for use in human patients in Japan for nearly two decades. It is now available in North America for general use in human patients.

Its physical characteristics were noted earlier in this chapter. However, it is important to point out here again that unlike other contemporary inhalation anesthetics sevoflurane is degraded in the presence of soda lime and Baralyme, commonly used CO_2 absorbents in anesthetic delivery circuits (Wallin et al. 1975; Liu et al. 1991; Strum et al. 1987; Frink et al. 1992a). Sevoflurane degrades to $CH_2F–O–C=CF_2$ (CF_3) (known as Compound A) that is lethal in 50% of animals (LD_{50}) at a concentration of 400 ppm (Morio et al. 1992). Mazze (1992) has discussed concerns of levels of Compound A in human patients.

The in vitro rate of defluorination of sevoflurane is about the same as for methoxyflurane (Cook et al. 1975a,b). In vivo, however, the serum F^- concentration associated with sevoflurane is much less than with methoxyflurane (Cook et al. 1975a; Holaday and Smith 1981; Baden and Rice 1994; Martis et al. 1981). Likely this difference is related to sevoflurane's reduced tissue solubility. Sevoflurane defluorination is increased by prior induction of microsomal enzymes with drugs such as phenobarbital (Cook et al. 1975b; Baden and Rice 1994).

Like desflurane and other commonly used inhalation anesthetics, sevoflurane decreases cerebral vascular resistance and cerebral metabolic rate, increases intracranial pressure in a dose-related manner (Drummond and Shapiro 1994; Manohar 1986; Scheller et al. 1988), and does not cause EEG or gross motor evidence of seizure activity in dogs (Wallin et al. 1975; Scheller et al. 1990).

Except for causing a higher heart rate, sevoflurane's actions on the circulatory and respiratory systems are qualitatively and quantitatively similar to those of isoflurane (Eger 1994). Sevoflurane does not increase the arrhythmogenicity of the heart (Wallin et al. 1975), and the arrhythmogenic dose of epinephrine in dogs anesthetized with sevoflurane is similar to that during isoflurane anesthesia (Hayashi et al. 1988).

Current information suggests that sevoflurane or its degradation products do not produce hepatic or renal injury. However, caution is warranted since the biodegradation of sevoflurane to F^- occurs and degradation by soda lime or Baralyme produces another renal toxic agent, Compound A. The concentration threshold for renal toxicity in rats can be reached in clinical practice (Eger 1993, 1994). Indeed, recognition of possible renal damage from Compound A led to the present package labeling for sevoflurane that warns physicians against its use for human patients at fresh gas flow rates (from the anesthetic delivery apparatus) of less than 2 L/min. Mazze and Jamison (1995) recommend that sevoflurane not be used in patients with impaired renal function.

Sevoflurane enhances the action of neuromuscular blocking drugs and can trigger malignant hyperthermia in susceptible animals (Gronert and Antognini 1994; Schulman et al. 1981).

DIETHYL ETHER. *Ether,* USP (diethyl ether; C_2H_5–O–C_2H_5), is a colorless volatile liquid with a characteristic odor. It has a vapor pressure of about 425 mm Hg (at 20° C) and boils at 35° C. Because of its ease of vaporization and wide margin of safety it can be used with simple vaporizers positioned within the patient breathing circuit.

Its blood/gas PC at 37° C is 12, very near that for methoxyflurane (Eger 1974). Its vapor is highly flammable and forms an explosive mixture with air. This, along with the introduction of halothane and methoxyflurane and the introduction of more electronic tools into the operating room, in large part accounted for its rapid decline from widespread clinical use in North America in the 1960s.

Ether is biodegraded in the body to CO_2 and nonvolatile urinary products. It is presumed that the ether linkage is cleaved by hepatic microsomal enzymes (mixed-function oxidase system), producing two-carbon by-products such as ethanol and acetic acid, which then enter the general metabolic pool and are further oxidized to CO_2 (Van Dyke et al. 1964; Green and Cohen 1971; Cohen 1971). From a metabolic viewpoint, ether is a very safe agent because it degrades into nontoxic products (Green and Cohen 1971). Most of the ether unaltered is eliminated via the expired air.

Ether is an excellent anesthetic and causes dose-related generalized CNS depression. The MAC for ether in dogs is 3.04% (Eger et al. 1965). The MACs for other species are summarized elsewhere (Eger 1974).

Ether at anesthetic concentrations is an irritant to the mucosa of the respiratory tree and as a result increases the amount of respiratory tract secretions. In humans and dogs ventilation is not severely depressed until deep levels of ether anesthesia are produced (Larson et al. 1969; Muallem et al. 1969).

In sympathetically denervated animals, ether depressed myocardial contractility (Brewster et al. 1953; Brown and Crout 1971). In the animal with intact sympathetic nervous system responses, diethyl ether is known to provide universally stable hemodynamic conditions. Cardiac output and heart rate usually increase, and arterial blood pressure remains stable. An increase in sympathetic nervous activity is the mechanism that compensates for the direct depressant action of ether (Jones et al. 1962; Price 1961; Skovsted and Price 1970; Eger et al. 1971).

Emesis is a common complication of low-dose ether and frequently occurs during anesthetic recovery in otherwise unmedicated dogs. Ether also provides profound skeletal muscle relaxation.

THE GASEOUS ANESTHETIC: NITROUS OXIDE. The pharmacology of N_2O and its scope in the clinical practice of anesthesiology (human and animal patients) have been reviewed by Eger, and readers are advised to consult his text as the next step for information beyond the brief summary given here (Eger 1985b).

Nitrous oxide, USP (N_2O), is a colorless, nonirritant, slightly sweet-smelling, nonflammable gas. Nitrous oxide is commercially available as a gas stored in steel cylinders at a pressure of about 50 atmospheres. Since its introduction into clinical practice more than 150 years ago, its use has formed the basis for more general anesthetic techniques of human patients than any other single inhalation agent. Its widespread use resulted from many desirable properties, including low blood solubility (Table 11.4), limited cardiovascular and respiratory system depression, and minimal toxicity (Eger 1985b). Its use in the anesthetic management of animals became a natural extension of its use for humans.

An overview of uptake and distribution (pharmacokinetics) of inhalation anesthetics including brief insight into some relatively unique ways the physical properties of N_2O influence its movement into, within, and from the body was given above and because of space limitations will not be further addressed here. Readers are referred to the works of Eger (Eger 1974, 1985b) for more information on such clinically important subjects as "the second gas effect," "diffusion hypoxia," and movement of N_2O into closed gas spaces.

BIOTRANSFORMATION. Nitrous oxide is metabolized (reductive pathway) by intestinal anaerobic bacteria to molecular nitrogen (N_2) and free radicals (Hong et al. 1980a,b). Unlike other inhalation anesthetics, N_2O is not believed to be directly metabolized by animal tissues.

CENTRAL NERVOUS SYSTEM. Nitrous oxide is not a potent anesthetic (Table 11.7) and under ambient conditions will not anesthetize a fit, healthy individual. Consequently, to get important benefits of N_2O it is necessary to use it in high inspired concentrations but at the same time remembering that as the concentration of N_2O is increased there is a change in the proportion and partial pressure of the various other constituents of the inspired breath, notably O_2. Consequently, to avoid hypoxemia, 75% of the inspired breath is the highest concentration that can be safely administered (at sea level to healthy individuals, less at altitude or in the face of, especially, cardiopulmonary disease). The potency of N_2O in animals important to clinical veterinary medicine is only about one-half the anesthetic potency of that found in humans. Thus, the value of N_2O in veterinary clinical practice is further compromised. When used it serves as an anesthetic adjuvant; that is, it is used in conjunction with an injectable and/or another inhalation anesthetic. Since its depression of other vital organs such as the heart, lungs, kidneys, etc., is small, its purpose in this case is to reduce the amount of the primary, more potent inhaled or injectable anesthetic drug for anesthesia to lessen overall harmful effects on vital organ function.

The effects of N_2O on the EEG are similar to those produced by the volatile anesthetics. At low subanesthetic levels (about 30%, inspired), N_2O increases EEG frequency and lowers voltage, and at higher subanesthetic concentrations (e.g., 60%), N_2O increases voltage. Adding N_2O to a light level of anesthesia produced by other drugs tends to increase voltage and decrease frequency (Frost 1985).

At subanesthetic doses N_2O causes an increase in cerebral blood flow and intracranial pressure. The magnitude of change seems to depend upon whether it is administered alone or in conjunction with other anesthetics. Dramatic increases in intracranial pressure occur in animals when N_2O is used alone (Theye and Michenfelder 1968; Pelligrino et al. 1984; Drummond and Shapiro 1994).

CARDIOVASCULAR AND RESPIRATORY SYSTEMS. Under ambient conditions the effects of N_2O on the cardiovascular and respiratory function (other than reducing the inspired O_2 concentration) are small compared to those of the other inhalation anesthetics. Nitrous oxide is a direct myocardial depressant. However, it also causes sympathetic nervous system stimulation and the release of catecholamines. The sympathetic stimulation, coupled with the mild, direct depressant properties of N_2O, results in comparatively little cardiovascular depression (Eisele 1985; Steffey et al. 1974a,b, 1975; Steffey and Howland 1978c; Dolan et al. 1974; Pavlin and Su 1994; Eger 1985b). This end result is one of the distinguishing factors of N_2O relative to the other inhalation anesthetics.

In some circumstances N_2O may contribute to an increased incidence of cardiac arrhythmias (Liu et al. 1982; Lampe et al. 1990a). There is some evidence to suggest that its use contributes to an increased incidence of myocardial ischemia in some circumstances (Philbin et al. 1985; Leone et al. 1988; Nathan 1988; Diedericks et al. 1993).

LIVER AND KIDNEY. Nitrous oxide has little or no effect on liver or kidney function in patients exposed under most clinical circumstances (Brodsky 1985; Lampe et al. 1990b,c). Nitrous oxide interferes with several vitamin B_{12} dependent reactions. The result is an irreversible inactivation of the enzyme methionine synthase that in turn results in a reduced amount of thymidine, an essential DNA base. The subsequent interference with DNA synthesis prevents production of both leukocytes and red blood cells by bone marrow. Similarly, exposure to N_2O can produce a polyneuropathy ("nitrous oxide neuropathy") that is indistinguishable from that associated with pernicious anemia, that is, subacute degeneration of the spinal cord (Baden and Rice 1994; Brodsky 1985). The bone marrow changes would be expected to be seen only in the sickest of patients and after about 10 hours or more of N_2O anesthesia (O'Sullivan et al. 1981). The neurologic disease is most commonly associated with rare, long-term exposure in a grossly contaminated work environment or with chronic abuse of N_2O (a potential consideration in the management of the veterinary practice) (Layzer et al. 1978; Layzer 1978; Baden and Rice 1994; Brodsky 1985). Both forms are described in humans and animals.

SKELETAL MUSCLE. Nitrous oxide is at best only a weak trigger to the development of malignant hyperthermia in susceptible subjects (Gronert and Antognini 1994).

TRACE CONCENTRATIONS OF INHALATION ANESTHETICS: OCCUPATIONAL EXPOSURE.

In 1968, Bruce and coworkers (Bruce et al. 1968) published a retrospective study of the causes of death among anesthesiologists over a 20-year period. Their work revealed a trend toward higher than normal incidences of death from reticuloendothelial and lymphoid malignancies. The possibility that chronic exposure to low levels of waste inhalation anesthetic agents constitutes a health hazard to medical personnel attracted worldwide interest among health workers (Cohen et al. 1971, 1975; Linde and Bruce 1969; Whitcher et al. 1971; Millard and Corbett 1974; Manley and McDonell 1980b; Milligan et al. 1980; Dreesen et al. 1981; Manley et al. 1982). Of particular concern are reports that inhalation anesthetics are potential mutagens, carcinogens, and/or teratogens and that fetal death, spontaneous abortion, birth defects, or cancer in exposed workers might result (Ad Hoc Committee on the Effect of Trace Anesthetics on the Health of Operating Room Personnel 1974; Cohen et al. 1971). To date, "the overwhelming conclusion from both animal and human studies is that there is no carcinogenic risk either from working in the operating or dental suite or from exposure to anesthetics" (Baden and Rice 1994). "[T]he overwhelming evidence from in vitro tests indicates that all currently used and most previously used anesthetics are not mutagens . . . [however,] two recent (1990 and 1992) studies have shown cytogenic damage in operating room personnel exposed to waste anesthetic gases (Natarajan and Santhiya 1990; Sardas et al. 1992)" (Baden and Rice 1994). Data to date regarding human reproduction effect remain equivocal; a firm cause-and-effect relationship between chronic exposure to trace levels of anesthetics and human health problems does not exist. Nevertheless, interest in this topic remains high and is fueled by, for example, a study in which reduced fertility was reported among dental assistants exposed to high levels of nitrous oxide

(Rowland et al. 1992). For more in-depth review of potential hazards to health care providers, readers are referred to Baden and Rice's (1994) updated chapter in Miller's *Anesthesia* (pp. 172–179).

The risk of long-term exposure to trace concentrations of inhalation anesthetics for those in operating-room conditions seems minimal. However, "even if anesthetics have low potential for causing long-term toxicity, exposure of a large population may represent a considerable public health hazard . . . surgeons, dental personnel, and *veterinarians and their technical assistants* have a variable but sometimes heavy exposure to [inhalation] anesthetics. The total number of occupationally exposed or potentially exposed persons in the United States each year is about 225,000 (National Institute for Occupational Safety and Health (NIOSH) 1977)" (Baden and Rice 1994, emphasis added). Accordingly, current knowledge is suggestive enough to cause concern and to encourage practices to reduce the contamination by inhalation anesthetics of operating-room personnel. More information on this subject is available in anesthesiology texts such as Miller's *Anesthesia* and elsewhere (Lecky 1977, 1980; Ad Hoc Committee on Effects of Trace Anesthetic Agents on Health of Operating Room Personnel 1983; Manley and McDonell 1980a; Dorsch and Dorsch 1984).

REFERENCES

Ad Hoc Committee on Effects of Trace Anesthetic Agents on Health of Operating Room Personnel. 1983. Waste Anesthetic Gases in Operating Room Air: A Suggested Program to Reduce Personnel Exposure. Park Ridge, Illinois: American Society of Anesthesiologists.

Ad Hoc Committee on the Effect of Trace Anesthetics on the Health of Operating Room Personnel. 1974. Occupational disease among operating room personnel: a national study. Anesthesiology 41:321–40.

Andrews, J. J. 1990. Inhaled anesthetic delivery systems. In R. D. Miller, ed., Anesthesia, 3rd ed., pp. 171–223. New York: Churchill Livingstone.

Andrews, J. J., and Johnston, R. V., Jr. 1993. The new tec 6 desflurane vaporizer. Anesth Analg 76:1338–41.

Baden, J. M., and Rice, S. A. 1994. Metabolism and toxicity. In R. D. Miller, ed., Anesthesia, 4th ed., pp. 157–83. New York: Churchill Livingstone.

Bagwell, E. E., and Woods, E. F. 1962. Cardiovascular effects of methoxyflurane. Anesthesiology 23:51–57.

Bahlman, S. H., Eger, E. I., II, Halsey, M. J., Stevens, W. C., Shakespeare, T. F., Smith, N. T., Cromwell, T. H., and Fourcade, H. 1972. The cardiovascular effects of halothane in man during spontaneous ventilation. Anesthesiology 36:494–502.

Barr, G. A., Cousins, M. J., Mazze, R. I., Hitt, B. A., and Kosek, J. C. 1974. A comparison of the renal effects and metabolism of enflurane and methoxyflurane in Fischer 344 rats. J Pharmacol Exp Ther 190:257–64.

Bassell, G. M., Cullen, B. F., Fairchild, M. D., and Kusske, J. A. 1982. Electroencephalographic and behavioral effects of enflurane and halothane anaesthesia in cats. Br J Anaesth 54:659–65.

Bednarski, R. M., and Majors, L. J. 1986. Ketamine and arrhythmogenic dose of epinephrine in cats anesthetized with halothane and isoflurane. Am J Vet Res 47:2122–26.

Bednarski, R. M., Majors, L. J., and Atlee, J. L. 1985. Epinephrine-induced ventricular arrhythmias in dogs anesthetized with halothane: potentiation by thiamylal and thiopental. Am J Vet Res 46:1829–32.

Bergman, N. A. 1976. New tests of pulmonary function. Anesthesiology 44:220.

Berl, T. 1990. Treating hyponatremia: what is all the controversy about? Ann Intern Med 113:417–19.

Bernard, J. M., Doursout, M. F., Wouters, P., Hartley, C. J., Cohen, M., Merin, R. G., and Chelly, J. E. 1991. Effects of enflurane and isoflurane on hepatic and renal circulations in chronically instrumented dogs. Anesthesiology 74:298–302.

Biermann, J. S., Rice, S. A., Gallagher, E. J., and West, J. A. 1986. Effect of diazepam treatment on hepatic microsomal anesthetic defluorinase activity. Arch Int Pharmacodyn Ther 283:181–93.

Boban, M., Stowe, D. F., Buljubasic, N., Bampine, J. P., and Bosnjak, Z. J. 1992. Direct comparative effects of isoflurane and desflurane in isolated guinea pig hearts. Anesthesiology 76:775–80.

Booth, N. H., and McDonald, L. E. 1988. Veterinary Pharmacology and Therapeutics, 6th ed., Ames: Iowa State Univ Press.

Brewster, W. R., Jr., Isaacs, J. P., and Waino-Andersen, T. 1953. Depressant effect of ether on myocardium of the dog and its modification by reflex release of epinephrine and nor-epinephrine. Am J Physiol 175:399–414.

Brodsky, J. B. 1985. Toxicity of nitrous oxide. In E. I. Eger, II, ed., Nitrous Oxide/N_2O, pp. 259–79. New York: Elsevier.

Brown, B. R., and Crout, J. R. 1971. A comparative study of the effects of five general anesthetics on myocontractility: I. Isometric conditions. Anesthesiology 34:236–45.

Brown, B. R., Jr., and Sipes, I. G. 1977. Biotransformation and hepatotoxicity of halothane. Biochem Pharmacol 26:2091–94.

Bruce, D. L., Eide, K. A., Linde, H. W., and Eckenhoff, J. E. 1968. Causes of death among anesthesiologists: a 20-year survey. Anesthesiology 29:565–69.

Butterworth, J. F., and Strichartz, G. R. 1990. Molecular mechanisms of local anesthesia: a review. Anesthesiology 72:711–34.

Cahalan, M. K., Johnson, B. H., and Eger, E. I., II. 1981. Relationship of concentrations of halothane and enflurane to their metabolism and elimination in man. Anesthesiology 54:3–8.

Caldwell, J. E., Laster, M. J., Magorian, T., Heier, T., Yasuda, N., Lynam, D. P., Eger, E. I., II, and Weiskopf, R. B. 1991. The neuromuscular effects of desflurane, alone and combined with pancuronium or succinylcholine in humans. Anesthesiology 74:412–18.

Calverley, R. K., Smith, N. T., Jones, C. W., Prys-Roberts, C., and Eger, E. I., II. 1978a. Ventilatory and cardiovascular effects of enflurane anesthesia during spontaneous ventilation in man. Anesth Analg 51:610–18.

Calverley, R. K., Smith, N. T., Prys-Roberts, C., Eger, E. I., II, and Jones, C. W. 1978b. Cardiovascular effects of enflurane anesthesia during controlled ventilation in man. Anesth Analg 57:619–28.

Caropreso, P. R., Gittleman, M. A., Reilly, D. J., and Patterson, L. T. 1975. Malignant hyperthermia associated with enflurane anesthesia. Arch Surg 110:1491–93.

Carpenter, R. L., Eger, E. I., II, Johnson, B. H., Unadkat, J. D., and Sheiner, L. B. 1986a. Pharmacokinetics of inhaled anesthetics in humans: measurements during and after the simultaneous administration of enflurane, halothane, isoflurane, methoxyflurane, and nitrous oxide. Anesth Analg 65:575–83.

———. 1986b. The extent of metabolism of inhaled anesthetics in humans. Anesthesiology 65:201–6.

———. 1987. Does the duration of anesthetic administration affect the pharmacokinetics or metabolism of inhaled anesthetics in humans? Anesth Analg 66:1–8.

Cascorbi, H. F., Blake, D. A., and Helrich, M. 1970. Differences in the biotransformation of halothane in man. Anesthesiology 32:119–23.

Chase, R. E., Holaday, D. A., Fiserova-Bergerova, V., Saidman, L. J., and Mack, F. E. 1971. The biotransformation of ethrane in man. Anesthesiology 35:262–67.

Clark, D. L., and Rosner, B. D. 1973. Neurophysiologic effects of general anesthetics. 1. The electroencephalogram and sensory evoked responses in man. Anesthesiology 38:564–82.

Cohen, E. N. 1971. Metabolism of the volatile anesthetics. Anesthesiology 35:193–202.

Cohen, E. N., Bellville, J. W., and Brown, B. W. 1971. Anesthesia, pregnancy, and miscarriage: a study of operating room nurses and anesthetists. Anesthesiology 35:343–47.

Cohen, E. N., Brown, B. W., Jr., Bruce, D. L., Cascorbi, H. F., Corbett, T. H., Jones, T. W., and Whitcher, C. E. 1975. A survey of anesthetic health hazards among dentists. J Amer Dental Assoc 90:1291–96.

Colgan, F. J. 1965. Performance of lungs and bronchi during inhalation anesthesia. Anesthesiology 26:778

Cook, T. L., Beppu, W. J., Hitt, B. A., Kosek, J. C., and Mazze, R. I. 1975a. Renal effects and metabolism of sevoflurane in Fischer 344 rats: an in-vivo and in-vitro comparison with methoxyflurane. Anesthesiology 43:70–77.

———. 1975b. Comparison of renal effects and metabolism of sevoflurane and methoxyflurane in enzyme-induced rats. Anesth Analg 54:829–35.

Coon, R. L., and Kampine, J. P. 1975. Hypocapnic bronchoconstriction and inhalation anesthetics. Anesthesiology 43:635–41.

Corbally, M. T., and Brennan, M. F. 1990. Noninvasive measurement of regional blood flow in man. Am J Surg 160:313–21.

Cousins, M. J., Mazze, R. I., Barr, G. A., and Kosek, J. C. 1973. A comparison of the renal effects of isoflurane and methoxyflurane in Fischer 344 rats. Anesthesiology 38:557–63.

Cousins, M. J., Greenstein, L. R., Hitt, B. A., and Mazze, R. I. 1976. Metabolism and renal effects of enflurane in man. Anesthesiology 44:44–53.

Crandell, W. B., Pappas, S. G., and Macdonald, A. 1966. Nephrotoxicity associated with methoxyflurane anesthesia. Anesthesiology 27:591–607.

Cromwell, T. H., Stevens, W. C., Eger, E. I., II, Shakespear, T. F., Halsey, M. J., Bahlman, S. H., and Fourcade, H. E. 1971. The cardiovascular effects of compound 469 (Forane) during spontaneous ventilation and CO2 challenge in man. Anesthesiology 35:17–25.

Cullen, B. F., and Eger, E. I., II. 1972. Diffusion of nitrous oxide, cyclopropane, and halothane through human skin and amniotic membrane. Anesthesiology 36:168–73.

Daunt, D. A., Steffey, E. P., Pascoe, J. R., Willits, N., and Daels, P. F. 1992. Actions of isoflurane and halothane in pregnant mares. J Am Vet Med Assoc 201:1367–74.

deGroot, H., Harnisch, U., and Noll, T. 1982. Suicidal activation of microsomal cytochrome P-450 by halothane under hypoxic conditions. Biochem Biophys Res Commun 107:885

De Jong, R. H., and Eger, E. I., II. 1975. MAC expanded: AD_{50} and AD_{95} values of common inhalation anesthetics in man. Anesthesiology 42:408–19.

Diedericks, J., Leone, B. J., Foex, P., Sear, J. W., and Ryder, W. A. 1993. Nitrous oxide causes myocardial ischemia when added to propofol in the compromised canine myocardium. Anesth Analg 76:1322–26.

Dobkin, A. B., and Fedoruk, S. 1961. Comparison of cardiovascular, respiratory and metabolic effects of methoxyflurane and halothane in dogs. Anesthesiology 22:355–62.

Dobkin, A. B., Kim, D., Choi, J. K., and Levy, A. A. 1973. Blood serum fluoride levels with enflurane (Ethrane) and isoflurane (Forane) anaesthesia during and following major abdominal surgery. Can Anaesth Soc J 20:494–98.

Doi, M., and Ikeda, K. 1987. Respiratory effects of sevoflurane. Anesth Analg 66:241–44.

Dolan, W. M., Stevens, W. C., Eger, E. I., II, Cromwell, T. H., Halsey, M. J., Shakespeare, T. F., and Miller, R. D. 1974. The cardiovascular and respiratory effects of isoflurane-nitrous oxide anaesthesia. Can Anaesth Soc J 21:557–68.

Dorsch, J. A., and Dorsch, S. E. 1984. Understanding Anesthesia Equipment: Construction, Care and Complications, 2nd ed. Baltimore: Williams & Wilkins.

Dreesen, D. W., Jones, G. L., Brown, J., and Rawlings, C. A. 1981. Monitoring for trace anesthetic gases in a veterinary teaching hospital. J Am Vet Med Assoc 179:797–99.

Drummond, J. C., and Shapiro, H. M. 1994. Cerebral physiology. In R. D. Miller, ed., Anesthesia, 4th ed., pp. 689–729. New York: Churchill Livingstone.

Drummond, J. C., Todd, M. M., Scheller, M. S., and Shapiro, H. M. 1986. A comparison of the direct cerebral vasodilating potencies of halothane and isoflurane in the New Zealand white rabbit. Anesthesiology 65(5):462–68.

Duncalf, D. 1982. Flammable anesthetics are nearing extinction. Anesthesiology 56:217–18.

Dunlop, C. I., Steffey, E. P., Miller, M. F., and Woliner, M. J. 1987. Temporal effects of halothane and isoflurane in laterally recumbent ventilated male horses. Am J Vet Res 48:1250–55.

Eger, E. I., II. 1974. Anesthetic Uptake and Action. Baltimore: Williams & Wilkins.

———. 1982. Isoflurane (Forane): A Compendium and Reference. Madison: Ohio Medical Products.

———. 1985a. Isoflurane: A Compendium and Reference, 2nd ed. Madison: Anaquest.

———. 1985b. Nitrous Oxide/N_2O. New York: Elsevier.

———. 1987. Partition coefficients of I-653 in human blood, saline, and olive oil. Anesth Analg 66:971–74.

———. 1990. Uptake and distribution. In R. D. Miller, ed., Anesthesia, 3rd ed., pp. 85–104. New York: Churchill Livingstone.

———. 1992. Desflurane animal and human pharmacology: aspects of kinetics, safety, and MAC. Anesth Analg 75:S3–S9.

———. 1993. Desflurane (Suprane): A Compendium and Reference. Rutherford: Healthpress Publishing Group.

———. 1994. New inhaled anesthetics. Anesthesiology 80:906–22.

Eger, E. I., II, and Johnson, B. H. 1987. Rates of awakening from anesthesia with I-653, halothane, isoflurane, and sevoflurane: A test of the effect of anesthetic concentration and duration in rats. Anesth Analg 66:977–982.

Eger, E. I., II, and Severinghaus, J. W. 1964. Effect of uneven pulmonary distribution of blood and gas on induction with inhalation anesthetics. Anesthesiology 25:620–26.

Eger, E. I., II, Brandstater, B., Saidman, L. J., Regan, M. J., Severinghaus, J. W., and Munson, E. S. 1965. Equipotent alveolar concentrations of methoxyflurane, halothane, diethyl ether, fluroxene, cyclopropane, xenon, and nitrous oxide in the dog. Anesthesiology 26:771–77.

Eger, E. I., II, Smith, N. T., Stoelting, R. K., Cullen, D. J., Kadis, L. B., and Whitcher, C. E. 1970. Cardiovascular effects of halothane in man. Anesthesiology 32:396–409.

Eger, E. I., II, Smith, N. T., Cullen, D. J., Cullen, B. F., and Gregory, G. A. 1971. A comparison of the cardiovascular effects of halothane, fluroxene, ether and cyclopropane in man: a resume. Anesthesiology 34:25–41.

Eger, E. I., II, White, A. E., Brown, C. L., Biava, C. G., Corbett, T. H., and Stevens, W. C. 1978. A test of the carcinogenicity of enflurane, isoflurane, halothane, methoxyflurane and nitrous oxide in mice. Anesth Analg 57:678–94.

Eger, E. I., II, Smuckler, E. A., Ferrell, L. D., Goldsmith, C. H., and Johnson, B. H. 1986. Is enflurane hepatoxic? Anesth Analg 65:21–31.

Eger, E. I., II, Johnson, B. H., Strum, D. P., and Ferrell, L. D. 1987. Studies of the toxicity of I-653, halothane, and isoflurane in enzyme-induced, hypoxic rats. Anesth Analg 66:1227–30.

Eger, R. R., and Eger, E. I., II. 1985. Effect of temperature and age on the solubility of enflurane, halothane, isoflurane, and methoxyflurane in human blood. Anesth Analg 64:640–42.

Eisele, J. H., Jr. 1985. Cardiovascular effects of nitrous oxide. In E. I. Eger II, ed., Nitrous Oxide/N_2O, pp. 125–56. New York: Elsevier.

Engelking, L. R., Dodman, N. H., Hartman, G., Valdez, H., and Spivak, W. 1984. Effects of halothane anesthesia on equine liver function. Am J Vet Res 45:607–15.

Englesson, S. 1974. The influence of acid-base changes on central nervous system toxicity of local anesthetic agents. I. An experimental study in cats. Acta Anaesth Scand 18:79.

Fassoulaki, A., Lockhart, S. H., Freire, B. A., Yasuda, N., Eger, E. I., II, Weiskopf, R. B., and Johnson, B. H. 1991. Percutaneous loss of desflurane, isoflurane, and halothane in humans. Anesthesiology 74:479–83.

Fleming, J. T., and Pedersoli, W. M. 1980. Serum inorganic fluoride and renal function in dogs after methoxyflurne anesthesia, tetracycline treatment, and surgical manipulation. Am J Vet Res 41:2025–29.

Fogdall, R. P., and Miller, R. D. 1975. Neuromuscular effects of enflurane, alone and combined with *d*-tubocurarine, pancuronium, and succinylcholine, in man. Anesthesiology 42:173–78.

Fourcade, H. E., Stevens, W. C., Larson, C. P. J., Cromwell, T. H., Bahlman, S. H., Hickey, R. F., Halsey, M. J., and Eger, E. I., II. 1971. The ventilatory effects of Forane, a new inhaled anesthetic. Anesthesiology 35:26–31.

Frink, E. J., Jr., Malan, T. P., Atlas, M., Dominquez, L. M., DiNardo, J. A., and Brown, B. R., Jr. 1992. Clinical comparison of sevoflurane and isoflurane in healthy patients. Anesth Analg 74:241-245.

Frink, E. J., Jr., Malan, T., Morgan, S., Brown, E., Malcomson, M., and Brown, B. R., Jr. 1992a. Quantification of the degradation products of sevoflurane in two CO_2 absorbents during low-flow anesthesia in surgical patients. Anesthesiology 77:1064–69.

Frink, E. J., Jr., Morgan, S. E., Coetzee, A., Conzen, P., and Brown, B. R., Jr. 1992b. The effects of sevoflurane, halothane, enflurane, and isoflurane on hepatic blood flow and oxygenation in chronically instrumented greyhound dogs. Anesthesiology 76:85–90.

Frost, E. A. M. 1985. Central nervous system effects of nitrous oxide. In E. I. Eger II, ed., Nitrous Oxide/N_2O, pp. 157–76. New York: Elsevier.

Gelman, S. 1987. General anesthesia and hepatic circulation. Can J Physiol Pharmacol 65:1762–79.

Gelman, S., Fowler, K. C., and Smith, L. R. 1984a. Liver circulation and function during isoflurane and halothane anesthesia. Anesthesiology 61:726–31.

———. 1984b. Regional blood flow during isoflurane and halothane anesthesia. Anesth Analg 63(6):557–66.

Giesecke, A. H., Jr., Beck, G. P., Jenkins, M. T., Kallus, F. T., and Tembridge, V. A. 1966. Hepatic effects of methoxyflurane in nutritionally deprived dogs. Anesth Analg 45:829–34.

Gopinath, C., and Ford, E. J. 1976. The influence of hepatic microsomal amidopyrine demethylase activity on halothane hepatotoxicity in the horse. J Pathol 119:105–12.

Gopinath, C., Jones, R. S., and Ford, E. J. H. 1970. The effect of repeated administration of halothane on the liver of the horse. J Pathol 102:107–14.

Grandy, J. L., Hodgson, D. S., Dunlop, C. I., Curtis, C. R., and Heath, R. B. 1989. Cardiopulmonary effects of halothane anesthesia in cats. Am J Vet Res 50:1729–32.

Green, K., and Cohen, E. N. 1971. On the metabolism of [^{14}C]-diethyl ether in the mouse. Biochem Pharmacol 20:393–99.

Gronert, G. A., and Antognini, J. F. 1994. Malignant hyperthermia. In R. D. Miller, ed., Anesthesia, 4th ed., pp. 1075–93. New York: Churchill Livingstone.

Hall, L.W. 1971. Wright's Veterinary Anaesthesia and Analgesia, 7th ed. London: Bailliere Tindall.

Harper, M. H., Collins, P., Johnson, B., Eger, E. I., II, and Biava, C. 1982a. Hepatic injury following halothane enflurane and isoflurane anesthesia in rats. Anesthesiology 56:14–17.

———. 1982b. Postanesthetic hepatic injury in rats: influence of alterations in hepatic blood flow, surgery and anesthesia time. Anesth Analg 61:79–82.

Haskins, S., and Sansome, A. L. 1979. A time-table for exhaustion of nitrous oxide cylinders using cylinder pressure. Vet Anesth 6:6–8.

Haskins, S. C., and Klide, A. M., eds. 1992. Opinions in small animal anesthesia. Vet Clin North Am Small Anim Pract 22:381–411.

Hayashi, Y., Sumikawa, K., Tashiro, C., Yamatodani, A., and Yoshiya, I. 1988. Arrhythmogenic threshold of epinephrine during sevoflurane, enflurane, and isoflurane anesthesia in dogs. Anesthesiology 69(1):145–47.

Hill, D. W. 1980. Physics Applied to Anaesthesia, 4th ed. London: Butterworth & Co.

Hirshman, C. A., and Bergman, N. A. 1978. Halothane and enflurane protect against bronchospasm in an asthma dog model. Anesth Analg 57:629–33.

Hirshman, C. A., Edelstein, H., Peetz, S., Wayne, R., and Kownes, H. 1982. Mechanism of action of inhalational anesthesia on airways. Anesthesiology 56:107–11.

Hodgson, D. S., Steffey, E. P., Woliner, M., and Grandy, J. 1985a. Ventilatory effects of isoflurane anesthesia in horses. Vet Surg 14:74(Abstr).

Hodgson, D. S., Steffey, E. P., Woliner, M. J., and Miller, M. F. 1985b. Alteration in breathing patterns of horses during halothane and isoflurane anesthetic induction. In J. Grandy, S. Hildebrand, W. McDonell, et al. Proceedings of the Second International Congress of Veterinary Anesthesia, pp. 195–96. Santa Barbara: Veterinary Practice Publishing Co.

Holaday, D. A., and Smith, F. R. 1981. Clinical characteristics and biotransformation of sevoflurane in healthy human volunteers. Anesthesiology 54:100–106.

Holaday, D. A., Rudofsky, S., and Treuhaft, P. S. 1970. Metabolic degradation of methoxyflurane in man. Anesthesiology 33:579–93.

Holaday, D. A., Fiserova-Bergerova, V., Latto, I. P., and Zumbiel, M. A. 1975. Resistance of isoflurane to biotransformation in man. Anesthesiology 43:325–32.

Holmes, M. A., Weiskopf, R. B., Eger, E. I., II, Johnson, B. H., and Rampil, I. J. 1990. Hepatocellular integrity in swine after prolonged desflurane (I-653) and isoflurane anesthesia: evaluation of plasma alanine aminotransferase activity. Anesth Analg 71:249–53.

Hong, K., Trudell, J. R., O'Neil, J. R., and Cohen, E. N. 1980a. Metabolism of nitrous oxide by human and rat intestinal contents. Anesthesiology 52:16–19.

———. 1980b. Biotransformation of nitrous oxide. Anesthesiology 53:354–55.

Horrigan, R. W., Eger, E. I., II, and Wilson, C. 1978. Epinephrine-induced arrhythmia during enflurane anesthesia in man: a nonlinear dose-response relationship and dose-dependent protection from lidocaine. Anesth Analg 57:547–50.

Hubbard, A. K., Gandolfi, A. J., and Brown, B. R., Jr. 1988. Immunological basis of anesthetic-induced hepatotoxicity. Anesthesiology 69:814–17.

Ingwersen, W., Allen, D. G., Dyson, D. H., Pascoe, P. J., and O'Grady, M. R. 1988. Cardiopulmonary effects of a halothane/oxygen combination in healthy cats. Can J Vet Res 52:386–92.

Iwatsuki, N., Shimosato, S., and Etsten, B. E. 1970. The effects of changes in time interval of stimulation on mechanics of isolated heart muscle and its response to Ethrane. Anesthesiology 32:11–16.

Joas, T. A., and Stevens, W. C. 1971. Comparison of the arrhythmic doses of epinephrine during Forane, halothane, and fluroxene anesthesia in dogs. Anesthesiology 35:48–53.

Joas, T. A., Stevens, W. C., and Eger, E. I., II. 1971. Electroencephalographic seizure activity in dogs during anaesthesia: studies with Ethrane, fluroxene, halothane, chloroform, divinyl ether, diethyl ether, methoxyflurane, cyclopropane and Forane. Br J Anaesth 43:739–45.

Johnston, R. R., Eger, E. I., II, and Wilson, C. 1976. A comparative interaction of epinephrine with enflurane, isoflurane and halothane in man. Anesth Analg 55:709–12.

Jones, R. E., Linde, H. W., Deutsch, S., Dripps, R. D., and Price, H. L. 1962. Hemodynamic actions of diethyl ether in normal man. Anesthesiology 23:299–305.

Jones, R. M. 1990. Desflurane and sevoflurane: inhalation anaesthetics for this decade? Br J Anaesth 65:527–36.

Jones, R. M., Koblin, D. D., Cashman, J. N., Eger, E. I., II, Johnson, B. H., and Damask, M. C. 1990. Biotransformation and hepato-renal function in volunteers after exposure to desflurane (I-653). Br J Anaesth 64:482–87.

Joyce, J. T., Roizen, M. F., and Eger, E. I., II. 1983. Effect of thiopental induction on sympathetic activity. Anesthesiology 59:19–22.

Julien, R. M., and Kavan, E. M. 1972. Electrographic studies of a new volatile anesthetic agent: enflurane (Ethrane). J Pharmacol Exp Ther 183:393–403.

———. 1974. Electrographic studies of isoflurane (Forane). Neuropharmacol 13:677–681.

Katz, R. L., and Epstein, R. A. 1968. The interaction of anesthetic agents and adrenergic drugs to produce cardiac arrhythmias. Anesthesiology 29:763–84.

Kavan, E. M., and Julien, R. M. 1974. Central nervous systems' effects of isoflurane (Forane). Can Anaesth Soc J 21:390–402.

Klide, A. M. 1976. Cardiovascular effects of enflurane and isoflurane in the dog. Am J Vet Res 37:127–31.

Klide, A. M., and Aviado, D. M. 1967. Mechanism for the reduction in pulmonary resistance induced by halothane. J Pharmacol Exp Ther 158:28–35.

Knill, R. L., and Gelb, A. W. 1978. Ventilatory responses to hypoxia and hypercapnia during halothane sedation and anesthesia in man. Anesthesiology 49:244–51.

Koblin, D. D. 1992. Characteristics and implications of desflurane metabolism and toxicity. Anesth Analg 75:S10–S16.

Koblin, D. D., Eger, E. I., II, Johnson, B. H., Collins, P., Terrell, R. C., and Speers, L. 1981. Are convulsant gases also anesthetics? Anesth Analg 60:464–70.

Koblin, D. D., Eger, E. I., II, Johnson, B. H., Konopka, K., and Waskell, L. 1988. I-653 resists degradation in rats. Anesth Analg 67:534–39.

Lampe, G. H., Donegan, J. H., Rupp, S. M., Wauk, L. Z., Whitendale, P., Fouts, K.E., Rose, B.M., Litt, L.L., Rampil, I. J., Wilson, C. B., and Eger, E. I., II. 1990a. Nitrous oxide and epinephrine-induced arrhythmias. Anesth Analg 71:602–5.

Lampe, G. H., Wauk, L. Z., Donegan, J. H., Pitts, L. H., Jackler, R. K., Litt, L. L., Rampil, I. J., and Eger, E. I., II. 1990b. Effect on outcome of prolonged exposure of patients to nitrous oxide. Anesth Analg 71:586–90.

Lampe, G. H., Wauk, L. Z., Whitendale, P., Way, W. L., Murray, W., and Eger, E. I., II. 1990c. Nitrous oxide does not impair hepatic function in young or old surgical patients. Anesth Analg 71:606–9.

Larson, C. P., Jr., Eger, E. I., II, Muallem, M., Buechel, D. R., Munson, E. S., and Eisele, J. H. 1969. The effects of diethyl ether and methoxyflurane on ventilation: II. A comparative study in man. Anesthesiology 30:174–84.

Laster, M. J., Fang, Z., and Eger, E. I., II. 1994. Specific gravities of desflurane, enflurane, halothane, isoflurane, and sevoflurane. Anesth Analg 78:1152–53.

Layzer, R. B. 1978. Myeloneuropathy after prolonged exposure to nitrous oxide. Lancet 2:1227–30.

Layzer, R. B., Fishman, R. A., and Schafer, J. A. 1978. Neuropathy following abuse of nitrous oxide. Neurology 28:504–6.

Lebowitz, M. H., Blitt, C. D., and Walts, L. F. 1970. Depression of twitch response to stimulation of the ulnar nerve during Ethrane anesthesia in man. Anesthesiology 33:52–57.

Lecky, J. H. 1977. The mechanical aspects of anesthetic pollution control. Anesth Analg 56:769–74.

———. 1980. Anesthetic pollution in the operating room: a notice to operating room personnel. Anesthesiology 52:157–59.

Leone, B. J., Philbin, D. M., Lehot, J. J., Foex, P., and Ryder, W. A. 1988. Gradual or abrupt nitrous oxide administration in a canine model of critical coronary stenosis induces regional myocardial dysfunction that is worsened by halothane. Anesth Analg 67:814–22.

Lerman, J., Schmitt-Bantel, B. I., Gregory, G. A., Willis, M. M., and Eger, E. I., II. 1986. Effect of age on the solubility of volatile anesthetics in human tissues. Anesthesiology 65(3):307–12.

Lewis, J. H., Zimmerman, H. J., Ishak, K. G., and Mullick, F. G. 1983. Enflurane hepatotoxicity: a clinicopathologic study of 24 cases. Ann Intern Med 98:984–92.

Linde, H. W., and Berman, M. L. 1971. Nonspecific stimulation of drug-metabolizing enzymes by inhalation anesthetic agents. Anesth Analg 50:656–67.

Linde, H. W., and Bruce, D. L. 1969. Occupational exposure of anesthetists to halothane, nitrous oxide and radiation. Anesthesiology 30:363–68.

Liu, J., Laster, M. J., Eger, E. I., II, and Taheri, S. 1991. Absorption and degradation of sevoflurane and isoflurane in a conventional anesthetic circuit. Anesth Analg 72:785–89.

Liu, W. S., Wong, K. C., Port, J. D., and Aridriano, K. P. 1982. Epinephrine-induced arrhythmia during halothane anesthesia with the addition of nitrous oxide, nitrogen or helium in dogs. Anesth Analg 61:414–17.

Lockhart, S. H., Rampil, I. J., Yasuda, N., Eger, E. I., II, and Weiskopf, R. B. 1991a. Depression of ventilation by desflurane in humans. Anesthesiology 74:484–88.

Lockhart, S. L., Yasuda, N., Peterson, N., Laster, M. J., Taheri, S., Weiskopf, R. B., and Eger, E. I., II. 1991b. Comparison of percutaneous losses of sevoflurane and isoflurane in humans. Anesth Analg 72:212–15.

Lowe, H. J., and Ernst, E. A. 1981. The Quantitative Practice of Anesthesia: Use of Closed Circuit. Baltimore: Williams & Wilkins.

Ludders, J. W., Rode, J., and Mitchell, G. S. 1989. Isoflurane anesthesia in sandhill cranes (*Grus canadensis*): minimal anesthetic concentration and cardiopulmonary dose-response during spontaneous and controlled breathing. Anesth Analg 68:511–16.

Lumb, W. V., and Jones, E. W. 1973. Veterinary Anesthesia. Philadelphia: Lea & Febiger.

Lutz, L. J., Milde, J. H., and Milde, L. N. 1990. The cerebral functional, metabolic, and hemodynamic effects of desflurane in dogs. Anesthesiology 73:125–31.

———. 1991. The response of the canine cerebral circulation to hyperventilation during anesthesia with desflurane. Anesthesiology 74:504–7.

Manley, S. V., and McDonell, W. F. 1980a. Recommendations for reduction of anesthetic gas pollution. J Am Vet Med Assoc 176:519–24.

———. 1980b. Anesthetic pollution and disease. J Am Vet Med Assoc 176:515–18.

Manley, S. V., Taloff, P., Aberg, N., and Howitt, G. A. 1982. Occupational exposure to waste anesthetic gases in veterinary practice. California Vet 36:14–19.

Manohar, M. 1986. Regional brain blood flow and cerebral cortical O2 consumption during sevoflurane anesthesia in healthy isocapnic swine. J Cardiovasc Pharmacol 8(6):1268–76.

Mapleson, W. W. 1989. Pharmacokinetics of inhalational anaesthetics. In J. F. Nunn, J. E. Utting, and B. R. Brown Jr., eds., General Anaesthesia, 5th ed., pp. 44–59. London: Butterworths.

Mapleson, W. W., Allott, P. R., and Steward, A. 1972. The variability of partition coefficients for halothane in the rabbit. Br J Anaesth 44:650

Marshall, C., Lindgren, L., and Marshall, B.E. 1984. Effects of halothane, enflurane and isoflurane on hypoxic pulmonary vasoconstriction in rat lungs in vitro. Anesthesiology 60:304–9.

Martis, L., Lynch, S., Napoli, M. D., and Woods, E. F. 1981. Biotransformation of sevoflurane in dogs and rats. Anesth Analg 60:186–91.

Matthews, K. A., Doherty, T., Dyson, D. H., Wilcock, B., and Valliant, A. 1990. Nephrotoxicity in dogs associated with methoxyflurane anesthesia and flunixin meglumine analgesia. Can Vet J 31:766–71.

Mazze, R. I. 1992. The safety of sevoflurane in humans. Anesthesiology 77:1062-1063.

Mazze, R. I., and Fujinaga, M. 1989. Biotransformation of inhalational anaesthetics. In J.F. Nunn, J.E. Utting, and B.R. Brown, eds., General Anaesthesia, 5th ed., pp. 73–85. London: Butterworths.

Mazze, R. I., and Jamison, R. 1995. Renal effects of sevoflurane (editorial). Anesthesiology 83:443-445.

Mazze, R. I., Cousins, M. J., and Kosek, J. C. 1972. Dose-related methoxyflurane nephrotoxicity in rats: a biochemical and pathologic correlation. Anesthesiology 36:571–87.

Mazze, R. I., Cousins, M. J., and Barr, G. A. 1974a. Renal effects and metabolism of isoflurane in man. Anesthesiology 40:536–42.

Mazze, R. I., Hitt, B. A., and Cousins, M. J. 1974b. Effect of enzyme induction with phenobarbital on the in vivo and in vitro defluorination of isoflurane and methoxyflurane. J Pharmacol Exp Ther 190:523–29.

Mazze, R. I., Calverley, R. K., and Smith, N. T. 1977. Inorganic fluoride nephrotoxicity: prolonged enflurane and halothane anesthesia in volunteers. Anesthesiology 46:265–71.

McMurphy, R. M., and Hodgson, D. S. 1994. Cardiopulmonary effects of desflurane in cats. Proceedings, Fifth International Congress of Veterinary Anesthesia 191 (Abstr).

Merin, R. G., and Borgstedt, H. H. 1971. Myocardial function and metabolism in the methoxyflurane depressed canine heart. Anesthesiology 34:562–68.

Merin, R. G., Kumazawa, T., and Luka, N. L. 1976. Enflurane depresses myocardial function perfusion and metabolism in the dog. Anesthesiology 45:501–7.

Merin, R. G., Bernard, J. M., Doursout, M. F., Cohen, M., and Chelly, J. E. 1991. Comparison of the effects of isoflurane and desflurane on cardiovascular dynamics and regional blood flow in the chronically instrumented dog. Anesthesiology 74:568–74.

Merkel, G., and Eger, E. I., II. 1963. A comparative study of halothane and halopropane anesthesia including method for determining equipotency. Anesthesiology 24:346–57.

Michenfelder, J. D., and Cucchiara, R. F. 1974. Canine cerebral oxygen consumption during enflurane anesthesia and its modification during induced seizures. Anesthesiology 40:575–80.

Miletich, D. J., Ivankovich, A. D., Albrecht, R. F., Reimann, C. R., Rosenberg, R., and McKissic, E. D. 1976. Absence of autoregulation of cerebral blood flow during halothane and enflurane anesthesia. Anesth Analg 55:100–109.

Millard, R. I., and Corbett, T. H. 1974. Nitrous oxide concentrations in the dental operatory. J Oral Surg 32:593–94.

Miller, E. D., Jr, and Greene, N. M. 1990. Waking up to desflurane: the anesthetic for the 90s? Anesth Analg 70:1–2.

Miller, R. D., Way, W. L., Dolan, W. M., Stevens, W. C., and Eger, E. I., II. 1972. The dependence of pancuronium- and *d*-tubocurarine-induced neuromuscular blockades on alveolar concentrations of halothane and Forane. Anesthesiology 37:573–81.

Milligan, J. E., Sablan, J. L., and Short, C. E. 1980. A survey of waste anesthetic gas concentrations in U.S. Air Force veterinary surgeries. J Am Vet Med Assoc 177:1021–22.

Moore, M. A., Weiskopf, R. B., Eger, E. I., II, Wilson, C., and Lu, G. 1993. Arrhythmogenic doses of epinephrine are similar during desflurane or isoflurane anesthesia in humans. Anesthesiology 79:943–47.

Morio, M., Fujii, K., Satoh, N., Imai, M., Kawakami, U., Mizuno, T., Kawai, Y., Ogasawara, Y., Tamura, T., Negishi, A., Kumagai, Y., and Kawai, T. 1992. Reaction of sevoflurane and its degradation products with soda lime: Toxicity of the byproducts. Anesthesiology 77:1155-1164.

Muallem, M., Larson, C. P. J., and Eger, E. I., II. 1969. The effects of diethyl ether on $PaCO_2$ in dogs with and without vagal, somatic and sympathetic block. Anesthesiology 30:185–91.

Muir, B. J., Hall, L. W., and Littlewort, M. C. G. 1959. Cardiac irregularities in cats under halothane anaesthesia. Br J Anaesth 31:488–89.

Muir, W. W., III, Werner, L. L., and Hamlin, R. L. 1975. Effects of xylazine and acetylpromazine upon induced ventricular fibrillation in dogs anesthetized with thiamylal and halothane. Am J Vet Res 36:1299–1303.

Munson, E. S., and Tucker, W. K. 1975. Doses of epinephrine causing arrhythmia during enflurane, methoxyflurane and halothane anesthesia in dogs. Can Anaesth Soc J 22:495–501.

Munson, E. S., Larson, C. P. J., Babad, A. A., Regan, M. J., Buechel, D. R., and Eger, E. I., II. 1966. The effects of halothane, fluroxene and cyclopropane on ventilation: a comparative study in man. Anesthesiology 27:716–28.

Natarajan, D., and Santhiya, S. T. 1990. Cytogenic damage in operating theatre personnel. Anaesthesia 45:574–77.

Nathan, H. J. 1988. Nitrous oxide worsens myocardial ischemia in isoflurane-anesthetized dogs. Anesthesiology 68:407–16.

National Institute for Occupational Safety and Health (NIOSH). 1977. Criteria for a recommended standard . . . occupational exposure to waste anesthetic gases and vapors. NIOSH Pub. No. 77–140.

Navarro, R., Weiskopf, R. B., Moore, M. A., Lockhart, S., Eger, E. I., II, Koblin, D., Lu, G., and Wilson, C. 1994. Humans anesthetized with sevoflurane or isoflurane have similar arrhythmic response to epinephrine. Anesthesiology 80:545–49.

Neigh, J. L., Garman, J. K., and Harp, J. R. 1971. The electroencephalographic pattern during anesthesia with Ethrane: effects of depth of anesthesia, $PaCO_2$ and nitrous oxide. Anesthesiology 35:482–87.

Ona, F. V., Portanella, H., and Ayub, A. 1980. Hepatitis associated with enflurane anesthesia. Anesth Analg 59:146–49.

Ossipou, M. H., and Gebhart, G. F. 1984. Light pentoarbital anesthesia diminishes the antinociceptive potency of morphine administered intracranially but not intrathecally in the rat. Eur J Pharmacol 97(1–2):137–41.

O'Sullivan, H., Jennings, F., Ward, K., McCann, S., Scott, J. M., and Weir, D. G. 1981. Human bone marrow biochemical function and megaloblastic hematopoiesis after nitrous oxide anesthesia. Anesthesiology 55:645–49.

Pagel, P. S., Kampine, J. P., Schmeling, W. T., and Warltier, D. C. 1991a. Influence of volatile anesthetics on myocardial contractility in vivo: desflurane versus isoflurane. Anesthesiology 74:900–907.

———. 1991b. Comparison of the systemic and coronary hemodynamic actions of desflurane, isoflurane, halothane, and enflurane in the chronically instrumented dog. Anesthesiology 74:539–51.

———. 1993. Evaluation of myocardial contractility in the chronically instrumented dog with intact autonomic nervous system function: effects of desflurane and isoflurane. Acta Anaesth Scand 37:203–10.

Pavlin, E. G., and Su, J. Y. 1994. Cardiopulmonary pharmacology. In R. D. Miller, ed., Anesthesia, 4th ed., pp. 125–56. New York: Churchill Livingstone.

Pedersoli, W. M. 1977a. Serum fluoride concentration, renal and hepatic function test results in dogs with methoxyflurane anesthesia. Am J Vet Res 38:949–53.

———. 1977b. Blood serum inorganic ionic fluoride tetracycline and methoxyflurane anesthesia in dogs. JAAHA 13:242–46.

———. 1980. Serum bromide concentrations during and after halothane anesthesia in dogs. Am J Vet Res 41:77–80.

Pelligrino, D. A., Miletich, D. J., Hoffman, W. E., and Albrecht, R. F. 1984. Nitrous oxide markedly increases cerebral cortical metabolic rate and blood flow in the goat. Anesthesiology 60:405

Philbin, D. M., Foex, P., Drummond, G., Lowenstein, E., Ryder, W. A., and Jones, L. A. 1985. Postsystolic shortening of canine left ventricle supplied by a stenotic coronary artery when nitrous oxide is added in the presence of narcotics. Anesthesiology 62:166–74.

Plummer, J. L., Beckwith, A. L. J., Bastin, F. N., Adams, J. F., Cousins, M. J., and Hall, P. 1982. Free radical formation in vivo and hepatotoxicity due to anesthesia with halothane. Anesthesiology 57:160–66.

Pohl, L. R., and Gillette, J. R. 1982. A perspective on halothane-induced hepatotoxicity. Anesth Analg 61:809–11.

Pohl, L. R., Satoh, H., Christ, D. D., and Kenna, J. G. 1988. The immunologic and metabolic basis of drug hypersensitivities. Annu Rev Pharmacol Toxicol 28:367–87.

Pohl, L. R., Kenna, J. G., Satoh, H., and Christ, D. 1989. Neoantigens associated with halothane hepatitis. Drug Metab Rev 20:203–17.

Price, H. L. 1961. Circulatory actions of general anesthetic agents and the homeostatic roles of epinephrine and norepinephrine in man. Clin Pharmacol Ther 2:163–76.

———. 1966. The significance of catecholamine release during anesthesia. Br J Anaesth 38:705–11.

Price, H. L., Skovsted, P., Pauca, A. L., and Cooperman, L. H. 1970. Evidence for β-receptor activation produced by halothane in man. Anesthesiology 32:389–95.

Purchase, I. F. 1966. Cardiac arrhythmias occurring during halothane anaesthesia in cats. Br J Anaesth 38:13–22.

Quasha, A. L., Eger, E. I., II, and Tinker, J. H. 1980. Determination and applications of MAC. Anesthesiology 52:315-334.

Rampil, I. J., Weiskopf, R. B., Brown, J. G., Eger, E. I., II, Johnson, B. H., Holmes, M. A., and Donegan, J. H. 1988. I-653 and isoflurane produce similar dose-related changes in the electroencephalogram of pigs. Anesthesiology 69:298–302.

Rampil, I. J., Lockhart, S. H., Eger, E. I., II, Yasuda, N., Weiskopf, R. B., and Cahalan, M. K. 1991. The electroencephalographic effects of desflurane in humans. Anesthesiology 74:434–39.

Raventos, J. 1956. The action of fluothane: a new volatile anaesthetic. Brit J Pharmacol 11:394–409.

Regan, M. J., and Eger, E. I., II. 1967. Effect of hypothermia in dogs on anesthetizing and apneic doses of inhalation agents: determination of the anesthetic index (apnea/MAC). Anesthesiology 28:689–700.

Rehder, K., Forbes, J., Alter, H., Hessler, O., and Stier, A. 1967. Halothane biotransformation in man: a quantitative study. Anesthesiology 28:711–15.

Rice, S. A., and Steffey, E. P. 1985a. Metabolism of three inhaled anesthetics by cow, dog, lamb and rat hepatic microsomes. In J. Grandy, S. Hildebrand, W. McDonell, et al. Proceedings of the Second International Congress of Veterinary Anesthesia, pp. 164–65. Santa Barbara: Veterinary Practice Publishing Co.

———. 1985b. Metabolism of halothane and isoflurane in horses. Vet Surg 14:76(Abstr).

Rice, S. A., Maze, M., Smith, C. M., Kosek, J. C., and Mazze, R. I. 1987. Halothane hepatotoxicity in Fischer 344 rats pretreated with isoniazid. Toxicol Appl Pharmacol 87:411–20.

Ross, W. T., and Cardell, R. R. 1978. Proliferation of smooth endoplasmic reticulum and induction of microsomal drug-metabolizing enzymes after ether or halothane. Anesthesiology 48:325–31.

Ross, W. T., Jr., and Daggy, B. P. 1981. Hepatic blood flow in phenobarbital pretreated rats during halothane anesthesia and hypoxia. Anesth Analg 60:306–9.

Rowland, A. S., Baird, D. D., Weinberg, C. R., Shore, D. L., Shy, C. M., and Wilcox, A. J. 1992. Reduced fertility among women employed as dental assistants exposed to high levels of nitrous oxide. N Engl J Med 327:993–97.

Sardas, S., Cuhruk, H., Karakaya, A. E., and Atakurt, Y. 1992. Sister-chromatic exchanges in operating room personnel. Mutat Res 279:117–20.

Scheller, M. S., Tateishi, A., Drummond, J. C., and Zornow, M. H. 1988. The effects of sevoflurane on cerebral blood flow, cerebral metabolic rate for oxygen, intracranial pressure, and the electroencephalogram are similar to those of isoflurane in the rabbit. Anesthesiology 68:548–52.

Scheller, M. S., Nakakimura, K., Fleischer, J. E., and Zornow, M. H. 1990. Cerebral effects of sevoflurane in the dog: comparison with isoflurane and enflurane. Br J Anaesth 65:388–92.

Schulman, M., Braverman, B., Ivankovich, A., and Gronert, G. 1981. Sevoflurane triggers malignant hyperthermia in swine (letter). Anesthesiology 54:259–60.

Sessler, D. I., Israel, D., Pozos, R. S., Pozos, M., and Rubinstein, E. H. 1988. Spontaneous post anesthetic tremor does not resemble thermoregulatory shivering. Anesthesiology 68:843–50.

Seyde, W. C., and Longnecker, D. E. 1984. Anesthetic influences on regional hemodynamics in normal and hemorrhaged rats. Anesthesiology 61:686–98.

Shingu, K., Eger, E. I., II, and Johnson, B. H. 1982a. Hypoxia per se can produce hepatic damage without death in rats. Anesth Analg 61:820–23.

———. 1982b. Hypoxia may be more important than reductive metabolism in halothane-induced hepatic injury. Anesth Analg 61:824–27.

Short, C. E. 1987. Inhalant anesthetics. In C.E. Short, ed., Principles and Practice of Veterinary Anesthesia, pp. 70–90. Baltimore: Williams & Wilkins.

Skovsted, P., and Price, H. L. 1970. Central sympathetic excitation caused by diethyl ether. Anesthesiology 32:202–9.

———. 1972. The effect of ethrane on arterial pressure, preganglionic sympathetic activity and barostatic reflexes. Anesthesiology 36:257–62.

Soma, L. R. 1971. Textbook of Veterinary Anesthesia. Baltimore: Williams & Wilkins.

Sommer, R. 1987. Preventing endotracheal tube fire during pharyngeal surgery. Anesthesiology 66:439

Staddon, G. E., Weaver, B. M. Q., and Webb, A. I. 1979. Distribution of cardiac output in anaesthetized horse. Res Vet Sci 27:38–45.

Steffey, E. P. 1978. Enflurane and isoflurane anesthesia: a summary of laboratory and clinical investigations in horses. J Am Vet Med Assoc 172:367–73.

———. 1991. Inhalation anesthetics and gases. In W.W. Muir III and J. A. E. Hubbell, eds., Equine Anesthesia: Monitoring and Emergency Therapy, pp. 352–79. St. Louis: Mosby Year Book.

———. 1994. Inhalation anesthesia. In L. W. Hall and P. Taylor, eds., Feline Anaesthesia, pp. 157–93. London: Bailliere Tindall.

———. 1996. Inhalation anesthetics. In J.C. Thurmon, W. Tranquilli, and G.J. Benson, eds., Veterinary Anesthesia. Baltimore: Lea & Febiger.

Steffey, E. P., and Howland, D., Jr. 1977. Isoflurane potency in the dog and cat. Am J Vet Res 38:1833–36.

———. 1978a. Cardiovascular effects of halothane in the horse. Am J Vet Res 39:611–15.

———. 1978b. Potency of enflurane in dogs: comparison with halothane and isoflurane. Am J Vet Res 39:673–77.

———. 1978c. Potency of halothane-N2O in the horse. Am J Vet Res 39:1141–46.

———. 1979. Halothane anesthesia in calves. Am J Vet Res 40:372–76.

———. 1980. Comparison of circulatory and respiratory effects of isoflurane and halothane anesthesia in horses. Am J Vet Res 40:821–25.

Steffey, E. P., Gillespie, J. R., Berry, J. D., and Eger, E. I., II. 1974a. Cardiovascular effects with the addition of N2O to halothane in stump-tailed macaques during spontaneous and controlled ventilation. J Am Vet Med Assoc 165:834–37.

Steffey, E. P., Gillespie, J. R., Berry, J. D., Eger, E. I., II, and Rhode, E. A. 1974b. Circulatory effects of halothane and halothane-nitrous oxide anesthesia in the dog: controlled ventilation. Am J Vet Res 35:1289–93.

———. 1974c. Cardiovascular effect of halothane in the stump-tailed macaque during spontaneous and controlled ventilation. Am J Vet Res 35:1315–19.

———. 1975. Circulatory effects of halothane and halothane-nitrous oxide anesthesia in the dog: spontaneous ventilation. Am J Vet Res 36:197–200.

Steffey, E. P., Howland, D., Jr., Giri, S., and Eger, E. I., II. 1977. Enflurane, halothane and isoflurane potency in horses. Am J Vet Res 38:1037–39.

Steffey, E. P., Zinkl, J., and Howland, D., Jr. 1979. Minimal changes in blood cell counts and biochemical values associated with prolonged isoflurane anesthesia of horses. Am J Vet Res 40:1646–48.

Steffey, E. P., Farver, T., Zinkl, J., Wheat, J. D., Meagher, D. M., and Brown, M. P. 1980. Alterations in horse blood cell count and biochemical values after halothane anesthesia. Am J Vet Res 41:934–39.

Steffey, E. P., Farver, T. B., and Woliner, M. J. 1984. Circulatory and respiratory effects of methoxyflurane in dogs: comparison of halothane. Am J Vet Res 45:2574–79.

Steffey, E. P., Wong, P., Hildebrand, S. V., Hodgson, D., Meagher, D. M., Pascoe, J. R., Wheat, J. D., et al. 1985. Halothane and isoflurane anesthesia in foals. In J. Grandy, S. Hildebrand, W. McDonell, et al. Proceedings of the Second International Congress of Veterinary Anesthesia, pp. 102–3. Santa Barbara: Veterinary Practice Publishing Co.

Steffey, E. P., Dunlop, C. I., Farver, T. B., Woliner, M. J., and Schultz, L. J. 1987a. Cardiovascular and respiratory measurements in awake and isoflurane-anesthetized horses. Am J Vet Res 48:7–12.

Steffey, E. P., Farver, T. B., and Woliner, M. J. 1987b. Cardiopulmonary function during 7 h of constant-dose halothane and methoxyflurane. J Appl Physiol 63:1351–59.

Steffey, E. P., Hodgson, D. S., Dunlop, C. I., Miller, M. F., Woliner, M. J., Heath, R. B., and Grandy, J. 1987c. Cardiopulmonary function during 5 hours of constant-dose isoflurane in laterally recumbent, spontaneously breathing horses. J Vet Pharmacol Ther 10:290–97.

Steffey, E. P., Kelly, A. B., and Woliner, M. J. 1987d. Time-related responses of spontaneously breathing, laterally recumbent horses to prolonged anesthesia with halothane. Am J Vet Res 48:952–57.

Steffey, E. P., Kelly, A. B., Hodgson, D. S., Grandy, J. L., Woliner, M. J., and Willits, N. 1990a. Effect of body posture on cardiopulmonary function in horses during five hours of constant-dose halothane anesthesia. Am J Vet Res 51:11–16.

Steffey, E. P., Woliner, M. J., and Dunlop, C. 1990b. Effects of five hours of constant 1.2 MAC halothane in sternally recumbent, spontaneously breathing horses. Equine Vet J 22:433–36.

Steffey, E. P., Willits, N., Wong, P., Hildebrand, S. V., Wheat, J. D., Meagher, D. M., Hodgson, D., Pascoe, J. R., Heath, R. B., and Dunlop, C. 1991. Clinical investigations of halothane and isoflurane for induction and maintenance of foal anesthesia. J Vet Pharmacol Ther 14:300–309.

Steffey, E. P., Dunlop, C. I., Cullen, L. K., Hodgson, D. S., Giri, S. N., Willits, N., Woliner, M. J., Jarvis, K. A., Smith, C. M., and Elliott, A. R. 1993a. Circulatory and respiratory responses of spontaneously breathing, laterally recumbent horses to 12 hours of halothane anesthesia. Am J Vet Res 54:929–36.

Steffey, E. P., Eisele, J. H., Baggot, J. D., Woliner, M. J., Jarvis, K. A., and Elliott, A. R. 1993b. Influence of inhaled anesthetics on the pharmacokinetics and pharmacodynamics of morphine. Anesth Analg 77:346–51.

Steffey, E. P., Giri, S. N., Dunlop, C. I., Cullen, L. K., Hodgson, D. S., and Willits, N. 1993c. Biochemical and haematological changes following prolonged halothane anaesthesia in horses. Res Vet Sci 55:338–45.

Stier, A., Alter, H., Hessler, O., and Rehder, K. 1964. Urinary excretion of bromide in halothane anesthesia. Anesth Analg 43:723–28.

Stoelting, R. K., and Eger, E. I., II. 1969. Percutaneous loss of nitrous oxide, cyclopropane, ether and halothane in man. Anesthesiology 30:278–83.

Stoelting, R. K., and R. D. Miller. 1989. Basics of Anesthesia. New York: Churchill Livingston.

Stover, S. M., Steffey, E. P., Dybdal, N. O., and Franti, C. E. 1988. Hematologic and biochemical values associated with multiple halothane anesthesias and minor surgical trauma of horses. Am J Vet Res 49:236–41.

Strum, D. P., and Eger, E. I., II. 1987. Partition coefficients for sevoflurane in human blood, saline, and olive oil. Anesth Analg 66:654–57.

Strum, D. P., Johnson, B. H., and Eger, E. I., II. 1987. Stability of sevoflurane in soda lime. Anesthesiology 67:779–81.

Theye, R. A., and Michenfelder, J. D. 1968. The effect of nitrous oxide on canine cerebral metabolism. Anesthesiology 29:1119–24.

Thurmon, J. C., Tranquilli, W., and Benson, G. J., eds. 1996. Lumb and Jones' Veterinary Anesthesia. Baltimore: Lea & Febiger.

Tinker, J. H., Gandolfi, A. J., and Van Dyke, R. A. 1976. Elevation of plasma bromide levels in patients following halothane anesthesia: time correlation with total halothane dosage. Anesthesiology 44:194–96.

Todd, M. M., and Drummond, J. C. 1984. A comparison of the cerebrovascular and metabolic effects of halothane and isoflurane in the cat. Anesthesiology 60:276–83.

Tranquilli, W. J., Thurmon, J. C., Benson, G. J., and Davis, L. E. 1986. Alteration in the arrhythmogenic dose of epinephrine (ADE) following xylazine administration to halothane-anesthetized dogs. J Vet Pharmacol Ther 9:198–203.

Tucker, W. K., Rackstein, A. D., and Munson, E. S. 1974. Comparison of arrhythmic doses of adrenaline, metaraminol, ephedrine, and phenylephrine, during isoflurane and halothane anesthesia in dogs. Br J Anaesth 46:392–96.

Van der Reis, L., Askin, S. H., Frecker, G. N., and Fitzgeralk, W. J. 1974. Hepatitis associated with enflurane anesthesia. JAMA 227:76

Van Dyke, R. A., and Wood, C. L. 1975. *In vitro* studies on irreversible binding of halothane metabolite to microsomes. Drug Metab Dispos 3:51–57.

Van Dyke, R. A., Chenoweth, M. B., and Van Poznak, A. 1964. Metabolism of volatile anesthetics. I. Conversion *in vivo* of several anesthetics to $^{14}CO_2$ and chloride. Biochem Pharmacol 13:1239–47.

Walker, J. A., Eggers, G. W. N., and Allen, C. R. 1962. Cardiovascular effects of methoxyflurane anesthesia in man. Anesthesiology 23:639–42.

Wallin, R. F., Regan, B. M., Napoli, M. D., and Stern, I. J. 1975. Sevoflurane: a new inhalational anesthetic agent. Anesth Analg 54:758–66.

Warltier, D. C., and Pagel, P. S. 1992. Cardiovascular and respiratory actions of desflurane: is desflurane different from isoflurane? Anesth Analg 75:S17–S31.

Warren, R. G., and Webb, A. I. 1986. Nasotracheal intubation of the rabbit. Am Coll Vet Anesth 1986 Scientific Meeting (Abstr).

Webb, A. I. 1985. The effect of species differences in the uptake and distribution of inhalant anesthetic agents. In J. Grandy, S. Hildebrand, W. McDonell, et al., Proceedings of the Second International Congress of Veterinary Anesthesia, pp. 27–32. Santa Barbara: Veterinary Practice Publishing Co.

Wedel, D. J., Iaizzo, P. A., and Milde, J. H. 1991. Desflurane is a trigger of malignant hyperthermia in susceptible swine. Anesthesiology 74:508–12.

Weiskopf, R. B., Holmes, M. A., Eger, E. I., II, Johnson, B. H., Rampil, I. J., and Brown, J. G. 1988. Cardiovascular effects of I-653 in swine. Anesthesiology 69:303–9.

Weiskopf, R. B., Eger, E. I., II, Holmes, M. A., Rampil, I. J., Johnson, B. H., Brown, J. G., Yasuda, N., and Targ, A. G. 1989a. Epinephrine-induced premature ventricular contractions and changes in arterial blood pressure and heart rate during I-653, isoflurane, and halothane anesthesia in swine. Anesthesiology 70:293–98.

Weiskopf, R. B., Holmes, M. A., Rampil, I. J., Johnson, B. H., Yasuda, N., Targ, A. G., and Eger, E. I., II. 1989b. Cardiovascular safety and actions of high concentrations of I-653 and isoflurane in swine. Anesthesiology 70:793–99.

Weiskopf, R. B., Cahalan, M. K., Eger, E. I., II, Yasuda, N., Rampil, I. J., Ionescu, P., Lockhart, S. H., Johnson, B. H., Freire, B., and Kelley, S. 1991. Cardiovascular actions of desflurane in normocarbic volunteers. Anesth Analg 73:143–56.

Weiskopf, R. B., Eger, E. I., II, Ionescu, P., Yasuda, N., Cahalan, M. K., Freire, B., Peterson, N., Lochhart, S. H., Rampil, I. J., and Laster, M. 1992. Desflurane does not produce hepatic or renal injury in human volunteers. Anesth Analg 74:570–74.

Whitcher, C. E., Cohen, E. N., and Trudell, J. R. 1971. Chronic exposure to anesthetic gases in the operating room. Anesthesiology 35:348–53.

Yasuda, N., Lockhart, S. L., Eger, E. I., II, Weiskopf, R. B., Liu, J., Laster, M. J., Taheri, S., and Peterson, N. A. 1991. Comparison of kinetics of sevoflurane and isoflurane in humans. Anesth Analg 72:316–24.

Young, W. L. 1992. Effects of desflurane on the central nervous system. Anesth Analg 75:S32–S37.

12 INJECTABLE ANESTHETICS

KEITH R. BRANSON

Indications for Injectable Anesthesia
Disadvantages of Injectable Anesthesia
Properties of an Ideal Injectable Anesthetic Drug
The Barbiturates
  Pentobarbital Sodium
  Thiopental Sodium
  Thialbarbital Sodium
  Thiamylal Sodium
  Methohexital Sodium
  Secobarbital Sodium
  Hexobarbital Sodium
Propofol
Etomidate
Chloral Hydrate
Chloral Hydrate and Magnesium Sulfate
Guaifenesin
Althesin
Dissociative Anesthetics
  Phencyclidine Hydrochloride
  Ketamine Hydrochloride
  Tiletamine Hydrochloride
Miscellaneous Agents
  Chloralose
  Urethane
  Propanidid
  Metomidate

Stages of anesthesia for central nervous system (CNS) depressants are similar in a patient whether anesthetic is injected intravenously or administered by inhalation. However, it is possible to proceed more rapidly through induction with IV anesthetics than with almost all of the inhalation anesthetics. Clinically, a rapid course of induction is desirable to avoid excitement and struggling.

Anesthetics administered intravenously appear to conform to the same laws of tissue distribution and the same theories of activity as discussed for other anesthetics. There is no anesthetic agent that produces ideal anesthesia under all circumstances. It is desirable to know advantages and disadvantages of different methods and drugs producing general anesthesia to select the kind most suited to a particular clinical condition.

INDICATIONS FOR INJECTABLE ANESTHESIA. There are many situations where injectable anesthesia has distinct advantages over inhalation anesthesia. Induction of general anesthesia and intubation are often accomplished most efficaciously by the IV injection of a short-acting anesthetic or, in the case of animals that are difficult to restrain, the intramuscular (IM) injection of an anesthetic agent. Some minor procedures require only a short time, and injectable anesthesia provides a safe and efficient means of providing short-duration anesthesia. The increased use of endoscopic upper airway examination has also increased the use of injectable anesthesia. The use of injectable anesthesia allows easy visualization of the larynx and proximal trachea as well as endoscopic examination of the distal airways without the difficulties of administering inhalation anesthesia concurrently. Large-animal surgical procedures (especially equine) are often done using injectable anesthesia since the equipment needed for inhalation anesthesia is not readily transportable. The capture and immobilization of wild animals rely almost exclusively on injectable anesthetics or related compounds. Finally, in situations where economy is the primary concern, the use of injectable anesthesia is attractive since there is no need to invest in the equipment required to administer inhalation anesthesia.

DISADVANTAGES OF INJECTABLE ANESTHESIA. Traditionally the depth, or level, of anesthesia has been thought to be less readily controlled with drugs injected intravenously or parenterally than with inhalation anesthetic agents. However, some of the agents currently available have such short durations of action that depth of anesthesia can be readily adjusted by changing the administration rate.

A major portion of inhalant anesthetics is rapidly eliminated unaltered in exhaled air after administration ceases, whereas an injectable anesthetic drug ceases to act only after it is metabolized and/or excreted. However, use of ultrashort-acting barbiturates and other even shorter acting agents, most notably propofol, have provided better control of IV anesthesia. These have made possible safe and satisfactory anesthesia without the use of inhalation agents. The concurrent use of other drugs such as opiates and tranquilizers improves the analgesia and muscle relaxation.

Many injectable anesthetic agents as well as agents commonly used concurrently with them are classified as controlled substances under the 1970 Controlled

Substances Act. This places restrictions on the purchase, storage, and use of these drugs.

PROPERTIES OF AN IDEAL INJECTABLE ANESTHETIC DRUG. There is no ideal injectable (or inhalation) anesthetic drug available at this time. One can, however, hypothesize what properties such a drug would have. These can be divided into physiological and pharmacological properties.

Ideal Physiological Properties. The ideal injectable anesthetic agent should provide physiological homeostasis. This means there should be no life-threatening changes in cardiovascular and respiratory function. There should be analgesia that is adequate for the procedure to be performed. Some degree of muscle relaxation should be produced. The amount of muscle relaxation needed certainly varies with the procedure. Finally, an injectable anesthetic needs to produce unconsciousness. Since pain is a psychological perception, anything that produces unconsciousness will provide some degree of analgesia by depressing the activity of the higher centers of the brain (Kitchell 1983).

Ideal Pharmacological Properties. An ideal injectable anesthetic should have a wide margin of safety in a variety of species. It should have a short duration of action with minimal cumulative effects so the duration of anesthesia could be easily controlled. The drug should be readily metabolized and/or excreted: ideally by more than one route. And finally a specific and complete reversal agent should be available.

THE BARBITURATES. Barbital sodium and phenobarbital were the first of the barbituric acid derivatives introduced into medicine. When used to produce anesthesia, the major limitation of the earlier barbiturates was their long period of action. In 1924 Somnifene was used intravenously to produce general anesthesia. Dial was introduced during the same year. Pentobarbital was introduced in 1926 by Page and Coryllos for animal experimental use; by 1930, it was used in clinical veterinary medicine. During 1928 amobarbital sodium was employed in animals.

In 1933 hexobarbital sodium was introduced and recognized as a marked advancement in IV anesthesia because of a very rapid hypnotic action of brief duration. In 1934 thiopental sodium was introduced and appeared to possess certain advantages over hexobarbital. In 1946 and 1948 respectively, new ultrashort-acting barbituric acid derivatives called thialbarbital sodium and thiamylal sodium were introduced into veterinary medicine.

There are many other barbituric acid derivatives (e.g., aprobarbital, butabarbital, mephobarbital, metharbital, probarbital, talbutal). These, however, are infrequently or seldom used in veterinary medicine; several of the most widely used barbituric acid derivatives are listed in Table 12.1, with generalizations regarding official status, duration of action, and chemical structure.

Intermediate- and long-acting barbiturates should be restricted to sedative or anticonvulsant use. Their long action precludes using them for general anesthetic purposes.

Chemistry. The barbiturates are bitter-tasting white powders except for those containing sulfur. These may have a yellowish tint. Barbiturates are hygroscopic and will decompose on exposure to air, heat, and light. They should be stored in dark bottles, sealed ampules, or colored capsules. Solutions of barbiturates decompose rapidly unless stabilized. Boiling of aqueous solutions quickly decomposes most barbiturates. Certain thiobarbiturates are relatively unsta-

TABLE 12.1—Major barbiturates used in veterinary medicine

	Official names and synonyms	Approximate duration of action	Radicals attached to carbon 5: R_1	R_2
←decreased-Duration-increased→	Phenobarbital Sodium (soluble phenobarbital, soluble phenobarbitone, luminal sodium), USP	Long	Ethyl	Phenyl
	Barbital Sodium (soluble barbital, soluble barbitone, veronal sodium), NF	Long	Ethyl	Ethyl
	Amobarbital Sodium (amytal sodium), USP	Intermediate	Ethyl	Isoamyl
	Pentobarbital Sodium (nembutal sodium), USP	Short	Ethyl	1-Methyl butyl
	Secobarbital Sodium (seconal sodium), USP	Short	Allyl	1-Methyl butyl
	Thiopental Sodium* (pentothal sodium), USP	Ultrashort	Ethyl	1-Methyl butyl
	Thiamylal Sodium* (surital sodium), USP	Ultrashort	Allyl	1-Methyl butyl
	Thialbarbital Sodium* (kemithal sodium), INN	Ultrashort	Allyl	Cyclohexenyl
	Methohexital Sodium† (Brevane), USP	Ultrashort	Allyl	1-Methyl-2-pentynyl

*Sulfur replaces oxygen on carbon 2.
†Methyl group replaces hydrogen on nitrogen 1.

ble; solutions of these may be entirely decomposed in 36 hours at room temperature but will last longer if refrigerated.

Barbiturates are derived from the nondepressant barbituric acid or malonylurea, which contains a pyrimidine nucleus. When the hydrogens on carbon 5 are substituted with an appropriate alkyl or aryl group, depressant activity on the CNS is possessed by the compound. A few barbituric acid derivatives contain a sulfur atom attached to carbon 2 in substitution for the oxygen (see Fig. 12.1).

Barbituric acid and its carbon 5 substituted derivatives are sparingly soluble in water. Aqueous solutions are weakly acid and will combine with sodium or other fixed alkalis to form water-soluble salts. The sodium atom joins the oxygen atom attached to carbon 2. These salts hydrolyze in water to form alkaline solutions with a pH usually between 9 and 10.

Conversion of barbituric acid derivatives into water-soluble salts made possible the IV injection of barbiturates that has been so widely and satisfactorily practiced in veterinary medicine.

Several hundred barbituric acid derivatives have been synthesized, but only a few have survived the rigors of clinical trial. From pharmacologic study of these compounds, certain relationships of chemical structure and pharmacologic response have become apparent, so certain generalities are justified:

1. To be hypnotically effective, both hydrogen atoms on carbon 5 must be replaced by an alkyl or aryl group.
2. To obtain optimal therapeutic results, the substituting radicals on carbon 5 should contain a minimum of 4 and a maximum of 9 carbons; addition of more leads to convulsant activity.
3. Unsaturated carbon chains are more readily oxidized and hence are short acting.
4. Short chains are more stable and hence are long acting.
5. Long chains are easily oxidized and are short acting.
6. Branched chains tend to be shorter in action than straight chains.
7. Only one aryl radical should be attached to carbon 5.
8. Replacement of the oxygen atom on carbon 2 by a sulfur atom increases potency and instability and shortens duration of action of the compound.
9. Attachment of an alkyl group to one of the N atoms (position 1 or 3) increases anesthetic potency and tends to stimulate the CNS. Substitution in both N atoms produces a convulsant.
10. Replacement of the oxygen on carbon 2 by an HN= group destroys the hypnotic activity of the molecule.

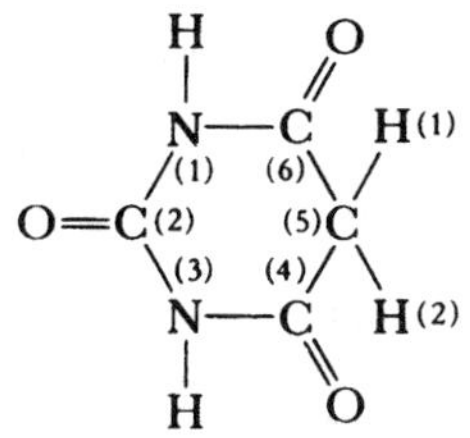

```
         H     O
         |    //
         N—C    H(1)
        /(1) (6)\  /
O=C(2)      (5)C
        \(3) (4)/  \
         N—C    H(2)
         |    \\
         H     O
```

Barbituric Acid (malonylurea)

FIG. 12.1

Central Nervous System. The major action of barbiturates is to depress the CNS. This effect is the reason for the extensive use of barbiturates in medicine. Effects upon other systems become important as toxic limitations to use of the drug are approached.

Each of the many barbiturates depresses the CNS. Clinically they differ in respect to effective dosage, time required for initial effect, duration of action, and method of administration. The degree of depression may vary from mild sedation and hypnosis to surgical anesthesia.

Barbiturates both enhance and mimic the action of the neurotransmitter γ-aminobutyric acid (GABA), the principal inhibitory neurotransmitter in the CNS (Olsen 1988). Barbiturates depress the cortex of the brain and probably the thalamus. They depress motor areas of the brain and thus can be used to control convulsive seizures. They also depress sensory areas and induce anesthesia. Relatively large dosages of barbiturates are necessary to deaden the physiological response to noxious stimuli. Pentobarbital plasma concentrations necessary to abolish the response to noxious stimuli in the dog is 23 ± 2.9 μg/mL (Frederiksen et al. 1983).

Numerous investigations have shown a decrease in oxygen uptake by the brain following barbiturate administration. Utilization of oxygen by the cortical areas of the brain is more depressed than by other regions of the CNS. In clinical concentrations, barbiturates are the most potent known depressants of cerebral oxygen consumption (Steen and Michenfelder 1979). As much as a 55% decrease in oxygen consumption may occur.

Barbiturate anesthetics, but not anticonvulsants, abolish the spontaneous activity of cultured spinal cord neurons; the anesthetics directly increase membrane conductance, an effect that is suppressed by GABA antagonists such as picrotoxin and penicillin (Macdonald and Barker 1978). Pentobarbital is GABA-mimetic; i.e., it interacts with GABA receptors to produce an increase in neuronal chloride conductance (Saunders and Ho 1990; Davies et al. 1998). A major action of GABA, an inhibitory neurotransmitter substance, is to increase chloride permeability in postsynaptic neurons (Enna 1981). The sedative and anesthetic properties of the barbiturates are a result of their interaction with the GABA receptor complex. When barbiturates bind to the barbiturate receptor portion of the GABA receptor complex, the rate of dissociation of GABA from its receptor is decreased and increased chloride conductance is maintained. This results in membrane hyperpolarization and reduced neuronal excitability. As the barbiturate concentration increases, barbiturates can directly activate chloride channels even without GABA present. The GABA-dependent increase in chloride conductance may be the mechanism for the sedative-hypnotic effects of the barbiturates while the GABA- independent increases result in "anesthesia" (Fragen and Avram 1994). It is becoming more apparent that there is a multiplicity of GABA, barbiturate, and benzodiazepine receptors that are associated or linked together in many ways.

Transmission of nerve impulses at synaptic as well as at neuroeffector junctions is normally decreased by barbiturates; blocking effects of decamethonium and *d*-tubocurarine upon skeletal muscle are increased. These effects occur because barbiturates decrease sensitivity of polysynaptic junctions to the depolarizing action of acetylcholine.

It has been demonstrated in animals, particularly cats, that barbiturates raise the threshold of spinal reflexes. Lowering of the threshold by strychnine can be overcome by barbiturates, even to the practical elimination of crossed reflexes. Barbiturates are used clinically with considerable success in treatment of strychnine poisoning and other convulsants.

Numerous investigators have directed their work toward the effect of barbiturates upon the reticular activating system of the CNS. This system is particularly sensitive to barbiturates (Harvey 1975). Animals are unable to be aroused or to maintain the wakeful state following administration of hypnotic to anesthetic dose levels of barbiturates.

Respiratory Center. With the exception of the cat, therapeutic doses of barbiturates depress respiration slightly, but no more than would be expected from the general sedation produced by the drug. In the cat the marked susceptibility of respiratory function following barbiturate administration, especially its marked blocking effect upon the reticular formation, may explain why this animal reacts adversely to barbiturates. The reticular formation of the cat apparently feeds signals or impulses into the medullary control centers governing respiration. In contrast to a single major mechanism in most other species, respiratory activity appears to be governed at two levels within the CNS.

In many animals, subanesthetic doses of barbiturates accelerate respiration rate (Borison 1978). Conversely, large doses are markedly depressant to the respiratory center in the medulla. Doses of barbiturates that induce deep surgical anesthesia severely depress frequency as well as tidal volume of respiration, resulting in a dangerous hypoxia and respiratory acidosis.

IV injection of a barbiturate produces a more severe depression of respiration than that following oral administration, probably as a result of production of a higher momentary concentration of drug effective upon the center. The blood concentration inhibiting the respiratory center is considerably less than that arresting the heart. Therefore, when respiratory arrest occurs during barbiturate anesthesia, attention should be devoted first to reestablishing respiration, since the heart continues to function for a brief period. According to Chenoweth and Van Dyke (1969), more animals are lost from failure to maintain an adequate airway than from any other single difficulty in anesthesia. In most species, insertion of an endotracheal tube can be accomplished so that oxygen and artificial ventilation may be given when depression of respiration results from an anesthetic overdose. Pentobarbital at a dose of approximately four times that producing respiratory arrest may be administered before cardiac arrest occurs in the artificially ventilated animal.

Cardiovascular System. Pentobarbital is probably the most widely used IV anesthetic by biomedical research laboratories in a dose of 25–30 mg/kg in the dog (Frederiksen et al. 1983). Although there is universal agreement that the anesthetic induces tachycardia (originally thought to be caused by its vagolytic activity in the above dose), reports of its effects on arterial pressure and cardiac output are divergent. An excellent study of pentobarbital anesthesia upon various hemodynamic parameters has been conducted in the dog by Manders and Vatner (1976); effects upon mean arterial pressure, systolic arterial pressure, cardiac output, total peripheral resistance, and heart rate are summarized in Fig. 12.2 for intact and denervated (bilateral sectioned carotid sinus and aortic nerves) dogs. Mean arterial pressure drops from a control of 91 ± 2 to 85 ± 3 mm Hg at 2.5 minutes; it returns to control at 7.5–10 minutes and then falls slightly below at 15–25 minutes. Systolic arterial pressure is significantly depressed for the entire measurement period. Cardiac output rises from 2.20 ± 0.16 to 2.73 ± 0.24 L/min at 2.5 minutes, then gradually declines. However, it is significantly reduced below the control only at 25–30 minutes. The total peripheral resistance drops significantly below control at 2.5 minutes, rises above the control at 15 minutes, and remains significantly elevated. Stroke volume falls from 33 ± 3.0 to 18 ± 2.8 mL ($P < 0.01$) and remains significantly depressed. Heart rate rises from 80 ± 3 to 160 ± 4 beats/min at 2.5 minutes, then drops gradually to 109 ± 5 beats/min at 30 minutes. Myocardial contractility in the dog falls significantly following pentobarbital anesthesia, as reflected by 30–40% decreases in myocardial force ($\Delta P/\Delta t$), myocardial velocity, and shortening velocity (Manders and Vatner 1976).

Following bilateral sectioning of the carotid sinus and aortic nerves, the role of arterial pressoreceptor reflexes in the dog has been determined during pentobarbital anesthesia (Manders and Vatner 1976). As anticipated, in denervated animals, arterial pressure drops by a significantly greater amount. The most surprising effect of denervation is absence of tachycardia after pentobarbital anesthesia. Inasmuch as heart rate does not remain elevated during anesthesia in denervated dogs, the mechanism for tachycardia appears to

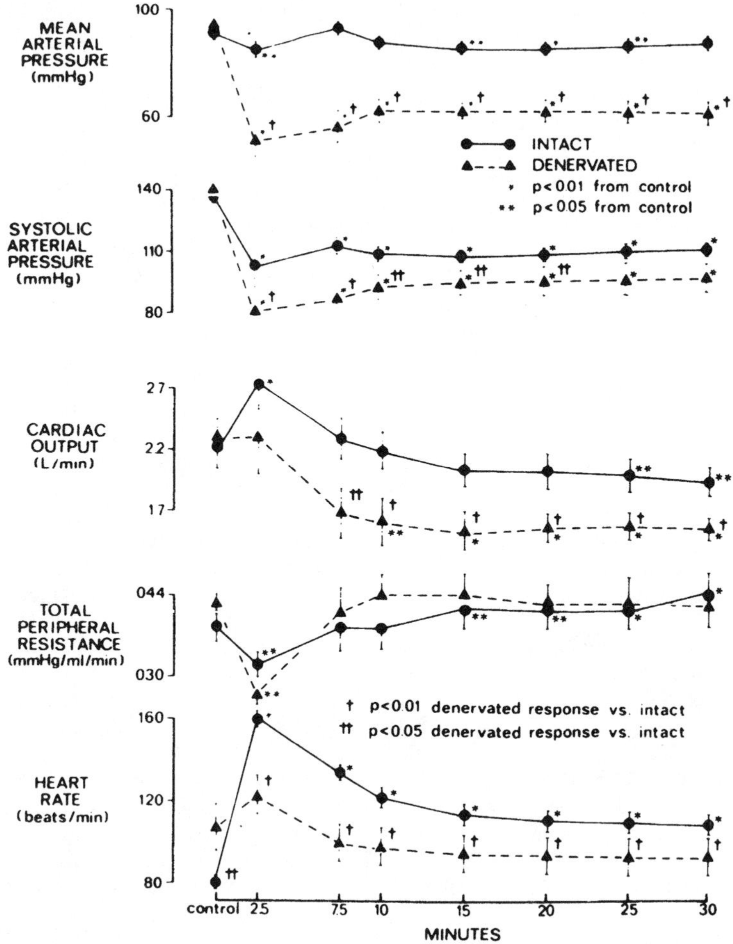

FIG. 12.2—Effects of pentobarbital, 30 mg/kg intravenously, on mean arterial pressure, systolic arterial pressure, cardiac output, total peripheral resistance, and heart rate of intact dogs (n = 9, solid lines) and denervated dogs (n = 7, dashed lines). * = changes significantly different from control. † = responses of denervated dogs that are significantly different from those of intact dogs. I = ± SEM. Intact dogs were able to maintain arterial pressure better than denervated dogs. In both cases systolic arterial pressure fell significantly. The heart rate response in the denervated dogs was qualitatively different from that of the intact ones, since heart rate failed to rise in the denervated dogs (Manders and Vatner 1976).

be mediated by arterial pressoreceptor reflexes rather than by a vagolytic effect of pentobarbital (Manders and Vatner 1976).

In the calf, cardiac output does not appear to change significantly following IV injection of a relatively small dose of pentobarbital (Anderson et al. 1972). However, a transient but significant effect upon pulmonary and systemic circulations may occur following administration of this anesthetic. A pressor response of the pulmonary circulation is observed, which may be attributable to a local vasoconstrictor effect on resistance vessels. In contrast to a pulmonary pressor effect produced by pentobarbital in cattle, it appears to have no effect upon the resistance vessels of pulmonary circulation in dogs. Pentobarbital appears to have a varying effect on systemic circulation (Anderson et al. 1972). These authors consistently observed tachycardia, which also has been seen in other species.

The incidence of ventricular fibrillation is increased, especially when animals are subjected to both anesthesia and hypothermia (Blair 1969). Ventricular fibrillation may occur in 100% of the hypothermic animals following administration of pentobarbital. It occurs in 50% of the animals following administration of thiopental.

In contrast to thiamylal-halothane anesthesia, the arrhythmogenic dose of epinephrine, dopamine, or dobutamine necessary to produce ventricular arrhythmia during pentobarbital anesthesia is greater in normothermic dogs (Bednarski and Muir 1985).

Consequently, pentobarbital does not sensitize the myocardium to catecholamine-induced arrhythmia.

The vascular system, especially the vasomotor center, is affected more by the concentration of barbiturate acting on it than by the total dose given. Rapid IV injection of a relatively safe dose of barbiturate causes a sharp but transitory fall in arterial pressure because of the high concentration briefly depressing the vasomotor center. Large IV doses depress the vasomotor center, resulting in peripheral vasodilation with a severe drop in arterial pressure. Excessive IV concentrations of barbiturates may injure capillary musculature directly to such an extent that sufficient capillary dilation occurs to induce vascular shock.

Pentobarbital and streptomycin interact to induce vasodilation in the perfused kidney and other vessels of the dog. Administration of Ca^{++} antagonizes the renal vascular effects of streptomycin (Wolf and Wigton 1971). IV injection of Ca^{++} antagonizes the hypotensive effects of streptomycin during pentobarbital anesthesia in dogs. Consequently, the inhibitory effects of aminoglycoside antibiotics on Ca^{++}-dependent vascular functions appear to contribute to their hypotensive activity in intact animals (Adams et al. 1976).

There is indication that pentobarbital also influences myocardial performance by Ca^{++}-dependent mechanisms; e.g., it appears to decrease binding availability of Ca^{++} at superficial membrane sites in cardiac cells (Nayler and Szeto 1972). Since aminoglycoside antibiotics such as streptomycin, neomycin, and possibly others also alter Ca^{++}-dependent functions, it is most likely that interaction with pentobarbital occurs. Such an interaction should induce a severe cardiodepressant effect, especially upon the myocardial contractile mechanism.

Intra-arterially, barbiturates, in particular thiopental, produce spasm of the arterial wall to the extent that massive gangrene occurs. Accidental intra-arterial injection of barbiturates has occurred on a number of occasions in humans and has resulted in the loss of fingers or the arm from thrombosis and gangrene. Thiopental has been shown to cause vasoconstriction in the perfused rabbit ear; this effect was associated with release of norepinephrine from the arterial wall. Under no circumstances should barbiturates, especially thiobarbiturates, be injected intra-arterially for induction of anesthesia. In humans, effects of an inadvertent, intra-arterial injection can be significantly minimized or completely prevented by using a solution of thiopental no greater than 2.5%.

A congenital porphyrin condition ("pink tooth") is sometimes observed in cattle. Porphyrin metabolism may be disturbed in normal animals from exposure to chemicals such as hexachlorobenzene, griseofulvin, and aminopyrine. In the liver, synthesis of porphyrin comes about by condensation of succinyl coenzyme A with glycine to form aminolevulinic acid. Formation of this acid occurs in the mitochondria of hepatic cells through enzymic activity (i.e., aminolevulinic acid synthetase). Barbiturates stimulate greater production of this enzyme, which increases porphyrin production. Death may occur in humans because the rise in porphyrin levels leads to neurologic disturbances from demyelination of peripheral and cranial nerves. Animals afflicted with a known or suspected disturbance in porphyrin metabolism should not be subjected to a barbiturate anesthetic.

Caution should be taken during administration of barbiturates in animals that have had extensive blood loss. The anesthetic induction dose may decrease from 28 to 38% after severe hemorrhage (Weiskopf and Bogetz 1985).

Gastrointestinal (GI) Tract. As a group, barbiturates appear to depress activity of intestinal musculature. However, after an initial depression, thiobarbiturates may increase both tonus and motility. After years of clinical use, no important effects such as diarrhea or intestinal stasis have been noted.

Kidney. The barbiturates appear to have no direct effect upon the kidney. Lack of renal function does not appear to alter the pharmacokinetics of pentobarbital (Davis et al. 1973). According to Davis and coworkers, the anesthetic can be used in dogs with impaired renal function. Pentobarbital elimination is normal in humans afflicted with renal failure (Reidenberg et al. 1976). However, sensitivity of animals to barbiturates may be increased by uremia; e.g., pentobarbital, hexobarbital sodium, and other barbiturate sleeping times are increased in uremic animals. This interesting phenomenon is due to a decreased capacity of the plasma protein for binding acidic drugs such as barbiturates.

By lowering blood pressure, barbiturates can indirectly produce oliguria or anuria. Only when prolonged, as in overmedication, does this effect become important. A drop in renal blood flow of as much as 42% may occur up to 1 hour following pentobarbital anesthesia.

There is some evidence that phenobarbital and occasionally pentobarbital inhibit water but not saline diuresis in dogs, possibly through an influence upon the antidiuretic hormone.

Barbital, a long-acting barbiturate, is excreted primarily unaltered in urine. The substituent group on carbon 5 of phenobarbital (also a long-acting barbiturate) is resistant to oxidation by the liver or other tissues. Unaltered long-acting barbiturates are excreted slowly over several days, which accounts for their prolonged periods of action. This slow excretion may lead to cumulative toxicity when an excessive dose is administered repeatedly. In the dog, about 20–25% of the total dosage of barbital is excreted in urine in the first 24 hours. A total of 85% is excreted in urine in 6 days.

In humans, as much as 50% of a dose of phenobarbital is excreted by the kidney in the unaltered form (Harvey 1975). Clearance of phenobarbital is considerably greater in alkaline than in acid urine. In carnivores, alkalinization of urine with sodium bicarbonate increases the elimination rate of long-acting barbiturates. Use of sodium bicarbonate and diuretics is clinically useful in treatment of intoxication from long-acting barbiturates.

Renal damage interferes with excretion of long-acting barbiturates. There is real danger of severe depression and death when these drugs are administered to a patient with impaired renal function.

Chickens will recover from pentobarbital anesthesia, but the avian kidney excretes barbital so slowly that they die in coma from respiratory failure. Since intermediate and long-acting barbiturates are detoxified over a prolonged period, they are not recommended for anesthetic use in avian or mammalian species.

Liver. Therapeutic doses of barbiturates have no significant effect upon liver function. In patients with liver damage, large doses of barbiturates may cause further injury. The detoxifying action of the liver has been discussed above under the fate of barbiturates.

Uterus and Fetus. Sedative doses of barbiturates do not influence uterine activity. Full anesthetic doses are believed, on the basis of in vitro studies, to depress uterine contractions during parturition. However, an equally if not more important consideration is the effect of barbiturates upon the fetus. Most barbiturates that have been studied can traverse the placenta with relative ease (Mirkin 1975). Equilibrium between maternal and fetal circulations is established within a few minutes in most circumstances.

Pentobarbital and thiopental in concentrations that fail to produce maternal anesthesia will completely inhibit fetal respiratory movements without maternal hypoxia prevailing. However, thiopental is not as depressant to the fetus as pentobarbital. Even though respiration is not completely depressed in a newborn animal following use of a barbiturate, there is no assurance that the animal will survive. A number of studies have revealed that the liver in the newborn of a number of animals lacks the microsomal enzyme system required to biotransform or metabolize drugs such as barbiturates. This important enzyme mechanism usually begins to develop during the 1st week following birth and does not attain maximal development until 8 weeks of age or older. Without this important enzyme mechanism to assist in degradation of barbiturates, the animal must depend primarily on renal elimination of the drugs. Even this route poses a problem because renal function in the newborn is less efficient than in the mature animal. Clinically, it is well known that a cesarean section performed solely under barbiturate anesthesia will depress the fetus and may produce up to 100% fetal mortality.

Hormone Release, Metabolism, and Clearance. In the rat, it is well established that the luteinizing hormone (LH) and follicle-stimulating hormone rise concomitantly on the afternoon of proestrus and that injection of pentobarbital just before onset of the spontaneous gonadotropin surge prevents this release from taking place. This phenomenon is referred to as pentobarbital-blockade (Chappel and Barraclough 1976). LH release is either suppressed or delayed in the normal, cycling female baboon (*Papio* sp.) by pentobarbital following IM injection of 35 mg/kg (Hagino 1979).

Pentobarbital anesthesia also depresses plasma LH concentration in the hamster and markedly elevates plasma concentrations of progesterone and cortisol in sheep. Use of pentobarbital in combination with halothane elevates progesterone and cortisol plasma levels in the ewe (Green and Moor 1977). Since barbiturates reduce both renal and hepatic blood flows, reduction in hepatic metabolism and renal excretion of steroids is partially if not principally responsible for the increase in plasma concentrations of progesterone and cortisol.

Metabolic Rate. Sedative doses of barbiturates do not significantly influence the basal metabolic rate. Doses producing surgical anesthesia depress basal metabolism so that less body heat is produced during anesthesia concurrently with excessive heat loss as a result of vasodilation. It is important that surgical patients anesthetized with barbiturates be kept warm while depressed, especially when overmedicated. Consequently, it is always wise to monitor the effect of barbiturate anesthesia upon body temperature (Chenoweth and Van Dyke 1969). With a decline in heat production during anesthesia and an increase in heat loss owing to peripheral vasodilation, the anesthetized animal drifts toward the temperature of the surrounding environment (Lutsky 1969). A definite hypothermic state is seen when the anesthetized dog is exposed to air temperatures below 27°C (Dale et al. 1968); rectal temperature decreases from 1 to 5° at an air temperature of 27°C to 10–18° at an air temperature of 10°C. This not only results in prolongation of recovery from pentobarbital anesthesia but deaths also occur. During winter energy shortages, lower room temperatures in operating and recovery rooms have been responsible for inducing hypothermia and delayed recovery from anesthesia in small animals (Waterman 1975).

Skeletal Muscle. Barbiturates (particularly pentobarbital) suppress sensitivity of the motor endplate of skeletal muscle to acetylcholine (Seyama and Narahashi 1975). However, barbiturates do not completely relax the abdominal musculature. If additional relaxation is required in surgery, curariform agents may be used. Since skeletal muscle relaxants are not analgesics or anesthetics, caution in using them under the guise of anesthesia must be avoided for humane reasons. The photomotor reflex should be checked to determine whether an animal is regaining consciousness when a skeletal muscle relaxant is used in conjunction with a barbiturate anesthetic.

In the horse, postanesthetic forelimb lameness believed to be due to muscular ischemia during the recumbent phase of anesthesia has been observed in animals subjected to barbiturate and inhalant anesthetics (Trim and Mason 1973).

Absorption. Barbiturates are absorbed readily from the GI tract. The rate of absorption varies but in general is faster for short-acting and slower for long-acting drugs. Although intrathoracic administration of barbiturates is not recommended, absorption following this route is quite rapid.

After IV injection, pentobarbital in plasma reaches distribution equilibrium in the brain within 3–4 minutes.

Distribution. Barbiturates are distributed more or less generally throughout the body. Values for the specific volume of distribution (V′d) have not been determined for many barbiturates. Not only would these values differ for different barbiturates but also among the various species. In the goat, the V′d for pentobarbital (30 mg/kg) administered intravenously is 0.72 L/kg; the first-order disappearance rate kinetic constant (Kd) is 0.76 hour and the half-life ($t_{1/2}$) is 0.91 hour (Boulos et al. 1972). In the dog, the elimination-phase half-life (8.2 ± 2.2 hr) of pentobarbital is considerably longer (Frederiksen et al. 1983).

Thiopental, a highly lipid soluble drug, passes readily through the blood-brain barrier. Soon after IV injection, its concentration in cerebrospinal fluid and plasma of the dog is found to be nearly equal. Phenobarbital and barbital have low partition coefficients and penetrate the blood-brain barrier much more slowly. CNS depression does not occur until 15 minutes or longer following IV administration of these compounds.

Thiobarbiturates are initially present in quite high concentrations in highly perfused tissues (e.g., the brain), resulting in rapid induction of general anesthesia. Thiobarbiturates then redistribute to the moderately perfused body tissues (such as muscle). This redistribution to moderately perfused tissues decreases the brain concentration to a level which allows the animal to regain consciousness. Further redistribution to adipose tissue from both highly and moderately perfused tissues results in the complete recovery from thiobarbiturate anesthesia. Since sighthounds (e.g., Greyhounds) have a lower percentage of adipose tissue, their complete recovery from the thiobarbiturates is delayed. Other patients with cachexia or with extremely low body fat would also be expected to have prolonged recoveries from thiobarbiturates (Price et al. 1960; Paddleford 1988).

Barbiturates diffuse through the placenta into fetal tissue and may occur in the milk in small amounts. It is possible to detect minute amounts of barbiturates in body fluids such as plasma and urine as low as 500 pg/mL using radioimmunoassay procedures (Flynn and Spector 1972).

Fate. Barbiturates are eliminated by renal excretion in urine and/or destroyed by oxidative activity of hepatic and extrahepatic tissues. Trace amounts may be excreted in milk of a lactating female.

TABLE 12.2—Degradation of barbiturates by liver, brain, and muscle brei (120 μg of appropriate barbiturate added to all samples)

Barbiturate	Percentage liver destruction	Percentage brain destruction	Percentage muscle destruction
Seconal	30	0	0
Pentothal*	53	10	0
Phenobarbital	0	0	0

Source: Dorfman and Goldbaum 1947.
*Thiopental sodium.

HEPATIC METABOLISM. Pentobarbital and many other barbiturates are metabolized principally by the hepatic microsomal enzyme system (Freudenthal and Carroll 1973). Disappearance of pentobarbital from plasma of dogs is attributed to biotransformation of the drug by the liver as well as redistribution to muscle and adipose tissue. Pentobarbital is 3-hydroxylated or oxidized by liver microsomes. Evidence indicates that oxidative metabolism is not necessarily impaired in patients with poor renal function (Reidenberg et al. 1976).

Approximately 50% of the dose of pentobarbital given is recovered in urine as the 3-hydroxy metabolite. The rate of hydroxylation or oxidation of pentobarbital is increased markedly by pretreatment with phenobarbital. Thiobarbiturates are destroyed by the liver and extrahepatic tissues, especially in brain and kidney. Their destruction in the extrahepatic tissues is more rapid than for any other barbiturates (see Table 12.2). Oxybarbiturates are metabolized by the liver.

The rate at which thiobarbiturates are metabolized is not as rapid as previously thought. Originally, their brief action was believed to parallel the rate of destruction by the liver and extrahepatic tissues. Metabolism of thiopental is too slow to account for its rapid disappearance from plasma. Later it became apparent that the systemic action of the thiobarbiturates was quickly terminated by redistribution from the brain to other body tissues.

Short-acting barbiturates are not recovered from urine following sedative doses and in only trace amounts at higher doses. Activity of these drugs is brief because of rapid tissue oxidation. Additional evidence of the importance of the liver in destruction of many barbiturates is the clinical finding that anesthesia with a short-acting barbiturate may be prolonged many times in the presence of hepatic injury or disease. The clinician should therefore avoid use of short-acting barbiturates in patients showing liver disturbances. A dose of thiopental or a comparable ultrashort-acting barbiturate producing anesthesia in a normal patient for only about 15 minutes may anesthetize a patient with impaired liver function for several hours.

Studies have shown that a number of drugs, including pentobarbital, are metabolized by hepatic microsomal enzymes (Conney 1967), which are located in the endoplasmic reticulum. Activity of drug-metabolizing

TABLE 12.3—Effects of certain barbiturates injected intravenously in dogs

Barbiturate	Number of dogs	Dose	Duration of anesthesia*	Down time†	Return to normal§	Average respiratory rate
		(mg/kg)	*(min)*	*(min)*	*(min)*	
Pentobarbital	8	25	200	252	358	11
Hexobarbital	12	40	69	183	340	19
Thiopental	12	26	50	69	137	15

Source: Hunt et al. 1948.
*anesthesia = absence of pad reflex.
†Down time = from onset of anesthesia until animal stood.
§Return to normal = from onset of anesthesia until the dog could climb stairs without ataxia.

enzymes in hepatic microsomes may be affected by several factors; e.g., newborn and young animals possess only a fraction of the capability of adult animals to metabolize drugs, and starving the animal significantly depresses the activity of hepatic microsomes to metabolize drugs. Liver microsomal activity may be accelerated by administration of various drugs (e.g., phenobarbital, phenytoin) to the degree that the same drug or others may be metabolized at a greater rate; e.g., phenobarbital has the capability of stimulating metabolism of other barbiturates. Consequently, animals become resistant or tolerant to these drugs because of a greater rate of metabolism of the barbiturate to inactive metabolites. This phenomenon has been noted in rats pretested with phenobarbital; they were anesthetized only 11 minutes by hexobarbital compared to 216 minutes for the control group. Chemical agents such as DDT and other chlorinated pesticides can affect duration of anesthesia produced by pentobarbital; DDT administered 2 days prior to pentobarbital reduces duration of anesthesia in animals by 25–50% (Conney and Burns 1972).

After exposure to phenobarbital, it may take up to 7 months for the complete disappearance of enzyme induction in the dog. Once initiated, it may continue for a long period.

SPECIES VARIATION. The rate of metabolism of barbiturates varies considerably between and among various species; e.g., the mouse metabolizes hexobarbital many times faster than humans. In general, most laboratory animals metabolize drugs more rapidly than humans. The cat, however, is an exception and requires a longer time to metabolize barbiturates. Pentobarbital is metabolized at a rate of 4%/hr in humans compared with 15%/hr in dogs and 50%/hr in horses. In ruminants, particularly sheep and goats, pentobarbital is metabolized at a rapid rate (Bryant 1969). In sheep, pentobarbital is cleared from plasma at the rate of about 49%/hr, and thiopental is cleared at about 17%/hr following tissue equilibrium. The mean biologic half-life of pentobarbital in the plasma of sheep is 66.8 ± 16 minutes (Santos and Bogan 1974). The difference in the rate of metabolism is the primary cause of the differences in the duration of action seen when pentobarbital is administered to various species. The reappearance of CNS reflexes occurs at similar plasma levels after pentobarbital anesthesia in goats and dogs, but the time for the return of those reflexes is much longer in dogs (Davis et al. 1973).

Pretreatment of sheep with phenobarbital does not influence in vitro metabolism of hexobarbital or pentobarbital (Shetty et al. 1972). Apparently, sheep are incapable of inducing a more rapid rate of metabolism in an already active microsomal enzyme system.

Tolerance. Dogs become tolerant to several barbiturates as determined by the reduction in anesthesia time of a given and frequently repeated dose. Cross-tolerance for all barbiturates occurs with a tolerance developed to one barbiturate. Tolerance is soon lost by withdrawal of the drug.

This is known as pharmacodynamic tolerance. As applied to barbiturates, this involves adaptation of nervous tissue to the presence of the drug (Harvey 1975).

Development of tolerance to barbiturates in dogs would be of interest only in clinical cases where sedative doses of barbital or phenobarbital have been given regularly for prolonged periods.

Stimulation or induction of microsomal enzyme activity in the liver markedly affects duration of action of barbiturates. The so-called development of tolerance that occurs after a brief exposure to barbiturates in low dosage is due to enhancement of microsomal enzyme activity.

Duration of Depressant Effect. Duration of action of two IV barbiturates (pentobarbital, thiopental) commonly used in veterinary medicine is illustrated in Table 12.3. The same depth of surgical anesthesia was obtained for all drugs, with a dosage carefully determined by previous trials.

Duration of the depressant actions of orally administered barbiturates is illustrated in Fig. 12.3, which is based on more than 1000 trials in dogs (Swanson 1944). Other factors to be considered are nutritional status, age, and individual variations in the animal. A starved animal is much more sensitive to barbiturates because of a reduced ability to metabolize them (Chenoweth and Van Dyke 1969). Neonates and young animals are less able to metabolize barbiturates than adults and therefore will be anesthetized much longer

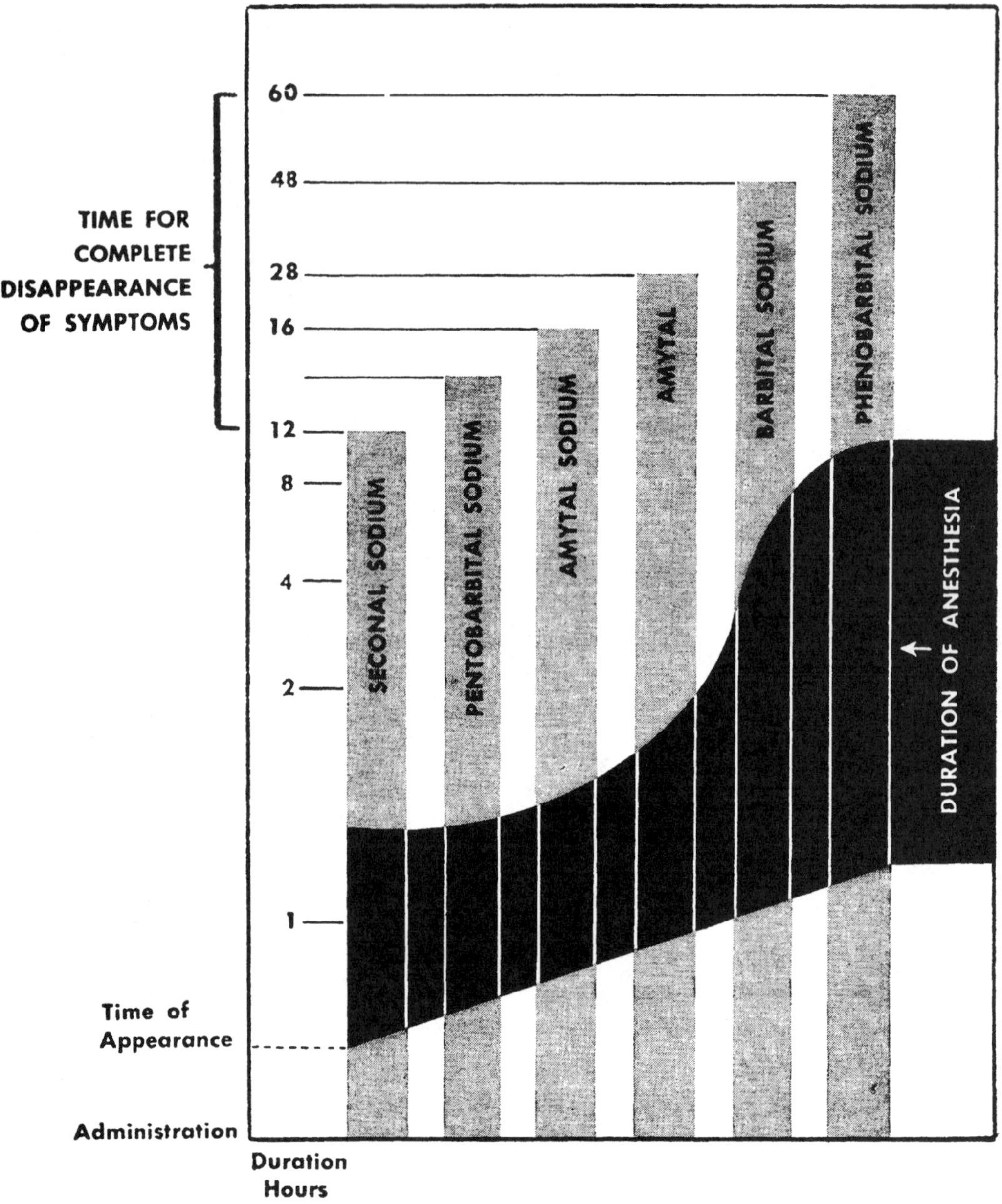

FIG. 12.3—Time of appearance, duration of anesthesia, and time needed for complete disappearance of symptoms after oral administration of equivalent single anesthetic doses in animals (Swanson 1944; courtesy of the Lilly Research Laboratories).

and recover more slowly from the depressant effects. Even the influence of circadian rhythm can appreciably affect the depth of depression and duration of anesthetic action (Simmons et al. 1974). In nocturnal animals such as laboratory rodents, the hazard of drug-induced mortality is increased at night and recovery is prolonged. Individual variations exist not only because of age, sex, weight, and nutritional status but also with respect to the degree that microsomal enzyme induction is affected; this may vary qualitatively and quantitatively among individuals as well as among species (Chenoweth and Van Dyke 1969).

In addition to species variation, there are differences within the breeds of animals with respect to duration of action of barbiturates. For example, thiobarbiturates induce longer anesthetic effects in Greyhound dogs than in mixed breeds (Sams et al. 1985). Methohexital, an oxybarbiturate, induces a shorter period of anesthesia in the Greyhound than thiobarbiturates such as thiopental or thiamylal.

As long ago as 1962, it was known that chloramphenicol could prolong the hypnotic action of hexobarbital in mice and slow its rate of biotransformation. Duration of the depressant effect of pentobarbital is prolonged by pretreatment or concurrent administration of chloramphenicol (a broad-spectrum antibacterial agent) in the mouse, rat, dog, cat, and monkey (Adams 1970; Adams and Dixit 1970; Teske and Carter 1971). Chloramphenicol suppresses or inhibits hepatic microsomal enzyme activity. If it is given immediately preceding administration of pentobarbital in the dog and cat, a 120% increase in duration of anesthesia occurs. This effect can be produced by relatively small quantities of chloramphenicol and can be detected as long as 24 days following the last administration of the antibiotic agent.

If an animal has had a recent history of being treated with chloramphenicol, pentobarbital should not be used for induction of anesthesia for at least 25 days following. Since duration of anesthetic action of thiobarbiturates does not appear to be affected by chloramphenicol (Adams and Dixit 1970), their use should be safer for induction of anesthesia, followed by maintenance of anesthesia with inhalant anesthetics. Nevertheless, it is advisable to use thiobarbiturates conservatively following administration of chloramphenicol. Studies in mice given chloramphenicol sodium succinate simultaneously with thiamylal indicate that sleep is about 10 times longer compared with sleeping time in animals given thiamylal alone (Azadegan et al. 1980).

The anesthetic action of barbiturates, but not of other common depressants, can be potentiated by IV or intraperitoneal injection of dextrose; fructose; intermediary metabolites such as lactate, pyruvate, and glutamate; and a few other substances of diverse nature. The lactate, pyruvate, and glutamate are known to increase the rate of entrance of barbital into the brain and thus increase cerebral depression. It is probable that dextrose, fructose, and other substances act similarly. This reaction can be inhibited by administration of acetylcholine, which decreases cell permeability and entrance of barbital into the cortex. Clinically, about one-fourth the dogs just recovering from pentobarbital anesthesia can be reanesthetized by IV injection of 550 mg/kg lactate; about one-half will give a partial response, and the remaining one-fourth are refractory.

Other studies reveal that doses of glucose of 200 to greater than 600 mg/kg administered intravenously in the dog fail to influence the mode of respiration or the electroencephalogram (EEG) shortly after induction of surgical anesthesia with pentobarbital (Hamlin et al. 1965). Fear of embarrassing ventilation or depression of cortical activity through a "glucose effect" should not contraindicate infusion of glucose. However, this conclusion may require some modification (Hatch 1966). According to Hatch's study, rapid IV administration of glucose in the dog that is regaining voluntary movement from thiopental anesthesia results in immobilization of 11% of the subjects. This period of apparent reanesthetization represents about a 50% increase in sleep time. Sodium lactate causes a similar reimmobilization in 39% of the dogs, with approximately 50% increase in sleep time. Epinephrine produces reimmobilization in about 85% of the animals with an extension of about 40% in total sleep time. Hatch (1966) concluded that the possibility of producing reanesthetization with glucose, sodium lactate, and epinephrine need be of no practical concern as long as these substances are used properly. Improper use of these compounds, especially in the presence of longer acting barbiturates, could lead to a dangerously prolonged period of incapacitation.

Influence of adrenergic agents upon recovery of dogs anesthetized with thiopental and methohexital sodium has been studied by Heavner and Bowen (1968). Administration of epinephrine and isoproterenol at the time dogs are recovering from thiopental anesthesia results in reanesthetization. This effect is not seen in animals recovering from methohexital anesthesia. Reanesthetization of dogs recovering from thiopental has not been associated with α- or β-adrenergic activity. Heavner and Bowen (1968) believe there is a possibility that epinephrine produces a peripheral analgesic action that is responsible for the reanesthetization because depression of the sensory electroneurogram of the superficial radial nerve is induced.

Reinduction of thiopental anesthesia is also induced by administration of high doses of aspirin and phenylbutazone in the rat (Chaplin et al. 1973). These nonsteroidal anti-inflammatory agents displace thiopental from rabbit plasma proteins in vitro. It is unlikely that reinduction of anesthesia by these agents is as marked in animals that have received pentobarbital because its binding to sheep plasma (36%) is less than the binding of thiopental (67%). Nevertheless, the sleep time of pentobarbital in small laboratory rodents can be significantly increased by sulfonamides (sulfanilamide, sulfamethazine, sulfaethylthiazol), salicylic acid, acetylsalicylic acid (aspirin), sodium salicylate, and doxycycline. All these drugs displace pentobarbital and other barbiturates from plasma proteins, which leads to an increased blood level of unbound barbiturate for further depressant effect upon the CNS. With the increasing number of pharmacologic agents used in therapeutic procedures, the clinician needs to be alert to these potential drug interactions.

Even the type of bedding upon which an animal is kept has a marked effect on anesthetic dosage and duration of anesthesia. Softwood bedding such as cedar or pine shavings induces drug-metabolizing enzymes in the liver, thus reducing the period or duration of anesthesia.

Duration of the depressant effect of barbiturates is also generally increased (except for barbital) by hypothermia (Blair 1969); the activity of pentobarbital is greatly enhanced, and sleeping time in the dog at a body temperature of 27°C is 3.5 times that of the normothermic sleeping time. Consequently, about one-third of the normal dose of pentobarbital is required to maintain a specified level of anesthesia at this temperature (Blair 1969). Inadvertent hypothermia can be avoided by frequent or continuous temperature monitoring and by employing warming boards, water mattresses, or other such devices (Lutsky 1969).

Use of thiobarbiturates in maintenance of anesthesia cannot be supported or condoned (Dodman et al. 1984). Their continuous use in maintenance of anesthesia will result in prolonged and unfavorable recovery.

Anesthetic-Antibiotic Interaction. In cats anesthetized with pentobarbital, administration of neomycin induces a complete neuromuscular paralysis (Adams and Mathew 1974), which is believed to be due to the persistent binding by neomycin of Ca^{++}-receptive sites at the motor end plate of skeletal muscle. Apnea and death have also occurred in a dihydrostreptomycin-treated dog that was originally breathing spontaneously during recovery from pentobarbital anesthesia (Adams and Bingham 1971). The above examples illustrate problems that may occur in a patient seemingly recovering uneventfully from anesthesia and surgery. The margin of safety of neuromuscular transmission should be considered when anesthetics, neuromuscular blocking agents, and antibiotics that depress neuromuscular function are employed in multiple drug regimens (Adams et al. 1976).

The effect of chloramphenicol upon suppression of microsomal enzyme activity and the depressant effect of pentobarbital anesthesia has been discussed.

Margin of Safety. All barbiturates seem to possess approximately the same margin of safety between the anesthetic dose and the median lethal dose (LD_{50}). Using recommended techniques of administration, 50–70% of the LD_{50} is needed to anesthetize an animal. Apparently no barbiturate possesses a markedly advantageous margin of safety over any other when the anesthetic dose and the LD_{50} are compared. However, fewer postanesthetic complications follow use of the shorter acting barbiturates because of the reduced incidence of hypostatic congestion, which often leads to cardiopulmonary as well as other complications.

Toxicology. Barbiturates produce death by depression of the respiratory center, which leads to cessation of respiration. As the severity of CNS depression progresses, respiration becomes shallow and slow. The pupils dilate as hypoxia develops. A weak and rapid pulse exists. Reflexes disappear and the skin is cold and cyanotic. Sometimes the respiration stops abruptly following too rapid IV injection of a barbiturate; following this, the heart continues to beat briefly until hypoxia and hypercarbia cause cardiac arrest. More often, breathing continues at a progressively depressed rate and amplitude until it stops within a few minutes after the drug is given. Mechanical obstruction of the airway must be avoided, especially in brachiocephalic breeds of dogs. Artificial respiration with 100% oxygen should be administered to prevent hypoxia. Although less reliable than use of oxygen, doxapram or other analeptic drugs may be used to stimulate the respiratory center.

Shorter-acting barbiturates such as pentobarbital are largely destroyed by the liver and therefore should not be administered to animals with hepatic disease. Patients suffering from shock and toxemia have a lesser margin of safety than normal animals. The newborn cannot metabolize barbiturates as readily as adults and consequently have a lesser margin of safety and are subject to more prolonged effect.

When barbiturates are injected intravenously, the lethal dose varies inversely with rate of injection. The more rapid injection results in a higher local blood concentration that is able to paralyze the vital medullary centers. The amount administered actually would not be a lethal dose if injected slowly. Fatal doses of pentobarbital cause some inflammation of the vital organs, congestion of the brain and meninges, and perivascular hemorrhage and edema.

A drug interaction has been reported in mice treated with cyclophosphamide, a potent antineoplastic agent of the mustard family, and barbiturates (hexobarbital, phenobarbital, pentobarbital). An increased lethality occurs when barbiturates are administered concurrently with cyclophosphamide (Rose et al. 1973). Since cyclophosphamide is being used increasingly as an antineoplastic agent in animals, the clinician must remember to omit use of all barbiturates in such cases.

Pentobarbital Sodium. Immediately after its introduction, *Pentobarbital Sodium,* USP (Nembutal sodium, Pentobarbitone sodium, Sagatal, Napental), was widely accepted in veterinary medicine as a surgical anesthetic. At one time it was the most widely used anesthetic agent in small animals.

The structure of pentobarbital is similar chemically to thiopental sodium. The presence of the oxygen atom in the pentobarbital molecule instead of a sulfur atom is the differentiating characteristic of the two barbiturates (see Fig. 12.4 for the comparative structural formulas). The human formulation (Nembutal) uses propylene glycol as a vehicle and has been associated with intravascular hemolysis when administered intravenously to animals at doses sufficient to produce anesthesia.

ADMINISTRATION AND ORAL DOSAGE. Pentobarbital can be administered orally to carnivora to produce sedation. If the stomach is empty, the drug may be given orally to produce surgical anesthesia in about 0.5 hour at a dose level of 28–30 mg/kg. Oral administration in food produced lateral recumbency in five of six dogs in an average of 59 minutes at an average dose of 63 mg/kg (Ramsay and Wetzel 1998).

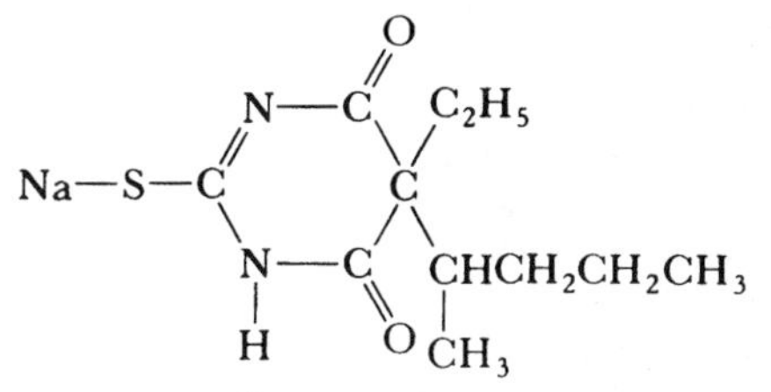

```
              O
             //
         N—C   C2H5
        //   \ /
Na—S—C       C
        \    / \
         N—C   CHCH2CH2CH3
         |  \\   |
         H   O  CH3
```

Thiopental Sodium

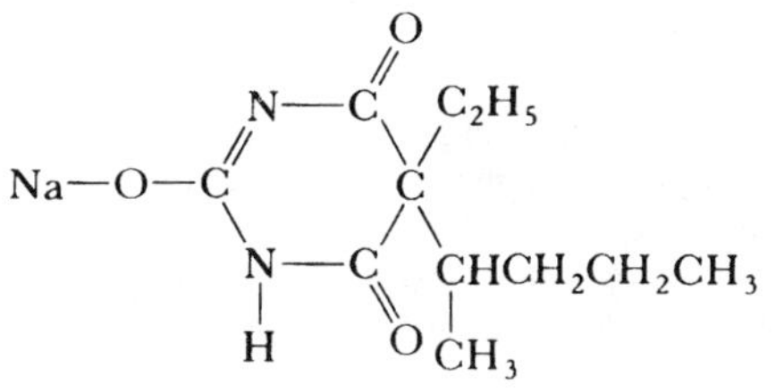

```
              O
             //
         N—C   C2H5
        //   \ /
Na—O—C       C
        \    / \
         N—C   CHCH2CH2CH3
         |  \\   |
         H   O  CH3
```

Pentobarbital Sodium

FIG. 12.4

INTRAPERITONEAL. Intraperitoneal injection of pentobarbital has been widely practiced in small animals but now is limited primarily to those difficult to restrain for IV injections, such as rodents and other small laboratory animals. The dose generally employed is 28–30 mg/kg up to 15–16 kg, but is reduced somewhat for heavier animals. Depression appears in about 15 minutes and persists in some measure 4–8 hours.

INTRAVENOUS. IV injection of pentobarbital is the most satisfactory method of administration for production of anesthesia. This route generally can be used in all species and is most often preferred in veterinary medicine where restraint of the patient is practicable. By this method the dose is not inflexibly set by weight but can be fitted to the individual susceptibility of the patient or administered "to effect" as judged by disappearance of normal reflexes.

The IV dose is determined by the response desired, and the drug is given until the desired effect is obtained. However, the anesthetic dose approximates 24–33 mg/kg. Once the anesthetic is injected, it cannot be removed. Duration of pentobarbital anesthesia in the dog is 1–2 hours (Leash 1969); 4 or more hours are usually required before an animal is ambulatory after an IV injection.

Injections should be made carefully to avoid accidental perivascular deposit of pentobarbital, since it irritates the tissues and occasionally causes sloughing. If a perivascular injection of the barbiturate inadvertently occurs, the area should be infiltrated with 1 or 2 mL 2% procaine hydrochloride or 2% lidocaine hydrochloride solution (Leash 1969). If these solutions are unavailable, infiltration with a physiologic saline solution may be of value in reducing tissue irritation and eventual sloughing.

An IV injection of a small dose of pentobarbital may be used to produce hypnosis or sedation to avoid the fright, excitement, and resistance to restraint that are so dangerous and objectionable in handling a patient. This sedation can be followed by a local or an inhalant anesthetic.

INTRAMUSCULAR. Pentobarbital has been suggested via the IM route in the dog (Leash 1969). Doses recommended are 20 mg/kg for basal anesthesia, 30 mg/kg for moderate anesthesia, and 40 mg/kg for general anesthesia. However, this route of administration is not recommended because of the likelihood of tissue irritation and variability in effect.

INTRATHORACIC. Barbiturates have been administered by the intrathoracic route to animals such as the cat. Since trauma, pleural irritation, and parenchymal necrosis of lung tissue can occur following the intrathoracic injection of barbiturates, this route is not recommended. This method is sometimes used for euthanasia of animals when IV or other routes are inaccessible.

CLINICAL USE. Although pentobarbital is used in a number of species, it is approved by the US Food and Drug Administration (FDA) for use only in the dog and cat.

DOGS AND CATS. Pentobarbital is frequently used as an anesthetic in the dog and cat. However, it is not without toxic effects that require constant alertness by the veterinarian. For brief anesthesia, pentobarbital is surpassed by the ultrashort-acting barbiturates of more recent introduction. For IV anesthesia in the dog, about 24–33 mg/kg of pentobarbital in about 3–6% aqueous solution should be used. The average IV dose for dogs is approximately 30 mg/kg. In the cat, the recommended IV dose is 25 mg/kg with an additional 10 mg/kg if the initial dose is inadequate (Strobel and Wollman 1969).

Approximately one-half the anticipated dose should be injected at a moderately fast rate so that stage II, or the excitement stage, of anesthesia is bypassed. A pause for a few seconds to 1 minute is recommended to allow the drug to exert its full effect. Thereafter, the pentobarbital must be injected to effect. It is administered slowly in repeated small amounts over a period of 2–4 minutes with continuous observation of reflexes and respiratory activity until the desired depth of surgical anesthesia is obtained. Induction of anesthesia intravenously is generally uneventful; however, delirium or excitement as seen in stage II may occur if the initial dose is inadequate.

Sometimes an IV injection must be stopped in the presence of shock or toxemia. A given level of anesthesia will persist for about half an hour, after which depression decreases, with complete recovery in 6–24 hours. Some dogs show considerable delirium or excitement during recovery, as manifested by whining, barking, attempts to stand or walk, and leg paddling movements. Narcotic analgesics or phenothiazine tranquilizers in combination with barbiturate anesthesia are often used to eliminate this undesirable behavior (Leash 1969).

Basically, the procedure for induction of pentobarbital anesthesia in the cat is similar to that described for the dog. The anesthetic dose of pentobarbital by the IV route is not appreciably different on a body weight basis than that of the canine species. Female cats (33 mg/kg) are more susceptible to action of pentobarbital than males (40 mg/kg). In the newborn kitten, pentobarbital is an inadequate anesthetic, since the depth of anesthesia is difficult to control and recovery time is extremely prolonged (Sis and Herron 1972). In the adult cat, recovery of the righting reflex after an IV dose of 30 mg/kg pentobarbital occurs in 270 ± 52 minutes; recovery of the corneal and flexor withdrawal reflexes occurs at 25 ± 8 minutes and 31 ± 11 minutes respectively (Child et al. 1972a).

Premedication. Sometimes it is difficult to intravenously inject an excitable dog or cat that has not been previously medicated with a depressant drug. Without administration of a preanesthetic agent, the average dog requires 28.6 mg/kg pentobarbital to become surgically anesthetized. Use of preanesthetic agents not only renders the animal easier to handle and treat but also decreases the amount of barbiturate up to 50% or more for surgical anesthesia and reduces the likelihood of excitement during recovery. Xylazine, used as a sedative preanesthetic agent, decreases the dose of pentobarbital necessary to induce anesthesia in dogs up to 78% (Hatch et al. 1983).

In severely toxic patients, pentobarbital alone should not be used to depress a patient beyond the beginning of light surgical anesthesia. It is much safer to use preanesthetics to reduce the amount of pentobarbital needed. In many instances the safest anesthesia in toxic patients is obtained by premedication with a narcotic analgesic or a short-acting barbiturate followed by an inhalant anesthetic. Atropine sulfate is an additional preparation that should be used routinely prior to barbiturate anesthesia.

Control of Convulsions. Pentobarbital is an important drug for relieving convulsive seizures, especially when caused by strychnine or other convulsants. IV administration is preferable because a better balance between convulsant and depressant influences can be obtained. In the dog, pentobarbital is antidotal to as much as 35 LD_{50} of strychnine.

Treatment with pentobarbital of convulsions induced by lidocaine hydrochloride in the dog results in a detrimental or lethal interaction (Caron and LeLorier 1979). It is quite well known that lidocaine, a local anesthetic, has general anesthetic properties. Studies in the late 1950s in humans revealed that IV lidocaine reduces the amount of barbiturate (thiopental) required to accomplish smooth anesthesia by 13%. Unlike phenobarbital, a dose of pentobarbital that will produce unconsciousness is needed to control seizures (Macdonald and Barker 1979).

Lethal Doses. The lethal dose of pentobarbital in the dog is 85 mg/kg orally and 40–60 mg/kg intravenously. Toxicosis, including death, has been reported in dogs fed uncooked meat from a horse euthanatized 8 days previously with pentobarbital (Polley and Weaver 1977). It is unlikely that cooking inactivates pentobarbital in meat, since the chemical is considered to be relatively stable. Animals euthanatized with pentobarbital and rendered in a steam-jacketed cooker for about 3 hours at 127–132°C show virtually no degradation of the drug (O'Connor et al. 1985).

Toxicosis in a bitch has been reported from ingesting a puppy euthanatized by pentobarbital (Fucci et al. 1986). Indiscriminate disposal of carcasses that contain large quantities of barbiturates should be avoided.

Euthanasia. Several barbituric acid derivatives may be used in euthanasia of small animals. Of the barbiturates, pentobarbital is most commonly used (Report of the AVMA Panel on Euthanasia 1993).

The lethal dose for dogs, administered intravenously, is generally regarded as 40–60 mg/kg or approximately double the dose used for surgical anesthesia. Both respiratory and cardiac arrest occur following successful euthanasia.

COWS AND HORSES. Pentobarbital will produce surgical anesthesia in the horse, mule, and cow as well as other large animals, but its use alone is not generally recommended. Some excitement may be noted, even with rapid induction. At the completion of IV injection of pentobarbital alone, the horse sometimes rears and falls over backward, injuring the poll. Pentobarbital produces prolonged periods of recumbency and usually excitement during recovery. Large animals make futile attempts to stand before they have recovered complete control of their locomotor activities, and dangerous struggling occurs.

Pentobarbital has been used with greater success in foals and small colts for sedation (e.g., while taking radiographs) and anesthesia. Minimal excitement occurs in some.

Pentobarbital can be used in large animals as a sedative, or it may be used preoperatively in combination with a local anesthetic. An IV dose of 1–4.4 mg/kg provides a marked sedative or hypnotic action, so with the aid of a local anesthetic, several standing operations can be performed if desired.

SWINE. Pentobarbital administered by IV injection provides reasonably good anesthesia in swine weighing less than 45 kg. Above this weight, pentobarbital appears to have a considerably lessened margin of safety. The tendency in the USA is to administer only sedative dosages of pentobarbital intravenously in heavy swine and to follow this with local anesthesia at the surgical site. Since respiratory depression is readily induced in swine following barbiturate anesthesia, hypoxia and hypoventilation can be prevented by use of oxygen.

IV dosages of pentobarbital should be fitted to each patient or administered to effect by observing the disappearance of reflexes. Slow injection of the solution is essential. Recovery generally requires 60–90 minutes. Pentobarbital appears to have a considerable margin of safety in pigs of 10–22.5 kg. It has been determined that 24 mg/kg produces anesthesia suitable for most kinds of surgery. For swine weighing over 99 kg, the IV dose should be no more than 19.8 mg/kg. For castration of a large boar where brief light anesthesia is required, only 9.9 mg/kg via the IV route is needed.

Pentobarbital is also administered intratesticularly to achieve anesthesia for castration procedures (Henry 1968). A dose of 1.5 mL (450 mg)/10 kg pentobarbital (300 mg/mL concentration or a 30% solution) is injected into each testicle with a maximum of 20 mL per testicle for a very large boar. Satisfactory anesthesia is achieved within 10 minutes after administration. It is recommended that the anesthetic solution be injected below the tail of the epididymis in the upper one-third of the testicle. After injection of the anesthetic, the animals become incoordinated in a few minutes. Recumbency occurs between 5 and 15 minutes following administration. As soon as no response is elicited upon pricking the scrotal skin with a needle, the castration procedure should be conducted as rapidly as possible. The unabsorbed anesthetic solution is eliminated with surgical removal of the testes, allowing for a more rapid and safe recovery. Recovery from anesthesia requires 20–40 minutes. To avoid fatal poisoning in dogs or other animals, the testes should be disposed of properly.

Preanesthetic medication not only reduces the amount of anesthetic required for major surgical procedures but facilitates handling of the pig prior to induction of anesthesia (Booth 1969). Preanesthetic medication in the pig consists of atropine (0.07–0.09 mg/kg), meperidine hydrochloride (1–2 mg/kg), and promazine hydrochloride (2 mg/kg). All preanesthetic preparations are injected intramuscularly in separate sites 45–60 minutes prior to administration of the anesthetic. It is often necessary to administer atropine at hourly intervals during anesthesia to prevent salivation and mucus formation in the respiratory tract.

IV pentobarbital (9 mg/kg) administered 2 minutes after IM ketamine (11 mg/kg) induces surgical anesthesia for 45 minutes in swine weighing up to 50 kg; atropine sulfate (0.05 mg/kg) and fentanyldroperidol (1 mL/13.7 kg) are administered intramuscularly as premedicants 10 minutes prior to administration of ketamine (Bauck 1984).

GOATS AND SHEEP. Pentobarbital has a short duration of action in ruminants compared to other species because of a more rapid microsomal oxidative metabolism. The initial IV anesthetizing dose (25 mg/kg) of pentobarbital in the goat should be administered slowly (Bryant 1969). Anesthesia will be deep for about 5 minutes and then become less until complete recovery occurs in 40–60 minutes. Duration of satisfactory anesthesia is about 20 minutes, which is sufficient time to catheterize the jugular vein for supplementary injections and to intubate the trachea. Compared to the dog, duration of anesthesia in the goat is much shorter for an equivalent level of anesthesia. It is preferable to use pentobarbital for induction of anesthesia in the goat and then to maintain it with an inhalant anesthetic after tracheal intubation.

In adult sheep, pentobarbital is rapidly metabolized, requiring additional increments to maintain anesthesia for more than 15–30 minutes. The drug is useful for induction of anesthesia; this permits intubation of the trachea and maintenance of anesthesia by use of inhalant anesthetics. The average dose of pentobarbital for induction of anesthesia is about 24 mg/kg, with a range of 11–54 mg/kg. In the lamb, the IV dose of pentobarbital ranges from 15 to 26 mg/kg; this usually maintains anesthesia for 15 minutes. An additional 5.5 mg/kg administered intravenously extends anesthesia a further 30 minutes. Recovery from anesthesia is rapid. Short et al. (1985) reported that an IV dose of 14.3 mg/kg pentobarbital produces anesthesia in sheep for about 5.39 ± 7.5 minutes; this time was from induction to return of the palpebral reflex.

RABBITS. Rabbits are considered to be one of the more difficult and unpredictable species of laboratory animals to anesthetize because they vary considerably in response to commonly used anesthetic agents, and the margin between surgical anesthesia and respiratory arrest is narrow (Murdock 1969). According to Murdock, the recommended IV dose of pentobarbital is generally 25–40 mg/kg. One-half to three-fourths of the calculated dose of 2% pentobarbital is injected slowly into the marginal ear vein until the animal becomes relaxed. Injection of more concentrated solutions is apt not only to lead to an overdose of the anesthetic but to cause severe injury to the vessel wall to the extent that thrombosis occurs. If this happens, vessel occlusion results, which will ultimately lead to necrosis and sloughing of the affected portion of the ear. Recovery from pentobarbital anesthesia is erratic in the rabbit, varying from 1 to 10 hours.

MINK. IV injection is not practical in vicious animals. Pentobarbital (22 mg/kg), injected subcutaneously, has been reported to produce a hypnosis suitable for examining mink and for artificial insemination procedures. The hypnotic state occurs in about 10 minutes and lasts for about 40 minutes, with complete recovery in about 1.5 hours.

Pentobarbital (35 or 40 mg/kg) has been used intraperitoneally in ranch mink (*Mustela vison*) without mortality (Graham et al. 1967). The use of diazepam, a neuroleptic agent, may be beneficial in mink prior to administration of anesthetics. Diazepam has been of value in calming aggressive and vicious animals prior to mating.

BIRDS. According to a number of literature sources, pentobarbital administered alone and intravenously has not been satisfactory as an anesthetic for the chicken because of the narrow margin of safety. The dose of pentobarbital varies greatly in chickens of the same strain, age, sex, and weight. Dose levels fatal for some birds produce only light anesthesia in others.

Pentobarbital readily depresses respiration or may paralyze respiratory activity of the chicken. However, it has been the experience of investigator, R. A. Herin, that pentobarbital (15 mg/kg) administered through the external thoracic vein provides safe anesthesia when oxygen is continuously administered to prevent hypoxia. Pentobarbital has been used in mature chicken hens for induction of light narcosis prior to inhalation of ether for maintenance anesthesia (Fussel 1969). The barbiturate is administered intraperitoneally in an average dose of 25 mg/kg; greater doses frequently produce respiratory and cardiac failure. Pentobarbital has a hypotensive action in fowl; soon after its administration there is a decline of 30–50 mm Hg in the arterial blood pressure, but this is followed by partial recovery in a few minutes.

Pentobarbital has also been satisfactorily used in the turkey by injecting 26 mg/kg via the radial or saphenous veins. It is recommended that birds be fasted 12–18 hours prior to anesthesia. Use of pentobarbital in the Aylesbury domestic duck by IV injection (30–60 mg/kg) produces unsatisfactory anesthesia (Desforges and Scott 1971).

An anticholinergic agent such as atropine sulfate (0.045 mg/kg intramuscularly) should be administered prior to use of barbiturates in birds to prevent bronchial secretion. Pentobarbital (1%) has been administered intramuscularly at a dose level of 0.01 mL (0.1 mg)/2 g to canaries, sparrows, parakeets, and chickens. Induction of anesthesia occurs in about 2 minutes; 5–9 minutes following the injection there is no skeletal muscle resistance to extension of the extremities. Surgical anesthesia lasts for approximately 30 minutes; the birds stand within 90 minutes after the injection.

Pentobarbital has been used for anesthesia in the Adelie penguin (*Pygoscelis adeliae*) (Andrews 1975). A dose of 50 mg/kg is recommended intraperitoneally for deep surgical anesthesia if it is a nonsurvival procedure. Induction of anesthesia is slow in the penguin, requiring an average time of 130 minutes. Up to 45% of body weight of the penguin consists of adipose tissue. What effect this may have upon anesthetic absorption and distribution is unclear. In addition, barbiturates appear to be metabolized very slowly in the penguin (Andrews 1975).

NONHUMAN PRIMATES. With introduction of ultrashort-acting barbiturates (thiopental, thiamylal), use of pentobarbital in primates has declined; however, pentobarbital is essentially safe and effective in monkeys. In the rhesus monkey (*Macaca mulatta*) most anesthetic failures in healthy animals following pentobarbital administration are attributable to an excessively rapid rate of injection or use of a highly concentrated solution (Domino et al. 1969). The commercially available pentobarbital solution containing 60 mg/mL is too concentrated and should be diluted 1:2 or 1:4 just prior to use. Moreover, the solution must be injected by slow, steady infusion at a rate not to exceed 2 mL/min until the corneal reflexes are abolished and respiration becomes slow, deep, and regular. Monkeys so treated can be expected to remain in surgical anesthesia for a minimum of 2 hours; recovery ordinarily does not occur in less than 6 hours (Domino et al. 1969).

Pentobarbital has been very useful as a restraint and anesthetic agent in the chimpanzee (*Pan troglodytes*) (Day 1965). The dose of pentobarbital recommended for mature and young chimpanzees is 24–29 mg/kg and 29–40 mg/kg respectively. A 5% pentobarbital solution is used in both age groups. Anesthesia occurs in most instances in 6–15 minutes. Complete recovery usually results within 6–8 hours, with the younger animals recovering in less time.

GUINEA PIGS AND GERBILS. Although the usual intravascular routes (IV and intracardiac) for administering anesthetics are available in the guinea pig, they are infrequently used (Hoar 1969); the intraperitoneal route is most common because of its easy and ready accessibility. A number of literature sources indicate that the anesthetic level for pentobarbital is 15–30 mg/kg administered intraperitoneally. However, an intraperitoneal dose of pentobarbital as high as 50 mg/kg is used in guinea pigs (McKay and Clement 1977). A heated operating board is recommended to prevent the severe hypothermia that occurs following this dose.

In the gerbil, pentobarbital in a dose of 5 mg/100 g (50 mg/kg) is recommended intraperitoneally (Stunkard and Miller 1974).

RATS AND MICE. Pentobarbital diluted in sterile physiologic saline solution is usually given intraperitoneally at a dose of 30–40 mg/kg to the adult albino male rat (Ben et al. 1969). However, Sprague-Dawley rats, both male and female, weighing 300–350 g are anesthetized with 60 mg/kg of pentobarbital intraperitoneally (Kawabori 1979).

Female rats are usually less capable of metabolizing pentobarbital and may require less than the male. Pentobarbital may be administered by the IV route in the rat; however, the dose level and rate of administration must be carefully observed (Ben et al. 1969). In mice, pentobarbital is the most commonly used parenteral anesthetic agent and is generally given intravenously or intraperitoneally in doses of 40–70 mg/kg (Taber and Irwin 1969). Intraperitoneally, this dose range induces anesthesia of 20–30 minutes following a latency interval of 5–10 minutes with less than 10% mortality. Literature sources indicate that male mice are more sensitive to the effect of barbiturates than females. In the neonatal subject (1–4 days old), an intraperitoneal dose of 5 mg/kg pentobarbital produces anesthesia of approximately 1 hour (Taber and Irwin 1969).

AMPHIBIANS AND REPTILES. Frogs (*Rana pipiens*) can be satisfactorily anesthetized with pentobarbital administered through the dorsal lymph sac at a dose of 60 mg/kg (Kaplan 1969). Surgical anesthesia is attained in about 0.5 hour and will last for as long as 9 hours. Turtles (*Pseudemys*) can also be anesthetized with pentobarbital by IV or intracardiac injection at a dose level of 15.5–17.5 mg/kg. Induction time of anesthesia is approximately 30–53 minutes by these routes; the animals may remain in deep anesthesia as long as 3 hours. Turtles may also be anesthetized by the intraperitoneal route with pentobarbital at a dose of 16 mg/kg (Kaplan 1969).

BEARS AND LARGE CATS. Pentobarbital has been used intravenously (37–59 mg/kg) in bears following IM administration of morphine sulfate (8.8 mg/kg) and promazine (4.4 mg/kg). For safe handling and minor surgery, a mean IV dose of 13.5 mg/kg pentobarbital is recommended in bears; supplemental increments will maintain the animals in anesthesia for up to 6 hours. The principal disadvantage in using pentobarbital in bears is the necessity for immobilizing them so that a venipuncture can be made; once this is achieved, pentobarbital (12–15 mg/kg) is administered as rapidly as possible (Day 1965). This is about 50–75% of the anesthetizing dose. The remaining portion is then given until an adequate level of anesthesia is reached.

Pentobarbital is contraindicated in any of the large zoo cats because of their apparent inability to metabolize it. Large cats may be anesthetized for 6 or 7 days following use of pentobarbital. When ultrashort-acting barbiturates (thiamylal or thiopental) are administered, these animals sleep 6–24 hours.

Thiopental Sodium. As the name indicates, *Thiopental Sodium,* USP (Pentothal sodium, Intraval sodium, Thiopentone sodium), is a sulfur-containing barbiturate or a thiobarbiturate. Instead of having the *R*-O-Na characteristic of most other sodium salts of the barbituric acid derivatives, thiopental possesses a sulfur atom, *R*-S-Na, in substitution for the oxygen atom. Except for the sulfur atom, thiopental is similar chemically to pentobarbital (see Fig. 12.4). Thiopental is classified as a Schedule III drug under the 1970 Controlled Substances Act.

Thiopental is a weak organic acid with a pK_a value of 7.6; it has a relatively low ionization (39%) at the pH of plasma (Brandon and Baggot 1981). High lipid solubility of the nonionizing moiety is the primary property of this anesthetic agent, permitting it to quickly penetrate the blood-brain barrier.

STORAGE AND STABILITY. Thiopental is available in sealed, evacuated or nitrogen-filled ampules as a powder buffered with sodium carbonate and should be stored away from light in a cool place. It is unstable in aqueous solution or when exposed to moisture. Steady deterioration occurs in proportion to the temperature of the solution. For maximum effect and safety, aqueous solutions of thiopental should be prepared just prior to use. When large amounts are used, as in a hospital, a bulk solution of thiopental may be prepared if careful attention is given to its expiration date. A 5% bulk solution can be stored in a refrigerator at 5–6°C until turbidity appears, but for no longer than 7 days. At room temperature at 18–22°C a solution should be kept no longer than 3 days. Solutions kept beyond these limits contain clinically active thiopental, but the progressive loss of action at any given period cannot be easily determined. When aged solutions are used, the same characteristic action of the drug is obtained by injecting larger volumes of solution. However, from the standpoint of maintaining a reliable anesthetic and surgical routine, it is desirable to use fully potent, fresh solutions.

PHARMACOLOGIC CONSIDERATIONS. Thiopental is not ordinarily associated with excitatory side effects and, even when administered in dosages sufficient to induce an isoelectric electroencephalogram (EEG), has no ostensible direct toxic effect on the CNS (Steen and Michenfelder 1979). In the dog, large doses have been given to produce an isoelectric EEG for 30 minutes or longer. Under these conditions, cerebral oxygen consumption is about 40% of normal; brain energy stores, i.e., adenosine triphosphate and phosphocreatine, are normal throughout this period as well as the concentration of brain lactate. Such findings in dogs are consistent with the clinical experience with barbiturate intoxication in humans. If respiratory and circulatory supports are instituted early enough and adequately maintained in reversal of the intoxication, cerebral recovery is expected even when EEG activity is initially absent (Steen and Michenfelder 1979).

In the horse, thiopental elevates the blood glucose level and induces a leukopenia. The cardiac rate increases, while cardiac output decreases. No significant change in arterial pressure or packed cell volume occurs in the horse following administration of thiopental. Respiration is slowed and frequently becomes irregular for brief periods. This leads to an elevated arterial P_{CO2} and concomitant decrease in blood pH. Plasma levels of thiopental do not correlate well with the clinical signs or EEG in the horse or other species.

Middleton et al. (1982) reported that 60% of the cats in a study developed apnea that lasted over 50 seconds after the beginning of an IV injection of 1.25% thiopental (20 mg/kg) at a rate of 0.5 mL/sec. Also, a mild arterial hypotension occurs between 5 and 10 minutes after injection.

In Greyhound dogs (22–25 kg), IV administration of 2.5% thiopental (10 mg/kg) reduces systemic arterial pressure about 40% immediately after injection (Smith et al. 1982). However, the pressure returns to near normal within 5 minutes after injection.

In the dog, thiopental has an arrhythmogenic effect with an incidence of about 40%. This is lower than the incidence (i.e., 85%) of arrhythmia produced in the dog by thiamylal (Pedersoli and Brown 1973).

IV thiopental-induced (20 mg/kg) anesthesia potentiates development of ventricular arrhythmia when epinephrine is administered to halothane-anesthetized dogs (Atlee and Malkinson 1982). This potentiation may last for at least 4 hours after the thiopental-induced anesthesia (Bednarski et al. 1985).

Anesthetics such as the ultrashort-acting barbiturates (thiopental, thiamylal, methohexital)that trigger cardiac arrhythmias set the stage for the heart to go into ventricular fibrillation, especially if endogenous or exogenous catecholamines appear at the right time.

Compared to IV thiopental (22 mg/kg) alone in the dog, the IV combination of thiopental (11 mg/kg) and lidocaine (8.8 mg/kg) induces no arrhythmia and produces less cardiopulmonary depression (Rawlings and Kolata 1983). Bigeminy, with alternating premature ventricular depolarization and normal sinus-initiated depolarizations, occurred after intubation of the trachea during 19 of 20 thiopental inductions; the bigeminies were preceded by tachycardia and an increase in arterial pressure during tracheal intubation. In contrast, 20 dogs given the thiopental-lidocaine combination did not develop cardiac arrhythmia. According to Rawlings and Kolata (1983), the thiopental-lidocaine combination would appear to be a good method of inducing anesthesia in animals with cardiopulmonary disease because it elicits less cardiopulmonary depressive effects and protects against arrhythmia.

Between 30 and 60 minutes of IV thiopental anesthesia (25 mg/kg) in the dog, there is a slight decrease in cardiac output and left ventricular work (Ahlgren et al. 1978). Blood flow is reduced to the lungs, kidneys, and liver. Between 60 and 90 minutes following administration of thiopental, a steady state in cardiovascular function is essentially attained. Only blood flow to the liver remains below normal.

METABOLISM AND DISTRIBUTION. Thiopental is metabolized primarily by the hepatic microsomal enzyme system. Studies in the monkey with thiopental containing labeled sulfur, S^{35}, indicate that at least 12 metabolic products are excreted in urine. Within 4 days after an IV injection of 35 mg/kg, the monkey excretes about 86% of the dose in urine. Additional small amounts are found in feces and tissues.

In humans, only about 0.3% of administered thiopental is excreted unchanged, indicating that the drug is almost totally transformed. Oxidation of one of the alkyl side chains yields thiopental carboxylic acid, a metabolite of thiopental, which is almost completely metabolized; only traces of this metabolite appear in urine. The metabolite has little if any anesthetic activity. In chronic renal failure patients (human), the rate of thiopental elimination is much the same as in normal individuals (Burch and Stanski 1982).

In clinical anesthesia a small dose of thiopental has a brief duration of action, not because of its rapid metabolic destruction but because of rapid distribution of the drug from plasma into the adipose tissues. Actually, the metabolic conversion of thiopental is slow (10–15%/hr). Since fat is capable of localizing thiopental, the plasma level of the anesthetic is below that required to maintain anesthesia, and the animal recovers soon after injection. Following large doses or repeated small doses of thiopental, the plasma level remains near that of the fat and tissues, and anesthesia persists for a longer period because of slow metabolism of the anesthetic.

Use of a thiobarbiturate such as thiopental in maintenance of anesthesia is not condoned (Dodman et al. 1984). Its continuous use in maintenance of anesthesia will result in prolonged and unfavorable recovery.

Since recovery depends on redistribution of thiopental from the brain to other tissues, animals that are severely cachexic will have prolonged recoveries.

In sheep, thiopental is cleared from plasma at the rate of 17%/hr after tissue equilibrium is reached. The half-life of thiopental in sheep (herbivore) is about one-half that of the carnivore (Baggot et al. 1984). Pentobarbital is cleared at a rate of approximately 49%/hr in sheep. Binding of the two barbiturates to sheep plasma proteins occurs to the extent of 67% for thiopental and 36% for pentobarbital. Only free (unbound) thiopental is able to cross the blood-brain barrier.

The phenomenon of microsomal enzyme induction has been demonstrated in calves pretreated with phenobarbital (Sharma et al. 1970). Plasma levels of thiopental are reduced at a more rapid rate as a result of enzyme induction. The development of enzyme induction should be considered while treating domestic animals because they are frequently exposed to potent inducers of microsomal enzymes such as halogenated pesticides and other compounds. Such induction may be responsible for wide variation in metabolism of certain drugs and may greatly affect an animal's response (Sharma et al. 1970).

PHARMACOKINETICS. After IV injection of thiopental (20 mg/kg) in a concentration of 2%, the apparent volume of distribution in sheep is 1005 ± 196 mL/kg (Toutain et al. 1983). Its body clearance is 3.5 ± 0.8 mL/kg/min and the plasma half-life is 196 ± 64 minutes.

In the dog, IV administrations of 2.5% thiopental results in a plasma half-life of 6.99 ± 2.18 hours, an apparent volume of distribution of 843 ± 194 mL/kg and a body clearance value of 1.51 ± 0.60 mL/kg/min (Brandon and Baggot 1981). The plasma half-life of thiopental in the dog is about 5–6 times longer than in sheep. According to Brandon and Baggot, the relatively short duration of thiopental anesthesia in sheep may be attributed primarily to biotransformation of the drug by hepatic metabolism and uptake by body fat.

Pharmacokinetic studies of thiopental have been made possible by development of a highly sensitive, rapid reverse phase, high-pressure liquid chromatographic (HPLC) method (Christensen and Andreasen 1979). The detection limit of thiopental in blood by HPLC is 90 ng/mL, or 90 ppb.

TOXICITY. The major toxic effect of thiopental is a marked depression of the respiratory centers; the rate is slowed and amplitude decreased. Ordinarily, the respiratory rate is a good indication of the condition of the animal and the dosage of drug. When given properly, thiopental has little toxic action upon the cardiovascular system, about 16 times as much is needed to stop the myocardium as to paralyze respiration. As long as the cardiovascular system functions well, there is every opportunity for recovery of a patient if proper oxygenation is maintained by artificial respiration.

An apparent lethal anaphylactic response to thiopental has been reported in the dog (Mason 1976). The reaction developed 10 days following a second administration in a 4-year-old Border Collie. Acepromazine and atropine premedication in conjunction with β-irradiation therapy as well as a corticosteroid were used during thiopental anesthesia. A survey of the veterinary medical literature failed to locate any evidence of anaphylactic reaction to thiopental. Anecdotal evidence suggests equine patients may occasionally develop urticaria after thiopental administration. In humans, an anaphylactic reaction to repeated administration of thiopental is recognized as a rare entity. Painful vesicular lesions (mouth, skin), referred to as fixed-drug eruptions, have been reported in the human several hours after conclusion of thiopental anesthesia (Butler et al. 1982).

In general, thiopental possesses a wide margin of safety. The twice daily injection of 20 mg/kg into dogs for 2–3 weeks results in only slight depression of liver function.

GENERAL USE. The brief duration of effect of thiobarbiturates can be employed advantageously for numerous conditions, including setting fractures; gynecologic, radiographic, and other kinds of examinations; short surgical procedures; and premedication to an inhalant anesthetic. The rapid, complete recovery permits quick return of the patient to the owner if hospitalization is undesirable. The minimal hypnotic dose of thiopental injected intravenously produces anesthesia for only about one-fourth as long as pentobarbital under the same conditions.

During World War II, thiopental came into wide use as a routine anesthetic in humans in front-line hospitals where equipment was limited.

ADMINISTRATION AND DOSAGE. Thiopental is administered only by IV injection. Subcutaneous or IM injections are irritating and may result in sloughing of tissue. The anesthetic is too irritant to inject into a body cavity. An equal volume of 1% procaine infiltrated into the perivascular tissue where the thiopental may have been injected by accident is claimed to obviate the usual tissue reaction. Thiopental is usually prepared as a 2.5% solution for IV injection in smaller animals. In larger animals the concentration should be increased to 5%, although 10% solutions have been used. It should be borne in mind that injection of the more concentrated solution (5 or 10%) will produce serious complications if the barbiturate anesthetic is accidentally administered intra-arterially. The "quick-shot" administration of thiopental in the horse via the external jugular vein may result in inadvertent injection of the anesthetic extravascularly. This often results in severe tissue reaction, including abscessation and necrosis of the involved tissue (Jones 1968). If thiopental is accidentally injected perivascularly, normal saline should be injected to dilute the drug; in addition, hyaluronidase should be added to normal saline to promote dispersion and absorption of the thiopental (Jones 1968).

The amount of thiopental needed varies with the disposition of the patient and the nature of the operation. Of the several factors seeming to influence depth and duration of anesthesia, the most important is rate of injection. When small animals are injected rapidly (i.e., within 0.5 min), onset of anesthesia is abrupt and sometimes alarming. It must not be forgotten that too rapid IV injection depresses the vasomotor center and results in a vascular dilation with sudden drop in blood pressure.

Rapid injection usually induces anesthesia in less than a minute and lowers the dosage needed, but the anesthesia is of brief duration. Duration is directly proportional to the time taken for injection of the anesthetic dose. The duration can vary from 2–3 minutes to 25–30 minutes, depending on the rate and amount of drug injected. At either extreme, the same depth of depression can be produced. Repeated injection of thiopental is not advised; recovery is prolonged with each additional dose administered. Barbiturate anesthesia in the horse should not be maintained for long periods; no more than a total of 5 g of any barbiturate should be administered intravenously even to horses of draft proportions (Heath 1977).

In the dog, the anesthetic IV dose of thiopental approximates 15–17 mg/kg; for the cat it is 9–11 mg/kg (Mark et al. 1968) up to 20 mg/kg (Middleton et al. 1982). However, each dose should be adjusted to the patient to compensate for individual differences. Regardless of the dose, the initial injection of a solution of thiopental in small animals should consist of about 13 mg/kg followed by a pause of 30–60 seconds. The remainder of the desired dose can be injected to effect during the next 1–2 minutes.

For brief anesthesia of 7–10 minutes (suitable for radiography, minor surgery, and examinations) a dose of 13–18 mg/kg is suggested. In myelography it is advisable to avoid use of barbiturates; sodium methiodal, a contrast medium, may displace bound thiopental and induce anesthetic complications (Bonhaus et al. 1981). For anesthesia of 10–15 minutes, as might be needed for reducing a fracture, a dose of 18–22 mg/kg is desirable. For anesthesia of 15–25 minutes to permit major surgery, a dose of 22–29 mg/kg is needed in most small animals. Thiopental is not recommended for extended periods of anesthesia. It may be used to induce anesthesia, followed then by safer agents such as inhalant anesthetics for prolonged effect. A small dose of thiopental injected rapidly produces anesthesia briefly.

If desired, morphine can be administered preanesthetically to thiopental as it is to pentobarbital. However, morphine does not cause a significant extension of thiopental-induced anesthesia in the dog. Prolongation by a therapeutic dose of the narcotic analgesics appears to be less significant than that observed with most of the phenothiazine tranquilizers. Atropine sulfate or glycopyrrolate should be routinely used preceding thiopental anesthesia to prevent parasympathetic side effects. Atropine sulfate, but not atropine methylnitrate, nonspecifically reduces the anesthetic dosage of thiopental plasma level at awakening (Hatch 1972).

RECOVERY. The recovery period varies with dosage from 15 minutes to 6–8 hours before full leg coordination appears and may not be complete in less than 24 hours in the dog following an IV dose (15–25 mg/kg) of thiopental (Chenoweth and Van Dyke 1969). With repeated administration of the drug, recovery time is prolonged to the extent that there is little advantage over the use of pentobarbital. According to Hatch (1966), rapid administration of glucose in the dog that is regaining voluntary movement from thiopental anesthesia results in reanesthetization of 11% of the animals. Sodium lactate and epinephrine also produce an increase in the sleep time. However, the possibility of producing reanesthetization with these substances is of little practical concern as long as they are administered properly.

Old animals may exhibit hindleg weakness for 1–2 days after thiopental anesthesia. Incoordination of the legs, especially the rear legs, causes the patient to stagger about for an hour or so when disturbed during recovery. If the patient is not disturbed, recovery ordinarily is uneventful. Complete recovery requires approximately 2 hours and is usually free from excitement. Vomiting or other signs of postanesthetic toxicity have seldom been noted.

RESUSCITATION. As with other barbiturates, excessive amounts of thiopental produce severe respiratory depression. Continuous administration of oxygen and artificial ventilation is more beneficial than any other therapeutic measure for combating the respiratory depression from barbiturate overdosage.

CLINICAL USE. Thiopental is approved by the FDA for use in the dog, cat, bovine, sheep, and swine.

SMALL ANIMALS. Anesthesia produced by thiopental in small animals is very similar to that by pentobarbital. Although muscular relaxation is fair, it is inferior to that produced by ether and other inhalant anesthetics. Respiration is regular but slow and shallow. The heart beat is fast but strong. Excitement is generally absent during induction and recovery if the patient is kept quiet. IV thiopental (10 mg/kg) is used for induction of anesthesia in the dog premedicated with atropine to permit endotracheal intubation for administration of an inhalant anesthetic (Cribb et al. 1977).

The anesthetic dose of thiopental for the dog is 15–20 mg/kg administered by the IV route; for the cat it is 9–11 mg/kg (Robinson et al. 1986; Sams et al. 1985; Turner and Ilkiw 1990; Quandt and Robinson 1992; Mark et al. 1968). These doses are generally considered to be on the conservative side; e.g., some authors recommend an IV dose of 25–30 mg/kg thiopental for both the dog and cat (Mitchell 1966; Strobel and Wollman 1969). Strobel and Wollman reported that 30 mg/kg of the drug will produce 10–20 minutes of anesthesia and 2 hours of somnolence. The use of preanesthetic agents such as xylaxine or acepromazine will reduce the dose of thiopental required to produce anesthesia (Ko et al. 1993; Hatch et al. 1985; Hatch 1972; Hatch 1973c). In the Greyhound, compared to other breeds of dogs, the recovery rate from thiopental anesthesia is more prolonged. The Greyhound can metabolize methohexital, an ultrashort-acting oxybarbiturate, much more rapidly than the thiobarbiturate anesthetics.

Doses of 12 and 24 mg/kg thiopental administered intravenously in the cat require 27 ± 8 minutes and 63 ± 6 minutes after the barbiturate is injected before recovery of the righting reflex (Child et al. 1972a). Because of considerable variability in the anesthetic dose level for the dog and cat, thiopental should be administered cautiously and to effect. In the cat, administration of increasing amounts of thiopental does not allow EEG patterns to be related to the clinical depth of anesthesia or plasma thiopental concentration (Hatch et al. 1970).

SWINE. Thiopental in 5% IV solution has been used satisfactorily in swine varying in weight from 4.5 to 270 kg. Although dose levels of thiopental generally used in clinical practice can differ considerably from those recommended by Muhrer (1950), the information is nevertheless useful for determining the initial amount of drug needed for induction (Table 12.4). Swine weighing 5–50 kg usually require doses of 10–11 mg/kg (Booth 1969). In pregnant sows weighing 165–323 kg, induction of anesthesia without premedication is accomplished by IV injection of thiopental (2.5–6.25 g) to effect; no reliable dose/weight relationship is observed (Cummings et al. 1972). After endotracheal intubation, a gas mixture of oxygen and nitrous oxide in a ratio of 1:1 or 1:2 can be delivered to the animal.

About 1 hour is required before swine can move about satisfactorily after thiopental administration. This period is ordinarily longer than in humans, dogs, rabbits, and some other animals where approximately 15 minutes are usually required for recovery. In general, swine show a slower recovery rate from the effects of any CNS depressant than other species. The obese condition of swine is apparently contributory to a slower recovery period because thiopental is known for its ability to localize in fat.

Hemorrhage or blood loss of 30% in the pig decreases the anesthetic induction dose of thiopental by

TABLE 12.4—Suggested IV dose of thiopental sodium in swine

Weight	Dose	Dose in 5% solution
(kg)	*(mg/kg)*	*(ml/kg)*
4.5–22.7	11.0	0.22
22.7–45.4	9.9	0.19
45.4–90.9	8.8	0.17
90.9–136.3	7.7	0.15
136.3–181.8	6.6	0.13
181.8–272.7	5.5	0.11

Source: Muhrer 1950.
Note: Unthrifty animals require less drug for a comparable effect.

33% (Weiskopf and Bogetz 1985). The resulting hypovolemia may alter the degree of binding of thiopental to serum albumin. Consequently, the presence of hypoproteinemia that accompanies blood loss and hypovolemia would mean that less anesthetic is bound to serum albumin. Thus the anesthetic effect may possibly increase due to less bound or more free circulating thiopental after hemorrhage.

Thiopental is best given intravenously via the cranial vena cava by an indwelling catheter (Booth 1969). Since respiratory depression readily occurs in swine, endotracheal intubation is necessary for oxygen administration and/or artificial respiration. In addition, intubation of the pig provides an excellent means for supplementing thiopental with inhalant anesthetics.

CATTLE. IV thiopental has been used to produce surgical anesthesia for laparotomy in calves under 2 weeks. A 6.5% solution (65 mg/mL) should be injected slowly during 4–5 minutes until complete muscular relaxation occurs. The total dose varies from 15 to 22 mg/kg. The stage of light surgical anesthesia usually lasts for 10–12 minutes. Partial recovery follows rapidly, with complete recovery of limb coordination in 2 hours. A transient stage of deep hypnosis or light surgical anesthesia results from rapid injection of a small dose of thiopental; 6.6 mg/kg injected intravenously within 10 seconds produces deep hypnosis in 270–360 kg steers. The full effect is apparent within 1–2 minutes and persists 5–10 minutes. Steers fall to the ground soon after the rapid injection and assume a normal recumbent position in about 0.5 hour and stand within 2–3 hours. The phlegmatic disposition of the bovine ordinarily results in quiet recovery and only slight incoordination when the animals stand. Thiopental (0.2%) and guaifenesin (5%) in 5% glucose is used intravenously (2.2 mL/kg) in Angus and Hereford bulls for induction of anesthesia (Garner et al. 1975). This is followed with halothane-oxygen for maintenance of anesthesia.

HORSES. Rapid IV injection of thiopental without benefit of preanesthetic agents or tranquilizers has been tried in horses. While anesthesia may occur briefly, the recovery period in the horse is so marked by excitement and incoordination that use of thiopental alone is contraindicated. Adverse effects may arise partly from action of the drug, but much of the difficulty undoubtedly results from the nervous and excitable disposition of the horse in comparison to the phlegmatic disposition of the bovine.

Frankland and Camburn (1977) have used IV xylazine hydrochloride (0.22 mg/kg) 10–15 minutes prior to induction of anesthesia with 10% IV thiopental (1 g/90 kg given evenly over 20 seconds). They have also used IV acepromazine (0.05 mg/kg) 15 minutes prior to thiopental induction or 30 minutes prior to induction of anesthesia when acepromazine is administered intramuscularly. The mean induction time of anesthesia following xylazine and acepromazine is 28.2 and 14.6 seconds respectively. Although induction time of anesthesia is shorter following acepromazine, xylazine usually provides a greater degree of tranquilization (Frankland and Camburn 1977). However, both these regimens are satisfactory clinically. According to Frankland and Camburn, it is still a matter of personal preference which of these preanesthetics is used.

Clinical experience with thiopental (10%) in the horse indicates that the rapid IV injection of a dose (10 mg/kg) that will induce anesthesia is accompanied by a moderate tachycardia, a slight reduction in arterial pressure, and a brief period of apnea lasting from 0.5 to more than 1 minute (Tavernor and Lees 1970). In addition, a transient reversal in the T wave of the electrocardiogram (ECG) is seen in some animals. Thiopental is considered to be relatively safe for anesthesia in the horse, providing the rate and character of respiration are carefully observed. It is often used intravenously for rapid ("crash" or "quick-shot") induction of anesthesia in the horse at the rate of 6.6 mg/kg in a tranquilized animal (Short 1974; Short and Brunson 1978). Without tranquilization, the dose of thiopental required to induce anesthesia may increase as much as 25%. Induction of anesthesia usually requires 0.5–1 minute after injection of the drug and corresponds to the speed or rate of injection of the anesthetic agent. A more gradual approach to induction of anesthesia may be preferred by use of thiopental in combination with guaifenesin. Three grams of thiopental are added to 1 liter of 5% guaifenesin. This mixture is rapidly administered through a 12-gauge IV catheter. Recumbency occurs after approximately 1 mL/kg has been administered. Additionally, an IV bolus of 2–4 mg/kg of thiopental can be administered when limb weakness is noted to speed induction and decrease the amount of guaifenesin-thiopental mixture needed. Premedication with xylazine (0.5–1.0 mg/kg IV) or acepromazine (0.03–0.06 mg/kg IV) is recommended (Benson and Thurmon 1990).

GOATS. Thiopental (5%) has been satisfactorily used in the goat for surgical procedures lasting about 2 hours. Since the animal detoxifies the anesthetic at a rapid rate, the dose required for anesthesia varies greatly. An initial IV dose of 20–22 mg/kg is usually effective in anesthetizing the goat.

Atropine is capable of controlling salivation in the goat following barbiturate anesthesia. However, larger preanesthetic IM doses (0.7 mg/kg) are required than customarily used in other species. To maintain control of salivation during surgical anesthesia, it is necessary to repeat the atropine, administered by the IV route, at 15-minute intervals at a dose of 0.1–0.2 mg/kg.

An endotracheal catheter is routinely used to protect the airway from possible regurgitated ruminal contents. Tracheal intubation is valuable for administration of oxygen in the event of respiratory depression or arrest from an overdose of anesthesia.

BIRDS. Thiopental is administered intravenously via the wing vein to geese, ducks, chickens, and pigeons for induction of anesthesia. Anesthetic doses are 13–22 mg/kg for native Chinese geese, 18–26 mg/kg for ducks, and 13–18 mg/kg for chickens and pigeons. Sudden death often occurs in pigeons during administration of the anesthetic. In the chicken, injection of 13 mg/kg of thiopental is without satisfactory results, and death occurs if the dose exceeds 18 mg/kg. The relative lack of safety and short duration of anesthesia make this agent unsatisfactory for poultry surgery.

NONHUMAN PRIMATES. When short-term surgical procedures are indicated and rapid recovery is preferred, thiopental is a useful anesthetic agent in nonhuman primates (Day 1965; Sawyer 1965a; Domino et al. 1969). In the chimpanzee, thiopental is the agent of choice for long-term (3–4 hr), light-stage anesthetic procedures and short-term (30–45 min) surgical procedures (Day 1965). According to Day, the initial dose of thiopental is 33 mg/kg, which produces light stage III anesthesia.

In the rhesus monkey, thiopental is administered intravenously at a dose level of 25–30 mg/kg (Sawyer 1965a; Domino et al. 1969). According to Sawyer, the excitatory phase during induction of anesthesia is not as turbulent as in the canine species, and the slow rate of administration of the barbiturate can be readily performed. This type of response during induction of anesthesia reduces the possibility of administering an overdose. Sawyer (1965a) advocates administration of atropine (0.04 mg/kg) prior to or at the time of anesthesia induction.

Duration of thiopental anesthesia from a single administration is not more than 10 minutes in the rhesus monkey, and recovery generally is complete within 45–60 minutes (Domino et al. 1969).

RABBITS. Thiopental (2.5%) is used as the IV anesthetic of choice in the rabbit (Sawyer 1965b). Sawyer recommends slow administration via the ear vein while the respiratory rate and oral and palpebral reflexes are observed. He also emphasizes that the pedal reflex should not be used to determine depth of anesthesia; when this reflex is severely depressed or absent, animals may be in the terminal stage of anesthesia. The IV dose level of thiopental recommended for the rabbit ranges from 30 to 50 mg/kg; this will produce anesthesia varying from 5 to 20 minutes. Full recovery usually occurs within 15 minutes (Murdock 1969; Wood 1978).

SNAKES. Experimentally, skin grafting procedures have been conducted in bull snakes (*Pituophis catenifer*) and Texas rat snakes (*Elaphe quadrivittata*) using thiopental and thiamylal 2–6 mg/kg intraperitoneally for induction of surgical anesthesia (Kraner et al. 1965). It is necessary to administer both in dosages near the lethal level to be effective. Moreover, recovery is observed to be extremely slow, taking 48–72 hours even when analeptic agents are used (Kraner et al. 1965). A large number of snakes fail to survive barbiturate-induced anesthesia. For this reason, Kraner et al. (1965) found the use of inhalant anesthetics more satisfactory than thiopental or thiamylal.

KANGAROOS. Small kangaroos (tammar, wallaby, quokka) are often anesthetized up to 2–3 hours for therapeutic or research purposes (Richardson and Cullen 1981). Thiopental (2.5%) given in an IV dose of 28.4 ± 6.2 mg/kg for wallabies and 27.8 mg/kg for quokkas provides an unconscious state satisfactory for tracheal intubation and maintenance with halothane.

Thialbarbital Sodium. *Thialbarbital Sodium,* INN (Thialbarbitone sodium), is a sulfur-containing barbiturate (Fig. 12.5). Its duration of action is intermediate between the short-acting and ultrashort-acting barbiturates. Thialbarbital has a potency of approximately one-half that of thiopental and has similar pharmacologic characteristics. It is classified as a Schedule III compound under the 1970 Controlled Substances Act.

CHEMISTRY. This compound is a sodium salt of 5-(2-cyclohexen-1-yl)-5-allyl-2-thiobarbituric acid. Thialbarbital is used in about a 10% buffered aqueous solution. Unbuffered solutions have a pH of 10.6. Thialbarbital is almost entirely detoxified by body tissues.

Thiamylal Sodium. *Thiamylal Sodium,* USP, is an ultrashort-acting thiobarbiturate (see Fig. 12.6) prepared for use in a mixture with sodium carbonate, a buffering agent. It consists of pale yellow, hygroscopic

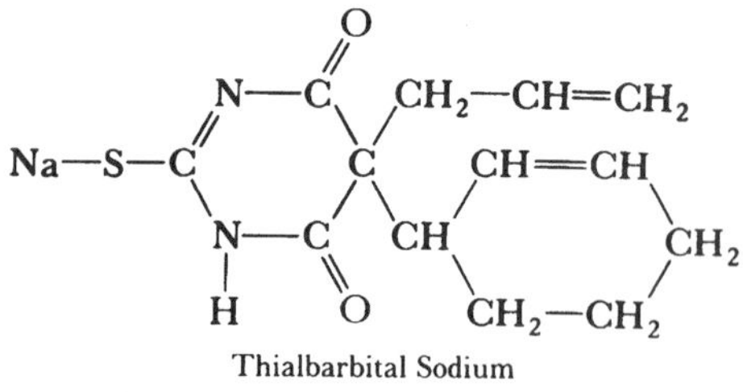

O
N—C CH$_2$—CH=CH$_2$
Na—S—C C CH=CH
N—C CH CH$_2$
H O CH$_2$—CH$_2$
Thialbarbital Sodium

FIG. 12.5

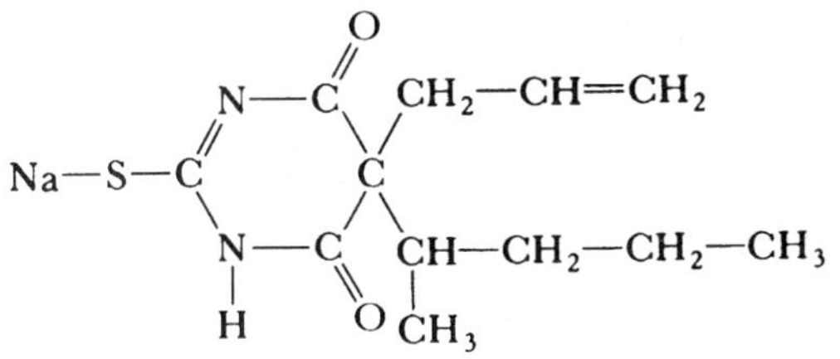

Thiamylal Sodium

FIG. 12.6

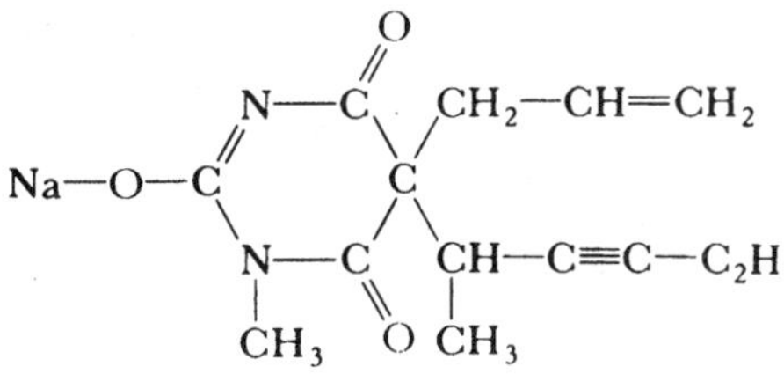

Methohexital Sodium

FIG. 12.7

masses of crystals. Thiamylal is classified as a Schedule III compound under the 1970 Controlled Substances Act. Thiamylal is not currently produced in the USA, although it was widely used when available.

CHEMISTRY. Thiamylal is the thiobarbiturate analog of secobarbital. It is freely soluble in water, with a pH of about 10.5. The solution is clear, bright, and yellow, with a pungent odor; the pH decreases slowly when carbon dioxide is absorbed from the atmosphere. Air should not be bubbled through the solution during preparation. It should be discarded if a precipitate forms.

STABILITY. Thiamylal is relatively stable as a dry powder mixed with sodium carbonate and stored in airtight vials. Solutions of thiamylal cannot be subjected to heat or sterilization because of deterioration. Refrigeration or storage in a cool, dark place is necessary once the preparation is in the form of a solution, and it should be used within 24 hours.

CLINICAL USE. The clinical use of thiamylal is very similar to that of thiopental. Thiamylal is slightly more potent than thiopental. This drug is discussed in greater detail in the 7th edition of this text.

Methohexital Sodium. Several hundred barbiturates have been synthesized in an effort to find an ultrashort-acting barbiturate with greater potency and shorter duration of action than the thiobarbiturates, viz., thiopental and thiamylal. As the result of this effort, an oxybarbiturate (methohexital sodium) was synthesized. *Methohexital Sodium,* USP (Brevane, Brietal, Brevital, Brevimytal), has been approved by the FDA for use only in the dog and cat. It is classified as a Schedule IV compound under the 1970 Controlled Substances Act.

CHEMISTRY. Chemically, methohexital is α-*dl*-1-methyl-5-(1-methyl-2-pentynyl)-5-allyl-barbituric acid sodium (see Fig. 12.7). This anesthetic agent resembles secobarbital and pentobarbital, the oxygen analogs of thiamylal and thiopental respectively.

Methohexital, with a methyl group on an N atom, is more potent than thiopental but has a higher incidence of CNS excitatory effects. When the anesthetic was first introduced in clinical trials, convulsions were commonly encountered in humans (Steen and Michenfelder 1979). Upon separation of the compound into its isomers and identification of those responsible for CNS excitation, the convulsant properties of methohexital were greatly reduced. However, CNS excitation including convulsions remains a possibility following its use. The excitatory activity of methohexital has been used to advantage in clinical diagnostic investigations of petit mal and temporal lobe epilepsy in humans. Methohexital activates abnormal EEG tracings in epilepsy-prone subjects.

STABILITY. Methohexital is stable in an aqueous solution at room temperature for at least 6 weeks at a pH of 11. It is readily dissolved in saline or distilled water.

ADMINISTRATION. Methohexital is administered as a 1% solution in the dog and cat by the IV route. Perivascular injection does not produce tissue irritation. Rate of administration of methohexital plays an important role in depth and duration of anesthesia. It is recommended that the drug be injected as rapidly as possible, consistent with safety, to reach a suitable plane of anesthesia. The 1% solution is injected at approximately 1 mL/sec. If a slow injection rate is used, muscular tremors frequently occur. Similar findings, including CNS excitation, have been reported in humans.

When methohexital is injected rapidly, induction of anesthesia is smooth and rapid. Dogs and cats are able to lift their heads or can sit up within 5–10 minutes. Complete recovery occurs within 30 minutes. When IM promazine (3.3 mg/kg) is administered preceding methohexital by 1 hour, duration of methohexital anesthesia is slightly prolonged but recovery is smoother.

In the Greyhound, recovery from thiobarbiturate (thiopental or thiamylal) anesthesia is prolonged compared to mixed-breed dogs (Sams et al. 1985). Recovery is over 2–3 times as long after thiobarbiturate anesthesia as from methohexital anesthesia.

The effective IV dose of methohexital for induction of anesthesia in the Greyhound is 9–11 mg/kg. The recommended rate of injection is about 25 mg/sec (1 mL/sec of a 2.5% solution). Inadvertent extravascular injection of this concentration does not result in any untoward effects when left untreated as compared to a

5% solution of thiopental, which causes swelling, lameness, and even sloughing of tissues.

In humans, the anesthetic is considered to be an ideal preparation for rapid induction of hypnosis when inhalation anesthesia such as halothane is used. Since the drug is rapidly metabolized, it does not interfere with use of inhalant anesthetics.

TOXICITY. It has been observed in humans that respiratory depression is more severe following use of methohexital than with thiamylal or thiopental at a comparable level of narcosis (Taylor and Stoelting 1960). Inasmuch as respiratory depression is prevalent throughout the course of anesthesia in the human subject, it is necessary to assist respiration by artificial means. In humans, pain at the injection site occurs in 60% of the patients.

In the normal, healthy dog and cat at least twice the calculated dose of methohexital can be given with safety.

CONTRAINDICATIONS. Methohexital should not be used as an anesthetic in known or suspected cases of epilepsy in animals. Its use for anticonvulsant purposes in treatment of strychnine poisoning, tetanus, or other conditions associated with increased CNS excitation is inadvisable.

DOSAGE. Clifford and Soma (1969) recommend a dose of 5.7 mg/kg for the cat. This dose of methohexital is slightly less than that (i.e., 7.3 mg/kg) formerly recommended. For dogs weighing up to 13.6 kg, an IV dose of 7.3 mg/kg methohexital is recommended; for dogs over 13.6 kg, the IV dose is 5.5 mg/kg.

CLINICAL USE. Comparison of the potency of methohexital and thiopental for several species has indicated that methohexital is twice as potent as thiopental (Turner and Ilkiw 1990). Table 12.5 gives the median anesthetic doses and average durations of anesthesia in the dog, cat, and monkey.

Methohexital is used in the horse as a 2.5% solution at a dose of 5 mg/kg. The anesthetic preparation is injected intravenously at a rapid rate. The horse falls to the ground within 15–20 seconds, with the period of anesthesia not exceeding 5 minutes. This permits enough time to insert an endotracheal catheter so that inhalant anesthetics can be administered.

Methohexital should not be used alone because excitation during recovery limits its use in the horse (Grono 1966). Premedication with neuroleptic agents (acepromazine, promazine) in conjunction with narcotic analgesics (meperidine, morphine) reduces the severity of excitation upon recovery.

Methohexital is used on occasion in swine for detusking boars, hoof trimming, foot inspection, and other minor procedures not requiring more than a few minutes. A dose of 5 mg/kg is recommended for these purposes (Emberton 1966).

This ultrashort-acting oxybarbiturate has also been used for performing a ventriculocordectomy in swine held in biomedical research facilities (Mackey et al. 1970). The recommended IV dose of methohexital is 8 mg/kg, which produces surgical anesthesia of approximately 10–15 minutes.

If additional anesthesia is necessary to complete surgery, inhalant anesthetic (ether) has been used. With this combination of anesthetic agents the animals are usually standing within 10 minutes following surgery.

The pig characteristically shakes its head vigorously during recovery from most barbiturates, including methohexital. The animals should recover in a well-padded area and not on concrete floors or other hard surfaces.

In the domestic duck, methohexital administered intravenously has no apparent effect when given in doses of 5–10 mg/kg initially or when followed with additional dosages every 3–4 minutes. It is unclear whether the large fat depots are responsible for this unresponsive effect or if a hyperactive hepatic microsomal enzyme system exists in ducks.

In the rabbit, IV methohexital is given rapidly at 10 mg/kg; it induces light anesthesia within 10 seconds for 2–5 minutes (Wood 1978).

Methohexital (10 mg/kg, IV bolus) has been used in captive and free-ranging muntjac (*Muntiacus reevesi*) for immobilization purposes (Cooper et al. 1986). Although it induces rapid induction of anesthesia, some animals manifest an excitatory behavior during recovery.

Secobarbital Sodium. *Secobarbital Sodium,* USP (Seconal sodium) (sodium 5-allyl-5-[1-methylbutyl]

TABLE 12.5—Median anesthetic dose and average duration of anesthesia in animals

	Methohexital sodium			Thiopental sodium		
Animal	Number of animals	AD50 ± S.E.*	Duration of anesthesia	Number of animals	AD 50 ± S.E.*	Duration of anesthesia
		(mg/kg)	*(min)*		*(mg/kg)*	*(min)*
Dog	15	9.74 ± 0.93	29	15	16.0 ± 0.97	142
Cat	20	5.78 ± 0.54	39	15	10.4 ± 0.92	58
Monkey	15	4.43 ± 0.21	15	15	9.95 ± 1.39	44

Source: Taylor and Stoelting 1960.
*Standard error.

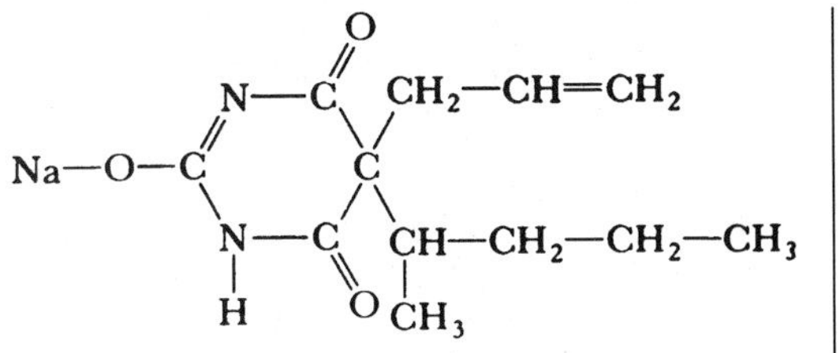

Secobarbital Sodium

FIG. 12.8

barbiturate), is a short-acting oxybarbiturate and the chemical analog of thiamylal sodium (see Fig. 12.8).

Secobarbital has been used in dogs as an IV anesthetic in combination with mephenesin, a skeletal muscle relaxant. However, this barbiturate appears to be better suited to preanesthetic, basal anesthetic, and sedative uses. Since abdominal relaxation is not satisfactory following mephenesin, its use in combination with barbiturate anesthetics has been virtually discarded. Secobarbital has been used as a sedative prior to EEG recordings because it is purported to have less neurophysiologic effect than many other barbiturates (Strobel and Wollman 1969). Secobarbital and its salts are subject to the 1970 Controlled Substances Act as Schedule II preparations. This drug is discussed in greater detail in the 7th edition of this text.

Hexobarbital Sodium. *Hexobarbital Sodium,* NF (Evipal sodium), is an ultrashort-acting oxybarbiturate infrequently used for clinical purposes. It is subject to the 1970 Controlled Substances Act as a Schedule III drug. A distinct disadvantage of hexobarbital is the uncontrollable excitement and ataxia exhibited during recovery in the dog. In the small laboratory animal, hexobarbital is occasionally used for short surgical procedures. For use in the rabbit, an IV dose of 40 mg/kg will produce anesthesia for 5–10 minutes, with complete recovery in 15 minutes (Murdock 1969). In the adult albino rat, hexobarbital is usually administered intraperitoneally at a dose of 100 mg/kg for induction of anesthesia (Ben et al. 1969). This drug is discussed in greater detail in the 7th edition of this text.

PROPOFOL. *Propofol,* USP ($C_{12}H_{18}O$, Diprivan, Rapinovet, Propoflo), is a chemically unique anesthetic agent used both as an induction agent and as a maintenance anesthetic agent delivered by continuous IV infusion or intermittent bolus (see Fig. 12.9). Propofol has been available for human use since 1989 and was recently labeled for veterinary use in the USA. It is available for both human and veterinary use in Europe. Propofol is insoluble in water so it is available as an emulsion. Initially it was prepared with Cremophor EL, but this was replaced with the currently available emulsion due to the anaphylactoid reactions associated with the Cremophor EL (Branson and Gross 1994; Reves et al. 1994).

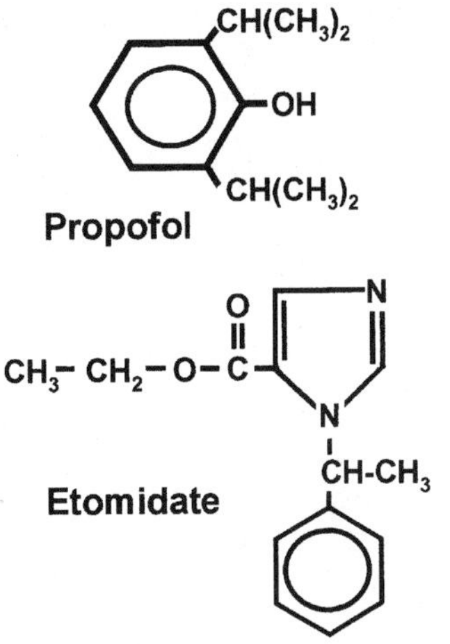

Propofol

Etomidate

FIG. 12.9

Chemistry. Propofol (2,6-diisopropylphenol) is an alkyphenol that is an oil at room temperature and water insoluble but highly lipid soluble. It is available as an aqueous emulsion containing propofol (10 mg/mL), soybean oil (100 mg/mL), glycerol (2.5 mg/mL), egg lecithin (12 mg/mL), and sodium hydroxide (to adjust pH). It is stable at room temperature and not light sensitive. The formulation available contains no preservatives and will support bacterial growth and endotoxin production (Arduino et al. 1991).

Pharmacokinetics. The pharmacokinetics of propofol in dogs is best described using a two-compartment open model (Zoran et al. 1993). Initially the drug is extensively taken up by the CNS, resulting in rapid inductions. It is then rapidly redistributed from the brain to other tissues and removed from the plasma by metabolism. Propofol's lipophilic nature results in a large apparent volume of distribution (Vd) (17.9 L/kg in mixed-breed dogs); the steady-state volume of distribution (Vd_{ss}) is also large (9.7 mL/kg). The initial distribution half-life ($t_{1/2\alpha}$) is short, as is the plasma disappearance ($t_{1/2\beta}$), due to rapid redistribution of the drug from the brain to other tissues and extensive metabolism. The Vd and Vd_{ss} are smaller in Greyhounds, 11.2 L/kg and 6.3 mL/kg respectively, suggesting sighthounds have slower recoveries, probably due to differences in body composition (Zoran et al. 1993). The pharmacokinetics of propofol in cats has not been determined; however, cats appear to have a similar response to and dose requirement for propofol (Geel 1991; Weaver and Raptopoulos 1991; Morgan and Legge 1989; Brearley et al. 1988).

Metabolism and Excretion. The total body clearance of propofol is rapid and exceeds hepatic blood flow, suggesting extrahepatic metabolism. Indeed, in one study done on human patients undergoing liver transplantation, the amount of propofol metabolite excreted did not decrease when the liver was excluded from the circulation (Veroli et al. 1992). The site of extrahepatic metabolism is not certain, but pulmonary tissue has been shown to contribute to propofol metabolism in cats (Matot et al. 1993) and sheep (Mather et al. 1989). However, there may be species differences in the site and amount of extrahepatic metabolism. Propofol is metabolized to glucuronide and sulfate conjugates, with only trace amounts of other compounds formed. The primary route of metabolite excretion is in the urine, with only small amounts found in the feces (Simons et al. 1991).

Cardiovascular System. Propofol can induce mild arterial hypotension in dogs but the changes are minimal and are due to dose-related vasodilation and decrease in myocardial contractility (Pagel and Warltier 1993). Even in hypovolemic dogs the propofol induced cardiovascular changes were minimal (Ilkiw et al. 1992). In Greyhounds propofol infusion did result in a decrease in the heart rate (Robertson et al. 1992). Propofol can enhance the ability of epinephrine to induce cardiac arrhythmias but does not appear to be inherently arrhythmogenic (Kamibayashi et al. 1991). Propofol can induce oxidative injuries to feline red blood cells if used repeatedly over several days. This can result in anorexia, diarrhea, and malaise (Day et al. 1993).

Respiratory System. The effect of propofol on the respiratory system is similar to that of the thiobarbiturates. Short periods of apnea are commonly seen with propofol administration in dogs. Mild hypercapnia and acidosis are also seen in spontaneously breathing dogs, but neither is severe (Ilkiw et al. 1992; Robertson et al. 1992).

Central Nervous System. Propofol induces CNS depression by enhancing the effects of GABA, an inhibitory neurotransmitter. The site of action is different from that of the benzodiazepines (Reves et al. 1994). Propofol will decrease the intracranial pressure (ICP) in patients with normal or elevated ICP. There is also a decrease in cerebral perfusion pressure associated with propofol administration, and the decrease in perfusion pressure is the major cause of the decrease in ICP (Reves et al. 1994; Wooten 1992). Propofol causes a decrease in intraocular pressure as well. The effect of propofol on seizure activity is not certain. It was initially considered to have no influence on seizure activity, but later studies have shown a dose-related anticonvulsant effect (Heavner et al. 1992). More recently there have been several anecdotal accounts of spontaneous movement and seizure activity during and after propofol anesthesia in humans and dogs. After low doses of propofol, the EEG shows an initial increase in α activity followed by a change to δ and θ frequencies. Increasing plasma propofol levels results in burst suppression (Reves et al. 1994).

Clinical Use. Propofol is used as an induction agent to be followed with inhalation anesthesia and as a maintenance anesthetic. It can be administered by intermittent IV bolus and continuous infusion. It can be diluted for continuous infusion in 5% dextrose, but it should not be diluted to a concentration less than 2 mg/mL. It should only be administered intravenously; pain on injection is regularly observed, especially if small peripheral veins are used. Propofol does cross the placenta and enter the fetal circulation, but it appears to be readily removed from the fetal circulation after birth and produces minimal effects on healthy, newborn, human infants (Dailland et al. 1989). Propofol is used almost exclusively in small animals for economic reasons; however, it has been evaluated in other species.

DOGS. Propofol can be used as a single IV bolus for induction. In unpremedicated dogs the mean dose required ranges from 5.0 to 6.9 mg/kg (Geel 1991; Weaver and Raptopoulos 1991). The induction dose will produce a short period of unconsciousness, usually no more than 2–4 minutes (Morgan and Legge 1989). Premedication with a tranquilizer or other CNS depressants will reduce the dose required by 25% or more. The induction dose required for Greyhounds was not different from that required for mixed-breed dogs; however, the recovery time was longer for Greyhounds. If propofol is to be used as the maintenance anesthetic, it can be delivered as an infusion or as intermittent boluses. A dose of 0.5–2.0 mg/kg is used for the incremental boluses, and they will need to be repeated at regular intervals. The infusion rate will vary somewhat depending on the other drugs used and the amount of surgical stimulation. Since propofol itself is a poor analgesic, an opiate or other analgesic is often used concurrently (Branson and Gross 1994). After premedication with acepromazine and atropine, an infusion rate of 0.4 mg/kg/min produced surgical anesthesia in all patients undergoing various procedures (Hall and Chambers 1987). Lower infusion rates are utilized if more-potent drugs are used concurrently. A propofol infusion rate of 0.25 mg/kg/min produces surgical anesthesia after premedication with xylazine (0.2 mg/kg), fentanyl (0.01 mg/kg), and glycopyrrolate (0.005 mg/kg) (Zoran et al. 1993).

CATS. The reported induction dose of propofol in cats ranges from 5.0 to 8.0 mg/kg (Weaver and Raptopoulos 1991; Morgan and Legge 1989). The reported effect of premedication with acepromazine is somewhat variable, with some reports showing no effect (Geel 1991; Weaver and Raptopoulos 1991; Brearley et al. 1988) and one showing a reduction in propofol requirements (Morgan and Legge 1989). As with dogs, anesthesia can be maintained using intermittent boluses (1.8

mg/kg) (Morgan and Legge 1989) or continuous infusion (0.5 mg/kg/min) (Brearley et al. 1988).

OTHER SPECIES. Propofol (2 mg/kg) was administered to horses following xylazine (0.5 and 1.0 mg/kg) premedication (Mama et al. 1994). The horses given the low dose of xylazine were recumbent for 25 minutes and those receiving 1.0 mg/kg of xylazine were recumbent for 33 minutes. In both regimens the quality of recovery was excellent. Unpremedicated horses were given 2, 4, or 8 mg/kg of propofol intravenously. Administration of 2 mg/kg did not always result in lateral recumbency. When 8 mg/kg was administered, the horses took approximately 48 minutes to stand up and exhibited a decrease in respiratory rate and $PaCO_2$ (Mama et al. 1993). Propofol has also been used in donkeys for induction (2 mg/kg IV) and maintenance of anesthesia after detomidine (0.015 mg/kg IV) premedication. The average maintenance infusion rate was 0.21 mg/kg/min (Hartsfield et al. 1993). In foals propofol (2.0 mg/kg IV) has been used for induction. After induction an infusion at an average rate of 0.33 mg/kg/min was used to maintain anesthesia. The foals were premedicated with xylaxine (0.5 mg/kg IV).

Propofol has been used in rabbits, and the "MAC equivalent" infusion rate has been determined to be approximately 1.2 mg/kg/min (Henderson et al. 1994). Propofol has been used as an induction agent in rabbits premedicated with acepromazine, medetomidine, or medetomidine and midazolam. The IV propofol doses were 10, 4, and 2 mg/kg, respectively (Evans and Eberhart 1992; Ko et al. 1992). In pigs infusions of 9–13 mg/kg/hr did produce anesthesia, but the animals still responded to painful stimuli even at the highest infusion rate. Also, at 13 mg/kg/hr the pigs were apneic (Mascias et al. 1992).

ETOMIDATE. Etomidate (Amidate, Hypnomidate) is a nonbarbiturate IV anesthesia induction agent that does not possess analgesic activity (Owen 1979) (see Fig. 12.9). Induction of anesthesia is rapid (like that of thiopental) (Famewo and Odugbesan 1978). Etomidate administration decreases plasma cortisol levels by slowing the formation of cortisol. This occurs as a result of the inhibition of the enzyme 11-β-hydroxylase. This has been a concern in surgical patients because of the potential for a decreased response to the stress of surgery (Reves et al. 1994). In both humans (Reves et al. 1994) and dogs (Dodam et al. 1990) the plasma cortisol levels are not below normal values.

Chemistry. Etomidate is an imidazole with a chemical formula of *R*-(+)-pentylethyl-1*H*-imidazole-5 carboxylate sulfate. There are two isomers but the (+) isomer is the only one with anesthetic properties. Etomidate is supplied as a 2% solution in 35% propylene glycol. It is not water soluble and is unstable in a neutral solution. The propylene glycol base has been associated with intravascular hemolysis (see Doenicke et al. 1997; Moon 1994; Ko et al. 1993).

Pharmacokinetics. Etomidate appears to fit a three-compartment pharmacokinetic model. The initial primary cause of the return to consciousness after administration of a bolus of etomidate is redistribution from the brain to other body tissues. It has a short redistribution half-life (29 minutes in humans; 21 minutes in cats) and a relatively large steady-state volume of distribution (2.5–4.5 L/kg in humans; 2.5–7 L/kg in cats). The elimination half-life varies from 2.9 to 5.3 hours in humans and is 3 hours in cats (Reves et al. 1994; Haskins 1992). Approximately 75% of etomidate is protein bound in the plasma (Haskins 1992). Because of its rapid redistribution and elimination it is administered both as a single bolus for short anesthesia and as an infusion for longer anesthetic times (Robertson 1992). The drug does cross the placenta but fetal blood levels are appreciably less than maternal blood levels (Esener et al. 1992).

Metabolism and Excretion. Etomidate undergoes hepatic hydrolysis to form a carboxylic acid as a major, inactive metabolite or secondarily undergoes *N*-dealkylation (Reves et al. 1994). The metabolites are excreted via the kidney and bile. Very little is excreted unchanged. Decreased hepatic function prolongs the half-life of etomidate.

Cardiovascular System. The lack of significant cardiovascular effect is etomidate's primary advantage. It has minimal cardiac or peripheral vascular effects in the normal patient (Robertson 1992; Suzer et al. 1998; Tassani et al. 1997). The cardiovascular stability seen in etomidate-anesthetized patients may be due to its lack of response to baroreceptor-mediated cardiovascular control mechanisms (Kissin et al. 1983). There is some evidence that patients with cardiomyopathy may not respond in the same way. An increase in peripheral resistance was seen in animals that had induced left ventricular myopathy (Pagel et al. 1998).

Respiratory System. Respiration is only slightly depressed by etomidate. A dose of 1.5 mg/kg in the dog did not produce significant changes in arterial blood gas values and a dose of 3.0 mg/kg produced only a mild decrease in arterial PO_2 and a mild respiratory acidosis (Nagel et al. 1979).

Central Nervous System. Etomidate's mechanism of action appears to be via an enhancement of the effect of GABA at its receptor site (Tomlin et al. 1998). This effect is limited to the R(+) isomer of etomidate. Etomidate significantly reduces cerebral blood flow and the cerebral metabolic oxygen requirement and produces a decrease in intracranial pressure in patients with elevated intracranial pressure. The effect on the EEG is similar to that of the barbiturates. It has been associated with an increase in EEG activity in epileptogenic foci and is associated with myoclonic movement, but the myoclonic activity is not associated with EEG changes associated with seizures (Reves et al. 1994).

Clinical Use. In animals, the drug has potent hypnotic action and a wider margin of safety than thiopental, methohexital, and propanidid (Janssen et al. 1975; Van Hamme et al. 1978). The therapeutic index of etomidate in the dog is 16. This means the lethal dose is 16 times the clinical dose. The therapeutic index for thiopental is 7 (Robertson 1992).

DOGS. In the dog, IV etomidate produces rapid and safe anesthesia that is hemodynamically safer than thiamylal (Nagel et al. 1979). Dogs given medetomidine (0.015 mg/kg) followed by etomidate given IV at a dose of 0.5 mg/kg and an infusion of etomidate at a rate of 0.05 mg/kg/min exhibited no significant cardiovascular changes related to the etomidate infusion (Ko et al. 1994). Even in hypovolemic dogs, the significant cardiovascular changes associated with etomidate administration are limited to a decrease in heart rate (Pascoe et al. 1992). Loss of consciousness occurs in 15–20 seconds; a small dose (1.5 mg/kg) induces anesthesia for 8 ± 5 minutes, and a large dose (3 mg/kg) produces anesthesia for 21 ± 9 minutes (Nagel et al. 1979).

CATS. Etomidate (0.8 mg/kg) is equipotent to ketamine (5 mg/kg), methohexital (2 mg/kg), and althesin (1.2 mg/kg) administered intravenously in awake cats (Inque and Arndt 1982). Etomidate has been used for anesthetic induction in cats at a dose of 1 mg/kg, after premedication with a tranquilizer (Ilkiw 1994).

OTHER SPECIES. In laboratory mice, etomidate (23.7 ± 1.5 mg/kg) given intraperitoneally permits surgical procedures up to 20 minutes after induction (Gomwalk and Healing 1981). Etomidate can be used as a maintenance anesthetic in pigs at a dose of 0.2 mg/kg with midazolam 0.1 mg/kg (Clutton et al. 1997).

CHLORAL HYDRATE. *Chloral Hydrate,* USP ($CCl_3CH[OH]_2$), was introduced into medicine as a hypnotic in 1869 by Liebrich because it released chloroform in vitro and was thought to do the same in vivo. Subsequent investigation revealed the error of this assumption. It was among the first CNS depressants to be used in veterinary surgery.

Chloral hydrate was first injected intravenously into experimental animals in 1872 by Oré. Three years later Humbert injected 30–70 g intravenously into horses. Chloral hydrate has since been injected intravenously to produce surgical anesthesia in large animals, especially horses.

The drug is classified as a Schedule IV compound under the 1970 Controlled Substances Act.

Chemistry. When acetic aldehyde is chlorinated, trichloroacetaldehyde (CCl_3CHO) is formed. The end product is chloral, a heavy, acrid oil. Chloral combines with one molecule of water to form chloral hydrate. It occurs as colorless, translucent crystals containing not less than 99.5% of $CCl_3CH(OH)_2$. Chloral hydrate volatilizes on exposure to air and has an aromatic, penetrating odor. It has a slightly bitter, caustic taste. One g is soluble in 0.25 mL water and in 1–2 mL of the common fat solvents.

Administration. Chloral hydrate in solution can be injected intravenously and is administered orally in solution or by capsule. Simple-stomached animals generally have little fluid in their stomachs, so the drug is better administered in dilute solution to these species to decrease local irritation to the gastric mucosa. Vomiting is often produced in carnivorous animals from irritation of the gastric mucosa. Presence of food in the stomach reduces irritant effects of the drug upon the mucosa and decreases the likelihood of vomiting.

Chloral hydrate is not a satisfactory anesthetic because it has low pain-relieving power. In addition, so-called anesthetic dosages severely depress the respiratory and vasomotor centers. The anesthetic dosage approaches the LD_{50} and therefore is hazardous.

Chloral hydrate is best employed in the horse for its hypnotic action or for general anesthesia as a basal narcotic with supplementation by thiopental (Crispin 1981). IV injection for hypnotic effect provides the advantage of almost immediate action compared to a delay of 15–30 minutes following oral administration. This drug is discussed in greater detail in the 7th edition of this text.

CHLORAL HYDRATE AND MAGNESIUM SULFATE. A mixture of 12% chloral hydrate and 6% magnesium sulfate in solution for IV injection has been advocated for anesthesia in large animals. This mixture is stable indefinitely. The solution is administered intravenously in horses at a rate not exceeding 30 mL/min to avoid excessive depression of the CNS. Administration is discontinued when the stage of surgical anesthesia appears, as indicated by slowing or absence of nystagmus and other significant reflexes. Anesthesia usually lasts over 30 minutes.

Addition of magnesium sulfate was originally thought to enhance depressant action of the drug mixture through its own depressant effect upon the CNS. It is now known that the magnesium ion exerts little if any direct depressant effect on the CNS (Bowen et al. 1970). The primary effect of magnesium is its neuromuscular blocking action, similar to the curariform agents. From this standpoint, magnesium is beneficial in producing skeletal muscle relaxation, which chloral hydrate does poorly. Inasmuch as magnesium sulfate alone produces only neuromuscular blockade and death due to asphyxia, it is considered inhumane to use it in euthanasia (Bowen et al. 1970).

The combination of chloral hydrate, magnesium sulfate, and pentobarbital sodium (originally marketed under the proprietary names of Chloropent and Equithesin) provides some of the desirable depressant actions of each compound without the individual pronounced toxicities. The original combination proposed by Millenbruck and Wallinga (1946) for anesthesia in horses and cattle consists of chloral hydrate, 30 g; magnesium sulfate, 15 g; and pentobarbital, 6.6 g dissolved in 1000 mL water.

Pentobarbital cannot be added to the solution of chloral hydrate and magnesium sulfate unless it is to be used within about 1 hour. After 2 hours a precipitate forms from exposure of chloral hydrate to the alkalinity of pentobarbital. Commercially, stable solutions are prepared by substituting the relatively insoluble pentobarbituric acid for the soluble sodium salt. Solubility of the acid compound has been increased by use of propylene glycol and ethyl alcohol in the solvent. This drug is discussed in greater detail in the 7th edition of this text.

GUAIFENESIN. *Guaifenesin,* USP (Gecolate, Guaiphenesin Guailaxin), formerly named glyceryl guaiacolate, has been used as a therapeutic agent for over 8 decades. An excellent review of the historical development of medical uses of guaifenesin has been written by Funk (1970). The drug was first used for its analgesic, antipyretic, and expectorant properties. Guaifenesin is chemically similar to mephenesin and meprobamate; it is designated as 3-(0-methoxyphenoxy)-1,2-propanediol (Fig. 12.10).

Guaifenesin has been used as an adjunct to anesthesia in the horse since 1949; in the USA it was first used in 1965. The compound increases the potency of preanesthetic agents and barbiturates. It is a central-acting skeletal muscle relaxant that selectively depresses or blocks nerve impulse transmission at the internuncial neuron level of the spinal cord, brainstem, and subcortical areas of the brain.

Guaifenesin is approved by the FDA as a muscle relaxant for use in the horse but must not be used in animals intended for human consumption. A 5% concentration of the compound is prepared by dissolving the powder (50 g/L) in sterile water.

Stability. Guaifenesin is a white powder with a bitter taste. It is not readily soluble and partially precipitates out of solution at 22°C or lower (Funk 1973). Heating and agitation usually eliminate the precipitate. Only freshly prepared solutions should be used. However, a

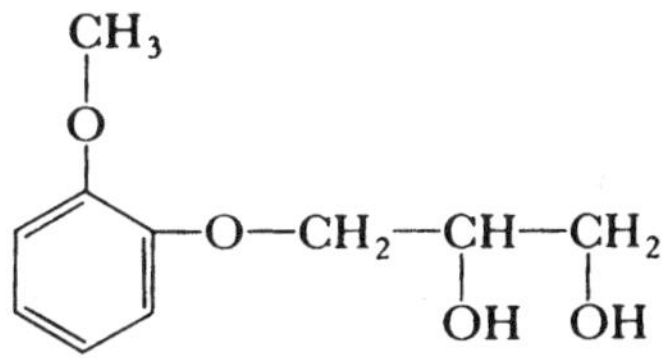

CH_3
O
$—O—CH_2—CH—CH_2$
OH OH

Guaifenesin

FIG. 12.10

10% solution of guaifenesin made in sterile distilled water can apparently be safely stored at room temperature for at least 1 week; the only problem is development of a precipitate (Grandy and McDowell 1980). Guaifenesin appears to possess some bactericidal and bacteriostatic properties.

In Australia, a stabilized solution of guaifenesin (Quilate Stabil) for horses has been commercially formulated in a concentration of 15% (Kalhoro and Rex 1984).

Administration and Duration of Action. Although guaifenesin has been administered by all parenteral routes, it is best administered intravenously. Orally, the drug must be administered in high dosages to produce a perceptible effect. Accidental perivascular injection of 5% guaifenesin does not result in severe tissue reaction. However, thrombophlebitis of the jugular vein occurs several days after anesthesia; this effect may be associated with use of guaifenesin (Schatzman 1974).

The primary disadvantage in the use of guaifenesin is the large volume of solution required parenterally to produce relaxation. The effect of the drug is brief (Tavernor and Jones 1970). Duration of action of a single muscle relaxant dose is 15–30 minutes (Pedersoli 1972).

Pharmacologic Considerations. Polysynaptic reflexes are more effectively blocked by guaifenesin than monosynaptic reflexes. A number of literature sources indicate that by itself guaifenesin has sedative, hypnotic, and analgesic effects. There is evidence that sedative and hypnotic effects of the drug are due to the depressant effect upon the reticular formation of the brainstem.

Side effects produced by the drug include a transient decline in systemic arterial pressure when used (200 mg/kg) intravenously in the dog with thiopental and halothane anesthesia (Tavernor and Jones 1970). When used alone in the dog, the effect upon systemic arterial pressure is slight. A tachycardia occurs after the drug is administered, but heart rate returns to normal within 5 minutes after injection.

Guaifenesin (50 mg/mL) in 5% dextrose in combination with xylazine (0.25 mg/mL) and ketamine (1 mg/mL) has been infused intravenously in dogs at the rate of 2.2 mL/kg/hr for over 2 hours without adverse effect (Benson et al. 1985). Continuous infusion of the guaifenesin-xylazine-ketamine mixture does not significantly alter the heart rate, arterial pressure, or systemic vascular resistance. The cardiac index is decreased significantly by the mixture, which may be due to a decrease in stroke volume. An increase in arterial carbon dioxide tension and lowered arterial pH occurs after IV infusion of these three drugs; this coincides concomitantly with hypoventilation that is induced by guaifenesin, xylazine, and ketamine. Benson et al. (1985) did not see ventricular dysrhythmias or ECG signs of myocardial hypoxia or ischemia during the infusion. However, sinus dysrhythmia was observed; it was abolished by IV administration of 0.011 mg/kg glycopyrrolate.

In the horse, IV administration of guaifenesin (160 mg/kg) produces recumbency; minor effects on cardiac and respiratory rates, along with a slight drop in mean systemic arterial pressure and arterial PO_2, occur (Tavernor 1970). In buffalo calves, guaifenesin induces a respiratory acidosis (Singh et al. 1981). Ataxia and muscle relaxation are produced in cattle after an IV dose (50 mg/kg) of guaifenesin; recumbency is induced after an IV dose of 100 mg/kg (Hubbell et al. 1986).

When guaifenesin (80 mg/kg) is administered intravenously in the horse with thiopental (3.5 mg/kg), recumbency and slight decline in mean systemic arterial pressure occur. IV administration of guaifenesin alone (134 ± 34 mg/kg), sufficient to produce lateral recumbency in adult horses, results in a significant ($P < 0.05$) drop in arterial pressure (Hubbell et al. 1980). However, changes in heart rate, respiratory rate, right atrial pressure, pulmonary arterial pressure, and cardiac output are insignificant following administration in horses.

Guaifenesin in therapeutic amounts does not lead to the hazard of paralysis of the muscles (intercostal and diaphragm) of respiration as peripheral-acting skeletal muscle relaxants do. Respiratory activity usually remains normal after a therapeutic dose. In the dog, an IV dose (200 mg/kg) has only a slight effect on arterial PO_2, indicating that alveolar ventilation is unaltered (Tavernor and Jones 1970). Only when doses greater than those recommended are used in therapeutics will respiratory paralysis become a problem. Approximately three to four times the quantity required to produce recumbency of the horse can be administered before death occurs (Funk 1973).

Hemolysis may be induced when concentrations of guaifenesin in excess of 5% are used. However, a few sources in the veterinary literature indicate that hemolysis is insignificant with guaifenesin solutions up to 15%.

Kinetics of disappearance of guaifenesin from blood plasma in the pony have been studied by Davis and Wolff (1970). Of particular interest is the sex difference in rate of disappearance of guaifenesin. Rate of disappearance ($t_{1/2}$ = 59.6 ± 4.8 min) in the female is more rapid than in the male ($t_{1/2}$ = 84.4 ± 7.9 min). This indicates that the drug would need to be administered more frequently to maintain effect in the female, and recovery would be more rapid.

Clinical Use. Guaifenesin has been used in humans, domestic animals, and various species of laboratory animals. The IV dose approved for use of 5% guaifenesin in the horse is at a fixed level of 2.2 mL/kg (110 mg/kg). Most clinical uses in the horse are in line with this dosage (Gertsen and Tillotson 1968; Heath and Gabel 1970; Coffman and Pedersoli 1971; Jackson and Lundvall 1972; Pedersoli 1972).

Guaifenesin (110 mg/kg) given alone and rapidly by the IV route induces recumbency in about 2 minutes for about 6 minutes of light, not quite surgical level restraint (Heath 1977). Premedication with a phenothiazine derivative followed by guaifenesin (110 mg/kg) produces recumbency more easily and rapidly. This provides about 12–14 minutes of light, almost surgical level restraint.

Preanesthetic preparations used intravenously and recommended prior to administration of guaifenesin offer a number of options (Pedersoli 1972): (1) chloral hydrate (4 g/50 kg), (2) promazine (300 mg/454 kg), or (3) acepromazine (0.08 mg/kg).

Usually, guaifenesin (5%) plus an ultrashort-acting barbiturate such as thiopental is administered rapidly by the IV route 10–15 minutes following a preanesthetic level of xylazine. Guaifenesin (60 g) has also been used with pentobarbital (3 g) and 50% dextrose (125 mL) in water up to 1 L (Keeran 1972). A total of 1 L of this preparation is used by rapid IV injection for ovariectomy in adult mares.

Horses may be premedicated with IM acepromazine (0.02–0.05 mg/kg) or an α_2 agonist such as sylazine or detomidine 30–90 minutes before a 10% guaifenesin solution is administered by the IV route through an indwelling catheter (Brouwer 1985). Guaifenesin is given to effect until relaxation of the hindquarters occurs. It is terminated when this effect develops. This is immediately followed by a rapid IV injection of thiopental at a dose of 5.6 mg/kg or 1 g/180 kg. Guaifenesin administered by the above infusion procedure amounts to 48.7 ± 7.7 mg/kg over 3–4 minutes (Brouwer 1985). When about one-half the dose of guaifenesin is administered, the head of the horse drops slightly and light sedation occurs. Continuance of the guaifenesin infusion ultimately leads to relaxation of the hindquarters and swaying. Recumbency occurs 20–30 seconds after the IV bolus of thiopental. According to Brouwer, the limbs and jaw are immediately relaxed, which makes it easy to intubate the trachea for administration of halothane-oxygen. The time of recovery until standing after halothane-oxygen anesthesia and induction with guaifenesin-thiopental is 35 ± 22 minutes (Brouwer 1985).

Guaifenesin as the sole induction agent followed by halothane anesthesia has been used successfully in the horse (Schatzman 1974). When used alone (i.e., not with an ultrashort-acting barbiturate for induction), a higher average respiration rate and a lower, more balanced pulse rate are noted. However, it requires a higher average concentration of halothane to induce and maintain anesthesia.

Administration of xylazine (1.1 mg/kg) intravenously 5 minutes prior to guaifenesin reduces the IV dose necessary to induce lateral recumbency to 88 ± 10 mg/kg in adult horses (Hubbell et al. 1980). Without prior administration of xylazine, the IV dose required to produce recumbency is 134 ± 34 mg/kg.

Guaifenesin, xylazine, and ketamine hydrochloride can be used as a safe method of restraint for casting the horse (Muir et al. 1978). This drug combination minimally depresses cardiopulmonary function even if anesthesia is to be maintained with halothane or enflurane. Moreover, the combination provides safe induction and recovery from anesthesia. Approximately 20 minutes prior to induction of anesthesia with IV guaifenesin (55 mg/kg) in 5% dextrose, xylazine (2.2 mg/kg) is administered intramuscularly. Immediately following induction of anesthesia with guaifenesin, ketamine (1.7 mg/kg) is administered intravenously (Muir et al. 1978). Anesthesia can be maintained with halothane or enflurane. Guaifenesin (50 mg/mL), xylazine (0.5 mg/mL), and ketamine (1 mg/mL) can be used as a continuous infusion for maintenance of anesthesia in horses. It is administered at the rate of 2.2 mL/kg/hr after an induction protocol using xylazine (1.1 mg/kg) IV followed in 5 minutes by ketamine (2.2 mg/kg) IV (Benson and Thurmon 1990). Guaifenesin has been combined with detomidine (40 μg/mL) and ketamine (4 mg/mL) and administered at a continuous infusion rate of 0.8 mL/kg/min (Taylor et al. 1998).

The combination of guaifenesin (50 mg/mL), ketamine (1 mg/mL), and xylazine (0.25 mg/mL) provides effective analgesia in the dog; it is infused intravenously at a rate of 2.2 mL/kg/hr (Benson et al. 1985). In swine a combination of guaifenesin (50 mg/mL), ketamine (1 mg/mL), and xylazine (1 mg/mL) can be used for induction and maintenance of anesthesia. An initial volume of 0.5–1.0 mL/kg is rapidly infused and then 2.2 mL/kg/hr is infused to maintain anesthesia (Thurmon 1986).

Guaifenesin has been used repeatedly at 4- to 8-week intervals in the horse; one animal received the drug 4 times without any adverse effect (Lindley 1976). In a mare with dystocia, guaifenesin (25 g/400 mL) has been used with xylazine (2 mg/kg) and pentobarbital (1 g in the initial 400 mL of solution) intravenously for cesarean section (Cohen 1975). This anesthetic procedure is recommended to save the mare when the fetus is not alive.

It has been shown that a 10% solution of guaifenesin made in sterile distilled water is most suitable for clinical equine anesthesia (Grandy and McDonell 1980). More than 500 horses have been given this concentration without clinical evidence of drug-related problems.

In the mature bull, 5% guaifenesin and 0.2% thiopental in 5% glucose solution is administered (2.2 mL/kg) intravenously for induction of anesthesia (Garner et al. 1975). This is followed with halothane-oxygen for maintenance of anesthesia.

An IV dose of guaifenesin (165 mg/kg) has been used alone in male buffalo calves (*Bubalus bubalis*) (Singh et al. 1981) and in a dose of 90 mg/kg with thiopental (3.6 mg/kg) (Agrawal et al. 1983). A marked arterial hypotension and tachycardia occur in the buffaloes after induction of anesthesia. Also, guaifenesin has been used in IV doses of 27–110 mg/kg in a variety of nondomestic ungulates such as the Przewalski's horse, oryx, eland, and waterbuck (Janssen and Oosterhuis 1984).

Guaifenesin (50 mg/mL) has been combined with ketamine (1 mg/mL) and xylazine (0.1 mg/mL) in 5% glucose for use in cattle and small ruminants. This combination is administered intravenously to produce recumbency (about 0.5 mL/kg); maintenance of anesthesia requires a flow rate of 2.2 mL/kg/hr.

ALTHESIN. Althesin (*Saffan,* CT 1341) is a steroidal preparation containing two pregnanediones for induction of anesthesia (Child et al. 1972a). The anesthetic properties of steroids have been known since the 1940s. A paper published by Hans Selye as long ago as 1941 began the saga of the use of steroids in anesthesiology.

Althesin is in use within Canada and the UK but has not been approved in the USA by the FDA for use in animals. The steroid anesthetic combination has been released for human use in Canada; it may become a useful anesthetic in outpatients undergoing minor surgery (Dunn et al. 1978).

Althesin produces immediate induction of anesthesia of short duration when it is administered intravenously into experimental animals; recovery is rapid and without complications. Anesthetic activity of althesin has been determined in mice, rats, rabbits, cats, dogs, and monkeys (Child et al. 1971).

Chemistry. Althesin contains two pregnanediones, alphaxalone and alphadolone acetate, referred to as steroid I and steroid II respectively (Fig. 12.11) (Child et al. 1972a). A polyoxyethylated castor oil, Cremophor EL, is the vehicle, or carrier substance, for these steroids. IV injection of the vehicle into cats and dogs induces a severe arterial hypotension (Lorenz et al. 1971); this effect is not produced in sheep, rabbits, pigs, or humans.

The anesthetic preparation contains 0.9% weight/volume (*W/V*) steroid I and 0.3% *W/V* steroid II. One mL of althesin contains 12 mg of both steroids, i.e., 9 mg steroid I and 3 mg steroid II. Dosage is expressed as mL formulated solution/kg or mg total steroids/kg.

Pharmacologic Activity. In the cat, 1.2–9 mg/kg althesin administered intravenously produces a transient drop in systemic arterial blood pressure and tachycardia within a few seconds after injection (Child et al. 1972a; Middleton et al. 1982). This is succeeded by a slight rise in blood pressure during recovery from anesthesia. A similar effect upon arterial pressure has been observed by Haskins et al. (1975). On comparing effects of althesin in the cat with ketamine and xylazine (all administered intramuscularly), althesin induces a sustained decrease in arterial systolic pressure of about 23%, while xylazine and ketamine elevate the pressure (Fig. 12.12).

Within 6–9 minutes following injection, Child and coworkers (1972a) reported that animals are able to stand and, after a period of ataxia, a rapid return to normal is observed. An IV dose of 7.2 mg/kg althesin

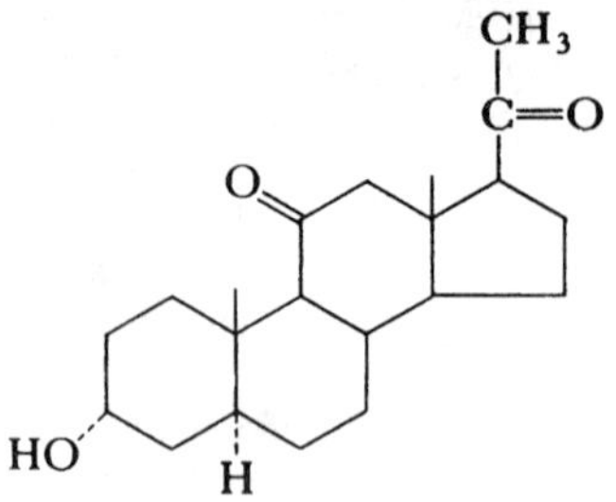

Steroid I (alphaxalone; 3α-hydroxy-5α-pregnane-11,20, dione)

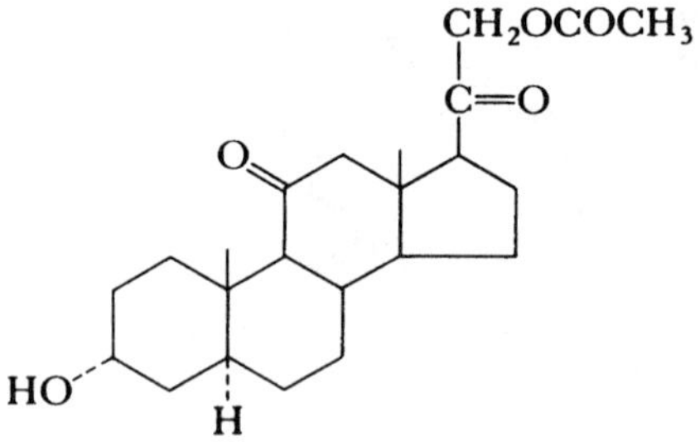

Steroid II (alphadolone; 21-acetoxy-3α-hydroxy-5α-pregnane-11,20, dione)

FIG. 12.11

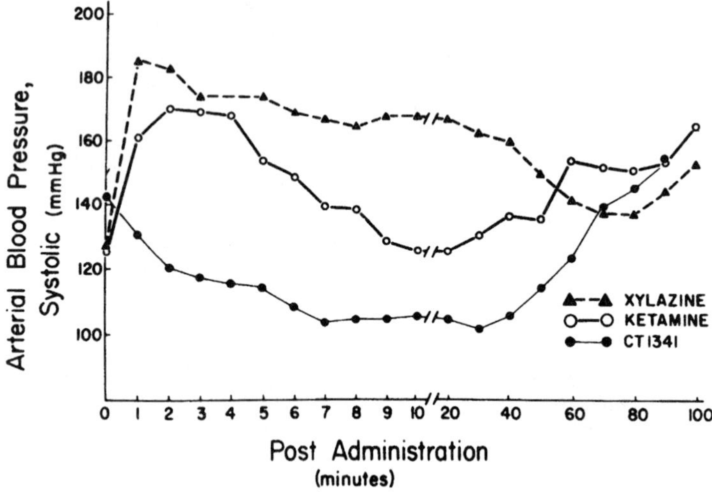

FIG. 12.12—Average systolic blood pressure responses of 4 cats anesthetized with althesin (15 mg/kg), ketamine (33 mg/kg), and xylazine (4.4 mg/kg) (Haskins et al. 1975).

administered 5–10 minutes prior to use of inhalant anesthetics has proved to be a compatible procedure. Cats are satisfactorily maintained for 50 minutes by inhalation agents (Child et al. 1972a). Neuromuscular agents such as succinylcholine, *d*-tubocurarine, or gallamine with althesin are compatible. Preanesthetic agents such as atropine (1 mg/kg) and meperidine (7.5 mg/kg) administered intramuscularly 1 hour before induction with althesin (7.2 mg/kg) are satisfactorily tolerated (Child et al. 1972a).

A dose (0.4 mg/kg) of althesin administered intravenously at a rate of 0.1 mL/kg/sec or 1.2 mg/kg/sec in the cat produces immediate loss of the righting reflex, which lasts for about 1 minute, with complete recovery from ataxia after about 7 minutes (Davis and Pearce 1972). Depth and duration of effect increases as dosage increases, until with 3.6 mg/kg the corneal reflex is absent for 3 minutes. Surgical anesthesia is achieved for 5–10 minutes with a dose of 7.2 mg/kg. Cats tolerate a dose of 19.2 mg/kg with only slight depression of respiration, but 32.4 mg/kg induces apnea, vascular collapse, and death (Davis and Pearce 1972).

Induction of anesthesia with althesin does not potentiate halothane-epinephrine dysrhythmias during halothane maintenance (Dodds and Twissell 1972). An increase in pulmonary vascular resistance in goats occurs following 0.11 mL/kg or 0.22 mL/kg of althesin (Foâx and Prys-Roberts 1972). Heart rate increases 23% with the low dose and only slightly (6%) with the higher dose. Cardiac output increases slightly with the low dose (0.11 mL/kg) and returns to near normal about 1 minute after IV administration of althesin. The higher dose (0.22 mL/kg) decreases cardiac output to almost 20%; it returns to near normal about 4–5 minutes following administration (Foâx and Prys-Roberts 1972). Althesin has less of a negative inotropic action on the myocardium of the cat than thiopental or propanidid (Gordh 1972).

The half-life of alphaxalone in plasma of rats after IV administration of althesin is approximately 7 minutes (Child et al. 1972b). A similar half-life exists in mice and monkeys. Neither alphaxalone nor alphadolone acetate is extensively protein bound in serum of rats, cats, horses, or humans; about 70% of the radiolabeled compounds are excreted in the bile within the first 3 hours after IV administration of althesin. Appreciable amounts of radioactivity appear in both urine (20–30%) and feces (60–70%) for up to 5 days after administration. Gunn rats, a strain deficient in glucuronyl transferase, sleep longer after althesin than normal rats. Apparently, glucuronide synthesis plays a part in metabolism and excretion of these steroids. Preliminary studies with radio-labeled alphaxalone indicate that the major biliary metabolite in the rat is a glucuronide of 2 α-hydroxyalphaxalone (Child et al. 1972b).

Irrespective of the dosage of althesin, Child and coworkers (1972a) observed no injury to the veins and no vomiting in the cat. The IM route of administration (15–18 mg/kg) is useful in kittens where venipuncture is difficult to perform (Hall 1972).

Hormonal effects of althesin have been evaluated in mice, rats, and rabbits (Child et al. 1971). Althesin possesses less than one-sixtieth the activity of betamethasone and is slightly less active than hydrocortisone. In adrenalectomized rats no evidence of mineralocorticoid activity occurs following administration of althesin. Moreover, it does not possess estrogenic or progestational activity in mice. Althesin is capable of antagonizing the uterotropic action of exogenous estradiol; consequently, it possesses weak antiestrogenic activity.

Clinical Use

CATS. Depth and duration of anesthesia with different dosages of althesin have been divided into four easily observable phases (Davis and Pearce 1972): (1) the cat is ataxic, (2) there is loss of the righting reflex and the cat is lying on its side, (3) the pedal withdrawal reflex is absent, and (4) the corneal reflex is absent.

For induction of anesthesia in the cat, a single IV dose of althesin (9 mg/kg or 0.75 mL/kg) has been used clinically for castration and dental surgery (Evan et al. 1972). Duration of anesthesia is 10–12 minutes; surgical procedures requiring more than 5–10 minutes may be extended by injection of additional small amounts of the anesthetic preparation. Even after 48 hours of intermittent administration of althesin, cats awaken within 30–45 minutes of the final injection (Hall 1976).

Althesin can be used to maintain surgical anesthesia for a prolonged period in the cat by repeated supplementary injections of one-half the IV induction dose without significant cumulative anesthetic or respiratory depressant effects (Dodds and Twissell 1973). However, isolated clinical reports have indicated that cessation of respiration occasionally occurs and efforts to revive these animals are unsuccessful.

Althesin may also be administered intramuscularly (9 mg/kg) for clinical procedures such as radiography, dematting, and examination of the mouth (Evan et al. 1972). This dose will produce sedation of the animal in approximately 7 minutes after injection and sedation will last for about 5 minutes. According to Evan and coworkers (1972), 12 mg/kg (1 mL/kg) althesin administered intramuscularly will result in deep sedation or light anesthesia that is sufficient to permit a number of minor surgical procedures such as drainage of an abscess or suturing small superficial wounds. The maximum response produced by this dose level occurs in 7–8 minutes and has a duration of action of about 15 minutes. Light sedation produced by an IV dose of 4 mg/kg has been suggested in premedication prior to induction of full anesthesia with althesin or other anesthetic agents (Evan et al. 1972).

RABBITS. Althesin administered intravenously in the healthy rabbit at 20 mg/kg (one-half rapidly and the remainder slowly to effect) will induce light anesthesia within 1 minute and lasts 6–7 minutes (Wood 1978). Additional althesin (4–6 mg/kg) can be administered intravenously to increase duration of anesthesia. Induction and recovery from althesin is without CNS excitation; full recovery occurs within 30 minutes.

AVIAN SPECIES. Cooper and Frank (1973) concluded that althesin is of value in the chicken when administered by the IV route. Analgesia, muscle relaxation, and speed of recovery were considered to be excellent at an IV dose level up to 14 mg/kg. However, they suggested an IV dose for birds of 10 mg/kg. Althesin appears to be a safe drug even in recently captured birds of prey unaccustomed to restraint. Given by IM and intraperitoneal routes, the drug is of limited value because large volumes are required to induce analgesia (Cooper and Frank 1973).

In the red-tailed hawk (*Buteo jamaicensis*), the dose of althesin should be 5 mg/kg or less intravenously (Cooper and Redig 1975; Cribb and Haigh 1977). Complete sinus arrest, followed in some cases by ectopic beats and then by tachycardia for several minutes, occurs after administration of althesin. Sinus arrest and transient bradycardia followed by tachycardia are seen in mallard ducks (*Anas platyrhynchos*) and Canada geese (*Branta canadensis*). With the high incidence of sinus arrest and tachycardia, it appears that althesin should be used cautiously in red-tailed hawks, mallards, and Canada geese (Cribb and Haigh 1977). Intubation of the trachea in birds is relatively easy because althesin abolishes the swallowing reflex (Harcourt-Brown 1978).

In the budgerigar (*Melopsittacus undulatus*) an IM dose of althesin (36 mg/kg) provides an average of 12 minutes of anesthesia (Curtis et al. 1977). This dose appears to be satisfactory for general use, since repeated dosages can be safely administered if the initial effect is insufficient for induction of anesthesia or if prolongation of anesthesia is necessary. Hypothermia is well recognized following anesthesia of small birds. Maintenance of the bird's normal body temperature during anesthesia and recovery contributes to the safety margin of anesthetics, including that of althesin (Curtis et al. 1977).

A combination of althesin (12–17 mg/kg), ketamine (5 mg/kg), and xylazine (1 mg/kg) injected into the jugular vein has been used to induce anesthesia in ostriches (*Struthio camelus*) (Gandini et al. 1986).

SHEEP. At least 1.65 mg/kg IV althesin is needed to induce anesthesia in sheep (Waterman 1981). The mean arterial pressure decreases 50% at 30 seconds after injection but lasts for only 10 minutes. Premedication with atropine or mepyramine fails to alter this hypotensive action. Injection of the carrier or vehicle Cremophor EL alone has no effect upon mean arterial pressure. Althesin in a mean IV dose of 3 mg/kg is most useful clinically. Infusion of a dilute solution (0.234 mg/kg/min) maintains anesthesia. Sheep recover rapidly from althesin anesthesia.

SWINE. Althesin (1–8 mg/kg) administered intramuscularly into the neck induces slight incoordination with mild sedation to a deep sedative effect and inability to stand in swine weighing 17–93 kg (Cox et al. 1975). Effects of althesin usually occur within 5 minutes of administration, are maximal between 10 and 90 minutes, and are inapparent after 90–180 minutes.

IV administration of althesin (2–3 mg/kg) is followed by loss of consciousness within 10–20 seconds (Cox et al. 1975). Apnea occurs in some animals for 15 seconds after IV administration of the drug. Muscular relaxation is excellent for 4–10 minutes, and endotracheal intubation can be performed during this time without difficulty. Some animals are given azaperone (4 mg/kg) intramuscularly as a preanesthetic 50 minutes prior to althesin.

Preliminary clinical studies indicate that althesin (6–8 mg/kg) induces an excellent sedative effect in swine when injected intramuscularly; in contrast to azaperone, sensory stimuli do not appear to elicit a marked arousal response (Cox et al. 1975). The large volumes of the anesthetic solution required to achieve anesthesia by this route of administration and the expense preclude such use at present. Conversely, according to Cox and coworkers (1975), smaller volumes produce a short period of anesthesia, with excellent muscular relaxation and minimal depression of respiration when the IV route is used. In this respect althesin is superior to combined use of etorphine and acepromazine (Immobilon). Additionally, recovery is rapid, with less struggling compared to use of the short-acting hypnotic (i.e., metomidate hydrochloride). The disadvantage of althesin for induction of anesthesia in the pig is its short duration of action (Cox et al. 1975).

HORSES. Althesin administered intravenously in horses and ponies is associated with CNS excitation for up to 30 seconds after recumbency (Eales 1976). Muscle relaxation is poor. Slight stimulation results in twitching and violent kicking for up to 15 minutes. Althesin does not appear to offer an advantage over presently used anesthetics in equine practice and has several disadvantages (Eales 1976).

BABOONS. Althesin is safe to administer as an IV infusion to baboons premedicated with ketamine (Cookson and Mills 1983). Induction is smooth and recovery is rapid.

REPTILES. Althesin has been used in 13 reptilian species (Lawrence and Jackson 1983). It appears to be an ideal agent for anesthesia in lizards and chelonians.

FISH. Althesin has been used in brown or rainbow trout following immersion in a solution of benzocaine (formerly ethyl aminobenzoate) (50 mg/L). Within 30 seconds fish are sufficiently sedated to permit weighing and subsequent injection of the calculated anesthetic dose (18–36 mg/kg) (Oswald 1978). Althesin is injected by the IP route or a combination of two thirds intraperitoneally and one-third intramuscularly. IM injections greater than 0.2–0.3 mL are not recommended because of reflux of anesthetic solution out of the injection site.

Doses of althesin 18 mg/kg and over produce anesthesia; lower doses only induce sedation. Duration of anesthesia ranges from 1–3 hours at 24 mg/kg to 4–6 hours at 36 mg/kg. Doses of 24 mg/kg and over always induce apnea. Recovery from anesthesia is characterized by a slight phase of excitement and is quickly followed by sedation. In most fish, recovery from althesin is complete within 2 hours (Oswald 1978).

Contraindications and Drug Interactions. Use of althesin in the dog is contraindicated because the nonionic surface active agent (i.e., Cremophor EL or polyoxyethylated castor oil) in the preparation causes release of histamine (Stock 1973), which results in cardiovascular collapse in this species. However, IV Cremophor EL may also liberate mast cell histamine in the cat and induce arterial hypotension, as in dogs (Lorenz et al. 1971). Allergic reactions such as scratching, peripheral edema, hyperemia of the ears, urination, and defecation are regularly seen in cats (Dodman 1980; Middleton et al. 1982). Anaphylactoid reactions may have been responsible for some of the unexpected deaths after administration of althesin (Edmonds 1973; Rheinberger et al. 1979). Moreover, respiratory failure after use of althesin has resulted in death (Ruben 1979).

Apart from barbiturates, any preoperative and postoperative medicant and inhalational agent can be used in conjunction with althesin (Stock 1973). Althesin *must not be used with barbiturates* (Tavernor 1977). Anesthetic adjuvants, including pressor agents, adrenergic blocking agents, and analeptics have been used without adverse effects (Stock 1973). Skeletal muscle–paralyzing drugs have also been used in the cat during althesin analgesia and anesthesia. Only a slight reduction in activity of succinylcholine chloride is noted during prolonged infusion of althesin. No effect on activity of other neuromuscular blocking agents has been observed.

DISSOCIATIVE ANESTHETICS. Three dissociative anesthetic drugs have current interest in veterinary medicine: phencyclidine hydrochloride and its congeners, ketamine hydrochloride, and tiletamine hydrochloride. With a high abuse record in humans, phencyclidine was banned in 1979 for use in the USA. It was moved from Schedule II to Schedule I under the Controlled Substances Act of 1970 but has been reclassified as a Schedule II drug.

A cataleptic-type state referred to as dissociative anesthesia is typical of phencyclidine and its derivatives and is accompanied by marked analgesia in most species (Thurmon et al. 1972). The term dissociative anesthetic originated from use of ketamine in human medicine, which causes the patient to feel dissociated from or unaware of the environment during induction (Price 1975). Ketamine is approved by the FDA for use in the cat and subhuman primates. Tiletamine in combination with zolazepam (Telazol) was approved by the FDA in 1982 for anesthetic use in dogs and cats.

Phencyclidine Hydrochloride. Chemically, phencyclidine hydrochloride (Sernylan, Sernyl, GP-121, CI-395) is 1-(1-phenylcyclohexyl) piperidine hydrochloride (Fig. 12.13). It is a white, glistening solid with a high degree of solubility in water. Phencyclidine is classified as a Schedule II drug under the Controlled Substances Act of 1970.

PHARMACOLOGIC CONSIDERATIONS. Phencyclidine differs greatly from general anesthetics in that absence of responses to nociceptive stimuli is not accompanied with loss of corneal, pupillary, and other reflexes. In most if not all species, phencyclidine in high dosages produces a generalized increase in skeletal muscular tone and catalepsy. It induces stages I and II anesthesia but not stage III anesthesia.

The primary pharmacologic effect of phencyclidine is depression or stimulation of the CNS or a combination of these (Stoliker 1965). According to Stoliker, the quality of the effect produced by phencyclidine is highly species-specific. In mice the principal initial effect is excitation and not depression. However, in the dog and other species, depression is produced by phencyclidine at low dosages; excitation leading to convulsive seizures may occur following large doses (Stoliker 1965).

IM administration of 2 mg/kg phencyclidine in the rhesus monkey results in significant decrease in heart rate about 3 minutes after the injection and lasts 2 hours (Popovic et al. 1972). A corresponding decrease in systolic and diastolic arterial pressures, along with a drop in central venous pressure, occurs. These changes are only significant for the initial 90 minutes. ECG irregularities, along with prominent changes in the QRS amplitude also occur.

The EEG of phencyclidine-treated monkeys is affected within 3 minutes following injection. Decreases in amplitude of α rhythm and, occasionally, δ waves appear to be reestablished (Popovic et al. 1972).

Three hours later, upon repeated administration of phencyclidine up to one-half the dose (i.e., 1 mg/kg) by the IV route, the drug produces an immediate but temporary decline in arterial pressure, change in the ECG, and catalepsy (Popovic et al. 1972).

A number of authors have referred to the effect of phencyclidine and other central-acting drugs upon behavioral qualities of offspring following use of these agents in pregnant animals. It is suggested by Tonge (1973) that the developing brain of neonates may be particularly susceptible to phencyclidine.

Ketamine Hydrochloride. *Ketamine Hydrochloride*, USP (Ketalar, Ketaset, Vetalar, Ketaject), is a congener of phencyclidine and is chemically designated as 2-(*o*-chlorophenyl)-2-(methylamino)-cyclohexanone hydrochloride (Fig. 12.14).

Ketamine is a unique general anesthetic first introduced into human medicine in 1965; in 1970 it was introduced for anesthesia in the cat. Its lack of cardiorespiratory depression is unequaled by any other general anesthetic currently available (Lanning and Harmel 1975). Ketamine is an extremely versatile agent because it can be administered by the IM or IV

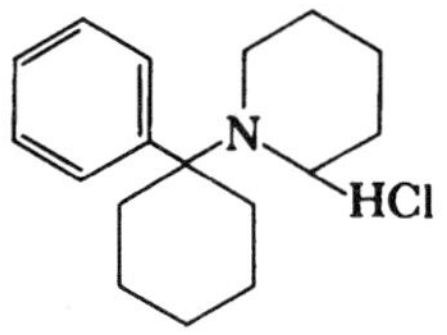

N HCl

Phencyclidine Hydrochloride

FIG. 12.13

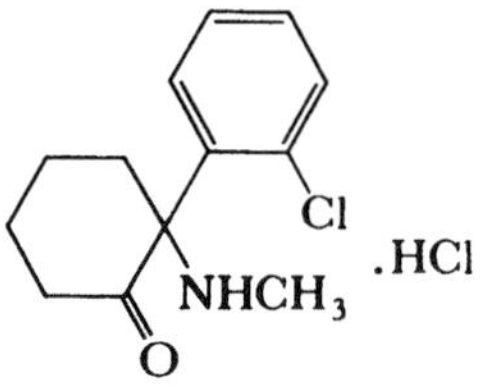

Cl .HCl NHCH$_3$ O

Ketamine Hydrochloride

FIG. 12.14

route without appreciable tissue irritation. Some irritation occurs during IM injection because the pH of an aqueous preparation of ketamine is 3.5.

Adverse effects produced by phencyclidine such as oculogyric activity, tremors, tonic spasticity, and convulsive seizures are ordinarily less pronounced with ketamine. Although ketamine has been approved by the FDA for use only in the cat and subhuman primates, it is being used in most of the other species (Wright 1982). It has not been approved for use in animals intended for human consumption.

Ketamine is classified as a Schedule III drug under the Controlled Substances Act of 1970.

Ketamine is more commonly used in combination with other anesthetic agents. Its use with nitrous oxide and skeletal muscle relaxants provides adequate anesthesia for intra-abdominal and thoracic surgery (Vaughan and Stephen 1974).

Ketamine appears to exert the majority of its CNS actions via its antagonistic effect at *N*-methyl-D-aspartate (NMDA) receptors (Orser et al. 1997). Other evidence suggests it may have effects at other receptors, such as glutamate (Moghaddam et al. 1997; Kress 1997; Sharp 1996; Lees et al. 1994; Goodchild 1993). Ketamine-induced analgesia is mediated at least in part via opiate receptors (Taylor and Kenny 1993; Finck and Ngai 1982).

PHARMACOLOGIC CONSIDERATIONS. In humans, ketamine has been used primarily in children for rapid induction of analgesia. According to Virtue and coworkers (1967), there is presently no more rapid method than IV administration of ketamine.

CNS effects of ketamine, as characterized by the EEG, indicate that depression of the thalamoneocortical system occurs in conjunction with activation of the limbic system. Even though limbic activation including epileptiform EEG patterns develop, there is no evidence that seizure activity spreads to the cerebral cortex (White et al. 1982). Paradoxically, studies have revealed that natural sleep is a more potent stimulant of convulsions than ketamine in the epileptic individual. Consequently, ketamine is not likely to induce convulsions in patients with seizure disorders. Actually, experimental studies indicate that ketamine may have anticonvulsant activity (Reder et al. 1980). However, some of the early and more recent literature refers to ketamine as an "epileptogenic anesthetic" (Oguchi et al. 1982). Until more information is available, ketamine probably should not be used in animals with a history of epileptic seizures. Because of the dual CNS action of ketamine, it is characterized as a dissociative anesthetic.

Ketamine induces anesthesia and amnesia by functional disruption (dissociation) of the CNS through marked CNS stimulation or induction of a cataleptoid state. It induces stages I and II anesthesia but not stage III anesthesia.

Ketamine generally stimulates the cardiovascular system. This effect is thought to be due to central effects that mimic the effect of sympathetic nervous system stimulation. This central stimulation overrides any direct peripheral cardiovascular depressant effects of ketamine (Reves et al. 1994).

Ketamine increases cardiac output, mean aortic pressure, pulmonary arterial pressure, central venous pressure, and heart rate. It has a variable effect upon peripheral vascular resistance. There is evidence that the adrenergic system must be intact for these cardiovascular responses to occur (Christ et al. 1997). Consequently, ketamine probably acts either directly by stimulating the central adrenergic centers or indirectly by inhibiting the neuronal uptake of catecholamines, especially norepinephrine (Adams 1997). These cardiac-stimulating properties, in addition to its antiarrhythmic action, make ketamine a good induction agent for poor-risk and hypovolemic patients (Lanning and Harmel 1975). However, for maintenance, ketamine may be a liability in subjects with severe coronary insufficiency, since it elevates myocardial oxygen consumption. Moreover, dogs made hypotensive by hemorrhaging develop a greater oxygen debt and deteriorate more rapidly with ketamine than with halothane or neuroleptanalgesia. In the isolated perfused rat heart, ketamine alters electrical activity by prolongation of the PR and Q-T intervals (Aronson and Hanno 1978). However, ketamine does not induce major alterations in the ECG pattern of nonhuman primates (Gonder et al. 1980).

Work in the cat has shown that ketamine inhibits efferent cardiac vagal drive by its central action independently of baroreflex function; this central vagolytic effect is believed to be responsible for the positive chronotropic effects of ketamine (Inque and Arndt 1982). Other anesthetics that induce a central vagolytic action leading to tachycardia are althesin and the barbiturates.

An interesting and important pharmacologic effect of ketamine is its effect upon ventilation. Many anesthetics are potent depressants of the ventilatory response to hypoxia, whereas ketamine is not. Ketamine decreases airway resistance in asthmatic patients (human); a bronchodilator such as aminophylline may also be administered before or during ketamine anesthesia without adverse effect (Stirt et al. 1982). In the dog anesthetized with thiopental, an IV combination of ketamine (5 mg/kg) and aminophylline (10, 25, and 50 mg/kg) does not induce cardiac arrhythmias.

When ketamine is used as a monoanesthetic, pharyngeal and laryngeal reflexes remain active (Lanning and Harmel 1975). Preservation of these reflexes, however, leads to increase of laryngospasm, bronchospasm, and coughing secondary to secretions or manipulation in the oropharynx. These complications make ketamine a poor drug for use in endoscopy or oropharyngeal surgery. Additionally, ketamine stimulates salivation, which must be blocked by a noncentrally active antisialagogue (e.g., glycopyrrolate) prior to induction of anesthesia. Also, ketamine increases tracheal-bronchial mucous gland secretions, which is additional justification for using an antisialagogue (White et al. 1982).

As with all general anesthetics, ketamine should be administered with the usual precautions when the stomach is full of ingesta. Nevertheless, presence of a patent airway and lack of respiratory depression make ketamine the general anesthetic of choice when intubation is impossible (Lanning and Harmel 1975). Despite the presence of protective laryngeal and pharyngeal reflexes, tracheal aspiration has been reported after induction of anesthesia by ketamine. Consequently, one should maintain a patent airway or intubate the trachea, as practiced with other anesthetic agents (White et al. 1982).

Clinical case reports in humans have suggested that an interaction occurs between thyroid hormones and ketamine. Human patients on thyroid replacement therapy have developed a severe hypertension and tachycardia following ketamine administration. If such an adverse action occurs, β-adrenergic blocking agents may be of value. Other interactions reported in humans have involved potentiation of respiratory depression and/or paralysis following use of succinylcholine and propanidid (Bovill et al. 1971).

Similar interactions between *d*-tubocurarine have been observed using the cat sciatic nerve–gastrocnemius muscle preparation (Cronnelly 1972; Cronnelly et al. 1973). Potentiation of skeletal muscle twitch of the cat by edrophonium chloride is antagonized by ketamine in IV doses of 1 and 2 mg/kg (Cronnelly 1972). However, ketamine alone produces no significant effect upon muscle twitch (Cronnelly et al. 1973). This is expected, since ketamine produces only a 30% reduction of end plate sensitivity.

Ketamine has been used safely in humans with myopathies and malignant hyperthermia (White et al. 1982). Use of ketamine in animals susceptible to malignant hyperthermia is controversial (Kirmayer et al. 1984).

The combination of IM ketamine (0.55 mg/kg) and acepromazine (11 mg/kg) provides good skeletal muscle relaxation in rhesus monkeys. According to Porter (1982), this combination is useful for surgery or orthopedic work.

Ketamine (2 mg/kg) administered intravenously, increases cerebral blood flow in the dog 80% and cerebral oxygen consumption 16%; EEG changes accompany those of increased cerebral oxygen consumption in that the wave frequency increases after injection of the drug (Dawson et al. 1971). Dawson and associates concluded that ketamine is a cerebral metabolic stimulant and a cerebral vasodilator. They were able to block these pharmacologic effects by prior administration of thiopental.

Ketamine and xylazine have been used in the horse to determine their effects upon intraocular pressure. A decrease in intraocular pressure occurs after an IV dose of 1.1 mg/kg xylazine. Ketamine (2.2 mg/kg) administered intravenously 8 minutes after the xylazine does not induce any further change in the pressure (Trim et al. 1985). The prevalence of nystagmus produced by this combination is considered to be a disadvantage that may complicate ocular surgery. However, maintenance of anesthesia with halothane after ketamine administration is a way to circumvent this complication (Trim et al. 1985).

Ketamine is rapidly distributed into all body tissues, primarily adipose tissue, liver, lung, and brain (Lanning and Harmel 1975). Plasma protein binding of ketamine in the horse averages 50% over the concentration range of 0.3–20 μg/mL (Kaka et al. 1979). Binding of ketamine to plasma and albumin is dependent upon the pH; it is decreased at a pH lower than 7.4 and increased at a higher pH (Dayton et al. 1983).

Biotransformation occurs in the liver by *N*-demethylation and hydroxylation of the cyclohexanone ring, with formation of water-soluble glucuronide derivatives that are eliminated in urine (White et al. 1982). In sheep, metabolites of ketamine have been identified (Waterman and Livingston 1978a). A demethylated metabolite and subsequent oxidation metabolites have been detected in plasma and urine of sheep.

An analytic method for ketamine is capable of detecting 0.1 μg/mL of the compound in blood and urine (Kochhar 1977). This method should be adaptable in detection of ketamine residues in tissue samples.

The apparent biologic half-life of ketamine in humans is 2–3 hours (White et al. 1982). In the horse the distribution (α phase) and elimination (β phase) half-lives of ketamine average 2.9 and 42 minutes respectively following IV injection of 2.2 mg/kg (Kaka et al. 1979).

The elimination half-life of ketamine in the calf is 60.5 minutes (Waterman 1984). Premedication with xylazine does not affect the half-life of ketamine significantly; however, the clearance rate of ketamine is reduced about 50%.

In the cat, a rapid distribution phase ($t_{1/2\alpha}$ = 3 min) is followed by a slower first-order elimination phase (Baggot and Blake 1976). The half-life of ketamine (66.9 ± 24.1 min) is independent of the route of parenteral administration. Absorption from the IM site of administration is rapid; peak plasma concentration is reached in 10 minutes (Baggot and Blake 1976). The elimination half-life of ketamine is prolonged and recovery from ketamine anesthesia is delayed by use of sedative premedicants such as diazepam or secobarbital (Lo and Cumming 1975).

Ketamine anesthesia does not appear to alter endocrine functions in the crab-eating macaque (*Macaca fascicularis*) or rhesus monkeys (Castro et al. 1981; Fuller et al. 1984).

As the result of extensive metabolization of ketamine by the liver, its duration of action is not prolonged in humans with renal impairment (Lanning and Harmel 1975).

Ketamine has a wide therapeutic index. In animals, a ketamine LD_{50}/ED_{50} ratio five times that of pentobarbital has been demonstrated. Repeated administration of ketamine does not lead to development of any significant tolerance or complications. However, ketamine induces the hepatic microsomal enzyme system (Marietta et al. 1977). Although less potent than phenobarbital, ketamine appears to act similarly in induction of hepatic microsomal metabolizing enzymes of rats.

In the cat, body temperature declines by an average of 1.6°C following clinical dosage of ketamine (Beck et al. 1971). Ketamine does not abolish pedal and pinnal reflexes; photic and corneal reflexes persist in the cat as well as laryngeal and pharyngeal reflexes. Skeletal muscle tone is also increased.

When ketamine (3–5 mg/kg) is used intravenously and as the only agent in cats, their eyes remain completely open with a fixed stare and the pupils are dilated. Other clinical signs are licking of the lips and profuse salivation. Increased salivation in cats is consistent with the drug's sympathomimetic action. Slow movements of the head are observed; rigidity or extension of the forelimbs is also seen, and opisthotonus occurs after an IV dose of 8–10 mg/kg. Convulsive seizures have been reported in 5.3% (Beck et al. 1971) and in 20% of the cats that receive clinical dosages of ketamine (Stock 1973). Diazepam has been used to abolish ketamine-induced convulsive seizures in the cat (Reid and Frank 1972). An IV dose of 0.44 mg/kg is used for this purpose. The benzodiazepines (diazepam, lorazepam, midazolam) appear to be most effective in reducing the psychic actions and cardiovascular responses of ketamine in humans upon emergence or recovery (White et al. 1982). In the cat, diazepam used alone induces irritability and aberrant behavior.

According to Beck et al. (1971), IM doses of ketamine less than 22 mg/kg produce basic chemical restraint without total analgesia but are satisfactory for physical examination and minor procedures. IM doses of 22–44 mg/kg produce cataleptoid anesthesia, a comatose state similar to decerebrate rigidity (Beck et al. 1971). This effect is adequate for performing short, simple diagnostic procedures and short surgical procedures; duration of surgical cataleptoid anesthesia ranges from 20 to 40 minutes. Although recovery from ketamine is frequently prolonged and may be accompanied by excitement, the cat is ordinarily able to attain the sitting position after 2 hours (Massey 1973).

The mechanism of ketamine-induced catalepsy has not been extensively investigated and consequently is not clearly understood. With the plethora of literature on catalepsy and other mobility disorders, there is indication that most of these may be due to a deficiency of dopamine function or an imbalance in cholinergic-dopaminergic function. Moreover, other neurotransmitting chemicals cannot be ignored from consideration in catalepsy; e.g., serotonin is also associated with the extrapyramidal system and can induce catalepsy when it is administered intracerebroventricularly in the cat.

When an antiserotonin neuroleptic agent (i.e., methiothepin maleate) is administered in the cat prior to ketamine, it is interesting that the ketamine-induced catalepsy is not observed (Hatch 1973a). Instead of muscle tonus and presence of limb rigidity, which typifies action of ketamine in the cat, muscle flaccidity is observed. Another agent that is an antidopamine neuroleptic (i.e., pimozide) was also employed by Hatch (1973a). The only effect of pimozide on ketamine is that it prevents the sporadic stimulus-induced paw twitch often seen in the cat. The blocking effect of methiothepin upon serotonin suggests that serotonergic mechanisms are involved in ketamine-induced catalepsy, whereas the blocking effect of pimozide suggests that dopamine is involved in the ketamine-induced sporadic movements of muscles and limbs.

The pharmacologic effects of ketamine can be antagonized or shortened almost immediately by administration of a mixture of *l*-amphetamine and yohimbine (Hatch and Ruch 1974). Because yohimbine has been classified as a specific α_2-adrenoceptor blocking agent upon presynaptic receptors (Hedler et al. 1981), antagonism of ketamine may occur from release of central neuronal dopamine and norepinephrine.

ADVERSE EFFECTS. A 2-year-old Giant Poodle with no previous history of respiratory or circulatory complications died of pulmonary edema 2 days after a combination of ketamine (9 mg/kg) and xylazine (1.4 mg/kg) were administered parenterally (Kommonen and Koskinen 1984). Until more clinical experience with this combination of drugs is attained, considerable caution needs to be taken in its use.

CONTRAINDICATIONS AND PRECAUTIONS. Ketamine must not be used in animals intended for human consumption. As the only agent for anesthesia, it is not recommended for use in cesarean section (Dodman 1979). Use of ketamine as the sole agent for abdominal and orthopedic surgery cannot be recommended; its use in major surgical procedures must be supplemented with general anesthesia. Moreover, it is contraindicated in subjects that have arterial aneurysms, uncontrolled arterial hypertension, and right or left heart failure.

Ketamine is contraindicated in animals afflicted with hepatic or renal dysfunction. It is also contraindicated in head injuries, since it elevates the cerebrospinal fluid pressure. Although ketamine is an unlikely agent to trigger generalized convulsions in human patients with seizure disorders (White et al. 1982), it probably should be used cautiously or not at all in animals subject to epileptic seizure.

For procedures involving the pharynx, larynx, or trachea, a probable or relative contraindication to its use is suggested. Also, relative contraindications are suggested in use of ketamine in the presence of increased intraocular pressure or open-globe injury to the eye and in subjects with a thyrotoxic condition (White et al. 1982).

Precautions should be taken to control hemorrhage after surgery because arterial hypertension from use of ketamine occurs; this precaution is especially important following declawing of mature cats, particularly if the paws are not bandaged (Evans et al. 1972).

It has been suggested that it may be prudent to avoid use of ketamine-xylazine in animals that have a reduced cardiopulmonary reserve (Kolata and Rawlings 1982). Use of ketamine alone in patients with respiratory complications is not considered to be contraindicated providing endotracheal intubation, supplemental oxygen, and artificial ventilation are available (Haskins et al. 1985). The combination of ketamine and acepromazine probably should not be used in dogs predisposed to arterial hypotension or respiratory depression (Farver et al. 1986).

Caution is advised in administration of ketamine in animals that have undergone severe hemorrhage. Blood loss of 30% of the total blood volume decreases the anesthetic induction dose of ketamine from 35 to 45% in animals (Weiskopf and Bogetz 1985). In myelographic procedures, ketamine should not be used in seizure-prone animals (Clark et al. 1982).

CLINICAL USE

CAT. Prior to administration of ketamine, atropine or glycopyrrolate should be given to prevent salivation and other autonomic nervous system effects. It is recommended that a bland ophthalmic ointment be used soon after the peak effect of ketamine to prevent drying and irritation of the cornea.

Ketamine is most valuable as an immobilizing agent for examinations, radiographic procedures, and prior to induction of general anesthesia with conventional agents (Glen 1973). The recommended IM dose is from 11 to 33 mg/kg. However, some clinicians use an IM dose as high as 44 mg/kg; 3–5 minutes are required for the animal to become anesthetized (DeYoung et al. 1972). Pain, apparently due to the low pH of the injectable formulation, is elicited during IM injection of ketamine at the dose of 11–44 mg/kg (Evans et al. 1972).

Duration of effects of ketamine following IM injection of 11–44 mg/kg may last 20–45 minutes (DeYoung et al. 1972) and can vary from 15 to 60 minutes (Evans et al. 1972). Recovery may not be complete for 10 hours after administration; however, most animals are able to stand within 2 hours (Evans et al. 1972).

According to Green et al. (1981), an optimum IM dose of ketamine for sedation or analgesia in the cat is 20 mg/kg. Its onset of action is 3 minutes; time to loss of the righting reflex is 10 minutes; time to reach peak effect is 20 minutes; duration of the peak effect is 35 minutes; time to recovery of the righting reflex is 60 minutes; and time to complete recovery is less than 5 hours.

Endotracheal intubation can be achieved during analgesia with ketamine followed by supplementation with an inhalant anesthetic such as methoxyflurane in conjunction with nitrous oxide and oxygen. Nitrous oxide significantly reduces the dose of ketamine required for surgical anesthesia and shortens the recovery period in humans (Wessels et al. 1973). It is the only inhalation agent recommended for use with ketamine in maintenance of anesthesia in humans (White et al. 1982). In the cat, ultrashort-acting barbiturates (thiamylal or thiopental) can also be used in small IV doses (4.4–8.8 mg/kg) to supplement ketamine. Since in the presence of halothane the brain and plasma half-lives of ketamine are longer and recovery from anesthesia is prolonged, caution should be exercised in use of this combination of drugs.

When ketamine is used without intervention of other pharmacologic agents, undesirable side effects occur in many animals (Reid and Frank 1972). By using a combination of oxymorphone (Numorphan) at a dose of 165 μg/kg and triflupromazine (1.1 mg/kg) prior to administration of ketamine, its side effects can be effectively blocked. The dosage of ketamine is reduced by 2.5–10% of the recommended IM dose and is not given until after the peak effect of oxymorphone and triflupromazine has been reached. Both oxymorphone and triflupromazine may be administered by the SC, IM, or IV route. Once the peak effect of these agents is attained, IV ketamine is administered at a dose of 1.1–2.2 mg/kg (Reid and Frank 1972). Ketamine (25 mg/kg) is commonly combined with acepromazine (0.2 mg/kg) and butorphanol (0.4 mg/kg) to provide anesthesia for elective procedures such as ovariectomy (Tranquilli et al. 1988). The addition of acepromazine and butorphanol, an opiate agonist-antagonist, provides improved muscle relaxation and visceral analgesia.

Xylazine has been used prior to ketamine in the cat to prevent muscular hypertonicity (Amend et al. 1972). An IM dose of 0.55–1.1 mg/kg xylazine effectively sedates the cat and renders it relatively insensitive to the subsequent injection of ketamine. Twenty minutes after administration of xylazine, 11–22 mg/kg of ketamine are given intramuscularly. Premedication with xylazine prolongs duration of analgesia, reduces the dose of ketamine required, and shortens recovery time. Disturbances of recovery often noted when ketamine is used alone are eliminated with the combined use of xylazine (Amend et al. 1972).

A combination of ketamine and xylazine is used to induce anesthesia for a number of clinical procedures in the cat (Cullen and Jones 1977). Xylazine (1.1 mg/kg) is administered intramuscularly along with atropine (0.3 mg) by the same route. After 20 minutes, ketamine (22 mg/kg) is administered intramuscularly. Onset of anesthesia occurs on an average of 6 minutes. The palpebral reflex persists during the period of ketamine anesthesia, which lasts about 30 minutes. Supplementation of ketamine anesthesia is achieved with nitrous oxide-oxygen, thiopental, or althesin.

Faulk (1978) reported the satisfactory use of xylazine and ketamine in cats for surgical procedures of less than 1 hour. Xylazine (2.2 mg/kg) is given about 10 minutes prior to ketamine (11 mg/kg); both drugs are administered intramuscularly.

The combination of ketamine and xylazine can induce negative cardiopulmonary changes that are severe (Kolata and Rawlings 1982). It has been suggested that it may be wise to avoid the use of ketamine-xylazine in animals recognized as having or suspected of having reduced cardiopulmonary reserves. In cats given IM injections of xylazine (1 mg/kg) and ketamine (10 mg/kg), the cardiac output is low for 2.5 hours; the prolonged duration of effect may overlap postsurgical complications that could lead to death (Dyson and Allen 1985).

Another clinical approach in reduction of ketamine side effects involves IM injection of acepromazine (0.11 mg/kg) and atropine (0.045–0.067 mg/kg) about 15–20 minutes prior to IM administration of 22 mg/kg ketamine (Rosin 1974). This procedure reduces the dosage of ketamine about 50%.

When ketamine is used in conjunction with meperidine or morphine in the cat, its effects are neither improved nor complicated by these agents (Hatch 1973b). Neither meperidine or morphine appear to have any value as sedative or anticataleptic agents given prior to administration of ketamine.

In fractious cats, ketamine (22 mg/kg) is administered by squirting the drug into the mouth with a syringe when the animal is hissing (Macy and Siwe 1977). This procedure is safe for immobilizing cats. Oral administration induces excessive salivation apparently from the bitter taste or low pH.

Ketamine (22 mg/kg) given intramuscularly interacts with the parenteral administration of chloramphenicol (55 mg/kg) by prolongation of sleep time (Bree et al. 1975). Following administration of dihydrostreptomycin sulfate and procaine penicillin G (Combiotic), relatively no change occurs in duration of sleep time.

NONHUMAN PRIMATES. Ketamine is recommended for restraint and minor surgical procedures in a number of subhuman primates (Beck and Dresner 1972). The usual therapeutic dose recommended for primates is 3–15 mg/kg administered intramuscularly. However, an IM dose as high as 20 mg/kg has been used in patas monkeys (*Erythrocebus patas*) (Britton et al. 1974). This produces safe and adequate sedation for 30 minutes, with minimal respiratory depression. The successful use of ketamine in the infant pigtail monkey (*Macaca nemestrina*) has been reported (Bowden et al. 1974). It is used at an IM dose level of 18 mg/kg prior to an IV injection of thiamylal (15 mg/kg). According to Bowden and coworkers (1974), IM administration of ketamine prior to thiamylal has three advantages: it simplifies the venipuncture procedure for administration of thiamylal, reduces the amount of thiamylal required for induction of anesthesia, and shortens the recovery time.

Parenteral use of 8–10 mg/kg ketamine in the rhesus monkey does not significantly alter length of the menstrual cycle nor lead to significant changes in estrogen or progesterone levels throughout the cycle (Channing et al. 1977). Also, in rhesus and *Macaca fascicularis* monkeys, ketamine anesthesia does not appear to alter endocrine functions (Castro et al. 1981; Fuller et al. 1984).

Heart rate, left ventricular systolic pressure, and respiratory rate decrease significantly in the rhesus monkey following IM injection of 10 mg/kg ketamine (Ochsner 1977). When ketamine (11 mg/kg) and acepromazine (0.55 mg/kg) are administered intramuscularly at the same time in rhesus monkeys, a smooth induction to anesthesia occurs in less than 5 minutes (Connolly and Quimby 1978). The average duration of anesthesia induced by the combination of drugs is slightly less than 1 hour.

Primates immobilized with ketamine have a near normal acid-base balance and are handled more easily than physically restrained animals (Bush et al. 1977). Repeated administration of ketamine on an every-other-day basis up to 60 days in howler monkeys (*Aloutta caraya*) does not lead to habituation (Colillas 1978). The minimum effective IM dose in the howler monkey is 6 mg/kg. After 5 minutes, this induces deep sedation lasting 20 minutes; the animals recover in 18 minutes. In the squirrel monkey (*Saimiri sciureus*), ketamine is satisfactory for chemical restraint at IM doses less than 13 mg/kg (Greenstein 1975). Doses of ketamine of 25 mg/kg and above intramuscularly induce surgical anesthesia in squirrel monkeys; deaths occur only at 350 mg/kg.

In the baboon (*Papio cynocephalus*), a combination of ketamine (11 mg/kg) and xylazine (0.5 mg/kg) administered intramuscularly in a single injection increases sleep time, decreases heart rate, provides good muscle relaxation, prevents voluntary muscle movement, and permits passage of an endotracheal tube (White and Cummings 1979). Ketamine has been used successfully for cesarean section in a 13-year-old gorilla weighing 100 kg (O'Grady et al. 1978). The animal had destroyed three successive infants. To avoid a repeat performance, the period of gestation was estimated by physical examination, radiography, amniocentesis, and ultrasonographic cephalometry. Ketamine (total of 800 mg, or 8 mg/kg) was initially given by injection dart. This was followed by 1 mg atropine intramuscularly. After intubation of the trachea, oxygen was administered along with 50% nitrous oxide. During the operative procedure, which lasted 100 minutes, additional doses of ketamine were given intravenously at 5- to 20-minute intervals. The total dose of ketamine was 2400 mg, or 24 mg/kg. Ketamine has been used as a maintenance anesthetic in the *Gorilla gorilla;* it is administered either by the IV route at 0.5–1 mg/kg or intramuscularly at 1–2 mg/kg (Ludders et al. 1982).

Work in rhesus monkeys indicates that the ketamine-xylazine combination leads to a decrease in alveolar ventilation, with subsequent changes in blood gas tensions, which are probably due to the ketamine content of the combination (Reutlinger et al. 1980). In the event the combination is used, caution must be taken because vital functions are compromised. According to Reutlinger and coworkers, the apparent beneficial effects of the combination that are seen clinically are detrimental physiologically. Presence of the small amount of xylazine in this combination dominates control of the cardiovascular system and abrogates the beneficial effect of ketamine. Conversely, the ketamine component of the combination dominates control mechanisms of the pulmonary system and eliminates to a lesser degree the beneficial effects of xylazine. The end result is that the physiologic effect of the combination has an unfavorable effect upon the cardiopulmonary system (Reutlinger et al. 1980).

DOGS. Ketamine has not been approved by the FDA for use in the dog. However, some practitioners feel that it can be used as safely and effectively in dogs as in cats. Ketamine in combination with xylazine is now commonly used in the dog for general anesthetic purposes. It is also used in combination with diazepam for general anesthesia (Haskins et al. 1986b).

In the discussion of the pharmacologic action of ketamine in the cat it was pointed out that serotonin may function in mediation of catalepsy and that dopamine may mediate ketamine-induced muscle jerking (Hatch 1973a). Studies in the dog indicate that brain mechanisms involved with the various effects of ketamine could be quite different and more complex than those suggested in the cat (Hatch 1974). It appears that dopaminergic and nicotinic chlolinoceptive receptors could be involved in mediation of ketamine anesthesia in the dog. This is particularly suggested because ketamine is antagonized by a subsequent dose of the antidopaminergic neuroleptic pimozide and is partly antagonized by the nicotinic cholinoceptor blocking agent mecamylamine (Hatch 1974). Ketamine-induced muscle jerking and emergent delirium are both enhanced by a subsedative dose of pimozide, by atropine, and by small doses of chlorpromazine. It is known that chlorpromazine possesses both antidopaminergic and anticholinergic actions. All these drug effects suggest that dopaminergic and muscarinic cholinoceptive receptors could have a role in modulating the myoclonic and deliriant effects of ketamine in the dog (Hatch 1974).

Clinically, ketamine (11–22 mg/kg) has been administered intramuscularly 10–15 minutes following atropine (0.045 mg/kg) and acepromazine (0.55 mg/kg) (Kaplan 1972). This has been followed by IV thiamylal (2.5%) administered to effect (usually 0.5–3 mL) about 5 minutes later. Results are less predictable when thiamylal is omitted in the anesthetic procedure. Adverse reactions include a 3.4% convulsion rate, evidence of transient local muscle pain at the site of ketamine injection, and moderate to marked salivation. The dose of atropine must be greater than 0.045 mg/kg to control salivation following use of ketamine. Some dogs with a previous epileptogenic history develop convulsive seizures 2–7 minutes after administration of ketamine and before administration of thiamylal (Kaplan 1972).

Ketamine in doses as low as 5–10 mg/kg given alone and intramuscularly in Beagle dogs induces excitation, apprehension, and, in some animals, tonoclonic convulsive seizures (Green et al. 1981). In IV doses of 10 mg/kg, ketamine administered alone does not produce satisfactory anesthesia for surgical purposes in the dog (Haskins et al. 1985).

Diazepam is used intravenously for alleviation of tonoclonic spasms induced by ketamine; it is used more often than acepromazine in combination with ketamine (Rucker 1976). IV diazepam (0.5 mg/kg) followed by IV ketamine (10 mg/kg) is commonly used to induce general anesthesia in dogs (Haskins et al. 1986a). Muscle hypertonicity related to use of ketamine alone is lessened by diazepam. However, vomiting is increased with this combination.

Acepromazine (0.22 mg/kg) and ketamine (11–17.6 mg/kg) are used in combination (presumably via the IM route) for restraint of aggressive dogs when it is impossible to give an IV anesthetic (Werner 1976). According to Farver et al. (1986), IV acepromazine (0.2 mg/kg) followed 5 minutes later by IV ketamine (10 mg/kg) probably should be avoided in dogs predisposed to arterial hypotension or respiratory depression.

When comparing the IM ketamine (22 mg/kg) and IV acepromazine (1.1 mg/kg) combination with IV xylazine (2.2 mg/kg) alone, it is considered to be superior to xylazine (Gelatt et al. 1976). Xylazine does not provide enough sedation, and during angiography dogs object to the rapid flash of the photo strobe.

Ketamine and xylazine have been used in combination for cesarean section (Navarro and Friedman 1975). Atropine (0.045 mg/kg) is administered intramuscularly and followed by IM xylazine in a dose of 0.55 mg/kg. Ketamine (22 mg/kg) is administered intravenously and given to effect 10–15 minutes following xylazine.

This drug combination is used for minor surgery, dentistry, and restraint during examinations, including radiography (Billiar 1976). Xylazine is given intramuscularly in a dose of 2.2 mg/kg. After approximately 10 minutes, ketamine (11 mg/kg) is administered intramuscularly. In dogs weighing over 22.7 kg, the dose of both drugs is reduced by about 25%. If the ketamine-xylazine anesthesia is insufficient, the animal is intubated so that methoxyflurane can be administered (Billiar 1976). IV xylazine (1 mg/kg) followed 5 minutes later with IV ketamine (10 mg/kg) is a common combination for induction of general anesthesia in the dog (Haskins et al. 1986b).

In the dog (and perhaps other species), the combination of ketamine and xylazine can produce adverse cardiopulmonary changes (Kolata and Rawlings 1982). It has been suggested that it may be prudent to avoid the use of ketamine-xylazine in animals that have or are suspected of having reduced cardiopulmonary reserves. Conversely, the IV infusion of guaifenesin, ketamine, and xylazine appears to provide safe analgesia in dogs, with minimal effect upon cardiopulmonary function (Benson et al. 1985).

A combination of atropine, xylazine, and ketamine in IM doses of 0.044 mg/kg, 1.1 mg/kg, and 22 mg/kg respectively has been used in the dog; xylazine is given 15 minutes postatropine and ketamine is given 5 minutes postxylazine (Clark et al. 1982). Analgesia and restraint with fair to good skeletal muscle relaxation are induced. All reflexes except the ocular are depressed. After administration of xylazine, ECG alterations such as sinus tachycardia, sinus arrest, first-degree heart block, second-degree heart block, and ventricular extrasystole occur. Ten minutes after ketamine is given, the only ECG effect noted is sinus tachycardia. Concurrent with cardiovascular stimulation, respiratory depression occurs, causing less favorable conditions for cardiac metabolism. Alterations in serum chemistry are not significant. One animal had CNS seizures 2 days after anesthesia and after a second anesthetic trial. According to Clark et al. (1982), dogs with cardiopulmonary problems may be at increased anesthetic risk from this drug combination. It is suggested that endotracheal intubation and withholding food prior to anesthesia will reduce the risk of inhalation pneumonia; use of oxygen will prevent myocardial hypoxic conditions that are induced by this drug combination. With these guidelines, clinicians should be able to reach a more informed decision regarding use of the atropine-xylazine-ketamine combination in the dog (Clark et al. 1982).

RABBITS. Ketamine in an IM dose of 44 mg/kg induces anesthesia for 15–30 minutes (Weisbroth and Fudens 1972). In an IM dose of 20 mg/kg, a cataleptoid condition occurs that permits endotracheal intubation (Lindquist 1972). According to Green et al. (1981), ketamine given alone in IM doses ranging from 10 to 60 mg/kg does not provide consistent sedation. Also, analgesia is poor because all rabbits respond to painful stimuli.

A combination of ketamine (75 mg/kg) and promazine hydrochloride (5.6 mg/kg) provides effective anesthesia for 50–60 minutes after a single IM injection (Mulder 1978b). The combined use of ketamine and xylazine in the rabbit has been employed for analgesia in surgical procedures (White and Holmes 1976). Ketamine (35 mg/kg) and xylazine (5 mg/kg) are given as a single IM injection. An optimum level of analgesia and anesthesia is attained after 10–20 minutes.

SHEEP AND SWINE. Although ketamine has not been approved for food-producing animals, it is used in animals such as sheep and swine that are maintained for experimental purposes.

In the use of ketamine in sheep, IM or IV doses of 22–44 mg/kg are adequate for short surgical and diagnostic procedures (Thurmon et al. 1973). Preanesthetic treatment with atropine (0.2 mg/kg) via the IM route is carried out 20–25 minutes before administration of ketamine. Acepromazine (0.55 mg/kg) is given intravenously 15 minutes following administration of atropine, and ketamine is administered 10 minutes later. Additionally, ketamine can be combined with guaifenesin and xylazine and administered intravenously for induction and maintenance of anesthesia (see section on guaifenesin in this chapter).

According to Thurmon et al. (1973), administration of atropine reduces the volume of saliva secreted in sheep. Acepromazine reduces the dosage of ketamine required for a given period of analgesia, increases skeletal muscle relaxation, and prevents reflex movement of the limbs. Conversely, the recovery period in sheep is longer with the use of acepromazine than with use of ketamine alone.

Effects and duration of anesthesia in sheep following IV administration of ketamine have been studied by Waterman and Livingston (1978b). Sheep become ataxic and settle into sternal recumbency following a dose of 2 mg/kg. The animals do not settle into lateral recumbency and appear to remain alert; moreover, there is no evidence of analgesia at this dosage. Respiration is shallow and rapid (30–70 min), and the pulse rate does not change from preinjection values. Animals are able to stand about 8 minutes after injection. At an IV dose of 5 mg/kg, ketamine produces analgesia and anesthesia (Waterman and Livingston 1978b). Pulse rate increases to 100–110/min but drops to the control value of 82 ± 4.5/min within 10 minutes. Respiration is altered to an apneustic pattern that ceases at the time of return of the animal to sternal recumbency. IV doses of ketamine (11.6 and 22 mg/kg) give longer periods of anesthesia (about 15 minutes and 20 minutes respectively) and have a marked effect upon pulse rate. The pulse rate increases to 114 ± 7/min at 1 minute following 11.6 mg/kg ketamine and is 110.7 ± 6.4/min at 5 minutes following injection. At 10 minutes the pulse rate is not significantly different from control levels (94 ± 7/min). An apneustic pattern of respiration persists until sternal recumbency is regained. This is followed by rapid, shallow respiration. Regurgitation of ruminal contents does not occur at any of these dosages of ketamine. Swallowing and palpebral reflexes are present throughout ketamine anesthesia in sheep. Salivation occurs in the unatropinized animal at all dosages of ketamine (Waterman and Livingston 1978b).

Pregnant ewes are successfully anesthetized with IV ketamine (2 mg/kg) followed by a drip infusion (0.2% ketamine in 5% glucose) given at a rate of 4 mL/min during the 1–2 hours of operative procedure (Taylor et al. 1972). Intubation of the trachea is not necessary when the animals are operated upon in the supine position. Moreover, premedication and fasting are not necessary. No vomiting occurred during or following ketamine anesthesia. The rumen did not become distended, and no saliva flowed from the mouth. Consequently, eructation and swallowing must have been present. Nystagmus was sometimes present during ketamine anesthesia. All ewes chewed hay within a few minutes and were standing within 10–15 minutes after removal from the surgical table. Death of one ewe from unknown causes occurred 24 hours after surgery (Taylor et al. 1972).

The experience of Green et al. (1981) with ketamine in sheep is in marked contrast to some of the reports in the literature. They considered that ketamine alone in sheep is not a satisfactory way to induce anesthesia. It is necessary to use xylazine or diazepam to achieve conditions approaching surgical anesthesia. IM xylazine at 0.1 mg/kg 10 minutes before IV ketamine

(4 mg/kg) or IV diazepam (2 mg/kg) about 15 minutes before an initial dose of IV ketamine (4 mg/kg) provides satisfactory anesthesia. This is followed by an IV infusion of ketamine to effect. The combination of xylazine or diazepam with ketamine has an advantage over barbiturate-induced anesthesia; normal eructive and swallowing reflexes are maintained with the ketamine-xylazine or ketamine-diazepam combination. This avoids the problem of ruminal bloating. Nevertheless, Green et al. (1981) found it necessary to intubate the trachea of sheep or goats whenever animals were anesthetized with either of the combinations.

In swine, ketamine has been used intramuscularly at a dose of 20.2 ± 0.92 mg/kg for surgical procedures lasting 10–20 minutes (Thurmon et al. 1972). In longer surgical procedures, ketamine is supplemented with local infiltration of the surgical site with 2% lidocaine, or thiopental is administered intravenously at a dose of 6.6–11 mg/kg.

IM administration of ketamine from 10 to 20 mg/kg alone in pigs induces a distressed or violent reaction in most animals (Green et al. 1981). Ataxia and muscle tremors, including extensor rigidity, panting, salivation, and erythema occur. Consequently, the use of ketamine alone is unsatisfactory in the pig.

A combination of ketamine and acepromazine has been used in miniature swine averaging 23.2 kg (Gray et al. 1978). Acepromazine (0.39 mg/kg) is administered intramuscularly 30 minutes prior to IM ketamine (15 mg/kg). Animals become recumbent 5 minutes following the injection of ketamine and recovery occurs 65–80 minutes later.

Ketamine (11 mg/kg) is used intramuscularly with droperidol-fentanyl (1 mL/13.6 kg) for surgical procedures in swine weighing up to 45 kg (Benson and Thurmon 1979). Droperidol-fentanyl and atropine (0.045 mg/kg) given intramuscularly precede administration of ketamine by 10–15 minutes. Surgical anesthesia is produced in 5–10 minutes and has a duration of 30–45 minutes.

For prolongation of anesthesia, supplemental ketamine is administered intramuscularly (2.2–6.6 mg/kg) or intravenously to effect. Additionally, ketamine can be combined with guaifenesin and xylazine and administered intravenously for induction and maintenance of anesthesia (see section on guaifenesin in this chapter). Pentobarbital (2.2–6.6 mg/kg) is given intramuscularly in larger pigs; it is used in animals with excessive muscle tone or movement and is effective for controlling reactions during recovery (Benson and Thurmon 1979). Ketamine (20 mg/kg) simultaneously with xylazine (2 mg/kg) have been used intramuscularly in swine weighing 20–45 kg (Kyle et al. 1979). The drugs are given following a 24-hour fast period. Sufficient depth of anesthesia is attained within 7–10 minutes.

Xylazine (1 mg/kg) and ketamine (10 mg/kg) have been injected intravenously in rapid succession in the pig (Trim and Gilroy 1985); atropine was not administered. According to Trim and Gilroy, this combination provides excellent immobilization for surgical procedures in healthy pigs weighing about 55 kg. Moreover, they observed that decreases in cardiac output and $P_{\alpha}O_2$ were tolerated, with recovery occurring rapidly and uneventfully.

Since more data on the safety and efficacy of the combined use of ketamine and xylazine are needed, caution is advised in their use.

CATTLE. Ketamine (2 mg/kg) for major and minor surgical procedures has been given by rapid IV injection (Fuentes and Tellex 1974). This dose produces rapid onset of dissociative analgesia with no loss of swallowing, palpebral, and anal reflexes. Moreover, there is no appreciable loss of consciousness. Dissociative analgesia is maintained by IV drip infusion of 0.2% ketamine in physiologic saline solution administered at the rate of 10 mL/min. The cattle did not receive preoperative care or premedication. They were fasted 24 hours prior to ketamine anesthesia. The rumen did not become distended, and no regurgitation or salivation occurred. With termination of the ketamine infusion, all animals could stand 30 minutes later. No deaths occurred from ketamine anesthesia (Fuentes and Tellez 1974).

In contrast to the dog, cat, and horse, there are reports in the literature that an additional pharmacologic agent such as xylazine is not required with ketamine to induce skeletal muscle relaxation in cattle (Wright 1982). However, IM administration of ketamine (2–5 mg/kg) is recommended with IM xylazine (0.05–0.1 mg/kg) in calves but not adult cattle; also, IV ketamine (2 mg/kg) may be used after guaifenesin (5%) is administered to effect (Ring and Muir 1982). Guaifenesin is used with ketamine and xylazine in adult cattle (see section under Guaifenesin in this chapter).

GOATS. Ketamine (5–15 mg/kg) given intramuscularly does not produce desirable anesthesia, sedation, or analgesia in the goat (Bowen 1977). According to Bowen, goats resist induction, salivate profusely throughout the 15-minute sedation period, and violently struggle and bleat during the 20-minute recovery period. A similar experience with IM ketamine (20 mg/kg) in the goat has been reported by Green et al. (1981). They considered that ketamine administered alone is unsatisfactory for anesthesia. Use of IM xylazine (0.1 mg/kg) 10 minutes before IV ketamine (4 mg/kg) or IV diazepam (2 mg/kg) about 15 minutes before an initial dose of IV ketamine (4 mg/kg) provides a satisfactory level of anesthesia. This is then followed up by an IV infusion of ketamine to effect. Normal eructive and swallowing reflexes are maintained with the ketamine-xylazine or ketamine-diazepam combination; the problem of ruminal bloating is avoided. Nevertheless, Green et al. (1981) found it necessary to intubate the trachea of goats or sheep whenever animals were anesthetized with either of the combinations. More information is needed on the safety and efficacy of these drug combinations in animals.

A combination of ketamine and xylazine has been used in domestic goats (Kumar et al. 1976); two procedures are described. One consists of administering xylazine (0.22 mg/kg) intramuscularly 8–10 minutes prior to IV injection of ketamine (11 mg/kg). Duration of anesthesia is 40–45 minutes and is prolonged by giving supplemental IM increments of ketamine (6 mg/kg). The second procedure consists of administering a mixture of xylazine (0.22 mg/kg) and ketamine (11 mg/kg), which is injected intramuscularly. For prolongation of anesthesia, a supplemental IM dose of ketamine (9 mg/kg) is administered. In both anesthetic procedures, food is withheld for 24 hours and water for 12. Atropine (0.4 mg/kg) is administered parenterally 20–25 minutes prior to xylazine or ketamine (Kumar et al. 1976). Until the safety and efficacy of the combined use of ketamine and xylazine has been established, caution in their use is recommended.

HORSES. Ketamine, guaifenesin, and xylazine have been used as a method of restraint for casting the horse (Muir et al. 1978). Approximately 20 minutes prior to IV anesthetic induction with guaifenesin (55 mg/kg) in 5% dextrose, xylazine (2.2 mg/kg) is administered intramuscularly. Immediately following induction of anesthesia with guaifenesin, ketamine (1.7 mg/kg) is administered intravenously (Muir et al. 1978). Anesthesia can be maintained with inhalant anesthetics such as halothane or enflurane. Since an interaction between halothane and ketamine has been demonstrated in the rat, the combination of these agents should be used conservatively and with caution until more information is available.

Ketamine (2.2 mg/kg) administered intravenously at the same time or following xylazine (1.1 mg/kg) provides analgesia and light anesthesia in the horse (Muir et al. 1977). Larger IV doses of ketamine (6.6 mg/kg) following sedation with IV xylazine (1.1 mg/kg) are accompanied by muscular tremor and rigidity, oculogyric movements, mydriasis, sweating, arterial hypertension, tachycardia, and elevated body temperature during recovery from anesthesia.

Xylazine (1.1 mg/kg) is administered intravenously about 4 minutes prior to IV ketamine (1.65 mg/kg for ponies, 2.2 mg/kg for horses). This combination provides induction anesthesia for tracheal intubation (Ellis et al. 1977). This anesthesia can be maintained using an infusion of ketamine, guaifenesin, and xylazine (see section on guaifenesin in this chapter).

A combination of ketamine (2 mg/kg) and promazine (1 mg/kg) administered intravenously and simultaneously is used to induce short-term anesthesia in the horse (Fuentes 1978). A state of dissociative anesthesia is induced with a mean duration of 17.1 ± 2 minutes.

A triple drug combination involving diazepam, xylazine, and ketamine provides anesthesia characterized by smooth induction and recovery periods, analgesia with excellent muscle relaxation, and stable cardiopulmonary function (Butera et al. 1978). Diazepam (0.22 mg/kg) is administered intramuscularly. After 20 minutes, xylazine (1.1 mg/kg) is given intravenously, with sedation and moderate ataxia occurring after 2 or 3 minutes. Ketamine (2.2 mg/kg) is given intravenously soon after xylazine has taken effect; about 2 minutes later, the horse becomes recumbent.

It has been reported that ketamine fails to induce analgesia in some horses after using the recommended dose of xylazine (Fisher 1984; Trim et al. 1987). Caution is suggested in the combined use of ketamine and xylazine. More information is needed on the safety and efficacy of this combination in animals.

AVIAN AND EXOTIC SPECIES. Use of ketamine alone in the domestic chicken does not produce satisfactory analgesia. Analgesia is not attained even with large doses of ketamine; this precludes its use as the only agent for inducing anesthesia for surgical procedures (McGrath et al. 1984).

In pigeons, ketamine alone does not produce a state of anesthesia even when used in doses of 400 mg/kg (Bree and Gross 1969). However, anesthesia is achieved by using pentobarbital (20 mg/kg), followed 10 minutes later with 16, 32, or 64 mg/kg ketamine. Both drugs are administered into the pectoral muscles. Induction of anesthesia is smooth and varies from 5 to 30 minutes after administration of ketamine. Mean duration of anesthesia following pentobarbital and ketamine (i.e., after 16, 32, and 64 mg/kg) is 20, 40, and 109 minutes respectively. Anesthesia is maintained for as long as 15 hours in some birds by successive administration of ketamine in doses of 32 mg/kg at 1- to 3-hour intervals. Recovery from anesthesia is uneventful (Bree and Gross 1969). Ketamine doses as low as 0.11–0.13 mg/g in the pigeon result in respiratory failure and death (Boever and Wright 1975).

In the parakeet, ketamine is considered to be a safe anesthetic (Mandelker 1973). A dose of 0.05 mg/g to 0.1 mg/g administered intramuscularly appears adequate. For parakeets and other small birds, ketamine in an IM dose of 2 mg/30 g induces surgical anesthesia in 3–5 minutes and lasts 5–20 minutes (Amand 1977). Anesthesia can be satisfactorily maintained with methoxyflurane (Mandelker 1972). The lethal dose of ketamine for the parakeet is approximately 0.5 mg/g (Mandelker 1973).

Ketamine (0.025 mg/g or 0.05 mg/g) and diazepam (0.0025 mg/g) administered together intramuscularly have been used in parakeets (Green et al. 1981). Onset of anesthesia occurs quickly and without struggling within seconds after the injection. Recovery is rapid after 30–60 minutes of anesthesia.

After induction of anesthesia with ketamine, endotracheal intubation is recommended for giving inhalant agents; most birds weighing more than 100 g can be intubated (Elkins and Herron 1982). Parakeets and canaries are too small for endotracheal intubation. Also, premedication with atropine (0.04–0.1 mg/kg or 0.00004–0.0001 mg/g) has been suggested.

Ketamine has also been used in wildfowl for immobilization purposes (Kittle 1971; Borzio 1973). The

TABLE 12.6—Intramuscular doses of ketamine hydrochloride recommended for exotic species

Species	Dose	References
	(mg/kg)	
Lion cub	4*	Cannon and Higgins 1972
Kangaroo	15–19	Denny 1973
Tiger	11–13†	Johnston 1974
Pinnipeds	4.5–11	Geraci 1973
Snakes	55–88§	Glenn et al. 1972
Opossum	20–25	Hughes et al. 1975; Jepson et al. 1984
Oryx	3††	Tadmor 1980
Northern elephant seal	2.5–3.5	Briggs et al. 1975
Agouti	63–83	Bacher et al. 1976
Raccoon	20	Speckmann 1975
Ferret	10–20	Janssens 1978; Green et al. 1981
Rattlesnakes	91–131	Harding 1977
European badger	14–26‖	Hunt 1976
Lizards	35–65	Jones 1977
East African reptiles	40–60	Cooper 1974 b
Mule deer	11#	Richter 1977
Mink	10–15‖	Hunt 1976
Nondomesticated cats	5–25**	Hime 1974
Pine marten	7	Wilson 1976
Aldabra turtle	20	Crane et al. 1980
Green sea turtle	38–71§§	Wood et al. 1982
Terrapins and turtles	60–80	Green et al. 1981
Striped skunk	10.5–15.5	Rosatte and Hobson 1983
Springbok	8–9##	Jacobson 1983
Water buffalo (calves)	2	Pathak et al. 1982
Camel (dromedary or Bactrian)	1–2***	Higgins and Kock 1984

*Administered in conjunction with acepromazine (0.25 mg/kg).
†Used in combination with acepromazine (0.22 mg/kg) and atropine in the same projectile syringe.
§Effects last 1–3 days.
‖Administered subcutaneously.
#Atropine (0.4 mg/kg) is given intramuscularly 15 minutes prior to ketamine; xylazine (0.22 mg/kg) is also given intramuscularly along with ketamine.
**Convulsions occur in some animals.
††Rapid IV injection; intubated for administration of halothane-oxygen anesthesia.
§§Administered intraperitoneally.
##Combined with IM xylazine (0.5 mg/kg).
***Combined with IM or IV xylazine (1–2 mg/kg).

recommended initial IM dose for most wildfowl is 15–20 mg/kg supplemented with increments of 10 mg/kg (Borzio 1973). Immobilization is produced in 1–5 minutes to 6 hours, depending upon the total dose administered.

Baseline values for IM ketamine dosages in various species of birds are as follows (Boever and Wright 1975): (1) birds weighing less than 100 g (canaries, finches, parakeets), 0.1–0.2 mg/g; (2) birds weighing between 250 and 500 g (parrots, pigeons), 0.05–0.1 mg/g; (3) birds weighing between 500 and 3000 g (chickens, owls, hawks), 0.02–0.1 mg/g; (4) birds weighing more than 3000 g (ducks, swans), 0.02–0.05 mg/g. The dose of ketamine is inversely proportional to body weight; larger birds require less ketamine per kilogram of body weight than smaller birds (Boever and Wright 1975).

Large adult birds such as the emu (*Dromiceius novaehollandiae*) that weigh 40 kg are successfully anesthetized with IM ketamine in an initial dose of 25 mg/kg (Grubb 1983). Additional ketamine (about 5–8 mg/kg) is injected intravenously until anesthesia is sufficient for surgical procedures. Ketamine is considered to be much safer in the emu than IV pentobarbital. In the ostrich, ketamine has been used in combination with xylazine and althesin for anesthesia (see section under althesin in this chapter).

For doses of ketamine recommended in exotic species, see Table 12.6.

In Weddell seals (*Leptonychotes weddelli*), deaths occur in some animals when doses of 5 and 6 mg/kg ketamine are administered intramuscularly (Hammond and Elsner 1977). IV or IM atropine (0.02–0.04 mg/kg) and IV diazepam (0.22 mg/kg) given 5–10 minutes prior to IV ketamine (4 mg/kg) provide chemical restraint and anesthesia in California sea lions, northern elephant seals, and harbor seals (Gage 1984).

Ketamine (17–30 mg/kg) and diazepam (0.32–0.58 mg/kg) have been used in combination for anesthetic purposes in river otter (*Lutra canadensis*) (Elmore et al. 1985). The route of administration was not given by Elmore et al. for this combination; the IM route was probably used.

LABORATORY ANIMALS. Anesthesia is achieved in inbred Fisher or Lewis strains of rats with 87 mg/kg ketamine and 13 mg/kg xylazine (Van Pelt 1977). The drugs are mixed together prior to use via the IM route. Anesthesia begins 10–15 minutes after administration and lasts 15–30 minutes; this is followed by a relatively long period of immobility (mean of 3.8 hr) and reduced responsiveness to stimuli.

Ketamine (100 mg/kg) administered intraperitoneally appears to be a suitable anesthetic for use in studies of prolactin secretion in male rats (Meltzer et al. 1978). The anesthetic is known to inhibit uptake of both dopamine and serotonin, two neurotransmitters that have a marked effect on rat prolactin secretion. Anesthetics such as ether, urethane, chloral hydrate, and pentobarbital increase plasma prolactin several-fold (Lawson and Gala 1974).

A combination of ketamine (100 mg/mL), promazine (7.5 mg/mL), and aminopentamide (6.25 μg/mL) provides effective anesthesia in the rat (Mulder and Johnson 1978). The IM dose is 0.75 mL/kg (75 mg/kg ketamine, 5.625 mg/kg promazine, and 46.875 μg/kg aminopentamide). Aminopentamide controls excessive salivation and has other anticholinergic activity. Duration of anesthesia ranges from 41 to 50 minutes, with recovery occurring within 26–34 minutes. About 10% of the animals manifest a transitory CNS excitation that consists of running and jumping during induction of anesthesia (Mulder and Johnson 1978).

IM ketamine (50 mg/kg) plus P diazepam (5 mg/kg) have been used in gerbils (Flecknell et al. 1983). However, anesthesia is not entirely satisfactory because occasional spontaneous limb movements occur.

In laboratory mice, the ketamine-promazine-aminopentamide combination in a dose of 1 mL/kg produces effective anesthesia for 30–50 minutes after a single IM injection (Mulder 1978a). Hyperexcitement is seen in some mice but is not considered to be a serious problem. IM ketamine given alone at 10–400 mg/kg does not induce analgesia even in mice that are heavily sedated; when combined with xylazine, analgesia is insufficient for surgery (Green et al. 1981).

Ketamine (100 mg/kg) given intramuscularly induces anesthesia in the hamster (Hughes et al. 1975). In the golden hamster, the combination of ketamine (50–200 mg/kg) and xylazine (10 mg/kg) administered intraperitoneally is acceptable for general anesthesia (Curl and Peters 1983).

Doses of 22–64 mg/kg and 128–256 mg/kg ketamine given intramuscularly provide tranquilization and anesthesia respectively in guinea pigs. In contrast, Green et al. (1981) reported that IM ketamine (10–150 mg/kg) produced only a mild sedation in guinea pigs. Additionally, the concurrent use of diazepam or xylazine improved skeletal muscle relaxation but did not prevent pain perception.

In the guinea pig (Hartley strain), ketamine (44 mg/kg) and diazepam (0.1 mg/kg) have been administered in combination by the IM route (Gilroy and Varga 1980). Loss of the righting reflex occurs in 1.96 ± 1.06 minutes, and duration of immobilization is 54.6 ± 9.3 minutes. Ketamine (25 mg/kg) and xylazine (5 mg/kg) have been used in combination via the IM route in guinea pigs (Gilroy and Varga 1980). Loss of the righting reflex occurs in 2.88 ± 1.39 minutes, and duration of immobilization is 77.3 ± 14.6 minutes. Although both combinations immobilize guinea pigs rapidly and safely, neither is recommended for general anesthesia because the extent of analgesia induced is uncertain (Gilroy and Varga 1980).

FISH. Ketamine has been used in rainbow trout following immersion in a solution of benzocaine (50 mg/L). Within 30 seconds the fish are sufficiently sedated to permit weighing and subsequent injection of the calculated anesthetic dose (130 or 150 mg/kg) of ketamine (Oswald 1978). Ketamine is injected by the IM route; no more than 0.2–0.3 mL is recommended because of reflux of the anesthetic solution out of the injection site. Ketamine anesthesia lasts only 20 minutes following 130 mg/kg and between 50–80 minutes after 150 mg/kg. Apnea is produced in some fish and requires ventilatory assistance. Recovery is prolonged, taking up to 90 minutes, and is characterized by CNS excitation and ataxia (Oswald 1978).

ANTAGONISM OF KETAMINE ANESTHESIA. In humans, physostigmine antagonizes ketamine; however, it is not antagonized in cats (Hatch and Ruch 1974). This species difference is not surprising because marked variations are known to exist in the concentrations of brain neurotransmitters.

Phencyclidine or its congeners (ketamine, tiletamine) are antagonized by adenosine receptor agonists, N^6-cyclohexyladenosine or 1-phenylisopropyladenosine, in the rat (Browne and Welch 1982). These agonists may possibly be useful in reversal of the CNS effects of ketamine in species other than rats.

In mule deer (*Odocoileus hemionus*), IV yohimbine hydrochloride (0.125 mg/kg) reverses the xyalzine-induced sedation of ketamine-xylazine anesthesia (Jessup et al. 1983).

IV tolazoline (0.5 mg/kg) has been used to reverse the xyalzine-induced sedation of the African elephant immobilized with a combination of IM xylazine (0.2 mg/kg) and IM ketamine (1–1.5 mg/kg) (Allen 1986).

Tiletamine Hydrochloride. *Tiletamine Hydrochloride,* INN (CI-634), like ketamine, is also a congener of phencyclidine. Adverse effects characteristic of phencyclidine are considered to be less pronounced following administration of tiletamine. Chemically, tiletamine is designated as 2-(ethylamino)-2-(2-thienyl) cyclohexanone hydrochloride (Fig. 12.15).

Tiletamine in combination with zolazepam hydrochloride (Telazol, CI-744) was approved by the FDA in 1982 for anesthetic use in dogs and cats. The drug combination is reconstituted in sterile distilled water; this provides both tiletamine and zolazepam with amounts equivalent to 50 mg/mL. Dosage of this preparation is expressed in milligrams of the drug combination.

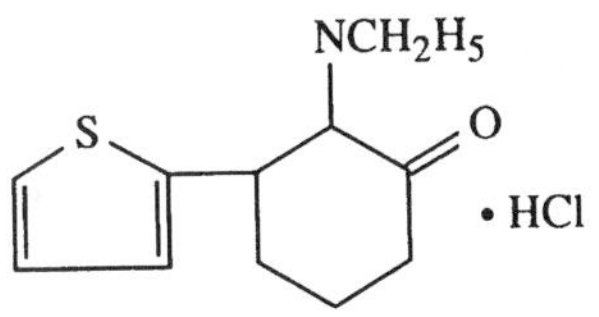

NCH_2H_5

S O

• HCl

Tiletamine Hydrochloride

FIG. 12.15

PHARMACOLOGIC ACTIVITY. Most of the pharmacologic characteristics of tiletamine are similar to those of ketamine. The duration of action of tiletamine is about 3 times longer than with ketamine.

Pharmacologic studies have been conducted with tiletamine alone in the mouse, rat, pigeon, guinea pig, rabbit, dog, cat, and monkey (Chen et al. 1967). In mice and rats, CNS excitation is observed; it is not as marked in other species. Tiletamine in large doses induces analgesia and general anesthesia in mice, rats, pigeons, cats, and monkeys. In the guinea pig and rabbit, only CNS depression occurs; anesthesia is not induced in these two species.

Tiletamine alone is more effective in induction of anesthesia in nonhuman primates and in cats than in other species. Increased CNS activity occurs in cats after IM administration of 10 mg/kg tiletamine (Garmer 1969); this includes clonic muscle spasms, particularly in the face and limbs. Administration of 30 mg/kg of tiletamine initiates muscle spasms that progress into a convulsive seizure; it is necessary to administer thiopental for control. A severe metabolic acidosis occurs in cats manifesting clonic muscular spasms. The body temperature drops from 38.5 to 36°C in animals following IM administration of 30 mg/kg tiletamine.

Although it has been reported (Bennett 1969) that tiletamine has moderate to no perceptible effect upon respiratory activity in the cat, Calderwood et al. (1971) are not in agreement with these findings. According to these authors, an irregular respiratory rate, frequently tending toward an inspiratory breath-holding pattern (i.e., apneustic-type pattern), is seen; conversion to a normal pattern may be attained by IV administration of a neuroleptic agent (prozamine or diazepam).

In the cat, a decrease in the heart rate and systemic arterial pressure occurs after an IM injection of tiletamine; it declines to a minimum level within 30 minutes, with a gradual return to normal thereafter. After an IV injection, an elevated arterial pressure and heart rate are observed; also, arrhythmias are frequent following IV administration of tiletamine. In the unanesthetized dog, an IV injection of 2 mg/kg tiletamine results in an increase of arterial pressure and heart rate that lasts about 30 minutes (Chen et al. 1967). A similar dose of tiletamine in dogs anesthetized with pentobarbital also produces arterial hypertension; at higher doses (4–8 mg/kg), hypotension occurs. Doses of 6.6–19.8 mg/kg administered intravenously to dogs awakening from isoflurane anesthesia produced an initial decrease in arterial blood pressure followed by a dose-related increase. Heart rate and cardiac output also increased in a dose-related manner. The highest dose produced a marked decrease in minute ventilation (Hellyer et al. 1989). Premedication with tiletamine does not potentiate the hypertensive response to norepinephrine. Also, no anticholinergic or antihistaminergic effects are seen when tiletamine is compared with the hypotensive effects produced by acetylcholine and histamine respectively. Tiletamine does not produce an emetic effect in cats (Chen and Ensor 1968).

ONSET, DURATION OF ACTION, AND RECOVERY. Tiletamine has an anesthetic induction time comparable to ketamine; it ranges between 1 and 3 minutes in the cat after an IM injection (Chen and Ensor 1968). Duration of the peak effect of tiletamine is about 1 hour, or about 3 times longer than ketamine.

Onset of action after IM injection of tiletamine in the cat begins with the appearance of akinesia; this is followed by motor paralysis of the rear limbs, then the forelimbs (Chen and Ensor 1968). Recovery from the effects of tiletamine varies from 1 to 5 hours in cats given doses of 10–40 mg/kg.

CLINICAL USE. Tiletamine hydrochloride in combination with zolazepam (diazepinone tranquilizer) is available in a 1:1 ratio. Undesirable side effects are seen when the components of the combination are administered alone or separately; combining these agents yields a compatible preparation with desirable anesthetic, analgesic, and ataractic properties (Booker et al. 1982).

DOGS. Tiletamine and zolazepam (6–13 mg/kg) given intramuscularly produce satisfactory anesthesia for surgical procedures lasting 30–60 minutes (Ward et al. 1974). An initial IM dose of the combined preparation approved by the FDA in healthy dogs is 6.6–9.9 mg/kg for diagnostic procedures; for surgery of short duration (30 minutes) requiring mild to moderate analgesia, such as repair of wounds and castrations, an IM dose of 9.9–13.2 mg/kg is approved. Additional doses of tiletamine-zolazepam, when required, should be less than the initial dose; the total IM dose should not exceed 26.4 mg/kg. The maximum safe IM dose is 29.9 mg/kg in dogs. IV administration of 9.9 mg/kg resulted in more rapid inductions and a similar duration (Tracy et al. 1988). Smaller doses administered intravenously (2 mg/kg and 4 mg/kg) produced slightly shorter anesthetic times (Donaldson et al. 1989). The quality of recovery is somewhat poorer in dogs than in cats. This is probably due to the relatively more rapid metabolism of zolazepam in dogs than in cats (Tracy et al. 1988). Interaction of tiletamine-zolazepam with chloramphenicol in the dog has no apparent effect upon duration of surgical anesthesia or time of recovery (Bree et al. 1976a). This is in contrast to the cat, in which duration of surgical anesthesia and time of recovery are increased by chloramphenicol (Bree et al. 1976b). Telazol (8.8 mg/kg) can be combined with xylazine (1.1 mg/kg) and butorphanol (0.22 mg/kg), all administered intramuscularly, to provide approximately 70 minutes of good muscle relaxation and anesthesia. Anticholinergics will effectively treat bradycardia, and minimal respiratory depression occurred (Benson et al. 1989).

CATS. IM doses of 6–13 mg/kg tiletamine and zolazepam provide satisfactory anesthesia for surgical interventions of 30–60 minutes (Ward et al. 1974). An initial dose of 8.8–11.9 mg/kg is approved by the FDA in healthy cats for dentistry, incision of abscesses, foreign-body removal, and other similar procedures; for surgery requiring mild to moderate analgesia, such as repair of lacerations, castration, and other procedures of short duration (30 minutes), an IM dose of 10.6–12.5 mg/kg is approved. Also, the FDA has approved an initial dose of 14.3–15.8 mg/kg tiletamine-zolazepam for ovariohysterectomy and onychectomy. Supplemental IM doses should be administered in increments that are less than the initial dose; the total dose (initial plus supplemental doses) should not exceed 71.9 mg/kg (the maximum safe dose). In cats, IV doses of 12.8 mg/kg produced anesthesia of approximately 30 minutes duration (Tracy et al. 1988).

Chloramphenicol therapy increases the mean duration of surgical anesthesia by approximately 30 minutes; it also increases the time to return of the righting reflex by about 2–2.5 hours and time to return to normal by about 3 hours (Bree et al. 1976b). This interaction with chloramphenicol can be avoided by not anesthetizing animals with tiletamine-zolazepam. Unlike the interaction with chloramphenicol, cats wearing flea collars do not have an apparent interaction after tiletamine-zolazepam anesthesia (Bree et al. 1977).

NONHUMAN PRIMATES. Dissociative anesthesia provided by tiletamine-zolazepam is suitable for surgical procedures and restraint, particularly for physiologic studies in the rhesus monkey (Booker et al. 1982). An IM dose of 3 mg/kg of the anesthetic combination produces anesthesia for minor surgical procedures.

Tiletamine-zolazepam has been used in 51 primate species (Eads 1976). Adverse reactions totaling 71 (2.9%) out of 2342 anesthetic procedures have been observed; this includes salivation (2.14%), respiratory depression (0.3%), prolonged recovery (0.26%), and emesis (0.21%). Also, 3 deaths resulted after administration of the anesthetic combination.

LABORATORY RODENTS. Tiletamine-zolazepam (20–30 mg/kg) given intramuscularly in the rat provides satisfactory anesthesia for surgical procedures of 30–60 minutes (Ward et al. 1974). The combination is not effective for mice or hamsters (Silverman et al. 1983).

GUINEA PIGS AND RABBITS. In the guinea pig and rabbit, lack of skeletal muscle relaxation and response to external stimuli make tiletamine-zolazepam unsatisfactory for surgical anesthesia (Ward et al. 1974).

OTHER SPECIES. Tiletamine-zolazepam has been administered intravenously in calves (4 mg/kg) with minimal cardiovascular and respiratory changes (Lin et al. 1989). This dose produced light anesthesia for approximately 50 minutes. The addition of xylazine (0.1 mg/kg) produced transient hypertension and a moderate decrease in cardiac output. The duration of anesthesia was also increased (Lin et al. 1991). Pigs receiving 6 mg/kg of tiletamine-zolazepam with 1.1 or 2.2 mg/kg of xylazine (all given IM) rapidly became recumbent and remained unresponsive to stimuli for an average of 47 (low dose) or 68 (high dose) minutes (Thurmon et al. 1988). Tiletamine-zolazepam has been administered to horses in combination with xylazine or detomidine. The dose of tiletamine-zolazepam ranged from 1.1 to 3.0 mg/kg and produced anesthesia of up to an hour duration with the high dose (Lin et al. 1992; Hubbell et al. 1989).

EXOTIC SPECIES. Tiletamine-zolazepam has been used in the chinchilla (Schulz and Fowler 1974). Surgical anesthesia is produced by IM dose levels of 22–110 mg/kg; however, some deaths occurred at doses of 66 mg/kg and above.

Clinical trials indicate that tiletamine-zolazepam has a wide margin of safety for restraint and immobilization of the red kangaroo (*Macropus rufus*); adequate anesthesia and muscle relaxation are obtained with IM doses of from 2 to 6.9 mg/kg (Boever et al. 1977). In lions and leopards, tiletamine-zolazepam has been used for induction of anesthesia; dosage is expressed in $mg/kg^{0.75}$ and related to duration of anesthesia by use of regression equations (King et al. 1977). Male lions and leopards are more susceptible to the CNS depressant effects of tiletamine-zolazepam than females; males are anesthetized 15 minutes longer for a given dosage.

Tiletamine-zolazepam (5 mg/kg) given intramuscularly has been used in polar bears (Haigh et al. 1984). It is considered to be an ideal immobilizing preparation for ear-tagging procedures.

In reptilian species, tiletamine-zolazepam provides suitable anesthesia for surgical procedures only in iguanas; IM doses of 33 and 44 mg/kg produce surgical anesthesia lasting about 16 hours (Boever and Caputo 1982). Use of IM tiletamine-zolazepam (22, 33, or 44 mg/kg) in snakes produces a deep CNS depression; it may be necessary to supplement with an inhalant agent to abolish reflex activity suitable for anesthesia. In turtles, tiletamine-zolazepam is not acceptable as a surgical anesthetic agent (Boever and Caputo 1982).

PRECAUTIONS AND CONTRAINDICATIONS. Tiletamine-zolazepam must not be used in pregnant animals or in those that have pancreatic, renal, cardiac, or pulmonary dysfunctions. The drug combination should be reduced in geriatric animals. The unused reconstituted solution of tiletamine-zolazepam must be discarded after 48 hours.

MISCELLANEOUS AGENTS

Chloralose. The family of compounds called chloraloses (α-chloralose, monochloral *d*-glucose) are prepared by condensing anhydrous glucose with chloraldehyde (chloral) in the presence of sulfuric acid. A mixture, 3 dichloralglucoses and 2 monoglucochloraloses (i.e., α-chloralose and β-chloralose), is formed. In the experimental laboratory α-chloralose is used more frequently than any of the other chloralose preparations. It is usually administered intravenously in 1% concentration. However, concentrations of 10% have been prepared by using an inert dispersing agent such as polyethylene glycol (Bass and Buckley 1966).

Chloralose is difficult to dissolve in an aqueous medium without simultaneous heating. Because of deterioration, chloralose solutions should not be boiled. After solution is accomplished, the preparation is allowed to cool to the approximate body temperature of the animal before IV injection.

Chloralose is metabolized to chloraldehyde or chloral, which is mainly transformed into trichloroethanol. Hypnosis and anesthesia produced by chloral hydrate and chloralose are quite similar because of formation of trichloroethanol.

Chloralose possesses the unique characteristic of altering the mental component of CNS activity while increasing reflex activity. Spinal reflex activity may increase to the degree that convulsions similar to those of strychnine develop in the dog and cat (Lees 1972). Functional disruption (dissociation) of the CNS through marked CNS stimulation or induction of a cataleptoid state typifies the action of chloralose (Winters 1976). It induces stage I and stage II anesthesia but not stage III.

The oral LD_{50} of chloralose for rats, cats, and dogs is 400–600 mg/kg (Balis and Monroe 1964). For the IV or IP routes, it is 120–150 mg/kg. In dogs and cats, 40–100 mg/kg IV injection may produce violent tonic convulsions resembling strychnine poisoning.

As an anesthetic agent, chloralose is restricted to laboratory animals in which recovery from anesthesia is not necessary. It is used primarily in physiologic experimentation because it purportedly does not interfere with respiratory and cardiac reflexes, e.g., baroceptor and chemoceptor activities.

Use of IV chloralose (100 mg/kg) in the dog has followed a sedative IV dose (1 mg/kg) of xylazine for myocardial function studies (Caffrey et al. 1985). Combination of xylazine with chloralose should lessen gross movements such as limb paddling that often occur with use of chloralose alone.

In the dog and cat, the IV dose of chloralose is between 40 and 100 mg/kg; anesthesia lasts 6–10 hours (Lees 1972). It is usually administered with ether to reduce spinal reflex activity and "convulsive-like" actions associated with use of chloralose. The cardiovascular responses following IV administration of chloralose (100 mg/kg) have been studied extensively in the dog (Cox 1972). With the exception of brief effects immediately after injection, which last about 15 minutes, there are no changes in systemic hemodynamics. In the cat, chloralose (75 mg/kg) is commonly used intravenously for anesthesia in the research laboratory.

Chloralose has been used in sheep at a dose of 48–55 mg/kg. Onset of action is delayed following administration and does not attain its full effect for at least 20 minutes. In swine, following premedication with a small dose of morphine, the IV dose of chloralose required to induce an effect is 55–86 mg/kg. Paddling movements of the limbs are observed in the pig similar to those seen in sheep.

In the UK, chloralose is employed for killing rats and is available to the general public (Lees 1972). Cases of suspected chloralose poisoning have been reported in the dog and cat (Copestake 1967). The drug apparently is also being illegally used in baits against crows, gulls, and foxes (Conder 1973). However, other birds (golden eagle, buzzard, hen harrier), whether intended or not, also receive the bait and have died from its use.

In the USA, chloralose has been used to capture wild turkeys and mourning doves (Cline and Greenwood 1972) and has been used with diazepam for capture of Canada geese.

Urethane. *Urethane,* NF ($NH_2COOC_2H_5$), is also known as ethyl carbamate. It is chemically related to urea and is readily soluble in water and alcohol. Urethane is used only occasionally as an anesthetic in laboratory animals and then only in nonsurvival or acute experiments. The drug can be administered intravenously (1 g/kg) or intraperitoneally (1–2 g/kg). In small laboratory animals such as the rat, urethane (1.25 g/kg) is administered intraperitoneally.

Urethane is not used clinically because there are safer anesthetics available. It produces anesthesia that lasts many hours. It is metabolized slowly into carbamic acid and ethyl alcohol. Liver injury is produced by urethane. The rate of elimination is so slow that pulmonary edema usually occurs before the animal fully recovers from anesthesia. In addition, urethane has a carcinogenic effect in several species.

Propanidid. Propanidid (Epontol, Fabantol, Fabontal) is a nonbarbiturate IV anesthetic used for inducing anesthesia in humans. It induces CNS excitatory side effects with either rigidity or uncontrolled movement (Steen and Michenfelder 1979). When given to epileptic patients, propanidid (like ketamine) triggers seizure activity.

Propanidid (17.7 mg/kg) given intravenously induces hypnosis in rats; an IV dose of 50 mg/kg is necessary to induce sleep for 2–5 minutes (Janssen et al. 1975). After administration of 50 mg/kg, recovery requires 9 minutes.

Metomidate. *Metomidate,* INN (Hypnodil), is a nonbarbiturate drug recommended for anesthesia in birds of prey (Cooper 1974a; Cadle and Martin 1976). It is administered intramuscularly into the leg using a 1 mL tuberculin syringe and a 25- or 23-gauge needle. Doses of metomidate range between 8.8 and 16 mg/kg for various species. Some deaths have occurred following repeated use at doses of 10 mg/kg and above. Duration of anesthesia ranges from 70 to 165 minutes. In birds, other drugs generally are not administered with metomidate; occasionally, maintenance of anesthesia may require supplemental use of an inhalant anesthetic. However, metomidate has been used with azaperone in swine.

Metomidate (50 mg/kg) plus fentanyl (0.05 mg/kg) given subcutaneously consistently produces surgical anesthesia in two species of gerbils (Flecknell et al. 1983). In the dog, IV metomidate (4 mg/kg) has been used in combination with xylazine and a phenothiazine tranquilizing agent (Holenweger et al. 1984).

Metomidate is not available for use in the USA. It is used primarily in the UK and other countries.

REFERENCES

Adams, H. A. 1997. Anaesthetist 46 (Suppl 1):S30.
Adams, H. R. 1970. J Am Vet Med Assoc 157:1908.
Adams, H. R., and Bingham, G. A. 1971. J Am Vet Med Assoc 159:179.
Adams, H. R., and Dixit, B. N. 1970. J Am Vet Med Assoc 156:902.
Adams, H. R., and Mathew, B. P. 1974. Arch Int Pharmacodyn Ther 210:288.
Adams, H. R., Teske, R. H., and Mercer, H. D. 1976. J Am Vet Med Assoc 168:409.
Agrawal, K. B. P., Prasad, B., and Sobti, V. K. 1983. Res Vet Sci 35:53.
Ahlgren, I., Aronsen, K. F., Bjorkman, I., et al. 1978. Acta Anaesth Scand 22:76.
Allen, J. L. 1986. Am J Vet Res 47:781.
Amand, W. B. 1977. In R. W. Kirk, ed., Current Veterinary Therapy, VI: Small Animal Practice, p. 705. Philadelphia: W. B. Saunders.
Amend, J. F., Klavano, P. A., and Stone, E. C. 1972. Vet Med Small Anim Clin 67:1305.
Anderson, F. L., Kralios, A. C., Tsagaris, T. J., et al. 1972. J Surg Res 13:182.
Andrews, C. J. H. 1975. J Small Anim Pract 16:515.
Arduino, M. J., Bland, L. A., McAllister, S. K., et al. 1991. Infect Control Hosp Epidem 12:535.
Aronson, C. E., and Hanno, E. R. S. 1978. Gen Pharmacol 9:249.
Atlee, J. L., and Malkinson, C. E. 1982. Anesthesiology 57:285.
Azadegan, A., Johnson, D. W., and Stowe, C. M. 1980. Am J Vet Res 41:976.
Bacher, J. D., Potkay, S., and Baas, E. J. 1976. Lab Anim Sci 26:195.
Baggot, J. D., and Blake, J. W. 1976. Arch Int Pharmacodyn Ther 220:115.
Baggot, J. D., Toutain, P. L., Brandon, R. A., et al. 1984. J Vet Pharmacol Ther 7:197.
Balis, G. U., and Monroe, R. R. 1964. Psychopharmacologia 6:1.
Bass, B. G., and Buckley, N. M. 1966. Am J Physiol 210:854.
Bauck, S. W. 1984. Can Vet J 25:162.
Beck, C. C., and Dresner, A. J. 1972. Vet Med Small Anim Clin 67:1082.
Beck, C. C., Coppock, R. W., and Ott, B. S. 1971. Vet Med 66:993.
Bednarski, R. M., and Muir, W. W. 1985. Cornell Vet 75:512.
Bednarski, R. M., Majors, L., and Atlee, J. L. 1985. Vet Surg 14:71.
Ben, M., Dixon, R. L., and Adamson, R. H. 1969. Fed Proc 28:1522.
Bennett, R. R. 1969. Am J Vet Res 30:1469.
Benson, G. J., and Thurmon, J. C. 1979. J Am Vet Med Assoc 174:594.
———. 1990. Vet Clinics of N Amer: Equine Pract 6:513.
Benson, G. J., Thurmon, J. C., and Tranquilli, W. J. 1985. Am J Vet Res 46:1896.
Benson, G. J., Wheaton, L. G., Thurmon, J. C., Tranquilli, W. J., and Olson, W. A. 1989. Proc Annu Meet ACVA. New Orleans.
Billiar, R. R. 1976. Mod Vet Pract 57:319.
Blair, E. 1969. Fed Proc 28:1456.
Boever, W. J., and Caputo, F. 1982. J Zoo Anim Med 13:59.
Boever, W. J., and Wright, W. 1975. Ved Med Small Anim Clin 70:86.
Boever, W. J., Stuppy, D., and Kane, K. K. 1977. J Zoo Anim Med 8:14.
Bonhaus, D. W., Sawyer, D. C., and Hook, J. B. 1981. Am J Vet Res 42:1612.
Booker, J. L., Erickson, H. H., and Fitzpatrick, E. L. 1982. Am J Vet Res 43:671.
Booth, N. H. 1969. Fed Proc 28:1547.
Borison, H. L. 1978. Pharmacol Ther (B) 3:377.
Borzio, F. 1973. Vet Med Small Anim Clin 68:1364.
Boulos, B. M., Jenkins, W. L., and Davis, L. E. 1972. Am J Vet Res 33:943.
Bovill, J. G., Coppel, D. L., Dundee, J. W., et al. 1971. Lancet 1:1285.
Bowden, D. M., Holm, R., and Morgan, M. K. 1974. Lab Anim Sci 24:675.
Bowen, J. M., Blackmon, D. M., and Heavner, J. E. 1970. J Am Vet Med Assoc 157:164.
Bowen, J. S. 1977. J Am Vet Med Assoc 171:1249.
Bowery, N. G., and Dray, A. 1978. Br J Pharmacol 63:197.
Brandon, R. A., and Baggot, J. D. 1981. J Vet Pharmacol Ther 4:79.
Branson, K. R., and Gross, M. E. 1994. JAVMA 204:1888.
Brearley, J. C., Kellagher, R. E., and Hall, L. W. 1988. J Small Anim Pract 29:315.
Bree, M. M., and Gross, N. B. 1969. Lab Anim Sci 19:500.
Bree, M. M., Park, J. S., and Short, C. E. 1975. Vet Med Small Anim Clin 70:1309.
Bree, M. M., Park, J. S., Beck, C. C., et al. 1976a. Vet Med Small Anim Clin 71:1243.
Bree, M. M., Park, J. S., Short, C. E., et al. 1976b. Vet Med Small Anim Clin 71:764.
Bree, M. M., Park, J. S., Moser, J. H., et al. 1977. Vet Med Small Anim Clin 72:869.
Briggs, G. D., Hendrickson, R. V., and LeBoeuf, B. J. 1975. J Am Vet Med Assoc 167:546.
Britton, B. J., Wood, W. G., and Irving, M. H. 1974. Lab Anim Sci 8:41.
Brouwer, G. J. 1985. Equine Vet J 17:133.
Brown, D. A., and Constanti, A. 1978. Br J Pharmacol 63:217.
Browne, R. G., and Welch, W. M. 1982. Science 217:1157.
Bryant, S. H. 1969. Fed Proc 28:1553.
Burch, P. G., and Stanski, D. R. 1982. Clin Pharmacol Ther 32:212.
Bush, M., Custer, R., Smeller, J., et al. 1977. J Am Vet Med Assoc 171:866.
Butera, T. S., Moore, J. N., Garner, H. E., et al. 1978. Vet Med Small Anim Clin 73:490.

Butler, J. M., Kazmierowski, J. A., Bruss, R. D., et al. 1982. Anesthesiology 57:51.
Buyniski, J. P., and Christie, G. J. 1977. Vet Med Small Anim Clin 72:559.
Cadle, D. R., and Martin, G. R. 1976. Vet Rec 98:91.
Caffrey, J. L., Gaugl, J. F., and Jones, C. E. 1985. Am J Physiol 248:H-382.
Calderwood, H. W., Klide, A. M., Cohn, B. B., et al. 1971. Am J Vet Res 32:1511.
Cannon, J. E., and Higgins, W. Y. 1972. Mod Vet Pract 53:40.
Caron, M., and LeLorier, J. 1979. Toxicol Appl Pharmacol 51:537.
Castro, M. I., Rose, J., Green, W., et al. 1981. Proc Soc Exp Biol Med 168:389.
Channing, C. P., Fowler, S., Engel, B., et al. 1977. Proc Soc Exp Biol Med 155:615.
Chaplin, M. D., Roszkowski, A. P., and Richards, R. K. 1973. Proc Soc Exp Biol Med 143:667.
Chappel, S. C., and Barraclough, C. A. 1976. Proc Soc Exp Biol Med 153:1.
Chen, G., and Ensor, C. R. 1968. Am J Vet Res 29:863.
Chen, G., Ensor, C. R., and Bohner, B. 1967. J Pharmacol Exp Ther 168:171.
Chenoweth, M. B., and Van Dyke, R. A. 1969. Fed Proc 28:1432.
Child, K. J., Currie, J. P., Davis, B., et al. 1971. Br J Anaesth 43:2.
Child, K. J., Davis, B., Dodds, M. G., et al. 1972a. Br J Pharmacol 46:189.
Child, K. J., Gibson, W., Harnby, G., et al. 1972b. Postgrad Med J (June Suppl):37.
Christ, G., Mundigler, G., Merhaut, C., Zehetgruber, M., Kratochwill, C., Heinz, G., and Siostrzonek, P. 1997. Anaesthesia and Intensive Care 25(3):255.
Christensen, J. H., and Andreasen, F. 1979. Acta Pharmacol Toxicol 44:260.
Christie, G. J., and Buyniski, J. P. 1977. Vet Med Small Anim Clin 72:383.
Clark, D. M., Martin, R. A., and Short, C. A. 1982. J Am Anim Hosp Assoc 18:815.
Clifford, D. H., and Soma, L. R. 1969. Fed Proc 28:1479.
Cline, D. R., and Greenwood, R. J. 1972. J Am Vet Med Assoc 161:624.
Clutton, R. E., Blissitt, K. J., Bradley, A. A., and Camburn, M. A. 1997. Vet Rec 141(6):140.
Code of Federal Regulations. 1974. Title 21, pts. 130–40. Washington, DC: US Government Printing Office.
Coffman, M. T., and Pedersoli, W. M. 1971. J Am Vet Med Assoc 158:1548.
Cohen, J. 1975. Vet Rec 97:369.
Colillas, O. J. 1978. Lab Anim Sci 28:101.
Conder, P. 1973. Vet Rec 92:325.
Conney, A. H. 1967. Pharmacol Rev 19:317.
Conney, A. H., and Burns, J. J. 1972. Science 178:576.
Connolly, R., and Quimby, F. W. 1978. Lab Anim Sci 28:72.
Cookson, J. H., and Mills, F. J. 1983. Lab Anim 17:196.
Cooper, J. E. 1974a. Vet Rec 94:437.
———. 1974b. Vet Rec 95:37.
Cooper, J. E., and Frank, L. 1973. Vet Rec 92:474.
Cooper, J. E., and Redig, P. T. 1975. Vet Rec 97:352.
Cooper, J. E., Harris, S., Forbes, A., et al. 1986. Br Vet J 142:150.
Copestake, P. 1967. Vet Rec 80:81.
Cox, J. E., Done, S. H., Lees, P., et al. 1975. Vet Rec 97:497.
Cox, R. H. 1972. Am J Physiol 223:660.
Crane, S. W., Curtis, M., Jacobson, E. R., et al. 1980. J Am Vet Med Assoc 177:945.
Cribb, P. H., and Haigh, J. C. 1977. Vet Rec 100:472.
Cribb, P. H., Hird, J. F. R., and Hall, L. W. 1977. Vet Rec 101:50.
Crispin, S. M. 1981. Equine Vet J 13:19.
Cronnelly, R. 1972. Surv Anesthesiol 16:372.
Cronnelly, R., Dretchen, K. L., Sokoll, M. D., et al. 1973. Eur J Pharmacol 22:17.
Cullen, L. K., and Jones, R. S. 1977. Vet Rec 101:115.
Cummings, J. N., Harris, W. H., and Agar, J. L. 1972. Can Anaesth Soc J 19:557.
Curl, J. L., and Peters, L. L. 1983. Lab Anim 17:290.
Curtis, R., Jemmett, J. E., and Hendy, P. G. 1977. J Small Anim Pract 18:465.
Dailland, P., Cockshott, I. D., Lirzin, J. D., et al. 1989. Anesthesiology 71:827.
Dale, H. E., Elefson, E. E., and Niemeyer, K. H. 1968. Am J Vet Res 29:1339.
Davies, M., Thuynsma, R. P., and Dunn, S. M. 1998. Can J Physiol Pharmacol 76(1):46.
Davis, B., and Pearce, D. R. 1972. Postgrad Med J (June Suppl):17.
Davis, L. E., and Wolff, W. A. 1970. Am J Vet Res 31:469.
Davis, L. E., Baggot, J. D., Davis, C. A. N., et al. 1973. Am J Vet Res 34:231.
Davis, L. E., Davis, C. H., and Baggot, J. D. 1973. In L. T. Harmison, ed., Research Animals in Medicine, p. 715. National Institutes of Health.
Dawson, B., Michenfelder, J. D., and Theye, R. A. 1971. Anesth Analg 50.443.
Day, P. W. 1965. In D. C. Sawyer, ed., Experimental Animal Anesthesiology, p. 289. Brooks Air Force Base, TX: USAF School of Aerospace Medicine.
Day, T. K., Andress, D. G., and Day, D. G. 1993. Proc Annu Meet ACVA, p. 15. Washington, DC.
Dayton, P. G., Stiller, R. L., Cook, D. R., et al. 1983. Eur J Clin Pharmacol 24:825.
Denny, M. J. S. 1973. Br Vet J 129:362.
Desforges, M. F., and Scott, H. H. 1971. Res Vet Sci 12:596.
DeYoung, D. W., Paddleford, R. R., and Short, C. E. 1972. J Am Vet Med Assoc 161:1442.
Dodam, J. R., Kruse-Elliot, K. T., Aucoin, D. P., and Swanson, C. R. 1990. Am J Vet Res 51:786.
Dodds, M. G., and Twissell, D. J. 1972. Postgrad Med J (June Suppl):17.
———. 1973. J Small Anim Pract 14:487.
Dodman, N. H. 1979. J Small Anim Pract 20:449.
———. 1980. Vet Rec 107:481.
Dodman, N. H., Seeler, D. C., and Court, M. H. 1984. Br Vet J 140:505.
Doenicke, A. Roizen, M. F., Hoernecke, R., Mayer, M., Ostwald, P., and Foss J. 1997. Br J Anaesth 79(3):386.
Domino, E. F., McCarthy, D. A., and Deneau, G. A. 1969. Fed Proc 28:1500.
Donaldson, L. L., McGrath, C. J., and Tracy, C. H. 1989. Vet Med 84:1201.
Dorfman, A., and Goldbaum, L. R. 1947. J Pharmacol Exp Ther 90:330.
Dunn, G. L., Houlton, P. J., Morison, D. H., et al. 1978. Can Anaesth Soc J 25:125.
Dyson, D. H., and Allen, D. G. 1985. Vet Surg 14:72.
Eads, F. E. 1976. Vet Med Small Anim Clin 71:648.
Eales, F. A. 1976. Vet Rec 99:270.
Edmonds, M. J. 1973. Vet Rec 92:243.
Elkins, A. D., and Herron, M. R. 1982. Vet Med Small Animal Clin 77:582.
Ellis, R. G., Lowe, J. E., Schwark, W. S., et al. 1977. J Equine Med Surg 1:259.
Elmore, R. G., Hardin, D. K., Balke, J. M. E., et al. 1985. Vet Med 80:55.
Emberton, G. A. 1966. Vet Rec 78:541.
Enna, S. J. 1981. Trends Pharmacol Sci 2:62.
Esener, Z., Sarihasan, B., Guven, H., and Ustun, E. 1992. Br J Anaesth 69(6):586.

Evan, J. M., Aspinall, K. W., and Hendy, P. G. 1972. J Small Anim Pract 13:479.
Evans, A. T., and Eberhart, S. 1992. Proc 8th Vet Midwest Anes Conf. Urbana, Ill.
Evans, A. T., Krahwinkel, D. J., and Sawyer, D. C. 1972. J Am Anim Hosp Assoc 8:371.
Famewo, C. E., and Odugbesan, C. O. 1978. Can Anaesth Soc J 25:130.
Farver, T. B., Haskins, S. C., and Patz, J. D. 1986. Am J Vet Res 47:631.
Faulk, R. H. 1978. Feline Pract 8:15.
Finck, A. D., and Ngai, S. H. 1982. Anesthesiology 56:291.
Fisher, R. J. 1984. Equine Vet J 16:176.
Flecknell, P. A., John, M., Mitchell, M., et al. 1983. Lab Anim 17:118.
Flynn, E. J., and Spector, S. 1972. J Pharmacol Exp Ther 181:547.
Foâx, P., and Prys-Roberts, C. 1972. Postgrad Med J (June Suppl):24.
Fragen, R. J., and Avram, M. J. 1994. Barbiturates. In R. D. Miller, ed., Anesthesia, 4th ed., p. 229. New York: Churchill Livingstone.
Frankland, A. L., and Camburn, M. A. 1977. Vet Rec 100:472.
Fredericksen, M. C., Henthorn, T. K., Ruo, T. I., et al. 1983. J Pharmacol Exp Ther 225:355.
Freudenthal, R. I., and Carroll, F. I. 1973. Drug Rev 2:265.
Fucci, V., Monroe, W. E., Riedesel, D. H., et al. 1986. J Am Vet Med Assoc 188:191.
Fuentes, V. O. 1978. Equine Vet J 10:78.
Fuentes, V. O., and Tellez, E. 1974. Vet Rec 94:482.
Fuller, G. B., Hobson, W. C., Reyes, F. I., et al. 1984. Proc Soc Exp Biol Med 175:487.
Funk, K. A. 1970. Equine Vet J 2:173.
———. 1973. Equine Vet J 5:15.
Fussell, M. H. 1969. Res Vet Sci 10:332.
Gage, L. J. 1984. Proc Annu Meet Am Assoc Zoo Vet, p. 31.
Gandal, C. P. 1969. Fed Proc 28:1533.
Gandini, G. C. M., Keffen, R. H., Burroughs, R. E. J. 1986. Vet Rec 118:729.
Garmer, N. L. 1969. Res Vet Sci 10:382.
Garner, H. E., Mather, E. C., Hoover, T. R., et al. 1975. Can J Comp Med 39:250.
Geel, J. K. 1991. Tydskr S Afr ver Ver 62:118.
Gelatt, K. N., Henderson, J. D., Jr., and Steffen, G. R. 1976. J Am Vet Med Assoc 169:980.
Geraci, J. R. 1973. J Am Vet Med Assoc 163:574.
Gertsen, K. E., and Tillotson, P. J. 1968. Vet Med Small Anim Clin 63:1062.
Gilroy, B. A., and Varga, J. S. 1980. Vet Med Small Anim Clin 75:508.
Glen, J. B. 1973. Vet Rec 92:65.
Glenn, J. L., Straight, L. R., and Snyder, C. C. 1972. Am J Vet Res 33:1901.
Gomwalk, N. E., and Healing, T. D. 1981. Lab Anim 15:151.
Gonder, J. C., Gard, E. A., and Lott, N. E. III. 1980. Am J Vet Res 41:972.
Goodchild, C. S. 1993. Anaes Pharmacol Rev 1:184.
Gordh, T. 1972. Postgrad Med J (June Suppl):31.
Graham, D. L., Dunlop, R. H., and Travis, H. F. 1967. Am J Vet Res 28:293.
Grandy, J. L., and McDonell, W. N. 1980. J Am Vet Med Assoc 176:619.
Gray, K. N., Raulston, G. L., Flow, B. L., et al. 1978. Southwest Vet 31:27.
Green, C. J., Knight, J., Precious, S., et al. 1981. Lab Anim 15:163.
Green, D., and Moor, R. M. 1977. Res Vet Sci 22:122.
Greenstein, E. T. 1975. Lab Anim Sci 25:774.
Grono, L. R. 1966. Aust Vet J 42:398.
Grubb, B. 1983. Vet Med Small Anim Clin 78:247.
Hagino, N. 1979. Horm Metab Res 11:296.
Haigh, J. C., Stirling, I., and Broughton, E. 1984. Proc Annu Meet Am Assoc Zoo Vet, p. 130.
Hall, L. W. 1972. Vet Rec 90:303.
———. 1976. J Small Anim Pract 17:661.
Hall, L. W., and Chambers, J. P. 1987. A clinical trial of propofol infusion anaesthesia in dogs. J Small Anim Pract 28:623.
Hamlin, R. L., Redding, R. W., Rieger, J. E., et al. 1965. J Am Vet Med Assoc 146:238.
Hammond, D., and Elsner, R. 1977. J Zoo Anim Med 8:7.
Harcourt-Brown, N. H. 1978. J Small Anim Pract 19:573.
Harding, K. A. 1977. Vet Rec 100:289.
Hartsfield, S. M., Matthews, N. S., Taylor, T. S., et al. 1993. Proc Annu Meet ACVA, p. 10. Washington, DC.
Harvey, S. C. 1975. In L. S. Goodman and A. Gilman, eds., The Pharmacological Basis of Therapeutics, 5th ed., p. 60. New York: Macmillan.
Haskins, S. C. 1992. Vet Clin North Am Small Animal Pract 22(2):245.
Haskins, S. C., Peiffer, R. L., and Stowe, C. M. 1975. Am J Vet Res 36:1537.
Haskins, S. C., Farver, T. B., and Patz, J. D. 1985. Am J Vet Res 46:1855.
———. 1986a. Am J Vet Res 47:795.
Haskins, S. C., Patz, J. D., and Farver, T. B. 1986b. Am J Vet Res 47:636.
Hatch, R. C. 1966. J Am Vet Med Assoc 158:135.
———. 1972. Am J Vet Res 33:365.
———. 1973a. Pharmacol Res Commun 5:311.
———. 1973b. J Am Vet Med Assoc 162:964.
———. 1973c. Am J Vet Res 34:1321.
———. 1974. Pharmacol Res Commun 6:289.
Hatch, R. C., and Ruch, T. 1974. Am J Vet Res 35:35.
Hatch, R. C., Currie, R. B., and Grieve, G. A. 1970. Am J Vet Res 31:291.
Hatch, R. C., Clark, J. D., Booth, N. H., et al. 1983. Am J Vet Res 44:2312.
Hatch, R. C., Wilson, R. C., Jernigan, A. D., et al. 1985. Am J Vet Res 46:1473.
Heath, R. B. 1977. Colo State Univ Clin Sci Newsl 1, No. 10.
Heath, R. B., and Gabel, A. A. 1970. J Am Vet Med Assoc 157:1486.
Heavner, J. E., and Bowen, J. M. 1968. Am J Vet Res 29:2133.
Heavner, J. E., Arthur, J., Zou, J., et al. 1992. Anesthesiology 77:A802.
Hedler, L., Stamm, G., Weitzell, R., et al. 1981. Eur J Pharmacol 70:43.
Hellyer, P., Muir, W. W., Hubbell, J. A., and Sally, J. 1989. Vet Surg 18:160.
Henderson, S., Gelb, A., and Craen, R. 1994. Proc 5th Int Cong of Vet Anesthesia, p. 107. Guelph, Canada.
Henry, D. P. 1968. Aust Vet J 44:418.
Higgins, A. J., and Kock, R. A. 1984. Br Vet J 140:485.
Hime, J. M. 1974. Vet Rec 95:193.
Hoar, R. M. 1969. Fed Proc 28:1517.
Holenweger, J. A., Tagle, R., Waserman, A., et al. 1984. Vet Med Rev (1):13.
Hubbell, J. A., Bednarski, R. M., and Muir, W. W. 1989. Am J Vet Res 50:737.
Hubbell, J. A. E., Muir, W. W., and Sams, R. A. 1980. Am J Vet Res 41:1751.
Hubbell, J. A. E., Hull, B. L., and Muir, W. W. 1986. Beef Cont Ed Art 8:F32.
Hughes, H. C., Jr., White, W. J., and Lang, C. M. 1975. Vet Anesth 2:19.
Hunt, P. S. 1976. Vet Rec 98:94.
Hunt, W. H., Fosbinder, R. J., and Barlow, O. W. 1948. J Am Pharm Assoc 37:1.

Ilkiw, J. E. 1994. In L. W. Hall and P. M. Taylor, eds., Anaesthesia of the Cat, p. 224. Philadelphia: Bailliere Tindall.
Ilkiw, J. E., Pascoe, P. J., Haskins, S. C., and Patz, J. D. 1992. Am J Vet Res 53:2323.
Inque, K., and Arndt, J. O. 1982. Br J Anaesth 54:1105.
Jackson, L. L., and Lundvall, R. L. 1972. J Am Vet Med Assoc 161:164.
Jacobson, E. R. 1983. J Am Vet Med Assoc 183:1260.
Janssen, D. L., and Oosterhuis, J. E. 1984. Proc Annu Meet Am Assoc Zoo Vet, p. 59.
Janssen, P. A. J., Niemegeers, C. J. E., and Marsboom, R. P. H. 1975. Arch Int Pharmacodyn 214:92.
Janssens, L. 1978. Vet Rec 102:350.
Jepsen, P., Lynch, B., and Woodard, A. 1984. Lab Anim 13:54.
Jessup, D. A., Clark, W. E., Gullett, P. A., et al. 1983. J Am Vet Med Assoc 183:1339.
Johnston, G. A. R., and Willow, M. 1982. Trends Pharmacol Sci 3:328.
Johnston, N. L. 1974. Vet Med Small Anim Clin 69:1243.
Jones, D. M. 1977. Vet Rec 101:340.
Jones, R. S. 1968. Br Vet J 124:72.
———. 1979. J Small Anim Pract 20:345.
Kaka, J. S., Klavano, P. A., and Hayton, W. L. 1979. Am J Vet Res 40:978.
Kalhoro, A. B., and Rex, M. A. E. 1984. Aust Vet J 61:49.
Kamibayashi, T., Hayashi, Y., Sumikawa, K., et al. 1991. Anesthesiology 75:1035.
Kaplan, B. 1972. Vet Med Small Anim Clin 67:631.
Kaplan, H. M. 1969. Fed Proc 28:1541.
Kawabori, I. 1979. Proc Soc Exp Biol Med 161:53.
Keeran, R. J. 1972. Proc Am Assoc Equine Pract, p. 41.
King, J. M., Bertram, B. C. R., and Hamilton, P. H. 1977. J Am Vet Med Assoc 171:894.
Kirmayer, A. H., Klide, A. M., and Purvance, J. E. 1984. Am Vet Med Assoc 185:978.
Kissin, I., Motomura, S., Aultman, D. F., and Reves, J. G. 1983. Anesth Analg 62:961.
Kitchell, R. L. 1983. In R. L. Kitchell, ed., Animal Pain, p. vii.Baltimore: Williams & Wilkins.
Kittle, E. L. 1971. Mod Vet Pract 52:40.
Ko, J. C., Thurmon, J. C., Tranquilli, W. J., et al. 1992. Proc 8th Vet Midwest Anes Conf. Urbana, Ill.
Ko, J. C., Thurmon, J. C., Benson, G. J., Tranquilli, W. J., and Hoffman, W. E. 1993. J Vet Anesth 20:92.
Ko, J. C., Thurmon, J. C., Benson, G. J., et al. 1994. Am J Vet Res 55:842.
Kochhar, M. M. 1977. Clin Toxicol 11:265.
Kolata, R. J., and Rawlings, C. A. 1982. Am J Vet Res 43:2196.
Kommonen, B., and Koskinen, L. 1984. Acta Vet Scand 25:346.
Kraner, K. L., Silverstein, A. M., and Parshall, C. J., Jr. 1965. In D. C. Sawyer, ed., Experimental Animal Anesthesiology, p. 374. Brooks Air Force Base, TX: USAF School of Aerospace Medicine.
Kress, H. G. 1997. Anaesthetist 46 (Suppl 1):S8.
Kumar, A., Thurmon, J. C., and Hardenbrook, H. J. 1976. Vet Med Small Anim Clin 71:1707.
Kyle, O. C., Novak, S., and Bolooki, H. 1979. Lab Anim Sci 29:123.
Lanning, C. F., and Harmel, M. H. 1975. Annu Rev Med 26:137.
Lawrence, K., and Jackson, O. F. 1983. Vet Rec 112:26.
Lawson, D. M., and Gala, R. R. 1974. J Endocrinol 62:75.
Leash, A. M. 1969. Fed Proc 28:1436.
Lees, G., Ortells, M. O., and Lunt, G. G. 1994. Anaes Pharmacol Rev 2:11.
Lees, P. 1972. Vet Rec 91:330.
Lin, H. C., Thurmon, J. C., Benson, G. J., et al. 1989. Vet Surg 18:328.
Lin, H. C., Thurmon, J. C., Tranquilli, W. J., et al. 1991. Am J Vet Res 52:1606.
Lin, H. C., Branson, K. R., Thurmon, J. C., et al. 1992. ACTA Vet Scand 33:109.
Lindley, W. H. 1976. Mod Vet Pract 57:121.
Lindquist, P. A. 1972. Lab Anim Sci 22:898.
Lo, J. N., and Cumming, J. F. 1975. Anesthesiology 43:307.
Lorenz, W., Meyer, R., Doenicke, A., et al. 1971. Nauyn-Schmiedeberg's Arch Pharmacol 269:417.
Ludders, J. W., Sedgewick, C. J., Manley, S. V., et al. 1982. J Zoo Anim Med 13:78.
Lutsky, I. 1969. Fed Proc 28:1477.
Macdonald, R. L., and Barker, J. L. 1978. Science 200:775.
———. 1979. Neurology 29:432.
McGrath, C. J., Lee, J. C., and Campbell, V. L. 1984. Am J Vet Res 45:531.
McKay, D. H., and Clement, J. G. 1977. Lab Anim Sci 27:1036.
Mackey, W. J., Anderson, W. D., and Kubicek, W. G. 1970. Lab Anim Sci 20:992.
Macy, D. W., and Siew, S. T. 1977. Feline Pract 7:44.
Mama, K. R., Steffey, E. P., and Pascoe, P. J. 1993. Evaluation of propofol in horses. Proc Annu Meet ACVA, p. 14. Washington, DC.
Mama, K., Steffey, E., and Pascoe, P. 1994. Proc 5th Int Cong of Vet Anesthesia, p. 113. Guelph, Canada.
Mandelker, L. 1972. Vet Med Small Anim Clin 67:55.
———. 1973. Vet Med Small Anim Clin 68:487.
Manders, W. T., and Vatner, S. F. 1976. Circ Res 39:512.
Marietta, M. P., Vore, M. E., Way, W. L., et al. 1977. Biochem Pharmacol 26:2451.
Mark, L. C., Perel, J. M., Brand, L., et al. 1968. Anesthesiology 29:1159.
Mascias, A., Pera, A. M., Santos, M. , et al. 1992. Proc Annu Meet ACVA, p. 14. New Orleans.
Mason, T. A. 1976. Vet Rec 98:136.
Massey, G. M. 1973. Aust Vet J 49:207.
Mather, L. E., Selby, D. G., Runciman, W. B., and McLean, C. F. 1989. Xenobiotica 19:1337.
Matot, I., Neely C. F., Katz R. Y., et al. 1993. Anesthesiology 78:1157.
Meltzer, H. Y., Stanisic, D., Simonovic, M., et al. 1978. Proc Soc Exp Biol Med 159:12.
Middleton, D. J., Ilkiw, J. E., and Watson, A. D. J. 1982. Res Vet Sci 32:157.
Millenbruck, E. W., and Wallinga, M. H. 1946. J Am Vet Med Assoc 108:148.
Mirkin, B. L. 1975. Anesthesiology 43:156.
Mitchell, B. 1966. Vet Rec 79 (Clin Suppl 3).
Moghaddam, B., Adams, B., Verma, A., and Daly, D. 1997. J Neurosci 17(8):2921.
Moon, P. F. 1994. Lab Anim Sci 44(6)590.
Morgan, D. W., and Legge, K. 1989. Vet Rec 124:31.
Muhrer, M. E. 1950. J Am Vet Med Assoc 117:293.
Muir, W. W., Skarda, R. T., and Milne, D. W. 1977. Am J Vet Res 38:195.
Muir, W. W., Skarda, R. T., and Sheehan, W. 1978. Am J Vet Res 39:1274.
Mulder, J. B. 1978a. Lab Anim Sci 28:70.
———. 1978b. Lab Anim Sci 28:321.
Mulder, J. B., and Johnson, H. B., Jr. 1978. J Am Vet Med Assoc 173:1252.
Murdock, H. R., Jr. 1969. Fed Proc 28:1510.
Nagel, M. L., Muir, W. W., and Nguyen, K. 1979. Am J Vet Res 40:193.
Navarro, J. A., and Friedman, J. R. 1975. Vet Med Small Anim Clin 70:1075.
Nayler, W. G., and Szeto, J. 1972. Am J Physiol 222:339.
Ochsner, A. J., III. 1977. Lab Anim Sci 27:69.

O'Connor, J. J., Stowe, C. M., and Robinson, R. R. 1985. Am J Vet Res 46:1721.
O'Grady, J. P., Davidson, E. C., Jr., Thomas, W. D., et al. 1978. J Am Vet Med Assoc 173:1137.
Oguchi, K., Arakawa, K., Nelson, S. R., et al. 1982. Anesthesiology 57:353.
Olsen, R. W. 1988. Int Anesthesiol Clin 26(4):254.
Orser, B. A., Pennefather, P. S., and MacDonald, J. F. 1997. Anesthesiology 86(4):903.
Oswald, R. L. 1978. Comp Biochem Physiol 60C:19.
Owen, R. T. 1979. Drugs Today 15:477.
Paddleford, R. R. 1988. In R. R. Paddleford, ed., Manual of Small Animal Anesthesia, p. 31. New York: Churchill Livingstone.
Pagel, P. S., and Warltier, D. C. 1993. Anesthesiology 78:100.
Pagel, P. S., Hettrick, D. A., Kersten, J. R., Tessmer, J. P., Lowe, D., and Warltier, D. C. 1998. Anesth Analg 86:932.
Pascoe, P. J., Ilkiw, J. E., Haskins, S. C., and Patz, J. D. 1992. Am J Vet Res 53:2178.
Pathak, S. C., Nigam, J. M., Peshin, P. K., et al. 1982. Am J Vet Res 43:875.
Pedersoli, W. M. 1972. Auburn Vet 29:6.
Pedersoli, W. M., and Brown, M. K. 1973. Vet Med Small Anim Clin 68:1286.
Polley, L., and Weaver, B. M. Q. 1977. Vet Rec 100:48.
Popovic, N. A., Mullane, J. F., Vick, J. A., et al. 1972. Am J Vet Res 33:1649.
Porter, W. P. 1982. Lab Anim Sci 32:373.
Price, H. L. 1975. In L. S. Goodman and A. Gilman, eds., The Pharmacological Basis of Therapeutics, p. 97. New York: Macmillan.
Price, H. L., Kovnat, P. J., Safer, B. S., et al. 1960. Clin Pharmacol Ther 1:16.
Quandt, I. E., and Robinson, E. P. 1992. Vet Surg 21:83.
Ramsay, E. C., and Wetzel, R. W. 1998. JAVMA 213(2):240.
Rawlings, C. A., and Kolata, R. J. 1983. Am J Vet Res 44:144.
Reder, B. S., Trapp, L. D., and Troutman, K. C. 1980. Anesth Analg (Cleve) 59:406.
Reid, J. S., and Frank, R. J. 1972. J Am Anim Hosp Assoc 8:115.
Reidenberg, M. M., Lowenthal, D. T., Briggs, W., et al. 1976. Clin Pharmacol Ther 20:67.
Report of the AVMA Panel on Euthanasia. 1993. JAVMA 202:229.
Reutlinger, R. A., Karl, A. A., Vinal, S. I., et al. 1980. Am J Vet Res 41:1453.
Reves, J. G., Glass, P. S., and Lubarsky, D. A. 1994. In R. D. Miller, ed., Anesthesia, 4th ed., p. 247. New York: Churchill Livingstone.
Rheinberger, R., Strakosch, M. R., and Pinney, C. M. 1979. Aust Vet Pract 9:228.
Richardson, K. C., and Cullen, L. K. 1981. J Am Vet Med Assoc 179:1162.
Richter, A. G. 1977. J Am Vet Med Assoc 171:988.
Ring, D. M., and Muir, W. W. 1982. Can J Comp Med 46:386.
Robertson, S. 1992. Vet Clin North Am Small Anim Pract 22(2):277.
Robertson, S. A., Johnston, S., and Beemsterboer, J. 1992. Am J Vet Res 53:1027.
Robinson, E. P., Sams, R. A., and Muir, W. W. 1986. Am J Vet Res 47:2105.
Rosatte, R. C., and Hobson, D. P. 1983. Can Vet J 24:134.
Rose, W. C., Munson, A. E., and Bradley, S. G. 1973. Proc Soc Exp Biol Med 143:1.
Rosin, E. 1974. Personal communication.
Ruben, J. M. 1979. Vet Rec 98:109.
Rucker, N. C. 1976. Mod Vet Pract 57:320.
Sams, R. A., Muir, W. W., Detra, R. L., et al. 1985. Am J Vet Res 46:1677.
Santos, M. D., and Bogan, J. A. 1974. Res Vet Sci 17:226.
Saunders, P. A., and Ho, I. K. 1990. Progress in Drug Res 34:261.
Sawyer, D. C. 1965a. In D. C. Sawyer, ed., Experimental Animal Anesthesiology, p. 321. Brooks Air Force Base, TX: USAF School of Aerospace Medicine.
———. 1965b. In D. C. Sawyer, ed., Experimental Animal Anesthesiology, p. 344. Brooks Air Force Base, TX: USAF School of Aerospace Medicine.
Schatzman, U. 1974. Equine Vet J 6:164.
Schulz, T. A., and Fowler, M. E. 1974. Lab Anim Sci 24:810.
Seeman, P. 1972. Pharmacol Rev 24:583.
Seyama, I., and Narahashi, T. 1975. J Pharmacol Exp Ther 192:95.
Sharma, R. P., Stowe, C. M., and Good, A. L. 1970. Toxicol Appl Pharmacol 17:400.
Sharp, J. W. 1996. Brain Res 728(2):215.
Shetty, S. N., Himes, J. A., and Edds, G. T. 1972. Am J Vet Res 33:935.
Short, C. E., and Brunson, D. B. 1978. Cornell Vet 68 (Suppl 7):276.
Short, C. R., Kappel, L. C., Ruhr, L. P., et al. 1985. J Vet Pharmacol Ther 8:234.
Silverman, J., Huhndorf, M., Balk, M., et al. 1983. Lab Anim Sci 33:457.
Simmons, D. J., Lesker, P. A., and Sherman, N. E. 1974. J Interdiscipl Cycle Res 5:71.
Simons, P. J., Cockshott, I. D., Douglas, E. J., et al. 1991. Xenobiotica 21:1243.
Singh, J., Sobti, V. K., Kohli, R. N., et al. 1981. Zentribl Veterinaermed (A) 28:60.
Sis, R. F., and Herron, M. A. 1972. Lab Anim Sci 22:746.
Smith, G., Thornburn, J. T., and Rogers, K. 1982. Acta Anaesth Scand 26:126.
Speckmann, G. 1975. J Zoo Anim Med 6:31.
Steen, P. A., and Michenfelder, J. D. 1979. Anesthesiology 50:437.
Stirt, J. A., Berger, J. M., Roe, S. D., et al. 1982. Anesth Analg (Cleve) 61:685.
Stock, J. E. 1973. Vet Rec 92:351.
Stoliker, H. E. 1965. In D. C. Sawyer, ed., Experimental Animal Anesthesiology, p. 158. Brooks Air Force Base, TX: USAF School of Aerospace Medicine.
Strobel, G. E., and Wollman, H. 1969. Fed Proc 28:1386.
Stunkard, J. A., and Miller, J. C. 1974. Vet Med Small Anim Clin 69:1181.
Suzer, O., Suzer, A., Aykac, Z., and Ozuner, Z. 1998. Eur J Anaesth 15(4):480.
Swanson, E. E. 1944. Therapy with Barbiturates. Indianapolis: Eli Lilly.
Taber, R., and Irwin, S. 1969. Fed Proc 28:1528.
Tadmor, A. 1980. J Am Vet Med Assoc 177:949.
Tassani, P., Martin, K., Janicke, U., and Ott, E. 1997. J Cardiothorac Vasc Anesth 11(5):562.
Tavernor, W. D. 1970. Res Vet Sci 11:91.
———. 1977. Vet Anesth 4:22.
Tavernor, W. D., and Jones, E. W. 1970. J Small Anim Pract 11:177.
Tavernor, W. D., and Lees, P. 1970. Res Vet Sci 11:45.
Taylor, C., and Stoelting, V. K. 1960. Anesthesiology 21:29.
Taylor, I. N., and Kenny, G. N. C. 1993. Non-opioid analgesics. Anaes Pharmacol Rev 1:152.
Taylor, P., Hopkins, L., Young, M., et al. 1972. Vet Rec 90:35.
Taylor, P. M., Kirby, J. J., Shrimpton, D. J., and Johnson, C. B. 1998. Equine Vet J 30(4):304.
Teske, R. H., and Carter, G. G. 1971. J Am Vet Med Assoc 159:777.
Thurmon, J. C. 1986. Vet Clinics of N Amer: Food Anim Pract 2:567.

Thurmon, J. C., Nelson, D. R., and Christie, G. J. 1972. J Am Vet Med Assoc 160:1325.
Thurmon, J. C., Kumar, A., and Link, R. P. 1973. J Am Vet Med Assoc 162:293.
Thurmon, J. C., Tranquilli, W. J., and Benson, G. J. 1985. Vet Surg 14:76.
Thurmon, J. C., Benson, G. J., Tranquilli, W. J., et al. 1988. Vet Med 83:841.
Tomlin, S. L., Jenkins, A., Lieb, W. R., and Franks, N. P. 1998. Anesthesiology 88(3):708.
Tonge, S. R. 1973. J Pharm Pharmacol 25:164.
Toutain, P. L., Brandon, R. A., Alvinerie, M. 1983. J Vet Pharmacol Ther 6:201.
Tracy, C. H., Short, C. E., and Clark, B. C. 1988. Vet Med 83:104.
Tranquilli, W. J., Thurmon, J. C., Speiser, J. R., et al. 1988. Vet Med 83:848.
Trim, C. M., and Gilroy, B. A. 1985. Res Vet Sci 38:30.
Trim, C. M., and Mason, J. 1973. Equine Vet J 5:71.
Trim, C. M., Colbern, G. T., and Martin, C. L. 1985. Vet Rec 117:442.
Trim, C. M., Adams, J. G., Hovda, L. R. 1987. J Am Vet Med Assoc 190:201.
Turner, D. M, and Ilkiw, J. E. 1990. Am J Vet Res 51:598.
Van Hamme, M. J., Ghoneim, M. M., and Ambre, J. J. 1978. Anesthesiology 49:274.
Van Pelt, L. F. 1977. J Am Vet Med Assoc 171:842.
Vaughan, R. W., and Stephen, C. R. 1974. Anesth Analg (Cleve) 53:271.
Veroli, P., O'Kelly, B., Bertrand, F., et al. 1992. Brit J Anaes 68:183.
Virtue, R. W., Alanis, J. M., Mori, M., et al. 1967. Anesthesiology 28:823.
Ward, G. S., Johnsen, D. O., and Roberts, C. R. 1974. Lab Anim Sci 24:737.
Waterman, A. 1975. Vet Rec 96:308.
Waterman, A., and Livingston, A. 1978a. J Vet Pharmacol Ther 1:141.
———. 1978b. Res Vet Sci 25:225.
Waterman, A. E. 1981. Res Vet Sci 30:114.
———. 1984. J Vet Pharmacol Ther 7:125.
Watney, G. C., and Pablo, L. S. 1992. Am J Vet Res 53:2320.
Weaver, B. M., and Raptopoulos, D. 1991. Vet Rec 126:617.
Weisbroth, S. H., and Fundens, J. H. 1972. Lab Anim Sci 22:904.
Weiskopf, R. B., and Bogetz, M. S. 1985. Br J Anaesth 57:1022.
Werner, R. E. 1976. Mod Vet Pract 57:319.
Wessells, J. V., Allen, G. W., and Slogoff, S. 1973. Anesthesiology 39:382.
White, G. L., and Cummings, J. F. 1979. Vet Med Small Anim Clin 74:392.
White, G. L., and Holmes, D. D. 1976. Lab Anim Sci 26:804.
White, P. F., Way, W. L., and Trevor, A. J. 1982. Anesthesiology 56:119.
Wilson, P. 1976. Vet Rec 98:302.
Winters, W. D. 1976. Annu Rev Pharmacol Toxicol 16:413.
Wolf, G. L., and Wigton, R. S. 1971. Arch Int Pharmacodyn Ther 194:285.
Wood, C. 1978. Vet Rec 102:304.
Wood, F. E., Critchley, K. H., and Wood, J. R. 1982. Am J Vet Res 43:1882.
Wooten, C. L. 1992. Vet Surg 21:85.
Wright, M. 1982. J Am Vet Med Assoc 180:1462.
Zoran, D. L., Riedesel, D. H., and Dyer, D. C. 1993. Am J Vet Res 54:755.

13 OPIOID AGONISTS AND ANTAGONISTS

KEITH R. BRANSON AND MARJORIE E. GROSS

Opioid Source and Composition
Opioid Receptors
Endogenous Opioids
Opioid Pharmacodynamics
  Full Agonists
  Full Antagonists
  Partial Agonists
  Agonist-Antagonists
Opioid Agonists
  Morphine Sulfate
  Codeine Phosphate
  Hydromorphone Hydrochloride
  Oxymorphone Hydrochloride
  Meperidine Hydrochloride
  Methadone Hydrochloride
  Fentanyl Citrate
  Sufentanil Citrate
  Alfentanil Hydrochloride
  Carfentanil Citrate
  Remifentanil Citrate
  Etorphine Hydrochloride
  Propoxyphene Hydrochloride
Opioid Antagonists
  Naloxone Hydrochloride
  Diprenorphine Hydrochloride
  Levallorphan Tartrate
  Naltrexone
  Nalmefene
Opioid Partial Agonists
  Buprenorphine Hydrochloride
  Tramadol Hydrochloride
Opioid Agonist-Antagonists
  Nalbuphine Hydrochloride
  Pentazocine Lactate
  Butorphanol Tartrate
  Nalorphine Hydrochloride
Opioids and Spinal Analgesia
Opioids and Peripheral Analgesia

The analgesic drugs play an important role in the clinical practice of veterinary medicine. Lloyd E. Davis (1983) succinctly described the correct role of analgesic therapy:

> One of the psychological curiosities of therapeutic decision making is the withholding of analgesic drugs, because the clinician is not absolutely certain that the animal is experiencing pain. Yet the same individual will administer antibiotics without documenting the presence of a bacterial infection. Pain and suffering constitute the only situation in which I believe that, if in doubt, one should go ahead and treat.

Pain management also is of increasing importance in laboratory animal medicine. Guidelines were issued in January 1975 by the US Department of Agriculture, which has the responsibility for enforcing the US Animal Welfare Act, to ensure appropriate use of pain-relieving drugs by biomedical research laboratories. Regulations of the act place considerable responsibility upon the attending doctor of veterinary medicine to ensure appropriate use of analgesic agents in experimental animals.

Although other classes of drugs produce analgesia, the primary type of drug used for analgesia has been, and will probably continue to be, the opioids. Since the 1960s, analgesic agents such as fentanyl, oxymorphone, etorphine, and others have been introduced for use in animals. These agents are important in alleviation of pain and are valuable in facilitating restraint and handling of animals.

In 1978, carfentanil citrate, a fentanyl analog, was introduced for use in human medicine; 2 years later another analog, named alfentanil hydrochloride, appeared on the scene. Carfentanil has been used in several species of wildlife for immobilization purposes. Another analog of fentanyl, sufentanil citrate, was introduced for human use in 1984. Its duration of action is shorter and about 10 times more potent than fentanyl in the dog (Reddy et al. 1980). The most recent fentanyl analog, remifentanil, became available for human use in 1996.

Numerous other synthetic opioids have also been developed in an attempt to minimize the undesirable effects of these drugs. These chemically diverse compounds take advantage of selective activity at opioid receptors.

The increasing practice of combining an analgesic agent with neuroleptic drugs (droperidol and the phenothiazine tranquilizers) or α_2 agonists has expanded the number of preparations the veterinarian can use for neuroleptanalgesic purposes.

OPIOID SOURCE AND COMPOSITION. Opium has been used in medicine since the dawn of history. It was recommended for relief of pain in the *Papyros Ebers,* written about 1500 BC. Greek, Arabian, and Roman physicians were well versed in the uses of opium. Arabian traders introduced it into the Orient. Opium has been widely used by physicians throughout the world from times of earliest record, through the Dark Ages in Europe, the Renaissance, and to the present day. During the eighteenth century, Portuguese merchant shippers promoted its use in China solely for economic exploitation. Armed conflict resulting from this and other exploitations led to international regulation of opium commerce by the former League of Nations and now by the United Nations.

Within the USA the Drug Enforcement Agency of the Justice Department maintains a large workforce to regulate and control importation, processing, sale, and dispensing of all opium and its alkaloids, since it is capable of producing addiction in humans. On May 1, 1971, the Controlled Substances Act of 1970 was implemented; it superseded the Harrison Narcotic Act of 1914. With the exception of heroin and some other opiate derivatives, morphine and all derivatives are classified as Schedule II drugs. Heroin is classified as a Schedule I drug because it has no accepted medical use in the USA.

The addictive property of morphine is of little direct importance in animal medicine because generally animals are not given the opportunity to develop drug dependence. However, development of addiction in humans has led to restrictions that have caused many veterinarians to forgo use of morphine and morphine substitutes in their practice. This is unfortunate because these drugs have valuable applications in veterinary medicine. Opium is the air-dried milky exudate obtained from the incised unripe seed capsules of the poppy plant, *Papaver somniferum,* which is indigenous to Asia Minor. The plant is cultivated in other countries, such as China, India, Iran, and Egypt. After the flower petals fall, the green seed capsule is incised. The milky juice dries on the capsule to form a brownish, gummy mass, which is collected, dried further, and powdered to make *Opium,* USP. Interestingly, morphine may be a ubiquitous component of plant-derived foods such as hay and lettuce. Its discovery has been reported in cow and human milk in concentrations of 200–500 ng/L (Hazum et al. 1981).

Pharmacologically, the active constituents of opium are alkaloids. Opium contains about 24 alkaloids but only 2, morphine and codeine, have much clinical use. The principal alkaloid of opium is morphine. A small fraction of opium contains thebaine (dimethylmorphine), another alkaloid, which has convulsant activity similar to strychnine.

OPIOID RECEPTORS. Opioid receptors have been identified within the central and autonomic nervous systems, the myenteric plexus of the gastrointestinal (GI) tract, heart, kidney, vas deferens, pancreas, fat cells, lymphocytes, and adrenal glands. These receptors are stimulated by opioids at the cell membrane surface in a stereospecific manner that has been described as a lock and key interaction. Opioid agonists have been described as "keys" that fit into a "lock," with only agonists being able to completely "turn in the lock" and produce a pharmacological response. A more complete description of the agonist-antagonist relationship is presented in the next section of this chapter.

The activation of the opioid receptor is coupled to changes in ion conductance and G-protein interaction. Opioid agonists with μ- or δ-receptor coupling will evoke G-protein-mediated inhibition of cAMP. This results in an increase in potassium conductance, hyperpolarization of neuronal membranes, and decreasing synaptic transmission. Kappa receptors have a similar G-protein-mediated mechanism, with resultant decreases in calcium influx and neurotransmitter mobilization and release. This decrease in calcium influx may partially explain the potentiation of opioid-induced analgesia by calcium entry blockers (Murkin 1991). It has been suggested that opioid agonists may produce a local anesthetic-like effect on the surface of excitable cells. Such an effect would not involve a stereospecific receptor (Frank 1985). Serotonergic pathways (Althaus et al. 1985) and GABA receptors (Bailey and Stanley 1994) may also play roles in the production of opioid-mediated analgesia. Opioids and α_2-adrenergic agonists are similar in their activation of inhibitory presynaptic adrenergic receptors on nociceptive fibers, but then exert their analgesic effects along different pathways. As a result, analgesia is enhanced and duration of analgesia is increased when α_2-adrenergic agonists and opioids are administered simultaneously.

Based upon studies in the chronic spinal dogs, W. R. Martin and coworkers in 1976 proposed the existence of three distinct types of opioid receptors. Each of these receptors was named for a drug that demonstrated high binding affinity for that receptor: μ (morphine), κ (ketacyclazocine), σ (SKF 10,047; *N*-allylnormetazocine). The δ receptor has since been identified, and subdivisions of the μ and κ receptors have been suggested. One of the κ subtypes may actually represent a new type of opioid receptor, the ε receptor (Nock et al. 1990). The μ, κ, and δ receptors are currently the most firmly recognized receptor classes (Pleuvry 1993).

Mu (μ) Opioid Receptor. Most of the effects of morphine-like drugs appear to be mediated by the μ opioid receptor. Two subtypes of this receptor have been identified (Wolozin and Pasternak 1981; Pasternak and Wood 1986; Itzhak 1988). The analgesic effects of morphine-like drugs are believed to be mediated by both the μ_1 and μ_2 subtypes, whereas the μ_2 subtype appears to mediate respiratory depression and inhibition of GI motility. The μ_1 subtype produces supraspinal analgesia and the μ_2 receptors produce spinal analgesia. Enkephalins appear to be the endogenous ligands for the μ_1 receptor, but endogenous ligands for the μ_2 receptor have not been identified.

Delta (δ) Opioid Receptor. The δ receptor shows the greatest selectivity for the enkephalin endogenous opioids. There are also opioid drugs that bind to δ receptors, and it has been suggested that the δ and μ receptors may exist as an interactive molecular complex (Vaught et al. 1982). The δ receptor appears to mediate analgesia primarily at the spinal level. There is some evidence to support two δ receptors; a δ_1, which is primarily involved in spinal pain modulation, and a δ_2, which is active supraspinally (Jiang et al. 1991; Mattia et al. 1991; Mattia et al. 1992)

Naloxone attenuates the decrease in blood pressure that occurs in shock, apparently by preventing δ-receptor activation by endogenous opioids released during shock (Holaday 1983a).

Large doses of naloxone are required to block δ receptors. Although naloxone is effective in reversal of shock, it also blocks the μ receptor, which mediates analgesia. This action of naloxone is not desirable in shock therapy because excruciating pain is intensified. A selective δ antagonist would be superior to naloxone in reversal of shock; such a selective antagonist, if it is eventually synthesized, will have the combined benefit of reversing the shock or cardiovascular depression without blocking opiate analgesia produced at non-δ receptors. Experimentally, a selective δ antagonist, ICI M 154129, will reverse such hypotension at doses that fail to antagonize morphine analgesia (Holaday 1983b).

Kappa (κ) Opioid Receptor. The κ receptor is involved in both spinal and supraspinal antinociception (Millan 1990). Both κ and μ receptors mediate analgesia, but the μ agonists produce euphoria and the κ agonists produce sedation and dysphoria. In addition, κ agonists produce naloxone-sensitive psychotomimetic effects (Millan 1990). The endogenous ligand for the κ receptor is probably dynorphin. Dynorphin is stored with vasopressin in the posterior pituitary. It appears to mediate an inhibitory feedback loop by activating κ receptors when released with vasopressin, preventing further release (Cox 1988). There is evidence of three κ-receptor subtypes. The κ_1 receptor is believed to mediate analgesia supraspinally, the κ_3 has spinal analgesic properties (Pasternak 1994), and it has been suggested that one of the subtypes may actually be the β-endorphin-specific ε receptor (Nock et al. 1990).

Sigma (σ) Opioid Receptor. The σ receptor was originally believed to mediate psychotomimetic effects of opioid agonist-antagonists, and opioids that produced such effects came to be known as sigma opioids. It is now understood that the drug originally used to characterize the σ receptor (SKF 10,047) is a racemic mixture of dextro- and levorotatory isomers that bind at least three types of receptors. The levorotatory isomers bind μ and κ opioid receptors, and the dextrorotatory isomers bind phencyclidine receptors and another receptor that was designated as σ (Musacchio 1990). The σ receptor exhibits a preference for dextrorotatory forms and is not sensitive to naloxone, which is a levorotatory form. The psychotomimetic effects of agonist-antagonists are mediated by levorotatory forms and can be antagonized by naloxone. This would apparently exclude the σ and phencyclidine receptors as mediators in production of opioid-related psychotomimetic effects. The σ receptors do not appear to mediate analgesic effects.

ENDOGENOUS OPIOIDS. Endogenous opioids are believed to exist in all vertebrate species and in many invertebrate species (Olson et al. 1981). Three families of endogenous opioids have been described: β endorphin, enkephalins, and dynorphin. The first, β endorphin, is produced from the precursor proopiomelanocortin, which cleaves to form adrenocorticotropic hormone (ACTH) and β lipotropin (Pasternak and Childers 1984). Beta lipotropin is devoid of opioid activity and cleaves further to yield β endorphin (Mains et al. 1977). The highest concentrations of β endorphin occur in the pituitary gland and in the medial, basal, and arcuate regions of the hypothalamus (Rossier et al. 1977). Beta endorphin also exists outside the central nervous system (CNS), in the small intestine, placenta, and plasma (Orwall and Kendall 1980; Houck et al. 1980). Proenkephalin is the precursor for methionine-enkephalin ([Met]enkephalin) and several other enkephalins (Gubler et al. 1981). Enkephalins are widely distributed in areas of the CNS which receive afferent nociceptive information (amygdala, globus pallidus, striatum, hypothalamus, thalamus, brain stem, and laminae I, II, and V of the dorsal horn of the spinal cord). [Met]enkephalin will rapidly depress ventilation and to a lesser extent heart rate and blood pressure when applied to the ventral surface of the brain stem in cats. These effects are naloxone-reversible (Florez et al. 1977). Enkephalins also exist in the peripheral nervous system (peripheral ganglia, autonomic nervous system, adrenal medulla), the GI tract, and plasma (Pasternak and Childers 1984). Dynorphin and leucine-enkephalin ([Leu]enkephalin) are derived from the precursor molecule prodynorphin. Dynorphins are believed to function primarily as neuromodulators in the CNS through interaction with μ, κ, and δ opioid receptors (Paquette and Young 1991) and may play a role in the central control of the cardiovascular system (Rochford et al. 1991). Dynorphin appears to be distributed throughout other areas of the CNS involved in nociception: periaqueductal gray, limbic system, thalamus, and laminae I and V of the dorsal horn of the spinal cord.

The endogenous opioids are part of a functional hierarchy that exists in nociception. Initial processing of afferent nociceptive information occurs from peripheral nerve endings to the dorsal horn of the spinal cord, areas in which both dynorphins and enkephalins are active. High concentrations of dynorphins, enkephalins, and β endorphin are found in key ascending and descending relay stations for nociception in the midbrain, brain stem, and thalamus. Dynorphin, enkephalin, and β endorphin are also associated with neurons in higher brain centers involved in the perception of pain (limbic system, amygdala, and cortex) (Bailey and Stanley 1994).

The greatest role of β endorphin is probably modulation of nociception during stress, midbrain periaqueductal gray stimulation, and acupuncture. Enkephalins act as inhibitory neurotransmitters and may elicit analgesia through the modulation of substance P release in the dorsal horn. Enkephalins may also play a role in acupuncture-mediated analgesia. Dynorphin may be more important in nociception at the spinal cord level through activation of κ receptors (Bailey and Stanley 1994), although current information suggests activity of κ receptors at both the spinal and supraspinal levels (Millan 1990). Other roles have been suggested for endogenous endorphins but are incompletely defined at this time.

OPIOID PHARMACODYNAMICS. When the pharmacodynamics of opioids is discussed, several terms must be defined and explained.

Affinity describes a drug's ability to bind to its receptor sites within the body. A drug with a high affinity will bind readily and strongly to those receptors. Conversely, a drug with no affinity for a specific receptor will not interact with that receptor at all.

The *activity* of a drug describes its ability to cause an action in or on the cell where its receptor resides. A drug with no activity will have no direct effect even if it is bound to a receptor for which it has a high affinity.

In the case of opioids the *potency* of a drug is often directly related to its affinity for opioid receptor sites. This means a drug can be described as very potent (high affinity) even if it exhibits little or no activity when bound to a receptor. This terminology can be confusing since the potency of an opioid is often assumed to be an indication of its analgesia-producing ability.

The *efficacy* of an opioid is a better indication of its analgesic properties. The efficacy of a drug can be illustrated using a dose-response curve (Fig. 13.1). On a dose-response curve the drug that produces the most analgesia, as evidenced by the height at the right end of the curve, is the most efficacious. If two drugs have equal activity at a receptor site, the drug with the higher affinity is the most potent. Alternatively, the opioid with the greater activity is the more efficacious when two drugs with equal affinity are compared.

If the activity of opioids was limited to one receptor type, the relationship between efficacy, activity, and potency would be straightforward, but this is not the case. The affinity and activity of an opioid can vary between receptor types, and this results in many variations in overall analgesic efficacy. In an attempt to describe this relationship, the opioids are often categorized as to their affinity and activity into full agonists, full antagonists, partial agonists, and agonist-antagonists.

Full Agonists. These opioids have both affinity for and activity at all the clinically relevant receptors. The full agonists are known for their ability to produce profound analgesia as well as significant side effects such as respiratory depression. Morphine is an example of a full agonist. The dose response curve for a full agonist is shown in Fig. 13.1A.

Full Antagonists. These opioids have affinity for but no activity at opioid receptors. The antagonists are used as reversal agents for agonists because they have no significant analgesic properties (Fig. 13.1B). To effectively reverse the agonists they must bind to the receptors and block access by the agonists. This can be done by using an antagonist with a higher receptor affinity than the agonist or using a larger dose of antagonist. Administration of an antagonist after an agonist results in a shift of the dose-response curve of the agonist to the right. This means the agonist dose needed to produce a specified level of analgesia is now greater. These drugs are often used clinically to reverse the effects of a full agonist. The goal is to reverse the agonist's undesirable effects, but unfortunately it is not possible to selectively leave the analgesia unaffected. Careful titration of the antagonist dose can, however, result in some residual analgesia. These drugs are competitive antagonists, meaning they are competing with the agonist for a limited number of receptor sites.

Partial Agonists. Partial agonists have affinity for only some opioid receptors, and they have significant activity for the receptors they do interact with. But there are other opioid receptors where they have no affinity or activity. The efficacy of these drugs is limited when compared to the full agonists since they cannot involve all the receptor types in pain control. As a result, the initial portion of their dose-response curve is similar to that of the full agonists, but the maximal analgesia produced is less (Fig. 13.1C).

Agonist-Antagonists. Classically, these opioids are described as having affinity for all opioid receptors but only demonstrating agonist behavior at some of them; they were thought to act as antagonists at the other opioid receptors. More recently there is increasing evidence that they may have some very weak agonist activity at the receptors where they were previously thought to be antagonists (Bowdle and Nelson 1994). But this activity is of such low magnitude that they are unable to produce the degree of analgesia associated with the full agonists. The dose-response curve of an agonist-antagonist indicates a lower maximal efficacy (Fig. 13.1D). The agonist-antagonists effectively act as antagonists at receptors where they show affinity but have little to no activity when they are administered with full agonists since they shift the dose-response

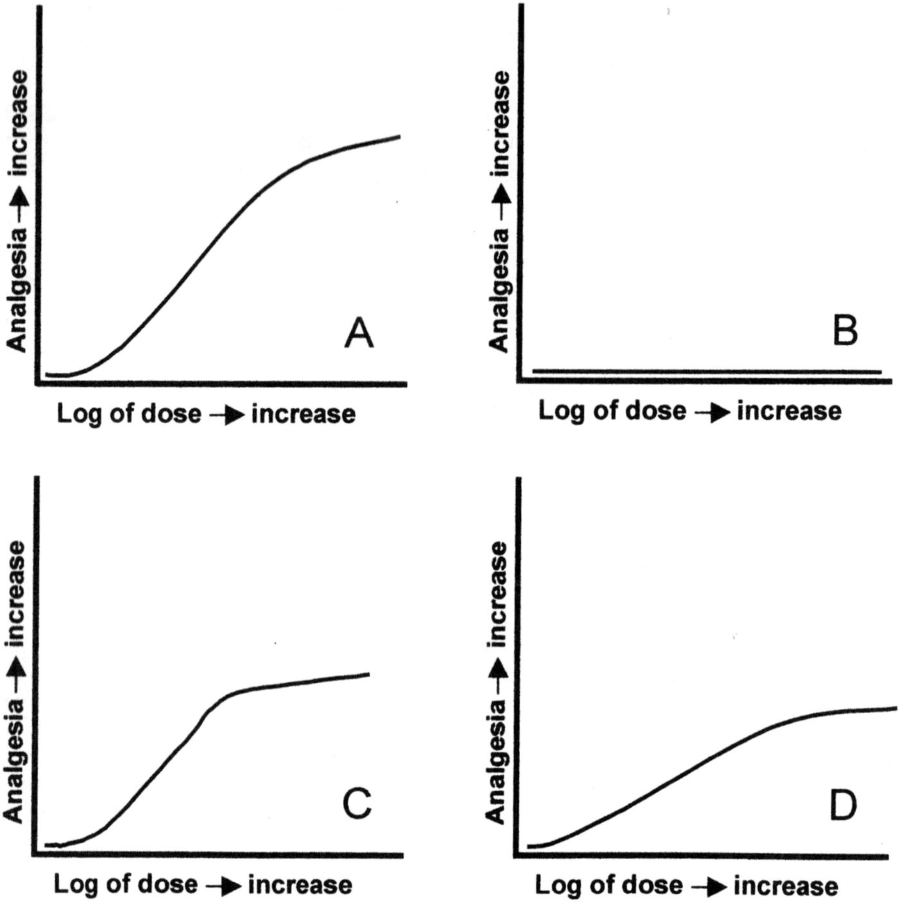

FIG. 13.1.—Four dose-response curves for different types of opioids. The horizontal axes are the log of the dose and the vertical axes are the amount of analgesia produced. (A) A full agonist type opioid such as morphine. (B) A full antagonist type opioid such as naloxone. (C) A partial agonist type opioid such as buprenorphine. (D) An agonist-antagonist type opioid such as butorphanol.

curve of the agonist to the right. Clinically, these agents can be used to partially reverse the effects of the full agonists. With them it is somewhat easier to provide partial reversal with some analgesia remaining because of their own, albeit weaker, intrinsic analgesic properties.

OPIOID AGONISTS

Morphine Sulfate. Morphine was the first of the plant alkaloids to be isolated. It was crystallized from crude opium by F. W. A. Sertürner in 1805. *Morphine Sulfate,* USP, is the principal salt of morphine. Pharmacopeias generally base the standard for opium upon its morphine content. The *United States Pharmacopeia* states that official powdered opium shall contain not less than 10% nor more than 10.5% of anhydrous morphine. In addition to the alkaloids, opium contains pharmacologically inert substances such as organic acids, resins, gums, and sugars, which constitute about 75% of the weight of dried powdered opium.

CHEMISTRY. The morphine molecule consists of a partially hydrogenated phenanthrene nucleus, an oxide link, and a nitrogen-containing structure (ethenamine, —CH_2CH_2—NCH_3). In addition, two hydroxy groups (alcoholic and phenolic; see Fig. 13.2) are important in maintaining the pharmacologic integrity of the morphine molecule.

Synthesis of morphine has been accomplished with considerable difficulty. Semisynthetic derivatives are relatively easy to manufacture by substitution of chemical radicals in place of the hydrogen atoms at one or both hydroxy positions of the morphine molecule. Chemical relationships of the natural and semisynthetic opiates are given in Table 13.1.

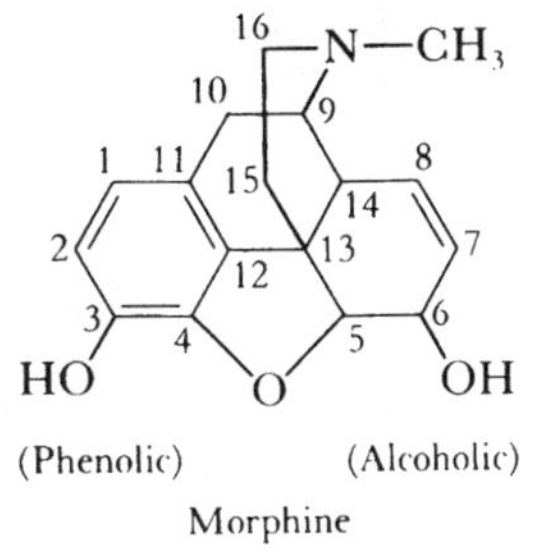

(Phenolic) (Alcoholic)

Morphine

FIG. 13.2

TABLE 13.1—Natural and semisynthetic opiates

Drug	Phenolic position	Alcoholic position
Morphine	H	H
Methylmorphine (codeine)	CH_3	H
Hydromorphone*	H	O
Diacetylmorphine (heroin)	$COCH_3$	$COCH_3$
Oxymorphone†	H	O

*Hydrogenation of carbons 7 and 8 occurs with the double bond being removed; an oxygen atom replaces the H and OH groups in position 6.

†With exception of an OH group replacing the H atom in carbon 14 position (opposite or to the left of carbon 8), the chemical structure is identical to hydromorphone.

When substitutions are made in place of one or both hydrogen atoms at the phenolic and alcoholic hydroxy position, pharmacodynamic activity of the morphine molecule is altered in an interesting manner. Alteration of the phenolic hydroxy group reduces analgesic potency, respiratory depression, and the likelihood of constipation. A stimulant activity upon the CNS is noted when substitution is made in this position. The lessened analgesic potency and increased stimulant effect typify the pharmacodynamic activity of codeine. If substitution is made at the alcoholic hydroxy position, narcotic and respiratory depression are enhanced. Consequently, hydromorphone hydrochloride is more potent as an analgesic agent than morphine. Substitution in either of the hydroxy positions lessens emetic activity of the parent molecule. As a result, both codeine and hydromorphone are less potent than morphine in producing emesis.

Other semisynthetic derivatives of morphine are apomorphine hydrochloride, a potent emetic agent, and naloxone hydrochloride, an antagonist of opiate-type drugs that has important clinical application.

To date thousands of opioid analgesics with diverse chemical structures have been synthesized and studied for their analgesic, antidiarrheal, antitussive, and addicting characteristics (Martin 1984). Consequently, many analgesics have been discovered that have been classified as either opiates or morphine-like drugs. The morphine-like drugs generally differ from morphine in their pharmacologic actions.

PHARMACOLOGIC ACTIONS. The pharmacologic actions of morphine are described below in great detail and are similar to the general effects of all the opioids. The specific organ effects of the other opioids are not described as thoroughly since they are generally similar to those of morphine.

BRAIN AND SPINAL CORD. The action of morphine upon the brain and entire CNS is irregular. It appears that the brain contains at least three distinct opioid nerve networks: an enkephalin system with components similar to those found in the adrenal medulla, a β-endorphin system, and a dynorphin system (Watson et al. 1982). The enkephalin system appears to be a separate entity from the β-endorphin and dynorphin systems. Immunochemically, dynorphin occurs in neurons, while enkephalin does not.

The basis of irregular action attributable to morphine can be better understood now that different types of opioid receptors have been identified. The major pharmacologic action of morphine is produced almost exclusively by the (−) enantiomer or isomer. The unnatural (+) enantiomer of morphine induces only minimal activity.

Early CNS effects of morphine administration in animals include changes in behavior (Simon and Hiller 1978). CNS depression is seen in the dog, monkey, and human, while CNS stimulation or excitatory behavior is elicited in the cat, horse, goat, sheep, pig, and cow following systemic administration of morphine. In an effort to ascertain whether the species difference in behavior induced by morphine is a reflection of the distribution pattern of opiate binding sites in the brain, Simon (1977) investigated binding of radiolabeled etorphine in various regions of the brain in a number of species. There is reasonably good reproducibility of binding level for any given anatomical region in the dog, monkey, human, sheep, cow, and cat. The only areas of the CNS that show consistent differences are the amygdala and frontal cortex. These regions are at least two times higher in receptor level for the species that show CNS depression than for the species that show CNS excitation to opiates (Simon 1977). These consistent differences between the two groups of mammals are most baffling. The amygdala and frontal cortex are components of the limbic system wherein most of the areas of high opiate binding in dog, monkey, and human are located (Simon 1977). Interestingly, monkeys become placid following bilateral amygdalectomy, whereas the cat displays a sustained aggression and ferocity. Consequently, amygdalectomy resembles the effects seen in acute morphine administration in these two species.

Considerable controversy has existed regarding whether morphine should be used in the cat because of its inability to consistently produce sedation. Studies indicate that morphine sulfate is effective in obtunding intense pain. According to Davis and Donnelly (1968), the excitatory response frequently observed in the cat may be the effect of overdosage with morphine. When doses of morphine hydrochloride of 5, 10, and 20 mg/kg are injected intraperitoneally in conscious cats, a manic response characterized by hyperexcitement and aggressive behavior is observed (Dhasmana et al. 1972). This response can be prevented by pretreatment with either CNS catecholamine depletors (i.e., reserpine, tetrabenazine) or central dopaminergic receptor blocking agents such as those produced by chlorpromazine hydrochloride and haloperidol, which also have α-adrenergic receptor blocking action. Another interesting action of morphine in the cat is the production of insomnia, which is reversible by naloxone. If β endorphin or morphine is injected intraventricularly, insomnia is produced (King et al. 1981).

The CNS excitation or manic effect induced by morphine in the cat may occur from alteration in the functioning of brain dopaminergic or noradrenergic systems. It is known that drugs that block dopamine receptors always increase striatal dopamine synthesis and turnover. This is also true with morphine (Lal 1975). Brain concentration of homovanillic acid, a metabolite of dopamine, increases following morphine, suggesting that an increase in catabolism occurs in brain dopamine. Conversely, morphine depresses noradrenergic activity in the locus ceruleus of the rat, and this effect appears to be related to the unavailability of norepinephrine at the receptor sites. It is possible that stimulatory action of morphine and related compounds, including fentanyl, is due to indirect action of these drugs, predominantly on noradrenergic cerebral functions (Fidecka et al. 1978). If this is correct, it may explain the inhibitory effect of reserpine on stimulatory actions of morphine and fentanyl. Reserpine does not inhibit synthesis of dopamine but does inhibit activity of dopamine-β-hydroxylase, making interaction between the enzyme and dopamine more difficult. Consequently, reserpine decreases the rate of synthesis of norepinephrine. Increased locomotor activity or persistent restlessness (stereotypy) seen after morphine administration appears to be due to release of norepinephrine and not dopamine.

As stated, swine, goats, sheep, cattle, and horses are generally stimulated by morphine. However, effects of morphine in the horse and the ox are somewhat irregular. In these species it may be that the dosages used are higher than required to produce analgesia similar to that observed in the cat. Moreover, increased turnover of dopamine or increased release of norepinephrine following morphine administration may also be involved in production of restlessness and CNS excitation in these species similar to that in the cat. If this is true, dopaminergic and noradrenergic blocking agents such as the phenothiazines or droperidol should effectively prevent excitation as it does in cats. Since the phenothazine-derivative tranquilizers such as chlorpromazine and acepromazine induce arterial hypotensive effects, their use for this purpose is potentially dangerous.

CNS depression does not necessarily need to occur prior to or concomitantly with development of the state of analgesia. Morphine is capable of producing a high degree of analgesia without accompanying CNS or respiratory depression in animals such as the hamster. Perhaps the hamster has few or lacks entirely the μ and δ opioid receptors that mediate the respiratory depressant effects of opiates. It is possible that the hamster could have a higher density of σ opioid receptors that mediate an increase in the respiratory rate.

In addition to known analgesic effects following intracerebral administration of enkephalins or morphine, long-lasting electrographic seizures occur in most animals. In the rat, analgesia occurs after injections of methionine-enkephalin into or near the ventral, caudal midbrain periaqueductal gray matter. Epileptiform seizures and other electroencephalographic disorders are seen with enkephalin injections into or near the forebrain dorsomedial nucleus of the thalamus. Seizures are accompanied by myoclonic twitches, catalepsy, muscular rigidity, and "wet-dog shakes" and are blocked by prior administration of naloxone (Frank et al. 1978). These effects suggest that enkephalin-induced analgesia and seizures are mediated by opioid receptors located in different regions of the brain that are pharmacologically different. Now that it is known that the σ opioid receptor mediates mania and that dynorphin induces a wide spectrum of motor effects via the κ receptors, these receptors may be involved.

Crib biting, often referred to as a vice in horses, probably is better described as a stereotypy (Dodman et al. 1987) or an aberrant type of motor behavior. It is interesting that Dodman and associates have found that narcotic antagonists (naloxone, naltrexone, others) will prevent crib biting. Its prevention by narcotic antagonists is evidence that this form of stereotypy involves activation of opioid receptors, possibly by release of endogenous opioids in the CNS (Dodman et al. 1987).

Interestingly, laboratory animals with only the spinal cord intact will show strychnine-like tetany following administration of morphine. This cord-stimulating activity, as well as increased central seizures, is the reason that morphine is strictly contraindicated in treatment of strychnine poisoning. The CNS and cord stimulant effects of morphine strongly suggest that it should be contraindicated in treatment and control of epilepsy in dogs and cats. The author has induced convulsive seizures in the dog and rabbit with large doses of morphine (500 mg/kg).

Ability of opiates to evoke generalized convulsive seizures is well recognized and, for the most part, has been considered to be an undesirable side effect (Martin 1984). Opioids appear to exert both convulsant and anticonvulsant activity through several modes of action and probably through a number of receptor mechanisms.

The dog shows a brief preliminary period of central excitement marked by restlessness, panting, salivation, nausea, vomiting, urination, and defecation. These symptoms gradually disappear and are followed by a stupor indicating depression of the cerebral cortex. Inasmuch as morphine induces CNS depression and accompanying analgesia in the dog, clinicians have used it almost entirely in this species. Of the opiate derivatives, morphine is preferred by clinicians primarily for preanesthetic medication in the dog over its use in other animals because the drug facilitates handling for induction of general anesthesia.

Information on effectiveness of morphine in relieving pain comes primarily from use of the drug in human patients because of the ease of noting the subjective response. Morphine will relieve pain without blocking motor activity or consciousness. The pain threshold is increased so that moderate pain disappears and sharp pain is dulled. Morphine is most useful in humans in relieving pain arising from the viscera and from trauma. Anxiety and alarm disappear. Sleep may be produced during the period of morphine analgesia. In human patients, morphine is used almost exclusively for relief of pain. These observations give some indication as to the probable effectiveness of morphine in relieving pain in animals.

EMETIC CENTER. Considerable species variation occurs with respect to effect of morphine upon vomiting in animals; e.g., swine and chickens do not respond to central-acting emetics (morphine, apomorphine) but do respond to local emetic agents (copper sulfate, zinc sulfate). It is interesting that apomorphine stimulates dopamine receptors (dopamine agonist), whereas morphine does not. Morphine blocks emetic action of apomorphine.

Both dogs and cats will respond to central- and local-acting emetics. However, the cat requires considerably higher doses of morphine or apomorphine to induce vomiting than the dog. For example, morphine and apomorphine dosages 740–2800 times greater are required in the cat over the level that stimulates vomiting in the dog (Brand and Perry 1966). Horses and ruminants do not vomit following administration of central- or local-acting emetics. The emetic center in the dog is readily stimulated by small to moderate dosages of morphine. Within 5–10 minutes after subcutaneous (SC) injection of morphine, most dogs will vomit profusely unless the stomach is empty, in which case only saliva and bile may be lost. The act of vomiting is preceded by salivation and nausea and is usually accompanied by defecation.

A trace of morphine applied directly to the floor of the fourth ventricle will produce simulated vomiting in dogs from which the entire GI tract has been removed. This effect would seem to exclude gastric irritation as a causative factor as has been previously believed.

COUGH CENTER. The cough center appears to be more susceptible to morphine than other medullary centers. Morphine is an excellent cough sedative, and were it not for its addictive properties to dogs as well as humans, the drug probably would be the most widely used and effective control available for dry, nonproductive coughs. Generally, morphine is used only in those patients for whom codeine previously was ineffective.

THERMOREGULATION. A variation in effect upon body temperature is seen in different species following administration of morphine. Hypothermia is the dominant body temperature response to morphine in rabbits, dogs, and monkeys, whereas hyperthermia usually occurs in cats, goats, cattle, and horses (Oka 1978). In guinea pigs, rats, and mice, low dosages of morphine elicit a hyperthermic effect, while higher dosages induce hypothermia. The hypothermic action of morphine wanes in rabbits following repeated or chronic administration. In monkeys and rats not only is the hypothermic action of morphine reduced following repeated administration but hyperthermia becomes the dominant response.

Morphine accelerates release of 5-hydroxytryptamine (serotonin) from the serotonergic neurons in the hypothalamus (Oka 1978). Release of serotonin stimulates warm-sensitive interneurons and/or inhibits cool-sensitive interneurons in the hypothalamus. Activation of warm-sensitive neurons stimulates heat-dissipation responses, and inhibition of cool-sensitive neurons depresses the heat-production responses. Stimulation of the heat-loss pathway and/or inhibition of the heat-production pathway result in a drop in body temperature (Oka 1978).

Morphine-induced hypothermia is abolished following serotonin depletion with parachlorophenylalanine (an inhibitor of tryptophan 5-hydroxylase). Administration of 5-hydroxytryptophan, a precursor of serotonin, to animals pretreated with parachlorophenylalanine restores the typical hypothermic response to morphine, meperidine, and methadone. Hypothermia (also catalepsy) induced by opiates is antagonized by thyrotropin-releasing hormone (TRH); TRH does not affect the analgesic effects of the opiate-type drugs (Zaloga et al. 1984). Although TRH does not bind to opioid receptors, it is referred to as a physiologic opiate antagonist (Bernton et al. 1985).

In the cat, IV injection of morphine (1–10 mg/kg) induces a dose-related hyperthermic response (Clark and Cumby 1978). Administration of metiamide (an H_2-histamine-receptor blocking agent) or indomethacin (prostaglandin synthetase inhibitor) does not antagonize morphine-induced hyperthermia in the cat. This indicates that histamine and prostaglandins are apparently not required for the hyperthermic effect induced by morphine (Clark and Cumby 1978).

The morphine antagonist (naloxone) does not prevent febrile responses in cats to leukocytic pyrogen (Clark and Harris 1978). This implies that endogenous opioid peptides (enkephalins) that are antagonized by naloxone are not likely to mediate febrile responses to pyrogens. The cerebral ventricular administration of methionine-enkephalin induces both hyperthermia and emesis in cats (Clark 1977). Pretreatment with naloxone reduces the hyperthermic response and prevents the emetic response of methionine-enkephalin in the cat.

Panting is noted initially in the dog after administration of morphine but finally stops with a decline in body temperature. Sweating and hyperglycemic response in the horse following administration of morphine is believed to be associated with increased circulating level of epinephrine.

Although apomorphine is a semisynthetic derivative of morphine, it induces hyperthermia in rabbits but not the hypothermia seen following administration of morphine. Apomorphine is well established as a dopaminergic agonist. Dopamine is one of a number of catecholamines found in the brainstem that have a thermoregulatory role in the rabbit. Experimental evidence exists indicating that central dopaminergic mechanisms are activated prior to a temperature response in animals following administration of *d*-amphetamine or apomorphine; both these drugs induce hyperthermia, and the hyperthermic response can be blocked by a dopaminergic receptor blocking agent such as pimozide or haloperidol.

In some species (mice, rats), apomorphine elicits hypothermia. Dopamine-receptor blocking agents such as pimozide and haloperidol are able to competitively antagonize hypothermia induced by apomorphine (DiChiara and Gessa 1978).

EYE. Morphine produces a variable effect upon the size of the pupil in animals. Morphine causes mydriasis in the monkey, cat, sheep, and horse and causes miosis in dogs, rats, rabbits, and humans. The dog is less sensitive to the miotic action of morphine than humans (Martin 1984). Over 2 mg/kg morphine administered parenterally is required to induce maximum miosis in the dog.

The iris of the bird is not affected because it contains nonresponsive skeletal muscles. Although morphine activates parasympathetic input (i.e., increases the spontaneous firing rate of light-sensitive neurons recorded from the anterior oculomotor nucleus) to the iris, the miotic effect is antagonized by increased catecholamine release from the adrenal glands; this results in mydriasis (Wallenstein and Wang 1979). Adrenalectomy or administration of phenoxybenzamine antagonizes the mydriasis induced by release of catecholamines in the cat, and miosis is observed.

Since the σ receptor mediates pupillary dilation, the variation in response induced by morphine upon the eye in different species may be related to the density or number of σ receptors within the oculomotor nucleus.

RESPIRATORY SYSTEM. The respiratory center of the dog is initially stimulated; panting is seen and is attributable to the initial rise in body temperature. As body temperature declines and CNS depression increases, respiratory activity is depressed by morphine, resulting in decreased minute volume of respired air. The threshold of response to carbon dioxide stimulation is increased and the alveolar concentration of carbon dioxide is higher. Respirations become slower and shallower. In deep sedation, Cheyne-Stokes type respiration may occur.

The agonistic effects of morphine upon μ_2 and σ opioid receptors can result respectively in either depression or stimulation of respiratory activity. Depressant or stimulatory activity upon respiration is dependent upon the dose of morphine administered and can also vary within the various animal species.

In normal, healthy dogs, small doses of morphine may not decrease respiratory minute volume and oxygen consumption by more than about 10%. Following large doses of morphine that lead to convulsive seizures, respiration rate is markedly increased. Eventually, depression and paralysis of the respiratory center develop, ostensibly from overstimulation. Moreover, moderate to large doses are known to produce bronchiolar constriction in the dog. Significant bronchoconstriction occurs following an IV dose of 1 mg/kg, and a more marked effect is produced following a dose of 2.5 mg/kg; a decrease in lung capacity at the latter dose averaged 24% (Shemano and Wendel 1965).

CARDIOVASCULAR SYSTEM. Although opiate peptides were initially associated with regulation of pain, they appear to have importance in regulation of the cardiovascular system. They are particularly important in its central neural control (Holaday 1983).

In the conscious dog, morphine (2 mg/kg) administered intravenously induces a substantial degree of coronary vasoconstriction, reduction in coronary blood flow, and increase in coronary vascular resistance (Vatner et al. 1975). Interestingly, coronary vasoconstriction is not seen after α-adrenergic blockade; morphine apparently has an indirect α-adrenergic stimulating action, since it stimulates release of catecholamines.

In the anesthetized dog, morphine (0.5 mg/kg) administered intravenously induces a transient drop in arterial pressure and a concomitant increase in heart rate (DeSilva et al. 1978a). Arterial pressure soon returns to base line or control levels following administration of morphine. As arterial pressure returns to normal to slightly elevated levels, heart rate decreases appreciably from increased pressoreceptor activity as well as from a vagotonic effect of morphine. Due to its vagotonic and sedative actions, morphine exerts significant protective effect on increased ventricular vulnerability to fibrillation (DeSilva et al. 1978b).

Effects of morphine in humans are in marked contrast to dogs. Coronary blood flow is increased and a slight coronary vasodilation occurs in humans (Leaman et al. 1978). Although morphine has been used satisfactorily for years in treatment of human patients with cardiac disease (e.g., acute pulmonary edema from left heart failure, pain relief following acute myocardial infarction), its use in the dog for treatment of cardiopulmonary complications (e.g., "cardiac dyspnea") may not, as originally thought, have therapeutic merit. Use of morphine in such cases may be imprudent.

URINARY TRACT. The initial effects of morphine along with salivation, nausea, vomiting, and defecation may also include urination. As the effect progresses, morphine can decrease urine secretion in the dog to 10% or less of normal by liberating an excess of the antidiuretic hormone from the pituitary gland. This hormone, in excess, stimulates intensive reabsorption of the glomerular filtrate by the cells of the renal tubules. To produce such a response, the dose of morphine must approach 2.4 mg/kg intravenously or 5 mg/kg subcutaneously.

There is evidence that dynorphin, an opioid peptide, may be released concomitantly from the pituitary with the antidiuretic hormone (i.e., vasopressin). With the presence of opioid receptors in the kidney, it is also logical to expect a direct action of inhibition of prostaglandin activity.

Morphine increases muscular tone of the bladder, which, among other effects, results in spasm of the sphincter, which may make urination difficult. Conversely, animals seem to be less affected and have less difficulty in this respect than humans.

GI TRACT. Emptying the GI tract is the dog's first response to morphine. Following the initial emptying, morphine causes constipation of the dog and other animals. The GI tract appears to contain both μ and δ opioid receptors. Activation or stimulation of either receptor results in inhibition of GI tract motility. This action is the basis for using opiate-type antidiarrheal agents for control of diarrhea.

Since it has been postulated that all peptide hormone-producing cells are derived embryologically from the neural ectoderm, it should not be too surprising to learn of the presence of brain peptides in the GI tract (Guillemin 1978); e.g., opioid receptors are present in the myenteric plexus of the GI tract. Enkephalins and substance P have also been identified in association with opioid receptors in the GI tract. Stimulation of opioid receptors in guinea pig ileum leads to constipation (Knoll 1977).

Morphine has a persistent spasmogenic effect upon intestinal smooth muscle by a direct action, partly by a cholinergic and partly by a histaminergic mechanism (Türker and Kaymakcalan 1971). Atropine partially inhibits the spasmogenic effect of morphine. Mepyramine partially blocks or antagonizes spasmogenic activity of morphine; apparently this is related to its histamine-releasing action. Release of serotonin occurs in the isolated intestine of the dog when it is perfused with morphine.

By virtue of the persistent spasmogenic action, the primary effect of morphine is to increase tonus of smooth muscles of the entire GI tract. The sphincters exhibit a spastic tonus. The propulsive motility of the tract is markedly depressed, apparently as a result of excessive tonus that interferes with normal peristaltic waves. The tonus may become great enough to close or constrict the intestinal lumen in the conscious dog. Thus passage of food through the tract is delayed. The delay results in increased absorption of water from the ingesta, which contributes to constipation. Tonus of the anal sphincter is increased by morphine. In addition, morphine depresses mental perception of ordinary sensory stimuli for the defecation reflex.

The effect of morphine upon enzyme secretions of the digestive tract of the dog is variable but slight. Biliary secretion appears to be reduced to one-third of normal. Morphine causes an initial delay in gastric secretion of HCl, which is later compensated by excessive secretion.

ENDOCRINE SYSTEM. Exogenous and endogenous opiates induce an array of effects upon pituitary hormone release in both animals and humans (Morley 1981). In the rat, opiates stimulate release of growth hormone, ACTH, and prolactin; they also inhibit release of glycoprotein hormones. In humans, endogenous opiates appear to be important in the physiologic regulation of ACTH and gonadotropin release. Paradoxically, the inhibitory release of ACTH in Cushing's disease suggests a potential use of specific and long-acting opiate antagonists in treatment of this condition (Morley 1981).

Opiates exert an important modulating action upon the hypothalamus; additional modulating effects may occur at the pituitary and upon target organs. Opiate-induced endocrine actions appear to be mediated through dopaminergic and/or serotoninergic mechanisms (Morley 1981).

IMMUNE SYSTEM. An interaction between the immune system and central neuroendocrine mechanisms has been suspected for a long time (Joseph et al. 1985). The nonspecific influence of the pituitary-adrenal axis upon the immune system by altering or increasing resistance to infectious diseases has been recognized from the time of the Hans Selye era of stress research.

Recent discoveries have resulted in identification of corticotropin-releasing factor (CRF), as well as the simultaneous secretion of ACTH and β endorphin, from the pituitary during stressful conditions (Plotnikoff and Murgo 1985). This has led to identification of interactions among the stress hormones (CRF and enkephalins-endorphins) as well as thymus hormones and even interferons, ACTH, and endorphins at the peripheral level of the lymphocyte. Viral infection of lymphocytes induces the cells to synthesize Ir ACTH and Ir endorphins (Blalock and Smith 1985).

In summary, it appears that the immune and neuroendocrine systems have the capability of signaling each other through common or related peptide hormones and receptors. Enkephalins and endorphins can be considered immunomodulators and modifiers of the physiologic response and may have important application in immunotherapy (Wybran 1985).

ABSORPTION, FATE, AND EXCRETION. Morphine is a weak acid; it has a pK_a of 8.0, which means it is poorly ionized at physiological pH. In humans it is 20–40% protein bound, the elimination half-life is 2–4 hours, the steady-state volume of distribution (Vd) is 3–5 L/kg, and the clearance rate is 15–30 mL/min/kg (Bailey and Stanley 1994).

Morphine is absorbed from the small intestine and some may be absorbed from the stomach. The absorption from the GI tract is somewhat variable, with a large individual variability (Dohoo and Tasker 1997). It is absorbed promptly following SC injection. Morphine is not absorbed through intact skin, but a scarified epithelium permits slow entrance to the circulation.

Biotransformation of morphine to morphine-3-glucuronide is the primary metabolic pathway for inactivation and eventual elimination of the drug (Sanchez and Tephly 1974). The principal catalyst in formation of morphine glucuronide is a hepatic microsomal uridine diphosphate (UDP)-glucuronyl transferase, which transfers a glucuronic acid moiety from UDP-glucuronic acid (UDPGA) to morphine. Other metabolites are formed as well, some of which are pharmacologically active. The most prevalent of these is morphine-6-glucuronide (Christrup 1997). With the exception of the cat, approximately 50% of morphine administered to most mammals appears in the urine as the glucuronide form. In the cat, a deficiency in UDPGA and its associated glucuronyl transferase enzyme does not favor glucuronidation of morphine. Increased toxicity of aspirin and salicylate drugs is linked to failure of the cat to conjugate the compounds with glucuronic acid. The biologic half-life of morphine would be expected to be longer in the cat because of its inability to form glucuronides. Surprisingly, the biologic half-life in plasma is only 3.05 hours in the cat following SC injection of morphine (1 mg/kg) (Davis and Donnelly 1968). The biologic half-life of morphine in other species is probably shorter than in the cat; these values were not located in the literature.

In humans, morphine was studied after a single IV dose (10 mg/70 kg); a rapid initial decline of morphine in the blood occurred during the first 6 hours after administration (Spector and Vesell 1971). After rapid initial decline of the drug, levels of morphine could be detected in blood for several hours; this may be attributable to enterohepatic recirculation, persistence of metabolites, or a combination of these and other factors. During the first 6 hours, the half-life of morphine ranged from 1.9 to 3.1 hours. Following this, disappearance of the drug was slow, with a half-life of 10–44 hours (Spector and Vesell 1971).

In horses, morphine can be found in serum samples for at least 24 hours after an IV injection of 0.1 mg/kg; it is present in urine for up to 144 hours (Combie et al. 1981).

TOXICITY. Newborn animals are known to be more sensitive to morphine than adults (Auguy-Valette et al. 1978). Morphine-induced toxicity decreases with maturity of the animal. This is associated with decrease in the capability of morphine to enter the brain commensurate with development of the blood-brain barrier.

The toxic dose of morphine for the dog appears to be variable. Subcutaneously or intravenously, the fatal dose is 110–220 mg/kg. Convulsive seizures quite similar to strychnine occur in most species following administration of higher doses of morphine. Thebaine (dimethylmorphine), a component of opium, is also well known for its strychnine-like seizures.

In the small rodent (mouse), acute toxicity and death from morphine are produced by IV administration of 221–311 mg/kg; an SC dose between 420 and 526 mg/kg produces death. Young swine apparently are quite susceptible to the stimulant action of morphine.

Addiction is rarely encountered in animals because narcotic drugs are not ordinarily administered for prolonged periods. There is a clinical report of addiction from prolonged (6–8 months) use of paregoric (camphorated tincture of opium) in the dog by an overzealous owner (Segall 1964).

With discovery of β-endorphin and opioid receptors, the most exciting outgrowth from this research could be the prospect that endorphin deficiency might play some role in narcotic addiction. A hypothesis has been advanced by Goldstein (1976) that classical hormonal feedback mechanisms might act to inhibit or suppress endogenous opioid synthesis (i.e., β endorphin) when receptors are occupied by an exogenous opiate like morphine. Sudden withdrawal of the exogenous substance can expose the deficiency in endogenous synthesis (compare the adrenal crisis if corticosteroid administration is abruptly stopped); thus induced endorphin deficiency might play a role in the immediate or protracted abstinence syndrome (addiction). It would be most interesting if this postulated disease entity proved to be an endorphin deficiency.

PRECAUTIONS AND CONTRAINDICATIONS. Morphine should be used with care in acutely uremic and toxemic dogs. By stimulating secretion of the antidiuretic hormone, morphine increases reabsorption of the renal filtrate. A large dose of morphine may decrease urine flow in the dog by 90%.

Morphine cannot be used to control convulsive disorders such as strychnine poisoning, tetanus, and epilepsy. It should not be administered to dogs suffering from traumatic shock because of its immediate hypotensive effect upon arterial pressure. This is important if provisions are not available to expand the blood volume and restore systemic arterial pressure.

Opiates must not be used in animals with head injury. This use results in an increase in intracranial pressure due to a decreased sensitivity to arterial carbon dioxide partial pressures (Heidrich 1985).

In large animals, opiates should be used cautiously. Overdoses can result in prolonged periods of restlessness and excitement.

CLINICAL USES. Morphine has been used for a wide variety of clinical conditions since the beginning of recorded history. Several of these uses are still valid. When an opiate is used to relieve pain or control diarrhea or coughs, only symptomatic therapy is administered. The underlying etiology and pathology are still present. Furthermore, unwise use of opiates may obscure symptomatic progress of disease.

DOGS. Morphine is important in canine surgery to relieve pain, facilitate handling the patient for local or general anesthesia, and decrease the amount of CNS depressants necessary to produce surgical anesthesia. The peak effect of morphine is usually reached between 30 and 45 minutes following SC injection. Duration of the analgesic effect has not been accurately determined but appears to last 1–2 hours. The SC doses of morphine recommended for preanesthetic medication vary from 0.1 to 2 mg/kg. For inducement of analgesia in the dog, an IV, IM, or SC dose of 0.25–0.5 mg/kg is generally recommended.

Onset of action after an IM or SC injection is within a few minutes. Atropine (0.045 mg/kg) is routinely administered by the SC or IM route at the same time as morphine to prevent salivation and bronchial secretions. Very young, aged, and debilitated dogs are more susceptible to morphine than normal, middle-aged, vigorous ones. A dog depressed by morphine should be handled gently and quietly because roughness and noise may awaken it and provoke delirium. The emetic actions of morphine may cause great inconvenience if it is not anticipated. Conversely, it is a definite advantage to have the stomach emptied in the event fasting was insufficient prior to anesthesia and surgery.

Premedication with sufficient morphine will decrease the total amount of general anesthetic required for surgical anesthesia to one-half or perhaps even to one-third. This supports the concept of balanced anesthesia and increases the safety of anesthetic procedures.

Oral administration could potentially be of value for the control of pain in dogs; however, the absorption, and therefore the efficacy, are variable. The use of oral sustained-release products does not prolong the duration of action in dogs (Dohoo and Tasker 1997).

Morphine is of value postoperatively for overcoming the recurring delirium observed in dogs recovering from anesthesia with pentobarbital. Without a depressant such as morphine, a dog may, by its struggles, induce hemorrhage, injury, or fracture or open a surgical incision.

Traditionally, morphine has been used cautiously in cesarean section of the dog because of fetal respiratory depression. It now appears that fetal respiratory movements are not abolished by doses of morphine that depress maternal respiration and produce maternal analgesia. However, they may be depressed by large doses of morphine. A large dose also interferes with uterine contraction and parturition.

By virtue of its morphine content as well as all the components in opium, *Paregoric,* USP, is used for its antidiarrheal effect. The oral dose recommended for the dog is 0.05–0.06 mL/kg administered every 8 or 12 hours (Chiapella 1980).

CATS. An effective SC analgesic dose of morphine in the cat is 0.1 mg/kg (Davis and Donnelly 1968). Other investigators have also found that SC administration of morphine (0.1 mg/kg) produces effective analgesia in the cat (Watts et al. 1973). Preanesthetic medication of cats with morphine (0.5 mg/kg) is probably valueless in ketamine anesthesia; morphine administered intramuscularly at this dose may induce respiratory depression (Hatch 1973).

For postoperative use, Heavner (1970) recommends morphine in the cat up to 0.1 mg/kg intravenously for management of pain. He noted that recovery from anesthesia is smoother, and upon awakening the animals lie quietly.

GUINEA PIGS, MICE, AND RATS. Morphine may be used subcutaneously or intramuscularly as a preanesthetic agent in the guinea pig and rat (Strobel and Wollman 1969) prior to parenteral or inhalant anesthetics; the recommended dose in these species is 2–5 mg/kg. According to Strobel and Wollman (1969), the usual analgesic and sedative doses of morphine exert an effect within 15 minutes of SC administration and last several hours. In the rat, mouse, and guinea pig, Wright et al. (1985) recommend a SC dose of 10 mg/kg morphine.

RABBITS. Morphine has a profound depressant effect in the rabbit. The IM use of morphine (8 mg/kg) is advocated 30 minutes prior to IV thiamylal (20 mg/kg) anesthesia. Atropine (0.2 mg/kg) is also administered intramuscularly at the same time as the morphine injection. A SC or IM dose of 5 mg/kg morphine is also recommended by Wright et al. (1985).

SWINE. Morphine has more CNS stimulant than depressant effects in the pig. However, it is used successfully for analgesic effect in the pig prior to chloralose and barbiturate anesthesia (Booth 1969); the recommended IM dose is 0.2–0.9 mg/kg. The mechanism of the excitatory effect produced by morphine in the pig is probably similar to that described in the cat.

SUBHUMAN PRIMATES. Comparatively large doses (1–3 mg/kg) of morphine are necessary for chemical restraint and sedation of the chimpanzee (Clifford 1971). The dosage for the dog is recommended for adequate sedation and safe management of the subhuman primate (Soma 1971). Wright et al. (1985) recommend 1–2 mg/kg morphine by the SC route in monkeys.

HORSES. Morphine and other opiates have been used in the horse for various ailments, but particularly to relieve acute pain of spasmodic colic. Morphine (0.22 mg/kg) is administered intramuscularly or slowly by the IV route (White 1981). For preanesthetic use, morphine is given in an IV dose of 0.12 mg/kg (Muir et al. 1978). Although some patients are relieved, many horses show undesirable and dangerous central stimulation and excitement. Loss of coordination occurs in the horse between 20 and 100 minutes after IV administration of 2.4 mg/kg morphine and lasts up to 7 hours (Combie et al. 1979). Horses walk, stagger, or bump into walls and appear to be unaware of their surroundings; they have the capability of making appropriate postural corrections in spite of coordination difficulties. Some clinicians contend that overdosing is the reason morphine has fallen into disrepute in treatment of spasmodic colic in the horse.

Morphine (0.1 mg/kg) can be detected in blood up to 48 hours and in urine for 144 hours after IV administration in the horse (Combie et al. 1983). A serum half-life for this dose is nearly 88 minutes.

Phaneuf et al. (1972) reported IV use of morphine chlorhydrate (1 mg/kg) in two ponies with classic forms of colic. The analgesic effect produced by the drug resulted in a hyperactive but uniform contraction of the jejunum. The jejunal spasms disappeared, motility of the colon became prominent, and the stomach remained quiescent.

Morphine has been used satisfactorily with xylazine for sedation and analgesia in the horse (Klavano 1975). Specific information on dosage and use is discussed under the section on xylazine in Chap. 14.

RUMINANTS. Morphine and other related derivatives have not been used in ruminants for clinical purposes. Experimentally, it is known that opioids inhibit cyclic forestomach motility in various ruminant species. Normal cyclic motility of the reticulorumen of sheep is inhibited by opioids that appear to act through central and peripheral mechanisms (Maas and Leek 1985). Central action leads to a reduced frequency and amplitude of the cyclic contractions. Both the central and peripheral inhibitory actions of the opioids upon the rumen can be antagonized by naloxone.

Codeine Phosphate. *Codeine Phosphate,* USP (methylmorphine), occurs in opium to the extent of around 0.5%. Most of it is produced semisynthetically from morphine. The phosphate salt is more widely used than codeine sulfate despite respective solubilities in water of 2.3 and 30 parts.

Codeine is metabolized rapidly by the tissues of humans, dogs, and rats. Metabolic alteration followed by rapid urinary excretion begins a few minutes after IM injection and after a slight delay following oral administration. About one-half an ordinary dose is eliminated within 6 hours and all within 24 hours. In the dog, about 50% of the dose is excreted in a conjugated (glucuronide) form in the urine. Limited conversion of codeine to morphine does not occur in the dog as in humans. Excretion products in humans include norcodeine, conjugated codeine, morphine, and traces of codeine in the feces. Interestingly, codeine is one-tenth as potent as morphine when administered to intact animals and only one-hundredth as potent in the isolated guinea pig ileum (Pert and Snyder 1973).

Codeine is widely used to depress the cough center. The dose of codeine should be increased proportionately over that of morphine to produce the desired depression of the cough reflex with less undesirable side action. Unfortunately, codeine possesses some of the constipating action of morphine; therefore, large doses or prolonged administration may result in constipation. Since the analgesic action of codeine is less than morphine, codeine is not commonly used in animals for control of severe pain. Addiction to codeine is uncommon.

Codeine is used in an expectorant and cough syrup mixture at 1.1–2.2 mg/kg to allay irritating coughs in dogs; this level is administered orally 3–4 times daily. For additional information on the cough-suppressant or antitussive action of codeine and related derivatives, see Chap. 54.

Analgesic dosages of codeine for laboratory animals are: rat, SC dose, 6.25–25 mg/kg; mouse, SC dose, 25.5 mg/kg; and rabbit, oral or IV dose, 10 mg/kg (Wright et al. 1985). Codeine can also be used as an orally administered analgesic in the dog. The dose is 0.5–2.0 mg/kg every 6–8 hours.

Hydromorphone Hydrochloride. *Hydromorphone Hydrochloride,* USP (Dilaudid), is about five times more potent as an analgesic than morphine. In the dog it produces less nausea, emesis, and GI disturbance than morphine. It is soluble in 3 parts of water. The SC dose for the dog is 1.1–2.2 mg/kg.

Oxymorphone Hydrochloride. *Oxymorphone Hydrochloride,* USP (Numorphan), is approximately 2.5 times as potent as hydromorphone and about 10 times more potent than morphine on an mg/mg basis. See Table 13.1 for its chemical relationships with morphine and other morphine substitutes.

This narcotic analgesic is potent when used alone or in combination with neuroleptic agents or barbiturates in the dog and cat. To avoid precipitation, oxymorphone must not be mixed with a barbiturate in the same syringe. Naloxone is an effective antagonist of oxymorphone. Oxymorphone is approved by the FDA for use in the dog and cat.

In the cat, a combination of oxymorphone (0.165 mg/kg) and triflupromazine (1.1 mg/kg) has proved satisfactory (Reid and Frank 1972). This neuroleptanalgesic mixture is followed with IV ketamine (1.1–2.2 mg/kg). According to Reid and Frank (1972), the combination of oxymorphone and triflupromazine can be administered by the SC, IM, or IV route. They recommend that ketamine not be administered until after oxymorphone and triflupromazine have taken effect because simultaneous administration of all three drugs induces prolonged apnea resembling the "locked chest" syndrome described in humans.

When used alone, preanesthetic effectiveness of oxymorphone is limited in the dog and cat because its CNS depressant effects are slight (Palminteri 1963). It produces a mild ataxia and hyperesthesia in the cat when used by itself. In combining the narcotic analgesic with a tranquilizer, such as acepromazine or valium, or with an α_2 agonist, such as xylazine, a greater degree of neurolepsia or tranquilization is achieved. Oxymorphone (1.5 mg/mL) is used in combination with triflupromazine (20 mg/mL) by mixing equal volumes of both drugs in the same syringe for IV, IM, or

TABLE 13.2—Parenteral doses of a mixture of equal volumes of oxymorphone (1.5 mg/ml) and triflupromazine (20 mg/ml) required to produce analgesia in small animals

Animal	Body weight	Volume of narcotic-tranquilizer mixture
	(kg)	*(ml)*
Dogs	0.9–2.3	1.0
	2.3–6.8	1.0–2.0
	6.8–13.6	2.0–4.0
	13.6–27.2	4.0–6.0
	27.2+	6.0–8.0
Cats	Small	0.5–1.0
	Large	1.0–2.0

Source: Palminteri 1963.

SC administration. For the dosage schedule recommended in the dog and cat, see Table 13.2.

In the dog, premedication with oxymorphone reduces the amount of thiamylal required to produce surgical anesthesia by one-third to two-thirds. Oxymorphone induces minimal cardiorespiratory changes in the dog. It produces mild respiratory depression with an increase in P_aCO_2 and decrease in tidal volume. Oxymorphone administration results in an increase in arterial blood pressure and stroke volume. Heart rate decreases along with slight decreases in cardiac output (Copeland et al. 1987; Haskins et al. 1991). Use of the analgesic agent prior to thiamylal requires IM or SC doses of oxymorphone varying from 0.065 to 0.44 mg/kg. The lower doses are administered to the large breeds. For all dogs, the average dose is 0.198 mg/kg. Thiamylal (2.5%) is administered intravenously to effect 45–90 minutes after administration of oxymorphone.

Oxymorphone doses approved by the FDA for IV, IM, or SC administration in the dog and cat are given in Table 13.3.

For postoperative pain, oxymorphone is recommended in an IV dose of 0.1 mg/kg every 4–6 hours for the cat and dog (Heidrich 1985). In the horse, it is recommended for postoperative pain in either an IV or IM dose of 0.2–0.3 μg/kg.

Although more work is needed to evaluate the safety and efficacy of oxymorphone, it has been used in equine colic intramuscularly or intravenously (10–15 mg/mature horse) (Hackett 1976). Oxymorphone (22 μg/kg) administered intramuscularly or slowly by the IV route has been recommended for alleviation of pain associated with equine colic (White 1981). For preanesthetic use, oxymorphone is recommended in an IV dose of 30 μg/kg (Muir et al. 1978).

Meperidine Hydrochloride. *Meperidine Hydrochloride,* USP (Demerol Pethidine, Dolantin) (Fig. 13.3), was synthesized in Germany during a search for an atropine-like drug having smooth muscle spasmolytic activity (Eisleb and Schaumann 1939). Meperidine is not only spasmolytic but also analgesic and sedative.

TABLE 13.3—Oxymorphone doses approved by the FDA for the dog and cat

Animal	Body weight	Dose
	(kg)	*(mg)*
Dogs	0.9–2.7	0.75
	2.7–6.8	0.75–1.5
	6.8–13.6	1.5–2.5
	13.6–27.2	2.5–4.0
	Over 27.2	4.0
Cats	Small	0.4–0.75
	Large	0.75–1.5

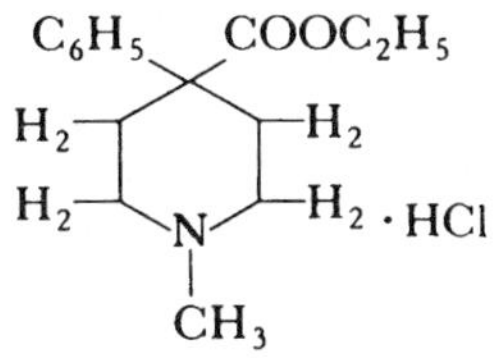

C_6H_5 $COOC_2H_5$ … $\cdot HCl$ … CH_3

Meperidine Hydrochloride

FIG. 13.3

The hydrochloride salt is used in medicine. It is a colorless crystalline powder with a neutral reaction, a slightly bitter taste, and ready solubility in water. The aqueous solution is not decomposed by a short period of boiling.

Meperidine and its related derivative *Diphenoxylate Hydrochloride,* USP, are Schedule II drugs subject to the Controlled Substances Act of 1970. Diphenoxylate, an antiperistaltic agent, in combination with atropine is classified as a Schedule V preparation.

ADMINISTRATION. Meperidine is best administered intramuscularly in animals. The absorption after IM administration can be somewhat variable (Waterman and Kalthum 1989, 1990). The SC route is not preferred because local irritation and pain may be produced. Oral administration is not advised in large animals because of the cost. If the drug contacts buccal mucosa, particularly in the cat, considerable irritation and salivation result. IV injection must be made slowly to avoid cardiovascular collapse. Following IM or SC administration in the cat, emesis does not occur, but defecation occurs in some animals.

METABOLISM AND FATE. Meperidine is absorbed rapidly following SC, IM, or oral administration. The drug is largely inactivated in the liver. This results in a low bioavailability of meperidine due to a first-pass effect after oral administration (Ritschel et al. 1987). A small amount is excreted unchanged in urine; the major part of a given dose is demethylated (normeperidine) and hydrolyzed before being excreted. Parahydroxymeperidine has also been identified in the rat. Both normeperidine and parahydroxymeperidine have been shown to possess less analgesic activity than meperidine (Dahlstrom et al. 1979). The metabolite normeperidine is more toxic and possesses greater convulsant activity than meperidine, the parent compound.

There is considerable species variation with respect to metabolism of meperidine (Caldwell et al. 1979). Biotransformation of meperidine in the rat is considerably different from that in humans and monkeys. Of the monkeys, the mangabey (*Cerecebus tarquinus*) provides a good metabolic model for humans, whereas the mona (*Cercopithecus mona*) and patas (*Erythrocebus patas*) monkeys are less acceptable in metabolism studies of meperidine.

In humans, only about 5% of meperidine administered is excreted unchanged; the remaining portion undergoes *N*-demethylation to normeperidine acid or conjugation with glucuronic acid. About 60% of meperidine administered in humans can be recovered (Greene 1968); 5% of the drug is unchanged, 5% is in the form of unbound normeperidine, 20% is meperidine acid, 7% is normeperidine acid, and 12% each is recovered as bound meperidine and normeperidine. Disposition of the remaining 40% of the parent compound is unknown. Biotransformation of meperidine in humans occurs at the rate of 10–20%/hour; *N*-demethylation occurs through hepatic microsomal enzyme activity together with nicotinamide adenine dinucleotide phosphate and oxygen. Only the unchanged meperidine molecule can be metabolized by the liver; all other metabolic changes or degradation occur to some degree in extrahepatic tissues.

When meperidine (22 mg/kg) is administered intravenously, Davis and Donnelly (1968) found the plasma half-life to be 0.7 hour in the cat. Despite the short half-life in plasma, the analgesic effect of 11 mg/kg of the drug given intramuscularly is apparent at 2 hours but not at 0.5 or 4 hours after administration. In the dog, the half-life of intravenously administered meperidine is 0.75 hours, the volume of distribution is 2.4 L/kg, and the total clearance is 42.5 mL/min/kg (Ritschel et al. 1987). Because duration of effective plasma levels of meperidine is short and the biotransformation is rapid, Davis and Donnelly (1968) stated that meperidine probably will serve better as a preanesthetic drug than in management of severe pain in cats.

Meperidine is rapidly cleared from pony plasma after IV administration (Alexander and Collett 1974). The estimated half-life of the drug is 66 ± 8.7 minutes. Alexander and Collett found that less than 5% of the administered dose (350 mg IV) is excreted unaltered in pony urine during the 48 hours after administration.

Pharmacokinetic studies in the pregnant ewe indicate that fetal blood levels of meperidine peak less than 10 minutes after an IV injection (Mirkin 1975). Serum concentrations in the fetus are generally greater than those in corresponding samples from maternal subjects. A single IV injection of meperidine (0.85–2.5 mg/kg) into the pregnant ewe is not associated with significant effects on maternal or fetal arterial blood pressure and heart rate (Jenkins and Dilts 1971).

THERMOREGULATORY EFFECT. In the cat, following SC injection of large doses (30–50 mg/kg) of meperidine, a marked rise to 40.5–41.6° C occurs in rectal temperature. This appears to be a dose-related phenomenon. Inasmuch as morphine induces a hyperthermic response in the cat, the mechanism of meperidine-induced hyperthermia may be similar to that of morphine.

CARDIOPULMONARY EFFECT. Following an IM dose of 10 mg/kg meperidine, reduction in heart rate and drop in the systemic arterial pressure occur in dogs. Generally, the fall in blood pressure is moderate, and occurs 10–20 minutes after IM injection, with return to the control level in 30 minutes. The decline in systemic arterial pressure is probably the result of peripheral vasodilation following release of histamine.

A significant degree of bronchoconstriction occurs in the dog following an IV dose of 0.5 mg/kg (Shemano and Wendel 1965). Also, meperidine administered at 2.5 mg/kg intravenously produces a 22% decrease in lung capacity. Shemano and Wendel suggested that the bronchoconstrictor effect of meperidine and morphine may be due to a combination of central vagal stimulation and histamine release.

ANALGESIC ACTION. The analgesic effect of meperidine is intermediate between codeine and morphine. In dogs, meperidine (4.4 mg/kg) administered intramuscularly every 3–6 hours has been used to depress the cough reflex and in treatment of cardial "asthma." In the horse, meperidine produces analgesia within a few minutes following IV administration and 15–25 minutes after an IM injection.

SPASMOLYTIC ACTION. The spasmolytic activity of meperidine is significant but considerably less than morphine and methadone. Meperidine will relax the intestine, bronchi, ureter, and, to some degree, uterus. Meperidine, morphine, and methadone depress intestinal peristalsis in the dog. This effect is capitalized upon in the use of paregoric, a compound containing morphine, or diphenoxylate hydrochloride, a meperidine derivative for antidiarrheal purposes.

The ratio of doses producing the same degree of intestinal inhibition is morphine 1 and meperidine 750. Because the ratio of doses producing a given analgesic effect is 1:10, meperidine has an advantage of 75 to 1 over morphine when an analgesic drug is needed that does not depress intestinal motility. It is apparent that meperidine possesses a marked advantage over morphine for relief of postoperative pain because it can be given in many times (up to 750) the dose of morphine before it depresses intestinal propulsion as much.

Diphenoxylate hydrochloride is combined with atropine as adjunctive therapy in management or control of severe diarrhea in humans. Control of diarrhea occurs by virtue of the antiperistaltic actions of both diphenoxylate and atropine.

TABLE 13.4—Effect of varying doses of meperidine in the cat

Dose	Number tested	Number showing excitation	Number showing muscular spasms	Number showing convulsions	Deaths
(mg/kg)					
5	10	0	0	0	0
10	25	5 (slight)	0	0	0
20	15	8	0	0	0
30	15	15	9	6*	0
40	15	15	13	11†	0
50	10	10	10	9§	0

Source: Booth and Rankin 1954.
Note: Pentobarbital (15–20 mg/kg) was used as an anticonvulsant in 3 cats,* 1 cat,† and 7 cats§ of these respective groups.

The diphenoxylate-atropine mixture (Lomotil) has been used in the UK for treatment of feline diarrhea. Not more than 0.5 mg/kg based upon the diphenoxylate content of the mixture is suggested by the oral route of administration (Ormerod et al. 1978). The mixture, in tablet form, contains diphenoxylate (2.5 mg) and atropine (0.025 mg). Toxicity induced by the drug preparation in cats results in extreme excitement, restlessness, and marked mydriasis with visual impairment. A goose-stepping gait, loss of balance, extension of claws, and leaping everywhere are additional signs seen following overdosages of the mixture. In the dog, an oral dose of diphenoxylate (2.5–5 mg total dose) is used every 6 or 8 hours for antidiarrheal purposes (Chiapella 1980).

Caution in the use of diphenoxylate with CNS depressant agents must be considered. It may potentiate the actions of barbiturates, tranquilizers, and other CNS depressants.

Naloxone reverses the action of diphenoxylate. In the USA, diphenoxylate-atropine has not been approved for use in animals by the FDA.

TOXICITY. SC doses in excess of 20–30 mg/kg can produce excitement and clonic convulsions in cats (see Table 13.4). Convulsions can be controlled by injection of pentobarbital. Barbiturates can be used successfully to antagonize lethal convulsive effects of meperidine. However, meperidine potentiates the depressant effect of the barbiturates upon respiration and will only increase the certainty of death if administered in barbiturate intoxication. Naloxone is an antagonist of the respiratory depressant and toxic effects of meperidine. However, naloxone does not antagonize CNS convulsions and other signs of CNS stimulation such as hyperreflexia and tremors (Dystra and Leander 1978).

Normeperidine is considered to be more toxic than the parent drug meperidine. Its accumulation may result in toxicologic consequences. However, prolonged administration of meperidine to dogs in amounts up to six times the recommended therapeutic dose produces no toxic effects other than slight anorexia and loss of weight. Although no addiction to meperidine has been demonstrated in animals, addiction manifested by withdrawal symptoms occurs in humans.

CLINICAL USE. In dogs and cats, meperidine given preanesthetically reduces the period of excitement and reduces the amount of anesthetic needed. There is individual variation in the depressant effects of meperidine.

DOGS AND CATS. In the dog, meperidine is used intramuscularly for preanesthetic medication varying from 2.5 to 6.5 mg/kg (Soma 1971). The postanalgesic dose recommended in the dog is 5–10 mg/kg intramuscularly. Duration of analgesia induced by meperidine is approximately 45 minutes. In contrast to morphine, meperidine does not produce miosis in the dog; parenteral administration (4 mg/kg) causes mydriasis (Martin 1984).

In the cat, the IM dose of meperidine is 2.2–4.4 mg/kg for preanesthetic medication (Chase 1977). Premedication of cats with meperidine is probably of no value in ketamine anesthesia; IM meperidine (5 mg/kg) may induce respiratory depression (Hatch 1973).

SWINE. Meperidine (10 mg/kg) administered subcutaneously in large sows and boars contributes little toward restraint. For preanesthetic medication in the pig, meperidine (1–2 mg/kg), promazine hydrochloride (2 mg/kg), and atropine (0.07–0.09 mg/kg) work satisfactorily prior to barbiturate and inhalant anesthesia (Booth 1969). All these preanesthetic preparations are administered intramuscularly in separate sites 45–60 minutes prior to induction of anesthesia.

HORSES AND CATTLE. Total IV and IM doses of meperidine recommended for the adult horse are 500 and 1000 mg respectively. It must be given slowly intravenously because dangerous arterial hypotension can occur.

In cattle an IM dose of 500 mg is recommended. Meperidine is used in the mare to relieve pain and discomfort following cesarean section (Cohen 1975). It has also been used to treat equine colic, especially acute spasmodic conditions. However, meperidine (2.2 mg/kg) administered intramuscularly produces only an

TABLE 13.5—Doses and indications of meperidine for use in laboratory animals

Species	Dose	Route of administration	Major indications	Reference
	(mg/kg)			
Mouse	20	SC,IM	Analgesia	Wright et al. 1985
Rate	20	SC,IM	Analgesia	Wright et al. 1985
Hamster	2	IM	Preanesthetic	—
Guinea pig	2	IM	Preanesthetic	Maykut 1958
Rabbit	10	SC,IM	Analgesia	Gardner 1964
Subhuman primates	2–4	IM	Analgesia	Wright et al. 1985

inconsistent and transient analgesia in the horse following experimentally induced colic; xylazine is a superior analgesic compared to meperidine, pentazocine, and dipyrone for treatment of induced colic (Lowe 1978). A dose of meperidine as high as 4 mg/kg administered intramuscularly or subcutaneously is recommended for control of pain in horses (Baggot and Cooper 1980).

Spontaneous locomotor activity is prominent in the horse after an IV dose of 5 mg/kg meperidine (Combie et al. 1979). For the first 14 minutes postinjection, meperidine induces incoordination, trembling, and immobility. However, the locomotor effect is relatively brief; it peaks at about 30 minutes and returns to normal by about 3 hours (Combie et al. 1979). An IV dose of 2.5 mg/kg elicits a modest increase in motor activity, whereas 1 mg/kg has no effect.

In cattle, the drug is used for calving to calm the nervous heifer and provide analgesia during parturition. Meperidine does not inhibit uterine contractions in cattle.

LABORATORY ANIMALS. Meperidine is useful as an analgesic in laboratory species. Doses are given in Table 13.5.

On a body weight basis, the rhesus monkey is twice as sensitive to meperidine as the squirrel monkey. According to Robinson and Janssen (1980), 10 mg/kg meperidine administered subcutaneously for postsurgical analgesia in a colobus monkey (*Colobus guereza kikuyensis*) is followed within several minutes by respiratory arrest. Administration of oxygen and an IV dose (0.04 mg/kg) of naloxone are effective resuscitative measures in reversal of respiratory arrest resulting from meperidine overdosage.

EXOTIC ANIMALS. Meperidine (2.2–4.4 mg/kg) has been used subcutaneously in bears and large cats for analgesia (Wright et al. 1985). For immobilization purposes in the elephant, an IM dose of 0.03 mg/kg is recommended (Tamas and Geiser 1983).

Methadone Hydrochloride. Two proprietary names for *Methadone Hydrochloride,* USP, are Amidone and Dolophine. Methadone was synthesized in Germany in 1941 as a result of the continuing search for a substitute for morphine (Fig. 13.4). In 1973, methadone was removed from general medical use. It has been reinstated as a Schedule II drug and is again available for veterinary medical use. Methadone is a bitter, white, crystalline compound that is readily soluble in water. The *l*-isomer has 25 times the analgesic potency of the *d*-isomer. This drug is discussed in greater detail in the 7th edition of this text.

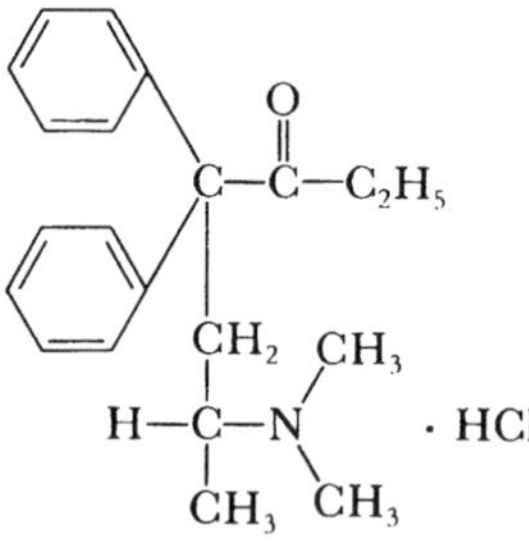

Methadone Hydrochloride

FIG. 13.4

CLINICAL USE. In the horse, methadone (0.11 mg/kg) and acepromazine (0.11 mg/kg) have been administered in combination by the IV route to provide analgesia and restraint for treatment of wounds, loading unruly animals into transporting vehicles, suturing of wounds, and various types of minor surgery (Schauffler 1969). CNS depression occurs within 30 seconds following injection; within 3 minutes, the effect is usually sufficient to carry out various treatments or surgical procedures. However, peak CNS depression may not be attained for 15 minutes following administration of methadone-acepromazine; duration of the effect is about 1 hour. Recovery occurs gradually over a 6- to 12-hour period. Occasionally, a horse may be slightly drowsy for up to 3 days after receiving this drug combination (Schauffler 1969).

Horses ordinarily do not become recumbent following methadone-acepromazine even at high dosages. The animals may appear somnolent but will usually retain their standing position (Schauffler 1969). Moreover, horses are sufficiently free of incoordination so there is little hazard of their falling upon, stepping upon, or otherwise injuring attending personnel. If the animals become recumbent, they can be returned to the standing position without difficulty.

Methadone (0.04 mg/kg) plus acepromazine (0.04 mg/kg) has been used intravenously in the horse prior to IV ketamine (2–2.5 mg/kg) (Parsons and Walmsley 1982). The mean time between administration of the premedication and ketamine was 15 minutes; time of standing from induction averaged 13 minutes. More data are needed to determine the safety and efficacy of using these drugs in combination.

Fentanyl Citrate. *Fentanyl Citrate,* USP (Sublimaze), is a phenylperadine derivative. It is more lipid soluble than morphine, which contributes to its rapid onset and short duration of action (Hug and Murphy 1981). Its analgesic properties are at least 100 times that of morphine. It is a full opioid agonist and is active at μ, κ, and δ receptors. It has a high abuse potential and is a Schedule II drug.

METABOLISM AND FATE. Fentanyl is metabolized by the liver by hydroxylation and dealkylation. The primary route of excretion for the metabolites is in the urine (McLain and Hug 1980). It is highly protein bound and undergoes significant tissue redistribution, which leads to some variability in the rate of excretion of the drug. It has a steady-state Vd of 3–5 L/kg, a clearance rate of 10–20 mL/min/kg, and an elimination half-life of 2–4 hours (Bailey and Stanley 1994).

CARDIOPULMONARY EFFECTS. In the dog, fentanyl given alone induces analgesic, respiratory, and cardiovascular effects within the same range of plasma concentrations. It does not produce respiratory arrest when injected intravenously at 2.5, 5, 20, 40, and 100 μg/kg at 5-minute intervals to a cumulative dose of 167.5 μg/kg given over 20 minutes. After these doses, spontaneous respiration is maintained in all animals; respiratory rate, P_aO_2, heart rate, and cardiac output are reduced to about one-half at the peak effect of fentanyl. Doses in excess of those required to produce complete analgesia do not interfere with adequacy of oxygenation (Arndt et al. 1984). Even doses up to 3 mg/kg failed to produce apnea or severe hypercapnia in spontaneously breathing dogs (Bailey et al. 1987). Fentanyl appears to have minimal direct cardiac depressant effect (other than bradycardia), although some negative inotropic effect is seen at excessive doses (Montomura et al. 1984). There is an overall sympatholytic effect seen with fentanyl administration (Tayeyama et al. 1993). The respiratory effect of fentanyl is similar to that of morphine in that it depresses the patient's response to increases in arterial carbon dioxide partial pressure. Its respiratory depressant effects are often of surprisingly long duration and may exhibit a biphasic pattern. This is probably due to the significant amount of fentanyl sequestered in peripheral tissues, which must then reenter the plasma before elimination (Bailey and Stanley 1994).

CLINICAL USE. In veterinary medicine fentanyl was most commonly used with droperidol (see Chap. 14) in the fixed drug combination Innovar-Vet, which is no longer available. Each milliliter contained 20 mg droperidol and 0.4 mg fentanyl.

Fentanyl (without droperidol) is used prior to general anesthesia or as part of a balanced anesthesia protocol, also termed neuroleptanalgesia (Sawyer 1985). In dogs it is often used with other tranquilizers such as medetomidine (20 or 40 μg/kg) IM and fentanyl (2 μg/kg) IV (England and Clarke 1989) or xylazine (0.2 mg/kg) IV, glycopyrrolate (0.01 mg/kg) IV, and fentanyl (10 μg/kg) IV. Fentanyl (55 μg/kg) and xylazine (1.1 mg/kg) have been used in the horse (Pippi and Lumb 1979).

Fentanyl is also available in a transdermal delivery system (Duragesic). The delivery system consists of a small reservoir with a semipermeable membrane that is applied to the skin over a hairless area. The reservoirs come in several sizes to adjust the dosage rate and are labeled to indicate the total administration rate in micrograms per hour. The sizes available are 25, 50, 75, and 100 μgrams/hr. The dose most commonly used in dogs and cats is 2–4 μg/kg/hr. In dogs the absorption rate is variable and it can take up to 24 hours for the plasma concentration to reach a steady state but the plasma concentrations obtained are highly variable (Kyles et al. 1996; Egger et al. 1998). The lipophilic nature of fentanyl allows successful transdermal administration since the rate-limiting step is diffusion through the lipophilic stratum corneum (Guy et al. 1987; Samir and Flynn 1989).

Sufentanil Citrate. *Sufentanil Citrate,* USP (Sufenta) is a phenylperadine derivative similar to fentanyl. It is 5–10 times more potent than fentanyl but has a safety margin over 6 times larger than fentanyl (Stoelting 1991). Sufentanil is more lipid soluble than fentanyl. It is a full opioid agonist and is a Schedule II drug because of its high abuse potential.

METABOLISM AND FATE. Sufentanil is metabolized by the liver primarily by dealkylation and demethylation. Most of the metabolites are excreted in the urine (60%) in dogs and in the feces (62%) in rats (Meuldermans et al. 1987). In plasma, sufentanil is highly protein bound. It has a steady-state Vd of 2.5–3.0 L/kg, a clearance rate of 10–15 mL/min/kg, and an elimination half-life of 2–3 hours (Bailey and Stanley 1994).

CARDIOPULMONARY EFFECTS. Equipotent doses of fentanyl and sufentanil produce similar cardiovascular and respiratory effects.

CLINICAL USE. Sufentanil is generally used when it is desirable to have an anesthetic protocol with excellent cardiovascular stability. It is administered as a continuous infusion with concurrent use of a tranquilizer or inhalation anesthetic. When a sufentanil infusion was administered in conjunction with lenperone, the sufentanil-induced cardiovascular changes were minimal (Benson et al. 1987).

Alfentanil Hydrochloride. *Alfentanil Hydrochloride,* USP (Alfenta), is a phenylperadine derivative similar to fentanyl. It is less potent than fentanyl and has a shorter half-life. The short duration of action makes it very appropriate for use as an infusion. It is more lipid soluble and exhibits greater protein binding than fentanyl (Stoelting 1991). It is a full opioid agonist and is a Schedule II drug because of its high abuse potential.

METABOLISM AND FATE. Alfentanil is metabolized by the liver primarily by dealkylation and demethylation. Most of the metabolites are excreted in the urine (75%) in both dogs and rats (Meuldermans et al. 1987). In plasma alfentanil is highly protein bound. It has a steady-state Vd of 0.4–1.0 L/kg, a clearance rate of 4–9 mL/min/kg, and an elimination half-life of 1–2 hours (Bailey and Stanley 1994). Its short duration of action is a result of redistribution from the brain to other tissues, and its rapid metabolism results in minimal accumulation.

CLINICAL USE. In dogs infusions of 8 μg/kg/min produced a 69% reduction in the minimum alveolar concentration (MAC) of enflurane (Hall et al. 1987). In humans, alfentanil can be used for induction of anesthesia (150–300 μg/kg IV) followed by an infusion of 25–150 μg/kg/hr with an inhalation anesthetic (Ausems et al. 1983). In the horse, doses of 20 and 40 μg/kg resulted in increased motor activity for a short period of time (Pascoe et al. 1989).

Carfentanil Citrate. *Carfentanil Citrate,* USP (Wildnil) is another phenylperadine derivative that is an extremely potent opioid agonist. It is approximately 10,000 times more potent than morphine (Mather 1983). It is currently labeled only for the immobilization of cervidae but it has been used on numerous other species. It is a Schedule II drug and requires special registration with the US Drug Enforcement Agency before it can be purchased. The normal dose used for capture is 0.005–0.02 mg/kg injected intramuscularly. Nielson (1996) has numerous doses for carfentanil as well as other capture drugs. Carfentanil can be dangerous to the user, and the manufacturer recommends the user takes every precaution to avoid human exposure. In addition, the user should never work alone, and an appropriate opioid agonist (such as diprenorphine) should be immediately available.

Remifentanil Citrate. *Remifentanil Citrate,* USP is the newest synthetic opioid. It is 20–30 times more potent than alfentanil. Remifentanil has the distinction of having a very large therapeutic index (33,000) and an extremely short half-life (7.5 min) (Stanley 1994). This drug is the first in a group of new opioids potentially able to safely function as anesthetic agents when used alone.

Etorphine Hydrochloride. *Etorphine Hydrochloride,* INN (M-99, Oripavine), is a semisynthetic opiate derivative having up to 10,000 times the analgesic potency of morphine (Harthoorn 1965a). Chemically, it is 6,14-endoetheno-7α-(2-hydroxy-2-pentyl)-tetrahydro-oripavine hydrochloride (Fig. 13.5). Etorphine binds to the opioid receptors in a number of regions within the CNS (see discussion on opioid receptors in this chapter).

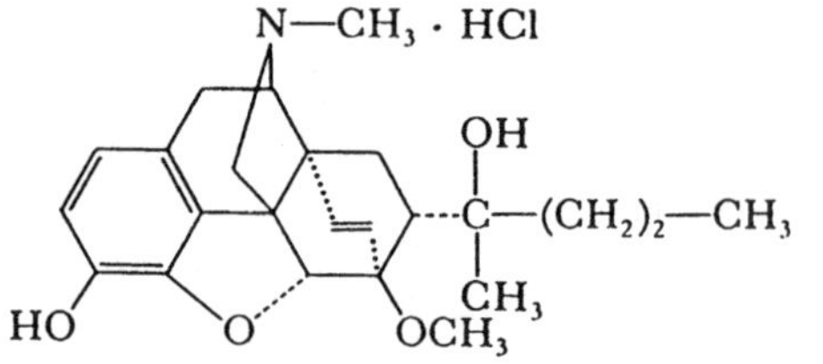

Etorphine Hydrochloride

FIG. 13.5

Etorphine is commonly used as a capture drug and it is generally recommended to dose heavily and then reverse as soon as possible with diprenorphine, the antagonists of etorphine. Insufficient dosage or underdosing with etorphine may result in hyperexcitability and other complications. It should never be used unless diprenorphine or other suitable antagonists are available.

FREE-RANGING WILD ANIMALS. Etorphine was used in the early 1960s for field investigations in the immobilization and capture of exotic species (Harthoorn 1965b); since then it has been used extensively in the field of animal conservation (Harthoorn 1972).

The potency of etorphine is extremely impressive. One milligram is capable of immobilizing a rhinoceros weighing approximately 2000 kg; this is equivalent to 0.5 μg/kg. A dose of 4 mg is capable of immobilizing an African elephant weighing about 5000 kg; this amounts to less than 1 μg/kg (Harthoorn and Bligh 1965).

The action of etorphine can be antagonized or reversed by diprenorphine. If the action is not antagonized, the immobilized state usually persists from 30 to 60 minutes. Used by itself in exotic species, the IM doses of etorphine that usually result in rapid immobilization, sedation, and analgesia are as follows (Alford et al. 1974):

Family	*Dose (mg/45 kg)*
Equidae (Mongolian horse, zebra)	0.44
Ursidae (black, grizzly, polar bear)	0.5
Cervidae (fallow deer, moose)	0.98
Bovidae (antelope, bighorn sheep)	0.09

According to Harthoorn (1966), the dose of etorphine for most exotic animals is about 1–2 mg (total dose); e.g., the zebra requires about 1.5 mg and the rhinoceros 1–1.5 mg (total dose). The IM dose of etorphine alone for chimpanzees is 0.66–1.76 μg/kg; for small primates it is 0.44–1.3 μg/kg (Wallach 1969).

Use of etorphine alone in the Asiatic working elephant at doses of 5–8 mg have also proved satisfactory for immobilization (Jainudeen et al. 1971). Etorphine has been successfully used for anesthesia in the two-stage castration of a 9-year-old Asian elephant; anesthesia was induced by an IM injection of 6 mg (Fowler and Hart 1973) and maintained by intermittent injections of 1 mg into an ear vein.

Etorphine has been used to immobilize the American alligator, red-ear turtle, and Galapagos tortoise (Wallach and Hoessle 1970). Immobilization of these poikilothermic animals was satisfactory. However, the total dose required to attain a desired affect is much greater on a body weight basis than those required in homeothermic species.

CAPTIVE WILD ANIMALS. Etorphine is used to immobilize many species of animals that are maintained in zoological establishments and circuses. It is used for diagnostic procedures and/or treatment in animals that are difficult and dangerous to approach.

In the camel (dromedary), etorphine (0.25–0.5 mg/45 kg) is administered by the IM route; IV administration is contraindicated (Higgins and Kock 1984). A maximum of 4 mg is suggested for the adult dromedary weighing 400–500 kg; for juvenile animals, a total IM dose of 0.5–2 mg is suggested.

Gatesman and Wiesner (1982) have found that the average effective IM dose for etorphine plus zylazine in bears is: polar bears, 7.312 μg/kg, with a maximum of 7.95 μg/kg; brown bears, 16.82 μg/kg. The IM dose of xylazine for bears is added to the etorphine; 10 mg xylazine is given to animals weighing 300 kg or more and 5 mg is used in animals weighing less than 300 kg. Hyaluronidase (150 IU) is also added to this mixture to increase the absorption rate. A blowpipe and dart system of 2 mL volume is used for delivering the drug mixture into the neck or shoulder musculature where body fat is thinnest. Other anatomic regions of the body may have up to 7.5 cm of subcutaneous fat; absorption of drugs is delayed and induction effects are much slower when the injection is made in body fat. For reversal of the effects of etorphine, IM and SC doses of diprenorphine are given. The lingual vein is also accessible in bears for administering the antagonist drug (Gatesman and Wiesner 1982).

Etorphine-xylazine has been used in a female greater kudu (*Tragelaphus strepsiceros*) for 14 immobilizations over a period of 9 months with satisfactory results (Kollias et al. 1983). Etorphine (7 μg/kg) and xylazine (130 μg/kg) are administered intramuscularly in the quadriceps femoris via projectile syringe. IV diprenorphine (14 μg/kg) reverses the effects of etorphine (after immobilization periods of 20–150 minutes) within a mean period of 2 minutes.

DOMESTIC SPECIES. Etorphine has been approved by the FDA in the USA for use only in wild or exotic species. Information is incomplete on tissue residue patterns as well as excretion of etorphine and its metabolites in food-producing animals. The use of etorphine in domestic species is discussed in greater detail in the 7th edition of this text.

PRECAUTIONS AND CONTRAINDICATIONS. Safe use of etorphine requires special precautions. Domestic animals should be properly controlled and restrained prior to IV or IM administration to avoid accidental self-injection. The lethal dose of etorphine for adult humans is small. It is estimated to be 30–120 μg (micrograms not milligrams!) (Haigh and Haigh 1980).

Accidental injections of small amounts of etorphine-acepromazine have led to serious respiratory depression and coma of a veterinary assistant (Firm 1973) and to death of a veterinarian (Vet Rec News and Reports 1976). Consequently, the manufacturer's license for production of the drug combination was temporarily suspended. The product was soon reinstated for use in animals following revised warnings by the manufacturer. In the event of an accidental injection of etorphine-acepromazine, warnings include immediate IV or IM administration of naloxone (0.8 mg); naloxone is to be repeated at 5-minute intervals if symptoms are not reversed. Reliance on the use of naloxone is emphasized by Ross (1986) rather than use of diprenorphine for antagonizing the effects of etorphine from accidental self-injection. If naloxone is unavailable, nalorphine hydrochloride should be administered intravenously or intramuscularly in a dose of 10 mg. Nalorphine can be repeated at 5-minute intervals if necessary up to a total of 4 mg. Adequate cardiopulmonary activity and/or resuscitation must be maintained until emergency medical assistance arrives.

Etorphine and its antagonist diprenorphine must not be used in domestic or wild animals intended for human consumption.

Propoxyphene Hydrochloride. The analgesic potency of *Propoxyphene Hydrochloride,* USP (Darvon), is less than that of codeine. Propoxyphene has weak analgesic potency and only 1/200 the affinity of morphine for receptor binding (Pert and Snyder 1973). It is structurally similar to the methadone molecule.

Because of hazards and potential toxicity of the drug, the FDA has considered the possibility of sharply curtailing or banning propoxyphene for human use (Smith 1979). A shift from Schedule IV to Schedule II has also been under consideration by the FDA and US Drug Enforcement Agency.

Propoxyphene has not been used to any great extent in clinical veterinary medicine. A dose of 2.2 mg/kg administered intramuscularly was found useful in obtunding experimentally induced pain (Davis and Donnelly 1968). Toxicity of propoxyphene has been studied in dogs and rabbits. Metabolization of the drug is rapid. Its major metabolite, norpropoxyphene, has a longer plasma half-life in the dog than propoxyphene (Page et al. 1979).

When dogs receive a single oral dose (40 mg/kg) of propoxyphene, signs of CNS toxicity develop (Page et al. 1979). Tremors, salivation, vomiting, and ataxia may occur. Convulsions develop following doses of 60 mg/kg and lethal effects are induced by 125 mg/kg.

Propoxyphene has been evaluated in three IV doses (0.5, 1, and 2.2 mg/kg) in the horse (Muir et al. 1980). Cardiopulmonary function is not altered by 0.5 or 1 mg/kg of the drug. Muscle fasciculation occurs in some animals following a dose of 0.5 mg/kg. A brief period of ataxia and muscle fasciculations develops after a dose of 1 mg/kg; increased motor activity also is seen and lasts about 30 minutes. The dose of 2.2 mg/kg is followed by increase in heart rate and arterial blood pressure; ataxia and disorientation also occur for a brief period and increase in locomotor activity that lasts several hours is observed. Naloxone (0.005 mg/kg) administered intravenously lessens increased locomotor activity or results in return of animals to a normal quiet behavior pattern.

In the rabbit, propoxyphene and norpropoxyphene produce cardiac arrhythmias and a number of electrocardiographic alterations (Lund-Jacobsen 1978).

Circulatory shock is induced in the pig by the IV infusion of 675–2025 mg propoxyphene administered at the rate of 15 mg/kg/min; a plasma concentration is attained between 9.6 and 15.3 μg/mL, which is a similar plasma concentration range considered to be lethal in humans (Sørenson et al. 1985).

Behavioral alterations in offspring of rats exposed to propoxyphene are known to occur (Vorhees et al. 1979). The drug appears to meet the criteria for being a pure behavioral teratogen.

Therapeutic efficacy of propoxyphene has not been determined in most species. Moreover, it has not been approved by the FDA for use in animals.

OPIOID ANTAGONISTS. Pure opioid antagonists of current importance in veterinary medicine include naloxone and diprenorphine.

Naloxone Hydrochloride. *Naloxone Hydrochloride,* USP (*N*–allylnoroxymorphone hydrochloride, Narcan), is approved by the FDA for use in the dog. Chemically, naloxone is 17-allyl-4,5α-epoxy-3,14-dihydroxymorphinan-6-one hydrochloride (Fig. 13.6).

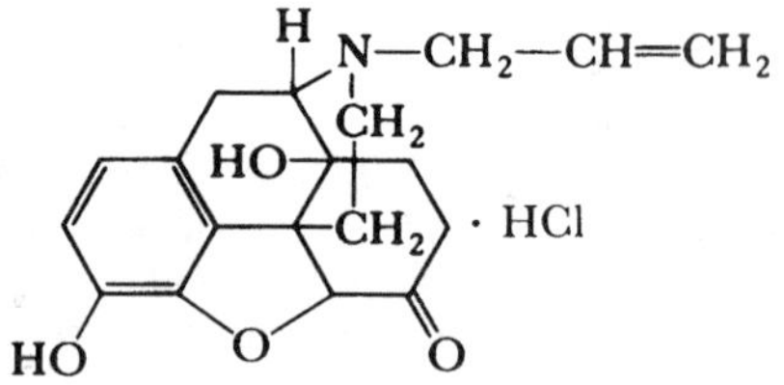

H N—CH_2—CH=CH_2 CH_2 HO CH_2 · HCl HO O O

Naloxone Hydrochloride

FIG. 13.6

Naloxone has a potency 10–30 times that of nalorphine. Unlike nalorphine, it lacks the agonistic effect that is highly desirable if the drug is to be depended on as an antagonist of narcotic analgesics. In general, naloxone is regarded as a virtually pure competitive antagonist. Consequently, it does not produce respiratory depression, which commonly occurs with other narcotic antagonists.

Naloxone is not subject to the Controlled Substances Act of 1970. This is an advantage over use of other narcotic antagonists that are subject to regulation under the act.

PHARMACOLOGIC ACTION. In low doses, naloxone has a high binding affinity for μ opioid receptors; both μ_1 and μ_2 receptors are blocked. Compared to μ receptors, large doses of naloxone are required to block δ opioid receptor activity. Moreover, κ opioid receptors, which have high binding affinity for ketocyclazocines, have a very low binding affinity for naloxone; extremely large doses of naloxone (20–30 times needed to block μ receptors) are necessary for blockade of κ receptors. The σ opioid receptor is insensitive to naloxone. Some of the functions of opioid receptors have been discussed previously in this chapter.

Although naloxone is considered to be a specific opiate antagonist, it also antagonizes the effects of nonopiate depressants, affects dopaminergic mechanisms, and antagonizes GABA. High doses of naloxone can initiate both biochemical and physiological effects (seizures or convulsions), mimicking those produced by GABA antagonists (Yaksh and Howe 1982). The prevalent idea that naloxone only induces an effect on specific opioid receptors needs revision. It is axiomatic that one should never accept the idea that a potent drug has but one action.

CARDIOVASCULAR SYSTEM. Naloxone has no effect upon arterial blood pressure in normotensive subjects (Zaloga et al. 1984). It acts upon sites (probably δ opioid receptors) within the CNS and/or at peripheral sites to improve cardiovascular function in experimental shock (Holaday and Faden 1980). Also, the protective action of naloxone depends on an intact pituitary-adrenal, medullary-sympathetic nervous system (Davis et al. 1984). The cardiovascular effects of naloxone in spinal shock are mediated by the parasympathetic nervous system and by release of dopamine. Additionally, other catecholamines (epinephrine and norepinephrine) are released by high doses of naloxone when administered after opioids. Apparently, opioid peptides modulate the release of catecholamines from the sympathetic nervous system by inhibiting their output (Mannelli et al. 1983).

Since naloxone also blocks the endogenous opiate ligand, β endorphin, it has been used experimentally in the dog for reversal of hypovolemic shock (Vargish et al. 1980). Beta endorphin, which is released during or following hemorrhagic shock, is blocked by naloxone from interacting with opioid receptors present in brain, heart, GI tract, kidney, adrenal glands, and possibly other tissues. An IV bolus of naloxone (2 mg/kg) and an infusion at 2 mg/kg/hr promptly increases systemic arterial pressure, left ventricular contractility, and cardiac output. This dose results in 100% survival, whereas untreated or control dogs die within 30 minutes. In canine endotoxic shock, naloxone also improves survival and cardiac performance; this indicates that endorphins or opioid receptors are involved in cardiovascular pathophysiology of endotoxic shock (Reynolds et al. 1980).

Since the studies of Vargish et al. (1980) and Reynolds et al. (1980) on shock, it has been established unequivocally that β-endorphin and ACTH concentrations in blood increase simultaneously in response to stress. Beta endorphin release has a potent arterial hypotensive effect that can be blocked by naloxone. It is also possible that naloxone may exert some of its protective effects in shock unrelated to its action as an opiate antagonist.

Administration of naloxone in the dog clearly indicates that it increases myocardial contractile force in a dose-dependent manner (Caffrey et al. 1985). Conversely, opiate peptides (endorphins) of circulating or myocardial origin appear to depress or decrease myocardial contractile force. The fact that naloxone releases catecholamines, thus increasing the contractile force of the myocardium, is compatible with the release of norepinephrine from sympathetic nerves within the myocardium. It has been suggested that one of the opioid receptors involved in the myocardium may be localized on presynaptic terminals or sympathetic neurons that innervate the myocardium (Caffrey et al. 1985). Excitation of these receptors in turn inhibits or blocks the release of norepinephrine and depresses myocardial contractility. Administration of naloxone would compete by binding or displacing the opiate peptides from the receptor sites; this would then result in immediate release of norepinephrine and an increase in myocardial contractility.

In the cat, IV naloxone (8 mg/kg/hr) significantly reduces the plasma myocardial depressant factor (MDF) in treatment of hemorrhagic shock (Curtis and Lefer 1980). In addition to decreasing MDF, naloxone also lowers circulating amino nitrogen concentrations and plasma cathepsin D. These findings indicate that naloxone lowers the release of lysosomal enzymes, hinders proteolysis, and prevents toxic factor formation (MDF and cathepsin D) during shock. It appears that naloxone has a dual protective effect through its nonspecific action as well as through its so-called specific opiate antagonist action.

Naloxone (2 mg/kg IV dose followed by continuous infusion of 2 mg/kg/hr) has been used in experimental endotoxemia 3 days postoperatively in the pig; severe metabolic derangement and increased mortality occur (Fettman et al. 1984). In the pony, IV naloxone (1 mg/kg/hr) administered in treatment of endotoxic shock failed to prevent hemodynamic and biochemical alterations (Moore et al. 1983). These studies differ from those that have shown a protective effect of naloxone in the rat, dog, and cat. There is a possibility that a species variation exists with respect to the responsive effects of naloxone in treatment of shock. It may also be possible that higher doses of naloxone are required in the pig and pony before the protective effects of naloxone can be achieved. Additional research will be necessary to clear up these differences.

Other vasoactive substances (histamine, bradykinin, adenosine, leukotrienes, and/or prostaglandin release) besides β-endorphin are involved in shock. Also, the buildup of hypoxanthine and its subsequent conversion to superoxide radicals by xanthine oxidase appear to be prominently involved in irreversible shock (McCord 1985).

A disadvantage in use of naloxone for treatment of traumatic shock is its blockade of the μ_1 opioid receptor, which mediates analgesia. Since the δ receptors are believed to mediate the arterial hypotensive effects of β endorphin, a selective δ-receptor antagonist would ideally be a more efficacious approach in treatment of painful shock; perhaps a selective antagonist for δ opioid receptors will eventually be synthesized for clinical use.

Another antagonist that appears to have potential value in reversing the adverse action of β endorphin upon blood pressure is TRH (Zaloga et al. 1984). Although TRH does not bind to opioid receptors, it is referred to as a physiologic opiate antagonist. It improves survival and reverses arterial hypotension produced by hemorrhagic and endotoxic shock. Synthesis of TRH analogs are now under study for possible use in shock therapy.

ENDOCRINE SYSTEM. Curiously, naloxone can alter expression of the estrogen-induced daily surge signal in ovariectomized rats (Sylvester et al. 1980). It appears that endogenous opioid peptides (enkephalins or endorphins) may possibly play a role in modulating steroid regulation of the neural surge signal for luteinizing hormone (LH) and follicle-stimulating hormone.

Opioid receptor blockade by naloxone elevates serum concentrations of LH in rats and humans. The effect of naloxone on LH secretions is opposite to that induced by morphine or exogenous opiate peptides. Consequently, naloxone appears to antagonize an inhibition of LH release that is mediated by opioid receptors (Blank and Mann 1981).

Injection of naloxone into mother rats just before suckling of their pups results in significant inhibition of growth hormone (GH) and prolactin release (Miki et al. 1981). Inhibition of prolactin release by naloxone is dose related. These findings suggest that the suckling stimulus induces release of endogenous opiate peptides, which in turn are involved in release of GH and prolactin.

In humans, naloxone does not alter basal GH, prolactin, or TRH release; however, it stimulates a significant elevation in cortisol and gonadotropins (Delitala et al. 1981). Infusion of naloxone increases the rate and amplitude of LH pulsatility. Naloxone does not alter the pituitary response to TRH and luteinizing-releasing hormone stimulation. Elevation of cortisol following naloxone administration suggests the presence of an inhibitory opioid influence upon basal ACTH release (Blankenstein et al. 1980). Consequently, it appears that ACTH release is under tonic inhibition by an opioid pathway.

MOTOR BEHAVIORAL EFFECT. In horses, crib biting is a repetitive behavioral characteristic that may involve activation of opioid and dopamine receptors in the CNS (Dodman et al. 1987). Naloxone administered in IV or IM doses (0.02–0.04 mg/kg) prevents crib-biting behavior for 20 minutes after a single injection. Other narcotic antagonists such as naltrexone, nalmefene, and diprenorphine prevent this stereotyped behavior for longer periods (Dodman et al. 1987).

CLINICAL USE. In the dog and cat, one part of naloxone will antagonize respiratory depression produced by 15–20 parts of oxymorphone (Palminteri 1966). The reversal of all actions of oxymorphone, including its analgesic effect, occurs when a ratio of 0.4 mg naloxone to 1.5 mg oxymorphone is administered. Effects of morphine and meperidine are reversed by naloxone to a lesser degree than those of oxymorphone. Naloxone does not antagonize the anesthetic effect of halothane (Harper et al. 1978). Barbiturates, procaine, and tranquilizers also are unaffected by naloxone. No adverse reactions in dogs and cats occur when naloxone is used with ether, methoxyflurane, pentobarbital, thiamylal, procaine, oxymorphone, morphine, meperidine, or many commercially available phenothiazine tranquilizers.

In the dog, naloxone will also adequately reverse the fentanyl component of droperidol-fentanyl (Paddleford and Short 1973). It has no effect in antagonizing the action of droperidol. However, 4-aminopyridine (0.5 mg/kg) administered intravenously in combination with naloxone (0.04 mg/kg) immediately reverses the actions of both droperidol and fentanyl (Booth et al. 1982).

A number of literature sources state that naloxone will reverse the emetic action of apomorphine, a dopamine agonist. Findings by Keith et al. (1981) indicate that naloxone has no therapeutic effect in reversal of apomorphine-induced emesis in the dog.

Naloxone can be administered by all of the parenteral routes; however, the IV route is preferred to attain immediate effect from the drug. Where it is difficult to locate veins, naloxone can be administered intramuscularly at high doses in wild herbivores without overdosages (Smuts 1975). In large wild species, 1 mg naloxone injected intravenously is sufficient to antagonize 1 mg etorphine or 10 mg fentanyl. According to Smuts, naloxone compares favorably with diprenorphine, the antagonist used to reverse action of etorphine; e.g., in the young adult elephant, 10 mg naloxone intravenously is sufficient to antagonize 8 mg etorphine used in combination with various tranquilizing agents.

Respiratory depressant effects of overdosages of oxymorphone in dogs and cats can be reversed with a ratio of 0.1 mg naloxone to 1.5 mg oxymorphone (Palminteri 1966). If the narcotic antagonist is administered intramuscularly or subcutaneously, onset of action occurs in 1–5 minutes; intravenously, onset is immediate and lasts 1–2 hours.

In reversal of narcotic effects of morphine and fentanyl in the dog, 0.016–0.1 mg/0.45 kg naloxone is used intravenously (Paddleford and Short 1973). This quantity of naloxone antagonizes effects of 0.02–0.03 mg/0.45 kg fentanyl administered intramuscularly and 0.01 mg/0.45 kg fentanyl administered intravenously. This same quantity of naloxone antagonizes the effect of 0.5 mg/0.45 kg morphine intravenously.

The parenteral dose of naloxone approved by the FDA for the dog is 0.04 mg/kg. When the drug is administered intravenously, this dosage may be repeated at 2- to 3-minute intervals to produce the desired effect.

Naloxone is available in concentrations of 0.02, 0.04, or 1 mg/mL.

Diprenorphine Hydrochloride. Chemically, diprenorphine hydrochloride (Nororipavine, Cyprenorphine, M-285, M50-50, Revivon) is *N*-(cyclopropylmethyl)-6,7,8,14-tetrahydro-7-α-(1-hydroxy-1-methylethyl)-6,14-endo-ethano-nororipavine hydrochloride (Fig. 13.7).

Diprenorphine at double the dosage of etorphine is capable of completely reversing the action of etorphine in wild animals (Alford et al. 1974). Diprenorphine (2 mg/mL) was approved by the FDA in 1973 for use in wild and exotic animals to specifically reverse the effects of etorphine. It is administered intravenously or intramuscularly. Diprenorphine must not be used 30 days before or during the hunting season in free-ranging animals that might be used for human consumption. The drug is subject to the Controlled Substances Act of 1970 (Schedule II).

ADMINISTRATION AND DOSAGE. Prior to administration of diprenorphine, every consideration must be given to dealing with a fully conscious animal in as soon as a few seconds up to 4 minutes after IV injec-

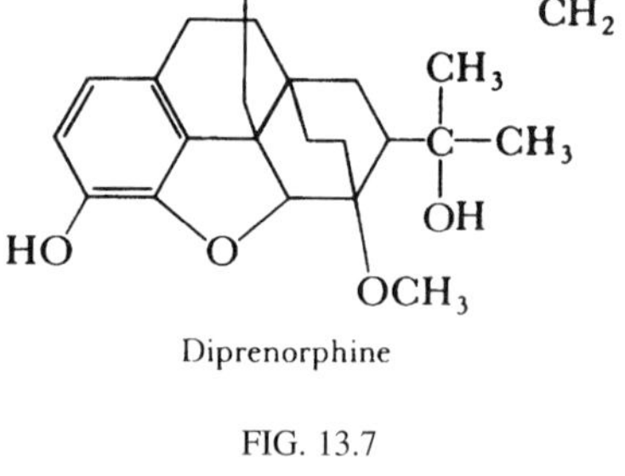

Diprenorphine

FIG. 13.7

tion. Consequently, a safe place should be available to avoid attacks by wild animals upon recovery from etorphine.

Most consistent results are obtained when an etorphine to diprenorphine ratio of 1:2 is used (i.e., 1 mg of etorphine is antagonized by 2 mg of diprenorphine). Reversal of narcotic effects of etorphine is obtained by IV administration of either diprenorphine or naloxone. Residual narcosis after administration of diprenorphine is less than that from nalorphine (Alford et al. 1974). If diprenorphine is administered intramuscularly to reverse the effect of etorphine, 5–20 minutes may be required before CNS depressant effects are reversed.

In horses, diprenorphine (0.02–0.03 mg/kg intramuscularly) prevents crib biting in horses for 4 hours or more (Dodman et al. 1987). Other narcotic antagonists (naloxone, naltrexone, nalmefene, TRH) also prevent this stereotypic behavioral effect in horses.

Diprenorphine (30 μg/kg) is also recommended intravenously for reversal of effects of etorphine (22 μg/kg) when employed in combination with acepromazine for immobilization of the horse (Jenkins 1972).

Diprenorphine rapidly reverses immobilizing effects of etorphine used in combination with acepromazine in the camel; complete recovery occurs 1.5–3 minutes following IV administration (Schels and Nowrouzian 1977). IV use of diprenorphine for reversal of the immobilizing effects of etorphine is usually followed by rapid recovery in most animal species.

Levallorphan Tartrate. *Levallorphan Tartrate,* USP (Lorfan), acts as an antagonist during CNS action of opiate and related analgesics. The CNS effects of these compounds are antagonized or reversed by levallorphan; however, if it is administered in the absence of opiate-derivative analgesics, it usually induces respiratory depression. Consequently, the partial agonist characteristics of the drug are seen.

Levallorphan is ineffective in antagonizing respiratory depressant actions of anesthetics, barbiturates, or nonnarcotic drugs and may even increase the respiratory and CNS depressant effects of these drug classes.

IV administration of levallorphan (0.022 mg/kg) has been used to relieve or prevent the excitable effects of morphine in the horse (Klavano 1975).

Naltrexone. *Naltrexone,* INN (Trexan), is a μ, κ, and δ opioid receptor antagonist (Bailey and Stanley 1994). It has been used experimentally for prevention of crib biting, an aberrant behavioral pattern in horses (Dodman et al. 1987). A single IV dose of 0.4 mg/kg naltrexone prevents biting for 6 hours after administration.

Nalmefene. *Nalmefene,* INN (previously named nalmetrene), is an opioid receptor antagonist similar to naltrexone, with greater preference for μ receptors than for κ or δ receptors (Michel et al. 1988). Nalmefene is also effective in preventing crib biting in horses for 4 hours or more in an IV or IM dose of 0.08 mg/kg (Dodman et al. 1987). The stereotyped biting can be prevented completely by nalmefene for up to 1 week by continuous IV administration of 5–10 mg/kg/hr; crib biting resumes when the infusion is stopped.

Other narcotic antagonists (naloxone, diprenorphine, TRH) will also interrupt or prevent crib biting behavior in horses. Use of narcotic antagonists in the neuropharmacologic management of other stereotypies in the horse and other species has potential value. According to Dodman et al. (1987), captive animals in zoos are potential sources of investigational material because pacing and other forms of repetitive behavior as a result of boredom or stress are commonly observed.

OPIOID PARTIAL AGONISTS

Buprenorphine Hydrochloride. *Buprenorphine Hydrochloride,* USP (Buprenex), is a partial agonist with a very high affinity for the μ opioid receptor but only partial activity. It is a thebaine derivative with a structure similar to morphine but has a lower abuse potential and is classed as a Schedule V drug. It is highly lipophilic but is slow to associate and dissociate from opioid receptors. This results in a slow onset and long duration of action (Bailey and Stanley 1994). The elimination half-life, total body clearance, and steady-state Vd are 2.8 hours, 23.2 mL/min/kg, and 4.2 L/kg, respectively, in the rat (Ohtani et al. 1994). In the dog it is metabolized primarily by glucuronidation, and the principal metabolite, buprenorphine glucuronide, is eliminated almost completely (92%) in the bile (Garrett and Chandran 1990). It is commonly used for postoperative analgesia because of its long duration of action and minimal adverse side effects. Buprenorphine is also often used for analgesia in laboratory animals. The doses (in mg/kg IV, IM, or SC) for various species are as follows: dog and cat, 0.01–0.02; ruminant and swine, 0.005–0.01; rat and mouse, 0.1–1; rabbit, guinea pig, and hamster, 0.05; and horse, 0.01–0.02. The usual dosing interval is 8–12 hours.

Tramadol. *Tramadol Hydrochloride,* USP (Ultram), is a new compound, and its exact mechanism of action is unclear. It appears to be a partial μ agonist. It exhibits very little respiratory depression and abuse potential. An additional analgesia mechanism may involve inhibition of reuptake of norepinephrine and serotonin (Raffa et al. 1992; Driessen and Reimann 1992; Kayser et al. 1992). Lintz et al. (1981) described its biotransformation and excretion in several species. The drug is well absorbed when administered orally and is metabolized via demethylation followed by conjugation. The metabolites are excreted primarily in the urine. Tramadol is metabolized more rapidly in animals than in humans.

OPIOID AGONIST-ANTAGONISTS

Nalbuphine Hydrochloride. *Nalbuphine Hydrochloride,* USP (Nubain), is a semisynthetic opioid with a

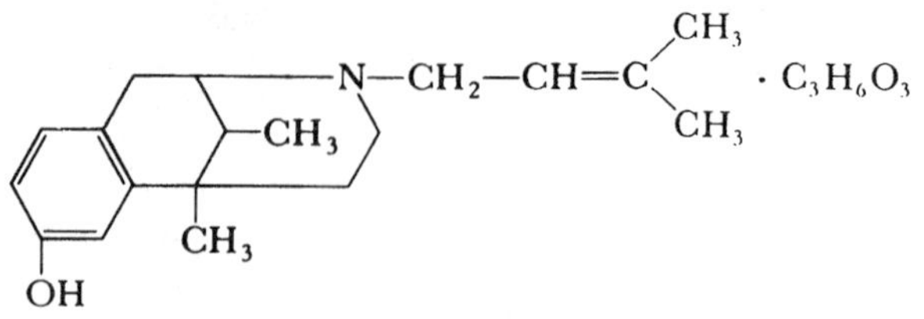

$N-CH_2-CH=C(CH_3)_2 \cdot C_3H_6O_3$

CH_3

CH_3

OH

FIG. 13.8

structure similar to oxymorphone. It is an agonist-antagonist that acts primarily as an antagonist at μ receptors and as an agonist at κ receptors. This results in limited analgesia as well as limited respiratory depression. It is metabolized by the liver. Nalbuphine produces minimal cardiovascular changes, leading to its use in human medicine as an analgesia for patients with heart disease and as a reversal agent for the respiratory depression associated with opioid agonist administration (Stoelting 1991). Its use in veterinary medicine has been somewhat limited. Nalbuphine has been shown to produce visceral analgesia in cats (Sawyer and Rech 1987).

Pentazocine Lactate. In the search for antagonists with a benzomorphan structure, pentazocine lactate (Talwin-V) emerged as an analgesic with few side effects. Consequently, it received considerable attention for use in humans because of its potential as a non-addicting and effective analgesic. However, addictive characteristics were uncovered that dictated placement of pentazocine on the Schedule IV list in 1979.

Chemically, pentazocine is 2′-hydroxy-5,9-dimethyl-2-(3,3-dimethylallyl)-6,7-benzomorphan (Fig. 13.8). Each milliliter of the commercially available preparation contains 30 mg pentazocine. The FDA has approved its use in the horse; in 1982, pentazocine was approved for use in the dog.

PHARMACOLOGIC CONSIDERATIONS. The pharmacologic characteristics of pentazocine are quite similar to those of the opiate compounds. Consequently, the principal effects of the analgesic agent are upon the CNS and smooth muscle. The analgesic potency is approximately one-half to one-fourth that of morphine and is about five times that of meperidine. Pentazocine is an agonist-antagonist, with its primary agonist effect at the κ receptors and weak antagonist activity at the μ receptors (Bailey and Stanley 1994).

FATE AND METABOLISM. The kinetics of disappearance of pentazocine from plasma following an IM injection of 3 mg/kg have been determined in ponies, goats, swine, dogs, and cats (Davis and Sturm 1970). This dose of pentazocine is higher than that employed in humans (i.e., 0.6 mg/kg). However, according to Davis and Sturm, the dosage used in their studies was considerably below the amount reported to induce toxic effects in animals. With exception of the dogs, disappearance of pentazocine from plasma follows first-order kinetics. The peak plasma concentrations after its administration occur at 15 minutes in dogs, goats, and swine; at 30 minutes in ponies; and at 1 hour in cats (Davis and Sturm 1970). The plasma half-life values range from 22 minutes in dogs to 97 minutes in ponies (see Table 13.6).

TABLE 13.6—Kinetic constants for disappearance of pentazocine from blood plasma of domesticated animals

Species	C_o	$t_{1/2}$	$K'd$	$V'd$
	(mg/L)	*(min)*	*(hr^{-1})*	*(L/kg)*
Ponies	0.59	97.1	0.0071	5.09
Goats	0.52	51.0	0.0136	5.77
Swine	0.63	48.6	0.0143	4.76
Dogs	0.85	22.1	0.0313	3.66
Cats	1.08	83.6	0.0083	2.78

Source: Davis and Sturm 1970.

Note: C_o = plasma concentration of drug at zero time; $t_{1/2}$ = plasma half-life; $K'd$ = apparent first-order disappearance rate constant; $V'd$ = apparent specific volume of distribution of drug.

After IV injection, pentazocine (1 mg/kg) distributes widely in the horse (V′d = 5.7 L/kg) and binds (80%) extensively to plasma proteins (Tobin and Miller 1979). Pentazocine has a relatively slow distribution in the horse. The α phase half-time is 27 minutes and the β phase half-time is about 138 minutes. Following an IM injection of 0.66 mg/kg pentazocine, peak plasma levels are attained in about 30 minutes (Tobin and Miller 1979).

In humans, the plasma half-life of pentazocine is about 2 hours after IV (20–25 mg/70 kg) or IM (45 mg/70 kg) administration (Berkowitz 1971). The peak analgesic effect occurs between 30 and 60 minutes after an IM dose and lasts 2–3 hours. The plasma half-life of pentazocine and duration of action in humans are longer than in domestic animals.

Pentazocine is metabolized in humans to a large degree with little of the unchanged (<5%) or parent compound appearing in the urine. The fate of pentazocine is probably quite similar to that of morphine and its derivatives. Its conjugation with glucuronic acid and excretion as a glucuronide have been established. Trace amounts of pentazocine and its metabolites can be detected in urine for several days after a single administration of the drug.

In the horse, about 30% of a dose of pentazocine is eliminated in urine as a glucuronide metabolite (Tobin et al. 1979). When urine is analyzed for this metabolite, pentazocine can be detected for up to 5 days after administration.

Pentazocine crosses the placenta less readily than meperidine (Mirkin 1975). Fetal blood concentrations of pentazocine/mL are attained in humans at 60% of those observed in maternal blood.

CLINICAL USE. Pentazocine has been restricted primarily to preanesthetic medication because of its lack of profound sedation in animals. According to Soma (1971), use of pentazocine for postanalgesic effect in both small-animal and equine anesthesia is inconclusive. Soma suggested an IM dose of pentazocine in the dog of 1.5–3 mg/kg. However, findings suggest pentazocine is unlikely to induce adverse side effects in dogs when administered intramuscularly at a dose of 2 mg/kg (Cooper and Organ 1977).

The FDA-approved dose of pentazocine in the dog is 1.65–3.3 mg/kg; it is approved for IM use only. According to Miner and Losacco (1984), this dosage produces analgesia for 3 hours in the dog.

In the cat, pentazocine (2.2–3.3 mg/kg by the SC, IM, or IV route) has been used for its analgesic action (Wright et al. 1985). For inducing analgesia in laboratory animals, it is used as follows: mouse, SC dose of 10 mg/kg; rat, SC dose of 10 mg/kg; rabbit, SC or IM dose of 2–5 mg/kg.

In the horse, Soma (1971) indicated that the total IV dose of pentazocine is 200–400 mg. Doses of 6–10 mg/kg in the dog (presumably via the IM route) produce tremors and convulsions reminiscent of morphine-like compounds (Soma 1971). Side effects are also observed in the pony when 2.2–4.4 mg/kg pentazocine are administered intravenously or intramuscularly (Lowe 1969). The side effects consist of incoordination, muscular tremors, hypertonicity of muscles, and hypersensitivity to noise. In one trial, a dose of 3 mg/kg by the IM route caused the animal to fall backward to the floor; it paddled its feet in the lateral recumbent position and in a few seconds returned to the standing position.

The analgesic action of pentazocine in the pony provides a more prolonged and consistent effect than meperidine; duration of analgesia for pentazocine is 48 minutes, and for meperidine it is 21 minutes (Lowe 1969). An IV dose of pentazocine (0.55–1.1 mg/kg) produces analgesia lasting 10–20 minutes; an IM or IV dose of 1.65–2.2 mg/kg produces an analgesic effect varying from 15 to 60 minutes (Lowe 1969).

Pentazocine is used for control of pain caused by colic in horses. The drug is slowly administered intravenously at 0.33 mg/kg. A second dose in the same amount is recommended intramuscularly 10–15 minutes after the first. Use of pentazocine in horses subjected to experimentally induced colic indicates that xylazine is a more effective analgesic (Lowe 1978). Pentazocine has also been used in conjunction with Cloropent and acepromazine for treatment of wounds in horses. For preanesthetic use in horses, an IV dose of 0.9 mg/kg pentazocine is recommended (Muir et al. 1978). It must not be used in horses intended for human consumption.

In the clinical evaluation of pentazocine and meperidine for relief of postoperative pain, a blind study was conducted in the dog by Short et al. (1971). It was concluded that meperidine was more effective than pentazocine for surgery of the extremities and thorax, whereas pentazocine was more effective for ocular surgery. In the case of both pentazocine and meperidine, relief of pain varied most in obtunding moderate pain, but both drugs were comparable in relief of severe pain (Short et al. 1971).

Butorphanol Tartrate. *Butorphanol Tartrate,* USP (Torbugesic, Torbutrol, Stadol), is a central-acting analgesic with both agonist and antagonist properties. It is a morphinan derivative and is chemically *l-N*–cyclobutylmethyl-6, 10αβ-dihydroxy-1,2,3,9,10, 10α-hexahydro-(4*H*)10, 4α-imino-ethanophenanthrene tartrate. The molecular formula is $C_{21}H_{29}NO_2 \cdot C_4H_6O_6$.

Butorphanol is an agonist-antagonist with affinity for both the μ and κ opioid receptors. Its primary effect at the μ receptor is as an antagonist, and at the κ receptor as an agonist.

Butorphanol has narcotic antagonist activity equivalent to that of nalorphine, 30 times that of pentazocine, and one-fortieth that of naloxone. As an analgesic, it is considered to be 4–7 times more potent than morphine, 20 times greater than pentazocine, and 40 times greater than meperidine (Pircio et al. 1976; Vandam 1980). However, these relative potencies must be evaluated in light of the ceiling effect of the agonist-antagonists. In addition to its analgesic action, butorphanol is a potent cough suppressant or antitussive agent.

In 1982, it was approved by the FDA for antitussive use in the dog. Butorphanol was later approved as an analgesic for equine use. It is classified as a Schedule IV drug under the 1970 Controlled Substances Act.

PHARMACOLOGIC CONSIDERATIONS. In the horse, the analgesic effects of butorphanol are dose related, with a duration of analgesia ranging from 15 to 90 minutes (Kalpravidh et al. 1984a). An IV dose of 0.2 mg/kg appears to produce optimal analgesia in the horse. Although side effects such as restlessness, ataxia, and shivering occur at this dosage, the combination of butorphanol with a sedative may be helpful in minimizing them (Kalpravidh et al. 1984a). Combinations containing butorphanol for use in the horse include xylazine 0.66 mg/kg IV with butorphanol 0.03 mg/kg IV or detomidine 2.5–5 μg/kg IV with butorphanol 0.03 mg/kg IV (Muir 1991).

When butorphanol is administered to healthy horses in IV doses of 0.1, 0.2, and 0.4 mg/kg, no significant alteration in heart rate, diastolic aortic pressure, diastolic pulmonary arterial pressure, or cardiac output occurs; however, the systolic arterial pressure significantly increases only in the horses given the 0.2 mg/kg dose (Robertson et al. 1981). Minimal effects upon cardiopulmonary functions also have been observed in the dog after IV doses of 0.1 and 0.4 mg/kg butorphanol (Trim 1983). According to Trim, the sedative effect of butorphanol resembles the sedation produced by equipotent doses of meperidine and pentazocine.

In ponies subjected to experimental pain as induced by superficial and visceral stimuli, butorphanol (0.22 mg/kg intramuscularly) has been compared with the analgesic and behavioral effects of IM doses of flunixin (2.2 mg/kg), levorphanol (0.033 mg/kg), morphine (0.66 mg/kg), and xylazine (2.2 mg/kg) (Kalpravidh et al. 1984b). Interestingly, xylazine produces the best analgesia; analgesic effects for superficial and visceral pain persist 3 and 4 hours respectively. Butorphanol is the next best drug after xylazine in obtunding visceral pain; its duration of effect for 4 hours is similar to that of xylazine in the horse. Flunixin, as anticipated, has no effect upon experimentally induced pain. Since flunixin, like aspirin, inhibits biosynthesis of prostaglandins in inflamed tissue to prevent superficial pain perception, it is more effective in blocking pain from pathologic origins. Levorphanol does not produce analgesia for superficial pain; moderate analgesia for visceral pain lasts for at least 4 hours. Morphine produces good analgesia for pain superficially induced for 30 minutes; a slight analgesic effect for visceral pain lasts for 60 minutes. Motor effects (restlessness as exhibited by pacing, pawing, body swinging, and/or head shaking) are produced by butorphanol, levorphanol, and morphine (Kalpravidh et al. 1984b). They do not occur with xylazine or flunixin.

Muir and Robertson (1985) also observed that xylazine (1.1 mg/kg intravenously) produces the most pronounced visceral analgesia in the horse; it lasts about 90 minutes. This is shorter than the 4 hours reported by Kalpravidh et al. (1984b). These differences are probably related to the dose of xylazine administered as well as to IV versus IM administration. According to Muir and Robertson (1985), butorphanol (0.2 mg/kg intravenously) is the best after xylazine for its analgesic effect (60 minutes) upon visceral pain. This is followed by meperidine (1 mg/kg intravenously) and pentazocine (0.99 mg/kg intravenously) with a duration of analgesia for 30–35 minutes.

In small animals butorphanol is often used as part of a preanesthetic regimen, with or without a tranquilizer, and to control mild to moderate pain. The dose usual ranges from 0.1 to 0.4 mg/kg and can be given SC, IM, or IV. It would appear that the analgesia lasts longer in the cat than in the dog (Hosgood 1990; Sawyer et al. 1991). One advantage of the use of butorphanol in cats is its lack of an excitatory effect. Large doses of butorphanol, infusions of 0.1–0.2 mg/kg/min, resulted in generally inadequate anesthesia and profound cardiovascular depression in dogs (Sederberg et al. 1981). Butorphanol can also be administered orally to small animals: the dose is 0.5–1.0 mg/kg 2–3 times daily (Tranquilli et al. 1989).

SC doses of butorphanol to induce analgesia in the mouse and rat are 5.4 and 23.3 mg/kg respectively (Flecknell 1984).

In humans, it is recommended that the dose of butorphanol be reduced when administered simultaneously with phenothiazine tranquilizers or other CNS depressants.

Much more pharmacologic, toxicologic, and clinical data are needed to determine the efficacy and safety of butorphanol before it can be approved for analgesic use in animals.

Nalorphine Hydrochloride. *Nalorphine Hydrochloride,* USP (*N*–allylnormorphine, Nalline, Lethidrone), is a morphine derivative in which an *N*–methyl group has been replaced with an *N*–allyl group. Although nalorphine is a partial agonist, it antagonizes many of the reactions of morphine and its congeners.

ADMINISTRATION. Nalorphine is available as a liquid (5 mg/mL) and is subject to the Controlled Substances Act of 1970 as a Schedule III drug. It is injected by the SC, IM, or IV route; however, the IV route is preferred to attain immediate effect of the drug. Nalorphine has been approved by the FDA for use in the dog.

ABSORPTION AND FATE. Nalorphine is relatively ineffective after oral administration but is promptly absorbed after SC or IM injection. Biotransformation of nalorphine probably is quite similar to that of morphine because it is also conjugated by liver tissue. The duration of action of nalorphine appears to be briefer than morphine.

ACTION. During the action or effect of narcotics, nalorphine usually acts as a narcotic antagonist. However, in their absence, nalorphine acts like a narcotic and may produce CNS depression and analgesia as a result of its partial agonist activity. Now that naloxone is available, there is practically no justification for use of partial agonists such as nalorphine and levallorphan. Nalorphine does not antagonize mild respiratory depression and may actually aggravate it. Very large doses will paralyze respiration in the dog, but lower dosages have little effect. Nalorphine is not constipative in the dog as morphine is. It has little effect upon the cardiovascular system.

The most prominent antagonist action of nalorphine is in preventing or relieving typical respiratory-depressant activity of morphine and all its derivatives, meperidine, and fentanyl. The analgesic and narcotic actions of diethylthiambutene are terminated by an IV injection of nalorphine. It is ineffective against respiratory depression of barbiturates, and inhalant anesthetics. Nalorphine may increase respiratory depressant effects on nonnarcotic CNS depressants. It does not antagonize the effects of xylazine, a nonnarcotic analgesic.

DOSAGE. One milligram nalorphine is recommended for every 10 mg morphine or 20 mg meperidine for reversal of narcotic effects. For reversal of the effects of etorphine, a ratio of 10–20 mg nalorphine to 1 mg etorphine is required (Alford et al. 1974). The IV route is recommended for administration.

The FDA-approved dose of nalorphine in the dog is 0.44 mg/kg by the IV, IM, or SC route.

TOXICITY. Nalorphine appears to possess about the same toxicity as morphine but provides less relief from pain. The SC injection of 11–22 mg/kg in the dog produces little analgesia.

Caution should be observed to ensure proper dosage of nalorphine. If the first dose fails to reverse or antagonize opioid-type agents, additional doses are contraindicated. In the event of an overdosage of nalorphine, respiratory supportive measures must be instituted, including establishment of a patent airway and oxygen administration. Although no data seem to be available, the partial agonist activity of nalorphine should be antagonized by naloxone.

OPIOIDS AND SPINAL ANALGESIA. Opioids can be administered in the epidural or intrathecal space in an attempt to provide analgesia while minimizing the adverse effects typically seen with opioids. When administered in this manner, they interact with opioid receptors within the spinal cord as well as having some systemic effects. The degree of systemic effect seen is a result of the lipophilicity of the opioid used. Epidural or intrathecal use of the more lipophilic agents has limited advantage over systemic use because the vascular uptake of a spinally administered drug is such that significant systemic effects are seen; the dose required is often similar to the systemic dose; and the short duration of actions necessitates frequent redosing or continuous infusion (Rawal 1993). The more lipophilic agents, such as fentanyl, have a rapid effect but a short duration of action. Less lipophilic agents (e.g., morphine) for example, have a slower onset but a much longer duration. The major difference between the epidural and intrathecal routes is dose. There is a 1:10 to 1:20 ratio in the dose of morphine for the intrathecal route versus the epidural route. In dogs 0.11 mg/kg of morphine administered epidurally gives 6 hours of analgesia (Branson et al. 1993). Epidural buprenorphine (0.001 mg/kg) has also been administered to dogs and cats for analgesia. Epidural morphine (0.11 mg/kg) has been used to control abdominal pain in horses.

OPIOIDS AND PERIPHERAL ANALGESIA. Opioid receptors have been demonstrated on primary afferent nerve fibers, but their function has not been determined (Fields et al. 1980). Recent evidence indicates they may modulate pain transmission via μ and κ receptors, especially when inflammation is present (Stein et al. 1988; Joris et al. 1987).

REFERENCES

Alexander, F., and Collett, R. A. 1974. Res Vet Sci 17:136.

Alford, B. T., Burkhart, R. L., and Johnson, W. P. 1974. J Am Vet Med Assoc 164:702.

Althaus, J. S., Miller, E. D., Moscicki, J. C., et al. 1985. Anes Analg 64:857.

Arndt, J. O., Mikat, M., and Parasher, C. 1984. Anesthesiology 61:355.

Auguy-Valette, A., Cros, J., Gouarderes, Ch., et al. 1978. Br J Pharmacol 63:303.

Ausems, M. E., Hug, C. C., and deLange, S. 1983. Anes & Anal 62:982.

Baggot, J. D., and Cooper, B. S. 1980. More Rational Use of Veterinary Drugs, p. 1. Palmerston North, N.A.: Nassey Univ.

Bailey, P. L., Port, J. D., McJames, S., et al. 1987. Anes & Anal 66:542.

Bailey, P. L., and Stanley, T. H. 1994. In R. D. Miller, ed., Anesthesia, 4th ed., p. 291. New York: Churchill Livingstone.

Beckman, A. L., Llados-Eckman, C., and Stanton, T. L. 1981. Science 212:1527.

Benson, G. J., Hartsfield, S. M., and Thurmon, J. C. 1977. Pract Vet (Spring-Summer):20.

Benson, G. J., and Thurmon, J. C. 1979. J Am Vet Med Assoc 174:594.

Benson, G. J., Thurmon, J. C., Tranquilli, W. J., and Corbin, J. E. 1987. Am J Vet Res 48:1372.

Berkowitz, B. 1971. Ann NY Acad Sci 179:269.

Bernton, E. W., Long, L. B., and Holaday, J. W. 1985. Fed Proc 44:290.

Blalock, J. E., and Smith, E. M. 1985. Fed Proc 44:108.

Blank, M. S., and Mann, D. R. 1981. Proc Soc Exp Biol Med 168:338.

Blankenstein, J., Reyes, F. I., Winter, J. S. D., et al. 1980. Proc Soc Exp Biol Med 164:363.

Booth, N. H. 1969. Fed Proc 28:1547.

Booth, N. H., Hatch, R. C., and Crawford, L. M. 1982. Am J Vet Res. 43:1227.

Booth, N. H., and Rankin, A. D. 1954. Vet Med 49:249.

Bowdle, T. A. 1993. Anaes Pharm Rev 2:135.

Bowdle, T. A., and Nelson, W. L. 1994. In T. A. Bowdle, A. Horita, and E. D. Kharasch, eds., The Pharmacologic Basis of Anesthesiology, p. 121. New York: Churchill Livingstone.

Brand, J. J., and Perry, W. L. M. 1966. Pharmacol Rev 18:895.

Branson, K. R., Ko, J. C., Tranquilli, W. J., et al. 1993. J Vet Pharm Therap 16:369.

Caffrey, J. L., Gaugh, J. F., and Jones, C. E. 1985. Am J Physiol 248:H-382.

Caldwell, J., Notarianni, L. J., Smith, R. L., et al. 1979. Toxicol Appl Pharmacol 48:273.

Chase, P. E. 1977. Feline Pract 7:24.

Chiapella, A. 1980. Am Vet Med Assoc Meet.

Christrup, L. L. 1997. ACTA Anaesthesiologica Scandinavica 41:116.

Clark, W. G. 1977. Proc Soc Exp Biol Med 154:540.

Clark, W. G., and Cumby, H. R. 1978. Br J Pharmacol 63:65.

Clark, W. G., and Harris, N. F. 1978. Eur J Pharmacol 49:301.

Clifford, D. 1971. In L. R. Soma, ed., Textbook of Veterinary Anesthesia, p. 385. Baltimore: Williams & Wilkins.

Cohen, J. 1975. Vet Rec 97:369.

Combie, J., Dougherty, J., Nugent, D., et al. 1979. J Equine Med Surg 3:377.

Combie, J., Blake, J. W., Ramey, B. E., et al. 1981. Am J Vet Res 42:1523.
Combie, J. D., Nugent, T. E., and Tobin, T. 1983. Am J Vet Res 44:870.
Cooper, J. E., and Organ, P. 1977. Vet Rec 101:409.
Copeland, V. S., Haskins, S. C., and Patz, J. D. 1987. Am J Vet Res 48:16260.
Cowan, A., Geller, E. B., and Adler, M. W. 1979. Science 206:465.
Cox, B. M. 1988. In G. W. Pasternak, ed., The Opiate Receptors. Clifton: Humana Press.
Curtis, M. T., and Lefer, A. M. 1980. Am J Physiol 239:H-416.
Dahlstrom, B. E., Paalzow, L. K., Lindberg, C., et al. 1979. Drug Metab Dispos 7:108.
Davis, L. E. 1983. In R. L. Kitchell, ed., Animal Pain, p. 161. Baltimore: Williams & Wilkins.
Davis, L. E., and Donnelly, E. J. 1968. J Am Vet Med Assoc 153:1161.
Davis, L. E., and Sturm, B. L. 1970. Am J Vet Res 31:1631.
Davis, S. D., McDonald, W. J., Kendall, J. W., et al. 1984. Proc Soc Exp Biol Med 175:380.
Delitala, G., Devilla, L., and Arata, L. 1981. Acta Endocrinol 97:150.
DeSilva, R. A., Verrier, R. L., and Lown, B. 1978a. Cardiovasc Res 12:167.
———. 1978b. Am Heart J 95:197.
Dhasmana, K. M., Dixit, K. S., Jaju, B. P., et al. 1972. Psychopharmacologia 24:380.
DiChiara, G., and Gessa, G. L. 1978. Adv Pharmacol Chemother 15:87.
Dodman, N. H., Seeler, D. C., and Court, M. H. 1984. Br Vet J 140:505.
Dodman, N. H., Shuster, L., Court, M. H., et al. 1987. Am J Vet Res 48:311.
Dohoo, S. E., Tasker, R. A. 1997. Can J vet Res 61:251.
Dorn, A. S. 1972. Aust Vet J 48:54.
Driessen, B., Reimann, W. 1992. Br J Pharmacol 105:147.
Dystra, L. A., and Leander, J. D. 1978. Pharmacol Biochem Behav 8:387.
Egger, C. M., Duke, T., Archer, J., Cribb, P. H. 1998. Vet Surg 27:159.
Eisleb, O., and Schaumann, O. 1939. Dtsch Med Wochenschr 65:967.
England, G. C., and Clarke, K. W. 1989. Acta Vet Scand Suppl 85:179.
Feldman, D. B., and Self, J. L. 1971. Lab Anim Sci 21:717.
Fettman, M. J., Hand, M. S., Chandrasena, L. G., et al. 1984. J Surg Res 37:208.
Fidecka, S., Malec, D., and Langwinski, R. 1978. Pol J Pharmacol Pharm 30:5.
Field, W. E., Yelnosky, J., Mundy, J., et al. 1966. J Am Vet Med Assoc 149:896.
Fields, H., Emson, P., Leigh, B., et al. 1980. Nature. 284:351.
Firn, S. 1973. Lancet 2:95.
Flecknell, R. A. 1984. Lab Anim 18:417.
Florez, J., Hurle, M. A., and Mediavilla, A. 1977. Life Sci 31:2189.
Fowler, M. E., and Hart, R. 1973. J Am Vet Med Assoc 163:539.
Frank, G. B. 1985. Can J Physiol Pharmacol 63:1023.
Frank, H., McCarty, B. C., and Liebeskind, J. C. 1978. Science 200:335.
Franklin, I. I., and Reid, J. S. 1965. Vet Med 60:927.
Gardner, A. F. 1964. Lab Anim Sci 14:214.
Garrett, E. R., and Chandran, V. R. 1990. Biopharmaceutics & Drug Disposition 11:311.
Gatesman, T., and Wiesner, H. 1982. J Zoo Anim Med 13:11.
Gingerich, D. A., Rourke, J. E., Chatfield, R. C., et al. 1985. Vet Med 80:72.
Goldstein, A. 1976. Science 193:1081.
Greene, N. M. 1968. Anesthesiology 29:327.
Gubler, U., Kilpatrick, D. L., Seeburg, P. H., et al. 1981. Proc Natl Acad Sci USA 789:5484.
Guillemin, R. 1978. Science 202:390.
Guy, R. H., Hadgraft, J., Bucks, D. A. 1987. Xenobiotica 17:325.
Hackett, R. P. 1976. Vet Anesth 3:100.
Haigh, J. C., and Haigh, J. M. 1980. Vet Hum Toxicol 22:1.
Hall, R. I., Szlam, F., and Hug, C. C. 1987. Anes & Anal 66:1287.
Harper, M. H., Winter, P. M., Johnson, B. H., et al. 1978. Anesthesiology 49:3.
Harthoorn, A. M. 1965a. Wildlife monographs. Application of pharmacological and physiological principles in restraint of wild animals, p. 40. Washington, DC: Wildlife Society.
———. 1965b. J S Afr Vet Assoc 36:45.
———. 1966. J Am Vet Med Assoc 149:875.
———. 1972. Vet Rec 91:63.
Harthoorn, A. M., and Bligh, J. 1965. Res Vet Sci 6:290.
Haskins, S. C., Copeland, V. S., and Patz, J. D. 1991. Vet Emergency and Critical Care 1:32.
Hatch, R. C. 1973. J Am Vet Med Assoc 162:964.
Hatch, R. C., Clark, J. D., Booth, N. H., et al. 1983. Am J Vet Res 44:2312.
Hatch, R. C., Jernigan, A. D., Wilson, R. C., et al. 1986. Can J Vet Res 50:251.
Hazum, E., Sabatka, J. J., Chang, K.-J., et al. 1981. Science 213:1010.
Heavner, J. E. 1970. J Am Vet Med Assoc 156:1018.
Heidrich, J. E. 1985. J Am Vet Med Assoc 187:513.
Higgins, A. J., and Kock, R. A. 1984. Br Vet J 140:485.
Holaday, J. W. 1983a. Biochem Pharmacol 32:573.
———. 1983b. Ann Rev Pharmacol Toxicol 23:541.
Holaday, J. W., and Faden, A. I. 1980. Brain Res 189:295.
Hosgood, G. 1990. JAVMA 196:135.
Houck, J. C., Kimball, C., Chang, C., et al. 1980. Science 207:78.
Hug, C. C., and Murphy, M. R. 1981. Anesthesiology. 55;369.
Itzhak, Y. 1988. In G. W. Pasternak, ed., The Opiate Receptors. Clifton: Humana Press.
Jainudeen, M. R., Bongso, T. A., and Perera, B. M. O. A. 1971. Vet Rec 89:686.
Järnberg, P.-O., Santesson, J., and Eklund, J. 1978. Acta Anaesth Scand 22:167.
Jiang, Q., Takemori, A. E., and Sultanta, P. S. 1991. J Pharmacol Exp Ther 257:1069.
Jenkins, J. T. 1972. Vet Rec 90:207.
Jenkins, V. R., II, and Dilts, P. V., Jr. 1971. Am J Obstet Gynecol 109:1005.
Jensen, J. M. 1982. J Zoo Anim Med 13:101.
Jones, J. B., and Simmons, M. L. 1968. Lab Anim Sci 18:642.
Joris, J. L., Dubner, R., Hargreaves, K. M. 1987. Anesth Analg 66:1277.
Joseph, S. A., Pilcher, W. H., and Knigge, K. M. 1985. Fed Proc 44:100.
Kalpravidh, M., Lumb, W. V., Wright, M., et al. 1984a. Am J Vet Res 45:211.
———. 1984b. Am J Vet Res 45:217.
Kayser, V., Besson, J. M., Guilbaud, G. 1992. Europ J Pharmacol 224:83.
Keith, J. C., Jr., Wilson, R. C., Booth, N. H., et al. 1981. J Vet Pharmacol Ther 4:315.
King, C., Masserano, J. M., Codd, E., et al. 1981. Sleep 4:259.
Klavano, P. A. 1975. Proc Am Assoc Equine Pract, p. 149.
Knoll, J. 1977. Pol J Pharmacol Pharm 29:165.
Kollias, G. V., Jr., Colahan, P. T., and Walsh, M. T. 1983. J Am Vet Med Assoc 183:1334.
Krahwinkel, D. J., Sawyer, D. C., and Evans, A. T. 1972. J Am Anim Hosp Assoc 8:368.

Kyles, A. E., Papich, M., Hardie, E. M. 1996. Am J Vet Res 57:715.
Lal, H. 1975. Life Sci 17:483.
Leaman, D. M., Nellis, S. H., Zelis, R., et al. 1978. Am J Cardiol 41:324.
Leash, A. M., Beyer, R. D., and Wilber, R. G. 1973. Lab Anim Sci 23:720.
Lewis, G. E., Jr., and Jennings, P. B., Jr. 1972. Lab Anim Sci 22:430.
Lintz, W., Erlacin, S., Frankkus, E., Uragg, H. 1981. Arzneimittel-Forschung 31:1932.
Lowe, J. E. 1969. Proc Am Assoc Equine Pract, p. 31.
———. 1978. J Equine Med Surg 2:286.
Lund-Jacobsen, H. 1978. Acta Pharmacol Toxicol 42:171.
Maas, C. L., and Leek, B. F. 1985. Vet Res Commun 9:89.
McCord, J. M. 1985. N Engl J Med 312:159.
McLain, D. A., and Hug, C. C. 1980. Clin Pharmacol Ther 22:106.
McPherson, R. W., and Traystman, R. J. 1984. Anesthesiology 60:180.
Mains, R. E., Eipper, B. A., and Ling, N. 1977. Proc Natl Acad Sci USA 74:3014.
Mannelli, M., Maggi, M., DeFeo, M. L., et al. 1983. N Engl J Med 308:654.
Martin, W. R. 1984. Pharmacol Rev 35:283.
Mather, L. E. 1983. Clin Pharmacol 8:442.
Mattia, A., Vanderah, T., Mosberg, H. I., and Porreca, I. 1991. J Pharmacol Exp Ther 258:583.
Mattia, A., Farmer, S. C., Takemore, A. E., et al. 1992. J Pharmacol Exp Ther 260:518.
Maykut, M. O. 1958. Can Anaesth Soc J 5:161.
Meuldermans, W., Hendrick, J., Lauwers, W., et al. 1987. Drug Metabolism & Disposition 15:905.
Michel, M. E., Bolgen, G., Weisman, B. A. 1988. Pharmacologist 26:201.
Miki, N., Sonntag, W. E., Forman, L. J., et al. 1981. Proc Soc Exp Biol Med 168:330.
Millan, M. J. 1990. Trend Pharmacol Sci 11:70.
Miner, W. S., and Losacco, C. L. 1984. Vet Med Small Anim Clin 79:183.
Mirkin, B. L. 1975. Anesthesiology 43:156.
Moller, A. W. 1968. In R. W. Kirk, ed., Current Veterinary Therapy III: Small Animal Practice, p. 421. Philadelphia: W. B. Saunders.
Montomura, S., Kissin, I., Aultman, D. F., and Reves, J. G. 1984. Anes Analg 63:47.
Moore, A. B., Roesel, O. F., Fessler, J. F., et al. 1983. Am J Vet Res 44:103.
Morley, J. E. 1981. Metabolism 30:195.
Muir, W. M. 1991. In W. M. Muir and J. A. Hubbell, eds., Equine Anesthesia, p. 247. St. Louis: Mosby Year-Book.
Muir, W. W., and Robertson, J. T. 1985. Am J Vet Res 46:2081.
Muir, W. W., Skarda, R. T., and Sheehan, W. 1978. In J. D. Powers and T. E. Powers, eds., Equine Pharmacology, p. 173. Proc 2nd Equine Pharmacol Symp. Golden, CO: American Association of Equine Practitioners.
Muir, W. W., Sams, R. A., and Huffman, R. 1980. Am J Vet Res 41:575.
Murkin, J. M. 1991. J Cardiothorac Vasc Anesth 5:268.
Musacchio, J. 1990. Neuropsychopharmacology 3:191.
Nielson, L. 1996. In J. C. Thurmon, W. J. Tranquilli, and G. J. Benson, eds., Veterinary Anesthesia, p. 736. Baltimore: Williams & Wilkins.
Nock, B., Giordano, A. L., Cicero, R. J., et al. 1990. J Pharmacol Exp Ther 48:412.
Ohtani, M., Kotaki, H., Uchine, K., et al. 1994. Drug Metab Dispos 22:2.
Oka, T. 1978. Gen Pharmacol 9:151.
Olson, G. A., Olson, R. E., Kastin, A. J., et al. 1981. Peptides 2:349.
Ormerod, E., Bogan, J. A., and Lauder, I. M. 1978. Vet Rec 102:110.
Orwall, E. S., Kendall, J. W. 1980. Endocrinology 107:438.
Paddleford, R. R., and Short, C. E. 1973. J am Vet Med Assoc 163:144.
Page, J. G., Sullivan, H. R., Due, S. L., et al. 1979. Toxicol Appl Pharmacol 50:505.
Palminteri, A. 1963. J Am Vet Med Assoc 143:160.
———. 1966. J Am Vet Med Assoc 148:1396.
Panerai, A. E., Massei, R., DeSilva, E., et al. 1985. Br J Anaesth 57:954.
Paquette, N. C., and Young, G. A. 1991. Eur J Pharmacol 196:61.
Parsons, L. E., and Walmsley, J. P. 1982. Vet Rec 111:395.
Pascoe, P. J., Black, W. D., Claxton, J. M., and Sansom, R. E. 1989. Proc Ann Meet ACVA. New Orleans.
Pasternak, G. W. 1994. In T. A. Bowdle, A. Horita, and E. D. Kharasch, eds., The Pharmacologic Basis of Anesthesiology, p. 19. New York: Churchill Livingstone.
Pasternak, G. W., and Childers, S. R. 1984. In W Shoemaker, ed., Critical Care: State of the Art, vol. V, p. F1. Fullerton, CA: Society of Critical Care Medicine.
Pasternak, G. W., and Wood, P. L. 1986. Life Sci 38:1889.
Pert, C. B., and Snyder, S. H. 1973. Science 179:1011.
Phaneuf, L. P., Grivel, M. L., and Ruckebusch, Y. 1972. Comp Med 36:138.
Pippi, N. L., and Lumb, W. V. 1979. Am J Vet Res 40:1082.
Pircio, A. W., Gylys, J. A., Cavanagh, R. I., et al. 1976. Arch Int Pharmacodyn 220:231.
Pleuvry, B. J. 1993. Anaes Pharmacol Rev 12:114.
Plotnikoff, N. P., and Murgo, A. J. 1985. Fed Proc 44:91.
Raffa, R. B., Friderichs, E., Reimann, W., et al. 1992. J Pharmacol Exp Ther 260:275.
Ragan, H. A., and Gillis, M. F. 1975. Lab Anim Sci 25:409.
Rawal, N. 1993. Anaes Pharmacol Review 1:168.
Reddy, P., Lui, W.-S., Port, D., et al. 1980. Can Anaesth Soc J 27:345.
Reid, J. S., and Frank, R. J. 1972. J Am Anim Hosp Assoc 8:115.
Reynolds, D. G., Gurll, N. J., Vargish, T., et al. 1980. Circ Shock 7:39.
Ritschel, W. A., Neub, M., and Denson, D. D. 1987. Methods & Findings in Exp Clin Pharmacol 9:811.
Robertson, J. T., Muir, W. W., and Sams, R. 1981. Am J Vet Res 42:41.
Robinson, P. T., and Janssen, D. L. 1980. J Am Anim Hosp Assoc 16:279.
Rochford, J., Godin, C., and Henry, J. L. 1991. Brain Res 565:67.
Ross, C. M. 1986. Vet Rec 119:22.
Rossier, J., Vargo, T. M., Minick, S., et al. 1977. Proc Natl Acad Sci USA 74:5162.
Rubright, W. C., and Thayer, C. B. 1970. Lab Anim Sci 20:989.
Samir, D. R., and Flynn, G. L. 1989. Pharm Res 6:825.
Sanchez, E., and Tephly, T. R. 1974. Drug Metab Dispos 2:248.
Sawyer, D. C. 1985. Neuroleptanalgesia and Anesthesia. Proc 2nd Int Congr Vet Anes 1985:1.
Sawyer, D. C., and Rech, R. H. 1987. J Am Anim Hosp Assoc 23:438.
Sawyer, D. C., Rech, R. H., Durham, R. A., et al. 1991. Am J Vet Res 1826.
Schauffler, A. F. 1969. Mod Vet Pract 50:46.
Schels, H. F., and Nowrouzian, I. 1977. Vet Rec 101:388.
Schwartz, R. H., and Riddle, M. 1985. J Am Vet Med Assoc 187:206.
Sederberg, J., Stanley, T. H., Reddy, P., et al. 1981. Anesth Analg 60:715.

Segall, S. 1964. J Am Vet Med Assoc 144:603.
Shemano, I., and Wendel, H. 1965. J Pharmacol Exp Ther 149:379.
Short, C. E., Hoppingardner, J., Bendick F., et al. 1971. Vet Med Small Anim Clin 66:586.
Simon, E. J. 1977. In J. R. Smythies and R. J. Bradley, eds., Receptors in Pharmacology, p. 257. New York: Marcel Dekker.
Simon, E. J., and Hiller, J. M. 1978. Ann Rev Pharmacol Toxicol 18:371.
Smith, R. J. 1979. Science 203:857.
Smuts, G. L. 1975. J Am Vet Med Assoc 167:559.
Soma, L. R., ed. 1971. Textbook of Veterinary Anesthesia, pp. 121, 621. Baltimore: Williams & Wilkins.
Soma, L. R., and Shields, D. R. 1964. J Am Vet Med Assoc 145:897.
Sørenson, M. B., HÑggmark, S., Nyhman, H., et al. 1985. Acta Anaesth Scand 29:130.
Spector, S., and Vesell, E. S. 1971. Science 174:421.
Stanley, T. H. 1994. Proc 5th Int Cong Vet Anes, pp. 49.
Stein, C., Millan, M. J., Yassouridis, A., and Herz, A. 1988. Europ J Pharmacol 155: 255.
Stoelting, R. K. 1991. In Pharmacology and Physiology in Anesthetic Practice, 2nd ed., p. 70. Philadelphia: J. B. Lippincott.
Strack, L. E., and Kaplan, H. M. 1968. J Am Vet Med Assoc 153:822.
Strobel, G. E., and Wollman, H. 1969. Fed Proc 28:1386.
Sylvester, P. W., Chen, C. T., and Meites, J. 1980. Proc Soc Exp Biol Med 164:207.
Tamas, P. M., and Geiser, D. R. 1983. J Am Vet Med Assoc 183:1312.
Tayeyama, C., Goto, H., Kohno, N., et al. 1993. Anes & Analg 77:44.
Thayer, C. B., Lowe, S., and Rubright, W. C. 1972. J Am Vet Med Assoc 161:665.
Tobin, T. T., 1978. J Equine Med Surg 2:397.
Tobin, T. T., and Miller, J. R. 1979. J Equine Med Surg 3:191.
Tobin, T. T., Combie, J., Miller, J. R., et al. 1979. Ir Vet J 33:169.
Tornetta, F. J., and Wilson, F. S. 1969. Anesth Analg 48:850.
Tranquilli, W. J., Fikes, L. L., and Raffee, M. R. 1989. Vet Med 84:692.
Trim, C. M. 1983. Am J Vet Res 44:329.
Türker, R. K., and Kaymakcalan, S. 1971. Arch Int Pharmacodyn Ther 193:397.
Vandam, L. D., 1980. N Engl J Med 302:381.
Vargish, T., Reynolds, D. G., Gurll, N. J., et al. 1980. Circ Shock 7:31.
Vatner, S. F., Marsh, J. D., and Swain, J. A. 1975. J Clin Invest 55:207.
Vaught, J. L., Rothman, R. B., and Westfall, T. C. 1982. Life Sci 30:1443.
Vet Rec News and Reports. 1976. Vet Rec 98:414.
Vorhees, C. V., Brunner, R. L., and Butcher, R. E. 1979. Science 205:1220.
Wallach, J. D. 1969. Vet Med Small Anim Clin 64:53.
Wallach, J. D., and Hoessle, C. 1970. Vet Med Small Anim Clin 65:163.
Wallenstein, M. C., and Wang, S. C. 1979. Am J Physiol 236:R292.
Waterman, A. E., and Kalthum, W. 1989. Vet Rec 124;12:293.
———. 1990.Res in Vet Sci 48:245.
Watson, S. J., Klachaturian, H., Akil, H., et al. 1982. Science 218:1134.
Watts, S. J., Slocombe, R. F., Harbison, W. D., et al. 1973. Aust Vet J 49:525.
White, S. L. 1981. Ga Vet 33:14.
Wolozin, B. L., Pasternak, G. W. 1981. Proc Natl Acad Sci USA 78:6181.
Wright, E. M., Jr., Marcella, K. L., and Woodson, J. F. 1985. Lab Anim 14:20.
Wybran, J. 1985. Fed Proc 44:92.
Yaksh, T. L., and Howe, J. R. 1982. Anesthesiology 56:246.
Zaloga, G. P., Hostinsky, C., and Chernow, B. 1984. Heart Lung 13:421.

14 TRANQUILIZERS, α_2-ADRENERGIC AGONISTS, AND RELATED AGENTS

MARJORIE E. GROSS

Phenothiazine Derivatives
- **The Dopamine Receptor**
- **General Pharmacologic Considerations**
- **Chlorpromazine Hydrochloride**
- **Promazine Hydrochloride**
- **Acepromazine Maleate**
- **Prochlorperazine Edisylate**
- **Trimeprazine Tartrate**

α_2-Adrenergic Agonists
- **The α_2 Adrenoceptor**
- **Xylazine Hydrochloride**
- **Detomidine Hydrochloride**
- **Medetomidine Hydrochloride**
- **New α_2-Adrenergic Agonists**
- **α_2-Adrenergic Antagonists**

Benzodiazepine Derivatives
- **The Benzodiazepine Receptor**
- **Diazepam**
- **Midazolam Maleate**
- **Chlordiazepoxide Hydrochloride**
- **Benzodiazepine Antagonists**

Butyrophenone Derivatives
- **Mechanism of Action**
- **Droperidol**
- **Azaperone**

In the 1950s, phenothiazine derivatives (chlorpromazine, promazine, and others) were introduced into clinical veterinary medicine as ataractics (tranquilizers). Their discoverers coined the term *neuroleptics* to indicate that their most prominent pharmacologic effects are on certain functions of the central nervous system (CNS).

Neuroleptic drugs of major importance in veterinary medicine are the phenothiazines, α_2-adrenergic agonists, and benzodiazepines. Butyrophenones are used infrequently in veterinary medicine. See previous editions of this book for a review of the pharmacology and clinical use of tranquilizers and related agents that are now rarely or no longer used in veterinary medicine.

PHENOTHIAZINE DERIVATIVES

The Dopamine Receptor. The principal central activity of the phenothiazine tranquilizers is blockade of the effects of dopamine, a catecholamine CNS neurotransmitter. Dopamine is believed to have primarily inhibitory activity in the brain, with the greatest concentrations in the basal ganglia and the limbic system. A deficiency of dopamine within the basal ganglia has been shown to be associated with a definite dysfunction of this neuroanatomical system, i.e., the Parkinsonian syndrome in humans and catalepsy in experimental animals (Hornykiewicz 1973).

Dopamine exerts its effects through interaction with specific receptors located on the neuronal membrane surface. Postsynaptic neuronal dopamine receptors have been described, but there is evidence suggesting that presynaptic dopamine receptors may also exist. Dopamine receptors are included in the family of G-protein-coupled receptors. Dopamine acts as a *first messenger* by interacting with the receptor proteins of the postsynaptic membrane. This interaction results in transduction of the signal by a guanine nucleotide-binding regulatory protein (G protein) to an appropriate intracellular effector system, or *second messenger.* Three major types of second messengers have been described in the CNS: adenylyl cyclase (cyclic AMP), guanylyl cyclase, and phospholipid hydrolysis (eicosanoid) systems (Cooper et al. 1991).

It was originally believed that stimulation of adenylyl cyclase activity was the principal effect of dopamine. However, inhibition of adenylyl cyclase activity has also been demonstrated with some dopaminergic agonists. This led to the initial classification of dopamine receptors into subtypes D_1 and D_2. Interaction with the D_1-receptor subtype stimulates adenylyl cyclase activity and increases intracellular levels of cyclic AMP; interaction with the D_2 receptor subtype inhibits adenylyl cyclase activity. At present, five mammalian dopamine receptor subtypes have been described and classified into D_1 and D_2 *subfamilies* of dopamine receptors (Lachowicz and Sibley 1997).

Based on hydropathy analysis, the dopamine receptor has been described structurally as seven hydrophobic domains that traverse the plasma membrane. The amino acids in these domains are believed to be in an α-helical configuration. The D_1-receptor subfamily has a relatively small third cytoplasmic loop, which is consistent with stimulatory G-protein-associated receptors. The D_2 receptor subfamily has large third cytoplasmic loops and short carboxyl termini, which are characteristic of inhibitory G-protein-associated receptors (Strader et al. 1989; Dohlman et al. 1991).

The D_1 subfamily includes the traditional D_1 subtype (also referred to as D_{1A}) and the D_5 receptor (also referred to as the D_{1B} receptor). Both the D_1 and D_5 receptors bind dopaminergic agonists and antagonists with similar affinity but differ in primary amino acid sequence and anatomical distribution (Lachowicz and Sibley 1997). There is a high degree of structural homology between the D_{1A}/D_1 and D_{1B}/D_5 receptor subtypes, although dopamine binds to the D_{1B}/D_5 receptors with a five- to tenfold greater affinity than to the D_1 receptor (Grandy et al. 1991; Monsma et al. 1991; Sunahara et al. 1991; Tiberi et al. 1991; Weinshank et al. 1991).

The D_2 subfamily includes D_3 and D_4 receptor subtypes, as well as the traditional D_2 receptor subtype, which has been isolated into short (D_{2S}) and long (D_{2L}) isoforms (Lachowicz and Sibley 1997). In addition to adenylyl cyclase inhibition (Neve et al. 1989), the D_2 receptors potentiate a variety of signal transduction pathways, including stimulation of arachidonic acid release (Kanterman et al. 1991), phosphatidylinositol hydrolysis and mobilization of calcium (Vallar et al. 1990), regulation of K^+ channels (Einhorn et al. 1990; Liu et al. 1994, 1996), and suppression of prolactin release (Albert et al. 1990). The D_2 long isoform receptor contains a 29 amino acid sequence that is missing from the D_2 short receptor. The two isoforms share similar pharmacological profiles and functional abilities, although they may act via different G proteins in mediating adenylyl cyclase inhibition (Dal Toso et al. 1989; Senogles 1994) and regulation of potassium channels (Einhorn et al. 1990; Liu et al. 1994, 1996). It has been suggested that the 29 amino acid sequence may function to direct the isoforms along different regulatory pathways (Lachowicz and Sibley 1997).

The pharmacological profile of the D_3 receptor is similar to that of the D_2 receptor (Sokoloff et al. 1990; Freedman et al. 1993; Malmberg et al. 1993; Mackenzie et al. 1994). D_3-receptor-mediated adenylyl cyclase inhibition has been reported to be minimal compared to that of the D_2 receptor (Castro and Strange 1993; Seabrook et al. 1992; Chio et al. 1993). However, other D_3-receptor-mediated effects have been identified, and it has been suggested that these effects may be mediated by a second-messenger system that has yet to be described (Lachowicz and Sibley 1997). Most dopaminergic agonists bind with greater affinity to the D_3 receptor, whereas most antagonists bind with greater affinity to the D_2 receptor (Sokoloff et al. 1990, 1992).

Binding properties of the D_4 receptor resemble those of the D_2 receptor, although most dopaminergic agonists and antagonists bind to the D_2 receptor with greater affinity than to the D_4 receptor (Van Tol et al. 1991; O'Malley et al. 1992; Asghari et al. 1994; Chabert et al. 1994; Tang et al. 1994). An exception is clozapine, a highly effective antipsychotic drug used in human patients. Clozapine is a dopaminergic antagonist that binds preferentially to D_4 receptors, with an affinity that is about tenfold greater than its affinity for D_2 receptors (Coward 1992). Clozapine is not associated with extrapyramidal effects that may occur with the blockade of D_2 receptors in the basal ganglia nuclei. As there appears to be a greater concentration of D_4 receptors in limbic nuclei than in the basal ganglia nuclei, this has led to the hypothesis that the D_4 receptor may be the therapeutic target for antipsychotic drugs (Lachowicz and Sibley 1997).

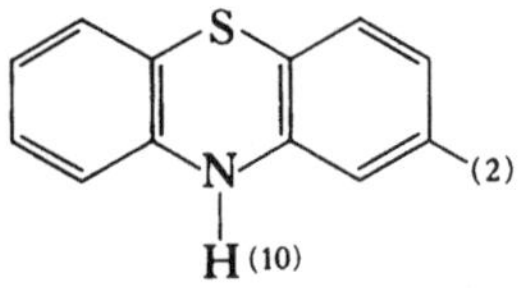

S
N
(2)
H (10)
Phenothiazine

FIG. 14.1

General Pharmacologic Considerations. Phenothiazine is the parent compound for all the derivatives in this group (Fig. 14.1). Substitution is made primarily in the phenothiazine nucleus at the 2 and 10 positions.

The majority of pharmacologic actions discussed for phenothiazines pertain to chlorpromazine hydrochloride. However, the mechanisms of action for other phenothiazines are similar to chlorpromazine except for variations primarily referable to potency and duration of action. In clinical practice, greater potency of a drug does not necessarily imply greater effectiveness. This is true of phenothiazines because controlled investigations have been unable to show any significant difference in effectiveness of these agents when administered in equipotent doses.

All phenothiazines exert a sedative action by depressing the brain stem and connections to the cerebral cortex but may vary in potency and duration of action. Unlike barbiturates, the sedative effect does not appreciably affect coordinated motor responses, and arousal is easily accomplished. If a piperazine structure is linked to position 10 of the molecule, reduced or no sedative action is observed (as with prochlorperazine).

All phenothiazines decrease spontaneous motor activity in animals. At high doses, cataleptic effects may be produced so that animals will remain immobile in a fixed position for long periods. Extrapyramidal symptoms (rigidity, tremor, akinesia) are also observed as prominent side effects of phenothiazines in animals administered high doses.

Most phenothiazine derivatives increase the rate of dopamine turnover (i.e., synthesis and destruction) in the brain (Hornykiewicz 1973; Matthysse 1973). Moreover, there is an increased turnover of norepinephrine. This effect may be related to the potency of these compounds in eliciting extrapyramidal symptoms (catalepsy) in animals. Chlorpromazine and other phenothiazines that have been observed to produce extrapyramidal symptoms also increase the synthesis and destruction of dopamine (Matthysse 1973); chlorpromazine increases the concentration of the dopamine metabolite homovanillic acid in the caudate nucleus of the cat and rabbit. Conversely, the prototype phenothiazine derivative, promethazine, has antihistaminic activity and does not increase the concentration of homovanillic acid or affect the synthesis and destruction of dopamine. Trimeprazine tartrate, a nonpsychotropic phenothiazine, produces a slight increase in the dopamine metabolite level within the corpus striatum of the rabbit.

In addition to blockade of the central effect of catecholamines (e.g., dopamine), phenothiazines are known to block peripheral actions of catecholamines. Chlorpromazine and other related compounds can prevent and reverse a number of actions of epinephrine (epinephrine reversal). Since α-adrenergic receptors are blocked by chlorpromazine and related derivatives, the β-adrenergic receptors are stimulated by the potent β component of epinephrine; this results in vasodilation and/or arterial hypotension and may induce shocklike conditions. Administration of epinephrine is contraindicated whenever phenothiazine derivatives are used. However, norepinephrine can be used without risk of aggravating arterial hypotensive effects of phenothiazines, because of its weak β-agonist action compared to epinephrine. It has been suggested that the major action of the phenothiazines may be stimulation of β_2 receptors (vasodilation) rather than blockade of α receptors. However, most pharmacologists indicate that phenothiazines block α-adrenergic receptors, which then results in vasodilation or hypotension. Regardless of mechanism, chlorpromazine and most other phenothiazine derivatives cause arterial hypotension. Phenothiazines are contraindicated in regional (epidural and intrathecal) anesthetic procedures because they potentiate the arterial hypotensive effects of local anesthetics.

Chlorpromazine and, to a lesser degree, acepromazine maleate prevent epinephrine-induced ventricular fibrillation during use of halogenated anesthetics (halothane, methoxyflurane, and others) similar to α-adrenergic blocking agents. Chlorpromazine has antidysrhythmic activity, implying that it protects the heart from the β_1-receptor stimulant effects of epinephrine and norepinephrine. However, the direct depressant effect of chlorpromazine upon the myocardium may be the actual mechanism that prevents the dysrhythmic effects of catecholamines.

Morphine-induced hyperexcitement and manic behavior in the cat can be prevented by pretreatment with chlorpromazine (Dhasmana et al. 1972). It is believed that morphine sulfate enhances release of dopamine in the CNS, which in turn stimulates central dopaminergic receptors to induce the manic response. Moreover, morphine appears to increase norepinephrine release, which may also result in CNS excitation in the cat.

Unlike morphine and its derivatives, the phenothiazine derivatives have little or no analgesic activity. Tranquilization must be supplemented with analgesics and/or general anesthetics to block nociceptive responses during painful procedures.

Hypothermic effects appear to be induced by phenothiazines as a result of depletion of catecholamine substances within the hypothalamus, where thermoregulation is controlled centrally.

Chlorpromazine affects pituitary activity only in quantities that exceed those required to induce depressant effects (de Wied 1967). At high doses, chlorpromazine appears to block release of the follicle-stimulating hormone and luteinizing hormone. Ovulation is blocked and the estrous cycle is suppressed. It has been shown that chlorpromazine, acepromazine, and perphenazine increase the plasma level of prolactin in a number of species (i.e., rat, sheep, goat, human) (Blackwell et al. 1973). An increase of plasma prolactin can result in galactorrhea. Other endocrine effects include inhibition of release of the melanocyte-stimulating hormone and antidiuretic hormone and inhibition of oxytocin release.

Hyperglycemia has been observed following administration of chlorpromazine and other phenothiazines in several species, including humans. The principal mechanism of phenothiazine-evoked hyperglycemia is believed to be release of epinephrine via the adrenal medulla; this in turn mobilizes liver glycogen. Inasmuch as the relative effectiveness of phenothiazines in elevating blood glucose does not correlate well with their capability to stimulate secretion of adrenal catecholamine, questions arise about the actual mechanism(s) involved. Phenothiazines do indeed elevate blood glucose through release of epinephrine from the adrenal medulla because extirpation of the adrenal medullae abolishes or reduces the glycemic responses. However, extra-adrenal mechanisms are also involved and appear to be more important in the overall effect upon blood glucose; e.g., inhibition or blockade of the effect of insulin is a major factor in determining the degree of hyperglycemic effect produced by certain phenothiazines (Proakis and Borowitz 1974).

Chlorpromazine and other phenothiazines have a paralyzing action upon skeletal muscle similar to that produced by *d*-tubocurarine. Chlorpromazine's action can be antagonized to some extent by eserine or neostigmine.

Amphetamine, an excitatory dopamine receptor agonist and many sympathomimetic compounds structurally similar to catecholamines are blocked centrally by phenothiazine derivatives. In amphetamine overdosage, chlorpromazine is recommended as one of the antidotes for treatment of CNS excitation and convulsions. Serotonin is also blocked by chlorpromazine. In addition, it blocks the locomotor hyperactivity and stereotyped motor behavior evoked in animals by apomorphine, a potent dopamine agonist (Hornykiewicz 1973). The antiemetic activity of chlorpromazine and other phenothiazines is related to blockade of dopamine receptors of the chemoreceptor trigger zone within the medulla (DiChiara and Gessa 1978). Emetic stimulant effects of ergot alkaloids are also inhibited by chlorpromazine.

Although phenothiazine tranquilizers will antagonize the CNS-stimulating effects of sympathomimetic amines (e.g., amphetamine and related drugs), they do not prevent the convulsive action of strychnine, pentylenetetrazol, and picrotoxin. Phenothiazines in therapeutic doses suppress conditioned avoidance behavior, inhibit spontaneous motor activity, and reduce aggressive behavior and hostility. At higher doses, interference with locomotor function is observed. Moderate doses produce sedation and drowsiness; in larger concentrations, phenothiazines induce ataxia and somnolence.

Clinical levels of phenothiazines ordinarily have little effect upon respiratory activity. If arterial hypotension occurs, respiratory activity may be reflexly accelerated through decreased activity of the carotid and aortic pressoreceptors. Large doses, however, will depress respiratory activity. Vasomotor activity controlled via the hypothalamus or at the medullary level is depressed by low levels of chlorpromazine.

Chlorpromazine and other phenothiazines markedly reduce the hematocrit of animals. At one time the mechanism was thought to be related to a hemodilution effect or an increased plasma volume. However, reduction in the hematocrit or packed-cell volume (PCV) by the phenothiazines is believed due to splenic sequestration of red blood cells, and blood samples drawn from phenothiazine-treated animals for diagnostic purposes should be interpreted accordingly.

Chlorpromazine Hydrochloride. Chemically, *Chlorpromazine Hydrochloride,* USP (Thorazine, Largactil), is 2-chloro-10-(3-dimethylaminopropyl)-phenothiazine (Fig. 14.2). In the hydrochloride salt form, it is a grayish white crystalline powder that is very soluble in water. Although it decomposes in light, it can be boiled without decomposition. Chemical synthesis of chlorpromazine soon followed the observation that an antihistaminic agent (i.e., promethazine), also a phenothiazine compound, produces CNS depression. Chlorpromazine has slight antihistaminic activity.

PHARMACOLOGIC CONSIDERATIONS. Interestingly, the stereochemical model of chlorpromazine is similar to the structures of epinephrine, norepinephrine, and dopamine. This similarity is inapparent when only the two-dimensional structures are compared. Thus, chlorpromazine interacts with both the dopamine and norepinephrine receptors.

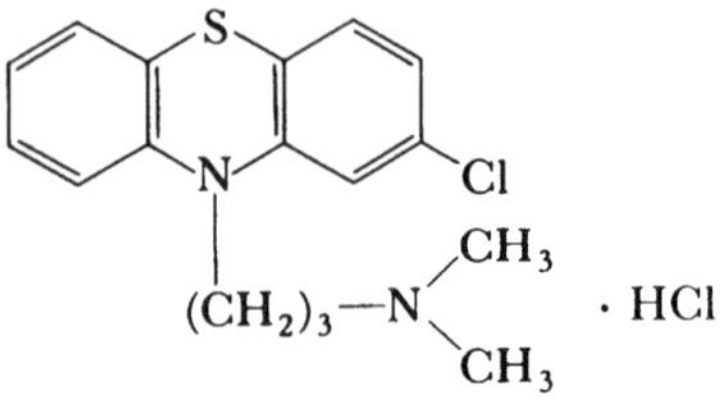

Chlorpromazine Hydrochloride

FIG. 14.2

The hypothermic mechanism and other effects of chlorpromazine are difficult to understand because the drug interferes with several neuronal pathways in the brain (Lin 1979); e.g., chlorpromazine blocks the central catecholamine receptors and elevates brain levels of these amines (dopamine, serotonin, norepinephrine). Additionally, the peripheral cholinergic-blocking activity, adrenergic-blocking activity, adrenergic activity, antihistaminic effects, and antitryptaminergic effects of chlorpromazine further complicate understanding of these mechanisms. Nevertheless, it appears that brain monoaminergic systems have a functional role in eliciting or modulating chlorpromazine-induced hypothermia; e.g., depletion of serotonin brain concentrations, as well as depression in activity of this neurotransmitter, appears to augment chlorpromazine-induced hypothermia (Lin 1979).

Other important effects of chlorpromazine apart from its central influences are its adrenergic blocking action in conjunction with weak anticholinergic, antihistaminic, and antispasmodic effects. Chlorpromazine also potentiates the effect of atropine sulfate, analgesics, hypnotics, and local and general anesthetics. Although the blocking effect of local anesthetics is enhanced by chlorpromazine, its use is contraindicated in regional (epidural and intrathecal) anesthetic procedures due to potentiation of arterial hypotensive effects of local anesthetics.

In the dog, but not in the cat, chlorpromazine is effective in antagonizing apomorphine-induced emesis. It also protects against vomiting induced by morphine but is ineffective against IV copper sulfate, digitalis glycosides, veratrum, and oral copper sulfate. The antiemetic effect of chlorpromazine in dogs is related to selective depression of the emetic chemoreceptor trigger zone located in the brain stem. Chlorpromazine in a dose of 0.5 mg/kg is used for antiemetic action in the dog; the route of administration was unspecified by Willard (1985). It was probably given parenterally (i.e., by the intramuscular or intravenous route).

Paradoxically, chlorpromazine is an antidysrhythmic agent by preventing the stimulant effects of epinephrine and norepinephrine upon the heart. However, cardiac dysrhythmias are induced in the unanesthetized and anesthetized dog by either chlorpromazine or promazine in parenteral doses ranging from 2.5 to 5 mg/kg (Santos-Martinez et al. 1972). Atropinization reverts the dysrhythmia to characteristic anticholinergic effects such as sinus and atrial tachycardia.

Effects of chlorpromazine upon metabolism and autonomic nervous activity under conditions of environmental temperature changes and other types of stress have been the target of many studies. In transportation of animals to abattoirs for slaughter, this so-called antistress effect of neuroleptics was investigated to reduce weight losses (shrinkage) and bruising in transport. This use is not approved by the US Food and Drug Administration (FDA) because of the possibility that tissue residues will persist above the accepted tolerance levels permitted in food for human consumption.

High doses of chlorpromazine in the cat produce tremors of one or more extremities or the head. Variable degrees of shivering, lethargy, relaxation of the anal sphincter, diarrhea, and diminution or loss of righting reflexes occur. Rigidity of extremities and trunk without evident alteration in postural and righting reflexes may also occur in the cat. Upon discontinuance of medication, rigidity and other side effects disappear within 10 days, and the cat appears to be fully recovered and normal.

In the horse, chlorpromazine produces undesirable effects in many animals and is no longer advocated in equine practice. After a few minutes of initial sedation following administration of the drug, the animal becomes unsteady, sinks backward on its hocks, and then lunges forward in an uncoordinated manner. The horse may stumble and fall, then stand and continue lunging and rearing. This violent reaction alternates with periods of sedation.

Experimentally, chlorpromazine induces significant antisecretory activity in the intestinal tract; it apparently inhibits intracellular calmodulin activity (Willard 1985). In piglets with experimental colibacillosis induced by *Escherichia coli* toxins, intramuscular (IM) chlorpromazine (1–5 mg/kg) significantly decreases intestinal fluid losses and shortens duration of diarrhea.

Administration. In most species, chlorpromazine is administered primarily by the IM and intravenous (IV) routes. IM injections are slower, somewhat irritating, and less reliable in action. In the rabbit, IM injection of chlorpromazine produces severe myositis, lameness, swelling, muscular atrophy, and paralysis. IM use of this drug is contraindicated in the rabbit for preanesthetic medication (Bree et al. 1971).

Metabolism and Elimination. Chlorpromazine is metabolized slowly in the dog. The biologic half-life is about 6 hours. In humans, and probably in the dog, hydroxylation in the 3 and 7 positions and conjugation with glucuronic acid represent the major metabolic pathways in degradation of chlorpromazine. Sulfoxide is the next important product of metabolic biotransformation of chlorpromazine. The sulfoxide form possesses about one-eighth the sedative action of the parent drug in the dog.

In mental patients, chlorpromazine and various metabolites may be detected in urine 6–18 months after termination of treatment (Jarvik 1970). In food-producing animals, drug residues may possibly persist in edible tissues for long periods; information on this subject is lacking.

Chlorpromazine stimulates hepatic microsomal enzyme activity in the rat (Aurori and Vesell 1974). Its administration for 3 days stimulates ethylmorphine *N*-demethylase activity to 135% of control values. Stimulation of both aniline hydroxylase activity and cytochrome P-450 content to levels of 150% of control values occurs following 3 days of treatment with chlorpromazine or promazine hydrochloride.

Little or no chlorpromazine is eliminated in urine of the dog. The primary excretory product is chlorpromazine sulfoxide, but only 10–15% of the dose is eliminated as such. In other species, there is little information about excretion patterns of chlorpromazine and its metabolites.

Limited studies of excretion patterns have been conducted in the horse following IM and oral administration of chlorpromazine (Weir and Sanford 1972). After IM injection, metabolites are detected in urine up to 96 hours. Following oral administration, metabolites are no longer detected after 80–96 hours. The percentage of the dose recovered in equine urine is low, with the average being 10% after IM and 27% after oral administration. Unconjugated metabolites excreted in the horse represented only 1–1.5% of the dose after either route of administration; these were excreted entirely as sulfoxide derivatives. Glucuronide-conjugated metabolites are predominantly excreted by the horse in a ratio to unconjugated metabolites of approximately 7:1 after IM injection and 18:1 after oral administration. Sulfate-conjugated metabolites make up about 5% of the total after oral administration but are detected only in trace amounts after IM injection. With use of spectroscopic analytical methodology, phenothiazine derivatives in the feces of horses are not detected (Weir and Sanford 1972).

In the goat, the concentration of chlorpromazine is higher in milk than in plasma (Nawaz and Rasmussen 1979). Renal clearance of chlorpromazine in goats is low due to extensive plasma protein binding (91–99%). The plasma elimination half-life of chlorpromazine (2.5 mg/kg) given as a single IV dose in the goat is 1.51 ± 0.48 hours (Nawaz 1981). It is suggested that a satisfactory IV regimen of chlorpromazine in the goat should be 2–3.5 mg/kg; this should produce a drug action lasting 5–6 hours.

Contraindications and Precautions. Administration of epinephrine is contraindicated whenever phenothiazines are used. Phenothiazine derivatives are contraindicated in epidural anesthetic procedures because they potentiate arterial hypotensive activity of local anesthetics. Their use in control of strychnine, pentylenetetrazol, and picrotoxin convulsive seizures is contraindicated because of their ineffectiveness. Additionally, phenothiazine derivatives lower the seizure threshold and increase intracranial pressure, particularly in patients with severe facial trauma (Short et al. 1984). Also, phenothiazines must not be used in patients with a history of seizures or if CNS excitation is present after traumatic episodes.

Package inserts of drug firms caution against use of phenothiazines when animals have been exposed to organophosphates because they may potentiate toxicity of the organophosphates. Repeated administration of chlorpromazine and promazine increases toxicity of parathion in the rat. The anthelmintic phenothiazine does not seem to potentiate toxic effects of organophosphates such as malathion, coumaphos, ronnel, crufomate, dichlorvos, and others (Schlinke and Palmer 1973). In addition, caution against use of phenothiazines in conjunction with procaine hydrochloride is listed on package inserts; the activity of procaine may also be potentiated.

Use of chlorpromazine alone in the horse is contraindicated because of violent incoordination and excitement that often occur following administration. In the air transport of horses, administration of phenothiazines appears to be contraindicated because of variable effects that may be produced, such as incoordination, anxiety, and excitement.

Precautions in use of phenothiazine derivatives include their careful use in debilitated and cardiac disease patients. Caution must be taken in animals suffering from hypovolemic shock as well as those that have sympathetic blockade following epidural anesthesia.

Mixing glycopyrrolate in the same syringe with phenothiazine derivatives or diazepam is contraindicated (Short et al. 1984).

TOXICITY. In the dog, a subcutaneous (SC) dose of 1.5 mg/kg chlorpromazine produces no gross signs of toxicity. However, when the dose is administered intravenously, moderate depression and ataxia occur, which last 6–12 hours. When an IV dose of 3 mg/kg is injected, marked CNS depression and ataxia are noted for 24–48 hours.

The toxicity of physostigmine and dichlorvos are increased by chlorpromazine (Michalek and Stavinoha 1978). Physostigmine is a carbamate anticholinesterase agent, and dichlorvos is an organophosphate compound that inhibits cholinesterase activity. In vitro, chlorpromazine is a weak inhibitor of specific acetylcholinesterase and a rather potent inhibitor of pseudocholinesterase. Inhibition of cholinesterase by phenothiazine derivatives is reversible; it is not reversible when the enzyme is inhibited by organophosphates.

In vivo, chlorpromazine potentiates toxicity of the herbicide paraquat (Siddik et al. 1979). The potentiating mechanism of increased toxicity remains unknown.

Chlorpromazine in high doses produces cleft lip and cleft palate in mouse fetuses (Walker and Patterson 1974). The mouse appears to be more susceptible than the rat or rabbit to teratogenic effects of phenothiazine derivatives (Szabo and Brent 1974). Of six phenothiazine derivatives administered to the rabbit, none induced teratogenic or structural malformations in fetuses. Pregnant mice treated with high doses of phenothiazines eat less and gain less weight. Interestingly, limitation in food and water consumption of pregnant mice to a similar degree while receiving phenothiazines leads to an even higher incidence of cleft palate. Maternal nutritional deprivation results in retardation of fetal growth and may also affect development of the palate adversely (Szabo and Brent 1974). This raises the possibility that other drugs capable of inducing teratogenic effects in the mouse act principally by reduction in food and water intake; thus the embryopathy may be a secondary effect.

Limited studies in the rhesus monkey indicate that phenothiazines do not induce cleft palate or any other congenital defect. In domestic animals, data are lacking regarding effects of phenothiazines on pregnancy and fetal development. Clinical experience in domestic animals indicates that phenothiazine derivatives do not produce structural anomalies during fetal development. However, caution should be exercised in use of these agents during pregnancy; e.g., behavioral teratogenic effects appear to be produced in offspring (rats) that have been exposed perinatally to chlorpromazine (Taub and Peters 1978). Chlorpromazine given to newborn rats produces long-lasting alterations in serotonin and 5-hydroxyindoleacetic acid levels in several brain regions. It is not known to what extent these alterations may affect temperament, learning ability, neurologic activity, or other functions in adulthood.

In the Beagle and American Foxhound, chlorpromazine given orally at 30 mg/kg/day produces ocular lesions within 73 days in both breeds, whether exposed to natural daylight or maintained under ultraviolet-free artificial light (Barron et al. 1972). In the Beagle, an irreversible retinopathy can be induced in less than 4 months following daily oral doses of 30 mg/kg chlorpromazine (Mason 1977). Granular corneal deposits are produced by chlorpromazine and persist for many weeks in the dog even after withdrawal or discontinuance of treatment.

In mice, ocular lesions (toxic retinopathy) are not seen in albino animals following chlorpromazine administration. The retinopathy is related to affinity of chlorpromazine for melanin structures of the eye. In pregnant mice, radiolabeled chlorpromazine rapidly crosses the placenta and accumulates in the eyes of both fetuses and mothers (Ullberg et al. 1970). Marked radioactivity remains in tissues of the eye for 5 months after the drug had been eliminated from other tissues.

Clinically, phenothiazines are used intermittently and usually do not entail a protracted period of therapeutic use in veterinary medicine. The likelihood that ocular lesions would develop under short-term therapeutic use is improbable.

Experimental phototoxicity can be induced in laboratory animals following administration of chlorpromazine in the presence of black-light irradiation (Akin et al. 1979). Although phototoxic reactions in animals do not appear to be an important clinical problem, those with scanty hair and white hair probably should not receive excessive exposure to sunlight during treatment with phenothiazines.

CLINICAL USE

DOGS AND CATS. Chlorpromazine is approved as a prescription item by the FDA for use only in the dog and cat. At one time, chlorpromazine was the most extensively used neuroleptic agent in these species; however, promazine and acepromazine are now preferred.

Clinically, chlorpromazine has been used in the dog and cat at 0.55–4.4 mg/kg by IV injection for immediate effect. The sedative effect is especially helpful in nervous or aggressive animals. By the IM route of administration, the dose recommended is 1.1–6.6 mg/kg. The oral dose recommended consists of 1 tablet containing 10 mg/3.2 kg or 1 tablet containing 25 mg/7.7 kg. For all routes of administration (IV, IM, oral), chlorpromazine is administered 1–4 times daily, depending on the size of the dose used within the ranges given and needs of the patients.

For preanesthetic purposes, chlorpromazine should be injected intramuscularly 1–1.5 hours prior to anesthesia for surgery at a dose not to exceed 1.1 mg/kg. Clinical effects are prominent for 4–5 hours, but total action may persist for 24 hours. Premedication with chlorpromazine decreases the amount of barbiturate anesthetic (thiopental sodium) required to produce anesthesia by approximately 50% but does not alter duration of anesthesia (Hatch 1967). However, the combination of atropine and chlorpromazine has been shown to reduce the amount of thiopental needed by about 50% but increases sleep time by 33%.

The most consistent clinical effects of chlorpromazine premedication include drowsiness and disinclination to move. When aroused, the animal takes a normal interest in its surroundings. Body temperature may fall several hours later. The pulse rate does not change appreciably nor is respiration markedly depressed.

A claim has been made that chlorpromazine has antiemetic action in the cat and dog. This is questionable in the cat because chlorpromazine fails to inhibit apomorphine-induced emesis; in the dog, chlorpromazine does prevent emesis induced by apomorphine. However, emesis is not prevented by chlorpromazine in animals that are subjected to vestibular stimulation.

FOOD-PRODUCING SPECIES. Use of phenothiazines in food-producing animals has not been approved by the FDA because of the possibility that residues may persist in edible tissues such as meat, milk, and eggs. A tissue tolerance level for chlorpromazine has not been published, but one has been published for promazine.

Chlorpromazine (0.2 mg/kg) administered intramuscularly is considered to be the drug of choice of the neuroleptic agents for preanesthetic use in cattle (Bowen 1976).

BREEDING ANIMALS. Chlorpromazine is sometimes used in animals not scheduled for food use or slaughter, e.g., for breeding. The pig is easily restrained for IV injections 45–60 minutes following IM administration (1.1 mg/kg). Prior to induction of anesthesia with barbiturates, an IM dose of 2–4 mg/kg has been used.

Chlorpromazine is recommended in excitable sows following farrowing, especially in those reluctant to accept their newborn. IV doses of 75–100 mg have been used in sows weighing 125–136 kg. If the drug is used immediately prior to parturition, the sow will farrow naturally. To prevent venous thrombosis, chlorpromazine should be given in dilute solution when it is used intravenously (Jones 1972). Chlorpromazine has been useful as an adjunct to treatment of agalactia, which is a frequent clinical problem following parturition in swine (Lewis and Oakley 1971).

EXOTIC SPECIES. Chlorpromazine has been used in capture of African lions and as an adjunct to restraint and anesthesia in lions (Harthoorn et al. 1971). For induction of neuroleptanalgesia in bears, the drug is administered via a projectile syringe dart in combination with analgesic preparations (Kuntze 1967). Neuroleptics are effective agents in zoo practice; IM doses of chlorpromazine recommended for several species are as follows:

Species	*Dose (mg/kg)*
Tiger	4.0
Jackal	2.0
Bear	2.5
Rhesus monkey	1.4–2.0
Dromedary	1.5–2.5
Water buffalo	2.5
Bison	2.5

Chlorpromazine has been used in reptiles intramuscularly (10 mg/kg) prior to barbiturate anesthesia (Calderwood 1971).

Promazine Hydrochloride. Chemically, *Promazine Hydrochloride,* USP (Sparine), is 10-(3-diethylaminopropyl) phenothiazine monohydrochloride (Fig. 14.3). It is used in the hydrochloride form, and 1 g is soluble in about 3 mL water. The drug is incompatible with alkalies, heavy metals, and oxidizing agents.

Although promazine has been used in nearly all domestic animals, monkeys, and small laboratory rodents, it is approved by the FDA for use only in the dog, cat, and horse. Promazine cannot be used in animals intended for food; a zero tolerance has been established in tissues of food-producing animals.

ADMINISTRATION. Following IV administration of promazine, the onset of action in the dog is generally within 5 minutes; following IM injection, about 20–30 minutes elapses before effective tranquilization results. Onset of action may be 5–10 minutes slower in large species. Duration of action is dose dependent and can vary within 4–6 hours.

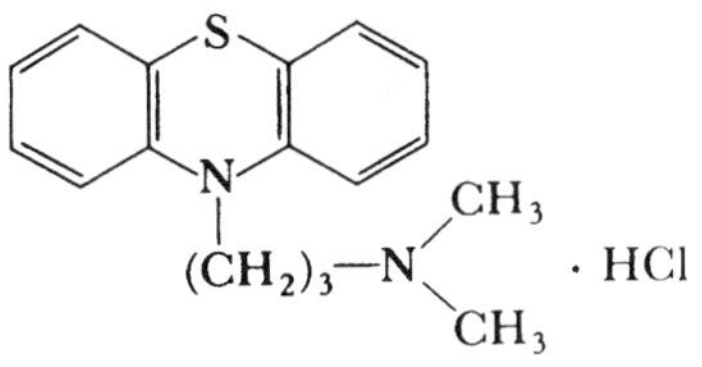

S
N
$(CH_2)_3$—N
CH_3
CH_3
· HCl

Promazine Hydrochloride

FIG. 14.3

METABOLISM AND ELIMINATION. Excretion patterns of promazine have been studied in the horse (Weir and Sanford 1972). When 10 mg/kg are given orally, the excretion rate reaches maximums of about 55 mg/hr within 8 hours of dosing and about 25 mg/hr between 16 and 24 hours. Metabolites cannot be detected in urine after 72 hours (Weir and Sanford 1972). The percentage of promazine recovered in urine averages 10%. Glucuronide-conjugated metabolites are predominant; conjugated metabolites are excreted almost entirely in the form of sulfoxide.

Following IM administration of 0.1–0.6 mg/kg promazine, Maylin (1978) detected four metabolites in urine of Standardbred mares; the metabolites were 2,3-hydroxypromazine, promazine *N*-oxide, promazine *N*-oxide sulfoxide, and 5,3-hydroxynorpromazine.

CONTRAINDICATIONS AND PRECAUTIONS. In general, contraindications described for chlorpromazine apply to promazine. However, unlike chlorpromazine, promazine can be administered to horses with less likelihood of producing excitation. Some animals may be unusually reactive to noise and may respond violently to disturbances.

Caution must be taken to avoid intracarotid injection of promazine; otherwise the horse may become violent and exhibit muscular tremors, stertorous respiration, and pupillary dilation; eventually recumbency and convulsions appear (Christian et al. 1974). Large-caliber needles, especially 14 or 16 gauge, favor pulsatile flow of arterial blood, whereas smaller-bore needles do not, with the result that walls of the external jugular vein are easily passed through and the external carotid artery is inadvertently penetrated with small-bore needles.

CLINICAL USE

DOGS. The major use of neuroleptics, including promazine, is as a preanesthetic agent to facilitate handling through its sedative action. This permits smoother induction of anesthesia and reduces the amount of anesthetic required by 30–50%. In the dog, the dose recommended by the parenteral routes (IM or IV) is 2–6 mg/kg. For antiemetic use, the above dose should be reduced by one-third to one-half (Leash 1969). Promazine may be repeated as necessary at 4- to 6-hour intervals.

Promazine is indicated in animals manifesting nervous behavior and excitability. It has value in alleviation of self-inflicted mutilation associated with otitis, pruritis, and eczemic conditions. The drug assists in handling of animals for radiographic diagnosis or therapy and in other procedures where restraint is required.

Promazine (6.6 mg/kg IV) has been used for cesarean section in 1- to 6-year-old Beagles in conjunction with infiltration of 6 mL 2% lidocaine hydrochloride or mepivacaine hydrochloride into the abdominal wall (Gupta et al. 1970). If this dose of promazine does not produce complete relaxation, more is given subcutaneously at the rate of 2.2–4.4 mg/kg for the latent effect during surgery. Of the puppies delivered by this procedure, Gupta et al. reported that 98% lived and nursed with no signs of tranquilization. The oral dose of promazine recommended in dogs and cats is 2.2–6.6 mg/kg every 4–6 hr.

CATS. Clinical indications and recommended parenteral dosage for the cat are similar to those for the dog. Compared to chlorpromazine, twice as much promazine is generally required to produce a comparable effect in the cat. Arterial hypotension and other cardiovascular effects produced by promazine in the cat are considerably less than those of chlorpromazine (Clifford and Soma 1969).

One of the therapeutic claims made for promazine is that its administration before a vermifuge will prevent emesis in the cat. This is debatable because studies have shown that a related congener, i.e., chlorpromazine, fails to antagonize emesis induced by apomorphine in cats.

A combination of promazine and ketamine hydrochloride has been advocated for use in the cat (see clinical use of ketamine in Chap. 12).

HORSES. The recommended dose of promazine in the horse is 0.44–1.1 mg/kg via the IV or IM route. When 0.88 mg/kg promazine is administered intramuscularly to a horse weighing 454 kg (total dose of 400 mg), the effect of the drug is apparent in 10–15 minutes and lasts about 0.5 hour (Fraser 1967). According to Fraser, promazine takes effect less rapidly than acepromazine.

Promazine is also useful in facilitating dental operations such as “floating the teeth” of horses. In loading and surface transportation of horses, promazine is valuable. Heath (1978) prefers not to give foals phenothiazines because they usually sleep all day before recovery occurs.

Promazine has been recommended for treatment of tetanus in horses. However, side effects of phenothiazines include stimulation of extrapyramidal neuronal pathways. It would seem that these effects of promazine and other phenothiazines would result in their contraindication as therapeutic agents for treatment of tetanus. Many clinicians now favor use of diazepam in treatment of tetanus.

Promazine has also been used as a treatment for equine colic. However, severe arterial hypotension may occur in the presence of devitalized bowel and impending shock.

Promazine is used in conjunction with chloral hydrate and ultrashort-acting barbiturates in the horse. The procedure consists of administering promazine intravenously in a dose of 0.7–1.1 mg/kg. Ten minutes following IV injection, 7% chloral hydrate is administered intravenously at a dose of 333 mL/454 kg. After casting the animal, a catheter is placed in the external jugular vein so that a barbiturate can be injected to maintain surgical anesthesia. Barbiturates should not be used intravenously in the horse without preanesthetic sedation. An IV dose of 0.55 mg/kg promazine is recommended for preanesthesia. Promazine has been used in combination with ketamine for induction of anesthesia in horses (see clinical use of ketamine in Chap. 12).

Promazine is also provided for oral use in the feed. The oral dose is 0.99–1.98 mg/kg. Promazine must not be used in horses intended for human food.

CATTLE. The granular form of promazine can be used in feed of nonlactating cattle (1.65–2.75 mg/kg). In the opinion of Garner et al. (1975), a smoother recovery from general anesthesia occurs when promazine is not used as a preanesthetic agent.

Unless the drug has been withdrawn from feed for at least 72 hours prior to slaughter, animals cannot be sold for human consumption. The established tolerance level for promazine in food is zero.

SWINE. Promazine (2 mg/kg) along with atropine (0.07–0.09 mg/kg) and meperidine hydrochloride (1–2 mg/kg) is useful as a preanesthetic in swine used for experimental surgical purposes (Booth 1969). Promazine provides a mild tranquilizing effect and assists in restraint of the pig prior to general anesthesia.

RABBITS. Promazine has been used in combination with ketamine for induction of anesthesia in rabbits (see clinical use of ketamine in Chap. 12).

LABORATORY ANIMALS. A combination of promazine and ketamine has been used in rats and mice for induction of short-term anesthesia (see clinical use of ketamine in Chap. 12).

EXOTIC SPECIES. Promazine has been used in tranquilizing bears. IM injection of 4.4 mg/kg promazine is effective in potentiating morphine. Promazine has been useful in combination with other drugs for immobilization of bears as well as other exotic species (Seal and Erickson 1969).

Preparturient and postparturient use of promazine has been successful in a hippopotamus weighing about 2273 kg (Graham-Jones 1962); 4.4 mg/kg, or a total of 10 g, were used in the feed and administered daily for 1 week prior to parturition, which occurred normally, with survival of the calf.

Acepromazine Maleate. *Acepromazine Maleate,* INN (Atravet, Notensil, Promace), formerly called acetylpromazine, is approved by the FDA for use in the dog, cat, and horse. This phenothiazine derivative is extensively used in veterinary medicine. Acepromazine is 2-acetyl-10-(3-dimethylaminopropyl) phenothiazine (Fig. 14.4). The drug is a yellow, odorless, crystalline powder with a bitter taste; the powder melts at 135–138° C.

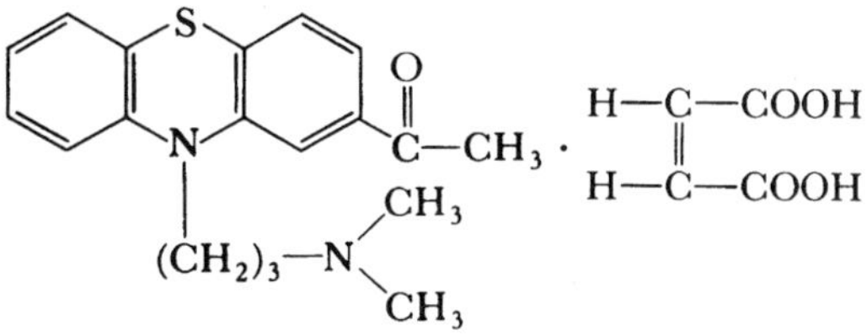

Acepromazine Maleate

FIG. 14.4

PHARMACOLOGIC CONSIDERATIONS. Most of the pharmacologic effects of acepromazine are similar to those of other phenothiazine derivatives. It is more potent than chlorpromazine and promazine and is effective parenterally in small doses. The contraindications are generally the same as those for promazine and chlorpromazine.

Experimentally, acepromazine decreases arterial blood pressure in the dog 3 minutes after 1 mg/kg is administered by the IM route (Popovic et al. 1972); this effect lasts 2 hours. A significant increase in central venous pressure occurs 90 minutes after administration of the drug and generally persists for the duration of its effect. Intermittent bradycardia also occurs (Popovic et al. 1972). Sinoatrial (SA) arrest occurs at 3.5 minutes following injection of acepromazine and lasts about 8 seconds; recovery is spontaneous, with no apparent permanent cardiac injury. Atropine (0.045 mg/kg) should be used in conjunction with acepromazine prior to administration of a general anesthetic to minimize or prevent vagal effects that may induce bradycardia or SA arrest. IV acepromazine (0.033 or 0.067 mg/kg) does not induce cardiac arrhythmia in horses anesthetized with halothane (Steffey et al. 1985).

Following IV administration of acepromazine in doses of 0.11, 0.55, and 1.1 mg/kg, decrease in arterial pressure occurs in the dog (Coulter et al. 1981). Interestingly, the decline in pressure was not dose related; the lowest IV dose (0.11 mg/kg) appeared to reduce arterial pressure as markedly as the highest dose (1.1 mg/kg). The results of Coulter et al. are in contrast to those found in the dog by Muir and Hubbell (1985); they found that an IV dose of acepromazine less than 0.4 mg/kg is not likely to produce significant changes in the arterial pressure of healthy dogs.

Doses (0.05, 0.125, and 0.25 mg/kg) of IV acepromazine in the dog decrease the mean arterial pressure from 2.3 ± 6.0 to 16.8 ± 14.2% (Ludders et al. 1983). Phenylephrine, an α-adrenergic agonist, antagonizes the hypotensive action of acepromazine; an IV dose of 0.088 mg/kg (a clinically recommended dose) or higher is necessary to increase the mean arterial pressure. Phenylephrine has a duration of 20 minutes after IV administration.

In the dog, acepromazine blocks or prevents arrhythmic and ventricular fibrillatory actions of epinephrine and halothane (Muir et al. 1975). It markedly decreases respiratory rate in the dog. Despite this, however, no significant alteration results in the P_aCO_2, pH, P_aO_2, and oxyhemoglobin saturation (Popovic et al. 1972). Significant drops in level of hemoglobin concentration are first observed 45 minutes after drug administration; this persists for at least 2 hours.

Administration of acepromazine (0.09 mg/kg) intravenously in the horse induces an insignificant decrease in heart rate and cardiac output when compared with baseline or control values (Muir et al. 1979). Mean pulmonary arterial pressure does not decrease significantly from control values following this dose. However, the mean central venous pressure, mean aortic pressure, and respiratory rate in the horse decrease significantly 15 minutes following injection. Although the respiratory rate is decreased by acepromazine, the arterial pH, P_aO_2, and P_aCO_2 are not significantly different from control values (Muir et al. 1979).

Acepromazine in an extremely low IV dose (0.002 mg/kg) produces a significant effect upon the hematocrit or PCV; this is the most sensitive pharmacologic response induced by acepromazine in the horse (Ballard et al. 1982). This is followed by changes in penile extension and depression of the respiratory rate, which are the next most sensitive responses to acepromazine in the horse.

In general, the effect of acepromazine upon reduction of the hematocrit in the horse is dose dependent. For example, an IV dose as low as 0.01 mg/kg reduces the hematocrit by 25% within 30 minutes after acepromazine administration (Ballard et al. 1982); higher doses may reduce the hematocrit as much as 50%. Duration of the effect upon the hematocrit may be 12 or more hours before the PCV recovers to normal; e.g., mean hematocrit values recover to control levels by 12 hours after IV doses of 0.05 mg/kg and 21 hours after 0.15 mg/kg (Parry and Anderson 1983). The decrease in hematocrit is primarily due to splenic sequestration of red blood cells.

The hypotensive action of acepromazine in the horse is related to both the dose and the route of administration (Parry et al. 1982). In healthy horses, the arterial pressure remains significantly below control values for more than 6 hours after an IM injection of 0.025 mg/kg. According to Parry et al. (1982), individual horses vary in responsiveness to acepromazine. For example, one horse decreased from a resting value of 112/82 to 91/55 mm Hg at 1 hour after IV administration of acepromazine (0.1 mg/kg) and returned to 111/79 mm Hg in 4 hours. In another animal after the same IV dose, the arterial pressure decreased from 132/94 to 61/45 mm Hg at 15 minutes after injection; the pressure remained below 87/67 mm Hg for 6 hours after injection and recovered to normal (125/90 mm Hg) at 15 hours.

In general, greater tranquilization induced by acepromazine results in greater arterial hypotension. Thus acepromazine is a dangerous drug in circumstances where circulatory embarrassment or acute circulatory failure is a possibility (Parry and Anderson 1983).

In treatment of equine colic, an adequate blood volume and arterial pressure are necessary before acepromazine or related derivatives can be safely used; most fatal colic cases are probably due to cardiovascular collapse. Considering the marked arterial hypotension and prolonged effect of acepromazine in healthy horses and the speed with which hypotension can occur in colic cases, use of acepromazine or other phenothiazines at any stage in treatment of equine colic is seriously questioned (Parry and Anderson 1983).

Arterial hypotension after administration of acepromazine also occurs in the healthy cat. When administered intramuscularly at 0.11 mg/kg, the arterial pressure declines 30% within the first 10 minutes postinjection (Colby and Sanford 1981). Acepromazine in combination with ketamine induces a shorter depressant effect upon the mean arterial pressure, heart, and respiratory rates than ketamine-xylazine combinations (Sanford and Colby 1982).

After IV injection, acepromazine is distributed extensively in the horse (Vd = 6.6 L/kg) and binds extensively (>99%) to plasma proteins (Ballard et al. 1982). Plasma concentrations of acepromazine (after an IV injection of 0.3 mg/kg) decline with an α-phase half-life of 4.2 minutes; the β-phase, or elimination, half-life is about 185 minutes.

Acepromazine in IM doses of 1.1 and 1.65 mg/kg respectively prevents occurrence of halothane-induced malignant hyperthermia in 40 and 73% of susceptible pigs (McGrath et al. 1981). For additional information on halothane-induced malignant hyperthermia, see Chap. 11.

Following IM administration of acepromazine (0.01–0.1 mg/kg) in mature Standardbred mares, metabolites are present in urine (Maylin 1978). The metabolites are 2-(1-hydroxyethyl) promazine sulfoxide, 2-(1-hydroxyethyl) promazine, 7-hydroxyacetylpromazine, and 2-(1-hydroxyethyl)-7-hydroxypromazine.

CONTRAINDICATIONS AND PRECAUTIONS. Clinically, a few case reports have revealed adverse reactions following administration of acepromazine in dogs (Garland and White 1968; White 1968). Within 5–10 minutes after IM injection of 0.55 mg/kg acepromazine, sudden collapse has been observed. Initially, animals manifested apnea, then a slow pulse and unconsciousness. A fatal interaction involving Diathal, thiamylal, and acepromazine has been reported in the dog (Webb et al. 1983). See discussion under the toxicity of thiamylal in Chap. 12 of the 7th edition of this text. Adverse behavioral alterations have been observed in use of acepromazine in the dog; aggressiveness and vicious behavior are sometimes manifested after administration (Waechter 1982).

According to Dodman et al. (1984), acepromazine can produce complications in certain conditions: (1) In most types of shock, use of acepromazine in low cardiac output states or hypervolemia can result in a critical drop in arterial pressure and venous return owing to its α-adrenergic blocking action. (2) CNS seizure threshold may be lowered by acepromazine, which can trigger seizures in susceptible animals. It should not be

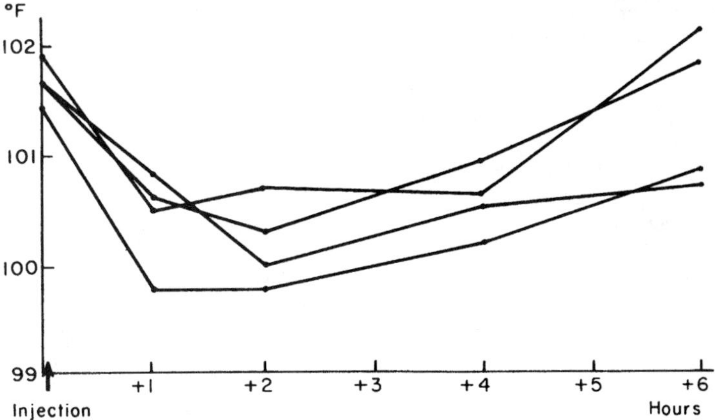

FIG. 14.5.—Changes in rectal temperature of four dogs following IM injection of acepromazine at a dose of 0.25 mg/kg (Pugh 1964).

used in these animals or animals undergoing myelographic procedures. (3) Acepromazine can cause syncope associated with high vagal tone and subsequent bradycardia; this occurs in brachycephalic breeds, particularly in Boxers. The response may be prevented by administering a low dose of acepromazine and a concomitant injection of an anticholinergic agent such as atropine.

Caution in administration of acepromazine to weak, debilitated, aged, and cardiac disease patients must be observed to minimize adverse effects. Also, a drug interaction with organophosphates must be avoided because toxicity of the phenothiazines is enhanced. Mixing glycopyrrolate in the same syringe with phenothiazines or diazepam is contraindicated (Short et al. 1984).

CLINICAL USE. The primary use of acepromazine has been as a preanesthetic agent in the dog, cat, and horse. It markedly potentiates barbiturates and facilitates handling and restraint of animals.

DOGS. Acepromazine may be administered by the IV, IM, SC, or oral route in the dog. For preanesthetic use, the IM dose (0.05–0.1 mg/kg) is considerably lower than that used for ordinary restraint purposes (Dodman et al. 1984) (see below). The recommended dose of acepromazine for the parenteral routes ranges from 0.55 to 1.1 mg/kg; for oral administration in tablet form, the recommended dose is 0.55–2.2 mg/kg. All doses may be repeated, depending on degree and duration of tranquilization required. Usually it is necessary to repeat the dose every 6–8 hours to maintain tranquilization. Because of the potent effect of acepromazine, most clinicians generally use dosages below those recommended above in the dog. Since there is individual variation in the responses induced by acepromazine, it is best to begin on the conservative side in dose administration. If necessary, more drug can always be given later.

According to Pugh (1964), oral administration of 1–3 mg/kg acepromazine in a single dose produces deep sedation in the dog. This is also accompanied by lethargy and reduced motor activity as evidenced by some posterior ataxia. Onset of the effect is noted by changes in facial expression. Skin overlying the frontal portion of the skull appears more pliable and wrinkled, the upper eyelid droops (ptosis), and the nictitating membrane is relaxed and protruded. The first indication of posterior ataxia is usually evident at this time. Recumbency soon follows, and the animal frequently goes into a somnolent state.

Clinical signs of acepromazine usually begin to regress after 3–4 hours but may be present after 7 hours (Pugh 1964). As in other species, a drop in rectal temperature occurs. This effect is shown in Fig. 14.5.

For preanesthetic use, the dose of acepromazine is 0.11 mg/kg intramuscularly (Rosin 1974). Also, atropine (0.045–0.066 mg/kg) is administered by the IM or SC route. After the peak effect (usually 15–20 minutes) of acepromazine has been attained, thiamylal is then administered to effect to produce general anesthesia; this permits endotracheal intubation so that inhalant anesthetics may be administered. The dose of thiamylal necessary to produce general anesthesia is reduced by about 50%. Like other phenothiazines (chlorpromazine, promazine), acepromazine produces a moderate degree of blockade of the α-adrenergic receptors. This effect is believed to assist in prevention of renal ischemia and maintenance of adequate kidney function during general anesthesia as well as in minimization of postsurgical uremia (Rosin 1974).

Adequate sedation is provided by 0.04 mg/kg acepromazine in the dog prior to induction with thiamylal; the route of administration was not specified (Rutherford 1983). It was probably given intramuscularly.

According to Rutherford, no more than a total of 3 mg acepromazine is given to any dog, and large dogs may be sensitive to a total of 2 mg.

Acepromazine in a large IM dose (0.3 mg/kg) has been used in dogs 20 minutes prior to euthanasia with carbon monoxide (Dallaire and Chalifoux 1985). It improves the esthetic aspects of the use of carbon monoxide in euthanasia by decreasing vocalization, agitation, and other effects in the dog.

An IV combination of acepromazine (0.2 mg/kg) and ketamine (10 mg/kg) is useful for clinical anesthesia in the dog if stimulation of cardiovascular function is not necessary or desirable (Farver et al. 1986; see clinical uses of ketamine in Chap. 12). This combination probably should not be used in dogs predisposed to arterial hypotension or respiratory depression.

For neuroleptanalgesic purposes, acepromazine (0.11 mg/kg) has been administered (route of administration unspecified, probably IM) in combination with oxymorphone (0.2 mg/kg). This permits intubation and use of halothane-oxygen for induction of anesthesia (Short et al. 1984).

Acepromazine (0.1 mg/kg) is recommended for antiemetic use in the dog. The route of administration was not specified by Willard (1985); it was probably by the IM or IV route to be effective immediately. This dose of acepromazine is ineffective in preventing apomorphine-induced emesis. An IM dose of 0.5 mg/kg does not block the emetic action of an IV dose of 0.04 mg/kg apomorphine in dogs (Keith et al. 1981).

Acepromazine in large doses has been recommended for treatment of metaldehyde poisoning in the dog. However, diazepam is preferable for control of convulsive seizures induced by metaldehyde. A side effect of phenothiazine neuroleptics, including acepromazine, is stimulation of extrapyramidal motor pathways. Thus acepromazine would lower the convulsive threshold and is not the drug of choice for treatment of metaldehyde toxicity.

CATS. Acepromazine may be administered by the IV, IM, SC, or oral route in the cat. The recommended dose for the parenteral and oral routes ranges from 1.1 to 2.2 mg/kg. It is usually necessary to repeat the dose every 8–12 hours to maintain tranquilization. Many of the drug effects produced in the dog are also seen in the cat (see above). Since acepromazine is a potent phenothiazine derivative, most clinicians generally use dosages below those recommended in the cat. It is best to begin on the conservative side of dose administration. Larger doses can always be given later to produce the desired effect.

Clinically, acepromazine is important as a preanesthetic agent in the cat. The dose successfully used in clinical practice is 0.11 mg/kg administered intramuscularly (Rosin 1974). Atropine (0.045–0.066 mg/kg) is also injected intramuscularly or subcutaneously. General anesthesia with an ultrashort-acting barbiturate or inhalant anesthetic may be administered 15–20 minutes after the peak effect of acepromazine has been reached. As in the dog, the amount of general anesthetic is reduced significantly.

IV acepromazine (0.11 mg/kg) has been used in the cat with IV ketamine (11 mg/kg) to provide skeletal muscle relaxation and a smoother recovery (Wright 1982). However, in a double-blind study, acepromazine did nothing to contribute to the effect of ketamine in the cat; according to Chase (1977), piperacetazine hydrochloride is more useful.

HORSES. Acepromazine must not be used in horses intended for human consumption. It may be administered intravenously or intramuscularly. The recommended preanesthetic dose ranges from 0.02 to 0.05 mg/kg.

Because of the potent effect of acepromazine, most clinicians use dosages below those specified by manufacturers. MacKenzie and Snow (1977) noted that the tranquilizing action of acepromazine may last for 24 hours in the horse; this is considerably longer than the responses (i.e., 8 hours) claimed by the manufacturers' recommended dosages.

According to Fraser (1967), acepromazine administered at an IM dose of 0.066 mg/kg is effective in 2–3 minutes. Clinical signs are drooping of the upper eyelid, slight protrusion of the nictitating membrane, and dropping of the head below its normal level. An overdose of the drug produces ataxia and may interfere with clinical procedures.

Acepromazine reduces excitability so that the animal can be easily handled; e.g., rectal examination and exploration of the genitalia are facilitated. Some clinicians have dispensed oral acepromazine tablets to provide tranquilization of horses for travel in a trailer. The dose for this purpose is 2–4 mg/45 kg; tablets of the drug are generally buried in a piece of apple and administered 30–45 minutes prior to loading.

Tranquilization of dangerous animals may lead to a false sense of security. Painful procedures should be avoided because phenothiazines provide little, if any, analgesic effect.

Horses medicated with acepromazine retain auditory and visual acuity; loud sounds or rapid movements should be avoided.

Acepromazine even in high therapeutic doses infrequently produces recumbency. Although horses may appear to be somnolent, they will usually remain standing. In the event the animal lies down, it can ordinarily be persuaded to stand. Risk of the animal stepping or falling on the attending veterinarian is minimal. Retention of coordination and alertness in the horse is important, since many diagnostic and surgical procedures must be conducted upon a standing animal (Ballard et al. 1982).

An important use of acepromazine is as a preanesthetic. A total dose of 15 mg/454 kg, or 0.033 mg/kg, is administered intravenously and followed 10 minutes later with an IV injection of thiamylal (2.5–3 g/454 kg) (Shideler 1971). This permits endotracheal intubation so that an inhalant anesthetic can be administered for maintenance of surgical anesthesia.

Acepromazine is being used in treatment of equine colic. An IV dose of 0.066 mg/kg brings about prompt relief (Frank 1970). This effect is due to its antispasmodic activity. Partial blockade of the α-adrenergic receptors may possibly explain this antispasmodic effect. Adequate blood volume and arterial pressure are necessary before acepromazine or related derivatives can be used safely; most fatal colic cases are probably due to cardiovascular collapse or shock. Considering the marked arterial hypotensive effect of acepromazine in healthy horses and the rapidity with which hypotension can occur in colic cases, use of acepromazine at any stage in treatment of equine colic is seriously questioned (Parry and Anderson 1983).

Acepromazine in combination with meperidine, an analgesic and antispasmodic drug, is considered to be an effective neuroleptanalgesic agent in the horse (Jones 1972). The IV dose of the mixture is 100 mg acepromazine and 50 mg meperidine for animals weighing 454 kg; nervous and highly bred or excited animals receive a higher dose; calm, less excitable animals receive less of the mixture (Schauffler 1968). Since these agents may induce severe arterial hypotension, extreme caution is necessary in their use. This is particularly true in the presence of shock.

Acepromazine-methadone in combination with ketamine has been used in the horse. For detailed information on this combination of drugs, see the discussion on methadone in Chap. 13.

A combination of acepromazine and another analgesic agent (etorphine hydrochloride) has been advocated in the horse and other domestic animals in the UK (see Chap. 13). Acepromazine in a concentration of 10 mg/mL is combined with 2.45 mg/mL etorphine; this neuroleptanalgesic preparation is sometimes used for minor surgery (Jenkins 1972).

Priapism or penile prolapse occurs occasionally following use of phenothiazine neuroleptic agents; acepromazine is associated with this condition in the horse (Pearson and Weaver 1978). IV doses (0.04 and 0.1 mg/kg) induce essentially complete penile protrusion within 30 minutes after administration; at the higher dose, protrusion remains maximally distended up to about 100 minutes following administration (Tobin and Ballard 1979). The duration and extent of penile protrusion are dose related; a dose of acepromazine as low as 0.01 mg/kg induces penile prolapse (Ballard et al. 1982). At 0.4 mg/kg, prolapse occurs for 4 hours and does not retract completely until 10 hours after administration of acepromazine. Acepromazine-induced prolapse of the penis in a 3-year-old Thoroughbred gelding was corrected by a slow IV injection of 8 mg *Benztropine Mesylate,* USP (Cogentin); within 30 minutes after administration, the penis appeared normal, flaccid, and retracted (Sharrock 1982). According to Sharrock, it may be necessary to increase or repeat the benztropine dose in stallions.

Penile prolapse may in part be due to relaxation of retractor penis muscles, which are innervated by adrenergic nerve fibers. Relaxation may occur from the α-adrenergic blocking effects of acepromazine. Etorphine in combination with acepromazine may also contribute to the development of priapism. Of 7 horses with priapism following use of acepromazine, 5 had also received etorphine in combination with the phenothiazine neuroleptic agent (Pearson and Weaver 1978). Inasmuch as the penis is prolapsed and turgid following the sole use of etorphine and is flaccid following the use of only acepromazine, elevated blood pressure induced by etorphine has been suspected to be a contributory factor leading to penile paralysis. However, it is highly improbable that etorphine would increase the arterial pressure high enough to induce paralysis. During coitus the pressure generated in the corpus cavernosum penis is several thousand mm Hg and that in the corpus spongiosum penis is usually greater than 700 mm Hg (Beckett et al. 1973, 1975). With administration of acepromazine and etorphine in a combined mixture, arterial pressure does not increase; instead it may become dangerously hypotensive. Thus priapism still occurs following hypotension induced by the drug mixture. Consequently, an elevated arterial pressure seen with use of etorphine alone would not appear to be a contributory factor in development of priapism. Since difficulties are encountered with use of acepromazine in stallions, the drug should not be used in stud or breeding animals.

CATTLE. Acepromazine has not been approved by the FDA in food-producing animals because of the potential risk of residues in meat and milk products.

In the opinion of Garner et al. (1975), a smoother recovery from general anesthesia in cattle occurs when acepromazine is not used as a preanesthetic agent. A sedative dose (0.05–0.01 mg/kg) of acepromazine has been used in cattle by the IV, IM, or SC route (Howard 1981). According to Hubbell et al. (1986), acepromazine in an IV dose of 0.01–0.02 mg/kg or an IM dose of 0.03–0.1 mg/kg produces mild sedation. It is useful for calming nervous cattle when used in conjunction with local anesthesia for surgical procedures. It fails to induce sufficient sedation in control of unmanageable or hyperexcited cattle. Arterial blood pressure may be decreased severely after use of acepromazine in sick or debilitated cattle. Acepromazine is not recommended as a preanesthetic in calm cattle, and it may have little effect in cattle that do not tolerate restraint (Hubbell et al. 1986).

Caution in use of acepromazine in cattle is advised; more data are needed to determine its safety and efficacy. Death has occurred in cattle injected with acepromazine after prolonged transit. Transit under stressful conditions (in cold or hot weather, without water or feed, for long distances) increases the susceptibility and risk of animals to the arterial hypotensive action of acepromazine.

SWINE. For tranquilization or sedation, Anderson (1973) recommends IV administration of 0.03–0.1 mg/kg. As a preanesthetic agent, Benson and Thurmon

(1979) use acepromazine intramuscularly in a dose of 0.11–0.22 mg/kg; they do not recommend a total dose of more than 15 mg in any pig. According to McGrath (1984), IM morphine (1–2 mg/kg) in combination with IM acepromazine (0.05–0.2 mg/kg) can be substituted for the combination of fentanyl-droperidol (Innovar-Vet) in depressed or toxemic sows.

Acepromazine is also used in combination with ketamine for induction of anesthesia in miniature swine (see clinical uses of ketamine in Chap. 12).

SHEEP AND GOATS. Acepromazine (0.05–0.1 mg/kg) has been used in conjunction with ketamine (2–5 mg/kg) by the IM or IV route (McGrath 1984). For more information on use of these drugs in combination, see Chap. 12.

RABBITS. Acepromazine administered intramuscularly at 1 mg/kg will tranquilize the rabbit in about 10 minutes for 1–2 hours (Wood 1978).

Prochlorperazine Edisylate. *Prochlorperazine Edisylate,* USP (Darbazine, Compazine), is a piperazine derivative of phenothiazine (Fig. 14.6). Extrapyramidal symptoms, especially at high dosages, are more characteristic of piperazines than of nonpiperazine derivatives (e.g., chlorpromazine, promazine, acepromazine). The antiemetic properties of piperazine phenothiazine derivatives are greater than those of nonpiperazine derivatives.

Pharmacologically, the sedative effect of prochlorperazine is moderate compared to chlorpromazine and triflupromazine hydrochloride. Consequently, only a slight effect upon consciousness is elicited by prochlorperazine. The hypotensive and respiratory effects are low compared to promazine.

Prochlorperazine has been approved as an injectable preparation by the FDA for use in combination with isopropamide iodide, which is a potent, long-acting anticholinergic drug that suppresses both gastrointestinal (GI) motility and secretions for about 12 hours after a single oral dose. This injectable combination has been approved for use in the dog and cat.

PRECAUTIONS AND CONTRAINDICATIONS. Precautions and contraindications previously described for the phenothiazine neuroleptic agents are essentially similar for prochlorperazine. It is contraindicated in cases of glaucoma, stenosis or obstruction of the pylorus, and prostatic hypertrophy. Since extrapyramidal effects are marked following use of prochlorperazine, caution should be used in administering this drug to animals subject to convulsive disorders. Capsules (Neo-Darbazine) that contain neomycin must not be used in dogs that have renal disorders.

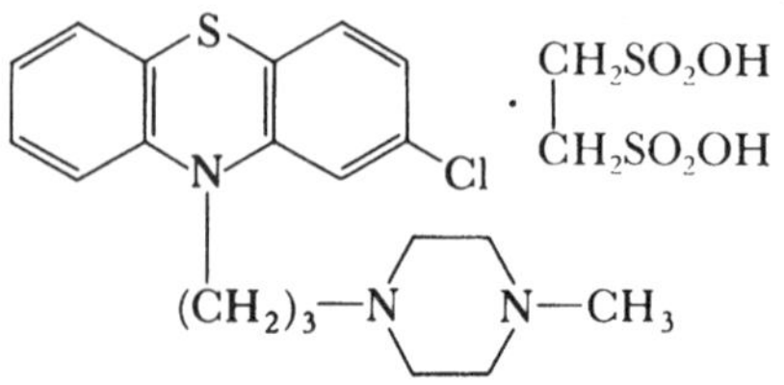

S, N, Cl, $(CH_2)_3$—N, N—CH_3, · CH_2SO_2OH | CH_2SO_2OH

Prochlorperazine Edisylate

FIG. 14.6

CLINICAL USE. In the dog (but not the cat) a sustained-release capsule for oral use has been approved by the FDA. The capsule contains prochlorperazine dimaleate and isopropamide to provide control of GI disturbances associated with emotional stress.

The injectable preparation contains 6 mg/mL of prochlorperazine edisylate or the equivalent of 4 mg prochlorperazine and 0.38 mg/mL isopropamide iodide or the equivalent of 0.28 mg isopropamide. The drug combination in the dog and cat is based on SC injection twice daily at a dosage as follows (Code of Federal Regulations 1974):

Animal weight (kg)	*Dose (mL)*
Up to 1.8	0.25
2.2–6.8	0.5–1
6.8–13.6	2–3
13.6–20.4	3–4
20.4–27.2	4–5
Over 27.2	6

If medication needs to be continued in the dog, a change to the oral form or sustained-release capsules can be made in 6–8 hours following the last injection. Two capsule sizes are available for dogs, the small size for animals weighing up to 13.6 kg and the large size for dogs weighing 13.6 kg and over. The small capsules contain 3.33 mg prochlorperazine dimaleate and 1.67 mg isopropamide; the dose is administered by the oral route twice daily as follows: less than 1 capsule or fraction thereof for animals weighing less than 1.8 kg, 1 capsule/1.8–6.8 kg, and 1–2 capsules/6.8–13.6 kg. The large capsules contain 10 mg prochlorperazine dimaleate and 5 mg isopropamide; the dose is administered by the oral route twice daily as follows: 1 capsule for animals weighing 13.6 kg and over.

Prochlorperazine and isopropamide have also been combined with neomycin sulfate to provide a product (Neo-Darbazine) for treatment of infectious enteritis in the dog. It is particularly indicated in cases of emotional stress that are associated with bacterial infections. In the small capsule, 35.7 mg/kg neomycin sulfate is added, which is equivalent to 25 mg neomycin base. Identical quantities of prochlorperazine and isopropamide are present in the small sustained-release capsule as described above. In the large capsule, 107 mg neomycin sulfate or the equivalent of 75 mg neomycin base is added; again, identical quantities of prochlorperazine and isopropamide are present in the large sustained-release capsule as described above. Each large capsule is equivalent to three small capsules in content.

The twice-daily oral dose schedule of the small, 25 mg neomycin-base capsule is as follows:

Animal weight (kg)	*No. of small capsules*
4.5–9	1
9–13.6	2
Over 13.6	3

The twice-daily oral dose schedule of the large, 75 mg neomycin-base capsule is as follows:

Animal weight (kg)	*No. of large capsules*
Over 13.6	1
Over 27	2

Medication should not last for more than 5 days. Most cases will respond favorably within this time. If not, the diagnosis and/or therapy must be reconsidered.

Prochlorperazine edisylate (1 mg/kg) without isopropamide has been suggested in the dog for antiemetic effects (Willard 1985). Administration was not specified; it was probably given by the SC or IM route.

Trimeprazine Tartrate. *Trimeprazine Tartrate,* USP (Temaril), chemically is (*dl*-10-[3-dimethylamino-2-methylpropyl]-phenothiazine) (Fig. 14.7). In addition to having a tranquilizing effect, it is antipruritic, antitussive, and antihistaminic.

Trimeprazine (5 mg) is combined with prednisolone (2 mg) in tablet form for oral administration in the dog, which is the only species in which this combination product (Temaril-P) has been approved by the FDA. Twice-daily oral doses are as follows:

Weight (kg)	*Tablets*
Up to 4.5	0.5
5–9	1.0
9.5–18	2.0
Over 18	3.0

Following 4 days of treatment, the dose is decreased to about one-half the initial dose, which is sufficient to prevent return of symptoms. Because of individual variation, doses will need to be regulated in accordance with the clinical response desired.

Trimeprazine-prednisolone is indicated for alleviation of pruritis, irrespective of etiology, and for reduction of inflammatory reactions associated with skin disorders such as eczema, otitis, and allergic dermatitis. The drug combination has been advocated as an adjunctive treatment in conditions such as kennel cough and various forms of bronchitis. Thus this product also has antitussive activity.

With incorporation of prednisolone into the tablet, the preparation must not be used in viral infections or ulceration of the cornea. Healing of the cornea will be delayed or inhibited. Moreover, prednisolone should not be used in the last trimester of pregnancy because it may induce premature parturition with dystocia, fetal death, retained placenta, and metritis.

α_2-ADRENERGIC AGONISTS

The α_2 Adrenoceptor. Alpha$_2$-adrenergic agonists have been used by veterinarians for over two decades to provide dose-dependent sedation, analgesia, and muscle relaxation. Xylazine was synthesized in Germany in 1962 and was the first α_2-adrenergic agonist to be used as a sedative and analgesic by veterinarians. Reports on the effectiveness of xylazine as an anesthetic adjunct began to appear in the 1970s, but it was not until 1981 that xylazine's anesthetic action was linked to the stimulation of central α_2-adrenergic receptors (adrenoceptors) (Hsu 1981; Clough and Hutton 1981). Alpha$_2$ adrenoceptors have been identified in the cardiovascular, respiratory, renal, endocrine, gastrointestinal, hematologic, and central nervous systems.

α adrenoceptors were originally classified into α_1 and α_2 subtypes based on the pharmacologic effects of yohimbine and prazosin (Cheung et al. 1982). The α_2-adrenoceptor belongs to the group of membrane receptors known as G-protein-coupled receptors (Gilman 1987). Transduction of a message carried by an α_2 agonist into cellular responses is referred to as transmembrane signaling and involves the coupling of at least three components: a receptor protein, a guanine nucleotide-binding regulatory protein (G protein), and an effector mechanism. When an α_2 agonist binds to the receptor, a conformational change occurs that facilitates contact with the G protein. The G proteins allow rapid stimulation of an effector system. Effector mechanisms are most often changes in transmembrane voltage and neuronal excitability. At least five separate

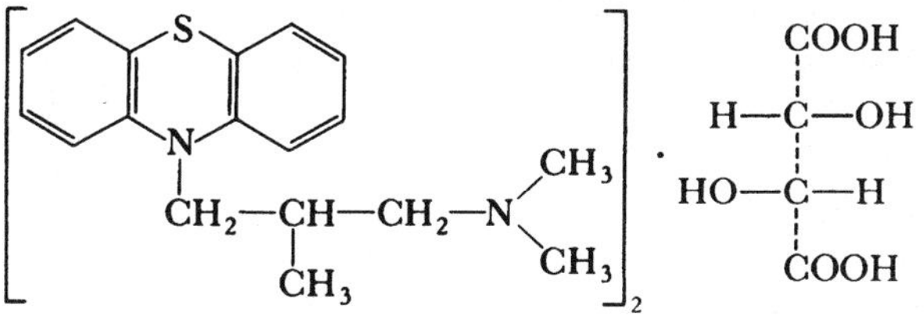

S N CH_2—CH—CH_2—N CH_3 CH_3 CH_3 · COOH H—C—OH HO—C—H COOH

Trimeprazine Tartrate

FIG. 14.7

effector mechanisms that are directly modulated by the activated α_2 adrenoceptor have been identified (Maze and Tranquilli 1991). For example, the reduction in anesthetic requirement demonstrated by the superselective α_2 agonist dexmedetomidine is probably mediated by a central α_2-adrenergic isoreceptor and involves a pertussis toxin–sensitive G protein and a 4-aminopyridine-sensitive potassium channel (Doze et al. 1989; Regan et al. 1989; Doze et al. 1990). Similarly, a pertussis toxin–sensitive G protein and a voltage-operated calcium channel appear to be involved in the analgesic response to an α_2 agonist (Hoehn et al. 1988; Dunlap and Fischbach 1981; Holz et al. 1986). Enhancement of the analgesic response may also occur as the result of a synergistic interaction between α_2-adrenergic agonists and opiates in the spinal cord (Ossipov et al. 1989; Drasner and Fields 1988).

The adrenoceptor has been described structurally as seven hydrophobic transmembranous domains consisting of 20–25 amino acids in an α-helical configuration. The hydrophobic domains are believed to determine the specificity of ligand recognition by forming binding sites for small ligands. The seven hydrophobic domains are separated by three intracellular and three extracellular loops of variable lengths comprising hydrophilic amino acids. The intracellular loops provide the site of interaction with G proteins.

Efforts are presently being directed toward classification of α_2-adrenoceptor subtypes (Aantaa et al. 1995; Kendall 1996; MacKinnon et al. 1994; Bylund 1988). Pharmacologic studies utilizing selective antagonists have identified four α_2-adrenoceptor subtypes: α_{2A}, α_{2B}, α_{2C}, and α_{2D}, although it has been suggested that the α_{2D} subtype may actually be a species homolog of the α_{2A} subtype. Although amino acid sequencing and chromosomal location support the existence of α_2-adrenoceptor subtypes, the functional significance, if any, of the α_2-adrenoceptor subtypes remains to be determined.

Xylazine Hydrochloride. *Xylazine Hydrochloride,* INN (Rompun, Bay Va 1470), was first synthesized in 1962 and given the code name Bay Va 1470. Chemically, xylazine is 2(2,6-dimethylphenylamino)-4*H*-5,6-dihydro-1,3-thiazine hydrochloride (Fig. 14.8); it is related to clonidine, a drug used to control arterial hypertension in humans. Pharmacologically, xylazine is classified as an analgesic as well as a sedative and skeletal muscle relaxant. It is not a neuroleptic or tranquilizer nor an anesthetic agent. Xylazine is approved by the FDA for use in the dog, cat, horse, deer, and elk.

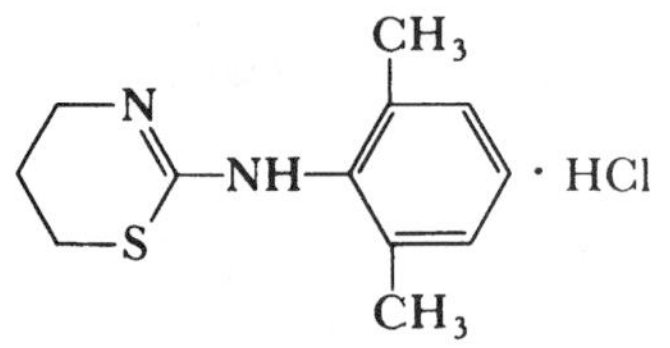

Xylazine Hydrochloride

FIG. 14.8

PHARMACOLOGIC CONSIDERATIONS. Xylazine is a potent α_2-adrenergic agonist. It acts upon the CNS by activation or stimulation of α adrenoceptors such as the α_2-adrenergic receptors; this decreases sympathetic discharge and reduces release of norepinephrine. Receptors that control central neuronal dopamine and norepinephrine storage and/or release are α_2 adrenoceptors (Hedler et al. 1981). Through its central stimulation of α_2-adrenegic receptors, xylazine has potent antinociceptive or analgesic activity. In addition to α_2-adrenergic activity, xylazine has α_1-adrenergic effects (Kobinger and Pichler 1982). Consequently, xylazine elicits both peripheral and central actions upon these adrenergic receptor subtypes.

Xylazine has a number of pharmacologic characteristics in common with morphine, but it will not substitute for morphine in dependent rats, and its effect is not antagonized by naloxone. Xylazine does not produce the CNS excitation usually induced by narcotic analgesics in mice, rats, and cats. Instead, it produces depression and sedation in these species.

Electroencephalographic studies in rabbits and cats suggest that xylazine activates central α adrenoceptors related but distinct from the peripheral α adrenoceptors (Loc et al. 1974). The antinociceptive action is antagonized effectively by yohimbine and piperoxan. Inasmuch as yohimbine has been classified as a specific α_2-adrenoceptor blocking agent upon presynaptic receptors, xylazine apparently induces its major effect at this target site.

Xylazine also produces skeletal muscle relaxation by inhibition of intraneuronal transmission of impulses at the central level of the CNS. Apparently because of direct stimulatory effect upon the emetic center, emesis is commonly induced by xylazine in the cat and occasionally in the dog. The chemoreceptor trigger zone of the area postrema is activated by xylazine to trigger emesis; its action may be mediated by an opiate type of molecular receptor (Colby et al. 1981). Alpha-adrenergic and dopaminergic blocking agents do not prevent xylazine-induced emesis. In contrast to the dog and cat, xylazine does not elicit emesis in cattle, sheep, goats, horses, and some other species.

Xylazine has a variable effect upon the cardiovascular system. In many species, IM or IV injections produce a short-lived arterial pressor effect followed by a longer period of hypotension and bradycardia. These contrasting actions upon the arterial pressure apparently are related to the α_1- and α_2-adrenergic actions of xylazine. For example, the peripheral α_1- and α_2-adrenergic actions of IV xylazine produce an acute arterial vasopressor effect in halothane-anesthetized dogs (Tranquilli et al. 1984). The longer period of arterial hypotension associated with xylazine appears to be related to its central α_2-adrenergic action or decrease in central sympathetic nervous system activity (Schmitt et al. 1970).

Since xylazine can induce arterial hypotension, it is logical to think that this effect would interact with other compounds that induce hypotension, such as acepromazine. According to Muir et al. (1979b), the combination of xylazine and acepromazine is a hemodynamically stable drug mixture in the horse. However, in animals with cardiopulmonary problems, considerable caution should be taken in use of this drug mixture.

Arterial hypotension may result from a depressant effect of xylazine upon cardiac contractility and an associated drop in cardiac output. In dogs given xylazine 20 minutes prior to anesthesia, ventricular arrhythmias, including ventricular fibrillation, are induced with much smaller doses of epinephrine than in nonpremedicated dogs (Muir et al. 1975). Thus xylazine appears to sensitize the heart to epinephrine. Tranquilli et al. (1986) indicate that xylazine does indeed significantly decrease the arrhythmogenic dose of epinephrine in halothane-anesthetized dogs. Recent work, however, suggests that this does not occur when administered in low preanesthetic doses (Lemke et al. 1992).

Cardiac output is decreased 5–10 minutes following IV injection of xylazine (0.66 mg/kg) in the pony and then returns to normal in 15 minutes (Garner et al. 1971a). No significant alteration in the systemic arterial pressure and cardiac rate occurs 2 minutes after administration in the pony. In the horse, atrioventricular (AV) nodal block of the second-degree type occurs (McCashin and Gabel 1975). Additionally, xylazine may induce first- and third-degree AV block in the horse; incomplete AV block generally occurs within 2 minutes of the beginning of IV injection and spontaneously disappears by 4 minutes after IV injection of xylazine (Tranquilli et al. 1984).

A transient second-degree AV block is induced by xylazine in the horse with IV doses of 0.55, 1.1, and 2.2 mg/kg (Kerr et al. 1972b). Atropine sulfate (0.011 mg or more/kg) administered intravenously and immediately before administration of xylazine prevents the heart block. In a clinical evaluation of xylazine in the horse, no cardiac alterations other than bradycardia were reported (Hoffman 1974). It is well known that horses have functional or second-degree heart block, especially young animals. Its incidence may be as high as 16%, and it is not considered a pathologic entity because it disappears following excitement and administration of atropine.

In the horse, bradycardia and second-degree AV block probably occur from increased vagal activity caused by the vasopressor effect of xylazine (Knight 1980). The systolic and diastolic pressures increase initially following IM injection of xylazine (2.2 mg/kg); bradycardia and a decrease in respiration occur. Additionally, the marked depressant effect of thiamylal sodium and halothane following xylazine administration is also obvious (see Fig. 14.9). General anesthetics must be cautiously administered and monitored following use of xylazine.

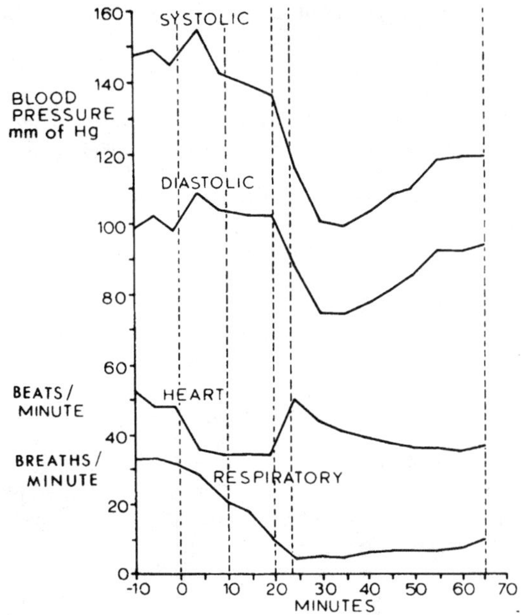

FIG. 14.9.—Mean blood pressure and heart and respiratory rates (determinations on 11 horses). Xylazine was injected at "0" time, thiamylal was injected at 20 minutes, and halothane inhalation was done from 23 to 65 minutes (McCashin and Gabel 1975).

In the dog, IV administration of xylazine (1.1 mg/kg) decreases heart rate and aortic blood flow; there is an initial increase in arterial pressure and peripheral resistance (Klide et al. 1975). Increase in arterial pressure is transient and is followed by decrease in pressure. Additionally, arterial pH, P_aO_2, and P_aCO_2 do not change from control values following this dose of xylazine in the dog (Klide et al. 1975).

IV injection of nifedipine (20 μg/kg), a slow-channel calcium-blocking agent, blocks the initial pressor action of IV xylazine (1.1 mg/kg) in the dog anesthetized with halothane; in addition to blockade of xylazine-induced acute vasoconstriction mediated by α_2-adrenergic receptors, nifedipine blocks the Ca^{++}-dependent action of xylazine but not its α_1-adrenergic receptor action. Also, sinus tachycardia and/or second-degree AV block induced by xylazine are blocked by nifedipine.

Cardiopulmonary effects of the combination xylazine-morphine have been evaluated in the horse (Muir et al. 1979a). In animals given xylazine (0.66 mg/kg) and morphine (0.12 or 0.66 mg/kg) intravenously, a decrease in heart rate, cardiac output, and respiratory rate occurs. Central venous, systemic arterial, and pulmonary arterial pressures also increase. Arterial P_aCO_2 and P_aO_2 as well as arterial pH remain unaltered following administration of the xylazine-morphine combination.

In the pony, no statistically significant alterations occur in arterial pH, P_aCO_2, or P_aO_2 following IV injection of xylazine (0.6–1 mg/kg); no significant change occurs in tidal and minute volumes at this dosage (Garner et al. 1971b).

There is little alteration in serum electrolytes following IV administration of xylazine (1.1 mg/kg) in the horse (Short et al. 1972). Electrolyte values are affected only by a decline in the potassium level. Serum protein levels remain unchanged.

In the horse, the visceral analgesic effects of xylazine were compared with butorphanol, meperidine, and pentazocine (Muir and Robertson 1985). Visceral pain (colic) was produced by inflation of a balloon in the cecum. Of the analgesics studied, xylazine induced the best analgesia. Moreover, the xylazine-induced analgesia was longest (about 90 minutes), followed by butorphanol (about 60 minutes) and then by meperidine and pentazocine (about 30–35 minutes). Similar results have been reported on the analgesic action of xylazine in ponies; obtundation of superficial and visceral pain by xylazine persisted 3 and 4 hours, respectively (Kalpravidh et al. 1984).

In cattle, urine volume or output is greatly increased for about 5 hours following administration of xylazine (Thurmon et al. 1978). Urine pH decreases in cattle during the first hour following administration and then increases. Glucose is detected in bovine urine of xylazine-treated animals 15–30 minutes after injection; it reaches a maximum in 2 hours and is undetectable at 5–6 hours. Additionally, plasma insulin concentrations decrease 25–33% in cattle that receive xylazine by the IM or IV route (Symonds and Mallinson 1978). Administration of insulin 20 minutes after injection of xylazine induces a rapid drop in blood glucose and reduces the rate of glucose production by the liver.

Ruminants are the most sensitive of the domestic animals to the action of xylazine. In cattle, doses that produce deep sedation and analgesia are one-tenth those required in horses, dogs, and cats (Hopkins 1972). Bradycardia and salivation are lessened or prevented in cattle by giving IM atropine (0.1 mg/kg) 10 minutes prior to injection of xylazine (Brown 1986).

In the young Hereford calf, hemodynamic effects of xylazine (0.22 mg/100 kg) administered intramuscularly are quite similar to those observed in other species in both anesthetized and unanesthetized states (Campbell et al. 1979). Effects include bradycardia and decline in the cardiac output and stroke volume as well as increased total peripheral resistance. In other species (but not in the calf) xylazine initially increases mean arterial pressure. Arterial pressure of the calf is markedly lower at 4 minutes after administration than that of control animals (Campbell et al. 1979). In the goat, IM administration of xylazine (0.22 mg/kg) results in significant reduction in respiratory rate (Kumar and Thurmon 1979). The mean arterial blood pressure and rectal temperature remain unaltered.

The pig is less affected than any of these species, and dose levels are reported to be 20–30 times greater than those required in cattle. According to Benson and Thurmon (1979), xylazine is not effective in swine.

Toxicity trials in cattle have shown that the median lethal dose of xylazine in adult cattle is three times the highest recommended dose of 0.3 mg/kg. According to Hopkins (1972), this is six times the dose rate indicated for the majority of clinical cases.

IM xylazine (0.08, 0.1, or 0.2 mg/kg) induces a dose-dependent inhibition of reticulorumen contractions in cattle (Ruckebusch and Toutain 1984). Its action is antagonized or quickly reversed by either the IV (0.2 mg/kg) or SC (0.5 mg/kg) administration of tolazoline. Interestingly, omasal activity is increased by xylazine in sheep (Brikas et al. 1986).

Apparently, the effect of xylazine on the body temperature of cattle is variable and may depend on the size of the dose administered. In one study, after IM xylazine (0.4 mg/kg) administration, the body temperature, pulse rate, and respiratory rate exhibited a decrease lasting for almost 24 hours (Dockal et al. 1975). In another study, the body temperature of cattle reached a peak increase (1.9° C) 4–5 hours after IM injection of 0.2 mg/kg xylazine (Young 1979). It remained elevated after 12 hours and did not return to preinjection values until 18 hours after injection (Fig. 14.10).

The type of sedation produced by xylazine in cattle closely resembles that produced by chloral hydrate (Clarke and Hall 1969). Moreover, analgesia is not present except in deeply sedated animals; supplementation with a general or local anesthetic is necessary to prevent movement in response to nociceptive stimuli. More information is needed to establish the efficacy and safety of xylazine in cattle.

METABOLISM AND ELIMINATION. After IM administration, absorption of xylazine is rapid, with a half-life of 2.8–5.4 minutes (Garcia-Villar et al. 1981). However, it is incompletely absorbed since its bioavailability ranges from 52 to 90% in the dog, 17–73% in sheep, and 40–48% in the horse. Distribution is rapid, with a half-life between 1.2 and 6 minutes. The apparent volume of distribution for xylazine is 1.9–2.7 L/kg in the dog, horse, sheep, and cow (Garcia-Villar et al. 1981).

The half-life of elimination after IV administration of a single dose of xylazine is 49.5 minutes in the horse, 36.5 minutes in cattle, 23 minutes in sheep, and 30 minutes in the dog. Plasma kinetics in cattle are difficult to relate to some of the sustained clinical effects of the drug. The short half-life of xylazine in cattle (36.5 minutes) contrasts with the duration of polyuria (5 hours), hyperthermia (18 hours), hypothermia (24 hours), prostration after a high dose (36 hours), and/or appearance of diarrhea (about 12–24 hours) after injection. Similar to the nonsteroidal anti-inflammatory agents, the plasma half-life or elimination half-life of xylazine cannot be related to these bizarre biochemical and physiologic effects.

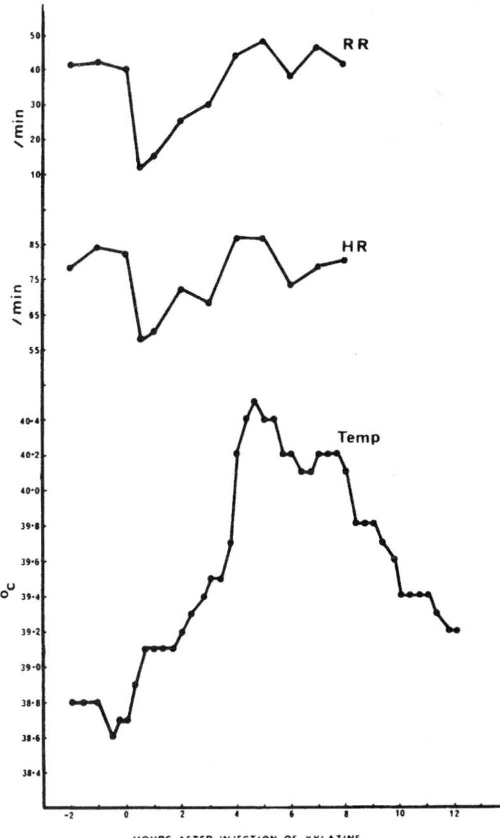

FIG. 14.10.—Effect of IM injection of 0.2 mg/kg xylazine on body temperature, heart rate, and respiratory rate (Young 1979).

In rats, only 8% of the intact, or unchanged, drug appears in urine, whereas in cattle less than 1% unchanged xylazine is eliminated 2 hours after administration (Duhm et al. 1969; Garcia-Villar et al. 1981). Xylazine undergoes rapid metabolism, yielding about 20 metabolites in rats. Peak excretion of metabolites occurs between 2 and 4 hours after administration of xylazine in cattle; this suggests that the drug is extensively metabolized. A metabolite that must form rapidly in cattle is 1,amino-2-6-dimethybenzene (ADB), which appears in urine within 4 hours after an IM dose (therapeutic level) is administered (Pütter and Sagner 1973). ADB probably forms from oxidative or hydrolytic breakdown of the thiazine ring.

Precautions and Contraindications. Xylazine must not be used in food-producing animals or exist as a drug residue in products (meat, milk, eggs) intended for human consumption. Since xylazine appears to sensitize the heart to epinephrine, administration of epinephrine is contraindicated.

Use of xylazine should be carefully considered when the following complications or conditions exist: (1) cardiac aberrations (xylazine induces arrhythmias and is also a direct depressant of the myocardium), (2) arterial hypotension and/or shock (further enhanced by the hypotensive action as well as reduced cardiac output effect of xylazine), (3) renal impairment (excreted via the kidney), (4) hepatic impairment (apparently the primary degradation of xylazine is dependent upon a functional liver), and (5) epilepsy (may possibly precipitate seizures in susceptible animals).

Animals should be handled carefully after xylazine is administered. A false sense of security may result in injury to personnel because animals can respond by kicking or reacting in other defensive ways. Intra-arterial injection of xylazine should be avoided. See Chap. 12 for discussion of problems associated with intra-arterial injection of anesthetic or tranquilizer agents.

Xylazine must be used cautiously in conjunction with neuroleptics or tranquilizers. Additive depressant effects occur from use of xylazine and barbiturates; use of barbiturates to induce anesthesia must be at a reduced dosage level, and barbiturates must be administered slowly when injected by the IV route. Use of xylazine in combination with ketamine must be carefully considered in animals with cardiopulmonary complications; see discussion in this chapter and Chap. 12.

Sudden death occurred in a nervous Arab stallion suffering from mild colic following IV administration of 1 mg/kg xylazine (Fuentes 1978). Instead of sedation, CNS excitation and convulsions developed (these symptoms are similar to those seen after an intra-arterial injection of xylazine). This was followed by collapse and death about 2 minutes after injection. The action of xylazine during stress and/or release of epinephrine in the horse apparently has not been studied. The effects or interaction of xylazine and epinephrine release in the equine species remain to be determined. A question has arisen about the possibility of epinephrine reversal or hypotension following xylazine. Conversely, xylazine has a hypotensive effect of longer duration than the initial pressor effect in the horse. Hypotensive action of the drug may be responsible for enhancement of the shocklike effect of colic. A cautious approach should be taken whenever xylazine is used in treatment of colic.

Toxicosis in a 6-year-old, 400 kg Standardbred gelding developed after IV injection of xylazine (200 mg) and reserpine (12.5 mg) (Lloyd et al. 1985). A number of side effects, including sporadic episodes of colic, occurred. It is obvious that an undesirable interaction between xylazine and reserpine occurs. This combination of drugs is contraindicated.

Ventricular fibrillation has been reported in one horse after receiving 0.5 mg/kg xylazine intravenously (Steffey et al. 1985). Although the incidence of this happening is considered to be rare, caution needs to be taken in administration of xylazine to animals with cardiac complications.

TABLE 14.1—Xylazine doses

Species	Intravenous	Intramuscular
	(mg/kg)	*(mg/kg)*
Horse	0.5–1.1	1–2
Cattle*	0.03–0.1	0.1–0.2
Sheep*	0.05–0.1	0.1–0.3
Goat*	0.01–0.5	0.05–0.5
Pig	. . .	2–3
Dog	0.5–1	1–2
Cat	0.5–1	1–2
Birds	. . .	5–10

*Lower dose should be used if sedation without recumbency is desired (Knight 1980).

In the dog, two precautions in the use of xylazine need to be emphasized. First, bradycardia, heart block, and severe arterial hypotension can occur; second, bloat (apparently from aerophagia) sometimes develops. Breeds such as the Basset Hound, Great Dane, and Irish Setter appear susceptible to bloat and may require emergency treatment several hours after administration of xylazine. For radiographic restraint, xylazine should be avoided as a sedative because gaseous distention of the stomach will occur; this makes radiographic interpretation more difficult (Folkers 1980).

Debilitated animals with depressed respiration, cardiac disease, renal and liver impairment, shock, or any other stress conditions should be carefully monitored whenever xylazine is administered. The drug is contraindicated in animals within the last month of pregnancy, since it precipitates an early parturition or abortion (Jones 1972). Xylazine should not be administered to dehydrated cattle or those with urinary obstruction (Brown 1986).

DOSAGE. Doses of xylazine recommended in domestic animals are summarized in Table 14.1.

EPIDURAL ADMINISTRATION. In ponies, xylazine has been found to produce more profound and longer-lasting epidural analgesia than lidocaine (Fikes et al. 1988). Xylazine-induced analgesia is not accompanied by the same motor blockade as with local anesthetics (LeBlanc et al. 1988), but xylazine has a significant local anesthetic effect (Aziz and Martin 1978). This effect cannot be blocked by an α_2-adrenergic antagonist, suggesting a membrane-stabilizing effect of locally applied xylazine (O'Regan 1989). In horses, duration of analgesia has been significantly lengthened by coadministration of xylazine and lidocaine (Grubb et al. 1992).

In cattle, the cardiopulmonary depressant effects of epidural xylazine, but not the sedation or regional analgesia, were antagonized with tolazoline, an α_2 antagonist (Skarda et al. 1990). Similar results have been reported in conscious sheep in which dose-dependent regional analgesia of the forelimbs was produced by intrathecally administered xylazine and abolished by intrathecal idazoxan, an α_2 antagonist (Waterman et al. 1988). This would suggest that at least part of the analgesic effect of xylazine is produced through activation of spinal cord α_2 adrenoceptors. This mechanism of analgesia is also supported by prolongation of epidural opioid analgesia with coadministration of other α_2 agonists, such as medetomidine (Branson et al. 1993).

CLINICAL USE

DOGS AND CATS. A commercial preparation containing 20 mg/mL xylazine is available for IV (1.1 mg/kg), IM, or SC (2.2 mg/kg) administration in the dog and cat. In dogs weighing over 22 kg, an IM dose of 1.1 mg/kg is usually recommended for sedation and analgesia. The analgesic effect produced is pronounced over head, neck, and body but is minimal in extremities. With IV barbiturates and inhalant anesthetics, smooth, rapid induction of anesthesia is achieved along with uneventful recovery. The amount of IV barbiturate needed to induce anesthesia is decreased by about one-half or more in the dog and cat. Inhalant anesthetics are also reduced but administered to effect.

Onset of action after IM or SC injection is within 10–15 minutes, and after IV administration it occurs within 3–5 minutes in dogs and cats (Newkirk and Miles 1974). A sedative or sleeplike effect occurs and appears to be dose dependent; this effect usually lasts 1–2 hours. The analgesic effect lasts only 15–30 minutes. Complete recovery from xylazine varies with the dose administered. Recovery is usually complete within 2–4 hours in the dog and cat.

For restraint of the dog in cystometry, an SC dose of xylazine (2.2 mg/kg) is the only drug that has proved adequate without interfering with the micturition reflex (Oliver and Young 1973). Xylazine significantly decreases (26–71%) the amount of pentobarbital required to induce general anesthesia in the dog (Lacuata and Subang 1973). Depth of analgesia produced by xylazine alone is insufficient to permit endotracheal intubation before administration of an inhalant anesthetic; after administration of xylazine, the inhalant anesthetic can be delivered easily with a face mask and then can be followed by intubation (Moye et al. 1973).

IV xylazine (1 mg/kg) and IV ketamine (10 mg/kg) administered 5 minutes afterward is a common combination used in the dog for general anesthesia (Haskins et al. 1986a).

Emesis occurs in the majority of cats 3–5 minutes following administration of xylazine (Moye et al. 1973). An IM dose of 1 mg/kg is considered an optimum level for inducement of emesis in the cat; however, analgesic effects are not observed at this dosage (Amend and Klavano 1973).

In the dog, emesis may also occur following xylazine administered in large doses. The emetic effect is clinically beneficial in emptying the stomach; this prevents the likelihood of vomitus being aspirated into the trachea prior to and during surgery. Xylazine can be used to perform cesarean section under local anesthesia without a depressant effect developing in puppies (Yates 1973). Ketamine hydrochloride has also been used in combination with xylazine for cesarean section and other procedures in the dog (see Chap. 12). Deaths have occurred in two German Shepherds within 24 hours following use of xylazine and ketamine (Kirkpatrick 1978). Both animals were ambulatory and were sent home; they were resting comfortably in the evening only to be found dead by morning. Until more information is available on the safety and efficacy of xylazine-ketamine, caution is suggested in use of these agents (see Chap. 12).

Xylazine premedication is recommended to eliminate muscular hypertonic effects in cats during ketamine anesthesia (Amend et al. 1972; Amend 1973). A combination in which IM xylazine (0.55–1.1 mg/kg) is given as a preanesthetic, followed 20 minutes later with an IM injection of ketamine (15–22 mg/kg), provides analgesia and relaxation in an average of 30 minutes. Xylazine renders the cat relatively insensitive to the pain often associated with injection of ketamine. Ketamine anesthesia in cats is significantly increased by xylazine (Waterman 1983). Additionally, it prolongs the plasma half-life of ketamine (almost doubled, to 69 minutes) and significantly delays formation of the primary metabolite of ketamine.

Also, xylazine (2.2 mg/kg) and ketamine (11 mg/kg) administered intramuscularly are used in cats for surgical procedures requiring general anesthesia of less than 1 hour (Faulk 1978). Since emesis usually follows xylazine injection in most cats within 4–8 minutes or less, ketamine is injected about 10 minutes following injection of xylazine. See Chap. 12 for other information on use of ketamine in combination with xylazine in cats.

HORSES. A commercial preparation containing 100 mg/mL xylazine is available for IV (1.1 mg/kg) or IM (2.2 mg/kg) use in the horse. Xylazine must not be used in horses or other animals intended for human food.

In the horse, doses of about 2 mg/kg xylazine have been given by IM injection 15–20 minutes prior to thiopental sodium or methohexital sodium anesthesia (Clarke and Hall 1969). Two to 3 mg/kg are reported to produce rapid, deep sedation lasting about 30 minutes, followed by rapid recovery. Other clinical reports in the horse pertaining to duration of effect are essentially in agreement with the observations of Clarke and Hall. After an IV injection of xylazine (1.1 mg/kg), onset of effect is noted in 1–1.5 minutes after injection; in 3 minutes the head droops; in 6–6.5 minutes the drug exerts its maximum effect and will continue 10–15 minutes (McCashin and Gabel 1971).

According to McCashin and Gabel (1971), xylazine is more dependable and has resulted in a higher percentage of quieter recoveries from surgical anesthesia in the horse than when promazine hydrochloride or acepromazine maleate is used for preanesthetic medication. They concluded that the most satisfactory dose of xylazine is 1.1 mg/kg intravenously or 2.2 mg/kg intramuscularly. However, weak or debilitated animals should be given a lower dose, particularly if the drug is administered intravenously. Considerably higher doses of xylazine than those recommended rarely produce recumbency in the horse; however, animals may become incoordinated so that it is difficult to work on them (McCashin and Gabel 1971).

Within a very short time after IV injection in the horse, the head characteristically drops or droops. The only disadvantage to this effect is the difficulty in examination of the mouth or passage of the endoscope (McCashin and Gabel 1971). Assisting personnel can hold up the head so that examination of the mouth can be conducted. Hypostatic congestion of nasal mucosa sometimes occurs in the head-down position. Muscle tone of the animal is decreased after administration of xylazine; difficulty in walking occurs soon after the drug is administered intravenously. In colts and geldings, prolapse of the penis sometimes occurs but paraphimosis does not; the effect upon the retractor muscle of the penis is less than that seen with promazine (McCashin and Gabel 1971).

Xylazine administered intravenously (1.1 mg/kg) or intramuscularly (2.2 mg/kg) prior to induction of anesthesia either with thiamylal or with thiamylal and halothane is a satisfactory preanesthetic agent in the horse; less respiratory depression and greater cardiovascular stability follow use of xylazine than with IV administration of 0.66 mg/kg acepromazine (Kerr et al. 1972a). Of the drugs evaluated in the horse, xylazine in the presence of epinephrine release is less likely to produce tachycardia than acepromazine (Aitken and Sanford 1972). For other information on the use of thiamylal with xylazine, see the 7th edition of this text.

For preanesthetic purposes in the horse, IV xylazine is administered at a dose of 0.55–1.1 mg/kg (Short 1974). In addition, atropine (0.045 mg/kg) is administered subcutaneously or intramuscularly.

Hoffman (1974) found the sedative and analgesic effects to be good to excellent in 88 and 81% of the horses respectively following IV administration of xylazine; the optimal dose is 1.1 mg/kg. The quantity of general anesthetic needed is the same as when promazine is used as a preanesthetic medication. Although recovery is rapid and smooth after general anesthesia of short duration, it is too rapid and often violent when anesthesia is prolonged for 45 minutes or more (Hoffman 1974).

Klein and Baetjer (1974) as well as Klavano (1975) have found that combined use of xylazine and morphine provides satisfactory sedation and analgesia in the standing horse. Xylazine (1.2 mg/kg) is administered intravenously; this is followed 5–10 minutes later with IV injection of morphine (0.75 mg/kg). These drugs are useful for suturing wounds and external surgical procedures. Aspiration or injection is possible into the joint of a horse that would otherwise not tolerate such a procedure. As effects of xylazine disappear, animals may become excitable and restless. IV administration of levallorphan tartrate (0.022 mg/kg) is recommended to relieve or prevent excitable effects of morphine (Klavano 1975). For preanesthethic purposes, xylazine (0.22 mg/kg) and morphine (0.12–0.6 mg/kg) have been used intravenously.

Xylazine (1.1 mg/kg) is administered intravenously about 4 minutes prior to IV ketamine (1.65 mg/kg for ponies and 2.2 mg/kg for horses). This combination provides satisfactory induction of anesthesia for tracheal intubation (Ellis et al. 1977).

Xylazine (1.1 mg/kg) given intravenously, followed in 2–3 minutes by IV ketamine (1.65–2.2 mg/kg) provides 12–15 minutes of surgical anesthesia in the horse (Heath 1977). An IV dose of 1.65 mg/kg ketamine results in about 10–12 minutes of recumbency, while 2.2 mg/kg intravenously provides 15 minutes and occasionally up to 20–25 minutes. Xylazine (2.2 mg/kg) is used intramuscularly 20 minutes prior to IV administration of guaifenesin (55 mg/kg) in 5% dextrose. Immediately after induction of anesthesia with guaifenesin, IV ketamine (1.7 mg/kg) is administered (Muir et al. 1978). Anesthesia can be maintained with inhalant anesthetics such as halothane or enflurane.

Xylazine has also been used in combination with ketamine and diazepam for short-term anesthesia in horses. Dosages of these drugs are covered in Chap. 12 under clinical uses of ketamine in horses. Since there is increased risk of using a combination of xylazine and ketamine in animals afflicted with cardiopulmonary complications, caution is advised whenever this combination of drugs is administered.

Xylazine (1.1 mg/kg) has been used prior to induction of thiopental (4.4 mg/kg) anesthesia in the horse (Butera et al. 1980). It is given intravenously 2.5 minutes before IV thiopental (10%). Within 1–2 minutes the horse quietly becomes recumbent. Approximately 15–20 minutes of effective analgesia appears to be provided by this combination of drugs. Minor surgical procedures such as castrations, suturing lacerations, and removal of cutaneous tumors can be carried out following administration of xylazine and thiopental. If necessary, inhalant anesthetics can be administered to maintain surgical anesthesia.

Xylazine (0.055 mg/kg) given intravenously is recommended for dental examination of the horse (Scoggins 1979). Doses in excess of this result in oversedation and cause an undesirable dropping of the head.

Xylazine also has been used successfully in supportive therapy for controlling seizures following *Clostridium tetani* infections in horses (Beroza 1980). A number of analgesics have been compared for their efficacy in an experimental colic model. Lowe (1982) has found that xylazine is the best analgesic agent for prompt effect in alleviating the pain of colic. Since xylazine has an arterial hypotensive component that possibly could enhance the shocklike effect of severe colic, a cautious approach is advised whenever it is used for this treatment.

CATTLE. Xylazine is not approved by the FDA for use in cattle and has been the subject of several malpractice suits in the USA (Ames 1979). It would be easy to overdose cattle, since they require only one-tenth the dose of xylazine on a body weight basis as horses, dogs, and cats.

Rickard et al. (1974) administered xylazine (0.22 mg/kg) and atropine (0.044 mg/kg) intramuscularly in bulls of mixed breeding; the ages of the animals were 15–24 months and body weights were 500–600 kg. Ten to 15 minutes after administration of xylazine, the animals became recumbent in the sternal position. They were then placed in lateral recumbency and restrained with a halter and leg ropes in preparation for electroejaculation and semen collection. In a fourth series of semen collections, xylazine in a dose of 0.22 mg/kg was observed to be less effective. Inasmuch as the animals attempted to stand during the electrostimulation, an additional 20–40 mg of the drug were administered to maintain restraint. With semen collection extending through a 3-week period that required repeated administration of xylazine, this additional dosage could possibly indicate that induction of microsomal enzyme activity had occurred. If so, a more rapid degradation and metabolism of the drug would result. Also, the decreased response could be due to xylazine or agonist-induced decreases in α_2-adrenergic cell receptors. A decrease in the cell receptor number is referred to as "down-regulation" by molecular pharmacologists.

An IM dose of xylazine (0.09–0.35 mg/kg) produces light to deep sedation in cattle (Hopkins 1972). Intravenously, xylazine (0.05–0.1 mg/kg) produces basal narcosis in cattle for 1–2 hours (Clarke and Hal 1969). Sedation and slight muscle relaxation with the animal in the standing position were reported following an IM dose of 0.05 mg/kg (Jones 1972). Xylazine (0.1 mg/kg) at increased IM dosages produces good sedation, marked muscle relaxation, and some analgesia; this dosage ordinarily allows the animal to remain in the standing position but may result in recumbency. At still higher IM doses of xylazine (0.2 mg/kg), deep sedation and a useful level of analgesia are induced, with the animal usually lying down. Following administration of this dose, the first effects are noted within 5 minutes and the maximum effect is induced 10 minutes later (Jones 1972).

Xylazine induces a marked degree of salivation in ruminants. Preanesthetic medication with atropine partially reduces this problem and is recommended when large doses of xylazine are used (Knight 1980).

Ruminal atony, bloating, and regurgitation with aspiration pneumonia may occur in cattle following use of xylazine. Cattle should be monitored for about 2 hours after xylazine administration for signs of bloat (Brown 1986). It is advisable to fast cattle for 24 hours before injection of xylazine to lessen the risk of regurgitation. Loose feces and liquid hemorrhagic diarrhea, including recumbency for about 1 hour, have occurred in large bulls following a sedative dose of xylazine (Knight 1980). Diarrhea may appear about 12–24 hours after injection. It is of a transitory type in most cases and believed to be due to ruminal and intestinal stasis during sedation. Also, xylazine induces a marked polyuria in many animals.

In lactating cows, IM doses (0.2 or 0.4 mg/kg) of xylazine do not result in detectable concentrations in milk at 5 and 21 hours after injection; cows ostensibly do not excrete xylazine in milk (Pütter and Sagner 1973). However, lactating animals must not receive xylazine, according to the FDA, when milk is sold for human consumption.

In the calf, use of xylazine-ketamine results in an undesirable and potentially dangerous reduction in P_aO_2. It is recommended that supplemental oxygen be given to calves receiving xylazine-ketamine anesthesia (Ring and Muir 1982).

SWINE. A xylazine-ketamine combination has been used in the pig (see Chap. 12). More data are needed in this species to determine the safety and efficacy of this combination of drugs.

GOATS. Xylazine (0.1 mg/kg) administered intravenously provides deep sedation in goats that lasts 30–35 minutes. It has been used in combination with ketamine for induction of anesthesia (see Chap. 12).

LABORATORY ANIMALS. A combination of xylazine and ketamine has been used in rats and rabbits to induce short-term anesthesia (see Chap. 12).

In the mouse, a combination of 1 mL xylazine (100 mg/mL) and 1 mL ketamine (100 mg/mL) is added to 4.6 mL sterile water (Mulder and Mulder 1979). The total volume of the mixture is 6.6 mL. An adult mouse averages about 30 g. For each 30 g of body weight, 0.1 mL (1.5 mg each of xylazine and ketamine) of the combination is used to provide 50 mg/kg of each drug. At this dosage, adequate anesthesia is maintained for 60–100 minutes after a single IM injection in C57BL and DBA mice. This length of anesthesia provides sufficient time to complete most surgical procedures.

FISH. Although xylazine is effective as an anesthetic in fish, it cannot be recommended because of its convulsant activity during induction and recovery (Ostwald 1978).

AVIAN AND EXOTIC SPECIES. Xylazine has been used in nine avian species (Levinger et al. 1973). Following IM injection, xylazine produces a marked sedative effect in birds. IM doses of 1–2 mg/kg xylazine produce no change in behavior. At doses above 5 mg/kg, signs of CNS depression occur. Light sedation is induced with xylazine in the chicken and turkey at 10 mg/kg administered intramuscularly (Levinger et al. 1973). Xylazine has been used in combination with ketamine and althesin to induce anesthesia in ostriches (see Chap. 12).

Xylazine has been used in a large number of exotic species (Bauditz 1972); however, in the past lack of a suitable antidote has been a serious shortcoming in reversal of its action. Recovery of immobilized animals requires 2–3 hours before ambulation is attained (Young and Whyte 1973). Experimental studies completed in dogs (Hatch et al. 1982) and cattle (Kitzman et al. 1982) have shown that xylazine can be antagonized by IV administration of 4-aminopyridine and yohimbine hydrochloride. It is possible that these antagonists will serve importantly in reversal of the immobilizing effects of xylazine in exotic species. For additional information on antagonists that reverse the action of xylazine, see Chap. 16.

The most important value of xylazine pertains to its excellent synergistic properties when used in combination with potent analgesics such as etorphine hydrochloride or fentanyl citrate. Moreover, it markedly potentiates the immobilizing action of ketamine.

Sedation and immobilization doses of xylazine administered by projectile syringe or intramuscularly are listed for some of the exotic species (Table 14.2). The drug has also been used in combination with ketamine for induction of anesthesia (see Chap. 12). Also refer to the precautions discussed for use of the combination of xylazine and ketamine.

Giraffes are extremely sensitive to xylazine, and its sole use does not permit safe manipulative procedures in this species (Bush et al. 1976). However, its use in conjunction with etorphine produces desirable restraint or immobilization.

In fallow deer, a fatal hyperthermia greater than 44° C occurred following use of xylazine and etorphine (Pertz and Sundberg 1978). It is not known whether other exotic species may be similarly affected by this combination. Hyperthermia in exotic animals has been seen chiefly following use of promazine tranquilizers alone and in combination with morphomimetic agents.

For restraint of Bactrian camels, IM xylazine (0.27–0.51 mg/kg) provides adequate sedation for tuberculin testing and other procedures (Custer et al. 1977). In an elephant weighing about 3500 kg, IM xylazine (400 mg) given into the triceps muscle induced immobilization (Robinson and Meier 1977).

Baby African elephants have been successfully sedated and immobilized by xylazine (Trembath 1984); IM doses are as follows:

Weight (kg)	*Light sedation (mg)*	*Immobilization (mg)*
180	20	40
300	80	120
450	120	160

Xylazine has been used in combination with etorphine for immobilization of polar and brown bears. For the dosages used, see Chap. 13.

Use of xylazine for immobilization of Reeves' muntjac (*Muntiacus reevesi*) is unpredictable in its effect (Cooper et al. 1986). Prolonged recovery of the animals limits its value for use under field conditions.

Detomidine Hydrochloride. *Detomidine hydrochloride* ([4-(5)-(2,3-dimethylbenzyl) imidazole hydrochloride]; Dormosedan) (Fig. 14.11) is a

TABLE 14.2—Sedative and immobilizing doses of xylazine for exotic species

Species	Dose	
	Sedation	Immobilization
	(mg/kg)	
Fallow deer (*Dama dama*)	1–2	5–8
Red deer (*Cervus nippon*)	2	3–4*
Roe deer (*Capreolus capreolus*)	0.5–1	1.5–3
White-tailed deer (*Odocoileus virginianus*)	0.5–1	3–4
Elk (*Alces alces*)	0.5	1.5
Reindeer (*Rangifer tarandus*)	0.5	2
Greater kudu (*Tragelaphus strepsiceros*)	1	3
Bushbuck (*Tr. spekei*)	1.5	3
Eland (*Taurotragus oryx*)	1	3
Sable antelope (*Hippotragus niger*)	1.5	3
Gazelle (*Gazella* sp.)	1	2–4
Water buffalo (*Bubalis arnee*)	0.5–1	1–2(?)
Yak (*Bos mutus*)	0.3	0.6–1
American bison (*Bison bison*)	0.1–0.3	0.6–1
Musk ox (*Ovibos moschatus*)	<0.5	0.5–1.5
Dromedary (*Camelus dromedarius*)	0.1	0.5
Llama (*Lama guanicoe glama*)	0.2–0.5	1–2
Bear (most species)	2–6	8–10
Striped hyena (*Hyaena striata*)	3–5	7–8
Wolf (*Canis lupus*)	3–5	7–8†
Puma (*Puma concolor*)	. . .	8
Jaguar (*Panthera onca*)	. . .	8
Lion (*P. leo*)	. . .	8–10
Leopard, spotted (*P. pardus*)	. . .	8–10
Cheetah (*Acinonyx jubatus*)	. . .	2(?)
Zebra (*Equus quagga*)	3–5	. . .
Subhuman primates (many species)	0.5–1	2–5

*If 3–4 mg/kg as recommended by the manufacturer is used in Isle of Rhum red deer off the west coast of Scotland, a coma lasting 6–9 hours occurs (Fletcher 1974). The correct dose for Rhum red deer is 0.1–0.2 mg/kg. The marked hypersensitivity of the animals to xylazine compared to mainland red deer may possibly be due to a high degree of inbreeding.

†The effective dose range for captive Arctic wolves is 3–6.8 mg/kg (Philo 1978).

FIG. 14.11.—Detomidine Hydrochloride

sedative-analgesic that was originally developed for use in horses and cattle (Virtanen et al. 1985). Detomidine is more potent than xylazine, with greater specificity at central α_2 adrenoceptors (Virtanen and MacDonald 1985), although very high concentrations will activate α_1 adrenoceptors (Virtanen and Nyman 1985).

Detomidine induces cardiovascular effects similar to xylazine. Decreased myocardial contractility, bradycardia, and a biphasic blood pressure response may occur after IV injection (Wagner et al. 1991). The bradycardia is commonly accompanied by first- or second-degree AV block. These effects may be alleviated by anticholinergic administration (Short et al. 1986).

Detomidine (10–60 μg/kg IV) produces cardiovascular changes in horses that are nearly identical to those produced by xylazine (1.1 mg/kg IV) (Sarazan et al. 1989). Sedation and analgesia produced by detomidine are of longer duration than those produced by xylazine in equivalent doses (Jochle and Hamm 1986; Clarke and Taylor 1986). Detomidine (20 μg/kg IV) induced 45 minutes of analgesia and sedation in a cecal balloon colic model, whereas the equianalgesic dose of xylazine (1.1 mg/kg IV) was effective for only 20 minutes (Lowe and Hifiger 1986). It is not uncommon to observe good sedation for 90–120 minutes and analgesia for 75–80 minutes after a 40 μg/kg IV dose of detomidine. For this reason, it has been suggested that detomidine is the analgesic of choice for relieving equine colic pain (Tranquilli and Maze 1993).

Detomidine is an effective preanesthetic for horses and cattle and can be used in combination with ketamine to induce short periods of anesthesia (Clarke and Taylor 1986; Clarke et al. 1986a). The combination of detomidine with Telazol (tiletamine and zolazepam, see Chap. 12) has proven to be an effective combination in horses and ponies (Wan et al. 1992; Lin et al. 1992). Recovery from inhalation anesthesia is usually uneventful in horses premedicated with detomidine. As with xylazine, hyperglycemia and increased urine output may occur after detomidine administration (Tranquilli and Maze 1993).

Concurrent administration of an α_2-adrenergic agonist may diminish or eliminate the excitation that occurs with opioid use in horses. Opioid stimulation was not observed when detomidine was combined with methadone, morphine, meperidine, or butorphanol (Clarke and Paton 1988). The combination of detomidine and butorphanol may provide the most effective sedation and analgesia while minimizing cardiopulmonary depression (Clarke and Paton 1988; LeBlanc 1991). Detomidine (10–15 μg/kg IV) injection precedes butorphanol (20–30 μg/kg IV) injection. The full effect should be allowed to develop prior to start of the procedure. Sedation is accompanied by ataxia, slight tremor of the face and lips, and a tendency to lean forward and head press (Tranquilli and Maze 1993). Detomidine is approved for use in horses in the USA.

Medetomidine Hydrochloride. Chemically, *Medetomidine hydrochloride* is (±)-4-[1-(2,3-dimethylphenyl)-ethyl]-1*H*-imidazole monohydro-chloride (Domitor) (Fig. 14.12). Medetomidine is the most potent α_2-adrenoceptor-selective agonist available for use in veterinary medicine. The α_2/α_1 receptor selectivity binding ratio for medetomidine is 1620, compared to 260 and 160 for detomidine and xylazine, respectively (Virtanen 1989). It produces sedation, muscle relaxation, and analgesia in a variety of domesticated species. Variability in effects among species seems to be less for medetomidine than for xylazine, a less-specific α_2 agonist.

Medetomidine induces dose-dependent sedation and analgesia in dogs and cats (Vainio 1989). As with xylazine and detomidine, administration of additional drug increases the duration of effect but does not result in more sedation.

Profound sedation and bradycardia consistently occur in dogs administered 40 μg/kg of medetomidine intramuscularly (Raiha, M. P., et al. 1989; Vainio and Palmu 1989). In dogs not premedicated with atropine, blood pressure decreases in a dose-dependent manner after administration of 10–60 μg/kg of medetomidine (Bergstrom 1988).

Prior administration of an anticholinergic may be more effective at preventing the bradycardia than reversing the bradycardia after it has occurred (Short 1991), but it may increase the initial hypertensive effect that occurs during onset of sedation (Vainio 1989; Bergstrom 1988). Duration of sedation in cats is dose dependent, although bradycardia is not (Stenberg 1989). When combined with ketamine, the bradycardic effect of medetomidine may be offset by the sympathomimetic properties of the dissociative (Verstegen et al. 1991).

Respiration rate decreases in a dose-dependent manner after administration of 10–60 μg/kg of medetomidine in dogs (Bergstrom 1988). A 20 μg/kg IV infusion of medetomidine results in less depression of the hypercapnic response curve in dogs than 1 minimum alveolar concentration (MAC) isoflurane (1.38%) anesthesia (Bloor et al. 1989)). End-tidal CO_2 and P_aCO_2 values were decreased significantly in dogs administered medetomidine versus those administered isoflurane anesthesia.

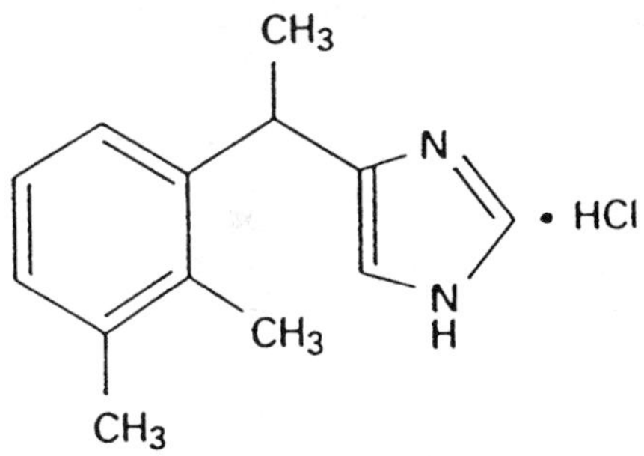

CH3 CH3 N • HCl N H CH3

FIG. 14.12.—Medetomidine Hydrochloride

IM or SC administration of medetomidine may result in vomiting in dogs and cats (Virtanen 1989). Diuresis occurs even with low doses (10 μg/kg), producing large amounts of dilute urine (Crighton 1990).

IM medetomidine at a dose of 30 μg/kg provides sedation and analgesia in dogs equivalent to a 2.2 mg/kg dose of xylazine. Combinations of medetomidine and ketamine have provided short periods of anesthesia and immobilization in dogs, cats, and many laboratory and exotic animal species (Vähä-Vahe 1989; Jalanka 1989, 1990; Nevalainen et al. 1989; Arnemo and Soli 1992; Van Heerden and Keffen 1991). Medetomidine (40 μg/kg) combined with 5.0 mg/kg of ketamine produces anesthesia in dogs comparable to that produced with 1 mg/kg xylazine and 15 mg/kg ketamine (Moens and Fargetton 1990). Dogs premedicated with medetomidine (20–40 μg/kg) have been administered propofol (2 mg/kg loading dose; 165 μg/kg/min), etomidate (0.5 mg/kg loading dose; 50 μg/kg/min), or ketamine (4 mg/kg IV) for maintenance of anesthesia (Thurmon et al. 1995; Ko et al. 1994; J. E. Raiha et al. 1989).

Medetomidine produces greater ataxia at equal sedative/analgesic doses in horses than xylazine or detomidine. Consequently, xylazine or detomidine may be the preferred α_2 agonists for use in horses (Kamerling et al. 1991; Bryant et al. 1991).

Medetomidine produces more predictable sedation and analgesia in swine than does xylazine (Sakaguchi et al. 1992). Medetomidine doses of 30–80 μg/kg produce sedation in pigs. As with dogs and cats, higher doses do not produce increased sedation.

Similar to xylazine and detomidine, the administration of medetomidine with an opioid may enhance sedation and analgesia beyond that expected with either drug alone (England and Clarke 1989). Medetomidine is approved for veterinary use in dogs and cats in the USA.

New α_2-Adrenergic Agonists. Romifidine is the newest α_2-adrenergic agonist assessed for sedative and analgesic activity in the horse. Romifidine (80 μg/kg) produces sedation similar to xylazine (1 mg/kg) or detomidine (20 μg/kg). Xylazine and detomidine produce greater ataxia and sedation of shorter duration than romifidine (England et al. 1992).

Dexmedetomidine is a very selective α_2-adrenoceptor agonist whose role as an anesthetic adjunct in veterinary medicine is still being defined.

α_2-Adrenergic Antagonists. The incidence of unfavorable reactions to α_2-adrenoceptor antagonists is rare when they are administered appropriately for reversal of α_2-adrenoceptor agonist-induced CNS depression. Deaths have been reported after rapid IV administration of high doses of tolazoline and yohimbine (Hsu et al. 1987). Acute and delayed death has occurred in llamas administered tolazoline. Profound hypotension and tachycardia may occur after rapid IV injection but may be prevented by slow administration to the desired effect. Anxiety, pacing, and panting in dogs, and hyperexcitement in cats or very young animals, have occurred with administration of yohimbine. Diarrhea and piloerection have occurred in dogs after administration of tolazoline. Other species differences in response to α_2-adrenoceptor antagonists have not yet been established.

YOHIMBINE. *Yohimbine* (17-hydroxyyohimban-16-carboxylic acid methyl ester; Yobine, Antagonil) (Fig. 14.13) is an α_2-adrenoceptor antagonist that is approximately 60 times more selective for the α_2 than the α_1 adrenoceptor (Clarke et al. 1986b). It antagonizes α_2-adrenoceptor-mediated depression and enhances the release of norepinephrine and other excitatory neurotransmitters (Tranquilli and Maze 1993). Yohimbine has been effective in antagonizing α_2-agonist-induced sedation and analgesia in many species (Holmberg and Gershon 1961; Lang and Gershon 1963; Delbarre and Schmitt 1971, 1973).

Yohimbine administered alone has proven effective in reversing the sedative-immobilizing effects of anesthetic combinations incorporating xylazine (Jessup et al. 1985; McGruder and Hsu 1985; Hsu 1985; Hsu et al. 1986; Jacobson et al. 1985; Hsu and Shulaw 1984; Jessup et al. 1983). Yohimbine administered in conjunction with 4-aminopyridine effectively induced anesthetic reversal in many domestic and wild species (Hatch et al. 1982; Kitzman et al. 1984; Wallner et al. 1982; Hatch et al. 1983a; Cronin et al. 1983a; Kitzman et al. 1982; Hatch et al. 1983b; Hatch et al. 1984). Yohimbine is approved for use in dogs (Yobine) and wild, exotic, and ranched deer (Antagonil). Antagonism of the effects of xylazine is also discussed in Chap. 16.

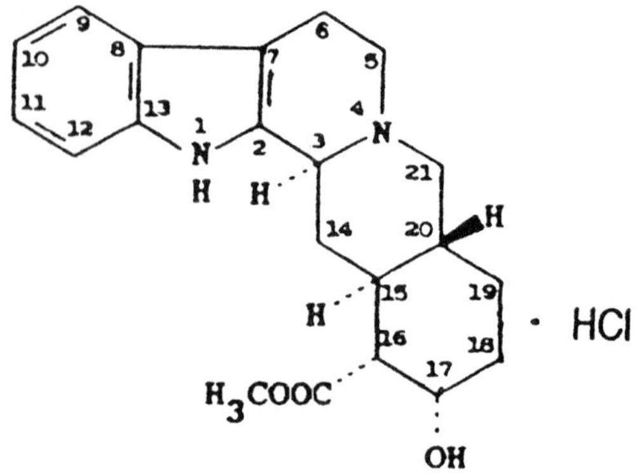

FIG. 14.13.—Yohimbine Hydrochloride

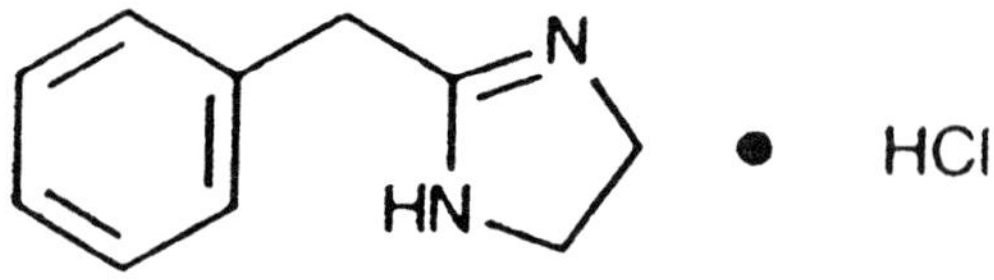

TOLAZOLINE. *Tolazoline* (2-benzyl-2-imidazoline; Priscoline) (Fig. 14.14) has been used in a number of species to reverse xylazine sedation or to partially reverse the depressant effects of xylazine when administered as part of an anesthetic regimen (Hsu et al. 1987; Allen and Oosterhuis 1986; Kreeger et al. 1986a; Kreeger et al. 1986b; Allen 1986; Tranquilli et al. 1984; Thurmon et al. 1989). Tolazoline is the least specific antagonist for α_2 adrenoceptors but may be more effective than yohimbine at antagonizing some of the effects of xylazine. In cats sedated with xylazine, tolazoline induced a calmer recovery (Hartsfield et al. 1986), and it was more efficient in decreasing the time to recovery in calves sedated with xylazine (Thurmon et al. 1989). Tolazoline also induces potent H_2-receptor agonist actions, and chronic use in humans has been associated with GI bleeding and other complications (Silverman et al. 1970). Sudden unexplained death, both acute and delayed, has occurred in llamas administered tolazoline. It has been suggested that the cause is a combination of hypotensive shock and bradycardia. Further investigation is necessary to define the use of tolazoline in llamas. Tolazoline has not been approved for veterinary use.

ATIPAMEZOLE. *Atipamezole hydrochloride* (4-(2-ethyl-2,3-dihydro-1*H*-inden-2-yl)-1*H*-imidazole hydrochloride; Antisedan) (Fig. 14.15) has greater α_2-adrenoceptor specificity and may be more effective in antagonizing the effects of α_2 agonists. It has an α_2/α_1 selectivity ratio that is 200–300 times greater than that of yohimbine and is devoid of activity at other types of receptors (Virtanen et al. 1989). Dosage recommendations for atipamezole vary among species and for various α_2 agonists (Tranquilli and Maze 1993). For example, a xylazine dose of 0.3 mg/kg in calves is reversed

FIG. 14.14.—Tolazoline Hydrochloride

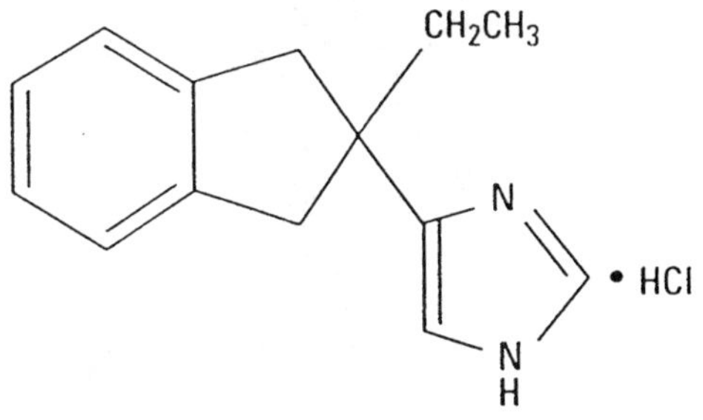

FIG. 14.15.—Atipamezole Hydrochloride

by an atipamezole dose of 30 μg/kg (Thompson et al. 1991, but a medetomidine dose of 40 μg/kg in a dog requires 160–240 μg/kg of atipamezole for reversal (Vähä-Vahe 1990).

In horses administered atipamezole at 10 times the administered dose of detomidine or medetomidine, mydriasis and analgesia were abolished, but bradycardia and sedation were only transiently influenced (Kamerling et al. 1991). The administration of atipamezole alone in horses produces mild sedation and myocardial depression without analgesia, as well as consistent dose-related changes in behavior and autonomic variables. Atipamezole-induced sedation in the dog or cat has not been reported. Atipamezole is approved for IM use in dogs.

BENZODIAZEPINE DERIVATIVES

The Benzodiazepine Receptor. Benzodiazepine derivatives used in veterinary medicine include diazepam, midazolam, zolazepam (in combination with tiletamine as Telazol, see Chap. 12), and chlordiazepoxide.

Based on electrophysiologic investigations, it is believed that benzodiazepines produce hypnotic, sedative, anxiolytic, anticonvulsant, and skeletal muscle–relaxant effects by enhancing the action of the neurotransmitter γ-aminobutyric acid (GABA) on its receptors (Polc 1988). GABA type A, or $GABA_A$, receptors are membrane-associated glycoproteins that exhibit some similarity to nicotinic acetylcholine, glycine, and 5-hydroxytryptamine type 3 receptors (Darlison and Albrecht 1995). The $GABA_A$ receptor comprises five (pentameric) protein subunits, of which several different types have been identified: six α, four β, three γ, one δ, and two ρ subunits (Sieghart 1994).

The benzodiazepine receptor is a modulatory site on the $GABA_A$ receptor that allosterically regulates the postsynaptic chloride channel gating that occurs with the interaction of GABA with $GABA_A$ receptors (Olsen and Tobin 1990; Sieghart 1994). Modulation of $GABA_A$-receptor activity occurs only at submaximal concentrations of GABA. That is, benzodiazepines have no modulating effect at the $GABA_A$ receptors when the GABA concentration reaches saturation level (Haefely 1989). The modulation of $GABA_A$-receptor activity may be either positive or negative (Polc et al. 1982). Positive modulation occurs with the binding of anxiolytic compounds such as benzodiazepine agonists. Negative modulation occurs with the binding of inverse agonists, which are anxiogenic. A third group of high-affinity ligands, the benzodiazepine-receptor antagonists, have only a weak or no intrinsic activity for modulating $GABA_A$ activity but are able to inhibit the effects of both benzodiazepine-receptor agonists and inverse agonists. Partial agonists and partial inverse agonists have also been identified (Haefely et al. 1985).

It has been demonstrated that only the combination of α, β, and γ subtypes results in $GABA_A$ receptors that may be modulated by benzodiazepines (Pritchett et al. 1989). In addition, the benzodiazepine pharmacology of the $GABA_A$ receptors is determined by the α and γ subunits that are present. The presence of the γ_2 subunit yields receptors with high-affinity binding for benzodiazepine agonists, the benzodiazepine antagonist flumazenil, and the inverse agonist DMCM (β-carboline methyl-4-ethyl-6,7-dimethoxy-β-carboline-3-carboxylate). The presence of the α_1 subunit allows binding of certain substances (triazolopyridazine compounds, β carbolines) with higher affinity than receptors possessing either an α_2 or α_3 subunit do (Pritchett et al. 1989).

Both central and peripheral benzodiazepine receptors have been described (Zisterer and Williams 1997). The central type is present exclusively in the CNS and is localized to neurons (Young and Kuhar 1979). At least two central benzodiazepine receptor subtypes have been described: the BZI receptor, located predominantly in the cerebellum; and the BZII receptor, located in the hippocampus and some other brain regions. $GABA_A$ receptors containing an α_1 subunit (together with the β_1 and γ_2 subunits) are associated with the BZI binding sites. Those $GABA_A$ receptors with either the α_2 or the α_3 subunit are associated with the BZII binding sites. The binding of benzodiazepines to the central benzodiazepine receptors is stimulated in the presence of GABA and other $GABA_A$ receptor agonists (Karobath et al. 1981). Reciprocally, the binding of GABA to $GABA_A$ receptors is enhanced by the presence of benzodiazepines (Bristow et al. 1990; Skerritt et al. 1982). The peripheral type benzodiazepine receptors were initially discovered in peripheral tissues (rat kidney, liver, lung) (Braestrup and Squires 1977), but later studies demonstrated their presence in the CNS also (Schoemaker et al. 1981). The peripheral receptors are pharmacologically distinct from and unrelated to the $GABA_A$-receptor-associated benzodiazepine receptors (Zisterer and Williams 1997; Sieghart 1994).

$GABA_A$ receptors are also associated with binding sites for other substances. In addition to benzodiazepine receptor binding sites, there are also binding sites for barbiturates, certain steroids and channel blockers, and the anthelmintic avermectin B1a

(McDonald and Olsen 1994; Sieghart 1992). Both barbiturates and benzodiazepines potentiate the effects of GABA, but the barbiturates prolong the open time of the chloride ion channel, whereas benzodiazepine agonists increase the frequency of channel opening (McDonald and Olsen 1994).

In 1977, Claus Braestrup and Richard Squires discovered that the brain has its own specific receptor for benzodiazepines. Use of radioactively labeled benzodiazepines has demonstrated that there are high-affinity binding sites in the mammalian brain (associated with synaptosomal membranes) that fulfill many of the criteria of pharmacologic receptors for these compounds. Benzodiazepine receptors appear to have widespread distribution in the brain. Interestingly, lack of receptors in white matter is a consistent finding in all species. In addition to the presence of benzodiazepine receptors in the brain, receptors are also present in peripheral tissues, including kidney, liver, heart, and lung (Gee et al. 1984).

Widespread distribution of benzodiazepine receptors in the CNS contrasts with the more discrete localization of other receptors (e.g., opiate receptors). This fits evidence from behavioral and electrophysiologic studies that benzodiazepines interact at many levels of the brain to elicit their effects (Tallman et al. 1980). It has also been suggested that different receptor subtypes mediate the different actions of the benzodiazepines. The anxiolytic, anticonvulsant, and muscle relaxation effects are believed to be mediated at the benzodiazepine $GABA_A$ receptor, whereas the hypnotic effects may be mediated by alterations in a potential-dependent calcium ion flux (Mendelson 1992). The different actions may also be a function of blood levels, with the anxiolytic effect occurring at lower levels, and sedation and unconsciousness occurring with increasing blood levels (Amrein et al. 1988).

Interactions between the benzodiazepine receptor and anions also occur. Chloride, bromide, iodide, nitrite, and thiocyanate (but not fluoride) enhance binding of diazepam. Sedative action of the once used and now obsolete drug sodium bromide may have induced its effect at this level.

Embryologically, the benzodiazepine receptor is present at 14 days of gestation in the rat, and the number of receptor sites increases in parallel with GABA-receptor recognition sites.

The benzodiazepine receptor is associated with the anxiolytic and anticonvulsant actions of benzodiazepines. Two strains of rats, bred for high and low fearfulness, have significantly different densities of brain benzodiazepine receptors. Inasmuch as these two strains differ in their emotionality, differences in receptor number may be physiologically important in regulation of anxiety or apprehension (Robertson et al. 1978). Binding of benzodiazepines is also altered in spontaneous epilepsy in the baboon (Squires et al. 1979), and an increase in the number of benzodiazepine receptors has been reported in rats following experimentally induced seizures (Paul and Skolnick

CH_3
N
O
N
Cl

Diazepam

FIG. 14.16

1978). These alterations in number of receptors are comparable to those seen in other CNS receptors after treatments designed to alter neuronal input (Skolnick et al. 1978). Rapid onset (within minutes) of alterations in benzodiazepine receptors and their return to control levels (within 1 hour) is rather remarkable (Tallman et al. 1980). Such alterations in other central CNS receptors generally occur over a time frame of days.

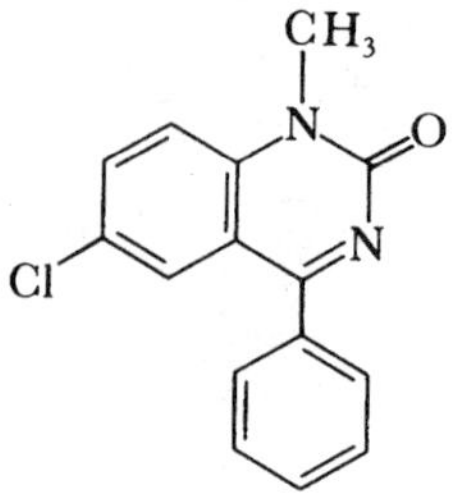

Diazepam. Chemically, *Diazepam,* USP (Valium), is 7-chloro-1,3-dihydro-1-methyl-5-phenyl-2*H*-1,4-benzodiazepin-2-one (Fig. 14.16). A major disadvantage of diazepam is its insolubility in water. Diazepam and other benzodiazepines are classified as Schedule IV agents under the 1970 Controlled Substances Act.

CENTRAL NERVOUS SYSTEM. Benzodiazepines are thought of as “disinhibitors” of suppressed behavior; they induce taming effects in animals. They modify behavior in both humans and animals. In humans, benzodiazepine derivatives (diazepam, chlordiazepoxide, and flurazepam, referred to as Dalmane) are used widely in clinical practice as muscle relaxants, anticonvulsants, anxiolytics, and hypnotics (especially flurazepam sleeping pills). Like most psychotropic agents, benzodiazepines produce undesirable effects (e.g., ataxia) that may or may not be related to their therapeutic effects (Tallman et al. 1980).

Of the benzodiazepine derivatives diazepam is about 20 times more potent than chlordiazepoxide in blocking decerebrate rigidity in animals. The principal site of CNS depression produced by diazepam is the brain stem reticular formation.

In decerebrate cats, polysynaptic reflexes elicited by sciatic nerve stimulation can be depressed to 50% or less by IV administration of diazepam (0.05–0.2 mg/kg), chlordiazepoxide (10–30 mg/kg), and pentobarbital (24 mg/kg); blockade of polysynaptic reflexes by these drugs is immediate and lasts up to 4 hours (Ngai et al. 1966). Diazepam and chlordiazepoxide do not significantly alter monosynaptic reflexes. Pentobarbital, cyclopropane, and nitrous oxide reduce monosynaptic reflexes. According to Ngai et al., these findings suggest that central depressants such as diazepam, chlordiazepoxide, and some anesthetics act upon supraspinal structures (most likely the reticular facilitatory system) in blockade of spinal polysynaptic reflexes.

It has been proposed that a number of neurotransmitter systems, including acetylcholine, catecholamines, serotonin, GABA, and glycine, participate in sedative, anxiolytic, muscle-relaxant, and anticonvulsant action of benzodiazepines (Costa and Guidotti 1979). The neurotransmitter dopamine may also be affected by benzodiazepines. Experimental evidence exists that diazepam (1–10 mg/kg) administered intraperitoneally in rats decreases synthesis of dopamine in the limbic and striatal areas of the brain (Biswas and Carlsson 1978). However, most evidence shows that GABA and benzodiazepines interact and that benzodiazepines potentiate GABA-mediated inhibition in the CNS.

In vitro binding of ^{3}H-strychnine and benzodiazepines has suggested that the inhibitor amino acid transmitter glycine may also be associated in mediation of benzodiazepine action. However, in vivo studies indicate that inhibitory response to glycine is unaffected by presence of benzodiazepines. Thus the glycinergic hypothesis for benzodiazepine action can be discounted, because benzodiazepines do not preferentially antagonize convulsions induced by strychnine (Costa and Guidotti 1979).

Existence of benzodiazepine receptors and failure of a wide variety of known transmitters to inhibit diazepam binding suggest that the brain may contain an unidentified endogenous ligand. To date, purines (inosine, hypoxanthine), nicotinamide, ethyl-β-carboline-3-carboxylate, and thromboxane A_2 are likely candidates as endogenous ligand substances. However, affinity of these substances, especially the purines, for the benzodiazepine receptor is many orders of magnitude lower than that of the benzodiazepines (Tallman et al. 1980). Nicotinamide appears to be the most likely candidate from the standpoint of benzodiazepine-like neuropharmacologic profile (Möhler 1981).

It is possible that the efficacy of benzodiazepines in long-term treatment of epilepsy may be improved by concurrent administration of centrally active drugs that mimic the effect of GABA (Tallman et al. 1980). Development of such agents could also advance knowledge of the mechanism of benzodiazepine binding and activity. One such compound has already been reported to enhance benzodiazepine binding and appears to modify behavior of animals (Beer et al. 1978; Williams and Risley 1979).

CARDIOPULMONARY SYSTEM. Diazepam produces minimal effects on the cardiovascular system and has some respiratory depressant effect. A transient arterial hypotensive effect occurs in the dog following IV injection (8 mg/kg), and doses as high as 15 mg/kg injected over 3 hours decrease mean arterial pressure (Randall et al. 1961). In human patients with ischemic heart disease, there is evidence that coronary blood flow is maintained or increased following induction of anesthesia with diazepam.

In the horse, IV doses (0.05, 0.1, 0.2, and 0.4 mg/kg) of diazepam have been administered to determine their effect upon cardiopulmonary function (Muir et al. 1982). No significant changes in heart rate; cardiac output; mean pulmonary arterial, aortic, and right atrial pressures; respiratory rate; and arterial pH or blood gas values were observed. According to Muir et al., use of commercially formulated diazepam in 40% propylene glycol does not alter cardiac rate or rhythm in horses. In humans, the solvent for diazepam periodically produces arterial hypotension and arrhythmias (Greenblatt and Koch-Wesser 1973).

PHARMACOKINETICS. The major metabolite of diazepam in the dog is *N*-desmethyl-diazepam (or nordiazepam) (Jeppsson 1976). Mean plasma half-lives of diazepam and nordiazepam in the dog after an IV injection of diazepam (1.25 mg/kg) are 142 ± 17 and 171 ± 8 minutes respectively. Administered at a higher IV dose (2 mg/kg), the elimination half-life of diazepam in the dog is 3.2 hours (Löscher and Frey 1981). The major metabolite, nordiazepam, appears rapidly in the plasma of the dog and can exceed the concentration of the parent drug. Other plasma metabolites of diazepam found in the dog are oxazepam and 3-hydroxydiazepam. Nordiazepam and oxazepam metabolites are active at an equivalent order of magnitude as diazepam upon the CNS.

Oral administration of diazepam (1 or 2 mg/kg) 3 times daily maintains steady-state plasma concentrations of 1–2 μg/mL nordiazepam and maximal diazepam concentrations of 0.1–0.8 μg/mL (Löscher and Frey 1981). Concentrations of oxazepam in plasma did not exceed 0.1–0.2 μg/mL. Also, this dose regimen does not appear to induce microsomal enzyme activity.

Pharmacokinetically, diazepam and nordiazepam have been studied in the cat after IV doses of 5, 10, and 20 mg/kg diazepam and 5 and 10 mg/kg nordiazepam (Cotler et al. 1984). Distribution or α phase of diazepam is rapid, with a harmonic mean half-life of 0.35 hour; the mean elimination half-life is 5.46 hours. For nordiazepam, a harmonic mean elimination half-life of 21.3 hours was obtained; this elimination rate in the cat is 4.3 times slower than diazepam (Colter et al. 1984). About 50% of an administered dose of diazepam is metabolized to nordiazepam in the cat.

In the horse, IV infusion of 80 mg diazepam/animal (0.17–0.19 mg/kg) over 5 minutes results in a plasma elimination half-life of 6.94–21.6 hours. These data were obtained from 3 horses (Muir et al. 1982).

Nordiazepam (*N*-desmethyldiazepam) is conjugated to glucuronic acid in the horse; this conjugate is the major urinary metabolite of diazepam (Muir et al. 1982). Interestingly, no nordiazepam is detected in the plasma of the horse. Apparently, the biotransformation of diazepam and formation of the glucuronide conjugate of nordiazepam are so rapid that neither the metabolite (i.e., nordiazepam) nor its conjugate can be detected in plasma. Additionally, other metabolites (oxazepam and *N*-methyloxazepam) are detectable in urine of the horse; diazepam is not detected (Muir et al. 1982).

At a serum concentration of 75 ng/mL, serum protein binding of diazepam averages 87% in the horse (Muir et al. 1982). After IM administration of diazepam (0.17–0.19 mg/kg), plasma concentrations increase rapidly and attain maximum levels at 1.5–2 hours; thereafter, plasma concentrations decline. In horses given this IM dose regimen, bioavailability averages 93% (Muir et al. 1982). In the dog, diazepam (1 or 2 mg/kg) administered orally 3 times daily resulted in bioavailability values ranging from 74 to 100% (Löscher and Frey 1981).

SKELETAL MUSCLE. The central muscle-relaxing action of diazepam and related benzodiazepines principally affects polysynaptic reflexes at the supraspinal level (Kanto and Klotz 1982). A spinal cord depressant action at the interneuronal level, as well as an inhibitory effect upon acetylcholine release at the presynaptic level, has been proposed.

Diazepam is capable of prolongation or potentiation of the muscle-relaxing action of nondepolarizing drugs such as *d*-tubocurarine and pancuronium. However, this interaction does not appear to be clinically significant. In the dog, diazepam does not reduce or attenuate the occurrence or severity of succinylcholine-induced muscle fasciculations (Raffe et al. 1982). This action would be anticipated, since succinylcholine is a depolarizing agent at the neuromuscular junction. According to Raffe et al., use of diazepam as a pretreatment for preventing succinylcholine-induced muscle fasciculation cannot be recommended.

TERATOGENESIS AND CARCINOGENESIS. Until more is learned about possible teratogenic effects of the benzodiazepines during gestation or pregnancy, diazepam and related drugs should not be used in breeding animals. Cleft palate has been associated with maternal intake of diazepam in humans (Saxen and Saxen 1975).

Inasmuch as benzodiazepines are extensively used in humans, concern about possible adverse effects have arisen because of reports that oxazepam induces liver neoplasms in mice. Moreover, there are indications that diazepam has neoplasm-promoting activity (Horobin 1981).

In the rat, studies were conducted upon six benzodiazepine tranquilizers to determine whether or not initiation or promotion of tumors can be induced in the liver (Remandet et al. 1984). Among those studied were diazepam, oxazepam, lorazepam, and clorazepate. No evidence could be found of initiating or promoting activity of benzodiazepines for rat liver. With respect to the importance and extensive use of the benzodiazepines, additional research is necessary to explore the suggestion of some investigators of a possible neoplasm-promoting effect in other organs.

BEHAVIORAL CHANGES. In the human, maintenance of verbal contact is an advantage when benzodiazepines are used in certain diagnostic or operative procedures. In outpatients they are useful as sedative-anxiolytic and amnesic agents.

In veterinary medicine, diazepam has been used in dosages that moderately sedate animals. However, the cat does not appear to respond as well as most species; aberrant behavior is sometimes seen. In the horse, the behavioral effects become more prominent as the IV doses (0.05, 0.1, 0.2, and 0.4 mg/kg) of diazepam are increased (Muir et al. 1982); increased CNS depression and muscle relaxation occur with increasing dosages. IV doses of diazepam greater than 0.2 mg/kg produce marked muscle-relaxant action and sternal or lateral recumbency. A fixed gaze and muscle tremors of the head, neck, and thorax occur after the IV injection of 0.2 mg/kg diazepam; ataxia occurs 2 minutes after its administration in horses. Other effects after this dose is administered have been described by Muir et al. (1982): (1) One animal collapsed and was recumbent for 3 minutes; however, it regained a standing position but remained ataxic. The ataxia was manifested by weaving from side to side, leaning against the stockade, or standing with crossed rear limbs. (2) None of the horses extended or lowered their heads; they appearead to be less aware of their surroundings. Ataxia and less awareness of their surroundings lasted for about 50 minutes in 4 of 7 horses. (3) Two hours after diazepam administration, all horses were calm but appeared to have recovered to normal.

ANTICONVULSANT ACTION. The anticonvulsant properties of the benzodiazepines are useful in treatment of status epilepticus (see Chap. 16), tetanus, convulsions caused by metaldehyde toxicity, and convulsions caused by overdoses of local anesthetics. Generally, diazepam and related benzodiazepines have been recommended as first aid agents in treatment of convulsions of different origin (Kanto and Klontz 1982). However, in the adroit hands of the clinician, the rapid and anticonvulsant effect of thiopental or thiamylal must also be considered.

DRUG INTERACTIONS. Diazepam and related derivatives potentiate the action of other CNS depressants such as the phenothiazines and barbiturates. Since diazepam binds to plasma proteins extensively, its use with other known compounds that bind heavily with plasma proteins should be carefully considered.

Although benzodiazepines potentiate the action of nondepolarizing skeletal muscle relaxants, this does not appear to be clinically significant. Cimetidine, an H_2-histamine-receptor blocking agent, impairs the hepatic microsomal oxidation of diazepam; this prolongs its clearance from the body and increases its elimination half-life (Greenblatt et al. 1984).

CLINICAL USE. Although the FDA has not approved use of benzodiazepines in animals, they are being used (especially diazepam) with increasing frequency in veterinary medicine. As a class of drugs the benzodiazepines are used as behavioral modifiers, premedicants, anesthesia induction agents, and adjuvants in neuroleptanalgesia and for their anticonvulsant effects (see Chap. 16 for details on anticonvulsant action of diazepam).

Diazepam is available in injectable and oral forms. The injectable preparation contains 5 mg/mL diazepam compounded with 40% propylene glycol, 10% ethyl alcohol, 5% sodium benzoate and benzoic acid as buffers, and 1.5% benzyl alcohol for preservative purposes. Extreme caution is necessary in administering this preparation; it is necessary to inject the IV drug form slowly. Small veins should not be used. Intra-arterial administration must be avoided. Diazepam and the vehicular organic solvents can irritate blood vessels and induce pain on injection. In humans, phlebitis and thrombosis after injection of diazepam can result in the loss of a limb (Schneider and Mace 1984).

DOGS AND CATS. In the dog there is considerable individual variation in response to the sedative effects of diazepam. It produces excitation in some dogs and does not induce sedation in others (Haskins et al. 1986b). Diazepam does not have a tranquilizing effect in the healthy dog and should not be used without benefit of an adjunct sedative (Haskins et al. 1986b).

A small IV dose of diazepam will produce unconsciousness in some animals, whereas others may not be drowsy after 2 mg/kg (Hall 1976).

In general, the recommended dose of diazepam in the dog and cat is 1 mg/kg administered intravenously or orally (Kirk 1977). A maximum of 20 mg and 5 mg for a single dose is suggested as the upper limit for the dog and cat respectively. In treatment of epileptic seizures, it may be necessary to exceed these upper limits (see Chap. 16).

Diazepam (5 mg) given intramuscularly and sodium penicillin G (600,000 units every 8 hours) administered intravenously were used in treatment of a 4-month old-Brittany Spaniel afflicted with tetanus (Bodily 1979). This treatment was followed with 10 mg diazepam and 30,000 units of tetanus antitoxin in an IV drip of lactated Ringer's solution; a few hours later, methocarbamol at 45 mg/kg was given intravenously to achieve muscle relaxation. Other pharmacologic agents (pentobarbital, procaine penicillin G, phenobarbital, ampicillin, and an expectorant-antihistamine-antitussive combination) were used up to discharge from the clinic on day 10.

Diazepam (1–2 mg/kg) has been used in the dog to treat convulsive seizures resulting from metaldehyde poisoning (Turner 1973). Diazepam (0.2–0.6 mg/kg) administered intramuscularly or intravenously is considered a very effective and safe premedicant, particularly in the aged dog with cardiac disease (Muir 1977).

In the dog, IV diazepam (0.27–0.44 mg/kg) followed by IV ketamine (11 mg/kg) is used to induce anesthesia (Wright 1982). Duration of anesthesia is 5–22 minutes; recovery is characterized by 10–15 minutes of ataxia and incoordination. However, this is followed by recovery soon thereafter (Wright 1982).

In humans, the combined use of benzodiazepines with ketamine is referred to as "ataranalgesia" or "ataranesthesia." This combination prevents side effects of ketamine such as cardiovascular complications, elevation in intracranial pressure, and psychomimetic responses. However, a longer recovery period must be accepted. Under field or primitive conditions, ketamine-diazepam infusions may be an optional method of choice.

In the dog, IV diazepam (0.5 mg/kg) followed by IV ketamine (10 mg/kg) is being used for general anesthesia (Haskins et al. 1986b). Until more data are available on the safety and efficacy of this drug combination, its use should be approached cautiously.

Use of diazepam for sedative, ataractic, or neuroleptic effect in the cat is apparently of questionable value. According to Chase (1977), diazepam induces irritability and aberrant behavior to such a degree that it cannot be used in cats. Diazepam (0.05–0.4 mg/kg) has been administered by the IV, IM, and oral routes to induce eating in debilitated and anorexic cats (Macy and Gasper 1985). After IV administration, eating begins in a few seconds. Benzodiazepines may increase the appetite by enhancing the negative GABA effect upon serotonin (Morely 1980).

HORSES. Use of diazepam in combination with ketamine and xylazine hydrochloride is characterized by smooth induction of and recovery from anesthesia. Dosages of diazepam, ketamine, and xylazine are described in Chap. 12 in the section on ketamine.

It has been alleged that there has been widespread use of diazepam and reserpine for their taming effects in competitive animals such as race and show horses (Ray et al. 1978). This unauthorized use creates problems in enforcement for both racing commissions and various horse show associations. Sensitive methods for quantitation of reserpine indicate that approximately 100 pg/mL of the drug can be detected in plasma; the lower limit of detection for diazepam is approximately 2 ng/mL plasma (Ray et al. 1978).

SWINE. In the opinion of Ragan and Gillis (1975), diazepam is the tranquilizing agent of choice in swine. An IM dose of 8.5 mg/kg produces excellent sedation in about 30 minutes and reduces the dose of pentobarbital by about 50%. For neuroleptic or tranquilizing action only, the recommended IM dose of diazepam is 5.5 mg/kg. The most noticeable side effect seen about 5 minutes following administration is a moderately severe posterior ataxia. This poses no serious problem because the animals usually become recumbent about 10 minutes after injection (Ragan and Gillis 1975).

For induction of anesthesia in swine, an IV combination of diazepam (0.55 mg/kg) and ketamine (11 mg/kg) has been used by R. B. Heath (Wright 1982). Duration of anesthesia is 15–35 minutes; recovery is smooth.

MINK. Diazepam has been used in mink to prevent conditions of anxiety and aggressiveness (Sandelien 1966). In white mink of the Hedlund strain, the animals are totally deaf and are extremely restless and excitable when handled. Pure breeding of this valuable strain is extremely difficult. The females frequently refuse to mate during normal estrus and may initiate vicious and even fatal fights. In reduction of this aberrant behavior, various drugs such as sedatives, hypnotics, bromines, morphine, ethanol, barbiturates, and phenothiazines, including chlorpromazine, have been used with variable success (Sandelien 1966). Trials with diazepam administered in the feed indicate that it is possible to improve mating and to prevent the females from killing their kits during whelping. For improvement of mating, the oral dose of diazepam consists of 1 mg/animal/day for 2 successive days followed by a maintenance level of 0.66 mg/animal/day. For use of diazepam in standard dark mink during whelping, 0.66 mg/animal/day is fed for 1 month or more.

GOATS. In the goat, IM atropine (0.44 mg/kg) has been used 15 minutes preceding the IM administration of diazepam (0.88 mg/kg); this is followed 10 minutes later by an IM injection of ketamine (22 mg/kg) for induction of analgesia (Kumar et al. 1983). Duration of analgesia is more than 22 minutes; time to standing without assistance is 70.8 minutes. Administration of diazepam prolongs the period of analgesia, increases muscle relaxation, and prevents reflex movements of limbs (Kumar et al. 1983). The IM dose of atropine (0.44 mg/kg) used in this study was 10 times greater than that recommended in the dog and cat on a milligram per kilogram basis; however, it must be remembered that the goat and ruminants in general require much higher doses of atropine to induce anticholinergic effects.

As in the cat, IV administration of diazepam (0.04 mg/kg) significantly stimulates feed intake in the goat; it is increased over animals that receive only IV normal saline (Anika 1985). The effect appears to be the most prominent within the first 15 minutes after administration; it is no longer evident between 30 and 45 minutes after the injection (Anika 1985).

In the goat, Bermuda grass toxicosis or tremors are suppressed for several hours by administration of diazepam (Strain et al. 1982). An IV dose of 0.8 mg/kg suppresses the tremors at the peak of toxicosis.

CATTLE. Diazepam is being studied for its sedative and appetite-stimulating effects in cattle. It induces sedation in calves with an IV dose of 0.4 mg/kg (Mirakhur et al. 1984). Additional studies are required to demonstrate the efficacy and safety of diazepam in cattle.

LABORATORY ANIMALS. Ketamine alone and combined with diazepam or xylazine has been used in a number of common laboratory animals (Green et al. 1981). Diazepam has been used in the rabbit with a number of analgesic agents for induction of neuroleptanalgesia (Flecknell et al. 1983a). In the gerbil (*Meriones unguiculatus*), IP diazepam (5 mg/kg) plus IM ketamine (50 mg/kg) has been used for induction of anesthesia (Flecknell et al. 1983b).

EXOTIC SPECIES. IV administration of ketamine (30–40 mg/kg) and diazepam (1–1.5 mg/kg) has been successfully used in diurnal raptors representing 11 species (Redig and Duke 1976). Ketamine and atropine are mixed together and administered into the brachial vein of the bird. Birds usually become immobilized within 15 seconds and anesthesia occurs within 1 minute. Five minutes after ketamine and atropine administration, diazepam is given intravenously. Owls are more sensitive to the anesthetic combination and require lower doses (10 mg/kg) of ketamine as well as greater attention during anesthetization. The anesthesia induced permits amputation of injured wings and legs, open reduction and intramedullary pinning of fractured long bones, laparotomies, and minor procedures such as radiography and repair of lacerations (Redig and Duke 1976).

For immobilization of wild mammals, doses of diazepam vary from 1 to 3.5 mg/kg depending on species and degree of excitement at the time of IM or IV injection (Fowler 1978). Oral administration is not recommended by Fowler for chemical restraint or immobilization procedures. Onset of action is within 1–2 minutes following IV administration; after IM injection, 15–30 minutes is generally required. Clinical effects of diazepam generally are gone within 60–90 minutes (Fowler 1978).

Diazepam in combination with ketamine has been used for anesthetic purposes in river otters (see Chap. 12).

In the leopard seal (*Hydrurga leptonyx*), a combination of IM diazepam (0.2 mg/kg) and IM ketamine (1 mg/kg) has been used to induce light sedation (Gales 1984). Administration of additional doses of ketamine and diazepam are necessary to induce anesthesia.

Harbor seals (*Phoca vitulina*) and gray seals (*Halichoerus grypus*) can be immobilized by a combination of IV or IM ketamine (1.5 mg/kg) and IV or IM diazepam (0.05 mg/kg) (Geraci et al. 1981). Induction and recovery with this combination of drugs are smoother than with use of ketamine alone.

In northern elephant seal pups (*Mirounga angustirostris*) weighing 50 kg or less, IV diazepam (2.5–5 mg/animal) is generally sufficient to induce sedation (Gage 1984). Larger animals need a 0.1–0.25 mg/kg IV dose (via the intravertebral extradural vein) for sedation to facilitate force feeding. Immobilization is required in California sea lions (*Zalophus californianus*), northern elephant seals, and harbor seals for surgical diagnostic procedures; a combination of IM or IV atropine (0.02–0.04 mg/kg), IM or IV diazepam (0.22 mg/kg), and IM ketamine (4–10 mg/kg) induces anesthesia for about 15 minutes. It is suggested that atropine and diazepam be administered 5–10 minutes before administration of ketamine. The lower dose

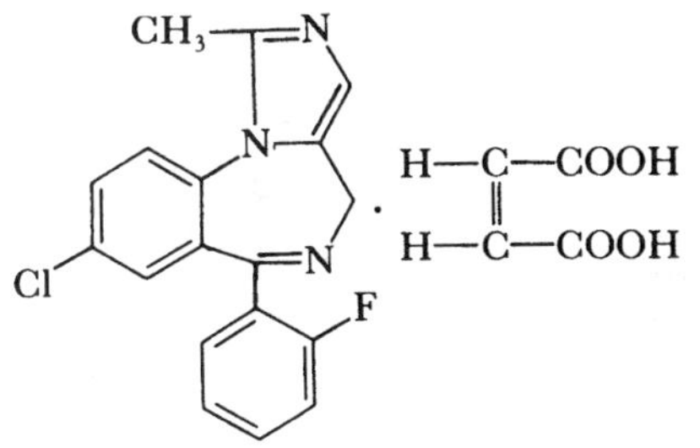

Midazolam Maleate

FIG. 14.17

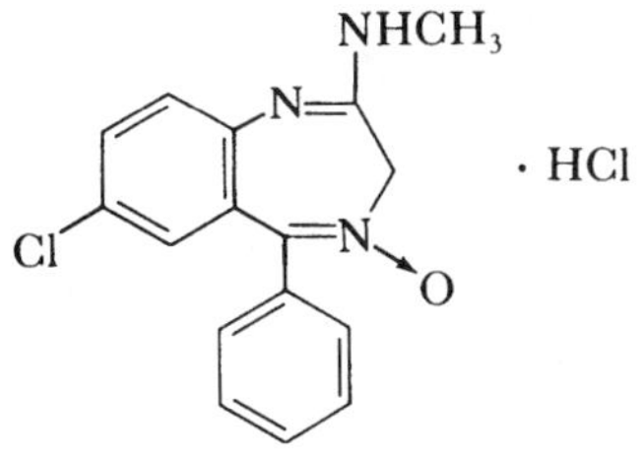

Chlordiazepoxide Hydrochloride

FIG. 14.18

given in the dose range above is suggested whenever ketamine is given intravenously. Animals may be intubated for halothane administration when procedures last more than 15 minutes (Gage 1984).

For restraint of the American alligator (*Alligator mississippiensis*), diazepam (mean dose of 0.37 mg/kg) is administered by the IM route; 20 minutes later, succinylcholine at a mean IM dose of 0.24 mg/kg is given (Spiegel et al. 1984). Muscle relaxation of the immobilized alligator facilitates examination for reproductive procedures.

Midazolam Maleate. *Midazolam Maleate,* INN (Versed), is a benzodiazepine with pharmacologic and chemical structural properties similar to those of diazepam (Fig. 14.17). It was synthesized in 1976.

Midazolam possesses all the properties characteristic of benzodiazepines. It is anxiolytic and anticonvulsant and will produce hypnosis, sedation, amnesia, and muscle relaxation. Unlike diazepam, midazolam is water soluble. High lipophilicity is reflected in the large volumes of distribution for midazolam and diazepam, although the relatively greater lipid solubility of midazolam results in a more rapid onset of action than diazepam. Midazolam is approximately 3–4 times as potent as diazepam, although relative potencies differ among the benzodiazepines with respect to each of the pharmacodynamic effects (Reves et al. 1994). The imidazole ring of midazolam is rapidly oxidized by the liver, accounting for its shorter duration of action when compared with diazepam. According to metabolism and plasma clearance, midazolam is classified as short lasting, whereas diazepam is classified as long lasting (Reves 1984; Greenblatt et al. 1981). Midazolam is biotransformed to hydroxymidazolams, which are relatively inactive metabolites (Ziegler et al. 1983).

Midazolam appears to be useful for induction of anesthesia in humans when a substitute for ultrashort-acting barbiturates is desired (Sarnquist et al. 1980). Ten mg midazolam is equivalent to 200 mg thiopental in duration of sleep induced. Apnea following IV administration of midazolam is less frequent and of shorter duration than after thiopental. In humans, midazolam appears to be a satisfactory agent for induction of anesthesia; it is about 20 times as potent as thiopental. However, it will not replace thiopental as an induction agent (Reves et al. 1985).

Midazolam cannot be used alone to maintain adequate anesthesia; nitrous oxide and halothane are effective agents for its maintenance (Reves et al. 1985). On June 1, 1986, midazolam was approved by the FDA for use in humans.

Midazolam dosages for use in veterinary patients have not been established. Suggested dosages are similar to those for diazepam: 0.045–0.1 mg/kg by IV or IM injection for the dog and cat; 0.0045–0.01 mg/kg by IV injection for the horse (Muir and Hubbell 1989).

Chlordiazepoxide Hydrochloride. Chemically, *Chlordiazepoxide Hydrochloride,* USP (Librium), is 7-chloro-2-methylamino-5-phenyl-3*H*-1,4-benzodiazepine 4-oxide monohydrochloride (Fig. 14.18). Its pharmacologic activity is comparable to that of diazepam; however, it has less overall potency. In treatment of anxiety and related conditions in humans, its long-term use is ordinarily free from most complications. Several publications report liver damage, including icterus, from long-term administration of chlordiazepoxide. In the rat, studies on the isolated perfused liver reveal that the drug decreases bile flow and biliary excretion of sulfobromophthalein (Abernathy et al. 1975). Most veterinary medical uses in animals do not extend over long periods. Development of liver impairment in animals following short-term treatment is unlikely.

In humans, data suggest the possibility that chlordiazepoxide may be teratogenic when administered during the first 6 weeks of pregnancy (Milkovich and Van Den Berg 1974). SC administration of high doses (50 and 200 mg/kg) 1 or more days prior to the time for normal palate closure in the mouse results in structural deformities (i.e., cleft palate) (Walker and Patterson 1974). Until more is learned about possible teratogenic effects of chlordiazepoxide during gestation or pregnancy, its use should be avoided in breeding animals.

Chlordiazepoxide is classified as a Schedule IV drug under the 1970 Controlled Substances Act.

TABLE 14.3—Dose of chlordiazepoxide used in zoological species

Species	Dose	Route	Effects
	(mg/kg)		
European lynx	6	Oral	Calm in 2–3 hr; drowsiness and ataxia noted for several hours
Dingo	3	Oral	Onset of action in about 2 hr; no ataxia noted; allowed petting
	7	Oral	Ataxia produced
Guinea baboon	13	Oral	Docile in 2.5 hr to allow IV pentobarbital
Sea lion	7	Oral	Lethargy and calmness noted 4 hr later
Burmese macaque	5	IM	Calmed for anesthesia
Red kangaroo	11	Oral	Calm in 1.5 hr for radiographs
Mule deer	2.2	IV	Calm within a few minutes
Gnu	4	IM	Calm in 45 min
Gerenuk	5	IM	Calm in 45 min

Clinical Use

SWINE. Chlordiazepoxide in an IM dose of 5–10 mg/kg has an onset of action about 1 hour following administration (Ragan and Gillis 1975). Sedative action of the drug is unpredictable; there is no advantage in its use over phenothiazine derivatives (Ragan and Gillis 1975).

EXOTIC ANIMALS. Although chlordiazepoxide produces a satisfactory effect in a number of exotic animals, it fails to produce a desired effect in the Sumatran tiger, Hensel's cat, tapir, and klipspringer (Heuschele 1961). However, the lynx and dingo are converted from hostile, aggressive animals to docile ones. Doses of chlordiazepoxide reported by Heuschele (1961) to have produced favorable responses in zoological species are summarized in Table 14.3.

Benzodiazepine Antagonists. Three different classes of benzodiazepine ligands have been identified: agonists, antagonists, and inverse agonists (Möhler and Richards 1988). The agonists alter the conformation of the $GABA_A$-receptor complex, with the resulting occurrence of the agonist effects (anxiolysis, hypnosis, anticonvulsant action, muscle relaxation). Antagonists occupy the benzodiazepine receptor but produce no activity, therefore blocking the actions of the agonists. The inverse agonists reduce the efficiency of the GABA inhibitory system, thereby resulting in CNS stimulation.

Flumazenil. In 1979, a specific benzodiazepine receptor antagonist, flumazenil (formerly R015-1788; Mazicon), was synthesized. *Flumazenil* (ethyl-8-fluoro-5,6-dihydro-5-methyl-6-oxo-4*H*-imidazo[1,5-a] benzodiazepine-3-carboxylate) (Fig. 14.19) was the first benzodiazepine antagonist approved for clinical use in human medicine (Brogden and Goa 1991). Flumazenil has high affinity and great specificity for the benzodiazepine receptor and minimal intrinsic effect (Haefely 1988; File and Pellow 1986). It is a competitive antagonist, interacting with the receptor in a concentration-dependent and reversible manner. Flumazenil is metabolized in the liver and rapidly cleared from the plasma. Compared to other benzodiazepines, flumazenil has the highest clearance and shortest elimination half-life. This results in the potential for resedation when a benzodiazepine agonist with a longer duration of action is administered (Reves et al. 1994). Similarly, agonists that are more potent than flumazenil, such as lorazepam, may require administration of additional antagonist (Dunton et al. 1988). Flumazenil has successfully reversed several benzodiazepine agonists, including midazolam and diazepam (Reves et al. 1994). Flumazenil is devoid of any inherent cardiovascular and respiratory effects but will reverse those effects of the agonists. Flumazenil has no anticonvulsant properties and will reverse the anticonvulsant properties of benzodiazepine agonists. There is evidence that flumazenil tends to reverse the hypnotic and respiratory effects more than the amnesic effects of benzodiazepine agonists (Weinbrum and Geller 1990; Ghoneim et al. 1989; Curran and Birch 1991). It will not reverse respiratory depression associated with opioid administration (Weinbrum and Geller 1990).

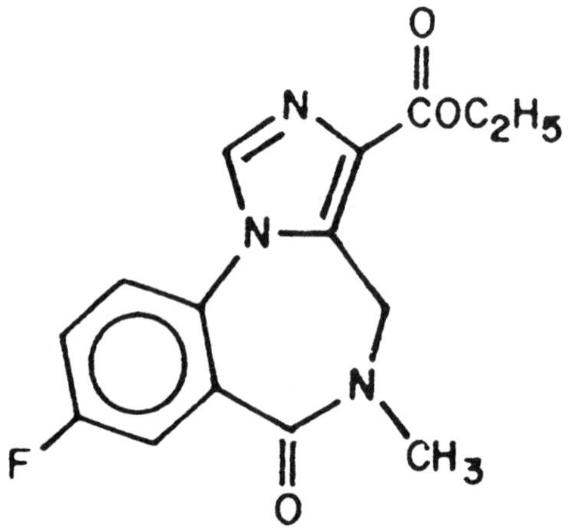

FIG. 14.19.—Flumazenil

A role for flumazenil in veterinary medicine has not been established. At present, the most likely use for flumazenil will be in human medicine to treat overdose with benzodiazepines or to reverse benzodiazepine sedation associated with anesthesia (Reves et al. 1994). Flumazenil has also increased the effectiveness of a benzodiazepine derivative that has been used to treat schistosomiasis in humans. Patients become profoundly sedated when administered 3-methylclonazepam to destroy the parasite. Flumazenil prevents the sedation of the benzodiazepine but does not interfere with the antiparasitic effects, because it is ineffective at benzodiazepine binding sites in schistosomes (Möhler et al. 1981).

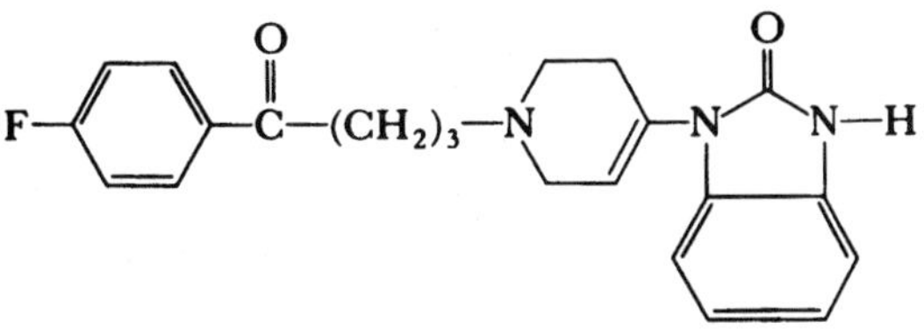

Droperidol

FIG. 14.20

BUTYROPHENONE DERIVATIVES

Mechanism of Action. The butyrophenones are neuroleptics similar to the phenothiazines, with the predominant effect of dopamine receptor blockade (see the section on the phenothiazine derivatives). The butyrophenones have selective affinity only for the dopamine D_2-receptor subfamily, whereas the phenothiazines have affinity predominantly for the D_1-receptor subfamily (Hyttel et al. 1985). Butyrophenones are often referred to as selective dopamine antagonists, but they also possess some affinity for 5-hydroxytryptamine (5-HT) and α_1 adrenoceptors. Although there is a high correlation between dopamine-receptor blockade and neuroleptic activity, it has been suggested that interaction with other receptor types may also play a part in neuroleptic effects or may be implicated in neuroleptic-associated side effects (Hyttel et al. 1985).

Droperidol. *Droperidol,* USP (Inapsine, Droleptan), also known as dehydrobenzperidol, has a complex chemical structure (Fig. 14.20). Droperidol was combined with fentanyl citrate and marketed under the proprietary name of Innovar-Vet, but the combination is no longer available (see Chap. 13). A combination of 4-AP and naloxone (0.5 mg/kg and 0.04 mg/kg respectively) administered rapidly by the IV route antagonizes the effects of droperidol-fentanyl in dogs (Booth et al. 1982). Droperidol-fentanyl-pentobarbital anesthesia in dogs is best antagonized by the IV combination of naloxone (1 mg/kg) and doxapram (5 mg/kg) (Hatch et al. 1986).

PHARMACOLOGIC CONSIDERATIONS. Droperidol is 400 times more active in dogs than chlorpromazine or chlorprothixene and 10 times more active than haloperidol. Droperidol has the shortest action of the butyrophenones. It is the most potent antiemetic known, being up to 1000 times more active than chlorpromazine and chlorprothixene. Droperidol-fentanyl in an IV dose of 1 mL/16 kg is capable of blocking the emetic effect of an IV dose of 0.04 mg/kg apomorphine in the dog (Keith et al. 1981).

As cataleptic immobility–producing drugs and inhibitors of spontaneous and conditioned learning behavior in rats, butyrophenones are several times more effective than chlorpromazine and chlorprothixene. They are also several times more effective as antagonists of amphetamine and apomorphine action in the rat than chlorpromazine and chlorprothixene. Quite unlike butyrophenones, phenothiazines are potent hypotensive and hypothermic agents as well as antagonists of epinephrine. Phenothiazines induce ataxia at much lower dosages and are quantitatively more toxic in action than butyrophenones. The wide safety margin of droperidol is related to its brief duration of action of about 2 hours. Droperidol as well as chlorprothixene may be classified among the most potent antitraumatic shock agents known. There seems to be an interrelationship between antitraumatic shock activity and ability of these agents to inhibit arterial vasoconstriction. In the dog, droperidol has a wide safety margin; tremors, muscle spasticity, and hyperirritability occur only after IV administration and at high doses (11–22 mg/kg). At an IV dose of 0.5 mg/kg, droperidol has little or no effect on cardiac output but decreases arterial pressure, total peripheral resistance, and heart rate. Adrenergic blockade is one of the principal pharmacologic actions of IV droperidol (0.125 mg/kg) in the dog. The slight hypotensive effect at this level is probably due to peripheral vasodilation caused at least in part by adrenergic blockade. IV droperidol (4 mg/kg) causes slowing of respiration and heart rate, hypotension, and a drop in cardiac output as well as a decrease in the force of myocardial contraction.

In the USA, droperidol is available as a single agent for use in humans. Its use in veterinary medicine is primarily in combination with fentanyl for neuroleptanalgesic purposes (see Chap. 13).

PRECAUTIONS AND CONTRAINDICATIONS. Since droperidol and related butyrophenones block α-adrenergic receptors, administration of epinephrine is contraindicated. In animals with severe cardiovascular disorders, the hypotensive action of droperidol may worsen the condition; cardiovascular collapse is possible. Plasma prolactin concentrations are increased by butyrophenone drugs by virtue of their blockade of dopamine receptors within the hypothalamus. Galactorrhea may occur as a side effect.

Azaperone. Azaperone (Stresnil, Suicalm) is a neuroleptic agent belonging to the butyrophenone derivatives. It has been used for nearly two decades in

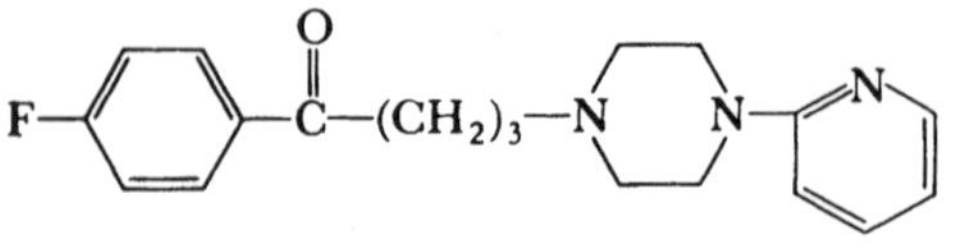

Azaperone

FIG. 14.21

European countries. In October 1983, azaperone was approved by the FDA for use as a tranquilizer in swine weighing up to 36.4 kg to control aggressiveness and fighting (Porter and Slusser 1985).

Azaperone chemically is 4′-fluoro-4-[4-(2-pyridyl)-1-piperazinyl]butyrophenone (Fig. 14.21).

Azaperone is commercially available in the USA as an injectable solution containing 40 mg/mL. It should be stored at 15–30° C.

PHARMACOLOGIC CONSIDERATIONS. Azaperone is a relatively nontoxic, short-acting drug that is rapidly detoxified and eliminated. It is active for 2–3 hours and is nearly eliminated from body tissues within 16 hours (Callear and Van Gestel 1973). Tissue residues of azaperone accumulate in kidney, liver, brain, and skeletal muscle, ranging from less than 20 to 80 ppm 1 hour after an IM injection of 0.4 mg/kg (Rauws and Olling 1978). The metabolite of azaperone (i.e., azaperol) is also present as a tissue residue. For more information on tissue residues, see Chap. 58.

Studies have been conducted on the hemodynamic and pulmonary effects of azaperone following IM and IV administration in swine (Clarke 1969). IM doses of 0.54–3.5 mg/kg reduce arterial pressure to between 70 and 84% of control values and reflexly stimulate respiration. The severity of the drop in blood pressure appears to be related to dose level and usually occurs within 5–10 minutes after administration. The skin of the pig becomes pink, ostensibly from cutaneous vasodilation (Clarke 1969), which may be related to the blockade of α-adrenergic receptors. Such blockade by azaperone occurs in the rat, cat, and dog (Hapke and Priggs 1972). In the pig, azaperone blocks the α-adrenergic action of phenylephrine (Gregory and Wilkins 1986). Additionally, azaperone has a moderate β-adrenergic blocking action and may suppress sympathetic reflexes.

Administration of 0.03 mg/kg azaperone by the IV route in the pig results in a greater drop in arterial pressure (42% of the control value). In addition, initial violent excitement occurs, with good sedation following later. Respiration rate becomes elevated during the period of sedation, and a fall in the P_aCO_2 is observed (Clarke 1969). Other cardiovascular effects include reduction in heart rate and cardiac output.

In the pony, mean arterial pressure is lowered for at least 4 hours by IM injection of azaperone (0.4 or 0.8 mg/kg) (Lees and Serrano 1976). This is about as long as the neuroleptic action of azaperone lasts. Arterial hypotension in the early stage of drug action is due to a drop in peripheral resistance, which is similar to the pharmacologic action of droperidol. Azaperone does not alter plasma protein concentrations; the packed-cell volume and hemoglobin concentration are lowered by 5–10% for at least 4 hours in the pony. Arterial pH, P_aCO_2, and P_aO_2 remain relatively stable throughout the action of azaperone (Lees and Serrano 1976).

Azaperone prevents halothane-induced malignant hyperthermia in susceptible swine (McGrath et al. 1985). The minimal IM protective dose of azaperone that protects 100% of the pigs is 0.5 mg/kg; the minimal IM dose that produces toxicity is 10 mg/kg.

Because azaperone has a number of other pharmacologic properties similar to droperidol, see the discussion above on droperidol.

CLINICAL USE

SWINE. Azaperone is used in swine to prevent population stress and aggressiveness and fighting that occur upon mixing litters (Symoens and Van Den Brande 1969). It is indicated in reduction of excitement during parturition and in prevention of sows from overt mistreatment and abuse of their young. In Pietrain pigs, azaperone is used for prevention of excitement and reduction of mortality from the "overloading of the heart" syndrome common to this breed. It is used prior to minor and major surgical procedures conducted under local, regional, and general anesthesia (Jones 1972).

The efficacy of azaperone against aggressiveness in the pig has been evaluated in animals brought together in small, unfamiliar groups (Symoens and Van Den Brande 1969). After an IM dose of less than 1.5 mg/kg, piglets and adult pigs lie down in 3 and 10 minutes respectively for 30–60 minutes. Despite the influence of azaperone, violent fighting follows whenever they are startled by inadvertent noise or disturbance in an adjacent pen. Some animals treated at doses lower than 1.5 mg/kg die following episodes of fighting (Symoens and Van Den Brande 1969). When IM doses of 1.5–3 mg/kg are administered, sedation is observed within 5–15 minutes. This effect lasts about 2 hours, after which the pigs move about without difficulty and without manifesting aggressiveness. Although occasional fighting occurs to establish a pecking order, it usually is of short duration and intensity. No deaths have occurred in animals treated at these dosages (Symoens and Van Den Brande 1969). Untreated or control animals fight more than twice as frequently and four times as long.

The remarkable action of azaperone in inhibiting aggressiveness in the pig not only occurs during sedation but appears to be permanent. Perhaps by the time sedative effects have waned or disappeared, animals have adapted to each other by exchange of sensory information (smell) and acceptance of one another occurs (Symoens and Van Den Brande 1969). In contrast to these findings, Blackshaw (1981) reported that 1 mL/20 kg or 2 mg/kg of injected azaperone (probably by the IM route) does not prevent fighting. Fighting in treated groups was seen as often upon recovery from the drug as in untreated groups. The different results of these investigators are unexplained.

In a field study involving a large number of pigs, azaperone use has been classified according to type of effect following IM administration (Callear and Van Gestel 1973): (1) low doses (0.4–1.2 mg/kg) for stress conditions such as anxiety and nervousness permit animals to remain ambulatory and calm; (2) median doses primarily for the socializing effect at a level of 2 mg/kg cause animals to eventually lie down and appear somnolent but allow them to move around if disturbed; and (3) when high doses of 4 mg/kg in adult pigs and 8 mg/kg in piglets are given for their knock-down effect for minor surgical procedures, animals become recumbent and are unable to stand.

To avoid untoward effects, it is recommended that 2 mg/kg not be exceeded in large boars (Callear and Van Gestel 1973).

Recommendations of the European manufacturers for use of azaperone in the pig intramuscularly are 1 mg/kg for production of sedation, 2.5 mg/kg for reduction of aggressiveness, and 5–10 mg/kg for knock-down or immobilization effect (Cox 1973). In the USA, an IM dose of azaperone (2.2 mg/kg) in the feeder pig is approved by the FDA.

Azaperone must be administered by the IM route or it will be ineffective. It must be given by deep IM injection either behind the ear and perpendicularly to the skin or in the gluteal region; injection into or near the sciatic nerve must be avoided. A disadvantage of azaperone for immobilization of adult swine is the large volume that must be administered.

According to Blackshaw (1981), azaperone does not reduce the aggressive interactions between pigs at weaning nor does it provide an added growth or weight gain advantage in the period after weaning. Moreover, Blackshaw stated that there appears to be no economic or commercial advantage to injecting azaperone into pigs placed together at weaning.

In boars, IM azaperone (1.5 mg/kg) reduces fighting but does not eliminate aggressive behavior (Pasco 1986). It is suggested that azaperone may be of value in transporting boars in close confinement for no more than 4 hours if they have been detusked.

Azaperone and a hypnotic drug, *Metomidate,* INN (Hypnodil), are used in combination to produce a condition resembling neuroleptanalgesia in the pig. Azaperone is given in an IM dose of 2 mg/kg and is immediately followed by metomidate intraperitoneally at 10 mg/kg (Cox 1973). As an alternative, azaperone (2.5 mg/kg) is given intramuscularly, and 20–30 minutes later metomidate (2.5 mg/kg) is administered intravenously (Jones 1972). This combination produces deep sedation for over 1 hour and is satisfactory for surgical procedures such as amputation of a digit or cesarean section in conjunction with regional or local anesthesia. If it is necessary to extend or increase the period of sedation, another dose of metomidate (1 mg/kg) may be administered intravenously. When general anesthesia is required, and to enable endotracheal intubation, 5 mg/kg metomidate are recommended following administration of azaperone (Jones 1972). Metomidate is a nonbarbiturate agent and is used in other species (see Chap. 12).

HORSES. Azaperone is an excellent ataractic agent in the horse (Hillidge et al. 1977; Mackenzie and Snow 1977). IV administration should be avoided because it can induce marked arterial hypotension. Azaperone (0.29–0.57 mg/kg) quite frequently evokes excitement or a panic reaction following IV administration (Dodman and Waterman 1979).

The sedative effect of 0.8 mg/kg azaperone is considered to be greater than that produced by 0.1 mg/kg acepromazine when administered intramuscularly. If azaperone is used prior to induction of anesthesia with thiopental, it is suggested that IV thiopental not exceed 7 mg/kg (Hillidge et al. 1977). Generally, the cardiovascular actions of azaperone are likely to have little effect in normal animals; however, caution needs to be taken when azaperone is administered to anemic, hypovolemic, or debilitated animals.

In the pony, an IM dose of 0.4 mg/kg azaperone induces a slight to excellent degree of neurolepsy (Lees and Serrano 1976). Following a higher dose (0.8 mg/kg), a good to excellent effect is obtained. Onset of action is generally seen within 10 minutes, reaching a peak after 10–70 minutes. Effects of azaperone in the pony decrease by 2 hours and usually disappear after 4 hours.

Limited studies with azaperone-metomidate have been conducted in the horse (Hillidge et al. 1973). Azaperone has been used in an IV dose of 0.2 mg/kg followed by IV metomidate (3.5 mg/kg); surgical anesthesia lasts 8 ± 3 minutes; the approximate time required to stand takes 35 ± 25 minutes (Crispin 1984).

Hemolysis occurs in samples of venous plasma collected between 5 minutes and 6 hours following administration of azaperone-metomidate. Until more information is gained about the hemolytic effect, this drug combination should not be used in the horse (Archer 1973).

Precautions and contraindications in the use of azaperone are generally the same as those discussed for droperidol in this chapter.

REFERENCES

Aantaa, R., Marjamaki, and A., Scheinin, M. 1995. Molecular pharmacology of α_2-adrenoceptor subtypes. Annals of Medicine 27:439–449.

Abernathy, C. O., Smith, S., and Zimmerman, H. J. 1975. Proc Soc Exp Biol Med 149:271.

Akin, F. J., Rose, A. P., III, Chamness, T. W., et al. 1979. Toxicol Appl Pharmacol 49:219.

Albert, P. R., Neve, K. A., Bunzow, J. R., et al. 1990. Coupling of a cloned rat dopamine-D_2 receptor to inhibition of

adenylyl cyclase and prolactin secretion. J Biol Chem 265:2098–2104.
Allen, J. L. 1986. Use of tolazoline as an antagonist to xylazine-ketamine-induced immobilization in African elephants. Am J Vet Res 47:781–783.
Allen, J. L., and Oosterhuis, L. E. 1986. Effect of tolazoline on xylazine-ketamine-induced anesthesia in turkey vultures. J Am Vet Med Assoc 189:1011–1012.
Amend, J. F., Klavano, P. A., and Stone, E. C. 1972. Premedication with xylazine to eliminate muscular hypertonicity in cats during ketamine anesthesia. Vet Med/Small Anim Clinician 67(12):1305–1307.
Amrein, R., Hetzel, W., Harmann, D., et al. 1988. Clinical pharmacology of flumazenil. Eur J Anaesthesiol 2:65.
Anderson, I. L. 1973. Aust Vet J 49:474.
Anika, S. M. 1985. Vet Res Commun 9:309.
Archer, R. K. 1973. Vet Rec 93:379.
Arnemo, J. M., and Soli, N. E. 1992. Immobilization of mink (*Mustela vison*) with medetomidine-ketamine and remobilization with atipamezole. Vet Res Commun 16:281–292.
Asghari, V., Schoots, O., Van Kats, S., et al. 1994. Dopamine D_4 receptor repeat: Analysis of different native and mutant forms of the human and rat genes. Mol Pharmacol 46:364–373.
Aurori, K. C., and Vesell, E. S. 1974. Drug Metab Disp 2:566.
Aziz, M. A., and Martin, R. J. 1978. Alpha agonist and local anesthetic properties of xylazine. Zentrablatt Vet Med 25:180–188.
Ballard, S., Shults, R., Kownacki, A. A., et al. 1982. J Vet Pharmacol Ther 5:21.
Barron, C. N., Rubin, L. F., and Steelman, R. L. 1972. Exp Mol Pathol 16:158.
Bauditz, R. 1972. Vet Med Rev 3/4:204.
Beckett, S. D., Hudson, R. S., Reynolds, T. M., et al. 1973. Am J Physiol 225:1072.
Beckett, S. D., Walker, D. F., Hudson, R. S., et al. 1975. Am J Vet Res 36:431.
Beer, B., Klepner, C. A., Lippa, A. S., et al. 1978. Pharmacol Biochem Behav 9:849.
Benson, G. J., and Thurmon, J. C. 1979. J Am Vet Med Assoc 174:594.
Bergstrom, K. 1988. Cardiovascular and pulmonary effects of a new sedative/analgesic (medetomidine) as a preanesthetic drug in the dog. Acta Vet Scand 29:109–116.
Beroza, G. A. 1980. J Am Vet Med Assoc 177:1152.
Biswas, B., and Carlsson, A. 1978. Arch Pharmacol 303:73.
Blackshaw, J. K. 1981. Aust Vet J 57:272.
Bloor, B. C., Abdul-Rasool, I., Temp, J., et al. 1989. The effects of medetomidine, an α_2 adrenergic agonist, on ventilatory drive in the dog. Acta Vet Scand 85:65–70.
Bodily, K. J. 1979. Auburn Vet 35:16.
Booth, N. H. 1969. Fed Proc 28:1547.
Booth, N. H., Hatch, R. C., and Crawford, L. M. 1982. Am J Vet Res 43:1227.
Bowen, J. M. 1976. Vet Anesth 3:100.
Braestrup, C., and Squires, R. F. 1977. Specific benzodiazepine receptors in rat brain characterized by high affinity [3H]diazepam binding. Proc Nat Acad Sci USA 74:1839–1847.
Branson, K. R., Ko, J. C. H., Tranquilli, W. J., et al. 1993. Duration of analgesia induced by epidurally administered morphine and medetomidine in the dog. J Vet Pharmacol Ther 16:369–372.
Bree, M. M., Cohen, B. J., and Abrams, G. D. 1971. J Am Vet Med Assoc 159:1598.
Brikas, P., Tsiamitas, C., and Wyburn, R. S. 1986. J Vet Med A33:174.
Bristow, D. R., Moratalla, R., and Martin, I. L. 1990. Flunitrazepam increases the affinity of the GABAA receptor in cryostat-cut rat brain sections. Eur J Pharmacol 184:339–340.
Brogden, R. N., and Goa, K. L. 1991. Flumazenil. Drugs 42:1061.
Brown, J. R. 1986. Mod Vet Pract 67:125.
Bryant, C. E., England, G. C., and Clarke, K. W. 1991. Comparison of the effects of medetomidine and xylazine in horses. Vet Rec 129:421–423.
Bush, M., Ensley, P. K., Mehren, K., et al. 1976. J Am Vet Med Assoc 169:884.
Butera, S. T., Garner, H. E., Moore, J. N., et al. 1980. Vet Med Small Anim Clin 75:765.
Bylund, D. B. 1988. Subtypes of α_2-adrenoceptors: pharmacological and molecular biological evidence converge. Trends Pharmacol Sci 9:356–361.
Calderwood, H. W. 1971. J Am Vet Med Assoc 159:1618.
Callear, J. F. F., and Van Gestel, J. F. E. 1973. Vet Rec 92:284.
Campbell, K. B., Klavano, P. A., Richardson, P., et al. 1979. Am J Vet Res 40:1777.
Castro, S. W., and Strange, P. G. 1993. Coupling of D_2 and D_3 dopamine receptors to G-proteins. FEBS Letts 315:223–226.
Chabert, C., Cavegn, C., Bernard, A., et al. 1994. Characterization of the functional activity of dopamine ligands at human recombinant dopamine D_4 receptors. J Neurochem 63:62–65.
Chase, P. E. 1977. Feline Pract 7:24.
Cheung, Y.-D., Barnett, D. B., and Nahorski, S. R. 1982. ^{3}H-rauwolscine and ^{3}H-yohimbine binding to rat cerebral and human platelet membranes: evidence for possible heterogeneity of α_2-adrenoceptors. Eur J Pharmacol 84:79–85.
Chio, C. L., Lajiness, M. E., and Huff, R. M. 1993. Activation of heterologously expressed D_3 dopamine receptors: comparison with D_2 dopamine receptors. Mol Pharmacol 45:51–60.
Christian, R. G., Mills, J. H. L., and Kramer, L. L. 1974. Can Vet J 15:29.
Clarke, K. W. 1969. Vet Rec 85:649.
Clarke, K. W., and Hall, L. W. 1969. Vet Rec 85:512.
Clarke, K. W., and Paton, B. S. 1988. Combined use of detomidine with opiates in horses. Equine Vet J 20:331–334.
Clarke, K. W., and Taylor, P. M. 1986. Detomidine: a new sedative for horses. Equine Vet J 18(5):366–370.
Clarke, K. W., Taylor, P. M., and Watkins, S. B. 1986a. Detomidine/ketamine anesthesia in the horse. Acta Vet Scand 82:167–179.
Clarke, R. D., Michel, A. D., and Whiting, R. L. 1986b. Pharmacology and structure-activity relationships of α_2-adrenoceptor antagonists. Prog Med Chem 23:1–39.
Clifford, D. H., and Soma, L. R. 1969. Fed Proc 28:1479.
Clough, D. P., and Hutton, R. 1981. Hypotensive and sedative effects of an adrenoceptor agonist: relationship to α_1 and α_2 adrenoceptor potency. Br J Pharmacol 73:595–604.
Code of Federal Regulations. 1974. 21 CFR 131.11. Washington, DC.: Government Printing Office.
Colby, E. D., and Sanford, T. D. 1981. Feline Pract 11:19.
Colby, E. D., McCarthy, L. E., and Borison, H. L. 1981. J Vet Pharmacol Ther 4:93.
Cooper, J. E., Harris, S., Forbes, A., et al. 1986. Br Vet J 142:350.
Cooper, J. R., Bloom, F. E., and Roth, R. H. 1991. The Biochemical Basis of Neuropharmacology. 6th ed. New York: Oxford Univ Press.
Costa, E., and Guidotti, A. 1979. Ann Rev Pharmacol Toxicol 19:531.
Cotler, S., Gustafson, J. H., and Colburn, W. A. 1984. J Pharm Sci 73:348.
Coulter, D. B., Whelan, S. C., Wilson, R. C., et al. 1981. Cornell Vet 71:76.

Coward, D. M. 1992. General pharmacology of clozapine. Brit J Psych Suppl 17:5–11.

Cox, J. E. 1973. Vet Rec 92:143.

Crighton, M. 1990. Diuresis following medetomidine. Vet Rec 126:201.

Crispin, S. M. 1984. Equine Vet J 13:19.

Cronin, M. F., Booth, N. H., Hatch, R. C., et al. 1983a. Acepromazine-xylazine combination in dogs: antagonism with 4-aminopyridine and yohimbine. Am J Vet Res 44:2037–2042.

———. 1983b. Am J Vet Res 44:2586.

Curran, H. V., and Birch, B. 1991. Differentiating the sedative, psychomotor and amnesic effects of benzodiazepines: a study with midazolam and the benzodiazepine antagonist, flumazenil. Psychopharmacology (Berlin) 103:519.

Custer, R., Kramer, L., Kennedy, S., et al. 1977. J Am Vet Med Asoc 171:899.

Dallaire, A., and Chalifoux, A. 1985. Can J Comp Med 49:171.

Dal Toso, R., Sommer B., Ewert, M., et al. 1989. The dopamine D_2 receptor: Two molecular forms generated by alternative splicing. EMBO J. 8:4025–4034.

Darlison, M. G., Albrecht, B. E. 1995. $GABA_A$ receptor subtypes: which, where, and why? The Neurosciences 7:115–126.

Delbarre, B., and Schmitt, H. 1971. Sedative effects of α-sympathomimetic drugs and their antagonism by adrenergic and cholinergic blocking drugs. Eur J Pharmacol 13:356–363.

———. 1973. A further attempt to characterize sedative receptors activated by clonidine in chickens and mice. Eur J Pharmacol 22:355–359.

de Wied, D. 1967. Pharmacol Rev 19:251.

Dhasmana, K. M., Dixit, K. S., Jaju, B. P., et al. 1972. Psychopharmacologia 24:380.

DiChiara, G., and Gessa, G. L. 1978. Adv Pharmacol Chemother 15:87.

Dockal, K., Hais, R., Hosek, J., et al. 1975. Acta Veta Brno 44:59.

Dodman, N. H., and Waterman, A. E. 1979. Equine Vet J 11:33.

Dodman, N. H., Seeler, D. C., and Court, M. H. 1984. Br Vet J 140:505.

Dohlman, H. G., Thorner, J., Caron, M. G., and Lefkowitz, R. J. 1991. Model systems for the study of seven-transmembrane-segment receptors. Ann Rev Biochem 60:653–688.

Doze, V. A., Chen, B.-X., and Maze, M. 1989. Dexmedetomidine produces a hypnotic-anesthetic action in rats via activation of central α_2 adrenoceptors. Anesthesiology 71:75–79.

Doze, V. A., Chen, B.-X., Tinklenberg, J. A., et al. 1990. Pertussis toxin and 4-aminopyridine differentially affect the hypnotic-anesthetic action of dexmedetomidine and pentobarbital. Anesthesiology 73:304–307.

Drasner, K., and Fields, H. L. 1988. Synergy between the antinociceptive effects of intrathecal clonidine and systemic morphine in rats. Pain 32:309–312.

Duhm, B., Maul, W., Medenwald, M., et al. 1969. Berl Munch Tieraerz Wochenschr 82:104.

Dunlap, K., and Fischbach, G. D. 1981. Neurotransmitters decrease calcium conductance activated by depolarization of embryonic sensory neurones. J Physiol (Lond) 317:519–535.

Dunton, A. W., Schwam, E., Pitman, V., et al. 1988. Flumazenil: U.S. clinical pharmacology studies. Eur J Anaesthesiol 2:81.

Einhorn, L. C., Falardeau, P., Caron, M. G., et al. 1990. Both forms of the D_2 dopamine receptor couple to a G protein–activated K^+ channel when expressed in GH4 cells. Soc Neurosci Abstr 16:382.

Ellis, R. G., Lowe, J. E., Schwark, W. S., et al. 1977. J Equine Med Surg 1:259.

England, G. C. W., and Clarke, K. W. 1989. The use of medetomidine/fentanyl combinations in dogs. Acta Vet Scand 85:179–186.

England, G. C., Clarke, K. W., and Goossen, S. L. 1992. A comparison of the sedative effects of three alpha 2-adrenoceptor agonists (romifidine, detomidine, xylazine) in horses. J Vet Pharmacol Ther 15(2):194–201.

Farver, T. B., Haskins, S. C., and Patz, J. D. 1986. Am J Vet Res 47:631.

Faulk, R. H. 1978. Feline Pract 8:15.

Fikes, L. W., Lin, H. C., and Thurmon, J. C. 1988. A preliminary comparison of xylazine and lidocaine as epidural analgesics in ponies. Vet Surg 18(1):85–86.

File, S. E., and Pellow, S. 1986. Intrinsic actions of the benzodiazepine receptor antagonist RO 15-1788. Psychopharmacology (Berlin) 88:I–II.

Flecknell, P. A., John, M., Mitchell, M., et al. 1983a. Lab Anim 17:104.

———. 1983b. Lab Anim 17:118.

Fletcher, J. 1974. Hypersensitivity of an isolated population of red deer (*Cervus elaphus*) to xylazine. Vet Rec 94:85–86.

Folkers, E. R. 1980. J Am Vet Med Assoc 176:956.

Fowler, M. E. 1978. Restraint and Handling of Wild and Domestic Animals, p. 49. Ames: Iowa State Univ Press.

Frank, C. J. 1970. Vet Rec 87:497.

Fraser, A. C. 1967. Vet Rec 80:56.

Freedman, S. B., Patel, S., Marwood, R, et al. 1993. Expression and pharmacological characterization of the human D_3 dopamine receptor. J Pharmacol Exp Therap 268:417–426.

Fuentes, V. O. 1978. Vet Rec 102:106.

Gage, L. J. 1984. Proc Annu Meet Am Assoc Zoo Vet, p. 31.

Gales, N. J. 1984. Aust Vet J 61:295.

Garcia-Villar, P. L., Toutain, M., Alvinerie, M., et al. 1981. J Vet Pharmacol Ther 4:87.

Garland, J. E., and White, K. B. 1968. Vet Rec 83:641.

Garner, H. E., Amend, J. F., and Rosborough, J. P. 1971a. Vet Med Small Anim Clin 66:1016.

———. 1971b. Vet Med Small Anim Clin 66:921.

Garner, H. E., Mather, E. C., Hoover, T. R., et al. 1975. Can J Comp Med 39:250.

Gee, K. W., Yamamura, S. H., and Roeske, W. R. 1984. Fed Proc 43:2767.

Geraci, J. R., Skirnisson, K., and St. Aubin, D. J. 1981. J Am Vet Med Assoc 179:1192.

Ghoneim, M. M., Dembo, J. B., and Block, R. I. 1989. Time course of antagonism of sedative and amnesic effects of diazepam by flumazenil. Anesthesiology 70:899.

Gilman, A. G. 1987. G proteins: transducers of receptor-generated signals. Annu Rev Biochem 56:615–649.

Gopal, T., Oehme, F. W., and St. Omer, V. 1976. Am J Vet Res 37:1143.

Graham-Jones, O. 1962. Vet Rec 74:1021.

Grandy, D. K., Zhang, Y., Bouvier, C., et al. 1991. Multiple human D_5 dopamine receptor genes: a functional receptor and two pseudogenes. Proc Nat Acad Sci USA 88:9171–9179.

Green, C. J., Knight, J., Precious, S., et al. 1981. Lab Anim 15:163.

Greenblatt, D. J., and Koch-Weser, J. 1973. Am J Med Sci 266:261.

Greenblatt, D. J., Shader, R. I., and Harmatz, J. S. 1981. Benzodiazepines: a summary of pharmacokinetic properties. Br J Clin Pharmacol 11:11.

Greenblatt, D. J., Abernethy, D. R., Morse, D. S., et al. 1984. N Engl J Med 310:1639.

Gregory, N. G., and Wilkins, L. J. 1986. J Vet Pharmacol Ther 9:164.

Grubb, T. L., Riebold, T. W., and Huber, M. J. 1992. Comparison of lidocaine, xylazine, and xylazine/lidocaine for caudal epidural analgesia in horses. J Am Vet Med Assoc 201(8):1187–1190.
Gupta, B. N., Moore, J. A., and Conner, G. H. 1970. Lab Anim Sci 20:474.
Haefely, W. 1988. The preclinical pharmacology of flumazenil. Eur J Anaesthesiol 2:25.
———. 1989. Pharmacology of the allosteric modulation of $GABA_A$ receptors by benzodiazepine receptor ligands. In E. A. Barnard and E. Costa, eds., Allosteric Modulation of Amino Acid Receptors: Therapeutic Implications, pp. 47–69. Fidia Research Foundation Symposium Series, vol. 1. New York: Raven Press.
Haefely, W., Kyburz, E., Gerecke, M., et al. 1985. Recent advances in the molecular pharmacology of benzodiazepine receptors and in the structure-activity relationships of their agonists and antagonists. In B. Testa, ed., Advances in Drug Research, vol. 14, pp. 165–322. London: Academic Press.
Hall, L. W. 1976. J Small Anim Pract 17:661.
Hapke, H. J., and Priggs, E. 1972. DTW 79:500.
Harthoorn, A. M., Harthoorn, S., and Sayer, P. D. 1971. Vet Rec 89:159.
Hartsfield, S. M., Thurmon, J. C., and Benson, G. H. 1986. Comparison of the effects of tolazoline, yohimbine, and 4-aminopyridine in cats medicated with xylazine (abstr). Vet Surg 15:459–460.
Haskins, S. C., Farver, T. B., and Patz, J. D. 1986b. Am J Vet Res 47:795.
Haskins, S. C., Patz, J. D., and Farver, T. B. 1986a. Am J Vet Res 47:636.
Hatch, R. C. 1967. J Am Vet Med Assoc 150:27.
Hatch, R. C., Booth, N. H., Clark, J. D., et al. 1982. Am J Vet Res 43:1009.
Hatch, R. C., Booth, N. H., Kitzman, J. V., et al. 1983a. Antagonism of ketamine anesthesia in cats by 4-aminopyridine and yohimbine. Am J Vet Res 44:417–423.
Hatch, R. C., Clark, J. D., Booth, N. H., et al. 1983b. Comparison of five preanesthetic medicaments in pentobarbital-anesthetized dogs: antagonism by 4-aminopyridine, yohimbine, and naloxone. Am J Vet Res 44:2312–2319.
Hatch, R. C., Kitzman, J. V., Clark, J. D., et al. 1984. Reversal of pentobarbital anesthesia with 4-aminopyridine and yohimbine in cats pretreated with acepromazine and xylazine. Am J Vet Res 45:2586–2590.
Hatch, R. C., Jernigan, A. D., Wilson, R. C., et al. 1986. Can J Vet Res 50:251.
Heath, R. B. 1977. Colo State Univ Clin Sci Newsl 1, No. 10.
———. 1978. In J. D. Powers and T. E. Powers, eds., Equine Pharmacology, p. 189. Golden, CO: American Association of Equine Practitioners.
Hedler, L., Stamm, G., Weitzell, R., et al. 1981. Eur J Pharmacol 70:43.
Heuschele, W. P. 1961. J Am Vet Med Assoc 139:996.
Hillidge, C. J., Lees, P., and Serrano, L. 1973. Vet Rec 93:307.
———. 1977. Vet Rec 101:174.
Hoehn, K., Reid, A., and Sawynok, J. 1988. Pertussis toxin inhibits antinociception produced by intrathecal injection of morphine, noradrenaline and baclofen. Eur J Pharmacol 146:65–72.
Holmberg, G., and Gershon, J. 1961. Autonomic and psychic effects of yohimbine hydrochloride. Psychopharmacology (Berlin) 2:93–106.
Holz, G. G., Rane, S. G., and Dunlap, K. 1986. GTP-binding proteins mediate transmitter inhibition of voltage-dependent calcium channels. Nature 319:670–672.
Hopkins, T. J. 1972. Aust Vet J 48:109.
Hornykiewicz, O. 1973. Br Med Bull 29:172.
Horobin, D. F. 1981. Lancet 1:277.
Howard, J. L. 1981. In J. L. Howard, ed., Current Veterinary Therapy: Food Animal Practice, p. 1204. Philadelphia: W. B. Saunders.
Hsu, W. H. 1981. Xylazine induced depression and its antagonism by alpha-adrenergic blocking agents. J Pharmacol Exp Ther 218:188–192.
———. 1985. Xylazine-pentobarbital anesthesia in dogs and its antagonism by yohimbine. Am J Vet Res 46:852–855.
Hsu, W. H., and Shulaw, W. P. 1984. Effect of yohimbine on xylazine-induced immobilization in whitetailed deer. J Am Vet Med Assoc 185:1301–1303.
Hsu, W. H., Bellin, S. I., Dellmann, H. D., et al. 1986. Xylazine-ketamine-induced anesthesia in rats and its antagonism by yohimbine. J Am Vet Med Assoc 189:1040–1043.
Hsu, W. H., Schaffer, D. D., and Hanson, C. E. 1987. Effects of tolazine and yohimbine on xylazine-induced central nervous system depression, bradycardia, and tachypnea in sheep. J Am Med Assoc 190(4):423–426.
Hubbell, J. A. E., Hull, B. L., and Muir, W. W. 1986. Beef Contin Educ Artic 8:F–92.
Hyttel, J., Larsen, J.-J., Christensen, A. V., et al. 1985. Receptor-binding profiles of neuroleptics. Psychopharm Suppl 2:9–18.
Jacobson, E. R., Allen, J., Martin, H., et al. 1985. Effects of yohimbine on combined xylazine-ketamine-induced sedation and immobilization in juvenile African elephants. J Am Vet Med Assoc 187:1195–1198.
Jalanka, H. 1989. The use of medetomidine, medetomidine-ketamine combinations and atipamezole at Helsinki Zoo—A review of 240 cases. Acta Vet Scand 85:193–197.
Jalanka, H. H. 1990. Medetomidine and medetomidine-ketamine induced immobilization in blue foxes (*Alopex lagopus*) and its reversal by atipamezole. Acta Vet Scand 31:63-71.
Jarvik, M. E. 1970. In L. S. Goodman and A. Gilman, eds., The Pharmacological Basis of Therapeutics, 4th ed., p. 163. New York: Macmillan.
Jenkins, J. T. 1972. Vet Rec 90:207.
Jeppsson, R. I. 1976. J Clin Pharmacol 1:181.
Jessup, D. A., Clark, W. E., Gullett, P. A., et al. 1983. Immobilization of mule deer with ketamine and xylazine, and reversal of immobilization with yohimbine. J Am Vet Med Assoc 183:1339–1340.
Jessup, D. A., Jones, K., Mohr, R., et al. 1985. Yohimbine antagonism to xylazine in free ranging mule deer and desert bighorn sheep. J Am Vet Med Assoc 187:1251–1253.
Jochle, W., and Hamm, D. 1986. Sedation and analgesia with Domosedan (detomidine hydrochloride) in horses: dose response studies on efficacy and its duration. Acta Vet Scand 82:69–84.
Jones, R. S. 1972. Vet Rec 90:613–617.
———. 1972. Vet Rec 90:613.
Kalpravidh, M., Lumb, W. V., Wright, M., et al. 1984. Am J Vet Res 45:217.
Kamerling, S., Keowen, M., Bagwell, C., et al. 1991. Pharmacologic profile of medetomidine in the equine. Acta Vet Scand 87:161–162.
Kanterman, R. Y., Mahan, L. C., Briley, E. M., et al. 1991. Transfected D2 dopamine receptors mediate the potentiation of arachidonic acid release in Chinese Hamster vary cells. Mol Pharmacol 39:364–369.
Kanto, J., and Klotz, U. 1982. Acta Anaesthesiol Scand 26:554.
Karobath, M., Supavilai, P., Placheta, P., et al. 1981. Interactions of anxiolytic drugs with benzodiazepine receptors. In B. Angrist, ed., Recent Advances in Neuropsychopharmacology, pp. 229–238. Advances in the Bio-sciences, vol. 31. New York: Pergamon Press.

Kendall, D. A. 1996. Classification of α_2-adrenoceptors. J Psychopharm Supp 10 3:2–5.
Kerr, D. D., Jones, E. W., Holbert, D., et al. 1972a. Am J Vet Res 33:777.
Kerr, D. D., Jones, E. W., Huggins, K., et al. 1972b. Am J Vet Res 33:525.
Kirk, R. W., ed. 1977. Current Veterinary Therapy, VI: Small Animal Practice, p. 1375. Philadelphia: W. B. Saunders.
Kirkpatrick, R. M. 1978. Canine Pract 5:53.
Kitzman, J. V., Booth, N. H., Hatch, R. C., et al. 1982. Am J Vet Res 43:2165.
Kitzman, J. V., Wilson, R. C., Hatch, R. C., et al. 1984. Antagonism of xylazine and ketamine anesthesia by 4-aminopyridine and yohimbine in geldings. Am J Vet Res 45:875–879.
Klavano, P. A. 1975. Proc Am Assoc Equine Pract, p. 149.
Klein, L. V., and Baetjer, C. 1974. Vet Anesth 1:2.
Klide, A. M., Calderwood, H. W., and Soma, L. R. 1975. Am J Vet Res 36:931.
Knight, A. P. 1980. J Am Vet Med Assoc 176:454.
Ko, J. C. H., Thurmon, J. C., Benson, G. J., et al. 1994. Hemodynamic and analgesic effects of etomidate infusion in medetomidine-premedicated dogs. Am J Vet Res 55:842–846.
Kobinger, W., and Pichler, L. 1982. J Cardiovasc Pharmacol 4(Suppl):S-81.
Kreeger, T. J., Seal, U. S., and Faggella, A. M. 1986a. Xylazine HCl-ketamine HCl immobilization of wolves and its antagonism by tolazoline HCl. J Wildl Dis 22:397–402.
Kreeger, T. J., Del-Giudice, G. D., Seals, U. S., et al. 1986b. Immobilization of whitetailed deer with xylazine HCl and ketamine HCl and antagonism by tolazoline HCl. J Wildl Dis 22:407–412.
Kumar, A., and Thurmon, J. C. 1979. Lab Anim Sci 29:486.
Kumar, A., Thurmon, J. C., Nelson, D. R., et al. 1983. Vet Med Small Anim Clin 78:955.
Kuntze, A. 1967. Vet Rec 80:278.
Lachowicz, J. E., and Sibley, D. R. 1997. Molecular characteristics of mammalian dopamine receptors. Pharmacol and Toxicol 81:105–113.
Lacuata, A. Q., and Subang, P. M. 1973. Philipp J Vet Med 12:143.
Lang, W. J., and Gershon, S. 1963. Effects of psychoactive drugs on yohimbine induced responses in conscious dogs. Arch Int Pharmacodyn 142:457–472.
Leash, A. M. 1969. Fed Proc 28:1436.
LeBlanc, P. H. 1991. Chemical restraint for surgery in the standing horse. Vet Clin North Am/Equine Pract 7:(3):521–533.
LeBlanc, P. H., Caron, J. P., Patterson, J. S., et al. 1988. Epidural injection of xylazine for perineal analgesia in horses. J Am Vet Med Assoc 193(11):1405–1408.
Lees, P., and Serrano, L. 1976. Br J Pharmacol 56:263.
Lemke, K. A., Tranquilli, W. J., Thurmon, J. C., et al. 1992. Alterations in the arrhythmogenic dose of epinephrine following xylazine and medetomidine administration in halothane anesthetized dogs with and without cholinergic blockade (abstr). Proc, Vet Midwest Anesth Conf.
Levinger, I. M., Kedem, J., and Abram, M. 1973. Br Vet J 129:296.
Lewis, C. J., and Oakley, G. A. 1971. Vet Rec 88:380.
Lin, H. C., Branson, K. R., Thurmon, J. C., et al. 1992. Ketamine, telazol, xylazine, and detomidine: a comparative anesthetic drug combinations study in ponies. Acta Vet Scand 33(2):109–115.
Lin, M. T. 1979. Can J Physiol Pharmacol 57:16.
Liu, L.-X., Monsma, F. J., Sibley, D. R., et al. 1994. D_2S and D_2L receptors couple to K^+ currents in NG108-15 cells via different signal transduction pathways. Soc Neurosci Abs 20:523.
———. 1996. D_2L, D_2S, and D_3 dopamine receptors, stably transfected into NG108-15 cells, couple to a voltage-dependent potassium current via distinct G proteins. Synapse 24:156–164.
Lloyd, K. C. K., Harrison, I., and Tulleners, E. 1985. J Am Vet Med Assoc 186:980.
Loc, T. Q., Tsoucaris-Kupfer, D., Bogaievsky, Y., et al. 1974. J Pharmacol (Paris) 5:51.
Löscher, W., and Frey, H.-H. 1981. Arch Int Pharmacodyn 254:180.
Lowe, J. E. 1982. Proc Equine Colic Res Symp, p. 30.
Lowe, J. E., and Hifiger, J. 1986. Analgesic and sedative effects of detomidine compared to xylazine in a colic model using IV and IM routes of administration. Acta Vet Scand 82:85–95.
Ludders, J. W., Reitan, J. A., Martucci, R., et al. 1983. Am J Vet Res 44:996.
Mackenzie, G., and Snow, D. H. 1977. Vet Rec 101:30.
MacKenzie, R. G., Vanleeuwen, D., Pugsley, T. A., et al. 1994. Characterization of the human dopamine D_3 receptor expressed in transfected cell lines. Eur J Pharmacol 266:79–85.
MacKinnon, A. C., Spedding, M., and Brown C. M. 1994. α_2-Arenoceptors: More subtypes but fewer functional differences. Trends in Pharm Sci 15:119–123.
Macy, D. W., and Gasper, P. W. 1985. J Am Anim Hosp Assoc 21:17.
Malmberg, A., Jackson, D. M., Eriksson, A., et al. 1993. Unique binding characteristics of antipsychotic agents interacting with human dopamine D_2A, D_2B, and D_3 receptors. Mol Pharmacol 43:749–754.
Mason, C. G. 1977. J Toxicol Environ Health 2:977.
Matthysse, S. 1973. Fed Proc 32:200.
Maylin, G. A. 1978. In J. D. Powers and T. E. Powers, eds., Equine Pharmacology, p. 193. Golden, CO: American Association of Equine Practitioners.
Maze, M., and Tranquilli, W. 1991. Alpha-2 adrenoceptor agonists: defining the role in clinical anesthesia. Anesthesiology 74:581–605.
McCashin, F. B., and Gabel, A. A. 1971. Proc 17th Annu Meet Am Assoc Equine Pract, p. 111.
———. 1975. Am J Vet Res 36:1421.
McDonald, R. L., and Olsen, R. W. 1994. $GABA_A$ receptor channels. Annu Rev Neurosci 17:569–602.
McGrath, C. J. 1984. Mod Vet Pract 65:522.
McGrath, C. J., Rempel, W. E., Addis, P. B., et al. 1981. Am J Vet Res 42:195.
McGrath, C. J., Lee, J. C., and Ashen, M. D. 1985. Vet Surg 14:75.
McGruder, J. P., and Hsu, W. H. 1985. Antagonism of xylazine-pentobarbital anesthesia by yohimbine in ponies. Am J Vet Res 46:1276–181.
Mendelson, W. B. 1992. Neuropharmacology of sleep induction by benzodiazepines. Neurobiology 16:221.
Michalek, H., and Stavinoha, W. B. 1978. Toxicology 9:205.
Milkovich, L., and Van Den Berg, B. 1974. N Engl J Med 291:1268.
Mirakhur, K. K., Khana, A. K., and Prasad, B. 1984. Agri-Practice 5:29.
Moens, Y., and Fargetton, X. 1990. A comparative study of medetomidine/ketamine and xylazine/ketamine anaesthesia in dogs. Vet Rec 127:567–571.
Möhler, H. 1981. Trends Pharmacol Sci 2:116.
Möhler, H., and Richards, J. G. 1988. The benzodiazepine receptor: a pharmacological control element of brain function. Eur J Anaesthesiol 2:15.
Möhler, H., Burkard, W. P., Keller, H. H., et al., 1981. J Neurochem 37:714.
Monsma, F. J., Shen, Y., Gerfen, C. R., et al. 1991. Molecular cloning of a novel D_{1B} dopamine receptor from rat kidney. Soc Neuro Abst 17:85.

Morley, J. E. 1980. Life Sci 27:355.
Moye, R. J., Pailet, A., and Smith, M. W., Jr. 1973. Vet Med Small Anim Clin 68:236.
Muir, W. 1977. In R. W. Kirk, ed., Current Veterinary Therapy, VI: Small Animal Practice, p. 388. Philadelphia: W. B. Saunders.
Muir, W. W., and Hubbell, J. A. E. 1985. J Am Anim Hosp Assoc 21:285.
———. 1989. Drugs used for preanesthetic medication. In Handbook of Veterinary Anesthesia, p. 20. St. Louis: C. V. Mosby Co.
Muir, W. W., and Robertson, J. T. 1985. Am J Vet Res 46:2081.
Muir, W. W., Werner, L. L., and Hamlin, R. L. 1975. Am J Vet Res 36:1299.
Muir, W. W., Skarda, R. T., and Sheehan, W. 1978. Am J Vet Res 39:1274.
———. 1979a. Am J Vet Res 40:1417.
———. 1979b. Am J Vet Res 40:1518.
Muir, W. W., Sams, R. A., Huffman, R. H., et al. 1982. Am J Vet Res 43:1756.
Mulder, K. J., and Mulder, J. B. 1979. Vet Med Small Anim Clin 74:569.
Nawaz, M. 1981. J Vet Pharmacol Ther 4:157.
Nawaz, M., and Rasmussen, F. 1979. J Vet Pharmacol Ther 2:39.
Nevalainen, T., PyhÑlÑl, L., Voipio, H. M., et al. 1989. Evaluation of anaesthetic potency of medetomidine-ketamine combinations in rats, guinea-pigs and rabbits. Acta Vet Scand 85:139–143.
Neve, K. A., Henningsen, R. A., Bunzow, J. R., et al. 1989. Functional characterization of a rat dopamine D_2 receptor cDNA expressed in a mammalian cell line. Mol Pharmacol 36:446–451.
Newkirk, H. L., and Miles, D. G. 1974. Mod Vet Pract 55:677.
Ngai, S. H., Tseng, D. T. C., and Wang, S. C. 1966. J Pharmacol Exp Ther 153:344.
Oliver, J. E., Jr., and Young, W. O. 1973. Am J Vet Res 34:665.
Olsen, R. W., and Tobin, A. J. 1990. Molecular biology of $GABA_A$ receptors. FASEB J 4:1469–1480.
O'Malley, K. L., Harmon, S., Tang, L., et al. 1992. The rat dopamine D_4 receptor: sequence, gene structure, and demonstration of expression in the cardiovascular system. Nature New Biol 4:136–146.
O'Regan, M. H. 1989. Xylazine evoked depression of rat cerebral cortical neurons: a pharmacologic study. Gen Pharmacol 20(4):469–474.
Ossipov, M. H., Suaarez, L. J., and Spaulding, T. C. 1989. Antinociceptive interactions between α_2-adrenergic and opiate agonists at the spinal level in rodents. Anes Analg 68:194–200.
Ostwald, R. L. 1978. Comp Biochem Physiol [C] 60:19.
Parry, B. W., and Anderson, G. A. 1983. J Vet Pharmacol Ther 6:121.
Parry, B. W., Anderson, G. A., and Gay, C. C. 1982. Aust Vet J 59:148.
Pascoe, P. J. 1986. Can Vet J 27:272.
Paul, S. M., and Skolnick, P. 1978. Science 202:892.
Pearson, H., and Weaver, B. M. Q. 1978. Equine Vet J 10:85.
Pertz, C., and Sundberg, J. P. 1978. J Am Vet Med Assoc 173:1243.
Philo, L. M. 1978. Evaluation of xylazine for chemical restraint of captive arctic wolves. J Am Vet Med Assoc 173:1163–1166.
Polc, P. 1988. Electrophysiology of benzodiazepine receptor ligands: multiple mechanisms and sites of action. Prog Neurobiol 31:349–424.
Polc, P., Bonetti, E. P., Schaffner, R., et al. 1982. A three-state model of the benzodiazepine receptor explains the interactions between the benzodiazepine antagonist Ro15-1788, benzodiazepine tranquilizers, β carbolines, and phenobarbitone. Naunyn-Schmiedeberg's Arch Pharmacol 321:260–264.
Popovic, N. A., Mullane, J. F., and Yhap, E. O. 1972. Am J Vet Res 33:1819.
Porter, D. B., and Slusser, C. A. 1985. Vet Med 80:88.
Pritchett, D. B., Sontheimer, H., Shivers, B. D., et al. 1989. Importance of a novel $GABA_A$ receptor subunit for benzodiazepine pharmacology. Nature 338:582–585.
Proakis, A. G., and Borowitz, J. L. 1974. Biochem Pharmacol 23:1693.
Pugh, D. M. 1964. Vet Rec 76:439.
Pütter, J., and Sagner, G. 1973. Vet Med Rev 2:145.
Raffe, M. R., Crimi, A. J., and Ruff, J. 1982. Am J Vet Res 43:510.
Ragan, H. A., and Gillis, M. F. 1975. Lab Anim Sci 25:409.
Raiha, J. E., Raiha, M. P., and Short, C. E. 1989. Medetomidine as a preanesthetic prior to ketamine-HCl and halothane anesthesia in laboratory beagles. Acta Vet Scand 85:103–110.
Raiha, M. P., Raiha, J. E., and Short, C. E. 1989. A comparison of xylazine, acepromazine, meperidine, and medetomidine as preanesthetics to halothane anesthesia in dogs. Acta Vet Scand 85:97–102.
Randall, L. V., Heise, G. A., Schallek, W., et al. 1961. Curr Ther Res 3:405.
Rauws, A. G., and Olling, M. 1978. J Vet Pharmacol Ther 1:57.
Ray, R. S., Sams, R. A., and Huffman, R. 1978. In J. D. Powers and T. E. Powers, eds., Equine Pharmacology, p. 209. Golden, CO: American Association of Equine Practitioners.
Redig, P. T., and Duke, G. E. 1976. J Am Vet Med Assoc 169:886.
Regan, J. W., Doze, V. A., Daniel, K., et al. 1989. Is dexmedetomidine's anesthetic activity dependent on isoreceptor selectivity? (Abstr) Anesthesiology 71:A579.
Remandet, B., Gouy, D., Berthe, J., et al. 1984. Fund Appl Toxicol 4:152.
Reves, J. G. 1984. Benzodiazepines. In C. Prys-Roberts and C. C. Hug, eds., Pharmacokinetics of Anaesthesia, p. 157. Boston: Blackwell Scientific Publications.
Reves, J. G., Corssen, G., and Holcomb, C. 1978. Can Anaesth Soc J 25:211.
Reves, J. G., Fragen, R. J., Vinik, H. R., et al. 1985. Anesthesiology 62:310.
Reves, J. G., Glass, P. S. A., and Lubarsky, D. A. 1994. Nonbarbiturate intravenous anesthetics. In R. D. Miller, ed., Anesthesia, 4th ed., p. 248. New York: Churchill Livingstone.
Rickard, L. J., Thurmon, J. C., and Lingard, D. R. 1974. Vet Med Small Anim Clin 69:1029.
Ring, D. M., and Muir, W. W. 1982. Can J Comp Med 46:386.
Robertson, H. A., Martin, I. L., and Candy, J. M. 1978. Eur J Pharmacol 50:455.
Robinson, P. T., and Meier, J. E. 1977. Vet Med Small Anim Clin 72:1638.
Rosin, E. 1974. Personal communication.
Ruckebusch, Y., and Toutain, P. L. 1984. Vet Med Rev 1:3.
Rutherford, J. J. 1983. J Am Vet Med Assoc 183:746.
Sakaguchi, M., Nishimura, R., Sasaki, N, et al. 1992. J Vet Med Sci 54:643–647.
Sandelien, H. 1966. Nord Vet Med 18:271.
Sanford, T. D., and Colby, E. D. 1982. Feline Pract 12:16.
Santos-Martinez, J., Aviles, T. A., and Laboy-Torres, J. A. 1972. Surv Anesth 16:373.
Sarazan, R. D., Starke, W. A., Krause, G. F., et al. 1989. Cardiovascular effects of detomidine, a new α_2 adrenoceptor agonist in the conscious pony. J Vet Pharmacol Ther 12:378–88.
Sarnquist, F. H., Mathers, W. D., Brock-Utne, J., et al. 1980. Anesthesiology 52:149.

Saxen, I., and Saxen, L. 1975. Lancet 2:498.
Schauffler, A. F. 1968. Mod Vet Pract 49:43.
Schlinke, J. C., and Palmer, J. S. 1973. J Am Vet Med Assoc 163:756.
Schmitt, H., Fournadjier, G., and Schmitt, H. L. 1970. Eur J Pharmacol 10:230.
Schneider, S., and Mace, J. 1984. Pediatrics 53:112.
Schoemaker, H., Bliss, M., and Yamamura, H. I. 1981. Specific high affinity saturable binding of [^{3}H]Ro5-4864 to benzodiazepine binding sites in rat cerebral cortex. Eur J Pharmacol 71:173–175.
Scoggins, R. D. 1979. J Am Vet Med Assoc 174:183.
Seabrook, G. R., Patel, S., and Marwoood, R. 1992. Stable expression human D_3 dopamine receptors in GH_4C1 pituitary cells. FEBS Letts 312:123–126.
Seal, U. S., and Erickson, A. W. 1969. Fed Proc 28:1410.
Senogles, S. E. 1994. The D_2 dopamine receptor isoforms signal through distinct G_i alpha proteins to inhibit adenylyl cyclase. J Biol Chem 37:23120–23127.
Sharrock, A. G. 1982. Aust Vet J 58:39.
Shideler, R. K. 1971. Proc Am Assoc Equine Pract, p. 119.
Short, C. E. 1974. Mod Vet Pract 55:393.
Short, C. E. 1991. Effects of anticholinergic treatment on the cardiac and respiratory systems in dogs sedated with medetomidine. Vet Rec 129:310–313.
Short, C. E., Tumbleson, M. E., and Merriam, J. G. 1972. Vet Med Small Anim Clin 67:747.
Short, C. E., Jones, R. S., and Tintle, L. M. 1984. Br Vet J 140:169.
Short, C. E., Matthews, N., Harvey, R., et al. 1986. Cardiovascular and pulmonary function studies of a new sedative/analgesic (Detomidine) for use alone in horses or as a preanesthetic. Acta Vet Scand 82:139–155.
Siddik, Z. H., Drew, R., and Gram, T. E. 1979. Toxicol Appl Pharmacol 50:443.
Sieghart, W. 1992. $GABA_A$ receptors: ligand-gated Cl^- ion channels modulated by multiple drug-binding sites. Trends Pharmacol Sci 13:446–450.
———. 1994. Pharmacology of benzodiazepine receptors: an update. J Psychiatr Neurosci 19:24–29.
Silverman, A. G., Wilner, H. I., and Okun, R. 1970. A case of gastrointestinal bleeding following the use of tolazoline. Toxicol Appl Pharmacol 16:318–320.
Skarda, R. T., St. Jean, G., and Muir, W. W. 1990. Influence of tolazoline on caudal epidural administration of xylazine in cattle. Am J Vet Res 51(4):556–560.
Skerritt, J. H., Willow, M., and Johnston, G. A. R. 1982. Diazepam enhancement of low affinity GABA binding to rat brain membranes. Neurosci Lett 29:63–66.
Skolnick, P., Stalvey, L. P., Daly, J. W., et al. 1978. Eur J Pharmacol 47:201.
Sokoloff, P., Andrieux M., Besancon, R., et al. 1990. Molecular characterization of a novel dopamine receptor (D_3) as a target for neuroleptics. Nature 347:146–151.
———. 1992. Pharmacology of human dopamine D_3 receptor expressed in a mammalian cell line: comparison with D_2 receptor. Eur J Pharmacol 225:331–337.
Spiegel, R. A., Lane, T. J., Larsen, R. E., et al. 1984. J Am Vet Med Assoc 185:1335.
Squires, R. F., Benson, D. I., Braestrup, C., et al. 1979. Pharmacol Biochem Behav 10:825.
Steffey, E. P., Kelly, A. B., Farver, T. B., et al. 1985. J Vet Pharmacol Ther 8:290.
Stenberg, D. 1989. Physiologic role of α_2-adrenoceptors in the regulation of vigilance and pain: Effect of medetomidine. Acta Vet Scand 85:21–28.
Strader, C., Sigal I. S., and Dixon, R. A. 1989. Structural basis of β-adrenergic receptor function. FASEB J 3:1825–1832.
Strain, G. M., Seger, C. L., and Flory, W. 1982. Am J Vet Res 43:158.
Sunahara, R. K., Guan, H. C., O'Dowd, B. F., et al. 1991. Cloning of the gene for a human dopamine D_5 receptor with higher affinity for dopamine than D_1. Nature 350:614–619.
Symoens, J., and Van Den Brande, M. 1969. Vet Rec 85:64.
Symonds, H. W., and Mallinson, C. B. 1978. Vet Rec 102:27.
Szabo, K. T., and Brent, R. L. 1974. Lancet 1:565.
Tallman, J. F., Paul, S. M., Skolnick, P., et al. 1980. Science 207:274.
Tang, L., Todd, R. D., Heller, A., et al. 1994. Pharmacological and functional characterization of D_2, D_3, and D_4 dopamine receptors in fibroblast and dopaminergic cell lines. J Pharmacol Exp Therap 268:495–502.
Taub, H., and Peters, D. A. V. 1978. Gen Pharmacol 9:97.
Thompson, J. R., Kersting, K. W., and Hsu, H. W. 1991. Antagonistic effect of atipamezole on xylazine-induced sedation, bradycardia, and ruminal atony in calves. Am J Vet Res 52:1265–1268.
Thurmon, J. C., Ko, J. C. H., Benson, G. J., et al. 1995. Clinical appraisal of propofol as an anesthetic in dogs premedicated with medetomidine. Canine Pract 20:21–25.
Thurmon, J. C., Lin, H. C., Tranquilli, W. J., et al. 1989. A comparison of yohimbine and tolazoline as antagonists of xylazine sedation in calves (abstr). Vet Surg 18:170.
Thurmon, J. C., Nelson, D. R., Hartsfield, S. M., et al. 1978. Aust Vet J 54:178.
Tiberi, M., Jarvie, K. R., Silvia, C., et al. 1991. Cloning, molecular characterization, and chromosomal assignment of a gene encoding a second D_1 dopamine receptor subtype: differential expression pattern in rat brain compared with the D_{1A} receptor. Proc Nat Acad Sci USA 88:7491–7495.
Tobin, T., and Ballard, S. 1979. J Equine Med Surg 3:460.
Tranquilli, W. J., and Maze, M. 1993. Clinical pharmacology and use of α_2-adrenergic agonists in veterinary anesthesia. Anaes Pharmacol Rev 1:297–309.
Tranquilli, W. J., Thurmon, J. C., Corbin, J. E., et al. 1984. J Vet Pharmacol Ther 7:23.
Tranquilli, W. J., Thurmon, J. C., Paul, A. J., et al. 1985. Am J Vet Res 46:1892.
Tranquilli, W. J., Thurmon, J. C., Benson, G. J., et al. 1986. J Vet Pharmacol Ther 9:198.
Trembath, P. R. 1984. Vet Med Rev 4:169.
Turner, T. 1973. Vet Rec 93:524.
Ullberg, S., Lindquist, N. G., and Sjostrand, S. E. 1970. Nature 227:1257.
Vähä Vahe, A. T. 1990. The clinical effectiveness of atipamezole as a medetomidine antagonist in the dog. J Vet Pharmacol Therap 132:198–205.
Vähä-Vahe, T. 1989. The clinical efficacy of medetomidine. Acta Vet Scand 85:151–153.
Vainio, O. 1989. Introduction to the clinical pharmacology of medetomidine.1989. Acta Vet Scand 85:85–88.
Vainio, O, and Palmu, L. 1989. Cardiovascular and respiratory effects of medetomidine in dogs and influence of anticholinergics. Acta Vet Scand 30:401–408.
Vallar, L., Muca, C. Magni, M., et al. 1990. Differential coupling of dopaminergic D_2 receptors expressed in different cell types. J Biol Chem 265:10320–10326.
Van Heerden, J., and Keffen, R.H. 1991. A preliminary investigation into the immobilising potential of a tiletamine/zolazepam mixture, metomidate, a medetomidine and azaperone combination and medetomidine in ostriches. J S Afr Vet Assoc 62:114–117.
Van Tol, H. H. M., Bunzow, J. R., Guan, H. C., et al. 1991. Cloning of the gene for a human dopamine D_4 receptor with high affinity for the antipsychotic clozapine. Nature 350:660–664.
Verstegen, J., Fargetton, X., Donnay, I., et al. 1991. An evaluation of medetomidine/ketamine and other drug combinations for analgesia in cats. Vet Rec 128:32–35.

Virtanen, R. 1986. J Vet Pharmacol Ther 9:286.
Virtanen, R. 1989. Pharmacologic profiles of medetomidine and its antagonist atipamezole. Acta Vet Scand 85:29–37.
Virtanen, R., and MacDonald, E. 1985. Comparison of the effects of detomidine and xylazine on some alpha 2 adrenoceptor-mediated responses in the central and peripheral nervous systems. Eur J Pharmacol 115(2):277–284.
Virtanen, R., and Nyman, L. 1985. Evaluation of the alpha 1- and 2-adrenoceptor effects of detomidine, a novel veterinary sedative analgesic. Eur J Pharmacol 108(2):163–169.
Virtanen, R., Ruskoaho, H., and Nyman, L. 1985. J Vet Pharmacol Ther 8:30.
Virtanen, R., Savola, J. M., and Saano, V. 1989. Highly selective and specific antagonism of central and peripheral alpha 2-adrenoceptors by atipamezole. Arch Int Pharmacodyn Ther 297:190–204.
Waechter, R. A. 1982. J Am Vet Med Assoc 180:73.
Wagner, A. E., Muir, W. W., and Hinchcliff, K. W. 1991. Cardiovascular effects of xylazine and detomidine in horses. Am J Vet Res 52(5):651–57.
Walker, B. E., and Patterson, A. 1974. Teratology 10:159.
Wallner, B. M., Hatch, R. C., Booth, N. H., et al. 1982. Complete immobility produced in dogs by xylazine-atropine: antagonism by 4-aminopyridine and yohimbine. Am J Vet Res 43:2259–2265.
Wan, P. Y., Trim, C. M., and Mueller, P. O. 1992. Xylazine-ketamine and detomidine-tiletamine-zolazepam anesthesia in horses. Vet Surg 21(4):312–318.
Waterman, A. E. 1983. Res Vet Sci 35:285.
Waterman, A., Livingston, A., and Bouchenafa, O. 1988. Analgesic effects of intrathecally applied alpha 2 agonists in conscious, unrestrained sheep. Neuropharmacology 27(2):213–216.
Webb, A. I., Warren, R. G., and Spencer, K. R. 1983. J Am Vet Med Assoc 182:691.
Weinbrum, A., and Geller, E. 1990. The respiratory effects of reversing midazolam sedation with flumazenil in the presence or absence of narcotics. Acta Anaesthesiol Scand 92:65.
Weinshank, R. L., Adham, N., Macchi, M., et al. 1991. Molecular cloning and characterization of a high affinity dopamine receptor (D_{1b}) and its pseudogene. J Biol Chem 266:22427–22435.
Weir, J. J. R., and Sanford, J. 1972. Equine Vet J 4:88.
White, K. 1968. Vet Rec 83:688.
Williams, M., and Risley, E. A. 1979. Life Sci 24:833.
Wood, C. 1978. Vet Rec 102:304.
Wright, M. 1982. J Am Vet Med Assoc 180:1462.
Yates, W. D. 1973. Vet Med Small Anim Clin 68:483.
Young, E., and Whyte, I. J. 1973. J S Afr Vet Assoc 44:177.
Young, P. L. 1979. Aust Vet J 55:442.
Young, W. S., and Kuhar, J. M. 1979. Autoradiographic localisation of benzodiazepine receptors in the brains of humans and animals. Nature 280:393–395.
Ziegler, W. H., Schalch, E., Leishman, B., et al. 1983. Comparison of the effects of intravenously administered midazolam, triazolam and their hydroxy metabolites. Br J Clin Pharmacol 16:63S.
Zisterer, D. M., and Williams, D. C. 1997. Peripheral-type benzodiazepine receptors: a review. Gen Pharmacol 29:305–314.

15 LOCAL ANESTHETICS

KHURSHEED R. MAMA AND EUGENE P. STEFFEY

History
Requirements of an Ideal Local Anesthetic
General Properties
  Chemical Structure
  Physicochemical Properties and Structure-Activity Relations
Pharmacokinetics
  Absorption
  Distribution
  Biotransformation and Excretion
Pharmacodynamics
  Mechanism of Action
  Toxicity and Complications
Clinical Pharmacology
  Anesthetic Potency
  Onset of Anesthetic Action
  Duration of Anesthetic Action
  Pregnancy
Uses of Local Anesthetics
Local Anesthetic Agents
  Aminoester Local Anesthetics
    Cocaine Hydrochloride
    Procaine Hydrochloride
    Chloroprocaine Hydrochloride
    Tetracaine Hydrochloride
    Benzocaine
    Proparacaine Hydrochloride
  Aminoamide Local Anesthetics
    Lidocaine Hydrochloride
    Prilocaine Hydrochloride
    Eutectic Mixture of Lidocaine and Prilocaine (EMLA)
    Mepivacaine Hydrochloride
    Bupivacaine Hydrochloride
    Etidocaine Hydrochloride
    Ropivacaine Hydrochloride

Local anesthetics are drugs that when applied locally to nerve tissue (endings or fibers) cause reversible blockade of nerve impulse conduction. At effective concentrations, local anesthetics block transmission of autonomic, somatic sensory, and somatic motor impulses. Thus, depending upon the nerve and the area innervated, autonomic nervous system blockade, anesthesia, and/or skeletal muscle paralysis may result. The action of local anesthetics is reversible. Recovery of nerve conduction occurs spontaneously without evidence of structural damage to nerve cells or fibers. This is in contrast to other compounds such as phenol that will also block neural conduction. However, in this case the action is irreversible because phenol causes cellular destruction.

HISTORY. The first clinically significant local anesthetic to be used was cocaine hydrochloride. It is an alkaloid and was first obtained from the leaves of *Erythroxylon coca,* a tree indigenous to Chile, Peru, and Bolivia. The native runners of this area chewed coca leaves to allay hunger and fatigue and produce psychic stimulation while they carried messages through the forests. The tree is cultivated now in several tropical countries. It was imported to Europe as a botanical curiosity. In 1860 Niemann isolated alkaloidal cocaine from leaves of the tree. The local anesthetic effect of the alkaloid was noted but not utilized until Koller used cocaine to anesthetize the eye in 1884. Thereafter, cocaine was accepted as a local anesthetic. It was used in dental and surgical procedures by the methods of infiltration and nerve blocking. In 1885 Corning injected cocaine intrathecally (into the subarachnoid space) in a dog and paralyzed posterior spinal nerves to produce spinal anesthesia. It was nearly 15 years later before the technique was successfully employed on humans. Also in 1885 McLean, a veterinarian of Meadville, Pennsylvania, first successfully used cocaine for nerve blocks of the limbs in the horse.

Willstatter completed the chemical structure and final synthesis of cocaine in 1902. It became apparent that cocaine possessed at least two undesirable properties, viz., a marked toxicity and drug addiction. Chemists began searching for substitutes that possessed the same local anesthetic properties. Three years later, Einhorn synthesized procaine hydrochloride. Many other compounds have been synthesized since then for use as local anesthetics. While they differ little in therapeutic efficacy, none is entirely free from undesirable properties.

The search for new and better local anesthetics continues. There are presently about 50 local anesthetic compounds of recognized clinical value. Only those of primary importance in veterinary medicine in North America will be covered here.

Requirements of an Ideal Local Anesthetic. The ideal local anesthetic should provide reversible sensory nerve blockade with no local (e.g., neural) or systemic (e.g., central nervous system [CNS] or cardiac) toxicity. The onset and duration of blockade should be predictable and consistent in all applications. As this ideal agent is not currently available, appropriate clinical selection of a local anesthetic agent must be based on an understanding of the physiology of neural conduction and the pharmacokinetics and pharmacodynamics of each individual drug.

GENERAL PROPERTIES

Chemical Structure. The typical local anesthetic molecule consists of an unsaturated aromatic group (usually a benzine ring) linked by an intermediate chain to a tertiary amine end (Fig. 15.1). The tertiary amine is a base (proton acceptor). The clinically important local anesthetics are divided into two distinct chemical groups based on their intermediate chain. The aminoesters are local anesthetics with an ester link between the aromatic and amine ends; procaine, chloroprocaine, and tetracaine are examples. Aminoamides are local anesthetics with an amide link between the aromatic and amine ends; lidocaine, mepivacaine, bupivacaine, and ropivacaine are examples (Fig. 15.2). *(Note:* a memory aid for differentiating modern, clinically important local anesthetics into the ester or the amide grouping is that [except for piperacaine, an ester not discussed in this review] amides have an "i" in the prefix [before "caine"] of the generic name of the anesthetic.)

Physicochemical Properties and Structure-Activity Relations

LIPOPHILIC-HYDROPHILIC BALANCE. The aromatic ring system and alkyl substitution to either the aromatic region or amine end of the basic local anesthetic molecule impart lipophilic characteristics to the molecule. The lipophilic nature of the molecule affects the tendency of a compound to associate with membrane lipids (lipid solubility, or hydrophobicity). Lipid solubility is related to anesthetic potency; the more lipid soluble, the greater the potency. Duration of action also increases with increased lipophilicity. For example, etidocaine has more carbon atoms on the amine end of the molecule than lidocaine and is four times more potent and has a longer duration of action (Fig. 15.2, Table 15.1). The dominance of aromatic ring substitution (over the amine substitution) in determination of lipophilicity is exemplified by comparing the actions of the two ester local anesthetics procaine and tetracaine. Although procaine has a greater amine substitution than tetracaine, the latter has a greater aromatic substitution (butyl) and is more potent and reported to have a longer clinical duration of action than procaine.

HYDROGEN ION CONCENTRATION. Local anesthetics are weak bases. In solution, local anesthetics exist in

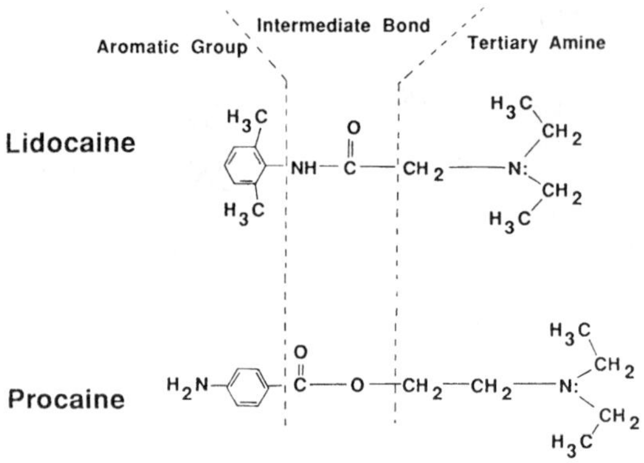

FIG. 15.1—Local anesthetics consist of hydrophilic and lipophilic (hydrophobic) ends connected by a hydrocarbon chain. The connecting chain is either an amide, as in lidocaine, or an ester, as in procaine. (From Strichartz and Berde 1994, reprinted with permission.)

chemical equilibrium between the uncharged base (the un-ionized form) and the cationic (the ionized) form. The relative proportion of these two forms is determined by the chemical nature of the compound (salt of acid or base), the pK_a (pH at which the concentrations of the ionized and un-ionized forms are equal) of the compound, and the pH of the environment into which the solution is injected. This relationship is described by the following modified version of the Henderson-Hasselbach equation:

$$\log\left(\frac{\text{ionized form}}{\text{un-ionized form}}\right) = pK_a - pH$$

Since local anesthetics are weak bases with pK_a values in the range of 7.5-9, the predominant form at physiologic pH is the ionized, or cationic, form (Table 15.1). While the cationic form is felt to be important for local anesthetic activity at the receptor site, it is the uncharged base that is especially important in the rapid penetration and diffusion through biological membranes (the local anesthetic receptor is likely not accessible from the external side of the cell membrane). Thus the amount in the base form strongly influences the onset of drug action and the drug's potency.

PROTEIN BINDING. The tertiary amine is relatively hydrophilic and bears some positive charge in the physiologic pH range. The degree of ionization has been positively correlated to protein binding. In general, the degree to which local anesthetics bind to proteins influences their duration of action; greater binding relates to prolonged duration of action. As discussed below, the conduction block caused by local anesthetics is believed to occur following interaction of the anesthetic with a protein receptor located within the sodium channel of the nerve membrane. If the agent has a greater affinity for the receptor and binds

Generic[a] and Common Proprietary Name	Chemical Structure	Approximate Year of Initial Clinical Use	Main Anesthetic Utility	Representative Commercial Preparation
Cocaine	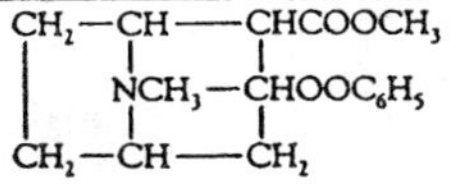 $CH_2-CH-CHCOOCH_3$; $NCH_3-CHOOC_6H_5$; $CH_2-CH-CH_2$	1884	Topical	Bulk powder
Benzocaine (Americaine)	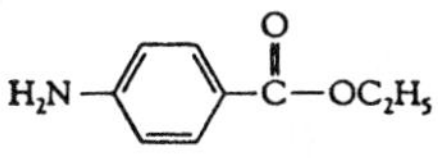 H_2N–(ring)–$C(=O)-OC_2H_5$	1900	Topical Topical	20% ointment 20% aerosol
Procaine (Novocain)	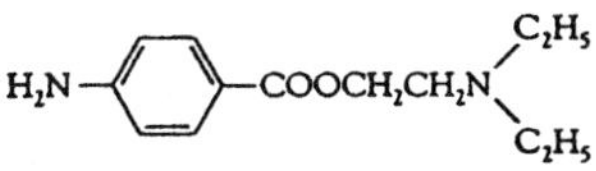 H_2N–(ring)–$COOCH_2CH_2N(C_2H_5)_2$	1905	Infiltration Spinal	10 & 20 mg/ml solutions 100 mg/ml solution
Tetracaine (Pontocaine)	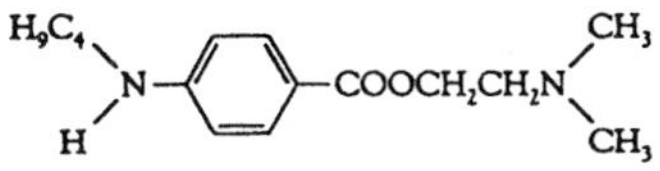 $H_9C_4(H)N$–(ring)–$COOCH_2CH_2N(CH_3)_2$	1930	Spinal Spinal	Niphanoid crystals—20 mg/ml 10 mg/ml solutions
Lidocaine (Xylocaine)	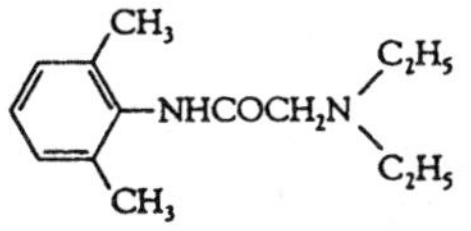 (ring, CH_3, CH_3)–$NHCOCH_2N(C_2H_5)_2$	1944	Infiltration Peripheral nerve blocks Epidural Spinal Topical Topical	5 & 10 mg/ml solutions 10, 15, & 20 mg/ml solutions 10, 15, & 20 mg/ml solutions 50 mg/ml solution 2.0% jelly, viscous 2.5%, 5.0% ointment
Chloroprocaine (Nesacaine)	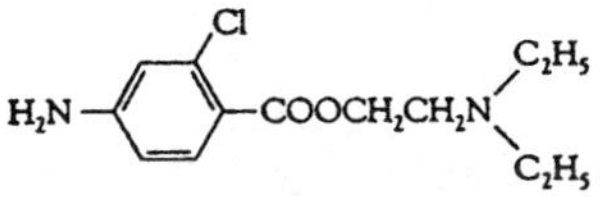 H_2N–(ring, Cl)–$COOCH_2CH_2N(C_2H_5)_2$	1955	Infiltration Peripheral nerve blockade Epidural	10 mg/ml solution 10 & 20 mg/ml solutions 20 & 30 mg/ml solutions
Mepivacaine (Carbocaine)	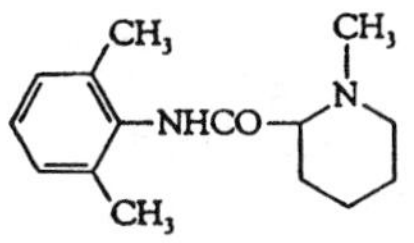 (ring, CH_3, CH_3)–NHCO–(piperidine, N–CH_3)	1957	Infiltration Peripheral nerve blockade Epidural	10 mg/ml solution 10 & 20 mg/ml solutions 10, 15, & 20 mg/ml solutions
Prilocaine (Citanest)	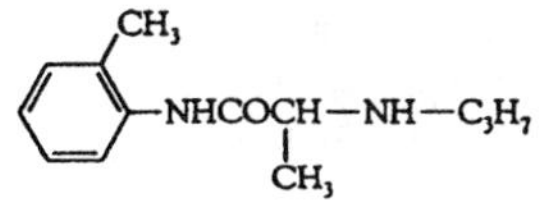 (ring, CH_3)–$NHCOCH(CH_3)-NH-C_3H_7$	1960	Infiltration Peripheral nerve blockade Epidural	10 & 20 mg/ml solutions 10, 20, & 30 mg/ml solutions 10, 20, & 30 mg/ml solutions
Bupivacaine (Marcaine)	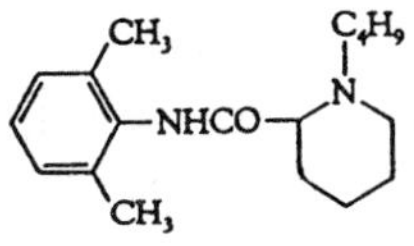 (ring, CH_3, CH_3)–NHCO–(piperidine, N–C_4H_9)	1963	Infiltration Peripheral nerve blockade Epidural Spinal	2.5 mg/ml solutions 2.5 & 5 mg/ml solutions 2.5, 5, & 7.5 mg/ml solutions 5 & 7.5 mg/ml solutions
Etidocaine (Duranest)	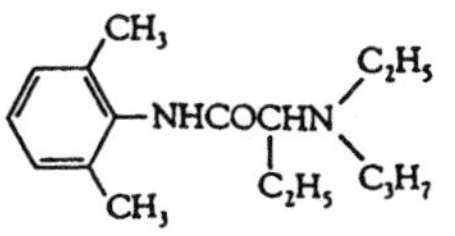 (ring, CH_3, CH_3)–$NHCOCH(C_2H_5)N(C_2H_5)(C_3H_7)$	1972	Infiltration Peripheral nerve blockade Epidural	2.5 & 5 mg/ml solutions 5 & 10 mg/ml solutions 5 & 10 mg/ml solutions
Ropivacaine (Noropin)	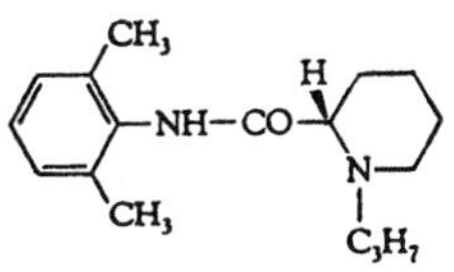 (ring, CH_3, CH_3)–NH–CO–(H)(piperidine, N–C_3H_7)	1990	Infiltration Peripheral nerve blockade Epidural Spinal	2 & 5 mg/ml solutions 2.5 & 7.5 mg/ml solutions 5, 7.5, & 10 mg/ml solutions 7.5 & 10 mg/ml solutions

[a]USP nomenclature.

FIG. 15.2—Representative local anesthetic agents in common clinical use. (Modified from Strichartz and Berde 1994.)

TABLE 15.1—Comparative pharmacology of commonly used local anesthetics

Classification	Potency*	Onset of action	Duration of action (min)	pK_a	Fraction nonionized (%) pH = 7.4	Protein binding (%)	Lipid solubility
Esters							
Procaine	1	Slow	45–60	8.9	3	6	0.6
Chloroprocaine	3	Rapid	30–45	8.7	5	—	—
Tetracaine	8	Slow	60–180	8.5	7	76	80
Amides							
Lidocaine	2	Rapid	60–120	7.9	25	70	2.9
Mepivacaine	1.5	Intermediate	90–180	7.6	39	77	1
Bupivacaine	8	Intermediate	180–480	8.1	15	95	28
Etidocaine	8	Slow	240–280	7.7	33	94	141
Prilocaine	1.8	Slow	60–120	7.9	24	55	0.9
Ropivacaine	~8	Intermediate	Similar to bupivacaine	8.1	Similar to bupivacaine	94	Between mepivacaine and bupivacaine

Source: Modified from Stoelting 1987 (Table 7-1) and Strichartz and Berde 1994 (Table 15-2).
*Blocking potency relative to procaine; data from isolated nerve studies (Strichartz and Berde 1994, Table 15-2).

more firmly to the receptor site, it presumably will remain within the channel for a longer period of time, and this condition will result in a more prolonged block. This explanation remains speculative since most of the information on local anesthetic protein binding has been obtained from studies of plasma protein binding. It is assumed that a relationship exists between plasma protein binding and the degree of local anesthetic binding to membrane proteins. Bupivacaine, etidocaine, and ropivacaine are examples of local anesthetic agents that are highly protein bound and have a longer duration of action than their amide or ester counterparts (Table 15.1).

It is important to remember that the action of local anesthetics relates in large part to their chemical and physical properties and that these have largely been determined in vitro. However, in vivo the actions of these agents may be markedly altered by other circumstances; some of these will be reviewed briefly later in this chapter.

PHARMACOKINETICS. Local anesthetic agents are usually injected into a localized area of the body to block specific nerves. The absorption of the drug from the site of injection, the drug's distribution kinetics, and the degree of biotransformation and excretion of drug and breakdown products from the body are of primary importance in determining the systemic disposition of the drug and potential for toxicity (side effects).

Absorption. The systemic absorption of local anesthetic agents is influenced by many factors, including the dosage (volume and concentration), site of injection, presence of a vasoconstrictor, and physicochemical and pharmacologic properties of the drug. Many of these factors also influence duration of effect of the drug at the site of action.

In general, while the effect on systemic absorption of varying either volume or concentration (at a constant dose) of local anesthetic administered is variable and generally not significant, the overall dose is correlated with increased systemic absorption and higher peak drug levels. Site of injection also significantly influences the peak drug concentrations in the blood. Local anesthetic deposited in a highly vascular area will be absorbed more rapidly and result in higher blood levels of drug than if injected into tissue of less blood flow.

The presence of vasoconstrictor substances such as epinephrine tends to reduce systemic absorption by reducing local blood flow. But this effect may vary somewhat depending on the nature of the local anesthetic. For example, compared to use of a local anesthetic alone, concurrent use of a vasoconstrictor such as epinephrine (e.g., at concentrations of 1:200,000) reduces the peak blood levels of the shorter acting drugs (e.g., lidocaine) but has a less pronounced effect on the more lipophilic and longer acting agents (e.g., etidocaine).

Distribution. Amide local anesthetic agents are widely distributed in the body following an intravenous bolus injection; a two- or three-compartment model (Table 15.2) usually describes their pharmacokinetic properties. Distribution of ester anesthetics in tissues is much more limited because their plasma half-lives are very short (within a few minutes) due to their rapid breakdown by plasma pseudocholinesterase.

Distribution of especially amide-type local anesthetics may be further influenced by anatomic and pathophysiologic factors. For example, the lung is capable of extracting at least some amide local anesthetics and thereby limits the amount of drug reaching the systemic circulation and downstream sensitive sites (Tucker 1986). Conversely, hypercapnia and resulting acidosis in the CNS will likely increase regional blood flow and as a result increase local anesthetic concentrations in the brain and increase the risk of toxicity.

Protein binding is another factor that may influence plasma drug concentrations, as it influences the free

Table 15.2—Pharmacokinetic properties in humans of selected amide local anesthetics

Agent	$t_{1/2\alpha}$ (min)	$t_{1/2\beta}$ (min)	$t_{1/2\gamma}$ (h)	Vd_{ss} (L)	Cl (L/min)
Prilocaine	0.5	5.0	1.5	261	2.84
Lidocaine	1.0	9.6	1.6	91	0.95
Mepivacaine	0.7	7.2	1.9	84	0.78
Bupivacaine	2.7	28.0	3.5	72	0.47
Ropivacaine	—	—	1.9	59	0.73
Etidocaine	2.2	19.0	2.6	133	1.22

Sources: Strichartz and Berde 1994; Lee et al. 1989.
Note: Vd_{ss} = volume of distribution at steady state; Cl = clearance.

drug available for both activity and clearance by the liver. Toxic plasma concentration is inversely proportional to degree of protein binding.

Biotransformation and Excretion. A major difference between the aminoamides and aminoesters is the pattern of metabolism. The esters are hydrolyzed primarily by plasma pseudocholinesterase, whereas the amides largely undergo enzymatic degradation in the liver. The difference in metabolism has implications for both clinical usefulness and observed toxicity for the two classes of compounds.

The principal metabolic pathway of local anesthetics with ester linkages is enzymatic hydrolysis. Derivatives of 4-amino-benzoic acid are primarily hydrolyzed in the plasma by nonspecific pseudocholinesterases. Cocaine is an atypical ester in that it undergoes significant hepatic metabolism and urinary excretion. The rate of plasma hydrolysis for the other ester compounds varies; chloroprocaine has the most rapid rate, followed by procaine, and tetracaine has the slowest. Toxicity is inversely related to the rate of hydrolysis.

Pregnancy, which reduces plasma cholinesterase activity, might prolong the clearance of the ester anesthetics and increase the potential for toxicity. Despite generally rapid systemic clearance of the ester anesthetics, subarachnoid administration of these drugs will result in a clinical effect until the drug is systemically absorbed. This is likely due to the lack of significant pseudocholinesterase activity in the cerebrospinal fluid. Products of hydrolysis either can be directly excreted (e.g., nearly 25% of diethylaminoethanol from degradation of procaine) by the kidney or, more commonly, can undergo metabolic transformation (Kolwas 1979). Para-aminobenzoic acid (PABA) is a breakdown product of the esters responsible for allergic reactions in some human patients.

Compared with the ester local anesthetics, the metabolism of the amide local anesthetics is more complex. Metabolism takes place primarily in the liver, although some plasma hydrolysis is thought to occur. Plasma hydrolysis may contribute to the rate of clearance of the different amide agents from the blood; prilocaine, etidocaine, and to a lesser extent lidocaine are all thought to undergo plasma hydrolysis. The amide bonds of mepivacaine and bupivacaine do not undergo hydrolysis by plasma esterases.

A common pathway in biotransformation of amide local anesthetics is dealkylation (Kolwas 1979). This chemical process involves alkyl groups either linked to nitrogen or oxygen atoms of the local anesthetic or in its products of hydrolysis. Dealkylation occurs primarily within the hepatic microsomes. Lidocaine, which has been studied extensively in human beings, undergoes oxidative *N*-dealkylation to monoethylglycinexylidide. This intermediate compound is then hydrolyzed to 4-hydroxy-2,6-xylidine, which is excreted in the urine.

Bupivacaine also undergoes hepatic dealkylation and hydrolysis but is thought to be at least partially detoxified by conjugation with glucuronic acid. This may be of clinical significance in cats since they have a limited ability to form glucuronide conjugates. The clearance of mepivacaine is reduced in neonates, which is likely due to immature enzyme system development, and hence is not recommended for use during cesarean section. Prilocaine is metabolized to ortho-toluidine, which is capable of oxidizing hemoglobin to methemoglobin, thereby limiting its clinical application.

In general, the order of clearance of amides is prilocaine (most rapid) > etidocaine > lidocaine > mepivacaine/ropivacaine > bupivacaine (least rapid). Since the amides undergo primary enzymatic degradation in the liver, changes in hepatic function and/or hepatic blood flow (as may be induced with hypotension during regional or general anesthesia and in certain disease states) will prolong the clearance of the drugs from the body and may increase the potential for side effects.

Similarly, changes in renal function might also influence clearance of local anesthetic metabolites (and to a far lesser extent the unaltered parent drugs), as they are eliminated almost entirely by the kidney. In general, because most local anesthetics contain alkaline amino radicals, excretion in an acid urine is greater because of increased ionization. In alkaline urine, renal elimination of local anesthetics is delayed or slower because the drug remains principally in the un-ionized state and may be easily reabsorbed.

PHARMACODYNAMICS

Mechanism of Action

PERIPHERAL NERVE ANATOMY. Nerve fibers are classified based on their size and myelination and have specific associated functions (Table 15.3). A typical peripheral nerve consists of individual nerve fibers, or axons, grouped together as fascicles within an outer sheath. Each of these layers has an associated connective tissue covering: axon, endoneurium; fascicle, perineurium; entire nerve, epineurium.

Peripheral nerves may be myelinated or nonmyelinated. Schwann cells form multiple myelin layers around each axon of myelinated nerves and only a single membrane layer around nonmyelinated axonal

TABLE 15.3—Nerve fibers and their susceptibility to block by local anesthetics

Fiber type	Fiber diameter (μm)	Myelination	Function	Sensitivity to block
Type A				
Alpha	12–20	Heavy	Proprioception and motor	+
Beta	5–12	Heavy	Touch and pressure	++
Gamma	3–6	Heavy	Muscle	++
Delta	2–5	Heavy	Pain and temperature	+++
Type B	<3	Light	Preganglionic autonomic	++++
Type C				
Dorsal root	0.4–1.2	None	Pain	++++
Sympathetic	0.3–1.3	None	Postganglionic	++++

Source: Modified from Stoelting and Miller 1987.

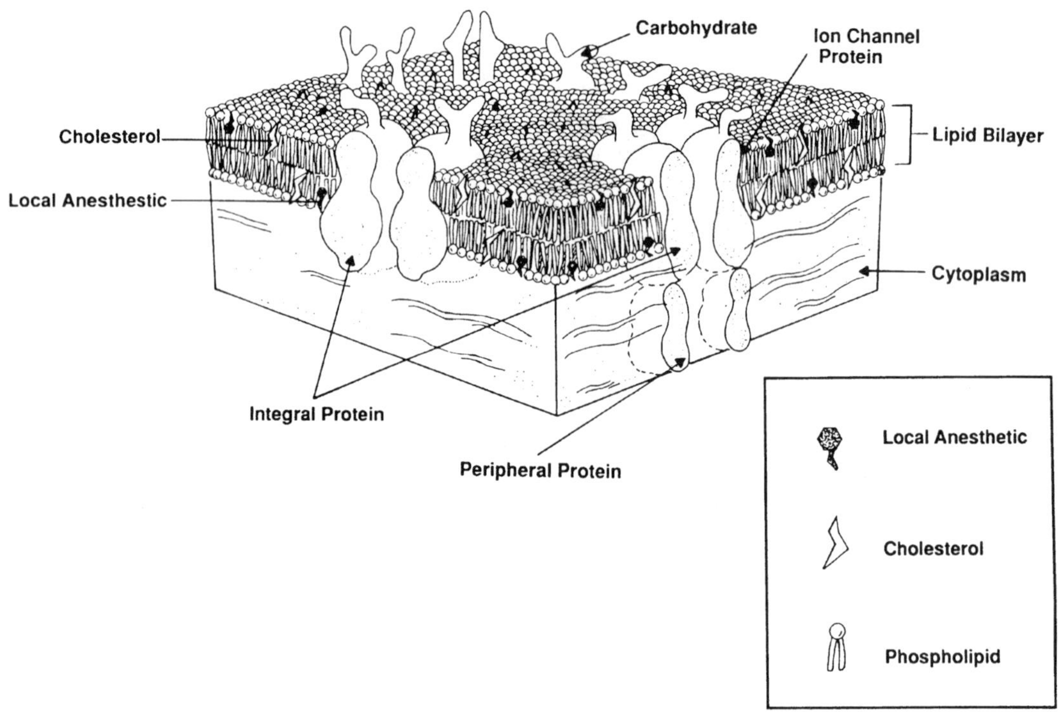

FIG. 15.3—Drawing of a typical plasma membrane showing the lipid bilayer. Probable sites for local anesthetic action are also shown. (From Strichartz and Berde 1994, reprinted with permission.)

fibers. In nonmyelinated nerves ion channels supporting propagation of the action potential are distributed all along the axon. This is in contrast to myelinated nerves, where these ion channels are concentrated at the nodes of Ranvier, which are periodic interruptions in the myelin sheath.

The axonal membrane structure is similar to that of other biologic membranes and consists of a phospholipid bilayer containing both surface and embedded proteins and carbohydrates (Fig. 15.3).

PHYSIOLOGY OF NERVE CONDUCTION AND ANESTHETIC ACTION. Local anesthetics inhibit the generation and propagation (conduction) of nerve impulses by blockage of voltage-gated sodium channels in the nerve membrane. Nerve signals are conducted by action potentials, which are rapid changes in the electrical gradients across the nerve membrane. Each action potential begins with a sudden change from the normal resting negative potential (of about –90 mV) to a positive membrane potential and then ends with a rapid shift back again to the negative potential. The action potential moves along the unmyelinated nerve fiber (conduction of the impulse) until it reaches the fiber's end. In myelinated nerves the impulse jumps from one node of Ranvier to the next (saltatory conduction). Repolarization resets the nerve membrane potential to resting conditions until it is again depolarized.

Depolarization is due to the rapid inward passage of sodium ions from the extracellular to the intracellular space via sodium channels in the membrane. Toward the end of the depolarization phase, sodium channels close and become inactivated. At the same time potassium channels slowly (compared to the sodium channels) open and allow potassium to exit from the cell. The outward flow of potassium repolarizes the membrane toward the potassium equilibrium potential (about −95 mV). The sodium channels are also returned to the resting state. At completion of this action potential, the transmembrane ionic equilibrium is reestablished by the membrane sodium-potassium pump (Guyton and Hall 1996).

Current knowledge indicates that the sodium ion channel in the nerve membrane (Fig. 15.3) is the site of action for local anesthetics. The most prominent hypothesis is that the anesthetic enters the lipoprotein membrane and binds to a receptor site in the sodium channel to impede or prevent sodium ion movement. Sodium-generated currents are reduced because the drug inhibits channel conformational changes, and thus drug-bound channels fail to open. This slows the rate of depolarization of the membrane, preventing attainment of the membrane's threshold potential. Thus, an action potential is not propagated. To a lesser extent movement through the channel is prevented also because of the bound drug's physical blockade of the ion-conducting pore. A sodium channel that is inhibited by a local anesthetic is functionally similar to an inactivated channel. If the sodium movement is blocked over a critical length of the nerve, propagation across the blocked area is not possible. The blockade of sodium channels by most local anesthetics is both voltage- and time- or frequency-dependent. For example, a higher frequency of stimulation (and depolarization) and more positive membrane potential (prolonged depolarization) facilitate a greater degree of anesthetic block. Clinically important rates of onset and duration of anesthetic block are related to the relatively slow diffusion of an agent to sites of action rather than to its faster binding to ion channels (Butterworth and Strichartz 1990; Strichartz and Berde 1994; Catterall and Mackie 1996).

DIFFERENTIAL NERVE BLOCK. Local anesthetics are capable of blocking all nerves; hence their action is not limited to the usually more desirable loss of sensation; motor loss also occurs. Nerve fibers differ substantially in their susceptibility to local anesthetic blockade due to size and presence or absence of myelination. In general the smaller fibers with higher firing rates and less distance over which such fibers can passively propagate an impulse (type B and C fibers) are blocked before larger (type A) fibers. Myelinated fibers are blocked before unmyelinated fibers of the same diameter. Thus, autonomic fibers, small unmyelinated C fibers (mediating pain sensations), and small myelinated Aδ fibers (also mediating pain and other sensations) are blocked before larger myelinated A (γ, β, α; in order of ease of block) fibers (Table 15.3). Preferential blockade also results from the state-dependent mechanism of action of local anesthetics noted above (i.e., many sensory fibers have a high firing rate and long action potential duration).

All things considered and with an eye toward practical application, a generalized (variation among individuals is large) summary of the disappearance of nervous function in response to local anesthetic blockade, in order of first to last, is as follows: pain, warmth, touch, deep pressure, and finally motor function. Such variation in neural sensitivity to local anesthetics has thus made it possible to clinically block sensory transmission in patients without also causing motor paralysis.

Anatomic considerations contribute exceptions to the size- and myelination-related blockade story. For example, in large peripheral nerve trunks, motor nerves are more circumferentially located and hence are exposed to the local anesthetic agent first. Therefore, motor blockade in this circumstance might occur prior to sensory blockade. It is also important to remember that in general the mantle of the peripheral nerve trunk contains sensory innervation to the proximal aspect of an extremity while the core contains distal sensory innervation. Hence anesthesia will develop proximally prior to distal areas becoming desensitized.

Toxicity and Complications. Local anesthetic agents are relatively free of harmful side effects when administered at an appropriate dose. Most harmful or potentially harmful reactions occur after accidental intravenous (IV) administration. However, since vascular absorption occurs, reactions may also follow regional administration of large amounts of anesthetic, especially in debilitated patients.

Side effects of local anesthetic agents are local and systemic in origin (Table 15.4). Systemic toxicity is due to elevated plasma concentration of local anesthetic, most specifically the free, or unbound, portion. The most prominent and potentially damaging systemic effects are those involving the CNS and cardiovascular system. Animal studies indicate that in general lower blood levels are required to cause CNS toxicity than to cause cardiovascular reactions. However, adverse effects involving the cardiovascular system tend to be more life threatening and difficult to manage than CNS effects.

SYSTEMIC TOXICITY

CENTRAL NERVOUS SYSTEM. Low systemic doses of local anesthetic administered to awake, unmedicated

TABLE 15.4—Side effects of local anesthetics

Local tissue irritation (damage)
Systemic toxicity
Central nervous system
Excitation
Depression
Cardiovascular system
Hypertension
Hypotension
Ventricular dysrhythmias
Cardiovascular collapse
Other
Allergy
Methemoglobinemia
Addiction (personnel, cocaine)

humans are reported to cause numbness of the tongue and oral cavity. Low systemic doses will also likely contribute to reduced anesthetic requirement during general anesthesia (DiFazio et al. 1976; Himes et al. 1977, 1979; Doherty and Frazier 1998). As plasma concentration increases, local anesthetics produce a predictable pattern of CNS excitement and then depression that may be accompanied by apnea and cardiovascular collapse. Initially, humans report restlessness and difficulty in focusing their eyes. As plasma levels increase further, slurred speech and skeletal muscle twitching (usually initially in the face and limbs) occur, which precede the onset of tonic-clonic seizures. Still further increases in plasma levels result in CNS depression, unconsciousness, and respiratory arrest (Scott 1986). If a sufficiently large dose or rapid injection of local anesthetic is given, brief mild signs of CNS excitation followed rapidly by generalized depression occur. If other CNS depressant drugs (e.g., barbiturates, benzodiazepines, inhalation anesthetics) are administered in conjunction with the local anesthetic, a preceding excitatory phase is usually not seen. CNS excitation has long been believed to be the result of a local anesthetic drug block of inhibitory pathways in the cerebral cortex (Wagman et al. 1967).

Plasma concentrations producing the various phases of overdose are drug-related (and perhaps species-related). For example, in cats, procaine is least potent in terms of CNS effects (convulsions at about 35 mg/kg), and bupivacaine is one of the most potent (convulsions beginning at about 5 mg/kg) (Englesson 1974). In dogs, the relative CNS toxicity of bupivacaine, etidocaine, and lidocaine is 4:2:1 (Liu et al. 1983). There is an inverse relationship between the arterial carbon dioxide partial pressure (and arterial pH) and seizure thresholds of local anesthetics. This may reflect increases in cerebral blood flow (which in turn increases the amount of drug delivered to the brain) and/or decreases in plasma protein binding of local anesthetics (Englesson 1974; Burney et al. 1978).

CARDIOVASCULAR SYSTEM. Local anesthetics can produce direct effects on both the heart and peripheral vascular smooth muscle and indirect effects via influence on autonomic nervous activity. Direct effects on the heart may be both electrophysiological (decrease in the rate of depolarization and bradycardia and other cardiac dysrhythmias) and mechanical (decrease in myocardial contractility). Both effects on the heart result in a decrease in cardiac output. Evidence indicates that the more potent the drug as a local anesthetic, the greater the ability of the agent to decrease contractility (Stewart et al. 1963). Bupivacaine and etidocaine may produce severe cardiac dysrhythmias, including ventricular fibrillation (Tanz et al. 1984; Kotelko et al. 1984; Bruelle et al. 1996).

The effect of local anesthetics on peripheral vascular smooth muscle may be biphasic. In low concentrations constriction may occur. The more usual clinical response, especially with increasing concentrations, is relaxation resulting in vasodilation. Both the vasodilation and decrease in cardiac output result in arterial hypotension. The pulmonary circulation may be especially sensitive to the stimulatory effects of local anesthetics, and both ester and amide agents can cause marked increases in pulmonary artery resistance and hypertension (Strichartz and Berde 1994). When administered via the epidural or intrathecal route, cardiovascular collapse may be further exacerbated by sympathetic nervous system blockade as the agent spreads cranially. See also the review of Reiz and Nath (1986) for additional, more in-depth information.

LOCAL TISSUE TOXICITY

NEURAL TOXICITY. Local anesthetics are rarely neurotoxic at clinically administered concentrations. However, irreversible conduction blockade in isolated nerves has been produced with high concentrations of these agents (Strichartz and Berde 1994). Occasional prolonged sensory and motor deficits have also been reported following epidural or subarachnoid administration of chloroprocaine. This is now believed to be related to the antioxidant sodium bisulfite and not to the parent drug itself.

SKELETAL MUSCLE TOXICITY. When properly used, local anesthetics rarely produce localized tissue damage. However, there are reports that even at clinical doses for local infiltration, there may be skeletal muscle damage (Basson and Carlson 1980). This effect is more commonly seen with the longer acting agents, and the effect is generally felt to be reversible. In higher concentrations local anesthetics may be more generally histotoxic (Benoit and Belt 1970, 1972; Carlson 1976; Hall-Craggs and Singh-Seyen 1975; Libelius et al. 1970; Vasseur et al. 1984).

OTHER EFFECTS

METHEMOGLOBINEMIA. Methemoglobinemia has been reported as developing following exposure to a number of local anesthetics (Lund and Cwik 1965; Paddleford et al. 1985; Ferraro et al. 1988; Davis et al. 1993), most notably prilocaine. A dose-response relationship exists between the amount of prilocaine administered and the incidence of methemoglobinemia. Breakdown products from the metabolism of the local anesthetic are likely responsible (Hjelm and Holmdahl 1965). In the case of prilocaine, oxidation of hemoglobin to methemoglobin is caused by *o*-toluidine, a product of prilocaine metabolism.

ALLERGIES. Although allergic-type reactions to the amide local anesthetics are rare, it is possible for the aminoester local anesthetics such as procaine to cause hypersensitivity or anaphylactic responses. Most commonly implicated is PABA, a product of ester metabolism. Other potential causes of allergic reactions are preservatives contained in local anesthetic solutions. Methylparaben is one such agent that is reported to be chemically similar to PABA.

ADDICTION. Since the use of cocaine in clinical veterinary practice is virtually nil, the issue of human abuse potential is not commonly discussed in texts focused on veterinary medicine. However, abuses of this drug both directly (i.e., by humans with access to the compound) and indirectly (e.g., administration to horses as a stimulant prior to a race) are still possibilities worthy of this brief mention and of further thought and consideration by the reader.

CLINICAL PHARMACOLOGY. Clinically important properties of local anesthetics include anesthetic potency, speed of onset of action, duration of anesthetic action (Table 15.1), and differential sensitivity to anesthetic action. These properties are influenced by a number of other factors, such as dose of drug, site of injection, addition of vasoconstrictor to the injectate, and carbonation and pH adjustment of the local anesthetic (Strichartz and Berde 1994).

Anesthetic Potency. Lipid solubility, or hydrophobicity, seems to be a primary determinant of intrinsic anesthetic potency. The smaller and more lipophilic the molecule, the faster the rate of interaction with the sodium channel receptor. However, the relationship is less clear clinically than in the studies of isolated nerve preparations. The relative potencies of agents as determined in in vivo preparations are highly dependent not only on intrinsic factors but also on anatomic and physiologic factors (Strichartz et al. 1990). Water solubility (hydrophilicity) is also important for diffusion to the site of local anesthetic action.

Onset of Anesthetic Action. In isolated nerves the onset of local anesthetic action is related to the agent's physicochemical properties. In the patient, onset of action is also influenced by agent dose or concentration. A larger number of molecules of anesthetic in the region of the nerve facilitates more rapid action (and prolongation of effect).

DOSE OF ANESTHETIC AGENT. Use of a greater volume of anesthetic or a more concentrated solution increases the number of agent molecules in the region of the nerve. This facilitates a more rapid anesthetic onset and increases the probability and duration of successful anesthesia. When injected in the epidural or intrathecal space, increased volume of local anesthetic solution will also influence the spread of the agent.

CARBONATION AND pH ADJUSTMENT. In the isolated nerve preparation, addition of bicarbonate to the local anesthetic solution results in a more rapid onset of nerve blockade at a reduced anesthetic concentration (Wong et al. 1993). Controversy exists concerning the merits of this practice under clinical conditions. The reasoning behind this practice is that by increasing the pH of the solution, the amount of drug in the uncharged base form is increased, which should increase the rate of anesthetic diffusion and modify the dose required and time of onset of action.

USE OF HYALURONIDASE. Addition of this mucolytic enzyme is thought to enhance the diffusion of local anesthetic agents to the site of action (e.g., peripheral nerve). However, it may also enhance systemic absorption (and so toxicity) and is currently not felt to be cost-effective.

Duration of Anesthetic Action. The duration of anesthetic action of local anesthetics varies (Table 15.1). In vivo duration of action is influenced not only by the anesthetic's intrinsic action on nerves but also by its action on local blood vessels. All agents except cocaine tend to have a biphasic effect on vascular smooth muscle. At low concentrations local anesthetics tend to cause vasoconstriction, whereas in clinical doses vasodilation is usually present. Consequently, the duration of block may be shorter in vivo than that determined in isolated nerve preparations.

SITE OF INJECTION. Duration of action is inversely related to the absorption of the drug from the injection site. This is generally independent of the agent used. Hence the shortest duration of action is usually seen following intrathecal administration and the longest duration following the peripheral nerve blocks (e.g., brachial plexus, sciatic).

USE OF A VASOCONSTRICTOR. Addition of a vasoconstrictor to the local anesthetic solution decreases local perfusion, delays the rate of vascular absorption of local anesthetic, and therefore prolongs anesthetic action. Epinephrine (5 μg/mL, or 1:200,000) is the agent most commonly added to the local anesthetic. Others, such as phenylephrine and norepinephrine, are also used but without substantial clinical advantage over epinephrine. A potential reason for the occasional failure of clinical benefit from the addition of epinephrine is related to the low pH of the epinephrine preparation; when added to the local anesthetic, the low pH has the potential to further reduce the free base available for diffusion through tissues, thus delaying the onset of the local anesthetic block.

INFLUENCE OF VARYING BARICITY. Although perhaps of less consequence in veterinary patients due to their horizontal posture (four-legged stance), varying the baricity of local anesthetic solutions will influence the spread of these agents within the spinal cord. Hypobaric solutions (i.e., with a specific gravity less than that of cerebrospinal fluid [CSF]) will tend to migrate to nondependent areas, whereas hyperbaric solutions (i.e., those with a specific gravity greater than that of CSF) will migrate from the site of injection to dependent areas. This is a frequently applied technique with human patients but rarely or at least infrequently considered in veterinary patients.

MIXTURES OF LOCAL ANESTHETICS. The basis of mixing local anesthetics is to enhance onset and prolong the duration of neural blockade. While this may indeed work in some clinical situations, it is not universally effective. This is likely due to drug interactions that negate these potentially beneficial effects. For example, in isolated nerve studies, it has been suggested that when chloroprocaine (short onset and duration) and bupivacaine (long onset and duration) are mixed, metabolites of chloroprocaine may inhibit the binding of bupivacaine to receptor sites. At present there appears to be little clinically significant benefit to the use of mixtures of local anesthetics.

Pregnancy. Plasma cholinesterase activity is reduced with pregnancy and, this will influence the duration of the ester local anesthetics. The spread and depth of epidural or spinal local anesthetic is also reported to be greater in pregnant patients. Mechanical factors (such as engorged epidural vasculature) causing a decrease in the size of the spinal and epidural space have been implicated, as have hormonal changes (higher progesterone levels) associated with pregnancy. It is therefore advisable to reduce the dose of local anesthetics administered via this route in these patients.

USES OF LOCAL ANESTHETICS. Local anesthetics are most often used to produce regional anesthesia (Table 15.5). Some may also occasionally be used to provide analgesia, supplement actions of IV and inhalation anesthetics, and prevent or treat cardiac dysrhythmias. Rarely, an agent such as lidocaine may be administered in low dose to suppress grand mal seizures and to prevent or treat increases in intracranial pressure.

Regional anesthesia is a term loosely used to refer to a variety of applications of local anesthetics for anesthetic purposes. The term implies that a region of the body is affected as opposed to the entire body as with general anesthesia. The region affected may be very limited or broad in scope. In terms of organization, regional anesthesia includes the subcategories listed below.

Topical Anesthesia. Surface, or topical, anesthesia results when the drug is applied to the skin or mucous membrane to cause loss of sensation by paralyzing sensory nerve endings. Local anesthetics are widely used on the mucous membranes of the eye, nose, and mouth. Most are ineffectively used on unbroken skin, because cornified epidermis limits penetration. The recent introduction of a combination of lidocaine and prilocaine in a eutectic mixture has overcome this problem and is now commonly used to provide dermal analgesia for venipuncture and catheterization (Gajraj et al. 1994).

Local Infiltration. Infiltration anesthesia is perhaps the most common method of regional anesthesia and consists of making numerous subcutaneous (SC) injections of small volumes of local anesthetic solution into the tissues. The drug diffuses into surrounding tissue from the site of injection and anesthetizes nerve fibers and endings. Large amounts of relatively dilute solutions are often infiltrated into operative sites.

Peripheral Nerve Block. Peripheral nerve block (conduction block) is produced by injection of local anesthetic in the immediate vicinity of individual peripheral nerves or a nerve plexus. Paravertebral nerve blocks in

TABLE 15.5—Uses of local anesthetics

Anesthetic	Topical anesthetic	Local infiltration	Peripheral nerve block	Intravenous block	Epidural block	Subarachnoid block
Procaine	No	Yes	Yes	No	No	Yes
Chloroprocaine	No	Yes	Yes	No	Yes	No
Tetracaine	Yes	No	No	No	No	Yes
Lidocaine	Yes	Yes	Yes	Yes	Yes	Yes
Mepivacaine	No	Yes	Yes	No	Yes	No
Bupivacaine	No	Yes	Yes	Yes	Yes	Yes
Etidocaine	No	Yes	Yes	No	Yes	No
Prilocaine	No	Yes	Yes	Yes	Yes	No
Ropivacaine	No	Yes	Yes	No	Yes	Yes

Source: Modified from Stoelting 1987.

cattle (Horney 1966) and horses (Moon and Suter 1993), intercostal nerve blocks, and the brachial plexus block are peripheral nerve blocks. Intrapleural anesthesia is an alternative to multiple intercostal nerve blocks and may be considered a regional peripheral nerve block.

Intra-articular Administration. Local anesthetics may be administered via the intra-articular route to facilitate diagnosis of lameness, as is commonly done in the horse. The technique may also be used to desensitize the affected joint prior to and following surgical intervention (e.g., arthroscopy).

Intravenous Block. Intravenous local or regional anesthesia is accomplished by IV injection of large volumes of dilute local anesthetic into an extremity isolated from the rest of the circulation by a tourniquet. The apparent mechanism of action is by diffusion of local anesthetic across blood vessels to local nerves. Normal nervous and muscle function returns quickly upon release of the tourniquet, which allows blood flow to dilute the regional local anesthetic concentration. The technique is frequently used for operations of the digit in cattle (Weaver 1972; Bogan and Weaver 1978; Skarda 1987).

Epidural Block. Injecting local anesthetic solution into the epidural space generally at the lumbosacral space (dog, pig) or first or second intercoccygeal space (horse, cow; sometimes referred to as caudal anesthesia) produces epidural or extradural anesthesia. The anesthetic acts upon the posterior spinal nerves before they leave the vertebral column. The extent of anesthetic action is dependent on the spread of the drug and diffusion to neural tissues from the site of injection.

Spinal (Subarachnoid) Block. Spinal block is produced by injecting local anesthetic into the subarachnoid space, generally (in veterinary patients, e.g., sheep, cat) at the lumbosacral space. Because the vertebral level of termination of the spinal cord varies among animal species, this form of anesthesia is technically more difficult than epidural injection. Readers are referred to Skarda 1987 and veterinary anesthesia textbooks such as Thurmon et al. 1996 for further information on these techniques in animals.

LOCAL ANESTHETIC AGENTS

Aminoester Local Anesthetics

COCAINE HYDROCHLORIDE. Although it was the first local anesthetic to be used clinically, cocaine is no longer used in veterinary practice due to its highly addictive nature. It is classified as a Schedule II drug, and its use is highly regulated. Despite minimal or no clinical use in veterinary medicine, information about cocaine is of interest historically because of its continued common use in human patients, its abuse by humans, and its potential for illicit use in performance animals.

Cocaine Hydrochloride, USP (Fig. 15.2), is a white crystalline substance readily soluble in water. The alkaloidal form is sparingly soluble in water but freely soluble in organic solvents. Alkaloidal cocaine is not used orally or parenterally. Local anesthetics chemically related to cocaine are esters of PABA, with the alkyl amine introduced into the alkyl group.

ADMINISTRATION. The primary route of administration is via direct application to mucous membranes, through which it penetrates rapidly. Because it penetrates the horny epidermis slowly, cocaine is not sufficiently effective when applied to the intact skin. Cocaine will anesthetize tissues into which it is infiltrated, but it is no longer employed in this manner because of its high tissue toxicity. Although it has been suggested that cocaine is destroyed or hydrolyzed by gastric secretions following ingestion, evidence indicates that cocaine is not inactivated and can be rapidly absorbed from the gastrointestinal tract (Van Dyke et al. 1978).

ACTION. Sensory nerve endings are completely and reversibly paralyzed upon local contact with cocaine. For a number of years this drug was looked upon as the most effective of the local anesthetics for production of surface anesthesia. However, local anesthetics with comparable potency and no addicting potential are now more commonly employed clinically.

Local vasoconstriction characteristically occurs following application of cocaine to tissue. Cocaine blocks uptake of catecholamines at adrenergic nerve endings and is the only common local anesthetic possessing this action. Consequently, it sensitizes the sympathetic effector mechanism so that effector cells give an exaggerated response to catecholamines. In addition to vasoconstrictor action, the pupil of the eye is dilated following topical use of cocaine. Ophthalmologists have found it useful for inducing mydriasis in eye examinations as well as for concurrent local anesthesia of the eye.

DURATION. Duration of local anesthesia from cocaine depends on concentration and site of application of the solution. Concentrations as low as 0.02% applied locally to susceptible tissues will produce fleeting anesthesia. Higher concentrations may produce local anesthesia lasting as long as 0.5 hour.

THERAPEUTIC USE. Cocaine should be used only for topical anesthesia. Cocaine solutions in concentrations of 5-10% are used to anesthetize mucous membranes of the nose, larynx, and buccal cavity in large animals. In smaller species, concentrations of 5% are adequate.

TOXICITY. Acute toxicity from cocaine can occur clinically due to a drug overdose, rapid absorption, or improper administration. Adverse or toxic effects from

SC use in the horse can occur at a dose as low as 600 mg. However, excitation has been reported when only 180 mg cocaine was injected hypodermically. Severe toxic effects without fatality occur in the horse following IV administration of cocaine at doses of 0.93-1.13 mg/kg. A dose as low as 120-180 mg (presumably injected by the IV route) can be lethal in the horse. On a body weight basis (i.e., mg/kg), the horse is more sensitive to cocaine than humans. The computed range of safety that should not be exceeded when cocaine is used on mucous membranes of the horse is 300-420 mg. Cocaine is cumulative upon repeated injection; no tolerance develops from its continued use. The cocaine LD_{100} for a variety of species is given in earlier editions of this text.

The first toxic effect of cocaine is stimulation of the CNS followed by violent convulsive seizures. If sufficient cocaine is given, stimulation is followed by a period of depression that may terminate in unconsciousness and death from respiratory paralysis. Cocaine also induces cardiotoxicity that may be associated with an overstimulation of the adrenergic system. Chronic poisoning or addiction to cocaine may occur in animals under unusual conditions, but addiction is generally limited to humans.

TREATMENT OF COCAINE TOXICITY. An antagonist to the cardiotoxic effect of cocaine has been experimentally achieved by use of *Nitrendipine* (INN) (Baypress), a calcium modulator and chemically a dihydropyridine (Trouve and Nahas 1986). It does not depress the myocardium and has a coronary vasodilator action.

When simultaneously administered intra-arterially with cocaine (2 mg/kg/min) in rats, nitrendipine (1.46 μg/kg/min) suppresses the cardiac arrhythmia produced by cocaine. It also increases the survival time about 4 times, and the dose of cocaine required to produce death is increased more than 4 times. It protects the heart from the acute morphologic lesions induced by cocaine administration and suppresses some of the CNS effects of cocaine (Trouve and Nahas 1986).

Fleming et al. (1990) have reviewed the pharmacology and therapeutic applications with regard to anesthetic management.

PROCAINE HYDROCHLORIDE. *Procaine Hydrochloride,* USP (Novocaine), is a white crystalline powder that dissolves in an equal weight of water. The chemical structure is given in Fig. 15.1. It is relatively stable while exposed to air and also in aqueous solution. A minor degree of deterioration in a solution of procaine is indicated by a yellowish tint. A distinct yellowing or a darkening of the solution indicates that it should be discarded.

Procaine was synthesized after cocaine was discovered to be habit forming and relatively toxic. Procaine is still a commonly used local anesthetic, although it is not very effective as a surface, or topical, anesthetic.

ACTION. The solution of procaine is nonirritant and promptly effective when injected subcutaneously. Anesthesia is relatively brief because the drug is absorbed rapidly and destroyed quickly by plasma cholinesterases. Anesthesia with procaine is commonly prolonged by addition of a vasoconstrictor to the solution to delay absorption from the site of injection.

METABOLISM AND EXCRETION. Procaine is hydrolyzed primarily in blood plasma by nonspecific pseudocholinesterases. Hydrolysis of procaine is rapid. For example, following rapid IV injection of procaine (1000 mg), the plasma concentration of the drug decreases with a half-life of about 25 minutes (Tobin et al. 1976).

Two products of procaine degradation are PABA and diethylaminoethanol. PABA exhibits no local anesthetic action, but diethylaminoethanol has a part of the full anesthetic activity of procaine. PABA inhibits the action of sulfonamide antibiotics and interferes with the chemical determination of sulfonamide concentration in biological fluids. As mentioned previously, allergic reactions to ester local anesthetic agents are attributed to this metabolite.

The kidney excretes procaine and PABA. The pK_a of procaine, a weak organic base, is 8.9 (Table 15.1). The nonionized form of procaine passes more readily through cell membranes than the ionized form. Consequently, an important factor in excretion of procaine is the urinary pH (Evans and Lambert 1974). In the horse, e.g., urinary pH may fluctuate diurnally from the alkaline to the acid side; the pH may also fluctuate depending upon whether the animal is at rest or exercising. A single dose of 60 mg procaine administered intramuscularly in the horse requires an elimination time of 27.5 hours after injection (Evans and Lambert 1974). Acidification of urine with ammonium chloride hastens excretion of ionized procaine; e.g., 600 mg, or 10 times the above dose, administered intramuscularly as a single dose requires only 10 hours for complete elimination.

TOXICITY. The greatest difference between the toxicities of procaine and a potent local anesthetic such as cocaine is rate of metabolism. Cocaine is slowly metabolized, whereas procaine is rapidly detoxified. An LD_{50} of procaine is detoxified in the cat within 20 minutes, whereas an LD_{50} of cocaine is metabolized in 60 minutes. Table 15.6 gives average LD_{50} data for procaine in four species of animals.

CLINICAL USES. Procaine is used in veterinary medicine for infiltration and nerve block (Table 15.5). For infiltration in small animals, a concentration of 1% is generally employed, whereas in larger animals, 2% is preferable. About 2-5 mL of a 2% solution are used for nerve block (conduction) anesthesia in small animals. In large animals, 5-10 mL of a 4% solution are most commonly used. Epinephrine solution may be added to give a concentration of 1:100,000, i.e., 1 mL epinephrine solution (1:1000) to each 99 mL anesthetic solution. Procaine is rarely used for surface

TABLE. 15.6—Average LD_{50} of procaine (g/kg)

	Route	
Species	SC	IV
Guinea pig	0.43	0.05
Rabbit	0.46	0.055
Cat	0.45	0.045
Dog	0.25	—

Source: Graubard and Peterson 1950.

anesthesia because it is not very effective via this route of administration.

The horse seems to be more sensitive to CNS stimulation by procaine than other species of domestic animals. Rapid IV injection of 1000 mg in Thoroughbred mares elicited variable signs of CNS excitation for as long as 4 minutes in a study by Tobin et al. (1976). Considerably larger doses are necessary to produce central stimulation in the cow, whereas the response by the pig is intermediate between that of the horse and cow. Because of its CNS stimulant and analgesic actions, procaine has been used illegally in racing animals to attempt to improve their performance and/or to mask lameness in track and racing events.

Procaine is sometimes combined with other drugs because in doing so a less soluble drug is produced, prolonging drug action. A combination of procaine with penicillin G results in an antibiotic that is absorbed very slowly and prolongs detectable (therapeutic) concentrations in plasma and urine. When using large doses of procaine-penicillin G, the side effects of procaine (see above) should be considered. This also has implications during drug testing for potential abuse in racing and performance animals.

CHLOROPROCAINE HYDROCHLORIDE. *Chloroprocaine Hydrochloride,* USP (Nesacaine) is characterized by a rapid onset and short duration of action. It has a low potency but may be used in higher concentrations (3%) due to its low systemic toxicity. This compound, which has the addition of a chlorine atom to the benzene ring of procaine, is hydrolyzed 3 times more rapidly than procaine. It is hydrolyzed by plasma cholinesterase to 2-chloroaminobenzoic acid and 2-diethylaminoethanol.

Chloroprocaine may be used for infiltration and IV anesthesia, but its main use is via the epidural route for obstetrical anesthesia. Thrombophlebitis following IV administration is reported and likely related to concentration of drug administered. When concentrations of less than 0.5% of preservative-free 2-chloroprocaine are used, this effect is negated. Prolonged neural deficits following its use have been reported, which are now believed to be caused by the preservative sodium bisulfite and not the parent drug itself.

TETRACAINE HYDROCHLORIDE. *Tetracaine Hydrochloride,* USP (Pontocaine), is a potent ester local anesthetic (Fig. 15.2, Table 15.1). It is used to provide topical anesthesia of the eye, nose, and throat and for spinal anesthesia when both sensory and motor blockade are desired. Its rapid absorption from mucosa to which it is applied increases the potential for systemic toxicity in light of its slower metabolism (than that of procaine) by plasma cholinesterase. Both a patch application system and a gel preparation have been evaluated for percutaneous analgesia with favorable results (McCafferty and Woolfson 1993).

BENZOCAINE. *Benzocaine,* USP (Americaine), previously referred to as ethyl aminobenzoate, is structurally similar to procaine except that it lacks a terminal diethyl amino group. It is available as a dusting powder or in oil as an ointment for surface application. It has been used to varying degrees in dentistry to provide anesthesia of the gums and buccal mucosa. Cutaneous application is also reported. Its low solubility allows it to remain localized in wounds to provide long-term analgesia. Benzocaine is also a component (as is tetracaine) in a topical local anesthetic mixture known as cetacaine, which is commonly used as a spray to anesthetize the larynx prior to intubation.

In fish, benzocaine (50 mg/L) induces sedation within 30 seconds after immersion (Oswald 1978). This permits weighing of the fish and injection of the calculated anesthetic doses of other anesthetic drugs.

Benzocaine is relatively nonirritating to tissues, and following absorption it is metabolized to PABA and acetyl PABA. It has been reported to cause methemoglobinemia in some species (e.g., sheep), which may limit its widespread use in clinical practice.

PROPARACAINE HYDROCHLORIDE. *Proparacaine Hydrochloride,* USP (Alcaine, AK-Taine, Ophthetic), is an ester-type local anesthetic about equal in potency to tetracaine. It is chemically distinct from procaine and exhibits little cross-sensitivity. Unlike some topical anesthetics, it produces little or no tissue irritation (Ritchie and Greene 1990). Because proparacaine induces little discomfort upon instillation into the human eye, it is widely used as an ophthalmic anesthetic.

Aminoamide Local Anesthetics

LIDOCAINE HYDROCHLORIDE. *Lidocaine Hydrochloride,* USP (Xylocaine, Lidocaine HCL) (α-diethylaminoaceto-2,6-xylidide), is a white or slightly yellow powder with a characteristic odor (Fig. 15.1). It is relatively stable but nearly insoluble in water. Lidocaine is available as a sterile aqueous solution from 0.5 to 5% with or without epinephrine and in a gel preparation from 2 to 5%.

Lidocaine is one of the most versatile and one of the most (if not the most) widely used of the local anesthetics in veterinary medicine. It is an amide-type local anesthetic and therefore an agent of choice for use with individuals sensitive to the ester-type agents (e.g., procaine).

METABOLISM AND FATE. Lidocaine is relatively quickly absorbed from the gastrointestinal tract and following injection (Boyes et al. 1971; Keenaghan and Boyes 1972). The rate of systemic absorption following parenteral administration is slowed and the duration of action is prolonged when lidocaine is used with a vasoconstrictor.

Lidocaine is metabolized in the liver by mixed-function oxidases at a rate nearly as rapid as that for procaine. The unchanged form is excreted in urine of the dog in a concentration of 10-20%. Two metabolites have been identified in the dog from hepatic *N*-deethylation of lidocaine (Wilcke et al. 1983). One of these, monoethylglycinexylidide, has significant pharmacologic activity; after a second *N*-dealkylation, glycinexylidide (4-hydroxy-2,6-dimethylaniline) is formed. Both compounds may be further hydroxylated to 4-hydroxy-2,6-xylidine, which is the major metabolite excreted in the urine.

Following administration of lidocaine (10 mg/kg) in pregnant guinea pigs, it rapidly crosses the placenta (Finster et al. 1972). High concentrations are found in the fetal liver, heart, and brain. The liver of the fetal guinea pig is the only organ in which lidocaine is found in higher concentration than in the maternal subject.

The kinetics and oral absorption rate of lidocaine have been determined in the dog (Boyes et al. 1970); 78% of the administered dose reaches the general circulation. Emesis occurs regularly at 2.5 hours after administration.

The pharmacokinetics of lidocaine in humans is given in Table 15.2. Pharmacokinetic data have also been reported for the dog after the IV and IM administration of single doses (6 mg/kg) of lidocaine hydrochloride (Wilcke et al. 1983). The mean elimination rate constant and mean specific clearance for IV lidocaine in the dog are 0.786/hr and 2.4 L/kg/hr, respectively. After IM administration, the mean absorption rate constant is 7.74/hr. Absorption is essentially complete (91.9%) after an IM injection of lidocaine (Wilcke et al. 1983).

In the dog, administration of an IV loading dose of 0.8 mg/kg/min over 10 minutes, followed by an infusion of 0.085 mg/kg/min over 3 hours, provides a steady-state plasma concentration of 3.5-5.5 µg/mL (DeRick et al. 1981). In a simulation of an IM dose schedule for lidocaine (6 mg/kg every 1.5 hours) in the dog, an average serum concentration of 1.48 µg/mL is expected, which is near the therapeutic range (Wilcke et al. 1983).

CLINICAL USES. Lidocaine is used for all forms of local anesthesia (Table 15.5). In addition to its use as a local anesthetic, it is used intravenously as an antiarrhythmic agent and also as a supplement to general anesthesia (Phillips et al. 1960). It decreases the requirement for inhalation and injectable anesthetics (DiFazio et al. 1976; Himes et al. 1977, 1979; Kissin and McGee 1982; Doherty and Frazier 1998).

PRILOCAINE HYDROCHLORIDE. *Prilocaine Hydrochloride,* USP (Citanest), is a local anesthetic of the amide type (Fig. 15.2) whose pharmacological properties resemble those of lidocaine (Table 15.1). However, it causes significantly less vasodilation and hence may be used without the addition of epinephrine to prolong the duration of effect. It is also reported to be the least toxic of the amide local anesthetics and so best suited for IV anesthesia. Methemoglobinemia is a side effect of overdose and accounts for its declining use, especially for human patients.

EUTECTIC MIXTURE OF LIDOCAINE AND PRILOCAINE (EMLA). A eutectic mixture of local anesthetics (EMLA) consisting of a 1:1 mixture of lidocaine and prilocaine is available commercially for transcutaneous application. It has been shown that when the base forms of these two compounds are mixed, an oil is formed at temperatures over 18° C (Brodin et al. 1984). This eutectic mixture is commercially available in a preparation containing arlacton as an emulsifier and carbapol as a thickening agent. Each gram (mL) contains 25 mg of lidocaine and 25 mg of prilocaine. The reported bioavailability is 3% for lidocaine and 5% for prilocaine (Klein et al. 1994). This may, however, vary with the site of application and skin pigmentation and condition.

EMLA has been evaluated as a percutaneous analgesic prior to venipuncture in dogs, cats, rabbits, and rats (Flecknell et al. 1990). Its efficacy following a 60-minute application was good in dogs, cats, and rabbits but questionable in study rats. In human adults, the efficacy is improved following a 90-120 minute application. Hence, in people the general recommendation is to apply the emulsion to the cutaneous tissue using an occlusive dressing for a minimum of 60-90 minutes prior to application of a noxious stimulus (Bjerring and Arendt-Nielsen 1990; Buckley and Benfield 1993). Analgesic benefits have been shown for at least 30 minutes following removal of the emulsion in human patients.

The toxicity of EMLA is related primarily to the metabolism of prilocaine to *o*-toluidine, which can result in methemoglobinemia, as mentioned previously. It is not recommended for use in human neonates due to the immature methemoglobin reductase enzyme. In 6- to 12-month-old human infants, a maximum dose of 2 grams is suggested (Engberg et al. 1987; Buckley and Benfield 1993). Blanching or hyperemia may be noticed in the area of application following removal of the occlusive bandage and is likely due to the relative vasoactivity of the two compounds.

MEPIVACAINE HYDROCHLORIDE. *Mepivacaine Hydrochloride,* USP (Carbocaine), is a local anesthetic of the amide type (Fig. 15.2). Its pharmacological properties are similar to those of lidocaine. Although actual potency figures vary, it is about equal (or slightly less) in local anesthetic potency to lidocaine (Table 15.1). It has a slightly longer duration of action, likely due to less intrinsic vasodilator activity than lidocaine. While its use in clinical practice is similar to that of lidocaine

(Table 15.5), mepivacaine is not recommended for obstetrical anesthesia, because its actions are markedly prolonged in the fetus. In the adult, the toxicity of mepivacaine is about 1.5-2 times that of procaine but slightly less than that of lidocaine.

BUPIVACAINE HYDROCHLORIDE. *Bupivacaine Hydrochloride,* USP (Sensorcaine, Marcaine), is an amide-type local anesthetic chemically related to mepivacaine (Fig. 15.2). Bupivacaine is a long-acting local anesthetic. It is about 4 times more potent than lidocaine (Table 15.1) and has a duration of action that ranges from 3 to 8 hours. It is used most commonly for regional and epidural nerve blocks and was the first local anesthetic agent to show significant separation of sensory and motor blockade, making it the drug of choice for obstetrical anesthesia. Central nervous system and cardiac toxicity result from lower doses and blood levels than those reported for lidocaine.

ETIDOCAINE HYDROCHLORIDE. *Etidocaine Hydrochloride,* USP (Duranest), is a long-acting derivative of lidocaine (amide type, Fig. 15.2). It is about equal in potency and toxicity to bupivacaine. Unlike bupivacaine, however, etidocaine shows little separation between sensory and motor blockade and hence, while valuable during surgical anesthesia, is less useful for obstetrics and postoperative pain management.

ROPIVACAINE HYDROCHLORIDE. *Ropivacaine Hydrochloride,* USP (Naropin) (1-propyl-2′6′-pipecoloxylidide hydrochloride monohydrate) is a new long-acting aminoamide local anesthetic that is structurally related to mepivacaine and bupivacaine (Fig. 15.2). Ropivacaine differs from mepivacaine and bupivacaine in that it is an *S*-isomer, whereas the latter agents are racemic mixtures (previous studies of isomers of local anesthetics suggested that the systemic toxicity of the *S*-isomer of various compounds may be less than that of racemic preparations). The physicochemical properties of ropivacaine are similar to those of bupivacaine with the exception of its lipid solubility (ropivacaine is substantially less lipid soluble) (Rosenberg and Heinonen 1983; Rosenberg et al. 1986). Its pharmacokinetic profile following IV administration is given in Table 15.2 (Arthur et al. 1988). At low concentrations ropivacaine has intrinsic vasoconstricting properties, whereas higher concentrations result in vasodilation.

Ropivacaine is used in a manner similar to bupivacaine (Table 15.5). Reports indicate that the motor block following epidural administration is less dense and of a shorter duration than for bupivacaine. This, along with ropivacaine's reduced cardiotoxic potential when compared to bupivacaine (Feldman et al. 1989; Reiz et al. 1989), offers advantages for clinical use when differential blockade is desired. Ropivacaine also reportedly caused fewer CNS symptoms in human volunteers and was at least 25% less toxic than bupivacaine with regard to the dose tolerated (Scott et al. 1989). See McClure 1996 for a recent review.

REFERENCES

Arthur, G. R. 1987. Pharmacokinetics. In G. R. Strichartz, ed., Handbook of Experimental Pharmacology: Local Anesthetics, Vol. 81, pp. 165-186. Berlin: Springer-Verlag.

Arthur, G. R., Feldman, H. S., and Covino, B. G. 1988. Comparative pharmacokinetics of bupivacaine and ropivacaine, a new amide local anesthetic. Anesth Analg 67:1053-1058.

Basson, M. D., and Carlson, B. M. 1980. Myotoxicity of single and repeated injections of mepivacaine (Carbocaine) in the rat. Anesth Analg 59:275-282.

Benoit, P. W., and Belt, W. D. 1970. Destruction and regeneration of skeletal muscle after treatment with a local anesthetic, bupivacaine (Marcaine). J Anat 107:547.

———. 1972. Some effects of local anesthetic agents on skeletal muscle. Exp Neurol 34:264-278.

Bjerring, P., and Arendt-Nielsen, L. 1990. Depth and duration of skin analgesia to needle insertion after topical application of EmLa cream. Br J Anaesth 64:173-177.

Bogan, J. A., and Weaver, A. D. 1978. Lidocaine concentrations associated with intravenous regional anesthesia of the distal limb of cattle. Am J Vet Res 39:1672-1673.

Boyes, R. N., Adams, H. J., and Duce, B. R. 1970. Oral absorption and deposition kinetics of lidocaine hydrochloride in dogs. J Pharmacol Exp Ther 174:1-8.

Boyes, R. N., Scott, D. B., Jebson, P. J., Godman, M. J., and Julian, D. G. 1971. Pharmacokinetics of lidocaine in man. Clin Pharmacol Ther 12:105-116.

Brodin, A., Nyqvist-Mayer, Wadsten, T., Forslund, B., and Bromberg, F. 1984. Phase diagram and aqueous solubility of the lidocaine-prilocaine binary system. J. Pharmaceut Sci 73:481-484.

Bruelle, P., Lefrant, J.-Y., de La Coussaye, J. E., Peray, P. A., Desch, G., Sassine, A., and Eledjam, J.-J. 1996. Comparative electrophysiologic and hemodynamic effects of several amide local anesthetic drugs in anesthetized dogs. Anesth Analg 82:648-656.

Buckley, M. M., and Benfield, P. 1993. Eutectic lidocaine/prilocaine cream: a review of the topical anesthetic/analgesic efficacy of a eutectic mixture of local anesthetics (EMLA). Drugs 46:126-151.

Burney, R. G., DiFazio, C. A., and Foster, J. A. 1978. Effects of pH on protein binding of lidocaine. Anesth Analg 57:478-480.

Butterworth, J. F., and Strichartz, G. R. 1990. Molecular mechanisms of local anesthesia: a review. Anesthesiology 72:711-734.

Carlson, B. M. 1976. A quantitative study of muscle fiber survival and regeneration in normal, predenervated, and marcaine-treated free muscle grafts in the rat. Exp Neurol 52:421-432.

Catterall, W., and Mackie, K. 1996. Local anesthetics. In J. G. Hardman, L. E. Limbird, P. B. Molinoff, R. W. Ruddon, and A. G. Gilman, eds., Goodman and Gilman's The Pharmacological Basis of Therapeutics, 9th ed., pp. 331-347. New York: McGraw-Hill.

Covino, B. G. 1987. Toxicity and systemic effects of local anesthetic agents. In G. R. Strichartz, ed., Handbook of Experimental Pharmacology: Local Anesthetics, vol. 81, pp. 187-213. Berlin: Springer-Verlag.

Davis, J. A., Greenfield, R. E., and Brewer, T. G. 1993. Benzocaine-induced methemoglobinemia attributed to topical application of the anesthetic in several laboratory animal species. Am J Vet Res 54:1322-1326.

DeRick, A., Rosseel, M.-T., Belpaire, F., and Bogaert, M. 1981. Lidocaine plasma concentrations obtained with standardized infusion in the awake and anaesthetized dog. J Vet Pharmacol Ther 4:129.

DiFazio, C. A., Niederlehner, J. R., and Burney, R. 1976. The anesthetic potency of lidocaine in the rat. Anesth Analg 55:818-821.

Doherty, T. J., and Frazier, D. L. 1998. Effect of intravenous lidocaine on halothane minimum alveolar concentration in ponies. Equine Vet J 30:300-303.
Engberg, G., Danielson, K., Henneberg, S., and Nilsonn, A. 1987. Plasma concentrations of prilocaine and lidocaine and methaemoglobin formation in infants after epicutaneous application of a 5% lidocaine-prilocaine cream (EMLA). Acta Anaesth Scand 31:624-628.
Englesson, S. 1974. The influence of acid-base changes on central nervous system toxicity of local anesthetic agents. I. An experimental study in cats. Acta Anaesth Scand 18:79-87.
Evans, J. A., and Lambert, M. B. T. 1974. Estimation of procaine in urine of horses. Vet Rec 95:316-318.
Feldman, H., Arthur, G., and Covino, B. 1989. Comparative systemic toxicity of convulsant and supraconvulsant doses of intravenous ropivacaine, bupivacaine, and lidocaine in the conscious dog. Anesth Analg 69:794-801.
Ferraro, L., Zeichner, S. G. G., and Groeger, J. S. 1988. Cetacaine-induced acute methemoglobinemia. Anesthesiology 69:614-616.
Finster, M., Morishima, H. O., Boyes, R. N., and Covino, B. G. 1972. The placental transfer of lidocaine and its uptake by fetal tissues. Anesthesiology 36:159-163.
Flecknell, P. A., Liles, J. H., and Williamson, H. A. 1990. The use of lidocaine-prilocaine local anesthetic cream for pain-free venipuncture in laboratory animals. Lab An 24:142-146.
Fleming, J. A., Byck, R., and Barash, P. G. 1990. Pharmacology and therapeutic applications of cocaine. Anesthesiology 73:518-531.
Gajraj, N. M., Pennant, J. H., and Watcha, M. F. 1994. Eutectic mixture of local anesthetics (EMLA) cream. Anesth Analg 78:574-583.
Gelatt, K. N. 1978. Veterinary Ophthalmic Pharmacology and Therapeutics, 2nd ed., p. 23. Bonner Springs, KS: Veterinary Medicine Publishing.
Graubard, D. J., and Peterson, M. C. 1950. Clinical Uses of Intravenous Procaine. Springfield, IL: Charles C. Thomas.
Guyton, A. C., and Hall, J. E. 1996. Textbook of Medical Physiology. 9th ed. Philadelphia: W. B. Saunders.
Hall-Craggs, E. C. B., and Singh-Seyen, H. 1975. Histochemical changes in innervated and denervated skeletal muscle fibers following treatment with bupivacaine (Marcaine). Exp Neurol 46:345-354.
Havener, W. H. 1983. Ocular Pharmacology, p. 72. 5th ed. St. Louis: C. V. Mosby.
Himes, R. S., Jr., DiFazio, C. A., and Burney, R. G. 1977. Effects of lidocaine on the anesthetic requirements of nitrous oxide and halothane. Anaesthesiology 47:437-440.
Himes, R. S., Jr., Munson, E. S., and Embro, W. J. 1979. Enflurane requirement and ventilatory response to carbon dioxide during lidocaine infusion in dogs. Anesthesiology 51:131-134.
Hjelm, M., and Holmdahl, M. H. 1965. Biochemical effects of aromatic amines. Acta Anaesth Scand 9:99-120.
Horney, F. D. 1966. Anesthesia in the bovine. Can Vet J 7:224-230.
Keenaghan, J. B., and Boyes, R. N. 1972. The tissue distribution, metabolism, and excretion of lidocaine in rats, guinea pigs, dogs, and man. J Pharmacol Exp Ther 180:454-463.
Kendig, J., and Cohen, E. N. 1977. Pressure antagonism to nerve conduction block by anesthetic agents. Anesthesiology 47:6-10.
Kissin, I., and McGee, T. 1982. Hypnotic effect of thiopental-lidocaine combination in the rat. Anesthesiology 57:311-313.
Klein, J., Fernandes, D., Gazarian, M., et al. 1994. Simultaneous determination of lidocaine, prilocaine, and the prilocaine metabolite *o*-toluidine in plasma by high-performance liquid chromatography. J Chromatography B 655:83-88.
Kotelko, D. M., Shnider, S. M., Dailey, P. A., Brizgys, R., and Levinson, G. 1984. Bupivacaine-induced cardiac arrhythmias in sheep. Anesthesiology 60:10-19.
Kolwas, J. 1979. Drugs Today 15:357.
Lee, A., Fagan, D., Lamont, M., Tucker, G. T., Halldin, M., and Scott, D. P. 1989. Disposition kinetics of ropivacaine in humans. Anesth Analg 69:736-738.
Libelius, R., Sonesson, B., Stamenovic, B. A., and Thesleff, A. 1970. Denervation-like changes in skeletal muscle after treatment with a local anesthetic (Marcaine). J Anat 106:297-309.
Liu, P. L., Feldman, H. S., Giasi, R., Patterson, M. K., and Covino, B. G. 1983. Comparative CNS toxicity of lidocaine, etidocaine, bupivacaine, and tetracaine in awake dogs following rapid IV administration. Anesth Analg 62:375-379.
Lund, P. G., and Cwik, J. G. 1965. Propitocaine (Citanest) and methemoglobinemia. Anesthesiology 26:569-571.
McCafferty, D. F., and Woolfson, A. D. 1993. New patch delivery system for percutaneous local anaesthesia. Br J Anaesth 71:370-374.
McClure, J. H. 1996. Ropivacaine. Br J Anaesth 76:300-307.
Metcalfe, J. C., and Burgen, A. S. V. 1968. Relaxation of anaesthetics in the presence of cyto-membranes. Nature 220:587-588.
Moon, P. F., and Suter, C. M. 1993. Paravertebral thoracolumbar anaesthesia in 10 horses. Equine Vet J 25:304-308.
Morishima, H. O., Pedersen, H., Finster, M., Hiraoka, H., Tsuji, A., Feldman, H. S., Arthur, H. R., and Covino, B. G. 1985. Bupivacaine toxicity in pregnant and nonpregnant ewes. Anesthesiology 63:134-139.
Oswald, R. L. 1978. Injection anaesthesia for experimental studies in fish. Comp Biochem Physiol (C) 60:19-26.
Paddleford, R. R., Krahwinkel, D. J., Fuhr, J. E., and Kitchen, H. 1985. Experimentally induced methemoglobinemia in the dog following exposure to topical benzocaine HCl. In J. Grandy, S. Hildebrand, W. McDonell, et al. Proc Second Internat Congr Vet Anesth, pp. 98-100. Santa Barbara: Veterinary Practice Publishing.
Phillips, O. C., Lyons, W. B., Harris, L. C., Nelson, A. T., Graff, T. D., and Frazier, T. M. 1960. Intravenous lidocaine as an adjunct to general anesthesia: a clinical evaluation. Anesth Analg 39:317-322.
Reiz, S., Haggmark, S., Johansson, G., and Nath, S. 1989. Cardiotoxicity of ropivacaine: a new amide local anaesthetic agent. Acta Anaesth Scand 33:93-98.
Reiz, S., and Nath, S. 1986. Cardiotoxicity of local anaesthetic agents. Br J Anaesth 58:736-746.
Ritchie, J. M., and Greene, N. M. 1990. In A. G. Goodman, L. S. Goodman, and A. Gilman, eds., The Pharmacological Basis of Therapeutics, 8th ed., p. 311. New York: Pergamon Press.
Rosenberg, P. H., and Heinonen, E. 1983. Differential sensitivity of A and C nerve fibres to long-acting amide local anaesthetics. Br J Anaesth 55:163-167.
Rosenberg, P. H., Kytta, J., and Alila, A. 1986. Absorption of bupivacaine, etidocaine, lignocaine and ropivacaine into *N*-haptane, rat sciatic nerve, and human extradural and subcutaneous fat. Br J Anesth 58:310-314.
Scott, D. B. 1986. Toxic effects of local anaesthetic agents on the central nervous system. Br J Anaesth 58:732-735.
Scott, D. B., Lee, A., Fagan, D., Bowler, G. M. R., Bloomfield, P., and Lundh, R. 1989. Acute toxicity of ropivacaine compared with that of bupivacaine. Anesth Analg 69:563-569.

Skarda, R. T. 1987. Local and regional analgesia. In C. E. Short, ed., Principles and Practice of Veterinary Anesthesia, pp. 91-153. Baltimore: Williams & Wilkins.

Stewart, D. M., Rogers, W. P., Mahaffrey, J. E., Witherspoon, S., and Woods, E. F. 1963. Effect of local anesthetics on the cardiovascular system in the dog. Anesthesiology 24:620-624.

Stoelting, R. K. 1987. Pharmacology and Physiology in Anesthetic Practice. Philadelphia: J. B. Lippincott.

———. 1991. Pharmacology and Physiology in Anesthetic Practice. 2nd ed. Philadelphia: J. B. Lippincott.

Stoelting, R. K., and Miller, R. D. 1987. Basics of Anesthesia. 2nd ed. New York: Churchill Livingstone.

Strichartz, G. R., and Berde, C. B. 1994. Local anesthetics. In R. D. Miller, ed., Anesthesia, 4th ed., pp. 489-521. New York: Churchill Livingstone.

Strichartz, G. R., Sanchez, V., Arthur, G. R., Chafetz, R., and Martin, D. 1990. Fundamental properties of local anesthetics. II. Measured octanol:buffer partition coefficients and pK_a values of clinically used drugs. Anesth Analg 71:158-170.

Tanz, R. D., Heskett, T., Loehning, W., and Fairfax, C. A. 1984. Comparative cardiotoxicity of bupivacaine and lidocaine in the isolated perfused mammalian heart. Anesth Analg 63:549-556.

Thurmon, J. C., Tranquilli, W. J., and Benson G. J., eds. 1996. Veterinary Anesthesia. 3rd ed. Baltimore: Williams & Wilkins.

Tobin, T., Blake, J. W., Tai, C. Y., and Arnett, S. 1976. Pharmacology of procaine in the horse: a preliminary report. Am J Vet Res 37:1107-1110.

Trouve, R., and Nahas, G. 1986. Nitrendipine: an antidote to cardiac and lethal toxicity of cocaine. Proc Soc Exp Biol Med 183:392-397.

Tucker, G. T. 1986. Pharmacokinetics of local anaesthetics. Br J Anaesth 58:717-731.

Van Dyke, C., Jatlow, P., Ungerer, J., Barash, P. G., and Byck, R. 1978. Oral cocaine: plasma concentrations and central effects. Science 200:211-213.

Vasseur, P. B., Paul, H. A., Dybdal, N., and Crumley, L. 1984. Effects of local anesthetics on healing of abdominal wounds in rabbits. Am J Vet Res 45:2385-2389.

Wagman, I. H., deJong, R. H., and Prince, D. A. 1967. Effects of lidocaine on the central nervous system. Anesthesiology 28:155-169.

Weaver, A. D. 1972. Intravenous local anesthesia of the lower limb in cattle. J Am Vet Med Assoc 160:55-57.

Wilcke, J. R., Davis, L. E., Neff-Davis, C. A., and Koritz, G. D. 1983. Pharmacokinetics of lidocaine and its active metabolites in dogs. J Vet Pharmacol Ther 6:49-57.

Wong, K., Strichartz, G. R., and Raymond, S. A. 1993. On the mechanism of potentiation of local anesthetics by bicarbonate buffer: drug structure-activity studies on isolated peripheral nerve. Anesth Anal 76:131-143.

16 ANTICONVULSANT DRUGS AND ANALEPTIC AGENTS

DAWN M. BOOTHE

Anticonvulsants
- Pathophysiology of Seizures
- Biochemical Aspects of Epilepsy
- General Mechanisms of Anticonvulsant Action
- General Pharmacokinetic Considerations of Anticonvulsant Drugs
- Phenobarbital Sodium
- Primidone
- Phenytoin Sodium
- Benzodiazepines: Diazepam, Clonazepam, and Clorazepate
- Bromide
- Pentobarbital Sodium
- Miscellaneous Antiepileptics
- Drugs Contraindicated in Epileptic Patients

CNS Stimulants
- Doxapram Hydrochloride
- Methylxanthine Derivatives
- Antagonists

ANTICONVULSANTS

Pathophysiology of Seizures. The normal resting membrane potential (RMP) of the neuronal cell is –70 mV. The electrical difference across the cell membrane is maintained by a Na^+,K^+-ATPase (adenosine triphosphatase) pump. Depolarization and the generation of an action potential occur when the RMP becomes sufficiently positive to reach threshold. As in other cells, the RMP of a neuron is determined by the concentration of negative and positive ions across the membrane. The concentration reflects ion flux and thus permeability of the cell membrane to the ions. Fluxes resulting in an increase in positive ions inside the cell relative to the outside hypopolarize the RMP, bringing it closer to threshold and subsequent depolarization. The tendency of a neuron to depolarize reflects, in part, the sum total effect of neurotransmitters (NTs) interacting with the cell membrane. Inhibitory NTs such as γ-aminobutyric acid (GABA) render the RMP more negative and less susceptible to depolarization. Excitatory NTs such as acetylcholine and glutamate elevate the RMP to a more positive status and thus make it more susceptible to reaching the threshold necessary for depolarization. Inappropriate depolarization may reflect a number of abnormalities, such as alteration of the Na^+,K^+ pump, permeability changes in the cell membrane (induced, e.g., by hypoxia, inflammation, or trauma), altered concentrations of excitatory (increased) or inhibitory (decreased) neurons, or altered cellular metabolism.

Seizures are the clinical results of rapid, excessive neuronal discharge in the brain. Seizures are classified as primary (i.e., genetic) or secondary (acquired) and as generalized or focal. Generalized seizures are much more common in small animals; the incidence is greater in dogs than in cats. With seizure onset of a generalized character, convulsive electroencephalographic activity begins simultaneously in all brain regions (Faingold 1985). Many seizures in epileptic subjects have been attributed to a cortical origin. However, there is increasing evidence that the brain stem can exhibit self-sustained seizure discharge, and this area of the brain may serve an important role in the generation and expression of generalized tonic convulsions (Browning 1985). Within the brain stem, the pontine reticular formation is believed to play a key role in the generation and/or expression of tonic convulsions. Studies indicate that the ability to depress reticular core activity is an essential characteristic of antiepileptic drugs, which suggests that the reticular formation is involved in the spread and generalization of clinical seizures (Fromm 1985).

In the dog, the most common form of epilepsy is generalized tonic-clonic, or grand mal, seizures (Cunningham 1984; Schwartz-Porsche et al. 1985). Epilepsy and other seizure disorders of the central nervous system (CNS) in the dog may be caused by an acquired organic lesion such as brain tumor, head trauma, toxicosis, electrolyte imbalance, hypoglycemia, renal failure, or hepatic disease (acquired, or secondary, epilepsy); or may be genetic or inherited ("true," idiopathic, or primary epilepsy). An autosomal gene associated with a sex-linked suppressor on the X chromosome may explain the higher incidence of seizures in male dogs.

Status epilepticus refers to failure of the patient to recover to a normal alert state between repeated tonic-clonic attacks or episodes that last at least 30 minutes (Delgado-Escueta et al. 1982). Convulsive, or tonic-clonic, status epilepticus is a medical emergency in which convulsive seizures must be terminated by treatment with anticonvulsant agents. In humans, epileptic seizures must not be allowed to persist more than 60 minutes if severe and permanent neurologic injury or death is to be avoided (Delgado-Escueta et al. 1982). The longer an epileptic seizure persists, the greater the incidence of mortality and morbidity. Hyperthermia due to continuous muscle contraction may become life threatening during continued seizure activity.

Biochemical Aspects of Epilepsy. Until the underlying biochemical mechanisms leading to genesis of epileptic seizures are better understood, all therapy administered for control of seizures will continue to be directed toward treatment of symptoms. Although experimentally induced CNS seizures have provided valuable information regarding some of the biochemical events preceding and following a seizure, the question always remains whether the induced seizure simulates those observed in the clinical setting.

In humans, amino acid analysis of plasma in subjects with epilepsy indicates much higher concentrations of taurine (2-aminoethanesulfonic acid) and glutamic acid than in normal subjects (van Gelder et al. 1975). Also, the glutamic acid in urine is elevated in subjects that are known epileptics. Oral administration of taurine does not appreciably affect concentrations of amino acids with the exception of glutamic acid. In human patients with an abnormal plasma concentration of glutamic acid, administration of taurine lowers the glutamic acid in the normal direction along with a drop in urinary excretion (van Gelder et al. 1975). Consequently, taurine administration appears to partially reverse these biochemical abnormalities. According to van Gelder and associates, there is little doubt that, in both the CNS and the periphery, taurine serves a major physiologic and biochemical function by regulating glutamic acid levels in the tissue. Moreover, the central role of glutamic acid in the metabolism of the cell (energy, protein synthesis, pH regulation, Ca^{++} retention) may explain why correcting its concentration with taurine has a beneficial effect on experimentally induced epilepsy.

Taurine is important in the maintenance of osmotic equilibrium across cell membranes (Thurston et al. 1981). In chronically hypernatremic animals, brain amino acids are significantly increased. The greatest increases in the brain are in GABA, glycine, glutamate, and taurine. Physiologically, GABA and glycine have well-known NT inhibitory roles in reduction of CNS excitability. Extensive research is needed to determine if other biochemical factors besides taurine are involved in modulation and/or reversal of the epileptiform seizure. The efficacy and safety of employing taurine in treatment and control of seizures remain to be established.

General Mechanisms of Anticonvulsant Action. Seizures can be initiated by four general mechanisms conducive to pharmacologic manipulation: (1) altered neuronal membrane function, which can lead to excessive depolarization; (2) decreased inhibitory NTs, such as GABA, the most potent inhibitory NT in the CNS; (3) increased excitatory NTs, such as glutamate; and (4) altered extracellular potassium and calcium concentration. An increase in extracellular potassium and a decrease in calcium, which occur during a seizure, increase neuronal excitability and facilitate the initiation and spread of the seizure. Once initiated, the seizure discharge may synchronize with other neurons and propagate to surrounding areas in the brain. Anticonvulsants block seizure initiation and propagation by blocking abnormal events in a single neuron or the synchronization of related neurons. Drugs acting at more than one point (e.g., phenobarbital) tend to be most effective. Drugs active at the GABA receptor also tend to be particularly efficacious. The GABA receptor interacts with several other drugs as well as with GABA. Response to anticonvulsant drugs may vary with the origin of the seizure. For example, using kindling-induced seizures in cats, Sumi (1993) demonstrated differences in response of temporal lobe epilepsy to phenobarbital, depending upon whether the seizure originated from the hippocampus or amygdaloid tissues.

General Pharmacokinetic Considerations of Anticonvulsant Drugs. Epilepsy is controlled, not cured; control of canine epilepsy is possible only in 60-70% of the cases (Parker 1982). Generally, treatment must be administered for the life of the animal (Frey 1986). The most common anticonvulsant drugs used in veterinary medicine are phenobarbital, primidone, diazepam, and potassium bromide. The disposition of each of the anticonvulsant drugs may impact the efficacy of the drug.

Absorption determines time to peak effect as well as magnitude of effect. Most anticonvulsants are given either orally or intravenously (IV). General statements regarding absorption are limited to the oral route. Most of the anticonvulsants are well absorbed following oral administration. An exception is phenytoin, which is so variable that bioavailability can be as little as 40%, varying dramatically among products. Phenobarbital is characterized by almost 100% bioavailability, although food will slow the rate of absorption of phenobarbital and probably other anticonvulsants. Peak plasma drug concentrations of anticonvulsants may occur as late as 4-6 hours after administration. Thus, when monitoring drug concentrations, peak samples should not be collected until 4-5 hours after administration. Fasting prior to sample collection is preferred.

Most anticonvulsant drugs are lipid soluble and are distributed to a volume that exceeds total body water (i.e., greater than 0.6 L/kg). Distribution into the CNS is important for all anticonvulsant drugs; at steady state, all anticonvulsant drugs sufficiently distribute into the CNS. The rate of CNS distribution following IV administration is of concern in a patient with status epilepticus. The drug must be sufficiently lipid soluble to be rapidly distributed into the CNS in therapeutic concentration. Diazepam is the most lipid soluble anticonvulsant and very rapidly distributes in the CNS. Phenobarbital is less lipid soluble, and therapeutic effects may take as long as 15 minutes to be achieved. Binding to serum proteins limits the amount of free drug and thus the rate and amount of drug distribution into the CNS. Diazepam is greater than 90% protein bound; however, its lipid solubility is so great that distribution into the CNS is sufficiently rapid in patients in status epilepticus. Phenytoin is also highly protein bound but is less lipid soluble; thus, it does not distribute rapidly into the CNS. Phenobarbital is less than 50% protein bound.

Because they are lipid soluble, most anticonvulsants must be eliminated by hepatic metabolism. Metabolism of anticonvulsant drugs can have a profound effect on therapeutic success. The effect in part depends upon the effects of phase I metabolism on the particular drug (i.e., inactivation, activation, or generation of toxic compounds). In general, most anticonvulsants are slowly metabolized. An exception is diazepam, which has a short half-life. In contrast to its action in humans, phenytoin is very rapidly metabolized in dogs (half-life less than 2 hr).

A consequence of phase I metabolism may be activation to a compound of equal, greater, or less anticonvulsant efficacy compared to the parent drug. Primidone must be metabolized in the liver to its active metabolite, phenobarbital, before it is effective in dogs. Clorazepate, a benzodiazepine, is also a prodrug, but it is converted in the stomach to its active metabolite. Although diazepam is rapidly metabolized, its duration of pharmacologic effect is prolonged since most of its metabolites have some degree of anticonvulsant effect. The half-lives of the metabolites may also be longer than that of the parent compound.

Safety of anticonvulsant drugs is profoundly affected by metabolism. Phase I metabolites, by their nature, are reactive. Although intended to progress to phase II metabolism, some reactive metabolites can interact with and damage surrounding tissues. Hepatotoxicity is a common side effect of long-term anticonvulsant use. The greater the amount of drug metabolized, the greater the potential toxicity.

The relationship between half-life and dosing interval is important to successful anticonvulsant therapy (see Table 16.1). Half-life will determine dosing interval and time to steady state. The relationship between dosing interval and half-life determines the rate of drug accumulation (or lack thereof). If the drug half-life is substantially smaller than dosing interval, plasma drug concentrations markedly fluctuate during the dosing interval, which may be undesirable. Toxic concentrations may occur postdosing, followed by subtherapeutic concentrations at the end of the dosing interval. If the patient misses a dose, seizures may occur. Because therapeutic concentrations are achieved with each dose, giving an extra dose to a seizuring patient may help control seizures during an episode. Shortening the interval may also help by decreasing fluctuations between peak and trough. When monitoring, both peak and trough samples should be collected in order to characterize the degree of fluctuation in plasma drug concentrations.

If the drug half-life of an anticonvulsant is substantially longer than the dosing interval, fluctuation in plasma drug concentrations is minimized. Since much of the previous dose(es) is still in the body at the administration of each new dose, plasma drug concen-

TABLE 16.1—Relationship between drug half-life and dosing interval in anticonvulsant therapy

Drug	Dose (mg/kg)[a]	Route	Dosing interval	$t_{1/2}$	Time to steady state[b]	Therapeutic range[b]
Clorazepate	0.5–1.0	PO	8 hr	<12 hr	<24 hr	150–400 ng/mL[c]
Diazepam	1–2	PO	8 hr	<3 hr	<24 hr	As above
	0.5–2.0[d]	IV	5–10 min			
	5–20[e]	IV inf	60 min			
Felbamate	15	PO	Divided 8–12 hr	<8 hr	<24 hr	—
Phenobarbital	2	PO	12 hr	56–102 hr	2–3 wk[g]	20–45 μg/mL
	3–6[f]	IM				
	3–16[f] total	IV inf	60 min			
	6–12[h]	IV slow				
Primidone	10[i]	PO	12 hr	56–102	hr 2–3 wk[g]	As above
Bromide	30	PO	12–24 hr	24 d	2–3 mo	1–3 mg/mL[j]

[a]Maintenance dose unless otherwise noted is starting dose; doses are dependent on patient response and serum drug concentrations.
[b]Extrapolated from human literature unless noted otherwise.
[c]Based on an ongoing clinical trial.
[d]Can be repeated up to 3 times for control of life-threatening seizures.
[e]Diluted in either 5% dextrose or 0.9% NaCl; first flush 50 mL through polyvinyl catheter to allow for binding of diazepam.
[f]Following diazepam for management of life-threatening seizures.
[g]Half-life is likely to shorten with chronic therapy.
[h]Loading dose as sole drug for management of life-threatening seizures.
[i]Based on phenobarbital as the active anticonvulsant.
[j]Lower concentrations may be effective when combined with phenobarbital.

trations accumulate until a steady state is reached. At this point, the amount eliminated during each dosing interval is equal to the amount dosed with each interval. Each daily dose represents only a small amount of drug in the animal. In this situation, giving an extra dose to the seizuring patient will do little to increase plasma drug concentrations and thus to stop seizures. Missing a dose will probably not result in seizures since little drug will be eliminated during that time period. Shortening the dosing interval in this scenario is also not likely to help. In contrast to drugs with a short half-life, only a single sample needs to be collected for monitoring of drugs with a long drug half-life since peak and trough samples are not likely to be substantially different during a single dosing interval.

Any drug metabolized by the liver can potentially induce drug-metabolizing enzymes, and drug interactions are a common sequela. The type of interaction is difficult to predict and varies with each drug combination. Phenobarbital is the most potent inducer of drug-metabolizing enzymes known. The rate of drug metabolism will increase clearance, and (assuming patient volume of distribution does not change) elimination half-life of many drugs will decrease. Phenobarbital increases its own rate of metabolism. Phenytoin is also a potent enzyme inducer. It can decrease the drug concentration of phenobarbital. However, it can also compete with phenobarbital for metabolism, resulting in an increase in the concentration of one or the other drug. These effects are not predictable. Clorazepate increases concentrations of phenobarbital (reason unknown).

Phenobarbital Sodium. *Phenobarbital Sodium,* USP (soluble phenobarbitone, Luminal sodium), was the second barbituric acid derivative of clinical importance to be developed. It was synthesized in 1912 in Germany and patented under the trade name of Luminal. Phenobarbital is only slightly soluble in water, so a readily soluble sodium salt was prepared.

MECHANISM OF ACTION. Phenobarbital sodium specifically depresses the motor centers of the cerebral cortex, giving it excellent anticonvulsant properties. Electroshock experiments in cats and other species have established phenobarbital as one of the most potent anticonvulsants available. It has the widest spectrum of activity in different convulsive seizure patterns. Most other antiepileptic agents have been synthesized as structural variants of phenobarbital (de Angelis 1979). For example, primidone is a close congener of phenobarbital.

Phenobarbital is the most effective anticonvulsant to inhibit the progressive intensification of seizure activity that may accompany epilepsy. Phenobarbital both increases the seizure threshold required for seizure discharge and decreases the spread of discharge to surrounding neurons. The primary means by which phenobarbital decreases seizure activity is by enhancing responsiveness to the inhibitory postsynaptic effects of GABA. Interaction of GABA with phenobarbital opens a chloride channel, resulting in higher intracellular concentrations of chloride and hyperpolarization of the RMP. However, phenobarbital also inhibits glutamate activity and probably calcium fluxes across the neuronal membrane. Phenobarbital can be considered a "broad-spectrum" anticonvulsant. Despite introduction of new antiepileptics, phenobarbital remains the anticonvulsant of choice in the cat and dog (Schwartz-Porsche et al. 1985). It is effective in all types of epileptic seizures observed in cats and dogs (Kay and Fenner 1977).

DISPOSITION. As a weak acid (pK_a 7.3), phenobarbital is absorbed well following oral administration, although peak plasma concentrations may not be reached for 4-6 hours after administration. The absorption half-life in dogs is 1.27 ± 0.21 hours (Pedersoli et al. 1987). About 6.4 hours is required for near complete absorption of phenobarbital from the gastrointestinal (GI) tract. Absorption is 88-95% complete. Phenobarbital is 45% bound to serum proteins in dogs (Frey and Löscher 1985). Its volume of distribution in dogs is 0.7 ± 0.15 L/kg. To attain steady-state serum concentrations, 8-15.5 days of multiple dosing is necessary. Maintenance doses of 1.8 mg/kg 3 times a day or 5.5 mg/kg once daily administered orally are required to reach an average serum concentration of 20 μg/mL (Ravis et al. 1984).

Through microsomal enzyme action, phenobarbital is metabolized by oxidative hydroxylation to form hydroxyphenobarbital. This metabolite has weak anticonvulsant activity and does not contribute significantly to the action of phenobarbital. In the dog, hydroxyphenobarbital is rapidly eliminated from blood by conjugation with glucuronide and excretion in urine. Up to 25% of the parent drug is eliminated renally in dogs. Alkalinization of urine accelerates excretion of unaltered phenobarbital because the process of back-diffusion (tubular reabsorption) is reduced appreciably by ionization of the drug (de Angelis 1979). Individual variability in the rate of phenobarbital elimination is marked due to differences in hepatic metabolism. Half-life varies not only between and within species but also in the same animal. Phenobarbital is a potent inducer of hepatic drug-metabolizing enzymes and is capable of increasing the rate of clearance of other drugs metabolized by the liver as well as increasing its own rate of metabolism (see Drug Interactions).

In the dog, phenobarbital (2 mg/kg) administered orally 3 times a day for 5 days results in an elimination half-life between 37 and 75 hours, with a mean elimination half-life of 53 ± 15 hours (Ravis et al. 1984). In dogs following a single 5 mg/kg IV dose, clearance is 5.6-6.6 mL/kg/hr, and elimination half-life is 92.6 ± 23.7 hours (Pedersoli et al. 1987). The effects of multiple doses of phenobarbital were documented by Ravis and coworkers. Following 90 days of treatment (5.5 mg/kg), mean elimination half-life decreased from 88.7 ± 19.6 to 47.5 ± 10.7 hours (Ravis et al. 1989).

Phenobarbital volume of distribution is 0.96 ± 0.060 L/kg in horses (Knox et al. 1992; Ravis et al. 1987; Duran et al. 1987). Following a single IV dose of 12 mg/kg (infused over 20 min), phenobarbital reached an extrapolated peak serum concentration of μg/mL and was characterized by a distribution half-life of 6 minutes. The elimination half-life of phenobarbital is short: 18 hours. The apparent volume of distribution at steady state was 0.8 L/kg, similar to that of other species, but total body clearance was rapid, at 0.03 L/hr/kg (Duran et al. 1987). Following single oral administration of 5.5 mg/kg, peak concentrations of μg/mL were achieved at 11 hours and the elimination half-life was 19 ± 4 hours and mean residence time was 37 hours (Ravis et al. 1987). Oral bioavailability was 101%, with a mean absorption time of 11 hours. A daily dose of 11 mg/kg administered once daily was recommended by the authors based on this dose. As in other species, multiple administration of phenobarbital results in changes in drug disposition. Mean elimination half-life of phenobarbital decreases from 24.2 ± 4.7 to 11.2 ± 2.3 hours, and clearance increases from 28.2 ± 5.1 to 57.3 ± 9.6 mL/hr/kg (Knox et al. 1992). In foals, IV phenobarbital (20 mg/kg) undergoes first-order elimination (Spehar et al. 1984); its elimination half-life is 12.8 ± 2.1 hours. Although foals are sedated by phenobarbital for the first 1-2 hours, they can walk but are ataxic. Additionally, some hyperexcitability occurs 3-8 hours after the phenobarbital infusion (Spehar et al. 1984).

Side Effects

BEHAVIOR. Polyphagia, polydipsia, and polyuria are side effects that occur in animals receiving clinical dosages of phenobarbital (Kay and Fenner 1977). The polyuric effect is apparently due to an inhibitory action in release of antidiuretic hormone. Identical sedative side effects are observed in the dog after treatment with phenobarbital or primidone (Schwartz-Porsche et al. 1985). Dogs appear fatigued and listless after receiving either drug; some are weak in the rear legs, and ataxia occurs. All of these effects may be long lasting and may persist in some cases for the duration of treatment.

HEPATOTOXICITY. At high plasma drug concentration doses (i.e., greater than 30-40 μg/mL), phenobarbital appears to be hepatotoxic. Animals whose livers are induced and thus require high doses of phenobarbital to maintain drug concentrations in the lower therapeutic range may also be more susceptible to toxicity because of increased formation of metabolites. Phenobarbital will also cause nonpathologic changes in hepatic clinical laboratory tests due to induction of enzymes. Serum alkaline phosphatase (SAP) and the transaminases are likely to increase with prolonged therapy (Chauvet et al. 1995). These are not necessarily indicative of liver disease. Changes associated with true hepatic pathology are more likely with primidone (see below). Moderate elevations in serum alanine transferase and SAP, coupled with changes in bile acids and bilirubin, are more indicative of hepatic pathology (i.e., liver disease). Serum albumin and cholesterol also may decrease (Chauvet et al. 1995). Hepatic function tests (e.g., serum bile acids) should be used to monitor the development and/or progression of liver disease. The incidence of serious liver toxicity can be reduced by avoiding combination therapy, using therapeutic monitoring to achieve adequate serum concentrations at the smallest dose possible, and evaluating clinical pathology changes every 4-6 months while the patient is on therapy. Note that, due to the effects of hypoxia, etc., liver enzymes are generally increased following a seizure.

NEUROENDOCRINE EFFECTS. Phenobarbital given orally and daily for 2 weeks to infant rats at 60 mg/kg and 15 mg/kg produces a 12 and 3%, respectively, reduction in brain growth (Diaz and Schain 1978). Although it is known that brief exposure of newborn animals to various drugs may result in behavior and brain alterations later in life, information is lacking on the short- or long-term effects of phenobarbital. In addition to alteration in the brain weight, phenobarbital fed to rats as 0.25% of their diet results in a reduced gain in body weight (Peraino et al. 1980). It is suggested that the lower weight gain in animals chronically exposed to phenobarbital occurs from alterations in hepatic metabolism; however, the effect of phenobarbital upon food intake may also be a factor in growth reduction.

In one study of 5 dogs receiving phenobarbital for 12 months, endogenous ACTH concentrations increased, although they remained within reference limits. Plasma ACTH-stimulated aldosterone concentration also increased over the course of the study (Chauvet et al. 1995).

REPRODUCTION. Administration of phenobarbital to pregnant rats from day 12 to day 19 of gestation suppresses weight gain and induces significant effects on reproductive function of their offspring (Gupta et al. 1980). Some of these effects are delay in onset of puberty, disorders in the estrous cycle, and infertility (Gupta and Yaffee 1982). Additionally, animals exposed to phenobarbital in utero have altered concentrations of sex steroids, gonadotropic hormones, and estrogen receptors. These studies suggest that phenobarbital exposure during prenatal growth can induce permanent changes in sexual development (Gupta et al. 1980). Pregnant animals treated with phenobarbital are more sensitive or responsive to its depressant effects than nonpregnant animals (Middaugh et al. 1983). Consequently, phenobarbital should be used cautiously during pregnancy and at a minimum therapeutic dose.

DRUG INTERACTIONS. Hepatic microsomal enzyme activity, especially mixed-function oxidase induction, is accelerated by phenobarbital. Enzyme induction by phenobarbital appears to be dose related (Tavernor et al. 1983). Long-acting barbiturates are better inducers of microsomal enzyme activity than are short-acting compounds. Compared on a molar basis, phenobarbital is the most potent enzyme stimulatory agent known (Valerino et al. 1974). Pentobarbital and thiopental sodium are less potent inducers of microsomal enzyme activity. Enzyme induction may take weeks to months and may occur with each dose increase. Induction has been documented in dogs (Aldridge and Neims 1979; Bekersky et al. 1977; Ciaccio and Halpert 1989; McKillop 1985). Once enzyme induction is initiated by exposure to phenobarbital, it may take up to 7 months for its complete disappearance in the dog after treatment has stopped. Phenobarbital does appear to induce its own elimination, although drug-metabolizing enzymes responsible for phenobarbital metabolism may not be as impacted as enzymes responsible for metabolism of other drugs (e.g., antipyrine) (Abramson 1988a). Antipyrine metabolism in dogs treated with phenobarbital increased up to 13-fold, potentially converting a "capacity-limited" drug to a "flow-limited" drug (Abramson 1988b).

In newborn rats, phenobarbital induces a long-term, perhaps permanent, alteration in hepatic mixed-function oxidase activity (Faris and Campbell 1981).

If rats are treated with phenobarbital, the weight of their livers is increased. An increase occurs in the amount of microsomal protein per gram of liver as well as in the content of cytochrome P-450. The result of the increased level of enzyme is a more rapid rate of drug metabolism in treated animals. In fetal rat livers, phenobarbital significantly increases the metabolic destruction of hexobarbital by 263% over controlled conditions (Sunouchi et al. 1984). Induction of drug-metabolizing enzymes is likely to necessitate a larger dose in order to maintain the same drug concentration.

Treatment with phenobarbital stimulates hepatic drug-metabolizing enzymes in several other animals, including swine, sheep, and cattle (Conney and Burns 1972). Administration of low doses of phenobarbital to lactating cows given DDT for several days results in a significant decline in the content of DDT metabolites in milk (Alary et al. 1971).

Phenobarbital is likely to increase the metabolism and clearance of other drugs cleared by the liver. The clinical sequelae depend on the role of hepatic metabolism in the disposition of the drug. The most clinically important sequelae are the generation of toxic metabolites and therapeutic failure due to decreased drug efficacy. Increased metabolism may also increase formation of an active drug from a prodrug; and it may promote tumors (Kitagawa et al. 1979).

In the dog, prolonged administration of phenobarbital (180 mg/day orally) decreases the bioavailability of propranolol, a β-adrenergic blocking agent, from 8 to 35% (Vu et al. 1983). Additionally, it alters the binding, metabolism, and pharmacokinetics of propranolol (Bai and Abramson 1983). Phenobarbital shortens the duration of β blockade by propranolol. The clearance of thiopental is increased in Greyhounds treated with phenobarbital for 14 days (Sams and Muir 1988). Duration of anesthetic effects of xylazine is decreased in dogs pretreated with phenobarbital for 4 days (Nossaman et al. 1990). Although phenobarbital had no effect on clorazepate concentrations in one study (Forrester et al. 1993), in our laboratory clorazepate concentrations decreased in patients receiving phenobarbital. Phenobarbital is likely to increase adverse response to toxins whose toxicity reflects reactive metabolites. A seven-to ninefold increase occurs in the toxicity of carbon tetrachloride after treatment of sheep with phenobarbital and DDT (Seawright et al. 1972). Phenobarbital pretreatment potentiates the toxic response of renal cortical slices of the rabbit to chloroform in vitro (Bailie et al. 1984). Cephaloridine nephrotoxicity in rabbits is potentiated by phenobarbital (Kuo et al. 1982).

Treatment of animals with phenobarbital increases activity of microsomal enzymes that metabolize endogenous hormones. Estrogens, androgens, progestational steroid, and adrenocortical steroid hydroxylation are increased. Thyroid hormones (e.g., thyroxine) are decreased due to increased hepatic metabolism and possibly increased deiodination. Animals may test as hypothyroid despite lack of clinical signs. Accelerated hydroxylation of steroidal hormones by microsomal enzymes is influenced in vivo by an increased metabolism and altered physiologic action of the steroids. Because it stimulates increased hepatic microsomal enzyme activity, phenobarbital may be a tumor-promoting agent (Kitagawa et al. 1979). In the presence of 2-methyl-*N, N*-dimethyl-4-amino-azobenzene, a noncarcinogen in rats, hepatocellular carcinomas develop by 72 weeks when animals have been treated simultaneously with phenobarbital.

An interaction involving phenobarbital, phenytoin, and vitamin D may lead to development of rickets or osteomalacia. An interaction between phenobarbital and griseofulvin may decrease griseofulvin blood levels by impairing absorption of the antifungal agent (de Angelis 1979).

Enzymes responsible for phenobarbital metabolism are subject to effects of drugs that inhibit drug-metabolizing enzymes. Ciaccio et al. (1987) demonstrated the inhibitory effects of chloramphenicol on phenobarbital metabolism.

TREATMENT OF PHENOBARBITAL TOXICOSIS. Artificial respiration with oxygen should be administered to prevent hypoxia from respiratory arrest induced by overdoses of phenobarbital. Although less effective than oxygen, doxapram or other analeptic drugs may be used to stimulate the respiratory center. Also, alkalinization of the urine accelerates renal excretion of phenobarbital via increased ionization of phenobarbital by this alkalinization (de Angelis 1979). Activated charcoal effectively accelerates the body clearance of phenobarbital (Berg et al. 1982). When charcoal is administered in the human, the biologic half-life of phenobarbital is decreased from 110 ± 8 to 45 ± 6 hours; it increases the total body clearance of phenobarbital from 4.4 ± 0.2 to 12.0 ± 1.6 mL/kg/hr (Berg et al. 1982).

PREPARATIONS. Phenobarbital is available as oral or injectable preparations. Oral tablets contain 1/4-, 1/2-, or 1-grain (15, 30, and 65 mg, respectively) phenobarbital. An elixir is also available (4 mg/mL) for treatment in very small animals. The injectable form is intended for IV use but can be given intramuscularly (IM). Under the 1970 Controlled Substances Act, phenobarbital is classified as a Schedule IV drug.

CLINICAL USE. Phenobarbital has a more specific depressant effect upon convulsive seizures than any other barbiturate. It can be an effective anticonvulsant at clinical dosages that produce minimal sedation (Macdonald and Barker 1978). Phenobarbital has long been used in the symptomatic or prophylactic control of convulsive seizures of epilepsy. It is effective in 60-80% of canine patients suffering from epilepsy if serum concentrations of the drug are maintained within recommended therapeutic ranges of 15-40 μg/mL. Patients are not considered refractory to phenobarbital therapy until concentrations reach 35 μg/mL. Due to a large individual variability in phenobarbital clearance, required dosages for dogs can be as little as 1 mg/kg to greater than 15 mg/kg every 12 hours to control seizures, although hepatotoxicity may be more likely at high doses and concentrations (Schwartz-Porsche et al. 1985). Therapeutic monitoring can be used to ascertain the dosage regimen necessary to achieve and maintain therapeutic serum concentrations in the individual patient. Marked variability in the elimination of this drug occurs between dogs and in the same animal depending on duration of therapy. In patients with a drug half-life of 36 hours or less, the same total dose at 8-hour intervals may be useful since plasma drug concentrations may drop below therapeutic ranges during a 12-hour dosing interval in some animals.

A loading dose of 12 mg/kg can be administered to avoid delay in therapeutic effects in the dog. With this dose range, the plasma concentrations of phenobarbital fall within the range of 20-40 μg/mL that has been proposed in treatment of human epilepsy. In animals where complete control of the seizure is not possible, Schwartz-Porsche and associates (1985) administered daily oral doses of phenobarbital up to 17 mg/kg.

In the cat, an oral dose (4 mg/kg) every 12 hours is suggested; the total daily IV dose in the cat was 15-60 mg in one study (Kay and Fenner 1977). More recently, following a single IV administration of 10 mg/kg, phenobarbital reached an extrapolated peak serum concentration of μg/mL that ranged from 8.8 to 12.7 in cats and was characterized by an apparent volume of distribution of 0.93 L/kg and an elimination half-life of 58 ± 4 hours. A single oral 10 mg/kg dose yielded a similar half-life, a peak serum concentration that ranged from 11.0 to 16.6 μg/mL, and a bioavailability of 120% (Cochrane 1990a). Following multiple oral administration of 5 mg/kg, peak concentrations were 5.7 to 7.2 μg/mL at the first dose and 18 to 22 μg/mL at 21 days, and elimination half-life was 43 ± 3 hours. Induction apparently occurs with chronic administration in cats, following administration of the same dose for 21 days (Cochran 1990b). For terminating status epilepticus in the cat, 60-120 mg phenobarbital has been recommended IM or to effect by the IV route. Phenobarbital at 10 mg/kg IV was effective in controlling experimentally induced (pentylenetrazol) interical spikes in 7 of 10 cats. At this dose, phenobarbital also slightly depressed the heart rate and blood pressure (by 10 mm Hg) of treated cats. Phenobarbitial was also useful for controlling seizures induced experimentally following injection of tetanus toxin in the hippocampus of cats (Darcey and Williamson 1992) and in kindling seizures induced in the hippocampus or amygdalus (Sumi 1993). Concentrations of 15-25 μg/mL were effective for generalized seizures of hippocampal origin, although concentrations up to 50 μg/mL were necessary to control afterseizures (Sumi 1993). Amygdaloid-induced seizures, in contrast, were much more resistant to phenobarbital. In equine neonatal seizure disorders, an IV loading dose of phenobarbital (20 mg/kg) diluted in 30-35 mL sterile saline and infused over 25-30 minutes is recommended; maintenance doses of 9 mg/kg at 8-hour intervals should also be infused slowly (Spehar et al. 1984). A phenobarbital serum concentration of 15-40 μg/mL should be achieved. In epileptic chickens, phenobarbital plasma concentrations between 12.6 and 17.1 μg/mL provide complete protection against intermittent photic stimulation-induced seizures for 6 hours (Johnson et al. 1977). Based upon required plasma concentrations, seizure processes in humans and epileptic fowl show comparable sensitivity to antiepileptic action of phenobarbital. Compared to use of phenytoin (Davis et al. 1978), phenobarbital provides complete protection from seizures in the chicken without signs of toxicity. When based on dosage requirements, the benzodiazepines (clonazepam, diazepam) are the most potent anticonvulsants in epileptic fowl (Johnson et al. 1979).

Primidone. *Primidone,* USP (Mylepsin, Mysoline) (*S*-phenyl-*S*-ethylhexahydropyrimidine-4,6-dione) (Fig. 16.1), is a close congener of phenobarbital. The drug is a white, crystalline, tasteless substance. Primidone is approved by the FDA for use in the dog for control of convulsions associated with "true" (primary) epilepsy, epileptiform seizures, virus encephalitis, distemper, and "hardpad" disease. It may be the most commonly used antiepileptic agent in veterinary medicine (Cunningham 1984). According to Schwartz-Porsche et al. (1982), only primidone and phenobarbital are effective in treatment of epilepsy in the dog. Although primidone therapy does not appear to have an advantage over phenobarbital therapy in control of seizure disorders, this does not exclude the possibility that a single animal may respond more favorably to one or the other (Farnbach 1984; Schwartz-Porsche et al. 1985). Primidone is less well tolerated than phenobarbital because of its potential for inducing hepatotoxicity (Schwartz-Porsche et al. 1985).

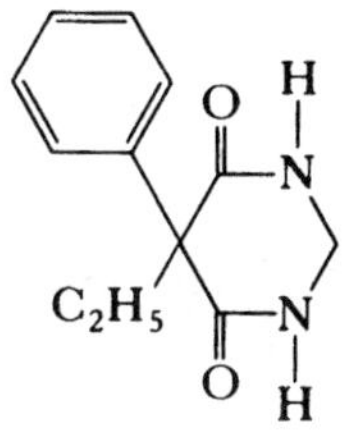

Primidone

FIG. 16.1

PHARMACOLOGIC ACTIVITY. In humans, approximately 60-90% of an oral dose of primidone is rapidly absorbed from the GI tract, with a peak serum level being attained in about 3 hours (de Angelis 1979). In animals, primidone is oxidized at carbon-2 (C-2) to phenobarbital and ring cleavage at C-2 to phenylethylmalondiamide (PEMA). Although all three compounds have anticonvulsant activity, most of primidone's anticonvulsant activity in dogs results from phenobarbital: as the compound with the longest half-life, it accumulates to the highest concentrations (Cunningham et al. 1983). The potency of primidone and PEMA is 1/30 of that of phenobarbital. The efficacy of primidone generally is equal to or less than that of phenobarbital, and anticonvulsant activity can be correlated to serum phenobarbital levels. Because of this relationship, serum phenobarbital concentrations can and should be used to guide design of primidone dosing regimens (Cunningham et al. 1983). Target therapeutic ranges are the same as for phenobarbital. Primidone continues to be used in patients which have proven refractory to phenobarbital at the maximum therapeutic drug concentration (i.e., 40 μg/mL). Note that its efficacy in this scenario has not been proven. Efficacy may simply reflect improved conversion to phenobarbital (i.e., animals that are induced may metabolize the drug to greater concentrations of phenobarbital than those generated from administration of phenobarbital alone). According to Farnbach (1984), there is no advantage in using primidone rather than phenobarbital for control of epilepsy in most dogs.

Although primidone is less potent than phenobarbital as a general CNS depressant, it is considered to be more potent in protection of animals against maximal seizures induced by electroshock and pentylenetetrazol. Primidone is more toxic in cats and rabbits than in rats or mice; it is not recommended for therapeutic use in cats. Cats metabolize primidone to phenobarbital to a lesser extent than dogs. This may be why it is far less effective in cats than in dogs (Frey 1986).

DISPOSITION. Primidone is well absorbed following oral administration. IV administration can be associated with undesirable side effects; in addition, as a prodrug, it is not preferred for emergency therapy. In dogs, 3.8 mg primidone is converted to 1 mg phenobarbital. In cats, the conversion of primidone to phenobarbital is less effective (Sawchuk et al. 1985). Peak plasma concentrations of primidone are much higher in cats than in dogs and peak plasma concentrations of phenobarbital are much lower (<50%) when the same dosing regimens are used in both species. Thus, while the drug may appear to be safe in cats, the recommended dose may not be sufficient to be effective.

SIDE EFFECTS. Identical sedative side effects are seen in the dog after treatment with phenobarbital and after treatment with primidone (Schwartz-Porsche et al. 1985); see the discussion on antiepileptic action of phenobarbital. Primidone will cause all of the side effects noted for phenobarbital. Primidone may induce nystagmus, nausea, drowsiness, and ataxia. According to Schwartz-Porsche et al. (1985), polydipsia is more common in dogs treated with primidone. In humans, it is recommended that therapeutic plasma concentrations of primidone and its metabolite phenobarbital not exceed 15 μg/mL and 30 μg/mL, respectively. Megaloblastic anemia is one of the more serious adverse effects of primidone in humans.

In the dog, primidone induces progressive hepatic injury as manifested by increases in liver enzyme values (Meyer and Noonan 1981). In a clinical study, signs of liver toxicity were reported in 14 of 20 dogs (Schwartz-Porsche et al. 1985). Hepatic cirrhosis associated with primidone and phenobarbital after 7 years of use has been reported in a dog (Poffenbarger and Hardy 1985). Dermatitis is a rarely reported side effect (Henricks 1987).

In humans, long-term (more than 2 years) treatment of epileptic patients with primidone has been associated with development of osteomalacia; subnormal serum calcium is seen in such patients. Primidone may induce or stimulate increased production of hepatic microsomal enzymes that increase the metabolism or degradation of vitamin D.

Primidone should not be used concurrently with chloramphenicol, which is a potent inhibitor of the microsomal enzyme system. Severe CNS depression and inappetence occur in the dog after concurrent use of these drugs (Campbell 1983).

CLINICAL USE. In the early 1950s, primidone was used in veterinary medicine for control of convulsive seizures in the dog soon after it was introduced into human medicine for clinical use (Chastain and Graham 1978). Primidone should be reserved for treatment of seizures in the dog that have not responded to phenobarbital administered at doses sufficient to achieve 30-40 μg/mL. Only 1/15 of dogs refractory to phenobarbital can be expected to respond to primidone. The recommended dose for primidone is 30-55 mg/kg/day (or 5-15 mg/kg every 8 hours). Because of gradual or progressive microsomal enzyme induction, complete control of seizures in the dog can sometimes be attained only with daily oral doses of 50 mg/kg;

however, daily oral doses as high as 107 mg/kg may fail to control seizure disorders in the dog (Schwartz-Porsche et al. 1982, 1985). When primidone is substituted for another antiepileptic agent, the dosage should be gradually increased while gradually withdrawing the dosage of the drug being replaced over a period of at least 15 days so that adequate seizure control is maintained (de Angelis 1979). If converting from phenobarbital to primidone, a conversion ratio of 250 mg primidone per 65 mg phenobarbital can be used. Therapeutic monitoring should be used to guide therapy. Toxicosis to primidone, manifested as temporary ataxia and signs of depression, has been reported in cats after administration of single doses ranging from 10 to 25 mg/kg. The safety of doses necessary to achieve therapeutic concentrations of phenobarbital has not been documented in the cat.

Primidone has been used in the Thoroughbred foal to control recurrent convulsive seizures (May and Greenwood 1977). Daily doses consisted of 1-1.5 g administered by stomach tube.

Phenytoin Sodium. *Phenytoin Sodium,* USP (Dilantin sodium, Epanutin), previously named diphenylhydantoin, depresses motor areas of the cortex (antiepileptic action) without depressing sensory areas. It is approved by the US Food and Drug Administration (FDA) for use in the dog for control of epileptiform convulsions.

Phenytoin is a hydantoin derivative (de Angelis 1979); others, of lesser importance, are mephenytoin and ethotoin. Hydantoins are five-membered ring structures, whereas barbiturates are six-membered structures. A major point of difference between the hydantoins and barbiturates is the absence of a C=O group. Phenytoin is not a general anticonvulsant, as is phenobarbital, and is not used for emergency treatment of poisoning by convulsant drugs or tetanic seizures.

Oral preparations are available in suspension, capsule, and tablet forms. Phenytoin (50 mg/mL) is also available for human use in a special solvent for IV administration. IV injection of the drug causes a marked drop in arterial pressure and is not advised in the dog (Pasten 1977). Absorption of phenytoin is erratic following IM administration. This may be related to crystallization of the drug at the injection site because of alteration in pH by tissues (de Angelis 1979). Administration of phenytoin by the IM route is not advised, because considerable necrosis and sloughing at the injection site occur (Pasten 1977). Absorption of the drug from the GI tract of the dog is poor (Sanders and Yeary 1978). Bioavailability of phenytoin from the tablet formulation averages 36% in the dog (Frey and Löscher 1980). In the horse, a bioavailability of 34.5 ± 8.6% has been reported (Kowalczyk and Beech 1983).

Phenytoin has declined in use for control of seizures in the dog because of lack of efficacy (Sanders and Yeary 1978), which may be related to decreased bioavailability and rapid clearance. Phenytoin is much less effective in the dog than either phenobarbital or primidone in control of epileptic seizures (Farnbach 1984). The half-life of phenytoin is too short in the dog to permit maintenance of adequate drug concentrations in plasma and the CNS (Schwartz-Porsche et al. 1985). When administered alone, phenytoin cannot be considered a satisfactory drug for treatment of epilepsy in the dog (Frey and Löscher 1980; Frey 1986). Due to drug interactions and enhanced hepatotoxicity, a combination of phenytoin with phenobarbital is not a viable alternative.

In the cat, phenytoin is relatively toxic and generally undesirable as an anticonvulsant (Kay and Fenner 1977). Studies are needed to determine the efficacy and safety of phenytoin in cats (Frey 1986).

Pharmacologic Activity. Phenytoin produces a stabilizing effect upon synaptic junctions that ordinarily allow nerve impulses to be readily transmitted at lower thresholds. Consequently, the level of synaptic excitability that permits impulses to be transmitted easily is reduced and/or stabilized. This effect appears to be associated with active extrusion of Na^+ from neurons and decrease of posttetanic potentiation or spread of nerve impulses to adjacent neurons. There is also a possibility that phenytoin reduces movement of calcium across cell membranes. Phenytoin may inhibit activation of protein phosphorylation by the calcium-calmodulin complex (Marx 1980). Phosphorylation and norepinephrine release in neurons require calmodulin.

Reduction in spread of the "burst" activity associated with epilepsy prevents genesis of the cortical seizure. The activity of phenytoin in stabilizing hyperexcitable neurons so that epileptic seizure does not develop occurs without causing general depression of the CNS (de Angelis 1979).

Disposition. Poor oral absorption and differences in product bioavailability (as little as 40% bioavailable) contribute to the difficulty in achieving effective serum levels of phenytoin. The generic preparations of phenytoin should not be used.

At therapeutic concentrations (10-20 μg/mL), phenytoin is highly bound (75-85%) to plasma proteins of animals and humans (Baggot and Davis 1973). The high degree of phenytoin binding predisposes this acidic drug to interaction with other drugs by a displacing effect at protein (albumin) binding sites. In uremic patients, there is a decrease in plasma protein binding of phenytoin. This accelerates renal clearance or elimination of the drug. Phenytoin readily crosses the placenta (Mirkin 1975). High concentrations are attained in the maternal liver and maternal and fetal hearts. The brain (ostensibly the primary target organ) contains nearly the lowest concentration of the drug.

Phenytoin is metabolized into meta- or parahydroxyphenytoin. These metabolites are then conjugated with glucuronic acid. In humans, about 60-75% of the daily dose of phenytoin is excreted in the glucuronide form (de Angelis 1979); the dog also converts a high percentage of phenytoin into this form. In addition, diphenylhydantoic acid, a minor metabolite in some laboratory animals, and dihydrodiol are formed. Interestingly, after treatment with phenytoin high concentrations of diphenylhydantoic acid are found in cat urine. The dihydrodiol metabolite is probably involved in formation of catechol metabolites; these are also formed in most animals (Glazko 1973). Epoxide metabolites are also speculated to be formed in humans. The combined used of phenytoin and phenobarbital or primidone may lead to increased formation of epoxide metabolites in animals. This could possibly result in cholestatic hepatic injury similar to that reported in 3 dogs (Bunch et al. 1987). If epoxide intermediates are formed, mercapturic acid should also be present; however, no such metabolites have yet been identified. Since phenytoin is not very soluble in water, little of the unmetabolized drug is excreted in urine.

Phenytoin has a long duration of action in the cat. The long plasma half-life (ca. 24-108 hours) (Tobin et al. 1973) and the prolonged effect of phenytoin observed in the cat over some of the other species may also be related to the cat's decreased ability to conjugate compounds with glucuronic acid. Phenytoin is excreted after formation of a hydroxylated derivative and conjugation with glucuronic acid or sulfate. A plasma half-life of 108 hours, following oral administration of phenytoin (10 mg/kg) in the cat, has been reported (Roye et al. 1973).

In the dog, despite relatively large single daily doses (50 mg/kg) administered orally, the plasma concentration of the drug is low. Paralleling this observation, the plasma half-life of a single 50 mg/kg dose in the dog is only 6-7.8 hours (Dayton et al. 1967). Roye et al. (1973) found the plasma half-life was 4-6 hours after an IM injection of phenytoin (50 mg/kg). The apparent discrepancy between results of these two studies may be due to pretreatment of the dogs for 9 days with phenytoin by Roye et al. (1973). Studies have shown that the half-life of phenytoin in the dog dramatically decreases after 7-9 days of treatment (Frey and Löscher 1980). Apparently, phenytoin is a potent inducer of the hepatic microsomal enzyme system in the dog (see "Drug Interactions"). Other biologic half-life data reported in the dog are the following: after a single IV dose (15 mg/kg), a value of 4.5 hours was obtained by Sanders et al. (1979b), and a half-life of 3.65 hours was determined by Pedersoli et al. (1981) after an IV bolus of 11 mg/kg.

CLINICAL USE. Recommended therapeutic doses of phenytoin administered orally every 8 hours for control of seizure disorders in the dog show considerable variation: 6.6-11 mg/kg (Pasten 1977), 11 mg/kg (Cunningham 1984), and 35 mg/kg (Sanders and Yeary 1978). In humans, clinical therapeutic effects and intoxication are related to the blood concentration of phenytoin. A reduction in the number of seizures occurs when phenytoin blood concentrations exceed 10 μg/mL.

Since the half-life of phenytoin in the dog is reduced considerably after use for 7-9 days (Frey and Löscher 1980), high oral doses up to 30 mg/kg every 8 hours may be required for satisfactory control of seizures (Cunningham 1984). Oral administration of 4.4 and 11 mg/kg phenytoin every 8 hours fails to achieve the assumed therapeutic level of the drug in serum at 10 μg/mL. The serum content of phenytoin in the dog after single or repeated oral doses of 10 mg/kg does not exceed a concentration of 2 μg/mL (Sanders and Yeary 1978). To achieve a serum concentration of approximately 10 μg/mL phenytoin, it appears that an oral dose of at least 35 mg/kg given 3 times daily is necessary for the adult dog (Sanders and Yeary 1978). Use of phenytoin for control of seizures has declined due to its lack of efficacy, which may be the result of inadequate dosage (Sanders and Yeary 1978). According to Pedersoli et al. (1981), an oral dosage schedule of 20 mg/kg every 8 hours of the phenytoin microcrystalline suspension should be sufficient to reach a serum concentration of 10 μg/mL or higher. However, this dose will only maintain a plasma therapeutic level for the first 2 or 3 days of treatment (Frey and Löscher 1980). The marked variation in the dosage of phenytoin needed to maintain a therapeutic level in the dog is attributable in large measure to its rapid biotransformation by the hepatic microsomal enzyme system.

In the horse, phenytoin administered orally at 8-hour intervals provides average serum steady-state concentrations of 5 and 10 μg/mL with doses of 2.83-8.22 and 5.67-16.43 mg/kg, respectively (Kowalcyzk and Beech 1983). After IV administration of 8.8 mg/kg phenytoin in the horse, the mean biologic half-life is 8 hours.

DRUG INTERACTIONS. Phenytoin must be considered a potent inducer of the hepatic microsomal enzyme system in the dog (Frey and Löscher 1980). Seven to 9 days after administration of phenytoin, its half-life may be reduced from 5.5 to 1.3 hours. In contrast, the half-life after oral administration in humans averages 22 hours, with a range of 7-42 hours. Phenytoin has moderate ability in the human to induce cytochrome P-450 mixed-function oxidase activity (microsomal enzyme induction). Consequently, it is a much more efficacious drug for control of epileptic seizures in humans than in dogs.

Phenytoin and phenobarbital have been used in combination for treatment of epilepsy in both humans and dogs. This combined use is considered optimal therapy for epilepsy in humans (Morselli et al. 1971). Use of both drugs is controversial in animals because both drugs induce hepatic microsomal enzyme activity. The metabolism (i.e., hydroxylation) of phenytoin is increased. Phenytoin likewise increases the metabolism of phenobarbital. This seesaw effect in metabolism of both drugs complicates successful therapy, and the combined use of the drugs is discouraged (Pasten 1977).

Inhibition of phenytoin metabolism by other drugs has been observed in humans. Prolongation of the effect has been reported following simultaneous administration of dicoumarol, chloramphenicol, phenylbutazone, and the phenothiazines. Also, in vitro inhibition of phenytoin metabolism has been seen in the presence of diazepam and propoxyphene hydrochloride. The significance of this in vivo has not been determined. In the dog, an interaction has been seen following clinical use of phenytoin and chloramphenicol (Sanders et al. 1979a). The serum half-life of IV phenytoin is increased from 3 to 15 hours. Increase in the serum half-life is best explained by reduction in rate of metabolism of phenytoin by hepatic microsomal enzymes. Interestingly, the signs of phenytoin toxicosis are reversed within 24 hours after cessation of chloramphenicol treatment (Sanders et al. 1979a). Phenylbutazone is also known to elevate plasma concentration of phenytoin through inhibition of metabolism of phenytoin (de Angelis 1979).

Metabolism of a number of chemicals or drugs is enhanced by phenytoin. These include digitoxin, dexamethasone, DDT, dieldrin, and cortisol (Conney and Burns 1972).

An interaction also exists between phenytoin and vitamin B_6. Serum phenytoin concentration drops after folic-acid therapy probably because the hydroxylase enzyme metabolizing phenytoin is folate dependent. In humans, the usual therapeutic concentration of phenytoin in plasma reduces the half-life of theophylline (a drug used in treatment of airway obstruction) and increases its body clearance about twofold (Marquis et al. 1982). A similar action of phenytoin upon the half-life of theophylline in animals would be expected.

Phenytoin may prolong the prothrombin time (Keith et al. 1983). Blood coagulation defects similar to that induced by vitamin K deficiency can occur in neonates exposed to phenytoin in utero. The coagulation defect can be reversed by treatment with vitamin K.

BLOOD CONCENTRATIONS AND ASSOCIATED TOXICITY. In humans, mild signs of intoxication such as nystagmus develop with blood levels of 20 µg/mL; patients with levels over 40 µg/mL have marked stagmus and are incoordinated and lethargic. Blood levels in the dog would probably have to increase a comparable 100-400% over therapeutic levels as in humans before serious signs of intoxication develop.

Hepatitis, jaundice, and death following clinical use of phenytoin have been reported for one animal (Nash et al. 1977). However, this animal had initially received primidone (500 mg daily) orally for the control of seizures. Toxic hepatopathy and intrahepatic cholestasis associated with phenytoin administration in combination with phenobarbital and/or primidone have been reported in 3 dogs (Meyer and Noonan 1981; Bunch et al. 1987). Induction of enzymes may increase the formation of toxic metabolites and contribute to hepatotoxicity. Hepatotoxicity due to phenytoin is more likely if phenytoin is used in combination therapy with either primidone or phenobarbital. Toxicity may be related to generation of toxic metabolites. Two forms of toxicity appear to occur with phenytoin therapy: a dose-independent chronic hepatitis which may progress to cirrhosis and which appears to be reversible following discontinuation of the drug early in the disease, and a dose-dependent intrahepatic cholestasis, which is accompanied by a poor prognosis.

SIDE EFFECTS. The side effects of phenytoin in a dog are moderate because it is rapidly metabolized (Cunningham 1984). Transient incoordination and oversedation may occasionally occur following administration of phenytoin. A moderate degree of polyphagia, polydipsia, and polyuria may be seen in animals medicated with this drug. Sialosis, weight loss, and vomiting have been reported following the use of phenytoin in the cat. In the horse, head twitching occurs 2-5 minutes after the end of an IV infusion of 8.8 mg/kg (Kowalczyk and Beech 1983). Inhibition of release of antidiuretic hormone accounts for the polyuria that develops after administration of phenytoin. There is also an inhibition of insulin secretion (de Angelis 1979).

In laboratory mice, a single dose of phenytoin administered to pregnant animals on the 9th-14th day of gestation produces various fetal anomalies (Harbison and Becker 1969; Millicovsky and Johnston 1981), including changes in fetal growth. Embryo lethal effects were also reported. However, the intraperitoneal (IP) dose required to produce this teratogenic effect in mice is exceedingly large (7-150 mg/kg). It has been postulated that teratogenesis occurs in mice as a result of formation of a phenytoin-epoxide complex and its covalent binding to gestational tissue. Studies indicate that the development of cleft palate by phenytoin has a common pathway with that produced by glucocorticoids (Katasumata et al. 1982). Both phenytoin and glucocorticoids inhibit ribonucleic acid and protein synthesis in mouse fetal palates. It has been hypothesized that phenytoin and glucocorticoids bind to a common cell receptor. Teratogenesis in the dog from use of phenytoin has not been identified or reported in the veterinary literature.

Rickets, hypocalcemia, decreased duodenal calcium transport, and reduction of calcium-binding protein have been produced in chickens treated with phenytoin (Villareale et al. 1974). These findings suggest that close attention should be given to the calciferol intake in patients requiring epileptic seizure treatment. Calciferol metabolism apparently is altered by phenytoin, which in turn leads to functional vitamin D deficiency. A similar effect in humans has been seen following long-term use of primidone (discussed above).

Benzodiazepines: Diazepam, Clonazepam, and Clorazepate

MECHANISM OF ACTION. Benzodiazepines enhance the inhibitory effects of GABA in both the brain and the spinal cord. Thus they not only decrease seizure spread but also block arousal and centrally depress spinal reflexes. Tolerance to anticonvulsant activity of diazepam develops within 1 week in the dog; thus, diazepam (Valium) is not an effective anticonvulsant for chronic therapy in dogs. However, IV diazepam is the drug of choice for the treatment of status epilepticus in both dogs and cats because it crosses the blood-brain barrier into the cerebral spinal fluid very rapidly. Diazepam (1-2 mg every 8 hr) is also the second-choice anticonvulsant for chronic control of seizures in the cat whose seizures do not respond to phenobarbital; efficacy is equal to phenobarbital. Tolerance to the anticonvulsant effects of clorazepate does not appear to develop in dogs as rapidly as it does to diazepam.

DISPOSITION. Diazepam is the prototype benzodiazepine used in small animals. The drug is well absorbed following oral administration but undergoes rapid and extensive hepatic metabolism once in the circulation. Although only 1-3% of diazepam is orally bioavailable, 74-100% of the drug and all active metabolites are available (Frey and Löscher 1985). Diazepam is generally administered intravenously. It can also be administered intramuscularly, although absorption is not predictable. In human pediatric patients, it has been administered rectally as well. The metabolites of diazepam (nordiazepam and oxazepam) are active, although less so (25-33%) than the parent compound. However, the half-lives of the metabolites are slightly longer than that of diazepam (4 to 6 and 5.2 hr, respectively). In horses, diazepam is characterized by an elimination half-life of 7.5-13 hours (0.05-0.08 mg/kg) and a clearance that ranges between 1.86 and 3.44 mL/min/kg (Shini et al. 1997). Diazepam is still present in plasma at 24 hours. The apparent volume of distribution approximates 2.0-2.25 L/kg. An earlier study (Muir et al. 1982) found elimination half-life to vary between 2.5 and 22 hours, clearance to range between 7 and 9.5 mL/min/kg, and apparent volume of distribution to vary between 1.6 and 3 L/kg. Diazepam is up to 98% protein bound (Klotz et al. 1976). Doses studied ranged from 0.05 to 0.4 mg/kg. Three major metabolites of diazepam detected in horses included n-desmethyldiazpeam, oxazepam, and n-methyloxazepam (Muir et al. 1982).

Following oral administration, metabolite concentration surpasses that of the parent compound. The generation of active metabolites complicates the utility of therapeutic monitoring as a guide to therapy since anticonvulsant activity will not necessarily be correlated with serum diazepam concentrations. All metabolites and parent drugs should be measured. Metabolism in the dog is rapid (half-life of 3.2 hr). Clorazepate is metabolized in the stomach to its active metabolite, nordiazepam (desmethyl diazepam), which is also a major, although less efficacious, metabolite of diazepam.

Diazepam has been studied following rectal administration in dogs (Papich and Alcorn 1995; Mealey and Boothe 1995). Rectal bioavailability of the parent compound approximated only 7.5% at 2 mg/kg and 2.5% at 0.5 mg/kg in one study. However, bioavailability of total metabolites was 79% and 66%, respectively, for each dose in one study and had a mean of 0.517% (range 14-81%) in another, suggesting efficacy following rectal administration (Mealey and Boothe 1995).

PREPARATIONS. Diazepam is available as both an IV and oral preparation; clorazepate is available as an oral preparation. Cautious IV use of the drug must be observed. Use of diazepam in animals has not been approved by the FDA. It is classified as a Schedule IV drug under the 1970 Controlled Substances Act.

SAFETY. Sedation is the most common direct side effect of the benzodiazepines. Adverse effects (sedation, ataxia, increased appetite, and in some cases hyperactivity) are likely to occur if concentrations reach 500 ng/mL. Drug interactions may result in indirect side effects with chronic administration of clorazepate. Phenobarbital concentrations may increase shortly after clorazepate therapy is begun if the two drugs are given simultaneously. Decreased phenobarbital dosing may be indicated. Clorazepate concentrations may decrease several months after combination therapy. Clinically important drug interactions resulting from chronic diazepam therapy have not been reported.

CLINICAL USE. Diazepam is the first drug of choice for status epilepticus in both the dog and the cat and is the second drug of choice for long-term control of seizures in the cat. Clorazepate can be used (generally in combination with phenobarbital) for long-term control in dogs. The therapeutic range of benzodiazepines (including metabolites) in dogs has been extrapolated from people and does not reflect combination therapy. Interactions between phenobarbital and clorazepate may necessitate dose modification. Monitoring (diazepam and its metabolites) is available through some laboratories. Since drug half-life is short, both peak and trough samples are recommended. The incidence of adverse affects may be reduced by using a smaller dose at 8-hour intervals.

USE IN TREATMENT OF STATUS EPILEPTICUS. Because of the efficacy and rapidity of its action and lack of toxicity, the IV use of diazepam is the drug of choice for control of status epilepticus in humans (de Angelis 1979). In the dog, diazepam is rapidly metabolized and tolerance to its antiepileptic effect develops rapidly (Frey 1986); thus it is not satisfactory for continued treatment and/or control of epilepsy. Diazepam is best suited and is the drug of choice for emergency IV use in control of status epilepticus (Frey and Löscher 1985). IV diazepam may be rivaled by clonazepam, a relatively new benzodiazepine, because tolerance to its anticonvulsant effects develops more slowly.

The onset of more than one seizure per hour is a medical emergency (Cunningham 1984). To terminate the seizures in dogs, various methods of administration have been recommended. Diazepam has been recommended in an IV dose of 5-20 mg and in an IV dose of

0.5-1 mg/kg (Frey and Löscher 1985). Because it has a short half-life, dosing may have to be repeated once or twice during the first 2 hours to stabilize the dog (Cunningham 1984). A comparable IM dose may be given for longer stabilization. Alternatively, IV phenobarbital may be given. If the seizures are not subdued by diazepam, it may be necessary to give a general anesthetic (see discussion below on pentobarbital). Another procedure for treatment of status epilepticus has been described by Averill (1970). A dose of 5 mg diazepam is administered slowly by the IV route. In the event this dose level does not abolish the seizure in 1-2 minutes, the dose is repeated. If a response has not occurred following the second dose of the drug, IV pentobarbital sodium (16.5 mg/kg) is slowly administered. Patients that respond to the first and/or second dosages of diazepam are carefully monitored, and if status epilepticus returns in 2-4 hours after the initial treatment, the regimen is repeated. An oral anticonvulsant is started as soon as seizures are abolished.

Diazepam is used in control of epileptic disorders in the cat regardless of etiology (Kay 1975). Generally, an IV dose (5-10 mg) is given to effect. A dose as high as 20 mg may be necessary; if high dosages are used, they must be injected slowly. The procedure commonly followed is to administer 2-10 mg IV and then wait 10 minutes. In the event seizures persist, Kay (1975) recommends IV administration of phenobarbital sodium (5-60 mg). Caution must be taken not to oversedate or depress the animal when these drugs are administered close together. Should the animal manifest refractoriness to diazepam and phenobarbital, pentobarbital anesthesia is then carefully administered to effect (see discussion below). Once the seizures have been brought under control, oral anticonvulsant therapy should be initiated. Phenobarbital (8-32 mg) is given orally 2-3 times daily; diazepam may be used in place of phenobarbital in animals that react unfavorably to barbiturate therapy. Diazepam is given orally in doses of 2-5 mg 2 or 3 times daily. Phenobarbital dosages may be adjusted by increasing or decreasing in 4-8 mg increments; diazepam may be increased or decreased in increments of 2 mg (Kay 1975).

CLONAZEPAM. *Clonazepam,* USP (Clonopin), is a benzodiazepine derivative and is chemically 5-(*o*-chlorophenyl)-1,3-dihydro-7-nitro-2*H*-1,4-benzodiazepin-2-one (Fig. 16.2). It is more potent than diazepam and is used only in the emergency treatment of status epilepticus in the dog (Frey and Löscher 1985). Clonazepam is given IV in a dose of 0.05-0.2 mg/kg. Accumulation occurs upon continued administration. However, tolerance develops due to hepatic enzyme induction within days to weeks after administration. Consequently, clonazepam, like diazepam, is unsatisfactory in long-term control of epilepsy.

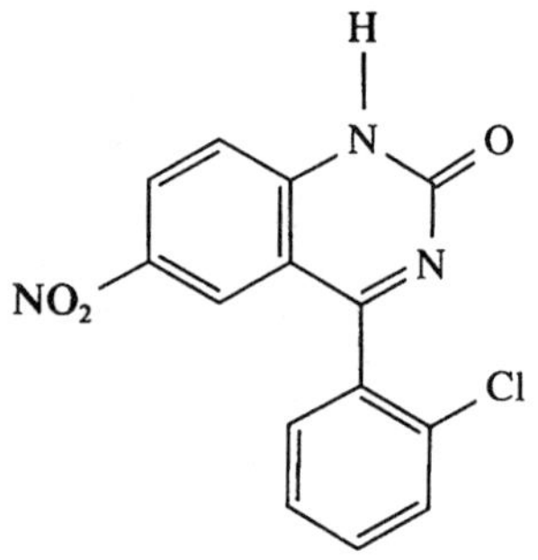

Clonazepam

FIG. 16.2

Bromide

MECHANISM OF ACTION. Bromide is an old anticonvulsant and sedative whose mechanism of action is not completely understood (Wuth 1927). Replacement of negatively charged chloride with bromide has been hypothesized as the mechanism; the neuron becomes hyperpolarized (i.e., the RMP becomes more negative in relation to the threshold potential). The anticonvulsant effects of bromide correlate with plasma concentration (Grewal 1954). Bromide is available in several salt forms (sodium, potassium, and ammonia). Differences among the products reflect solubility (thus ease of compounding) in water and the amount of bromide per gram of compound (i.e., more bromide in NaBr than in KBr because Na weighs less than K).

DISPOSITION. The pharmacokinetics of bromide has not been well established. The half-life in dogs may be 24 days. Steady-state concentrations are not achieved for 3-6 months. Distribution is to extracellular fluid. Bromide is eliminated slowly (perhaps due to marked reabsorption) in the kidney. Its rate of elimination changes with salt administration. Increased dietary salt will increase the rate of elimination of bromide (perhaps due to preferential reabsorption?), and decreased salt will cause the opposite (Rauws and van Logeten 1975; Shaw et al. 1996). Bromide has not been studied in cats.

SIDE EFFECTS. Adverse reactions to bromide are usually neurological and include ataxia, grogginess, and sedation (Nichols et al. 1996; Yohn et al. 1992). Skin reactions have been reported and are probably more likely in patients that already have skin disease (e.g., flea bite dermatitis). Vomiting is not unusual and probably reflects the hyperosmolality of the drug. In the case of acute bromide toxicity, NaCl administration (0.9% NaCl) is the treatment of choice. Hepatotoxicity is not a concern with this drug.

CLINICAL USE. In humans, bromide has been used to treat intractable seizures in pediatric patients (Woody 1990; Podell and Fenner 1993). In dogs bromide is most commonly used as an "add-on" anticonvulsant in epileptic patients who have not sufficiently responded to or cannot tolerate phenobarbital (especially due to hepatotoxicity) (Pearce 1990; Schwarze-Porsche and Jurgens 1991; Boothe 1998). Because steady state may require 2-3 months, a loading dose is recommended to achieve therapeutic concentrations more rapidly. Therapeutic efficacy cannot be fully evaluated for several months following the start of administration unless a loading dose is administered. The loading dose should establish steady-state concentrations immediately and is based on a volume of distribution of 0.3 L/kg and a target concentration of 1.5 mg/mL: 450-600 mg/kg over 5 days plus the recommended daily dose. The 5-day duration of dosing reduces the likelihood of emesis postadministration. Plasma drug levels should be measured after loading to evaluate the efficacy of the loading dose.

Bromide is not available in a medicine grade and must be purchased from a chemical company (request ACS grade). Some companies will not sell the chemical if a medicinal use is planned. Application to the FDA for regulatory discretion will avoid illegalities associated with the use of bromide for seizure control.

Bromide can be mixed to a convenient concentration in water (administer 44 mg/kg every 24 hr orally) or administered in a gelatin capsule. Twice daily administration may be necessary because of the bitter taste and its tendency to induce vomition. Its primary indication is probably in combination with phenobarbital in refractory epileptics. Decreasing phenobarbital doses may be possible once therapeutic concentrations have been reached and may be indicated if animals become groggy or ataxic. Recommended target ranges are controversial and depend on whether phenobarbital is also being given. Our laboratory uses 0.8-2 mg/mL if in combination with phenobarbital or, if sole agent, up to 3 mg/mL.

Pentobarbital Sodium. *Pentobarbital Sodium,* USP (Nembutal sodium, Pentobarbitone sodium, Sagatal, Napental), administered IV is considered the most efficacious procedure for abolishing refractory status epilepticus in the dog (Redding 1969). Pentobarbital is also valuable in terminating refractory status epilepticus in other species. Extreme care, however, is required not to overdose. The dose of the anesthetic varies considerably from one animal within a species to the next. Consequently, pentobarbital is carefully given to effect.

In humans, tonic-clonic status epilepticus that is refractory to phenobarbital, phenytoin, and diazepam may respond to an IV infusion of pentobarbital given continuously for several days. Then it is discontinued, and oral phenobarbital along with other anticonvulsants is advocated to control recurring epileptic episodes. Respiratory and myocardial depression necessitate EEG and cardiopulmonary monitoring and support (Jagoda and Riggio 1993).

Miscellaneous Antiepileptics. Other antiepileptic agents, infrequently used in veterinary medicine, are available in human medicine for treatment of various CNS seizure disorders. Their safety and effectiveness in clinical veterinary medicine have not been determined in most instances. Additionally, the biologic half-lives for some (e.g., valproic acid, carbamazepine) of these compounds are too short in the dog to permit maintenance of adequate drug concentrations in plasma and the CNS (Frey 1986). Valproic acid (valproate) and carbamazepine have found established places in treatment of human seizure disorders (Eadie 1991). The benzodiazepine derivatives, primarily clonazepam, have proven useful and effective in treatment of human epilepsy. The use of anticonvulsants such as paramethadione, aloxidone, and troxidone (of the oxazolidinedione family) have declined extensively for control and/or treatment of epilepsy in humans. They have been essentially replaced by the less toxic and more effective succinimide derivatives (notably ethosuximide) and more recently by clonazepam and valproate. New hydantoins (albutoin, methoin) have been synthesized in an attempt to find a better antiepileptic than phenytoin; to date this effort has been unsuccessful.

Drugs Contraindicated in Epileptic Patients. Reserpine and phenothiazine and butyrophenone tranquilizers are contraindicated in epileptic patients because they can induce seizures. Other drugs capable of inducing seizures in selected patients include metaclopramide and fluorinated quinolones. Morphine sulfate and related compounds as well as CNS stimulants such as the methylxanthines should be avoided. Chloramphenicol also activates the CNS and should not be used in dogs known to be subject to epileptiform seizures.

CNS STIMULANTS. A large number of drugs possess the ability to stimulate the CNS. Stimulant, or convulsant, drugs vary markedly in their total pharmacologic action. Some can be used for therapeutic stimulation within narrow limits of dosage; others are only poisons. Some, such as ephedrine, influence the function of the CNS only secondarily while primarily affecting another system of the body. Toxic drugs, such as nicotine and strychnine, stimulate the CNS as a manifestation of poisoning. Many of these are considered poisons and are discussed accordingly.

Some drugs affecting the CNS have a specific action that limits their clinical application. Apomorphine hydrochloride, for example, stimulates the emetic center in the medulla more than other parts of the brain, so it is used clinically to induce emesis in species sensitive to its action. Stimulants of the CNS such as caffeine and other methylxanthines used by humans stimulate sensory areas of the brain to combat mental fatigue. Compared to other stimulants, the methylxanthines have been less important in veterinary medicine. However, the discovery of the adenosine receptors should increase interest in use of methylxanthines such as theophylline.

Other drugs that stimulate the CNS act directly on the respiratory center to counteract respiratory collapse. These are employed in treatment of barbiturate poisoning, drowning, neonatal asphyxia, heat or lightning shock, and threatened respiratory collapse during anesthesia. Doxapram is an example.

The term "respiratory analeptic" refers to drugs that stimulate a depressed respiratory center to produce increased respiratory exchange. In addition to restoring respiratory function, analeptics may restore depressed vasomotor and cerebral functions, including consciousness (Wang and Ward 1977).

Drugs used for analeptic effect, with the exception of carbon dioxide, exert an arousal effect characterized by a partial return of consciousness of the patient. Animals often do not return to a state of normal cerebration or locomotion. Animals may become traumatized during this stimulation period. The period of stimulation is brief. Generally, the best therapy for respiratory paralysis is to apply artificial ventilation using oxygen. The introduction of safer and much more specific antagonists such as naloxone for the opioid agents and yohimbine for α agonists and the discovery of other compounds with specific antagonist activity have increased the number of drugs available to treat selected causes of respiratory depression.

Doxapram Hydrochloride. *Doxapram Hydrochloride,* USP (Dopram), is approved by the FDA for use in the dog, cat, and horse. It has not been approved for use in animals intended for human consumption. Chemically, doxapram is l-ethyl-4-(2-morpholinoethyl)-3,3-diphenyl-2-pyrrolidinone hydrochloride.

PHARMACOLOGIC CONSIDERATIONS. Doxapram is primarily used to stimulate respiratory activity in the postanesthetic, recovery period. Doxapram directly stimulates chemoreceptors of the carotid and aortic regions (Wang and Ward 1977). It may also stimulate the medullary respiratory center (Severinghaus et al. 1976). Tidal volume increases as a result. Stimulation of other portions of the CNS occurs only when high dose levels are used. Convulsions or alterations in electroencephalographic (EEG) patterns are not seen with therapeutic levels (Soma and Kenny 1967). The convulsant dose of doxapram is 70-75 times the dose that stimulates respiratory center activity.

Doxapram is considered superior to all combinations of analeptic agents evaluated. The respiratory minute volume is increased 200% within 1 minute after administration of doxapram in the dog (Klemm 1966). When doxapram (2 mg/kg) is administered intravenously, the change in expired minute volume is marked and rapid (Soma and Kenny 1967). The ventilatory and cardiovascular stimulatory effects occur within one circulation time of the drug. The initial marked increase in expired minute volume is due to an increase in tidal volume and respiration rate. However, the increase in tidal volume is not maintained and diminishes in 5-6 minutes. Overall improvement in ventilation is reflected by changes in the acid-base status of the blood as well as in the oxygen tension of arterial blood.

The pressor response of doxapram occurs rapidly and concurrently with respiratory effects (Soma and Kenny 1967) and is believed to be mediated through activation of the sympathetic nervous system. An arterial hypotensive effect of brief duration occurs after IV administration of a large dose (4 mg/kg); this effect does not occur when a dose of 2 mg/kg or less is administered. The pressor and respiratory responses occur when the dose of doxapram is not higher than 2 mg/kg (Soma and Kenny 1967).

Studies in cats anesthetized with pentobarbital sodium have determined the effects of bilateral and unilateral pneumotaxic center ablation upon doxapram-induced respiratory changes (St. John et al. 1973). In these ablated animal preparations, doxapram stimulation of respiration caused only minor changes in tidal volume, but frequency of respiratory activity increased. IV doses of doxapram (1-2.5 mg/kg) were adequate to stimulate effects through peripheral chemoreceptor and medullary respiratory area activation. Doxapram-induced stimulatory influences arising from one or both these areas (i.e., chemoreceptor and/or medullary respiratory center) are integrated by the pontile pneumotaxic center.

Doxapram has also been experimentally used in the pig, rabbit, sheep, and chicken; sheep and rabbits appear to be far less sensitive than other species to effects of analeptic agents (Beretta et al. 1973). Although there are variations in the degree of responses produced by different analeptics in various species, doxapram, when used alone or in combination with other analeptics, usually elicits marked improvement in respiratory activity.

CLINICAL USE. Use of doxapram in clinical practice is specified for reversal of central respiratory depression from barbiturates and inhalant anesthetics. In neonatal puppies, doxapram can be administered subcutaneously or sublingually (topically on mucous membrane) at a total dose of 1-5 mg. It may also be administered in the umbilical veins of puppies at the time of birth to stimulate respiration. It may be given to neonatal kittens subcutaneously or sublingually (topically on mucous membrane) at a total dose of 1-2 mg.

Table 16.2 lists some of the clinical uses and recommended IV doses of doxapram. Doses of doxapram can be repeated within 15-20 minutes and should be decreased or increased to achieve the desired effect. Efficacy decreases with subsequent doses (Jensen and Klemm 1967).

Experimentally, IV doxapram (1 mg/kg) is capable of antagonizing subcutaneous (SC) xylazine (3 mg/kg) in the dog (Dendi 1979). Immediately after administration of doxapram, dogs are able to walk without difficulty. Dogs given IV xylazine (2.2 mg/kg), followed by IV doxapram (5.5 mg/kg) about 15 minutes later, were able to walk within 3-5 minutes (Short et al. 1982). Those treated with normal saline required 30-120 minutes to recover from xylazine. To reverse the sedative action of 1.1 mg/kg IV xylazine in the dog, an IV dose

Table 16.2—Clinical uses and recommended IV doses of doxapram

Species	Dose (mg/kg)	Clinical use
Dog and cat	5.5–11	Barbiturate depression
Dog and cat	1.1	Depression from inhalant anesthetics
Horse	0.55	Depression from chloral hydrate and/or pentobarbital
Horse	0.44	Depression from inhalant anesthetics

Caffeine

Theophylline

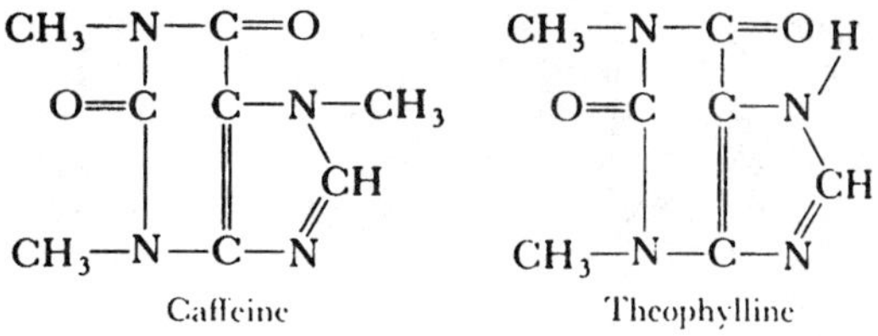

FIG. 16.3

of 1.1 mg/kg doxapram is sufficient in most cases (Sodikoff 1982).

In the dog, IV doxapram (5.5 mg/kg) administered 15-20 minutes after IM acepromazine (1.1 mg/kg) induces walking within 2-10 minutes in 5 of 6 animals studied; the 6th dog began to walk after 30 minutes (Short et al. 1982). In control dogs treated with normal saline, more than 2 hours elapsed before any of the animals given acepromazine could begin walking.

Doxapram is the most effective antagonist of thiopental-acepromazine-anesthetized dogs (Hatch et al. 1985b). However, yohimbine is the most effective antagonist of thiopental anesthesia in xylazine-treated dogs. Droperidol-fentanyl-pentobarbital anesthesia in the dog is best reversed by IV doxapram (5 mg/kg) plus a IV dose of naloxone (1 mg/kg) (Hatch et al. 1986).

In the horse, clinical evaluation of doxapram (0.55 mg/kg) as a respiratory stimulant was conducted during and after general anesthesia with IV injections of chloral hydrate alone and chloral hydrate in combination with pentobarbital and magnesium sulfate (Short and Cloyd 1970). The arousal time was reduced; respiratory volume and rate increased immediately following administration of the drug. No toxic or adverse effects were noted. A clinical evaluation of doxapram (0.46 mg/kg) in the horse during and after general anesthesia with halothane and methoxyflurane indicated that doxapram improved ventilation in horses anesthetized with halothane soon after administration of the drug (Short and Cloyd 1970). However, studies in humans revealed that halothane anesthesia virtually abolishes the respiratory stimulant effect of doxapram (Knill and Gelb 1978). Previous studies indicated that peripheral chemoreceptor-mediated reflexes are relatively durable and resistant to depressant effects of anesthetic agents. However, work on the hypoxic chemoreflex in dogs anesthetized with halothane, isoflurane, or enflurane contradicts this viewpoint (Weiskopf et al. 1974; Hirshman et al. 1977). Additional work is needed to reexamine the pharmacologic action of doxapram in horses and other species anesthetized with halothane and possibly with other inhalant anesthetics.

Doxapram (100-160 mg) is used intravenously to facilitate endoscopic examination of laryngeal motion in the horse; hyperpnea is induced in about 20 seconds following injection of the drug (Marks 1973). Hypoxic respiratory activity induced by an etorphine-acepromazine mixture is only partially reversed by doxapram, so there is no overall advantage in using doxapram to reverse etorphine-induced hypoxia (Hillidge 1976).

In cattle, IV doxapram (0.46-0.6 mg/kg) is capable of reversing the action of IV xylazine (0.2 mg/kg) (Dendi and Parada 1981). IV doxapram (1 mg/kg) followed immediately by IV 4-aminopyridine (0.3 mg/kg) has proven to be effective in antagonizing large IM doses of xylazine (0.3-0.4 mg/kg) in steers (Zahner et al. 1984).

Methylxanthine Derivatives. Caffeine, theophylline, and theobromine are closely related alkaloids, all containing the xanthine nucleus (Fig. 16.3). Theobromine is of interest primarily as a toxicant. These drugs have important pharmacologic properties in addition to CNS stimulation.

Caffeine is found in coffee beans to the extent of about 1%. Theophylline and caffeine are present in tea leaves to around 3%. The methylxanthine compounds affect the same organs but to a varying degree. They all stimulate the CNS, dilate the coronary blood vessels, and promote diuresis. However, caffeine is primarily a CNS stimulant. Theophylline is better for promoting diuresis and relaxation of bronchial smooth muscle.

CAFFEINE. *Caffeine,* USP, is primarily used in human medicine. Discovery of more potent CNS stimulants has essentially made caffeine obsolete as an analeptic agent. Therapeutic use of caffeine is limited in animals. It has been used experimentally as a test of hepatic function since its plasma elimination reflects activity of drug-metabolizing enzymes in the liver (Boothe et al. 1994).

ACTION. Caffeine increases irritability of the sensory cortex, which results in increased mental alertness. Caffeine is a potent cerebral stimulant that may superimpose exceptional muscular activity over fatigue and temporarily increase capacity for muscular work. Large doses cause an increased motor activity that may lead to exaggerated responses to normal stimuli.

Caffeine will stimulate respiratory centers directly when they are depressed by CNS depressant drugs. It has been suggested that caffeine may act by rendering respiratory centers more sensitive to carbon dioxide. The mechanism of action of the methylxanthines is controversial. Proposed mechanisms include translocation of intracellular calcium, accumulation of cyclic nucleotides (e.g., cyclic adenosine 3′,5′-monophosphate, or cAMP), and blockade of adenosine receptors. The last may be the most important. There are known cellular mechanisms through which methylxanthines may cause their varied pharmacologic effects. Caffeine and other methylxanthines inhibit phosphodiesterase, an enzyme that degrades cAMP. Cardiac acceleration (from β-adrenergic stimulation) occurs with an increase in cAMP. Arrhythmia may be induced following administration of caffeine. Drinking one cup of coffee can induce arrhythmia in some human subjects.

METABOLISM. Caffeine is readily absorbed from the digestive tract or from the site of injection in small animals. It is partially demethylated to theophylline and theobromine and other metabolites before it is excreted in urine. In dogs, caffeine distributes rapidly to a volume of 0.8 L/kg and is minimally (83% ± 16% at 20 μg/mL) bound to serum proteins. It is characterized by a clearance of 2.05 ± 0.1 mL/min/kg and an elimination half-life of 255 ± 76 minutes (Boothe et al. 1994). Liver disease results in decreased clearance and an increased elimination half-life (750 ± 450 hr) (Boothe et al. 1994).

In the horse, following oral administration of 3 g caffeine, about 3% of the dose is eliminated unaltered in urine during the first 24 hours (Tobin et al. 1979). There is no evidence that caffeine is conjugated in horses as either glucuronides or arylsulfates. However, traces of theobromine are found in horse urine for up to 10 days after a dose of caffeine. Theobromine is found in sufficient quantities to make urine test positive for caffeine. Use of caffeine in the competitive racing animal is illegal.

TOXICITY. Caffeine has a wide margin of safety. An excessive dose can produce convulsions, but the amount is of such magnitude as to render clinical occurrence unlikely. At first the convulsions are epileptiform, but later they become tonic as the effect of caffeine descends to the spinal cord. The convulsive effect may be counteracted by administration of a barbiturate. A lethal dose of caffeine administered parenterally in the dog and cat is 110-175 mg/kg and 80-150 mg/kg, respectively.

AMINOPHYLLINE. *Aminophylline,* USP (theophylline ethylenediamine), is one of the more soluble salt forms of theophylline. It has a brief but potent action in stimulating diuresis. In laboratory animals, theophylline has been shown to dilate coronary blood vessels. This effect is highly beneficial because the increased blood flow that it brings to the myocardium increases mechanical efficiency of the heart. Theophylline is an inhibitor of phosphodiesterase, an enzyme that destroys cAMP.

In addition to inhibitory action upon phosphodiesterase, the methylxanthines block the action of adenosine (A_1 and A_2 receptors; also referred to in some literature sources as purinoceptors or P_1 and P_2 receptors) in a competitive manner (Kulkarni and Mehta 1984). Adenosine is believed to be a neuromodulator in the brain, because it modifies adrenergic neurotransmission by inhibiting norepinephrine release in various tissues. It is also recognized as having sedative and anticonvulsant activity. Consequently, the effects of adenosine are opposite to those of theophylline or caffeine.

The CNS depressant activity of adenosine is believed to be potentiated by diazepam and related benzodiazepines; e.g., it has been suggested that this action is due to an inhibition of adenosine uptake in the brain. Purine nucleosides related to adenosine (e.g., inosine and hypoxanthine) may be endogenous ligands for benzodiazepines. Thus, benzodiazepines such as diazepam may exert their pharmacologic actions by displacement or by mimicking these ligands. In humans, aminophylline is a potent antagonist to the sedative and CNS depressant actions of diazepam (Arvidsson et al. 1984; Marrosu et al. 1985).

Interestingly, morphine enhances the release or efflux of adenosine from brain tissue. It is believed that some of the action of morphine may be mediated through adenosine receptors (purinoceptors) as a result of adenosine release. Methylxanthines, adenosine antagonists, have been reported to antagonize the inhibitory effect of morphine upon release of acetylcholine (ACh) and other NTs (Kulkarni and Mehta 1984). Additionally, morphine-induced deaths and inhibition of electrically induced contractions of the guinea pig ileum can be antagonized by theophylline. Also, pretreatment with naloxone (an antagonist of morphine) potentiates the toxicity of theophylline.

TOXICITY. Generally, large doses of methylxanthines are required to produce toxic effects in animals. There is no specific antidote for the methylxanthines.

Compared to the dog, the horse appears to be more sensitive to the CNS action of theophylline and other methylxanthine derivatives. Side effects such as agitation, tremors, hyperesthesia, sweating, polypnea, and tachycardia occur in the horse after an IV dose of 15 mg/kg theophylline (Errecalde et al. 1985). CNS effects are moderate at 10 mg/kg and mild or absent at 5 mg/kg following its IV administration in horses. A plasma theophylline concentration of 15 mg/mL is considered to be the upper safe limit in horses (Errecalde et al. 1985).

A clinical case of aminophylline toxicity occurred in swine from the inadvertent packaging of this product by a manufacturer. The owner believed he was administering piperazine adipate to his pigs for anthelmintic purposes. After administering the recommended dose, 5 out of a total of 8 pigs died. Some of the clinical signs of the survivors were intense excitement and incoordination. They staggered as they walked and then lay down to thrash or paddle their feet.

CLINICAL USE. Methylxanthines are rarely used for their CNS stimulant activity in animals. Their effects as CNS stimulants are of clinical interest primarily as a sign of toxicity when used therapeutically (e.g., as bronchodilators) or diagnostically (e.g., caffeine as a test of hepatic function).

Antagonists

4-AMINOPYRIDINE. *4-Aminopyridine* (4-AP) has potent CNS stimulant activity. In overdosages it is a convulsive agent. 4-AP has been used clinically in humans for several years in Europe as an antagonist to *d*-tubocurarine. It appears to facilitate neuronal Ca^{++} uptake and enhance ACh release in its antagonism of *d*-tubocurarine and other nondepolarizing skeletal muscle relaxants. In addition to its probable action upon Ca^{++}, 4-AP produces a selective block of K^{+} channels in excitable membranes (Glover 1982).

4-AP is also effective in reversal of intercostal and diaphragmatic paralysis induced by aminoglycoside antibiotics, such as neomycin and dihydrostreptomycin. Because of its cholinergic activity involving the neuromuscular junction, 4-AP has been used effectively in treatment of *Clostridium botulinum* paralysis.

The action of 4-AP upon the CNS is not well understood. A number of NTs apparently are released by it in the brain. Consequently, 4-AP is capable of antagonizing several CNS depressants partially or completely.

In humans, 4-AP in the same IV dose (0.3 mg/kg) that safely antagonizes effects of *d*-tubocurarine and pancuronium increases the rate of recovery from diazepam-ketamine anesthesia (Agoston et al. 1980). In veterinary medicine, 4-AP appears to have considerable potential as an antagonistic agent for accelerating recovery from a number of CNS depressants.

Studies in the dog have revealed that IV 4-AP (0.5 mg/kg) combined with naloxone (0.04 mg/kg) will immediately reverse the neuroleptanalgesic action of a droperidol-fentanyl combination (Booth et al. 1982). Moreover, it is effective in combination with yohimbine as an antagonist of xylazine sedation in the dog (Hatch et al. 1982). IV 4-AP (0.3 mg/kg) plus IV yohimbine (0.125 mg/kg) antagonizes the standard clinical IM dose of xylazine (2.2 mg/kg) as well as the 5 times overdose of 11 mg/kg. The combination of 4-AP and yohimbine is also effective in reversal of xylazine used with a large dose of atropine (Wallner et al. 1982) and in reversal of acepromazine-xylazine in the dog (Cronin et al. 1983).

In the cat, IV 4-AP (0.6 mg/kg) plus IV yohimbine (0.25 mg/kg) appears to be a safe and effective partial antagonist of IM ketamine (20 mg/kg) anesthesia (Hatch et al. 1983a). Cats pretreated with IM acepromazine (0.25 mg/kg) and anesthetized by IV pentobarbital (16.8 ± 3.8 mg/kg) can be aroused by an IV combination of 4-AP (0.5 mg/kg) and yohimbine (0.4 mg/kg); yohimbine enhances the antagonistic action of 4-AP (Hatch et al. 1984a).

Thiopental anesthesia is antagonized rapidly and permanently in atropinized (IM dose of 0.05 mg/kg) cats pretreated with IM xylazine (2.2 mg/kg) and given IV 4-AP (0.15 mg/kg) with IV yohimbine (0.125 mg/kg) (Hatch et al. 1984b). Meperidine-acepromazine-pentobarbital anesthesia can be smoothly and permanently reversed within minutes with IV 4-AP (0.5 mg/kg) plus IV yohimbine (0.4 mg/kg) in the cat (Hatch et al. 1984c).

In cattle, the combination of 4-AP plus doxapram is considered the most efficacious antagonist of xylazine sedation (see discussion in this chapter on doxapram). The pharmacokinetic characteristics of 4-AP have been determined in cattle (Kitzman et al. 1984b). After an IV injection of 0.3 mg/kg, the distribution half-life is 12 minutes and the elimination half-life is 129 minutes.

In the horse, 4-AP alone is the best antagonist of xylazine-ketamine anesthesia (Kitzman et al. 1984c). An IV dose of 0.2 mg/kg reverses IV xylazine (1.1 mg/kg) plus ketamine (2.2 mg/kg) anesthesia. The pharmacokinetic parameters of 4-AP have been determined in horses (Hendricks et al. 1984). After a bolus IV injection of 0.2 mg/kg, the distribution half-life is 7 minutes and the elimination half-life is 259 minutes. The elimination half-life of 4-AP in the horse is twice that of cattle (Kitzman et al. 1984b). Also, the horse has a longer elimination half-life than the dog (2.1 hr, Rupp et al. 1983) and the human (3.6 hr, Uges et al. 1982). From a toxicity standpoint, the horse appears to be quite sensitive to 4-AP; the lethal dose is estimated at 2-3 mg/kg (Ray et al. 1978). Methodology for detecting 4-AP in horse plasma as low as 25 ng/mL has been developed (Hendricks et al. 1984).

In the goat, IM xylazine (0.5 mg/kg) administered at 2.5 times the standard dosage for this species along with 0.5 mg/kg atropine is antagonized by an IV dose of 4-AP (0.3 mg/kg) plus yohimbine (0.125 mg/kg) (Jensen et al. 1983). Also, 4-AP plus yohimbine has been used to antagonize the combination of xylazine-atropine in white-tailed deer, North American otters, striped hyenas, and giraffes (Jensen et al. 1983).

In moose *(Alces alces),* mule deer *(Odocoileus hemionus),* and white-tailed deer *(Odocoileus virginianus),* successive IV administration of 4-AP (0.26 mg/kg, moose; 0.29 mg/kg, deer) plus yohimbine (0.15 mg/kg) markedly enhances the speed of recovery from xylazine-induced immobilization (Renecker and Olsen 1985).

4-AP has not been approved for use in animals by the FDA. Studies on its safety and efficacy will first need to be conducted, as well as tissue residue studies in food-producing animals.

YOHIMBINE HYDROCHLORIDE. Yohimbine hydrochloride is an old drug alleged to have aphrodisiac characteristics. An indolealkylamine alkaloid, it is found in rauwolfia root and is structurally similar to reserpine. It is a competitive α_2 antagonist. It disappeared from clinical use and became an obsolete drug many years ago. However, yohimbine is again serving as an important pharmacologic tool as a preferred α_2-adrenergic blocking agent (Starke et al. 1975).

In the 1960s, a number of investigators proposed that activation of central α-adrenergic receptors induces sedation in sleep. Agents such as xylazine and its related derivative clonidine induced sedation and/or sleep. It was learned that yohimbine could antagonize the sedative or sleeplike effects of clonidine in mice and chickens (Delbarre and Schmitt 1973). Moreover, it was discovered that yohimbine antagonized the analgesic activity of xylazine, an α-sympathomimetic agent, in the rat (Schmitt et al. 1974). The sedative, sleep, and analgesic actions produced by xylazine were attributed to its agonist effect upon α_2-adrenergic receptors in the brain. Consequently, yohimbine, piperoxan, and tolazoline, which preferentially block α_2-adrenergic receptors, are capable of antagonizing the actions of xylazine and clonidine. Additionally, yohimbine partially antagonizes other CNS depressants that affect synaptic mechanisms, such as barbiturates (Hatch 1973), ketamine (Hatch and Ruch 1974), and benzodiazepines (Lang and Gershon 1963). Thus, by binding on the same preferential, or primary (α_2-adrenergic), and secondary (cholinergic, serotonergic, GABAergic) receptor sites as some of the CNS depressants, yohimbine serves as an effective antagonist of a number of CNS agents. Xylazine, in particular, is antagonized quite effectively by yohimbine.

In the dog, yohimbine is more effective than 4-AP or doxapram in antagonizing the effects of xylazine (Hatch et al. 1985a). An IV dose (0.2 mg/kg) reverses the effect of a standard IM dose of 2.2 mg/kg xylazine. IM xylazine (11 mg/kg) 5 times the standard dose can be antagonized rapidly and completely by an IV dose of 0.4 mg/kg yohimbine (Hatch et al. 1985a). An IV combination of yohimbine (0.25 mg/kg) and 4-AP (0.5 mg/kg) can reverse pentobarbital anesthesia in atropinized dogs that are given IM xylazine (2.2 mg/kg) premedication; this dose of xylazine decreases the required dosage of pentobarbital about 80% (Hatch et al. 1983b). Hsu (1985) also observed that xylazine-pentobarbital anesthesia can be antagonized by yohimbine. Yohimbine also antagonizes the cardiovascular effects of jing songling, a xylazine analog (Hsu et al. 1985a).

The hypertensive, hypotensive, and cardiac slowing actions of IV xylazine (1 mg/kg) are antagonized in the dog by an IV dose of 0.1 mg/kg yohimbine (Hsu et al. 1985a). Yohimbine, administered as a single IV dose at 0.1 mg/kg in dogs anesthetized with pentobarbital, increases systolic arterial pressure, heart rate, and cardiac performance (Andrejak et al. 1983).

In cats treated with IM acepromazine (0.25 mg/kg), an IV combination of yohimbine (0.4 mg/kg) plus 4-AP (0.5 mg/kg) is the most effective antagonist in reversal of anesthesia induced by pentobarbital (Hatch et al. 1984a). Yohimbine enhances the antagonistic actions of 4-AP. In cats anesthetized with pentobarbital and premedicated with IM xylazine (2.2 mg/kg), IV yohimbine (0.4 mg/kg) is effective by itself. Yohimbine and 4-AP will partially reverse the anesthesia, but not the cataplexy, associated with ketamine (Hatch et al. 1983a). Jensen (1985) has reported treating an overdose of xylazine in a cat with yohimbine. An IV injection of 0.1 mg/kg yohimbine exerted its effect in about 2 minutes; the cat regained consciousness and was clinically normal within 10 minutes.

In the pony, IV yohimbine (0.1 mg/kg) reverses anesthesia induced by a combination of xylazine and thiopental (Hsu et al. 1985b). Also, IV yohimbine (0.1 mg/kg) is effective in reversing anesthesia induced by xylazine and pentobarbital (McGruder and Hsu 1985).

Yohimbine has been used to reverse the immobilizing effects of xylazine and xylazine-ketamine combinations in exotic species. In the African elephant tranquilized with ketamine (0.3 mg/kg) and xylazine (0.1 mg/kg), arousal occurs within 2-3 minutes after an IV injection of 0.125 mg/kg yohimbine (Jacobson and Kollias 1984). In African elephants, dromedary camels, sika deer, Père David deer, Barbary sheep, and springbok immobilized with xylazine or xylazine-ketamine, IV yohimbine (0.125 mg/kg) alone or in combination with doxapram (0.4 mg/kg) produces standing within 4 minutes after injection.

In mule deer, ketamine (9.2 mg/kg) and xylazine (0.73 mg/kg) anesthesia have been reversed in an average of 8.2 minutes by IV yohimbine (0.125 mg/kg); although unspecified, administration of ketamine and xylazine was probably by the IM route (Gullet 1984). Mule deer given xylazine alone at 0.75-1 mg/kg regain ambulatory ability 3 minutes or less after administration of IV yohimbine (0.125 mg/kg). Yohimbine has also been used in a few elk and bighorn sheep. According to Gullet (1984), the drug has potential for increasing anesthetic safety and human handler safety and for saving wildlife agencies hundreds of hours of labor.

Pretreatment with IV yohimbine (0.1 mg/kg) prevents sedation, bradycardia, sinus arrhythmia, and arterial hypertension induced by amitraz (Hsu et al. 1986). Amitraz apparently has α_2-adrenergic agonist activity.

Use of yohimbine in animals has not been approved by the FDA. Before it can be approved for use in food-producing animals, tissue residue studies must be conducted.

TOLAZOLINE HYDROCHLORIDE. *Tolazoline Hydrochloride,* USP (Priscoline), is chemically 2-benzyl-2-imidazoline. It has a wide range of pharmacologic effects, including adrenergic blocking, sympathomimetic, antihistaminic, and antihypertensive actions. Tolazoline has been used primarily in human medicine.

Since tolazoline is an α_2-adrenergic blocking agent, it has been used in the reversal of xylazine sedation. In the dog, IV tolazoline (5 mg/kg) reverses IV xylazine (1.1 mg/kg) (Tranquilli et al. 1984). Animals anesthetized with xylazine-halothane require increased concentration of halothane after tolazoline blocks the action of xylazine.

In sheep, IV tolazoline (2 mg/kg) antagonizes 2-4 times the recommended dose of xylazine (Hsu et al. 1987). It reverses the bradycardia and tachypnea induced by xylazine.

Tolazoline (0.5 mg/kg) by the IV route has been used to antagonize xylazine-ketamine immobilization of the juvenile African elephant (Allen 1986). Its administration induces rapid arousal and return to mobility.

In dogs, IV tolazoline (5 mg/kg) antagonizes the apparent α_2-adrenergic agonist action of amitraz (Hsu et al. 1986).

Tolazoline is less potent than yohimbine as an α_2-adrenergic blocking agent. It has not been approved by the FDA for use in animals. Data are needed to determine its safety and efficacy as an antagonist of xylazine and of other drugs that have α_2-adrenergic agonist activity.

REFERENCES

Abramson F. P. Autoinduction of phenobarbital elimination in the dog. 1988a. J Pharmaceut Sci 77(9):768–70.

———. The effect of induction with phenobarbital on the kinetics and bioavailability of antipyrine in the dog. 1988b. Eur J Drug Metab Pharmacokin 13(2):123–27.

Agoston, S., Salt, P. J., Erdmann, W., Hilkemeijer, T., Bencini, A., and Langrehr, D. 1980. Antagonism of ketamine-diazepam anaesthesia by 4-aminopyridine in human volunteers. Br J Anaesth 52:367-70.

Alary, J. G., Guay, P., and Brodeur, J. 1971. Effect of phenobarbital pretreatment on the metabolism of DDT in the rat and the bovine. Toxicol Appl Pharmacol 18:457-68.

Aldridge, A., and Neims, A. H. 1979. The effects of phenobarbital and beta-naphthoflavone on the elimination kinetics and metabolite pattern of caffeine in the Beagle dog. Drug Metab Dispos 7(3):378-82.

Allen, J. L. 1986. Use of tolazoline as an antagonist to xylazine-ketamine-induced immobilization in African elephants. Am J Vet Res 47:781-83.

Andrejak, M., Ward, M., and Schmitt, H. 1983. Cardiovascular effects of yohimbine in anaesthetized dogs. Eur J Pharmacol 94:219-28.

Arvidsson, S., Niemand, D., Martinell, S., and Ekstrom-Jodal, B. 1984. Aminophylline reversal of diazepam sedation. Anesthesiology 39:806-9.

Averill, D. R., Jr. 1970. Treatment of status epilepticus in dogs with diazepam sodium. J Am Vet Med Assoc 156:432-34.

Baggot, J. D., and Davis, L. E. 1973. Comparative study of plasma protein binding of diphenylhydantoin. Comp Gen Pharmacol 4:399-404.

Bai, S. A., and Abramson, F. P. 1983. Interaction of phenobarbital with propranolol in the dog. 3. Beta blockade. J Pharmacol Exp Ther 224:62-67.

Bailie, M. B., Smith, J. H., Newton, J. F., and Hook, J. B. 1984. Mechanism of chloroform nephrotoxicity. IV. Phenobarbital potentiation of in vitro chloroform metabolism and toxicity in rabbit kidneys. Toxicol Appl Pharmacol 74:285-92.

Bekersky, I., Maggio, A. C., Mattaliano, V., Jr., et al. 1977. Influence of phenobarbital on the disposition of clonazepam and antipyrine in the dog. J Pharmacokinet Biopharm 5(5):507-12.

Beretta, C., Faustini, R., and Gallina, G. 1973. Analeptic medication in domestic animals: species differences observed with doxapram and combinations of it with other stimulants. Vet Rec 92:217-21.

Berg, M. J., Berlinger, W. G., Goldberg, M. J., et al. 1982. Acceleration of the body clearance of phenobarbital by oral activated charcoal. N Engl J Med 307:642-44.

Booth, N. H., Hatch, R. C., and Crawford, L. M. 1982. Reversal of the neuroleptanalgesic effect of droperidolfentanyl in the dog by 4-aminopyridine and naloxone. Am J Vet Res 43:1227-31.

Boothe, D. M. 1998. Anticonvulsant therapy in small animals. Vet Clin N Am Small Anim Pract 28(2):411–48.

Boothe, D. M., Collen, J. M., Calvin, J. A., et al. 1994. Antipyrine and caffeine dispositions in clinically normals dogs and dogs with progressive liver disease. Am J Vet Res 55:254-61.

Browning, R. A. 1985. Fed Proc 44:2425.

Bunch, S. E., Conway, M. B., Center, S. A., et al. 1987. J Am Vet Med Assoc 190:194.

Campbell, C. L. 1983. Primidone intoxication associated with concurrent use of chloramphenicol. J Am Vet Med Assoc 182:992-93.

Carnel, S. B., Schraeder, P. L., and Lathers, C. M. 1985. Effect of phenobarbital pretreatment on cardiac neural discharge and pentylenetetrazolinduced epileptogenic activity in the cat. Pharmacology 30(4):225–40.

Chastain, C. B., and Graham, C. L. 1978. Xanthomatosis secondary to diabetes mellitus in a dog. J Am Vet Med Assoc 172:1209-11.

Chauvet, A. E., Feldman, E. C., and Kass, P. H. 1995. Effects of phenobarbital administration on results of serum biochemical analyses and adrenocortical function tests in epileptic dogs. J Am Vet Med Assoc 207(10):1305–7.

Ciaccio, P. J., Duignan, D. B., and Halpert, J. R. 1987. Selective inactivation by chloramphenicol of the major phenobarbital–inducible isozyme of dog liver cytochrome P–450. Drug Metab Disp 15(6):852–56.

Ciaccio, P. J., and Halpert, J. R. 1989. Characterization of a phenobarbital inducible dog liver cytochrome P450 structurally related to rat and human enzymes of the P450IIIA (steroid-inducible) gene subfamily. Arch Biochem Biophys 271:284-99.

Cochrane, S. M., Black, W. D., Parent, J. M., Allen, D. G., and Lumsden, J. H. 1990a. Pharmacokinetics of phenobarbital in the cat following intravenous and oral administration. Can J Vet Res 54(1):132–38.

Cochrane, S. M. Parent, J. M., Black, W. D., Allen, D. G., and Lumsden, J. H. 1990b. Pharmacokinetics of phenobarbital in the cat following multiple oral administration. Can J Vet Res 54(3):309–12.

Conney, A. H., Burns, I. J. 1972. Metabolic interactions among environmental chemicals and drugs. Science 178:576-86.

Cronin, M. F., Booth, N. H., Hatch, R. C., Brown, J. 1983. Acepromazine-xylazine combination in dogs: antagonism with 4-aminopyridine and yohimbine. Am J Vet Res 44:2037-42.

Cunningham, J. G. 1984. Canine Pract 11:39.

Cunningham, J. G., Haidukewych, D., and Jensen, H. A. 1983. Therapeutic serum concentrations of primidone and its metabolites, phenobarbital and phenylethylmalonamide, in epileptic dogs. J Am Vet Med Assoc 182:1091-94.

Darcey, T. M., and Williamson, P. D. 1992. Chronic/semichronic limbic epilepsy produced by microinjection of tetanus toxin in cat hippocampus. Epilepsia 33(3):402–19.

Davis, H. L., Johnson, D. D., and Crawford, R. D. 1978. Epileptiform seizures in domestic fowl. VII. Plasma phenytoin concentrations and anticonvulsant activity. Can J Physiol Pharmacol 56:310-15.

Dayton, P. G., Cucinell, S. A., Weiss, N., and Perel, J. M. 1967. Dose-dependence of drug plasma level decline in dogs. J Pharmacol Exp Ther 158:305-16.

de Angelis, L. 1979. Drugs Today 15:107.

Delbarre, B., and Schmitt, H. 1973. A further attempt to characterize sedative receptors activated by clonidine in chickens and mice. Eur J Pharmacol 22:355-59.

Delgado-Escueta, A. V., Wasterlain, C., Treiman, D. M., et al. 1982. Current concepts in neurology: management of status epilepticus. N Engl J Med 306:1337-40.

Dendi, J. A. H. 1979. Vet Med Rev 2:103.
Dendi, J. A. H., and Parada, H. L. 1981. Vet Med Rev 4:1.
Diaz, J., and Schain, R. J. 1978. Science 199:90.
Duran, S. H., Ravis, W. R., Pedersoli, W. M., and Schumacher, J. 1987. Pharmacokinetics of phenobarbital in the horse. Am J Vet Res 48(5):807–10.
Eadie, M. J. 1991. Formation of active metabolites of anticonvulsant drugs. Clin Pharmacol Int 21:27-41.
Errecalde, J. O., Button, C., Mulders, M. S. 1985. Some dynamic and toxic effects of theophylline in horses. J Vet Pharmacol Ther 8:320-27.
Faingold, C. L. 1985. Fed Proc 44:2412.
Faris, R. A., and Campbell, T. C. 1981. Exposure of newborn rats to pharmacologically active compounds may permanently alter carcinogen metabolism. Science 211:719-21.
Farnbach, G. C. 1984. Serum concentrations and efficacy of phenytoin, phenobarbital, and primidone in canine epilepsy. J Am Vet Med Assoc 184:1117-20.
Forrester, S. D., Wilcke, J. R., Jacobson, J. D., et al. 1993. Effects of a 44-day administration of phenobarbital on disposition of clorazepate in dogs. Am J Vet Res 54:1136-38.
Frey, H.-H. 1986. Vet Rec 118:484.
Frey, H.-H., and Löscher, W. 1980. Clinical pharmacokinetics of phenytoin in the dog: a reevaluation. Am J Vet Res 41:1635-38.
———. 1985. Pharmacokinetics of anti-epileptic drugs in the dog: a review. J Vet Pharmacol Ther 8:219.
Fromm, G. H. 1985. Fed Proc 44:2432.
Glazko, A. J. 1973. Diphenylhydantoin metabolism. A prospective view. Drug Metab Dispos 1:711-14.
Glover, W. W. 1982. Gen Pharmacol 13:259.
Grewal, M. S. 1954. Correlation between anticonvulsant activity and plasma concentration of bromide. J Pharmacol Exp Ther 112:109-15.
Gullet, P. A. 1984. Proc Annu Meet Am Assoc Zoo Vet, p. 58.
Gupta, C., Sonawane, B. R., Yaffe, S. J., et al. 1980. Phenobarbital exposure in utero: alterations in female reproductive function in rats. Science 208:508-10.
Gupta, C., and Yaffee, S. J. 1982. Prenatal exposure to phenobarbital permanently decreases testosterone and causes reproductive dysfunction. Science 216:640-42.
Harbison, R. D., and Becker, B. A. 1969. Relation of dosage and time of administration of diphenylhydantoin to its teratogenic effect in mice. Teratology 2:305-11.
Hatch, R. C. 1973. Experiments on antagonism of barbiturate anesthesia with adrenergic, serotonergic, and cholinergic stimulants given alone and in combination. Am J Vet Res 34:1321-31.
Hatch, R. C., and Ruch, T. 1974. Experiments on antagonism of ketamine anesthesia in cats given adrenergic, serotonergic, and cholinergic stimulants alone and in combination. Am J Vet Res 35:35-39.
Hatch, R. C., Booth, N. H., Clark, J. D., Crawford, L. M., Jr., Kitzman, J. V., and Wallner, B. 1982. Antagonism of xylazine sedation in dogs by 4-aminopyridine and yohimbine. Am J Vet Res 43:1009-14.
Hatch, R. C., Booth, N. H., Kitzman, J. V., Wallner, B. M., and Clark, J. D. 1983a. Antagonism of ketamine anesthesia in cats by 4-aminopyridine and yohimbine. Am J Vet Res 44:417-23.
Hatch, R. C., Clark, J. D., Booth, N. H., and Kitzman, J. V. 1983b. Comparison of five preanesthetic medicaments in pentobarbital-anesthetized dogs: antagonism by 4-aminopyridine, yohimbine, and naloxone. Am J Vet Res 44:2312-19.
Hatch, R. C., Jernigan, A. D., Wilson, R. C., Lipham, I. B., Booth, N. H., Clark, J. D., and Brown, J. 1986. Prompt arousal from fentanyl-droperidol-pentobarbital anesthesia in dogs: a preliminary study. Can J Vet Res 50:251-58.
Hatch, R. C., Kitzman, J. V., Clark, J. D., Zahner, J. M., and Booth, N. H. 1984a. Reversal of pentobarbital anesthesia with 4-aminopyridine and yohimbine in cats pretreated with acepromazine and xylazine. Am J Vet Res 45:2586-90.
Hatch, R. C., Kitzman, J. V., Zahner, J. M., et al. 1984b. Am J Vet Res 45:2322.
Hatch, R. C., Zahner, J. M., Booth, N. H. 1984c. Meperidine-acepromazine-pentobarbital anesthesia in cats: reversal by 4-aminopyridine and yohimbine. Am J Vet Res 45:2658-62.
Hatch, R. C., Kitzman, J. V., Zahner, J. M., and Clark, J. D. 1985a. Antagonism of xylazine sedation with yohimbine, 4-aminopyridine, and doxapram in dogs. Am J Vet Res 46:371-75.
Hatch, R. C., Wilson, R. C., Jernigan, A. D., Clark, J. D., and Brown, J. 1985b. Reversal of thiopental-induced anesthesia by 4-aminopyridine, yohimbine, and doxapram in dogs pretreated with xylazine or acepromazine. Am J Vet Res 46:1473-78.
Hendricks, H. L., Bush, P. B., Kitzman, J. V., and Booth, N. H. 1984. Determination of 4-aminopyridine in horse plasma using gas-liquid chromatography. J Chromatogr 287:429-32.
Henricks, P. M. 1987. Dermatitis associated with the use of primidone in a dog. J Am Vet Med Assoc 191(2):237–38.
Hillidge, C. J. 1976. The use of Dopram as a respiratory stimulant following Immobilon in the pony. Equine Vet J 8:173-75.
Hirshman, C. A., McCullough, R. E., Cohen, P. J., Weil, and J. V. 1977. Depression of hypoxic ventilatory response by halothane, enflurane and isoflurane in dogs. Br J Anaesth 49:957-63.
Hsu, W. H. 1985. Xylazine-pentobarbital anesthesia in dogs and its antagonism by yohimbine. Am J Vet Res 46:852-55.
Hsu, W. H., Lu, Z.-X., and Hembrough, F. B. 1985a. Effect of xylazine on heart rate and arterial blood pressure in conscious dogs, as influenced by atropine, 4-aminopyridine, doxapram, and yohimbine. J Am Vet Med Assoc 186:153-56.
Hsu, W. H., McGruder, J. P., and Lu, Z.-X. 1985b. Vet Med 90:69.
Hsu, W., and Lu, Z.-X. 1986. Effect of amitraz on heart rate and aortic blood pressure in conscious dogs: influence of atropine, prazosin, tolazoline, and yohimbine. Toxicol Appl Pharmacol 84:418-22.
Hsu, W. H., Schaffer, D. D., and Hanson, C. E. 1987. Effects of tolazoline and yohimbine on xylazine-induced central nervous system depression, bradycardia, and tachypnea in sheep. J Am Vet Med Assoc 190:423-26.
Jagoda, A., and Riggio, S. 1993. Refractory status epilepticus in adults. Annals of Emerg Med 22:129-140.
Jacobson, E. R., and Kollias, G. V. 1984. Proc Annu Meet Am Assoc Zoo Vet, p. 58.
Jensen, E. C., and Klemm, W. R. 1967. Clinical evaluation of the analeptic, doxapram, in dogs and cats. J Am Vet Med Assoc 150:516-25.
Jensen, J., Tamas, P., and McNeil, B. 1983. Proc Annu Meet Am Assoc Zoo Vet, p. 65.
Jensen, W. A. 1985. J Am Vet Med Assoc 187:627.
Johnson, D. D., Davis, H. L., Bailey, D. G., et al. 1977. Epileptiform seizures in domestic fowl. VI. Plasma phenobarbital concentrations and anticonvulsant activity. Can J Physiol Pharmacol 55:848-54.
Johnson, D. D., Davis, H. L., and Crawford, R. D. 1979. Pharmacological and biochemical studies in epileptic fowl. (Review.) Fed Proc 38:2417-23.
Katasumata, M., Gupta, C., Baker, M. K., et al. 1982. Diphenylhydantoin: an alternative ligand of a glucocorti-

coid receptor affecting prostaglandin generation in A/J mice. Science 218:1313-15.
Kay, W. J. 1975. J Am Anim Hosp Assoc 11:77.
Kay, W. J., and Fenner, W. R. 1977. In R. W. Kirk, ed., Current Veterinary Therapy VI: Small Animal Practice, p. 853. Philadelphia: W. B. Saunders.
Keith, D. A., Gundberg, C. M., Japour, A., et al. 1983. Vitamin K-dependent proteins and anticonvulsant medication. Clin Pharmacol Ther 34:529-32.
Kitagawa, T., Pitot, H. C., Miller, E. C., et al. 1979. Promotion by dietary phenobarbital of hepatocarcinogenesis by 2-methyl-N,N-dimethyl-4-aminoazobenzene in the rat. Cancer Res 39:112-15.
Kitzman, J. V., Wilson, R. C., Booth, N. H., et al. 1984b. Pharmacokinetics of 4-aminopyridine in cattle. Am J Vet Res 45:2625-27.
Kitzman, J. V., Wilson, R. C., Hatch, R. C., and Booth, N. H. 1984c. Antagonism of xylazine and ketamine anesthesia by 4-aminopyridine and yohimbine in geldings. Am J Vet Res 45:875-79.
Klemm, W. R. 1966. Evaluation of effectiveness of doxapram and various analeptic combinations in dogs. J Am Vet Med Assoc 148:894-99.
Klotz, U., Antonin, K. H., and Bieck, P. R. 1976. Pharmacokinetics and plasma binding of diazepam in man, dog, rabbit, guinea pig and rat. J Pharmacol Exp Therap 199(1):67–73.
Knill, R. L., and Gelb, A. W. 1978. Ventilatory responses to hypoxia and hypercapnia during halothane sedation and anesthesia in man. Anesthesiology 49:244-51.
Knox, D. A., Ravis, W. R., Pedersoli, W. M., et al. 1992. Pharmacokinetics of phenobarbital in horses after single and repeated oral administration of the drug. Am J Vet Res 53:706-10.
Kowalczyk, D. F., and Beech, J. 1983. Pharmacokinetics of phenytoin (diphenylhydantoin) in horses. J Vet Pharmacol Ther 6:133-40.
Kulkarni, S. K., and Mehta, A. K. 1984. Drugs Today 20:217.
Kuo, C.-H., Braselton, W. E., and Hook, J. B. 1982. Effect of phenobarbital on cephaloridine toxicity and accumulation in rabbit and rat kidneys. Toxicol Appl Pharmacol 64:244-54.
Lang, W. J., and Gershon, S. 1963. Arch Int Pharmacodyn 142:457.
Macdonald, R. L., and Barker, J. L. 1978. Different actions of anticonvulsant and anesthetic barbiturates revealed by use of cultured mammalian neurons. Science 200:775-77.
Marks, D. 1973. Mod Vet Pract 54:43.
Marquis, J.-F., Carruthers, S. G., Spence, J. D., et al. 1982. Phenytoin-theophylline interaction. N Engl J Med 307:1189-90.
Marrosu, F., Marchi, A., DeMartino, M. R., Saba, G., Gessa, G. L. 1985. Aminophylline antagonizes diazepam-induced anesthesia and EEG changes in humans. Psychopharmacology 85:69-70.
Marx, J. L. 1980. Science 208:274.
May, Greenwood, 1977.
McGruder J. P., Hsu, W. H. 1985. Antagonism of xylazine-pentobarbital anesthesia by yohimbine in ponies. Am J Vet Res 46:1276-81.
McKillop, D. 1985. Effects of phenobarbitone and beta-naphthoflavone on hepatic microsomal drug metabolising enzymes of the male Beagle dog. Biochem Pharmacol 34(17):3137-42.
Mealey, K. L., and Boothe, D. M. 1995. Bioavailability of benzodiazepines following rectal administration of diazepam in dogs. J Vet Pharmacol Therap 18(1):72–74.
Middaugh, L. D., Zemp, J. W., and Boggan, W. O. 1983. Pregnancy increases reactivity of mice to phenobarbital. Science 220:534-36.
Millicovsky, G., and Johnston, M. C. 1981. Maternal hyperoxia greatly reduces the incidence of phenytoin-induced cleft lip and palate in A/J mice. Science 212:671-72.
Mirkin, B. L. 1975. Perinatal pharmacology: placental transfer, fetal localization, and neonatal disposition of drugs. Anesthesiology 43:156-70.
Morselli, P. L., Rizzo, M., and Garattini, S. 1971. Interaction between phenobarbital and diphenylhydantoin in animals and in epileptic patients. Ann NY Acad Sci 179:88-107.
Muir, W. W., Sams, R. A., Huffman, R. H., and Noonan, J. S. 1982. Pharmacodynamic and pharmacokinetic properties of diazepam. American Journal of Veterinary Research. 43(10):17561762.
Nash, A. S., Thompson, H., and Bogan, J. A. 1977. Phenytoin toxicity: a fatal case in a dog with hepatitis and jaundice. Vet Rec 100:280-81.
Nichols, E. S., Trepanier, L. A., and Linn, K. 1996. Bromide toxicosis secondary to renal insufficiency in an epileptic dog. J Am Vet Med Assoc 208(2):231–33.
Nossaman, B. C., Amouzadeh, H. R., and Sangiah, S. 1990. Effects of chloramphenicol, cimetidine and phenobarbital on and tolerance to xylazine-ketamine anesthesia in dogs. Vet Hum Tox 32(3):216-19.
Papich, M. G., and Alcorn, J. 1995. Absorption of diazepam after its rectal administration in dogs. Am J Vet Res 56(12):1629–36.
Parker, A. J. 1982. Mod Vet Pract 63:460.
Pasten, L. J. 1977. J Am Anim Hosp Assoc 13:247.
Pearce, L. K. 1990. Potassium bromide as an adjunct to phenobarbital for the management of uncontrolled seizures in dogs. Probl Vet Neurol 1(1):95-101.
Pedersoli, W. M., Redding, R. W., and Nachreiner, R. F. 1981. J Am Anim Hosp Assoc 17:271.
Pedersoli, W. M., Wike, J. S., and Ravis, W. R. 1987. Pharmacokinetics of single doses of phenobarbital given intravenously and orally to dogs. Am J Vet Res 48:679-83.
Peraino, C., Ehret, C. F., Groh, K. R., et al. 1980. Phenobarbital effects on weight gain and circadian cycling of food intake and body temperature. Proc Soc Exp Biol Med 165:473-79.
Podell, M., and Fenner, W. R. 1993. Bromide therapy in refractory canine idiopathic epilepsy. J Vet Int Med 7:318-27.
Poffenbarger, E. M., and Hardy, R. M. 1985. J Am Vet Med Assoc 186:978.
Rauws, A. G., van Logeten, M. J. 1975. The influence of dietary chloride on bromide excretion in the rat. Toxicology 3:29-32.
Ravis, W. R., Nachreiner, R. F., Pedersoli, W. M., et al. 1984. Am J Vet Res 45:1283.
Ravis, W. R., Duran, S. H., Pedersoli, W. M., and Schumacher, J. 1987. A pharmacokinetic study of phenobarbital in mature horses after oral dosing. J Vet Pharmacol Therap 10(4):283–89.
Ravis, W. R., Pedersoli, W. M., and Wike, J. S. 1989. Pharmacokinetics of phenobarbital in dogs given multiple doses. Am J Vet Res 50(8):1343-47.
Ray, A. C., Dwyer, J. N., Fambro, G. W., and Reagor, J. C. 1978. Clinical signs and chemical confirmation of 4-aminopyridine poisoning in horses. Am J Vet Res 39:329-31.
Redding, R. W. 1969. J Am Anim Hosp Assoc 5:79.
Renecker, L. A., and Olsen, C. D. 1985. Use of yohimbine and 4-aminopyridine to antagonize xylazine-induced immobilization in North American Cervidae. J Am Vet Med Assoc 187:1199-201.
Roye, D. B., Serrano, E. E., Hammer, R. H., and Wilder, B. J. 1973. Plasma kinetics of diphenylhydantoin in dogs and cats. Am J Vet Res 34:947-50.
Rupp, S. M., Shinohara, Y., Fisher, D. M., Miller, R. D., and Castagnoli, N., Jr. 1983. Pharmacokinetics and

pharmacodynamics of 4-aminopyridine in anesthetized dogs. J Pharmacol Exp Ther 225:351-54.

Sams, R. A., and Muir, W. W. 1988. Effects of phenobarbital on thiopental pharmacokinetics in Greyhounds. Am J Vet Res 49(2):245-49.

Sanders, J. E., and Yeary, R. A. 1978. Serum concentrations of orally administered diphenylhydantoin in dogs. J Am Vet Med Assoc 172:153-56.

Sanders, J. E., Yeary, R. A., Fenner W. R., et al. 1979a. Interaction of phenytoin with chloramphenicol or pentobarbital in the dog. J Am Vet Med Assoc 175:177-80.

Sanders, J. E., Yeary, R. A., Powers, J. D., et al. 1979b. Relationship between serum and brain concentrations of phenytoin in the dog. Am J Vet Res 40:473-76.

Sawchuck, S. A., Parker, A. J., Neff-Davis, C., and Davis, L. 1985. Primidone in the cat. J Am Anim Hosp Assoc 21:647-50.

Schmitt, H., LeDouarec, J.-C., and Petillot, N. 1974. Antagonism of the antinociceptive action of xylazine, an alpha-sympathomimetic agent, by adrenoceptor and cholinoceptor blocking agents. Neuropharmacology 13:295-303.

Schwartz-Porsche, D., Löscher, W., and Frey, H.-H. 1982. Treatment of canine epilepsy with primidone. J Am Vet Med Assoc 181:592-95.

———. 1985. J Vet Pharmacol Ther 8:113.

Schwartz-Porsche, D., and Jurgens, U. 1991. Effectiveness of bromide in therapy resistant epilepsy of dogs. Tierarztliche Praxis 19(4):395–401.

Seawright, A. A., Steele, D. P., Mudie, A. W., and Bishop, R. 1972. The effect of diet and drugs on hepatic microsomal amino pyridine N-demethylase activity in vitro and susceptibility to carbon tetrachloride in sheep. Res Vet Sci 13:245-56.

Severinghaus, J., Ozanne, G., and Massuda, Y. 1976. Measurement of the ventilatory response to hypoxia: a step hypoxia three-minute test. Chest 70:121-24.

Shaw, N., Trepanier, L. A., Center, S. A., and Garland, S. 1996. High dietary chloride content associated with loss of therapeutic serum bromide concentrations in an epileptic dog. J Am Vet Med Assoc 208(2):234–36.

Shini, S., Klaus, A. M., and Hapke, H. J. 1997. Kinetics of elimination of diazepam after intravenous injection in horses. DTW—Deutsche Tierarztliche Wochenschrift. 104(1):22–25.

Short, C. E., and Cloyd, G. D. 1970. The use of doxapram hydrochloride with inhalation anesthetics in horses. II. Vet Med Small Anim Clin 65:260-61.

Short, C. E., Cloyd, G. D., and Ward, J. W. 1970. An evaluation of doxapram hydrochloride to control respiration in dogs during and after inhalation anesthesia. Vet Med Small Anim Clin 65:787-90.

Short, C. E., Gleed, R. D., Bristol, D., et al. 1982. Vet Med Small Anim Clin 80:1761.

Sodikoff, C. 1982. Mod Vet Pract 63:563.

Soma, L. R., and Kenny, R. 1967. Am J Vet Res 28:191.

Spehar, A. M., Hill, M. R., Mayhew, I. G., et al. 1984. Preliminary study on the pharmacokinetics of phenobarbital in the neonatal foal. Equine Vet J 16:368-71.

Starke, K., Borowski, E., and Endo, T. 1975. Preferential blockade of presynaptic alpha-adrenoceptors by yohimbine. Eur J Pharmacol 34:385-88.

St. John, W. M., Cunningham, M. H., Johnson, J. W., and Glasser, R. L. 1973. Pontile pneumotaxic center regulation of doxapram-induced respiratory alterations. Proc SocExp Biol Med 142:1215-21.

Sumi, T. 1993. Different effects of chronically administered phenobarbital on amygdaloid– and hippocampal–kindled seizures in the cat. Hokkaido Igaku Zasshi—Hokkaido J Med Sci 68(2):177–89.

Thurston, J. H., Hauhart, R. E., and Naccarato, E. F. 1981. Taurine: possible role in osmotic regulation of mammalian heart. Science 214:1373-74.

Tobin, T., Dirdjosudjono, S., and Baskin, S. I. 1973. Pharmacokinetics and distribution of diphenylhydantoin in kittens. Am J Vet Res 34:951-54.

Tobin, T. T., Combie, J., and Shults, 1979. J Equine Med Surg 3:102.

Tranquilli, W. J., Thurmon, J. C., Corbin, J. E., Benson, G. J., and Davis, L. E. 1984. Halothane-sparing effect of xylazine in dogs and subsequent reversal with tolazoline. J Vet Pharmacol Ther 7:23-28.

Uges, D. R., Sohn, Y. J., Greijdanus, B., Scaf, A. H., and Agoston, S. 1982. 4-Aminopyridine kinetics. Clin Pharmacol Ther 31:587-93.

Valerino, D. M., Vesell, E. S., Aurori, K. C., and Johnson, A. O. 1974. Effects of various barbiturates on hepatic microsomal enzymes: a comparative study. Drug Metab Dipos 2:448-57.

van Gelder, N. M., Sherwin, A. L., Sacks, C., and Anderman, F. 1975. Biochemical observations following administration of taurine to patients with epilepsy. Brain Res 94:297-306.

Villareale, M., Gould, L. V., Wasserman, R. H., Barr, A., Chiroff, R. T., and Bergstom, W. H. 1974. Diphenylhydantoin: effects on calcium metabolism in the chick. Science 183:671-73.

Vu, V. T., Bai, S. A., and Abramson, F. P. 1983. Interactions of phenobarbital with propranolol in the dog. 2. Bioavailability, metabolism and pharmacokinetics. J Pharmacol Exp Ther 224:55-61.

Wallner, B. M., Hatch, R. C., Booth, N. H., Kitzman, J. V., Clark, J. D., and Brown, J. 1982. Complete immobility produced in dogs by xylazine-atropine: antagonism by 4-aminopyridine and yohimbine. Am J Vet Res 43:2259-65.

Wang, S. C., and Ward, J. W. 1977. Analeptics. Pharmacol Ther (B)3:123-65.

Weiskopf, R. B., Raymond, L. W., and Severinghaus, J. W. 1974. Effects of halothane on canine respiratory responses to hypoxia with and without hypercarbia. Anesthesiology 41:350-60.

Woody, R. C. 1990. Bromide therapy for pediatric seizure disorder intractable to other antiepileptic drugs. J Child Neurology 5:65-67.

Wuth, O. 1927. Rational bromide treatment. JAMA 88:2013-17.

Yohn, S. E., Morrison, W. B., and Sharp, P. E. 1992. Bromide toxicosis (bromism) in a dog treated with potassium bromide for refractory seizures. J Am Vet Med Assoc 201(3):468–740.

Zahner, J. M., Hatch, R. C., Wilson, R. C., Booth, N. H., Kitzman, and J. V., Brown, J. 1984. Antagonism of xylazine sedation in steers by doxapram and 4-aminopyridine. Am J Vet Res 45:2546–51.

17 DRUGS AFFECTING ANIMAL BEHAVIOR

DAWN M. BOOTHE[1]

PHYSIOLOGY AND PATHOPHYSIOLOGY OF BEHAVIOR DISORDERS
DRUGS USED TO MODIFY BEHAVIOR
Antipsychotic Drugs
Structure-Activity Relationship
Pharmacologic Effects
Disposition
Side Effects and Toxicity
Drug Interactions
Clinical Indications
Antidepressant Drugs
Tricyclic Antidepressants
Selective Serotonin-Reuptake Inhibitors
Monoamine Oxidase Inhibitors
Anxiolytics
Anxioselective Drugs: Azapirones (Buspirone)
Miscellaneous (Nonspecific) Drugs Used to Modify Behavior
Progestins
Anticonvulsants
Narcotic Agonists and Antagonists
Antihistamines
Beta Blockers
Stimulants

PHYSIOLOGY AND PATHOPHYSIOLOGY OF BEHAVIOR DISORDERS

Little is known regarding the cellular mechanisms of abnormal behavior in humans or animals. The most likely neurotransmitters associated with abnormal behavior are assumed to be those targeted by drugs used to modify the behaviors. These include the biogenic amines, serotonin and histamine (H_1 subtype); the monoamine dopamine; the catecholamine norepinephrine; acetylcholine; γ-aminobutyric acid (GABA); and excitatory amino acids (Overall 1997; Simpson and Simpson 1996).

The drugs most effective in modifying behavior tend to be selective for serotonin (e.g., fluoxetine, clomipramine). Some studies support serotonin as the most likely neurotransmitter associated with abnormal behavior. For example, in cats, activation of serotonin receptor subtypes 5-HT_{1A} and 5-$HT_{2/1C}$ in the hypothalamus modulates the expression of rage behavior (Shaikh et al. 1997). Serotonin is synthesized in the brain from tryptophan. Of at least nine serotonin (5-hydroxytryptamine, 5-HT) receptor subtypes found in the body, four appear to be particularly important (Simpson and Simpson 1996). Serotonin receptors differ in anatomical location and behavioral roles. The 5-HT_1 receptors, located primarily in the brain, are predominantly inhibitory (inhibition of adenyl cyclase), both pre- and postsynaptically. They appear to affect mood and behavior (Overall 1997). Regulation of serotonin action is complex, involving both pre- and postsynaptic mechanisms (Simpson and Simpson 1996).

Norepinephrine, the end product of dopamine oxidation, is inactivated primarily by active transport, i.e., reuptake from the synaptic-cleft presynaptic vesicles. It is deaminated by mitochondrial monoamine oxidases. Norepinephrine is located predominantly in the gray matter of the pons and in the medulla. Norepinephrine interacts with α_1 (via G-protein-mediated activation of phospholipase C and subsequent formation of inositol triphosphate) and β receptors (via activation of adenylyl cyclase) postsynaptically. Interaction with α_2 receptors (also via G proteins) occurs presynaptically. Norepinephrine appears to affect arousal, functional reward systems, and mood. The last effect may reflect a decrease in depression and an increase in mania.

Dopamine is synthesized from L-dopa in presynaptic vesicles; L-dopa is produced from dietary tyrosine (Simpson and Simpson 1996). Tyrosine is first oxidated (by tyrosine oxidase), then decarboxylated. Dopamine is metabolized by monamine oxidases (MAO) and catechol-*O*-methyltransferase (COMT). Dopamine receptors are distributed throughout the brain, but less so than norepinephrine. Dopamine appears to be largely located in the midbrain, hypothalamus, and limbic system (the part of the brain thought to control emotions) (Simpson and Simpson 1996). Dopamine receptors (at least five subtypes) also are found in portions of the extrapyramidal system responsible for coordinated movement (Overall 1997). At least four dopamine receptors are affected by mood disorders and stereotypies; increased dopamine appears to stimulate these abnormal behaviors (Overall 1997).

GABA is a major inhibitory neurotransmitter, being active at 30% of the synapses in the human central nervous system (CNS). It is formed from glutamate, which is widely distributed throughout the brain. Two primary receptor types, $GABA_A$ and $GABA_B$, appear to cause postsynaptic inhibition by facilitating chloride ion influx into the neuron. Several drugs, including benzodiazepines and barbiturates (such as phenobarbital), interact with the receptor in an agonistic fashion, causing neuronal inhibition (Overall 1997). The physiologic and behavioral effects of GABA and its receptors have not yet been well characterized (Simpson and Simpson 1996).

Excitatory neurotransmitters may increase and cause or be associated with several abnormal behaviors, including aggressive, impulsive, and schizophrenic disorders in humans. Among the more important excitatory neurotransmitters is glutamate. Glutamate is preformed and stored in synaptic vesicles that are released by calcium-mediated endocytosis. Barbiturates and progesterone modulate behavior, in part, by inhibiting calcium uptake and thus the release of glutamate at the neurotransmitter (Overall 1997).

Acetylcholine is the most widely distributed neurotransmitter in the brain (Simpson and Simpson 1996). It is produced from choline and rapidly metabolized by acetylcholinesterase. It tends to be an excitatory neurotransmitter. Like glutamate, it is preformed and stored at the terminal end of the synapse in vesicles that are stimulated by calcium to release the neurotransmitter by exocytosis. The primary significance of acetylcholine and behavior-modifying drugs is the likelihood of adverse reactions occurring when M_1 receptors are antagonized (Overall 1997).

Because neurotransmitters tend to be formed and degraded locally, both formation and inhibition offer pharmacologic targets. A number of drugs result in an increase in the presence of neurotransmitters in the synaptic cleft by inhibiting either the metabolism (e.g., dopamine) or the reuptake (e.g., serotonin, norepinephrine) of the neurotransmitter following release (Fig. 17.1).

DRUGS USED TO MODIFY BEHAVIOR

Drugs that modify behavior include the antipsychotic drugs (predominantly antidopaminergic in action), anxioselective drugs such as the azapirones (primarily antiserotonergic in action), drugs used to treat affective or mood disorders (antidepressants, lithium, and selected anticonvulsant drugs), and drugs used to treat anxiety and related disorders (anxiolytics, minor tranquilizers, benzodiazepines). Other drugs include antihistamines, beta blockers, progestins, anticonvulsants, and opioid antagonists. Many of these drugs are also used to treat other disorders and may be discussed elsewhere in this book. Only drugs that have veterinary application are discussed.

Care must be taken to distinguish behavior that is perceived to be abnormal by the pet owner from normal behavior. Pharmacologic management of abnormal behavior should be approached as an adjunct, and specifically as a facilitator, to normalizing behavior rather than as a cure. A number of nondrug techniques have been recommended by many animal behaviorists (Landsberg 1994; Voith 1985a,b, 1992; Houpt 1997a,b). Abnormal behaviors that require drug therapy should be simultaneously managed with behavioral modification training (e.g., decreasing arousal and fear can facilitate learning a new behavior; Juarbe-Diaz 1997a,b). The use of behavior-modifying drugs is not well studied in cats and dogs, and recommended indications are rarely based on well-controlled clinical trials. In addition, many of the drugs used to modify behavior can cause serious side effects, and the unpredictability of plasma or tissue drug concentrations increases the likelihood of adverse reactions. Many of the side effects may not be readily observed by the pet owner, further increasing the risk. Finally, slow response to therapy may lead to unsupervised manipulation of dosing regimens by the pet owner, again predisposing the animal to adverse reactions. Owners should be well counseled regarding the risks and benefits of behavior-modifying drugs, including potential changes in behavior that may be less desirable than the behavior targeted by the drug. Although many drugs recommended for use in dogs and cats are approved for human but not veterinary use, behavior-modifying drugs stand out as potential adverse risks (Johnson 1990). Obtaining informed owner consent is prudent prior to implementing therapy with these drugs. Caution should also be taken to prevent substance abuse by pet owners.

Monitoring serum drug concentrations may be of benefit for selected drugs. However, monitoring must be performed in conjunction with clinical response, including both efficacy and safety. Antidepressants should be used cautiously or not at all in patients suffering from metabolic illnesses. Adequate time must be given before a drug or a dosing regimen is considered to have failed. At least two drug elimination half-lives should elapse. In general, combinations of behavior-modifying drugs should be avoided. One drug should be withdrawn, often slowly, before another is begun. A drug-free period of two drug elimination half-lives is recommended in humans before a new drug is begun. Generally, 10–20 days should elapse for a short-acting drug and up to 6–8 weeks for longer acting drugs (Overall 1997).

The descriptions of drug therapy for selected behaviors that follow (see also Table 17.1) are not intended to be used as a "cookbook" approach to managing abnormal behavior in dogs and cats. Rather, clinicians should familiarize themselves with the assumed behavior and its proper nondrug behavioral modification management. Clinicians should be thoroughly familiar with the drug to be used. Because indications are less clear with these drugs, emphasis should be placed on side effects, drug interactions, and contraindications. Consultation with a veterinary animal behaviorist is strongly recommended prior to implementing any drug therapy.

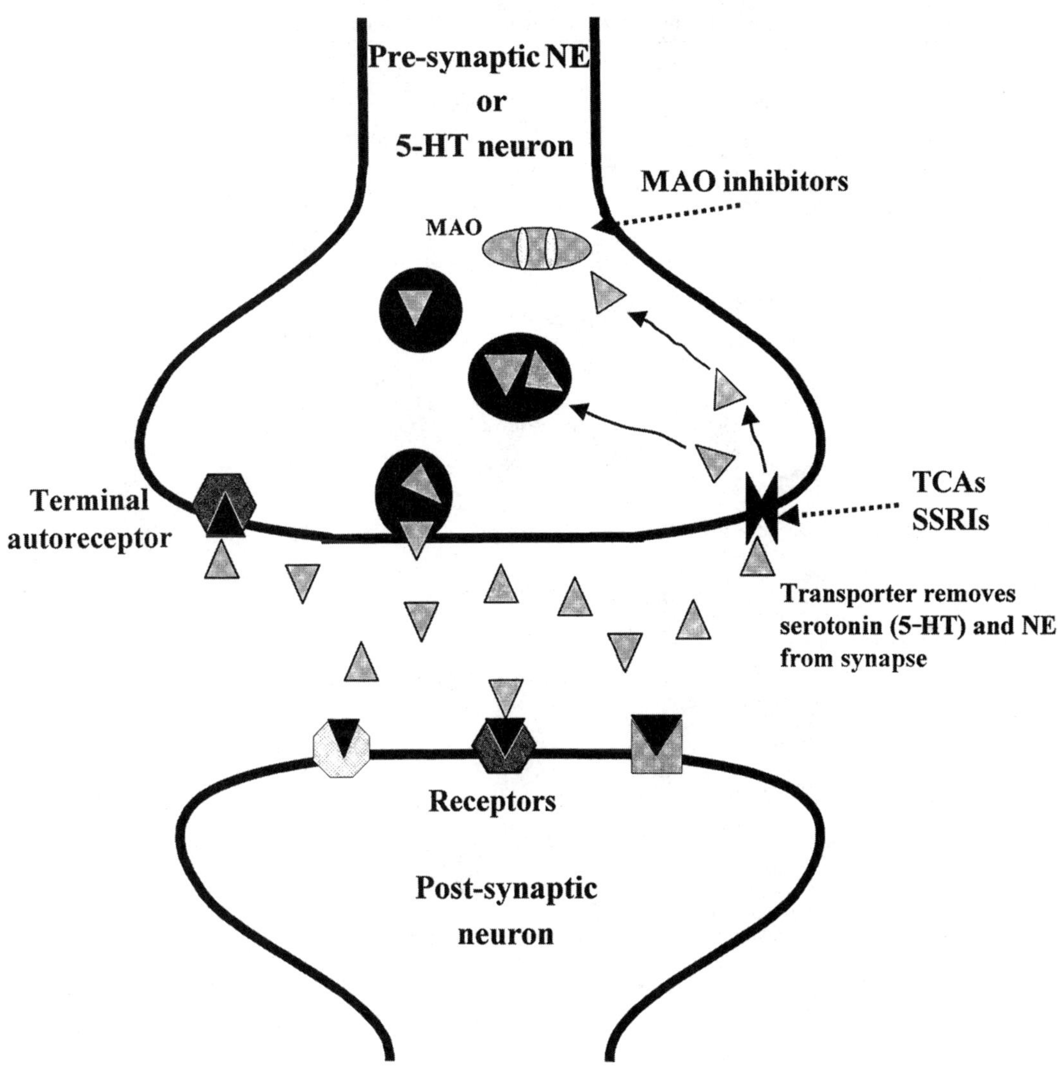

FIG. 17.1—Mechanism of action of selected behavior-modifying drugs. Neurotransmitters responsible for behavior are released from the presynaptic neuron into the synaptic cleft and interact with postsynaptic receptors. Following exocytosis, inactivation of the transmitter occurs primarily by reuptake into the presynaptic neuron, the site of action of most behavior-modifying drugs (TCAs = tricyclic antidepressants; SSRIs = selective serotonin reuptake inhibitors; NE = norepinephrine). Activation also may involve metabolic degradation, as in the case of the monamine oxidases (MAO).(Reprinted, with permission, from Boothe in press.)

ANTIPSYCHOTIC DRUGS. Psychotic disorders in humans involve a severe disturbance of brain function characterized by thought and speech disruption and hallucinations or delusions (Simpson and Simpson 1996). Although psychotic disorders do not occur in veterinary medicine, drugs developed for their management in humans have proven efficacious for a number of veterinary applications. Antipsychotic drugs (also called neuroleptics or major tranquilizers) include the phenothiazines, thioxanthenes (structurally related to the phenothiazines), heterocyclic dibenzepines, butyrophenones, and diphenylbutylpiperidines (Baldessarini 1996a) (Fig. 17.2).

Structure-Activity Relationship. Antipsychotic drugs are categorized by structure and by potency. Low-potency drugs (chlorpromazine, acepromazine, promazine) are characterized by greater sedation and more cardiac and anticholinergic side effects than their high-potency counterparts. High-potency drugs (e.g., haloperidol, fluphenazine, trifluoperazine, prochlorperazine, and thiothixene) are administered at lower doses

TABLE 17.1—Doses of drugs used to modify behavior in small animals

Drug	Class	Dose	Route	Interval (hr)
Acepromazine	Phenothiazine	1–2 mg/kg	PO	8
	Sedative	0.05–0.1 mg/kg	IV, IM	8
Alprazolam	Benzodiazepine	0.01–0.1 mg/kg [D] (not to exceed 4 mg)	PO	As needed
	Anxiolytic	0.125–0.25 mg/kg [C]	PO	12
Amitriptyline	TCA	1–4.4 mg/kg [D]	PO	12–24
		0.5–2.0 mg/kg [C]	PO	12–24
Buspirone	Azaperone	2.5–10 mg [D] (not to exceed 2 mg/kg)	PO	24
	Anxioselective	1 mg/kg [D]	PO	8–12
		0.5–1 mg/kg [C]	PO	8–12
Carbamazepine	Anticonvulsant	400–1600 mg	PO	Divided every 8–12 hr
		4–8 mg/kg [D]	PO	8-12
Clomipramine	TCA	1–3 mg/kg [D] (not to exceed 200 mg/day)	PO	12–24, increasing dose at 14-d intervals
		0.5 mg/kg [C]	PO	24
Clonazepam	Benzodiazepine	1–10 mg [D]	PO	6–24
	Anxiolytic	0.5–1.5 mg/kg [D]	PO	
Clorazepate	Benzodiazepine Anxiolytic	0.5–1 mg/kg	PO	12–24
	Benzodiazepine sustained delivery Anxiolytic	11.25––22.5 mg/dog	PO	12–24
Dextrometamphetamine	Stimulant	2.5–5 mg (medium-sized dog)	PO	12-24
Diazepam	Benzodiazepine Anxiolytic	0.25–1 mg/kg	PO	6–12
	Benzodiazepine sustained delivery Anxiolytic	0.5–1 mg/kg	PO	12–24
Doxepin	TCA (antihistaminergic)	3–5 mg/kg [D]	PO	12
Fluoxetine	SSRI	1 mg/kg [D]	PO	12–24
	Antidepressant	0.5–1 mg/kg [C]	PO	24
Haloperidol	Tranquilizer Butyrophenone	1–4 mg [D]	PO	12
Hydrocodone	Opioid agonist	0.25 mg/kg [D]	PO	8
		0.25–1 mg/kg [C]	PO	8–12
Hydroxyzine	Antihistamine (H_1)	2.2 mg/kg	PO	8
Imipramine	TCA	2.2–4.4 mg/kg [D]	PO	12–24
Lorazepam	Benzodiazepine Anxiolytic			
Medroxyprogesterone acetate	Progestin	11 mg/kg	IM, SC	As needed (3–6 mo)
Megestrol acetate	Progestin	1–2 mg/kg (up to 4 mg/kg; see text)	PO	24 for 7–14 d then decreasing doses by ½ until discontinued at 3–6 wk
Methylphenidate	Stimulant	0.25 mg/kg [D]	PO	12–24?
Nalfeme	Opioid antagonist	1–4 mg/kg	IM	As needed
Naloxone	Opioid antagonist	11–22 µg/kg	IV, SC, IM	As needed
Naltrexone	Opioid antagonist	1–4 mg/kg	PO	12–24
Nortryptiline	TCA (metabolite of amitriptyline)	1–2 mg/kg [D]	PO	12
Oxazepam	Anxiolytic Benzodiazepine	0.2–0.5 mg/kg [C]	PO	12–24
Paroxetine	SSRI	1 mg/kg	PO	24
Perphenazine	Phenothiazine Tranquilizer	0.88 mg/kg	PO	8–12
Pindolol	Beta blocker	0.124–0.25	PO 24	
Propranolol	Beta blocker	0.5–2 mg/kg	PO	8
Protriptyline	TCA	5 mg [D]	PO	24, at bedtime
Thioridazine	Phenothiazine	1.1–2.2 mg/kg [D]	PO	12–24

Note: [D] = dog; [C] = cat; TCA = tricyclic antidepressant; SSRI = selective serotonin-reuptake inhibitor.

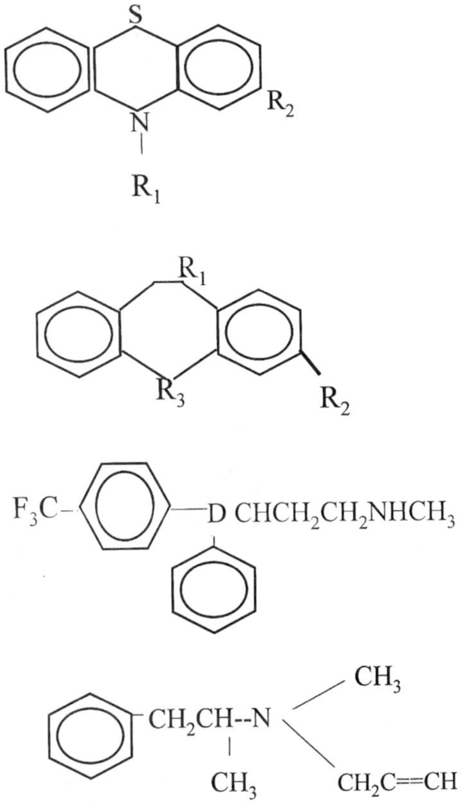

Phenothiazines

Chlorpromazine
Acepromazine

Tricyclic Antidepressants

Amitriptyline
Clomipramine
Doxepin
Imipramine

Selective Serotonin-Reuptake Inhibitor

Fluoxetine

Monoamine Oxidase Inhibitor

Selegiline

FIG. 17.2—Structures of selected behavior-modifying drugs. (Reprinted, with permission, from Boothe in press.

and are associated with less sedation and fewer anticholinergic and cardiac side effects. However, they have a greater incidence of extrapyramidal side effects. The largest structural class of antipsychotics is composed of the phenothiazines, or tricyclic antipsychotics (not to be confused with the tricyclic antidepressant drugs) (Baldessarini 1996a).

Tricyclic antipsychotic drugs are represented by phenothiazine, a three-ring structure containing a sulfur and a nitro group in the ring connecting two benzene rings. Substitutions on one of the benzene rings yield different drugs (e.g., chlorpromazine, promazine), which differ in efficacy (Fig. 17.2). The pharmacology is also impacted by substitutions on the nitro groups such that potency (but not efficacy) is reduced by an aliphatic side chain (e.g., chlorpromazine, thorazine, acepromazine, and trifluopromazine) (Baldessarini 1996a). The length of the side chain also determines antihistaminergic properties, with two-carbon side chains such as that occurring in promethazine being more antihistaminergic. Drugs with higher potency have a piperazine side chain, including fluphenazine and rifluoperazone. Esterification with long-chain fatty acids results in long-acting (due to slow hydrolysis and absorption) drugs (e.g., fluphenazine enanthate and decanoate) (Baldessarini 1996a). The use of these long-acting drugs in veterinary medicine has yet to be established.

The butyrophenone antipsychotics include haloperidol (the prototype) and droperidol. The latter is very short acting and highly sedative; thus its use is limited to anesthetic regimens (Baldessarini 1996a).

Pharmacologic Effects. The pharmacologic effects of antipsychotic drugs generally are similar in human beings and animals (Baldessarini 1996a). Phenothiazines are also categorized as tranquilizers. As tranquilizers, the phenothiazines are calming in nature, causing a decrease in spontaneous activity and generally a decrease in response to external stimuli (Overall 1997). The predominant antipsychotic action of the phenothiazines is neuroleptic, a term derived from the effect of the drugs on human psychiatric patients and intended to indicate the difference from signs typical of CNS depression (Baldessarini 1996a). The neuroleptic effects are attributed (but not conclusively) to antidopaminergic effects at D_2 dopamine receptors (Baldessarini 1996a). Some of the neuroleptics (e.g., phenothiazines) have high affinity for and thus also antagonize D_1 receptors, although pharmacologic effects at these receptors appear to be minimal. Phenothiazines also block D_3 and D_4 (which are D_2-like) receptors. Selected "atypical" antipsychotic drugs (e.g., clozapine) have a low affinity for D_2 receptors and are not characterized by extrapyramidal effects. However, they are characterized by α_1-adrenergic antagonism. Some of the antipsychotic drugs also have affinity for serotonergic (5-HT_2) receptors (e.g., clonazpine). Cholinergic and histaminergic (H_1) receptors also are targeted by some of the drugs, resulting in unique pharmacologic effects among the neuroleptics. Variable interactions with different receptor types lead to unpredictable effects on the autonomic nervous system (ANS). Among the neuroleptics, chlorpromazine has significant α-adrenergic antagonistic actions. In general, the antimuscarinic actions of neuroleptics are weak.

Neuroleptic effects include suppression of spontaneous movements or complex behaviors but minimal effects on spinal reflexes and unconditioned nociceptive avoidance behaviors. Interest in the environment is minimized as are manifestations of emotion. Patients are easily aroused; ataxia or incoordination should not be evident at appropriate doses (Baldessarini 1996a). Aggressive or impulsive behavior should gradually diminish. As a result, conditioned avoidance (but not unconditioned escape or avoidance) behavior and exploratory behavior are minimized. Feeding and emesis also are inhibited. At high doses, cataleptic immobility is evident (particularly in cats; Simpson and Simpson 1996), resulting in increased muscle tone (and the ability to place animals in an abnormal posture) and ptosis. Akathisia, an increase in restless activity, is an undesirable side effect that occurs in human beings but apparently not in animals. Akathisia occurs as adaptive responses to phenothiazines increase in extrapyramidal tissues (Baldessarini 1996a).

The effects of phenothiazines occur throughout the CNS. Cortical effects are responsible for many of the neuroleptic actions. Many of these sites appear to be spared from the adaptive changes of tolerance (Baldessarini 1996a). Neuroleptics have been associated with an increased incidence of seizures. Many of these drugs lower seizure threshold as well as induce discharges typical of epileptic seizures. Aliphatic, low-potency phenothiazines are particularly characterized by this effect (Baldessarini 1996a). Although the effect is more likely to occur in patients who are epileptic or are predisposed to seizures, the effect is also characterized by dose dependency in some drugs. Thus, these drugs should not be used in epileptic patients or patients undergoing withdrawal from central depressants (Baldessarini 1996a). Increasing doses slowly and accompanying anticonvulsant therapy are indicated if the drugs must be used in epileptic patients. Antagonism of D_2 receptors is largely responsible for the various extrapyramidal effects of the drugs.

The neuroleptic drugs have a number of effects in the limbic system. Although D_2 antagonism occurs in the limbic system, attempts are being made to identify D_3-selective drugs for treatment of psychoses because D_3 receptor stimulation may be responsible for many of the behaviors targeted by neuroleptics (Baldessarini 1996a). Neuroleptics stimulate prolactin secretion in human beings. Indeed, the potency of neuroleptic action and ability to cause prolactin secretion are well correlated for most drugs. Tolerance to this effect is not likely to develop. In humans, prolactin secretion caused by neuroleptics is also responsible for breast engorgement and galactorrhea. Releases of growth hormone and corticotropin-releasing hormone (especially chlorpromazine) occur in response to stress; neuroleptics also interfere with the release of growth hormone, although apparently not sufficient for treatment of acromegaly. Impaired release of serotonin may result in weight gain (particularly low-potency drugs), and glucose tolerance and insulin release may be impaired in prediabetic patients (especially chlorpromazine) (Baldessarini 1996a).

In the brain stem, the neuroleptics have little effect, even in cases of acute overdosing. Life-threatening coma is rare. In contrast, most neuroleptics protect against nausea and emesis at the chemoreceptor trigger zone in the medulla. These effects occur at low doses. Potent piperazines and butyrophenones are also often effective against nausea stimulated by the vestibular system (Baldessarini 1996a).

Phenothiazines characterized by lower potency have a predominant sedative effect that is more apparent initially but tends to decline as tolerance develops. The phenothiazines are characterized by anxiolytic effects, but more specific anxiolytic drugs are available. In addition, the risk of either autonomic (e.g., low-potency drugs) or extrapyramidal effects (e.g., highly potent drugs) increases the likelihood of causing anxiety (Baldessarini 1996a).

The neuroleptic drugs impart physiologic (especially cardiovascular) effects due to peripheral actions. However, the effects are complex because the neuroleptics interact with a number of receptor types that have cardiovascular effects. Hypotension induced by phenothiazines (low potency in particular) reflects direct effects on the blood vessels, indirect actions in the CNS and autonomic receptors, and a direct negative inotropic effect on the heart. Chlorpromazine has antiarrhythmic effects on the heart, similar to quinidine.

Disposition. The antipsychotics are characterized by variable bioavailability, high lipophilicity, high protein binding, and accumulation in a number of tissues. Elimination occurs primarily through hepatic metabolism. In humans, the elimination half-life is long, ranging from 20 to 40 hours. Biologic effects persist for longer than 24 hours, allowing once-daily therapy in people (Baldessarini 1996a). Metabolites can be detected in urine for several months.

Side Effects and Toxicity. Despite the variety of potential side effects, the antipsychotic drugs tend to be very safe. Lethal ingestion is rare in human patients.

Side effects tend to reflect the pharmacologic actions of the drugs and include CNS, cardiovascular, endocrine, and autonomic effects (Baldessarini 1996a). In human patients, other effects include dry mouth, blurry vision, and constipation. Urinary retention may occur in male patients with prostatitis. Extrapyramidal neurologic side effects occur in people but have not been reported in animals. However, some animals have exhibited signs of hyperactivity after treatment with acepromazine (Simpson and Simpson 1996). In addition, at least one report cites increased agitation and irritability following treatment of aggression with acepromazine (Marder 1991). Jaundice has occurred in people following administration of chlorpromazine and may resolve with continued treatment. Blood dyscrasias, including leukopenia, eosinophilia, and leukocytosis, occur but are less common with low-potency phenothiazines. Skin reactions tend to be common in people, again more often with low-potency phenothiazines.

Drug Interactions. Chlorpromazine is used in combination anesthetic regimens because of its ability to potentiate central depressants. Effects of analgesics and sedatives also can be enhanced. Interactions with antihypertensive drugs can be unpredictable and are more likely to be adverse with low-potency products (Baldessarini 1996a). Selected phenothiazines can antagonize the positive inotropic effects of digoxin.

Clinical Indications. In general, the use of phenothiazines for treatment of aggressive behavioral abnormalities is inappropriate because they blunt normal, as well as abnormal, behavior. Acepromazine is particularly problematic. Restraint of aggressive dogs with the drug renders dogs more likely to be reactive to noises and more easily startled (Overall 1997). In addition, because the degree and duration of tranquilization vary, reactions in dogs are unpredictable. Phenothiazines are not selective as antianxiety drugs but can reduce responsiveness in general and thus be useful in some cases of episodic anxiety (Simpson and Simpson 1996). Thioridazine has been used in one case of aberrant motor behavior (Jones 1987).

ANTIDEPRESSANT DRUGS. Much of the information regarding the use of mood-modifying drugs in animals has been extrapolated from human use. These drugs are characterized by clinical pharmacology and mechanisms of action that are likely to markedly differ among animals. Nevertheless, little scientific information is available to guide their use in animals. Currently, none of these drugs are approved for use in animals.

In people, affective (behavior) disorders targeted by tricyclic antidepressants range from depression to manic-depressive disorders. In animals, the list of targeted disorders is much greater and often appears to include any type of behavior deemed "unacceptable" by pet owners. Among the human drugs that have been used in animals are the tricyclic antidepressants, the MAO inhibitors (selegiline), and selective serotonin-reuptake inhibitors (SSRIs, fluoxetine). To best understand the pharmacologic actions (intended and undesirable) of these drugs, it is necessary to appreciate the extent to which neurotransmitters targeted by these drugs are active in the brain. Among the most commonly targeted neurotransmitters is the biogenic amine system, with norepinephrine, 5-hydroxytryptamine (5-HT, serotonin), and dopamine serving as primary targets. However, acetylcholine and histamine are common, although generally secondary, targets. In addition, α-adrenergic receptors may be stimulated by some of these drugs. The pharmacologic effects (and side effects) of these drugs vary with the neurotransmitter targeted. Drugs that are more specific in their actions tend to be safer. The inability to predict the effect of antidepressant drugs on behavior reflects, in part, the inability to predict effects at the synapse, as well as a lack of knowledge regarding the impact of neurotransmission on behavior. In general, blockade of dopamine transport appears to be stimulatory rather than antidepressant. Inhibition of serotonin reuptake appears to be antidepressant. Inhibition of norepinephrine reuptake consistently yields antidepressant actions.

Tricyclic Antidepressants

Structure-Activity Relationship. The tricyclic antidepressants (TCA) are among the most frequently prescribed drugs in human behavior medicine. Their name reflects their chemical structure (Fig. 17.2). The TCAs were identified as a group of potentially useful drugs for the modification of behavior in the 1940s following the generation of a number of drugs with antihistaminergic, sedative, analgesic, and antiparkinsonian effects. Imipramine was selected based on its hypnotic and sedative effects. Imipramine differs from phenothiazines only by the replacement of sulfur with an ethylene bridge, yielding a seven-member ring. This compound proved ineffective in quieting agitated psychotic patients but was very effective for selected mood disorders (Baldessarini 1996b). The search for chemically related compounds yielded a number of additional drugs. Clomipramine, amitriptyline, and doxepin are all derivatives of imipramine (Baldessarini 1996b). Each contains a tertiary amine at one of the substitution sites on the seven-member ring. Desipramine, a major metabolite of imipramine, and nortriptyline, the *N*-demethylated metabolite of amitriptyline, are secondary amine tricyclics. Proptriptylline and trimipramine are other TCAs but have few veterinary applications (Simpson and Simpson 1996; Shores and Redding 1987). The effects of neurotransmitter reuptake vary with the different amine structures (Baldessarini 1996b).

Mechanism of Action. The mechanism of action of the TCAs (and of the MAO inhibitors and the SSRIs) is blockade of the mechanisms of physiologic inactivation. For the TCAs, the mechanism is inhibition of reuptake at presynaptic biogenic amine neurotransmitter receptors in the brain. As reuptake is inhibited, the concentration of neurotransmitters increases, prolonging their actions (CNS stimulation). The chemical structure of the TCAs determines, in part, which neurotransmitters are affected (Baldessarini 1996b). Imipramine and its derivatives with a tertiary-amine side chain block norepinephrine reuptake but have little effect on dopamine reuptake. The secondary amine derivatives of imipramine are potent and highly selective inhibitors of norepinephrine reuptake; however, they are characterized by fewer autonomic and anticholinergic effects. Tertiary amines that are metabolized in the patient to secondary amines will exhibit the effects on norepinephrine reuptake. Clomipramine has marked effects on serotonin reuptake. Doxepin is characterized by greater antihistaminergic actions (thus explaining its frequent recommendation for chronic pruritus). Although amitriptyline has been the most commonly prescribed drug in animals, clomipramine has recently been approved for use in dogs and may be more appropriate for clinical studies because of its relative selectivity for serotonin.

Pharmacologic Effects

ADAPTATION TO PHARMACOLOGIC EFFECTS. The effect of TCAs at pre- and postsynaptic receptors and autoregulation result in complex responses that are not well understood. Although inhibition of reuptake occurs very rapidly, peak effects still take several weeks. This prolonged time to maximal effect reflects in part disposition (see section on clinical pharmacology) but also appears to reflect adaptation in the CNS to changes in neurotransmitter concentrations at the synapse. Administration of a TCA results in an immediate decrease in the synthesis and release of norepinephrine or serotonin (depending on the major target of the TCA) in selected areas of the brain. The effects appear to be mediated presynaptically through autoreceptors (α_2 or serotonin, respectively). However, turnover gradually normalizes within 1–3 weeks. Autoreceptors appear to be down-regulated and become desensitized to the presence of the TCA (Baldessarini 1996b). The number and sensitivity of postsynaptic adrenergic receptors do not appear to be impacted by continued use of TCAs.

Adaptive responses appear to influence the pharmacologic properties of TCAs at adrenergic receptor sites. The TCAs have a moderate affinity for α_1 receptors and only limited affinity for α_2 and β receptors. Changes in serotonin receptors following repeated treatment with TCAs are complex. Although the impact is not clear, the general effect appears to be increased sensitivity to serotonin. This may be an important component in the outcome of prolonged treatment (Baldessarini 1996b). The TCAs also appear to impact the effect of other neurotransmitters and their receptors, including GABA (unknown significance) and dopamine (D_2; desensitization of autoreceptors, resulting in mood elevation). Other factors to consider regarding adaptation to TCA effects include changes in cyclic-AMP-dependent protein kinases and potential changes at the level of gene expression (Baldessarini 1996b).

In addition to tolerance (to sedative and autonomic effects), physical dependence can develop to the TCA. Physical dependence following acute withdrawal is manifested in human patients as malaise, chills, coryza, and muscle aches (Baldessarini 1996b). Slow discontinuation of the drug is recommended.

AUTONOMIC NERVOUS SYSTEM. The predominant effect of TCAs on the ANS appears to reflect inhibition of norepinephrine transport into adrenergic nerve terminals and antagonism of muscarinic, cholinergic, and α_1-adrenergic responses to the neurotransmitters. Blurred vision, dry mouth, constipation, and urinary retention at therapeutic doses (documented in humans) appear to reflect anticholinergic effects (Baldessarini 1996b).

CARDIOVASCULAR SYSTEM. Cardiovascular effects of TCAs occur at therapeutic doses and can become life-threatening with overdosing. Postural hypotension occurs in human beings due to α-adrenergic blockade. Mild sinus tachycardia occurs due to inhibition of norepinephrine uptake and muscarinic (M_1) blockade (Baldessarini 1996b). Conduction time is prolonged, especially at concentrations above 200 ng/mL. The TCA also can directly suppress the myocardium (Baldessarini 1996b). The myocardial depressant effects are greater in the presence of underlying cardiac disease.

CLINICAL PHARMACOLOGY. The disposition of the TCA favors adverse reactions in that the characteristics of disposition tend to vary greatly among animals and extrapolation between species is complicated. Unfortunately, the disposition of the drugs has not been scientifically studied in animals and information is extrapolated from human beings. The TCAs are very lipophilic. As such, they are well absorbed following oral administration. However, they can undergo marked first-pass metabolism. High doses can cause anticholinergic effects on the gastrointestinal tract, slowing absorption or making it erratic. Absorption in humans can result in peak concentrations as rapidly as 2 hours or as long as 12 hours after administration (Baldessarini 1996b). The drugs are very highly protein bound, but unbound drug is characterized by a very large volume of distribution (10–15 L/kg in human patients), contributing to a long elimination half-life. Drug may bind avidly to selected tissues. Drugs are eliminated by hepatic (oxidative) metabolism. Metabolism is variable among human patients, accounting for plasma concentrations that differ by 10- to 30-fold. Metabolism yields active and inactive metabolites. It is not clear what percentage of the antidepressant activity of the TCA is associated with the metabolites. Metabolites generally have an elimination half-life that is at least twice that of the parent compound (Baldessarini 1996b). Thus, accumulation of the metabolites can result in a marked proportion of the pharmacologic effect of TCAs.

SIDE EFFECTS. Up to 5% of human patients receiving a TCA react adversely. Sedation is common (Simpson and Simpson 1996), although clomipramine generally is associated with less sedation than the other TCAs (Juarbe-Diaz 1997a). The most common reactions are due to the antimuscarinic effect or overdosing. Cardiac toxicity is a less frequently reported but serious toxicity. Side effects include dry mouth, gastric distress, constipation, dizziness, tachycardia or other arrhythmias, blurred vision, and urinary retention (particularly problematic in the presence of prostatitis hypertrophy) (Baldessarini 1996b). Weakness and fatigue reflect CNS effects. Cardiac toxicity is more likely in patients that start therapy with cardiac disease. In healthy patients, the most likely cardiac response is hypotension due to α-adrenergic blockade.

An undesirable side effect of antidepressant drugs in people is referred to as the "switch process." Patients undergo a transition from depression to hypomanic or manic excitement (Baldessarini 1996b). This effect has not been reported in animals. Confusion and delirium are behavior aberrations that occur commonly in human patients, with the incidence of 10% in all patients increasing to greater than 30% in patients over 50 (Baldessarini 1996b). Miscellaneous toxic effects in human patients include leukopenia, jaundice, and skin rashes. Weight gain occurs, particularly with the drugs that are selective for serotonin reuptake. Reports addressing the side effects of TCAs in dogs are uncommon. Goldberger and Rapoport (1991) reported side effects in 5 of 13 dogs receiving clomipramine for lick granuloma. Clinical signs included lethargy, anorexia, diarrhea, and growling.

Acute poisoning with TCAs is common in human patients (accidental or intentional) and appears to be a significant problem in animals (Johnson 1990). Symptoms in humans vary and are complex. Excitement and restlessness may be accompanied by myoclonus or tonic-clonic seizures. Coma may rapidly develop, associated with depressed expiration, hypoxia, hypothermia, and hypotension (Baldessarini 1996b). Anticholinergic effects include mydriasis, dry mucosa, absent bowel sounds, urinary retention, and cardiac arrhythmias, including tachycardia. Clinical signs reported following accidental ingestion in animals (Johnson 1990) include hyperexcitement and vomiting as early manifestations, followed by ataxia, lethargy, and muscular tremors. Bradycardia and other cardiac arrhythmias occur later. These later signs occurred shortly before death in experimental animal models of TCA toxicoses (Johnson 1990).

Treatment for TCA toxicoses is supportive, including respiratory (intubation) and cardiovascular support. Gastric lavage with activated charcoal can be used early. Emetics probably should be avoided because of the risk of aspiration pneumonia in seizuring animals (emetics may further predispose the animal to seizures). Short-acting barbiturates (or similar drugs) without preatropinization are preferred for anesthetic control during gastric lavage. Cathartics (sorbitol or sodium sulfate–Glauber's salt) can be of benefit. Magnesium sulfate should not be used because impaired gastrointestinal motility can facilitate absorption of magnesium. Resolution of coma may require several days; the threat of cardiac arrhythmias likewise persists for several days. Pharmacologic interventions for cardiac arrhythmias have not been well established. Alkalinization (sodium bicarbonate sufficient to maintain blood pH above 7.5: 2–3 mEq/kg over 15–30 minutes IV) may prevent death by increasing protein binding and cardiac automaticity (due to potassium shifts) (Johnson 1990). Cardiac drugs, including antiarrhythmics and digoxin, are contraindicated in human patients. Phenytoin may provide antiarrhythmic effects and in human patients is useful for treatment of seizures (Baldessarini 1996b). This latter effect is not likely to occur safely in animals. Diazepam is indicated for acute management of seizures. Beta-adrenergic receptor antagonists and lidocaine may be useful (Baldessarini 1996b). The risk of tonic-clonic seizures increased in human patients, particularly at high doses.

CLINICAL INDICATIONS. The TCAs have been recommended by animal behaviorists for most abnormal behaviors manifested in dogs and cats. These include, but are not limited to, behaviors associated with fear and aggression (Juarbe-Diaz 1997a,b; Overall 1997; Haupt 1997; Marder 1991), stereotypies, obsessive-compulsive or self-mutilation disorders, and excessive barking. Clomipramine recently has been approved for use in dogs (ClomCalm®, Novartis Animal Health) for treatment of separation anxiety. Protriptyline is a nonsedative TCA that has been used successfully in human narcoleptic patients. The drug has been used successfully in one dog whose narcolepsy was manifested as hyperinsomnia (Shores and Redding 1987).

CONTRAINDICATIONS. The TCAs should be avoided in animals with metabolic diseases. Specific contraindications include a history of cardiac or hepatic disease, seizures, glaucoma, hyperthyroidism, or thyroid hormone supplementation (Juarbe-Diaz 1997a).

DRUG INTERACTIONS. The TCAs can interact with a number of other drugs. Competition for protein-binding sites with other highly protein-bound drugs can result in increased drug concentrations. Drugs that impact drug-metabolizing enzymes, through either inhibition or induction, will impact the clearance of TCAs. The sequelae of the impact are difficult to predict since active metabolites similarly will be impacted. However, in general, drugs that inhibit metabolism are likely to result in greater drug accumulation and increased risk of toxicity. Other antidepressants and TCAs can also compete with other compounds for metabolism. The drugs themselves may impact metabolism of other drugs. Clomipramine inhibits the metabolism of other drugs (Baldessarini 1996b). Antidepressants potentiate the effects of sedative drugs. In general, TCAs should not be used in combination with other drugs that modify CNS neurotransmitters, such as MAO inhibitors and amitraz (Juarbe-Diaz 1997a). In human patients, a potentially lethal interaction has been reported when a TCA, particularly one that inhibits serotonin uptake, is combined with a MAO (Baldessarini 1996b). The term "serotonin syndrome" has been applied to the interaction, which is characterized by restlessness, muscle twitches, hyperreflexia, shivering, tremors, etc.

CLINICAL USE. Most antidepressant drugs require 2–3 weeks for clinical efficacy to be realized. The exception might be amitriptyline, which may cause response within 3–5 days (Juarbe-Diaz 1997a). Therapeutic drug monitoring may facilitate the safe and effective use of the drugs. In human patients, plasma concentrations that range from 100 to 250 ng/mL are most likely to cause satisfactory antidepressant effects; toxicity can be expected at concentrations above 500 ng/mL, with fatal consequences likely as concentrations approach 1000 ng/mL (Baldessarini 1996b). Variability among human patients (and presumably among animals) supports the use of monitoring to guide therapy. However, monitoring to avoid toxicity is complicated because serum concentrations by themselves are not reliable predictors of toxic responses.

Because of the risk of withdrawal due to physical dependence, discontinuation of TCAs should occur over a week or longer if therapy has been prolonged (Baldessarini 1996b).

Selective Serotonin-Reuptake Inhibitors

STRUCTURE-ACTIVITY RELATIONSHIP AND MECHANISM OF ACTION. The SSRIs enhance CNS serotonin by blocking presynaptic neuronal uptake. They may also increase postsynaptic receptor sensitivity (Simpson and Simpson 1996). Drugs currently approved in humans include fluoxetine, paroxetine, sertraline, and fluvoxamine. Because of their selectivity for serotonin uptake, the diverse effects characterizing TCAs are generally absent with SSRIs.

CLINICAL PHARMACOLOGY. The clinical pharmacology of the SSRIs is similar to that of the TCAs. Oral absorption, lipophilicity, protein-binding, and volume of distribution are similar. Like the TCAs, fluoxetine is metabolized by the liver to active (norfluoxetine) and inactive metabolites (Baldessarini 1996b). The active metabolite is very long acting. In addition, it interferes with the metabolism of other antidepressants (including the TCAs), prolonging metabolite elimination even when the parent drug is no longer present. The elimination half-life of norfluoxetine is 150–200 hours in people, compared to 50 hours for the parent compound. Thus, based on accumulation alone, the metabolite can have a profound impact on therapeutic effect. Paroxetine and fluvoxamine have no active metabolites (in human patients). The time to efficacy of SSRIs (which is up to 3 weeks in human patients) reflects, in part, the time for maximum accumulation of the parent drug and its metabolites.

The use of monitoring to guide therapy was addressed with the TCAs. As with the TCAs, effective concentrations have not been established in animals but must be extrapolated from people. The relationship between plasma drug concentrations and therapeutic efficacy has not been well established (Simpson and Simpson 1996). Plasma concentrations thought to be effective in human patients range from 100 to 300 ng/mL for fluoxetine (and its active metabolites). Effective concentrations for paroxetine are 30–100 ng/mL; for sertraline, 25–50 ng/mL (Baldessarini 1996b).

DRUG INTERACTIONS. The SSRIs can inhibit the metabolism of other drugs; the order of potency of inhibition is paroxetine > norlouoxetine > fluoxetine = sertraline. Because of the risk of drug interactions, SSRIs should not be used in combination with other antidepressants (see discussions on serotonin syndrome and on drug interactions of TCAs and MAO inhibitors) (Baldessarini 1996b).

SIDE EFFECTS. Compared to the TCAs, SSRIs appear to be safe. Unlike the TCAs, SSRIs have minimal effects on the cardiovascular system (Baldessarini 1996b). However, the safety of their use in patients with underlying cardiac disease has not been established. Sedation is not a common side effect, being least likely with fluoxetine (Simpson and Simpson 1996). In humans, gastrointestinal side effects are the most common, occurring in as many as 25% of patients receiving the drug (Simpson and Simpson 1996). Their incidence is minimized by starting with a low dose and gradually increasing the dose until efficacy is evident. Side effects have been reported in animals. In a report of 14 dogs in which fluoxetine was used for the treatment of lick granuloma (Raboport 1992), side effects in 4 dogs included lethargy, anorexia, and hyperactivity. Another study (Melman 1995) reported these same side effects as well as polydypsia, diarrhea, and increased or decreased appetite. At least 50% of animals appeared to develop some type of side effect, although side effects were described as "mild." Side effects reported by owners in a study of fluoxetine for treatment of canine dominance-related aggression included fatigue, lethargy, and decreased appetite (Dodman and Mertens 1995).

CLINICAL INDICATIONS. Probably no behavior-modifying drug has received more attention in the veterinary and lay literature than fluoxetine (Kauffman 1994; Marder 1995). Despite the plethora of opinions and testimonials regarding the efficacy of this drug for treatment of animal behavioral disorders, few scientific studies exist. Efficacy for treatment of lick granulomas is supported by a double-blinded crossover study (Rapoport et al. 1992). One-third of the animals studied did not repeat the abnormal behavior when fluoxetine was discontinued. Fluoxetine also has been studied in an open (nonblinded) study in dogs afflicted with a variety of behavioral problems (Melman 1995). Approximately 65% of dogs with lick granuloma, 100% of animals with separation anxiety, and 85% of animals with tail mutilation disorders responded to fluoxetine. Unfortunately, data were not controlled for other treatments, making interpretation of the success of fluoxetine in this study difficult. Fluoxetine has also been used successfully to treat psychogenic alopecia in a cat (Hartmann 1995) and dominance aggression in dogs (Dodman and Mertens 1995; Dodman et al. 1996).

Monoamine Oxidase Inhibitors

STRUCTURE-ACTIVITY RELATIONSHIP. The recognition that the antitubercular drug isoniazid tended to elevate the mood of patients receiving the drug for treatment of tuberculosis led to further discovery of drugs that inhibit monoamine oxidase. The first drugs used were structurally related to hydrazine and associated with marked hepatotoxicity. An attempt was made to synthesize CNS stimulant compounds unrelated to hydrazine but similar to amphetamine. Ultimately, this later effort yielded selegiline (Baldessarini 1996b).

The MAO inhibitors potentially impact a variety of monamines by inhibiting mitochondrial MAO and preventing the subsequent degradation of monoamines, most notably dopamine. Most of the clinically relevant drugs are nonselective toward two major enzyme groups (Baldessarini 1996b), which are characterized by different substrate specificities. MAO-A prefers serotonin and is inhibited by clorgyline, whereas MAO-B prefers phenylethylamine and is inhibited by selegiline. Selegiline is the only currently used MAO inhibitor characterized by selectivity. Because it targets MAO-B, it is relatively selective for dopamine. It is approved for use in dogs for treatment of pituitary-dependent hyperadrenocorticism (purported to be a dopamine deficiency). Binding to the MAO is irreversible, and recovery from effects requires synthesis of new enzyme. In human patients, this appears to require 1–2 weeks. Metabolism occurs more slowly in geriatric patients (Baldessarini 1996b).

PHARMACOLOGIC EFFECTS. The effects of the MAO inhibitors occur on systems affected by sympathomimetic amines and serotonin. Although as a class MAO inhibitors affect a number of other enzyme systems, generalizations to the class do not necessarily apply to selegiline. Selegiline potentiates dopamine in selected neurons and has been approved to treat Parkinson's disease in humans and cognitive dysfunctions in animals, conditions assumed to be associated with dopamine deficiency. Selegiline also scavenges oxygen radicals and reduces neuronal damage due to reactive products of oxidative metabolism of dopamine and other compounds (Baldessarini 1996b). A delay in the therapeutic effect up to 2 or more weeks characterizes the use of selegiline. Reasons for the delay are not known (Baldessarini 1996b).

CLINICAL PHARMACOLOGY. The MAO inhibitors are readily absorbed following oral administration. Maximal inhibition occurs within 5–10 days. Despite a long biological activity, efficacy appears to decrease in human patients if the drugs are administered at an interval longer than 24 hours (Baldessarini 1996b).

SIDE EFFECTS AND DRUG INTERACTIONS. Selective MAO inhibitors appear to be safe. However, severe and potentially fatal interactions have been described when MAO inhibitors have been combined with other antidepressants. Particularly problematic is the combination of MAO inhibitors with drugs that inhibit the reuptake of serotonin (see the discussion on the serotonin syndrome of TCAs). Other drugs with which MAO inhibitors may interact include meperidine and precursors of biogenic amines. Selective MAO inhibitors such as selegiline are not necessarily safer than the older or nonselective inhibitors when combined with other drugs. Hypertensive crisis, a serious side effect that occurs when aged cheeses containing tyramine (a bacterial monoamine by-product) are ingested in the presence of nonselective MAO inhibitors, does not occur with selective MAO inhibitors such as selegiline.

Anxiolytics

PHARMACOLOGY. The primary anxiolytics used in veterinary medicine are the benzodiazepines (Chap. 16), including diazepam, its metabolite oxazepam, clorazepate (metabolized in the stomach to *N*-desmethyl diazepam, a major metabolite of diazepam), lorazepam, alprazolam, and clonazepam. The assumed mechanism of action of these drugs is GABA-minergic through interaction with the $GABA_A$ receptor. The anxiolytic effects are separate from the general CNS depressant effects caused by these drugs. Their central effects are somewhat dose dependent. Sedative effects occur at low doses; as a result, excitement is tempered. Antianxiety effects are evident at moderate doses and are beneficial to social interactions. At high doses, hypnotic effects become evident. Sedation becomes profound at high doses and ataxia is evident and sleep is facilitated (Overall 1997). Decreased skeletal muscle activity (particularly of value in seizuring animals) is central in nature and is independent of sedative effects. Cats appear to be more prone than dogs to muscle relaxation (Overall 1997). Benzodiazepines may distribute differently in cats, with extensive binding of diazepam and its major metabolite, desmethyldiazepam, in the brain (Placidi et al. 1976).

The effects of the benzodiazepines reflect in part metabolism to active, inactive, and potentially toxic metabolites. If efficacy reflects formation of an active metabolite (e.g., desmethyldiazepam), accumulation may be necessary before maximum effects are seen. Lorazepam and oxazepam have short elimination half-lives in human patients and are metabolized by phase II (glucuronidation) enzymes. Thus, metabolites of these drugs are not likely to be active or toxic.

The elimination half-life of many benzodiazepines in general is short. Efficacy can be prolonged by metabolism to active metabolites. The drugs are categorized by their duration of effect in humans, although it is not clear if the same categorization will apply to animals. Clorazepate is available as a sustained-release product that can be administered less frequently.

Tolerance develops to the anticonvulsant and sedative effects of many benzodiazepines. However, tolerance to the anxiolytic effects of these drugs appears less likely to develop (Simpson and Simpson 1996). In contrast, withdrawal can accompany rapid discontinuation of the drug. Thus, doses should be gradually tapered (e.g., 25% per week) as the drug is discontinued (Simpson and Simpson 1996; Overall 1997).

SIDE EFFECTS. In addition to changes in behavior, the benzodiazepines have been associated with a number of side effects in human patients. Reaction may be to the parent drug or a metabolite. Long-term use in human patients has been associated with neutropenia and liver disease. Recently, acute fulminating hepatotoxicity has been reported in cats receiving diazepam orally (Center 1996). Clinical signs include anorexia, vomiting, lethargy, hypothermia, and jaundice. The adversity appears to be dose dependent (and thus may be idiosyncratic), occurring in most animals within 5–11 days after therapy is begun. Mortality is high (8 out of 11 cats in one report) despite intensive therapy. Histology revealed severe acute to subacute lobular to massive hepatic necrosis, suppurative cholangitis, and biliary hyperplasia. Baseline hepatic function data might be collected in cats prior to starting therapy and 3–5 days after therapy is begun in order to minimize the damage induced by diazepam administered to cats at risk. Any evidence of illness (or evidence of prolonged elimination) should lead to discontinuation of the drug.

CLINICAL INDICATIONS. The benzodiazepines are less desirable as behavior-modifying drugs because of their nonspecific nature (Overall 1997). Thus, a notable disadvantage of the long-term use of benzodiazepines is their tendency to interfere with the ability to learn in animals undergoing behavior modification as part of their treatment program (Lindell 1997). An exception can be made for chlordiazepoxide, which appears to facilitate operant conditioning in nervous (Pointer) dogs (Simpson and Simpson 1996). Paradoxical reactions may occur in some animals, including rage, hyperexcitability, and anxiety. In addition, the risk of substance abuse by pet owners should lead to close scrutiny of drug needs and use.

Benzodiazepines are indicated for the treatment of anxiety. Alprazolam and clonazepam may be associated with fewer side effects and might be preferred (Overall 1997); however, fewer reports exist regarding their use in animals. The benzodiazepines are contraindicated in aggressive patients (Overall 1997). Simpson and Simpson (1996) notes that the contraindication may depend on the cause of aggression. If aggression is a manifestation of an underlying fear or anxiety, then the benzodiazepines may reduce aggression. If, however, anxiety or fear is masking aggression, benzodiazepines may increase aggression. Other indications for benzodiazepines include treatment of inappropriate elimination (Overall 1997), noise phobias, and selected anxieties such as visits to the veterinarian (Simpson and Simpson 1996; Overall 1997).

Anxioselective Drugs: Azapirones (Buspirone)

STRUCTURE-ACTIVITY RELATIONSHIP. Buspirone is referred to as a nonspecific anxiolytic. Azapirones were specifically developed for atypical depressions, nonspecific generalized anxiety disorders, and selected obsessive-compulsive disorders. Buspirone is the first nonsedating antianxiety drug to be marketed (Simpson and Simpson 1996). Its effects appear to reflect blockade of 5-HT_1 receptors at both pre- and postsynaptic sites. Presynaptic inhibition increases low serotonergic activity, whereas postsynaptic control reduces high (Simpson and Simpson 1996). Buspirone causes downregulation of 5-HT receptors. In addition, it acts as a dopamine agonist throughout the brain (Simpson and Simpson 1996).

SIDE EFFECTS. In contrast to benzodiazepine anxiolytic drugs, buspirone has no sedative, muscle relaxant, or anticonvulsant actions. It does not impair motor performance (Simpson and Simpson 1996). Side effects to buspirone manifested in cats include increased aggressiveness (toward other household cats), increased affection toward owners, mild sedation, and agitation (Cooper 1997). Vomiting and tachycardia also have been reported (Cooper 1997). In contrast to the anxiolytic drugs and TCAs, buspirone is associated with a low abuse potential. Withdrawal following discontinuation of the drug apparently does not occur (Overall 1997).

CLINICAL INDICATIONS. Buspirone has been used to treat canine aggression, canine and feline stereotypic behaviors, self-mutilation, obsessive-compulsive disorders, thunderstorm phobias, and feline spraying (Hart et al. 1993; Overall 1997). Buspirone apparently has been particularly useful for treatment of anxiety associated with social situations such as aggression or marking behaviors (Overall 1997). However, treatment for anxiety is more likely to be successful short term rather than long term, perhaps because of the slow onset of action characterizing the drug.

MISCELLANEOUS (NONSPECIFIC) DRUGS USED TO MODIFY BEHAVIOR

Progestins. Progestin interaction with GABA receptors is 10–50 times more potent than that of barbiturates (Overall 1997). This may account for the nonspecific calming effects of the drugs observed in veterinary medicine. The advent of newer behavior-modifying drugs (e.g., TCAs, SSRIs) and the incidence of side effects largely limit their use to animals that have not responded to other medications and are faced with euthanasia.

Several side effects have been well documented in animals receiving progestins long term. Among the more notable because of their magnitude or life-threatening nature are gynecomastia, mammary gland neoplasia, diabetes mellitus, aplastic anemia, and pyometra (Juarbe-Diaz 1997a). Animals should be frequently monitored for evidence of adversities.

Progestins are most wisely reserved for adjuvant short-term therapy (until the second drug takes affect, i.e., 4–6 weeks), and only the oral form is recommended. The progestins are an alternative for animals for whom euthanasia is being considered; in such cases, a high dose (4 mg/kg orally every 24 hours) has been recommended in order to stimulate a rapid response (Juarbe-Diaz 1997a).

Anticonvulsants. A number of anticonvulsant drugs have been used to treat behavioral abnormalities. The most notable of those used in animals include the barbiturate phenobarbital, its congener primidone, and phenytoin, a hydantoin derivative. They have been somewhat efficacious for treatment of overactive or aggressive behaviors (which actually may have been an expression of psychomotor epilepsy) (Overall 1997). However, efficacy is generally dependent on sedative (and, with long-term use, potentially toxic) effects. They have largely been replaced by the TCAs and SSRIs. The side effects of these drugs (discussed in Chap. 16) limit their long-term use, although monitoring (as with anticonvulsant therapy) may help prevent toxicity.

Phenytoin has been useful for the treatment of explosive aggression in human patients. Phenobarbital may prove useful for controlling excessive feline vocalization during car travel (Overall 1997) and canine aggression (Dodman and Shuster 1994). Carbamazepine (an iminodiabenzyl derivative of imipramine) also has been used to treat explosive aggression in humans. Valproic acid may be useful for treatment of aggression (Dodman and Shuster 1994).

Narcotic Agonists and Antagonists. These drugs are discussed in depth in Chap. 13. The antagonists in particular have proven useful in the treatment of selective obsessive-compulsive disorders in humans. Efficacy also has been reported when used to treat selected self-mutilation disorders in dogs (e.g., acral lick dermatitis or lick granuloma) (Overall 1997; Dodman et al. 1988; Dodman and Shuster 1994; Simpson and Simpson 1996). Pure antagonists, including naloxone and naltrexone (the latter an orally bioavailable product), and mixed agonists/antagonists such as pentazocine appear effective. These drugs block μ and κ receptors. The assumed mechanism of action is blockade of self-reward mediated by endogenous opioid release that may accompany self-destructive behavior. Hydrocodone also has proven effective in selective self-destructive behaviors in both the dog and the cat.

Antihistamines. The mildly sedative (e.g., hydroxyzine) or hypnotic (e.g., diphenhydramine) effects caused by H_1-receptor blockade can be of benefit for treatment of some behavioral disorders. These drugs are discussed in depth in Chap. 51 as antiemetics at the vestibular apparatus. Indications as behavior-modifying drugs might include the treatment of chronic pruritus, late-night activity, problems during car travel, and selected transient behaviors accompanied by pacing and vocalization (Overall 1997).

Beta Blockers. Beta-adrenergic blockers (e.g., propranolol, pindolol) have been used in human medicine for the treatment of aggressive outburst associated with self-mutilation or injury problems, intermittent explosive behaviors, conduct disorders, dementia, and schizophrenia (Overall 1997). However, the use of these drugs for similar disorders in animals has not been very successful (Overall 1997). Nonselective beta blockers also have been used to treat anxiety in human beings. One animal behaviorist reports success with the use of propranolol or pindolol (the latter also affecting serotonin receptors) for the treatment of fear aggression in dogs (Dodman and Shuster 1994).

Stimulants. Stimulants include dextroamphetamine, methylphenidate (Ritalin®), and pemoline. Stimulants are characterized by paradoxical effects in that they cause excitement in the normal patient but have a calming effect on the hyperactive patient. Their indication in human patients is for the treatment of attention deficits. Conditions of hyperactivity are rare in veterinary medicine. Proper diagnosis is imperative for successful therapy with stimulants. They increase sympathomimetic stimulation. Side effects include increased heart and respiratory rate and anorexia. Tremors and hyperthermia may occur. The drugs are contraindicated in patients with cardiovascular disease, glaucoma, and hyperthyroidism. The drugs should not be used in combination with other behavior-modifying drugs (Overall 1997).

NOTE

1. Portions of this chapter are reprinted from Dawn Merton Boothe, *Small Animal Clinical Pharmacology and Therapeutics,* Philadelphia: WB Saunders Company; copyright © 2000 Mosby, Inc., a Harcourt Health Series Company. All rights reserved.

REFERENCES

Baldessarini, R. J. 1996a. Drugs and the treatment of psychiatric disorders: apsychosis and anxiety. In J. G. Hardman, L. E. Limbird, P. B. Molinoff, R. W. Ruddon, and A. G. Gilman, eds., Goodman and Gilman's The Pharmacological Basis of Therapeutics, 9th ed., pp. 402–419. New York: McGraw-Hill.

———. 1996b. Drugs and the treatment of psychiatric disorders: depression and mania. In J. G. Hardman, L. E. Limbird, P. B. Molinoff, R. W. Ruddon, and A. G. Gilman, eds., Goodman and Gilman's The Pharmacological Basis of Therapeutics, 9th ed., pp. 431–446. New York: McGraw-Hill.

Boothe, D. M. 2000. Small Animal Clinical Pharmacology and Therapeutics. Philadelphia: W. B. Saunders.

Center, S. A., Elson, T. H., Rowland, P. H., et al. 1996. Fulminant hepatic failure associated with oral diazepam in 11 cats. J Am Vet Med Assoc 190:618–625.

Cooper, L. L. 1997. Feline inappropriate elimination. Vet Clin N Am: Sm Anim Pract 27(3):569–600.

Cooper, L., and Hart, B. L. 1992. Comparison of diazepam with progestin for effectiveness in suppression of urine spraying behavior in cats. J Am Vet Med Assoc 200:797–801.

Dodman, N. H., and Mertens, P. A. 1995. Fluoxetine (Prozac) for the treatment of dominance-related aggression in dogs (abstr). Newslet Am Vet Soc Anim Behav 17:3.

Dodman, N. H., and Shuster, L. 1994. Pharmacologic approaches to managing behavior problems in small animals. Vet Med, Oct:960–969.

Dodman, N., Shuster, L., White, S. D., et al. 1988. Use of narcotic antagonists to modify stereotypic self-licking, self-chewing, and scratching behavior in dogs. J Am Vet Med Assoc 193:815–819.

Dodman, N. H., Donnelly, R., Shuster, L., et al. 1996. Use of fluoxetine to treat dominance aggression in dogs. J Am Vet Med Assoc 209:1585–1587.

Goldberger, E., and Rapoport, J. L. 1991. Canine acral lick dermatitis: response to the antiobsessional drug clomipramine. J Am Anim Hosp Assoc 27:179–182.

Hart, B. L., Eckstein, R. A., Powell, K. L., et al. 1993. Effectiveness of buspirone on urine spraying and inappropriate urination in cats. J Am Vet Med Assoc 203:254–258.

Hartmann, L. 1995. Cats as possible obsessive-compulsive disorder and medications models (letter). Am J Psychiatry 152: 1236.

Houpt, K. A. 1997a. Sexual behavior problems in dogs and cats. Vet Clin N Am: Sm Anim Pract 27(3):601–616.

———, ed. 1997b. Progress in Companion Animal Behavior. Philadelphia: W. B. Saunders.

Johnson, L. R. 1990. Tricyclic antidepressant toxicosis. Vet Clin N Am: Sm Anim Pract 20(2):393–403.

Jones, R. D. 1987. Use of thioridazine in the treatment of aberrant motor behavior in a dog. J Am Vet Med Assoc 191:89–90.

Juarbe-Diaz, S. V. 1997a. Social dynamics and behavior problems in multiple dog households. Vet Clin N Am: Sm Anim Pract 27(3):497–514.

———. 1997b. Assessment and treatment of excessive barking in the domestic dog. Vet Clin N Am: Sm Anim Pract 27(3):515–532.

Kauffman, S. 1994. Problem pets may now get Prozac. Raleigh News-Observer, Aug 1:1B–5B.

Landsberg, G. 1994. Products for preventing or controlling undesirable behavior. Vet Med, Oct:970–983.

Lindell, E. M. 1997. Diagnosis and treatment of destructive behavior in dogs. Vet Clin N Am: Sm Anim Pract 27(3):533–534.

Marder, A. R. 1991. Psychotropic drugs and behavioral therapy. Vet Clin N Am: Small Anim Pract 21:329–342.

———. 1995. The promise of Prozac. Vet Product News, May/June(1):45.

Melman, S. A. 1995. Use of Prozac in animals for selected dermatological and behavioral conditions. Vet Forum 12:19–27.

Neville, W. H., Scott, D. W., and Wellington, J. R. 1992. Nonsteroidal management of canine pruritus with amitriptyline. Cornell Vet 82:53–57.

Overall, K. L. 1994a. Use of clomipramine to treat ritualistic stereotypic motor behavior in three dogs. J Am Vet Med Assoc 205:1733–1741.

———. 1994b. Commentary on Buspirone for use in treating cats. Adv Small Anim Med Surg 7:4.

———. 1997. Pharmacologic treatments for behavior problems. Vet Clin N Am: Sm Anim Pract 27(3):637–666.

Placidi, G. F., Togoni, G., Pacifici, G. M., et al. 1976. Regional distribution of diazepam and its metabolites in the brain of cats after chronic treatment. Psychopharmacology 48:133.

Rapoport, J. L., Ryland, D. H., and Kriete, M. 1992. Drug treatment of canine acral lick: an animal model of obsessive-compulsive disorder. Arch Gen Psychiatry 49:517–521.

Shaikh, M. B. De Lanerolle, N. C., and Siegel, A. 1997. Serotonin 5-HT1A and 5-HT2/1C receptors in the midbrain periaqueductal gray differentially modulate defensive rage behavior elicited from the medial hypothalamus of the cat. Brain Res 765(2):198–207.

Shores, A., and Redding, R. W. 1987. Narcoleptic hypersomnia syndrome responsive to protriptyline in a Labrador Retriever. J Am Anim Hosp Assoc 23:455–458.

Simpson, B. S., and Simpson, D. M. 1996. Behavioral pharmacotherapy. In V. L. Voith, and P. L. Borchelt, eds., Readings in Companion Animal Behavior, pp. 100–115. Veterinary Learning Systems.

Voith, V. L. 1992. Behavioral Disorders. In S. J. Ettinger, ed., Textbook of Veterinary Internal Medicine, pp. 227–238. Philadelphia: W. B. Saunders.

Voith, V. L., and Borchelt, P. L. 1985a. Separation anxiety in dogs. Comp Cont Educ Small Anim Pract 7:42–53.

———. 1985b. Fears and phobias in companion animals. Comp Cont Educ Small Anim Pract 7:209–218.

18 EUTHANIZING AGENTS

EUGENE P. STEFFEY

Agent Evaluation Criteria
Agent Category and Mode of Action
Inhaled Vapors and Gases
Carbon Monoxide
Carbon Dioxide
Hydrogen Cyanide
Inhalation Anesthetics
Nitrogen
Injectable Agents
Barbiturates
Chloral Hydrate
Ethanol
T-61 Euthanasia Solution
Neuromuscular Blocking Drugs
Miscellaneous Injectable Drugs
Agents for Aquatic Animals

Euthanasia (literally a "good death") is the act of inducing humane death. Euthanasia can be performed using physical or chemical means. Information in this chapter is limited to chemical agents of euthanasia. The subject has been reviewed over the past few decades in five published reports by American Veterinary Medical Association (AVMA) Panels on Euthanasia. A new panel will be commissioned soon, and likely a published (the sixth) report of this sixth panel will appear before the next edition of this text. The fourth and fifth AVMA Panel reports (Smith et al. 1986; Andrews et al. 1993) and "Recommendations for Euthanasia of Experimental Animals," parts 1 and 2, prepared by a working party for the European Commission (Close et al. 1996, 1997), serve collectively as an informational focus for this chapter and a source of animal species–specific information. The present review also draws information from an earlier edition of this text (Hatch 1988).

AGENT EVALUATION CRITERIA. Several criteria should be used in evaluating agents for animal euthanasia. These include (1) ability to induce death without causing pain; (2) time required to induce loss of consciousness; (3) time required to produce death; (4) reliability; (5) safety of personnel; (6) potential for minimizing undesirable psychological stress on the animal (i.e., anxiety, apprehension, or distress); (7) nonreversibility; (8) compatibility with requirement and purpose; (9) emotional effect upon observers or operators; (10) economic feasibility; (11) compatibility with histopathologic evaluation; and (12) drug availability and personnel abuse potential. The ideal euthanizing agent should have the following properties:

1. The agent should produce death without causing pain or meet this condition as closely as possible under the circumstances of the moment.
2. The agent should not cause or require restraint that causes undue anxiety, struggling, vocalization, or clinical signs of autonomic activation.
3. The agent should be fast acting; unconsciousness and death should be instantaneous or occur within minutes of agent administration.
4. The agent's effects should be reliably and consistently produced.
5. The agent should be safe for properly trained personnel to use.
6. The agent should be easy to administer and not require complicated administration methods.
7. The agent should not be a drug with potential for abuse by humans.
8. The agent's operation should be aesthetically acceptable to those people observing the event.
9. The agent should be compatible with the overall reason and purpose of euthanizing the animal(s).
10. The agent and its method of delivery should be economical.
11. The agent should not be a threat to the environment or pose a sanitation problem.
12. The agent should not cause tissue changes that complicate necropsy results, including histopathologic inspection of tissues or toxicologic evaluation of body components. There should be no agent or agent-related tissue residues in animals intended for consumption.

AGENT CATEGORY AND MODE OF ACTION. Chemical agents that are used to euthanize animals can be categorized as injectable drugs or inhaled vapors or gases. A list is given in Table 18.1.

Chemical agents ultimately end life by decreasing the delivery of oxygen to cells to a level incompatible with sustained cellular function. The specific mechanism of individual agents varies. Adequate delivery of oxygen is a function of the respiratory and circulatory

TABLE 18.1—Chemical agents currently used as euthanizing agents

Inhalation agents
Carbon monoxide
Carbon dioxide
Inhalation anesthetics (diethyl ether, enflurane, halothane, isoflurane, methoxyflurane)
Nitrogen
Injectable agents
Barbiturates
Chloral hydrate and adjuvants
Ethanol
Miscellaneous injectable general anesthetics (used as adjuvants to other, primary agents in selected circumstances)

TABLE 18.2—Mechanism of action of euthanizing agents

Agent	Action	Comments
Inhalation agents		
Carbon monoxide	Combines with hemoglobin, lowering oxygen content of blood	Unconsciousness occurs rapidly; motor activity may persist after unconsciousness
Carbon dioxide	Direct depression of CNS and other vital organs; anesthetic effects	Unconsciousness occurs rapidly; possible involuntary motor activity after unconsciousness
Hydrogen cyanide	Direct inhibition of cellular utilization of oxygen	Unconsciousness occurs rapidly; involuntary motor activity after unconsciousness; dangerous to personnel; recently removed from lists of acceptable methods of euthanasia
Inhalation anesthetics	Direct depression of CNS and other vital organs	Used largely for individual animals in selected specific circumstances
Nitrogen	Displaces oxygen in the inspired breath; lowers oxygen content of blood	Unconsciousness occurs rapidly; involuntary motor activity may persist after unconsciousness
Injectable agents		
Barbiturates	Direct depression of CNS; anesthetic effects	Unconsciousness occurs rapidly when given by IV route
Chloral hydrate and combinations	Direct depression of CNS; anesthetic effects	Unconsciousness occurs rapidly; generally reserved for large domestic animals
Ethanol	Direct depression of CNS	Use with small laboratory animals only
T61	Direct depression of CNS	Transient struggling may occur before unconsciousness; objectionable tissue damage may occur; recently withdrawn from US market
Neuromuscular blocking drugs	Paralysis of respiratory muscles	Unacceptable for use as a sole agent

Sources: Modified from AVMA Panel reports on euthanasia (Smith et al. 1986; Andrews et al. 1993).

systems and their own associated regulatory mechanisms (central, peripheral, and autonomic nervous systems). Euthanizing agents can and often do influence the process of oxygen delivery at one or multiple stages. Table 18.2 lists the sites of action of frequently used euthanizing agents.

Inhaled Vapors and Gases

CARBON MONOXIDE. Carbon monoxide (CO) comes from natural sources such as forest fires and atmospheric oxidation of methane and from human activity. The greatest source from human activity is as a byproduct of internal combustion engines. It also can be produced chemically (Klaassen 1990). It has a high affinity for hemoglobin—more than 200 times that of oxygen for hemoglobin (Nunn 1987). Its toxicity is largely due to its combination with hemoglobin to form carboxyhemoglobin. This form of hemoglobin cannot carry oxygen. As a result, the partial pressure of oxygen may not change from normal but the oxygen content of blood and therefore the amount of oxygen available to the tissues decrease markedly. By its presence it also accounts for a shift to the left in the dissociation curve of remaining hemoglobin combined with oxygen. This means that it is more difficult to unload oxygen from hemoglobin at the tissue level. Therefore, less oxygen is available to tissues by yet a different mechanism. Carbon monoxide also exerts a direct toxic effect by binding to cellular cytochromes.

Carbon monoxide is odorless, tasteless, nonirritating, and causes no increase in ventilation or cyanosis (blood is cherry red). The tissues most affected by CO and other euthanizing agents that directly influence oxygen delivery are those most sensitive to oxygen deprivation, like the brain and the heart. Unconsciousness occurs without pain or apparent appreciable discomfort. A concentration of 6% or greater is usually desired for purposes of euthanasia. Agitation and vocalization may occur before loss of consciousness, but this can be minimized by pretreatment with tranquilizers (Chalifoux and Dallaire 1983; Dallaire and Chalifoux 1985).

Carbon monoxide used for individual or mass euthanasia is considered acceptable for small animals, including dogs and cats, providing appropriate precautions are taken. These are discussed further in recent panel reports (Smith et al. 1986; Andrews et al. 1993; Close et al. 1996). Because of its insidious nature, personnel safety is of particular concern with its use.

CARBON DIOXIDE. Carbon dioxide (CO_2) has been and continues to be used widely to euthanize small laboratory animals, but there is debate about which method and concentration should be used: i.e., rapid immersion in a gas mixture of high CO_2 concentration versus gradual induction with increasing CO_2 concentrations (Dannemann et al. 1997; Smith and Harrap 1997; Andrews et al. 1993; Close et al. 1996). It has also been used for preslaughter narcosis of some food animals (Smith et al. 1986; Andrews et al. 1993; Gregory et al. 1987), but use for euthanasia of large laboratory animals is not common (Ewbank 1983).

Time to anesthesia and death are inversely related to CO_2 concentration (Dannemann et al. 1997). At low concentrations (5-8%) CO_2 elevates the pain threshold (Stokes et al. 1948), and at higher concentrations (<30%) it has a rapid anesthetic effect (Nunn 1987; Leake and Waters 1929; Mattsson et al. 1972; Klemm 1964; Simonsen et al. 1981; Glen and Scott 1973; Hansen et al. 1991). Eisele et al. (1967) showed in dogs that an arterial CO_2 partial pressure greater than 95 mm Hg (alveolar concentration of about 13% at sea level) is associated with arterial and cerebrospinal fluid pH of less than 7.10 and is increasingly anesthetic; a basal level of general anesthesia (1.0 minimum alveolar concentration) is produced by an arterial CO_2 partial pressure of about 245 mm Hg (an alveolar concentration of about 35%). The major effect of CO_2 on the central nervous system is likely caused by alteration of the intracellular pH with consequent derangements of metabolic processes (Woodbury and Karler 1960). The work of Eisele et al. (1967) showed that the degree of CO_2 narcosis correlated better with cisternal cerebrospinal fluid pH than with arterial CO_2 partial pressure. Adverse reactions such as involuntary muscle activity and convulsions may occur in some animals, but this is usually after the animals are unconscious (Leake and Waters 1929; Hansen et al. 1991; Smith et al. 1986; Forslid 1987). Hemorrhaging from the nose and pulmonary hemorrhage and edema are also observed on histologic examination of some animals (Dannemann et al. 1997).

Carbon dioxide is available as a compressed gas in cylinders. Oxygen can be added in low concentrations (15-20%) if desirable to minimize or prevent hypoxic conditions during CO_2 inhalation (Coenen et al. 1995). Carbon dioxide is nonflammable and nonexplosive and thus represents little hazard to personnel. Additional information on the pharmacologic effects of CO_2 can be found in Chap. 10.

HYDROGEN CYANIDE. Hydrogen cyanide (HC) induces rapid death because it blocks mitochondrial utilization of oxygen. Cellular respiration is thus inhibited and cytotoxicity results (Klaassen 1990). Convulsions may occur, usually following unconsciousness, and are presumably related to cellular hypoxic conditions in the brain. Use poses a substantial risk for harm to animal handlers. Hydrogen cyanide has been removed from the AVMA Panel's list of acceptable methods of euthanasia (AVMA 1992; Andrews et al. 1993). Therefore, its action will not be further discussed here. Additional information can be found in the panel's reports (Smith et al. 1986; Andrews et al. 1993) and elsewhere (Klaassen 1990).

INHALATION ANESTHETICS. The inhalation anesthetics, including diethyl ether, halothane, methoxyflurane, enflurane, isoflurane, and the recently introduced sevoflurane and desflurane, may be used to euthanize animals via overdose. With small animals, any of these agents can be delivered by placing an animal or animals in a closed receptacle containing gauze pledget soaked with the anesthetic liquid. Alternatively, the anesthetic can be delivered under more controlled circumstances by introducing the anesthetic along with carrier gas into a chamber or chambers from a flowmeter-vaporizer assembly, equipment similar to that used in the clinical delivery of inhaled anesthetics to patients. The inhalation anesthetics are generally less desirable than other techniques because the prolonged time to death may be excessive, especially with the more soluble agents such as ether and methoxyflurane. The species is also a factor in this decision (Blackshaw et al. 1988).

The anesthetic potency of nitrous oxide is too low to be used by itself as a euthanizing agent under this category. At inspired concentrations of nitrous oxide greater than 80% (sea level conditions) hypoxemic conditions exist. Human abuse is a potential with this drug.

The long-term adverse effects on health from occupational exposure to trace concentrations of waste anesthetic gases is a controversial subject. Present information indicates that inhaled anesthetics have no more than a low potential for causing long-term toxicity (Baden and Rice 1990). However, until definitive information is available, it is best to consider that all of the inhaled anesthetics are potentially hazardous to personnel who are chronically exposed.

NITROGEN. Nitrogen (N_2) is a colorless, odorless, inert gas that constitutes about 79% of normal atmospheric air. It is readily available commercially as a compressed gas stored in cylinders.

Euthanasia is induced by rapidly replacing the air within a sealed chamber with pure N_2 at ambient pressure. The N_2 displaces oxygen within the chamber and hypoxic conditions result. Unconsciousness occurs rapidly, but gasping, yelping, muscle tremors, or convulsions may precede death. Newborn animals are not euthanized by this method as rapidly as older animals; therefore, N_2 is not recommended for euthanasia of these animals (Smith et al. 1986). Nitrogen gas is considered an acceptable agent for mass euthanasia, but in many situations other methods are considered preferable (Andrews et al. 1993).

Injectable Agents. Noninhalation agents can be administered via a variety of routes. In the past, intravenous, intracardiac, intraperitoneal, intrathecal, intramuscular, intrathoracic, subcutaneous, rectal, and oral routes have been used. Preference is given to the intravenous route because the effect is most rapid and predictable. Contemporary opinion does not support the routine use of intra cardiac, intrathoracic, and intrathecal routes, especially in unsedated healthy animals (Andrews et al. 1993). Administration of drugs for euthanasia via the oral, rectal, or subcutaneous routes is generally inadvisable because of prolonged onset of action (Smith et al. 1986; Grier 1991).

BARBITURATES. The barbiturates are used extensively for euthanasia. They may be administered by a variety of routes but intravenous is preferred for speed of unconsciousness and lack of trauma. There is a rapid progression from unconsciousness to deep general anesthesia, respiratory arrest, and finally cardiac arrest.

Pentobarbital alone or in combination with other depressant drugs is most commonly used to euthanize individual animals. It is not suitable for mass euthanasia because of the technical expertise required and the need to handle individual animals regardless of their temperament or the available facilities. Barbiturates require professional supervision and are listed as Schedule II drugs under current Drug Enforcement Administration (DEA) regulations. Human abuse potential is of concern. Meat from barbiturate-euthanized animals should not be used for animal (or human) consumption.

CHLORAL HYDRATE. This drug, like the barbiturates, causes progressive dose-related central nervous system depression. However, because some of its accompanying actions (e.g., slower onset of action vs. barbiturates, gasping, vocalizations) in otherwise unmedicated animals are considered by some objectionable, it is not recommended by the AVMA Panel for routine use with dogs, cats, and other small animals (Andrews et al. 1993).

Chloral hydrate and mixtures of chloral hydrate, magnesium sulfate, and pentobarbital have long been in use as an anesthetic for large domestic animals, especially horses. Intravenous overdose of these chloral hydrate mixtures is suitable for euthanasia of individual large animals.

Chloral hydrate and its mixtures are classed as Schedule IV drugs under DEA regulations.

ETHANOL. Ethanol is a widely available drug with potent hypnotic and sedative effects. It has recently been advocated as an alternative and effective method of euthanasia for small laboratory animals (e.g., mice) (Prien et al. 1988).

Ethanol is a primary central nervous system depressant. As blood ethanol concentration is increased, general impairment of nervous function occurs followed by general anesthesia and ultimately coma and death via respiratory arrest, conditions not unlike actions related to increasing doses of barbiturates. In one study of mice, 70% ethanol injected intraperitoneally reportedly caused death in 2.68 minutes with no discomfort observable in any individual (Prien et al. 1988).

T-61 EUTHANASIA SOLUTION. T-61 is an injectable drug mixture marketed as a non-DEA-controlled alternative to barbiturate solutions. It is a mixture of an agent with general anesthetic properties (*N*-2-[methoxyphenyl]-2-ethylbutyl-1-hydroxybutyramide), a muscle relaxant (4,4′-methylene *bis*-cyclohexyl-tri-methyl ammonium iodide), and a local anesthetic (tetracaine hydrochloride). Each milliliter of T-61 contains 200, 50, and 5 mg of these components, respectively.

The agent has been recently withdrawn from the market in the US but is available in Canada (Andrews et al. 1993). There is no human abuse potential.

Because it causes discomfort when administered extravascularly, T-61 should only be administered intravenously. The agent is unsuitable in many cases in which postmortem tissue studies are desirable because of widespread undesirable effects on structure and biochemistry of tissues and body fluid (Prien et al. 1988; Hellebrekers et al. 1990; Doughty and Stuart 1995).

NEUROMUSCULAR BLOCKING DRUGS. Neuromuscular blocking drugs, also referred to as curariform or peripheral-acting muscle relaxant drugs, must never be used by themselves for euthanasia. Drugs in this classification include curare (*d*-tubocurarine), succinylcholine, pancuronium, and atracurium. They induce death by immobilizing the respiratory muscles, causing fatal suffocation. There is no central nervous system depression. Animals are immobile but fully conscious and sensitive to their immediate surroundings and body part manipulations. The use of these drugs as sole agents for euthanasia is unacceptable.

MISCELLANEOUS INJECTABLE DRUGS. A wide variety of anesthetic and anesthetic adjuvant drugs (Chap. 9) may be useful in allaying animal apprehension and facilitating control of animals presented for euthanasia. Readers are encouraged to review pharmacological advantages and disadvantages in appropriate sections elsewhere in this text.

A number of drugs have been used alone in the past to euthanize animals but are now considered undesirable. These include strychnine and nicotine (Smith et al. 1986). In addition, drugs such as digitalis and calcium, magnesium, and potassium ions act directly on heart muscle and cause death by stopping the heart. They have no effect on consciousness and are not analgesic. Therefore, they too should not be used alone to purposely end life.

AGENTS FOR AQUATIC ANIMALS. Discussion in this chapter has focused on chemicals for mammals and birds. Some of these agents may also be used for causing humane death in aquatic animals, e.g., pentobarbital via injection. In addition, agents may be placed in the water environment for absorption through the skin and gills (Andrews et al. 1993; Close et al. 1996). For example, inhalation anesthetic agents may be bubbled into the water environment. Benzocaine dissolved in acetone before adding to tank water is an effective and humane method of killing fish and amphibians. Death occurs subsequent to generalized CNS depression. Tricaine methane sulphonate (MS-222), a dose-related CNS depressant, is commonly used as a general anesthetic for fish and like barbiturates may be used in overdose for a euthanasia agent.

Euthanasia of a pet animal is a very sensitive situation for the client-veterinarian relationship (Edney 1989; Cohen and Sawyer 1991; Kay et al. 1988) and must satisfy humane and ethical tests. It is a procedure that is common to varying degrees in most companion animal health care facilities (Gorodetsky 1997) and its conduct requires careful consideration and empathy on the part of the veterinarian (Randolph 1994).

Laboratory animal euthanasia also must satisfy scientific criteria. For example, euthanasia per se might alter cellular architecture (Feldman and Gupta 1976; Port et al. 1978; Prien et al. 1988) or components of host immune defenses (Howard et al. 1990; Lord et al. 1991) or other aspects of laboratory study. Accordingly, agent selection is multifactorial and complex. In many cases, information on which to base a sound decision is lacking.

REFERENCES

Andrews, E. J., Bennett, B. T., Clark, J. D., Houpt, K. A., Pascoe, P. J., Robinson, G. W., and Boyce, J. R. 1993. Report of the AVMA Panel on Euthanasia (1993). J Am Vet Med Assoc 202:230-49.

AVMA. 1992. Euthanasia panel to hold public session in Boston. J Am Vet Med Assoc 200:1605-6.

Baden, J. M., and Rice, S. A. 1990. Metabolism and toxicity. In R. D. Miller, ed., Anesthesia, 3rd ed., pp. 135-70. New York: Churchill Livingstone.

Blackshaw, J. K., Fenwick, D. C., Beattie, A. W., and Allan, D. J. 1988. The behaviour of chickens, mice and rats during euthanasia with chloroform, carbon dioxide and ether. Lab Anim 22:67-75.

Chalifoux, A., and Dallaire, A. 1983. Physiologic and behavioral evaluation of CO euthanasia of adult dogs. Am J Vet Res 44:2412-17.

Close, B., Banister, K., Baumans, V., Bernoth, E.-M., Bromage, N., Bunyan, J., Erhardt, W., Flecknell, P., Gregory, N., Hackbarth, H., Morton, D., and Warwick, C. 1996. Recommendations for euthanasia of experimental animals: Part 1. Lab Anim 30:293-316.

———. 1997. Recommendations for euthanasia of experimental animals: Part 2. Laboratory Animals 31:1-32.

Coenen, A. M. L., Drinkenburg, W. H. I. M., Hoenderken, R., and van Luijtelaar, E. L. J. M. 1995. Carbon dioxide euthanasia in rats: oxygen supplementation minimizes sighs of agitation and asphyxia. Lab Anim 29:262-68.

Cohen, S. P., and Sawyer, D. C. 1991. Suffering and euthanasia. Problems Vet Med 3:101-9.

Dallaire, A., and Chalifoux, A. 1985. Premedication of dogs with acepromazine or pentazocine before euthanasia with carbon monoxide. Can J Comp Med 49(2):171-78.

Dannemann, P. J., Stein, S., and Walshaw, S. O. 1997. Humane and practical implications of using carbon dioxide mixed with oxygen for anesthesia or euthanasia. Lab An Sci 47:376-85.

Doughty, M. J., and Stuart, D. 1995. Quantification of the hemolysis associated with use of T-61® as a euthanasia agent in rabbits: a comparison with Euthanyl® (pentobarbital sodium) and the impact on serum hexosaminidase measurements. Can J Physiol Pharmacol 73:1274-80.

Edney, A. T. B. 1989. Killing with kindness. Vet Rec 124:320-22.

Eisele, J. H., Eger, E. I., and Muallem, M. 1967. Narcotic properties of carbon dioxide in the dog. Anesthesiology 28:856-65.

Ewbank,R. 1983. Is CO_2 euthanasia humane? Nature 305:268.

Feldman, D. B., and Gupta, B. N. 1976. Histopathologic changes in laboratory animals resulting from various methods of euthanasia. Lab Anim Sci 26:218-21.

Forslid, A. 1987. Transient neocortical, hippocampal and amygdaloid EEG silence induced by one minute inhalation of high concentration CO_2 in swine. Acta Physiol Scand 130:1-10.

Glen, J. B., and Scott, W. N. 1973. Carbon dioxide euthanasia of cats. Br Vet J 129:471-79.

Gorodetsky, E. 1997. Epidemiology of dog and cat euthanasia across Canadian prairie provinces. Can Vet J 38:649-652.

Gregory, N. G., Moss, B. W., and Leeson, R. H. 1987. An assessment of carbon dioxide stunning in pigs. Vet Rec 121:517-18.

Grier, R. L. 1991. Administration of euthanasia agents—a letter in reply. J Am Vet Med Assoc 198:1102-3.

Hansen, N. E., Creutzberg, A., and Simonsen, H. B. 1991. Euthanasia of mink (*Mustela vison*) by means of carbon dioxide (CO_2), carbon monoxide (CO) and nitrogen (N_2). Br Vet J 147:140-46.

Hatch, R. C. 1988. Euthanatizing agents. In N. H. Booth and L. E. McDonald, eds., Veterinary pharmacology and therapeutics, 6th ed., pp. 1143-48. Ames: Iowa State University Press.

Hellebrekers, L. J., Baumans, V., Bertens, A. P. M., and Hartman, W. 1990. On the use of T61 for euthanasia of domestic and laboratory animals: an ethical evaluation. Lab Anim 24:200-204.

Howard, H. L., McLaughlin-Taylor, E., and Hill, R. L. 1990. The effect of mouse euthanasia technique on subsequent lymphocyte proliferation and cell mediated lympholysis assays. Lab Anim Sci 40:510-14.

Kay, W. J., Cohen, S. P., Nieburg, H. A., Fudin, C. E., Grey, R. E., Kutscher, A. H., and Osman, M. M., eds. 1988. Euthanasia of the Companion Animal. Philadelphia: Charles Press.

Klaassen, C. D. 1990. Nonmetallic environmental toxicants: air pollutants, solvents and vapors, and pesticides. In A. G. Gilman, T. W. Rall, A. S. Nies, et al., eds., The Pharmacological Basis of Therapeutics, 8th ed., pp. 1615-39. New York: Pergamon Press.

Klemm, W. R. 1964. Carbon dioxide anesthesia in cats. Am J Vet Res 25:1201-5.

Leake, C. D., and Waters, R. M. 1929. The anesthetic properties of carbon dioxide. Anesth Analg 8:17-19.

Lord, R., Jones, G. L., and Spencer, L. 1991. Ethanol euthanasia and its effect on the binding of antibody generated against an immunogenic peptide construct. Res Vet Sci 51:164-68.

Mattsson, J. L., Stinson, J. M., and Clark, C. S. 1972. Electroencephalographic power-spectral changes coincident with onset of carbon dioxide narcosis in rhesus monkey. Am J Vet Res 33:2043-49.

Nunn, J. F. 1987. Applied Respiratory Physiology. 3rd ed. Boston: Butterworths.

Port, C. D., Garvin, P. J., Ganote, C. E., and Sawyer, D. C. 1978. Pathologic changes induced by an euthanasia agent. Lab Anim Sci 28:448-50.

Prien, T., Traber, D. L., Linares, H. A., and Davenport, S. L. 1988. Haemolysis and artifactual lung damage induced by an euthanasia agent. Lab Animal 22:170-72.

Randolph, J. W. 1994. Learning from your own pet's euthanasia. JAVMA 205:544-55.

Simonsen, H. B., Thordal-Christensen, A., and Ockens, N. 1981. Carbon monoxide and carbon dioxide euthanasia of cats: duration and animal behaviour. Br Vet J 137:274-78.

Smith, A. W., Houpt, K. A., Kitchell, R. L., Kohn, D. F., McDonald, L. E., Passaglia, M., Jr., Thurmon, J. C., and Ames, E. R. 1986. Report of the AVMA Panel on Euthanasia. J Am Vet Med Assoc 188:252-68.

Smith, W. and Harrap, S. B. 1997. Behavioural and cardiovascular responses of rats to euthanasia using carbon dioxide gas. Lab Anim 31:337-46.

Stokes, J., III, Chapman, W. P., and Smith, L. H. 1948. Effects of hypoxia and hypercapnia on perception of thermal cutaneous pain. J Clin Invest 27:299-304.

Woodbury, D. M., and Karler, R. 1960. The role of carbon dioxide in the nervous system. Anesthesiology 21:686-91.

SECTION 4

Autacoids and Anti-inflammatory Drugs

19 HISTAMINE, SEROTONIN, AND THEIR ANTAGONISTS

H. RICHARD ADAMS

Histamine
- **H_1, H_2, and H_3 Histamine Receptors**
- **Endogenous Histamine**
- **Histamine Release**
- **Role in Health and Disease**
- **Pharmacologic Effects**
- **Biotransformation**
- **Medical Use**

Antihistamines
- **Development**
- **Chemistry**
- **Pharmacologic Effects**
- **Side Effects and Interactions**
- **Toxicity**
- **Therapeutic Uses**

Serotonin
- **Chemistry**
- **Pharmacologic Effects**
- **Role in Physiologic and Pathologic Processes**
- **Antagonists**

HISTAMINE. Histamine is a biogenic amine detected in the early 1900s as a common bacterial-source contaminant of ergot extracts (Dale and Laidlaw 1910). Because histamine evoked a contractile response in smooth muscles and also lowered blood pressure, attention was drawn to similarities between its actions and anaphylactic-type reactions. Histamine was discovered in mammalian tissues and found to be released upon cellular trauma, leading to the theory of histamine as an endogenous mediator of cell injury. Subsequent studies have provided a wealth of physiologic and pathophysiologic roles for histamine quite apart from simple cellular trauma (Barnes et al. 1990; Falus and Meretey 1992). This amine is involved in inflammations, anaphylaxis, allergies, and certain types of drug reactions, and it regulates gastric secretion (Obrink 1991; Morris 1992; Mitsuhashi and Payan 1992). Histamine itself is not used therapeutically, but antihistaminic agents are commonly used to inhibit effects of endogenous histamine.

H_1, H_2, and H_3 Histamine Receptors. Histamine contracts several types of smooth muscles, including those of the bronchi, gut, and large blood vessels. In contrast, small arterioles are relaxed by histamine to the extent that peripheral vascular resistance and blood pressure fall. Capillary permeability is increased. Gastric secretion of hydrochloric acid is stimulated, as are secretory activities of other exocrine glands. In humans, flushing of the facial skin and burning and itching sensations also are evoked. With large doses of histamine, blood pressure progressively falls and is accompanied by hemoconcentration caused by extravasation of plasma. "Histamine shock" may terminate in death (Pearce 1991).

Responses to histamine can be explained by activation of specific histamine receptors on various target cells. Analysis of histamine-receptor interactions was advanced by Bovet and Staub (1937), who described the first antihistamine. This type of drug competitively inhibits several biologic effects of histamine and protects guinea pigs from the high lethality of anaphylactic shock. Ash and Schild (1966) subsequently pointed out the likelihood for two types of histamine receptors in mammalian tissue. This theory was based on the knowledge that conventional antihistaminic drugs available at that time, such as pyrilamine and diphenhydramine, blocked only certain actions of histamine. Other activities, most notably stimulation of gastric secretion, were not amenable to inhibition by such drugs and were therefore thought to be mediated by a second type of receptor.

The existence of two general types of histamine receptors was confirmed by Black et al. (1972), who conducted a systematic pharmacologic study of compounds derived from the basic structural components of histamine. Based on this investigation, histamine receptors were designated as histamine type 1 (H_1) and histamine type 2 (H_2). Histamine-induced contraction of bronchial and intestinal smooth muscle is mediated through H_1 receptors and inhibited by pyrilamine and other standard antihistamines (now called H_1 blockers). In contrast, histamine-induced stimulation of gastric secretion is mediated by H_2 receptors and inhibited by the newly available H_2 blockers burimamide, metamide, and cimetidine. Different histamine receptor agonists likewise display preferential action at receptor subtypes. For example, 2-methylhistamine evokes rather selective agonist action at H_1 receptors; whereas, 4-methylhistamine acts preferentially at H_2 receptors.

Studies have also indicated yet a third class of histamine receptors. These H_3 receptors are believed to be linked to inhibition of adenylyl cyclase through an inhibitory G_i protein (Arang et al. 1987). H_3 receptors may be localized to the central nervous system (CNS), and their therapeutic relevance to veterinary medicine remains to be discovered.

Endogenous Histamine. Histamine is 2-(4-imidazolyl) ethylamine (Fig. 19.1); it is derived from the decarboxylation of an amino acid, histidine. Conversion of histidine to histamine is catalyzed in mammalian tissues by a specific enzyme, histidine decarboxylase; this enzyme is present in all cell types that contain histamine.

Histamine is widely distributed throughout mammalian tissue, but concentrations vary considerably in different species; e.g., quantities of circulating histamine are relatively high in the goat and rabbit but low in the horse, dog, cat, and human. It is generally accepted that most of the histamine stored within the body is derived locally from enzymatic decarboxylation of histidine. Dietary histamine and histamine produced by enteric bacteria are disposed of rapidly after absorption into the portal circulation and contribute little or nothing to tissue storage sites.

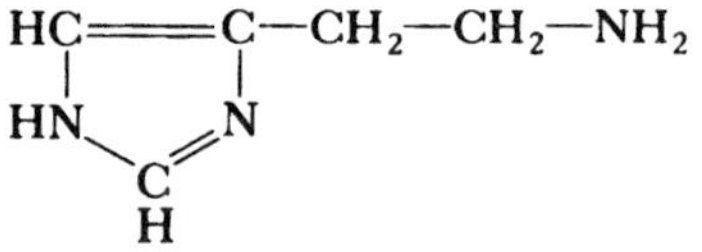

HC═C—CH_2—CH_2—NH_2
HN N
C
H

Histamine

FIG. 19.1

Two general stores of histamine can be identified in mammalian species: the mast cell pool made up of mast cells and basophils and the non-mast cell pool localized in the gastrointestinal (GI) tract, CNS, dermis, and other organs. These two pools differ not only in cellular locale but also in responsiveness to physiologic and pharmacologic stimuli.

The mast cell pool of highly concentrated histamine is distributed in connective tissue throughout the body. Circulating basophils, free counterparts of fixed-tissue mast cells, also contain high concentrations of histamine and are grouped with the mast cell because of basic similarities. Within these two cell types, histamine is synthesized rather slowly and stored tenaciously in secretory granules; hence, turnover rate is low. Experimental drugs such as compound 48/80 have the interesting capability of liberating histamine from storage granules. Because of the slow turnover rate, mast cell stores are replenished slowly after exposure to a histamine-releasing agent. The mast cell pool represents the histamine that participates in inflammatory responses, allergic phenomena, shock, some adverse drug reactions, and other forms of cellular insult.

The precise cellular localizations and physiologic functions of the non-mast cell pool of histamine within the gastric mucosa, brain, and skin are not known with certainty. Histamine in these regions, in contrast to the mast cell pool, undergoes a rapid turnover rate; it is synthesized and released continuously rather than being stored. Functional roles of this newly synthesized or nascent histamine are under considerable investigation. Portions of this histamine are present within neural elements, and neurotransmitter functions have been proposed. In the gastric mucosa, a "local hormone" action of histamine controls gastric secretion. Interestingly, non-mast cell histamine is generally resistant to the histamine-releasing drugs such as compound 48/80.

Histamine Release. Histamine is highly concentrated in mast cell granules, where it is stored with a heparin-protein complex, proteolytic enzymes, and other autacoids. Release of histamine basically is a two-step process: sudden exocytotic extrusion of granules from the cell and release of histamine from the granules into the interstitial milieu. The latter occurs as an ionic exchange reaction between extracellular cations and molecules of granular histamine. Release can be initiated by a variety of stressful stimuli, including anaphylaxis-allergy, different drugs and chemicals, and physical injury.

ANAPHYLAXIS AND ALLERGY. Hypersensitivity phenomena associated with antigen-antibody reactions evoke active release of histamine from the mast cell pool. Free histamine then plays an important role in mediating physiologic manifestations of such reactions as vasodilation, itching, smooth muscle contraction, and edema. Other autacoids also participate in tissue responses to hypersensitivity reactions. Signs of histamine involvement in systemic anaphylaxis vary in different species. In carnivores, histamine and anaphylaxis produce pronounced hypotension and hepatomegaly. In rabbits, pulmonary arterioles constrict and the right heart dilates in response to either histamine injection or exposure of a sensitized individual to the appropriate antigen. In guinea pigs, dominant manifestations are bronchial constriction and death by asphyxiation. Humans seem to respond like guinea pigs and dogs in that severe hypotension, bronchial constriction, and laryngeal edema are principal signs of anaphylaxis.

The mast cell pool of histamine represents a major target for acute types of hypersensitivity-allergy reactions. Expulsion of the granular contents of mast cells and basophils is initiated by interaction of specific antigen and cell-bound reaginic (IgE) antibody. This interaction increases permeability of the cell to calcium ions (Ca^{++}). The resulting influx of Ca^{++} from the interstitium then evokes release of histamine in a manner basically analogous to the secretory responses of various endocrine and exocrine cells to their respective secretagogues (Douglas 1974). Release is an active process, requiring metabolic energy as well as Ca^{++}, and should be distinguished from simple release secondary to cell destruction and cytolysis.

The ubiquitous cyclic adenosine 3′,5′-monophosphate (cAMP) system may be involved in histamine release evoked by antigen-antibody interactions. Studies indicate that an increase in cAMP concentration suppresses histamine release (Lichtenstein and Margolis 1968). Agents that activate adenylyl cyclase (e.g., catecholamines) or inhibit phosphodiesterase (e.g., xanthines) can be anticipated to inhibit the release of histamine. The beneficial effects of drugs widely used in treating allergic disorders, such as the catecholamines and theophylline, may therefore involve inhibition of histamine release in addition to their well-known and more important physiologic antagonism of histamine actions on target cells.

DRUGS AND CHEMICALS. Many drugs and chemicals produce direct degranulation of mast cells with release of histamine independently from development of allergy. This characteristic action represents an untoward side effect associated either with intravenous (IV) administration of a relatively large dose or direct intradermal injection. Conversely, certain chemicals have as their dominant property the ability to release histamine from the mast cell pool.

The curare-alkaloids are used clinically as neuromuscular blocking agents (Chap. 8), but they also are notorious for releasing histamine as an adverse side effect; in some species, IV injection of these agents can be followed by histamine-induced bronchospasm and hypotension. Other clinically used drugs that may release histamine include morphine, codeine, papaverine, meperidine, polypeptide antibiotics (polymyxin), atropine, and, under some conditions, even sympathomimetic amines. Histamine release usually is significant with most of these agents only when large doses are used.

Certain other chemicals have been classified simply as histamine-releasing agents because this particular activity supersedes their other pharmacologic properties. The best known and most active is an organic base called compound 48/80, a condensation product of *p*-methoxyphenylethylmethylamine with formaldehyde (Goth and Johnson 1975). Injection of compound 48/80 or other similar agents evokes classic pharmacologic signs of histamine release that are susceptible to blockade by antihistaminic drugs. Tachyphylaxis to repeated injections is characteristic of these chemicals, presumably because of decreased availability of releasable stores of histamine. Other substances such as dextran, ovomucoid (from egg white), histones, and lysosomal enzymes also can release histamine, depending upon the species. Endogenous substances that provoke histamine release and may be involved in physiologic release mechanisms include bradykinin, kallidin, and substance P. Cellular reactions to many venoms and toxins also involve histamine release.

The basis for species-dependent actions of different releasing agents has not been clarified, and little is known about cellular mechanisms of drug-induced histamine release phenomena. Compound 48/80 not only elicits release of histamine but causes complete discharge of all the granular contents of mast cells. This process is Ca^{++} and energy dependent, but it is not known if such drugs act like pseudoantigens at cell membranes or directly mobilize cellular calcium instead (Douglas 1974; Goth and Johnson 1975).

PHYSICAL INJURY. When the skin is scratched or pricked, the characteristic redness and urtication that result are due to histamine. This response is quite pronounced in humans. Dermal reactions to severe cold or heat stress likewise depend on histamine liberated by local mast cells. Physical injury of virtually any type sufficiently intense to damage the cells will also evoke release of histamine.

Role in Health and Disease

GASTRIC SECRETION. Histamine is a potent stimulant of hydrochloric acid secretion by the gastric mucosa. This finding led early investigators to portray endogenous histamine as the final common mediator of gastric secretion, irrespective of whether stimulation arises from chemical, mechanical, or nervous elements. Full acceptance of this theory was delayed for over 50 years because conventional antihistaminic drugs available at the time (i.e., the H_1 blockers) failed to prevent gastric effects of histamine. This impediment was surmounted when Black et al. (1972) reported that the new H_2-blocking agents are quite efficacious in inhibiting gastric stimulant activities of histamine and its congeners. H_2-blocking drugs also reduce the gastric secretory response evoked by ingestion of a meal or administration of either the gastric hormone gastrin or its synthetic derivative pentagastrin.

NEURONS. Locally released or injected histamine stimulates sensory nerve endings, thereby evoking the classic symptoms of itching and pain. Histamine also is present in the brain, where it is concentrated in the hypothalamus; subcellular distribution studies have localized histamine to some nerve endings. These and related studies, in conjunction with the obvious CNS effects of histamine blockers, have prompted the suggestion that histaminergic neurons are present in the brain and that histamine released from these fibers functions as a neurotransmitter. Some investigators have proposed the existence of peripheral efferent histaminergic nerves; these fibers are envisioned as subserving vasodilation and participating as active components of reflex vasodilation in conjunction with the passive withdrawal of sympathetic vasoconstrictor tone in this reflex.

OTHERS. A variety of biologic roles have been proposed for endogenous histamine in addition to those previously addressed, including local regulation of the microcirculatory response to injury and inflammation, some type of anabolic activity in rapidly growing or repairing tissues, systemic signs associated with excessive numbers of mast cells or basophils, and involvement in different types of headaches in humans. In domestic animals, histamine released from damaged tissue has been suggested as a mediator in several pathologic states, including allergic reactions to drugs, venoms, and other antigens; ruminant bloating; overeating and other GI disorders of ruminants; laminitis; azoturia; retained placenta; pneumonia; gut edema of the pig; and various types of circulatory shock syndromes (e.g., septic shock). Except for allergic phenomena, however, the role of histamine in these conditions usually is more empirically based than experimentally founded.

Pharmacologic Effects. Histamine administered orally has essentially no effect because it is destroyed rapidly by the GI tract and liver. When injected intravenously, histamine produces a spectrum of characteristic effects. These activities include smooth muscle contraction, hypotension, increased gastric secretion, dermal reactions, and others.

Difficulties are encountered when attempts are made to designate H_1- or H_2-receptor responsibility for each action of histamine. In some tissues, H_1 and H_2 receptors are complementary and subserve similar tissue responses. In contrast, distinct and even opposing functions of the two receptor types have been identified in some tissues. Species differences are formidable and in most cases await further study for classification. In the following paragraphs, only the more representative examples of H_1- or H_2-receptor involvement, when known, are discussed.

CARDIOVASCULAR SYSTEM. The principal circulatory effects of histamine are dilation of terminal arterioles and other vessels of the microcirculation, edema formation caused by increased capillary permeability, and contraction of large arteries and veins. Relative dominance of the different actions varies in different species so that net circulatory response to histamine changes as the zoologic scale is ascended; e.g., arterioles are contracted strongly by histamine in rodents, less so in cats, and actually are dilated in dogs, nonhuman primates, and humans.

In rabbits, histamine is a pressor agent as a result of pronounced constriction of large blood vessels. This constrictor activity is feeble in carnivores where vasodilation of the microcirculation dominates instead. Thus the blood pressure response to histamine in cats, dogs, and primates is hypotension caused by a sharp fall in peripheral vascular resistance. The fall in blood pressure is dose dependent but is usually short-lived because of compensatory reflexes and inactivation of histamine.

The striking effects of histamine on the microcirculation can be demonstrated quite convincingly in the human subject. When this agent is administered intradermally, a characteristic triple response is produced, which includes localized redness at the injection site, developing within a few seconds and attaining maximal hue within a minute; localized edema fluid, forming a wheal in about 90 seconds; and diffuse redness or "flare," extending about 1 cm from the original red spot. The central redness and edema are from the dilation and increased permeability of local microcirculatory vessels (terminal arterioles, capillaries, and venules). The surrounding flush, which is accompanied by itching and perhaps pain, is due to dilation of neighboring arterioles brought about by a poorly understood axonal reflex mechanism. The triple response of human skin may be similar to manifestations of urticaria in animals.

Vascular actions of histamine formerly were believed to be mediated solely by H_1 receptors; however, it now seems that both types of histamine receptors are involved. The vasodilator response to H_1-receptor activation occurs at low doses of histamine and is rapid in onset and of brief duration. The H_2-receptor vasodilator response is evoked with larger doses and is slower in onset and of longer duration. The small-vessel permeability changes evoked by histamine are clearly mediated by H_1 receptors, while the role of H_2 events is uncertain. The precise ratio of H_1- and H_2-receptor involvement in vascular responses to histamine varies in domestic animal species; some of the more important species differences were reviewed by Hirschowitz (1979).

Cardiac effects of histamine are minimal when compared to vascular actions. In the intact animal, slight tachycardia is a common finding. This response is mainly secondary to baroreceptor reflexes activated by the depressor effect. In isolated heart muscle, histamine can elicit positive inotropic and chronotropic effects that are due partly to release of norepinephrine from nerve endings and also to direct activation of H_2 receptors in the heart muscle. There is some evidence that in vivo cardiac responses to histamine injection may partially reflect activation of cardiac H_2 receptors (Hirschowitz 1979).

NONVASCULAR SMOOTH MUSCLE. Histamine contracts bronchial smooth muscle via H_1 receptors in numerous mammals including the guinea pig, rabbit, dog, goat, calf, pig, horse, and human (Chand and Eyre 1975). Guinea pigs are exceptionally sensitive, and even minute doses of histamine can evoke bronchoconstriction leading to death. Humans with bronchial asthma likewise demonstrate increased sensitivity to bronchial effects of histamine and other bronchial smooth muscle stimulants. In contrast, histamine can mediate relaxation of respiratory smooth muscle in some species. Histamine-induced tracheal relaxation in cats involves both H_1 and H_2 receptors, while bronchial relaxation in sheep seems to be mediated by H_2 receptors (Hirschowitz 1979).

Relaxation of the rat uterus by histamine is mediated by H_2 receptors, but uterine muscle of other species is generally contracted by histamine. Responses of intestinal muscle also vary with species and region, but the classic effect is a contractile response caused by H_1 receptors. Although an indirect component mediated by neural elements may be involved, smooth muscle effects of histamine chiefly involve direct actions on the muscle itself.

EXOCRINE GLANDS. The following exocrine glands are listed in descending order of response to histamine: gastric, salivary, pancreatic, bronchial, and lacrimal. Gastric secretion of hydrochloric acid and, to a lesser degree, pepsinogen is unquestionably the most important; this response is mediated by H_2 receptors.

MECHANISM OF ACTION. The H_1 receptors in some cell types are linked to activation of phospholipase C and the resulting increase in inositol triphosphate and intracellular Ca^{++}. This process most likely involves a G protein, as discussed in Chap. 5 (Lambert 1993). The H_2 receptors also utilize G proteins linked to activation of adenylyl cyclase and its increased synthesis of cAMP, culminating in activation of the latter's intracellular receptor, protein kinase A. Interestingly, the vasodilator response elicited by endothelial H_1 receptors involves activation of nitric oxide synthase and release of endothelium-derived nitric oxide. The vasodilatory H_2 receptors, on the other hand, are localized on the vascular smooth muscle itself.

Biotransformation. Histamine administered orally is poorly absorbed, but absorption is virtually complete after parenteral injection. Pharmacologic actions are brief because of rapid metabolism and distribution into tissues. Exogenous histamine can be incorporated into storage granules to some extent; however, this pathway is probably unimportant to endogenous storage pools of the amine.

Biotransformation of histamine involves methylation and oxidation, as shown in Fig. 19.2. Histamine is acted upon by the enzyme histamine-*N* methyltransferase (imidazole-*N*-methyltransferase) to form methylhistamine; most of this metabolite is oxidized to methylimidazole acetic acid by the enzyme monoamine oxidase (>50%). The second pathway is oxidative deamination catalyzed by the enzyme diamine oxidase (histaminase) to form imidazoleacetic acid, which is conjugated with ribose as riboside (>25%). Only a small percentage of the primary amine can be acetylated in the GI tract, absorbed, and excreted in urine (1%). Some free histamine is also excreted in urine (2-3%).

Medical Use. Clinical applications in humans involve use of histamine as a test agent for achlorhydria, in diagnosis of pheochromocytoma, and for production of the triple response to evaluate the integrity of sensory innervations and circulatory competency. The polypeptide pentagastrin and histamine analogs such as the H_2-selective agonist impromidine have been used as alternative means of evaluating gastric secretory function because of less objectionable H_1-mediated side effects. Repeated injections of histamine in an attempt to desensitize patients with allergies has not met with general acceptance.

Cromolyn is an interesting drug used in human medicine as a prophylactic treatment of bronchial asthma. Cromolyn exerts this activity by inhibiting the release of histamine and other autacoids that participate in the asthmatic syndrome. The application of cromolyn to animal medicine remains untested.

ANTIHISTAMINES. Although the pharmacologic effects of histamine can be antagonized by several types of drugs, the term antihistamine should be restricted to agents that act on histamine receptors. The receptors are not activated by such interaction, but their occupancy by the antihistamine limits accessibility to

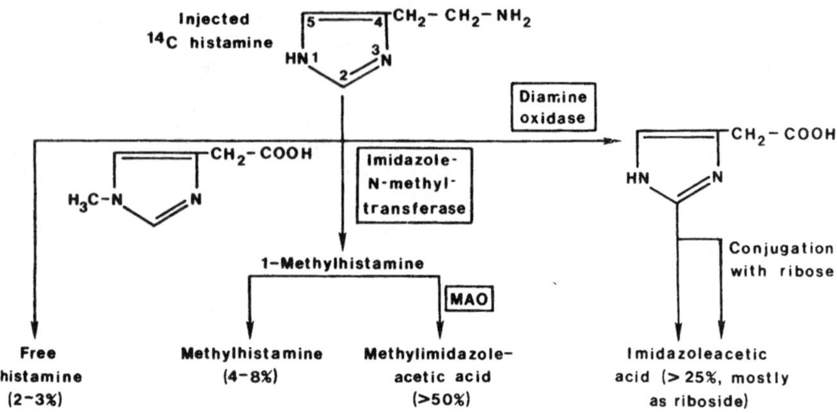

FIG. 19.2—Synthesis, metabolism, and urinary metabolites of histamine recovered in 12 hours following intradermal injection of ^{14}C-histamine in a human male (% values from Schayer and Cooper 1956).

histamine and thereby prevents the latter from exerting its cellular actions. Other agents such as catecholamines and xanthines exhibit pharmacologic activities that are, among other things, antagonistic to actions of histamine. However, these opposing actions are mediated by different receptors and cellular pathways; they represent physiologic antagonism.

Development. Bovet and Staub (1937) of the Pasteur Institute in Paris first demonstrated that two phenolic esters possessed antihistaminic activity. One of these compounds, 929F (thymoxyethyldiethylamine), protected guinea pigs against several lethal doses of histamine. Although the original drugs were too toxic for therapeutic use, their discovery led to development of many modern antihistaminic agents. Such compounds are now referred to as H_1 and H_2 antihistamines, based on the previously described differentiation of histamine receptors into H_1 and H_2 subtypes (Ash and Schild 1966; Black et al. 1972).

Chemistry. Some of the more frequently used H_1 antihistamines are listed in Table 19.1. The chemical structure of nearly all the H_1 antihistaminic drugs can be depicted by the structural formula shown in Fig. 19.3. The nucleus of the structure is ethylamine (CH_2CH_2N), which is also present in histamine. This moiety is thought to be the molecular component necessary for competition with histamine for specific cell receptors.

Three types of H_1 antihistaminics are known in which the element X (as depicted in Fig. 19.3) is nitrogen, oxygen, or carbon. The X represents a nitrogen for the ethylenediamine class (e.g., pyrilamine, Neoantergan), oxygen for the ethanolamine class (e.g., diphenhydramine, Benadryl), and carbon for the alkylamine class (e.g., Teldrin). The fourth class of antihistaminics contains a piperazine in place of the conventional ethylenediamine linkage (e.g., cyclizine, Marezine). The representative of the fifth class (e.g., promethazine, Phenergan) is not related directly to the previous drugs, since it is a phenothiazine derivative. The sixth class comprises the peperidines terfenadine and astemizole; these agents have aromatic ring moieties on either end of the ethylamine chain. These different chemical substitutions influence the potency of H_1-antihistaminic action as well as producing a variety of side effects.

The H_2 antihistamines differ from the H_1 blockers in their chemistry, pharmacokinetics, and pharmacodynamics. The imidazole ring structure of histamine is modified extensively or replaced by other substituents in the H_1 antagonists. In the H_2-blocking agents, however, the side chain is modified extensively, while the imidazole moiety is preserved. In contrast to the H_1 antihistaminics, the H_2 antagonists are somewhat less lipid soluble and do not effectively penetrate the blood-brain barrier. Hence the H_2 antagonists do not cause sedation, a prominent side effect of most of their H_1 counterparts.

Burimamide was the first H_2 antagonist, but it was absorbed too poorly to be effective after oral administration. Metiamide was subsequently synthesized; it was absorbed effectively from the GI tract, but several human patients treated with the drug developed agranulocytosis. A newer H_2 blocker, cimetidine, was then introduced into clinical medicine and so far has not been associated with hematologic toxicity. Ranitidine, famotidine, and nizatidine are some of the newer H_2 blockers.

Pharmacologic Effects. Antihistaminics of the H_1 subtype are absorbed satisfactorily after oral administration in monogastic animals but not in ruminants. Effects are usually expected within 20-45 minutes after oral administration, and the duration of action ranges from 3 to 12 hours (Table 19.1). IV administration elicits immediate effects, but this route is not often recommended because of resulting stimulation of the CNS and other side effects. The intramuscular

TABLE 19.1—Preparations and doses of some H_1 antihistamines in veterinary use

Generic name	Trade name	Single dose and route (in mg/kg unless indicated otherwise)	Preparation	Special properties
Diphenhydramine Hydrochloride, USP	Benadryl, Caladryl (lotion)	LA: 0.5–1 SA: 1–2 PO, IV/12 hr	Inj. 10, 25, 50 mg/mL Elix. 10 mg/4 mL	Marked sedation; anti-motion sickness
Pyrilamine Maleate, NF	Histosol,[a] Neoantergan	LA, SA: 1–2 IM, IV, SC	Inj. 20–25 mg/mL Tab. 25–50 mg	Prominent sedation
Tripelennamine Hydrochloride, USP	Pyribenzamine	LA: 1–2 PO, IV SA: 1–1.5 PO, q8h	Inj. 20 mg/mL Tab. 25–50 mg Bolus 500 mg	Sedation; if overdose, ataxia; convulsions
Chlorpheniramine Maleate, NF	Telodron,[b] Teldrin	SA: 1 span. for dogs >3.6–18 kg/12 hr 2 span. for dogs >18 kg/12 hr	Span. 8 mg., sustained-release form	Moderate sedation
Dimenhydrinate, USP	Dramamine	LA, SA: 1–1.5 PO, IM, SC	Inj. 50 mg/mL Tab. 50mg Liquid 12.5 mg/4 mL	Prominent anti-motion sickness
Promethazine Hydrochloride, USP	Phenergan	LA, SA: 0.2–1 IM, IV, PO, q8h	Inj. 25–50 mg/mL Tab. 25, and 50 mg Also available as cream for topical use	Long acting, marked sedation; anti-motion sickness
Clemastine	Tavist 1	SA: 0.5–1 PO, q12h	Tab.	Few side effects
Hydroxyzine	Atarax	SA: 2 PO, q8h	Tab.	Sedation
Trimeprazine	Temaril	SA: 0.5–2 PO, q12h	Tab.	Sedation
Astemizole	Hismanal	SA: 2.5–10 PO, q24h	Tab.	Nonsedative
Terfenadine	Seldane		Tab.	Nonsedative
Amitriptyline	Eleva	SA:1.0–2 PO, q12h	Tab.	Tricyclic

Abbreviations: LA = large animal, SA = small animal, PO = oral, SC = subcutaneous, IM = intramuscular, IV = intravenous, inj. = injection, elix. = elixer, tab. = tablet, span. = spansule, q8h = every 8 hr.

[a]Also available: Pyrazine with ephedrine (injectable and oral); Antiphrine with ephedrine (injectable and granules to administer in feed); Novahistine with phenylephrine hydrochloride.

[b]Metrevet and Predmaton with prednisone for oral use in dogs and cats.

```
R1         |   |       R
   \       |   |     /
    X  —  C  —  C  — N
   /       |   |     \
R2         |   |       R
```

FIG. 19.3—General formula of most H_1 antihistaminic agents.

route rarely gives rise to side effects and is commonly used. Topical application may be suitable in certain skin conditions.

Antihistamines act as competitive antagonists for specific histamine receptors in the tissue cells; their binding to the cell receptors evokes no direct cellular action. This mechanism of action is based on quantitative considerations; therefore, histamine in excess may displace antihistaminics. Generally, antihistaminics are more effective against exogenously administered histamine than against endogenously released histamine. They are also more effective in preventing actions of histamine than in reversing them.

H_1 antihistaminics are useful in countering action of histamine on bronchial, intestinal, uterine, and vascular smooth muscle. They antagonize both the vasoconstrictor effects of histamine and the more important vasodilator effects as well as the increase in capillary permeability produced by this agent. These antihistaminic effects counteract urticaria, whealing, and other types of edema formation in response to injury, antigens, allergens, or histamine-liberating drugs in many species. H_1 antihistaminics also suppress itching and flare in humans and greatly reduce itching associated with allergic reaction.

H_1 antihistaminics only partially antagonize histamine-induced arterial hypotension because portions of this response are associated with H_2 receptors. Similarly, H_1 antagonists do not block the stimulant effect of histamine on gastric secretion, which is an H_2-dependent function. Importantly, neither H_1 nor H_2 antihistamines prevent histamine release; some antihistaminics possess histamine-liberating properties. This latter action may be of clinical significance in therapeutic use of these drugs.

H_2 antagonists block the gastric stimulating effects of histamine as well as other actions of histamine that have been defined as H_2 receptor dependent (e.g., stimulation of rat uterus, cardiac excitatory effects, and some vascular effects).

Side Effects and Interactions. Each antihistaminic produces certain side effects. Those of clinical importance for the H_1 blockers include sedation or CNS excitement, GI disturbances, parasympatholytic action, local anesthetic properties, allergenic properties, and teratogenic effects.

In therapeutic doses, H_1 antihistaminics elicit a sedative effect, which is expressed by drowsiness or ataxia. In higher doses they produce irritability, convulsions, hyperpyrexia, and even death. Intestinal disorders involve anorexia, nausea, vomiting, constipation, or diarrhea when antihistamines are administered orally for a prolonged period. The anticholinergic effects are expressed by a dry mouth, pupillary dilation, blurred vision, and tachycardia. Local anesthetic properties are of value when these agents are used as antipruritic drugs in topical application. Paradoxically, antihistaminics also can be allergenic when applied to the skin. The teratogenic effects of certain of these agents suggest caution in their use during pregnancy. These drugs possess antiserotonin properties as well as cocainelike effects on catecholamine uptake. The newer H_1-antihistamines terfenadine and astemizole are largely excluded from the CNS when given in therapeutic doses (Janssens and Howart 1993). Their lack of sedation as a side effect is a distinct advantage in human medicine. Study is needed in veterinary medicine to determine their clinical efficacy and whether lack of sedation is an important attribute in animals (Miller et al. 1989).

Toxicity. In recommended doses H_1 antihistaminics are relatively nontoxic; however, overdosage or combinations with the above potentiating agents can elicit toxic effects, which are expressed by hyperexcitability and even convulsions. Treatment of acute toxicity is symptomatic; sedative or ultrashort-acting barbiturates may be of value, but caution is indicated because additive effects are possible.

Therapeutic Uses. Clinically, H_1 antagonists are used to prevent participation of endogenous histamine in the body's reaction to certain allergic disorders and anaphylactic syndromes. However, the clinician must be aware that autacoids other than histamine also play important roles in allergy-anaphylaxis disorders. Eyre and Burka (1978) reviewed this field and listed the following compounds as primary or secondary mediators of hypersensitivity reactions: histamine, serotonin, dopamine, kinins, slow-reacting substance of anaphylaxis, platelet activating factor, eosinophil chemotactic factor of anaphylaxis, prostaglandins, complement, and lymphokines. Thus it is not surprising that antihistamines alone are often ineffective in treating allergic-type reactions in animals.

Clinical signs of allergy vary with different species. The most frequently observed signs are restlessness, anorexia, yawning, salivation, lacrimation, nasal discharge, coughing, edema, urticaria, eczema, necrosis, hemorrhage, inflammation of the mucous membranes and eyes, contraction of smooth muscle (bronchoconstriction), and cardiovascular disturbances. In acute or delayed anaphylaxis, clinical signs occur quickly and, if not treated, are followed by collapse and death in minutes.

Diagnosis is dependent on anamnesis, specific signs, feed tests, eosinophil count, and skin tests; in large animals, skin tests are of questionable value. Eosinophilia is evident in several allergic conditions; some authorities believe that in parasitic diseases it may also be allergy related.

Treatment consists of further avoidance of allergens, emergency measures, administration of antihistaminics, and prophylactic desensitization. Anaphylactic syndrome requires emergency treatment because it progresses rapidly to irreversible cardiovascular collapse. The drug of choice is epinephrine; this catecholamine does not directly inhibit mediators of anaphylaxis but reverses their effects. Thus epinephrine acts as a physiologic antagonist (Chap. 6). Other sympathomimetic drugs (ephedrine and isoproterenol) have been used in a variety of acute and chronic allergic reactions. Aminophylline may be beneficial (especially in small animals) as a smooth muscle relaxant in bronchoconstriction and in edema of the bronchial mucosa. Other emergency treatment may include oxygen or even tracheotomy in the presence of laryngeal edema. Corticosteroids are used as suppressants of allergic inflammation, especially in pruritus in dogs. Although corticosteroids have less indication in emergency treatment, their use may prevent late development of skin reactions.

Nonallergic but suspected histamine-related phenomena, which in empirical experience respond to antihistaminic therapy in animals, include many pathologic conditions. Those in which H_1 antihistaminics are reported to be of therapeutic value are pruritus, urticaria, various types of dermatitis, moist eczema, acute eczematous otitis, insect stings, nutritional types of laminitis, pregnancy laminitis, paroxysmal myoglobinuria or azoturia, periodic ophthalmia, and pulmonary emphysema in horses. Antihistamines also are considered to be of value in treatment of bovine asthma (pulmonary emphysema), some types of bloat and acetonemia in ruminants, acute septic and gangrenous mastitis, septic metritis and retained placenta, pregnancy toxemia, and gut edema of pigs. These agents are also helpful in some types of asthma and motion sickness.

The action of antihistaminics is symptomatic in character, and the important involvement of other autacoids in the pathologic conditions and allergic phenomena limit the effectiveness of antihistamines. These drugs are not a panacea, and removal of etiologic factors must be a primary goal of therapy. H_1 antihistaminics frequently used in animals and representative doses are given in Table 19.1.

H_2 antagonists are used extensively in treatment of gastric ulceration and other gastric hypersecretory states in humans. H_2 blockers also are utilized commonly in animal patients when suppression of gastric hyperacidity and prevention of gastric mucosal ulceration are indicated. H_2 antagonists should not be used indiscriminately in an attempt to provide complete protection from histamine release and hypersensitivity reactions.

SEROTONIN. Rapport et al. (1948) isolated a vasoconstrictor substance from serum and gave it the name serotonin. These investigators discovered that, chemically, serotonin was 5-hydroxytryptamine (5-HT). Independently, another group of researchers studying histochemical properties of the intestinal mucosa discovered an active agent in enterochromaffin cells and gave it the name enteramine (Erspamer and Asero 1952). After discovery of 5-HT in blood, it was soon confirmed that enteramine had the same chemical structure.

Chemistry. 5-HT is synthesized from dietary tryptophan in a two-stage chemical reaction. First, tryptophan is hydroxylated by the enzyme tryptophan 5-hydroxylase to give 5-hydroxytryptophan (5-HTP). The latter is then decarboxylated to yield 5-HT, as shown in Fig. 19.4.

Like histamine, 5-HT is widely distributed in animals and plants. It occurs in high concentration in some fruits such as bananas, pineapples, and plums; it also is present in stings (common stinging nettle) and venoms. Endogenous 5-HT is synthesized from about 1% of the dietary tryptophan. It is formed and localized in three essential pools; enterochromaffin cells of the intestine (about 90%), a small number of neurons in the CNS, and mast cells of rodents (rats, mice, hamsters) along with histamine and heparin. Although 5-HT is concentrated in blood platelets, it is not synthesized there because of lack of decarboxylase. It appears to be bound within cytoplasmic granules and is also continually produced and destroyed in the pool of the intestine and brain. In platelets it appears to be released only upon their destruction.

Most 5-HT is metabolized by oxidative deamination to form 5-hydroxyindoleacetic acid (5-HIAA); the enzyme catalyzing this reaction is monoamine oxidase. The end product of metabolism, 5-HIAA, is excreted in urine. However, in the pineal gland, *N*-acetylation and 5-methylation of 5-HT form the hormone melatonin.

Pharmacologic Effects. 5-HT exerts multiple actions with great variation in different species. Its essential effects are on smooth muscle and central and peripheral nerves, including afferent nerve endings. Given orally, it is quickly degraded and produces no effect.

Rapid IV injection of 5-HT produces a triphasic response: an initial fall of systemic arterial pressure accompanied by paradoxical bradycardia, caused mainly by reflex chemoreceptor stimulation (Bezod-Jarisch effect); a short period of pressor effect (similar to epinephrine effect); and a prolonged fall in systemic blood pressure attributed to a vasodilator effect in the vascular bed of skeletal muscle. 5-HT also causes a fall in pulmonary arterial pressure (pulmonary depressor reflex). A continuous infusion of 5-HT, which most closely resembles endogenous release of this agent, causes a prolonged fall in arterial pressure as a result of vascular bed dilation. Only in rodents does this agent increase small vessel permeability similar to effects of histamine.

The nonvascular smooth muscle of the bronchi and intestines is stimulated by 5-HT. Intestinal effects are both direct and indirect; the latter is mediated via excitation of ganglion cells in the myenteric plexus. In some species, it causes contraction of the ureter and uterus (rodent). After repeated doses, tachyphylaxis is a common phenomenon.

When 5-HT is injected, it has no effect on the brain or spinal cord because it is strongly polar and cannot effectively cross the blood-brain barrier. However, 5-HTP can penetrate into the brain and be decarboxylated to 5-HT; this may produce behavioral changes. 5-HT can also stimulate afferent nerve endings, ganglion cells, and adrenal medullary cells.

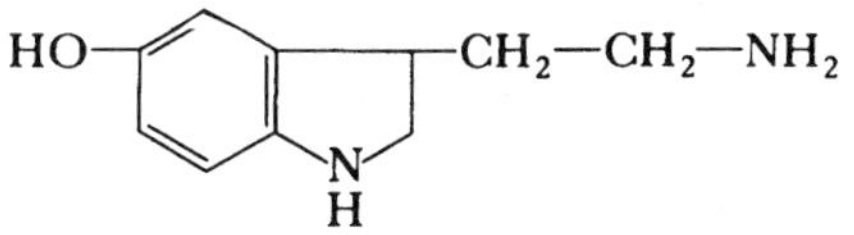

Role in Physiologic and Pathologic Processes. The finding that 5-HT is present in the CNS, the hypothalamus, and other areas and that reserpine releases it from these areas led to the hypothesis of its role as a central neurotransmitter. 5-HT influences sleep, intestinal motility, and temperature regulation and affects the mood and behavior of humans. It seems that an excess of this agent brings about stimulation and that a deficiency produces depression. Its role in platelets is related to the mechanism of hemostasis via vasoconstriction and platelet aggregation.

Evidence exists that 5-HT exerts an inhibitory effect on a variety of behaviors (Green and Harvey 1974) and plays a role in some mental disorders of humans. The only disease in which 5-HT probably plays an important role is the carcinoid syndrome, which is characterized by widespread development of a serotonin-producing tumor in the GI tract. Symptoms are related to action on smooth muscle of the blood vessels and digestive and respiratory tracts. The 5-HT in the blood of a carcinoid subject is 0.5-2.7 μg/mL, while the normal amount is 0.1-0.3 μg/mL. The urinary metabolite has significant diagnostic value; excretion of 5-HIAA has been reported as 76-850 mg in 24 hours (normal is 2-8 mg). This results in 60% of the dietary intake of tryptophan being converted to 5-HT. Consequently, a deficiency may develop, producing symptoms of pellagra and negative nitrogen balance.

Antagonists. Different types of 5-HT receptors have been identified (Derkach et al. 1989). Actions of 5-HT are countered by two general groups of antagonists. Neural effects in smooth muscle of the digestive tract

HO— —CH_2—CH_2—NH_2
N
H

Serotonin

FIG. 19.4

are antagonized by morphine, atropine, and cocaine; the direct effects on smooth muscle are antagonized by phenoxybenzamine and two derivatives of ergot alkaloids, LSD and methysergide. An antihistamine, cyproheptadine, is also a powerful antiserotonin agent. Chlorpromazine and phenoxybenzamine are weak blocking agents. Reserpine and compound 48/80 are examples of drugs that deplete serotonin in the brain. Another antagonist frequently used experimentally is *p*-chlorphenylamine, but this agent acts by inhibition of serotonin synthesis. For clinical use in humans, methysergide (oral dose 2-4 mg 3 times daily) and cyproheptadine (oral dose 4 mg 3 times daily) are the available effective antagonists. Ketanserin is a new 5-HT antagonist that acts preferentially at the 5-HT_2 receptor subtype without significant action at the 5-HT_1 receptors. The relevance of 5-HT receptor subtypes and 5-HT antagonists to clinical veterinary medicine is unknown.

REFERENCES

Arang, J. M., Garbarg, M., Lancelot, J. C., Lecomte, J. M., Pollard, H., Robba, M., Schunack, W., Schwartz, J. C. 1987. Highly potent and selective ligands for histamine H_3-receptors. Nature 327:117-23.

Ash, A. S., Schild, H. O. 1966. Receptors mediating some actions of histamine. Br J Pharmacol 27:427-39.

Barnes, P. J., Belvisi, M. G., Rogers, D. F. 1990. Modulation of neurogenic inflammation: novel approaches to inflammatory disease. TIPS 11:185-89.

Black, J. W., Duncan, W. A., Durant, C. J., et al. 1972. Definition and antagonism of histamine H2-receptors. Nature 236:385-90.

Bovet, D., Staub, A. M. 1937. Action protectrice des ethers phenoliques au cours de l'intoxication histaminique. CR Soc Biol (Paris) 124:547-49.

Chand, N., Eyre, P. 1975. Classification and biological distribution of histamine receptor subtypes. Agents Actions 5:277-95.

Dale, H. H., Laidlaw, P. P. 1910. The physiological action of β-iminazolylethylamine. J Physiol (Lond) 41:318-44.

Derkach, V., Surprenant, A., North, R. A. 1989. 5-HT_3 receptors are membrane ion channels. Nature 339:706-9.

Douglas, W. W. 1974. Involvement of calcium in exocytosis and the exocytosis-vesiculation sequence. Biochem Soc Symp 39:1-28.

Erspamer, V., Asero, B. 1952. Identification of entermine, a specific hormone of enterochromaffin cell system, as 5-hydroxytryptamine. Nature 169:800-801.

Erye, P., Burka, J. F. 1978. Hypersensitivity in cattle and sheep: A pharmacological review. J Vet Pharmacol Ther 1:97-109.

Eyre, P., Wells, P. W. 1973. Histamine H2-receptors modulate systemic anaphylaxis: a dual cardiovascular action of histamine in calves. Br J Pharmacol 49:364-67.

Falus, A., Meretey, K. 1992. Histamine: an early messenger in inflammatory and immune reactions. Immunol Today 13:154-56.

Goth, A., Johnson, A. R. 1975. Current concepts on the secretory function of mast cells. Life Sci 16:1201-13.

Green, T. K., Harvey, J. A. 1974. Enhancement of amphetamine action after interruption of ascending serotonergic pathways. J Pharmacol Exp Ther 190:109-17.

Hirschowitz, B. I. 1979. H-2 histamine receptors. Annu Rev Pharmacol 19:203-44.

Janssens, M. M. L., Howart, P. H. 1993. The antihistamines of the nineties. Clin Rev Allergy 11:111-53.

Lambert, D. G. 1993. Signal transduction: G proteins and second messengers. Br J Anaesthesia 71:86-95.

Lichtenstein, L. M., Margolis, S. 1968. Histamine release in vitro: Inhibition by catecholamines and methylxanthines. Science 161:902-3.

Miller, W. H., Jr., Griffin, G. E., Scott, D. W., et al. 1989. Clinical trial of DVM DermCaps in the treatment of allergic disease in dogs: a nonblinded study. J Am Anim Hosp Assoc 25:163.

Mitsuhashi, M., Payan, D. G. 1992. Functional diversity of histamine and histamine receptors. J Invest Dermatol 98:8S-11S.

Morris, A. I. 1992. The success of histamine-2 receptor antagonists. Scand J Gastroenterol 27(Suppl 194):71-75.

Obrink, K. J. 1991. Histamine and gastric acid secretion. Scand J Gastroenterol 26(Suppl 180):4-8.

Pearce, F. L. 1991. Biological effects of histamine: an overview. Agent Actions 33:4-7.

Rapport, M. M., Green, A. A., Page, I. H. 1948. Serum vasoconstrictor (serotonin); isolation and characterization. J Biol Chem 176:1243-51.

Schayer, R. W., Cooper, J. A. D. 1956. Metabolism of C14 histamine in man. J Appl Physiol 9:481-83.

Schror, K. 1992. Role of prostaglandins in the cardiovascular effects of bradykinin and angiotensin-converting enzyme inhibitors. J Cardiovasc Pharmacol 20(Suppl 9):S68-S73.

Schwieler, J. H., Hjemdahl, P. 1992. Influence of angiotensin-converting enzyme inhibition on sympathetic neurotransmission: possible roles of bradykinin and prostaglandins. J Cardiovasc Pharmacol 20(Suppl 9):S39-S46.

20 PEPTIDES: ANGIOTENSIN AND KININS

H. RICHARD ADAMS

Angiotensin
Endogenous Renin-Angiotensin System
Pharmacology of the Renin-Angiotensin System
Kinins
Kinin Formation: Components and Chemistry
Pharmacologic Effects of Kinins
Role of Endogenous Kinins
Other Peptides

ANGIOTENSIN. Discovery of angiotensin has its origins in the old observation that renal extracts contain a pressor substance that early investigators named renin (Tigerstedt and Bergman 1898). Subsequent researchers found that systemic hypertension could be produced by constriction of the renal artery, and they suggested that a circulating pressor agent released by the ischemic kidney acted as the mediator of the hypertensive response (Goldblatt et al. 1934). The pressor substance, identified as renin, is an enzyme that acts on a plasma substrate, resulting in formation of a peptide with exceptional vasoconstrictor potency. The peptide was called "hypertensin" and "angiotonin" until 1958 when the compromise term angiotensin was adopted (Braun-Menendez and Page 1958).

Angiotensin is a blood-borne polypeptide that serves as a circulating link between the kidney and systemic hemodynamic control systems (Matsusaka and Ichikawa 1997). This peptide is not manufactured directly by the kidney but is formed within the blood by a complex series of reactions initiated by the renal enzyme renin. Release of renin by the kidney is accelerated when this organ is subjected to physiologic stimuli associated with hypovolemia and hypotension (Bernstein 1993).

The renin-angiotensin relationship was complicated by the discovery that, after entering the bloodstream, renin and its substrate (angiotensinogen) yielded an inactive precursor, the decapeptide angiotensin I, which was then converted by other enzymes to the active octapeptide angiotensin II. The latter is an exceptionally potent vasoconstrictor agent and a stimulant of aldosterone secretion. Angiotensin II evokes an increase in peripheral vascular resistance and a reduction of urine and salt output, thereby tending to restore blood pressure and blood volume to more normal values. Pharmacologic manipulation of this system has recently gained considerable importance in clinical medicine. The angiotensin-converting enzyme inhibitors are now one of the most commonly used drugs to treat heart failure and hypertension (Dietz et al. 1993; Holtz 1993). Because angiotensin modulates cardiac cellular growth and hypertrophy, angiotensin-converting enzyme inhibitors are also being evaluated in treatment of cardiac hypertrophic states (Matsusaka and Ichikawa 1997).

The biologic half-life of angiotensin II was found to be quite brief because of the presence in plasma and tissues of proteolytic enzymes, collectively referred to as angiotensinases. A heptapeptide fragment of angiotensin II, originally thought to be an inactive metabolite, was found to possess considerable pharmacologic activity. The active fragment is now referred to as angiotensin III. In the following discussion, the term angiotensin is used to refer to angiotensin II unless otherwise noted.

Endogenous Renin-Angiotensin System

RENIN RELEASE. Renin is a proteolytic enzyme synthesized and stored within cytoplasmic granules of modified smooth muscle cells that line the afferent arteriole of the glomerulus. Both the afferent and efferent arterioles are associated anatomically and functionally with the macula densa, a group of specialized cells localized at the origin of the distal tubule of the nephron. The entire structure is referred to as the juxtaglomerular apparatus (Oparil and Haber 1974; Johnston 1992).

Renin is released from the juxtaglomerular apparatus in response to several stimuli associated with hypotension, hypovolemia, or both. Factors that reduce blood volume, renal perfusion pressure, or plasma sodium concentration tend to stimulate release of renin, while factors that increase these parameters tend to lower it (Gibbons et al. 1984; Bernstein 1993). Actual secretion of renin is regulated by an intrarenal baroreceptor mechanism of the afferent arteriole, an intrarenal chemoreceptor mechanism of the macula densa, the renal sympathetic nerves, and several humoral agents. These factors often interact with each other, resulting in considerable complexity. Basic aspects are summarized below and in Fig. 20.1.

An intrarenal baroreceptor mechanism detects and responds to changes in wall tension or transmural

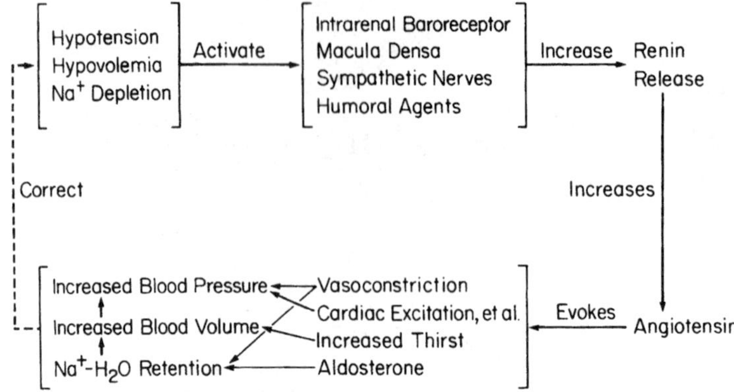

FIG. 20.1—Hemodynamic interrelationships of the renin-angiotensin system.

pressure gradients in the afferent arteriole of the glomerulus. Renin release from the juxtaglomerular apparatus is increased when renal blood flow and, especially, renal blood pressure are decreased. There is evidence that intrarenal prostaglandins serve as a chemical link between pressure changes and the resulting increase in renin secretion, at least within the autoregulatory range of renal blood flow (Schror 1992; Schwieler and Hjemdahl 1992).

The macula densa serves as a Na^+-sensitive and perhaps Cl^- sensitive chemoreceptor that detects these ions in renal tubular fluid. If Na^+ and/or Cl^- concentrations are reduced, renin release is increased.

Activation of the renal sympathetic nerves evokes release of renin. This response is mediated by an intrarenal β-adrenergic receptor. An α-adrenergic receptor that subserves an inhibitory effect on renin release seems to be present within the kidney, but its importance is not known.

Several circulating humoral agents and electrolytes influence renin release. Angiotensin itself can feed back to inhibit renin release; vasopressin is also inhibitory. Since angiotensin acts on the brain to increase release of vasopressin, there seems to be a vasopressin-angiotensin feedback loop. Other agents that can influence renin release include catecholamines, prostaglandins, cyclic nucleotides, K^+, Mg^{++}, Ca^{++}, serotonin, adenosine, and others. The importance of all these factors to normal control of renin release has not been determined (Keeton and Campbell 1981). There may be species differences in which scheme is dominant.

ANGIOTENSIN FORMATION. The known amino acid sequence of renin substrate, angiotensinogen, is limited to a 14 amino acid segment at the amino terminus of a larger protein. Once in the blood, renin cleaves the bond that joins the *N*-terminal 10 amino acid sequence to the remainder of angiotensinogen. The released decapeptide is angiotensin I; it can be considered as a circulating and essentially inactive prohormone to angiotensin II (Ardaillou 1997).

After the decapeptide angiotensin I is formed, two amino acids are removed from its *C*-terminus by converting enzyme to yield the octapeptide angiotensin II. The sequential formation of angiotensin is summarized in Fig. 20.2. Converting enzymes are present in endothelial cells throughout the body, but especially the lungs. Virtually all the circulating angiotensin I can be converted to angiotensin II by a single passage through the pulmonary vascular circuit. The angiotensin-converting enzyme is also known as kininase II, the enzyme responsible for inactivating bradykinin.

Angiotensin II is metabolized rapidly by plasma and tissue angiotensinases. The best characterized of the plasma enzymes are an aminopeptidase (angiotensinase A) and a less important endopeptidase (angiotensinase B). A heptapeptide fragment of angiotensin II is des-Asp^1 angiotensin II or, as it is now named, angiotensin III. This peptide shares many of the pharmacologic actions of its parent molecule, especially the ability to stimulate aldosterone secretion. However, the physiologic significance of angiotensin III in the intact animal is not known.

CARDIOVASCULAR EFFECTS. Angiotensin II exerts a wide spectrum of effects that are directed toward maintenance of blood pressure and volume (Cody 1997; Matsusaka and Ichikawa 1997). First and foremost, angiotensin produces a pronounced vasoconstriction as a result of direct stimulation of vascular smooth muscle cells (Berk and Corson 1997). This effect is most prominent on arteries and, especially, small arterioles, with less influence on veins. The vasoconstrictor action of angiotensin is most pronounced in the kidney, skin, and splanchnic tissues and less pronounced in the brain, heart, and skeletal muscle. The net result is an increase in peripheral vascular resistance and hence in blood pressure (Griendling and Alexander 1990).

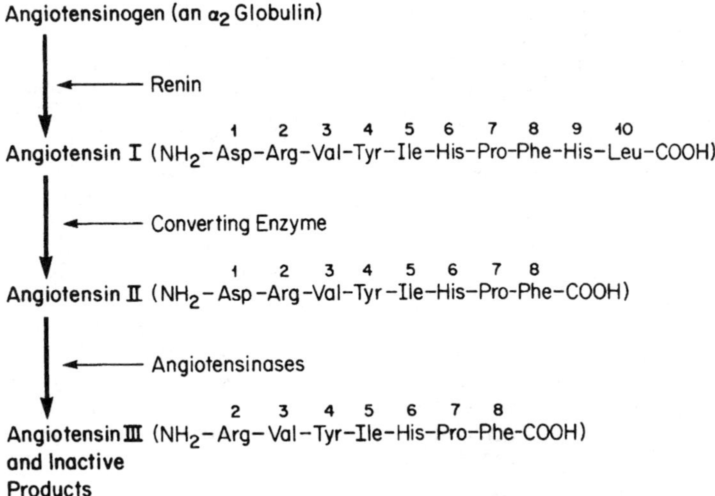

FIG. 20.2—Sequential formation of angiotensins I, II, and III. The structure of angiotensin shown is that found in the rat, pig, horse, and human. Bovine angiotensin contains valine in position 5.

Angiotensin also increases cardiac output by direct stimulation of the heart and action on the sympathetic nervous system. By an effect on the brain, angiotensin elicits an increase in sympathetic discharge to the heart and blood vessels. This contributes further to increases in cardiac output and vascular resistance. Angiotensin also provokes release of norepinephrine and epinephrine from the adrenal medulla, facilitates release of norepinephrine from postganglionic sympathetic neurons, stimulates sympathetic ganglia, and decreases uptake of norepinephrine into adrenergic axons. Thus angiotensin produces a state of cardiovascular excitation through several pathways (Peart 1975; Cody 1997; Matsusaka and Ichikawa 1997).

Aside from its direct cardiovascular effects, angiotensin accelerates steroidogenesis in the adrenal cortex. This action results in increased synthesis and release of the mineralocorticoid aldosterone, which acts in turn on the distal tubule of the kidney to increase reabsorption of Na^+ and, subsequently, water (Vecsei et al. 1978). Angiotensin also releases vasopressin (antidiuretic hormone) from the brain and produces a marked dipsogenic effect. All these actions help to expand or restore blood volume and hence assist in maintaining normal blood pressure and circulatory function.

From the above description, it is obvious that the renin-angiotensin system can play an important role in electrolyte-water balance and hemodynamics. Disruptions of this system contribute to certain pathophysiologic states such as renovascular hypertension and aldosteronism. In states of low cardiac output, angiotensin is believed to contribute to maintenance of blood pressure. The physiologic functions of extrarenal renins (the "isorenins" found in blood vessels, the brain, and other tissues) are under considerable study (Ganong 1984; Lee et al. 1993).

Pharmacology of the Renin-Angiotensin System. Several drugs interact with the renin, angiotensin, and associated enzyme system (Keeton and Campbell 1981; Csajka et al. 1997). The amide of angiotensin II (1-*l*-asparaginyl-5-*l*-valyl angiotensin octapeptide, Hypertensin) activates angiotensin receptors throughout the body. This drug is diluted and administered by slow intravenous infusion for its pressor actions; blood pressure should be monitored continuously.

Different types of angiotensin receptors have been identified, e.g., angiotensin-1 (AT_1) and angiotensin-2 receptors (Matsusaka and Ichikawa 1997), but the clinical value of such differentiation is unknown. Saralasin acetate (1-sar-8-ala angiotensin II, Sarenin) is the prototype for drugs defined as angiotensin receptor blockers. These agents interact with the receptors, thereby preventing angiotensin from eliciting its physiologic-pharmacologic actions. Saralasin and other angiotensin receptor blockers are used experimentally in attempts to define biologic roles of angiotensin, and clinically in humans as antihypertensive agents (Csajka et al. 1997).

The proline derivative captopril (Capoten) and the related drug enalapril (Vasotec) are inhibitors of angiotensin-converting enzyme. They prevent transformation of angiotensin I to angiotensin II. They also inhibit the inactivation of bradykinin and kallidin. Converting enzyme inhibitors are used to diagnose and treat certain forms of hypertension in humans. Converting enzyme inhibitors also are being used increasingly in human and veterinary medicine to relieve vasoconstriction and lessen fluid retention in patients with congestive heart failure (Knowlen et al. 1983; Dietz et al. 1993; Holtz 1993). An important part of the endogenous compensatory attempt in heart failure syndrome involves increased formation of angiotensin and aldosterone, leading in turn to peripheral vasoconstriction and enhanced urinary reabsorption of salt and water respectively. By inhibiting angiotensin formation, converting enzyme inhibitors evoke vasodilation and reduced cardiac workload as well as lessen aldosterone-mediated fluid retention and the propensity for edema formation (Cody 1997; Matsusaka and Ichikawa 1997; Berk and Corson 1997).

A large number of drugs used for other therapeutic purposes also influence the renin-angiotensin system; e.g., vasodilators indirectly cause renin release resulting from a reflex increase in sympathetic nervous system discharge to the kidney. General anesthetics also provoke nonspecific increase in renin release. Propranolol inhibits renin secretion by blocking the intrarenal β-adrenergic receptors that subserve release of renin from the juxtaglomerular apparatus (Schwieler and Hjemdahl 1992).

KININS. Discovery of the mammalian kallikrein-kinin system can be traced to the old observation that urine produces a fall in blood pressure when injected intravenously. The urinary principle responsible for the hypotensive activity is an enzyme called kallikrein. However, kallikrein itself does not affect blood pressure directly but converts an inactive α-2 globulin in the plasma, kininogen, into bradykinin, the active depressor substance. Bradykinin and other related polypeptide kinins such as kallidin are exceptionally potent vasodilators. The kinins also increase permeability of the microcirculation, cause contraction of several nonvascular smooth muscles, and evoke pain.

Because the kallikrein enzymes are present in various glandular tissues and bodily fluids of mammals, the kinins have been proposed as endogenous mediators of cellular responses to certain types of physiologic and pathophysiologic stimuli. Many aspects remain unresolved, however, and pharmacologic control of the kallikrein-kinin system is still in its infancy.

Early studies of kinins were carried out independently by two groups of scientists. The resulting terminology was confusing because of the development of different nomenclatures. One group called their plasma enzyme kallikrein; it formed the active peptide kallidin from the inactive precursor kallidinogen. Other workers reported that trypsin released an active peptide (bradykinin) from a plasma globulin substrate (bradykininogen) (Rocha e Silva et al. 1949).

Similarities between the trypsin-bradykininogen-bradykinin system and the kallikrein-kallidinogen-kallidin system soon became apparent. Schachter and Thain (1954) subsequently introduced the generic term kinin to encompass both bradykinin and kallidin, since these two polypeptides exert essentially identical pharmacologic actions. Bradykinin and kallidin are now recognized as members of a group of closely related kinin peptides occurring naturally in wasp, hornet, and other venoms or released from mammalian plasma substrate by kallikreins, trypsin, and certain snake venoms.

Current terminology for the kinin system uses kallikrein-kininogen-kinin as general terms for designating the enzymes, the inactive precursors (substrates), and the active polypeptides respectively (Schachter 1980).

Kinin Formation: Components and Chemistry. A schematic representation of the contributions of kallikrein, kininogen, and other factors to kinin formation is depicted in Fig. 20.3.

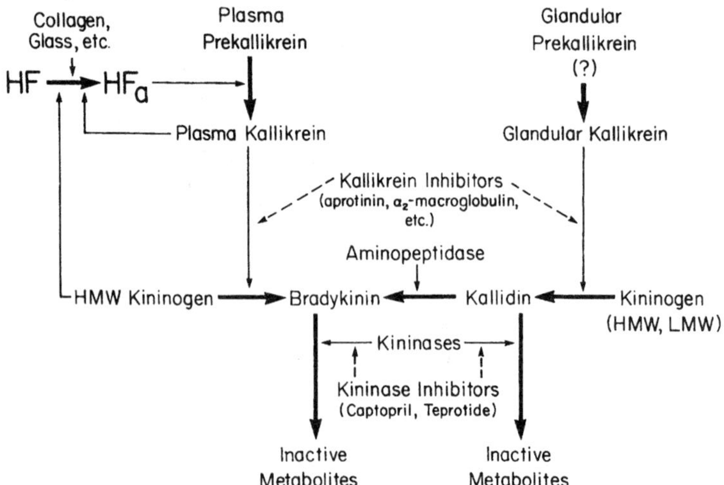

FIG. 20.3—Formation and inactivation of kinins. HF = Hageman factor, HF_a = activated HF, HMW and LMW = high and low molecular weight. Wide solid lines represent conversion of substrate to product. Narrow solid lines represent enzyme acceleration of substrate conversion to product. Dashed lines represent sites of inhibitory actions.

KALLIKREINS, PREKALLIKREINS, AND KALLIKREIN INHIBITORS

KALLIKREINS. The term kallikreins denotes the endogenous serine protease enzymes that liberate kinins from specific kininogen substrates by limited proteolysis. The term kininogenase encompasses the kallikreins and other serine proteases such as trypsin, some snake venoms, thrombin, fibrinolysin, and other enzymes that share the common property of releasing kinins from kininogen (Schachter 1980).

Mammals have two basic kallikrein types: plasma and glandular. The latter is localized in exocrine glands and their secretions and has been isolated from porcine pancreas; guinea pig coagulation gland; intestine of the rat, pig, dog, and human; urine from the horse, rat, and human; and saliva from humans. Structurally, the kallikreins are glycoproteins with molecular weights between 24,000 and 43,000 for those of glandular origin and at least 100,000 for the plasma form.

In general, the glandular kallikreins yield kallidin, from which bradykinin is formed rapidly by aminopeptidase activity in plasma and tissue (Erdös 1976). Bradykinin is formed directly by plasma kallikrein and also by trypsin, fibrinolysin, and snake venom (Fig. 20.3).

PREKALLIKREINS. Kallikrein is present in some tissues (especially the pancreas, intestines, and plasma) in inactive or prekallikrein forms (referred to formerly as kallikreinogens). Prekallikreins are converted to the active mode by various factors that disrupt plasma homeostasis (Fig. 20.3). These include pH changes; organic solvents; trypsin; and contact with glass, collagen, skin, or damaged tissue. The major plasma activators of prekallikreins are the Hageman factor and its fragments, i.e., blood clotting factor XII.

KALLIKREIN INHIBITORS. Once kallikrein is activated, its capability to form kinins is short-lived because of rapid inhibition by several plasma protease inhibitors. These include α_2 macroglobulin, α_1 antitrypsin, antithrombin III, and C,1 esterase inhibitor (Fig. 20.3).

In addition, a polyvalent kallikrein-trypsin inhibitor called aprotinin has been isolated from bovine tissues where it is localized in mast cells (Fritz et al. 1979). This inhibitor is a low molecular weight protein; it is prepared commercially as Trasylol. Aprotinin has been used outside the USA with varying success in treatment of acute pancreatitis and the carcinoid syndrome in humans.

KININOGENS. The kinin precursors, kininogens, are acidic glycoproteins of the α-2 globulin fraction of plasma; they have been isolated from human, bovine, equine, and rabbit blood.

At least two plasma kininogens have been identified, the high-molecular-weight (HMW) and the low-molecular-weight (LMW) forms. Both types have been isolated from different species, and the HMW and LMW

Kallidin

Lys—Arg—Pro—Gly—Phe—Ser—Pro—Phe—Arg

Bradykinin

FIG. 20.4—Amino acid sequence of bradykinin and kallidin

kininogens of bovine origin have molecular weights of 76,000 and 48,000 respectively. The HMW form, also referred to as substrate 1, is a good substrate for both plasma and glandular kallikrein. Substrate 2, the LMW type, is a good substrate for glandular kallikrein only (Fig. 20.3).

KININS AND KININ INHIBITORS

KININS. The amino acid sequence of the two most important plasma kinins, bradykinin and kallidin, is shown in Fig. 20.4. Bradykinin is a nonapeptide, whereas kallidin is a decapeptide identical to the former except for the addition of an *N*-terminal lysine. Thus kallidin also is referred to as lysylbradykinin. Addition of methionine to the *N*-terminal lysine of kallidin yields a third biologically active kinin called methionyl-kallidin or methionyl-lysylbradykinin.

KININ INHIBITORS. Specific inhibitors or antagonists of kinin actions on effector cells have not yet been satisfactorily identified. Accordingly, little is known about kinin-specific receptors, although they have been divided into a series of subtypes (Drouin et al. 1979; Burch et al. 1990; Farmer et al. 1989). Analgesic and anti-inflammatory drugs such as aspirin and indomethacin reduce pain and inflammatory responses to kinins. However, these drugs probably act by blocking synthesis of prostaglandins, which mediate or modulate certain activities of kinins (Marceau et al. 1983).

KININASES AND KININASE INHIBITORS

KININASES. Plasma and other tissues contain enzymes, collectively called kininases, that rapidly inactivate kinins (Fig. 20.3). The most important kininases have been named simply kininase I and II.

Kininase I is a carboxypeptidase probably synthesized by the liver, but it can be recovered from the lungs and, possibly, the skin. More attention has been directed to kininase II, a peptidyl dipeptide hydrolase. Kininase II also converts angiotensin I to angiotensin II and in this context is commonly referred to as angiotensin-converting enzyme. It is present in many tissues but is extremely active in the lungs (Erdös 1975).

KININASE INHIBITORS. Captopril and teprotide are new drugs that inhibit kininase activity, thereby retarding inactivation of bradykinin. As discussed earlier in this chapter, the kininase inhibitors also reduce the conversion of angiotensin I to angiotensin II (Erdös 1976).

Although captopril and teprotide are increasingly being used to diagnose and treat forms of hypertension in humans, the importance of the kininases to normal and abnormal circulatory function remains uncertain (Mills 1979; Bhoola et al. 1992).

Pharmacologic Effects of Kinins. Kinins are extremely potent vasodilators, being about 10 times as active as histamine. They act directly on vascular smooth muscle, but the net effect in different vascular beds varies with species and dose. Smooth muscle of the microcirculation (i.e., of terminal arterioles and small venules) is relaxed by the kinins, yielding a marked decrease in systemic vascular resistance. Blood pressure falls accordingly, but a reflex increase in heart rate and cardiac output may occur. Large arteries and veins, in contrast to the microcirculatory vessels, tend to contract upon exposure to kinins. Permeability of the microcirculation is increased by the kinins, resulting in edema formation similar to the wheal and flare response seen with histamine (Chap. 19). Bradykinin is believed to act in part through activation of the phospholipase C-inositol trisphosphate-Ca^{++} triad (Fasolato et al. 1988).

Intestinal and uterine smooth muscle generally is contracted by kinins, but the duodenum in the rat is relaxed. Bronchoconstriction by kinins is prominent in the guinea pig and in some asthmatic humans but is generally unremarkable in other species.

Kinins are potent algesic substances, and they evoke pain when applied topically to exposed blisters or when injected intra-arterially. These responses are thought to be associated with stimulation of sensory nerve endings. Since aspirin and other inhibitors of prostaglandin synthesis reduce kinin-induced pain, prostaglandins may mediate or modulate the algesic activities of the kinins (Marceau et al. 1983). Kinins also can stimulate autonomic ganglia and release catecholamines from the adrenal medulla.

Role of Endogenous Kinins. Considerable speculation has centered on the possible roles of kinins in physiologic and pathophysiologic processes. Pathologic conditions in which kinins may participate include acute inflammations, arthritic states, carcinoid syndrome, pancreatitis, migraine headache, allergic reactions, endotoxin shock, and anaphylactic shock. Kinins most likely interact with other autacoids in some of these pathologic states, but their precise involvement remains speculative in most cases (Schror 1992).

The physiologic roles of the kallikreins-kinins, even in tissues where they exist in large concentrations (e.g., pancreas, plasma, and parotid gland), also remain uncertain. There is evidence that kallikreins-kinins influence blood flow in exocrine glands and even participate in reproductive activities and cell proliferation (Schachter 1980).

Studies have focused on the roles of plasma kallikrein and HMW kininogen in blood coagulation independently from their involvement in kinin formation. There is considerable evidence that plasma kallikrein activates the Hageman factor (factor XII). Activated Hageman factor and its fragments in turn accelerate conversion of prekallikrein to kallikrein. This establishes a local positive feedback system for sustained activation of clotting factor XII for the coagulation cascade (Fig. 20.3). In addition, the HMW kininogen may participate in the coagulation process by increasing the activation of factor XII, prekallikrein, factor XI, and plasminogen activator. Since plasma kallikrein and plasminogen activator are chemotactic for leukocytes, there seem to be functional interactions between blood coagulation, kallikreins and other kininogenases, and inflammation (Cochrane et al. 1973; Mandle et al. 1976; Ratnoff and Saito 1979).

Studies also have suggested that renal kallikrein may be of significance in regulating fluid and electrolyte balance and, perhaps, renal hemodynamics. In contrast to the renin-angiotensin system, however, kallikrein and bradykinin are diuretic and natriuretic agents; i.e., they increase urine volume and salt excretion. Part of the physiologic actions of the kinins seems to be mediated or modulated by prostaglandins and other autacoids (Busse and Fleming 1996), but the contribution of kinins to the regulation of renal blood flow and nephron function remains speculative (Margolius 1978; Mills 1979). The exact physiologic roles of the kinins probably will not be delineated until specific blockers of kinin receptors are identified (Regoli et al. 1996).

OTHER PEPTIDES. Several other vasoactive peptides, of which the actions in pathophysiologic states are less known, are substance P, vasoactive intestinal polypeptide (VIP), eledoisin, physalaemin, coerulein, colostrokinin, urokinin, and the kinins of wasp and hornet venoms. VIP is present in the small intestine and also widely distributed in peripheral nerves and the central nervous system. Although VIP exerts multiple pharmacologic actions in different tissues, its physiologic relevance remains questionable. Substance P was first extracted from horse intestine and brain; it is an endecapeptide structurally similar to eledoisin and physalamin. Substance P has some bradykininlike action and is a potent stimulant of the gut. Eledoisin (from the octopus) and physalamin (from the skin of an amphibian) are endecapeptides with bradykinin-like activity. Coerulein, a related decapeptide, is an extremely potent stimulator of pancreatic and other exocrine secretions.

Atrial natriuretic factor is released from the right atrial musculature of the heart in response to blood volume overload and cardiac stretch. This peptide promotes sodium excretion and diuresis and may have future application in the therapy of congestive heart failure.

Other vasoactive peptides such as oxytocin and vasopressin are discussed in the chapters on hormones, and the cytokines are addressed in Chap. 21 along with the eicosanoids.

REFERENCES

Ardaillou, R. 1997. Active fragments of angiotensin II: enzymatic pathways of synthesis and biological effects. Current Opinion in Nephrology and Hypertension 6:28-34.

Berk, B. C., Corson, M. A. 1997. Angiotensin II signal transduction in vascular smooth muscle. Circ Res 80:607-16.

Bernstein, K. E. 1993. The renin-angiotensin system: a biological machine. Ann Med 24:113-15.

Bhoola, K. D., Figueroa, C. D., Worthy, K. 1992. Bioregulation of kinins: kallikreins, kininogens, and kininases. Pharmacol Rev 44:1-80.

Braun-Menendez, E., Page, I. H. 1958. Suggested revision of nomenclature—angiotensin. Science 127:242.

Burch, R. M., Farmer, S. G., Steranka, L. R. 1990. Bradykinin receptor antagonists. Med Res Rev 10:143-75.

Busse, R., Fleming, I. 1996. Molecular responses of endothelial tissue to kinins. Diabetes 45:S58-S13.

Cochrane, C. G., Revak, S. D., Wuepper, K. D. 1973. Activation of Hageman factor in solid and fluid phases: a critical role of kallikrein. J Exp Med 138:1564-83.

Cody, R. J. 1997. The integrated effects of angiotensin II. Amer J Cardiol 79(5A):9-11.

Csajka, C., Buclin, T., Brunner, H. R., Biollaz, J. 1997. Pharmacokinetic-pharmacodynamic profile of angiotensin II receptor antagonists. Clin Pharmacokinet 32(1):1-29.

Dietz, R., Waas, W., Susselbeck, T., Willenbrock, R., Osterziel, K. J. 1993. Improvement of cardiac function by angiotensin converting enzyme inhibition: sites of action. Circulation 87 (Suppl IV):108-16.

Drouin, J. N., St. Pierre, S. A., Regoli, D. 1979. Receptors for bradykinin and kallidin. Can J Physiol Pharmacol 57:375-79.

Erdös, E. G. 1975. Angiotensin I converting enzyme. Circ Res 36:247-55.

———. 1976. The kinins: a status report. Biochem Pharmacol 25:1563-69.

Farmer, S. G., Burch, R. M., Meeker, S. A., Wilkins, D. E. 1989. Evidence for a pulmonary B_3 bradykinin receptor. Mol Pharmacol 36:1-8.

Fasolato, C., Pandiella, A., Meldolesi, J., Pozzan, T. 1988. Generation of inositol phosphates, cytolsolic Ca^{2+}m and ionic fluxes in Pc12 cells treated with bradykinin. J Biol Chem 263:17350-59.

Fritz, H., Kruck, J., Russe, I., et al. 1979. Immunofluorescence studies indicate that the basic trypsin-kallikrein-inhibitor of bovine organs (Trasylol) originates from mast cells. Hoppe Seylers Z Physiol Chem 360:437-44.

Ganong, W. F. 1984. The brain renin-angiotensin system. Annu Rev Physiol 46:17-31.

Gibbons, G. H., Dzau, V. J., Farhi, E. R., et al. 1984. Interaction of signals influencing renin release. Annu Rev Physiol 46:291-308.

Goldblatt, H., Lynch, J., Hanzal, R. F., et al. 1934. Studies on experimental hypertension: production of persistent elevation of systolic blood pressure by means of renal ischemia. J Exp Med 59:347-79.

Griendling, K. K., Alexander, R. W. 1990. Angiotensin, other pressors, and the transduction of vascular smooth muscle contraction. In J. H. Laragh and B. N. Brenner, eds., Hypertension: Pathophysiology, Diagnosis and Management, Vol. 1, pp. 583-600. New York: Raven Press.

Holtz, J. 1993. The cardiac renin-angiotensin system: physiological relevance and pharmacological modulation. Clin Investig 71:S25-S34.

Johnston, C. I. 1992. Renin-angiotensin system: a dual tissue and hormonal system for cardiovascular control. J Hypertens 10(Suppl 7):S13-S26.

Keeton, T. K., Campbell, W. B. 1981. The pharmacologic alteration of renin release. Pharmacol Rev 32(2):81-227.

Knowlen, G. G., Kittleson, M. D., Nachreiner, R. F., et al. 1983. Comparison of plasma aldosterone concentration among clinical status groups of dogs with chronic heart failure. J Am Vet Med Assoc 183:991-96.

Lee, M. A., Bohm, M., Paul, M., Ganten, D. 1993. Tissue renin-angiotensin systems: their role in cardiovascular disease. Circulation 87 (Suppl IV):7-13.

Mandle, R. J., Colman, R. W., Kaplan, A. P. 1976. Identification of prekallikrein and high-molecular-weight kininogen as a complex in human plasma. Proc Natl Acad Sci USA 73:4179-83.

Marceau, F., Lussier, A., Regoli, D., et al. 1983. Pharmacology of kinins: their relevance to tissue injury and inflammation. Gen Pharmacol 14:209-29.

Margolius, H. S. 1978. Kallikrein, kinins, and the kidney: what's going on in there? J Lab Clin Med 91:717-20.

Matsusaka T., Ichikawa I. 1997. Biological functions of angiotensin and its receptors. Annu Rev Physiol 59:395-412.

Mills, I. H. 1979. Kallikrein, kininogen and kinins in control of blood pressure. Nephron 23:61-71.

Oparil, S., Haber, E. 1974. The renin-angiotensin system (first of two parts). N Engl J Med 291:389-401.

Peart, W. S. 1975. Renin-angiotensin system. N Engl J Med 292:302-6.

Proud, D., Kaplan, A. P. 1988. Kinin formation: mechanisms and role in inflammatory disorders. Annu Rev Immunol 6:49-83.

Ratnoff, O. D., Saito, H. 1979. Interactions among Hageman factor, plasma prekallikrein, high molecular weight kininogen, and plasma thromboplastin antecedent. Proc Natl Acad Sci USA 76:958-61.

Regoli, D., Calo, G., Rizzi, A., Bogoni, G., Gobeil, F., Campobasso, C., Mollica, G., Beani, L. 1996. Bradykinin receptors and receptor ligands (with special emphasis on vascular receptors). Regulatory Peptides 65:83-89.

Rocha e Silva, M., Bernaldo, W. T., Rosenfeld, G. 1949. Bradykinin, hypotensive and smooth muscle stimulating factor released from plasma globulin by snake venom and by trypsin. Am J Physiol 156:261-73.

Schachter, M. 1980. Kallikreins (kininogenases)—a group of serine proteases with bioregulatory actions. Pharmacol Rev 31:1-17.

Schachter, M., Thain, E. M. 1954. Chemical and pharmacological properties of potent, slow contracting substance (kinin) in wasp venom. Br J Pharmacol 9:352-59.

Schror, K. 1992. Role of prostaglandins in the cardiovascular effects of bradykinin and angiotensin-converting enzyme inhibitors. J Cardiovasc Pharmacol 20(Suppl 9):S68-S73.

Schwieler, J. H., Hjemdahl, P. 1992. Influence of angiotensin-converting enzyme inhibition on sympathetic neurotransmission: possible roles of bradykinin and prostaglandins. J Cardiovasc Pharmacol 20(Suppl 9):S39-S46.

Tigerstedt, R., Bergman, P. G. 1898. Niere und kreislauf. Skand Arch Physiol 8:223-71.

Vecsei, P., Hackenthal, E., Ganten, D. 1978. The renin-angiotensin-aldosterone system: past, present and future. Klin Wochenschr 56(Suppl I):5-21.

21 PROSTAGLANDINS, RELATED FACTORS, AND CYTOKINES

H. RICHARD ADAMS

History
Chemistry and Terminology of Prostaglandins
Biosynthesis of Eicosanoids
Cyclooxygenase
Lipoxygenase
Inhibition of Biosynthesis of Eicosanoids
Physiologic-Pharmacologic Aspects of Eicosanoids
Reproductive System
Cardiovascular System
Blood
Kidney
Inflammation
Others
Mechanism of Action
Clinical Aspects
Platelet-Activating Factor
Cytokines
Tumor Necrosis Factor-α
Interleukin-1
Interleukin-6

Prostaglandins, thromboxanes, and leukotrienes are principal members of a diverse family of endogenous fatty acid derivatives synthesized from cell membrane phospholipids by virtually all types of mammalian cells. These compounds and their relatives are referred to collectively as the eicosanoids, because their fatty acid precursors share "eicosa" as the prefix in their chemical nomenclatures. Eicosanoids and other related fatty acid derivatives such as platelet-activating factor (PAF) have a remarkable spectrum of biologic activities. These substances represent some of the most important autacoids involved in homeostatic regulation. The breadth of biologic effects of the eicosanoids is believed to encompass practically every bodily activity, including various reproductive functions, blood pressure control, renal function, thrombus formation, inflammation, and many more. Interaction with the prostaglandin system is now recognized as an important mechanism of pharmacologic action of certain therapeutic agents such as aspirin and other nonsteroidal anti-inflammatory drugs (Masferrer and Kulkarni 1997; de Brum-Fernandes 1997; Donnelly and Hawkey 1997).

In addition to eicosanoids and PAF, this chapter briefly addresses another group of endogenous proinflammatory mediators, the cytokines. These agents are not chemically related to the eicosanoids or other fatty acid derivatives; rather, the cytokines are proteins secreted by a variety of cell types in response to inflammation and other stimuli that often concomitantly promote increased synthesis of the eicosanoids.

HISTORY. Recognition of the eicosanoids can be traced to the early 1930s. Two American gynecologists reported that human semen contained a substance affecting the contractile activity of human uterine strips (Kurzrok and Lieb 1930). Extracts of seminal fluid and accessory reproductive glands affected systemic blood pressure and smooth muscle contractile function. The active substance was distinct from the then known autacoids and was identified as a lipid-soluble acid and was named prostaglandin (PG).

Continuing investigations revealed that PG actually comprised a large family of closely related acidic lipids with unique chemical structure. The basic structural unit of the PG compounds proved to be a 20-carbon unsaturated carboxylic acid (Bergström and Samuelsson 1968); the initial PGs were named according to chemical structure and were designated by the letters A-F. $PGF_{2\alpha}$ continues to receive the most attention relative to animal reproductive problems, which represent the most important clinical uses of PG compounds in veterinary medicine (Schultz 1980; Seguin 1980). Recent advancements have shifted emphasis away from the classic PGs (i.e., PGA-PGF) and toward newer compounds such as the cyclic endoperoxides PGG_2 and PGH_2, prostacyclin, thromboxane A_2, leukotrienes, other eicosanoids, and the related PAF (Campbell 1990; Baird and Morrison 1993).

CHEMISTRY AND TERMINOLOGY OF PROSTAGLANDINS. Common to the structure of naturally occurring PGs is the unnatural fatty acid named prostanoic acid; this compound is a 20-carbon carboxylic acid with a cyclopentane ring (Fig. 21.1). The primary or classic PGs are individually named according to substituents on the cyclopentane ring; these are PGA, PGB, PGC, PGD, PGE, and PGF, as shown in Fig. 21.1. This figure also pictures the ring moieties of the newer PG-related compounds: PGG, PGH, prostacyclin (PGI), and thromboxane (Fig. 21.1).

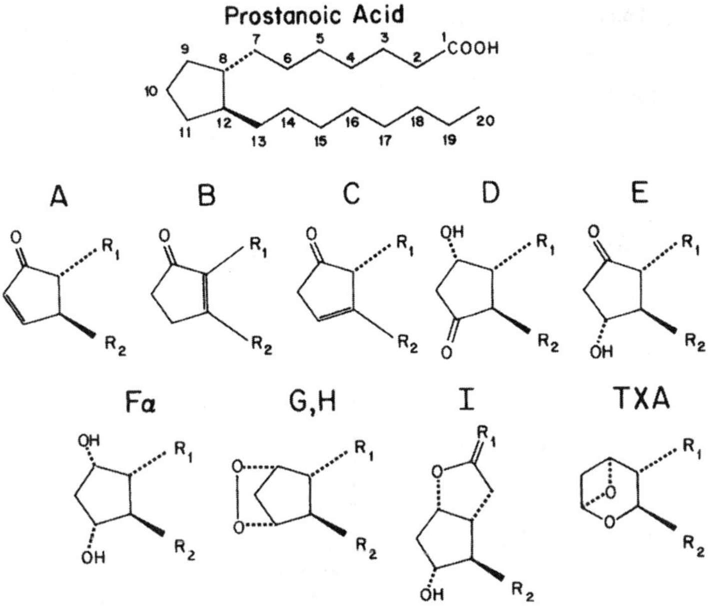

FIG. 21.1—Structures of prostanoic acid and the ring moieties of the six primary PGs (A-F), the cyclic endoperoxides (G, H), prostacyclin (I), and thromboxane A (TxA). In the stereochemical convention used in this and subsequent illustrations, the substituents indicated by the triangle lie in front of the plane of the ring structure, whereas those indicated by the dashed line lie behind it.

The PGs and related substances are further categorized as mono-, di-, or triunsaturated depending on the number of carbon-carbon double bonds in the side chains. This classification appears as a subscript to the letter; e.g., a PG_1 has one double bond between C-13 and C-14, a PG_2 has an additional double bond between C-5 and C-6, and a PG_3 has an additional double bond between C-17 and C-18. As an example, the structural formulas of PGE_1, PGE_2, and PGE_3 are compared in Fig. 21.2.

Biosynthetically, the PGs are derived from 20-carbon polyunsaturated fatty acids that contain a total of three, four, or five double bonds. These acids are 8, 11, 14-eicosatrienoic acid (dihomo-γ-linolenic acid); 5, 8, 11, 14-eicosatetraenoic acid (arachidonic acid); and 5, 8, 11, 14, 17-eicosapentaenoic acid respectively (Fig. 21.3). These essential fatty acids yield PGs with one, two, or three double bonds remaining in the side chains respectively, which account for the previously described classification as mono- (PG_1), bis- (PG_2), or trienoic (PG_3) PGs (see Fig. 21.3) (Wolfe 1982).

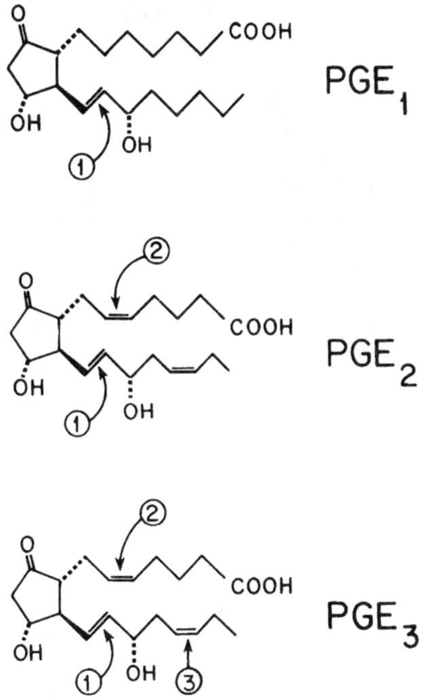

FIG. 21.2—Structures of PG E_1, E_2, and E_3.

BIOSYNTHESIS OF EICOSANOIDS. The eicosanoids, in contrast to many other autacoids, are not localized or stored in tissue pools. Instead, release of these compounds from cellular components reflects increased rate of their synthesis from available fatty acid precursors. Arachidonic acid, the precursor of the bisenoic PGs, is believed to be the most important

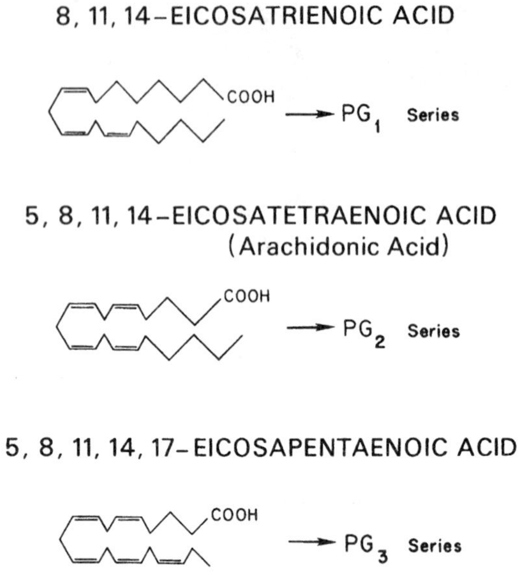

8, 11, 14-EICOSATRIENOIC ACID

COOH → PG_1 Series

5, 8, 11, 14-EICOSATETRAENOIC ACID
(Arachidonic Acid)

COOH → PG_2 Series

5, 8, 11, 14, 17-EICOSAPENTAENOIC ACID

COOH → PG_3 Series

FIG. 21.3—Structures of fatty acid precursors of the 1, 2, and 3 series PGs.

source of the PG compounds found in higher mammalian species. The trienoic PGs may be important in marine animals, where the eicosapentaenoic acid seems to be the predominant fatty acid precursor.

Arachidonic acid is an essential fatty acid. It is incorporated by ester linkage into phospholipids of cell membranes and may be contained in other complex lipids such as the triglycerides. Cellular phospholipids release arachidonic acid in response to phospholipase A_2. This enzyme is activated by a wide array of physiologic, pharmacologic, and pathologic stimuli. Hormones, neurohormones, and other autacoids can participate in initiation of this process; e.g., potent, vasoactive kinins and angiotensin activate tissue phospholipase A_2 and thereby accelerate PG synthesis. This activity in turn results in changes in intensity and range of action of bradykinin and angiotensin, since PG can also modulate the biologic effects of these polypeptides (McGiff 1979). Thus complex feedback systems exist, which regulate PG synthesis relative to the physiologic status of the animal and the resulting activities of other biologically active compounds. Even simple mechanical agitation or trauma of tissues can result in phospholipase activation with release of arachidonic acid (Moncada and Vane 1978).

After its liberation from phospholipids, arachidonic acid is subject to rapid oxidative catabolism by two separate enzymatic pathways involving a cyclooxygenase and a lipoxygenase. Transformation of arachidonic acid to some of its more important PG derivatives is illustrated in Fig. 21.4 and summarized below.

Cyclooxygenase. Synthesis of PG compounds begins with the oxygenation and cyclization of arachidonic acid; these events are catalyzed by the enzyme known as fatty acid cyclooxygenase (Fig. 21.4). This enzyme is widely distributed in mammals, and arachidonic acid can be metabolized to its PG derivatives by virtually all tissue types that have been tested. The immediate product of cyclooxygenase and arachidonic acid is the cyclic endoperoxide PGG_2, which is transformed to the closely related cyclic endoperoxide PGH_2 (Fig. 21.4).

Endoperoxides PGG_2 and PGH_2 are quite unstable, with biologic half-lives of 5 minutes at physiologic pH and body temperature. The endoperoxides undergo enzymatic or nonenzymatic transformation, yielding different PG products (i.e., PGD_2, PGE_2, and $PGF_{2\alpha}$) (Fig. 21.4). PGA, PGB, and PGC compounds are formed from the corresponding PGE during chemical extraction procedures and may not occur biologically. $PGF_{2\alpha}$ can be transformed from PGE_2 in some tissues by a 9-keto-reductase enzyme, but the presence of this enzyme under biologic conditions is somewhat debatable. In addition, enzymelike activity called PG endoperoxide $F_{2\alpha}$ reductase, which can form $PGF_{2\alpha}$ from the endoperoxides, has been detected in the bovine uterus (Kindahl 1980).

In addition to yielding PGs of the D, E, and F series, endoperoxide PGH_2 also is metabolized into two other compounds called thromboxane A_2 and prostacyclin. These substances are highly active but possess structures that differ somewhat from those of the primary PGs (Fig. 21.4).

Studies have shown that there are two major isoforms of cyclooxygenase: cyclooxygenase-1 (COX-1) and cyclooxygenase-2 (COX-2). The former enzyme is constitutively expressed in most cells under basal conditions, and it serves to synthesize the small amounts of PGs that participate in normal physiologic functions. COX-1 is especially important in producing those eicosanoids that have protective actions on gastrointestinal mucosa. Inhibition of COX-1 activity can therefore be detrimental to the patient because of loss of gastrointestinal protection of mucosal epithelial cells (Masferrer and Kulkarni 1997).

The other isoform of cyclooxygenase, COX-2, is not constitutively present; it is nondetectable under basal nonstimulated conditions. However, when cells are exposed to bacterial lipopolysaccharide and certain inflammatory cytokines and growth factors, the synthesis of COX-2 is induced. The inducible COX-2 results in increased concentrations of PGs that participate in inflammatory reactions (de Brum-Fernandes 1997).

THROMBOXANE A_2. An enzyme first isolated from equine and human thrombocytes was found to convert PGH_2 into a compound containing an oxane ring instead of the cyclopentane ring of the PGs. This substance was named thromboxane A_2 (TxA_2), and the responsible enzyme was named thromboxane synthase (Fig. 21.4).

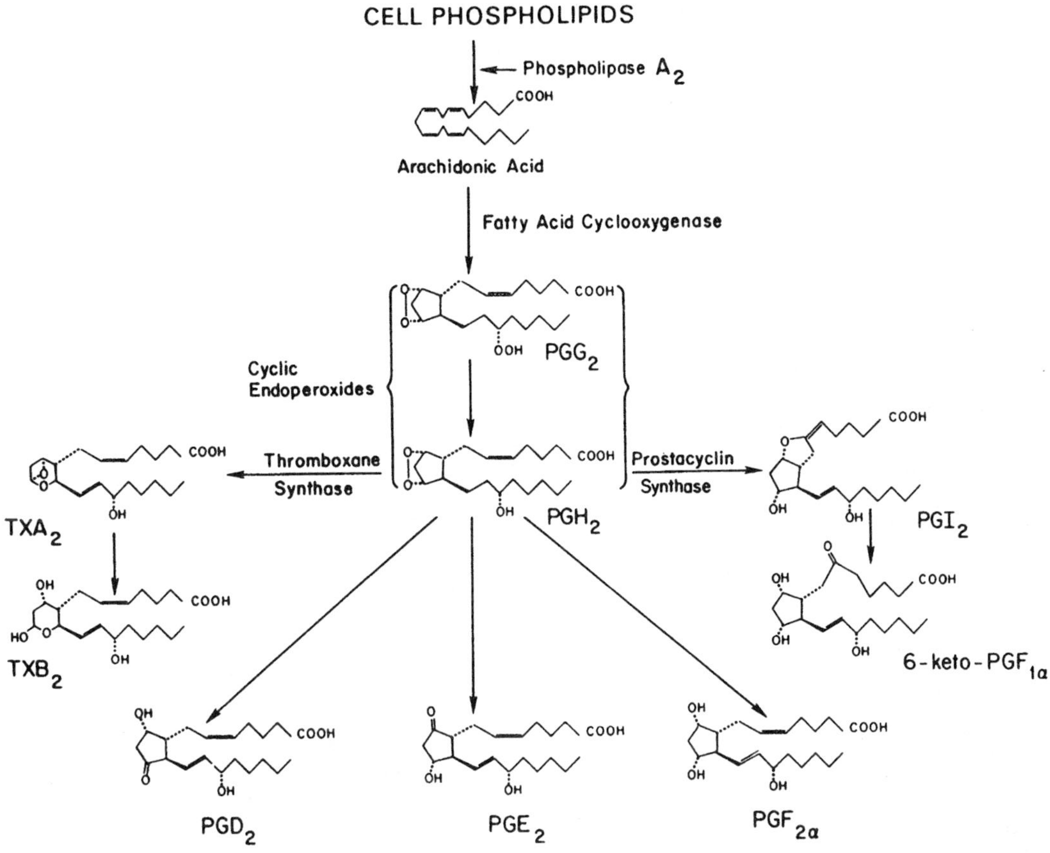

FIG. 21.4—Cyclooxygenase-catalyzed conversion of arachidonic acid to major PG compounds.

TxA_2 has a brief half-life of about 30 seconds under physiologic conditions, and it degrades into the stable compound thromboxane B_2 (Fig. 21.4). As will be discussed subsequently, TxA_2 plays an important physiologic role as a vasoconstrictor and proaggregate in thrombus formation (see Chap. 28).

PROSTACYCLIN. An enzyme localized in vascular tissue was found to convert PGH_2 into yet another highly active metabolite called prostacyclin or PGI_2 (Fig. 21.4). The enzyme was named prostacyclin synthase (Fig. 21.4).

PGI_2 has a double-ring component rather than the single cyclopentane ring (Figs. 21.1, 21.4). The biologic half-life of PGI_2 is quite short, between 2 and 3 minutes; it is converted nonenzymatically into a relatively inactive but stable product, 6-keto-$PGF_{1\alpha}$ (Fig. 21.4). PGI_2 is a potent vasodilator and exerts antiaggregatory activity on blood platelets (see below and Chap. 28).

Lipoxygenase. Although fatty acid cyclooxygenase is widely distributed, lipoxygenases have so far been found mainly in lung, platelets, and white blood cells. Metabolism of arachidonic acid via lipoxygenase pathways yields unstable hydroperoxides, which then break down to the stable hydroxyacids or are further transformed into other derivatives such as the leukotrienes. Selected products of lipoxygenases are shown in Fig. 21.5; these include 12-hydroperoxyarachidonic acid (HPETE) and its stable metabolite 12-hydroxyarachidonic acid (HETE). The breadth of physiologic actions of these compounds remains uncertain, but they are chemotactic for leukocytes and participate in inflammatory responses.

The name leukotriene has been proposed for a group of noncyclized, 20-carbon, carboxylic acid products of arachidonic acid formed by 5-lipoxygenase activity (Fig. 21.5). The trivial name leukotriene was chosen because these compounds were discovered in leukocytes and shared a common structural feature as conjugated trienes (Samuelsson 1983). The initial reaction of the 5-lipoxygenase pathway is the formation of 5-HPETE (Fig. 21.5); 5-HPETE is converted either to 5-HETE or to leukotriene A_4, a 5,6 epoxide. Leukotriene A_4 is converted in turn either to leukotriene B_4 or C_4. The latter is a glutathionyl derivative, formed by the

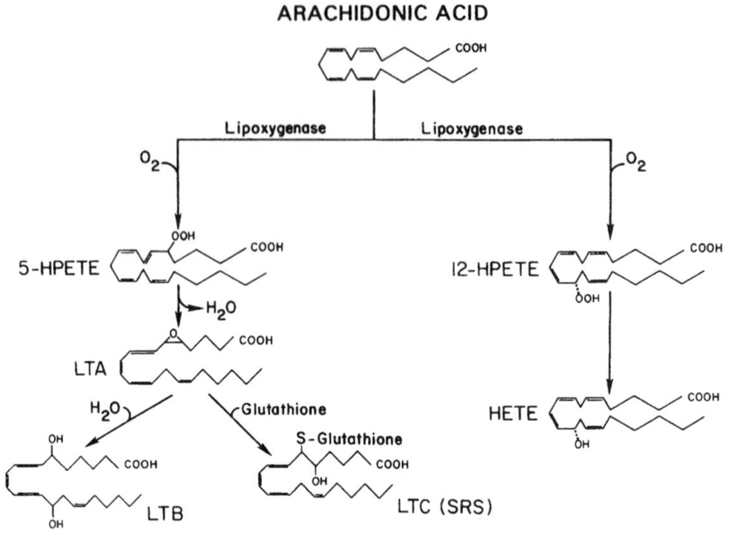

FIG. 21.5—Lipoxygenase-catalyzed conversion of arachidonic acid to hydroperoxyarachidonic acids (HPETE), hydroxyarachidonic acid (HETE), and leukotriene (LT) A_4, B_4, and C_4. SRS = slow-reacting substance of anaphylaxis.

enzyme glutathione-*S*-transferase (Fig. 21.5). Leukotriene D_4 is formed via the cleavage of the glycine moiety from leukotriene C_4, while E_4 is synthesized by the subsequent removal of glycine. The biologic importance of the leukotrienes is under intensive investigation; there is considerable evidence that these substances participate in inflammatory reactions, and a combination of the cysteine-containing leukotrienes (i.e., C_4, D_4, and E_4) is now believed to compose the slow-reacting substance of anaphylaxis (Samuelsson 1983; Samuelsson et al. 1980). As a general rule, the dihydroxy acids are chemotactic for leukocytes but have minimal smooth muscle-stimulating properties, whereas the sulfur linkage and amino acid residues at C-6 are required for smooth muscle-stimulating properties (Piper 1983).

INHIBITION OF BIOSYNTHESIS OF EICOSANOIDS. Tissue distribution of the different enzymes involved in PG biosynthesis is important to medicine. These enzymes currently represent the most vulnerable targets for pharmacologic manipulation of the PG system.

Cyclooxygenase seems to be rather ubiquitous, because most tissues are able to convert arachidonic acid to the intermediate endoperoxides PGG_2 and PGH_2. However, the fate of the latter compounds varies considerably in different tissues.

Reproductive organs of several species are able to synthesize PGE_2 and $PGH_{2\alpha}$, whereas the spleen and lung can produce the whole range of PG compounds. The major PG formed by blood vessel endothelial cells is PGI_2; hence, prostacyclin synthase is of major importance in this tissue. On the other hand, thromboxane synthase is dominant in blood platelets; TxA_2 is a primary PG product of this cell type. Various drugs have been studied in attempts to regulate the PG system via effects on the participating enzymes.

Starting with Vane's work in 1971, the rather pronounced influence of aspirin-like drugs on the PG system became apparent. Aspirin and other anti-inflammatory agents of the nonsteroidal type disrupt the cellular release of PGs by interfering with their biosynthesis. The site of inhibitory action of these drugs is localized high in the PG cascade, at the cyclooxygenase level (Fig. 21.4). By inhibiting cyclooxygenase, aspirin prevents conversion of arachidonic acid to the endoperoxides PGG_2 and PGH_2. Accordingly, the formation of PG products below PGG_2 and PGH_2 in the metabolic pathway is likewise retarded by the action of aspirin (Vane 1971).

Other nonsteroidal anti-inflammatory agents that inhibit cyclooxygenase include other salicylates, indomethacin, phenylbutazone, naproxen, flunixin, and meclofenamic acid (see Chap. 22). The anti-inflammatory, antipyretic, and analgesic actions of such drugs are mediated principally by inhibition of PG biosynthesis at the cyclooxygenase level (Moncada and Vane 1978). The side effects of this group of drugs also depend on inhibition of PG synthesis (see Chap. 22). Aspirin-like drugs are not inhibitors of the lipoxygenase enzymes that participate in other metabolic pathways of arachidonic acid.

Traditional nonsteroidal anti-inflammatory agents are nonselective inhibitors of both the constitutive COX-1 and the inducible COX-2 isoenzymes. Inhibition of COX-2 results in therapeutically useful reductions in the synthesis of proinflammatory eicosanoids, but inhibition of COX-1 would at the same time result in loss of protective and other physiologic functions of PGs necessary for normal cellular functions (de Brum-Fernandes 1997; Donnelly and Hawkey 1997). Drugs with greater inhibitory action on COX-2 than on COX-1 would be therapeutically beneficial because they would selectively reduce synthesis of inflammatory PGs while sparing cellular protective actions of COX-1 products. Newer nonsteroidal anti-inflammatory agents with selective COX-2 inhibitory actions are addressed in Chap. 22.

Corticosteroids interfere with PG biosynthesis by inducing the synthesis of a protein inhibitor of phospholipase activity, thereby retarding release of arachidonic acid from cellular phospholipids (Wolfe 1982). Corticosteroids also modulate expression of the inducible COX-2 enzyme, thereby decreasing its formation (Masferrer and Kulkarni 1997; de Brum-Fernandes 1997; Donnelly and Hawkey 1997).

Considerable interest is directed toward characterization of selective inhibitors of the PG-synthesizing enzymes; e.g., imidazole and certain of its analogs preferentially inhibit thromboxane synthase. Certain analogs of PGG_2 and PGH_2 also exert selective inhibitory actions on this enzyme. Conversely, prostacyclin synthase is inhibited by lipid peroxides such as 15-HPETE. Clinical application of the above enzyme inhibitors is unproven, but potential advantages over the aspirin-like cyclooxygenase inhibitors reside in the possibility of selectively reducing production of one PG derivative without affecting others.

PHYSIOLOGIC-PHARMACOLOGIC ASPECTS OF EICOSANOIDS. Although a multitude of biologic activities has been assigned to the different eicosanoids, the physiologic value of all such effects and relative importance of individual derivatives undergo almost continual reappraisal as new discoveries are unfolded. Artifactual conversion of one PG to another during tissue isolation has delayed attempts to designate biologic responsibility. In addition, data obtained from one animal species may not apply to others because there are formidable species differences in responsiveness to many members of the eicosanoid complex. In the following paragraphs, some of the better defined physiologic and pharmacologic aspects of the biologic activities of this system are summarized.

Reproductive System. The involvement of PGs in reproductive physiology is covered later in this volume. Briefly, PG compounds have been associated with luteolysis, abortion, and parturition.

Interest is focused mainly on $PGF_{2\alpha}$, which is believed to be the long-sought luteolytic hormone produced by the uterus in some nonprimate species (e.g., mare, cow, sow, ewe, and guinea pig). This factor is believed to control the life span of the corpus luteum; e.g., in nonpregnant cows the luteolytic hormone or $PGF_{2\alpha}$ is released about day 14 or 15 of the estrous cycle. The corpus luteum degenerates, which evokes the return of estrus. Pregnancy inhibits release of the luteolytic factor, hence the corpus luteum persists and the fetus develops.

In addition to producing luteolysis, $PGF_{2\alpha}$ also causes contraction of uterine smooth muscle. Since blood concentrations of PG increase during labor, $PGF_{2\alpha}$ release is viewed as important for prepartum lysis of the corpus luteum, which removes the progesterone block, and for evoking uterine contractions during parturition. Increased PG production has also been associated with abortion and premature labor. In support of these concepts, aspirin was found to delay parturition, reduce uterine contractions during labor, retard premature labor, and delay abortion. The participation of PG in reproductive events has been reviewed by Schultz (1980), Seguin (1980), and Stabenfeldt et al. (1980).

Cardiovascular System. Systemic administration of PGs can evoke pronounced hemodynamic responses, depending upon the individual compound and animal species tested (Camu et al. 1992). Blood pressure effects of all the PG derivatives mainly reflect changes in peripheral vascular resistance; these agents affect smooth muscle contractile activity in large arteries, arterioles, precapillaries, venules, and large veins. Primary PGs of the E and A series, particularly PGE_2, are potent vasodilators in most species. Conversely, vascular smooth muscle is generally contracted by $PGF_{2\alpha}$. Vasodilator effects of the latter and vasoconstrictor effects of PGE_2 have been seen in certain vascular beds (McGiff 1979).

TxA_2 is a potent stimulant of vascular smooth muscle and has produced vasoconstriction in all blood vessel systems yet tested. TxA_2 was originally detected as rabbit aorta-contracting substance released from guinea pig lungs during anaphylaxis (Piper and Vane 1969). As opposed to TxA_2, PGI_2 is an exceptional vasodilator. It is several times more potent than PGE_2. Pronounced vasodilator effects of PGI_2 have been demonstrated in several regions, including the coronary, renal, skeletal muscle, and omental vascular beds.

A systemic depressor response is evoked by the vasodilators PGI_2, PGE_2, and PGE_1, whereas a pressor response is produced by the vasoconstrictors $PGF_{2\alpha}$ and TxA_2. Interestingly, PGI_2 is equipotent as a vasodilator whether administered intravenously or intra-arterially. This is an important difference from PGE_1 or PGE_2, which are much less active when given intravenously. These differences were explained when it was discovered that PGE_1 and PGE_2 undergo almost complete metabolism during a single passage through the pulmonary vascular circuit, whereas PGI_2 is not metabolized rapidly by the lungs. In fact, the lungs seem able to release PGI_2 into the circulation. Persistence of PGI_2 in the blood contributed to the suggestion that this agent may be a circulating PG with more hemodynamic responsibility than the rapidly inactivated PGE_2 (Moncada and Vane 1978).

The intermediate endoperoxides PGG_2 and PGH_2 exert variable effects on vascular smooth muscle; both vasoconstriction and vasodilation have been reported. This scope of activity reflects some intrinsic vasoconstrictor actions of the endoperoxides as well as their rapid conversion to other potent agents such as PGI_2. Similarly, injection of arachidonic acid can elicit circulatory effects that are mediated by its metabolites; such effects are inhibited by aspirin.

Cardiac output is increased slightly by PGs of the A, E, and F series, but cardiac responses to PG in intact subjects are mainly a result of reflex adjustment to systemic blood pressure changes. Only weak inotropic effects are seen with isolated heart muscle preparations. The heart can release endogenously produced PGI_2 upon exposure to certain stimuli, but this activity reflects PG synthesis by the coronary vasculature and not by the cardiac muscle cell (Sivakoff et al. 1979).

There is increasing evidence that different eicosanoids participate in the pathogenicity of circulatory depressant effects associated with gram-negative endotoxicosis. Most studies have focused on TxA_2 and PGI_2, and the concentrations of both increase during endotoxin shock in dogs and horses (Moore et al. 1986).

Although leukotrienes C_4 and D_4 exert potent cardiovascular effects, differences exist relative to animal species and to route of administration. Both agents cause an initial hypertensive response followed by long-lasting hypotension when injected intravenously. When given arterially, the pressor phase is reduced, while the depressor response is prolonged. Interestingly, at least a portion of the cardiovascular response to the leukotrienes may be secondary to release of PGs, because cyclooxygenase inhibitors attenuate the prolonged hypotensive response to the leukotrienes. Piper (1983) has reviewed the cardiovascular profile of the leukotrienes.

Since certain fetal and maternal blood vessels can synthesize PGI_2, this agent may participate in circulatory adjustments to pregnancy and parturition (Terragno and Terragno 1979). Locally synthesized PGI_2 has been implicated in maintenance of the patency of the ductus arteriosus. This concept was based in part on the observation that aspirin could produce closure of the ductus in neonates. Indomethacin has proven superior to aspirin in this respect, but mixed results have been seen in clinical trials.

Blood. Compared to most cell types, erythrocytes lack the capacity to generate significant amounts of PG. In contrast, blood platelets are prolific producers of the endoperoxides PGG_2 and PGH_2 and of TxA_2. These compounds, especially the more active TxA_2, are potent aggregating agents; their involvement in thrombus formation is contrasted with the antiaggregating action of PGI_2 in Fig. 28.1.

Briefly, the platelet-aggregating effects of TxA_2 are believed to be important to the thrombus-forming and thus hemostatic mechanisms provoked by damage to blood and blood vessels. Conversely, the antiaggregating action of PGI_2 may serve to modulate thrombus formation. Indeed, PGI_2 is the most potent endogenous inhibitor of platelet aggregation yet discovered. It is 1000 times more potent than adenosine and 30-40 times more active than PGE_1. Also, PGI_2 disaggregates platelets in vitro, in vivo in the circulatory system, and in extracorporeal circuits where platelet clumping has occurred.

It has been suggested that small amounts of PGI_2 are present in the circulation, circulating PGI_2 is responsible for lack of aggregation of normal platelets, locally produced PGI_2 is involved in providing vascular endothelium with its smooth-surfaced characteristics, and vascular endothelium may even scavenge endoperoxides from platelets for use in production of PGI_2. The latter activity is envisioned to serve as a control mechanism to prevent spread of thrombi onto normal vascular endothelium when adjacent injuries have evoked TxA_2 formation and platelet aggregation. Thus platelet TxA_2 and vascular PGI_2 serve as biologically opposite regulators of interactions between platelets and blood vessels (Gorman 1979; Moncada and Vane 1978).

The antiaggregating action of PGI_2, PGE_1, and PGD_2 has been associated with an increase in the concentration of cyclic adenosine monophosphate (cAMP). Although different PG receptors may be involved, it seems that adenylyl cyclase is activated by each of the antiaggregating PG compounds. Conversely, the endoperoxides and TxA_2 inhibit the stimulatory effect of PGI_2 on adenylyl cyclase, thereby lowering cAMP concentration. Drugs that increase cAMP concentration, such as the phosphodiesterase inhibitor dipyridamole (Persantine), enhance the antiaggregating effects of PGI and antagonize the proaggregating effects of TxA_2.

Kidney. Although cyclooxygenase is present in various regions of the kidney, the major products of arachidonic acid metabolism are thought to be tissue-specific in this organ (McGiff and Wong 1979). PGI_2 is synthesized within the kidney primarily by the vascular smooth muscle compartment. Small quantities of this PG cause renal vasodilation and thereby lower vascular resistance and increase blood flow in the kidney. Urinary excretion of sodium, potassium, chloride, and water is increased by PGI_2; these changes may reflect direct effects on tubular transport mechanisms or secondary effects caused by redistribution of blood flow. There is increasing evidence that PGI_2 also regulates release of renin through actions exerted at the vascular pole of the glomerulus, and PG formation may be involved in certain types of hypertension (Oates et al. 1979).

The major PG derivative of renal medullary interstitial cells seems to be PGE_2. Collecting ducts also are capable of generating PGE_2. This PG can increase salt and water excretion independently of blood flow changes, an effect caused in part by inhibition of the action of antidiuretic hormone on permeability of collecting ducts. There is increasing evidence that effects of PGE_2 and also $PGF_{2\alpha}$ on salt and water excretion involve interaction with the kallikrein-kinin system within the renal urinary compartment (McGiff and Wong 1979; Moncada and Vane 1978).

TxA_2 is believed to be synthesized by the kidney only under pathologic conditions, e.g., after ligation or other obstructions of the ureter. Pathophysiologic stimuli such as hemorrhage or laparotomy can also increase synthesis of renal PG, especially PGE_2, which then contributes to maintenance of renal blood flow. The physiologic value of PG to renal blood flow in normal nonstressed animals remains unclear.

Inflammation. PGs and other eicosanoids are released from soft tissues in response to a variety of noxious stimuli such as infection and mechanical, thermal, and chemical trauma. Once liberated from irritated or damaged cells, PG contributes importantly to different phases of the local inflammatory reaction. Large concentrations of PG elicit pain by direct stimulation of sensory nerve endings. More typically, PGs in quite small concentrations sensitize sensory nerve endings to other pain-provoking stimuli such as bradykinin, histamine, and other mediators of inflammation. Edema-inducing and hyperemic effects of kinins and other autacoids are likewise enhanced by certain PGs, e.g., PGE_2 and PGI_2. These PGs do not seem to directly affect vascular permeability but facilitate leukocyte infiltration and edema formation through vasodilation-induced increase in blood flow. Metabolites of the lipoxygenase pathway also contribute to the inflammatory process, and increasing evidence has linked these compounds and certain PG derivatives with immunologic phenomena.

The peptide leukotrienes increase vascular permeability and contribute further to inflammation by their chemotactic effect on leukocytes. Leukotriene B_4 is especially active as a chemoattractant for polymorphonuclear leukocytes. Other lipoxygenase products such as 5-HPETE and 5-HETE may facilitate the release of histamine and other inflammatory autacoids from mast cells.

Others. PGs affect contractile activity of several smooth muscles besides those of the reproductive and vascular systems. Many species differences exist, and the net effect in each tissue is influenced by the age, health, sex, and endocrine status of the test subject. PGs of the F series, especially $PGF_{2\alpha}$, generally contract tracheal and bronchial smooth muscle in several species. Members of the E series generally relax respiratory muscle. In asthmatic humans, $PGF_{2\alpha}$ has induced intense bronchospasm, while PGE_1 and PGE_2 are potent bronchodilators. TxA_2, PGG_2, and PGH_2 contract tracheal muscle and induce bronchospasm.

PGI_2 affects smooth muscle motility and fluid transport mechanisms in the intestine, where it exerts an antidiarrheal effect. In contrast, PGE_2 produces diarrhea, which is an important limitation to therapeutic use of this agent.

PGI_2 is a major product of the gastric mucosa of several species. It is a potent vasodilator in this tissue, where it also inhibits the acid secretion evoked by pentagastrin. Thus PGI_2 may serve as a suppressant modulator of gastric acid secretion and as a participant in functional hyperemia of the stomach. The untoward ability of aspirin-like drugs to induce gastric irritation and ulceration has been attributed to inhibition of PGI_2 synthesis.

Numerous central nervous system effects have been attributed to PG, but large concentrations are generally needed to demonstrate such actions. Several PG derivatives depress release of norepinephrine from adrenergic neurons of the autonomic nervous system, but physiologic significance remains questionable.

Mechanism of Action. Membrane receptors for PG have been identified in certain tissues, and smooth muscle-stimulating effects of PG have been associated with alterations in calcium movement induced by cell membrane depolarization. Changes in cellular metabolism of calcium may also be involved in other actions of PG, secondary to changes in various enzyme activities. Certain of the PGs increase cAMP concentrations by stimulating adenylyl cyclase activity, e.g., PGI_2 in platelets. Others are inhibitory to such relationships, e.g., TxA_2 in platelets. In certain tissues, however, cAMP can inhibit PG biosynthesis.

The biological complexity of the eicosanoids is exemplified by the complexity of PG receptors and their associated signal-transduction mechanisms. The G-protein-adenylyl cyclase-cAMP system is linked with some PG receptors (Smith 1992), whereas the phospholipase C-inositol trisphospate-Ca^{++} system is linked with others (Mitchell and Trautman 1993). This area was reviewed by Campbell (1990), and Table 21.1 summarizes some of the PG receptor types and their affiliated receptor mechanisms. Although antagonists for PG receptors are under intense investigation, inhibition of biosynthetic enzymes in the eicosanoid cascades (Figs. 21.4 and 21.5) is the most viable therapeutic mechanism for altering eicosanoid actions.

Clinical Aspects. Bell et al. (1980) compiled lengthy lists of possible therapeutic uses of different members of the PG group in veterinary medicine. Disorders that were listed as potentially responsive to PG or to anti-PG treatment varied from such diverse disorders as equine laminitis and feline cardiomyopathies to paralytic ileus and porcine gastric ulceration. Use of PG in treating such pathophysiologic states may well prove to have clinical value in the future. Currently, pharmacologic manipulation of the PG complex involves mainly the cardiovascular system, reproductive functions, and inflammation.

The capability of $PGF_{2\alpha}$ and synthetic analogs to influence reproductive performance represents the most important clinical application of PG compounds in veterinary medicine. Use of aspirin-like cyclooxygenase inhibitors for analgesic, anti-inflammatory, and antipyretic effects is discussed elsewhere in this volume.

TABLE 21.1—Classification of some eicosanoid receptors and their affiliated signal-transduction pathways in vascular smooth muscle and platelets

Receptor type	Endogenous agonist	Transduction mechanism	Vascular effect	Platelet aggregation
DP	PGD_2	cAMP	—	Inhibit
EP_1	PGE_2; $PGF_{2\alpha}$	IP_3–Ca^{++}	Vasoconstrict	—
EP_2	PGE_2; PGE_1	cAMP	Vasodilate	Inhibit
FP	$PGF_{2\alpha}$	IP_3–Ca^{++}	Vasoconstrict	—
IP	PGI_2; PGE	cAMP	Vasodilate	Inhibit
TP	TxA_2; PGH_2	IP_3–Ca^{++}	Vasoconstrict	Enhance

Source: Campbell 1990; Smith 1992; Mitchell and Trautman 1993.

Note: P = prostaglandin; cAMP = the $G_s$protein-adenylyl cyclase-cAMP-protein kinase A pathway; IP_3-Ca^{++} = the phospholipase C-IP_3-diacylglycerol–protein kinase C–Ca^{++} pathway. The — designates unknown or vasoconstriction and vasodilation depending on tissues. cAMP = cyclic adenosine monophosphate.

Pharmacologic manipulation of the PG system also has application in treating or preventing disorders of the cardiovascular system, but such uses are mainly experimental; e.g., PGI_2 has been used to retard platelet aggregation and thromboembolism in several systems of extracorporeal circulation such as renal dialysis and cardiopulmonary bypass. PGI_2 and its analogs may also become important in controlling thromboembolism in the intact circulation. Intra-arterial infusions of the vasodilators PGE_2 and PGI_2 were reported to increase blood flow, reduce pain, and accelerate healing of ulcers in human patients with peripheral vascular disease (Szczeklik et al. 1979).

Platelet cyclooxygenase is more sensitive to the inhibitory action of aspirin than the cyclooxygenase of blood vessels. Aspirin irreversibly inhibits cyclooxygenase by acetylating its active site. Since platelets cannot synthesize new protein during their sojourn in the bloodstream, the inhibitory effect of aspirin persists for several days, i.e., until new platelets are produced by the bone marrow. Thus small doses of aspirin preferentially inhibit platelet production of the proaggregating TxA_2 without marked reduction of vascular production of the antiaggregating PGI_2. The net result is expressed as an antithrombotic effect with increased bleeding time. Aspirin therefore is an antithrombotic agent used for prevention of conditions characterized by excessive platelet aggregation. However, large doses also inhibit vascular cyclooxygenase, resulting in loss of preferential block of TxA_2 synthesis. The clinical application of such interrelationships in animals remains to be clearly defined.

PLATELET-ACTIVATING FACTOR. Platelet-activating factor (PAF) is another autacoid derived from membrane phospholipids rich in arachidonic acid and other precursors of polyunsaturated fatty acids, and is therefore chemically related to the ubiquitous eicosanoid family. Whereas the eicosanoids are formed from a wide variety of cell types, PAF is synthesized principally by platelets, endothelial cells, and circulating leukocytes. The wide distribution of these cells throughout the body ensures PAF the opportunity to affect a host of tissue and cellular functions.

PAF not only provokes platelet aggregation, as its name implies, but it also modulates smooth muscle activity in blood vessel walls and promotes leakage of vascular fluid across endothelial surfaces. Although PAF lowers blood pressure due to its relaxing effect on vascular smooth muscle, it markedly contracts smooth muscle of the gut, stomach, uterus, and peripheral airways of the lungs. PAF can promote the synthesis and release of thromboxane A_2 and therefore exerts both direct and indirect effects on blood pressure. Since some of the smooth muscle and proinflammatory effects of PAF can be prevented by cyclooxygenase inhibitors, PAF is considered to be one of the most active endogenous activators of prostaglandins and related eicosanoids. In this regard, PAF and cyclooxygenase products are commonly activated concomitantly in response to inflammatory stimuli such as bacterial infection. This type of cohort relationship is exemplified in Fig. 21.6, wherein the response of a mammalian cell membrane to bacterial lipopolysaccharide (endotoxin) is schematized. Endotoxin lipopolysaccharide interacts with cellular constituents, culminating in activation of the cell membrane enzyme phospholipase A_2. Not only does the latter release arachidonic acid for eicosanoid biosynthesis through the cyclooxygenase (Fig. 21.4) and lipoxygenase pathways (Fig. 21.5), but this same reaction also yields a lysophospholipid that can be formed into PAF (Fig. 21.6). Thus, biological roles for PAF are often linked to those exhibited by the eicosanoid family. Despite the wealth of physiologic and pathophysiologic activities proposed for PAF (Campbell 1990), pharmacologic manipulation of PAF synthesis and receptors is at a preliminary stage. The clinical significance of PAF antagonists is currently unknown for veterinary medicine.

CYTOKINES. In response to certain inflammatory and immunologic stimuli, many types of mammalian cells produce one or more of a variety of small proteins termed cytokines. Cytokines include tumor necrosis factor-α (TNF-α), gamma interferon, and the interleukins (IL). Currently, monoclonal antibodies raised against these specific proteins represent the primary pharmacotherapeutic intervention relevant to the area

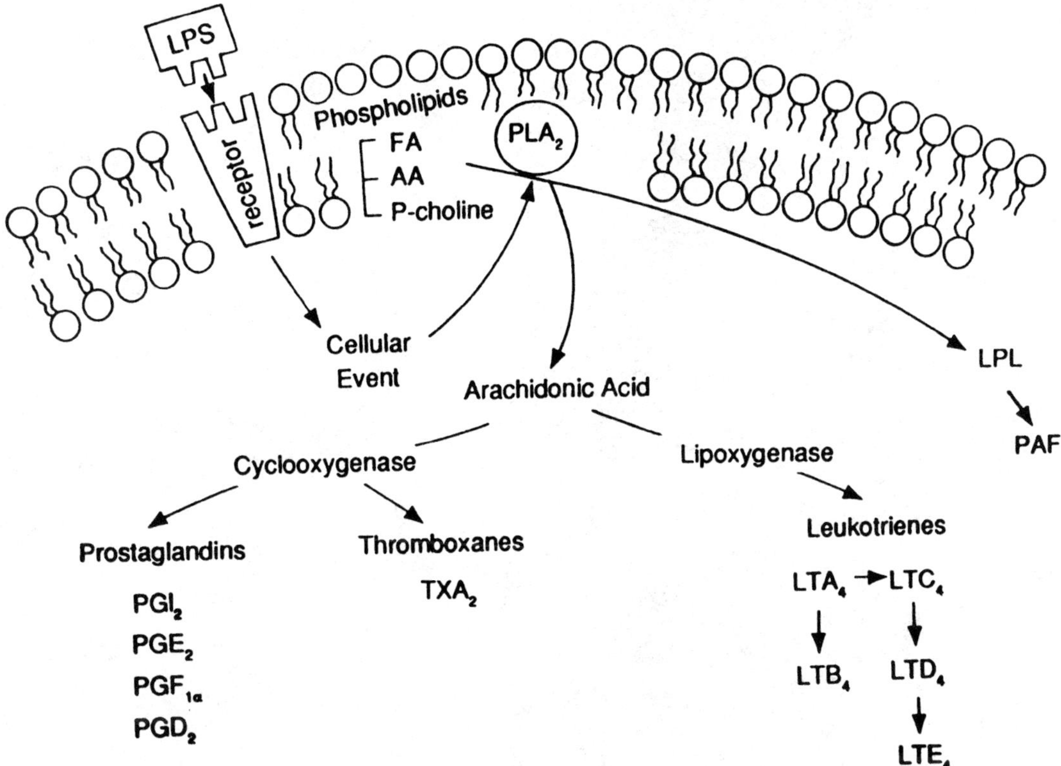

FIG. 21.6—Schematic diagram of endotoxin (lipopolysaccharide, LPS)-induced activation of phospholipase A_2 (PLA_2). Activated PLA_2 results in the release of arachidonic acid from the 2-acyl position of membrane phospholipids, leaving a lysophospholipid (LPL) that can be used to form platelet-activating factor (PAF). Arachidonic acid is metabolized to prostaglandins (PG), thromboxanes (TX), and leukotrienes (LT). FA = fatty acid; AA = arachidonic acid; and P-choline = phosphatidylcholine. (Source: Bottoms and Adams 1992.)

of cytokines. However, because of the likely future importance of cytokines to pharmacologic management of bacterial invasion and other inflammatory conditions, the following discussion briefly summarizes key aspects about TNF-α and the interleukins.

Tumor Necrosis Factor-α. The polypeptide cytokine TNF-α occupies a prominent and perhaps central role as proximal mediator of endotoxic shock (Tracey et al. 1989; Morris et al. 1990). Macrophages exposed to endotoxin and related stimuli release large quantities of TNF-α. On reaching the circulation, TNF-α binds to high-affinity receptors in normal tissues and triggers a wide array of biological effects. The infusion of recombinant TNF-α from human beings can induce lethal shock and tissue injury in animals, closely simulating key elements of the pathophysiologic derangements characteristic of endotoxemia (Tracey et al. 1986; Tracey et al. 1987a,b).

The production and release of other cytokines, eicosanoids, and humoral factors are elicited by TNF-α (Fig. 21.7). In addition to induction of IL-1, IL-4, and IL-6 synthesis, other biological activities attributed to TNF-α include T-cell activation, endogenous pyrogen activity, induction of eicosanoid synthesis, activation of osteoclastic bone resorption, inhibition of bone collagen synthesis, induction of acute-phase reactant synthesis and granulocyte/monocyte colony-stimulating factor, and inhibition of lipoprotein lipase and other enzymes of lipid metabolism (Grunfield and Palladino 1990; Beutler and Cerami 1989; Rosonblum and Donato 1989). In neutrophils, TNF-α stimulates activation, respiratory burst, degranulation, and adherence to the vascular endothelium.

At low concentrations, TNF-α exerts its primary effects locally as a paracrine and autocrine regulator of leukocytes and endothelial cells. These actions are critical for the containment of infection. However, when TNF-α gains access to the systemic circulation, signs of septicemia develop and high concentrations of TNF-α can be lethal. Cyclooxygenase inhibitors can block the rapid-onset monophasic fever that is induced by TNF-α. Lethal effects of endotoxin and TNF-α can be reduced under certain conditions by the administration

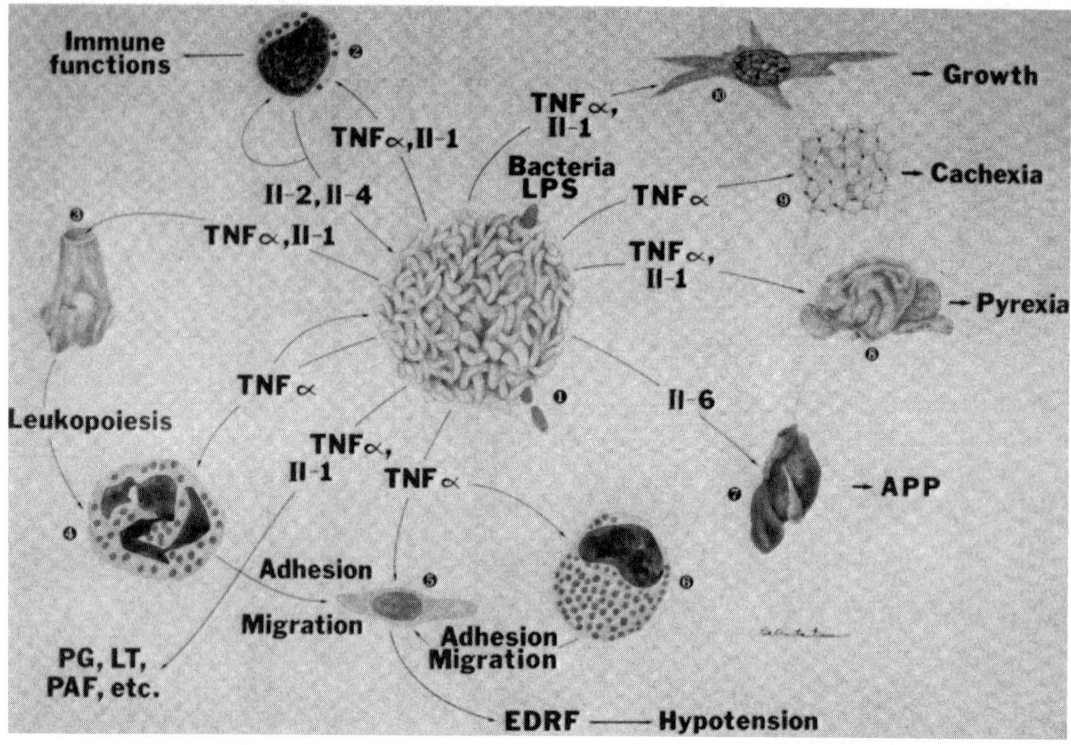

FIG. 21.7—Reaction of macrophage to gram-negative bacteria and endotoxin and representative responses of tissues to liberation of tumor necrosis factor-α (TNF-α) and interleukin (IL) cytokines from macrophages. The following numbered items refer to corresponding numbers in the figure: (1) macrophage: recognizes and assimilates bacteria and endotoxin (lipopolysaccharide, LPS), resulting in macrophage activation and release of cytokine mediators such as TNF-α and IL-1; (2) T and B lymphocytes: TNF-α and IL-1 enhance immunoregulatory functions, and lymphocytes release IL-4 and IL-2, which can affect macrophage function in an autocrine manner; (3) bone marrow: cytokines increase leukopoiesis; (4) neutrophils: activated by TNF-α to enhance migration and adhesion to vascular endothelium; (5) endothelium: TNF-α enhances adhesion and modulates release of hypotensive agents such as endothelium-derived relaxing factor (EDRF); (6) eosinophils: TNF-α promotes migration and adhesion; (7) liver: cytokines promote synthesis of acute-phase proteins (APP); (8) brain: cytokines modulate thermoregulatory functions, resulting in pyrexia; (9) adipocytes: TNF-α modulates metabolic regulatory enzymes, yielding cachexia; and (10) fibroblasts: cytokines enhance proliferation and growth. Cytokines also modulate the release of other mediators, such as prostaglandins (PG), leukotrienes (LT), and platelet-activating factor (PAF). (This figure was modeled after the illustration in Old 1988 and was drawn by Dr. Gheorghe M. Constantinescu, Department of Veterinary Biomedical Sciences, University of Missouri, Columbia. Source: Green and Adams 1992.)

of neutralizing TNF-α antiserum (Tracey et al. 1987a,b; Shimamoto et al. 1988). Long-term exposure to TNF-α results in cachexia, which accounts for its synonym, cachectin.

Interleukin-1. The polypeptide IL-1 has been termed lymphocyte activating factor, because it enhances T-cell responses during antigen presentation, and endogenous pyrogen, because it induces fever. Production of IL-1, primarily by mononuclear phagocytes (Fig. 21.7), is stimulated by endotoxin, other macrophage-derived cytokines such as TNF-α, other microbial products, and antigens. Although they are structurally distinct, IL-1 performs many of the same biological activities as TNF-α (Dinarello 1985). The principal biological function of IL-1 is believed to be mediation of the host response in natural immunity; IL-1 interacts with antigen-stimulated T cells to induce the release of IL-2 by T cells and synthesis of IL-2 receptors. By direct effect on B cells, IL-1 invokes B-cell activation, proliferation, and antibody synthesis. Natural killer cell activity is enhanced by synergism of IL-1 with other cytokines. Arachidonic acid metabolism, secretion of inflammatory proteins, neutrophil chemoattraction, and fibroblast proliferation are stimulated by IL-1. With TNF-α and IL-6, IL-1 participates in the acute-phase response, which is characterized by fever, hepatic production of acute-phase proteins, neutrophilia, procoagulant activity, and hypoferremia. Endothelial cells are stimulated by IL-1 to synthesize prostacyclin, procoagulant activity, PAF, and neutrophil adherence protein. Evidence suggests that IL-1 and TNF-α interact synergistically to induce many of the tissue reactions associated with endotoxemia.

Interleukin-6. The phosphoglycoprotein IL-6 is produced and secreted by macrophages, monocytes, fibroblasts, vascular endothelial cells, T lymphocytes, and mast cells (Kishimoto 1989). Cells are stimulated to produce IL-6 by various inflammatory stimuli, including IL-1 and, to a lesser extent, endotoxin, TNF-α, platelet-derived growth factor, and viral infection. The primary inflammatory action of IL-6 is the induction of hepatic production of acute-phase proteins (Fig. 21.7), such as fibrinogen, C-reactive protein, serum amyloid A, haptoglobin, ferroxidase, α-1-antitrypsin, and complement. Growth and differentiation of B cells are enhanced by IL-6, and IL-6 serves as a costimulator of T cells. High concentrations of IL-6 have been measured in serum and body fluids in human beings after the administration of endotoxin, TNF-α, and IL-1, and during acute bacterial infection and sepsis. Whereas the effects of TNF-α and IL-1 may be detrimental, IL-6 appears to be beneficial. Acute-phase reactants protect the host nonspecifically against microorganisms, and IL-6 does not cause tissue injury and vascular thrombosis characteristic of endotoxin and TNF-α.

The wide spectrum of biological actions of TNF-α and IL-1 are illustrated in Fig. 21.7. Despite the wealth of physiologic activities ascribed to cytokines, the clinical significance of their pharmacologic manipulation remains unclear (Green and Adams 1992).

REFERENCES

Baird, N. R., Morrison, A. R. 1993. Amplification of the arachidonic acid cascade: Implications for pharmacologic intervention. Am J Kidney Dis 21:557-64.

Bell, T. G., Smith, W. L., Oxender, W. D., Maciejko, J. J. 1980. Biologic interaction of prostaglandins, thromboxane, and prostacyclin: potential nonreproductive veterinary clinical applications. J Am Vet Med Assoc 176(10 Spec No):1195-200.

Bergström, S., Samuelsson, B. 1968. The prostaglandins. Endeavour 27(102):109-13.

Beutler, B., Cerami, A. 1989. The biology of cachectin/tumor necrosis factor-α primary mediator of the host response. Ann Rev Immunol 7:625-55.

Bottoms, G. D., Adams, H. R. 1992. Involvement of prostaglandins and leukotrienes in the pathogenesis of endotoxemia and sepsis. J Am Vet Med Assoc 200:1842-48.

Campbell, W. B. 1990. Lipid-derived autacoids: eicosanoids and platelet-activating factor. In A. G. Gilman, T. W. Rall, A. S. Nies, P. Taylor, eds., Pharmacological Basis of Therapeutics, 8th ed., pp. 600-617. New York: Pergamon Press.

Camu, F., VanLersberghe, C., Lauwers, M. H. 1992. Cardiovascular risks and benefits of perioperative nonsteroidal anti-inflammatory drug treatment. Drugs 44 (Suppl 5):42-51.

de Brum-Fernandes, A. J. 1997. New perspectives for nonsteroidal antiinflammatory therapy. J Rheumatol 24:246-48.

Dinarello, C. A. 1985. An update on human IL-1: From molecular biology to clinical relevance. J Clin Immunol 5:287-97.

Donnelly, M. T., Hawkey, C. J. 1997. Review article: COX-II inhibitors—a new generation of safer NSAIDs? Aliment Pharmacol Ther 11:227-36.

Gorman, R. R. 1979. Modulation of human platelet function by prostacyclin and thromboxane A_2. Fed Proc 38(1):83-88.

Green, E. M., Adams, H. R. 1992. New perspectives in circulatory shock: pathophysiologic mediators of the mammalian response to endotoxemia and sepsis. J Am Vet Med Assoc 200:1834-41.

Grunfield, C., Palladino, M. A. 1990. Tumor necrosis factor immunologic, antitumor, metabolic, and cardiovascular activities. Adv Intern Med 35:45-72.

Kindahl, H. 1980. Prostaglandin biosynthesis and metabolism. J Am Vet Med Assoc 176(10 Spec No):1173-77.

Kishimoto, T. 1989. The biology of interleukin-6. Blood 74:1-10.

Kurzrok, R., Lieb, C. C. 1930. Proc Soc Exp Biol Med 28:268.

Masferrer, J. L., Kulkarni, P. S. 1997. Cyclooxygenase-2 inhibitors: a new approach to the therapy of ocular inflammation. Surv Ophthalmol 41:S35-S40.

McGiff, J. C. 1979. Prostaglandins in circulatory disorders. Triangle 18(4):101-7.

McGiff, J. C., Wong, P. Y. 1979. Compartmentalization of prostaglandins and prostacyclin within the kidney: Implications for renal function. Fed Proc 38(1):89-93.

Mitchell, M. D., Trautman, M. S. 1993. Molecular mechanisms regulating prostaglandin action. Mol Cell Endocrinol 93:C7-C10.

Moncada, S., Vane, J. R. 1978. Pharmacology and endogenous roles of prostaglandin endoperoxides, thromboxane A_2, and prostacyclin. Pharm Rev 30(3):293-331.

Moore, J. N., Hardee, M. M., Hardee, G. E. 1986. Modulation of arachidonic acid metabolism in endotoxic horses: Comparison of flunixin meglumine, phenylbutazone, and a selective thromboxane synthetase inhibitor. Am J Vet Res 47(1):110-13.

Morris, D. D., Crowe, N., Moore, J. N. 1990. Correlation of clinical and laboratory data with serum tumor necrosis factor activity in horses with experimentally induced endotoxemia. Am J Vet Res 51:1935-40.

Oates, J. A., Whorton, A. R., Gerkens, J. F., Branch, R. A., Hollifield, J. W., Frolich, J. C. 1979. The participation of prostaglandins in the control of renin release. Fed Proc 38(1):72-74.

Old, L. J. 1988. Tumor necrosis factor. Sci Am 258:59-75.

Piper, P. J. 1983. Pharmacology of leukotrienes. Br Med Bull 39(3):255-59.

Piper, P. J., Vane, J. R. 1969. Release of additional factors in anaphylaxis and its antagonism by anti-inflammatory drugs. Nature 223(201):29-35.

Rosonblum, M. G., Donato, N. J. 1989. Tumor necrosis factor-alpha: A multifaceted peptide hormone. Crit Rev Immunol 1:21-44.

Samuelsson, B. 1983. Leukotrienes: Mediators of immediate hypersensitivity reactions and inflammation. Science 220(4597):568-75.

Samuelsson, B., Hammarstrom, S., Murphy, R. C., Borgeat, P. 1980. Leukotrienes and slow reacting substance of anaphylaxis (SRS-A). Allergy 35(5):375-81.

Schultz, R. H. 1980. Experiences and problems associated with usage of prostaglandins in countries other than the United States. J Am Vet Med Assoc 176(10 Spec No):1182-86.

Seguin, B. E. 1980. Role of prostaglandins in bovine reproduction. J Am Vet Med Assoc 176 (10 Spec No):1178-81.

Shimamoto, Y., Chen, R. L., Bollon, A., et al. 1988. Monoclonal antibodies against human recombinant tumor necrosis factor: Prevention of endotoxic shock. Immunol Lett 17:311-18.

Sivakoff, M., Pure, E., Hsueh, W., Needleman, P. 1979. Prostaglandins and the heart. Fed Proc 38(1):78-82.

Smith, W. L. 1992. Prostanoid biosynthesis and mechanisms of action. Am J Physiol 263:F181-F191.

Stabenfeldt, G. H., Hughes, J. P., Neely, D. P., Kindahl, H., Edqvist, L. E., Gustafsson, B. 1980. Physiologic and pathophysiologic aspects of prostaglandin F2 alpha during the reproductive cycle. J Am Vet Med Assoc 176(10 Spec No):1187-94.

Szczeklik, A., Nizankowski, R., Skawinski, S., Szczeklik, J., Gluszko, P., Gryglewski, R. J. 1979. Successful therapy of advanced arteriosclerosis obliterans with prostacyclin. Lancet 1(8126):1111-14.

Terragno, N. A., Terragno, A. 1979. Prostaglandin metabolism in the fetal and maternal vasculature. Fed Proc 38(1):75-77.

Tracey, K. J., Beutler, B., Lowry, S. F., et al. 1986. Shock and tissue injury induced by recombinant human cachectin. Science 234:470-74.

Tracey, K. J., Cerami, A., Morris, D. D., Crowe, N., Moore, J. N. 1989. Cachectin/tumor necrosis factor and other cytokines in infectious disease. Curr Opin Immunol 1:454-64.

Tracey, K. J., Fong, Y., Hesse, D. G., et al. 1987a. Anti-cachectin/TNF monoclonal antibodies prevent septic shock during lethal bacteremia. Nature 330:662-64.

Tracey, K. J., Lowry, S. F., Fahey, T. F., et al. 1987b. Cachectin/tumor factor necrosis factor induces shock and stress hormone responses in the dog. Surg Gynecol Obstet 164:415-22.

Vane, J. R. 1971. Inhibition of prostaglandin synthesis as a mechanism of action for aspirin-like drugs. Nature 231(25):232-35.

Wolfe, L. S. 1982. Eicosanoids: Prostaglandins, thromboxanes, leukotrienes, and other derivatives of carbon-20 unsaturated fatty acids. J Neurochem 38(1):1-14.

22 THE ANALGESIC, ANTIPYRETIC, ANTI-INFLAMMATORY DRUGS

DAWN M. BOOTHE

The Pathophysiology of Inflammation
The Role of Chemical Mediators in the Inflammatory Response
Nonsteroidal Anti-inflammatory Drugs
Chemistry
Mechanism of Action
Pharmacokinetics
Pharmacologic Effects
Drug Interactions
Adverse Reactions
Aspirin
Phenylbutazone
Flunixin Meglumine
Carprofen
Naproxen
Ibuprofen
Meclofenamic Acid
Ketoprofen
Piroxicam
Indomethacin
Acetominophen
Treatment of Osteoarthritis
Orgotein
Polysulfated Glycosaminoglycan
Hyaluronic Acid
Dimethylsulfoxide

THE PATHOPHYSIOLOGY OF INFLAMMATION. Inflammation can occur in any vascularized tissue in the body. The sequelae of inflammation are manifested as five cardinal signs: redness, heat, swelling or edema, pain, and loss of function. Vasoconstriction of small vessels in the area of injury is the initial vascular response to damage. Vascular occlusion serves to control hemorrhage. However, within 5-10 minutes, vasodilation and increased vascular permeability of small venules occur. Leukocytes, platelets, and erythrocytes in the injured vessels become "sticky" and adhere to the endothelium. Leakage of cells and of plasma-derived protein-rich fluid is followed by platelet aggregation and fibrin formation. Initially, the predominant cell type infiltrating damaged tissues is the polymorphonuclear leukocyte (PMN)—in part, because it predominates in circulation. As the short-lived PMNs die, macrophages become the predominant cell type. The migration to and concentration of PMNs at the site of injury are facilitated by chemical mediators that act as chemotactic agents. As PMNs die, the contents of the lysed cells accumulate to form the component of inflammatory exudate commonly referred to as pus.

The Role of Chemical Mediators in the Inflammatory Response. The mediators released during the inflammatory process perpetuate the inflammatory response and are responsible for the clinical signs associated with inflammation, including pain and fever (Vane and Botting 1987). Mediators of inflammation (Table 22.1) are derived from both the cells and the fluid which reach the site of tissue damage from blood. Although there are quantitative differences between species, and tissue concentrations of the mediators vary, the effect of each mediator and its role in the pathophysiology of inflammation are predominantly the same in all species. Leukocytes are a rich source of a variety of chemical mediators of inflammation (Fig. 22.1). These cells, as well as cells of other tissues that are injured and dying following either the initial damage or subsequent inflammation, perpetuate the inflammatory response. Mediators include lysosomal and other enzymes, granular mediators such as histamine and serotonin, eicosanoids (products of arachidonic acid metabolism: prostaglandins, leukotrienes, and related compounds), platelet-activating factor, oxygen radicals, and cytokines. The role of each of these mediators in the perpetuation of the inflammatory response varies, in part, according to the phase of inflammation during which the mediator is released.

Plasma-derived mediators are also important contributors to the inflammatory process. Examples include kinins (e.g., bradykinin), released from their precursor form following appropriate physiologic or pathologic stimulation; complement and complement-derived peptides, released following activation of either the classic or an alternative pathway; and fibrinopeptides, released during the conversion of fibrinogen to fibrin during the clotting process and subsequent proteolysis of fibrin by plasmin.

Pharmacological control of inflammation is oriented toward preventing the release of various chemical or plasma mediators, inhibiting their actions, and/or treating pathophysiological responses to them. Drugs useful for modulating the activity of chemical

TABLE 22.1—Mediators important in the course of inflammation

Mediator	Source	Action	Pharmacologic modulator
Lysosomal contents	Phagocytes	Vessel permeability Membrane degradation Chemotactic factors Collagen, fibrin, cartilage, etc., degradation	Glucocorticoids Dimethylsulfoxide Organic gold compounds
Histamine	Granulocytes	Vasodilation Capillary permeability Pain	Antihistamines (particularly H_1 and possibly H_2 blockers)
Serotonin	Platelets	Vasodilation/constriction Capillary permeability Pain	
Eicosanoids Prostaglandins Leukotrienes Lipoxygenases	All cells	Chemotaxis Vascular permeability Vasodilation Pain	Glucocorticoids Nonsteroidal anti-inflammatory drugs
Platelet-activating factor	Platelets	Platelet aggregation Chemotaxis Oxygen radical production	Glucocorticoids
Oxygen radicals	Damaged tissues Leukocytes	Destruction of a number of cellular constituents, particularly lipid membranes	Superoxide dismutase Vitamine E Ascorbic acid Dimethylsulfoxide Xanthine oxidase inhibitors
Kinins	Plasma	Vasodilation Capillary permeability Pain	Nonsteroidal anti-inflammatory drugs
Complement	Plasma	Lysis of cells Histamine release Vascular permeability Release of lysosomal contents Chemotaxis	Glucocorticoids Dimethylsulfoxide Antihistamine
Fibrinopeptides	Plasma	Enhancement of kinins Vascular permeability Chemotaxis	Nonsteroidal anti-inflammatory drugs

mediators derived from cells and plasma are summarized in Table 22.2.

NONSTEROIDAL ANTI-INFLAMMATORY DRUGS

Chemistry. Although nonsteroidal anti-inflammatory drugs (NSAIDs) have been variably defined, the term is used here to describe compounds that are not steroidal and that suppress inflammation. Generally, the classification is restricted to those drugs that inhibit one or more steps in the metabolism of arachidonic acid (AA) (Boynton et al. 1988). The NSAIDs vary in their ability to influence inflammation. The mechanism of action of some of these drugs is not limited to inhibition of AA metabolism (Hochberg 1989).

Aspirin, one of the earliest components of herbal therapy, is the progenitor NSAID, and terms such as "aspirin-like" and "aspirin and related drugs" are commonly used to refer to this group of drugs (Boynton et al. 1988). Structurally, NSAIDs can be broadly classified into salicylate or carboxylic acid derivatives, including the indoles (indomethacin), propionic acids (ibuprofen and naproxen), fenamates (meclofenamic acid), oxicams (piroxicam), or the pyrazolones or enolic acids (phenylbutazone and dipyrone) (Boynton et al. 1988).

Mechanism of Action. Eicosanoids, such as prostaglandins and leukotrienes, are 20-carbon-chain derivatives of cell membranes. These compounds are synthesized when oxygen reacts with the polyunsaturated fatty acids of cell membrane phospholipids (Fig. 22.1). The most important of these fatty acids is AA, which is released into the cell from damaged cell membranes. Once inside the cell, AA serves as a substrate for enzymes which generate intermediate and end (eicosanoid) products (Fig. 22.1) (Weissmann 1991; D. R. Robinson 1989). Cyclooxygenases (prostaglandin synthase or prostaglandin H synthase), located in all cells except mature red blood cells, add oxygen to AA, generating unstable prostaglandin endoperoxides (PGG_2). Subsequent peroxidase reactions convert PGG_2 to PGH_2, the precursor of all other prostaglandins and thromboxane. The final prostaglandin product depends on the presence of specific isomerase enzymes (D. R. Robinson 1989). While all tissues have the capacity to produce cyclooxygenase end products, the concentration varies with the type

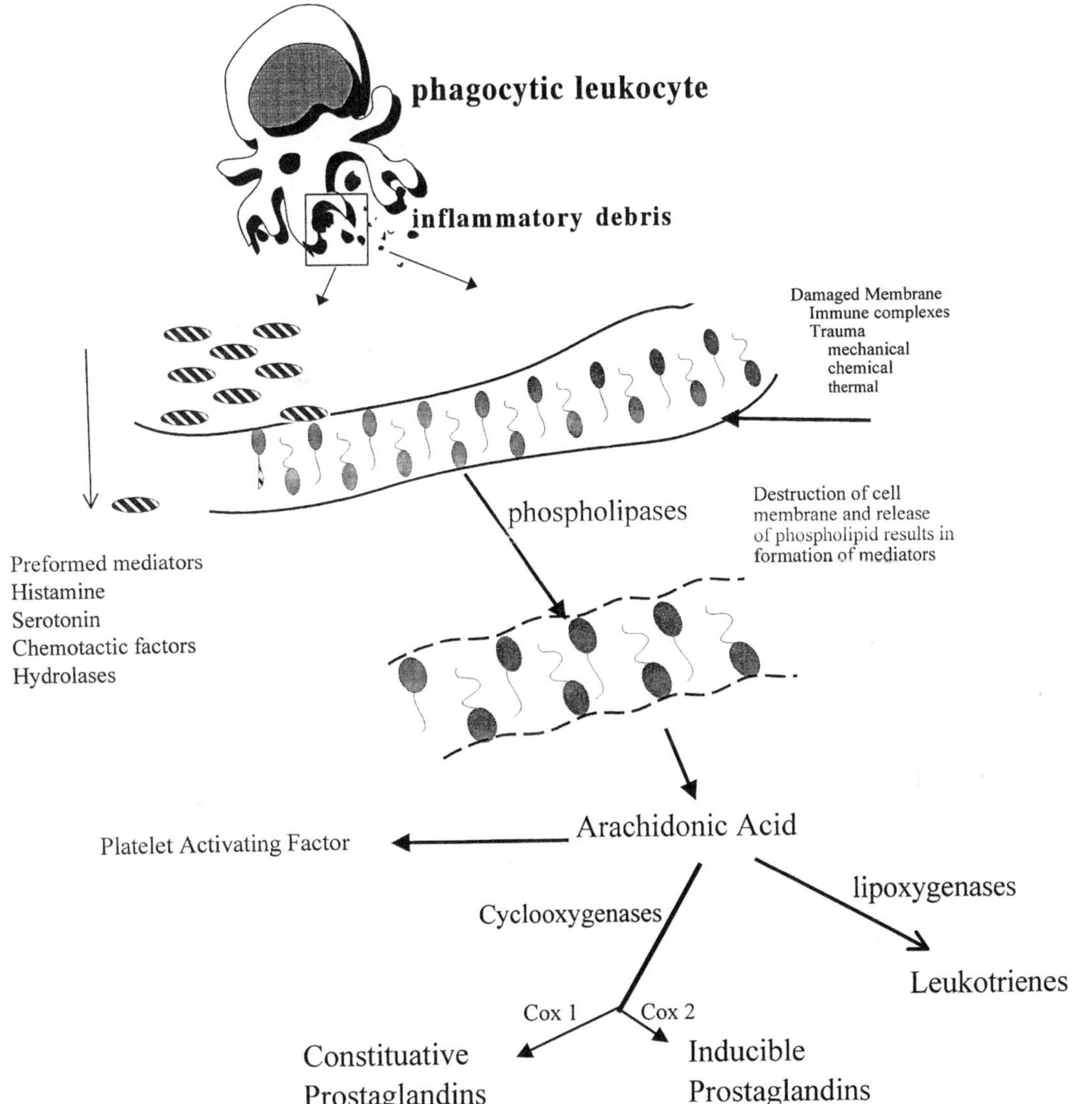

FIG. 22.1—Leukocytes are an important source of inflammatory mediators that perpetuate the inflammatory response. Cellular mediators of inflammation include those preformed in granules or lysosomes and those formed in situ from arachidonic acid released by phospholipases in the cell membrane. Although the phagocytic cell is intimately involved in the inflammatory reaction, it is not the only cell type capable of generating mediators of inflammation. The mediators of cellular origin interact with plasma-derived mediators, further compounding the response. Drugs used to control inflammation target specific mediators (Table 22.1).

and amount of the individual isomerases (D. R. Robinson 1989).

Prostaglandins have important roles in normal physiology that might best be described as protective in nature. Prostaglandin formation is mediated by either one of two isoforms of cyclooxygenase (Fig. 22.1) (Williams 1996; Griswold and Adams 1996; Vane et al. 1998; Pairet and Engelhardt 1996). Cyclooxygenases 1 (COX 1) mediate the formation of constitutive prostaglandins produced by many tissues, including gastrointestinal (GI) cells, platelets, endothelial cells, and renal cells. Prostaglandins generated from COX 1 are constantly present and impart a variety of normal physiologic effects. These include protection of the GI mucosa, hemostasis, and the kidney when subjected to hypotensive insults. Cyclooxygenases 2 (COX 2)

TABLE 22.2—Doses for analgesic, antipyretic, and anti-inflammatory drugs

Aspirin	
Cows	100 mg/kg PO 12 hr
Dogs	10 mg/kg PO 8–24 hr
	10 mg/kg PO 24 hr (endarteritis)
	10 mg/kg 12 hr (antipyresis)
	25-35 mg/kg PO 8 to 12 hr (autoimmune diseases)
	25-35 mg/kg PO 24 hr (preoperative ocular surgery)
	40 mg/kg PO every 18 hr (anti-inflammatory)
	3 mg/kg every 6 days (antithrombotic)
Cats	10 mg/kg PO 48 hr
	75 mg/kg 48 hr (antithrombotic)
Carprofen	
Dogs	2.2 mg/kg PO 12 hr
Dimethylsulfoxide	
Horses	0.25-1.0 g/kg IV 6–24 hr
	90% gel solution topical 8–12 hr
Dipyrone	
Dogs	25 mg/kg IM, SQ 8–12 hr
Cats	10–25 mg/kg IM, SQ 24 hr
Flunixin meglumine	
Cows	2.2 mg/kg, then 1.1 mg/kg 8 hr (limited analgesia, effective PG inhibition)
Dogs	0.5-1.0 mg/kg IV 24 hr; IM × 1-3 hr (analgesic)
	0.25 mg/kg IV 24 hr × 5 days (uveitis)
Ketoprofen	
Horses	2.2 mg/kg IV 24 hr
Dogs	1.1 mg/kg [D] IV, PO 24 hr
	0.5 mg/kg [C] PO 24 hr
Naproxen	
Horses	10 mg/kg PO 12 hr
Dogs	1–2 mg/kg PO 24-48 hr
Phenylbutazone	
Cows	10-20 mg/kg PO, then 2.5-5.0 mg/kg 24 hr
Bulls	24 mg/kg, then 6 mg/kg 48 hr
Horses	4 g/450 kg PO 24 hr
	2 g/horse maximum IV
	15 mg/kg IV, then 10 mg/kg at 6 and 12 hr
	8.8 mg/kg maximum
Dogs	10 mg/kg PO 8-12 hr
	10-15 mg/kg IV 12 hr (not to exceed 4 doses)
	22 mg/kg PO 8 hr (not to exceed 800 mg)
Piroxicam	
Dogs	0.3 mg/kg 48 hr
Meclofenamic acid	
Cows	2 mg/kg IV
	10 mg/kg intraruminal (oral) or 20 mg/kg IM
Acetaminophen	10-15 mg/kg PO 6-8 hr
Hyaluronic acid	
Horses	20-40 mg intra-articular (remove equal volume of synovial fluid)

Note: IV = intravenous; IM = intramuscular; PO = per os.

catalyze the formation of inducible prostaglandins, which are needed only intermittently (Williams 1996; Griswold and Adams 1996; Vane et al. 1998; Pairet and Engelhardt 1996; Cashman 1996; Donnelly and Hawkey 1997). Prostaglandins that mediate inflammation are an example. Inflammation is mediated or perpetuated by inducing vasodilation, changes in capillary permeability, and chemotaxis, all of which can be caused by inflammatory prostaglandins. They also potentiate the effects of other chemical mediators of inflammation such as histamine and bradykinin and are capable of inducing a state of hyperalgesia. Although specific points remain controversial, the role of prostaglandins in the inflammatory process have been described (D. R. Robinson 1989). Prostaglandins (PGE) also modify both T- and B-cell function, in part by inhibition of interleukin-2 secretion (D. R. Robinson 1989).

Eicosanoids are potent mediators of inflammation and are particularly important in the later stages (D. R. Robinson 1989). NSAIDs block the first step of prostaglandin synthesis by binding to and inhibiting cyclooxygenase (D. R. Robinson 1989). This action is both dose and drug dependent. The precise site at which cyclooxygenase is inhibited is not known. The planar form that characterizes these drugs is thought to facilitate their binding to cyclooxygenase (Boynton et al. 1988; Higgins 1985). Several investigators have shown that some NSAIDs (e.g., phenylbutazone and flunixin meglumine) also reduce formation of prostaglandin E_2 in inflammatory exudate at therapeutic doses (Lees et al. 1986). The major therapeutic and toxic effects of NSAIDs have been correlated extensively to their ability to inhibit prostaglandin synthesis (D. R. Robinson 1989). Their potency as anti-inflammatory agents relates to their relative potency of inhibition of prostaglandin synthesis (D. R. Robinson 1989).

The differential effect of NSAIDs on the isoforms of cyclooxygenase offers some insight as to the differential pharmacologic and toxic effect of this class of drugs. As a class, NSAIDs appear to inhibit both COX 1 and COX 2. The amount of drug necessary to inhibit each of the two isoforms provides a basis for assessing the relative safety and efficacy of each drug. The ratio of COX 2 to COX 1 describes the amount of drug necessary to inhibit the respective isoforms of the cyclooxygenase enzyme. A drug that inhibits COX 2 at a lower concentration than that necessary to inhibit COX 1 is probably safer since COX 2 prostaglandins (inducible) are inhibited at lower drug concentrations than COX 1 (constitutive) prostaglandins. A COX 2/COX 1 ratio of less than 1 (which indicates that COX 2 is inhibited by less drug than COX 1) is desirable (Griswold and Adams 1996; Williams and DuBois 1996; Cashman 1996; Donnelly and Hawkey 1997). Carprofen, etodolac, and meloxicam appear to be NSAIDs with a favorable COX 2/COX 1 ratio because they preferentially inhibit COX 2.

Lipoxygenase enzymes located within cells can also metabolize AA to inflammatory mediators (Hochberg 1989; Newcombe 1988). Among these enzymes, 5-lipoxygenase appears to be the most important (D. R. Robinson 1989). This enzyme adds oxygen to AA to form 5-hydroperoxyeicosatetraenoic acid (HPETE). Leukotriene (LT) C_4, LTD_4, and LTE_4 result from addition of glutathione to LTA_4 by glutathione-*S*-transferase. These are potent mediators of inflammation. In addition, LTA_4 can also be converted to LTB_4, a potent chemotactic agent (D. R. Robinson 1989). Leukotrienes and other selected lipoxygenase products modulate lymphocyte function (D. R. Robinson 1989). Lipoxygenases are not as ubiquitous as prostaglandins and are found predominantly in the lungs, white blood cells, platelets, and liver. Although lipoxygenases are formed primarily by leukocytes, the end products of lipoxygenase activity, leukotrienes and lipoxins, are also potent mediators of local inflammation (Hochberg 1989). Originally, studies indicated that NSAIDs were not capable of inhibiting leukotriene synthesis. A potential consequence of cyclooxygenase blockade by NSAIDs is increased production of leukotrienes from AA, which would otherwise have been metabolized to prostaglandin products (D. R. Robinson 1989). Aspirin hypersensitivity is associated with the diversion of AA from the prostaglandin to the leukotriene (5-lipoxygenase) pathway and the production of mediators that are more inflammatory than the products of prostaglandin H synthase (Weissmann 1991). Thus, NSAIDs may cause undesirable effects by augmenting leukotriene synthesis (D. R. Robinson 1989). More recently, the anti-inflammatory efficacy of some of these drugs has been ascribed to inhibition of lipoxygenases and thus prevention of leukotriene formation (Boynton et al. 1988), but their ability to inhibit 5-lipoxygenase is controversial (D. R. Robinson 1989).

Inhibition of cyclooxygenase as the sole anti-inflammatory mechanism of action of NSAIDs has recently been scrutinized and criticized. These drugs also appear to alter cellular and humoral immune responses and may suppress inflammatory mediators other than prostaglandins (Hochberg 1989). Connective tissue metabolism may also be affected (Hochberg 1989). As a group, all NSAIDs are planar and anionic and are able to partition into lipid environments, including neutrophil cell membranes. As a result, cell membrane viscosity is altered, even at low concentrations (Weissmann 1991). At higher concentrations, NSAIDs appear to uncouple protein-protein interactions within the plasma membrane and thus interfere with a variety of cell membrane processes such as oxidative phosphorylation and cellular adhesion (Weissmann 1991). The drugs appear to disrupt the response of inflammatory cells to extracellular signals by affecting signal-transduction proteins (G proteins) (Weissmann 1991). Thus, at low doses, prostaglandin H synthase appears to be the target of NSAIDs, whereas membrane-bound signal-processing complexes appear to be the target at higher doses (Weissmann 1991).

Studies using in vitro systems have shown that NSAIDs alter the inflammatory response by inhibiting activation of neutrophils and thus the subsequent release of inflammatory cellular enzymes such as collagenase, elastase, hyaluronidase, and others (Hochberg 1989). NSAIDs interfere with multiple aspects of neutrophil function, including adherence. Some NSAIDs inhibit several neutrophil functions, while others inhibit few. The extent of inhibited neutrophil activation varies with the individual drug. For example, piroxicam inhibits both the generation of superoxide ions and the release of lysosomal enzymes, whereas ibuprofen does neither (Weissmann 1991). All NSAIDs appear to inhibit adhesion. Several NSAIDs, including phenylbutazone, oxyphenylbutazone, and flunixin, inhibit leukocyte cell movement. Of these drugs, flunixin is the most potent inhibitor in vitro at concentrations achieved in equine plasma and inflammatory exudate (Dawson and Sedgwick 1987).

NSAIDs are also capable of immunomodulation. Several prostaglandins and leukotrienes are important immunomodulators (D. R. Robinson 1989). NSAIDs indirectly influence lymphocyte activity through altered prostaglandin formation (Hochberg 1989). Certain NSAIDs appear to enhance cellular immunity by inhibiting prostaglandin E_2, a mediator which dampens the immune response (Hochberg 1989). This effect appears to be more important in the immunosuppressed animal.

NSAIDs have been shown to inhibit proteoglycan synthesis in vitro, and for the salicylates, this is supported by in vivo studies (Brandt 1991). This effect has been attributed to inhibition of uridine diphosphate-glycose dehydrogenase, an enzyme important in proteoglycan synthesis (Brandt 1991). However, hyaluronic acid synthesis, which is also dependent on this enzyme, does not appear to be affected. The effects of NSAIDs on cartilage are controversial. More recent evidence indicates that they may, in fact, favorably modify the metabolism of proteoglycans, collagen, and matrix and may decrease the release of proteases or toxic oxygen metabolites (Brandt 1991).

Pharmacokinetics. The NSAIDs share a number of pharmacokinetic properties. As weak acids, the NSAIDs tend to be well absorbed following oral administration. Bioavailability can vary between animals but has not been established for many NSAIDs because of the lack of intravenous (IV) preparations (Brater 1988). Food can impair the oral absorption of some NSAIDs, or contribute to drug interactions for others (e.g., phenylbutazone in the horse) (Tobin et al. 1986; Munsiff et al. 1988). Solutions of injectable preparations tend to be alkaline and can cause necrosis or pain if perivascular leakage occurs. The drugs are lipid soluble but are characterized by a small volume of distribution (approximately 10%) due to binding to serum albumin, which can exceed 99% in some species. Unbound drug is distributed to extracellular fluid. Only a small portion of pharmacologically active drug reaches peripheral tissues. Displacement from albumin due to competition with other substrates for binding sites or due to decreased serum albumin concentrations initially can result in higher than expected concentrations of pharmacologically active drug and thus predispose the patient to drug-induced adverse effects. This increase, however, is only transient due to increased clearance of unbound drug (Brater 1988).

Clearance of the NSAIDs is variable, differing among drugs and species. Differences in clearance rates are largely responsible for differences in drug half-life among animals (Brater 1988). Most NSAIDs are eliminated primarily by hepatic metabolism. Both phase I and phase II hepatic drug-metabolizing enzymes are important. Conjugated metabolites are predominantly eliminated through the urine, although several drugs undergo extensive enterohepatic circulation in some species (e.g., naproxen and meclofenamic acid in dogs) (Aitken and Sanford 1975). For some drugs, a portion may be eliminated unchanged from the kidneys by active tubular secretion. Age and species differences in drug clearance should lead to caution when extrapolating doses from one animal to another. Although most pharmacokinetic studies measure total, rather than unbound, drug, clearance of unbound drug is substantially less in geriatric patients, whereas clearance of bound drug does not differ. The volume of distribution of unbound drug in adult animals is half that of pediatric patients. Because of these differences in NSAID disposition, geriatric and pediatric patients may require much smaller doses of the NSAIDs (Brater 1988). Species differences in the elimination of the NSAIDs have been well documented and are responsible for some of the adverse reactions commonly associated with the use of these drugs. Recently, stereoselective metabolism has become an additional important consideration when extrapolating doses in human beings (Brater 1988).

Pharmacologic Effects. The pharmacologic effects of this class of drugs include analgesia, antipyresis, and control of inflammation. The mechanisms by which NSAIDs inhibit (interact with) cyclooxygenase are responsible, in part, for the variable anti-inflammatory effect of these drugs. Aspirin binds reversibly to the cyclooxygenase activity site on prostaglandin H synthase and then inactivates the enzyme irreversibly by acetylating a serine residue (Weissmann 1991). The effects of aspirin on platelet activity remain for the life of the platelet because the platelet apparently cannot produce additional thromboxane synthase enzyme. In contrast, endothelial cells are able to synthesize more prostacyclin synthase and are less susceptible to the inhibitory effects of low doses of aspirin (Weissmann 1991). In contrast to irreversible binders of cyclooxygenase, ibuprofen binds reversibly with cyclooxygenase and thus competes with AA. In laboratory animals and humans, relative potency has been established for the NSAIDs: meclofenamic acid > indomethacin > naproxen > phenylbutazone > aspirin (Lee and Higgins 1985). A similar pattern occurs in domestic animals: the relative potency of the NSAIDs in horses has been reported to be flunixin meglumine > meclofenamic acid > phenylbutazone > naproxen > aspirin (Lee and Higgins 1985). However, potency does not necessarily confer therapeutic advantage. Rather, these compounds may be equally effective simply by adjusting the dose appropriately.

Along with inhibition of prostaglandins, disruption of cellular signaling is responsible for all the pharmacologic effects of all NSAIDs. These effects are dose and drug dependent and are antithrombosis, occurring at the lowest doses; analgesia and antipyresis; and control of inflammation, which occurs at the highest doses (Weissmann 1991). Although several NSAIDs are characterized by a short plasma elimination half-life, the clinical response may last for over 24 hours following a single dose or up to 72 hours following multiple doses. Irreversible binding to cyclooxygenase has been postulated as an explanation for the discrepancy between plasma half-life and biological response (Lee and Higgins 1985). Alternatively, prolonged elimination of NSAIDs from inflammatory exudate compared to plasma has also been suggested (Lee and Higgins 1985; Tobin et al. 1986).

Drug Interactions. The NSAIDs can be involved in a variety of drug interactions during any phase of drug disposition. Displacement of only a small percentage of bound drug from albumin can increase the concentration of pharmacologically active drug in tissues. Few, if any, adverse reactions resulting from drug displacement have been reported, in part because the increase in pharmacologically active drug is only transient: clearance of the unbound drug by both the liver and kidneys will increase (Bater 1988). Several NSAIDs can induce or inhibit drug-metabolizing enzymes and thus the clearance and half-life of other drugs cleared by the liver (Bater 1988). Phenylbutazone can both increase and inhibit certain drug-metabolizing enzymes, whereas salicylates increase metabolism (Bater 1988). Renal competition with other organic acids for active renal tubular secretion in the proximal tubule has been documented for aspirin and other drugs.

Adverse Reactions. All NSAIDs induce undesirable and potentially life-threatening side effects. The most commonly consumed NSAIDs in accidental poisoning include ibuprofen, acetaminophen, aspirin, and indomethacin (Jonnes et al. 1992). The most common clinical signs of toxicosis in one study were vomiting, diarrhea, CNS depression, and circulatory manifestations (Jonnes et al. 1992). The majority of adverse reactions reflect the inhibitory effects of NSAIDs on prostaglandin activity. In addition, acute intoxication by several drugs can be fatal. The major toxicities associated with NSAIDs affect the GI, hematopoietic, and renal systems. Miscellaneous side effects associated with use of NSAIDs include hepatotoxicity (Lewis 1984), aseptic meningitis (Clemmons and Meyers 1984; Berliner et al. 1985; Syvlia et al. 1988), diarrhea, and CNS depression (Jonnes et al. 1992).

GASTROINTESTINAL. GI damage is the most common and serious side effect of the NSAIDs. Although not completely understood, several mechanisms have been hypothesized (McCormack and Brune 1987). Gastroduodenal erosion and ulceration reflect inhibition of prostaglandin E_2-mediated bicarbonate and mucus secretion, epithelization, and blood flow (Chastain 1987). Control of gastric acid secretion is consequently decreased as is mucus and bicarbonate secretion, epithelization of the mucosa, and mucosal blood flow. Breakdown of small blood vessels due to a deficiency of mucus may be the initiating lesion (Mazué et al. 1983). Direct irritation by acidic drugs may be important (Chastain 1987). In addition, salicylates cause local damage due to "back-diffusion" of acid, which causes injury to mucosal cells and submucosal capillaries. Impaired platelet activity may contribute to mucosal bleeding. Oral ulceration has been reported in horses receiving oral phenylbutazone (Tobin et al. 1986). There appears to be no chemical characteristic that can be used to predict the likelihood of GI toxicity by a particular NSAID (Chastain 1987; Mazué et al. 1983). Drugs that undergo enterohepatic circulation may be associated with a greater incidence of GI upset. Treatment for GI toxicity should include prostaglandin (PGE) replacement (i.e., misoprostol) and a cytoprotectant such as sucralfate (Collins and Tyler 1985).

HEMATOPOIETIC. All NSAIDs are able to impair platelet activity due to impaired thromboxane synthesis. At pharmacologic doses, aspirin selectively and irreversibly acetylates a serine residue of a platelet cyclooxgenase (Jackson 1987). The platelet form of this enzyme is up to 250 times more sensitive to acetylation by aspirin compared to cyclooxygenases (prostacyclin synthase) in vascular endothelial cells. Although platelets cannot regenerate more cyclooxygenase, endothelial cells apparently are able to rapidly synthesize and replace impaired cyclooxygenase (Jackson 1987). Platelet aggregation defects caused by aspirin can last up to 1 week. In addition to their antiplatelet effects, some NSAIDs (e.g., phenylbutazone) have also been associated with bone marrow dyscrasias (Martin et al. 1984; Carlisle et al. 1968; Watson et al. 1980; Markel 1986).

RENAL. Analgesic nephropathy is a relatively common adverse effect of NSAIDs in human beings (Dunn et al. 1988). However, it does not occur as frequently in domestic animals, in part because the drugs are not used as chronically. In the kidney, vasodilatory prostaglandins are protective, ensuring that medullary vasodilation and urinary output continue during states of renal arterial vasoconstriction. The loss of this protective effect becomes important in patients with compromised renal function (Dunn et al. 1988). Patients who are predisposed to analgesic nephropathy include geriatric patients, patients suffering from cardiac, renal, or liver disease, patients in hypovolemic states such as shock and dehydration, and patients receiving nephrotoxic (i.e., aminoglycosides, amphotericin B, or other antiprostaglandin drugs) or nephroactive (e.g., diuretics) drugs.

Aspirin. Aspirin, the salicylic acid ester of acetic acid, is the prototype of the salicylate drugs, which include sodium salicylate and bismuth subsalicylate. In addition to inhibition of cyclooxygenase enzyme activity, salicylates inhibit the formation and release of kinins, stabilize lysosomes, and remove energy necessary for inflammation by uncoupling oxidative phosphorylation. Aspirin is available in a variety of different preparations, including plain, film coated, buffered, time-release, and enteric coated tablets. Capsules and suppositories are also available (Chastain 1987).

Oral bioavailability of aspirin products may vary due to differences in disintegration, drug formulation, stomach content, and gastric pH (Conlon 1988). Although buffered aspirin is more soluble than plain aspirin, a larger proportion is ionized and less rapidly absorbed. The amount absorbed of both products is the same (Chastain 1987). Aspirin undergoes rapid metabolism to the hydrolyzed active product, salicylic acid. This metabolite is not as potent an analgesic or anti-inflammatory drug because of the loss of the acetyl group, which is able to acetylate key proteins (Chastain 1987). Salicylic acid is between 50 and 70% bound to serum albumin among species (Davis and Westfall 1972). Hypoalbuminemia may result in transient increases in plasma drug concentrations, with associated adverse effects. Distribution of salicylic acid into extracellular fluid is rapid and includes synovial and peritoneal fluid, saliva, and milk. Salicylic acid is eliminated by hepatic conjugation with glucuronide and glycine and by renal excretion by glomerular filtration and tubular secretion (Davis and Westfall 1972; Short et al. 1990). Species differences in the biotransformation and elimination of salicylate are dramatic. Plasma half-lives among species studied range from 1.0 (ponies) to 37.6 (cats) hours (Davis and Westfall 1972). Excretion is more rapid in alkaline urine; therefore, elevation of urine pH can be used therapeutically to treat acute aspirin intoxication.

Aspirin is characterized by a wide safety margin in most species. The recommended therapeutic range in humans is 100-250 μg/mL (Beasley and Buck 1980). Toxicity occurs if serum salicylate concentrations exceed 300 μg/mL; however, analgesia and antipyresis require concentrations of only 20-50 μg/mL (Chastain 1987). Control of inflammation may require concentrations that exceed 50 μg/mL; rheumatoid arthritis in human beings requires concentrations of about 200 μg/mL. Although drug concentrations necessary to achieve an antithrombotic effect have not been established for aspirin in animals, small doses are recommended. Toxic (acute) overdose is usually manifested in depression, vomition, hyperthermia, electrolyte imbalances, convulsions, coma, and death. Acute toxicity includes serious acid-base disturbances due to uncoupling of oxidative phosphorylation. Hyperventilation due to direct stimulation of the respiratory center may be followed by depression at high doses. Bleeding disorders may also be evident (Larson 1963; Chastain 1987). Dose-dependent hepatotoxicity may also occur.

Oral salicylates such as sulfasalazine have been used to treat chronic inflammatory conditions of the bowel.

Although their mechanism of action is unclear, they cause splitting of the diazo bond by colonic bacteria to yield sulfapyridine and 5-aminosalicylic acid (5-ASA). The 5-ASA is considered to be the active moiety (M. G. Robinson 1989). Both the sulfapyridine and the sulfasalazine (up to 25%) are absorbed from the small intestine, but the majority of the 5-ASA remains in the colon. That absorbed (approximately 20% in humans) is rapidly acetylated and inactivated by either the colonic mucosa or liver. Newer products composed principally of 5-ASA are being investigated for the treatment of chronic inflammatory bowel diseases (M. G. Robinson 1989).

RUMINANTS. Although orally bioavailable (70%), salicylate absorption following administration of aspirin is slow in ruminants (absorption half-life of 3 hours) (Gingerich et al. 1975) while elimination is very rapid (elimination half-life of 32 minutes) (Gingerich et al. 1975). The drug is distributed to a volume of 0.24 L/kg. Thus, compared to other species, much larger oral doses (100 mg/kg) of aspirin must be given to achieve and maintain therapeutic concentrations (30 μg/mL) in the cow. Salicylate elimination in goats appears to be similar to that in cows. In both species, salicyluric acid is the sole metabolite detected in urine following oral or IV administration. In cows, a significantly larger portion of administered drug is eliminated as the glycine conjugate rather than as the parent drug. Glucuronide and sulfate conjugates are not detectable in goats or cows (Short et al. 1990). Aspirin has been used to treat acute mastitis in cows (Moore 1986).

HORSES. Aspirin is characterized by a very short half-life (less than 1 hour) in horses, in part because urinary pH is basic (Tobin 1979; Davis and Westfall 1972). Effective doses must be very large and given frequently (Pasargiklian and Bianco 1986). Prolonged bleeding time and decreased platelet stickiness have been reported in horses receiving a single oral dose (20 mg/kg) of aspirin. While it may prove clinically useful as an antithrombotic, aspirin may potentiate epistaxis in some training or exercising horses (Lee and Higgins 1985). Salicylate is a normal constituent of horse urine, thus making it difficult to detect therapeutic use (Tobin 1979).

DOGS. In dogs, aspirin is distributed to a volume ranging from 0.4 to 0.6 L/kg. Bioavailability probably varies with the manufacturer as well as preparation and ranges from 68 to 76% (Morton and Knottenbelt 1989). Bioavailability of plain, buffered, and enteric coated aspirin (25 mg/kg) does not appear to vary markedly, although plasma salicylate concentrations were most variable for the enteric coated preparation (Lipowitz et al. 1986). Following several doses of 25 mg/kg at 12-hour intervals, the biological half-life of aspirin is 7.5 hours in dogs. However, this time increased to a mean of 12.2 hours when the dosing interval was decreased to 8 hours (Konturek 1986). In another study, the elimination half-life of aspirin varied following IV injection of 36-60 mg/kg, ranging from 2.2 to 8.7 hours. The dose necessary to maintain clinical control of various lamenesses in dogs in one study ranged from 23 to 86 mg/kg twice daily, resulting in plasma drug concentrations ranging from 71 to 281 μg/mL (Jezyk 1983). Marked individual variability in drug elimination among animals suggests that therapeutic drug monitoring may be useful to ensure that therapeutic drug concentrations have been achieved and toxic concentrations (>300 μg/mL) are avoided (Morton and Knottenbelt 1989). One study in clinical patients found that plasma salicylate concentrations correlated with response (Morton and Knottenbelt 1989). When 25 mg/kg is administered at 8-hour intervals, therapeutic concentrations can be expected to be maintained throughout the dosing interval. GI side effects of aspirin in dogs appear to be dose and preparation related. Doses of 25 mg/kg of plain aspirin caused mucosal erosions in 50% of dogs which received plain aspirin, while there was minimal damage in animals receiving buffered and enteric coated preparations (Lipowitz et al. 1986).

CATS. As a phenol, aspirin is a compound that cats glucuronidate poorly (Larson 1963; Yeary and Swanson 1973). Plasma elimination half-life of aspirin in cats is 37.6 hours (Davis et al. 1973). The elimination of aspirin may be dose dependent: the half-life is 22-27 hours following doses of 5-12 mg/kg but 45 hours following administration of 25 mg/kg (Hochberg 1989). No clinical signs of toxicosis occurred in one study in which cats were treated with 25 mg/kg every 48 hours (Yeary and Swanson 1973).

Phenylbutazone. Phenylbutazone is a weakly acidic, lipophilic NSAID approved by the FDA for use in horses and dogs. Inhibition of the AA cascade occurs after conversion to reactive intermediate at prostaglandin H synthase and prostacyclin synthase. Prostanoid-dependent swelling, edema, erythema, and associated pain are reduced (Tobin et al. 1986). Phenylbutazone has been associated with some attenuation of some of the clinical signs associated with endotoxic shock in experimental models (Moore et al. 1986; Jarlov et al. 1992).

Bioavailability following intramuscular (IM) administration of phenylbutazone is less than that following oral administration in most species studied because of precipitation in the neutral pH of muscle (Williams 1988; De Backer et al. 1980; Tobin et al. 1986). Phenylbutazone is metabolized by the liver, with less than 2% of the drug being excreted as parent compound in the urine in some species. Its major metabolites are oxyphenylbutazone, which is less active than phenylbutazone, and inactive γ-hydroxyphenylbutazone (Tobin et al. 1986). Reported adverse reactions caused by phenylbutazone include bleeding dyscrasias, hepatopathy, and nephropathy (Tobin et al. 1986; Carlisle et al. 1968; Murray 1985; Tandy and Thorpe 1967).

RUMINANTS. Phenylbutazone is absorbed slowly following oral administration in ruminants (mean absorption half-life hours) and is only approximately 66% bioavailable, although this varies among animals (range, 41.9-95.5%). Peak plasma drug concentration following oral administration is 36 ± 1.9 μg/mL (De Backer et al. 1980). Bioavailability of phenylbutazone following IM administration in cows is 89% (Williams 1988; Eberhardson et al. 1979). Phenylbutazone is cleared more slowly in ruminants (1.24 ± 0.14 mL/kg/hr) than in horses and carnivores. Following a single IV administration of 5 mg/kg, phenylbutazone elimination half-life ranges from 30 to 82 hours (mean 55 ± 6) (De Backer et al. 1980). The apparent volume of distribution (total drug measured) is 0.09 L/kg. Phenylbutazone is 93% bound to plasma proteins in the cow, with unbound drug distributing to extracellular fluid (Williams 1988; Eberhardson et al. 1979). Following repeated administration, drug concentrations in milk are less than 1% of plasma drug concentrations, although total drug concentration increases with increased plasma drug concentration (Martin et al. 1984). Tissue binding of phenylbutazone is minimal.

Dosing once daily or every other day has been recommended in cows in order to achieve and maintain plasma drug concentrations within the therapeutic range recommended in human beings (60-90 μg/mL). Administration of a single loading dose can be used to achieve steady-state drug concentrations rapidly (De Backer et al. 1980). If an appropriate dosing regimen is used, peak plasma drug concentrations of 70 μg/mL can be expected (Williams 1988). In contrast to horses and dogs, elimination of phenylbutazone is not dose dependent in cows. In fact, steady-state plasma drug concentrations following repetitive doses (9 days) may be lower than predicted (Martin et al. 1984). Increased elimination probably reflects an increase in the fraction of unbound drug, with subsequent distribution into tissues (increased volume of distribution). The induction of hepatic drug-metabolizing enzymes is also likely to be responsible for the decrease (Martin et al. 1984). Phenylbutazone has been associated with decreased peripheral leukocyte count and serum bilirubin in cows (Martin et al. 1984). Phenylbutazone is recommended in cows for long-term analgesia and to control inflammation associated with arthritis, spondylitis, and laminitis (Williams 1988).

HORSES. Phenylbutazone is approved for use in horses as an oral tablet, paste, or gel or as an IV preparation. As in other species, bioavailability of phenylbutazone in horses is less following IM, compared to oral, administration. Bioavailability varies with drug preparation and product and feeding schedule (Tobin et al. 1986; Maitho et al. 1986). Among oral preparations, paste preparations are more bioavailable than powder (Tobin et al. 1986). Food reduces both peak plasma drug concentration and time to reach peak concentration (Tobin et al. 1986; Munsiff et al. 1988). Adsorption of the drug on hay in the GI tract contributes to decreased bioavailability and delayed absorption. In Welsh ponies, mean time to peak plasma drug concentration was 13 hours in animals fed before and after dosing compared to 1.3-5.8 hours in fasted animals (Maitho et al. 1986). Drug adsorbed to hay is subsequently released by fermentative processes in the colon and cecum and can cause a second peak in plasma drug concentration (Maitho et al. 1986). Ulceration of the cecum and colon may occur.

In horses, 96-99% of phenylbutazone in plasma is bound to plasma proteins (Tobin et al. 1986). Unbound drug is distributed to a volume of 0.25 L/kg. After IV administration, elimination half-life ranges from 3 to 10 hours and appears to be dose dependent, although apparently not within therapeutic concentrations (Tobin et al. 1986). Mean residence time is 1.7 hours (Mealey et al. 1997). Phenylbutazone is eliminated by hepatic metabolism, with less than 2% of the drug being excreted in the urine as the parent compound (Tobin et al. 1986). Clearance of phenylbutazone may be influenced by age, being twice as fast in 3-year-old ponies as in 8- to 10-year-old ponies (Tobin et al. 1986; Traub et al. 1983).

Although increasing urinary pH up to 8.5 increases the concentration of parent compound and selected metabolites (most notably oxyphenylbutazone) in the urine, plasma drug concentration and elimination half-life are not affected (Tobin et al. 1986). Approximately 77 elimination half-lives, or up to 26 days, must elapse in horses before 99% of a dose of phenylbutazone is eliminated. Although plasma concentrations apparently are not affected by urinary pH (little of the parent drug is eliminated in urine), the detection of the drug in urine can be enhanced by increasing urinary pH. As urinary pH increases, the amount of phenylbutazone and its metabolites in urine also increases. Depending on the sensitivity of the assay used for detection, the drug can still be detected in urine 24-96 hours following a dose. Detection time can be prolonged as much as threefold by altering urine pH (Tobin et al. 1986).

Phenylbutazone is characterized by a narrow therapeutic index in horses. The recommended therapeutic concentration of phenylbutazone in horses is 5-20 μg/mL, which is much lower than the concentration recommended in humans (50-150 μg/mL). This may reflect lower plasma protein binding and thus a greater proportion of active drug in horses (Lee and Higgins 1985). Alternatively, the drug may persist longer in exudative tissue than in plasma, which may explain prolonged efficacy despite subtherapeutic plasma drug concentrations (Tobin et al. 1986).

Drug accumulation predisposes animals with longer drug half-life to drug-induced toxicity. In general, toxicity seems most likely when manufacturer's recommended doses are exceeded. Although oral administration may increase the likelihood of GI toxicity, lesions also occur following IV administration (Tobin et al. 1986). In one study, horses receiving 8-14 mg/kg for 7-14 days showed evidence of toxicity, with 3 of 8 horses dying (Tobin et al. 1986). In a more recent study, phenylbutazone was compared with two other NSAIDs (flunixin meglumine and ketoprofen) and was cited as the most potentially toxic, causing GI ulceration in horses treated with 4.4 mg/kg phenylbutazone IV every 8 hours for 12 days (MacAllister et al. 1993). Ponies may be more susceptible to toxicity than horses (Tobin et al. 1986). Lesions predominate in the GI tract and range from shallow erosions to massive ulcerations of the cecum and colon. Renal papillary necrosis has also been reported. Initial signs of GI toxicity include inappetence, depression, and weight loss. With progression, classic signs of hypovolemic shock occur. Toxicity can occur weeks after drug administration has discontinued. Decreased serum total protein secondary to protein-losing enteropathy appears to be the most sensitive indicator of toxicity (Tobin et al. 1986). Some clinical evidence of renal disease may also occur (Tobin et al. 1986). One study also documented neutropenia, bone marrow suppression, and a toxic left shift in horses receiving large doses of phenylbutazone (Murray 1985). Necrotizing phlebitis occurs in portal veins following oral administration and in jugular veins following IV administration. Finally, one study provided evidence that phenylbutazone can produce a dose-dependent hepatotoxicity in horses (Tobin et al. 1986). Despite its relatively low safety margin, phenylbutazone remains the most widely used drug for the treatment of osteoarthritic and osteoporotic conditions. Large IV doses are necessary for treatment of equine colic (Lee and Higgins 1985).

DONKEYS. Phenylbutazone has been studied in donkeys (Mealey et al. 1997). Clearance in donkeys was greater (up to fivefold) than in horses, and the appearance of the metabolite oxyphenbutazone in serum was more rapid in donkeys than in horses, indicating that hepatic metabolism of phenylbutazone is more rapid in donkeys than in horses. Dosing intervals subsequently may need to be shorter in donkeys than in horses.

CATS. Although phenylbutazone has been used in cats, a high incidence of toxicity suggests extreme caution. In one study, 100% of cats treated with 44 mg/kg daily became anorectic at 2-3 days, with 80% mortality at 2-3 weeks. Toxicity occurs primarily in the bone marrow and is characterized by decreased erythroblastic activity and possible interference with myeloid maturation. GI toxicity, nephrotoxicity, and hepatotoxicity also occur (Carlisle et al. 1968).

DOGS. Despite FDA approval of the oral preparation for use in dogs, there is little information regarding the use of phenylbutazone. Dogs apparently are more tolerant of phenylbutazone than humans are. Toxicity manifested as hemorrhage, biliary stasis, and renal failure has been reported in one dog receiving close to recommended doses (Tandy and Thorpe 1967). For reasons not explained, the package insert notes a total maximum dose and requires the drug to be discontinued slowly.

Flunixin Meglumine. Flunixin meglumine is a nicotinic acid derivative approved for use in the horse. Described as a potent analgesic agent, it has been used to control pain that might otherwise respond only to opioids. It is particularly useful for visceral pain. In addition to its analgesic effects, flunixin meglumine has been studied and cited for its antiendotoxic effects in experimental models of septic shock in several species (Hardie et al. 1983; Moore et al. 1986; Templeton et al. 1987; Jarlov et al. 1992; Davidson et al. 1992).

RUMINANTS. Flunixin meglumine elimination half-life in cows is 8.12 hours, which is significantly longer than that reported in either horses (1.6-2.5 hours) (Semrad et al. 1985; Lee and Higgins 1985) or dogs (3.67 hours). Flunixin has been used to treat acute mastitis. However, a study comparing phenylbutazone and flunixin meglumine for treatment of acute mastitis found no differences among treatment groups (Dascanio et al. 1995). Flunixin megulmine acts as an antipyretic in cows given intramammary endotoxin (Anderson et al. 1986a,b; Jarlov et al. 1992). Although it is not approved for use in cows, flunixin has been recommended for treatment of acute bovine pulmonary emphysema in lieu of corticosteroids, which often cause abortion.

HORSES. Flunixin meglumine is FDA approved for use in horses following IV or oral paste or granule administration. Oral and IM absorption of flunixin meglumine is rapid in horses, with peak plasma drug concentrations occurring within 30 minutes. Onset of action occurs within 2 hours, with peak effect between 2 and 16 hours. Oral bioavailability is approximately 80% (Semrad et al. 1985; Lee and Higgins 1985). Elimination does not appear to be dose dependent in horses. Following IV administration of 0.25-1.1 mg/kg, the drug is distributed to a volume of 0.2-0.3 L/kg and is cleared at a rate of 0.76-0.98 mL/min/kg. Drug concentrations at the recommended dose peak at 1.6 μg/mL. Reported elimination half-life is short, ranging from 1.6 to 2.5 hours (Semrad et al. 1985; Lee and Higgins 1985). Renal excretion appears to contribute significantly to elimination of flunixin in horses (Lee and Higgins 1985).

Toxicity to flunixin meglumine appears to be rare in horses. Oral administration at 3 times the recommended dose for 10 days failed to induce signs of toxicity in one study (Lee and Higgins 1985). However, hypoproteinemia was reported in one Shetland pony. In a more recent study, GI ulceration/erosion occurred in 80% of horses receiving 1.1 mg/kg IV every 8 hours for 12 days (MacAllister et al. 1993). While more potent than phenylbutazone in an experimental model of equine pain, improved efficacy was not demonstrated. However, in another study, flunixin improved lameness in horses by 55% and swelling by 34% compared to 52% and 23%, respectively, for phenylbutazone (Tobin 1979). The wider margin of safety for flunixin compared to phenylbutazone may justify the former as the preferred musculoskeletal anti-inflammatory (Lee and Higgins 1985). The duration of response that characterizes flunixin may be an additional advantage. Onset of efficacy is rapid. Although peak response may take as long as 12 hours after the dose, duration of effect is up to 30 hours (Tobin 1979). Although the mode of action has not been documented, flunixin is specifically recommended as an analgesic in the treatment of colic. It also appears useful for the treatment (and especially pretreatment) of endotoxic shock (Lee and Higgins 1985). It prevents many of the adverse effects caused by administration of endotoxin, thromboxane A_2, and prostaglandin I_2 (Hardie et al. 1985).

DOGS. Following an IV dose of 1.1 mg/kg in healthy dogs, the elimination half-life of flunixin meglumine is 3.67 ± 1.2 hours and its clearance is 0.064 ± 0.01 L/hr/kg. Its volume of distribution is 0.18 ± 0.08 L/kg (Hardie et al. 1985). Flunixin meglumine appears to modulate response to septic shock in dogs (Hardie et al. 1983; Davidson et al. 1992; McKellar et al. 1989). In dogs, a dose of 1.1 mg/kg flunixin meglumine blocks prostaglandin I_2 production, and 2.2 mg/kg improves survival times of septic dogs (Hardie et al. 1985). The pharmacokinetics of flunixin in septic dogs does not appear to differ from that of control dogs (Hardie et al. 1985). Toxicity, most commonly manifested as GI upset, limits use of this drug in dogs to 2-3 days. Doses at 3-5 times that recommended caused GI disturbances in one study. Thomas et al. (1997) have documented that phenylbutazone can be detected in the urine of greyhounds following topical administration in a commercially available cream.

Carprofen. Carprofen is approved for use in dogs in the US and both dogs and cats in selected countries outside the US. The mechanism of action of this NSAID appears to involve specific inhibition of COX 2. The physiologic or protective actions of prostaglandins appear to be minimally inhibited with no loss of anti-inflammatory efficacy. Other proposed mechanisms of carprofen include inhibition of phospholipase and impaired release of AA. Like other NSAIDs, carprofen is highly protein bound. Carprofen is metabolized by the liver and in dogs is characterized by a half-life of 10 hours. Carprofen is equally or more effective than most other NSAIDs studied in the control of inflammation and presumably the pain associated with inflammation of osteoarthritis. Its safety is supported by the lack of GI side effects in dogs dosed with more than 10 times the dose necessary to achieve therapeutic concentrations. A clinical trial of 70 dogs found that 6 of 36 carprofen-treated dogs developed clinical signs indicative of GI upset; 3 placebo dogs also developed GI signs (Vasseur et al. 1995).

Carprofen is approved for use in the treatment of osteoarthritis in dogs (Vasseur et al. 1995). Effects of carpofen on cartilage synthesis appear to be concentration dependent. At lower concentrations (<10 μg/mL), in vitro studies reveal no inhibitory effects of carprofen on cartilage synthesis and an increase in polysulfated glycosaminoglycan (GAG) synthesis. However, at 10 μg/mL, carprofen inhibited GAG and protein synthesis (Benton et al. 1997). Concentrations that occur in dog synovial fluid following administration of a therapeutic dose of carprofen have not been determined. Thus, the most likely effect of carprofen on cartilage is not apparent.

Since carprofen's release in 1999, GI upset typical of NSAIDs has been reported in a number of dogs. Although the drug still is among the safest of the NSAIDs used in dogs, precautions must still be discussed with owners when contemplating the use of this drug in dogs. Hepatotoxicity reflecting acute hepatic necrosis has been reported as an unexpected adverse effect of carprofen in dogs (MacPhail et al. 1998). Although death has occurred in some animals, discontinuation of the drug can lead to complete resolution of biochemical abnormalities. Animals with liver disease in one study also had evidence of renal tubular disease (MacPhail et al. 1998). In addition, acute hepatopathy (perhaps idiosyncratic) has been described in a number of dogs receiving the drug. Older dogs appear to be predisposed, as might animals receiving drugs that induce drug-metabolizing enzymes (e.g., phenobarbital).

Carprofen has been studied in cats and is characterized by a small volume of distribution but long half-life. Cats, like humans, do not appear to benefit from the same level of safety of carprofen as do dogs, and carprofen should be used only short term in cats.

Carprofen is such an effective analgesic that it shows potential for control of postoperative pain (Lascelles et al. 1995). Carprofen appears to be an effective postoperative analgesic in cats (4 mg/kg SC) (Balmer et al. 1998) and dogs (Welsh et al. 1997) when administered short term preoperatively.

A number of studies with carprofen have been performed in large animals. A tissue cage model of inflammation in calves demonstrated that carprofen was effective for control of inflammation (Lees et al. 1996).

Naproxen

HORSES. Naproxen is FDA approved for use in horses as an oral granular preparation. As a granule, naproxen is approximately 50% bioavailable in horses (Pasargiklian and Bianco 1986). Peak plasma drug concentrations of 25 μg/mL occur 2-3 hours following administration of 10 mg/kg. Elimination half-life from plasma is 46 hours (Tobin 1979). Easily detected in urine, the approximate half-life of naproxen and its major metabolite is 6 hours in urine (Tobin 1979). The drug appears to have a relatively wide margin of safety in horses. Toxicity does not occur following oral administration of 3 times the recommended dose for 6 weeks (Lee and Higgins 1985). Naproxen was proved more efficacious than either phenylbutazone or placebo for the treatment of experimentally induced myositis (Lee and Higgins 1985; Tobin 1979). The drug appears to be particularly efficacious for the treatment of soft tissue inflammation.

DOGS. In dogs, naproxen is rapidly absorbed following oral administration, with maximal plasma drug concentrations occurring at 0.5-3 hours. Bioavailability ranges from 68 to 100%. Naproxen is 99% bound to serum proteins in dogs, resulting in a volume of distribution of 0.13 L/kg. Total body clearance is 0.021 mg/kg/min. Notably, compared to 12-15 hours in humans and 5 hours in horses, the elimination half-life of naproxen following IV administration in dogs ranges from 45 to 92 hours (Frey and Rieh 1981). Extensive enterohepatic circulation has been credited as the cause for prolonged elimination in dogs. Because of its long half-life, naproxen need only be given once daily in dogs, and a loading dose is indicated. The dog has been described as the animal most sensitive to naproxen (Frey and Rieh 1981). GI toxicity occurs at doses of 5 mg/kg daily. Bleeding and GI toxicities have been reported. Toxicity appears most likely when plasma drug concentrations exceed 50 μg/mL. Bleeding dyscrasias have also been reported in dogs receiving large doses of naproxen (Frey and Rieh 1981; Roudebush and Morse 1981; Gfeller and Sandors 1991).

Ibuprofen. Ibuprofen is a propionic acid derivative which has been used in dogs. Ibuprofen is less effective as an analgesic compared to aspirin, perhaps due to differences in binding of cyclooxygenase (reversible for ibuprofen and irreversible for aspirin). Ibuprofen is a popular drug in human medicine because its use is associated with a low incidence of GI side effects. However, GI erosions consistently occur in dogs receiving therapeutic doses for 2-6 weeks.

Ibuprofen is rapidly absorbed following oral administration in dogs, with peak plasma drug concentrations occurring between 0.5 and 3 hours and bioavailability ranging from 60 to 80% (mean, 77%). Volume of distribution is 0.164 L/kg. Plasma elimination half-life following oral or IV administration is 4.6 ± 0.8 hours, and clearance is 0.49 mL/min/kg. Pharmacokinetics are similar at doses of 5 and 10 mg/kg (Scherkl and Frey 1987). However, a dose of 12-15 mg/kg is necessary to achieve therapeutic concentrations as reported in humans (Scherkl and Frey 1987). Following repetitive administration of this dose, plasma drug concentrations decrease despite no change in drug half-life (Scherkl and Frey 1987).

Vomition commonly occurs following 2-6 days following ibuprofen therapy in dogs with either the gelatin or enteric coated capsules (Scherkl and Frey 1987). GI inflammation and gastric erosions have been documented following administration of 8 mg/kg daily despite the lack of clinical signs of toxicity (Scherkl and Frey 1987). Because gastric lesions occur at doses less than those necessary to achieve therapeutic concentrations, ibuprofen is not recommended for use in dogs.

Meclofenamic Acid

RUMINANTS. Meclofenamate is an anthranilic NSAID available as a palatable granular preparation intended to be mixed with food. Among the NSAIDs, it is noted for its slow onset of action. Sodium meclofenamate, which is more water soluble than meclofenamic acid, has been studied in calves. Following oral administration of 2 mg/kg, peak plasma concentrations of 0.54-1.43 μg/mL occurred at 0.5 hours. Decline in plasma drug concentrations is followed by a second (and, in some animals, higher) peak at 4-6 hours. The second peak likely reflects enterohepatic circulation. Plasma half-life after the second peak is 4 hours. A similar pattern occurs following IV injection, although peak concentrations are approximately 10 times higher. Slower absorption in calves following intraruminal administration suggests that oral administration is characterized by passage directly into the abomasum (Aitken and Sanford 1975).

HORSES. Little information regarding the safety and clinical efficacy is available for the use of meclofenamic acid in horses. There appears to be a narrow therapeutic window, and strict adherence to the manufacturer's recommended dosing regimen is indicated (Lee and Higgins 1985). Decreased plasma protein concentration has been documented following 10 days of 2.2 mg/kg in ponies, although no adverse effects were documented following over 2 months of administration in stallions and mares (Lee and Higgins 1985). Symptoms of toxicosis, when they occur, are similar to those induced by phenylbutazone. Despite a plasma elimination half-life of 2.5 hours, once-a-day dosing is sufficient for the treatment of acute and chronic inflammatory conditions in horses. Although peak plasma drug concentrations of 1 μg/mL are attained within 0.5-4 hours following oral administration of meclofenamic acid, onset of action is slow, requiring 36-96 hours. Thus, clinical efficacy requires 2-4 days of dosing (Lee and Higgins 1985). Less than 15% of the drug is eliminated in the urine, suggesting that elimination in the bile may be important (Tobin 1979). However, the drug is detectable in urine for up to 96 hours (Tobin 1979). Clinical experience suggests that this drug is particularly effective for the treatment of acute and chronic laminitis and skeletal conditions (Lee and Higgins 1985). One clinical trial reported a 78% response rate in cases with navicular disease, 76% in cases with laminitis, and 61% in cases with osteoarthritis (Tobin 1979).

Ketoprofen. Ketoprofen is a propionic acid NSAID approved for use in humans and horses. Because ketoprofen is a strong inhibitor of cyclooxygenase, it has powerful anti-inflammatory, analgesic, and antipyretic properties. In human patients suffering from rheumatoid arthritis, ketoprofen has been shown to be as efficacious as aspirin, naproxen, indomethacin, ibuprofen, diclofenac, and piroxicam (Avouac and Teule 1988).

Similar results occurred in cancer patients receiving either aspirin-codeine combinations or ketoprofen (Stambough and Drew 1988). In control of postoperative pain, ketoprofen has proven as effective as pentazocine and meperidine (Avouac and Teule 1988) and as effective as but longer lasting than acetaminophen-codeine combinations (Turek and Baird 1988). Although not firmly established, the efficacy of ketoprofen has also been attributed to its ability to inhibit some lipoxygenases and thus formation of leukotrienes (Williams and Upton 1988). Ketoprofen is also a powerful inhibitor of bradykinin (Williams and Upton 1988).

Ketoprofen is rapidly absorbed from the GI tract. Although peak plasma drug concentrations are lower in dogs following oral, compared to IV, administration, mean residence times (4.59 vs. 3.81 hours, respectively) were very similar (Schmitt and Guentert 1990). Although peak drug concentrations may be decreased, bioavailability does not seem to be impaired by food. As with other NSAIDs, ketoprofen is approximately 99% protein bound, principally to albumin. Elimination is via metabolism to inactive metabolites by the liver and excretion as the glucuronide conjugate in the urine (Williams and Upton 1988). Drug interactions involving ketoprofen have not yet been documented (Cailleteau 1988).

About 30% of the human patients studied reported adverse reactions to ketoprofen (Beaver 1988; Stambough and Drew 1988). The most frequent complaint was upper GI upset. Other commonly encountered side effects were CNS reactions, such as headaches and dizziness, and nephritis. Side effects were severe enough in one report that therapy was discontinued in approximately 13% of patients (Cailleteau 1988). In a comparison of phenylbutazone, flunixin meglumine, and ketoprofen in horses, ketoprofen was determined to be the least potentially toxic of the drugs, although all three drugs were administered at doses that exceeded those recommended on the drug labels (MacAllister et al. 1993). Anorexia, evident with the other two drugs, did not occur in horses receiving ketoprofen. Erosions or ulcers of the tongue and of both glandular and nonglandular portions of the stomach occurred in all horses receiving ketoprofen. Alternative preparations, such as rectal suppositories, have been formulated for ketoprofen to reduce the incidence of GI toxicity (Schmitt and Guentert 1990). Ketoprofen is approved for IV use in horses and is currently being considered for approval for use in dogs.

Piroxicam. Piroxicam is an oxicam NSAID approved for use in humans that has been used to treat osteoarthritis in dogs. More recently, it has received attention for its ability to reduce the size of tumors (transitional cell tumors and others) in dogs (Knapp et al. 1992). This latter effect may result from immunomodulation, but more likely it results from decreased inflammation at the tumor site. Piroxicam is a potent anti-inflammatory in musculoskeletal conditions. Oral absorption is rapid, with 100% bioavailability (Galbraith and McKellar 1991). Distributed to a volume of 0.34 L/kg, its half-life of 40-45 hours in dogs is similar to that in humans. Although the LD_{50} of piroxicam is greater than 700 mg/kg in dogs, gastric lesions and renal papillary necrosis have occurred in dogs receiving 1 mg/kg daily (Galbraith and McKellar 1991; Knapp et al. 1992). However, little evidence of toxicity (GI or bleeding) was noted after administration of 0.3 mg/kg every other day (Galbraith and McKellar 1991; Knapp et al. 1992). Extrapolation from use in humans to dogs should be done cautiously because of possible differences in volume of distribution, therapeutic concentrations, or safety margin.

Indomethacin. Indomethacin is a NSAID that was developed specifically to abate the inflammatory response to the indolic hormones serotonin and tryptophan (Boynton et al. 1988). As a powerful anti-inflammatory, it became a standard for comparison. In humans, toxicities are not serious but CNS side effects are undesirable (Boynton et al. 1988). The incidence of GI hemorrhage following administration of indomethacin at doses of 2-5 mg/kg precludes its clinical utility in dogs. In one study, all dogs developed melena within 1 week of receiving 2 mg/kg daily; 60% of these animals had gastric ulcers (Ewing 1972).

Acetaminophen. Acetaminophen (paracetamol) is a coal tar analgesic used in human medicine as an effective alternative to aspirin for control of fever and pain. It has been assumed to have poor anti-inflammatory activity, although this view has recently become more controversial (Mburu et al. 1988). Although often classified as a NSAID, its mechanism does not involve inhibition of cyclooxygenase. Rather, acetaminophen interferes with the endoperoxide intermediates of AA conversion. Its relatively weak anti-inflammatory activity has been attributed to the high concentration of peroxides occurring in peripheral inflammatory lesions. Acetaminophen may be more effective against inflammatory conditions in the CNS.

The major disadvantage to the use of acetaminophen in veterinary patients is the narrow safety margin that characterizes its use in cats. The drug is normally conjugated with glucuronide and to a lesser degree with sulfate. Drug that is not conjugated is metabolized by phase I microsomal enzymes to cytotoxic oxidative metabolites. Intracellular glutathione normally scavenges the metabolites, but in the case of overdose or glucuronide deficiency (as with the cat), the formation of toxic metabolites overwhelms the glutathione scavenging system. In cats, methemoglobinemia is the most common indication of toxicity, although centrolobular hepatic necrosis may also occur.

Treatment of acetaminophen toxicity includes administration of antioxidants, including *N*-acetylcysteine, a precursor of glutathione, and ascorbic acid (vitamin C) (St. Omer and McKnight 1980; Cullison 1984; Savides et al. 1985). The administration of cimetidine, a microsomal enzyme inhibitor, will reduce the formation of toxic metabolites and will result in clinical improvement if given within 48 hours of acetaminophen administration (Jackson 1982; Ruffalo and Thompson 1982).

Acetaminophen may be as effective as aspirin for the control of postoperative pain and inflammation in dogs. At daily doses of 0.5 g every 8 hours (average weight 18 kg) acetaminophen causes no clinical signs of adverse drug effects (Mburu et al. 1988). However, other studies have shown that adverse reactions (depression, methemoglobinemia, and vomiting) can occur at higher (0.1 g/kg) doses (Hjelle and Grauer 1986; Savides and Oehme 1983). In another study, 0.9 g/kg IV caused fulminant hepatic failure in dogs (Francavilla et al. 1989).

TREATMENT OF OSTEOARTHRITIS. Recent advances in the pathophysiology of degenerative joint disease (DJD; osteoarthritis) have provided new therapeutic foci. The progressive degeneration of articular cartilage which characterizes this disease reflects an imbalance between cartilage matrix synthesis and breakdown. The role of inflammation in the pathophysiology of DJD is controversial. Mechanisms of therapeutic drugs designed to retard DJD deterioration include inhibition of synovial cell-derived cytokines and chondrocyte-derived degradative enzymes, inactivation of superoxide radicals, stimulation of matrix synthesis, and enhancement of synovial fluid lubrication (Pinals 1992; Altman et al. 1989). The impact of NSAID therapy is apparently either harmful or beneficial, depending on the drug. The primary effect of NSAIDs on the disease is probably analgesic rather than anti-inflammatory (Pinals 1992). A number of other anti-inflammatory drugs have been studied for their efficacy in the treatment of DJD.

Orgotein. Orgotein, or superoxide dismutase, is a copper- and zinc-containing metalloprotein that can be an effective anti-inflammatory. As an endogenous intracellular enzyme, it occurs at very low concentrations in many tissues, but particularly the liver, where it scavenges tissue-damaging oxygen radicals. Phagocytic cells (neutrophils and macrophages) generate large amounts of cytotoxic superoxides during the inflammatory process. The half-life of phagocytic cells is prolonged in the presence of superoxide dismutase (Salin and McCord 1975; Tobin 1979). Approximately 2-6 weeks of therapy may be required before therapeutic benefits are realized. Orgotein is characterized by a wide margin of safety, with the lethal dose being over 40,000 times the therapeutic dose. As a large molecule, efficacy via any route other than intra-articular is questionable due to poor absorption. However, the drug has also been administered clinically both IM and orally (Breshears et al. 1974). Molecular size limits renal elimination of the drug. Following intra-articular administration, orgotein was 94% effective in horses lame for less than 2 months, compared to only 49% in horses lame for greater than 2 months prior to treatment (Ahlengard et al. 1978).

Polysulfated Glycosaminoglycan. Recent efforts in the treatment of osteoarthritis have focused on drugs that favorably shift the balance between degradation and synthesis of cartilage matrix.

CHEMISTRY. Polysulfated glycosaminoglycan (PSGAG; Adequan; Arteparon) is a polymeric chain of repeating units of hexosamine and hexuronic acid. Considered a hypersulfated compound, approximately 14% of the drug is sulfated. It is extracted and purified from bovine tracheal tissues (White 1988). Normal cartilage matrix is composed of proteoglycan complexes, collagen, and water. Side chains of glycosaminoglycans (keratin and chondroitin) are attached to the core protein of the proteoglycan molecule by a strand of hyaluronate. Water trapped in between these complexes accounts for the resiliency of cartilage. PSGAG closely mimics the proteoglycan complexes found in normal articular cartilage.

PHARMACOLOGIC EFFECT. PSGAG appears to be chondroprotective in both in vitro and in vivo models. In vivo models have included chemically and traumatically induced cartilage damage (Francis et al. 1989; Hannan et al. 1987). Cartilage degradation is retarded in the presence of PSGAG. Although the mechanisms of these protective actions are not known, chondrocyte proliferation and matrix biosynthesis appear to be important (Hannan et al. 1987). Collagen, proteoglycan, and hyaluronic acid synthesis increases (Nethery et al. 1992). In addition, proteolytic enzymes such as collagenase (Halverson et al. 1987; Nethery et al. 1992), leukocyte elastase (Rao et al. 1990), proteases (White 1988; Montefiori et al. 1990), and lysosomes are inhibited (Montefiori et al. 1990), although these actions are likely to be complex (Nethery et al. 1992). Complement activity is also inhibited; the degree of inhibition appears to be related to the sulfate load of the chondroitin sulfate matrix (Biffoni and Paroli 1991). PSGAG appears to have no effect on the ability of interleukin-1 to stimulate metalloproteinase activity in cartilage (Arsenis and McDonnell 1989).

DISPOSITION AND SAFETY. Deposition of PSGAG in normal and damaged cartilage has been demonstrated after parenteral administration. Drug that is not retained in cartilage is excreted primarily by the kidneys with minimal degradation of the parent compound. Toxicity is limited in all species studied. In dogs, the LD_{50} is 1000 mg/kg. In horses, the reported rate of adverse reaction (0.02%) has been much lower than the expected reaction rate of 1.8% (White 1988). Heparin and PSGAG are chemically similar. Adverse effects related to the anticoagulant activity of PSGAG have been suggested but not reported. However, heparin-associated thrombocytopenia, a decrease in circulating platelets presumably immunologically mediated, has been reported in human patients receiving PSGAG (Greinacher et al. 1992).

Clinical Use. PSGAG (Adequan) is approved for use in the horse with intra-articular administration, but it has been widely used as an antiarthritic in both horses (White 1988) and dogs with IM administration. However, the disposition of PSGAG following IM administration has not been reported, and the current label is for intra-articular use only. The drug is currently being considered for approval for use in dogs.

Hyaluronic Acid. Hyaluronic acid is an essential component of synovial fluid, where it is chemically linked to proteoglycans in articular cartilage. Its mode of action is not certain, but it is assumed to function as a lubricant (Pinals 1992). Following intra-articular injection, the drug persists in joints for several days. High molecular weight hyaluronic acid inhibits phagocytosis and lymphocyte migration and synovial permeability. Prior treatment with glucocorticosteroids or bony changes limits response (Tobin 1979). Intra-articular injection of the drug has met with variable success in horses (Asheim and Lindblad 1976) and dogs.

Dimethylsulfoxide. Dimethylsulfoxide (DMSO) is a hygroscopic solvent derived from wood pulp. It is used as a drug vehicle because of its ability to dissolve drugs not soluble in water. Because of its chemical characteristics, DMSO is variably categorized (Brayton 1986; Alsup 1984).

Pharmacologic Effect. As an anti-inflammatory, DMSO is a scavenger of free oxygen radicals. Anti-inflammatory effects have been reported in acute musculoskeletal injuries, CNS inflammatory processes, and CNS trauma (Wong and Reinertson 1984; Spitzer 1991). Chronic diseases are less responsive to the anti-inflammatory effects of DMSO. Immunomodulation may be responsible for some of its anti-inflammatory effects. The drug inhibits white blood cell migration, antibody production, and fibroblast proliferation. The analgesic effects of DMSO have been compared to those of narcotic analgesics. Analgesia has been reported in a variety of situations, including acute and chronic musculoskeletal disorders and postoperative pain. Although nerve blockade has been reported in vitro, it is unlikely that sufficient concentrations occur in vivo to effect this response. Opiate receptors also do not seem to be involved. Other pharmacologic effects include inhibition or stimulation of enzymes, vasodilation (due to histamine release), inhibition of platelet aggregation, radioprotection, cryopreservation, and antimicrobial (antifungal, bacterial, and viral) activity (Wong and Reinertson 1984; Brayton 1986). Diuresis occurs after topical, oral, or parenteral administration, probably due to its hygroscopic nature and ability to pull water into the tubules. DMSO (3.0 mg/kg in 20% solution) has been reported to protect the kidneys against ischemic insults to the kidneys. A sedative effect has also been reported in several species (Brayton 1986).

Disposition. Following oral administration of 1 g/kg, peak plasma drug concentrations occur within 4-6 hours, and detectable levels persist in the plasma for 400 hours (Wong and Reinertson 1984). Within 20 minutes of topical application, DMSO penetrates the skin and can be detected in all organs of the body (Brayton 1986). Peak plasma drug concentrations occur 2 hours after topical administration (Wong and Reinertson 1984). Its ability to penetrate the skin is believed to reflect exchange and interchange with water in biological membranes. Mucous membranes, lipid membranes of cells and organelles, and the blood-brain barrier are similarly penetrated without irreversible membrane damage (Brayton 1986). Tooth enamel and keratin appear to be the only tissues that DMSO does not penetrate (Wong and Reinertson 1984). DMSO facilitates penetration of other substances across membranes; cutaneous penetration of steroids, sulfadiazine, phenylbutazone, and other drugs has been documented (Brayton 1986; Alsup 1984). Enhanced absorption of therapeutic drugs can lead to toxicity, particularly for anesthetic, cardioactive, and anticholinesterase drugs.

DMSO is partially metabolized by hepatic microsomal enzymes (Brayton 1986), but the primary route of elimination appears to be in the urine as the parent compound (Wong and Reinertson 1984). Although a significant amount of DMSO may be eliminated in the bile, most undergoes enterohepatic circulation (Wong and Reinertson 1984). Hepatic metabolism of a small amount of DMSO (3-6%) to dimethylsulfide and subsequent pulmonary excretion of this metabolite account for the halitosis which occurs regardless of the route of administration (Wong and Reinertson 1984).

Adverse Effects. DMSO has a large safety margin. Signs associated with near lethal IV doses include sedation, diuresis, intravascular hemolysis, and hematuria. Death is preceded by hypotension, prostration, convulsions, and respiratory distress characterized by dyspnea, tachypnea, and pulmonary edema. Phlebitis and venous obstruction may occur with IV dosing. Intravascular hemolysis is concentration and rate dependent, and concentrations less than 10% are recommended for IV administration. Susceptibility to hemolysis will vary with species due to differences in erythrocyte fragility. Nephrotoxicity has been reported in some species. Necropsy lesions include hematuria, hemoglobinuria, and mild tubular nephrosis. Chronic toxicity studies in laboratory animals have documented hepatotoxicity, which may be due to its metabolism by the liver to toxic metabolites. DMSO may also enhance hepatotoxicity of other drugs as well as hepatic binding and metabolism of selected carcinogens. Teratogenicity has also been reported in some animals. Ocular toxicity occurs with daily, long-term administration and develops more rapidly in young animals. Lesions occur in the lens and appear as altered relucency, making animals myopic. Histologic abnormalities are not apparent. Such a response was reported in one horse which received 0.6 g/kg daily, cutaneously, for 2 months. Skin reactions are common, particularly at higher concentrations, and are manifested as erythema, warmth, and local vasodilation. A wheal-and-flare response and pruritus may also occur. Repeated application may result in drying and desquamation of the epithelium (Brayton 1986).

CLINICAL USE. DMSO is FDA approved for topical application in horses suffering from acute swelling due to trauma and in the treatment of acute or chronic otitis. In humans, DMSO is approved for interstitial cystitis. Although not approved, DMSO has been recommended for therapy in male cats suffering from urinary tract obstruction (Brayton 1986). Other reported applications of DMSO include facilitation of healing of skin wounds (including habronemiasis of horses), acral lick dermatitis in dogs, postoperative fibrous adhesions, acute CNS trauma, inflammation, edema or ischemia, intervertebral disk disease, fibrocartilaginous embolization, ischemic insults, postoperative myositis, rheumatic diseases, myasthenia gravis, and chronic musculoskeletal conditions. DMSO also inhibits alcohol dehydrogenase and thus has been recommended for the treatment of ethylene glycol toxicity (Brayton 1986).

REFERENCES

Ahlengard, S., Tufvesson, G., Pettersson, H., et al. 1978. Treatment of traumatic arthritis in the horse with intra-articular orgotein (Palosein). Equine Vet J 10:122-24.

Aitken, M. M., and Sanford, J. 1975. Plasma levels following administration of sodium meclofenamate by various routes. Res Vet Sci 19:241-44.

Alsup, E. M. 1984. Dimethyl sulfoxide. J Am Vet Med Assoc 185:1011-14.

Altman, R. D., Kapila, P., Dean, D. D., et al. 1989. Future therapeutic trends in osteoarthritis. Scand J Rheumatol Supp 77:37-42.

Anderson, K. L., Smith, A. R., Shanks, R. D., et al. 1986a. Efficacy of flunixin meglumine for the treatment of endotoxin-induced bovine mastitis. Am J Vet Res 47:1366-72.

———. 1986b. Endotoxin-induced bovine mastitis: immunoglobulins, phagocytosis, and effect of flunixin meglumine. Am J Vet Res 47:2405-10.

Arsenis, C., and McDonnell, J. 1989. Effects of antirheumatic drugs on the interleukin-1α induced synthesis and activation of proteinases in articular cartilage explants in culture. Agents and Actions 27:261-64.

Asheim, A., and Lindblad, G. 1976. Intra-articular treatment of arthritis in race-horses with sodium hyaluronate. Acta Vet Scand 17:379-94.

Avouac, B., and Teule, M. 1988. Ketoprofen: the European experience. J Clin Pharmacol 28:S2-S7.

Balmer, T. V., Irvine, D., Jones, R. S., Roberts, M. J., Slingsby, L., Taylor, P. M., Waterman, A. E., and Waters, C. 1998. Comparison of carprofen and pethidine as postoperative analgesics in the cat. J Small Anim Pract 39(4):158-64.

Bater, D. C. 1988. Clinical pharmacology of NSAIDs. J Clin Pharmacol 28:518-23.

Beasley, V. R., and Buck, W. B. 1980. Acute ethylene glycol toxicosis: a review. Vet Hum Tox 22:255.

Beaver, W. T. 1988. Ketoprofen: a new nonsteroidal anti-inflammatory analgesic. J Clin Pharmacol 28:S1.

Benton, H. P., Vasseur, P. B., Broderick-Villa, G. A., and Koolpe, M. 1997. Effect of carprofen on sulfated glycosaminoglycan metabolism, protein synthesis, and prostaglandin release by cultured osteoarthritic canine chondrocytes. Am J Vet Res 58(3):286-92.

Berliner, S., Weinberger, A., Shoenfeld, Y., et al. 1985. Ibuprofen may induce meningitis in (NZB X NZW) mice. Arthritis Rheum 28:104-7.

Biffoni, M., and Paroli, E. 1991. Complement in vitro inhibition by a low sulfate chondroitin sulfate (matrix). Drugs Exptl Clin Res 27:35-39.

Boynton, C. S., Dick, C. F., and Mayor, G. H. 1988. NSAIDs: an overview. J Clin Pharmacol 28:512-17.

Brandt, K. D. 1991. The mechanism of action of nonsteroidal anti-inflammatory drugs. J Rheumatol 18:120-21.

Brater, D. C. 1988. Clinical pharmacology of NSAIDs. J Clin Pharmacol 28:518-23.

Brayton, C. F. 1986. Dimethyl sulfoxide (DMSO). Cornell Vet 76:61-90.

Breshears, D. E., Brown, C. D., Riffel, D. M., et al. 1974. Evaluation of orgotein in treatment of locomotor dysfunction in dogs. Mod Vet Pract 55:85-93.

Budsberg, S., Johnston, S., Schwarz, P., et al. 1996. Evaluation of etodolac for the treatment of osteoarthritis of the hip in dogs: a prospective multicenter study (abstract). Vet Surg 25:420.

Cailleteau, J. G. 1988. Ketoprofen in dentistry: a pharmacologic review. Oral Surg Oral Med Oral Pathol 66:620-24.

Carlisle, C. H., Penny, R. H. C., Prescott, C. W., et al. 1968. Toxic effects of phenylbutazone on the cat. Br Vet J 124:560-66.

Cashman, J. N. 1996. The mechanisms of action of NSAIDs in analgesia drugs. Drugs 52(Suppl 5):13-23.

Chastain, C. B. 1987. Aspirin: new indications for an old drug. Compendium Small Animal 9:165-70.

Clemmons, R. M., and Meyers, K. M. 1984. Acquisition and aggregation of canine blood platelets: basic mechanisms of function and differences because of breed origin. Am J Vet Res 45:137-44.

Collins, L. G., and Tyler, D. E. 1985. Experimentally induced phenylbutazone toxicosis in ponies: description of the syndrome and its prevention with synthetic prostaglandin E2. Am J Vet Res 46:1605-15.

Conlon, P. D. 1988. Nonsteroidal drugs used in the treatment of inflammation. Vet Clin North Am Small Anim Pract 18:1115-31.

Cullison, R. F. 1984. Acetaminophen toxicosis in small animals: clinical signs, mode of action, and treatment. Compendium on Cont Educ 6:315-21.

Dascanio, J. J., Mechor, G. D., Grohn, Y. T., Kenney, D. G., Booker, C. A., Thompson, P., Chiffelle, C. L., Musser, J. M., and Warnick, L. D. 1995. Effect of phenylbutazone and flunixin meglumine on acute toxic mastitis in dairy cows. Am J Vet Res 56(9):1213-18.

Davidson, J. R., Lantz, G. C., Salisbury, S. K., et al. 1992. Effects of flunixin meglumine on dogs with experimental gastric dilatation-volvulus. Vet Surg 21:113-20.

Davis, L. E., and Westfall, B. A. 1972. Species differences in biotransformation and excretion of salicylate. Am J Vet Res 33:1253-62.

Davis, L. E., Westfall, B. A., and Short, C. R. 1973. Biotransformation and pharmacokinetics of salicylate in newborn animals. Am J Vet Res 34:1105-8.

Dawson, J., and Sedgwick, A. D. 1987. Actions of nonsteroidal anti-inflammatory drugs on equine leucocyte movement in vitro. J Vet Pharmacol Therap 10:150-59.

De Backer, P., Braeckman, R., Belpaire, F., et al. 1980. Bioavailability and pharmacokinetics of phenylbutazone in the cow. J Vet Pharmacol Therap 3:29-33.

Donnelly, M. T., and Hawkey, C. J. 1997. Review article: COX-II inhibitors—a new generation of safer NSAIDs? Alimentary Pharmacol Therap 11(2):227-36.

Dunn, M. J., Simonson, M., Davidson, E. W., et al. 1988. Nonsteroidal anti-inflammatory drugs and renal function. J Clin Pharmacol 28:524-29.

Eberhardson, B., Olsson, G., Appelgren, L.-E., et al. 1979. Pharmacokinetic studies of phenylbutazone in cattle. J Vet Pharmacol Therap 2:31-37.

Ewing, G. O. 1972. Indomethacin-associated gastrointestinal hemorrhage in a dog. J Am Vet Med Assoc 161:1665-68.

Francavilla, A., Makowka, L., Polimeno, L., et al. 1989. A dog model for acetominophen-induced fulminant hepatic failure. Gastroenterology 96:470-78.

Francis, D. J., Forrest, M. J., Brooks, P. M., et al. 1989. Retardation of articular cartilage degradation by glycosaminoglycan polysulfate, pentosan polysulfate, and DH-40J in the rat air pouch model. Arthritis Rheum 32:608-16.

Frey, H. H., and Rieh, B. 1981. Pharmacokinetics of naproxen in the dog. Am J Vet Res 42:1615-17.

Galbraith, E. A., and McKellar, Q. A. 1991. Pharmacokinetics and pharmacodynamics of piroxicam in dogs. Vet Rec 128:561-65.

Gfeller, R. W., and Sandors, A. D. 1991. Naproxen-associated duodenal ulcer complicated by perforation and bacteria- and barium sulfate-induced peritonitis in a dog. J Am Vet Med Assoc 198:644-46.

Gingerich, D. A., Baggot, J. D., and Yeary, R. A. 1975. Pharmacokinetics and dosage of aspirin in cattle. J Am Vet Med Assoc 167:945-48.

Greinacher, A., Michels, I., SchÑfer, M., et al. 1992. Heparin associated thrombocytopenia in a patient treated with polysulphated chondroitin sulphate: evidence for immunological crossreactivity between heparin and polysulphated glycosaminoglycan. Br J Haematol 81:252-54.

Griswold, D. E., and Adams, J. L. 1996. Constitutive cyclooxygenase (COX-1) and inducible cyclooxygenase (COX-2): rationale for selective inhibition and progress to date. Medicinal Res Rev 16(2):181-206.

Halverson, P. B., Cheung, H. S., Struve, J., et al. 1987. Suppression of active collagenase from calcified lapine synovium by arteparon. J Rheumatol 14:1013-17.

Hannan, N., Ghosh, P., Bellenger, C., et al. 1987. Systemic administration of glycosaminoglycan polysulphate (arteparon) provides partial protection of articular cartilage from damage produced by meniscectomy in the canine. J Orthoped Res 5:47-59.

Hardie, E. M., Kolata, R. J., and Rawlings, C. A. 1983. Canine septic peritonitis: treatment with flunixin meglumine. Circ Shock 11:159-73.

Hardie, E. M., Hardee, G. E., and Rawlings, C. A. 1985. Pharmacokinetics of flunixin meglumine in dogs. Am J Vet Res 46:235-37.

Hendricks, H. L., Bush, P. B., Kitzman, J. V., and Booth, N. H. 1984. Determination of 4-aminopyridine in horse plasma using gas-liquid chromatography. J. Chromatogr. 287(2):429-32.

Higgins, A. J. 1985. The biology, pathophysiology and control of eicosanoids in inflammation. J Vet Pharmacol Therap 8:1-18.

Hjelle, J. J., and Grauer, G. F. 1986. Acetominophen induced toxicosis in dogs and cats. J Am Vet Med Assoc 188:742-46.

Hochberg, M. C. 1989. NSAIDs: mechanisms and pathways of action. Hos Pract 15:185-98.

Jackson, J. E. 1982. Cimetidine protects against acetaminophen toxicity. Life Sci 31:31-35.

Jackson, M. L. 1987. Platelet physiology and platelet function: inhibition by aspirin. Compendium on Continuing Education 9:627-38.

Jarlov, N., Andersen, H. P., and Hesselholt, M. 1992. Pathophysiology of experimental bovine endotoxicosis: endotoxin induced synthesis of prostaglandins and thromboxane and the modulatory effect of some non-steroidal anti-inflammatory drugs. Acta Vet Scand 33:1-8.

Jezyk, P. F. 1983. Metabolic diseases: an emerging area of veterinary pediatrics. Compendium on Continuing Education 5:1026-31.

Jonnes, R. D., Baynes, R. E., and Nimitz, C. T. 1992. Nonsteroidal anti-inflammatory drug toxicosis in dogs and cats: 240 cases. J Am Vet Med Assoc 201:475-77.

Knapp, D. W., Richardson, R. C., Bottoms, G. D., et al. 1992. Phase I. Trial of piroxicam in 62 dogs bearing naturally occurring tumors. Cancer Chemother Pharmacol 29:214-18.

Konturek, S. J. 1986. Physiology and pharmacology of prostaglandin. Dig Dis Sci 31:6S-19S.

Larson, E. J. 1963. Toxicity of low doses of aspirin in the cat. J Am Vet Med Assoc 143:837-40.

Lascelles, B. D., Cripps, P., Mirchandani, S., and Waterman, A. E. 1995. Carprofen as an analgesic for postoperative pain in cats: dose titration and assessment of efficacy in comparison to pethidine hydrochloride. J Small Anim Pract 36(12):535-41.

Lee, P., and Higgins, A. J. 1985. Clinical pharmacology and therapeutic uses of non-steroidal anti-inflammatory drugs in the horse. Equine Vet J 17:83-96.

Lees, P., Taylor, J. B. O., Higgins, A. J., et al. 1986. Phenylbutazone and oxyphenbutazone distribution into tissue fluids in the horse. J Vet Pharmacol Therap 9:204-12.

Lees, P., Delatour, P., Foster, A. P., Foot, R., and Baggot, D. 1996. Evaluation of carprofen in calves using a tissue cage model. Br Vet J 152(2):199-211.

Lewis, J. H. 1984. Hepatic toxicity of nonsteroidal anti-inflammatory drugs. Clin Pharm 3:128-38.

Lipowitz, A. J., Boulay, J. P., and Klausner, J. S. 1986. Serum salicylate concentrations and endoscopic evaluation of the gastric mucosa in dogs after oral administration of aspirin-containing products. Am J Vet Res 47:1586-89.

MacAllister, C. G., Morgan, S. J., Borne, A. T., et al. 1993. Comparison of adverse effects of phenylbutazone, flunixin meglumine, and ketoprofen in horses. J Am Vet Med Assoc 202:71-77.

MacPhail, C. M., Lappin, M. R., Meyer, D. J., Smith, S. G., Webster, C. R., and Armstrong, P. J. 1998. Hepatocellular toxicosis associated with administration of carprofen in 21 dogs. J Am Vet Med Assoc 212(12):1895-901.

Maitho, T. E., Lees, P., and Taylor, J. B. 1986. Absorption and pharmacokinetics of phenylbutazone in Welsh Mountain ponies. J Vet Pharmacol Therap 9:26-39.

Markel, M. D. 1986. What is your diagnosis? J Am Vet Med Assoc 188:307-8.

Martin, K., Andersson, L., Stridsberg, M., et al. 1984. Plasma concentration, mammary excretion and side-effects of phenylbutazone after repeated oral administration in healthy cows. J Vet Pharmacol Therap 7:131-38.

Mazué, G., Richez, P., and Berthe, J. 1983. Pharmacology and comparative toxicology of non-steroidal anti-inflammatory agents. In Y. Ruckebusch, P. L. Toutain, and G. D. Koritz, eds., Veterinary Pharmacology and Toxicology, pp. 321-31. Boston: MTP Press.

Mburu, D. N., Mbugua, S. W., Skoglund, L. A., et al. 1988. Effects of paracetamol and acetylsalicylic acid on the post-operative course after experimental orthopaedic surgery in dogs. J Vet Pharmacol Therap 11:163-71.

McCormack, K., and Brune, K. 1987. Classical absorption theory and the development of gastric mucosal damage associated with the non-steroidal anti-inflammatory drugs. Arch Toxicol 60:261-69.

McKellar, Q. A., Galbraith, E. A., Bogan, J. A., et al. 1989. Flunixin pharmacokinetics and serum thromboxane inhibition in the dog. Vet Rec 24:651-54.

Mealey, K. L., Matthews, N. S., Peck, K. E., Ray, A. C., and Taylor, T. S. 1997. Comparative pharmacokinetics of phenylbutazone and its metabolite oxyphenbutazone in clinically normal horses and donkeys. Am J Vet Res 58(1):53-55.

Montefiori, D. C., Robinson, W. E., Modliszewski, A., et al. 1990. Differential inhibition of HIV-1 cell binding and HIV-1-induced syncytium formation by low molecular weight sulphated polysaccharides. J Antimicrob Chemother 25:313-18.

Moore, J. N. 1986. Treatment of equine colic and endotoxemia. In International Symposium on Nonsteroidal Anti-inflammatory Agents, pp. 11-14. Trenton, NJ: Veterinary Learning Systems Co.

Moore, J. N., Hardee, M. M., and Hardee, G. E. 1986. Modulation of arachidonic acid metabolism in endotoxic horses: comparison of flunixin meglumine, phenylbutazone, and a selective thromboxane synthetase inhibitor. Am J Vet Res 47:110-13.

Morton, D. L., and Knottenbelt, D. C. 1989. Pharmacokinetics of aspirin and its application in canine veterinary medicine. J S Afr Vet Assoc 60:191-94.

Munsiff, I. J., Koritz, G. D., McKiernan, B. C., et al. 1988. Plasma protein binding of theophylline in dogs. J Vet Pharmacol Therap 11:112-14.

Murray, M. J. 1985. Phenylbutazone toxicity in a horse. Compendium on Continuing Education 7:S389-S394.

Nethery, A., Giles, I., Jenkins, K., et al. 1992. The chondroprotective drugs, arteparon and sodium pentosan polysulphate, increase collagenase activity and inhibit stromelysin activity in vitro. Biochem Pharmacol 44:1549-53.

Newcombe, D. S. 1988. Leukotrienes: regulation of biosynthesis, metabolism, and bioactivity. J Clin Pharmacol 28:530-49.

Pairet, M., and Engelhardt, G. 1996. Distinct isoforms (COX-1 and COX-2) of cyclooxygenase: possible physiological and therapeutic implications. Fundamental & Clin Pharmacol 10(1):1-17.

Pasargiklian, M., and Bianco, S. 1986. Perspectives in the treatment of reversible airway obstruction. Respiration 50:131-365.

Pinals, R. S. 1992. Pharmacologic treatment of osteoarthritis. Clin Ther 14:336-46.

Rao, N. V., Kennedy, T. P., Rao, G., et al. 1990. Sulfated polysaccharides prevent human leukocyte elastase-induced acute lung injury and emphysema in hamsters. Am Rev Respir Dis 142:407-12.

Robinson, D. R. 1989. Eicosanoids, inflammation, and antiinflammatory drugs. Clin Exp Rheumatol 7:155-61.

Robinson, M. G. 1989. New oral salicylates in therapy of chronic idiopathic inflammatory bowel disease. Gastroenterol Clin North Am 18:43-50.

Roudebush, P., and Morse, G. E. 1981. Naproxen toxicosis in a dog. J Am Vet Med Assoc 179:805-6.

Ruffalo, R. L., and Thompson, J. F. 1982. Cimetidine and acetylcysteine as antidote for acetaminophen overdose. South Med J 75:954-58.

Salin, M., and McCord, J. M. 1975. Free radicals and inflammation: protection of phagocytosing leukocytes by superoxide dismutase. J Clin Invest 56:1319-23.

Savides, M. C., and Oehme, F. W. 1983. Acetaminophen and its toxicity. J Appl Toxicol 3:96-111.

Savides, M. C., Oehme, F. W., and Leipold, H. W. 1985. Effects of various antidotal treatment on acetaminophen toxicosis and biotransformation in cats. Am J Vet Res 46:1485-89.

Scherkl, R., and Frey, H. H. 1987. Pharmacokinetics of ibuprofen in the dog. J Vet Pharmacol Therap 10:261-65.

Schmitt, M., and Guentert, T. W. 1990. Biopharmaceutical evaluation of ketoprofen following intravenous, oral, and rectal administration in dogs. J Pharm Sci 79:614-16.

Semrad, S. D., Hardee, G. E., Hardee, M. M., et al. 1985. Flunixin meglumine given in small doses: pharmacokinetics and prostaglandin inhibition in healthy horses. Am J Vet Res 46:2474-79.

Short, C. R., Hsieh, L. C., Malbrough, M. S., et al. 1990. Elimination of salicylic acid in goats and cattle. Am J Vet Res 51:1267-70.

Spitzer, W. O. 1991. Drugs as determinants of health and disease in the population. J Clin Epidemiol 44:823-30.

Stambough, J., and Drew, J. 1988. A double-blind parallel evaluation of the efficacy and safety of a single dose of ketoprofen in cancer pain. J Clin Pharmacol 28:S34-S39.

St. Omer, V. V., and McKnight, E. D. 1980. Acetylcysteine for treatment of acetaminophen toxicosis in the cat. J Am Vet Med Assoc 176:911-13.

Syvlia, L. M., Forlenza, S. W., and Brocavich, J. M. 1988. Aseptic meningitis associated with naproxen. DICP: Annals of Pharmacotherapy 22:399-401.

Tandy, J., and Thorpe, E. 1967. A fatal syndrome in the dog following administration of phenylbutazone. Vet Rec 81:398-99.

Taylor, P. M., Delatour, P., Landoni, F. M., Deal, C., Pickett, C., Shojaee Aliabadi, F., Foot, R., and Lees, P. 1996. Pharmacodynamics and enantioselective pharmacokinetics of carprofen in the cat. Res Vet Sci 60(2):144-51.

Templeton, C. B., Bottoms, G. D., Fessler, J. F., et al. 1987. Endotoxin-induced hemodynamic and prostaglandin changes in ponies: effects of flunixin meglumine, dexamethasone, and prednisolone. Circ Shock 23:231-40.

Thomas, A. D., Bowater, I. C., Vine, J. H., and McLean, J. G. 1997. Uptake of drugs from topically applied anti-inflammatory preparations applied to racing animals. Aust Vet J 75(12):897-901.

Tobin, T. 1979. Pharmacology review: the nonsteroidal anti-inflammatory drugs. II. Equiproxen, meclofenamic acid, flunixin and others. J Equine Med Surg 6:298-302.

Tobin, T., Chay, S., Kamerling, S., et al. 1986. Phenylbutazone in the horse: a review. J Vet Pharmacol Therap 9:1-25.

Traub, J. L., Paulsen, L. M., and Reed, S. M. 1983. The use of phenylbutazone in the horse. Compendium on Cont Educ 5:S320-S327.

Turek, M. D., and Baird, W. M. 1988. Double-blind parallel comparison of ketoprofen, acetaminophen plus codeine, and placebo in postoperative pain. J Clin Pharmacol 28:S23-S28.

Vane, J. R., and Botting, R. 1987. Inflammation and the mechanism of action of antiinflammatory drugs. FASEB J 1:89-96.

Vane, J. R., Bakhle, Y. S., and Botting, R. M. 1998. Cyclooxygenases 1 and 2. Ann Rev Pharmacol Toxicol 38:97-120.

Vasseur, P. B., Johnson, A. L., Budsberg, S. C., Lincoln, J. D., Toombs, J. P., Whitehair, J. G., and Lentz, E. L. 1995. Randomized, controlled trial of the efficacy of carprofen, a nonsteroidal anti-inflammatory drug, in the treatment of osteoarthritis in dogs. J Am Vet Med Assoc 206(6):807-11.

Watson, A. D. J., Wilson, J. T., Turner, D. M., et al. 1980. Phenylbutazone-induced blood dyscrasias suspected in three dogs. Vet Rec 107:239-41.

Weissmann, G. 1991. The actions of NSAIDs. Hos Pract 15:60-76.

Welsh, E. M., Nolan, A. M., and Reid, J. 1997. Beneficial effects of administering carprofen before surgery in dogs. Vet Rec 141(10):251-53.

White, G. W. 1988. Adequan: a review for the practicing veterinarian. Vet Review 8:463-67.

Williams, C. S., and DuBois, R. N. 1996. Prostaglandin endoperoxide synthase: why two isoforms? Am J Physiol 270(3, pt. 1):G393-400.

Williams, R. J. 1988. Pharmacokinetics of phenylbutazone in mature bulls. Proc ACVIM 6:458-60.

Williams, R. L., and Upton, R. A. 1988. The clinical pharmacology of ketoprofen. J Clin Pharmacol 28:S13-S22.

Wong, L. K., and Reinertson, E. L. 1984. Clinical considerations of dimethyl sulfoxide. Iowa St Vet 46:89-95.

Yeary, R. A., and Swanson, W. 1973. Aspirin dosages for the cat. J Am Vet Med Assoc 163:1117-78.

SECTION 5

Drugs Acting on the Cardiovascular System

23

DIGITALIS AND VASODILATOR DRUGS

H. RICHARD ADAMS

Basic Aspects of Cardiac Function
- **Intrinsic Regulation**
- **Regulation by the Nervous System**
- **Cellular Concepts**

Digitalis and Related Cardiac Glycosides
- **Chemistry and Sources**
- **Cardiovascular Effects**
- **Extracirculatory Effects**
- **Pharmacokinetics**
- **Digitalis Toxicity**
- **Therapeutic Indications for Digitalis**
- **Clinical Procedures**
- **Preparations**

Amrinone and Milrinone

Vasodilator Drugs
- **Prazosin**
- **Hydralazine Hydrochloride**
- **Captopril and Enalapril Maleate**
- **Calcium Channel Blocking Drugs**
- **Other Vasodilators**

Ancillary Therapy in Congestive Heart Failure
- **Oxygen Demand and Delivery**
- **Diuretics**
- **Morphine**
- **Other Procedures**

An understanding of the clinical pharmacodynamics of cardiac drugs is essential to veterinary medicine for two important reasons. First, the indispensable pumping function of the heart in maintaining circulation rules that life-threatening events are often present when pharmacologic agents are needed to control the heart. Second, cardiac dysfunctional states that are amenable to drug therapy are common in some species. This chapter considers the more important drugs used in therapeutic management of cardiac disorders, with focus on basic aspects of cardiac function, digitalis and related cardiac glycosides, bipyridine inotropic drugs, and vasodilator agents. Antiarrhythmic drugs are covered in Chap. 24. Other classes of drugs that elicit prominent cardiac responses (e.g., adrenergic and cholinergic agents) are addressed specifically in appropriate chapters.

BASIC ASPECTS OF CARDIAC FUNCTION. The heart, blood, lungs, and blood vessels compose an integrated physiologic system that supplies oxygen and other nutrients to tissues and removes carbon dioxide and other waste products. Efficiency of the heart muscle and of tissue functions throughout the body is critically dependent on adequate supplies of oxygenated blood. This necessitates a series of sensitive and dynamic control mechanisms to ensure that cardiac output is sufficient to supply cellular demands.

The three primary pathways by which the heart can increase its cardiac output in response to body needs for increased blood flow are: an intrinsic response of the muscle to changes in muscle length, changes in heart rate, and adjustments in contractility. These physiologic control systems are of considerable importance to pharmacology because the net response of the heart to drugs is controlled by these mechanisms.

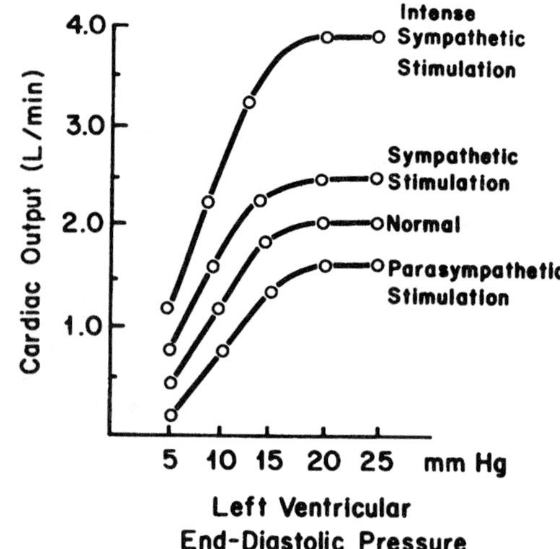

FIG. 23.1—Frank-Starling law of the heart. As end-diastolic ventricular volume increases, the myofiber is stretched, enhancing the contractile state of the muscle; cardiac output is thus increased. The cardiac output curve can be influenced by different degrees of sympathetic and parasympathetic stimulation.

Intrinsic Regulation. Contractile response of cardiac muscle to a change in its own length is the primary mechanism whereby the heart adjusts its pumping activity under normal physiologic conditions (Fozzard 1976). In the whole heart, the volume of blood returning to cardiac chambers from the veins controls resting muscle length. Individual myofibers are stretched as the intraventricular diastolic volume expands to accommodate increased venous return. The stretched muscle responds in turn with enhanced contractile strength, thereby pumping the increased volume of blood into the arterial circuits.

The fundamental capability of the heart to autoregulate its pumping capacity in response to end-diastolic filling, and thus muscle length, is referred to as the Frank-Starling law of the heart (Frank 1895; Starling 1918). This length-force relationship is the result of stretching the sarcomere to a more optimal interdigitating arrangement of the actin and myosin elements. The relationship between end-diastolic filling and cardiac output under basal conditions and under dominance by the sympathetic and parasympathetic nervous systems is shown in Fig. 23.1.

Regulation by the Nervous System. The autonomic nervous system regulates the heart mainly by adjusting cardiac rate and myocardial contractility. Details concerning cardiac effects and mechanisms of action of the sympathetic neurotransmitter norepinephrine and the parasympathetic neurotransmitter acetylcholine (ACh) are presented in Chaps. 5-7.

Sympathetic stimulation of cardiac muscle markedly increases the force of contraction irrespective of end-diastolic muscle length. A change in contractile strength that is independent of muscle length is referred to as a change in contractility (inotropy). In the presence of inotropic stimulation by the sympathetic system, cardiac output at each level of ventricular filling is enhanced considerably over the basal state (Fig. 23.1). Conversely, parasympathetic nerves exert their primary influences on cardiac output, not by changing the inotropic state, but by adjusting heart rate. Vagal discharge produces bradycardia; with fewer heartbeats per unit of time, less blood can be pumped and cardiac output is decreased at all levels of venous return (Fig. 23.1). In contrast, sympathetic stimulation produces marked tachycardia and, within physiologic limits, cardiac output is increased proportionately. Coronary blood flow increases in response to sympathetic stimulation, but much of this change is secondary to increased metabolic-oxygen demands of the heart muscle.

Myocardial oxygen demand varies directly with three main factors: heart rate, myocardial wall tension, and inotropic state. Myocardial wall tension is directly proportional to ventricular radius (cardiac size) and intraventricular pressure, i.e., the law of Laplace. Primary determinants of ventricular wall tension are preload (i.e., end-diastolic volume and stretch) and afterload (aortic blood pressure). By reducing preload or afterload, certain drugs can elicit marked reduction in cardiac work without direct inotropic action on a heart muscle cell.

Cellular Concepts. The basic contractile unit of a heart muscle cell is the sarcomere, composed of the interdigitating protein filaments actin (thin filament) and myosin (thick filament). Activation of the filaments is regulated by a protein assembly unit composed of tropomyosin and troponin and associated with actin molecules. Availability of ionized calcium (Ca^{++}) in the vicinity of troponin is the obligate modulator of the relaxation-contraction cycle.

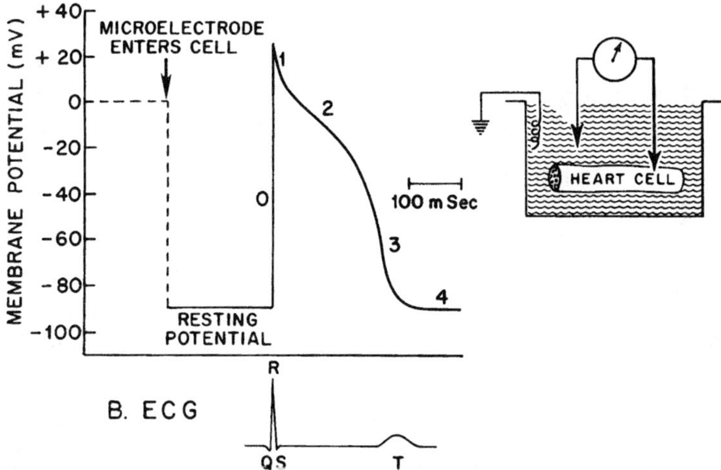

FIG. 23.2—(A) Cardiac action potential recorded from a single myocardial cell. The following phases are listed: 0 = rapid depolarization upstroke, 1 = rapid repolarization, 2 = plateau, 3 = delayed repolarization, and 4 = diastolic potential. The plateau phase is due partly to a slow current representing entry of Ca^{++} into the cell during excitation-contraction coupling. (B) Electrocardiogram (ECG) of the ventricle correlating with the respective phases above (Parker and Adams 1977).

Binding of Ca^{++} to a high-affinity subunit of the troponin molecule evokes the movement of tropomyosin from its diastolic blocking position on actin. Cross-linkages or "cross-bridges" are formed between projections of the myosin molecules and exposed sites on actin. As cross-bridges are formed, the thick and thin filaments move laterally in relation to one another, and contraction occurs. Calcium delivery to the myofibrils is initiated by bioelectric events at the cell membrane, represented by the cardiac action potential.

CARDIAC ACTION POTENTIAL. The diastolic (resting) membrane potential in heart cells is maintained at about –90 mV (negative inside in relation to outside the cell), primarily as a result of uneven distribution of potassium ions (K^+) inside, $(K^+)_i$, and outside, $(K^+)_o$, the cell. The cell membrane (sarcolemma) is selectively permeable to K^+ during diastole compared to other electrolytes like sodium ions (Na^+), and yet an active ion transport system maintains high $(K^+)_i$ relative to $(K^+)_o$, and low $(Na^+)_i$ relative to $(Na^+)_o$. The high permeability of the cell membrane to K^+ allows a net outward leakage of this positively charged ion. This outward current, in combination with impermeate organic anions within the cell, yields a negatively charged intracellular space. When the cell is stimulated, selective permeability characteristics of the sarcolemma to K^+ are lost. The resulting change in ion distribution can be recorded as an action potential by using a microelectrode capable of penetrating a single myocardial cell (Fozzard and Gibbons 1973).

The action potential of a ventricular muscle cell contains two basic components, depolarization and repolarization, which can be differentiated into five phases (Fig. 23.2). The rapid upstroke, phase 0, is similar to the depolarization spike seen in skeletal muscle and neurons; it represents a rapid flux of Na^+ into the cell. As the permeability characteristics of the cell membrane are reestablished, rapid (phase 1) and delayed (phase 3) repolarization occur, restoring the membrane potential to its diastolic level (phase 4).

The plateau (phase 2) is due partly to a slow inward current that is carried by Ca^{++} through membrane passageways (channels or pores) that are distinct from those participating in the rapid Na^+ upstroke phase of the action potential. The plateau phase is critically important because the slow inward Ca^{++} current is believed to be the link in heart muscle that couples membrane excitation with activation of the contractile apparatus (Reuter 1979, 1985; see Chap. 24).

EXCITATION-CONTRACTION COUPLING. Although Ca^{++} enters the cell during the plateau phase of the action potential, the amount of Ca^{++} that enters by this slow-current pathway is insufficient by itself for optimal activation of the contractile apparatus (Solaro et al. 1974). Instead, the small amount of Ca^{++} entering the cell during the plateau of the action potential fills sarcoplasmic reticulum stores of Ca^{++} and also acts as a trigger to cause a regenerative release of additional amounts of this cation that have been previously sequestered at the sarcoplasmic reticulum (Fabiato and Fabiato 1979).

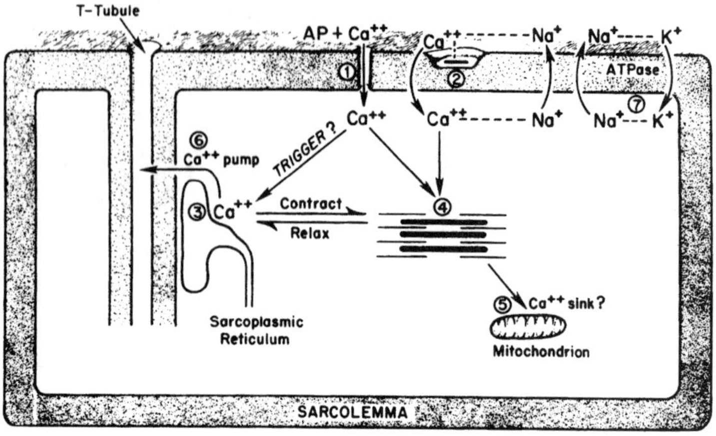

FIG. 23.3—Schematic representation of cellular ion movements controlling excitation-contraction coupling in heart muscle. An action potential (AP) instigates the inward movement of Ca^{++} through slow Ca^{++} channels of the sarcolemma (1). Inward-moving calcium fills sarcoplasmic reticulum stores of the cation and also serves as a trigger to release additional Ca^{++} from storage sites of the sarcoplasmic reticulum (3). These Ca^{++} sources and that resulting from Na^+–Ca^{++} exchanges across the sarcolemma (2) activate the contractile proteins (4). Relaxation occurs as calcium is sequestered at storage sites of sarcoplasmic reticulum (3). Mitochondrion (5). Ca^{++} is pumped out of the cell (6). Altered sodium pump activity (7) may also affect sodium concentrations available from Na^+–Ca^{++} exchange (Parker and Adams 1977).

At least a portion of the contractile-dependent Ca^{++} in heart muscle is in rapid equilibrium with extracellular Ca^{++} and is derived from superficial binding sites on the cell membrane. Two separate pathways of movement of superficial Ca^{++} are believed to be involved (Langer 1976, 1980; Parker and Adams 1977). The primary electrogenic route is associated with the previously discussed plateau phase of the action potential. An additional influx of Ca^{++} is linked with a Ca^{++}-Na^+ exchange across the sarcolemma. In this system, an increase in the amount of Na^+ at the interior surface of the cell membrane would activate a membrane carrier molecule that would translocate three Na^+ across the sarcolemma in an outward direction and in return carry one Ca^{++} into the cell. The Na^+-Ca^{++} exchange system is a bidirectional transporter, and during diastole it seems to move Ca^{++} into the interstitium, thus facilitating relaxation (Reuter 1985). A schematic representation of excitation-contraction coupling in mammalian heart muscle is shown in Fig. 23.3.

RELAXATION. During repolarization, Ca^{++} is actively sequestered by the sarcoplasmic reticulum, which avidly binds and stores myoplasmic Ca^{++} with affinity greater than troponin. Relaxation occurs as Ca^{++} moves to the sarcoplasmic reticulum from troponin binding sites on the myofibrils, and the cytoplasmic Ca^{++} concentration decreases below the threshold required to trigger actin-myosin cross-bridge formation (Fig. 23.3).

MAINTENANCE OF ELECTROLYTE GRADIENTS. There is a net influx of Na^+ and Ca^{++} and efflux of K^+ with each action potential. Membrane-bound enzymes that act as pumps to relocate ions and prevent their improper accumulation have been identified (Gadsby 1984). Sodium-potassium-activated adenosine triphosphatase (Na^+,K^+-ATPase) localized in the cell membrane propels Na^+ out of and K^+ into the cell, against their respective concentration gradients. Excess intracellular Ca^{++} is pumped out of the cell by systems believed to be localized in regions of the sarcoplasmic reticulum that are in close approximation to the sarcolemma (Fig. 23.3). A sarcolemmal Ca^{++}-ATPase also contributes to extrusion of Ca^{++}.

Although many aspects of the actual processes involved in excitation-contraction coupling are unresolved, the necessity of an adequate supply of superficial membrane-bound Ca^{++} in heart muscle is unequivocal. Superficial Ca^{++} sources are now known to be causally involved in the mechanism of action of many clinically useful drugs, including the digitalis glycosides.

DIGITALIS AND RELATED CARDIAC GLYCOSIDES. Digitalis and several closely allied chemicals are derived from the purple foxglove plant (*Digitalis purpurea*), other related species of the figwort family, and some plant species unrelated to digitalis. Medicinal use of plant extracts containing cardioactive principles has a long and colorful history, dating to ancient times of the Greeks and Romans.

Application of digitalis to modern medicine can be traced to 1785, when William Withering, a physician of Birmingham, England, reported his account of the therapeutic use of foxglove. This remarkable story starts with an old woman from Shropshire who for many years had concocted an herbal folk remedy purported to be efficacious in treating dropsy (edema). Although the remedy was a family secret and included at least 20 different herbs, Withering correctly ascribed beneficial therapeutic results to the foxglove ingredient. After 10 years of study, Withering was convinced of the therapeutic value of the plant and published his now classic monograph, "An Account of the Foxglove and Some of Its Medical Uses: With Practical Remarks on Dropsy and Other Diseases."

Withering recognized that only some types of dropsy were improved with digitalis, but he apparently failed to distinguish congestive heart failure from other edema-producing conditions. Because of the often pronounced diuretic response, the kidney was thought to be the primary target organ of foxglove; however, Withering stated, "It has the power over the motion of the heart, to a degree yet unobserved in any other medicine, and this power may be converted to salutary ends."

Subsequent studies by numerous investigators clearly identified the heart as the focus of digitalis action in congestive failure patients and designated a positive inotropic effect on the myocardium as the relevant mechanism of action. These agents also exert important antiarrhythmic action that has therapeutic application whether or not congestive failure is present. Thus the principal indications for therapeutic use in veterinary medicine are congestive failure and certain forms of cardiac dysrhythmias.

Chemistry and Sources. Chemical and structure-activity relationships of the digitalis glycosides are quite complex, but several basic similarities are retained in the different compounds. The nomenclature is interesting, since it is not derived from specific chemical structures but is based instead on botanical origins.

Official digitalis is the dried leaf of the purple foxglove plant; 100 mg of this material is equivalent to 1 USP Digitalis Unit. Three cardiac glycosides are derived from the leaves: digitoxin, which is used in clinical medicine, and the less well known gitoxin and gitalin. Digitoxin, digoxin (another glycoside used therapeutically), and gitoxin also can be extracted from the leaf of a related plant, *D. lanta,* the woolly foxglove. Strophanthidin and ouabain are important glycosides contained in the seeds of *Strophanthus* sp.; *S. gratus,* the source of ouabain, is an African tree. Acetylstrophanthidin is a semisynthetic derivative of strophanthidin used experimentally. Of toxicologic interest, several cardioactive glycosides are found in the skin of some toads (*Bufo vulgaris, B. maritimus*), in certain oleander plants, and in a large number of other unrelated botanical species.

Although 300 or more cardioactive principals of vegetable origin have been identified, the three compounds most important to veterinary therapeutics are digoxin, digitoxin, and ouabain. Because of considerable pharmacologic similarities between the different

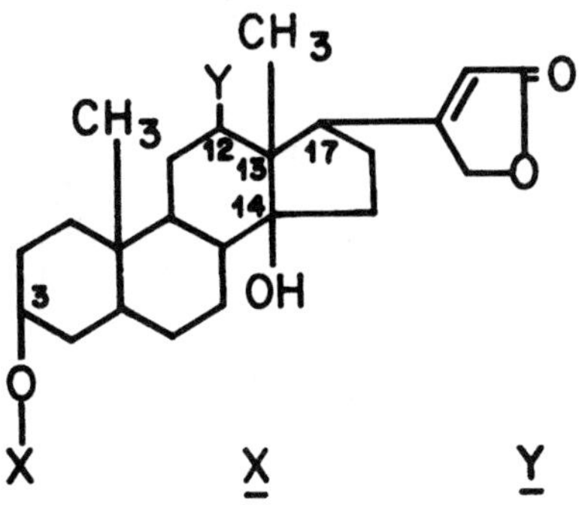

	X	Y
Digitoxigenin	H	H
Digitoxin	Digitoxose (3)	H
Digoxin	Digitoxose (3)	OH
Digoxigenin	H	OH

FIG. 23.4—Structural arrangements of digoxin and digitoxin and the aglycones digoxigenin and digitoxigenin.

glycosides, the collective term digitalis is used to designate the entire group rather than referring only to the dried leaf.

The term "glycoside" in general refers to a compound linked by an oxygen atom to a sugar molecule(s). Plant-derivative digitalis glycosides with the most intense pharmacologic activity consist of an aglycone (genin) moiety combined with one to four sugar molecules. Aglycones are structurally related to sterols, bile acids, and sex and adrenocorticosteroid hormones. The basic steroid-type nucleus is a cyclopentanoperhydrophenanthrene to which is attached an unsaturated lactone ring at carbon atom 17 (C-17). The sugar molecules usually are attached at C-3; they influence water solubility, cell penetrability, duration of action, and other pharmacokinetic characteristics.

Cardioactivity of the molecule resides principally in the aglycone moiety, but the positive myocardial actions of these entities are somewhat less potent and of briefer duration than the parent glycoside. In modern medicine, the pure glycosides are increasingly being used instead of the older powdered leaf or other impure admixtures that required biologic assay. Bioassay techniques depended on lethal potency of an unknown preparation in cats, frogs, and pigeons or emetic effects in pigeons. Pure glycosides can now be measured spectrophotometrically.

The structures of digitoxin, digoxin, and the aglycones digitoxigenin and digoxigenin are shown for comparative purposes in Fig. 23.4; some chemical aspects of several important compounds are summarized in Table 23.1.

Cardiovascular Effects. The therapeutic response to digitalis in congestive heart failure patients entails a

TABLE 23.1—Plant sources and chemical composition of selected digitalis glycosides

Plant	Glycoside	Sugar	Aglycone
Digitalis purpurea (leaf)	Digitoxin*	Digitoxose (3)	Digitoxigenin
	Gitoxin	Digitoxose (3)	Gitoxigenin
	Gitalin	Digitoxose (3)	Gitoxigenin hydrate
D. lanta (leaf)	Digitoxin*	Digitoxose (3)	Digitoxigenin
	Digoxin*	Digitoxose (3)	Digoxigenin
	Gitoxin	Digitoxose (3)	Gitoxigenin
Strophanthus kombé (seed)	Strophanthin	Glucose and cymarose	Strophanthidin
S. gratus (seed)	Ouabain* (G-Strophanthin)	Rhamnose	Ouabagenin (G-Strophanthidin)

Source: Moe and Farah 1975.
*Clinically important to veterinary medicine.

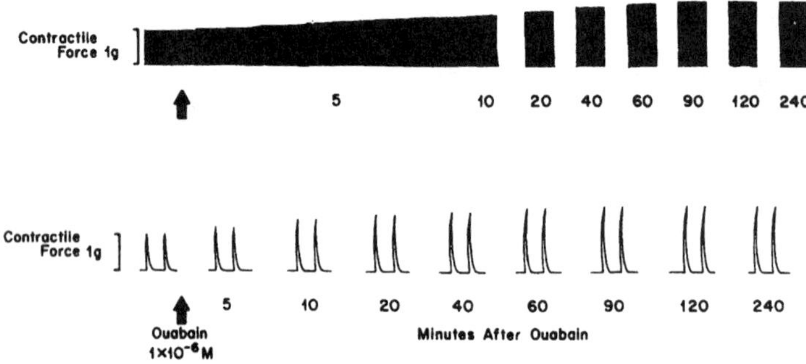

FIG. 23.5—Myographic recordings from a heart muscle before and after exposure to the cardiac glycoside ouabain. Top tracings were taken at a slow recording speed; bottom tracings show individual muscle contractions at designated intervals after addition of ouabain. Notice that contractile force increased by almost 100% and that this effect lasted for the 4-hour measurement period.

broad scope of hemodynamic adjustments: augmented myocardial contractility; increased cardiac output; diuresis and diminution of edema; control of cardiac arrhythmias; and reductions in blood volume, venous pressures, heart size, and heart rate. Improved myocardial contractility undoubtedly is the most important; it is the primary action on which other effects depend.

MYOCARDIAL CONTRACTILITY. The ability of cardiac glycosides to increase contractile vigor of the heart has been demonstrated in a multitude of experimental preparations. Heart muscle suspended at constant external length responds to digitalis with an increase in isometric systolic force; studied under isotonic conditions, muscle shortening is enhanced. Intravenous (IV) infusion of the drug augments intraventricular pressure development in intact subjects even when heart rate, venous return, and blood pressure are maintained constant by experimental means. These results validate a direct effect on contractile strength independent of changes in resting fiber length, heart rate, or afterload. A typical response of heart muscle to the cardiac glycoside ouabain is shown in Fig. 23.5.

The positive inotropic action of cardiac glycosides is particularly pronounced in the hypodynamic or failing heart. However, this should not be construed as evidence that digitalis selectively corrects the specific biochemical defect in the chronically failing heart. This defect has yet to be identified in a satisfactory manner. Digitalis, by increasing Ca^{++} availability in the myocardial fiber (see section on cellular mechanisms of inotropic action), increases contractility of the normal as well as the failing heart. Thus cardiac glycosides may increase contractile strength by way of a cellular pathway that bypasses or only partially involves the spontaneous defect (Aranow 1992).

CELLULAR MECHANISMS OF INOTROPIC ACTION. The mechanism of digitalis action that is helpful in congestive failure is a positive inotropic effect on the heart muscle. However, what is the cellular mechanism of action whereby cardiac glycosides enhance inotropy of the individual muscle fibers in heart failure patients (Feldman 1993)? Only portions of this question can be answered without controversy.

LACK OF DEPENDENCE ON ADRENERGIC MECHANISMS. The inotropic response to digitalis is not prevented by reserpine (which depletes endogenous catecholamines) or propranolol (which blocks β-adrenergic receptors). Digitalis drugs do not increase intracellular concentration of cyclic 3′,5′-adenosine monophosphate (cAMP), an effect closely associated with positive inotropic action of catecholamines (Ezrailson et al. 1977) (see Chap. 5). Thus a preponderance of data clearly has established that the positive inotropic action of digitalis does not depend on release of norepinephrine from adrenergic nerve terminals and that these two agents exert contractile effects through dissimilar receptors and cellular pathways.

CONTRACTILE PROTEINS. Cardiac glycosides do not appear to act by directly modifying energy production or storage, nor is there convincing evidence for improved energy utilization at the level of the contractile proteins and associated enzymes. Similarly, most studies indicate unremarkable effects of cardiac glycosides on isolated actomyosin and the troponin-tropomyosin complex. Thus an intact cell is a prerequisite to the inotropic action of digitalis, and considerable evidence linking this activity with ionic changes is now available.

INHIBITION OF NA^+,K^+-ATPASE. Total cellular Ca^{++} is increased by the glycosides; this net gain reflects an augmented Ca^{++} influx. However, phase 2 of the cardiac action potential, which depends partly on electrogenic influx of Ca^{++}, does not seem to be affected remarkably by therapeutic amounts of digitalis. These data have led investigators to propose an increased influx of Ca^{++} across the cell membrane in exchange for Na^+ as a mechanism of inotropic action of digitalis. This change in Ca^{++} movement as well as modifications of Na^+ and K^+ locations are explained by the well-known inhibitory effect of digitalis glycosides on the Na^+-K^+ pump of the sarcolemma (Fozzard and Sheets 1985; Katz 1985).

The Mg^{++}-dependent Na^+,K^+-ATPase of the cell membrane supplies energy for the active pumping of Na^+ outward and K^+ inward against their large concentration gradients (Fig. 23.3). Beginning with experiments on erythrocytes by Schatzmann (1953), the ability of cardiac glycosides to inhibit membrane transport of Na^+ and K^+ has been confirmed in several tissues, including the heart. The Na^+,K^+-ATPase is believed to be the cellular receptor for digitalis glycosides (Schwartz 1977; Akera and Ng 1991).

Inhibition of Na^+,K^+-ATPase results in progressive reduction of $(K^+)_i$ as the ability of the pump to transport K^+ inward and Na^+ outward progressively fails. A decrease in $(K^+)_i$ and/or an increase in $(K^+)_o$ reduces resting membrane potential to a less negative value, which can lead to increased automaticity and eventually impaired conduction and excitability. Inhibition of ATPase and resulting depletion of $(K^+)_i$ are responsible for many toxic arrhythmogenic activities of digitalis.

The inotropic effect involves activation of a Na^+-Ca^{++} exchange mechanism through accumulation of $(Na^+)_i$. Baker et al. (1969) demonstrated with the giant squid axon that an increase in $(Na^+)_i$ enhanced the uptake of Ca^{++} by a Na^+-Ca^{++} exchange process. This mechanism seems to be operative in other excitable tissues and has been evoked as the link between inhibition of Na^+,Ka^+-ATPase and digitalis inotropy in the heart (Langer 1977). The sequence of events can be visualized to include the following progression: digitalis interacts with and inhibits cell membrane Na^+,K^+-ATPase, outward pumping of Na^+ is slowed, $(Na^+)_i$ accumulates, increased $(Na^+)_i$ augments transmembrane exchange of intracellular Na^+ for extracellular Ca^{++}, $(Ca^{++})_i$ is increased, and Ca^{++} delivery to the contractile proteins is increased; thus the positive inotropic effect is gained. A schematic that illustrates the dominance of Na^+-K^+ exchange in the normal state and the putative augmentation of Na^+-Ca^{++} exchange after inhibition of ATPase by digitalis is shown in Fig. 23.6.

CARDIAC OUTPUT. Digitalis glycosides exert a fundamentally similar action on the normal and failing myocardium, an increase in contractility. However, changes in cardiac output are influenced by the functional status of the cardiovascular system at the time of digitalis administration.

NORMAL HEART. Output of the normal heart increases minimally and may even decrease slightly after treatment with digitalis (Braunwald 1985). Total peripheral resistance is increased by digitalis in the normal subject as a result of a centrally mediated increase in sympathetic vasomotor tone and direct vasoconstrictor effect. Impedance of the arterial circuit to ventricular ejection is thereby increased, which opposes the trend toward increased output produced by positive inotropic response to the drug. Increased outflow impedance and increased cardiac contractility tend to counteract each other, yielding little net change in cardiac output in normal populations.

FAILING HEART. The work capacity of the failing ventricle at any given end-diastolic volume or pressure is inadequate to generate a normal stroke volume (Fig. 23.7). The ejection fraction is diminished accordingly, which increases residual blood in the ventricle after systole (Moalic et al. 1993). If diastolic filling continues at a near normal rate, the ventricle will dilate to accommodate increased end-diastolic volume. After digitalization, the above processes are reversed. Digitalis-increased contractile vigor of the heart muscle augments work capacity of the ventricle at any given end-diastolic filling pressure, as illustrated in Fig. 23.7, where ventricular function curves derived in the pre-failure state (normal) are compared with curves derived from congestive failure patients prior to and after digitalis therapy. Digitalis shifts the complete ventricular function curve upward in the direction of improved contractility (Mason 1973; Braunwald 1985). Systolic emptying is now more complete, and residual ventricular volume is diminished. Cardiac output increases and

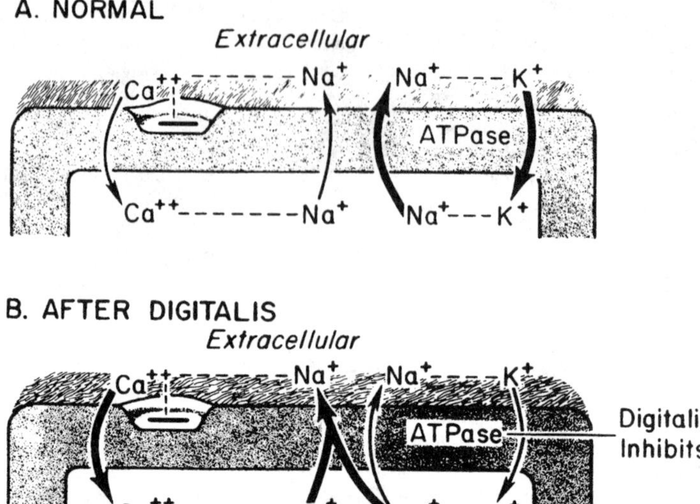

FIG. 23.6—Schematic representation of a proposed mechanism for the positive inotropic action of cardiac glycosides. Inhibition of Na^+,K^+–ATPase (sodium pump) by digitalis results in increased intracellular concentrations of sodium available for exchange with calcium. Heavy arrows designate the dominant pathway of ion exchange during normal conditions (A) and after inhibition by digitalis of Na^+,K^+–ATPase (B). (After Langer 1976; from Parker and Adams 1977.)

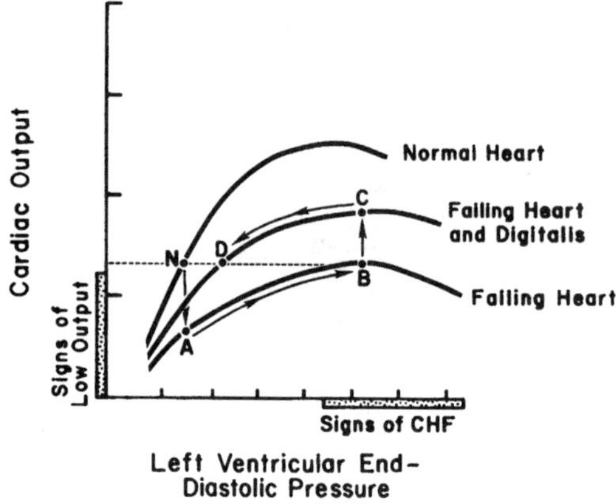

FIG. 23.7—Diagrammatic representation of how changes in left ventricular filling influence cardiac output by the Frank-Starling mechanism in a normal heart and in a failing heart before and after digitalis. The points N to D represent in sequence: N–A, normal cardiac output falls to A because of initial contractile depression from congestive heart failure (CHF); A–B, shift to higher end-diastolic filling and thus higher cardiac output in accord with the Frank-Starling law; B–C, increase in contractility after digitalization; C–D, reduction in use of Frank-Starling compensation, which digitalis allows. N, B, and D: identical cardiac output on the vertical axis but achieved at different end-diastolic filling pressure on the horizontal axis. Levels of cardiac output and end-diastolic filling associated with signs of low output (e.g., fatigue) or CHF (e.g., dyspnea, edema) are represented by the dotted areas. (Modeled after Mason 1973.)

size of the heart is reduced as ventricular filling volume is lowered.

Subsequent hemodynamic adjustments evoke other responses that contribute to maintenance of improved cardiac output in the congestive failure patient; e.g., sympathetically mediated vasoconstriction and its attending increase in peripheral vascular resistance are already in progress in these individuals as part of the compensatory response to their pathophysiologic condition; increased impedance to ventricular ejection is in force. After digitalis, however, the pronounced augmentation of myocardial contractility and stroke volume set into motion a reflex withdrawal of vasomotor tone. This in turn evokes peripheral vasodilation, reduced peripheral resistance, and diminished outflow impedance. This sequence of events continues to dominate as peripheral perfusion and tissue oxygenation improve, and it more than compensates for the direct vasoconstrictor effect of digitalis. The increase in cardiac output persists as long as the state of myocardial compensation prevails.

CARDIAC ENERGY METABOLISM. Early studies provided evidence that the positive inotropic response to cardiac glycosides was unique, when contrasted to catecholamine activity, because digitalis increased contractile strength without a commensurate increase in oxygen consumption. Later studies with nonfailing muscle, however, showed that cardiac glycosides increased oxygen consumption proportionately with increased contractile force (Lee and Klaus 1971).

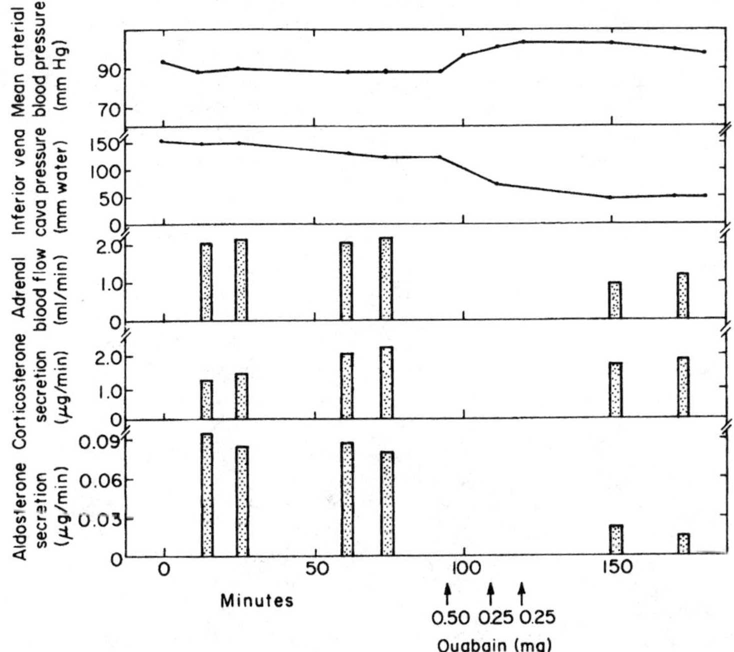

FIG. 23.8—The effects of IV ouabain injection (total dose 0.05 mg/kg) in an 8-year-old, 20 kg male Pointer with naturally occurring congestive heart failure. Following injection, mean arterial blood pressure increased from 88 mm Hg to a maximum of 110 mm Hg, and inferior vena cava pressure fell from a control value of 150-140 mm water to a minimum of 38 mm water; these changes started within 5 minutes after beginning the ouabain injection and reached a maximum 40-50 minutes postinjection. Following drug administration, there was also a marked fall in adrenal corticosterone and aldosterone secretion (Carpenter et al. 1962).

These seemingly contradictory data can be reconciled by comparing the cardiodynamics of digitalis in normal and failing hearts. The heart with a normal ventricular volume responds to digitalis with increase in oxygen consumption commensurate with increase in contractility. Increased oxygen consumption is the direct result of increased contractility, in accordance with the concept that myocardial oxygen demand (MVO_2) is influenced directly by the inotropic state, heart rate, and wall tension. Ventricular wall tension is directly proportional to ventricular pressure and radius (tension $\approx$ pressure $\times$ radius; Laplace relation); tension will decrease if either pressure or radius is reduced. In the failing and dilated heart, reduction in cardiac size secondary to the inotropic action of digitalis therapy leads to a significant reduction in wall tension, which in turn leads to decreased MVO_2.

That is, increased contractility at constant fiber length increases oxygen consumption (response of normal heart); however, decreased fiber length reduces wall tension and thus oxygen consumption (response of dilated heart). If the latter processes dominate enough in the failing heart to yield a net reduction in oxygen consumption in the presence of positive inotropic action of digitalis, this agent can indeed increase mechanical efficiency of the failing heart.

BLOOD PRESSURE. Adjustments in blood pressure after cardiac glycoside therapy are secondary to cardiodynamic improvement in the congestive failure patient, and systemic pressure tends to normalize (Fig. 23.8).

CARDIAC RATE AND RHYTHM. The principal effects of digitalis therapy on heart rate and rhythmicity in congestive failure patients are a decrease in sinus rate and a slowing of atrioventricular (AV) impulse conduction. These responses are gained by complex mechanisms involving direct action on cardiac fibers and, especially, readjustments in autonomic nervous system traffic to the heart (Gillis and Quest 1980; Watanabe 1985).

SYMPATHETIC TONE. Reflex sinus tachycardia is not an uncommon finding as part of the compensatory effort in congestive failure. Circulatory improvement after digitalization tends to remove the stimuli responsible for reflex increments in heart rate, allowing sinus rate to return toward normal. Thus slowing of heart rate by digitalis is mainly secondary to hemodynamic improvement and the resulting reflex decrease in sympathetic tone and increase in vagal tone to the heart.

VAGAL DEPENDENT ACTION. The portion of the digitalis-induced decrease in heart rate and slowing of AV conduction that is blocked by atropine is referred to as the vagal-dependent or atropine-sensitive action of the cardiac glycosides. By releasing ACh, vagal discharge evokes characteristic effects in the atria: slowing of sinus rate, decreased action potential duration and refractory period, and slowed impulse conduction. Cholinergic stimulation also slows impulse conduction in the AV node but lengthens the refractory period in this tissue. Thus vagal discharge can slow sinus rate and exacerbate atrial tachyarrhythmias but can effectively slow AV impulse conduction at the same time. Digitalis, by evoking vagal-dependent actions, can accomplish similar effects.

The vagal component of cardiac glycoside action has been attributed to at least three mechanisms: direct stimulation of vagal centers in the brain, sensitization of carotid sinus baroreceptors to blood pressure, and enhancement at the myocardial level of the pacemaker response to ACh (Gillis and Quest 1980).

EXTRAVAGAL ACTIONS. Extravagal actions are unmasked by pretreatment with atropine or large doses of digitalis that overwhelm indirect (nervous system) effects. In the atropinized or denervated heart, the ability of digitalis to slow AV conduction is somewhat reduced compared to intact hearts. Duration of the atrial refractory period, although abbreviated by vagal action, is actually prolonged by digitalis after atropine. Direct effects are mediated in part by disruption of cellular electrolyte gradients associated with ATPase inhibition. A portion of the nonvagal effect is reflected by an antagonism of the cardiac response to adrenergic stimulation; e.g., the facilitatory effect of sympathetic stimulation on pacemaker discharge and AV conduction is reduced in dogs by acetyldigoxin (Mendez et al. 1961a,b). This activity has been designated as a sympatholytic or antiadrenergic action of digitalis. Paradoxically, toxic doses of digitalis may also increase sympathetic nerve traffic to the heart (Gillis and Quest 1980; Watanabe 1985).

BIOELECTRIC CHANGES IN THE HEART. As stated, the principal rhythm adjustments beneficial to the patient treated with digitalis are slowing of sinus rate and AV conduction, which are mediated by direct and, especially, indirect mechanisms. Direct and indirect electrophysiologic effects of digitalis can be demonstrated throughout the heart (Gillis and Quest 1980). In the following discussion and in Table 23.2, only the more important aspects of digitalis-evoked actions on electrophysiologic activities of the heart are summarized. Remember that the positive inotropic response to digitalis can occur before transmembrane potential changes are produced.

EXCITABILITY. The reduced intracellular K^+ and increased intracellular Na^+ resulting from inhibition of Na^+,K^+-ATPase yield a partial depolarization of the cell; i.e., negativity of the cell interior is diminished. The resulting decrease in diastolic potential brings this value closer to threshold, thus tending to enhance excitability. Increased excitability can be observed in atria and ventricles with a small dose of digitalis; however, excitability becomes depressed with progressively larger amounts of the drug as diastolic depolarization progresses beyond a critical limit.

AUTOMATICITY. Pacemaker cells are characterized by phase 4 spontaneous depolarization, which lowers diastolic potential to the threshold potential required for activation of phase 0, thereby firing automatically (see Chap. 24). Therapeutic doses of cardiac glycosides produce a decrease in the slope of spontaneous depolarization of the sinoatrial pacemaker, which yields a reduced firing rate. This effect, however, is secondary to increased vagal tone and decreased sympathetic tone. After pretreatment with atropine, or with relatively high doses of digitalis, the nonvagal effects dominate, and an increase in automaticity is observed; this response is prevalent in the specialized conducting systems of atria and, especially, ventricles. A typical transmembrane potential recording of a subsidiary pacemaker cell prior to and after digitalis is shown in Fig. 23.9.

Increased automaticity evoked by cardiac glycosides is due to an accelerated rate of spontaneous diastolic depolarization (Fig. 23.9). The normally latent pacemaker activities of cells within the ventricular conducting system are thereby magnified, leading to ectopic ventricular beats as an important early sign of digitalis toxicity. In contrast, muscle fibers in atria and ventricles can be depolarized to the extent of inexcitability without demonstrating spontaneous impulse generation. If excitability of ventricular muscle falls below normal concomitantly with increased frequency of ectopic impulses from specialized conduction fibers, the tendency for ventricular fibrillation is promoted.

The clinical significance of the unusual "delayed afterdepolarizations" that can be seen with digitalis toxicity is not completely resolved. These secondary depolarizations of the transmembrane potential initially are subthreshold and appear spontaneously during diastole after a usual action potential. The afterdepolarizations can reach threshold as toxicity worsens; the resulting extrasystoles contribute to ectopic arrhythmias associated with digitalis intoxication.

IMPULSE CONDUCTION AND REFRACTORY PERIODS. Conduction in atrial and ventricular muscle fibers may be enhanced slightly by low doses of digitalis if excitability is increased. However, the dominant effect of digitalis on impulse conduction is to slow conduction velocity by both vagal and nonvagal mechanisms. This response is particularly prevalent in the AV transmission system and contributes importantly to the beneficial effects of digitalis in controlling ventricular rate during atrial fibrillation and flutter.

TABLE 23.2—Characteristic effects of digitalis on electrophysiologic properties of the heart

Electrophysiologic property	Cardiac region	Effects	Response
Automaticity	SA node	Decreases as a result of vagal-dependent actions and sympathic withdrawal (may increase after atrophine)	Decreases sinus rate
	Atrial specialized conducting fibers	Little change; increases with toxicity	Increases ectopic pacemakers
	AV junction tissues	Variable; increases with larger doses	Increases AV junctional rhythms
	Purkinje fibers	Variable; increases with larger doses	Increases ectopic pacemakers
	Atrial and ventricular muscle	Usually little change; rarely increases with toxic doses	
Excitability	Atrial and ventricular muscle	Variable; progressively decreases with larger doses; severe decrease with toxicity	
	Purkinje fibers	Variable; progressively decreases with larger doses	
Conduction	Atrial and ventricular muscle	Increases slightly; decreases with larger doses	Promotes atrial fibrillation
	AV junctional tissues	Decreases as a result of vagal-dependent actions; progressively decreases with toxicity	Decreases ventricular rate in atrial fibrillation; AV block
	Purkinje fibers	Decreases; further decrease with toxicity	Promotes ventricular reentry forms of arrhythmias
Refractoriness	Atrium	Decreases as a result of vagal-dependent actions; (increase after atropine)	Promotes atrial fibrillation
	Ventricle	Decreases	Favors reentry forms of arrhythmias
	AV junctional tissues	Increases as a result of vagal-dependent actions	Contributes to ventricular rate decreases in atrial fibrillation; AV block with toxicity
	Purkinje fibers	Increases; progressively decreases with larger doses	Favors reentry forms of arrhythmias

Note: SA = sinoatrial; AV = atrioventricular.

Refractory periods also are influenced by cardiac glycosides through direct and indirect mechanisms. Vagal-dependent actions in the intact animal shorten the refractory period of atrial fibers, which tends to exacerbate atrial fibrillatory rhythms. In contrast, the refractory period of the AV conduction system is prolonged markedly by the vagal mechanisms. Digitalis shortens the refractory period in the ventricle, which contributes to reentrant arrhythmias (Table 23.2).

COMBINED EFFECTS DURING ATRIAL FIBRILLATION AND FLUTTER. During atrial fibrillation, the ventricular rate is rapid and dysrhythmic as a result of rapid but irregular transmission of impulses through the AV node. This contributes further to heart failure syndrome by promoting incomplete ventricular filling and ejection. Because digitalis prolongs the refractory period and delays impulse conduction through the AV junction, the ventricle will be bombarded by fewer impulses effectively traversing the junction. Thus the ventricular rate is adjusted to a slower, more physiologic level (Meijler 1985).

Similar benefits are gained during atrial flutter. Digitalis can convert this rhythm to atrial fibrillation (or increase the frequency of the latter) by vagal-dependent mechanisms, evoking a reduction in the atrial refractory period. Ventricular rate is still decreased, however, through prolonged AV refractoriness and slowed impulse conduction. Conversion of atrial flutter to fibrillation by digitalis is viewed optimistically because ventricular rate is controlled more easily during fibrillation than during flutter.

EFFECTS ON THE ELECTROCARDIOGRAM. The multiplicity of electrophysiologic effects of cardiac glycosides in myocardial tissues can be expressed as equally complex changes in the electrocardiogram (ECG). Most types of conduction disturbances and dysrhythmias detected in diseased animals can be reproduced in normal individuals by the cardiac glycosides. Most of these changes are more important to diagnosis of digitalis toxicosis than to therapy.

Congestive failure patients with sinus tachycardia or other supraventricular tachyarrhythmias usually demonstrate return toward more normal ECG patterns after digitalization. Rapid ventricular rates associated with atrial fibrillation or flutter should be reduced as the AV depressing action of digitalis is manifested.

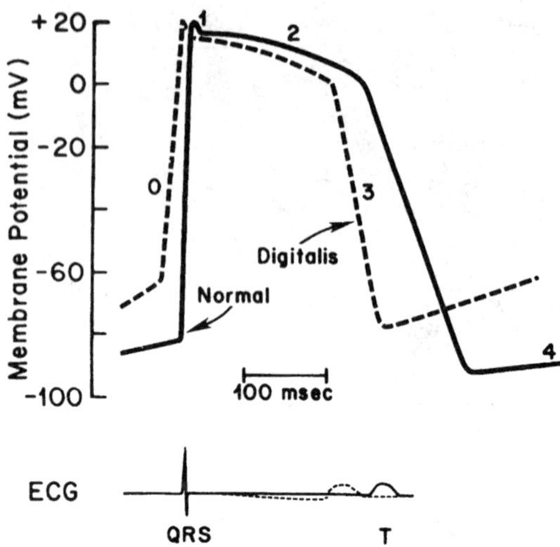

FIG. 23.9—Electrophysiologic effects of digitalis on transmembrane potential of a subsidiary pacemaker cell. Digitalis (*a*) decreases (less negative) the maximal diastolic potential, (*b*) decreases the maximal rate of depolarization of phase 0, V_{max}, and (*c*) enhances automaticity by increasing the slope of phase 4 spontaneous depolarization.(*a*) and (*b*) lead to decreased conduction velocity and, in conjunction with (*c*), can lead to arrhythmias of both impulse formation and impulse conduction. (Modeled after Mason et al. 1971.)

Prolonged PR intervals, reflecting delayed AV conduction, are relatively common ECG features of digitalized dogs. Conversely, a lengthened PR interval is not necessarily a prerequisite for the therapeutic response. Some cardiologists believe that prolongation of the PR interval can be a borderline sign of digitalis toxicity (Tilley 1979).

Different types of ECG abnormalities can appear if therapeutic response to digitalis degenerates into intoxication. The following progression of ECG signs has been recognized as evidence of digoxin action (Detweiler 1977): (1) signs occasionally observed in normal dogs but also characteristic of digoxin effects (first degree AV block or AV block with dropped beats), (2) signs unlikely to occur spontaneously in normal resting dogs (sinus bradycardia less than 50 beats/min or sinus tachycardia exceeding 200 beats/min), and (3) signs not occurring in normal dogs (AV dissociation, paroxysmal atrial tachycardia with or without block, ectopic atrial beats, fusion beats, intraventricular block, or ventricular ectopic beats).

KIDNEYS AND DIURESIS. Compensatory mechanisms that participate in an attempt to restore blood flow in congestive failure include reflex increases in sympathetic vasoconstrictor tone. Arteriolar constriction in the kidney is particularly crucial because diminished renal blood flow reduces glomerular filtration rate, resulting in sodium and water retention. Renal underperfusion also activates a kidney-dependent humoral mechanism that further promotes salt and water reabsorption. This sequence involves the following progressive pathway: diminished cardiac output, hypotension, baroreceptor reflexes, increased sympathetic activity, renal arteriolar constriction, reduced renal flow, release of renin, increased formation of angiotensin, increased release of aldosterone, sodium retention, water retention, and blood volume expansion.

Increased blood volume tends to increase cardiac output; however, a detrimental consequence is increased interstitial fluid volume, which promotes edema formation. As blood volume expands and intravascular pressures increase, likelihood for edema increases proportionately. Edema forms in the lungs and more peripheral tissue respectively if left and right ventricular failure progressively worsens.

After digitalization, the above processes are reversed. Reflex vasoconstriction withdraws as cardiac output and hemodynamics are improved; renal blood flow and glomerular filtration rate increase and stimuli for increased release of aldosterone are diminished. A remarkable fall in aldosterone secretion can be measured after digitalization in the dog with naturally occurring congestive failure (Fig. 23.8). Profuse diuresis results as salt and water retention by the kidneys is decreased. Diuresis and a lowering of capillary hydrostatic pressure move tissue water from the interstitial compartment into the vascular space, providing relief from edema. Diuresis is not a prominent feature of digitalis therapy if edema does not accompany the congestive failure syndrome. Similarly, digitalis does not evoke diuresis if edema is not cardiogenic. Thus the diuretic response to digitalis is secondary to circulatory improvement and is not from a direct effect on the kidney.

Extracirculatory Effects. Cardiac glycosides can affect cellular functions throughout the body, apparently by inhibiting the ubiquitous Na^+,K^+-ATPase; e.g., these agents can affect skeletal muscle function, thyroid gland activity, hematologic parameters, and numerous other functions. Such activities are believed to have little therapeutic importance except for overt toxicosis and generally require quantities of the drug in excess of those that should be administered.

Vomiting reactions after digitalis are due mainly to a central action and occur even after parenteral administration in the eviscerated animal. Both the chemoreceptor trigger zone and the medullary emetic center seem to be involved; local irritation of the gastric mucosa also may participate in the emetic response after oral administration.

Administration of a subtherapeutic dose of digitalis through a catheter in one renal artery results in sodium and water diuresis only in that kidney. This and other related findings were interpreted as evidence that Na^+,K^+-ATPase is involved in urine concentration mechanisms and that by inhibiting this enzyme, digitalis could evoke a direct diuretic effect on the kidney

(Robinson 1972). However, this experimental observation is believed to be unimportant in relation to diuresis achieved by circulatory improvement in congestive failure patients after effective digitalization.

Pharmacokinetics. In general, absorption across biologic membranes and the extent of protein binding and biotransformation of the individual glycosides are related directly to their lipid solubility and thus inversely to their polarity. The number of hydroxyl groups on the steroid nucleus basically determines polarity. Digitoxin has only one steroidal hydroxyl group and is therefore relatively nonpolar; it is well absorbed after oral administration, is highly bound to plasma proteins, and undergoes metabolic degradation. Digoxin, with two hydroxyl groups, is absorbed somewhat less effectively than digitoxin; the former also undergoes less protein binding and biotransformation. Ouabain, with five hydroxyl groups, is absorbed inefficiently across the gastrointestinal (GI) mucosa; it is not bound extensively to plasma proteins and is excreted unchanged by the kidneys (Moe and Farah 1975).

The small intestine is the principal site of digitalis absorption after oral administration, but the rate and extent of this process vary with different compounds and their formulations. Ouabain is absorbed inefficiently after the oral route, only 5-10% in dogs and cats. Absorption of digoxin and digitoxin after oral administration of an elixir usually is uniform, up to 75-90%, with peak serum concentrations attained in 45-60 minutes (Krasula et al. 1976). The peak serum value is smaller and occurs somewhat later (90 minutes) when the tablet form is used. Depending on the pharmaceutical methods used in formulating tablets, absorption of digitalis glycosides can be erratic and inefficient to the extent that therapeutically useful serum concentrations are not gained.

After IV administration, the maximal positive inotropic responses to digitoxin and digoxin were obtained within 60 minutes after injection (Hamlin et al. 1971). There is an initial fall in serum concentration as the drug mixes in the vascular compartment and distributes through the tissues; a slower exponential decline follows. Biologic half-life values for digitalis glycosides in dogs remain somewhat uncertain because of variable results obtained from laboratory to laboratory and even within the same one. Breznock (1973) reported that the plasma half-life value for digoxin and digitoxin was 38.9 hours and 48.6 hours respectively. In a later study, Breznock (1975) reported almost the opposite, 55.9 hours for digoxin and 37.9 hours for digitoxin. Other approximate values include digoxin, 27 hours (Barr et al. 1972), 30 hours (Hahn 1977), 24 hours (Doherty 1973), and 31 hours (De Rick et al. 1978); digitoxin, 14 hours (De Rick et al. 1978), and 21 hours (Beck 1969). Differences can be attributed to analytical problems, perhaps, but remarkable interpatient variability is also observed; e.g., the half-life for digoxin in dogs after therapy for 13 days varied from 14.4 to 46.5 hours (De Rick et al. 1978). These variables strengthen the need for adoption of individual dosage regimens depending on the patient's response.

Approximately 70-90% of digitoxin can be bound to plasma proteins, whereas digoxin is bound perhaps 25% (Breznock 1973). There is some biotransformation of digitoxin by the liver, whereas urinary excretion seems to be the more important route of elimination for digoxin. Digitalis glycosides and their biotransformation products can follow an enterohepatic cycle in which compounds are excreted by the liver into bile and some parent glycoside and metabolites are subsequently reabsorbed. The importance of this cyclic pathway varies from one species to another. In humans, digitoxin undergoes relatively slow hepatic biotransformation and is extensively recycled and slowly eliminated by both renal and biliary routes; the plasma half-life may be as long as 5-7.5 days. Digoxin undergoes insignificant metabolism in humans and is minimally recycled and eliminated mainly by renal excretion; the half-life is generally 1.5-3 days. In dogs, both digoxin and digitoxin undergo some hepatic biotransformation, but their recycling is less important and their biologic half-life values are shorter than in humans.

Cardiac glycosides are not concentrated selectively in the heart but are distributed in numerous organs. Highest concentrations, as with many drugs, are found in excretory tissues such as liver, bile, intestinal tract, and kidneys. Moderate concentrations are localized in lungs, spleen, and heart, while lower concentrations are found in blood, skeletal muscle, and nervous system.

Digitalis Toxicity

PLASMA CONCENTRATIONS. Development of an accurate radioimmunoassay for measuring quantities of digoxin and digitoxin in biologic fluids is an important advancement in the field of pharmacology. The clinical application of this method permits correlation of serum concentrations of the drugs with therapeutic or toxic effects (Haber 1985).

Digitoxin plasma concentrations of 14-26 ng/mL are considered to be within the therapeutic range in humans, whereas values higher than 34 ng/mL are considered toxic. Therapeutic concentrations of digitoxin in dogs with spontaneous cardiac failure are not available, but values of 26-77 ng/mL are associated with signs of toxicity; plasma concentrations less than 15 ng/mL are nontoxic in normal dogs. In humans, therapeutic and toxic plasma concentrations of digoxin usually are set at 0.8-1.6 ng/mL and greater than 2.4 ng/mL respectively (Moe and Farah 1975). Similar numbers have been derived from studies with animals; e.g., digoxin plasma concentrations of 0.5-2 ng/mL were nontoxic in horses (Button et al. 1980c); 2.3 ng/mL were not toxic in cats (Ericksen et al. 1980). Plasma digoxin concentrations up to 2.5 ng/mL were reported to be essentially nontoxic in healthy dogs and in dogs with spontaneous cardiac failure; importantly, values from 0.8 to 1.9 ng/mL may have been therapeutically effective in the latter group. Concentrations of digoxin greater than 2.5-3 ng/mL were associated with increased probability of toxicosis in these animals (De Rick et al. 1978).

The acute toxic IV dose of digoxin in dogs was determined in one study as approximately 0.177 mg/kg (Beck 1969). Subacute digoxin toxicosis could be induced and maintained in healthy Beagle dogs by an IV loading dose of 0.125-0.150 mg/kg given in increments at 0, 1, 4, and 24 hours, followed by a daily IV maintenance dose of 0.015-0.025 mg/kg (Fillmore and Detweiler 1973; Teske et al. 1976). Signs of toxicity were generally mild or absent when serum digoxin concentrations were less than 2.5 ng/mL. Moderate signs of intoxication were associated with concentrations of 2.5-6 ng/mL, whereas severe toxicosis and some deaths occurred when levels exceeded 6 ng/mL. The highest digoxin concentrations were associated with mild hypothermia (0.6-1.7° C reduction), increased blood urea nitrogen (BUN), and increased serum creatinine. The unexpected increase in serum creatinine and BUN concentrations was interpreted as evidence that digoxin toxicity compromised renal function.

CLINICAL SIGNS. Digitalis intoxication is characterized by several clinical signs varying from mild GI upset to chronic weight loss and life-threatening arrhythmias (Detweiler 1977; Tilley 1979). Initial anorexia and loose stools are common side effects; if they do not progressively worsen, a reduction in dose may not be necessary. Vomiting after IV administration of cardiac glycosides is a relatively common reaction and usually not cause for alarm. Vomiting in dogs receiving oral digitalis preparations is viewed more seriously, especially if protracted diarrhea is an accompaniment; these individuals should be examined for additional evidence of toxicity. GI disturbances are certainly troublesome and may debilitate the patient; however, the lethal outcome of digitalis intoxication is due to cardiac arrhythmias.

A variety of abnormalities can appear in the ECG as digitalis toxicity develops. The reduced sinus rate and slowed AV conduction attained with digitalis therapy can progress to incomplete or complete heart block with dropped beats and ST segment changes as intoxication supervenes. AV block in turn may progress to junctional escape rhythms and ventricular premature systoles. If an extra QRS complex recurs after each regular systole, then digitalis has evoked ventricular bigeminy (coupled ventricular systoles). Ventricular bigeminal rhythm can appear prior to, with, or after development of other arrhythmias that may be associated with digitalis intoxication. Paroxysmal ventricular or atrial tachycardia with block and multifocal premature ventricular systoles are further evidence of serious cardiac disturbances. Occurrence of these or any other important ECG abnormalities necessitates complete withdrawal of digitalis therapy; treatment with smaller doses should not be instituted until the ECG is free of such arrhythmias.

Large therapeutic and toxic doses of digitalis drugs have been associated with various neurologic disturbances in humans, including central nervous system depression, ataxia, psychotic episodes, mental confusion, restlessness, hallucinations, delirium, and coma. These problems are not commonly detected in dogs receiving digitalis, but their presence could be masked by the generalized weakness and malaise that may accompany cardiac toxicity.

Species differences in sensitivity to acute toxic effects of digitalis glycosides were reviewed by Detweiler (1967). The relative median lethal dose in several species, taking the cat as unity, are: cat, 1; rabbit, 2; various frogs, 28; various toads, >400; and rat, 671. Resistance to digitalis toxicity seems to reside in the heart and may be a reflection of the relative sensitivity of the Na^+,K^+-ATPase to glycoside inhibition.

ELECTROLYTE INVOLVEMENT. Cardiac toxicity of digitalis is affected by availability of electrolytes, especially K^+ and Ca^{++}. Potassium has considerable influence on arrhythmias and conduction disturbances evoked by digitalis but less effect on inotropic activity of the drug. In essence, reduced K^+ potentiates digitalis arrhythmogenicity, whereas excess K^+ antagonizes arrhythmogenic activity. The antiarrhythmic activity of K^+ in digitalis intoxication is probably related to direct effects of K^+ and an inhibition by the cation of glycoside binding to the Na^+,K^+-ATPase. The intracellular-extracellular ratio of K^+ seems to be a primary determinant of the interaction between this ion and digitalis rather than interstitial concentrations of K^+ alone. Digitalis-induced dysrhythmia can occur in the presence of normal K^+ plasma concentration because of the intracellular depletion of this cation that accompanies Na^+,K^+-ATPase inhibition (Rosen 1985).

Intoxication with digitalis can be precipitated by intervals of hypoxemia, hypomagnesemia, disturbances in acid-based balance, and hypercalcemia. Digitalis cardiac toxicosis provoked by hypoxia and acidosis may be due in part to further depletion of myocardial K^+. Hypokalemia can be secondary to malnutrition, corticosteroid therapy, hemodialysis, and too vigorous use of diuretics that do not spare K^+. All these factors should be considered when a differential diagnosis is made between an absolute digitalis overdosage and a relative overdosage caused by K^+ disturbances.

Cardiac actions of Ca^{++} are similar in certain ways to those evoked by digitalis in this tissue, and there is considerable concern by clinicians that excess Ca^{++} augments digitalis intoxication. In canine experiments a synergistic or additive interaction between Ca^{++} and digitalis could be demonstrated with concentrations of each agent that were toxic or near toxic even when given alone (Lown et al. 1960). In an effort to exploit Ca^{++}-digitalis interaction, Ca^{++} chelating agents such as ethylenediaminetetraacetic acid (EDTA) and sodium citrate have been used to lower serum Ca^{++} and thereby control digitalis-induced arrhythmias. Whether the antiarrhythmic action of chelating agents under these circumstances are specific or nonspecific remains unclear.

The divalent cation magnesium (Mg^{++}) depresses cardiac contractility and excitability when present in excessively high concentrations. This substance has only a transient and inconstant protective effect against digitalis arrhythmias, but there is some evidence that Mg^{++} depletion may sensitize the heart to cardiac glycosides (Lown et al. 1960).

TREATMENT. Although radioimmunoassay techniques can distinguish obviously subtherapeutic and toxic plasma concentrations of digitalis, considerable overlap occurs; a therapeutic concentration in one patient may be toxic to another. Clinical experience and judgment must still be exercised when digitalis intoxication is differentiated from exacerbation of cardiac failure with its attending dysrhythmias.

When digitalis intoxication is diagnosed, the first procedure is to withdraw glycoside therapy; the patient's progress should then be followed closely with frequent ECG monitoring. These conservative measures in conjunction with cage rest often are effective in controlling cardiac arrhythmias and other signs of intoxication; however, appropriate therapy should be instituted if arrhythmias worsen or fail to revert spontaneously.

Potassium chloride (KCl) has been administered in an attempt to increase plasma K^+ concentrations to upper limits of the normal range and thereby suppress glycoside arrhythmias. Conversely, if plasma K^+ is already high in the digitalis-intoxicated dog, administration of exogenous K^+ can actually cause further deterioration of ECG patterns. Obviously, considerable care should be exerted when K^+ therapy is employed in managing digitalis toxicity. In dogs, the dosage schedule for KCl has included 0.6-1 g orally as the initial dose, followed by 0.3-0.5 g every 1-2 hours for 2 doses, and continued at 4-hour intervals as necessary to control arrhythmias (Detweiler 1977). Slow IV infusion of KCl with frequent monitoring of the ECG and serum K^+ concentrations may be attempted (Ettinger and Suter 1970). However, too rapid an infusion of potassium salts may precipitate other arrhythmias, including ventricular fibrillation.

Cholestyramine Resin, USP, is an exchange resin that binds glycoside within the digestive tract; it has been used experimentally in attempts to interrupt the enterohepatic cycle and thereby hasten elimination of the digitalis compound. The use of specific antiglycoside antibodies is another therapy (Haber 1985; Kurowski et al. 1992). Agents such as Mg^{++}, procainamide, quinidine, EDTA, sodium citrate, saturated lactones, and salts of canrenoate have received little clinical use in animals. Of the antiarrhythmic agents, lidocaine, propranolol, and, especially, phenytoin are the most useful in controlling digitalis-induced arrhythmias (see Chap. 24). Atropine may be helpful in cases with severe sinus bradycardia. In the presence of AV block, antiarrhythmic agents and K^+ therapy should be avoided. Use of antiarrhythmic interventions so that the dose of digitalis can be increased in the hope of attaining a larger inotropic response is dangerous and unwarranted. Quinidine may actually cause an increase in plasma concentrations of digoxin (see Chap. 24).

Therapeutic Indications for Digitalis

CONGESTIVE HEART FAILURE. The most important indication for digitalis therapy in veterinary medicine, as in human medicine, is congestive heart failure. However, while there are considerable data available from experimental studies in animals and clinical studies in humans, there is remarkably less information about clinical use of digitalis in animals with spontaneous heart disease. Accordingly, controversy exists relative to the actual survival benefits of digitalis glycosides in the long-term therapeutic management of cardiac disease in animal patients (Hamlin et al. 1973; Patterson et al. 1973). Nevertheless, many, if not most, clinicians and cardiologists believe firmly that digitalis remains a mainstay of therapy for congestive heart failure (Braunwald 1985).

In a study of 10 large-breed dogs with idiopathic congestive cardiomyopathy, Kittleson et al. (1985a) reported that only 4 dogs showed echocardiographic evidence of a positive inotropic response to digoxin (0.22 mg/m^2 body surface area, twice a day). The average survival time for the 4 digoxin-responsive patients was almost 10 months, and 3 of these lived for 2-7 years. Survival time of the 6 nonresponders ranged only from 1 to 12 weeks. These studies suggest that only a portion of large dogs with congestive cardiomyopathy respond to digoxin but that survival may be prolonged in this subset of patients. Alternatively, as the authors point out, perhaps the 4 responsive dogs simply had reversible heart disease and with the aid of digoxin therapy reverted to normal function. These types of clinical pharmacologic studies are needed in veterinary medicine, and they should be expanded to include larger numbers of patients and drug withdrawal study periods.

Cardiac glycosides are indicated in congestive failure irrespective of whether it is predominantly of the left ventricle, right ventricle, or both. Heart failure resulting from an absolute or relative chronic overload in which the supply of energy to the heart is uncompromised is especially responsive to digitalis therapy. These types of problems include valvular lesions, hypertension, passive outflow impedance (e.g., dirofilariasis), and idiopathic dilated cardiomyopathy. Cardiac dysrhythmias can affect the response to digitalis glycosides, but they do not alter the indication for the drug if congestive failure is present.

ATRIAL ARRHYTHMIAS. Digitalis often is considered the most useful drug in treatment of atrial fibrillation or flutter, whether or not congestive heart disease is present. However, the drug should not be employed for abolition of the arrhythmic pattern. The goal of digitalis therapy in either of these states is to reduce ventricular rate by slowing AV conduction, eliminate the pulse deficit if present, and improve cardiac efficiency (Meijler 1985). Subsequently, quinidine can be used to abort atrial dysrhythmia. (However, see Chap. 24.) The potential involvement of latent or hidden congestive heart failure in pathogenesis of atrial fibrillation in some animals should not be discounted; the beneficial results from digitalis in treating what seems to be uncomplicated atrial fibrillation may well involve such complexities.

PROPHYLACTIC DIGITALIZATION. Digitalis pretreatment may be of some value in patients scheduled for unusual cardiac strain, as in open-heart surgery, if there is evidence of reduced cardiac reserve. Experimentally, the positive inotropic effect of the drug provides some protection to the heart against depressant effects of anesthetics. Early studies indicated that prophylactic digitalization protected dogs from myocardial weakening in experimental hemorrhagic shock and thus prolonged survival time (Braunwald and Kahler 1964). However, routine clinical use of digitalis in such situations is not recommended and actually may be contraindicated. As stated earlier, digitalis therapy can cause peripheral vasoconstriction in the normal patient without congestive failure syndrome. Splanchnic arteriolar constriction can intensify tissue hypoxia in shock. An obvious major hazard of prophylactic therapy with digitalis is inadvertent attainment of intoxication rather than digitalization. In most situations, therefore, digitalis should be reserved for therapy of congestive heart failure and should not be used in attempts to prevent cardiac failure in seemingly normal patients.

PRECAUTIONS. Digitalis is not indicated in cases of circulatory shock, renal failure, hepatic failure, ventricular premature contractions, ventricular tachycardia, or heart block unless the abnormality is associated with congestive heart failure. Digitalis therapy in congestive failure patients with heart block or ventricular tachycardia should be supervised in a particularly intensive manner, and digitalization should be monitored closely with an ECG. Digitalis can accentuate AV block and a serious decrease in ventricular rate may result. Digitalis treatment can also transform ventricular tachyarrhythmias to fibrillation.

Although digitalis slows sinus rate in congestive heart disease, this activity is complex and has no application in attempts to reduce heart rate when sinus tachycardia is present without evidence of congestive failure. Tachycardia associated with other conditions such as fever, thyrotoxicosis, constrictive pericarditis, or cardiac tamponade is not amenable to digitalis therapy. Hypertrophic cardiomyopathies and ruptured chorda tendinae constitute other nonindications for digitalis therapy.

Digitalis toxicosis can simulate certain aspects of cardiac disease, especially serious arrhythmias. Clinicians should always ascertain that any patient scheduled for cardiac glycoside treatment has not recently received any digitalis preparation; otherwise, an attempt to produce therapeutic digitalization in a patient actually suffering from unrecognized digitalis intoxication can have negative results.

Clinical Procedures

SELECTION OF DIGITALIS GLYCOSIDE. Ouabain is the most potent of the three glycosides, it acts most rapidly, and its effect dissipates most quickly. Ouabain is absorbed too poorly to be effective if given orally, and its use has been reserved for IV administration during emergencies. Currently, however, ouabain is rarely used in clinical veterinary medicine because digoxin is also effective when parenterally administered and is believed to be relatively less toxic than ouabain. Both digoxin and digitoxin are suitable for oral and parenteral digitalization and maintenance therapy. Digoxin often is preferred over digitoxin when a more rapid effect with oral administration is desired (Detweiler 1977). It should be emphasized, however, that well-controlled clinical comparisons between digitoxin and digoxin are lacking. Some clinicians believe that digoxin is more effective, more reliable, and less toxic than digitoxin. Conversely, some clinicians advocate that digitoxin is just as dependable and less toxic than digoxin. Additional documentation of clinical results is needed to resolve these differences.

DIGITALIZATION. A basic procedure followed in the past by many clinicians involves initial administration of a large amount of digitalis in several divided doses over a relatively short period (24-48 hours) to quickly achieve the desired therapeutic effect. Treatment is then continued daily with smaller doses to maintain therapeutic efficacy. The quantity of drug necessary to achieve the initial response is commonly designated as the digitalization or loading dose, whereas the daily dose needed to maintain this level of therapeutic action is called the maintenance dose. The digitalization and even the maintenance dose cannot be precalculated with absolute precision because of marked interpatient variation in response to therapeutic and toxic actions of the glycosides. Thus digitalization of each patient should be considered an individual and separate project subject somewhat to trial and error as the search is made for an efficacious dose without inducing toxic side effects.

To achieve this objective, an estimate of the digitalization dose is based on the standard range of loading doses for the selected glycoside and severity of the physiologic status of the patient (e.g., age, phase of cardiac disease, renal function). An estimate of the maintenance dose is based in turn on the standard maintenance dose range of the drug and, most importantly, the patient's response to the loading dose regimen. In essence, the goal is to determine the smallest amount of glycoside that will effectively maintain the patient in a state of cardiac compensation without inducing signs of intoxication.

ORAL SCHEDULES AND MAINTENANCE DOSES. Techniques used for achieving oral digitalization can be placed into three general time courses: slow, rapid, and intensive. The slow method is generally used when mild failure is presented; the total estimated loading dose is administered in 5 equal parts over 48 hours until salutary effects are gained or toxicity supervenes. With the rapid technique, the loading dose is divided into 3 equal amounts given at intervals of 6 hours. The intensive schedule is usually not selected unless an emergency or near emergency exists; one-half the loading dose is given initially, one-fourth is given 6 hours later, and one-eighth is given at 4- to 6-hour intervals. After digitalization is achieved with the above schedules, the maintenance dosage regimen is then instituted (Detweiler 1977).

In actual practice, the precise schedule selected can be less important than the care taken in monitoring patient response during implementation. In all cases, a predetermined dose should not be administered indiscriminately until toxic effects are seen. Careful supervision of the patient should allow detection of therapeutic benefits before toxicity is evoked. Nevertheless, if signs of intoxication supervene early in the digitalization schedule before salutary effects are attained, treatment must be halted and resumed at a lower dose after signs of toxicosis are absent. Similarly, if toxicity develops during maintenance therapy, the dose must be readjusted to a lower level. Conversely, the dose may have to be increased or administered at shorter intervals if therapeutic effects are not achieved with the predetermined schedule. Thus semantics about rigid time schedules should be interpreted in the clinic in accordance with needs of the individual patient. Unquestionably, as pointed out below, many clinicians now believe that loading dose digitalization techniques are unnecessary and may lead to intoxication.

A listing of average dose levels of digitalis glycosides is provided in Table 23.3. An approximate total loading dose for digoxin in dogs is 0.11-0.22 mg/kg; this amount can be divided into 5 equal doses of 0.022-0.044 mg/kg and each dose administered at 12-hour intervals for 48 hours. The daily maintenance dose of digoxin is 0.022 mg/kg; this can be divided into 2 equal doses of 0.011 mg/kg and each dose administered at 12-hour intervals after initial digitalization has been achieved (Table 23.3).

Modifications of the above procedure have been proposed. Data published by De Rick et al. (1978) indicated that administration of 0.025 mg/kg digoxin every 12 hours for 36 hours (i.e., a total digitalization dose of 0.1 mg/kg), followed by a maintenance dose of 0.01 mg/kg every 12 hours, was associated with less toxicity than larger loading dose techniques. The digoxin data presented in Fig. 23.10 show that this schedule leads to therapeutic blood levels, whereas a larger loading dose results in initial plasma concentrations associated with toxicosis.

Harris (1974) and Hahn (1977) advocated that a loading dose of digoxin is not necessary in dogs and that daily maintenance doses of 0.022 mg/kg given in 2 equal amounts at 12-hour intervals should be implemented as the original procedure. This would reduce the likelihood of intoxication associated with the larger loading dose techniques. Using complex pharmacokinetic calculations based on individual animals, Button et al. (1980a,b) found that the standard 0.022 mg/kg was a likely daily maintenance dose of digoxin in dogs.

Kittleson (1983) pointed out that because of its high toxic/therapeutic dose ratio, digitalis should be administered according to body surface area rather than body weight. Thus, since the body surface area/body weight ratio generally decreases as the size of the dog

TABLE 23.3—Guidelines for approximating doses and dosage schedules for digitalis glycosides in dogs

	Loading dose technique		
Drug	Total dose	Administration schedule	Daily maintenance dose and schedule
Oral			
Digitoxin*	0.11–0.22 mg/kg	0.022–0.044 mg/kg q12h for 48 hr	0.011 mg/kg q12h
Digoxin†	0.066 mg/kg	Three divided doses on day 1 of therapy	0.022 mg/kg daily
Digoxin§	0.1 mg/kg	0.025 mg/kg q12h for 36 hr	0.011 mg/kg q12h
Digoxin‖	. . .	. . .	0.011 mg/kg q12h
Digitoxin*	0.022–0.044 mg/kg	0.0044–0.0088 mg/kg q12h	0.0022–0.0044 mg/kg q12h
Digitoxin#	0.44 mg/kg	Divided doses over 48 hr	0.11 mg/kg daily
Parental			
Ouabain	0.022–0.033 mg/kg	Three divided doses over 24 hr	Oral digoxin 0.011 mg/kg q12h
Digoxin	0.022–0.044 mg/kg	Three divided doses over 24 hr	Oral digoxin 0.011 mg/kg q12h

Sources: *Drug companies and others, †Detweiler and Knight 1977; §De Rick et al. 1978; ‖Harris 1974; Hahn 1977; #Ettinger 1996.
Note: q12h = every 12 hours.

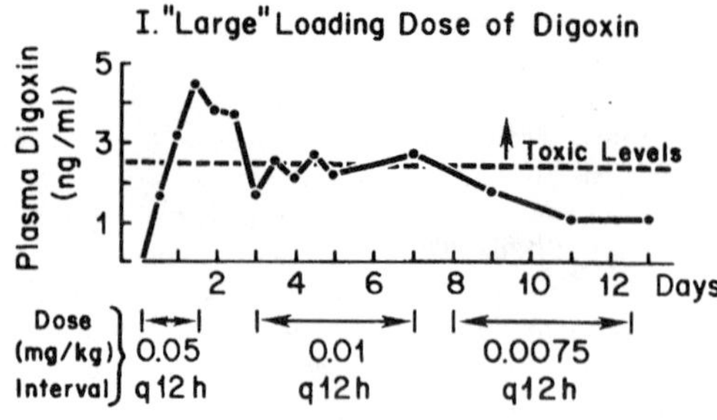

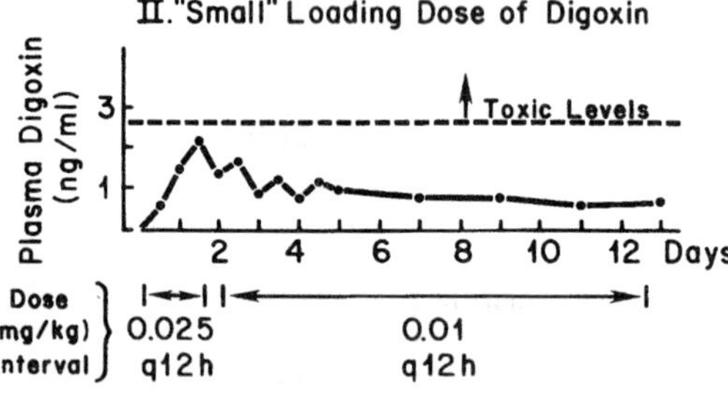

FIG. 23.10—Dosage schedules and plasma concentrations of digoxin after oral digitalization with a "large" (I) or "small" (II) loading dose. Notice in the top graph that with a large loading dose technique (0.05 mg/kg every 12 hr), plasma concentrations initially were in the toxic range (>2.5 ng/mL), whereas in the bottom graph with the smaller loading dose technique (0.025 mg/kg/12 hr), plasma concentrations did not exceed toxic levels and remained within presumed therapeutically effective concentrations. (Modeled after De Rick et al. 1978.)

increases, larger canine breeds would require less digitalis per kilogram of body weight than the small breeds. According to a recommended twice-a-day digoxin dose of 0.22 mg/m^2 body surface area (Kittleson 1983), dogs weighing 10, 20, 30, 40, and 50 kg would receive 0.011, 0.009, 0.008, 0.007, and 0.006 mg digoxin/kg respectively twice daily. Clinical trials support the merit of this approach (Kittleson et al. 1985a).

One pharmaceutical company that produces digitoxin suggested a loading dose of 0.022-0.044 mg/kg, followed by a maintenance dose of 0.0044-0.0154 mg/kg every 24 hours in dogs. Another company proposed a loading dose of 0.044 mg/kg divided into 10 equal doses, each dose given every 8 hours, followed by a daily maintenance dose of one-fifth of the digitalization dose (i.e., 0.0088 mg/kg) (Table 23.3). Much larger amounts of digitoxin have been used and advocated by clinicians (Ettinger 1966; Detweiler 1977). Differences may well relate to product formulations, routes of administration, bioavailability, and technical methods. These problems validate the need for the clinician to become thoroughly familiar with use of a few preparations rather than attempting to use a wide variety of the different products now available.

Cats are generally much more sensitive to digitalis than are dogs, and digitalis is not commonly used in cats. Tilley and Weitz (1977) indicated that an average maintenance dose of digoxin in cats is 0.008-0.01 mg/kg/day, divided into 2 equal doses.

Body weight resulting from edema fluid should be discounted in estimating the digitalis dose. Because of the importance of renal and hepatic function in eliminating digitalis glycosides, dose levels also should be reduced in animals with kidney or liver disease. Otherwise, toxicosis may develop unexpectedly following usual loading doses. As outlined earlier, dogs weighing more than 12-15 kg generally require less digitalis per kilogram of body weight than smaller dogs.

PARENTERAL SCHEDULES. IV administration of cardiac glycosides is indicated when the patient does not retain oral medications or has acute cardiac decompensation or respiratory distress.

Dose schedules for routine parenteral digitalization with digoxin and ouabain are included in Table 23.3. IV administration increases the likelihood for toxic arrhythmias, and this limitation should be considered. Intramuscular injection reduces the danger, but pain and swelling at the injection site limits patient acceptance of this method. Oral maintenance doses should be substituted if feasible.

The positive inotropic response to digoxin and digitoxin can be detected within 15-30 minutes after IV administration in dogs (Hamlin et al. 1971), somewhat sooner with ouabain. The rapid hemodynamic effects of ouabain in a dog with congestive failure are illustrated in Fig. 23.8. When an emergency is presented, the total IV loading dose for both ouabain and digoxin is approximately 0.044 mg/kg (Ettinger and Suter 1970). These two drugs are administered somewhat differently based on their dissimilar durations of action. With both ouabain and digoxin, 25-50% of the total dose is administered initially by slow IV injection; an additional 25% is given every 30-60 minutes (ouabain) or 60-120 minutes (digoxin). Patients treated with these techniques should be closely examined for signs of intoxication and monitored continuously for ECG abnormalities. Other emergency procedures are covered later.

LARGE ANIMALS. Loading or digitalization dose ranges for several digitalis preparations used in horses and cattle are given in Table 23.4. The daily maintenance dose is generally set at one-eighth to one-fifth of the loading dose. Actually, however, relatively little clinical work has been done with digitalis in these species, and dosage recommendations should be considered provisional (Detweiler and Patterson 1963). Parenteral administration is used in cattle and other ruminants because ruminal microorganisms can inactivate a large portion of digitalis.

Based on experimental pharmacokinetic data derived from normal horses, Button et al. (1980c) proposed the following schedule for digoxin: an IV loading dose of

TABLE 23.4—Approximate digitalization doses for horses and cattle

Preparation	Route	Total dose
Horses		
Digitalis powder	Oral	33–66 mg/kg
Digitalis tincture	Oral	0.33–0.66 ml/kg
Digitoxin	Oral	0.033–0.066 mg/kg
Digoxin	Oral	0.066 mg/kg
Digoxin	Parenteral	0.022–0.033 mg/kg
Ouabain	Parenteral	0.0132–0.022 mg/kg
Cattle		
Digitoxin	Intramuscular	0.031 mg/kg
Digoxin	Intravenous	0.0088 mg/kg
Ouabain	Intravenous	0.0132–0.022 mg/kg

Source: Detweiler 1977.

0.014 mg/kg, an IV maintenance dose of 0.007 mg/kg/24 hr, an oral loading dose of 0.07 mg/kg, and an oral maintenance dose of 0.035 mg/kg/24 hr. When these doses were given to horses, plasma digoxin concentrations measured 12 and 24 hours after administration were mostly in the assumed therapeutic range of 0.5-2 ng/mL.

Preparations. *Digitalis,* USP—*Digitalis purpurea;* potency of digitalis (100 mg) should be equivalent to but not less than 1 USP Digitalis Unit.

Powdered Digitalis, USP.

Digitalis Tablets, USP—tablets, 60 and 100 mg.

Digitoxin, USP—cardiotonic glycoside from *D. purpurea, D. lanata,* and other suitable species of the genus *Digitalis.*

Digitoxin Injection, USP—digitoxin in 5-50% alcohol; injections, 0.2 mg digitoxin/1 mL.

Digitoxin Tablets, USP—tablets, 0.1 and 0.5 mg.

Digoxin, USP—cardiotonic glycoside from *D. lanata.*

Digoxin Injection, USP—digoxin in 10% alcohol; injections, 0.5 mg/2 mL.

Digoxin Tablets, USP—tablets, 0.25 and 0.5 mg.

Digoxin Elixir—digoxin, 0.05 or 0.15 mg/mL in 30% alcohol.

Ouabain, USP—G-strophanthin.

Ouabain Injection, USP—injections, 0.25 mg/mL and 0.5 mg/2 mL.

AMRINONE AND MILRINONE. Amrinone and milrinone are bipyridine derivatives commonly referred to as nonglycoside, noncatecholamine inotropic drugs. These compounds were discovered during an investigative search for cardiac stimulant agents that could be used to replace digitalis in the therapy of heart failure (Alousi et al. 1979). Numerous studies have now confirmed that amrinone and milrinone evoke both a positive inotropic action in the heart and a peripheral vasodilator effect. The mechanism of action of the bipyridines is dissimilar from that of digitalis and does not involve adrenergic or other cell surface receptors. Rather, the cardiac inotropic and peripheral vasodilator actions of amrinone and milrinone involve inhibition of the type III cyclic nucleotide phosphodiesterase enzyme. This enzyme is responsible for the selective metabolism of cAMP; hence, inhibition of type III phosphodiesterase by amrinone or milrinone results in the accumulation of intracellular cAMP in cardiac and vascular tissues. Cyclic AMP subserves a positive inotropic response in myocardium and a vasodilatory response in blood vessels. Because of concurrent inotropic and vasodilator actions, considerable attention has been focused first on amrinone and more recently on milrinone as alternatives for digitalis in managing congestive heart failure patients (Mancini et al. 1985; Colucci et al. 1986a,b).

Amrinone. IV administration of amrinone (1-10 mg/kg) to anesthetized and unanesthetized dogs increased cardiac contractile force and left ventricular pressure with relatively small changes in heart rate and blood pressure. Administered orally to dogs, amrinone (2-10 mg/kg) produced a positive inotropic effect with rapid onset (within 15 minutes) and long duration of action (approximately 5 hours). Acute hemodynamic response to amrinone also has been studied extensively in human patients with refractory heart failure. Amrinone by oral or IV administration consistently enhanced cardiac contractile indexes while decreasing ventricular filling pressure/volume (preload) and systemic vascular resistance (afterload). Heart rate and blood pressure were affected slightly by therapeutic doses. Importantly, amrinone also decreased myocardial oxygen consumption of the failing heart. Thus reductions in cardiac preload and afterload represent important aspects of amrinone's hemodynamic profile because they apparently offset the metabolic cost of the drug's positive inotropic action. Because of this beneficial spectrum of cardiovascular effects, parenterally administered amrinone was approved for use in the short-term therapy of heart failure in humans.

Despite obvious beneficial actions of amrinone in managing acute exacerbation of heart failure, studies in humans have questioned whether long-term oral administration of amrinone is clinically effective in therapy of chronic congestive heart failure (Massie et al. 1985). These results illustrate the potential pitfalls of trying to extrapolate results from acute studies to the exceedingly more complex situation of chronic therapy of heart failure. Moreover, adverse side effects occurred in 83% of these amrinone-treated patients after long-term therapy, necessitating drug withdrawal in 34%. Thrombocytopenia is a serious side effect of amrinone in about 15% of human patients chronically treated. This untoward reaction does not seem to be a problem in dogs.

Milrinone. Milrinone is a structural congener of amrinone, and the former is 20-30 times more potent than the latter. Initial studies suggested that milrinone might be relatively free of adverse side effects in reasonable doses and could be helpful in the management of heart failure patients in human medicine (Colucci et al. 1986a, b). However, studies with human patients with moderately severe heart failure indicated that milrinone was less effective than digoxin, and the combination of milrinone and digoxin was no more effective than digoxin alone. Moreover, milrinone administration was associated with an increased incidence of both ventricular and supraventricular tachyarrhythmias as adverse side effects (DiBianco et al. 1989).

Tachyarrhythmias could have been predicted as an adverse side effect of milrinone and other phosphodiesterase inhibitors inasmuch as their mechanism of action depends upon accumulation of cAMP. The latter not only subserves positive inotropic actions in the heart but also increases cardiac automaticity in sinoatrial pacemaker cells and other cardiac tissues that carry spontaneous automaticity. Emergence of latent pacemakers and associated ectopic beats and tachyarrhythmias can be expected as limiting side effects of drugs that affect the heart through the cAMP system. Hence, the initial enthusiasm for cardiac uses of milrinone and other type III phosphodiesterase inhibitors has decreased (Massie et al. 1985; DiBianco et al. 1989).

A collaborative investigation involving three teaching veterinary hospitals provided evidence that milrinone may be effective in dogs with spontaneous heart failure (Kittleson et al. 1985b). This study included a randomized blinded evaluation of milrinone (0.5-1.0 mg/kg) versus placebo for a 4-week period in a total of 14 dogs, 11 with left ventricular failure and 3 with right ventricular failure. All dogs in this study with echocardiographic evidence of mild-to-severe myocardial failure and clinical evidence of poor-to-good compensation for their heart failure responded favorably to treatment with milrinone as the sole therapeutic agent, as determined by echocardiography. This salutary effect was sustained for the 4 weeks of the study; it was not due to spontaneous remission of the disease because heart failure worsened when milrinone was withdrawn and improved when the drug was reinstituted. The only apparent adverse reactions were asymptomatic ventricular dysrhythmias in 2 dogs. The improved ventricular performance observed in this study was attributed to a direct increase in myocardial contractility owing to milrinone's positive inotropic action, to a decrease in cardiac work load owing to milrinone's vasodilator effects or, more likely, to a combination of both. These investigators concluded that milrinone may be an effective drug for treating myocardial failure in the dog when administered orally twice daily in 0.5-1 mg/kg doses.

The biologic half-life of milrinone is about 2 hours in dogs; the onset of action occurs within 30 minutes of oral administration and the duration of effect has been reported to be about 6 hours. However, the maximal response to milrinone in dogs with spontaneous heart failure develops about 1.5-2 hours after administration and dissipates rather quickly thereafter. Kittleson et al. (1985b) suggested, therefore, that dogs with severe decompensation of their heart failure may benefit from 3-4 daily doses of milrinone to take advantage of the maximal effects of the drug.

Milrinone was advanced as either a primary drug of choice in congestive heart failure or as an alternative in congestive failure patients who become refractory to digitalis. Additional controlled clinical trials with milrinone are needed to determine whether the beneficial results observed by Kittleson et al. (1985b) during their 4-week study are sustained over longer intervals without limiting side effects. It is unclear if arrhythmogenic side effects will be a limiting factor for milrinone in dogs, as it is in humans (DiBianco et al. 1989).

VASODILATOR DRUGS. Careful use of peripheral vasodilator drugs has been developed extensively as treatment in congestive failure to "unload" the failing heart (Hamlin 1977; Zelis et al. 1979; Remme 1993). The rationale for this treatment is the idea that decreasing the work load of the heart is better for the patient than administering a positive inotropic agent with considerable toxic potential (i.e., digitalis). If systemic arterial pressure (i.e., left ventricular afterload) is reduced by a vasodilator drug, the left ventricle will be ejecting blood into a circuit with lowered resistance. Further, peripheral venodilation will divert blood volume from the pulmonary to the systemic vasculature. This response is antagonistic to the formation of pulmonary edema and also tends to restrict venous return to the heart (i.e., ventricular preload). Left ventricular size and wall tension decrease in response to reduction in ventricular preload and afterload. Myocardial oxygen demands decrease accordingly as the workload of the heart is reduced; cardiac output and hemodynamics should improve (Packer 1984; Abrams 1985).

Before resorting to vasodilator therapy in treating congestive failure in animals, the clinician should be aware of potential problems; e.g., it has been assumed that drug-induced vasodilation would automatically increase peripheral perfusion and thereby increase oxygen availability to all tissues. However, vasodilator agents of the nitroglycerin type exert a predominant reduction in peripheral venous resistance as compared to arteriolar resistance. Pooling of blood in the venous capacitance beds in no way ensures increased perfusion of all tissues. Vasodilators are beneficial to the failing heart because they decrease cardiac workload, not by directly improving peripheral perfusion because of vascular dilation. Furthermore, if arterial pressure is critically decreased, blood flow through the coronary and renal vascular beds may be compromised further. Reflex tachycardia accompanied by increased myocardial oxygen demand is another potential problem associated with fall in systemic blood pressure.

Prazosin. Atwell (1979) indicated that peripheral vasodilation induced by prazosin hydrochloride (Minipress), an α_1-adrenergic selective blocking agent (Chap. 6), was effective in 4 dogs with congestive failure that were refractory to digoxin. However, digoxin was actually continued in 3 of the 4 dogs at reduced dosage levels. Thus the beneficial response may well have resulted from a combination of mechanisms involving both a positive inotropic action on the heart (digoxin) and peripheral vasodilation (prazosin).

Hydralazine Hydrochloride. *Hydralazine Hydrochloride,* USP (Apresoline), is an arteriolar dilator that has undergone limited clinical trial in dogs with volume-overload heart failure (Kittleson et al. 1983). Because of its vasodilator action in systemic arterial beds, hydralazine reduces peripheral vascular resistance and lowers impedance to left ventricular ejection. Stroke volume and cardiac output increase proportionately, thereby initiating hemodynamic improvement.

Beneficial effects of hydralazine are manifested mainly in congestive heart failure that is secondary to mitral valve insufficiency. In this pathophysiologic state, forward left ventricular stroke volume is reduced owing to a regurgitant fraction being pumped backward through the incompetent AV valve into the left atrium. By lowering systemic impedance to left ventricular ejection, hydralazine increases forward stroke volume and thereby reduces the regurgitant fraction. End-systolic volume and cardiac size are reduced because more blood is pumped out of the cardiac chambers per beat. Reduction in cardiac size leads to commensurate decreases in wall tension and myocardial oxygen consumption and, also importantly, to reduction of the orifice of the incompetent mitral valve. The latter contributes in turn to further diminution of the regurgitant fraction. This cycle leads to hemodynamic improvement and, it is hoped, pharmacologically supported compensation of the heart failure patient. Indeed, clinical studies indicate that hydralazine therapy is effective in dogs with volume-overload congestive failure caused by mitral valve insufficiency (Kittleson et al. 1983). Hydralazine may be similarly effective in aortic valvular insufficiency.

Hydralazine is absorbed rapidly after oral administration in dogs; its onset of action develops within 1 hour, and peak response occurs at 3-5 hours. The drug undergoes extensive hepatic metabolism during its initial passage through the liver in the portal blood. There is evidence that uremia in some way affects biotransformation of hydralazine, so that blood concentrations may increase in uremic patients. A recommended dose schedule for hydralazine in dogs involves the initial oral administration of 1 mg/kg; this dose can be adjusted upward, depending upon evidence of clinical improvement, but should not exceed 3 mg/kg. Average-size adult cats may require an initial oral dose of 2.5 mg, which may be adjusted upward to 10 mg. The therapeutic response generally lasts 11-13 hours; thus twice daily administration is suggested as the standard (Kittleson 1983).

Important side effects of hydralazine therapy in humans are tachycardia and hypotension. It was reported that hypotension was not a problem in dogs when hydralazine dosage was titrated carefully against signs of clinical improvement; however, tachycardia does seem to be a common untoward development in congestive-failure dogs treated with hydralazine (Kittleson et al. 1983). Since tachycardia increases myocardial oxygen consumption and may therefore lead to cardiac decompensation, heart rate should be monitored during therapeutic implementation with hydralazine or any other vasodilating drug.

Concomitant administration of a β-blocking drug might reduce the reflex tachycardia produced by hypotensive reactions to hydralazine. On the other hand, the potential negative inotropic response to β-receptor blockade in the heart may exacerbate heart failure (see Chap. 6).

Captopril and Enalapril Maleate. Recognition of the contribution of the renin-angiotensin-aldosterone axis to the pathophysiology of congestive heart failure led to development of a new group of vasodilator agents. These compounds are the angiotensin-converting enzyme (ACE) inhibitors such as captopril and enalapril maleate (Holtz 1993; Dietz et al. 1993).

Reduced perfusion of the kidneys during heart failure evokes release into the circulation of the renal enzyme renin. As detailed in Chap. 20, renin synthesizes the formation of angiotensin I. The latter is relatively inactive; however, it is metabolized by ACE into the potent vasoconstrictor angiotensin II. Thus, by inhibiting ACE, captopril and enalapril decrease the formation of angiotensin II and through this mechanism evoke peripheral vasodilation in the heart failure patient. Angiotensin II-mediated release of aldosterone also is decreased by ACE inhibitors, thus facilitating sodium excretion and diuresis. Captopril improves hemodynamics in dogs with experimental heart failure (Kittleson et al. 1993), and reduces blood concentrations of aldosterone and improves clinical status in dogs with naturally occurring heart failure (Knowlen et al. 1983); 1-2 mg/kg orally 3 times daily has been suggested as a successful dose for captopril in congestive failure in dogs (Kittleson 1983).

Recent studies with ACE inhibitors in human medicine have indicated that these agents exert substantial beneficial effects in heart failure patients (Dietz et al. 1993; Swedberg 1993). Enalapril and other ACE inhibitors improve exercise tolerance, decrease signs and symptoms of heart failure, and prolong life. Because of the rapidly expanding role of ACE inhibitors in cardiovascular therapeutics in human medicine, these drugs also are being tested in animals with spontaneous cardiac disease.

The therapeutic efficacy of the ACE inhibitor enalapril was examined in a carefully controlled study involving over 400 dogs with naturally occurring dilated cardiomyopathy or chronic valvular heart disease (Ettinger et al. 1994). Some of the dogs were subjected to invasive monitoring of cardiodynamic functions, while other dogs were observed for signs of clinical improvement or mortality. Nearly all of the dogs continued to receive conventional therapy for heart failure involving diuretics (usually furosemide) without or with digoxin. Thus, this multicenter trial actually examined the ability of ACE inhibition to augment digitalis and diuretic therapy of heart failure, rather than therapeutic benefits from enalapril alone. Nevertheless, this study yielded convincing evidence that inhibition of ACE with enalapril can improve quality of life and delay mortality in dogs with heart failure.

Enalapril reduced the following variables in dogs with heart failure: pulmonary capillary wedge pressure, heart rate, mean blood pressure, and pulmonary arterial pressure (Sisson 1992). Similar results were also seen in experimental studies with captopril (Kittleson et al. 1993). Improvements in cardiovascular functions were evident over the first 24 hours of treatment with enalapril. After 3-4 weeks of enalapril plus conventional therapy, improvement was detected in several clinical markers of hemodynamic function. These included increased exercise capacity and resulting reduction in class of heart failure, reduced signs of pulmonary edema, and overall improvement in well being. Mortality was lower in the dogs treated with enalapril, and fewer of these patients exhibited progressive worsening of heart failure (Ettinger et al. 1994).

In a subset of 148 dogs, the long-term efficacy of enalapril was evaluated by measuring when the patients died or when they had to be removed from the study because of clinical deterioration. Dogs treated with enalapril (plus standard heart failure therapy) remained in the trial for 169 ± 14 days, compared to 90 ± 17 days for dogs receiving placebo (plus standard heart failure therapy). A group of 17 Doberman Pinschers treated with enalapril and standard therapy remained in the study for 80 ± 11 days, compared to only 38 ± 8 days in the placebo cohort group of 19 Dobermans. All other breeds of dogs treated with enalapril remained in the trial 189 ± 15 days, compared to 110 ± 14 days for the placebo group. When the dogs that died from congestive heart failure or died suddenly were analyzed separately, dogs treated with enalapril lived approximately 50% longer than placebo-treated dogs. Although these studies did not evaluate enalapril alone, they clearly indicate that enalapril is markedly beneficial in the management of heart failure when added to conventional therapy with diuretics and digoxin (Ettinger et al. 1994).

Because of the importance of angiotensin in maintaining renal perfusion in heart failure and other low cardiac output conditions, renal function should be monitored during therapy with ACE inhibitors. However, results from the multicenter trial with enalapril in dogs indicated that sporadic episodes of azotemia (elevated BUN and/or serum creatinine) were seen with approximately the same frequency in the enalapril and placebo groups. Furthermore, regression analysis indicated that BUN was correlated with the dose of furosemide but not with the dose of either digoxin or enalapril. Based on these data, Ettinger et al. (1994) supported the position that the dose of furosemide should be decreased first should azotemia occur in a dog with heart failure receiving furosemide and enalapril with or without digoxin. Nevertheless, the potential for renal failure should be closely followed whenever ACE inhibitors are used.

Based on results from the multicenter study with enalapril, Ettinger et al. (1994) proposed the following guidelines for pharmacologic treatment of dogs with chronic valvular heart disease or dilated cardiomyopathy. Treatment programs should be customized to the severity of the patient's disease.

1. Dogs with Class I heart disease do not have clinical evidence of heart disease except in response to exceptionally powerful exercise or other severe cardiovascular challenges. In general, these patients do not require drugs. High-salt diets should be avoided to prevent water retention and hypervolemia. Both chronic valvular disease and idiopathic dilated cardiomyopathy are progressive and usually irreversible conditions. Their rate of progression may be abated by therapeutic intervention; however, currently there are no reliable measures that will cease progressive deterioration of the heart in these pathologic entities.

2. Dogs with Class II heart disease exhibit signs of insufficient cardiac function upon mild or moderate exercise. Enalapril at a dosage of 0.5 mg/kg once daily should be considered along with a restricted-salt diet. Renal function should be monitored regularly as signs of clinical improvement are followed.

3. Dogs with Class III heart disease have overt signs of heart failure during mild exercise; signs include dyspnea, orthopnea, cardiac cough, and episodes of pulmonary edema. Exercise tolerance is markedly diminished. Ascites and other evidence of right side heart failure commonly appear. Aggressive drug therapy should be implemented along with restriction of physical activity and dietary salt. A diuretic such as furosemide is usually started first for 2-4 days, followed by institution of enalapril at 0.5 mg/kg once daily. The dose of enalapril may be increased to a total of 1 mg/kg per day in two divided doses, depending upon clinical response. Digoxin may also be prescribed at a standard dosage and concomitantly with the diuretic, depending on signs of heart failure and cardiac tachyarrhythmias.

4. Dogs with Class IV heart failure are in acute decompensation and usually require aggressive emergency therapy with oxygen, morphine, cardiac inotropes, IV diuretics, and preload reducers. ACE inhibitors should be reserved until the patient is out of danger from acute pulmonary edema and cardiac decompensation.

ACE inhibitors such as enalapril truly represent a major new addition to drug therapy of heart failure. However, renal function should be monitored to ensure adequate perfusion of the kidneys. Furthermore, despite the impressive results of the multicenter trial with enalapril (Ettinger et al. 1994), it should be remembered that enalapril was studied only as an adjunct to conventional therapy with digoxin and diuretics. The results with these combined therapies will most likely be improved upon as additional studies examine the full therapeutic spectrum for ACE inhibitors such as enalapril.

Calcium Channel Blocking Drugs. These agents suppress calcium ion (Ca^{++}) influx through plasma membrane channels in cardiac tissues, vascular smooth muscle, and other excitable cell types (Katz 1985; Allert and Adams 1987; Opie 1984). The resulting decrease in intracellular Ca^{++} concentration leads to characteristic changes in physiologic activity of affected tissues, including reduction in myocardial contractility, vasodilation in coronary and peripheral arterial beds, lowered impedance to left ventricular ejection, reduced myocardial oxygen demand, and slowed AV impulse conduction. Because of this diverse pharmacologic profile, Ca^{++} channel blockers have been studied extensively for therapeutic application in a wide spectrum of cardiovascular disorders. Drugs of this group have been approved for the management of ischemic heart disease, hypertension, and some forms of cardiac dysrhythmias in human medicine. Other indications in people include obstructive cardiomyopathies, asthma, and cerebral ischemia (Stone and Antmann 1983; Conti et al. 1985).

Although Ca^{++} channel blockade has become a therapeutic mainstay in human medicine (Katz 1985), less is known about the clinical application of this concept in veterinary medicine (Adams 1986a; Novotny and Adams 1986; Johnson 1985; Bright 1992). The present discussion is an overview of this topic and addresses the pharmacodynamic rationale for Ca^{++} channel blocking drugs in cardiovascular therapeutics in animals, as summarized by Allert and Adams (1987). The use of verapamil and diltiazem as Class IV antiarrhythmics in treating supraventricular tachyarrhythmias is addressed in Chap. 24.

HISTORY AND TERMINOLOGY. Discovery of Ca^{++} channel blocking drugs can be traced to 1964, when the German cardiologist Fleckenstein reported that the newly synthesized drug verapamil mimicked the cardiac effects of Ca^{++} withdrawal (Fleckenstein 1983). Verapamil was being developed as a coronary vasodilator, but it also inhibited myocardial contractile strength while leaving the cardiac action potential essentially intact. Importantly, the cardiodepressant effects of verapamil could be antagonized promptly and completely by excess Ca^{++}. Fleckenstein coined the term "Ca^{++} antagonists" to describe verapamil and other drugs that exerted this basic Ca^{++}-dependent inhibitory effect as their predominant pharmacologic property (Fleckenstein 1983). Dozens of drugs that share this action subsequently have been identified, and several have been approved for clinical use in human medicine, including nifedipine, verapamil, and diltiazem. Only the last two have found useful application in veterinary medicine.

The term "Ca^{++} antagonist" is used commonly in the scientific literature. Others have questioned its pharmacologic appropriateness, however, because these drugs are not Ca^{++} analogs and they do not act by inhibiting Ca^{++} binding to cellular Ca^{++}-binding receptors such as calmodulin or troponin (Katz 1985). Rather, these agents interfere with the function of plasma membrane channels that mediate Ca^{++} entry into excitable cells. For these reasons, the terms "Ca^{++} antagonists," "Ca^{++} entry blockers," "Ca^{++} channel antagonists," and other nomenclatures are sometimes used interchangeably. Regardless of terminology, the pharmacologic rationale for therapeutic use of these drugs resides in the fundamental importance of Ca^{++} influx as an intracellular messenger system in cardiovascular tissues (Schramm and Towart 1985; Janis and Triggle 1984).

FUNDAMENTALS OF Ca^{++} CHANNEL BLOCKADE

PHARMACOLOGIC CONCEPTS. The essential roles of Ca^{++} in coupling cell membrane excitation to intracellular functions in cardiac and vascular muscle have been reviewed in detail (Janis and Triggle 1984; Reuter 1985). In essence, Ca^{++} influxing through specific plasma membrane channels gains access to intracellular organelles and through this pathway leads to activation of Ca^{++}-dependent cellular functions.

The molecular architecture and biophysical operation of the cell membrane Ca^{++} channels are incompletely understood. The channel structures are protein moieties embedded within and spanning the permeability barrier of the phospholipid plasma membrane bilayer, as illustrated in Fig. 23.11. Some of the Ca^{++} channel blocking drugs interact with specific ligand binding sites of channel elements, others seem to "plug" the outer orifice of the channel pore, whereas others may have to gain access to the cytosolic face of the cell membrane to interfere with channel operation (Schramm and Towart 1985; Janis and Triggle 1984). Despite dissimilar molecular mechanisms, the Ca^{++} channel blockers share a common pharmacodynamic property: they all inhibit Ca^{++} influx and the associated Ca^{++}-dependent physiologic responses of affected cells.

PHYSIOLOGIC CONCEPTS. A schematic representation of excitation-contraction coupling in heart muscle cells and the importance of Ca^{++} channels in this physiologic process are presented in Fig. 23.11. Cardiac excitation initially involves a rapid influx of sodium ions (Na^+) through plasma membrane passageways referred to as "fast Na^+ channels." Rapid Na^+ influx depolarizes the cell membrane. Depolarization then leads to a voltage-dependent opening of another type of plasma membrane channel referred, to as "slow Ca^{++} channels" or simply as "Ca^{++} channels" (Reuter 1985). Calcium moves inward through these open channels and serves two critical interconnected functions on a beat-to-beat basis. It replenishes sarcoplasmic reticulum stores of Ca^{++} and triggers the release of additional amounts of Ca^{++} from sarcoplasmic reticulum storage sites into the

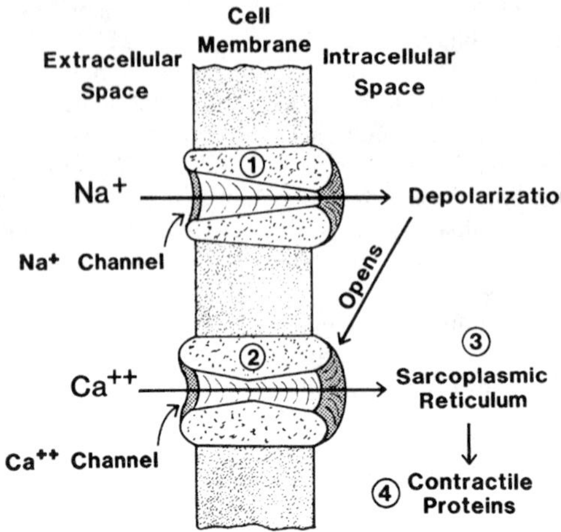

FIG. 23.11—Schematic representation of cell membrane Ca^{++} channel involvement in excitation-contraction coupling in mammalian heart. Na^{+} channels (1) open during cell excitation, and the inward Na^{+} current depolarizes the cell membrane. Depolarization opens Ca^{++} channels (2), and Ca^{++} influx triggers shift of additional Ca^{++} from sarcoplasmic reticulum (3) to contractile proteins (4). Calcium channel blocking drugs reduce Ca^{++} influx through the Ca^{++} channels (2) (Allert and Adams 1987).

cytosol. The resulting increase in intracellular Ca^{++} concentration ($[Ca^{++}]_i$) proportionately activates the contractile proteins of the cardiac myocyte (Fig. 23.11), and the heart contracts. Diastolic relaxation develops as the sarcoplasmic reticulum avidly resequesters Ca^{++} away from the contractile apparatus. Thus, Ca^{++} channel blocking drugs induce negative inotropic effects in the heart by reducing trans-sarcolemmal influx of activator Ca^{++} (Fig. 23.11).

Contraction of vascular smooth muscle is mediated by Ca^{++} and depends on the influx of Ca^{++} through cell membrane channels (Somlyo 1985). Therefore, Ca^{++} channel blockade in vascular smooth muscle evokes vascular smooth muscle relaxation and vasodilatory responses in different vascular beds. The resultant peripheral vasodilation and accompanying decrease in peripheral vascular resistance lower impedance to left ventricular ejection, thereby reducing ventricular wall tension during stroke volume ejection. Diminution of ventricular wall tension during systole (i.e., reduced cardiac afterload), coupled to direct negative inotropic actions of Ca^{++} channel blockade in the heart muscle, proportionately lowers myocardial oxygen demand. Hence, and this is an important aspect, Ca^{++} channel blocking drugs can preserve cardiac integrity by hemodynamically lowering myocardial oxygen demand. Certain Ca^{++} channel blocking drugs also have pronounced coronary vasodilator effects, which further improve tissue perfusion-metabolic demand relationships in the heart. This complex pharmacologic spectrum probably explains the salutary effects of Ca^{++} channel blockade in managing coronary artery-ischemic heart disease and the resulting anginal pain in people (Katz 1985; Nayler 1980; Opie 1984; Stone and Antmann 1983; Conti et al. 1985).

ELECTROPHYSIOLOGIC CONCEPTS. The importance of slow inward Ca^{++} currents to normal and abnormal rhythmicity mechanisms in the heart is reviewed in Chap. 24 (Adams 1986b; Novotny and Adams 1986). Briefly, usual electrophysiologic mechanisms of the sinoatrial (SA) and AV nodes involve Ca^{++} influx through the plasma membrane Ca^{++} channels in these tissues. Calcium channel blockade can suppress these normal mechanisms, reduce sinus rate, and slow AV conduction velocity. There also is evidence that aberrant Ca^{++} currents can arise from injured cardiac tissue and lead to reentry and automaticity forms of arrhythmias that are responsive to Ca^{++} channel blockade. Because of their unique Ca^{++}-dependent antiarrhythmic mechanism, the Ca^{++} channel blockers are considered Class IV antiarrhythmic agents (Adams 1986b; Novotny and Adams 1986; Vaughn Williams 1984) (see Chap. 24).

PATHOPHYSIOLOGIC CONCEPTS. Cellular Ca^{++} influx-efflux control mechanisms are set awry during ischemia and perhaps in many other fundamental forms of cellular injury (Trump et al. 1982; White et al. 1984). During ischemic and hypoxemic conditions, the failure of oxidative metabolism results in progressive depletion of cellular energy stores. The ability of the cell to maintain energy-dependent ionic gradients is impaired, leading to intracellular potassium ion (K^{+}) depletion and concomitant intracellular Na^{+} and Ca^{++} overloads. One consequence of increased $[Ca^{++}]_i$ is activation of Ca^{++}-regulated catabolic and lysosomal enzyme systems (Trump et al. 1982; White et al. 1984). These degradative enzymes disrupt cellular regulatory functions with further compromise of cell membrane integrity and further loss of ion permeability barriers. The $[Ca^{++}]_i$ progressively overloads the cell via this putative pathway and sequentially inhibits mitochondrial oxidative phosphorylation, impairs Ca^{++} uptake-release functions of sarcoplasmic reticulum, and eventually culminates in cell death and necrosis. Evidence for this or an analogous series of pathophysiologic processes funneling to the common event of intracellular Ca^{++} overload has been derived from studies with various types of tissue, including heart, vascular muscle, and neurons (Trump et al. 1982; White et al. 1984). Calcium channel blocking drugs reduce the increase in $[Ca^{++}]_i$ by lowering the quantity of Ca^{++} influx, at least that component occurring through the Ca^{++} channels. Decreased $[Ca^{++}]_i$ then should reduce activation of Ca^{++}-dependent degradative enzymes, thereby preserving cell viability after ischemic-related injuries (Trump et al. 1982; White et al. 1984).

CLINICAL PRECAUTIONS. On the basis of the foregoing schema of physiologic and pathophysiologic roles for Ca^{++}, it is now possible to discuss three basic types of pharmacodynamic pathways incorporating Ca^{++} channel blocking drugs into cardiovascular therapeutics in veterinary medicine. First, by evoking arteriolar dilatation and lowering total peripheral vascular resistance, these drugs should improve blood flow-oxygen demand relationships during hypodynamic circulatory conditions such as heart failure. Second, these drugs should be able to restore hemodynamic stability in patients with cardiac arrhythmias caused by abnormal Ca^{++} influx patterns. Third, these drugs should directly prolong cell viability in various tissues during ischemic-related syndromes by modulating the cellular Ca^{++} overload cascade. Some essential issues remain unresolved, however, and several important precautions should be considered by the clinician before these drugs are accepted for routine therapeutic use.

PHARMACOLOGIC HETEROGENEITY. Although the Ca^{++} channel blockers share common cellular effects, they comprise chemically unrelated subgroups with somewhat disparate tissue and systemic pharmacologic profiles (Spedding 1985; Defeudis 1985). Nifedipine, e.g., directly reduces myocardial contractile strength and slows AV conduction in isolated cardiac tissues. However, these direct cardiodepressant effects of nifedipine may not be manifested in patients with normal myocardial contractile reserves, owing to more potent vasodilator actions and the resulting baroreflex-induced cardiac stimulation. In contrast, verapamil can induce direct myocardial contractile depression and antiarrhythmic responses at dosages that induce peripheral vasodilatation. Diltiazem is a potent vasodilator that also directly decreases sinus firing rate in dosages that usually spare cardiac contractile mechanisms. Dissimilarities in systemic pharmacologic profiles have clinical relevance because they indicate that the various Ca^{++} channel blockers should not be construed as being therapeutically interchangeable.

CARDIOVASCULAR SIDE EFFECTS. Because of the essential physiologic roles for Ca^{++} influx in activation of cardiovascular tissues, the Ca^{++} channel blocking agents can be likened to a "double-edged sword" relative to benefit-risk relationships. On the one hand, the negative inotropic effects and vasodilator actions of Ca^{++} channel blockade can benefit hemodynamics by reducing cardiac workload. On the other hand, if unexpected or unabated, these same cardiovascular depressant responses obviously carry the risk of exacerbating underlying abnormalities of the circulatory system.

Adverse circulatory side effects of Ca^{++} channel blockade include contractile depression of the heart, with reduced cardiac output and hypotension. This combination of effects can result in decompensation of preclinical or compensated heart failure, precipitation of pulmonary edema, and worsening of the primary ailment. Other potential side effects are sinus bradycardia and heart block attributable to direct depression of SA firing rate and AV conduction, respectively. The propensity for cardiovascular depression should be considered whenever Ca^{++} channel blocking drugs are used. This precaution is especially valid in patients with preexisting or suspected myocardial contractile failure.

Clinical Applications

SUPRAVENTRICULAR TACHYARRHYTHMIAS. The clinical antiarrhythmic applications for Ca^{++} channel blockade mainly involve the use of verapamil and diltiazem for treatment of supraventricular tachyarrhythmias (Kittleson et al. 1986; Hamlin 1986; Johnson 1985; Adams 1986a; Novotny and Adams 1986). Verapamil and diltiazem are used for conversion of paroxysmal atrial tachycardia to sinus rhythm. Atrial fibrillation and flutter constitute other important indications (Wasman et al. 1981; Smith et al. 1981). Verapamil and diltiazem usually do not convert these high-frequency atrial patterns to sinus rhythm but effectively reduce AV conduction and thereby lower the ventricular rate response, as discussed in Chap. 24.

HEART FAILURE SYNDROMES. Initial studies with nifedipine, verapamil, and diltiazem indicated favorable results in human beings with chronic myocardial contractile failure, valvular insufficiencies, or obstructive cardiomyopathies (Katz 1985; Conti et al. 1985; Lorell 1985; Rosing et al. 1979). Beneficial effects were attributed to reduced cardiac workload; improved aortic blood flow, with reduced regurgitant fraction in valvular insufficiencies; enhanced diastolic compliance, with increased ventricular filling in obstructive heart disease; or a combination of these effects. The therapeutic use of Ca^{++} channel blockade in congestive cardiomyopathies with severe cardiac contractile failure is controversial (Colucci et al. 1985; Josephson and Singh 1985; Brooks et al. 1980; Packer 1985). Josephson and Singh (1985) suggested caution in the use of these agents in patients with impaired ventricular performance and stated that available data do not support the use of calcium antagonists as afterload-reducing agents in chronic heart failure. Packer (1985) cautioned that both verapamil and nifedipine may exert notable depressant effects on right ventricular performance in patients with impaired right ventricular function. Colucci et al. (1985) similarly warned that Ca^{++} channel blockade in the setting of severe left ventricular dysfunction can result in abrupt decompensation and development of overt pulmonary edema. In contrast, treatment with verapamil or nifedipine seemed particularly effective in human patients with hypertrophic cardiomyopathy (Lorell 1985; Rosing et al. 1979). Because of shared pathophysiologic similarities between human and feline obstructive hypertrophic heart conditions (Tilley et al. 1977), it is not surprising that Ca^{++} channel blocking drugs are useful in cats with hypertrophic heart disease.

HYPERTROPHIC CARDIOMYOPATHY. In contrast to the lack of clinical interest for Ca^{++} channel blockers in dilated cardiomyopathy, verapamil and especially diltiazem are being used increasingly in dogs and cats with hypertrophic cardiomyopathy (Bright 1992). Because of reduced propensity for side effects associated with cardiac contractile depression, diltiazem is commonly the preferred drug for this condition. Recommended doses range from 1.75 to 2.5 mg/kg orally BID to TID. As with any highly active cardiovascular drug, therapy with diltiazem or other Ca^{++} channel blocker should be implemented with careful patient monitoring.

CIRCULATORY SHOCK AND TRAUMA. Calcium channel blocking drugs have been tested for salutary pharmacologic effects in experimental models of hemorrhagic shock, traumatic shock, cerebral ischemia, cardiopulmonary resuscitation, and endotoxemic shock. Studies have involved various representatives of this drug group, including verapamil, diltiazem, lidoflazine, nimodipine, nisoldipine, nivadipine, and nitrendipine (Adams 1986a). Initial data favored the general conclusion that Ca^{++} channel blocking drugs can improve the short-or long-term outcome of various induced forms of shock and trauma. Other studies, however, have indicated that Ca^{++} channel blocking effects were not helpful in some forms of induced shock and ischemia (Denis et al. 1985; Lanza et al. 1984) and could result in further reductions in blood pressure and cardiac output. Ca^{++} channel blocking drugs are not used in emergency medicine dealing with circulatory shock and trauma (Adams 1986a).

Investigators in human medicine caution that higher than "optimal" dosages of Ca^{++} channel blocking drugs can nonspecifically alter Ca^{++}-dependent hemodynamic control mechanisms and thereby exacerbate the circulatory instability already underway in a patient with compromised cardiac function (Colucci et al. 1985; Josephson and Singh 1985; Brooks et al. 1980; Packer 1985). Because of the potential for serious cardiovascular side effects associated with Ca^{++} channel blocking drugs, the patient should be under diligent monitoring or hospitalized conditions during initial determination of therapeutic response. With this conservative approach, patients with preclinical, occult, or compensated heart failure will have the advantage of immediate care if cardiovascular depressant side effects intervene. These complexities should be assessed judiciously by the clinician when the Ca^{++} channel blocking agents are considered for use in veterinary medicine. Verapamil and especially diltiazem are rapidly finding a useful niche in veterinary therapeutics dealing with supraventricular tachyarrhythmias and hypertrophic cardiomyopathies.

Other Vasodilators. Several other vasodilator drugs have been studied and employed therapeutically in humans with heart failure, including nitroprusside, nitroglycerin, isosorbide dinitrate, and Ca^{++} entry-blocking drugs. Clinical trials with these compounds are lacking in veterinary medicine. Indeed, with the notable exception of a few outstanding studies (Kittleson et al. 1983, 1985a,b; Knowlen et al. 1983; Ettinger et al. 1994), controlled clinical drug trials in spontaneous congestive heart failure in animal patients are almost nonexistent. This is in sharp contrast to human medicine, where literally dozens of double-blind, placebo-controlled drug trials appear almost annually in the cardiovascular literature. Until such studies are done in animals with spontaneous cardiac disease, cardiovascular drug therapy in veterinary internal medicine will involve a somewhat empiric approach and should be implemented carefully, with close supervision of each patient.

ANCILLARY THERAPY IN CONGESTIVE HEART FAILURE. The basic goal of therapeutic management of patients with congestive heart failure is to adjust cardiac output to meet bodily needs and, importantly, vice versa. In addition to improving mechanical performance of the heart with digitalis, other procedures helpful in attaining this goal include reducing oxygen demand by the tissues, improving oxygen uptake into the pulmonary capillary bed, decreasing pulmonary capillary pressure, reducing respiratory froth, and reducing salt intake. Except for dietary changes, all these goals theoretically can be achieved by effective drug therapy and its attendant hemodynamic improvement; however, other interventions may be necessary. This is particularly relevant in emergency situations when time may not be available for the full effects of digitalis to become manifested. Several clinical aspects concerning emergency management of congestive failure patients have been reviewed by Adams (1981).

Oxygen Demands and Delivery. In animals with mild stages of congestive failure to be treated as outpatients, severe restriction of physical exertion may be adequate to decrease oxygen needs. The owner of the animal should be advised that reduced physical activity will in all likelihood be necessary throughout the remainder of the animal's life. Initial therapy of severe cases of congestive failure includes complete inactivity in a well-oxygenated cage, especially if acute cardiac decompensation is presented. An oxygen mask, nasal catheter, or even endotracheal tube may be necessary in severe episodes of cardiogenic pulmonary edema; intermittent positive pressure ventilation is sometimes required if fluid accumulation in the lungs is overwhelming.

Diuretics. Use of potent loop-acting diuretics usually is indicated in congestive failure, and some clinicians believe these agents are drugs of choice in this condition (Hamlin et al.. 1973). However, sole therapy with diuretics alone should be carefully monitored. Pronounced diuresis could reduce blood volume to the extent that ventricular filling would be inadequate. A reduced ventricular filling pressure is good on the one hand because it reduces wall tension and myocardial oxygen demand and propensity for edema. Conversely, excessive loss of venous return without concurrent positive inotropic effects may well lead to reduced cardiac output. Most cardiologists advocate the use of diuretics in conjunction with positive inotropic drugs.

Morphine. Morphine has been advocated as an agent of choice, second only to effective delivery of oxygen, in managing pulmonary edema (Davis 1979). Morphine purportedly exerts beneficial effects by three actions: sedation and relief of anxiety; conversion of rapid, violent ventilatory patterns to slow, deep respirations by depressing the respiratory centers; and dilation of splanchnic vasculature, thereby diverting blood volume from the pulmonary to the systemic circuit. IV administration of small quantities of morphine (0.05-0.1 mg/kg) can be made every 3-6 minutes while the patient's progress is monitored closely.

Inasmuch as morphine substantially reduces coronary blood flow in the dog, the question arises whether it is efficacious in treatment of cardiac dyspnea.

Other Procedures. Bronchodilating drugs (e.g., aminophylline) have been strongly advocated in treatment of congestive failure (Bolton 1977). Aminophylline and other xanthines are potent bronchodilators, but they also have direct stimulatory activity on the heart, some diuretic activity, and vasodilator effects. A usual dose of aminophylline is 10 mg/kg given orally or parenterally 2 to 3 times a day. IV administrations should be infused slowly, preferably in dilute solution. A large number of bronchodilatory antitussive-expectorant preparations have been used in congestive failure, but the potential for unexpected drug interactions should be considered. Nebulization of a 20% solution of ethanol into the respiratory tract may be of some help in reducing foaming of respiratory fluids in acute cases. Sodium intake should be restricted on a long-term basis to reduce the potential for edema formation. Low-salt dog foods are available commercially.

REFERENCES

Abrams, J. 1985. Vasodilator therapy for chronic congestive heart failure. J Am Med Assoc 254:3070-74.

Adams, H. R. 1981. Cardiovascular emergencies: drug and resuscitative principles. Vet Clin North Am 11:77-102.

———. 1986a. Ca^{++} channel blocking drugs in shock and trauma: new approaches to old problems? Am J Emerg Med 15:1457-60.

———. 1986b. New perspectives in cardiology: pharmacodynamic classification of antiarrhythmic drugs. J Am Vet Med Assoc 189:525-32.

Akera, T., Ng, Y. C. 1991. Digitalis sensitivity of Na^+,K^+-ATPase, myocytes and the heart. Life Sci 48:97-106.

Allert, J. A., Adams, H. R. 1987. New perspectives in cardiovascular medicine: the calcium channel blocking drugs. J Am Vet Med Assoc 190:573-78.

Alousi, A. A., Farah, A. E., Lesher, G. Y., et al. 1979. Cardiotonic activity of amrinone—Win 40680 [5-amino-3,4′-bipyridine-6(1H)-one]. Circ Res 45:666-77.

Aranow, W. S. 1992. Clinical use of digitalis. Comp Ther 18:38-41.

Atwell, R. B. 1979. The use of alpha blockade in the treatment of congestive heart failure associated with dirofilariasis and mitral valvular incompetence. Vet Rec 104:114-16.

Baker, P. F., Blaustein, M. P., Hodgkin, A. L., et al. 1969. The influence of calcium on sodium efflux in squid axons. J Physiol (Lond) 200:431-58.

Barr, I., Smith, T. W., Klein, M. D., et al. 1972. Correlation of the electrophysiologic action of digoxin with serum digoxin concentration. J Pharmacol Exp Ther 180:710-22.

Beck, A. M. 1969. M.S. thesis, Univ. of Pennsylvania.

Bolton, G. R. 1977. In R. W. Kirk, ed., Veterinary Therapy, VI: Small Animal Practice, p. 340. Philadelphia: W. B. Saunders.

Braunwald, E. 1985. Effects of digitalis on the normal and the failing heart. J Am Coll Cardiol 5:51A-59A.

Braunwald, E., Kahler, R. L. 1964. The mechanism of action of cardiac drugs. Physiol Physicians 2:1-5.

Breznock, E. M. 1973. Application of canine plasma kinetics of digoxin and digitoxin to therapeutic digitalization in the dog. Am J Vet Res 34:993-99.

———. 1975. Effects of phenobarbital on digitoxin and digoxin elimination in the dog. Am J Vet Res 36:371-73.

Bright, J. M. 1992. Update: diltiazem therapy of feline hypertrophic cardiomyopathy. In Kirk's Current Veterinary Therapy XI, Ed. R. W. Kirk, J. D. Bonagura, p. 766-73.

Brooks, N., Cattell, M., Pidgeon, J., et al. 1980. Unpredictable response to nifedipine in severe cardiac failure. Br Med J 281:1324.

Button, C., Gross, D. R., Allert, J. A. 1980b. Application of individualized digoxin dosage regimens to canine therapeutic digitalization. Am J Vet Res 41:1238-42.

Button, C., Gross, D. R., Johnston, J. T., et al. 1980a. Pharmacokinetics, bioavailability, and dosage regimens of digoxin in dogs. Am J Vet Res 41:1230-37.

Button, C., Gross, D. R., Johnston, J. T., et al. 1980c. Digoxin pharmacokinetics, bioavailability, efficacy, and dosage regimens in the horse. Am J Vet Res 41:1388-95.

Carpenter, C. C., Davis, J. O., Wallace, C. R., et al. 1962. Acute effects of cardiac glycosides on aldosterone secretion in dogs with hyperaldosteronism secondary to chronic right heart failure. Circ Res 10:178-87.

Colucci, W. S., Fifer, M. A., Lorell, B. H., et al. 1985. Calcium channel blockers in congestive heart failure: theoretic considerations and clinical experience. Am J Med 78(Suppl 2B):9 -17.

Colucci, W. S., Wright, R. F., Braunwald, E. 1986a. New positive inotropic agents in the treatment of congestive heart failure: mechanisms of action and recent clinical developments, 1. N Engl J Med 314:290-99.

———. 1986b. New positive inotropic agents in the treatment of congestive heart failure: mechanisms of action and recent clinical developments, 2. N Engl J Med 314:349-58.

Conti, C. R., Pepine, C., Feldman, R. L., et al. 1985. Calcium antagonists. Cardiology 72:297-321.

Davis, L. E. 1979. Management of acute pulmonary edema. J Am Vet Med Assoc 175:97-98.

Defeudis, F. V. 1985. Calcium antagonist subgroups. Trends Pharmacol Sci 6:237-38.

Denis, R., Lucas, C. E., Ledgerwood, A. M., et al. 1985. The beneficial role of calcium supplementation during resuscitation from shock. J Trauma 25:594-600.

De Rick, A., Belpaire, F. M., Bogaert, M. G., et al. 1978. Pharmacokinetics of digoxin. Am J Vet Res 39:811-18.

Detweiler, D. K. 1967. Comparative pharmacology of cardiac glycosides. Fed Proc 26:1119-24.

———. 1977. In L. M. Jones, N. H. Booth, and L. E. McDonald, eds., Veterinary Pharmacology and Therapeutics, 4th ed. Ames: Iowa State Univ. Press.

Detweiler, D. K., Knight, D. H. 1977. Congestive heart failure in dogs: therapeutic concepts. J Am Vet Med Assoc 171:106-14.

Detweiler, D. K., Patterson, D. F. 1963. In J. F. Bone, ed., Equine Medicine and Surgery. Wheaton, Ill.: American Veterinary Publications.

DiBianco, R., Shabetai, R., Kostuk, W., Moran, J., Schlaut, R. C., Wright, R. 1989. A comparison of oral milrinone, digoxin, and their combination in the treatment of patients with congestive heart failure. N Eng J Med 320:677-83.

Dietz, R., Waas, W., Susselbeck, T., Willenbrock, R., Osterziel, K. J. 1993. Improvement of cardiac function by angiotensin converting enzyme inhibition: sites of action. Circulation 87 (Suppl IV):108-16.

Doherty, J. E. 1973. Digitalis glycosides: pharmacokinetics and their clinical implications. Ann Int Med 79:229-38.

Erichsen, D. F., Harris, S. G., Upson, D. W. 1980. Therapeutic and toxic plasma concentrations of digoxin in the cat. Am J Vet Res 41:2049-58.

Ettinger, S. J., Benitz, A. M., Ericsson, G. F. 1994. Relationships of enalapril with other CHF treatment modalities. In Proc 12th Amer Col Vet Int Med Forum, pp. 251-53.

Ettinger, S. J., Suter, P. F. 1970. Canine Cardiology, p. 237. Philadelphia: W. B. Saunders.

Ezrailson, E. G., Potter, J. D., Michael, L., et al. 1977. Positive inotropy induced by ouabain, by increased frequency, by X537A (RO2-2985), by calcium and by isoproterenol: the lack of correlation with phosphorylation of TnI. J Mol Cell Cardiol 9:693-98.

Fabiato, A., Fabiato, F. 1979. Calcium and cardiac excitation-contraction coupling. Ann Rev Physiol 41:473-84.

Feldman, A. M. 1993. Modulation of adrenergic receptors and G-transduction proteins in failing human ventricular myocardium. Circulation 87(Suppl IV):27-34.

Fillmore, G. E., Detweiler, D. K. 1973. Maintenance of subacute digoxin toxicosis in normal beagles. Toxicol Appl Pharmacol 25:418-29.

Fleckenstein, A. 1983. History of calcium antagonists. Circ Res 52(Suppl 1):3-16.

Fozzard, H. A. 1976. In M. Vassale, ed., Cardiac Physiology for the Clinician, p. 61. New York: Academic Press.

Fozzard, H. A., Gibbons, W. R. 1973. Action potential and contraction of heart muscle. Am J Cardiol 31:182-92.

Fozzard, H. A., Sheets, M. F. 1985. Cellular mechanism of action of cardiac glycosides. J Am Coll Cardiol 5:10A-15A.

Frank, O. 1895. Z Biol 32:370.

Gadsby, D. C. 1984. The Na/K pump of cardiac cells. Ann Rev Biophys Bioeng 13:373-98.

Gillis, R. A., Quest, J. A. 1980. The role of the nervous system in the cardiovascular effects of digitalis. Pharmacol Rev 31:19-97.

Haber, E. 1985. Antibodies and digitalis: the modern revolution in the use of an ancient drug. J Am Coll Cardiol 5:111A-117A.

Hahn, A. W. 1977. In R. W. Kirk, ed., Veterinary Therapy, VI: Small Animal Practice, p. 329. Philadelphia: W. B. Saunders.

Hamlin, R. L. 1977. New ideas in the management of heart failure in dogs. J Am Vet Med Assoc 171:114-18.

———. 1986. Clinical and experimental studies with verapamil in the dog. In Proc 5th Symp Am Acad Vet Pharm Therap., pp. 89-96.

Hamlin, R. L., Dutta, S., Smith, C. R. 1971. Effects of digoxin and digitoxin on ventricular function in normal dogs and dogs with heart failure. Am J Vet Res 32:1391-98.

Hamlin, R. L., Pipers, F. S., Carter, K. L., et al. 1973. Treatment of heart failure in dogs without use of digitalis glycosides. Vet Med Small Anim Clin 68:349-50.

Harris, S. G. 1974. In R. W. Kirk, ed., Veterinary Therapy, V: Small Animal Practice, p. 320. Philadelphia: W. B. Saunders.

Holtz, J. 1993. The cardiac renin-angiotensin system: physiological relevance and pharmacological modulation. Clin Investig 71:S25-S34.

Jacobs, A. S., Nielsen, D. H., Gianelly, R. E. 1985. Fatal ventricular fibrillation following verapamil in Wolff-Parkinson-White syndrome with atrial fibrillation. Ann Emerg Med 14:159-60.

Janis, R. A., Triggle, D. J. 1984. 1,4-Dihydropyridine Ca^{++} channel antagonists and activators: a comparison of binding characteristics with pharmacology. Drug Dev Res 4:257-74.

Johnson, J. T. 1985. Conversion of atrial fibrillation in two dogs using verapamil and supportive therapy. J Am Anim Hosp Assoc 21:429-34.

Josephson, M. A., Singh, B. N. 1985. Use of calcium antagonists in ventricular dysfunction. Am J Cardiol 55:81B-88B.

Kae, A. M., Hager, W. D., Messineo, F. C., et al. 1985. Cellular actions and pharmacology of the calcium channel blocking drugs. Am J Med 77(Suppl 2B):2-10.

Katz, A. M. 1985. Effects of digitalis on cell biochemistry: sodium pump inhibition. J Am Coll Cardiol 5:16A-21A.

Kittleson, M. D. 1983. In R. W. Kirk, ed., Veterinary Therapy, VIII: Small Animal Practice, p. 285. Philadelphia: W. B. Saunders.

Kittleson, M. D., Eyster, G. E., Knowlen, G. G., et al. 1985a. Efficacy of digoxin administration in dogs with idiopathic congestive cardiomyopathy. J Am Vet Med Assoc 186:162-65.

Kittleson, M. D., Eyster, G. E., Olivier, M. B., et al. 1983. Oral hydralazine therapy for chronic mitral regurgitation in the dog. J Am Vet Med Assoc 182:1205-9.

Kittleson, M. D., Johnson, L. E., Pion, P. D., Mekhamer, Y. E. 1993. The acute hemodynamic effects of captopril in dogs with heart failure. J Vet Pharmacol Therap 16:1-7.

Kittleson, M. D., Keene, B., Woodfield, J. A. 1986. The acute therapy of supraventricular tachycardia with verapamil. In Proc 5th Symp Am Acad Vet Pharm Therap., p. 97-102.

Kittleson, M. D., Pipers, F. S., Knauer, K. W., et al. 1985b. Echocardiographic and clinical effects of milrinone in dogs with myocardial failure. Am J Vet Res 46:1659-64.

Knowlen, G. G., Kittleson, M. D., Nachreiner, R. F. 1983. Comparison of plasma aldosterone concentration among clinical status groups of dogs with chronic heart failure. J Am Vet Med Assoc 183:991-96.

Krasula, R. W., Gardella, L. A., Zaroslinsk, J. F., et al. 1976. Comparative bioavailability of four dosage forms of digoxin in dogs. Fed Proc 35:327(abst.).

Kurowski, V., Iven, H., Djonlagic, H. 1992. Treatment of a patient with severe digitoxin intoxication by Fab fragments of anti-digitalis antibodies. Intensive Care Med 18:439-42.

Langer, G. A. 1976. Events at the cardiac sarcolemma: localization and movement of contractile-dependent calcium. Fed Proc 35:1274-78.

———. 1977. Relationship between myocardial contractility and the effects of digitalis on ionic exchange. Fed Proc 36:2231-34.

Langer, G. A. 1976. Events at the cardiac sarcolemma: localization and movement of contractile-dependent calcium. Fed Proc 35:1274-78.

———. 1980. The role of calcium in the control of myocardial contractility: an update. J Mol Cell Cardiol 12:231-39.

Lanza, R. P., Cooper, D. K. C., Barnard, C. N. 1984. Lack of efficacy of high-dose verapamil in preventing brain damage in baboons and pigs after prolonged partial cerebral ischemia. Am J Emerg Med 2:481-85.

Lee, K. S., Klaus, W. 1971. The subcellular basis for the mechanism of inotropic action of cardiac glycosides. Pharmacol Rev 23:193-261.

Lorell, B. H. 1985. Use of calcium channel blockers in hypertrophic cardiomyopathy. Am J Med 78(Suppl 2B):43-54.

Lown, B., Black, H., Moore, F. D. 1960. Digitalis, electrolytes and the surgical patient. Am J Cardiol 6:309-37.

Mancini, D. M., Keren, G., Aogaichi, K., et al. 1985. Inotropic drugs for the treatment of heart failure. J Clin Pharmacol 25:540-54.

Mason, D. T. 1973. Regulation of cardiac performance in clinical heart disease: interactions between contractile state mechanical abnormalities and ventricular compensatory mechanisms. Am J Cardiol 32:437-48.

Mason, D. T., Zelis, R., Lee, G., et al. 1971. Current concepts and treatment of digitalis toxicity. Am J Cardiol 27:546-59.

Massie, B., Bourassa, M., DiBianco, R., et al. 1985. Long-term oral administration of amrinone for congestive heart failure: lack of efficacy in a multicenter controlled trial. Circulation 71:963-71.

Meijler, F. L. 1985. An "account" of digitalis and atrial fibrillation. J Am Coll Cardiol 5:60A-68A.

Mendez, C., Aceves, J., Mendez, R. 1961a. The anti-adrenergic action of digitalis on the refractory period of the A-V transmission system. J Pharmacol Exp Ther 131:199-204.

———. 1961b. Inhibition of adrenergic cardiac acceleration by cardiac glycosides. J Pharmacol Exp Ther 131:191-98.

Moalic, J. M., Charlemagne, D., Mansier, P., Chevalier, B., Swynghedauw, B. 1993. Cardiac hypertrophy and failure—a disease of adaptation. Circulation 87(Suppl IV):21-26.

Moe, G. K, Farah, A. E. 1975. In L. S. Goodman and A. Gilman, eds., The Pharmacological Basis of Therapeutics, 5th ed., p. 653. New York: Macmillan.

Nayler, W. G. 1980. Calcium antagonists. Eur Heart 1:225-37.

Novotny, M. J., Adams, H. R. 1986. New perspectives in cardiology: recent advances in antiarrhythmic drug therapy. J Am Vet Med Assoc 189:533-39.

Opie, L. H., ed. 1984. Calcium antagonists and cardiovascular disease. New York: Raven Press.

Packer, M. 1984. Conceptual dilemmas in the classification of vasodilator drugs for severe chronic heart failure: advocacy of a pragmatic approach to the selection of a therapeutic agent. Am J Med 76:3-13.

———. 1985. Therapeutic application of calcium channel antagonists for pulmonary hypertension. Am J Cardiol 55:81B-88B.

Parker, J. L., Adams, H. R. 1977. Drugs and the heart muscle. J Am Vet Med Assoc 171:78-84.

Patterson, D. F., Abt, D. A., Detweiler, D. K., et al. 1973. On digitalis glycosides in treatment of heart failure: Criticism and reply. Vet Med Small Anim Clin 68:708.

Pion, P. D., Batish, J., Schwark, W., et al. 1986. Pharmacokinetics and electrocardiographic effects of verapamil in the cat. In Proc 5th Symp Am Acad Vet Pharm Therap., pp. 141-53.

Remme, W. J. 1993. Vasodilator therapy for heart failure: early, late, or not at all? Circulation 87(Suppl IV):97-107.

Reuter, H. 1979. Properties of two inward membrane currents in the heart. Ann Rev Physiol 41:413-24.

———. 1985. Calcium movements through cardiac cell membranes. Med Res Rev 5:427-40.

Rick, A. D., Belpaire, F. M., Bogaert, M. G., et al. 1978. Plasma concentrations of digoxin and digitoxin during digitalization of healthy dogs and dogs with cardiac failure. Am J Vet Res 39:811-15.

Robinson, J. W. 1972. The inhibition of glycine and beta-methyl glucoside transport in dog kidney cortex slices by ouabain and ethacrynic acid: contribution to the understanding of sodium-pumping mechanisms. Com Gen Pharmacol 3:145-59.

Rosen, M. R. 1985. Cellular electrophysiology of digitalis toxicity. J Am Coll Cardiol 5:22A-34A.

Rosing, D. R., Kent, K. M., Borer, J. S., et al. 1979. Verapamil therapy: a new approach to the pharmacologic treatment of hypertrophic cardiomyopathy, 1. Hemodynamic effects. Circulation 60:1201-7.

Schatzmann, H. J. 1953. Herzglykoside als Hemmstoffe für den aktiven kalium-und natriumtransport durch die erythrocytenmembran. Helv Physiol Pharmacol Acta 11:346-54.

Schramm, M., Towart, R. 1985. Modulation of calcium channel function by drugs. Life Sci 37:1843-60.

Schwartz, A. 1977. New aspects of cardiac glycoside action: introduction. Fed Proc 36:2207-8.

Sisson, D. D. 1992. Hemodynamic, echocardiographic, radiographic, and clinical effects of enalapril in dogs with chronic heart failure. In Proc 10th Amer Col Vet Int Med Forum, pp. 589-91.

Smith, W. J., Wenger, T. L., Grant, A. O., et al. 1981. The antiarrhythmic spectrum of verapamil. Drug Ther (Hosp) 6:63-75.

Solaro, R. J., Wise, R. M., Shiner, J. S., et al. 1974. Calcium requirements for cardiac myofibrillar activation. Circ Res 34:525-30.

Somlyo, A. P. 1985. Excitation-contraction coupling and the ultrastructure of smooth muscle. Circ Res 57:497-507.

Spedding, M. 1985. Calcium antagonists subgroups. Trends Pharmacol Sci 6:109-14.

Starling, E. H. 1918. The Linacre Lecture on the Law of the Heart. London: Longmans, Green.

Stone, P. H., Antmann, E. M, eds. 1983. Calcium channel blocking agents in the treatment of cardiovascular disorders. New York: Fritina Publishing Co.

Swedberg, K. 1993. Reduction in mortality by pharmacological therapy in congestive heart failure. Circulation 87(Suppl IV):126-29.

Teske, R. H., Bishop, S. P., Righter, H. F., et al. 1976. Subacute digoxin toxicosis in the beagle dog. Toxicol Appl Pharmacol 35:283-301.

Tilley, L. P. 1979. Essentials of Canine and Feline Electrocardiography. St. Louis: C. V. Mosby.

Tilley, L. P., Liusk, Gilbertson, S. R., et al. 1977. Primary myocardial disease in the cat: a model for human cardiomyopathy. Am J Pathol 86:493-513.

Tilley, L. P., Weitz, J. 1977. Pharmacologic and other forms of medical therapy in feline cardiac disease. Vet Clin North Am 7:415-28.

Trump, B. F., Berezesky, I. K., Cowley, R. A. 1982. The cellular and subcellular characteristics of acute and chronic injury with emphasis on the role of calcium. In R. A. Cowley, B. F. Trump, eds., Pathophysiology of Shock, Anoxia, and Ischemia, p. 646. Baltimore: Williams & Wilkins.

Vaughn Williams, E. M. 1984. Classification of antiarrhythmic actions reassessed after a decade of new drugs. J Clin Pharmacol 24:129-47.

Wasman, H. L., Myerburg, R. J., Appel, R., et al. 1981. Verapamil for control of ventricular rates in paroxysmal supraventricular tachycardia and atrial fibrillation or flutter. Ann Intern Med 94:1-6.

Watanabe, A. M. 1985. Digitalis and the autonomic nervous system. J Am Coll Cardiol 5:35A-42A.

White, B. C., Aust, S. D., Arfors, K. E., et al. 1984. Brain injury by ischemic anoxia: hypothesis extension—a tale of two ions? Ann Emerg Med 13:862-67.

Withering, W. 1785. Reprinted 1937. Account of foxglove, and some of its medical uses; with practical remarks on dropsy, and other diseases. Med Classics 2:305-443.

Zelis, R., Flaim, S. F., Moskowitz, R. M., et al. 1979. How much can we expect from vasodilator therapy in congestive heart failure? Circulation 59:1092-97.

24

ANTIARRHYTHMIC AGENTS

H. RICHARD ADAMS

Rhythmicity of the Heart
Electrophysiologic Properties of Cardiac Cells
Classification of Arrhythmogenic Mechanisms
Fast and Slow Responses and Conduction
Antiarrhythmic Drugs
Classification
Autonomic Drugs
Digitalis
Quinidine Sulfate
Procainamide Hydrochloride
Phenytoin Sodium
Lidocaine Hydrochloride
Propranolol Hydrochloride
Verapamil and Diltiazem
Newer Drugs
Clinical Indications

An arrhythmia is an abnormality in the rate, regularity, or site of origin of the cardiac impulse or a disruption in impulse conduction such that the normal sequence of atrial and ventricular activation is changed. Although numerous drugs have been identified that suppress cardiac rhythm disturbances, relatively few antiarrhythmic drugs have found strong clinical use in veterinary medicine. This chapter focuses on the more common antiarrhymic agents along with their principal pharmacodynamic actions on cardiac rate and rhythm.

RHYTHMICITY OF THE HEART. Normal cardiac rhythmicity is maintained by (1) dominance of a single pacemaker discharging regularly with the highest frequency, (2) rapid and uniform conduction through normal routes of impulse conduction, and (3) long and uniform duration of the action potential and refractory period of cardiac myofibers. In addition, duration of the Purkinje fiber action potential normally outlasts that of the ventricular muscle, thus providing a safety factor preventing reentry and reexcitation of the Purkinje system by the muscle action potential. A disturbance in any of the preceding factors can be arrhythmogenic, e.g., an inappropriate increase in automaticity of normally latent pacemaker cells, abbreviation of the refractory period, slowing of conduction velocity, or disparate refractory periods of adjacent fibers.

Arrhythmias often are associated with imbalance of the parasympathetic and sympathetic branches of the autonomic nervous system; changes in serum electrolyte concentrations, especially potassium and calcium ions (K^+ and Ca^{++}); hypoxemia; acidosis; changes in concentration of carbon dioxide; excessive stretch of cardiac tissue; mechanical trauma; myocardial disease states such as congestive heart failure and viral myocarditis; numerous drugs; and ischemia and infarction of the heart muscle.

Hemodynamic instability occurring during cardiac arrhythmias results from alterations in heart rate, changing the regularity of heartbeats, and losing atrial assistance in ventricular filling. Electromechanical synchrony of the cardiac chambers is thereby lost, culminating in ineffectual filling and ejection of the ventricles and hemodynamic deterioration of the patient. Antiarrhythmic drugs suppress arrhythmias and help restore hemodynamic stability by altering basic electrophysiologic processes in the heart.

Electrophysiologic Properties of Cardiac Cells. The classification system for clinically useful antiarrhythmic drugs is based mainly on the predominant pharmacologic effects of a drug on the action potential of cardiac cells (Vaughn Williams 1984; Adams 1986). Accordingly, a useful understanding of antiarrhythmic drug actions and affiliated nomenclature depends first on a good comprehension of basic bioelectric properties of the heart. An overview of salient features of this topic is outlined below relative to action potentials of cardiac cells and types of cardiac arrhythmogenesis.

Action Potentials of Cardiac Cells. The electrical activity of individual heart muscle cells can be recorded with a microelectrode capable of entering the intracellular space of a single cell, as shown schematically in Fig. 24.1. Some of the common terms used to describe the configuration and ionic determinants of cardiac action potential components are defined below (Adams 1986):

1. Membrane potential is the voltage difference across the cell membrane, i.e., the difference in electrical voltage between the intracellular and extracellular spaces. By convention, the resting membrane potential is defined as the charge inside the cell relative to the extracellular side, in which case the resting potential is a negative charge. An increase in resting membrane

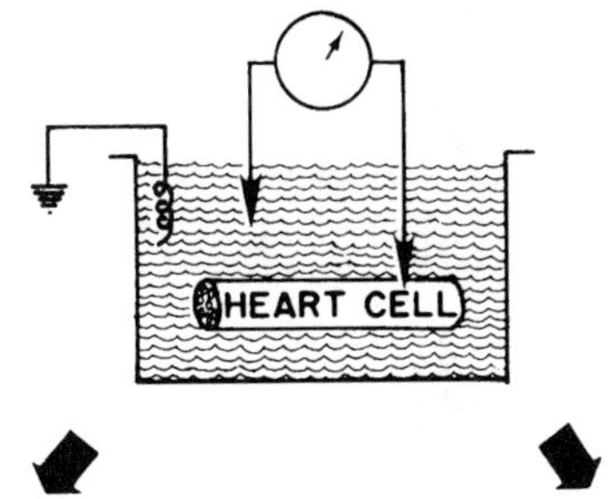

A. WORKING MUSCLE CELL

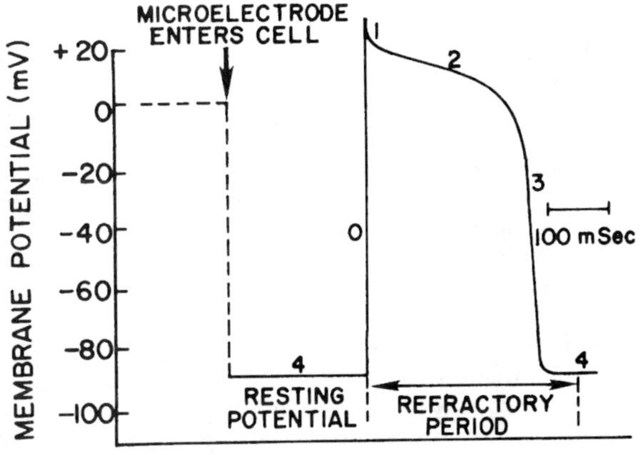

B. SINOATRIAL NODE CELL

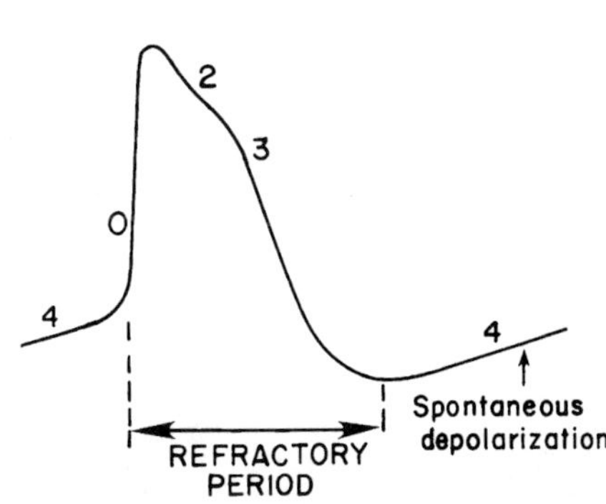

FIG. 24.1—Cardiac action potentials recorded from a working myocardial cell (A) and a sinoatrial pacemaker cell (B). The nonautomatic working muscle cell (A) exhibits a constant phase 4 resting potential during diastole, whereas the automatic cell (B) undergoes spontaneous depolarization during phase 4, leading to threshold and spontaneous excitation. The cell is inexcitable or poorly responsive to additional stimuli during much of the action potential, and this refractory period helps prevent premature excitation. See text for further details. (Source: Adams 1986.)

potential would therefore designate a more negative intracellular charge (e.g., an increase from –70 to –90 mV), while a decrease in resting membrane potential would designate a less negative intracellular charge (e.g., a decrease from –70 to –50 mV).

2. Depolarization is the loss or decrease in electronegativity of the intracellular space, e.g., a decrease in membrane potential from –90 to –50 mV (partial depolarization) or from –90 to 0 mV (complete depolarization).

3. Hyperpolarization is an increase in electronegativity of the intracellular space.

4. Inward current is the change in electrical charge across the cell membrane that results from influx of positively charged ions or, alternatively, from efflux of negatively charged ions.

5. Spontaneous depolarization of automatic cells is a physiologic and progressive decrease in resting potential during diastole, leading spontaneously to threshold and automatic firing.

6. Threshold potential is the membrane potential required for excitation of the cell, initiating the action potential and affiliated cellular responses.

7. Phase 0 is the rapid depolarization phase of the action potential of the excited cell, mediated by a rapid inward current carried by Na^+ through fast sodium channels of the cell membrane.

8. Phase 1 is the initial early repolarization phase of the action potential.

9. Phase 2 is the plateau phase of the action potential, mediated in part by a slow inward current carried by Ca^{++} through slow calcium channels of the cell membrane.

10. Phase 3 is the rapid repolarization phase of the action potential, returning membrane potential to the diastolic level.

11. Phase 4 is the membrane potential during diastole; it is constant in working muscle cells but undergoes spontaneous depolarization in cells with automaticity.

12. Refractory period is that early and late interval of the action potential during which excitability of the cell is essentially absent (functional refractory period) or depressed (relative refractory period) respectively.

13. Depressed fast sodium ion (Na^+) responses are slowly rising phase 0 depolarizations due either to

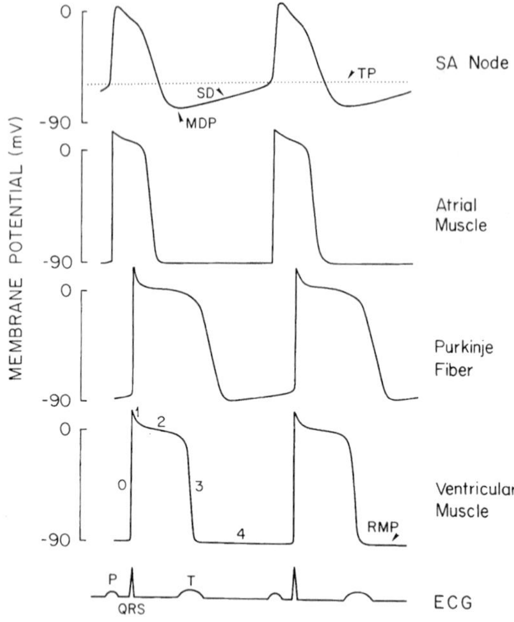

FIG. 24.2—Schematic diagrams demonstrating the temporal relationships between transmembrane action potentials recorded from cells of the sinoatrial node (SA), atrial muscle, Purkinje fibers, and ventricular muscle (see text for discussion). (Modeled after Trautwein 1963. Source: Adams 1986.)

premature excitation during the relative refractory period of normal cells or excitation of sick cells with low diastolic potentials; depressed fast Na^+ response action potentials develop cardiac impulses that propagate poorly with reduced conduction velocity.

14. Slow Ca^{++} responses are analogous to the slow inward Ca^{++} current during phase 2; this term is used to describe the very slowly rising phase 0 depolarizations mediated by Ca^{++} when the fast Na^+ channels are inoperative. Slow Ca^{++} action potentials develop cardiac impulses that propagate poorly with extremely slow conduction.

When a cardiac cell is stimulated, the electrical potential measured across the cell membrane undergoes a depolarization and repolarization cycle that can be differentiated into five interconnected components. These components are referred to as phases 0, 1, 2, 3, and 4 (Fig. 24.1). The precise morphology of the 5 phases of the cardiac action potential varies with the anatomic region of the heart. A schematic diagram illustrating the configuration of action potentials derived from SA tissue, atrial muscle (AM), Purkinje fibers (PF), and ventricular muscle (VM) is depicted in Fig. 24.2 along with corresponding waveforms of the electrocardiogram (ECG). Action potentials of a sinoatrial pacemaker cell (Fig. 24.1B) and a typical working heart muscle cell (Fig. 24.1A) will be addressed as examples of cardiac tissue with and without normal automaticity respectively.

WORKING HEART MUSCLE CELLS. Electrical diastole is designated by phase 4 of the action potential (Fig. 24.1A); during this period, the resting membrane potential of heart muscle cells is steady at about –90 mV. The interior of the cell is charged negatively relative to the extracellular space; this state of polarization across the cell membrane is maintained primarily because of the unequal distribution of K^+ inside and outside the cell. The Na^+,K^+-adenosine triphosphatase transport system maintains high intracellular K^+ relative to extracellular K^+, and the cell membrane is selectively permeable to K^+ during phase 4 diastole when compared to other ions such as Na^+ or Ca^{++}. When the cell is stimulated to its particular threshold level, however, the selective permeability characteristics of the cell membrane to K^+ are momentarily lost. Other ions now cross the sarcolemma and produce the typical depolarization-repolarization cycle that comprises the action potential (Fig. 24.1).

Phase 0 of the action potential reflects the extremely rapid depolarization spike produced by Na^+ rushing into the cell through specific "fast Na^+ channels" or passageways of the sarcolemma. As the permeability characteristics of the sarcolemma are reestablished, phase 0 is terminated as early (phase 1) and delayed (phase 3) repolarization occur, restoring the membrane potential to its resting diastolic level of phase 4 (Fig. 24.1). The cell is inexcitable or nonresponsive to additional stimuli during the early and intermediate phase of the action potential cycle; it is only partially responsive if stimulated prior to complete repolarization and return to normal phase 4 diastolic potential. This period of refractoriness provides a safety factor, preventing reexcitation by the initiating cardiac impulse itself.

Phase 2 is the plateau of the action potential (Fig. 24.1); it partially represents a brief anomalous delay in restoration of K^+ permeability. In addition, a critically important component of phase 2 comprises an influx of Ca^{++} through specific "slow Ca^{++} channels" or "slow cation channels" of the cell membrane. The plateau phase is important because this slow inward Ca^{++} current is the mechanism whereby membrane excitation is coupled to activation of the contractile elements of heart muscle cells (Parker and Adams 1977). The influx of Ca^{++} during phase 2 triggers a release of greater amounts of Ca^{++} from intracellular storage sites. The increased availability of cytosolic Ca^{++} directly and proportionately activates the contractile machinery of the myocardial cells. As will be addressed subsequently, the slow inward Ca^{++} current participates also in certain types of automaticity mechanisms and conduction disturbances.

SINOATRIAL PACEMAKER CELLS. Unlike working myocardial cells, automatic cells do not exhibit a clearly definable resting membrane potential during phase 4. Instead, phase 4 is characterized by a slow spontaneous depolarization to threshold potential (Fig. 24.1B), thereby discharging automatically and leading into the more rapid depolarization of phase 0. However, the slope of phase 0 depolarization of SA pacemaker cells is much less than that of working muscle cells (Figs. 24.1, 24.2). This distinction may be explained by a component of slow Ca^{++} influx in the genesis of phase 0 depolarization in these types of automatic cells (Adams 1986). In addition to SA pacemaker tissue, cells with normal automaticity (i.e., spontaneous phase 4 depolarization) also are found in specialized atrial conduction tracts, the distal region of the AV node, AV valves, and PF. Although working muscle cells do not normally develop spontaneous depolarization during phase 4 (Fig. 24.1A), they may generate aberrant automaticity during heart disease and thereby mediate or contribute to associated arrhythmogenic events.

Classification of Arrhythmogenic Mechanisms. Theories on the basic mechanisms involved in genesis of cardiac arrhythmias focus on abnormalities of impulse formation (i.e., arrhythmias caused by changes in automaticity), impulse conduction (i.e., arrhythmias caused by reentry phenomena), and a combination of automaticity and reentry (Singh et al. 1980; Binah and Rosen 1984; Boyden and Wit 1985).

DISTURBANCES IN AUTOMATICITY. The action potential from the SA node, AM, PF, and VM are shown in Fig. 24.2. The five phases of the action potential (0, 1, 2, 3, 4) are numbered in the first complex of VM. Notice spontaneous depolarization (SD), maximal diastolic potential (MDP), and threshold potential (TP) in the automatic cells of SA and PF. The resting membrane potential (RMP) is shown in the nonautomatic cells of the AM and VM. The P wave of the ECG corresponds to depolarization of SA and AM, while the QRS complex and T wave correspond to depolarization and repolarization respectively of ventricular cells (Fig. 24.2).

Automatic cells of the SA node normally are the dominant pacemaker, reaching threshold first with the resultant propagating impulse exciting all other potential pacemaker cells before they spontaneously attain threshold values (Fig. 24.2). If automaticity of the SA node is depressed or the spontaneous firing rate in some other tissue (latent pacemaker) is accelerated, regions of the heart other than the SA node may serve as the pacemaker and initiate ectopic impulses. Examples are shown in Fig. 24.3.

Automaticity is enhanced when the slope of phase 4 SD is increased (e.g., from a to b in I of Fig. 24.3); this decreases the time required to reach TP, thereby increasing the frequency of spontaneous discharge. The result is an increase in heart rate when the SA pacemaker is involved or emergence of ectopic beats if a normally latent pacemaker is involved. By decreasing the slope of spontaneous depolarization (e.g., from b to a or from a to c in I of Fig. 24.3), drugs can depress ectopic foci and restore normal sinus rhythm without affecting MDP or TP. If a drug raises TP to less negative values (e.g., from TP-a to TP-b in II of Fig. 24.3), additional time will be required to reach TP, thereby depressing automaticity. By increasing the MDP (e.g., from MDP-a to MDP-b in III of Fig. 24.3), a drug can suppress automaticity since additional time would be required before TP is attained.

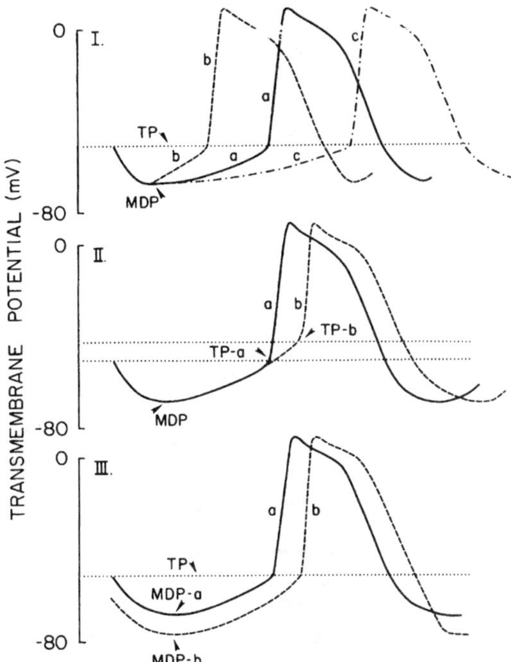

FIG. 24.3—Schematic representations of transmembrane action potentials of cardiac cells with the property of automaticity and potential mechanisms whereby antiarrhythmic drugs can influence automaticity (see text for discussion). (Modeled after Hoffman and Cranefield 1960; Mason et al. 1973.)

DISTURBANCES IN IMPULSE CONDUCTION. Arrhythmias caused by disturbances in impulse conduction are thought to be associated with a phenomenon of reentry or circus movement. The concept of reentry is based on very slow conduction velocity, an area of the heart demonstrating unidirectional block of impulse conduction and perhaps an abnormally brief refractory period (Schmidt and Erlanger 1929; Wit et al. 1972, 1974). This theory holds that a cardiac impulse can travel circuitously around an anatomic loop of fibers in which slowed conduction velocity and brief refractoriness permit the impulse to arrive at cells that are no longer refractory, thereby permitting perpetual reexcitation.

A schematic demonstration of impulse reentry at a junctional region between PF and ventricular muscle is shown in Fig. 24.4 (Adams 1986). Acceptance of this

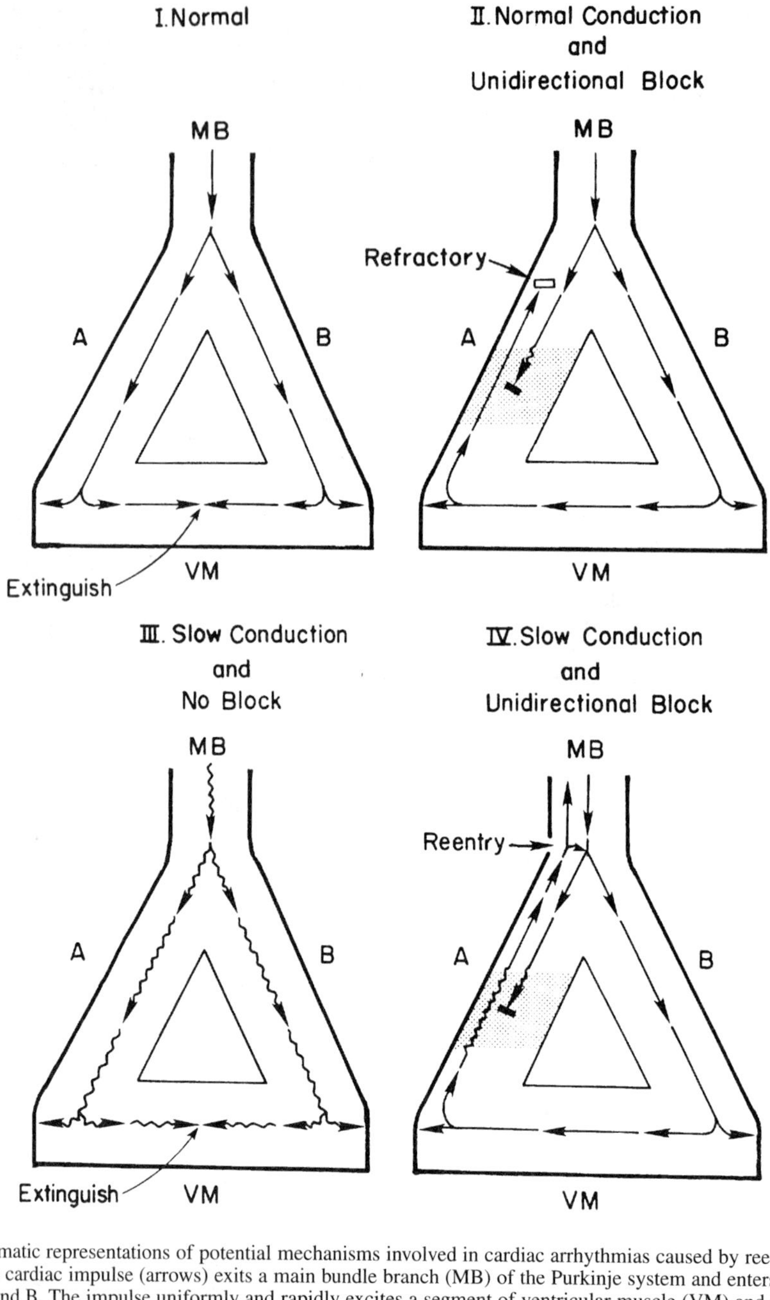

FIG. 24.4—Schematic representations of potential mechanisms involved in cardiac arrhythmias caused by reentry phenomena.

I. Normal. The cardiac impulse (arrows) exits a main bundle branch (MB) of the Purkinje system and enters terminal Purkinje branches A and B. The impulse uniformly and rapidly excites a segment of ventricular muscle (VM) and would be extinguished within the VM due to refractoriness of the cells just excited.

II. Normal conduction and unidirectional block. Because of an area of damaged tissue (shaded area) that blocks antegrade conduction in branch A, the impulse traversing branch B and the VM will excite branch A. The impulse will traverse branch A and the area of unidirectional block through a retrograde pathway; however, since it is conducted at a normally fast speed, it will encounter refractory cells (open square) and be extinguished.

III. Slow conduction velocity and no block. Although the cardiac impulse may be conducted at an abnormally slow velocity (wavy arrows), the lack of unidirectional conduction block causes the impulse to arrive at refractory cells and extinguish.

IV. Slow conduction and unidirectional block. Same as II but the speed of impulse conduction through the area of unidirectional block (wavy arrows), and perhaps through B and VM as well, is so slow that the impulse encounters cells after their refractory period. Thus the impulse can reenter the conduction pathway, thereby establishing perpetual reexcitation. (Modeled after Cranefield 1973; Mason et al. 1973. Source: Adams 1986.)

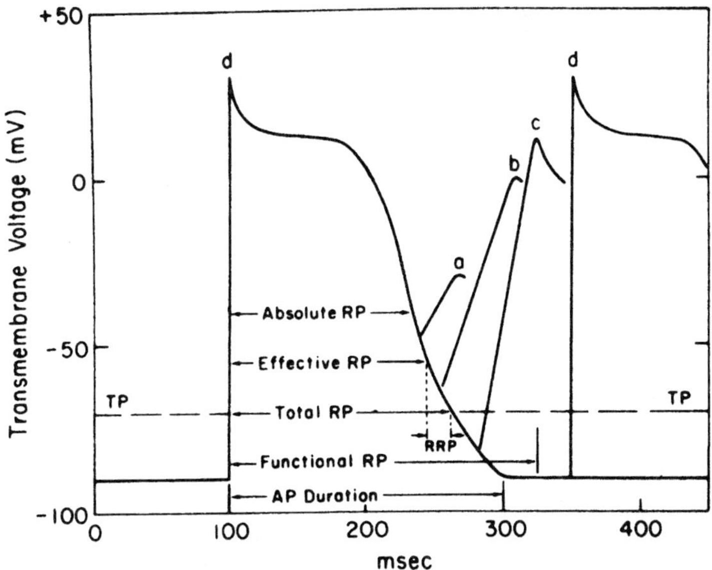

FIG. 24.5—Schematic diagram of transmembrane potentials (TMP) of a working ventricular muscle cell. The maximal rate of rise of phase 0 depolarization of the action potentials labeled a, b, c, and d depends on the magnitude of the TMP at the time of excitation. Thus the rate of depolarization is least at low levels of membrane potential (a), becomes progressively greater as TMP increases (b, c), and finally reaches a maximum at the resting potential (d). RP = refractory period, RRP = relative refractory period, AP = action potential, TP = threshold potential (Mason et al. 1973).

theory was delayed by difficulty in visualizing a decrease in conduction velocity adequate to comply with the value deemed necessary for establishing reentry phenomena. After all, the normal conduction velocity in PF can be as high as 2-4 m/sec, thus displaying a high safety factor for impulse propagation. As will be discussed in the following section, however, the velocity of impulse conduction can be diminished to as low as 0.01-0.1 m/sec by pathologic emergence of action potentials that demonstrate activation-deactivation kinetics that are remarkably slower than the normal fast responses.

Reentry theoretically could be controlled by a drug that either creates bidirectional block or bidirectional conduction through the region of cells causing the unidirectional block; accelerates speed of impulse conduction, thus returning the impulse to the site of reentry when cells are still inexcitable; prolongs action potential duration of normal cells, thereby extending their refractory period; or exhibits a combination of the above actions.

It should be appreciated also that other forms of cardiac electrophysiologic disturbances, in addition to primary abnormalities of impulse conduction and automaticity, may be important. Examples would include abnormal excitability, early afterdepolarizations, delayed afterdepolarizations, triggered electrical activities, and perhaps others. However, genesis of these types of abnormalities may overlap mechanistically with disturbances of automaticity and impulse conduction. Thus arrhythmias arising from primary automaticity and conduction abnormalities are adequate for modeling the classes of antiarrhythmic drugs relative to their effects on cardiac action potential characteristics and arrhythmogenesis.

FAST AND SLOW RESPONSES AND CONDUCTION. Phase 0 depolarization of a spontaneously active PF, and also of nonautomatic muscle cells in the atria and ventricles, represents the transmembrane potential change caused by a rapid influx of Na^+ through "fast Na^+ channels" of the cell membrane (see Figs. 24.1A, 24.2). There is increasing evidence that phase 0 of automatic SA and AV nodal cells is dependent upon a slow influx of Ca^{++} through "slow cation channels" of the cell membrane that are quite distinct from the fast Na^+ passageways. Under pathophysiologic influences, cells that normally exhibit fast Na^+ currents can develop slow Ca^{++}-dependent currents leading to conduction disturbances.

Conduction of a cardiac impulse through the different regions of the heart is dependent upon bioelectric characteristics of the individual cells in each region. The velocity of impulse conduction varies directly with magnitude of the maximal rate of depolarization of the cardiac cell (V_{max}), which is determined in turn by magnitude of the transmembrane voltage at the instant of excitation (Fig. 24.5). If the intracellular potential is reduced to less negative voltages, $\dot{V}_{max}$ and conduction velocity decrease proportionately (Fig. 24.5).

TABLE 24.1—Comparison of properties of fast Na^+ and slow Ca^{++} inward currents in cardiac muscle

Electrophysiologic property	Fast current (fast response)	Slow current (slow response)
Activation-inactivation kinetics	Rapid	Slow
Dependent on extracellular concentration of:	Na^+	Ca^{++}
Blocked by:	Tetrodotoxin	Verapamil, D600
Threshold	−60 to −70 mV	−30 to −40 mV
Diastolic membrane potential	*−80 to −90 mV*	*−40 to −70 mV*
Conduction velocity	*0.5 to 3.0 m/sec*	*0.01 to 0.1 m/sec*
Overshoot	+20 to +35 mV	0 to +15 mV
V_{max}	*100 to 1000 V/sec*	*1 to 10 V/sec*
Safety factor for conduction	*High*	*Low*
Relationship to nodal tissues	Probably none	May mediate pacemaker potentials
Catecholamines	Little effect	Significant enhancement

Source: Singh et al. 1980.
Note: Particularly important differences are italicized.

It now seems that many cardiac diseases and disturbances can cause the diastolic potential of myocardial cells to become less negative, i.e., they become partially depolarized (Boyden and Wit 1985). As the diastolic potential approaches about −60 mV, the fast Na^+ channels normally responsible for the rapid influx of Na^+ during phase 0 depolarization become progressively inactivated. If the fast Na^+ channels are completely inoperative owing to a resting potential less than −60 to −55 mV, cells may generate action potentials with an extremely slow rate of depolarization (i.e., a low $\dot{V}_{max}$) caused entirely by a slow current flowing through the slow cation channels of the cell membrane. Such an action potential is called a slow response and thought to be carried predominantly by Ca^{++}. It is now believed that slow responses and associated irregularities of impulse conduction may be involved in the genesis of different types of arrhythmias (Cranefield 1975). Some comparisons between fast and slow inward currents and their associated electrophysiologic properties are provided in Table 24.1.

ANTIARRHYTHMIC DRUGS

Classification. Investigators have attempted to classify antiarrhythmic drugs according to their electrophysiologic actions, but disagreements have arisen owing to lack of consensus over which drug-induced changes in the transmembrane potential are responsible for antiarrhythmic activity. The classification system advocated by Vaughn Williams (1984) and co-workers has become the standard nomenclature model for antiarrhythmic drugs. This system is rather straightforward; it is based on the observation that most antiarrhythmic drugs have one dominant electrophysiologic action on the myocardial cell, which may be influenced by the drug's subsidiary myocardial effects as well as its extracardiac activities (Adams 1986). Antiarrhythmic drugs are divided into Class I to IV in this system, as summarized in Table 24.2.

CLASS I DRUGS. Class I drugs are potent local anesthetics for nerves as well as the myocardial cell membrane, but this activity is generally more pronounced in the heart than in nerve fibers. The dominant electrophysiologic action of this group is a reduced maximal rate of depolarization of cardiac fibers. This decrease occurs without a significant change in the resting membrane potential. This activity is associated in turn with an increase in the threshold of excitability, a decrease in conduction velocity, and in some instances prolongation of the effective refractory period. These alterations invariably are associated with an inhibition of the spontaneous diastolic depolarization in automatic cells. The effect on pacemaker cells, especially ectopically active ones, seems to be more prevalent than effects on conduction velocity or excitability. Thus by inhibiting spontaneous diastolic depolarization, Class I drugs can control arrhythmias caused by enhanced automaticity. Also, by prolonging the refractory period, these agents are likely to be effective in abolishing reentrant tachyarrhythmias.

Since quinidine is the original and prototypical Class I drug, compounds in this group often are referred to collectively as the "quinidine-like" antiarrhythmic agents. Some important dissimilarities exist, however, relative to the precise effects of the different Class I drugs on phase 0 depolarization in normal and abnormal cells, action potential duration, and length of refractoriness. These differences prompted Keefe et al. (1981) to place Class I agents into three subdivisions: Class IA, IB, and IC.

Class IA includes quinidine, procainamide, and disopyramide. Their distinguishing features include a consistent reduction of the rate of phase 0 depolarization in normal and injured cardiac cells. Class IA agents also uniformly prolong the cardiac action potential duration and especially the affiliated refractory period.

Class IB drugs include lidocaine, phenytoin, tocainide, mexiletine, and aprindine. Although some controversy exists, a distinguishing feature of Class IB

TABLE 24.2—Classification and mechanisms of action of antiarrhythmic drugs

Class	Drug	Depression of fast Na^+ $\dot{V}_{max}$	Action potential duration	β–Blockade	Depression of slow responses	Extracardiac effects
I *Local anesthetic agents—membrane stabilizers*						
	Quinidine	4+	Lengthen +	Slight	0	Anticholinergic
	Procainamide	4+	Lengthen +	0	0	Anticholinergic
	Lidocaine	4+[a]	Shorten +	0	0	Local anesthetic
	Phenytoin	4+[a]	Shorten +	0	0	Anticonvulsant
	Disopyramide	4+	Lengthen	0	0	Anticholinergic
	Aprindine	4+	0	0	0	Anticonvulsant
	Tocainide	4+	0	0	0	Local anesthetic
II *β blockers*						
	Propranolol	+	Shorten +	4+	0[b]	Slight
	Oxyprenolol	+	Shorten +	4+	0[b]	Slight
	Alprenolol	+	Shorten +	4+	0[b]	Slight
III *Agents that prolong action potential duration*						
	Bretylium	0	Lengthen 4+	Neuron blockade	0	Hypotension
	Amiodarone	0	Lengthen 4+	0	0	Coronary vasodilator
IV *Ca^{++} channel blockers*						
	Verapamil	0	Lengthen phase 1 and 2+	0	4+	Coronary vasodilator

Source: Singh et al. 1980; Vaughn Williams 1984.
Note: 4+ = principal electrophysiologic action; + = subsidiary action; 0 = little or no effect in presumed therapeutic plasma concentrations.
[a]May decrease Na^+ conductance in injured, rather than normal, cells (see text for subclassification of IA, IB, and IC).
[b]May indirectly inhibit slow responses that are initiated by catecholamines.

drugs pertains to their reduction of phase 0 depolarization and conduction velocity in injured cardiac tissue but much less effect on these variables in normal cells (Table 24.2). Another feature of the Class IB compounds is their minimal shortening effect on action potential duration and refractory period (Table 24.2). This is quite different from quinidine and other Class IA drugs that reliably prolong action potential duration and refractoriness.

Three principal members of Class IC are encainide, lorcainide, and flecainide. These drugs, like the quinidine Class IA group, markedly depress the maximal rate of phase 0 depolarization in normal as well as abnormal cardiac cells. The Class IC agents, however, exert little effect on refractoriness and action potential.

Although the antiarrhythmic drug classification system facilitates an understanding of the various agents, the clinical importance of the subdivision of Class I drugs remains to be established.

CLASS II DRUGS. Class II drugs are defined as agents that exert antiadrenergic activity in the heart. Clinically useful Class II drugs are β-blocking agents; these compounds are discussed in Chap. 6. Propranolol is the prototype of Class II; newer agents include oxyprenolol, alprenolol, metoprolol, timolol, and pindolol. The basis for classifying agents that block cardiac sympathetic stimulation into a separate category derives from the fact that hyperactivity of the sympathetic nervous system is an important factor in pathogenesis of different types of arrhythmias, especially tachyarrhythmias associated with ectopic pacemaker foci. By reducing sympathetic input, β-blocking drugs obviously would be effective in controlling arrhythmias associated with sympathoadrenal discharge.

In addition, propranolol and some other β-blocking agents exert local anesthetic activity. They have been classified by some investigators as quinidine-like agents rather than being placed in a separate antiadrenergic category. At this time, however, it seems that β-adrenoceptor blocking agents in therapeutically effective concentrations act primarily and perhaps exclusively by β-adrenergic blockade; their local anesthetic properties, apparent in high concentrations, may be unimportant in control of cardiac arrhythmias (Singh et al. 1980).

CLASS III DRUGS. Class III drugs produce a "pure" prolongation of the action potential, thereby extending the refractory period. Development of this concept is based on the observation that cardiac arrhythmias are frequent in hyperthyroid states, which exhibit brief action potentials, but infrequent in hypothyroid conditions, which exhibit prolonged action potential duration. An antianginal drug, amiodarone, was found to exert antiarrhythmic activity associated with a prolonged action potential duration without effect on resting membrane potential. Bretylium, an adrenergic neuronal-blocking agent (Chap. 6), has Class III activity.

CLASS IV DRUGS. Class IV drugs are generally classified as calcium antagonists or Ca^{++} channel blockers; they exert little local anesthetic activity on fast Na^{+} responses but have relatively specific inhibitory effects on Ca^{++}-dependent slow responses. Because of slow Ca^{++} current participation in AV nodal conduction, Ca^{++} blockers slow AV conduction and thereby have application for controlling supraventricular arrhythmias that involve AV reentry pathways (Allert and Adams 1987). Action potentials may also arise from cells with pacemaker activity on the basis of slow Ca^{++} inward currents. Thus blockade of slow Ca^{++} responses may control both ectopic and reentry arrhythmias when such disturbances are dependent on slow response activity. Verapamil is the prototype drug of Class IV.

Autonomic Drugs. With exception of the β-adrenoceptor blocking agents, autonomic drugs usually are not included in classic groupings of antiarrhythmics. However, the clinician should not overlook the fact that during the actual practice of medicine, drugs other than the classic antiarrhythmic agents generally are preferred in controlling arrhythmias associated with uncomplicated autonomic imbalance. Atropine, e.g., would be an obvious choice when severe sinus bradycardia or sinus arrest is presented secondary to vagal discharge and accumulation of acetylcholine (ACh). Epinephrine is indicated in attempts to restart the heart after cardiac arrest, isoproterenol is useful in reversing AV block, and both can be effective in increasing heart rate if sinus bradycardia associated with impaired sympathetic drive is diagnosed (Adams 1981; Tilley 1985). Pharmacologic actions of the autonomic drugs are covered in Chaps. 5-7.

Digitalis. The pharmacologic action of digitalis, a quite useful antiarrhythmic agent for controlling ventricular rate in atrial tachyarrhythmias, is discussed in Chap. 23. It should be remembered that irrespective of the presenting arrhythmia, digitalis glycosides generally are the agents of choice if congestive heart failure is involved.

Quinidine Sulfate. *Quinidine Sulfate,* USP (Quinidex, Quinicardine), is the dextrorotatory isomer of quinine. Both compounds are present in cinchona bark, and their use as antiarrhythmic drugs can be traced to Wenckebach in 1914. This Viennese cardiologist learned that quinine, used to treat malaria, could also control irregular pulse rates in patients with atrial fibrillation. Subsequent investigation indicated that quinidine was more effective than quinine, and the former became a drug of choice in controlling atrial fibrillation.

Quinidine has both direct and indirect effects on cardiac rhythmicity. Like other Class I agents (Table 24.2), quinidine decreases the maximal rate of phase 0 depolarization of cardiac cells. This activity is demonstrable in atrial, ventricular, and Purkinje fibers; it reflects a direct depressant effect on Na^{+} permeability or the relationship between resting membrane potential and Na^{+} conductance (see Fig. 24.5). Quinidine also decreases the slope of spontaneous depolarization of Purkinje fibers but usually spares automaticity of the SA node except when excessive amounts are administered. Thus careful use of quinidine can control ectopic automaticity with less effect on firing frequency of normal pacemaker cells.

Clinically useful doses of quinidine prolong the effective refractory period of atrial and ventricular muscle with relatively less effect on the refractory period of normal pacemaker cells. Quinidine is subtyped as a Class IA drug owing to its characteristic prolongation of the refractory period. The capability of quinidine to directly prolong the refractory period of atrial fibers is thought to account for its effectiveness in converting atrial fibrillation to sinus rhythm.

As a subsidiary action, quinidine exerts an atropine-like vagolytic effect and therefore antagonizes the cardiac actions of vagally released ACh. This activity contributes to the effectiveness of quinidine in controlling atrial tachyarrhythmias because the action of ACh to shorten the atrial refractory period would be antagonized. Thus quinidine not only directly lengthens the refractory period, it also acts indirectly to lengthen this parameter by its anticholinergic action (Moss and Patton 1973). An adverse result of the atropine-like activity of quinidine, however, is improved AV conduction. Accordingly, an untoward effect of quinidine in treating supraventricular tachyarrhythmias is a sometimes pronounced increase in ventricular rate before the atrial dysrhythmia itself is controlled. This characteristic seems to be particularly prevalent when quinidine is administered by the intravenous (IV) route.

To avoid the potentially dangerous acceleration of ventricular rate by quinidine, it is traditional to first pretreat with a digitalis glycoside. The latter slows AV conduction and can thereby provide control of ventricular rate in atrial fibrillation and flutter (see Chap. 23). However, care should be exercised in the concomitant use of digoxin and quinidine, since the latter may substantially increase the plasma concentration of the former (Leahey et al. 1978).

Acute quinidine toxicoses is characterized by hemodynamic changes due largely to nonselective depression of various electromechanical functions of the heart. Impulse conduction through the AV node can be depressed to the extent that AV block develops. SA block and even ventricular fibrillation may also occur. Hypotension, decreased cardiac output, decreased myocardial contractility, and prolongation of the PR, QRS, and QT intervals of the ECG can result if large amounts of quinidine are administered intravenously. IV administration is not advocated because of potential dangers. Quinidine and other Class I agents usually are considered to be contraindicated in AV block or intraventricular block.

Quinidine is absorbed efficiently and rapidly when administered by the oral or intramuscular (IM) route. After IV administration, quinidine rapidly passes from the blood and distributes in tissues; distribution equilibrium is complete within 30 minutes (Neff et al. 1972). Approximate plasma half-life values in hours are: dogs (5.5), swine (5.5), ponies (4.4), cats (1.9), and goats (0.9). Protein binding varies from 82 to 92%. A large portion of quinidine undergoes metabolic degradation in the liver, and less than 40% is excreted in urine. Dissimilar rates of biotransformation and elimination probably account for species differences with this drug.

CLINICAL ASPECTS. Quinidine has generally been less successful in treatment of atrial fibrillation in small breeds of dogs (Detweiler 1957) than in large breeds such as the Great Dane, St. Bernard, and Newfoundland (Pyle 1967; Bohn et al. 1971). Apparently, atrial fibrillation can occur in large dogs with less extensive cardiac pathology than in small breeds.

Some of the inconsistencies about the effectiveness of quinidine in controlling supraventricular tachyarrhythmias in dogs may be explained partially by the differences in doses used by different investigators. Detweiler (1977) indicated that 50-100 mg may be given orally as a test dose in dogs with atrial fibrillation, followed several hours later or on the following day by 6.6-13.2 mg/kg every 2 hours for 4-5 doses daily. Hilwig (1976), in contrast, listed 3-10 mg quinidine by mouth 2-3 times daily in managing supraventricular tachycardias, without designating body weight of the patient. Tilley (1979) listed 6-20 mg/kg by the oral route every 6-8 hours. Suggested doses for IM injection of quinidine also have varied: 2-6 mg/kg every 6-8 hours (Tilley 1979) and 0.6-2 mg/kg every 6-8 hours (Hilwig 1976). In view of the limited amount of well-controlled data actually available about clinical use of quinidine in treating spontaneous arrhythmias in animals, dosage recommendations are somewhat provisional. Care is necessary in individual management of each patient, and dosage should be adjusted according to initial results after institution of a conservative regimen.

Quinidine has been used in the treatment of atrial fibrillation in horses (Detweiler and Patterson 1963); the following dose schedule for oral administration by capsule or stomach tube has been recommended (Detweiler 1977):day 1, 5 g (test dose); day 2, 10 g 3 times daily at 3-hour intervals; day 3, 10 g 4 times daily at 2-hour intervals; day 4, 10 g 4 times daily at 2-hour intervals.

Adverse effects of quinidine in horses include urticarial wheals, digestive disturbances, inflammation of the nasal mucosa with respiratory difficulty, laminitis, cardiovascular dysfunction, and even sudden death (Detweiler 1977). IV administration of quinidine has been employed by some clinicians, but this route is more hazardous than oral therapy. An IV preparation is available (*Quinidine Gluconate,* USP), but none of the quinidine products have been approved by the U.S. Food and Drug Administration for use in animals.

Procainamide Hydrochloride. *Procainamide Hydrochloride,* USP (Pronestyl), is a derivative of procaine containing an amide linkage in place of the ester linkage in the procaine molecule. This structural modification prolongs the biologic half-life of procainamide to 3-4 hours, making it more useful than the shorter lasting procaine.

The pharmacologic actions of procainamide, a Class IA agent, are qualitatively similar to those of quinidine (Table 24.2). In general, procainamide is considered more effective in controlling ventricular arrhythmias than atrial arrhythmias.

Huisman and Teunissen (1963) recommended IV infusion of procainamide at the rate of 100 mg/min when used in controlling dangerous ventricular tachycardias in dogs. Ettinger and Suter (1970) employed doses of 250 mg injected intramuscularly as frequently as every 2 hours in dogs weighing 11-16 kg (i.e., about 15-20 mg/kg). Hilwig (1976) listed the dose of procainamide as 4-8 mg/kg when given by IV injection or 25-50 mg/min by IV drip. Tilley (1979) listed an oral dose of procainamide as 125-500 mg every 6-8 hours (not to exceed 33 mg/kg/day), an IM dose as 8-16 mg/kg every 3-6 hours, and an IV dose as 1-2 mg/kg every 5 minutes to effect or to signs of intoxication (not to exceed 1 g).

Signs of procainamide toxicosis include greater than 50% widening of the QRS complex of the ECG, additional arrhythmias, bradycardia, tachycardia, or hypotension. Ideally, the ECG and blood pressure should be monitored during administration of procainamide, especially if given by a parenteral route.

Phenytoin Sodium. *Phenytoin Sodium,* USP (Dilantin, Diphenytoin), originally referred to as diphenylhydantoin, is a primary anticonvulsant drug used in humans and animals for control of epileptic seizures (see Chap. 16). Phenytoin also exerts antiarrhythmic activity in the heart, but this characteristic has a narrow spectrum of therapeutic application. Studies in isolated cardiac tissues have shown convincingly that phenytoin exerts direct antiarrhythmic actions similar in some respects to those of quinidine. Thus phenytoin usually is classified as a "local anesthetic-like" antiarrhythmic belonging in the Class I group (Table 24.2). Because it minimally shortens the refractory period, phenytoin is subtyped as a Class IB drug. Under some circumstances, phenytoin actually may enhance membrane responsiveness and increase conduction velocity, thereby improving impulse conduction through damaged tissue; however, the clinical significance of these activities is uncertain (Singh et al. 1980).

In general, phenytoin is considered to be effective in controlling digitalis-induced arrhythmias of all types; it also is useful in treating ventricular arrhythmias from other causes but is relatively ineffective in abolishing atrial dysrhythmias unless they are related to digitalis toxicosis (Hayes 1972). When administered slowly by the IV route, the usual dose of phenytoin for dogs is approximately 5-10 mg/kg at an infusion rate of about 25-50 mg/min. This appears to be effective in treatment of digitalis-induced arrhythmias without depressant effect on myocardial contractile function (Helfant et al. 1967; Scherlag et al. 1968; Damato 1969). Tilley (1979) and Hilwig (1976) have used 4 mg/kg phenytoin for slow IV administration in dogs. Data pertaining to phenytoin use in cats are lacking; in view of the remarkably long plasma half-life of phenytoin in this species (Roye et al. 1973), much smaller doses than those used in dogs should be considered.

The complete pharmacokinetic disposition of phenytoin has not been determined, but studies in dogs indicate that the drug is absorbed somewhat poorly from the gastrointestinal (GI) tract (approximately 40%) and has a short serum half-life (approximately 3 hours) (Sanders and Yeary 1978). Furthermore, an oral dose of 10 mg/kg phenytoin in this same study yielded serum concentrations that did not exceed 2 μg/mL. If therapeutically effective serum concentrations of phenytoin are accepted as approximately 10 μg/mL, the oral dose of phenytoin may have to be increased over the usual recommendations of approximately 5-10 mg/kg. Sanders and Yeary (1978) proposed that 35 mg/kg of phenytoin administered three times daily (i.e., a total daily dose of 105 mg/kg) may be necessary to achieve plasma concentrations likely to be therapeutically effective in controlling convulsions or cardiac arrhythmias in dogs.

Phenytoin is metabolized in dogs by the microsomal enzymes of the liver, and pharmacokinetic-based drug interactions are likely. Dogs receiving phenytoin were reported to develop signs of phenytoxin toxicosis (postural ataxia and hypermetric gait) when chloramphenicol was added to the therapeutic regimen; this adverse drug interaction was attributed to the inhibitory effect of chloramphenicol on phenytoin metabolism (Adams 1975; Sanders et al. 1979).

Lidocaine Hydrochloride. *Lidocaine Hydrochloride,* USP (Xylocaine), is a local anesthetic drug found to exert antidysrhythmic action that has therapeutic application in treating ventricular tachyarrhythmias. Lidocaine is classified as a Class IB agent. Lidocaine is not recommended for controlling supraventricular arrhythmias but is considered to be useful primarily in reverting ventricular dysrhythmias that develop during general anesthesia, surgery, ischemia, and other forms of trauma. In humans it also is used following myocardial infarction. Lidocaine has been advocated in cardiac emergencies to antagonize the profibrillatory activity of epinephrine (Clark 1977). Experimentally, lidocaine shares an efficacy similar to phenytoin in controlling digitalis-induced arrhythmias, but it has received little clinical use for this purpose.

Therapeutic assets of lidocaine in emergency situations are its rapid onset and short duration of action after IV injection. However, it is not useful for maintenance therapy because of ineffective absorption after oral administration and short duration of action. In large doses, lidocaine can produce hypotension and exert negative chronotropic and inotropic actions on the heart.

Tilley (1979) lists the following dose schedules for IV administration of lidocaine in dogs: 2-4 mg/kg over 1-2 minutes, 0.5-2 mg/kg every 20-60 minutes by slow injection, or 0.025-0.060 mg/kg/min by constant infusion with ECG monitoring. Rapid IV administration of more than approximately 4 mg/kg lidocaine is likely to cause CNS seizures.

Propranolol Hydrochloride. Drugs that exhibit β-adrenoceptor blocking properties have an established place in treating and preventing cardiac dysrhythmias in humans but have received less clinical use in animals. In view of the effectiveness of β-blocking agents in controlling a wide variety of dysrhythmias, it seems likely that these drugs will be used increasingly in animals with spontaneous cardiac arrhythmias.

Propranolol Hydrochloride, USP (Inderal), is the prototype; newer agents include oxprenolol, metoprolol, timolol, alprenolol, pindolol, and practolol. Experimental evidence in animals and clinical studies in humans support the view that β blockade is the primary determinant of the antiarrhythmic activity of this group of drugs. Their local anesthetic or quinidine-like activities currently are considered to be less important (perhaps unimportant) in most clinical situations (Table 24.2). The efficacy of β-blocking agents in preventing various cardiac dysrhythmias emphasizes the importance of autonomic imbalance, particularly sympathetic overactivity, in the genesis of different rhythm disturbances in the heart.

Propranolol slows the rate of spontaneous discharge of the SA and ectopic pacemakers and slows both antegrade and retrograde conduction through anomalous pathways of the heart. Thus propranolol can provide relief from arrhythmias associated with disturbances of automaticity, reentry phenomena, or both. Propranolol increases the refractory period of the AV node, which has therapeutic application in slowing ventricular rate during atrial fibrillation or flutter. During the latter conditions, propranolol usually does not slow the fibrillatory or flutter frequency of the atria and only rarely does it restore sinus rhythm. However, the slowing of ventricular rate by propranolol often is effective and is reported to be useful in some cases that are refractory to other antiarrhythmic agents.

Propranolol and other β blockers are effective in reducing frequency of paroxysmal supraventricular tachycardia, especially in the Wolff-Parkinson-White syndrome (Singh and Jewitt 1974). Tachyarrhythmias associated with digitalis intoxication and physical exertion respond well to β-blocking agents. Arrhythmias evoked during inhalation anesthesia with halogenated hydrocarbon anesthetics often can be prevented or reversed by propranolol administration prior to or during anesthesia respectively.

Propranolol is well absorbed from the gut and is eliminated largely from portal blood by the liver before it reaches the systemic circulation. Because of this large "first-pass effect," six to ten times larger doses are necessary when propranolol is administered by mouth as compared to the IV route (Weidler et al. 1979). The order of plasma clearance for propranolol in different species is: rat > dog > cat > human > monkey.

In a study in cats, a two-step IV infusion technique was found to be more effective in attaining and maintaining steady-state plasma concentrations of propranolol than IV bolus injection. The two-step technique involved the following schedule: continuous IV infusion first at a rapid rate of approximately 8-11 μg/kg/min for 15 minutes, than a slow rate of approximately 1-4 μg/kg/min for 4 hours (Weidler et al. 1979). Steady-state plasma concentrations of propranolol achieved with this schedule were 60-80 ng/mL. Application of such techniques to clinical management of arrhythmias probably would be useful depending upon severity of the dysrhythmia and whether the animal is ill enough or tractable enough to allow prolonged IV infusions.

In the dog, suppression of catecholamine-induced arrhythmias by propranolol requires smaller IV doses (0.1-1 mg/kg) than abolition of ouabain-induced arrhythmias (3-5 mg/kg). Relatively large IV doses of propranolol (3 and 5 mg/kg) are toxic in dogs subjected to myocardial infarction after ligation of the anterior descending branch of the left coronary artery (Shanks and Dunlop 1967). Care must be exercised when β-blocking agents are administered to animals with reduced cardiac reserve.

Importantly, rapid bolus injections of large amounts of propranolol can produce nonspecific cardiovascular depressant effects. Ideally, blood pressure and the ECG should be monitored closely when β blockers are administered intravenously. Oral doses of propranolol in animals vary from approximately 2 mg/kg to as high as 40 mg/kg 2 or 3 times daily (Hilwig 1976; Tilley 1979).

Metoprolol Tartrate, USP (Lopressor), is considered to be a cardioselective β-blocking agent; i.e., it is relatively more effective in blocking $β_1$ receptors of the heart than $β_2$ receptors of vascular and bronchiolar smooth muscles (see Chap. 6). This selectivity is important, because a limiting side effect of propranolol and other nonselective β blockers is airway obstruction owing to a block of adrenergically regulated dilation of bronchioles. Thus metoprolol or other $β_1$ selective blockers may well be the β-blocking agents of choice in patients with a history of chronic obstructive airway disease.

PRECAUTIONS. Beta-blocking agents should be administered with caution in patients with reduced cardiac reserve (e.g., congestive heart failure). Under such pathophysiologic conditions, cardiac function is characterized by increased dominance of the sympathetic nervous system as part of the compensatory attempt to maintain cardiac output (see Chap. 23). Blockade of sympathetic input to the heart by propranolol, particularly if sudden, can precipitate cardiac decompensation and all the associated problems that entails (Kittleson and Hamlin 1981). This warming is valid despite the suggestion that propranolol, by reducing myocardial oxygen consumption, is a potential adjunct to treating aged dogs with heart failure (Hamlin 1977).

Verapamil and Diltiazem. Verapamil (Isoptin) is a systemic and coronary vasodilator that also exerts important antiarrhythmic action (Allert and Adams 1987). Early data were interpreted as evidence that verapamil either blocked β-adrenergic receptors (i.e., a Class II propranolol action) or exerted quinidine-like local anesthetic properties (i.e., Class I). However, verapamil and its methoxy derivative D600 were discovered to inhibit transmembrane fluxes of Ca^{++} in various excitable tissues. In the heart, studies demonstrated that verapamil has a unique cellular action in selectively inhibiting transmembrane influx of Ca^{++} (and perhaps Na^{+}) through the aforementioned slow cation channels of the cardiac sarcolemma. Since this action seems crucial to the antiarrhythmic effects of these drugs, verapamil and diltiazem are placed in a separate category (i.e., the calcium antagonists or Ca^{++} channel blockers of Class IV) (Table 24.2).

Arrhythmias caused by disturbances in either impulse formation (automaticity) or impulse conduction (reentry) are theoretically amenable to verapamil if their origin is associated with the emergence of slow response depolarizations (see Table 24.1). In addition, verapamil depresses SA and AV nodal discharge rates and conduction velocity, because slow Ca^{++}-dependent events are normal characteristics of automaticity in these tissues (Spedding 1985). Thus verapamil has application in certain types of atrial arrhythmias and in aborting supraventricular tachycardias that depend on continuous reentry of impulses utilizing the AV node as part of the reentrant pathway (Singh et al. 1980).

In veterinary medicine the clinical antiarrhythmic applications for Ca^{+} channel blockade mainly involve use of verapamil and diltiazem for treatment of supraventricular tachyarrhythmias (Allert and Adams 1987; Kittleson et al. 1988). Verapamil is used in human medicine for short-term conversion of paroxysmal atrial tachycardia to sinus rhythm. Atrial fibrillation and flutter constitute other important indications. Verapamil and diltiazem usually do not convert these high-frequency atrial patterns to sinus rhythm but effectively reduce AV conduction and thereby lower the ventricular rate response. Primary ventricular arrhythmias generally are unresponsive to Ca^{++} channel blockade, unless they are secondary to myocardial ischemia. Nifedipine has little clinical antiarrhythmic utility because reflex cardiac stimulation evoked by this drug's systemic vasodilator effects usually nullifies any direct Ca^{++}-dependent antiarrhythmic properties.

Few clinical trials have examined the antiarrhythmic efficacy of Ca^{++} channel blockade in animals with cardiac disease. Verapamil was reported to be effective in converting paroxysmal or chronic atrial fibrillation to sinus rhythm in only 3 of 7 dogs tested (Johnson 1985). Further, one of the 3 responding dogs developed ventricular tachycardia within 1 day after verapamil treatment was started. Verapamil was discontinued and replaced effectively by combination therapy with quinidine and propranolol. Clinical details were presented for only 2 dogs in the study, and apparently other cardioactive agents (e.g., digoxin, milrinone) were routinely administered along with verapamil. Thus it is difficult to determine whether improvement or lack of improvement in cardiac rhythmicity could be ascribed solely to verapamil.

Results from two additional clinical studies with verapamil use in dogs have been presented (Kittleson et al. 1988; Hamlin 1986). In one study, verapamil was successful in terminating supraventricular tachycardia in 12 of 14 dogs when administered intravenously in 1 to 3 doses at the rate of 0.05 mg/kg (Kittleson et al. 1988). One nonresponding dog developed a transient hypotensive crisis after a total verapamil dose of 0.15 mg/kg.

A second study involved 27 dogs with either atrial tachycardia (17 dogs) or atrial fibrillation with rapid ventricular rate responses (10 dogs) (Hamlin 1986). A qualification for subjects in that study was the absence of overt heart failure, as evidenced by lack of dyspnea and severe cardiomegaly. Verapamil was administered orally at a dose of 0.5 mg/kg every 6 hours, but greater doses were used for some dogs at the beginning of the study. Seven dogs retained their arrhythmia after verapamil, 5 dogs with atrial fibrillation had a reduction in ventricular rate of more than 50 beats/min, and 9 dogs with supraventricular tachycardia converted to sinus rhythm (Hamlin 1986). Thus about 50% of the dogs with supraventricular tachyarrhythmia responded favorably to verapamil. Importantly, however, 6 dogs died within 2-3 hours after the initial dosing of verapamil. Five of these dogs were treated at the rate of 1.5-2.5 mg/kg. Because the deaths occurred so rapidly, they probably were attributable to verapamil rather than to natural progression of the disease. Cardiovascular depressant effects resulting from these relatively large doses of verapamil may have exacerbated underlying cardiac dysfunction, thus evoking acute decompensation of preexisting subclinical heart failure.

A combination of Wolff-Parkinson-White syndrome and atrial fibrillation may constitute a serious precaution or even a contraindication to verapamil treatment. Clinical reports in human medicine have indicated that when these conditions exist simultaneously, verapamil may paradoxically evoke an increase in ventricular rate and lead to fatal ventricular fibrillation (Jacobs et al. 1985). Perhaps episodes of ventricular tachycardia or mortality associated with verapamil therapy in dogs with atrial fibrillation (Johnson 1985; Hamlin 1986) might have involved occult Wolff-Parkinson-White or analogous syndromes.

Adverse circulatory side effects of Ca^{++} channel blockade include contractile depression of the heart, with reduced cardiac output and hypotension. This combination of effects can result in decompensation of preclinical or compensated heart failure, precipitation of pulmonary edema, and worsening of the primary ailment. Other potential side effects are sinus bradycardia and heart block attributable to direct depression of SA firing rate and AV conduction respectively. The propensity for cardiovascular depression should be considered whenever Ca^{++} channel blocking drugs are used. This precaution is especially valid in patients with preexisting or suspected myocardial contractile failure (Allert and Adams 1987).

Newer Drugs. Data are generally insufficient to provide information about clinical use in animals of most of the newer antidysrhythmic drugs. Practical applications are likely in the future, however, because some of these offer potential advantages over the older agents, as summarized below.

BRETYLIUM. Bretylium tosylate (Bretylol) is a bromobenzyl quaternary ammonium compound originally introduced as an antihypertensive agent in humans. This drug is broadly classified as an adrenergic neuronal-blocking agent because it inhibits release of norepinephrine from adrenergic nerve endings (see Chap. 6). Although bretylium is no longer considered useful as an antihypertensive agent, subsequent studies have shown that it exerts direct antiarrhythmic actions in the heart. This characteristic is thought to reside with a relatively "pure" prolongation of action potential duration. Thus bretylium is designated a Class III agent (Table 24.2).

Bretylium lengthens the action potential duration as well as the refractory period in ventricular muscle cells and PF in a homogeneous manner; however, this characteristic effect is not manifested in the atria. Accordingly, bretylium is particularly effective in controlling ventricular arrhythmias, but supraventricular tachycardias are poorly responsive to the drug. Bretylium has received little clinical application in animals, but it has been approved for management of refractory and recurrent ventricular tachycardia or fibrillation in humans (Koch-Weser 1979; Singh et al. 1980).

Bretylium has been reported to bring about defibrillation in clinical episodes of ventricular fibrillation in humans and in experimental episodes in dogs (Koch-Weser 1979). Conflicting data have been presented, however, as Breznock et al. (1977) reported that bretylium (6-24 mg/kg) did not induce chemical defibrillation in dogs when administered by the IV or intracardiac route. Furthermore, bretylium did not seem to stabilize ventricular irritability nor facilitate resuscitation by electrical defibrillation. Additional work is needed in both the clinic and laboratory before therapeutic applications of bretylium are identified in animals with spontaneous cardiac dysrhythmias.

Administration of bretylium to animals anesthetized with halogenated hydrocarbon anesthetics may be contraindicated, since a study demonstrated severe and long-lasting ventricular arrhythmias under such circumstances in cats (Condouris et al. 1979). These anesthetics are known to sensitize the heart to the arrhythmogenic activities of the catecholamines. Because bretylium initially causes a release of catecholamines from adrenergic nerves prior to neuronal blockade, the ventricular arrhythmias evoked by the drug may have been secondary to release of norepinephrine.

The pharmacokinetics of bretylium are not fully elucidated, but it is effective after parenteral (IM, IV) or oral administration. Absorption from the GI tract is somewhat poor and erratic; bretylium is not biotransformed to a significant extent and is excreted essentially unchanged in urine, accounting for its long elimination half-life (Hurley et al. 1960).

DISOPYRAMIDE. Disopyramide is a Class IA agent. The spectrum of electrophysiologic actions and the range of therapeutic effectiveness of disopyramide basically resemble respective characteristics of the other two Class IA drugs, procainamide and quinidine (Novotny and Adams 1986). Although efficacy in controlling supraventricular arrhythmias has been reported, most data indicate that disopyramide is therapeutically effective mainly against tachyarrhythmias of ventricular origin. In this respect, clinical applications for disopyramide more closely resemble those for procainamide than for quinidine.

Although disopyramide was approved recently for antiarrhythmic therapy in humans, adverse side effects and pharmacokinetic characteristics may limit the use of this drug in veterinary medicine. First, disopyramide is absorbed quickly after oral administration, but it undergoes metabolism and clearance almost as rapidly. The biological half-life in dogs is only 2-3 hours, which would necessitate multiple daily administrations (Bonagura and Muir 1985). Second, disopyramide has pronounced atropine-like side effects and can elicit an alarming increase in ventricular rate responses in patients with atrial fibrillation or flutter. Last, and perhaps most important, disopyramide exerts rather potent negative inotropic effects in the heart. The latter characteristic is a potentially critical limitation because it is especially pronounced in patients with preexisting myocardial disease. Indeed, disopyramide was reported to exacerbate congestive heart failure in over one-half of human patients who had preexistent left ventricular dysfunction. Because of pharmacokinetic disadvantages and limiting side effects, Bonagura and Muir (1985) indicated that disopyramide may prove to have limited application in veterinary medicine.

TOCAINIDE. Tocainide is a Class IB antiarrhythmic drug; it was discovered as a structural congener of lidocaine that shared basic electrophysiologic and antiarrhythmic actions with the parent compound. Tocainide has distinct pharmacokinetic advantages because it is effective after oral administration and has a long duration of action. Like lidocaine, tocainide is a narrow spectrum antiarrhythmic drug with clinical efficacy against ventricular arrhythmias.

Patients that respond to parenterally administered lidocaine usually respond to oral tocainide. Reports in the human literature often concern patients whose arrhythmias were refractory to other antiarrhythmic agents before tocainide was tried, so the actual efficacy of tocainide as an initial antiarrhythmic drug may be higher than some studies would indicate.

Tocainide may have clinical usefulness in veterinary medicine. It has potential application in cases where ventricular arrhythmias are initially responsive to IV lidocaine or tocainide, but refractory to the older oral antiarrhythmic agents such as quinidine or procainamide. Lidocaine itself is inappropriate for oral therapy because it is rapidly metabolized after absorption from the GI tract. Plasma concentrations of tocainide in the dog are maintained in the therapeutic range for up to 12 hours after oral administration, making tocainide suitable for administration only 2 times a day.

A slightly different chemical structure from lidocaine protects tocainide from rapid first-pass hepatic metabolism, markedly improving its bioavailability when compared to lidocaine. Metabolism occurs in the liver, but in humans as much as 50% of the drug can be excreted unchanged in the urine. Similar hepatic and renal mechanisms of drug elimination are believed to be found in dogs. The side effects anticipated with tocainide are similar to those seen with lidocaine, but in studies in humans the side effects are usually minor, well tolerated, and generally eliminated by dosage adjustment.

MEXILETINE. Mexiletine is a Class IB drug that exerts electrophysiologic and antiarrhythmic actions similar to those of lidocaine and tocainide (Novotny and Adams 1986). As with tocainide, mexiletine was developed for its lidocaine-like effectiveness in treating serious ventricular arrhythmias in a formulation suitable for oral administration. Mexiletine undergoes minimal first-pass metabolism by the liver after nearly complete absorption from the GI tract. As with tocainide, mexiletine may find its greatest clinical utility in controlling ventricular arrhythmias that are found to be lidocaine-sensitive and when continued outpatient therapy by the oral route is desirable. In one clinical study involving a small group of dogs (Bonagura and Muir 1985), success was limited when mexiletine was administered orally 2 or 3 times daily at doses of 1-2 mg/kg, but as with tocainide, more extensive clinical trials are necessary.

APRINDINE. Aprindine is a Class I agent that shares basic electrophysiologic actions with lidocaine, except that aprindine seems to have a somewhat broader spectrum of antiarrhythmic efficacy. Aprindine is effective against premature ventricular beats and ventricular tachycardias but also has potential for suppressing supraventricular premature beats. Aprindine is less effective and is not used in the settings of atrial fibrillation, atrial flutter, or supraventricular paroxysmal

TABLE 24.3—Suggested antiarrhythmic drugs of choice in treating canine arrhythmias

	Supraventricular				Ventricular			
Treatment	Sinus bradycardia	Atrial tachycardia	Atrial flutter	Atrial fibrillation	Ventricular premature complexes	Ventricular tachycardia	Ventricular fibrillation	Symptomatic second- and third-degree AV block
Drugs								
Atropine	+ + +	0	0	0	0	0	0	+ + +
Digoxin	0	+ + +	+ + +	+ + +	0	0	0	0
Isoproterenol	+ +	0	0	0	0	0	0	+ +
Lidocaine	0	0	0	0	+ + +	+ + +	0	0
Phenytoin	0	+	0	0	+ +	+ +	0	0
Procainamide	0	+ +	+ +	+	+ + +	+ + +	0	0
Propranolol	0	+ +	+ +	+ +	+	+	0	0
Quinidine	0	+	+ +	+	+ + +	+ +	0	0
Electrical methods								
Cardioversion	0	+	+ + +	+ +	0	+ + +	+ + +	0
Pacing	+	+	+	0	0	+	0	+ + +

Source: Tilley 1979, 1985.

Note: For each arrhythmia the drug or procedure of first choice (response excellent) is indicated by + + +; of second choice (response good) by + +; of third choice (response fair and rarely indicated) by +; and contraindicated by 0. Combination antiarrhythmic therapy is often based on this table, with first- and second-choice therapies used concurrently.

tachycardia. Aprindine may accelerate AV conduction and precipitate increased ventricular rate responses. Aprindine's usefulness in humans has been somewhat limited, owing to a rather narrow toxic-therapeutic ratio; leukopenia, agranulocytosis, and hepatotoxicosis are potential side effects. Dose-related and reversible untoward reactions include hypotension, ataxia, nausea, seizures, transient depression of myocardial contractile function, and prolongation of the PR, QRS, and QT intervals (Novotny and Adams 1986).

Aprindine underwent clinical trial in 20 dogs with spontaneous ventricular arrhythmias (Muir and Bonagura 1982); 17 of the dogs had failed to respond to treatment with quinidine, procainamide, lidocaine, propranolol, or a combination of these drugs. Aprindine was administered by IV infusion at a dose of 0.1 mg/kg/min for 5 minutes and repeated at 10-minute intervals until the arrhythmia was controlled or signs of intoxication intervened. The subsequent oral dose was 1-2 mg/kg, 3 times daily. Aprindine was effective with this schedule in converting ventricular tachycardia to sinus rhythm in 15 of the dogs and in slowing ventricular rate in 4 others; one dog had an increased ventricular rate. Antiarrhythmic efficacy in 19 of 20 dogs is an impressive success rate. Aprindine likewise was effective in controlling ventricular tachycardia in another clinical trial involving Doberman Pinschers with congestive cardiomyopathy (Calvert et al. 1982).

These findings suggest that aprindine may be an alternate strategy for controlling ventricular arrhythmias in dogs resistant to standard antiarrhythmic therapy. Further study is warranted to substantiate the utility of aprindine, and to evaluate therapeutic-toxic ratios in animals. Because of the potential of aprindine for leukopenia and hepatotoxicosis, this drug may be reserved for ventricular arrhythmias resistant to other drugs. Interestingly, indecainide is a new aprindine congener purported to have fewer side effects and six times the potency of aprindine.

ENCAINIDE, FLECAINIDE, AND LORCAINIDE. Encainide, flecainide, and lorcainide are Class I members discovered and characterized during a search for drugs with efficacy against arrhythmias resistant to standard treatment regimens. They share basic Na^+ conductance-blocking properties with quinidine; however they are distinct from other quinidine-like drugs because they do not prolong the refractory period. Because of this spectrum of electrophysiologic actions, encainide, flecainide, and lorcainide are subgrouped as Class IC antiarrhythmic drugs (Novotny and Adams 1986).

As a general rule, Class IC agents seem to be effective against ventricular tachycardias and premature beats of either ventricular or atrial origin. These compounds are less effective and perhaps clinically ineffective in controlling atrial fibrillation and flutter. Encainide, flecainide, and lorcainide are absorbed after oral administration, but more work is needed with each compound before clinical recommendations can be made relative to their use as alternative approaches to drug-resistant ventricular arrhythmias in animals. Indeed, recent clinical studies in human medicine have indicated these drugs may increase the incidence of serious ventricular arrhythmias after myocardial infarction.

AMIODARONE. Amiodarone has been in clinical use in human medicine for several years in Europe and more recently in the United States. Few reports are available about the use of amiodarone in animals with heart disease. As a Class III antiarrhythmic agent, amiodarone selectively prolongs the action potential and refractory period; this is expressed clinically as a prolongation of

TABLE 24.4—Dose recommendations for drugs used to treat cardiac arrhythmias in dogs

Drug	Dose and route of administration	Indications
Atropine sulfate, 1/200 g tablets; 0.4 mg/ml injectable	Oral: 0.04 mg/kg every 6–8 hours SC, IM, IV: 0.04 mg/kg every 4–6 hours	Sinus bradycardia, AV block, SA arrest
Calcium chloride*	IV, IC: 0.05–0.10 ml/kg of 10% solution	Ventricular asystole (to increase cardiac irritability), electrical-mechnical dissociation
Digoxin (Lanoxin), 0.125, 0.25, and 0.50 mg tablets; 0.05 mg/ml oral elixir; 0.25 mg/ml IV	Oral: 0.1–0.2 mg/kg in 4 divided doses over 48 hours or to effect (rapid method); 0.02 mg/kg average daily maintenance divided into 2 doses IV: 0.02–0.03 mg/kg in 4 divided doses over 4 hours or to effect	Congestive heart failure, APCs, atrial tachycardia, atrial fibrillation, atrial flutter, sick sinus syndrome (after pacemaker insertion)
Epinephrine hydrochloride* (Adrenalin), 1:1000 solution; 1 mg/ml injectable	IC: 6–10 μg/kg IV: 0.1–0.3 mg of 1:10,000 dilution	Ventricular asystole, changing fine ventricular fibrillition to coarse fibrillation
Isoproterenol (Proternol), 15 and 30 mg tablets; (Isuprel), 0.2 mg/ml injectable	Oral: 15–30 mg 4–6 times daily SC, IM: 0.1–0.2 mg every 4 hours IV: 1 mg/500 ml 5% dextrose/water and titrate to effect	Sinus bradycardia, complete AV block, to initiate heartbeat
Lidocaine (2% without epinephrine) (Xylocaine), 20 and 40 mg/ml injectable	IV: 2–4 mg/kg as bolus over 1–2 min, 0.5–2.0 mg/kg every 20–60 min (slow injection), 25–60 μg/kg/min with monitoring (constant infusion)	Ventricular tachycardia, ventricular premature complexes (especially multiform)
Phenytoin (diphenylhydantoin) (Dilantin), 30 and 100 mg capsules; 125 mg/5 ml syrup; 50 mg/ml injectable	Oral: 4–8 mg/kg divided 3–4 times daily IV: 4 mg/kg slowly once	Ventricular arrhythmias, digitalis-induced arrhythmias
Procainamide (Pronestyl), 250, 375, and 500 mg capsules or tablets; 100 mg/ml injectable	Oral: 125–500 mg every 6–8 hr (not to exceed 33 mg/kg day) IM: 8–16 mg/kg every 3–6 hr IV: 1–2 mg/kg/5 min to effect or toxicity (>50% widening of QRS), not to exceed 1 g	Ventricular premature complexes, ventricular tachycardia
Propranolol (Inderal), 10, 20, and 40 mg tablets; 1 mg/ml injectable	Oral: 2.5–40 mg 2–3 times daily unless desired effect at lower dose or toxicity IV: 0.05 to 0.15 mg/kg slowly to effect or toxicity	Sinus tachycardia, digitalis-induced atrial arrhythmias, supraventricular tachycardias and ventricular arrhythmias, preexcitation arrhythmias, and with digoxin for atrial fibrillation
Quindine sulfate (short-acting form) 3 g tablets; quinidine sulfate (Quinidex Extentabs) (long-acting form), 300 mg tablets; quinidine gluconate injectable (IM), 80 mg/ml; quinidine gluconate (Quinaglute Duratabs) (long-acting form), 5 g tablets; quinidine polygalacturonate (Cardioquin) (long-acting form), 3 g tablets	Oral: 6–20 mg/kg every 6–8 hours (short-acting form), 8–12 hours (long-acting form) IM: 2.0–6.0 mg/kg every 6–8 hours	Ventricular premature complexes, ventricular tachycardia, maintenance therapy after electroconversion of atrial fibrillation and/or flutter, Wolff-Parkinson-White syndrome

Source: Tilley 1979, 1985. See text for other recommendations.
Note: IV = intravenous, IM = intramuscular, SC = subcutaneous, IC = intracardiac, AV = atrioventricular, SA = sinoatrial, APC = atrial premature contraction.
*Drugs for cardiac arrest.

AV nodal conduction time and an increase in atrial and ventricular refractory periods (Novotny and Adams 1986). Its use in human medicine has been largely in patients with conditions refractory to other antiarrhythmic agents, including conditions such as paroxysmal atrial tachycardia, atrial flutter and fibrillation, and a recurrent ventricular tachycardia and fibrillation. Amiodarone has a long biologic half-life; days to weeks may be required to gain steady-state plasma concentrations with oral administration.

Clinical Indications. Important clinical uses of antiarrhythmic drugs were summarized when appropriate in the preceding sections on individual drugs. Data shown in Table 24.3 provide a listing of drugs of choice for several common arrhythmias and also point out relevant contraindications (Tilley 1979, 1985). Tables 24.4 and 24.5 provide schedules for approximating doses of several drugs in dogs and cats respectively. The fact remains, however, that although several antiarrhythmic drugs routinely are advocated for control of

TABLE 24.5—Dose recommendations for drugs used to treat cardiac arrhythmias in cats

Drug	Dose and route of administration	Indications
Atropine sulfate, 0.4 mg/ml injectable	SC, IM, IV: 0.04 mg/kg every 4–6 hours	Sinus bradycardia, AV block
Calcium chloride*	IC, IV: 0.05–0.10 ml of 10% solution/kg	Ventricular asystole (to increase cardiac irritability), electrical-mechanical dissocation
Digoxin (Lanoxin), 0.125 mg tablets; 0.25 mg/ml IV	Oral: 0.008–0.01 mg/kg, average daily maintenance divided into 2 doses (e.g., ¼ of a 0.125 mg tablet twice daily for 6 kg cat) IV: 0.02–0.03 mg/kg in 4 divided doses over 4 hours or to effect	Congestive heart failure, APC, atrial tachycardia, atrial fibrillation, atrial flutter
Epinephrine hydrochloride* (Adrenalin), 1:1000 solution; 1 mg/ml injectable	IC: 6–10 μg/kg IV: 0.05–0.1 mg of 1:10,000 dilution	Ventricular asystole, changing fine ventricular fibrillation to coarse fibrillation
Isoproterenol (Isuprel), 0.2 mg/ml injectable	IV: 0.5 mg/250 ml 5% dextrose/water and titrate to effect	Sinus bradycardia, complete AV block
Propranolol (Inderal), 10 mg tablets; 1 mg/ml injectable	Oral: 2.5 mg every 8–12 hours for average 5 kg cat; higher doses to effect IV: 0.25 mg diluted in 1 ml of saline, given as 0.2 ml boluses to effect	Sinus tachycardia, supraventricular tachycardia and ventricular arrhythmias, preexcitation arrhythmias, and with digoxin for atrial fibrillation

spontaneous arrhythmias in animals, well-controlled clinical data on the subject generally are lacking. Dosage recommendations by different investigators often vary widely in the same species, necessitating careful judgment in the clinical setting.

The clinician should integrate basic knowledge about the pharmacologic control of arrhythmias into a rational clinical approach to managing cardiac dysfunction in patients. A precise classification of individual drugs is of less importance to the clinician than a basic understanding of their pharmacodynamic and therapeutic applications. Initial therapy should be directed at correcting specific etiologies; e.g., if serum electrolyte abnormalities are responsible, obviously these should be corrected before a potent antiarrhythmic drug is introduced into the animal. Arrhythmias secondary to congestive heart failure may respond to restitution of cardiac compensation, and initial treatment with a primary antiarrthythmic drug may intensify rather than reverse the disease. Use of physical maneuvers such as ocular pressure, massage of the carotid sinus region, or a blow to the chest should not be disregarded (Ettinger and Suter 1970; Hilwig 1976; Tilley 1979, 1985).

REFERENCES

Adams, H. R. 1975. Acute adverse effects of antibiotics. J Am Vet Med Assoc 166:983-87.

———. 1981. Cardiovascular emergencies: drug and resuscitative principles. Vet Clin North Am 11:77-102.

———. 1986. New perspectives in cardiology: pharmacodynamic classification of antiarrhythmic drugs. J Am Vet Med Assoc 189:525-32.

Allert, J. A., Adams, H. R. 1986. New perspectives in cardiovascular medicine: the calcium channel blocking drugs. J Am Vet Med Assoc 190:573-78.

Binah, O., Rosen, M. R. 1984. The cellular mechanisms of cardiac antiarrhythmic drug action. Ann NY Acad Sci 432:31-44.

Bohn, F. K., Patterson, D. F., Pyle, R. L. 1971. Atrial fibrillation in dogs. Br Vet J 127:485-96.

Bonagura, J. D., Muir, W. W. 1985. In L. D. Tiley, ed., Essentials of Canine and Feline Electrocardiography, 2nd ed., p. 266. Philadelphia: Lea & Febiger.

Boyden, P. A., Wit, A. L. 1985. In L. D. Tiley, ed., Essentials of Canine and Feline Electrocardiography, 2nd ed., p. 266. Philadelphia: Lea & Febiger.

Breznock, E. M., Kagan, K., Hibser, N. K. 1977. Effects of bretylium tosylate on the in vivo fibrillating canine ventricle. Am J Vet Res 38:89-94.

Calvert, C. A., Chapman, W. L., Jr., Toal, R. L. 1982. Congestive cardiomyopathy in Doberman pinscher dogs. J Am Vet Med Assoc 181:598-602.

Clark, D. R. 1977. Recognition and treatment of cardiac emergencies. J Am Med Assoc 171:98-106.

Clark, D. R., Knauer, K. 1980. Personal communication.

Condouris, G. A., Ortiz, J., Lyness, W. 1979. Cardiac arrhythmias produced by bretylium in cats anesthetized with halothane. Eur J Pharmacol 55:93-97.

Cranefield, P. F. 1973. Ventricular fibrillation. N Engl J Med 289:732-36.

———. 1975. The Conduction of the Cardiac Impulse, p. 1. Mt. Kisco, N.Y.: Futura.

Damato, A. N. 1969. Diphenylhydantoin: pharmacological and clinical use. Prog Cardiovasc Dis 12:1-15.

Detweiler, D. K. 1957. Electrocardiographic and clinical features of spontaneous auricular fibrillation and flutter (tachycardia) in dogs. Zntralbl Veterinaermed 4:509-56.

———. 1977. In L. M. Jones, N. H. Booth, and L. E. McDonald, eds., Veterinary Pharmacology and Therapeutics, 4th ed., p. 496. Ames: Iowa State Univ. Press.

Detweiler, D. K., Patterson, D. F. 1963. In J. F. Bone, ed., Equine Medicine and Surgery. Wheaton, Ill.: American Veterinary Publications.

Ettinger, S. J., Suter, P. F. 1970. Canine Cardiology, p. 237. Philadelphia: W. B. Saunders.

Hamlin, R. L. 1977. New ideas in the management of heart failure in dogs. J Am Vet Med Assoc 171:114-18.

———. 1986. Clinical and experimental studies with verapamil in the dog. In Proc 5th Symp Am Acad Vet Pharm Therap, pp. 89-96.
Hayes, A. H., Jr. 1972. The actions and clinical use of the newer antiarrhythmic drugs. Ration Drug Ther 6:1-6.
Helfant, R. H., Scherlag, B. J., Damato, A. N. 1967. Protection from digitalis toxicity with the prophylactic use of diphenylhydantoin sodium: an arrhythmic-inotropic dissociation. Circulation 36:119-24.
Hilwig, R. W. 1976. Cardiac arrhythmias in the dog: detection and treatment. J Am Vet Med Assoc 169:789-98.
Hoffman, B. F., Cranefield, P. F. 1960. Electrophysiology of the Heart. New York: McGraw-Hill.
Huisman, G. H., Teunissen, G. H. B. 1963. Paroxysmal ventricular tachycardia in the dog. Zentralbl Veterinaermed 10:273-85.
Hurley, R. E., Page, I. H., Dustan, H. R. 1960. Bretylium tosylate as an antihypertensive drug. J Am Med Assoc 172:2081-83.
Jacobs, A. S., Nielsen, D. H., Gianelly, R. E. 1985. Fatal ventricular fibrillation following verapamil in Wolff-Parkinson-White syndrome with atrial fibrillation. Ann Emerg Med 14:159-60.
Johnson, J. T. 1985. Conversion of atrial fibrillation in two dogs using verapamil and supportive therapy. J Am Anim Hosp Assoc 21:429-34.
Keefe, D. L., Kates, R. E., Harrison, D. C. 1981. New antiarrhythmic drugs: their place in therapy. Drugs 22:363-400.
Kittleson, M. D., Hamlin, R. L. 1981. Hydralazine therapy for severe mitral regurgitation in a dog. J Am Vet Med Assoc 179:903-5.
Kittleson, M. D., Keene, B. W., Pion, P. 1988. Verapamil administration for acute termination of supraventricular tachycardia in dogs. J Am Vet Med Assoc 193:1525-30.
Koch-Weser, J. 1979. Drug therapy: bretylium. N Engl J Med 300:473-77.
Leahey, E. B., Jr., Reiffel, J. A., Drusin, R. E., et al. 1978. Interaction between quinidine and digoxin. J Am Med Assoc 240:533-34.
Mason, D. T., Demaria, A. N., Amsterdam, E. A., et al. 1973. Antiarrhythmic agents. I. Mechanisms of action and clinical pharmacology. Drugs 5:261-91.
Moss, A. J., Patton, R. D. 1973. Antiarrhythmic Agents. Springfield, Ill.: Charles C. Thomas.
Muir, W. W., Bonagura, J. D. 1982. Aprindine for treatment of ventricular arrhythmias in the dog. Am J Vet Res 43:1815-19.
Neff, C. A., Davis, L. E., Baggot, J. D. 1972. A comparative study of the pharmacokinetics of quinidine. Am J Vet Res 33:1521-25.
Novotny, M. J., Adams, H. R. 1986. New perspectives in cardiology: recent advances in antiarrhythmic drug therapy. J Am Vet Med Assoc 189:533-39.
Parker, J. L., Adams, H. R. 1977. Drugs and the heart muscle. J Am Vet Med Assoc 171:78-84.
Pyle, R. L. 1967. Conversion of atrial fibrillation with quinidine sulfate in a dog. J Am Vet Med Assoc 151:582-89.
Roye, D. B., Serrano, E. E., Hammer, R. H., et al. 1973. Plasma kinetics of dephenylhydantoin in dogs and cats. Am J Vet Res 34:947-50.
Sanders, J. E., Yeary, R. A. 1978. Serum concentrations of orally administered diphenylhydantoin in dogs. J Am Vet Med Assoc 172:153-56.
Sanders, J. E., Yeary, R. A., Fenner, W. R., et al. 1979. Interaction of phenytoin with chloramphenicol or pentobarbital in the dog. J Am Vet Med Assoc 175:177-80.
Scherlag, B. J., Helfant, R. H., Ricciutti, M. A., et al. 1968. Dissociation of the effects of digitalis on myocardial potassium flux and contractility. Am J Physiol 215:1288-91.
Schmitt, F. O., Erlanger, J. 1929. Directional differences in conduction of impulse through heart muscle and their possible relation to extrasystolic and fibrillary contractions. Am J Physiol 87:326-47.
Shanks, R. G., Dunlop, D. 1967. Effect of propranolol on arrhythmias following coronary artery occlusion. Cardiovasc Res 1:34-41.
Singh, B. N., Collett, J. T., Chew, C. Y. 1980. New perspectives in the pharmacologic therapy of cardiac arrhythmias. Prog Cardiovasc Dis 22:243-301.
Singh, B. N., Jewitt, D. E. 1974. Beta-adrenergic receptor blocking drugs in cardiac arrhythmias. Drugs 7:426-61.
Spedding, M. 1985. Calcium antagonist subgroups. Trends Pharmacol Sci 6:109-14.
Tilley, L. P., ed. 1979. Essentials of Canine and Feline Electrocardiography. St. Louis: C. V. Mosby.
———, ed. 1985. Essentials of Canine and Feline Electrocardiography, 2nd ed. Philadelphia: Lea & Febiger.
Trautwein, W. 1963. Generation and conduction of impulses in the heart as affected by drugs. Pharmacol Rev 15:277-332.
Vaughn Williams, E. M. 1984. A classification of antiarrhythmic actions reassessed after a decade of new drugs. J Clin Pharmacol 24:129-47.
Weidler, D. J., Jallad, N. S., Garg, D. C., et al. 1979. Pharmacokinetics of propranolol in the cat and comparisons with humans and three other species. Res Commun Chem Pathol Pharmacol 26:105-14.
Wit, A. L., Hoffman, B. F., Cranefield, P. F. 1972. Slow conduction and reentry in the ventricular conducting system. I. Return of extrasystole in canine Purkinje fibers. Circ Res 30:1-10.
Wit, A. L., Rosen, M. R., Hoffman, B. F. 1974. Electrophysiology and pharmacology of cardiac arrhythmias. II. Relationship of normal and abnormal electrical activity of cardiac fibers to the genesis of arrhythmias B. Re-entry. Section I. Am Heart J 88:664-70.

SECTION 6

Drugs Affecting Renal Function and Fluid-Electrolyte Balance

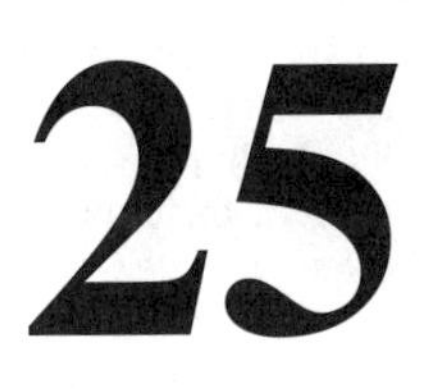

PRINCIPLES OF ACID-BASE BALANCE: FLUID AND ELECTROLYTE THERAPY

DEBORAH T. KOCHEVAR

Composition and Distribution of Body Fluids
- **Units of Measure**
- **Body Fluid Compartments**
- **Fluid and Electrolyte Distribution**

Water, Sodium, and Chloride
- **Homeostasis**
- **Renal Regulation of Sodium, Chloride, and Water Excretion**
- **Disorders of Water, Sodium, and Chloride Balance**
  - **Types of Dehydration**
  - **Hypernatremia**
  - **Hyponatremia**
  - **Hyperchloremia**
  - **Hypochloremia**

Potassium
- **Homeostasis**
- **Renal Regulation of Potassium Excretion**
- **Disorders of Potassium Balance**
  - **Hyperkalemia**
  - **Hypokalemia**

Principles of Acid-Base Metabolism
- **Homeostasis**
- **Regulation of Hydrogen Ion, Carbon Dioxide, and Bicarbonate**
- **Assessment of Acid-Base Disturbances**
- **Anion Gap**
- **Nontraditional (Stewart's) Acid-Base Analysis**

Disorders of Acid-Base Metabolism
- **Metabolic (Nonrespiratory) Acidosis**
  - **Lactic Acidosis**
  - **Ketoacidosis and Other Causes**
- **Metabolic (Nonrespiratory) Alkalosis**
- **Respiratory Acidosis**
- **Respiratory Alkalosis**
- **Mixed Acid-Base Disturbances**

Practical Aspects of Fluid Therapy
- **Diagnosis and Monitoring**
- **Fluid Volume and Type**
- **Rates and Routes of Administration**

Products for Fluid Therapy
- **Crystalloids**
- **Colloids**
- **Hypertonic Solutions**

Special Topics
- **Horses**
- **Cattle**
- **Anesthetic and Surgical Effects**

TABLE 25.1—Units of measure and conversions commonly used in fluid therapy

Term	Abbreviation	Description and conversion
Molecular (formula) weight	MW	Sum of atomic weights of all elements in a chemical formula
Millimole	mmol (mM)	Molecular (formula) weight of a substance in mg, equals 1 mM
Milliequivalent	mEq	Weight, in mg, of an element that combines or replaces 1 mg (1 mmol) of hydrogen (H^+)
Milliosmole	mOsm	Always contains 6.0×10^{23} molecules and equals 1 mmol of a nondissociable substance
Milliequivalent per liter	mEq/L	= mmol/L × valence = [(mg/dL × 10)/MW] × valence

COMPOSITION AND DISTRIBUTION OF BODY FLUIDS

Units of Measure. The units of measure commonly utilized in discussion of fluid balance are presented in Table 25.1. Ions or electrolytes combine according to valence (charge) rather than molecular weight. Hence in the case of univalent ions, 1 mM = 1 mEq. One mM of a divalent ion provides 2 mEq. By expressing most electrolyte concentrations in milliequivalents per liter (mEq/L), and comparing the concentration of cations to anions in the body, it becomes clear that electroneutrality exists. Although extracellular cations are often more completely documented in the course of clinical investigations, anions, particularly chloride and bicarbonate, are the electrical counterbalance. Some electrolytes are measured in millimoles per liter (mM/L) because they exist in variable states of protein binding or valence. An example is total calcium, because protein binding confounds any simple assessment of ionized fraction. Phosphorus exists in variable proportions of phosphate and monohydrogen and dihydrogen phosphate, so no valence can be assigned and calculation of milliequivalence is therefore inaccurate. Since mEq/L are the most common and informative unit of comparison for most electrolytes, conversion formulas are also provided in Table 25.1.

Solutes exert an osmotic effect in solution that is dependent only on the number of particles in solution, not on molecular weight or valence. Hence for nondissociable substances, 1 osmole contains 1 mole of substance. If a substance dissociates in solution, the number of osmoles is increased according to the number of particles generated per mole of dissociated substance. For example, each mmol of a completely dissociated NaCl solution yields 2 mOsm. Osmolarity refers to the number of osmoles per liter, and osmolality indicates the number of osmoles per kilogram of solvent (Rose 1989). In physiological systems the difference between these two is usually small. The concept of osmolality explains why solutions of diverse chemical and electrical composition (e.g., 5% dextrose, 0.9% NaCl, and 1.3% sodium bicarbonate) can all be considered isotonic. For mammals, isotonic solutions equal approximately 300 mOsm.

Body Fluid Compartments. Semipermeable membranes separate most body compartments, allowing the free passage of water and selected solutes. The effective osmolality, or tonicity, of a solution is related to the ability of a solute to attract water and to sustain an increase in osmotic pressure as a result of water movement. For example, two substances with equal ability to attract water down a concentration gradient and across a semipermeable membrane may have very different effects on osmotic pressure, depending upon the movement of the substance itself through the semipermeable membrane. While the measured osmolality of a solution includes all osmoles, whether effective or ineffective, tonicity of a solution relates only to effective osmolality. For example, a solution containing 300 mOsm of nonpenetrating NaCl and 100 mOsm of urea, which can cross plasma membranes, would have a total osmolarity of 400 mOsm and would be hyperosmotic. However, if one put red blood cells in this solution, they would not shrink or swell, because the urea would diffuse into the cells and reach equilibrium inside and outside the cells. Thus, both extracellular and intracellular solutions would have the same osmolarity. There would be no difference in the water concentration across the membrane and no change in cell volume. The solution is therefore considered isotonic.

Ultimately all fluids within the body are in dynamic equilibrium, but it is helpful during fluid therapy to consider body water as existing in several compartments since critical fluid shifts can and do occur. Determination of the volumes of these compartments is problematic, as can be deduced from the large number of different methods that have been used to estimate these volumes (Kohn and DiBartola 1992). The most common method for assessment of volume in body fluid compartments depends upon intravenous administration of a known amount of a dye or radioisotope-tagged substance that distributes only in the compartment of interest. This is followed by assessment of dye or radioisotope concentration in the compartment. Ideally, the indicator substance must distribute rapidly and homogeneously, remain in the space to be measured, not be metabolized or bound, and be nontoxic. The volume of distribution (Vd) of a drug, or in this case a volume marker, may be derived according to the same principles of pharmacokinetics described elsewhere in this text.

Total body water (TBW) is approximated at 60% of body weight, but this figure varies from 50 to 75% depending upon age, lean body mass, and individual

TABLE 25.2—Approximate volumes of selected fluid compartments in the dog

Compartment	% Body weight (BW)	Method
Total body water (TBW)	60	Indicator substance
ECF	20–27	Indicator substance
Red blood cells (RBC)	3	Counted + calculations
Plasma volume (PV)	5	Indicator substance
Total blood volume (BV)	5.7–10	Calculated: RBC volume + PV
Interstitial lymph fluid	15	Calculated: ECF – BV
Transcellular fluid	1–6	Estimated
Bone and dense connective tissue	5	Estimated
ICF	33–40	TBW – ECF

Source: Estimated from data collected in multiple studies as detailed in Kohn and DiBartola 1992, 5–7.

animal variations. Since fat is lower in water content than lean tissue, obesity is associated with decreased TBW (approximately 50%). To avoid overhydration of obese patients, fluid requirements are best estimated based on lean body mass. Very young animals are about 70–75% water, with TBW declining with advancing age. Table 25.2 provides estimates of selected volumes in dogs. TBW is broadly divided into two types: intracellular (ICF) and extracellular fluid (ECF). The ECF is further divided into four subcompartments: plasma volume, interstitial lymph fluid, transcellular fluid, and fluid present in dense connective tissue and bone. Table 25.3 provides experimentally derived blood volumes as percentages of body weight for various species.

Transcellular fluid is found in diverse locations, including cerebrospinal fluid, pleural cavity, gastrointestinal tract, bladder, synovia, aqueous humor, and peritoneal cavity. Transcellular volumes vary greatly from monogastrics (1–6%) to horses and ruminants (10–15%), dependent largely upon the amount of fluid sequestered in the gastrointestinal tract. Transcellular volumes are not readily mobilized during volume deficits but are of importance in terms of drug disposition and equilibrium. In certain disease processes, transcellular fluids may accumulate, causing ascites, hydropericardium, hydrothorax, synovitis, or other conditions, depending on the location of fluid accumulation.

Fluid and Electrolyte Distribution. Body solutes are not distributed homogeneously throughout TBW. Like drugs, every solute has a defined space or volume of distribution that can be assessed experimentally. As with estimation of body compartment volumes, determination of solute distribution is limited by the features of the labeled solute used. Because normal vascular endothelium is largely impermeable to formed blood elements and plasma protein, these cells and solutes are usually limited to the plasma. Vascular endothelium is freely permeable to ionic solutes, and the concentration of these ions is almost the same in interstitial as in plasma fluid. Table 25.4 provides estimations of ion composition in plasma of normal mammals.

The volume of ICF and ECF compartments is determined by the number of osmotically active particles in each space. ECF osmolality can be estimated from the following formula:

TABLE 25.3—Approximate values for blood volumes of various animals expressed as percentages of body weight

Species	Total blood volume	Plasma volume	RBC volume
Dogs	8.5	4.5	4.0
Cats	6.7	4.7	2.0
Chickens	6.5	4.5	2.0
Cattle	5.7	3.8	1.9
Goats	7.0	5.4	1.6
Horses			
Draft	7.0	4.0	3.0
Thoroughbred	10.0	6.0	4.0
Saddle	7.7	5.2	2.5
Pigs	7.5	4.8	2.7
Sheep	6.5	4.5	2.0

Source: Smith 1970. Values represent averages from approximately 30 references.

$$\text{ECF osmolality (mOsm/kg)} = 2\left(\left[Na^+\right]+\left[K^+\right]\right) + \frac{\text{glucose}}{18} + \frac{\text{blood urea nitrogen (BUN)}}{2.8}$$

(Rose 1989). Because cell membranes are permeable to urea and K^+, these substances contribute only ineffective osmoles, as described earlier. At normal blood glucose concentrations, Na^+ is the primary determinant of effective ECF osmolality. Because Na^+ is the most abundant and osmotically active ECF cation, maintenance of an extracellular-to-intracellular sodium gradient is critical and is accomplished by the cell membrane Na^+,K^+-adenosine triphosphatase (ATPase) pump. This pump is also responsible for maintaining appropriate concentrations of intracellular K^+. Because K^+ is the most abundant intracellular cation, the ratio of intracellular-to-extracellular K^+ concentration is the major determinant of the resting cell membrane potential (–70 to –90 mV). Because all body fluid spaces are isotonic with one another, the effective osmolality of the ICF, and indeed TBW, must be equal to that of the ECF. Acute addition or loss of fluid and/or solutes from the body inevitably results in alterations in

TABLE 25.4—Approximate average concentrations of cations and anions in plasma in normal mammals

Cations	mEq/L	Anions	mEq/L
Sodium	135–160	Chloride	110–125
Potassium	3–5	Bicarbonate	18–22
Calcium (total calcium 5–10 mM/L)	4–6	Phosphate	1–3*
Magnesium	1–3	Sulfate	1–2
Trace elements	1	Lactate	1–2
		Other organic acids	3–5
		Protein	10–16
Total	144–175		144–175

Source: Gross 1994.
*Phosphate exists in variable proportions of phosphate and monohydrogen and dihydrogen phosphate, so no valance can be identified and the number of mEq/L is therefore an estimate (Gross 1994).

compartment volumes and tonicity. Homeostatic shifts of fluid between compartments must then occur to return the system to isotonicity.

The critical distribution of water between the plasma and the interstitium is maintained by the colloidal osmotic pressure of plasma protein (oncotic pressure). This is the force that draws water into the capillaries and balances the hydrostatic pressure driving water out. These so-called Starling forces describe the capillary balance between forces that favor filtration of water from plasma and those that retain vascular volume:

$$\text{Net filtration (NF)} = K_f\,[(P_{cap} - P_{if}) - (\pi_p - \pi_{if})]$$

where K_f represents permeability of the capillary wall, P represents hydrostatic pressure in the capillaries (P_{cap}) (blood) or tissues (P_{if}) (interstitial fluid), and π represents oncotic pressure generated by plasma protein (π_p) or filtered proteins and glycosaminoglycans in the interstitium (π_{if}). Applying Starling's relationships yields the prediction that hypoproteinemia (decreased π_p) will increase loss of vascular fluid and that water depletion (with a relative increase in π_p and a decrease in P_{cap}) will promote reabsorption of interstitial fluid into the vasculature (Kohn and DiBartola 1992). The volume of intracellular water in a given tissue is maintained by intracellular protein. As plasma water decreases, plasma protein competes with intracellular protein for water, resulting in cellular dehydration. Clinical alterations in plasma osmolality may be assessed by comparing measured osmolality in a patient to calculated serum osmolality as determined using Na^+, K^+, glucose, and BUN measurements (see the ECF osmolality equation provided above). Observed changes in the osmolal gap (difference between measured osmolality and the osmolality calculated from normal concentrations) may be useful in determining the presence of unmeasured osmoles associated with toxic substances such as ethylene glycol. The osmolal gap may also be useful in assessing shifts in plasma sodium concentration (Kohn and DiBartola 1992).

The number of cations in the ECF must equal the number of anions in order to maintain electroneutrality. In practice, only selected cations and anions are routinely measured in a clinical setting. Calculation of the difference between the commonly measured cations and anions in ECF yields the unmeasured anions, or anion gap (Oh and Carrol 1977; Emmett and Narins 1977). The anion gap calculation can be useful in assessing the etiology of metabolic acidosis and will be discussed in this context subsequently.

WATER, SODIUM, AND CHLORIDE

Homeostasis. Daily intake of water, nutrients, and minerals is normally balanced by daily excretion of these substances. *Water turnover* is the term used to describe input and output of body water over a given period of time. Values for water turnover, per 24 hours, in various domestic animals resting in cages or stalls range from about 40 to 132 mL/kg/day. The range is influenced by species, age, and physiologic state (Adolph 1939; Smith 1970). Extremes of temperature, psychologic state, disease, and other variables may change water demands markedly. Water turnover in mature dogs is approximated as 40–60 mL/kg/day, while immature and lactating animals may turn over approximately twice this amount (Muir and DiBartola 1983). Maintenance fluid needs are defined as the volume of fluid required daily to maintain an animal in zero fluid balance, that is, no net gain or loss of water.

Normal water intake occurs in response to thirst, which is stimulated by plasma hypertonicity and/or contracted ECF volume. Plasma hypertonicity, the primary stimulus, prompts osmoreceptors in the supraoptic and paraventricular nuclei of the hypothalamus to release vasopressin, also called antidiuretic hormone (ADH), which is released into the circulation at the level of the pituitary neurohypophysis. Binding of vasopressin to receptors in the distal nephron and renal collecting duct cells activates adenylyl cyclase and increases intracellular cyclic AMP. A protein kinase cascade initiated by activation of protein kinase A results in opening of luminal water pores in the tubule cell. Permeability of the collecting duct to water and reabsorption of water increase. Sustained release of vasopressin depends additionally upon calcium cycling across the plasma membrane and activation of protein kinase C–dependent pathways. Prostaglandins inhibit the renal response to vasopressin. Drugs with anticyclooxygenase activity that inhibit prostaglandin synthesis thereby enhance the action of endogenous vasopressin. Fig. 25.1 summarizes the effects of selected drugs and electrolytes on vasopressin release and action.

If ECF volume and renal perfusion decrease, volume receptors in the renal juxtaglomerular apparatus respond, causing the secretion (or release) of renin, which converts angiotensinogen to angiotensin I. This is the rate-limiting step in the renin-angiotensin sys-

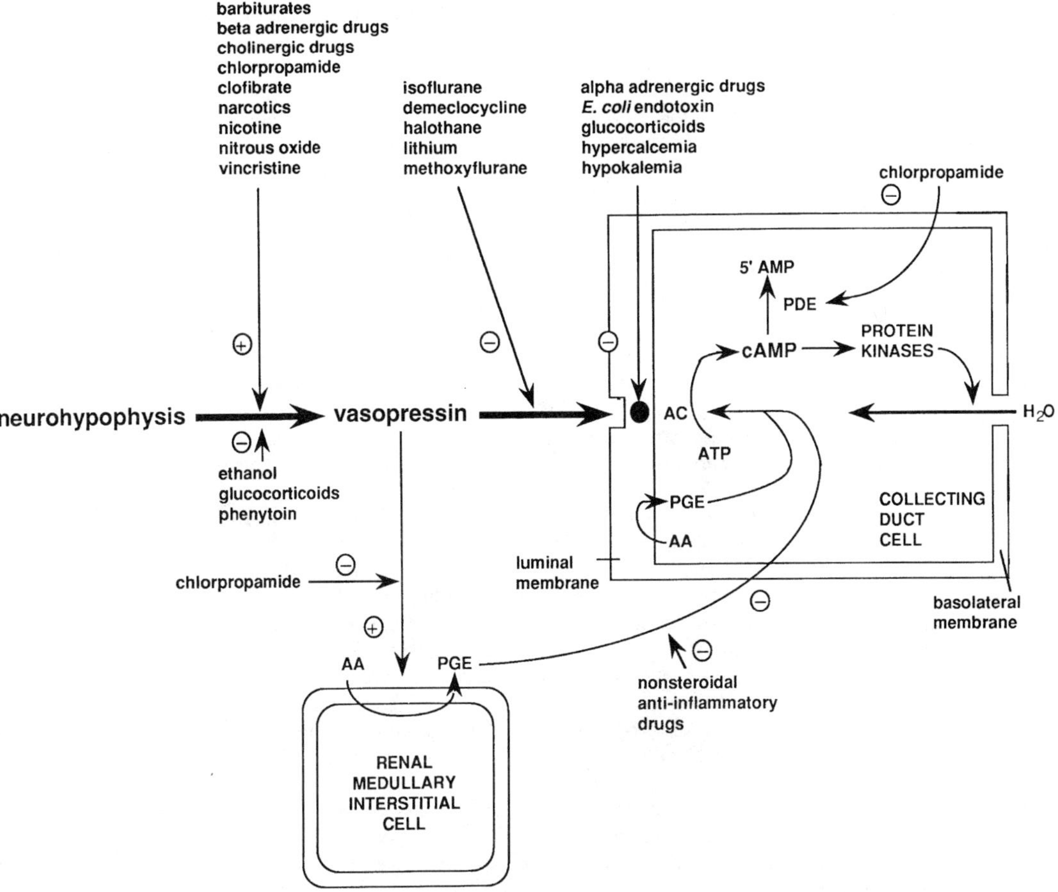

FIG. 25.1—Effects of drugs and electrolytes on vasopressin release and mechanisms of cellular action. AA = arachidonic acid; AC = adenylyl cyclase; ATP = adenosine triphosphate; cAMP = cyclic adenosine monophosphate; PDE = phosphodiesterase; PGE = prostaglandin E. (Adapted from DiBartola 1992c, Fig. 3-3.)

tem. Angiotensin I is activated to the potent vasoconstrictor angiotensin II in the lung and in endothelial cells throughout the body by angiotensin-converting enzyme (ACE). Angiotensin II stimulates the zona glomerulosa of the adrenal cortex to secrete aldosterone, which, in turn, causes increased reabsorption of sodium from the distal nephron with excretion of K^+ and H^+. Due to the increased concentration of sodium, plasma becomes hypertonic, causing vasopressin release and water retention.

Water intake occurs in response not only to thirst but also to hunger. Water content of food may be as low as 10% (dry food) or as high as 90% (succulent green pasture). Canned pet foods generally contain more than 70% water, and semimoist foods are intermediate (20–40% water) (Lewis and Morris 1987). Intake of dietary water is governed centrally by appetite control mechanisms rather than by fluid and electrolyte homeostasis. In addition to water intake related to eating and drinking, metabolic water is produced endogenously by catabolism of proteins, fats, and carbohydrates (approximately 5 mL/kg/day) and represents about 10–15% of total water intake in dogs and cats (Anderson 1983).

Normal water loss occurs via urine, fecal water, and saliva (sensible loss), with insensible losses occurring via evaporation from cutaneous and respiratory epithelia. Insensible losses account for TBW elimination of about 15–30 mL/kg/day in healthy, sedentary animals in a thermoneutral environment (Kohn and DiBartola 1992).

Metabolic rate, and therefore a portion of daily water turnover, are directly proportional to the ratio of body surface area to total volume. For example, the surface area to volume ratio in a puppy is much larger than in an adult dog and the puppy has a higher basal metabolic rate. Both lead to a much greater evaporative loss of water from the skin per unit volume. Hence, daily water turnover per unit body weight may be nearly twice that of the adult animal. Small, immature animals are therefore at greater risk for insensible water loss than large, mature animals.

The most important and predictable loss of water in healthy, sedentary animals, in a thermoneutral environment, occurs via the urine. Urinary losses can vary from 2 to 20 mL/kg/day. Daily urinary water losses may be divided into obligatory water loss and free water loss (Kohn and DiBartola 1992). Obligatory water loss represents water eliminated in order to excrete the daily renal solute load. The renal solute load is derived from dietary sources of protein and minerals and consists of urea, Na^+, K^+, Ca^{++}, Mg^{++}, NH_4^+, and other cations; and PO_4^{3-}, Cl^-, SO_4^{2-}, and other anions. Hence, daily renal solute load is a function of the quantity and composition of food ingested. Urea accounts for two-thirds of the urinary solute load in dogs (O'Connor and Potts 1969).

In normal animals increased urine solute load is eliminated by an increase in urine volume (obligatory water loss) rather than a marked increase in urine osmolality. Hence, urine osmolality is not generally maximized in order to accomplish steady-state elimination of solutes. Obligatory renal water loss is clinically important for removal of renal solutes but also because this type of water loss will continue even in states of relative water deficit. Free water loss represents water excreted unaccompanied by solute. Excretion of free water is controlled by vasopressin and increases during relative water excess or hypotonicity and decreases during water deficit or hypertonicity. Obligatory fecal water loss occurs in order to excrete fecal solutes. Fecal losses ordinarily account for 2–5% of TBW losses and vary with the species. Feces typically contain 50–80% water (Kohn and DiBartola 1992).

Renal Regulation of Sodium, Chloride, and Water Excretion. Elimination or conservation of body water and solutes via the kidneys depends upon the processes of glomerular filtration and renal tubular reabsorption and secretion. A major mechanism for conservation of water is urine concentration. The canine kidney can concentrate urine to as much as 2400 mOsm, compared to 1200–1400 mOsm achieved in human urine. Elimination of substances via the urine depends upon renal clearance of each substance from the plasma. The volume of plasma that must be filtered each minute to account for the amount of substance appearing in the urine each minute under steady-state conditions defines renal clearance of that substance.

As much as 20% of cardiac output is directed to the kidneys, with blood entering a renal glomerulus through an afferent arteriole and leaving through an efferent arteriole. Resistance changes in afferent and efferent capillaries regulate glomerular filtration rate (GFR). For discussions of normal and abnormal renal physiologic function the reader is referred to any standard physiology text. An understanding of the complexities of renal function is crucial to the understanding of water, acid-base, and electrolyte balances.

As glomerular filtrate flows through the tubules, most of the water (greater than 90%) and varying amounts of solute are reabsorbed into the peritubular capillaries. The composition of the tubular reabsorbate closely approximates that of ECF. Reabsorption is largely achieved by transport of electrolytes and other solutes in two steps: (1) absorption of solutes from tubular fluid into tubular cells and (2) movement of solutes from tubular cells into the ECF. Several types of transport account for tubular reabsorption of solutes, including passive transport (simple diffusion), facilitated diffusion, active transport, and cotransport. These mechanisms are discussed in more detail in the context of diuretic drugs (Chap. 26) and summarized in Fig. 26.2. Fig. 25.2 depicts some of the functional processes for regulation of salt and water transport in different segments of the nephron.

As much as 60–65% of filtered solute is reabsorbed in the proximal tubule accompanied by osmotically proportional amounts of water. The tubular fluid at the distal portion of the proximal tubule becomes slightly hypoosmotic. Passive reabsorption of substances, especially sodium and chloride, continues in the thin segment of the loop of Henle. The thick ascending limb of the loop of Henle and the distal convoluted tubule are relatively impermeable to water but actively reabsorb solute. Sodium and chloride enter tubular cells in the thick ascending limb of Henle's loop by crossing the luminal membrane coupled to potassium in a proportion of 1 Na^+:1 K^+:2 Cl^-. Sodium is then actively extruded across the basolateral membrane to maintain intracellular sodium at low levels. Potassium and chloride leave the tubular cell passively. Two consequences of this are decreased concentration of sodium and chloride in the tubular lumen and increased concentration of each in interstitial fluid. A concentration gradient across the tubular epithelium is established, and this becomes multiplied in a longitudinal direction by the countercurrent mechanism. The collecting ducts are responsive to vasopressin, and in its presence the ducts become highly permeable to water. Tubular fluid equilibrates with hyperosmotic interstitium, and hypertonic (concentrated) urine results. In the absence of vasopressin, the ducts are relatively impermeable to water. In this case, sodium and chloride have been reabsorbed proximally to the collecting ducts, tubular fluid is hypoosmotic, and voided urine is dilute (Thier 1987).

Renal reabsorption of sodium in the distal nephron is increased by aldosterone, a mineralocorticoid synthesized in the zona glomerulosa of the adrenal cortex. Aldosterone is produced and released in response to stimulation by angiotensin II, hyperkalemia, and by a decrease in dietary sodium intake. Adrenocorticotropic hormone (ACTH) and hyponatremia play permissive roles in promoting aldosterone secretion. Increased dietary sodium and atrial natriuretic peptide (ANP) decrease aldosterone production. ANP is a polypeptide released from atrial and ventricular myocytes in response to atrial distention asso-

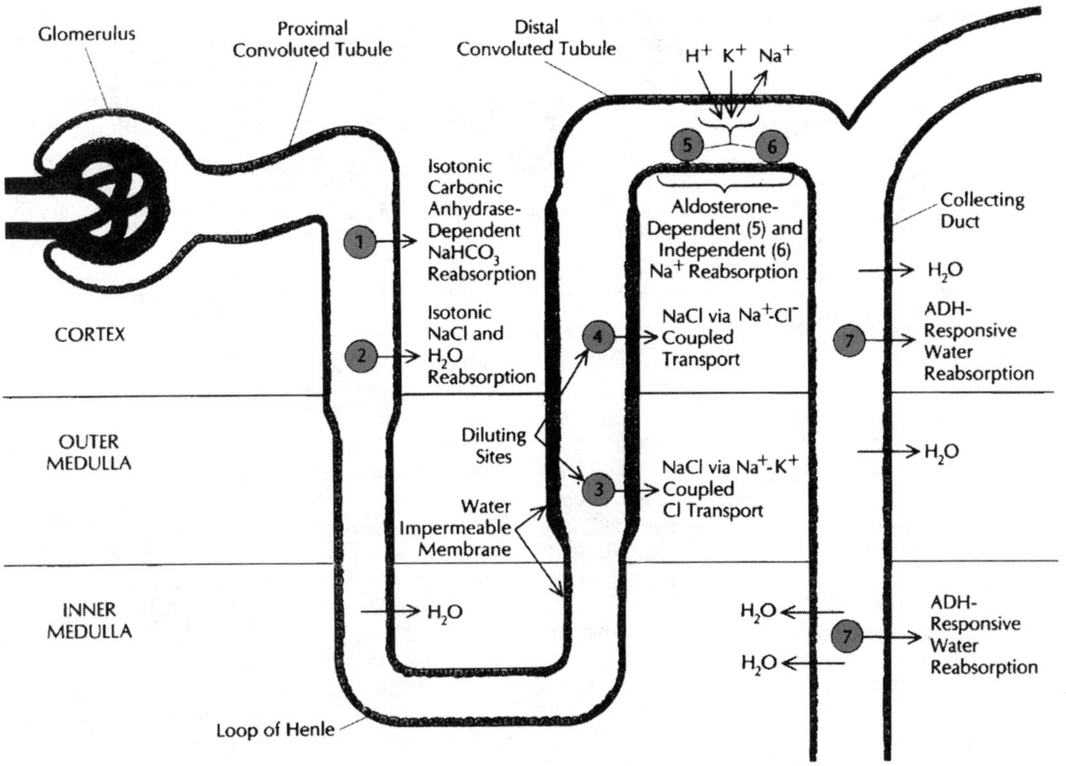

FIG. 25.2—Functional processes for regulation of salt and water transport in a nephron. (Reprinted from Thier 1987, 83, Fig. 1.)

ciated with volume expansion. ANP causes vascular smooth muscle relaxation, inhibits production of aldosterone in the adrenal glands, and blocks the production of angiotensin II. Study results suggest that parathyroid hormone (PTH) is required for augmented ANP secretion in response to acute volume loading in rats. PTH may play an important role in the regulation of fluid homeostasis via control of ANP (Geiger et al. 1992).

In general, chloride is reabsorbed with sodium throughout the nephron. As previously noted, chloride is exchanged in a ratio of 1 Na^+:1 K^+:2 Cl^- in the thick ascending limb of Henle's loop during sodium reabsorption. Because the cotransporter in this exchange has a very high affinity for both Na^+ and K^+, luminal Cl^- concentration is normally the rate-limiting step in NaCl entry into the cell (Gregor and Velazquez 1987). Additional active and passive processes contribute to proximal Cl^- reabsorption in the renal tubules. Chloride exchange for formate appears to occur via an anion exchanger in the luminal membrane. Low concentrations of filtered formate combine with H^+ to form formic acid (HF) in the tubular lumen. Because HF is uncharged, it moves freely into the tubular cell. Two additional mechanisms set the stage for conversion of HF back to formate and H^+. First, basolateral Na^+,K^+-ATPase pumps maintain a low intracellular sodium concentration, and this, in turn, allows for the continued exchange of Na^+-H^+ across the luminal membrane. As Na^+ is reabsorbed and H^+ is secreted, the interior of the cell is left with a lower [H^+] than the tubular lumen. Under these conditions HF is converted back to H^+ and formate, providing for continued chloride-formate exchange. Reabsorbed chloride is returned to the ECF across the basolateral membrane by selective Cl^- channels and a K^+-Cl^- cotransporter (Rose 1994). Additional transport mechanisms in type B intercalated cells in the cortical collecting tubule may exchange bicarbonate for chloride. The favorable inward concentration gradient for chloride (lumen concentration greater than inside the cell) presumably provides the energy for bicarbonate secretion via this mechanism (Bastani et al. 1991).

Disorders of Water, Sodium, and Chloride Balance

TYPES OF DEHYDRATION. Dehydration may be considered in three general categories: hypertonic, isotonic, and hypotonic. Pure water loss and loss of hypotonic fluid lead to hypertonic dehydration. As pure water is lost from the ECF, fluid shifts from the intra- to the extracellular compartment in response to increased osmolality. The resulting proportionate distribution of volume loss results in fewer clinically detectable signs of volume depletion in the patient. Causes of dehydration associated with pure water deficit include

TABLE 25.5—Physical findings in dehydration

Percent dehydration	Clinical signs
4 or less	History of fluid loss, mucous membranes still moist, evidence of thirst
5–6	Subtle loss of skin elasticity, slight delay in return of skin to normal position, hair coat dull, mucous membranes slightly dry but tongue still moist
7–8	Definite delay in return of skin to normal position, both mucous membranes and tongue may be dry, eyeballs may be soft and sunken, slight prolongation of capillary refill time
9–11	Tented skin does not return to normal position, definite prolongation of capillary refill time, eyes definitely sunken in orbits, all mucous membranes dry, may be signs of shock such as tachycardia, cool extremities, rapid and weak pulses
12–15	Definite signs of shock and circulatory collapse, death is imminent.

hypodypsia due to neurologic disease, diabetes insipidus, respiratory losses during exposure to elevated temperatures, fever, and inadequate access to water.

Loss of hypotonic fluid, as compared to pure water, results in a greater depletion of ECF volume since there is less osmotic drive to pull volume from the intracellular space. Hypotonic fluid losses are common and have been subclassified as extrarenal and renal. Extrarenal losses could include gastrointestinal (e.g., vomiting or diarrhea) or third-space loss (e.g., pancreatitis, peritonitis, as a result of surgery or cutaneous injury). *Third spacing* is a term used to describe extravasation of fluid from the vascular compartment into extravascular spaces. As tonicity of lost fluid approaches or exceeds normal plasma osmolality (about 300 mOsm/kg), disproportionate depletion of ECF causes more evident clinical signs of dehydration. Volume depletion would likely be the most clinically apparent in cases of hypertonic fluid loss.

Estimations of percent dehydration based on clinical signs are given in Table 25.5. Skin elasticity is a useful indicator of hydration status. However, age of the animal, body condition, and the technique used for evaluating elasticity may affect hydration assessment. With advancing age or cachexia, loss of fat and protein may account for decreased skin elasticity unrelated to hydration. Conversely, obese animals are likely to retain skin elasticity longer in the face of dehydration. Possibly as a result of variations in elastin content of skin, some species display smaller changes in elasticity for a given degree of dehydration. This may be clinically important in the horse. While dry mucous membranes can indicate dehydration, open-mouthed breathing associated with respiratory disease may cause misleading mucous membrane dryness. Degree of enopthalmos is considered a very useful parameter in assessment of dehydration in large animals. For example, the measured gap between the eyeball and orbit has been included as a guideline for assessment of dehydration in neonatal calves. A gap less than 0.5 cm is correlated with 9–10% dehydration, and a gap greater than 0.5 cm suggests 11–12% loss of hydration (Naylor 1996). A recent study evaluated several clinical and laboratory parameters to determine which were most useful in assessment of dehydration in diarrheic calves. Factors assessed included extent of enophthalmos, skin-tent duration on neck, thorax, and upper and lower eyelids, heart rate, mean central venous pressure, peripheral (extremities) and core temperatures, packed-cell volume, and hemoglobin and plasma protein concentration. The best predictors of degree of dehydration were extent of enophthalmos, skin elasticity on neck and thorax, and plasma protein concentration (Constable et al. 1998). Laboratory parameters such as hematocrit, plasma protein, and osmolality are often useful, but assessment should include consideration of possible preexisting derangements, such as anemia or hypoproteinemia, that could confound interpretation. If an accurate previous body weight is known, serial changes in weight are considered a very useful and accurate measurement in determining degree of dehydration.

HYPERNATREMIA. As the most important and abundant ECF cation, sodium is essential for proper maintenance of membrane potentials, initiation of action potentials, and, according to strong ion difference theory, maintenance of acid-base balance. Plasma sodium concentration and plasma osmolality generally vary in parallel since sodium and its associated anions account for greater than 95% of plasma osmolality. Plasma sodium concentration reflects the ratio of body sodium ion concentration to TBW. Total body sodium content, however, is independent of plasma sodium concentration and may be increased, decreased, or unchanged in the presence of hyper- or hyponatremia.

Clinical signs associated with alterations in serum sodium are more related to the rapidity of change rather than to the magnitude of sodium increase or decrease. Hypernatremia (e.g., >155 mEq sodium/L in dogs) and ECF hypertonicity can be caused by a loss of pure water, a loss of hypotonic fluid (extrarenal or renal), or a gain of impermeable sodium-containing solute (see Fig. 25.3). Clinical signs of hypernatremia are usually observed in dogs and cats as sodium concentration approaches and exceeds 170 mEq/mL. The signs seen are related to the osmotic movement of water out of cells. Negative effects of cellular dehydration are most pronounced in the brain and lead to the characteristic neurologic deficits associated with hypernatremia. These deficits include abnormal behavior and mentation, ataxia, seizures, and coma. The more rapidly water shifts out of brain cells, the greater the chance that decreased brain volume will lead to rupture of

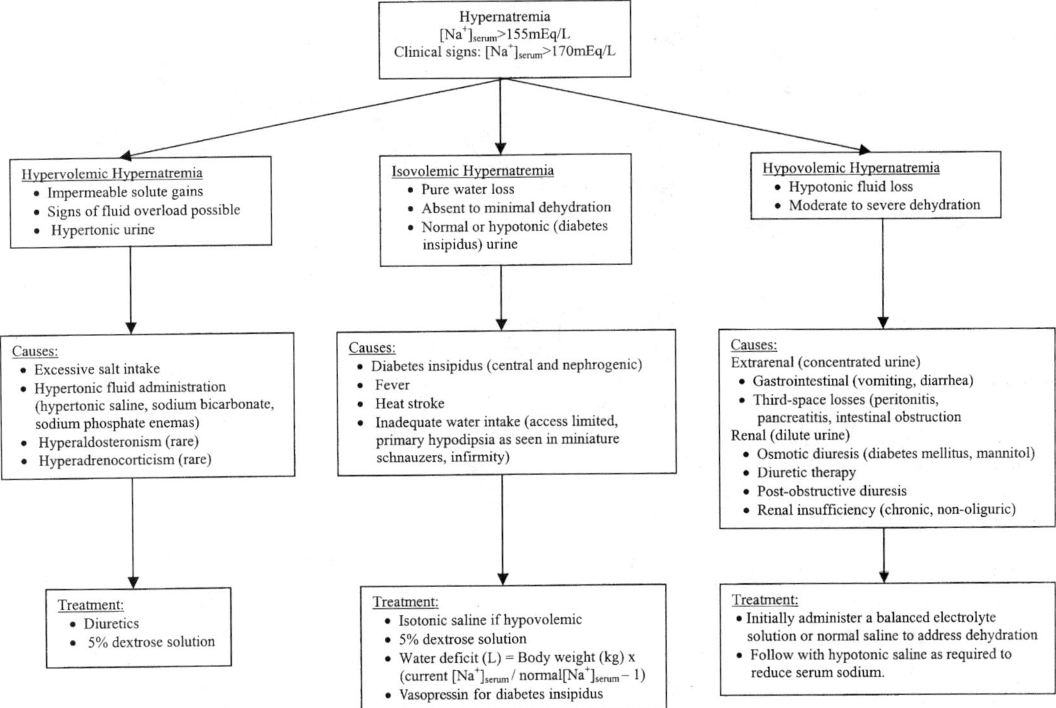

FIG. 25.3—Summary of classification, causes, and treatment of hypernatremia. See text for additional details of treatment.

cerebral vessels and focal hemorrhage (Arieff and Guisado 1976). If sodium concentration or concentration of sodium-containing impermeable solute increases slowly, the brain attempts to adapt to the hypertonic state by production of intracellular solutes (e.g., sugars, amino acids) known as "idiogenic" osmoles. Production of these osmotically active substances protects the cell by retaining intracellular volume and preventing cellular dehydration. In addition to neurologic deficits, other clinical signs of hypernatremia include thirst, anorexia, lethargy, vomiting, and muscle weakness. If hypernatremia is related to hypotonic fluid loss, then clinical signs of dehydration (as previously described) may be present. If a gain of sodium has caused the hypernatremia, volume overload may be a problem, especially in patients with cardiac disease.

Restoration of ECF volume and tonicity is of primary importance in treatment of hypernatremia. Volume replacement must be accomplished slowly to avoid rapid shifts in plasma osmolality. In general, the rate of fluid administration is determined by the rate of onset of the hypernatremia. When treating chronic hypernatremia, the serum sodium concentration should drop at a rate that does not exceed 0.7 mEq/L/hr (O'Brien 1995). If plasma osmolality drops quickly, water may be attracted intracellularly by idiogenic osmoles, resulting in development of cerebral edema. In the case of pure-water loss, volume can be replaced with 5% dextrose in water over a 48- to 72-hour period. Since the dextrose ultimately enters cells and is metabolized, 5% dextrose administration is essentially replacement with pure water. Use of a 1:1 mixture of normal saline with 5% dextrose solution yields an isotonic solution of 2.5% dextrose, 0.45% saline that has also been utilized. This solution decreases plasma tonicity more slowly and decreases the chance for cerebral edema. Hypotonic fluid losses should generally be replaced with an isotonic crystalloid solution. If hypernatremia has resulted from addition of sodium or sodium-containing impermeable solute, then administration of 5% dextrose and water should be accomplished cautiously to avoid pulmonary edema. Diuretics may be useful in promoting saluresis (sodium excretion) as ECF volume is restored (Marks 1998).

HYPONATREMIA. Causes of hyponatremia (<135–140 mEq sodium/L) are best categorized if two additional variables, osmolality and hydration, are also considered. As indicated in Fig. 25.4, the more common causes of hyponatremia are accompanied by decreased plasma osmolality (<290 mOsm/kg) with or without volume depletion. If volume depletion exists with hyponatremia, then loss of body sodium has exceeded water loss. Physiologic responses to hypovolemia lead to impaired water excretion and a relative dilution of

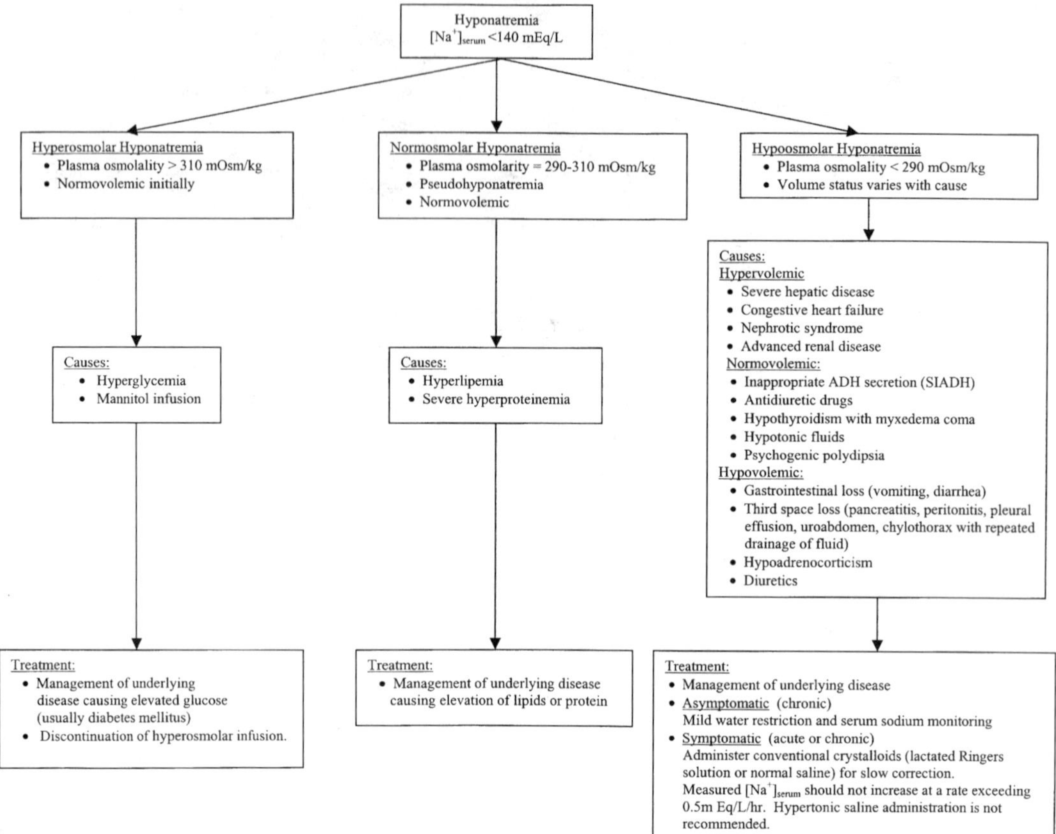

FIG. 25.4—Summary of classification, causes, and treatment of hyponatremia. See text for additional details of treatment.

the sodium remaining in body fluids. Hypovolemia causes decreased renal perfusion and GFR, leading to a decline in water excretion. Slower movement of filtrate through renal tubules enhances isosmotic reabsorption of salt and water in the proximal tubules and decreases presentation of tubular fluid at distal diluting sites. Additionally, hypovolemia prompts vasopressin release, further impairing water elimination. Finally, thirst related to hypovolemia results in consumption of low-sodium fluids that also dilute existing plasma sodium (DiBartola 1992c).

Hyponatremia accompanied by hypervolemia and low plasma osmolality occurs in clinical disorders where there is a physiological perception of volume depletion by in vivo volume detectors. The physiological response is volume expansion. For example, in congestive heart failure, decreased cardiac output is sensed as volume depletion by baroreceptors. Release of vasopressin impairs water excretion, leading to expanded vascular volume. Decreased effective circulating volume and decreased renal perfusion also lead to activation of the renin-angiotensin-aldosterone system. Enhanced renal retention of sodium contributes to expanded vascular volume. In cirrhosis and the nephrotic syndrome, hypoalbuminemia and decreased oncotic pressure may contribute to decreased effective circulating volume and, ultimately, vasopressin release and volume expansion. Other features of hepatic and renal disease also contribute to decreased circulating volume and/or impaired water excretion (DiBartola 1992c).

Hyponatremia is relatively less common when associated with increased plasma osmolality. The most frequent cause of sodium decreases in the presence of increased plasma osmolality is the increased circulating glucose levels associated with diabetes mellitus. Each 100 mg/dL increase in glucose results in a measured decrease of serum sodium by 1.6 mEq/L (Katz 1973). In response to the increased concentration of serum glucose, water shifts from the intracellular to the extracellular compartment, resulting in dilution of measured sodium. Serum osmolality remains high due to elevated glucose concentrations.

Hyponatremia associated with normal plasma osmolality is referred to as pseudohyponatremia. The decreased sodium concentrations are spurious and are almost universally related to technical difficulties in sodium measurement when plasma lipid or protein concentrations are high.

As with hypernatremia, clinical signs of hyponatremia are more severe if sodium concentration changes rapidly than if it changes over a more prolonged period of time. If sodium concentrations and plasma osmolality decrease quickly, water shifts out of the ECF and into cells. The central nervous system (CNS) is most affected by a rapid fluid shift, which, in hyponatremia, results in development of cerebral edema. If onset of hyponatremia is slow, the brain can adjust cell volume by decreasing intracellular osmolality and preventing influx of water from the ECF. Patients with chronic hyponatremia will also adjust intracellular osmolality to an extent that clinical signs may not be obvious even though sodium concentrations are quite low.

Treatment of hyponatremia varies with etiology of the disorder. The goals of therapy are to manage the underlying disease and, if necessary, to increase serum sodium and osmolality. Infusion with conventional crystalloid solutions (e.g., normal saline or lactated Ringer's solution) is reported to accomplish sodium and volume replacement in hyponatremic, hypovolemic patients (DiBartola 1992c). Use of hypertonic saline solutions is not recommended since overly rapid correction of hyponatremia may do more harm than good. Chronic hyponatremia, in which the brain has adjusted to the decrease in osmolality and sodium, must be handled cautiously to avoid brain dehydration and injury, including osmotic demyelination syndrome. This syndrome, often occurring several days after correction of hyponatremia, results from areas of demyelination caused by treatment-induced increases in serum sodium concentration. Dogs with asymptomatic chronic hyponatremia are best treated by mild water restriction and monitoring of serum sodium. Chronic, symptomatic dogs should be treated such that the rate of increase of serum sodium does not exceed 10–12 mEq/L/day (0.5 mEq/L/hr) (DiBartola 1998). Again, the most important therapeutic goal in management of hyponatremia should be treatment of the underlying disease.

HYPERCHLOREMIA. Fluid loss associated with small bowel diarrhea often results in greater loss of HCO_3^- than chloride due to loss of alkaline pancreatic secretions and bile and HCO_3^- secretion in exchange for Cl^- in the ileum. The resulting hyperchloremic metabolic acidosis is characterized by a normal anion gap. Additional causes and treatment for hyperchloremic metabolic acidosis will be considered subsequently under the heading of metabolic acidosis. Please refer to the discussion of hypernatremia for treatment of hyperchloremia associated with loss of free water.

HYPOCHLOREMIA. Hypochloremia may be seen in patients with fluid losses due to vomiting or excessive diuretic administration. Hypochloremic metabolic alkalosis may develop in these cases because an excess of chloride is lost, leading to decreased filtered Cl^- in the renal tubules. As previously noted, activity of the Na^+-K^+-$2Cl^-$ cotransporter in the luminal membrane of the macula densa cell is primarily determined by the availability of Cl^-. In hypochloremia, less Cl^- is delivered, resulting in less NaCl reabsorption, promotion of renin release leading to secondary hyperaldosteronism, and increased distal H^+ secretion. If further Na^+ reabsorption does occur, then Na^+ must be accompanied by an anion other than chloride, usually bicarbonate, or must be exchanged for a secreted cation, either H^+ or K^+. In addition, bicarbonate secretion in exchange for chloride, which is thought to occur in intercalated cells of the cortical collecting tubule, will decrease since this process is presumably driven by a favorable inward gradient for Cl^-. As luminal $[Cl^-]$ decreases, the gradient is dissipated and bicarbonate is retained in the system. All of the foregoing mechanisms promote retention of base and excretion of H^+, leading to a hypochloremic metabolic alkalosis (Rose 1994). Treatment with chloride-replete fluid such as normal saline is usually adequate to resolve chloride-responsive alkalosis. As will be discussed below, potassium depletion may also promote a metabolic alkalosis and should be addressed as needed by addition of potassium chloride to fluids.

POTASSIUM

Homeostasis. As the major intracellular cation, potassium concentrations inside (145 mEq/L) and outside (3.5–5.5 mEq/L) the cell are maintained by the Na^+,K^+-ATPase pump. Under normal circumstances each pump actively transports three sodium ions out of and two potassium ions into the cell, but the ratio can change depending upon the circumstances. The ratio of intra- to extracellular concentration of potassium ($[K^+]_i/[K^+]_o$) is the major determinant of resting membrane potential. Resting membrane potential is crucial to normal membrane excitability associated with cardiac conduction, muscle contraction, and nerve impulse transmission.

The normal dietary intake of potassium is much more than the body requires. About 90% of this intake is excreted in the urine, with the remainder of what is not required eliminated in the stool. Plasma potassium concentration is determined by the movement of potassium into or out of cells. Two important factors stimulating the transport of potassium into cells are insulin and β-adrenergic stimulation (Clausen and Flatman 1987). Aldosterone is the primary determinant of potassium secretion across renal tubular epithelial surfaces.

Renal Regulation of Potassium Excretion. Most filtered potassium (60–80%) is reabsorbed in the proximal tubule. In the early proximal tubule, potassium enters the tubular cell at the luminal surface by active transport. The intracellular concentration of potassium is high, and the lumen of the tubule is negatively charged relative to the interior of the early proximal tubular cell. Potassium passively exits the basolateral membrane of the tubular cell down a favorable chemical concentration gradient. In the mid-to-late proximal tubule, the tubular lumen is relatively more positively charged than the tubular cell interior. This favors the passive reabsorption of potassium. Potassium again exits on the basolateral side of the tubular cell down a concentration gradient. Potassium reabsorption by intercalated cells in the distal nephron is similar to the process in the early proximal tubule and involves active transport at the luminal cell membrane followed by passive diffusion from the cell at the basolateral membrane.

Tubular secretion of potassium is aldosterone mediated and occurs in the distal nephron (late distal tubule or connecting tubule of the collecting duct system) primarily in the "principal" cells of the collecting tubules. Additional information on mechanisms of collecting duct system reabsorption and secretion is given in Chap. 26 (Fig. 26.2). Principal cells are rich in Na^+,K^+-ATPase and respond to aldosterone by increasing the number and activity of Na^+,K^+-ATPase pumps in the basolateral membrane. The increasing luminal membrane permeability to sodium causes greater lumen negativity relative to the tubular cell interior and increases luminal permeability to potassium. This facilitates potassium secretion into the tubule lumen. Aldosterone-stimulated Na^+,K^+-ATPase actively pumps potassium out of the peritubular fluid through the basolateral tubular cell membrane. Movement of potassium from the tubular cell through the luminal membrane and into the tubule lumen is favored by relative negativity of the lumen compared to the interior of the distal tubule cell (Black 1993).

When plasma potassium concentration is low, secretion of potassium by the principal cells is reduced while hydrogen ion secretion may be increased. Active potassium reabsorption by intercalated cells in the distal nephron is also stimulated by a potassium deficit. An additional factor affecting the movement of potassium across tubular cells is related to tubular flow rate. A rapid flow of filtrate through the tubules maximizes the potassium concentration gradient between the tubular cell interior and the lumen of the tubule and enhances potassium excretion. A reduction of tubular flow slows secretion by allowing a relatively greater concentration of potassium to be maintained in the lumen of the distal tubule (DiBartola and Autran de Morais 1992).

Disorders of Potassium Balance. Disorders of potassium balance have marked effects on excitable membranes. The difference between the resting membrane potential and the membrane potential required for depolarization (threshold potential) determines the excitability of a cell. Hypokalemia makes the resting membrane potential more negative, thereby hyperpolarizing the cell and increasing the difference between resting and threshold potentials. Hyperkalemia causes the resting membrane potential to become more positive, hypopolarizing the cell and causing hyperexcitability. In hyperkalemia, if the resting potential decreases to less than the threshold potential, the cell depolarizes but is incapable of repolarizing, resulting in loss of cell excitability (DiBartola and Autran de Morais 1992). In cardiac muscle this results in diastolic arrest; in vascular smooth muscle hyperkalemia causes vasoconstriction.

Changes in pH affect the distribution of potassium between the ICF and the ECF. When acidosis is present, potassium moves out of cells in exchange for hydrogen, which moves intracellularly. In the distal tubule more hydrogen, and relatively less potassium, may be exchanged for sodium at the luminal membrane, leading to decreased potassium excretion. Based on these general principles, a clinical rule of thumb predicts that each 0.1 unit decrease in pH will be accompanied by a 0.6 mEq/L increase in serum potassium concentration.

Conversely, in alkalosis potassium tends to move into cells in exchange for extracellular movement of hydrogen. Hypokalemia has been thought to promote alkalosis because less potassium is available to be exchanged for sodium in the distal tubule. Instead, sodium exchanges for hydrogen at the luminal membrane, leading ultimately to reclamation of bicarbonate and increased systemic pH. At the same time that systemic pH is increasing, secreted hydrogen ions exchanged for sodium cause the urine pH to decline.

Although the principles outlined above are commonly stated and widely applied clinically, it is not clear that these explanations are adequate. In acidosis, the effect of pH changes on potassium translocation varies with the nature of the acid anion, blood pH and HCO_3^- concentration, osmolality, hormonal activity, and liver and renal function (DiBartola and Autran de Morais 1992). Although changes in serum potassium have been documented during acute mineral acidosis caused by HCl or NH_4Cl (Adrogue and Madias 1981), acute metabolic acidosis caused by organic acids did not increase serum potassium as predicted (Oster et al. 1980; Adrogue and Madias 1981). In certain conditions (e.g., diabetic ketoacidosis), hyperkalemia may be more directly associated with hyperosmolality and insulin deficiency than with the acidosis itself. In lactic acidosis, increased serum potassium concentration may be the result of release of intracellular potassium caused by cell breakdown associated with decreased peripheral perfusion (Black 1993). Metabolic acidosis associated with both mineral and organic acids may directly or indirectly stimulate aldosterone secretion. The effects of aldosterone facilitate excretion of the acid load and, presumably, potassium, although one study failed to show any changes in serum potassium concentration (Perez et al. 1980).

Early studies of the effects of hypokalemia on acid-base balance may have overlooked the key role of chloride depletion in causing metabolic alkalosis (DiBartola and Autran de Morais 1992). When pure potassium depletion is created iatrogenically in rats, metabolic alkalosis results. However, in dogs, potassium deficit with normal chloride levels leads to metabolic acidosis due, presumably, to a distal renal tubular acidification defect (Garella et al. 1979).

HYPERKALEMIA. Total body potassium may be normal, decreased, or increased with hyperkalemia. Clinical signs of hyperkalemia (>7.5 mEq/L) are generally associated with changes in membrane excitability and are more severe if the increase in potassium has been rapid. Muscle weakness, twitching, and irritability may occur. Electrocardiographically determined cardiac effects may include extrasystoles, intraventricular conduction blocks, high-peaked T waves, altered QT interval, widened QRS interval, decreased amplitude or disappearance of P waves, depressed ST segment, ventricular asystole, or fibrillation.

Causes of hyperkalemia are summarized in Table 25.6. The more common causes are related to decreased urinary potassium excretion. Pseudohyperkalemia related to hemolysis can occur in species that have high red cell potassium concentrations similar to humans. Dogs, sheep, and cattle can be divided into two groups based on Na^+,K^+-ATPase activity in red cell membranes. Those animals with high activity and high intracellular potassium concentrations are at risk for hyperkalemia caused by hemolysis. Animals with genetically determined low activity and low intracellular concentrations of potassium are unlikely to suffer from pseudohyperkalemia since the concentration of potassium in red cells resembles the concentration in the ECF (DiBartola and Autran de Morais 1992).

The effects of several different drugs may impact serum potassium concentration. Since potassium uptake by cells is mediated in part by catecholamines at β receptors, β blockers decrease intracellular potassium movement and increase ECF potassium concentrations. Angiotensin-converting enzyme (ACE) inhibitors may cause hyperkalemia by interfering with angiotensin II–mediated aldosterone secretion. Prostaglandin inhibitors, heparin, and selected potassium-sparing diuretics (e.g., spironolactone) increase serum potassium by decreasing the secretion of aldosterone or by blocking its activity. In many cases drugs alone may not have a marked effect on serum potassium concentration but if combined with a potassium load or decreased renal function may cause clinically significant hyperkalemia.

Treatment of hyperkalemia varies with the severity of the condition in terms of magnitude and rapidity of onset. Emergency treatment is indicated if potassium rises quickly and exceeds 6.0–8.0 mEq/L (Phillips and Polzin 1998). Serum potassium concentrations less than these do not typically induce life-threatening cardiotoxicity and can usually be managed with administration of potassium-free fluids. More aggressive treatment is necessary if electrocardiographic signs suggest toxicity. Additional measures that may be taken in treatment of severe hyperkalemia are summarized in Table 25.7. Some are directed toward increasing movement of potassium from the extracellular to the intracellular compartment (i.e., glucose, insulin, and sodium bicarbonate), while others are intended to decrease potassium from the ECF by enhanced renal excretion (e.g., diuretics) or decreased gastrointestinal absorption (i.e., orally administered potassium-binding resins such as sodium polystyrene sulfonate). Therapy with calcium gluconate is included as part of the emergency treatment of hyperkalemia because changes in membrane excitability associated with alterations in potassium may be exacerbated by abnormalities in

TABLE 25.6—Causes of hyperkalemia

Decreased excretion
- Urethral obstruction
- Ruptured bladder
- Anuric or oliguric renal failure
- Hypoadrenocorticism
- Gastrointestinal diseases (e.g., trichuriasis, salmonellosis, perforated duodenal ulcers)
- Chylothorax with repeated drainage of the pleural effusion
- Drugs
  - ACE inhibitors (e.g., captopril, enalapril)
  - Potassium-containing drugs (e.g., potassium chloride)
  - Potassium-sparing diuretics (e.g., spironolactone, amiloride, triamterene)
  - Nonsteroidal anti-inflammatory agents
  - Heparin

Translocation from the ICF to ECF
- Acute mineral acidosis (e.g., HCl or NH_4Cl administration)
- Insulin deficiency (e.g., diabetic ketoacidosis)
- Ischemia reperfusion
- Drugs (e.g., propranolol)
- Acute tumor lysis syndrome
- Hyperkalemic periodic paralysis (rare)

Increased intake (rare)

Pseudohyperkalemia
- Thrombocytosis
- Hemolysis

Source: Adapted from DiBartola and Autran de Morais 1992, 108, Table 4.6.

TABLE 25.7—Therapeutic considerations in the management of severe hyperkalemia

- Establish venous access and administer potassium-deficient fluids
- Discontinue potassium intake, including drugs that may promote hyperkalemia
- Administer the following as needed:
  - $NaHCO_3$ (0.5–1 mEq/kg, slowly IV) if animal is acidotic
  - Calcium gluconate (10% solution; 0.5–1 mL/kg slowly IV up to 10 mL maximum)
  - Glucose (20% solution; 0.5–1.0 g/kg IV)
  - Insulin (0.5 IU/kg) and glucose (20% solution; 1 g/kg; half given IV bolus and the remainder infused over 2 hours)
- Potassium-wasting diuretics (furosemide, chlorothiazide, hydrochlorothiazide)
- Sodium polystyrene (20 g with 100 mL 20% sorbitol) per os or 50 g in 100–200 mL tap water (retention enema)
- Peritoneal dialysis (last resort)

ionized calcium. Ionized calcium affects the threshold potential of a membrane and, when calcium is decreased, brings threshold closer to resting membrane potential, resulting in greater membrane excitability. An increase in ionized calcium has an opposing effect on membrane excitability by increasing the threshold potential and making depolarization more difficult. Hence, hypocalcemia exacerbates hyperkalemia while hypercalcemia counteracts hyperkalemia.

HYPOKALEMIA. Since 97% of total body potassium is intracellular, depletion can occur with no change in plasma potassium concentration or even with an increase if acidosis is present. Clinical signs of hypokalemia (<2.5–3.0 mEq/L) can include weakness of skeletal and respiratory muscles and intestinal smooth muscle loss of tone. As in hyperkalemia, cardiac changes occur as potassium concentration changes. Supraventricular and ventricular arrhythmias are most commonly observed in animals. ECG hallmarks of hypokalemia in humans are flattened or inverted T waves, depressed S-T segment, and the appearance of U waves. Prolongation of the QT interval and U waves have been reported in dogs but are not as consistently seen as they are in humans. Hypokalemia is increasingly recognized as an important clinical problem in cats, especially in association with chronic renal failure and geriatric animals (Phillips and Polzin 1998). Feline hypokalemic polymyopathy syndrome, characterized by generalized muscle weakness associated with hypokalemia, is often manifest in cats as ventroflexion of the head and a stiff, stilted gait.

Increased loss associated with the gastrointestinal or the urinary system is a common cause of hypokalemia, as indicated in Table 25.8. Differentiating gastrointestinal from urinary causes of hypokalemia is largely accomplished by clinical signs and physical exam, but fractional potassium excretion rates (FE_K) may also be useful. Fractional potassium excretion can be calculated using the following formula:

$$FE_K = (U_K/S_K)/(U_{CR}/S_{CR}) \times 100$$

where U indicates the urine concentration of potassium (K^+) or creatinine (CR), and S indicates the serum concentration.

Treatment of hypokalemia is indicated if significant potassium loss is expected based on history and clinical signs (e.g., vomiting, diarrhea, overzealous use of diuretics) or if clinical signs of hypokalemia are present. Appropriate potassium administration is often required with prolonged fluid therapy. If feasible, oral potassium supplementation is most desirable since this is the safest route of administration. If intravenous potassium supplementation is warranted, the amount administered should be based on clinical status of the animal and measured serum potassium values. Oral and parenteral products for potassium supplementation are discussed later in this chapter. Table 25.9 provides approximate potassium dosages for treatment of hypokalemia in small animals. Alternatively, a rule of thumb may be applied in which 20 mEq/L of potassium is supplemented with careful monitoring of changes in serum potassium. An important admonition in the administration of intravenous potassium is not to exceed a rate of 0.5 mEq/kg/hr. Parenteral potassium administration should always be monitored to ensure that rate of potassium addition does not exceed rate of potassium movement into cells.

TABLE 25.8—Causes of hypokalemia

Increased loss
- Gastrointestinal (FE_K < 4–6%)
  - Persistent vomiting of stomach contents
  - Diarrhea
- Urinary (FE_K > 4–6%)
  - Chronic renal failure in cats
  - Diet-induced hypokalemic nephropathy in cats
  - Renal tubular acidosis
  - Postobstructive diuresis
- Excess circulating mineralocorticoid
  - Hyperadrenocorticism
  - Primary hyperaldosteronism (hyperplastic or neoplastic)
- Iatrogenic (drug induced)
  - Diuretics (loop acting, thiazides and osmotic)
  - Antibiotics (penicillins, amphotericin B, aminoglycosides)

Translocation from ECF to ICF
- Alkalemia
- Overadministration of insulin and glucose-containing fluids
- Hyperthyroidism
- Hypokalemic periodic paralysis
- Possible complication of hypothermia

Decreased intake
- Unlikely as sole cause

Source: Adapted from DiBartola and Autran de Morais 1992, 99, Table 4.3.

TABLE 25.9—Potassium supplementation in treatment of hypokalemia

Serum potassium concentration (mEq/L)	Supplement fluids (mEq/L)*
3.5 to 4.5	20
3.0 to 3.5	30
2.5 to 3.0	40
2.0 to 2.5	60
<2.0	80

*Quantity of potassium to add per liter of fluid. Do not exceed administration rate of 0.5 mEq K^+/kg/hr.

PRINCIPLES OF ACID-BASE METABOLISM

Homeostasis. Blood pH is highly regulated and is normally maintained between 7.38 and 7.42. Pulmonary and renal functions are necessary for precise regulation of pH of all body fluids, blood, and extravascular tissues. An acid is defined by Bronsted and Lowry as a substance that can supply H^+ (protons), and a base is defined as a substance that can accept H^+. In aqueous solutions, H^+ are hydrated; therefore, H_3O^+ is considered an acid and is implied by the symbol H^+. Blood pH is the negative logarithm of the hydrogen ion concentration. Although hydrogen ion concentration cannot be measured directly, hydrogen ion activity is measured chemically using a pH electrode. In body fluids, the difference between activity of hydrogen ions and concentration of hydrogen ions is negligible; hence hydrogen ion concentration and pH are commonly referred to in acid-base discussions. The hydrogen ion concentration of blood at pH 7.4 is 40 nmol/L (nanoequivalents per L) and is therefore approximately a million-fold lower than the blood concentration of electrolytes such as sodium and potassium. Appropriate hydrogen ion concentration is critical in order to maintain body proteins in configurations required for enzymatic and structural function. An increase in hydrogen ion concentration with a decrease in blood pH is termed acidemia and can be caused by pathophysiologic processes that cause accumulation of acids in the body. As the concentration of hydrogen ions decreases, and blood pH increases, alkalemia occurs and can be associated with pathophysiologic processes that cause accumulation of alkali in the body. The disordered processes leading to acidemia and alkalemia are termed acidosis and alkalosis, respectively.

On a daily basis, an excess of acid (70–100 mEq) is generated in the body as a result of dietary intake and intermediary metabolism. Catabolism of carbohydrate, fat, and protein account for most of this as a result of oxidation of sulfur-containing amino acids to sulfuric acid; oxidation of phosphoproteins to phosphoric acid; incomplete oxidation of fats and carbohydrates to organic acid; production of lactate/lactic acid during anaerobic glycolysis; and conversion of carbon dioxide and water produced in the tricarboxylic acid cycle to carbonic acid. Buffers throughout the body minimize changes in blood pH associated with alterations of acid-base balance. The most effective physiological buffers have pK_a values between 6.1 and 8.4, with buffering capacity being maximal within one pH unit of the pK_a. Important extracellular buffers include bicarbonate, inorganic phosphates, and plasma proteins.

Most extracellular buffering occurs as a result of the bicarbonate-carbonic acid buffer pair ($pK_a = 6.1$). Equilibrium of this buffer pair is indicated below:

$$CO_2 + H_2O \leftrightarrow H_2CO_3 \leftrightarrow H^+ + HCO_3^-$$

The hydration of CO_2 is a rapid reaction in the presence of the enzyme carbonic anhydrase (CA), which is found primarily in red blood cells and renal tubular cells. The dissociation of any acid, in this case carbonic acid, can be described utilizing the concept that the velocity of a reaction is proportional to the product of the concentration of the reactants. In the case of the bicarbonate buffer system, the carbonic anhydrase–catalyzed hydration of CO_2 to form H_2CO_3 reaches equilibrium almost instantaneously, with the number of dissolved CO_2 molecules far exceeding the number of carbonic acid molecules. By defining dissociation constants and rearranging, the useful Henderson-Hasselbalch form of the dissociation equilibrium equation can be derived:

$$pH = pK_a + \log [HCO_3^-]/[H_2CO_3]$$

Gaseous CO_2 produced in the tissues, primarily via the tricarboxylic acid cycle, is soluble in water; the concentration of dissolved CO_2 in body fluids can be related to the partial pressure of CO_2 in the gas phase, PCO_2, by the following expression:

$$[\text{dissolved } CO_2] = 0.03 \times PCO_2$$

Hence the clinically useful form of this equation for the bicarbonate–carbonic acid buffer system becomes

$$pH = 6.1 + \log [HCO_3^-]/(0.03 \times PCO_2)$$

The bicarbonate–carbonic acid system is the most physiologically important extracellular buffer system because it is present in relatively high concentrations in the blood and because it can effectively buffer by rapid regulation of PCO_2 through alveolar ventilation. As carbonic acid is formed from the buffering of excess H^+ by HCO_3^-, this drives the dissociation equation of carbonic acid to the left, causing an increase in PCO_2. An increase in ventilation enhances CO_2 excretion and lowers the PCO_2.

Intracellular buffers also contribute to maintenance of body pH. The primary intracellular buffers are proteins, organic and inorganic phosphates, and, in the red cell, hemoglobin. Hemoglobin is an especially important buffer for carbonic acid since the primary extracellular buffer, the bicarbonate system, cannot buffer this acid. Bone also acts as a tissue-based buffer by exchanging surface Na^+ and K^+ for H^+ under conditions of acid load. Additionally, dissolution of bone mineral results in release of buffer compounds into the ECF.

Regulation of Hydrogen Ion, Carbon Dioxide, and Bicarbonate. Pulmonary and renal control of dissolved CO_2 and bicarbonate concentrations, respectively, is responsible for maintenance of body pH. The "tail" of the Henderson-Hasselbalch equation for the bicarbonate system (i.e., HCO_3^-/dissolved CO_2) provides a simplistic but useful means to consider pulmonary and renal adjustments during simple acid-base disturbances. Under normal physiological conditions, the ratio of HCO_3^- to dissolved CO_2 is 20:1. This ratio can be disturbed by addition or loss of CO_2 or bicarbonate to the system. Table 25.10 depicts changes in the tail of the bicarbonate–carbonic acid dissociation equation that might occur during simple acid-base disturbances. The respiratory component of acid-base regulation (the denominator of the tail, or dissolved CO_2) involves changes in respiratory rate and volume prompted by changes in PCO_2. Initiation of these processes requires only minutes.

The renal component of acid-base regulation (the numerator of the tail, or HCO_3^-) involves selective absorption of bicarbonate and secretion of H^+. During periods of acidosis, relatively more H^+ are secreted, while relatively more K^+, Na^+, and HCO_3^- are retained.

TABLE 25.10—Examples of changes in the "tail" of the Henderson-Hasselbalch equation occurring during simple acid-base disturbances

Respiratory acidosis (↓ CO_2 elimination) associated with inadequate ventilation:										
$\frac{20\ HCO_3^-}{1\ CO_2}$	+	$2\ CO_2$	→	$\frac{20\ HCO_3^-}{3\ CO_2}$	+	$40\ HCO_3^-$	→	$\frac{60\ HCO_3^-}{3\ CO_2}$	=	$\frac{20}{1}$
(Normal)		(↓ Ventilation)		(Uncompensated)		(Renal production)		(Compensated)		
Respiratory alkalosis (↑ CO_2 elimination) associated with hyperventilation:										
$\frac{20\ HCO_3^-}{1\ CO_2}$	-	$0.5\ CO_2$	→	$\frac{20\ HCO_3^-}{0.5\ CO_2}$	-	$10\ HCO_3^-$	→	$\frac{10\ HCO_3^-}{0.5\ CO_2}$	=	$\frac{20}{1}$
(Normal)		(↑ Ventilation)		(Uncompensated)		(Renal excretion)		(Compensated)		
Metabolic acidosis (bicarbonate deficit) associated with diarrhea:										
$\frac{20\ HCO_3^-}{1\ CO_2}$	-	$10\ HCO_3^-$	→	$\frac{10\ HCO_3^-}{1\ CO_2}$	-	$0.5\ CO_2$	→	$\frac{10\ HCO_3^-}{0.5\ CO_2}$	=	$\frac{20}{1}$
(Normal)		(Loss in feces)		(Uncompensated)		(Eliminated by ↑ ventilation)		(Compensated)		
Metabolic alkalosis (bicarbonate excess) associated with administration of alkali:										
$\frac{20\ HCO_3^-}{1\ CO_2}$	+	$20\ HCO_3^-$	→	$\frac{40\ HCO_3^-}{1\ CO_2}$	+	$1\ CO_2$	→	$\frac{40\ HCO_3^-}{2\ CO_2}$	=	$\frac{20}{1}$
(Normal)		(Alkali) administration)		(Uncompensated)		(Eliminated by ↓ ventilation)		(Compensated)		

During alkalosis, K^+ is secreted, while relatively more H^+ and less Na^+ and HCO_3^- are retained. This process requires hours to days to produce an effect. The kidney regulates acid-base balance by maintaining the appropriate HCO_3^- in the plasma. The kidney accomplishes this by reclaiming virtually all filtered HCO_3^- and excreting an amount of acid that equals the amount of ingested or endogenously generated nonvolatile acid. In the proximal tubule of the kidney, cytoplasmic carbonic anhydrase catalyzes the formation of H^+ and bicarbonate from cellular carbon dioxide and water, controlling the rate of hydrogen secretion and bicarbonate reabsorption. In the luminal membrane, carbonic anhydrase converts carbonic acid to carbon dioxide and water, increasing net bicarbonate reabsorption (Fig. 25.5, panel A). In the distal nephron, intercalated cells specialized for hydrogen secretion contain large quantities of carbonic anhydrase, again yielding hydrogen and bicarbonate. In this case, secreted H^+ serves to titrate buffers in the urine (phosphate buffering is shown in Fig. 25.5, panel B) and lower urinary pH. As titratable acidity of the urine reaches a maximum, another adaptation, increased ammonia (NH_3) production by tubular cells, contributes to excretion of acid loads. Fig. 25.5, panel C, shows production of freely diffusable NH_3 from glutamine moving into the tubular lumen, where it combines with H^+ to form ammonium (NH_4^+). Ammonium, in turn, combines with chloride for excretion as ammonium chloride. While this is an oversimplification of the physiological events, it is acceptable to consider ammonium chloride as a flexible mechanism for H^+ secretion based on the ability of the kidney to generate ammonia.

Assessment of Acid-Base Disturbances. Disorders of acid-base equilibrium can result from a primary disturbance in pulmonary regulation of the concentration of H_2CO_3 in body fluids via changes in alveolar ventilation and PCO_2 levels, from metabolic changes in concentration of bicarbonate, or from a combination of these mechanisms.

The partial pressure of CO_2 (PCO_2) is generally accepted as the best measure of respiratory disturbances. Assessment of PCO_2 depends upon availability of a blood gas analyzer and proper arterial sample collection. A blood gas analysis provides three measured parameters (pH, PCO_2, PO_2) and typically two calculated values (actual bicarbonate and base excess). Acidemia and alkalemia (using pH), eucapnia, hypercapnia or hypocapnia (using PCO_2), and hypoxemia (using PO_2 if the sample is arterial) may be directly assessed. In-house blood gas and electrolyte analyzers have become much more common in practice, making assessment of these parameters practical and economical. Results obtained with one hand-held analyzer appropriate for in-house testing were similar to those obtained from a standard chemistry analyzer with the exception of sodium concentration in canine samples and hematocrit in equine samples (Looney et al. 1998).

Actual bicarbonate values are useful in assessment of nonrespiratory disorders, but these values will vary with compensatory changes in alveolar ventilation and PCO_2. Bicarbonate values are derived using the Henderson-Hasselbalch equation and measured values for pH and PCO_2. Plasma bicarbonate values may also be estimated by measurement of total CO_2. Total CO_2 combines measurement of both the numerator and the

A

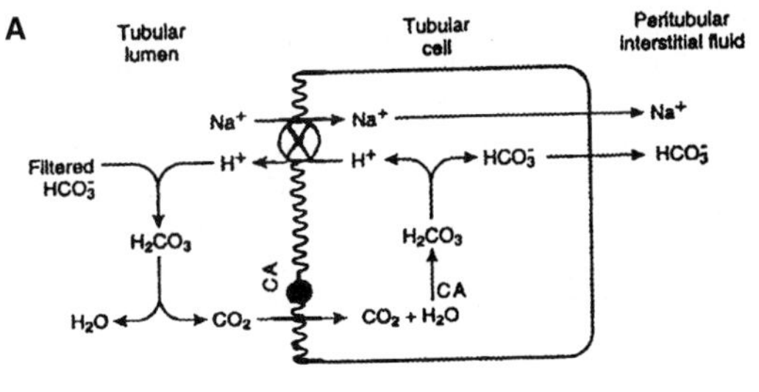

B

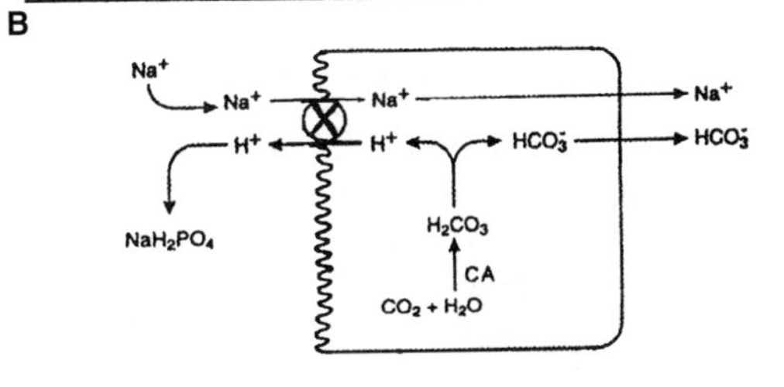

C

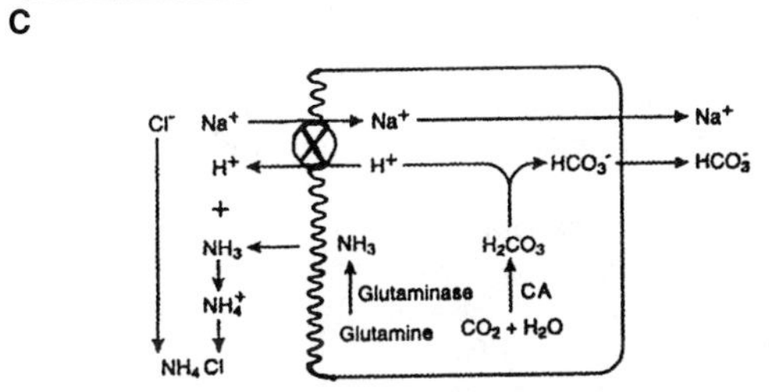

FIG. 25.5—Renal mechanisms for H^+ excretion. See text for explanation of each panel.

denominator of the tail of the Henderson-Hasselbalch equation ($[HCO_3^-]/[H_2CO_3]$) by converting both to measurable CO_2. Total CO_2 and plasma bicarbonate are used interchangeably in reporting plasma bicarbonate concentrations even though total CO_2 is actually plasma bicarbonate plus 1.1–1.3 mEq of H_2CO_3. As compared to actual plasma bicarbonate, standard bicarbonate is defined as the concentration of bicarbonate after fully oxygenated whole blood has been equilibrated with CO_2 at a PCO_2 of 40 mm Hg at 38° C; this measurement eliminates the influence of respiration on plasma HCO_3^-.

Standard base excess (BE) is the concentration of titratable base of ECF; this value may be calculated using a Siggaard-Anderson alignment nomogram that interrelates BE and total CO_2 and HCO_3^- when pH and PCO_2 are measured. Because this calculation is based on a constant oxygen saturation, error may be introduced by inclusion of air bubbles in a poorly handled blood sample. In veterinary medicine, error may also be inherent because the nomogram is based on human blood and excludes the effects of plasma protein and electrolytes on acid-base equilibrium. BE is useful because it accounts for the effects of CO_2 on carbonic acid equilibrium and identifies nonrespiratory causes of acid-base derangement. Base deficit is defined as the negative of base excess (Bailey and Pablo 1998).

Anion Gap. Further analysis, beyond pH, PCO_2, HCO_3^-, and BE, may be useful in assessment of complex acid-base disturbances. The anion gap (AG) is defined as the difference between the quantity of unmeasured cations (UCs) and unmeasured anions (UAs) in the blood. Major UAs include phosphates, sulfates, and organic acids (e.g., lactate, citrate, ketones), with chloride and bicarbonate being the measured anions. Major UCs include calcium and magnesium, with sodium and potassium being the measured cations. Calculation of the AG according to the following equations reflects the law of electroneutrality, according to which total cations must equal total anions (DiBartola 1992d).

$$[Na^+] + [K^+] + [UC] = [Cl^-] + [HCO_3^-] + [UA]$$

$$\text{Anion gap} = UC - UA = ([Na^+] + [K^+]) - ([Cl^-] + [HCO_3^-])$$

The normal AG varies with the species but is approximately 13–25 mEq/L in dogs and cats. AG is most often used to identify causes of metabolic acidosis. In organic acidoses, HCO_3^- buffers hydrogen ions that are generated from dissociation of organic acid (e.g., lactic acid). In theory, the measured $[HCO_3^-]$ should decrease as the concentration of the UA (the organic acid) increases. As long as $[Cl^-]$ remains unchanged (normochloremic metabolic acidosis), the gap will increase proportionately with the increase in acid. Several factors that may confound this simple relationship include the following: (1) other buffers besides HCO_3^- also respond to the influx of organic acid; (2) the volume of distribution of HCO_3^- may be different from that of the acid; and (3) the patient's AG baseline (prior to the presenting illness) is often not known. Hence the AG is useful but not fully predictable.

Increased AG often occurs in lactic acidosis, diabetic ketoacidosis, azotemic renal failure (due to increased phosphates and sulfates), and poisoning (ethylene glycol, salicylate). A recent study (Constable and Morin 1997) demonstrated a useful correlation between AG and serum creatinine concentration in calves with experimentally induced diarrhea and adult cattle with abomasal volvulus. Although the AG was not a useful predictor of all anion-associated changes (e.g., no correlation was found between AG and blood lactate levels), the AG could alert clinicians to the potential presence of uremic acidosis.

A normal AG usually occurs in metabolic acidosis related to diarrhea, renal tubular acidosis, excessive use of carbonic anhydrase inhibitors, or ammonium chloride administration and in iatrogenic expansion acidosis caused by excessive normal saline administration. The two most common causes of a decreased AG are hypoalbuminemia or dilution of plasma proteins caused by infusion of crystalloid solutions. In both cases the gap decreases as a result of a decreased concentration of net negative charges associated with plasma proteins. Each 1.0 g/dL decrease in albumin is associated with an approximately 2.4 mEq/L decrease in the AG (Gabow 1985).

Nontraditional (Stewart's) Acid-Base Analysis. An understanding of the traditional interrelationships between H^+, CO_2, and HCO_3^- is adequate to explain the behavior of aqueous solutions; however, it does not account for the effects of plasma proteins and electrolytes, particularly sodium and chloride, on acid-base status in biological systems. Stewart described a new approach to understanding acid-base physiology based on three fundamental concepts of electrolyte chemistry (Stewart 1978, 1983). First, electroneutrality must always be maintained. Hence, as with the concept of the AG, the sum of all positive charges must equal the sum of all negative charges. Second, mass must be conserved even though it may change in form within a solution. Finally, the dissociation or ionization of a substance in water is determined by its dissociation constant. Weak electrolytes relevant to acid-base physiology include proteins, water, and CO_2. In contrast, sodium and chloride are considered strong electrolytes because they are fully dissociated in water. Evaluation of acid-base status using the Stewart approach requires assessment of independent, or primary, variables; dependent, or unknown, variables; and dissociation constants of all variables. Values of independent variables are controlled externally and cannot be changed by processes occurring within the solution. Independent variables dictate the acid-base status of a solution.

The independent variables controlling acid-base status in biological solutions are strong ion difference (SID), PCO_2, and total weak acid concentration (A_{TOT}). The first variable, SID, is the sum of the strong cation concentrations minus the sum of the strong anion concentrations:

$$SID = ([Na^+] + [K^+]) - ([Cl^-] + [lactate^-] + [ketoacid])$$

Unless lactic acidosis or ketoacidosis is suspected in a given case, these terms may be eliminated from the equation since their values would be quite small. Likewise, $[K^+]$ is often dropped from the equation since it contributes a relatively small number to the total cation population. If PCO_2 and A_{TOT} remain constant, increases in SID suggest nonrespiratory alkalosis and decreases suggest nonrespiratory acidosis. Mean normal SID values are derived by each laboratory based on their reference population, and these values vary across species. The second independent variable, PCO_2, is an indication of the amount of CO_2 dissolved in plasma. As in traditional acid-base theory, an increase in PCO_2 shifts the dissociation equation for carbonic acid to the right, increasing the $[H^+]$ and making the solution more acidic. The final independent variable, $[A_{TOT}]$, is accounted for by plasma proteins (95%), primarily albumin, and inorganic phosphates (5%). A_{TOT} has been calculated for horses (Constable 1997) using the formula

$$[A_{TOT}]\ (mEq/L) = 2.25\ [albumin]\ (g/dL) + 1.4\ [globulin]\ (g/dL) + 0.59\ [phosphate]\ (mg/dL)$$

These three independent variables influence several dependent, or unknown, variables. Dependent variables are affected by processes occurring within the solution and do not change unless independent variables change. Values for dependent variables are thus the result, not the cause, of events in solution. Dependent variables include $[H^+]$, $[HCO_3^-]$, carbonate ion concentration ($[CO_3^{2-}]$), $[OH^-]$, concentration of dissociated weak acids ($[A^-]$), and concentration of nondissociated weak acids ([AH]). Values of dependent variables are not affected by the values of other dependent variables. Because the values for $[CO_3^{2-}]$ and $[OH^-]$ are so small, they are not measured or evaluated in a clinical setting. The variables for dissociated and nondissociated weak acids reflect the dynamic relationship between acid-base balance and protein ionization. The ability of proteins to function as enzymes, cell membrane pumps, ion channels, receptors, etc., depends upon their state of ionization, and this is directly affected by changes in independent variables (PCO_2, SID, and A_{TOT}). Likewise, the ratio of ionized to unionized calcium depends upon protein binding, which changes with alterations of A_{TOT} and pH.

Independent variables are controlled via respiration (PCO_2) and renal function (SID). As in traditional acid-base theory, rate and depth of respiration control retention or elimination of CO_2, which may lead to respiratory acidosis or alkalosis, respectively. Control of SID is primarily accomplished by the kidney with a smaller contribution from the gastrointestinal tract. Changes in SID via the kidneys are achieved much more slowly than respiratory changes and are on the order of hours to days. The kidney regulates SID by differential reabsorption of Na^+ and Cl^-. Since Na^+ reabsorption is strongly related to renal regulation of ECF volume, net Cl^- excretion relative to net Na^+ excretion is the primary mechanism for renal regulation of acid-base balance. Control of PCO_2 and SID is the primary determinant of acid-base balance because there is no evidence that the body alters the third independent variable, protein concentration $[A_{TOT}]$, in order to regulate acid-base balance.

In summary, the most important premise of Stewart's approach is that concentrations of HCO_3^- and H^+ are dependent on concentrations of primary, or independent, variables, notably CO_2, Na^+, and Cl^-. The complex equations derived by Stewart address the changes induced by independent variables and quantitate each potential influence by solving for the dependent variables. Much simplified versions of Stewart's formula have been adopted on a limited basis by clinicians who value Stewart's theories and believe that they provide a more complete picture of acid-base derangements. Table 25.11 summarizes the equations being applied for nontraditional analysis of nonrespiratory acid-base status (Russell et al. 1996). In brief, increases in SID suggest nonrespiratory alkalosis, whereas decreases

TABLE 25.11—Formulas for quantitative analysis of nonrespiratory acid-base status

I. Estimation of [SID]. (All values expressed as mEq/L.)

$[\text{SID approx.}] = [Na^+_{\text{mean normal}}] - [Cl^-_{\text{corrected}}]$

$[Cl^-_{\text{corrected}}] = [Cl^-_{\text{patient}}] \times ([Na^+_{\text{mean normal}}] / [Na^+_{\text{patient}}])$

II. Alterations in acid-base balance

A. Changes in acid-base balance due to weak acids

Δ albumin (mEq/L) = $3.7 \times ([alb_{\text{mean normal}}]\ (\text{mg/dL}) - [alb_{\text{patient}}]\ (\text{mg/dL}))$

Δ phosphorus:

$[phos_{\text{adjusted}}]\ (\text{mg/dL}) = [phos_{\text{mean normal}}]\ (\text{mg/dL}) - [phos_{\text{patient}}]\ (\text{mg/dL})$

$phos_{adj}\ (\text{mg/dL}) \times 0.3229 = phos\ (\text{mmol/L})$

effective phos (mEq/L) = $1.8 \times$ phos (mmol/L)

B. Changes in acid-base balance due to alterations in [SID]. (All values expressed in mEq/L.)

Δ free water = $z([Na^+_{\text{patient}}] - [Na^+_{\text{mean normal}}])$

where $z = [\text{SID}] / [Na^+_{\text{mean normal}}]$

Δ chloride = $[Cl^-_{\text{mean normal}}] - [Cl^-_{\text{corrected}}]$

Δ unmeasured anions (UA) = BE – (Δ free water + Δ Cl^- + Δ phos + Δ albumin)

TABLE 25.12—Characteristics of primary acid-base disturbances

Disorder	pH	$[H^+]$	Primary disturbance	Compensatory response
Metabolic acidosis	↓	↑	↓ $[HCO_3^-]$, ↓ [SID]	↓ PCO_2
Metabolic alkalosis	↑	↓	↑ $[HCO_3^-]$, ↑ [SID]	↑ PCO_2
Respiratory acidosis	↓	↑	↑ PCO_2	↑ $[HCO_3^-]$, ↑ [SID]
Respiratory alkalosis	↑	↓	↓ PCO_2	↓ $[HCO_3^-]$, ↓ [SID]

Source: Adapted from Rose 1994, 506.

suggest nonrespiratory acidosis. Negative values for Δ albumin suggest hyperproteinemic acidosis, whereas positive values reflect hypoproteinemic alkalosis. Negative values for Δ phosphorus suggest hyperphosphatemic acidosis. Negative changes in free water point to dilutional acidosis, and positive values suggest concentration alkalosis. Positive values for Δ chloride suggest hypochloremic alkalosis, and negative values suggest hyperchloremic acidosis.

While most clinicians still favor the traditional approach to evaluation of acid-base balance, modified applications of Stewart's theories broaden this scope and lend useful quantitative insights into the complexities of acid-base disturbances (Constable 1999).

DISORDERS OF ACID-BASE METABOLISM. Disorders of acid-base equilibrium can result from a primary disturbance in pulmonary regulation of the concentration of CO_2, from metabolic changes in strong ions and, dependently, bicarbonate, or from a combination of these mechanisms. An acid-base disturbance is considered simple if it is limited to a primary disturbance and an appropriate secondary or compensatory response. Primary disturbances and expected compensatory responses are modeled using the tail of the Henderson-Hasselbalch equation in Table 25.10 and summarized in Table 25.12. Mixed acid-base disturbances are suspected when the compensatory response to a primary disorder is not as expected or when the pH is changing in a direction opposite that predicted by the primary disorder. Mixed acid-base disturbances are characterized by two or more primary disturbances in the same patient.

Metabolic (Nonrespiratory) Acidosis. Metabolic acidosis may be characterized by a decrease in plasma HCO_3^- concentration, decreased pH, increased concentration of strong anions (such as chloride, lactic acid, or ketoacids), and decreased plasma sodium concentration associated with renal disease or diarrhea. The clinical signs most commonly associated with metabolic acidosis are hyperpnea and CNS depression. Laboratory analysis of blood and urine reveals a lowered urine and blood pH, decreased serum HCO_3^- (<20 mEq/L), decreased [SID], and a variable serum PCO_2 depending upon the degree of respiratory compensation. Fig. 25.6 summarizes causes of metabolic acidosis and provides general principles of treatment. Metabolic acidosis is the most common acid-base disorder in dogs, cats, and

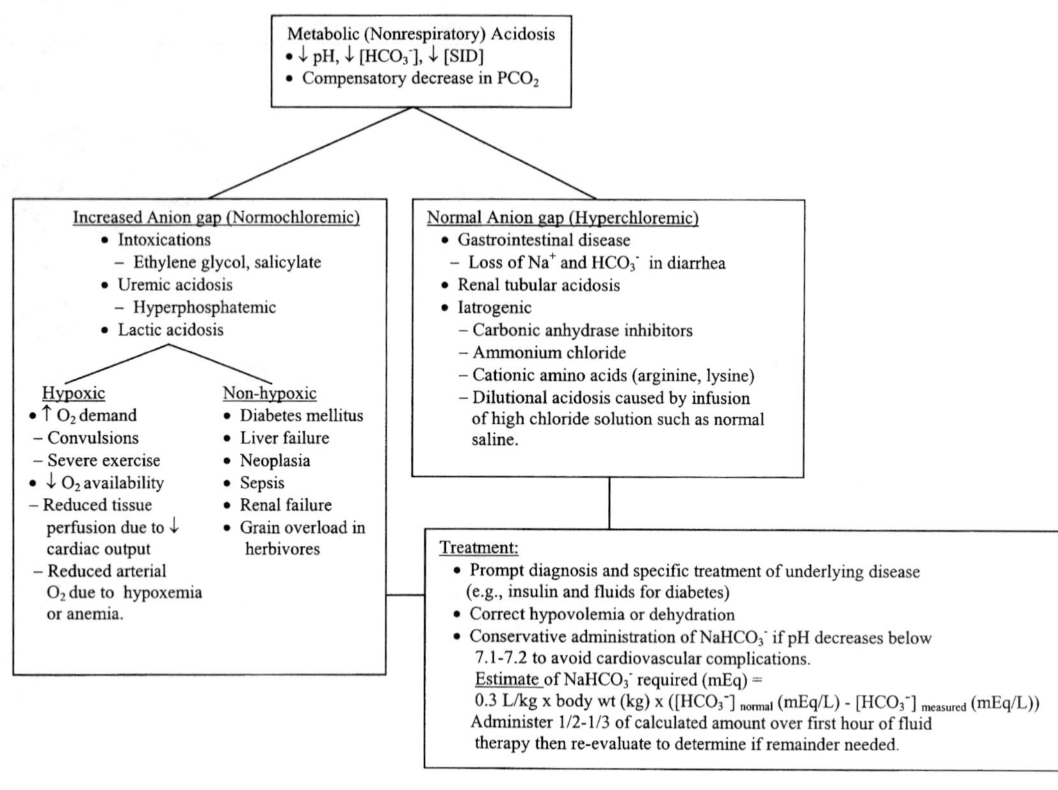

FIG 25.6—Causes of metabolic acidosis and general treatment principles.

horses, and causes may be usefully subdivided into those conditions that increase the AG and those that do not.

Loss of Na^+ and HCO_3^- associated with diarrhea is the most common cause of normal AG (hyperchloremic) metabolic acidosis. Intestinal secretions replete in Na^+ and HCO_3^- may also be sequestered in lower obstructive bowel disease and paralytic ileus. Hypoadrenocorticism may also present with a non-gap metabolic acidosis, but these patients usually have hypochloremia as a result of impaired water excretion, lack of aldosterone, and poor renal function.

LACTIC ACIDOSIS. Production of lactic acid and accumulation of lactate, an unmeasured anion, decrease the [SID], resulting in a high AG metabolic acidosis. Lactic acid is the final product of anaerobic glycolysis in eukaryotic cells and is formed by the action of lactate dehydrogenase (LDH) on pyruvic acid with NADH as a cofactor.

$$CH_3COO^- + NADH + H^+ \leftrightarrow CH_3CHOHCOO^- + NAD^+$$

(pyruvate) LDH (lactate)

The direction of the LDH reaction depends upon the relative intracellular concentrations of pyruvate and lactate and on the ratio of reduced (NADH) to oxidized (NAD^+) nicotinamide adenine dinucleotide cofactor. Newly produced lactic acid is partially buffered by HCO_3^-, resulting in rapid generation of sodium lactate, which dissociates to lactate and sodium ions. Under aerobic conditions in the liver and the kidney, lactate is converted back to pyruvate, and pyruvate is metabolized through the tricarboxylic acid (TCA) cycle to yield HCO_3^-, CO_2, and H_2O. Alternatively, hepatic uptake of lactate and conversion to pyruvate can feed gluconeogenesis, a process that also regenerates HCO_3^-. In either case, the net result of aerobic lactate metabolism is production of alkalinizing equivalents in the form of HCO_3^-:

Conversion via the TCA cycle:

$$lactate^- + 3O_2 \rightarrow HCO_3^- + 2CO_2 + 2H_2O$$

Conversion via gluconeogenesis:

$$2\ lactate^- + 2H_2O + 2CO_2 \rightarrow 2HCO_3^- + glucose$$

If the ratio of $NADH/NAD^+$ in the cell shifts toward accumulation of NADH (e.g., in exercising muscle or poorly oxygenated tissues), more lactic acid accumulates, decreasing cellular pH. In the case of poorly oxygenated tissues, inability to oxidize NADH via the respiratory chain blocks oxidative phosphorylation and production of ATP. ATP depletion in lactic acidosis causes leaky ATP-dependent K^+ channels, leading to hyperpolarized membranes and decreased Ca^{++} influx via voltage-dependent Ca^{++} channels. Decreased intracellular Ca^{++} produces smooth muscle relaxation, vasodilation, and a potential decline in systemic blood pressure (Landry and Oliver 1992).

Causes of the two types of lactic acidosis, hypoxic (type A) and nonhypoxic (type B), are listed in Fig. 25.6. (Only L-lactate is metabolized by animals; hence the discussion that follows refers only to L-lactic acidosis and not D-lactic acidosis, a condition described in humans and associated with small bowel resection or short bowel syndrome.) Reduced tissue perfusion and hypoxia caused by cardiac arrest/cardiopulmonary resuscitation, shock, hypovolemia, left ventricular failure, low cardiac output, and acute pulmonary edema limit oxygen availability and force cells into anaerobic glycolysis. As NADH accumulates, the LDH reaction is pushed to the right, resulting in lactic acid accumulation. Successful management of most of these conditions involves returning tissue perfusion and oxygenation to normal, often with the aid of parenteral fluid administration. Reversal of circulatory failure decreases further lactate accumulation and, if the liver is well perfused, will result in conversion of accumulated lactate to HCO_3^-.

Administration of $NaHCO_3^-$ to animals suffering from lactic acidosis is controversial. Benefits could include improved tissue perfusion related to reversal of acidemia-induced vasodilation and an increase in [SID] (associated with Na^+ administration). Potential risks include overshoot metabolic alkalosis caused by the cumulative effect of $NaHCO_3^-$ administration and metabolism of the accumulated lactate into HCO_3^-. A recent study in rats (Halperin et al. 1996) concluded that $NaHCO_3^-$ therapy extended the period of survival during acute, hypoxic L-lactic acidosis. Hypoxia was induced in anesthetized, paralyzed rats ventilated with a lowered (5.5%) oxygen concentration, which was sufficient to cause a severe degree of L-lactic acidosis. Survival in rats receiving $NaHCO_3^-$ was close to twofold longer than in rats receiving no sodium bicarbonate or NaCl only. The rate of $NaHCO_3^-$ infusion was titrated to equal the rate of L-lactic acid appearance in the ECF of control hypoxic rats. Part of the benefit of alkali treatment was hypothesized to be increased anaerobic glycolysis, causing enhanced ATP and L-lactic acid production and a decreased oxygen consumption. Despite continued accumulation of L-lactic acid and a decrease in cardiac output that was greater than in control rats, availability of ATP for vital organs was considered critical to prolonged survival in alkali-treated animals. While results using this controlled model are not directly clinically applicable, they suggest that continued consideration of the advantages and disadvantages of alkali supplementation in L-lactic acidosis may be merited. Many clinicians favor a conservative therapeutic approach in which small amounts of $NaHCO_3^-$ are administered to keep the arterial pH above 7.1–7.2 and to avoid progressive decline in cardiovascular function (Rose 1994). In the absence of severely elevated concentrations of lactate, and in the presence of a well-perfused liver, the use of lactate-containing alkalinizing solutions is effective for volume restoration. Alternatives to lactate-containing solutions include $NaHCO_3^-$, sodium gluconate, sodium acetate, and an equimolar mixture of sodium carbonate and sodium bicarbonate. The latter product, referred to as "Carbicarb" (Cohen 1995), has been promoted as a method of preventing the increased CO_2 production and paradoxical intracellular acidosis that has been reported as a complication of $NaHCO_3$ treatment. It has been found, using a canine model of severe hemorrhagic shock, that Carbicarb, $NaHCO_3$, and hypertonic saline all possess similar abilities to improve hemodynamics, despite the buffering properties of $NaHCO_3$ and Carbicarb. However, correction of arterial pH did not appear to improve the responses to blood retransfusion in this model (Benjamin et al. 1994).

KETOACIDOSIS AND OTHER CAUSES. Metabolic acidosis associated with ketonemia and ketonuria occurs when the rate of formation of ketone bodies is greater than the rate of their use. This occurs most often in two conditions, diabetes mellitus and starvation. Excess acetyl coenzyme A (CoA) derived from fatty acid or pyruvate oxidation is diverted, primarily in the liver, to production of ketone bodies (acetoacetate, beta-hydroxybutyrate, acetone). Ketones can be transported in the blood and utilized as an energy source by peripheral tissues. In diabetes the lack of insulin increases lipolysis, and an excess of glucagon indirectly increases fatty acyl CoA entry into hepatic mitochondria for conversion to ketones. An elevation of ketones in the blood results in acidemia because the carboxyl group of the ketone body has a pK_a of about 4. At physiological pH the ketoacid is fully dissociated, losing a proton (H^+), which lowers blood pH. Addition of a UA, the ketoacid, decreases the [SID] driving an acidosis. Ketoacidosis is often complicated by dehydration associated with osmotic (glucose-driven) diuresis. The use of alkali to treat diabetic ketoacidosis is controversial and not generally recommended. Rehydration (usually with normal saline) and administration of insulin is the treatment of choice since circulating ketoacids will subsequently be metabolized to HCO_3^- and move plasma pH toward normal.

Renal failure typically produces a normochloremic, high-AG metabolic acidosis due to accumulation of phosphates, sulfates, and other organic anions, altered handling of chloride, and an inability to excrete the daily dietary acid load. Enhanced generation of ammonia by the renal tubular cells allows the kidney to respond, up to a point, to the chronic retention of fixed acid. Use of alkali to treat metabolic acidosis associated with renal failure is controversial. Three reasons cited in support of treatment are that treatment (1) spares depletion of bone serving as a H^+ buffer, (2) prevents the potentially catabolic effects of acidosis on muscle protein, and (3) limits complement-mediated tubulointerstitial damage that may occur in concert with increased ammoniagenesis. Oral administration of $NaHCO_3$ (0.5–1.0 mEq/kg/day) with the goal of maintaining plasma HCO_3^- at 15 mEq/L may be effective if the associated sodium load does not encourage fluid retention.

Metabolic (Nonrespiratory) Alkalosis. Metabolic alkalosis is characterized by an excess of HCO_3^- caused by a deficit of H^+ in the ECF. This state may be caused by excessive vomiting (especially from gastrointestinal obstruction), excessive alkaline therapy or use of diuretics that can create iatrogenic metabolic alkalosis, or excessive loss of potassium caused by hyperadrenocorticism or administration of large quantities of K^+-free solutions. Clinical signs of metabolic alkalosis are depressed breathing (slow and shallow), nervous excitement, including tetany, and even convulsions and muscular hypertonicity. Respiratory compensation is not as effective as respiratory compensation for metabolic acidosis.

Values for serum electrolytes usually reveal elevated [HCO_3^-], lowered [Cl^-], and variable [Na^+]. There is usually a low serum [K^+] in this condition. A relationship exists between K^+ loss and metabolic alkalosis in that each can result in the other (positive feedback). In ruminants the situation is much more complex, and unlike in small animals, metabolic alkalosis is much more common. Compensation for metabolic alkalosis requires the kidneys to excrete HCO_3^- and retain H^+. Therapy for metabolic alkalosis involves treatment of the underlying disease and, potentially, use of acidifying solutions such as NaCl (0.9%), NH_4Cl (1.9%) (NH_3^+ is conjugated to urea in the liver, which frees H^+ and Cl^-), and Ringer's solution, which supplies Na^+, K^+, Ca^{++}, and Cl^-.

Respiratory Acidosis. Respiratory acidosis (Table 25.13) involves retention of CO_2 as a consequence of alveolar hypoventilation. The fall in pH is predictable from the Henderson-Hasselbalch equation. Impaired respiration can be caused by pneumonia, pulmonary edema, emphysema, pneumothorax, respiratory muscle paralysis, morphine, barbiturate, or anesthetic poisoning, airway occlusion, or, most commonly, hypoventilation during positive pressure ventilation (iatrogenic). Clinical signs include respiratory distress and CNS depression with progressive disorientation, weakness, and finally coma (CO_2 narcosis). Cyanosis is often present in the advanced stages. Laboratory analysis of blood and urine will show a decreased urine pH, decreased blood pH, increased serum HCO_3^- (from tissue buffers and renal reabsorption of HCO_3^-), and a decrease in serum Cl^- because of renal excretion. Hypoventilation results in CO_2 retention, an excess of H_2CO_3, and thereby an excess of H^+. The compensatory mechanism is for the kidneys to conserve HCO_3^- and excrete H^+. The most important treatment for this condition is proper ventilation of the animal. Use of alkalinizing solutions may aid in cases of lung disease when ventilation alone will not correct the condition.

TABLE 25.13—Causes of respiratory acidosis

- Inadequate mechanical ventilation
- Airway obstruction
- Respiratory center depression
  - Neurologic disease
  - Drugs (e.g., anesthetic agents, narcotics, sedatives)
- Cardiopulmonary arrest
- Neuromuscular defects
  - Myasthenia gravis
  - Tetanus
  - Botulism
  - Polyradiculoneuritis
  - Polymyositis
  - Tick paralysis
  - Hypokalemic periodic paralysis in Burmese cats
  - Hypokalemic myopathy in cats
  - Drugs (e.g., succinylcholine, pancuronium, aminoglycosides with anesthetics, organophosphates)
- Restrictive defects
  - Diaphragmatic hernia
  - Pneumothorax
  - Pleural effusion
  - Hemothorax
  - Chest wall trauma
  - Pulmonary fibrosis
  - Pyothorax
  - Chylothorax
- Pulmonary disease
  - Respiratory distress syndrome
  - Pneumonia
  - Severe pulmonary edema
  - Diffuse metastatic disease
  - Smoke inhalation
  - Pulmonary thromboembolism
  - Chronic obstructive pulmonary disease
  - Pulmonary fibrosis

Source: Adapted from DiBartola 1992a, 267, Table 10.3.

Whenever possible, therapy should be directed at removal of the causative factor.

Respiratory Alkalosis. Causes of respiratory alkalosis are indicated in Table 25.14. The most common cause of this disease in animals is overactive positive pressure ventilation during anesthesia (iatrogenic). Other causes include fever, stimulation of respiratory centers by encephalitis, salicylate intoxication, a deficiency of O_2 (hypoxia), heat prostration, hysteria, or conditions causing chronic hyperventilation (excessive blowing off of CO_2). Clinical signs include hyperpnea (with or without panting), hyperactive tendon reflexes, and CNS stimulation with or without convulsions. Laboratory analysis reveals increased urine pH, increased blood pH, and decreased serum HCO_3^-. Serum Cl^- is usually normal to slightly increased, and pathogenesis of the condition relates to excessive blowing off of CO_2. Compensation occurs by renal excretion of HCO_3^- and retention of H^+. Treatment for this condition should involve correcting the hyperventilation, when feasible, and use of the same acidifying solutions used for metabolic alkalosis. Underlying etiologic factor(s) must be eliminated.

Mixed Acid-Base Disturbances. The preceding discussion of acidosis and alkalosis has purposely dealt

TABLE 25.14—Causes of respiratory alkalosis

- Overzealous mechanical ventilation
- Hypoxemia (stimulation of peripheral chemoreceptors by decreased oxygen delivery):
  - Right-to-left shunts
  - Decreased PO_2 (e.g., high altitude)
  - Congestive heart failure
  - Severe anemia
  - Hypotension
  - Pulmonary diseases resulting in ventilation-perfusion mismatching:
    - Pneumonia
    - Pulmonary embolism
    - Pulmonary fibrosis
    - Pulmonary edema
  - Pulmonary disease resulting in stimulation of nociceptive receptors independent of hypoxemia:
    - Pneumonia
    - Pulmonary embolism
    - Interstitial lung disease
    - Pulmonary edema
- CNS-mediated hypocapnia with direct stimulation of medullary respiratory center:
  - Liver disease
  - Gram-negative sepsis
  - Drugs (e.g., salicylate intoxication, progesterone, xanthines)
  - Recovery from metabolic acidosis
  - Central neurologic disease
  - Heat stroke

Source: Adapted from DiBartola 1992a, 269, Table 10.4.

TABLE 25.15—Examples of potential causes of mixed respiratory and metabolic disorders

- Respiratory acidosis and metabolic acidosis
  - Hypoadrenocorticism-like syndrome in dogs with gastrointestinal disease
  - Cardiopulmonary arrest
  - Severe pulmonary edema
  - Thoracic trauma with hypovolemic shock
  - Low-cardiac-output heart failure with pulmonary edema
  - Advanced septic shock
  - Gastric dilatation volvulus
  - Acute tumor lysis syndrome
- Respiratory acidosis and metabolic alkalosis
  - Pulmonary edema and diuretics
  - Gastric dilatation volvulus
- Respiratory alkalosis and metabolic acidosis
  - Hypoadrenocorticism-like syndrome in dogs with gastrointestinal disease
  - Septic shock
  - Salicylate toxicity
  - Heat stroke
  - Gastric dilatation volvulus
  - Liver disease (renal tubular acidosis and impaired metabolism of lactate)
  - Lactic acidosis with excessive hyperventilation
  - Pulmonary edema
  - Parvovirus gastroenteritis and septicemia
  - Severe exercise
  - Acute tumor lysis syndrome
  - Cardiopulmonary resuscitation
- Respiratory alkalosis and metabolic alkalosis
  - Gastric dilatation volvulus
  - Hyperadrenocorticism with pulmonary thromboembolism
  - Ventilator-induced mixed alkalosis (too rapid correction of abnormal arterial PCO_2)
  - Congestive heart failure and diuretics
  - Hepatic disease and diuretics
  - Vomiting or hypoproteinemia
  - Parvovirus gastroenteritis and septicemia

Source: Adapted from DiBartola 1992a, 287, Table 11.9.

with idealized, single etiologic processes in the genesis of acid-base abnormalities. Such states rarely exist in real life. Mixed disturbances usually occur, and treatment will often convert one type of acid-base disturbance into another. Proper therapy must include careful appraisal of repeated laboratory determinations and close observation of the clinical situation. Using these techniques, mixed disturbances can be identified, evaluated, and managed successfully. Examples of potential causes of mixed respiratory and metabolic disorders are noted in Table 25.15.

PRACTICAL ASPECTS OF FLUID THERAPY

Diagnosis and Monitoring. When fluid therapy is under consideration, the practitioner must ask the following six questions: (1) When should fluid therapy be instituted? (2) What kind(s) of solution(s) should be used? (3) How much fluid should be administered? (4) How fast should the solution be given? (5) What route of administration should be used? (6) How will the success of the therapy be evaluated? The answers to these questions are individual in character and are critically dependent on a knowledge and understanding of normal homeostatic mechanisms. They are also dependent on the history of the patient, a basic understanding of how a particular disease affects water and electrolyte balance, and a correct diagnosis.

The purpose of fluid and electrolyte therapy is to correct dehydration or overhydration and electrolyte imbalance and/or acid-base imbalance. It may also be indicated to correct a condition of acidosis or alkalosis, treat shock, give parenteral nourishment, or even stimulate organ function (i.e., the kidneys). Causes of fluid, electrolyte, and/or protein loss include situations wherein substances are not available because of lack of supply or condition of the animal; for example, an animal with a fractured mandible may be unable to take in food or liquid, or an animal with a CNS disturbance may be unable to eat or drink because of the primary disease state. Other causes of fluid, electrolyte, and/or protein imbalances may involve excessive elimination.

The following information must be provided by questioning the owner, observation of the patient, and/or clinical examination: duration and frequency of vomiting and/or diarrhea, consistency of stools, frequency of urination, color of urine, presence and character of thirst, fluid and dietary intake, dryness or elasticity (turgor) of the skin, nature and color of the mucous membranes and sclera, presence of excessive salivation or panting, odor of the breath, and weight loss or gain.

In combination with clinical signs, laboratory examination of the blood provides a rational basis for estimating patient fluid and electrolyte needs and monitoring treatment success. Measurements should include hematocrit, plasma protein, blood gases (PO_2, PCO_2, base excess, HCO_3^-, or total CO_2) and electrolytes (Na^+, K^+, Cl^-), blood urea nitrogen, and creatinine. Because red blood cells and plasma protein are largely limited to the vascular space, the concentration of both tends to increase with dehydration. It is best to assess both hematocrit and plasma protein since results of one or the other test alone can be misleading if preillness values are out of the normal range. For example, preexisting anemia, hypoproteinemia, or physiologic events such as splenic contraction can confound interpretation of either parameter if considered alone.

Collection, measurement, and analysis of urine are important for proper care of the critically ill patient. Urinalysis should include tests for specific gravity, glucose, acetone, pH, and albumin and microscopic sediment examination. During a state of dehydration, if the kidneys are functioning normally, specific gravity will increase and urine volume will decrease. If the specific gravity of urine is unchanged or lowered and the animal shows clinical signs of dehydration, the kidneys are probably not functioning properly, and more sophisticated renal function tests must be employed. Specific gravity of urine should be monitored during the treatment period. A decrease in this parameter indicates that hydration is taking place. If the animal has not yet received treatment with a solution containing glucose and it is found in the urine, diabetic acidosis is possibly the cause of dehydration. The urine glucose should also be monitored during treatment. If the animal is receiving glucose and the urine glucose reaches +3 or +4, the dosage must be lowered. Acetone in the urine is a frequent finding during dehydration and/or carbohydrate starvation. If the pH of the urine in species with normally acid urine tests alkaline, a diagnosis of alkalosis may be indicated if no kidney or urinary tract disease is present. The presence of urinary albumin and sediment may be an indication of renal disease. If the kidneys are functioning properly, they can adjust markedly to insult. However, in the presence of renal impairment, therapy must be specific or the treatment may be fatal.

Diligent assessment of clinical signs and laboratory parameters is essential to successful diagnosis and monitoring of fluid and electrolyte imbalances. Useful parameters are summarized in Table 25.16.

TABLE 25.16—Parameters to be monitored during fluid therapy

- Normal bronchovesicular lung sounds on auscultation
- Packed-cell volume
- Total protein
- Electrolytes: Na^+, Cl^-, Ca^{2+}, HCO_3^-
- Arterial pH
- Arterial PCO_2
- Urine output
- Hemodynamics
    - Central venous pressure
    - Pulmonary capillary wedge pressures
    - Mean arterial pressure
    - Mean pulmonary arterial pressure

Source: Adapted from DiBartola 1992a, 503, Table 20.9.

Fluid Volume and Type. A standard approach to estimating fluid volume needs should be used. Replacement of adequate volume is often the single most important key to improved clinical status of animals with multiple fluid and electrolyte disturbances. Volume replacement should have three specific aims: correct existing deficits, satisfy maintenance needs, and replace continuing loss. Initial volume deficits are addressed by administration of replacement fluids. Calculation of the amount of fluid needed is based on clinical and laboratory assessment of percent of dehydration. See Table 25.5 for a summary of signs correlated to degree of dehydration. The volume needed to address the initial deficit is estimated according to the following equation:

$$\text{Replacement volume (L)} = \text{body weight (kg)} \times \%\ \text{dehydration}$$

Clinicians working with both small and large animals should become comfortable with the large differences in volume that will be required to address deficits in different animals. For example, the replacement volume needed to address an 8% fluid deficit in a dehydrated mare weighing 500 kg is 100 times greater than that needed for a similarly dehydrated cat weighing 5 kg. Forty liters of fluid would initially be administered to the mare versus 400 mL to the cat. In general, the composition of replacement fluids should reflect the composition of the volume of fluid lost. For example, if the volume deficit is related to loss of electrolyte-rich gastrointestinal fluid, then a balanced replacement solution containing Na^+, K^+, Cl^-, and bicarbonate equivalents would likely be selected. Table 25.17 details the compositions of commonly utilized replacement fluids.

In addition to replacing existing deficits, maintenance fluid needs must be calculated. Maintenance fluids are needed when a patient does not voluntarily ingest sufficient food and water to replace normal losses occurring via urine, feces, respiratory tract, and skin. The average resting animal at standard conditions of humidity and temperature has a rather constant rate of water turnover. For practical purposes, 40–65 mL/kg/24 hr (30 mL/lb/day is often used as a rule of thumb) for mature animals and 130 mL/kg/24 hr for immature animals serve as average water turnovers for all mammalian species. Based on these assumptions, an average mature dog weighing 20 kg requires about 1.3 L for a daily maintenance supply of water, while a horse weighing 450 kg would require about 29 L/day. Maintenance needs may be modified under conditions of severe stress or fever, extreme environmental conditions, or in the presence of various disease processes. Older animals may need more or less maintenance volume depending upon the presence of polyuria or com-

Table 25.17—Composition of selected fluid therapy solutions

		Characteristics		Ion composition (mEq/L)						
Type	Solution	pH	Osmolarity (mOsm/L)	Na^+	K^+	Cl^-	Ca^{++}	Mg^{++}	Glucose (g/L)	Alkalinizing equivalents (mEq/L)
Replacement										
Acidifying BES	Ringer's	5.4	309	147	4	155	4	0	0	0
Acidifying BES	Normal saline (0.9%)	5.0	308	154	0	154	0	0	0	0
Alkalinizing BES	Lactated Ringer's	6.6	273	130	4	109	3	0	0	28 (lactate)
Alkalinizing BES	Normosol-R	6.6	294	140	5	98	0	3	0	27 (acetate) 23 (gluconate)
Alkalinizing BES	Plasma-Lyte A	7.4	294	140	5	98	0	3	0	27 (acetate) 23 (gluconate)
Maintenance										
Acidifying	2.5% dextrose/water in 0.45% saline plus potassium addition (16 mEq/L)	4.5	280	77	16	77	0	0	25	0
	Equal volumes 5% dextrose/water and lactated Ringer's plus potassium addition (16 mEq/L)	5.0	309	65.5	18	55	1.5	0	25	14 (lactate)
	Normosol-M with 5% dextrose	5.0	363	40	13	40	0	3	50	16 (acetate)
	Plasma-Lyte M with 5% dextrose	5.5	377	40	16	40	5	3	50	12 (lactate) 12 (acetate)
Other Solutions	5% dextrose/water	4.0	252	0	0	0	0	0	5	0
	50% dextrose/water	4.2	2780	0	0	0	0	0	50	0
	7.5% saline	—	2566	1283	0	1283	0	0	0	0
	8.4% $NaHCO_3$	—	2000	1000	0	0	0	0	0	1000
	14.9% KCl	—	4000	0	2000	2000	0	0	0	0

Note: BES = balanced electrolyte solution.

promised cardiovascular function, respectively. Administration of various drugs (e.g., glucocorticoids, diuretics) will also affect maintenance needs. The electrolyte composition of fluids used for maintenance differs from that of replacement fluids used to address initial deficits. Because of the composition of fluid lost daily in urine and as insensible loss from the skin and respiratory tract, maintenance fluids are typically lower in sodium (approximately 40 mEq/L) and higher in potassium (approximately 10–16 mEq/L) than replacement fluids. Table 25.17 details the composition of both commercial maintenance fluids and maintenance fluids that can be prepared using other commonly available fluid components.

If the animal being treated continues to lose water during the treatment period (e.g., due to continued vomiting, diarrhea, polyuria) this additional amount must be estimated and added to the replacement and maintenance volumes. The volume required to replace continued loss is based on clinical observation (e.g., frequency of defecation, character and volume of feces in the case of diarrhea). Like the volume used to address the initial deficit, the type of fluid selected to replace continuing loss should, in general, resemble the fluid lost. More often than not, balanced electrolyte solutions such as lactated Ringer's are chosen.

Application of the principles outlined above may be appreciated using the following case example. A 2-year-old, 20 kg mixed-breed dog presents with a chief complaint of diarrhea of two days' duration. A physical exam reveals a loss of skin elasticity and a definite delay in return of skin to normal position when tented. Both mucous membranes and tongue are dry and the eyeballs feel soft and slightly sunken. Capillary refill time is slightly prolonged. Based on these clinical signs, dehydration is assessed at 8%. The dog is continuing to pass semifluid stools every 2–3 hours, resulting in an estimated ongoing loss of 150 mL/day. The owner reports that the dog is not eating or drinking. Calculation of the volume of fluid to be administered to this dog over the next 24 hours would include:

Replacement of initial deficit:	20 kg × 0.08 =	1.6 L
Maintenance needs:	65 mL/kg/day × 20 kg =	1.3 L
Continued loss:		0.15 L
Total estimated fluid needs:		3.05 L

This volume is considered an estimate because it is based on clinical signs and average maintenance losses. Despite the importance of good data collection and appropriate application of fluid therapy principles, at some level adjusting volume is dependent upon a "guess and reassess" process driven by diligent and thorough patient observation (Roussel 1990).

Rates and Routes of Administration. The rate of fluid and/or electrolyte replacement should parallel the severity of dehydration and electrolyte or acid-base imbalance. Fluids should be administered rapidly at first and then at decreasing rates until the condition is corrected. Most investigators report that rates of about 15 mL/kg/hr are reasonable. Cornelius et al. (1978) have shown that rates of 90 mL/kg/hr are well tolerated in moderately dehydrated, unanesthetized normal dogs. No deaths occurred, but clinical signs of severe overhydration were evident in dogs given fluids at 360 mL/kg/hr. At 90 mL/kg/hr, pulmonary artery wedge pressures and central venous pressures were increased in dogs with normally functioning hearts. It can be presumed that a seriously ill dog, with compromised cardiac muscle contractility, could be injured by infusion rates that result in acute volume overload. If central venous pressures are being monitored, the infusion rate can be individually adjusted for each patient. This technique is simple and inexpensive. The attending veterinarian should monitor this parameter in the critically ill patient and adjust the rate of fluid administration according to individual needs.

Conservative and reasonable practice would dictate infusion rates of about 50 mL/kg/hr in severely dehydrated cases. Less severe cases should tolerate rates of 15–30 mL/kg/hr. In all cases the rate of infusion should be slowed after the first hour of administration and should be slowed considerably if no urine flow is established. After 4 or more hours of fluid administration without urine flow, the rate of administration should be 2 mL/kg/hr or less. Every attempt must be made to establish renal function if no urine flow is detected after 2 hours of fluid administration. To accurately monitor urine flow, all critically ill animals should have a urinary bladder catheter in place.

Common sense and clinical judgment must be exercised. If an animal is severely dehydrated and in shock, it is difficult to administer fluids too fast during the initial stages of treatment. If, however, an animal is almost normally hydrated and the aim is only to maintain hydration, the rate should be slowed considerably. The importance of renal function has been repeatedly emphasized. A commonly used method of determining if the kidneys are capable of functioning is to inject a small bolus (1–25 mL, depending on size of the animal) of 50% glucose. Urine from the catheterized bladder is then checked every 5 minutes for the presence of glucose, which indicates glomerular filtration is occurring.

The route of fluid administration depends on the type of illness being dealt with and the severity of the condition, degree of dehydration, condition of the patient, type of electrolyte imbalance, organic functions of the patient, and time and equipment available. Probably the easiest, most physiologic, and most overlooked route of administration of fluid and electrolytes is oral or nasogastric. The oral route is the least dangerous, since the solution can be administered without strict attention to tonicity, volume, and asepsis. Oral replacement of electrolytes by using combinations of electrolyte salts, glycine, and dextrose has been especially successful (Hamm and Hicks 1975). Proper technique for oral fluid administration should preclude complications associated with fluid aspiration or administration of excessive amounts of air.

A relatively unused route of administration that might be considered, especially in very young animals, is per rectum. Warm water, K^+, Na^+, and Cl^- are well absorbed via this route. It may be difficult, however, to get the animal to retain material given in this manner, especially in the presence of gastrointestinal disease. Rectal infusion of fluids in birds has been suggested as an effective alternative route to intravenous, intraosseous, oral, or subcutaneous (Ephrati and Lemeij 1997).

The most commonly used and perhaps most practical routes of fluid and electrolyte administration are the parenteral routes: intravenous (IV), subcutaneous (SC), or intraperitoneal (IP). The IV route is the most versatile. Severe disturbances of fluid and electrolyte balance demand it. Nearly all the toxicity of solutions administered in this manner is more related to rate than volume or composition. No indications for hypotonic solutions have been found, but indications for isotonic and hypertonic solutions exist, and some of these have been discussed previously. Some of the problems associated with IV administration include those associated with maintenance and asepsis of indwelling catheters, clotting, and hematomas, as well as the location of a vein on very small or very ill animals. Obviously, the fluids administered and equipment used must be sterile. Large volumes of fluid administered too rapidly may overload the circulatory system, causing pulmonary edema and even death, especially in severely ill or toxic cases. This is the preferred route for blood, blood plasma, and plasma volume expanders.

Subcutaneous administration of fluid is referred to as hypodermoclysis. This technique is convenient for correction of mild to moderate deficits in small animals. Fluids are absorbed more slowly than by the IV route, but if the animal is not in critical condition, this is of no real consequence. Only isotonic solutions should be used in this manner. Dextrose of any tonicity or any solutions lacking electrolytes in isotonic levels are contraindicated because they may produce an initial rapid diffusion of major extracellular electrolytes to the area. This can result in severe reactions, including death, especially if the animal is already in shock. Hypodermoclysis is extremely valuable in very young or very small animals. If the animal is difficult to restrain long enough for a prolonged IV infusion, this is a useful technique. When edema is present, absorption will not occur, and this route of administration is contraindicated. If the animal is chilled by a cold environment or a cold fluid is injected, absorption by this route will be delayed, and it is recommended that fluids be prewarmed to body temperature when feasible. Administration of fluids in one anatomical location should be limited to amounts that are readily absorbed (approximately 10–12 mL/kg) (Greco 1998). Fluid should be deposited dorsally along the area bordered by the scapulae anteriorly and the iliac crests posteriorly. Hypodermoclysis is not commonly used as a route of administration in large animals.

IP infusion of fluids has the same restrictions as those for hypodermoclysis. The technique may predispose to peritonitis, so aseptic procedures must be used. The fluids are mobilized faster than in SC administration, but this route is potentially more hazardous (puncture of abdominal organs). Nevertheless, this is a good route for electrolyte and water absorption. Plasma and a large percentage of red blood cells administered using this technique are rapidly absorbed. In large animals it can be a very practical method of treatment, since a large quantity of fluid can be administered rapidly with few adverse effects. Perhaps the greatest application of this technique is with peritoneal lavage.

PRODUCTS FOR FLUID THERAPY. Major categories of parenteral fluids include crystalloids, colloids, blood replacements, and nutritional solutions. Blood replacement products (whole blood, blood components, and red blood cell substitutes) and nutritional solutions (amino acids and fat emulsions) are considered elsewhere. The composition and characteristics of selected crystalloid solutions and additives used to spike parenteral solutions are listed in Table 25.17. Types and recommended dosages of synthetic colloids are listed in Table 25.18.

Crystalloids. As detailed in Table 25.17, crystalloid solutions are polyionic but differ in the amount of each ion and in tonicity. As discussed previously, the tonicity of parenteral fluids partially dictates distribution of volume into interstitial and intracellular spaces. Fluids that most closely resemble the ECF are isotonic, high in sodium, and low in potassium and may be acidifying or alkalinizing. These replacement fluids, also referred to as balanced electrolyte solutions (BES), may be given in large volumes at a rapid rate to patients in shock in an attempt to reestablish effective perfusion without severely altering electrolyte concentrations. Alkalinizing solutions depend upon metabolism of various substrates (e.g., lactate, acetate, gluconate) to alkalinizing equivalents in order to reduce acidemia. Lactate and acetate are metabolized in the liver and muscle, respectively, while gluconate is metabolized widely in the body. Perfusion and function of the liver are required for generation of alkalinizing equivalents from the most commonly used replacement fluid, lactated Ringer's solution. A large percentage of veterinary patients that require fluid therapy suffer from nonrespiratory acidosis and are treated with alkalinizing balanced electrolyte solutions. These fluids are generally indicated for animals suffering from diarrhea, vomiting (assuming vomitus contains bile), renal disease, trauma, and shock and those requiring pre- and postsurgical support. To avoid calcium precipitation, calcium-containing balanced electrolyte solutions, such as lactated Ringer's solution, should not be coadministered through the same port with whole blood or sodium bicarbonate.

Normal saline and Ringer's solution are considered acidifying solutions and are used to treat the relatively small percentage of small-animal patients that present with metabolic alkalosis. Both solutions are high in chloride and promote renal excretion of bicarbonate. Normal saline is also commonly used in treatment of patients with electrolyte disorders such as hyperkalemia or hypercalcemia in which absence of electrolytes in parenteral fluids is desirable. Assuming appropriate insulin therapy is instituted, normal saline is also considered the fluid of choice for treatment of diabetic ketoacidosis.

Colloids. The critical distribution of water between plasma and interstitial fluid is maintained in part by the colloid osmotic pressure (COP) of plasma protein. COP includes the osmotic pressure exerted by plasma proteins and their associated electrolyte molecules. This force draws water into capillaries and balances the hydrostatic pressure driving water out (see Starling relationships described earlier in this chapter). Although the basic concept of Starling relationships is straightforward, in vivo application of these concepts is complicated by the heterogeneity of Starling forces within different tissues and the complexity of transvascular fluid dynamics. Despite these caveats, it is practical to say that the balance between intravascular COP and capillary hydrostatic pressure drives net fluid extravasation and forms the basis for intravenous colloid therapy.

Therapeutic colloids may be of two types: natural and synthetic. Natural colloids include whole blood, plasma, and albumin. Synthetic colloids, the focus of this discussion, include dextran 40, dextran 70, hetastarch, pentastarch, and oxypolygelatin. Therapeutic colloid solutions contain large particles and are retained within the vascular space more readily than crystalloids. As a result, smaller volumes of colloids cause greater volume expansion than crystalloids do. Initial tissue perfusion has been found to be better after volume expansion with colloids or combinations of colloids and crystalloids than with crystalloids alone (Funk and Baldinger 1995). The duration of this effect varies and is dependent upon many variables, including the species of animal, dose, specific colloid formulation, preinfusion intravascular volume status, and microvascular permeability (Hughes 2000).

The osmotic effect of colloid solutions is related to the number of particles rather than the size of particles in a solution. However, heterogeneity of particle size causes considerable complexity in the pharmacokinetics of these solutions. Synthetic colloids contain

Table 25.18—Indications, dosages, administration, and side effects associated with use of selected colloids in dogs

Type of colloid	Indications	Dosage and administration	Side effects and contraindications
Plasma	Coagulopathies; disseminated intravascular coagulation; low antithrombin; acute hypoalbuminemia.	20–30 mL/kg/day administered: (a) continuously over 24 hr, (b) as a 2–4 hr infusion, (c) 6–10 mL/kg in 1 hr infusions every 8 hr, or (d) until plasma albumin is over 2.0 g/dL. Approximately 22.5 mL/kg of plasma needed to increase patient albumin by 5 g/L.	Rapid volume expansion may be detrimental to patients with oliguric or anuric renal failure or congestive heart failure.
Dextran 40	Rapid, short-term intravascular volume resuscitation from hypovolemic shock; rapid improvement of microcirculatory flow by lowering blood viscosity; prophylaxis of deep vein thrombosis and pulmonary emboli.	10–20 mL/kg/day IV bolus to effect; with distributive shock due to SIRS dextran can be followed by a CRI of hetastarch to maintain MAP of at least 80 mm Hg.	*See* plasma. Dilutional effect on serum coagulation factors in addition to possible direct effects on these factors. May be of limited clinical relevance except in patients with preexisting coagulopathies. Contraindicated in patients with severe coagulopathies. Sludging of RBCs in microcirculation in dehydrated patients may occur if sufficient crystalloids are not administered. Anaphylaxis reported in humans. ARF has been reported.
Dextran 70	Rapid, intravascular volume resuscitation from hypovolemic, traumatic, or hemorrhagic shock.	*See* dextran 40.	*See* dextran 40. Dextran 70 is thought to impair coagulation more than dextran 40. No ARF reported.
Hetastarch (hydroxyethyl starch or HES)	Rapid, intravascular volume resuscitation from all forms of shock; small-volume resuscitation; volume replacement and maintenance in SIRS patients.	10–40 mL/kg/day IV bolus to effect; with cardiogenic shock, pulmonary contusions, or head injury, 5 mL/kg boluses are administered to effect, using the smallest volume possible to maintain MAP of 80 mm Hg.	*See* dextran 40. Anaphylaxis has not been reported with hetastarch, but pruritus possibly associated with deposits of HES in cutaneous nerves has been reported in up to 33% of patients treated with long-term infusions. No ARF reported.
Pentastarch (PEN)	Rapid, intravascular volume resuscitation from hypovolemic, traumatic, or hemorrhagic shock.	10–25 mL/kg/day; terminal half-life shorter than HES.	*See* dextran 40. Anaphylaxis and ARF have not been reported with pentastarch.
Oxypolygelatin	Rapid, short-term intravascular volume resuscitation from hypovolemic shock.	5 mL/kg over 15 min; titrate to effect; do not exceed 15 mL/kg total dose. If more volume required, follow with another synthetic colloid.	*See* dextran 40. No ARF reported.

Source: Modified from Rudloff and Kirby1998. Other sources for information in table include Mathews 1998 and Hughes 2000.

Note: ARF = acute renal failure; CRI = constant-rate infusion; MAP = mean arterial pressure; SIRS = systemic inflammatory response syndrome.

molecules that vary in molecular weight more than the molecules in a solution of a natural colloid such as albumin. After synthetic colloids are administered, the smaller molecules pass rapidly into the urine and are eliminated or move to the interstitium, negating their ability to attract water into the vasculature. Larger molecules remain in the circulation to exert COP until they are hydrolyzed by amylase or removed by the monocyte phagocytic system. Because of differences in particle behavior and in pharmacokinetic study design (e.g., duration of study, volume status of study subjects, volumes and rates of colloid administration), specific half-lives reported for colloids may vary considerably (Mathews 1998). Such variation may pose therapeutic problems since actual duration of action of colloids may not coincide with manufacturer estimates of the same.

Indications for colloid use include perfusion deficits, hypooncotic states, deficiency of blood components, and diseases that lead to systemic inflammatory response syndrome (SIRS). SIRS is a generalized inflammatory process with evidence of decreased organ perfusion. Sepsis may be the source of SIRS but other conditions may also result in generalized systemic pathophysiology (e.g., heat stroke, acute pancreatitis, neoplasia). Hallmarks of SIRS include alterations in temperature, heart rate, respiratory rate, PCO_2, and white blood cell count. Peripheral vasculature dilates, capillary permeability increases, and plasma proteins leak from affected vessels. The resulting hypoalbuminemia leads to a reduction in COP, loss of vascular volume, and hypoperfusion of tissues. High molecular weight colloids administered to SIRS patients are retained more effectively in leaky vessels and force retention of volume. Approximately 20–25% of crystalloid remains within the vasculature 1 hour after infusion into normal animals compared with 100% of the volume of infused colloid. Hence, colloids may initially expand the volume of the intravascular space approximately fourfold more than crystalloids (Hughes 2000).

Colloids are often included in fluid regimens for small-volume resuscitation (e.g., during traumatic, hypovolemic, or cardiogenic shock), improvement of microcirculatory flow and capillary integrity (e.g., SIRS), and management of ongoing hemorrhage. While colloids are useful in reestablishing vascular integrity, replenishment of interstitial and intracellular fluid deficits depends upon appropriate use of colloids and crystalloids in combination. Colloid administration typically reduces the required amount of crystalloid fluid by as much as 40–60% (Rudloff 1998). Care must be taken to adjust amounts and rates of all fluids administered to prevent intravascular volume overload and subsequent interstitial edema. Monitoring of colloid therapy ideally includes direct measurement of COP with a membrane osmometer in addition to measurement of traditional indices of perfusion and hydration.

Problems associated with colloid therapy may include dilutional effects caused by expansion of the intravascular space. Packed-cell volume, albumin concentration, serum potassium concentration, and amount of circulating coagulation factors typically decline following administration of synthetic colloids. Rapid volume expansion may be of greatest concern in patients with oliguric or anuric renal failure or congestive heart failure. Precipitation of acute renal failure has been reported in humans with dextran 40 (Ferraboli et al. 1997). Impairment of coagulation as a result of dilution of coagulation factors is thought to be of limited clinical relevance in veterinary medicine except in patients with preexisting coagulopathies. Anaphylactic or anaphylactoid reactions associated with colloids have been reported in humans. Concern has also been raised over the effects of selected colloids on reticuloendothelial function (Hughes 2000). Because cats are more likely to show signs of allergic reactions, especially when synthetic colloids are administered quickly, only small volumes infused at slow rates (5 mL/kg increments given over 5–10 minutes, repeated to effect up to 20 mL/kg) are recommended for use in this species.

Table 25.18 lists indications, dosages, and administration details for colloids commonly used to treat dogs. Albumin (66,000–69,000 daltons) accounts for 80% of the COP of the only natural colloid listed, plasma. Each gram of albumin can retain as much as 18 mL of fluid in the intravascular space, assuming infused albumin does not leak from damaged vessels. The intravascular half-life of albumin in plasma is approximately 16 hours (Mathews 1998). The three major categories of synthetic colloids are dextrans, hydroxyethyl starches, and gelatins. Dextrans are prepared from a macromolecular polysaccharide produced by bacterial fermentation of sucrose. Because these products represent a range of molecules with different molecular weights, they are described by a weight average molecular weight (MWw). MWw is defined as the sum of the number of molecules at each molecular weight times their mass divided by the total weight of the molecules. Dextran 70 (MWw = 70,000 daltons) is more commonly used and is available as a 6% solution in either 0.9% saline or 5.0% dextrose. Hydroxyethyl starches are derived from plant amylopectin and are modified by hydroxyethylation to reduce hydrolysis by amylase. The most commonly used product in this category, hetastarch (Hespan®), has a MWw of 100,000–300,000 daltons and is available as a 6% (6 g/dL) solution in 0.9% saline. Pentastarch has a narrower range of molecular weights, a shorter duration of action than hetastarch, and is only approved in this country for leukapheresis. Only one gelatin product, oxypolygelatin (Vetaplasma®) derived from bovine bone gelatin, is approved in this country as a plasma substitute for fluid resuscitation.

Hypertonic Solutions. For several decades, resuscitation of experimental and clinical animals suffering from shock has been attempted using hypertonic saline (HSS). Throughout the 1900s, studies have generally supported the benefits of HSS for transient restoration of cardiovascular function. Although a full understanding of the mechanism of action has been elusive, there is agreement that the primary benefits of HSS infusion result from plasma volume expansion. High circulating concentrations of sodium attract water into the vasculature from the interstitial and intracellular spaces and help to restore capillary flow and tissue perfusion. Cardiac output has been reported to increase as a result of increased preload, decreased afterload related to systemic and pulmonary vasodilation (Constable et al. 1995), increased adrenergic activity through release of catecholamines, and improved oxygen delivery to the heart (Tobias et al. 1993). Positive inotropy has also been reported but this remains a controversial point (Cambier et al. 1997). In vitro studies have shown that, at least during the initial treatment period, negative inotropy may predominate (Constable et al. 1994). All of the above effects are short-lived (peak occurs within approximately 1 hour) but resuscitative benefits may be prolonged by combination of HSS with colloids such as dextran 70. Ideally, rapid recovery of cardiovascular parameters occurs with administration of smaller volumes of HSS or HSS plus dextran (HSD) compared to crystalloids, thus decreasing the risk of edema related to volume overload. In addition to primary volume expansion, HSS is thought to invoke a lung vagal reflex important to circulatory control during hypovolemia. How much this reflex contributes to the cardiovascular effects of HSS infusion remains controversial. HSS may also have immunomodulatory effects that protect organs from oxidative injury and enhance cell-mediated immunity (Coimbra et al. 1996).

HSS use is indicated in the treatment of shock associated with hemorrhage (Bauer et al. 1993), trauma (Schertel et al. 1996), gastric-dilatation volvulus (Schertel et al. 1997), acute pancreatitis (Horton et al. 1989), burns (Horton et al. 1990), and sepsis (Fantoni et al. 1999; Maciel et al. 1998). The evidence for use of HSS in the first three of these is most compelling, with fewer studies unequivocally demonstrating advantage under specific study conditions associated with the other disorders. HSS has also been utilized in treatment of head injury since, like mannitol, HSS draws interstitial and intracellular water away from edematous tissues and into the vasculature (Prough and Zornow 1998). Regardless of the indication, HSS effects are transient, necessitating combination with crystalloids or colloids to achieve long-term resuscitative goals. Effects of HSS should be monitored by improvement in cardiovascular parameters correlated with increased perfusion as well as by assessment of mean arterial blood pressure, electrocardiogram, and electrolytes. Monitoring is aimed at preventing volume overload and electrolyte imbalances that may occur as a result of therapy.

HSS use is contraindicated in hypernatremic patients or those with increased plasma osmolality. Use in dehydrated animals is controversial since these patients frequently suffer from increases in both parameters. Studies that support HSS use in the presence of dehydration include those in which resuscitation with HSD of hypovolemic, diarrheic calves found this method to be at least as effective as others (Constable et al. 1996; Walker et al. 1998). In animals suffering from shock related to trauma and hemorrhage, two additional problems, hypokalemia and increased risk of rehemorrhaging, may be of concern. Rehemorrhage—bleeding caused by breakdown of clots in areas where hemorrhage has previously occurred—may be related to the sudden increase in cardiac output and arterial blood pressure associated with HSS resuscitation (Schertel and Tobias 2000). HSS may also dilute circulating coagulation factors and affect platelet function. As with colloids, these concerns may only be of practical significance if the patient suffers from preexisting coagulopathies or thrombocytopenia. Using a swine model of hemorrhagic shock, Dubick et al. (1993) demonstrated that the combination of 7.5% NaCl/6% dextran 70 did not significantly affect various measures of coagulation and platelet aggregation in their model. Studies continue to address the pros and cons of HSS use in various animal models and in clinical patients (Krausz 1995). Variation across species lines, differences in physiological circumstances of each study, and different views of cost versus benefit ratios may account for differing conclusions on the overall value of HSS treatment.

HSS is administered most effectively in combination with colloids or crystalloids in order to optimize resuscitative effects. 5% HSS, at a dose of 6–10 mL/kg, and 7–7.5% HSS, at a dose of 4–8 mL/kg, are administered at a rate of 1 mL/kg/min. Similar dosages may be used for HSD. More rapid administration rates may invoke a vagal-mediated hypotension, decreased heart rate, bronchoconstriction, and rapid, shallow breathing. To prepare 7% saline in 6% dextran 70, 33.0 g of anhydrous sodium chloride is added to a 500 mL bag of 6% dextran 70 in 0.9% saline. Half of the sodium chloride crystals are placed into the barrel of a 35 mL syringe and an adequate volume of dextran 70 solution is drawn into the syringe to dissolve the crystals. This solution is filtered through a 0.22 μm filter and is injected back into the bag of dextran 70. The procedure is repeated a second time to dissolve the remaining half of the sodium chloride (Schertel and Tobias 2000). Although a reported advantage of HSS is presumed sterility due to hypertonicity, St. Jean et al. have demonstrated the ability of bacteria to adapt and survive in the hypertonic environment of HSS (St. Jean et al. 1997). Hence, aseptic technique consistent with handling of all intravenous fluids should be followed.

SPECIAL TOPICS

Horses. Horses present some special problems in acid-base management. In cases of severe diarrhea, shock, and intestinal obstruction, the horse seems predisposed to rather severe metabolic acidosis (Waterman 1977). Respiratory acidosis is a very common sequel to closed-circuit inhalation anesthesia in the horse. An abnormally low concentration of Na^+ is a common problem in dehydrated horses. Severe hypokalemia, with blood K^+ values less than 2.5–3 mEq/L, may require treatment with solutions high in K^+. Dangerous hyperkalemia, with blood levels greater than approximately 7 mEq/L, may be associated with acidosis in foals. Prompt correction of the acidosis will usually correct the hyperkalemia.

Cattle. Ruminants also present special fluid and electrolyte management problems. When a diagnosis of abomasal disease is coupled with an obvious fluid balance disorder, hypochloremia, hypokalemia, and alkalosis are usually present. These should be confirmed by appropriate laboratory tests. Grain overloading will result in severe dehydration and metabolic acidosis. Calf diarrhea also results in severe dehydration and metabolic acidosis, with dangerous hyperkalemia in some cases. If hyperkalemia exists, one must guard against administration of even more K^+. When dealing with herbivores, it is important to remember that normal feed contains high levels of K^+. When these animals are anorexic, they frequently become K^+ depleted.

The best way to replace K^+ deficits is by consumption of hay or grass, but K^+ must be added parenterally when the situation dictates. A wide variety of electrolyte mixtures containing K^+ are available for oral administration.

Anesthetic and Surgical Effects. General anesthesia may exert several effects on water, electrolyte, and acid-base balance. Almost all general anesthetics induce some degree of Ca^{++} channel blockade, resulting in some degree of vasodilation and myocardial depression. The end effect can be a reduction in cardiac output and/or alterations in organ blood flow. Arterial pressures are frequently lowered in a dose-dependent manner, and GFR may be affected. The commonly used inhalation anesthetic agents (halothane, enflurane, and isoflurane) all cause direct systemic vasodilation. Narcotics and some muscle relaxants also can cause vasodilation. As a result of the vasodilation, fluid requirements may be increased during the course of the surgical procedure to maintain adequate blood pressure and cardiac output. After recovery from the general anesthetic, when vascular tone is normalized, the patient may be volume overloaded and hypertensive. Fluid loss may also increase during general anesthesia as a result of tracheal intubation and/or artificial ventilation. Normal mechanisms for the humidification of inspired air are bypassed, and the cold, dry gases from the anesthesia machine can cause a considerable amount of fluid loss. Open body cavities allow for evaporative losses. Third spacing may occur with extravasation of fluid from the vascular to the extravascular, extracellular spaces. If extravasated fluid is replaced to maintain adequate circulatory volumes, the patient with inadequate cardiac reserve or poor renal function may suffer fluid overload and congestive heart failure when postoperative redistribution of the fluid back into the circulation occurs (Gold 1992).

Surgical injury can result in significant reductions in serum albumin, total proteins, and total lymphocyte counts. These decreases are typically greater following abdominal surgery. The decreases have been found to be primarily caused by the volume of IV fluids frequently required for resuscitation and to compensate for blood loss.

REFERENCES

Adolph, E. F. 1939. Measurements of water drinking in dogs. Am J Physiol 125:75–86.

Adrogue, H. J., and Madias, N. E. 1981. Changes in plasma potassium concentration during acute acid-base disturbances. Am J Med 71:456–467.

Anderson, R. S. 1983. Fluid balance and diet. In Proceedings of the Seventh Kal Kan Symposium, pp. 19–25. Kal Kan Foods, Inc.

Arieff, A. I., and Guisado, R. 1976. Effects on the central nervous system of hypernatremic and hyponatremic states. Kidney Int 10:104–116.

Astrup, P., Jorgensen, K., Andersen, O. S., and Engel, K. 1960. The acid-base metabolism. Lancet 1:1035–1039.

Bailey, J. E., and Pablo, L. S. 1998. Practical approach to acid-base disorders. Vet Clin N Am, Small Anim Pract 28:645–662.

Bastani, B., Purcell, H., Hemken, P., et al. 1991. Expression and distribution of renal vacuolar proton-translocating adenosine triphosphatases in response to chronic acid and alkali loads in the rat. J Clin Invest 88:126.

Bauer, M., Marzi, I., Ziegenfuss, T., et al. 1993. Comparative effects of crystalloid and small volume hypertonic hyperoncotic fluid resuscitation on hepatic microcirculation after hemorrhagic shock. Circ Shock 40:187–193.

Benjamin, E., Oropello, J. M., Abalos, A. M., et al. 1994. Effects of acid-base correction on hemodynamics, oxygen dynamics, and resuscitability in severe canine hemorrhagic shock. Crit Care Med 22:1616–1623.

Black, R. M. 1993. Disorders of acid-base and potassium balance. In E. Rubenstein and D. D. Federman, eds., Scientific American Medicine, pp. 1–25. New York: Scientific American.

Brown, L. W., and Feigin, R. D. 1994. Bacterial meningitis: fluid balance and therapy. Pediatric Annals 23:93–98.

Button, C. 1979. Metabolic and electrolyte disturbances in acute canine babesiosis. JAVMA 175:475–479.

Cambier, C., Ratz, V., Rollin, F., Frans, A., Clerbaux, T., and Gustin, P. 1997. The effects of hypertonic saline in healthy and diseased animals. Vet Res Commun 21:303–316.

Clausen, T., and Flatman, J. A. 1987. Effect of insulin and epinephrine on Na^+-K^+ and glucose transport in soleus muscle. Am J Physiol 252:E492–499.

Cohen, R. D. 1995. New evidence in the bicarbonate controversy. Appl Cardiopul Pathophysiol 5:135–138.

Coimbra, R., Junger, W. G., and Hoyt, D. B. 1996. Hypertonic saline resuscitation restores hemorrhage induced immunosuppression by decreasing prostaglandin E_2 and interleukin 4 production. J Surg Res 64:203–209.

Constable, P. D. 1997. A simplified strong ion model for acid-base equilibria: application to horse plasma. J Appl Physiol 83:297–311.

———. 1999. Clinical assessment of acid-base status: strong ion difference theory. Vet Clin N Am, Food Anim Pract 15:447–471.

Constable, P. D., Gohar, H. M., Morin, D. E., and Thurmon, J. C. 1996. Use of hypertonic saline-dextran solution to resuscitate hypovolemic calves with diarrhea. Am J Vet Res 57:97–104.

Constable, P. D., Muir, W. W., III, and Binkley, P. F. 1994. Hypertonic saline is a negative inotropic agent in normovolemic dogs. Am J Physiol 267:H667–H677.

———. 1995. Effect of hypertonic saline solution on left ventricular afterload in normovolemic dogs. Am J Vet Res 56:1513–1521.

Constable, P. D., Streeter, R. N., Koenig, G., Perkins, N. R., Gohar, H. M., and Morin, D. E. 1997. Determinants and utility of the anion gap in predicting hyperlactatemia in cattle. J Vet Int Med 11:71–79.

Constable, P. D., Walker, P. G., Morin, D. E., and Foreman, J. H. 1998. Clinical and laboratory assessment of hydration status of neonatal calves with diarrhea. JAVMA 212:991–996.

Cornelius, L. M., Finco, D. R., and Culver, D. H. 1978. Physiologic effects of rapid infusion of Ringer's lactate solution into dogs. Am J Vet Res 39:1185–1190.

DiBartola, S. P., ed. 1992a. Fluid Therapy in Small Animal Practice. Philadelphia: W. B. Saunders.

———. 1992b. Renal physiology. In S. P. DiBartola, ed., Fluid Therapy in Small Animal Practice, pp. 35–56. Philadelphia: W. B. Saunders.

———. 1992c. Disorders of sodium and water: hypernatremia and hyponatremia. In S. P DiBartola, ed., Fluid Therapy in Small Animal Practice, pp. 57–88. Philadelphia: W. B. Saunders.

———. 1992d. Introduction to acid-base disorders. In S. P. DiBartola, ed., Fluid Therapy in Small Animal Practice, pp. 207–209. Philadelphia: W. B. Saunders.

———. 1998. Hyponatremia. Vet Clin N Am, Small Anim Pract 28:515–532.
DiBartola, S. P., and Autran de Morais, H. S. 1992. Disorders of potassium: hypokalemia and hyperkalemia. In S. P. DiBartola, ed., Fluid Therapy in Small Animal Practice, pp. 89–115. Philadelphia: W. B. Saunders.
Dubick, M. A., Kilani, A. F., Summary, J. J., et al. 1993. Further evaluation of the effects of 7.5% sodium chloride/6% Dextran-70 (HSD) administration on coagulation and platelet aggregation in hemorrhaged and euvolemic swine. Circ Shock 40:200–205.
Emmett, M., and Narins, R. G. 1977. Clinical use of the anion gap. Medicine 56:38–54.
Ephrati, C., and Lemeij, T. 1997. Rectal fluid therapy in birds: an experimental study. J Avian Med and Surg 11:4–6.
Fantoni, D., Auler, J., Futema, F., Cortopassi, S., Migliati, E., Faustino, M., deOliveira, C. 1999. Intravenous administration of hypertonic sodium chloride solution with dextran or isotonic sodium chloride solution for treatment of septic shock secondary to pyometra in dogs. JAVMA 215:1283–1287.
Ferraboli, R., Malheiro, P. S., and Abdukader, R. C. 1997. Anuric acute renal failure caused by dextran 40 administration. Ren Fail 19:303–306.
Funk, W., and Baldinger, V. 1995. Microcirculatory perfusion during volume therapy: a comparative study using crystalloid or colloid in awake animals. Anesthesiology 82:975–982.
Gabow, P. A. 1985. Disorders associated with an altered anion gap. Kidney Int. 27:472–483.
Garella, S., Chang, B., and Kahn, S. I. 1979. Alterations of hydrogen ion homeostasis in pure potassium depletion: studies in rats and dogs during the recovery phase. J Lab Clin Med 93:321–331.
Geiger, H., Hahner, U., Meissner, M., et al. 1992. Parathyroid hormone modulates the release of atrial natriuretic peptide during acute volume expansion. Am J Nephrol 12:259–264.
Gold, M. S. 1992. Perioperative fluid management. Crit Care Clinics 8:409–421.
Greco, D. S. 1998. The distribution of body water and general approach to the patient. Vet Clin N Am, Small Anim Pract 28:473–482.
Gregor, R., and Velazquez, H. 1987. The cortical thick ascending limb and early distal convoluted tubule in the urine concentrating mechanism. Kidney Int 31:590.
Gross, D. R. 1994. Animal models in cardiovascular research. Dordrecht: Kluwer.
Halperin, F. A., Cheema-Dhadli, S., Chen, C. B., and Halperin, M. L. 1996. Alkali therapy extends the period of survival during hypoxia: studies in rats. Am J Physiol 271 (Regulatory Integrative Comp Physiol 40):R381–R387.
Hamm, D., and Hicks, W. J. 1975. A new oral electrolyte in calf scours therapy. Vet Med Small Anim Clin 70:279–282.
Hardy, R. M. 1989. Hypernatremia. Vet Clin N Am, Small Anim Pract 19:231–240.
Horton, J. W., Dunn, C. W., Burnweit, C. S., and Wlaker, P. B. 1989. Hypertonic saline-dextran resuscitation of acute canine bile-induced pancreatitis. Am J Surg 158:48–56.
Horton, J. W., White, J., and Baxter, C. R. 1990. Hypertonic saline dextran resuscitation of thermal injury. Ann Surg 211:301–311.
Hughes, D. 2000. Fluid therapy with macromolecular plasma volume expanders. In S. P. DiBartola, ed., Fluid Therapy in Small Animal Practice, 2nd ed., pp. 483–495. Philadelphia: W. B. Saunders.
Katz, M. A. 1973. Hyperglycemia-induced hyponatremia: calculation of expected serum sodium depression. N Engl J Med 289:843–844.
Kohn, C. W., and DiBartola, S. P. 1992. Composition and distribution of body fluids in dogs and cats. In S. P. DiBartola, ed., Fluid Therapy in Small Animal Practice, pp. 1–34. Philadelphia: W. B. Saunders.
Krausz, M. M. 1995. Controversies in shock research: hypertonic resuscitation, pros and cons. Shock 3:69–72.
Landry D. W., and Oliver, J. A. 1992.The ATP-sensitive K^+ channel mediates hypotension in endotoxemia and hypoxic lactic acidosis in the dog. J Clin Invest 89:2071.
Lewis, L. D., and Morris, M. L. 1987. Small Animal Clinical Nutrition, 3rd ed., pp. 2–22. Topeka: Mark Morris Assoc.
Looney, A. L., Ludders, J., Erb, H. N., Gleed, R., and Moon, P. 1998. Use of a handheld device for analysis of blood electrolyte concentrations and blood gas partial pressures in dogs and horses. JAVMA 213:526–530.
Maciel, F., Mook, M., Zhang, H., and Vincent, J.-L. 1998. Comparison of hypertonic with isotonic saline hydroxyethyl starch solution on oxygen extraction capabilities during endotoxic shock. Shock 9:33–39.
Marks, S. L. 1998. Hypernatremia and hypertonic syndromes. Vet Clin N Am, Small Anim Pract 28:533–543.
Mathews, K. A. 1998. The various types of parenteral fluids and their indications. Vet Clin N Am, Small Anim Pract 28:483–513.
McEvoy, G. K. 1997. Electrolyte solutions. In G. K. McEvoy, ed., American Hospital Formulary Service Drug Information, pp. 1991–1994. Bethesda: American Society of Health-System Pharmacists.
Monafo, W. W. 1993. The second quinquennium: 1974–1978. J Burn Care Rehabil 14:236–237.
Muir, W. W., and DiBartola, S. P. 1983. Fluid therapy. In R. W. Kirk, ed., Current Veterinary Therapy VIII, pp. 28–40. Philadelphia: W. B. Saunders.
Naylor, J. M. 1996. Neonatal ruminant diarrhea. In B. P. Smith, ed., Large Animal Internal Medicine, 2nd ed., p. 403. St. Louis: Mosby Yearbook.
O'Brien, D. 1995. Metabolic dysfunction and the CNS. In Proc 13th Ann Vet Med Forum, American College of Veterinary Internal Medicine, Lake Buena Vista, FL, p. 447.
O'Connor, W. J., and Potts, D. J. 1969. The external water exchanges of normal laboratory dogs. Q J Exp Physiol 54:244–265.
Oh, M. S., and Carrol, J. H. 1977. The anion gap. N Engl J Med 297:814–817.
Oster, J. R., Perez, G. O., Castro, A., et al. 1980. Plasma potassium response to acute metabolic acidosis induced by mineral and nonmineral acids. Miner Electrolyte Metab 4:28–36.
Perez, G. O., Kem, D. C., Oster, J. R., et al. 1980. Effect of acute metabolic acidosis on the renin-aldosterone system. J Lab Clin Med 96:371–378.
Phillips, S. L., and Polzin, D. J. 1998. Clinical disorders of potassium homeostasis. Vet Clin N Am, Small Anim Pract 28:545–564.
Prough, D. S., and Zornow, M. H. 1998. Mannitol: an old friend on the skids? Crit Care Med 26:997–998.
Rose, B. D. 1989. Clinical Physiology of Acid-Base and Electrolytes, 3rd ed., pp. 248–260. New York: McGraw-Hill.
———. 1994. Clinical Physiology of Acid-Base and Electrolytes, 4th ed., pp. 73–75, 500–560, 651–694. New York: McGraw-Hill.
———. In press. Clinical Physiology of Acid-Base and Electrolytes. 5th ed. New York: McGraw-Hill.
Roussel, A. J. 1990. Fluid therapy in mature cattle. Vet Clin N Am, Food Anim Pract 6:111–123.
Rudloff, E., and Kirby, R. 1998. The critical need for colloids: administering colloids effectively. Compend Contin Educ Pract Vet 20:27–43.
Russell, K. E., Hansen, B. D., and Stevens, J. B. 1996. Strong ion difference approach to acid-base imbalances with clinical applications in dogs and cats. Vet Clin N Am, Small Anim Pract 26:1185–1201.

Schertel, R. R., Allen, D. A., Muir, W. W, Bourman, J. D., and DeHoff, W. D. 1997. Evaluation of a hypertonic saline-dextran solution for treatment of dogs with shock induced by gastric dilatation-volvulus. JAVMA 210:226–230.
Schertel, R. R., Allen, D. A., Muir, W. W., and Hansen, B. D. 1996. Evaluation of a hypertonic sodium chloride/dextran solution for treatment of traumatic shock in dogs. JAVMA 208:366–370.
Schertel, E. R., and Tobias, T. A. 2000. Hypertonic fluid therapy. In S. P. DiBartola, ed., Fluid Therapy in Small Animal Practice, 2nd ed., pp. 496–506. Philadelphia: W. B. Saunders.
Smith, C. R. 1970. Unpublished data.
Stewart, P. A. 1978. Independent and dependent variables of acid-base control. Respir Physiol 33:9–26.
———. 1983. Modern quantitative acid-base chemistry. Can J Physiol Pharmacol 61:1444–1461.
St. Jean, G., Chengappa, M. M., and Staats, J. 1997. Survival of selected bacteria and fungi in hypertonic (7.2%) saline. Aust Vet J 75:137–138.
Sun, X., Iles, M., and Weissman, C. 1993. Physiologic variables and fluid resuscitation in the post-operative intensive care unit patient. Crit Care Med 21:555–561.
Thier, S. O. 1987. Diuretic mechanisms as a guide to therapy. Hospital Pract 22:81–100.
Tobias, T. A., Schertel, E. R., Schmall, L. M., et al. 1993. Comparative effects of 7.5% NaCl in 6% Dextran 70 and 0.9% NaCl on cardiorespiratory parameters after cardiac output-controlled resuscitation from canine hemorrhagic shock. Circ Shock 398:139–146.
Vander, A. J., Sherman, J. H., and Luciano, D. S. 1994. Human Physiology: The Mechanisms of Body Function. 6th ed. New York: McGraw-Hill.
Wachtel, T. L., McCahan, G. R., and Monafo, W. W. 1977. Fluid resuscitation in a porcine burn shock model. J Surg Res 23:405–414.
Walker, P. G., Constable, P. D., Morin, D. E., Foreman, J. H., Drackley, J. K., and Thurmon, J. C. 1998. Comparison of hypertonic saline-dextran solution and lactated Ringer's solution for resuscitating severely dehydrated calves with diarrhea. JAVMA 213:113–121.
Waterman, A. 1977. A review of the diagnosis and treatment of fluid and electrolyte disorders in the horse. Equine Vet J 9:43–48.

26 DIURETICS

DEBORAH T. KOCHEVAR

Renal Physiology
- **Nephron Function**
- **Renal Epithelial Transport and Secretion**

Principles of Diuretic Use
- **Overview**
- **Edema Formation**
- **Diuretic Tolerance**

Inhibitors of Carbonic Anhydrase
- **Chemistry/Formulations**
- **Mechanisms and Sites of Action**
- **Absorption and Elimination**
- **Toxicity, Adverse Effects, Contraindications, and Drug Interactions**
- **Therapeutic Uses**

Osmotic Diuretics
- **Chemistry/Formulations**
- **Mechanisms and Sites of Action**
- **Absorption and Elimination**
- **Adverse Effects and Drug Interactions**
- **Contraindications**
- **Therapeutic Uses**

Inhibitors of Na^+-K^+-$2Cl^-$ Symport (Loop, or High-Ceiling, Diuretics)
- **Chemistry/Formulations**
- **Mechanisms and Sites of Action**
- **Absorption and Elimination**
- **Toxicity, Adverse Effects, Contraindications, and Drug Interactions**
- **Therapeutic Uses**

Inhibitors of Na^+-Cl^- Symport (Thiazide and Thiazide-like Diuretics)
- **Chemistry/Formulations**
- **Mechanisms and Sites of Action**
- **Absorption and Elimination**
- **Toxicity, Adverse Effects, Contraindications, and Drug Interactions**
- **Therapeutic Uses**

Inhibitors of Renal Epithelial Sodium Channels (K^+-Sparing Diuretics)
- **Chemistry/Formulations**
- **Mechanisms and Sites of Action**
- **Absorption and Elimination**
- **Toxicity, Adverse Effects, Contraindications, and Drug Interactions**
- **Therapeutic Use**

Antagonists of Mineralocorticoid Receptors (Aldosterone Antagonists and K^+-Sparing Diuretics)
- **Chemistry/Formulations**
- **Mechanisms and Sites of Action**
- **Absorption and Elimination**
- **Toxicity, Adverse Effects, Contraindications, and Drug Interactions**
- **Therapeutic Uses**

Aquaretics

Chapter 25 presents the physiological basis for fluid and electrolyte balance, including discussion of selected renal mechanisms for regulation of water, sodium, chloride, potassium, hydrogen, and bicarbonate. In this chapter these concepts will be extended in order to understand the mechanism of action, therapeutic uses, and side effects of diuretic agents. The history of diuretics dates back to consumption by Paleolithic humans of caffeine-containing plants. Besides xanthine derivatives such as caffeine, osmotic diuretics were clinically important prior to the 20th century. The use of mercurial diuretics, now therapeutically obsolete, began in the early 1900s and was followed by introduction of the first modern diuretic, acetazolamide, in the mid-1950s. By the late 1950s and early 1960s the formulary of modern diuretics included chlorothiazide, furosemide, and potassium-sparing diuretics (Morrison 1997). These drugs and their relatives constitute the mainstays of diuretic treatment. Although not currently available for clinical veterinary use, a new class of diuretic agents, aquaretics, have recently emerged and will likely become clinically relevant.

RENAL PHYSIOLOGY

Nephron Function. Knowledge of renal anatomy and physiology is essential to understanding the mechanism of action of diuretic drugs. Although a thorough review of these topics is beyond the scope of this text, a brief overview of nephron function is provided. The basic functional unit of the kidney is the nephron, which consists of a filtering apparatus, the glomerulus, connected to an extended tubular structure that reabsorbs and conditions the glomerular ultrafiltrate to produce urine. Each kidney is composed of thousands of nephron units. Fig. 26.1 is a schematic drawing of a single nephron unit, indicating the broad subdivisions of nephron segments and the sites of action of diuretic

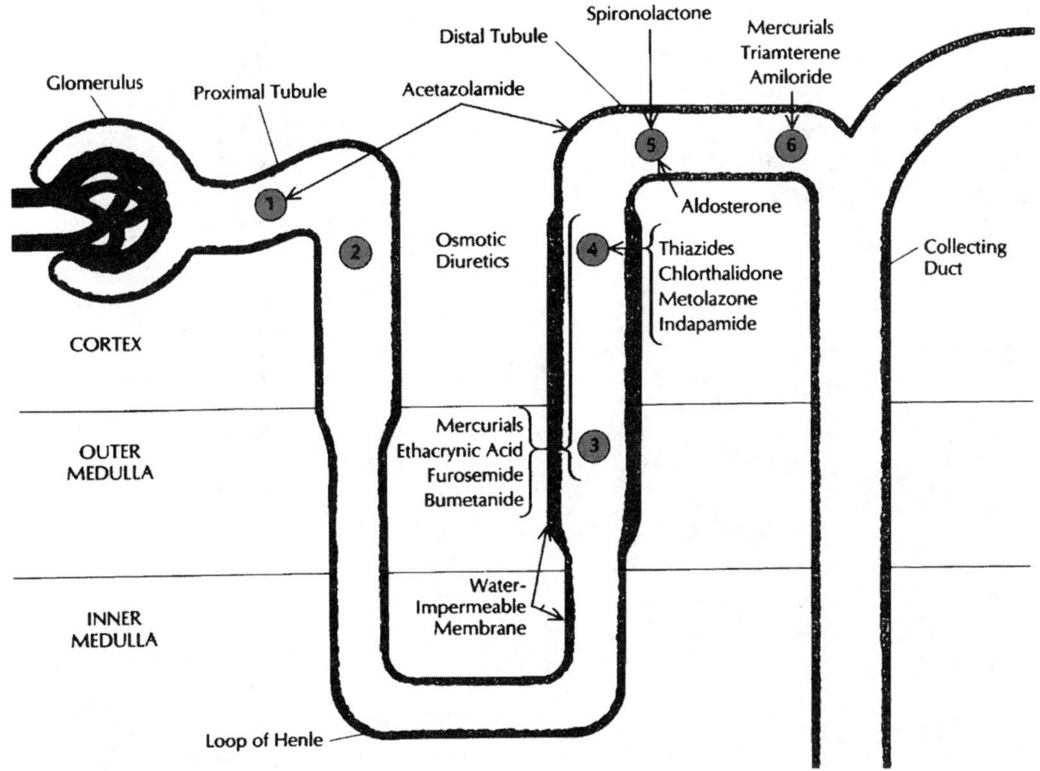

FIG. 26.1—Locations within the nephron where diuretic agents exert their effects.

agents. This diagram provides the simplest nomenclature for nephron segments. As knowledge of the function and epithelial morphology of each segment has increased, the tubular portion of the nephron has been subdivided into approximately 14 shorter segments referred to by a standardized nomenclature (Kriz and Kaissling 1992).

Formation of urine starts in the glomerulus, where a portion of plasma water is filtered through fenestrated glomerular capillary endothelial cells, a basement membrane, and, finally, filtration slit diaphragms formed by the visceral epithelial cells that cover the basement membrane on its urinary space side. The filtrate collects in Bowman's space, a double-walled invagination that forms a cup around the glomerular capillaries. From Bowman's capsule the filtered fluid passes into the proximal tubule and begins its passage through the renal tubular system. Small solutes are actively filtered with plasma water while larger elements, such as protein and macromolecules, are retained by the glomerular filter. The rate of filtration in each nephron (referred to as the single-nephron glomerular filtration rate, SNGFR) is a function of hydrostatic pressure in the glomerular capillaries (P_{GC}), hydrostatic pressure in Bowman's space or the proximal tubule (P_T), mean colloid osmotic pressure in the glomerular capillaries (Π_{GC}), colloid osmotic pressure in the proximal tubule (Π_T), and the ultrafiltration coefficient (K_f). The relationship between these forces is summarized by the following equation:

$$\text{SNGFR} = K_f[(P_{GC} - P_T) - (\Pi_{GC} - \Pi_T)]$$

This equation is usually simplified by defining $P_{GC} - P_T$ as the transcapillary hydraulic pressure difference (ΔP) and eliminating Π_T since little protein is filtered. Hence the equation below becomes the most useful expression:

$$\text{SNGFR} = K_f(\Delta P - \Pi_{GC})$$

Whereas K_f is determined by the properties of the filtering membrane, ΔP is primarily determined by the proportion of arterial pressure conveyed to the glomerular capillaries. As resistance changes in pre- and postglomerular vessels, ΔP varies. The pressure Π_{GC} depends upon the concentration of protein in arterial blood as well as the actual flow of blood to the nephron. SNGFR is an important parameter that may affect, or be affected by, the action of diuretic drugs.

Ultrafiltrate from the glomerulus enters the proximal tubule from Bowman's capsule. By the time urine exits the distal tubule and collecting duct, better than 99% of ultrafiltrate volume will be reabsorbed. Fig. 26.2 (left

Nephron Segment	Transport Systems
Proximal tubule • Isotonic reabsorption • Reabsorbs the bulk (approximately 65%) of filtered water and solute.	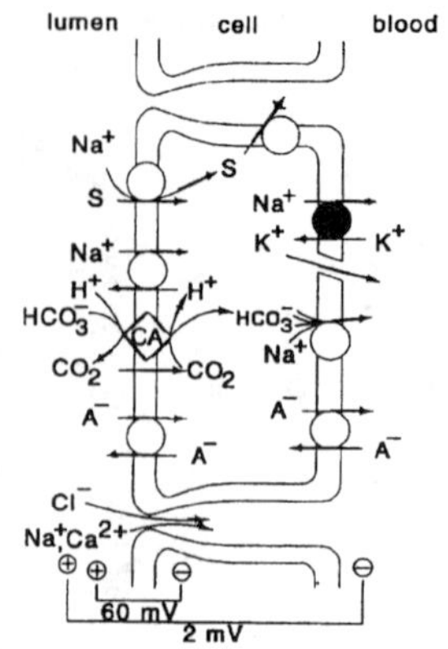 lumen cell blood Na^+ S S Na^+ K^+ K^+ Na^+ H^+ H^+ HCO_3^- CA HCO_3^- Na^+ CO_2 CO_2 A^- A^- A^- A^- Cl^- Na^+ Ca^{2+} ⊕ ⊕ ⊖ ⊖ 60 mV 2 mV
Thick ascending limb of Henle's loop • Actively transports sodium but effectively impermeable to water. • Location of macula densa that senses NaCl concentration in filtrate.	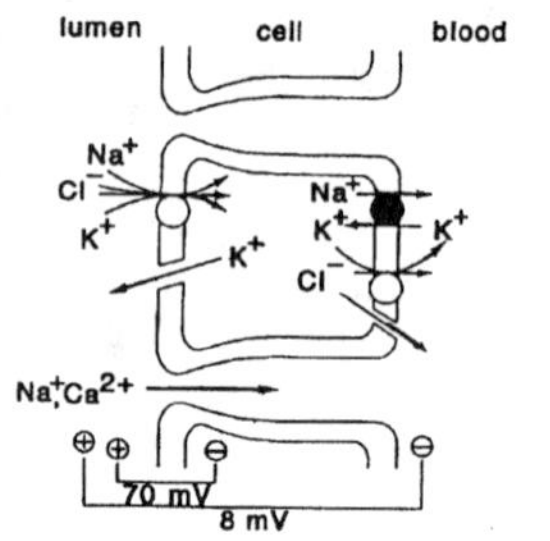 lumen cell blood Na^+ Cl^- K^+ K^+ Na^+ K^+ K^+ Cl^- Na^+ Ca^{2+} ⊕ ⊕ ⊖ ⊖ 70 mV 8 mV
Distaltubule cell • Actively transports sodium but effectively impermeable to water.	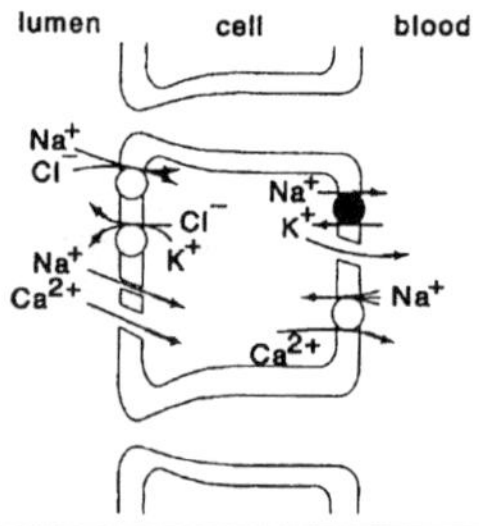 lumen cell blood Na^+ Cl^- Na^+ K^+ Cl^- K^+ Na^+ Ca^{2+} Na^+ Ca^{2+}
Collecting duct system (includes connecting tubule and collecting duct) • Principal cell (top) • Intercalated cells Type A (middle) Type B (bottom) • Principal cells of connecting tubule are responsive to aldosterone. • Collecting ducts are responsive to vasopressin.	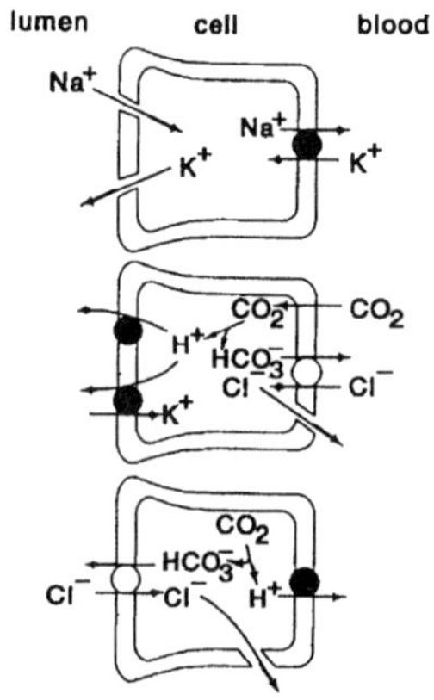 lumen cell blood Na^+ Na^+ K^+ K^+ CO_2 CO_2 H^+ HCO_3^- Cl^- Cl^- K^+ CO_2 HCO_3^- Cl^- Cl^- H^+

FIG. 26.2—Reabsorption in the nephron. General characteristics of segmental tubular reabsorption *(left)* and details of transport mechanisms in each segment *(right)*. Six of seven basic mechanisms for transport of solutes across renal epithelial membranes are shown. Channel-mediated diffusion (shown as an *interrupted cell membrane)* allows solutes to move passively through the membrane. Carrier-mediated, or facilitated, transport *(unfilled circle, single arrow)* (also referred to as a uniport) allows a single substance to move with, but not against, an electrochemical gradient. ATP-driven primary active transport *(filled circles)*, usually in the form of Na^+,K^+-ATPase, mediates the bulk of renal transport and can move solutes against an electrochemical gradient. Secondary active transport utilizes the potential energy stored in electrochemical gradients to move solutes across membranes against their gradients. Two types of secondary active transport are shown. Cotransport of solutes (S), such as glucose, inorganic phosphate, and amino acids, with sodium in the same direction occurs through symports *(unfilled circles, two arrows, each pointing in the same direction across the cell membrane)*. Countertransport of solutes in the opposite direction occurs through antiports *(unfilled circles, two arrows, each pointing in a different direction across the cell membrane)*. Simple diffusion down a concentration gradient can occur through cell membranes if the solute is lipid soluble. Simple diffusion that occurs between cells (paracellular) is shown *(arrows directed between cells)*. A final transport mechanism, solvent drag, can occur across membranes through aqueous pores or between cells *(not shown)*. A^- = organic acid (anion).

TABLE 26.1—Approximate renal tubular reabsorption (%) of filtered substances

	Proximal tubule	Thick ascending limb of Henle's loop	Distal tubule	Total reabsorption (all segments)
H_2O	60	20	19	99
Na^+	60	34	6	100
Cl^-	55	38	6	99
K^+	60	25	−5	80
HCO_3^-	90	0	10	100
Ca^{++}	60	30	9	99
HPO_4^{--}	70	10	0	80
Mg^{++}	30	60	0	90
Urea	Reabsorbed	Secreted	Reabsorbed	—

column) summarizes the characteristics of reabsorption in broad sections of the renal tubules. The thick ascending limb of the loop of Henle is of particular importance since this is the site of action of the most potent diuretic drugs. Approximately 25% of filtered solutes are reabsorbed in the loop of Henle, and most of this reabsorption occurs in the thick ascending limb. The thick ascending limb also makes a critical contact with the afferent arteriole through a cluster of specialized epithelial cells referred to as the macula densa. The macula densa monitors the NaCl concentration in filtrate leaving the loop of Henle. Together with extraglomerular mesangial cells and renin-producing cells of the glomerular arterioles, these components form the juxtaglomerular apparatus. A high concentration of salt in tubular fluid prompts a signal to the afferent arteriole causing constriction and decreased SNGFR. This, in combination with other responses, constitutes the tubuloglomerular feedback mechanism that protects the animal from salt and water wasting. Alternatively, excessive volume expansion causes the macula densa to inhibit renin release from the juxtaglomerular cells, leading to dilatation of the afferent arteriole. Because the ascending loop of Henle is poorly water permeable, tubular fluid at the end of this segment is dilute despite the presence of renal interstitial tissues with increasing osmolality toward the medulla. The renal interstitial concentration gradient, amplified by the countercurrent mechanism, provides the driving force for passive water reabsorption later in the nephron. The collecting duct system described in Fig. 26.2 includes the connecting tubule (also referred to as the late distal tubule), which is responsive to aldosterone. If extracellular fluid (ECF) sodium concentrations are too low, aldosterone is secreted, causing increased sodium reabsorption in the connecting tubule. Vasopressin, also referred to as arginine vasopressin (AVP) and antidiuretic hormone, is secreted when plasma osmolality is elevated or ECF volume contracts. Stimulation by vasopressin leads to receptor-mediated opening of water channels in the collecting ducts with subsequent retention of water and expansion of ECF volume. In general, modification of filtrate as it passes through the nephron is controlled at two different levels. Systemic regulatory mechanisms and effector hormones such as renin-angiotensin-aldosterone, natriuretic peptides, and vasopressin ensure the balance of salt and water metabolism. Cellular feedback loops and glomerulotubular balance modify tubular function and influence single-cell homeostasis. Diuretics may interfere at either or both levels to cause increases in salt and water excretion.

Renal Epithelial Transport and Secretion. Just as knowledge of functional renal anatomy has increased, so has understanding of cellular mechanisms for transport of solutes across renal epithelium. Since the early 1990s, many ion transporters and cotransporters that serve as targets for diuretic drugs have been cloned and characterized at the molecular level (Xu et al. 1994; Gamba et al. 1993, 1994). Fig. 26.2 (right column) summarizes the general mechanisms for renal epithelial transport in different segments of the renal tubules. Table 26.1 provides approximations of percent renal tubular reabsorption of selected substances by nephron segment.

In addition to ion transport mechanisms, the kidney also has highly effective and separate transport systems for movement of organic acids and bases. Energy from ATP-driven active transport is used to establish gradients for secondary active transport of both anions and cations. Families of proteins representing both anion and cation transporters move a wide variety of related substances. While these transporters have flexible stereospecificity, structural features of anions and cations that are efficiently transported have been identified (Jackson 1996). The presence of anion and cation transporters is essential for most highly protein-bound diuretic drugs to gain access to their site of action, the lumen of the renal tubule. Loop and thiazide diuretics and acetazolamide are secreted through the organic acid pathway, and amiloride and triamterene via an organic base transporter (Brater 1998). Renal insufficiency accompanied by reduced creatinine clearance decreases delivery of diuretic drugs to their secretory site and hence to their site of action. Accumulation of endogenous organic acids during chronic renal failure may result in competition with diuretics for transport at proximal tubule secretion sites (Brater 1993).

PRINCIPLES OF DIURETIC USE

Overview. The current therapeutic goal of diuretic use is increased excretion of sodium followed by water. The degree of sodium loss in the urine (referred to as natriuresis or, in combination with chloride, saluresis) varies with the mechanism of action of the drug. All except osmotic diuretics inhibit specific enzymes, transport proteins, hormone receptors, or ion channels that function, directly or indirectly, in renal tubular sodium reabsorption. Although saluresis is the primary clinical goal, diuretics also alter elimination of other ions to varying degrees (e.g., K^+, H^+, Ca^{2+}, Mg^{2+}, Cl^-, HCO_3^-, phosphates) and may affect renal hemodynamics. Diuretic-induced depletion of circulating blood volume may lead to adverse effects if therapy is not well monitored. For example, in patients with chronic hepatic disease hypoalbuminemia leads to a decrease in plasma colloidal osmotic pressure and shifts in fluid to other spaces. Even a small diuretic-induced decrease in arterial perfusion under these circumstances may lead to severe exacerbation of disease. Older animals and those with cardiac or renal disease are also at increased risk for adverse effects if diuretic-induced hypovolemia goes untreated. Because these groups are also the primary target groups for diuretic use, rational use of diuretic drugs is essential. Table 26.2 summarizes selected features of diuretic drugs most commonly used in veterinary medicine.

Edema Formation. The most common indication for diuretic use is mobilization of tissue edema. Understanding the physiological principles underlying edema formation depends upon an understanding of net capillary filtration (see Chap. 25 and the equation above for SNGFR). Net capillary filtration (NF), or fluid flux out of a capillary, is dependent upon Starling forces inside and outside the vessel. NF is determined by the difference between ΔP, which represents the hydrostatic pressure inside the capillary lumen minus the hydrostatic pressure in the interstitial fluid, and $\Delta\Pi$, representing the oncotic pressure inside the capillary minus the oncotic pressure in the interstitial fluid. This value multiplied by a filtration coefficient (K_f), representing the permeability of the capillary wall, predicts the movement of fluid into and out of the vascular compartment.

Normally the flux of fluid out of capillaries is equaled by the lymph flow away from the site. If flux exceeds flow, edema results. A simplistic explanation of edema formation starts with a decrease in plasma oncotic pressure that leads to loss of intravascular volume to the interstitial space. The loss of intravascular fluid leads to decreased plasma volume, which leads to renal salt and water retention. Eventually salt and water retention causes increased plasma volume, increased plasma hydrostatic pressure, and increased flux of fluid out of the capillary, resulting in accumulation of edema in the interstitium. In veterinary medicine the most

TABLE 26.2—Summary of diuretic drugs commonly used in veterinary medicine.

Drug	Indications, dosages, route of administration	Mechanism of action, route of elimination	Adverse effects
Mannitol	*Oliguric renal failure:* 0.25–0.5 gm/kg IV over 15–20 min. If diuresis occurs, may repeat every 4–6 hr up to a dose of 1.5 gm/kg in 12–24 hr. Monitor for urine production and dehydration. *Acute glaucoma:* 1–2 gm/kg IV over 15–20 min; withhold water for 30–60 min after dosing. *Increased intracranial pressure:*	Osmotic diuretic Renal elimination 1.5 gm/kg IV once.	Hyper- or hypo-osmolality Hypokalemia Acute hypotension associated with hyponatremia
Furosemide	*Edema of cardiac, hepatic or renal origin:* SMALL ANIMALS: 1– 3 mg/kg every 8–24 hr PO for chronic use; 2–5 mg/kg every 4–6 hr IV, IM, SC (dogs); 1–2 mg/kg every 12 hr up to 4 mg/kg every 8–12 hr IV, IM, SC, PO (cats). LARGE ANIMALS: 0.5–1.0 mg/kg twice daily or to effect. *Other uses:* Decrease bleeding in horses with EIPH (controversial). Establish diuresis in renal failure. Promote excretion of other substances (e.g.,other drugs, elevated electrolytes).	Inhibits Na+-K+-2Cl- symport. Referred to as loop or high ceiling diuretic. Primarily renal excretion of unchanged drug with remainder biotransformed by glucuronidation and renally excreted.	Hypokalemia Hypochloremic alkalosis Ototoxicity Hyperglycemia GI irritation Enhances aminoglycoside nephrotoxicity
Acetazolamide	Primarily ophthalmic use. Adjunctive therapy of glaucoma in dogs and cats: 10–30 mg/kg divided and administered 2–3 times daily orally. 50 mg/kg IV once.	Carbonic anhydrase inhibitor. Renal elimination.	Hypokalemia Acidosis Urinary tract calculi Hepatic encephalopathy

common causes of edema are cardiac (usually congestive heart failure; CHF), hepatic and renal disease.

CHF causes decreased cardiac output and decreased renal blood flow, leading to activation of the renin-angiotensin-aldosterone system followed by renal retention of salt and water. High baroreceptor activity causes increased peripheral vascular resistance and increased vasopressin, which lead to further salt and water retention by the kidneys. Increased central venous pressure caused by increased left ventricular end-diastolic pressures cause increased capillary hydrostatic pressure. All of these factors lead to greater fluid flux out of vessels, resulting in edema related to cardiac disease.

Diuretic Tolerance. This phenomenon has been best described in humans and can occur following short- or long-term administration of diuretics. Short-term tolerance, or diuretic braking, refers to a decrease in response to diuretics following administration of the first dose. Although the mechanism for braking is unclear, it may be mediated by sympathetic responsiveness and activation of the renin-angiotensin-aldosterone system, both of which act to restore circulating volume. Other mechanisms may include decreased arterial blood pressure, which reduces pressure-natriuresis, or alterations in atrial natriuretic peptide. Braking can be prevented by restoration of diuretic-induced volume loss. Long-term use of loop diuretics may cause hypertrophy of distal nephron segments that are continually flooded with higher-than-normal concentrations of sodium in tubular fluid. As distal segments hypertrophy and expression of renal epithelial transporters increases, more sodium is reabsorbed distally, blunting the initial saluretic effect achieved at the level of the loop of Henle. This form of tolerance can often be overcome by combinations of thiazides and loop diuretics that effectively block sodium reabsorption in both the loop of Henle and the distal nephron.

INHIBITORS OF CARBONIC ANHYDRASE

Chemistry/Formulations. This class of drugs was discovered as a result of the observation that sulfanilamide chemotherapeutic agents were capable of causing metabolic acidosis by inhibition of carbonic anhydrase (CA). Screening of sulfanilamides resulted in identification of compounds whose predominant mechanism of action was CA inhibition. These drugs have been used sparingly in veterinary medicine as diuretics and are more commonly used for ophthalmic purposes (see Chap. 55). The prototype drug in this class, acetazolamide (Diamox®, Dazamide®), is available in tablets (125 and 250 mg), extended-release capsules (500 mg), and injectable (500 mg per vial). Other CA inhibitors include preparations for oral use, dichlorphenamide (Daranide®) and methazolamide (Neptazane®), and a recently approved topical drug, dorzolamide (Trusopt®), for ophthalmic use.

Mechanisms and Sites of Action

RENAL MECHANISMS. Drugs in this class are active in the CA-rich segments of the nephron, in particular the proximal tubule. Noncompetitive, reversible inhibition of CA located in the luminal and basolateral membranes (type IV CA) as well as in the cytoplasm (type II CA) results in decreased formation of carbonic acid from CO_2 and H_2O (see Fig. 26.2 and equation below):

$$HCO_3^- + H^+ \leftrightarrow H_2CO_3 \leftrightarrow H_2O + CO_2$$

Reduction in the amount of carbonic acid yields fewer H^+ within proximal tubular cells. Because H^+ is normally exchanged for Na^+ from the tubular lumen, less Na^+ is reabsorbed and more is available to combine with urinary HCO_3^-. Diuresis is established when water is excreted with sodium bicarbonate. As sodium bicarbonate is trapped in the urine and eliminated, less HCO_3^- is returned to plasma, and a systemic acidosis eventually develops. As a result of the systemic acidosis, H^+ becomes available, Na^+ reabsorption is reestablished, and diuresis decreases. Continual use of CA inhibitors is therefore self-limiting in terms of diuretic action. Diuresis induced by CA inhibitors is mild due to incomplete inhibition of CA, redundancy of Na^+ transporting systems in the proximal tubule, and rescue of Na^+ by reabsorption later in the distal tubule. Because intracellular K^+ can, to some extent, substitute for H^+ in the Na^+ reabsorption step, CA inhibitors cause enhanced K^+ excretion. As more Na^+ is presented to the distal tubule, the potential for K^+ wasting increases. CA inhibitors also decrease secretion of titratable acids and ammonia in the collecting duct (Jackson 1996). For this reason, and due to the increased excretion of sodium bicarbonate, urine pH increases despite the decreasing systemic pH associated with CA-inhibitor-induced acidosis. This class of drugs has little, if any, effect on excretion of Ca^{2+} and Mg^{2+} but does enhance phosphate elimination.

EXTRARENAL ACTIONS. Other actions of CA inhibitors are related to the wide distribution of CA in body tissues including the eye, gastric mucosa, pancreas, central nervous system (CNS), and red blood cells. The most important therapeutic consequence is associated with CA inhibition in the eye. The ciliary processes of the eye mediate the formation of aqueous humor, which contains an abundance of HCO_3^-. This process is CA dependent and, when inhibited, leads to a decreased rate of formation of aqueous humor and subsequent reduction in intraocular pressure. Although not therapeutically relevant in veterinary medicine, CA inhibition in the CNS has been associated with anticonvulsant actions attributed to this class of drugs.

Absorption and Elimination. Limited information is available regarding pharmacokinetics of CA inhibitors in animals. Acetazolamide gains access to the renal tubules via the organic acid secretion pathway. A dose of 22 mg/kg is reported to have an onset of action of

30 minutes, maximal effects in 2–4 hours, and a duration of action of 4–6 hours in small animals (Roberts 1985). Oral absorption of drugs in this class is good. Acetazolamide is eliminated primarily through the kidneys.

Toxicity, Adverse Effects, Contraindications, and Drug Interactions. Because CA inhibitors are sulfonamide derivatives, side effects commonly associated with sulfonamides can occur. CNS drowsiness and disorientation may occur as a result of inhibition of CA in the CNS. Because CA inhibitors decrease ammonia excretion, the severity of preexisting hepatic disease may be worsened and hepatic encephalopathy can be induced. Use is also contraindicated in patients with electrolyte disturbances (due to K^+ and Na^+ wasting) and those with metabolic or respiratory acidosis. Use in patients with severe pulmonary disease who cannot respond to drug-induced metabolic acidosis with respiratory compensation is also contraindicated. Because CA inhibitors alkalinize the urine, calcium phosphate calculi formation is enhanced, and excretion of weak organic bases is reduced. Rare blood dyscrasias associated with CA inhibitors have also been reported in the human, but not the veterinary, literature.

Therapeutic Uses. The primary indication for use of CA inhibitors is to inhibit production of aqueous humor and reduce intraocular pressure. In veterinary medicine, acetazolamide (10–30 mg/kg divided and given three times daily) and methazolamide (2–10 mg/kg given 2–3 times daily) are used in dogs for management of glaucoma. A one-time IV dose of acetazolamide (50 mg/kg) has been reported for management of acute glaucoma. Methazolamide is often preferred over acetazolamide for long-term glaucoma therapy due to fewer side effects. CA inhibitors are also used preoperatively to lower ocular pressure.

A recently approved topical CA inhibitor, dorzolamide (previously referred to as MK-507), offers several advantages for treatment of increased intraocular pressure (Mindel 1997). Although systemic CA inhibitors are effective at decreasing intraocular pressures, use of these drugs is often accompanied by undesirable side effects (see above). Compared to other CA inhibitors, one drop of a 2% ophthalmic solution of dorzolamide administered three times daily has limited systemic effects. Ocular side effects may include a stinging or burning sensation in the eye as reported in human medicine and development of an allergic response to the drug. Dorzolamide lacks the cardiovascular and pulmonary side effects that can occur with other treatments for increased intraocular pressure associated with glaucoma (e.g., beta blockers, cholinergic agonists). Dorzolamide has been used in the contralateral eye of dogs with primary glaucoma to prevent development of bilateral disease and has been used to treat secondary glaucoma in dogs and cats. Dorzolamide is probably not effective in acute closed-angle glaucoma. A frequent side effect reported in humans medicated with topical dorzolamide is the presence of a bitter or metal-like taste postmedication. This is apparently associated with drug-laden lacrimal fluid draining into the oropharynx and causing inhibition of CA and accumulation of bicarbonate (Mindel 1997).

In human medicine, CA inhibitors have been used as an adjunctive therapy for epilepsy and in management of acute mountain (high-altitude) sickness. In both human and veterinary medicine, the use of CA inhibitors as diuretics has limited effectiveness due to the rapid development of tolerance. Theoretically, acetazolamide could be used to manage metabolic alkalosis, but this is not a typical clinical practice in veterinary medicine.

OSMOTIC DIURETICS

Chemistry/Formulations. Solutions used as osmotic diuretics contain simple solutes of low molecular weight that have an increased osmolarity relative to plasma. These substances are typically freely filtered by the glomerulus, undergo limited tubular reabsorption, and are pharmacologically inert. The most common osmotic diuretic is mannitol, a six-carbon nonmetabolizable polyalcohol with a molecular weight of 182. Other agents include glycerin, isosorbide, urea, and hypertonic saline solutions. Because mannitol is the most commonly used osmotic diuretic in both human and veterinary medicine, subsequent discussion will focus primarily on this drug. Concentrated mannitol (15–25%) may crystallize at cooler temperatures, in which case the drug can often be resolubilized by warming the solution. Prior to administration, the solution should be cooled and any remaining crystals removed using an in-line intravenous (IV) filter. Veterinary-approved mannitol, USP, for IV use in dogs contains 180 mg/mL (990 mOsm/L); human products (Osmitrol®, Resectisol®) ranging from 5% (275 mOsm/L) to 25% (1375 mOsm/L) are available for IV administration.

Mechanisms and Sites of Action. Hyperosmolar solutions exert part of their effects by establishing an osmotic gradient between plasma and tissue water compartments. Acute effects of this gradient include decreases in hematocrit, blood viscosity, plasma sodium, plasma pH, and, to some degree, the volume of solid organs. Hence, parenchymal dehydration and acute hemodilution are theoretically related as long as the osmotically active particles are effectively separated by a relatively solute-impermeable barrier.

RENAL MECHANISMS. Initially osmotic diuretics were thought to act primarily at the level of the proximal tubule by limiting the movement of water from the lumen into the interstitial space. Water retained in the tubular lumen diluted concentrations of sodium and other ions, reduced ion reabsorption, and promoted diuresis. It is now held that osmotic diuretics, in particular mannitol, have effects throughout the length of the tubule, with the most prominent action occurring in the loop of Henle. Sodium reabsorption is markedly reduced in the descending and thin limbs of the loop of Henle, as determined by studies in dogs and rats. Sodium load to the thick ascending limb of the loop of Henle and to the distal tubule is consequently increased, but the nephron fails to recapture the increased loads of salt and water. As demonstrated in the dog, sodium reabsorption is also thought to be directly inhibited in medullary collecting ducts (Better et al. 1997).

Other reported renal effects of mannitol include increases in cortical and medullary blood flow due to a decrease in renal vascular resistance, impairment of urinary concentration, dilution by dissipation of medullary hypertonicity, an increase in GFR during renal hypoperfusion (may vary according to species), and an increase in urinary excretion of other electrolytes (e.g., K^+, Ca^{2+}, Mg^{2+}, phosphate, bicarbonate) (Better et al. 1997). Mannitol may also prompt the release of atrial natriuretic factor (ANF) and vasodilatory prostaglandins. Inhibition of renin release by mannitol has also been described.

EXTRARENAL MECHANISMS. The actions of mannitol extend beyond the renal effects and include changes in blood rheology, direct transient effects on vascular tone, and increases in cardiac output. In addition to decreasing the hematocrit by hemodilution, mannitol decreases the volume, rigidity, and cohesiveness of red blood cell membranes. The combination of reduced viscosity and reduced mechanical resistance presumably leads to enhanced blood flow. Mannitol-induced increases in cardiac output are thought to be related to reduced peripheral resistance and reduced afterload, a transient increase in preload, and mild positive inotropy. Mannitol may also exert a cytoprotective effect by acting as an oxygen-free radical scavenger (Paczynski 1997).

Absorption and Elimination. Mannitol is not metabolized and is handled as an inert substance by the body. Studies in dogs and humans indicate that mannitol distribution and elimination follow a two-compartment model (Cloyd et al. 1986; Rudehill et al. 1993). The distribution half-life of intravenously administered mannitol is measured in minutes. Elimination half-life is dose dependent and ranges from 0.5 to 1.5 hours for doses between 0.25 and 1.5 g/kg. Mannitol is eliminated rapidly by the kidneys unless renal function is impaired. As a result, penetration of mannitol into tissues is limited by rapidly falling plasma concentrations. Mannitol and urea are administered intravenously in a slow bolus over 15–30 minutes. Glycerin and isosorbide are administered orally. Of the available osmotic diuretics, only glycerin is eliminated by biotransformation.

Adverse Effects and Drug Interactions

ACUTE ADVERSE EFFECTS. Pulse pressure and mean arterial blood pressure usually increase transiently with mannitol administration. However, acute hypotensive, hyponatremic effects of mannitol administration have been reported, especially subsequent to rapid infusion in dehydrated individuals. The mechanism for this acute vasodilatory effect is not well understood, but the problem can largely be prevented by appropriate rates of administration (0.25–1.5 g/kg over 15–30 min). Acute hyponatremia may account for the nausea and vomiting that are sometimes observed with mannitol infusion. Rapid expansion of plasma volume related to attraction of fluid into the vascular compartment may precipitate CHF or pulmonary edema in certain patient populations. However, because the drug is cleared rapidly this problem is not common unless renal function is impaired.

DEHYDRATION AND ELECTROLYTE DISTURBANCES. Because the ratio of the volume of fluid eliminated in urine to the volume of mannitol administered is high, care should be taken to avoid hypertonic dehydration. Circulating plasma volume tends to be preserved as hypertonic dehydration develops, making it harder to clinically detect that a problem exists. The presence of dehydration and significant hypernatremia should be closely monitored using body weight, urine output, and other clinical parameters. In addition to hypertonic dehydration, loss of other electrolytes, including potassium, phosphate, and magnesium, can lead to clinically significant cardiac arrhythmias and neuromuscular complications.

HYPEROSMOLAR STATE AND OSMOTIC COMPENSATION. The phenomenon of osmotic compensation occurs when cells respond to prolonged treatment with a hyperosmolar agent by increasing the presence of intracellular, idiogenic osmoles. Compensation is thought to occur rapidly when the osmolality of plasma is increased by 25 mOsm/kg or more above normal. Newly generated, osmotically active intracellular particles counteract the dehydrating effect of hyperosmolar plasma. Osmotic compensation can limit therapeutic effectiveness by decreasing the osmotic gradient from tissue to plasma. Increased intracellular osmolarity may also promote conditions, especially in the brain, where iatrogenic edema may occur. The risk of edema formation is increased if a hyperosmolar state is reversed rapidly, leaving the intracellular osmoles as the most osmotically active site. To prevent this complication, the duration of return of plasma to normal osmolality should be approximately equal to the duration of the hyperosmolar state.

REBOUND PHENOMENON. Rebound intracranial hypertension has been defined as a significant increase in tension of cerebrospinal fluid following a period of reduction in cerebrospinal fluid tension caused by administration of hypertonic solutions. The rebound phenomenon is thought to be caused by penetration of osmotically active particles into brain tissue, thus creating an osmotic gradient favoring the inward movement of water and edema formation. In the case of the blood-brain barrier (BBB), tonicity, or osmotic effectiveness, can be expressed using an osmotic reflection coefficient for a given solute. The ideal osmotic agent has a value of 1, and a fully permeable agent exerts no osmotic force and has a value of 0. It is relevant to note that the BBB is much less permeable to sodium, chloride, and mannitol and relatively more permeable to glucose and urea (Paczynski 1997). Hence if urea penetrates brain tissue and the concentration of urea in the plasma subsequently decreases, tissue urea becomes the most attractive osmotic draw and a likely site for iatrogenic edema formation. The incidence of true rebound phenomena is unclear and, as with other adverse effects of osmotherapy, may often be prevented by cautious use of hyperosmolar agents in patients with renal impairment or fluid imbalances.

Contraindications. The use of mannitol in patients with ongoing intracranial hemorrhage, anuric renal failure, severe dehydration, or pulmonary congestion or edema is contraindicated.

Adequate fluid therapy should be administered to dehydrated animals prior to administration of mannitol. Mannitol should not be added to whole-blood products unless at least 20 mEq/L of sodium chloride is added to the solution; otherwise, pseudoagglutination may occur.

Therapeutic Uses. Mannitol is used in the prophylaxis and treatment of renal failure, for the reduction of intracranial and intraocular pressure, and with other diuretics to mobilize edema. For reasons already discussed, short-term use of mannitol is most effective to prevent adverse effects and decreased therapeutic efficacy.

PROPHYLAXIS OF ACUTE RENAL FAILURE. Anuric patients should not be routinely treated with mannitol, although a small (0.25–0.5 g/kg), single test dose may be used to try and induce diuresis. Administration of mannitol to patients with renal dysfunction must be done cautiously to prevent problems associated with decreased elimination and prolonged hyperosmolality. Acute renal failure (ARF) may be caused extrinsically (pre- and postrenal failure) or intrinsically, often associated with acute renal tubular necrosis (ATN). Mannitol has been found to be effective in limiting the decrease in GFR caused by ATN if administered before the ischemic insult or exposure to nephrotoxins. Protection of tubules from necrosis may be due to dilution of nephrotoxic substances, reduction of swelling of tubular elements, or removal of tubular casts that are obstructing urine flow. In human medicine, mannitol has been shown to be clearly beneficial in the preservation of kidneys for transplant and for decreasing the incidence of posttransplant ARF. Fewer data are available to support the general value of mannitol for treatment of ARF outside the area of transplantation (Better et al. 1997). In vascular and open-heart surgery, prophylactic mannitol maintains urine flow but not GFR. Some evidence suggests that mannitol administration in patients with established ATN may increase the conversion of oliguric to nonoliguric patients (Levinsky and Bernard 1988).

REDUCTION OF INTRACRANIAL PRESSURE. Osmotherapy has been used for decades to decrease intracranial pressure (ICP). Reduction in ICP is rapid and usually appears within minutes of completion of administration, with maximum effects within the hour. Several theories have been formulated to account for the effectiveness of mannitol in reducing ICP. The osmotic theory holds that brain shrinkage occurs as a result of osmotically driven movement of fluid from tissue and into the vascular compartment. Sensitive, high-resolution imaging methods seem to support the significance of osmotically induced changes in brain water content (Betz et al. 1989). The hemodynamic theory of ICP reduction states that cerebral blood volume is decreased as a result of decreased blood viscosity and increased cerebral perfusion pressure, both of which act to enhance oxygen delivery to the brain. Increased oxygen delivery to the brain is thought to trigger a compensatory reduction in vascular caliber and secondarily a reduction in cerebral blood volume. Detractors of this idea suggest that mannitol is just as likely to decrease blood viscosity as a result of hemoconcentration secondary to hypertonic dehydration. While attention to fluid replacement should prevent dehydration, it has recently been suggested that alternative agents, such as hypertonic saline, are safer and equally effective at reducing ICP. Hypertonic saline has been shown to establish a strong transendothelial osmotic gradient but without the tendency to reduce intravascular volume (Prough and Zornow 1998). Finally, the diuretic theory of ICP reduction suggests that mannitol-induced decreases in central venous pressure translate directly to decreases in ICP due to the valveless communication between the central venous system and the jugular drainage system. This effect may be more important in sustaining, rather than inducing, a decrease in ICP (Paczynski 1997). Regardless of the theory, mannitol has been used for temporary reduction of ICP in patients with a variety of intracranial lesions as well as those with spinal cord trauma and edema. Evidence of ongoing intracranial hemorrhage is considered a contraindication for mannitol administration.

OTHER USES. Osmotic diuretics have also been used successfully to control intraocular pressure during acute glaucoma attacks and to reduce intraocular pressure before or after ophthalmic surgery. Decreases in intraocular pressure occur by loss of intraocular water to hyperosmolar plasma. As the vitreous shrinks, the lens moves posteriorly and the iridocorneal angle opens, improving drainage from the eye. The duration of action depends upon the degree to which the osmotic diuretic is excluded from ocular fluids. Mannitol is reported to increase retinal oxygen tension and is used at a dose of 1–2 g/kg at a rate of 1 mL/kg/min to reduce intraocular pressure in dogs.

INHIBITORS OF NA^+-K^+-$2CL^-$ SYMPORT (LOOP, OR HIGH-CEILING, DIURETICS). Drugs belonging to this class are among the most potent and the most commonly prescribed diuretics, and all share a common mechanism of action. By blocking a key sodium transport mechanism in the thick ascending limb of the loop of Henle (hence the name loop diuretic), these drugs inhibit reabsorption of approximately 25% of the filtered sodium load. Nephron segments distal to the thick ascending limb (TAL) are incapable of reabsorbing the additional solute, leading to a marked (or high-ceiling) natriuresis and diuresis. Because furosemide (Lasix®) is by far the most commonly used diuretic in veterinary medicine, the remaining discussion will focus primarily on this drug (also referred to as frusemide). Other drugs in this class include ethacrynic acid (Edecrin®), bumetanide (Bumex®), and the most recent addition approved in the United States, torsemide (Demadex®).

Chemistry/Formulations. Except for ethacrynic acid, the structurally diverse drugs in this class are sulfonamide derivatives. Furosemide is light sensitive and stable under alkaline conditions; the veterinary injectable preparations (Lasix®, Diuride®, or generic; 50 mg/mL) have a light yellow color, whereas the human injectable (Lasix®; 10 mg/mL) should not be used if it appears yellow. A wide range of veterinary preparations of furosemide are available, including oral tablets approved for use in dogs and cats (12.5 mg, 50 mg), oral solution approved for use in dogs (10 mg/mL), large-animal boluses approved for use in cattle (2 g/bolus), and injectable (5%) approved for use in dogs, cats, horses not intended for food, and cattle. Milk and slaughter withdrawal time for both oral and injectable formulations for cattle is 48 hours.

Mechanisms and Sites of Action

RENAL EFFECTS. Drugs in this class block the Na^+-K^+-$2Cl^-$ symporter in the TAL by binding to the Cl^- binding site of the transporter protein. All of these drugs must be actively secreted into the tubular lumen by an organic acid pathway in order to reach and inhibit the luminal symporter. A high degree of protein binding (>95%) limits glomerular filtration of furosemide and other loop diuretics, making tubular secretion essential. The mechanism involved in Na^+ reabsorption in the TAL depends upon Na^+,K^+-ATPase activity in the basal membrane of tubular cells (see Table 26.1). The transmembrane Na^+ gradient generated by ATPase drives the Na^+-K^+-$2Cl^-$ symporter in the luminal membrane. Basolateral Cl^- conductance and luminal K^+ conductance determine membrane voltage. The polarity of K^+ and Cl^- conductances results in a lumen-positive transepithelial voltage. This voltage drives cations between tubular cells via the paracellular shunt pathway. When loop diuretics block the Na^+-K^+-$2Cl^-$ symporter, Cl^- concentrations in the cell fall, the cell becomes hyperpolarized, transepithelial voltage is disrupted, and paracellular cation reabsorption is blocked (Bleich and Gregor 1997). Because renin-producing cells in the area of the macula densa generate part of their membrane voltage via Cl^- channels, the new Cl^- equilibrium also depolarizes these cells and enhances the secretion of renin. Loop diuretics interfere with establishment of a hypertonic medullary interstitium and disrupt the countercurrent mechanism. Hence, these drugs block the kidney's ability to concentrate and dilute urine appropriately. Inhibitors of the Na^+-K^+-$2Cl^-$ symporter also inhibit Ca^{2+} and Mg^{2+} reabsorption in the TAL by disruption of the transepithelial potential difference. Some loop diuretics, notably furosemide, also have weak CA-inhibiting activity that leads to enhanced urinary excretion of HCO_3^- and phosphate. All Na^+-K^+-$2Cl^-$ symporter inhibitors increase the urinary excretion of K^+ and H^+ by presenting a greater load of Na^+ to the distal tubule. Sodium is reabsorbed while K^+ and H^+ are excreted.

Nonsteroidal anti-inflammatory drugs (NSAIDs) inhibit the diuretic, natriuretic, and chloruretic responses to furosemide. Furosemide enhances production of prostaglandin E_2 (PGE_2), which in turn inhibits chloride and sodium reabsorption in the TAL. In the presence of NSAIDs, PGE_2 production is blocked, and furosemide-induced diuresis is prevented (Kirchner 1987). In the absence of volume depletion, loop diuretics generally increase and redistribute total renal blood flow. The mechanism for this effect is thought to be related to prostaglandins, and the effect is diminished or blocked in the presence of NSAIDs (Data et al. 1978). Furosemide-induced hemodynamic changes correlate with an increase in urinary excretion of PGE_2.

EXTRARENAL EFFECTS. Furosemide causes extrarenal hemodynamic effects that include increased venous compliance and decreased right atrial pressure, pulmonary artery pressure, pulmonary artery wedge pressure, and pulmonary blood volume (Hinchcliff and Muir 1991). Prostaglandins are thought to account for the acute increase in systemic venous capacitance and subsequent decrease in left ventricular filling pressure. All of these effects are dependent upon the presence of a functional kidney and the uninhibited production of prostaglandins. In the isolated rabbit heart, furosemide has also been reported to exert a mild negative inotropic effect that is prostaglandin dependent (Feldman et al. 1987). Inhaled furosemide in humans has been shown to protect against the early response to inhaled allergens and to prevent exercise-induced bronchoconstriction (Bianco et al. 1988, 1989). Furosemide may prevent bronchoconstriction in part by inhibiting release of inflammatory mediators from lung cells (Anderson et al. 1991). Pulmonary gas exchange is reportedly improved by furosemide in experimental pulmonary edema. Furosemide also reduces the rate of pulmonary transvascular fluid filtration through a reduction in pulmonary vein pressure (Demling and Will 1978).

Absorption and Elimination. Furosemide is approximately 77% bioavailable in dogs and has an elimination half-life of about 1 hour following an IV dose of 5 mg/kg (Hirai et al. 1992). The absorption of orally administered furosemide takes place mainly in the upper parts of the canine alimentary tract, decreasing rapidly across the jejunum. Due to variable oral bioavailability and rapid elimination in the dog, a prolonged-release furosemide formulated in hydroxypropyl methylcellulose matrix tablets has been investigated (Smal et al. 1996). Peak effects of an IV dosage of furosemide in the dog are reported at approximately 30 minutes and following oral dosing at about 1–2 hours. The rate of urinary furosemide excretion, more so even than the concentration of plasma furosemide, has been found to closely correlate with diuretic response in dogs. As in humans, the relation between the natriuretic response and the concentration of diuretic in the urine (at the site of action) is represented by a sigmoidal curve (Fig. 26.3). The shape of the curve suggests that a threshold quantity of drug must be achieved at the site of action in order to elicit a response and that a maximal dose can be identified that yields a maximal response. Beyond that maximal dose, the curve plateaus, and limited additional benefits are derived from dose increases (Brater 1998; Hirai et al. 1992).

Elimination half-life of IV furosemide in the horse is similar to that in the dog and, in the absence of renal impairment, is slightly less than 1 hour. Preventing renal elimination of the drug in horses by bilateral ureteral ligation increases elimination half-life by approximately 3-fold to an average of 164 minutes. This result demonstrates that furosemide elimination in the horse is primarily, but not exclusively, renal (Dyke et al. 1998). The hemodynamic effects of furosemide in this model are prevented by ureteral ligation, suggesting that these effects are diuresis dependent (Hinchcliff et al. 1996).

In humans and other animals, including the dog and horse, approximately 50–60% of a furosemide dose is excreted unchanged in the urine, and the remaining drug is conjugated to glucuronic acid in either the kidney, the liver, or other extrahepatic site (Brater 1998; Dyke et al. 1998).

Plasma half-life in patients with renal insufficiency is prolonged, and dosage adjustments should be made. Binding of furosemide to excessive amounts of albumin (>4g/L) in the urine decreases the amount of unbound, active drug and diminishes the diuretic response. In human patients with nephrotic syndrome, doses of two to three times normal are recommended to provide sufficient amounts of active drug to block the Na^+-K^+-$2Cl^-$ symporter.

In humans bumetanide and torsemide are metabolized in large part by the liver, and so dosage generally

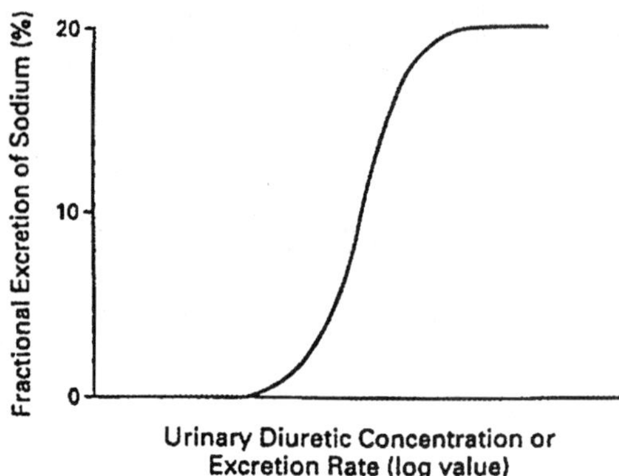

Figure 26.3—Pharmacodynamics of a loop diuretic. The relation between the natriuretic response and the amount of diuretic reaching the site of action is represented by a sigmoidal curve.

does not need to be adjusted for renal disease. Oral bioavailability of these drugs is much more predictable than that of furosemide and in humans ranges from 80 to 100% (Brater 1998).

Toxicity, Adverse Effects, Contraindications, and Drug Interactions. Most adverse effects of furosemide administration are related to abnormalities of fluid and electrolyte balance. Extracellular volume depletion and hyponatremia may lead to reduced blood pressure and diminished organ perfusion. Most at risk for adverse effects related to volume depletion are patients with renal disease (may decrease GFR, increase prerenal azotemia, and, possibly, cause tubular necrosis), cardiac disease (stroke volume and cardiac output may decrease), and hepatic disease (precipitation of hepatic encephalopathy). As noted previously, Na^+-K^+-$2Cl^-$ symporter inhibitors deliver an increased load of Na^+ to the distal tubules, resulting in a renin-angiotensin-aldosterone-driven increase in excretion of K^+ and H^+ in exchange for Na^+. Hypochloremic alkalosis and hypokalemia may result. Risk factors for cardiac dysrhythmias related to diuretic-induced hypokalemia include inadequate dietary intake of K^+, concurrent administration of cardiac glycosides, and additional electrolyte imbalances. A common cause of anorexia in CHF patients is digitalis toxicity, and risk of arrhythmias is increased in these patients if hypokalemia is present. Deficiencies in Mg^{2+} and Ca^{2+} may also be caused by diuretic-enhanced excretion of these substances. Serum electrolyte levels should be monitored in patients receiving ongoing diuretic therapy, especially if risk factors exist related to appetite, diuretic dosage, or severity of disease.

Ototoxicity that is usually transient has been described primarily with ethacrynic acid and less often with all other loop diuretics. In veterinary medicine, ototoxicity may be of greatest concern in treatment of cats with high-dose IV regimens. Other adverse effects reported with use of loop diuretics include gastrointestinal disturbances, bone marrow depression, and hyperglycemia. Hyperglycemia may be related to impairment of proinsulin-to-insulin conversion associated with diuretic-induced decreases in K^+ levels. Patients hypersensitive to sulfonamides may also be hypersensitive to furosemide since this drug contains a sulfonamide moiety. Diuretic-induced depletion of water-soluble vitamins may occur, and supplementation of B-complex vitamins has been recommended for animals receiving continuous diuretic therapy (Keene and Rush 1995).

Loop diuretics are contraindicated in animals with severe fluid and electrolyte disturbances or anuria that does not respond to test doses of diuretics.

Drug interactions may occur when furosemide is administered with theophylline (enhanced effects), aminoglycosides or cisplatin (enhanced ototoxicity and, if volume depleted, nephrotoxicity), digitalis glycosides (diuretic-induced hypokalemia may increase risk of arrhythmias), aspirin or other anticoagulants (anticoagulant activity increased), neuromuscular blockers (alteration in extent of muscle relaxation), corticosteroids (enhanced potassium wasting), insulin (alteration of insulin requirements associated with hyperglycemic effects), lithium and propranolol (increased plasma levels), probenecid (competition for secretion of diuretic into tubular lumen leading to decreased diuretic effect), NSAIDs (as previously described, decreased diuretic effects), and thiazides (synergistic diuretic activity).

Therapeutic Uses. Furosemide is used in small animals for treatment of edema of cardiac, hepatic, or renal origin. In general, the dose of drug in dogs (1–3 mg/kg every 8–24 hours PO for chronic use; 2–5 mg/kg every 4–6 hours IV, IM, SC) is higher than that used in cats (1–2 mg/kg every 12 hours up to 4 mg/kg every 8–12 hours IV, IM, SC, PO) (Ware 1998). Furosemide is also used to establish diuresis in renal failure and to promote excretion of other substances, including elevated electrolytes such as Ca^{2+} and K^+. In large animals, furosemide has been used to treat edema in cattle and edema and exercise-induced pulmonary hemorrhage (EIPH) in horses. A general dose of 0.5–1 mg/kg twice daily or as needed to control edema has been recommended in large animals (Reef and McGuirk 1996). Benefits of furosemide use for treatment of EIPH remain controversial (see below). Specific state guidelines should be consulted for details of furosemide use (dose, frequency, allowable levels) in racing animals.

RENAL INSUFFICIENCY. Decreased GFR and decreased delivery of drug to the tubular site of action and site of elimination in renal insufficiency results in decreased efficacy and increased half-life of furosemide. A sufficiently high dose of drug must be administered to attain an effective amount of drug at the site of action. For the dog, furosemide doses starting at 2 mg/kg IV and increasing in 2 mg/kg increments every hour for 3 hours may be used to try and induce diuresis in severe renal insufficiency. Once a maximal dosage is reached (approximately 6–8 mg/kg), exceeding this amount is not advantageous based on the sigmoidal shape of the fractional sodium excretion curve (Fig. 26.3). In all cases, fluid deficits should be addressed prior to furosemide therapy.

CARDIOGENIC OR PULMONARY EDEMA. Furosemide has been widely used to reduce extracellular volume and minimize venous and pulmonary congestion in chronic and acute CHF. Human patients with CHF do not require large dosages since furosemide is adequately delivered to the tubular fluid. However, because renal responsiveness to loop diuretics appears to be decreased in these patients, increased frequency of administration has been recommended (Brater 1998). Diuretics have traditionally been considered front-line therapy for the treatment of chronic CHF in small animals, and furosemide is reported to be the most frequently used drug for this purpose (Goodwin and Hamlin 1993; Watson and Church 1995). Despite the popularity of furosemide, human studies have revealed that CHF patients controlled on loop diuretics alone deteriorate more quickly than those treated with either angiotensin-converting enzyme (ACE) inhibitors or digoxin. Use of furosemide alone is thought to enhance early activation of the renin-angiotensin-aldosterone system, with detrimental effects on long-term prognosis (Svedberg et al. 1990). Current recommendations include furosemide for treatment of more advanced stages of heart failure in patients already receiving ACE inhibitors, digoxin, or both. Furosemide remains a drug of choice for treatment of acute cardiogenic pulmonary edema. Within the context of severity and chronicity of disease, the lowest effective dosage and frequency of furosemide administration should be determined by observation of clinical signs and consideration of owner observations.

EXERCISE-INDUCED PULMONARY HEMORRHAGE (EIPH). EIPH, or bleeding from the lungs as a consequence of exercise, occurs in horses engaged in a variety of athletic activities. The problem has been best studied in racing horses, particularly Thoroughbreds. In general, EIPH is thought to occur because systemic arterial pressures during maximal exercise are higher than pulmonary arterial pressures. As a result, pulmonary capillaries are subjected to rapid increases in transmural pressures sufficient to cause vascular disruption. Transmural pressures are calculated by subtracting pulmonary capillary pressure from alveolar pressure. Pulmonary capillary pressure can be estimated as the mean between left atrial and pulmonary arterial pressure. Alveolar pressure is approximated indirectly using transpulmonary pressure. This value is estimated by measurement of changes in esophageal pressures. Another parameter relevant to assessment of EIPH is pulmonary wedge pressure, defined as the back-pressure opposing pulmonary perfusion. This parameter increases with exercise and is considered an index of pulmonary venous pressure. In addition to changes in pulmonary pressures, other factors implicated in the pathophysiology of EIPH include concurrent small airway disease, upper airway obstruction, exercise-induced hyperviscosity, and environmental effects (Lester et al. 1999).

In most studies, furosemide has been found to reduce right atrial, pulmonary arterial, and pulmonary wedge pressures in exercising horses. Some studies suggest that changes in pulmonary pressures caused by furosemide are due to reduction in plasma and blood volume and not to direct effects of the drug on the pulmonary vasculature. Furosemide produces a rapid reduction in blood and plasma volume, which has been shown in the horse to be essential for subsequent reduction in pulmonary pressures (Hinchcliff et al. 1996). Furthermore, administration of polyionic fluids in an amount equal to the volume lost in urine restores furosemide-induced decreases in right atrial pressure and blood volume in the horse (Rivas and Hinchcliff 1997).

Data from additional studies leave open the question of direct effects of furosemide on pulmonary pressures and mechanics in EIPH. In one study horses treated with NSAIDs (phenylbutazone and flunixin) prior to administration of furosemide followed by exercise did not show reductions in pulmonary and right atrial pressures (Olsen et al. 1992). In a subsequent study these effects could not be reproduced (Manohar 1994). Differences in the studies may be related to drug dosages, time of administration, amount of diuresis, and degree of cyclooxygenase inhibition. While it is accepted that NSAIDs decrease the diuretic response to furosemide, it is as yet unresolved whether these drugs mitigate furosemide-induced reductions in pulmonary and right atrial pressures. It is also not clear whether the magnitude of reduction of pulmonary capillary transmural pressure with furosemide is sufficient to prevent capillary rupture in exercising horses (Soma and Uboh 1998). This is consistent with clinical observations that furosemide reduces, but does not completely eliminate, pulmonary hemorrhage in exercising horses.

Administration of furosemide to racing animals is thought to enhance their performance, although this conclusion remains somewhat controversial. Use of furosemide in racing Thoroughbreds, Quarter Horses, and Standardbreds is estimated at 74.3, 19, and 22.5%, respectively (Hinchcliff 1999). A recent cross-sectional study concluded that Thoroughbreds receiving furosemide raced faster, earned more money, and were more likely to win or finish in the top three positions than unmedicated horses (Gross et al. 1999). Early studies showed increases in racing times when EIPH was diagnosed and a subsequent improvement of racing times upon administration of furosemide (Soma et al. 1985). Treadmill studies have not consistently shown furosemide-induced changes in maximal O_2 consumption, time to fatigue, or the speed at which fatigue occurred in exercising horses (Hinchcliff et al. 1993). However, in these and later studies, the loss of weight associated with furosemide administration did reduce carbon dioxide production, the respiratory exchange ratio, and plasma lactate. Furosemide-induced gains in performance were reversed by addition of a weight equal to the weight of the volume lost. These results suggest that performance benefits associated with furosemide administration to EIPH horses may be unrelated to reduction in hemorrhage and more related to changes in body weight (Soma and Uboh 1998). Based on human studies, this interpretation should not be extended to circumstances in which the race distance is long and exertion prolonged. In these cases, the detrimental effects of dehydration would rapidly offset the advantage of running under reduced weight.

A final issue related to use of furosemide in racing animals involves the regulation of administration of furosemide and other drugs to equine athletes. Doses of 250–500 mg furosemide per horse (0.5–1.0 mg/kg) administered IV no later than 4 hours prior to post time are permitted for medication of horses with EIPH in most jurisdictions in the United States. Specific regulations at a given track should be consulted. The regulation of furosemide administration according to track rules has been approached in a variety of ways. Some jurisdictions use a combination of urine specific gravity of 1.015 or 1.010 and a plasma concentration of greater than 60 or 100 ng/mL as an indication of a violation of the rules. The combination of these two parameters, low specific gravity and high plasma concentration, will suggest that an irregularity related to dose, time, or route of furosemide administration occurred (Soma and Uboh 1998).

Widespread use of furosemide in racing animals also presents problems related to screening of urine for presence of regulated substances. The urinary concentration of coadministered drugs may be diluted as a function of furosemide-enhanced diuresis. Urinary excretion rates of some drugs, especially those that are water-soluble acids, may be altered as a result of furosemide competition for the organic anion tubular secretion pathway. Furosemide has been shown to decrease the urinary concentration of phenylbutazone through both of these mechanisms. In comparison, the excretion rate of other agents, notably fentanyl, procaine, and methylphenidate, is increased by furosemide. Faster clearance of these substances may make it more difficult to detect illegal use prior to a race (Hinchcliff and Muir 1991).

OTHER USES. Furosemide has been shown to decrease pulmonary resistance and increase dynamic compliance in ponies with chronic obstructive pulmonary disease. In this case, the rapidity of the response and the finding that the response could be blocked by NSAIDs suggested a cyclooxygenase-mediated event rather than an effect dependent upon loss of body fluid (Broadstone et al. 1991). Immediate changes in pulmonary pressures in other species (e.g., dogs with pulmonary edema) are thought to be related to direct effects of furosemide on the pulmonary vasculature. Similar to use in small animals, furosemide is indicated for treatment of CHF and associated pulmonary edema by decreasing cardiac preload and plasma volume. Furosemide is also recommended to increase urine flow in acute renal failure in horses.

INHIBITORS OF NA^+-CL^- SYMPORT (THIAZIDE AND THIAZIDE-LIKE DIURETICS)

Chemistry/Formulations. Thiazide diuretics are benzothiadiazines or analogs and are derivatives of CA-inhibiting sulfonamides. Compared to loop diuretics, thiazides promote renal excretion of chloride, rather than bicarbonate, with sodium, producing a true saluretic effect. Two of the first thiazides synthesized, and the two drugs most commonly used in veterinary medicine, are chlorothiazide (Diuril®, human-approved 250 and 500 mg tablets, 50 mg/mL suspension, and 500 mg/vial injectable available) and hydrochlorothiazide (Hydrozide®, veterinary-approved 25 mg/mL injectable; HydroDiuril®, human-approved 25, 50, and 100 mg tablets and 10 mg/mL oral suspension). Both drugs are derivatives of benzothiadiazine and are water soluble. Hydrozide® is the only veterinary-approved product for use in cattle and has a 72-hour milk withholding time for lactating dairy cattle; no meat withholding time has been reported. Newer generation, more lipid-soluble benzothiadiazine derivatives include cyclothiazide and methychlothiazide.

Nonbenzothiadiazine derivatives have thiazide-like effects, and these drugs also promote excretion of sodium with chloride. Quinazolinone derivatives are in this class and include metolazone and chlorthalidone. These drugs are not commonly used in veterinary medicine but are examples of thiazide-like diuretics.

Mechanisms and Sites of Action. The primary site of action of thiazides is the distal convoluted tubule, with some secondary activity, possibly CA-related, in the proximal tubule. In the distal tubule, NaCl reabsorption is mediated by an electroneutral cotransport (symport) system (see Fig. 26.2). The driving force for Cl^- entry is the transmembrane Na^+ gradient established by the activity of basolateral Na^+,K^+-ATPase. The apical NaCl cotransporter is reversibly inhibited by thiazides. Basolateral movement of Cl^- out of the cell is possibly mediated by a KCl cotransport system. The lumen-negative transepithelial potential generated by the polarity of K^+ and Cl^- exit may drive anion reabsorption via a paracellular shunt pathway. Ca^+ reabsorption is enhanced by thiazides, perhaps by increasing distal tubule Ca^{2+}-binding proteins. Because 90% of filtered Na^+ is reabsorbed prior to the distal tubule, the peak diuresis caused by thiazides is moderate compared to loop diuretics. Like loop diuretics, thiazides enhance excretion of K^+ by increasing the delivery of Na^+ to the distal tubule.

Absorption and Elimination. Thiazide and thiazide-like diuretics are absorbed slowly and incompletely from the gastrointestinal tract. Most drugs in this class are highly protein bound and are excreted renally (chlorothiazide and hydrochlorothiazide) or by a combination of renal and biliary routes (thiazide-like drugs). Hydrochlorothiazide is less protein bound (40%) than others in the class and partitions and accumulates in red blood cells (Velazquez et al. 1995). All drugs in this class gain access to the lumen of the renal tubule via an organic acid secretory pathway. Hence effectiveness of these drugs is decreased if renal blood flow diminishes.

Toxicity, Adverse Effects, Contraindications, and Drug Interactions. Similar to loop diuretics, most problems associated with administration of thiazides are related to fluid and electrolyte disturbances. Potassium wasting, especially with concurrent use of digitalis, increases the risk of cardiac arrhythmias. Low K^+ may secondarily affect conversion of proinsulin to insulin, leading to hyperglycemia. Enhanced calcium reabsorption can lead to hypercalcemia, and mild magnesuria may cause magnesium deficiency. Depletion of extracellular volume, hyponatremia, hypochloremia, and hypochloremic metabolic alkalosis may occur as adverse effects with prolonged or aggressive thiazide use. Because thiazides block solute reabsorption at nephron sites involved in dilution of urine, these agents increase the risk of hyponatremia under conditions of increased consumption of hypotonic fluids. CNS and gastrointestinal effects may occur but are not common.

Sensitivity to sulfonamides limits use of thiazide diuretics because of the structural similarity between these two classes of drugs. Patients with severe renal disease, hypovolemia, or electrolyte disturbances are poor candidates for thiazide therapy. Impaired hepatic function that may be worsened by volume contraction (leading to hepatic encephalopathy) is a contraindication for thiazide use. Diabetic patients are at risk for thiazide-induced derangements of glucose and insulin.

Drug interactions include decreased effects of anticoagulants and insulin and increased effects of some anesthetics, diazoxide, digitalis glycosides, lithium, loop diuretics, and vitamin D. Combination therapy using low-dose thiazides with front-line antihypertensives (e.g., ACE inhibitors) is currently considered to be an effective alternative strategy for management of human hypertension (Neutel et al. 1996). At low doses, side effects of thiazides are decreased, making their use in combination regimens particularly appealing.

Thiazides are reported to prolong the half-life of quinidine. In the face of thiazide-induced hypokalemia, an elevated plasma quinidine level increases the risk of polymorphic ventricular tachycardia (*torsades de pointes*), a condition that can deteriorate into ventricular fibrillation (Jackson 1996). NSAIDs may reduce the effectiveness of thiazides and loop diuretics by increasing solute reabsorption at the TAL of the loop of Henle (Brater 1998).

Therapeutic Uses. Thiazides may be used to treat edema of cardiac, hepatic, or renal origin. Typical oral dosages in the dog and cat are 20–40 mg/kg every 12 hours (chlorothiazide) and 2–4 mg/kg every 12 hours (hydrochlorothiazide). Effects of both chlorothiazide and hydrochlorothiazide peak at 4 hours and last up to 12 hours, with hydrochlorothiazide typically having a longer duration (12 hr) than chlorothiazide (6–12 hr). Cattle may be treated for udder edema with hydrochlorothiazide (125–250 mg IV or IM once or twice daily). Oral chlorothiazide (not a veterinary-approved product) at a dose of 4–8 mg/kg once or twice daily has been substituted for injectable hydrochlorothiazide following the first or second day of parenteral treatment.

Thiazides have previously been used in veterinary medicine in management of the early stages of CHF. As mentioned previously, early use of loop and thiazide diuretics in CHF activates aldosterone-mediated mechanisms that eventually lead to cardiac deterioration. For this and other reasons, the use of thiazides in treatment of CHF is not common in veterinary medicine. In general, furosemide is more commonly used in veterinary medicine to treat edema, whether it be cardiac, hepatic, or renal in origin. In human medicine, thiazides are commonly used in the management of hypertension. Because thiazides increase reabsorption of calcium, they may also be beneficial in treatment of calcium nephrolithiasis in humans and animals.

Thiazides are used effectively to reduce the volume of urine in patients with nephrogenic diabetes insipidus. Diuretic-induced volume contraction leads to increased proximal tubule reabsorption and a decrease in urine volume of 30–50%. Although dosages are individualized in these patients, starting ranges of 10–20 mg/kg twice daily (chlorothiazide) or 2.75–5.5 mg/kg (hydrochlorothiazide) twice daily have been suggested (Nichols and Thompson 1995).

INHIBITORS OF RENAL EPITHELIAL SODIUM CHANNELS (K^+-SPARING DIURETICS)

Chemistry/Formulations. The two relevant drugs in this class, triamterene (Dyrenium®) and amiloride (Midamor®), both belong to the class of cyclic amidine diuretics. Triamterene is a pteridine ring with amino groups at the 2, 4, and 7 positions. It was originally synthesized as a folic acid antagonist. Amiloride consists of a substituted pyrazine ring with a carbonylguanidinium side chain. A number of analogs of this basic structure have been synthesized and have been useful tools in elucidating mechanisms of sodium transport. Both triamterene and amiloride are organic bases and are secreted into the proximal tubule by an organic base transport system. Although neither of these drugs is used with frequency in veterinary medicine, triamterene is the more commonly used and hence will be the focus of these discussions. No parenteral forms of the drug are available; oral preparations are available in 50 and 100 mg capsules.

Mechanisms and Sites of Action. Triamterene and amiloride cause a mild increase in excretion of NaCl and a retention of K^+. Both drugs slightly augment diuresis and are used in combination with loop diuretics or thiazides to decrease K^+ excretion (hence the term *K^+-sparing*). Both drugs act at the late distal tubule (or connecting tubule) and collecting duct to block the electrogenic transport of Na^+ (see Fig. 26.2). As with other diuretics, the basolateral Na^+,K^+-ATPase creates an electrochemical gradient that drives events at the luminal surface of the tubular cell. In this case, the principal cells of the connecting tubule contain a Na^+ channel in their luminal membrane that provides a pathway for entry of Na^+ and sets up a lumen-negative transepithelial potential. The transepithelial voltage is the key force involved in driving K^+ out of the principal cell and into the tubular lumen. Blockade of Na^+ channels by triamterene or amiloride hyperpolarizes the luminal membrane, reduces the lumen–negative potential difference, and decreases the excretion of K^+, H^+, Ca^{2+}, and Mg^{2+}. It has been speculated that effects of both of these drugs may also be mediated by inhibition of a Na^+-H^+ antiport located in the late distal tubule and collecting duct. Additional, direct effects on Mg^{2+} excretion may also occur.

Triamterene has been shown to exert cardiac effects that are not secondary to alterations in renal function. Early studies documented a prolongation of the cardiac action potential duration and functional refractory period and an increase in myocardial contractile force. Triamterene has also been shown to decrease digitalis-induced K^+ loss from the heart and increase the dose of digitalis necessary to induce toxic effects in dogs (Palmer and Kleyman 1995; Netzer et al. 1995). Neither triamterene nor amiloride has been shown to affect renal hemodynamics, and neither acts as an aldosterone antagonist.

Absorption and Elimination. Both amiloride and triamterene are administered orally; triamterene is up to 70% bioavailable. Amiloride is renally excreted. The pharmacokinetics of triamterene are complex. The parent drug is converted in the liver to an active metabolite, 4-hydroxytriamterene sulfate, which is actively secreted into the renal tubules. Hence renal or hepatic disease could impair elimination of triamterene. The peak onset of action of triamterene is 6–8 hours, with effects persisting up to 12–16 hours.

Toxicity, Adverse Effects, Contraindications, and Drug Interactions. The most important potential side effect of these drugs is hyperkalemia. The presence of diseases or circumstances that may increase the risk of hyperkalemia (e.g., renal failure, coadministration of other drugs with K^+-sparing properties, including ACE inhibitors and K^+ supplements) should be noted and these patients treated with other diuretic combinations.

Triamterene may decrease GFR and, in combination with NSAIDs, has been shown to increase the likelihood of hyperkalemia and renal dysfunction. Triamterene-induced renal casts may be responsible for increased risk of interstitial nephritis and renal stones. Both triamterene and amiloride may induce hypersensitivity reactions that include rash and photosensitivity in humans. CNS, gastrointestinal, and hematological side effects have also been reported. As with most other diuretics, use in patients with severe hepatic disease or renal disease is contraindicated. In human patients with hepatic disease, the mild folic acid antagonism inherent in triamterene may increase the risk of megaloblastosis.

Therapeutic Use. Because these drugs have relatively weak diuretic properties, they are clinically important primarily because of their K^+-sparing properties in combination with loop and thiazide diuretics. Both have been used in this capacity for treatment of edema associated with CHF, liver cirrhosis, nephrotic syndrome, steroid-induced edema, and idiopathic edema. Triamterene is administered at a dose of 2–4 mg/kg/day orally to dogs with food to avoid gastrointestinal side effects.

ANTAGONISTS OF MINERALOCORTICOID RECEPTORS (ALDOSTERONE ANTAGONISTS AND K^+-SPARING DIURETICS)

Chemistry/Formulations. Spironolactone is a 17-spirolactone and is the only aldosterone antagonist approved in the United States. Canrenone, an active metabolite of spironolactone, and potassium canrenoate are closely related structurally and are available in other countries. All of these drugs share a four-ring, steroid structure similar to the mineralocorticoid aldosterone. Spironolactone is available as a human-approved oral preparation (Aldactone®) in 25, 50, and 100 mg tablets.

Mechanisms and Sites of Action. Aldosterone is a steroid hormone that binds to mineralocorticoid receptors (MRs) located in the cytoplasm of target cells. The inactive MR complex is bound to heat shock protein 90 (HSP90), a protective chaperon protein, and is incapable of binding to target DNA sequences. Upon binding of aldosterone, HSP90 dissociates from the receptor-hormone complex, allowing movement of the activated receptor into the nucleus. The complex binds to target sequences of DNA referred to as mineralocorticoid-response elements (also termed hormone-responsive elements) that regulate transcription of downstream, mineralocorticoid-responsive genes. Protein products of these responsive genes, aldosterone-induced proteins (AIPs), cause Na^+ reabsorption and increase excretion of K^+ and H^+ in the late distal tubule and collecting duct. AIPs are thought to have multiple effects, including activation, redistribution, and de novo synthesis of Na^+ channels and Na^+,K^+-ATPase, changes in permeability of tight junctions, and increased mitochondrial production of ATP. These effects combine to cause an increase in Na^+ conductance of the luminal membrane and increased Na^+ pump activity in the basolateral membrane. As a result, NaCl transport is increased across tubular epithelial cells, and the lumen-negative transepithelial voltage is increased. Secretion of K^+ and H^+ into the tubular lumen increases with increasing voltages.

Aldosterone antagonists act by binding to the MR and facilitating the release of HSP90 from the steroid-binding subunit of the receptor. The unprotected MR complex is thought to be inactivated by proteases. In the absence of activated MRs, gene transcription is not induced, AIPs are not produced, and the physiological effects of aldosterone are blocked.

In addition to antagonism of aldosterone, spironolactone is thought to act in a manner similar to calcium channel blockers to cause direct vasodilation. By binding to plasma membrane sites, spironolactone may inhibit inward slow calcium channels and depress contractions dependent on release of calcium from the sarcoplasmic reticulum. Aldosterone antagonists have also been shown to increase circulating levels of atrial natriuretic peptide as evaluated in the dog. Hence direct and aldosterone-mediated effects of the drug may contribute to its usefulness in treatment of cardiac disease (Endou and Hosoyamada 1995).

Absorption and Elimination. In humans, spironolactone is absorbed moderately well (60–90%), is highly protein-bound, and is extensively biotransformed in the liver, exhibiting a first-pass effect. An active metabolite, canrenone, has a longer half-life than the parent drug and extends the biological effects of spironolactone to about 16 hours in humans. Peak diuresis occurs as late as 2–3 days after initiation of therapy. Aldosterone antagonists do not require secretion into the renal tubule to induce diuresis.

Toxicity, Adverse Effects, Contraindications, and Drug Interactions. Hyperkalemia, dehydration, and hyponatremia are the most common side effects of aldosterone antagonists. When used alone, these drugs can also cause hyperchloremic metabolic acidosis. In humans, sexual side effects limit the use of spironolactone in some patients. The most likely explanation for these effects relates to the binding of drug not only to renal aldosterone receptors but also to progesterone and dihydrotestosterone receptors. This lack of receptor specificity drives continued efforts to identify a more MR-specific antagonist for use in human medicine.

As previously noted, combination of any K^+-sparing diuretic with ACE inhibitors must be accomplished cautiously to avoid hyperkalemia. This is a clinically significant scenario that merits patient monitoring of plasma K^+ concentrations. Because both spironolactone and digoxin have steroid-like structures, the former is thought to compete with digoxin for renal clearance, thus prolonging the half-life of digoxin (Hedman et al. 1992). The presence of spironolactone in plasma may also confound therapeutic drug monitoring of digoxin if a cross-reactive antidigoxin antibody is used in the assay. Aspirin apparently blocks spironolactone-induced natriuresis (Endou and Hosoyamada 1995).

Therapeutic Uses. The effectiveness of aldosterone antagonists in promoting diuresis is largely dependent upon elevated concentrations of endogenous aldosterone. Aldosterone secretion increases upon activation of the renin-angiotensin-aldosterone system, which, in turn, responds to reductions in serum sodium, effective blood volume, and cardiac output, and decreases in serum K^+. Secondary hyperaldosteronism and edema are associated with cardiac failure, hepatic cirrhosis, nephrotic syndrome, and severe ascites. Spironolactone is used in veterinary medicine at a dose of 2–4 mg/kg/day orally in management of refractory edema associated with these conditions and is considered the diuretic of choice in management of hepatic cirrhosis. In both human and veterinary medicine, aldosterone antagonists are commonly administered with a thiazide or loop diuretic to increase peak diuresis and to spare K^+.

Elevated aldosterone levels have been shown to be a useful prognostic indicator in heart failure, with higher levels correlated with a poorer prognosis. Activation of the renin-angiotensin-aldosterone system in arterial hypertension is thought to lead to remodeling of the myocardial collagen network with progressive cardiac interstitial fibrosis. As fibrosis increases, diastolic function deteriorates and pathologic cardiac hypertrophy occurs. When aldosterone-mediated effects are blocked by spironolactone, progression of myocardial failure is presumably slowed. A clinical study recently supported this contention by showing significant delays in progression of CHF in human patients treated with spironolactone (Pitt et al. 1999). Despite the potential side effect of hyperkalemia associated with coadministration of spironolactone and ACE inhibitors, this combination with appropriate dosages has been deemed effective in management of CHF. Patient monitoring for K^+ derangements is critical to safe implementation of this approach. In veterinary medicine, spironolactone may be useful in patients with CHF secondary to chronic valvular heart disease or dilated cardiomyopathy that become unresponsive to therapy with ACE inhibitors, digoxin, and furosemide.

AQUARETICS. Vasopressin (or arginine vasopressin, AVP) regulates water and solute excretion in the kidney by binding to V_2 receptors in the principal cells of the renal collecting duct system. As one of three G-protein-coupled AVP receptor subtypes (V_{1a}, V_{1b}, V_2), V_2 receptors mediate the antidiuretic effects of AVP. V_2 receptor antagonists, so-called aquaretic agents, promote solute-free water excretion. These antagonists hold considerable promise for treatment of edematous states associated with heart failure, liver cirrhosis, nephrotic syndrome, and syndrome of inappropriate secretion of antidiuretic hormone. An orally active, nonpeptide, selective V_2 receptor antagonist, OPC-31260, has been shown to induce aquaresis in humans and is currently in clinical development in Japan. This drug has been shown to significantly increase urine volume and decrease urine osmolality and body weight without affecting urinary sodium excretion (Orita and Nakahama 1998). Another promising V_2 antagonist, SR 121463A, has been shown to be highly selective for V_2 receptors and effective at induction of aquaresis in several species. Like OPC-31260, urinary electrolytes are unaltered by drug administration (Serradeil-Le Gal 1998).

Although vasopressin antagonists represent the most promising area of drug development for induction of aquaresis, drugs that interfere with secretion of AVP from the neurohypophysis and drugs that directly inhibit water channels in the collecting ducts are also of interest. Aquaporin-CD, the water channel of the principal cell of the cortical and medullary collecting duct, has been cloned and provides an attractive site for drugs intended to inhibit diuresis.

REFERENCES

Anderson, S., He, W., and Temple, D. 1991. Inhibition by furosemide of inflammatory mediators from lung fragments. N Engl J Med 324:131.

Better, O. S., Rubinstein, I., Winaver, J. M., and Knochel, J. P. 1997. Mannitol therapy revisited (1940–1997). Kidney International 51:886–894.

Betz, A. L., Ianotti, F., and Hoff, J. T. 1989. Brain edema: a classification based on blood-brain barrier integrity. Cerebrovasc Brain Metab Rev 1:133–154.

Bianco, S., Robuschi, M., and Vaghi, A. 1988. Prevention of exercise-induced bronchoconstriction by inhaled furosemide. Lancet 2:252–255.

Bianco, S., Pieroni, M., and Refini, R. 1989. Protective effect of inhaled furosemide on allergen-induced early and late asthmatic reactions. N Engl J Med 321:1069–1073.

Bleich, M., and Greger, R. 1997. Mechanism of action of diuretics. Kidney International 51 (Suppl 59):S11–S15.

Brater, D. C. 1993. Resistance to diuretics: mechanisms and clinical implications. Adv Nephrology 22:349–369.

———. 1998. Diuretic therapy. New Engl J Med 339:387–395.

Broadstone, R. V., Robinson, N. E., and Gray, P. R. 1991. Effects of furosemide on ponies with recurrent airway obstruction. Pulmonary Pharmacol 44:203–208.

Cloyd, J. C., Snyder, B. D., and Cleermans, B. 1986. Mannitol pharmacokinetics and serum osmolality in dogs and humans. J Pharmacol Exp Ther 236:301–306.

Data, J., Rane, A., and Gerkens, J. 1978. The influence of indomethacin on the pharmacokinetics, diuretic response, and hemodynamics of furosemide in the dog. J Pharmacol Exp Ther 206:431–438.

Demling, R., and Will, J. 1978. The effect of furosemide on the pulmonary transvascular fluid filtration rate. Crit Care Med 6:317–319.

Dormans, T. P. J, Pickkers, P., Russel, F. G. M. and Smits, P. 1996. Vascular effects of loop diuretics. Cardiovascular Res 32:988–997.

Dyke, T., Hubel, J., Grosenbaugh, D., Beard, W., Mitten, L., Sams, R., and Hinchcliff, K. 1998. The pharmacokinetics of furosemide in anaesthetized horses after bilateral ureteral ligation. J Vet Pharmacol Therap 21:298–303.

Endou, H., and Hosoyamada, M. 1995. Potassium-retaining diuretics: aldosterone antagonists. In R. F. Greger, H. Knauf, and E. Mutschler, eds., Handbook of Experimental Pharmacology, vol. 117, Diuretics, pp. 335–355. Berlin: Springer-Verlag.

Feldman, A., Levine, M., and Gerstenblith, G. 1987. Negative inotropic effects of furosemide in the isolated rabbit heart: a prostaglandin-mediated event. J Cardiovasc Pharmacol 9:493–499.

Gamba, G., Slatzberg, S. N., Lombardi, M., et al. 1993. Primary structure and functional expression of a cDNA encoding the thiazide-sensitive, electroneutral sodium-chloride cotransporter. Proc Natl Acad Sci USA 90:2749–2753.

Gamba, G., Miyanoshita, A., Lombardi, M., et al. 1994. Molecular cloning, primary structure, and characterization of two members of the mammalian electroneutral sodium- (potassium-) chloride cotransporter family expressed in kidney. J Biol Chem 269:17713–17722.

Goodwin, J., and Hamlin, R. 1993. Preferences of veterinarians for drugs used to treat heart disease in dogs and cats: a 20-year follow-up study. J Vet Intern Med 7:118.

Gross, D. K., Morley, P. S., Hinchcliff, K. W., and Wittum, T. E. 1999. Effect of furosemide on performance of Thoroughbreds racing in the United States and Canada. JAVMA 215:670–675.

Hedman, A., Angelin, B., Arvidsson, A., and Dahogvist, R. 1992. Digoxin interactions in man: spironolactone reduces renal but not biliary digoxin clearance. Eur J Clin Pharmacol 42:481–485.

Hinchcliff, K. W. 1999. Effects of furosemide on athletic performance and exercise-induced pulmonary hemorrhage in horses. JAVMA 215:630–635.

Hinchcliff, K. W., and Muir, W. 1991. Pharmacology of furosemide in the horse: a review. J Vet Int Med 5:211–218.

Hinchcliff, K. W., McKeever, K. H., and Muir, W. W. 1993. Effect of furosemide and weight carriage on energetic responses of horses to incremental exertion. Amer J Vet Res 54:1500–1504.

Hinchcliff, K. W., Hubbell, J., Grosenbaugh, D., Mitten, L., and Beard, W. 1996. Hemodynamic effects of furosemide are dependent on diuresis. Proc Am Assoc Equine Practitioners, 42:229–230.

Hirai, J., Miyazaki, H., and Taneike, T. 1992. The pharmacokinetics and pharmacodynamics of furosemide in the anaesthetized dog. J Vet Pharmacol Therap 15:231–239.

Jackson, E. K. 1996. Diuretics. In J. G. Hardman and L. E. Limbird, eds., Goodman and Gilman's The Pharmacological Basis of Therapeutics, 9th ed., pp. 685–713. New York: McGraw-Hill.

Keene, B., and Rush, J. 1995. Therapy of heart failure. In S. Ettinger and E. Feldman, eds., Textbook of Veterinary Internal Medicine, 4th ed., pp. 878–881. Philadelphia: W. B. Saunders.

Kirchner, K. 1987. Indomethacin antagonizes furosemide's intratubular effects during loop segment microperfusion. J. Pharmacol Exp Ther 243:881–886.

Kriz, W., and Bankir, L. 1988. A standard nomenclature for structures of the kidney. Am J Physiol 254:F1–F8.

Kriz, W., and Kaissling, B. 1992 In D. W. Seldin and G. Giebisch, eds., The Kidney: Physiology and Pathophysiology, 2d ed., pp. 707–777. New York: Raven Press.

Lang, F., and Busch, A. 1995. Basic concepts of renal physiology. In R. F. Greger, H. Knauf, and E. Mutschler, eds., Handbook of Experimental Pharmacology, vol. 117, Diuretics, pp. 67–114. Berlin: Springer-Verlag.

Lester, G., Clark, C., Rice, B., Steible-Hartless, C., and Vetro-Widenhouse, T. 1999. Effect of timing and route of administration of furosemide on pulmonary hemorrhage and pulmonary arterial pressure in exercising Thoroughbred racehorses. Am J Vet Res 60:22–28.

Levinsky, N. G., and Bernard, D. B. 1988. Mannitol and loop diuretics in acute renal failure. In B. M. Brenner and J. M. Lazarus, eds., Acute Renal Failure, 2nd ed., pp. 841–856. New York: Churchill Livingstone.

Manohar, M. 1994. Pulmonary vascular pressures of strenuously exercising Thoroughbreds after administration of flunixin meglumine and furosemide. Am J Vet Res 55:1308–1312.

Mindel, J. S. 1997. Dorzolamide: development and clinical application of a topical carbonic anhydrase inhibitor. Survey of Ophthalmology 42:137–151.

Morrison, R. T. 1997. Edema and principles of diuretic use. Med Clin N Am 81:689–704.

Netzer, T., Ullrich, R., Knauf, H., and Mutschler, E. 1995. Potassium-retaining diuretics: triamterene. In R. F. Greger, H. Knauf, and E. Mutschler, eds., Handbook of Experimental Pharmacology, vol. 117, Diuretics, pp. 396–421. Berlin: Springer-Verlag.

Neutel, J., Black, H., and Weber, M. 1996. Combination therapy with diuretics: an evolution of understanding. Am J Med 101 (Suppl 3A):61S–70S.

Nichols, R., and Thompson, L. 1995. Pituitary-hypothalamic disease. In S. Ettinger, and E. Feldman, eds., Textbook of Veterinary Internal Medicine, 4th ed., p. 1432. Philadelphia: W. B. Saunders.

Olsen, S. C., Coyne, C. P., and Lowe, B. S. 1992. Influence of cyclooxygenase inhibitors on furosemide-induced hemodynamic effects during exercise in horses. Am J Vet Res 53:1562–1567.

Orita, Y., and Nakahama, H. 1998. Vasopressin receptor antagonists. Internal Med 37:219–221.

Paczynski, R. 1997. Osmotherapy: basic concepts and controversies. Crit Care Clin 13:105–129.

Palmer, L. G., and Kleyman, T. R. 1995. Potassium-retaining diuretics: amiloride. In R. F. Greger, H. Knauf, and E. Mutschler, eds., Handbook of Experimental Pharmacology, vol. 117, Diuretics, pp. 363–388. Berlin: Springer-Verlag.

Pfeiffer, N. 1997. Dorzolamide: development and clinical application of a topical carbonic anhydrase inhibitor. Suv Ophthalmol 42:137–151.

Pitt, B., Zannad, F., Remme, W. J., et al. 1999. The effect of spironolactone on morbidity and mortality in patients with severe heart failure. New Engl J Med 341:709–717.

Prough, D. S., and Zornow, M. H. 1998. Mannitol: an old friend on the skids? Crit Care Med 26:997–998.

Reef, V., and McGuirk, S. 1996. Diseases of the cardiovascular system. In B. Smith, ed., Large Animal Internal Medicine, 2nd ed., p. 531. St. Louis: Mosby Year Book.

Rivas, L. J., and Hinchcliff, K. W. 1997. Effect of furosemide and subsequent intravenous fluid administration on right atrial pressure of splenetomized horses. Am J Vet Res 58:632–635.

Roberts, S. E. 1985. Assessment and management of the ophthalmic emergency. Compend Cont Ed 7:739–752.

Rudehill, A., Gordon, E., and Ohman, G. 1993. Pharmacokinetics and effects of mannitol on hemodynamics, blood, and cerebrospinal fluid electrolytes, and osmolality during intracranial surgery. J Neurosurg Anesthesiol 5:4–12.

Serradeil-Le Gal, C. 1998. Nonpeptide antagonists for vasopressin receptors. In Zingg et al., eds., Vasopressin and Oxytocin, pp. 427–438. New York: Plenum Press.

Smal, J., Marvola, M., Liljequist, C., and Happonen, I. 1996. Prolonged-release hydroxypropyl methylcellulose matrix tablets of furosemide for administration to dogs. J Vet Pharmacol Therap 19:482–487.

Soma, L. R., and Uboh, C. E. 1998. Review of furosemide in horse racing: its effects and regulation. J Vet Pharmacol Therap 21:228–240.

Soma, L. R., Laster, L., and Oppenlander, F. 1985. Effects of furosemide on the racing times of horses with exercise-induced pulmonary hemorrhage. Am J Vet Res 46:763–768.

Svedberg, K., et al. 1990. Hormones regulating cardiovascular function in patients with severe congestive heart failure and their relation to mortality: Consensus Trial Study Group. Circulation 82:1730.

Velazquez, H., Knauf, H., and Mutschler, E. 1995. Thiazide diuretics. In R. F. Greger, H. Knauf, and E. Mutschler, eds., Handbook of Experimental Pharmacology, vol. 117, Diuretics, pp. 275–321. Berlin: Springer-Verlag.

Ware, W. 1998. Disorders of the cardiovascular system. In R. Nelson and C. G. Couto, eds., Small Animal Internal Medicine, 2nd ed., pp. 58–59. St. Louis: Mosby.

Watson, A., and Church, D. 1995. Preferences of veterinarians for drugs to treat heart disease in dogs and cats. Aus Vet J 72:401–403.

Xu, J. C., Lytle, C., Zhu, T. T., Payne, J. A., Benz, E., Jr., and Forbush, B., III. 1994. Molecular cloning and functional expression of the bumetanide-sensitive Na-K-Cl cotransporter. Proc Natl Acad Sci USA 91:2201–2205.

SECTION 7

Drugs Acting on Blood and Blood Elements

27 ANTIANEMIC AGENTS

MARTIN J. FETTMAN AND H. RICHARD ADAMS

Erythropoiesis
- **Erythrocyte Kinetics**
- **Erythroid Bone Marrow**
- **Tissue Oxygenation as a Stimulus**
- **Erythropoietin**

Micronutrients Required for Erythropoiesis
- **Hemoglobin Synthesis**
- **The Iron Cycle**
- **Nutrient Deficiencies Affecting Hemoglobin Synthesis**
- **Nutrient Deficiencies Affecting Division of Erythroid Precursor Cells**

Anemia
- **Classification of Anemia**
- **Blood Loss Anemia**
- **Chronic Hemorrhage and Iron Deficiency Anemia**
- **Hemolytic Anemia**
- **Nonregenerative (Hypoplastic) Anemia**
- **Primary Dietary Iron Deficiency Anemia**

Polycythemia

Treatment of Anemia
- **Blood Loss Anemia**
- **Baby Pig Anemia**
- **Hemolytic Anemia**
- **Nonregenerative (Hypoplastic) Anemia**
- **Anemia of Chronic Renal Disease**

Nutrients as Hematinic Drugs
- **Iron**
- **Vitamin and Mineral Preparations**

Blood can be considered a bodily organ comprising several different cell types suspended in a fluid medium, or plasma. Blood volume is typically about 8% of body weight; approximately 40% of this consists of cellular elements (erythrocytes, leukocytes, and thrombocytes), and about 60% consists of plasma. More than 99% of the blood cells are erythrocytes, and their principal function is to transport hemoglobin, which in turn carries oxygen from the lungs to the tissues. Erythrocytes have other activities besides transport of hemoglobin-bound oxygen, including carbon dioxide transport from tissues to the lungs for excretion and buffering of acids produced in the normal course of cellular respiration. Although small in number relative to erythrocytes, leukocytes play an indispensable role in the processing of antigens, defense against microorganisms, reparation of wounds, and propagation of the inflammatory response. Likewise, thrombocytes are participants in many inflammatory and reparative processes and are absolutely essential for normal coagulation of blood. However, inadequate tissue oxygenation is the principal pathophysiologic event and is caused by the selective depletion of circulating erythrocyte numbers, i.e., anemia.

The clinical effects of anemia depend upon the severity of reduction in erythrocyte numbers, the time over which this depletion has occurred, and whether this loss is accompanied by a comparable loss of plasma, which affects circulating blood volume. Acute depletion of 25–40% of blood volume can lead to hypovolemic shock. The loss of large numbers of erythrocytes is better tolerated when the loss is of sufficient duration to allow compensatory physiologic adaptations. Thus, depletion of erythrocyte numbers can result in acute illness and death or chronic debilitating illness characterized by unthriftiness and poor performance. Antianemic agents, also referred to as hematinic or hematopoietic drugs, are potentially useful adjuncts to the therapeutic management of such patients if drug selection is based on timely identification of specific causative factors. Certain hematinic drugs may be used nonspecifically to support erythropoiesis irrespective of etiology, whereas other agents are specifically for particular causes of anemia. It is, therefore, important to understand the process of erythropoiesis and affiliated laboratory indices employed in the classification of erythrocyte disorders.

ERYTHROPOIESIS

Erythrocyte Kinetics. The total mass of circulating erythrocytes (the erythron) is regulated in the normal animal within very narrow limits so that sufficient amounts of hemoglobin are available to provide adequate oxygenation of tissues, but without erythrocytes becoming so concentrated in plasma that they impede the flow of blood through small vessels. A small percentage of the erythron is renewed on a continual basis, as senescent erythrocytes are removed from the circulation and new erythrocytes are released from hematopoietic organs as replacements (Jain 1986). The principal site for erythropoiesis in healthy, adult animals is the bone marrow, whereas "extramedullary hematopoiesis" may also occur in the spleen and liver in utero, in neonates, and in anemic adults when the bone marrow regenerative response is inadequate. The "preprogrammed" demise of older erythrocytes is determined largely by their inability to undergo self-repair, wherein certain cellular enzymes gradually lose activity, with subsequent deterioration of cellular metabolic properties (Table 27.1). In mammalian erythrocytes, new enzymes can no longer be produced, owing to lack of the nucleus and ribosomes required for protein synthesis. In avian and reptilian species, which have nucleated mature erythrocytes, the life span of red blood cells can reach 600–1400 days (Lee et al. 1999). Shortening of erythrocyte life span may occur when extracellular events accelerate oxidation of the cell membrane or denaturation of intracellular proteins, principally hemoglobin (Harvey 1997). Conversely, the activity of intracellular reparative pathways that normally defend against such damage may also be altered by specific nutrients or toxicants. The principal mechanisms of erythrocyte destruction include fragmentation, osmotic lysis, erythrophagocytosis, complement-induced cytolysis, and hemoglobin denaturation (Lee et al. 1999). The principal sites of erythrocyte destruction are extravascular and depend on the actions of the mononuclear phagocyte system (formerly called the reticuloendothelial system), which is located predominantly in the spleen and liver. No more than about 10% of the normal destruction of effete erythrocytes occurs intravascularly, but this can increase significantly in certain pathologic states.

TABLE 27.1—Erythrocyte life span in adults of various mammalian species

Species	Mean life span (days)
Human	117–127
Cattle	157–162
Dog	119–122
Cat	86–106
Goat	160–165
Horse	140–150
Pig	62–71
Sheep	70–153

Source: Modified from Jain 1986.

Erythroid Bone Marrow. Erythropoiesis is a function of rapidly dividing precursor cells located in the hematopoietic tissues. It can be characterized by a model wherein pluripotent stem cells serially give rise to lineage-restricted stem cells, which in turn divide and change into morphologically recognizable erythroid precursor cells (Beutler et al. 2000; Weiser 1995) (Fig. 27.1). Characteristic changes in cell size, morphology, antigenic markers, humoral responsiveness, and function occur through predictable stages of cell proliferation and differentiation, until relatively mature erythrocytes are released into the circulation. The rate and integrity of erythropoiesis can be evaluated in most animals by the enumeration and morphologic evaluation of erythroid precursors in the bone marrow. Erythropoiesis is also reflected in the appearance of erythrocytes newly released into the circulation. These cells are characterized in most species (Equidae are notable exceptions) by cytosolic remnants of ribosomal ribonucleic acid and can be estimated by enumeration of specially stained peripheral blood "reticulocyte" counts (Jain 1986). Likewise, they are typically somewhat larger than more mature cells and may also be identified by various methods to determine their greater

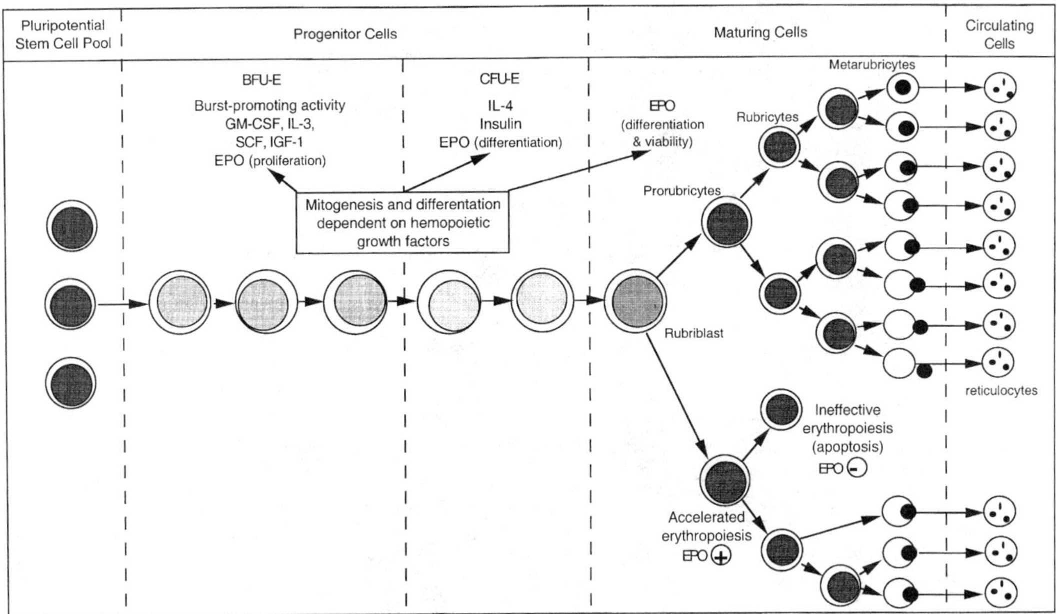

FIG. 27.1—Model of erythropoiesis. BFU-E = burst-forming units—erythroid, CFU-E = colony-forming units—erythroid, GM-CSF = granulocyte–macrophage–colony-stimulating factor, IL-3 = interleukin-3, SCF = stem cell factor, IGF-1 = insulin-like growth factor-1, EPO = erythropoietin, (+) = stimulatory, (–) = inhibitory. (Modified from Beutler 2000 and Weiser 1995.)

cell volume or their effect on mean corpuscular volume of the total erythrocyte population (Radin et al. 1986).

Tissue Oxygenation as a Stimulus. The rate of erythrocyte production is typically increased by conditions that decrease the quantity of oxygen delivered to tissues (Lee et al. 1999). When an animal becomes anemic or hypoxemic, the bone marrow is stimulated to accelerate production of large numbers of erythrocytes for release into the circulation. Chronic pathologic states that result in diminished blood flow through peripheral tissues, and especially those conditions that interfere with oxygen uptake by the blood as it passes through the pulmonary circulation, also cause an acceleration of erythropoiesis. Heart failure and lung diseases, in particular, result in cellular hypoxia, which can trigger increased production of erythrocytes. These examples represent compensatory adjustments by the erythropoietic system to improve the capability of blood to provide adequate delivery of oxygen to the tissues. This increase in erythrocyte production is initiated quite rapidly in response to inadequate tissue oxygenation but only becomes apparent after approximately 48 hours (Weiser 1995). After 3–5 additional days, the rate of erythropoiesis is maximized and may become as much as 8–10 times normal. Erythrocytes continue to be released at an accelerated rate as long as the animal is subjected to the pathophysiologic condition that initially reduced oxygen delivery. Thus, the erythrocyte mass would have to increase to levels sufficient to compensate for a reduction in their numbers or hemoglobin content. Alternatively, the oxygen content of blood and its release in peripheral tissues would have to increase to levels sufficient to compensate for a reduction in inspired oxygen tension, a decrease in oxygen uptake by blood in the pulmonary circulation, or impairment of oxygen delivery by hemoglobin to the peripheral tissues. Upon resolution of the abnormality, transport of oxygen to the tissues will normalize, and the stimulus for increased erythrocyte production is thereby lost. Consequently, erythropoiesis decelerates, and control of the number of circulating erythrocytes is returned to the usual servomechanism for replacing senescent cells.

Erythropoietin. Inadequate oxygenation of the erythropoietic centers of the bone marrow is not a *direct* stimulus for increased erythrocyte production; i.e., the bone marrow does not detect or respond directly to hypoxia itself. Instead, hypoxia promotes release into the circulation of a humoral factor synthesized and secreted predominantly by the kidneys, and it is this factor (erythropoietin) that subsequently stimulates proliferation and differentiation of erythroid precursors in hematopoietic tissues (Erslev and Besarab 1997; Sawyer 1994). Hypoxia increases expression of erythropoietin (EPO) mRNA in interstitial cortical cells located near the base of the renal proximal tubular cells (Fig. 27.2). Hepatocytes, macrophages, and even some erythroid precursor cells may also be capable of

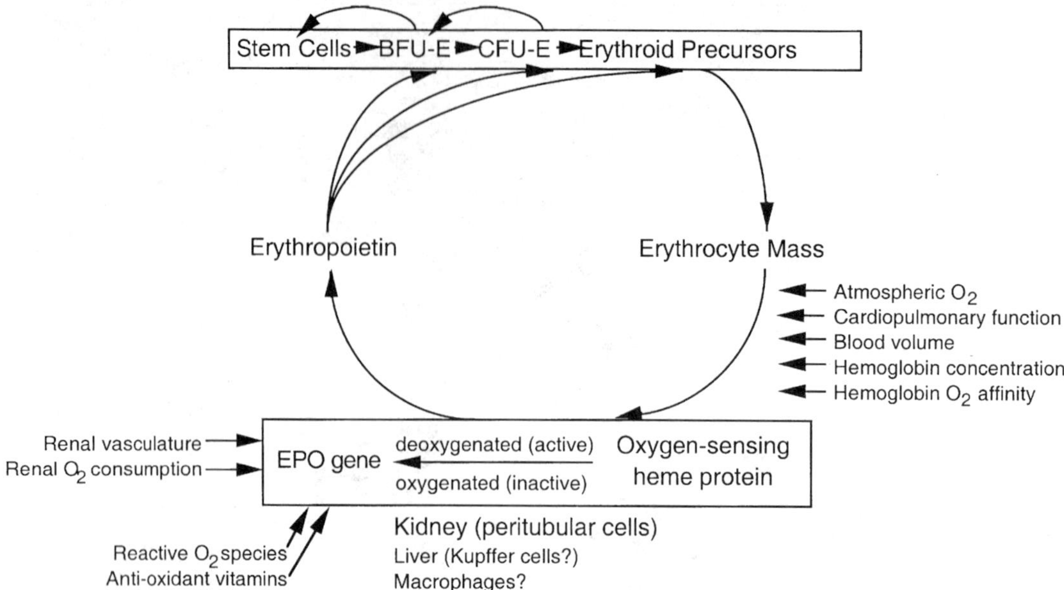

FIG. 27.2—Model of feedback loop controlling erythropoietin production. BFU-E = burst-forming units—erythroid), CFU-E = colony-forming units—erythroid, EPO = erythropoietin. (Modified from Beutler 2000.)

producing small amounts of EPO. Although oxygenation is the key effector in EPO synthesis, various agonists (such as androgens, interleukin-4, and insulin-derived growth factors) and antagonists (such as tumor necrosis factor-α, interleukin-1, and transforming growth factor-β) also influence its production (Erslev and Besarab 1997; Sawyer 1994; Jelkmann et al. 1994). Experimental findings, including the inhibition of EPO production at low partial pressures of oxygen by carbon monoxide, provide evidence that a heme protein is intimately involved in the oxygen-sensing mechanism (Goldberg et al. 1988). During hypoxia, this heme protein is in its active deoxy conformation, which through binding to specific ligands triggers expression of the EPO gene. When oxygen tension is sufficiently high, the heme protein sensor is converted to its inactive, oxygenated form and no longer stimulates EPO production. Potential therapeutic implications of this mechanism will be discussed later.

EPO appears to exert its trophic effects principally during the progenitor cell stages of erythropoiesis (Erslev and Besarab 1997; Sawyer 1994). Mitogenesis and differentiation of both the pluripotential and unipotential burst-forming units—erythroid and colony-forming units—erythroid cells are stimulated by EPO, in conjunction with other humoral factors, including granulocyte–macrophage–colony-stimulating factor, interleukin-3, interleukin-4, stem cell factor, insulin, and insulin-like growth factor-1 (DeMartino et al. 1994; Kelley et al. 1993; Kurtz et al. 1983). EPO may also play a supporting role in promoting the differentiation and viability of maturing erythroid cells, including induction of globin mRNA transcription and suppression of apoptosis in later erythroid precursors (DeMartino et al. 1994; Sawyer 1994; Silva et al. 1996). Heterogeneity in responsiveness to EPO among early erythroid progenitors and later erythroid precursor cells appears to be related to differences in target cell EPO receptor numbers, affinity for EPO, and/or structure-function interactions with second messengers (Kelley et al. 1994). A dose-response relationship between the concentration of EPO and the inhibition of apoptosis in erythroid precursors has been linked to selective expression of a full length or a truncated form of the EPO receptor in target cells (Nakamura et al. 1992).

Erythrocyte production may be inadequate despite maximal stimulation by EPO. This may occur if release of other erythropoietic humoral factors is insufficient to support normal erythropoiesis, as may be the case in diseases characterized by microenvironmental changes in the bone marrow due to inflammation or neoplasia (Fuchs et al. 1994). Likewise, a hormonal milieu conducive to erythropoiesis may result in ineffectual erythrocyte production when specific nutrients are lacking (e.g., iron, copper, pyridoxine, vitamin B_{12}, folic acid) or when erythroid precursor cells are prematurely destroyed prior to maturation and release of erythrocytes from the bone marrow (e.g., immune-mediated destruction). In addition to the production of decreased numbers of mature erythrocytes, ineffectual erythropoiesis may be characterized by the appearance of incomplete, immature, or morphologically and functionally abnormal cells in the circulation.

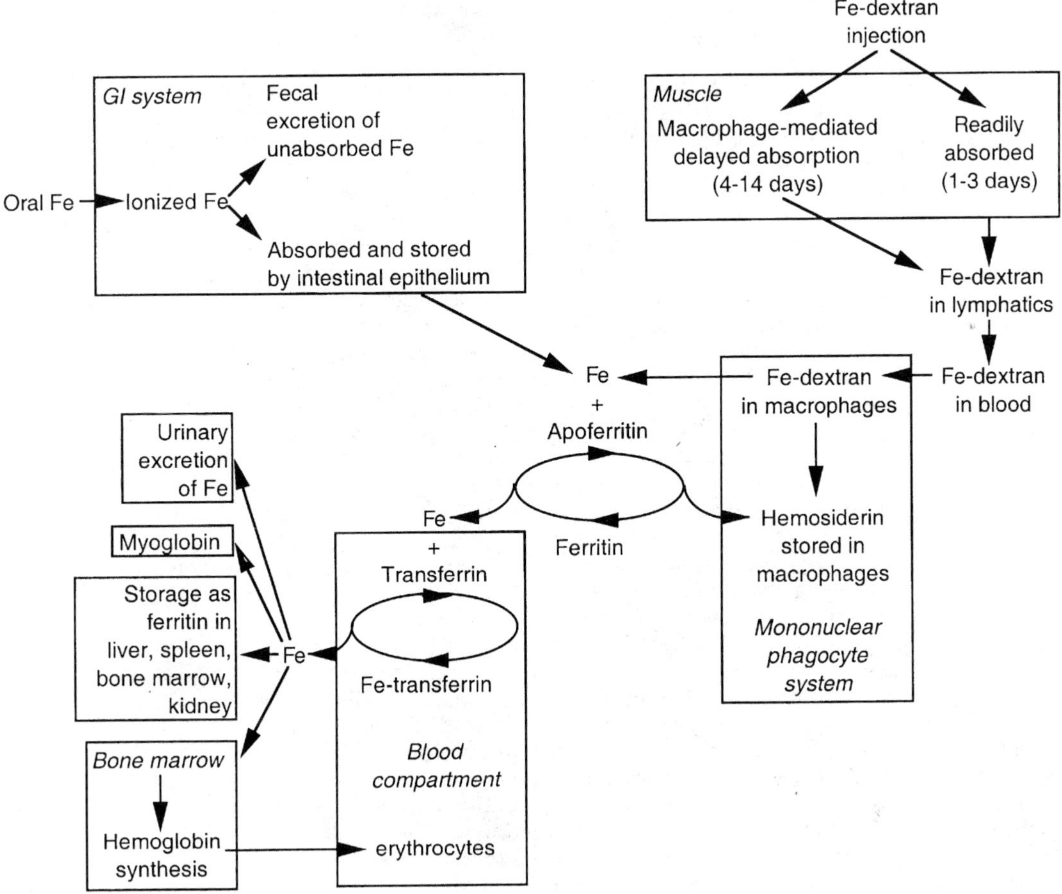

FIG. 27.3—Model of iron metabolism. GI = gastrointestinal, Fe = iron. (Modified from Adams 1995.)

MICRONUTRIENTS REQUIRED FOR ERYTHROPOIESIS

Hemoglobin Synthesis. Hemoglobin synthesis is initiated in the early stages of erythrocyte production, becomes microscopically visible in Wright's stained preparations during the rubricyte (or polychromatophilic normoblast) stage, and continues until the nucleus (in mammals) undergoes pyknotic degeneration in the metarubricyte (or orthochromatic normoblast) stage (Lee et al. 1999). Production of *d*-aminolevulinic acid (ALA) from glycine and succinyl-CoA in the mitochondria is the first, and rate-limiting, step of heme synthesis (Kaneko 1997). This reaction requires pyridoxal phosphate as a cofactor, and a dietary deficiency of vitamin B_6 can result in an anemia morphologically and functionally characteristic of decreased hemoglobin synthesis (see section on iron deficiency anemia below). ALA is transported to the cytosol, where through a series of reactions it is converted into coproporphyrinogen III, which is then transported back into the mitochondria for derivation of protoporphyrin IX. Insertion of ferrous iron into protoporphyrin IX is catalyzed by heme synthetase (ferrochelatase) to produce the heme molecule, which is transferred from the mitochondria to the cytosol for condensation with globin chains to produce hemoglobin. During this process, the iron moiety of heme becomes oxidized to the ferric state, and the ferriheme thus formed is inserted into an α- or β-globin chain. The ferriheme-containing globin chains spontaneously combine to form α-β dimers, two of which combine, in turn, to produce mature hemoglobin tetramers.

The Iron Cycle. Iron is required not only for the formation of hemoglobin but also for myoglobin and ferroenzymes such as the cytochromes, cytochrome oxidases, catalase, and others. Because of the essential participation of iron-containing substances in normal cellular functions throughout the body, it is not surprising that iron is conserved and recycled in a highly efficient manner (Fig. 27.3) (Smith 1997). Approximately two-thirds of total body iron is contained in hemoglobin, which is distributed throughout the erythron in circulating cells and in immature erythrocytes in the hematopoietic tissues. When aged erythrocytes are removed from the circulation, their hemoglobin is rapidly metabolized by cells of the mononuclear phagocyte system. Most of the iron released from this process is recirculated and made available to newly forming erythrocytes within the bone marrow. Thus, little iron is wasted, and only a small portion of dietary iron need normally be absorbed on a daily basis to maintain adequate body stores and normal synthesis of hemoglobin for erythropoiesis. The amount of iron assimilated daily by normal animals, usually only a few milligrams or less, balances the small amount of iron normally lost from the body in hair, nails, and desquamation of cells.

The small intestine proximal to the midjejunum is the principal absorptive and excretory organ for iron. Absorption of iron across the intestinal mucosa is the rate-limiting step in controlling body stores of this element. Iron is absorbed in the ferrous (reduced) state through the intestinal epithelial cells in a process regulated by enterocyte mitochondrial activity and cytosolic iron-chelating proteins such as transferrin and apoferritin. Small quantities of excess iron are stored in the intestinal epithelial cells after oxidation to the ferric form and combination with apoferritin to form ferritin. This iron may subsequently be excreted from the body when the ferritin-containing enterocytes are shed from their villous tips into the intestinal lumen. The circulating form of iron, bound to transferrin, is transported throughout the body and utilized by the bone marrow in the synthesis of hemoglobin. Iron can also be placed in storage as ferritin in most cells of the body, especially the hepatocytes. Excess iron may form intracellular aggregates with proteins and polysaccharides to form poorly soluble complexes of hemosiderin. When body iron stores are increased, circulating levels of ferritin are increased, blood transferrin becomes saturated, and, in turn, the transfer of iron from intestinal mucosal cells becomes limited. This "mucosal block" of iron absorption is thought to be an important limiting factor that prevents the body from accumulating excess iron under normal conditions. The capacity of the mucosal block mechanism can be exceeded if excessive amounts of iron are ingested, thereby leading to iron toxicosis.

Nutrient Deficiencies Affecting Hemoglobin Synthesis. Intestinal iron absorption can increase up to 15-fold in dogs with chronic blood loss anemia and maximally stimulated erythropoiesis. This no doubt occurs because of a reversal of the mucosal block as binding sites for iron become increasingly available in both the transferrin and apoferritin pools. Dietary iron deficiency is uncommon in adult animals (Fulton et al. 1988) but is routinely observed in neonates that are born with limited iron reserves and that principally consume milk or milk substitutes low in iron content (Fettman et al. 1987; Weiser and Kociba 1983). Iron deficiency in adults is most often associated with chronic blood loss, resulting in a deficit between the rate of iron loss and the rate of dietary iron intake (Weiser and O'Grady 1983). Iron deficiency is manifested initially as a normocytic, hypochromic anemia, owing to impaired hemoglobin synthesis. As iron stores are depleted and hemoglobin synthesis is further handicapped, the anemia typically becomes microcytic and hypochromic. Iron deficiency anemia may also be due to increased removal of erythrocytes from the circulation. Iron deficiency appears to increase erythrocyte fragility, thereby shortening their life span, perhaps due to decreased erythrocytic glutathione peroxidase activity and decreased capacity to prevent oxidative damage to the cell membrane and/or hemoglobin (Weiser and O'Grady 1983).

It is thought that the concentration of hemoglobin in maturing erythroid precursor cells determines the number of cell divisions prior to release from the bone marrow. Thus, impaired hemoglobin synthesis leads to both decreased cell hemoglobin content and additional cell divisions, resulting in smaller mature erythrocytes. Dietary vitamin B_6 deficiency likewise results in a microcytic, hypochromic anemia, owing to impaired hemoglobin synthesis. Ceruloplasmin, the principal copper-binding protein in the body, also functions as a ferrooxidase. In this role, it is responsible for the oxidation of ferrous iron from ferritin to ferric iron for transport in transferrin and subsequent incorporation into heme proteins. A deficiency of copper and of ferrooxidase activity will therefore effectively result in an iron deficiency and also produce a microcytic, hypochromic anemia.

Nutrient Deficiencies Affecting Division of Erythroid Precursor Cells

VITAMIN B_{12}. Cyanocobalamin (vitamin B_{12}) is a cobalt-containing vitamin required by cells throughout the body for conversion of ribose nucleotides into deoxyribose nucleotides, a major step in the formation of deoxyribonucleic acid (DNA). Thus, it is an essential nutrient for nuclear maturation and cell division, and deficiency of this vitamin results in generalized depression of cellular development and tissue growth. Because the erythropoietic centers of the bone marrow are among the most rapidly growing and proliferating tissues, inadequate amounts of cyanocobalamin are especially manifested by decreases in erythrocyte production.

Erythrocytic precursors fail to mature properly under conditions of vitamin B_{12} deficiency, and cell proliferation is inhibited (Lee et al. 1999). Instead of repeated divisions yielding numerous progressively smaller progeny, the more primitive cells of the erythroid series undergo fewer cell divisions, continue to synthesize hemoglobin, and remain larger than normal. The enlarged cells typically retain an immature nucleus and develop malformed and fragile cell membranes. The affected precursor cells are termed "megaloblasts," and the corresponding anucleate mature erythrocytes are termed "macrocytes." The latter contain normal concentrations of hemoglobin and are capable of transporting oxygen after entering the circulation. However, immaturity of both the megaloblasts and the macrocytes results in increased cellular fragility, causing the cells to have a shortened life span. Thus, both decreased rates of erythropoiesis and increased rates of erythrocyte senescence contribute to the development of the macrocytic, normochromic anemia characteristic of a vitamin B_{12} deficiency. This should not be confused with the normo- or hypochromic, macrocytic changes typical of many regenerative anemias, wherein larger and less mature anucleate erythrocytes are released into the circulation (Jain 1986).

A major cause of maturation failure of erythrocytes in humans is a defect in intestinal absorption of vitamin B_{12}, resulting in "pernicious anemia" (Lee et al. 1999). This condition is associated most commonly with failure of the gastric mucosa to produce "intrinsic factor," a glycoprotein substance that combines with dietary vitamin B_{12} to protect it from digestive enzymes and to promote its uptake by pinocytosis into intestinal epithelial cells. Absorbed vitamin is then released into the blood and stored in the liver. The large quantity and long biological half-life of B_{12} in the liver may result in a lag time of many months between insufficient intake of the vitamin and expression of deficiency as a maturation failure in circulating erythrocytes.

Naturally occurring anemia due to vitamin B_{12} deficiency is infrequently recognized in domestic animals. A hereditary defect in intestinal cobalamin absorption has been identified in dogs, but intestinal malabsorption associated with exocrine pancreatic insufficiency or small intestinal bacterial overgrowth is more common (see Chap. 36). Nevertheless, a vitamin B_{12}–responsive macrocytic anemia is rarely observed. Adult ruminants are not dependent on a dietary source of this vitamin because ruminal microflora synthesize all the required supplies of cyanocobalamin. However, a dietary source of cobalt is required by ruminal organisms to synthesize vitamin B_{12}, and cobalt shortage can result in an indirect deficiency of the vitamin. Enteric bacteria of many nonruminant species can also synthesize cyanocobalamin, thereby reducing the need for a dietary source. However, vitamin B_{12} deficiencies may still result from inadequate absorption of the vitamin from the digestive tract.

FOLIC ACID. Pteroylglutamic acid (folic acid), like cyanocobalamin, is an obligate participant in the synthesis of nucleoproteins involved in erythrocyte division and maturation (Lee et al. 1999). Anemias associated with a lack of folic acid are, therefore, also characterized as megaloblastic and macrocytic. Folic acid deficiency anemias are considered rare in most species; however, naturally occurring folate antagonists in moldy feeds can block intestinal microbial synthesis of folacin in herbivores. Folic acid–responsive anemias may occur in animals treated with synthetic folate antagonists for their antineoplastic (methotrexate) or antimicrobial (sulfonamides) activities. Likewise, the anticonvulsants phenytoin and primidone may also have folate-antagonistic activity.

PROTEIN. Protein in adequate amounts is important for a normal rate of hemoglobin synthesis and erythrocyte production. A primary deficiency of protein in the diet, or a secondary deficiency subsequent to intestinal or urinary protein loss, can contribute to the development of anemia. Nevertheless, protein deficiency, by itself, has not been demonstrated as an important cause of anemia in domestic animals, and treatment with protein alone will not correct anemia of any cause. As a supportive measure, protein supplementation may be of benefit to the patient convalescing from anemia, particularly if hypoproteinemia is a concurrent problem.

OTHER NUTRIENTS. Production of normal erythrocytes is influenced directly or indirectly by several nutrients that act as coenzymes or cofactors in the synthesis of hemoglobin, metabolic enzymes, or other important structural and functional proteins. These include riboflavin, niacin, pantothenic acid, thiamin, biotin, and ascorbic acid. Antioxidant vitamins A, E, and C play an important role in protecting erythrocytes against oxidative damage from free radicals, and their deficiency can contribute to shortened erythrocyte survival in the circulation. Recent studies have also shown that vitamin A exerts a specific effect to stimulate EPO production by quenching reactive oxygen species, thereby enhancing the production of a ligand termed "hypoxia-inducible factor-1," which activates an enhancer element in the EPO gene (Jelkmann et al. 1997). It is possible that supplementation with vitamin A or its carotenoid precursors may be useful as adjunctive therapy for the anemia of chronic renal disease, by increasing intrinsic EPO production. Primary deficiencies of most nutrient cofactors are rarely seen in domestic animals; exceptions will be noted in subsequent paragraphs when different types of anemias are considered. Details about vitamins and trace minerals are provided in Section 9.

ANEMIA

ANEMIA. Inadequate erythrocyte mass is usually a secondary condition rather than a primary disorder. Anemia is best regarded as an important clinical sign indicative of an underlying pathophysiologic process that must be identified and corrected if hematopoietic therapy is to be successful; e.g., it would be irrational to administer iron to an animal with iron deficiency anemia due to gastrointestinal parasitism if the parasite burden is not also reduced. Knowledge about hematinic drugs should be integrated into a rational approach to management of anemia that depends upon identification and treatment of etiologic factors.

Classification of Anemia. Several classification systems have been used to describe different forms of

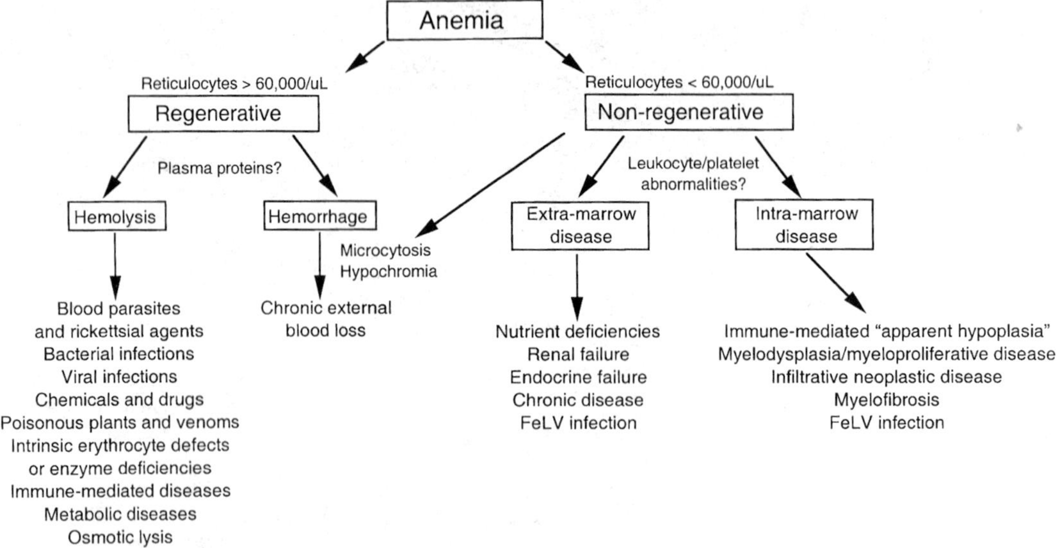

FIG. 27.4—Flowchart of approach to classification of anemia. FeLV = feline leukemia virus.(Modified from Weiser 1995.)

anemia (Fig. 27.4). These systems are based on several variables, including etiology, changes in erythrocyte morphology, and degree of bone marrow regenerative response (Beutler et al. 2000; Weiser 1995). The classification scheme involving the bone marrow regenerative response is necessary to determine the integrity of the erythropoietic response, and observation of changes in morphology is useful in refining the etiologic diagnosis (Table 27.2).

In a regenerative anemia, there is no problem intrinsic to erythrocyte production by hematopoietic tissues. The erythroid marrow responds to inadequate erythrocyte mass by accelerating erythropoiesis, which is reflected in peripheral blood by the appearance of polychromasia in Wright's stained blood films, reticulocytosis >60,000/mL in new methylene blue or brom cresol green stained blood films, and perhaps even the appearance of nucleated erythrocytes (Weiser 1995). Chronic blood loss from the body or increased rates of erythrocyte destruction are the principal causes of regenerative anemias (Fig. 27.4).

In a nonregenerative anemia, the erythropoietic response is insufficient relative to the required rate of replacement of senescent, damaged, or lost erythrocytes. Both extra- and intramarrow diseases can be responsible for the decreased production or maturation abnormalities characteristic of nonregenerative anemias (Fig. 27.4). Peripheral blood demonstrates none of the typical features of accelerated erythropoiesis expected in a regenerative anemia. There is an absence of sufficient polychromasia and a decrease, or negligible increase, in the reticulocyte count (<60,000/mL). Instead, there is a reduction in the circulating numbers of morphologically normal erythrocytes (normocytic, normochromic anemia) or the appearance of morphologically abnormal cells (macrocytic or microcytic anemias), which may have abnormal hemoglobin content (hypochromic anemia) (Table 27.2).

Blood Loss Anemia. Loss of blood from the vascular space, whether to the exterior of the body or to extravascular regions within the tissues, can be acute or chronic. The principal pathophysiologic effect of acute hemorrhage is hypovolemia rather than inadequate erythrocyte mass; e.g., the patient with acute, massive blood loss will more likely die of hemorrhagic shock before an anemia is manifested. If the animal survives acute hemorrhage, and especially if blood loss continues chronically, anemia may occur as erythropoietic capabilities are exceeded. Erythrocyte parameters such as packed-cell volume (PCV) and hemoglobin content can be normal for up to 18 hours after acute blood loss. In fact, the PCV and hemoglobin content may transiently increase following sympathetic activation, splenic contraction, and release of "residual" erythrocytes from the spleen. Hemodilution then occurs as a result of mobilization of extravascular fluids following changes in the balance of capillary hydrostatic pressure and interstitial oncotic pressure. The erythropoietic response is initiated shortly thereafter, owing to detection of hypoxia by the kidney, release of EPO, and stimulation of erythroid stem cell and precursor cell division and differentiation. A maximal erythropoietic response may require approximately 5 days after the hemorrhagic event, and restoration of normal erythrocyte mass can be complete within 7–10 days following a single hemorrhagic episode.

TABLE 27.2—Morphologic and etiologic classifications of anemia

Morphologic classification		
Erythrocyte size	Hemoglobin content	Etiologic classification
Macrocytic	Normochromic	Cobalt or vitamin B_{12} deficiency Folic acid deficiency FeLV-associated myelodysplasia Congenital erythropoietic porphyria Infrequent, asymptomatic characteristic of toy and miniature Poodles
Macrocytic	Hypochromic	Transient condition occurring during the active phase of erythroid regeneration following erythrocyte destruction or acute blood loss: Hemolysis blood parasites and rickettsial agents bacterial infections viral infections chemicals and drugs poisonous plants and venoms intrinsic erythrocyte defects/enzyme deficiencies immune-mediated metabolic diseases osmotic lysis Hemorrhage external internal
Normocytic	Normochromic	Acute blood loss prior to onset of regenerative response Anemia of chromic inflammatory disease Myelodysplasia/myeloproliferative disease Infiltrative neoplastic disease Myelofibrosis FeLV-associated myelodysplasia Immune-mediated destruction of erythroid progenitor cells resulting in "apparent erythroid hypoplasia" Anemia of chronic renal failure Anemia of certain endocrinopathies: hypoadrenocorticism hypothroidism panhypopituitarism hypoandrogenism hyperestrogenism Lead poisoning Cytotoxic marrow damage radiation chemicals bracken fern poisoning
Normocytic	Hypochromic	Early iron deficiency
Microcytic	Normochromic	Iron deficiency in progression Normal, asymptomatic characteristic of Japanese Akitas
Microcytic	Hypochromic	Iron deficiency congenital anemia of neonates chronic external blood loss chronic gastrointestinal blood loss infestation with hematophagous parasites Copper deficiency Pyridoxine deficiency Molybdenum toxicity

Source: Modified from Adams 1995 and Jain 1986.

Chronic Hemorrhage and Iron Deficiency Anemia. If blood loss continues, sufficient iron eventually will be lost from the body to produce an iron-depleted state even with continued ingestion of the usual quantities of dietary iron and increased efficiency of iron absorption. Under these conditions, the rate of hemoglobin loss exceeds that of iron absorption, so that the animal experiences a negative iron balance. The shortage of iron may severely impede erythropoiesis, and the typical microcytic, hypochromic anemia develops if blood loss continues. This is the type of iron deficiency anemia most commonly encountered in companion animals, and typically occurs with chronic gastrointestinal blood loss due to parasitism, bleeding ulcers, inflammatory bowel disease, or hemorrhaging tumors.

Hemolytic Anemia. Destruction of erythrocytes occurs in various disease states in domestic animals. Various blood parasites (*Anaplasma, Babesia, Hemobartonella, Eperythrozoon, Cytauxzoon*), rickettsia (*Ehrlichia*), bacteria (*Leptospira, Clostridium*), and viruses (feline leukemia virus, equine infectious anemia) have been associated with hemolytic anemias. A variety of chemical agents (saponins, snake venoms, phenothiazines), trace elements (lead, copper), and toxicants from poisonous plants (red maple, onion) are additional potential extrinsic causes of hemolysis (Harvey 1997). Immune-mediated hemolytic anemia following pharmaceutical administration, vaccination, or blood transfusion or of idiopathic origin has also been observed in all species. This is typically characterized by the observation of spherocytes in peripheral blood films. These cells have normal volume but appear to be smaller and without the usual biconcave disk appearance of healthy erythrocytes (Weiser 1995). Following opsonization by antibody and/or complement, it is thought that portions of the damaged cell membrane are removed by cells of the mononuclear phagocyte system, thereby reducing the ratio of cell surface area to cell volume. Cross-linking of erythrocytes by antibodies can result in microscopic or macroscopic autoagglutination, which may in some cases be temperature sensitive (cold vs. warm "hemagglutinins").

In cattle, hemolytic anemia has been associated with hypophosphatemic, postparturient hemoglobinuria (Harvey 1997). Congenital porphyria in cattle, pigs, cats, and humans resulting from genetically defective hemoglobin metabolism leads to accumulation of abnormal porphyrins in erythrocytic precursors, which results in hemolysis (Kaneko 1997). The human types of hereditary hemolytic anemias such as sickle cell disease and the thalassemias are not well documented in animals. Erythrocytic enzyme deficiencies, including glucose-6-phosphate dehydrogenase, phosphofructokinase, and pyruvate kinase, have been identified in animals with hereditary forms of hemolytic anemia (Harvey 1997).

Intact erythrocytes remaining in the blood may contain normal amounts of hemoglobin during hemolytic anemia. In the case of iron or copper deficiency, predisposition to oxidative hemolysis may be coupled with the traditional findings of hypochromic microcytosis. Erythroid centers of the bone marrow are usually hyperplastic, and iron from destroyed erythrocytes undergoes rapid recycling to support accelerated erythropoiesis. The appearance of immature erythrocytes in the peripheral blood is common, resulting in a regenerative hypo- or normochromic macrocytosis, polychromasia, and reticulocytosis.

Hemolytic anemia with Heinz body formation is characteristic of exposure of erythrocytes to agents that mediate oxidative damage and induce denaturation of hemoglobin (Harvey 1997). These include methylene blue (urinary antiseptic), phenothiazines (tranquilizers), doxorubicin (antineoplastic), propylene glycol (dietary humectant), benzyl alcohol (preservative), and allyl disulfides (phytochemicals). Because of low hepatic conjugative enzyme activities, cats have decreased capacity relative to other mammals to deactivate oxidative toxicants (Fettman 1991). In addition, feline hemoglobin is uniquely susceptible to oxidative damage, leading to a propensity for Heinz body formation in oxidatively damaged feline erythrocytes (Fettman 1991). Christopher (1989) studied the relationships between disease in 120 cats and the occurrence of Heinz bodies. Diabetes mellitus was most commonly associated with Heinz bodies (15.8% of the cases), followed by hyperthyroidism (12.5%), lymphoma (10.8%), and nonhemic cancer (10.8%).

Nonregenerative (Hypoplastic) Anemia. Anemia associated with bone marrow dysfunction may or may not be accompanied by defective production of other cell lines when granulocyte and thrombocyte production is also affected. Hypoplastic anemia occurs rarely as an idiopathic disorder. Potential extramarrow causes include exposure to bone marrow–suppressive chemicals (pesticides, insecticides, antineoplastic agents), endocrine failure affecting cell division and erythropoiesis (EPO, insulin, thyroid hormones), chronic inflammation/infection, feline leukemia virus infection, and nutrient deficiencies as described earlier (Fig. 27.4). Potential intramarrow causes include primary myelodysplastic and myeloproliferative diseases, infiltrative neoplastic diseases, and feline leukemia virus infection. A particular form of "apparent erythroid hypoplasia" has been associated with immune-mediated destruction of erythroid precursor cells (Jonas et al. 1987; Holloway et al. 1990). There may appear to be hyperplasia of early nucleated erythrocytes, but a "maturation arrest" of the erythroid line occurs, owing to phagocytosis and destruction of antibody/complement-fixated precursors. The peripheral blood is devoid of polychromatophilic erythrocytes or reticulocytes, and so the anemia appears to be hypoplastic.

Primary Dietary Iron Deficiency Anemia. Iron-responsive, microcytic, hypochromic anemia is relatively common in neonates of all species (Weiser and Kociba 1983) but is especially important in the swine industry (Hubbard et al. 1952). Pigs are born with limited body stores of iron (and copper), and sow's milk provides only one-seventh the daily requirement of iron for growth (Smith 1997). The incidence and susceptibility of suckling pigs to iron deficiency anemia have increased in parallel with an increase in intensification of modern husbandry techniques aimed at increasing weaning weight. Rapidly growing pigs are the most susceptible. In the past, pigs raised on natural dirt surfaces had free access to considerable amounts of iron in the soil. Pigs ingest only a limited amount of iron from their environment when kept on clean concrete floors. Clinical signs of anemia can develop by 3 weeks of age if preventive therapy with iron is omitted. Approximately 300 mg of iron must be absorbed by the baby pig during the first 3 weeks of life, but only ~21 mg (1 mg/day) is acquired by ingestion of sow's milk, and perhaps only 100 mg may be obtained from the environment during this time period. Thus, pigs raised in this manner are apt to be lacking nearly 200 mg of iron in their first 3 weeks. Supplementation is needed for approximately the first 5 weeks of life, until baby pigs can consume creep feed to provide the required iron.

Anemia of baby pigs is hypochromic and microcytic, typical of iron deficiency. Some pigs may seem fairly well nourished, but problems develop, exhibited in poor growth, listlessness, rough hair coat, wrinkled skin, and drooping ears and tails. The pigs may exhibit dyspnea, fatigue, pale skin, pale mucous membranes, and increased susceptibility to disease. Sudden death is not uncommon, and the mortality rate may be high.

POLYCYTHEMIA. A relative or absolute increase in the concentration of circulating erythrocytes is termed "polycythemia" (Campbell 1990). An increase in erythrocyte numbers is usually associated with a corresponding increase in the hemoglobin concentration of the blood as well. Relative polycythemia, or "erythrocytosis," results from loss of the fluid component of blood, or "hemoconcentration." This is often a transient state secondary to dehydration as a result of prolonged vomiting, persistent diarrhea, polyuria, excessive sweating, or loss by exudation and evaporation from burns and large wounds. Because this loss of fluid may be superimposed upon a deficiency of erythrocytes, it is possible that hemoconcentration may obscure the detection of anemia. If fluid loss is accompanied by protein loss as well, it may not be possible to use hyperproteinemia as an index of hemoconcentration. Thus, evaluation of physical signs of hypovolemia (skin resiliency, capillary refill time, enophthalmos, etc.) is essential in identifying concurrent hemoconcentration and anemia.

Absolute polycythemia is characterized by an increase in the total erythron. It may be transient, due to release of stored cells following sympathetically mediated splenic contraction but is usually associated with hyperplasia of erythropoietic elements of the bone marrow. It can be idiopathic as a primary disorder termed "polycythemia vera," wherein no other diseases may be found, and EPO levels are normal or decreased (Cook and Lothrop 1994; Hasler and Giger 1996). Absolute polycythemia can also result from a physiologically inappropriate increase in erythrogenesis, stimulated by excessive release of erythropoietic humoral factors such as EPO. Tumor-associated polycythemia has been observed with many types of neoplasia in humans, including renal cell carcinoma, hepatoma, pheochromocytoma, and adrenocortical tumors. It has been reported in dogs with carcinoma, fibrosarcoma, or lymphosarcoma of the kidneys (Gorse 1988; Nelson and Hager 1983; Peterson and Zanjani 1981). Physiologically appropriate absolute polycythemia can also develop secondary to diseases associated with chronic hypoxia that stimulate EPO release from the kidneys. Examples include "right-to-left" circulatory shunts, chronic pulmonary disease, or residence at high altitude, causing decreased partial pressure of inspired oxygen.

Clinical signs of polycythemia include plethora (ruddy mucous membranes), central nervous system disorders (seizures, ataxia, lethargy, dementia, blindness), and episodes of bleeding (epistaxis, hematemesis, hematochezia, and hematuria) (Campbell 1990). Many of these signs stem from increased blood viscosity that impedes blood flow, distends small capillaries, and predisposes to thrombosis and rupture of small vessels.

Treatment of secondary polycythemia should be directed at the primary disease and improvement of oxygen delivery to tissues. Likewise, paraneoplastic syndromes of absolute polycythemia may respond to removal of the tumor. Phlebotomy may be indicated for patients whose absolute polycythemia is responsible for clinical signs, before treatment can be directed at the tumor or myeloproliferative disorder responsible for excessive erythropoiesis. Various myelosuppressive drugs have been used to decrease erythropoiesis in patients with idiopathic polycythemia. These include chlorambucil, busulfan, melphalan, hydroxyurea, and radiophosphorus (^{32}P) (Campbell 1990; Peterson and Randolph 1982; Smith and Turrel 1989).

TREATMENT OF ANEMIA

Blood Loss Anemia

ACUTE HEMORRHAGE. The life-threatening problem in animals experiencing a single, acute episode of blood loss is hypovolemia leading to the onset of hemorrhagic shock. Blood volume repletion is the main therapeutic goal in these patients, usually on an emergency basis accompanied by other cardiopulmonary resuscitative procedures. Transfusion of whole blood is not always necessary under these conditions because the remaining endogenous erythrocyte mass generally is sufficient for hemoglobin-oxygen transport if volume repletion is sufficient. A balanced crystalloid solution, comparable in composition to normal extracellular fluid, may be adequate. When the source of hemorrhage has been controlled, additional use of a hypertonic crystalloid solution, such as 7.2% sodium chloride, may be indicated to promote fluid redistribution from extravascular tissues to the vascular compartment, as well as for its positive inotropic effects on the heart (Fettman 1985). If there is significant hypoproteinemia, vascular fluid loss to the extravascular tissues, or insufficient restoration of blood pressure following crystalloid fluid administration, synthetic colloid-containing solutions may be indicated (Rudloff and Kirby 1997). These include 0.9% saline solutions with 6–10% Dextran-40, Dextran-70, pentastarch, or hetastarch, but caution is urged for patients with preexisting dehydration, underlying renal disease, or coagulation abnormalities. Plasma transfusions may also be effective, but they do carry some risk of adverse immunologic reactions or occult infectious disease transmission.

If an acute bleeding episode continues for a lengthy interval (e.g., in a major surgical procedure), erythrocyte mass may become inadequate for oxygen transport despite blood volume maintenance with crystalloid or colloid solutions. At this point, hemoglobin replacement therapy is indicated through whole-blood transfusion, packed red blood cell transfusion, or administration of a cell-free, chemically modified hemoglobin solution. Whole-blood or packed-cell transfusions require ready accessibility to blood type–matched donors and/or the means for processing, storing, and replenishing supplies of fresh blood products (Callan et al. 1996; Harrell et al. 1997a,b; Kerl and Hohenhaus 1993; Wardrop et al. 1997). Transfusion reactions are a significant concern even when cross-match tests have been performed, because antibodies to other blood components or small amounts of antibodies to erythrocytes may not be detected. Because of the complexity and cost of maintaining an acceptable blood transfusion program, cell-free polymerized hemoglobin solutions have recently received increased attention in the human and veterinary medical communities. Only one polymerized, ultrapurified bovine hemoglobin preparation has received FDA approval for veterinary use, but chemically modified hemoglobin solutions that have been studied include polymerized, pyridoxylated, stroma-free human hemoglobin, fumaryl-ββ-cross-linked bovine hemoglobin, and polyethylene glycol-polymerized bovine hemoglobin (Gilroy and Odling-Smee 1990; Migita et al. 1997; Sprung et al. 1995; Ulatowski et al. 1996). These solutions have a colloid osmotic pressure similar to that of whole blood, a *P*50 for oxygen lower than that of whole blood but adequate for efficient oxygen delivery in clinical situations, and an extended shelf life compared to fresh blood products. They have been shown to be more effective than colloid solutions in restoring blood volume, oxygen transport, and cardiovascular performance in experimental models of hemorrhagic shock in rats, cats, dogs, and sheep. There are indications that some cell-free, polymerized hemoglobin solutions may also exert erythropoietic effects on the bone marrow, though the mechanism remains vague.

CHRONIC HEMORRHAGE. Successful therapy for chronic blood loss anemia requires the diagnosis and treatment of the inciting ailment as the principal objective. Severe anemia may require transfusion of whole blood or blood products. In addition to general supportive care and adequate nutrition, prolonged therapy with iron or other erythropoietic nutrients may be indicated. Because patients with chronic anemia are principally deficient in erythrocytes, plasma components may not be necessary. However, it is not unusual for anemic animals to be dehydrated as well; this may lead to circulatory shock and seems to be associated with packed-cell volumes of less than 15% in dogs and less than 12% in cats. Blood volume expansion is indicated under these circumstances, for which whole blood or cell-free, polymerized hemoglobin, crystalloid, and/or colloid solutions may be beneficial.

Baby Pig Anemia. Anemia of newborn pigs can be prevented by a variety of methods. Because of the labor involved in repeated oral administrations, a single intramuscular injection of an iron compound (e.g., 100–150 mg elemental iron as iron dextran) on the second or third day of life is often the preferred method of treatment. Within 3 days of iron administration, blood hemoglobin concentrations increase markedly (Fig. 27.5), and recipients respond by ingesting more milk and growing more rapidly than untreated pigs. Because copper deficiency may also participate in the pathogenesis of baby pig anemia, application of iron-copper preparations to the sow's udder has also proven effective in preventing this form of anemia.

Iron dextrans are frequently used iron supplements in newborn pigs; these compounds are absorbed into the lymphatic system within 3 days following intramuscular injection. The process of absorbing and transferring this iron from the injection site into the lymphatic system is achieved predominantly by macrophages. A variable portion of the iron dextran remains in the connective tissue at the injection site as a continuing, but less available, depot of iron. Iron dextran passes rapidly from the lymphatics into the blood and readily enters cells of the mononuclear phagocyte system throughout the body. Separation of the free iron from the polysaccharide occurs in these cells, and the dextran is largely excreted in the urine or metabolized

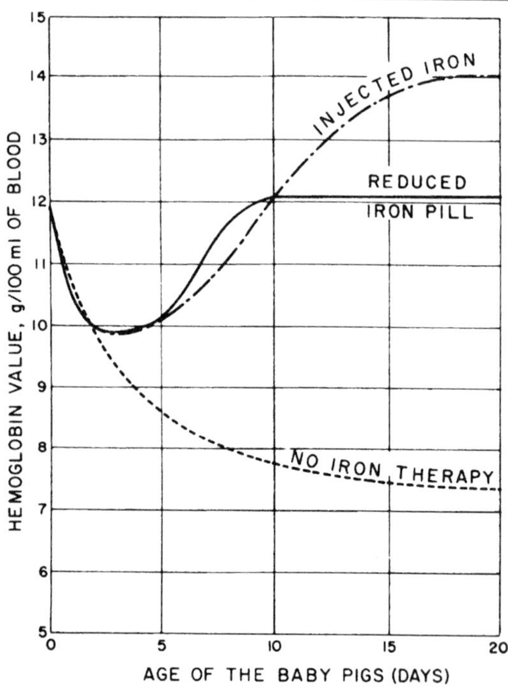

FIG. 27.5—Influence of iron therapy upon the hemoglobin value of newborn pigs. (From Hubbard et al. 1952.)

to glucose. The free iron enters the blood and combines with transferrin for transport throughout the body.

There is no established indication for iron therapy in pigs weighing 20 kg or more. Should anemia occur in older swine, it is more likely associated with an infectious agent or chronic blood loss than with a simple dietary deficiency of iron. Administration of iron preparations to prevent tail biting and other social vices induced by confinement is not indicated and has been associated with discoloration and condemnation of meat at slaughter.

Hemolytic Anemia. This condition is often a direct result of specific chemical, infectious, or antigenic agents that elicit oxidative or immunological damage to erythrocytes. Supportive therapy includes transfusion of whole blood or blood products if tissue oxygenation is sufficiently compromised. Specific treatment should focus on identification and elimination of the etiologic agents (Table 27.2), as discussed in detail elsewhere in this book. Existing oxidative damage to erythrocytes is difficult to reverse, but continued injury may be ameliorated by antioxidants or substances that promote endogenous free-radical-scavenging mechanisms. Intravenous *N*-acetylcysteine has been employed as a glutathione precursor in subduing the actions of oxidative drugs, including acetaminophen, propofol, and doxorubicin (Fettman 1991). Dietary cysteine supplementation has also been used to promote glutathione synthesis, as a preventative against oxidative damage by mycotoxins and plant alkaloids (Fettman 1991). Vitamins with antioxidant properties (A, E, and C) may also be beneficial. Infectious agents should be eliminated by treatment with appropriate antimicrobial agents. Immunologically mediated erythrocyte damage is also difficult to reverse, but continued injury may be prevented by administration of immunosuppressive drugs (corticosteroids, cyclophosphamide, azathioprine). Intravenous administration of human immune globulin has been useful for short-term stabilization of some dogs with immune-mediated hemolytic anemia but does not appear to have affected long-term survival (Scott-Montcrieff et al. 1997).

Nonregenerative (Hypoplastic) Anemia. The nonregenerative form of immune-mediated anemia, characterized by erythroid precursor phagocytosis within the bone marrow and subsequent abrogation of the erythropoietic response, may respond to immunosuppressive drugs or human γ globulin (Scott-Montcrieff et al. 1995). These cases usually are more refractory to treatment and may require immunosuppression of greater intensity and duration than do those with only immune-mediated destruction of mature erythrocytes. Systemic endocrinopathies such as hypothyroidism or hyperestrogenism that result in hypoplastic anemia must be treated by addressing the primary disorder. However, treatment with lithium carbonate (11 mg/kg per os, twice daily) has been associated with improved hematopoiesis in dogs with estrogen-induced bone marrow suppression (Hall 1992).

Anemia of Chronic Renal Disease

GENERAL APPROACH. Loss of endogenous EPO resulting from chronic renal disease culminates in a nonregenerative anemia (Cowgill 1992). In addition, uremia can be associated with reduced erythrocyte survival, platelet dysfunction, gastrointestinal bleeding, uremic inhibitors of erythropoiesis, myelofibrosis, and nutritional deficiencies that contribute to anemia. Therapy directed at slowing the progression of chronic renal failure or ameliorating the adverse consequences of uremia not only improve clinical performance but also promote erythropoiesis. Reducing circulating levels of uremic toxins removes inhibitory influences on bone marrow responsiveness to EPO and other erythropoietic hormones. Modification of the dietary intake of water, protein, essential fatty acids, phosphorus, sodium, water-soluble vitamins, antioxidants, trace minerals (including iron), alkalinizing agents, and other nutrients limits future renal damage and maintains or restores glomerular filtration.

SECONDARY HYPERPARATHYROIDISM. Secondary hyperparathyroidism is a fundamental component of chronic renal failure, and its management is associated with amelioration of further renal damage and improved mineral homeostasis (Polzin and Osborne 1995; Cowgill 1995). In addition, it has been proposed that increased parathyroid hormone (PTH) concentrations mediate several uremic changes, including suppression of EPO release and bone marrow responsiveness. Although serum PTH levels correlate poorly with the degree of uremia in dogs with chronic renal failure, most anemic patients have significantly higher PTH values than do nonanemic animals (King et al. 1992). Dietary phosphorus restriction and/or calcitriol supplementation have both been demonstrated to alleviate renal secondary hyperparathyroidism, and calcitriol has been shown to improve anemia and reduce the need for erythropoietin in human dialysis patients (Goicoechea et al. 1998).

IRON DEFICIENCY. Because gastrointestinal hemorrhage is a frequent complication of uremia, histamine H_2-receptor antagonists (cimetidine, ranitidine) and mucosal protectants (sucralfate) should be considered for the prevention and treatment of gastric ulceration associated with blood loss (Polzin and Osborne 1995; Cowgill 1995). Because this can result in iron deficiency, it is essential that renal disease patients be evaluated for iron status prior to institution of other pharmacotherapies for anemia. Treatment with iron supplements is the same as described for other causes of iron deficiency anemia below.

ANABOLIC STEROIDS. Treatment with exogenous erythropoietic hormones such as androgenic steroids is used to support the erythron in chronic renal disease patients (Shahidi 1973). However, evidence supporting the use of anabolic steroids to treat the anemia of chronic renal disease in veterinary patients has been equivocal. Following experimental nephrectomy in one study, dogs treated for 6 weeks with 3-oxo-D1,4-androstadiene-17β-ol-undecylenate experienced no significant improvement in food intake, lean body mass, nitrogen balance, or PCV (Finco et al. 1984). In another study of surgically-induced chronic renal failure, dogs who received 2 mg stanozolol orally, twice each day for six weeks experienced a significant increase in lean body mass and nitrogen balance, but effects on the erythron were not reported (Cowan et al. 1997). Longer duration therapy has been necessary to demonstrate beneficial effects in studies of human patients, who also have received maintenance hemodialysis. Based upon the definitive success of anabolic steroids in experimental animal models and in human patients, androgens have become a common, although not wholly proven, adjunct to the therapy for anemia of chronic renal disease in veterinary medicine (Cowgill 1995). Three classes of androgens have been used in uremic humans, including testosterone esters (propionate, enanthate, or cypionate), nortestosterone esters (nandrolone phenylpropionate, decanoate), and 17α-alkylated androgens. Androgens may improve erythropoiesis by directly stimulating erythroid precursors in the bone marrow and by stimulating EPO production by the remnant kidneys. Potential adverse effects of androgenic steroids include masculinization of females, fluid retention, hepatic toxicity, and, in males, prostatic hyperplasia or neoplasia.

ERYTHROPOIETIN. The clinical efficacy of endogenous EPO replacement with a recombinant human erythropoietin (rhEPO) has been documented in human patients (Erslev and Besarab 1997). Because the structure of EPO molecules has been relatively well conserved across many species, rhEPO can also be quite effective in restoring erythropoiesis to normal levels in uremic veterinary patients (Cowgill 1995; Cowgill et al. 1998). Patients with mild anemia of chronic renal disease may not require rhEPO treatment, but for those with moderate to marked anemia (PCV <30% in dogs and PCV <25% in cats), the benefits of rhEPO treatment often outweigh potential adverse effects. Therapy is initiated at 100 units/kg body weight by subcutaneous injection three times per week. This will initiate a regenerative response characterized by the appearance of reticulocytes in the peripheral blood (up to ~4.5% of total erythrocyte numbers in dogs and ~3.0% in cats) within a few days. PCV typically increases rapidly (up to ~1% per day during the first month) and returns to normal values within 2–3 weeks. When target erythrocyte numbers are attained, the dosage interval is reduced to twice, or even once, weekly, to avoid induction of erythrocytosis. If target values are not attained within 8–12 weeks, the dose is increased by 25–50 units/kg of body weight. Failure to respond to rhEPO can be attributed to many factors. It is essential that the patient's uremia is controlled, nutrient intake and body weight are stabilized, potential gastrointestinal bleeding is prevented, and iron status is normalized. Refractoriness to rhEPO has been observed in a significant number of treated animals and can be attributed to the development of anti-rhEPO antibodies in 20–50% of patients (Cowgill 1995). Recombinant canine EPO (rcEPO) has recently become available. Because rcEPO does not seem to cause erythroid hypoplasia in dogs, it may represent an improved alternative to rhEPO treatment in canine renal failure (Randolph et al. 1999). Potential adverse effects of rhEPO include polycythemia, systemic hypertension, vomiting, seizures, injection site discomfort, allergic mucocutaneous reactions, and, rarely, acute anaphylactic reactions. Severe, life-threatening anemia due to development of anti-rhEPO antibodies has been reported in horses and may resolve following cessation of rhEPO administration (Piercy et al. 1998).

NUTRIENTS AS HEMATINIC DRUGS

Iron. Therapeutic use of iron is indicated only in treatment and, in specific situations, prevention of iron deficiency anemia. Administration of iron in an attempt to correct anemia associated with other ailments is strictly empirical and has no proven clinical value. This limitation should be recognized by the clinician despite the fact that iron is included in a large number of commercial supplements intended to improve appetite, increase breeding efficiency, promote growth, and more. It should also be recognized that indiscriminate administration of iron preparations is accompanied by the danger of iron toxicosis or iron storage disease in healthy, as well as in unhealthy, animals.

Absorption, distribution, metabolism, and excretion of iron was summarized earlier (also see Fig. 27.3). Iron is distributed in several pools throughout the body: the hemoglobin pool in erythrocytes (60–70%), intracellular deposits of ferritin and hemosiderin (25%), the myoglobin pool in muscle (3–7%), the circulating pool of plasma transferrin (0.1%), and the respiratory enzyme pool (0.1%).

When administered orally, organic iron sources are better absorbed than inorganic sources, and ferrous salts are absorbed more efficiently than ferric salts. Many dietary components influence iron absorption from the intestine. Intraluminal factors that enhance absorption by increasing iron solubility include sugars (fructose and sorbitol), some amino acids, and a number of other organic acids, including ascorbic, succinic, lactic, and citric. Factors that depress iron absorption include calcium, phosphates, oxalate, bicarbonate, and phytic acid. Iron salts are chemically incompatible with many drugs, and mixing preparations is not advised; e.g., chelation of iron from ferrous sulfate by tetracycline limits the absorption of both compounds.

Extraluminal factors that affect iron absorption include the level of erythropoietic activity, body iron stores, and anemia. Hypoxic stimuli that promote erythropoiesis also increase iron absorption. Iron absorption is also increased when body stores of this element are low, even when hemoglobin content and oxygen transport are normal. Iron-deficient dogs will absorb up to 60% of orally administered iron, whereas less than 10% of dietary iron is absorbed under normal circumstances. Erythrocytosis following multiple transfusions, a return to normal oxygen tension after episodes of reduced oxygen availability, or large doses of antiproliferative chemotherapeutic agents or radiation will diminish erythropoiesis and iron absorption.

Severe iron deficiency paradoxically causes intestinal malabsorption of iron in dogs and humans (Kimber and Weintraub 1968). Thus, iron deficiency of sufficient intensity or duration may result in refractoriness to oral iron therapy for anemia. Thus, it is recommended that iron deficiency be treated first by administration of a parenteral preparation, followed by continued oral iron supplementation for approximately 1 month or for as long as the cause of iron imbalance might otherwise continue. In dogs, iron dextran should be administered intramuscularly at a dose of 10–20 mg/kg (Weiser and Kociba 1983). For neonatal cats, a single injection of 50 mg iron dextran is administered intramuscularly at approximately 18 days of age to prevent congenital iron deficiency anemia (Weiser and O'Grady 1983). The daily dose for ferrous sulfate is 100–300 mg/kg for adult dogs and 50–100 mg/kg for adult cats. Although little is known regarding an efficacious dose for iron dextran in adult large animals, doses for ferrous sulfate have been derived. They include 8–15 g per os per day for 2 weeks or more in cattle, 2–8 g per os per day for 2 weeks or more in horses, and 0.5–2 g per os per day for 2 weeks or more in swine and sheep.

ADVERSE EFFECTS. Mucosal block of iron absorption can be superseded by excessive doses of the element, especially if administered for prolonged periods of time. Iron overload and toxicosis can result. The usual concentration of iron in plasma is about 100 mg/dL, which is approximately one-third the binding capacity of the circulating transferrin pool. Transferrin can become completely saturated during iron overload. Accumulation of iron in the body may be expressed by two known conditions: hemosiderosis and hemochromatosis. Hemosiderosis refers to a localized process of abnormal iron pigmentation caused by increased amounts of hemosiderin in the tissues. This usually occurs after hemorrhage into tissues or a body cavity. Hemochromatosis is a systemic disease characterized by widespread hemosiderosis and micronodular hepatic cirrhosis. The former is due to systemic iron accumulation by tissue macrophages, and the latter is due to iron accumulation and toxicity of hepatocytes and Kupffer cells. Hemochromatosis can be found in association with intravascular hemolysis following exceptionally abundant destruction of erythrocytes due to immune-mediated hemolytic anemia or transfusion reactions, and after prolonged ingestion or large doses of iron. In addition, hemochromatosis is an inherited disease in humans and Salers cattle that is characterized by idiopathically increased gastrointestinal iron absorption and abnormal deposition of iron in parenchymal tissues (House et al. 1994).

All iron preparations probably have equal potential toxicity per unit of elemental iron. Orally administered iron is known to be relatively safe for humans and animals, provided excessive amounts are not administered acutely. Clinical signs of iron toxicosis in baby pigs include erosion, ulceration, and hemorrhage of the gastrointestinal mucosa, followed by melena and/or hematochezia and signs of acute blood loss, including pale skin, tachycardia, hypotension, dyspnea, lethargy, and circulatory shock. Animals treated with commercial parenteral iron preparations intended for other species are particularly prone to toxicosis. Twenty of 36 Simmental heifers treated with a large dose of a commercial iron preparation intended for horses died within 72 hours following treatment. Iron toxicity was evidenced by petechial hemorrhages in multiple organs, severe centrolobular necrosis of the liver, and >500 mg/dL elemental iron in the serum. Caution must be exercised when administering parenteral iron supplements, because the body does not have an efficient extraintestinal mechanism for iron excretion.

Treatment of oral iron poisoning is directed at preventing absorption by intestinal mucosal cells and is facilitated by use of a gastrointestinal adsorbent or an emetic agent as long as hemorrhagic vomiting is not occurring. Sodium bicarbonate (6% solution) can be used as a lavage, followed by oral administration of deferoxamine mesylate, a specific iron-chelating drug (Pitt et al. 1979; Klaassen 1996). For systemic treatment, the most effective means of removing iron is by chelation. Deferoxamine is administered intramuscularly (20 mg/kg every 4 hours). If circulatory shock is evident, the preparation can be administered intravenously (40 mg/kg over a 4-hour period, followed by 20 mg/kg every 12 hours). Deferoxamine promotes the urinary excretion of chelated iron so that several days of therapy are required to eliminate the entire toxic dose. Continued appearance of a reddish discoloration of the urine indicates that iron is still undergoing excretion and that deferoxamine chelation treatment should continue.

Vitamin and Mineral Preparations. The general indications and limitations of therapeutic use of vitamins and minerals are discussed in Section 9. The only established clinical use of these substances as hematinic agents is in the treatment of anemias caused by specific vitamin or mineral deficiencies. Successful therapy with these substances depends upon a clear understanding of their normal participation in the erythropoietic process and identification of the specific cause of anemia. Indiscriminate administration of vitamins or minerals can complicate the anemic state and be harmful in certain situations; e.g., in humans, therapy with folic acid can temporarily correct the hematologic manifestations of vitamin B_{12} deficiency while

TABLE 27.3—Representative iron preparations for veterinary use

Oral preparations	
Ferrous sulfate*	*E-Kwine®* vitamin B complex, cobalt
	Feosol® elixir, tablets, or sustained release capsules
	Fer-In-Sol® drops or exissicated capsules
	Fer-Iron® drops
	Fero-Gradumet Filmtabs® timed release tablets
	Ferospace® timed release capsules
	Ferralyn Lanacaps® timed release capsules
	Ferra-TD® timed release capsules
	Ferratin® arsenic, strychnine, copper, cobalt
	Ferro-Folic-500® folic acid, controlled release
	Ironate® vitamin B complex, vitamin C, copper
	Mol-Iron® tablets
	Livibron® vitamin B complex, manganese
	Vi-Natura® vitamin B complex
Ferrous lactate	*Ferro drops®* 25 mg/ml; for small animals
Ferrous gluconate	*Triple A & N Tab®* strychnine, arsenic, nucleic acids
	V-L-I-B® desiccated liver, vitamin B complex; for small animals
	Livolex® vitamin B complex
Ferrous fumarate	*V-Sorbits®* vitamin B complex, vitamins A, D, E
	Livitamin® vitamin B complex, vitamin C, desiccated liver
Ferrous sulfate	*Lib®* copper, cobalt, desiccated liver
Ferric pyrophosphate	*Vi-Sorbin®* vitamin B complex, sorbitol
Ferric ammonium citrate:	*Ferrisol, Iron-Plus Mineral Supplement®* vit. B complex, copper, cobalt
	Allane® vitamin B complex
Ferric chloride	*Caco-Copper®* arsenic, copper
Ferric citrochloride	*Ferrogen®* strychnine, cobalt, copper
Ferric hydroxide	*Purina Oral Pigemia®* dextran complex
Ferric methionine	*Ferrodex®* vegetable oil paste
Ferric proteinate	*Lixotinic®* vitamin B complex, copper, beef liver
	Duriron® copper proteinate, dried yeast
Parenteral preparations	
Iron dextran	*Ferrextran®, Ferrodex®, Nonemic®, Dexiron®*
Iron hydrogenate dextran	*Iron-Gard®*
Ferric hydroxide	*Iro-Jex®, Iron-Gard®*

*Dose (as ferrous sulfate septahydrate, providing 200 mg elemental iron per gram), daily for 2 weeks or more: horse, 2–8 g; cattle, 8–15 g; sheep and swine, 0.5–2 g; dog, 100–300 mg; cat, 50–100 mg.

allowing the serious neurological damage associated with the latter to progress.

A large number of multivitamin-multimineral "shotgun" admixtures are available for use in animals. Many of these preparations are advocated as hematinics; some examples are listed in Table 27.3. The antianemic efficacy of these remedies has not been established by carefully controlled studies. Clinicians should be aware of unsubstantiated claims in regard to vitamin-mineral mixtures. Typical effects that have been claimed for some preparations include strengthening of convalescing animals, increasing food intake, improving feed efficiency, and enhancing growth and production. If a deficiency is diagnosed, the clinician is best advised to administer only the deficient substance rather than rely on a multicomponent preparation that contains unnecessary and potentially toxic ingredients.

REFERENCES

Adams, H. R. 1995. Antianemic agents. In H. R. Adams, ed., Veterinary Pharmacology and Therapeutics, 7th ed., pp. 531–543. Ames: Iowa State University Press.

Beutler, E., Seligsohn, U., Lichtman, M. A. 2000. Williams' Hematology. 6th[h] ed. New York: McGraw-Hill.

Callan, M. B., Oakley, D. A., Shofer, F. S., and Giger, U. 1996. Canine red blood cell transfusion practice. J Am Anim Hosp Assoc 32:303–311.

Campbell, K. L. 1990. Diagnosis and management of polycythemia in dogs. Comp Cont Educ Prac Vet 12:543–550.

Christopher, M. M. 1989. Relation of endogenous Heinz bodies to disease and anemia in cats: 120 cases (1978–1987). J Am Vet Med Assoc 194:1089–1095.

Cook, S. M., and Lothrop, C. D. 1994. Serum erythropoietin concentrations measured by radioimmunoassay in normal, polycythemic, and anemic dogs and cats. J Vet Int Med 8:18–25.

Cowan, L.A., McLaughlin, R., Toll, P. W., Brown, S. A., Moore, T. L., Butine, M. D., Milliken, G. 1997. Effect of stanozolol on body composition, nitrogen balance, and food consumption in castrated dogs with chronic renal failure. J Am Vet Med Assoc 211:719–722.

Cowgill, L. D. 1995. Medical management of the anemia of chronic renal failure. In C. A. Osborne and D. R. Finco, eds., Canine and Feline Nephrology and Urology, pp. 539–554. Baltimore: Williams & Wilkins.

Cowgill, L. D., James, K. M., Levy, J. K., Browne, J. K., Miller, A., Lobingier, R. T., Egrie, J. C. 1998. Use of recombinant human erythropoietin for management of anemia in dogs and cats with renal failure. J Am Vet Med Assoc 212:521–528.

DeMartino, J., Carroll, M., Mathey-Prevot, B., et al. 1994. Erythropoietin receptor contains both growth-promoting

activity and differentiation-promoting activity. Ann NY Acad Sci 718:213–222.
Erslev, A. J., and Besarab, A. 1997. Erythropoietin in the pathogenesis and treatment of the anemia of chronic renal failure. Kidn Intl 51:622–630.
Fettman, M. J. 1985. Hypertonic crystalloid solutions for the treatment of hemorrhagic shock. Comp Cont Educ Prac Vet 7:915–923.
———. 1991. Comparative aspects of glutathione metabolism affecting individual susceptibility to oxidant injury. Comp Cont Educ Prac Vet 13:1079–1091.
Fettman, M. J., Brooks, P. A., and Phillips, R. W. 1987. Antimicrobial alternatives for calf diarrhea: Sera trace element responses to *Escherichia coli*-, deferoxamine-, or gallium-induced diarrhea. Am J Vet Res 48:703–711.
Finco, D. R., Barsanti, J. A., and Adams, D. D. 1984. Effects of an anabolic steroid on acute uremia in the dog. Am J Vet Res 45:2285–2288.
Fuchs, D., Zangerle, R., Denz, H., and Wachter, H. 1994. Inhibitory cytokines in patients with anemia of chronic disorders. Ann NY Acad Sci 718:344–346.
Fulton, R., Weiser, M. G., Freshman, J. L., et al. 1988. Electronic and morphologic characterization of erythrocytes of an adult cat with iron deficiency anemia. Vet Pathol 25:521–523.
Gilroy, D., and Odling-Smee, W. 1990. Oxygen transport by a modified haemoglobin solution (PPSFH) in a dog model of acute anemia following hypovolaemia. Intensive Care Med 16:237–241.
GoicoecheaM., VazquezM. I., RuizM. A., Gomez-Campdera, F., Perez-Garcia, R., Valderrabano, F. 1998. Intravenous calcitriol improves anaemia and reduces the need for erythropoietin in haemodialysis patients. Nephron 78:23–27.
Goldberg, M. A., Dunning, S. P., and Bunn, H. F. 1988. Regulation of the erythropoietin gene: evidence that the oxygen sensor is a heme protein. Science 242:1412–1415.
Gorse, M. J. 1988. Polycythemia associated with renal fibrosarcoma in a dog. J Am Vet Med Assoc 192:793–794.
Hall, E. J. 1992. Use of lithium for treatment of estrogen-induced bone marrow hypoplasia in a dog. J Am Vet Med Assoc 200:814–816.
Harrell, K., Parrow, J., and Kristensen, A. 1997a. Canine transfusion reactions. Part I. Causes and consequences. Comp Cont Educ Prac Vet 19:181–190.
———. 1997b. Canine transfusion reactions. Part II. Prevention and treatment. Comp Cont Educ Prac Vet 19:193–200.
Harvey, J. W. 1997. The erythrocyte: physiology, metabolism, and biochemical disorders. In J. J. Kaneko, J. W. Harvey, and M. L. Bruss, eds., Clinical Biochemistry of Domestic Animals, 5th ed., pp. 157–203. San Diego: Academic Press.
Hasler, A. H., and Giger, U. 1996. Serum erythropoietin values in polycythemic cats. J Am Anim Hosp Assoc 32:294–301.
Holloway, S. A., Meyer, D. J., and Mannella, C. 1990. Prednisolone and danazol for treatment of immune-mediated anemia, thrombocytopenia, and ineffective erythroid regeneration in a dog. J Am Vet Med Assoc 197:1045–1048.
House, J. K., Smith, B. P., Maas, J., et al. 1994. Hemochromatosis in Salers cattle. J Vet Int Med 8:105–111.
Hubbard, E. D., Bauriedel, W. R., Picken, J. C., et al. 1952. Nutritional Anemia of Suckling Pigs. Ames: Iowa State University Press.
Jain, N. C. 1986. Schalm's Veterinary Hematology. 4th ed. Philadelphia: Lea & Febiger.
Jelkmann, W. E. B., Fandrey, J., Frede, S., et al. 1994. Inhibition of erythropoietin production by cytokines. Ann NY Acad Sci 718:300–311.
Jelkmann, W., Pagel, H., Hellwig, T., et al. 1997. Effects of antioxidant vitamins on renal and hepatic erythropoietin production. Kidn Intl 51:497–501.
Jonas, L. D., Thrall, M. A., and Weiser, M. G. 1987. Nonregenerative form of immune-mediated hemolytic anemia in dogs. J Am Anim Hosp Assoc 23:201–204.
Kaneko, J. J. 1997. Porphyrins and the porphyrias. In J. J. Kaneko, J. W. Harvey, and M. L. Bruss, eds., Clinical Biochemistry of Domestic Animals, 5th ed., pp. 205–221. San Diego: Academic Press.
Kelley, L. L., Koury, M. J., Bondurant, M. C., et al. 1993. Survival or death of individual proerythroblasts results from differing erythropoietin sensitivities: A mechanism for controlled rates of erythrocyte production. Blood 82:2340–2352.
Kelley, L. L., Green, W. F., Hicks, G. G., et al. 1994. Apoptosis in erythroid progenitors deprived of erythropoietin occurs during the G_1 and S phases of the cell cycle without growth arrest or stabilization of wild-type p53. Mol Cell Biol 14:4183–4192.
Kerl, M. E., and Hohenhaus, A. E. 1993. Packed red blood cell transfusions in dogs: 131 cases (1989). J Am Vet Med Assoc 202:1495–1499.
Kimber, C., and Weintraub, L. R. 1968. Malabsorption of iron secondary to iron deficiency. New Engl J Med 279:453–459.
King, L. G., Giger, U., Diserens, D., and Nagode, L. A. 1992. Anemia of chronic renal failure in dogs. J Vet Int Med 6:264–270.
Klaassen, C. D. 1996. Heavy metals and heavy metal antagonists. In J. G. Hardman, L. E. Limbird, P. B. Molinoff, R. W. Ruddon, and A. G. Gilman, eds., Goodman and Gilman's The Pharmacological Basis of Therapeutics, 9th ed., pp. 1649–1671. New York: McGraw-Hill.
Kurtz, A., Jelkmann, W., and Bauer, C. 1983. Insulin stimulates erythroid colony formation independently of erythropoietin. Brit J Haematol 53:311–316.
Lee, G. R., Foerster, J., Lukens, J., Paraskevas, F., Greer, J. P., Rodgers, G. M. 1999. Wintrobe's Clinical Hematology. 10th ed. Philadelphia: Williams and Wilkins.
Migita, R., Gonzales, A., Gonzales, M. L., et al. 1997. Blood volume and cardiac index in rats after exchange transfusion with hemoglobin-based oxygen carriers. J Appl Physiol 82:1995–2002.
Nakamura, Y., Komatsu, N., and Nakauchi, H. 1992. A truncated erythropoietin receptor that fails to prevent programmed cell death of erythroid cells. Science 257:1138–1141.
Nelson, R. W., and Hager, D. 1983. Renal lymphosarcoma with inappropriate erythropoietin production in a dog. J Am Vet Med Assoc 182:1396–1397.
Peterson, M. E., and Randolph, J. F. 1982. Diagnosis of canine primary polycythemia and management with hydroxyurea. J Am Vet Med Assoc 180:415–418.
Peterson, M. E., and Zanjani, E. D. 1981. Inappropriate erythropoietin production from a renal carcinoma in a dog with polycythemia. J Am Vet Med Assoc 179:995–996.
Piercy, R. J., Swarson, C. J., Hinchcliff, K. W. 1998. Erythroid hypoplasia and anemia following administration of recombinant human erythropoietin to two horses. J Am Vet Med Assoc 212:244–247.
Pitt, C. G., Gupta, G., Estes, W. E., et al. 1979. The selection and evaluation of new chelating agents for the treatment of iron overload. J Pharmacol Exptl Ther 208:12–18.
Polzin, D. J., and Osborne, C. A. 1995. Conservative medical management of chronic renal failure. In C. A. Osborne and D. R. Finco, eds., Canine and Feline Nephrology and Urology, pp. 508–538. Baltimore: Williams & Wilkins.
Radin, M. J., Eubank, M. C., and Weiser, M. G. 1986. Electronic measurement of erythrocyte volume and volume

heterogeneity in horses during erythrocyte regeneration associated with experimental anemias. Vet Pathol 23:656–660.

Randolph, J. F., Stokol, T., Scarlett ,J. M., MacLeod ,J. N. 1999. Comparison of biological activity and safety of recombinant canine erythropoietin with tat of recombinant human erythropoietin in clinically normal dogs. Am J Vet Res 60:636–642.

Rudloff, E., and Kirby, R. 1997. The critical need for colloids: selecting the right colloid. Comp Cont Educ Prac Vet 19:811–825.

Sawyer, S. T. 1994. The erythropoietin receptor and signal transduction. Ann NY Acad Sci 718:185–190.

Scott-Moncrieff, J. C., Reagan, W. J., Glickman, L. T., et al. 1995. Treatment of nonregenerative anemia with human γ-globulin in dogs. J Am Vet Med Assoc 206:1895–1900.

Scott-Moncrieff, J. C., Reagan, W. J., Snyder, P. W., et al. 1997. Intravenous administration of human immune globulin in dogs with immune-mediated hemolytic anemia. J Am Vet Med Assoc 210:1623–1627.

Shahidi, N. T. 1973. Androgens and erythropoiesis. N Engl J Med 289:72–80.

Silva, M., Grillot, D., Benito, A., et al. 1996. Erythropoietin can promote erythroid progenitor survival by repressing apoptosis through Bcl-X_L and Bcl-2. Blood 88:1576–1582.

Smith, J. E. 1997. Iron metabolism and its disorders. In J. J. Kaneko, J. W. Harvey, and M. L. Bruss, eds., Clinical Biochemistry of Domestic Animals, 5th ed., pp. 223–239. San Diego: Academic Press.

Smith, M., and Turrel, J. M. 1989. Radiophosphorus (^{32}P) treatment of bone marrow disorders in dogs: 11 cases (1970–1987). J Am Vet Med Assoc 194:98–102.

Sprung, J., Mackenzie, C. F., Barnas, G. M., et al. 1995. Oxygen transport and cardiovascular effects of resuscitation from severe hemorrhagic shock using hemoglobin solutions. Crit Care Med 23:1540–1553.

Ulatowski, J. A., Nishikawa, T., Matheson-Urbaitis, B., Bucci, E., Traystman, R. J., and Koehler, R. C. 1996. Regional blood flow alterations after bovine fumaryl bb-crosslinked hemoglobin transfusion and nitric oxide synthase inhibition. Crit Care Med 24:558–565.

Wang, L. M., Myers, M. G., Sun, X. J., et al. 1993. IRS-1: essential for insulin- and IL-4-stimulated mitogenesis in hematopoietic cells. Science 261:1591–1594.

Wardrop, K. J., Tucker, R. L., and Mugnai, K. 1997. Evaluation of canine red blood cells stored in a saline, adenine, and glucose solution for 35 days. J Vet Int Med 11:5–8.

Weiser, M. G. 1995. Erythrocyte responses and disorders. In S. J. Ettinger and E. C. Feldman, eds., Textbook of Veterinary Internal Medicine, 4th ed., chap. 142. Philadelphia: W. B. Saunders.

Weiser, M. G., and Kociba, G. J. 1983. Sequential changes in erythrocyte volume distribution and microcytosis associated with iron deficiency anemia in kittens. Vet Pathol 20:1–12.

Weiser, M. G., and O'Grady, M. 1983. Erythrocyte volume distribution analysis and hematologic changes in dogs with iron deficiency anemia. Vet Pathol 20:230–241.

28

HEMOSTATIC AND ANTICOAGULANT DRUGS

H. RICHARD ADAMS

Hemostasis
- **Vascular and Platelet Phases**
- **Coagulation Phase**
- **Fibrinolysis Phase**
- **Natural Anticoagulants**
- **Coagulopathies and Drugs**

Hemostatic Drugs
- **Topical Hemostatics**
- **Systemic Hemostatics**

Anticoagulants
- **In Vitro Anticoagulants**
- **Systemic Anticoagulants**
- **Vitamin K Antagonists**

Fibrinolytic Agents
- **Clinical Aspects**
- **Tissue Plasminogen Activator**

Antiplatelet Drugs
- **Aspirin**
- **Ticlopidine**
- **Dipyrimadole**

Several drugs and animal tissue extracts exert pronounced effects on hemostatic and blood coagulative mechanisms. Some of these substances promote hemostasis and have clinical value in control of blood oozing from small vessels. Hemostatic agents include thrombin, thromboplastin, fibrin, and fibrinogen. In contrast, drugs such as heparin and sodium citrate retard hemostasis by impeding clot formation. These anticoagulant agents are employed in the laboratory to prevent clotting of blood used in diagnostic tests or stored for transfusion. Heparin also is used in vivo, as are the coumarin-derivative anticoagulants, in treatment and prevention of thromboembolic disorders. Additional approaches involve the enzymes streptokinase and urokinase, which activate fibrinolytic breakdown of formed clots and clotting factors. Thrombus formation also is reduced by inhibitors of platelet aggregation such as aspirin and ticlopidine.

An overview of local factors involved in control of bleeding will first be presented as an aid to understanding how hemostatic and anticoagulant drugs affect hemostasis-related mechanisms.

HEMOSTASIS. The term hemostasis refers to prevention or control of hemorrhage. Physiologic control systems operate to ensure fluidity of blood under normal conditions, yet opposing systems promote coagulation when the circulatory system is invaded. Hemostasis is achieved through a series of interdependent mechanisms, including vascular spasm of the injured artery or vein, local aggregation of platelets into a plug, coagulation of the blood into a clot, and dissolution of the formed clot by fibrinolysis. The basic process of hemostasis can be separated into the vascular, platelet, coagulation, and fibrinolysis phases. The phases overlap considerably, and events in one step promote and even cause development of subsequent phases (Chart and Sanderson 1979).

Vascular and Platelet Phases. The vascular and platelet phases are closely allied. Until recently the central role of vascular endothelium in hemostasis was not appreciated. The endothelium has a multitude of anticoagulant and procoagulant functions (Nawroth et al. 1986). The inability to reproduce the effects of the endothelium on hemostasis helps explain why in vitro coagulation assays sometimes fail to properly reflect in vivo pathophysiologic events.

Immediately after a blood vessel is cut or otherwise traumatized, the vascular wall contracts and platelets start adhering to the injured site. The local vasoconstrictor response, or vascular spasm, mechanically retards the flow of blood escaping from the vessel. Vascular spasm may be partly a local reflex or myogenic response and partly humoral owing to vasoactive agents released from platelets and nearby cells. Local vasoconstriction lasts as long as 20-30 minutes, during which the ensuing phases of platelet aggregation and blood coagulation take place (Weiss 1978; Moncada and Vane 1979).

Damage to a blood vessel results in exposed subendothelial collagen. Collagen and other proteins localized to the subendothelium are strong stimuli for platelet adherence. For platelets to properly attach to a traumatized area, von Willebrand factor (vWf) must be present because the platelets express a vWf receptor that facilitates adherence. Once adhesion has occurred, the platelets undergo a change in shape and release diverse substances that recruit further platelets to the clot and promote the coagulation cascade. This process is termed aggregation. The substances released include adenosine diphosphate (ADP), adenosine triphosphate (ATP), serotonin, platelet factor 3 and 4, thromboxane A_2, and platelet-derived growth factor. This aggregation yields a rather loosely formed plug or platelet thrombus at the injury site.

INVOLVEMENT OF PROSTAGLANDINS. Adenosine diphosphate is a potent chemical activator of platelet aggregation, which in turn activates a phospholipase that acts on membrane phospholipid to yield arachidonic acid. The latter is transformed by a platelet cyclooxygenase into short-lived but potent aggregating compounds called cyclic endoperoxides (prostaglandins [PGs] G_2 and H_2). These endoperoxides are converted by platelet thromboxane synthase to a potent aggregating compound called thromboxane A_2. Thus platelet clumping initiates formation of chemical agents that promote further platelet aggregation. In contrast, prostacyclin (PGI_2) is a PG that inhibits platelet aggregation and may act as a counterbalance to thromboxane. PGI_2 is formed from arachidonic acid and intermediate cyclic endoperoxides. Prostacyclin synthase, the enzyme responsible for transformation of PGI_2 from the cyclic endoperoxides, is localized in the vascular wall rather than in platelets. The platelet activation sequence is shown in Fig. 28.1.

Vascular spasm and platelet adhesion, aggregation, and release of chemical agents are initiated within seconds after vascular trauma. During subsequent events, the platelet plug becomes more tightly bound and organized by incorporation of fibrin strands formed during coagulation.

Coagulation Phase. Blood clotting results from a complex series of interdependent events. Clotting ingredients normally exist as inactive factors in blood vessels, perivascular tissue, and the blood itself. Upon injury to the circulatory system, the inactive or procoagulant substances are transformed to active clotting factors. Activation of all factors does not occur simultaneously. Rather, the activated form of one factor activates a subsequent factor in a sequential series of reactions, yielding a cascade or "waterfall" effect. Biochemically, the activation process is accomplished for most of the clotting factors by the proteolytic splitting off of a small moiety of the inactive procoagulant factor.

Blood clotting factors generally are designated by Roman numerals I-V and VII-XIII, as listed in Table 28.1. Nomenclature of the factors has undergone considerable revision over the years. The terminologies used by Guyton (1976), Erslev and Gabuzda (1979), and Platt (1979) are basically followed in this discussion. Factors V and VII-XIII usually are designated by

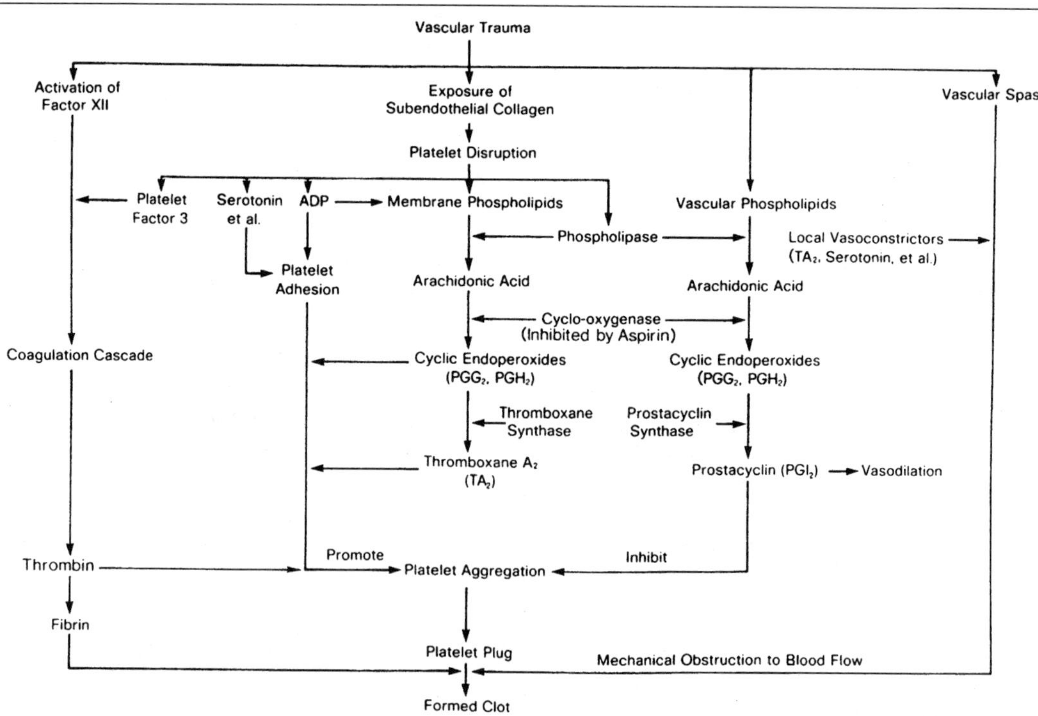

FIG. 28.1—Vascular and platelet phases of hemostasis. PG = prostaglandin; ADP = adenosine diphosphate.

TABLE 28.1—Blood coagulation factors and their synonyms

Factor	Synonym
Factor I	Fibrinogen
Factor II	Prothrombin
Factor III	Tissue thromboplastin
Factor IV	Calcium
Factor V	Proaccelerin
Factor VII	Proconvertin; serum prothrombin conversion accelerator
Factor VIII	Antihemophilic factor
Factor IX	Plasma thromboplastin component; Christmas factor
Factor X	Stuart-Prower factor
Factor XI	Plasma thromboplastin antecedent
Factor XII	Hageman factor
Factor XIII	Fibrin stabilizing factor

their numbers, whereas factors I and II are referred to more commonly as fibrinogen and prothrombin respectively. Tissue thromboplastin is factor III and should not be confused with platelet factor 3. There is no factor VI. Important synonyms for the major clotting factors are included in Table 28.1.

Although clotting factors participate in coagulation through different pathways, the overall coagulation process can be divided into three major events: (1) a substance called prothrombin activator or complete thromboplastin is formed in response to trauma to blood vessels, extravascular tissues, or the blood itself; (2) prothrombin activator catalyzes the transformation of prothrombin to thrombin; and (3) thrombin rapidly catalyzes conversion of fibrinogen into threads of fibrin, which in turn enmesh platelets, plasma, and erythrocytes to form a clot.

The initial step, formation of prothrombin activator, is the most complex and least understood. This substance can be produced by two basic routes: the intrinsic pathway instigated by trauma to the blood itself and the extrinsic pathway that begins with damage to the vessel wall and extravascular tissues. In vivo the coagulation factors involved in the intrinsic and extrinsic coagulation pathways interact with each other. The strict separation of the intrinsic and extrinsic coagulation pathways is based upon the in vitro coagulation assays.

INTRINSIC PATHWAY. Blood taken by venipuncture and placed in a glass container clots normally within 5-10 minutes because all factors required for coagulation are present within the blood (Fig. 28.2). This pathway is initiated because trauma to the blood directly affects two important coagulation factors within the blood itself, the platelets and factor XII. Platelets damaged by contact with a wettable surface like glass (or collagen in vivo) release the phospholipid commonly referred to as platelet factor 3. In addition, factor XII is transformed into activated factor XII when disturbed by trauma to the blood. The activated form of factor XII in turn activates factor XI and forms kallikrein. Factor XI converts factor IX to an activated form. The activated factor IX interacts with factor VIII in conjunction with the platelet phospholipid to convert factor X to activated factor X. Finally, activated factor X interacts with factor V and platelet phospholipids to yield the complex called prothrombin activator (intrinsic thromboplastin system). Prothrombin activator immediately catalyzes the cleavage of prothrombin to thrombin, which converts fibrinogen into fibrin (Fig. 28.2).

EXTRINSIC PATHWAY. When tissue extract is added to whole blood, clotting occurs rapidly in about 10-15 seconds. The extrinsic factor that sets the coagulation cascade into motion is released from traumatized tissues (Fig. 28.2). Referred to as tissue thromboplastin, the extrinsic factor includes a combination of a proteolytic enzyme simply called tissue factor and tissue phospholipids that are probably derived from cell membrane components. First, the tissue factor interacts with clotting factor VII; this complex converts factor X to activated factor X in the presence of the tissue phospholipids. In addition, factor IX is activated, which can also lead to further factor X activation. The subsequent step is essentially the same as the last step in the intrinsic pathway; i.e., activated factor X interacts with factor V and tissue phospholipid to form prothrombin activator (extrinsic thromboplastin system). The difference is that tissue phospholipids are used in the extrinsic system while platelet phospholipids are used in the intrinsic system (Fig. 28.2).

FIBRIN FORMATION. Prothrombin activator, whether derived from the intrinsic or extrinsic pathway, converts the α_2-globulin prothrombin into thrombin. Thrombin in turn acts as a proteolytic enzyme and cleaves two low molecular weight peptides from each molecule of fibrinogen, forming a molecule of fibrin monomer. Thrombin also promotes platelet aggregation and activates factors XIII, XII, VIII, and V. Fibrin monomers immediately polymerize with each other, forming long fibrin threads that act as the reticulum network for the clot. The fibrin chains initially are somewhat loosely bound. However, clotting factor XIII (fibrin-stabilizing factor) quickly acts as an enzyme to cause covalent bonding between fibrin monomers and between adjacent fibrin threads. This process stabilizes and strengthens the meshwork of the clot. The clot comprises the interlocking fibrin chains and the entrapped blood cells, platelets, and plasma. Final clot retraction and serum extrusion are caused by a contractile protein thrombosthenin that is released from platelets (Fig. 28.2).

INVOLVEMENT OF CALCIUM. Calcium ions (Ca^{++}), referred to as clotting factor IV (Table 28.1), are required for all coagulation reactions except the first two steps in the intrinsic pathway. This dependency is exploited in the laboratory; Ca^{++}-complexing agents such as citrate are used as in vitro anticoagulants.

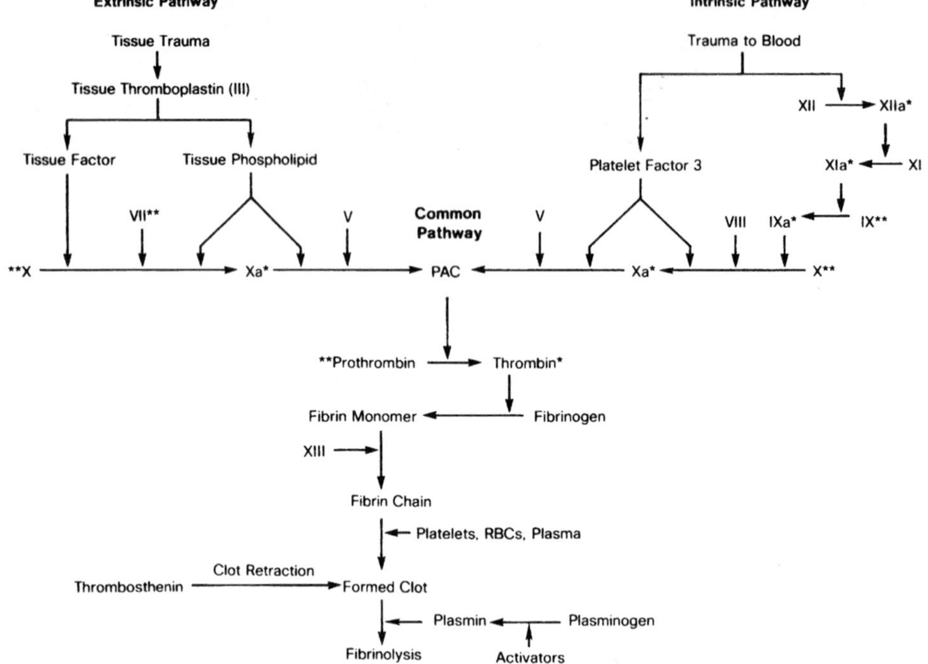

FIG. 28.2—Blood coagulation, clot formation, and fibrinolysis. PAC = prothrombin activator complex (also referred to as complete thromboplastin, prothrombinase, prothrombinase complex, and intrinsic or extrinsic thromboplastin); a = activated forms of clotting factors; * = factors inhibited by heparin; ** = factors inhibited by coumarin derivatives. Calcium is required in most reactions.

Availability of calcium generally is not a limiting factor in the body except rarely after massive transfusion of citrated blood. Usually, death from tetany and respiratory failure would result from hypocalcemia before the calcium concentration was low enough to significantly affect coagulation.

INVOLVEMENT OF KALLIKREIN-KININ SYSTEM. A deficiency of prekallikrein or high molecular weight kininogen prolongs the partial thromboplastin time of blood in vitro and thus slows the intrinsic clotting pathway. Kallikrein amplifies activation of factor XII, which in turn further increases conversion of prekallikrein to kallikrein (Donaldson et al. 1976).

Fibrinolysis Phase. A plasma β globulin called plasminogen is bound to fibrin and incorporated into the clot along with other plasma constituents. Fibrinolysis is initiated when plasminogen is activated by local agents to plasmin. Tissue-type plasminogen activator is produced by endothelial cells and fibroblasts and utilizes fibrin as a cofactor in the conversion of plasminogen to plasmin. Plasmin is a proteolytic enzyme that digests the fibrin chains into soluble polypeptides, thereby preventing further fibrin polymerization. Plasmin also digests other substances in the clot and surrounding blood, e.g., prothrombin; fibrinogen; and clotting factors V, VIII, and XII. Formation of plasmin results in dissolution of the clot and also in hypocoagulability of the blood because of loss of clotting factors. Thus fibrinolysis represents the physiologic converse of the coagulation process. It serves as a defense mechanism against overactivity of the coagulation mechanism. The long-term patency of the vascular tree no doubt depends on a balanced equilibrium between coagulation and fibrinolysis (Fig. 28.2).

Natural Anticoagulants. The sensitivity of the coagulation cascade to hematologic disruptions necessitates equally sensitive control systems to prevent indiscriminate clotting. As stated so colorfully by Erslev and Gabuzda (1979), the clotting factors "stand poised as the parts of a loaded gun with trigger cocked, aimed at fibrinogen." Physiologic systems are available that either "clean up" the clotted target after the thrombin bullet is shot or act as "safeties" to prevent the gun from discharging needlessly.

First, the vascular endothelium is exceptionally smooth surfaced, thereby preventing contact activation of platelets and factor XII. Prompt removal of activated factors from the circulation is attained physically by rapid blood flow that washes local concentrations away from the site of thrombus formation. The liver rapidly clears the activated factors with a half-life of only a few

TABLE 28.2—Selected hemostatic diseases in animals

I. Vascular defects (vasculitis)
II. Platelet defects
   A. Thrombocytopenia
      1. Idiopathic immune-mediated destruction
      2. Immune-mediated destruction secondary to drug administration, vaccination, and various diseases
      3. Bone marrow suppression (chemotherapeutics, estrogens)
      4. Increased consumption (disseminated intravascular coagulation, microangiopathy associated with neoplasia)
   B. Thrombocytopathy
      1. Inherited (Otterhounds, Basset Hounds, cattle)
      2. Acquired (drug administration [e.g., aspirin, antibiotics, lidocaine] gammopathy associated, uremia)
III. Von Willebrand disease (inherited deficiency of von Willebrand factor leading to defective platelet adhesion; found in humans, swine, dogs, and rabbits)
IV. Coagulation defects
   A. Inherited
      1. Hemophilia A (lack of functional factor VIII; found in humans, horses, cats, and dogs)
      2. Hemophilia B (lack of factor IX; found in humans, dogs, and cats)
      3. Hagemann factor deficiency (lack of factor XII; will produce significant prolongation of APTT and ACT results but is rarely related to a clinical bleeding disorder)
   B. Acquired
      1. Deficiency of vitamin K activity (vitamin K-antagonist rodenticide poisoning, malabsorption)
      2. Decreased hepatic synthesis (neoplasia, cirrhosis, infection)
      3. Increased consumption (disseminated intravascular coagulation)
V. Thrombotic diseases
   A. Disseminated intravascular coagulation (neoplasia, severe generalized inflammation, pancreatitis, hemolysis)
   B. Deficiency of AT III (nephrotic syndrome, heartworm adulticide treatment)
   C. Circulatory abnormalities (cardiomyopathy in cats)

minutes. Fibrinolytic dissolution of formed clots has been discussed.

Humoral inhibitors of intermediate products of coagulation play a vital role in limiting coagulatory processes. Substances with inhibitory effects include heparin, plasmin, antithrombin III, and tissue factor inhibitor (extrinsic pathway inhibitor, lipoprotein-associated coagulation inhibitor). Antithrombin III (AT III) is the most vital of these factors. It is a globulin with a molecular weight of 65,000 and has the ability to inactivate factors Xa, IXa, XIa, and XIIa and thrombin. Binding to heparin markedly increases the rate of inactivation of factor Xa and thrombin. In addition, the surface of the vascular endothelium serves as the site of the thrombomodulin/protein C/protein S anticoagulant system. Thrombomodulin is an integral membrane protein, and protein C and protein S are circulating vitamin K-dependent proteins. Thrombomodulin has a receptor site for thrombin. Once thrombin has been bound, its ability to form fibrin and aggregate platelets is nullified. Additionally, it becomes a powerful activator of protein C. Protein C has anticoagulation effects through inactivation of factors Va and VIIIa (Marlar et al. 1982) and promotes fibrinolysis (Roemisch et al. 1991). Protein S increases the rate of inactivation of factor V.

Humoral inhibitors of intermediate products of coagulation include heparin, antithromboplastin, plasmin, and antithrombin III (not to be confused with clotting factor III or platelet factor 3). Antithrombin III also is called the heparin cofactor. This enzyme is a thrombin antagonist, but it additionally inhibits activated forms of factors IX, X, XI, and XII. Antithrombin III combines in a stable manner with the enzymatically active binding sites of these factors, thereby preventing their accessibility to subsequent substrates in the clotting cascade. The combination of heparin with antithrombin III increases approximately 100-fold the affinity of the latter for the activated clotting factors. The anticoagulant activity of heparin is due to its interaction with antithrombin III; without the latter, heparin does not prevent clot formation (see discussion of heparin later in this chapter).

Fibrin itself is an effective antithrombin factor, because it removes from the circulation approximately 90% of the thrombin formed during the clotting process. This action assists in localizing the clot to the target site and retarding its spread to other regions of the vasculature.

Coagulopathies and Drugs. Clinically, a large number of pathophysiologic states influence hemostatic events in animals. Abnormalities of one or more of the vascular, platelet, coagulation, and fibrinolytic phases are not uncommon; some of these disorders are summarized in Table 28.2. Drugs can be helpful in managing certain types of coagulopathies, but identification of etiologic factors is important. Some of the more commonly used hemostatic, anticoagulant, fibrinolytic, and antiplatelet drugs are discussed below. Commonly used tests of hemostatic function are listed in Table 28.3.

HEMOSTATIC DRUGS

Topical Hemostatics. Several locally applied substances can provide assistance in control of persistent capillary bleeding if blood coagulation mechanisms are otherwise intact. The ideal topical hemostatic substance should provide good hemostasis, have minimal

TABLE 28.3—Hemostatic assays and their clinical relevance

1. **One-step prothrombin time (OSPT):** Screening test of the extrinsic and common pathway. It is most sensitive to factor VII deficiency. First assay to be prolonged with vitamin K deficiency.
2. **Activated partial thromboplastin time (APTT):** Screening test of the intrinsic and common pathway. Will be prolonged with hemophilia and with prolonged vitamin K deficiency.
3. **Activated coagulation test (ACT):** Screening test for the intrinsic pathway, with less sensitivity than APTT.
4. **Buccal mucosal bleeding time:** Screening test for primary hemostasis. Will be prolonged with platelet dysfunction, thrombocytopenia, vWf deficiency, or vasculitis.

tissue reactivity, and be easy to sterilize and handle. If hemostatic or fibrinolytic defects are present, however, topical agents are of little or no value; replacement therapy is indicated (Chap. 29). Although lyophilized concentrates of several clotting factors are available for investigational use, most clinically useful topical hemostatic preparations contain thrombin or collagen. These compounds control bleeding by providing artificial clotting material or forming a structural matrix for coagulation events and clot formation. Because most topical hemostatics are absorbed gradually over varying intervals, they commonly are referred to as the absorbable hemostatics.

The clinician must recognize that locally applied hemostatics are indicated only in the combat of capillary oozing from minute vessels of denuded or superficially bleeding surfaces. These compounds will not effectively prevent loss of blood from arteries or veins where there is appreciable pressure.

THROMBOPLASTIN. Thromboplastin (thrombokinase) is produced naturally by platelets and tissues in response to trauma. The commercial preparation is a powder extracted from bovine brains or from acetone-extracted lung and/or brain of rabbits. *Thromboplastin,* USP, aids hemostasis by promoting conversion of prothrombin to thrombin, thereby accelerating the coagulation process. It is employed as a local hemostatic in surgery when applied by spray or direct application in a sponge. Thromboplastin is used in measurement of prothrombin time and activity of blood in vitro, an important guide in anticoagulant drug therapy.

THROMBIN. *Thrombin,* USP, is a white sterile powder prepared by interaction of thromboplastin and calcium with prothrombin of bovine origin. It is standardized on the basis of National Institutes of Health (NIH) units; one NIH unit is the amount of thrombin required to clot 1 mL standard fibrinogen solution in 15 seconds. In control of bleeding, thrombin converts endogenous fibrinogen to fibrin for clot formation. It is useful where there is bleeding from parenchymatous tissues, cancellous bone, dental sockets, laryngeal and nasal surgery, and reconstructive surgery. Thrombin is particularly valuable as an adhesive agent for fixation of skin grafts. It can be applied topically as a powder or as a solution in sterile distilled water or isotonic saline (approximately 1000 units/mL); it can also be used in conjunction with absorbable gelatin sponge or fibrin foam. After neutralization of stomach acid, thrombin may be of some value in bleeding of the upper gastrointestinal (GI) tract.

Thrombin must not be injected or otherwise allowed to enter large blood vessels. Extensive intravascular clotting and even death may result. Local ischemia can result from subcutaneous or intramuscular (IM) injection. Thrombin is antigenic, but allergic reactions are encountered rarely when it is applied topically.

FIBRINOGEN. *Human Fibrinogen,* USP (Fibrogen, Parenogen), is a concentrated fraction of normal human plasma and is available as sterile white powder. It is readily soluble in normal saline and is used principally on denuded mucous membranes and as an adhesive in skin grafts (as a 2% solution). Fibrinogen also is used for restoring normal plasma fibrinogen concentrations in the treatment of hemorrhagic complications arising from massive blood loss or acute hypofibrinogenemia. Adequate amounts of endogenous thrombin are required for conversion of fibrinogen into fibrin.

FIBRIN FOAM. Fibrin foam is a spongelike material prepared by action of thrombin on human fibrinogen. It is an insoluble substance marketed as strips of fine white sponge. Fibrin foam may be applied directly, with pressure, to the hemorrhagic area or after presoaking it in thrombin solution. This preparation acts as a preformed network to trap blood oozing from the surface area.

ABSORBABLE GELATIN SPONGE. *Absorbable Gelatin Sponge,* USP (Gelfoam), is a sterile, water-insoluble, gelatin-base sponge. It is nonantigenic and will absorb several times its weight of whole blood. This denaturized gelatin usually is soaked in bovine thrombin and left in the bleeding area following closure of operative wounds. When applied to the surface of the body or mucosal membranes, it liquefies within 3-5 days. Gelatin sponge is completely absorbed in 4-6 weeks, usually without inducing a reaction or excessive scar tissue formation. It is used primarily for capillary or venous bleeding.

OXIDIZED CELLULOSE. *Oxidized Cellulose,* USP (Surgicel, Oxycel, Hemo-Pak), is a specially treated form of surgical gauze or sponge that aids coagulation by reaction between hemoglobin and cellulosic acid. Upon interaction with blood and tissue fluids, oxidized cellulose facilitates formation of a gummy matrix for clot formation. It should be used only as temporary packing because its permanent implantation in tissues and fractures interferes with bone regeneration and may result in cyst formation. Oxidized cellulose also interferes with epithelialization and hence should not be used as a topical dressing except for short-term control of bleeding. Complete absorption of large amounts may require weeks. Also, oxidized cellulose should not be used in conjunction with thrombin since the latter is inactivated by the former's acidity. Oxidized cellulose is available as sterile cotton pledgets and gauze pads and strips.

MICROCRYSTALLINE COLLAGEN. Microcrystalline collagen is a surface hemostatic agent. A valuable property of this substance is its affinity for wet surfaces, to which it quickly adheres. Microcrystalline collagen is absorbed in about 6 weeks with minimal tissue reaction. It may be effective in the presence of clotting factor deficiencies but is less effective in thrombocytopenia. It has also been shown to be effective in systemically heparinized patients (Abbott 1974). Surface hemostasis obtained with this agent appears to be most effective and reliable in such cases as venoarterial anastomoses or surgery of the spleen and liver.

EPINEPHRINE AND NOREPINEPHRINE. Topically applied, *Epinephrine,* USP, and *Norepinephrine Bitartrate,* USP, produce an immediate but transitory vasoconstriction, which may be of some value in local control of bleeding from small vessels. See Chap. 6 for indications and limitations.

MISCELLANEOUS TOPICAL HEMOSTATICS. The locally acting hemostatics known as styptics are the oldest blood-clotting drugs. Styptics include such agents as ferric chloride, ferric sulfate, ferric subsulfate, alum, tannic acid, chromium trioxide, silver nitrate, zinc chloride, cotarnine chloride, and a variety of other astringent substances. Some of these drugs are used locally in full strength as powders dusted onto a bleeding area; in solution they are used in concentrations from 1 to 20%. Action of these drugs depends upon precipitation of the protein of blood and soft tissue, and they supposedly seal off the ruptured vessel. However, many of these agents, especially if used in high concentration, may damage tissues, resulting in sloughing and even recurrence of hemorrhage. Thus they should be used carefully and only on superficial lesions.

Systemic Hemostatics

BLOOD. Fresh whole blood or blood components are indicated for emergency treatment of acute hemorrhagic syndromes associated with deficiency of clotting factors or platelets (see Chap. 29).

VITAMIN K. Vitamin K is a fat-soluble vitamin that is found in a variety of plants and is produced by microorganisms. It occurs as a viscous clear liquid that is very sensitive to light. Its main therapeutic usage is in the treatment of vitamin K antagonist rodenticide intoxication.

CHEMISTRY AND MECHANISM OF ACTION. Vitamin K exists in three main forms. Vitamin K-1 (phytonadione) is present in plants, vitamin K-2 (menaquinone) is produced by microorganisms, and vitamin K-3 (menadione) is a synthetic derivative (Fig. 28.3). All of these compounds are naphthoquinone derivatives. Vitamin K aids in the production of functional clotting factors II, VII, IX, and X by postribosomal carboxylation of glutamyl residues. It also is vital for the production of active protein C and protein S, both of which have anticoagulatory effects.

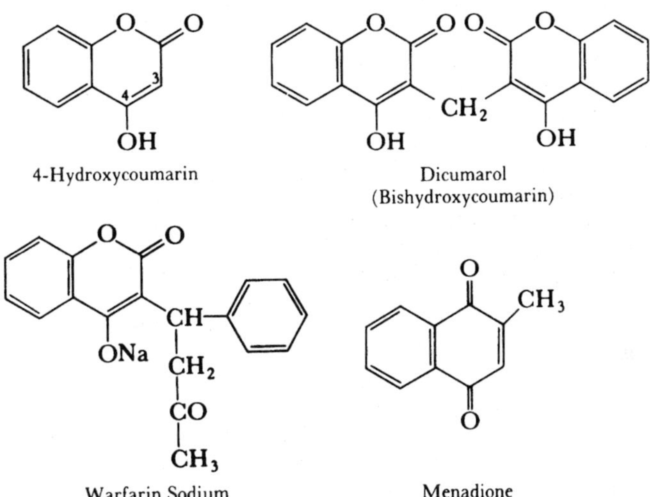

FIG. 28.3—Structures of 4-hydroxycoumarin, dicumarol (bishydroxycoumarin), warfarin, and synthetic vitamin K (menadione).

Vitamin K-1 is actively absorbed in the small intestine. Vitamins K-2 and K-3 are passively absorbed in the ileum and colon. Solubilization by bile acids is required for absorption of vitamins K-1 and K-2. Biotransformation in the organism is required for vitamin K-3 to become active (Mount 1982).

CLINICAL USE. Deficiency of vitamin K activity will lead to a hypocoagulable state. The major cause of this syndrome in veterinary medicine is the ingestion of vitamin K antagonists. Antagonists can occur naturally (dicumarol, sweet clover poisoning) or as commercial rodenticides (coumarin, warfarin, indandiones, brodifacoum). Occasionally disorders in fat absorption can lead to decreased vitamin K absorption. Coagulopathies have been documented with lymphocytic-plasmacytic enteritis, exocrine pancreatic insufficiency, and bile duct obstruction (Perry et al. 1991; Edwards and Russell 1987; Neer and Hedlund 1987). In birds prolonged administration of sulfonamides for the treatment of coccidiosis can lead to vitamin K deficiency by destroying the intestinal microorganisms. In swine porcine hemorrhagic syndrome in weaned pigs is believed to be related to low vitamin K levels in feed (Liggett 1989). A heritable multifactor vitamin K-dependent coagulopathy has been documented in Devon Rex cats (Soute et al. 1992).

Hypocoagulability is documented clinically by prolongation of the coagulation times (activated coagulation test [ACT], prothrombine time [PT], activated partial thromboplastin time [APTT]). Factor VII is the vitamin K-dependent clotting factor with the shortest half-life and is also the factor predominantly measured by PT. As a result, PT values will change before APTT or ACT values will. This makes PT a good test to detect and monitor the therapy of a vitamin K-deficient state.

The therapeutic agent of choice is vitamin K-1. Vitamin K-3 has demonstrated poor efficacy in veterinary patients as well as toxic side effects (Alstad et al. 1985; Fernandez et al. 1984). Subcutaneous injection or oral administration are the preferred modes of administration. Intramuscular injections have been recommended; however, such an injection in an animal with a coagulopathy may lead to extensive life-threatening hemorrhage. Intravenous administration has been associated with anaphylactoid reactions. Most protocols recommend giving the initial dose of vitamin K by subcutaneous injection to ensure that therapeutic levels are reached. Thereafter, the drug can be given orally. A fatty meal will enhance oral absorption. Duration of treatment and dosage used will vary depending upon the clinical indication. Poisoning from first-generation vitamin K-antagonist rodenticides (coumarin, warfarin) should be treated for 4-6 days with 0.25-2.5 mg/kg divided BID in small animals, 300-500 mg TID in horses (Byars et al. 1986), and 1.1-3.3 mg/kg in cattle (Alstad et al. 1985). For second-generation vitamin K-antagonist rodenticides (diphacinone, brodifacoum), the treatment period should be extended to 14 days and a loading dose of 5 mg/kg should be given initially, followed by 2.5 mg/kg daily (Woody et al. 1992). Determination of PT 48 hours after cessation of therapy is recommended to detect residual toxicity. Substitution of vitamin K will begin to normalize PT values in 12-24 hours.

DESMOPRESSIN ACETATE (DDAVP). Desmopressin is a synthetic analog of vasopressin, and is used in the treatment of central diabetes insipidus and to transiently elevate levels of vWf. The elevation in vWf allows surgical procedures to be performed and aids in the control of capillary bleeding from wounds in animals with von Willebrand disease. In comparison to vasopressin, DDAVP has minimal pressor effects. Administration of this drug leads to the release of stored vWf from endothelial cells and macrophages. When DDAVP is given, a rapid rise in vWf levels occurs, with larger, more-active multimeres predominating (Kraus et al. 1987; Johnstone and Crane 1986). This effect is reduced if the drug is given repeatedly, since the storage pools will be depleted. The duration of elevation is approximately 2 hours (Mansell and Parry 1991). Though the elevation in vWf levels found in dogs is considerably lower than in humans, clinically a decrease in buccal mucosal bleeding time was seen (Kraus et al. 1989). In some dogs only a minimal response was noted. The recommended dosages for dogs is 0.4 μg/kg given subcutaneously.

PROTAMINE SULFATE. *Protamine Sulfate,* USP, is a low molecular weight protein found in the sperm of certain fish. It is strongly basic and combines with acidic heparin to form a stable salt that prevents any further anticoagulant activity of heparin. Protamine is used as an antagonist only to heparin-evoked hemorrhages. It also arrests action of heparin in vitro. Protamine itself has anticoagulant properties probably caused by interference with the reaction of thrombin and fibrinogen. This would imply that the clinician must take care not to overneutralize the action of heparin.

Protamine is available as a 1-2% solution. It is administered slowly by the IV route at a rate no greater than 50 mg over a 10-minute period. The average dose is 1-1.5 mg to antagonize each 1 mg heparin. The dose is related to the lapse of time from administration; e.g., 30 minutes after heparin injection only 0.5 mg protamine may be required to antagonize each 1 mg heparin.

ANTICOAGULANTS. The principal uses of anticoagulant agents are in vitro to prevent clotting of blood for transfusion or diagnostic use and in vivo to prevent development and enlargement of thrombi.

In Vitro Anticoagulants. A variety of chemicals have been used to prevent coagulation of shed blood. Essentially two categories of chemicals are used: those employed as anticoagulants in samples of blood intended for physical or chemical examination and those employed to preserve blood for transfusion. Certain of these agents can be used to prevent clotting both in vitro and in vivo (heparin), while others may be good for use in vitro but are not practical in vivo because of their toxicity (oxalates).

Anticoagulant agents used in laboratory examination of blood include (1) sodium oxalate in a concentration of 20% at the level of 0.01 mL/mL (2 mg/mL) blood; (2) *Sodium Citrate,* USP, in a concentration of 25% at the rate of 0.01 mL/mL (2.5 mg/mL) blood; (3) *Edetate Disodium,* USP (Endrate, Sodium Versenate), to prevent coagulation when used in a concentration of 1 mg/5 mL blood, the anticoagulant property being related to its ability to chelate calcium; and (4) heparin sodium to prevent coagulation (75 units to each 10 mL whole blood).

Any of these anticoagulants may be added to sample tubes in the desired amounts and evaporated to dryness. Sterile vacuum tubes that contain appropriate anticoagulants and double needles for ease in blood collection are available.

Anticoagulants used for blood and blood component transfusions ideally should maintain the function of the individual components and have preservative effects. Anticoagulant agents used for blood and blood plasma transfusion include (1) *Acid Citrate Dextrose,* USP (ACD solution), consisting of sodium citrate 25 g, citric acid 8 g, dextrose 24.5 g, and distilled water to make a total volume of 1000 mL, given at the level of 15 mL/100 mL blood. Several commercial firms prepare vacuum bottles containing these or comparable ingredients. The toxicity of citrated blood injected intravenously varies with rate of injection and total dose. The lethal dose of sodium citrate for the dog is estimated to be about 132 mg/kg after extensive hemorrhage; in the normal intact dog the lethal dose is about 286 mg/kg. (2) Citrate-phosphate-dextrose-adenine (CPDA-1) is now the most commonly used anticoagulant in human and veterinary transfusion medicine. It can maintain a high level of erythrocyte posttransfusion viability for up to 20 days in dogs (Price et al. 1988).

Other means also may prevent or retard coagulation. These are cold, at 2-5° C, and collection of blood into a receptacle having smooth and unwettable walls, e.g., paraffin or silicone coated. Silicone coating is the most effective method for many types of mechanical devices used for implantation, transfusion, and dialysis.

Systemic Anticoagulants. Two types of anticoagulants are used therapeutically for preventing enlargement of thrombi. Heparin used parenterally has a direct and almost instantaneous action on the coagulation process, whereas the coumarin derivatives (for oral administration) have an indirect anticoagulant effect by acting as vitamin K antagonists in the hepatic synthesis of certain coagulation factors. Therefore, action by the coumarin derivatives is delayed for several hours. For emergency treatment, heparin is used first and then may be followed by the coumarin derivatives.

Other anticoagulants include edetate sodium, sodium oxalate, and sodium citrate, which hinder coagulation by combining with calcium. However, these agents are not effective in vivo because lowering ionized calcium to the anticoagulant level is incompatible with life. Dextran sulfate has anticoagulant properties but its activity is variable; its use is limited to a plasma expander.

Both categories of the systemic anticoagulants act by inhibition of the action of formation of one or more clotting factors (see Fig. 28.2). This implies that these drugs exert their action by evoking a clotting defect similar to that of clinical diseases. Consequently, there is a relatively narrow therapeutic ratio, since hemorrhage can occur as a result of individual susceptibility or an interaction with other drugs used simultaneously (Szabuniewicz and McCrady 1977).

HEPARIN. Heparin (Heparin sodium, USP; Heparin calcium, Calciparine) is the only parenteral anticoagulant available and is also the most commonly used anticoagulant in veterinary medicine. It can be used in vivo and in vitro. Heparin has both antithrombotic and anticoagulatory effects, which are not necessarily dependent on each other. Heparin is prepared from bovine lung tissue or porcine intestinal mucosa. Both calcium and sodium salts of heparin are available for therapeutic use and occur as a white hygroscopic powder that is easily soluble in water. In human medicine recent research has focused on synthetic heparinoids and the clinical applicability of heparin fractions of various molecular weights.

CHEMISTRY AND MECHANISM OF ACTION. Pharmaceutical-grade heparin is a heterogeneous mixture of anionic sulfated mucopolysaccharides with molecular weights ranging from 1200 to 40,000 daltons. Relative antithrombotic and anticoagulatory activity is related to molecular size. The variability in both molecular composition and biologic activity necessitates standardization of drug concentration by bioassay of anticoagulant activity (expressed as units).

The reversible binding of heparin to antithrombin III (AT III), a protease inhibitor, is responsible for most of the anticoagulatory effect of heparin. Affinity for AT III is dependent upon molecular size (Fareed et al. 1985). Binding to AT III causes a conformational change in the AT III molecule that significantly enhances its inhibitory effect on various activated coagulation factors, especially thrombin and activated factor X (Xa). The rate of inactivation can increase 2000- to 10,000-fold. After inactivation has occurred, the heparin molecule dissociates from the complex and is available for further interactions. In a pharmaceutical heparin preparation, only 30-50% of the heparin molecules present will bind to AT III. Heparin acts as a template to which thrombin and AT III can bind and thereby interact to form an inactive compound. Simultaneous binding of factor Xa to AT III and heparin is not required for inactivation. Low-molecular-weight (LMW) fractions of heparin inactivate only factor Xa because they are not large enough to bind thrombin and AT III concurrently. The additional inactivation of thrombin by high-molecular-weight (HMW) fractions of heparin increases their anticoagulatory ability. At higher dosages heparin can also bind to heparin cofactor II, which inhibits only thrombin. Heparin also binds to endothelial cell walls, imparting a negative charge, affects platelet aggregation and adhesion, and increases levels of plasminogen activator (Hirsh et al. 1992a). In addition, it recently has been found that heparin administration leads to an increase in the levels of tissue factor inhibitor (Ostergaard et al. 1993). These effects all contribute to the anticoagulatory and antithrombotic action of heparin and vary with the individual heparin fractions. An additional effect of heparin that does not seem to be related to hemostasis is the ability to liberate lipoprotein lipase, which lowers serum triglyceride levels. This characteristic can be used to detect lipoprotein lipase deficiency.

The pharmacokinetics and pharmacodynamics of heparin are very complex. Most of an administered dose of heparin is bound extensively to endothelial cells, macrophages, and plasma proteins, which act as storage pools. Once these pools have been saturated, free heparin appears in the plasma and is excreted slowly by the kidney. Heparin is metabolized by the liver and also by the reticuloendothelial system (RES). Clearance of LMW fractions is slower than that of HMW fractions, which leads to their cumulation in the organism. All of these factors cause the kinetics of heparin to be highly variable between individuals and within the individual. A fixed dose cannot be expected to produce a uniform level of anticoagulation or antithrombotic effect. In addition, since most of heparin efficacy is dependent on AT III, low levels of this protein will result in reduced anticoagulant activity. Biologic half-life is variable and depends upon the dosage administered and the route of administration. Subcutaneous administration leads to slow release of heparin and has been found to have an effect equivalent to intravenous heparin for the prophylaxis of thrombosis. Intravenous administration leads to high initial levels with a short half-life.

CLINICAL USE. Heparin has a variety of uses in veterinary medicine. In humans it is used widely, especially in the prevention of venous thrombosis. Its use in the treatment of established thrombi is also advocated. The predominant use of heparin in veterinary medicine has been in the management of disseminated intravascular coagulation (DIC) and other potentially hypercoagulable states (Cushing's disease, nephrotic syndrome, cardiomyopathy). Low-dose heparin has been reported to decrease the complications associated with heartworm adulticide treatment (Vezzoni and Genchi 1989). It may also be of benefit in the treatment of severe pancreatitis (Wright and Goodhead 1970).

The major adverse side effect in animals is excessive anticoagulation leading to hemorrhage. Intramuscular administration is contraindicated, as it may lead to extensive hematoma formation. In horses, treatment for several days with doses of heparin that were believed to produce therapeutically desired levels of anticoagulation led to a significant (50%) drop in red blood cell (RBC) mass. This may have been associated with increased RBC removal by the RES (Duncan et al. 1983). Erythrocyte agglutination has also been associated with heparin therapy in horses (Mahaffey and Moore 1986).

Guidelines for heparin dosage vary widely. Both high-dose and low-dose regimens have been developed, their applicability will depend upon the clinical indication. High-dose heparin therapy aims to increase APTT 1.5-2.5 times baseline or ACT 1.2-1.4 times baseline. Its main clinical indication is the treatment of established thromboemboli. The amount of heparin required to achieve this goal will vary with each individual and, since the pharmacokinetics are nonlinear, will vary with each dose administered. In dogs 150-250 U/kg TID and in cats 250-375 U/kg TID will usually suffice to achieve this goal. A higher loading dose may be of benefit. Regular and frequent monitoring of clotting times is essential. Severe anemia was detected in horses administered dosages that led to the desired prolongation of clotting times after several days of treatment. Low-dose regimens are generally 75 U/kg TID in small animals and 25-100 U/kg TID in horses. This regimen is especially useful in the management of DIC. The effect on APTT should be minimal with low-dose heparin therapy, yet antithrombotic efficacy should be maintained. Bleeding tendencies also are reduced.

Vitamin K Antagonists

COUMARIN DERIVATIVES. Vitamin K antagonists are administered orally; the most important group of the oral anticoagulants are the coumarin derivatives. Coumarin, normally present in some species of sweet clover, has no anticoagulant action. However, bishydroxycoumarin, a derivative of moldy or spoiled sweet clover, is responsible for a hemorrhagic disease in cattle. This compound was synthesized by Link (1943-44). Other drugs have been synthesized with the 4-hydroxycoumarin structure. Of the several coumarin derivatives, bishydroxycoumarin (*Dicumarol,* USP) was the first oral anticoagulant and 3-(α-acetonylbenzyl)-4-hydroxycoumarin (*Warfarin Sodium,* USP; Panwarfin, Coumodin) was the second compound used.

CHEMISTRY. Dicumarol is a colorless, crystalline solid; it is relatively insoluble in water but forms soluble salts with strong alkalies. The chemical structures of coumarin, dicumarol, warfarin, and menadione are shown in Fig. 28.3. The structure of vitamin K suggests the competitive relation between the vitamin and these inhibitors. Bioavailability of warfarin is much greater than dicumarol because it is approximately 75,000 times more soluble in aqueous media. Warfarin is extensively used as a rodenticide because it produces fatal internal bleeding. Domestic animals also may be poisoned accidentally.

ACTION. Coumarin derivatives share one major pharmacologic action: in vivo inhibition of blood coagulative mechanisms. This activity is achieved not by direct depression of preformed components of the coagulation cascade but by inhibition of hepatic synthesis of vitamin K-dependent clotting factors, i.e., prothrombin and factors VII, IX, and X (Fig. 28.2). Unlike heparin, therefore, coumarin compounds are inactive in vitro. Their in vivo anticoagulant activity is apparent only after a latent period of at least 8-12 hours, which accounts for the time required for natural breakdown of circulating factors already present in the blood. After cessation of administration, anticoagulant effects can last for several days. This reflects the time necessary for reappearance of newly synthesized clotting factors.

The formation of functional clotting factors II, VII, IX, and X is dependent upon the presence of vitamin K. After the precursor proteins of these clotting factors have been synthesized in the liver, they must undergo carboxylation of terminal glutamic acid residues. The carboxylation results in the oxidative inactivation of vitamin K. The resulting vitamin K epoxide is then recycled by epoxide reductase so that it can again participate in the conversion of precursor proteins to functional clotting factors. Vitamin K antagonists exert their effect by inhibiting epoxide reductase. This results in a rapid depletion of vitamin K stores. The coagulation factors are still produced but are not functional.

Experimental evidence indicates that vitamin K and dicumarol are mutually antagonistic (O'Reilly 1972). Administration of vitamin K can reverse hypoprothrombinemia produced by coumarin compounds. This action is clinically important where there is an unusual response to dicumarol, as in overdosage or accidental ingestion. The antidotal effect of vitamin K and its clinical use have been discussed. The characteristics of coumarin derivatives and those of heparin are shown in Table 28.4.

ABSORPTION AND METABOLISM. Dicumarol, as other coumarin derivatives, is absorbed from the GI tract; over 90% is bound to plasma protein and some is stored in the liver. This binding is reversible and is in part responsible for the long plasma half-life of these drugs. Despite this property, the drug displays great variability in action. This may be due to variable metabolic transformation, GI absorption, a possible influence of diet (amount of vitamin K), and interaction with other drugs. Dicumarol is hydroxylated by hepatic enzymes to inactive compounds that are excreted in urine; the metabolites have no anticoagulant effect. Variations in rate of metabolism are due in part to genetic factors. A small quantity, if any, appears unchanged in urine. However, coumarins cross the placenta and are probably secreted in milk (Szabuniewicz and McCrady 1977).

LABORATORY CONTROL. Because of variability in individual and species response to dicumarol, laboratory monitoring of prothrombin activity is essential in its clinical use. The most widely used method for regulating dosage of the drug is the Quick test, or the one-stage prothrombin time. The prothrombin time for a patient on oral anticoagulant therapy should be two to two and one-half times the control value for that individual.

CLINICAL USE. Clinical use of dicumarol in humans has been rated as effective for prophylaxis and treatment of venous thrombosis. All coumarin derivatives can cause one principal side reaction, hemorrhage. However, bleeding rarely occurs if the dose is regulated in relation to prothrombin test results. Contraindications include bleeding from any cause, purpura of any type, or a severe state of malnutrition. The coumarin drugs have received little clinical use in animals.

DRUG INTERACTION. Drug interactions may be associated with the process of absorption, distribution, binding, metabolism, and excretion. A large number of interactions may potentiate or inhibit the anticoagulant action of the coumarin group of drugs. The most important prescribed drugs that may increase the response are phenylbutazone, heparin, salicylates, quinine, broad-spectrum antibiotics, and anabolic steroids. Among those that may decrease response are barbiturates (by induction of liver microsomal enzymes), chloral hydrate, and griseofulvin. Experimentally, it has been shown that the hypoprothrombinemic activity of orally administered dicumarol is nullified in sheep pretreated with phenobarbital (Shetty et al. 1972).

TABLE 28.4—Pharmacologic characteristics of heparin and coumarin derivative anticoagulants

Characteristic	Heparin	Coumarin derivatives
Mechanism of action	Antagonist to thrombin and activated factors IX, X, XI, and XII	Inhibit hepatic synthesis of vitamin K-dependent clotting factors (II, VII, IX, and X)
Onset of action	Immediate	Delayed 12–24 hr
Duration of action	4 hr	2–5 days
Route of administration	Parenteral	Oral
Laboratory control test	Clotting time, partial thromboplastin time	Prothrombin time
Antidotal therapy	Protamine, fresh blood	Vitamin K, fresh blood or plasma
In vitro activity	Yes	No

Coumarins may inhibit metabolism of phenytoin. Some physiologic factors may increase the action of coumarins; e.g., hepatic dysfunction, hypermetabolism, and vitamin K deficiency resulting from poor absorption. Other physiologic factors may decrease response to anticoagulants, e.g., pregnancy and diuresis.

ADMINISTRATION. The dosage of oral anticoagulants in dogs is based on the schedule used in humans. Dicumarol is given on the first day at 5 mg/kg; the average daily maintenance is one-third to two-thirds the first day's dose and is dependent on daily prothrombin time determinations. When prothrombin activity is reduced to less than 25%, the drug must be discontinued.

Dicumarol is available in 25, 50, and 100 mg capsules and tablets. Warfarin is available in tablet form (2-25 mg) and for parenteral use (25 mg/mL).

OTHER ORAL ANTICOAGULANTS. In addition to dicumarol and warfarin, other oral anticoagulants have been developed. These include phenprocoumon, acenocoumarol, and the indandione derivatives. These compounds have little if any clinical use in animals.

FIBRINOLYTIC AGENTS. The basic event of fibrinolysis is abstracted in Fig. 28.2. Pharmacologic acceleration of this process involves drugs that enhance the conversion of the inactive precursor plasminogen to the active fibrinolytic enzyme plasmin (Sherry and Gustafson 1985). Plasminogen exists in two phases, the plasma or soluble phase found in the circulating blood and the gel phase bound to fibrin in the formed clot. Thus when a plasminogen-activating agent comes in contact with the clot, fibrin-bound gel-phase plasminogen is activated to plasmin locally with selective fibrinolysis. There is increased tendency for systemic bleeding if, instead, soluble-phase plasminogen is also activated. Plasmin formation would then occur throughout the circulation rather than being localized to the formed clot. Indeed, the presence of plasmin in peripheral blood indicates a pathologic fibrinolytic state. Such a condition reflects overactivation of plasminogen, which overcomes the neutralizing capacity of an endogenous antagonist to plasmin called α_2-antiplasmin.

Fibrinolytic activity can be activated or inhibited by several additional endogenous and exogenous agents. Common activators are hormones (androgens, corticosteroids, growth hormone), enzymes (streptokinase, staphylokinase), epinephrine (exercise, stress), and agents from the body fluids (urokinase, thrombin). Inhibition may result by preventing activation of plasminogen (ε-aminocaproic acid, calcium, and antibodies to streptokinase or staphylokinase) or prevention of action of plasmin (antiplasmin α_1, α_2-globulin) (Szabuniewicz and McCrady 1977).

Clinical Aspects. Overactivity or underactivity of the fibrinolytic mechanism may result in hemorrhage or vascular thrombi respectively. Overactive fibrinolysis has been recognized in a variety of pathologic conditions in humans (e.g., shock, blood disorders, hepatic cirrhosis, snakebite, and following lung surgery). In these conditions, excessive fibrinolytic activity may be present in association with rapid digestion of prothrombin by plasmin or inhibition of other factors (V, VII, and VIII). Two drugs are available for treatment of hyperfibrinolytic conditions: *Aminocaproic Acid,* USP (Amicar, Caprocid), and a biologic inhibitor, aprotinin (Transylol). Aprotinin is a kallikrein or protease enzyme inhibitor. In humans, underactive fibrinolysis is postulated to play a role in occlusive vascular disease, as in myocardial infarction, pulmonary thromboembolic disease, massive postsurgical adhesions, and such unrelated processes as inflammation and malignancy. It appears possible to enhance fibrinolytic activity with drugs. Those undergoing clinical trials for human use are sulfonylurea in nondiabetic subjects (tolbutamide, chlorpropamide), anabolic steroids (ethylestrol, methenolone), clofibrate (Atromid-S), and biguanidine (phenformin, metformin).

Experimentally, postoperative adhesions have been successfully prevented in the dog with urokinase (Gervin et al. 1973). Anticoagulants (heparin or coumarins) are effective only in prevention of thrombi and have little or no effect on fibrin already formed.

Streptokinase is available for clinical use. It is a stable, vacuum-dried powder containing streptococcal enzymes. Streptokinase activates human plasminogen to the humoral proteolytic enzyme plasmin. Plasmin liquefies fibrin or clotted blood. The conversion of animal plasminogens to plasmins by streptokinase is variable. Local use is indicated whenever removal of fibrin or a viscous exudate is desired and drainage can be achieved. Clinical trials have demonstrated its usefulness in treatment of wounds not responding to antibacterial therapy, such as burns, ulcers, chronic eczema, ear hematoma, otitis externa, sinusitis, cysts, fractures with fistulous tracts, and osteomyelitis. Locally, it can be administered as a powder or wet pack by infusion or irrigation. Liquefaction of blood clots and fibrinous exudates may occur in 30 minutes to 12 hours.

Parenteral administration has been used in treatment of ulcers, eczema, dermatitis, edema, cellulitis, hematoma, trauma, and pneumonia. For parenteral use, the solution may be administered intramuscularly or intravenously. The daily dose for large animals is 5000-10,000 units/45 kg. The recommended total daily dose for small animals is 5000-10,000 units. Therapy may be given 1 or 2 times daily for up to 5 days.

Streptokinase-streptodornase is available in vials containing 100,000 streptokinase units, 25,000 streptodornase units, and 500 plasminogen units. It is recommended that antibacterial agents be administered simultaneously with the enzyme preparation. Anaphylactic reactions may occur following parenteral use. The product is contraindicated in the presence of a blood dyscrasia.

Fibrinolysin (Thrombolysin, Actase) is an enzyme preparation derived from a fraction of human plasma. It is prepared by action of streptokinase on human profibrinolysin and is potentially useful in treatment of thrombosis and embolism. The drug has several unpleasant side effects. In humans a dose of 50,000-100,000 units/hr by IV drip for 1-6 hr/day is recommended; this dose may be given 3-4 days. An effective antagonist of fibrinolysin is aminocaproic acid.

Urokinase (Win-Kinase, Abbokinase, Breokinase), excreted in human urine, is an activator of plasminogen. It is believed that this preparation may have some advantages over streptokinase. It purportedly prevents serosal postoperative adhesions in 80% of the dogs when administered as a lavage in a dose of 5000-10,000 units/kg into the peritoneal cavity.

Bisorbin lactate (EN 1661) is a synthetic fibrinolytic drug in the investigational phase; it resembles urokinase in action.

Tissue Plasminogen Activator. Tissue-type plasminogen activator (t-PA) predominantly exerts its effect in association with fibrin clots. Its specificity for clots is therapeutically attractive. Unlike other plasminogen activators, t-PA does not induce a systemic proteolytic state. Though the commercial product is recombinant DNA produced human-type tissue plasminogen activator, its efficacy has been demonstrated in cats (Pion 1988). In addition, the local application of t-PA has been found efficacious in reducing intraocular fibrin deposition (Gerding et al. 1992). The major clinical use to date has been the lysis of aortic thromboemboli in cats. Intravenous administration of t-PA resulted in a rapid return to function. However, 50% of the animals treated died acutely after treatment. This was attributed to the rapid reperfusion of the rear extremities, which resulted in hyperkalemia and heart failure. A factor that may limit the use of t-PA is the expense of the drug.

ANTIPLATELET DRUGS. Platelets have a central role in the initiation and propagation of thrombus formation. They release a variety of substances that promote coagulation, and they also form the initial platelet plug. Platelets begin to adhere and aggregate in response to a myriad of stimuli. The central process in aggregation is alteration of cAMP levels in the platelet. Increased cAMP is inhibitory, while decreased cAMP is proaggregatory. It is important to remember that a variety of stimuli influence platelet function in vivo, but many of the in vitro methods used to assess platelet reactivity and the effectiveness of antiplatelet drugs suffer from the inability to truly recreate the in vivo environment. Another factor that leads to difficulties in assessing clinical efficacy based on experimental work is that platelet reactivity varies between individuals and with health status.

A variety of drugs are used to reduce platelet function. Clinically this should be beneficial in the prevention of thrombotic disease, especially if affecting arteries. In humans the efficacy of some of these drugs in the prevention of myocardial infarction and stroke has been proven. The most common indications in veterinary medicine are to prevent thrombi associated with feline cardiomyopathy and to reduce the severity of pulmonary endarteritis associated with heartworm disease. The efficacy of antiplatelet drugs in alleviating the proliferative changes in arteries associated with heartworm infestation remains controversial (Boudreaux et al. 1991a; Keith et al. 1983; Schaub et al. 1983). Platelet inhibition may also be beneficial in membranous glomerulonephritis, mild DIC, and pulmonary thromboembolism as well as in the reduction of metastasis. In horses platelet inhibition may be of benefit in the treatment of thrombotic disorders such as laminitis and navicular disease.

Aspirin. The only commonly used antiplatelet drug in veterinary medicine is aspirin (acetylsalicylic acid, ASA). Aspirin is a nonsteroidal anti-inflammatory drug (NSAID) that inhibits the activity of cyclooxygenase. Other NSAIDs, such as phenylbutazone and flunixin meglumine, share the same mechanism of action, yet aspirin is unique in that even at low doses it causes irreversible inhibition of platelet cyclooxygenase. Aspirin acetylates this enzyme, which leads to decreased production of eicosanoids by the platelet. The most pivotal eicosanoids for hemostasis are prostacyclin (PGI_2) and thromboxane A_2 (TA_2). PGI_2 is a potent vasodilator and inhibitor of aggregation, while TA_2 is a vasoconstrictor and a strong aggregatory stimulus.

Aspirin is rapidly absorbed after oral administration. Hydrolysis of the acetylsalicylic acid yields salicylate and acetic acid. In the liver the salicylate is conjugated with glucuronic acid, which can then be excreted by the kidney. Animals, such as cats, with a relative deficiency of glucuronyl transferase activity will have prolonged ASA half-lives, which can lead to cumulation and toxicity.

Once ASA has been administered, rapid and irreversible inhibition of platelet cyclooxygenase occurs. Since platelets do not produce appreciable amounts of new enzymes, this results in decreased platelet aggregation response because of lower TA_2 levels throughout the life span of the platelet. Aggregation response will return to normal as new platelets enter the bloodstream. Endothelial cell cyclooxygenase activity is also inhibited but recovers more rapidly. This inhibition is considered deleterious since endothelial cells produce PGI_2, which is antithrombotic. Proposed explanations for the more rapid recovery of endothelial cell cyclooxygenase activity include reduced sensitivity to ASA of the endothelial cell cyclooxygenase, ability to synthesize new cyclooxygenase, and the pharmacologic distribution of ASA (Hirsh et al. 1992b). The last theory postulates that platelets are exposed to ASA in the enterohepatic circulation before ASA is hydrolyzed. At low doses endothelium will primarily be exposed to circulating salicylate rather than ASA. Higher doses will result in circulating ASA leading to endothelial cell cyclooxygenase inhibition. The differential inhibition of platelet and endothelial cell cyclooxygenase has resulted in research efforts to find an ideal dose of ASA that will maximally limit proaggregatory platelet TA_2 and minimally decrease levels of antithrombotic PGI_2. In addition, low dosages should minimize the gastrointestinal side effects seen with ASA. The goal of finding an optimum low ASA dose has proven elusive. In healthy dogs individual variation in the amount of ASA required to inhibit aggregation in vitro is marked. Experimental infestation and embolization with heartworms lead to a pronounced increase in the amount of ASA needed to maintain this level of inhibition (Boudreaux et al. 1991a).

Dosage recommendations for platelet inhibition vary widely. In healthy dogs a dose of 0.5 mg/kg BID was found to be more effective than higher doses (Rackear et al. 1988). A dose of 10 mg/kg has been recommended to reduce the sequelae of heartworm infestation and adulticide treatment (Keith et al. 1983). In cats 25 mg/kg twice weekly has been found to inhibit platelet aggregation without evidence of toxicity (Greene 1985). Experimental studies in horses showed that oral ASA (12 mg/kg) significantly increased bleeding times for 48 hours posttreatment (Trujillo et al. 1981). A lower dose (4 mg/kg) prolonged bleeding times for 4 hours posttreatment (Cambridge et al. 1991).

Ticlopidine. Ticlopidine is an antiplatelet drug that is undergoing extensive testing for use in the prevention of thrombotic diseases. In humans it has been proven to be as effective as ASA in the prevention of stroke. The mechanism of action of ticlopidine is unclear. It is postulated that the drug affects platelet membranes, possibly by inhibiting the formation of fibrinogen receptors (Di Minno et al. 1985). The drug limits platelet aggregation response to a variety of stimuli. Cyclooxygenase is not inhibited, so endothelial PGI_2 levels are not affected. Inhibition of aggregation persists for the life span of the platelet. Onset of antiplatelet effect is approximately 2-5 days after treatment is initiated, possibly indicating that an intermediate breakdown product is the agent actually responsible for the clinical response. Experience with ticlopidine in veterinary medicine is limited. In healthy animals 62 mg/kg daily inhibited platelet aggregation responses. In heartworm-infected and heartworm-embolized dogs, higher dosages were necessary (Boudreaux et al. 1991b). Ticlopidine administration was associated with a reduction of pulmonary lesions caused by the heartworms.

Dipyrimadole. Originally marketed as a vasodilator, dipyrimadole has been shown to have a synergistic effect with ASA. It inhibits cAMP phosphodiesterase, which leads to increased cAMP levels in the platelet. If used alone, its effect on platelets is minimal (Boudreaux et al. 1991a).

REFERENCES

Abbot, W. M., Austen, W. G. 1975. The effectiveness and mechanism of collagen-induced topical hemostasis. Surgery 78:723-29.

Alstad, A. D., Casper, H. H., Johnson, L. J. 1985. Vitamin K treatment of sweet clover poisoning in calves. J Am Vet Med Assoc 187:729-31.

Boudreaux, M. K., Dillon, A. R., Ravis, W. R., Sartin, E. A., Spano, J. S. 1991a. Effects of treatment with aspirin or aspirin/dipyrimadole combination in heartworm-negative, heartworm-infected, and embolized heartworm-infected dogs. Am J Vet Res 52:1992-99.

Boudreaux, M. K., Dillon, A. R., Sartin, E. A., Ravis, A. R., Spano, J. S. 1991b. Effects of treatment with ticlopidine in heartworm-negative, heartworm-infected, and embolized heartworm-infected dogs. Am J Vet Res 52:2000-2006.

Byars, T. D, Greene, C. E., Kemp, D. T. 1986. Antidotal effect of vitamin K_1 against warfarin induced anticoagulation in horses. Am J Vet Res 47:2309-12.

Cambridge, H., Lees, P., Hooke, R. E., Russell, C. S. 1991. Antithrombotic actions of aspirin in the horse. Equine Vet J 23:123-27.

Chart, I. S., Sanderson, J. H. 1979. General aspects of the blood coagulation system. Pharmacol Ther 5:229-33.

Di Minno, G., Cerbone, A. M., Mattioli, P. L., Turco, S., Lovine, C., Mancini, M. 1985. Functionally thrombasthenic state in normal platelets following the administration of ticlopidine. J Clin Invest 75:328-38.

Donaldson, V. H., Glueck, H. I., Miller, M. A., Movat, H. Z., Habul, F. 1976. Kininogen deficiency in Fitzgerald trait: role of high molecular weight kininogen in clotting and fibrinolysis. J Lab Clin Med 87:327-37.

Duncan, S. G., Meyers, K. M., Reed, S. M. 1983. Reduction of the red blood cell mass of horses: toxic effect of heparin anticoagulant therapy. Am J Vet Res 44:2271-76.

Edwards, D. F., Russell, R. G. 1987. Probable vitamin K-deficient bleeding in two cats with malabsorption syndrome secondary to lymphocytic-plasmacytic enteritis. J Vet Intern Med 1:97-101.

Erslev, A. J., Gabuzda, T. G. 1979. Pathophysiology of Blood, 2nd ed. Philadelphia: W. B. Saunders.

Fareed, J., Walenga, J. M., Williamson, K., Emanuele, R. A., Kumar, A., Hoppensteadt, D. A. 1985. Studies on the antithrombotic effects and pharmacokinetics of heparin fractions and fragments. Sem in Thromb and Hemostasis 11:56-74.

Fernandez, F. R., Davies, A. P., Teachout, D. J., Krake, A., Christopher, M. M., Perman, V. 1984. Vitamin K-induced heinz body formation in dogs. J Am Anim Hosp Assoc 20:711-20.

Gerding, P. A., Essex-Sorlie, D., Yack, R., Vasaune, S. 1992. Effects of intracameral injection of tissue plasminogen activator on corneal endothelium and intraocular pressure in dogs. Am J Vet Res 53:890-93.

Gervin, A. S., Puckett, C. L., Silver, D. 1973. Serosal hypofibrinolysis: a cause of post-operative adhesions. Am J Surg 125:80-88.

Greene, C. E. 1985. Effects of aspirin and propranolol on feline platelet aggregation. Am J Vet Res 46:1820-23.

Guyton, A. C. 1991. Medical Physiology, 8th ed. Philadelphia: W. B. Saunders.

Hass, W. K., Easton, J. D., Adams, H. P., Pryse-Phillips, W., Molony, B. A., Anderson, S., Kamm, B. 1984. A randomized trial comparing ticlopidine hydrochloride with aspirin for the prevention of stroke in high-risk patients. N Engl J Med 321:501-7.

Hirsh, J., Dalen, J. E., Deykin, D., Poller, L. 1992a. Heparin: mechanism of action, pharmacokinetics, dosing considerations, monitoring, efficacy and safety. Chest 102:337S-351S.

Hirsh, J., Dalen, J. E., Fuster, V., Harker, L. B., Salzman, E. W. 1992b. Aspirin and other platelet-active drugs: the relationship between dose, effectiveness, and side effects. Chest 102:327S-336S.

Jain, N. C. 1993. Essentials of Veterinary Hematology. Philadelphia: Lea & Febiger.

Johnstone, I. B., Crane, S. 1986. The effects of desmopressin on hemostatic parameters in the normal dog. Can J Vet Res 50:265-71.

Keith, J. C., Rawlings, C. A., Schaub, R. G. 1983. Pulmonary thromboembolism during therapy of dirofilariasis with thiacetarsamide: modification with aspirin or prednisolone. Am J Vet Res 44:1278-83.

Kraus, K. H., Turrentine, M. A., Jergens, A. E., Johnson, G. S. 1989. Effect of desmopressin acetate on bleeding times and plasma von Willebrand factor in Doberman Pinscher dogs with von Willebrand's disease. Vet Surg 18:103-9.

Kraus, K. H., Turrentine, M. A., Johnson, G. S. 1987. Multimeric analysis of von Willebrand factor before and after desmopressin acetate (DDAVP) administration intravenously and subcutaneously in male Beagle dogs. Am J Vet Res 48:1376-79.

Liggett, A. D. 1989. Porcine hemorrhagic syndrome in recently weaned pigs. Comp Cont Ed 11:1409-11.

Link, K. P. 1943-44. The anticoagulant from spoiled sweet clover hay. Harvey Lect 39:162-216.

Mahaffey, E. A., and Moore, J. N. 1986. Erythrocyte agglutination associated with heparin treatment in three horses. J Am Vet Med Assoc 189:1478-80.

Mansell, P. D., and Parry, B. W. 1991. Changes in factor VII: coagulant activity and von Willebrand factor antigen concentration after subcutaneous injection of desmopressin in dogs with mild hemophilia A. J Vet Intern Med 6:191-94.

Marlar, R. A., Kleiss, A. J., Griffin, J. H. 1982. Mechanism of action of human activated protein C, a thrombin-dependent anticoagulant enzyme. Blood 59:1067-72.

Moncada, S., Vane, J. R. 1979. Arachidonic acid metabolites and the interactions between platelets and blood-vessel walls. N Engl J Med 300:1142-47.

Mount, M. E. 1982. Vitamin K and its therapeutic importance. J Am Vet Med Assoc 180:1354-56.

Nawroth, P. P., Handley, D., Stern, D. M. 1986. The multiple levels of endothelial cell-coagulation factor interactions. Clinics in Haematology 15:293-321.

Neer, T. M., Hedlund, C. S. 1987. Vitamin K-dependent coagulopathy in a dog with bile and cystic duct obstructions. J Am Anim Hosp Assoc 25:461-64.

Ostergaard, P., Nordfang, O., Petersen, L. C., Valentin, S., Kristensen, H. 1993. Is tissue factor pathway inhibitor involved in the antithrombotic effect of heparins. Haemostasis 23:107-11.

Perry, L. A., Williams, D. A., Pidgeon, G. L., Boosinger, T. R. 1991. Exocrine pancreatic insufficiency with associated coagulopathy in a cat. J Am Anim Hosp Assoc 27:109-14.

Pion, P. D. 1988. Feline aortic thromboemboli and the potential utility of thrombolytic therapy with tissue plasminogen activator. Vet Clin North Am: Sm Anim Pract 18:79-86.

Platt, W. R. 1979. Color Atlas and Textbook of Hematology, 2nd ed. Philadelphia: J. B. Lippincott.

Price, G. S., Armstrong, P. J., McLeod, D. A., Babineau, C. A., Metcalf, M. R., Sellett, L. C. 1988. Evaluation of citrate-phosphate-dextrose-adenine as a storage medium for packed canine erythrocytes. J Vet Int Med 2:126-32.

Rackear, D., Feldman, B., Farver, T., Lelong, L. 1988. The effect of three different dosages of acetylsalicylic acid on canine platelet aggregation. J Am Anim Hosp Assoc 24:23-26.

Roemisch, J., Diehl, K. H., Reiner, G., Paques, E. P. 1991. Activated protein C: antithrombotic properties and influence on fibrinolysis in an animal model. Fibrinolysis 5:191-96.

Schaub, R. G., Keith, J. C., Rawlings, C. A. 1983. Effect of acetylsalicylic acid on vascular damage and myointimal proliferation in canine pulmonary arteries subjected to chronic injury by *Dirofilaria immitis.* Am J Vet Res 44:449-54.

Sherry, S., Gustafson, E. 1985. The current and future use of thrombolytic therapy. Ann Rev Pharmacol Toxicol 25:413-31.

Shetty, S. N., Himes, J. A., Edds, G. T. 1972. Effect of phenobarbital on bishydroxycoumarin plasma concentration and hypoprothrombinemia responses in sheep. Am J Vet Res 33:825-34.

Soute, B. A., Ulrich, M. M., Watson, A. D., Maddison, J. E., Ebberink, R. H., Vermeer, C. 1992. Congenital deficiency of all vitamin K-dependent blood coagulation factors due to a defective vitamin K-dependent carboxylase in Devon Rex cats. Thrombosis and Hemostasis 68:521-25.

Szabuniewicz, M., McCrady, J. D. 1977. Hemostasis, hemostatic, anticoagulant and fibrinolytic agents. In L. M. Jones, N. H. Booth, L. E. McDonald, eds., Veterinary Pharmacology and Therapeutics, 4th ed. Ames: Iowa State Univ. Press.

Trujillo, O., Rios, A., Maldonado, R., Rudolph, W. 1981. Effect of oral administration of acetylsalicylic acid on haemostasis in the horse. Equine Vet J 13:205-6.

Vairel, E. G., Bouty-Boye, H., Toulemonde, F., Doutremepuich, C., Marsh, N. A., Gaffney, P. J. 1983. Heparin and a low molecular weight fraction enhances thrombolysis and by this pathway exercises a protective effect against thrombosis. Thrombosis Research 30:219-24.

Vezzoni, A., Genchi, C. 1989. Reduction of post-adulticide thromboembolic complications with low dose heparin therapy. Proc Heartworm Symposium 1989:73-83.

Woody, B. J., Murphy, M. J., Ray, A. C., Green, R. A. 1992. Coagulopathic effects and therapy of brodifacoum toxicosis in dogs. J Vet Intern Med 6:23-28.

Wright, P. W., Goodhead, B. 1970. Prevention of hemorrhagic pancreatitis with fibrinolysin or heparin. Arch Surg 100:42-46.

29

BLOOD AND BLOOD COMPONENTS

DAWN M. BOOTHE

Blood Groups
- **Antigens**
- **Isoantibodies**

Donors
Collection
- **Materials**
- **Collection Procedure**

Storage and Blood Components
- **Whole Blood and Packed Red Blood Cells**
- **Plasma**
- **Platelets**
- **Cryoprecipitate**

Clinical Use
- **Blood**
- **Plasma**
- **Transfusion Reactions**

Autotransfusion
Blood Substitutes
Bone Marrow Transplantation

BLOOD GROUPS

Antigens. Blood cells of each species are grouped according to antigens located on the red blood cell (RBC) surface, which determine the immunological specificity of the cell. The number of antigens that have been detected varies among species. Although canine blood has been characterized by at least 11 blood groups (Stormont 1982), 8 are generally recognized and are designated as DEA (dog erythrocyte antigen) 1.1,1.2, and 3 through 8 (Dodds 1985). Of these, DEA 1.1, 1.2, and 7 are the most common clinically significant antigens. The cat has 3 blood groups, designated A, B, and AB. Types A and B are unrelated to human blood groups. Both are allelic, with the A allele expressing dominance over B. The incidence of each blood type is characterized by marked geographic differences both outside and in the United States. Type A is by far the most common, with an incidence ranging from 99% in the United States to 70% in Australia (Cotter 1991; Giger et al. 1989; Auer and Bell 1981). A very low incidence of type AB (0.4%) has been reported (Auer and Bell 1981; Giger and Bucheler 1991; Authement et al. 1987). In the United States, only 0.1% or fewer cats have been identified as having type AB blood. Type A is also the most common in purebred cats; approximately 10% have type B blood. Breeds such as Abyssinians, Persians, Himalayans, and Rex appear to have a higher incidence of type B (Norsworthy 1992). Some catteries have exclusively type B cats. No Siamese cats have been reported to have type B. Cats lacking both type A and B antigens have not been identified. Ferrets thus far have not proven to have demonstrable blood groups that correspond to human or animal typing.

Large animals have numerous blood groups. Bovine blood has 11 phenogroups in the A system, 1000 in the B system, and 100 in the C system. While blood group variation in the horse is smaller, at least 30 factors have been segregated into 8 genetic systems (Stormont 1982).

Isoantibodies. Plasma contains isoantibodies whose activity is directed toward antigens on RBCs from animals of the same species. Naturally occurring isoantibodies are genetically determined and are present when an animal receives its first blood transfusion. A transfusion reaction may occur with the first transfusion if the recipient plasma contains isoantibodies directed toward the donor RBC antigens. A less severe reaction can occur if the donor plasma contains isoantibodies directed toward the recipient RBC antigens. However, the incidence of clinically important natural isoantibodies is low, and incompatible antigen-antibody reactions are uncommon with initial blood transfusions (Stormont 1982; Dodds 1985). Anti-DEA 7 is the most common isoantibody in dogs, present in about 50% of the canine population. About 45% of the blood tested in dogs contains DEA 7 (Cotter 1991). Shortened survival of DEA 7 blood following transfusion into DEA 7-negative dogs has been documented (Cotter 1991). However, routine cross-matching procedures generally do not test for this reaction (Cotter 1991). Cats with either A or B types have naturally occurring isoantibodies, but the anti-A antibody is stronger and responsible for most of the serious incompatibility reactions. In Australia, the blood of approximately 35% of type A cats contains isoantibodies against type B cells. However, these antibodies are only weakly agglutinating when the titer is less than 1:2, and thus transfusion reactions are absent or mild (Auer and Bell 1981; Giger and Bucheler 1991). Destruction occurs extravascularly due to IgM and IgG. In contrast, approximately 70% of type B cats have strong isoagglutinins (titers > 1:8) to type A. Thus, cats with type B blood are at a greater risk for serious transfusion reactions (Auer and Bell 1981; Giger and Bucheler 1991). Cats with type AB blood apparently do not have isoantibodies to either type A or B. Destruction of RBCs occurs intravascularly and is complement- and IgM-mediated (Giger and Bucheler 1991). In cows, anti-J are the most important isoantibodies. Bovine RBCs do not agglutinate easily, but isohemolysins are important. Anti-R isoantibodies are most important in sheep, for which both isoagglutinins and lysins exist (Hunt and Moore 1990).

In addition to naturally occurring isoantibodies, administration of whole donor blood containing antigens foreign to the recipient will stimulate formation of new isoantibodies directed against donor RBCs. Antigens DEA 1.1 and 1.2 (often referred to as type A) (Cotter 1991) are the most likely canine antigens to sensitize a recipient, and cross-matching procedures concentrate on these antigens (Cotter 1991). For example, administration of blood containing DEA 1.1 antigens to a DEA 1.1-negative recipient will result in the formation of anti-DEA 1.1 antibodies in the recipient. Formation of new antibodies will take 10-14 days. Approximately 25% of random primary (i.e., first) transfusions in dogs cause DEA 1 antibody formation (Tangner 1982). As a result, the recipient may develop a delayed transfusion reaction to the first transfusion, or severe immunological reactions can develop upon subsequent readministration of DEA 1 blood. The incidence of transfusion reactions following a random second blood transfusion has been estimated to be 15% in the dog (Stormont 1982; Dodds 1985). A foreign antigen's potential for stimulating antibody production varies with each antigen. DEA 1.1 and 1.2, which together occur in about 60% of the canine population, are the most likely to stimulate antibody production in canine recipients. Thus, the administration of blood from DEA 1.1 or 1.2 dogs should be avoided, particularly in animals that may require a second transfusion at a later date. Destruction of transfused RBCs is accelerated when transfused into incompatible animals. In cats, mean survival time (time when one-half of the transfused cells have been removed from the circulation) of autologous (from the same animal) washed RBCs is 38 ±2 days. Mean survival time of same-type transfusions (e.g., type A cat receiving type A) is 30 days, and that of different-type transfusions is less than 15 days. If type A blood is transfused into a type B cat, the survival time is less than 2 hours (Norsworthy 1992). Repeated transfusions are characterized by an even shorter RBC mean survival time of less than 5 days (Marion and Smith 1983a; Turnwald 1985). In cows, horses, and goats, the short survival times characterizing RBCs from seemingly compatible animals have been attributed to naturally occurring isoantibodies (Cotter 1991).

Cross-matching detects the presence of both natural and induced isoantibodies in plasma of either the recipient (major cross-match) or the donor (minor cross-match) (Authement et al. 1987). It does not prevent sensitization; rather, it detects what has already occurred (Cotter 1991). The major cross-match is the most important of the two and can be relatively easily performed on fresh blood. Cross-matching is particularly essential for animals that have received a transfusion within the past 4 days (Dodds 1985; Lees 1985; Marion and Smith 1983b; Cotter 1991). Feline typing reagents are not readily available. However, major cross-matching may detect incompatible transfusions (Cotter 1991). Cross-matching may be of limited value in horses and cows. Shortened RBC survival has been documented at days 3 and 4 posttransfusion in cross-matching compatible animals of both species (Hunt and Moore 1990). Nonetheless, major and minor cross-matching is frequently performed for horses (Hunt and Moore 1990; Morris 1983).

The life span of compatible, transfused, nonstored RBCs should be similar to that of normal RBCs. Transfusion of incompatible cells can result in immediate destruction or delayed destruction, depending on rapidity of antibody production. Decreased survival as early as 3-4 days posttransfusion has been noted for several large animal species (Cotter 1991); increased destruction at 2-21 days posttransfusion has been noted for dogs and cats (Tangner 1982; Marion and Smith 1983a). Prolonged storage of RBCs will also reduce survivability (Marion and Smith 1983b).

DONORS. Canine donors should be young, healthy, and cooperative, with no history of a blood transfusion. Blood collection is easier in shorthaired, lean animals. Dogs should weigh at least 20 kg and cats 4 kg (Pichler and Turnwald 1985; Authement et al. 1987). Cats should have a packed cell volume (PCV) of at least 35% (Homeida et al. 1986). Dogs preferably should be DEA 1- and 7-negative. Greyhounds are often considered to be the ideal canine donor choice because their incidence of these antigens is low (Authement et al. 1987). Female donors should be neutered. Donor animals should be free of blood-transmitted infections. Dogs should be tested for ehrlichiosis, brucellosis, microfilaremia, hemobartonellosis, and babesia; cats should be tested for leukemia, immunodeficiency and infectious peritonitis virus, toxoplasmosis, and hemobartonellosis. Splenectomy of donor animals to cause recrudescence of blood-borne diseases to enhance detection is controversial. Routine care for donor animals should include vaccinations and internal and external parasiticide treatment. Supplemental care for small-animal donors should include adequate dietary intake of vitamins (particularly B_{12}, folic acid, and pyridoxine), minerals (iron), and proteins of meat origin. Records should be kept on donors, particularly with regard to date and amount of collections (Pichler and Turnwald 1985; Lees 1985).

Equine donors should be negative for A, C, and Q RBC antigens (Morris 1983). Male ponies with no previous history of blood transfusion are reasonable alternative donors in the event that cross-matching cannot be performed; these animals generally are negative for clinically important antigens. Bovine donors should not be pregnant and should be free of bovine leukosis virus, anaplasmosis, brucellosis, tuberculosis, noncytopathic bovine virus, diarrhea virus, salmonellosis, *Sarcocystis bovicanis,* and other indigenous blood parasites (Hunt and Moore 1990). Donors should not have been vaccinated for Johne's disease, anaplasmosis, or adult-age brucellosis (Hunt and Moore 1990).

COLLECTION

Materials

RECEPTACLES. Two types of containers are available for collection of blood (Authement et al. 1987; Norsworthy 1992). Vacuum bottles are simple to use because the vacuum allows collection from the jugular vein in small animals. However, the bottle is penetrated during collection, which may allow bacterial contamination of collected blood. Other disadvantages of glass-bottle collection include (1) inability to separate blood components (e.g., plasma or platelets); (2) activation of platelets and some coagulation factors; (3) potential for air embolism; and (4) breakage of the bottle. In contrast, plastic bags remain sterile, separation of components is easy if units with satellite bags (in which the components can be collected) are purchased, and activation of blood components is not as likely as with glass. Plastic bags for single-unit, small-animal, whole-blood collection are less expensive than glass bottles. However, collection is more difficult into plastic bags than into glass bottles because (1) sedation may be needed in small animals; (2) the time necessary for collection is longer; (3) clotting is more likely to occur in the collection tubing; and (4) arterial hemorrhage may complicate femoral arterial collection. Materials designed for blood collection can be purchased from several commercial sources (e.g., Baxter). Products specifically designed for collection from small animals (including small collection bags) can be purchased from Animal Blood Bank, PO Box 6211, Vacaville, CA, 95696 (916-678-3009). A vacuum apparatus is also available (Animal Blood Bank, California) that precludes the need to use arterial sites for collection into plastic bags in dogs. Small plastic bags designed for collection of blood from cats can also be purchased; however, anticoagulant must be added to these bags. Syringes can be used to collect blood from small animals or pediatric animals (Pichler and Turnwald 1985; Lees 1985). For large animals, 1-3 liter plastic transfer bags are available for direct-transfer transfusion of large quantities of whole blood (Eicker and Ainsworth 1984). Anticoagulant-flushed extension sets are used when harvesting multiple units of blood (Hunt and Moore 1990). Blood can also be collected in open-mouthed containers if bags or bottles are not available (Hunt and Moore 1990).

ANTICOAGULANTS. Anticoagulants used for blood collection include ACD (acid, citrate, and dextrose), CPD (citrate, phosphate, and dextrose), heparin, and sodium citrate (Oberman et al. 1981; Authement et al. 1987; Norsworthy 1992). Each has its advantages and disadvantages. Maintenance of normal RBC physiology is an important consideration in selection of the most appropriate anticoagulant. The RBC undergoes significant changes in physiology during storage. The oxygen-carrying capacity of RBCs will change as adenosine triphosphate (ATP) and 2,3-diphosphoglycerate (2,3-DPG) content decline. The oxygen dissociation curve thus shifts to the left, and delivery of oxygen to tissues by the transfused blood is decreased. However, these metabolic changes are largely reversible. Up to 50% of depleted 2,3-DPG is replaced within 24 hours of transfusion, although replacement occurs at the expense of host RBCs (Oberman et al. 1981; Lees 1985). In addition to pH and related changes, stored RBCs may become spherical and rigid and thus less deformable. Once the cells are transfused, their destruction by the host is accelerated if they maintain their abnormal shape (Auer et al. 1982). ACD (14 mL/100 mL blood) will preserve blood for up to 3 weeks. However, CPD (14 mL/100 mL blood) will preserve canine RBCs better and longer (4-6 weeks) due to enhanced preservation of pH, ATP, 2,3-DPG, and RBC deformability (Pichler and Turnwald 1985; Lees 1985). Feline blood can be stored in ACD for at least 30 days (Marion and Smith 1983b). ACD can be prepared by diluting a mixture of 1.8 g (3.6 mL) of 50% dextrose, 1.6 g sodium citrate, and 0.5 g citric acid with enough distilled water to make 50 mL. After sterilization by autoclave, the solution will be sufficient for collection of 450 mL blood. ACD is also commercially available in prepackaged quantities (Blynco Development Company, Sherburn, MN), which can be dissolved in sterile water and used to collect 1 gallon of blood (Hunt and Moore 1990).

Heparin (250-625 units/mL) (Authement et al. 1987) is limited to collection of small quantities of blood (50 mL), such as that needed for pediatric patients or cats. Blood collected with heparin cannot be stored (Authement et al. 1987) since heparin contains no preservatives and will be inactivated within 24-48 hours. Heparin also activates platelets, rendering them nonfunctional, an undesirable effect if the host is deficient in platelets. Sodium citrate (1 part 3.5% solution to 9 parts blood) can also be used for collection of small quantities of blood in dogs and cats. It is the anticoagulant generally used for collection of blood from large animals (Hunt and Moore 1990). Although sodium citrate contains no preservatives or energy sources, it is rapidly metabolized and excreted and therefore safe to the recipient. Collected blood can be refrigerated up to 35 days prior to use.

Collection Procedure. A total of 20-25 mL blood can be collected per kilogram weight of donor dog every 14-21 days. Up to 6 mL per pound, up to a maximum of 50 mL, is recommended for collection from cats (Pichler and Turnwald 1985; Authement et al. 1987; Norsworthy 1992). Up to 20% of a donor's body weight (10-15 mL/kg) can be collected safely at 2- to 4-week intervals (Hunt and Moore 1990). This total can be divided into multiple withdrawals during the prescribed time period, as long as intervals are at least 7 days in dogs and 10 days in cats. The jugular vein is the safest and most efficient site of collection in all animals, but in the dog and cat, suction or vacuum is needed (Pichler and Turnwald 1985). The placement of a sterile jugular catheter is recommended in large ruminants (Hunt and Moore 1990). The femoral artery can also be used for plastic-bag collection in dogs, but this route requires moderate sedation and added care to avoid hemorrhage. Cardiac puncture as a means to collect blood is contraindicated except in terminal (euthanasia) cases or in ferrets (Pichler and Turnwald 1985).

Regardless of the site of blood collection, a sterile preparation is necessary. The puncture must be "clean" to avoid activation of platelets and factors. Blood should be gently mixed throughout collection to equally disperse the anticoagulant. Collected blood should be labeled and dated prior to refrigeration, and the collection should be recorded in the donor's record. The amount of blood collected can be measured by weighing (1 g = 1 mL).

STORAGE AND BLOOD COMPONENTS

Whole Blood and Packed Red Blood Cells. Whole blood contains all blood constituents with the exception of coagulation proteins. Fresh whole blood is whole blood that is administered within 6 hours of collection; coagulation proteins remain active until that time. Packed RBCs are collected from whole blood that either has undergone centrifugation or has been stored at 10° C until red cells have settled by sedimentation. Blood-collection units with integral transfer containers should be used if preparation of RBCs is anticipated. The removal of 225-250 mL of plasma from 500 mL of whole blood will generally result in residual RBCs with a hematocrit between 70 and 80%. As with whole blood, packed RBCs must be refrigerated at 1-6° C and, when stored properly, will have the same expiration date as whole blood. However, packed cells with a hematocrit greater than 80% undergo accelerated aging during storage and have a decreased mean survival time following transfusion. Whole blood or packed RBCs must be maintained (Oberman et al. 1981).

Collected whole blood or packed RBCs should be either used within 24 hours or, in the case of ACD- or CPD-anticoagulated blood, stored at refrigerator temperatures (1-6° C) for the previously described period. Preservation of RBCs can be enhanced by gentle mixing at intervals throughout the storage period and by uniform temperatures. Blood stored in a standard refrigerator should be placed as far back on the shelf as possible to minimize temperature fluctuations, which decrease RBC life span. Refrigerated blood that is subsequently warmed to greater than 10° C should be used within 24 hours (Auer et al. 1982; Lees 1985; Authement et al. 1987; Turnwald 1985). Methods for collection and preparation of component parts have been described by Authement et al. (1987).

Plasma. Storage requirements for blood component parts (e.g., plasma, cryoprecipitate) are different from those for whole blood and packed RBCs. Plasma that has been separated from RBCs can be prepared and stored in several ways. Fresh plasma must be separated from RBCs and administered within 6 hours of collection. Frozen plasma (which contains electrolytes and proteins such as albumin and fibrinogen) can be separated from whole blood at any time following collection up to the expiration date of the whole blood. However, the viability of factors depends on the rapidity with which the blood is frozen after collection, as well as the duration of freezing and the storage temperature. The vitamin K-dependent factors (II, VII, IX, and X) remain stable in frozen plasma (Cotter 1991). Fresh frozen plasma differs from frozen plasma in that coagulation factors V and VIII remain stable; however, it must be frozen within 6 hours after collection, preferably at –40 to –80° C. It can be stored at these temperatures for 1 year or in a household freezer for 3 months, at which time it becomes frozen plasma (Cotter 1991; Authement et al. 1987). Units should be stored individually in boxes. A rubber band should be placed around the plasma bag so that a crease is formed during freezing. The rubber band is removed when the unit is frozen. The loss of the crease prior to administration indicates the unit has been inadvertently thawed (Authement et al. 1987).

Platelets. Platelets and platelet-rich plasma require centrifugation within 6 hours of collection. Platelet yield is greatest when centrifugation occurs at high speeds (1200 G) for a short time (2.5 minutes) at 20° C. After preparation, platelets which are not immediately used should be continuously rocked or intermittently mixed for up to 72 hours at room temperature. Platelets can be stored at 1-6° C without agitation for 48 hours (Authement et al. 1987). However, refrigerated platelets do not maintain their function or viability as well as those stored at room temperature. Platelet products cannot be stored (Marion and Smith 1983b).

Cryoprecipitate. Cryoprecipitate contains concentrated sources of coagulation factor VIII, von Willebrand factor (vWf), fibrinogen, and fibronectin (Cotter 1991). It is the white foamy precipitate formed following centrifugation of partially thawed (slurry consistency) fresh frozen plasma that has been frozen for 6 months or less (Authement et al. 1987). When frozen immediately after collection in a satellite bag, the component can be stored for another year at –40 to –80° C.

CLINICAL USE

Blood. Blood transfusion in small animals is indicated in cases of acute hemorrhage or anemia in which the PCV is less than 20%. Packed cells are preferred in the normovolemic animal so that the administration of isoantibodies and other foreign protein can be avoided.

Blood for therapy of chronic anemia generally is limited to animals with a PCV of less than 10%. Component therapy is indicated for special cases.

ADMINISTRATION. Blood administration requires sterile preparation at the site. Blood should be gently mixed prior to administration. A blood administration set should be used to remove clots and large particles. Filters do not remove microaggregates that may accumulate during storage (Marion and Smith 1983b). An infusion set with a side-arm lever connector is available for the administration of blood collected in a syringe for small animals (Marion and Smith 1983b). A large-gauge intravenous catheter should be used (20 ga in dogs, 22 ga in cats, 23 ga in pediatrics). Larger needles should be used for administration of packed cells; forcing blood through small-gauge needles results in turbulence, which causes hemolysis of RBCs. Whole blood or packed cells may be mixed with normal saline to reduce viscosity (Turnwald 1985). Coadministration of other fluids should be avoided (Authement et al. 1987; Turnwald 1985).

The site of administration is partially dependent on patient size. A large vein is preferred. Intraperitoneal administration may be used for pediatrics. Up to 40% of administered blood will be absorbed in 24 hours, and 82% in 1 week (Turnwald 1985), although the life span of the RBC is probably reduced. Intramedullary administration is also recommended in pediatric patients. Usually the femur—but often the humerus—is the site of administration. Absorption is rapid, with 93% of administered blood absorbed in 5 minutes. Regardless of the site of administration, a filter (80 or 170 μm) should be used to remove macroaggregates which form in blood during storage. Filters can be purchased as part of a blood administration set (straight-type [4C2116] or Y-type [4C2197] blood recipient sets; Fenwal Laboratories, Division of Travenol, Deerfield, IL) or separately but adaptable to a syringe for transfusion of smaller volumes (Hemo-nate Filter).

Blood can be warmed in a 40° C water bath up to 37° C to avoid hypothermia and cardiac arrhythmias in the host animal. Commercially available blood-warming baths and coils are also available (V5420, McGaw Laboratories, Inc., Sabana Grande, Puerto Rico).

The dose of blood necessary to change the PCV can be calculated based on the patient's body weight and the present PCV. Generally, patient PCV and protein do not change until more than 20 mL of blood/kg recipient weight have been transfused. Accurate calculations of total blood volumes necessary to achieve a specific posttransfusion PCV in the recipient can be made from the following formula, in which

$$1 \text{ mL donor blood} = \text{recipient weight (kg)} \times 90 \text{ mL/kg} \times \frac{\text{desired PCV} - \text{recipient PCV}}{\text{PCV of donor}}$$

where 90 mL/kg for dogs (or 70 mL/kg for cats) is the blood volume. Finally, the amount of blood needed for a transfusion can be roughly but rapidly estimated, assuming a donor PCV of 40%, by the formula

milliliters donor blood = 1 mL whole blood
per pound body weight of recipient
per 1% change in PCV desired

(Turnwald 1985). For example, to obtain a PCV of 25% in a 30 lb dog with a PCV of 15%, one would need to transfuse 30 × (25 – 15), or 300 mL, whole blood.

RATE. Regardless of the amount of blood to be transfused, baseline vital signs should be measured and the initial rate of administration should be slow: 0.25 mL/kg during the first 10-30 minutes. In large ruminants, particularly in instances where cross-matching is not feasible, 200 mL can be injected intravenously and a period of 10 minutes allowed to elapse before administering the remaining blood (Hunt and Moore 1990). During this time, the patient should be monitored for volume overload (particularly if it is a cardiac patient) and transfusion reactions. For the remaining period, the rate should be 1-5 mL/kg/hr, although a rate of 22 mL/kg/hr may be used in hypovolemic patients. Fluid therapy is also indicated in hypovolemic (including shock) patients. A rate of 4 mL/kg/hr should be used to administer blood in cardiac patients (Turnwald 1985).

Plasma. Plasma therapy may be indicated for patients whose serum albumin is less than 1.5 g/dL; and fresh frozen plasma may be indicated for patients whose clotting factors are deficient. Cryoprecipitate is indicated for hemophilia, von Willebrand's disease, and other specific syndromes. Plasma and related products containing foreign proteins should be administered cautiously. A total dose of 5-10 mL/kg is recommended with each transfusion. Since plasma contains the majority of donor proteins (including antibodies), transfusion reactions are not uncommon and, as with whole blood, may occur with the initial transfusion. Thus, administration should probably be slower than 2-5 mL/kg/hr.

Transfusion Reactions. When reactions between donor and recipient cells/antibodies are moderate to severe, the reaction is considered to be a transfusion reaction (Authement et al. 1987). Adverse reactions to blood transfusions can be either immunologically or nonimmunologically (Lees 1985; Turnwald 1985) mediated. Immunological responses include immediate (acute) or delayed (chronic) transfusion reactions. *Acute hemolysis* is due to an immediate reaction between donor and recipient antigens and isoantibodies. It can occur with an initial transfusion, but it is more likely to follow subsequent transfusions. The signs of an acute reaction due to hemolysis include nausea, vomition, salivation, tachycardia, hypovolemia, prostration, urticaria, and fever. The use of DEA 1- and 7-negative blood will reduce the incidence of acute transfusion reactions in dogs. *Delayed transfusion reactions* are likely if an unexplained decrease in the PCV occurs 2-21 days after the transfusion. These usually occur within 7-10 days following transfusion and are more likely with repeated transfusions due to sensitization of the donor to recipient RBC antigens. Jaundice may be present. Cross-matching can help reduce the incidence of acute and delayed transfusion reactions. Reactions can also result from white blood cell antigen/antibody reactions.

Nonimmunological adverse reactions to blood transfusion include fever, which indicates bacterial contamination of the blood; vascular overload, indicated by clinical signs of coughing, dyspnea, vomition, and pulmonary edema; energy expenditure in the very debilitated recipient following massive transfusion of energy-depleted blood (i.e., following prolonged storage); and air embolism if glass bottles are used (Lees 1985; Marion and Smith 1983b). Overdosage of the anticoagulant used in the donor blood may also occur following massive transfusion, thus impairing the recipient's coagulation system. Citrate toxicity has been reported following transfusions of blood using ACD or CPD. This results from the chelation of recipient calcium by the anticoagulant in the donor blood and is manifested as hypocalcemic tetany. Liver disease in the recipient may exacerbate this problem (Lees 1985; Authement et al. 1987).

AUTOTRANSFUSION. Autotransfusion involves collection of blood and readministration to the same patient (Niebauer 1991; Zenoble and Stone 1978). Blood can be collected from a healthy patient in anticipation of a future need for blood (within 3 weeks). When using this technique, 3-6 collections should be made over a 10-14 day period. Autotransfusions may also be used in patients suffering hemorrhage into a body cavity from which the blood can be efficiently collected for readministration. Such blood is immediately available and is minimally physiologically affected, and transfusion reactions are avoided. Blood collected from body cavities requires filtering to remove clots and other materials. No anticoagulant is necessary if the blood has been in contact with a peritoneal or pleural surface for longer than 45 minutes. Blood can be simultaneously collected and administered using a butterfly catheter, stopcock, in-line transfusion filter, and syringes (Turnwald 1985). The major disadvantage of this method is that biogenic amines released by defibrination will not be removed from the blood and can cause severe reactions.

BLOOD SUBSTITUTES. Two types of blood substitutes are currently being developed for their ability to carry and deliver substantial amounts of oxygen to tissues: free hemoglobin and fluorocarbons (Lowe 1986; Gould et al. 1985). Free hemoglobin solutions are characterized by a short half-life (20 minutes) and oxygen saturation lower than blood, both of which will decrease oxygen availability in tissues. Fluorocarbons are chemicals which are miscible with blood and can carry as much as 5.25 mL of oxygen per 100 mL of blood, depending upon oxygen tension. While the oxygen-carrying capacity of these compounds is not adequate for total blood replacement, their low viscosity makes them potentially useful in disorders characterized by abnormalities in microcirculation. In addition, the use of these agents in nonvascular tissue (such as the peritoneal cavity) may help supplement oxygen exchange in tissues during respiratory failure.

Oxyglobin® (Biopure Corporation: www.oxyglobin.com) is a hemoglobin-based oxygen-carrying fluid derived from polymerized bovine hemoglobin. Oxyglobin has an average molecular mass of 180 kDa, with 50% of the hemoglobin polymers between 65 and 130 kDa. As such, it has colloidal properties similar to dextran 70 and hetastarch. However, because it is a polymerized hemoglobin, the molecules are much larger than those of hemoglobin, and the compound is not likely to be filtered by the kidney (thus, avoiding renal side effects of hemoglobinuria).

Oxyglobin® increases plasma and total hemoglobin concentration and thus increases arterial oxygen content. Because it is a free solution (rather than in RBCs), antibody formation generally associated with administration of intact RBCs is avoided. However, antigenicity to bovine hemoglobin may result in antibodies, and caution is recommended with repeat administration 10 or more days apart. Repeated administration of the product apparently has not been studied. Because it is a foreign protein, anaphylactic reactions are possible.

Oxyglobin® is eliminated similarly to hemoglobin by reticuloendothelial cells. Its elimination half-life in dogs is estimated to range between 30 and 40 hours. As such, 90% of the drug will be gone within 5-7 days after infusion. As a protein, the compound provides oncotic pressure (draw), and its use in patients already suffering from volume overload (e.g., congestive heart failure) or accidental overdose (>10 mL/kg/hr) can be associated with circulatory overload and its negative sequelae (e.g., pulmonary edema, pleural effusion, increased central venous pressure, dyspnea, or coughing).

Oxyglobin® will mildly decrease PCV immediately postinfusion and will increase total and plasma hemoglobin concentration for at least 24 hours. PCV and RBC counts will not be accurate measures of anemia for 24 hours following administration. Adequate hydration is important, but overhydration should be avoided because of the plasma-expanding properties of Oxyglobin. Administration of other colloidal solutions should be avoided. The most likely side effect is circulatory volume overload. Central venous pressure (CVP) or clinical signs indicative of circulatory overload should be monitored during and immediately following administration of Oxyglobin.

Transient changes or side effects reported by Biopure Corporation following administration of Oxyglobin® include yellow-orange discoloration of the skin, sclera, and gums; red–dark green discoloration of feces; brown-black discoloration of urine; vomiting; diarrhea; and decreased skin elasticity within 48 hours of dosing. The frequency and/or intensity of these clinical signs were dose dependent. The product is intended for one-time use only at a recommended dosage of Oxyglobin® dose of 30 mL/kg IV at a rate of up to 10 mL/kg/hr.

Conditions studied in controlled canine clinical trials included immune-mediated hemolysis (n = 30), blood loss (gastrointestinal, traumatic, surgical, rodenticide intoxication) (n = 25), and ineffective erythropoiesis (idiopathic, RBC aplasia, ehrlichiosis) (n = 9). Relative to pretreatment, plasma hemoglobin concentration significantly increased ($p = 0.001$), and clinical signs associated with anemia (lethargy/depression, exercise intolerance, and increased heart rate) significantly improved ($p = 0.001$) following treatment with Oxyglobin®. Treatment success was defined as the lack of need for additional oxygen-carrying support (i.e., blood transfusion) for 24 hours following the completion of infusion with Oxyglobin®. Success in the treatment group was 95%, compared with 32% in untreated control dogs.

Oxyglobin® may be warmed to 37° C prior to administration. It cannot be frozen but is stable for 24 months. It is approved for use in dogs but apparently has been studied in and is safe in cats. The price will be about $30/kg, although animals may not need the full 30 mL/kg; according to the manufacturer, 10 mL/kg may be sufficient in some cases. Oxyglobin has been used in a number of other species with no apparent adverse effects. Care should be taken to use or dispose of any opened product within 4-5 days. The foil wrap in which the product is enclosed is an oxygen barrier. Exposure to oxygen following removal of the wrap will result in methemoglobin formation of the hemoglobin, which can be detected by brown discoloration of the solution.

BONE MARROW TRANSPLANTATION. Although this technique is not yet clinically practical, it has proven successful and may provide an avenue of therapy for cases of aplastic anemia or pancytopenia in future (Harris and Beck 1986). Transplantation requires matching of donor and recipient major histocompatibility gene complex. The recipient must be "conditioned" to receive the graft by total body irradiation so that the tendency to reject the graft is decreased. Bone marrow is collected from the donor by multiple bone marrow aspirations from long bones using heparin as the anticoagulant. Dimethyl sulfoxide is used as the preservative. The marrow is then transfused intravenously. The cell numbers needed for a successful transplantation depend on the degree of donor-recipient gene matching. Complications include host-versus-graft rejection (the host rejects the transplant) and graft-versus-host rejection, in which the graft is so successful that it rejects (and kills) the host.

REFERENCES

Auer, L., and Bell, K. 1981. The AB blood group system of cats. Animal Blood Group and BiochemicalGenetics 12:287-97.

Auer, L., Bell, K., and Coates, S. 1982. Blood transfusion reactions in the cat. J Am Vet Med Assoc 180:729-30.

Authement, J. M., Wolfsheimer, K. J., and Catchings, S. 1987. Canine blood component therapy: Product preparation, storage, and administration. J Am Anim Hos Assoc 23:483-93.

Cotter, S. M. 1991. Clinical transfusion medicine. Adv Vet Sci Comp Med 36:187-223.

Dodds, W. J. 1985. Canine and feline blood groups. In D. H. Slatter, ed., Textbook of Small Animal Surgery, pp. 1195-98. Philadelphia: W. B. Saunders Co.

Eicker, S. W., and Ainsworth, D. M. 1984. Equine plasma banking: collection by exsanguination. J Am Vet Med Assoc 182:772-74.

Giger, U., and Bucheler, J. 1991. Transfusion of type-A and type-B blood to cats. J Am Vet Med Assoc 198:411-18.

Giger, U., Kilrain, C. G., Filippich, L. J., et al. 1989. Frequencies of feline blood groups in the United States. J Am Vet Med Assoc 195:1230-32.

Gould, S. A., Sehgal, L. R., Rosen, A. L., et al. 1985. Red cell substitutes: an update. Ann Emerg Med 14:798-803.

Harris, C. K., and Beck, E. R. 1986. Bone marrow transplantation in the dog. Compendium on Continuing Education 8:337-45.

Homeida, M. M. A., Daneshmend, T. K., Ali, E. M., et al. 1986. Assessment of oxidative metabolism in adults with hepatocellular carcinoma in the Sudan. Gut 27:382-85.

Hunt, E., and Moore, J. S. 1990. Use of blood and blood products. Vet Clin Morth Am Food Anim Pract 6:133-47.

Lees, G. E. 1985. Blood transfusion. In D. H. Slatter, ed., Textbook of Small Animal Surgery, pp. 74-81. Philadelphia: W. B. Saunders Co.

Lowe, K. C. 1986. Blood transfusion or blood substitution. Vox Sang 51:257-63.

Marion, R. S., and Smith, J. E. 1983a. Survival of erythrocytes after autologous and allogenic transfusion in cats. J Am Vet Med Assoc 183:1437-39.

———. 1983b. Posttransfusion viability of feline erythrocytes stored in acid-citrate-dextrose solution. J Am Vet Med Assoc 183:1459-60.

Morris, P. 1983. Blood transfusions. In N. E. Robinson, ed., Current Therapy in Equine Medicine, pp. 325-28. Philadelphia: W. B. Saunders Co.

Niebauer, G. W. 1991. Autotransfusion for intraoperative blood salvage: a new technique. Compendium on Continuing Education 13:1105-21.

Norsworthy, G. D. 1992. Clinical aspects of feline blood transfusions. Compendium on Continuing Education North American Edition 14:469-75.

Oberman, H. A., Barnes, B., Beattie, K. M., et al. 1981. Blood storage and shipment. In F. K. Widmann, ed., Technical Manual of the American Association of Blood Banks, 8th ed., pp. 52-59. Philadelphia and Toronto: J. B. Lippincott Co.

Pichler, M. E., and Turnwald, G. H. 1985. Blood transfusion in the dog and cat. Part I. Physiology, collection, storage, and indications for whole blood therapy. Compendium on Continuing Education 7:64-72.

Stormont, C. J. 1982. Blood groups in animals. J Am Vet Med Assoc 181:1120-23.

Tangner, C. H. 1982. Transfusion therapy for the dog and cat. Compendium on Continuing Education 4:521-28.

Turnwald, G. H. 1985. Blood transfusion in dogs and cats. Part II. Administration, adverse effects, and component therapy. Compendium on Continuing Education 7:115-26.

Zenoble, R. D., and Stone, E. A. 1978. Autotransfusion in the dog. J Am Vet Med Assoc 172:1411-14.

SECTION 8
Endocrine Pharmacology

30 HYPOTHALAMIC AND PITUITARY HORMONES

DUNCAN C. FERGUSON AND MARGARETHE HOENIG

ANTERIOR PITUITARY AND ASSOCIATED REGULATORY HORMONES
- **Corticotropin and Related Peptides**
  - **Corticotropin-Releasing Hormone**
  - **Adrenocorticotropin**
  - **Diagnostic Uses of CRH and ACTH**
- **Glycoprotein Hormones and Associated Releasing Hormones**
  - **Thyrotropin-Releasing Hormone**
  - **Thyrotropin**
- **Somatomammotropins and Regulatory Hormones**
  - **Growth Hormone–Releasing Hormone**
  - **Somatostatin (Growth Hormone Release–Inhibiting Hormone)**
  - **Somatotropin (Growth Hormone)**
  - **Prolactin**

POSTERIOR PITUITARY HORMONES
- **Antidiuretic Hormone**
  - **Structure**
  - **Stimuli for Release**
  - **Mechanism of Action**
  - **Absorption, Metabolism, and Excretion**
  - **Preparations**
  - **Diagnostic Use**
  - **Therapeutic Uses**
  - **Toxicity**
  - **Other Drugs for Treatment of Central Diabetes Insipidus**
  - **Treatment of Nephrogenic Diabetes Insipidus**
- **Oxytocin**

The hypothalamus and pituitary control the function of the thyroid, adrenal glands, and gonads. Neurons and endocrine gland cells share the characteristics of being able to secrete chemical mediators and being electrically excitable. Chemical messengers can be secreted as a neurotransmitter or as a hormone. The neuroendocrine systems consist of clusters of peptide- and monoamine-secreting cells in the anterior and middle portions of the ventral hypothalamus. Their fibers project via nerve fibers to terminals in the outer layer of the median eminence. The capillary plexus of the median eminence is proximate to the nerve terminals of the hypophysiotropic neurons which make corticotropin-releasing hormone (CRH), thyrotropin-releasing hormone (TRH), gonadotropic hormone–releasing hormone (GnRH), and growth hormone–releasing hormone (GHRH). The concentrations of the releasing and inhibitory hormones in the median eminence are 10–100 times as great as in other parts of the hypothalamus because the hormones are stored in the nerve terminals (Rijnberk 1996). The process of neurosecretion is characteristic of the hypothalamic nuclei, which release releasing hormones into the portal hypophysial vessels, which mediate the release of the anterior pituitary hormones such as growth hormone (GH), prolactin (PRL), thyrotropin (TSH), follicle-stimulating hormone (FSH), luteinizing hormone (LH), and the proopiomelanocortin (POMC)-derived peptides adrenocorticotropic hormone (ACTH), β lipotropin (β LPH), α melanotropin (α MSH), and the opioid β endorphin (β END). For each of the anterior lobe hormone systems (ACTH, LH, FSH, TSH, GH, and PRL) there is a closed-loop feedback system. Anterior lobe hormone and hypophysiotropic hormone secretions are suppressed by hormonal products of the respective end-organs, such as thyroid, gonadal, and adrenal glands. Some hormones, like PRL, regulate their own secretion by inhibition via short-loop feedback on the hypothalamus. The somatotropes account for 50% or more of the anterior pituitary lobe cells, while other types of anterior lobe cells account for between 5 and 15% of the gland (Rijnberk 1996). Table 30.1 outlines the location of neuroendocrine substances in the nervous system and endocrine organs. Tables 30.2–30.4 show the key features of the structure and function of the hypothalamic regulatory and pituitary hormones. Many of these peptides find their clinical use as agents used for diagnostic tests of pituitary or endocrine end-organ function. Therefore, the related hypothalamic and anterior pituitary hormones will be discussed concomitantly.

The supraoptic (SO) nuclei and periventricular (PV) neurons of the hypothalamus terminate in the posterior

TABLE 30.1—Location of hypothalamic and pituitary peptides

Substance	Neurotransmitter in nerve endings	Hormone secreted by neurons	Hormone secreted by endocrine cells
GnRH	+	+	+
TRH	+	+	
CRH	+	+	+
GHRH	+	+	+
Somatostatin	+	+	+
POMC derivatives	+		+
TSH	+		+
FSH	+		+
LH	+		+
GH	+		+
PRL	+		+
Oxytocin	+	+	+
Vasopressin (ADH)	+	+	+

TABLE 30.2—Hypothalamic regulatory hormones

Hormone	Action	Structure	Precursor	Target organ
TRH	Elevates TSH, PRL	Blocked tripeptide (pGlu-His-Pro-NH_2)	29-kDa precursor containing five copies of TRH	Pituitary thyrotroph
GnRH	Elevates LH, FSH	Blocked decapeptide (pGlu . . . Gly-NH_2)	Amino terminus of 90-amino-acid precursor	Pituitary gonadotroph
Somatostatin	Decreases GH	14-amino-acid peptide with disulfide bond between residues 3 and 14	Carboxy-terminus of 92-amino-acid precursor	Pituitary somatotroph
CRH	Elevates ACTH	41-amino-acid peptide with amidated carboxy-terminus	Carboxy-terminus of 196-amino-acid precursor	Pituitary corticotroph
GHRH	Elevates GH	44-amino-acid peptide with amidated carboxy-terminus	Residues 32-75 from a 108-amino-acid precursor	Pituitary somatotroph
Dopamine	Decreases PRL, increases GHRH or GH, decreases CRH or ACTH	Catechol		Pituitary lactotroph, somatotroph, corticotroph

TABLE 30.3—Anterior pituitary hormones

Hormone	Molecular weight	Amino acids	Other
ACTH-LPH			
ACTH	4,500	39	
β LPH	11,200	91	Derived from POMC
β END	4,000	31	
Glycoproteins			
LH	29,000	α subunit: 89 β subunit: 115	α subunits are identical within a species; β subunits confer biologic specificity
FSH	29,000	α subunit: 89 β subunit: 115	
TSH	28,000	α subunit: 92–96 β subunit: 110–118	
Somatomammotropins			
GH	21,500	191	Common ancestral hormone
PRL	22,000	198	

Source: Adapted from Tyrell et al. 1994, 74.

TABLE 30.4—Hormones of the hypothalamus and the pituitary gland

Hormone	Site of action (target organ)	Biologic activity
Hypothalamus		
Gonadotropin-releasing hormone	Anterior pituitary (AP)	Release LH and FSH
Thyrotropin-releasing hormone	AP	Release TSH
Corticotropin-releasing hormone	AP	Release ACTH
Somatotropin-releasing hormone	AP	Release somatotropin
Somatotropin-inhibitory hormone	AP	Inhibit somatotropin output
Prolactin-inhibitory hormone	AP	Inhibit prolactin output
Prolactin-releasing hormone	AP	Release prolactin
Adenohypophysis		
Pars distalis (anterior lobe)		
Somatotropin (growth hormone)	General soma	Body growth (bone, muscle, organs), protein synthesis, carbohydrate metabolism, regulation of renal functions (glomerular filtration rate) and water metabolism; increases cell permeability to amino acids; favors lactation
Adrenocorticotropic hormone (ACTH, corticotropin)	Adrenal cortex	Maintenance of structural integrity of adrenal cortex; regulation of glucocorticoid secretion by zona fasciculata
Thyroid-stimulating hormone (TSH; thyrotropin)	Thyroid	Maintenance of normal structure and function of the thyroid gland; production of thyroxin and analogs
Prolactin (lactogenic hormone)	Mammary gland	Possibly favors lactation
Gonadotropins		
Follicle-stimulating hormone (FSH)	Ovary Testis seminiferous tubules	Growth and maturation of ovarian follicles; germ-cell production (spermatogenesis)
Interstitial cell-stimulating, or luteinizing, hormone (LH)	Ovary	Synergistically with FSH causes estrogen secretion, follicle maturation, and ovulation; corpus luteum development in some species
	Testis Leydig cells	Stimulation of interstitial tissue, androgen secretion
Pars intermedia		
Intermedin (melanocyte-stimulating hormone)	Melanophore cells of amphibia and reptiles	Melanophore-expanding activity with resultant maintenance of skin color (of negligible importance in mammals)
Neurohypophysis		
Antidiuretic hormone (vasopressin)	Renal tubules (distal convoluted)	Regulation of water excretion by resorption of water, pressor effect only in high doses
Oxytocin	Mammary myoepithelium	Letdown of milk by contraction of myoepithelium
	Uterine myometrium	Contraction of uterine musculature to aid parturition and sperm transport

Source: McDonald 1988, 583.

pituitary lobe and secrete vasopressin (antidiuretic hormone; ADH) and oxytocin into the circulation.

ANTERIOR PITUITARY HORMONES AND ASSOCIATED REGULATORY HORMONES

The anterior pituitary hormones can be classified into three general categories: ACTH-LPH, glycoproteins (LH, FSH, and TSH), and somatomammotropins (GH, PRL) (see Table 30.3).

CORTICOTROPIN AND RELATED PEPTIDES

Corticotropin-Releasing Hormone (CRH). CRH-secreting neurons are found in the anterior part of the paraventricular nuclei, and their nerve endings terminate in external layers of the median eminence. CRH is synthesized as part of a 196-amino-acid prohormone and undergoes enzymatic modification to an amidated 41-amino-acid peptide that is identical in humans, dogs, rats, and horses (Mol et al. 1994; Rijnberk 1996). CRH stimulates synthesis and secretion of ACTH i.e., POMC, by pituitary corticotrophs. CRH has receptors in both the cytoplasm (matrix and secretory granules) and the nucleus of corticotrophs, but its mechanism of action at the plasma membrane or nucleus remains to be established. CRH appears to exert its ACTH-releasing activity through both the adenylate cyclase and calcium-calmodulin signal transduction systems (Klonoff and Karam 1992; Tyrell et al. 1994).

Adrenocorticotropin

BIOSYNTHESIS. Adrenocorticotropin (ACTH) is a 39-amino-acid peptide hormone (molecular weight = 4500) that is one of several products from the metabolism of the 267-amino-acid precursor molecule POMC (Fig. 30.1; molecular weight = 28,500; Rijnberk 1996: p. 63, Fig. 4-5). Between species there is significant sequence homology in the ACTH amino acid structure. Canine ACTH differs by only one C-terminal amino acid from ACTH of other species (Mol et al. 1991). The other fragments of POMC with biological activity include β-lipotropin (β-LPH), α-melanocyte-stimulating hormone (α-MSH), β-MSH, and the opioid β-endorphin, as well as the N-terminal fragment (see Rijnberk 1996: p. 63, Fig. 4-5). ACTH is metabolized to $ACTH_{1\text{-}13}$, which is identical to α MSH, and to corticotropin-like intermediate-lobe peptide (CLIP), which represents $ACTH_{18\text{-}39}$. These fragments are observed in species with developed intermediate lobes, such as the rat and horse, as well as fish, reptiles, and amphibians. Beta LPH is secreted in equimolar amounts to ACTH. The 91 amino acids of β LPH include the amino acid structure for β MSH (41–58), γ LPH (1–58), and β endorphin (61–91). The first (N-terminal) 23 amino acids of ACTH, which are identical in humans, cattle, pigs, and sheep, produce all of its biological effects (Klonoff and Karam 1992; Tyrell et al. 1994). The sequence of the remaining amino acids varies among species (Chastain and Ganjam 1986). MSH causes pigment granules in melanocytes to disperse so that skin will darken. Although genetic factors associated with skin color are more important in the higher vertebrates, MSH may cause transiently increased pigment synthesis in mammals.

STRUCTURE. ACTH is a peptide that contains 39 amino acids in a straight-chain molecule in sheep, pigs, cows, and humans. The first 24 and last 7 amino acids are identical and there are minor differences in amino acids 25 through 32 (see Fig. 30.2). The amino acid sequence of canine β-END differs from the human sequence by 4 amino acids (Young and Kemppainen 1994). The distribution of molecular forms of β-END in the canine intermediate lobe and anterior pituitary more closely resembles the distribution in rats than that in other species such as sheep or horses, in which acetylated and shortened forms exist in substantial amounts. In all species studied to date, ACTH and related peptides are synthesized and cleaved from the common precursor molecule POMC. Posttranslational processing of POMC differs in the pars distalis and pars intermedia of the pituitary gland. In the pars distalis, POMC is processed to form ACTH, β-LPH, some γ LPH, and β endorphin. In the pars intermedia, however, POMC is processed to ACTH and β-LPH; ACTH is then further processed to α MSH and CLIP, and β-LPH is further processed to β-MSH, β-END, and β-END metabolites. As a result, ACTH and β-LPH are intermediates to α MSH and the opiate β-END. The pattern of POMC-derived peptide secretion from the pars intermedia has been characterized in rats, horses, pigs, sheep, dogs, and cats. The plasma POMC peptide concentrations found in cats is similar to that in rats but is markedly different from that in dogs, in which the secretion of POMC peptides in the pars intermedia is normally low (Peterson et al. 1994b). The role of N-POMC1-48 is now known to promote adrenocortical cell replication.

REGULATION OF SECRETION. Beta LPH and β END are secreted in a pattern similar to ACTH, increasing in response to stress and paralleling ACTH in a variety of disease conditions. The regulation of ACTH is most directly influenced by the hypothalamic hormone CRH, which stimulates ACTH in a pulsatile fashion. Arginine-vasopressin (ADH) is also a potent stimulus for ACTH secretion (van Wijk et al. 1994). The pulsatility of ACTH release appears to occur in most species. Although a diurnal variation of cortisol was postulated by older studies, more recent studies with sampling at 30-minute intervals for 48 hours have not confirmed a diurnal variation in ACTH in dogs or cats (Peterson et al. 1994c).

Four mechanisms that regulate ACTH secretion have been identified: (1) episodic secretion and possible

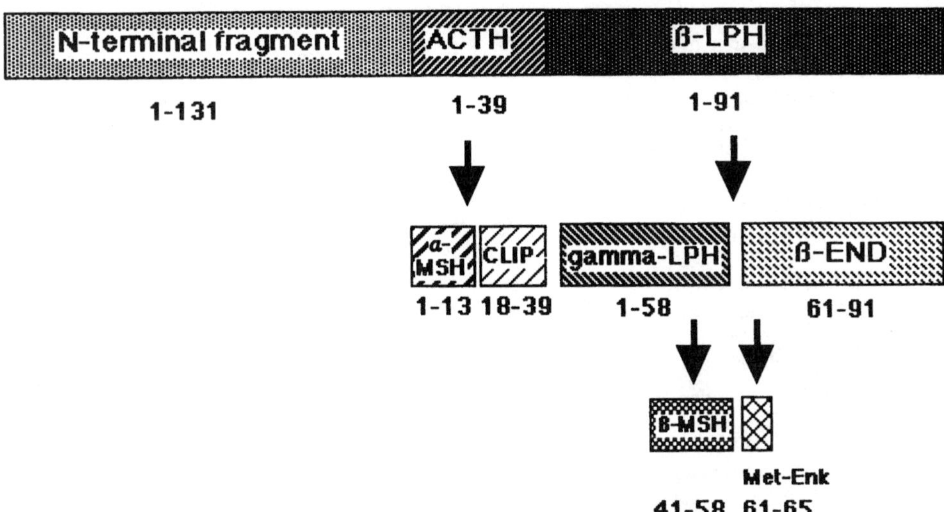

FIG. 30.1—Relationships of peptides derived from proopiomelanocortin (POMC). Following synthesis in the anterior or intermediate lobe of the pituitary, POMC is cleaved to form adrenocorticotropin (ACTH) and β lipotropin (β LPH). ACTH is further degraded, particularly in the intermediate lobe, to α-melanocyte stimulating factor (α MSH) and corticotropin-like intermediate-lobe peptide (CLIP). β-LPH is cleaved to produce γ LPH and the endogenous opiate β endorphin (β END). γ LPH is cleaved to produce β MSH, and β END is further processed to produce another opioid, Met-enkephalin (Met-Enk).

1	2	3	4	5	6	7	8	9	10	11	12	13	-------	25	26	27	28	29	30	31	32	33	34	35	36	37	38	39
Ser	Tyr	Ser	Met	Glu	His	Phe	Arg	Trp	Gly	Lys	Pro	Val	(human)	Asp	Ala	Gly	Glu	Asp	Gln	Ser	Ala	Glu	Ala	Phe	Pro	Leu	Glu	Phe
Ser	Tyr	Ser	Met	Glu	His	Phe	Arg	Trp	Gly	Lys	Pro	Val	(pig)	Asp	Gly	Ala	Glu	Asp	Gln	Leu	Ala	Glu						
Ser	Tyr	Ser	Met	Glu	His	Phe	Arg	Trp	Gly	Lys	Pro	Val	(beef)	Asp	Gly	Glu	Ala	Glu	Asp	Ser	Ala	Gln						
Ser	Tyr	Ser	Met	Glu	His	Phe	Arg	Trp	Gly	Lys	Pro	Val	(sheep)	Ala	Gly	Glu	Asp	Asp	Glu	Ala	Ser	Glu						

FIG. 30.2—Amino acid sequences of human, pig, cattle, and sheep ACTH. Amino acids 1–13 are also present in α MSH. Note areas of species homology in shaded boxes. (Reprinted from Klonoff and Karam 1992: Fig. 36.2.)

diurnal variation, mediated by the central nervous system (CNS) and hypothalamus; (2) response to stress (cats are much more sensitive than dogs), also CNS and hypothalamus mediated; (3) feedback inhibition by cortisol at both the hypothalamus and pituitary; and (4) immunological factors (IL-1, IL-6, tumor necrosis factor, etc.) which act at the hypothalamus to increase CRH (Rijnberk 1996).

Facilitatory and inhibitory pathways, involving GABAergic, cholinergic, adrenergic, dopaminergic, and serotoninergic systems, are all involved in hypothalamic regulation of ACTH and therefore cortisol secretion. Drugs manipulating these systems have been used to pharmacologically manage pituitary-dependent hyperadrenocorticism in the dog and horse. Ergot alkaloids (dopamine agonists) and serotonin antagonists (cyproheptadine) have been utilized to manipulate ACTH release without much clinical success. The monoamine oxidase B inhibitor L-deprenyl is currently under study in pituitary-dependent Cushing's disease due to its ability to decrease the degradation of dopamine, which has been postulated to be depleted in canine pituitary-dependent hyperadrenocorticism (Cushing's disease) (Klonoff and Karam 1992).

Many factors stimulate ACTH: pain trauma, hypoxia, hypoglycemia, surgery, cold, pyrogens, and ADH. CRH is often used to release ACTH from the pars distalis, and the drug haloperidol can be used to stimulate pars intermedia secretion, with pars distalis effects being removed by dexamethasone. In cultured canine anterior pituitary cells, it appears that CRH stimulates ACTH secretion, but arginine-vasopressin, oxytocin, and angiotensin II do not (Kemppainen et al. 1992).

NEGATIVE-FEEDBACK SYSTEMS. Exogenous corticosteroids suppress the ACTH response to stress. Negative feedback of cortisol occurs via both the hypothalamus and pituitary. Feedback occurs in three ways:

1. Fast feedback is sensitive to the rate of change in cortisol and probably occurs via a nonnuclear receptor.
2. Slow feedback is sensitive to the cortisol concentration in plasma. This feedback loop is tested by the low-dose dexamethasone suppression test.
3. Short-loop feedback by ACTH occurs on the release of CRH by neurons in the hypothalamus and corticotrope receptors in the corticotropic cells of the anterior pituitary. The feedback is mediated through a type I mineralocorticoid-preferring receptor (MR) and a type II glucocorticoid-preferring receptor (GR). The highest levels of GR in the dog brain are found in the septohippocampal complex and the anterior lobe of the pituitary (Reul et al. 1990; Keller-Wood 1990; Klonoff and Karam 1992; Tyrell et al. 1994).

FUNCTION. ACTH stimulates the secretion of glucocorticoids, mineralocorticoids, and adrenal androgens by increasing the activity of cholesterol desmolase, the enzyme that is rate limiting for steroid production and converts cholesterol to pregnenolone. ACTH also stimulates adrenal hypertrophy and hyperplasia. Steroids are not stored in the adrenal cortex but are immediately released upon stimulation of the zona fasciculata. ACTH causes growth of both the zona fasciculata and glomerulosa. The biological activity is conveyed by the amino terminal end of the molecule. ACTH stimulates adrenocortical growth and steroidogenesis by increasing cellular cAMP (Tyrell et al. 1994).

LPH induces lipolysis in adipocytes of some species, but its function, other than serving as a precursor peptide for the endogenous opiate β END, is unknown for most species (Klonoff and Karam 1992; Kuret and Murad 1990).

Diagnostic Uses of CRH and ACTH. The most important applications of CRH and ACTH are as diagnostic agents to test adrenocorticotroph and adrenal functional reserve.

CRH STIMULATION TEST. The CRH stimulation test is used mainly as a research tool to assess pituitary ACTH secretory capacity. In animals administered exogenous glucocorticoids, the ACTH and cortisol response to CRH is diminished. In dogs and cats, ovine CRH is administered at 1 μg/kg intravenously and plasma is sampled for ACTH measurement at 0 and 0.5 hours for peak effect (see Table 30.5). Other sampling times have been employed in research reports (Crager et al. 1994; Moore and Hoenig 1992; Peterson et al. 1994b,c). Studies of normal dogs and dogs with pituitary-dependent hyperadrenocorticism have shown that ACTH secretion is less sensitive to CRH than it is to lysine vasopressin (LVP). It was also found that adrenocortical tumors develop an aberrant sensitivity to LVP, with adrenal tissue appearing to directly respond to LVP (van Wijk et al. 1994).

TABLE 30.5—Dosage protocols for CRH stimulation test

Preparation	Horses and cattle	Dogs	Cats
Ovine CRH (μg/kg IV)	NA	1	1
Sampling times (hr)	NA	0, 0.5	0, 0.5

Sources: Crager et al. 1994; Moore and Hoenig 1992; Peterson et al. 1994b,c; Peninsula Laboratories.
Note: NA = not available.

PREPARATIONS OF ACTH. Synthetic human $ACTH_{1\text{-}24}$ is called cosyntropin. Repositol ACTH gel from animal (porcine) sources is no longer available commercially. However, when comparing dosage protocols, 1 unit of porcine ACTH is approximately equal to 10 μg of cosyntropin. Synthetic ACTH is well absorbed by the intramuscular (IM) route. The biological half-life of all forms of ACTH is 10–20 minutes, and the effect on the adrenal cortex lasts for 12–48 hours.

ACTH STIMULATION TEST. The main use of ACTH is for the differential diagnosis of adrenocortical hyperplasia from adrenocortical neoplasia (primary) in dogs, cats, and horses (see Table 30.6) and for the definitive diagnosis of primary adrenal hypofunction. ACTH is well absorbed following IM injection. Following injection of aqueous synthetic ACTH, plasma cortisol concentrations peak at 30–90 minutes, largely because of the short half-life of ACTH. Therefore, most sampling protocols with aqueous ACTH in dogs and cats recommend sampling times at 1 hour after administration for a peak effect. The administration of 250 μg synthetic ACTH to dogs resulted in similar cortisol patterns whether the dose was given IV or IM, despite the fact that there were much higher peak ACTH concentrations with the IV dose. The peak cortisol concentration was at 60–90 minutes (Hansen et al. 1994). However, in cats, the IV dose of synthetic ACTH appeared to provide a greater response than the IM dosage (Peterson et al. 1994b,c).

GLYCOPROTEIN HORMONES AND ASSOCIATED RELEASING HORMONES. Only the thyroid-related peptides TRH and TSH will be discussed in this chapter. Gonadotropin-releasing hormone (GnRH), luteinizing hormone (LH), placental (human) chorionic gonadotropin (HCG), and pregnant mare serum gonadotropin (PMSG) are discussed in Chapter 31 on reproductive hormones.

Thyrotropin-Releasing Hormone. Thyrotropin-releasing hormone (TRH) is a tripeptide: PyroGlu-His-Pro NH_2. Neurons secreting TRH are located in the medial portion of the paraventricular nuclei, and their

TABLE 30.6—Dosage protocol for ACTH stimulation test

Preparation	Horses and cattle	Dogs	Cats
Synthetic: Cosyntropin (μg IV, IM) (Cortrosyn, Organon Pharmaceuticals)	NA	250	125 (IV preferred)
Sampling times (hr)	NA	0, 1	0, 1

Sources: Hansen et al. 1994; Moore and Hoenig 1992; Peterson et al. 1994b,c.
Note: NA = not applicable or available.

axons terminate in medial portions of the external lamina of the medial eminence. TRH is present extensively in the brain outside the classic "thyrotropic area" of the hypothalamus. An intact amide and the cyclized glutamic acid terminus are essential for activity. TRH is synthesized as a large 242-amino-acid precursor that contains five repeating sequences in the rat and six in the human called preprothyrotropin-releasing hormone (preproTRH) (Jackson 1982; Johnannson et al. 1981; Lechan et al. 1984; Yamada et al. 1990). The prohormone undergoes extensive posttranslational processing, including enzymatic cleavage, cyclization of NH_2-terminal glutamic acid, and exchange of an amide for the COOH-terminal glycine. TRH binds to specific receptors on the plasma membrane of the pituitary cell (Halpern and Hinkle 1981). TRH was thought to act by activating membrane adenylate cyclase with the formation of cAMP and increase in cAMP stimulates TSH secretion. However, cAMP may not increase under all conditions of TRH-induced TSH release, and increased intracellular cAMP is not always associated with an increase in TSH secretion. There is increasing evidence that the TRH-induced increase in cAMP levels is a secondary event. It is now widely accepted that TRH action is mediated mainly through activation of phospholipase C. It causes hydrolysis of phosphatidyl-inositol into 1,4,5-biophosphate and 1,2-diacylglycerol (DAG). DAG then activates protein kinase C. TRH induces an immediate and rapid increase in intracellular free calcium that decays rapidly, followed by an extended plateau of elevated calcium. The first phase reflects increased release of intracellular calcium stores, whereas the second phase represents calcium influx. This biphasic action correlates with electrical charges, induction of Ca^{++} fluxes, and secretory activity in pituitary cells (Geras and Gershengorn 1981; Gershengorn et al. 1980; Tashjian et al. 1987; Vale et al. 1977; Winiger and Schlegel 1988).

TRH Stimulation Test

DIAGNOSING HYPOTHYROIDISM IN THE DOG. The TRH stimulation test, as it is used diagnostically in the diagnosis of human pituitary and thyroid disease, is designed to evaluate the pituitary's responsiveness to TRH as manifested by the change in serum TSH concentration. In primary thyroid gland failure, the pituitary response to TRH is increased, and in hyperthyroidism, it is decreased. Because an immunoassay for TSH only became available for the dog in 1997, serum thyroxine (T_4) concentrations were most commonly measured until that time. Fig. 30.3 shows the theoretical response of serum T_4 to TRH and TSH administration. In theory, the administration of TRH should lead to an increase in T_4 only if the pituitary-thyroid axis is intact. Therefore, responsiveness to TRH should be observed only in tertiary (hypothalamic) thyroid insufficiency, a condition not yet documented in the dog (Ferguson 1984, 1994). Since the availability of the canine TSH assay in 1997, more has been learned about regulation of TSH secretion. However, evaluation of TRH-stimulated TSH responsiveness has not proved to be of much more diagnostic value than baseline canine TSH concentrations (Scott-Moncrieff et al. 1998; Hoenig and Ferguson 1997).

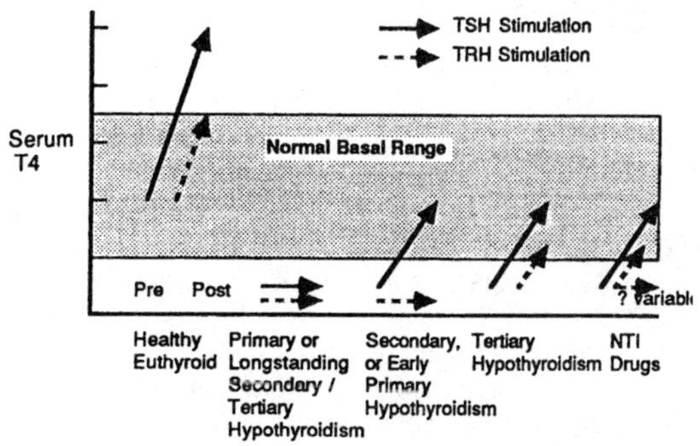

FIG. 30.3—Diagnostic classifications based on TRH and TSH stimulation tests in dogs. The arrows represent in a schematic fashion the classic response of serum T_4 concentrations to optimal doses of TRH and TSH. The actual magnitude of response will, in part, be determined by the dosage of TRH and TSH and the time of serum sampling post-TRH or post-TSH. The shaded area represents the normal baseline serum T_4 concentrations. Note the lower relative response to even maximal dosages of TRH compared to TSH. The left-hand arrow *(solid line)* represents the response to TSH, and the right-hand arrow *(broken line)* represents the response to TRH. NTI = nonthyroidal illness. (Reprinted from Peterson and Ferguson 1989: Fig. 95-5.)

A variety of TRH dosages have been proposed for use in the dog. In general, regardless of the species, increasing the TRH or TSH dose increases the duration of the serum T_4 response. In the dog, side effects were

TABLE 30.7—Protocols for TRH stimulation test

	Dose	Route	Sampling times (hr)
Dogs	100 μg/kg (or 200 μg)	IV	0, 4 (6)
Cats	100 μg/kg	IV	0, 4
Horses	1000 μg	IV	0, 4

Sources: Ferguson 1984, 1994; Lothrop and Nolan 1986; Lothrop et al. 1984; Peterson and Ferguson 1989; Peterson et al. 1994a,c.

Note: Preparations used are Relefact TRH (Rhone-Poulenc Rorer), Thypinone (Abbott Diagnostic), and TRH (Peninsula Laboratories).

more significant at dosages greater than 100 μg/kg; salivation, urination, defecation, vomition, miosis, tachycardia, and tachypnea were observed (see Table 30.7). The recommended protocol for the TRH stimulation test is the administration of 100 μg TRH/kg (Relefact TRH, Rhone-Poulenc Rorer; Thypinone, Abbott Diagnostic) intravenously with the collection of serum for T_4 measurement at 0 and 6 hours post-TRH. Using this protocol in normal dogs, at least a 50% increase in serum T_4 was observed in 90% of dogs, and all dogs had an increase of at least 0.5 μg/dL (6.4 nmol/L) above baseline (see Fig. 30.3). With the lower dose of 200 μg TRH per dog, serum T_4 was shown to be maximal 4 hours after TRH administration. Because of the small increments following TRH, the successful application of the TRH stimulation test requires the use of a T_4 assay with extremely good internal reproducibility or, preferentially, measurement of canine TSH.

DIAGNOSING HYPOTHYROIDISM IN THE HORSE. TRH has been evaluated in horses as an alternative for establishing the pituitary thyrotrope and thyroid functional reserve. Intravenous administration of 1000 μg of TRH increases serum concentrations of T_4 and T_3, peaking at 4 hours post-TRH (see Table 30.7) (Lothrop and Nolan 1986).

DIAGNOSING MILD HYPERTHYROIDISM IN THE CAT. In some instances, thyroid hormone concentrations (T_4 and T_3) are normal, borderline, or even fluctuate into and out of the normal range in cats with mild hyperthyroidism. TRH stimulation has been studied as a test of thyroid autonomy. In euthyroidism, the thyroid gland of the cat responds significantly to IV TRH, but the response in the hyperthyroid cat is considerably less, implying that thyroid function is not under the influence of endogenous TSH. The dosage of 100 μg/kg TRH administered intravenously is followed by serum sampling at 4 hours after injection. Serum T_4 concentrations increased by >50% in all normal cats and cats with nonthyroidal disease, whereas only 11% of hyperthyroid cats showed a >50% increase in serum T_4 concentration after TRH administration. Adverse side effects in the cat associated with administration of TRH were common and included transient vomiting, salivation, tachypnea, and defecation. As a diagnostic test, the TRH stimulation test compares favorably with the T_3 (see suppression test but requires less time and is more convenient to perform (Peterson et al. 1994a,c).

The biological activity of freshly reconstituted TRH is maintained for 1–5 weeks when frozen at –20° C (Rosychuk et al. 1988).

Thyrotropin

CHEMISTRY. Thyrotropin (TSH) is a glycoprotein (molecular weight = 28,000) that is synthesized by thyrotrope cells of the anterior pituitary (see Table 30.3). It is chemically related to LH, FSH, and HCG.

LH, FSH, and TSH all share similarities in tertiary structure conferred by the evolutionary preservation of cysteine residues, particularly those involved in the "cysteine knot" motif identified by recent crystallographic information about HCG. Furthermore, sites of N-glycosylation also appear to be preserved during evolution. As described below, glycoproteins contribute to the tertiary structure as well as the functional and immunogenic characteristics of the dimers (Zerfaoui and Ronan 1996).

TSH is a heterodimer composed of two noncovalently bound subunits, α and β. The α subunits are approximately 20–22 kD, have 92–96 amino acid residues, and contain two N-linked carbohydrate groups. The human, cow, mouse, horse, and rat α-subunit genes are similar. All species have a single mRNA species that is between 730 and 800 bases long. The mRNA encodes the precursor of the α subunit and a leader sequence of an average of 24 amino acids. TSH, like other mammalian pituitary hormones, consists presumably of a canine-specific α subunit common to all canine pituitary hormones noncovalently associated with a β subunit with a structure specific to the hormone and species. The α-subunit peptide is more abundant than the unique β subunit of the peptides. Free serum α subunits are secreted and are present in concentrations equivalent to the combined concentration of TSH, LH, and FSH. Free serum β-subunit concentrations are lower, usually below the level of detectability. Overabundance of the α subunit suggests that regulation of β-subunit synthesis is the rate-limiting step in modulating the levels of TSH, LH, and FSH (Yang et al. 2000b).

The subunits are synthesized as separate peptides from distinct mRNAs (Vamvakopoulos and Kourides 1979). The α subunit is common to all three hormones, but the β subunit is unique for each hormone and confers biological specificity. For all four glycoproteins within each species, the amino acid sequence of the α subunit is common. However, the carbohydrate structure may vary. Microheterogeneity of the carbohydrate constituents of the individual hormones causes heterogeneity in receptor affinity, biological potency, and metabolic clearance (Pierce and Parson 1981; Wondisford et al. 1988).

The alpha subunits are approximately 20 to 22 kD, have 92 to 96 amino acid residues, and contain two N-linked carbohydrate groups. The human, cow, mouse, dog, and rat α-subunit genes are similar (Yang et al. 2000b). All species have a single mRNA species that is between 730 and 800 bases long. The mRNA encodes the precursor of the α subunit and a leader sequence of an average of 24 amino acids.

The TSH β subunit is approximately 18 kD, consists of approximately 110–118 amino acids, and contains one N-linked complex carbohydrate (Green and Baenzinger 1988). TSH, like LH, contains sulfate groups that terminate certain chains; such sulfation is found only to a small extent in FSH and not at all in HCG. The genes for the β subunit of TSH of mouse, cow, human, dog, and horse have been cloned, and recombinant canine TSH has been expressed in vitro (Yang et al. 2000a,b). Each mRNA is approximately 700 bases in length with minor variations. The TSH β mRNA encodes the precursor TSH β subunit with a 20-amino-acid leader sequence and a 117- or 118-amino-acid coding region.

ACTION. TSH binds to specific receptors on the thyroid plasma membrane. TSH receptors from dog, pig, human, and rat have been completely cloned. The extracellular domain of the receptor contains 398 amino acids with five sites for N-linked glycosylation. The intracellular domain has 346 amino acids with seven putative transmembrane segments. The stimulatory guanine nucleotide regulatory protein binds to the third intracellular loop. The receptor has a glycoprotein component and a ganglioside that may be involved in TSH activation of adenylate cyclase. Only intact TSH binds to the receptor, and the β subunit does not possess biological activity (Chan et al. 1987; Field 1975). Binding of TSH to its receptor activates adenylate cyclase and subsequent accumulation of cAMP but is not dependent on the interaction of the TSH from that species with the receptor. This results in the stimulation and dissociation of the regulatory and catalytic subunits of cAMP-dependent protein kinase (protein kinase A) with subsequent phosphorylation of various cellular proteins resulting in an increase in thyrocyte iodide uptake, thyroid hormone organification, and thyroid hormone secretion. This cAMP-mediated pathway appears to be important in both thyroid hormone secretion and thyroid glandular growth (Chayoth et al. 1985).

The binding of TSH is also known to activate the phospholipase C signaling system. Activation of phospholipase C results in hydrolysis of phosphotidylinositol 4,5-biphosphate (PIP_2) with formation of diacylglycerol (DAG) and inositol-1,4, 5-triphosphate (IP_3). The former activates a Ca^{++}-phospholipid-dependent protein kinase (protein kinase C) and the latter increases intracellular Ca^{++} concentrations. The effect of TSH on phospholipase C is slower and requires larger amounts of the hormone than its activation of adenylate cyclase, suggesting a high-capacity and low-affinity TSH binding site. The physiological significance of activation of PIP_2 hydrolysis by TSH is not known but is suspected to be involved in thyroid glandular proliferation (Chayoth et al. 1985; Taguchi and Field 1988).

PREPARATIONS. Biochemically purified native TSH is purified from bovine pituitary glands and is stored in a lyophilized form for reconstitution and parenteral administration. A study evaluated the effects of freezing reconstituted bovine TSH and demonstrated that bioactivity remained intact for at least 3 months at –20° C (Kobayashi et al. 1990).

Two bovine thyrotropin products have been available in the past. Currently, recombinant human TSH has replaced the bovine products in human clinical use in the United States and there are no approved veterinary thyrotropin products on the market.

TSH STIMULATION TEST. The administration of exogenous bovine TSH followed by the measurement of serum T_4 and/or T_3 provides important information in the diagnosis of hypothyroidism, used primarily in the dog, cat, and horse, because it tests thyroid secretory reserve. Although the variable availability and high cost of bovine TSH has made this test less practical, the TSH stimulation test continues to be the most definitive noninvasive test for the diagnosis of primary hypothyroidism.

Protocols for this test vary widely in the dog; they are summarized in Table 30.8. Although the TSH dose and serum sampling times are often dictated by practical and economic considerations, increasing the TSH dose administered generally delays the time of the T_4 peak and, up to a limit, results in a higher serum T_4 response and a plateau that is maintained for a longer period of time. The route of administration may be intravenous, intramuscular, or subcutaneous; however, the most consistent and rapid response is seen after intravenous dosing. For the dog, the suggested protocol is to draw a baseline blood sample for serum T_4 determination and then administer 0.1 IU/kg TSH intravenously (maximum dose 5 IU), followed by a blood sample at 4 hours post-TSH (Ferguson 1984, 1994; Peterson and Ferguson 1989). Studies using 1 IU of bovine TSH per dog have indicated that the mean increase in serum T_4 and T_3 above baseline at 6 hours

TABLE 30.8—Protocols for TSH stimulation test

	Dose	Route	Sampling times (hr)
Dogs	0.1 IU/kg IV (max. 5 IU)	IV	0, 4
	1 IU/dog	IV	0, 4
Cats	1 IU/kg	IV	0, 6
	1 IU/cat	IV	0, 4
Horses	5–10 IU	IV	0, 4, 6

Sources: Beale et al. 1990; Chen and Li 1987; Ferguson 1984, 1994; Peterson and Ferguson 1989.

Note: Preparation used is bovine TSH (Thytropar, Rhone-Poulenc Rorer). For older protocols in the dog, see Ferguson 1984 for a review.

post-TSH was significantly lower following TSH at 1 IU than TSH at 5 IU but was not significantly different at 4 hours post-TSH for the two doses of TSH evaluated. Based on the criteria for adequate response to TSH, TSH at 1 IU led to classification of 35% of the dogs as having a decreased response to TSH at 4 hours and 35% at 6 hours. TSH at 5 IU resulted in no dogs having a decreased response at 4 hours and 1 dog in 20 (5%) at 6 hours (Beale et al. 1990).

Assuming a pharmacological dosage of TSH is used, the diagnosis of hypothyroidism in the dog is usually confirmed when the post-TSH serum T_4 concentration is below the normal range for basal T_4 (usually <1.0 μg/dL or <13 nmol/L in the dog) and rarely increases greater than 0.2 μg/dL (2.6 nmol/L) above the baseline. In pituitary forms of hypothyroidism, the thyroid gland should remain responsive to TSH. The rare cases of long-standing secondary (pituitary) or tertiary (hypothalamic) hypothyroidism with subsequent thyroid atrophy may require 2 or 3 consecutive daily doses of TSH to eventually demonstrate thyroid responsiveness (Fig. 30.3; Ferguson 1984, 1994).

A study of normal dogs evaluated the predictive value of blood sampling times after 5 IU of IV TSH: in 80% of the animals, a doubling of the serum T_4 concentration was not achieved by 4 hours but was achieved in all cases by 6 hours post-TSH. Animals that responded favorably to thyroid replacement therapy have on average virtually no increase in serum T_4 concentration following TSH. An advantage of the TSH stimulation test is that post-TSH T_4 concentrations tend to be less variable because the thyroid is maximally stimulated.

STRUCTURAL HOMOLOGY AMONG SPECIES. There is 80–90% homology at the amino acid level among the sequences of most of the mammalian TSH β molecules. As an example of avian species, the amino acid sequence of the quail TSH β subunit shows homologies of about 70% to that of mammalian species, about 60% to that of amphibians, and about 50% to that of teleost fish. There is evidence that the functional domains of the TSH β subunit and the TSH receptor have diverged cooperatively during evolution. Many regions of identical sequences are apparent in various β subunits of glycoprotein hormones and the regions around residues 51–57 and 75–80 in the β structures are suggested to be involved in interaction with the common α subunit (Maurer et al. 1984; Lawrence et al. 1997; Kato et al. 1997; Nagai et al. 1998).

TSH RECEPTORS AND BIOLOGICAL ACTION. Thyroidal TSH receptors from dog, pig, rat, mouse, and human have been cloned and sequenced. The extracellular domain of the receptor contains 398 amino acids with five sites for N-linked glycosylation. The intracellular domain has 346 amino acids with seven putative transmembrane segments, similar to other G-protein-coupled receptors. The stimulatory guanine nucleotide regulatory protein binds to the third intracellular loop. The receptor has a glycoprotein component and a ganglioside that may be involved in TSH activation of adenylate cyclase. Only intact TSH binds to the receptor and the β subunit alone does not possess biological activity. Binding of TSH to its receptor activates adenylate cyclase and subsequent accumulation of cAMP, but the interaction is not species specific, as the long-standing use of bovine TSH in human and veterinary medicine demonstrates. The binding results in the stimulation and dissociation of the regulatory and catalytic subunits of cAMP-dependent protein kinase (protein kinase A) with subsequent phosphorylation of various cellular proteins resulting in an increase in thyrocyte iodide uptake, thyroid hormone organification, and thyroid hormone secretion. This cAMP-mediated pathway appears to be important in both thyroid hormone secretion and thyroid glandular growth.

The binding of TSH is also known to activate the phospholipase C signaling system. Activation of phospholipase C results in hydrolysis of phosphotidylinositol 4,5-biphosphate (PIP_2) with formation of diacylglycerol (DAG) and inositol-1,4, 5-triphosphate (IP_3). The former activates a Ca^{++}-phospholipid-dependent protein kinase (protein kinase C) and the latter increases intracellular free calcium concentrations. The effect of TSH on phospholipase C is slower and requires larger amounts of the hormone than its activation of adenylate cyclase, suggesting a high-capacity and low-affinity TSH binding site. The physiological significance of activation of phosphoinositide hydrolysis by TSH is not known but is suspected to be involved in thyroid glandular proliferation.

GLYCOSYLATION PATTERNS: RELEVANCE TO BIOACTIVITY AND IMMUNOREACTIVITY. The pituitary glycoproteins LH, FSH, and TSH are produced and secreted in multiple molecular forms. In vivo, microheterogeneity of the carbohydrate constituents of the individual hormones causes heterogeneity in affinity for the receptor and in metabolic clearance of the hormone. In vitro, immunoreactivity is affected by this heterogeneity. Much has been learned from studies of human and equine chorionic gonadotropin because of the use of these agents as pharmaceuticals. For example, highly sialylated human FSH variants exhibit lower receptor binding, bioactivity, and immunoactivity compared to less sialated counterparts. Each isoform appears to have a different affinity for the receptor. For example, FSH glycosylation variants appear to induce or stabilize distinct receptor conformations that result in different degrees of activation or inhibition of a given signal transduction pathway.

The oligosaccharide chains of pituitary glycoprotein hormones such as human thyroid-stimulating hormone (hTSH) have been shown to be important in biosynthesis, subunit association, secretion, and bioactivity. However, the exact biological significance of these glycosylation isoforms remains controversial. Human TSH glycosylation variants more basic in isoelectric point were found to be significantly more active than acidic ones in stimulating cAMP formation; however, there were no differences in stimulation of inositol phosphate release. In support of efforts to develop recombinant pituitary glycoproteins as pharmaceuticals, the bioactivity of glycoproteins produced in vitro appears to be as great or, in some cases, greater than that of the pituitary-derived form (Zerfaoui and Ronan 1996; Papandreou et al. 1990).

EFFECTS OF DRUGS ON TSH CONCENTRATIONS. A recent study by Daminet et al. (1999) suggested that serum TSH concentrations do not appear to change significantly with glucocorticoid administration. However, as the authors discuss, the currently available TSH assay is not capable of reliably detecting TSH changes within the normal range. Future studies might examine the impact of glucocorticoid administration in animals with elevated TSH values, or following TRH stimulation.

Two recent studies have examined the effects of phenobarbital on thyroid function tests. Daminet and coworkers (1999) prospectively examined the effect of a 3-week course of phenobarbital on TT_4, FT_4D, and TSH and observed no significant alteration of these values over this time frame. Gaskill and coworkers (1999), in an effort to dissect out the effects of phenobarbital, documented TT_4 and TSH in 78 dogs receiving phenobarbital and compared them with 48 untreated epileptic dogs. Of the dogs on phenobarbital, 40% had low TT_4 and 7% had elevated TSH, while only 8% of untreated dogs had low TT_4 and none had elevated TSH. Of the latter group, only dogs with recent seizure activity had low TT_4 values. The investigators found no effect of phenobarbital on serum binding of T_4. The mean serum TT_4 was significantly lower and mean serum TSH was significantly higher in the phenobarbital-treated group. As with the subacute study (Daminet et al. 1999), there did not appear to be a correlation between phenobarbital dosage or duration of treatment and the serum TT_4 and TSH concentrations.

SOMATOMAMMOTROPINS AND REGULATORY HORMONES. Growth hormone (GH) and prolactin have similarities in amino acid structure and also share some biological activities. As a result they are called somatomammotropic or somatolactotropic hormones.

Growth Hormone–Releasing Hormone (GHRH). GHRH is secreted by neurons located in the arcuate nuclei with their axons terminating in the external lamina of the median eminence. GHRH is synthesized from a precursor of 108 amino acids. Initially, two peptides of 44 and 40 amino acids with GH-releasing activity were isolated. Synthetic peptides that contain only the first 29 amino acid residues of GHRH are as potent as natural GHRH. GHRH stimulates synthesis and secretion of GH by somatotrophs. GHRH binds to specific cell surface receptors that are coupled to adenylyl cyclase though G proteins. Cyclic AMP mediates the GHRH effect on GH gene transcription and GH secretion. GHRH also has a mitogenic effect on somatotrophs (Brazeau et al. 1982; Guillemin et al. 1981; Mayo et al. 1983; Michel et al. 1983; Rivier et al. 1982).

Somatostatin (Growth Hormone Release–Inhibiting Hormone). Somatostatin-producing neurons within the CNS are concentrated mainly in the anterior periventricular region of the hypothalamus with nerve terminals in the external lamina of the median eminence. However, somatostatin-producing neurons are also distributed in other regions of the CNS and outside the CNS in epithelial cells (D cells) of the gastric mucosa, small intestine, kidney, islets of Langerhans of the pancreas, and parafollicular cells of the thyroid. Somatostatin (GHRIH) is synthesized as a precursor of 116 amino acids that is processed proteolytically to peptides with 14 or 28 amino acids. Somatostatin exerts its effects by binding to specific receptors on the surface of target cells which interact with G proteins. G proteins mediate a number of intracellular events, including inhibition of adenyl cyclase activity, leading to suppression of cAMP accumulation, and inhibition of calcium fluxes, leading to enhanced K^+ conductance and hyperpolarization. The fall in intracellular calcium reduces hormone secretion. GHRIH also exerts a direct antiproliferative effect; it inhibits DNA synthesis and cell replication by blocking epidermal growth factor induced centrosomal separation. This action might occur by interfering with movement of microfilaments and by preventing microtubule disassembly by inhibiting calcium influx. Table 30.9 summarizes the wide biological effects of somatostatin (Brazeau et al. 1973; Lamberts 1986; Montminy et al. 1984; Reichlin 1983; Schonbrunn 1990).

TABLE 30.9—Actions of somatostatin (GHRIH)

Inhibits hormone secretion by:
Pituitary gland (TSH, GH, PRL, ACTH)
Gastrointestinal tract
Gastrin
Secretin
GIP
Motilin
Enteroglucagon
VIP
Pancreas
Insulin
Glucagon
Somatostatin
Genitourinary tract
Renin
Inhibits other gastrointestinal actions:
Gastric acid secretion
Gastric emptying
Pancreatic enzyme and bicarbonate secretion
Intestinal absorption
Gastrointestinal blood flow
AVP-stimulated water transport
Bile flow

OCTREOTIDE. Somatostatin has limited clinical utility because of its short half-life (2–3 minutes) and its multiple effects. The somatostatin analog octreotide has been used to help manage pituitary disorders (Klonoff and Karam 1992). Octreotide (Sandostatin®; Sandoz) has been employed in the management of acromegaly, gastrinoma, pancreatic beta-cell tumors, and glucagonoma in the dog.

Somatotropin (Growth Hormone)

STRUCTURE AND SECRETION. Somatotropin (GH) is a polypeptide hormone with a molecular weight of approximately 22 kD. The principal form of human somatotropin is a single-chain, 191-amino-acid hormone and was published in 1969 by Li. There is considerable species specificity for somatotropin, and human, bovine, and porcine somatotropin used clinically are now commercially produced by recombinant techniques (Kostyo and Reagan 1976; Wallis 1975). Porcine somatotropin has not been approved yet for use in the United States. The sequence of canine growth hormone was first identified in 1994 (Ascacio-Martinez and Berrera-Saldana 1994).

Somatotropin is synthesized and released under the influence of growth hormone–releasing hormone, a 44-amino-acid peptide. The secretion of somatotropin occurs in a pulsatile fashion, which results from the asynchronous release of GHRH and somatostatin, a potent inhibitor of somatotropin release (Müller 1987). Pulsatile release of somatotropin appears to be the effect of GHRH pulsatile secretion, whereas between-pulse concentrations are largely determined by somatostatin (somatotropin-release inhibiting factor; SRIF) (Rijnberk 1996). Many physiologic, pharmacologic, and pathologic factors influence the secretion of somatotropin, including exercise and hypoglycemia, which increase somatotropin secretion as do α-adrenergic agonists, β-adrenergic antagonists, and dopamine agonists. Glucocorticoids, α-adrenoceptor blockers, and β-adrenergic agonists decrease somatotropin secretion, as do hyperglycemia and obesity. See Table 30.10 for a review of regulatory factors for somatotropin release.

FUNCTION. Somatotropin's effects can be divided into two main categories: rapid or metabolic actions, and slow or hypertrophic actions (Rijnberk 1996). Acute catabolic effects are mediated by somatotropin's decrease of carbohydrate utilization and impairment of glucose uptake into cells, which results in glucose intolerance and secondary hyperinsulinism (Lean et al. 1992). The slower, anabolic effects are mediated via insulin-like growth factors (IGFs). These hormones are produced in many tissues, particularly liver, in response to somatotropin. Via IGF-1, somatotropin increases protein synthesis and decreases protein catabolism by mobilizing fat. This protein-sparing effect is important for linear growth and development.

TABLE 30.10—Factors influencing somatotropin (GH) secretion

Factors
Factors stimulating secretion:
Sleep
Exercise
Stress
Amino acids
Hypoglycemia
GHRH
ACTH
ADH
α_1-adrenergic agonists (clonidine)
β-adrenergic antagonists
Dopamine or agonists
GABA or agonists
Factors inhibiting secretion:
Hyperglycemia
Free fatty acids
Somatostatin
Progesterone
Glucocorticoids
α–adrenergic antagonists
β–adrenergic agonists
Dopamine antagonists (phenothiazines)

THERAPEUTIC USE

SMALL-ANIMAL APPLICATIONS. In young dogs, somatotropin deficiency can occur as a primary endocrine abnormality resulting in pituitary dwarfism. It may be treated with bovine, porcine, or human somatotropin. Porcine somatotropin is structurally identical to canine somatotropin and may be preferred for treatment in the dog once it becomes available in the United States (Ascacio-Martinez and Barrera-Saldana 1994).

It has been recommended to administer somatotropin at 0.1 IU/kg subcutaneously three times weekly for 4–6 weeks (Eigenmann 1982). If ACTH and TSH secretion are also abnormal, the animal needs to be treated with replacement doses of glucocorticoids and thyroid hormone. Growth hormone-responsive dermatosis has been treated successfully with 0.15 IU/kg two times weekly for 6 weeks (Schmeitzel and Lothrop 1990).

LARGE-ANIMAL APPLICATIONS. Bovine somatotropin has been used in cattle for several reasons. Somatotropin improves feed efficiency and leads to an effective increase in protein and reduction of fat, thus providing a desirable carcass in terms of degree of fatness and meat quality (Groenwegen et al. 1990; Schwarz et al. 1993). This has also been seen when bovine somatotropin was administered in finishing lambs (McLaughlin et al. 1993). In the pig, porcine somatotropin also leads to increased growth rates and improved meat quality (Campbell et al. 1988; Etherton et al. 1987). In addition to improvements in meat quality, somatotropin has been used to increase milk production in the cow. Somatotropin also has an effect on milk composition, resulting in fewer short- and medium-chain fatty acids and more long-chain fatty acids (Bauman 1992; Lean et al. 1992). Administration of somatotropin increases IGF-1 concentrations in bovine milk, the public health effects of which are still under study. Somatotropin itself is degraded by the gastric acid when ingested orally.

Several formulations of bovine somatotropin (BST) are or will be available on the market. These include a daily dose and 7-, 14-, and 28-day prolonged-release preparations. The 14- and 28-day preparations are methionyl BST preparations. Exogenous BST must be present every day in order to continue an augmented milk response. The reason is that the BST peptide is rapidly cleared from the body. When given to cattle daily, maximum milk response is achieved with BST doses of 30–40 mg/day, and no further increase is observed with higher doses. Most production trials have employed doses between 10 and 50 mg/day. POSILAC® (Monsanto) is 500 mg of met^{-1}. . .leu^{126} bovine somatotropin (Sometribove, USAN) in a 14-day prolonged-release preparation that is administered every 14 days. Milk yield generally increases the first few days of BST treatment, reaching the maximum about the sixth day. In swine, prolonged release (4–6 week) injectables or ear tags are products in development (Bauman 1992; Lean et al. 1992).

ADVERSE EFFECTS. In dogs, diabetes mellitus is the major potential side effect of somatotropin administration; therefore, fasting blood glucose concentrations should be determined before and at weekly intervals while on somatotropin therapy. Hypersensitivity reactions might also occur after treatment with somatotropin (Schmeitzel and Lothrop 1990).

In the bovine species, treatment with somatotropin has been reported to cause an initial decrease in food intake; however, after a few weeks an increase is seen. It has also been suggested that somatotropin treatment increases the incidence of mastitis, which may be a function of the increase in milk production (Bauman 1992; Lean et al. 1992); however, in a multinational study involving over 900 cows, no effect on incidence of clinical mastitis was seen (White et al. 1994). There are no indications that somatotropin administration leads to an increase in metabolic diseases in this species (Bauman 1992; Lean et al. 1992).

Prolactin

STRUCTURE AND BIOSYNTHESIS. Prolactin (PRL) is a 198-amino-acid polypeptide hormone with a molecular weight of 22,000 and is synthesized and secreted by the lactotrophs of the anterior pituitary. It is classified as a somatomammotropic hormone, and about 10–15% of the molecule represents glycosylation. Although glycosylated PRL is less potent, the glycosylation appears to stabilize the molecule to degradation in the body. In the species for which its structure has been identified, PRL has 3 intrachain disulfide bridges. The amino acid sequences of canine and feline PRL have not yet been identified (Rijnberk 1996). There are no pharmaceutical preparations of this hormone and few, if any, therapeutic applications. PRL regulation is relevant to the reproductively cycling animal in a variety of species. PRL evolved from a hormone common to somatotropin and human placental lactogen (hPL), but it now shares only a minority of residues (13 and 16%, respectively) with these hormones. The precursor molecule for PRL is a 227-amino-acid precursor with a molecular weight of 40,000–50,000 and contributes to some of the plasma PRL immunoreactivity (Klonoff and Karam 1992; Tyrell et al. 1994).

FUNCTION. PRL stimulates lactation in the postpartum period. It appears to have functions related to reproduction, particularly related to the care, feeding, and protection of offspring, even in fish and birds. PRL seems to have effects on salt and water metabolism and is important in the ability of the salmon, for example, to change from a saltwater to a freshwater environment. In mammals, the increasing concentrations of prolactin during pregnancy, combined with the hormonal effects of estrogens and progestins, induce the development of mammary tissue. In rodents, PRL prolongs the life of the corpus luteum but does not perform this function in humans or domestic mammals. The secretion of PRL with suckling in certain species, most notably humans, is also likely to inhibit ovarian function and prevent ovulation and fertility (Klonoff and Karam 1992; Tyrell et al. 1994).

REGULATION OF SECRETION. Secretion of PRL by the pituitary is normally under inhibitory control by the hypothalamus, specifically by the neurotransmitter dopamine. Therefore, dopamine agonists inhibit PRL secretion. Factors influencing secretion of somatotropin often have similar effects on PRL: sleep, stress, hypoglycemia, and exercise all increase PRL and somatotropin. Other PRL-releasing hormones include TRH, which may explain galactorrhea in some hypothyroid bitches. Also, the dopamine antagonists phenothiazine and metoclopramide, as well as butyrophenones, increase PRL secretion. The half-life of PRL in plasma is only 15–20 minutes. A PRL-inhibiting hormone (PRIH) of peptide nature has been investigated in rats. In humans, heavy athletic training, likely through opioid release, may inhibit PRL production and result in reproductive alterations, specifically amenorrhea in women (Kuret and Murad 1990).

THERAPEUTIC USES. There are no applications of clinical relevance. Milk production in cattle does not seem to be limited by the usual concentrations of circulating PRL. However, research has focused upon the ability of somatotropin to be galactopoietic.

POSTERIOR PITUITARY HORMONES

There are two known pituitary hormones: vasopressin (antidiuretic hormone; ADH) and oxytocin. Both hormones differ from vasotocin, which is found in nonmammalian vertebrates, by only one amino acid. Posterior pituitary hormones are synthesized in the hypothalamus and transported to the posterior pituitary, where they are released into the circulation.

ANTIDIURETIC HORMONE. Two 9-amino-acid peptides are secreted by the neurohypophysial system: ADH and oxytocin. They are synthesized by the magnocellular neurons of the supraoptic nuclei and the lateral and superior parts of the paraventricular nuclei. ADH regulates the water permeability of the distal tubules and collecting duct of the nephron. It also is a vasoconstrictor and influences cardiovascular function.

Structure. ADH has a molecular weight of 1084 and is characterized by a 6-amino-acid ring and a 3-amino-acid side chain with a disulfide linkage. The prohormone for ADH includes the ADH sequence and neurophysin II, which binds to ADH. Following synthesis of the peptide, secretory granules containing the prohormone move down the axon to the nerve terminal in the posterior lobe of the pituitary. Upon exocytosis, equimolar amounts of the neurophysin and ADH are released. The neurons also project to the choroid plexus, where they also release ADH into the cerebrospinal fluid.

Stimuli for Release. The primary physiological stimulus for ADH release is an increase in plasma osmolality. However, hypovolemia, pain, exercise, and some drugs may stimulate ADH release.

Mechanism of Action. ADH binds to two types of receptors. V_1 receptors are found on vascular smooth muscle cells and cause vasoconstriction. V_2 receptors are found on the renal tubule cells and are involved in the mediation of antidiuresis through increased water permeability and water reabsorption in the collecting ducts. ADH increases cAMP in the tubule, which increases water permeability at the luminal surface, resulting in increased urine osmolality and decreased urine volume. V_2 receptors outside the kidney also mediate the release of the coagulation factor VII and von Willebrand factor. Desmopressin acetate (DDAVP; 1-desamino-8-L-arginine vasopressin) is a long-acting synthetic analog of predominately V_2 or antidiuretic activity. Table 30.11 summarizes the actions of ADH and the respective ADH receptors (V_1 and V_2) mediating the actions.

Absorption, Metabolism, and Excretion. ADH must be administered parenterally and has a very short half-life of about 20 minutes.

Preparations. Natural and synthetic ADH are available commercially for the diagnosis and treatment of diabetes insipidus. Natural ADH (Pitressin) from cows and pigs is available as a water-soluble product. Dogs, cats, horses, and humans produce arginine ADH and pigs produce lysine ADH.

Diagnostic Use. Diabetes insipidus (DI) is caused by the deficiency of ADH (central DI) or by absence of a renal response to this anterior pituitary hormone (nephrogenic DI). The main presenting signs, in the absence of other conditions, are polyuria and polydipsia.

Central DI is due to the absolute deficiency of ADH. In partial central DI, some endogenous ADH secretion remains. These conditions are the result of the destruction of the supraoptic and paraventricular nuclei of the hypothalamus, which have axons terminating in the posterior pituitary. The damage may be due to head trauma, surgical transection of the pituitary stalk (usually only transient DI), or primary or metastatic tumors, or, most commonly in veterinary medicine, the cause is not known (idiopathic DI).

Nephrogenic DI results when the renal tubule is insensitive to ADH. In this condition, ADH does not increase intratubular cAMP concentrations, a necessary prerequisite to the increased water permeability normally induced by ADH. This abnormality of ADH responsiveness may also be partial or total. Primary causes of nephrogenic diabetes are rare. However, secondary nephrogenic DI may result from pyometra, liver

TABLE 30.11—Actions of antidiuretic hormone

Target organ	Receptor type	Action
Renal glomerulus	V_1	Mesangial cell contraction
Vasa recta	V_1	Decrease medullary blood flow
Juxtaglomerular cells	V_1	Suppress renin release
Arterioles	V_1	Constriction
Liver	V_1	Increase glycogenolysis
Anterior pituitary	V_1	Increase ACTH release
Baroreceptors	?	Desensitization of baroreflex
Cortical and medullary collecting tubules	V_2	Increase H_2O permeability
Papillary collecting ducts	V_2	Increase H_2O permeability
Thick ascending loop of Henle	V_2	Increase Na^+, K^+, Cl^- reabsorption
Baroreceptors	?	Sensitization of baroreflex

disease, hyperadrenocorticism, hyperthyroidism, hypercalcemic disorders, renal failure, and pyelonephritis.

DI is diagnosed if the urine specific gravity is dilute (<1.008) in the face of dehydration and/or an elevated plasma osmolality. However, it is not infrequent for the animal to present in a hydrated state and to have a normal or only slightly elevated plasma osmolality. A modified water deprivation test is recommended to confirm that endogenous ADH and urine osmolality will not rise in the face of moderate dehydration. Following carefully monitored gradual water withdrawal over three days, water is completely withdrawn on the fourth day and the urine osmolality and plasma osmolality are monitored. If greater than 5% dehydration is achieved and no urine concentration is observed, then exogenous ADH is administered to test the ability to respond to exogenous hormone.

ADH can be administered in two ways in this test:

1. 0.55 units per kg intramuscular aqueous ADH (Pitressin Synthetic, Parke-Davis; Vasopressin USP, Quad) up to a maximum of 5 units. Urine volume and osmolality (or specific gravity) should be measured at 30, 60, and 120 minutes after administration.
2. The administration of 1 milliunit/mL of aqueous ADH (Pitressin Synthetic, Parke-Davis; Vasopressin USP, Quad) in lactated Ringer's or 5% dextrose. This solution is then administered over 1 hour at the rate of 10 mL/kg body weight. Urine samples should be obtained at 15-minute intervals for 90 minutes following ADH administration.

In an animal with complete central DI, the urine osmolality will not have risen above isoosmolality (300 mOsm/kg) with dehydration; and subsequent ADH administration will increase urine osmolality at least 50%. In an animal with partial central DI, the urine osmolality will increase above isoosmolality but will increase an additional 10–50% following exogenous ADH. Animals with nephrogenic DI do not concentrate their urine upon dehydration above isoosmolality and also do not respond to exogenous ADH.

Therapeutic Uses. Aqueous ADH or ADH analogs are currently the only formulations available for the treatment of total and partial central DI. The synthetic ADH analogs DDAVP (Desmopressin acetate, Rorer, injectable and nasal, USV Laboratories) and LVP (Lysine-8-vasopressin, Diapid Nasal Spray®, Sandoz Pharmaceuticals) are the most commonly used. Both of these preparations can be administered intranasally or into the conjunctival sac. The latter route appears to be better tolerated by the animals. Ocular or conjunctival irritation is a rare problem.

DDAVP is a drug with greater potency and slower metabolism than the natural ADH molecule. Administration of 5–20 μg of DDAVP (2–4 drops) in single or divided doses controls polyuria in most animals. The peak drug action is seen at 2–6 hours, and its duration may last from 10 to 27 hours. The clear advantage of this medication is that it does not require parenteral administration. However, the conjunctival route results in variable amounts of drug reaching the bloodstream and variable duration of effect even in the same patient. DDAVP is also quite expensive, and therefore it might be prudent to use the drug only when polyuria is observed or to prevent excessive nocturnal urine production.

LVP (Lysine-8-vasopressin) is another product which is available for managing DI via nasal or conjunctival administration. However, its duration of action is shorter and its expense is greater than the other products. As a result, it has not found much application in veterinary medicine (Chastain and Ganjam 1986; Ferguson et al. 1992).

DDAVP has also been used for bleeding disorders (von Willebrand's disease and hemophilia A). In pharmacologic doses, it increases plasma levels of factor VIII:C and von Willebrand factor, by preferentially increasing levels of larger von Willebrand factor multimers and by increasing platelet adhesion. Controlled studies on the use of DDAVP in dogs are lacking, but the clinical impression is that DDAVP is beneficial in some but not all von Willebrand dogs (Nichols and Hohenhaus 1994).

Toxicity. Immediately following a dose, in order to prevent water intoxication, dogs should not be given unlimited quantities of water. The transiently high levels of ADH will prevent the excretion of a free water load by the kidney and result in overhydration and possible neurological sequelae such as cerebral edema. Cerebral edema may be manifest by depression, vomiting, salivation, ataxia, muscle tremors, and convulsions. Animals with central or nephrogenic DI disease may also be successfully managed by providing free access to water at all times and by housing the animals outdoors. Another inexpensive maneuver which reduces the urine output is the restriction of dietary sodium using homemade diets or the commercial diets designed for use in congestive heart failure (e.g., Hill's H/D). Such products generally contain less than 0.1% sodium on a dry weight basis (Ferguson et al. 1992).

Other Drugs for Treatment of Central Diabetes Insipidus. Oral agents have also been used primarily as adjuncts to ADH therapy of central DI. Chlorpropamide (Diabinese®, Pfizer), a sulfonylurea hypoglycemic agent used to treat non-insulin-dependent diabetes in humans, has produced inconsistent antidiuretic effects in the dog and cat. Chlorpropamide's effect is to enhance the effect of ADH on the renal tubules and collecting duct by increasing intracellular cAMP. It may also stimulate pituitary ADH release. As a result, it is only effective in the presence of sufficient endogenous (partial central DI) or exogenously administered ADH. Careful dosage studies for chlorpropamide have not been performed in the dog. Reported doses include 250 mg every 12 hours and 10–40 mg/kg/day. Reduction in urinary volumes ranging from 18 to 50% have been reported. Maximal antidiuretic effects take 1–2 weeks to develop. Side effects of hypoglycemia can be minimized by frequent feedings and periodic monitoring of blood glucose concentrations.

Carbamazepine (Tegretol®, Geigy Pharmaceuticals), an antiepileptic, and clofibrate (Atromid®, Ayerst Laboratories), an antihyperlipidemic drug, are also effective in some cases of central DI. In contrast to the other drugs, these agents may increase the secretion of ADH and therefore would be rational therapy only in partial central DI. However, there have been no reports in the veterinary literature of the use of these drugs for the successful treatment of DI.

Thiazide diuretics when used together with salt restriction may serve to potentiate the effect of exogenous or endogenous ADH (see below) (Ferguson et al. 1992; Klonoff and Karam 1992; Tyrell et al. 1994).

Treatment Of Nephrogenic Diabetes Insipidus. Treatment for nephrogenic DI should, if possible, start with correction of the underlying cause of the nephrogenic DI (hypercalcemia, renal infection, hyperadrenocorticism without a compressive pituitary tumor). Except for institution of a low-sodium diet, the thiazide diuretics are the only agents that have been shown to be effective in the treatment of nephrogenic DI.

Thiazide diuretics have a paradoxical antidiuretic effect in central and nephrogenic DI. These agents may reduce the reabsorption of sodium in the ascending loop of Henle, resulting in enhanced urinary sodium loss, mild reduction in plasma osmolality, and, therefore, diminished thirst. The reduction in water intake causes contraction of the extracellular volume, and proximal tubular sodium reabsorption is increased and the glomerular filtration rate decreased. The urine volume is thereby reduced without overt concentration of the urine osmolality. Hydrochlorothiazide (Hydrodiuril®, Merck, Sharp, and Dohme) at a dosage of 2.5–5 mg/kg has succeeded in reducing water intake by 50–85% in cases of ADH-resistant polyuria. Due to the kaliuretic effect of the thiazides, serum potassium should be monitored and oral potassium (Kaon Elixir®, Adria) administered if the animal becomes anorexic (Ferguson et al. 1992).

OXYTOCIN. Oxytocin induces contraction of smooth muscle, most importantly of the myoepithelial cells of the mammary gland, which result in milk ejection. Furthermore, it also results in uterine smooth muscle contraction, an effect that increases during pregnancy. Its clinical use in the management of milk letdown and uterine contraction (induction of parturition and treatment of pyometra) is described in detail in Chap. 31.

Oxytocin affects the transmembrane ionic currents in uterine smooth muscle cells, resulting in sustained uterine contraction. Oxytocin-induced myometrial contractions can be inhibited by tocolytic agents such as β-adrenergic agonists, magnesium sulfate, and inhalation anesthetics (Klonoff and Karam 1992; Tyrell et al. 1994).

REFERENCES

Ascacio-Martinez, J. A., and Barrera-Saldana, H. A. 1994. A dog growth hormone cDNA codes for a mature protein identical to pig growth hormone. Gene 143:277–280.

Bauman, D. E. 1992. Bovine somatotropin: review of an emerging animal technology. J Dairy Sci 75:3432–3451.

Beale, K. M., Helm, L. J., and Keisling, K. 1990. Comparison of two doses of aqueous bovine thyrotropin for thyroid function testing in dogs. J Am Vet Med Assoc 197:865.

Bilezikian, L. M., and Vale, W. 1983. Glucocorticoids inhibit corticotropin-releasing factor–induced production of adenosine 3′,5′-mono-phosphate in cultured anterior pituitary cells. Endocrinology 113:657–662.

Bitman, J. L., Tyrell, H. F., Bauman, D. E., et al. 1984. Blood and milk responses induced by growth hormone administration in lactating cows. J Dairy Sci 67:2873–2880.

Bolander, F. F. 1989. Molecular Endocrinology, pp. 21–27. San Diego: Academic Press.

Brazeau, P., Ling, N., Esch, F., et al. 1982. Somatocrinin (growth hormone–releasing factor) in vitro bioactivity: Ca^{++} involvement, cAMP mediated action and additivity of effect with PGE_2. Biochem Biophys Res Commun 109:588–594.

Brazeau, P., Vale, W., Burgus, R., et al. 1973. Hypothalamic polypeptide that inhibits the secretion of immunoreactive pituitary growth hormone. Science 179:77–79.

Campbell, R. G., Steele, N. C., Caperna, T. J., McMurtry, J. P., and Solomon, M. B., and Mitchell, A. D. 1988. Interrelationships between energy intake and endogenous porcine growth hormone administration on the performance, body composition and protein and energy metabolism of growing pigs weighing 25–55 kilograms live weight. J Anim Sci 66:1643.

Chan, J., Sandisteban, P., Deluca, M., Isozedi, E., Grollman, E., and Kohn, L. 1987. TSH receptor structure. Acta Endocrinol (Copenh) 281(suppl):166.

Chastain, C. B., and Ganjam, V. K. 1986. The endocrine brain and clinical tests of its function. In Clinical Endocrinology of Companion Animals, pp. 37–68. Philadelphia: Lea & Febiger.

Chayoth, R., Arem, R., Yoshimura, Y., and Field, J. B. 1985. The role of calcium in the induction of refractoriness to cyclic AMP stimulation by TSH. Metabolism 34:1128.

Chen, D. C. L., and Li, O. W. 1987. Hypothyroidism. In N. E. Robinson, ed., Current Therapy in Equine Medicine 2, pp. 185–187. Philadelphia: W. B. Saunders.

Crager, C. S., Dillon, A. R., Kemppainen, R. J., Brewer, W. G., and Angarano, D. W. 1994. Adrenocorticotropic hormone and cortisol concentrations after corticotropin-releasing hormone stimulation tests in cats administered methylprednisolone. Am J Vet Res 44(5):704–709.

Daminet, S., Paradis, M., Refsal, K. R., and Price, C. 1999. Short-term influence of prednisone and phenobarbital on thyroid function in euthyroid dogs. Can Vet J 40(6):411–415.

Eigenmann, J. E. 1982. Diagnosis and treatment of pituitary dwarfism in dogs. Proceedings of the 6th KalKan Symposium. Columbus, Ohio, p. 81.

Esch, F., Ling, N., Bohlen, P., et al. 1984. Isolation and characterisation of bovine hypothalamic corticotropin-releasing factor. Biochem Biophys Res Commun 122:899–905.

Etherton, T. D., Wiggins, J. P., Chung, C. S., Evock, C. M., Rebhun, J. F., Walton, P. E., and Steele, N. C. 1987. Stimulation of pig growth performance by porcine growth

hormone: determination of the dose-response relationship. J Anim Sci 64:433.
Ferguson, D. C. 1984. Thyroid function tests in the dog. Vet Clin N Amer 14:783–808.
———. 1994. Update on the diagnosis of canine hypothyroidism. Vet Clin No Am 24(3):515–540.
Ferguson, D. C., Hoenig, M., and Cornelius, L. M. 1992. Endocrinologic disorders. In M. D. Lorenz, L. M. Cornelius, and D. C. Ferguson, eds., Small Animal Medical Therapeutics, pp. 85–148. Philadelphia: J. B. Lippincott.
Field, J. B. 1975. Thyroid stimulating hormone and cyclic adenosine 3′,5′-monophosphate in the regulation of thyroid gland function. Metabolism 24:381.
Gaskill, C. L., Burton, S. A., Gelens, H. C. G., Ihle, S. E., Miller, J. B., Shaw, D. H., Brimacombe, M. B., and Cribb, A. E. 1999. Effects of phenobarbital treatment on serum thyroxine and thyroid-stimulating hormone concentrations in epileptic dogs. J Am Vet Med Assoc 215(4):489–496.
Geras, E. J., and Gershengorn, M. D. 1981. Evidence that TRH stimulates secretion of TSH by two calcium-mediated mechanisms. Am J Physiol 242:109.
Gershengorn, M. C., Rebecchi, M. J., Geras, E., and Arelvalo, C. O. 1980. Thyrotropin releasing hormone (TRH) action in mouse thyrotropic tumor cells in culture: evidence against a role for adenosine, 3′,5′-monophosphate as a mediator of TRH-stimulated thyrotropin release. Endocrinology 207:665.
Giguere, V., Labrie, F., Cote, J., et al. 1982. Stimulation of cyclic AMP accumulation and corticotropin release by synthetic ovine corticotropin-releasing factor in rat anterior pituitary cells: site of glucocorticoid action. Proc Natl Acad Sci USA 79:3466–3469.
Green, E. D., and Baenzinger, J. U. 1988. Asparagine-linked oligosaccharides on lutropin, follitropin, and thyrotropin. I. Structural elucidation of the sulfated and sialylated oligosaccharides on bovine, ovine, and human pituitary glycoprotein hormones. J Biol Chem 263(1):25–35.
Groenwegen, P. P., McBride, B. W., Burton, J. J., and Elsasser, T. H. 1990. Effect of bovine somatotropin on the growth rate, hormone profiles and carcass composition in Holstein bulls. Domest Anim Endocrinol 7:43.
Guillemin, R., Barazeau, P., Bohlen, P., et al. 1981. Growth hormone–releasing factor from a human pancreatic tumor that caused acromegaly. Science 218:585–587.
Halpern, J., and Hinkle, P. M. 1981. Direct visualization of receptors for thyrotropin releasing hormone with a fluorescein-labeled analog. Proc Natl Acad Sci USA 78:587–591.
Hansen, B. L., Kemppainen, R. J., and MacDonald, J. M. 1994. Synthetic ACTH (Cosyntropin) stimulation tests in normal dogs: comparison of intravenous and intramuscular administration. J Am An Hosp Assoc 30:38–41.
Hoenig, M., and Ferguson, D. C. 1997. Comparison of TRH-stimulated thyrotropin (cTSH) to TRH- and TSH-stimulated T4 in euthyroid, hypothyroid, and sick dogs. Proceedings, Annual Forum, American College of Veterinary Internal Medicine.
Jackson, I. M. D. 1982. Thyrotropin releasing hormone. N Engl J Med 306:145–155.
Johnansson, O., Hokfelt, T., Pernov, B., et al. 1981. Immunohistochemical support for three putative transmitters in one neuron: coexistence of 5-hydroxytryptamine, substance P, and thyrotropin releasing hormone-like immunoreactivity in medullary neurons projecting to the spinal cord. Neuroscience 6:1857–1881.
Kato, Y., Kato, T., Tomizawa, K., and Iwasawa, A. 1997. Molecular cloning of quail thyroid-stimulating hormone (TSH) beta subunit. Endocr J 44(6):837–840.
Keller-Wood, M. 1990. Fast feedback control of canine corticotropin by cortisol. Endocrinology 126(4):1959–1966.
Kemppainen, R. J., Clark, T. P., Sartin, J. L., and Zerbe, C. A. 1992. Regulation of adrenocorticotropin secretion from cultured anterior pituitary cells. Am J Vet Res 53(12):2355–2358.
Klonoff, D. C., and Karam, J. H. 1992. Hypothalamic and pituitary hormones. In B. C. Katzung, ed., Basic and Clinical Pharmacology, 5th ed., pp. 513–528. East Norwalk: Appleton & Lange.
Kobayashi, D. L., Nichols, R., and Peterson, M. E. 1990. Serum thyroid hormone concentrations in clinically normal dogs after administration of freshly reconstituted vs. previously frozen and stored thyrotropin. J Am Vet Med Assoc 197(5):597–599.
Kostyo, J. L., and Reagan, R. C. 1976. The biology of somatotropin. Pharmacol Theriogenol 2:591.
Kuret, J. A., and Murad, F. 1990. Adenohypophyseal hormones and related substances. In The Pharmacological Basis of Therapeutics, pp. 1334–1360. New York: Pergamon Press.
Lamberts, S. W. J. 1986. Non-pituitary actions of somatostatin: a review on the therapeutic role of SM 201-995 (Sandostatin). Acta Endocrinol 276(suppl):41–55.
Lawrence, S. B., Vanmontfort, D. M., Tisdall, D. J., McNatty, K. P., and Fidler, A. E. 1997. The follicle-stimulating hormone beta-subunit gene of the common brushtail possum (*Trichosurus vulpecula*). analysis of cDNA sequence and expression. Reprod Fertil Dev (RAI)9(8):795–801.
Lean, I. J., Troutt, H. F., Bruss, M. L., and Baldwin, R. L. 1992. Bovine somatotropin. Vet Clinics North Amer 8:147–163.
Lechan, R. M., Adelman, L. S., Forte, S., et al. 1984. Organization of thyrotropin releasing hormone immunoreactivity in the human spinal cord. Soc Neurosci Abstr, p. 431.
Lewin, M. J., Reyl-Desmars, F., and Ling, N. 1983. Somatocrinin receptor coupled with cAMP-dependent protein kinase on anterior pituitary granules. Proc Natl Acad Sci USA 80:6538–6541.
Li, C. H. 1969. Recent studies on the chemistry of human growth hormone. In M. Fontaine, ed., La specificite zoologique des hormones hypophysaires et de leurs activites. Paris: Centre National de la Recherche Scientifique.
Lothrop, C. D., Jr., and Nolan, H. L. 1986. Equine thyroid function assessment with the thyrotropin-releasing hormone response test. Am J Vet Res 47(4):942–944.
Lothrop, C. D., Tamas, P. M., and Fadok, V. A. 1984. Canine and feline thyroid function assessment with the thyrotropin-releasing hormone response test. Am J Vet Res 45:2310–2313.
Maurer, R. A., Croyle, M. L., and Donelson, J. E. 1984. The sequence of a cloned cDNA for the beta-subunit of bovine thyrotropin predicts a protein both NH_2- and COOH-terminal extensions. J Biol Chem 259:5024–5027.
Mayo, K. E., Vale, W., Rivier, J., et al. 1983. Expression-cloning and sequence of a cDNA encoding human growth hormone-releasing factor. Nature 306:86–88.
McDonald, L. E. 1988. Hormones of the pituitary gland. In N. H. Booth and L. E. McDonald, eds., Veterinary Pharmacology and Therapeutics, 6th ed., pp. 581–592. Ames: Iowa State Univ Press.
McLaughlin, C. L., Byatt, J. C., Hedrick, H. B., Veenhuizen, J. J., Curran, D. F., Hintz, R. L., Hartnell, G. F., Kasser, T. R., Collier, R. J., and Baile, C. A. 1993. Performance, clinical chemistry, and carcass responses of finishing lambs to recombinant bovine somatotropin and bovine placental lactogen. J Anim Sci 71:3307–3318.
Michel, D., Lefevre, G., and Labrie, F. 1983. Interactions between growth hormone–releasing factor, prostaglandin

E_2 and somatostatin on cyclic AMP accumulation in rat adenohypophysial cells in culture. Mol Cell Endocrinol 33:255–264.

Mol, J. A., Van Mansfeld, D. M., Kwant, M. M., Van Wolferen, M., and Rothuizen, J. 1991. The gene encoding proopiomelanocortin in the dog. Acta Endocrinol 125(Suppl 1):77–83.

Mol, J. A., Van Wolferen, M., Kwant, M., and Meloen, R. 1994. Predicted primary and antigenic structure of canine corticotropin releasing hormone. Neuropeptides 27:7–13.

Montminy, M. R., Goodman, R. H., Horovitch, S. J., et al. 1984. Primary structure of the gene encoding rat pre-prosomatostatin. Proc Natl Acad Sci USA 81:3337–3340.

Moore, G. E., and Hoenig, M. 1992. Duration of pituitary and adrenocortical suppression after long-term administration of anti-inflammatory doses of prednisone in dogs. Am J Vet Res 53(5):716–720.

Müller, E. E. 1987. Neural control of somatotropic function. Physiol Rev 67:962–1053.

Murakami, K., Hashimoto, K., and Ota, Z. 1985. Calmodulin inhibitors decrease the CRF and AVP-induced ACTH release in vitro: interaction of calcium-calmodulin and cyclic AMP system. Neuroendocrinology 41:7–12.

Nagai, T., Okuda, K., Kato, T., and Ueda, S. 1998. Expression and purification of biologically active porcine follicle-stimulating hormone in insect cells bearing a baculovirus vector. J Mol Endocrinol 20(1):55–65.

Nichols, R., and Hohenhaus, A. E. 1994. Use of the vasopressin analogue desmopressin for polyuria and bleeding disorders. J Am Vet Med Assoc 205(2):168–173.

Papandreou, M. J., Sergi, I., Benkirane, M., and Ronan, C. 1990. Carbohydrate-dependent epitope mapping of human thyrotropin. Mol Cell Endocrinol 73(1):15–26.

Peterson, M. E., Broussard, J. D., and Gamble, D. A. 1994a. Use of the thyrotropin releasing hormone stimulation test to diagnose mild hyperthyroidism in cats. J Vet Int Med 8(4):279–286.

Peterson, M. E., and Ferguson, D. C. 1989. Thyroid diseases. In S. J. Ettinger, ed., Textbook of Veterinary Internal Medicine, vol. 2, pp. 1632–1675. Philadelphia: W. B. Saunders.

Peterson, M. E., Kemppainen, R. J., and Orth, D. N. 1994b. Plasma concentrations of immunoreactive proopiomelanocortin peptides and cortisol in clinically normal cats. Am J Vet Res 55(2):295–300.

Peterson, M. E., Randolph, J. F., and Mooney, C. T. 1994c. Endocrine diseases. In R. G. Sherding, ed., The Cat: Diseases and Clinical Management, 2d ed., vol. 2, pp. 1403–1506. New York: Churchill Livingstone.

Pierce, J. G., and Parson, T. F. 1981. Glycoprotein hormones: structure and function. Ann Rev Biochem 50:465–495.

Reichlin, S. 1983. Somatostatin. N Engl J Med 309:1495–1501, 1556–1563.

Reul, J. M. H. M., DeKloet, E. R., Van Sluijs, F. J., Rijberk, A., and Rothuizen, J. 1990. Binding characteristics of mineralocorticoid and glucocorticoid receptors in dog brain and pituitary. Endocrinology 127:907–915.

Rijnberk, A. 1996. Clinical Endocrinology of Dogs and Cats.

Rivier, J., Speiss, J., Thorner, M., et al. 1982. Characterization of a growth hormone–releasing factor from a human pancreatic islet tumor. Nature 300:276–278.

Rosychuk, R. A. W., Freshman, J. L., Olson, P. N., Olson, J. D., Husted, P. W., and Crowder-Sousa, M. E. 1988. Serum concentrations of thyroxine and 3,5,3′-triiodothyronine in dogs before and after administration of freshly reconstituted or previously frozen thyrotropin-releasing hormone. Am J Vet Res 49(10):1722–1725.

Sauve, F., and Paradis, M. 2000. Use of recombinant human thyroid-stimulating hormone for thyrotropin stimulation test in euthyroid dogs. Can J Vet 41(3):215–219.

Schmeitzel, L. P., and Lothrop, C. D. 1990. Hormonal abnormalities in Pomeranians with normal coat and in Pomeranians with growth hormone–responsive dermatosis. J Am Vet Med Assoc 197:1333–1341.

Schonbrunn, A. 1990. Somatostatin action in pituitary cells involve two independent transduction mechanisms. Metabolism 39(suppl 2):96–100.

Scott-Moncrieff, J. C. R., Nelson, R. W., Bruner, J. M., and Williams, D. A. 1998. Comparison of serum concentrations of thyroid stimulating hormone in healthy dogs, hypothyroid dogs, and euthyroid dogs with concurrent disease. J Am Vet Med Assoc 212(3):387–391.

Schwarz, F. J., Schams, D., Röpke, R., Kirchgessner, M., Kögel, J., and Matzke, P. 1993. Effects of somatotropin treatment on growth performance, carcass traits, and the endocrine system in finishing beef heifers. J Anim Sci 71:2721–2731.

Shen, L. P., and Rutter, W. J. 1984. Sequence of human somatostatin I gene. Science 224:168–171.

Taguchi, M., and Field, J. B. 1988. Effect of thyroid stimulating hormone, carbachol, norepinephrine and cAMP on polyphosphatidylinositol phosphate hydrolysis in dog thyroid slices. Endocrinology 123:2019.

Tashjian, A. H., Jr., Heslop, J. P., and Berridge, M. J. 1987. Subsecond and second changes in inositol polyphosphates in GH4C1 cells induced by thyrotropin releasing hormone. Biochem J 243:305–308.

Tyrell, J. B., Findling, J. W., and Aron, D. C. 1994. Hypothalamus and pituitary. In F. S. Greenspan and J. D. Baxter, eds., Basic and Clinical Endocrinology, pp. 64–127. East Norwalk: Appleton & Lange.

Vale, W., Rivier, C., and Brown, M. 1977. Pharmacology of thyrotropin releasing factor (TRF) and somatostatin. In J. C. Porter, ed., Hypothalamic Peptide Hormones and Pituitary Regulation, pp. 123–156. New York: Plenum.

Vale, W., Spiess, J., Rivier, C., et al. 1981. Characterization of a 41-residue ovine hypothalamic peptide that stimulates secretion of corticotropin and β-endorphin. Science 213:1394–1397.

Vamvakopoulos, N. C., and Kourides, I. A. 1979. Identification of separate mRNAs coding for the alpha and beta subunits of thyrotropin. Proc Natl Acad Sci USA 76:3809–3813.

van Wijk, P. A., Rijnberk, A., Croughs, R. J. M., Wolfswinkel, J., Selman, P. J., and Mol, J. A. 1994. Responsiveness to corticotropin-releasing hormone and vasopressin in canine Cushing's syndrome. Eur J Endocrinol 130:410–416.

Wallis, M. 1975. The molecular evolution of pituitary hormones. Biol Rev 50:35.

White, T. C., Madsen, K. S., Hintz, R. L., et al. 1994. Clinical mastitis in cows treated with sometribove (recombinant bovine somatotropin) and its relationship to milk yield. J Dairy Sci 77:2249–2260.

Willemse, T., Vroom, M. W., Mol, J. A., and Rijnberk, A. 1993. Changes in plasma cortisol, corticotropin, and a-melanocyte stimulating hormone concentrations in cats before and after physical restraint and intradermal testing. Am J Vet Res 54:69–72.

Winiger, B. P., and Schlegel, W. 1988. Rapid transient elevations of cytosolic calcium triggered thyrotropin releasing hormone in individual cells of pituitary line GH3B6. Biochem J 255:161–167.

Wondisford, F. E., Radovic, S., Moates, J. M., et al. 1988. Isolation and characterization of the human thyrotropin beta-subunit gene: differences in gene structure and promoter function from murine species. J Biol Chem 263:12538–12542.

Wynn P. C., Aguilera, G., Morell, J., and Catt, K. J. 1983. Properties and regulation of high affinity pituitary receptors for corticotropin releasing factor. Biochem Biophys Res Commun 110:602–608.

Yamada, M., Radovick, S., Wondisford, F. E., et al. 1990. Cloning and structure of human genomic DNA and hypothalamic cDNA encoding human preprothyrotropin-releasing hormone. Mol Endocrinol 4:551–556.

Yang, X., McGraw, R. A., Su, X. Su, Katakam, P., Grosse, W. M., Li, O.W., and Ferguson, D.C. 2000a. Canine thyrotropin α-subunit gene: cloning and expression in *Escherichia coli,* generation of monoclonal antibodies, and transient expression in the Chinese hamster ovary cells. Domestic Anim Endocrinol, 18:363–378.

Yang, X., McGraw, R. A., and Ferguson, D. C. 2000b. cDNA cloning of canine common α gene and its co-expression with canine thyrotropin β gene in baculovirus expression system. Domestic Anim Endocrinol, 18:379–393.

Young, D. W., and Kemppainen, R. J. 1994. Molecular forms of β-endorphin in the canine pituitary gland. Am J Vet Res 55(4):567–571.

Zerfaoui, M., and Ronan, C. 1996. Glycosylation is the structural basis for changes in polymorphism and immunoreactivity of pituitary glycoprotein hormones. Eur J Clin Chem Clin Biochem 34(9):749–753.

31 HORMONES AFFECTING REPRODUCTION

FREDERICK N. THOMPSON

Reproductive Endocrinology
General Effects and Utility of Reproductive Drugs
Progestins
Gonadotropins and Gonadotropin-Releasing Hormone
Prostaglandin $F_{2\alpha}$
Gonadal Steroids, Ergonovine, Oxytocin, Glucocorticoids, and Melatonin
Specific Drug Usage in Large Animals
Induction of Ovarian Activity in the Pig
Use of Melatonin to Advance the Breeding Season
Use of Testosterone in the Cow
Use of Altrenogest in the Mare
Use of Altrenogest in Swine
Progestins
Use of GnRH and Analogs
Prostaglandin F and Analogs
Induced Parturition
Postpartum Usages of Oxytocin, Estrogen, and Prostaglandin
Induction of Superovulation
Induction of Lactation in the Cow
Specific Drug Usage in Small Animals
Drugs to Stimulate the Gonads
Drugs for Abortion and Evacuation of the Uterus in the Bitch and Queen
Postponement of Estrus
Treatment of Pseudopregnancy, Uterine Inertia, Cryptorchidism, and Prostatic Hypertrophy

REPRODUCTIVE ENDOCRINOLOGY. The ultimate control of reproduction rests in neural processes. Gonadotropin-releasing hormone (GnRH) secreted from the hypothalamus is transported by the portal system to the pituitary, where it increases secretion of the gonadotropins—follicle-stimulating hormone (FSH) and luteinizing hormone (LH)—in both sexes. Frequent administration of GnRH may result in decreased LH and FSH secretion via down-regulation (tachyphylaxis) of pituitary GnRH receptors. The gonadotropins stimulate the secretion of gonadal steroids (testosterone in the male and estrogens and progesterone in the female). During the estrous cycle ovarian follicles produce estradiol, an estrogen, predominately in response to pulsatile secretion of the gonadotropins. Following ovulation mediated by a surge secretion of LH, progesterone is secreted from one corpus luteum or several corpora lutea (CL). The CL requires pituitary hormones for support (luteotropic factors). The luteotropic factor(s)—LH and prolactin—and estradiol are species-specific. A decrease in luteotropic factor secretion will result in decreased CL function and abortion in the pregnant animal. The life span of the CL is lengthened with pregnancy, resulting in continued progesterone secretion, which is necessary for pregnancy maintenance. Late in diestrus in the cycling (nonpregnant) large animal, prostaglandin $F_{2\alpha}$ ($PGF_{2\alpha}$) released from the endometrium mediates CL regression (luteolysis). Estrus follows CL regression within a few days. Such utero-ovarian relationships whereby uterine $PGF_{2\alpha}$ results in luteolysis do not exist in the bitch.

Gonadal steroids in the female, estrogen and progesterone, have prominent stimulatory effects upon the endometrium and the mammary gland, while increased circulating concentrations may result in pathological changes in target organs. Gonadal steroids mediate reproductive behavior and gametogenesis in both sexes. Ovarian steroids generally decrease gonadotropin secretion (negative feedback). The exception to this is a positive feedback effect of estradiol, in the relative absence of progesterone, upon gonadotropin secretion immediately prior to ovulation that results in a surge secretion of both gonadotropins. LH mediates ovulation. Exogenously administered gonadal steroids may inhibit gonadotropin secretion, result in uterine and mammary gland pathology, and interrupt gonadal function.

Testosterone in the male mediates behavior and stimulates male sex accessory glands. Increased circulating testosterone from either an exogenous or endogenous source may result in prostatic hypertrophy and hyperplasia. Additionally, testosterone administration results in decreased gonadotropin secretion and interruption of spermatogenesis.

GENERAL EFFECTS AND UTILITY OF REPRODUCTIVE DRUGS

Progestins. The sources of progesterone include the CL in animals undergoing estrous cycles (cycling) and the placenta in certain species. Progesterone and its synthetic analogs (progestins) mimic the effects of a CL and thereby inhibit estrus during administration. Following withdrawal there is a shortened interval to estrus, with synchrony of that event in large animals. These effects are mediated by increased gonadotropin (FSH and LH) secretion. Synchronization of estrus in large animals by progestins or other drugs facilitates artificial insemination and thereby genetic improvement. Progestins are effective both in the cycling female and also in the prepubertal and postpartum anestrus animal; following withdrawal, ovarian activity is increased, especially in conjunction with gonadotropin administration. Progesterone itself will inhibit estrus but must be given at least daily. This short half-life discourages usage in the production setting. Progestins are used to inhibit the onset of the reproductive cycle in dogs and cats.

Gonadotropins and Gonadotropin-Releasing Hormone. Stimulation of the gonad in either sex is achieved via use of GnRH; the nonpituitary gonadotropins, human chorionic gonadotropin (HCG) and pregnant mare serum gonadotropin (PMSG, also known as equine chorionic gonadotropin); or pituitary gonadotropin preparations themselves (FSH and equine pituitary extract, EPE).

GnRH is a hypothalamic decapeptide that increases LH and FSH secretion. In some instances GnRH therapy may be appropriate to achieve ovulation or luteinization of an ovarian cyst. The effects of GnRH in elevating gonadotropin secretion are brief, lasting generally only several hours.

HCG and PMSG are large-molecular weight glycoproteins secreted during pregnancy in the woman and mare, respectively. These nonpituitary gonadotropins mediate a long-lasting biological effect (> 24 hr); only a single injection is necessary. PMSG is secreted from the endometrial cups of pregnant mares in early pregnancy in order to maintain a luteotropic (CL stimulatory) effect upon the primary and secondary CL in the mare. Its gonadotropic activity is primarily FSH-like activity to increase ovarian follicular growth. PMSG is frequently used to stimulate ovarian follicular growth in the anestrous sheep or goat. Because of difficulty in standardizing PMSG, this drug is frequently not available in the USA. HCG is secreted from the chorionic portion of the placenta of the woman. HCG, in contrast to PMSG, has biologic activity that is primarily LH-like, and it, therefore, induces ovulation. HCG can be used, e.g., to induce ovulation in the mare after an appropriate follicular size has been documented. Such treatment in the mare shortens the period of estrus and allows more accurate prediction of the time of ovulation. HCG is also used in a diagnostic manner to assess the presence of a testicle. A HCG test challenge (10,000 IU) IV will result in increased testosterone secretion in the presence of a testicle as soon as 30 minutes postinjection. This may be desirable to ascertain the status of a supposedly gelded horse. The various uses of GnRH, HCG, and PMSG are described later in this chapter.

The pituitary gonadotropins are extracted from animal pituitaries. FSH and EPE are used to stimulate follicular growth and superovulation in animals that will serve as embryo donors.

Prostaglandin $F_{2\alpha}$. The primary source of $PGF_{2\alpha}$ is the endometrium in large domestic animals, where it is released late in diestrus in the cycling animal and near term in the pregnant animal. $PGF_{2\alpha}$ mediates a decrease in circulating progesterone via luteolysis (CL regression) and decreased placental progesterone production. The mechanism of $PGF_{2\alpha}$-mediated luteolysis involves an antisteroidogenic effect via activation of protein kinase C and a cell death effect mediated by increased intracellular free calcium (Niswender et al. 1994). $PGF_{2\alpha}$ and its analogs are used to decrease estrous cycle length and thereby hasten the onset of estrus and to induce abortion and parturition. In the cow $PGF_{2\alpha}$ is used to stimulate uterine contractions to facilitate placental delivery or for another ecbolic effect. As a luteolytic agent, $PGF_{2\alpha}$ shortens the life span of the CL and, therefore, decreases the interestral interval. Used strategically, in most large animal species except the pig, $PGF_{2\alpha}$ results in synchrony of estrus in a group of animals. Since $PGF_{2\alpha}$ does not result in luteolysis in the pig until after day 14 or 15 of the cycle, it has limited utility in this species to synchronize estrus, but it is used in the pig to induce parturition. In the bitch $PGF_{2\alpha}$ is used to treat uterine infections via luteolytic and ecbolic effects.

Gonadal Steroids, Ergonovine, Oxytocin, Glucocorticoids, and Melatonin. The use of gonadal steroids, such as estrogen and testosterone, in large animals is now limited. Testosterone is used to androgenize cows in order to produce a "teaser" animal to identify cows in estrus. A variety of esters of estradiol (benzoate, propionate, cypionate, and valerate) that increase duration of activity are available. These products will induce estrus but generally not ovulation. Estrogens are used as abortifacient agents in early pregnancy in the cow and for antinidatory activity in the bitch. Administration of estrogen to the postpartum cow is advocated as an adjunct to treatment of mild uterine infections because it promotes uterine blood flow and contractility. Estradiol valerate is used along with a progestin (norgestomet) for estrous synchronization in ruminants. Estradiol valerate mediates luteolysis via $PGF_{2\alpha}$ release.

Ergonovine has a direct effect on the uterus and increases uterine contractions and vasoconstriction (Brazeau 1975). It is used in the postpartum animal to enhance involution and placental expulsion.

Oxytocin is synthesized in the hypothalamus and stored in the posterior pituitary. Following secretion, this hormone mediates contractility of the estrogen-dominated myometrium during parturition and contractility of the myoepithelial cells surrounding the alveoli in the mammary gland. As a result, milk ejection is mediated with no effect upon milk synthesis. Following intravenous (IV) bolus administration, its effect is immediate but brief (20 minutes or less). The time to onset of activity following intramuscular (IM) administration is 5 minutes. Oxytocin is used to induce labor in the mare, to combat uterine inertia during delivery in all species, and to stimulate milk letdown in animals agalactic for this reason.

Glucocorticoids will induce parturition in ruminants via an endocrine cascade involving $PGF_{2\alpha}$. Finally, melatonin, a product of the pineal gland secreted in response to darkness, will advance the onset of the breeding season in species that respond to decreasing photoperiod (environmental lighting) with an onset of estrous cycles (deer, goats, and sheep).

SPECIFIC DRUG USAGE IN LARGE ANIMALS

Induction of Ovarian Activity in the Pig. PG-600 (Intervet of America, Inc.) is a combination of 400 IU of PMSG and 200 IU of HCG used to induce estrus in the prepubertal gilt (Britt et al. 1989). PG-600 increased the percentage of peripubertal gilts in estrus at both 7 and 28 days after treatment with no alteration in farrowing rate or pigs per litter. The implication is that PG-600 would allow for the maintenance of fewer gilts, resulting in greater efficiency in a swine operation.

Anestrus sometimes occurs during late summer and autumn in the pig in conjunction with elevated environmental temperatures and humidity. This delays the onset of puberty in the gilt and the return to estrous behavior in the weaned sow. A single injection of PMSG (725 or 1088 IU) IM was effective in induction of puberty in gilts in the adverse environment (Britt et al. 1986). Similarly, a single dose of PMSG (1200 IU) given to sows the day after weaning was effective in bringing about a return to estrus.

Use of Melatonin to Advance the Breeding Season. A melatonin implant (18 mg), Regulin (Hoechst Veterinaer, Munich), advanced the breeding season in ewes, goats, and deer with an increased ovulation rate early in this induced period (Staples et al. 1992). Increased plasma melatonin levels via this implant result in increased gonadotropin secretion in short-day breeders. This treatment advanced the onset of the breeding season by up to 100 days, with a lag phase from treatment of approximately 50-70 days in a variety of sheep breeds. Introduction of the ram has the similar effect of hastening the onset of the breeding season, but simultaneous use of Regulin resulted in increased ovulation rates.

Use of Testosterone in the Cow. Exposure of postpartum cows to a bull or testosterone-treated cows shortened the interval from calving to estrus (Burns and Spitzer 1992). The biostimulation effect of bulls and of testosterone-treated cows was similar. By decreasing postpartum anestrum, more animals conceive early in the breeding season and wean heavier calves. Testosterone-treated cows received testosterone (2 g) 2 weeks before use and booster dosages at 2-week intervals. Treatment of cows with testosterone has also been used to enhance the detection of other cows in estrus (Kiser et al. 1977). Testosterone-treated cows were as effective in estrous detection as surgically altered bulls. Cows used for this purpose were given testosterone propionate (200 mg) IM on alternate days for 20 days as an induction procedure, followed by testerone enanthate (1.0 g) every 2 weeks.

Use of Altrenogest in the Mare. Altrenogest (Regumate; Hoechst-Roussel) is a synthetic orally administered progestin approved for controlling the estrous cycle of the mare. This drug also appears in the literature as allyl-trenbolone. The manufacturer recommends that altrenogest (0.044 mg/kg) be given orally for 15 days to suppress estrus and allow for a predictable occurrence of estrus. The drug is used to manage the prolonged periods of estrus observed during the transitional period into the breeding season and to schedule breeding of mares during the physiological breeding season.

Altrenogest feeding for 15 days during the breeding season resulted in estrus in most mares within 3.5-5 days and ovulation 9-11 days after treatment (Lofstedt 1988). When altrenogest was given for 12 days after daily environmental photoperiod had been extended to 16 hours for approximately 56 days, more treated mares exhibited estrus and ovulated within 12 days of treatment withdrawal compared to controls (Squires et al. 1979). It has been recommended that to have a smooth transition from winter anestrum to the breeding season mares be exposed first to a 16-hour photoperiod beginning the first two weeks of December (Colbern et al. 1987). Once follicular activity has been noted, altrenogest is given for 12 days. To hasten ovulation, HCG (3300 IU) may be given when ovarian follicles are larger than 40 mm.

During the breeding season, use of altrenogest for 12 days beginning either at estrus or during diestrus resulted in good control of estrus; however, the interval from treatment to estrus was shorter for those treated during diestrus versus those treated during estrus (Squires et al. 1979). In both cases the mean interval to estrus was 2.8-4.8 days. Fertility was not altered. Control of estrus has been achieved following administration of altrenogest for 7 days, with control of ovulation being achieved by administration of HCG (2500 IU) 5-7 days after withdrawal (Bristol 1986). Use of altrenogest in the lactating mare has resulted in good fertility with 15 days of treatment beginning on the day of parturition (Sigler et al. 1989). In this research, controls were inseminated at the second estrus postpartum, and the treated mares were inseminated at the first estrus after altrenogest withdrawal. Estrus occurred at a mean interval of 26 and 36 days postpartum and conception rate was 67 and 100% for controls and treated, respectively.

In some mares altrenogest does not suppress follicular growth; consequently, ovulation occurs during treatment or ovulation occurs sooner than expected after treatment (Lofstedt and Patel 1989). An apparent explanation is found in the fact that altrenogest has only a minimum effect on LH secretion (Squires et al. 1983). Therefore, some mares have CLs at the end of the altrenogest treatment period, and a luteolytic dose of prostaglandin may be required to achieve the desired effect.

Although not approved for the maintenance of pregnancy, altrenogest has been administered with this objective. Experimentally, 6 out of 7 control mares aborted following administration of endotoxin, but abortion did not occur in the altrenogest-treated mares (Daels et al. 1991). To ascertain if altrenogest has an adverse effect on pregnancy and subsequent events, the drug was given from day 30 to day 320 of pregnancy. No adverse effect was detected on periparturient events, viability and growth of the offspring, or subsequent reproductive performance of the mares (Shoemaker et al. 1989). Similarly, reproductive performance of offspring from mares given altrenogest during gestation was not affected in either sex (Squires et al. 1989).

Use of Altrenogest in Swine. Swine producers are particularly interested in synchronizing estrus in gilts in order to reduce the number of replacement gilts. This also allows for more efficient use of labor and facilities. Although altrenogest is not approved for use in the pig in the US, it is effective in synchronizing estrus in the gilt (Kraeling et al. 1981; Webel and Day 1982). When gilts that had been previously observed in estrus were fed 15-20 mg altrenogest daily for 18 days, approximately 95% expressed estrus 4-7 days after treatment. Only approximately 75-85% of the gilts with unknown reproductive histories were so synchronized. Farrowing rate and litter size in gilts was unaltered in most trials; however, an increase in cystic follicles (Redmer and Day 1981) and a decreased farrowing rate in a commercial situation have been noted (Wood et al. 1992).

Progestins

SYNCRO-MATE B IN CATTLE. Syncro-Mate B (SMB; Merial Limited, Athens, GA) treatment is composed of an ear implant containing the progestin norgestomet (6.0 mg) and an injectable solution of norgestomet (3.0 mg) and estradiol valerate (5.0 mg). This treatment synchronizes estrus in heifers and postpartum cows. Animals are given an ear implant for 9 days, and norgestomet and estradiol valerate are injected IM at the time of implantation. The estradiol is intended to bring about luteolysis via prostaglandin release. Norgestomet inhibits LH secretion and thereby inhibits CL function. Insemination without respect to estrous detection is recommended by the manufacturer beginning 48 hours after implant removal. A high percentage (77-100%) of cattle exhibit estrus after treatment but first-service conception rates are variable (33-68%) (Odde 1990). This variability in conception rates is a function of the percentage of the animals in a herd undergoing estrous cycles before treatment. Herds with fewer than 50% of the animals cycling before treatment had reduced conception rates. A 30% conception rate was found in noncycling heifers treated with SMB, compared with a 48% conception rate in cycling heifers (Brown et al. 1988).

Reasons for failure to conceive after SMB include luteal dysfunction due to insufficient LH secretion after implant removal (Hixon et al. 1981) and stage of the cycle when implanted (Brink and Kiracofe 1988). Those implanted prior to day 11 of the cycle had a 47% conception rate compared to 37% for those implanted after day 11. Separation of calves from suckled beef cows at the time of implant removal increased conception rates (Kiser et al. 1980). Some cows treated during metestrus do not experience CL regression during treatment (Burns et al. 1993). Therefore, synchrony of estrus is not achieved. Increasing the norgestomet dose to 6.0 mg when animals were implanted during metestrus resulted in more pregnancies (Fanning et al. 1992). The use of GnRH in conjunction with SMB has increased pregnancy rates. Suckled beef cows that received 250 μg GnRH 30 hours after norgestomet implant removal had increased pregnancy rates after a timed insemination (Troxel et al. 1993). Another adjunct to SMB treatment has been the use of $PGF_{2\alpha}$. When beef heifers treated with SMB for 7 days were given $PGF_{2\alpha}$ on either day 6 or 7, a good estrus and pregnancy response occurred (Heersche et al. 1979). Similarly, injection of $PGF_{2\alpha}$ 2 days before implant removal has resulted in a good synchrony of estrus (Odde et al. 1984).

SYNCRO-MATE B IN GOATS. SMB treatment during the breeding season resulted in a good synchrony of estrus in dairy goats (Bretzlaff et al. 1992). Goats were implanted with half of the cattle implant for norgestomet and given an IM injection with 0.375 mg norgestomet plus 0.625 mg estradiol valerate. Implants were removed after 9 days. Those implanted early in the cycle responded less with respect to synchrony of estrus than those implanted later in the cycle.

MELENGESTROL ACETATE IN CATTLE. Melengestrol acetate (MGA; Upjohn Co., Kalamazoo, MI) is an orally active progestin supplied as a premix which is fed at 0.5 mg daily for 14 days. Estrus is expected 16-20 days after the start of 14 days of MGA feeding. The advantages of MGA include ease in administration, lower relative costs, and the potential to induce estrus in noncycling animals. Since fertility at the first estrus after MGA is reduced (Zimbelman et al. 1970), $PGF_{2\alpha}$ is given 17 days after MGA withdrawal (Brown et al. 1986). $PGF_{2\alpha}$ induces luteolysis in the MGA-synchronized animals. Use of MGA without $PGF_{2\alpha}$ in natural mating situations has resulted in desired results (Patterson et al. 1990). In this case bulls were joined with heifers 15-18 days after MGA withdrawal. It was determined that 83% of the animals conceived within the first 30 days of the breeding season. Calf removal for 48 hours on days 16-17 after a 14-day MGA regimen has facilitated the estrous response (Patterson et al. 1990). In this case, $PGF_{2\alpha}$ was administered on day 31.

MELENGESTROL ACETATE IN SHEEP. MGA has been used to induce estrus in anestrous ewes (Safranski et al. 1992). MGA (0.125 mg twice daily) was fed for 9 days beginning in the spring. This treatment resulted in a significant increase in the percentage of ewes lambing and the number of lambs born per ewe exposed to rams. The administration of PG-600 in addition to MGA did not further enhance ewe productivity.

RELEASE OF PROGESTERONE INTRAVAGINALLY

CONTROLLED INTERNAL DRUG RELEASE (CIDR) DEVICE CONTAINING PROGESTERONE. These intravaginal progesterone-releasing devices are marketed for cattle (CIDR-Bovine, Eazi Breed), sheep (CIDR-S), and goats (CIDR-G) by AHI Plastic Co., Hamilton, New Zealand. The CIDR-B has 10% progesterone (1.9 g) incorporated. These devices remain in place for 7 days, with $PGF_{2\alpha}$ given at the time of removal in cycling animals or administration of 400 IU PMSG in anestrous animals. Placement of the CIDR-B for 15 days in cows and heifers resulted in 87% of the animals being mated by 96 hours and pregnancy rates were 50% over a 4-day period (Mcmillan and Macmillan 1989).

PROGESTERONE-RELEASING INTRAVAGINAL DEVICE (PRID). The PRID is composed of stainless steel coils coated with silicone rubber containing 6.75% progesterone. Estradiol benzoate (10 mg) in a gelatin capsule is sometimes attached to the PRID (Peters and Ball 1987). The PRID is efficacious in synchronizing estrus and ovulation in cattle. Placement for either 6 or 7 days, with $PGF_{2\alpha}$ administration either the day before PRID removal or the day of removal, resulted in good estrous synchrony of and pregnancy rates in heifers (Smith et al. 1984). PRID placed in beef cows for 12 days beginning the first eight days of the estrous cycle along with an injection of estradiol valerate (5.0 mg) resulted in good estrous synchrony (Sprott et al. 1984).

Polyurethane sponges impregnated with a variety of progestins (flurogestone acetate, FGA, Cronolone; chlorgestone acetate, CAP, Chlormadinone; medroxyprogesterone acetate, MAP, Provera) have been used to synchronize estrus in cycling ewes or in combination with PMSG to induce estrus in prepubertal or anestrous ewes (McDonald 1986). Puberty induction in lambs has utilized a progestin sponge for 10-14 days followed by 400-600 IU of PMSG. The same scheme is utilized in seasonally anestrous ewes, with 500-800 IU of PMSG at the time of progestin withdrawal.

Use of GnRH and Analogs

GENERAL. There are three GnRH preparations. Gonadorelin (Cystorelin®, Merial Limited; Factel®, Fort Dodge) is a hypothalamic decapeptide that stimulates the secretion of both FSH and LH. GnRH analogs include fertirelin acetate (Fertagyl®; Takeda Chemical Industries, Ltd., Osaka, Japan) and buserelin (Receptal®; Hoechst-Roussel Agri-Vet Co., Bucks., UK). A comparison of the biological activity of these products in terms of FSH/LH secretion in heifers has been reported (Chenault et al. 1990). Fertirelin acetate was 2.5-10 times more potent than gonadorelin, whereas buserelin was approximately 10-20 times more potent than fertirelin acetate. The use of GnRH around the time of insemination to increase fertility in cattle has yielded mixed results. Buserelin (10 µg) given to dairy cows at the time of insemination did not improve fertility. However, pregnancy rates were significantly improved when buserelin was given 12 days postinsemination (Drew and Peters 1994).

FOLLICULAR CYSTS. Ovarian follicular cysts in cows are defined as follicle-like structures that persist rather than ovulate. These are more than 25 mm in diameter and have been present for 10 days or more in the absence of a CL (Kesler and Garverick 1982). Occurrence is frequent in the postpartum dairy cow but rare in beef cows. Treatment recommendations are either HCG 5000 IU IV or 10,000 IU IM (Youngquist 1990). Most cows respond with the establishment of an estrous cycle within 3-4 weeks. Alternatively, this condition may be treated with 100 µg GnRH, which generally results in luteinization of the cystic structure, with estrus occurring in 18-23 days. The administration of $PGF_{2\alpha}$ 9 days after GnRH will often shorten the interval to estrus.

INDUCTION OF OVARIAN ACTIVITY IN THE MARE. The administration of the GnRH agonist buserelin to anestrous mares resulted in follicular growth, with ovulation induced by HCG (McCue et al. 1992). Mares received twice daily subcutaneous (S/Q) injections of buserelin (10 µg) beginning midwinter for a maximum of 28 days, with 2,500 IU HCG IV given when follicle size was more than 35 mm. This resulted in induction of estrus in 72% of the mares. Pregnancy rate and embryonic mortality were not altered.

Prostaglandin F and Analogs

CATTLE. $PGF_{2\alpha}$ administration results in luteolysis in cattle beginning on day 5 of the estrous cycle (Lauderdale 1972). Because of this effect, $PGF_{2\alpha}$ is followed by estrus 2-5 days postinjection. There are three prostaglandin products available for cattle: dinoprost tromethamine ($PGF_{2\alpha}$ tham salt) (Lutalyse®; Upjohn Co., Kalamazoo, MI), and two $PGF_{2\alpha}$ analogs, cloprostenol (Estrumate®; Mobay Corp., Shawnee, KS) and fenprostalene (Bovilene®; Syntex Animal Health, Inc., West Des Moines, IA). Dosages are 25 mg dinoprost tromethamine, 500 µg cloprostenol, and 1.0 mg fenprostalene.

$PGF_{2\alpha}$ given twice 10-12 days apart to a herd will result in the majority of the animals expressing estrus

3-5 days after the second injection (Lauderdale 1979). Pregnancy rates were not altered by breeding in estrus compared to a timed insemination 80 hours after the second injection. However, such a scheme of two injections may result in only 70% of the animals expressing estrus at the expected time (Burfening et al. 1978). The reason for this less-than-perfect synchrony is that animals injected during days 10-15 of the cycle were more likely to express estrus compared to those injected during days 5-9 of the cycle (MacMillan and Henderson 1984). A single $PGF_{2\alpha}$ injection scheme is satisfactory whereby animals are inseminated as they are observed in estrus for 4 days and then $PGF_{2\alpha}$ is injected on day 5, with breeding continuing on days 5-9 (Lauderdale et al. 1980).

MARE. Prostaglandins are used in mares to control the estrous cycle by induction of estrus because of diagnostic or therapeutic considerations, to synchronize with the stallion, or because of a missed breeding date (Meyers and LeBlanc 1991). Other reasons for control of estrus include shortening the first cycle postpartum to avoid breeding on foal heat, treatment for a persistent CL, synchronization of mares for embryo transfer, and ensuring that luteal structures are regressed following use of progestins to suppress estrus. Two products are approved for the mare: dinoprost tromethamine (Lutalyse®) 10 mg IM and fluprostenol (Equimate®; Miles) 250 μg IM.

Most mares will respond to the luteolytic effects of $PGF_{2\alpha}$ by day 5 of the cycle. The follicular status of the mare affects the interval from $PGF_{2\alpha}$ to estrus and ovulation (Neely 1983). When a large follicle is present at the time of $PGF_{2\alpha}$ administration, the mare will generally express estrus and ovulate within 6 days; however, the mare may ovulate within 24-72 hours and not show estrus. In contrast, if $PGF_{2\alpha}$ is administered when follicles are regressing, there may be a delay in expressing estrus because a longer period is required for follicular growth with sufficient estrogen secretion to elicit estrus. Ovulation during diestrus, not an infrequent event in the mare, could negate any intended effect of $PGF_{2\alpha}$.

Two injections of $PGF_{2\alpha}$ 14-18 days apart results in good synchrony of estrus in mares (Bristol 1987). Approximately 60% of the treated mares expressed estrus by 4 days after the second $PGF_{2\alpha}$ injection, and about 90% were in estrus by 6 days. The duration of estrus (3-10 days), as well as the time of ovulation (2-12 days), is highly variable. $PGF_{2\alpha}$ can be combined with HCG to decrease the variability in time of ovulation. An injection of 2000-3300 IU HCG IV when follicles are larger than 35 mm will generally induce ovulation within 24-48 hours (Ginther and Pierson 1989). GnRH is not effective in this regard unless it is given on a daily basis beginning on day 2 of estrus (Brinsko 1991).

GOAT. The use of $PGF_{2\alpha}$ in this species allows for planned breeding to a superior buck and facilitates estrous synchronization. A total of 2.5 mg $PGF_{2\alpha}$ is effective in mediating luteolysis in goats weighing up to 65 kg, although 8 mg $PGF_{2\alpha}$/doe has been used in some studies (Ott 1986). Estrus can be expected on an average of 50 hours after $PGF_{2\alpha}$ in those animals injected between days 4 and 16 of the estrous cycle. Two injections of 8 mg $PGF_{2\alpha}$ 11 days apart during the breeding season resulted in good synchrony of estrus and fertility.

Induced Parturition

CATTLE. Parturition may be induced in cattle by glucocorticoids and $PGF_{2\alpha}$. The reasons for induced parturition include allowance for more time postpartum before the next breeding season, an attempt to reduce calf size and therefore dystocia, prevention of excessive udder edema in dairy cattle, and to take advantage of available forage for milk production, as in New Zealand (Barth 1986). Generally, induction of parturition 1-2 weeks prematurely does not alter dystocia scores even though calf size has been reduced and does not adversely affect the calves. Some large European beef breeds calve up to 2 weeks beyond the normally accepted gestation lengths and consequently beef producers may elect to induce parturition in cows that have not calved when expected. This procedure generally results in placental retention, but subsequent fertility is not affected (Wagner et al. 1974).

Dexamethasone (20-30 mg) or flumethasone (8-10 mg) IM is 80-90% effective in parturition induction, with calving occurring 24-72 hours posttreatment. Calves can be expected to attain normal levels of immunoglobulins when induction is done within 2 weeks of term. Retention of placental membranes has exceeded 75% in some cases. Long-acting glucocorticoids (dexamethasone trimethylacetate, 20 mg; triamcinolone acetonide, 30 mg; flumethasone suspension, 10 mg; and betamethasone, 20 mg) are used primarily in New Zealand (Barth 1986). Treatment is given once IM approximately 1 month before calving. The mean interval to parturition is 15 days. The incidence of retained placentas is decreased relative to the short-acting glucocorticoids, but calf mortality is high (17-45%).

Calving may be induced with $PGF_{2\alpha}$ (25-30 mg) or cloprostenol (500 μg) IM with results similar to that found with short-acting glucocorticoids. The interval from injection to calving is 24-72 hours (Barth 1986). A combination of treatments with dexamethasone and cloprostenol has resulted in a shorter interval from treatment to delivery and a greater percentage induced compared to either drug alone or two injections of cloprostenol.

Reasons for terminating a pregnancy in this species include pregnancy in young heifers, reduced feed efficiency in pregnant feedlot heifers and cows, and pathologic pregnancies such as hydropic conditions (hydramnios and hydrallantois) and fetal mummification (Barth 1986). Prevention of the establishment of a pregnancy can be mediated by administration of 8 mg of estradiol 24-48 hours after an unwanted service. Estradiol cypionate (10-20 mg) IM will induce abortion up to 5 months. Abortion occurs within 3-7 days in 60-80% of heifers. A second injection 4-7 days after the first may be required. A single luteolytic dose of $PGF_{2\alpha}$ or its analog will induce abortion in cattle up to 5 months of gestation. Pregnancy may be terminated in hydropic conditions following single or multiple treatments with 20-40 mg dexamethasone, or prostaglandins may be used at twice the luteolytic dose.

MARE. Reasons for parturition induction in the mare are to permit a convenient observation and professional assistance at foaling. Clinical situations that warrant this are prolonged gestation, preparturient colic, and impending rupture of the prepubic tendon (Jeffcott and Rossdale 1977). Additionally, mares that previously foaled and experienced soft-tissue damage may be candidates to prevent recurrence. Mares that are experiencing preparturient loss of colostrum and those that are destined to be nurse mares are also candidates.

The ability of the foal to survive induction of parturition is assessed by the following criteria: the mare's mammary glands should be developed and contain colostrum, gestation length should be greater than 320-330 days, and the cervix should be softened (Meyers and LeBlanc 1991). The readiness for birth can be estimated by measuring the electrolyte concentrations in the mammary secretions. During the last 9-10 days of gestation, the sodium concentration in the mammary secretions decreases from more than 130 mmol/L to less than 30 mmol/L. Calcium and potassium concentrations increase during this period, with the increase in calcium being a change most correlated with neonatal survivability (Leadon et al. 1984). A calcium concentration of less than 3 mmol/L is associated with poor neonatal survival. Premature separation of the placenta may occur during induction. This appears as a red velvety chorioallantoic membrane and should be treated as an emergency to expedite delivery.

Oxytocin is the most widely used drug for induction of parturition in the mare. Delivery is usually complete within 90 minutes of administering oxytocin but may occur as soon as 10 minutes (Meyers and LeBlanc 1991). Oxytocin may be delivered via several schemes. The greater oxytocin dose produces a more rapid onset of parturition but results in more discomfort to the mare. One method involves the administration of 60-100 U oxytocin IM. Second-stage labor is generally experienced within 30-60 minutes, with delivery complete within 45-90 minutes. Another way to administer oxytocin is to place 100 U into 250-500 mL of physiologic saline and give by IV drip. The advantage of this method is the ability to administer the drug to effect (approximately 1 U/min). In case of colic, the drug delivery may be slowed or stopped. Frequently, parturition can be induced with 20-50 U oxytocin via IV drip. A final method of oxytocin delivery is to administer small oxytocin (10-20 U) boluses IV at 15- to 20-minute intervals. Foaling induced by this method results in less severe colic signs, but foaling is slightly prolonged. This method usually requires 2-4 injections, with delivery complete within 60 minutes.

The normal luteolytic dose of $PGF_{2\alpha}$ increased by 20-30% will terminate equine pregnancies between days 12 and 35 with estrus 4-5 days after treatment (Lofstedt 1986). After development of the endometrial cups (days 35-120), it is more difficult to abort a mare. Once the endometrial cups are developed, there frequently is a long delay in return to estrus; the mare may not return to estrus again that season. Repeated daily doses of $PGF_{2\alpha}$ of 1.0 mg/45 kg will abort mares after 4 months of pregnancy. Approximately 70% will abort during the first week and the remainder within 21 days.

SWINE. Induced farrowing in the pig is a practical management aid to allow for increased supervision of the event and to improve utilization of labor. The optimal farrowing response to $PGF_{2\alpha}$ is achieved by administration within 2 days of normal delivery for a herd (Dial et al. 1987). When oxytocin is administered 16-24 hours after $PGF_{2\alpha}$, farrowing is initiated in most sows within 3-6 hours. Administration of 10 mg of $PGF_{2\alpha}$ IM on day 112, 113, or 114 of gestation followed 20 hours later by 30 U of oxytocin IM resulted in the greatest synchrony of farrowing. The mean onset of farrowing was 2.1 hours after oxytocin. The number of interventions necessary to remove retained pigs was increased by the addition of oxytocin compared to $PGF_{2\alpha}$ alone. Inclusion of β-adrenergic blocking agents to the induction scheme in swine has shortened the duration of the parturient event and reduced obstetric complications (Holtz et al. 1990).

Postpartum Uses of Oxytocin, Estrogen, and Prostaglandin. Research data are conflicting regarding the effectiveness of oxytocin for treatment or prevention of retained placentas and uterine infections in the cow (Hemeida et al. 1986). Oxytocin (20 U) IM given immediately after calving and repeated 2-4 hours later reduces the incidence of retained placentas in cows that experienced difficult calving. Oxytocin doses for retained placenta in the mare are 30-40 U IM at 60- to 90-minute intervals (Plumb 1991). Alternatively, 80-100 U oxytocin may be added to 500 mL normal saline and given IV according to the mare's reaction in terms of abdominal pain. Placentas are generally expelled in 30 minutes. In order for oxytocin to mediate uterine contractions the uterus must be estrogen-dominated, as occurs at term. In the situation of a uterine infection in the cow or mare, 20 U oxytocin IM 3-4 times daily for 2-3 days has been recommended. The dose for small ruminants and sows is 5-10 U oxytocin. See Table 31.1.

Treatment of the postpartum cow with estrogen has been advocated to prevent and to treat uterine infections as a sole agent and to hasten uterine involution (Hemeida et al. 1986). Estrogen doses for the cow are 3-10 mg of estradiol benzoate, valerate, or cypionate. Conflicting data exist on the value of $PGF_{2\alpha}$ as an alter-

TABLE 31.1—Oxytocin doses (U)

Species	Obstetrics and gynecological uses	Milk letdown
Bitch	Augment contractions:[a] 1-5 S/Q or IM Primary inertia: 5-20 IM or IV infusion Manual reduction uterine prolapse: 5-20 IM	Oxytocin nasal spray[b] (Syntocinon®) tid
Cow	Augment contractions:[c] 30 IM, repeat at 30 min if necessary	10-20
Mare	Augment contractions: 20 IM For induction, see text	
Sow	Augment contractions:[a] 10 IM, repeat at 30 min if necessary	5-20 IV[a] 20-50 IM or 5-10 IV[d] as adjunct with agalactia
Ewe, doe, and goat	Retained placenta:[a] 10-20 IM Control uterine bleeding[a] in goats: 10-20 IV, repeat at 20 min S/Q	

[a]Plumb 1991. [b]Loar 1992. [c]Hemeida et al. 1986. [d]Einarsson 1986.

native treatment for metritis in the cow (Wichtel 1991). An advantage to $PGF_{2\alpha}$ treatment is that milk withdrawal is not necessary. $PGF_{2\alpha}$ (for doses, see the section on PGF and analogs) is the appropriate treatment to achieve luteolysis in cases of pyometra. Research data support the recommendation of whole-herd prostaglandin (25 mg dinoprost tromethamine or 500 μg cloprostenol) treatment of postpartum dairy cows once or twice between days 14 and 40 in herds with poor reproductive performance or a high incidence of uterine infections. Such treatment has resulted in decreased intervals from parturition to conception and increased first-service conception rates (Young and Anderson 1986; Etherington et al. 1988). This is attributed to either hastened uterine involution or the luteolytic effect that is helpful to eventual fertility.

TABLE 31.2—Superovulation in the cow

Day of cycle	Time	Treatment 1[a]	Treatment 2
10	A.M.	2500 IU PMSG	6 mg FSH
	P.M.		6 mg FSH
11	A.M.		4 mg FSH
	P.M.	Recipients receive $PGF_{2\alpha}$	4 mg FSH
12	A.M.	Donors receive $PGF_{2\alpha}$	2 mg FSH
	P.M.		2 mg FSH
13	A.M.		2 mg FSH
	P.M.		2 mg FSH
14	A.M.		
	P.M.	AI[b]	AI
15	A.M.	AI	AI
	P.M.	AI	AI

[a]Mapletoft 1986. [b]Artificial insemination.

Induction of Superovulation

CATTLE. Valuable cattle may be induced to ovulate multiple follicles (superovulation) so that embryos can be transferred to recipient animals to increase the number of progeny. In cattle, superovulation results in about 10 ovulations, compared to the normal, single ovulation (Seidel and Seidel 1991). Superovulation, on the average, results in about 6 usable embryos. The ideal response is 5-12 embryos from one-third of the donors. The donor superovulation injection program is begun between day 9 and 14 of the estrous cycle with FSH given over 4 days and $PGF_{2\alpha}$ given on days 3 and 4 (Mapletoft 1986) (Table 31.2). A problem with FSH products has been contamination with LH, which results in a decreased number of transferable embryos. FSH products include FSH-P (Schering-Plough), derived from pituitaries of domestic animals, and Super-Ov (Ausa International, Inc., Tyler, TX), derived from pig pituitaries. The Super-Ov product contains a controlled level of LH (Donaldson and Ward 1986), which results in a more uniform number of transferable embryos.

SWINE. The major reason for performing embryo transfer in swine is disease prevention (Martin 1986). Sows may be superovulated with an injection of PMSG (1200-1500 IU) at weaning. Alternatively, PMSG (1200-1500 IU) may be given 24 hours after the first injection of $PGF_{2\alpha}$ in sows that were either pregnant (16-45 days) or pseudopregnant. Pseudopregnancy is created by the use of estradiol injections on days 11-15 of the cycle (Kraeling et al. 1975).

Estrogen is luteotropic in the sow, resulting in CL maintenance. Pseudopregnant and pregnant sows are given $PGF_{2\alpha}$ twice (15 mg followed by 10 mg) at a 12-hour interval to bring about synchrony of estrus. Estrus can be expected within 4-7 days. The superovulatory response to PMSG has averaged between 30 and 45 ovulations.

GOATS AND SHEEP. The drug regime for superovulation in these species depends upon the reproductive status (Amoah and Gelaye 1990). During the breeding season, $PGF_{2\alpha}$ is used to mediate luteolysis, and gonadotropins are given to increase the ovulatory rate. The anestrous animal is given a progestin followed by gonadotropin treatment. Dairy goats were superovulated successfully during the breeding season by placement of an intravaginal sponge (MAP; 60 mg) for 11 days, 125 μg cloprostenol IM on days 1 and 9 of sponge treatment, and twice daily injections of FSH-P

(2.5 mg) IM for 3 days beginning on day 9 of sponge treatment (Nuti et al. 1987). Ewes were superovulated during the nonbreeding season with a progestin-impregnated sponge inserted for 12 days (Ryan et al. 1992). At 48 hours before sponge removal, 400 IU PMSG IM was given along with 12 mg FSH-P given twice daily over a 3-day period in a decreasing dose regime (3, 3; 2, 2; 1, 1 mg/ewe).

Induction of Lactation in the Cow. This procedure is performed in order to salvage milk from subfertile dairy cows. It should be recognized that drugs (estradiol 17β, progesterone, dexamethasone, and reserpine) used in induction of lactation may temporarily interrupt ovarian function and result in prolonged periods of estrus. The mean interval to the first estrus following treatment was 43 days (Collier and Davis 1986). Use of reserpine in the cow, while not approved, is used to stimulate prolactin secretion and has resulted in greater milk yields. Results generally indicate that approximately 70% of the animals treated will lactate greater than 9 kg/day. A greater milk production results from lactation induced in the spring compared to the fall. In order to obviate twice-daily injections, vaginal delivery of estradiol 17β (500 mg) and progesterone (1000 mg) via an impregnated sponge has been used (Davis et al. 1983). The sponge was left in place for 10 days. Six days after sponge insertion, a long-acting dexamethasone (20 mg) preparation was given IM. Reserpine (2.5 mg) IM was given on days 6, 8, and 10 after sponge insertion. In this study a 96% success rate was claimed.

SPECIFIC DRUG USAGE IN SMALL ANIMALS

Drugs to Stimulate the Gonads

GONADOTROPIN-RELEASING HORMONE (LIBIDO, CYSTIC FOLLICLES, AND DIAGNOSTIC USAGES). GnRH increased libido in the male dog and tomcat (Purswell 1994). A dose of 2.2 μg/kg IM once weekly for a month is recommended for this purpose prior to a breeding. Administration of GnRH results in peak LH secretion within 10-15 minutes, with testosterone subsequently increased. Testosterone facilitates male behavior. GnRH (2.2 μg/kg IM daily for 3 days) has also been effective in treating cystic ovarian disease in bitches (Olson et al. 1989). It should be recognized that cystic ovaries like granulosa cell tumor are manifested by persistent estrus. An increase in serum progesterone (>1.0 ng/mL) several days posttherapy indicates either ovulation or luteinization has occurred.

GnRH can be used diagnostically to assess the secretory ability of the pituitary-gonadal axis in cases of suspected deficiencies in the release of LH and gonadal steroids (Kemppainen et al. 1983). In this regard a GnRH (100 μg) is given either IM or IV, and serum or plasma LH and testosterone are measured over time.

INDUCTION OF ESTRUS IN THE BITCH. This procedure has often met with variable and disappointing results (Concannon 1989). Induction of estrus should not be attempted unless either the serum progesterone is less than 1.0 ng/mL or the previous estrus occurred 4-5 months previously. Moses and Shille (1988) were successful in inducing estrus followed by pregnancy and whelping in the bitch using diethylstilbestrol (DES) followed sequentially by LH and FSH. This order of gonadotropins is reversed with regard to conventional usage. Since LH is no longer commercially available, and substitution of LH with either FSH, HCG, or GnRH was not successful, their methodology currently cannot be replicated.

DES alone induced estrus and conception in 5 out of 5 bitches, with a resultant normal mean litter size (Bouchard et al. 1993). Anestrous mongrel bitches were given DES 5.0 mg/day orally until proestrus, with treatment continuing for 2 additional days. The mean duration of DES treatment was 7.4 days (range 6-9). GnRH administered either in a pulsatile manner or via continuous infusion resulted in the induction of estrus and ovulation (Cain et al. 1989). Pulsatile administration requires special equipment, so it is not practical in most clinical settings. Continuous administration of GnRH (2.3-14.0 ng/kg/min for approximately 7-9 days) resulted in 2 out of 4 bitches ultimately ovulating. Estrus occurred 24-27 days after the start of treatment in those that ovulated. A noncommercially available GnRH agonist (D-Trp 6) given by constant infusion was most successful in this regard (Concannon 1989).

Drugs for Abortion and Evacuation of the Uterus in the Bitch and Queen

ABORTION OF THE BITCH AND QUEEN. $PGF_{2\alpha}$, while not approved for use in the bitch, has been successfully used in the treatment of uterine infections and to induce abortion. $PGF_{2\alpha}$ is considered to be the only safe abortifacient for the bitch (Romagnoli et al. 1991). Due to its short half-life, $PGF_{2\alpha}$ requires frequent administration. $PGF_{2\alpha}$ exerts its effect via luteolysis and stimulation of uterine smooth muscle contractions. The CL in the bitch is most susceptible to luteolysis by $PGF_{2\alpha}$ after midgestation or day 30 after ovulation (Lein 1986). However, $PGF_{2\alpha}$ administration will first mediate luteolysis in the bitch after day 5 of cytologic diestrus (day 13 from the first rise in serum progesterone, or 5 days with less than 50% of the vaginal cells cornified) (Oettle et al. 1988). The natural $PGF_{2\alpha}$ (Lutalyse®) has been recommended for use in small animals as opposed to PG analogs with increased potency (Purswell 1994). However, others have terminated pregnancy safely using analogs (Vickery and McRae 1980; Shille et al. 1984). A large-scale clinical report with pregnant bitches (30-35 days) utilizing abdominal ultrasonography to monitor the abortifacient effects of PG defined acceptable $PGF_{2\alpha}$ abortifacient regimens. The following three $PGF_{2\alpha}$ regimens were effective: 0.1 mg/kg every 8 hours; 0.25 mg/kg every 12 hours; or 0.1 mg/kg every 8 hours for 2 days and then 0.2 mg/kg every 8 hours afterward) (Feldman et al. 1993). Treatment continued until abortion was complete. All bitches aborted within 9 days of beginning treatment. Early in pregnancy (beginning day 5 of diestrus) a $PGF_{2\alpha}$ dosage of 250 µg/kg S/Q twice a day for 4 consecutive days is recommended (Romagnoli et al. 1991). This treatment was 80% effective in Beagle bitches (Oettle et al. 1988). Failures were attributed to the refractoriness of CL due to their transitional status.

Bitches treated on or before days 8 or 9 of diestrus did not have a vaginal discharge associated with the loss of pregnancy; loss occurred before implantation. Those treated on days 12-14 of diestrus had a bloody-mucoid discharge around day 28 (Romagnoli et al. 1991). The interestrous interval may be shortened by this treatment, particularly when $PGF_{2\alpha}$ is given early in diestrus. A bitch given $PGF_{2\alpha}$ between diestrus days 10 and 12, e.g., was in estrus 42 days later (Johnston 1990).

Significant side effects are noted in the bitch given $PGF_{2\alpha}$; a median lethal dose is 5 mg/kg (Sokolowski and Geng 1977). Side effects are emesis, ataxia, anxiety, abdominal cramping, hyperpnea, diarrhea, and hypersalivation. Vomition resulted from the administration of 0.5 mg/kg $PGF_{2\alpha}$, and only one- fourth this dose was required to elicit defecation (Moncada et al. 1985). A transient hypothermic effect occurs for approximately 3 hours post-$PGF_{2\alpha}$. Generally, side effects are observed within 5 minutes after administration and persist for 20-40 minutes. Atropine administration prior to $PGF_{2\alpha}$ and walking the animal after $PGF_{2\alpha}$ administration have reduced side effects (Braakman et al. 1993). These effects tend to diminish after 4 or 5 injections. Because of the adverse effects, $PGF_{2\alpha}$ should only be administered to healthy young bitches.

Pregnancy has been terminated in queens after day 40 of pregnancy following either 0.50 or 1.00 mg/kg $PGF_{2\alpha}$ once or twice (Lein 1986). Abortion followed 8-24 hours post-$PGF_{2\alpha}$. Luteolysis occurred in pseudopregnant queens after day 21-25 in response to either 220 or 440 µg/kg $PGF_{2\alpha}$.

MECHANISMS TO EVACUATE THE INFECTED CANINE UTERUS. Uterine infections (metritis/pyometra) most commonly occur a few weeks postovulation during diestrus and shortly after whelping. Administration of either estrogenic or progestogenic preparations increases the incidence. $PGF_{2\alpha}$, in addition to causing luteolysis, results in cervical dilatation and uterine contractions (Burke 1982; Nelson et al. 1982; Sokolowski 1980). $PGF_{2\alpha}$ (25-1000 µg/kg S/Q or IM) is recommended twice daily for 3-5 days or until the vaginal discharge is scant and uterine size is considerably reduced (Lein 1986). Antibiotics are also used. In a large study, the successful $PGF_{2\alpha}$ dose varied from 26.8 to 258 µg/kg twice a day for 2-26 days (Gilbert et al. 1989). Clinical cure from symptoms was achieved in 33 of 40 bitches. It has been recommended that a further dose of $PGF_{2\alpha}$ be given 3-5 days after the intensive $PGF_{2\alpha}$ regimen to ensure that the uterus is not filling again with exudate (Burke 1982). Bitches should be bred at the next opportunity since pyometra may develop after the next nonpregnant cycle. Queens with pyometra may be similarly treated.

Oxytocin (2-3 U/45.5 kg) IM and ergonovine (0.2 mg/13.5 kg) PO or IM have been used to evacuate the uterus in the postpartum bitch with metritis (Johnston 1993). Oxytocin may be repeated at 30- to 40-minute intervals. Prior administration of estradiol cypionate (0.25 mg) IM enhances the effectiveness of oxytocin and ergonovine.

ANTINIDATORY ACTIVITY OF ESTROGENS IN THE BITCH AND QUEEN. Diethylstilbestrol (DES), a nonsteroidal compound with estrogenic activity, has been recommended as being antinidatory in the bitch (Shille 1982). However, DES given daily (0.075 kg) orally for 7 days during estrus did not interrupt pregnancy (Bowen et al. 1985). Benzoate, valerate, and cypionate estradiol delay absorption and metabolism of estradiol; consequently, they have a longer duration of action. Estradiol benzoate has been recommended (0.01 mg/kg) S/Q twice daily on days 3 and 5 postcoitum (Braakman et al. 1993). Estradiol cypionate given at 44 µg/kg IM during estrus or early diestrus prevented pregnancy (Bowen et al. 1985). Estradiol cypionate, however, resulted in a 25% incidence of pyometra when given during diestrus. Administration of 250 µg estradiol cypionate to queens 40 hours after coitus resulted in delayed ovum transport with degeneration of ova in 3 of 4 cats (Herron and Sis 1974).

Dogs are susceptible to estrogen toxicity (Bowen et al. 1985; Legendre 1976; Schalm 1978; Teske 1986). One problem with estrogens in the bitch has stemmed from the administration of estradiol cypionate, a long-acting (21-28 days) preparation (Shille 1982). The effects were more frequently noted with higher dosages in older dogs. Exogenous estrogen or that elaborated from tumors in the dog causes bone marrow depression characterized by thrombocytopenia followed by hemorrhages and pancytopenia. Cystic endometrial hyperplasia and pyometra are also sequelae. The queen is regarded as more tolerant of estrogens; however, estrogens potentially may suppress bone marrow activity in this species as well. Estrogen treatment also extends the period of estrus. The antinidatory mechanism of estrogens is via altered embryo tubal transport (Shille 1982) and biochemical environment of the uterus and the oviduct (Makler and Morris 1971).

MIFEPRISTONE (PROGESTERONE RECEPTOR ANTAGONIST). Mifepristone (RU-486, Roussel-Uclaf) is a synthetic steroid that interacts with the progesterone receptor and blocks the effect of progesterone upon the myometrium. Mifepristone is not available in the US. This is an effective abortifacient in the bitch without direct side effects (Concannon et al. 1990, Lavoud 1989). Administration of mifepristone (5-10 mg/kg) IM during the second half of pregnancy for 5-7 days resulted in abortion 5-7 days later (Taverne et al. 1989).

Mifepristone given early in pregnancy (days 6-23) at 5 mg/kg IM for 3 days aborted all animals (Lavaud 1989). In some cases there was a considerable delay in the occurrence of abortion (15-21 days). A temporary purulent vaginal discharge was noted in a minority of animals.

BROMOCRIPTINE AND CABERGOLINE (ERGOLINE DERIVATIVES). Prolactin is luteotropic during the second half of diestrus in the bitch (Concannon 1991). Ergoline derivatives are dopaminergic agents that suppress serum prolactin, and consequently progesterone secretion decreases. This sequence leads to abortion (Concannon et al. 1987; Conley and Evans 1984). Bitches given 20-30 μg/kg bromocriptine (Parlodel, Sandoz) orally twice daily for 4 days beginning day 42 of pregnancy aborted 3-5 days later (Conley and Evans 1984). Transient vomition, nausea, and anorexia were noted. Fewer side effects were noted when one-half the dosage was used several days prior to giving the full dose. Fewer side effects have been attributed to cabergoline than to bromocriptine (Post et al. 1988). Cabergoline (5-15 μg/kg) orally daily for 5 days after day 42 of pregnancy resulted in abortion (Post et al. 1988; Jöchle et al. 1989).

Postponement of Estrus

PROGESTINS. Megestrol acetate (Ovaban; Schering Plough), a synthetic progestin, prevents the occurrence of estrus in the bitch when treatment is begun during anestrus. This agent is given daily (0.55 mg/kg/day) for up to 32 days beginning 1 week before expected proestrus. More than two consecutive treatment periods is considered inappropriate. Care should be given not to administer this drug to pregnant bitches (Concannon and Meyers-Wallen 1991). Megestrol acetate is not recommended prior to the first estrus, although it is effective and safe in this regard (Bigbee and Hennessy 1977). Treatment once proestrus has begun should be initiated within the first 3 days of proestrus. The dosage then is 2.2 mg/kg/day for 8 days. Proestrus should be suppressed within 3-8 days after onset of treatment. Return to estrus is expected 4-6 months later. This increased dose may result in cystic endometrial hyperplasia and pyometra. Contraindications for use are diabetes mellitus, liver disease, and mammary tumors (Concannon and Meyers-Wallen 1991).

Megestrol acetate is not approved for use in cats in the US, although it is marketed for this species in the UK. It prevents estrus in queens when given at a dosage of 5 mg/cat/day for 3 days and then continued at 2.5-5.0 mg once a week for 10 weeks (Housdell and Hennessey 1977) or as long as 18 months for maintenance of anestrus (Concannon and Meyers-Wallen 1991). Side effects of progestin usage in the cat are adrenal suppression and diabetes mellitus (Mansfield et al. 1986).

Progestins given as injectable depot preparations (crystalline suspensions) are used to prevent estrus in bitches in Europe (Jöchle 1991). These preparations are chlormadinone acetate, delmadinone acetate, medroxyprogesterone acetate, and proligestone. These compounds are regarded as having central and peripheral progesterone-like effects with antigonadotropic, antiestrogenic, and antiandrogenic activity. Chlormadinone acetate and delmadinone acetate are the most potent; proligestone has the least activity. This may be the reason proligestone has fewer side effects such as pyometra and pseudopregnancy following withdrawal. The administration of these compounds at the correct time (anestrus) and at the recommended lower dosage greatly reduces side effects. Medroxyprogesterone acetate was marketed in the US until 1969 as a canine contraceptive until it was associated with an appreciable incidence of uterine cystic endometrial hyperplasia that sometimes resulted in pyometra. The minutesimal effective dose of medroxyprogesterone acetate is approximately 2 mg/kg every 3 months or 3 mg/kg every 4 months (Concannon and Meyers-Wallen 1991). These long-acting progestins have also resulted in diabetes mellitus and acromegaly in the bitch (Eigenmann et al. 1983).

MIBOLERONE. Mibolerone (Cheque Drops; Upjohn Co.) is an androgenic steroid used to prevent estrus in the bitch. Treatment is to be initiated 30 days before the onset of estrus but not prior to the first estrus. Treatment beginning in late anestrus may be ineffective as estrus may begin within the first 30 days. The maximal duration of administration recommended is 2 years; however, it is effective in preventing proestrus for up to 5 years (Concannon and Meyers-Wallen 1991). This drug is not recommended in bitches which will be bred. The dosage depends on body weight and breed (0.5-12 kg: 30 μg/d; 12-23 kg: 60 μg/d; 23-45 kg: 120 μg/d; >45 kg: 180 μg/d; and any German Shepherd or Alsatian-derived bitch: 180 μg/d). Mibolerone is not recommended for use in Bedlington Terriers. This drug is contraindicated with perianal adenoma or carcinoma. A vaginal discharge and clitoral enlargement have been found in 15-20% of the treated bitches. Mibolerone is regarded as effective in treating bitches with short interestrous intervals (less than 4 months) and hence are infertile (Purswell 1994). This drug is not approved for use in cats.

TESTOSTERONE. Weekly testosterone propionate (110 mg) IM has been used to prevent estrus in Greyhounds (Gannon 1976). Oral dosing with 25 mg methyltestosterone tablets (Goldline Laboratories) twice a week also prevents estrus in the Greyhound (Purswell 1994). Testosterone enanthate (Steris Laboratories) or testosterone cypionate (Goldline Laboratories) has been used (0.5 mg/kg) IM at 5-day intervals successfully. Side effects of testosterone include clitoral enlargement, prolonged interestrous intervals, and reduced fertility following withdrawal.

Treatment of Pseudopregnancy, Uterine Inertia, Cryptorchidism, and Prostatic Hypertrophy

PSEUDOPREGNANCY. Overt pseudopregnancy frequently occurs in the bitch at the end of diestrus and is manifested in behavioral and/or physical changes, including congestion of the mammary glands and inappropriate lactation. These signs may also be associated with withdrawal of progestin therapy. Spontaneous remission will occur without treatment; however, treatment may be desired. Ergoline derivatives and other dopamine agonists reduce prolactin secretion and thus seem appropriate. Bromocriptine (Parlodel, Sandoz) tablets orally at either 30 μg/kg daily for 16 days or 10 μg/kg for 10 days have been effective (Janssens 1986). Vomiting occurred in about 25% of the animals. The owners were instructed to mix the bromocriptine in the food and to give 0.5 mg/kg metoclopramide, a dopamine antagonist and antiemetic, a half an hour before the meal if the first dose of bromocriptine elicited vomition. Cabergoline, another ergoline derivative, was found to be effective at 5 μg/kg/day IM for 7 days (Jöchle et al. 1989). Vomition again was a significant side effect. Testosterone has also been used to treat pseudopregnancy (Purswell 1994). A single dose of either testosterone cypionate or enanthate (0.66 mg/kg) has been effective and without side effects. Mibolerone has been recommended at 0.016 mg/kg orally daily for 5 days (Brown 1984).

UTERINE INERTIA. Oxytocin results in myometrial contractions during delivery. The dosage for uterine inertia in the dog is 5-20 U/dog IM (Table 31.1). This dosage may be repeated at 30- to 40-minute intervals, although the bitch may become refractory (Johnston 1993). Postpartum oxytocin promotes uterine involution and milk letdown.

CRYPTORCHIDISM. Cryptorchidism is the failure of one or both testes to be present in the scrotum of the dog by 6-8 weeks of age (Feldman and Nelson 1987). The testes migrate from the caudal pole of the kidney to the scrotum via guidance from the gubernaculum testis. At birth the testes in the dog are usually within the abdomen near the internal inguinal ring (Jones and Joshua 1982). The testes move through the inguinal canal and are in the scrotum by 10-14 days of age. Because this condition has a genetic basis, dogs with this condition should not be used for breeding purposes. The ethics of medical management of this condition should be considered by the veterinarian and the owner (Feldman and Nelson 1987). The most common method of treatment is serial injections of HCG. Dogs younger than 16 weeks of age are the best candidates. The IM injection of 100-1000 IU HCG 4 times in a 2-week period resulted in descent in 21 of 22 dogs. None of the 28 controls had complete descent.

BENIGN PROSTATIC HYPERTROPHY. Benign prostatic hypertrophy occurs in dogs over 5 years of age with an incidence thought to be at least 80%. Signs associated with this problem are constipation, blood in the urine or semen, and increased frequency of urination. The treatment of choice is castration; however, if this is declined there are medical alternatives. Megestrol acetate (Ovaban) decreases 5 α-reductase in prostate tissue, thereby interfering with the conversion of testosterone to dihydrotestosterone, the agent that mediates the hypertrophy. Megestrol acetate (0.55 mg/kg) given orally to dogs for 8 weeks inhibited the hematuria and blood in the ejaculate (Olson et al. 1987). This drug is not recommended to be given for more than 32 days and undoubtedly will interfere with sperm production. The antiandrogen finasteride (Proscar®; Merck) at a dose of 1.0 mg/kg daily is recommended (Johnston 1993).

REFERENCES

Amoah, E. A., and Gelaye, S. 1990. Small Rumin Res 3:63.
Arbeiter, K., Brass, W., Ballabio, R., and Jöchle, W. 1988. J Small Anim Pract 29:781.
Barth, A. D. 1986. In D. A. Morrow, ed., Current Therapy in Theriogenology, 2nd ed., p. 205. Philadelphia: W. B. Saunders Co.
Bigbee, H. J., and Hennessy, P. W. 1977. Vet Med Sm Anim Clin 72:1727.
Bouchard, G. F., Gross, S., Ganjam, V. K., Youngquist, R. S., Concannon, P. W., Krause, G. F., and Reddy, C. S. 1993. J Reprod Fertil 1(Suppl 47):515.
Bowen, R. A., Olson, P. N., Behrendt, M. D., Wheeler, S. L., Husted, P. W., and Nett, T. M. 1985. J Am Vet Med Assoc 186:783.
Braakman, A., Okkens, A. C., and Haaften, B. 1993. The Compendium 15:1505.
Brazeau, P. 1975. In L. S. Goodman and A. G. Gilman, The Pharmacological Basis of Therapeutics, 5th ed., p. 874. New York: Macmillan.
Bretzlaff, K. N., Nuti, L. C., Elmore, R. G., Meyers, S. A., Rugila, J. N., Brinsko, S. P., Blachard, T. L., and Weston, P. G. 1992. Am J Vet Res 53:930.
Brink, J. T., and Kiracofe, G. H. 1988. Theriogenology 29:513.
Brinsko, S. P. 1991. Vet Med 86:1112.
Bristol, F. 1986. In D. A. Morrow, ed., Current Therapy in Theriogenology, 2nd ed., p. 661. Philadelphia: W. B. Saunders Co.
———. 1987. In N. E. Robinson, ed., Current Therapy in Equine Medicine, 2nd ed., p. 495. Philadelphia: W. B. Saunders Co.
Britt, J. H., Day, B. N., Webel, K. K., and Brauer, M. A. 1989. J Anim Sci 67:1148.
Britt, J. H., Esbenshade, K. L., and Heller, K. 1986. Theriogenology 26:697.
Brown, J. M. 1984. J Am Vet Med Assoc 184:1467.
Brown, L. N., Odde, K. G., King, M. E., LeFever, D. E., and Neubauer, C. J. 1988. Theriogenology 30:1.
Brown, L. N., Odde, K. G., LeFever, D. E., King, M. E., and Neubauer, C. J. 1986. J Anim Sci 63(Suppl 1):383.
Burfening, P. J., Anderson, D. C., Kinkie, R. A., Williams, J., and Friedrick, R. L. 1978. J Anim Sci 47:999.
Burke, T. J. 1982. Vet Clin N Am: Small Anim Pract 12:107.
Burns, P. D., and Spitzer, J. C. 1992. J Anim Sci 70:358.
Burns, P. D., Spitzer, J. C., Bridges, W. C., Jr., Henricks, D. M., and Plyler, B. B. 1993. J Anim Sci 71:983.
Cain, J. L., Lasley, B. C., Cain, G. R., Feldman, E. C., and Stabenfeldt, G. H. 1989. J Reprod Fertil Suppl 39:143.
Chenault, J. R., Kratzer, D. D., Rzepkowski, R. A., and Goodwin, M. C. 1990. Theriogenology 34:81.
Colbern, G. T., Squires, E. L., and Voss, J. L. 1987. Theriogenology 7:69.
Collier, R. J., and Davis, S. R. 1986. In D. A. Morrow, ed., Current Therapy in Theriogenology, 2nd ed., p. 379. Philadelphia: W. B. Saunders Co.

Concannon, P. W. 1989. J Reprod Fertil Suppl 39:149.
———. 1991. In P. T. Cupps, ed., Reproduction in Domestic Animals, p. 518. San Diego: Academic Press.
Concannon, P. W., and Meyers-Wallen, V. N. 1991. J Am Vet Med Assoc 198:1214.
Concannon, P. W., Weinstein, R., Whaley, S., and Frank, D. 1987. J Reprod Fertil 81:175.
Concannon, P. W., Yeager, A., Frank, D., and Iyampillai, A. 1990. J Reprod Fertil 88:99.
Conley, A. J., and Evans, L. E. 1984. In Proc 10th International Congress on Animal Reproduction and Artificial Insemination (Abs 504). Champaign-Urbana, IL, June 10-14.
Daels, P. F., Stabenfeldt, G. H., Hughes, J. P., Odensvik, K., and Kindahl, H. 1991. Am J Vet Res 52:282.
Davis, S. R., Welch, R. A. S., Pearce, M. C., and Peterson, A. J. 1983. J Dairy Sci 66:450.
Dial, G. D., Almond, G. W., Hilley, H. D., Repasky, R. R., and Hagan, M. S. 1987. Am J Vet Res 48:966.
Donaldson, L. E., and Ward, D. N. 1986. Theriogenology 25:747.
Drew, S. B., and Peters, A. R. 1994. Vet Rec 134:267.
Eigenmann, J. E., Eigenmann, R. Y., Rijnberk, A., van der Gaag, I., Zapf, J., and Froesch, E. R. 1983. Acta Endocrinologica 104:167.
Einarsson, S. 1986. In D. A. Morrow, ed., Current Therapy in Theriogenology, 2nd ed., p. 935. Philadelphia: W. B. Saunders Co.
Etherington, W. G., Martin, S. W., Bonnett, B., Johnson, W. H., Miller, R. B., Savage, N. C., Walton, J. S., and Montgomery, M. E. 1988. Theriogenology 29:565.
Fanning, M. D., Spitzer, J. C., Burns, G. L., and Plyler, B. B. 1992. J Anim Sci 70:1352.
Feldman, E. C., Davidson, A. P., Nelson, R. W., Nyland, T. G., and Munro, C. 1993. J Am Vet Med Assoc 202:1855.
Feldman, E. C., and Nelson, R. W. 1987. Canine and Feline Endocrinology and Reproduction, p. 494. Philadelphia: W. B. Saunders Co.
Gannon, U. 1976. Racing Greyhound 1:12.
Gilbert, R. O., Nöthling, J. O., and Oettle, E. E. 1989. J Reprod Fertil Suppl 39:225.
Ginther, I. J., and Pierson, R. A. 1989. J Eq Vet Sci 9:4.
Heersche, G., Jr., Kiracofe, G. H., DeBennedett, R. C., Wen, S., and McKee, R. M. 1979. Theriogenology 11:197.
Hemeida, N. A., Gustafsson, B. J., and Whitmore, H. L. 1986. In D. A. Morrow, ed., Current Therapy in Theriogenology, 2nd ed., p. 45. Philadelphia: W. B. Saunders Co.
Herron, M. A., and Sis, R. F. 1974. Am J Vet Res 35:1277.
Hixon, D. L., Kesler, D. J., Troxel, T. R., Vincent, D. L., and Wiseman, B. S. 1981. Theriogenology 16:219.
Holtz, W., Schmidt-Baulain, R., Meyer, H., and Welp, C. 1990. J Anim Sci 68:3967.
Houdeshell, J. W., and P. W. Hennessey. 1977. Vet Med Small Anim Clin 72:1013.
Janssens, A. A. 1986. Vet Rec 119:172.
Jeffcott, L. B., and Rossdale, P. D. 1977. Eq Vet J 4:208.
Jöchle, W. 1991. J Am Vet Med Assoc 198:1225.
Jöchle, W., Arbeiter, K., Post, K., Ballabio, R., and D'Ver, A. S. 1989. J Reprod Fertil Suppl 39:199.
Johnston, S. 1993. Canine Theriogenology Short Course, March 5-7, University of Georgia, p. 136.
Johnston, S. D. 1990. In Proc Annu Meeting Soc Theriogenology, p. 264. Toronto.
Jones, D. E., and Joshua, J. O. 1982. Reproductive Clinical Problems in the Dog, p. 122. Bristol, England: John Wright and Sons.
Kemppainen, R. J., Thompson, F. N., and Lorenz, M. D. 1983. J Endocrinol 96:293.
Kesler, D. J., and Garverick, H. A. 1982. J Anim Sci 55:1147.
Kiser, T. E., Britt, J. H., and Ritchie, H. D. 1977. J Anim Sci 44:1030.
Kiser, T. E., Dunlap, S. E., Benyshek, L. L., and Mares, S. E. 1980. Theriogenology 13:381.
Kraeling, R. R., Barb, C. R., and Davis, B. J. 1975. Prostaglandins 9:459.
Kraeling, R. R., Dziuk, P. J., Pursel, V. G., Rampacek, G. B., and Webel, S. K. 1981. J Anim Sci 52:831.
Lauderdale, J. W. 1972. J Anim Sci 35:246.
———. 1979. Proc Lutalyse Symp., p. 17. Kalamazoo, MI: Upjohn Co.
Lauderdale, J. W., McAllister, J. F., Moody, E. L., and Kratazer, D. D. 1980. J Anim Sci 51(Suppl 1):296.
Lavoud, J. 1989. Prat Med Chir 24:253.
Leadon, D. P., Jeffcott, L. B., and Rossdale, P. D. 1984. Eq Vet J 16:256.
Legendre, A. M. 1976. J Am Anim Hosp Assoc 12:525.
Lein, D. H. 1986. In D. A. Morrow, ed., Current Therapy in Theriogenology, 2nd ed., p. 481. Philadelphia: W. B. Saunders Co.
Loar, A. S. 1992. In R. V. Morgan, ed., Handbook of Small Animal Practice, 2nd ed., p. 675. New York: Churchill Livingstone.
Lofstedt, R. M. 1986. In D. A. Morrow, ed., Current Therapy in Theriogenology, 2nd ed., p. 715. Philadelphia: W. B. Saunders Co.
———. 1988. Vet Clin N Amer (Eq. Pract) 4:177.
Lofstedt, R. M., and Patel, J. H. 1989. J Am Vet Med Assoc 194:361.
MacMillan, K. L., and Henderson, H. V. 1984. Anim Reprod Sci 6:245.
Makler, A., and Morris, J. M. 1971. Fertil Steril 22:204.
Mansfield, P. D., Kemppainen, R. J., and Sartin, J. L. 1986. J Am Anim Hosp Assoc 22:515.
Mapletoft, R. J. 1986. In D. A. Morrow, ed., Current Therapy in Theriogenology, 2nd ed., p. 54. Philadelphia: W. B. Saunders Co.
Martin, P. A. 1986. In D. A. Morrow, ed., Current Therapy in Theriogenology, 2nd ed., p. 66. Philadelphia: W. B. Saunders Co.
McCue, P. M., Warren, R. C., Appel, R. D., Stabenfeldt, G. H. Hughes, J. P., and Lasley, B. L. 1992. J Eq Vet Sci 12:21.
McDonald, M. F. 1986. In D. A. Morrow, ed., Current Therapy in Theriogenology, 2nd ed., p. 887. Philadelphia: W. B. Saunders Co.
McMillan, W. H., and MacMillan, K. L. 1989. In Proc New Zealand Soc of Anim Prod 49:85.
Meyers, S. A., and LeBlanc, M. M. 1991. Vet Med 86:1117.
Moncada, S., Flower, R. J., and Vane, J. R. 1985. In L. S. Goodman, A. G. Gilman, T. W. Rall, and F. Murad, eds., The Pharmacological Basis of Therapeutics, 7th ed., p. 660. New York: Macmillan.
Moses, D. C., and Shille, V. M. 1988. J Am Vet Med Assoc 192:1541.
Myers, P. J. 1991. Vet Med 86:1106.
Neely, D. P. 1983. In J. P. Hughes, ed., Hormone Therapy, p. 24. Trenton: Veterinary Learning Systems.
Nelson, R. W., Feldman, E. C., and Stabenfeldt, G. H. 1982. J Am Vet Med Assoc 181:899.
Niswender, G. D., Juengel, J. L., McGuire, W. J., Belfiore, C. J., and Wiltbank, M. C. 1994. Biol Reprod 50:239.
Nuti, L. C., Minhas, B. S., Baker, W. C., Capehart, J. S., and Marrack, P. 1987. Theriogenology 28:481.
Odde, K. G. 1990. J Anim Sci 68:817.
Odde, K. G., LeFevar, D. G., Anderson, R. S., and Taylor, R. E. 1984. Colorado State Univ Beef Program Rep., p. 34, Fort Collins.
Oettle, E. E., Bertschinger, H. J., Botha, A. E., and Marais, A. 1988. Theriogenology 29:757.

Olson, P. N., Wrigley, R. H., Husted, P. W., Bowen, R. A., and Nett, T. M. 1989. In S. J. Ettinger, ed., Textbook of Veterinary Internal Medicine, vol. 2, 3rd ed., p. 1792. Philadelphia: W. B. Saunders Co.
Olson, P. N., Wrigley, R. H., Thrall, M. A., and Husted, P. W. 1987. Comp Cont Edu Pract Vet 9:613.
Ott, R. S. 1986. In D. A. Morrow, ed., Current Therapy in Theriogenology, 2nd ed., p. 583. Philadelphia: W. B. Saunders Co.
Patterson, D. J., Corah, L. R., and Brethour, J. R. 1990. Theriogenology 33:661.
Peters, A. R., and Ball, P. J. H. 1987. In A. R. Peters and P. J. H. Ball, eds., Reproduction in Cattle, p. 75. London: Butterworth.
Plumb, D. C. 1991. Veterinary Drug Handbook, p. 301.
Post, K., Evans, L. E., and Jöchle, W. 1988. Theriogenology 29:1233.
Purswell, B. J. 1994. Semin Vet Med Surg (Small Anim) 9:54.
Redmer, D. A., and Day, B. N. 1981. Theriogenology 16:195.
Romagnoli, S. E., Cela, M., and Camillo, F. 1991. Vet Clin N Am (Small Anim Pract) 21:487.
Ryan, J. P., Hunton, J. R., and Maxwell, M. C. 1992. Reprod Fertil Dev 4:91.
Safranski, T. J., Lamberson, W. R., and Keisler, D. H. 1992. J Anim Sci 70:2935.
Schalm, O. W. 1978. Canine Pract 5:57.
Seidel, G. E., and Seidel, S. M. 1991. In Training Manual for Embryo Transfer in Cattle, p. 27. Rome: Food and Agriculture Organization of the U.N.
Shille, V. M. 1982. Vet Clin N Am 12:99.
Shille, V. M., Dorsey, D., and Thatcher, M.-J. 1984. Am J Vet Res 45:1295.
Shoemaker, C. F., Squires, E. L., and Shideler, R. K. 1989. J Eq Vet Sci 9:69.
Sigler, D. H., Ericson, D. E., Gibbs, P. G., Kiracofe, G. H., and Stevenson, J. S. 1989. J Anim Sci 67:1154.
Smith, R. D., Pomerantz, A. J., Beal, W. E., McCann, J. P., Pilbeam, T. E., and Hansel, W. 1984. J Anim Sci 58:792.
Sokolowski, J. H. 1980. J Am Anim Hosp Assoc 16:119.
Sokolowski, J. H., and Geng, S. 1977. J Am Vet Med Assoc 170:536.
Sprott, L. R., Wiltbank, J. N., Songster, W. N., and Webel, S. 1984. Theriogenology 21:349.
Squires, E. L., Hesseman, C. P., Webel, S. K., Shideler, R. K., and Voss, J. L. 1983. J Anim Sci 56:901.
Squires, E. L., Shideler, R. K., and McKinnon, A. O. 1989. J Equ Vet Sci 9:73.
Squires, E. L., Stevens, W. B., McGlothlin, D. E., and Pickett, B. W. 1979. J Anim Sci 49:729.
Staples, L. D., McPhee, S., Kennaway, D. J., and Williams, A. H. 1992. Anim Reprod Sci 30:185.
Taverne, M. A. M., Weyden, G. C., vander Oovd, H. A. 1989. In L. J. Christiansen, ed., Proc Symp on Reproduction in the dog, p. 71. Royal Veterinary and Agricultural University, Copenhagen, Denmark.
Teske, E. 1986. In R. W. Kirk, ed., Current Veterinary Therapy IX, p. 495. Philadelphia: W. B. Saunders Co.
Troxel, T. R., Cruz, L. C., Ott, R. S., and Kesler, D. J. 1993. J Anim Sci 71:2579.
Vickery, B. H., and McRae, G. 1980. Biol Reprod 22:438.
Wagner, W. C., Willham, R. L., and Evans, L. E. 1974. J Anim Sci 38:485.
Webel, S. K., and Day, B. N. 1982. In D. J. A. Cole and G. R. Foxcroft, eds., Control of Pig Reproduction, p. 197. London: Butterworth Scientific.
Wichtel, J. J. 1991. Vet Med 86:647.
Wood, C. M., Kornegay, E. T., and Shipley, C. F. 1992. J Anim Sci 70:1357.
Young, I. M., and Anderson, D. B. 1986. Vet Rec 118:212.
Youngquist, R. S. 1990. In B. P. Smith, ed., Large Animal Internal Medicine, p. 1364. St. Louis: CV Mosby Co.
Zimbelman, R. G., Lauderdale, J. W., Sokolowski, J. H., and Schalk, T. G. 1970. J Am Vet Med Assoc 157:1528.

32 THYROID HORMONES AND ANTITHYROID DRUGS

DUNCAN C. FERGUSON

Introduction
- **Hypothyroidism**
- **Hyperthyroidism**

Thyroid Physiology
- **Iodine Metabolism**
- **Thyroid Hormone Synthesis**
- **Thyroid Hormone Secretion**
- **Hypothalamic-Pituitary-Thyroid-Extrathyroid Axis**
- **Metabolism of Thyroid Hormone**
- **Plasma Hormone Binding of Thyroid Hormone**
- **Tissue Thyroid Hormone Uptake: The "Free Hormone" Hypothesis**
- **Metabolic Clearance Rates**

Extrathyroidal Factors Altering Thyroid Hormone Metabolism
- **Effect of Illness and Malnutrition**
- **Effect of Drugs**

Mechanisms of Thyroid Hormone Action
- **Nuclear Receptor–Mediated Effects of Thyroid Hormone**
- **Extranuclear Actions of Thyroid Hormone**
- **Physiologic and Possible Pharmacologic Effects of Thyroid Hormone**

Thyroid Hormone Preparations
- **Crude Thyroid Products**
- **Synthetic L-Thyroxine**
- **Synthetic L-Triiodothyronine**
- **Effects of Thyroid Hormone Overdose (Iatrogenic Thyrotoxicosis)**
- **Therapeutic Trial for Diagnosis of Hypothyroidism**
- **Monitoring Therapy**
- **Therapeutic Failure**
- **Treatment of Myxedema Coma**

Antithyroid Drugs
- **Goitrogens**
- **Thioureylenes (Thionamides)**
- **Nonthioureylene Antithyroid Agents**

Thyroid Imaging

INTRODUCTION

Hypothyroidism. Hypothyroidism is the most common endocrinopathy of the dog and is diagnosed with some frequency in the horse, but spontaneous hypothyroidism is rare in the cat and other domestic species. Less commonly, hypothyroidism can be caused by iodine deficiency or by the ingestion of goitrogenic substances (compounds that interfere with thyroid hormone synthesis by the thyroid gland) in the environment or food.

Clinical signs of hypothyroidism common to most species generally reflect the reduction in basal metabolic rate of the body and include lethargy, mental depression, weakness, inability to train, and/or nonpruritic hair loss (Feldman and Nelson 1987b; Ferguson, 1989a, 1993; Ferguson and Hoenig 1991b; Ferguson et al. 1992; Peterson and Ferguson 1990).

Hyperthyroidism. Hyperthyroidism is now the most common endocrine disorder in the cat and is only occasionally seen in other domestic species. Hyperthyroidism, or thyrotoxicosis, is caused by excessive concentrations of the circulating thyroid hormones, thyroxine (T_4) and triiodothyronine (T_3), most commonly the result of hyperplastic or benign adenomatous malignant thyroid glands in cats and adenocarcinomas in dogs. Hyperthyroidism occurs most frequently in middle-aged to geriatric cats, and discussion of therapeutic agents will focus on those used in this species. The most common clinical signs associated with hyperthyroidism that can be directly related to thyroid hormone excess are weight loss in spite of ravenous appetite, hyperactivity, polydipsia, polyuria, diarrhea, intermittent fever, vomiting, and symptoms of cardiovascular disease such as tachycardia and dyspnea. Often the cats shed excessive amounts of hair, or the coat may be matted. Rarely, hyperthyroid cats present in a way similar to what has been called "apathetic hyperthyroidism," when the cats are lethargic and often anorectic, perhaps representing an end-stage form of the disease (Feldman and Nelson 1987b; Ferguson and Hoenig 1991a; Peterson and Ferguson 1990).

THYROID PHYSIOLOGY

Iodine Metabolism. Thyroid hormones are the only iodinated organic compounds in the body. The two major secretory products of the thyroid gland, thyroxine (L-T_4) and 3,5,3′-triiodothyronine (L-T_3), contain 65% and 59% iodine, respectively. The minimum iodine requirement of most animals is unknown, but the daily amount needed in the ration to prevent goiter in all animals is generally accepted to be 1 μg/kg body weight. The daily recommended amount of iodine in the dog is 15 μg/kg and, while it has not been carefully studied in the cat, is believed to be about 100 μg/cat/day. Although true nutrient requirements for this micronutrient are not well established, most commercial dog and cat food preparations include at least three to five times this minimum requirement for iodine when fed in recommended amounts. As a result, iodine deficiency has become a rare condition in domestic animals. During pregnancy, the recommended minimum daily requirement for iodine is increased fourfold. Areas of iodine deficiency in North America include the Great Lakes region and eastern British Columbia (Belshaw et al. 1974; Kaptein et al. 1994; Peterson and Ferguson 1990).

Ingested iodine is converted to iodide in the gastrointestinal tract and absorbed into the circulation. The dog has plasma iodide concentrations of 5–10 μg/dL, which are 10–20 times the levels in human plasma. In the thyroid gland, iodide is concentrated or "trapped" by active transport mechanisms of the basolateral plasma membrane of the thyroid follicular cell, resulting in intracellular iodide concentrations that are 10–200 times that of serum. This process is stimulated by the interaction of thyrotropin (thyroid-stimulating hormone; TSH) with follicular cell surface receptors leading to the stimulation of cyclic AMP (cAMP) (see Fig. 32.1). Other tissues, including the salivary glands, gastric mucosal cells, renal proximal tubule cells, placenta, ciliary body, choroid plexus, and mammary glands, can take up considerable amounts of radioiodide in a TSH-independent fashion.

Diagnostically, radioactive iodide, or pertechnetate (TcO_4^-), which, unlike iodine, cannot be organified, can be used to assess the anion transport function (uptake) by the thyroid gland. Iodide trapping can be inhibited by other anions, such as thiocyanate (SCN^-), NO_3^-, and ClO_4^-. Thiocyanate is a metabolic product of some naturally occurring compounds in plants and may result in goitrogenic (antithyroid) activity of the plant. Oral administration of perchlorate following the administration of a tracer dose of radioiodine can be used to diagnose congenital defects in the thyroidal organification of iodide (perchlorate discharge test) (Greenspan 1994; Taurog 1971).

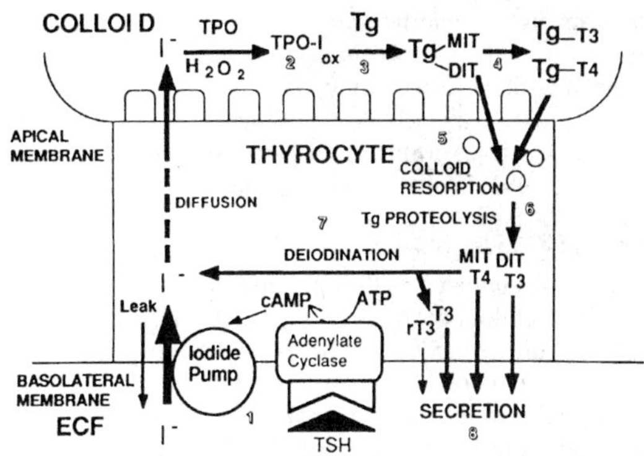

FIG. 32.1—Iodide uptake, organification, and secretion by the thyroid cell. Step 1: Iodide uptake. Inorganic iodide (I^-) is actively translocated into the thyrocyte from the extracellular fluid (ECF) to the cytosol of the follicular cell. The maintenance of the sodium gradient via the Na^+,K^+-ATPase pump appears to be important for this process. This step is stimulated by thyrotropin (TSH) interaction with a plasma TSH receptor and activation of adenylate cyclase. Steps 2 and 3: Oxidation and organification. After diffusion to the apical plasma membrane, the iodide is oxidized by the thyroid peroxidase enzyme (TPO) (step 2) and organified onto tyrosine residues of preformed thyroglobulin (Tg) (step 3) to form monoiodotyrosine (MIT) and diiodotyrosine (DIT). Step 4: Coupling. The MIT and DIT residues on Tg couple to form T_3, and two DIT residues couple to form T_4. Step 5: Colloid resorption. Under the stimulus of TSH, follicular colloid containing Tg is resorbed into the thyrocyte. Step 6: Tg proteolysis. Thyroid hormones, MIT, and DIT are released from Tg under the stimulus of TSH. Step 7: Deiodination. Also stimulated by TSH at the time of secretion, deiodinase enzymes convert T_4 to T_3 and reverse T_3 (rT_3), and iodotyrosines are deiodinated to allow recycling of iodide. Step 8: Secretion. T_4, T_3, and rT_3 are released into the bloodstream. (Reprinted from Peterson and Ferguson 1990, Fig. 95-1.)

Thyroid Hormone Synthesis. Thyroglobulin (Tg), an iodinated glycoprotein with a molecular weight of 660,000, serves as a synthesis and storage site for thyroid hormones and their precursors in the thyroid follicle. After synthesis within the endoplasmic reticulum of the thyroid follicular cell, membrane vesicles containing noniodinated Tg fuse with the apical membrane and are released (by exocytosis) into the follicular cell lumen, where Tg is stored as colloid.

Once inside the thyroid cell, iodide diffuses down a concentration gradient to the apical surface of the cell, where it is oxidized by the enzyme thyroid peroxidase (TPO) to iodine (Fig. 32.1). It is then incorporated into tyrosine residues of Tg in a process called organification, forming monoiodotyrosine (MIT) and diiodotyrosine (DIT). Thyroxine (T_4) is then formed by coupling two DIT molecules, and 3,5,3′-triiodothyronine (T_3) is formed by coupling one MIT molecule with one DIT molecule (Burrow et al. 1989; Greenspan 1994; Peterson and Ferguson 1990; Taurog 1991).

When iodine intake is adequate, production of T_4 is favored. However, in iodine-deficient states and impending thyroid failure, the intrathyroidal synthesis of T_3 is preferred over that of T_4. By this autoregulation, the thyroid gland produces the most active thyroid hormone (T_3 is 3–10 times more potent than T_4) while using less iodide. Conversely, chronic iodine excess may lead to excessive storage of thyroidal hormone.

The *Wolff-Chaikoff effect,* another intrathyroidal regulatory mechanism, is key to understanding the potential acute antithyroid effect of large amounts of ingested iodide. Mediated via inhibition of the TPO enzyme, iodide decreases the rate of its own relative and absolute organification. In humans, this effect is transient, and "escape" is seen within several weeks. This inhibitory effect may be a mechanism through which the organism is protected from massive thyroid hormone release following a large dietary iodine load (Taurog 1991; Wolff 1989).

Thyroid Hormone Secretion. Thyroid hormone secretion is initiated as the epithelial follicular cells take up Tg in colloid droplets by a process called pinocytosis. Simultaneously, lysosomes (containing proteases and hydrolytic enzymes) migrate from the basal region of the cell and fuse with the colloid droplets (Fig. 32.1). Degradation of Tg by the lysosomal proteolytic enzymes produces both the iodotyrosines (MIT and DIT) and iodothyronines (T_4 and T_3). Little of the released MIT and DIT enters the circulation, because the iodine is removed from these substances by a specific dehalogenase enzyme (Fig. 32.1). Some of this iodine is recycled internally for iodination of new tyrosine residues in Tg, but in carnivores, much iodine is released to the circulation (Belshaw et al. 1974; Kaptein et al. 1994). This inefficient thyroidal reutilization of iodine may help explain the high daily iodine requirements of the dog and cat compared to humans.

Proteolysis of Tg, as described above, liberates relatively large amounts of T_4, but only small quantities of T_3, into the cytosol. Enzymes present within the thyroid gland, however, can deiodinate T_4 to either T_3 or 3′,5′,3-T_3 (reverse T_3). As a result, although the T_4:T_3 ratio stored in the gland is 12:1 in the canine thyroid, the ratio of secreted products is 4:1. Production rates of the thyroid hormones in the dog have been estimated to be 8 µg/kg/day for T_4 and 0.8–1.5 µg/kg/day for T_3. These production rates are greater than twice those for T_4 and greater than three times the rate for T_3 in humans (Kaptein et al. 1993, 1994).

Hypothalamic-Pituitary-Thyroid-Extrathyroid Axis. Thyrotropin (TSH), a glycoprotein produced in the thyrotropes of the pituitary pars distalis, has a stimulatory effect on thyroid hormone synthesis and secretion. In addition, TSH stimulates thyroid growth, probably in conjunction with actions of the insulin-like growth factors (IGF-I and -II). TSH has a molecular weight of about 30,000 and consists of an α subunit (identical to a subunit of the other glycoprotein pituitary hormones LH and FSH) and a β subunit, which is specific to the TSH molecule (see Chap. 30). The structure of the canine β subunit of TSH has been reported (Su et al. 1995). TSH binds to a specific TSH receptor on the thyroid follicular cell membrane and stimulates adenylate cyclase, the production of cyclic AMP, and the active uptake of inorganic iodide (Fig. 32.1). The TSH receptor in dogs and humans has been cloned and expressed. TSH also stimulates the synthesis of Tg, its release into the colloid, and its iodination by TPO (i.e., organification). As a final step in the delivery of hormone into plasma, TSH stimulates Tg resorption and proteolysis to release T_3 and T_4. The thyroidal enzymes deiodinating T_4 to T_3 and reverse T_3 are also stimulated by TSH (Magner 1990; Rapaport and Nagayama 1992; Shupnick et al. 1989).

A detailed study of the hypothalamic-pituitary-thyroid-extrathyroid axis is only possible with the availability of a valid TSH radioimmunoassay (RIA) for each species. In recent years, an immunoassay for canine TSH has allowed further study of this axis in the dog. There is now direct and indirect evidence for an increase in TSH following administration of thyrotropin-releasing hormone (TRH), which suggests that the hypothalamic-pituitary regulation in the dog is similar to that in rat and human (see Fig. 32.2). The canine TSH assays have not had sufficient sensitivity, and TSH is elevated in only about one-fourth of clinical cases of otherwise confirmed hypothyroidism. Although it is possible that some of these cases have TSH deficiency, it is also possible that some forms of the glycosylated TSH peptide are not detected by the assay. Availability of this assay has helped to demonstrate that most of the replacement dosages of L-T_4 recommended for the dog are well in excess of those needed for suppression of endogenous TSH into the normal range. The currently available assays do not reliably distinguish between normal and low TSH con-

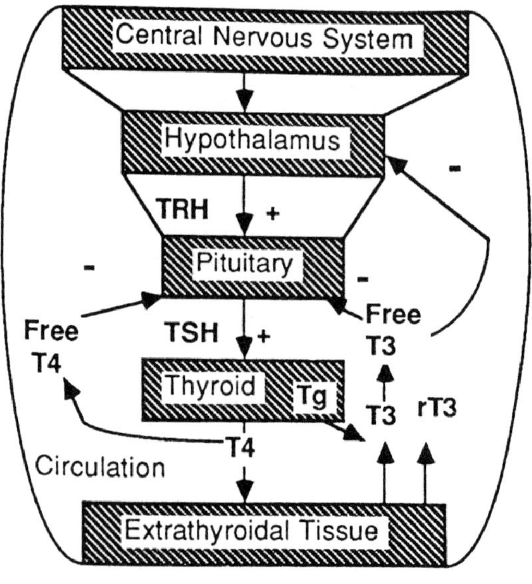

FIG. 32.2—Hypothalamic-pituitary-thyroid-extrathyroid axis. TRH = thyrotropin-releasing hormone; TSH = thyrotropin; Tg = thyroglobulin. TRH has a stimulatory effect on pituitary TSH synthesis and release. TSH stimulates thyroidal hormone synthesis and secretion. The free forms of T_4 and T_3 have a negative-feedback effect on the pituitary and the hypothalamus, decreasing TSH and TRH secretion, respectively. Extrathyroidal tissue takes up T_4, the main secretory product of the thyroid, and produces T_3, a more active hormone, or rT_3, a thyromimetically inactive compound. (Reprinted from Peterson and Ferguson 1990, Fig. 95-4.)

centrations, making it more difficult to confirm an overdosage (Braverman and Utiger 1991; Ferguson 1984; Greenspan 1994; Quinlan and Michaelson 1981; Williams et al. 1996; Bruner et al. 1998).

The tripeptide TRH is produced in the paraventricular nucleus of the hypothalamus and transported to the pituitary pars distalis by the hypophyseal portal system in the pituitary stalk. In the pituitary gland, TRH binds to specific receptors on the thyrotrope cell and stimulates TSH secretion (Fig. 32.2). In the dog, as in other species, TRH also stimulates the secretion of prolactin. The hypothalamic hormone somatostatin acts to inhibit TSH secretion and may function as a thyrotropin inhibitory factor (Reichlin 1986).

NEGATIVE-FEEDBACK REGULATION. The negative-feedback effect of thyroid hormones (in the free or unbound form) is the principal mechanism regulating TSH secretion. Tonic stimulation by TRH has a permissive role in TSH secretion. The pituitary thyrotrope cell completely deiodinates T_4 (derived from the plasma) to T_3, which subsequently inhibits TSH synthesis and secretion through alteration of nuclear receptor binding, mRNA transcription, and protein synthesis. Circulating T_4 taken up by the pituitary is the preferred source of T_3 in the pituitary, at least in the rat (Larsen et al. 1981). In human patients with hypothyroidism, thyroid replacement therapy with L-T_4 normalizes serum TSH concentrations only when the serum T_4 value is high-normal to slightly high; serum T_3 concentrations usually remain within normal range in these patients (Fish et al. 1987; Larsen et al. 1981).

There is also evidence that thyroid hormones may have a direct negative-feedback effect on the hypothalamus to inhibit the release of TRH (Fig. 32.2). Also, TSH and TRH may have "short-loop" and "ultrashort-loop" negative-feedback effects, respectively, upon the hypothalamus to inhibit TRH release. Although pulses of TSH secretion and an evening rise in serum TSH have been described in humans (possibly resulting from a fall in circadian circulating cortisol concentrations), studies in the dog and cat have failed to demonstrate such a circadian rhythm in circulating thyroid hormone concentrations (Fish et al. 1987; Larsen et al. 1981; Magner 1990; Reichlin 1986; Bruner et al. 1998).

Metabolism of Thyroid Hormone. The metabolically active thyroid hormones are the iodothyronines L-thyroxine (L-T4) and 3,5,3′-L-triiodothyronine (L-T_3) (see Fig. 32.3). Thyroxine is the main secretory product of the normal thyroid gland. However, T_3, which is about 3–10 times more potent than T_4, as well as smaller amounts of 3,3′,5′-L-triiodothyronine (reverse T_3; a thyromimetically inactive product) and other deiodinated metabolites are also secreted by the thyroid gland of most mammals (Figs. 32.2 and 32.3) (Belshaw et al. 1974; Ferguson 1984; Inada et al. 1975; Kaptein et al. 1993, 1994; Laurberg 1980).

Although all T_4 is secreted by the thyroid, a considerable amount (40–60% in the dog) of T_3 is derived from extrathyroidal enzymatic 5′-deiodination of T_4. Therefore, although it also has intrinsic metabolic activity, T_4 has been called a "prohormone," and its

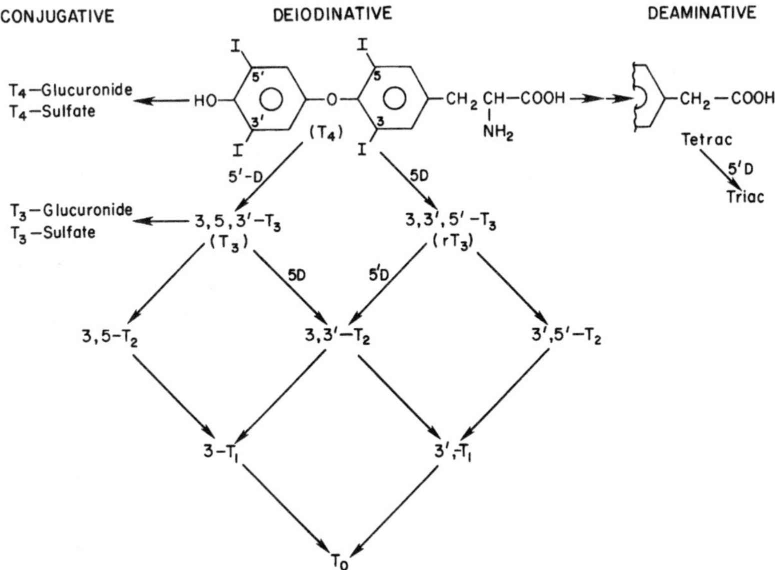

FIG. 32.3—Pathways of metabolism of thyroid hormones. 5′-D = 5′-deiodinase. 5-D = 5-deiodinase (Reprinted from Ferguson 1984.)

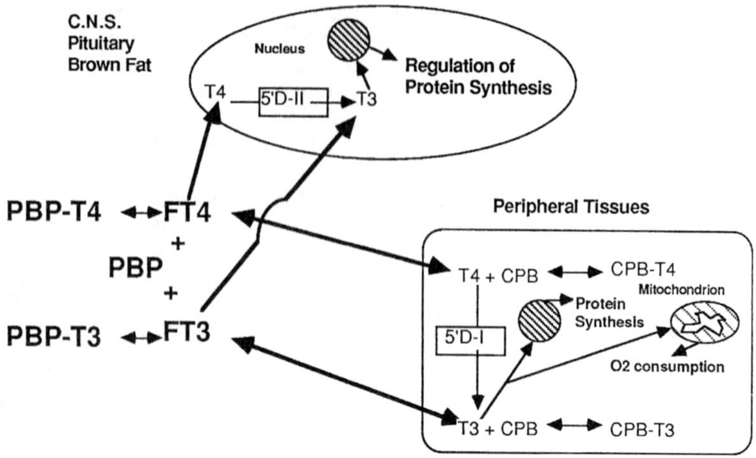

FIG. 32.4—Peripheral action of thyroid hormones. T_4 and T_3, in amounts proportional to their free forms (FT_4 and FT_3) in plasma at equilibrium with plasma binding proteins (PBP), are taken up by peripheral tissues such as liver and kidney, which have the type I 5′-deiodinase enzyme (5′-D-I). T_3 from the plasma (or that derived from T_4) interacts with mitochondrial receptors to rapidly increase oxygen consumption and with nuclear receptors to initiate protein synthesis. Cytosolic binding proteins (CBP) buffer the effects of intracellular hormones and provide a relatively unsaturable hormone reservoir. In the brain, pituitary, and brown fat, another isoenzyme of the 5′-deiodinase enzyme (5′-D-II) converts T_4 to T_3. This enzyme is regulated very differently from the type I enzyme. (Reprinted from Peterson and Ferguson 1990.)

"activation" to the more potent T_3 is a step regulated individually by peripheral tissues (see Figs. 32.3 and 32.4). The vast majority (approximately 90%) of reverse T_3 (rT_3) is derived from extrathyroidal sources in the dog (Belshaw et al. 1974; Kaptein et al. 1993, 1994; Larsen et al. 1981).

TYPES AND REGULATION OF 5′-DEIODINASE ENZYME. The identification of three distinct types of 5′-deiodinase (5′-D) enzymes has underscored the importance of the regulation of T_3 production in individual tissues from T_4. Type I 5′-D is found in most peripheral tissues but has its highest activity in liver, kidney, muscle, and thyroid gland. This enzyme is now known to be a selenoenzyme requiring trace quantities of selenium for optimal activity. Muscle, although it has low enzyme activity, may produce a significant amount (approximately 60% in the rat) of the body's T_3 solely because of its large mass. The physiological role of type I 5′-D is the provision of *circulating* T_3. This enzyme is capable of "outer-ring" and "inner-ring" deiodination and can deiodinate T_4 with a high capacity and is sensitive to the thionamide antithyroid agent, propylthiouracil (PTU). Type II 5′-D is found in the central nervous system (CNS), pituitary, brown fat, and placenta, and its physiological role is provision of *intracellular* T_3. This enzyme acts upon T_4 and other compounds with outer-ring iodine at concentrations within the physiological range and is resistant to PTU. The type III 5′-D is present in placenta, CNS, skin, and fetal liver and has as its physiological role *inactivation* of T_4 and T_3 through *inner-ring* (ring with amino acid moiety) deiodination, with preference for T_3 as a substrate. The rationale for L-T_4 therapy in hypothyroidism is based on the disorder's dramatic reduction of the activity of the type I and III 5′-deiodinases and its increase of the activity of the type II enzyme. Through this regulation, the brain may continue to obtain cellular T_3 levels necessary to prevent or delay neurologic dysfunction resulting from T_4 deficiency, while the liver reduces its production of T_3, thereby leading to decreased systemic metabolism (see Fig. 32.4) (Burrow et al. 1989; Ferguson 1988; Larsen et al. 1981; Peterson and Ferguson 1990).

The process of deiodination continues until the thyroid hormone nucleus is stripped of its remaining iodine molecules, thereby allowing iodine to recycle for hormone resynthesis (Fig. 32.3). These further deiodinated metabolic products (other than T_3 and T_4) do not have thyromimetic activity. A number of nonthyroidal illnesses and drugs may affect the local tissue regulation of thyroid hormone deiodination. Other pathways of thyroid hormone metabolism include conjugation to form soluble glucuronides and sulfates for biliary or urinary excretion as well as cleavage of the ether linkage of the iodothyronine molecule (Braverman and Utiger 1991; Burrow et al. 1989; Ferguson 1984, 1988; Kaptein et al. 1994).

With oral administration of thyroid hormone preparations, the first-pass effect must be considered, as a large quantity of hormone can be conjugated and secreted into the bile, where the hormone may either be deconjugated and reabsorbed by bacteria in the large intestine or eliminated in the feces. The intestinal pool of thyroid hormone is known to be very large. In the dog, over 50% of the T_4 and about 30% of the T_3 produced each day are lost in the feces. In both the dog and cat, the extrathyroidal body stores of T_4 are eliminated and replaced in about 1 day, whereas stores of T_3 are lost and replaced twice daily (Kaptein et al. 1993, 1994). Such fecal wastage is responsible, in part, for the higher daily replacement doses of thyroid hormone required on a per body weight basis in dogs and cats. It is possible, but not proven, that, in some animals, dividing the daily oral replacement dose may serve to reduce the loss of hormone due to the hepatic first-pass effect, resulting in a more consistent clinical response.

Plasma Hormone Binding of Thyroid Hormone. Thyroid hormones are water-insoluble lipophilic compounds. Their ability to circulate in plasma is dependent upon binding by specific binding proteins, thyroxine-binding globulin (TBG) and thyroxine-binding prealbumin (TBPA; transthyretin), as well as by albumin itself. Thyroid hormone–binding proteins provide a hormone reservoir in the plasma and "buffer" hormone delivery into tissue (Fig. 32.4). TBPA and possibly albumin also may serve as intermediary carriers for specific tissue uptake of the hormone by tissues (Mendel 1989; Pardridge 1981). The dog has a high-affinity thyroid hormone–binding protein comparable to TBG in the human, but plasma concentrations of TBG in the dog are only 25% of those in the human. In addition to TBG, TBPA, and albumin, circulating T_4 in canine plasma appears to bind to certain plasma lipoproteins. These include a high-density lipoprotein (HDL_2) that migrates in the α_1 region on the electrophoretic pattern and a very low density lipoprotein (VLDL) that migrates in the β region. At normal serum T_4 concentrations in the dog, about 60% of T_4 is bound to TBG, 17% to TBPA, 12% to albumin, and 11% to the HDL_2. Thyroxine-binding globulin in the dog is not saturated until the total T_4 concentration is six times the normal serum T_4 values, whereas the other serum proteins are virtually unsaturable (Inada et al. 1975). The cat does not appear to have a high-affinity thyroid hormone–binding protein (such as TBG) but has only TBPA and albumin as serum thyroid hormone–binding proteins. Partly as a result of weaker serum protein binding, total T_4 concentrations are lower, the unbound, or free, fraction of circulating T_4 is higher, and hormone metabolism is more rapid in most domestic animals than in humans (Bigler 1976; Kaptein et al. 1994; Larsson et al. 1985; Larsson 1987).

Tissue Thyroid Hormone Uptake: The "Free Hormone" Hypothesis. The free hormone hypothesis, proposed by Robbins and Rall 40 years ago and restated by Mendel, states that it is the unbound fraction of hormone which is available to tissues and therefore proportional to the action, metabolism, and elimination of that hormone (Robbins and Rall 1960; Mendel 1989). This hypothesis has stood the clinical test of the past 40 years; direct or indirect measurements of free T_4 have been a mainstay in the diagnosis of thyroid disease in human medicine. There is also strong evidence that certain cell types actively transport or exchange thyroid hormone from the plasma into the cytosol. The presence of a plasma membrane protein specific for thyroid hormone transport certainly reflects the premium the cell is willing to pay to facilitate entry and possibly concentration of thyroid hormone. However, some investigators would argue that the serum binding proteins, particularly albumin and TBPA, may serve to distribute hormones to specific tissues. Most theories of thyroid hormone exchange have assigned a passive "reservoir" role to cytosolic thyroid hormone–binding proteins (CTBP; CBP in Fig. 32.4), the proteins that retain thyroid hormone in a predominantly bound state inside the cell. Little is known about the regulation of these proteins, which are often called "intracellular albumin" because of their low specificity, low affinity, and high capacity. However, in renal cytosol, the affinity of CTBP may be acutely regulated by cellular redox potential, increasing when nicotinamide adenine dinucleotide phosphate (NADPH) levels are high (Burrow et al. 1989; Hashizume et al. 1987; Kaptein et al. 1994; Mendel 1989; Pardridge 1981).

Irrespective of the mechanisms, the following observations in the clinical patient must be recognized:

1. The linear correlation between the serum free T_4 concentration, rate of hormonal degradation, and basal metabolic rate in humans.
2. The inverse correlation between the serum free T_4 concentration and the cellular distribution volume of T_4, which exists in all subjects regardless of thyroid state.
3. The positive correlation between the in vitro perfused organ free T_4 concentration and tissue T_4 uptake and T_3 production in vivo and in vitro. Most researchers agree that the steady-state tissue concentrations of hormone are the driving force for thyroid hormone metabolism and action (Mendel 1989).

In the healthy euthyroid dog or cat, about 0.1% of total concentration of serum T_4 is free (i.e., not bound to thyroid hormone–binding proteins), whereas about 1% of circulating T_3 is free (Ferguson and Peterson 1992; Kaptein et al. 1994). The proportion of free hormone may change in response to drug administration or illness. For example, plasma compounds in uremia (possibly free fatty acids) compete for hormone binding, resulting in a transient increase in free serum thyroid hormone concentrations but decreased total hormone values (Ferguson 1988, 1989b, 1994). However, it appears that the thyroid status of the animal does not change, since the absolute level of the free hormone concentrations tends to soon return to within normal range or remains relatively constant (Ferguson 1988, 1989b, 1994).

Most evidence suggests that the thyroid hormone uptake by tissues is proportional to but not limited to the free, or unbound, fraction of circulating hormone. Approximately 50–60% of the body's T_4 and 90–95%

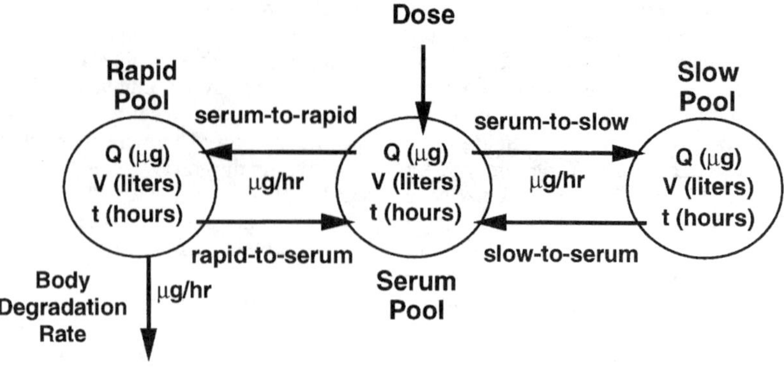

FIG. 32.5—Compartmental model of thyroid hormone metabolism.

of the body's T_3 are located in the intracellular compartment (Fish et al. 1997). Certain organs, particularly the liver and kidney, can concentrate thyroid hormones and exchange hormone rapidly with the plasma. In humans, about 60% of the intracellular T_4 is in these *rapidly equilibrating* tissues (liver and kidney), whereas only 6% of the intracellular T_3 is in these tissues. About 80% of all extrathyroidal T_3 is located in the *slowly equilibrating* tissues (e.g., muscle, skin), while only 20% of intracellular T_4 is in this compartment. As a result, most of the body's T_4 is located in plasma, interstitial fluid, liver, and kidney. The majority of the body's extrathyroidal T_3 is in the cells of the muscle and skin and in a conjugated form in the intestinal tract. Kaptein et al. have used a three-pool model to describe the distribution and metabolism of thyroid hormone metabolites and iodide (see Fig. 32.5). Table 32.1 compares the model parameters for T_4, T_3, rT_3, and iodide in dogs, cats, and humans (Kaptein et al. 1994).

Metabolic Clearance Rates. The plasma half-life of T_4 has been estimated to be 8 hours (Kaptein et al. 1993, 1994) or 10–16 hours in the dog (Fox and Nachreiner 1981) and 11 hours in the cat (Kaptein et al. 1994), compared to a plasma half-life of about 7 days in humans (see Table 32.2). The plasma half-life of T_3 in the dog has been estimated to be 5–6 hours, compared to 24–36 hours in humans. Studies in the normal cat indicate that the plasma half-lives of T_4 and T_3 are similar to those of the dog (Fox and Nachreiner 1981; Kaptein et al. 1994). It should be emphasized that these figures reflect plasma disappearance rates and do not necessarily indicate extent or duration of biological action.

EXTRATHYROIDAL FACTORS ALTERING THYROID HORMONE METABOLISM

Effect of Illness and Malnutrition. In humans, a wide range of clinical conditions such as chronic starvation or malnutrition, surgery, diabetes mellitus, hepatic and renal disease, and chronic systemic illness may result in decreased serum T_3 concentrations together with elevated serum rT_3 values. This "low T_3" syndrome results from inhibition of 5′-deiodinase, the enzyme necessary for conversion of T_4 to T_3 and the conversion of rT_3 to 3,3′-T_2 (Braverman and Utiger 1991; Burrow et al. 1989; Kaptein et al. 1994; Kaptein 1986).

The reduction in the production of T_3, the most potent thyroid hormone, appears to be a beneficial adaptive mechanism by which the body serves to limit the loss of protein and perhaps lower the metabolic rate during illness. Maintenance of serum T_3 concentrations (with T_3 replacement therapy) in euthyroid fasting humans leads to excessive nitrogen excretion and blunting of the pituitary's TSH response to TRH, as if there was a state of hyperthyroidism. At this time, the body of evidence does not support the contention that lowering of serum T_3 during malnutrition and illness is associated with "tissue" hypothyroidism. Also, other than these regulatory mechanisms, there is, as yet, no evidence that an isolated 5′-deiodinase deficiency exists in animals or in specific tissues (Braverman and Utiger 1991; Ferguson 1984, 1988; Kaptein et al. 1993, 1994; Kaptein 1986).

In acute and severe illnesses in humans, serum T_4 and T_3 concentrations may also fall, in what is called the "low-T_4 state of medical illness." Impaired serum protein binding of T_4 caused by inhibitors of binding (such as free fatty acids) or a reduction in binding-protein concentration results in reduced total serum T_4 concentrations and increased free fractions of T_4. In most cases, however, the absolute free T_4 concentrations remain normal. A fall in serum TSH concentrations may also contribute to the subnormal serum T_4 concentrations, especially in human patients treated with dopamine or glucocorticoids, drugs that inhibit TSH release. No studies have examined systematically the benefit or detriment of thyroid hormone therapy in domestic animals; however, studies of critically ill patients with low

TABLE 32.1—Thyroid hormone and iodide kinetics in normal dogs, cats, and humans using a three-pool model

	Dogs	Cats	Humans
T_4			
Plasma concentration (μg/dL)	2.8	1.68	6.8
Free fraction (%)	0.102	0.056	0.030
Total mean residence time (d)	0.54	0.69	6.8
Clearance rate (L/[kg·d])	0.24	0.38	0.017
Degradation rate (μg/[kg·d])	6.81	6.2	1.14
Total pool size (μg/kg)	3.7	4.3	7.8
Distribution (%)			
Plasma pool	46	13	32
Rapidly equilibrating pool	23	19	26
Slowly equilibrating pool	31	68	42
T_3			
Plasma concentration (ng/dL)	43	32	140
Free fraction (%)	1.426	0.48	0.299
Total mean residence time (d)	0.40	0.62	1.50
Clearance rate (L/[kg·d])	1.99	1.77	0.32
Degradation rate (μg/[kg·d])	0.84–0.89	0.52–2.2	0.43–0.46
Total pool size (μg/kg)	0.34	0.30	0.66
Distribution (%)			
Plasma pool	7	3.6	9
Rapidly equilibrating pool	29	18	19
Slowly equilibrating pool	64	79	73
Reverse T_3			
Plasma concentration (ng/dL)	22	—	13
Free fraction (%)	0.560	—	0.111
Total mean residence time (d)	0.12	—	0.16
Clearance rate (L/[kg·d])	1.44	—	1.78
Degradation rate (μg/[kg·d])	0.32–0.42	—	0.23–0.33
Total pool size (μg/kg)	0.039	—	0.036
Distribution (%)			
Plasma pool	31	—	15
Rapidly equilibrating pool	29	—	29
Slowly equilibrating pool	40	—	55
Inorganic iodide[a]			
Plasma mass (μg/kg)[b]	21	—	1.67
Total mean residence time (d)	1.07	0.82	0.35–0.36[c]
Clearance rate (L/[kg·d])	0.43	0.63	1.00–1.01
Total distribution volume (L/kg)	0.46	0.44	0.35–0.36
Distribution (%)			
Plasma pool	19	11	13[c]
Rapidly equilibrating pool	9	32	38
Slowly equilibrating pool	72	57	50

Source: Kaptein et al. 1994. Dog and human data from Kaptein et al. 1990; Kaptein et al. 1993. Cat data from Hays et al. 1988.

Note: Parameter values were estimated using a three-pool model. Only mean values are presented. Conversion to SI units: Total T_4 in μg/dL × 12.87 = nmol/L; total T_3 and reverse T_3 in ng/dL × 0.01536 = nmol/L.

[a]Thyroid gland unblocked for all species.

[b]Dog data from Belshaw et al. 1974.

[c]Data from Hays and Solomon 1965 (reanalyzed in three-pool model); Belshaw et al. 1974.

serum T_4 and T_3 concentrations have revealed that T_4 therapy is not beneficial and fails to improve survival (Kaptein 1986; Kaptein et al. 1993, 1994).

The effects of nonthyroidal illness on thyroid hormone metabolism in the dog are less well characterized than in humans. In the dog, depressed serum T_4 concentrations have been reported in various nonthyroidal illnesses such as hyperadrenocorticism (e.g., Cushing's syndrome), diabetes mellitus, hypoadrenocorticism (e.g., Addison's disease), chronic renal failure, hepatic disease, as well as a variety of other critical medical illnesses requiring intensive care (Ferguson 1984, 1988, 1994; Ferguson and Peterson 1992).

Effect of Drugs. A variety of drugs may impair plasma or tissue binding of the thyroid hormones or alter thyroid hormone metabolism. Drugs used in veterinary medicine that are most likely to alter circulating thyroid hormone concentrations include the glucocorticoids, anticonvulsants, quinidine, salicylates, phenylbutazone, and radiocontrast agents. The mechanisms by which these drugs exert their effect vary. Quinidine and other membrane-stabilizing drugs may inhibit 5′-deiodinase. Salicylates, furosemide, and oleic acid may directly displace thyroid hormone from plasma binding sites. Phenylbutazone appears to have a direct antithyroid (goitrogenic) effect in some species,

TABLE 32.2—Thyroxine kinetics in dogs, cats, and humans following intravenous, subcutaneous, and oral L-thyroxine administration

	Dogs	Cats	Humans
T_4 degradation rate (µg/[kg·day])	6.81	6.2	1.14
Intravenous			
Time to peak (hr)	0.02–0.03	0.02–0.03[a]	0.02–0.03
Total mean residence time (hr)	13.0	16.6[a]	164
Terminal half-life (hr)	7.6	10.7[b]	168
Subcutaneous			
Dosage (µg/[kg·day])	5–7	—	—
Absorption (%)	100[c]	—	81
Time to peak (hr)	1.5–1.8	—	72
Terminal half-life (hr)	14.7	—	120
Oral			
Dosage (µg/[kg·day])	20–40[c]	20–30[c]	2.11
Absorption (%)	10–50[c]	10.5[c]	50–80
Time to peak (hr)	—	3–4[c]	2–4
Terminal half-life (hr)	7.6	10.7[c]	168

Source: Kaptein et al. 1994. Data on dogs and humans from Kaptein et al. 1993.
Note: Conversion to SI units: Total T_4 in µg × 1.287 = nmol.
[a]Data from Hays et al. 1988.
[b]Data from Hays et al. 1992.
[c]Data from Hulter et al. 1984.

having been shown to decrease total and free T_4 in the horse (Ramirez et al. 1997). In vitro, it appears to decrease serum hormone binding. Radiocontrast agents (e.g, diatrizoate, iopanoic acid, ipodate, tyropanoate, and metrizamide) may act by preventing the uptake of T_4 by tissue, by directly inhibiting 5′-deiodinase or by releasing the iodine they contain to exert an antithyroid effect on the thyroid gland. No studies have been reported in domestic animals to evaluate the influence of these iodine-containing drugs on thyroid function tests or on subsequent radioiodine uptake (Ferguson 1984, 1989b, 1994).

Exogenous glucocorticoids have also been shown to have a profound effect on thyroid function tests in the dog, but similar studies have demonstrated only a small effect on serum T_4 levels in the cat and horse. A single high immunosuppressive dose of glucocorticoid (2.2 mg/kg prednisone, 0.6 mg/kg dexamethasone) will lower serum T_3 but not serum T_4 concentrations in the dog (Kemppainen et al. 1983; Laurberg and Boye 1984). Serum T_3 concentrations may be decreased because of glucocorticoid inhibition of 5′-deiodinase or simply because of a reduced availability of plasma T_4, the substrate for the enzyme. Most dogs on chronic, high-dose, daily glucocorticoid therapy will have very low or undetectable serum T_4 concentrations, as well as subnormal serum T_3 values (Ferguson and Peterson 1992; Kaptein et al. 1992; Kemppainen et al. 1983; Moore et al. 1993; Torres et al. 1992). Based upon electron microscopic examination of thyroid tissue, it was postulated that glucocorticoids may interfere with thyroid hormone secretion by inhibiting lysosomal hydrolysis of colloid in the follicular cell (Woltz et al. 1983). Because the thyroid retains its responsiveness to TSH during chronic glucocorticoid excess, suppression of pituitary TSH secretion is probably the primary and most important mechanism by which serum T_4 concentrations are suppressed. Measurement of TSH values after TRH administration have not confirmed a state of secondary hypothyroidism caused by glucocorticoids (Ferguson 1984, 1994; Moore et al. 1993).

The ability of a variety of other drugs to alter thyroid hormone metabolism or serum or tissue binding of the thyroid hormones has been well documented in the dog. The anticonvulsants diphenylhydantoin and phenobarbital, which are mixed-function oxidase inducers, consistently decrease serum T_4 concentrations to subnormal values, possibly by enhancing its rate of deiodinative metabolism and biliary excretion. It appears that free T_4 values also are slightly depressed (Kantrowitz et al. 1999).

A study evaluated the effect of a standard dosage of trimethoprim/sulfamethoxazole on thyroid function tests in dogs with pyoderma and normal baseline serum T_4 concentrations. The average serum T_4, but not T_3, concentration fell significantly during the treatment period of 6 weeks. The TSH response also fell in several dogs and radionuclide imaging suggested that the preparation (likely the sulfa component) interfered with iodine metabolism by the thyroid gland (Hall et al. 1993). The thyroid carcinogenic potential of sulfonamides, which has resulted in restriction of some forms in food animals, is likely due to its goitrogenic potential, chronic elevation of serum TSH, and subsequent stimulation of thyroid growth (Hall et al. 1993).

MECHANISMS OF THYROID HORMONE ACTION. Thyroid hormones (T_4 and/or T_3) act on many different cellular processes via specific ligand-receptor interactions with the nucleus, the mitochondria, and the plasma membrane (Fig. 32.4). The effects of thyroid hormone are seen in most tissues throughout the body. Although both L-T_4 and L-T_3 have intrinsic

TABLE 32.3—Relative nuclear binding affinity of thyroid hormone analogs to T_3

	Relative binding affinity (T_3 = 1)	
Analog	In vitro	In vivo
L-T_3	1.0	1.0
D-T_3	0.6	0.7
Triiodothyroacetic acid (triac)	1.6	1.0
Isopropyl T_2	1.0	1.0
L-T_4	0.1	0.1
Tetraiodothyroacetic acid (tetrac)	0.16	0.05
3,3′,5′-T_3 (reverse T_3)	0.001	0
Monoiodotyrosine	0	0
Diiodotyrosine	0	0

Source: Oppenheimer 1983.

metabolic activity, L-T_3 is 3–10 times more potent in binding to the nuclear receptors and similarly more potent in stimulating oxygen consumption (see Table 32.3). Except for the deaminated forms of T_4 and T_3 (tetraiodothyroacetic acid [Tetrac] and triiodothyroacetic acid [Triac], respectively), most thyroid hormone metabolites have little thyromimetic activity.

The effects of thyroid hormone can generally be divided into those that are rapid and evident within minutes to hours of administration, such as stimulation of amino acid transport and mitochondrial oxygen consumption, and those that require protein synthesis and a longer period of time (usually no sooner than six hours) to be manifested. Of course, the clinical manifestations may require weeks to months to clearly appreciate. About one-half of the increment in oxygen consumption produced by thyroid hormone has been related to activation of the plasma membrane-bound Na^+,K^+-ATPase, which, at least in the kidney and liver, is secondary to increases in passive K^+ fluxes caused directly and primarily by thyroid hormone via as yet undetermined mechanisms. These changes have been linked directly to the calorigenic effect of thyroid hormone. The rapid hormone effects can be observed clinically in the hypothyroid patient starting on thyroid replacement therapy by signs such as increased physical and mental activity (Braverman and Utiger 1991; Burrow et al. 1989; Greenspan 1994).

Nuclear Receptor–Mediated Effects of Thyroid Hormone. Chronic effects of thyroid hormone invariably are related to the cellular actions of the hormone requiring interaction with nuclear T_3 receptors followed by an increase in protein synthesis. Clinically, these are effects such as growth, differentiation, proliferation, and maturation. A common clinical presentation of thyroid insufficiency is bilateral symmetrical alopecia, the result of diminished turnover of shafts of hair within the hair follicle, resulting in greater numbers of telogen (inactive) hairs. Such changes are slow in onset and, upon treatment, slow to resolve.

Free thyroid hormone is translocated by passive diffusion or specific plasma membrane carriers to bind to

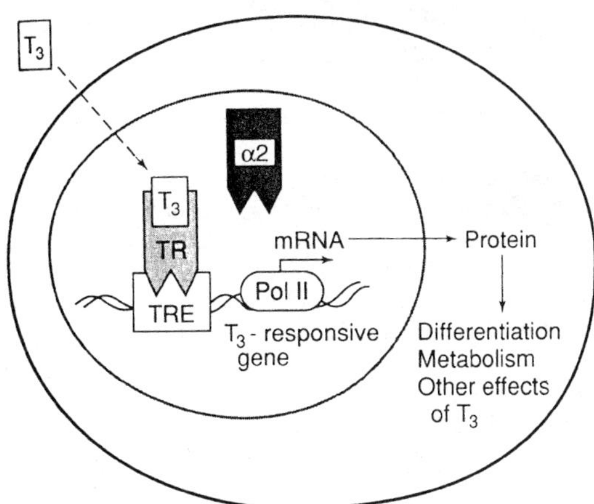

FIG. 32.6—Model of the mediation of T_3 action by nuclear thyroid hormone receptors (TR). T_3 either enters the cell (as depicted) or is derived from intracellular deiodination of T_4. Nuclear interaction between a T_3-bound TR and a thyroid hormone–responsive element (TRE) results in increased or decreased activity of RNA polymerase II (Pol II) on a T_3-responsive gene. The TRE is indicated as containing two half-sites, and the TR may bind as a dimer. Effects on mRNA levels are translated into increased or decreased cellular concentrations of proteins so as to promote differentiation, metabolic processes, and other cell-specific effects of T_3. In the absence of T_3, the TRE-bound TR may repress basal transcription. c-*erb*A_a2 (α2), the non-T_3-binding splice variant, can inhibit the effects of T_3-bound TRs by a mechanism that has not yet been established, probably involving heterodimer formation or competition for the TRE. A similar mechanism is likely to explain the dominant negative effect of the v-*erb*A oncoprotein and mutated TRs, as in the syndromes of generalized resistance to T_3. (Reprinted from Lazar and Chin 1990, Fig. 4-29.)

CTBP as a form of intracellular hormone storage, all in equilibrium with specific nuclear thyroid hormone receptors (see Fig. 32.6). The nuclear receptor for T_3 has been cloned and is a member of a family of receptors that is similar to the v-*erb* A receptor (which is a receptor for the avian erythroblastosis virus) and includes the nuclear glucocorticoid, mineralocorticoid, estrogen, progestin, vitamin D-3, and retinoic acid receptors. The human thyroid hormone receptor (hTR) exists in at least three forms: hTR-α1, hTR-α2, and hTR-β1. The α1 and β1 forms are associated with biological effects. Each receptor contains three domains: an amino terminal sequence that enhances receptor activity, a central DNA-binding domain, and a carboxyl-terminal hormone-binding domain. The thyroid hormone receptors are the specific thyroid hormone–responsive element (TRE) sites on the DNA in the absence of T_3. L-T_3 binding to the receptor results in stimulation or, in some cases, inhibition of the transcription of the genes, with changes in messenger RNA levels encoding the protein product of the genes that mediate the ultimate thyroid hormone biological response. When an action is mediated via the nuclear T_3 receptor, the binding affinity of thyroid analogs directly predicts the biological activity of that analog (see Table 32.3).

Extranuclear Actions of Thyroid Hormone. Some of the actions of thyroid hormone occur in the absence of new protein synthesis. There are direct nongenomic effects of thyroid hormone, such as the reduction of pituitary type II 5′-deiodinase enzyme, as well as stimulation of glucose and amino acid transport and Ca^{++}-ATPase activity in the red blood cell membranes of some species. A mitochondrial T_3 receptor has also been identified and has been postulated to mediate the activity of the mitochondrial ATP/ADP translocase, indirectly stimulating oxygen consumption (Greenspan et al. 1994).

Physiologic and Possible Pharmacologic Effects of Thyroid Hormone. Thyroid hormones, in physiological quantities, are anabolic. Working in conjunction with growth hormone and insulin, protein synthesis is stimulated and nitrogen excretion is reduced. However, in excess (i.e., hyperthyroidism), they can be catabolic, with an increase in gluconeogenesis, protein breakdown, and nitrogen wasting. Table 32.4 summarizes the multiple organ effects of thyroid hormones and the clinical manifestations of hormone deficit (hypothyroidism).

CALORIGENESIS AND THERMOREGULATION. Thyroid hormones increase oxygen consumption and heat production to a large extent by stimulating Na^+,K^+-ATPase in all tissues except the brain, spleen, and testis. As such, thyroid hormones determine the basal (resting) metabolic rate (BMR) of the animal. A reduced BMR results in mental dullness, lethargy, an unwillingness to exercise, hypothermia, and the tendency for the animal to seek heat (Greco et al. 1998). Once-daily administration of 0.022 mg/kg was sufficient to normalize BMR when measured by indirect calorimetry. Clinical signs in 93% of the dogs either improved or were completely resolved. This dosage was also shown to suppress TSH values to undetectable levels in most thyroidectomized dogs (Ferguson and Hoenig 1997).

EFFECTS ON GROWTH AND MATURATION. The fetus in most mammals is dependent on its own thyroid secretion. Thyroid hormones are crucial for growth and development of the skeleton and CNS. Therefore, in addition to the well-recognized signs of adult-onset hypothyroidism, prominent signs of congenital and juvenile-onset hypothyroidism are disproportionate dwarfism and impaired mental development (cretinism). With primary congenital hypothyroidism, enlargement of the thyroid gland (goiter) is also often observed. Puppies, kittens, and foals with this condition are behaviorally dull and less active and may have a shuffling gait and a poor appetite. On neurological

TABLE 32.4—Physiological effects of thyroid hormone

Site of action	Effect of hormone	Effects of deficit
Calorigenesis	Increase in BMR	Lethargy, weakness
Thermoregulation	O_2 consumption	Distal extremity hypothermia, heat-seeking
Growth and maturation	Normal CNS development	Mental retardation of cretin and dullness in adults; neuropathies
Carbohydrate metabolism	Increase in glycogenolysis and glycolysis, anti-insulin effects	Obesity despite normal or decreased appetite
Protein metabolism	Increased synthesis and degradation	Muscle weakness, poor hair coat and regrowth
Dermatologic	Normal maintenance of anagen hairs, maintenance of fatty acid turnover in skin, normal keratin turnover rates	Bilateral symmetrical alopecia, hyperkeratosis, myxedema
Cardiovascular	Stimulation of myosin ATPase, stimulation of Na^+,K^+-ATPase, increased β-receptor numbers	Decreased heart rate, pulse, pressure, and cardiac output
Neuromuscular	Normal myelin production, maintenance of balance between slow-twitch and fast-twitch fibers	Polyneuropathy, muscle atrophy, weakness, stiffness, myotonia
Gastrointestinal	Maintenance of normal electrical activity of GI smooth muscle, normal segmentation	Diarrhea or constipation
Reproductive	Maintenance of normal protein synthetic rates	*Female:* anestrus, irregular cycles, galactorrhea, stillbirth *Male:* azospermia, lack of libido
Immunologic	Stimulus of humoral and cell-mediated immunity	Recurrent infections (especially pyodermas)
Hematologic	Bone marrow stimulation, factor VIII and VIIIAg production, normal platelet synthesis and function	Nonresponsive anemia, possible bleeding tendency
Endocrine	Normal secretion of growth hormone, gonadotropins, cortisol; inhibition of secretion of prolactin	Secondary growth hormone deficiency, galactorrhea

Source: Modified from Ferguson 1989a.
Note: BMR = basal metabolic rate; CNS = central nervous system; GI = gastrointestinal.

examination, the animal is often weak and hyporeflexic or hyperreflexic (if there is muscle tremor or spasticity) and may lack conscious proprioception. Angular deformities have been observed in foals. Radiographic signs of underdeveloped epiphyses, shortened vertebral bodies, and delayed epiphyseal closure are common.

EFFECTS ON LIPID AND CARBOHYDRATE METABOLISM. Thyroid hormones increase gluconeogenesis and glycogenolysis, contributing to their insulin-antagonistic properties. Cholesterol synthesis and degradation are both increased by thyroid hormones and are mediated by an increase in hepatic low-density lipoprotein (LDL) receptors. Therefore, hypercholesterolemia is a common finding in hypothyroidism. Thyroid hormones stimulate lipolysis, releasing fatty acids and glycerol. Obesity may develop in some hypothyroid animals despite a normal appetite and caloric intake.

DERMATOLOGIC EFFECTS. Thyroid hormones in physiological quantities are necessary for normal hair and skin turnover. Thyroid insufficiency results in an increased percentage of telogen (inactive) hair follicles and an increase in keratin and sebum production. Dryness of the hair coat, excessive shedding, and retarded regrowth of hair are early signs of hypothyroidism in dogs. Alopecia, present in about two-thirds of affected dogs, is usually bilateral and symmetrical in distribution and is most obvious over points of friction, such as the ventral trunk and neck, axilla, and tail ("rat-tail" appearance), but also is common in the perineal area and the dorsum of the tail and nose. The alopecia is classically nonpruritic unless secondary seborrhea or dermatitis has developed. Thickening of the skin and/or the development of myxedema (subcutaneous accumulation of glycosaminoglycans) develop in some cases. Myxedema is most prominent in the facial features, which may take on a puffy or "tragic" appearance. The type and distribution of dermal fatty acids can even be stimulated by replacement dosages of thyroid hormone in euthyroid animals. It is possible that this effect is truly a pharmacological effect of thyroid hormones and might explain the improvement in hair coat that some dogs experience following thyroid hormone administration even when diagnostic tests fail to confirm hypothyroidism.

CARDIOVASCULAR EFFECTS. The major physiologic effects of thyroid hormones on the myocardium are (1) a direct positive inotropic effect, (2) stimulation of myocardial hypertrophy, and (3) increased responsiveness to adrenergic stimulation. Thyroid hormones increase the sarcolemmal Na^+,K^+-ATPase activity and favor the transcription of the α, or "fast-twitch," form of the cardiac myosin ATPase, improving cardiac contractility. In addition, myocardial contractility is improved by increasing the number of L-type calcium channels and enhancing sarcoplasmic reticulum calcium uptake and release.

Thyroid hormones increase the number of β-adrenergic receptors in the heart, skeletal muscle, adipose tissue, and lymphocytes. In hyperthyroidism, tachycardia often results from this mechanism. Thyroid hormones also decrease α-adrenergic receptors in cardiac and vascular tissue. In hypothyroidism, the sensitivity to catecholamines in the peripheral vasculature is increased and may lead to peripheral hypothermia.

NEUROMUSCULAR EFFECTS. Thyroid hormones stimulate the synthesis of many proteins associated with normal nerve and muscle activity. For example, nerve Na^+,K^+-ATPase and fast forms of the myosin ATPase in muscle are stimulated by thyroid hormones. Myopathies have also been associated with hypothyroidism in domestic animals. Severe muscle weakness and delayed reflexes may be the clinical manifestation, or the signs may be vague, such as stiffness, reluctance to move, and muscle wasting. Facial muscle and eyelid weakness (lip and lid droop) attributable to cranial nerve VII paralysis or paresis has been observed in dogs. Also, head tilt may be observed consistent with vestibular nerve disruption. These changes are likely due to the swelling of and around the dural sheath of the facial, vestibular, and cochlear nerves as they pass through bony foramina in the facial bones. Bilateral laryngeal paralysis has been associated with hypothyroidism in dogs as well. The pathophysiology of polyneuropathies associated with hypothyroidism is poorly understood but may be due to altered neuronal metabolism. Segmental demyelination and axonopathy have also been shown. Alternatively, compressive neurologic abnormalities may be the result of tissue swelling (myxedema) around the spinal cord or peripheral nerve. Clinically and electrodiagnostically, the polyneuropathy is indistinguishable from those caused by other diseases with hyporeflexia, slow nerve conduction velocities, fibrillation potentials, and positive sharp waves on electromyography. Although extremely rare, CNS signs of seizures, disorientation, and circling also have been reported in hypothyroid dogs with cerebrovascular atherosclerosis caused by the hyperlipidemia associated with hypothyroidism. Severe mental obtundation can also be observed in the syndromes of cretinism and myxedema coma.

GASTROINTESTINAL EFFECTS. Studies in hypothyroid dogs have demonstrated a decrease in the intestinal and gastric electrical and motor activity. Although hypothyroid dogs usually have normal bowel movements, constipation and diarrhea have also been observed.

REPRODUCTIVE EFFECTS. Normal thyroid hormone concentrations appear to be important for normal reproductive cycling of mammals. Hypothyroidism has been associated with a variety of reproductive disturbances in dogs and horses. In breeding bitches, persistent or sporadic anestrus, infertility, abortion, and high puppy mortality have been observed. Galactorrhea is a rare sign of hypothyroidism that develops in some intact female dogs whose mammae have been primed for lactation. Hyperprolactinemia, perhaps resulting from the excessive stimulation of prolactin-secreting pituitary cells by TRH, appears to be the cause of galactorrhea in susceptible bitches and may be at least partially responsible for the infertility associated with canine hypothyroidism. Lack of libido, testicular atrophy, hypospermia, and infertility have been suspected in the male with hypothyroidism, but studies of thyroidectomized dogs showed no changes in sperm count or motility. It is possible that there are components of autoimmune orchitis coexisting with autoimmune thyroiditis in the spontaneously developing form of hypothyroidism.

IMMUNOLOGIC EFFECTS. Any dog with a recurrent infection, particularly of the skin, should be evaluated for hypothyroidism. Pyoderma that is unresponsive or only temporarily responsive to appropriate antibacterial agents may be exacerbated by the reduced phagocytic function of white blood cells in hypothyroidism.

HEMATOLOGIC EFFECTS. The increased cellular demand for oxygen stimulated by thyroid hormones leads to increased production of erythropoietin and increased red blood cell production by the bone marrow. Thyroid hormones also increase the 2,3-diphosphoglycerate content of erythrocytes, allowing increased oxygen dissociation from hemoglobin and increased availability to tissues.

A cause-and-effect relationship between canine hypothyroidism and the development of an acquired coagulation defect (von Willebrand's disease) has been postulated, but controlled studies in hypothyroid dogs have not confirmed a relationship. Similarly, in dogs with von Willebrand's disease treated with thyroid hormone, a rise in factor VIII antigen has been described even when little evidence of primary hypothyroidism exists. The mechanism of action of T_4 in these circumstances is uncertain but may reflect the nonspecific action of thyroid hormone on protein synthesis. Since the breed incidence of von Willebrand's disease and hypothyroidism overlap (e.g., Doberman Pinscher, Golden Retriever, Miniature Schnauzer), it is critical to rule out the coexistence of these conditions in individual dogs where hypothyroidism may unmask a subclinical bleeding tendency. Platelet number and function can be decreased in hypothyroidism.

ENDOCRINE EFFECTS. Thyroid hormones influence the normal secretion and metabolism of a variety of hormones and xenobiotics. Secretion of growth hormone, gonadotropins, and cortisol is stimulated by thyroid hormones, and prolactin secretion is inhibited. Hypothyroidism may cause galactorrhea due to the subsequent increase in prolactin secretion in this condition (Braverman and Utiger 1991; Burrow et al. 1989; Ferguson 1989a, 1990, 1993; Ferguson and Hoenig 1991b; Greenspan 1994; Panciera and Johnson 1994, 1996; Johnson et al. 1999).

THYROID HORMONE PREPARATIONS. Thyroid hormone preparations can be classified into the following groups: (1) crude hormones prepared from animal thyroid gland, (2) synthetic L-thyroxine (L-T_4), and (3) synthetic L-triiodothyronine (L-T_3). The available products and dosage ranges are listed in Table 32.5.

Crude Thyroid Products. Thyroid hormone products derived from thyroid tissue from hogs, sheep, or cattle are available in the forms of desiccated thyroid (thyroglobulin). There are no good reasons to continue to use these products for replacement therapy in small animals; however, due to decreased cost, these products still have some utility in large animals. Problems with desiccated thyroid products include a highly variable content of T_4 and T_3, unphysiologically low ratios of T_4/T_3 (2:1 to 4:1), and short shelf life; these drawbacks outweigh the lower cost of these products. The newer standards set by the US Pharmacopoeia (USP) for control of hormone content may have improved the reproducibility of these products but are unlikely to eliminate the other disadvantages. A recent study compared the administration of T_4 to humans with replacing 50 μg of the normal T_4 dose with 12.5 μg of T_3. Neuropsychological methods were used for evaluation and revealed that the T_3-treated individuals showed improved cognitive performance (Bunevicius et al. 1999).

Synthetic L-Thyroxine. Thyroxine (L-T_4) is the thyroid hormone replacement compound of choice in all species. It is generally formulated and used as levothyroxine sodium for oral administration. Injectable forms are also available (for the rare indication of myxedema coma). Thyroxine is recommended for the following reasons:

1. L-T_4 is the main secretory product of the thyroid gland.
2. L-T_4 is the physiological "prohormone"; administration of L-T_4 does not bypass the cellular regulatory processes controlling the production of the more potent T_3 from T_4 (5′-deiodination).
3. In human patients with untreated hypothyroidism, serum TSH concentrations correlate inversely with serum T_4 concentrations and, to a lesser extent, with serum T_3 concentrations. However, as mentioned previously, recent evidence suggests that there might be some clinical benefits associated with administration of a small amount of T_3 in humans, and studies in rodents have long shown that normalization of TSH values with T_4 monotherapy often results in T_4 values that are in the high normal or high range.
4. The therapeutic goal should be to normalize both tissue and serum T_4 and T_3 concentrations, and this is accomplished in all tissues only with exogenous T_4 administration.
5. The CNS and pituitary derive a large proportion of their intracellular T_3 from local 5′-deiodination of T_4. With administration of T_3, the serum T_3 concentrations must be higher than normal to normalize serum TSH (see Fig. 32.7).

TABLE 32.5—Thyroid hormone replacement products

Drug	Product names	Dosage range and routes: Dog	Cat	Horse
L-Thyroxine	**Veterinary products:** Soloxine (Daniels); Nutrived Chewable Tablets (Vedco); Thyro-Tab (Vet-A-Mix); Thyro-Form (Vet-A-Mix); Thyro-L powder (Vet-A-Mix); ThyroSyn (Vedco); Levo-Tabs and Levo-Powder (Vetus); Thyroxine-L Tablets (Butler); Thyrozine (Phoenix); Thyroxine (W.V.S.); Chewable Thyroid Supplement (Heska): also includes vitamins D and E; Equisyn-T_4 (Eudaemonic); **Human products:** Levothroid (Forest); Levoxyl (Daniels); Synthroid (Knoll); Levo-T (Lederle)	0.02–0.04 mg/kg q24h or divided q12h PO or 0.5 mg/m^2 body surface area q24h or divided q12h PO; **Rarely necessary to exceed:** 1 mg/d	0.02–0.04 mg/kg q24h or divided q12h PO; **Rarely necessary to exceed:** 0.2 mg/d	0.01–0.1 mg/kg q24h or divided q12h PO; **Rarely necessary to exceed:** 100 mg/d
L-Thyroxine sodium for injection	Synthroid (Knoll); Levothroid (Forest)	100–200 µg IV or SC once	NA	NA
L-Triiodothyronine	Cytobin (Daniels) (veterinary); Cytomel (SK Beecham) (human)	4–6 µg/kg q8h PO	4.4 µg/kg q8–12h PO	NA
L-Triiodothyronine sodium for injection	Triostat Injection (SK Beecham) (human)	NA	NA	NA
Combination T_4/T_3 products	Thyrolar (Forest) (human) 4:1 T_4/T_3 ratio	Based on T_4 dose: see above	NA	NA
Desiccated thyroglobulin (human)	Thyroid USP (various generics); S-P-T (Fleming); Thyrar (Rhone Poulenc Rorer); Armour Thyroid (Forest); Thyroid Strong (Jones Medical)	NA	NA	15 grains/d/horse (~0.5–1.5 mg T_4/0.08–0.4 mg T_3)

Note: NA = not appropriate, applicable, or available. Products are listed in *Compendium of Veterinary Products,* 5th ed. (Port Huron, MI: North American Compendiums, Inc., 1999); *Physicians' Desk Reference,* 53rd ed. (Montvale, NJ: Medical Economics Data Production Co., 1999); *Facts and Comparisons,* CD-ROM (Wolters Kluwer, 1999).

6. In general, variability in bioavailability of synthetic T_4 preparations is less than for the crude products.
7. L-T_4 is less expensive than other synthetic preparations.

QUALITY CONTROL OF THYROID HORMONE PRODUCTS. In 1982, the USP adopted a new method for the assay of hormone content in thyroid hormone preparations. The old, less accurate determinations based upon iodine content were replaced by high-pressure liquid chromatographic (HPLC) determination. Recent studies of brand-name and generic L-T_4 preparations showed that the hormonal content of some generic tablets may be as little as 30% of the amount stated on the label. Therefore, when starting an animal on a thyroid replacement product, it is recommended to start with a brand-name product (or proven generic product) with which broad experience has been obtained and use this product until a distinct clinical response has been seen. If no response is seen at a reasonable dose after a period of at least 4–6 weeks, and normal serum T_4 concentrations are achieved after administration, then the

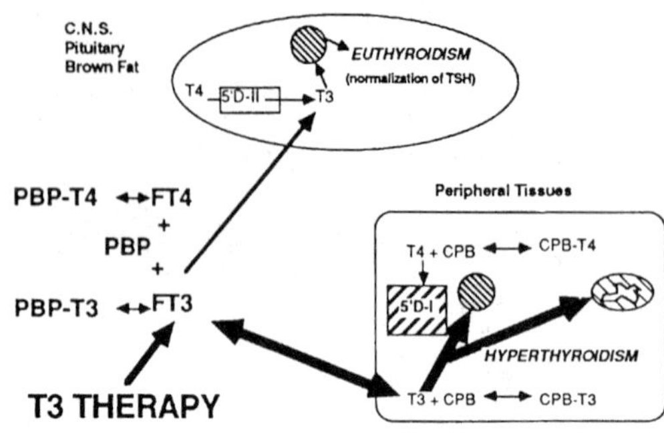

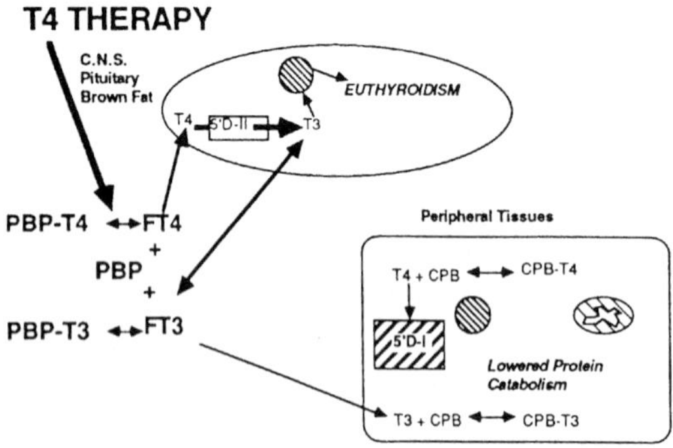

FIG. 32.7—Thyroid replacement therapy of hypothyroidism with L-T_3 (*top*) or L-T_4 in supervening nonthyroidal illness. *Top,* L-T_3 therapy during nonthyroidal illness bypasses the individual tissue regulation of the 5′-deiodinase enzymes. Shown is the scenario when the amount of T_3 administered is sufficient to re-create euthyroidism in the pituitary, brown fat, or CNS. In the pituitary, TSH secretion would be reduced to normal. This amount of T_3 would be excessive for tissues such as the liver and kidney, which are trying to limit protein catabolism during illness. A state of tissue hyperthyroidism results. *Bottom,* In contrast to therapy with L-T_3, L-T_4 therapy allows individual tissues to regulate T_3 production. Therefore, the brain, pituitary, and brown fat continue to produce adequate amounts of T_3 derived from plasma T_4, but the liver, kidney, and other tissues reduce local T_3 production, allowing a lowering of protein catabolism in illness. PBP = plasma binding protein, CBP = cytosolic binding protein, FT_3 = free triiodothyronine, FT_4 = free thyroxine. (Reprinted from Peterson and Ferguson 1990, Fig. 95-7.)

diagnosis should be reevaluated. Except for financial reasons, the concern about mild overreplacement is minimal in most cases since the dog (as well as the cat) are very resistant to the development of thyrotoxic signs, requiring 10–20 times the replacement dose chronically in order to demonstrate signs. This is likely the result of the dog's and cat's capacity to efficiently clear thyroid hormone via biliary and fecal excretion (Ferguson 1986; Kaptein et al. 1994).

DOSAGE CONSIDERATIONS FOR L-THYROXINE. Thyroid hormone replacement therapy is almost always indicated for the remainder of the dog's life. Therefore, careful initial diagnosis and tailoring of treatment is essential. A variety of dosage regimens for T_4 therapy have been recommended. This probably reflects the variation between animals in hormone absorption and metabolism, the variable degree of remaining endogenous hormone secretion by the failing thyroid, the possible effect of circulating anti-T_4 antibodies in a subgroup of animals, the resistance to the development of thyrotoxicosis with overdoses in the dog, and the vague and variable criteria by which clinical improvement is judged. With the advent of the canine TSH assay, objective analysis of the body's (at least the pituitary's) response to exogenous hormone replacement is now possible.

In addition to the mentioned effects of concomitant drug therapy on thyroid hormone metabolism, increased doses of T_4 appear to be necessary in hypothyroid humans during the colder months of winter. While similar studies have not been performed in animals, it is possible that an animal housed outdoors might require a higher dose of T_4 than an animal predominantly in the house, particularly during the colder months. In the dog, as in humans, basal serum concentrations of T_4 decrease with age. It has been observed in humans that older hypothyroid patients require lower doses of T_4 for adequate replacement and are more apt to develop the adverse effects of slight thyroid hormone overdoses (Ferguson 1986; Rosychuk 1982).

L-THYROXINE DOSAGES FOR THE DOG. Based upon isotopic kinetic studies, L-thyroxine is produced and degraded at the rate of 7 μg/kg/day in dogs (see Table 32.2) (Kaptein et al. 1993, 1994). In general, reported oral replacement doses for T_4 in the dog range from a total dose of 0.02 mg/kg to 0.04 mg/kg daily. Based upon this indirect evidence and studies by Ferguson and Hoenig (1997) of the oral bioavailability of common brand names of L-T_4, the fraction of oral absorption of L-T_4 products may range between 10 and 50%, averaging 35%, in part explaining the variation in oral dosage necessary to attain clinical euthyroidism. It has also been proposed that the dosage might be calculated according to body surface area (0.5 mg/m^2), reasoning that it is proportional to the metabolic rate. When the L-T_4 dosage is determined on a body weight basis, large-breed dogs have a greater tendency to develop thyrotoxicosis or, at least, elevated serum T_4 concentrations. For example, according to body surface area, a 5 kg (0.29 m^2 BSA) dog would start on a dose of 0.15 mg L-T_4 daily, or 0.03 mg/kg. A 50 kg dog (1.36 m^2 BSA) would start on 0.70 mg/day, or less than half the dose according to body weight, 0.014 mg/kg. There are no published experimental studies, however, to confirm the validity of this dosing method. It is rarely necessary to exceed 1 mg of L-T_4 per day in dogs, but some experts place the upper dosage at 1.6 mg per day (Ferguson 1986; Ferguson and Hoenig 1991b; Ferguson et al. 1992; Rosychuk 1982).

As thyroid replacement therapy is initiated, a common practice is to divide the total daily dosage into two separate doses given at 12-hour intervals. Because of the significant intracellular capacity for storage of T_4, particularly in rapidly exchanging pools like liver and kidney, the initial oral doses of thyroid hormone may be substantially distributed into tissue stores. As previously outlined, hypothyroidism reduces the deiodinative and conjugative rate of thyroid hormone metabolism. Division of the daily dose reduces the metabolic effect of a bolus of thyroid hormone on hypothyroid tissues and decreases the "one-pass" effect (i.e., hepatic metabolism and excretion of a portion of a bolus dose of hormone before ever reaching the systemic circulation). During the initial days to weeks of replacement therapy in a hypothyroid animal, the hormone stores of the liver and kidney are repleted to euthyroid levels and then can serve to "buffer" serum concentrations when the circulating hormone "store" bound to binding proteins begins to be depleted. The clinical result is that many hypothyroid animals can be maintained on once-daily T_4 therapy despite the fact that the serum half-life is much shorter. In humans, it seems that clinical improvement and suppression of serum TSH can be maintained by any replacement regimen that, over the course of a day, leads to a normal average serum concentration without leading to the acute toxic effects of thyroid hormone. Although the serum T_4 concentration might be high at one time of the day and low at another, the tissue response "integrates" the serum concentration throughout the day, thereby reflecting the average concentration. Once-daily administration also leads to greater compliance by owners. In an animal that has responded to twice-daily therapy, the reappearance of clinical signs of hypothyroidism on a once-daily regimen should be a signal to return to the successful twice-daily regimen. Because the metabolism of thyroid hormone changes with correction of hypothyroidism, dosage regimes should be reassessed by clinical and laboratory criteria after at least 4 weeks of initial therapy.

L-THYROXINE DOSAGES FOR THE CAT. As in the dog, the recommended treatment for feline hypothyroidism is daily administration of L-T_4, using an initial dose of 0.1–0.2 mg/day. This dosage should subsequently be adjusted on the basis of the cat's clinical response and postpill serum T_4 evaluation (as described below under Monitoring Therapy). Complete resolution of clinical signs can usually be expected in cats with adult-onset iatrogenic hypothyroidism. However, the mental dullness and dwarfism that develop in kittens with hypothyroidism usually persist because of the time elapsed between onset and diagnosis in these cats (Peterson and Ferguson 1990; Rosychuk 1982).

L-THYROXINE DOSAGES FOR THE HORSE. There is little published information establishing therapeutic criteria for L-T_4 dosing in the horse. The oral L-T_4 dosage required clinically appears to depend largely on the form of hormone (crude vs. synthetic) used for replacement therapy.

Synthetic L-Triiodothyronine. Although T_3 is the active intracellular hormone, there are few valid reasons to use this product for replacement therapy and some good reasons not to use it. T_3 therapy is not physiological, as it bypasses the final cellular regulatory step of 5′-deiodination of T_4 (see Fig. 32.7). T_4 does have intrinsic thyromimetic activity. Its role is particularly important in the CNS and pituitary, tissues in which normalization of the intracellular T_3 concentration depends upon the normalization of both serum T_4 and T_3. Treatment with T_3 alone may provide amounts sufficient for organs like the liver, kidney, and heart, which derive a high proportion of T_3 from plasma. However, the brain and pituitary, which derive a majority of their T_3 from T_4 intracellularly, may then be deficient in thyroid hormone. Conversely, T_3 therapy adequate for the brain and pituitary may be excessive for the liver, kidney, and heart (see Fig. 32.7, top).

At present, it cannot be recommended that T_3 therapy be instituted in the "low-T_3 syndrome" associated with nonthyroidal illness. Because of its higher oral bioavailability, it may be used to improve the clinical response in a dog with demonstrated or suspected poor T_4 absorption in which posttherapy serum T_4 and T_3 concentrations remain low despite increases in the oral daily T_4 dose. T_3 therapy may be indicated when thyroid replacement is necessary because of the simultaneous administration of drugs, such as glucocorticoids, that inhibit the conversion of T_4 to T_3.

Anecdotal reports suggest that a small fraction of hypothyroid dogs convert T_4 to T_3 poorly in the absence of obvious nonthyroidal illness and, therefore, do not respond to L-T_4 therapy. T_3 therapy has been recommended in these cases as an adjunct to T_4 or as sole therapy. The most likely cause of apparently low serum T_3 concentrations and normal or high T_4 concentrations following T_4 therapy is the presence of anti-T_3 antibodies, which, in certain T_3 radioimmunoassays, will result in an extremely low reading for the T_3 concentration. This observation is an in vitro artifact that has no relevance to the choice of replacement therapy products. Because the binding capacity of antithyroid hormone antibodies is easily overcome in most cases, it is recommended that usual dosages of L-T_4 be administered and the dose increased (if needed) until a clinical response is seen. The posttreatment serum T_3 concentration should be ignored in these dogs with T_3 autoantibodies (Ferguson 1986; Rosychuk 1982).

TRIIODOTHYRONINE (T_3) SUPPRESSION TEST IN THE CAT. As part of a workup for hyperthyroidism in cats, the administration of L-T_3 is utilized to evaluate the autonomy of thyroid secretion from the influence of pituitary TSH. L-T_3 is administered at a dose of 25 μg every 8 hours for 2 days, giving a seventh dose on the morning of the third day. A blood sample for serum T_4 measurement is taken before T_3 administration and again at 4 hours after the last dose. Presumably mediated via a fall in pituitary TSH, serum T_4 is depressed by at least 50% in normal cats, whereas little suppression is seen in cats with hyperthyroidism because TSH is already depressed. The advantages of this test are that the doses of T_3 can be given at home on an outpatient basis, with an office visit 4 hours after the last dose (Graves and Peterson 1994; Peterson and Ferguson 1990).

Effects of Thyroid Hormone Overdose (Iatrogenic Thyrotoxicosis). Except for financial reasons, the concern about mild overreplacement is minimal in most cases because the dog is very resistant to the development of thyrotoxic signs. This resistance to iatrogenic thyrotoxicosis is the result of the dog's capacity to efficiently clear thyroid hormone via biliary and fecal excretion. Animals on replacement therapy, particularly with a T_3-containing product, can develop signs of thyrotoxicosis; however, the incidence at recommended doses is rare. Animals should be monitored for signs suggesting an overdose, including polyuria, polydipsia, nervousness, weight loss, increase in appetite, panting, and fever. Diagnosis is confirmed by elevated serum T_4 and/or T_3 concentrations and the amelioration of signs by temporary discontinuation of therapy. Following accidental ingestion of massive amounts of L-T_4, dogs should be treated with activated charcoal within several hours of ingestion, possibly managed with β-adrenergic blockers if tachycardic, and heart rate and body temperature should be carefully monitored. Clinical experience has generally shown that dogs survive intoxication with few side effects despite considerable elevations in serum T_4 and T_3 concentrations.

Therapeutic Trial for Diagnosis of Hypothyroidism. Thyroid replacement therapy, without confirmatory laboratory evidence of hypothyroidism, has been suggested as a valid diagnostic step in a dog suspected to be hypothyroid. Although the major factor cited in defense of this practice is the cost of the diagnostic testing for the owner, it should be emphasized to an owner that replacement therapy is generally necessary for the remainder of the animal's life. Therefore, an incorrect diagnosis (and unnecessary long-term thyroid hormone treatment) can also be quite expensive. In one study of normal dogs given L-T_4 at the dosage of 0.5 mg/m^2 twice daily, the mean serum T4 response to exogenous TSH had suppressed to 56% and 46% of the pretreatment value when retested at 4 and 8 weeks on treatment, respectively. Four weeks after cessation of L-T_4 therapy, the serum T_4 response to TSH was still slightly suppressed, indicative of residual thyroid atrophy (Panciera et al. 1990). Therefore, if TSH stimulation testing is used to confirm the diagnosis of hypothyroidism in a dog that has recently been receiving thyroid hormone, TSH testing should not be performed for at least four weeks following discontinuation of thyroid hormone replacement therapy.

Monitoring Therapy. The most important indicator of the success of thyroid replacement therapy is the progress made toward ameliorating clinical signs. Before therapy is begun, the clinician and owner should have a clear idea of the goals of therapy and the time frame in which these goals can reasonably be achieved. The reversal of changes in hair coat and body weight should be assessed no sooner than after 2 months of therapy. In cases in which clinical improvement is marginal or signs of thyrotoxicosis are seen, the clinical observations can be supported by therapeutic monitoring of serum thyroid hormone concentrations ("postpill testing"). Clearly, the documentation of distinctly elevated serum T_4 concentrations following T_4 administration and elevated serum T_3 concentrations following T_3 administration, concomitant with signs of thyrotoxicosis, confirms an overdose. The interpretation of postpill serum thyroid hormone concentrations in cases of suspected underdosing can be more complicated because the timing of sampling may be critical to the proper interpretation. Ideally, therapeutic monitoring should not be attempted until steady-state conditions are reached, minimally 1 week after the initiation of therapy from a pharmacokinetic standpoint, but probably 1 month after initiation of therapy from a pharmacodynamic and clinical standpoint. With once-daily T_4 administration, the peak serum concentrations of T_4 generally should be in the high normal to slightly high range 4–8 hours after dosing and should be low normal to normal 24 hours after dosing. Given the dog's resistance to signs of thyrotoxicosis, it may be reasonable and adequate to check the serum T_4 concentration 24 hours after the previous day's dose. This is the method of choice of the author. In this situation, serum T_4 concentrations should still be in the normal range. Some endocrinologists prefer to measure "peak" T_4 concentrations at 4 or 6 hours after once-daily dosing, and some measure at "peak" and "trough" times. Animals on twice-daily administration probably can be checked at any time, but peak concentrations can be expected at the middle of the dosing interval (4–8 hours) and the nadir just prior to the next dose. Once the dog's dose is stabilized, once- or twice-yearly checks of serum T_4 (with or without T_3) concentrations are recommended.

With the advent of the canine TSH assay, monitoring therapy became possible by measurement of suppression of serum TSH. With the current generation of assay, TSH concentrations are elevated only in about 75% of cases. In those cases where it is elevated, suppression of TSH into the normal range or even lower to the undetectable range is evidence that the body has adequate amounts of thyroid hormone in the serum. Unfortunately, the assay sensitivity does not allow the distinction of normal values from low values, so establishment of overtreatment and hyperthyroidism is not yet possible. In a study of treatment of thyroidectomized dogs, it was shown that dosages as little as 0.02 mg/kg once a day will almost always suppress endogenous TSH concentrations into the normal or undetectable range. This observation establishes that the biological half-life of thyroid hormone exceeds by far the serum half-life (Ferguson and Hoenig 1997).

Although not recommended routinely, serum T_3 measurements following L-T_4 administration should be interpreted together with the serum T_4 results and, most important, the clinical response. Low serum T_3 and T_4 concentrations, together with a poor clinical response, suggest an underdose or inadequate bioavailability (absorption). With T_3 administration, serum concentrations are reported to peak 2–3 hours after administration. Serum T_4 concentrations are routinely low or undetectable in dogs receiving T_3 therapy. Any remaining endogenous thyroidal T_4 secretion will be inhibited because of the suppression of pituitary TSH secretion by T_3 (Ferguson 1986; Peterson and Ferguson 1990; Rosychuk 1982).

Therapeutic Failure. If clinical signs of hypothyroidism remain despite the use of reasonable doses of thyroid hormone, the following possibilities must be considered: (1) the dose or frequency of administration is improper, (2) the owner is not complying with instructions or is not successfully administering the product, (3) the animal may not be absorbing the product well or is metabolizing and/or excreting it too rapidly, (4) the product is outdated, or (5) the diagnosis is incorrect. A syndrome of tissue resistance to thyroid hormone, while described in humans, has not yet been documented in the dog or cat.

Treatment of Myxedema Coma. Myxedema coma is a rare condition in domestic animals (only described in dogs to date) caused by severe untreated hypothyroidism. Often induced by an anesthetic episode, it results in severe mental obtundation or coma and hypothermia. Because of the extremely high mortality associated with this condition, it is essential that treatment be instituted promptly and vigorously as soon as the diagnosis is made. Treatment should include an intravenous dose of L-T_4 prepared for injection (100–200 μg), passive rewarming (wrapping in blankets, etc.), and mechanical respiratory support as needed. Therapy for shock must include glucocorticoids and fluid and electrolyte replacement. Oral T_4 therapy can be instituted when the animal stabilizes.

ANTITHYROID DRUGS

Goitrogens. With the isolation and purification of thyroid peroxidase (TPO) enzyme of the thyroid gland, it became apparent that most compounds with antithyroid (goitrogenic) activity are inhibitors of TPO-catalyzed iodination. Plants of the genus *Brassica,* such as rutabaga, cabbage, and turnip, contain a compound called *goitrin* (see structure in Fig. 32.8), which has antithyroid activity. In addition, plants such as broccoli and rapeseed include glucosinolates, which are metabolized to thiocyanate, an inhibitor of thyroid iodide uptake and organification. The so-called cyanogenic glucosides, found in foods such as cassava, lima beans, and sweet potatoes, can be a source of cyanide, which then is detoxified to thiocyanate. Substituted phenols, such as resorcinol, phloroglucinol, and 2,4,dihydroxybenzoic acid, which may be found as contaminants in the water supply near coal conversion plants and may arise from degradation of flavonoids in plant material, also have goitrogenic activity (Taurog 1991; Brucker-Davis 1998).

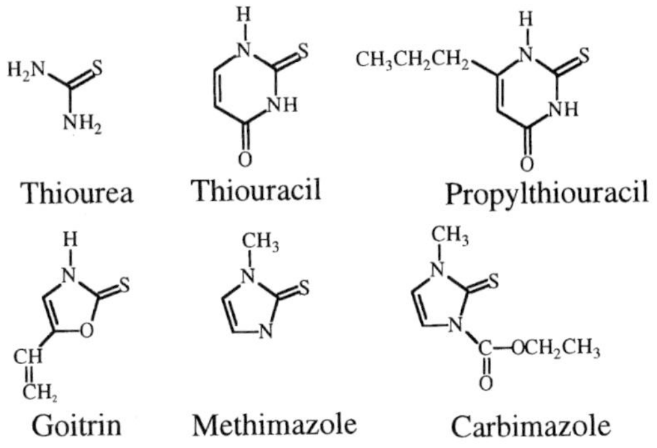

Thiourea Thiouracil Propylthiouracil

Goitrin Methimazole Carbimazole

FIG. 32.8—Thioureylene antithyroid drugs.

Thioureylenes (Thionamides). The thyroid organification and coupling steps are sensitive to inhibition by the antithyroid thioureylene (thionamide) drugs, which act to block thyroid hormone secretion. Fig. 32.8 shows the structure of thiourea, goitrin, and the antithyroid drugs thiouracil, propylthiouracil (PTU), methimazole (MMI), and carbimazole. After administration, these drugs are actively concentrated by the thyroid gland, where they act to inhibit the synthesis of thyroid hormones through the following mechanisms: (1) by blocking the incorporation of iodine into the tyrosyl groups in thyroglobulin; (2) by preventing the coupling of iodotyrosyl groups (mono- and di-iodotyrosines) to form the ether linkage of T_4 and T_3; and (3) through direct interactions with the thyroglobulin molecule (Fig. 32.1). Processes 1 and 2 are mediated by inhibition of the enzyme TPO. Thioureylene antithyroid drugs do not interfere with the thyroid gland's ability to concentrate, or "trap," inorganic iodine, do not block the release of stored thyroid hormone into the circulation, and do not damage the thyroid glandular tissue.

The thioureylene drugs PTU and MMI are the most commonly used antithyroid drugs in veterinary clinical practice (see Table 32.6 for products and dosages). Following initiation of treatment with MMI or PTU there is usually a slight delay in the fall of serum thyroid hormone concentrations as glandular hormone stores become depleted. PTU has the additional beneficial effect of blocking the conversion of T_4 to the more active T_3 in peripheral tissues like the liver and kidney. Therefore, serum T_4 may fall following both PTU and MMI therapy, but with MMI, due to autoregulatory mechanisms in the peripheral tissues, serum T_3 is usually maintained within the normal range even when T_4

TABLE 32.6—Antithyroid drugs

Drug	Product name	Dosage range and route (cats only)
Methimazole	Tapazole (Daniels Pharmaceuticals)	*Initial:* 2.5–5 mg q8–24h PO *Maintenance:* 2.5–20 mg q12–24h
Carbimazole	Available in Europe	Same as methimazole
Propylthiouracil	Propylthiouracil USP generics (Daniels Pharmaceuticals): e.g., Barr, Geneva, Major, Rugby, Schein	50 mg q8–12h PO
Ipodate	Orografin (Squibb)	*Initial:* 15 mg/kg q12h PO *Maintenance:* as needed up to 400 mg/cat/d (Note: dosage lowers serum T_3 only)
Potassium iodine (Lugol's)		50 mg q12–24h PO

is quite low. As a result of this mechanism, it is rare to see a cat on MMI develop clinical signs of hypothyroidism. In some elderly hyperthyroid cats, elevations in serum creatinine with occasional overt renal failure develop. In cases where pretreatment renal function is in question, the use of MMI has gained favor because it provides a reversible and more gradual mode of therapy for returning the animal to euthyroidism. It is not yet known whether the changes in renal function parameters are associated with the correction of hyperthyroidism to euthyroidism or rather to the transient development of hypothyroidism.

PROPYLTHIOURACIL. Despite its apparent additional therapeutic effects, the use of PTU has fallen out of favor because of its potential for serious side effects. Like MMI, it can cause anorexia, vomiting, lethargy, and the development of positive antinuclear antibody titers, and it has also been associated with the development of autoimmune hemolytic anemia and immune-mediated thrombocytopenia. Because of the latter two complications, which are a particular problem in the animal being prepared for surgery, PTU can no longer be recommended for routine use in the hyperthyroid cat (Ferguson and Hoenig 1991a; Ferguson et al. 1992; Kintzer 1994; Peterson and Ferguson 1990).

METHIMAZOLE. MMI is now the antithyroid medication of choice in the cat. The use of this drug in the cat has been well documented by a study of a 3-year experience with the drug in almost 300 cats. The administration of 5 mg three times daily will generally bring the serum T_4 concentrations down into the normal range by 2–3 weeks. From there, the daily dose of MMI should be adjusted upward or downward in 2.5 mg (1/2 tablet) intervals until the serum T_4 concentration falls within the normal range. As mentioned, even cats with low serum T_4 may not become hypothyroid because the serum T_3 concentration is normal. Once a satisfactory therapeutic effect is seen, many cats can be maintained on once-daily therapy, a major advantage for owner compliance. However, if a daily dose is missed, the serum T_4 concentration may rise rapidly. Cats on chronic MMI therapy should be checked every 3–6 months to draw blood for serum T_4 measurement and to monitor for signs of drug toxicity (see below) (Peterson et al. 1988).

PHARMACOKINETICS AND PHARMACODYNAMICS. Despite a serum half-life for MMI of only 4–6 hours, studies in human hyperthyroid patients have shown that the drug has an intrathyroidal residence time of approximately 20 hours. Since antithyroid drugs inhibit thyroid hormone synthesis only after they are concentrated within the thyroid gland, serum half-life of these drugs is of lesser importance than the intrathyroidal drug concentration for adequate control of the hyperthyroid state. A study of the pharmacokinetics of methimazole in normal cats has demonstrated that the bioavailability of the drug is highly variable (45–98%), as is the volume of distribution (0.12–0.84 L/kg). After oral dosing, the plasma elimination half-life ranges from 2.3 to 10.2 hours. There is usually a 1–3 week lag time between starting the drug and significant reductions in serum T_4 (Trepanier et al. 1989).

ADVERSE EFFECTS. MMI has been associated with the following adverse effects: anorexia (11.1%), vomiting (10.7%), lethargy (8.8%), excoriations (2.3%), bleeding (2.3%), hepatopathy (1.5%), thrombocytopenia (2.7%), agranulocytosis (1.5%), leukopenia (4.7%), eosinophilia (11.3%), lymphocytosis (7.2%), positive antinuclear antibodies (21.8%), positive direct antiglobulin test (1.9%). The gastrointestinal adverse effects generally developed within the first month of treatment and usually resolved even with continued therapy.

Mild clinical side effects associated with MMI treatment are relatively common (approximately 15% of cats) and include anorexia, vomiting, and lethargy. In most cats, these adverse signs are transient and resolve despite continued administration of the drug. Severe gastrointestinal signs persist in some cats, however, necessitating discontinuation of the drug. Self-induced excoriations of the face and neck also may develop in a few cats within the first 6 weeks of therapy. Although these cutaneous lesions tend to be partially responsive to treatment with systemic glucocorticoids, cessation of MMI administration is usually required for complete resolution of these excoriations. Finally, hepatic toxicity is an uncommon but serious reaction that can develop during drug treatment. MMI-induced hepatopathy is characterized by the development of marked increases in serum concentrations of ALT, AST, SAP, and total bilirubin. Clinical improvement, with resolution of anorexia, vomiting, and lethargy, usually occurs within a few days after cessation of MMI, but jaundice and abnormal serum biochemical tests indicative of liver disease may not resolve for several weeks. Rechallenge with the drug will again induce clinical signs and serum biochemical abnormalities indicative of hepatic disease within a few days. A variety of hematologic abnormalities may develop in cats during treatment with MMI. Those abnormalities that do not appear to be associated with any adverse effects include eosinophilia, lymphocytosis, and transient leukopenia with a normal differential count. As with PTU treatment, more serious hematologic reactions which develop in a few cats treated with MMI include severe thrombocytopenia (platelet count $< 75{,}000$ cells/mm^3) and agranulocytosis (severe leukopenia with a total granulocyte count < 250 cells/mm^3). Most cats that develop severe thrombocytopenia also show concomitant overt bleeding (i.e., epistaxis, oral hemorrhage). Development of agranulocytosis during MMI treatment predisposes to severe bacterial infections, systemic toxicity, and fever. If serious hematologic reactions develop during MMI therapy, the drug should be stopped and supportive care given; these adverse reactions should resolve within 5 days after MMI is withdrawn. Since most life-threatening side effects (e.g., hepatopathy, thrombocytopenia, agranulocytosis) caused by MMI treatment usually develop quickly again after rechallenge with the drug, alternative therapy with either surgery or radioiodine should be considered in these cases.

During MMI therapy, serum antinuclear antibodies (ANA) develop in a high percentage of cats. The risk of developing ANA appears to increase with the duration of MMI treatment, with ANA developing in approximately half of cats treated for longer than 6 months. The risk of developing serum ANA also appears to be greater for cats treated with higher daily MMI doses, since most cats that develop ANA are receiving doses ≥15 mg/day. ANA will disappear in most cats after the dosage is decreased. Despite the high prevalence of ANA development during long-term treatment with MMI, clinical signs associated with a lupus-like syndrome (i.e., dermatitis, polyarthritis, glomerulonephritis, hemolytic anemia, or fever) have not been observed in any of these cats. The daily drug dosage should therefore be decreased to as low as possible (while still maintaining serum T_4 values within the low-normal range), since ANA tests will become negative in many cats when the MMI dosage is decreased.

CARBIMAZOLE. The antithyroid drug carbimazole is a carbethoxy derivative of MMI that is rapidly and completely metabolized to the parent compound, which is responsible for its antithyroid activity. It is commonly used in treatment of feline hyperthyroidism outside North America. Carbimazole is a larger molecule than MMI; 10 mg of carbimazole is equimolar to 6 mg MMI. To achieve the same effect with carbimazole as with MMI, approximately twice the dosage of carbimazole is required. Clinical experience in Europe describes fewer gastrointestinal side effects for this medication. It is not apparent from the similar pharmacokinetics and the conversion of carbimazole to MMI why fewer serious side effects apparently occur with the use of carbimazole for treatment of hyperthyroidism (Peterson and Becker 1984).

Nonthioureylene Antithyroid Agents

IPODATE. Ipodate, a biliary radiographic contrast agent, has proven in both experimental hyperthyroidism and in spontaneously hyperthyroid cats to be an alternative medical treatment for patients not tolerating MMI or PTU. The structure of this iodinated compound is compared with L-T_3 in Fig. 32.9. In a study of cats in which hyperthyroidism was experimentally induced by the administration of T_4, ipodate significantly reduced the serum T_3 concentrations and was well tolerated by otherwise healthy cats. At the dose of 15 mg/kg BID orally, some cats with spontaneous hyperthyroidism anecdotally have shown improvement of clinical signs associated with a fall in serum T_3, even when serum T_4 concentrations do not fall. Although not yet studied, higher doses may result in a fall in serum T_4. Because ipodate contains 62% organic iodine, it should not be used immediately prior to radioiodine therapy. A withdrawal period of 3–6 months before definitive radioiodine therapy is recommended in human patients. Although not yet studied in the cat, a considerably shorter period off of medication is likely sufficient to allow washout of the drug and excess iodide. In addition to blocking thyroidal and peripheral hormone synthesis and deiodination like PTU, ipodate may also interfere with the action of thyroid hormone at the cellular level (Chopra et al. 1984; Ferguson et al. 1988; Murray and Peterson 1997).

RADIOACTIVE IODINE (^{131}I) THERAPY. Although only available in specialty referral centers, radioiodine

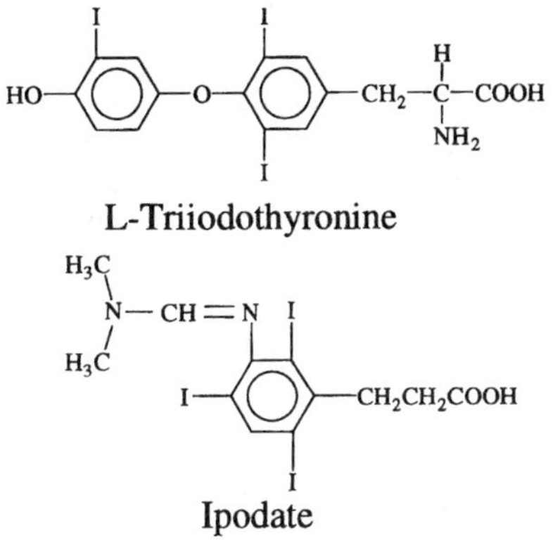

L-Triiodothyronine

Ipodate

FIG. 32.9—Comparison of ipodate and L-triiodothyronine structures.

treatment is the most effective and appropriate cure for toxic goiter in the cat because it selectively destroys the functioning thyroid tissue after being selectively taken up and incorporated into thyroid hormone precursors in the thyroid gland. There is rarely, if ever, damage to the nearby tissue responsible for regulating serum calcium by the secretion of parathyroid hormone and calcitonin. Iodine-131 has a half-life of 8 days and produces both gamma and beta radiation. The beta particles, with a short pathlength, produce most of the local tissue destruction. Radioiodine is also used in much higher doses in an attempt to ablate thyroid adenocarcinomas in cats and dogs. Following a therapeutic dose (generally 1–5 millicuries) of ^{131}I, the serum T_4 and T_3 concentrations will normalize within 1–2 weeks. The efficacy of radioiodine is reduced by recent antithyroid medical therapy, as these drugs reduce the long-term incorporation of iodine into the thyroid gland and reduce radioiodine's therapeutic effect. The major disadvantage of radioiodine therapy is that certain radiation safety precautions must be taken. Radioiodine is secreted in saliva and excreted in urine and feces. As such, handling of the cat's hair coat or waste may result in contamination. Unlike human patients, who may receive therapeutic doses on a outpatient basis, radioiodine-treated cats must be hospitalized for periods of 1–4 weeks, depending upon the dose administered and the radiation safety regulations. Despite these drawbacks, radioiodine therapy is the least invasive cure for bilateral adenomatous goiter, has no hypoparathyroidism or toxicity associated with it, and can be implemented without anesthesia or sedation, an important consideration in the elderly cat with other medical complications (Kintzer and Peterson 1991, 1994; Meric et al. 1986).

THYROID IMAGING. Thyroid imaging is performed using radioactive iodine or $^{99m}TcO_4^-$ (pertechnetate), which is taken up by mechanisms similar to iodide but is not incorporated into iodothyronines on thyroglobulin. Because of its rapid uptake and increased safety, technetium can be given in higher diagnostic doses and provides a better image than radioiodine. A semiquantitative comparison of technetium uptake to that of the salivary glands, which also take up iodide, can be used to assess increased uptake. Thyroid imaging also aids the diagnosis when an obvious enlargement of one thyroid lobe exists. Imaging is particularly useful in the diagnosis of the 30% of cases that are unilateral, as the function of the contralateral lobe is suppressed and not apparent on the scan. Thyroid imaging is also useful in cats with adenomas that have slipped into the mediastinum or the 1–2% of cats with adenocarcinomas that have a tendency to metastasize by extension into the mediastinum (Kintzer and Peterson 1991, 1994).

REFERENCES

Belshaw, B. E., Barandes, M., and Becker, D. V. 1974. A model of iodine kinetics in the dog. Endocrinology 95:1078–1093.

Bigler, B. 1976. Thyroxine-binding serum proteins in the cat: a comparison with dog and man. Schweiz Archiv Tierheilkd 118(12):559–662.

Braverman, L. E., and Utiger, R. D. (eds). 1991. Werner and Ingbar's The Thyroid: A Fundamental and Clinical Text, 6th ed. Philadelphia: Lippincott.

Brent, G. A., Moore, D. D., and Larsen, P. R. 1991. Thyroid hormone regulation of gene expression. Ann Rev Physiol 53:17–35.

Brucker-Davis, F. 1998. Effects of environmental synthetic chemicals on thyroid function. Thyroid 8:827–856.

Bruner, J. M., Scott-Moncrieff, C. R., and Williams, D. A. 1998. Effect of time of sample collection on serum thyroid-stimulating hormone concentrations in euthyroid and hypothyroid dogs. J Am Vet Med Assoc 212:1572–1575.

Bunevicius, R., Kazanavicius, G., Zalinkevicius, R., and Prange, A. J., Jr. 1999. Effects of thyroxine as compared with thyroxine plus triiodothyronine in patients with hypothyroidism. N Engl J Med 340(6):424–429.

Burrow, G. N., Oppenheimer, J. H., and Volpé, R. 1989. Thyroid Function and Disease. Philadelphia: W. B. Saunders.

Chopra, I. J., Huang, T. S., Hurd, R. E., and Solomon, D. H. 1984. A study of the cardiac effects of thyroid hormone: evidence of amelioration of the effects of thyroxine by sodium ipodate. Endocrinology 114:2039–2045.

Dong, B. J., Hauck, W. W., Gambertoglio, J. G., Gee, L., White, J. R., Bubp, J. L., and Greenspan, F. S. 1997. Bioequivalence of generic and brand-name levothyroxine products in the treatment of hypothyroidism. J Am Med Assoc 227:1205–1213.

Feldman, E. C., and Nelson, R. W. 1987a. Hypothyroidism. In E. C. Feldman and R. W. Nelson, eds., Canine and Feline Endocrinology and Reproduction, pp. 55–90. Philadelphia: W. B. Saunders.

———. 1987b. Hyperthyroidism and thyroid tumors. In E. C. Feldman and R. W. Nelson, eds., Canine and Feline Endocrinology and Reproduction, pp. 91–136. Philadelphia: W. B. Saunders.

Ferguson, D. C. 1984. Thyroid function tests in the dog. Vet Clin N Amer 14:783–808.

———. 1986. Thyroid hormone replacement therapy. In R. W. Kirk, ed., Current Veterinary Therapy IX, pp. 1018–1025. Philadelphia: W. B. Saunders.

———. 1988. Effect of nonthyroidal factors on thyroid function tests in the dog. Compendium for Cont Educ (Small Anim) 10(12):1365–1377.

———. 1989a. Hypothyroidism: many presentations, one treatment. In Small Animal Geriatrics: Viewpoints in Veterinary Medicine. Proc Alpo Symp on Geriatrics, pp. 30–36.

———. 1989b. Influence of common drugs on the free thyroxine fraction in canine serum. Proc Annual Forum of the ACVIM, San Diego, 5:1032 (abstract).

———. 1993. An internal medical perspective of hypothyroidism. Daniels Pharmaceuticals, Inc., Monograph, pp. 3–9.

———. 1994. Update on the diagnosis of canine hypothyroidism. Vet Clin N Am 24(3):515–540.

Ferguson, D. C., and Hoenig, M. E. 1991a. Feline hyperthyroidism. In D. G. Allen, ed., Small Animal Medicine, pp. 831–843. Philadelphia: J. B. Lippincott.

———. 1991b. Canine hypothyroidism. In D. G. Allen, ed., Small Animal Medicine, pp. 845–865. Philadelphia: J. B. Lippincott.

———. 1997. Re-examination of dosage regimens for L-thyroxine (T_4) in the dog: bioavailability and persistence of TSH suppression. Proc 15th ACVIM Forum, abstract 72, p. 668.

Ferguson, D. C., Hoenig, M., and Cornelius, L. 1992. Endocrinologic disorders. In M. D. Lorenz, L. M. Cornelius, and D. C. Ferguson, eds., Small Animal Medical Therapeutics, pp. 85–148. Philadelphia: J. B. Lippincott.

Ferguson, D. C., Jacobs, G. J., and Hoenig, M. 1988. Ipodate as an alternative medical treatment for hyperthyroidism: preliminary results in experimentally induced disease. Proc Am Coll Vet Med Annual Forum, Washington, DC, abstract 3, p. 718.

Ferguson, D. C., and Peterson, M. E. 1992. Serum free and total iodothyronine concentrations in dogs with spontaneous hyperadrenocorticism. Am J Vet Res 53:1636–1640.

Fish, L. H., Schwartz, H. L., Cavanagh, J., Steffens, M. W., and Bantle, J. P. 1997. Replacement dose, metabolism, and bioavailability of levothyroxine in the treatment of hypothyroidism: role of triiodothyronine in pituitary feedback in humans. N Engl J Med 316:764–770.

Fox, L. E., and Nachreiner, R. F. 1981. The pharmacokinetics of T_3 and T_4 in the dog. Proc 62nd Conf Res Workers in Anim Dis, p. 13.

Graves, T. K., and Peterson, M. E. 1994. Diagnostic tests for feline hyperthyroidism. Vet Clin N Am 24(3):567–576.

Greco, D. S., Rosychuk, R. A. W., Ogilvie, G. K., Harpold, L. M., and Van Liew, H. 1998. The effect of levothyroxine treatment on resting energy expenditure of hypothyroid dogs. J Vet Intern Med 12:7–10.

Greenspan, F. S. 1994. The thyroid gland. In F. S. Greenspan and J. D. Baxter, eds., Basic and Clinical Endocrinology, 4th ed., pp. 160–226. Norwalk: Appleton and Lange.

Hall, I. A., Campbell, K. L., Chambers, M. D., et al. 1993. Effect of trimethoprim/sulfamethoxazole on thyroid function in dogs with pyoderma. J Am Vet Med Assoc 202:1959–1962.

Hashizume, K., Takahide, M., Nishiano, Y., and Kobayashi, M. 1987. Evidence for the presence of active and inactive forms of cytosolic triiodothyronine (T_3) binding protein in the rat kidney: cooperative action of Ca^{++} in NADPH activation. Endocrinol Jpn 34:379.

Hays, M. T., Broome, M. R., and Turrel, J. M. 1988. A multicompartmental model for iodide, thyroxine, and triiodothyronine metabolism in normal and spontaneously hyperthyroid cats. Endocrinol 122:2444.

Hays, M. T., Hsu, L., and Kohatsu, S. 1992. Transport of the thyroid hormones across the feline gut wall. Thyroid 2:45.

Hays, M. T., and Solomon, D. H. 1965. Influence of the gastrointestinal iodide cycle on the early distribution of radioactive iodide in man. J Clin Invest 44:117.

Hoenig, M., and Ferguson, D. C. 1983. Assessment of thyroid functional reserve in the cat by the thyrotropin-stimulation test. Am J Vet Res 44:1229–1232.

Hulter, H. N., Gustafson, L. E., Bonner, E. L., et al. 1984. Thyroid replacement in thyroparathyroidectomized dogs. Miner Electrolyte Metab 10:228.

Inada, M., Kasagi, K., Kurata, S., Kazama, Y., Takayama, H., Torizuka, K., Fukase, M., and Soma, T. 1975. Estimation of thyroxine and triiodothyronine distribution and of the conversion rate of thyroxine to triiodothyronine in man. J Clin Invest 55:1337–1348.

Johnson, C., Olivier, B., Nachreiner, R., and Mullaney, T. 1999. Effect of ^{131}I-induced hypothyroidism on indices of reproductive function in adult male dogs. J Vet Intern Med 13:104–110.

Kantrowitz, L. B., Peterson, M. E., Trepanier, L. A., Melian, C., and Nichols, R. 1999. Serum total thyroxine, total triiodothyronine, free thyroxine, and thyrotropin concentrations in epileptic dogs treated with anticonvulsants. J Am Vet Med Assoc 214:1804–1808.

Kaptein, E. M. 1986. Thyroid hormone metabolism in illness. In G. Henneman, ed., Thyroid Hormone Metabolism, p. 297. New York: Marcel Dekker.

Kaptein, E. M., Hays, M. T., and Ferguson, D. C. 1994. Thyroid hormone metabolism: a comparative evaluation. Vet Clin N Am 24(3):431–466.

Kaptein, E. M., Hoopes, M. T., Ferguson, D. C., et al. 1990. Comparison of reverse triiodothyronine distribution and metabolism in normal dogs and humans. Endocrinol 126:2003.

Kaptein, E. M., Moore, G. M., Ferguson, D. C., and Hoenig, M. 1992. Effects of prednisone on thyroxine and 3,5,3′-triiodothyronine metabolism in normal dogs. Endocrinology 130(3):1669–1679.

———. 1993. Thyroxine and triiodothyronine distribution and metabolism in thyroxine-replaced athyreotic dogs and normal humans. Am J Physiol 264:E90–E100.

Kemppainen, R. J., Thompson, F. N., Lorenz, M. D., et al. 1983. Effects of prednisone on thyroid and gonadal endocrine function in dogs. J Endocrinol 96:293–302.

Kintzer, P. P. 1994. Considerations in the treatment of feline hyperthyroidism. Vet Clin N Am 24(3):577–585.

Kintzer, P. P., and Peterson, M. E. 1991. Thyroid scintigraphy in small animals. Semin Vet Med Surg (Small Anim) 6:131.

———. 1994. Nuclear medicine of the thyroid gland. Vet Clin N Am 24(3):587–605.

Larsen, P. R., et al. 1981. Relationships between circulating and intracellular thyroid hormones: physiological and clinical implications. Endocr Rev 2:87.

Larsson, M. 1987. Diagnostic methods in canine hypothyroidism and influence of non-thyroidal illness on thyroid hormones and thyroxine-binding proteins. PhD thesis, Uppsala, Sweden.

Larsson, M., Pettersson, T., and Carlstrom, A. 1985. Thyroid hormone binding in serum of 15 vertebrate species: isolation of thyroxine-binding globulin and prealbumin analogs. Gen Comp Endocrinol 58:360.

Laurberg, P. 1980. Iodothyronine release from the perfused canine thyroid. Acta Endocrinol (Suppl) 236:1.

Laurberg, P., and Boye, N. 1984. Propylthiouracil, ipodate, dexamethasone, and periods of fasting induce different variations in serum rT_3 in dogs. Metabolism 33:323.

Lazar, M. A., and Chin, W. W. 1990. Nuclear thyroid hormone receptors. J Clin Invest 86:1777.

Magner, J. A. 1990. Thyroid-stimulating hormone: biosynthesis, cell biology and bioactivity. Endocr Rev 11:354.

Mendel, C. M. 1989. The free hormone hypothesis: a physiologically based mathematical model. Endocrine Rev 10:232.

Meric, S. M., Hawkins, E. C., Washabau, R. J., Turrel, J. M., and Feldman, E. C. 1986. Radioactive iodine therapy in cats with hyperthyroidism. JAVMA 188:1038–1040.

Moore, G. E., Ferguson, D. C., and Hoenig, M. 1993. Effects of oral administration of anti-inflammatory doses of prednisone on thyroid hormone response to thyrotropin-releasing hormone and thyrotropin in clinically normal dogs. Am J Vet Res 54(1):130–135.

Murray, L. A. S., and Peterson, M. E. 1997. Ipodate treatment of hyperthyroidism in cats. JAVMA 211:63–67.

Oppenheimer, J. H. 1983. The nuclear receptor–triiodothyronine complex: relationship to thyroid hormone distribution, metabolism and biological action. In J. H. Oppenheimer and H. H. Samuels, eds., Molecular Basis of Thyroid Hormone Action, pp. 1–35. New York: Academic Press.

Panciera, D. L., and Johnson, G. S. 1994. Plasma von Willebrand factor antigen concentration in dogs with hypothyroidism. J Am Vet Med Assoc 205:1550–1553.

———. 1996. Plasma von Willebrand factor antigen concentration and buccal mucosal bleeding time in dogs with experimental hypothyroidism. J Vet Intern Med 10(2):60–64.

Panciera, D. L., MacEwen, E. G., Atkins, C. E., Bosu, W. T. K., Refsal, K. R., and Nachreiner, R. F. 1990. Thyroid function tests in euthyroid dogs treated with L-thyroxine. Am J Vet Res 51:22–26.

Pardridge, W. M. 1981. Transport of protein-bound hormones into tissues in vivo. Endocrine Rev 2:103.

Peterson, M. E., and Aucoin, D. P. 1993. Comparison of the disposition of carbimazole and methimazole in clinically normal cats. Res Vet Sci 54:351–355.

Peterson, M. E., and Becker, D. V. 1984. Radionuclide thyroid imaging in 135 cats with hyperthyroidism. Vet Radiol 25:23–27.

Peterson, M. E., and Ferguson, D. C. 1990. Thyroid diseases. In S. J. Ettinger, Textbook of Veterinary Internal Medicine, vol. 2, pp. 1632–1675. Philadelphia: W. B. Saunders.

Peterson, M. E., et al. 1984. Effects of spontaneous hyperadrenocorticism on serum thyroid hormone concentrations in the dog. Am J Vet Res 45:2034–2038.

Peterson, M. E., Kintzer, P. P., and Hurvitz, A. I. 1988. Methimazole treatment of 262 cats with hyperthyroidism. J Vet Int Med 2:150–157.

Plumb, D. C. 1999. Veterinary Drug Handbook. White Bear Lake, MN: PharmaVet Publishing.

Quinlan, W. J., and Michaelson, S. 1981. Homologous radioimmunoassay for canine thyrotropin: response of normal and x-irradiated dogs to propylthiouracil. Endocrinology 108:937–942.

Ramirez, S., Wolfsheimer, K. J., Moore, R. M., Mora, F., Bueno, A. C., and Mirza, T. 1997. Duration of effects of phenylbutazone on serum total thyroxine and free thyroxine concentrations in horses. J Vet Intern Med 11:371–374.

Rapaport, B., and Nagayama, Y. 1992. The thyrotropin receptor 25 years after its discovery: new insights after molecular cloning. Mol Endocrinol 6:145.

Reichlin, S. 1986. Neuroendocrine control of thyrotropin secretion. In S. H. Ingbar and L. E. Braverman, eds., The Thyroid, 5th ed., p. 241. Philadelphia: J. B. Lippincott.

Robbins, J. R., and Rall, J. E. 1960. Proteins associated with the thyroid hormones. Physiol Rev 40:415.

Rosychuk, R. A. W. 1982. Thyroid hormones and antithyroid drugs. Vet Clin N Am 12(1):111–148.

Shupnick, M. A., Ridgeway, E. C., and Chin, W. W. 1989. Molecular biology of thyrotropin. Endocr Rev 4:459.

Su, X., Katakam, P., Yang, X., Grosse, W. M., Li, O. W., McGraw, R. A., and Ferguson, D. C. 1995. Cloning, expression, and development of monoclonal antibodies against the beta subunit of canine thyrotropin, J Vet Int Med 9(3):185 (abstract).

Taurog, A. 1991. Hormone synthesis: thyroid iodine metabolism. In L. E. Braverman and R. D. Utiger, eds., Werner and Ingbar's The Thyroid: A Fundamental and Clinical Text, 6th ed. Philadelphia: Lippincott.

Torres, S. M. F., McKeever, P. J., and Johnstone, S. D. 1992. Effect of oral administration of prednisolone on thyroid function in dogs. Am J Vet Res 52:416.

Trepanier, L. A., Peterson, M. E., and Aucoin, D. A. 1989. Methimazole pharmacokinetics in the normal cat. J Vet Int Med 3(2):1256 (abstract).

Weinberger, C., Thompson, C. L., Ong, E. S., Lebo, R., Gruol, D. J., and Evans, R. M. 1986. The c-*erb*-A gene encodes a thyroid hormone receptor. Nature 324:641–646.

Williams, D. A., Scott-Moncrieff, C., Bruner, J., Sustarsic, D., Panosian-Sahakian, N., and el Shami, A. S. 1996. Validation of an immunoassay for canine thyroid-stimulating hormone and changes in serum concentration following induction of hypothyroidism in dogs. J Am Vet Med Assoc 209(10):1730–1732.

Wolff, J. 1989. Excess iodide inhibits the thyroid gland by multiple mechanisms. In R. Eckholm, L. D. Kohn, and S. H. Wollman, eds., Control of the Thyroid Gland. New York: Plenum.

Woltz, H. H., et al. 1983. Effect of prednisone on thyroid gland: morphology and plasma thyroxine and triiodothyronine concentrations in the dog. Am J Vet Res 44:2000–2003.

33

GLUCOCORTICOIDS, MINERALOCORTICOIDS, AND STEROID SYNTHESIS INHIBITORS

DUNCAN C. FERGUSON AND MARGARETHE HOENIG

Glucocorticoids
- **Management of Hypoadrenocorticism**
- **Management of Nonadrenal Disorders: Inflammatory, Allergic, and Autoimmune Disorders**
- **Review of Physiology**
- **Physiological Effects**
- **Pharmacologic Effects**
- **Chemistry**
- **Toxicity**
- **Principles of Rational Glucocorticoid Therapy**
- **Classes of Glucocorticoid Usage**

Mineralocorticoids
- **History**
- **Secretion and Mechanism of Action**
- **Preparations and Properties**
- **Therapeutic Use**
- **Side Effects**

Adrenolytic Drugs and Steroid Synthesis Inhibitors
- **Therapy for Hyperadrenocorticism**
- **Mitotane (*o,p′*-DDD)**
- **Ketoconazole**
- **L-Deprenyl**

GLUCOCORTICOIDS. Glucocorticoids are among the most widely used (and misused) class of drugs in veterinary medicine. Despite this, scientific information on glucocorticoid therapy in most domestic species is scarce, particularly with respect to optimal dosages and dosage intervals, physical and endocrine side effects, and efficacy in clinical applications. Therefore, therapeutic protocols are often the product of clinical experience, common sense, and information from human medicine. Though the following discussion emphasizes systemic use of glucocorticoids, it should be recognized that local application (ophthalmic, otic, intra-articular, topical, intralesional) also has similar systemic effects.

Management of Hypoadrenocorticism. Spontaneous glucocorticoid deficiency without concomitant mineralocorticoid deficiency is a relatively rare occurrence in dogs, the species that most commonly suffers from Addison's disease (gluco- and mineralocorticoid deficiency). The underlying cause is suspected to be an immune-mediated destruction of the adrenal cortex, making replacement of the physiological hormones aldosterone and cortisol (in most domestic animals) to be the primary clinical goal. Spontaneous selective glucocorticoid deficiency is rare; however, exogenous glucocorticoids may themselves induce selective atrophy of the glucocorticoid-producing part of the adrenal cortex (zonae fasciculata and reticularis) (Addison 1855; Feldman and Nelson 1987; Ferguson 1985a; Ferguson et al. 1978; Hoenig and Ferguson 1991b).

Management of Nonadrenal Disorders: Inflammatory, Allergic, and Autoimmune Disorders. Glucocorticoids are potent anti-inflammatory and immunosuppressant agents. The majority of therapeutic applications for these agents fall into these classifications. However, the adverse metabolic effects, as described below, are difficult to separate pharmacologically from the therapeutic benefits, making glucocorticoids potent, yet potentially dangerous, compounds.

Review of Physiology

BIOSYNTHESIS OF STEROIDS. The adrenal cortex synthesizes a variety of steroids from cholesterol and releases them into the circulation. Those steroids with effects on intermediary metabolism are termed "glucocorticoids" and are produced mainly in the layers of the adrenal gland called the zonae fasciculata and reticularis. The steroids with primarily salt-retaining activity are called mineralocorticoids and are synthesized in the zona glomerulosa. The adrenal gland is also capable of synthesizing steroids with androgenic and estrogenic activity. The major glucocorticoid in most domestic animals is cortisol, and in most mammals, the most important mineralocorticoid is aldosterone. In some species (e.g., the rat), corticosterone is the major glucocorticoid. It is less firmly bound to protein and therefore metabolized more rapidly. Quantitatively, dehydroepiandrosterone (DHEA) is the major androgen, with part of it being sulfated to DHEA-sulfate. Both DHEA and androstenedione are very weak androgens. A small amount of testosterone is secreted by the adrenal gland and may be of greater importance as an androgen. Little is known about the estrogens secreted by the adrenal gland. However, the adrenal androgens such as testosterone and androstenedione can be converted to estrone in small amounts by nonendocrine tissues (Aron and Tyrrell 1994; Tyrrell et al. 1994).

HYPOTHALAMIC-PITUITARY-ADRENAL AXIS. The major glucocorticoid in most domestic species is cortisol (hydrocortisone). It is synthesized from cholesterol and released into the circulation under the influence of adrenocorticotropic hormone (ACTH). The conversion of cholesterol to pregnenolone is the rate-limiting step of adrenal steroidogenesis. This step occurs via activity of the enzyme P-450sc and involves two hydroxylations and then side-chain cleavage of cholesterol. In most domestic species, as in humans, cortisol is the main glucocorticoid produced by the adrenal glands under the influence of ACTH. Production of ACTH is stimulated by corticotropin-releasing hormone (CRH), which is a hypothalamic hormone (see also Chap. 30); production of ACTH is also influenced by vasopressin (antidiuretic hormone; ADH), particularly during stress. There is also central nervous system (CNS) input into hypothalamic hormone secretion. A "short-loop" feedback system of ACTH on the corticotrophs (ACTH-producing cells) in the pituitary has also been described (see Fig. 33.1). In humans, cortisol is secreted in response to pulsatile ACTH release with diurnal variation. In humans, single daily doses of exogenous glucocorticoids are most commonly recommended to be given in the morning to mimic the adrenal gland's secretory pattern (Tyrrell et al. 1994). Although older reports claimed the existence of a diurnal cortisol variation in dogs and cats, with plasma cortisol level peaking in the morning in dogs and in the evening in cats (Feldman and Nelson 1987), more recent studies have not confirmed these observations (Kemppainen 1986). Under basal (nonstressful) conditions, the adrenal gland produces cortisol (hydrocortisone) at about 1 mg/kg body weight daily in most species.

Negative feedback of glucocorticoids on ACTH secretion occurs at both the hypothalamic and pituitary levels via two mechanisms:

1. "Fast-feedback" is sensitive to the rate of change of cortisol levels and likely occurs without interaction with nuclear steroid receptors.

2. "Slow-feedback" is sensitive to the absolute cortisol concentration and is a nuclear receptor–mediated effect which results in a decrease in ACTH synthesis. The clinical test for spontaneous hyperadrenocorticism, called the dexamethasone suppression test, is mediated by this mechanism of feedback (Keller-Wood 1990; Tyrrell et al. 1994).

Pharmacologic doses of glucocorticoids have a profound effect on endogenous glucocorticoid regulation, suppressing both hypothalamic and pituitary hormone production (Fig. 33.1). Cortisol inhibits ACTH secretion and CRH secretion through negative feedback at both hypothalamic and pituitary levels, a point that is important when considering recovery of the hypothalamic-pituitary-adrenal axis (HPAA) from exogenous glucocorticoid administration. Glucocorticoids with anti-inflammatory effects but no effects on the HPAA have not been identified to date. As a result, long-term use of supraphysiologic doses may lead to adrenocortical atrophy and decreased adrenal secretory reserve (Chastain et al. 1981; Chastain and Graham 1979; Hench 1952; Kemppainen et al. 1982; Moore and Hoenig 1992).

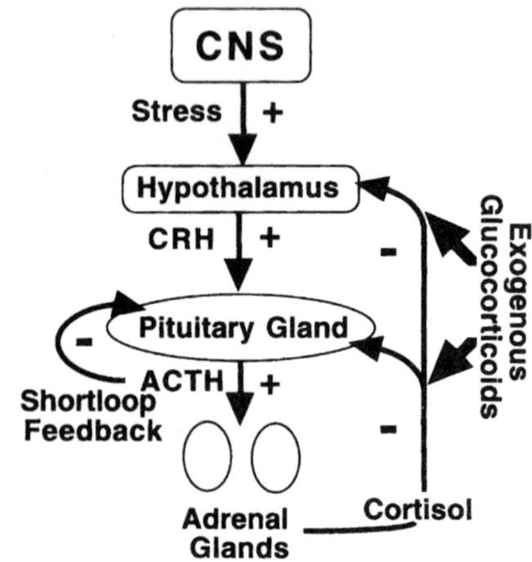

FIG. 33.1—Hypothalamic-pituitary-adrenal axis. Exogenous glucocorticoids inhibit the hypothalamic and pituitary function in a negative-feedback fashion. ACTH, through "short-loop" feedback, inhibits its own production. Therefore, recovery of the entire hypothalamic-pituitary-adrenal axis requires withdrawal of glucocorticoid and is not enhanced by the administration of exogenous ACTH. CNS = central nervous system; CRH = corticotropin-releasing hormone; ACTH = adrenocorticotropic hormone; + represents stimulation; – represents inhibition.

PLASMA BINDING, METABOLISM, AND EXCRETION. In plasma, cortisol is over 90% bound to plasma proteins. The remaining 10% free hormone is the active moiety according to the free-hormone hypothesis. Corticosteroid-binding globulin (CBG), an α_2 globulin synthesized by the liver, binds the majority of circulating hormone under normal circumstances. The remainder is free or loosely bound to albumin and is available to exert its effect on target cells. Cortisol is removed from the circulation by the liver, where it is reduced and conjugated to form water-soluble glucuronides and sulfates, which are excreted into the urine (Aron and Tyrrell 1994; Grote et al. 1993; Hammond 1990; Tyrrell et al. 1994).

MOLECULAR MECHANISM OF ACTION: STEROID RECEPTORS. The majority of steroid hormone actions are mediated by interaction with specific receptors in and on the target cell (see Fig. 33.2). The steroid hormone receptors are specific to the class of steroids (such as glucocorticoids, mineralocorticoids, androgens, estrogens). However, at very high concentrations, nonspecific effects due to direct interaction with the

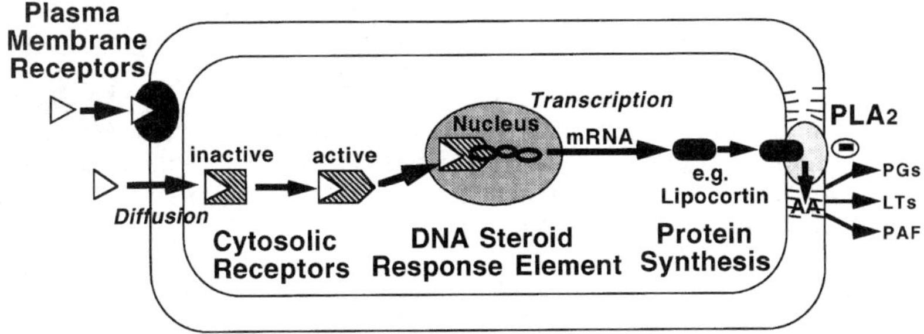

FIG. 33.2—Sites of cellular action of glucocorticoids. Glucocorticoids exert their cellular action via binding to plasma membrane and cytosolic receptors. The activated cytosolic receptors subsequently are translocated to the nucleus, where they bind to the steroid response element on nuclear DNA and result in specific expression of proteins, such as lipocortin, which can inhibit phospholipase A_2 (PLA_2) activity and thereby the production of prostaglandins (PG), leukotrienes (LT), and platelet-activating factor (PAF). Glucocorticoids also influence the synthesis of a variety of other proteins.

cell membrane lipid may occur. The classic mechanism of steroid hormone action begins with membrane permeation of the steroid and subsequent binding to cytosolic receptors. These proteins probably originate from the nucleus but then migrate into the cytosol when glucocorticoids are present. In binding, a protein known as "heat-shock" protein (hsp90) is released and may play a role in the actions of the hormone. The hormone-receptor complex is then transported into the nucleus, where it binds to glucocorticoid response elements (GREs) on various genes and alters their expression. The DNA binding domain of the receptor is characterized by cysteine-rich regions called "zinc fingers." The hormone facilitates the receptor protein's binding to DNA. In certain tissues, other proteins also must bind to the gene to allow expression of particular GREs. Most nuclear-mediated actions have an onset of pharmacologic effects of steroids that requires minimally several hours to occur.

The anti-inflammatory effects are mediated either by direct binding of the glucocorticoid/glucocorticoid-receptor complex to GREs in the promoter region of genes or by an interaction of this complex with other transcription factors, in particular activating protein-1 or nuclear factor kappaB (NF kappaB). Glucocorticoids inhibit many inflammation-associated molecules, such as cytokines, chemokines, arachidonic acid metabolites, and adhesion molecules. In contrast, anti-inflammatory mediators often are up-regulated by glucocorticoids (van der Velden 1998).

The rapid effects of steroids on ion fluxes and vascular permeability are likely independent of protein synthesis (Muller and Rankawitz 1991; Reull et al. 1990). Specific membrane-associated receptors for glucocorticoids have been identified and may be involved in the rapid effects of these agents in shock conditions (Gametchu et al. 1991; Grote et al. 1993; Liposits and Bohn 1993). These effects occur too rapidly to be explained by gene expression mechanisms (e.g., fastfeedback inhibition). The possible mechanisms for these actions are steroid hormone acting on receptors on plasma membranes (Fig. 33.2), changes in membrane fluidity via regulation of $GABA_A$ receptors on plasma membranes, and activation of steroid receptors by factors such as EGF, insulin-like growth factor-I (IGF-I), and dopamine. Receptor-mediated insertion of steroid hormones into DNA may also take place, with the steroid acting as a transcription factor. These diverse modes of action provide for integrated rapid and/or prolonged effects to address the physiological needs of the individual (Brann et al. 1995).

Glucocorticoids significantly inhibit multiple aspects of T-cell immunity largely through inhibition of cytokine expression at the transcriptional and posttranscriptional levels. The activated glucocorticoid-receptor complex can bind to and inactivate key proinflammatory transcription factors (e.g., AP-1, NF kappaB). This takes place at the promoter-responsive elements of these factors but has also been reported without the presence of DNA, via GREs up-regulating the expression of cytokine inhibitory proteins or via reduction of the half-life of cytokine mRNAs. Glucocorticoids also have been reported to act indirectly by inducing transforming growth factor (TGF)-β expression, which in turn blocks T-cell immunity. In contrast to their inhibitory effects on cytokine expression, glucocorticoids up-regulate cytokine receptors (Almawi et al. 1996). In vitro, glucocorticoids strongly diminish the production of the initial-phase cytokines interleukin (IL)-1β and tumor necrosis factor-α (TNF-α) and the immunomodulatory cytokines IL-2, IL-3, IL-4, IL-5, IL-10, IL-12, and IFN-γ, as well as of IL-6, IL-8, and the growth factor GM-CSF (granulocyte-macrophage colony stimulating factor). The production of the anti-inflammatory IL-10 is also inhibited. The exceptions of steroid down-regulatory activity on cytokine expression seem to affect repair-phase cytokines like TGF-β and PDGF. These are even reported to be up-regulated, which may explain the rather weak steroid dampening action on healing and fibrotic processes (Bratts and Linden 1996).

The induction of cell death in lymphoid cells by glucocorticoids is one of the earliest and most thoroughly studied models of apoptosis. Although the exact mechanism by which apoptosis occurs in lymphocytes is unknown, many biochemical and molecular changes have been shown to occur in these cells in response to glucocorticoids. The role of chromatin degradation and endonucleases in the apoptotic process has been closely studied, as well as the involvement of several oncogenes in glucocorticoid-induced cell lysis. In addition, the clinical importance of glucocorticoid-induced apoptosis in the treatment of lymphoid neoplasms has recently received increased attention (Schwartzman and Cidlowski 1994).

Glucocorticoids inhibit the release of arachidonic acid and platelet-activating factor (PAF) from lung and macrophages by enhancing the production of a protein called lipocortin, which inhibits the enzyme phospholipase A_2 in the cell membrane, thereby inhibiting the formation of prostaglandins, leukotrienes, and PAF (see Fig. 33.3). Glucocorticoids also may inhibit other phospholipases, such as phospholipase C (Barragry 1994; Goldfien 1992; Sorenson et al. 1988). Lipocortin-1, a 37 kDa member of the annexin superfamily of proteins, is now known to play a major regulatory role in systems as diverse as cell growth regulation and differentiation, neutrophil migration, CNS responses to cytokines, neuroendocrine secretion, and neurodegeneration (Flower and Rothwell 1994).

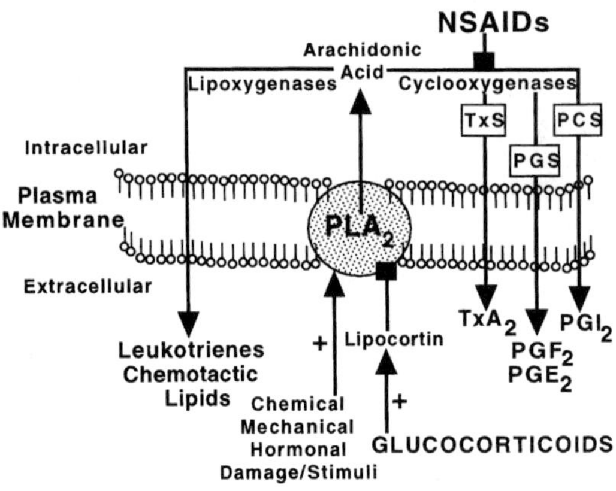

FIG. 33.3—Comparison of the effects of glucocorticoids and nonsteroidal anti-inflammatory drugs (NSAIDs) on arachidonic acid–derived mediators of inflammation. Glucocorticoids stimulate the production of lipocortin, which inhibits the activity of plasma phospholipase A_2 (PLA_2) and thereby inhibits the release of arachidonic acid and indirectly the production of newly formed inflammatory mediators of the cyclooxygenase pathway as well as the lipoxygenase pathway. The net result is a reduction in production of leukotrienes and chemotactic compounds, as well as less formation of thromboxane A_2 (TxA_2) by thromboxane synthase (TxS), of prostaglandins E_2 and $F_{2\alpha}$ by prostaglandin synthase (PGS), and of prostacyclin (PGI_2) by prostacyclin synthase (PCS).

Physiological Effects. A principal role of glucocorticoids is the maintenance of fluid homeostasis by regulation of volume and composition of body fluids and by being permissive for essential cellular metabolism. Without glucocorticoids, an animal cannot survive a stressful incident. The glucocorticoids have widespread effects because they influence the function of most cells in the body. Glucocorticoids in physiological quantities are essential for the dilution of the renal filtrate into the hyposthenuric range.

Other physiological roles of glucocorticoids are to increase gluconeogenesis, decrease protein synthesis, and increase lipolysis with the release of glycerol and free fatty acids (an insulin-antagonistic effect). Although many of the effects are dose related, glucocorticoids may also act in a permissive manner to optimize certain cellular reactions such as the gluconeogenesis stimulated by glucagon and catecholamines. The physiological effects of glucocorticoids in the fed state are not very significant; however, during fasting, glucocorticoids contribute to the maintenance of glucose concentrations by increasing the release of glucose by the liver and increasing gluconeogenesis and glycogen deposition by stimulating glycogen synthase. The effect on muscle is catabolic because glucose uptake decreases and amino acid release (gluconeogenesis) increases. Glucocorticoids also are permissive for activity of the hormone-sensitive lipase which is responsible for mobilization of free fatty acids from adipose stores. Lipolysis is stimulated; therefore, when insulin is lacking or being greatly antagonized, ketogenesis may result (Aron and Tyrrell 1994; Feldman and Nelson 1987; Ferguson 1985a; Goldfien 1992; Haynes 1990; Melby 1974; Wilcke and Davis 1982). Glucocorticoids also maintain microcirculation, normal vascular permeability, and stability of lysosomal membranes and suppress inflammatory reactions, although these functions are more commonly associated with the pharmacologic effects of glucocorticoids. Glucocorticoids play a physiological role in the development of pulmonary surfactant in the near-term fetus, allowing an adaptation to air breathing (Aron and Tyrrell 1994; Tyrrell et al. 1994).

Pharmacologic Effects

ENERGY METABOLISM. Glucocorticoids have an antagonistic effect to that of insulin, leading to increased glucose production from amino acids (gluconeogenesis) and reduced incorporation of amino acids into protein. As stated above, glucocorticoids enhance lipolysis; however, glucocorticoid excess (pharmacologic amounts) or spontaneous hyperadrenocorticism may result in redistribution of fat because glucocorticoids stimulate appetite, thereby stimulating hyperinsulinemia, which results in lipogenesis. As a result, diabetes mellitus may result from prolonged glucocorticoid use at high dosages in animals with diminished insulin secretory capacity (prediabetics). Muscle wasting and weakness are not uncommon with glucocorticoid excess; although glucocorticoids stimulate protein and RNA synthesis in the liver, they have catabolic effects in lymphoid and connective tissue, muscle, fat, and skin. While not usually a recognizable clinical problem in domestic animals, osteoporosis may result in people with Cushing's syndrome or on chronic glucocorticoid administration. The problem likely is most significant in areas of healing bone; glucocorticoids directly inhibit bone formation by inhibiting osteoblast proliferation and the synthesis of bone matrix while stimulating osteoclast activity. In addition, glucocorticoids potentiate the action of parathyroid hormone (PTH) and 1,24-dihydroxycholecalciferol ($1,25(OH)_2$-D_3) and inhibit the gut absorption of calcium, an effect which can be used to advantage in hypercalcemic states. In the young animal, the catabolic effects of excessive amounts of glucocorticoid reduce growth. In children, this reduced growth is not prevented by growth hormone (Aron and Tyrrell 1994; Tyrrell et al. 1994).

WATER AND ELECTROLYTE BALANCE. Glucocorticoid use invariably leads to polyuria and polydipsia via inhibition of ADH release and action, as well as alteration of the animal's psyche, resulting in increased water intake. No glucocorticoid given in large doses is completely devoid of mineralocorticoid (salt-retaining and K^+-losing) activity; therefore, excessive use may precipitate or exacerbate hypertension and induce hypokalemia. In part by increasing extracellular fluid volume, glucocorticoids increase the glomerular filtration rate and are required in physiologic amounts for maximal dilution of urine (Ferguson 1985a; Melby 1974; Nakamoto et al. 1992).

IMMUNE AND HEMATOLOGIC EFFECTS. Often the desired result of a therapeutic application, anti-inflammatory effects of glucocorticoids are primarily seen at pharmacologic doses. Glucocorticoids result in alterations in the concentration, distribution, and function of peripheral leukocytes and in inhibition of phospholipase A_2 activity in the plasma membranes of these cells. Glucocorticoids act indirectly by inducing lipocortin synthesis, which in turn inhibits arachidonic acid release from membrane-bound stores, and also by inducing TGF-β expression that subsequently blocks cytokine synthesis and T-cell activation. In addition to contributing to maintenance of the microcirculation and cell membrane integrity, glucocorticoids interfere with progressive dissolution and disruption of connective tissue and cells, possibly by stabilizing lysosomal membranes (Aron and Tyrrell 1994; Aucoin 1982; Barragry 1994). Although lysosomal stabilization by glucocorticoids has been demonstrated experimentally, it is hard to know what benefit these effects have in clinical situations. Glucocorticoids also decrease formation of induced histamine (histamine produced by cells during injury), the action of which is not blocked by antihistamines. They also antagonize toxins and kinins, reducing the resultant inflammation. It is important to realize, however, that most of their effects are *nonspecific;* that is, they have profound metabolic effects regardless of the initial insult.

Glucocorticoids are used to advantage to suppress both the number of cells and the actions of the immune system. The suppressive effects on cell-mediated immunity predominate over those on humoral immunity. Antibody production is generally unaffected by moderate dosages of glucocorticoids and is inhibited only at high dosages and with long-term therapy. They cause lymphopenia and eosmopenia, an effect secondary to cell redistribution and/or lysis, and lead to increased vascular demargination of neutrophils from the vascular bed to lymphoid tissue. Glucocorticoids inhibit virus-induced interferon synthesis and diminish the functional capacity of monocytes, macrophages, and eosinophils through inhibition of the formation of ILs such as IL1 (macrophages), IL2 (lymphocytes), IL3, and IL6 and other chemotactic factors (Barragry 1994; Ehrich et al. 1992; McDonald and Langston 1994; Melby 1974; Tyrrell et al. 1994).

Glucocorticoids can induce apoptosis on normal lymphoid cells and play a key role in the physiology of thymic selection. In clinics these molecules are also used for their potencies in inducing apoptosis of malignant lymphoid cells. The mechanisms of apoptosis induced by glucocorticoids fall roughly in two categories, depending on the type of lymphocytes: induction of "death genes" such as I kappa B and *c-jun* or repression of survival factors such as AP-1 and *c-myc.* By inhibiting the production of Th1 cytokines, glucocorticoids may enhance Th2 cell activity and generate a long-lasting state of tolerance (Pallardy and Biola 1998).

CARDIORESPIRATORY EFFECTS. In addition to indirect effects on electrolyte metabolism, glucocorticoids have direct positive chronotropic and inotropic actions on the heart. They appear to block the increased permeability of capillaries induced by acute inflammation, reducing transport of protein into damaged areas and maintaining microcirculation. Because glucocorticoids are necessary for maximal catecholamine sensitivity, they contribute to maintenance of vascular tone (Ferguson et al. 1978; Nakamoto et al. 1992). In shock, production of vasoactive products of lipid peroxidation (arachidonic acid cascade), such as the vasoconstrictor thromboxane A_2, may be decreased by glucocorticoids, but probably only in the early stage of cell disruption. Glucocorticoids cause vasoconstriction when applied directly to vessels. They decrease capillary permeability by inhibiting the activity of kinins and bacterial endotoxins and by reducing the amount of histamine released by basophils.

Glucocorticoids may induce hypertension in animals and humans through the following mechanisms: (1) activation of the renin-angiotensin (R-A) system due to an increase in plasma renin substrate (PRS), (2) reduced activity of the hypotensive kallikrein-kinin (K-K) system, prostaglandins (PGs), and the endothelium-derived relaxing factor (EDRF), nitric oxide (NO), and

(3) increased pressor responses to angiotensin II (Ang II) and norepinephrine. Furthermore, the number of Ang II type 1 receptors of vascular smooth muscle cells is significantly increased by glucocorticoids (Saruta 1996).

Glucocorticoids increase the number and affinity of β-adrenergic receptors. Glucocorticoids prevent receptor down-regulation and therefore tachyphylaxis, resulting in potentiation of the effects of β-adrenergic agonists on bronchial smooth muscle, an important effect in the asthmatic patient (Sprung et al. 1984; Tyrrell et al. 1994; Wilcke and Davis 1982).

CNS EFFECTS. Although rarely described in domestic animals, glucocorticoids (or lack of them) have marked effects on the psyche, resulting in a form of mental, as well as physical, dependence (Ferguson 1985a; Metz et al. 1982).

It is known that pretreatment of neonatal rats with dexamethasone provides protection against hypoxic-ischemic brain damage. This effect is likely mediated via glucocorticoid receptors, because glucocorticoid receptor antagonist RU38486 reverses the benefit. The neuroprotection also appears to be related to alterations in cerebral metabolism. Glucose utilization is reduced prior to hypoxia-ischemia by dexamethasone and is better maintained during hypoxia-ischemia. High-energy phosphates in the brain are higher in dexamethasone-treated animals. Thus, glucocorticoids may provide their protection against hypoxic-ischemic damage by decreasing basal metabolic energy requirements and/or increasing the availability or efficiency of use of energy substrates (Tuor 1997).

ENDOCRINE EFFECTS. Glucocorticoids, in addition to being diabetogenic, also have marked effects on hypothalamic and pituitary function. ACTH, β-lipotropin, thyroid-stimulating hormone (TSH), follicle-stimulating hormone (FSH), and growth hormone (GH) synthesis and secretion are all suppressed; however, β-endorphin levels are unaffected. Glucocorticoids, even at "physiological" dosages (0.22 mg/kg prednisolone once daily orally in the dog), result in HPAA suppression, as indicated by reduction in the ACTH-stimulated cortisol concentration increment and by reduction of the ratio of the zona fasciculata and reticularis to zona glomerulosa in the adrenal gland. Anti-inflammatory dosages of prednisolone (0.5 mg/kg q12h orally) resulted in adrenal suppression within 2 weeks of therapy (Chastain and Graham 1979). In another study in dogs, 1 month of the same dosage of prednisolone orally resulted in profound suppression of endogenous plasma ACTH and cortisol concentrations, CRH-stimulated ACTH release, and ACTH-stimulated cortisol release. However, following withdrawal of the prednisolone, the HPAA returned to normal within 2 weeks (Moore and Hoenig 1992). A similar ability to recover from exogenous glucocorticoids was seen in the cat. A dosage of 2 mg/kg q12h of methylprednisolone given orally for 7 days resulted in suppression of ACTH-stimulated cortisol and CRH-stimulated ACTH, but these changes completely reversed by 7 days after withdrawal of the exogenous glucocorticoid (Crager et al. 1994). Higher dosages and long-acting preparations (dexamethasone, triamcinolone, depot products) may result in more pronounced HPAA suppression (Kemppainen and Sartin 1984; Kemppainen 1986; Kemppainen et al. 1982).

The effect of glucocorticoids on glucose metabolism is time- and dose-dependent: insulin and glucose concentrations, or glucose tolerance, were not significantly altered by the administration for 28 days of an anti-inflammatory dosage of oral prednisone (Moore and Hoenig 1993). However, daily administration of high dosages of dexamethasone and growth hormone is a reliable model for induction of diabetes mellitus in the cat (Hoenig et al. 2000). There also have been case reports of diabetes mellitus induced in dogs after administration of corticosteroids and methylprednisolone pulse therapy (Jeffers et al. 1991).

Pharmacologic doses of glucocorticoids generally reduce serum thyroid hormone concentrations, presumably through suppression of pituitary TSH. These effects have been well documented in the dog, are not as significant in the cat, and are not well studied in other domestic species (Ferguson and Peterson 1992; Kaptein et al. 1992; Moore et al. 1993). The metabolic consequences of these lowered concentrations of thyroid hormones are not known in the dog; however, a state of hypothyroidism is not believed to be the result (Jennings and Ferguson 1984).

In humans, large doses of glucocorticoids stimulate excessive production of acid and pepsin in the stomach and may cause peptic ulcer. They facilitate fat absorption and appear to antagonize the effect of vitamin D on calcium absorption. Therefore, glucocorticoids are employed in chronic hypercalcemic states in an attempt to inhibit gastrointestinal calcium absorption (Aron and Tyrrell 1994; Tyrrell et al. 1994).

Chemistry

SOURCE. Although the natural corticosteroids can be obtained from animal adrenal glands, they are usually synthesized from cholic acid or steroid sapogenins found in plants of the Liliaceae and Dioscoreaceae families. Further modifications of these steroids have led to the marketing of a large group of synthetic steroids with special characteristics that are pharmacologically and therapeutically important (see Tables 33.1–33.2 and Figs. 33.4–33.5).

STRUCTURE-ACTIVITY RELATIONSHIPS. The actions of the synthetic steroids are similar to those of cortisol (see above). They bind to the specific intracellular receptor proteins and produce the same effects but have different ratios of glucocorticoid-to-mineralocorticoid potency (see Table 33.1).

STEROID BASE. Figs. 33.4 and 33.5 show the steroid base, or carbon skeleton, of glucocorticoids. The struc-

TABLE 33.1—Characteristics of various glucocorticoid bases

	Potency			
Drug	Glucocorticoid[a]	Mineralocorticoid	HPAA suppression[b]	Alternate-day therapy possible?
Short-acting (duration of action: <24 hr)				
Hydrocortisone	1	++	+	No (too short)
Cortisone	0.8	++	+	Yes (not ideal)
Prednisone	4	+	+	Yes
Prednisolone	4	+	+	Yes
Methylprednisolone	5	+	+	Yes
Intermediate-acting (duration of action: 24–48 hr)				
Triamcinolone	5	0	++	No
Long-acting (duration of action: >48 hr)				
Flumethasone	15	0	+++	No
Dexamethasone	30	0	+++	No
Betamethasone	30	0	+++	No

Note: Effective anti-inflammatory time equals the HPAA suppression time in most cases. However, the therapeutic success and fewer side effects with alternate-day therapy stem from the fact that some preparations have slightly longer anti-inflammatory or immunosuppressive action than their action to suppress the HPAA.

[a]Compared with hydrocortisone on a mg-for-mg basis.

[b]HPAA = hypothalamic-pituitary-adrenal axis.

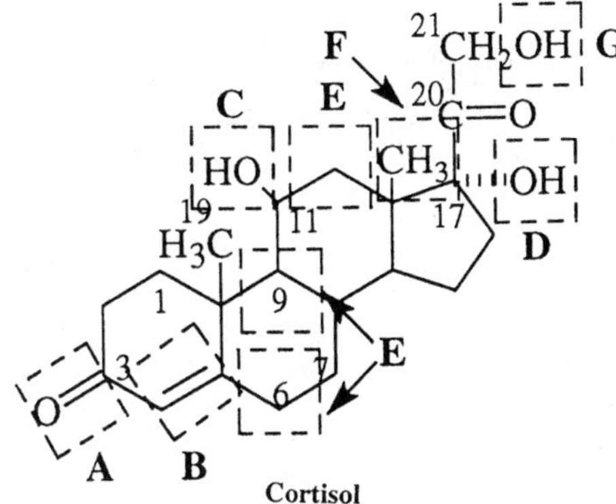

FIG. 33.4—Structure-activity relationships of glucocorticoids. Shown on the structure of the compound cortisol are the important structural sites determining the activity of a glucocorticoid base. *A:* 3 keto group essential for glucocorticoid activity; *B:* 4,5 double bond essential for glucocorticoid activity; *C:* 11 hydroxyl essential for optimal glucocorticoid activity; *D:* 17 α hydroxyl is important for glucocorticoid activity; *E:* 16 methylation or fluorination reduces mineralocorticoid activity considerably and increases glucocorticoid activity; *F:* 20 keto group is important for glucocorticoid activity; *G:* 21 hydroxyl is essential for mineralocorticoid activity and is the site of esterification.

ture of the base determines the *anti-inflammatory (glucocorticoid) potency, mineralocorticoid potency,* and the *duration of action once at the site of action.*

Alterations in the steroid base structure influence its affinity for glucocorticoid and mineralocorticoid receptors, as well as its protein-binding avidity, side-chain stability, rate of reduction, and metabolic products. Certain structures on the steroid base are essential for glucocorticoid activity (Figs. 33.4–33.5). An 11-ketol is essential for glucocorticoid activity, and compounds like cortisone and prednisone must first be reduced in the liver from the 11-carbon ketone to the ketol before full activity is seen. The 1,2 double bond provides a fourfold increase in glucocorticoid activity. The C-3 and C-20 ketone groups are also essential for glucocorticoid activity. The addition of 16-α-methyl 9-α-fluoro groups results in compounds with enhanced anti-inflammatory activity. Further substitution at the 17 ester position results in a new group of extremely potent steroids (e.g., beclomethasone and betamethasone) that are effective when applied topically for skin diseases and by inhalation for treating asthma. Modifications of the glucocorticoid molecular structure also alter the tendency for the molecule to bind with CBG in the plasma. An increase in binding to CBG results in a lower tendency for the hormone to be metabolized. Halogenation at the 9 position, unsaturation of the 1,2 bond, and methylation at the 2 or 16 position will prolong the half-life by more than 50–70%. The 11-hydroxyl group also appears to inhibit destruction, since the half-life of 11-deoxycortisol is half that of cortisol. In some cases, the agent administered is a prodrug: prednisone is rapidly reduced to prednisolone, and cortisone is rapidly converted to cortisol by the liver. The synthetic corticosteroids for oral use are in most cases rapidly and completely absorbed when given by mouth.

ESTER. Esterification of the alcohol at C-21 serves a number of potential purposes. The ester moiety determines to a significant extent the water/lipid solubility ratio and also influences the duration of action of the base compound's release from subcutaneous or intramuscular sites. Tissue esterases cleave the ester, resulting in free base, which then is distributed via the

TABLE 33.2—Glucocorticoid formulations commonly used in veterinary practice

Parenteral Glucocorticoid Preparations

Rapid Onset (<1 min) and Short Duration ($t_{1/2}$: 1–2 hr)

Applications and characteristics: Emergency situation, hemorrhagic shock, anaphylaxis
Products:
Hydrocortisone sodium succinate (Solu-CORTEF, Upjohn; A-hydroCort, Abbott)
Hydrocortisone sodium phosphate (Hydrocortone, Merck)
Hydrocortisone acetate (Hydrocortone Acetate, Merck)
Dosages
Dogs and cats: Shock: 150 mg/kg IV once
Anti-inflammatory: 4.4 mg/kg IV once
Horses: Anti-inflammatory: 1–4 mg/kg once
Cattle: 100–600 mg in 1 liter 10% dextrose/saline IV or SC
Prednisolone sodium succinate (Solu-Delta-CORTEF, Upjohn)
Prednisolone acetate injection (Key-Pred 25, Hyrex; Predalone 50, Forest; Predcor-50, Hauck)
Prednisone suspension for injection (generics and compounded)
Dosages
Dogs and cats: Replacement: 0.2 mg/kg IV or IM q24h
Anti-inflammatory: 0.2–0.5 mg/kg q12h IV or IM
Immunosuppressant: 1–3 mg/kg q12h IV or IM
Shock: 50–150 mg/kg IV or IM
Horses: Gluconeogenesis: 0.25–1 mg/ kg IV or IM
Anti-inflammatory/antiallergic: 1–2 mg/kg IV or IM
Cattle: Gluconeogenesis: 0.2–1 mg/kg IV or IM
Anti-inflammatory/antiallergic: 1–4 mg/kg IV
Methylprednisolone sodium succinate (Solu-Medrol, Upjohn)
Dosages
Dogs: Anti-inflammatory: 1–2 mg/kg/day divided q8–12h
Immunosuppressant/acute neurological: 11–30 mg/kg in 250 mL D5W infused IV × 3d
Shock: 30–35 mg/kg IV
Horses: Anti-inflammatory: 0.5 mg/kg IV or IM
Shock: 10–20 mg/kg IV
Methylprednisolone acetate (Depo-Medrol, Upjohn)
Dosages
Dogs: Anti-inflammatory: 1.1 mg/ kg SC or IM q3–4 wks
Intralesional (sublesional) use: 10–40 mg total dose%
Cats: 5.5 mg/kg SC or IM prn (q1 wk to q6 mo)
Horses: 200 mg IM repeated as necessary

Rapid Onset (within 5–45 min) and Intermediate Duration ($t_{1/2:}$ 3–4 hr)

Applications and characteristics: Emergency situations
Products:
Dexamethasone sodium phosphate (Azium SP Injection, Schering; Dex-A-Vet Injection, Anthony)
Dexamethasone in propylene glycol (Azium solution, Schering)
Dexamethasone 21-isonicotinate Injection (Voren; BioCeutic)
Dosages
Dogs and cats: Anti-inflammatory/antiallergic: 0.125–1 mg total dose/day IV, IM, or SC
Immunosuppressive: 0.2–1 mg/ kg IV or SC q12h
Shock or acute adrenocortical collapse: 4–6 mg/ kg IV
Horses: Anti-inflammatory/antiallergic: 0.05–0.2 mg/ kg once daily IV or IM or 2.5–20 mg IV or IM
Cattle: Anti-inflammatory/antiallergic: 5–40 mg IV or IM (also gluconeogenesis for primary ketosis)
Shock: 1–4 mg/kg IM or IV q4h

Slow Onset and Long Duration

Applications and characteristics: Skin disease, arthritis; less polyphagia, little Na^+ loss; intralesional therapy, topical therapy
Products:
Triamcinolone acetonide injectable (Vetalog, Fort Dodge)
Dosages
Dogs and cats: Anti-inflammatory/anti-allergic: 0.11–0.22 mg/kg IM or SC
Intralesional: 1.2–1.8 mg not more than 0.6 mg per site or more than 6 mg total dose
Horses: Anti-inflammatory/antiallergic: 0.02–0.2 mg/kg IM
Intra-articular: 6–18 mg total
Cattle: Anti-inflammatory/antiallergic: 0.02–0.04 mg/kg IM
Intra-articular: 6–18 mg total
Methylprednisolone acetate (Depo-Medrol)
Dosages
Dogs: 1.1 mg/kg SC or IM q2–3 wk
Cats: 5.5 mg/kg IM or SC prn
Horses: 2–4 mg/kg IM or 20–240 mg intra-articularly
Cattle: 20–240 mg intra-articularly

TABLE 33.2—*Continued*

Betamethasone diproprionate/sodium phosphate (Betasone aqueous suspension, Schering)
Dosages
Dogs: Anti-inflammatory/antiallergic: 1.75–3.5 mg as betamethasone per 10 kg IM × 3 wk (average); relief averages 3 wk in duration. Not more than 4 injections.
Flumethasone injection (Flucort Solution, Syntex)
Dosages
Dogs: Parenteral: 0.0625–0.25 mg IV, IM, SC q24h
Intra-articular: 0.166–1 mg as needed
Intralesional: 0.06–1 mg q24h
Cats: 0.03–0.125 mg IV, IM, or SC q24h
Horses: Anti-inflammatory/antiallergic: 1.0–2.5 mg/450 kg IV or IM
Intra-articular: 1.25–2.5 mg daily

Oral Glucocorticoid Preparations

Rapid Onset and Short Duration

Applications and characteristics: Acute and chronic conditions (alternate-day therapy); used mainly for replacement gluocorticoid therapy; relatively expensive
Products:
Hydrocortisone (base) (Cortef, Upjohn; Hydrocortone, Merck)
Cortisone (base) and **Cortisone acetate**
Hydrocortisone cypionate oral suspension (Cortef, Upjohn)
Dosages
Dogs and cats: Replacement: 1 mg/kg q24h PO
Anti-inflammatory: 4.4 mg/kg q12h PO
Horses: Not practical
Cattle: Not practical
Applications and characteristics: Mimics diurnal cortisol production, Na^+ retention not significant in dogs or cats, generally twice-daily doses given
Products:
Prednisolone (Delta-Cortef, Upjohn; generic; Prednisolone Oral Syrup, Prelone, Muro)
Prednisone: Prednisone Tablets (Meticorten, Schering; Orasone, Reid-Rowell; Deltasone, Upjohn; generic); Prednisone Oral Solution
Methylprednisolone (Medrol, Upjohn; generic)
Dosages
Dogs and cats: Replacement: 0.2 mg/kg q24h PO
Anti-inflammatory/antiallergic: 0.2–0.5 mg/kg q12h PO
Immunosuppressant: 1–3 mg/kg q12h PO
Horses: Anti-inflammatory/antiallergic: Initially, 600–800 mg PO in a 450-kg horse; then 200 mg q48h if possible
Cattle: Anti-inflammatory/antiallergic: 0.2–1 mg/kg PO

Rapid Onset and Short-to-Intermediate Duration

Applications and characteristics: Duration between 24–48 hr as base
Triamcinolone acetonide tablets, oral powder (Vetalog, Fort Dodge)
Dosages
Dogs and cats: Anti-inflammatory/antiallergiic: 0.05–0.22 mg/kg q24h PO
Immunosuppressive/acute neurologic: 0.5–1.0 mg/kg q24h PO
Horses: 0.011–0.022 mg/kg q24h PO
Cattle: Not approved

Slow Onset and Long Duration

Applications and characteristics: Extended duration; topical and parenteral preparations are well absorbed from joint, eye, skin, etc.
Products:
Dexamethasone (Azium Tablets, Schering; generic)
Dosages
Dogs and cats: 0.25–1.25 mg daily q12-24h
Horses: 0.02–0.2 mg/kg q24h PO
Cattle: Anti-inflammatory/gluconeogenic: 5–10 mg PO
Betamethasone oral solution or tablets (Celestone, Schering)
Dosages
Dogs and cats: Anti-inflammatory/antiallergic: 0.02–0.04 mg/kg q24–72h PO
Flumethasone (Flucort Tablets, Syntex)
Dosages
Dogs and cats: Anti-inflammatory/antiallergic: 0.03–0.12 mg q12h

Source: Plumb 1999.

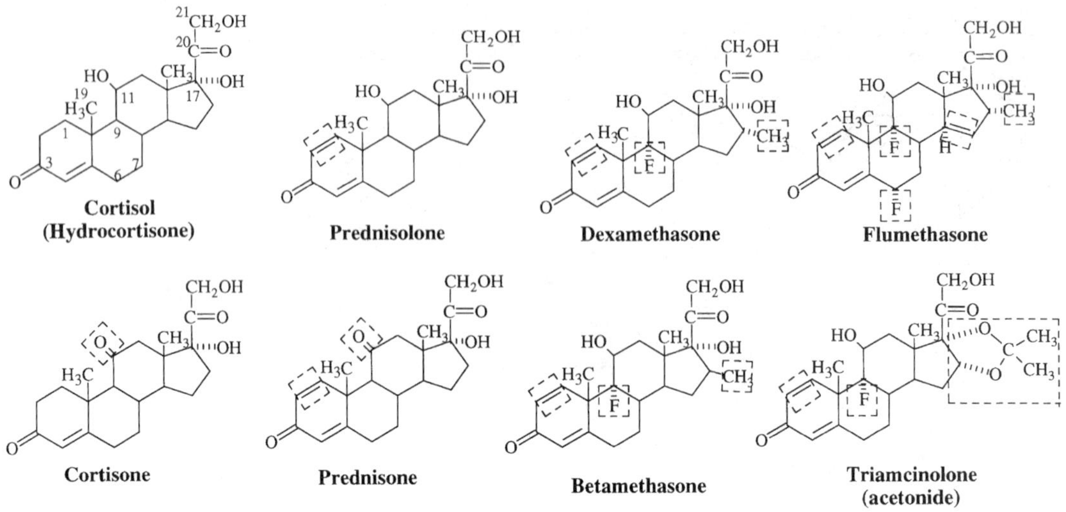

Cortisol (Hydrocortisone) **Prednisolone** **Dexamethasone** **Flumethasone**

Cortisone **Prednisone** **Betamethasone** **Triamcinolone (acetonide)**

FIG. 33.5—Structures of common glucocorticoids used in veterinary medicine. The key elements of structure differing from cortisol are identified by the outlined areas.

circulation to tissue sites of action. Routes of administration and duration of release are given for the following esters:

1. Phosphate and hemisuccinate: IV or IM, rapid action and metabolism.
2. Acetate, diacetate, tebutate: subcutaneous or IM depots, 2–14 days.
3. Acetonide: subcutaneous or IM depots, poorly H_2O soluble.
4. Pivalate: subcutaneous or IM depots; weeks to months.

The ability of a formulation to suppress the HPAA is determined by the *dosage,* the *potency of the base,* and the *duration of action of the formulation* (base + ester). The products used most commonly in veterinary medicine are listed in Table 33.2 with dosages for small animals, horses, and ruminants.

Toxicity. The main limiting factors for glucocorticoid administration are the global toxic effects of these agents. Table 33.3 lists most of the reported side effects as described in the dog, the species in which glucocorticoids are most widely used. Of course, there is variability from species to species. The following discussion highlights the basis for some of these effects.

METABOLIC/ENDOCRINE EFFECTS. The endocrine manifestations of glucocorticoid administration can be severe. Iatrogenic Cushing's syndrome may develop with adrenal insufficiency on withdrawal of the medication. The gluconeogenic effects may unmask or exacerbate diabetes and polyuric and polydipsic states and may induce hypertension.

CNS EFFECTS. In animals, the effects on mental status are difficult to assess or compare with those in humans; however, glucocorticoids likely induce a state of well-being. Neurologically, there is also evidence that glucocorticoids may decrease the threshold for seizures. Lethargy and panting occasionally develop in dogs and cats. Rapid withdrawal of glucocorticoids can induce depression and irritability (Ferguson 1985a,b; McDonald and Langston 1994).

GASTROINTESTINAL AND HEPATIC EFFECTS. The gastrointestinal and hepatic effects of glucocorticoids are among the most limiting regarding chronic administration. Glucocorticoids clearly induce a form of micronodular cirrhosis and stimulate the steroid-specific isozyme of alkaline phosphatase. In addition to hepatopathy and hepatomegaly, glucocorticoid excess may result in increased gastric acid and gastric ulceration, but more commonly high doses of potent glucocorticoids cause colonic perforation in dogs. Of course, glucocorticoids may stimulate appetite, an effect occasionally used to advantage in some therapeutic situations. Rarely, the animal will respond with anorexia. It has been postulated that glucocorticoids may also cause pancreatitis.

MUSCULOSKELETAL EFFECTS. Chronic glucocorticoid administration induces excessive catabolism and muscle atrophy. Animals may become clinically weak and be unable to exercise optimally. Bone growth may be inhibited and antagonism of vitamin D activity may result in osteoporosis with chronic administration of glucocorticoids.

TABLE 33.3—Reported side effects of glucocorticoid treatment (with emphasis on dogs)

Blood and blood chemistry	**Gastrointestinal**
Increases in:	Polyphagia
Neutrophils	Anorexia (rare)
Erythrocytes	Diarrhea (may be bloody)
Monocytes	Increased gastric acid secretion
Platelets	Hepatomegaly
Alkaline phosphatase*	Hepatopathy
Cholesterol	Pancreatitis
Glucose	Colonic perforation
Alanine aminotransferase	**Renal**
Decreases in:	Polyuria with secondary polydipsia*
Eosinophils*	Increased urinary calcium excretion
Lymphocytes	**Musculoskeletal**
Blood urea nitrogen	Muscle atrophy
Central nervous system	Weakness, exercise intolerance
Behavioral and mood changes (depression, increased irritability)	Myotonia (rare)
Lethargy	Osteoporosis
Panting	**Skin**
Endocrine	Calcinosis cutis
Iatrogenic Cushing's disease, HPAA suppression*, secondary adrenocortical insufficiency	Thin skin
Reduced thyroid hormone (T_4 and T_3) levels	Bilateral hair loss
Reduced gonadotropin and sex steroid levels	Increased bruising
Anestrus, testicular atrophy, reduced libido	**Other**
Elevated insulin levels, carbohydrate intolerance	Increased risk of infection
Reduced vitamin D levels	Enhanced spread of infection
Elevated parathyroid hormone levels	Poor wound healing
	Redistribution of body fat
	Reduced growth

Source: Summarized from Kemppainen 1986.
*Relatively common finding in dogs.

DERMATOLOGIC EFFECTS. Glucocorticoids reduce collagen synthesis and thereby reduce the rate of wound healing. The skin becomes thin and more easily stretched and bruised due to increased capillary fragility. Dogs on large dosages of glucocorticoids often develop bilateral symmetrical alopecia, known as a "Cushingoid" appearance. Cats tend to be less susceptible to these effects. Occasionally, exogenous glucocorticoid administration will induce calcium deposition in the dystrophic epidermis; however, the incidence in dogs appears to be less than with spontaneous hyperadrenocorticism (Scott 1982).

IMMUNOLOGIC EFFECTS. Although immune suppression is often the desired therapeutic effect of glucocorticoids, these agents are notorious for exacerbation of clinical or latent infectious disease processes. Animals on chronic glucocorticoid therapy have a higher incidence of bacterial infections; in one study, 75% of dogs on glucocorticoids for allergic skin disease had clinical or subclinical urinary tract infections. Of course, by inhibiting the cell-mediated immune response to an infection, glucocorticoids slow the function of immune cells that help contain an infection (Aucoin 1982; Fauci 1976; Feldman and Nelson 1987; Ferguson 1985a,b; Siegel 1985).

REPRODUCTIVE EFFECTS. High doses of glucocorticoids induce parturition during the latter part of pregnancy in ruminants and horses (Barragry 1994). There is also now evidence that dexamethasone can cause abortion in the dog. Glucocorticoids generally have teratogenic effects during early pregnancy and should be avoided in the breeding animal if possible.

FATAL SEQUELA IN THE DOG. As an example of the severe consequences of glucocorticoid excess in the dog, the following clinical case, reported in the veterinary literature (Bellah et al. 1989), is provided:

A dog was given multiple doses of glucocorticoids for treatment of intervertebral disk disease over a 25-day period: methylprednisolone acetate (Depo-Medrol)—20 mg IM; dexamethasone sodium phosphate—2 mg IM; flumethasone—0.5 mg and 1 mg IM; dexamethasone—0.25 mg q8h orally as needed; triamcinolone diacetate—40 mg IM (60 times the manufacturer's recommended dose).

The dog presented to the examining clinician with historical and physical findings of polyuria/polydipsia, fever, murmur, pendulous abdomen, marked hepatomegaly, hindlimb paraparesis, midlumbar hyperpathia, and normal pain perception in the hindlimbs. Initial laboratory findings included anemia; leukocytosis; neutrophilia; hyperalbuminemia; increased serum alkaline phosphatase (SAP), alanine aminotransferase (ALT), and glucose; increased bromsulfophthalein (BSP) retention; isosthenuria; bacteriuria (staphylococci); and low baseline and post-ACTH stimulation plasma cortisol levels.

Subsequently, laboratory findings demonstrated a deteriorating state of anemia, hypoproteinemia, leukocytosis, neutrophilia, thrombocytopenia, hyperglycemia, hyperbilirubinemia, and increased SAP and ALT. Radiographic findings included cardiomegaly, hepatomegaly, and a herniated intervertebral disk at L5-L6. Needle biopsy of the liver revealed a micronodular cirrhosis, changes consistent with glucocorticoid hepatopathy. Despite extensive supportive treatment, the dog succumbed following the development of *Haemobartonella*-induced hemolytic anemia, more vomiting, depression, anorexia, melena, and multiple cutaneous abscesses. The dog was euthanatized and necropsy revealed generalized atrophy, icterus, and thinning of the skin; hepatomegaly; severe adrenocortical atrophy; hepatic vacuolization; and pancreatic fibrosis with foci of necrosis and inflammation. Although this case represents an extreme overdosage, it illustrates the severe and potentially fatal toxicity that can result from excessive dosage or duration of glucocorticoid administration (Bellah et al. 1989).

LAMINITIS IN THE HORSE. High-dose glucocorticoids can induce or exacerbate laminitis in the horse. Steroids appear to potentiate the action of catecholamines in the equine digit. Because this constriction is more pronounced on venous beds than on arteriolar beds, the net result is often digital congestion and edema (Barragry 1994).

Principles of Rational Glucocorticoid Therapy. Because of their wide-ranging and nonspecific effects, reports of the clinical use of glucocorticoids are replete with pragmatic recommendations regarding dosage, duration of therapy, and severity of side effects. Much has been adopted from clinical use in humans, and much more is known about the fine points of glucocorticoid therapy in dogs and cats than in other species. In the following discussion, most of the specific comments will apply to the use of glucocorticoids in the dog; however, when available, appropriate information for other species will be mentioned. It is important to recognize that glucocorticoids rarely cure disease. With the possible exception of spontaneous glucocorticoid deficiency, they are used to try to suppress clinical signs long enough for a condition to run its natural course (Fauci 1976; Ferguson 1985a,b; Melby 1974; Wilcke and Davis 1982).

A well-known endocrinologist named Thorn proposed in 1966 that physicians ask themselves the following questions *before using* glucocorticoid therapy (Hench 1952). A similar approach is proposed for use in animals:

1. How serious is the underlying disorder?
2. How long will therapy be required?
3. Is the patient predisposed to any complications of glucocorticoid therapy?
4. What is the anticipated glucocorticoid *dosage?*
5. Which glucocorticoid preparation should be used?
6. Have *other types* of treatment been used to minimize glucocorticoid dosage and side effects?
7. Is an *alternate-day* regimen indicated?

These questions may help develop guidelines for practical and rational glucocorticoid therapy.

HOW SERIOUS IS THE UNDERLYING DISORDER? HOW LONG WILL THERAPY BE REQUIRED? The following general principles should be considered when glucocorticoid therapy is employed:

Diagnose the disease first, if possible. Glucocorticoids are generally only palliative and do not provide a true cure for any disease. In addition, if used before all reasonable diagnostic tests have been completed, they may mask signs of underlying disease and complicate specific diagnosis and therapy. Though a definitive diagnosis is not always possible, a presumptive diagnosis should be proposed (Ferguson 1985a,b).

Classify the disorder into one of the following categories of glucocorticoid therapy, according to a definitive or presumptive diagnosis: *physiologic replacement; intensive short-term; anti-inflammatory and antiallergic; immunosuppressive;* and *chronic palliative.* Each of these usage classifications will be discussed in more detail. By using these classifications, the clinician clearly defines the goal of therapy and can choose a starting dose and formulation appropriate for the disorder.

Use glucocorticoids to accomplish specific objectives. It is important to decide on the therapeutic end point *before* therapy is started in order to objectively assess efficacy and determine the smallest effective dose. For example, in treatment of a dog with autoimmune hemolytic anemia, the goal for initial glucocorticoid therapy might be to raise the hematocrit from 10% to 25%. In a horse with chronic obstructive pulmonary disease ("heaves"), the goal might be to suppress the allergic reaction for 1–2 weeks in order to allow the owners to change the feeding regimen to eliminate the offending allergen. By defining a therapeutic objective, the clinician can then judge the efficacy of a treatment protocol and decide when the glucocorticoid dose should be altered or alternative therapy chosen.

The length of therapy should also be anticipated. For example, immunosuppressive therapy generally requires several months of glucocorticoid use. Accordingly, a plan for instituting and later decreasing the dose should be considered from the outset. In such a case, intermittent or alternate-day therapy would not be appropriate, and an intermediate- or long-acting glucocorticoid could be used.

IS THE PATIENT PREDISPOSED TO ANY COMPLICATIONS OF GLUCOCORTICOID THERAPY? Because many of the therapeutic effects of glucocorticoids are nonspecific, clinicians should anticipate the impact on the patient of the previously outlined complications of glucocorticoid use. In doing so, the risk/benefit ratio of using these potent agents is considered.

WHAT IS THE ANTICIPATED GLUCOCORTICOID DOSAGE? WHAT GLUCOCORTICOID PREPARATION SHOULD BE USED? It is important to understand the relative potency and, perhaps more important, the relative *duration of action* of a glucocorticoid preparation, because the duration of anti-inflammatory effects usually parallels the duration of effects on the HPAA. Success with alternate-day therapy, more commonly applied in small-animal practice, depends on selecting a glucocorticoid preparation with slightly longer anti-inflammatory or immunosuppressive (beneficial) actions than HPAA-suppressive effects. *Dosages of glucocorticoids are derived by trial and error and should be constantly reevaluated.* Due to the aforementioned hazards of long-term daily glucocorticoid use, intermittent or alternate-day therapy is preferred when long-term use is necessary. As shown in Table 33.1, short- or intermediate-acting formulations, generally given orally, are most appropriate and safe for long-term use and alternate-day therapy. The goal of rational therapy is to maintain a condition in remission at the lowest effective glucocorticoid dosage (Fauci 1976; Feldman and Nelson 1987; Ferguson 1985a,b; Wilcke and Davis 1982).

Classes of Glucocorticoid Usage

PHYSIOLOGICAL REPLACEMENT THERAPY. Replacement therapy involves use of glucocorticoids in amounts similar to those of the naturally occurring glucocorticoids (cortisol in virtually all domestic species) from the adrenal gland. Ideal replacement therapy should mimic the adrenal gland's hormonal output under basal conditions, with doses increasing if the animal is stressed by illness or surgery.

Practically, this ideal is never achieved; however, the following regimens have been used successfully in adrenalectomized and Addisonian dogs and cats. As a general rule, animals produce approximately 1 mg/kg of cortisol (hydrocortisone) every day. It is not rational to employ alternate-day or intermittent glucocorticoid replacement therapy in a glucocorticoid-deficient animal, because the animal's metabolic well-being depends upon the presence of glucocorticoids *every day.* Therefore, physiological replacement therapy is aimed at providing a small daily amount of glucocorticoid. Physiological replacement therapy is rarely indicated or applied in large animals. In small animals, hydrocortisone or cortisone at 0.2–1 mg/kg/day or, more commonly, equipotent amounts of prednisolone or prednisone at 0.1–0.2 mg/kg/day once daily orally are indicated. There have been reports that the diurnal variation of cortisol results in a peak in the morning in dogs and in the evening in cats; however, more-recent studies have not confirmed this pattern (Kemppainen 1986; Scott 1982). Therefore, the timing of the single daily dosage would not appear to be critical, other than that it be provided approximately the same time each day. Because stress results in higher adrenal output of glucocorticoids, this pattern should be mimicked; in general, in moderate stress, give 2–5 times the physiologic dosage, and in severe stress (e.g., surgery), administer 5–20 times this dosage until the stressful experience has ended (Ferguson 1985a,b).

INTENSIVE SHORT-TERM AND SHOCK THERAPY. The effects of glucocorticoids in all forms of shock are still controversial; however, some evidence suggests that early treatment (probably about 4 hours postinduction in dogs) may lead to increased survival, particularly in hemorrhagic and septic shock. The nature of the formulation (particularly the ester) may affect the speed of cellular entry of glucocorticoids during shock; however, other conclusions have also been reached (Ferguson 1985a,b; Ferguson et al. 1978; Sprung et al. 1984; Wilcke and Davis 1982; Wilson 1979).

Glucocorticoids improve hemodynamics and enhance survival in canine models of endotoxic and hemorrhagic shock. However, therapy for shock should also include aggressive fluid therapy. Septic (endotoxic) shock is the most responsive form to glucocorticoid therapy; however, although human trials have shown improved short-term survival, most patients succumbed to chronic septicemia later (Sprung et al. 1984). Suspected endotoxic shock should be treated with fluid therapy and a broad-spectrum antimicrobial, with or without glucocorticoids. Glucocorticoids and antibiotics were synergistic when given within 2 hours of induction of septic shock in baboons.

The potential detrimental effects of massive doses of glucocorticoids should always be considered. However, proponents of glucocorticoid therapy for shock point out that short-term (~48 hr) glucocorticoid therapy has few negative effects, and the positive effects far outweigh the risks. Most human patients with sepsis survive beyond the acute stages of endotoxemia but succumb later to chronic septicemia (Sprung et al. 1984). Certainly, the immunosuppressive effects of glucocorticoids make their use contraindicated during chronic sepsis, and those supporting glucocorticoid use in septic shock do not generally advocate use other than during the early acute hypotensive state. Opponents to glucocorticoid use generally are not convinced that experimental studies in anesthetized animals adequately duplicate clinical situations and do not believe even short-term treatment to be innocuous, because of immunosuppressive effects (Wilcke and Davis 1982).

ANTI-INFLAMMATORY AND ANTIALLERGIC THERAPY. A large proportion of glucocorticoid use in veterinary practice is designed to combat inflammation or allergy. Unfortunately, many such diseases are difficult to definitively diagnose. Therefore, misuse of glucocorticoids is not uncommon in this category. Examples of anti-inflammatory and antiallergic use of glucocorticoids include symptomatic treatment of pruritic dermatoses, allergic pulmonary disease, and allergic gastroenteritis. Guidelines for anti-inflammatory and antiallergic dosages vary from species to species. Prednisolone or prednisone is most commonly used in small animals at 0.55 mg/kg q12h given orally for induction, then at 0.55–2.2 mg/kg every other day for maintenance. Although all dosages should be adjusted according to effect, a general, but undocumented, observation has been that cats require approximately twice the glucocorticoid dosage that dogs require to manage a similar condition. Methylprednisolone acetate may also be administered subcutaneously or intramuscularly at 1.1 mg/kg every 1–3 weeks; however, use of depot products brings the distinct disadvantage that the drug dosage cannot be stopped or reduced. Other long-acting injectable products and their duration include prednisolone acetate, 1–2 days; dexamethasone in propylene glycol, 1–7 days; triamcinolone acetonide, 3–7 days; and betamethasone valerate, 7–60 days.

For practical reasons of cost and potency, dexamethasone is the most commonly used glucocorticoid in large animals.

IMMUNOSUPPRESSIVE THERAPY. Protracted glucocorticoid use generally is required for immunosuppression. Therefore, use of a glucocorticoid with well-documented side effects and efficacy is recommended. It is important to use the highest recommended dosage until clinical signs abate. After that point, the dosage may be decreased in increments. In general, in small animals, the dosage may be decreased until the equivalent prednisolone dosage of 1.1 mg/kg is being given on alternate days (Aucoin 1982; Ferguson 1985a,b).

Long-term side effects of alternate-day therapy are few, and the dosage rarely must be decreased further. Therapy should not be discontinued until the autoimmune disease is in remission for 2–3 months; otherwise, signs are likely to recur (Aucoin 1982; Fauci 1978; Ferguson 1985a,b).

Glucocorticoids provide very nonspecific protective benefits: "The hormone appears not to extinguish the fire or to act like a carpenter to repair the damage of the fire. Instead, it appears to 'dampen the fire,' or to provide, as it were, an asbestos suit behind which the patient, like some Biblical Shadrach, Meshach or Abednego, protects his tissues from the fire. If this protection is removed prematurely, before the fire has spent itself, the patient and his tissues will react again to the burning. But, if the protection is not discarded until the natural duration of the fire is over, the patient remains largely free of symptoms and apparently 'well'" (Hench 1952).

Unlike other immunosuppressants, glucocortioids do not significantly inhibit antibody production by B lymphocytes. If glucocorticoids provide incomplete remission of an immune-mediated disorder, other immunosuppressant agents such as the alkylating agent cyclophosphamide may be added to complement the effects of glucocorticoids. Furthermore, if side effects of the glucocorticoids are too great, other immunosuppressants may be added to the regimen. If no clinical response is obtained with glucocorticoid therapy alone, addition of other immunosuppressants is less likely to succeed. Immune-mediated thrombocytopenia and autoimmmune hemolytic anemia are examples of diseases treated with immunosuppressive doses of glucocorticoids.

In small animals, immunosuppression is generally accomplished with prednisolone at 2.2–6.6 mg/kg or the equipotent dosage of dexamethasone at 0.33–1.1 mg/kg ql2h for induction, and prednisolone at 1.0–2.2 mg/kg every other day for maintenance. Note that, because its duration of action exceeds 24 hours, dexamethasone is acceptable for induction but not for alternate-day maintenance therapy (Ferguson 1985a,b).

The adverse effects of chronic immunosuppressive doses of glucocorticoid use can be serious. Therefore, clinicians should eventually attempt to maintain a satisfactory therapeutic result with the smallest possible dose of glucocorticoids on alternate days if possible. Nonsteroidal drugs (e.g., aspirin for inflammation or cyclophosphamide for immunosuppression) may be used as adjunctive therapy if necessary.

CHRONIC PALLIATIVE THERAPY. Glucocorticoids are commonly used in conjunction with nonsteroidal anti-inflammatory therapy, as in treating such conditions as chronic arthritis in most species or hip dysplasia in dogs. If nonsteroidal analgesics are not satisfactory, glucocorticoids may be used on an intermittent or alternate-day basis. Conversely, when intermittent glucocorticoid therapy alone leads to signs of disease on "off" days, nonsteroidal analgesics can be supplemented. It is important not to administer glucocorticoids erratically, as rapid withdrawal may itself precipitate signs of lameness or stiffness ("pseudorheumatism") (Fauci 1976, 1978; Ferguson 1985a,b).

ALTERNATE-DAY THERAPY. Side effects of long-term glucocorticoid use can be dramatically reduced by alternate-day therapy. Allowing the HPAA to recover on "off" days provides greater safety if therapy should suddenly be discontinued. Successful use of alternate-day therapy depends upon the therapeutic effects lasting longer than suppressive effects. As a result, this approach is not successful for all diseases. Also, true alternate-day therapy is rarely applied to large-animal cases because it is less practical to give large animals agents with low or intermediate potency like prednisolone. Weaning of more-potent agents such as dexamethasone often is accomplished by extending the between-dose interval to as long as 3–4 days in large animals; however, this is technically not considered alternate-day therapy, because full recovery of the HPAA is not allowed on alternate days (Barragry 1994; Ferguson 1985a,b).

Several common pitfalls of alternate-day therapy should be avoided. Alternate-day therapy is rarely, if ever, effective as primary therapy. It is usually first necessary to use daily therapy to achieve the desired clinical effect. Alternate-day therapy with long-acting glucocorticoids is not rational. The change to alternate-day glucocorticoid use ideally should be gradual, particularly after prolonged high-dosage therapy. Rapid change to alternate-day use may result in signs of glucocorticoid withdrawal. Finally, alternate-day glucocorticoid therapy may fail if used exclusively; supplemental use of nonsteroidal therapy should be considered, particularly on "off" days (Fauci 1978; Ferguson 1985a,b).

In inflammatory joint disease caused by infectious or immune-mediated conditions, early aggressive therapy is usually necessary to limit subsequent joint dysfunction. Of course, the primary therapy for immune-mediated arthritis, immunosuppression, can jeopardize the health of patients with infectious arthropathies. So before initiating immunosuppressive therapy, follow a thorough diagnostic plan to exclude infectious causes (Michels and Carr 1997).

CHANGING TO ALTERNATE-DAY THERAPY. Because glucocorticoid administration to dogs for longer than 2 weeks generally results in significant loss of adrenal functional reserve, for the sake of this discussion, administration of greater than 0.5 mg/kg/day of prednisolone or an equipotent dosage of a more potent drug for longer than 2 weeks should be considered chronic therapy (Chastain and Graham 1979). However, when 0.5 mg/kg ql2h (an anti-inflammatory dosage) was administered to dogs for 35 days and stopped abruptly, it took less than 2 weeks for the HPAA to totally recover (Moore and Hoenig 1992). This contrasts drastically with the experience in humans, where normalization of cortisol secretion and pituitary function may take as long as 6–9 months (Fauci 1976, 1978). Similar studies have not been performed in large-animal species.

There is no "correct" way to taper an animal from glucocorticoids. The following guidelines are suggested. If the glucocorticoid dosage is large (>1 mg/kg/day prednisolone or an equivalent) or therapy prolonged (>2 weeks in duration), some process of gradually reducing the steroid dosage (i.e., weaning) is indicated. One highly conservative approach is to double the glucocorticoid dose for "on" days and taper the dose for "off" days by 25% per cycle (a cycle may vary from 1 day to several weeks). Another conservative method includes increasing the dose for "on" days by the same amount as the dose for "off" days is decreased. Practical experience indicates that, in many canine patients, rapid tapering has few recognizable side effects unless the animal is severely stressed. Subtle adverse effects may be missed unless the owners and clinician are vigilant. Patient tolerance defines the success of any change. If therapy is for less than 2 weeks, it is probably safe to rapidly taper the dog and have no therapy on "off" days. If clinical signs are observed on "off" days, supplement with a replacement dose of glucocorticoids on those days, or add nonsteroidal therapy. If alternate-day therapy is ineffective, use of a single dose each morning (to mimic diurnal variation) may also minimize adverse effects. Examples of two conservative approaches to weaning a dog from prednisolone and application of alternate-day therapy are shown in Table 33.4.

WITHDRAWAL FROM GLUCOCORTICOIDS. The identification of clinical signs of glucocorticoid deficiency may be very difficult. Animals cannot complain of minor aches and pains or of mood swings as do people being withdrawn from glucocorticoids. Signs of glucocorticoid withdrawal may include dullness, depression, decreased exercise tolerance, incoordination, unthriftiness and weight loss, loose stools, and behavioral changes. Significant adrenocortical suppression occurs

TABLE 33.4—Examples of alternate-day therapy and weaning a dog from prednisolone

Example of alternate-day glucocorticoid therapy, initiated after 3 weeks of daily treatment, for a 20-kg dog being treated for autoimmune hemolytic anemia:

Week 1: 20 mg prednisolone q12h
Week 2: 15 mg prednisolone q12h
Week 3: 10 mg prednisolone q12h

Three different methods for weaning from week 4 onward:

	Milligrams of prednisolone orally per day					
	Method A (most conservative)		Method B (intermediate)		Method C (least conservative)	
	Day "on"	Day "off"	Day "on"	Day "off"	Day "on"	Day "off"
Week 4	40	15	20	15	20	0
Week 5	40	10	20	10	15	0
Week 6	40	5	20	5	10	0
Week 7	40	0	20	0	5	0
Week 8	30	0	15	0	off	
Week 9	20	0	10	0		
Week 10	10	0	5	0		
Week 11	5	0	off			
Week 12	off					

Note: Supplement during stress 1–2 months after discontinuation is probably indicated.

in dogs within 2 weeks of initiating daily glucocorticoid therapy. Therefore, it is reasonable to assume that dogs and cats may require supplementation of glucocorticoids during episodes of stress, such as illness or surgery, particularly if signs of glucocorticoid withdrawal are present. It should be emphasized that short-term use of glucocorticoids in physiological amounts has few risks despite the evidence that these "physiological" quantities significantly suppress the HPAA, resulting in adrenal atrophy (Byyny 1976; Chastain and Graham 1979).

TEST OF ADRENAL RESERVE. Laboratory tests usually are not necessary to diagnose most cases of iatrogenic adrenal insufficiency; a good history usually indicates the cause of the problem. Occasionally, in the absence of an accurate history or when surgery is considered for a dog with suspected adrenal insufficiency, an ACTH stimulation test is performed to test adrenal functional reserve.

ACTH STIMULATION TEST. A venous blood sample is collected in heparin tubes and centrifuged within 15 minutes, with the plasma immediately frozen for later plasma cortisol determination. A dose of 0.25 mg (25 units or an entire vial, though less will work, regardless of the animal's size) of synthetic ACTH (Cortrosyn, Organon) is given intravenously or intramuscularly. For the dog or horse, a postinjection venous blood sample, handled as for the preinjection sample, is collected 1 hour after IV Cortrosyn injection. If cost is a concern, valuable information on adrenal secretory reserve can be obtained by giving ACTH and collecting a blood sample only at the appropriate time after injection. Blood samples are then assayed by a clinical pathology laboratory for plasma cortisol levels. In cats, peak cortisol concentrations should be measured 30 minutes after intravenous ACTH administration (Feldman and Nelson 1987).

INTERPRETATION OF TEST RESULTS. Healthy unstressed animals have basal plasma cortisol levels in the normal range that increase by 50–100% after ACTH stimulation. Some dogs, after chronic glucocorticoid treatment, may have normal basal cortisol levels but a post-ACTH increase of less than 50%. Such dogs do well until stressed and then require glucocorticoid supplementation (see below). Other dogs may have low basal levels as well as low post-ACTH cortisol levels, indicating a need for continued regular glucocorticoid supplementation as well as additional glucocorticoids during periods of stress (Ferguson 1985a,b).

GLUCOCORTICOID SUPPLEMENTATION DURING STRESS. Animals with marginally adequate or deficient adrenal function require supplementation of glucocorticoids during periods of stress. In situations of minor stress such as minor surgery, general anesthesia, a minor illness, or even a visit to the veterinarian, glucocorticoid can be given to avoid collapse and other complications. For example, hydrocortisone or cortisone can be given at 2–5 mg/kg or prednisolone or prednisone at 0.4–1.0 mg/kg. In severely stressful situations, such as in severe illness or major surgery, higher dosages may be necessary. In preparing an animal for major surgery (including adrenalectomy), prednisolone acetate can be given intramuscularly at 0.4–2 mg/kg the night before and the morning of surgery. Alternatively, or in addition, 100–300 mg hydrocortisone can be given by IV drip. These large doses should be gradually reduced within 3–5 days to maintenance levels unless there are complications (Ferguson 1985a,b).

MISCELLANEOUS OR SPECIAL USAGES

TOPICAL AND INTRALESIONAL USAGE. Topical and intralesional glucocorticoid administration is occasionally used to manage localized lesions of the skin. Despite the route of administration, systemic effects, including suppression of the HPAA, should be expected. Acute inflammatory conditions such as pyotraumatic dermatitis and urticaria are usually managed with nonocclusive, nonheating glucocorticoid preparations. However, chronic conditions are most commonly managed with penetrating glucocorticoid creams and ointments. The potent fluorinated bases such as betamethasone, dexamethasone, triamcinolone, and fluocinolone are the most commonly preferred. The topical, intralesional, or intra-articular use of compounds (e.g., prednisone, cortisone) requiring hepatic activation is of questionable value (Coppoc 1984; Glaze et al. 1988; Kemppainen 1986; McDonald and Langston 1994; Scott 1982; Scott and Greene 1974; Wilcke and Davis 1982).

INTRA-ARTICULAR ADMINISTRATION. Intra-articular glucocorticoids have been utilized to manage the orthopedic conditions of traumatic arthritis, myositis, bursitis, and tendinitis. Used primarily in equine medicine to manage joint inflammation and pain, the practice of intra-articular glucocorticoid therapy is controversial and potentially dangerous. Glucocorticoids tend to reduce the pain for a working animal but also diminish chondrocyte collagen and synovial fluid production. The benefits cited for this practice include the reduction of proteolytic enzymes in joint fluid and reduction of joint swelling and discomfort. The hazards include encouragement of further mechanical damage, loss of joint proteoglycan, development of septic arthritis, and inhibition of chondrocyte and osteoblast activity with the end result being joint or bone breakdown. Intra-articular administration of glucocorticoids leads to systemic absorption and HPAA suppression. Furthermore, glucocorticoid administration has been considered a risk factor for laminitis. In summary, the intra-articular route of administration must be used judiciously (Barragry 1994).

OPHTHALMIC APPLICATIONS. Glucocorticoids are used topically and subconjunctivally to manage inflammatory conditions of the eye, including retinitis, choroiditis, optic neuritis, and orbital cellulitis. These agents stabilize the blood-aqueous and blood-retinal barriers, reducing the leakage of protein into the aqueous that accompanies edema and inflammation. Topical ophthalmic administration of glucocorticoid preparations is also employed to minimize neovascularity and, by inhibiting fibroblast activity, to inhibit corneal scarring, pigmentation, and the formation of synechia.

Topical glucocorticoids are available in solutions, ointments, and suspensions. Penetration, therefore, is determined by two factors: the chemical composition of the base and the vehicle. Except for prednisolone acetate, the alcoholic forms of cortisone, hydrocortisone, and prednisone penetrate the cornea more readily than the acetate ester forms.

Subconjunctival administration of glucocorticoids is used to manage conjunctivitis, keratitis, scleritis, and anterior uveitis. However, it is not the route of choice for diseases of the posterior segment. High concentrations of glucocorticoids can be achieved with subconjunctival administration because the sclera is very permeable to steroids.

Glucocorticoids are contraindicated in corneal ulcers because they slow the process of reepithelialization of the cornea. Furthermore, glucocorticoids enhance the activity of collagenase, which is produced by bacteria like *Pseudomonas* and by leukocytes, and may contribute to the development of "melting" corneal ulcers (Brightman 1982; Glaze et al. 1988; McDonald and Langston 1994). Iatrogenic Cushing's syndrome has resulted from topical ophthalmic preparations (Murphy et al. 1990).

NEUROLOGICAL APPLICATIONS. Neurological applications of glucocorticoid therapy are numerous. Potent anti-inflammatory action is often necessary to manage acute spinal or CNS trauma, acute cervical or lumbar pain, vestibular disease, acute traumatic and some chronic peripheral neuropathies, polymyositis, and CNS neoplasia (Ferguson 1985a,b; McDonald and Langston 1994; Metz et al. 1982; Wilcke and Davis 1982; Meintjes et al. 1996).

MINERALOCORTICOIDS

History. In 1855, Thomas Addison first described the clinical manifestations of primary adrenal insufficiency (Addison 1855); however, it was not until 1929 that crude extracts of adrenal cortex were used in clinical treatment trials of patients with Addison's disease (glucocorticoid and mineralocorticoid deficiency) (Rogoff and Stewart 1969). In 1937, the adrenocortical steroid 11-desoxycorticosterone was finally produced and made available for treatment of Addison's disease (Thorn et al. 1942). It was able to prevent the urinary sodium loss and was the major therapy for the treatment of Addison's for several years. It was not until the early 1950s that aldosterone was discovered, and it was established that this hormone was involved in water and electrolyte balance (Luetscher 1956; Simpson et al. 1954). Aldosterone was isolated and synthesized in the mid-1950s (Ham et al. 1955; Simpson et al. 1954). It is by far the most potent of the naturally occurring corticosteroids with regard to water and electrolyte balance.

Secretion and Mechanism of Action. Almost all naturally occurring and synthetically derived corticoids have both mineralocorticoid and glucocorticoid activity but are usually designated on the basis of their predominant activity. Mineralocorticoid hormones are secreted by both the zona glomerulosa and zona fasciculata. The zona glomerulosa produces aldosterone and 18-hydroxycorticosterone under the major control of angiotensin II, while the zona fasciculata produces mainly desoxycorticosterone, 18-hydroxydeoxycorticosterone, and corticosterone under ACTH regulation (Mantero et al. 1990). Most of our knowledge of mineralocorticoid action is derived from studies on the classical target organ for mineralocorticoids, the kidney. Mineralocorticoids bind to a specific receptor, the mineralocorticoid receptor (MR). The human MR was cloned in 1987 by Arriza (Arriza et al. 1987), and its mRNA was demonstrated in various tissues such as kidney, hippocampus, pituitary, heart, and spleen. The naturally occurring MR ligands are predominantly aldosterone and deoxycorticosterone, although other steroids such as progesterone show a high-affinity binding to MR. Aldosterone is the most potent regulator of electrolyte excretion and is essential for life (Sutanto and deKloet 1991). It is believed to exist in at least 5 isoforms, which may have different biological activity. Deoxycorticosterone is also a naturally occurring mineralocorticoid with similar binding patterns to MR as aldosterone. Mineralocorticoids exert their effect in target tissues through interaction with the MR receptor. Hormone-receptor complex binds to chromatin and induces transcription of mRNA, which is subsequently translated to generate proteins. All physiological actions of mineralocorticoids depend on gene activation and new protein synthesis (Johnson 1992). A two-step model for mineralocorticoid action has been proposed. Changes in membrane electrolyte transport in the kidney are fast (within minutes) and involve the stimulation of Na^+,K^+-ATPase and activation of the Na^+/H^+ exchanger, which leads to Na^+ influx into the cell at the expense of H^+ and K^+, while de novo synthesis of Na^+,K^+-ATPase is a late response (within hours or days). The net effect of mineralocorticoid action is, therefore, Na^+ retention, proton excretion, and K^+ excretion (Wehling et al. 1991; Wehling et al. 1992). The Addisonian patient typically has hypernatremia, hyperkalemia, and metabolic acidosis.

Preparations and Properties. The following preparations are currently available for the treatment of mineralocorticoid deficiency:

1. Desoxycorticosterone pivalate (DOCP), a long-acting ester of desoxycorticosterone acetate (DOCA),

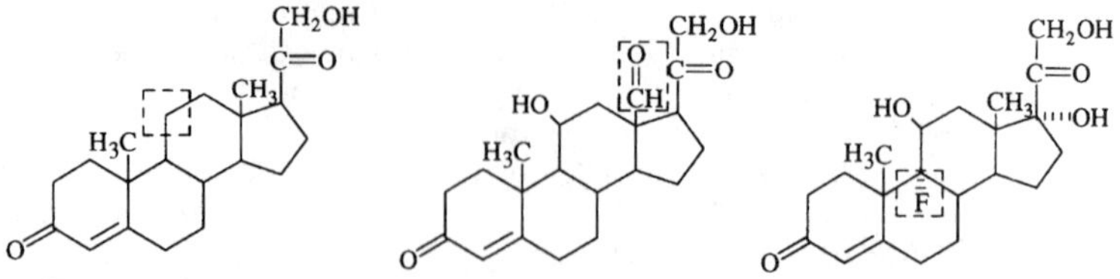

Deoxycorticosterone Aldosterone Fludrocortisone

FIG. 33.6—Structures of common mineralocorticoid drugs used in veterinary medicine. The key elements of structure differing from cortisol are identified by the outlined areas.

is available as a sterile suspension for intramuscular injection (Percorten™-V, Novartis). It has been approved for use in the dog.

2. Fludrocortisone acetate (Florinef acetate®, Squibb) is available for oral use as 0.1 mg tablets. It has a half-life of approximately 8 hours in humans. Fludrocortisone also has substantial glucocorticoid activity.

Note: Aldosterone is only available for research, not for therapeutic use. The structures of the mineralocorticoid compounds are shown in Fig. 33.6.

Therapeutic Use. Historically, DOCA was the treatment of choice for the mineralocorticoid deficiency in acute primary adrenal failure. However, this short-acting product is no longer on the US human or veterinary market. In animals that are not vomiting, fludrocortisone acetate may be used. It is administered orally at a dose of 0.1–0.5 mg/dog twice daily (Hoenig and Ferguson 1991b).

For maintenance therapy either DOCP or fludrocortisone acetate may be used. An initial starting dose of DOCP is 2.2 mg/kg of body weight every 25 days has been recommended (Lynn et al. 1993). In the cat a dose of 12.5 mg every 3–4 weeks has been recommended (Greco and Peterson 1989). These doses and the time intervals of injections may be adjusted depending on the response to therapy as measured by serum Na^+ and K^+ concentrations.

Fludrocortisone acetate must be administered daily for the treatment of hypoadrenocorticism. In the dog the dose is 0.1–0.5 mg orally twice daily or 0.01 mg/kg divided every 12 hours orally. In the cat the dose is 0.1–0.2 mg divided every 12 hours orally. The dose may have to be adjusted based on weekly electrolyte measurements. Once the animal is stable, rechecks including serum Na^+ and K^+ measurement should be made on a monthly basis. Dogs metabolize this drug rapidly and high doses may be necessary even for less-than-optimal results (Hoenig and Ferguson 1991b).

Side Effects. Adverse effects of mineralocorticoid replacement therapy are rare but may include hypokalemia, hypernatremia, muscle weakness, and hypertension, particularly in patients with borderline renal disease (Hoenig and Ferguson 1991b). Because fludrocortisone also has glucocorticoid activity, animals on large doses may show signs of glucocorticoid excess (Lynn et al. 1993). It is important that any fluid deficits be corrected prior to treatment with mineralocorticoids.

ADRENOLYTIC DRUGS AND STEROID SYNTHESIS INHIBITORS

Therapy for Hyperadrenocorticism. Spontaneous hyperadrenocorticism is characterized by excess secretion of the glucocorticoid cortisol. In 85–90% of cases in the dog and the majority of cases in the horse, the primary species suffering from this condition, the cause is excess ACTH production by the pituitary. The term "Cushing's disease" is the term used when the adrenal glands are bilaterally hypertrophied and producing excess cortisol in response to overproduction of ACTH by the pituitary corticotrophs. In the horse, an intermediate lobe pituitary tumor is the most common cause. Accordingly, in dog and horse, there have been attempts to reduce ACTH production with dopaminergic compounds like bromergocryptine or the antiserotoninergic agent cyproheptadine. The experience with these agents has largely been unsatisfactory in the dog due to toxicity and lack of efficacy, and the use of bromergocryptine in the horse is expensive and toxic as well.

Low hypothalamic dopamine concentrations have been observed in dogs with pituitary-dependent hyperadrenocorticism. As such, dopamine deficiency has been proposed as an underlying etiology for this condition. L-Deprenyl (Anypril®, Pfizer Animal Health), a monoamine oxidase B enzyme inhibitor that inhibits the breakdown of dopamine, has recently been approved for the treatment of pituitary-dependent hyperadrenocorticism in the dog.

Medical therapy for hyperadrenocorticism in the dog has been primarily aimed at reducing glucocorticoid production by the adrenal cortex. The two most frequently used drugs are mitotane and ketoconazole (Feldman and Nelson 1987; Ferguson et al. 1991; Hoenig and Ferguson 1991a). Both drugs are used for hyperadrenocorticism regardless of etiology. This is not true for L-deprenyl. Because it influences dopamine concentrations, it is only approved for

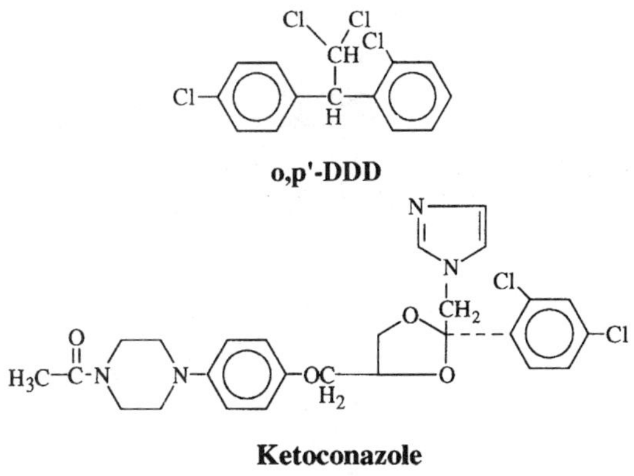

o,p'-DDD

Ketoconazole

FIG. 33.7—Structures of steroid synthesis inhibitors.

pituitary-dependent hyperadrenocorticism. The response of cats to medical therapy is inconsistent.

Mitotane (*o,p′*-DDD)

CHEMISTRY AND MECHANISM OF ACTION. Mitotane (1-(*o*-chlorophenyl)-1-(*p*-chlorophenyl)-2,2-dichlorethane; *o,p′*/4-DDD) (Fig. 33.7) is a compound that is chemically similar to the insecticides DDD and DDT and leads to a relatively selective destruction of the zonae fasciculata and reticularis by an unknown mechanism.

METABOLISM. Clinical studies in human patients indicate that approximately 40% of orally administered mitotane is absorbed, while the remainder is recovered in the feces. Similar studies are not available for the dog or cat.

PREPARATIONS AND PROPERTIES. Mitotane (Lysodren; Bristol-Myers Oncology Division) is available in 500 mg scored tablets.

THERAPEUTIC USES. The cytotoxic effect of mitotane to the dog adrenal cortex was first described in 1959 (Vilar and Tullner 1959); however, it was not until 1973 that mitotane was used therapeutically in veterinary medicine (Lorenz et al. 1973; Schechter et al. 1973). It is now the most commonly used form of treatment for pituitary-dependent hyperadrenocorticism (Peterson 1983) but has also proven to be efficacious in cases with adrenal neoplasia (Kintzer and Peterson 1989). Usually 50 mg/kg are given daily or divided twice daily for 7–10 days. The goal of this so-called loading period is to decrease the capacity of the adrenal cortex to the point that cortisol secretion becomes minimal and the animal is unable to respond to exogenous ACTH with an increase in cortisol secretion. If, after the loading period, the ACTH stimulation test indicates little or no response of the adrenal glands to ACTH and cortisol concentrations are low, the dog is kept on the same dose of mitotane, and a maintenance dose is given once weekly. To reduce side effects, it is advisable to divide the dose and give it over a 2-day period. If the ACTH stimulation test indicates a normal or even exaggerated response, the treatment with mitotane is continued and the dog retested at 5- to 10-day intervals until the desired response is obtained. In some cases, the mitotane dose needs to be increased to 75 mg/kg or 100 mg/kg to obtain the desired response. Higher doses are generally necessary to decrease cortisol concentrations in dogs with adrenal neoplasia. Cortisol-secreting tumors seem to be more resistant and sometimes even unresponsive to the adrenolytic effect of mitotane.

Diabetic animals need to be monitored carefully while on mitotane treatment because the decrease in cortisol concentrations makes the animal more sensitive to insulin. For that reason, some clinicians prefer to use 25–35 mg/kg of mitotane instead of 50 mg/kg in the diabetic. Dogs on maintenance treatment need to be reevaluated regularly. An ACTH stimulation test is the most accurate assessment of adrenal functional reserve. If the ACTH test shows normal or exaggerated cortisol response, the animal should undergo "loading" again for several days, with an increase in the maintenance dosage. Mitotane has not proven to have any therapeutic value in the Cushingoid cat (Hoenig and Ferguson 1991a; Kintzer and Peterson 1989; Schechter et al. 1973).

SIDE EFFECTS. The side effects of mitotane at routine therapeutic doses are usually mild and may consist of gastrointestinal problems such as vomiting and anorexia, mild hypoglycemia, CNS depression, and mild liver damage with increases in alkaline phosphatase. However, in some cases the rapid fall in cortisol levels may lead to weakness, diarrhea, and lethargy. In rare cases, the zona glomerulosa is affected by mitotane, and electrolyte abnormalities compatible with Addison's disease are seen (Kintzer and Peterson 1989; Schechter et al. 1973).

Ketoconazole

CHEMISTRY AND MECHANISM OF ACTION. Ketoconazole (*cis*-1-acetyl-4-[4-[[2-(2,44-dichlorophenyl)-2-(1H-imidazol-1-ylmethyl)-1,3-dioxolan-4-yl] methoxyl]phenyl]piperazine) is an imidazole derivative whose major effect is to inhibit sterol synthesis in fungi (Schecter et al. 1973). In mammalian cells, it inhibits the conversion of lanosterol to cholesterol by inhibition of cytochrome P_{-450}–dependent enzyme systems (Loose et al. 1983). Ketoconazole also inhibits the synthesis of hormones from cholesterol such as cortisol, estradiol, and testosterone (Pont et al. 1940 ; Pont et al. 1982; Willard et al. 1986). In male dogs it greatly increases serum progesterone concentrations (Willard 1989).

PREPARATIONS AND PROPERTIES. Ketoconazole (Nizoral®, Janssen) is available in tablet form, each containing 200 mg ketoconazole base, for oral administration. It is soluble in acids.

METABOLISM. Ketoconazole requires an acidic environment for the dissolution of the drug. Its bioavailability is therefore decreased in patients on antacids. After oral ketoconazole administration, maximal blood concentrations occur 1–2 hours later. There is considerable variation in the bioavailability of the drug in dogs (Baxter et al. 1986). Approximately 50% of ketoconazole is excreted unchanged in the feces, and the rest is metabolized mainly by the liver. Inactive metabolites are excreted primarily in the feces; a small amount is excreted in the urine.

THERAPEUTIC USES. Ketoconazole is used to decrease cortisol concentrations in dogs with pituitary-dependent hyperadrenocorticism and cortisol-secreting adrenal neoplasms. The drug is expensive but is a valuable alternative in those cases where mitotane is ineffective or as initial therapy prior to adrenalectomy in order to control the hyperadrenocorticism and reduce the risk of anesthesia and surgery. The recommended dose is 15 mg/kg twice daily. As ketoconazole inhibits cortisol synthesis only reversibly, it should be given on a daily basis.

No consistent therapeutic effect of ketoconazole has been demonstrated in the Cushingoid cat. The dose in the cat is 10 mg/kg twice daily.

SIDE EFFECTS. The main side effects are vomiting and anorexia. Hepatic enzymes can transiently increase. In rare cases, a reversible hepatopathy with icterus may be seen (Willard 1989). Gynecomastia and azoospermia have been reported in human patients (DeFelice et al. 1981). Ketoconazole is teratogenic and should not be used in pregnant animals.

L-Deprenyl

CHEMISTRY AND MECHANISM OF ACTION. L-Deprenyl hydrochloride (selegiline hydrochloride) is phenylisopropyl-*N*-methylpropinylamine and is an irreversible inhibitor of monoamine oxidase B. L-Deprenyl is thought to decrease the metabolism of dopamine and also other catecholamines, to inhibit the re-uptake of dopamine, and to increase its synthesis. It is hypothesized that the increase in dopamine concentrations decreases ACTH secretion from the pituitary and in turn cortisol secretion from the adrenal gland. In a study by Milgram and coworkers (1995), however, brain levels of dopamine were unaffected when dogs were given L-deprenyl for 3 weeks at different doses. The authors concluded that although dopamine was not increased, L-deprenyl could still affect dopaminergic transmission through one of its metabolites, phenylethylamine, whose levels were increased in dogs on L-deprenyl.

PREPARATIONS AND PROPERTIES. L-Deprenyl (Anipryl®, Pfizer Animal Health) is available for oral administration as white, convex tablets containing 2, 5, 10, 15, or 30 mg.

METABOLISM. The metabolism of L-deprenyl in the dog is unknown. In humans, L-deprenyl is metabolized to amphetamine and metamphetamine; amphetamine concentrations also were increased in dogs on L-deprenyl (Reynolds et al. 1978). Pharmacokinetic analysis in 4 dogs indicated that the drug had a short half-life, which was attributed to high clearance and large volume of distribution of the drug. After oral administration, the bioavailability of the drug was less than 10% (Mahmood et al. 1994).

THERAPEUTIC USES. L-Deprenyl is used for the treatment of uncomplicated Cushing's disease. In 125 cases with naturally occurring pituitary-dependent hyperadrenocorticism, L-deprenyl was shown to be effective in controlling clinical signs associated with the disease such as panting, polyuria, polydipsia, obesity, reduced activity, abdominal distention, and others. The initial dose is 1 mg/kg body weight once daily; this dose might have to be increased if a response is not seen after 4 weeks. The maximum dose is 2 mg/kg body weight per day. It is recommended that the drug be administered for a 2- to 3-month period to allow sufficient time to assess its clinical usefulness. Should the dog's condition deteriorate during that time or should the dog show complications due to high cortisol levels, L-deprenyl should be discontinued and treatment with mitotane initiated. Although the company claims that 80% of dogs with hyperadrenocorticism respond favorably to L-deprenyl treatment, a recent study in a very small group of dogs suggests that only about 20% show an improvement of the clinical signs associated with the disease (Reusch et al. 1999). It has been argued that only Cushingoid dogs with pituitary pars intermedia tumors might respond to this treatment. Pars intermedia tumors account for approximately 30% of pituitary tumors in dogs with Cushing's disease (Peterson 1999). More clinical studies are needed to evaluate the efficacy of this drug.

SIDE EFFECTS. L-Deprenyl is a very safe drug. The following adverse effects were noted infrequently in dogs on long-term treatment: vomiting, diarrhea, hyperactivity, anorexia, diminished hearing, weight loss, anemia, polydipsia, and weakness.

REFERENCES

Addison, T. 1855. On the Constitutional and Local Effects of Disease of the Suprarenal capsules. London: Highley.

Almawi, W. Y., Beyhum, H. N., Rahme, A. A., and Rieder M. J. 1996. Multiplicity of glucocorticoid action in inhibiting allograft rejection. J Leukoc Biol 60(5):563–572.

Almawi, W. Y., Hess, D. A., and Rieder, M. J. 1998. Regulation of cytokine and cytokine receptor expression by glucocorticoids. Cell Transplant 7(6):511–523.

Aron, D. C., and Tyrrell, J. B. 1994. Glucocorticoids and adrenal androgens. In F. S. Greenspan, and J. D. Baxter, eds., Basic and Clinical Endocrinology, pp. 307–346. Norwalk: Appleton & Lange.

Arriza, J. L., Weinberger, C., Cerelli, G., Glaser, T. M., Handelin, B. L., Housman, D. E., and Evans, R. M. 1987.

Cloning of human mineralocorticoid receptor complementary DNA: structural and functional kinship with the glucocorticoid receptor. Science 237:268–275.

Aucoin, D. P. 1982. Treatment of immune-mediated disease. Vet Clin No Am 12(l):61–66.

Barragry, T. B. 1994. Veterinary Drug Therapy, pp. 530–545. Philadelphia: Lea & Febiger.

Baxter, J. G., Brass, C., Schentag, J. J., and Slaughter, R. L. 1986. Pharmacokinetics of ketoconazole administered intravenously to dogs and orally as tablet and solution to humans and dogs. J Pharmaceut Sci 75:443–447.

Bellah, J. R., Lothrop, C. D., and Helman, R. G. 1989. Fatal iatrogenic Cushing's syndrome in a dog. J Am Anim Hosp Assoc 25(6):673–676.

Brann, D. W., Hendry, L. B., and Mahesh, V. B. 1995. Emerging diversities in the mechanism of action of steroid hormones. J Steroid Biochem Mol Biol 52(2):113–133.

Bratts, R., and Linden, M. 1996. Cytokine modulation by glucocorticoids: mechanisms and actions in cellular studies. Aliment Pharmacol Ther 10 (Suppl 2):81–90.

Brightman, A. H. 1982. Ophthalmic use of glucocorticoids. Vet Clin No Am 12(l):33–40.

Byyny, R. L. 1976. Withdrawal from glucocorticoid therapy. New Engl J Med 295:30–32.

Chastain, C. B., and Graham, C. L. 1979. Adrenocortical suppression in dogs on daily and alternate-day prednisone administration. Am J Vet Res 40:936–941.

Chastain, C. B., Graham, C. L., and Nichols, C. E. 1981. Adrenocortical suppression in cats given megestrol acetate. Am J Vet Res 42:2029–2035.

Coppoc, G. L. 1984. Relationship of dosage form of a corticosteroid to its therapeutic efficacy. J Am Vet Med Assoc 186(10):1098.

Crager, C. S., Dillon, A. R., Kemppainen, R. J., Brewer, W. G., and Angarano, D. W. 1994. Adrenocorticotropic hormone and cortisol concentrations after corticotropin-releasing hormone stimulation testing in cats administered methylprednisolone. Am J Vet Res 55:704–709.

DeFelice, R., Johnson, D. G., and Galgiani, J. N. 1981. Gynecomastia with ketoconazole. Antimicrob Agents Chemother 19:1073–1074.

Ehrich, E., Lambert, E. R., and McGuire, J. L. 1992. Rheumatic disorders. In K. L. Melmon, H. F. Morrelli, B. B. Hoffman, and D. W. Nierenberg, eds., Clinical Pharmacology: Basic Principles in Therapeutics, 3rd ed., pp. 469–485. New York: McGraw-Hill.

Eyre, P., and Elmes, P, J. 1980. Corticostero-idinduced laminitis: further observations on the isolated perfused hoof. Vet Res Commun 4:13.

Fauci, A. S. 1976. Glucocorticosteroid therapy: mechanisms of action and clinical considerations. Annals Int Med 84:304–315.

———. 1978. Alternate-day corticosteroid therapy. Am J Med 64:729–731.

Feldman, E. C., and Nelson, R. W. 1987. Glucocorticoid therapy. In E. C. Feldman and R. W. Nelson, eds., Canine and Feline Endocrinology and Reproduction, pp. 218–228. Philadelphia: W. B. Saunders.

Ferguson, D. C. 1985a. Rational steroid therapy. 1. Principles. Mod Vet Prac (Feb):101–105.

———. 1985b. Rational steroid therapy. 2. Therapeutic protocols. Mod Vet Prac (Mar):175–179.

Ferguson, D. C., and Peterson, M. E. 1992. Serum free and total iodothyronine concentrations in dogs with spontaneous hyperadrenocorticism. Am J Vet Res 53(9):1636–1640.

Ferguson, D. C., Hoenig, M., and Cornelius, L. 1991. Endocrinologic disorders. In M. D. Lorenz, L. M. Cornelius, and D. C. Ferguson, eds., Small Animal Medical Therapeutics, pp. 85–157. Philadelphia: J. B. Lippincott.

Ferguson, J. L., Roesel, O. F., and Bottoms, G. D. 1978. Dexamethasone treatment during hemorrhagic shock: blood pressure, tissue perfusion, and plasma enzymes. Am J Vet Res 39:817–824.

Flower, R. J., and Rothwell, N. J. 1994. Lipocortin-1: cellular mechanisms and clinical relevance. Trends Pharmacol Sci 15(3):71–76.

Gametchu, B., Watson, C. S., Shih, C. C., and Dashew, B. 1991. Studies on the arrangement of glucocorticoid receptors in the plasma membrane of S-49 lymphoma cells. Steroids 56(8):411–419.

Glaze, M. B., Crawford, M. A., Nachreiner, R. F., Casey, H. W., Nafe, L. A., and Kearney, M. T. 1988. Ophthalmic corticosteroid therapy: systemic effects in the dog. J Am Vet Med Assoc 192(l):73–75.

Goldfien, A. 1992. Adrenocorticosteroids and adrenocortical antagonists. In B. G. Katzung, ed., Basic and Clinical Pharmacology, 5th ed., pp. 543–558. Norwalk: Appleton & Lange.

Greco, D. S., and Peterson, M. E. 1989. Feline hypoadrenocorticism. In R. W. Kirk, ed., Current Veterinary Therapy X, pp. 1042–1045. Philadelphia: W. B. Saunders.

Grote, H., Ioannou, I., Voigt, J., and Sekeris, C. E. 1993. Localization of the glucocorticoid receptor in rat liver cells: evidence for plasma membrane bound receptor. Int J Biochem 25(11):1593–1599.

Ham, E. A., Harman, R. E., Brink, N. G., and Sarett, L. H. 1955. Studies on the chemistry of aldosterone. J Am Chem Soc 77:1637.

Hammond, G. L. 1990. Molecular properties of corticosteroid binding globulin and the sex-steroid binding proteins. Endocr Rev 11:65.

Haynes, R. C. 1990. Adrenocorticotropic hormone; adrenocortical steroids and their synthetic analogs; inhibitors of the synthesis and actions of adrenocortical hormones. In A. G. Gilman, T. W. Rall, A. S. Nies, and P. Taylor, The Pharmacological Basis of Therapeutics, pp. 1431–1462. New York: Pergamon Press.

Hench, P. S. 1952. Quoted in J. C. Krantz and C. J. Carr, Pharmacological Principles of Medical Practice, 5th ed., p. 1287. Baltimore: Williams & Wilkins, 1961.

Hoenig, M., and Ferguson, D. C. 1991a. Hyperadrenocorticism. In D. G. Allen, ed., Small Animal Medicine, pp. 807–820. Philadelphia: J. B. Lippincott.

Hoenig, M., Hall, G., Ferguson, D.C., Jordan, K., Henson,M., Johnson, K.H., and O'Brien , T.D. In press. A feline model of experimentally induced islet amyloidosis. Am J Pathol.

———. 1991b. Hypoadrenocorticism. In D. G. Allen, ed., Small Animal Medicine, pp. 821–830. Philadelphia: J. B. Lippincott.

Jeffers, J. G., Shanley, K. J., and Schick, R. O. 1991. Iatrogenic Cushing's syndrome in a dog caused by topical ophthalmic medications. J Am Vet Med Assoc 199:77–80.

Jennings, A. S., and Ferguson, D. C. 1984. Effect of clexamethasone on triiodothyronine production in perfused rat liver and kidney. Endocrinology 114:3136.

Johnson, J. P. 1992. Cellular mechanisms of action of mineralocorticoid hormones. Pharm Ther 53:1–29.

Kaptein, E. M., Moore, G. E., Ferguson, D. C., and Hoenig, M. 1992. Effects of prednisone on thyroxine and 3,5,3′-triiodothyronine metabolism in normal dogs. Endocrinology 130(3):1669–1679.

Keller-Wood, M. 1990. Fast feedback control of canine corticotropin by cortisol. Endocrinology 126(4):1959–1966.

Kemppainen, R. J. 1986. Principles of glucocorticoid therapy in nonendocrine disease. In R. W. Kirk, ed., Current Veterinary Therapy IX, pp. 954–962. Philadelphia: W. B. Saunders.

Kemppainen, R. J., and Sartin, J. L. 1984. Effects of single intravenous doses of dexamethasone on base-line plasma cortisol concentrations and responses to synthetic ACTH in healthy dogs. Am J Vet Res 45:742.

Kemppainen, R. J., Lorenz, M. D., and Thompson, F. N. 1982. Adrenocortical suppression in the dog given a single intramuscular dose of prednisone or triamcinolone acetonide. Am J Vet Res 42:204.

Kintzer, P. P., and Peterson, M. E. 1989. Mitotane (*o,p′*-DDD) treatment of cortisol-secreting adrenocortical neoplasia. In R. W. Kirk, ed., Current Veterinary Therapy X, pp. 1034–1037. Philadelphia: W. B. Saunders.

Kuhlenschmidt, M. S., Hoffmann, W. E., and Rippy, M. K. 1991. Glucocorticoid hepatopathy: effect on receptor mediated endocytosis of asialoglycoproteins. Biochem Med Metab Biol 46(2):152–168.

Liposits, Z., and Bohn, M. C. 1993. Association of glucocorticoid receptor immunoreactivity with cell membrane and transport vesicles in hippocampal and hypothalamic neurons of the rat. J Neurosci Res 35(l):14–19.

Loose, D. S., Kan, P. B., Hirst, M. A., Marcus, R. A., and Feldman, D. 1983. Ketoconazole blocks adrenal steroidogenesis by inhibiting cytochrome P450–dependent enzymes. J Clin Invest 7:1495–1499.

Lorenz, M. D., Scott, D. W., and Pulley, L. T. 1973. Medical treatment of canine hyperadrenocorticoidism with *o,p′*-DDD. Cornell Vet 63:646.

Luetscher, J. A. 1956. Studies of aldosterone in relation to water and electrolyte balance in man. Recent Prog Horm Res 12:175–184.

Lynn, R. C., Feldman, E. C., and Nelson, R. W. 1993. Efficacy of microcrystalline desoxycorticosterone pivalate for treatment of hypoadrenocorticism in dogs. J Am Vet Med Assoc 202:392–396.

Mahmood, I., Peters, D. K., and Mason, W. D. 1994. The pharmacokinetics and absolute bioavailability of selegiline in the dog. Biopharm Drug Disp 15:653–664.

Mantero, F., Armanini, D., Biason, A., Boscaro, M., Carpene, G., Fallo, F., Cipocher, G., Rocco, S., Scarom, C., and Sonino, N. 1990. New aspects of mineralocorticoid hypertension. Horm Res 34:175–180.

McDonald, R. K., and Langston, V. C. 1994. Use of corticosteroids and nonsteroidal antiinflammatory agents. In S. Ettinger and E. C. Feldman, eds., Textbook of Veterinary Internal Medicine, pp. 284–293. Philadelphia: W. B. Saunders.

Meintjes, E., Hosgood, G., and Daniloff, J. 1996. Pharmaceutic treatment of acute spinal cord trauma. Compend Contin Educ Pract Vet 18(6):625–635.

Melby, J. C. 1974. Systemic corticosteroid therapy: pharmacology and endocrinology considerations. Annals Int Med 81:505–512.

Metz, S. R., Taylor, S. R., and Kay, W. J. 1982. The use of glucocorticoids for neurological disease. Vet Clin No Am 12(l):41–60.

Michels, G.M., and Carr, A.P. 1997. Treating immune-mediated arthritis in dogs and cats. Vet Med 92(9):811–814.

Milgram, N. W., Ivy, G. O., Murphy, M. P., Head, E., Wu, P. H., Ruehl, W. W., Yu, P. H., Durden, D. A., Davis, B. A., and Boulton, A. A. 1995. Effects of chronic oral administration of L-deprenyl in the dog. Pharm Biochem Behav 51:421–428.

Moore, G. E., and Hoenig, M. 1992. Duration of ACTH and adrenocortical suppression following long-term anti-inflammatory doses of prednisone in the dog. Am J Vet Res 53:716–720.

———. 1993. Effects of orally administered prednisone on glucose tolerance and insulin secretion in clinically normal dogs. Am J Vet Res 54(l):126–129.

Moore, G. E., Ferguson, D. C., and Hoenig, M. 1993. Effects of oral administration of anti-inflammatory doses of prednisone on thyroid hormone response to thyrotropin-releasing hormone and thyrotropin in clinically normal dogs. Am J Vet Res 54(1):130–135.

Moore, G. E., Mahaffey, E. A., and Hoenig, M. 1992. Hematologic and biochemical effects of long-term anti-inflammatory doses of prednisone in the dog. Am J Vet Res 53:1033–1037.

Muller, M., and Rankawitz, R. 1991. The glucocorticoid receptor. Biochim Biophys Acta 1088:171.

Murphy, C. J., Feldman, E., and Bellhorn, R. 1990. Iatrogenic Cushing's syndrome in a dog caused by topical ophthalmic medications. J Am Anim Hosp Assoc 26(6):640–642.

Nakamoto, H., Suzuki, H., Kageyama, Y., Murakami, M., Ohishi, A., Naitoh, M., Ichihara, A., and Saruta, T. 1992. Depressor systems contribute to hypertension induced by glucocorticoid excess in dogs. J Hypertens 10(6):561–569.

Pallardy, M., and Biola, A. 1998. Induction de l'apoptose par les glucocorticoides dans les lymphocytes: entre physiologie et pharmacologie. C R Seances Soc Biol 192(6):1051–1063.

Peterson, M. E. 1983. *o,p′*-DDD (Mitotane) treatment of canine pituitary dependent hyperadrenocorticism. J Am Vet Med Assoc 182:527.

———. 1999. Medical treatment of pituitary-dependent hyperadrenocorticism in dogs: should L-deprenyl (Anipryl) ever be used? J Vet Int Med 13:289–290.

Peterson, M. E., Ferguson, D. C., Kintzer, P. P., and Drucker, W. D. 1984. Effects of spontaneous hyperadrenocorticism on serum thyroid hormone concentrations in the dog. Am J Vet Res 45(10):2034–2038.

Plumb, D. C. 1999. Veterinary Drug Handbook. 3rd ed. Ames: Iowa State Univ Press.

Pont, A., Williams, P. L., Azhar, S., Reitz, R. E., Bochra, C., Smith, E. R., and Stevens, D. A. 1940. Ketoconazole blocks testosterone synthesis. Arch Intern Med 142:2137–2140.

Pont, A., Williams, P. L., Loose, D. S., Feldman, D., Reitz, R. E., Bochra, C., and Stevens, D. A. 1982. Ketoconazole blocks adrenal steroid synthesis. Ann Intern Med 97:370–372.

Restrepo, A., Stevens, D. A., and Utz, J. P., eds. 1980. First International Symposium on Ketoconazole. Rev Infect Dis 2:519–699.

Reull, J. M., de Kloet, E. R., van Sluijs, F. J., Rijnberk, A., and Rothuizen, J. 1990. Binding characteristics of mineralocorticoid and glucocorticoid receptors in dog brain and pituitary. Endocrinology 127(2):907–915.

Reusch, C. E., Steffen, T., and Hoerauf, A. 1999. The efficacy of L-deprenyl in dogs with pituitary-dependent hyperadrenocorticism. J Vet Int Med 13:291–301.

Reynolds, G. P., Elsworth, J. D., Blau, K., Sandler, M., Lees, A. J., and Stern, G. M. 1978. Deprenyl is metabolized to metamphetamine and amphetamine in man. Br J Clin Pharm 6:542–544.

Rogoff, J. M., and Stewart, G. N. 1969. Suprarenal cortical extracts in suprarenal insufficiency (Addison's disease). J Am Med Assoc 92:1569.

Saruta, T. 1996. Mechanism of glucocorticoid-induced hypertension. Hypertens Res 19(1):1–8.

Schechter, R. D., Stabenfeldt, G. H., Gribble, D. H., and Ling, G. 1973. Treatment of Cushing's syndrome in the dog with an adrenocorticolytic agent, *o,p′*DDD. J Am Vet Med Assoc 162:629.

Schwartzman, R. A., and Cidlowski, J. A. 1994. Glucocorticoid-induced apoptosis of lymphoid cells. Int Arch Allergy Immunol 105(4):347–354.

Scott, D. W. 1982. Dermatologic use of glucocorticoids: systemic and topical. Vet Clin No Am 12(l):19–32.

Scott, D. W., and C. E. Greene. 1974. Iatrogenic secondary adrenocortical insufficiency in dogs. JAAHA 10:555–564.

Siegel, S. C. 1985. Corticosteroid agents: overview of corticosteroid therapy. J Allergy Clin Immunol 76:312.

Simpson, S. A., Tait, J. F., and Bush, I. E. 1952. Secretion of a salt-retaining hormone by the mammalian adrenal gland. Lancet 263:226–227.

Simpson, S. A., Tait, J. F., Wettstein, A., Neher, R., von Euw, J., Schindler, O., and Reichstein, T. 1954. Constitution of aldosterone, a new mineralocorticoid. Experientia 10:132.

Solter, P. F., Hoffmann, W. E., Hungerford, L. L., Peterson, M. E., and Dorner, J. L. 1993. Assessment of corticosteroid-induced alkaline phosphatase isoenzyme as a screening test for hyperadrenocorticism in dogs. J Am Vet Med Assoc 203(4):534–538.

Sorenson, D. K., et al. 1988. Corticosteroids stimulate an increase in phospholipase A2 inhibitor in human serum. J Steroid Biochem 2:271.

Sprung, C. L., Caralis, P. V., Marcial, E. H., Pierce, M., Gelbard, M. A., Long, W. M., Duncan, R. C., Tendler, M. D., and Karpf, M. 1984. The effects of high-dose corticosteroids in patients with septic shock. N Engl J Med 311:1137.

Streeten, D. H. P. 1975. Corticosteroid therapy. 1. Pharmacological properties and principles of corticosteroid use. JAMA 232:1046–1049.

Sutanto, W., and deKloet, E. R. 1991. Mineralocorticoid receptor ligands: biochemical, pharmacological, and clinical aspects. Med Res Rev 11:617–639.

Thorn, G. W., Dorrance, S. S., and Day, E. 1942. Addison's disease: evaluation of synthetic desoxycorticosterone acetate therapy in 158 patients. Ann Intern Med 16:1053.

Tuor, U. I. 1997. Glucocorticoids and the prevention of hypoxic-ischemic brain damage. Neurosci Biobehav Rev 21(2):175–179.

Tyrrell, J. B., Aron, D. C., and Forsham, P. H. 1994. Glucocorticoids and adrenal androgens. In F. S. Greenspan and J. D. Baxter, eds., Basic and Clinical Endocrinology, pp. 307–346. Norwalk: Appleton & Lange.

van der Velden, V.H. 1998. Glucocorticoids: mechanisms of action and anti-inflammatory potential in asthma. Mediators Inflamm 7(4):229–237.

Vilar, O., and Tullner, W. W. 1959. Effects of *o,p′*-DDD on the histology and 17-hydroxy corticosteroid output in the dog adrenal cortex. Endocrinology 65:80.

Ward, D. A., Ferguson, D. C., Ward, S. L., Green, K., and Kaswan, R. L. 1992. Comparison of the blood-aqueous barrier stabilizing effects of steroidal and non-steroidal anti-inflammatory agents in the dog. Prog in Vet and Comp Ophthalmology 2(3):117–124.

Wehling, M., Eisen, C., and Christ, M. 1992. Aldosterone-specific membrane receptors and rapid non-genomic actions of mineralocorticoids. Mol Cell Endocrinology 90:C5–C9.

Wehling, M., Kaesmayr, J., and Theisen, K. 1991. Rapid effects of mineralocorticoids on sodium-proton exchanger: genomic or non-genomic pathway? Am J Physiol 260:E719–E726.

Wilcke, J. R., and Davis, L. E. 1982. Review of glucocorticoid pharmacology. Vet Clin No Am 12(1):3–18.

Willard, M. D. 1989. Treatment of fungal and endocrine disorders with imidazole derivatives. In R. W. Kirk, ed., Current Veterinary Therapy X, pp. 82–84. Philadelphia: W. B. Saunders.

Willard, M. D., Nachreiner, R., and Roudebush, P. 1986. Hormonal and clinical pathologic changes with long-term ketoconazole therapy in the dog and cat. Washington, DC: ACVIM Scient Proc.

Wilson, J. W. 1979. Cellular localization of ^{3}H-labeled corticosteroids by electron microscopic autoradiography after hemorrhagic shock. In Upjohn Proc Symp on Steroids and Shock, pp. 275–299.

34 DRUGS INFLUENCING GLUCOSE METABOLISM

MARGARETHE HOENIG

Insulin
Oral Hypoglycemic Agents
  Sulfonylureas
  Metformin
  Thiazolidinediones
  Acarbose
Glucagon
Somatostatin
Miscellaneous
  Diazoxide

INSULIN

History. Diabetes mellitus has been recognized for centuries as a debilitating disease, characterized by the excretion of "sweet urine" (mellituria), polydipsia, wasting of tissue, and the development of ketoacidosis, hyperosmolar coma, and death. The role of the pancreas in the development of diabetes was first recognized in 1886 when Minkowski and von Mering produced diabetes by total pancreatectomy in the dog. In 1921 Banting and Best extracted the active compound from pancreas that was able to control hyperglycemia in diabetic dogs and humans. Insulin was prepared for the first time in crystalline form in 1926 by Abel, and it took 34 more years until its amino acid sequence was demonstrated by Sanger. Finally, in 1963 insulin was synthesized by Meyenhofer and coworkers, and in 1964 by Katsoyannis and coworkers. In 1967, Steiner discovered that insulin was synthesized as a larger precursor, proinsulin. An even larger molecule, named preproinsulin, was identified as a precursor for proinsulin in 1976 by Chan and coworkers (for a detailed review see Bliss 1983). These research efforts have culminated in the biosynthesis of human insulin by recombinant DNA techniques, allowing large-scale production of the hormone in 1983 (Frank and Chance 1983; Johnson 1983).

Spontaneous diabetes has been reported in many species. Diabetes is a major health problem and one of the leading causes of death in humans. In animals, it occurs most frequently in the dog and cat, with an incidence of approximately 0.2–0.5%. Diabetes is rare in horses, cattle, and sheep. Isolated cases have been reported in mules, ferrets, pigs, newts, buffalos, monkeys, and fish (Stogdale 1986). Diabetes also has been reported in several breeds of birds (Stogdale 1986). Diabetes in humans has been classified into two major categories which are of interest to veterinary medicine: type 1 diabetes, previously called insulin-dependent diabetes mellitus or juvenile onset diabetes, and type 2 diabetes, previously called non-insulin-dependent diabetes mellitus or maturity onset diabetes. Based on glucose-tolerance testing (Kaneko et al. 1977; O'Brien et al. 1985), it has been determined that most diabetic dogs and cats are insulin deficient.

Chemistry and Biosynthesis. Insulin is produced in the beta cells of the islets of Langerhans in the endocrine pancreas. The islet also contains glucagon-secreting, somatostatin-secreting delta cells and PP or F cells, which secrete pancreatic polypeptide. The beta cells compose about 60–80% of the islet. The endocrine cells are arranged in a nonrandom distribution, with beta cells forming a central core surrounded by a mantle of the other three cell types in some animals and humans (Bonner-Weir and Orci 1982). In the cat, the beta cells are located in the periphery (O'Brien et al. 1986), while in the horse, the alpha cells form a central core (Helmstaedter et al. 1976).

Insulin exists initially as preproinsulin, which is cleaved to proinsulin in the endoplasmic reticulum. Proinsulin is a large polypeptide consisting of an A and B chain and a connecting peptide (Fig. 34.1). By proteolytic cleavage, four basic amino acids and the connecting peptide are removed, and proinsulin is converted to insulin (Steiner et al. 1969). This reduces the molecular weight from 9000 (proinsulin) to one of 6000 (insulin) and one of 3000 (C-peptide). This conversion occurs soon after proinsulin is transported to the Golgi complex, where it is packaged into secretory granules. These granules therefore contain an equimolar amount of insulin and C-peptide. In the secretory granules, insulin is complexed with zinc and stored.

The amino acid sequence of insulin shows little species variation. Human insulin differs from porcine and rabbit insulin by a single amino acid, whereas dog insulin is identical to porcine insulin. Bovine insulin differs from human insulin by three amino acids (Neubauer and Schoene 1978; Porte and Halter 1981). Antiserum directed against insulin of one species usually cross-reacts with insulin of other species. Antiinsulin serum generally also cross-reacts with heterologous proinsulin, while C-peptides have no immunore-

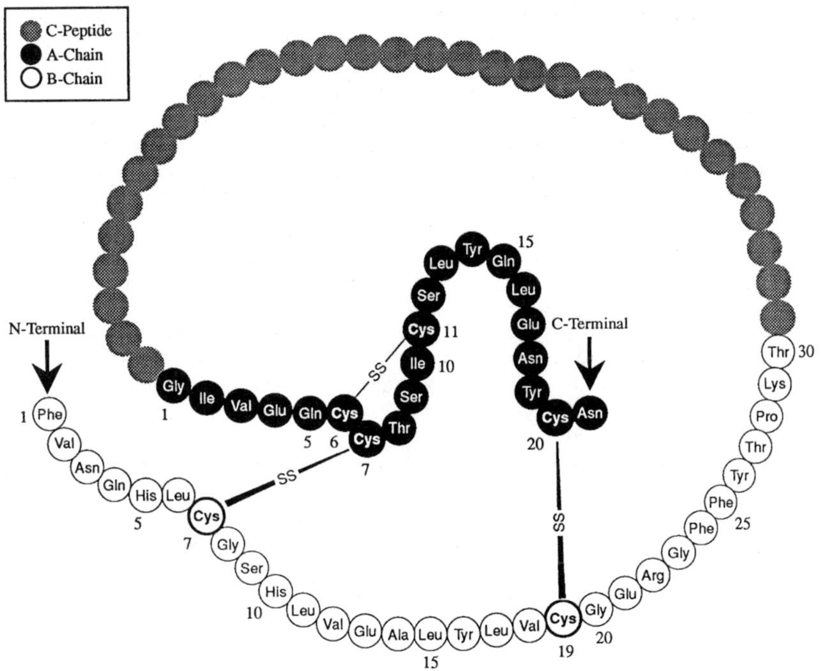

FIG. 34.1—Proinsulin

activity against insulin antiserum. The biological activity of proinsulin, however, is much less than that of insulin.

Secretion. The secretion of insulin from the beta cell occurs through the process of exocytosis in which there is fusion of the secretory granule with the plasma membrane. Insulin secretion is highly regulated primarily by glucose, but also by other fuels, hormones, and neurotransmitters (Porte and Halter 1981). On a cellular level, insulin release stimulated by glucose and other fuels is thought to be initiated by closure of ATP (adenosine triphosphate)-dependent K channels, which leads to depolarization of the beta cell and influx of calcium into the cytosol through voltage-gated calcium channels (Arkhammar et al. 1987; Cook et al. 1988). The increase in cytosolic free calcium may lead to activation of calcium-calmodulin-responsive protein kinases and other target systems. Insulin is released from the beta cell in a pulsatile fashion. It is currently thought that these rapid oscillations are generated through intra-islet mechanisms, because they can be seen even in isolated islets and beta cells (Berman et al. 1993). The underlying mechanism is not understood at this time.

In both type 1 and type 2 diabetes, islet function and insulin secretion are abnormal. It is now clear that in both types a loss of beta-cell mass has occurred and that the fundamental difference between the two major types of diabetes lies in the etiology of the beta-cell dysfunction and its severity but not its presence or absence (Porte 1991). Insulin resistance (frequently caused by obesity or other factors) is an important concomitant factor in type 2 diabetes and puts an additional stress on the beta cell. The beta cell tries to overcome the resistance by increasing the insulin output. Islet dysfunction in type 2 diabetes is therefore an essential element in the development of hyperglycemia. In some of the dogs and cats that are obese, the hyperglycemia, as in the human counterpart, can be alleviated, at least in part, by dietary manipulations resulting in weight loss. In some species (rat, cat, and human) the increase in insulin release from a reduced beta-cell mass in the type 2 form is associated with release and deposition of islet amyloid polypeptide, leading to further loss of beta cells (Porte and Kahn 1989). In type 1 the loss of beta cells is caused by immune-mediated destruction (MacLaren et al. 1989). About 50% of dogs have beta-cell antibodies, and the pathogenesis of the disease may therefore be similar to that in humans (Hoenig and Dawe 1992). Beta-cell antibodies have not been demonstrated in diabetic cats (Hoenig et al., in press).

Insulin secretion can also become autonomous, resulting in hyperinsulinemia associated with hypoglycemia. Insulin-secreting tumors (adenomas or carcinomas; also called insulinomas) occur infrequently and have been described in the dog, cat, ferret, cattle, and a pony (Capen 1990). The diagnosis of an insulinoma can be difficult, but frequently it can be made on the basis of an inappropriately high serum insulin concentration.

Mechanism of Action. Insulin is the most potent physiological anabolic agent. In insulin-responsive tissues, it facilitates cellular uptake and metabolism of glucose. Insulin promotes the synthesis of glycogen, protein, and fat and is involved in the uptake of ions such as K into the cell. Insulin exerts its effect by binding to specific receptors on the plasma membrane of cells. The insulin receptor is a tetrameric structure consisting of two subunits: an alpha and a beta subunit. Two of each of these subunits are joined together via disulfide bonds. Both subunits are glycosylated and exposed to the extracellular milieu; only the beta subunit is exposed to the intracellular environment. The insulin receptor has tyrosine kinase activity, which is enhanced by the binding of insulin. Not only does binding of insulin lead to receptor autophosphorylation, but the insulin receptor will also phosphorylate other cellular proteins (Goldfine 1987; White 1997). Once the insulin receptor kinase is activated, the presence of insulin is not necessary for its continued activity. The receptor is inactivated by dephosphorylation.

Despite our knowledge of insulin-receptor interaction, our understanding of molecular events that link the insulin-receptor interactions to the regulation of cellular metabolism is poor. Some, but not all, of the actions are due to the phosphorylation or dephosphorylation of target proteins on serine and threonine residues.

Metabolism. The existence of a relatively specific insulin-degrading enzyme (IDE, insulinase, insulin-specific protease) has been reported by several investigators (for a review see Duckworth 1990). Insulin-degrading activity has been found in essentially all tissues examined, and high activity has been seen in liver, kidney, muscle, brain, fibroblasts, and red blood cells. The enzyme seems to be located predominantly in the cytoplasm but can be found in other subcellular compartments. Plasma membrane preparations also contain this enzyme. Some receptor-bound insulin is degraded on the membrane, while some insulin is released intact from the receptor, and some is internalized with the receptor, and insulin degradation is then initiated in endosomes. The degradation of insulin via this process is rapid. Other enzymes may also be involved in the degradation of insulin, and further studies are needed to assess their role and to examine factors controlling insulin-degrading activity in various tissues and disease states.

Preparations and Properties. The biological activity of insulin preparations is documented using a bioassay that is based on the capacity of insulin to lower blood glucose concentrations. All but one insulin preparation have been standardized at 100 U/mL several years ago; a U 500 (500 U/mL) regular insulin preparation is available from Eli Lilly (Regular Iletin II). Protamine zinc insulin (PZI, Idexx Laboratories), a beef-pork insulin mixture, is currently under investigation for use in diabetic dogs and cats. This insulin contains 40 U/mL. For correct dosage, insulin preparations are administered with syringes that are calibrated for the appropriate standardization (e.g., U 100 syringes, U 40 syringes). All commercially available insulins in the United States contain no more than 25 parts per million of proinsulin. The insulin preparations currently available are summarized in Table 34.1.

In general, based on action profiles, insulin preparations can be divided into fast, intermediate, and long-acting. The onset, peak, and duration of action listed in Table 34.1 for the insulin preparations from Novo Nordisk pertain to human patients. The Lilly Company recognizes that the insulin responses are individually variable and does not publish fixed action times.

There is considerable species and individual variation in the insulin action profiles. For example, in the cat, it was found that Lente insulin peaks between 2 and 6 hours after insulin administration and has a duration of 8–14 hours (Bertoy et al. 1993). This would predict that once-daily Lente insulin would be sufficient therapy in some cats, while in other cats it would need to be given twice daily for adequate control. Ultralente in recombinant form seems to have a greater effect than the beef-pork combination (Broussard et al. 1993). In the dog, it was found that NPH insulin reaches peak action after approximately 1 hour and has a duration of approximately 9 hours (Goeders et al. 1987). However, it is important for the practitioner to realize that the time course of action of any insulin preparation may vary considerably between different individuals, or in the same individual from day to day (Hoenig and Ferguson 1991; Church 1981). It is also important to realize that the pharmacokinetics change with different doses. The time periods listed should therefore only be considered as initial guidelines for the treatment of a diabetic. Individual responses to insulin and the "fine-tuning" of insulin therapy have to be assessed by measuring blood glucose concentrations at frequent intervals, yielding what is often called a "glucose curve."

Insulin thus far needs to be injected for the effective treatment of diabetes. Although studies of oral and nasal administration of insulin have been published, results have been inconsistent (Saffran et al. 1991; Edmonds 1976). The most promising results in humans have been seen in clinical trials of therapy with inhaled human insulin (Cefalu et al. 1998). It remains to be seen whether this application could ever be used in the cat and dog. Although the short-acting regular insulin preparations can be injected intravenously, intramuscularly, and subcutaneously, the intermediate and long-acting insulins are for subcutaneous injection. The preferred injection site is the flank for those injections. Intermediate and long-acting insulin preparations are suspensions and need to be gently mixed before administration.

TABLE 34.1

Trademark	Common Name	Species	Strength	Composition	Onset of Action*	Maximum Effect*	End Effect*	To Increase Initial effect, Add...	Route of Administraiton	pH	Buffer	Preservative	Retarding Agent	Modifying Protein Salt	Amount of Modifying Protein Salt (mg/100 units)	Appearance	Can be Mixed With...	Company
Humulin® R	*R* REGULAR Insulin Injection		U-100						External pump	Neutral		M-Cresol		—	—	Clear solution		Lilly
Regular Iletin II			U-100 U-500						Subcutaneous intramuscular intravenous	Neutral		M-Cresol		—	—	Clear solution		Lilly
Novolin® *R* Regular	Regular, Human Insulin Injection (recombinant DNA origin) USP		U-100	Solution of human insulin	0.5 hr.	2.5-5 hrs.	8 hrs.	Not applicable	Subcutaneous intramuscular intravenous	Neutral	None	M-Cresol	None					Nordisk
R Regular	Regular Insulin Injection USP		U-100	Solution of porcine insulin	0.5 hr.	2.5-5 hrs.	8 hrs.	Not applicable	Subcutaneous intramuscular intravenous	Neutral	None	Phenol	None‡					Nordisk
Velosulin® Human	Human Insulin Injection (semi-synthetic)		U-100	Solution of human insulin	0.5 hr.	1-3 hrs.	8 hrs.		Subcutaneous intramuscular intravenous	Neutral	Sodium Phosphate	M-Cresol	None				Insulatard® NPH Human & Mixtard® 70/30 Human	Nordisk
Humulin N	*N* NPH Insulin Isophane Suspension		U-100						Subcutaneous	Neutral	Phosphate	M-Cresol Phenol		Protamine sulfate		Cloudy suspension		Lilly
NPH Iletin II			U-100						Subcutaneous	Neutral	Phosphate	M-Cresol Phenol		Protamine sulfate		Turbid or cloudy suspension		Lilly
Novolin® *N* NPH	NPH, Human Insulin Isophane Suspension (recombinant DNA origin)		U-100	Suspension of human protamine particles	1.5 hrs.	4-12 hrs.	24 hrs.	Novolin® R	Subcutaneous	Neutral	Phosphate	Phenol/ M-Cresol	Protamine- approx. 0.35 mg/ 100 units					Nordisk
N NPH	NPH Isophane Insulin Suspension USP		U-100	Suspension of pork insulin with protamine and zinc	1.5 hrs.	4-12 hrs.	24 hrs.	Regular	Subcutaneous	Neutral	Phosphate	Phenol/ M-Cresol	Zinc– approx. 0.02 mg/100 units Protamine– approx. 0.43mg/100 units					Nordisk
Humulin L	*L* LENTE® Insulin Zinc Suspension		U-100						Subcutaneous	Neutral	Acetate	Methylparaben		—	—	Turbid or cloudy suspension		Lilly
Lente Iletin II			U-100						Subcutaneous	Neutral	Acetate	Methylparaben		—	—	Turbid or cloudy suspension		Lilly
L Lente®	Lente® Insulin Zinc Suspension USP		U-100	Suspension of 30% amorphous & 70% crystalline pork insulin	2.5 hrs.	7-15 hrs.	24 hrs.	Regular Semilente®	Subcutaneous	Neutral	Acetate	Methylparaben	Zinc– approx. 0.15 mg/100 units					Nordisk
Novolin® *L* Lente®	Lente®, Human Insulin Zinc Suspension (recombinant DNA origin)		U-100	Suspension of human insulin; 30% is present in amorphous form & 70% in crystalline form	2.5 hrs.	7-15 hrs.	22 hrs.	Novolin® R	Subcutaneous	Neutral	Acetate	Methylparaben	Zinc– approx. 0.15 mg/100 units					Nordisk
Humulin U	*U* ULTRALENTE® Extended Insulin Zinc Suspension		U-100						Subcutaneous	Neutral	Acetate	Methylparaben		—	—	Turbid or cloudy suspension		Lilly
Humulin 70/30	70/30 70% Human Insulin Isophane Suspension 30% Human Insulin Injection		U-100						Subcutaneous	Neutral	Phosphate	M-Cresol Phenol		Protamine sulfate	0.22-0.26	Cloudy suspension		Lilly
Novolin® 70/30	70% NPH, Human Insulin Isophane Suspension & 30% Reg., Human Insulin Injection (recombinant DNA origin)		U-100	Suspension of human insulin protomine particles & solution of human insulin	0.5 hrs.	2-12 hrs.	24 hrs.	Not recommended	Subcutaneous	Neutral	Phosphate	Phenol/ M-Cresol	Protamine- approx. 0.25 mg/ 100 units					Nordisk
Humulin 50/50	50/50 50% Human Insulin Isophane Suspension 50% Human Insulin Injection		U-100						Subcutaneous	Neutral	Phosphate	M-Cresol Phenol		Protamine sulfate	0.16-0.18	Cloudy suspension		Lilly

Therapeutic Uses

TREATMENT OF DIABETES MELLITUS IN DOGS AND CATS. Insulin deficiency is characterized by increased catabolism. The breakdown of glycogen and the decreased utilization of glucose in peripheral tissues lead to hyperglycemia. There is increased protein breakdown, and the increased release of amino acids fuels gluconeogenesis. Finally, lipolysis leads to an increase in free fatty acids, which are transferred to the liver, where they are either reesterified or oxidized, resulting in fatty liver and ketoacidosis.

Treatment of diabetes must be adjusted to the clinical presentation of the animal. Usually two forms can be differentiated: uncomplicated and complicated diabetes mellitus. For practical purposes, complicated diabetics are those that cannot take food orally, such as the vomiting ketoacidotic patient or the comatose hyperosmolar patient (Hoenig and Ferguson 1991).

The goal of treatment of any diabetic animal is to maintain blood glucose concentrations in a *mild* hyperglycemic state; i.e., the blood glucose should stay between 150 and 200 mg/dL for most of the day and should not drop into the low-normal range. The practical therapeutic goal in diabetic animals is more conservative than the goal in a human diabetic, where tight control of normoglycemia has been demonstrated to prevent diabetic complications such as retinopathy, neuropathy, nephropathy, and other chronic sequelae. In the diabetic animal, one has to be more concerned with avoiding the dangers of hypoglycemia in a patient that cannot convey the more subtle signs of low blood glucose. In addition, the complications of persistent hyperglycemia play a lesser role in animals due in part to the shorter life span of the animal.

The fast-acting insulin preparations are used for the complicated diabetic patient. These animals can be treated with low-dose insulin infusions or several intramuscular insulin injections during the day while their blood glucose is maintained with a 2.5 or 5% dextrose infusion (see Tables 34.2 and 34.3 for treatment protocols).

The intermediate and long-acting insulin preparations are used in the diabetic that is able to eat and drink without vomiting. Treatment protocols are shown in Tables 34.4 and 34.5 and can serve as guidelines. Food is given before the insulin peak, which is characterized by the glucose nadir, and should not be given after insulin action has waned. As stated above, it is important to realize that each animal reacts differently to a given insulin preparation. As an example, in some animals NPH has to be given twice daily to achieve adequate control; in others, it can be given once daily. It is prudent to maintain a treatment regimen for 2–3 days before trying to regulate the time and dose of insulin or the time of feeding. It may take several weeks before an animal shows a consistent response to a given preparation.

TREATMENT OF KETOSIS IN CATTLE. Insulin is a powerful antiketogenic agent and has been used as

TABLE 34.2—Low-dose, continuous IV infusion protocol for the treatment of diabetic ketoacidosis

1. Place intravenous catheter.
2. Start fluid therapy (0.9% NaCl; consider replacement and maintenance fluid requirements).
3. [Insert urinary catheter and attach to a closed monitoring system.]
4. Add regular insulin to the saline solution (0.5 units/kg/day). Use pediatric infusion set or infusion pump for accurate administration.
5. Monitor blood glucose concentrations every 2 hours. If no change after 4 hours, increase insulin by 25%. Repeat if necessary.
6. Monitor urinary output.
7. Monitor electrolytes. Adjust if necessary.
8. Change saline solution to 2.5% dextrose in 0.45% saline or in lactated Ringer's when blood glucose reaches 250 mg/dL (13.8 mmol/L). Continue to administer regular insulin. Supplement K. Adjust glucose or insulin (glucose may have to be increased to 5%).
9. Keep animals on this regimen until they are able to eat without vomiting.
10. Stop insulin infusion in the evening. Start treatment of the uncomplicated diabetic the next morning.

TABLE 34.3—Alternative treatment of the complicated diabetic: intramuscular low-dose method

Initial dose of regular insulin: 0.25 units/kg
Followed by injections of 0.1 units/kg as needed (i.e., when blood glucose >250 mg/dL).

TABLE 34.4—Suggested initial protocol for the uncomplicated diabetic animal assuming BID insulin administration

7:50	Check blood glucose
7:55	Feed one-half of caloric needs
8:00	Administer insulin, 0.5 units/kg subcutaneously[a]
10:00–4:00	Check blood glucose every 2–4 hr
5:50	Check blood glucose
5:55	Feed one-half of caloric needs
6:00	Administer NPH insulin, 0.5 units/kg subcutaneously[b]
8:00	Check blood glucose
10:00	Check blood glucose

Note: As soon as the veterinarian has established a consistent response, the animal can be discharged. The owner should monitor and record urine glucose and ketones at home. In addition, weekly blood glucose checks by the veterinarian should be performed initially at the time of insulin peak.

Insulin dose can be increased 10–25% per day if necessary. Feeding time can be adjusted to optimize response if needed.

[a]Insulin is not administered if the blood glucose is 200 mg/dL.

[b]The second insulin injection is administered after 10 hours to allow the owner to observe the animal's reaction to insulin at a reasonable time. Usually, if insulin is metabolized fast enough to warrant a BID administration, the peak insulin action is approximately 4 hr after the injection.

TABLE 34.5—Suggested initial protocol for the uncomplicated diabetic animal assuming SID insulin administration

7:50	Check blood glucose
7:55	Feed one-half of caloric needs
8:00	Administer insulin, 0.5 units/kg subcutaneously
10:00	Check blood glucose
noon	Check blood glucose
2:00	Feed one-half of caloric needs
4:00–24:00	Check blood glucose every 2–4 hr

Note: Blood glucose concentrations only need to be monitored until glucose concentrations start rising after the insulin peak action has been seen.

As soon as the veterinarian has established a consistent response, the animal can be discharged. The owner should monitor and record urine glucose and ketones at home. In addition, weekly blood glucose checks by the veterinarian should be performed initially at the time of insulin peak.

Insulin dose can be increased by 10–25% per day. Feeding time can be adjusted to optimize response if needed.

adjunct treatment in ketosis therapy. It has been suggested that insulin therapy is particularly beneficial in those cases of ketosis that occur within the first week of lactation and are nonresponsive to glucose or glucocorticoid therapy alone (Herdt and Emery 1992). A dose of 200–300 IU of protamine zinc insulin per animal repeated as necessary at 24- to 48-hour intervals was administered.

Adverse Effects. Acute hypoglycemia may result from excessive insulin dose or inadequate food intake. The brain is particularly sensitive to glucose deficiency, and nervous system dysfunction is seen. Initially, confusion, nervousness, trembling, or hyperexcitability may be seen, which progress to convulsions if the hypoglycemia is not treated. Karo® syrup or other glucose-containing solutions can be used orally; however, the intravenous administration of dextrose solutions may be necessary to alleviate the hypoglycemic symptoms. Glucagon may also be used intramuscularly (see below).

The body itself combats hypoglycemia through the release of insulin-antagonistic hormones, primarily catecholamines, glucagon, glucocorticoids, and growth hormone. This frequently leads to hypoglycemia-induced hyperglycemia, also called Somogyi rebound (Cryer and Gerich 1990).

Antibody formation has been documented in diabetic dogs (Harb-Hauser et al. 1998) and diabetic cats (Hoenig et al. 2000). While this has not been examined in dogs, in cats the insulin dose was not different in the presence or absence of antibodies, and the clinical significance therefore seems to be minor.

ORAL HYPOGLYCEMIC AGENTS

Sulfonylureas

HISTORY. During World War II, Janbon and colleagues (1942) found that certain sulfonamide derivatives being used to treat typhoid fever caused hypoglycemia. After the end of the war, derivatives of these antibiotics were first used to treat patients with diabetes. Studies by Loubatieres showed that sulfonylureas did not alter blood glucose concentrations in pancreatectomized dogs and juvenile diabetics (i.e., type I), which suggested that sulfonylureas stimulated the pancreas to secrete insulin (Loubatieres 1946). Indeed, sulfonylureas have become the major therapeutic agent used to treat type 2 diabetes in humans until recently. In type 2 diabetics insulin secretion is still present although insufficient to control blood glucose concentrations. In most diabetic animals the insulin-secretory capacity of the beta cells is lost, and they require insulin for treatment.

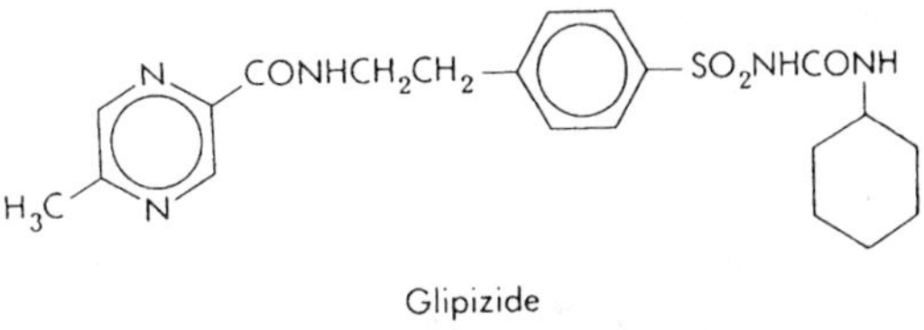

FIG. 34.2—Chemical structure of the sulfonylurea glipizide.

TABLE 34.6—Oral sulfonylurea agents available in the United States

Tolbutamide: Orinase (Upjohn) and generics
Tolazamide: Tolinase (Upjohn) and generics
Chlorpropamide: Diabinese (Pfizer) and generics
Acetohexamide: Dymelor (Lilly) and generics
Glyburide: Micronase (Upjohn) and DiaBeta (Hoechst-Roussel)
Glipizide: Glucotrol (Pfizer)
Glimepiride: Amaryl (Hoechst Marion Roussel)

CHEMISTRY. The chemical structure of the most commonly used sulfonylurea in veterinary medicine, glipizide, is shown in Fig. 34.2. Oral sulfonylurea agents available in the United States are listed in Table 34.6. Sulfonylureas differ in potency, duration of action, metabolism, and side effects.

GLIPIZIDE

MECHANISM OF ACTION. In the pancreatic beta cells, sulfonylureas inhibit ATP-dependent potassium (K^+) channels in the plasma membrane. This results in depolarization and release of insulin (Antomarchi et al. 1987). Because ATP-sensitive K^+ channels also exist in other tissues, sulfonylureas exert tissue-specific responses through the activation of the channels. The extrapancreatic effects of sulfonylureas have been described in detail by Gerich (1989). Sulfonylurea therapy augments the ability of insulin to inhibit hepatic glucose production and to stimulate glucose utilization. It is unclear if these effects are direct effects of the drugs or secondary to the reduced hyperglycemia caused by improved insulin secretion.

METABOLISM. In people, sulfonylureas are readily absorbed from the gastrointestinal tract and are highly protein-bound. Glipizide has a half-life in plasma of approximately 2–4 hours, but its hypoglycemic effects may persist for up to 24 hours. It is metabolized in the liver, and its inactive metabolites are excreted in the urine (Gerich 1989). Sulfonylureas should not be administered in patients with renal or hepatic insufficiency.

No studies on the pharmacokinetics of glipizide have been done in the cat or dog. Studies in healthy cats showed an immediate release of insulin after oral administration. Peak insulin concentrations were achieved 15 minutes later, and baseline concentrations were reached again after 60 minutes (Miller et al. 1992). In our own studies, the insulin concentration peaked 30 minutes after glipizide administration and did not return to baseline levels until several hours later (Hoenig, unpublished).

PREPARATIONS AND PROPERTIES. The preparation used in veterinary medicine is glipizide (Glucotrol®; Pfizer). It is marketed as 5 and 10 mg tablets.

THERAPEUTIC USES. Glipizide has been advocated as an antidiabetic agent for the cat (Miller et al. 1992; Nelson et al. 1991). The drug seemed to be effective in some cats; however, these cats were also on a high-fiber diet, which might have influenced the therapeutic response. A dose of 5 mg BID was given to each cat.

For glipizide to be effective, it is necessary for beta cells to still have the capacity to release insulin. Therefore, in theory, this drug should only be administered in those cases in which insulin secretion has been documented (with glucose/glucagon stimulation tests, etc.). However, it has recently been shown that glipizide accelerates amyloid deposition in cat islets (Hoenig and O'Brien 1998), which confirmed evidence in rats that these drugs may actually be harmful (Kahn et al. 1993). It is therefore prudent to treat all diabetic cats with insulin at this time until other oral antihypoglycemic agents have been evaluated and shown to be effective: the insulin-deficient patient whose beta cells no longer can secrete insulin and the patient who still has insulin but whose secretion rate is insufficient to control blood glucose concentrations. In the latter, the use of insulin will alleviate the overstimulation of the beta cells and amyloid formation.

ADVERSE EFFECTS. Hypoglycemia is the most frequently observed side effect of sulfonylureas in humans; however, severe life-threatening hypoglycemic reactions are rare. The hypoglycemic reactions may be potentiated by drugs which are highly protein-bound. Hepatotoxicity has been reported in dogs after tolbutamide administration. In cats, vomiting, hypoglycemia, and an increase in alanine aminotransferase (ALT) has been reported (Nelson et al. 1991). Other side effects seen in humans include increased cardiovascular mortality, gastrointestinal disturbances, allergic skin reactions, and hematologic changes (Gerich 1989).

Metformin. Metformin (*N,N*-dimethylbiguanide; Glucophage®, Bristol-Myers Squibb) is an oral antihyperglycemic agent used primarily in the management of type 2 diabetes in people. Metformin reduces blood glucose concentrations primarily by reducing hepatic glucose output and by improving peripheral sensitivity to insulin without affecting insulin secretion. It does not cause hypoglycemia at therapeutic doses (Michels et al., in press). Although the pharmacokinetics of metformin has been established in the cat (Michels et al. 1999) and is similar to that in people, data on the efficacy of the drug in clinical diabetes cases are not yet available. Since the drug is eliminated primarily by renal clearance in the cat (Michels et al., in press), it should not be used in cats with significant renal dysfunction.

Thiazolidinediones. Thiazolidinedione compounds have been developed to counteract the insulin resistance that is seen in type 2 diabetes. The exact mechanism by which they enhance the peripheral sensitivity to insulin is not well understood at this time. Thiazolidinediones are high-affinity ligands of PPAR γ (peroxisome-proliferator-activated receptor γ), a subtype of the nuclear receptor superfamily of ligand-activated transcription factors that is involved in the differentiation of adipose tissue. It is thought that the action of thiazolidinediones is through PPAR γ but probably not exclusively (Lehmann et al. 1995).

Among the thiazolidinedione compounds, troglitazone (Rezulin®, Parke Davis) was the first to become widely available (Nolan et al. 1994). The serious liver side effects have forced the discontinuation of the use of this drug. Other thiazolidinedione compounds are being developed.

There are no reports about the efficacy of this drug in the diabetic dog or cat. The pharmokinetics in the cat is similar to that in people (Michels et al., 2000).

Acarbose. Acarbose (Precose®, Bayer) is an alpha glucosidase inhibitor, a term applied to inhibitors of alpha amylase, which digests starch, and of brush border oligo- and disaccharidases, which cleave off glucose. Acarbose delays and reduces postprandial hyperglycemia after a carbohydrate meal. It has been used in human diabetic patients in combination with insulin and oral antihyperglycemic agents but also as monotherapy. Gastrointestinal disturbances such as diarrhea, flatulence, and abdominal pain are the major side effects (Scheen and Lefebvre 1998). The pharmacokinetics of acarbose has been established in the dog (Ahr et al. 1989), and a small number of diabetic dogs needed less insulin when treated with acarbose (Robertson et al. 1998). Because of the high cost of this drug, it remains to be seen if the clinical effect justifies its use.

GLUCAGON

History. Although the existence of a pancreatic hyperglycemic hormone was postulated in 1923 by Kimball and Murlin (1923), it was not until 1955 that Staub and coworkers succeeded in purifying glucagon (Staub et al. 1955). In 1957, Bromer and coworkers identified its amino acid sequence (Bromer et al. 1957).

Chemistry and Biosynthesis. Glucagon is a polypeptide hormone containing 29 amino acids. Its structure is highly preserved in different species, and the different glucagons differ usually only by 1 or 2 amino acids. Glucagon is synthesized in the alpha cells of the islets of Langerhans as a prohormone with a molecular mass of 18 kilodaltons. The exact mechanism of glucagon secretion into the blood is still controversial (Unger and Orci 1989). However, it seems that glucagon is co-released with two major proglucagon fragments. Glucagon-like immunoreactive peptides are also synthesized in the gastrointestinal tract. Glucagon bears striking structural similarity to secretin, gastric inhibitory peptide, and vasoactive intestinal peptide.

Secretion. Glucagon is a hyperglycemic hormone and as such is antagonistic to the action of insulin. The special arrangement of beta and alpha cells in the islet makes a close interaction of both hormones possible, and both, glucagon and insulin, exert a major regulatory function on metabolism. It seems that for many metabolic effects, the ratio of insulin to glucagon is important for the regulation of cellular responses (Smith 1989). In general, glucagon secretion is stimulated by low glucose concentrations, by protein intake, and by lowered fatty acid concentrations. Glucagon secretion is also under control of intestinal hormones and neurotransmitters (Unger and Orci 1989).

Mechanism of Action. Glucagon is a major antagonist of insulin action. Glucagon stimulates glycogenolysis, gluconeogenesis, and lipolysis. Administration of glucagon leads to a rapid increase in intracellular cyclic adenosine monophosphate (cAMP) concentrations, which is followed by activation of cAMP-dependent protein kinase and subsequent substrate phosphorylation (Smith 1989).

Metabolism. Glucagon is degraded in liver, kidney, plasma, and at its receptor on the plasma membrane. Its half-life in plasma is approximately 3–6 minutes (Unger and Orci 1989).

Preparations and Dosage. Glucagon is extracted from beef and pork pancreases. *Glucagon for injection* (Eli Lilly) contains glucagon as the hydrochloride and is dispensed in 1 or 10 mg vials. It is packaged with diluent containing glycerin and phenol. One mg is usually administered to dogs for insulin-induced hypoglycemia.

Therapeutic Uses. Glucagon can be used for the treatment of insulin-induced hypoglycemia when dextrose is unavailable. It is only useful as a hyperglycemic agent in those patients that have sufficient hepatic glycogen. Glucagon should not be used in hypoglycemia due to insulinoma or in patients with pheochromocytoma, because it can induce hormone release from the tumors. In humans it is also used for radiographic and endoscopic examination of the gastrointestinal tract, because it acts as a smooth muscle relaxant. Glucagon has been used in small animals for double-contrast gastroscopy (Evans and Biery 1983); however, a recent study could not confirm a beneficial effect for endoscopic examinations in the dog (Matz et al. 1991).

Adverse Effects. Glucagon is relatively free of adverse effects. Generalized allergic reactions have been reported in human patients after glucagon administration.

SOMATOSTATIN

History. Somatostatin was isolated from ovine hypothalamus in 1973 by Brazeau and coworkers (Brazeau et al. 1973). Soon it became evident that somatostatin was not only present in hypothalamus but also in other tissues, including the pancreas (Hökfeldt et al. 1975; Arimura et al. 1975). It became apparent that the islet D cells, first described by Bloom (1931), secreted this hormone, which inhibited insulin and glucagon secretion (Koerker et al. 1974).

Chemistry and Biosynthesis. Somatostatin is synthesized as a high-molecular weight precursor, which is differently processed in a tissue-specific manner. In the pancreas and hypothalamus it is cleaved mainly to a 14-residue peptide containing an internal disulfide bridge, whereas in the gastrointestinal tract the predominant form is a 28-residue peptide. Very little is yet known about the regulation of its biosynthesis.

Secretion. Much still needs to be learned about the regulation of somatostatin secretion. In the pancreas, somatostatin may act in a paracrine or endocrine manner when released from the delta cells.

Mechanism of Action. The mechanism of action by which somatostatin inhibits insulin and glucagon release from the islet cells is not well understood. It has recently been shown that somatostatin inhibits insulin gene expression through a posttranslational mechanism, however, at concentrations well above those measured in the peripheral blood. Somatostatin release is stimulated by most nutrients, including glucose, amino acids, and a fat-protein meal. Somatostatin also inhibits growth hormone release and a variety of gastrointestinal hormones (for a review see Long 1987).

Metabolism. It is unknown how somatostatin is metabolized. It has an apparent half-life of 3–5 minutes.

Preparations and Dosage. The only preparation available with pharmacologic actions similar to somatostatin is the synthetic agent octreotide acetate (L-cysteinamide; Sandostatin® Injection, Sandoz Pharmaceuticals), a cyclic octapeptide prepared as a clear solution of octreotide acetate in buffered saline for deep subcutaneous injection. In humans, peak concentrations are reached within 0.4 hours; the half-life is approximately 1.5 hours in humans and approximately 75 minutes in dogs (for a review see Long 1987). The duration of action of octreotide is variable but can extend up to 12 hours.

Therapeutic Uses. In humans, octreotide acetate is used most frequently in patients with VIP(vasoactive intestinal polypeptide)oma and carcinoid.

In dogs, the use of octreotide has been used for the treatment of some insulinomas and for gastrinomas. Not all of the tumors treated responded to octreotide, likely because of the absence of specific receptors. Octreotide has not proven to be useful in the treatment of acromegaly. The dose for the treatment of insulinomas is 10–20 μg BID to TID; in gastrinomas 20–60 μg TID have been recommended (Lothrop 1991).

Adverse Effects. In humans, gastrointestinal problems are most frequently encountered after octreotide administration. Side effects in dogs have not been described.

MISCELLANEOUS

Diazoxide. Diazoxide (Proglycem®; Schering) is 7-chloro-3-methyl-2*H*-1,2,4-benzothiadiazine 1,1-diazoxide. It is a white powder practically insoluble in water. This nondiuretic benzothiadiazine inhibits insulin release from the beta cell by increasing the permeability to potassium, thereby hyperpolarizing the cell membrane (Trube et al. 1986). It also has extrapancreatic effects and promotes hepatic glycogenolysis and decreases glucose uptake in the liver (Altzuler et al. 1977). It is used in the treatment of insulin-secreting tumors. The initial dose of diazoxide is 10 mg/kg body weight divided into two daily doses. This dose can be increased gradually but should not exceed 40 mg/kg daily. Diazoxide is available as 50 mg capsules or as a suspension containing 50 mg/mL diazoxide.

REFERENCES

Altzuler, N., Hampshire, J., and Moraru, E. 1977. On the mechanism of diazoxide-induced hyperglycemia. Diabetes 26:931–935.

Ahr, H.J, Boberg, M., Krause, H.P., Maul, W., Muller, F.O., Ploschke, H.J., Weber, H., Wunsche, C. 1989. Pharmacokinetics of acarbose. Part I: Absorption, concentration in plasma, metabolism and excretion after single administration of [14C]acarbose to rats, dogs and man. Arzneimittelforschung 39:1254–1260.

Antomarchi, S. H., Weille, J. D., Fosset, M., and Lazdunski, M. 1987. The receptor for antidiabetic sulfonylureas controls the activity of the ATP-modulated K channel in insulin-secreting cells. J Biol Chem 262:15840–15844.

Arimura, A., Sata, H., Dupont, A., et al. 1975. Abundance of immunoreactive hormone in rat stomach and pancreas. Science 189:1007.

Arkhammar, P., Nilsson, T., Rorsman, P., and Berggren, P.-O. 1987. Inhibition of ATP-regulated K channels precedes depolarization-induced increase in cytoplasmic free Ca concentration in pancreatic beta cells. J Biol Chem 262:5448–5454.

Berman, N., Chou, H.-F., Berman, A., et al. 1993. A mathematical model of oscillatory insulin secretion. Am J Physiol 264:R839–851.

Bertoy, E., Nelson, R., and Feldman, E. 1993. Lente insulin for the treatment of feline diabetes mellitus. ACVIM Proc 11, 925.

Bliss, M. 1983. The Discovery of Insulin. Chicago: Univ Chicago Press.

Bloom, W. 1931. A new type of granular cell in the islets of Langerhans of man. Anat Rec 49:363.

Bonner-Weir, S., and Orci, L. 1982. New perspectives on the microvasculature of the islets of Langerhans in the rat. Diabetes 31:883–889.

Brazeau, P., Vale, W., Burgus, R., et al. 1973. Hypothalamic peptide that inhibits the secretion of immunoreactive pituitary growth hormone. Science 179:77–79.

Bromer, W. W., Sinn, L. G., and Behrens, O. K. 1957. Amino acid sequence of glucagon. V. Location of amide groups, acid-degradation studies, and summary of sequential evidence. J Am Chem Soc 79:2807.

Broussard, J. D., Peterson, M. E., and Wallace, M. S. 1993. Comparison of absorption kinetics of PZI and ultralente insulin preparations in normal cats. ACVIM Proc 11, 926.

Capen, C. C. 1990. Tumors of the pancreatic islets. In J. E. Moulton, ed., Tumors in Domestic Animals, pp. 616–622. Berkeley: Univ California Press.

Cefalu, W. T., Gelfand, R. A., and Kourides, I. 1998. Treatment of type 2 diabetes mellitus with inhaled human insulin: a 3-month, multicenter trial. Diabetes 47(Suppl 1):A237.

Church, D. B. 1981. The blood glucose response to three prolonged duration insulins in canine diabetes mellitus. J Small Anim Pract 22:301–310.

Cook, D. L., Satin, L. S., Ashford, L. J., et al. 1988. ATP-sensitive K channels in pancreatic beta cells: spare channel hypothesis. Diabetes 37:495–498.

Cryer, P. E., and Gerich, J. E. 1990. Hypoglycemia in insulin dependent diabetes mellitus: insulin excess and defective glucose counterregulation. In H. Rifkin and D. Porte, eds., Ellenberg and Rifkin's Diabetes Mellitus: Theory and Practice, 4th ed., pp. 526–546. New York: Elsevier.

Diem, P., and Robertson, R. P. 1991. Preventive effects of octreotide (SMS 201-995) on diabetic ketogenesis during insulin withdrawal. J Clin Pharm 32:563–567.

Duckworth, W. C. 1990. Insulin-degrading enzyme. In P. Cuatrecasas and S. Jacobs, eds., Insulin, pp. 143–165. New York: Springer Verlag.

Edmonds, T. 1976. Evaluation of the effects of topical insulin on wound healing in the distal limb of the horse. VM/SAC, 451–457.

Evans, S. M., and Biery, D. N. 1983. Double contrast gastroscopy in the cat. Vet Rad 4:3–5.

Frank, B. H., and Chance, R. E. 1983. Two routes for producing human insulin utilizing recombinant DNA technology. Münch Med Wochenschr 125(Suppl 1):14–20.
Gerich, J. 1989. Oral hypoglycemic agents. N Engl J Med 321:1231–1245.
Goeders, L. A., Esposito, L. A., and Peterson, M. E. 1987. Absorption kinetics of regular and isophane (NPH) insulin in the normal dog. Domestic Anim Endocrinol 4:43–50.
Goldfine, I. D. 1987. The insulin receptor: molecular biology and transmembrane signalling. Endocrine Rev 8:235–255.
Harb-Hauser, M., Nelson, R., Gershwin, L., and Neal, L. 1998. Prevalence of insulin antibodies in diabetic dogs. Proc. 16th ACVIM Forum, A61.
Helmstaedter, V., Feurle, G. E., and Forssmann, W. G. 1976. Insulin-glucagon- and somatostatin-immunoreactive endocrine cells in the equine pancreas. Cell Tiss Res 172:447–454.
Herdt, T. H., and Emery, R. S. 1992. Therapy of diseases of ruminant intermediary metabolism. Vet Clin North Am 8(Appl Pharm Therap II):91–106.
Hoenig, M., and Dawe, D. L. 1992. A qualitative assay for beta cell antibodies: preliminary results in dogs with diabetes mellitus. Vet Immunol Immunopathol 32:195–203.
Hoenig, M., and Ferguson, D. C. 1991. Diabetes mellitus. In D. G. Allen, ed., Small Animal Medicine, pp. 795–805. Philadelphia: Lippincott.
Hoenig, M., and O'Brien, T. D. 1998. Glipizide leads to amyloidosis in a cat model of type 2 diabetes. Diabetologia 41(Suppl 1):648.
Hoenig, M., Reusch, C., and Peterson, M. In press. Beta cell and insulin antibodies in treated and untreated diabetic cats. Vet Immunol Immunopathol.
Hoenig, M., Reusch, C., and Peterson, M. E. 2000. Prevalence of antibodies against insulin in diabetic cats. Proceedings 18th ACVIM Forum.
Hökfeldt, T., Efendic, S., and Hellerström, C. 1975. Cellular localization of somatostatin in endocrine-like cells and neurons of the rat with special reference to the A_1-cells of the pancreatic islets and to the hypothalamus. Acat Endocrinol 80(Suppl 200):5.
Johnson, I. S. 1983. Human insulin from recombinant DNA technology. Science 219:632–637.
Kahn, S. E., Verchere, C. B., D'Alessio, D. A., Cook, D. L., and Fujimoto, W. Y. 1993. Evidence for selective release of rodent islet amyloid polypeptide through the constitutive secretory pathway. Diabetologia 36:570–573.
Kaneko, J. J., Mattheeuws, D., Rottiers, R. P., and Vermeulen, A. 1977. Glucose tolerance and insulin response in diabetes mellitus of dogs. J Small Anim Pract 18:85.
Kelly, K. L., Mato, J. M., Merida, I., and Jarett, L. 1987. Glucose transport and antilipolysis are differentially regulated by the polar head group of an insulin-sensitive glycophospholipid. Proc Nat Acad Sci USA 84:6404–6407.
Kimball, C. B., and Murlin, J. R. 1923. Aqueous extracts of pancreas: some precipitation reactions of insulin. J Biol Chem 58:337.
Koerker, D. J., Ruch, W., Chideckel, E., et al. 1974. Somatostatin: hypothalamic inhibitor of the endocrine pancreas. Science 184:482.
Lehmann, J. M., Moore, L. B., Smith-Oliver, T. A., Wilkinson, W. O., Willson, T. M., and Kliewer, S. A. 1995. An antidiabetic thiazolidinedione is a high affinity ligand for peroxisome-proliferator-activated receptor γ. J Biol Chem 270:12953–12956.
Long, R. G. 1987. Review: long-acting somatostatin analogues. Aliment Pharmacol Therap 1:191–200.
Lothrop, C. D. 1991. Octreotide treatment in canine and feline endocrine tumors. Proc 9th ACVIM Forum, 755–757.
Loubatieres, A. 1946. Etude physiologique et pharmacodynamique de certains derives sulfamides hypoglycemiants. Arch Int Physiol 54:174–177.
MacLaren, N., Schatz, D., Drash, A., et al. 1989. Initial pathogenic events in IDDM. Diabetes 38:534–538.
Matz, M. E., Leib, M. S., Monroe, W. E., Davenport, D. J., Nelson, L. P., and Kenny, J. E. 1991. Evaluation of atropine, glucagon, and metoclopramide for facilitation of endoscopic intubation of the duodenum in dogs. Amer J Vet Res 52:1948–1950.
Michels, G. M., Boudinot, F. D., Ferguson, D. C., and Hoenig, M. 1999. Pharmacokinetics of the antihyperglycemic agent, metformin, in cats. Am J Vet Res 60:738 n742.
Michels, G.M., Boudinot, F.D., Ferguson, D.C., Hoenig, M. 2000. Pharmacokinetics of the insulin-sensitizing agent, troglitazone, in cats. Am J Vet Res. 61:775-778.
Miller, A. B., Nelson, R. W., Kirk, C. A., Neal, L., and Feldman, E. C. 1992. Effect of glipizide on serum insulin and glucose concentrations in healthy cats. Res Vet Sci 52:177–181.
Nelson, R., Feldman, E., and Ford, S. 1991. Glipizide therapy for feline diabetes mellitus. Proc 9th ACVIM, p. 880, A46.
Neubauer, H. P., and Schoene, H. H. 1978. The immunogenicity of different insulins in several animal species. Diabetes 27:8–15.
Nolan, J. J., Ludvik, B., Beerdsen, P., Joyce, M., and Olefsky, J. 1994. Improvement in glucose tolerance and insulin resistance in obese subjects treated with troglitazone. N Engl J Med 331:1188–1193.
O'Brien, T. D., Hayden, D. W., Johnson, K. H., and Stevens, J. B. 1985. High-dose intravenous glucose-tolerance test and serum insulin and glucagon levels in diabetic and non-diabetic cats: relationship to insular amyloidosis. Vet Path 22:250.
O'Brien, T. D., Hayden, D. W., Johnson, K. H., et al. 1986. Immunohistochemical morphometry of pancreatic endocrine cells in diabetic, normoglycaemic glucose-intolerant and normal cats. J Comp Path 96:357–369.
Porte, D., Jr. 1991. Beta cells in type 2 diabetes mellitus. Diabetes 40:1660–1680.
Porte, D., Jr., and Halter, J. B. 1981. The endocrine pancreas and diabetes mellitus. In R. H. Williams, ed., Textbook of Endocrinology, 6th ed., p. 716. Philadelphia: W. B. Saunders.
Porte, D., Jr., and Kahn, S. E. 1989. Hyperproinsulinemia and amyloid in NIDDM: clues to etiology of islet beta cell dysfunction? Diabetes 38:1333–1336.
Robertson, J., Nelson, R., Feldman, E., and Neal, L. 1998. Effect of α-glucosidase inhibitor acarbose in healthy and diabetic dogs. Proc 16th ACVIM Forum, A54.
Saffran, M., Field, J. B., Pena, J., et al. 1991. Oral insulin in diabetic dogs. J Endocrinol 131:267–278.
Saltiel, A. R., Sherline, P., and Fox, J. A. 1987. Insulin-stimulated diacylglycerol production results from the hydrolysis of a novel phosphoinositol glycan. J Biol Chem 262:1116–1121.
Scheen, A. J., and Lefebvre, P. J. 1998. Oral antidiabetic agents: a guide to selection. Drugs 55(2):P225–236.
Smith, R. J. 1989. Biological actions and interactions of insulin and glucagon. In L. J. DeGroot, ed., Endocrinology, vol. 2, pp. 1333–1345. Philadelphia: W. B. Saunders.
Staub, A., Sinn, L., and Behrens, O. K. 1955. Purification and crystallization of glucagon. J Biol Chem 214:619.
Steiner, D. F., Clark, J. L., Nolan, D., et al. 1969. Proinsulin and the biosynthesis of insulin. Recent Prog Horm Res 25:207.
Stogdale, L. 1986. Definition of diabetes. Cornell Vet 76:156–174.

Trube, G., Rorsman, P., and Ohno-Sahosaku, T. 1986. Opposite effects of tolbutamide and diazoxide on the ATP-dependent K-channel in mouse pancreatic beta cells. Pflügers Arch 407:493–499.

Unger, R. H., and Orci, L. 1989. Glucagon secretion and metabolism in man. In L. J. DeGroot, ed., Endocrinology, vol. 2, pp. 1318–1332. Philadelphia: W. B. Saunders.

White, M. F. 1997. The insulin signaling system and the IRS proteins. Diabetologia 40:S2–S17.

SECTION 9
Nutritional Pharmacology

35 FAT-SOLUBLE VITAMINS

MARTIN J. FETTMAN

Vitamin A
Vitamin D
Vitamin E
Vitamin K

The chapters in Section 9 are concerned with quantitatively minor but essential dietary constituents that are required for optimal health, growth, and performance in animals. Included in this list of essential nutrients with prominent metabolic roles are the fat-soluble vitamins, water-soluble vitamins, macroelements, trace elements, and miscellaneous nutrients, including the essential fatty acids derived from linoleic and linolenic acid and the sulfur-containing amino acid, taurine. These substances have diverse biochemical and structural actions which are sometimes buried in the depths of complex physiological functions of the body, but all serve vital roles irrespective of species differences in dietary requirements or reciprocity of functions. Most of these nutrients are provided in adequate amounts by the natural diets of animals living in their usual environments. However, imposition of unusual environmental conditions or performance demands can alter the physiological requirements for many of these substances, and formulation of diets from alternative feed sources can change the bioavailability and interactions of these nutrients. In addition, particular diseases can influence the absorption, metabolism, or excretion of certain dietary constituents so that conditional deficiencies or excesses may develop. It is under these unusual conditions that one must consider, in addition to their nutritional properties, the pharmacological attributes of those nutrients.

Prevention of dietary deficiencies or excesses, rather than the treatment of dietary imbalances, should be a goal of veterinary medical practice. Thus, in this and the following chapters, emphasis will be placed on an understanding of the dietary interactions and biochemical functions of individual nutrients which are integral to their *normal* physiological roles, and on approaches to limit the incidence of imbalances that may impair health or impede performance. Where adequate information regarding the signs of dietary imbalance is available, recognition of those features and the treatment necessary for their correction will be discussed. Finally, information concerning the use of particular nutrients in "supraphysiological" quantities will be presented with due attention to the potential consequences of their injudicious use. Unsubstantiated use of vitamin-mineral supplements in animal dietetics and veterinary therapeutics has the potential to create conditions of dietary imbalance more deleterious than those of the presenting complaints and further emphasizes the necessity of a comprehensive understanding of nutritional pharmacology and its limitations.

Unless specifically stated to the contrary, all daily dietary requirements are based on the current recommendations of the National Academy of Sciences, National Research Council Committee on Animal Nutrition. Individual publications by this body give the nutrient requirements for all major species. They are regularly revised and present usual feed compositions and normal requirements, as well as textual and photographic illustrations of deficiency syndromes. These publications are a valuable addition to the practicing veterinarian's library and for a nominal fee may be acquired from the Printing and Publishing Office, National Academy of Sciences, 2101 Constitution Avenue NW, Washington, DC 20418.

VITAMIN A

Chemical Structure. Vitamin A, or retinol, is a fat-soluble, long-chain, unsaturated alcohol with five (vitamin A_1) or six (vitamin A_2) double bonds (Fig. 35.1). The former is found predominantly in tissues of mammals and marine fish, and the latter has been isolated from freshwater fish and possesses approximately half the biological activity of vitamin A_1. Vitamin A has several isomeric forms, depending on the configuration about its double bonds, including the all-*trans* form, which possesses the greatest biological activity, and several *cis* forms, which are less active. Replacement of the alcohol group on carbon 15 by an aldehyde group produces retinal, and replacement by an acid group produces retinoic acid. Vitamin A does not occur in plants, but its precursor, the carotenoids, do (Fig. 35.1). Of these, β-carotene possesses the greatest provitamin A activity; α-carotene, γ-carotene, and cryptoxanthin are only about one-fourth as potent (McDowell 1989a). Because only one molecule of vitamin A is produced from each molecule of β-carotene, pure vitamin A has twice the potency of β-carotene.

Sources and Chemical Properties. Carotenoids are the main source of vitamin A for herbivores, and many factors affect their availability, their potency as vitamin A precursors, and the efficiency of conversion to active vitamin A following consumption. All green parts of plants contain carotenoids and thus high potential provitamin A activity. Considerable provitamin A activity may be lost during hay-making, ensiling, dehydrating, processing, and storage of crops.

Animal-fat products, particularly fish oils and liver, contain large amounts of vitamin A, largely as retinyl palmitate, the esterified form. Animal by-products such as tankage, meat scraps, and fish meals often have little if any vitamin A activity, by virtue of composition and processing. Because the carotenoid content of legume hay is so high, dehydrated alfalfa remains one of the best natural sources of provitamin A activity. Yellow corn is the only concentrate containing significant amounts, with only about one-eighth that of good roughage (NRC 1982). Commercial sources of supplemental vitamin A are produced primarily from fish oils and from industrial chemical synthesis. Commercial sources are usually all-*trans* retinyl palmitate or acetate. Natural sources may be highly variable in potency owing to differences in conditions during growth, processing, or storage. Oxidation of vitamin A upon exposure to heat and oxygen is a prominent concern.

Several methods are available to determine carotenoid or vitamin A content in biological specimens. Physicochemical methods are quantitative and include colorimetric reactions, thin-layer chromatography, gas chromatography, and high-performance liquid chromatography (HPLC). Vitamin A activity is expressed in international units (IU) or in micrograms (μg) of retinol equivalents. An IU has the biological activity of 0.3 μg of retinol or 0.55 μg of retinyl palmi-

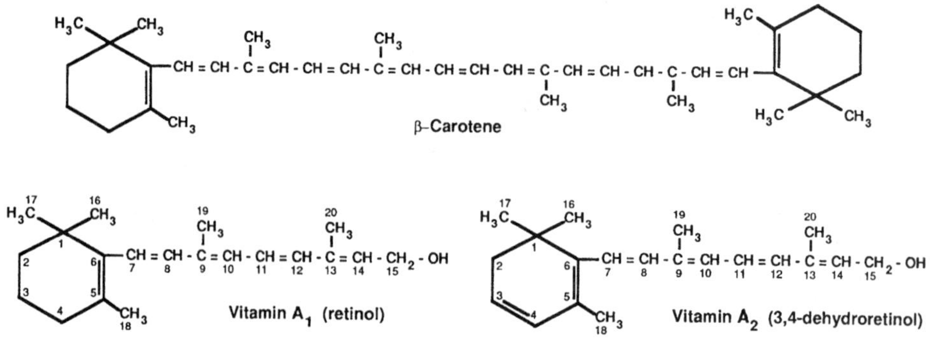

β-Carotene

Vitamin A_1 (retinol)

Vitamin A_2 (3,4-dehydroretinol)

FIG. 35.1

tate. One IU of provitamin A activity is equal to 0.6 μg of β-carotene. One retinol equivalent is equal to 1 μg or 3.33 IU of retinol, and 6 μg or 10 IU of β-carotene.

Biological Characteristics. The conversion of ingested carotenoids into vitamin A occurs in the small-intestinal mucosa and involves two enzymes. The first is β-carotene-15,15′-dioxygenase, which catalyzes the cleavage of β-carotene at the central double bond to produce two molecules of retinaldehyde. The second enzyme is retinaldehyde reductase, which reduces the retinaldehyde to retinol for uptake by the enterocytes. Because the cleavage enzyme is not present in the cat or mink, these species cannot utilize carotenoids, and they must be provided with a dietary source of active vitamin A (McDowell 1989a). There are species differences in the ability to absorb carotenoids; rats, pigs, goats, sheep, rabbits, buffaloes, and dogs cleave virtually all dietary carotenoids in the intestine; whereas, humans, cattle, horses, and carp absorb significant quantities for storage in the liver and adipose tissues. Breed differences in the absorption of carotenoids are also seen; the Guernsey and Jersey breeds of cattle readily absorb carotenoids and have yellow adipose tissue and milk fat, while Holsteins are efficient at cleavage and conversion to vitamin A and have white body fat and milk fat.

Similar to vitamin A derived from carotenoids, vitamin A as the palmitate or acetate ester in animal or industrial sources is absorbed predominantly as retinol, thus requiring its hydrolysis by pancreatic retinyl ester hydrolase. Lipid micelles from the intestinal contents facilitate the uptake of retinol by enterocytes, whereupon the retinol is esterified predominantly to palmitate, incorporated into chylomicrons, and taken up by the lymphatic system for transport to the liver. When vitamin A is released from the liver, the ester is hydrolyzed, retinol is released to the blood, and it is transported by retinol-binding protein (RBP), a specific carrier molecule synthesized by the hepatocytes (Goodman 1980). Nutritional status of the animal influences the synthesis of RBP; protein malnutrition reduces RBP synthesis, and vitamin A deficiency blocks RBP secretion by the liver. The liver contains approximately 90% of total body vitamin A; polar bear livers are so rich in vitamin A that their consumption may result in vitamin A toxicity. Measurement of hepatic vitamin A content may provide more accurate information regarding an animal's vitamin A status than blood levels, which may be maintained through long periods of dietary insufficiency by release from hepatic stores.

METABOLIC FUNCTIONS. Vitamin A is required for at least five distinct physiological processes: normal vision, maintenance of epithelial integrity, reproductive function, bone development, and immune competency (McDowell 1989a). Retinoic acid cannot replace retinol for visual or reproductive function and cannot support rapid epithelial cell division or differentiation, but can otherwise maintain normal growth and health.

VISION. For normal vision, the aldehyde form of vitamin A, 11-*cis*-retinal, combines with the protein opsin to produce rhodopsin, or visual purple, which reacts with light and in the process initiates the activation of the visual neural pathways (Fig. 35.2). Light converts 11-*cis*-retinal to the all-*trans* retinaldehyde, which cannot sustain a stable complex with opsin and is subsequently hydrolyzed from the protein (Fig. 35.2). The energy derived from this reaction is converted to a neural impulse which travels along the optic nerve to the brain, thereby mediating the visual process. Because some of the retinal is lost during this process and must be replaced by vitamin A from the blood, nutritional vitamin A deficiency results in progressive depletion of rhodopsin, which is manifested by slower dark adaptation, progressing to night blindness, and by rod degeneration, leading eventually to complete loss of sight. As part of its function in maintaining epithelial integrity, vitamin A is also required for normal conjunctival and corneal function. Vision may thus become impaired as a result of xerophthalmia, a manifestation of vitamin A deficiency in which the conjunctiva are dehydrated and the cornea becomes cloudy, ulcerated, inflamed, and keratinized. In cows, sheep, horses, and dogs, excessive lacrimation may also result.

EPITHELIAL INTEGRITY. In vitamin A deficiency, the epithelial lining of the respiratory, gastrointestinal, and genitourinary systems may undergo morphologic changes progressing through columnar-to-cuboidal and cuboidal-to-stratified squamous epithelial metaplasia, as well as loss of mucus-secreting capacity. In addition to loss of these systems' normal functions, impairment of the epithelial barriers to microorganisms may significantly reduce an animal's resistance to stress and disease. Vitamin A-responsive dermatoses have been reported in dogs fed commercial diets deficient in vitamin A but otherwise adequate (Ihrke and Goldschmidt 1983). Some of these disorders were histologically compatible with human phrynoderma, a disease thought to be associated with vitamin A deficiency,

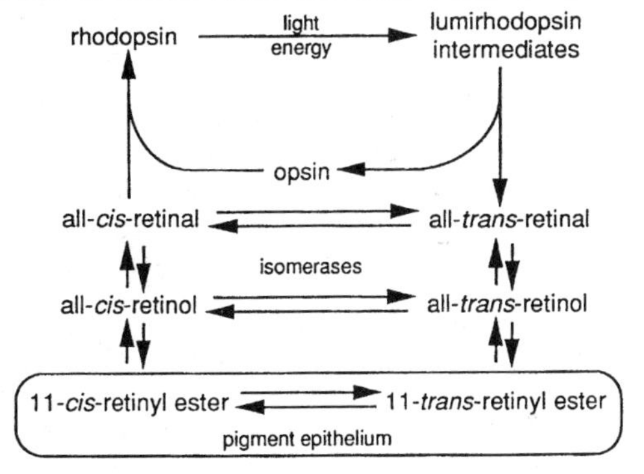

FIG. 35.2—Vitamin A participation in retinal photochemistry. (Adapted from Guyton 1981.)

while others may have responded to the nonspecific epitheliotropic effects of the vitamin.

REPRODUCTION. Vitamin A is required for normal reproductive function in both males and females. Deficiency in the male produces decreased sexual activity and failure of spermatogenesis. In the female, abnormal estrous cycles, resorption of the fetus, abortion, retained placentas, or birth of dead offspring may result (Hemken and Bremel 1982). Dietary supplementation with β-carotene beyond nutritional requirements has had variable effects on female reproductive function, although in some cases, fewer supplemented cows required treatment for clinical mastitis (Wang et al. 1988). A comparison of high-level dietary vitamin A supplementation in dairy cows (1-2 million IU/day versus 100,000 IU/day) revealed no significant effects on several reproductive parameters, including circulating progesterone and gonadotropin-releasing hormone levels, rate of estrus detection, first-service conception efficiency, postpartum interval, or placental retention (Tharnish and Larson 1992). In fact, very high dietary carotene intake has been associated with some adverse effects on fertility in dairy cows, including a higher number of days open, a higher number of inseminations per conception, and a lower overall pregnancy rate (Folman et al. 1987). Gilts injected with vitamin A and β-carotene had larger litters of greater birth weight than those that were made deficient, and their piglets had higher plasma immunoglobulin levels (Brief and Chew 1985). The effects on reproductive function of supplementing dietary vitamin A or β-carotene beyond established requirements have been quite variable, so recommendations can be made with certainty only for those animals with documented deficiencies.

BONE DEVELOPMENT. Normal bone development is dependent on vitamin A, through effects on osteoclast and osteoblast activity. These effects may account in part for locomotory changes observed in deficient animals. Growing ponies fed a vitamin A-deficient diet experienced lesser gains in body weight, heart girth, and height at the withers than normally fed controls. Hypovitaminosis A in feedlot cattle has been characterized by a gaunt and unthrifty appearance, anorexia, slow weight gain, changes in gait, and ataxia (Booth et al. 1987). Blindness or deafness in neonates and growing animals may result from pressure necrosis of the optic or auditory nerves, respectively, owing to inadequate growth of the foramina through which these nerves pass through the skull to the brain (Paulsen et al. 1989).

IMMUNE FUNCTION. Vitamin A deficiency has been associated with an increased frequency and severity of many infectious diseases, related both to alterations in epithelial barrier function and to loss of immune system responsiveness (Chew 1987; Chew et al. 1984; Butera and Krakowka 1986). Vitamin A deficiency has resulted in reduced lymphocyte transformation in response to various mitogens, decreased intestinal secretory IgA release, and impaired neutrophil phagocytic and bactericidal functions. Both in vivo and in vitro supplementation with retinol have resulted in enhanced mitogen-stimulated lymphocyte proliferation, delayed-type hypersensitivity, cell-mediated toxicity, natural killer cell activity, and enhanced humoral immunity to antigenic challenges. In some studies, β-carotene itself has been shown to promote phagocytic and/or bactericidal function of neutrophils and macrophages isolated from the mammary glands of lactating cows, where vitamin A had no effect (Daniel et al. 1991a). Beta-carotene has likewise been shown to potentiate bovine peripheral blood lymphocyte transformation induced by concanavalin A, a potent mitogen (Daniel et al. 1991b). In other studies, retinol or retinoic acid has been shown to depress in vitro phagocytosis and bactericidal capacity of isolated blood neutrophils (Tjoelker et al. 1988). Although there are some conflicting data, it is generally thought that dietary supplementation with vitamin A and/or β-carotene, beyond nutritional requirements, may afford some advantages in the immunological defense against certain infectious diseases.

HEMATOPOIESIS. Vitamin A deficiency in growing rats and chicks has been associated with the secondary development of an iron deficiency anemia which is unresponsive to supplemental dietary iron (Hodges et al. 1978). Gastrointestinal absorption of iron, estimates of whole-body iron turnover, and clearance rates for radioactively labeled iron from the plasma in these animals appear to be normal (Mejia et al. 1979). However, incorporation of iron into erythrocytes is markedly reduced, hepatic and splenic iron levels are increased, and plasma iron concentrations are decreased. In addition to its possible effects on iron release from storage sites or incorporation into hemoglobin, vitamin A deficiency may result in erythrocyte membrane abnormalities that lead to abnormal fragility and hemolysis. Epidemiological evidence from Third World countries also associates vitamin A deficiency in humans with iron deficiency anemia in the absence of dietary iron imbalance.

ANTIOXIDANT ACTIVITY AND CANCER PREVENTION. Epidemiologic studies have shown that the risk in humans for cancer of a variety of tissues may be significantly lower in individuals with an above-average intake of β-carotene (Weisburger 1991; Ziegler 1991). Beta-carotene is purported to have anticancer activity by virtue of its antioxidant function, wherein it quenches free radicals and inhibits lipid peroxidation and oxidative damage to key cellular macromolecules, including DNA (Burton and Ingold 1984). In experimental models of chemically induced carcinogenesis in rats and mice, and in cultured fibroblasts, carotenoids have inhibited the conversion of procarcinogens into active carcinogens by cytochrome P-450-linked hepatic biotransformation enzymes (Tan and Chu 1991). Vitamin A may also act as an anticarcinogen at the level of cell differentiation, thereby preventing loss of control of tissue growth. Studies have shown that vitamin A has no effect on the incidence of cardiovascular disease or cancer in humans (Greenberg et al. 1996; Hennekens et al. 1996; Kushi et al. 1996). Other studies of human smokers and of workers occupationally exposed to asbestos have indicated the possibility that supplemental β-carotene may actually be associated with as much as an 18% increase in the incidence of lung cancer and a 16-26% increase in mortality due to lung cancer or cardiovascular disease (Alpha-Tocopherol, Beta Carotene Cancer Prevention Study Group 1994; Albanes et al. 1996; Omenn et al. 1996). Safe and efficacious levels of dietary carotenoids and/or retinoids for the chemoprevention of cancer remain theoretical and await objective experimental verification.

Signs of Deficiency. In cattle, the signs of vitamin A deficiency include reduced feed intake, slow growth, nyctalopia, xerophthalmia, lacrimation, diarrhea, reproductive abnormalities, and increased susceptibility to infectious diseases. Signs in sheep are similar, with abnormalities in wool fiber structure and strength. In pigs, reproductive performance is impaired, including a variety of developmental abnormalities in term fetuses. In adults, nervous signs predominate, including ataxia, limb trembling, clonic spasms, and paralysis. Vitamin A deficiency in poultry reduces disease resistance, causes neuromuscular incoordination, decreases growth, and reduces egg production and hatchability. Horses develop eye lesions and visual abnormalities similar to those in ruminants, reproductive abnormalities, anorexia, and progressive weakness. In all species, vitamin A deficiency of sufficient severity and/or duration will result in death, either due directly to lesions attributable to retinoid deficiency or due to infectious diseases developed secondarily to impaired immunity.

Assessment of Status. Criteria used to evaluate vitamin A status have included biological response to supplementation, determination of hepatic vitamin A content, and analysis of blood vitamin A concentrations. Because blood vitamin A is maintained by release from the liver, in some species these values may be maintained until hepatic stores are depleted. Thus, low blood levels indicate deficiency, but normal values must be interpreted with caution. For adult dairy cattle, liver vitamin A values less than 1 IU/kg are representative of a deficiency (NRC 1978a). Plasma vitamin A concentrations less than 20 μg/dL in calves and less than 40 μg/dL in adult cattle suggest a deficiency (McDowell 1989a). Vitamin A values below 10 μg/g in the liver or below 10 μg/dL in the plasma indicate a deficiency in pigs (McDowell 1989a).

Dietary Requirements, Indications, and Use

INTRINSIC FACTORS. There are significant species differences in the efficiency of conversion of β-carotene to vitamin A, which in turn affects dietary requirements for both carotenoids and retinoids. Rats and poultry possess the greatest ability for conversion, while cats and mink possess no conversion capacity (NRC 1986). Ruminants generally have approximately one-fourth the conversion ability of rats; horses, one-third the capacity of rats; and dogs, one-half the capacity of rats. In any species, the efficiency of β-carotene conversion to vitamin A decreases with increasing dietary intake of β-carotene. Requirements for β-carotene and vitamin A are greatest during pregnancy, lactation, and rapid growth. Deficiency during these phases of life in herbivores can be caused by feeding large quantities of concentrates that are poor sources of provitamin A activity. It has been suggested that dietary requirements for growth in horses may be 1.5-5 times higher than those previously published (Donoghue et al. 1981; NRC 1978b).

EXTRINSIC FACTORS. Stressful environmental conditions and disease have been shown to depress β-carotene conversion ability. Gastrointestinal diseases may impair both β-carotene conversion and absorption of vitamin A. In young calves who are at risk for development of vitamin A deficiency owing to limited reserves at birth, infection with *Cryptosporidium parvum* has resulted in intestinal mucosal pathology sufficient to result in significant impairment of absorption of orally administered vitamin A (Holland et al. 1992). Seasonal effects on vitamin A status have been observed in horses owing to differences in feed carotenoid content, accumulated effects of storage on carotenoid stability, and changes in dietary requirements associated with changes in environment and reproductive status (Maenpaa et al. 1988a,b).

Other dietary constituents may have significant influences on β-carotene or vitamin A stability in feeds, absorption from the gut, or disposition in the body. Because both β-carotene and vitamin A are destroyed by oxidation, the unsaturated fat content of feed may affect their stability, particularly under adverse conditions of storage or handling. Transition elements, including iron, zinc, and copper, may act as catalysts in oxidative chemical reactions and thereby be detrimental to β-carotene and vitamin A stability. Dietary antioxidants such as vitamin E may both protect β-carotene and vitamin A from oxidative breakdown and improve gastrointestinal absorption or utilization. On the other hand, in some studies the combined supplementation of both vitamin A and E provided less protection against bacterial infection than either vitamin alone, implying there may be antagonistic effects at certain dietary levels (Tengerdy and Nockels 1975).

Preparations. Vitamin A is available in natural fish oils and as a synthetic ester of acetate, propionate, or palmitate. Injectable and oral preparations may be obtained singly or as part of a multivitamin preparation. Simple, aqueous solutions are indicated for injection, but because of oxidative instability, chemically stabilized forms of vitamin A are preferred for feed supplementation. Retinyl esters may be stabilized by protective coating with gelatin and antioxidants, included as part of a free-choice mineral mixture, or added with antioxidants to liquids such as oils or molasses that are sprayed onto the feed during processing. Single large doses may be given as intramuscular injections in the prophylaxis or therapy of specific conditions or diseases which increase vitamin A requirements. Large doses may also be included in drinking water or parenteral fluid preparations in the resuscitation of diseased or convalescent animals.

Toxicity. Of all the vitamins, vitamin A is most likely to be supplemented at toxic levels, and signs of toxicity have been demonstrated in most species. Upper safe limits are between 4 and 10 times the nutritional requirements for most nonruminants, and up to 30 times the requirements for ruminants (NRC 1987). Nevertheless, the inappropriate rationale "If a little bit helps, more is better" persists, and toxicity remains a concern. Hypervitaminosis A is characterized by adverse effects caused directly by the retinoids and indirectly by interference with the metabolism of other fat-soluble vitamins, including vitamins D, E, and K. Direct effects may be mediated by changes in cell and organelle membrane integrity caused by excess retinol permeation. Indirect effects may include changes in other fat-soluble vitamin-dependent functions, including bone formation, blood coagulation, and antioxidant functions. Clinical signs of chronic toxicity may include skeletal malformations and fractures, reduced growth and dwarfism, weight loss, dermatoses, anemia, reproductive problems, and enteritis. Acute toxicity, as has been seen in humans consuming polar bear liver or excessive "over-the-counter" supplements, may include drowsiness or insomnia, lethargy or restlessness, headache, and gastrointestinal disturbances. Significant elevations in plasma vitamin A concentrations (often greater than 200 μg/dL) are diagnostic of toxicity.

VITAMIN D

Chemical Structure. Vitamin D activity is derived from a group of sterols of plant or animal origin that undergo transformation by ultraviolet (UV) light and subsequent modification by animal tissues to produce the active vitamin (Fig. 35.3). Hormonal properties of vitamin D are essential to calcium and phosphorus metabolism. Ergocalciferol (vitamin D_2) is derived from ergosterol, a plant sterol, and is the most common dietary source. Cholecalciferol (vitamin D_3) is produced from 7-dehydrocholesterol, an animal sterol, and possesses 2-30 times the biological activity of vitamin D_2, depending on the species studied (McDowell 1989b).

Sources and Chemical Properties. Ergosterol is the main source of provitamin D activity for herbivores, and many factors affect its availability to animals, potency as a vitamin D precursor, and the efficiency of conversion to active vitamin D following consumption. Grains, roots, and oilseeds contain only small amounts of vitamin D activity (NRC 1982). All green parts of plants contain ergosterol and thus high potential provitamin D activity. Fresh green fodder contains little active ergocalciferol until it has been sufficiently exposed to UV light from the sun so that ergosterol becomes activated. Thus, unlike other fat-soluble vitamins, vitamin D activity increases with maturity, owing to an increase in the number of dead, UV-exposed leaves. Artificially dried and barn-cured hay contains less vitamin D than hay that has been cured in the sun. Of the animal sources for vitamin D, meat, unfortified milk and butter, and animal by-products contain little

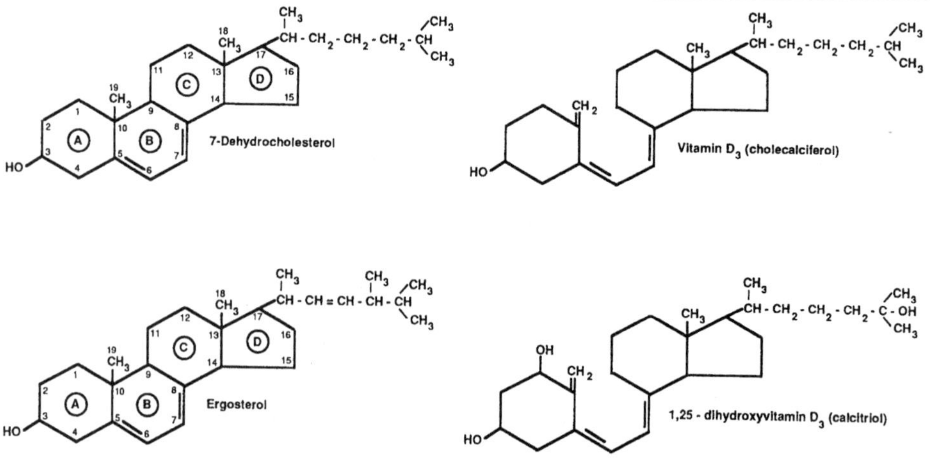

FIG. 35.3

activity. Saltwater fish, including salmon, sardines, and herring, contain high amounts of vitamin D, and the fish liver oils are likewise excellent sources of cholecalciferol. Provitamin D activity can be lost following overexposure to UV light, and several overirradiation products may be toxic or antagonistic to vitamin D activity. Vitamin D in a water-soluble crystalline form or in solution with oil and protected from UV light is highly stable. Oxidation may also occur under adverse environmental conditions, influenced by moisture, heat, light, and other feed constituents, including transition metals and rancid polyunsaturated fats.

Several methods are available for the determination of the vitamin D content in biological specimens. Physicochemical methods are quantitative and include colorimetric reactions, UV absorption spectroscopy, fluorescence spectroscopy, gas chromatography, HPLC, competitive protein-binding assay, radioimmunoassay, and enzyme-linked immunosorbent assay (ELISA) (Lind et al. 1997). Because there are so many closely related isomers and so many compounds with potential provitamin D activity, none of the physicochemical methods compare in sensitivity to the biological assays for actual vitamin D activity. Vitamin D activity is expressed in international units (IU) or in micrograms (μg) of cholecalciferol equivalents. An IU has the biological activity of 0.025 μg of cholecalciferol. For poultry, the international chick unit (ICU) is used to discriminate between the activities of D_2 and D_3 (NRC 1984).

Biological Characteristics. Dietary vitamin D absorption in the small intestine is in association with fats and is thus facilitated by biliary and pancreatic secretions. Absorbed vitamin D is incorporated with other lipids into the chylomicrons for transport via the lymphatics to the circulatory system. Cholecalciferol produced by UV irradiation of 7-dehydrocholesterol in the epidermis and absorbed into the blood is transported bound to an α-globulin for delivery to other sites for further metabolism (Allen and Weingand 1985). The conversion of ingested ergocalciferol or native cholecalciferol into active vitamin D occurs in two steps, involving enzymatic reactions in the liver and kidneys. The first is hydroxylation of carbon 25 in the side chain by a microsomal enzyme in the liver to produce 25-OH vitamin D. Following transport of 25-OH vitamin D in the blood to the kidneys in association with a binding globulin, a second hydroxylation takes place on carbon 1 of the A ring (Fig. 35.3). This reaction occurs in the mitochondria and is catalyzed by a mixed-function oxidase, 25-OH vitamin D 1α-hydroxylase, in association with nicotinamide adenine dinucleotide phosphate (NADPH), O_2, a flavoprotein, and cytochrome P-450 (Kumar 1986). In addition to 1,25-$(OH)_2D$, other hydroxylated metabolites of 25-OH vitamin D are produced, some of which have little if any biological activity (such as 25,26-$(OH)_2D$), are predominantly excretory products (such as 1,24,25-$(OH)_3D$), or have regulatory roles in the control of parathyroid hormone secretion and bone mineralization (such as 24,25-$(OH)_2D$). Because ergosterol and 7-dehydrocholesterol are hydroxylated at carbon 3, as are all of their metabolites, 1,25-$(OH)_2D$ is also referred to as calcitriol, a convenient term for activated vitamin D. Calcitriol and other 25-(OH) vitamin D metabolites are transported in the blood bound to the same binding protein for delivery to target organs.

There are species differences in the ability to store vitamin D, and most mammals do not store appreciable amounts in any tissue. However, the slow turnover rate of skin and adipose tissue may contribute to blood levels during periods of deprivation, and placental transfer of vitamin D may provide enough to support the neonate through weaning, particularly if the mother is provided additional prepartum supplementation.

METABOLIC FUNCTIONS. Vitamin D is predominantly concerned with regulation of parathyroid hormone secretion and homeorrhetic control of calcium (Ca) and phosphorus (P) metabolism, being essential to normal intestinal absorption, renal excretion, and bone mineralization of these elements. It has also been shown to participate in immune system regulation and has been hypothesized to have a role in hematopoiesis.

ENDOCRINE CONTROL OF CA AND P METABOLISM. Vitamin D activation and calcitriol's subsequent effects on Ca and P metabolism are intimately related to the functions of parathyroid hormone (PTH) and thyrocalcitonin (TCT) (Fig. 35.4; Allen and Weingand 1985; Kurokawa 1987). Calcitriol's cellular mechanism of action parallels that of other steroid hormones in that it circulates bound to a specific binding globulin, traverses target cell membranes to interact with a specific cytosolic receptor, and enters the nucleus bound to that receptor, and its ensuing actions are mediated by alterations in DNA transcription (Kumar 1986). Thus, one can consider Ca and P metabolism to be controlled by a triad of hormones: PTH, which has

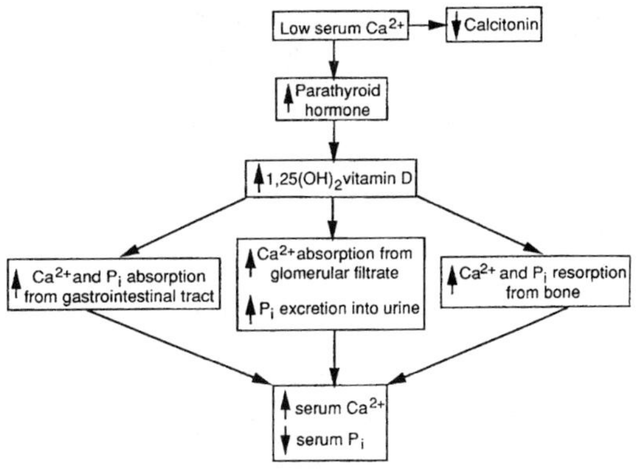

FIG. 35.4—Homeostatic response to hypocalcemia. (Adapted from Stewart and Broadus 1987.)

both direct effects on bone and kidney and indirect effects through its regulation of vitamin D activation; TCT, which has direct effects on bone and kidney; and calcitriol, which has direct effects on bone, kidney, and intestine, as well as indirect effects through its reciprocal regulation of PTH release. A decrease in blood ionized Ca concentration stimulates release of PTH by the parathyroid gland. PTH, in turn, promotes Ca mobilization from bone, renal tubular reabsorption of Ca from the glomerular filtrate (thereby reducing its renal excretion), and activation of renal 25-OH vitamin D 1α-hydroxylase (thereby increasing the rate of calcitriol production). An increase in blood ionized Ca concentration has the opposite effect and, in addition, stimulates TCT release by the perifollicular cells of the thyroid gland. TCT, in turn, antagonizes the bone and renal actions of PTH. Central to this regulatory triad are the functions of calcitriol.

INTESTINAL EFFECTS. Calcitriol stimulates Ca and P absorption by the small intestine through its regulation of the synthesis of several proteins essential to their transepithelial uptake and transport to the blood. The most important of these are intestinal membrane Ca-binding protein and intracellular Ca-binding protein, which facilitate Ca uptake from the intestinal lumen and its delivery to the basilar surface for transfer into the blood. Through mechanisms that have not been completely elucidated, calcitriol also stimulates P uptake by small-intestinal epithelial cells.

RENAL EFFECTS. PTH acts directly on the proximal tubules of the kidneys to inhibit solute reabsorption, including sodium, bicarbonate, calcium, and phosphorus. Because this is the only site for P reabsorption in the nephron, increased urinary excretion of P is effected by this action. In the loop of Henle, PTH stimulates active Ca absorption through a cyclic adenosine 3′,5′-monophosphate (cAMP)-mediated process, and Ca uptake throughout the distal nephron is further promoted by synthesis of intracellular Ca-binding protein, under the influence of calcitriol, as occurs in the intestinal mucosa. The net result of the interactive effects of PTH and calcitriol is increased Ca reclamation from the glomerular filtrate (Kurokawa 1987).

BONE EFFECTS. Normal bone development is dependent on vitamin D, through effects on osteoclast, osteocyte, and osteoblast activity, as well as normal matrix biosynthesis. These effects account for the development of rickets in deficient, growing animals, and osteomalacia in deficient, adult animals. In the process of bone growth, calcitriol is necessary for normal lysyl oxidase activity and collagen cross-linking of matrix and for normal mineralization of the organic matrix (Kumar 1986; Gonnerman et al. 1976). In the process of bone resorption for remodeling and maintenance of Ca and P homeostasis, calcitriol synergizes with PTH to promote mineral reabsorption.

IMMUNE FUNCTION. An increase in frequency and severity of infectious diseases in children with rickets has been observed historically and is related both to alterations in phagocytic cell function and to loss of lymphocyte proliferation regulatory responsiveness. Studies of vitamin D-deficient rats, mice, and children have shown that calcitriol supplementation reduces the frequency and severity of naturally and experimentally acquired infections (Reinhardt and Hustmeyer 1987). Calcitriol promotes monocyte differentiation into macrophages and enhances the chemotactic, phagocytic, and/or bactericidal function of neutrophils and macrophages isolated from the blood of deficient individuals. Administration of $1,25(OH)_2D_3$ to mice increased secretion of IL-6, IL-1, and tumor necrosis factor in mice infected with *Mycobacterium paratuberculosis,* thereby significantly reducing bacterial growth (Stabel and Goff 1996). Vitamin D inhibits the production of interleukin-2 (IL-2) by mitogen-stimulated lymphocytes, thereby suppressing lymphocyte proliferation, has direct inhibitory effects on T-cell-dependent, antigen-induced antibody production by B cells, and decreases the development of cytotoxic and helper-inducer T cells (Tsoukas et al. 1984; Reinhardt and Hustmeyer 1987). In human patients with end-stage renal disease, impaired monocyte superoxide generation and bactericidal activity were improved following 4 weeks of oral calcitriol supplementation (Hubel et al. 1991). Continuous infusion of calcitriol by osmotic pump promoted concanavalin A-stimulated lymphocyte mitogenesis in young calves (Hustmeyer et al. 1994). Although there are some conflicting data, it is hypothesized that dietary supplementation with vitamin D, beyond nutritional requirements, may afford some advantages in the immunological defense against certain infectious diseases.

HEMATOPOIESIS. Rickets in growing rats, chicks, and children has been associated with the secondary development of a nonregenerative anemia and decreased bone marrow cellularity. These conditions are responsive to calcitriol supplementation. Vitamin D analogs have also been used experimentally to induce cellular differentiation in myeloid leukemias, thereby reducing neoplastic proliferation (Reinhardt and Hustmeyer 1987).

Signs of Deficiency. The predominant signs of vitamin D deficiency relate to skeletal abnormalities associated with the clinical condition of rickets (McDowell 1989b). Failure of matrix formation, chondrocyte differentiation, and mineralization leads to abnormal proliferation and degeneration of the cartilage, weak and deformed bones, stiff and enlarged joints, pathologic fractures, and locomotory abnormalities. It is now thought that vitamin D deficiency is the primary cause of hypophosphatemic rickets in growing camelids less than 7 months of age. This disorder is identified by a serum P concentration of <4.5 mg/dL and serum $25(OH)D_3$ of <15 nmol/L and is readily treated with intramuscular vitamin D administration (Van Saun et al. 1996). Accessory signs of vitamin D deficiency in adults may include lethargy, anorexia, hypogalactia, and neuromuscular dysfunction. In poultry, vitamin D deficiency and subsequent abnormalities in Ca and P metabolism can lead to decreased eggshell thickness and increased fragility, or reduced hatchability due to mandibular anomalies in the chicks that impair their ability to crack the shell (McDowell 1989b).

Assessment of Status. Criteria used to evaluate vitamin D status have included biological response to supplementation, radiography of skeletal abnormalities, and histological observation of bone lesions consistent with rickets or osteomalacia. Determination of blood vitamin D concentrations and/or the presence of low blood calcium concentrations and high serum alkaline phosphatase activity may also be used in the diagnosis. Blood levels of 25-OH vitamin D provide an index of dietary intake and UV light exposure, whereas levels of 1,25-$(OH)_2D$ evaluate both supply and renal activation capacity.

Dietary Requirements, Indications, and Use

INTRINSIC FACTORS. Healthy animals allowed sufficient exposure to sunlight do not have a dietary requirement for vitamin D, given sufficient dietary Ca and P intake. Differences in skin pigmentation, hair coat or skin thickness due to age, and skin diseases may affect the penetration of UV light and subsequent activation of 7-dehydrocholesterol. Published dietary requirements for vitamin D are intended to meet metabolic needs for different physiological states in the absence of sunlight but are often included in feed formulations to cover any contingency.

EXTRINSIC FACTORS. Many extrinsic factors beyond that of exposure to sunlight can influence the dietary requirement for vitamin D. These include the amount and ratio of dietary Ca and P, as well as their availability for absorption from the gastrointestinal tract. Reductions in the dietary content of either of these minerals or divergence from an optimal dietary ratio will increase the vitamin D requirement. Dietary acidification favors Ca and P uptake from the intestinal tract. Metabolic acidosis promotes bone resorption of mineral, enhances PTH's effects on bone, and increases blood ionized Ca concentration. However, acidosis also inhibits PTH's renal effects and inhibits the activity of renal 25-OH vitamin D 1α-hydroxylase (thereby decreasing the rate of calcitriol production) (Ching et al. 1989; Reddy et al. 1982). This may result in reduced gastrointestinal Ca absorption and increased urinary Ca excretion, resulting in negative dietary balance. Other dietary components can form insoluble precipitates with Ca or P, thereby affecting their availability and the vitamin D requirement (Sheikh et al. 1987; Cook et al. 1991).

Diseases which interfere with hepatic or renal hydroxylation steps in the activation of vitamin D may adversely affect dietary requirements. Of particular note is chronic renal disease, in which renal 25-OH vitamin D 1α-hydroxylase activity may be directly suppressed by rising blood P concentrations or developing acidosis. Furthermore, loss of functional renal parenchyma also results in reduced synthesis of the 25-OH vitamin D 1α-hydroxylase (Satomura et al. 1988). Studies have demonstrated many beneficial effects of calcitriol supplementation in chronic renal disease (Voigts et al. 1983a,b; Nagode and Chew 1991). This replaces 1,25-$(OH)_2D$ no longer produced by the diseased kidneys, suppresses PTH release by virtue of improved Ca homeostasis and direct feedback on the parathyroid gland, and in turn minimizes the degree of renal secondary hyperparathyroidism and uremic signs thereof.

Prepartum supplementation of dairy cows with vitamin D as 1α-OH vitamin D_3 (Sachs et al. 1977), 1,25-$(OH)_2D_3$ (Hove and Kristiansen 1982), or 24F-1,25-$(OH)_2D_3$ (Goff et al. 1988) has been used to prevent parturient paresis (milk fever), predominantly by enhancing gastrointestinal Ca absorption but also through enhanced mobilization of Ca from bone reserves (Horst et al. 1994). Furthermore, in hypophosphatemic, recumbent cows with periparturient hypocalcemia who do not respond to calcium replacement therapy alone, 1α-$(OH)D_3$ (1 mg/kg body weight; one-half intravenously and one-half intramuscularly) rapidly restores serum P and is associated with a rapid clinical recovery (Barlet and Davicco 1992).

Preparations. Vitamin D is available as ergocalciferol (D_2) and cholecalciferol (D_3) in natural sources and as resins, gelatin beadlets, emulsions, and dried powders. Injectable and oral preparations may be obtained singly or as part of a multivitamin preparation. Simple, aqueous solutions are indicated for injection, but because of oxidative instability, chemically stabilized forms of vitamin D are preferred for feed supplementation. Vitamin D may be stabilized by protective coating with gelatin and antioxidants, included as part of a free-choice mineral mixture, or added with antioxidants to liquids such as oils or molasses that are sprayed onto the feed during processing. Single large doses may be given as intramuscular injections in the prophylaxis or therapeusis of specific conditions or diseases which increase vitamin D requirements. Large doses may also be included in drinking water or parenteral fluid preparations in the resuscitation of diseased or convalescent animals.

Toxicity. Following vitamin A, vitamin D is the next most likely to be supplemented at toxic levels, and signs of toxicity have been demonstrated in most species studied to date. Certain plants, including *Cestrum diurnum* and *Solanum* spp., naturally contain a toxic concentration of 1,25-$(OH)_2D$ (calcitriol) as a glycoside, which can result in toxicity once consumed (Krook et al. 1975). In addition, the use of cholecalciferol rodenticides has increased the occurrence of accidental vitamin D intoxications in domestic animals (Gunther et al. 1988). Upper safe limits for acute exposure are approximately 100 times the nutritional requirements for most animals, but only about 10 times the requirements when considering chronic exposure (NRC 1987). The median lethal dose of cholecalciferol is approximately 44 mg/kg of body weight for rodents and has been reported to be 88 mg/kg of body weight for dogs, although lethal intoxications have been reported with significantly lower exposures (Bahri 1990).

Hypervitaminosis D is characterized by adverse effects caused directly by calcitriol on Ca and P metabolism and indirectly by interference with the metabolism of other fat-soluble vitamins, including vitamins A, E, and K (Littledike and Horst 1982). Direct effects are mainly due to excessive Ca mobilization from storage sites and deposition as dystrophic mineralization in soft tissues, as well as acute necrosis of active osteocytes (Haschek et al. 1978). Hypercalcemia also produces vasoconstriction (leading to hypertension and ischemic tissue damage), polyuria, polydipsia, lethargy, vomiting, cardiac arrhythmias, and neurologic disturbances. Indirect effects may include changes in other functions dependent on fat-soluble vitamins, including blood coagulation and antioxidant functions. Significant elevations in plasma vitamin D metabolite concentrations are diagnostic of toxicity; values of 25-OH vitamin D in pigs exceeding 1000 ng/mL (Long 1984) and values of 1,25-$(OH)_2$D in horses exceeding 50 ng/mL have been reported (Harrington and Page 1983).

VITAMIN E

Chemical Structure. Vitamin E activity in plants is derived from two groups of compounds, the tocopherols and the tocotrienols, the latter differing from the former by the presence of three double bonds in the side chain (Fig. 35.5). There are, as well, several forms of vitamin E, depending on the placement of methyl groups on carbon 5, 7, or 8 of the side chain, resulting in the α, β, γ, or δ forms of tocopherol and tocotrienol. Of these, *d*-α-tocopherol (the principal naturally occurring compound) possesses the greatest vitamin E activity, *dl*-α-tocopherol is slightly less potent, *d*-β-tocopherol and *d*-α-tocotrienol have approximately one-half the activity, and the other forms are only about one-tenth as potent or less (McDowell 1989c).

Sources and Chemical Properties. Tocopherols and tocotrienols are highly susceptible to oxidation, which may be promoted by exposure to heat along with moisture, rancid fat, or transition metals. Oxidation of vitamin E in concentrates increases with grinding, pelleting, and mixing with minerals unless antioxidants are also included (McDowell 1989c). Animal products are generally poor sources of vitamin E activity, whereas plants, particularly the cereal grains and young, green, leafy plants, are the greatest sources (NRC 1982). Wheat germ oil is the most concentrated natural source, and other oils such as that from soybeans, peanuts, and cottonseeds are also rich sources.

Several methods are available for the determination of tocopherol or tocotrienol content in biological specimens. Physicochemical methods are quantitative and include colorimetric reactions, thin-layer chromatography, paper chromatography, gas chromatography, and HPLC. Vitamin E activity is expressed in international units (IU) or in milligrams (mg) of tocopherol equivalents, using *dl*-α-tocopheryl acetate as the standard (1 mg = 1 IU). Synthetic, free, *dl*-α-tocopherol has a potency of 1.1 IU/mg, naturally occurring *d*-α-tocopherol is 1.49 IU/mg, and *d*-α-tocopheryl acetate is 1.36 IU/mg.

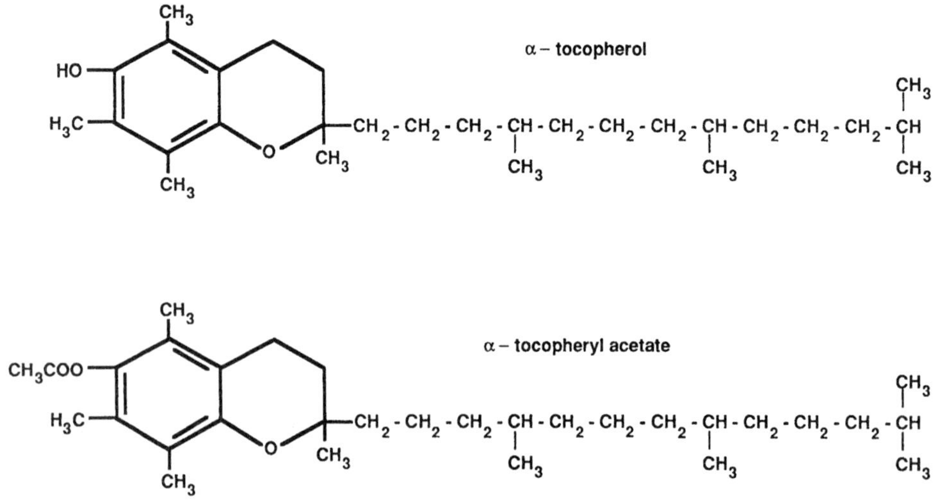

α – tocopherol

α – tocopheryl acetate

FIG. 35.5

Biological Characteristics. Absorption of vitamin E is dependent on fat digestion and is therefore facilitated by biliary and pancreatic secretions. Dietary vitamin E esters are hydrolyzed in the intestinal mucosa, and most vitamin E is absorbed as the free alcohol into the lymphatics for transport to the circulation. The efficiency of vitamin E absorption is less than that for vitamin A, with α-tocopherol being best absorbed and other forms being less well absorbed, in general correspondence with their lesser biological activities. A standardized, oral vitamin E absorption test used widely in humans has been adapted for use in horses to assess gastrointestinal handling of dietary vitamin E (Craig et al. 1991). Vitamin E is stored by all body tissues but predominantly by the liver. However, these stores are less than those for vitamin A and are more rapidly depleted by dietary deficiency.

METABOLIC FUNCTIONS. Vitamin E is required principally for its antioxidant effects, which in turn modulate several physiological processes, including membrane structure and prostaglandin biosynthesis, blood coagulation, reproductive function, and immune competency (McDowell 1989c). Some signs of vitamin E deficiency can be averted by dietary supplementation with other antioxidants, the most important of which is selenium, a cofactor for the free radical-quenching enzyme glutathione peroxidase.

ANTIOXIDANT EFFECTS AND MEMBRANE INTEGRITY. Vitamin E functions as an antioxidant by neutralizing free radicals and preventing membrane lipid peroxidation (Fig. 35.6). At the ultrastructural level, this spares membrane microarchitecture and enzyme activity and prevents the accumulation of oxidative reaction byproducts which may perpetuate the cascade of free radical damage. Gross evidence of these functions includes maintenance of erythrocyte membrane stability and capillary blood vessel integrity, inhibition of platelet aggregation, and prevention of nutritional muscular dystrophy and encephalomalacia. Its effects include promotion of prostaglandin E synthesis, rather than thromboxanes or leukotrienes, from arachidonic acid in a variety of tissues, which may in turn affect many systems' functions. In human subjects, erythrocyte susceptibility to oxidative damage correlates well with erythrocyte vitamin E content (Simon et al. 1997). In rats, free-radical-mediated lipid peroxidation associated with hyperthyroidism is ameliorated by vitamin E supplementation (Seven et al. 1996). However, dietary vitamin E supplementation in horses does not appear to reduce the severity of exercise-induced oxidative damage, as indicated by changes in gluteal muscle thiobarbituric-acid reactive substances and conjugated diene concentrations (Siciliano et al. 1997). Likewise, vitamin E supplementation had no effect on symptoms associated with experimental aflatoxicosis in growing swine (Harvey et al. 1994) or endophyte-infested tall fescue toxicosis in lactating dairy cows (Jackson et al. 1997).

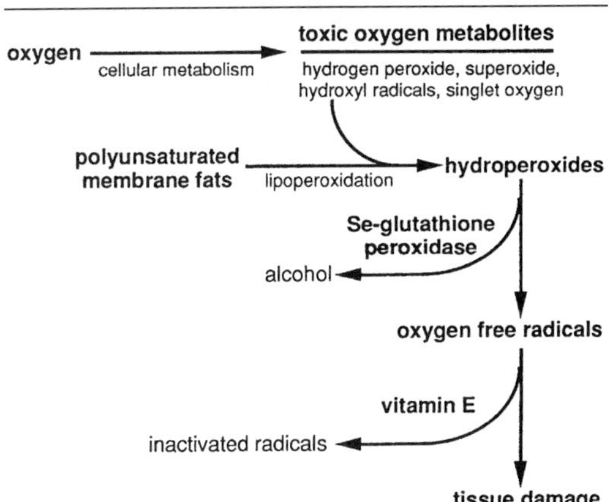

FIG. 35.6—The pathogenesis of lipoperoxidation and the roles of selenium and vitamin E in its control. (From Moore and Kohn 1991.)

REPRODUCTION. Vitamin E and selenium are thought to be required for normal reproductive function, and dietary supplementation has improved fertility and reduced the incidence of some reproductive disorders in several species. In cattle, injection with selenium and oral vitamin E supplementation have been found to reduce the incidence of retained placenta, metritis, and cystic ovaries (Harrison et al. 1984). It has been proposed that the incidence of retained fetal membranes in cows may be related to prepartum oxidative stress, which is responsive to vitamin E supplementation (Brzezinska-Slebodzinska et al. 1994). In sheep, long-term injections with vitamin E and selenium had no effect on fertility or prolificacy but did increase preweaning survival of lambs significantly (Kott et al. 1983).

IMMUNE FUNCTION. Vitamin E deficiency has been associated with an increased frequency and severity of many infectious diseases, because of alterations in immune system responsiveness. Stress alone can depress serum and tissue concentrations of vitamin E, and supplementation of stressed cattle with vitamin E can ameliorate other stress-induced chemical changes (Nockels et al. 1996). Vitamin E deficiency has resulted in reduced lymphocyte transformation and proliferation in response to various mitogens, and impaired neutrophil phagocytic and bactericidal functions (Langweiler et al. 1983; Lessard et al. 1991). Both in vivo and in vitro supplementation with vitamin E have resulted in enhanced mitogen-stimulated lymphocyte proliferation, cell-mediated toxicity, and natural killer cell activity (Reddy et al. 1987). Likewise, concanavalin A-stimulated mononuclear cells from vitamin E-supplemented steers expressed 55% higher interleukin-1 mRNA in vitro than cells from unsupplemented animals (Stabel et al. 1992).

Dietary vitamin E supplementation has enhanced the secondary humoral immune response of lambs challenged with parainfluenza$_3$ virus by increasing the serum IgM response to virus challenge (Reffet et al. 1988). In pigs, prepartum vitamin E and selenium injection beyond nutritional requirements has resulted in higher serum IgM and IgG concentrations in the sows, higher colostral IgM levels, increased serum IgM concentrations, and improved cell-mediated immune responses to phytohemagglutinin and concanavalin A in the piglets (Hayek et al. 1989; Nemec et al. 1994; Wuryastuti et al. 1993). Dietary supplementation of gilts with α-tocopherol resulted in an enhanced antibody response to ovalbumin immunization in their piglets (Babinsky et al. 1991). In yearling Holstein heifers, oral supplementation with *dl*-α-tocopheryl acetate increased serum IgM concentrations, phytohemagglutinin-stimulated in vitro lymphocyte blastogenesis, and in vitro serum inhibition of infectious bovine rhinotracheitis viral replication (Reddy et al. 1986). Dietary vitamin E supplementation of periparturient cows results in a more rapid influx of neutrophils into milk, improved neutrophil chemotaxis properties, and increased intracellular kill of ingested bacteria following intramammary bacterial challenge (Smith et al. 1997; Politis et al. 1996; Politis et al. 1995). When periparturient cows are given vitamin E with Freund's adjuvant in an *Escherichia coli* J5 vaccine, peak serum and milk immunoglobulin titers are increased significantly (Hogan et al. 1993). Supplementation of elderly human subjects with vitamin E for four months improved several indices of immune function, including both cell-mediated and antibody responses to challenge antigens (Meydani et al. 1997). Although there are some conflicting data, it is generally thought that dietary supplementation with vitamin E and/or selenium, beyond nutritional requirements, may afford some advantages in the immunological defense against certain infectious diseases.

HEMATOPOIESIS. Vitamin E deficiency in neonatal, suckling, and weaned pigs has been associated with the development of anemia, leukocytosis, multinucleation of erythrocytic precursor cells, and increased numbers of megakaryocytes in the bone marrow (Niyo et al. 1980). Multinucleation of erythroid precursors was likewise observed in experimentally induced vitamin E deficiency in rhesus macaques. In addition to its possible effects on erythrocytic precursor cell maturation, vitamin E deficiency may result in erythrocyte membrane abnormalities which lead to abnormal fragility and hemolysis (Brady et al. 1982). Experimental evidence from humans with anemia caused by glucose-6-phosphate dehydrogenase or glutathione synthetase deficiencies also indicates a nonspecific hematinic effect of vitamin E supplementation.

ANTIOXIDANT ACTIVITY AND CANCER PREVENTION. Several functions of vitamin E may play a role in the chemoprevention of cancer. Foremost of these is its function as an antioxidant, interrupting the cascades of oxidative free radical damage initiated by activated metabolites of several polycyclic hydrocarbons and aromatic amines (Gould et al. 1991; Ngah et al. 1991). Vitamin E's ability to enhance immune responsiveness may promote anticancer sentinel activities of the immune system. In addition, vitamin E may act as a scavenger of nitrite compounds, thereby inhibiting their conversion to carcinogenic nitrosamines. Epidemiologic evidence in humans indicates an inverse relationship between serum antioxidant concentrations and subsequent cancer risk, which may be particularly important in individuals with a high dietary polyunsaturated fatty acid intake (Packer 1991). Supplemental vitamin E has been associated in humans with as much as a 60% reduction in risk of death from cardiovascular disease (Kushi et al. 1996), but was without effect on risk for incidence of lung cancer (Alpha-Tocopherol, Beta Carotene Cancer Prevention Study Group 1994; Albanes et al. 1996). Safe and efficacious levels of dietary tocopherols for the chemoprevention of cancer remain theoretical and await objective experimental verification.

RELATIONSHIP WITH OTHER DIETARY ANTIOXIDANTS. Dietary oxidants like polyunsaturated fatty acids can increase vitamin E requirements, but other dietary antioxidants can have a reciprocal, sparing effect. Vitamin E prevents fatty acid hydroperoxide formation and inhibits free radical generation, sulfur amino acids are precursors of glutathione, which can quench free radicals and undergo conjugation with oxidative chemicals, and selenium is a necessary component of glutathione peroxidase, which catalyzes the reduction of free radicals by glutathione (Fettman 1991). Thus, many of the disturbances associated with vitamin E deficiency may be prevented and/or treated with selenium or other antioxidants, and vitamin E may ameliorate the signs of dietary selenium insufficiency.

Signs of Deficiency. Naturally occurring deficiencies of vitamin E are rare in adult animals, and most deficiency syndromes are observed in young, growing animals fed a diet deficient in vitamin E and/or selenium. Nutritional muscular dystrophy, or white muscle disease, occurs in young rats, rabbits, poultry, dogs, pigs, cattle, sheep, goats, and horses (McDowell 1989c). This disease is characterized clinically by generalized weakness, stiffness, motor disturbances, and heart failure (Moore and Kohn 1991). Muscle lesions occur bilaterally and are characterized grossly by a pale and mottled appearance. Microscopic findings include hyaline degeneration, fragmentation, and lysis of muscle fibers, followed by coagulative necrosis and dystrophic mineralization (Dill and Rebhun 1985). In pigs, hepatosis dietetica and dietetic microangiopathy may also be seen (Van Vleet and Kennedy 1989; Rice and Kennedy 1989). The former is characterized by a swollen, mottled liver with lobular hemorrhage and coagulative necrosis. The latter, also known as mulberry heart disease, is characterized by fibrinoid degeneration of arterioles, thrombi in myocardial arteries and capillaries, and subendocardial hemorrhages. Vitamin E deficiency in poultry produces two syndromes in addition to muscular dystrophy: exudative diathesis, characterized by lethargy, anorexia, and severe subcutaneous edema, and encephalomalacia, in which chicks from 2-6 weeks of age develop ataxia due to cerebellar hemorrhages and edema (McDowell 1989c). Horses with a particular, apparently heritable form of degenerative myeloencephalopathy appear to be vitamin E deficient, although gastrointestinal absorption tests are normal (Blythe et al. 1991).

Assessment of Status. Criteria used to evaluate vitamin E status have included biological response to supplementation and analysis of blood vitamin E concentrations. Because blood vitamin E is maintained by release from the liver (although not as well as vitamin A), in some species these values may be maintained until hepatic stores are depleted. Thus, low blood levels indicate deficiency, but normal values must be interpreted with caution. Sample-handling procedures which may have marked effects on serum or plasma tocopherol concentrations include temperature, light exposure, hemolysis, freezing, and freeze-thaw cycling (Craig et al. 1992). These variables may result in 2-33% decreases in vitamin E concentration assayed by HPLC (Craig et al. 1992). Plasma tocopherol concentrations of 0.5-1.0 μg/mL are considered low in most species, and values less than 0.5 μg/mL generally indicate a deficiency. Selenium concentrations in liver, renal cortex, and blood give indications of selenium status, as does erythrocyte glutathione peroxidase activity.

Dietary Requirements, Indications, and Use

INTRINSIC FACTORS. Requirements for vitamin E are greatest during pregnancy, lactation, and rapid growth. The potential for deficiency during these phases of life is increased by concurrent extrinsic factors relating to other dietary oxidants and antioxidants, environmental stress, and infectious diseases.

EXTRINSIC FACTORS. Stressful environmental conditions and disease have been shown to increase dietary vitamin E requirements. Gastrointestinal diseases may impair absorption of vitamin E. Seasonal effects on vitamin E status have been observed in horses owing to differences in feed content, accumulated effects of storage on tocopherol stability, and changes in dietary requirements associated with changes in environment and reproductive status (Maenpaa et al. 1988a,b). Other dietary constituents may have significant influences on vitamin E stability in feeds, absorption from the gut, or disposition in the body. Vitamin E requirements in dogs have been reported to increase fivefold with higher dietary polyunsaturated fat intakes (NRC 1985). Because vitamin E is destroyed by oxidation, the unsaturated fat content of feed may affect its stability, particularly under adverse conditions of storage or handling. Transition elements, including iron, zinc, copper, or manganese, may act as catalysts in oxidative chemical reactions and thereby be detrimental to vitamin E stability (Dove and Ewan 1991). Dietary selenium deficiency may adversely affect free radical scavenging capacity by reducing glutathione peroxidase activity, thereby increasing the dietary requirement for vitamin E and other antioxidants. Dietary antioxidants such as vitamin C may both protect vitamin E from oxidative breakdown and spare its utilization in the animal's defense against oxidative damage.

Preparations. Vitamin E is available in green plant materials and seed oils and as a synthetic acetate ester. Injectable and oral preparations may be obtained singly, in combination with selenium, or as part of a multivitamin preparation. Simple, aqueous solutions of free *dl*-α-tocopherol are best absorbed following parenteral injection, and the free form and the acetate ester are better absorbed from aqueous solutions than from oil-based ones. Because of oxidative instability, chemically stabilized forms of tocopherol with polyethylene glycol or tocopheryl esters of acetate, succinate, or nicotinate are preferred for feed supplementation (Anderson et al. 1995; Hidiroglou et al. 1992; Ochoa et al. 1992; Roquet et al. 1992). Tocopheryl acetate may be stabilized by protective coating with gelatin and antioxidants and included as part of a free-choice mineral mixture or added with antioxidants to liquids such as oils or molasses that are sprayed onto feed during processing. Single large doses may be given as intramuscular or intraperitoneal injections in the prophylaxis or therapeusis of specific conditions or diseases which increase vitamin E requirements (Hidiroglou 1996; Toutain et al. 1995; Njeru et al. 1992). Intramuscular injection of cows with 3000 IU of vitamin E at 10 days and 5 days prior to anticipated calving resulted, in one study, in significantly greater concentrations in the plasma, erythrocytes, and neutrophils than did 60 days of dietary supplementation at 1000 IU/day (Weiss et al. 1992). Injectable combination products of vitamin E and selenium contain approximately 50 IU of vitamin E and 5 mg of selenium per mL and are dosed at about 1 mL per 100 kg of body weight. Parenteral doses of up to 25 IU/kg of body weight and oral doses of up to 40 IU/kg body weight have been recommended to treat vitamin E deficiency in domestic animals. Large doses may also be included in drinking water or parenteral fluid preparations in the resuscitation of diseased or convalescent animals.

Toxicity. Compared with vitamin A or vitamin D, most studies have shown vitamin E to be relatively nontoxic. Upper safe limits are approximately 100 times the nutritional requirements for most species studied to date (NRC 1987). Nevertheless, extremely high doses are not entirely devoid of untoward effects. Excessive doses of vitamin E in rats, chicks, dogs, and humans have induced coagulation defects or exacerbated those associated with vitamin K deficiency. High dietary levels of vitamin E depress growth in rats and chicks and exacerbate abnormalities in bone calcification associated with dietary calcium or vitamin D deficiency. Large doses of vitamin E in anemic children were reported to suppress the hematological response to supplemental iron administration. In some studies the combined supplementation of both vitamin A and E provided less protection against bacterial infection than either vitamin alone, implying there may be antagonistic effects at certain dietary levels (Tengerdy and Nockels 1975).

VITAMIN K

Chemical Structure. Vitamin K is the term given to a group of fat-soluble compounds whose basic structure is that of a naphthaquinone with various side-chain modifications (Fig. 35.7). Vitamin K activity in plants is attributed to phylloquinone, or vitamin K_1. Activity produced through bacterial fermentation is attributed to menaquinone, or vitamin K_2. There are many natural analogs of vitamin K_2 that contain an unsaturated side chain on carbon 3 of the quinone core, with varying numbers of isoprenyl groups. None of these side-chain modifications affect vitamin K activity, and the synthetic and simplest molecular form is menadione, or vitamin K_3 (McDowell 1989d).

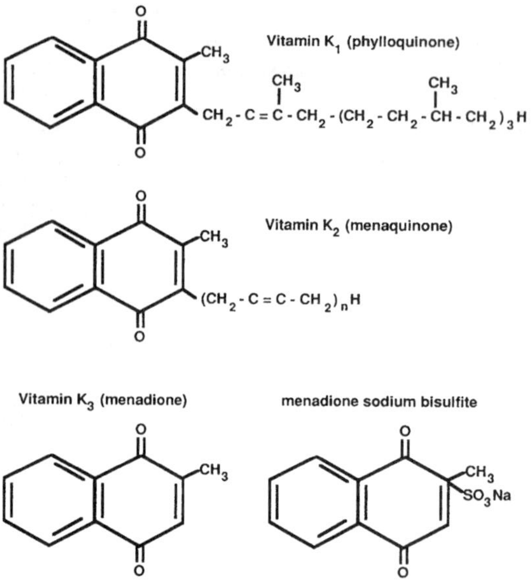

Sources and Chemical Properties. Vitamin K from natural sources is a yellow oil which is fat soluble and heat stable; some synthetic forms are water soluble. Vitamin K may be lost through oxidation under adverse environmental conditions, influenced by moisture, heat, light, and other plant constituents (McDowell 1989d). In addition, a number of vitamin K antagonists may be present in feedstuffs, particularly coumarins, which undergo conversion to active dicumarols following mold infestation or spoiling.

The two major sources of vitamin K are plants (phylloquinones) and gastrointestinal bacterial flora (menaquinones). All green parts of plants contain phylloquinone, whereas cereals and oilseed meals contain little vitamin K (NRC 1982). Liver and fish meals are good sources of vitamin K, and fish meals and fish liver oils are much higher in vitamin K following extensive bacterial putrefaction. Dehydrated alfalfa leaf meal remains one of the best natural sources of vitamin K activity. Commercial sources of supplemental vitamin K are produced primarily from fish oils and from industrial chemical synthesis. Natural sources may be highly variable in potency owing to differences in conditions during growth, processing, or storage.

Physicochemical methods for the determination of carotenoid or vitamin K content in biological specimens are quantitative and include colorimetric reactions, direct spectroscopy, and HPLC. Vitamin K activity is expressed in milligrams (mg) per unit of material assayed.

Vitamin K_1 (phylloquinone)

$CH_2-C=C(CH_3)-CH_2-(CH_2-CH_2-CH(CH_3)-CH_2)_3H$

Vitamin K_2 (menaquinone)

$(CH_2-C=C-CH_2)_nH$

Vitamin K_3 (menadione)

menadione sodium bisulfite

FIG. 35.7

Biological Characteristics. Similar to vitamins A, D, and E, vitamin K is absorbed predominantly in association with dietary fats and therefore requires biliary and pancreatic secretions. Lipid micelles from the intestinal contents facilitate the uptake of vitamin K by enterocytes, whereupon it is incorporated into chylomicrons and taken up by the lymphatic system for transport to the liver and other target organs. Phylloquinone is concentrated rapidly by the liver but does not have a long retention time. Menadione is poorly accumulated by the liver, distributes to all tissues, and is rapidly excreted. Measurement of conjugated metabolites of vitamin K in the urine may provide additional information regarding an animal's vitamin K status, beyond that of blood levels.

METABOLIC FUNCTIONS. Several vitamin K-dependent carboxylase enzyme systems are responsible for posttranslational modification of both structural proteins and enzymes, including some of the clotting factors synthesized in the liver.

BLOOD COAGULATION. Normal hemostasis is dependent on adequate vitamin K, owing to its participation in the synthesis of the active blood coagulation factors II (prothrombin), VII (proconvertin), IX (Christmas factor), and X (Stuart factor) (Fig. 35.8; Dodds 1989). Vitamin K does not become part of these molecules, nor does it function as an enzymatic cofactor; rather, it is required for the carboxylation reaction that converts their glutamic acid groups into active γ-carboxyglutamic acid residues. Hepatic microsomal enzymes oxidize vitamin K to its 2,3-epoxide and reduce the epoxide back to the nascent vitamin. The epoxide apparently

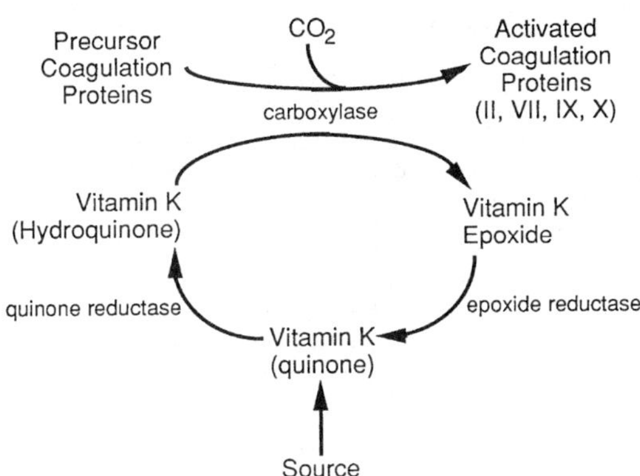

FIG. 35.8—Vitamin K participation in the activation of coagulation proteins. (Adapted from Mount et al. 1982.)

functions to labilize the γ-hydrogen, which is subsequently carboxylated by CO_2 (Bell 1978). Vitamin K-deficient animals continue to produce the coagulation factors, but the factors are not active in hemostasis.

CALCIUM METABOLISM. In addition to the vitamin K-dependent coagulation factors, several other proteins with γ-carboxyglutamic acid residues that are presumed to be dependent on vitamin K for their synthesis have been identified, including osteocalcin, which is necessary for normal bone formation (Gallop et al. 1980). Tissues with dystrophic mineralization and calcium-containing kidney stones have also been shown to contain proteins with γ-carboxyglutamic acid residues, leading to the hypothesis that these groups are central to protein interactions with calcium or other divalent cations (McDowell 1989d).

Signs of Deficiency. The predominant clinical sign of vitamin K deficiency in all species is impaired hemostasis, resulting in uncontrolled hemorrhaging and physical signs related to blood loss anemia or blood accumulation in body cavities, which impairs normal function (in the thorax, impeding respiration; in the joints, causing locomotory disturbances; etc.). Deficiency is usually seen only under conditions where enteric microbial synthesis is impaired, such as when oral antibiotics are used, or when metabolic antagonists are consumed, such as dicumarol from moldy sweet clover or warfarin from rodenticides (Osweiler 1978; Mount et al. 1982).

Assessment of Status. Criteria used to evaluate vitamin K status have included biological response to supplementation, determination of activated blood clotting time or prothrombin time (Dodds 1989), and analysis of blood vitamin K concentrations (Mount and Kass 1989). When coagulation times are abnormally prolonged in the absence of liver disease, a vitamin K deficiency should be suspected.

Dietary Requirements, Indications, and Use

INTRINSIC FACTORS. As for the other fat-soluble vitamins, the requirements for vitamin K are greatest during pregnancy, lactation, and rapid growth. The potential for deficiency during these phases of life is increased by the superimposition of other conditions which affect vitamin K assimilation and metabolism. Vitamin K deficiency may also result when fat digestion and absorption are abnormal, as in biliary obstruction or inflammatory bowel diseases.

EXTRINSIC FACTORS. Other dietary constituents may have significant influences on vitamin K stability in feeds, absorption from the gut, or disposition in the body. Because vitamin K is destroyed by oxidation, unsaturated fat content of the feed may affect its stability, particularly under adverse conditions of storage or handling. Transition elements, including iron, zinc, and copper, may act as catalysts in oxidative chemical reactions and thereby be detrimental to vitamin K stability. Dietary antioxidants such as vitamin E may protect vitamin K from oxidative breakdown. In coprophagous animals, vitamin K deficiency may result when their access to feces (and hence to microbially derived menaquinones) is blocked. Exposure to vitamin K antagonists must always be considered in the evaluation of potential vitamin K-dependent alterations in hemostasis (Dodds 1989; Byars et al. 1986; Green et al. 1979).

Preparations. If provided with natural dietary sources and/or if enteric microbial synthesis is functional, supplementary vitamin K is not necessary. For animals that are exposed to vitamin K antagonists, receive oral antibiotics, or have impaired gastrointestinal absorption, injectable and oral preparations of menadione may be obtained singly or as part of a multivitamin preparation. Simple, aqueous solutions are indicated for injection, but because of oxidative instability, chemically stabilized forms of vitamin K are preferred for feed supplementation. Water-soluble derivatives or menadione in combination with sodium bisulfite or dimethyl-pyrimidinol bisulfite are more stable and may be further protected by coating with gelatin and antioxidants, included as part of a free-choice mineral mixture, or added with antioxidants to liquids such as oils or molasses that are sprayed onto the feed during processing (McDowell 1989d). Single large doses of menadione may be given as intramuscular injections in the prophylaxis or therapeusis of specific conditions or diseases which increase vitamin K requirements. Large doses may also be included in drinking water or parenteral fluid preparations in the resuscitation of diseased or convalescent animals.

Toxicity. The natural forms of vitamin K, phylloquinone and menaquinone, are relatively nontoxic even at high doses. The toxic dietary level of menadione is approximately 1000 times the nutritional requirement for most animals (NRC 1987). The median lethal dose for a single parenteral injection of menadione in chicks, mice, rats, rabbits, and dogs is in the range of 75-200 mg/kg body weight, and at least 3-4 times that for a single oral dose. Clinical signs of intoxication may include hemolytic anemia and hemoglobinuria, and in horses a single parenteral dose of menadione bisulfite in the range of 2.1-8.3 mg/kg body weight produced acute renal failure (Rebhun et al. 1984). Significant elevations in plasma vitamin K concentrations are diagnostic of toxicity.

REFERENCES

Albanes, D., Heinonen, O. P., Taylor, P. R., Virtamo, J., Edwards, B. K., Rautalahti, M., Hartman, A. M., Palmgren, J., Freedman, L. S., et al. 1996. α-Tocopherol and β-carotene supplements and lung cancer incidence in the alpha-tocopherol, beta-carotene cancer prevention study: effects of base-line characteristics and study compliance. J Natl Cancer Inst 88:1560-1570.

Allen, T. A., Weingand, K. 1985. The vitamin D (cholecalciferol) system. Comp Cont Educ 7:482-88.

Alpha-Tocopherol, Beta Carotene Cancer Prevention Study Group. 1994. The effect of vitamin E and beta carotene on the incidence of lung cancer and other cancers in male smokers. New Engl J Med 330:1029-1035.

Anderson, L. E., Myer, R. O., Brendemuhl, J. H., McDowell, L. R. 1995. Bioavailability of various vitamin E compounds for finishing swine. J Anim Sci 73:490-495.

Babinsky, L., Langhout, D. J., Verstegen, M. W. A., den Hartog, L. A. , Joling, P., Nieuwland, M. 1991. Effect of vitamin E and fat source in sows' diets on immune response of suckling and weaned piglets. J Anim Sci 69:1833-42.

Bahri, L. E. 1990. Poisoning in dogs by vitamin D_3-containing rodenticides. Comp Cont Educ 12:1414-18.

Barlet, J. P., Davicco, M. J. 1992. 1α-hydroxycholecalciferol for the treatment of the downer cow syndrome. J Dairy Sci 75:1253-1256.

Bell, R. G. 1978. Metabolism of vitamin K and prothrombin synthesis: anticoagulants and the vitamin K-epoxide cycle. Fed Proc 37:2599-2604.

Blythe, L. L., Craig, A. M., Lassen, E. D., Rowe, K. E., Appell, L. H. 1991. Serially determined plasma α-tocopherol concentrations and results of the oral vitamin E absorption test in clinically normal horses and in horses with degenerative myeloencephalopathy. Am J Vet Res 52:908-11.

Booth, A., Reid, M., Clark, T. 1987. Hypovitaminosis A in feedlot cattle. J Am Vet Med Assoc 190:1305-8.

Brady, P. S., Sehgal, P. K., Hayes, K. C. 1982. Erythrocyte characteristics in vitamin E-responsive anemia of the owl monkey (*Aotus trivirgatus*). Am J Vet Res 43:1489-91.

Brief, S., Chew, B. P. 1985. Effects of vitamin A and β-carotene on reproductive performance in gilts. J Anim Sci 60:998-1004.

Brzezinska-Slebodzinska, E., Miller, J. K., Quigley, J. D., Moore, R., Madsen, F. C. 1994. Antioxidant status of dairy cows supplemented prepartum with vitamin E and selenium. J Dairy Sci 77:3087-3095.

Burton, G. W., Ingold, K. U. 1984. β-carotene: an unusual type of lipid antioxidant. Science 224:569-73.

Butera, S. T., Krakowka, S. 1986. Assessment of lymphocyte function during vitamin A deficiency. Am J Vet Res 47:850-55.

Byars, T. D., Greene, C. E., Kemp, D. T. 1986. Antidotal effect of vitamin K_1 against warfarin-induced anticoagulation in horses. Am J Vet Res 47:2309-12.

Chew, B. P. 1987. Vitamin A and β-carotene on host defense. J Dairy Sci 70:2732-43.

Chew, B. P., Luedecke, L. O., Holpuch, D. M. 1984. Effect of dietary vitamin A on resistance to experimental staphylococcus mastitis in mice. J Dairy Sci 67:2566-70.

Ching, S. V., Fettman, M. J., Hamar, D. W., Nogade, L. A., Smith, K. R. 1989. The effect of chronic dietary acidification using ammonium chloride on acid-base and mineral metabolism in the adult cat. J Nutr 119:902-915.

Cook, J. D., Dassenko, S. A., Whittaker, P. 1991. Calcium supplementation: effect on iron absorption. Am J Clin Nutr 53:106-11.

Craig, A. M., Blythe, L. L., Rowe, K. E., Lassen, E. D., Walker, L. L. 1991. Evaluation of the oral vitamin E absorption test in horses. Am J Vet Res 52:912-16.

Craig, A. M., Blythe, L. L., Rowe, K. E., Lassen, E. D., Barrington, R., Walker, K. C. 1992. Variability of alpha-tocopherol values associated with procurement, storage, and freezing of equine serum and plasma samples. Am J Vet Res 53:2228-2234.

Daniel, L. R., Chew, B. P., Tanaka, T. S., Tjoelker, L. W. 1991a. β-carotene and vitamin A effects on bovine phagocyte function in vitro during the peripartum period. J Dairy Sci 74:124-31.

———. 1991b. In vitro effects of β-carotene and vitamin A on peripartum bovine peripheral blood mononuclear cell proliferation. J Dairy Sci 74:911-15.

Dill, S. G., Rebhun, W. C. 1985. White muscle disease in foals. Comp Cont Educ 7:S627-S636.

Dodds, W. J. 1989. In J. J. Kaneko, ed., Clinical Biochemistry of Domestic Animals, pp. 274-315. New York: Academic Press.

Donoghue, S., Kronfeld, D. S., Berkowitz, S. J., Copp, R. L. 1981. Vitamin A nutrition of the equine: growth, serum biochemistry and hematology. J Nutr 111:365-74.

Dove, C. R., Ewan, R. C. 1991. Effect of trace minerals on the stability of vitamin E in swine grower diets. J Anim Sci 69:1994-2000.

Fettman, M. J. 1991. Comparative aspects of glutathione metabolism affecting individual susceptibility to oxidant injury. Comp Cont Educ Prac Vet 13:1079-91.

Folman, Y., Ascarelli, I., Kraus, D., Barash, H. 1987. Adverse effects of β-carotene in diet on fertility of dairy cows. J Dairy Sci 70:357-66.

Gallop, P. M., Lian, J. B., Hauschka, P. V. 1980. Carboxylated calcium-binding proteins and vitamin K. New Engl J Med 302:1460-66.

Goff, J. P., Horst, D. L., Beitz, D. C., Littledike, E. T. 1988. Use of 24-F-1, 25-dihydroxyvitamin D_3 to prevent parturient paresis in dairy cows. J Dairy Sci 71:1211-19.

Gonnerman, W. A., Toverud, S. V., Ramp, W. K., Mechanic, G. L. 1976. Effects of dietary vitamin D and calcium on lysyl oxidase activity in chick bone metaphyses. Proc Soc Exptl Biol Med 151:453-56.

Goodman, D. S. 1980. Vitamin A metabolism. Fed Proc 39:2716-22.

Gould, M. N., Haag, J. D., Kennan, W. S., Tanner, M. A., Elson, C. E. 1991. A comparison of tocopherol and tocotrienol for the chemoprevention of chemically-induced rat mammary tumors. Am J Clin Nutr 53:1068S-1070S.

Green, R. A., Roudebush, P., Barton, C. L. 1979. Laboratory evaluation of coagulopathies due to vitamin K antagonism in the dog: three case reports. Am Anim Hosp Assoc 15:691-97.

Greenberg, E. R., Baron, J. A., Karagas, M. R., Stukel, T. A., Nierenberg, D. W., Stevens, M. M., Mandel, J. S., Haile, R. W. 1996. Mortality associated with low plasma concentration of beta carotene and the effect of oral supplementation. J Am Med Assoc 275:699-703.

Gunther, R., Felice, L. J., Nelson, R. K., Franson, A. M. 1988. Toxicity of vitamin D_3 rodenticide to dogs. J Am Vet Med Assoc 193:211-14.
Guyton, A. C. 1981. In Textbook of Medical Physiology, 6th ed., pp. 736-747. Philadelphia: W. B. Saunders.
Harrington, D. D., Page, E. H. 1983. Acute vitamin D_3 toxicosis in horses: case reports and experimental studies of the comparative toxicity of vitamins D_2 and D_3. J Am Vet Med Assoc 182:1358-69.
Harrison, J. H., Hancock, D. D., Conrad, H. R. 1984. Vitamin E and selenium for reproduction of the dairy cow. J Dairy Sci 67:123-32.
Harvey, R. B., Kubena, L. F., Elissalde, M. H. 1994. Influence of vitamin E on aflatoxicosis in growing swine. Am J Vet Res 55:572-577.
Haschek, W. M., Krook, L., Kallfelz, F. A., Pond, W. G. 1978. Vitamin D toxicity: initial signs and mode of action. Cornell Vet 68:324-64.
Hayek, M. G., Mitchell, G. E., Harmon, R. J., Stahly, T. S., Cromwell, G. L., Tucker, R. E., Barker, K. B. 1989. Porcine immunoglobulin transfer after prepartum treatment with selenium or vitamin E. J Anim Sci 67:1299-1306.
Hemken, R. W., Bremel, D. H. 1982. Possible role of beta-carotene in improving fertility in dairy cattle. J Dairy Sci 65:1069-73.
Hennekens, C. H., Buring, J. E., Manson, J. E., Stampfer, M., Rosner, B., Vook, N. R., Belanger, C., LaMotte, F., Gaziano, J. M., Ridker, P. M., Willett, W., Peto, R. 1996. Lack of effect of long-term supplementation with beta-carotene on the incidence of malignant neoplasms and cardiovascular disease. New Engl J Med 334:1145-1149.
Hidiroglou, M. 1996. Pharmacokinetic profile of plasma tocopherol following intramuscular administration of acetylated a-tocopherol to sheep. J Dairy Sci 79:1027-1030.
Hidiroglou, N., McDowell, L. R., Papas, A. M., Antapli, M., Wilkinson, N. S. 1992. Bioavailability of vitamin E compounds in lambs. J Anim Sci 70:2556-2561.
Hodges, R. E., Sauberlich, H. E., Canham, J. E., Wallace, D. L., Rucker, R. B., Mejia, L. A., Mohanram, M. 1978. Hematopoietic studies in vitamin A deficiency. Am J Clin Nutr 31:876-885.
Hogan, J. S., Weiss, W. P., Smith, K. L., Todhunter, D. A., Schoenberger, P. S. 1993. Vitamin E as an adjuvant in an *Escherichia coli* J5 vaccine. J Dairy Sci 76:401-407.
Holland, R. E., Boyle, S. M., Herdt, T. H., Grimes, S. D., Walker, R. D. 1992. Malabsorption of vitamin A in preruminating calves infected with *Cryptosporidium parvum*. Am J Vet Res 53:1947-1952.
Horst, R. L., Goff, J. P., Reinhardt, T. A. 1994. Calcium and vitamin D metabolism in the dairy cow. J Dairy Sci 77:1936-1951.
Hove, K., Kristiansen, T. 1982. Prevention of parturient hypocalcemia: effect of a single dose of 1,25-dihydroxyvitamin D_3. J Dairy Sci 65:1934-40.
Hubel, E., Kiefer, T., Weber, J., Mettang, T., Kuhlmann, U. 1991. In vivo effect of 1,25-dihydroxyvitamin D_3 on phagocyte function in hemodialysis patients. Kidn Intl 40:927-33.
Hustmeyer, F. G., Beitz, D. C., Goff, J. P., Nonnecke, B. J., Horst, R. L., Reinhardt, T. A. 1994. Effects of in vivo administration of 1,25-dihydroxyvitamin D_3 on in vitro proliferation of bovine lymphocytes. J Dairy Sci 77:3324-3330.
Ihrke, P. J., Goldschmidt, M. H. 1983. Vitamin A-responsive dermatosis in the dog. J Am Vet Med Assoc 182:687-90.
Jackson, J. A., Harmon, R. J., Tabeidi, Z. 1997. Effect of dietary supplementation with vitamin E for lactating dairy cows fed tall fescue hay infected with endophyte. J Dairy Sci 80:569-572.
Kott, R. W., Ruttle, J. L., Southward, G. M. 1983. Effects of vitamin E and selenium injections on reproduction and preweaning lamb survival in ewes consuming diets marginally deficient in selenium. J Anim Sci 57:553-58.
Krook, L., Wasserman, R. H., Shively, J. N., Tashjian, A. H., Brokken, T. D., Morton, J. F. 1975. Hypercalcemia and calcinosis in Florida horses: implication of the shrub *Cestrum diurnum* as the causative agent. Cornell Vet 65:26-56.
Kumar, R. 1986. The metabolism and mechanism of action of 1,25-dihydroxyvitamin D_3. Kidn Intl 30:793-803.
Kurokawa, K. 1987. Calcium-regulating hormones and the kidney. Kidn Intl 32:760-77.
Kushi, L. H., Folsom, A. R., Prineas, R. J., Mink, P. J., Wu, Y., Bostick, R. M. 1996. Dietary antioxidant vitamins and death from coronary heart disease in postmenopausal women. New Engl J Med 334:1156-1162.
Langweiler, M., Sheffy, B. E., Schultz, R. D. 1983. Effect of antioxidants on the proliferative response of canine lymphocytes in serum from dogs with vitamin E deficiency. Am J Vet Res 44:5-7.
Lessard, M., Yang, W. C., Elliott, G. S., Rebar, A. H., Van Vleet, J. F., Deslauriers, N., Brisson, G. J., Schultz, R. D. 1991. Cellular immune responses in pigs fed a vitamin E and selenium-deficient diet. J Anim Sci 69:1575-82.
Lind, C., Chen, J., Byrjalsen, I. 1997. Enzyme immunoassay for measuring 25-hydroxyvitamin D_3 in serum. Clin Chem 43:943-949.
Littledike, E. T., Horst, R. L. 1982. Vitamin D_3 toxicity in dairy cows. J Dairy Sci 65:749-59.
Long, G. G. 1984. Acute toxicosis in swine associated with excessive dietary intake of vitamin D. J Am Vet Med Assoc 184:164-70.
Maenpaa, P. H., Koskinen, T., Koskinen, E. 1988a. Serum profiles of vitamins A, E, and D in mares and foals during different seasons. J Anim Sci 66:1418-23.
Maenpaa, P. H., Pirhonen, A., Koskinen, E. 1988b. Vitamin A, E, and D nutrition in mares and foals during the winter season: effect of feeding two different vitamin-mineral concentrates. J Anim Sci 66:1424-29.
McDowell, L. R. 1989. In Vitamins in Animal Nutrition: Comparative Aspects to Human Nutrition. New York: Academic Press. a: chapter 2, pp. 10-54; b: chapter 3, pp. 55-92; c: chapter 4, pp. 93-131; d: chapter 5, pp. 132-154.
Mejia, L. A., Hodges, R. E., Rucker, R. B. 1979. Role of vitamin A in the absorption, retention, and distribution of iron in the rat. J Nutr 109:129-37.
Meydani, S. N., Meydani, M., Blumberg, J. B., Leka, L. S., Siber, G., Loszewski, R., Thompson, C., Pedrosa, M. C., Diamond, R. D., Stollar, B. D. 1997. Vitamin E supplementation and in vivo immune response in healthy elderly subjects. J Am Med Assoc 277:1380-1386.
Moore, R. M., Kohn, C. W. 1991. Nutritional muscular dystrophy in foals. Comp Cont Educ 13:476-90.
Mount, M. E., Feldman, B. F., Buffington, T. 1982. Vitamin K and its therapeutic importance. J Am Vet Med Assoc 180:1354-56.
Mount, M. E., Kass, P. H. 1989. Diagnostic importance of Vitamin K_1 and its epoxide measured in serum of dogs exposed to an anticoagulant rodenticide. Am J Vet Res 50:1704-9.
Nagode, L. A., Chew, D. J. 1991. The use of calcitriol in treatment of renal disease in the dog and cat. Proc Purina Intl Symposium, Eastern States Veterinary Conference, pp. 39-49.
Nemec, M., Butler, G., Hidiroglou, M., Farnworth, E. R., Nielsen, K. 1994. Effect of supplementing gilts' diets with different levels of vitamin E and different fats on the

humoral and cellular immunity of gilts and their progeny. J Anim Sci 72:665-676.

Ngah, V. Z. W., Jarien, Z., San, M. M., Marzuki, A., Top, G. M., Shamaan, N. A., Kadir, K. A. 1991. Effect of tocotrienols on hepatocarcinogenesis induced by 2-acetylaminofluorene in rats. Am J Clin Nutr 53:1076S-1081S.

Niyo, Y., Glock, R. D., Ledet, A. E., Ramsey, F. K., Ewan, R. C. 1980. Effects of intramuscular injections of selenium and vitamin E on peripheral blood and bone marrow of selenium-vitamin E deficient pigs. Am J Vet Res 41:474-78.

Njeru, C. A., McDowell, L. R., Wilkinson, N. S., Linda, S. B., Williams, S. N., Lentz, E. L. 1992. Serum α-tocopherol concentration in sheep after intramuscular injection of DL-α-tocopherol. J Anim Sci 70:2562-2567.

Nockels, C. F., Odde, K. G., Craig, A. M. 1996. Vitamin E supplementation and stress affect tissue α-tocopherol content of beef heifers. J Anim Sci 74:672-677.

NRC. 1978a. Nutritional Requirements of Domestic Animals: Nutrient Requirements of Dairy Cattle. 5th ed. Washington, DC: National Academy of Sciences—National Research Council.

———. 1978b. Nutritional Requirements of Domestic Animals: Nutrient Requirements of Horses. 4th ed. Washington, DC: National Academy of Sciences—National Research Council.

———. 1982. United States—Canadian Tables of Feed Composition. 3rd ed. Washington, DC: National Academy of Sciences—National Research Council.

———. 1984. Nutritional Requirements of Domestic Animals: Nutrient Requirements of Poultry. 8th ed. Washington, DC: National Academy of Sciences—National Research Council.

———. 1985. Nutritional Requirements of Domestic Animals: Nutrient Requirements of Dogs. 2nd ed. Washington, DC: National Academy of Sciences—National Research Council.

———. 1986. Nutritional Requirements of Domestic Animals: Nutrient Requirements of Cats. Rev. ed. Washington, DC: National Academy of Sciences—National Research Council.

———. 1987. Vitamin Tolerance of Animals. Washington, DC: National Academy of Sciences—National Research Council.

Ochoa, L., McDowell, L. R., Williams, S. N., Wilkinson, N., Boucher, J., Lentz, E. L. 1992. α-Tocopherol concentrations in serum and tissues of sheep fed different sources of vitamin E. J Anim Sci 70:2568-2573.

Omenn, G. S., Goodman, G. E., Thornquist, M. D., Balmes, J., Gullen, M. R., Glass, A., Keogh, J. P., Meyskens, F. L., Valanis, B., Williams, J. H., Barnhart, S., Hammar, S. 1996. Effects of a combination of beta carotene and vitamin A on lung cancer and cardiovascular disease. New Engl J Med 334:1150-1155.

Osweiler, G. D. 1978. Hemostatic function in swine as influenced by warfarin and an oral antibacterial combination. Am J Vet Res 39:633-38.

Packer, L. 1991. Protective role of vitamin E in biological systems. Am J Clin Nutr 53:1050S-1055S.

Paulsen, M. E., Johnson, L., Young, S., Norrdin, R. W., Severin, G. A., Knight, A. P., King, V. 1989. Blindness and sexual dimorphism associated with vitamin A deficiency in feedlot cattle. J Am Vet Med Assoc 194:933-37.

Politis, I., Hidiroglou, M., Batra, T. R., Gilmore, J. A., Gorewit, R. C., Scherf, H. 1995. Effects of vitamin E on immune function of dairy cows. Am J Vet Res 56:179-184.

Politis, I., Hidiroglou, N., White, J. H., Gilmore, J. A., Williams, S. N., Scherf, H., Frigg, M. 1996. Effects of vitamin E on mammary and blood leukocyte function, with emphasis on chemotaxis in periparturient dairy cows. Am J Vet Res 57:468-471.

Rebhun, W. C., Tennant, B. C., Dill, S. G., King, J. M. 1984. Vitamin K_3-induced renal toxicosis in the horse. J Am Vet Med Assoc 184:1237-39.

Reddy, G. S., Jones, G., Kooh, S. W., Fraser, D. 1982. Inhibition of 25-hydroxyvitamin D_3-1-hydroxylase by chronic metabolic acidosis. Am J Physiol 243:E265-E272.

Reddy, P. G., Morrill, J. L., Minocha, H. C., Morrill, M. B., Dayton, A. D., Frey, R. A. 1986. Effect of supplemental vitamin E on the immune system of calves. J Dairy Sci 69:164-171.

Reddy, P. G., Morrill, J. L., Minocha, H. C., Stevenson, J. S. 1987. Vitamin E is immunostimulatory in calves. J Dairy Sci 70:993-999.

Reffett, J. K., Spears, J. W., Brown, T. T. 1988. Effect of dietary selenium and vitamin E on the primary and secondary immune response in lambs challenged with parainfluenza virus. J Anim Sci 66:1520-1528.

Reinhardt, T. A., Hustmeyer, F. G. 1987. Role of vitamin D in the immune system. J Dairy Sci 70:952-962.

Rice, D. A., Kennedy, S. 1989. Vitamin E, selenium, and polyunsaturated fatty acid concentrations and glutathione peroxidase activity in tissues from pigs with dietetic microangiopathy (mulberry heart disease). Am J Vet Res 50:2101-2107.

Roquet, J., Nockels, C. F., Papas, A. M. 1992. Cattle blood plasma and red blood cell α-tocopherol levels in response to different chemical forms and routes of administration of vitamin E. J Anim Sci 70:2542-2550.

Sachs, M., Bar, A., Cohen, R., Mazur, Y., Mayer, E., Hurxiwtz, S. 1977. Use of 1α-hydroxycholecalciferol in the prevention of bovine parturient paresis. Am J Vet Res 38:2039-2041.

Satomura, K., Seino, Y., Yamaoka, K., Tanaka, Y., Ishida, M., Yabuuchi, H., Tanaka, Y., DeLuca, H. F. 1988. Renal 25-hydroxyvitamin D_3-1-hydroxylase in patients with renal disease. Kidn Intl 34:712-716.

Seven, A., Seymen, O., Hatemi, S., Hatemi, H., Yigit, G., Candan, G. 1996. Lipid peroxidation and vitamin E supplementation in experimental hyperthyroidism. Clin Chem 42:1118-1119.

Sheikh, M. S., Sant Ana, C. A., Nicar, M. J., Schiller, L. R., Fordtran, J. S. 1987. Gastrointestinal absorption of calcium from milk and calcium salts. New Engl J Med 317:532-536.

Siciliano, P. D., Parker, A. L., Lawrence, L. M. 1997. Effect of dietary vitamin E supplementation on the integrity of skeletal muscle in exercised horses. J Anim Sci 75:1553-1560.

Simon, E., Paul, J. L., Soni, T., Simon, A., Moatti, N. 1997. Plasma and erythrocyte vitamin E content in asymptomatic hypercholesterolemic subjects. Clin Chem 43:285-289.

Smith, K. L., Hogan, J. S., Wiss, W. P. 1997. Dietary vitamin E and selenium affect mastitis and milk quality. J Anim Sci 75:1659-1665.

Stabel, J. R., Goff, J. P. 1996. Influence of vitamin D_3 infusion and dietary calcium on secretion of interleukin 1, interleukin 6, and tumor necrosis factor in mice infected with *Mycobacterium paratuberculosis*. Am J Vet Res 57:825-829.

Stabel, J. R., Reinhardt, T. A., Stevens, M. A., Kehrli, M. E., Nonnecke, B. J. 1992. Vitamin E effects on in vitro immunoglobulin M and interleukin-1β production and transcription in dairy cattle. J Dairy Sci 75:2190-2198.

Stewart, A. F., Broadus, A. E. 1987. Mineral metabolism. In P. Felig, J. D. Baxter, A. E. Broadus, and L. A. Fruhman, eds., Endocrinology and Metabolism, 2nd ed., pp. 1317-1453. New York: McGraw-Hill.

Tan, B., Chu, F. L. 1991. Effects of palm carotenoids in rat hepatic cytochrome P450-mediated benzo(a)pyrene metabolism. Am J Clin Nutr 53:1071S-1075S.

Tengerdy, R. P., Nockels, C. F. 1975. Vitamin E or vitamin A protects chickens against *E. coli* infection. Poultry Sci 54:1292-1296.

Tharnish, T. A., Larson, L. L. 1992.Vitamin A supplementation of Holsteins at high concentrations: progesterone and reproductive responses. J Dairy Sci 75:2374-2381.

Tjoelker, L. W., Chew, B. P., Tanaka, T. S., Daniel, L. R. 1988. Bovine vitamin A and β-carotene intake and lactational status. 1. Responsiveness of peripheral blood polymorphonuclear leukocytes to vitamin A and β-carotene challenge in vitro. J Dairy Sci 71:3112-3119.

Toutain, P. L., Hidiroglou, M., Charmley, E. 1995. Pharmacokinetics and tissue uptake of D-α-tocopherol in sheep following a single intraperitoneal injection. J Dairy Sci 78:1561-1566.

Tsoukas, C. D., Provvedini, D. M., Manolagas, S. C. 1984. 1,25-Dihydroxyvitamin D_3, a novel immunoregulatory hormone. Science 224:1438-1440.

Van Saun, R. J., Smith, B. B., Watrous, B. J. 1996. Evaluation of vitamin D status of llamas and alpacas with hypophosphatemic rickets. Am J Vet Res 209:1128-1133.

Van Vleet, J. F., Kennedy, S. 1989. Selenium-vitamin E deficiency in swine. Comp Cont Educ 11:662-668.

Voigts, A. L., Felsenfeld, A. J., Llach, F. 1983a. The effects of calciferol and its metabolites on patients with chronic renal failure. I. Calciferol, dihydrotachysterol, and calcifediol. Arch Int Med 143:960-963.

———. 1983b. The effects of calciferol and its metabolites on patients with chronic renal failure. II. Calcitriol, 1-alphahydroxyvitamin D_3, and 24,25-dihydroxyvitamin D_3. Arch Int Med 143:1205-1211.

Wang, J. Y., Owen, F. G., Larson, L. L. 1988. Effect of betacarotene supplementation on reproductive performance of lactating Holstein cows. J Dairy Sci 71:181-186.

Weisburger, J. 1991. Nutritional approach to cancer prevention with emphasis on vitamins, antioxidants, and carotenoids. Am J Clin Nutr 53:226S-237S.

Weiss, W. P., Hogan, J. S., Smith, K. L., Todhunter, D. A., Williams, S. N. 1992. Effect of supplementing periparturient cows with vitamin E on distribution of α-tocopherol in blood. J Dairy Sci 75:3479-3485.

Wuryastuti, H., Stowe, H. D., Bull, R. W., Miller, E. R. 1993. Effects of vitamin E and selenium on immune responses of peripheral blood, colostrum, and milk leukocytes of sows. J Anim Sci 71:2464-2472.

Zeigler, R. G. 1991. Vegetables, fruits, and carotenoids and the risk of cancer. Am J Clin Nutr 53:251S-259S.

36 WATER-SOLUBLE VITAMINS

MARTIN J. FETTMAN

Thiamine (Vitamin B_1)
Riboflavin (Vitamin B_2)
Niacin (Vitamin B_3)
Vitamin B_6
Pantothenic Acid
Biotin
Folacin
Vitamin B_{12}
Choline
Vitamin C

THIAMIN (VITAMIN B_1)

Chemical Structure. Thiamin, or vitamin B_1, was the first of the B vitamins to be isolated and consists of a pyrimidine and a thiazole moiety joined by a methylene bridge (Fig. 36.1). Most of the thiamin in animal tissues occurs as phosphoric acid esters: approximately 80% as thiamin pyrophosphate (TPP), 10% as thiamin triphosphate (TTP), and 10% as thiamin monophosphate (TMP) and free thiamin (McDowell 1989a).

Sources and Chemical Properties. Brewer's yeast is the richest natural source of thiamin. Cereal grains, their by-products (particularly the germ and seed coats), and oilseed meals are also relatively rich sources, the content dependent on the level of protein (NRC 1982). Thiamin content in forages is related to leafiness, greenness, and protein content and decreases with maturity. Reasonable animal sources include liver, kidney, egg yolk, and dried skim milk. Commercial sources of supplemental thiamin are produced primarily from yeast and from industrial chemical synthesis. They are available as the hydrochloride and mononitrate salts, the latter having lower water solubility and greater stability. Natural sources may be highly variable in potency owing to differences in conditions during growth, processing, or storage, and hydrolysis upon exposure to heat and moisture is a prominent concern.

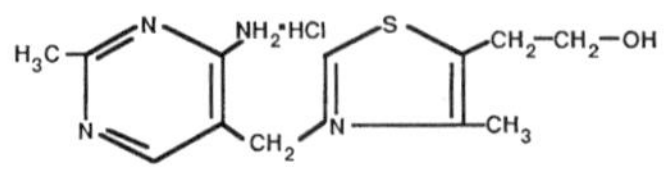

Heat-labile substances with thiaminase activity occur in certain types of raw fish, shellfish, bacteria, and molds (McDowell 1989a). Thiaminase activity develops with putrefaction and has been attributed in fish to a breakdown product of hemoglobin which splits thiamin at its methylene bridge. Thiamin occurs in many species of fresh- and saltwater fish, where it is found predominantly in the spleen, liver, intestines, and heart, and can be destroyed by cooking. Its production by ruminal bacteria appears to be induced by rapid changes to high-concentrate diets (Haven et al. 1983). Substances with antithiamin activity occur naturally, such as the phenolic acid derivative responsible for bracken fern poisoning in horses (Somogyi 1973), and are synthesized industrially, such as the avian and bovine coccidiostat, amprolium. Thiamin deficiency has been described in cats and dogs fed fresh, minced meat preserved with sulfur dioxide as a sulfiting agent, which is capable of cleaving thiamin into its constituent pyrimidine and thiazole moieties (Studdert and Labuc 1991). Physicochemical methods for the determination of thiamin content in biological specimens are quantitative and include fluorometric spectroscopy, thin-layer chromatography, and high-performance liquid chromatography (HPLC). Thiamin content is expressed as milligrams (mg) per unit dry matter of the substance assayed.

Biological Characteristics. Given adequate hydrochloric acid production in the stomach, thiamin from natural sources is readily digested and absorbed. Phosphoric acid esters are hydrolyzed in the small intestine; free thiamin is absorbed by both passive diffusion and active transport processes and is transported in the blood to the tissues bound to a carrier protein. Organs with higher metabolic activity, such as liver, kidneys, heart, and brain, maintain the highest levels, though little is stored for times of deficiency, with the exception of the pig, in which muscle levels are quite high (Blair and Newsome 1985).

METABOLIC FUNCTIONS. Thiamin functions mainly in its TPP form as the coenzyme cocarboxylase, which is required for oxidative decarboxylations of α-keto acids (McDowell 1989a). Thiamin is therefore neces-

Thiamin hydrochloride

FIG. 36.1

sary for the conversion of pyruvate to acetyl-coenzyme A (CoA), for entry of carbon units into the tricarboxylic acid (TCA) cycle, and for decarboxylation of α-ketoglutaric acid to succinyl-CoA, for progression of the TCA cycle. TPP is also the coenzyme for transketolase reactions in the oxidative pentose phosphate pathway, wherein 2-carbon units are transferred from ribulose-5-phosphate to ribose-5-phosphate, producing sedoheptulose-7-phosphate and glyceraldehyde-3-phosphate. This is essential for ribonucleotide synthesis and nicotinamide adenine dinucleotide phosphate, reduced (NADPH), production for fatty acid synthesis.

NEUROPHYSIOLOGY. Because many of the signs of thiamin deficiency are associated with neural dysfunction, several specific roles have been proposed for thiamin in nervous tissue (Read and Harrington 1986; McDowell 1989a). Through its role as cocarboxylase, it would be required for derivation of energy from oxidative decarboxylation of substrates in this highly metabolically active tissue. Through its role as coenzyme for transketolase, it would be necessary for normal fatty acid and cholesterol production, thereby affecting neuronal membrane synthesis and integrity. In addition, it is also necessary for the synthesis of the principal neurotransmitter, acetylcholine, and for the passive transport of sodium across excitable membranes.

Signs of Deficiency. Thiamin deficiency in animals is principally mediated by thiamin antagonists, or thiaminases, and is thus associated most with feeding of raw fish viscera to carnivores, fern poisoning in nonruminant herbivores, dietary changes to concentrates in ruminants, or coccidiostat overdosage in poultry and cattle. In ruminants, thiamin deficiency is characterized by weakness, ataxia, paresis, anorexia, and diarrhea, followed by signs characteristic of polioencephalomalacia, including blindness, head-pressing, convulsions, paralysis, and opisthotonos (Edwin et al. 1982; Haven et al. 1983). Deficiency in pigs progresses from inappetence and poor growth to sudden death due to myocardial inflammation and necrosis, cardiac arrhythmias, heart failure, and circulatory decompensation (Blair and Newsome 1985). In horses, clinical signs include lethargy, anorexia, weight loss, ataxia, cardiac arrhythmias, muscle tremors, and convulsions (Cunha 1991a). Thiamin deficiency in dogs produces anorexia, emesis, depression, paraparesis, torticollis, circling, and convulsions, progressing to death (Read and Harrington 1982, 1983, 1986). In poultry, neuromuscular effects predominate, including anorexia, paresis, opisthotonos, convulsions, and signs of polyneuritis (Gries and Scott 1972). A syndrome of severe lactic acidosis and circulatory shock in humans maintained with total parenteral nutrition lacking in thiamin has been described, and animals should be monitored for this condition as well (Oriot et al. 1991). Experimental induction of hydrogen sulfide-induced polioencephalomalacia in cattle by feeding high-sulfur, high-concentrate diets has confounded the issue of etiology and thiaminase participation in naturally occurring cases of what was previously thought to be thiamin deficiency in feedlot and range cattle (Sager et al. 1990; Gould et al. 1991).

Assessment of Status. Criteria used to evaluate thiamin status have included biological response to supplementation, determination of products of intermediate metabolism that are dependent on thiamin's function as a coenzyme (such as blood pyruvate or lactate levels), and analysis of enzyme activities for which thiamin is a cofactor (such as erythrocytic transketolase activity). Analysis of blood and urine thiamin concentrations offers a direct indication of status, but techniques have not been widely standardized, and the detection sensitivity for the various thiamin esters varies with the method employed.

Dietary Requirements, Indications, and Use

INTRINSIC FACTORS. There are significant species differences in the availability of thiamin synthesized by intestinal microflora, which in turn affects dietary requirements. Animals with functional rumens do not have a dietary requirement for supplemental thiamin, although growing calves and lambs are as susceptible to deficiency as simple-stomached animals. Adult horses are thought to absorb up to 25% of the free thiamin produced in the cecum and probably have no additional dietary requirement. Animals which practice coprophagy likewise are supported by intestinal microbial thiamin synthesis. Thiamin requirements increase with gestation, lactation, growth, or egg production. Increases in thyroid hormone release and metabolic rate induced by environment, disease, or neoplasia increase thiamin requirements, as does increasing age, owing to decreased efficiency of thiamin utilization. The urinary excretion of thiamin increases in polyuric renal diseases, thereby increasing the dietary requirement.

EXTRINSIC FACTORS. Stressful environmental conditions and disease have been shown to depress thiamin utilization. Gastrointestinal diseases may impair both enteric flora thiamin synthesis and subsequent absorption. Gastrointestinal parasites have been shown to compete with the host animal for thiamin, thereby increasing dietary requirements. Other dietary constituents may have significant influences on thiamin stability in feeds, absorption from the gut, or disposition in the body. Because thiamin is destroyed by heat and moisture, environment may affect its stability, particularly under adverse conditions of storage or handling. Spoiled or moldy feeds may contain thiamin antagonists or develop thiaminase activity. The need for thiamin increases dramatically with increasing dietary carbohydrate intake (McDowell 1989a). Conversely, dietary fats and proteins apparently have a "thiamin-sparing" effect. There is some evidence that thiamin may be effective in the treatment of lead toxicity, although its mechanism of action is uncertain (Bratton et al. 1981).

Preparations. Thiamin is available in yeast extracts and as a synthetic ester of hydrochloric or nitric acid. Injectable and oral preparations may be obtained singly or as part of a multivitamin preparation. Single large doses may be given as parenteral injections in the prophylaxis or therapeutics of specific conditions or diseases which increase thiamin requirements, such as for nonaffected ruminants in herd outbreaks of polioencephalomalacia or for carnivores when as little as 10% of their diet is uncooked fish like carp. Large doses may also be included in drinking water or parenteral fluid preparations in the resuscitation of diseased or convalescent animals.

Toxicity. Oral and parenteral thiamin in large doses is usually not toxic. For most animals, upper safe limits are approximately 1000 times their nutritional requirements (NRC 1987). Large intravenous doses in animals have caused vasodilation, bradycardia, hypotension, respiratory depression, and death, but this may have been due to hydrochloride-induced acid-base abnormalities rather than to thiamin itself.

RIBOFLAVIN (VITAMIN B_2)

Chemical Structure. Riboflavin, or vitamin B_2, was the second of the B vitamins to be isolated and consists of a dimethylisoalloxazine core with a ribose side chain (Fig. 36.2). Riboflavin occurs as the free alcohol, as flavin mononucleotide (FMN; riboflavin-5-phosphate), and as flavin adenine dinucleotide (FAD) (McDowell 1989b).

Sources and Chemical Properties. Brewer's yeast is one of the richest natural sources of riboflavin. Cereal grains and their by-products are low in riboflavin, oilseed meals are fair sources, and rapidly growing, green, leafy forages are very good sources (NRC 1982). Commercial sources of supplemental riboflavin are produced primarily from yeast and from industrial bacterial synthesis. They are available as the hydrochloride and mononitrate salts, the latter having lower water solubility and greater stability. Natural sources may be highly variable in potency owing to differences in conditions during growth, processing, or storage, and hydrolysis upon exposure to light and alkalinity is a prominent concern.

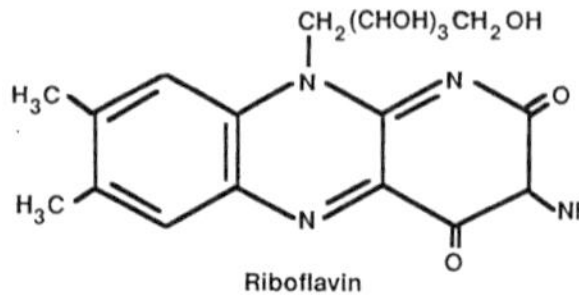

Up to one-fourth of riboflavin present in pet foods may be lost during the extrusion process. Physicochemical methods for the determination of riboflavin in biological specimens are quantitative and include fluorometric spectroscopy, thin-layer chromatography, and HPLC. Riboflavin content is expressed as milligrams (mg) per unit dry matter of the substance assayed.

$CH_2(CHOH)_3CH_2OH$

Riboflavin

FIG. 36.2

Biological Characteristics. Following hydrolysis of riboflavin nucleotides by phosphatases in the small intestine, free riboflavin is absorbed by both passive diffusion and active transport processes and is phosphorylated back to FMN in the enterocytes. FMN is transported in the blood to the liver bound to albumin and is converted to FAD in hepatocytes, where about one-third of the body's minimal supplies are stored for release upon demand. Organs with higher metabolic activity, such as liver, kidneys, heart, and brain, maintain the highest levels, though little is stored for times of deficiency.

METABOLIC FUNCTIONS. Riboflavin functions mainly as FMN and FAD, the prosthetic groups for flavoprotein enzymes which participate in the transfer of electrons in biological redox reactions. (McDowell 1989b). Some example flavoproteins are the aerobic dehydrogenases (amino acid oxidases, glucose oxidase), anaerobic dehydrogenases (lipoyl dehydrogenase, succinic dehydrogenase), and oxidases (xanthine oxidase; nicotinamide adenine dinucleotide, reduced [NADH]-cytochrome reductase). Thus, riboflavin plays a key role in the metabolism of carbohydrates, amino acids, and fats and is central to the processes of mitochondrial respiration and oxidative phosphorylation.

Signs of Deficiency. Riboflavin deficiency in animals is characterized by nonspecific signs related to its universal role in cellular metabolism. Because ruminal fermentation produces adequate riboflavin for the adult, its deficiency has only been characterized in young, growing ruminants, in which anorexia, diarrhea, poor growth, loss of hair, circumoral skin lesions, and excessive lacrimation and salivation have been observed. Deficiency in growing pigs produces anorexia, poor growth, dermatitis, alopecia, ataxia, emesis, and visual deficits. In gestating swine, riboflavin deficiency causes abortion, premature parturition, stillbirths, and greater postnatal mortality of piglets (Frank et al. 1984; Blair and Newsome 1985). Intestinal fermentation supplies all that is required for adult horses, but clinical signs produced by experimentally induced deficiency included lethargy, anorexia, severe weight loss, and poor growth (Cunha 1991b). It has been hypothesized that riboflavin deficiency might contribute to the development of periodic ophthalmia, but this has never been confirmed (Cunha 1991b). Riboflavin deficiency in dogs produces anorexia, reduced rates of growth, flaky dermatitis, erythema, muscle weakness, ataxia, and ocular lesions

(NRC 1985; Cline et al. 1996). In cats, riboflavin deficiency may cause hepatic lipidosis and alopecia as well (NRC 1986). In poultry, neuromuscular effects are observed in growing chicks as "curled toe paralysis," and in laying hens as reproductive failure (NRC 1984).

Assessment of Status. Criteria used to evaluate riboflavin status have included biological response to supplementation and analysis of enzyme activities for which riboflavin is a cofactor (such as erythrocytic glutathione reductase activity) (Frank et al. 1984, 1988; Cline et al. 1996). Analysis of blood and urine riboflavin concentrations offers a direct indication of status but first requires hydrolytic treatment to release free riboflavin from its esters.

Dietary Requirements, Indications, and Use

INTRINSIC FACTORS. Animals with functional rumens do not have a dietary requirement for supplemental riboflavin, although growing calves and lambs are as susceptible to deficiency as are simple-stomached animals. Adult horses are thought to absorb adequate riboflavin from that produced in the cecum and probably have no additional dietary requirement. Animals that practice coprophagy likewise are supported by intestinal microbial thiamin synthesis. The riboflavin requirement of adult dogs for maintenance has recently been demonstrated to be higher (~67 μg vs. 50 μg/kg body weight/day) than previously accepted (Cline et al. 1996). Riboflavin requirements increase with gestation, lactation, growth, or egg production. Increases in thyroid hormone release and metabolic rate induced by environment, disease, or neoplasia enhance the rate of riboflavin conversion into its mononucleotide and dinucleotide esters. Pregnant animals produce riboflavin-binding proteins whose synthesis is dependent on estrogen levels, which may facilitate placental transfer of riboflavin to the fetus. The urinary excretion of riboflavin increases in polyuric renal diseases, thereby increasing the dietary requirement.

EXTRINSIC FACTORS. Stressful environmental conditions like low temperature and disease have been shown to increase riboflavin requirements (McDowell 1989b). Gastrointestinal diseases may impair both enteric flora riboflavin synthesis and subsequent absorption. Other dietary constituents may have significant influences on riboflavin stability in feeds, absorption from the gut, or disposition in the body. Because riboflavin is destroyed by light and alkali, adverse conditions of storage or handling and alkalinizing feed additives like sodium bicarbonate may affect its stability. High-concentrate feeding increases riboflavin production by ruminal microflora (Miller et al. 1986a), and antibiotic feeding decreases it (Miller et al. 1986b). Supplemental nicotinamide also prevents the decrease in milk protein observed when diets of high-producing cows are supplemented with calcium salts of fatty acids (Cervantes et al. 1996).

Preparations. Riboflavin is available in yeast extracts, as crystalline riboflavin produced by chemical synthesis or bacterial fermentation, and as the water-soluble phosphate ester. Injectable and oral preparations may be obtained singly or as part of a multivitamin preparation. Single large doses may be given as parenteral injections in the prophylaxis or therapeusis of specific conditions or diseases which increase riboflavin requirements. Large doses may also be included in drinking water or parenteral fluid preparations in the resuscitation of diseased or convalescent animals. Differences exist in the gastrointestinal absorption and subsequent metabolism of nicotinic acid and nicotinamide. Nicotinamide is absorbed more rapidly, but rapid deamidation in the rumen may negate this effect in ruminants (Campbell et al. 1994). However, some source effects on niacin metabolism, such as effects on cellulose digestion, remain to be explained (Campbell et al. 1994; Cervantes et al. 1996).

Toxicity. Oral and parenteral riboflavin in large doses is usually not toxic. For most animals, upper safe limits are approximately 10-20 times, and possibly 100 times, their nutritional requirements (NRC 1987). Very large parenteral doses in laboratory animals have caused reproductive abnormalities and death, but adverse effects have not been reported in domestic species.

NIACIN (VITAMIN B_3)

Chemical Structure. Niacin, or vitamin B_3, is simply a modified pyrimidine synthesized from tryptophan; 3-pyridine carboxylic acid is nicotinic acid, and 3-pyridine amide is nicotinamide, or niacinamide (Fig. 36.3). Most of the niacin in animal tissues occurs as phosphoric acid esters with adenine, nicotinamide adenine dinucleotide (NAD), and nicotinamide adenine dinucleotide phosphate (NADP) (McDowell 1989c).

Sources and Chemical Properties. Niacin is ubiquitous in its distribution among plants and animals, and because of its stability when subjected to many of the usual environmental stresses, much activity is maintained during the pelleting process of feeds by steam and pressure or following cooking. Commercial sources of supplemental niacin are produced primarily from yeast and from industrial chemical synthesis and are available as the acid and the amide. Natural sources may be highly variable in potency owing to differences

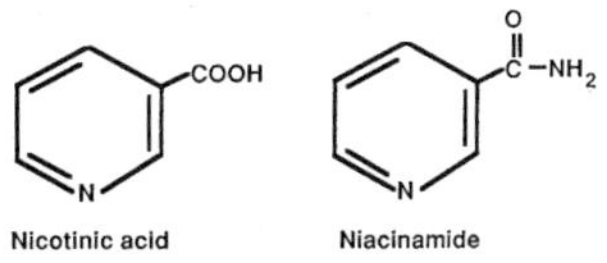

COOH
N
Nicotinic acid

O
C-NH_2
N
Niacinamide

FIG. 36.3

in conditions during growth, processing, or storage and to hydrolysis of bound forms upon processing (roasting, boiling, or alkali treatment) or digestion.

Substances with antiniacin activity have been synthesized, including 3-acetyl pyridine and pyridine sulfonic acid. Niacin is often present in feeds in a bound form that is virtually unavailable to simple-stomached animals and often unavailable to ruminal microorganisms as well. These are the niacinogens, in which niacin is linked to polysaccharides, peptides, or glycopeptides. Physicochemical methods for the determination of niacin content in biological specimens are quantitative and include colorimetric spectroscopy, thin-layer chromatography, and HPLC. Niacin content is expressed as milligrams (mg) per unit dry matter of the substance assayed.

Biological Characteristics. Unbound niacin from natural sources is readily digested and absorbed from the stomach and small intestine. Nicotinamide is hydrolyzed in the small intestine; nicotinic acid is then absorbed by both passive diffusion and active transport processes, is reconverted to the amide in the enterocytes, and is transported in the blood to the tissues, mostly in association with erythrocytes. The amino acid tryptophan is a precursor for synthesis of niacin in most animal species, depending on their conversion efficiency. Humans require approximately 60 mg of tryptophan to produce just 1 mg of niacin, whereas rats require half that amount. Poultry are less efficient converters than rats, and cats are virtually incapable of niacin production from tryptophan and thus have an absolute requirement for niacin in their diet (NRC 1986). Organs with higher metabolic activity, such as liver, kidneys, heart, and brain, maintain the highest levels, though little is stored for times of deficiency.

METABOLIC FUNCTIONS. Niacin functions mainly in its coenzyme forms (NAD and NADP), which act as hydrogen transfer agents in biological redox reactions (McDowell 1989c). As NAD, niacin is therefore necessary for the transfer of hydrogen atoms to O_2 in oxidative metabolism; and as NADP, niacin is necessary for hydrogen transfer in synthetic reactions, including the reductive steps of lipogenesis. In carbohydrate metabolism, the coenzyme forms are required for glycolysis and the TCA cycle. They function in lipid metabolism for glycerol synthesis and breakdown, fatty acid synthesis and oxidation, and steroid synthesis. For protein metabolism, they are necessary in the breakdown and synthesis of amino acids, and their carbon skeletons are oxidized in the TCA cycle.

Signs of Deficiency. Niacin deficiency in animals is characterized predominantly by metabolic disorders, particularly of the integumentary and digestive systems. Niacin deficiency per se is uncommon in ruminants, owing to adequate dietary tryptophan and enteric microbial synthesis to support their needs. However, supplemental niacin in ruminants improves nitrogen utilization and growth rate in growing animals (Brent and Bartley 1984) and rumen microbial protein synthesis and milk production in lactating animals (Riddell et al. 1980; Riddell et al. 1981). Large doses of niacin (6-12 g daily) have also been shown to significantly reduce the incidence and/or severity of ketosis in lactating cows (Fronk and Schultz 1979; Dufva et al. 1984). Potential deficiency in pigs is a concern, owing to the low available niacin and tryptophan content of corn, which composes a large part of many swine diets. Signs include inappetence, poor growth, nonregenerative anemia, stomatitis, vomiting, diarrhea, exfoliative dermatitis, and alopecia (Blair and Newsome 1985). Niacin deficiency has not been documented in horses, presumably due to adequate endogenous synthesis and production by intestinal microflora (Cunha 1991c). Niacin deficiency in dogs resembles that of humans most, and was first used to model pellagra. Signs of "blacktongue" in dogs include anorexia, depression, loss of body weight, cheilosis, glossitis, gingivitis, and bloody diarrhea, progressing to death (NRC 1985; McDowell 1989c). In poultry, signs of niacin deficiency include bowing of the legs and thickening of the hock joints (similar to that seen with biotin deficiency), as well as oral and gastrointestinal lesions of "blacktongue" (McDowell 1989c).

Assessment of Status. Criteria used to evaluate niacin status have included biological response to supplementation and analysis of urinary metabolites. Analysis of urinary Nμ-methylnicotinamide concentrations following a test dose of niacin offers an indirect measure of functional status.

Dietary Requirements, Indications, and Use

INTRINSIC FACTORS. There are significant species differences in the availability of bound niacin ingested in the feed or synthesized by intestinal microflora, which in turn affects their dietary requirement. As long as the dietary tryptophan level is at least 0.2% of the dry matter, niacin deficiency in growing calves is unlikely to occur. In adult ruminants, niacin synthesis by ruminal microflora and by host tissues is adequate under resting conditions, but requirements increase with stress, growth, gestation, or lactation, thereby necessitating supplementation. The urinary excretion of niacin may increase in polyuric renal diseases, thereby increasing the dietary requirement.

EXTRINSIC FACTORS. Stress can increase niacin requirements by 25% in poultry and by 100% in swine (McDowell 1989c). Other dietary factors increase niacin requirements, including excess leucine, arginine, or glycine, high-energy content, fat rancidity, or oral antibiotics. Gastrointestinal diseases may impair both enteric flora niacin synthesis and subsequent absorption. High-concentrate feeding increases niacin production by ruminal microflora (Miller et al. 1986a), whereas antibiotic feeding has little effect (Miller et al. 1986b).

Preparations. Niacin is available in yeast extracts, and both injectable and oral preparations may be obtained singly or as part of a multivitamin preparation. Single large doses may be given as parenteral injections in the prophylaxis or therapeusis of specific conditions or diseases which increase niacin requirements. Large doses may also be included in drinking water or parenteral fluid preparations in the resuscitation of diseased or convalescent animals.

Toxicity. High levels of niacin cause vasodilation, itching, heat sensations, nausea, emesis, headaches, and skin lesions in humans (NRC 1987). In laboratory rodents, high niacin intake has been shown to increase the activity of hepatic mixed-function oxidase and other xenobiotic metabolizing enzymes, which can affect the metabolism of a variety of drugs and toxicants. In dogs, 2 g/day of nicotinic acid produced bloody feces, convulsions, and death. Upper safe limits are approximately 350 mg nicotinamide/kg body weight/day, representing 10-1000 times the nutritional requirement, depending on species, and nicotinic acid may be tolerated at up to 4 times this level (NRC 1987).

VITAMIN B_6

Chemical Structure. Vitamin B_6 activity is attributed to three substituted pyridine compounds with equal biological activity in animals: the alcohol form, pyridoxol (pyridoxine); the aldehyde form, pyridoxal; and the amine form, pyridoxamine (Fig. 36.4; McDowell 1989d). Pyridoxol occurs mostly in plants, while the aldehyde and amine predominate in animal tissues. There are, in addition, two coenzyme forms of the vitamin: pyridoxal phosphate and pyridoxamine phosphate.

Sources and Chemical Properties. Vitamin B_6 is ubiquitous in its distribution among plants and animals (NRC 1982). Vitamin B_6 availability is greater from animal sources than from plant sources, perhaps due to differences in tissue protein binding. Because of susceptibility to breakdown upon processing or storage, much activity may be lost during the pelleting process of feeds by steam and pressure or following cooking. Commercial sources of supplemental vitamin B_6 are produced primarily from yeast and from industrial chemical synthesis and are most often available as the hydrochloride salt of pyridoxine. Natural sources may be highly variable in potency owing to differences in conditions during growth, processing, or storage.

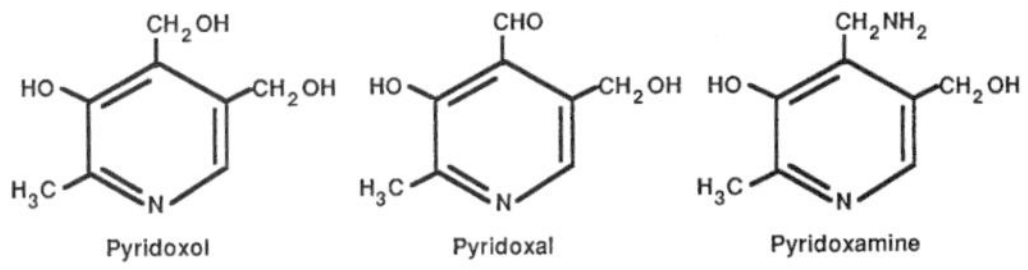

CH_2OH HO CH_2OH H_3C N Pyridoxol

CHO HO CH_2OH H_3C N Pyridoxal

CH_2NH_2 HO CH_2OH H_3C N Pyridoxamine

FIG. 36.4

Substances with anti-vitamin B_6 activity have been synthesized, including deoxypyridoxine, the antitubercular drug isonicotinic acid hydrazide (isoniazid), the antihypertensive drug hydralazine, and L-dopa. Physicochemical methods for the determination of vitamin B_6 content in biological specimens are quantitative and include fluorometric spectroscopy, thin-layer chromatography, gas chromatography, and HPLC. Vitamin B_6 content is expressed as milligrams (mg) per unit dry matter of the substance assayed.

Biological Characteristics. Free vitamin B_6 from natural sources is readily digested and absorbed, predominantly from the small intestine. Phosphoric acid esters are hydrolyzed by alkaline phosphatases in the small intestine, absorbed by passive diffusion, and transported in the blood to the liver, where most is converted to pyridoxal phosphate. Both niacin, as NADP, and riboflavin, as flavoprotein pyridoxamine phosphate oxidase, are necessary for phosphorylation of vitamin B_6 to form the active coenzymes. Organs with higher metabolic activity, such as liver, muscle, kidneys, heart, and brain, maintain the highest levels, though little is stored for times of deficiency. Pyridoxal phosphate is transported in the blood primarily in association with albumin and inside erythrocytes.

METABOLIC FUNCTIONS. Vitamin B_6 functions mainly in its coenzyme form of pyridoxal phosphate as a codecarboxylase for reactions involved in transamination, decarboxylation, deamination, desulfhydration, hydrolysis, and synthesis of amino acids (McDowell 1989d). Synthesis of niacin from tryptophan requires a vitamin B_6-dependent enzyme, kynureninase. Vitamin B_6 is required for the first step in porphyrin synthesis, wherein succinyl-CoA and glycine condense to form δ-aminolevulinic acid. Vitamin B_6 also plays a role in the synthesis of arachidonic acid from linoleic acid, hydrolysis of glycogen to glucose-1-phosphate, synthesis of the biogenic amines, and incorporation of iron into hemoglobin.

Signs of Deficiency. Vitamin B_6 deficiency is uncommon in adult ruminants, whose needs are provided by ruminal microorganisms. However, clinical signs of deficiency in growing calves have been documented, including anorexia, diarrhea, poor growth, vomiting, diarrhea, visual impairment, microcytic, hypochromic anemia, and nervous disorders due to demyelinization of peripheral nerves followed by axonal degeneration (Blair and Newsome 1985). Vitamin B_6 deficiency has not been documented in horses, presumably due to adequate endogenous synthesis and production by intestinal microflora (Cunha 1991d). Vitamin B_6 deficiency in dogs and cats causes inappetence, weight loss or growth depression, ataxia, convulsive seizures, cardiomyopathy, and microcytic, hypochromic anemia (NRC 1985, 1986; McDowell 1989d). Experimental pyridoxine deficiency in growing cats also induces renal lesions, characterized by tubular atrophy and dilatation, fibrosis, and calcium oxalate nephrolithiasis (Gershoff et al. 1959). In poultry, vitamin B_6 deficiency causes trembling, stiff and jerky movements, convulsions, and a squatting posture (McDowell 1989d). In elderly (>61 years of age) adult humans, vitamin B_6 deficiency impairs in vitro indices of immunity, including total number of peripheral blood lymphocytes, mitogenic responses to both T- and B-cell mitogens, and interleukin-2 (IL-2) production by peripheral blood mononuclear cells (Meydami et al. 1991).

Assessment of Status. Criteria used to evaluate vitamin B_6 status have included biological response to supplementation, measurement of plasma or urine concentrations, and analysis of changes in apoenzyme activity following incubation with added pyridoxal phosphate. Enzymes used for this assay have included tyrosine aminotransferase, tyrosine decarboxylase, aspartate aminotransferase, and alanine aminotransferase (McDowell 1989d). Analysis of urinary xanthurenic acid or kynurenic acid concentrations following a test dose of tryptophan offers an indirect measure of the functional status of pyridoxal phosphate as the cofactor for niacin synthesis.

Dietary Requirements, Indications, and Use

INTRINSIC FACTORS. Vitamin B_6 requirements increase with increasing dietary protein intake. Thus, species with higher dietary protein requirements, like cats, may likewise require more vitamin B_6 (Lewis et al. 1987; NRC 1986). In fact, studies have shown that the vitamin B_6 requirement of growing kittens is directly related to the level of dietary protein consumed and is approximately 1.0-2.0 mg/kg diet for kittens fed a 30% casein diet (Bai et al. 1991). In adult ruminants and horses, vitamin B_6 synthesis by gastrointestinal microflora is adequate under resting conditions, but as is the case for other species, requirements increase with stress, growth, gestation, or lactation, thereby necessitating supplementation. The urinary excretion of vitamin B_6 increases in polyuric renal diseases, thereby increasing the dietary requirement. In subtotally nephrectomized, chronically uremic rats, secondary vitamin B_6 deficiency was associated with greater reductions in glomerular filtration rate and augmentation of renal histologic lesions. Conversely, dietary supplementation with vitamin B_6 significantly improved renal function and may be indicated in naturally occurring renal diseases to mitigate progression (Wolfson et al. 1991).

EXTRINSIC FACTORS. Stress and other dietary factors increase vitamin B_6 requirements. Recent work with feedlot calves has demonstrated significant reductions in plasma concentrations of vitamin B_6 and pantothenic acid following short-term feed deprivation and transport stress (Dubeski et al. 1996a). Subsequent infection with bovine herpesvirus-1 (BHV-1) further decreased concentrations of vitamin B_6, vitamin B_{12}, pantothenic acid, and vitamin C (Dubeski et al. 1996a), and parenteral administration of a vitamin B complex significantly improved the serum immunoglobulin response to BHV-1 challenge (Dubeski et al. 1996b). Dietary amino acid imbalances caused by increased intake of tryptophan, methionine, and certain other amino acids also increase requirements. Gastrointestinal diseases may impair enteric flora vitamin B_6 synthesis and subsequent absorption. Because niacin and riboflavin are required for vitamin B_6 phosphorylation and activation, deficiencies in these vitamins may induce secondary vitamin B_6 deficiency. Antibiotics and other drugs, including penicillamine and estrogen, that act as vitamin B_6 antagonists also increase its dietary requirement.

Preparations. Vitamin B_6 is available in yeast extracts and as a synthetic hydrochloride salt. Injectable and oral preparations may be obtained singly or as part of a multivitamin preparation. Single large doses may be given as parenteral injections in the prophylaxis or therapeusis of specific conditions or diseases which increase vitamin B_6 requirements, such as for animals with chronic renal disease. Large doses may also be included in drinking water or parenteral fluid preparations in the resuscitation of diseased or convalescent animals.

Toxicity. The natural forms of vitamin B_6 are relatively nontoxic even at higher doses. For most animals, the toxic dietary level of vitamin B_6 is approximately 1000 times their nutritional requirements (NRC 1987). Rats, rabbits, and dogs have tolerated up to 1 g/kg of diet without effect (NRC 1987). In dogs, higher doses have caused anorexia, ataxia, muscle weakness, and incoordination due to demyelinization and axonal degeneration, much like vitamin B_6 deficiency (Phillips et al. 1978).

PANTOTHENIC ACID

Chemical Structure. Pantothenic acid is the amide of β-alanine and pantoic acid and is present predominantly in two coenzymes involved in intermediary metabolism: coenzyme A (CoA) and acyl carrier protein (Fig. 36.5; McDowell 1989e).

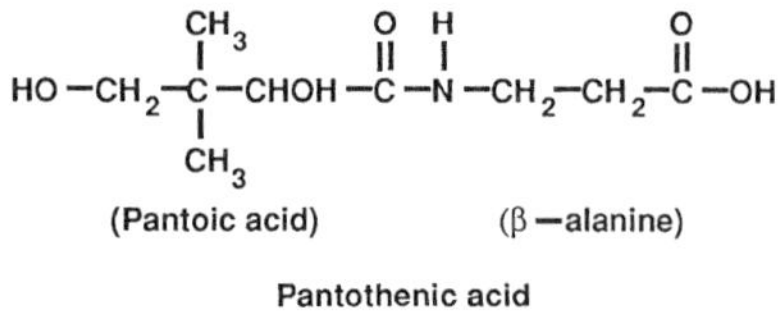

$$HO{-}CH_2{-}C(CH_3)_2{-}CHOH{-}C(=O){-}NH{-}CH_2{-}CH_2{-}C(=O){-}OH$$

(Pantoic acid) (β—alanine)

Pantothenic acid

FIG. 36.5

Sources and Chemical Properties. Pantothenic acid is found widely in both animal and plant sources. Pantothenic acid in grains like rice and wheat is present principally in the bran (NRC 1982). Stability in processed feedstuffs is relatively good. Commercial sources of supplemental pantothenic acid are produced primarily from yeast and from industrial chemical synthesis and are most often available as the calcium salt. Calcium pantothenate is produced industrially as a racemic mixture of both the *d*- and *l*-isomers. One gram of *d*-calcium pantothenate is equivalent in activity to 0.92 g of *d*-pantothenic acid, whereas 1 g of *dl*-calcium pantothenate has the activity of 0.46 g of *d*-pantothenic acid. Natural sources may be highly variable in potency owing to differences in conditions during growth, processing, or storage.

Substances with antipantothenate activity have been synthesized that contain alkyl or aryl ureide and carbamate moieties in the amide, but none are of practical concern. Physicochemical methods for the determination of pantothenic acid content in biological specimens are quantitative and include fluorometric spectroscopy, thin-layer chromatography, radioimmunoassay, and HPLC. Pantothenic acid content is expressed as milligrams (mg) per unit dry matter of the substance assayed.

Biological Characteristics. Pantothenic acid from natural sources is readily digested and absorbed, predominantly from the small intestine. Forms bound as CoA or acyl carrier protein are hydrolyzed by alkaline phosphatases in the small intestine, absorbed by passive diffusion, and transported in the blood to the tissues, where most is converted back to these enzymes. Organs with higher metabolic activity, such as liver, muscle, kidneys, heart, and brain, maintain the highest levels, though little is stored for times of deficiency. Pantothenic acid is transported in the blood primarily as CoA in erythrocytes and as the free acid in the plasma.

METABOLIC FUNCTIONS. Pantothenic acid functions mainly as CoA, which facilitates reactions of carboxylic acids catalyzed by such enzymes as pyruvate dehydrogenase, α-ketoglutarate dehydrogenase, fatty acid synthetase, propionyl CoA carboxylase, and acyl CoA synthetase (McDowell 1989e). It is necessary for the activation of acetic acid, as acetyl CoA for entry of carbon skeletons into the TCA cycle, synthesis of fatty acids and cholesterol, and the production of the neurotransmitter acetylcholine. As acyl carrier protein, it functions as a carrier for intermediate-chain acyl groups in the synthesis of fatty acids (McDowell 1989e).

Signs of Deficiency. Pantothenic acid deficiency in animals is characterized predominantly by disorders related to its prominent role in intermediary metabolism. Pantothenic acid deficiency is uncommon in adult ruminants and horses, whose needs are provided by ruminal and large-intestinal microorganisms, respectively (Cunha 1991e). Clinical signs of deficiency in growing calves have been produced experimentally, including anorexia, poor growth, diarrhea, rough hair coat, and particularly a scaly dermatitis around the eyes and muzzle. Many practical swine diets, particularly those based on corn or soybean meal, contain marginal levels of pantothenic acid. Deficiency in pigs is characterized by anorexia, poor growth, hemorrhagic diarrhea, dermatitis, and locomotor disorders, particularly affecting the hindlimbs (McDowell 1989e). The hindlimbs progressively show tremors, spasticity, and an exaggerated gait ("goose-stepping"), due to demyelinization of nerves in the dorsal root ganglia (Blair and Newsome 1985). Pantothenate deficiency causes inappetence, weight loss or growth depression, lowered antibody responses, and hindlimb spasticity in dogs, and hepatic lipidosis in kittens (NRC 1985, 1986; McDowell 1989e). Pantothenic acid deficiency in poultry produces dermatitis, hyperkeratosis, broken feathers, and decreased growth rates, as well as reduced egg production and hatchability (McDowell 1989e).

Assessment of Status. Criteria used to evaluate pantothenic acid status have included biological response to supplementation and measurement of plasma or urine concentrations. In humans, blood pantothenic acid concentrations less than 80 μg/dL and urinary pantothenate excretion less than 1 mg per day suggest a deficiency, but reference values for animals have not been established (McDowell 1989e).

Dietary Requirements, Indications, and Use

INTRINSIC FACTORS. Breed and strain differences in pantothenic acid requirements have been documented in pigs, resulting in the need for up to 50% increases in supplementation (McDowell 1989e). In adult ruminants and horses, pantothenic acid synthesis by gastrointestinal microflora is adequate under resting conditions, but as is the case for other species, requirements increase with stress, growth, gestation, or lactation, thereby necessitating supplementation. The urinary excretion of pantothenate may increase in polyuric renal diseases, thereby increasing the dietary requirement.

EXTRINSIC FACTORS. Dietary fat and protein intake can affect pantothenic acid requirements, as can ascorbic acid, biotin, and vitamin B_{12} levels (McDowell 1989e). Increased fat intake necessitates greater pantothenate for CoA synthesis and lipid metabolism, while high dietary protein apparently has a sparing effect on pantothenate requirements. Vitamin B_{12} deficiency increases pantothenate requirements, perhaps by trapping more as CoA-conjugated intermediates in the aberrant metabolism of propionic acid. Stress and other dietary factors increase pantothenic acid requirements as well. Gastrointestinal diseases may impair enteric flora pantothenate synthesis and subsequent absorption. Oral antibiotics also increase its dietary requirement, by inhibiting normal enteric microflora production.

Preparations. Pantothenic acid is available in yeast extracts and as a synthetic calcium salt. Injectable and oral preparations may be obtained singly or as part of a multivitamin preparation. Single large doses may be given as parenteral injections in the prophylaxis or therapeusis of specific conditions or diseases which increase pantothenate requirements. Large doses may also be included in drinking water or parenteral fluid preparations in the resuscitation of diseased or convalescent animals.

Toxicity. Pantothenic acid is relatively nontoxic even at higher doses. For most animals, the toxic dietary level is approximately 1000 times their nutritional requirements (NRC 1987). Rats have tolerated up to 10 g/kg body weight administered orally without effect, although the LD_{50} for a parenteral injection in rats was established as 1 g/kg body weight, and 80 mg/kg body weight administered intravenously produced some liver damage (NRC 1987). It is assumed that most species can tolerate a dietary level of at least 20 g/kg body weight (NRC 1987).

BIOTIN

Chemical Structure. Biotin is 2-keto-3,4-imidazilido-2-tetrahydrothiophenevaleric acid, a monocarboxylic acid with sulfur in a thioether linkage (Fig. 36.6; McDowell 1989f). Of the eight different isomers possible for this molecule, only *d*-biotin contains vitamin activity; the *l*-isomer possesses none.

Sources and Chemical Properties. Biotin is found widely in both animal and plant sources. The content and availability in crops are affected by seasonal factors, and processing and storage affect both plant and animal by-products (NRC 1982). Biotin is produced commercially primarily from yeast and from industrial chemical synthesis and is perhaps the most expensive of all the B vitamins to supplement.

Oxidation of biotin serially produces a sulfoxide, a sulfone, an oxybiotin (where oxygen replaces the sulfur), and desthiobiotin (in which the thioether is completely cleaved). Oxybiotin has minimal activity in rats and chicks, while the sulfone and desthiobiotin have activity only for some microorganisms. Substances with antibiotin activity have been isolated, best known of which is avidin, an albumin-like protein produced in poultry by oviductal mucosa and present in the egg white. Avidin can bind biotin and render it unavailable to animals consuming raw egg white or whole eggs; cooking destroys avidin's binding capacity (McDowell 1989f). Biotin in egg yolk is bound to a large, undialyzable protein which is similar to avidin but which releases biotin at 41° C. Release from the yolk binding protein is not complete, however, until denaturation at a temperature of 70° C. It has been estimated that at normal body temperatures in some species, as little as 20% of the biotin bound by this yolk protein may be available to the animal for gastrointestinal absorption (Wehr et al. 1980). Coupled with rapid intestinal transit time in mink, which reduces time for biotin absorption, feeding of unheated, dried, whole egg has resulted in biotin deficiency (Wehr et al. 1980). It has been stated that feeding of raw, whole eggs is unlikely to produce biotin deficiency in animals because the yolk biotin content is high enough to make up for the binding of biotin by avidin in the egg white, but this does not take into account other dietary and physiological effects on biotin absorption that may come into play and should not be assumed. Physicochemical methods for the determination of biotin content in biological specimens are quantitative and include fluorometric spectroscopy, thin-layer chromatography, and HPLC. Biotin content is expressed as milligrams (mg) per unit dry matter of the substance assayed.

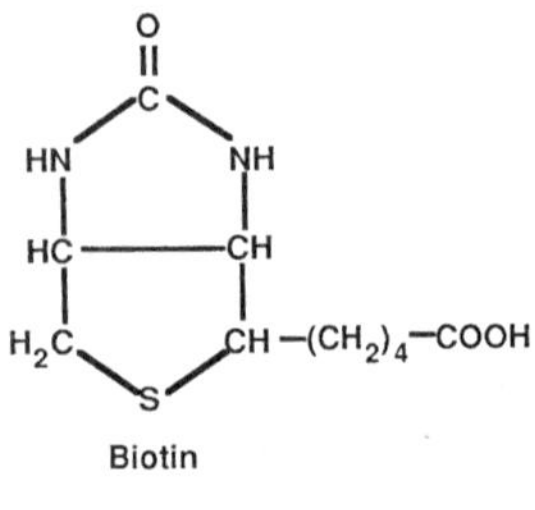

O
C
HN NH
HC CH
H_2C $CH-(CH_2)_4-COOH$
S

Biotin

FIG. 36.6

Biological Characteristics. Unbound biotin from natural sources is readily digested and absorbed, predominantly from the small intestine. Protein-bound forms are virtually unavailable, and in some cases less than one-half of the microbiologically determined biotin in feeds is available to animals (McDowell 1989f). Organs with higher metabolic activity, such as liver, muscle, kidneys, heart, and brain, maintain the highest levels, though little is stored for times of deficiency. Biotin is transported in the blood primarily as the free compound in the plasma.

METABOLIC FUNCTIONS. Biotin is a component of many carboxylating enzymes, in which it transports carboxyl moieties and facilitates the fixation of carbon dioxide to organic molecules (McDowell 1989f). Biotin is necessary for the carboxylation of pyruvic acid to form oxaloacetic acid in gluconeogenesis and for the interconversion of propionic acid and succinic acid and of succinic acid and α-ketoglutaric acid. Biotin is also required for the transcarboxylation and degradation of various amino acids and, in lipid metabolism, for the production of malonyl-CoA from acetyl-CoA, the first step in fatty acid synthesis (McDowell 1989f). In essential fatty acid metabolism, biotin facilitates the synthesis of arachidonic acid from linoleic acid, and its deficiency increases linolenic acid production and alters ω-6/ω-3 fatty acid ratios.

Signs of Deficiency. Biotin deficiency in animals most characteristically produces significant changes in the integumentary system. Its deficiency is uncommon in adult ruminants and horses, whose needs are provided by ruminal and large-intestinal microorganisms, respectively (Cunha 1991f). However, resolution of brittle hoof lesions has been reported in some horses supplemented with biotin (Comben et al. 1984). Many practical swine diets, particularly those based on corn or soybean meal, contain marginal levels of available biotin. Deficiency produces anorexia, poor growth, a dermatitis characterized by dryness, roughness, and ulceration, inflammation of the oral mucosa, and cracking of the soles and tops of hooves (McDowell 1989f). The feet become soft and rubbery and are prone to abrasive damage, particularly on rough flooring (Blair and Newsome 1985). Biotin deficiency in dogs and cats is uncommon but is characterized by inappetence, weight loss, dermatitis, and alopecia (NRC 1985, 1986; McDowell 1989f). Biotin deficiency in poultry reduced growth rates and caused dermatitis, hyperkeratosis, brittle and broken feathers, and severe foot disorders, as well as chondrodystrophy and perosis (McDowell 1989f). Signs of biotin deficiency in poults resemble those for pantothenic acid deficiency. In foxes and mink, biotin deficiency occurs whenever diets containing raw egg products are fed and is characterized by lethargy, scaly dermatitis of the paws, exudation from the eyes, and discoloration and loss of hair (Wehr et al. 1980). Experimental biotin deficiency in mice has resulted in skeletal malformations of the developing fetus, including cleft palate, micrognathia, micromelia, syndactyly, and deformities of the cervical vertebral arch (Watanabe and Endo 1991).

Assessment of Status. Criteria used to evaluate biotin status have included biological response to supplementation and measurement of blood or urine concentrations. However, the latter have proved unreliable and have been replaced by measures of pyruvate carboxylase activity (a biotin-dependent enzyme) in the plasma or erythrocytes in poultry and by liver biopsies in mammals (McDowell 1989f).

Dietary Requirements, Indications, and Use

INTRINSIC FACTORS. In adult ruminants and horses, biotin synthesis by gastrointestinal microflora is adequate under resting conditions, but as is the case for other species, requirements increase with stress, growth, gestation, or lactation, thereby necessitating supplementation. The urinary excretion of biotin may increase in polyuric renal diseases, thereby increasing the dietary requirement.

EXTRINSIC FACTORS. Dietary polyunsaturated fat content can increase biotin requirements in poultry and in rats, whereas inclusion of additional antioxidants like ascorbic acid or α-tocopherol protects against oxidative damage and reduces the required dietary level (McDowell 1989f). Stress and other dietary factors may increase biotin requirements, and gastrointestinal diseases may impair enteric flora biotin synthesis and subsequent absorption. Oral antibiotics also increase its dietary requirement, by inhibiting normal enteric microflora production.

Preparations. Biotin is available in yeast extracts and as a synthetic 100% crystalline product. Injectable and oral preparations may be obtained singly or as part of a multivitamin preparation. Single large doses may be given as parenteral injections in the prophylaxis or therapeusis of specific conditions or diseases which increase biotin requirements. Large doses may also be included in drinking water or parenteral fluid preparations in the resuscitation of diseased or convalescent animals.

Toxicity. Biotin is nontoxic even at higher doses. In rats levels of about 4-10 times the nutritional requirement caused reproductive abnormalities in gestating females, but tolerances have not otherwise been adequately evaluated in other species (NRC 1987). Because a high proportion of administered biotin appears rapidly in the urine for excretion, it is thought to be tolerated even at relatively high doses (NRC 1987).

FOLACIN

Chemical Structure. Folacin activity is attributed to a group of compounds based on folic (pteroylglutamic) acid (McDowell 1989g). Pure folic acid is pteroylmonoglutamic acid, which consists of a pteridine nucleus linked to *p*-aminobenzoic acid and one glutamic acid moiety (Fig. 36.7). Most of the folacin in natural sources occurs as pteroyl-γ-L-polyglutamates with from one to nine glutamic acid residues. Changes in the state of reduction of the pteridine group and addition of various 1-carbon substituents can produce modified folacin compounds such as 5,6,7,8-tetrahydrofolic acid, the principal coenzyme form, or

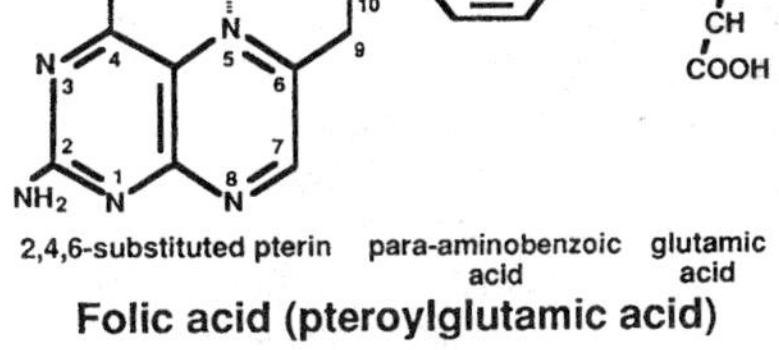

2,4,6-substituted pterin | para-aminobenzoic acid | glutamic acid

Folic acid (pteroylglutamic acid)

FIG. 36.7

N^5-methyltetrahydrofolic acid, the principal storage form of the vitamin.

Sources and Chemical Properties. Folacin is found widely in both animal and plant sources, mainly as tetrahydrofolic acid and polyglutamate derivatives (NRC 1982). Because of its sensitivity to light and heat, much folacin activity is lost upon cooking or processing of feeds. Folate analogs have been synthesized, predominantly for antimicrobial and anticancer therapy. They may act by binding to dihydrofolate reductase and blocking the conversion of pteroylmonoglutamic acid to tetrahydrofolic acid, or by blocking the transfer of methyl groups from tetrahydrofolic acid to acceptor compounds in metabolism. Sulfonamide antibiotics are analogs of *p*-aminobenzoic acid and competitively inhibit folacin synthesis by microorganisms. Naturally occurring folate antagonists identified in moldy feeds can block intestinal microbial synthesis of folacin. Physicochemical methods for the determination of folacin content in biological specimens are quantitative and include anion exchange, paired-ion reverse phase, conventional reverse phase, and fluorometric HPLC. A nonisotopic, cloned enzyme donor immunoassay system has been developed for the automated assay of folates in serum (van der Weide et al. 1992). Folacin content is expressed as milligrams (mg) per unit dry matter of the substance assayed.

Biological Characteristics. Polyglutamate forms of folacin must be hydrolyzed to pteroylmonoglutamate prior to absorption by the intestinal mucosa (McDowell 1989g). The intestinal conjugase responsible for this reaction is a zinc-dependent enzyme, and its activity is inhibited by acid conditions and drugs that lower intraluminal pH. Pteroylmonoglutamate is absorbed by active transport in the proximal small intestine, and the polyglutamate forms are reconstructed and transported to the tissues for storage, principally in the polyglutamate forms. Folacin-binding proteins facilitate intestinal mucosal uptake, transport in the blood, and uptake and storage by peripheral tissues. Liver contains up to half of body stores, and adult requirements can be met from stored folates for a prolonged period of time. Vitamin B_{12} deficiency can impair both the conversion of pteroylpolyglutamates to pteroylmonoglutamate and the transfer of methyl groups from methyltetrahydrofolate by methionine synthetase, thereby leading to a secondary folacin deficiency.

METABOLIC FUNCTIONS. Folacin, as 5,6,7,8-tetrahydrofolic acid, is essential to the transfer of single-carbon moieties in metabolism (McDowell 1989g). In its role as a methyl-group donor, it is responsible for the synthesis of purines and pyrimidines, the interconversion of serine and glycine, histidine degradation, and the transfer of methyl groups to homocysteine to form methionine, and to ethanolamine to form choline (McDowell 1989g). Because of its central role in nucleic acid synthesis, it is essential for cell division in rapidly growing tissues such as intestinal mucosa and bone marrow. By virtue of its effect on rapidly dividing cell populations, folacin deficiency has been linked to immune system dysfunction as well (Blair and Newsome 1985).

Signs of Deficiency. Folacin deficiency in animals is characterized principally by effects on tissues with rapid rates of cell division. Macrocytic anemia and leukopenia develop because inadequate nucleic acid precursors are available for normal hematopoiesis. Cytoplasmic maturation and hemoglobinization of erythroid precursors continue in the absence of normal cell division, and macrocytic or megaloblastic erythrocytes are produced. Epithelial linings of the gastrointestinal tract and epidermis are also affected. Its deficiency is uncommon in adult ruminants and horses, whose needs are provided by ruminal and large-intestinal microorganisms, respectively (Cunha 1991g). Experimental deficiency in growing lambs fed a semisynthetic diet has been characterized by leukopenia, diarrhea, and pneumonia. In gestating early-lactation dairy cows, large decreases in serum folate levels have been prevented by intramuscular administration of folacin, suggesting that supplementation might increase folacin availability to the fetus and improve neonatal performance (Girard et al. 1989). Studies in growing dairy heifers have documented an increase in weight gain, feed efficiency, hematocrit, and blood hemoglobin concentration following weekly intramuscular injections of 40 mg of folacin from 10 days to 16 weeks of age (Dumoulin et al. 1991). Inadequate folic acid intake in growing pigs and feeding of sulfa drugs to adult swine, thereby inhibiting normal microbial synthesis of folacin in the gut, result in a deficiency characterized by anemia, leukopenia, diarrhea, and a reduced growth rate (Blair and Newsome 1985). Folacin deficiency in dogs and cats has been characterized by inappetence, weight loss, anemia, leukopenia, and glossitis (NRC 1985, 1986; McDowell 1989g). In dogs, decreased antibody responses to infectious canine hepatitis virus and canine distemper virus have been documented (NRC 1985). Folacin deficiency in poultry is characterized by megaloblastic anemia, poor growth, poor feather development, depigmentation of feathers, perosis, reduced egg production and hatchability, and spastic cervical paralysis (McDowell 1989g).

A growing body of literature has associated hyperhomocysteinemia, caused by dietary folate deficiency, with increased risk for occlusive vascular disease in humans (Ueland and Refsum 1989; Clarke et al. 1991; Kang et al. 1992). Homocysteine is a normal constituent of body tissues and fluids and is derived by the cleavage of *S*-adenosylhomocysteine, which is produced from *S*-adenosylmethionine when it donates a methyl group for other synthetic reactions. Hyperhomocysteinemia arises from a deficiency of cystathionine β-synthase activity (which catalyzes the synthesis of cysteine from homocysteine and serine) in the hereditary disease homocystinuria or from a deficiency of folic acid, which is required for the re-methylation of homocysteine by 5-methyltetrahydrofolate-homocysteine methyltransferase (methionine synthase). As little as a 5 μmol/L increase in plasma homocysteine concentration elevates the risk for coronary artery disease by as much as a 20 mg/dL increase in serum cholesterol (Boushey et al. 1995). The risk for atherosclerotic vascular disease in folate deficiency-related hyperhomocysteinemia relative to euhomocysteinemic individuals is estimated to be approximately 2.2 (Graham et al. 1997). Consumption of 5 mg folic acid twice daily for one week, followed by once daily for two weeks, resulted in a decrease in plasma homocysteine levels of approximately 4 μmol/L in mildly hyperhomocysteinemic subjects (Rasmussen et al. 1996). Folic acid supplementation of as little as 400 μg/day has produced similar homocysteine-lowering effects (Boushey et al. 1995). Whether naturally occurring folate-responsive hyperhomocysteinemia or its associated vascular diseases occur in animals is unknown.

Assessment of Status. Criteria used to evaluate folacin status have included biological response to supplementation and measurement of serum and erythrocyte concentrations. Because signs of vitamin B_{12} deficiency may mimic those of folacin deficiency, concentrations of the former should be simultaneously evaluated. In folacin deficiency, the degradation of histidine into glutamic acid is interrupted, producing increased levels of formiminoglutamic acid (FIGLU), an intermediate acid. The amount of FIGLU excreted in the urine following a histidine challenge corresponds well with erythrocytic folate levels and offers a means of assessing functional stores of folacin in the body. In humans, plasma total homocysteine concentrations 6 hours after a standardized methionine loading test (100 mg/kg body weight per os) stress the pathway for irreversible degradation of homocysteine and serve as a marker of folate status (Graham et al. 1997).

Dietary Requirements, Indications, and Use

INTRINSIC FACTORS. In adult ruminants and horses, folacin synthesis by gastrointestinal microflora is adequate under resting conditions, but as is the case for other species, requirements increase with stress, growth, gestation, or lactation, thereby necessitating supplementation. Supplementation of sows with folic acid throughout gestation has consistently produced an increased litter size, apparently as a result of improved embryonic or fetal survival in utero (Lindemann 1993). The more rapid the rate of growth in young animals, or the greater the level of production, the greater the need for folacin. Whereas the supply of folates in the diet and by rumen microbial synthesis is adequate to maintain gestation and lactation, the requirement in multiparous or high-producing lactating cows may exceed natural supplies, necessitating supplementation during the first 6-8 weeks of lactation (Girard et al. 1995). The urinary excretion of folacin may increase in polyuric renal diseases, thereby increasing the dietary requirements.

EXTRINSIC FACTORS. Dietary deficiencies of choline, vitamin B_{12}, iron, and ascorbic acid have all been reported to increase folacin requirements (McDowell 1989g). Increased dietary fiber intake as xylan, wheat bran, and beans has increased intestinal microflora synthesis of folacin (Keagy and Oace 1984). Stress may increase folacin requirements, and gastrointestinal diseases may impair both enteric microbial folacin synthesis and subsequent absorption. Oral antibiotics, particularly sulfonamides, also increase its dietary requirement, by inhibiting normal enteric microflora production. Elevated serum folate concentrations are commonly observed in dogs with exocrine pancreatic insufficiency (Williams 1996). This may be explained by secondary small-intestinal overgrowth with bacteria that either synthesize or release folate and/or by enhanced folate absorption as a result of reduced pancreatic bicarbonate secretion and decreased duodenal pH (Rutgers et al. 1995; Williams 1996).

Preparations. Folacin is available in yeast extracts and as a synthetic 100% crystalline product. Injectable and oral preparations may be obtained singly or as part of a multivitamin preparation. Single large doses may be given as parenteral injections in the prophylaxis or therapeusis of specific conditions or diseases which increase folacin requirements. Large doses may also be included in drinking water or parenteral fluid preparations in the resuscitation of diseased or convalescent animals.

Toxicity. Folacin is nontoxic even at higher doses. In rats, single parenteral doses greater than 1000 times the nutritional requirement have induced epileptic seizures, and in rabbits, intraperitoneal injection with 50 mg/kg/day for 10 weeks induced renal lesions, but toxicity has not otherwise been observed in species studied to date (NRC 1987; Campbell 1996).

VITAMIN B_{12}

Chemical Structure. Vitamin B_{12} activity is attributed to a group of compounds whose structure resembles a porphyrin ring consisting of four pyrrole nuclei coupled together so that the inner nitrogen atom of each moiety is coordinated with a central atom of cobalt (McDowell 1989h). The coordinated pyrrole structure is also called a corrin nucleus, and a nucleotide is coupled to the cobalt atom by its nitrogen, and to a propionic acid moiety of the corrin nucleus D ring by a phosphate ester. When cyanide (CN) is attached to the cobalt atom, above the planar ring of the molecule, it is called cyanocobalamin, the most common and most stable form of the vitamin (Fig. 36.8). The CN moiety may be replaced by H_2O (aquacobalamin), OH (hydroxycobalamin), NO_2 (nitrocobalamin), or CH_3

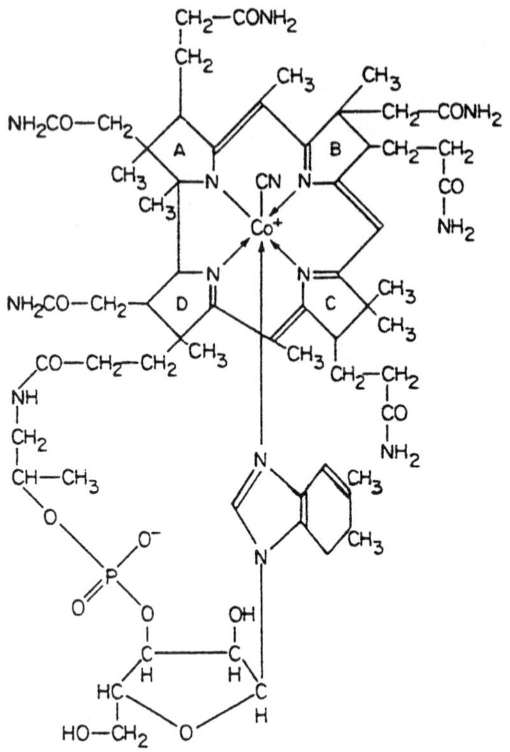

FIG. 36.8—Vitamin B_{12} (cyanocobalamin). (From McDowell 1989h.)

(methylcobalamin), and various nucleotide modifications may produce adenosylcobalamin or deoxyadenosylcobalamin, which along with hydroxy- and methylcobalamin are the predominant forms in animal tissues (McDowell 1989h).

Sources and Chemical Properties. Vitamin B_{12} in nature arises solely from bacterial synthesis and not from yeast or fungi. Vitamin B_{12} is found widely in animal sources, mainly as cyanocobalamin. Plant materials contain virtually no vitamin B_{12} (NRC 1982). Vitamin B_{12} analogs have been identified, predominantly consisting of intermediates in the biosynthesis of cyanocobalamin. They have little or no activity and do not act as vitamin B_{12} antagonists. Physicochemical methods for the determination of vitamin B_{12} content in biological specimens are quantitative and include colorimetric procedures wherein released cyanide is complexed with a chromogen and competitive protein-binding methods wherein cyanocobalamin in test materials displaces radioactively labeled cyanocobalamin in the reaction. A nonisotopic, cloned enzyme donor immunoassay system has been developed for the automated assay of vitamin B_{12} in serum (Kuemmerle et al. 1992). Vitamin B_{12} content is expressed as milligrams (mg) per unit dry matter of the substance assayed.

Biological Characteristics. Vitamin B_{12} in feed is bound to proteins, from which it is released through the action of gastric acidity and peptic digestion, and following which it is bound by a nonintrinsic factor protein until it reaches the proximal small intestine (McDowell 1989h). In the small intestine, trypsin degrades the nonintrinsic factor proteins, facilitating the binding of vitamin B_{12} to intrinsic factor, a glycoprotein which mediates vitamin B_{12} absorption. Vitamin B_{12} is absorbed almost exclusively in the ileum, in a carrier-mediated process with a specific receptor protein located on the microvillus border of the enterocytes. Defective brush border expression of the intrinsic factor-cobalamin receptor has been identified in a heritable syndrome of canine cobalamin malabsorption (Fyfe et al. 1991a,b). Following its transport from the enterocytes to the portal blood, vitamin B_{12} is bound to proteins called transcobalamins, which are synthesized by the liver and facilitate transport and storage of the vitamin. Liver contains much of the body's stores, and half-life has been reported to be as long as 1 month (McDowell 1989h). Vitamin B_{12} is converted to adenosylcobalamin, the coenzyme for mutase, or to methylcobalamin, the coenzyme for methyltransferase, in order to be metabolically active.

METABOLIC FUNCTIONS. As the methylcobalamin coenzyme for methyltransferase, vitamin B_{12} is essential, along with folacin, for the transfer of methyl groups in the synthesis of methionine and choline and for the production of purines and pyrimidines. Vitamin B_{12} deficiency impairs the removal of the methyl group from methyltetrahydrofolic acid, thereby trapping the folate in a nonutilizable form and producing an effective folate deficiency. Vitamin B_{12} is required for the incorporation of serine, methionine, and phenylalanine into proteins, and as the adenosylcobalamin coenzyme for mutase or methylmalonyl-CoA isomerase, it is required for the conversion of propionate to succinyl-CoA. Because methionine synthase activity is also impaired by a methylcobalamin deficiency, hyperhomocysteinemia, as described for folate deficiency, may also be responsive to vitamin B_{12} supplementation (Kang et al. 1992), though the effect is not as marked as for folate supplementation (Rasmussen et al. 1996).

Signs of Deficiency. Vitamin B_{12} deficiency in animals is characterized principally by effects on tissues with rapid rates of cell division and by neurological lesions. Megaloblastic anemia similar to that seen with folacin deficiency develops because inadequate nucleic acid precursors are available for normal hematopoiesis. Its deficiency is uncommon in adult ruminants and horses provided with adequate dietary cobalt, whose needs are provided by ruminal and large-intestinal microorganisms, respectively (Cunha 1991h). Signs attributable to cobalt deficiency are essentially those of vitamin B_{12} deficiency in these species. They include inappetence, anemia, dermatitis, rough hair coat, wasting, and death (McDowell 1989h). Subclinical cobalt (and, hence, vitamin B_{12}) deficiency is thought to have tremendous economic impact on production in areas with cobalt-deficient soils. A report in sheep indicated that reproductive performance and lamb viability in subclinically deficient ewes were significantly affected and could only be completely reversed by cobalt supplementation throughout the period of breeding, gestation, and lactation (Fisher and MacPherson 1991). Cobalt and vitamin B_{12} deficiency was at one time thought to play a role in ketosis and low milk fat syndromes in lactating dairy cows, due to its deleterious effects on propionate metabolism, to reduction in the rate of gluconeogenesis, and to methylmalonate-mediated inhibition of fatty acid synthesis (Elliot et al. 1979; Croom et al. 1981; Peters and Elliot 1983). Although cobalt and/or vitamin B_{12} supplementation of subclinically deficient animals can improve feed efficiency, growth rate, and production, these metabolic diseases have not been linked conclusively to vitamin B_{12} deficiency as yet. Vitamin B_{12} deficiency in pigs is characterized by a normocytic anemia, vomiting, diarrhea, rough hair coat, reduced growth rate, and neurological lesions of increased excitability, unsteady gait, and ataxia (Blair and Newsome 1985). Vitamin B_{12} deficiency has been described in dogs only in a family of Giant Schnauzers with inherited selective intestinal malabsorption of cobalamin. Abnormal findings included inappetence, lethargy, failure to grow, a chronic nonregenerative anemia with anisocytosis and poikilocytosis, and neutropenia with hypersegmentation (Fyfe et al. 1989). Vitamin B_{12} deficiency in kittens has been characterized by slow growth and increased methylmalonic acid excretion (NRC 1985, 1986; McDowell 1989h). A 9-month-old cat with methylmalonic acidemia secondary to a defect in intestinal cobalamin absorption expressed clinical signs including lethargy, fever, anorexia, and poor growth unless fed a restricted protein diet or treated with vitamin B_{12} (Vaden et al. 1992). A congenital disorder of intestinal cobalamin absorption may have been observed in a nine-month-old male cat characterized clinically by lethargy and poor growth, from which serum cobalamin concentrations were virtually nil and hepatic methylmalonyl-CoA-mutase activity was hyperresponsive to cobalamin supplementation in vitro (Vaden et al. 1992). Vitamin B_{12} deficiency in poultry is characterized by poor growth, reduced feed efficiency, perosis, reduced egg production and hatchability, limb weakness, and ataxia (McDowell 1989h).

Assessment of Status. Criteria used to evaluate vitamin B_{12} status have included biological response to supplementation and measurement of serum and tissue concentrations. Because signs of folacin deficiency overlap those of vitamin B_{12} deficiency, concentrations of the former should be simultaneously evaluated (McDowell 1989h). As for folate deficiency, in vitamin B_{12} deficiency, the degradation of histidine into glutamic acid is interrupted, producing increased levels of FIGLU acid, an intermediate, and offers a means of assessing functional stores of vitamin B_{12} in the body. Urinary excretion of methylmalonic acid is also elevated with vitamin B_{12} deficiency and may be used as an index of functional status. Finally, one may evaluate liver cobalt or vitamin B_{12} concentrations in ruminants, wherein concentrations of cobalt less than 0.07 ppm or of cobalamin less than 0.10 μg/g wet weight are diagnostic of deficiency.

Dietary Requirements, Indications, and Use

INTRINSIC FACTORS. In adult ruminants and horses, vitamin B_{12} synthesis by gastrointestinal microflora is adequate under resting conditions, but as is the case for other species, requirements increase with stress, growth, gestation, or lactation, thereby necessitating supplementation. The more rapid the rate of growth or the greater the level of production, the greater the need for vitamin B_{12}. The urinary excretion of vitamin B_{12} may increase in polyuric renal diseases, thereby increasing the dietary requirement. In humans, the condition of pernicious anemia occurs when there is a defect in vitamin B_{12} absorption by the gastrointestinal tract, owing to abnormalities in gastric acid production, pancreatic exocrine insufficiency, intrinsic-factor secretion, enterocyte receptor synthesis, or inflammatory bowel disease (McDowell 1989h). Exocrine pancreatic insufficiency (EPI) in dogs is commonly associated with severely subnormal serum cobalamin concentrations, pursuant to defects in intestinal cobalamin absorption (Simpson et al. 1989; Williams 1996). Replacement with exogenous canine pancreatic juice reverses the defect in experimental canine EPI (Simpson et al. 1989). However, it is unclear whether deficiencies of pancreatic proteases or pancreatic intrinsic factor, secondary small-intestinal bacterial overgrowth (SIBO), or some combination of effects is responsible for the cobalamin malabsorption and deficiency (Williams 1996). Serum cobalamin levels are also significantly depressed in some cases of SIBO, whether EPI coexists or not, and this may be due to cobalamin-binding by bacteria or mucosal damage and subsequent malabsorption (Rutgers et al. 1995).

EXTRINSIC FACTORS. Dietary deficiencies of choline, methionine, folacin, and, of course, cobalt have all been reported to increase vitamin B_{12} requirements (McDowell 1989h). Dietary supplementation with propionate increases vitamin B_{12} requirements (Hogue and Elliot 1964), but dietary factors which increase propionic acid production, such as supplementation with ionophores, have had little effect (Daugherty et al. 1986). Stress may increase vitamin B_{12} requirements, and gastrointestinal diseases may impair enteric microbial vitamin B_{12} synthesis and subsequent absorption. Oral antibiotics may also increase its dietary requirement, by inhibiting normal enteric microflora production.

Preparations. Vitamin B_{12} is available commercially as cyanocobalamin, produced by fermentation. Injectable and oral preparations may be obtained singly or as part of a multivitamin preparation. Single large doses may be given as parenteral injections in the prophylaxis or therapeusis of specific conditions or diseases which increase vitamin B_{12} requirements. Large doses may also be included in drinking water or parenteral fluid preparations in the resuscitation of diseased or convalescent animals. For ruminants, cobalt deficiency can be cured or prevented by treatment of soils with cobalt-containing fertilizers or by oral treatment of animals with cobalt salts or cobalt oxide pellets that remain in the rumen for long periods of time.

Toxicity. Vitamin B_{12} is nontoxic even at higher doses. In mice, a single parenteral dose of up to 1600 mg/kg body weight induced no adverse effects. Amounts greater than 1000 times the nutritional requirement are thought to be safe in most species (NRC 1987). Cobalt toxicity at dietary levels greater than 5 ppm has been documented in ruminants and is characterized by polycythemia, excessive salivation, respiratory difficulties, and decreased growth rates or milk production.

CHOLINE

Sources and Chemical Properties. Choline (Fig. 36.9) in nature occurs in virtually all sources of fat, including oilseed meals, cereal germs, glandular organ by-products, and fish (NRC 1982). Although choline is an essential nutrient, it differs from the true B vitamins in that it is required in much larger amounts, may be endogenously synthesized, and serves as a structural component rather than as a metabolic catalyst (McDowell 1989i). Choline chloride and choline bitartrate, the forms produced by chemical synthesis for supplementation, are white crystalline substances with solubility in water and alcohol. Choline itself is stable through processing and storage in pelleted and extruded feeds, but it decreases the stability of a number of other vitamins in commercial premixes. Choline content is expressed as milligrams (mg) per unit dry matter of the substance assayed.

Biological Characteristics. Choline availability from feeds is generally high, being present mostly in the form of lecithin (phosphatidylcholine) and, in a smaller amount, as sphingomyelin (McDowell 1989i). In the small intestine, approximately one-half of the lecithin consumed is absorbed intact into the lymph. From the remainder, choline is released by hydrolysis and is absorbed by both passive and active transport processes, predominantly in the ileum.

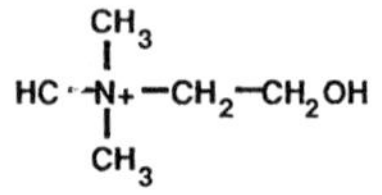

METABOLIC FUNCTIONS. Choline is essential as a component of lecithin, a key phospholipid for maintaining cell membrane structure and function. It is a "lipotrophic factor," and in the form of lecithin, it plays an important role in lipid metabolism, facilitating lipoprotein synthesis by the liver and preventing hepatic lipidosis. Choline is required for the synthesis of the neurotransmitter acetylcholine and serves as a methyl-group donor in the synthetic reactions for methionine from homocystine and for creatine from guanidoacetic acid. The severity of hyperhomocysteinemia from folate deficiency is amplified by concomitant dietary choline restriction (Kang et al. 1992).

Signs of Deficiency. Choline can be synthesized by most animals in amounts adequate to meet metabolic requirements. However, a number of other dietary, environmental, and physiological factors can increase the metabolic demand for choline beyond the synthetic capacity of the animal, resulting in a deficiency that may be characterized principally by effects on lipid metabolism, liver function, and neurologic functions. Signs attributable to choline deficiency in ruminants are restricted to those with heavy growth or lactational demands (McDowell 1989i). Neurologic and respiratory difficulties have been observed in young calves fed a synthetic milk replacer with inadequate choline (McDowell 1989i). Feed efficiency and rate of gain improved in feedlot steers fed supplemental choline (Swingle and Dyer 1970), and feed intake and milk fat percentage were increased following choline supplementation in lactating dairy cows (Erdman et al. 1984). However, supplementation of dairy cow diets with choline-rich feedstuffs can only marginally increase the postruminal passage of choline; rates of rumen degradation of choline from barley, cottonseed meal, fish meal, soybean meal, choline stearate, and choline chloride were all greater than about 80% (Sharma and Erdman 1989). When fed a choline product, however, lactating dairy cows responded with a significant increase in daily milk production, though no effect was observed on milk fat (Erdman and Sharma 1991). Choline deficiency in pigs is characterized by reduced growth rate, poor conformation, incoordination, joint rigidity, reproductive problems, and hepatic lipidosis (Blair and Newsome 1985). A characteristic "spraddled leg" conformation occurs in growing piglets (McDowell 1989i). Choline deficiency in puppies and kittens has been characterized by decreased growth and hepatic lipidosis (NRC 1985, 1986; McDowell 1989i). Choline deficiency in poultry causes growth retardation, perosis, fatty liver, and decreased egg production (McDowell 1989i).

Assessment of Status. Criteria used to evaluate choline status have included biological response to supplementation and measurement of plasma or tissue

CH_3
$HC \cdot N^{+} - CH_2 - CH_2OH$
CH_3

Choline

FIG. 36.9

concentrations of choline, acetylcholine, or phosphatidylcholine. Deficiency results in reduced acetylcholine levels in the brain and decreased phosphatidylcholine/phosphatidylethanolamine ratios in the liver.

Dietary Requirements, Indications, and Use

INTRINSIC FACTORS. In adult ruminants and horses, choline synthesis by gastrointestinal microflora is adequate under resting conditions, but as is the case for other species, requirements increase with stress, growth, gestation, or lactation, thereby necessitating supplementation. The more rapid the rate of growth or the greater the level of production, the greater the need for choline. Males appear to be more sensitive to choline deficiency than females, glucocorticoids appear to be capable of ameliorating signs of choline deficiency, and growth hormone increases choline requirements independent of its effects on growth (McDowell 1989i).

EXTRINSIC FACTORS. Dietary deficiencies of other nutrients affecting methyl-group transfer, such as methionine, folacin, or vitamin B_{12}, can increase choline requirements (McDowell 1989i). Choline, in turn, can spare dietary methionine requirements if adequate sulfate is also provided. Increased dietary fat or protein levels can increase the requirement for choline, while oral antibiotics appear to decrease the requirement, owing to reduced degradation by intestinal microflora. Stress may increase choline requirements, and gastrointestinal diseases may impair lipid digestion and subsequent lecithin or choline absorption.

Preparations. Choline is available commercially as choline chloride, choline bitartrate, or choline dihydrogen citrate, produced by chemical synthesis. Injectable and oral preparations may be obtained singly or as part of a multivitamin preparation. Single large doses may be given as parenteral injections in the prophylaxis or therapeusis of specific conditions or diseases which increase choline requirements. Large doses may also be included in drinking water or parenteral fluid preparations in the resuscitation of diseased or convalescent animals.

Toxicity. The maximum tolerable doses for choline vary with route of administration and among species. In mice, the LD_{50} for a single oral dose of choline chloride is 3900 mg/kg body weight, whereas it is only 53 mg/kg body weight when administered intravenously. The maximum tolerable level for rats is between 3.4 and 6.1 g/kg body weight when administered orally in a single dose. Choline supplementation up to 1000 ppm of the diet appears to improve growth in swine, whereas levels of 2000 or 4000 ppm reduced growth and feed efficiency (Southern et al. 1986). Dogs and poultry appear to be quite sensitive to choline; dogs develop an anemia when fed levels only 3 times the recommended dietary requirement, while growth depression was noted in broilers fed only twice the dietary requirement (NRC 1987).

VITAMIN C

Chemical Structure. Vitamin C activity is attributed to the *l*-isomer of ascorbic acid (reduced) and dehydroascorbic acid (oxidized) (Fig. 36.10). The reversible oxidation and reduction of these two forms is the basis for vitamin C's role as an antioxidant in biological systems (McDowell 1989j).

Sources and Chemical Properties. Fruits and vegetables are the principal natural sources of vitamin C, although some animal by-products, including fish meal and organs like liver and kidney, have activity comparable to some fruits and grains. The sodium salt of ascorbic acid is highly water soluble, and stabilized crystalline forms with ethylcellulose microcoating are available. It is highly susceptible to oxidative damage, which is accelerated by transition metal elements. Physicochemical methods for the determination of vitamin C content in biological specimens are quantitative and include colorimetric spectroscopy, gas chromatography, and HPLC. Vitamin C content is expressed as milligrams (mg) per unit dry matter of the substance assayed.

Biological Characteristics. Vitamin C is absorbed by sodium-dependent active transport processes in the small intestine similar to those for monosaccharides. Vitamin C absorbed from the diet, as well as that produced endogenously in those species capable of synthesis, is distributed widely in tissues. It accumulates in highest concentrations in the pituitary and adrenal glands and increases in concentration in areas of active fibroplasia, such as around wounds undergoing healing. Vitamin C is excreted in the urine as ascorbic acid itself or is metabolized first to oxalic acid when nutritional requirements are exceeded.

METABOLIC FUNCTIONS. Vitamin C is not incorporated into any coenzymes, but is required for many biochemical reactions, particularly those of oxidation. Enzymatic hydroxylation of proline and lysine during the synthesis of collagen requires ascorbic acid, probably to protect the hydroxylase enzymes from oxidative damage by ferrous ions and mixed disulfides. It is

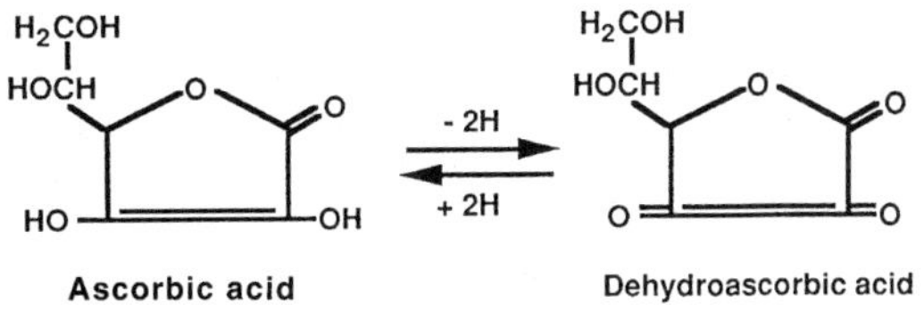

Ascorbic acid ⇌ (−2H / +2H) Dehydroascorbic acid

FIG. 36.10

likely that ascorbic acid plays an important role in other oxidative reactions, including those catalyzed by ascorbic acid oxidase, cytochrome oxidase, and peroxidase. Carnitine synthesis from lysine and methionine requires ferrous ion and ascorbic acid-dependent hydroxylases, and corticosteroid synthesis by the adrenal glands is dependent on ascorbic acid-related hydroxylations. The role of dietary ascorbic acid in promoting mineral absorption from the gut has received closer attention for its facilitation of supplemental calcium and nonheme iron uptake in adult women.

Vitamin C can inhibit the formation of nitrosamines from nitrates and, through its free radical-scavenging activity, probably plays additional roles in preventing chemical carcinogenesis induced by a number of xenobiotics that undergo activation by mixed-function oxidases. Although reports are conflicting, ascorbic acid appears to stimulate both T and B lymphocyte functions, as well as enhancing chemotactic, phagocytic, and bactericidal functions of neutrophils and macrophages (Leibovitz and Siegel 1980). It has also been reported to have direct antiviral properties and to stimulate interferon production by virus-infected cells in culture (Leibovitz and Siegel 1980). In one report, calves supplemented daily from 3 days through 4 weeks of age with 10 g of vitamin C/kg of dry milk replacer expressed lower levels of neutrophil-mediated phagocytosis and antibody-dependent cellular cytotoxicity than unsupplemented calves (Eicher-Pruiett et al. 1992). Concurrent dietary supplementation with 57 international units (IU) of vitamin E/kg of dry milk replacer reversed this effect and enhanced mitogen-induced lymphocyte proliferation (Eicher-Pruiett et al. 1992). Supplementation with vitamin C (1 g daily) also significantly enhances cytokine (tumor necrosis factor-α, interleukin-1β, interleukin-6) production by peripheral blood mononuclear cells in humans (Jeng et al. 1996).

Signs of Deficiency. Vitamin C deficiency is best known for the alterations in basement membrane collagen production, capillary fragility, periodontal disease, and bone deformities that characterize scurvy. Although ruminants can synthesize vitamin C, scurvy in growing calves fed insufficient milk has been characterized by oral mucosal lesions, dermatitis, hair loss, and general unthriftiness (McDowell 1989j). Some studies have suggested that young calves cannot synthesize adequate ascorbic acid and that resistance to infectious disease may be highly responsive to vitamin C supplementation (McDowell 1989j). Confinement housing of 1- to 2-month-old dairy calves has been shown to significantly decrease plasma ascorbic acid levels, resting IgG levels, and antibody titers following keyhole limpet hemocyanin challenge (Cummins and Brunner 1991). Piglets can synthesize ascorbic acid within the first week of life, and supplemental dietary vitamin C had no effect on bone metabolism, fecal rotavirus shedding, hematologic, or serum biochemical parameters (Mahan and Saif 1983); dietary supplementation also had no effect on humoral immunity or growth performance in cold-stressed weanling pigs (Kornegay et al. 1986). Periparturient supplementation of gilts with additional vitamin C similarly had no effect on gestational or lactational performance (Yen and Pond 1983). Under conditions of environmental temperature stress, rapid growth, or infectious disease, poultry appear to respond favorably to supplemental dietary vitamin C (McDowell 1989j). Guinea pigs are incapable of synthesizing ascorbic acid and, when fed a deficient diet, develop signs of scurvy, including reduced feed intake, weight loss, widespread hemorrhaging, anemia, gingivitis, and abnormal bone growth (McDowell 1989j). In human beings, vitamin C deficiency, as assessed by a low plasma ascorbic acid concentration, has been shown to be an independent risk factor for coronary artery disease (Nyyssonen et al. 1997), presumably due to increased low-density lipoprotein oxidation and subsequent atherosclerotic vascular damage (Kristenson et al. 1997). Vitamin C requirements in other species have not been extensively studied, owing to their presumed capability for adequate endogenous synthesis.

Assessment of Status. Criteria used to evaluate vitamin C status have included biological response to supplementation, analysis of serum, leukocyte, or liver ascorbic acid content, and measurement of urinary excretion following a loading test.

Dietary Requirements, Indications, and Use. Intrinsic differences in the ability to synthesize ascorbic acid de novo account for species or age differences in dietary requirement. Production, performance, environmental, and disease stresses can all increase the requirement for vitamin C. An all-inclusive example of increased needs is that of the neonatal calf, who must rely on endogenous stores and minimal intake in milk until endogenous synthesis begins. Environmental stress and exposure to infectious agents under these conditions of limited supply and rapid growth can increase the need for supplementation significantly. Other dietary factors, including polyunsaturated fat content, vitamins E and A, selenium, sulfur-containing amino acids, and transition metals, may influence oxidative susceptibility and vitamin C requirements as well.

Preparations. Vitamin C is available as free *l*-ascorbic acid and as sodium ascorbate in crystalline and ethylcellulose microencapsulated forms. Injectable and oral preparations may be obtained singly or as part of a multivitamin preparation. Single large doses may be given as parenteral injections in the prophylaxis or therapeusis of specific conditions or diseases which increase vitamin C requirements. Large doses may also be included in drinking water or parenteral fluid preparations in the resuscitation of diseased or convalescent animals. Because ascorbic acid is unstable when exposed to oxygen or transition elements, protection can be achieved by coating the vitamin with 2.5% ethylcellulose or by bonding it with Mg and P as magnesium-L-ascorbyl-2-phosphate (Mahan et al. 1994).

Toxicity. Although ascorbic acid is generally nontoxic, even at the supraphysiological levels promoted for improved disease resistance, signs of toxicity have been noted in some animal models (NRC 1987). These have included hyperoxaluria (and predisposition to oxalate urolithiasis), excessive absorption of iron, diarrhea, allergic responses, destruction of vitamin B_{12}, and interference with the hepatic mixed-function oxidase systems (NRC 1987). However, intakes as high as 3.3 g/kg of feed for swine have produced no adverse effects. Dogs given up to 9 g per day and horses given up to 10 g per day intravenously experienced no adverse effects. For most animals, upper safe limits are assumed to be perhaps 1000 times the nutritional requirements (NRC 1987).

REFERENCES

Bai, S. C., Sampson, D. A., Morris, J. G., Rogers, Q. R. 1991. The level of dietary protein affects the vitamin B6 requirement of cats. J Nutr 121:1054-1061.

Blair, R., Newsome, F. 1985. Involvement of water-soluble vitamins in diseases of swine. J Anim Sci 60:1508-1517.

Boushey, C. J., Beresford, A. A., Omenn, G. S., Motulsky, A. G. 1995. A quantitative assessment of plasma homocysteine as a risk factor for vascular disease. J Am Med Assoc 274:1049-1057.

Bratton, G. R., Zmudki, J., Kincaid, N., Joyce, J. 1981. Thiamin treatment of lead poisoning in ruminants. Modern Vet Pract 62:441-446.

Brent, B. E., Bartley, E. E. 1984. Thiamin and niacin in the rumen. J Anim Sci 59:813-822.

Campbell, J. M., Murphy, M. R., Christensen, R. A., Overton, T. R. 1994. Kinetics of niacin supplements in lactating dairy cows. J Dairy Sci 77:566-575.

Campbell, N. R. C. 1996. How safe are folic acid supplements? Arch Int Med 156:1638-1644.

Cervantes, A., Smith, T. R., Young, J. W. 1996. Effects of nicotinamide on milk composition and production in dairy cows fed supplemental fat. J Dairy Sci 79:105-113.

Clarke, R., Daly, L., Robinson, K., Naughten, E., Cahalane, S., Fowler, B., Graham, I. 1991. Hyperhomocysteinemia: an independent risk factor for vascular disease. New Engl J Med 324:1149-1155.

Cline, J. L., Odle, J., Easter, R. A. 1996. The riboflavin requirement of adult dogs at maintenance is greater than previous estimates. J Nutr 126:984-988.

Comben, N., Clark, R. J., Sutherland, D. J. B. 1984. Clinical observations on the response of equine hoof defects to dietary supplementation with biotin. Vet Record 15:642-645.

Croom, W. J., Bauman, D. E., Davis, C. L. 1981. Methylmalonic acid in low-fat milk syndrome. J Dairy Sci 64:649-654.

Cummins, K. A., Brunner, C. J. 1991. Effect of calf housing on plasma ascorbate and endocrine and immune function. J Dairy Sci 74:1582-1588.

Cunha, T. J. 1991. In Horse Feeding and Nutrition. 2nd ed. New York: Academic Press. a: pp. 64-66; b: pp. 66-67; c: pp. 69-70; d: pp. 72-73; e: pp. 70-71; f: pp. 76-79; g: pp. 74-76; h: pp. 67-69; i: pp. 73-74; j: pp. 62-64.

Daugherty, M. S., Galyean, M. L., Hallford, D. M., Hageman, J. H. 1986. Vitamin B_{12} and monensin effects on performance, liver and serum vitamin B_{12} concentrations, and activity of propionate metabolizing hepatic enzymes in feedlot lambs. J Anim Sci 62:452-463.

Dubeski, P. L., Owens, F. N., Song, W. O., Coburn, S. P., Mahuren, J. D. 1996a. Effects of B vitamin injections on plasma B vitamin concentrations of feed-restricted beef calves infected with bovine herpesvirus-1. J Anim Sci 74:1358-1366.

Dubeski, P. L., d'Offay, J. M., Owens, F. N., Gill, D. R. 1996b. Effects of B vitamin injection on bovine herpesvirus-1 infection and immunity in feed-restricted beef calves. J Anim Sci 74:1367-1374.

Dufva, G. S., Bartley, E. E., Nagaraja, T. G., Dayton, A. D., Frey, R. A. 1984. Effect of dietary niacin supplementation on phlorizin and 1,3-butanediol-induced ketonemia and hypoglycemia in steers. Am J Vet Res 45:1835-1837.

Dumoulin, P. G., Girard, C. L., Matte, J. J., St.-Laurent, C. J. 1991. Effects of a parenteral supplement of folic acid and its interaction with level of feed intake on hepatic tissues and growth performance of young dairy heifers. J Anim Sci 69:1657-1666.

Edwin, E. E., Markson L. M., Jackman, R. 1982. The aetiology of cerebrocortical necrosis: the role of thiamine deficiency and of deltapyrrolinium. Brit Vet J 138:337-349.

Eicher-Pruiett, S. D., Morrill, J. L., Blecha, F., Higgins, J. J., Anderson, N. V., Reddy, P. G. 1992. Neutrophil and lymphocyte response to supplementation with vitamins C and E in young calves. J Dairy Sci 75:1635-1642.

Elliot, J. M., Barton, E. P., Williams, J. A. 1979. Milk fat as related to vitamin B_{12} status. J Dairy Sci 62:642-645.

Erdman, R. A., Sharma, B. K. 1991. Effect of dietary choline in lactating dairy cows. J Dairy Sci 74:1641-1647.

Erdman, R. A., Sharmer, R. D., Vandersall, J. H. 1984. Dietary choline for the lactating cow: possible effects on milk synthesis. J Dairy Sci 67:410-415.

Fisher, G. E. J., MacPherson, A. 1991. Effect of cobalt deficiency in the pregnant ewe on reproductive performance and lamb viability. Res Vet Sci 50:319-327.

Frank, G. R., Bahr, J. M., Easter, R. A. 1984. Riboflavin requirement of gestating swine. J Anim Sci 59:1567-1572.

———. 1988. Riboflavin requirement of lactating swine. J Anim Sci 66:47-52.

Fronk, T. J., Schultz, L. H. 1979. Oral nicotinic acid as a treatment for ketosis. J Dairy Sci 62:1804-1807.

Fyfe, J. C., Giger, U., Hall, C. A., Jezyk, P. F., Klumpp, S. A., Levine, J. S., Patterson, D. F. 1991a. Inherited selective intestinal cobalamin malabsorption and cobalamin deficiency in dogs. Pediatric Res 29:24-31.

Fyfe, J. C., Jezyk, P. F., Giger, U., Patterson, D. F. 1989. Inherited selective malabsorption of vitamin B_{12} in giant schnauzers. J Amer Anim Hosp Assoc 25:533-539.

Fyfe, J. C., Ramanujam, K. S., Ramaswamy, K., Patterson, D. F., Settharam, B. 1991b. Defective brush-border expression of intrinsic factor-cobalamin receptor in canine inherited cobalamin malabsorption. J Biol Chem 266:4489-4494.

Gershoff, S. N., Faragalla, F. F., Nelson, D. A., Andrus, S. B. 1959. Vitamin B6 deficiency and oxalate nephrocalcinosis in the cat. Am J Med 27:72-80.

Girard, C. L., Matte, J. J., Tremblay, G. F. 1989. Serum folates in gestating and lactating dairy cows. J Dairy Sci 72:3240-3246.

———. 1995. Gestation and lactation of dairy cows: a role for folic acid? J Dairy Sci 78:404-411.

Gould, D. H., McAllister, M. M., Savage, J. C., Hamar, D. W. 1991. High sulfide concentrations in rumen fluid associated with nutritionally induced polioencephalomalacia in calves. Am J Vet Res 52:1164-1169.

Graham, I. M., Daly, L. E., Refsum, H. M., Robinson, K., Brattstrom, L. E., Ueland, P. M., Palma-Reis, R. J., Boers, G. H. J., Sheahan, R. G., et al. 1997. Plasma homocysteine as a risk factor for vascular disease. J Am Med Assoc 277:1775-1781.

Gries, C. L., Scott, M. L. 1972. The pathology of thiamin, riboflavin, pantothenic acid, and niacin deficiencies in the chick. J Nutr 102:1269-1285.

Haven, T. R., Caldwell, D. R., Jensen, R. 1983. Role of predominant rumen bacteria in the cause of polioencephalomalacia (cerebrocortical necrosis) in cattle. Am J Vet Res 44:1451-1455.

Hogue, D. E., Elliot, J. M. 1964. Effect of propionate on the dietary vitamin B_{12}, biotin, and folic acid requirement of the rat. J Nutr 83:171-175.

Jeng, K. C., Yang, C. S., Siu, W. Y., Tsai, Y. S., Liao, W. J., Kuo, J. S. 1996. Supplementation with vitamins C and E enhances cytokine production by peripheral blood mononuclear cells in healthy adults. Am J Clin Nutr 64:960-965.

Kang, S. S., Wong, P. W. K., Malinow, M. R. 1992. Hyperhomocysteinemia as a risk factor for occlusive vascular disease. Ann Rev Nutr 12:279-298.

Keagy, P. M., Oace, S. M. 1984. Folic acid utilization from high fiber diets in rats. J Nutr 114:1252-1259.

Kornegay, E. T., Meldrum, J. B., Schurig, G., Lindemann, M. D., Gwazdauskas, F. C. 1986. Lack of influence of nursery temperature on the response of weanling pigs to supplemental vitamins C and E. J Anim Sci 63:484-491.

Kristenson, M., Zieden, B., Kucinskiene, Z., Elinder, L. S., Bergdahl, B., Elwing, B., Abaravicius, A., Razinkoviene, L., Calkauskas, H., Olsson, A. G. 1997. Antioxidant state and mortality from coronary heart disease in Lithuanian and Swedish men: concomitant cross sectional study of men aged 50. Brit Med J 314:629-633.

Kuemmerle, S. C., Boltinghouse, G. L., Delby, S. M., Lane, T. L., Simondsen, R. P. 1992. Automated assay of vitamin B_{12} by the Abbott IMx analyzer. Clin Chem 38:2073-2077.

Leibovitz, B., Siegel, B. V. 1980. Ascorbic acid and the immune response. Adv Expt Med Biol 135:1-25.

Lewis, L. D., Morris, M. L., Hand, M. S. 1987. In Small Animal Clinical Nutrition III, chapter 4. Topeka: Mark Morris Associates.

Lindemann, M. D. 1993. Supplemental folic acid: a requirement for optimizing swine reproduction. J Anim Sci 71:239-246.

Mahan, D. C., Lepine, A. J., Dabrowski, K. 1994. Efficacy of magnesium-L-ascorbyl-2-phosphate as a vitamin C source for weanling and growing-finishing swine. J Anim Sci 72:2354-2361.

Mahan, D. C., Saif, L. J. 1983. Efficacy of vitamin C supplementation for weanling swine. J Anim Sci 56:631-639.

McDowell, L. R. 1989. In Vitamins in Animal Nutrition: Comparative Aspects to Human Nutrition. New York: Academic Press. a: chapter 6, pp. 155-182; b: chapter 7, pp. 183-209; c: chapter 8, pp. 210-235; d: chapter 9, pp. 236-255; e: chapter 10, pp. 256-274; f: chapter 11, pp. 275-297; g: chapter 12, pp. 298-322; h: chapter 13, pp. 313-346; i: chapter 14, pp. 347-364; j: chapter 15, pp. 365-387.

Meydami, S. N., Ribaya-Mercado, J. D., Russell, R. M., Shyoun, N., Morrow, F. D., Gershoff, S. N. 1991. Vitamin B_6 deficiency impairs interleukin-2 production and lymphocyte proliferation in elderly adults. Am J Clin Nutr 53:1275-1280.

Miller, B. L., Meiske, J. C., Goodrich, R. D. 1986a. Effects of grain source and concentrate level on B-vitamin production and absorption in steers. J Anim Sci 62:473-483.

———. 1986b. Effects of dietary additives on B-vitamin production and absorption in steers. J Anim Sci 62:484-496.

NRC. 1982. United States—Canadian Tables of Feed Composition. 3rd ed. Washington, DC: National Academy of Sciences—National Research Council.

———. 1984. Nutrient Requirements of Domestic Animals: Nutrient Requirements of Poultry. 8th ed. Washington, DC: National Academy of Sciences—National Research Council.

———. 1985. Nutritional Requirements of Domestic Animals: Nutrient Requirements of Dogs. 2nd ed. Washington DC: National Academy of Sciences—National Research Council.

———. 1986. Nutritional Requirements of Domestic Animals: Nutrient Requirements of Cats. Rev. ed. Washington, DC: National Academy of Sciences—National Research Council.

———. 1987. Vitamin Tolerance of Animals. Washington, DC: National Academy of Sciences—National Research Council.

Nyyssonen, K., Parviainen, M. T., Salonen, R., Tuomilehto, J., Salonen, J. T. 1997. Vitamin C deficiency and risk of myocardial infarction: prospective population study of men from eastern Finland. Brit Med J 314:634-638.

Oriot, D., Wood, C., Gottesman, R., Huault, G. 1991. Severe lactic acidosis related to acute thiamine deficiency. J Parent Entr Nutr 15:105-109.

Peters, J. P., Elliot, J. M. 1983. Effect of vitamin B_{12} status on performance of the lactating ewe and gluconeogenesis from propionate. J Dairy Sci 66:1917-1925.

Phillips, W. E. J., Mills, J. H. L., Charbonneau, S. M., Tryphonas, L., Hatina, G. V., Zawidzka, Z., Bryce, F. R., Munro, I. C. 1978. Subacute toxicity of pyridoxine hydrochloride in the beagle dog. Toxicol Appl Pharmacol 44:323-332.

Rasmussen, K., Moller, J., Lyngbak, M., Pedersen, A. M. H., Dybkjaer, L. 1996. Age- and gender-specific reference intervals for total homocysteine and methylmalonic acid in plasma before and after vitamin supplementation. Clin Chem 42:630-636.

Read, D. H., Harrington, D. D. 1982. Experimentally induced thiamine deficiency in beagle dogs: clinical observations. Am J Vet Res 42:984-991.

———. 1983. Experimentally induced thiamine deficiency in beagle dogs: clinicopathologic findings. Am J Vet Res 43:1258-1267.

———. 1986. Experimentally induced thiamine deficiency in beagle dogs: pathologic changes of the central nervous system. Am J Vet Res 47:2281-2289.

Riddell, D. O., Bartley, E. E., Dayton, A. D. 1980. Effect of nicotinic acid on rumen fermentation in vitro and in vivo. J Dairy Sci 63:1429-1436.

———. 1981. Effect of nicotinic acid on microbial protein synthesis in vitro and on dairy cattle growth and milk production. J Dairy Sci 64:782-791.

Rutgers, H. C., Batt, R. M., Elwood, C. M., Lamport, A. 1995. Small intestinal bacterial overgrowth in dogs with chronic intestinal disease. J Am Vet Med Assoc 206:187-193.

Sager, R. L., Hamar, D. W., Gould, D. H. 1990. Clinical and biochemical alterations in calves with nutritionally-induced polioencephalomalacia. Am J Vet Res 51:1969-1974.

Sharma, B. K., Erdman, R. A. 1989. In vitro degradation of choline from selected feedstuffs and choline supplements. J Dairy Sci 72:2772-2776.

Simpson, K. W., Morton, D. B., Batt, R. M. 1989. Effect of exocrine pancreatic insufficiency on cobalamin absorption in dogs. Am J Vet Res 50:1233-1236.

Somogyi, J. C. 1973. Toxicants Occurring Naturally in Foods. 2nd ed. Washington, DC: National Academy of Sciences.
Southern, L. L., Brown, D. R., Werner, D. D., Fox, M. C. 1986. Excess supplemental choline for swine. J Anim Sci 62:992-996.
Studdert, V. P., Labuc, R. H. 1991. Thiamin deficiency in cats and dogs associated with feeding meat preserved with sulphur dioxide. Aust Vet J 68:54-57.
Swingle, R. S., Dyer, I. A. 1970. Effects of choline on rumen microbial metabolism. J Anim Sci 31:404-408.
Ueland, P. M., Refsum, H. 1989. Plasma homocysteine, a risk factor for vascular disease: plasma levels in health, disease, and drug therapy. J Lab Clin Med 114:473-501.
Vaden, S. L., Wood, P. A., Ledley, F. D., Cornwell, P. E., Miller, R. T., Page, R. 1992. Cobalamin deficiency associated with methylmalonic acidemia in a cat. J Am Vet Med Assoc 200:1101-1103.
van der Weide, J., Homan, H. C., Cozijnsen-van Rheenen, E., Vivie-Kipp, Y., Poortman, J., Kraaijenhagen, R. J. 1992. Nonisotopic binding assay for measuring vitamin B_{12} and folate in serum. Clin Chem 38:766-768.
Watanabe, T., Endo, A. 1991. Biotin deficiency per se is teratogenic in mice. J Nutr 121:101-104.
Wehr, N. B., Adair, J., Oldfield, J. E. 1980. Biotin deficiency in mink fed spray-dried eggs. J Anim Sci 50:877-885.
Williams, D. A. 1996. The pancreas. In W. G. Guilford, S. A. Center, D. R. Strombeck, D. A. Williams, and D. J. Meyer, eds., Small Animal Gastroenterology, 3rd ed., pp.367-380.
Wolfson, M., Cohen, A. H., Kopple, J. D. 1991. Vitamin B_6 deficiency and renal function and structure in chronically uremic rats. Am J Clin Nutr 53:935-942.
Yen, J. T., Pond, W. G. 1983. Response of swine to periparturient vitamin C supplementation. J Anim Sci 56:621-624.

37 CALCIUM, PHOSPHORUS, AND OTHER MACROELEMENTS

MARTIN J. FETTMAN

Calcium and Phosphorus
Sodium and Chloride
Potassium
Magnesium
Sulfur

CALCIUM AND PHOSPHORUS

Source and Occurrence. Calcium (Ca) and phosphorus (P) are widely distributed in soil, and in general, hays contain more Ca than grains, and legume hays contain more than grass hays (Minson 1990a,b; NRC 1982). The P content of grains is higher than that of forages, although the same factors affecting forage Ca content seem to affect P concentrations as well. The true availability of Ca and P from plant materials depends on their chemical forms. Much of the P present is often in the form of phytic acid (inositol hexaphosphate), which not only reduces its availability but also binds cations, including Ca, magnesium, and zinc, thereby forming insoluble and unavailable complexes. Commercial sources of Ca and P include a wide variety of salts such as dicalcium phosphate, monocalcium phosphate, calcium carbonate (limestone), and calcium chloride, as well as animal by-products like bonemeal and oyster shell.

Chemical Forms and Distribution. Most of the Ca (approximately 98%) and most of the P (approximately 85%) in the body is present in bone. The remaining small amounts play critical roles in a variety of metabolic functions throughout all tissues of the body. A pH-dependent equilibrium exists between ionized Ca, inorganic phosphate ions, and calcium phosphate salts in the body fluids. In the blood plasma, approximately 45% of the Ca is in the free and ionized form, about 5% exists in salts with phosphate and other anions, and the remaining 50% is bound to anionic sites on plasma proteins. The degree of Ca binding to these proteins is influenced by pH, which likewise affects the disposition of Ca in the gastrointestinal (GI) tract, kidneys, and other organs. Much of the extra-osseous P occurs in the form of phosphate esters of organic acid intermediates in metabolism and as the "high-energy" phosphate bonds of adenosine triphosphate (ATP), guanosine triphosphate (GTP), etc.

Several methods are available for the determination of the Ca and P content in biological specimens. Ashed preparations or acid extracts of tissues may be analyzed by atomic absorption spectroscopy for Ca and by colorimetric reactions for P. Ca in blood and urine may be determined by atomic absorption or flame emission spectroscopy and by fluorescent or visible light spectrophotometry of chromogenic complexes, such as Ca-cresolphthalein (Welch et al. 1990; Farrell 1987a). Non-protein-bound (ultrafiltrable) Ca may be determined by any of these methods following mechanical or centrifugal filtration through an ultrafilter. Because ionized Ca is the physiologically active form and may vary independently of total Ca concentrations in biological fluids like blood, its direct and rapid measurement by ion-specific electrode potentiometry has found increasing clinical utility (Toffaletti 1987). P in blood and urine may be analyzed by ultraviolet or visible light spectrophotometry of chromogenic complexes formed directly, such as phosphomolybdate, or indirectly, following coupled enzymatic reactions with purine nucleoside phosphorylase, xanthine oxidase, and peroxidase (Farrell 1987b).

Biological Characteristics. As described in Chap. 35, one may consider Ca and P metabolism to be controlled by a triad of hormones: parathyroid hormone (PTH), which has both direct effects on bone and kidney and indirect effects through its regulation of vitamin D activation; thyrocalcitonin (TCT), which has direct effects on bone and kidney; and calcitriol (1,25-$(OH)_2$ vitamin D), which has direct effects on bone, kidney, and intestine, as well as indirect effects through its reciprocal regulation of PTH release (Fig. 37.1). Ingested Ca and P are predominantly absorbed in the small intestine by both active and passive processes. Intestinal Ca and P uptake is promoted by calcitriol, which is particularly important for the synthesis of calcium-binding proteins (CaBP) that facilitate Ca absorption and transfer to the blood. In the kidneys, Ca reabsorption from the glomerular filtrate is dependent on positive influences by both PTH and calcitriol. In the proximal nephron, PTH inhibits carbonic anhydrase activity; decreases sodium, bicarbonate, and water absorption; and thereby decreases the concentration gradients necessary for Ca and P reabsorption. Because P is not actively secreted by the nephron, this is the only means of increasing its excretion into

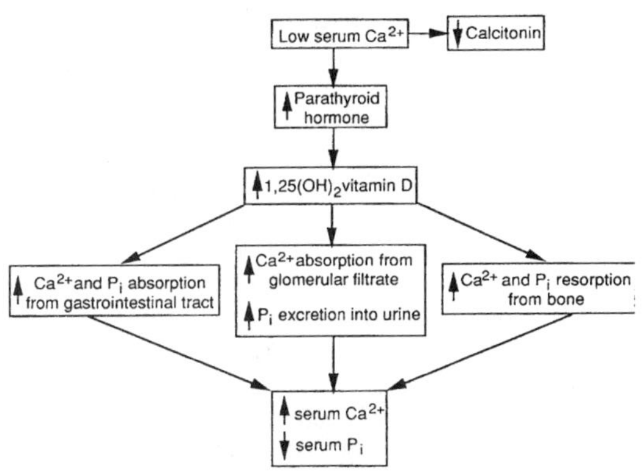

FIG. 37.1—Homeostatic response to hypocalcemia. (Adapted from Stewart and Broadus 1987.)

the urine. Proximal tubular loss of Ca is more than compensated for by PTH-stimulated increases in active Ca transport across the loop of Henle in a cyclic AMP-dependent process, and by calcitriol-dependent reuptake of Ca by the distal nephron in CaBP-mediated processes. In the bones, calcitriol facilitates both Ca and P resorption and deposition, the former being stimulated by PTH and the latter by TCT. Ionized Ca levels in the blood determine the release of PTH and TCT; PTH and blood inorganic phosphate concentrations exert reciprocal control over the rate of 25-OH vitamin D activation to calcitriol; and calcitriol, in turn modulates PTH release and affects interorgan Ca and P kinetics.

EFFECTS OF ACID-BASE METABOLISM. Because pH exerts an important influence on Ca binding to proteins and precipitation of salts of Ca and P, alterations in systemic acid-base metabolism can have profound effects on the disposition of these minerals in the body (Fredeen et al. 1988a,b). Changes in acid-base status also may have profound effects on the activity of PTH and calcitriol, which in turn may affect Ca and P balance. In general, acidosis increases the ionization of Ca, thereby increasing the resorption of Ca and P from bone, reducing mineral deposition in eggshells, and augmenting the proportion of ionized Ca in the blood (Peoples 1988). Conversely, alkalosis decreases Ca ionization and promotes bone deposition and eggshell formation. Metabolic acidosis has also been shown to alter bone remodeling through cellular effects. Decreased bicarbonate concentrations reduce osteoblast activity and stimulate osteoclast activity, in addition to the physicochemical effects noted above (Krieger et al. 1992; Bushinsky 1995). There is controversy in the literature regarding the relative "potency" of respiratory versus metabolic acidosis in altering bone mineral deposition (Sprague et al. 1994; Arnett et al. 1994). While acidosis promotes PTH's effects on bone, it apparently inhibits its renal tubular effects and directly suppresses the activity of renal 1α-hydroxylase, thereby inhibiting calcitriol production (Beck et al. 1986; Reddy et al. 1982). The net result is decreased GI absorption of Ca, increased bone mineral resorption, and increased urinary Ca excretion. This has resulted in negative Ca balance in cats (Ching et al. 1989), impaired growth in pigs (Golz and Crenshaw 1991), and bone demineralization in dogs (Burnell and Teubner 1971). The effect of acidification may be employed positively in the prevention of parturient paresis in lactating cows (see below), whereas purposeful alkalinization may be used to reverse demineralization in uremia and to promote eggshell quality in poultry.

It has been hypothesized that the usual daily load of acid produced through metabolism might have similar effects on calcium metabolism and bone turnover, even in the absence of overt disturbances in acid-base balance. In humans, daily oral intake of $KHCO_3$ (but not $NaHCO_3$) to neutralize endogenous acid production significantly improves calcium balance, reduces bone resorption, and increases bone formation in healthy adult males (Lemann et al. 1989) and in postmenopausal females (Sebastian et al. 1994).

METABOLIC FUNCTIONS

BONE DEVELOPMENT. Bone mineralization occurs through the process of calcification of an organic matrix produced by chondroblasts (endochondral ossification) or osteoblasts (intramembranous bone formation), and bone may subsequently be remodeled or serve as a source of Ca and P for the body through the additional actions of osteoclasts and osteocytes. Dietary Ca and P intake must be adequate and in the appropriate relative ratio to support bone mineralization. A deficiency of Ca or P or an otherwise adequate Ca intake in conjunction with an excess of dietary P can result in nutritional secondary hyperparathyroidism with the development of rickets in deficient growing animals and of osteomalacia in deficient adult animals. Conversely, excessive Ca intake over prolonged periods of time can lead to the development of hypercalcitoninism and osteopetrosis (NRC 1980).

NEUROMUSCULAR FUNCTION. Ca has two opposing effects on neural function. It blocks sodium channels in the neuronal membrane, making it less excitable, and it is required for the normal secretion of neurotransmitters like acetylcholine. Thus, hypocalcemia makes membranes more excitable but decreases neurotransmitter secretory capacity. In most species, enough neurotransmitter is released under conditions of hypocalcemia so that because of their enhanced excitability, muscles exhibit increased activity. Signs of hypocalcemia in most species thus include muscle fasciculations, seizures, and tetany, as seen in lactation tetany of horses and in puerperal tetany of dogs. It has been hypothesized that ruminants normally secrete much less neurotransmitter at the myoneural junction, so with hypocalcemia, not enough is released to elicit a response, and flaccid paralysis results. Signs of hypocalcemia in early-lactation cows with "milk fever" thus progress from an early stage of hypersensitivity and tetany to one of weakness and paresis and ultimately paralysis.

Muscle contractions are regulated by the concentration of ionized calcium in the sarcoplasm. Sarcoplasmic reticulum membranes contain an ATP-dependent Ca pump that maintains low concentrations in resting myocytes. Upon stimulation, Ca is rapidly released from the terminal cisternae of the sarcoplasmic reticulum and binds to the troponin component of the actin filaments. Troponin undergoes a conformational change that moves tropomyosin, which in turn uncovers myosin-binding sites on F-actin. This binding promotes the formation of cross-links between the actin and myosin filaments, which causes them to be drawn toward the center of the sarcomere, resulting in shortening of the myocyte and muscular contraction. This basic process is central to contraction of all smooth and striated muscle, including that of the heart. Hypocalcemia can produce significant electrocardiographic changes, arrhythmias, and even cardiac arrest. At a lesser order of magnitude, ciliary and flagellar contractions and movement of intracellular contractile elements such as microtubules and microfilaments similarly require Ca to function. Secretion of peptide hormones is dependent on mobilization and exocytosis of intracellular secretory granules in calcium-dependent processes. Peptide hormone action is also influenced by target cell Ca levels, which in conjunction with cyclic AMP, acts as a second messenger in the regulation of postreceptor functional responses.

Because of its central role in the intermediary metabolism of nutrients required for energy-yielding and synthetic processes, P is also necessary for all of the above actions attributed to Ca in the control of neuromuscular and other bodily functions.

HEMOSTASIS. Both the intrinsic and extrinsic systems of blood coagulation are dependent on Ca as a cofactor for activation of coagulation factors (Dodds 1989). The conversions of vitamin K-dependent factors II, VII, IX, and X to their active forms require ionic Ca. In addition to the procoagulant factors, other regulators of hemostasis depend on Ca, including protein C, which inactivates factors Va and VIIIa, and factor XIII, the fibrin-stabilizing factor which facilitates polymerization of fibrin monomers activated by the common pathway of coagulation.

PRODUCTION. Ca and P are the principal mineral components of milk and obviously account for the structure of eggshells. The dietary Ca and P requirements for lactation and egg production are the greatest of any period of life, and a deficiency of either, or otherwise adequate Ca intake in conjunction with an excess of dietary P, can result in marked decreases in milk production or eggshell quality and production. The concentrations of Ca and P in milk will remain relatively constant through periods of significant dietary deficiency or imbalance, which result rather in decreases in production corresponding to the degree of deficiency.

Signs of Deficiency. The signs of chronic Ca deficiency, or adequate Ca but excessive P intake, relate mostly to skeletal abnormalities associated with the clinical condition of rickets (Call et al. 1986; McDowell 1989; Cunha 1991a). Failure of mineralization leads to abnormal proliferation and degeneration of the cartilage, weak and deformed bones, stiff and enlarged joints, pathologic fractures, and locomotory abnormalities. Accessory signs may include lethargy, anorexia, weight loss, hypogalactia, and neuromuscular dysfunction (Call et al. 1986, 1987; Shupe et al. 1988). In poultry, Ca or P deficiency can lead to decreased eggshell thickness, increased fragility, and reduced hatchability (McDowell 1989). In cattle, dietary P deficiency can produce a periparturient syndrome characterized by hypophosphatemia, intravascular hemolysis, hemoglobinemia, and hemoglobinuria, apparently as a result of impaired ATP production and subsequent effects on erythrocyte viability (Ogawa et al. 1989a,b). There is little evidence that dairy cows exhibit a specific appetite for Ca- or P-containing mineral supplements even after 9-12 weeks of deficient intake (Coppock et al. 1976). It has been suggested that dietary Ca and/or P imbalances may be contributory factors in developmental orthopedic diseases of growing horses (Thatcher 1991). While their association with lesions characteristic of rickets is clear, their relationship to physitis and limb deformities is less so. In one study, mild to moderate physitis and flexure limb deformities were observed in 37 of 42 light horse weanlings studied for over 30 weeks and fed high-forage or high-concentrate rations, irrespective of low (~0.30% dry matter [DM]), medium (~0.70% DM), or high (~1.10%) P content; all lesions resolved before the end of the study (Cymbaluk and Christison 1989). Signs of acute Ca deficiency relate predominantly to neuromuscular and cardiovascular abnormalities, most notable among which are the syndromes of parturient paresis in lactating cows and of puerperal tetany, lactation tetany, or eclampsia in other species, as described earlier.

Assessment of Status. Criteria used to evaluate Ca and P status have included biological response to supplementation, analysis of blood Ca and P concentrations, measurement of urinary and/or fecal excretion of Ca and P (Ching et al. 1989), assessment of bone mineral density by noninvasive densitometric methods (Ching et al. 1990; Cummings et al. 1990), histomorphometric analysis of fluorescent-labeled bone turnover (Ching et al. 1990), and evaluation of indirect indices of bone turnover, including serum alkaline phosphatase activity, serum or urine osteocalcin concentrations, and urinary hydroxyproline excretion (Taylor et al. 1990; Ching et al. 1989; Maenpaa et al. 1988). Because blood Ca and P are maintained by release from bone stores, as well as by GI absorption and urinary excretion, these values may be maintained through long periods of imbalance. Thus, low blood levels may indicate deficiency, but normal values must be interpreted with caution. Because approximately one-half of blood Ca circulates bound to plasma proteins like albumin, hypoproteinemia can result in significant decreases in total serum Ca values, which must then be evaluated by correcting for hypoalbuminemia and/or by directly measuring ionized Ca levels. The former is used routinely in dogs but has not proved useful in cats (Meuten et al. 1982; Flanders et al. 1989). In addition, because blood pH influences the Ca-protein binding relationship, alterations in acid-base status may have profound, sometimes unpredictable effects on measured Ca levels (Kohn and Brooks 1990; Ching et al. 1989; Chew et al. 1989). Reference values for each species should be consulted in the interpretation of each parameter of Ca and P metabolism.

Dietary Requirements, Indications, and Use

INTRINSIC FACTORS. There are significant individual differences in the utilization of Ca and P from different dietary sources, in tolerance to discrepancies from the ideal Ca:P ratio, and in the utilization of Ca and P for nonmaintenance purposes, which in turn affects the requirement for both minerals. Requirements for Ca and P are greatest during pregnancy, lactation, and rapid growth. The potential for deficiency or imbalance during these phases of life is increased in herbivores fed large quantities of concentrates that are poor sources of Ca but very high in P. Growing horses fed such diets and not supplemented with Ca may develop the disorder known as "big head" or "miller's disease," wherein not only is Ca intake low, but excess dietary P depresses Ca availability, resulting in nutritional secondary hyperparathyroidism (Cunha 1991a). Young pigs and calves are likewise sensitive to wide Ca:P ratios (Mahan 1982; Miller et al. 1987). Conversely, older swine, mature horses, and lactating cows appear to be more tolerant to discrepant dietary Ca:P ratios, as long as minimum dietary requirements are met and vitamin D supply is adequate, although high dietary Ca or P fed during the dry period may predispose the latter to parturient paresis (Minson 1990a,b; Barton et al. 1987; Reinhart and Mahan 1986; Belyea et al. 1976).

Other intrinsic factors may affect Ca and P metabolism, including GI diseases, in which absorption is depressed. In chronic renal disease, excessive P is retained owing to decreased rates of glomerular filtration, insufficient 25-OH vitamin D is hydroxylated to calcitriol by the diseased kidneys, and GI and renal handling of Ca is impaired, resulting in renal secondary hyperparathyroidism. Although studies in partially nephrectomized dogs have not conclusively demonstrated a specific renoprotective effect of lower dietary P intake, survival was definitely enhanced, and the effects of restricted P intake were greater than those of restricted dietary protein (Finco et al. 1992).

EXTRINSIC FACTORS. In addition to the adverse effects of dietary P as phytic acid on Ca availability from feeds, oxalic acid may also chelate Ca and make it unavailable for GI absorption (Emanuele and Staples 1990; Ward et al. 1979). In horses, wheat bran phytate phosphorus availability is only about 30%, as opposed to 58% availability from inorganic mineral supplements (Cunha 1991a). Because ruminal microflora produce phytases which are capable of releasing P from phytic acid, natural feed sources of P, including those of phytic acid, are generally better utilized by ruminants than horses, whose large-intestinal flora produce only some phytases, or than simple-stomached animals who cannot utilize such chelated P at all (Morse et al. 1992a). Both a microbial-derived phytase and a recombinant phytase are now commercially available. When these products are fed to growing-finishing pigs, 15-30% of the unavailable P in a corn-soybean meal diet is made available (Cromwell et al. 1995a,b). In other studies, an equation was derived to predict the amount of dietary P released per unit of supplemented phytase (Yi et al. 1996). Phytase supplementation has also been shown to increase bone mineral content and density in a dose-related fashion in pigs fed a pearl millet-soybean meal-based diet (Murry et al. 1997). Some minerals, including magnesium, zinc, and iron, may depress Ca uptake, and high dietary aluminum markedly inhibits dietary P uptake by calves, resulting in reduced feed intake and weight gain and abnormal bone formation (Crowe et al. 1990). On the other hand, certain dietary constituents, like lactose, have been shown to enhance Ca uptake, even when lactose-induced maldigestion adversely affects protein or fat assimilation (Schuette et al. 1991). For cats, the mineral form (acid vs. alkaline salt) of dietary P affects its digestibility and subsequent excretory routes (Fettman et al. 1992), whereas for lactating cows, dietary P concentration has affected the amount and route (urine vs. feces vs. milk) of excretion (Morse et al. 1992b).

Preparations and Therapy. Ca and P are available in combination mineral products, including mono and dibasic calcium phosphate, as well as individually in Ca salts like calcium chloride, calcium carbonate, or calcium hydroxide and in P salts like magnesium, sodium, or potassium phosphates, defluorinated rock phosphates, and as phosphoric acid. Injectable and oral preparations may be obtained singly or as part of a multimineral preparation. Simple, aqueous solutions are indicated for injection, but because of acid-base interactions, large quantities should be used with caution. Likewise, Ca and bicarbonate salts cannot be combined in aqueous solution, where they will precipitate as calcium carbonate. Single large doses of calcium gluconate or calcium borogluconate may be given as intravenous, intramuscular, or subcutaneous injections in the prophylaxis or therapeusis of specific conditions or diseases which increase Ca requirements. A 20-33% calcium borogluconate solution is recommended for the treatment of parturient paresis in cattle and sheep, and a 10% solution is recommended for parturient eclampsia in dogs and cats. Intravenous administration of calcium gluconate to conscious horses at 0.1-0.4 mg/kg/min increases serum total and ionized calcium concentrations and improves cardiac index, stroke index, and cardiac contractility, without adverse effects (Grubb et al. 1996). Rapid administration of such solutions should be avoided, as cardiac arrhythmias and complete heart block can result.

For parturient paresis, the basic dysfunction appears to be an inability of the cow to adequately mobilize bone Ca or increase GI and renal absorption of Ca to meet the suddenly increased demands of early lactation. One prophylactic approach is to reduce dietary Ca intake during the last couple of weeks of the dry period, so that PTH and/or calcitriol responsiveness of these systems is primed in advance. Effective suggested levels for low Ca intake are in the range of 6-8 g/100 kg body weight/day. Following parturition, dietary intake should be increased to meet lactational needs. Because of their higher Ca content, legume hays should not be fed during the dry period, and nonlactating cows should certainly not be fed the same concentrate or mineral supplements as their lactating herdmates. Alternative prophylactic measures have included supplementation with oral or parenteral vitamin D preparations for defined periods of time immediately prior to parturition. Particularly when calcitriol is used and when the exact date of parturition cannot be accurately predicted, there is danger of toxicity due to overdosage. One approach with greater efficacy and reduced risk for adverse effects has been manipulation of dietary cation-anion balance as a means of effecting changes in acid-base metabolism that can modulate bone Ca release. It has further been suggested that dietary Ca concentration, per se, is not a risk factor for parturient paresis, but rather that dietary strong cations, especially K, induce metabolic alkalosis in the prepartum dairy cow and impair Ca homeostasis (Goff and Horst 1997). Dietary acidification during the dry period, through the addition of calcium chloride, calcium sulfate, magnesium chloride, ammonium chloride, or ammonium sulfate, have all been shown to induce a metabolic acidosis of sufficient magnitude to promote mechanisms of Ca mobilization that may protect against the development of parturient hypocalcemia (Block 1984; Oetzel et al. 1991; Tucker et al. 1991). Periparturient prophylactic treatment of dairy cattle with a calcium chloride-containing gel has also been shown to be effective in reducing the incidence of parturient paresis (Oetzel 1996). Administration of one tube (355 g) of the commercial product, containing 54 g of elemental calcium, 12 hours before expected calving, at calving, and 12 and 24 hours after calving completely prevented parturient paresis from occurring.

A new role for dietary P treatment has been reported for the use of sodium hexametaphosphate to inhibit dental calculus formation in dogs. Dental calculus is calcified dental plaque, covered by an unmineralized bacterial layer, and is composed of inorganic material (75-80%) and organic matter (20-25%). The inorganic portion in dogs is predominantly calcium carbonate, with small amounts of calcium phosphate. It was proposed that hexametaphosphate is incorporated into dental plaque and forms soluble calcium complexes so that plaque calcification cannot occur (Stookey et al. 1995). Dietary concentrations of sodium hexametaphosphate as low as 0.59%, added as a surface coating to dry dog food, were shown to reduce calculus formation by as much as 81% over 4 weeks, with no adverse side effects.

Toxicity. Animals appear to have a tolerance for widely differing dietary levels of Ca, as homeostatic mechanisms tend to protect them against excessive absorption. However, the addition of excessive Ca to a diet can produce other mineral deficiencies by interfering with their GI absorption. Among these are P, magnesium, iron, iodine, zinc, and manganese (NRC 1980). In growing pigs, when low dietary P is fed, Ca:P ratios above 1.3:1 resulted in decreased growth and impaired bone development (Reinhart and Mahan 1986). In addition, the form of Ca added to the diet may be important: addition of calcium chloride to the diet of growing pigs at a level of 4% DM resulted in suppressed appetite and reduced growth rate that were attributed to its acidifying effects (Yen et al. 1981). Rapid administration of calcium borogluconate solution can induce cardiac arrest in cows. If dietary levels of P are adequate, the following dietary Ca levels (DM basis) can be tolerated (although performance may be reduced): cattle, 2%; sheep, 2%; swine, 1%; poultry, 1.2%; laying hens, 4%; horses, 2%; and rabbits, 2% (NRC 1980).

Supplemental phosphates are not usually considered to be toxic, because single, large doses induce only minimal effects of abdominal distress and diarrhea. An exception to this is in cats, who may experience hyperphosphatemia and other electrolyte and acid-base abnormalities following injudicious use of phosphate-containing enemas or overdosage with phosphate-containing urinary acidifiers (Jorgensen et al. 1985; Fulton and Fruechte 1991). Chronic consumption of excessive dietary P, particularly when dietary Ca intake is low, will induce nutritional secondary hyperparathyroidism. Chronic, high dietary P has been associated with struvite urolithiasis in ruminants and with dystrophic renal calcification in laboratory rodents (NRC 1980). If dietary levels of Ca are adequate, the following dietary P levels (DM basis) can be tolerated (although performance may be reduced): cattle, 1%; sheep, 0.6%; swine, 1.5%; poultry, 1%; laying hens, 0.8%; horses, 1%; and rabbits, 1% (NRC 1980).

SODIUM AND CHLORIDE

Source and Occurrence. Sodium (Na) and chloride (Cl) content in plant materials varies greatly (Minson 1990c; NRC 1982). Forages are classified into two broad categories: Na accumulators and nonaccumulators (which includes all legumes), containing >2 g Na/kg DM or <2 g Na/kg DM, respectively. For Na accumulators, high soil potassium (K) levels can depress Na uptake, while high soil nitrogen can increase it (Minson 1990c). Commercial sources of Na and Cl include a wide variety of salts such as sodium chloride (common salt), sodium bicarbonate (a widely used dietary buffer), calcium chloride (used to alter dietary cation-anion balance), sodium phosphates (as P supplements), and magnesium chloride (as magnesium supplement). Salt (NaCl) is often added to diets as a matter of tradition, despite the provision of adequate levels from other sources, leading to increased water consumption, an increase in excreta volume, and, subsequently, increased NaCl deposition in soils, which in some locales can adversely affect soil fertility (Coppock et al. 1988). Conversely, the use of sodium bicarbonate as a dietary buffer may satisfy the Na requirement, but unless Cl is specifically included in the dietary formulation calculations, an inadequacy in Cl may result (Coppock 1986).

Chemical Forms and Distribution. Sodium is the principal cation and Cl is the main anion in the extracellular fluid. A large portion of body Na is located in bone as phosphate and carbonate salts, but the free Na and Cl ions play crucial roles in osmotic and acid-base homeostasis and in maintaining electrical potentials across intercompartmental barriers within the body. Because of significant bone stores, dietary Na deficiency can take a long time to develop, but because there are no major reserves of Cl in the body, dietary deficiency of Cl may become manifest in as little as 1-2 weeks.

Several methods are available for the determination of the Na and Cl content in biological specimens. Ashed preparations or acid extracts of tissues may be analyzed by atomic absorption spectroscopy for Na and by coulometric titration reactions for Cl. Na in blood and urine may be determined by atomic absorption or flame emission spectroscopy and by ion-specific electrode potentiometry (Korzun and Miller 1987). Cl in blood and urine may be analyzed by visible light spectrophotometry of chromogenic complexes such as mercuric/ferric cyanate, by coulometric titration with silver, or by ion-specific electrode potentiometry (Anderson and Miller 1987).

Biological Characteristics. The renin-angiotensin-aldosterone system plays a central role in control of Na (and K) balance and is, in part, dependent on Cl for normal function (Coppock and Fettman 1977). Decreases in blood pressure, volume, and/or Na concentration activate the juxtaglomerular apparatus of the kidneys to secrete renin. This enzyme catalyzes the conversion of angiotensinogen to angiotensin I, which is subsequently hydrolyzed by a converting enzyme to angiotensin II. Angiotensin II, in concert with adrenocorticotrophic hormone (ACTH) and K, increases aldosterone synthesis and release by the zona glomerulosa of the adrenal cortex. Aldosterone increases Na absorption (and K secretion) by the salivary glands, sweat glands, intestinal mucosa, and distal nephron of the kidneys. Cl is a required cofactor for the activity of the angiotensin-converting enzyme, as well as for a dipeptidyl aminopeptidase responsible for terminating the activity of angiotensin II. The processes that control Na and Cl distribution across cell barriers throughout the body are frequently dependent on energy consumption (active transport) and the coupled unidirectional transit of Na and Cl together. Thus, a deficiency of one element can impede the handling of the other, thereby leading to secondary imbalances. Likewise, because the movement of water across intercompartmental barriers frequently occurs along osmotic gradients established secondary to active Na and Cl transport, their deficiency can lead to abnormal water handling by the GI tract or kidneys and clinically significant disorders of hydration.

Metabolic Functions

GASTROINTESTINAL FUNCTION. Absorption of Na from the lumen of the GI tract is frequently coupled with the absorption of nutrients like amino acids and monosaccharides or with anions like bicarbonate or Cl. Coupled, active transport of Na and Cl is critical to ion and fluid absorption across the ruminal wall and small intestine and simultaneously regulates the balance of bicarbonate at these sites (Coppock and Fettman 1977). Following exposure to pathophysiologically important secretagogues like choleragen or *E. coli* enterotoxin, small-intestinal epithelial cells are stimulated to secrete Cl, following which Na and other ions and water are lost, resulting in the secretory diarrhea characteristic of cholera or neonatal scours syndromes. Cl is the requisite conjugate anion of gastric (hydrochloric) acid secretion and must be reabsorbed in later segments of the GI tract in order to maintain normal fluid and electrolyte homeostasis. In conditions of luminal obstruction, particularly in ruminants with a displaced abomasum, pathologic retention of Cl, protons, other ions, and water in the GI tract results in a significant electrolyte and acid-base disorder characteristic of this condition (Smith 1978; Garry et al. 1988; Constable et al. 1991). This is one example of a "third-space" syndrome (so called because the fluid and electrolytes are retained in the physical confines of the body but not in the usual intra-or extracellular spaces), which is characterized by hypochloremia and metabolic alkalosis. Secondary disturbances in renal handling of water and electrolytes may lead to hypokalemia, hyponatremia, and significant dehydration (see below).

RENAL FUNCTION. Active Na absorption in the proximal nephron creates an electrical gradient favorable to the concomitant absorption of bicarbonate, Cl, and other anions, as well as facilitating absorption of important nutrients like glucose and amino acids from the glomerular filtrate. The osmotic gradient established by this process governs water reabsorption and the subsequent absorption of solutes like Ca and P along their concentration gradients. In the thick ascending limb of the loop of Henle, active transport of Cl creates an electrogenic gradient necessary for coupled absorption of Na and other cations. In the distal nephron, active Na absorption is coupled to proton or K secretion by mineralocorticoid-regulated processes that are central to normal fluid, electrolyte, and acid-base homeostasis. A deficiency of Cl in the glomerular filtrate leads to preferential absorption of bicarbonate by the proximal tubules along the Na-generated electrical gradient, impairs normal ion transport by the loop of Henle, and increases the delivery of Na to the distal nephron (Fettman et al. 1984a,b). This activates the renin-angiotensin-aldosterone axis and can lead to excessive urinary K excretion or paradoxic urinary acidification in the face of metabolic alkalosis. Nephrogenic diabetes insipidus may also result, owing to depletion of the NaCl-dependent renal medullary concentration gradient necessary for water reclamation from the collecting tubules. Thus, either dietary Cl depletion, third-space retention, or pathologic losses in the sweat or excreta may lead to tertiary disorders of renal function and a vicious cycle of propagated fluid and electrolyte abnormalities.

CELL MEMBRANE ELECTRICAL POTENTIALS. The cell membranes of all cells have an ATP-dependent Na,K pump which pumps three Na ions to the exterior for every two K ions pumped to the interior of the cell. The handling of Na and K by this pump not only helps to maintain osmotic equilibrium across the cell membrane but also plays a central role in the propagation of electrical impulses across the membranes of "excitable" cells, including those of the nerves, heart, skeletal muscle, and numerous endocrine tissues. Because the resting cell membrane is many times more permeable to K than to Na, the resting electrical potential described by the Nernst equation (approximately –90 mV) is predominantly attributable to K. When an action potential is elicited, the membrane becomes much more permeable to Na, Na rapidly enters the cell, and the membrane potential rises to that described by the Nernst equation for Na (approximately +45 mV). This depolarization is responsible for transmission of nerve impulses, elicitation of muscle contraction, and stimulation of endocrine cell secretion. Repolarization is initiated via an increase in membrane permeability to K and its extracellular diffusion and is maintained by the subsequent return to normal membrane permeability for Na and K and reactivation of the Na,K-ATPase pump. Changes in Na balance are evidenced clinically by alterations in neuromuscular, cardiovascular, and endocrine functions similar to those described for K (see below).

LACTATION. As is the case for most nutrients, dietary requirements for Na and Cl increase significantly during lactation. Even during times of significant dietary deficiency, lactating cows seem unable to decrease milk Na concentrations appreciably (Smith and Aines 1959), although Cl levels may decrease by up to about 50% (Fettman et al. 1984a,b). Burkhalter et al. (1979) estimated the maintenance requirement for Cl to be quite low (approximately 0.04% DM). Coppock (1986) has estimated that a 600 kg cow producing 30 kg milk/day would secrete 33 g/day of Cl in the milk; for a production level of 40 kg/day, this would increase to 44 g/day lost in the milk. This would require an increased intake to a level of approximately 0.20-0.25% of the diet dry matter. The corresponding dietary requirement for Na would be approximately 0.15-0.20% DM (Minson 1990c). Dietary deficiencies of either Na or Cl have been reported to result in substantial decreases in feed intake, body weight, and milk production (Aines and Smith 1957; Fettman et al. 1984b,c).

SALT AND HYPERTENSION. Most studies in human subjects have definitively demonstrated a significant association between dietary salt consumption and hypertension. The "Intersalt" study of over 10,000 individuals demonstrated that a 24-hour urinary Na excretion higher by 100 mmol was associated with systolic blood pressure higher by 3-6 mm Hg (Elliott et al. 1996). A meta-analysis of 56 trials that had randomized allocation to control and dietary sodium intervention groups demonstrated a mean reduction of –3.7 mm Hg in systolic pressure and –0.9 mm Hg in diastolic pressure for a 100 mmol/day reduction in daily Na excretion in hypertensive patients (Midgley et al. 1996). In contrast, decreases in blood pressure in response to dietary sodium restriction were negligible in individuals who were normotensive (Midgley et al. 1996).

Studies of the prevalence of hypertension in dogs are few, and the associated risk factors, including dietary salt, have not been well studied. Approximately 10% of 102 apparently healthy dogs observed in one study were found to be hypertensive: systolic pressure > 202 mm Hg, and diastolic pressure > 116 mm Hg (Remillard et al. 1991). In a study of over 1900 pet dogs, hypertension was not defined, but increased systemic blood pressure was associated with specific breeds, advancing age, diabetes, obesity, hyperadrenocorticism, and hepatic disease (Bodey and Michell 1996). A modest increase in mean blood pressure was associated with chronic renal disease only in those dogs with substantial reductions in glomerular filtration rate. Although dietary sodium intake was not assessed, it appeared that consumption of home-made diets was associated with lower systolic pressure than was eating commercial food.

In another report, spontaneous systemic hypertension was identified in five dogs but was diagnosed as essential hypertension (no apparent causative disorder) in only one subject (Littman et al. 1988). None responded to dietary Na restriction alone. In healthy dogs, increasing dietary Na intake from 5 to 24[illegible] mmol/day caused no significant changes in mean arterial pressure, and even at a Na intake of 495 mmol/day, mean pressure increased only 7 mm Hg (Hall et al. 1980). Dogs fed a high-fat diet for 6 weeks in order to induce a weight gain of ~3 kg experienced increased sodium retention, higher plasma volume, and ~20 mm Hg increase in mean arterial pressure (Rocchini et al. 1989). Hyperinsulinemia pursuant to obesity-induced target cell insulin insensitivity can promote Na retention and sympathoadrenal hyperactivity, contributing to hypertension. Likewise, diet-induced obesity in dogs is associated with 50-70% degradation in urinary elimination of an intravenous saline load, thereby leading to volume expansion and increased blood pressure (West et al. 1992).

Partially nephrectomized dogs subjected to 4-week crossover trials of low (0.18% DM) and high (1.3% DM) Na diets experienced no differences in glomerular filtration rate (Greco et al. 1994a). However, those sequentially fed the low, high, and low Na diets experienced significantly higher systolic pressures (175 vs. 156 mm Hg) than those sequentially fed the high, low, and high Na diets (Greco et al. 1994b). Thus, low dietary Na intake in this study was paradoxically associated with moderate systolic hypertension in dogs with experimentally induced renal disease.

Finally, dogs with congestive heart failure that are fed a Na-restricted diet and treated with a diuretic may be predisposed to functional renal insufficiency and the development of azotemia when angiotensin-converting enzyme inhibitor therapy is also employed (Roudebush et al. 1994). Blood pressure, volume, and renal perfusion may be restored in these patients by replenishing body Na and reducing the diuretic dose.

Signs of Deficiency. The signs of chronic Na or Cl deficiency have been well documented in cattle and include lethargy, anorexia, weight loss, hypogalactia, neuromuscular and cardiovascular dysfunction, and a depraved appetite (Aines and Smith 1957; Fettman et al. 1984a,b,c). Impaired renal concentration capacity has been documented following both nutritional Na and nutritional Cl deficiency (Whitlock et al. 1975; Fettman et al. 1984b,c). Induced Cl deficiency in calves and lactating cows has been associated with the development of a hypochloremic, hypokalemic, hyponatremic, metabolic alkalosis, which responded well to oral electrolyte replacement (Blackmon et al. 1984; Fettman et al. 1984b,c). Beef cattle similarly have low maintenance NaCl requirements (perhaps 0.06-0.08% Na in the diet dry matter), but it increases with lactation to a smaller extent than seen in dairy cows (to 0.1% Na DM) (Morris 1980). Dietary Na and Cl intake has been shown to affect feed intake, feed efficiency, basic amino acid metabolism, and K balance (Honeyfield et al. 1985).

Na and Cl levels for optimal weight and feed efficiency were estimated to be 0.13% DM and 0.17% DM, respectively, in growing-finishing pigs fed a corn and soybean meal-based diet (Honeyfield et al. 1985). Although the NRC (1988) recommends a total dietary level of 0.10% Na and 0.08% Cl for young pigs (<10 kg body weight), recent studies with high-salt, dried whey-containing diets indicate that weanling pigs may respond favorably to levels twice this amount (Mahan et al. 1996).

In horses, Na deficiency will result in anorexia, dehydration, weight loss, depraved appetite, muscular incoordination, and rough hair coat (Cunha 1991b). It has been suggested that dietary Na and/or Cl imbalances may be contributory factors in the development of the syndrome of anhidrosis in horses exercised in hot climates (Correa and Calderin 1966; Mayhew and Ferguson 1987). Clinicopathologic findings in affected horses include hypochloremia and/or reduced urinary Cl excretion, and signs resolve following oral or parenteral NaCl administration. Horses will voluntarily consume large amounts of NaCl from salt blocks but consistently prefer diets containing lesser amounts of NaCl when given a choice (Schryver et al. 1987). In addition to the consistent development of a depraved appetite, there is some evidence that Na- or Cl-deficient animals will exhibit a specific appetite for Na- or Cl-containing mineral supplements (Denton and Sabine 1961; Fettman et al. 1984a,b; Cunha 1991b).

Assessment of Status. Criteria used to evaluate Na and Cl status have included biological response to supplementation, analysis of blood Na and Cl concentrations, measurement of urinary and/or fecal excretion of Na and Cl, and determination of salivary Na and Cl concentrations (Fettman et al. 1984a,b,c). Because blood Na is maintained to some degree by release from bone stores, in addition to GI absorption and urinary excretion, these values may be maintained through long periods of imbalance. Thus, low blood levels of Na may indicate deficiency, but normal values must be interpreted with caution. On the other hand, blood Cl concentrations appear to reflect the degree of body Cl depletion fairly well and, coupled with values for urinary and fecal Cl excretion, can help identify the source of pathologic losses and/or insufficient dietary intake. Salivary Na, but not Cl, concentration decreases significantly with dietary deficiency and has been used to detect Na deficiency (Morris 1980; Fettman 1984b; Cunha 1991b). Urinary Na and Cl excretion may also be indexed to urinary creatinine and plasma electrolyte and creatinine concentrations as the fractional excretion value (FE_{Na} and FE_{Cl}) for a gross indication of urinary loss. This value is particularly elevated in acute renal tubular diseases and is decreased with dietary depletion or extrarenal losses (Zarich et al. 1985; Anderson et al. 1984). Reference values for each species should be consulted in the interpretation of each parameter of Na and Cl metabolism.

Dietary Requirements, Indications, and Use

INTRINSIC FACTORS. Requirements for Na and Cl are greatest during pregnancy, rapid growth, and particularly during lactation. The potential for deficiency or imbalance during these phases of life is increased in herbivores fed large quantities of concentrates during these phases that are poor sources of Na and Cl. Other intrinsic factors may affect Na and Cl metabolism, including GI diseases, in which absorption is depressed, and in secretory diarrhea, where losses are increased. In acute renal disease, excessive Na and Cl may be lost owing to tubular damage and mineralocorticoid nonresponsiveness. In hypoadrenocorticism (Addison's disease), a deficiency in aldosterone secretion results in excessive urinary Na loss, K retention, metabolic acidosis, nephrogenic diabetes insipidus, and dehydration (Tyler et al. 1987).

EXTRINSIC FACTORS. The Na and Cl content of drinking water may significantly affect the necessity for dietary supplementation (Coppock et al. 1988). The temperature and humidity of the environment have important effects. In horses, heat and humidity affect Na and Cl excretion in the sweat. In all animals potential increases in water consumption may increase urinary losses. Lactating cows maintained in a hot, humid environment respond adversely to acidogenic Cl-containing salts like calcium chloride and appear to benefit from alkalinizing Na-containing salts like sodium bicarbonate (Coppock et al. 1982a,b; West et al. 1991; Shalit et al. 1991).

Preparations and Therapy. Na and Cl are available in a variety of mineral products, including common salt (NaCl), sodium phosphates, sodium bicarbonate, calcium chloride, and magnesium chloride. Injectable and oral preparations may be obtained singly or as part of a multimineral preparation. Simple, aqueous solutions are indicated for injection, and isotonic saline (0.9% NaCl) serves as the base for most extracellular fluid replacement solutions used in clinical practice. Single large doses of NaCl may be given as intravenous, intramuscular, or subcutaneous injections in the treatment of depletion disorders. Single large doses of sodium bicarbonate may be administered parenterally in the treatment of metabolic acidosis, but rapid administration of such solutions should be avoided, because paradoxic cerebrospinal fluid acidosis, impaired hemoglobin-oxygen dissociation, cranial hemorrhage, and other unwanted effects may result. Adverse effects on central nervous system function have been observed in hyponatremic human patients treated with Na-containing solutions either at too high a dose or at too great a rate of replenishment (Berl 1990). Frequent monitoring of blood and urine Na concentrations, coupled with a reasonable rate of replenishment, can prevent these potential problems (Berl 1990).

Toxicity. Animals appear to tolerate fairly high dietary levels of Na and Cl, because homeostatic mechanisms tend to protect them against excessive absorption. However, the addition of excessive NaCl to a diet can produce adverse effects, including polydipsia, polyuria, anorexia, weight loss, edema, nervousness, paresis, paralysis, and death (NRC 1980). In cattle, levels of salt below approximately 5% of the diet dry matter have little effect on general health, feed intake, weight gain, or milk production (NRC 1980). Fattening steers have tolerated as much as 9.33% DM without effect, but swine experience neuromuscular signs characteristic of salt poisoning with diets containing 6-8% DM as NaCl, and lactating ewes exhibit increased weight loss and decreased lamb survivability when fed 13.1% DM (NRC 1980). Poultry may tolerate NaCl up to 2% DM, and horses and rabbits up to 3% DM (NRC 1980). The major factor affecting NaCl toxicity is the availability of nonsaline drinking water during the consumption of excess salt. Although oral administration of water is effective in alleviating signs of acute toxicity, its rate of administration must be carefully regulated to avoid unwanted effects associated with reestablishment of osmotic equilibria, particularly across the blood-brain interface.

POTASSIUM

Source and Occurrence. Potassium (K) is widely distributed in the soil and found in high concentrations in most plant species (NRC 1982). Because the K content of feeds usually parallels that of protein, the substitution of purified protein or nonprotein nitrogen sources for natural protein sources may increase the potential for inadequate K intake in high-concentrate diets for producing, growing, or lactating animals (Ward 1978). Commercial sources of K include potassium chloride, carbonate, bicarbonate, sulfate, and phosphate salts.

Chemical Forms and Distribution. K is the principal cation of the intracellular fluid compartment and, after Ca and P, the third most abundant mineral in the body. Some K is located in bone as phosphate and carbonate salts, but the majority is found as the free ion in extraosseous tissues, where it plays a central role in osmotic and acid-base homeostasis and in maintaining cell membrane electrical potentials, in concert with Na. Despite its high body levels and critical role in metabolism, body reserves are limited and some excretory losses are obligatory, so dietary deficiency may become evident in as little as 1-2 weeks.

Several methods are available for the determination of K in biological specimens. Blood, urine, and ashed preparations or acid extracts or tissues may be analyzed by atomic absorption or flame emission spectroscopy. Fluid samples may also be analyzed by ion-specific electrode potentiometry. Chromogenic dye-binding methods have also been implemented for K determination by colorimetric spectrophotometry (Wong et al. 1985).

Biological Characteristics. As was described for Na, the renin-angiotensin-aldosterone system plays an important role in maintaining K homeostasis

Hypokalemia inhibits, and hyperkalemia stimulates, aldosterone release by the adrenal cortex. Aldosterone promotes K secretion (coupled to Na absorption) at a number of sites in the body, particularly in the GI tract and kidneys. The distribution of K between the intra- and extracellular fluid compartments is influenced by a number of humoral and metabolic factors (Fettman 1989). Thus, one must interpret extracellular fluid K concentrations (as in the blood plasma) with caution, in order to differentiate true K deficits caused by an imbalance between intake and excretion from apparent K deficits caused by redistribution of extracellular K to the intracellular compartment. Catecholamines, insulin, and metabolic or respiratory alkalosis all promote cellular K uptake and thereby induce hypokalemia without necessitating any change in total body K content. Conversely, dopamine, muscular activity, cell death, and metabolic or respiratory acidosis can cause K efflux from cells, producing hyperkalemia without change in total body K content. True potassium deficits may arise from inadequate dietary intake, increased extrarenal losses, or increased renal loss. Extrarenal routes include sweating, wound exudation, vomiting, and diarrhea. Renal losses may result from intrinsic renal disease or extrinsic factors affecting renal handling of K, including disturbances in glomerulotubular balance or acid-base metabolism and diseases which result in increased secretion of mineralocorticoids.

Metabolic Functions

GASTROINTESTINAL FUNCTION. Absorption of K from the GI tract occurs mainly in the small intestine by active transport processes. K secretion by intestinal epithelial cells is influenced by K intake, Na and Cl balance, acid-base status, and the level of mineralocorticoids released by the adrenal gland. Increases in fecal K loss are common in diarrheal diseases, where increased transit of water and ions (particularly Na) from the small to the large intestine stimulates colonic Na absorption, which is coupled to K secretion.

RENAL FUNCTION. Absorption of K from the glomerular filtrate occurs mainly in the proximal renal tubules and thick ascending limb of the loop of Henle. The former is driven by changes in electrical and concentration gradients which follow active Na transport, while the latter is coupled to active Cl absorption in a manner analogous to that described for Na. The kidney is the principal organ for fine-tuning the balance of K in the body. In the distal nephron, K secretion is coupled to Na absorption in an aldosterone-dependent process that is also regulated by acid-base balance, renal tubular flow rate, and the load of non-reabsorbable anions presented to the distal tubules (Fettman 1989). Reduced intracellular proton concentrations in alkalosis, faster tubular flow rates which decrease the luminal K concentration gradient, and increased luminal electronegativity accompanying higher concentrations of anions that have escaped proximal tubular reabsorption all promote K secretion by the distal tubular cells. Disorders resulting in Cl depletion, including third-space syndromes, dietary deficiency, or secretory diarrhea, can result in secondary K depletion through the impairment of normal renal tubular Na reabsorption, increase in renin-angiotensin-aldosterone activity, and subsequent stimulation of distal tubular K secretion.

Through effects that are not entirely clear, K depletion and hypokalemia can induce significant renal dysfunction, as well as morphological damage. The so-called kaliopenic nephropathy syndrome is characterized by reduced renal blood flow caused by increased release of humoral vasoconstrictors (including angiotensin II and thromboxane), nephrogenic diabetes insipidus due to impaired vasopressin responsiveness by collecting tubule cells, and tubulointerstitial injury apparently caused by pathologic increases in renal ammoniagenesis and complement activation (Fettman 1989). Although moderate reductions in renal function appear to be reversible, more severe changes may be followed by permanent renal dysfunction.

CARDIAC FUNCTION. As was described for the role of Na in maintaining cell membrane electrical potentials, K distribution across the intracellular-extracellular compartment interface is primarily responsible for the resting membrane potential of all cells and for the initiation of repolarization of excitable membranes following the elicitation of an action potential. K is particularly important in the electrophysiological control of cardiac function, where its relative distribution across cardiocyte membranes influences not only the rate and rhythm but also the force of cardiac contraction. As described by the Nernst equation, the relative concentrations of K in the intra- and extracellular fluid determine the resting membrane potential of the cardiocyte, which is usually approximately –90 mV. Hypokalemia increases the resting membrane potential (hyperpolarization), thereby increasing the threshold necessary to initiate an action potential (Bolton 1975). Conversely, hyperkalemia causes hypopolarization and decreases that threshold, making the cardiocyte more excitable. However, the amplitude of the resting membrane potential also determines the force of contraction once an action potential is elicited and the ease of repolarization once it is terminated, so that hypokalemia is associated with spastic contraction, and hyperkalemia is associated with flaccidity and dilatation (Bolton 1975). The latter effects can be alleviated to some extent by treatment with Ca, which can block K channels in the cardiocyte membrane and restore more normal electrical conductivity.

BLOOD PRESSURE REGULATION. Many studies have suggested a relationship between dietary K intake and blood pressure in humans, yet the role of K supplementation in treating or preventing systemic hypertension has remained controversial. In a recent meta-analysis of

33 randomized, controlled trials of K supplementation as the sole difference between intervention and control conditions, K was associated with a significant mean reduction in systolic and diastolic blood pressure of –3.11 mm Hg and –1.97 mm Hg, respectively (Whelton et al. 1997). In individual studies, systolic pressure was reduced by as much as –41.0 mm Hg (Obel 1989). These effects were achieved following daily supplementation with 60 mmol K/day or more in all but two of the trials and appeared to be enhanced when subjects concurrently consumed a diet high in Na.

Although not as well studied in veterinary patients, hypertension has been identified in cats with naturally occurring, chronic renal disease (Jensen et al. 1997). Although only 3 of 12 hypertensive subjects were hypokalemic, 10 of 12 were hyperaldosteronemic, which would contribute to impaired K balance. Given the association between kaliopenia and chronic renal disease in cats (Fettman 1989; Dow et al. 1990), it is possible that the occurrence of hypertension in feline chronic renal failure may be responsive to dietary K supplementation.

SKELETAL MUSCLE FUNCTION. The K gradient across muscle cell membranes influences cell volume, protein synthesis, enzyme activity, electrical conductivity, and changes in blood flow during exercise (Fettman 1989). K depletion can result in impaired myocytic carbohydrate metabolism, muscular paresis, followed by paralysis, myocytic swelling and rhabdomyolysis, and exercise-associated ischemic myonecrosis (Fettman 1989). Animals affected with so-called kaliopenic myopathy have generalized appendicular muscle weakness, an abnormal gait, and are reluctant to move. Cats so affected demonstrate a characteristic, persistent ventroflexion of the neck (Fettman 1989).

ACID-BASE METABOLISM. K ions and protons in the body are integrally related, owing to their ability to undergo exchange across interfaces between the intra- and extracellular fluid compartments (Fettman 1989). Acute alkalosis is often associated with hypokalemia, owing to exchange of intracellular protons for extracellular K ions and the relative replacement of K ion secretion by that of protons during the process of Na reabsorption by the distal renal tubules. The resulting redistribution allows intracellular acid reserves to buffer the extracellular proton deficiency, while altered renal excretion limits unwanted acid loss in the urine. Conversely, acidosis is often associated with hyperkalemia, in which intracellular uptake of extracellular protons for buffering is electrically counterbalanced by release of intracellular K ions. Urinary excretion of K ions is likewise decreased to facilitate coupling of distal renal tubular Na absorption to proton secretion. Paradoxically, chronic metabolic acidosis may result in K depletion, predominantly through stimulation of adrenal cortical aldosterone release by protons and subsequent stimulation of K excretion by the GI tract and kidneys. Chronic K depletion can likewise result in metabolic acidosis through an acquired syndrome of hypoadrenocorticism secondary to the chronic understimulation of mineralocorticoid release by low circulating K levels (Fettman 1989).

EFFECTS OF GROWTH AND LACTATION AND SIGNS OF DEFICIENCY. Because of the high K content of muscle tissue and the large amounts present in milk, growth and lactation are associated with the highest dietary requirements for K. Maintenance requirements for K range from as little as 0.20% of the diet dry matter for rodents and chickens to 0.40% DM in horses; requirements for growth or lactation may double or triple these values (Ward 1978). Growing pigs and calves require as much as approximately 0.60% DM (Golz and Crenshaw 1990; Weil et al. 1988). However, Leibholz et al. (1966) showed that increasing the dietary protein content for growing pigs increased the K requirement from 0.60% to approximately 1.20% DM. Likewise, although maintenance requirements for cats are approximately 0.35% DM, growth and increasing dietary protein intake can increase this to as much as 0.50% with 68% protein in the diet of growing kittens (Hills et al. 1982). Feeding trials have indicated that as much as 0.80% DM may be required to maximize feed efficiency and rate of gain in steers; 100% DM is required for horses (Devlin et al. 1969; Stowe 1971). A dietary K content of 0.70% DM appears to be adequate for cows in mid- to late lactation, and high-producing cows in early lactation may require 0.80-1.00% DM (Dennis and Hemken 1978).

The signs of chronic K deficiency include anorexia, depressed growth, dull and coarse hair or wool, pica, hypogalactia, lethargy, muscular weakness, stiffness or paralysis, and neurologic dysfunction. Because of changes in pancreatic β-cell electrical potential, insulin secretory responsiveness to glucose challenge may be impaired, resulting in carbohydrate intolerance. In pigs and in chickens, dietary basic amino acid requirements may increase during K deficiency, because their intracellular concentrations increase to maintain cation balance (Ward 1978).

Assessment of Status. Criteria used to evaluate K status have included biological response to supplementation, analysis of plasma and erythrocytic K concentrations, and measurement of urinary and/or fecal excretion of K (Dow et al. 1987a,b, 1990; Pradham and Hemken 1968). Because K is located principally within the intracellular fluid compartment, measurement of extracellular fluid K levels, as in blood plasma, can often be misleading as to the actual status of K in the whole body. One alternative is to measure K content in erythrocytes in those species where these levels parallel those of other tissues, which is not the case in dogs or cats (Harvey 1989). Urinary K excretion may also be indexed to urinary creatinine and plasma K and creatinine concentrations as the fractional excretion value (FE_K) for a gross indication of urinary loss. This value may be affected by dietary intake, by renal tubular dysfunction, and by creatinine clearance rate and should be interpreted with caution. Reference values for each species should be consulted in the interpretation of each parameter of K metabolism.

Dietary Requirements, Indications, and Use

INTRINSIC FACTORS. As discussed above, requirements for K are greatest during pregnancy, growth, and lactation. The potential for imbalance during these phases of life is increased in animals fed large quantities of concentrates during these phases that are poor sources of K. K availability from most feeds is relatively high, and its absorption may increase with increasing dietary content, although actual retention may be unaffected (Combs and Miller 1985a,b; Grings and Males 1987). GI disease may both depress absorption of K and increase its secretion, thereby rapidly depleting the animal of K. In acute renal disease, excessive K may be lost in the urine owing to tubular damage and impaired reabsorption from the glomerular filtrate. In disorders causing relative hyperadrenocorticism—including third-space syndromes, dietary NaCl depletion, and chronic metabolic acidosis—increased aldosterone secretion may result in excessive K excretion (Fettman 1989). Cats with underlying chronic renal dysfunction fed an acidified diet marginally sufficient in K have developed a clinically significant polymyopathy/nephropathy syndrome (Dow et al. 1987a,b, 1988, 1989).

EXTRINSIC FACTORS. Other dietary minerals have little effect on K availability from feeds (Erdman et al. 1980). Transport stress may increase dietary K requirements, and in feeder calves, blood parameters indicative of stress and weight gains following shipping were improved by increasing dietary K by 20% more than that required by nonstressed animals (Hutcheson et al. 1984). Milk yields in lactating cows exposed to heat stress have been increased significantly by increasing dietary K intake. In one study, a change from 0.66% to 1.08% DM increased milk yield by 7.4% (Mallonee et al. 1985), while in another a change from 1.3% to 1.8% DM increased milk production by 4.5% (Schneider et al. 1986). Dietary acidification in cats has reduced GI K absorption, increased urinary K excretion, and resulted in negative K balance (Ching et al. 1989; Dow et al. 1990). Primary K deficiency in cats appears to result in secondary taurine depletion, and earlier work in rats and dogs indicates that supplemental dietary taurine may ameliorate the cardiotoxic effects of K deficiency (Dow et al. 1992).

Preparations and Therapy. K is available in a variety of mineral products, including potassium chloride (lite salt), potassium carbonate, potassium bicarbonate, potassium citrate, potassium gluconate, and potassium monohydrogen or dihydrogen phosphate. Injectable and oral preparations may be obtained singly or as part of a multimineral preparation. Simple, aqueous solutions are indicated for injection, and lactated Ringer's solution (4 mmol/L K) serves as a base for many extracellular replacement solutions used in clinical practice. Single large doses of K salts in solution should be administered parenterally with a great deal of caution, because the rapid increase in blood K concentrations can be cardiotoxic. Single large oral doses of K salts in solution are much safer, as their absorption is regulated by the animal and takes place over a longer period of time. K concentration in intravenous solutions should be adjusted according to the estimated deficit of K in the patient, but because these calculations rely on blood plasma levels, they should be used conservatively. Generally speaking, K concentrations in intravenous solutions should not exceed 80 mmol/L or be administered in excess of 0.5 mmol/kg body weight/hour. Exceptions to this include cows with severe third-space syndromes following GI obstruction and cats with severe kaliopenic polymyopathy/nephropathy syndrome. For the latter, up to 10 mmol may be required to restore K levels, although most cats respond with oral supplementation of 2-4 mmol/day (Fettman 1989). Frequent monitoring of blood and urine K concentrations, coupled with reasonable rates of replenishment, should prevent unwanted effects.

Toxicity. K toxicosis is unlikely under most conditions, resulting only when supplemented dietary or parenteral levels of K-containing salts are excessive (NRC 1980). Lower levels of increased dietary K (2-4% DM) decrease diet palatability, feed intake, and rate of gain in growing animals (NRC 1980; Neathery et al. 1980). Higher levels of K (greater than 0.58 g/kg body weight) administered orally to young calves produced excess salivation, muscular tremors of the limbs, excitability, metabolic acidosis, and hemoconcentration (Neathery et al. 1979). Intravenous administration of large amounts of K results, in all species, in cardiotoxicity characterized by such electrocardiographic changes as increased T-wave amplitude, decreased P-wave amplitude, prolonged QT interval, and ventricular fibrillation or asystole (Bolton 1975). Chronic consumption of high dietary K can depress GI magnesium absorption significantly. Feeding 0.68 g K per 100 g body weight resulted in clinical signs of magnesium deficiency in rats, while in sheep 2-3% DM is tolerated before magnesium depletion results (NRC 1980; Grings and Males 1987; Greene et al. 1983). Contrary to previous reports (NRC 1980), the addition of Na to high-K diets in sheep did not improve magnesium homeostasis (Poe et al. 1985). Maximum tolerable dietary levels are assumed to be approximately 3% DM for most species (NRC 1980).

MAGNESIUM

Source and Occurrence. The magnesium (Mg) concentration of plants is affected by soil type, climate, light intensity, temperature, and stage of growth, as well as by the interacting effects of other minerals and organic constituents (Minson 1990d; NRC 1982). Increasing the K, Ca, or aluminum supply to plants has been shown to reduce plant Mg uptake (Grunes and Welch 1989; Minson 1990d). An increase in the rate of plant growth through nitrogen fertilization, seasonal changes, or increased light intensity also decreases Mg uptake (Grunes and Welch 1989; Minson 1990d). Winter wheat and other cereal grasses often contain extremely low levels of Mg. Commercial sources include a variety of Mg salts such as chloride, oxide, hydroxide, carbonate, and citrate.

Chemical Forms and Distribution. Approximately 60% of the Mg in the body is located in bone. Most of the rest is located intracellularly, particularly in muscle tissue. Approximately 1% of body Mg is located in the extracellular fluid. In the blood plasma, one-third is bound to proteins (25% to albumin and 8% to globulins) (Kroll and Elin 1985). Of the ultrafiltrable plasma Mg, about 20% is complexed to phosphates, citrate, and other anions, and 80% is the free ion.

Several methods are available for the determination of Mg content in biological specimens. Ashed preparations or acid extracts of tissues may be analyzed by atomic absorption spectroscopy. Mg in blood and urine may be determined by atomic absorption, fluorometric, or visible light spectrophotometry of chromogenic complexes, such as methylthymol blue (Farrell 1987c). Free Mg in biological fluids can be determined by mechanical or centrifugal ultrafiltration or by equilibrium dialysis. Ionized Mg concentrations may be analyzed with the metallochromic dye Eriochrome Blue SE or by ion-specific electrode potentiometry (Elin 1987; Rehal et al. 1996).

Biological Characteristics. Mg absorption in nonruminants is predominantly from the small intestine, while in ruminants it is primarily from the reticulorumen (Reinhart 1988; Fontenot et al. 1989). Whereas absorption of Mg from the rumen appears to be an active, Na-linked process, its absorption from the small intestine is mostly passive. The proportion of ingested Mg absorbed is inversely related to the amount ingested, and little or no Mg absorption occurs in the large intestine. Hence, large oral doses of Mg salts are frequently used as cathartics. Mg availability is influenced by a number of dietary factors discussed below. The kidney is the principal regulator of body Mg content. Non-protein-bound Mg is freely filtered through the glomerulus, and little if any Mg is secreted by the renal tubules. Approximately 25-30% of the filtered load of Mg is reabsorbed in the proximal renal tubules by a passive process that is dependent on active Na and water reabsorption and the subsequent development of an electrical and concentration gradient conducive to its uptake (Dirks 1983). The thick ascending limb of the loop of Henle is the principal site of Mg reabsorption from the glomerular filtrate, in a process dependent on the electronegative gradient created by active Cl absorption in this segment. PTH appears to promote this process, and by way of a negative feedback mechanism, hypomagnesemia stimulates PTH release, and hypermagnesemia inhibits it (Reinhart 1988). However, severe hypomagnesemia can inhibit PTH release and perhaps also depress 1α-hydroxylation of 25-OH vitamin D, which may explain the frequently concurrent finding of hypocalcemia in hypomagnesemic tetany of ruminants (Fontenot et al. 1989; Reinhart 1988). Pharmacological doses of calcitriol have been shown to increase intestinal Mg absorption in both vitamin D-deficient and vitamin D-replete animals and also to increase its urinary excretion, although the mechanisms are not known (Hardwick et al. 1991).

METABOLIC FUNCTIONS AND SIGNS OF DEFICIENCY. All enzymatic reactions involving the utilization or formation of ATP have an absolute requirement for Mg. It is necessary for all phosphate transfer reactions, stabilizes the anionic charges on ATP, ADP, and AMP, serves as a cofactor for thiamin pyrophosphate-requiring reactions, and participates in the synthesis of nucleic acids and the utilization of acetyl-coenzyme A (CoA). Through its interactions with phosphoryl groups of membrane phospholipids, its modulation of ATP metabolism, and its effects on transcellular Ca ion gating, Mg exerts many regulatory effects on cell membrane function, electrical conductivity, and hormonal signaling of intracellular processes.

Mg deficiency manifests itself predominantly through neuromuscular and cardiovascular disorders, characterized by muscular weakness, twitching, or tremor, hyperreflexia, tetany, opisthotonos, delirium, convulsions, and coma (Haggard et al. 1978; Reinhart 1988; Hoffsis et al. 1989). Electrocardiographic changes may include premature ventricular contractions, prolongation of the PR and QT intervals, T-wave flattening, and atrial fibrillation. Pathologic findings include widespread ecchymotic hemorrhages; calcification and fragmentation of elastic fibers in the heart, arteries, spleen, and lungs; focal interstitial nephritis; and dystrophic mineralization of the kidneys (Haggard et al. 1978; Fontenot et al. 1989). Magnesium depletion in rats has been associated with significant reductions in both cytochrome P-450 and glucuronosyl transferase-catalyzed drug biotransformations, which may alter therapeutic drug pharmacokinetics and predispose deficient individuals to toxic effects of xenobiotics (Brown and Bidlack 1991). In humans, Mg deficiency has been identified as a cause of refractory K depletion, which may be characterized predominantly by signs routinely associated with kaliopenia (Whang et al. 1985). A recent prospective, double-blind, randomized, placebo-controlled trial of magnesium sulfate supplementation in hypokalemic human critical-care patients demonstrated, within 30 hours, a significant reversal of net negative K balance and subsequently a lower requirement for supplemental K to restore serum K concentrations in the Mg-treated patients (Hamill-Ruth and McGory 1996). In milk-fed calves, dietary Mg deficiency may result in "milk tetany." In adults it results in a syndrome known as "grass tetany," "grass staggers," "winter tetany," and "wheat pasture poisoning." Although Mg deficiency may result from inadequate dietary intake of Mg, many factors can reduce its bioavailability from natural feedstuffs, thereby producing a relative deficiency.

Assessment of Status. Criteria used to evaluate Mg status have included biological response to supplementation, analysis of blood plasma, erythrocyte, and leukocyte Mg concentrations, and measurement of urinary and/or fecal excretion of Mg (Elin 1987). Because of its frequent association with hypokalemia, hypophosphatemia, hyponatremia, or hypocalcemia in humans, finding any of these abnormalities in a routine serum chemistry screening panel alerts the physician to the possibility of abnormalities in Mg balance (Whang et al. 1984; Boyd et al. 1983). Similar observations in animals have not yet been reported. Because so little of body Mg is distributed in the extracellular fluid, analysis of blood plasma levels is not reliable in interpreting whole-body Mg status. Thus, low blood levels may indicate deficiency, but normal values must be interpreted cautiously. The feasibility of a short-term Mg-loading test to identify functional Mg deficiency in critically ill human patients has recently been demonstrated (Hebert et al. 1997). Patients received 30 mmol/day of magnesium sulfate intravenously for each of 3 days, during which 24-hour urine collections were performed. Nineteen of 44 patients were identified as being functionally Mg deficient, even though only 4 had low serum ionized Mg concentrations.

Dietary Requirements, Indications, and Use

INTRINSIC FACTORS. Requirements for Mg are, as for other minerals, greatest during pregnancy, lactation, and periods of rapid growth. The potential for deficiency or imbalance may be exacerbated in ruminants fed large quantities of Mg-poor or Mg-antagonist-rich feeds during these phases of life. Except for lactating animals, herbivorous and omnivorous species obtain sufficient Mg if the diet contains 0.6 g/kg DM. This is adequately supplied by most natural sources. Lactating cows should receive a diet containing approximately 2 g/kg DM. As alluded to earlier, changes in PTH (or calcitonin) secretion may affect not only Ca and P metabolism but that of Mg as well. GI diseases may impair Mg uptake, and renal disease may impair its excretion.

EXTRINSIC FACTORS. In addition to their adverse effects on plant Mg uptake, high dietary K, Ca, P, or aluminum can suppress Mg absorption by the GI tract (Fontenot et al. 1989; Neathery et al. 1990; Hardwick et al. 1991). High nitrogen fertilization reduces plant Mg accumulation. High crude protein levels apparently depress Mg absorption by ruminants, perhaps through increased ruminal ammoniagenesis and alkalinization, resulting in the formation of insoluble magnesium ammonium phosphate salts. On the other hand, dietary supplementation with readily fermentable carbohydrates improves Mg uptake, perhaps by depressing ruminal ammonia levels (Giduck and Fontenot 1987). Dietary ionophores such as monensin and lasalocid, which facilitate the passage of ions across cell membranes, have been shown to enhance Mg uptake and even to overcome the adverse effects of high dietary K on ruminal Mg transport (Greene et al. 1986). Conversely, there appears to be an additive interaction between dietary Mg supplementation (0.32% vs. 0.16% DM) and treatment with laidlomycin propionate (11 ppm vs. 0 ppm DM) on ruminal starch digestion, dietary net energy value, and average daily gain in feedlot cattle (Zinn et al. 1996). The site and extent of Mg absorption by sheep and cattle have been shown to differ widely with the source of supplemental Mg fed (Hurley et al. 1990; Davenport et al. 1990; Lough et al. 1990).

Preparations and Therapy. Mg is available in a variety of mineral salts, including chloride and sulfate (also used as dietary acidifiers) and oxide, hydroxide, and carbonate (also used as dietary alkalinizers). Injectable and oral preparations may be obtained singly and as part of a multimineral preparation. Simple, aqueous solutions are indicated for injection, but because of acid-base interactions, large quantities should be used with caution. Mg and bicarbonate salts cannot be combined in aqueous solutions, where they may precipitate as magnesium carbonate. Single, large doses of magnesium sulfate, chloride, or lactate may be administered parenterally in the immediate treatment of hypomagnesemic tetany in ruminants. For an adult cow, approximately 200-300 ml of a 20% solution of magnesium sulfate can be used (Hoffsis et al. 1989). Parenteral treatment should be followed by oral therapy as described below for prophylaxis. Because all Mg-containing salts are unpalatable, they will not be consumed free-choice and must be mixed well into the feed or purposefully administered. The supplement should provide approximately 30 g Mg/day for large ruminants and 3.0 g Mg/day for small ruminants (Hoffsis et al. 1989). Dietary prophylaxis of hypomagnesemic tetany in ruminants may be accomplished by provision of Mg salt-supplemented concentrates, treatment of hay or silage with Mg salts as an afterdressing, oral drenching or rectal administration of suspensions or solutions of Mg salts, oral administration of Mg-containing gelatin capsules, or bolusing with a Mg alloy bullet for slow intraruminal release (Minson 1990d; Bacon et al. 1990; Robinson et al. 1989; Stuedemann et al. 1984). Because of its frequent association with other electrolyte abnormalities, treatment may also be required for these accompanying disorders. Thus, parenteral treatment of cattle with magnesium sulfate solutions is often followed by slow intravenous injection of 100-200 g Ca-Mg borogluconate, prepared by mixing 23% calcium borogluconate with 6% magnesium chloride solutions. Adverse effects on neuromuscular function have been observed in patients treated too rapidly with Mg-containing solutions, so caution should be exercised during rapid intravenous Mg replenishment.

Toxicity. Mg toxicosis has not been reported following consumption of natural feedstuffs and has been associated with excessive supplementation only from commercial sources. Chronic ingestion of low toxic levels of Mg has been associated with diarrhea, depressed nutrient utilization, and lower rates of growth in chicks, guinea pigs, calves, and sheep (NRC 1980; Chester-Jones et al. 1990a). Higher levels can cause anorexia, weight loss, severe diarrhea, impaired bone mineralization, lethargy, and progressive degeneration of the stratified squamous epithelium of the rumen papillae (NRC 1980; Chester-Jones et al. 1990b). Acute overdosage with Mg results in impaired motor function in horses, cattle, and dogs. In sheep and horses, respiratory paralysis, cyanosis, and cardiac arrest have also been observed (NRC 1980). Maximum tolerable dietary levels for Mg are approximately 0.50% in cattle and sheep and 0.30% in poultry and swine (NRC 1980). Intravenous administration of 0.028 g/kg body weight in horses, dogs, cattle, and sheep has produced clinical signs, recumbency, and death (NRC 1980). Oral administration of 1.5-2 times the recommended laxative dose of magnesium sulfate to horses with suspected intestinal impactions resulted in Mg toxicosis and may have been predisposed by renal insufficiency, hypocalcemia, and/or damaged intestinal integrity caused by vascular compromise or concurrent administration of dioctyl sodium sulfosuccinate (Henninger and Horst 1997). Minerals and other factors which depress GI Mg absorption will increase the tolerable limit of dietary Mg, and acute Mg intoxication can be alleviated by treatment with Ca salts such as calcium borogluconate.

Until recently a strong association was presumed between dietary Mg intake and the occurrence of feline lower urinary tract diseases (FLUTD), heretofore known under the catchall term of "feline urologic syndrome," or FUS. Experimental studies indicated a direct dose relationship between dietary Mg level and formation of magnesium ammonium phosphate (struvite) crystals, uroliths, and lower urinary tract obstruction (Lewis et al. 1978). Reassessment of this work revealed that the salt form of Mg used to supplement the experimental diets was magnesium oxide, a potent dietary alkalinizer. Subsequent studies have shown that dietary effects on urinary pH are substantially more important than the dietary intake and ensuing urinary excretion of Mg in predisposing cats to lower urinary tract disorders (Buffington et al. 1985). While the predominant form of crystal observed in naturally occurring cases of FLUTD is struvite, not all cases of FLUTD are associated with crystalluria or with any abnormalities of routine urinalysis (Buffington et al. 1997). Although dietary Mg and effects on acid-base metabolism are significant risk factors for FLUTD, other risk factors have included age, gender, season, weather, activity levels, and consumption of dry foods, and important findings have included mucus plug formation, urethral spasm, and viral or bacterial infections, none of which may be responsive to dietary manipulation, but all of which may interact to increase the relative risk for development of FLUTD (Buffington et al. 1997; Jones et al. 1997).

SULFUR

Source and Occurrence. Sulfur (S) in plants varies widely. Because sulfur-containing amino acids (SAA) are important, although minimal, components of all proteins, organic S levels tend to vary with nitrogen or crude protein content (NRC 1982). Thus, legumes contain more S than grasses, the leaf fraction contains more S than the stem, and total concentration decreases with plant maturity (Minson 1990e). SAA are produced by plants from inorganic sources of S absorbed from the soil. Plant S is found as SAA, elemental S, and sulfate salts of various cations. Commercial sources of S include those used for soil fertilization, food and pharmaceutical preservatives, dietary mineral supplements, fungicides, paper bleaches, fumigants, and sulfuric acids for industrial manufacture (NRC 1980).

Chemical Forms, Distribution, and Biological Characteristics. S is required for the synthesis of many S-containing compounds found in the body, including SAA (methionine, cysteine, cystine, taurine), some B vitamins (biotin, thiamine), structural compounds (chondroitin sulfate, proteins, glycosaminoglycans), and antioxidants (glutathione, cystathionine, cysteinylglycine). Disulfide bonds in some proteins play an important role in maintaining tertiary structure necessary for structural protein integrity or enzymatic activity. Conversely, oxidation of key sulfhydryl groups in other proteins produces mixed disulfide bridges, denaturation, and loss of function, as is seen in Heinz body formation from hemoglobin and membrane destabilization following oxidative free radical damage.

By virtue of microbial incorporation of inorganic S into amino acids, ruminants are capable of using a wide variety of dietary sources of S. Elemental sulfur, sodium sulfate, and DL-methionine were shown to result in similar increases in S retention in heifers fed a tall-fescue-based diet, although predominant routes of S excretion differed among treatments (Front et al. 1990). In sheep, dietary supplementation with sodium sulfate to approximately 2 g S/day resulted in approximately 50% absorbed and recycled through plasma sulfate (Kandylis and Bray 1987). In fact, it has been suggested that during dietary S deprivation, plasma sulfate recycled to the rumen via the saliva can significantly affect S balance in ruminants (Kandylis 1983). Monogastrics, on the other hand, must obtain all of their organic S in the form of exogenous SAA. However, all animals are capable of utilizing inorganic sulfates to some extent for the esterification of mucopolysaccharides and conjugation of xenobiotic metabolites for excretion. Sulfate ions are absorbed by a very efficient active transport mechanism in the small intestine, predominantly located in the ileum, and excess absorbed sulfate is predominantly excreted in the urine.

Several methods are available for the determination of S content in biological specimens. Ashed preparations or acid extracts of tissues and biological fluids may be analyzed by atomic absorption spectroscopy. Specific quantitation of sulfate ions can be done indirectly by turbidimetric spectrophotometry following precipitation with barium chloride, and directly by ion exchange chromatography or ion-specific electrode potentiometry. Reduced S, as sulfide, can be detected by paper chromatography or high-performance liquid chromatography following reaction with *p-N,N*-dimethylphenylenediamine to form methylene blue (Savage and Gould 1990).

Signs of Deficiency. S deficiency is most commonly manifest as a deficiency of SAA. Calves fed an elemental S-deficient diet for 1-2 months developed negative S balance, lower nitrogen balance, and significant weight loss compared to controls supplemented with elemental S (Slyter et al. 1988). Plasma levels of SAA, citrulline, and many nonessential amino acids decreased markedly, and GI and liver weights were reduced by dietary S deficiency. Similar findings were reported for sheep (Slyter et al. 1988). Studies of ruminal microflora in S-deficient calves and sheep have also found reduced rates of methanogenesis, fewer cellulolytic bacterial numbers, and increased numbers of facultative anaerobic bacteria (Slyter et al. 1986). Beef cattle grazed on oat-wheat small grain pastures following ammonium sulfate fertilization consumed greater amounts of dietary S and experienced marginally higher average daily rates of gain, although the economic analysis revealed lesser cost-effectiveness compared to urea fertilization without S (Hardt et al. 1991). S deprivation as dietary SAA deficiency has adverse effects on virtually every organ system, owing to negative nitrogen balance and reduced rates of protein synthesis, which affects all aspects of metabolism. Specific deficiency of taurine in cats, who are unique in their inability to synthesize this amino acid from other SAA, produces central retinal degeneration and dilatative cardiomyopathy and may adversely affect cellular K metabolism (Schmidt et al. 1976; Pion et al. 1987; Dow et al. 1992). Short-term fasting in healthy humans decreases the excretion of total S, inorganic sulfate, ester sulfate, methionine, cystathionine, cysteine, taurine, thiosulfate, and thiocyanate (Martensson 1982).

Dietary Requirements, Indications, and Use

INTRINSIC FACTORS. Requirements for S parallel those for protein and are greatest during pregnancy, growth, and lactation. Likewise, dietary requirements for S by Angora goats (0.27% DM) for the production of mohair appears to be similar to that of Alpine goats (0.26%) for the support of lactation (Qi et al. 1992a,b). Individual species differences are great in the amount required and form utilized. For example, ruminants utilize inorganic sources of S well, and nonruminants require most of their S as SAA. Cats have a much greater requirement for SAA than other animals and in addition require a dietary source of taurine (MacDonald et al. 1984). Other intrinsic factors that may affect the S requirement include GI diseases, in which absorption is depressed (or in ruminants where S fixation in proteins may be reduced); systemic diseases which increase the rate of protein catabolism and subsequent SAA elimination; oxidative stress due to inflammatory, neoplastic, or other toxic exposures which increase the rate of glutathione consumption for free radical quenching and xenobiotic biotransformation; and, in cats, K depletion due to chronic renal disease, which appears to increase dietary taurine requirements (Fettman 1991; Dow et al. 1992).

EXTRINSIC FACTORS. Considerable site and species-specific differences in plant S content can have significant effects on supplemental dietary S requirements in ruminants. Likewise, marked variation in biological value of proteins from both plant and animal sources can affect SAA content and subsequent supplemental dietary requirements for nonruminants, particularly in the case of carnivores. In ruminants, other dietary minerals like copper and molybdenum can form insoluble and unavailable complexes with S, thereby increasing these minerals' dietary requirements (Lesperance et al. 1985; Boila and Golfman 1991; Suttle 1991). Dietary levels of nonprotein nitrogen, like urea or ammonium salts, also increase the requirement for S in ruminants (Grieve et al. 1973a,b; Minson 1990e).

Preparations and Therapy. S is available in a variety of sulfate salts of ammonium, K, Na, etc., for use in crop fertilization but is unlikely to be administered either enterally or parenterally to individual animals for the sole purpose of replenishing a dietary S deficiency. Sulfate salts may be included in dairy rations to alter cation-anion balance to produce a greater degree of acidification in the prophylaxis of parturient hypocalcemia (Oetzel et al. 1991). A more common means of therapeutic administration of S would be as individual SAA or in high-quality protein sources in the nutritional support of critical-care patients who may require enteral hyperalimentation for maintenance or to replace losses incurred through accelerated protein catabolism. Immoderate SAA supplementation may have adverse effects owing to intestinal microbial conversion to encephalotoxic mercaptans, excessive systemic acidification through desulfuration and deamination processes, or through the toxic effects from metabolically derived sulfide, as described below (Maede et al. 1987).

Toxicity. S toxicity is highly dependent on the form and route of administration. Elemental S is relatively nontoxic, whereas hydrogen sulfide is as dangerous as cyanide, owing to its inhibitory effects on mitochondrial electron transport (NRC 1980). However, S toxicosis was reported in a large flock of sheep pastured on an alfalfa field 16 hours after the field had been sprayed with an aqueous 35% suspension of elemental S (Bulgin et al. 1996). Antemortem signs included obtundancy, convulsions, and prostration. Postmortem findings included a strong ruminal odor of rotten eggs and pulmonary edema, acutely, and polioencephalomalacia, chronically; consistent with sulfide toxicosis. Chronic, excessive dietary intake of S in ruminants as elemental S, sulfate salts, or as SAA decreases feed intake, depresses rumen microbial fermentation, and can reduce production performance (Kandylis 1984; NRC 1980). Dietary S in excess of 0.20% DM has been shown to have a detrimental effect on average daily gain, feed intake, and net energy value of the diet in finishing yearling heifers (Zinn et al. 1997).

Fermentative reduction of dietary S by ruminal microorganisms can produce signs of either acute or chronic sulfide toxicosis (Bulgin et al. 1996; Kandylis 1984; NRC 1980). Acute sulfide toxicosis may be seen as respiratory distress, central nervous depression, convulsions, and death. However, it has been suggested that rumen microorganisms must usually adapt to higher dietary sulfate content before they are capable of generating potentially toxic concentrations of sulfide (Cummings et al. 1995a,b). Chronic sulfide toxicosis may be characterized by depressed rumen motility, respiratory disease, anorexia, weight loss, and central nervous dysfunction. Much of this may be attributed to sulfide-induced polioencephalomalacia which resembles that produced by thiamine deficiency (Low et al. 1996; McAllister et al. 1992; Gould et al. 1991). Other dietary factors may influence susceptibility to S toxicity. Higher dietary levels of transition metal elements may afford some protection against sulfide toxicosis through precipitation as metal sulfide complexes (Gould et al. 1991; NRC 1980). In ruminants it appears that 0.40% of the diet dry matter is the maximum tolerable level for dietary S, other interacting factors aside (NRC 1980). Because high environmental temperatures will promote evaporative water loss and subsequent water consumption, it is likely that hot weather may precipitate sulfide toxicosis in regions where high-sulfate water is exclusively available to livestock. Up to 0.28% S has been fed to dogs as ammonium persulfate for 16 weeks without adverse effects, while rats have tolerated up to 0.69% total dietary S without effect (NRC 1980).

REFERENCES

Aines, P. D., Smith, S. E. 1957. Sodium versus chloride for the therapy of salt-deficient dairy cows. J Dairy Sci 40:682-688.

Anderson, F. P., Miller, G. W. 1987. Methods in Clinical Chemistry, pp. 73-77. St. Louis: C. V. Mosby.

Anderson, R. J., Gabow, P. A., Gross, P. A. 1984. Urinary chloride excretion in acute renal failure. Miner Electrolyte Metab 10:92-97.

Arnett, T. R., Boyde, A., Jones, S. J., Taylor. 1994. Effects of medium acidification by alteration of carbon dioxide or bicarbonate concentrations on the resorptive activity of rat osteoclasts. J Bone Miner Metab 9:375-379.

Bacon, J. A., Bell, M. C., Miller, J. K., Ramsey, N., Mueller, F. J. 1990. Effect of magnesium administration route on plasma minerals in Holstein calves receiving either adequate or insufficient magnesium in their diets. J Dairy Sci 73:470-473.

Barton, B. A., Jorgensen, N. A., DeLuca, H. F. 1987. Impact of prepartum dietary phosphorus intake on calcium homeostasis at parturition. J Dairy Sci 70:1186-1191.

Beck, N., Kim, H. P., Kim, K. S. 1975. Effect of metabolic acidosis on renal action of parathyroid hormone. Am J Physiol 228:1483-1488.

Belyea, R. L., Coppock, C. E., Lake, G. B. 1976. Effects of a low calcium diet on feed intake, milk production, and response to blood calcium challenge in lactating Holstein cows. J Dairy Sci 59:1068-1077.

Berl, T. 1990. Treating hyponatremia: damned if we do and damned if we don't. Kidn Intl 37:1006-1018.

Blackmon, D. M., Neathery, M. W., Miller, W. J., Brown, S. R., Crowell, W. A., McGurien, S. O., Gentry, R. P. 1984. Clinical aspects of experimentally induced chloride deficiency in Holstein calves. Am J Vet Res 45:1638-1640.

Block, E. 1984. Manipulating dietary anions and cations for prepartum dairy cows to reduce incidence of milk fever. J Dairy Sci 67:2939-2948.

Bodey, A. R., Michell, A. R. 1996. Epidemiological study of blood pressure in domestic dogs. J Sm Anim Pract 37:116-125.

Boila, R. J., Golfman, L. S. 1991. Effects of molybdenum and sulfur on digestion by steers. J Anim Sci 69:1626-1635.

Bolton, G. R. 1975. Handbook of Canine Electrocardiography, pp. 65-70. Philadelphia: W. B. Saunders.

Boyd, J. C., Bruns, D. E., Wills, M. R. 1983. Frequency of hypomagnesemia in hypokalemic states. Clin Chem 29:178-179.

Brown, R. C., Bidlack, W. R. 1991. Altered glucuronyl transferase activity in magnesium depleted rats. In L. S. Hurley, C. L. Keen, B. Lonnerdal, R. B. Rucker, eds., Trace Elements in Man and Animals, vol. 6, pp. 471-472. New York: Plenum Press.

Buffington, C. A., Chew, D. J., Kendall, M. S., Scrivani, P. V., Thompson, S. B., Blaisdell, J. L., Woodworth, B. E. 1997. Clinical evaluation of cats with nonobstructive urinary tract diseases. J Am Vet Med Assoc 210:46-50.

Buffington, C. A., Rogers, Q. R., Morris, J. G., Cook, N. E. 1985. Feline struvite urolithiasis: magnesium effect depends on urinary pH. Feline Pract 15:29-33.

Bulgin, M. S., Lincoln, S. D., Mather, G. 1996. Elemental sulfur toxicosis in a flock of sheep. J Am Vet Med Assoc 208:1063-1065.

Burkhalter, D. L., Neathery, M. W., Miller, W. J., Whitlock, R. H., Allen, J. C. 1979. Effects of low chloride intake on performance, clinical characteristics and chloride, sodium, potassium and nitrogen metabolism in dairy calves. J Dairy Sci 62:1895-1901.

Burnell, J. M., Teubner, E. 1971. Changes in bone sodium and carbonate in metabolic acidosis and alkalosis in the dog. J Clin Invest 50:327-331.

Bushinsky, D. A. 1995. Stimulated osteoclastic and suppressed osteoblastic activity in metabolic but not respiratory acidosis. Am J Physiol 268:C80-C88.

Call, J. W., Butcher, J. E., Shupe, J. L., Blake, J. T., Olson, A. E. 1986. Dietary phosphorus for beef cows. Am J Vet Res 47:475-481.

Call, J. W., Butcher, J. E., Shupe, J. L., Lamb, R. C., Bowman, R. L., Olson, A. E. 1987. Clinical effects of low dietary phosphorus concentrations in feed given to lactating dairy cows. Am J Vet Res 48:133-136.

Chester-Jones, H., Fontenot, J. P., Veit, H. P. 1990a. Physiological and pathological effects of feeding high levels of magnesium to steers. J Anim Sci 68:4400-4413.

Chester-Jones, H., Fontenot, J. P., Veit, H. P., Webb, K. E. 1990b. Physiological effects of feeding high levels of magnesium to sheep. J Anim Sci 67:1070-1081.

Chew, D. J., Leonard, M., Muir, W. 1989. Effect of sodium bicarbonate infusions on ionized calcium and total calcium concentrations in serum of clinically normal cats. Am J Vet Res 50:145-150.

Ching, S. V., Fettman, M. J., Hamar, D. W., Nogade, L. A., Smith, K. R. 1989. The effect of chronic dietary acidification using ammonium chloride on acid-base and mineral metabolism in the adult cat. J Nutr 119:902-915.

Ching, S. V., Norrdin, R. W., Fettman, M. J., LeCouteur, R. A. 1990. Trabecular bone remodeling and bone mineral density in the adult cat during chronic dietary acidification with ammonium chloride. J Bone Min Res 5:547-556.

Combs, N. R., Miller, E. R. 1985a. Development of an assay to determine the bioavailability of potassium in feedstuffs for the young pig. J Anim Sci 60:709-714.

———. 1985b. Determination of potassium availability in K_2CO_3, $KHCO_3$, corn, and soybean meal for the young pig. J Anim Sci 60:715-719.

Constable, P. D., St. Jean, G., Hull, B. L., Rings, D. M., Hoffsis, G. F. 1991. Preoperative prognostic indicators in cattle with abomasal volvulus. J Am Vet Med Assoc 198:2077-2085.

Coppock, C. E. 1986. Mineral utilization by the lactating cow—chlorine. J Dairy Sci 69:595-603.

Coppock, C. E., Everett, R. W., Belyea, R. L. 1976. Effect of low calcium or low phosphorus diets on free choice consumption of dicalcium phosphate by lactating dairy cows. J Dairy Sci 59:571-580.

Coppock, C. E., and Fettman, M. J. 1977. Chloride as required nutrient for lactating cows. Proc Cornell Nutr Conf, pp. 43-52.

Coppock, C. E., Grant, P. A., Portzer, S. J., Charles, D. A., Escobosa, A. 1982b. Lactating dairy cow responses to dietary sodium, chloride, and bicarbonate during hot weather. J Dairy Sci 65:566-576.

Coppock, C. E., Grant, P. A., Portzer, S. J., Escobosa, A., Wehrly, T. E. 1982a. Effect of varying dietary ratio of sodium and chloride on the responses of lactating dairy cows in hot weather. J Dairy Sci 65:552-565.

Coppock, C. E., Windle, L. M., Wilks, D. L., Woelfel, C. G., Greene, L. W. 1988. Addition of salt to cattle diets based on sodium and chloride in feedstuffs and drinking water. J Anim Sci 66:1592-1597.

Correa, J. E., Calderin, G. G. 1966. Anhidrosis, dry coat syndrome in the Thoroughbred. J Am Vet Med Assoc 149:1556-1560.

Cromwell, G. L., Coffey, R. D., Monegue, H. J., Randolph, J. H. 1995a. Efficacy of low-activity, microbial phytase in improving bioavailability of phosphorus in corn-soybean meal diets for pigs. J Anim Sci 73:449-456.

Cromwell, G. L., Coffey, R. D., Parker, G. R., Monegue, H. J., Randolph, J. H. 1995b. Efficacy of a recombinant-derived phytase in improving bioavailability of phosphorus in corn-soybean meal diets for pigs. J Anim Sci 73:2000-2008.

Crowe, N. A., Neathery, M. W., Miller, W. J., Muse, L. A., Crowe, C. T., Varnadoe, J. L., Blackmon, D. M. 1990. Influence of high dietary aluminum on performance and phosphorus bioavailability in dairy calves. J Dairy Sci 73:808-818.

Cummings, BA, Caldwell, DR, Gould, DH, Hamar, DW. 1995a. Identity and interactions of rumen microbes associated with dietary sulfate-induced polioencephalomalacia in cattle. Am J Vet Res 56:1384-1389.

Cummings, B. A., Gould, D. H., Caldwell, D. R., Hamar, D. W. 1995b. Ruminal microbial alterations associated with sulfide generation in steers with dietary sulfate-induced polioencephalomalacia. Am J Vet Res 56:1390-1395.

Cummings, S. R., Black, D. M., Nevitt, M. C., Browner, W. S., Cauley, J. A., Genant, H. K., Mascioli, S. R., Scott, J. C., Seeley, D. G., Steiger, P., Vogt, T. M., and the Study of Osteoporotic Fractures Research Group. 1990. J Amer Med Assoc 263:665-668.

Cunha, T. J. 1991a. Horse Feeding and Nutrition, pp. 98-113. 2nd ed. New York: Academic Press.

———. 1991b. Horse Feeding and Nutrition, pp. 113-19. 2nd ed. New York: Academic Press.

Cymbaluk, N. F., Christison, G. I. 1989. Effects of dietary energy and phosphorus content on blood chemistry and development of growing horses. J Anim Sci 67:951-958.

Davenport, G. M., Boling, J. A., Gay, N. 1990. Bioavailability of magnesium in beef cattle fed magnesium oxide or magnesium hydroxide. J Anim Sci 68:3765-3772.

Dennis, R. J., Hemken, R. W. 1978. Potassium requirement of dairy cows in early and mid-lactation. J Dairy Sci 61:757-761.

Denton, D. A., Sabine, J. R. 1961. The selective appetite for Na shown by Na-deficient sheep. J Physiol 157:97-116.

Devlin, T. J., Roberts, W. K., St. Osmer, V. V. 1969. Effects of dietary potassium upon growth, serum electrolytes, and intrarumen environment of finishing beef steers. J Anim Sci 28:557.

Dirks, J. H. 1983. The kidney and magnesium regulation. Kidn Intl 23:771-777.

Dodds, W. J. 1989. Hemostasis. In J. J. Kaneko, ed., Clinical Biochemistry of Domestic Animals, 4th ed., pp. 274-315. New York: Academic Press.

Dow, S. W., Fettman, M. J., Curtis, C. R., LeCouteur, R. A. 1989. Hypokalemia in cats: 186 cases (1984-1987). J Am Vet Med Assoc 194:1604-1608.

Dow, S. W., Fettman, M. J., LeCouteur, R. A. 1988. Muscle weakness syndrome of cats: results of an owner and veterinarian questionnaire. Comp Anim Pract 2(10):11-14.

Dow, S. W., Fettman, M. J., LeCouteur, R. A., Hamar, D. W. 1987b. Potassium depletion in cats: renal and dietary influences. J Am Vet Med Assoc 191:1569-1575.

Dow, S. W., Fettman, M. J., Smith, K. R., Ching, S. V., Hamar, D. W., Rogers, Q. R. 1992. Dietary potassium depletion and acidification induces taurine depletion and cardiovascular disease in adult cats. Am J Vet Res 53:402-405.

Dow, S. W., Fettman, M. J., Smith, K. R., Hamar, D. W., Nogade, L. A., Refsal, K., Wilke, W. L. 1990. Effects of dietary acidification and potassium depletion on acid-base balance, mineral metabolism, and renal function in adult cats. J Nutr 120:569-578.

Dow, S. W., LeCouteur, R. A., Fettman, M. J., Spurgeon, T. L. 1987a. Potassium depletion in cats: hypokalemic polymyopathy. J Am Vet Med Assoc 191:1563-1568.

Elin, R. J. 1987. Assessment of magnesium status. Clin Chem 33:1965-1970.

Elliott, P., Stamler, J., Nichols, R., Dyer, A. R., Stamler, R., Kesteloot, H., Marmot, M. 1996. Intersalt revisited: further analyses of 24 hour sodium excretion and blood pressure within and across populations. Brit Med J 312:1249-1253.

Emanuele, S. M., Staples, C. R. 1990. Ruminal release of minerals from six forage species. J Anim Sci 68:2052-2060.

Erdman, R. A., Hemken, R. W., Bull, L. S. 1980. Effect of dietary calcium and sodium on potassium requirement for lactating dairy cows. J Dairy Sci 63:538-544.

Farrell, E. C. 1987. Methods in Clinical Chemistry. St. Louis: C. V. Mosby. a: chapter 130, pp. 1003-1009; b: chapter 134, pp. 1038-1042; c: chapter 132, pp. 1021-1026.

Fettman, M. J. 1989. Feline kaliopenic polymyopathy/nephropathy syndrome. Vet Clin N Amer Sm Anim Pract 19:415-432.

———. 1991. Comparative aspects of glutathione metabolism affecting individual susceptibility to oxidant injury. Comp Cont Educ Prac Vet 13:1079-1091.

Fettman, M. J., Chase, L. E., Bentinck-Smith, J., Coppock, C. E., Zinn, S. A. 1984a. Effects of dietary chloride restriction in lactating dairy cows. J Am Vet Med Assoc 185:167-172.

———. 1984b. Restricted dietary chloride with sodium bicarbonate supplementation for Holstein cows in early lactation. J Dairy Sci 67:1457-1467.

———. 1984c. Nutritional chloride deficiency in early lactation Holstein cows. J Dairy Sci 67:2321-2335.

Fettman, M. J., Coble, J. M., Hamar, D. W., Norrdin, R. W., Seim, H. B., Kealy, R. D., Rogers, Q. R., McCrea, K., Moffat, K. 1992. Effect of dietary phosphoric acid supplementation on acid-base balance and mineral and bone metabolism in adult cats. Am J Vet Res 53:2125-2135.

Finco, D. R., Brown S. A., Crowell, W. A., Groves, C. A., Duncan, J. R., Barsanti, J. A. 1992. Effects of Pi/calcium-restricted and Pi/calcium-replete 32% protein diets in dogs with chronic renal failure. Am J Vet Res 53:157-163.

Flanders, J. A., Scarlett, J. M., Blue, J. T., Neth, S. 1989. Adjustment of total serum calcium concentration for binding to albumin and protein in cats: 291 cases (1986-1987). J Am Vet Med Assoc 194:1609-1611.

Fontenot, J. P., Allen, V. G., Bunce, G. E., Goff, J. P. 1989. Factors influencing magnesium absorption and metabolism in ruminants. J Anim Sci 67:3445-3455.

Fredeen, A. H., DePeters, E. J., Baldwin, R. L. 1988a. Characterization of acid-base disturbances and effects on calcium and phosphorus balances of dietary fixed ions in pregnant or lactating does. J Anim Sci 66:159-173.

———. 1988b. Effects of acid-base disturbances caused by differences in dietary fixed ion balance on kinetics of calcium metabolism in ruminants with high calcium demand. J Anim Sci 66:174-184.

Front, M. J., Boling, J. A., Bush, L. P., Dawson, K. A. 1990. Sulfur and nitrogen metabolism in the bovine fed different forms of supplemental sulfur. J Anim Sci 68:543-552.

Fulton, R. B., Fruechte, L. K. 1991. Poisoning induced by administration of a phosphate-containing urinary acidifier in a cat. J Am Vet Med Assoc 198:883-885.

Garry, F. B., Hull, B. L., Rings, D. M., Hoffsis, G. 1988. Comparison of naturally occurring proximal duodenal obstruction and abomasal volvulus in dairy cattle. Vet Surg 17:226-233.

Giduck, S. A., Fontenot, J. P. 1987. Utilization of magnesium and other macrominerals in sheep supplemented with different readily fermentable carbohydrates. J Anim Sci 65:1667-1673.

Goff, J. P., Horst, R. L. 1997. Effects of the addition of potassium or sodium, but not calcium, to prepartum rations on milk fever in dairy cows. J Dairy Sci 80:176-186.

Golz, D. I., Crenshaw, T. D. 1990. Interrelationships of dietary sodium, potassium, and chloride on growth in young swine. J Anim Sci 68:2736-2747.

———. 1991. The effect of dietary potassium and chloride on cation-anion balance in swine. J Anim Sci 69:2504-2515.

Gould, D. H., McAllister, M. M., Savage, J. C., Hamar, D. W. 1991. High sulfide concentrations in rumen fluid associated with nutritionally induced polioencephalomalacia in calves. Am J Vet Res 52:1164-1169.

Greco, D. S., Lees, G. E., Dzendzel, G. S., Komkov, A., Carter, A. B. 1994a. Effect of dietary sodium intake on glomerular filtration rate in partially nephrectomized dogs. Am J Vet Res 55:152-159.

Greco, D. S., Lees, G. E., Dzendzel, G. S., Carter, A. B. 1994b. Effects of dietary sodium intake on blood pressure measurements in partially nephrectomized dogs. Am J Vet Res 55:160-165.

Greene, L. W., Fontenot, J. P., Webb, K. E. 1983. Effect of dietary potassium on absorption of magnesium and other macroelements in sheep fed different levels of magnesium. J Anim Sci 56:1208-1213.

Greene, L. W., Schelling, G. T., Byers, F. M. 1986. Effects of dietary monensin and potassium on apparent absorption of magnesium and other macroelements in sheep. J Anim Sci 62:1960-1967.

Grieve, D. G., Coppock, C. E., Merrill, W. G., Tyrrell, H. F. 1973a. Sulfur supplementation of urea-containing silages and concentrates. I. Feed intake and lactation performance. J Dairy Sci 56:218-223.

Grieve, D. G., Merrill, W. G., Coppock, C. E. 1973b. Sulfur supplementation of urea-containing silages and concentrates. II. Ration digestibility, nitrogen, and sulfur balances. J Dairy Sci 56:224-228.

Grings, E. E., Males, J. R. 1987. Effects of potassium on macromineral absorption in sheep fed wheat straw-based diets. J Anim Sci 64:872-879.

Grubb, T. L., Foreman, J. H., Benson, G. J., Thurmon, J. C., Tranquilli, W. J., Constable, P. D., Olson, W. O., Davis, L. E. 1996. Hemodynamic effects of calcium gluconate administered to conscious horses. J Vet Int Med 10:401-404.

Grunes, D. L., Welch, R. M. 1989. Plant contents of magnesium, calcium, and potassium in relation to ruminant nutrition. J Anim Sci 67:3485-3494.

Haggard, D. L., Whitehair, C. K., Langham, R. F. 1978. Tetany associated with magnesium deficiency in suckling beef calves. J Amer Vet Med Assoc 172:495-497.

Hall, J. E., Guyton, A. C., Smith, M. J., Coleman, T. G. 1980. Blood pressure and renal function during chronic changes in sodium intake: role of angiotensin. Am J Physiol 239:F271-F280.

Hamill-Ruth, R. J., McGory, R. 1996. Magnesium repletion and its effect on potassium homeostasis in critically ill adults: results of a double-blind, randomized, controlled trial. Crit Care Med 24:38-45.

Hardt, P. F., Ocumpaugh, W. R., Greene, L. W. 1991. Forage mineral concentration, animal performance, and mineral status of heifers grazing cereal pastures fertilized with sulfur. J Anim Sci 69:2310-2320.

Hardwick, L. L., Jones, M. R., Brautbar, N., Lee, D. B. N 1991. Magnesium absorption: mechanisms and the influence of vitamin D, calcium, and phosphate. J Nutr 121:13-23.

Harvey, J. W. 1989. In J. J. Kaneko, ed., Clinical Biochemistry of Domestic Animals, pp. 204-205. New York: Academic Press.

Hebert, P., Mehta, N., Wang, J., Hindmarsh, T., Jones, G., Cardinal, P. 1997. Functional magnesium deficiency in critically ill patients identified using a magnesium-loading test. Crit Care Med 25:749-755.

Henninger, R. W., Horst, J. 1997. Magnesium toxicosis in two horses. J Am Vet Med Assoc 211:82-85.

Hills, D. L., Morris, J. G., Rogers, Q. R. 1982. Potassium requirement of kittens as affected by dietary protein. J Nutr 112:216-222.

Hoffsis, G. F., Saint-Jean, G., Rings, D. M. 1989. Hypomagnesemia in ruminants. Comp Cont Educ Prac Vet 11:519-526.

Honeyfield, D. C., Froseth, J. A., Barke, R. J. 1985. Dietary sodium and chloride levels for growing-finishing pigs. J Anim Sci 60:691-698.

Hurley, L. A., Greene, L. W., Byers, F. M., Carstens, G. E. 1990. Site and extent of apparent magnesium absorption by lambs fed different sources of magnesium. J Anim Sci 68:2181-2187.

Hutcheson, D. P., Cole, N. A., McLaren, J. B. 1984. Effects of pretransit diets and post-transit potassium levels for feeder calves. J Anim Sci 58:700-707.

Jensen, J., Henik, R. A., Brownfield, M., Armstrong, J. 1997. Plasma renin activity and angiotensin I and aldosterone concentrations in cats with hypertension associated with chronic renal disease. Am J Vet Res 58:535-540.

Jones, B. R., Sanson, R. L., Morris, R. S. 1997. Elucidating the risk factors of feline lower urinary tract disease. New Zeal Vet J 45:100-108.

Jorgensen, L. S., Center, S. A., Randolph, J. F., Brum, D. 1985. Electrolyte abnormalities induced by hypertonic phosphate enemas in two cats. J Am Vet Med Assoc 187:1367-1368.

Kandylis, K. 1983. Transfer of plasma sulfate from blood to rumen: a review. J Dairy Sci 66:2263-2270.

———. 1984. Toxicology of sulfur in ruminants: review. J. Dairy Sci 67:2179-2187.

Kandylis, K., Bray, A. C. 1987. Effects of variation of dietary sulfur on movement of sulfur in sheep rumen. J Dairy Sci 70:40-49.

Kohn, C. W., Brooks, C. L. 1990. Failure of pH to predict ionized calcium percentage in healthy horses. Am J Vet Res 51:1206-1210.

Korzun, W. J., Miller, W. G. 1987. Methods in Clinical Chemistry, pp. 86-93. St. Louis: C. V. Mosby.

Krieger, N. S., Sessler, N. E., Bushinsky, D. A. 1992. Acidosis inhibits osteoblastic and stimulates osteoclastic activity in vitro. Am J Physiol 262:F442-F448.

Kroll, M. H., Elin, R. J. 1985. Relationships between magnesium and protein concentrations in serum. Clin Chem 31:244-246.

Leibholz, J. M., McCall, J. T., Hays, V. W., Speer, V. C. 1966. Potassium, protein, and basic amino acid relationships in swine. J Anim Sci 25:37.

Lemann, J., Gray, R. W., Pleuss, J. A. 1989. Potassium bicarbonate, but not sodium bicarbonate, reduces urinary calcium excretion and improves calcium balance in healthy men. Kidn Intl 35:688-695.

Lesperance, A. L., Bohman, V. R., Oldfield, J. E. 1985. Interaction of molybdenum, sulfate, and alfalfa in the bovine. J Anim Sci 60:791-802.

Lewis, L. D., Chow, F. H. C., Taton, G. F., Hamar, D. W. 1978. Effect of various dietary mineral concentrations on the occurrence of feline urolithiasis. J Am Vet Med Assoc 172:559-563.

Littman, M. P., Robertson, J. L., Bovee, K. C. 1988. Spontaneous systemic hypertension in dogs: five cases (1981-1983). J Am Vet Med Assoc 193:486-494.

Lough, D. S., Beede, D. K., Wilcox, C. J. 1990. Lactational response to and in vitro ruminal solubility of magnesium oxide or magnesium chelate. J Dairy Sci 73:413-424.

Low, J. C., Scott, P. R., Howie, F., Lewis, M., FitzSimmons, J., Spence, J. A. 1996. Sulphur-induced polioencephalomalacia in lambs. Vet Rec 138:327-329.

MacDonald, M. L., Rogers, Q. R., Morris, J. G. 1984. Nutrition of the domestic cat, a mammalian carnivore. Ann Rev Nutr 4:521-562.

Maede, Y., Hoshino, T., Inaba, M., Namioka, S. 1987. Methionine toxicosis in cats. Am J Vet Res 48:289-292.

Maenpaa, P. H., Pirskanen, A., Koskinen, E. 1988. Biochemical indicators of bone formation in foals after transfer from pasture to stables for the winter months. Am J Vet Res 49:1990-1992.

Mahan, D. C. 1982. Dietary calcium and phosphorus levels for weanling swine. J Anim Sci 54:559-564.

Mahan, D. C., Newton, E. A., Cera, K. R. 1996. Effect of supplemental sodium chloride, sodium phosphate, or hydrochloric acid in starter pig diets containing dried whey. J Anim Sci 74:1217-1222.

Mallonee, P. G., Beede, D. K., Collier, R. J., Wilcox, C. J. 1985. Production and physiological responses of dairy cows to varying dietary potassium during heat stress. J Dairy Sci 68:1479-1487.

Martensson, J. 1982. The effects of short-term fasting on the excretion of sulfur compounds in healthy subjects. Metabolism 31:487-492.

Mayhew, I. G., Ferguson, H. O. 1987. Clinical, clinicopathologic, and epidemiologic features of anhidrosis in central Florida Thoroughbred horses. J Vet Int Med 1:136-141.

McAllister, M. M., Gould, D. H., Hamar, D. W. 1992. Sulphide-induced polioencephalomalacia in lambs. J Comp Path 106:267-278.

McDowell, L. R. 1989. Vitamins in Animal Nutrition: Comparative Aspects to Human Nutrition, pp. 55-92. New York: Academic Press.

Meuten, D. J., Chew, D. J., Capen, C. C., Kociba, G. J. 1982. Relationship of serum total calcium to albumin and total protein in dogs. J Am Vet Med Assoc 180:63-67.

Midgley, J. P., Matthew, A. G., Greenwood, C. M. T., Logan, A. G. 1996. Effect of reduced dietary sodium on blood pressure: a meta-analysis of randomized controlled trials. J Am Med Assoc 275:1590-1597.

Miller, W. J., Neathery, M. W., Gentry, R. P., Blackmon, D. M., Crowe, C. T., Ware, G. O., Fielding, A. S. 1987. Bioavailability of phosphorus from defluorinated and dicalcium phosphates and phosphorus requirement of calves. J Dairy Sci 70:1885-1892.

Minson, D. J. 1990. Forage in Ruminant Nutrition. New York: Academic Press. a: chapter 7, pp. 208-229; b: chapter 8, pp.230-264; c: chapter 10, pp. 291-309; d: chapter 9, pp. 265-290; e: chapter 6, pp. 162-207.

Morris, J. G. 1980. Assessment of sodium requirements of grazing beef cattle: a review. J Anim Sci 50:145-152.

Morse, D., Head, H. H., Wilcox, C. J. 1992a. Disappearance of phosphorus in phytate from concentrates in vitro and from rations fed to lactating dairy cows. J Dairy Sci 75:1979-1986.

Morse, D., Head, H. H., Wilcox, C. J., van Horn, H. H., Hissem, C. D., Harris, B. 1992b. Effects of concentration of dietary phosphorus on amount and route of excretion. J Dairy Sci 75:3039-3049.

Murry, A. C., Lewis, R. D., Amos, H. E. 1997. The effect of microbial phytase in a pearl millet-soybean meal diet on apparent digestibility and retention of nutrients, serum mineral concentration, and bone mineral density of nursery pigs. J Anim Sci 75:1284-1291.

Neathery, M. W., Crowe, N. A., Miller, W. J., Crowe, C. T., Varnadoe, J. L., Blackmon, D. M. 1990. Effect of dietary aluminum and phosphorus on magnesium metabolism in dairy calves. J Anim Sci 68:1133-1138.

Neathery, M. W., Pugh, D. G., Miller, W. J., Gentry, R. P., Whitlock, R. H. 1980. Effects of sources and amounts of potassium on feed palatability and on potassium toxicity in dairy calves. J Dairy Sci 63:82-85.

Neathery, M. W., Pugh, D. G., Miller, W. J., Whitlock, R. H., Gentry, R. P., Allen, J. C. 1979. Potassium toxicity and acid-base balance from large oral doses of potassium to young calves. J Dairy Sci 62:1758-1765.

NRC. 1980. Mineral Tolerance of Animals. Washington, DC: National Academy of Sciences—National Research Council.

———. 1982. United States—Canadian Tables of Feed Composition. 3rd ed. Washington, DC: National Academy of Sciences—National Research Council.

———. 1988. Nutrient Requirements of Swine. 9th ed. Washington, DC: National Academy of Sciences—National Research Council.

Obel, A. O. 1989. Placebo-controlled trial of potassium supplements in black patients with mild essential hypertension. J Cardiovasc Pharmacol 14:294-296.

Oetzel, G. R. 1996. Effect of calcium chloride gel treatment in dairy cows on incidence of periparturient diseases. J Am Vet Med Assoc 209:958-961.

Oetzel, G. R., Fettman, M. J., Hamar, D. W., Olson, J. D. 1991. Screening of anionic salts for palatability effects on acid-base status, and urinary calcium excretion in dairy cows. J Dairy Sci 74:965-971.

Ogawa, E., Kobayashi, K., Yoshiura, N., Mukai, J. 1989a. Bovine postparturient hemoglobinemia: hypophosphatemia and metabolic disorder in red blood cells. Am J Vet Res 48:1300-1303.

———. 1989b. Hemolytic anemia and red blood cell metabolic disorder attributable to low phosphorus intake in cows. Am J Vet Res 50:388-392.

Peoples, J. B. 1988. The role of pH in altering serum ionized calcium concentration. Surgery 104:370-374.

Pion, P. D., Kittleson, M. D., Rogers, Q. R., Morris, J. G. 1987. Myocardial failure in cats associated with low plasma taurine: a reversible cardiomyopathy. Science 237:764-768.

Poe, J. H., Greene, L. W., Schelling, G. T., Byers, F. M., Ellis, W. C. 1985. Effects of dietary potassium and sodium on magnesium utilization in sheep. J Anim Sci 60:578-582.

Pradham, K., Hemken, R. W. 1968. Potassium depletion in lactating dairy cows. J Dairy Sci 51:1377.

Qi, K., Lu, C. D., Owens, F. N. 1992a. Sulfate supplementation of Alpine goats: effects on milk yield and composition, metabolites, nutrient digestibilities, and acid-base balance. J Anim Sci 70:2828-2837.

Qi, K., Lu, C. D., Owens, F. N., Lupton, C. J. 1992b. Sulfate supplementation of Angora goats: metabolic and mohair responses. J Anim Sci 70:3541-3550.

Reddy, G. S., Jones, G., Kooh, S. W., Fraser, D. 1982. Inhibition of 25-hydroxyvitamin D_3-1-hydroxylase by chronic metabolic acidosis. Am J Physiol 243:E265-E271.

Rehal, N. N., Cecco, S. A., Niemela, J. E., Hristova, E. N., Elin, R. J. 1996. Linearity and stability of the AVL and Nova magnesium and calcium ion-selective electrodes. Clin Chem 42:880-887.

Reinhart, G. A., Mahan, D. C. 1986. Effect of various calcium:phosphorus ratios at low and high dietary phosphorus for starter, grower, and finishing swine. J Anim Sci 63:457-466.

Reinhart, R. A. 1988. Magnesium metabolism. Arch Int Med 148:2415-2420.

Remillard, R. L., Ross, J. N., Eddy, J. B. 1991. Variance of indirect blood pressure measurements and prevalence of hypertension in clinically normal dogs. Am J Vet Res 52:561-565.

Robinson, D. L., Kappel, L. C., Boling, J. A. 1989. Management practices to overcome the incidence of grass tetany. J Anim Sci 67:3470-3484.

Rocchini, A. P., Moorehead, C. P., DeRemer, S., Bondie, D. 1989. Pathogenesis of weight-related changes in blood pressure in dogs. Hypertension 13:922-928.

Roudebush, P., Allen, T. A., Kuehn, N. F., Magerkurth, J. H., Bowers, T. L. 1994. The effect of combined therapy with captopril, furosemide, and a sodium-restricted diet on serum electrolyte concentrations and renal function in normal dogs and dogs with congestive heart failure. J Vet Int Med 8:337-342.

Savage, J. C., Gould, D. H. 1990. Determination of sulfide in brain tissue and rumen fluid by ion-interaction reversed phase high performance liquid chromatography. J Chromatography 526:540-545.

Schmidt, S. Y., Berson, E. L., Hayes, K. C. 1976. Retinal degeneration in cats fed casein. I. Taurine deficiency. Invest Ophthalmol 15:47-52.

Schneider, P. L., Beede, D. K., Wilcox, C. J. 1986. Responses of lactating cows to dietary sodium source and quantity and potassium quantity during heat stress. J Dairy Sci 69:99-110.

Schryver, H. F., Parker, M. T., Daniluk, P. D., Pagan, K. I., Williams, J., Soderholm, L. V., Hintz, H. F. 1987. Salt consumption and the effect of salt on mineral metabolism in horses. Cornell Vet 77:122-131.

Schuette, S. A., Yasillo, N. J., Thompson, C. M. 1991. The effect of carbohydrates in milk on absorption of calcium by postmenopausal women. J Am Coll Nutr 10:132-139.

Sebastian, A., Harris, S. T., Ottaway, J. H., Todd, K. M., Morris, R. C. 1994. Improved mineral balance and skeletal metabolism in post-menopausal women treated with potassium bicarbonate. New Engl J Med 330:1776-1781.

Shalit, U., Maltz, E., Silanikove, N., Berman, A. 1991. Water, sodium, potassium, and chlorine metabolism of dairy cows at the onset of lactation in hot weather. J Dairy Sci 74:1874-1883.

Shupe, J. L., Butcher, J. E., Call, J. W., Olson, A. E., Blake, J. T. 1988. Clinical signs and bone changes associated with phosphorus deficiency in beef cattle. Am J Vet Res 49:1629-1636.

Slyter, L. L., Chalupa, W., Oltjen, R. R. 1988. Response to elemental sulfur by calves and sheep fed purified diets. J Anim Sci 66:1016-1027.

Slyter, L. L., Chalupa, W., Oltjen, R. R., Weaver, J. M. 1986. Sulfur influences on rumen microorganisms in vitro and in sheep and calves. J Anim Sci 63:1949-1959.

Smith, D. F. 1978. Right-side torsion of the abomasum in dairy cows: classification of severity and evaluation of outcome. J Am Vet Med Assoc 173:108-111.

Smith, S. E., Aines, P. D. 1959. Salt Requirements of Dairy Cows. Cornell Univ Agricultural Experiment Station Bull 938.

Sprague, S. M., Krieger, N. S., Bushinsky, D. A. 1994. Greater inhibition of in vitro bone mineralization with metabolic than respiratory acidosis. Kidn Intl 46:1199-1206.

Stewart, A. F., Broadus, A. E. 1987. Mineral metabolism. In P. Felig, J. D. Baxter, A. E. Broadus, L. A. Fruhman, eds., Endocrinology and Metabolism, 2nd ed., pp. 1317-1453. New York: McGraw-Hill.

Stookey, G. K., Warrick, J. M., Miller, L. L. 1995. Effect of sodium hexametaphosphate on dental calculus formation in dogs. Am J Vet Res 56:913-918.

Stowe, H. D. 1971. Effects of potassium in a purified equine diet. J. Nutr 101:629.

Stuedemann, J. A., Wilkinson, S. R., Lowrey, R. S. 1984. Efficacy of a large magnesium alloy rumen bolus in the prevention of hypomagnesemic tetany in cows. Am J Vet Res 45:698-702.

Suttle, N. F. 1991. The interactions between copper, molybdenum, and sulphur in ruminant nutrition. Ann Rev Nutr 11:121-140.

Taylor, A. K., Linkhart, S., Mohan, S., Christenson, R. A., Singer, F. R., Baylink, D. J. 1990. Multiple osteocalcin fragments in human urine and serum as detected by a midmolecule osteocalcin radioimmunoassay. J Clin Endo Metab 70:467-472.

Thatcher, C. D. 1991. Nutritional aspects of developmental orthopedic disease in growing horses. Vet Med, July:743-747.

Toffaletti, J. G. 1987. In Methods in Clinic Chemistry, pp. 1010-20. St. Louis: C. V. Mosby.

Tucker, W. B., Xin, Z., Hemken, R. W. 1991. Influence of calcium chloride on systemic acid-base status and calcium metabolism in dairy heifers. J Dairy Sci 74:1401-1407.
Tyler, R. D., Qualls, C. W., Heald, R. D., Cowell, R. L., Clinkenbeard , K. D. 1987. Renal concentrating ability in dehydrated hyponatremic dogs. J Am Vet Med Assoc 191:1095-1100.
Ward, G., Harbers, L. H., Blaha, J. J. 1979. Calcium-containing crystals in alfalfa. J Dairy Sci 62:715-723.
Ward, G. M. 1978. Nutrient deficiencies in animals: potassium. In CRC Handbook of Nutrition and Food, pp. 245-257.
Weil, A. B., Tucker, W. B., Hemken, R. W. 1988. Potassium requirement of dairy calves. J Dairy Sci 71:1868-1872.
Welch, M. M., Hamar, D. W., Fettman, M. J. 1990. Method comparison for calcium determination by flame atomic absorption spectrophotometry in the presence of phosphate. Clin Chem 36:351-354.
West, D. B., Wehberg, K. E., Kieswetter, K., Granger, J. P. 1992. Blunted natriuretic response to an acute sodium load in obese hypertensive dogs. Hypertension 19(Suppl):I96-I100.
West, J. W., Mullinix, B. G., Sandifer, T. G. 1991. Changing dietary electrolyte balance for dairy cows in cool and hot environments. J Dairy Sci 74:1662-1674.
Whang, R., Flink, E. B., Dyckner, T., Wester, P. O., Aikawa, J. K., Ryan, M. P. 1985. Magnesium depletion as a cause of refractory potassium repletion. Arch Int Med 145:1686-1689.
Whang, R., Oei, T. O., Aikawa, J. K., Watanabe, A., Vannatta, J., Fryer, A., Markanich, M. 1984. Predictors of clinical hypomagnesemia. Arch Int Med 144:1794-1796.
Whelton, P. K., He, J., Cutler, J. A., Brancati, F. L., Appel, L. J., Follmann, D., Klag, M. J. 1997. Effect of oral potassium on blood pressure: meta-analysis of randomized controlled clinical trials. J Am Med Assoc 277:1624-1632.
Whitlock, R. H., Kesler, M. J., Tasker, J. B. 1975. Salt (sodium) deficiency in dairy cattle: polyuria and polydipsia as prominent clinical features. Cornell Vet 65:512-526.
Wong, S. T., Spoo, J., Kerst, K. C., Spring, T. G. 1985. Colorimetric determination of potassium in whole blood, serum, and plasma. Clin Chem 31:1464-1467.
Yen, J. T., Pond, W. G., Prior, R. L. 1981. Calcium chloride as a regulator of feed intake and weight gain in pigs. J Anim Sci 52:778-782.
Yi, Z., Kornegay, E. T., Ravindran, V., Lindemann, M. D., Wilson, J. H. 1996. Effectiveness of Natuphos® phytase in improving the bioavailabilities of phosphorus and other nutrients in soybean meal-based semipurified diets for young pigs. J Anim Sci 74:1601-1611.
Zarich, S., Fang, L. S. T, Diamond, J. R. 1985. Fractional excretion of sodium. Arch Int Med 145:108-112.
Zinn, R. A., Alvarez, E., Mendez, M., Montano, M., Ramirez, E., Shen, Y. 1997. Influence of dietary sulfur level on growth performance and digestive function in feedlot cattle. J Anim Sci 75:1723-1728.
Zinn, R. A., Shen, Y., Adam, C. F., Tamayo, M., Rosalez, J. 1996. Influence of dietary magnesium level on metabolic and growth-performance responses of feedlot cattle to laidlomycin propionate. J Anim Sci 74:1462-1469.

38

TRACE ELEMENTS AND MISCELLANEOUS NUTRIENTS

MARTIN J. FETTMAN

Chromium
Cobalt
Copper
Fluorine
Iodine
Iron
Manganese
Molybdenum
Selenium
Vanadium
Zinc
Essential Fatty Acids
Taurine
Glutamine

CHROMIUM

Source and Occurrence. Chromium (Cr) occurs in three valency states as Cr(II), Cr(III), and Cr(VI). The trivalent and hexavalent forms are most stable, while Cr(II) is rapidly oxidized to Cr(III). Meats, grains, and brewer's yeast contain chromium, principally as Cr(III) (NRC 1982). Cr bioavailability appears to be greater from natural sources or supplemental $CrCl_3$ than from other salt forms such as chromium acetate but is nevertheless poorly absorbed from the gastrointestinal(GI) tract regardless of nutritional status or dosage. Recent work indicates that GI Cr absorption may be enhanced significantly by pretreatment with nonsteroidal anti-inflammatory drugs like indomethacin or aspirin (Kamath et al. 1997). This effect may be mediated by an increase in mucosal permeability, by inhibition of GI prostaglandin synthesis, or by the presence of a more acidic luminal environment and is reversed by replacement with an exogenous prostaglandin E_2 analog. Concurrent treatment of pigs with porcine pituitary somatotropin does not appear to affect assimilation of, or physiological response to, supplemental dietary Cr picolinate (Anderson et al. 1997).

Biological Characteristics and Signs of Deficiency. In animal tissues, Cr(III) is bound to plasma proteins and distributed predominantly in liver, kidney, and spleen. Cr(III) is the biologically active form, incorporated into a low molecular weight ligand consisting of nicotinic acid, glutamic acid, glycine, and cysteine (NRC 1980; Offenbacher and Pi-Sunyer 1988). This compound is known as "glucose tolerance factor" (GTF) and is required, together with insulin, for normal glucose utilization by peripheral tissues (Sargent et al. 1979). The GTF enhances the reactions between insulin and its cell membrane receptors via sulfhydryl groups, thereby facilitating insulin's actions. Rats consuming a Cr-free diet develop a syndrome indistinguishable from diabetes mellitus (Schroeder 1966; Wooliscroft and Barbosa 1977). Because of this biological function for Cr and declining tissue Cr levels with age in humans, it has been proposed that some forms of adult onset or non-insulin-dependent diabetes mellitus may be associated with nutritional Cr deficiency. In growing Holstein calves fed corn-cottonseed hull diets containing 370 mg Cr/kg dry matter (DM), glucose clearance during an intravenous glucose tolerance test (IVGTT) was improved by about 27%, and serum cholesterol decreased by about 10% (Bunting et al. 1994). Other studies have found that dietary Cr supplementation in humans may increase serum HDL (high-density lipoprotein) cholesterol concentrations, which may in turn reduce the risk for coronary heart disease (Roeback et al. 1991). Likewise, dietary supplementation of growing-finishing pigs with 200 mg/kg DM Cr as Cr picolinate or Cr tripicolinate has decreased serum cholesterol significantly (Page et al. 1993), as well as improved glucose disappearance by about 30% during an IVGTT (Amoikon et al. 1995). Fat thickness over the ribs was decreased, and nitrogen absorption, dry-matter digestibility, daily gain, longissimus muscle area, and percentage of muscling were increased in pigs (Page et al. 1993; Kornegay et al. 1997), while fat thickness over the ribs and serum cholesterol were each decreased by almost 20% in growing lambs (Kitchalong et al. 1995).

Studies have indicated that steer calves fed a corn silage diet may be Cr deficient, based on an increase in average daily gain and feed efficiency following dietary supplementation with 0.4 ppm Cr as a high-Cr yeast product (Chang and Mowat 1992). Following supplementation with 0.2 ppm Cr as high-Cr yeast, transport-stressed feeder calves experienced not only an increase in dry-matter intake, feed efficiency, and gain but also significant decreases in serum cortisol and increases in serum immunoglobulin concentrations and hemagglutinating antibody titers to human red blood cells (Moonsie-Shageer and Mowat 1993; Chang and

Mowat 1992). Dietary Cr supplementation with 0.5 ppm improved the peak antibody response to an infectious bovine rhinotracheitis (IBR) vaccine challenge in 8-month-old calves (Burton et al. 1994) and increased both the humoral response to ovalbumin and mitogen-stimulated blastogenic response of peripheral blood mononuclear cells in early-lactation dairy cows (Burton et al. 1993). When neonatal calves were fed a milk replacer diet containing 0.4 ppm supplemental Cr from $CrCl_3$ or a Cr-nicotinic acid complex, both in vitro and in vivo indices of cell-mediated immune function were enhanced, as was the response to an intranasal challenge with IBR (Kegley et al. 1996). However, in another study, supplemental dietary Cr (0.14 ppm) from yeast had no effect on antibody titers following vaccination in stressed feeder calves against IBR, parainfluenza-3 (PI_3), bovine respiratory syncitial virus (BRSV), or bovine viral diarrhea (BVD), and Cr from an amino acid-chelated source improved the response to BVD vaccination only (Chang et al. 1996). Likewise, 6- to 8-week-old calves supplemented with a high-Cr yeast product (3 mg Cr/day) exhibited no changes in the secretion of adrenocorticotropic hormone (ACTH), cortisol, and plasma tumor necrosis factor-α or in lymphocyte proliferative response to mitogen stimulation following challenge with bovine herpesvirus-1 (BHV-1) (Arthington et al. 1997). Although supplementation of weanling pigs with 0.2 ppm Cr as $CrCl_3$, Cr-picolinate, or Cr-nicotinic acid complex improved rate of gain, feed intake, and in vitro cellular immune response, it had no effect on in vivo immune challenge with lipopolysaccharide (van Heugten and Spears 1997). In another study, 0.3 ppm supplemental dietary Cr as Cr-picolinate did significantly decrease the plasma tumor necrosis factor-α response to lipopolysaccharide challenge in growing pigs (Myers et al. 1997).

Dietary Requirements, Indications, Use, and Toxicity. Few specific indications for Cr supplementation have been identified for domestic animals. It has been suggested that Cr, like iron and zinc, may be sequestered during infections, thereby increasing its requirements, but this has not been thoroughly studied. Newer studies cited above on growing calves and pigs and lactating cows indicate that typical feeds may not be adequate in Cr and that supplemental Cr, up to 0.4-0.5 ppm, may have beneficial effects on growth and immune function.

Some Cr salts (trioxide, chromates, and dichromates) are potent cytotoxins by virtue of their protein-precipitating and oxidizing properties. Signs of acute oral Cr toxicity have been infrequently observed. In young calves, gastric congestion and inflammation and ruminal and abomasal ulceration were seen following a single dose of 30-40 mg Cr(VI)/kg body weight (NRC 1980). Signs of chronic oral Cr toxicosis have included skin contact dermatitis, respiratory passage irritation, ulceration of the nasal septum, and lung cancer. Maximal tolerable dietary levels for Cr are approximately 3000 ppm in the oxide form and 1000 ppm as the chloride salt (NRC 1980).

COBALT

Source and Occurrence. Cobalt (Co) content of plants varies with soil content and pH, as well as with rate of plant growth. Australia, New Zealand, Great Britain, and portions of Africa have Co-deficient areas. In North America, low-Co soils are found around the Great Lakes and in New England and Florida. Uptake of Co is low by forages grown in alkaline soils or following the use of lime fertilizers (NRC 1982). Co content is also lower during periods of rapid plant growth.

Biological Characteristics and Signs of Deficiency. The principal function of Co is as a component of vitamin B_{12} (cyanocobalamin). Thus, nonruminants have not been shown to require elemental Co in their diets, since they receive vitamin B_{12} preformed. In ruminants, and possibly other herbivores, dietary Co is required to support enteric microbial synthesis of vitamin B_{12}. Supplemental sources of Co include cobalt oxide, cobalt chloride, and cobalt sulfate; however, much of an orally administered dose of elemental Co is not absorbed—in rats, 80% is excreted in the feces (NRC 1980).

As a vital component of biologically active vitamin B_{12}, Co is required for those metabolic functions described for cyanocobalamin. These include erythropoiesis (as a cofactor for purine and pyrimidine synthesis); histidine, methionine, and choline metabolism (as a cofactor for methyl group transfers); and propionic acid conversion to succinyl CoA (as a cofactor for methylmalonyl CoA isomerase). Marginal Co deficiency in ruminants may be associated with impaired reproductive function, reduced appetite, decreased growth rate, and reduced milk production. More obvious signs of chronic Co deficiency may include frank inappetence, progressive weight loss, emaciation, anemia, and death (NRC 1980).

Dietary Requirements, Indications, and Use. In areas of endemic deficiency, top dressing of soil with 100-150 g Co per acre is sufficient to prevent deficiency. Cobalt iron oxide pellets or cobalt oxide/ferruginous clay "bullets" may be administered intraruminally to provide for slow release. Problems associated with these pellets include regurgitation by the animal and coating with calcium phosphate, which reduces the bioavailability. Co salts may be included in trace mineral premixes and salt blocks or can be added to loose salt at a ratio of 15 g/100 kg for sheep and 50 g/100 kg for cattle. Evaluation of cobalt glucoheptonate to enhance in vitro fiber digestion in ruminal fluid obtained from steers fed a Co-sufficient diet indicates that increasing dietary Co above the minimum requirement recommended by the NRC (1989) has no additional effect (Hussein et al. 1994).

Toxicity. Co toxicosis is uncommon and in most species results in reduced feed intake and body weight, emaciation, and anemia (much like the signs for deficiency). In simple-stomached animals, larger amounts of Co may induce a polycythemia, accompanied by erythroid hyperplasia of the bone marrow, reticulocytosis, and increased blood volume. In dogs, an experimental Co-induced congestive cardiomyopathy has been characterized by tachycardia, decreased ejection fraction and increased end-diastolic pressure, significant endocardial and epicardial fibrosis, and reduced systemic vascular resistance (Unverferth et al. 1983). Toxic levels appear to be 300 times the dietary requirement for Co—at least 10 ppm in the diet for most species (NRC 1980).

COPPER

Source and Occurrence. Copper (Cu) content in the majority of forages and grains is below the dietary requirement for most animal species, particularly when one considers the negative interactive effects of other dietary constituents on Cu absorption from the GI tract (NRC 1980; Minson 1990a). Immature forages and leaf fractions are usually higher in Cu than stem fractions, so that with selective grazing by animals, actual Cu intake may be improved over apparent intake based on whole-plant concentrations (Minson 1990a). Cu-deficient soils have been identified in western Australia, lower areas of western Europe, and in the southeastern United States. Where soils may contain adequate Cu levels, bioavailability may be greatly reduced by high sulfur (S) and/or molybdenum (Mo) levels, which reduce GI Cu absorption. Areas high in Mo have been identified in the United States, including parts of Florida, California, Colorado, Idaho, Montana, Nevada, Oregon, Washington, and Wyoming (Minson 1990a).

Chemical Forms, Distribution, and Biological Characteristics. Cu is relatively available to ruminants from a variety of sources, including elemental Cu and insoluble salt forms, which are solubilized in the abomasum for absorption. Water-soluble, inorganic salts of Cu, including the sulfate, nitrate, and chloride, are readily available in all species following oral administration (NRC 1980). Chelated dietary forms of Cu, complexed as proteinates or with methionine or lysine have been purported to enhance bioavailability (Kincaid et al. 1986a; Ward et al. 1996; Du et al. 1996a,b). However, numerous studies have reported equivalent bioavailability among Cu-proteinate, Cu-lysine, Cu-oxide, and Cu-sulfate in both cattle and pigs (Ward and Spears 1993; Kegley and Spears 1994; Coffey et al. 1994; Apgar and Kornegay 1996; Du et al. 1996a,b). Dietary Mo and S levels strongly influence the absorption and retention of dietary Cu, and low absorption coefficients are common (Minson 1990a). However, it is possible that Mo may have deleterious effects on calf performance that are independent of secondary alterations in Cu status (Gengelbach et al. 1994). Absorbed Cu first appears bound to circulating plasma proteins like albumin and is subsequently stored in specific tissues in association with Cu-binding proteins: cerebrocuprein for brain, erythrocuprein for erythrocytes, and hepatocuprein for liver (NRC 1980). These storage proteins are predominantly metallothioneins and superoxide dismutases (Brewer 1987). Ceruloplasmin is an α2-macroglobulin produced by the liver, which is responsible for binding up to 95% of the Cu in plasma in most species (Brewer 1987). Interleukin-1 (IL-1), released during inflammatory disorders and particularly during bacterial infections or endotoxemia, induces hepatic ceruloplasmin synthesis, leading to mobilization of Cu from storage tissues, including liver and kidneys, and induction of hypercupremia (Pekarek et al. 1972). While this response may enhance the oxygen free radical-related bactericidal functions of phagocytic cells, it may also increase the auto-oxidative damage done to the host itself.

METABOLIC FUNCTIONS

CUPROENZYMES. Cu functions as a necessary cofactor for many metalloenzymes, most of which function as oxidases (Brewer 1987; Sanders 1983; NRC 1980). Cu deficiency is thus characterized by the loss of these particular enzymes' activities and the metabolic aberrations which follow.

Ceruloplasmin functions as a ferrooxidase and is responsible for the oxidation of ferrous iron stored in ferritin to ferric iron for transport in transferrin and incorporation in heme proteins. A deficiency of Cu and of ferrooxidase activity will, therefore, effectively result in an iron deficiency and microcytic, hypochromic anemia. Cytochrome c oxidase is a cuproenzyme necessary for electron transport in the mitochondria. Cu deficiency and loss of cytochrome c oxidase activity may result in uncoupling of mitochondrial respiration and disturbances in energy metabolism and ATP-requiring biosynthetic reactions. Prominent among these is the synthesis of specific phospholipids required for neuronal myelination, so that Cu deficiency is often manifested in lambs and calves in a syndrome known as neonatal ataxia, a result of hypomyelinization. Cu-containing amine oxidases are necessary for deamination of biogenic amines, including histamine, and polyamines, including spermine and putrescine. Dopamine β-hydroxylase catalyzes the conversion of dopamine to norepinephrine, diamine oxidase catalyzes the conversion of carotene to retinal, and tyrosinase catalyzes the synthesis of melanin. A deficiency of the last leads to achromotrichia, or hypopigmentation of hair or wool. Lysyl oxidase is necessary for normal collagen and elastin synthesis. Cu deficiency may result in signs similar to those of ascorbic acid deficiency, related to instability of connective tissues. These include neonatal cardiomyopathies, large-artery aneurysms, and developmental bone anomalies (thin cortices, broadened epiphyses, cartilage erosions, and osteoporosis).

IMMUNOLOGIC FUNCTION AND FREE RADICAL METABOLISM. Cu deficiency has been associated with impaired mitogen-stimulated T and B lymphocyte blastogenesis, reduced antibody production following challenge with certain antigens, and impaired cell-mediated immunity (Prohaska and Lukasewycz 1981; Koller et al. 1987; Failla et al. 1988; Bala et al. 1992). Cu deficiency has also been shown to impair respiratory burst activity (owing to loss of cytochrome c oxidase activity) and to suppress candidacidal activity (owing to loss of Cu, Zn-superoxide dismutase activity) in isolated rat peritoneal macrophages (Babu and Failla 1990a). Moreover, the respiratory burst and microbicidal activity of rodent and bovine neutrophils were likewise significantly impaired by Cu deficiency (Babu and Failla 1990b; Boyne and Arthur 1981 1986). Dietary Cu depletion of Holstein steers resulted in significant depressions in neutrophil superoxide dismutase activity and killing capacity for *Staphylococcus aureus* even when no other signs of Cu deficiency were apparent (Xin et al. 1991a). Copper deficiency in Holstein steers also impaired the immune responses generated against *Pasteurella hemolytica* and IBR virus challenge (Stabel et al. 1993). Abnormalities in Cu, Zn-superoxide dismutase activity in Cu-deficient laboratory rodents may have also resulted in increased free radical-mediated lipid peroxidation (Prohaska 1991; Lawrence and Jenkinson 1987; Balevska et al. 1981). In addition, simultaneous Cu deficiency-induced decreases in hepatic activities of Se-dependent glutathione peroxidase and non-Se-dependent glutathione transferase may have impaired alternative mechanisms for free radical quenching (Prohaska 1991; Allen et al. 1988). Thus, host defenses against both microbial and chemical insults may be impaired by Cu deficiency.

Signs of Deficiency. As indicated by its metabolic functions, Cu deficiency may result in dysfunction of several body systems. Clinical manifestations include a hypochromic, microcytic anemia similar to that seen with dietary iron deficiency, bone disorders, neonatal ataxia, hair or wool depigmentation, impaired keratinization (resulting in uncrimped, "steely" wool), infertility, cardiovascular disorders, diarrhea ("peat scours" in New Zealand due to dietary Mo excess), and immunosuppression (Lofstedt et al. 1988; Sanders 1983; Mills et al. 1976). In human patients maintained for longer than 1 year with enteral or parenteral feeding, Cu deficiency was associated with anemia, neutropenia, or pancytopenia, which were responsive to Cu supplementation (Tamura et al. 1994; Wasa et al. 1994). In the absence of other obvious signs of deficiency, a Cu-deficient, high-Mo diet fed to feedlot cattle has resulted in depressed feed intake, feed efficiency, and growth (Irwin et al. 1979). Other studies have shown that neonatal ataxia in calves may appear without other signs of Cu deficiency in the dams (Sanders and Koestner 1980). Likewise, lower plasma Cu levels in lactating cows have been associated with lower milk production, lower hematocrits, and impaired fertility without other, more obvious signs of Cu deficiency (Kappel et al. 1984). In another study, only combined supplementation with both Cu and Mg salts improved fertility in Holstein cows, while individual mineral supplementation alone had no effect (Ingraham et al. 1987).

In an epidemiologic study of osteochondrosis in Thoroughbred foals, 7 of 8 animals had subnormal serum Cu and ceruloplasmin concentrations, and pathologic lesions in the zones of endochondral ossification were similar to those observed in experimental Cu deficiency-induced lysyl oxidase dysfunction (Bridges et al. 1984). Three of those foals may have been exposed to excessive Zn, thereby suppressing dietary Cu availability. Foals fed 1000 ppm or more of dietary Zn developed a secondary Cu deficiency and cartilaginous disease characteristic of osteochondritis dissecans (Bridges and Moffitt 1990). Foals fed an experimental, low-Cu (1.7 ppm) liquid milk replacer diet also developed cartilaginous lesions, including focal fragmentation of articular cartilage, metaphyseal physis separation, and widespread chondrocytic hypoplasia and necrosis (Bridges and Harris 1988).

Assessment of Status. Plasma Cu levels may be determined by atomic absorption spectroscopy; lower-than-normal levels may indicate Cu deficiency. Conversely, increased plasma Cu levels may occur with inflammation (due to IL-1 effects) or with Cu toxicosis. Unfortunately, plasma Cu concentrations do not necessarily reflect storage levels in organs like liver or kidney. Thus, plasma Cu levels may be normal in the face of impending deficiency or toxicosis. Ashed preparations or acid extracts of biopsies of these storage tissues may also be analyzed by atomic absorption spectroscopy. Owing to wide variability among animals in a given herd, the minimal sample size for determination of blood Cu status in cattle has ranged from 1 to 22% of the herd (3-55 cattle sampled/herd) (Tanner et al. 1988). In horses, significant breed and age effects have been identified with respect to both plasma Cu and ceruloplasmin levels (Cymbaluk et al. 1986). The use of serum ceruloplasmin levels as an indicator of Cu status in cattle and sheep has been limited, as it appears to correlate better with plasma Cu concentrations than with corresponding liver Cu content (Blakeley and Hamilton 1985). Finally, as a result of Cu and cuproprotein consumption during the process of blood coagulation, Cu and ceruloplasmin levels in serum are lower than in plasma, and following storage of blood samples on ice for extended periods (Kincaid et al. 1986b).

Dietary Requirements, Indications, and Use

INTRINSIC FACTORS. Dietary Cu requirements are integrally related to the dietary intakes of competing elements, including Zn, Mo, and inorganic S. Under otherwise optimal dietary conditions, swine and poultry require approximately 4-5 ppm Cu in the diet, while ruminants require 8-10 ppm. Physiologic states of growth, pregnancy, and lactation increase the Cu requirement accordingly. GI disease, which may affect Cu absorption, and renal disease, which may affect Cu loss in the urine, are examples of disorders affecting the dietary Cu requirement.

EXTRINSIC FACTORS. Factors affecting Cu absorption include dietary levels, presence in the diet of minerals that may compete for transport (Fe, Zn, Ca, and Cd), and interfering substances that may bind Cu (phytate, fiber, chelating agents) (Fischer et al. 1981; Prince et al. 1984). The actual mechanisms responsible for the inhibitory effects of Mo and S on Cu absorption and metabolism have not been completely elucidated but may include GI precipitation of Cu as insoluble thiomolybdates, antagonism of Cu transport by enterocytes, and, if sufficient thiomolybdates are absorbed, chelation of Cu from plasma albumin and tissue metallothioneins, resulting in increased fecal and urinary Cu excretion (Kincaid and White 1988; Suttle 1991). Nomograms and equations describing the effects of dietary Mo and S on Cu absorption have been published to predict their effects on dietary Cu requirements (Minson 1990a). In addition, Cu availability may be affected by curing or storage of plant materials; Cu in fresh forage is generally less available than that in the same dried forage, owing to greater ruminal sulfide generation by fresh forages. Likewise, low-roughage, high-concentrate diets, which promote ruminal sulfide production, may interfere with Cu availability. Although interactions have been observed between dietary Cu source (CuO vs. $CuSO_4$) and acid-base metabolism, dietary cation-anion balance has not been shown to have any effect on dietary Cu availability (Xin et al. 1991b).

Preparations and Therapy. In deficient areas, Cu in the form of cupric sulfate can be added to salt at a rate of 0.5%. Soil fertilization with Cu has been used in Australia and New Zealand but may be ineffective in areas of the western United States where soil Mo levels are high. Oxidized copper wire, broken into small rods of 10 mm or less in length and referred to as copper oxide needles (CuO_n), may be administered to ruminants in gelatin capsules. Following their intraruminal deposition, they slowly pass to the abomasum for long-term release following the action by gastric acidity to solubilize the Cu (Cameron et al. 1989). A single oral dose of copper oxide needles at the start of the grazing season has been shown to provide adequate Cu supplementation for sheep and cattle for several months (Cameron et al. 1989; Suttle 1987). In sheep, a dose of 0.1 g/kg body weight (approximately 5.0 g/animal) appears to be adequate to maintain liver and serum Cu levels for at least 2 months (Suttle 1987). In cattle, as little as 5.0 g of copper oxide needles can maintain liver Cu stores for 240 days, and a dose-related increase in liver Cu is observed following administration of up to 20 g (Suttle 1987). Copper oxide wire also appears to have an anthelmintic action in sheep, with a 5.0 g bolus reducing parasite burdens by as much as 96% for *Haemonchus contortus* burdens and 56% for *Ostertagia cincta* (Bang et al. 1990). Another approach is the use of controlled-release copper oxide-impregnated glass boluses—17 g boluses for sheep and 75 g boluses for cattle, containing approximately 18% by weight of Cu (Allen et al. 1984). Sustained-release methods of Cu administration provide longer-term protection against Cu deficiency and a greater margin of safety against Cu toxicity, which is otherwise a concern with mineral salt supplementation.

Toxicity. Cu toxicosis may be either acute or chronic in chronology, but the signs of chronic Cu poisoning are usually evoked peracutely, thereby confusing its interpretation. Acute Cu toxicosis may occur following accidental overdosage or consumption of Cu-containing anthelmintics, foot baths, fungicides, or feed additives (NRC 1980). Clinical signs include nausea, vomiting, salivation, abdominal discomfort, convulsions, paralysis, collapse, and death (NRC 1980). Pathologic lesions include widespread organ congestion, extravascular fluid exudation, and hepatic and renal degeneration and necrosis. Chronic Cu toxicosis progresses through two phases. The first is the long-term accumulation phase, during which abnormally high levels of Cu are accumulated by the liver (Soli 1980). This results in a subclinical period of organ damage due to excessive Cu accumulation, which may be characterized by hepatocellular degeneration, elevations in serum levels of hepatic enzymes, and spongy degeneration of parts of the brain. The second phase may represent an acute culmination of this subclinical period or may be precipitated by some acute stress that results in lysosomal degeneration, Cu release, and a hemolytic crisis (Ishmael et al. 1971; Gopinath et al. 1974; Soli 1980). Three basic mechanisms have been identified for hepatic Cu accumulation: simple chronic Cu poisoning in response to excessive dietary intake; hepatogenous chronic Cu poisoning following injury by toxic plant alkaloids (such as from *Heliotropium europaeum* or *Senecia* spp.) and Cu accumulation by damaged hepatocytes; and phytogenous chronic Cu poisoning following consumption of plants grown under high-sulfate and/or excess-Mo conditions, which facilitate Cu accumulation to toxic levels (Bostwick 1982). Sheep are particularly sensitive to chronic Cu toxicosis, accumulating excessive hepatic levels following consumption of otherwise moderate levels of Cu in their feed. The hemolytic crisis may be caused by direct oxidative effects by Cu or lysosomally derived free radicals on hemoglobin, leading to Heinz body formation, and on erythrocyte membranes, leading to membrane instability (NRC 1980). In either case, red blood cell membrane rigidity increases their fragility and precipitates in hemolysis. Sheep appear to be the most sensitive species to chronic Cu toxicosis. Other species are affected only at much higher dietary intakes.

Subclinical effects of the chronic accumulation of toxic amounts of Cu by sheep may follow consumption of as little as 26 ppm Cu in the feed over 4-5 months, and include depressions in feed efficiency and growth rates. In calves, weight gains and feed efficiency are maintained from 3 to 45 days of age with consumption of up to 50 ppm dietary Cu (Jenkins and Hidiroglou 1989). At 200 ppm and beyond, subclinical effects result, but the acute hemolytic crisis is only evident following consumption of 1000 ppm (Jenkins and Hidiroglou 1989; Jenkins 1989).

Swine appear to be much more tolerant to chronic high dietary levels of Cu. Dietary levels of 200-300 ppm Cu have been fed to pigs as an antimicrobial and growth stimulant without adverse effects (Kornegay et al. 1989; Shurson et al. 1990). In fact, weanling pigs supplemented with 250 ppm dietary Cu as $CuSO_4$ expressed slower jejunal mucosal turnover rates, which may have contributed to lower observed energy requirements and improved growth rates with fat-supplemented, high-energy diets (Dove and Haydon 1992; Radecki et al. 1992). Levels of 400 ppm have been shown to depress the immune response to phytohemagglutinin and lysozyme and to reduce blood hemoglobin concentrations (Kornegay et al. 1989). Levels higher than this can cause chronic Cu toxicosis, evidenced by reduced feed intake, retarded growth, increased liver and serum Cu levels, elevated hepatic enzyme activities in the serum, and an anemia resembling that of iron deficiency, presumably due to Cu interference with GI iron absorption (Hatch et al. 1979a; NRC 1980).

In llamas, a dietary Cu intake of 36 ppm, in conjunction with dietary Mo of 2.2 ppm, resulted in chronic Cu toxicosis characterized by the usual antecedent increase in hepatic and serum Cu levels and in hepatic enzyme activities, followed by a hemolytic crisis (Junge and Thornburg 1989). Because concurrent dietary levels of Fe, Zn, Mo, and inorganic S can all affect Cu uptake from the GI tract, one cannot predict the occurrence of Cu toxicity by dietary Cu intake alone. When the dietary intakes of these minerals are "normal," the maximum tolerable levels of dietary Cu appear to be 25 ppm for sheep, 100 ppm for cattle, 250 ppm for swine, 800 ppm for horses, and 1000 ppm for rats (NRC 1980).

Wilson's disease is an autosomal recessive, inherited disorder associated with abnormal accumulation of Cu in the liver, kidneys, brain, and other tissues, pursuant to a defect in hepatic excretion of Cu into the bile (Su et al. 1982a). A similar disorder has been well documented in Bedlington terriers, which appears to follow an autosomal recessive pattern of inheritance as well (Twedt et al. 1979; Su et al. 1982b; Johnson et al. 1980). A less severe form of hepatic Cu accumulation has also been identified in West Highland White terriers, but only some of those animals eventually accumulate hepatotoxic levels of Cu (>2000 ppm) (Thornburg et al. 1996). A Cu hepatopathy resembling the human and canine disorders has also been described in juvenile sibling ferrets (Fox et al. 1994). The excess Cu is sequestered in lysosomes until excessive quantities induce lysosomal enzyme release and autodigestion of tissues. In the liver, this is characterized by progressive signs of functional disturbances in hepatic function, as well as by focal hepatitis, chronic hepatitis, and, ultimately, cirrhosis. The prophylaxis and treatment of copper toxicosis are achieved with cupriuretic agents like penicillamine and 2,3,2-tetramine tetrahydrochloride, which promote Cu excretion (Allen et al. 1987), as well as with zinc acetate to block intestinal absorption of dietary and endogenously recycled Cu (Brewer et al. 1992a,b).

FLUORINE

Source and Occurrence. Fluorine (F) occurs widely in nature, predominantly in deposits of fluorspar (CaF_2), cryolite ($NaAlF_6$), and fluorapatite ($Ca_{10}F_2(PO_4)_6$). Higher soil concentrations are found in particular areas of the United States, including Idaho and Tennessee. Plants do not accumulate significant quantities of F, even when exposed to high-F environments, although surface contamination from air and waterborne F may be important.

Biological Characteristics and Dietary Requirements. Under practical field conditions, no deficiency of F has ever been documented in domestic animals, although F toxicity is a potential problem. The essentiality of F as a nutrient has been controversial. Studies in laboratory rodents have documented its necessity for normal growth and reproduction and perhaps in the amelioration of neonatal iron deficiency anemia. Many studies have demonstrated an important role for F in preventing dental caries in laboratory rodents and in humans, and F may be beneficial in reducing age-associated bone demineralization and the onset or progression of senile osteoporosis.

F is absorbed throughout the GI tract by both passive and active transport processes, with digestibilities from soluble mineral sources as high as 90%. Conversely, dietary Ca, Al, and Cl depress F absorption by complexation or competitive inhibition of transport. Bone has the greatest affinity for F, where it is complexed with hydroxyapatite to form fluorapatite. Little F crosses the placenta or is secreted in milk of lactating animals, but sufficiently high maternal dietary intake may have significant adverse effects on fetal development and neonatal health in newborn calves.

Toxicity. Principal sources of excessive F levels capable of causing intoxication include F-contaminated water, plant leaves and stems contaminated by emissions from industrial sources, and dietary mineral supplements containing high levels of F, such as unprocessed (nondefluorinated) rock phosphates. Though uncommon, lesions of acute F toxicity may include restlessness, stiffness, anorexia, excessive salivation, nausea, vomiting, weakness, depression, and convulsions (NRC 1980). The principal lesions of chronic F toxicity, denoted as fluorosis, are predominantly due to effects on developing teeth and bones. Dental fluorosis results in discoloration, mottling, and staining of the enamel, followed by hypoplasia, pitting, and complete loss of enamel (Shupe and Olson 1971; Shearer et al. 1978; Shupe 1980; Krook et al. 1983; Maylin et al. 1987). Osteofluorosis is characterized by bilaterally symmetrical, hyperostotic, chalky-white bone lesions, which are most severe in those bones under the greatest mechanical stress. Changes may include osteosclerosis, osteoporosis, hyperostosis, and osteomalacia. Although intra-articular structures are not primarily involved, periosteal hyperostosis and osteophytosis may cause periarticular spurring and bridging lesions, leading to degenerative osteoarthrosis, calcification of periarticular structures, and subsequent stiffness and lameness. Nonskeletal lesions may include anorexia, weight loss, hypogalactia, ruminal microbial abnormalities, anemia, and hypothyroidism (Hillman et al. 1979).

Cattle are most sensitive to F toxicity, and maximum tolerable dietary F levels are generally lower for young, growing animals; 20 ppm for young cattle, 40 ppm for dairy cattle, 50 ppm for finishing beef cattle, and 100 ppm for breeding cattle (NRC 1980). Maximum tolerable dietary levels are 60 ppm for horses and breeding sheep, 150 ppm for swine, turkeys, and finishing sheep, and 200 ppm for chickens (NRC 1980). However, several studies have observed significantly lower tolerances for dietary F. For instance, as little as 7 ppm fed to growing-finishing pigs adversely affected bone integrity (Burnell et al. 1986). In addition, dietary levels of other nutrients, particularly P, can protect against F toxicity by interfering with its GI absorption (Suttie 1980).

IODINE

Source and Occurrence. Iodine (I) is found widely in nature but, with the exceptions of some marine products, only in very low concentrations. There are I-deficient areas throughout the world. In North America, the principal region extends from New England westward to areas around the Great Lakes and through the upper Midwest and Pacific Northwest.

Biological Characteristics and Signs of Deficiency. Iodine occurs in plant materials predominantly as inorganic iodide, which is absorbed throughout the GI tract and rapidly distributed in the body, principally to the kidneys and thyroid gland. Iodide is accumulated in the thyroid by active transport, activated by peroxidation, and organified by addition to tyrosine. The principal products of this process are the thyroid hormones, tetraiodothyronine (thyroxine, T4) and triiodothyronine (T3). Monodeiodination of T4 by peripheral tissues generates most of the biologically active T3 and is a necessary step in thyroxine's interactions with its target tissues. Thyroid hormones are responsible for maintenance of normal thermoregulation, intermediary metabolism, reproduction, growth, hematopoiesis, and integumentary function. Signs of I deficiency are principally those of hypothyroidism, although I probably also functions in the bactericidal activity of inflammatory cells, as a participant in free radical generation through the action of myeloperoxidase and generation of hypoiodous acid.

Dietary Requirements, Indications, and Use. Exact dietary requirements for I have not been ascertained for all animals, but diets containing 0.1-0.2 mg/kg are generally adequate. Requirements may generally be met by feeding iodized salt containing approximately 0.007% I. Lactating animals require increased dietary I because much is secreted in the milk. Thus, excessive dietary I fed to lactating dairy cows can result in excessive I levels in milk for consumption, thereby potentially contributing to thyrotoxicosis in humans or depressed performance in milk-fed calves (Berg et al. 1988; Swanson et al. 1990). Iodized salt is the safest and most practical means of providing supplemental dietary I. Other sources include calcium iodate, calcium iodibehenate, cuprous iodide, ethylenediaminedihydroiodide (EDDI), and iodide or iodate salts of potassium or sodium (NRC 1980). Nonnutrient uses for I include iodophor teat dips to prevent mastitis, EDDI to prevent or treat foot rot, and iodide salts for the treatment of actinomycosis or as an expectorant (Olson et al. 1980).

Toxicity. Iodine in high quantities may be toxic, but this is usually only encountered in artificial situations of excessive I supplementation. In dairy cows, clinical signs of I toxicosis may include lacrimation, alopecia, dermatitis, nasal discharge, salivation, coughing, and abortion (Hillman and Curtis 1980; Olson et al. 1980). Herd complaints may include a marked increase in disease incidence, decreased milk production, depressed feed consumption, and reduced weight gains (Olson et al. 1980). In calves, in addition, I toxicosis is associated with impaired cell-mediated and humoral immune functions, increased incidence of bronchopneumonia, and squamous metaplasia of the tracheal mucosa and parotid salivary gland ducts (Jenkins and Hidiroglou 1990; Mangkoewidjojo et al. 1980; Haggard et al. 1980). The maximum tolerable level of dietary I for cattle and sheep is 50 ppm, although this may result in high levels of I in the milk (NRC 1980). Pigs appear to tolerate 400 ppm, and for poultry, 300 ppm is safe. Horses are most sensitive to excess I, and a maximal tolerable dietary level is estimated to be only 5 ppm (NRC 1980).

IRON

Source and Occurrence. Iron (Fe) occurs widely in soil and is actually more abundant than many of the macroelements, although required in trace quantities. Legumes tend to contain more Fe than grasses, and forages generally contain more iron than cereal grains (NRC 1982). Mineral sources used to supply macroelements like Ca or P often contain Fe as well (NRC 1980).

Chemical Forms, Distribution, and Biological Characteristics. Most Fe in plant products is in the oxidized, ferric form in combination with organic compounds and must be released in the GI tract for absorption to occur. Sources like iron oxide, which is sometimes used as a coloring agent in feeds, are much less available owing to insolubility. In calves, Fe from ferrous sulfate has higher bioavailability than ferrous carbonate, which in turn affects not only the dietary requirement but also predisposition to toxicity and antagonistic effects on the intestinal absorption of other minerals, such as Zn and Cu (McGuire et al. 1985; Miller et al. 1991).

There are three main phases to Fe absorption from the GI tract (Narasinga 1981). During the intraluminal phase, food undergoes digestion and Fe is released in a soluble form. This is followed by the mucosal phase, during which ferrous Fe is taken up by enterocytes and transported transcellularly to the serosal surface. This phase appears to involve the interaction of Fe-binding proteins like ferritin and transferrin, as well as intercompartmental exchange between cellular organelles and cytosolic carriers (Furugouri 1977; Narasinga 1981). Finally, ferric Fe is delivered to the blood by transfer to circulating proteins, predominant among which is transferrin. Hydrochloric acid secreted in the stomach plays a vital role in facilitating Fe absorption by the intestinal mucosa. Acid conditions promote the solubilization of both inorganic and organic forms of Fe and reduce ferric Fe to the ferrous form, which is less likely to precipitate under the alkaline conditions of the upper small intestine and is more readily absorbed by the enterocytes. Nonheme iron is predominantly absorbed in the duodenum and proximal jejunum by a brush border receptor-mediated process, while heme Fe appears to enter the cells directly, perhaps by endocytosis.

Fe absorption from the GI tract appears to be regulated by body Fe stores, through an active process mediated by the synthesis of Fe-binding proteins like ferritin and transferrin, which are central to Fe absorption and distribution (Narasinga 1981). Increased metabolic demand for Fe facilitates its uptake from the circulating transferrin-bound pool, which is subsequently replenished by mobilization of Fe from ferritin-bound stores (in the bone marrow, liver, kidneys, spleen, and cells of the reticuloendothelial system). Depletion of Fe from circulating transferrin and body stores leads to induction of new transferrin synthesis and an increase in circulating iron-binding capacity. This facilitates Fe transfer from GI mucosal cells and, in turn, mucosal uptake of Fe from the intestinal lumen. Conversely, increased Fe stores result in increased apoferritin synthesis, increased circulating levels of ferritin, saturation of plasma transferrin with Fe, and reduced mucosal transfer and/or uptake of ingested Fe. Inflammatory disorders are often associated with tissue Fe sequestration and hypoferremia, owing to induction of apoferritin synthesis by IL-1. While this may have a beneficial bacteriostatic effect, deprivation of Fe to the host also may impair hemoglobin synthesis and erythropoiesis, resulting in the anemia of chronic disease (Weinberg 1974; Feldman et al. 1981).

Evaluation of body Fe status may be done directly by analysis of tissue (predominantly liver) biopsies or indirectly by analysis of serum Fe and iron-binding capacity. Several methods are available for the determination of Fe content in biological specimens. Biological fluids and ashed preparations or acid extracts of tissues may be analyzed by atomic absorption spectroscopy, by a colorimetric method using the chromogenic substrate ferrozine, and by a semiautomated coulometric method (Smith et al. 1981). For determination of unbound or total iron-binding capacity in serum, the sample may be incubated with excess Fe or an Fe-exchange resin, following which one of the above methods is repeated. Fe deficiency is generally associated with a decrease in serum Fe concentration and an increase in unbound iron-binding capacity (UIBC). This may be alternatively expressed as a decrease in percent saturation of transferrin. Induction of transferrin synthesis may also result in an increase in total iron-binding capacity (TIBC), while reduced apoferritin synthesis may result in decreased serum ferritin concentrations. Radioimmunoassay and enzyme-linked immunoassay procedures have been validated for determination of serum ferritin in humans (Polson et al. 1988), horses (Smith et al. 1984; Harvey et al. 1987), dogs (Weeks et al. 1989), cats (Andrews et al. 1994), and cows and calves (Furugouri et al. 1982; Miyata et al. 1984). Serum ferritin appears to offer a sensitive means of detection of Fe deficiency (decreased concentration) or overload (increased concentration) but is also an acute-phase reactant protein whose synthesis is induced by IL-1 released during inflammation (Weeks et al. 1989).

Signs of Deficiency. The most prominent manifestation of Fe deficiency is an ineffectual regenerative anemia, characterized by reticulocytosis and erythrocytic microcytosis in most species, and hypochromasia in some (Harvey et al. 1982; Weiser and O'Grady 1983). Congenital Fe-deficiency anemia is common in neonates of most species, owing to their negligible Fe stores at birth and consumption of a milk-based, Fe-deficient diet postpartum (Tennant et al. 1975; Weiser and Kociba 1983; Harvey et al. 1984). Fe-deficiency anemia is due not only to reduced rates of effective erythropoiesis but also to increased removal of red blood cells from the circulation. Fe deficiency appears to increase erythrocyte fragility, thereby shortening their life span, perhaps through adverse effects on erythrocytic glutathione peroxidase activity and the capacity to quench free radicals (Weiser and O'Grady 1983).

Fe deficiency has also been shown to impair cortisol secretion in humans (Saad et al. 1991), to cause intestinal malabsorption of Fe in dogs and humans (Kimber and Weintraub 1968), and to impair conversion of thyroxine to triiodothyronine in rats, thereby producing hypothermia (Dillman et al. 1980). With regard to immunologic function, Fe-deficiency anemia in mice has been associated with an impaired delayed cutaneous hypersensitivity reaction to dinitrofluorobenzene and an impaired blastogenic response of splenic lymphocytes to concanavalin A or phytohemagglutinin (Kuvibidila et al. 1981 1983). In rats, maternal Fe deficiency during certain pre- and postnatal growth periods has resulted in long-term impairment of humoral immunity (Kochanowski and Sherman 1985). It is also possible that Fe deficiency might reduce the pro-oxidant activity of transferrin in leukocytes or lactoferrin in milk, thereby reducing microbicidal activities (Klebanoff and Waltersdorph 1990). On the other hand, Fe supplementation of human infants and of neonatal piglets appears to increase their susceptibility to bacterial infections, by counteracting the bacteriostatic effects of IL-1-induced Fe sequestration (Becroft et al. 1977; Knight et al. 1983; Kadis et al. 1984).

Dietary Requirements, Indications, and Use

INTRINSIC FACTORS. Requirements for Fe are greatest during growth and with increased rates of erythropoiesis. Individual species differences are great in the amount required and form that may be utilized. For instance, insoluble salts of Fe have greater bioavailability in ruminants, owing to greater residence time and dissolution, than in nonruminants.

EXTRINSIC FACTORS. Certain dietary constituents may affect Fe availability by altering its solubility and/or oxidation state. Ascorbic acid, dicarboxylic acids, some sugars, and amino acids can form chelates with Fe which enhance its solubility (Narasinga 1981; Leigh and Miller 1983). Although pigs raised under normal conditions may have no dietary requirement for supplemental vitamin C in and of itself, supplemental dietary ascorbic acid has been shown to enhance feed intake and weight gain through a mechanism that appears to involve redistribution of absorbed Fe (Yen and Pond 1981). Phosphates, phytates, tannins, and fiber can precipitate Fe, thereby reducing its absorption (Narasinga 1981; Leigh and Miller 1983). Although the average iron content of vegetarian diets may be comparable to that of nonvegetarian diets, bioavailability of nonheme iron may be reduced significantly by phytates, fibers, and soybean protein. Median plasma ferritin concentration of vegetarians consuming a diet rich in soybean products in one study was approximately one-half the level of nonvegetarian cohorts (Shaw et al. 1995). Studies have also demonstrated an inhibitory effect of dietary Ca on Fe absorption. Calcium citrate, chloride, and phosphate appear to have a greater inhibitory effect than calcium carbonate, and the mechanism may be one of competitive antagonism of mucosal Fe transport processes (Cook et al. 1991; Hallberg et al. 1991).

Preparations and Therapy. Fe is available in a variety of salts of carbonate, chloride, sulfate, etc., for use either enterally or parenterally in individual animals for the purpose of repleting a dietary Fe deficiency. Iron dextran is often administered parenterally to neonates in the prophylaxis of congenital Fe deficiency anemia, and to adults following large, quantifiable losses of blood in the prophylaxis of blood loss-induced Fe-deficiency anemia. Supplementary dietary Fe may improve hematological status but has little effect on performance in Cu-supplemented growing pigs or beef calves (Dove and Haydon 1991; Reece et al. 1984). In growing lambs, additional dietary Fe may have the beneficial effect of decreasing dietary Cu availability, thereby reducing the potential for Cu toxicity (Prabowo et al. 1988).

Toxicity. Chronic, low-level Fe toxicosis may be manifested in reduced feed intake, growth rate, and efficiency of feed conversion (NRC 1980). Other signs may include those of secondary Cu or P deficiency, owing to Fe-induced inhibition of their GI absorption (NRC 1980). Signs of acute Fe toxicosis include anorexia, oliguria, diarrhea, hypothermia, metabolic acidosis, and death (NRC 1980). High dietary Fe increases lipid peroxidation and may increase the requirement for dietary antioxidants such as vitamin E (Jenkins and Kramer 1988). Fe-containing hematinics have been shown to induce acute iron toxicity when administered to species for which they are not intended (Ruhr et al. 1983). Pigs appear to tolerate higher dietary Fe levels than other species. Depending on the bioavailability of dietary sources, maximum tolerable dietary levels are approximately 3000 ppm for swine, 1000 ppm for cattle and poultry, and 500 ppm for sheep. Hemochromatosis is an inherited disease in humans that is characterized by increased GI Fe absorption and abnormal deposition of Fe in parenchymal tissues. A syndrome similar to this human disease has been identified in Salers cattle and was characterized by micronodular hepatic cirrhosis with marked deposition of hemosiderin in hepatocytes and Kupffer cells and increased hepatic Fe content, as well as hemosiderin deposition in lymph nodes, spleen, kidney, brain, pancreas, thyroid, and other glandular tissues (House et al. 1994).

MANGANESE

Source and Occurrence. Manganese (Mn) concentration in plant sources varies widely, depending on soil characteristics, water content, and plant growth rate (NRC 1982). Animal by-products are particularly low in Mn, with liver containing much lower amounts than other transition elements which are actively accumulated (NRC 1980).

Biological Characteristics and Dietary Requirements. Mn is absorbed throughout the GI tract, but especially in the small intestine, by a two-step process similar to that for iron, including mucosal uptake from the GI lumen and transepithelial transfer of Mn for delivery to the blood (NRC 1980). High dietary levels of Ca and P have been shown to reduce the availability of Mn in ruminants. Dietary phytates and fiber may also bind Mn and reduce its absorption. Other transition elements like Fe, Cu, and Zn may competitively inhibit its absorption by enterocytes. In rats, lactose inhibits Mn absorption, whereas in calves with a functionally developing rumen, it has no effect (King et al. 1980a,b).

Manganese oxide and manganese sulfate are the most commonly used dietary supplements, and in poultry, bioavailabilities of Mn from salts of sulfate, chloride, carbonate, and dioxide are equal (NRC 1980). However, in sheep, relative bioavailabilities of Mn from $MnSO_4$, MnO, MnO_2, and $MnCO_3$ are about 100, 58, 33, and 28% (Wong-Valle et al. 1989). In a study of bioavailability of different dietary Mn sources in lambs, a Mn-methionine complex was found to have approximately 20% greater availability than $MnSO_4$ (Henry et al. 1992). Estimated relative bioavailabilities of Mn in crossbred wether lambs were 100%, 121%, 71%, and 53% for $MnSO_4$-H_2O, Mn-methionine complex, and two types of feed grade MnO, respectively, suggesting the potential superiority of an amino acid complex (Henry et al. 1992).

Mn functions as the preferred cofactor for glycosyltransferases involved in mucopolysaccharide synthesis for organic matrix in normal skeletal growth (Hidiroglou et al. 1979). Additional functions for Mn include its roles as a cofactor for pyruvate carboxylase, which catalyzes the conversion of pyruvate to oxaloacetate for gluconeogenesis, and as a cofactor for superoxide dismutase, which catalyzes the conversion of superoxide to hydrogen peroxide for free radical quenching (NRC 1980). Intravenous administration of $MnCl_2$ to horses has resulted in dose-related increases in the superoxide-scavenging ability of blood plasma, although concomitant adverse reactions included defection, hyperexcitability, and sweating (Singh et al. 1992).

Mn deficiency is relatively uncommon in domestic animals, with the exception of poultry. Deficiency in growing birds results in malformation of the tibial condyles, leading to displacement of the gastrocnemius tendon and a clinical syndrome of perosis, similar to that induced by dietary choline deficiency (Hidiroglou 1979). Skeletal abnormalities attributed to Mn deficiency in neonatal animals include limb deformities in kids, enlarged joints and twisted limbs in calves, and joint pain and "bunny-hopping" in lambs (Hidiroglou 1979). Significant alterations in epiphyseal plate concentrations of uronic acid, sulfur-amino acids, dibasic amino acids, and hexosamines were observed in Mn-deficient newborn lambs (Hidiroglou et al. 1979).

Toxicity. In calves, high but nontoxic dietary Mn levels (up to 125-1000 ppm) do not cause alterations in organ Mn content or induce Mn toxicosis but do antagonize Fe absorption from the small intestine (Ho et al. 1984). Dietary Mn levels of up to 300 ppm have had no effect in sheep (Ivan and Hidiroglou 1980), but higher amounts which would not normally be encountered under field conditions (3000-9000 ppm) depressed feed intake and resulted in increased hepatic Cu and decreased hepatic Zn levels (Black et al. 1985a,b). Feeding 5000 ppm to cows depressed rumen microbial fermentation, and in pigs, 500 ppm dietary Mn retarded growth and induced limb stiffness and a stilted gait (NRC 1980). The maximum tolerable dietary limit for poultry is approximately 2000 ppm (NRC 1980).

MOLYBDENUM

Source and Occurrence. Molybdenum (Mo) concentrations in plants vary principally with the Mo content of the soil in which they are grown. Mo is present as both water-soluble (Na_2MoO_4, $(NH_4)_2MoO_4$) and insoluble (MoO_3, $CaMoO_4$, MoS_2) salts (NRC 1980, 1982). Contamination from industrial sources can cause marked elevations in plant Mo content, thereby promoting Mo toxicity.

Biological Characteristics and Dietary Requirements. Most mineral forms of Mo are readily absorbed from the GI tract, and absorption is influenced by dietary Cu, Zn, Fe, Pb, ascorbic acid, sulfur-amino acids, and protein. The most prominent dietary effect on Mo uptake is that of inorganic sulfate (SO_4) (NRC 1980). Inhibitory effects of other nutrients on GI Mo absorption primarily include complexation in the lumen and competitive inhibition of mucosal transport.

Mo-containing metalloenzymes include aldehyde oxidase, sulfide oxidase, and xanthine dehydrogenase/oxidase. The last is perhaps the most prominent biochemical role for Mo. Xanthine oxidase catalyzes the conversion of purines to uric acid for excretion and is responsible, in part, for the generation of oxygen free radicals in tissues during inflammation or ischemia. Natural deficiencies of Mo have not been documented in domestic animals and dietary requirements have not been well defined.

Toxicity. Lesions of dietary Mo toxicosis relate principally to its inhibitory effects on GI Cu absorption and to induction of a secondary nutritional deficiency of Cu. Subsequent deficiency of Cu-containing metalloenzymes may induce integumentary changes (due to loss of tyrosinase activity), anemia (due to loss of ferrooxidase activity), and skeletal or collagen disorders (due to loss of lysyl oxidase activity) (NRC 1980). Clinical findings of Mo toxicosis may include diarrhea, emaciation, anemia, achromotrichia, bone malformations, and, in neonates, enzootic ataxia (NRC 1980). It has been suggested that some forms of rickets in foals may result from Mo intoxication from pasture or dam's milk and subsequent deficiency of Cu and its enzymes. Maximum tolerable dietary levels of Mo are as low as 5-10 ppm for cattle and young horses, and as high as 1000 ppm for mule deer and swine (NRC 1980). Much higher dietary levels of Mo are tolerated by animals consuming diets that are also higher in inorganic sulfate, Cu, or other Mo antagonists.

SELENIUM

Source and Occurrence. Selenium (Se) concentrations in plants vary widely with soil content and plant species. In the United States there are several areas of Se-deficient soils, including the Southeast, Northeast, Great Lakes region, and Northwest (NRC 1980). There are also areas of seleniferous soils from which toxic levels may be accumulated in forages. In addition, there are several species of Se-accumulator plants, including *Astragalus, Machaeranthera, Haplopappus,* and *Stanleya;* when grown on seleniferous soils, levels in excess of 300 mg Se/kg DM may be produced (NRC 1980). Increased rates of plant growth resulting from nitrogen and phosphate fertilization result in lower concentrations of Se, and sandy soils produce lower Se concentrations in forages than heavier soils (Minson 1990b).

Chemical Forms, Distribution, and Biological Characteristics. Se occurs in several valence states (–2, 0, +4, and +6) and has chemical properties similar to those of sulfur (NRC 1980). As Se^{-2}, it occurs as hydrogen selenide, an unstable and toxic gas. In its elemental form, Se is insoluble and relatively nonreactive. Se^{+4} in inorganic selenites and Se^{+6} in selenates are highly water soluble, biologically available, and toxic. Even though selenite may be readily adsorbed to food particles or reduced to insoluble elemental Se or selenides in the acid gastric environment, bioavailability of Se from either Se^{+4} or Se^{+6} is similar in sheep and horses and only marginally better from selenate for cattle (Podoll et al. 1992). There was little difference in serum Se concentration or glutathione peroxidase activity in pigs fed up to 0.5 ppm DM of Se as sodium selenite versus Se-enriched yeast (Mahan and Kim 1996; Mahan and Parrett 1996). However, more Se was retained in muscle when the Se-enriched yeast source was fed. In contrast, Se from sodium selenite was 30% more available than Se from a yeast product in sheep fed a forage diet, and 15% more available in sheep fed a concentrate-based diet (Koenig et al. 1997).

Several methods are available for the determination of Se content in biological specimens (Minson 1990b). Ashed preparations or acid extracts of tissues and biological fluids may be analyzed by atomic absorption spectroscopy. Serum Se concentrations in female llamas was correlated to dietary Se supplementation and are predictive of Se status in the cria at birth (Herdt 1995). It has been recommended that both maternal blood and fetal liver Se concentrations be determined in order to accurately evaluate herd Se status of cattle (Kirk et al. 1995). The concentration of Se in whole blood is low but is highly correlated with the activity of erythrocytic glutathione peroxidase, providing a more rapid and economical means of determining Se status. A sandwich enzyme-linked immunosorbent assay (ELISA) using a monoclonal antibody to bovine erythrocytic glutathione peroxidase has been developed as a simple, rapid, and accurate method for estimating Se concentration in whole blood (Kinoshita et al. 1996). Subclinical muscular dystrophy resulting from Se deficiency may result in elevations in serum creatine phosphokinase activity, which although not specific, can be used as a screening test in suspect herds and to follow the clinical course of individual patients. Because Se is stored in liver, hepatic concentrations are indicative of nutritional status. In lambs, a concentration of 0.21 mg/kg DW is reportedly near the minimal requirement.

Se and other dietary antioxidants are closely related in their metabolic functions of free radical quenching and modulation of oxidative injury. Vitamins E and C act directly as free radical scavengers, sulfur-containing amino acids serve as precursors for glutathione synthesis, and Se functions as a necessary cofactor for the enzyme glutathione peroxidase. The interrelationship between Se and vitamin E is perhaps best documented, and although they cannot completely replace each other's dietary requirements, they appear to function synergistically in protecting against oxidative damage and in alleviating the multisystemic signs of their deficiencies.

Signs of Deficiency. Whole-blood Se concentrations have been used to identify the geographic distribution of Se deficiency among beef cows and heifers (Dargatz and Ross 1996). There was a higher prevalence of severe (18.6%) or marginal (23.8%) Se deficiency in cattle from southeastern states, and severe deficiency was mostly, but not completely, prevented by dietary or parenteral Se supplementation. Overt Se deficiency may result in a nutritional muscular dystrophy indistinguishable from that seen in vitamin E deficiency (see Chap. 35). It may be characterized by an acute onset of respiratory distress and musculoskeletal stiffness. Lesions may be found in cardiac and/or skeletal muscles consisting of pale, necrotic areas of Zenker's necrosis (Niyo et al. 1977; Maylin et al. 1980; Norton and McCarthy 1986). Less obvious signs of Se deficiency in adults may be increased incidence of infectious disease and myodegenerative disorders (Maas 1983; Braun et al. 1991). Reproductive disorders are more frequent, including decreased conception rates, irregular estrus cycles, retained placenta, abortions, and stillbirths (Harrison et al. 1984; Eger et al. 1985; Weiss et al. 1990). Lactating cows are predisposed to coliform and staphylococcal mastitis, and their milk neutrophils have impaired bactericidal activity (Erskine et al. 1989 1990; Grasso et al. 1990). Neonates may experience weakness, diarrhea, and decreased feed efficiency and have an unthrifty appearance (Niyo et al. 1980; Weiss et al. 1983; Moore and Kohn 1991). Se deficiency has been associated with significant derangements of both humoral and cell-mediated immunity in weanling pigs, beef calves, and lambs (Kott et al. 1983; Reffet et al. 1988; Swecker et al. 1989; Lessard et al. 1991). Prepartum treatment of sows with Se or vitamin E has resulted in higher colostral IgM levels and improved immune transfer to their offspring (Hayek et al. 1989). Dairy cows treated at 3 and 1.5 weeks before calving with Se as sodium selenite (5 mg/100 kg body weight) and *d,l*-α-tocopheryl acetate (25 IU/100 kg of body weight) produced 22% more colostrum during the first 36 hours postpartum and 10% more milk during the first 12 weeks of lactation than nonsupplemented cows (Lacetera et al. 1996). While blood glutathione peroxidase activities at birth and 28 days of age were higher in their calves, there was no effect on plasma immunoglobulin concentration or body weight.

Dietary Requirements, Indications, and Use

INTRINSIC FACTORS. Requirements for Se are greatest during pregnancy, growth, and lactation. Other intrinsic factors which may affect the Se requirement include systemic diseases which increase oxidative stress due to inflammatory, neoplastic, or other toxic effects, thereby increasing the need for free radical quenching and xenobiotic biotransformation (Fettman 1991; Pence 1991). Significant reductions in plasma Se concentrations of hospitalized human patients with euthyroid sick syndrome have been attributed to their hypercatabolic state (Van Lente and Daher 1992).

EXTRINSIC FACTORS. The considerable site- and species-specific differences in plant Se content can have significant effects on supplemental dietary Se requirements in ruminants. Likewise, variation in vitamin E content of both plant- and animal-source dietary components can affect supplemental dietary Se requirements. Regardless of the source of Se supplementation used, dietary Se appears to be more available to sheep fed a predominantly concentrate versus a predominantly forage diet (Koenig et al. 1997). Although dietary levels of transition elements may influence oxidative changes in feeds, neither Cu, Fe, or Zn have been shown to affect GI Se absorption (Minson 1990b; Dove and Ewan 1990). Diets for growing and finishing heifers and steers should probably contain at least 0.10 mg Se/kg DM, and those for breeding bulls and pregnant or lactating cows should contain 0.05-0.10 mg/kg DM (Minson 1990b). For dairy cows, GI Se absorption is linear over a range of approximately 0.4-3.1 mg/day, and the daily requirement is estimated at 2-2.5 mg/day (Harrison and Conrad 1984; Stowe et al. 1988). Reference values for serum Se (ng/mL) are 70-100 for cattle, 120-150 for sheep, 130-160 for horses, and 180-220 for swine (Stowe and Herdt 1992). Hepatic Se concentrations are normally between 1.2 and 2.0 μg/g DW, for all species and ages (Stowe and Herdt 1992).

Preparations and Therapy. Se fertilization of marginal soils is effective in raising plant Se content. Selenate salts appear to be more available than selenite salts, and in New Zealand, sodium selenate-containing granules with 1% Se have been used to apply approximately 10 g Se/hectare each year as a means of increasing forage Se levels (Minson 1990b). In the United States, the Food and Drug Administration allows up to 0.3 ppm Se in complete feeds for cattle, sheep, swine, chickens, turkeys, and ducks. Salt and mineral mixtures for free-choice feeding may contain up to 120 ppm for beef cattle and 90 ppm for sheep. Total daily intake should not exceed 3 mg for beef cattle and 0.7 mg for sheep. In breeding ewes, it is reported that oral doses of 5 mg Se one month before mating and one month before lambing may improve reproductive performance. Sustained-release pellets containing elemental Se in an iron matrix, as well as Se-containing osmotic pump boluses, are available for intraruminal administration (Maas et al. 1994). An alternative intraruminal slow-release device is a glass bolus impregnated with elemental Se. Injectable combination products of vitamin E and selenium contain approximately 50 IU of vitamin E and 5 mg of selenium per milliliter and are dosed at about 1 mL per 100 kg of body weight. Parenteral doses of approximately 5 mg/100 kg of body weight have been recommended to treat Se deficiency in domestic animals (Maas 1983; Van Vleet 1989; Moore and Kohn 1991). However, some more work indicates that a single label dose of injectable Se does not result in prolonged blood Se concentrations or glutathione peroxidase activity which is normally considered to be adequate (Maas et al. 1993). Blood Se was shown to peak at 5 hours postinjection and to decrease below normal levels thereafter, while blood glutathione peroxidase activity peaked at 28 days and never attained normal values. More work may be indicated to determine the optimal dose of this parenteral product, and/or alternative methods of Se supplementation may be required for long-term prevention of dietary deficiency.

Toxicity. Acute, high-level Se toxicosis may occur under pasture conditions, following consumption of sufficient quantities of Se-accumulator plants, and following overdosage with a Se supplement to prevent or treat deficiency. In pigs, as little as 3 mg Se/kg body weight produced fatal Se toxicosis manifested by vomiting, respiratory distress, weakness, central nervous system (CNS) depression, coma, and death (Hatch et al. 1979b; NRC 1980). Dietary levels of greater than 20 ppm have also induced toxicity in feeder pigs (Casteel et al. 1985). In young lambs, 10 mg sodium selenite administered orally resulted in depression, ataxia, dyspnea, pollakiuria, cyanosis, dilated pupils, tympany, and death. Pathologic lesions included edema, hyperemia, hemorrhages, and necrosis in several body systems (Morrow 1968). Selenium intakes as sodium selenite of up to 50 mg/day for 90 days or 100 mg/day for 28 days by adult Holstein cows had no adverse effects (Ellis et al. 1997). The minimum lethal dose for Se administered by intramuscular injection to dogs is approximately 2.0 mg/kg (Janke 1989). The minimum, single lethal doses of oral sodium selenite for horses, cattle, and pigs are 3.3, 10, and 17 mg/kg body weight, respectively (Traub-Dargatz and Hamar 1986).

Chronic Se poisoning resulting from prolonged intake of lower toxic levels of Se results in the clinical syndromes of "blind staggers" or "alkali disease" (NRC 1980). Blind staggers is a chronic clinical syndrome that has been linked to the consumption of Se-accumulator plants and has been characterized with the paradoxically acute onset of blindness, head pressing, circling, dysphagia, and paralysis (NRC 1980; O'Toole et al. 1996). However, it has been suggested that many field cases of "blind staggers" may have actually been sulfate intoxication-related polioencephalomalacia, and that others may have actually been malignant catarrhal fever, swainsonine intoxication (from the Se-accumulator *Astragalus* spp.), or pyrrolizidine alkaloid intoxication (*Senecio* spp.) (O'Toole et al. 1996). Alkali disease has been observed following the consumption of feeds containing 5-40 ppm Se over several weeks or months. Signs include lameness, hoof malformations, loss of hair (especially from the mane and tail), depression, anorexia, emaciation, and recumbency followed by death (NRC 1980; Traub-Dargatz and Hamar 1986). Approximately 2 ppm Se in the diet is considered the maximum tolerable level for all species.

VANADIUM

Source and Occurrence. Vanadium (V) occurs in four valency states as V(II), V(III), V(IV), and V(V). The pentavalent salts are vanadates, and the quadrivalent forms are vanadites. Vanadium is widely distributed in nature at low levels but on occasion may occur at toxic levels in rock phosphates which are used as phosphorus sources for animal diets (NRC 1980). Although less than 1% of ingested elemental V is actually absorbed from the GI tract, it is considered a nutritionally essential trace element, and definitive biological effects can be demonstrated following repletion of deficient animals.

Biological Characteristics and Signs of Deficiency. The exact metabolic pathways for V transport and incorporation into tissues have not been extensively studied. Absorbed V is taken up by most tissues of the body but is principally directed to growing bone, as well as liver, kidneys, and spleen. Supplementation of rat diets with 0.1 ppm V as sodium orthovanadate (Na_3VO_4) enhances growth significantly (NRC 1980). Diets containing less than 10 ppb retard feather growth in chicks (NRC 1980). Feeding 0.1 mg sodium metavanadate per kilogram body weight to calves increases growth rate and erythrocyte production (NRC 1980). Interest in V has increased in recent years because of the insulin-like actions it can exert on a variety of tissues. Following the first demonstration of insulin-like stimulation of glucose oxidation in isolated rat adipocytes by Na_3VO_4 (Schecter and Karlish 1980), further studies were initiated to determine whether vanadate might ameliorate some of the abnormalities observed in diabetes mellitus. When fed 70-100 mg Na_3VO_4 per kilogram body weight per day for 4 weeks, rats with streptozotocin-induced diabetes mellitus experienced significant improvements in blood glucose concentrations and dynamic cardiac performance compared to controls (Heyliger et al. 1985). Neither peroxyvanadate nor vanadate exerts any effects on insulin binding or insulin sensitivity in isolated human adipocytes, yet peroxyvanadate was as effective as insulin in inhibiting isoproterenol-mediated lipolysis (Lonnroth et al. 1993). In human patients with non-insulin-dependent diabetes mellitus (NIDDM), twice daily oral treatment with 50 mg vanadyl sulfate for 3 weeks significantly improved glycemic control during both oral glucose tolerance tests and euglycemic hyperinsulinemic clamps (Cohen et al. 1995). Adverse side effects of vanadyl sulfate (50 mg twice daily per os) in humans have included diarrhea, flatulence, nausea, and abdominal cramps, all of which disappeared after 1-2 weeks of treatment (Boden et al. 1996). Increased insulin-stimulated hepatic glycogen synthesis accounted for most of the nearly 90% increase in systemic glucose disposal, while hepatic glucose output was nearly completely suppressed by vanadium treatment. In another study, oral treatment with sodium metavanadate (125 mg/day) for 2 weeks improved glucose utilization by approximately 30-40% in human NIDDM patients, reduced exogenous insulin requirements by approximately 14% in insulin-dependent diabetics, and decreased serum cholesterol significantly in both groups (Goldfine et al. 1995).

Dietary Requirements, Indications, Use, and Toxicity. No specific indications for V supplementation have been identified for healthy domestic animals. It has been suggested that V, like iron and zinc, may be sequestered during infections, thereby increasing its requirements, but this has not been thoroughly studied. Vanadium exerts its toxic effects through inhibition of cell enzymes, including Na,K-ATPase (NRC 1980). In vitro ruminal fluid dry-matter digestibility is reduced by as little as 5-7 ppm in the inoculum (NRC 1980). However, sheep have tolerated up to 200 ppm in the diet, and cattle have been fed up to 7.5 mg/kg body weight without adverse effects (NRC 1980). Rats fed up to 20 ppm V in the diet exhibit no adverse effects, but progressively higher amounts can reduce growth, induce diarrhea, and ultimately cause death (NRC 1980). Supplemental dietary Cr has been shown to alleviate V toxicity, perhaps by antagonizing V-induced uncoupling of oxidative phosphorylation (NRC 1980). No specific recommendations may be made regarding a safe and efficacious dose for the treatment of NIDDM in animals.

ZINC

Source and Occurrence. Zinc (Zn) concentrations are generally higher in plant leaves than stems, so that legumes contain more than grasses, and immature plants contain more than mature ones (Minson 1990c; NRC 1982). Zn concentrations in fish and meat meals are higher than in plants, particularly because of higher Zn levels in certain organ tissues (liver, kidney).

Chemical Forms, Distribution, and Biological Characteristics. Zinc is relatively available from a variety of sources, including elemental zinc and insoluble salt forms, which are solubilized by gastric acids for absorption by the small-intestinal mucosa. Inorganic salts of Zn, including the oxide, carbonate, acetate, chloride, and sulfate, are readily available following oral administration (Neathery et al. 1975; NRC 1980; Wedekind and Baker 1990). Chelated dietary forms of Zn, complexed with methionine or lysine, have been purported to enhance bioavailability, and in one study improved immune responsiveness noticeably (Chirase et al. 1991). Most studies have found little difference in Zn bioavailability between $ZnSO_4$ and Zn-methionine or Zn-lysine complexes, although they both have greater availability than ZnO in pigs, cattle, and sheep (Swinkels et al. 1996; Schell and Kornegay 1996; Rojas et al. 1995; Wedekind et al. 1994). Oral administration of diiodohydroxyquinolein, a Zn-chelating compound, has been shown to enhance Zn bioavailability in rats and in hypozincemic human patients with chronic renal failure (Paniagua et al. 1995). Endogenous factors that play a role in Zn absorption include prostaglandin E_2, which may facilitate its mucosal transport, and metallothioneins, which are induced during inflammation and mediate changes in interorgan distribution of Zn (Sobocinski et al. 1978; Starcher et al. 1980). IL-1, released during inflammatory disorders and particularly during bacterial infections or endotoxemia, induces hepatic and renal metallothionein synthesis, leading to sequestration of Zn in these tissues and induction of hypozincemia (Etzel et al. 1982; Klasing 1984). While this response may deprive proliferating bacteria of Zn, thereby suppressing their growth, it is also possible that lower Zn levels may adversely affect host metabolic and immune responses as well.

Metabolic Functions

APOENZYME AND MEMBRANE INTERACTIONS. Zn functions as a necessary cofactor for many metalloenzymes, including alcohol, lactic acid, malic acid, and glutamic acid dehydrogenases, alkaline phosphatases, pancreatic carboxypeptidases A and B, carbonic anhydrase, deoxythymidine kinase, DNA- and RNA-polymerases, and superoxide dismutase. Zn binds to many organic molecular moieties, including sulfhydryl, amino, imidazole, and phosphate groups, thereby facilitating its interactions with a plethora of biologically important compounds. Zn has a direct stabilizing effect on cellular membranes and may alter membrane fluidity, thereby affecting ion gating, hormone-receptor interactions, cytoskeletal activity, membrane-bound enzyme activation, and membrane lipid participation in free radical reactions. In addition, the expression of several genes for the synthesis of hepatic proteins, including transthyretin and retinol-binding protein, is regulated by Zn and results in up-regulation of expression during Zn deficiency (Kimball et al. 1995).

IMMUNOLOGIC MODULATION. Zn-deficient mice demonstrate impaired cell-mediated immune responses to allogeneic tumor cell inoculations and reduced delayed-type hypersensitivity reactions to dinitrofluorobenzene, both of which are corrected following Zn supplementation (Frost et al. 1981; Fraker et al. 1982). Similarly, the humoral immune response to sheep red blood cells is reduced in Zn-deficient mice, predominantly through interference with T-helper cell proliferation and function, leading to reduced B-cell and plasmacyte development (Fraker et al. 1977; Luecke et al. 1978; Luecke and Fraker 1979). Zn deficiency in laboratory rodents increases their susceptibility to infection by bacteria (Sobocinski et al. 1977), as well as to yeast like *Candida albicans* (Salvin and Rabin 1984). Pretreatment with Zn increases survival following intravenous administration of *Salmonella typhimurium* in rats, through effects on host immunity and on developing endotoxemia (Tocco-Bradley and Kluger 1984). In fact, lethality in endotoxin-treated mice has been reduced significantly by pretreatment with Zn, through effects that appear to include stabilization of lysosomal membranes and moderation of cellular proteolytic reactions (Snyder and Walker 1976). In rhesus monkeys, Zn deficiency induces an intrinsic neutrophil defect that specifically affects chemotaxis, although phagocytosis of opsonized yeast was not affected (Vruwink et al. 1991).

Zn deficiency has likewise been linked to immune dysfunction in humans, including impaired T-cell mitogenic responses and decreased natural killer cell activity and monocyte cytotoxicity (Pekarek et al. 1979; Allen et al. 1981; Allen et al. 1983; Duchateau et al. 1981a). Oral Zn supplementation in humans over 70 years of age has resulted in increased circulating levels of T lymphocytes, improvement in the delayed cutaneous hypersensitivity reaction to Candidin and streptokinase-streptodornase, and increased IgG antibody response to tetanus vaccination (Duchateau et al. 1981b). Zn supplementation of human peripheral blood lymphocytes in vitro stimulates B-lymphocyte mitogenic responses (Cunningham-Rundles et al. 1980). Human patients who consumed Zn-gluconate-containing throat lozenges regularly throughout a cold experienced a significant reduction in duration of symptoms from 7.6 to 4.4 days and had fewer days with coughing, headache, hoarseness, nasal congestion and drainage, or sore throat (Mossad et al. 1996). In a study of stressed feeder calves, dietary Zn supplementation with either zinc oxide or zinc methionine increased feed intake but not average daily gain (Spears et al. 1991). However, zinc methionine appeared to have enhanced antibody titer formation following bovine herpesvirus-1 vaccination.

Dietary Zn deficiency in 5-week-old puppies resulted in lymphocyte depletion of T-cell-dependent areas of the lymph nodes, spleen, and thymus (Sanecki et al. 1985), and serum globulin concentrations were depressed in Zn-deficient Hampshire ewes (Nelson et al. 1984). In feedlot steers challenged with infectious bovine rhinotracheitis virus, dietary supplementation with Zn-methionine returned rectal temperature, feed intake, and body weight gains to normal more rapidly than no Zn supplementation or Zn oxide supplementation (Chirase et al. 1991).

NEOPLASIA. Because Zn is required for cell proliferative processes, as a cofactor for nucleic acid polymerases and deoxythymidine kinase, it may also play an important role in tumor growth. For instance, growth of Walker 256 carcinosarcoma implants was reduced in rats fed a Zn-deficient diet (McQuitty et al. 1970). On the other hand, because of its vital role in the host immune response, Zn deficiency might compromise immunologically mediated tumor rejection mechanisms. Voyatzoglou et al. (1982) demonstrated hyperzincuria and hypozincemia in human patients with lung cancer, and those with more severe abnormalities of Zn balance had a shorter life expectancy. Another study documented in human patients with lung cancer the association between higher urinary Zn excretion, lower serum Zn levels, and depressed T-cell phytohemagglutinin response, and reversal following dietary Zn supplementation, although the question of potential beneficial effects of Zn supplementation on tumor rejection was not addressed (Allen et al. 1985).

Signs of Deficiency. All-forage diets for sheep are considered marginal in Zn content but support normal growth, dry matter intake and digestibility, and Zn balance (Reid et al. 1987). In lactating dairy cattle, dietary Zn supplementation from 135 to 1386 ppm induced no differences in body weight change, milk yield, milk fat, or milk protein concentrations (Gaynor et al. 1988). However, Zn deficiency can cause depressions in growth, milk production, and reproductive function (Minson 1990c). Zn-deficient ewes gained less weight during pregnancy, experienced more abortions and difficulty at delivery, and produced smaller lambs with lower neonatal survival rates than Zn-supplemented ewes (Apgar and Fitzgerald 1985).

Zn deficiency in growing puppies results in skin lesions characterized by parakeratosis, hyperkeratosis, erosions, ulcerations, vesiculation, alopecia, and epidermitis, which are reversed following Zn supplementation (Sanecki et al. 1982). In sheep and goats fed Zn-deficient rations, integumentary lesions are further characterized by wool loosening, abnormal hoof growth, postural kyphosis, and testicular hypoplasia in males (Nelson et al. 1984). In sheep, both dietary supplementation of 0.5-0.75 g $ZnSO_4$/day and daily immersion in a 10% $ZnSO_4$ foot bath have been shown to be effective in controlling foot rot (Cross and Parker 1981a,b). Zn deficiency in foals also results in integumentary abnormalities and, in particular, leads to facial lesions and predisposes limb abrasions to infection (Cunha 1991).

Bovine hereditary Zn deficiency (lethal trait A46) is an autosomal recessive disorder that has been reported in Black Pied Friesian and Angus cattle and resembles acrodermatitis enteropathica in humans (Machen et al. 1996; Vestweber et al. 1994). The basic defect is an inability to absorb Zn from the GI tract, resulting in refractory Zn deficiency and clinical signs including diarrhea, hyperkeratotic skin lesions, perioral lesions which impair suckling in the young, delayed wound healing, and respiratory infections.

Dietary Requirements, Indications, and Use

INTRINSIC FACTORS. Requirements for Zn may parallel those for protein and are greatest during pregnancy, growth, and lactation (Prasad 1979). GI disease can lead to both decreased absorption of dietary Zn and increased loss of endogenous Zn complexed to protein in exudations or shed, diseased mucosal cells. Liver disease can impair Zn metabolism, and human patients with cirrhosis often have low serum and hepatic Zn and hyperzincuria. Proteinuria during renal disease can result in loss of Zn-protein complexes and a conditioned Zn deficiency. Similarly, protein exudation from major burns and accelerated cell desquamation from diseased skin can lead to Zn depletion.

EXTRINSIC FACTORS. Factors affecting Zn absorption include dietary levels, presence in the diet of minerals that compete for transport (Fe, Cu, Ca), and interfering substances that may bind Zn (phytate, fiber, chelating agents). When adequate Zn is fed to calves, varying levels of dietary P have little effect on Zn's bioavailability (LaFlamme et al. 1985). However, lower dietary P intake in calves has been associated with higher dietary Zn absorption and hepatic Zn levels (Neathery et al. 1990). Dietary supplementation in pigs with microbial-derived phytase significantly improves bioavailability of Zn, as well as P, Mg, and Cu (Adeola et al. 1995). Addition of 1500 phytase units/kg of feed was roughly as effective in improving feed efficiency in pigs as addition of 100 mg/kg diet Zn as $ZnSO_4$ (Adeola et al. 1995). High dietary aluminum intake has been associated with reduced dietary assimilation and organ Zn levels (Neathery et al. 1990). High levels of dietary Ca suppress feed efficiency and increase the incidence of parakeratosis in calves fed a Zn-deficient diet but have no effect when Zn intake is adequate (Minson 1990c).

Toxicity. Dietary Zn levels of up to approximately 600 ppm have produced no adverse effects in most species studied (NRC 1980). Levels of 1000 ppm or more may result in reduced feed intake and weight gains, anemia, impaired bone mineralization, bone and cartilage abnormalities, and decreased tissue levels of Fe, Mn, and Cu (NRC 1980). In adult, lactating cows, dietary Zn intake of 2000 ppm decreased feed intake, milk yield, and calf weight but had no long-term effects (Miller et al. 1989). Horses fed 25-186 mg Zn/kg body weight developed severe epiphyseal swelling, became lame, and grew more slowly (NRC 1980). Clinical signs of toxicity in calves developed after 23 days of being fed a milk replacer containing approximately 700 ppm Zn (Graham et al. 1987), although up to 500 ppm Zn has been tolerated for a period of 5 weeks (Jenkins and Hidiroglou 1991). These signs included pneumonia, ocular lesions, diarrhea, anorexia, bloating, cardiac arrhythmias, convulsions, and death. Zn toxicity was associated with pancreatic acinar cell necrosis, fibrosis, and atrophy in piglets receiving total parenteral nutrition containing 50 μg Zn/mL (Gabrielson et al. 1996). Heinz body hemolytic anemia has been associated with acute Zn toxicosis in dogs following ingestion of objects high in elemental Zn (nuts, bolts, US pennies), while chronic Zn toxicosis may cause anemia by interfering with Fe and Cu utilization, thereby inducing abnormalities in erythropoiesis (Luttgen et al. 1990). Interference with dietary Cu absorption and metabolism is one of the principal effects of prolonged, excessive dietary Zn intake, resulting in abnormalities in superoxide dismutase activity, alterations in serum lipoprotein profiles, depressed immune function, and other more specific signs of Cu deficiency (Fosmire 1990). On the other hand, an oral dosage of 50-100 mg Zn per day as zinc acetate has been successfully used for the long-term treatment of hepatic Cu toxicosis in Bedlington Terriers and West Highland White Terriers with heritable Cu toxicosis syndromes (Brewer et al. 1992a,b).

ESSENTIAL FATTY ACIDS

Chemical Structure. Fatty acids are denoted by a series of numbers which describe the position of the double bonds, the number of carbon atoms, the number of double bonds, and the location of the last double bond relative to the methyl group. For instance, docosahexaenoic acid (4,7,10,13,16,19-C22:6;ω-3) is a fatty acid with 22 carbon atoms and six double bonds, with the last double bond located at C-19, three away from the terminal methyl group. There are three families of unsaturated, 18-carbon fatty acids, differentiated by their omega (ω) number. The ω-9 family can be derived from endogenous stearic acid (18:0; ω-9), much as the family of unsaturated, 16-carbon fatty acids may be produced from endogenous palmitoleic acid (16:1;ω-7). The ω-6 family is derived from linoleic acid (9,12-C18:2;ω-6), and the ω-3 series from α-linolenic acid (9,12,15-C18:3;ω-3). All mammalian species have a dietary requirement for the *cis*-polyunsaturated 18-carbon fatty acids, which thus compose the group of essential fatty acids (EFAs).

Chemical Properties. The EFAs are liquids at room temperature, soluble in nonpolar solvents, and insoluble in water. Susceptibility to oxidative damage depends on the number of double bonds in each fatty acid. The oxidized forms, in turn, may propagate oxidative damage in other unsaturated fatty acids and electrophilic molecules, thereby potentially leading to consumption of antioxidants like vitamins E, A, and C and glutathione. When antioxidant reserves are depleted, lipid peroxidation, protein denaturation, or nucleic acid adduction may occur. This free radical damage may also be promoted by transition metal elements like iron and copper. EFAs are analyzed in vitro by gas-liquid chromatography and in vivo by bioassay of the growth response of deficient weanling rats (McDowell 1989).

Source and Occurrence. The EFAs are found in various plant oils, including corn oil, soybean oil, and cottonseed oil, of which about 50% are linoleic acid. Alpha-linolenic acid is found in higher amounts in oils from forages and green, leafy vegetables (McDowell 1989; Neuringer et al. 1988). Longer, more unsaturated derivatives of linoleic and α-linolenic acid are found predominantly in animals, where they are produced through the activities of chain elongation and desaturation enzymes, but the ω-3 and ω-6 series cannot be interconverted, and dietary requirements for each family are absolute (Figs. 38.1-38.3). Some confusion has existed on this point, however, because historical studies showed that α-linolenic acid could ameliorate some signs of linoleic acid deficiency. Although the tissue concentration of arachidonic acid is not altered in humans by changing dietary linoleic acid intake, tissue eicosapentaenoic acid concentrations are linearly responsive to increasing dietary levels of α-linolenic acid (Mantzioris et al. 1995).

The cat is exceptional among mammals for its inability to convert linoleic acid to arachidonic acid; the cat may also be unable to produce some longer-chain derivatives of α-linolenic acid (MacDonald et al. 1984; McLean and Monger 1989). The Δ6-desaturase enzyme is the rate-limiting enzyme in the metabolism of linoleic and α-linolenic acids in most mammals (Figs. 38.1 and 38.2) and is virtually nondetectable in the cat. Modifications of linoleic and α-linolenic acid can occur by an alternative pathway through the sequential activities of a Δ8- and Δ5-desaturase, which can produce arachidonic and eicosapentaenoic acid, respectively (Figs. 38.1 and 38.2). However, these alternative pathways' rates of activity are too low to support the cat's metabolic requirements, thus necessitating a dietary source of arachidonic acid and perhaps also of eicosapentaenoic or docosahexaenoic acid (McLean and Monger 1989). Until recently, the conversion of eicosapentaenoic acid (20:5;ω-3) was presumed to be catalyzed by a Δ4-desaturase. However, it

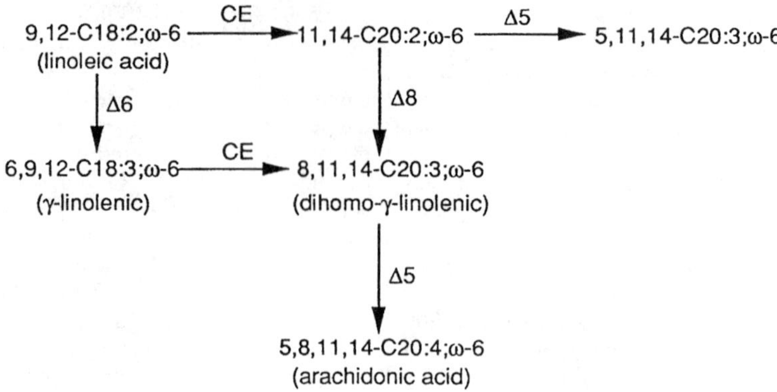

FIG. 38.1—Derivation of ω-6 fatty acids from linoleic acid. (Adapted from McLean and Monger 1989.)

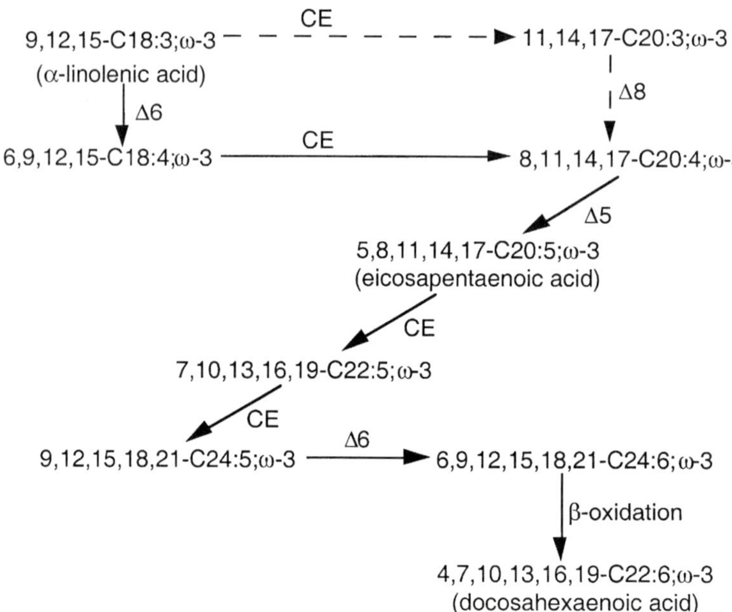

FIG. 38.2—Derivation of ω-3 fatty acids from α-linolenic acid. (Adapted from McLean and Monger 1989 and Sprecher et al. 1995.)

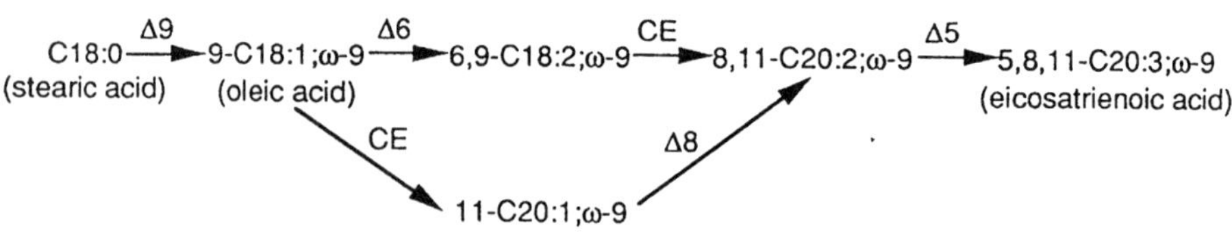

FIG. 38.3—Derivation of ω-9 fatty acids from stearic acid. (Adapted from McLean and Monger 1989.)

is now known that this enzyme does not exist, and that docosahexaenoic acid is derived by the sequential chain elongation of 20:5;ω-3 to 22:5;ω-3 and 24:5;ω-3, followed by Δ6-desaturation to 24:6;ω-3 and β-oxidation to 22:6;ω-3 (Sprecher et al, 1995; Figure 38.2).

Interest in the potential health benefits of the ω-3 family has increased in recent years, in large part due to epidemiological studies of societies consuming large amounts of marine fish. This led to the identification of marine fish oils as major sources of ω-3 fatty acids, which are synthesized de novo by phytoplankton at the base of the aquatic food chain and subsequently accumulated by the fish at the peak of that chain (Logas et al. 1991; McDowell 1989; Neuringer et al. 1988).

Biological Characteristics. The EFAs are absorbed along with other dietary lipids in the small intestine by a process dependent on biliary and pancreatic secretions. The preliminary hydrolysis by pancreatic lipase of ω-3 fatty acids from dietary triglycerides may not be as efficient as for other fats (Nestel 1990). In addition, pancreatic lipase preferentially splits the fatty acids in the 1-C and 3-C positions of dietary triglycerides. Because most of the ω-3 fatty acids in marine fish oil are in the C-2 position of the triglycerides, these would be absorbed predominantly as monoglycerides, which may influence their subsequent metabolism. The ω-3 fatty acids are more readily absorbed when specific synthetic triacylglycerols are administered with eicosapentaenoic acid (20:5;ω-3) or docosahexaenoic acid (22:6;ω-3) predominantly in the C-2 position and a medium-chain fatty acid, decaenoic acid, in the C-1 and C-3 positions (Christensen et al. 1995). Fatty acyl-binding proteins in the small-intestinal epithelial cells appear to facilitate intracellular transport and distribution of EFA either to local cellular organelles or to chylomicra for transport via the lymphatics to distant sites. In humans, chronic ingestion of oils containing high concentrations of ω-3 fatty acids results in incorporation of long-chain ω-3 fatty acids, in a dose-dependent manner, in adipose tissue (Leaf et al. 1995) and in plasma phospholipids (Andersen et al. 1996).

METABOLIC FUNCTIONS. Absorbed EFAs are interconverted to other fatty acids of the same ω series. Arachidonic acid (20:4;ω-6) derived from dietary linoleic acid (18:2;ω-6) and docosahexaenoic acid (22:6;ω-3) derived from dietary α-linolenic acid (18:3;ω-3) serve an important role in cell membrane structure and are the principal precursors for the biologically active ω-6 (bienoic, or 2-series) and ω-3 (trienoic, or 3-series) eicosanoids, respectively (Fig. 38.4). Arachidonic acid accounts for 5-15% of total fatty acids in most tissue phospholipids, while docosahexaenoic acid is present predominantly in the retina, cerebral cortex, testes, and sperm (Neuringer et al. 1988). In the cerebral gray matter, docosahexaenoic acid composes up to one-third of the fatty acids of phosphatidyl ethanolamine and phosphatidyl serine.

A deficiency of one series may lead to a complementary increase in tissue levels of another series. When completely deprived of ω-6 fatty acids, tissue levels of all ω-6 derivatives are lower than normal, whereas levels of ω-9 fatty acids like oleic (18:1;ω-9) and eicosatrienoic (20:3;ω-9) and of ω-7 fatty acids like palmitoleic (16:1;ω-7) are increased (McDowell 1989). Docosapentaenoic acid (22:5;ω-6) is normally very low in most tissues but replaces docosahexaenoic acid (22:6;ω-3) when there is an ω-3 EFA deficiency. Conversely, because the enzymes responsible for chain elongation and desaturation interact with all series of

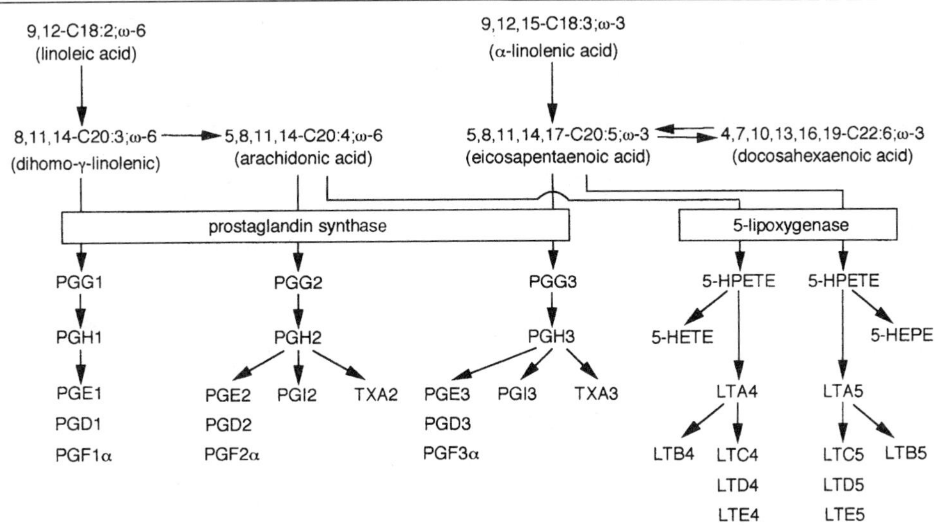

FIG. 38.4—Derivation of eicosanoids from ω-6 and ω-3 fatty acids. (Adapted from Barcelli 1991.)

polyunsaturated fatty acids, one series can suppress the metabolism of another. The ω-3 series tends to suppress the interconversion of the ω-6 series, and the ω-6 series tends to suppress the derivation of longer ω-9 fatty acids from oleic acid (McDowell 1989). Supplementation of diets with one series of EFA will also lead to replacement of other series in tissues.

ω-3 DOSE VERSUS ω-3:ω-6 RATIO. The exact mechanisms whereby ω-3 EFAs exert their various metabolic effects have not been clearly established. However, it is apparent that eicosapentaenoic and docosahexaenoic acids can inhibit the synthesis of arachidonic acid from linoleic acid, compete with arachidonate for the 2-acyl position in membrane phospholipids, and are preferentially metabolized by cyclooxygenase and lipoxygenase to eicosanoids and leukotrienes with differing biological activities from those of the ω-6 series (Fig. 38.4; Lefer 1989). It is unclear whether the absolute dietary amount of ω-3 fatty acids is of more or less biological importance than the ratio of ω-3:ω-6 fatty acids in the diet. It has been shown that dose-responsive suppression of eicosanoid synthesis from arachidonic acid by dietary ω-3 fatty acids is lost when the ratio of ω-3 to ω-6 fatty acids is maintained at a constant level by simultaneous dietary safflower oil addition (Boudreau et al. 1991). Thus, it appears that mechanisms for ω-3 effects relying on membrane fatty acid replacement depend on relative, rather than absolute dietary amounts of the various EFA classes. Studies in piglets and neonatal rats have shown that increasing brain and retina levels of arachidonic acid and docosahexaenoic acid result with increasing dietary intakes of linoleic and α-linolenic acid, respectively, until a plateau is reached at about 2.4% of dietary energy for linoleic acid and 0.7% of dietary energy for α-linolenic acid (Rioux et al. 1997). Further increases in the 18-carbon precursors do not affect plasma or tissue levels of their elongated counterparts. However, increased consumption of the long chain metabolites appear to continue increasing circulating plasma phospholipid levels without dose limitations (Rioux et al. 1997). Thus, effects of ω-3 fatty acid dose versus ω-3:ω-6 fatty acid ratio may depend on independent factors, including dietary energy density, fatty acid chain length, and biological availability of supplements. In dogs supplemented for 12 weeks with increasing ratios of ω-6:ω-3 fatty acids, manipulated by altering dietary menhaden, flaxseed, and safflower oil content, ratios of 5:1 and 10:1 significantly altered isolated neutrophil synthesis of leukotriene B_4 (30-33% less) and B_5 (370-500% more), whereas ratios of 25:1, 50:1, and 100:1 were without effect (Vaughn et al. 1994). Fatty acid dose and ratio of these diets were without clinically important effects on platelet function and blood coagulation pathways (Boudreaux et al. 1997).

ω-3 FATTY ACID WASHOUT KINETICS. The optimum intake of ω-3 fatty acids is also determined by their metabolic fate once incorporated into the tissues. Subsequent to enrichment of adipose tissue stores and membrane phospholipids, polyunsaturated fatty acids undergo differential rates of elution which are dependent on the metabolic activity of tissue as well as structural modifications of the fatty acids themselves. Studies with crossover designs require a washout period suitable for the species, tissue, and fatty acids of interest, and washout periods have varied from 4 to 10 weeks (Hansen et al. 1998). In rats, ω-3 fatty acids are selectively mobilized from fat stores in the following decreasing relative order: 20:5;ω-3 > 18:4;ω-3 > 22:6;ω-3 > 22:5;ω-3 (Raclot and Groscolas 1994). In humans, 2-3 months are required for effects of dietary ω-3 fatty acid supplementation on erythrocyte membrane composition and fluidity to dissipate (Prisco et al. 1996). Concomitant changes in susceptibility of erythrocyte membranes to oxidative damage and the relative availability of antioxidants like α-tocopherol may also accelerate membrane ω-3 fatty acid turnover (Palozza et al. 1996). In dogs fed a menhaden oil-supplemented diet for 8 weeks, serum docosahexaenoic acid and eicosapentaenoic acid concentrations remained elevated for 7 weeks and 3 weeks, respectively, following cessation of treatment (Hansen et al. 1998). The effect of washout must be closely evaluated in any study that includes a crossover design, as results may be suspect when washout periods of inadequate duration are employed (Clark et al. 1993; Wallace et al. 1995). This has made it difficult to conclusively determine whether specific dietary fatty acid therapies evaluated in crossover trials for canine atopy are effective (Bond and Lloyd 1992; Sture and Lloyd 1995; Scott et al. 1997).

LIPID METABOLISM. In the liver, ω-3 fatty acids appear to have some unique effects on lipid metabolism. They suppress fatty acid synthesis and esterification, increase fatty acid oxidation, promote phospholipid synthesis, and inhibit the activity of hydroxymethylglutaryl (HMG)-CoA reductase, thereby reducing cholesterol synthesis (Nestel 1990; Geelen et al. 1995). Circulating levels of triglyceride-rich very low-density lipoproteins (VLDL) and intermediate density lipoproteins (IDL) are reduced, with the average degree of reduction increasing in proportion to the initial level of triglycerides in the blood. At dietary intakes of ≥2 g/day, VLDL may decrease by 25% in normal humans and by 50% in hypertriglyceridemic patients (Nestel 1990). Chylomicron clearance by peripheral tissues also increases, although this effect does not appear to be due to increased lipoprotein lipase or hepatic triglyceride lipase activities. Plasma cholesterol levels respond variably to higher dietary ω-3 fatty acid intakes, depending on the balance of decreases in cholesterol synthesis, with decreases in clearance due to reduced hepatic LDL receptor levels (Nestel 1990). It also appears that the relative potencies of docosahexaenoic acid and eicosapentaenoic acid differ in their effects on the activities of hepatic lipid metabolic pathways and circulating lipid levels (Ikeda et al. 1994).

MEMBRANE FUNCTION. Polyunsaturated acids generally increase membrane fluidity, compliance, and permeability, but specific properties may be attributed to different ω-3 fatty acids owing to particular molecular configurations (Neuringer et al. 1988). For instance, substitution of arachidonic acid (20:4;ω-6) or docosahexaenoic acid (22:6;ω-3) for linoleic acid (18:2;ω-6) in artificial phosphatidylcholine membranes did not additively increase fluidity as expected but may have promoted tighter phospholipid packing and reduced deformability. In the retina, where docosahexaenoic acid predominates, this may afford a better configuration for interaction with the visual pigment rhodopsin (Neuringer et al. 1988). Studies in ω-3 EFA-deficient rats which have shown impaired exploratory behavior, maze-learning, and brightness discrimination may indicate some effects on central nervous function as well, which may be attributed to changes in neural membrane function. Reductions in vessel wall-induced blood coagulation and platelet aggregation in individuals fed higher levels of ω-3 EFAs may reflect changes in cell membrane reactivity and membrane-bound mediators like thromboplastin and platelet-activating factor, as well as alterations in thromboregulatory eicosanoid metabolism (Henry et al. 1991).

EICOSANOID METABOLISM. Cyclooxygenase and lipoxygenase-derived metabolites of the ω-3 fatty acids have different biologic activities from those of metabolites derived from the ω-6 family (Lefer 1989). Bienoic eicosanoids of the 2-series derived from ω-6 EFAs have counterregulatory effects on blood coagulation and vasoreactivity. Prostaglandins E_2 and I_2 tend to inhibit platelet aggregation and to promote vasodilation, whereas thromboxane A_2 promotes aggregation and vasoconstriction. In contrast, the trienoic products, prostaglandin E_3 and thromboxane A_3, may both have vasodilatory properties (Lefer 1989). The 5-series of leukotrienes and lipoxins derived from eicosapentaenoic acid is less active than the 4-series produced from arachidonic acid and competes against the 4-series metabolites for receptor sites in target organs. While leukotrienes B_4 and D_4, and lipoxin A_4, may increase microvascular permeability and enhance leakiness, their 5-series counterparts have little such activity (Lefer 1989). Dietary enrichment with ω-3 EFAs increases their levels in the tissues and reduces the production of ω-6 EFA-derived eicosanoids under inflammatory, vasoreactive, or procoagulant conditions, thereby effecting numerous changes in metabolism as described below (Lefer 1989; Barcelli 1991). Subsequent modulation of the production of cytokines, including interleukin-1, interleukin-6, and tumor necrosis factor-α, may contribute further to clinical improvements in inflammatory conditions as diverse as rheumatoid arthritis, psoriasis, atopic dermatitis, colitis, systemic lupus erythematosus, and endotoxemia (Blok et al. 1996; Meydani 1996).

HEMOSTASIS AND CARDIOVASCULAR DISEASE. Epidemiological studies of Greenland Eskimos first indicated a relationship between dietary ω-3 EFA consumption and reduced risk for cardiovascular disease (Fisher et al. 1986; Herold and Kinsella 1986). Compared to those living in Denmark and consuming a diet lower in ω-3 EFAs, these Eskimos had lower blood triglyceride, cholesterol, LDL, and VLDL levels; higher HDL levels; decreased ability of platelets to aggregate; and a much lower incidence of cardiac disease. Other studies have shown that Europeans consuming as little as 30 g of marine fish daily had a 50% lower rate of mortality due to coronary artery disease than non-fish-consuming cohorts. Experimental studies in rats, rabbits, pigs, dogs, and horses have demonstrated effects of supplementary ω-3 EFAs, including changes in tissue lipid composition, lipid metabolism, platelet aggregability, monocyte-derived procoagulant activity, and platelet survival, all of which may reduce the occurrence of arterial lesions (Herold and Kinsella 1986; Levine et al. 1989). Dietary fish oil supplementation attenuates the myocardial dysfunction caused by ischemia-reperfusion injury in the rat (Yang et al. 1993) and reduces the vulnerability of normal or ischemic myocardium to induced arrhythmias in nonhuman primates (McLennan et al. 1993). Studies in humans have, in addition, demonstrated a significant blood pressure-lowering effect of dietary ω-3 EFA supplementation in both middle-aged and elderly hypertensive patients (Radack et al 1991; Margolin et al. 1991), without adverse effects on glucose metabolism (Toft et al. 1995). Effects have been observed with as little as 2 g ω-3 EFA per day.

CHRONIC RENAL DISEASE. Studies of the effects of dietary modification on the progression of chronic renal disease have turned to the particular role of dietary lipids on renal function (Barcelli 1991). Early studies indicated that rats fed a diet high in linoleic acid experienced lesser degrees of azotemia and proteinuria following partial renal ablation than those fed a low-linoleic acid diet (Heifets et al. 1987). Feeding a high-linoleic acid diet resulted in increased renal cortical and medullary linoleic and arachidonic acid content and apparently reduced the degree of systemic hypertension, the loss of glomerular permselectivity, and the development of glomerular lesions. Conversely, dietary supplementation of partially nephrectomized rats with ω-3 EFA-rich menhaden fish oil produced more rapid progression of remnant renal dysfunction, characterized by lower glomerular filtration rates, higher degrees of proteinuria, and accelerated death rates due to renal failure (Scharschmidt et al. 1987). In contrast, studies of renal dysfunction in a uninephrectomized, obese Zucker rat model found that dietary ω-3 supplementation reduced the degrees of hypercholesterolemia, proteinuria, and focal glomerulosclerosis (Kasiske et al.

1991; Wheeler et al. 1991). Glomeruli from ω-3 EFA-supplemented rats produced smaller amounts of the 2-series eicosanoids and presumably benefited by improved intraglomerular hemodynamics. Unlike the earlier studies in 5/6-nephrectomized Sprague-Dawley rats, dietary ω-3 EFAs ameliorated the progression of chronic renal injury. In human patients, beneficial effects of dietary ω-3 EFAs on systemic blood pressure in hypertensive chronic renal disease, on inflammatory reactivity in immunologically mediated chronic renal disease, and on tolerance to cyclosporin in renal-transplant recipients appear to support specific indications for ω-3 EFAs in certain patients (Bilo et al. 1991). In general, dietary ω-3 EFAs appear to ameliorate the degrees of hyperlipidemia, glomerulosclerosis, and proteinuria observed in both experimentally induced and naturally occurring nephrotic syndrome (Barcelli 1991). It is possible that contrasting effects of ω-3 and ω-6 fatty acids in different models of renal disease depend on whether inflammatory or vascular mechanisms mediate the progression of pathological changes in that model. More recently, when dogs with 15/16 nephrectomy were fed a diet enriched with fish oil, they maintained higher creatinine clearance rates, demonstrated better renal histological scores, and experienced significantly longer survival times than dogs fed a safflower oil-supplemented diet (Brown et al. 1998). Dietary preconditioning in dogs with a fish oil-containing diet (5.7:1 of ω-6:ω-3 fatty acids) was also moderately effective in reducing acute, gentamicin-induced nephrotoxicosis, though not as effective as specific thromboxane synthesis inhibition (Grauer et al. 1996).

CIRCULATORY SHOCK AND ENDOTOXEMIA. Eicosanoid and leukotriene derivatives of arachidonic acid are important mediators of much of the inflammatory, vascular, and metabolic changes associated with circulatory shock and with endotoxemia (Larsson-Backstrom et al. 1990; Lefer 1989). Numerous studies have demonstrated beneficial effects of selective blockade of vasoconstrictor, procoagulant, and phlogistic arachidonic acid metabolites (Lefer 1989). Likewise, some studies have demonstrated a protective effect of dietary supplementation with ω-3 EFAs prior to experimental induction of circulatory shock or endotoxemia, presumably owing to their replacement of ω-6 derivatives in cell membranes and preferential production of trienoic eicosanoids and 5-series leukotrienes (Henry et al. 1991). In rats, dietary EFA deficiency leads to tissue accumulation of eicosatrienoic acid (5,8,11-20C:3;ω-9), which inhibits the lipoxygenase pathway of arachidonic acid metabolism and produces less potent 3-series sulfidopeptide leukotrienes (Li et al. 1990). In one study, endotoxin-induced changes in microvascular permeability, degree of hemoconcentration, and systemic blood pressure were less severe in EFA-deficient rats (Li et al. 1990). Endotoxin-stimulated monocytes from horses fed a diet enriched with α-linolenic acid produced less procoagulant activity and thromboxane B_2 in vitro than those from controls (Henry et al. 1990). Horses supplemented with α-linolenic acid had longer activated partial thromboplastin times than controls but did not experience any differences in clinical response to intravenous endotoxin administration (Henry et al. 1991). The degree of lactic acidosis and hypoxia induced by endotoxin infusion was ameliorated in guinea pigs receiving an ω-3 EFA-supplemented total parenteral nutrition formula (Pomposelli et al. 1990). Likewise, prior dietary enrichment with ω-3 EFAs improved lactic acid levels, microvascular tissue perfusion, and lung morphology in endotoxemic guinea pigs as compared to those receiving ω-6 EFA supplementation (Pomposelli et al. 1991). In addition to effects by ω-3 EFAs on eicosanoid and leukotriene synthesis, it is possible that inflammatory cytokine release is also affected by these treatments. The synthesis of IL-1 and tumor necrosis factor by human mononuclear cells is suppressed following dietary supplementation with ω-3 EFA-rich fish oil concentrate (Endres et al. 1989).

CANCER INCIDENCE AND CANCER CACHEXIA. Several studies have now suggested a role for dietary EFAs in the development and progression of cancer in experimental models. Following treatment with the colon carcinogen azoxymethanol, mice fed a diet high in ω-3 EFAs developed fewer focal areas of colonic dysplasia than those fed an ω-6 EFA-supplemented diet (Deschner et al. 1990). In rats treated with azoxymethane, dietary ω-3 EFA supplementation with menhaden oil reduced colon tumor incidence and multiplicity at both the initiation and postinitiation phases of carcinogenesis (Reddy et al. 1991). Replacing dietary medium-chain triglycerides with marine fish oil high in ω-3 EFAs significantly reduced tumor growth rate, host weight loss, and toxicity of both cyclophosphamide and 5-fluorouracil in a murine transplantable colon carcinoma model (Tisdale and Dhesi 1990). In vitro studies with a human breast cancer cell line have demonstrated enhanced cell growth following addition of ω-6 EFAs to the medium, and inhibition of cell growth following ω-3 EFA additions (Rose and Connolly 1990), as well as a reduction in the frequency and severity of metastases in vivo when transplanted to nude mice supplemented with dietary eicosapentaenoic and docosahexaenoic acids (Rose et al. 1995, 1996). In those studies, docosahexaenoic acid was more effective than eicosapentaenoic acid, and the effect was attributed predominantly to alterations in leukotriene synthesis rather than to eicosanoids. Dietary linseed oil supplementation in rabbits, to increase ω-3 EFA intake, was shown to stimulate cell-mediated immunity, as measured by the in vitro T-cell proliferative response to the mitogens phytohemagglutinin and concanavalin A (Kelley et al. 1988). However, in humans, dietary flaxseed oil (and ω-3 EFA) supplementation had the opposite effect, although indices of humoral immunity were improved (Kelley et al. 1991).

In one study of canine lymphoma patients, dogs were fed isocaloric amounts of a diet supplemented with menhaden fish oil and arginine (experimental diet) or an otherwise identical diet supplemented with corn oil (control diet) before and after remission was attained with up to 5 dosages of doxorubicin (Ogilvie et al. 2000). The ω-3 content of the experimental diet was 7.3% DM, with an ω-6/ω-3 ratio of 0.3:1, vs. the control diet with an ω-3 content of 1.6% DM and ω-6/ω-3 ratio of 7.7:1. Dogs fed the experimental diet had significantly higher serum levels of ω-3 fatty acids and arginine when compared to controls. Higher serum levels of docosahexaenoic acid and eicosapentaenoic acid were associated with lesser plasma lactic acid responses to intravenous glucose and diet tolerance testing. Increasing docosahexaenoic acid levels were significantly associated with longer disease-free interval and survival time for dogs with Stage III lymphoma fed the experimental diet.

Potential Adverse Effects of Dietary ω-3 Supplementation. Naturally occurring sources of ω-3 fatty acids are expensive and oxidatively unstable. Diet production is more sensitive to commercial processing conditions related to temperature and moisture. Unfavorable diet texture, odor, or palatability may affect acceptance of ω-3-supplemented diets by the diseased patient. Shelf life of commercial products may be limited by higher ω-3 fatty acid content, due to rancidity.

Increased dietary ω-3 intake may be associated with hemostatic abnormalities when coagulation or platelet aggregation is desirable, with reduced immune reactivity when inflammation and pathogen elimination is advantageous, or with deficiency of antioxidant nutrients in conditions otherwise prone to vitamin E, A, or C depletion. There may be specific phases of growth wherein competitive exclusion of ω-6 fatty acids by supplementary ω-3 fatty acids may be harmful to nervous system development (Neuringer et al. 1988). Dietary supplementation with ω-3 fatty acids may also retard the fibroplastic and maturational phases of wound healing (Albina et al. 1993). Because some canine atopy patients may require much higher levels of ω-3 fatty acids to control their pruritus than is provided by some commercial dietary supplements (Scott et al. 1997), it is possible that relatively greater doses may be instituted to achieve clinical management of certain disorders, only to induce untoward side effects in other body systems over time. Clearly, more information is needed regarding ω-3 fatty acid metabolism in pet species before widespread changes in dietary management are instituted.

Signs of Deficiency. An EFA deficiency is extremely difficult to induce experimentally and occurs only rarely under natural conditions where there is insufficient dietary fat intake, or in cats, when dietary arachidonic acid is not provided. Historically, experimentally induced EFA deficiency was predominantly an ω-6 deficiency, as only small amounts of ω-3 EFAs are required, and depletion is difficult to produce. Clinical signs most often include reduced growth rates, epidermal changes such as parakeratosis, increased dermal water loss, increased susceptibility to bacterial infection, reproductive failure, and organ malfunctions related to impaired eicosanoid biosynthesis (McDowell 1989). In calves, reduced growth rate, limb weakness, muscular twitching, dermatitis, hair loss, and diarrhea have been observed. Signs of EFA deficiency in pigs include slower growth rate, delayed sexual maturity, scaly dermatitis and epidermal necrosis, and hair loss. In poultry, EFA deficiency may produce a fatty liver, testicular degeneration, generalized edema, susceptibility to respiratory infections, and increased mortality. In dogs and cats, dietary EFA deficiency results in poor growth, lethargy, dermatitis, dull hair coat, hepatic lipidosis, and increased susceptibility to infections (NRC 1985 1986; McLean and Monger 1989). EFA deficiency in humans has primarily been observed in infants fed low-fat milk replacers. However, stressed and septic surgical patients supported with continuous total parenteral nutrition have been shown to be particularly prone to develop a deficiency of ω-6 EFAs that is only partially responsive to linoleic acid supplementation, owing to increased rates of docosapentaenoic acid (C22:5;ω-6) production (Alden et al. 1986).

Assessment of Status. The biochemical changes associated with EFA deficiency are the same across all species and are characterized by alterations in the tissue and body fluid levels of various EFA and non-EFA metabolites. Most prominent are the decreased levels of linoleic acid (18:2;ω-6) and arachidonic acid (20:4;ω-6), or α-linolenic acid (18:3;ω-3) and docosahexaenoic acid (22:6;ω-3), and the increased levels of eicosatrienoic acid (20:3;ω-9) and docosatrienoic acid (22:3;ω-9). This results from the "compensatory" increase in oleic acid (18:1;ω-9) desaturation by EFA-deficient tissues (McDowell 1989; McLean and Monger 1989). Another way to express these changes is by the triene:tetraene ratio of oleic acid metabolites relative to arachidonic acid. Values ≤ 0.4 are considered normal, which correspond in most species to a dietary linoleic acid content of approximately 1% of total caloric intake (McDowell 1989). Specific recommendations for dietary intake of α-linolenic acid or any of the ω-3 series have not yet been established.

Dietary Requirements. The specific requirements for dietary linoleic and α-linolenic acids vary with species, metabolic requirements of a particular physiological state, and the ability of the individual to utilize these precursors efficiently. In addition to their dietary requirement for arachidonic acid, cats require linoleic acid for its specific metabolic roles which can apparently alleviate many of the dermal signs and fatty liver associated with EFA deficiency (McLean and Monger 1989). Additional specific factors which may influence dietary EFA requirements include age and growth rate, which increase the requirement for new tissue synthesis; sex, in that males generally have a higher requirement than females; environment, wherein low humidity and high temperature may accentuate evaporative water loss and the development of dermal signs; and exposure to toxicants and carcinogens, which may increase the EFA requirement (McDowell 1989). The presence of other dietary polyunsaturated fatty acids and oxidative agents may affect the stability of the EFAs, thereby altering the apparent requirement.

Preparations, Treatment, and Toxicity. Diets based on corn, soybean meal, and animal by-products are unlikely to be deficient in EFAs. Diets suspected of being deficient may be supplemented with plant oils rich in either ω-3 EFAs (linseed, flaxseed) or ω-6 EFAs (safflower, rice bran). Elemental diets used in enteral hyperalimentation and total parenteral nutrition may be supplemented with commercial lipid supplements derived from these enriched plant oils as well. As the purported benefits of dietary ω-3 EFA supplementation become better documented, commercial products derived from marine fish and their oils will become more available. One potential concern with the use of products like menhaden fish oil, owing to their susceptibility to oxidative damage, is stability under standard storage conditions. Likewise, increased dietary EFA intake may require increases in dietary antioxidants such as tocopherol, β-carotene, retinol, ascorbic acid, selenium, or sulfur-containing amino acids. Signs of EFA toxicity most likely are related to those associated with excessive dietary fat (such as depressed ruminal cellulolytic activity in ruminants), oxidative damage (such as predisposition to vitamin E and selenium-responsive white muscle disease), or imbalances in ω-3/ω-6 EFA ratio, which adversely affect membrane structure, eicosanoid metabolism, and organ functions.

TAURINE

Chemical Structure and Properties. Taurine (2-aminoethanesulfonic acid) is a β-amino acid, existing as a colorless tetragonal crystal in pure form. It is highly soluble in water and, like many amino acids, behaves as an amphoteric electrolyte in solution. The latter property allows taurine to form complexes with cationic mineral elements, as well as to react with carboxylic acids to form amide linkages, as in the conjugation of bile acids and certain xenobiotics (Wright et al. 1986). Heat processing of foods reduces the taurine content and, in cats, also has marked effects on the GI disposition of dietary taurine through increases in taurine degradation by lower intestinal bacteria (NRC 1986; Hickman et al. 1990).

Source and Occurrence. Taurine is synthesized by most animals predominantly in the liver, from dietary sulfur-containing amino acids (SAA), and is found in highest concentrations in excitable tissues, including the heart, retina, CNS, and skeletal muscle (Pion and Kittleson 1990). There are three possible routes for the synthesis of taurine from SAAs: (1) oxidation of cysteine to cysteine sulfinic acid, followed by decarboxylation to hypotaurine and oxidation to taurine, (2) serial oxidations of cysteine through cysteine sulfinic acid and cysteic acid, followed by decarboxylation to taurine, and (3) condensation of cysteine with phosphopantothenic acid, followed by decarboxylation and cleavage to cysteamine, and serial oxidations through hypotaurine to taurine (Wright et al. 1986; Morris et al. 1990). The first pathway appears to be quantitatively most important (Morris et al. 1990). Raw clams, oysters, mussels, scallops, and squid are reported to contain very high concentrations of taurine, followed by animal muscle and liver (NRC 1986; Laidlaw et al. 1990). Most mammals' milk contains some taurine, but the amounts are generally low, and concentrations decrease during lactation (Wright et al. 1986).

Biological Characteristics. Dietary taurine is absorbed predominantly in the small intestine and merges with the pool of endogenously synthesized taurine (Miyamoto et al. 1989). Conjugation with bile acids is quantitatively the single largest pathway of taurine metabolism. A portion of the cholyltaurine secreted in the bile may undergo deconjugation by intestinal microflora, leading either to bacterial degradation or to enterohepatic recycling and lower small-intestinal reabsorption of taurine (Morris et al. 1990). Unlike other mammals, cats cannot substitute glycine for bile acid conjugation when taurine is deficient. In addition, the hepatic activity of cysteine sulfinic acid decarboxylase, the rate-limiting enzyme for the principal taurine-synthetic pathway, is much lower in cats than in other mammals. Thus, obligatory losses of taurine through bile acid conjugation and excretion, coupled with insufficient rates of endogenous synthesis, result in a much higher dietary requirement for taurine in cats than in other animals.

Metabolic Functions

PLATELET FUNCTION. Platelets contain very high concentrations of taurine, and although its exact functions are unclear, alterations in platelet taurine content have been associated with a variety of disorders. Platelets from human patients with congestive heart disease have been reported to accumulate taurine at slower rates, although their taurine concentrations tend to be higher than in normal platelets (Wright et al. 1986). Cats with taurine deficiency-associated cardiomyopathy often develop systemic thrombi, but experimentally induced dietary taurine deficiency produced inconsistent changes in coagulation pathway activity and platelet function (Welles et al. 1993). Taurine deficiency in cats induced increased antithrombin III activity, no change in fibrinolytic activities, decreased adenosine diphosphate (ADP)-induced platelet aggregation, increased collagen-induced platelet aggregation, and did not induce thrombus formation experimentally (Welles et al. 1993).

IMMUNE FUNCTION. Taurine represents over 60% of the free amino acid pool of human lymphocytes in vivo and in culture (Wright et al. 1986). Human lymphocytes grown in taurine-deficient media continue to multiply, but with decreased cell viability, which is reversible following resupplementation with taurine. Taurine's role as an antioxidant may help regulate phagocytic cell oxidative pathways, and both lymphocyte and neutrophil function are impaired in taurine-deficient animals (Pion and Kittleson 1990). Because oligotaurinemia in human trauma patients persists longer than other hypoaminoacidemias and is not fully corrected even after 7 days of supplementation, it is possible that taurine depletion plays a critical role in immune suppression following injury (Paauw and Davis 1994).

RETINAL FUNCTION. Taurine occurs in exceptionally high concentrations in the photoreceptor cells of the outer nuclear layer of the retina (Wright et al. 1986; Pion and Kittleson 1990). The retinas of some animals can synthesize significant quantities of taurine in situ, but most is accumulated by a sodium-dependent, energy-consuming, high-affinity transport system located in the retinal pigmented epithelium (Wright et al. 1986). Taurine thus accumulated is transferred to the neural layer by a passive process that is facilitated by taurine-specific binding proteins located in the inner retina. Taurine may (1) act as an inhibitory neurotransmitter, (2) regulate osmotic pressure in the rods, (3) regulate retinal ionic calcium concentrations, and (4) control phosphorylation-dependent functions of the neural retina. Taurine has also been shown to affect retinal phagocytic function and to scavenge free radicals, thereby playing an important role as an antioxidant to prevent lipid peroxidation in this light-sensitive region (Wright et al. 1986).

BRAIN FUNCTION. Taurine is actively accumulated by brain cells and appears to play important roles in CNS development and as a neuromodulatory agent (Pion and Kittleson 1990). Taurine-deficient kittens display numerous neurological abnormalities, including cerebellar dysfunction which has been linked to abnormal division and migration of cells into the external granular cell layer. Likewise, neuroblasts in the ventricular and pial zones undergo incomplete differentiation and migration into the molecular layer (Wright et al. 1986). As a poorly diffusible, zwitterionic molecule, its presence in high concentrations in the CNS may assist in osmotic regulation, ionic balance, and membrane depolarization (Pion and Kittleson 1990). Taurine has anticonvulsant properties and has been shown to protect the brain against osmotic stress during hypernatremia and diabetic hyperglycemia (Pion and Kittleson 1990).

MYOCARDIAL FUNCTION. Pion et al. (1987) reported that low plasma taurine concentrations in cats are associated with echocardiographic evidence of myocardial failure that is reversible following oral supplementation of taurine to restore plasma levels to normal. Dietary taurine supplementation (500-1000 mg/day) of cats with moderate-to-severe dilatative cardiomyopathy has resulted in marked improvements in clinical response to standard pharmaceutical treatment, as well as significant increases in survival rate (Pion et al. 1992). Because myocardial taurine content is directly related to plasma taurine concentrations, a direct link between taurine deficiency and myocardial failure is proposed. Subsequent studies have shown that compared to normal cats, taurine-deficient cats with cardiomyopathy also have 20% lower plasma tocopherol levels, 40% higher retinol concentrations, 36% lower cholesterol, and 100% higher triglyceride concentrations (Fox et al. 1993). Thus, nutrients other than taurine may affect the expression of dilated cardiomyopathy. The mechanisms whereby taurine affects cardiac function remain unclear. Taurine is present in high concentrations in mammalian myocardium (100-200 times that found in plasma), which are additionally maintained by active transport processes. Zwitterionic taurine may retard cardiocytic potassium (K) efflux associated with body K depletion, catecholamine-induced arrhythmias, or digoxin toxicity. Taurine addition to rat cardiac tissue slices in vitro, and taurine administered to rats and dogs in vivo, has been shown to restore cardiac K content and to reverse drug-induced arrhythmias. Dietary K depletion was hypothesized to adversely affect taurine efflux across the cell membranes or to affect its metabolism (Dow et al. 1992). Thus, there appears to be a reciprocal relationship between cellular K and taurine content, which may explain the induction of taurine deficiency secondary to K depletion and the concurrence of epidemiological findings in cats with taurine-responsive congestive cardiomyopathy and those with kaliopenic nephropathy-polymyopathy syndrome (Dow et al. 1987 1992).

Signs of Deficiency. The effects of naturally occurring taurine deficiency have almost exclusively been noted in domestic cats, although some studies in humans have documented taurine depletion in preterm infants (who have low cysteine sulfinic acid decarboxylase activity) fed low-taurine milk replacement formulas (Rassin et al. 1983; Watkins et al. 1983), in patients with chronic renal failure (Bergstrom et al. 1989), and in critically injured patients inadequately maintained by total parenteral nutrition (Paauw and Davis 1990).

The earliest reports of the effects of dietary taurine deficiency in cats related specifically to the occurrence of the syndrome of "feline central retinal degeneration" (Hayes et al. 1975). Degenerative changes begin as small foci in the area centralis, followed by band-shaped horizontal lesions which progressively enlarge to involve the entire retina and are characterized histologically by vesiculation and disintegration of the photoreceptor cells and degeneration of the underlying tapetum (Morris et al. 1990; da Costa and Hoskins 1990).

Taurine deficiency has important effects on reproduction, including abortion, reduced live births, decreased birth weight, and decreased neonatal survival, and on fetal development, including hydrocephalus, anencephaly, kyphosis, and limb anomalies (Morris et al. 1990). Taurine deficiency in kittens also impairs postnatal growth rate (Sturman et al. 1985) and may reduce auditory brain stem evoked potentials, indicating hearing loss (Morris et al. 1990).

Assessment of Status. Chemical analysis of taurine in biological specimens may be accomplished by colorimetric, fluorometric, radiometric, and enzymatic methods (Wright et al. 1986). Chromatographic procedures are most accurate and include amino acid analyzers, high-performance liquid chromatographs, gas chromatographs (GC), and GC-mass spectrometer methods.

The most direct means of assessing taurine status would be by analysis of taurine concentrations in tissue biopsies from organs of interest. The most practical alternative is by determining taurine concentration in whole blood or plasma. Of the total taurine in whole blood, more than 80% is located in the erythrocytes, leukocytes, and thrombocytes (Morris et al. 1990). Food deprivation and meal feeding lead to substantial fluctuations in plasma taurine concentration, whereas whole-blood levels remain relatively constant (Pion et al. 1991). Furthermore, significant leakage of taurine from blood cells into plasma can occur if samples are not processed immediately or kept on ice until centrifugal separation of plasma from cells (Morris et al. 1990). Thus, while plasma obtained under appropriate conditions may be safely evaluated, it has become apparent that whole blood may provide a more accurate indication of actual taurine status (Trautwein and Hayes 1990). It appears that the critical value for plasma taurine in cats, below which risk for congestive cardiomyopathy may increase, is about 20 nmol/mL. Cats with plasma levels less than 40 nmol/mL should be considered marginal and receive appropriate treatment (Pion and Kittleson 1990). Corresponding blood levels appear to be 10-20 nmol/mL higher than these plasma concentration cutoff values but have not been confirmed (Morris et al. 1990).

Dietary Requirements, Indications, and Use. There are significant species differences in the efficiency of synthesis of taurine from SAAs, which in turn affects their dietary requirement for exogenous sources. Historical studies of taurine requirements in cats indicated that a dietary level of approximately 400 mg/kg DM would be sufficient to prevent feline central retinal degeneration in adults and to support growth in kittens (NRC 1986). A level of 500 mg taurine/kg DM was recommended for reproduction (NRC 1986). Based on studies of the effects of food processing on bioavailability and GI absorptive kinetics (Hickman et al. 1990) and the incidence of taurine-responsive congestive heart failure in cats (Pion et al. 1987), it now appears that much higher dietary levels are required. Heat processing of natural food ingredients increases the amount of dietary taurine that reaches the lower intestine, which subsequently is degraded at increased rates by intestinal microflora (Hickman et al. 1990). Diets that have lower protein digestibilities may mediate increased intestinal secretion of cholecystokinin and, in turn, promote increased taurine-conjugated bile acid secretion and subsequent taurine depletion (Backus et al. 1995). Compared to isonitrogenous amounts of dietary casein, soybean protein increases fecal total bile acid and total taurine excretion and significantly reduces plasma taurine concentrations in cats (Kim et al. 1995). Douglass et al. (1991) have reported that commercial processing of canned diets has a much greater effect on taurine metabolism than that used in extruded, dry food production, so that dietary taurine requirements for cats are dependent on dietary form as well. Furthermore, dietary antibiotics can decrease fecal taurine loss in cats through changes in intestinal bacterial populations that may be involved in deconjugation of cholyltaurine and/or degradation of taurine (Kim et al. 1996). It is presently recommended that cats receive a dietary taurine level for maintenance of 1000-1200 mg/kg DM of dry diets, and 2200-2500 mg/kg DM for canned diets (Douglass et al. 1991; Morris et al. 1990). Based on studies in human patients, it appears that additional taurine may be required for chronic renal failure patients and critically injured individuals (Bergstrom et al. 1989; Paauw and Davis 1990). Because inflammatory cytokines like IL-1 and tumor necrosis factor-α alter tissue uptake of taurine, it is possible that many debilitated patients may benefit from taurine supplementation (Hashiguchi et al. 1997). In fact, in vitro studies have shown that supplemental taurine can exert a beneficial effect on the prevention of human endothelial cell apoptosis and necrosis during hypoxic conditions and may be indicated as a therapeutic agent in many inflammatory diseases (Wang et al. 1996). Following the association between potassium deficiency and secondary taurine depletion, additional taurine supplementation of kaliopenic cats appears to be warranted as well (Dow et al. 1987 1992).

Preparations, Treatment, and Toxicity. Commercial cat foods should be evaluated for taurine content when a deficiency is suspected based on clinical findings. Crystalline taurine is available from chemical supply companies and may be used to supplement diets that may be deficient, but a more economical means of dietary taurine supplementation is inclusion of a natural foodstuff whose taurine content is known to be relatively high (NRC 1986; Laidlaw et al. 1990). Although raw clam meat contains relatively high taurine levels, clam juice is relatively dilute (500 mg taurine/L as fed), and the volume necessary to meet a cat's dietary requirement would be excessive (Remillard 1989). Immoderate SAA supplementation, including that of taurine, may have adverse effects owing to intestinal microbial conversion to encephalotoxic mercaptans, excessive systemic acidification through desulfuration and deamination processes, or toxic effects from metabolically derived sulfide.

GLUTAMINE

Chemical Structure and Properties. Glutamine (α-aminoglutaramic acid) is the amide derivative of glutamic acid, existing as a colorless needle-shaped crystal in pure form. It is insoluble in most alcohols, has limited solubility in water (~3 g/100 mL at 20° C), and is unstable during heat sterilization and storage (Tremel et al. 1994). Synthetic dipeptides of glutamine, made with alanine (alanyl-glutamine) and glycine (glycyl-glutamine), exhibit greater water solubility and chemical stability and have received attention as supplements for parenteral solutions (Tremel et al. 1994; Petersson et al. 1994).

Source and Occurrence. Glutamine is synthesized from glutamic acid by all animals predominantly in the skeletal muscle, lungs, and adipose tissue, and is found in highest concentrations in these tissues, as well as liver, kidney, small intestine, and lymphocytes (Curthoys and Watford 1995). Glutamine comprises more than 60% of free α-amino acids in the body and has traditionally been considered a nonessential amino acid because it is readily derived from glutamic acid in healthy animals. Glutamic acid is derived from ammonium (NH_4^+) and α-ketoglutaric acid, a tricarboxylic acid (TCA) cycle intermediate, in a reaction catalyzed by glutamic acid dehydrogenase. An additional ammonium ion is incorporated into glutamic acid by the action of glutamine synthetase, to form glutamine in an amidation reaction driven by ATP hydrolysis. Glutamine is present in concentrations of 0.5-0.8 mM in plasma and up to 20 mM in the intracellular water of tissues like skeletal muscle. The plasma glutamine pool turns over very rapidly, and although some dietary glutamine is absorbed intact from the GI tract, the abdominal viscera usually exhibit net uptake, so that the majority of circulating glutamine is derived from de novo synthesis in extraspanchnic tissues.

Biological Characteristics. Glutamine synthetase is found in most tissues, but as a result of its large mass, skeletal muscle is the major site of glutamine production in the body. The lungs are the next most important site of glutamine production, and more recent studies indicate that adipose tissue is capable of significant rates of glutamine synthesis as well (Curthoys and Watford 1995). Glutamine has many unique metabolic functions in the body, which are met in healthy animals by its de novo endogenous synthesis. In critically ill, "hypercatabolic states," glutamine is released from muscle and lung tissue, intracellular glutamine levels decrease markedly, and plasma glutamine concentrations increase. However, glutamine turnover increases significantly as well, due to increased uptake for metabolism by liver, intestines, and kidneys. Elevated rates of glutamine synthesis may not be sufficient to meet the body's disease requirements, and so glutamine is now considered a "conditionally essential" amino acid in disorders as diverse as metabolic acidosis, starvation, cancer, sepsis, trauma, and diarrhea.

Metabolic Functions

GASTROINTESTINAL FUNCTION. The GI tract is the principal organ of glutamine utilization, accounting for extraction of up to 25% of circulating glutamine (Souba 1991). Although the small-intestinal epithelial cells require large amounts for synthetic purposes (e.g., purines and pyrimidines for nucleic acid synthesis), owing to their high rate of turnover, the majority of extracted glutamine serves as the principal respiratory fuel in these cells (Curthoys and Watford 1995). Glutamine undergoes oxidative deamidation to glutamate, and glutamate undergoes oxidative deamination to α-ketoglutarate for entry into the TCA cycle. Alternatively, glutamate undergoes transamination with pyruvate to produce alanine and α-ketoglutarate, or with oxaloacetate to produce aspartate and α-ketoglutarate. Much of the glutamine undergoes only partial oxidation to 3-carbon intermediates, including pyruvate, lactate, and alanine. These are utilized by other tissues, and the ammonia released during glutamine's catabolism contributes to urea synthesis in the liver.

During starvation, intestinal disease, as well as systemic diseases associated with hypercatabolism, intestinal glutaminase activity increases significantly, and glutamine extraction may more than double. Gluco-counterregulatory "stress" hormones, including glucocorticoids and glucagon, have been demonstrated to increase the specific activity of glutaminase in the small-intestinal mucosa while simultaneously diminishing glucose uptake and oxidation (Souba 1991; Colomb et al. 1997). Supplementation of parenteral feeding formulas with glutamine or glutamyl dipeptides (25-30% of amino acid nitrogen) has repeatedly been shown to spare villous morphology and ameliorate intestinal mucosal atrophy associated with deprivation of enteral nutrition (Schroder et al. 1995; Wiren et al. 1995; Burrin et al. 1994). Parenteral nutrition-associated increases in intestinal permeability, which may result in gut bacterial translocation and sepsis, are also prevented by supplementation of parenteral formulas with glutamine (2-4% w/w) (Gianotti et al. 1995; Li et al. 1994; Barber et al. 1990). A high-calorie oral rehydration solution supplemented with glutamine (30 mmol/L) was recently shown more effective in correcting plasma and extracellular fluid volumes in neonatal calves with enterotoxigenic *Escherichia coli* diarrhea than similar glutamine-free solutions (Brooks et al. 1997).

LIVER FUNCTION. The liver principally uses glutamine for gluconeogenesis and ureagenesis. Ammonia released by hepatic deamidation of glutamine is preferentially routed to urea synthesis, while the carbon skeleton (α-ketoglutarate) serves as a precursor to oxaloacetate, the key metabolic intermediate in new glucose synthesis (Fig. 38.5). Following deamidation, glutamine also serves as a precursor for the synthesis of ornithine, the rate-limiting substrate in the urea cycle.

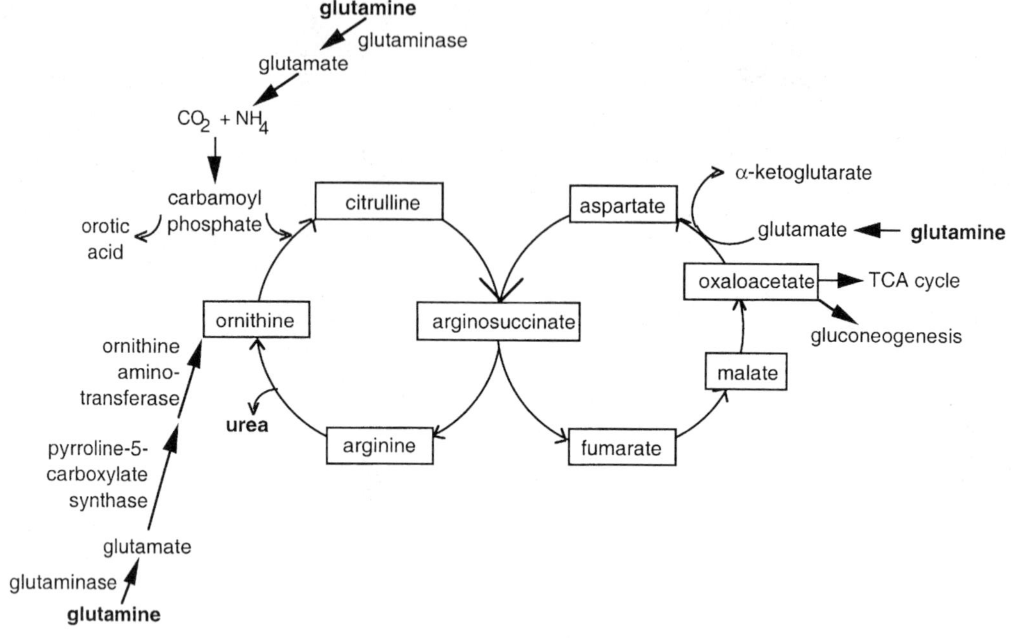

FIG. 38.5—The role of glutamine in the urea cycle.

This occurs via the serial actions of pyrroline-5-carboxylate synthase and ornithine aminotransferase on glutamate (Fig. 38.5). Catabolic illnesses, such as sepsis or trauma, result in increased circulating levels of glucocounterregulatory hormones, including glucocorticoids, glucagon, and the catecholamines, as well as inflammatory cytokines derived from activated mononuclear cells, including tumor necrosis factor, interleukin-1, and interleukin-6 (Fischer et al. 1995) (Fig. 38.6). These humoral factors are responsible for the hypercatabolism characterized by peripheral tissue lipid mobilization, muscle proteolysis, and associated increases in hepatic gluconeogenesis, ureagenesis, and acute-phase reactant protein synthesis. This results in systemic repartitioning of substrates to provide fuel for hypercatabolic tissues, to eliminate nitrogenous waste products, and to facilitate the synthesis of plasma proteins integral to host defense during infections or endotoxemia.

KIDNEY FUNCTION. Metabolic acidosis stimulates the activities of renal glutaminase and glutamic acid dehydrogenase (Preuss 1971; Shrock and Goldstein 1981). These enzymes, in turn, facilitate renal uptake of glutamine and glutamic acid, which then serve as sources of carbon skeletons for gluconeogenesis and of ammonia to facilitate renal tubular acidification of the urine (Curthoys and Watford 1995; Vinary et al. 1980). The latter process represents an interesting integrated adaptation by the kidneys to the metabolic effects of fasting. Fasting results in increased rates of hepatic ketogene-

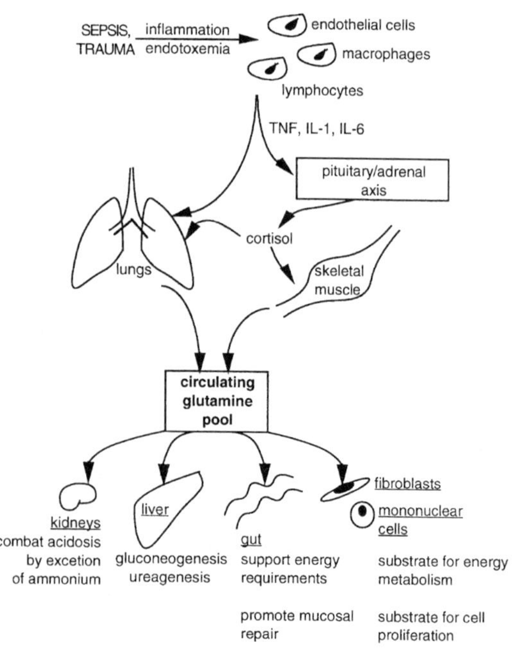

FIG. 38.6—Central role of glutamine as a conditionally essential nutrient in critical illness. TNF = tumor necrosis factor; IL-1 = interleukin-1; IL-6 = interleukin-6. (Adapted from Dudrick and Souba 1993.)

sis, following mobilization of fatty acids from peripheral tissues in excess of the oxaloacetate available for the liver to completely oxidize acetyl CoA in the TCA cycle. The resulting ketoacidosis stimulates renal glutamine extraction, as described above. This facilitates an increase in gluconeogenesis by the kidneys (which may supply up to 10% of glucose needs in the postabsorptive state), so that they can supply up to 40% of the body's glucose needs during prolonged starvation. The glucose thus produced supports glucose needs throughout the body (for glucose-requiring tissues and as oxaloacetate precursors for fatty acid and ketoacid metabolism), while the ammonia produced can buffer protons secreted into the renal tubules, thereby increasing urinary acid elimination to counteract the accumulation of ketoacids during fasting.

MUSCLE FUNCTION. As described earlier, the humoral response to systemic disease results in accelerated rates of lipolysis and proteolysis in muscle tissues. Deamination and transamination of amino acids lead to increased rates of muscle glutamine synthesis and release into the blood and supply carbon skeletons for local oxidative metabolism (Fig. 38.6). Carbon skeletons derived from glucogenic amino acids, and particularly from branched-chain amino acids, undergo markedly increased rates of oxidation, perhaps in part to provide oxaloacetate to facilitate fatty acid and ketoacid utilization by muscle under these conditions. Increased turnover of glutamine facilitates nitrogenous waste excretion via hepatic ureagenesis and renal ammoniagenesis. Likewise, these metabolic pathways are linked to accelerated rates of hepatic and renal gluconeogenesis to supply substrate for critical glucose-dependent tissues, including the central nervous system. Particularly during sepsis, glutamine supplementation (0.28-0.36 g/kg body weight/24 hr or as 30% of amino acid nitrogen) of enteral or parenteral nutrition appears to ameliorate adverse catabolic changes, increase fractional protein synthesis in the liver and skeletal muscle, restore muscle glutamine levels, and improve overall nitrogen balance, as well as improving recovery from illness (Naka et al. 1996; Long et al. 1995; Petersson et al. 1994; Hammarqvist et al. 1989; Stehle et al. 1989).

IMMUNE FUNCTION. Mononuclear cells (lymphocytes and macrophages) constitute another principal tissue for net glutamine extraction in the body (Curthoys and Watford 1995). This may be related to glutamine's role as a precursor for purine and pyrimidine synthesis during the course of phagocytic cell activation, antigen-presenting cell stimulation, lymphocyte blastogenesis, and antibody production (Fig. 38.6). In addition to its direct beneficial effects on intestinal mucosa to restore gut permselectivity, glutamine supplementation (2% w/w) of parenteral feeding formulas has also been shown to increase GI and biliary secretory IgA production (Burke et al. 1989). This would be expected to contribute to improved host defenses against bacterial translocation from the gut to distant sites, which is otherwise observed in critically ill patients. In addition, supplemental glutamine (1.1 g/dL or as ~23% of amino acid nitrogen) has been shown to improve bacterial clearance by peritoneal and hepatic macrophages, perhaps through enhanced phagocytosis, or killing function (Furukawa et al. 1997). Furthermore, peripheral blood T-lymphocyte function in human patients fed a glutamine-supplemented parenteral nutrition formula (0.18 g/kg body weight/day) was improved compared to individuals not receiving glutamine (O'Riordan et al. 1994). Likewise, in experimental tumor-bearing rats, enteral glutamine supplementation (1 g/kg body weight/day) significantly reduced tumor growth by improving natural killer (NK) cell activity (Fahr et al. 1994). It has been proposed that glutamine supplementation of cancer patients may offer the dual benefit of normalizing host catabolic changes and improving immune-mediated suppression of tumor growth (Souba 1993).

Assessment of Status, Dietary Requirements, Indications, and Use. Chemical analysis of glutamine in biological specimens may be accomplished by colorimetric, fluorometric, radiometric, and enzymatic methods (Wright et al. 1986). Chromatographic procedures are most accurate and include amino acid analyzers, high-performance liquid chromatographs, gas chromatographs (GC), and GC-mass spectrometer methods.

The most direct means of assessing glutamine status would be by analysis of glutamine concentrations in tissue biopsies from organs of interest. The most practical alternative is by determining glutamine concentration in whole blood or plasma. Critical values for determining glutamine requirements in ill animals have not been characterized. Because glutamine is relatively nontoxic and readily metabolized by many tissues, the approach used thus far experimentally has been to attempt nutritional supplementation in critical-care situations without regard for baseline glutamine concentrations in tissues or blood. Typical doses employed in published studies have been 25-30% of amino acid nitrogen in an enteral or parenteral formula, or 2-4% w/w of the formula, or 0.18-0.36 g/kg body weight/24 hours.

Preparations, Treatment, and Toxicity. Glutamine is available in crystalline form from a number of chemical suppliers and may be safely added to enteral formulas for nutritional support at the dosages cited above. Incorporation of glutamine into a formula intended for parenteral use requires special handling to ensure sterility of the preparation. Glutamine itself is not stable under typical conditions used for heat sterilization of liquids. An alternative is the use of heat-stable glutamine dipeptides (alanyl-glutamine or glycyl-glutamine) as reviewed earlier. However, these compounds are expensive and still require precautions to ensure sterility of the prepared formula. As is the case for other amino acids or protein supplements, caution should be exercised in individuals for which dietary protein restriction may be indicated, including certain forms of renal failure, hepatic dysfunction, or behavioral disorders.

REFERENCES

Adeola, O., Lawrence, B. V., Sutton, A. L., Cline, T. R. 1995. Phytase-induced changes in mineral utilization in zinc-supplemented diets for pigs. J Anim Sci 73:3384-3391.

Albina, J. E., Gladden, P., Walsh, W. R. 1993. Detrimental effects of an ω-3 fatty acid-enriched diet on wound healing. J Parent Ent Nutr 17:519-521.

Alden, P. B., Svingen, B. A., Johnson, S. B., Konstantinides, F. N., Holman, R. T., Cerra, F. B. 1986. Partial correction by exogenous lipid of abnormal patterns of polyunsaturated fatty acids in plasma phospholipids of stressed and septic surgical patients. Surgery 100:671-677.

Allen, J. I., Bell, E., Boosalis, M. G., Oken, M. M., McClain, C. J., Levine, A. S., Morley, J. E. 1985. Association between urinary zinc excretion and lymphocyte dysfunction in patients with lung cancer. Am J Med 79:209-215.

Allen, J. I., Kay, N. E., McClain, C. J. 1981. Severe zinc deficiency in humans: Association with a reversible T-lymphocyte dysfunction. Ann Int Med 95:154-157.

Allen, J. I., Perry, R. T., McClain, C. J., Kay, N. E. 1983. Alterations in human natural killer cell activity and monocyte toxicity induced by zinc deficiency. J Lab Clin Med 102:577-589.

Allen, K. G. D., Arthur, J. R., Morrice, P. C., Nicol, F., Mills, C. F. 1988. Copper deficiency and tissue glutathione concentration in the rat. Proc Soc Exptl Biol Med 187:38-43.

Allen, K. G. D., Twedt, D. C., Hunsaker, H. A. 1987. Tetramine cupruretic agents: a comparison in dogs. Am J Vet Res 48:28-30.

Allen, W. M., Sansom, B. F., Gleed, P. T., Mallinson, C. B., Drake, C. F. 1984. Boluses of controlled release glass for supplementing ruminants with copper. Vet Rec 115:55-57.

Amoikon, E. K., Fernandez, J. M., Southern, L. L., Thompson, D. L., Ward, T. L., Olcott, B. M. 1995. Effect of chromium tripicolinate on growth, glucose tolerance, insulin sensitivity, plasma metabolites, and growth hormone in pigs. J Anim Sci 73:1123-1130.

Andersen, L. F., Solvoll, K., Drevon, C. A. 1996. Very-long-chain ω-3 fatty acids as biomarkers for intake of fish and ω-3 fatty acid concentrates. Am J Clin Nutr 64:305-311.

Anderson, R. A., Bryden, N. A., Evock-Clover, M., Steele, N. C. 1997. Beneficial effects of chromium on glucose and lipid variables in control and somatotropin-treated pigs are associated with increased tissue chromium and altered tissue copper, iron, and zinc. J Anim Sci 75:657-661.

Andrews, G. A., Chavey, P. S., Smith, J. E. 1994. Enzyme-linked immunosorbent assay to measure serum ferritin and the relationship between serum ferritin and nonheme iron stores in cats. Vet Pathol 31:674-678.

Apgar, J., Fitzgerald, J. A. 1985. Effect on the ewe and lamb of low zinc intake throughout pregnancy. J Anim Sci 60:1530-1538.

Apgar, G. A., Kornegay, E. T. 1996. Mineral balance of finishing pigs fed copper sulfate or a copper-lysine complex at growth-stimulating levels. J Anim Sci 74:1594-1600.

Arthington, J. D., Corah, L. R., Minton, J. E., Elsasser, T. H., Blecha, F. 1997. Supplemental dietary chromium does not influence ACTH, cortisol, or immune responses in young calves inoculated with bovine herpesvirus-1. J Anim Sci 75:217-223.

Babu, U., Failla, M. L. 1990a. Respiratory burst and candidacidal activity of peritoneal macrophages are impaired in copper-deficient rats. J Nutr 120:1692-1699.

———. 1990b. Copper status and function of neutrophils are reversibly depressed in marginally and severely copper-deficient rats. J Nutr 120:1700-1709.

Backus, R. C., Rogers, Q. R., Rosenquist, G. L., Calam, J., Morris, J. G. 1995. Diets causing taurine depletion in cats substantially elevate postprandial plasma cholecystokinin concentrations. J Nutr 125:2650-2657.

Bala, S., Lunney, J. K., Failla, M. L. 1992. Effects of copper deficiency on T-cell mitogenic responsiveness and phenotypic profile of blood mononuclear cells from swine. Am J Vet Res 53:1231-1235.

Balevska, P. S., Russanov, E. M., Kassabova, T. A. 1981. Studies on lipid peroxidation in rat liver by copper deficiency. Int J Biochem 13:489-493.

Bang, K. S., Familton, A. S., Sykes, A. R. 1990. Effect of copper oxide wire particle treatment on establishment of major gastrointestinal nematodes in lambs. Res Vet Sci 49:132-137.

Barber, A. E., Jones, W. G., Minei, J. P., Fahey, T. J., Moldwater, L. L., Rayburn, J. L., Fischer, E., Keogh, C. V., Shires, G. T., Lowry, S. F. 1990. Glutamine or fiber supplementation of a defined formula diet: impact on bacterial translocation, tissue composition, and response to endotoxin. J Parent Enter Nutr 14:335-343.

Barcelli, U. O. 1991. Effect of dietary prostaglandin precursors on the progression of renal disease in animals. Kidn Intl 39(suppl 31):S57-S64.

Becroft, D. M., Dix, O. M. R., Farmer, K. 1977. Intramuscular iron dextran and susceptibility of neonates to bacterial infections. Arch Dis Child 52:778-781.

Berg, J. N., Padgitt, D., McCarthy, B. 1988. Iodine concentrations in milk of dairy cattle fed various amounts of iodine as ethylenediamine dihydroiodide. J Dairy Sci 71:3283-3291.

Bergstrom, J., Alvestrand, A., Furst, P., Lindholm, B. 1989. Sulphur amino acids in plasma and muscle in patients with chronic renal failure: Evidence for taurine depletion. J Internal Med 226:189-194.

Bilo, H. J. G., Van der Heide, J. J. H., Gans, R. O. B., Donker, A. J. M. 1991. Omega-3 polyunsaturated fatty acids in chronic renal insufficiency. Nephron 57:385-393.

Black, J. R., Ammerman, C. B., Henry P. R. 1985a. Effect of quantity and route of administration of manganese monoxide on feed intake and serum manganese in ruminants. J. Dairy Sci 68:433-436.

———. 1985b. Effects of high dietary manganese as manganese oxide or manganese carbonate in sheep. J Anim Sci 60:861-866.

Blakeley, B. R., Hamilton, D. L. 1985. Ceruloplasmin as an indicator of copper status in cattle and sheep. Can J Comp Med 49:405-408.

Blok, W. L., Katan, M. B., van der Meer, J. W. M. 1996. Modulation of inflammation and cytokine production by dietary (ω-3) fatty acids. J Nutr 126:1515-1533.

Boden, G., Chen, X., Ruiz, J., van Rossum, G. D. V., Turco, S. 1996. Effects of vanadyl sulfate on carbohydrate and lipid metabolism in patients with non-insulin-dependent diabetes mellitus. Metab 45:1130-1135.

Bond, R., Lloyd, D. H. 1992. A double-blind comparison of olive oil and a combination of evening primrose oil and fish oil in the management of canine atopy. Vet Rec 131:558-560.

Bostwick, J. L. 1982. Copper toxicosis in sheep. J Am Vet Med Assoc 180:386-387.

Boudreau, M. D., Chanmugan, P. S., Hart, S. B., Lee, S. H., Hwang, D. H. 1991. Lack of dose response by dietary ω-3 fatty acids at a constant ratio of ω-3 to ω-6 fatty acids in suppressing eicosanoid biosynthesis from arachidonic acid. Am J Clin Nutr 54:111-117.

Boudreaux, M. K., Reinhart, G. A., Vaughn, D. M., Spano, J. S., Mooney, M. 1997. The effects of varying dietary ω-6 to ω-3 fatty acid ratios on platelet reactivity, coagulation screening assays, and antithrombin III activity in dogs. J Am Anim Hosp Assoc 33:235-243.

Boyne, R., Arthur, J. R. 1981. Effects of selenium and copper deficiency on neutrophil function in cattle. J Comp Path 91:271-276.

———. 1986. Effects of molybdenum or iron induced copper deficiency on the viability and function of neutrophils from cattle. Res Vet Sci 41:417-419.

Braun, U., Forrer, R., Furer, W., Lutz, H. 1991. Selenium and vitamin E in blood sera of cows from farms with increased incidence of disease. Vet Rec 128:543-547.

Brewer, G. J., Dick, R. D., Schall, W., Yuzbasiyan-Gurkan, V., Mullaney, T. P., Pace, C., Lindgren, J., Thomas, M., Padgett, G. 1992a. Use of zinc acetate to treat copper toxicosis in dogs. J Am Vet Med Assoc 201:564-568.

Brewer, G. J., Dick, R. D., Schall, W., Yuzbasiyan-Gurkan, V., Mullaney, T. P., Pace, C., Lindgren, J., Thomas, M., Padgett, G. 1992b. Use of zinc acetate to treat copper toxicosis in dogs. J Am Vet Med Assoc 201:564-568.

Brewer, N. R. 1987. Comparative metabolism of copper. J Am Vet Med Assoc 190:654-658.

Bridges, C. H., Harris, E. D. 1988. Experimentally induced cartilaginous fractures (osteochondritis dissecans) in foals fed low-copper diets. J Am Vet Med Assoc 193:215-221.

Bridges, C. H., Moffitt, P. G. 1990. Influence of variable content of dietary zinc on copper metabolism of weanling foals. Am J Vet Res 51:275-280.

Bridges, C. H., Womack, J. E., Harris, E. D., Scrutchfield, W. L. 1984. Considerations of copper metabolism in osteochondrosis of suckling foals. J Am Vet Med Assoc 185:173-178.

Brooks, H. W., White, D. G., Wagstaff, A. J., Michell, A. R. 1997. Evaluation of a glutamine-containing oral rehydration solution for the treatment of calf diarrhoea using an *Escherichia coli* model. Vet J 153:163-170.

Brown S. A., Brown C. A., Crowell W. A., Barsanti J. A., Allen T., Cowell C., Finco D. R. 1998. Beneficial effects of chronic administration of dietary ω-3 fatty acids in dogs with renal insufficiency. J Lab Clin Med 131:447-455.

Bunting, L. D., Fernandez, J. M., Thompson, D. L., Southern, L. L. 1994. Influence of chromium picolinate on glucose usage and metabolic criteria in growing Holstein calves. J Anim Sci 72:1591-1599.

Burke, D. J., Alverdy, J. C., Aoys, E., Moss, G. S. 1989. Glutamine-supplemented total parenteral nutrition improves gut immune function. Arch Surg 124:1396-1399.

Burnell, T. W., Peo, E. R., Lewis, A. J., Crenshaw, J. D. 1986. Effect of dietary fluorine on growth, blood, and bone characteristics of growing-finishing pigs. J Anim Sci 63:2053-2067.

Burrin, D. G., Shulman, R. J., Langston, C., Storm, M. C. 1994. Supplemental alanylglutamine, organ growth, and nitrogen metabolism in neonatal pigs fed by total parenteral nutrition. J Parent Enter Nutr, pp. 313-319.

Burton, J. L., Mallard, B. A., Mowat, D. N. 1993. Effects of supplemental chromium on immune responses of periparturient and early lactation dairy cows. J Anim Sci 71:1532-1539.

———. 1994. Effects of supplemental chromium on antibody responses of newly weaned feedlot calves to immunization with infectious bovine rhinotracheitis and parainfluenza 3 virus. Can J Vet Res 58:148-151.

Cameron, H. J., Boila, R. J., McNichol, L. W., Stanger, N. E. 1989. Cupric oxide needles for grazing cattle consuming low-copper, high-molybdenum forage and high-sulfate water. J Anim Sci 67:252-261.

Casteel, S. W., Osweiler, G. D., Cook, W. O., Daniels, G., Kadlec, R. 1985. Selenium toxicosis in swine. J Am Vet Med Assoc 186:1084-1085.

Chang, G. X., Mallard, B. A., Mowat, D. N., Gallo, G. F. 1996. Effect of supplemental chromium on antibody responses of newly arrived feeder calves to vaccines and ovalbumin. Can J Vet Res 60:140-144.

Chang, X., Mowat, D. N. 1992. Supplemental chromium for stressed and growing feeder calves. J Anim Sci 70:559-565.

Chirase, N. K., Hutcheson, D. P., Thompson, G. B. 1991. Feed intake, rectal temperature, and serum mineral concentrations of feedlot cattle fed zinc oxide or zinc methionine and challenged with infectious bovine rhinotracheitis virus. J Anim Sci 69:4137-4145.

Christensen, M. S., Hoy, C. E., Becker, C. C., Redgrave, T. G. 1995. Intestinal absorption and lymphatic transport of eicosapentaenoic (EPA), docosahexaenoic (DHA), and decanoic acids: dependence on intramolecular triacylglycerol structure. Am J Clin Nutr 61:56-61.

Clark, W. F., Parbtani, A., Naylor, C. D., Leventon, C. M., Muirhead, N., Spanner, E., Huff, M. W. 1993. Fish oil in lupus nephritis: clinical findings and methodological implications. Kidn Intl 44:75-86.

Coffey, R. D., Cromwell, G. L., Monegue, H. J. 1994. Efficacy of a copper-lysine complex as a growth promotant for weanling pigs. J Anim Sci 72:2880-2886.

Cohen, N., Halberstram, M., Shlimovich, P., Chang, C. J., Shamoon, H., Rossetti, L. 1995. Oral vanadyl sulfate improves hepatic and peripheral insulin sensitivity in patients with non-insulin-dependent diabetes mellitus. J Clin Invest 95:2501-2509.

Colomb, V., Darcy-Vrillon, B., Jobert, A., Guihot, G., Morel, M. T., Corriol, O., Ricour, C., Duee, P. H. 1997. Parenteral nutrition modifies glucose and glutamine metabolism in rat isolated enterocytes. Gastroenterol 112:429-436.

Cook, J. D., Dassenko, S. A., Whittaker, P. 1991. Calcium supplementation: Effect on iron absorption. Am J Clin Nutr 53:106-111.

Cross, R. F., Parker, C. F. 1981a. Oral administration of zinc sulfate for control of ovine foot rot. J Am Vet Med Assoc 178:704-705.

———. 1981b. Zinc sulfate foot bath for control of ovine foot rot. J Am Vet Med Assoc 178:706-707.

Cunha, T. J. 1991. In Horse Feeding and Nutrition. 2nd ed. Academic Press, Inc. New York. pp. 124-131.

Cunningham-Rundles, S., Cunningham-Rundles, C., DuPont, B., Good, R. A. 1980. Zinc-induced activation of human B lymphocytes. Clin Immunol Immunopathol 16:115-122.

Curthoys, N. P., Watford, M. 1995. Regulation of glutaminase activity and glutamine metabolism. Ann Rev Nutr 15:133-159.

Cymbaluk, N. F., Bristol, F. M., Christensen, D. A. 1986. Influence of age and breed of equid on plasma copper and zinc concentrations. Am J Vet Res 47:192-195.

da Costa, P. D., Hoskins, J. D. 1990. The role of taurine in cats: Current concepts. Comp Cont Educ Pract Vet 12:1235-1240.

Dargatz, D. A., Ross, P. F. 1996. Blood selenium concentrations in cows and heifers on 253 cow-calf operations in 18 states. J Anim Sci 74:2891-2895.

Deschner, E. E., Lytle, J. S., Wong, G., Ruperto, J. F., Newmark, H. L. 1990. The effect of dietary omega-3 fatty acids (fish oil) on azoymethanol-induced focal areas of dysplasia and colon tumor incidence. Cancer 66:2350-2356.

Dillman, E., Gale, C., Green, W., Johnson, D. G., Mackler, B., Finch, C. 1980. Hypothermia in iron deficiency due to altered triiodothyronine metabolism. Am J Physiol 239:R377-R381.

Douglass, G. M., Fern, E. B., Brown, R. C. 1991. Feline plasma and whole blood taurine levels as influenced by commercial dry and canned diets. J Nutr 121:S179-S180.

Dove, C. R., Ewan, R. C. 1990. Effect of excess dietary copper, iron, or zinc on the tocopherol and selenium status of growing pigs. J Anim Sci 68:2407-2413.

Dove, C. R., Haydon, K. D. 1991. The effect of copper addition to diets with various iron levels on the performance and hematology of weanling swine. J Anim Sci 69:2013-2019.

———. 1992. The effect of copper and fat addition to the diets of weanling swine on growth performance and serum fatty acids. J Anim Sci 70:805-810.

Dow, S. W., LeCouteur, R. A., Fettman, M. J., Spurgeon, T. L. 1987. Potassium depletion in cats. Hypokalemic polymyopathy. J Am Vet Med Assoc 191:1569-1575.

Dow, S. W., Fettman, M. J., Smith, K. R., Ching, S. V., Hamar, D. W., Rogers, Q. R. 1992. Dietary potassium depletion and acidification induces taurine depletion and cardiovascular disease in adult cats. Am J Vet Res 53:402-405.

Du, Z., Hemken, R. W., Harmon, R. J. 1996a. Copper metabolism of Holstein and Jersey cows and heifers fed diets high in cupric sulfate or copper proteinate. J Dairy Sci 79:1873-1880.

Du, Z., Hemken, R. W., Jackson, J. A., Trammell, D. S. 1996b. Utilization of copper in copper proteinate, copper lysine, and cupric sulfate using the rat as an experimental model. J Anim Sci 74:1657-1663.

Duchateau, J., Delespesse, G., Vereecke, P. 1981a. Influence of oral zinc supplementation on the lymphocyte response to mitogens of normal subjects. Am J Clin Nutr 34:88-93.

Duchateau, J., Delespesse, G., Vrijens, R., Collet, H. 1981b. Beneficial effects of oral zinc supplementation on the immune response of old people. Am J Med 70:1001-1004.

Dudrick, P. S., Souba, W. W. 1993. Special fuels in parenteral nutrition. In J. L. Rombeau and M. D. Caldwell, eds., Clinical Nutrition–Parenteral Nutrition, 2nd ed., p. 214, Philadelphia: WB Saunders Company.

Eger, S., Drori, D., Kadoori, I., Miller, N., Schindler, H. 1985. Effects of selenium and vitamin E on incidence of retained placenta. J Dairy Sci 68:2119-2122.

Ellis, R. G., Herdt, T. H., Stowe, H. D. 1997. Physical, hematologic, biochemical, and immunologic effects of supranutritional supplementation with dietary selenium in Holstein cows. Am J Vet Res 58:760-764.

Endres, S., Ghorbani, R., Kelley, V. E., Georgilis, K., Lonneman, G., van der Meer, J. W. M., Cannon, J. G., Rogers, T. S., Klempner, M. S. Weber, P. C., Schaefer, E. J., Wolff, S. M., Dinarello, C. A. 1989. The effect of dietary supplementation with ω-3 polyunsaturated fatty acids on the synthesis of interleukin-1 and tumor necrosis factor by mononuclear cells. New Engl J Med 320:265-271.

Erskine, R. J., Eberhart, R. J., Grasso, P. J., Scholz, R. W. 1989. Induction of *Escherichia coli* mastitis in cows fed selenium-deficient or selenium-supplemented diets. Am J Vet Res 50:2093-2100.

Erskine, R. J., Eberhart, R. J., Scholz, R. W. 1990. Experimentally-induced Staphylococcus aureus mastitis in selenium-deficient and selenium-supplemented dairy cows. Am J Vet Res 51:1107-1111.

Etzel, K. R., Swerdel, M. R., Swerdel, J. N., Cousins, R. J. 1982. Endotoxin-induced changes in copper and zinc metabolism in the Syrian hamster. J Nutr 112:2363-2373.

Fahr, M. J., Kornbluth, J., Blossom, S., Schaeffer, R., Klimberg, V. S. 1994. Glutamine enhances immunoregulation of tumor growth. J Parent Enter Nutr 18:471-476.

Failla, M. L., Babu, U., Seidel, K. E. 1988. Use of immunoresponsiveness to demonstrate that the dietary requirement for copper in young rats is greater with dietary fructose than dietary starch. J Nutr 118:487-496.

Feldman, B. F., Keen, C. L., Kaneko, J. J., Farver, T. B. 1981. Anemia of chronic inflammatory disease in the dog: Measurement of hepatic superoxide dismutase, hepatic nonheme iron, copper, zinc, and ceruloplasmin and serum iron, copper, and zinc. Am J Vet Res 42:1114-1117.

Fettman, M. J. 1991. Comparative aspects of glutathione metabolism affecting individual susceptibility to oxidant injury. Comp Cont Educ Prac Vet 13:1079-1091.

Fischer, C. P., Bode, B. P., Abcouwer, S. F., Lukaszewicz, G. C., Souba, W. W. 1995. Hepatic uptake of glutamine and other amino acids during infection and inflammation. Shock 3:315-322.

Fischer, P. W. F., Giroux, A., L'Abbe, M. R. 1981. The effect of dietary zinc on intestinal copper absorption. Am J Clin Nutr 34:1670-1675.

Fisher, M., Levine, P. H., Weiner, B. H. 1986. The potential benefits of fish consumption. Arch Int Med 146:2322-2333.

Fosmire, G. J. 1990. Zinc toxicity. Am J Clin Nutr 51:225-227.

Fox, J. G., Zeman, D. H., Mortimer, J. D. 1994. Copper toxicosis in sibling ferrets. J Am Vet Med Assoc 205:1154-1156.

Fox, P. R., Trautwein, E. A., Hayes, K. C., Bond, B. R., Sisson, D. D., Mosie, N. S. 1993. Comparison of taurine, α-tocopherol, retinol, selenium, and total triglycerides and cholesterol concentrations in cats with cardiac disease and in healthy cats. Am J Vet Res 54:563-569.

Fraker, P. J., Haas, S. M., Luecke, R. W. 1977. Effect of zinc deficiency on the immune response of the young adult A/J mouse. J Nutr 107:1889-1895.

Fraker, P. J., Zwickl, C. M., Luecke, R. W. 1982. Delayed type hypersensitivity in zinc deficient adult mice: Impairment and restoration of responsivity to dinitrofluorobenzene. J Nutr 112:309-313.

Frost, P., Rabbani, P., Smith, J., Prasad, A. 1981. Cell-mediated cytotoxicity and tumor growth in zinc-deficient mice. Proc Soc Exptl Biol Med 167:333-337.

Furugouri, K. 1977. Iron binding substances in the intestinal mucosa of neonatal piglets. J Nutr 107:487-494.

Furugouri, K., Miyata, Y., Shijimaya, K. 1982. Ferritin in blood serum of dairy cows. J Dairy Sci 65:1529-1534.

Furukawa, S., Saito, H., Inaba, T., Lin, M. T., Inoue, T., Naka, S., Fukatsu, K., Hashiguchi, Y., Han, I., Matsuda, T., Ikeda, S., Muto, T. 1997. Glutamine-enriched enteral diet enhances bacterial clearance in protracted bacterial peritonitis, regardless of glutamine form. J Parent Enter Nutr 21:208-214.

Gabrielson, K. L., Remillard, R. L., Huso, D. L. 1996. Zinc toxicity with pancreatic acinar necrosis in piglets receiving total parenteral nutrition. Vet Pathol 33:692-696.

Gaynor, P. J., Montgomery, M. J., Holmes, C. R. 1988. Effect of zinc chloride or zinc sulfate treatment of protein supplement on milk production. J Dairy Sci 71:2175-2180.

Geelen, M. J. H., Schoots, W. J., Bijleveld, C., Beynen, A. C. 1995. Dietary medium-chain fatty acids raise and (ω-3) polyunsaturated fatty acids lower hepatic triacylglycerol synthesis in rats. J Nutr 125:2449-2456.

Gengelbach, G. P., Ward, J. D., Spears, J. W. 1994. Effect of dietary copper, iron, and molybdenum on growth and copper status of beef cows and calves. J Anim Sci 72:2722-2727.

Gianotti, L., Alexander, J. W., Gennari, R., Pyles, T., Babcock, G. F. 1995. Oral glutamine decreases bacterial translocation and improves survival in experimental gut-origin sepsis. J Parenter Enter Nutr 19:69-74.

Goldfine, A. B., Simonson, D. C., Folli, F., Patti, M. E., Kahn, C. R. 1995. Metabolic effects of sodium metavanadate in humans with insulin-dependent and noninsulin-dependent diabetes mellitus in vivo and in vitro studies. J Clin Endocrinol Metab 80:3311-3320.

Gopinath, C., Hall, G. A., Howell, J. M. 1974. The effect of chronic copper poisoning on the kidneys of sheep. Res Vet Sci 16:57-69.

Graham, T. W., Thurmond, M. C., Clegg, M. S., Keen, C. L., Holmberg, C. A., Slanker, M. R., Goodger, W. J. 1987. An epidemiologic study of mortality in veal calves subsequent to an episode of zinc toxicosis on a California veal calf operation using zinc sulfate-supplemented milk replacer. J Am Vet Med Assoc 190:1296-1301.

Grasso, P. J., Scholz, R. W., Erskine, R. J., Eberhart, R. J. 1990. Phagocytosis, bactericidal activity, and oxidative metabolism of milk neutrophils from dairy cows fed selenium-supplemented and selenium-deficient diets. Am J Vet Res 51:269-274.

Grauer, G. F., Greco, D. S., Behrend, E. N., Fettman, M. J., Mani, I., Getzy, D. M., Reinhart, G. A. 1996. Effects of dietary ω-3 fatty acid supplementation versus thromboxane synthetase inhibition on gentamicin-induced nephrotoxicosis in healthy male dogs. Am J Vet Res 57:948-956.

Haggard, D. L., Stowe, H. D., Conner, G. H., Johnson, D. W. 1980. Immunologic effects of experimental iodine toxicosis in young cattle. Am J Vet Res 41:539-543.

Hallberg, L., Brune, M., Sandberg, A., Rossander-Hulten, L. 1991. Calcium: Effect of different amounts on nonheme-and heme-iron absorption in humans. Am J Clin Nutr 53:112-119.

Hammarqvist, F., Wernerman, J., Ali, R., von der Decken, A., Vinnars, E. 1989. Addition of glutamine to total parenteral nutrition after elective abdominal surgery spares free glutamine in muscle, counteracts the fall in muscle protein synthesis, and improves nitrogen balance. Ann Surg 209:455-461.

Hansen, R. A., Ogilvie, G. K., Davenport, D., Gross, K, Walton, J. A., Richardson, K. L., Mallinckrodt,, C., Hand, M. S., Fettman, M. J. 1998. Prolonged elevation of eicosapentaenoate and docosahexaenoate levels in canine serum following cessation of menhaden fish oil supplementation. Am J Vet Res 59:864-868.

Harrison, J. H., Conrad, H. R. 1984. Effect of selenium intake on selenium utilization by the nonlactating dairy cow. J Dairy Sci 67:219-223.

Harrison, J. H., Hancock, D. D., Conrad, H. R. 1984. Vitamin E and selenium for reproduction of the dairy cow. J Dairy Sci 67:123-132.

Harvey, J. W., Asquith, R. L., McNulty, P. K., Kivipelto, J., Bauer, J. E. 1984. Haematology of foals up to one year old. Eq Vet J 16:347-353.

Harvey, J. W., Asquith, R. L., Sussman, W. A., Kivipelto, J. 1987. Serum ferritin, serum iron, and erythrocyte values in foals. Am J Vet Rers 48:1348-1352.

Harvey, J. W., French, T. W., Meyer, D. J. 1982. Chronic iron deficiency anemia in dogs. J Amer Anim Hosp Assoc 18:946-960.

Hashiguchi, Y., Fukushima, R., Saito, H., Naka, S., Inaba, T., Lin, M. T., Muto, T. 1997. Interleukin-1 and tumor necrosis factor alter plasma concentration and interorgan fluxes of taurine in dogs. Shock 7:147-153.

Hatch, R. C., Blue, J. L., Mahaffey, E. A., Jain, A. V., Smalley, R. E. 1979a. Chronic copper toxicosis in growing swine. J Am Vet Med Assoc 174:616-619.

Hatch, R. C., Clark, J. D., Jain, A. V., Mahaffey, E. A. 1979b. Treatment of induced acute selenosis in rats and weanling pigs. Am J Vet Res 40:1808-1811.

Hayek, M. G., Mitchell, G. E., Harmon, R. J., Stahly, T. S., Cromwell, G. L., Tucker, R. E., Barker, K. B. 1989. Porcine immunoglobulin transfer after prepartum treatment with selenium or vitamin E. J Anim Sci 67:1299-1306.

Hayes, K. C., Carey, R. E., Schmidt, S. Y. 1975. Retinal degeneration associated with taurine deficiency in the cat. Science 188:949-951.

Heifets, M., Morrissey, J. J., Purkerson, M. L., Morrison, A. R., Klahr, S. 1987. Effects of dietary lipids on renal function in rats with subtotal nephrectomy. Kidn Intl 32:335-341.

Henry, M. M., Moore, J. N., Feldman, E. B., Fischer, J. K. 1991. Influence of an ω-3 fatty acid-enriched ration on in vivo responses of horses to endotoxin. Am J Vet Res 52:523-532.

Henry, M. M., Moore, J. N., Feldman, E. B., Fischer, J. K., Russell, B. 1990. Effect of alpha-linolenic acid on equine monocyte procoagulant activity and eicosanoid synthesis. Circ Shock 32:173-188.

Henry, P. R., Ammerman, C. B., Littell, R. C. 1992. Relative bioavailability of manganese from a manganese-methionine complex and inorganic sources for ruminants. J Dairy Sci 75:3473-3478.

Herdt, T. H. 1995. Blood serum concentrations of selenium in female llamas (*Lama glama*) in relationship to feeding practices, region of United States, reproductive stage, and health of offspring. J Anim Sci 73:337-344.

Herold, P. M., Kinsella, J. E. 1986. Fish oil consumption and decreased risk of cardiovascular disease: A comparison of findings from animal and human feeding trials. Am J Clin Nutr 43:566-598.

Heyliger, C. E., Tahiliani, A. G., McNeill, J. H. 1985. Effect of vanadate on elevated blood glucose and depressed cardiac performance of diabetic rats. Science 227:1474-1477.

Hickman, M. A., Rogers, Q. R., Morris, J. G. 1990. Effect of processing on fate of dietary [^{14}C]taurine in cats. J Nutr 120:995-1000.

Hidiroglou, M. 1979. Manganese in ruminant nutrition: A review. Can J Anim Sci 59:217-236.

Hidiroglou, M., Williams, C. J., Siddiqui, I. R., Khan, S. U. 1979. Effects of Mn-deficit feeding to ewes on certain amino acids and sugars in cartilage of their newborn lambs. Am J Vet Res 40:1375-1377.

Hillman, D., Bolenbaugh, D. L., Convey, E. M. 1979. Hypothyroidism and anemia related to fluoride in dairy cattle. J Dairy Sci 62:416-423.

Hillman, D., Curtis, A. R. 1980. Chronic iodine toxicity in dairy cattle: Blood chemistry, leukocytes, and milk iodide. J Dairy Sci 63:55-63.

Ho, S. Y., Miller, W. J., Gentry, R. P., Neathery, M. W., Blackmon, D. M. 1984. Effects of high but nontoxic dietary manganese and iron on their metabolism by calves. J Dairy Sci 67:1489-1495.

House, J. K., Smith, B. P., Maas, J., Lane, V. M., Anderson, B. C., Graham, T. W., Pino, M. V. 1994. Hemochromatosis in Salers cattle. J Vet Int Med 8:105-111.

Hussein, H. S., Fahey, G. C., Wolf, B. W., Berger, L. L. 1994. Effects of cobalt on in vitro fiber digestion of forages and by-products containing fiber. J Dairy Sci 77:3432-3440.

Ikeda, I., Wakamatsu, K., Inayoshi, A., Imaizumi, K., Sugano, M., Yazawa, K. 1994. α-linolenic, eicosapentaenoic, and docosahexaenoic acids affect lipid metabolism differently in rats. J Nutr 124:1898-1906.

Ingraham, R. H., Kappel, L. C., Morgan, E. B., Srikandakumar, A. 1987. Correction of subnormal fertility with copper and magnesium supplementation. J Dairy Sci 70:167-180.

Irwin, M. R., Bergin, W. C., Sawa, T. R., McKinney, L. B., Kimura, H. 1979. Poor growth performance associated with hypocupremia in Hawaiian feedlot cattle. J Am Vet Med Assoc 174:590-593.

Ishmael, J., Gopinath, C., Howell, J. M. 1971. Experimental chronic copper toxicity in sheep. Res Vet Sci 12:358-366.

Ivan, M., Hidiroglou, M. 1980. Effect of dietary manganese on growth and manganese metabolism in sheep. J Dairy Sci 63:385-390.

Janke, B. H. 1989. Acute selenium toxicosis in a dog. J Am Vet Med Assoc 195:1114-1115.

Jenkins, K. J. 1989. Effect of copper loading of preruminant calves on intracellular distribution of hepatic copper, zinc, iron, and molybdenum. J Dairy Sci 72:2346-2350.

Jenkins, K. J., Hidiroglou, M. 1989. Tolerance of the calf for excess copper in milk replacer. J Dairy Sci 72:150-156.

———. 1990. Effects of elevated iodine in milk replacer on calf performance. J Dairy Sci 73:804-807.

———. 1991. Tolerance of the preruminant calf for excess manganese or zinc in milk replacer. J Dairy Sci 74:1047-1053.

Jenkins, K. J., Kramer, J. K. G. 1988. Effect of excess dietary iron on lipid composition of calf liver, heart, and skeletal muscle. J Dairy Sci 71:435-441.

Johnson, G. F., Sternlieb, I., Twedt, D. C., Grushoff, P. S., Scheinberg, I. H. 1980. Inheritance of copper toxicosis in Bedlington terriers. Am J Vet Res 41:1865-1866.

Junge, R. E., Thornburg, L. 1989. Copper poisoning in four llamas. J Am Vet Med Assoc 195:987-989.

Kadis, S., Udeze, F. A., Polanco, J., Dreesen, D. W. 1984. Relationship of iron administration to susceptibility of newborn pigs to enterotoxic colibacillosis. Am J Vet Res 45:255-259.

Kamath, S. M., Stoecker, B. J., Davis-Whitenack, M. L., Smith, M. M., Adeleye, B. O., Sangiah, S. 1997. Absorption, retention and urinary excretion of chromium-51 in rats pretreated with indomethacin and dosed with dimethylprostaglandin E_2, misoprostol, or prostacyclin. J Nutr 127:478-482.

Kappel, L. C., Ingraham, R. H., Morgan, E. B., Babcock, D. K. 1984. Plasma copper concentration and packed cell volume and their relationships to fertility and milk production in Holstein cows. Am J Vet Res 45:346-350.

Kasiske, B. L., O'Donnell, M. P., Lee, H., Kim, Y., Keane, W. F. 1991. Impact of dietary fatty acid supplementation on renal injury in obese Zucker rats. Kidn Intl 39:1125-1134.

Kegley, E. B., Spears, J. W. 1994. Bioavailability of feed-grade copper sources (oxide, sulfate, or lysine) in growing cattle. J Anim Sci 72:2728-2734.

Kegley, E. B., Spears, J. W., Brown, T. T. 1996. Immune response and disease resistance of calves fed chromium nicotinic acid complex or chromium chloride. J Dairy Sci 79:1278-1283.

Kelley, D. S., Branch, L. B., Love, J. E., Taylor, P. C., Riviera, Y. M., Iacono, J. M. 1991. Dietary α-linolenic acid and immunocompetence in humans. Am J Clin Nutr 53:40-46.

Kelley, D. S., Nelson, G. J., Serrato, C. M., Schmidt, P. C., Branch, L. B. 1988. Effects of type of dietary fat on indices of immune status of rabbits. J Nutr 118:1376-1384.

Kim, S. W., Morris, J. G., Rogers, Q. R. 1995. Dietary soybean protein decreases plasma taurine in cats. J Nutr 125:2831-2837.

Kim, S. W., Rogers, Q. R., Morris, J. G. 1996. Dietary antibiotics decrease taurine loss in cats fed a canned heat-processed diet. J Nutr 126:509-515.

Kimball, S. R., Chen, S. J., Risica, R., Jefferson, L. S., Leure-duPree, A. E. 1995. Effects of zinc deficiency on protein synthesis and expression of specific mRNAs in rat liver. Metabolism 44:126-133.

Kimber, C., Weintraub, L. R. 1968. Malabsorption of iron secondary to iron deficiency. New Engl J Med 279:453-459.

Kincaid, R. L., Blauwiekel, R. M., Cronrath, J. D. 1986a. Supplementation of copper as copper sulfate or copper proteinate for growing calves fed forages containing molybdenum. J Dairy Sci 69:160-163.

Kincaid, R. L., Gay, C. C., Krieger, R. I. 1986b. Relationship of serum and plasma copper and ceruloplasmin concentrations of cattle and the effects of whole blood sample storage. Am J Vet Res 47:1157-1159.

Kincaid, R. L., White, C. L. 1988. The effects of ammonium tetrathiomolybdate intake of tissue copper and molybdenum in pregnant ewes and lambs. J Anim Sci 66:3252-3258.

King, B. D., Lassiter, J. W., Neathery, M. W., Miller, W. J., Gentry, R. P. 1980a. Effect of a purified corn-skim milk diet on retention and tissue distribution on manganese-54 in calves. J Dairy Sci 63:86-90.

———. 1980b. Effect of lactose, copper, and iron on manganese retention and tissue distribution in rats fed dextrose-casein diets. J Anim Sci 50:452-458.

Kinoshita, C., Saze, K. I., Kumata, S., Mastuki, T., Homma, S. 1996. A simplified method for the estimation of glutathione peroxidase activity and selenium concentration in bovine blood. J Dairy Sci 79:1543-1548.

Kirk, J. H., Terra, R. L., Gardner, I. A., Wright, J. C., Case, J. T., Maas, J. 1995. Comparison of maternal blood and fetal liver selenium concentrations in cattle in California. Am J Vet Res 56:1460-1464.

Kitchalong, L., Fernandez, J. M., Bunting, L. D., Southern, L. L., Bidner, T. D. 1995. Influence of chromium tripicolinate on glucose metabolism and nutrient partitioning in growing lambs. J Anim Sci 73:2694-2705.

Klasing, K. C. 1984. Effect of inflammatory agents and interleukin-1 on iron and zinc metabolism. Am J Physiol 247:R901-R904.

Klebanoff, S. J., Waltersdorph, A. M. 1990. Prooxidant activity of transferrin and lactoferrin. J Exp Med 172:1293-1303.

Knight, C. D., Klasing, K. C., Forsyth, D. M. 1983. E. coli growth in serum of iron dextran-supplemented pigs. J Anim Sci 57:387-395.

Kochanowski, B. A., Sherman, A. R. 1985. Decreased antibody formation in iron-deficient rat pups—effect of iron repletion. Am J Clin Nutr 41:278-284.

Koenig, K. M., Rode, L. M., Cohen, R. D. H., Buckley, W. T. 1997. Effects of diet and chemical form of selenium on selenium metabolism in sheep. J Anim Sci 75:817-827.

Koller, L. D., Mulhern, S. A., Frankel, N. C., Steven, M. G., Williams, J. R. 1987. Immune dysfunction in rats fed a diet deficient in copper. Am J Clin Nutr 45:997-1006.

Kornegay, E. T., van Heugten, P. H. G., Lindemann, M. D., Blodgett, D. J. 1989. Effects of biotin and high copper levels on performance and immune response of weanling pigs. J Anim Sci 67:1471-1477.

Kornegay, E. T., Wang, Z., Wood, C. M., Lindemann, M. D. 1997. Supplemental chromium picolinate influences nitrogen balance, dry matter digestibility, and carcass traits in growing-finishing pigs. J Anim Sci 75:1319-1323.

Kott, R. W., Ruttle, J. L., Southward, G. M. 1983. Effects of vitamin E and selenium injections on reproduction and preweaning lamb survival in ewes consuming diets marginally deficient in selenium. J Anim Sci 57:553-558.

Krook, L., Maylin, G. A., Lillie, J. H., Wallace, R. S. 1983. Dental fluorosis in cattle. Cornell Vet 73:340-362.

Kuvibidila, S., Baliga, S., Suskind, R. M. 1981. Effects of iron deficiency anemia on delayed cutaneous hypersensitivity in mice. Am J Clin Nutr 34:2635-2640.

Kuvibidila, S., Nauss, K. M., Baliga, S., Suskind, R. M. 1983. Impairment of blastogenic response of splenic lymphocytes from iron-deficient mice: in vivo repletion. Am J Clin Nutr 37:15-25.

Lacetera, N., Bernabucci, U., Ronchi, B., Nardone, A. 1996. Effects of selenium and vitamin E administration during a late stage of pregnancy on colostrum and milk production in diary cows, and on passive immunity and growth of their offspring. Am J Vet Res 57:1776-1780.

LaFlamme, D. P., Miller, W. J., Neathery, M. W., Gentry, R. P., Blackmon, D. M., Logner, K. R., Fielding, A. S. 1985. The effect of low to normal dietary phosphorus levels on zinc metabolism and tissue distribution in calves. J Anim Sci 61:525-531.

Laidlaw, S. A., Grosvenor, M., Kopple, J. D. 1990. The taurine content of common feedstuffs. J Parent Ent Nutr 14:183-188.

Larsson-Backstrom, C., Arrhenius, E., Sagge, K., Lindmark, L., Paprocki, J., Svensson, L. 1990. Sequential changes in lipid metabolism and the fatty acid profiles in liver lipids during fasting and sepsis. Circ Shock 30:331-347.

Lawrence, R. A., Jenkinson, S. G. 1987. Effects of copper deficiency on carbon tetrachloride-induced lipid peroxidation. J Lab Clin Med 109:134-140.

Leaf, D. A., Connor, W. E., Barstad, L., Sexton, G. 1995. Incorporation of dietary ω-3 fatty acids into the fatty acids of human adipose tissue and plasma lipid classes. Am J Clin Nutr 62:68-73.

Lefer, A. M. 1989. Significance of lipid mediators in shock states. Circ Shock 27:3-12.

Leigh, M. J., Miller, D. D. 1983. Effects of pH and chelating agents on iron binding by dietary fiber: Implications for iron availability. Am J Clin Nutr 38:202-213.

Lessard, M., Yang, W. C., Elliott, G. S., Rebar, A. H., Van Vleet, J. F., Deslauriers, N., Brisson, G. J., Schultz, R. D. 1991. Cellular immune responses in pigs fed a vitamin E and selenium deficient diet. J Anim Sci 69:1575-1582.

Levine, P. H., Fisher, M., Schneider, P. B., Whitten, R. H., Weiner, B. H., Ockene, I. S., Johnson, B. F., Johnson, M. H., Doyle, E. M., Riendeau, P. A., Hoogasian, J. J. 1989. Dietary supplementation with omega-3 fatty acids prolongs platelet survival in hyperlipidemic patients with atherosclerosis. Arch Int Med 149:1113-1116.

Li, E. J., Cook, J. A., Spicer, K. M., Wise, W. C., Rokach, J., Halushka, P. V. 1990. Resistance of essential fatty acid-deficient rats to endotoxin-induced increases in vascular permeability. Circ Shock 31:159-170.

Li, J., Langkamp-Henken, B., Suzuki, K., Stahlgren, L. H. 1994. Glutamine prevents parenteral nutrition-induced increases in intestinal permeability. J Parent Enter Nutr 18:303-307.

Lofstedt, J., Jakowski, R., Sharko, P. 1988. Ataxia, arthritis, and encephalitis in a goat herd. J Am Vet Med Assoc 193:1295-1298.

Logas, D., Beale, K. M., Bauer, J. E. 1991. Potential clinical benefits of dietary supplementation with marine-life oil. J Am Vet Med Assoc 199:1631-1636.

Long, C. L., Nelson, K. M., DiRienzo, D. B., Weis, J. K., Stahl, R. D., Broussard, T. D., Theus, W. L., Clark, J. A., Pinson, T. W., Geiger, J. W., Laws, H. L., Blakemore, W. S., Carraway, R. P. 1995. Glutamine supplementation of enteral nutrition: impact on whole body protein kinetics and glucose metabolism in critically ill patients. J Parent Enter Nutr 19:470-476.

Lonnroth, P., Eriksson, J. W., Posner, B. I., Smith, U. 1993. Peroxyvanadate but not vanadate exerts insulin-like effects in human adipocytes. Diabetologia 36:113-116.

Luecke, R. W., Fraker, P. J. 1979. The effect of varying dietary zinc levels on growth and antibody-mediated response in two strains of mice. J Nutr 109:1373-1376.

Luecke, R. W., Simonel, C. E., Fraker, P. J. 1978. The effect of restricted dietary intake on the antibody-mediated response of the zinc deficient A/J mouse. J Nutr 108:881-887.

Luttgen, P. J., Whitney, M. S., Wolf, A. M., Scruggs, D. W. 1990. Heinz body hemolytic anemia associated with high plasma zinc concentration in a dog. J Am Vet Med Assoc 197:1347-1350.

Maas, J. P. 1983. Diagnosis and management of selenium-responsive diseases in cattle. Comp Cont Educ Prac Vet 5:S393-S400.

Maas, J., Peauroi, J. R., Tonjes, T., Karlonas, J., Galey, F. D., Han, B. 1993. Intramuscular selenium administration in selenium-deficient cattle. J Vet Int Med 7:342-348.

Maas, J., Peauroi, J. R., Weber, D. W., Adams, F. W. 1994. Safety, efficacy and effects on copper metabolism of intrareticularly placed selenium boluses in beef heifer calves. Am J Vet Res 55:247-250.

MacDonald, M. L., Anderson, B. C., Rogers, Q. R., Buffington, C. A., Morris, J. G. 1984. Essential fatty acid requirements of cats: Pathology of essential fatty acid deficiency. Am J Vet Res 45:1310-1317.

Machen, M., Montgomery, T., Holland, R., Braselton, E., Dunstan, R., Brewer, G., Yuzbasiyan-Gurkan, V. 1996. Bovine hereditary zinc deficiency: lethal trait A46. J Vet Diagn Invest 8:219-227.

Mahan, D. C., Kim, Y. Y. 1996. Effect of inorganic or organic selenium at two dietary levels on reproductive performance and tissue selenium concentrations in first-parity gilts and their progeny. J Anim Sci 74:2711-2718.

Mahan, D. C., Parrett, N. A. 1996. Evaluating the efficacy of selenium-enriched yeast and sodium selenite on tissue selenium retention and serum glutathione peroxidase activity in grower and finisher swine. J Anim Sci 74:2967-2974.

Mangkoewidjojo, S., Sleight, S. D., Convey, E. M. Pathologic features of iodide toxicosis in calves. Am J Vet Res 41:1057-1061.

Mantzioris, E., James, M. J., Gibson, R. A., Cleland, L. G. 1995. Differences exist in the relationships between dietary linoleic and α-linolenic acids and their respective long-chain metabolites. Am J Clin Nutr 61:320-324.

Margolin, G., Huster, G., Glueck, C. J., Speirs, J., Vandegrift, J., Illig, E., Wu, J., Steicher, P., Tracy, T. 1991. Blood pressure lowering in elderly subjects: A double blind crossover study of ω-3 and ω-6 fatty acids. Am J Clin Nutr 53:562-572.

Maylin, G. A., Eckerlin, R. H., Krook, L. 1987. Fluoride intoxication in dairy calves. Cornell Vet 77:84-98.

Maylin, G. A., Rubin, D. S., Lein, D. H. 1980. Selenium and vitamin E in horses. Cornell Vet 70:272-289.

McDowell, L. R. 1989. Chapter 17 in Vitamins in Animal Nutrition: Comparative Aspects to Human Nutrition, pp. 400-421. Academic Press, New York.

McGuire, S. O., Miller, W. J., Gentry, R. P., Neathery, M. W., Ho, S. Y., Blackmon, D. M. 1985. Influence of high dietary iron as ferrous carbonate and ferrous sulfate on iron metabolism in young calves. J Dairy Sci 68:2621-2628.

McLean, J. G., Monger, E. A. 1989. Factors determining the essential fatty acid requirements of the cat. In I. H. Burger and J. P. W. Rivers, eds., Nutrition of the Dog and Cat, pp. 329-342. New York: Cambridge Univ Press.

McLennan, P. L., Bridle, T. M., Abeywardena, M. Y., Charnock, J. S. 1993. Comparative efficacy of ω-3 and ω-6 polyunsaturated fatty acids in modulating ventricular fibrillation threshold in marmoset monkeys. Am J Clin Nutr 58:666-669.

McQuitty, J. T., DeWys, W. D., Monaco, L., Strain, W. H., Rob, C. G., Apgar, J., Pories, W. J. 1970. Inhibition of tumor growth by dietary zinc deficiency. Cancer Res 30:1387-1390.

Meydani, S. N. 1996. Effect of (ω-3) polyunsaturated fatty acids on cytokine production and their biologic function. Nutrition 12:S8-S14.

Miller, W. J., Amos, H. E., Gentry, R. P., Blackmon, D. M., Durrance, R. M., Crowe, C. T., Fielding, A. S., Neathery, M. W. 1989. Long-term feeding of high zinc sulfate diets to lactating and gestating dairy cows. J Dairy Sci 72:1499-1508.

Miller, W. J., Gentry, R. P., Blackmon, D. M., Fosgate, H. H. 1991. Effects of high dietary iron as ferrous carbonate on performance of young dairy calves. J Dairy Sci 74:1963-1967.

Mills, C. F., Dalgarno, A. C., Wensham, G. 1976. Biochemical and pathological changes in tissues of Friesian cattle during experimental induction of copper deficiency. Brit J Nutr 35:309-330.

Minson, D. J. 1990. In Forage in Ruminant Nutrition. Academic Press, Inc., New York. a: chapter 11, pp. 310-332; b: chapter 15, pp. 369-381; c: chapter 13, pp. 346-358.

Miyamoto, Y., Tiruppathi, C., Ganapathy, V., Liebach, F. H. 1989. Active transport of taurine in rabbit jejunal brush-border membrane vesicles. Am J Physiol 257:G65-G72.

Miyata, Y., Furugouri, K., Shijimaya, K. 1984. Developmental changes in serum ferritin concentration of dairy calves. J Dairy Sci 67:1256-1263.

Moonsie-Shageer, S., Mowat, D. N. 1993. Effect of level of supplemental chromium on performance, serum constituents, and immune status of stressed feeder calves. J Anim Sci 71:232-238.

Moore, R. M., Kohn, C. W. 1991. Nutritional muscular dystrophy in foals. Comp Cont Educ Prac Vet 13:476-490.

Morris, J. G., Rogers, Q. R., Pacioretty, L. M. 1990. Taurine: An essential nutrient for cats. J Sm Anim Pract 31:502-509.

Morrow, D. A. 1968. Acute selenite toxicosis in lambs. J Am Vet Med Assoc 152:1625-1629.

Mossad, S. B., Mackinin, M. L., Mebendorp, S. V., Mason, P. 1996. Zinc gluconate lozenges for treating the common cold: a randomized double-blind, placebo-controlled study. Ann Int Med 125:81-88.

Myers, M. J., Farrell, D. E., Evock-Clover, C. M., McDonald, M. W., Steele, N. C. 1997. Effect of growth hormone or chromium picolinate on swine metabolism and inflammatory cytokine production after endotoxin challenge exposure. Am J Vet Res 58:594-600.

Naka, S., Saito, H., Hashiguchi, Y., Lin, M. T., Furukawa, S., Inaba, T., Fukushima, R., Wada, N., Muto, T. 1996. Alanyl-glutamine-supplemented total parenteral nutrition improves survival and protein metabolism in rat protracted bacterial peritonitis model. J Parent Enter Nutr 20:417-423.

Narasinga, B. S. 1981. Physiology of iron absorption and supplementation. Brit Med Bull 37:25-30.

Neathery, M. W., Crowe, N. A., Miller, W. J., Crowe, C. T., Varnadoe, J. L., Blackmon, D. M. 1990. Influence of dietary aluminum and phosphorus in zinc metabolism in dairy calves. J Anim Sci 68:4326-4333.

Neathery, M. W., Lassiter, J. W., Miller, W. J., Gentry, R. P. 1975. Absorption, excretion and tissue distribution of natural organic and inorganic zinc-65 in the rat. Proc Soc Exptl Biol Med 149:1-4.

Nelson, D. R., Wolff, W. A., Blodgett, D. J., Luecke, B., Ely, R. W., Zachary, J. F. 1984. Zinc deficiency in sheep and goats: Three field cases. J Am Vet Med Assoc 184:1480-1485.

Nestel, P. J. 1990. Effects of ω-3 fatty acids on lipid metabolism. Ann Rev Nutr 10:149-167.

Neuringer, M., Anderson, G. J., Connor, W. E. 1988. The essentiality of ω-3 fatty acids for the development and function of the retina and brain. Ann Rev Nutr 8:517-541.

Niyo, Y., Glock, R. D., Ledet, A. E., Ramsey, F. K., Ewan, R. C. 1977. Effects of intramuscular injections of selenium and vitamin E on selenium-vitamin E deficiency in young pigs. Am J Vet Res 38:1479-1484.

———. 1980. Effects of intramuscular injections of selenium and vitamin E on peripheral blood and bone marrow of selenium-vitamin E deficient pigs. Am J Vet Res 41:474-478.

Norton, S. A., McCarthy, F. D. 1986. Use of injectable vitamin E and selenium-vitamin E emulsion in ewes and suckling lambs to prevent nutritional muscular dystrophy. J Anim Sci 62:497-508.

NRC. 1980. Mineral Tolerance of Animals. Washington, DC: National Academy of Sciences—National Research Council.

———. 1982. United States—Canadian Tables of Feed Composition. 3rd ed. Washington, DC: National Academy of Sciences—National Research Council.

———. 1985. Nutritional Requirements of Domestic Animals: Nutrient Requirements of Dogs. 2nd ed. Washington, DC: National Academy of Sciences—National Research Council.

———. 1986. Nutritional Requirements of Domestic Animals: Nutrient Requirements of Cats. Rev. ed. Washington, DC: National Academy of Sciences—National Research Council.

———. 1989. Nutritional Requirements of Domestic Animals: Nutrient Requirements of Dairy Cattle. 6th rev. ed. Washington, DC: National Academy of Sciences—National Research Council.

Offenbacher, E. G., Pi-Sunyer, F. X. 1988. Chromium in human nutrition. Ann Rev Nutr 8:543-563.

Ogilvie G. K., Fettman M. J., Mallinckrodt C.H., Walton J.A., Hansen R. A., Davenport D. J., Gross K. L., Richardson K. L., Rogers Q. R., Hand M. S. 2000. Effect of fish oil, arginine, and doxorubicin chemotherapy on remission and survival time in dogs with lymphoma. Cancer 88:1916-1928.

Olson, W. G., Stevens, J. B., Haggard, D. W. 1980. Iodine: A review of dietary requirements, therapeutic properties, and assessment of potential toxicity. Comp Cont Educ Pract Vet 2:S164-S168.

O'Riordan, M. G., Fearon, K. C. H., Ross, J. A., Rogers, P., Falconer, J. S., Bartolo, D. C. C., Garden, O. J.., Carter, D. C. 1994. Glutamine-supplemented total parenteral nutrition enhances T-lymphocyte response in surgical patients undergoing colorectal resection. Ann Surg 220:212-221.

O'Toole, D., Raisbeck, M., Case, J. C., Whitson, T. D. 1996. Selenium-induced "blind staggers" and related myths: a commentary on the extent of historical livestock losses attributed to selenosis on western US rangelands. Vet Pathol 33:104-116.

Paauw, J. D., Davis, A. T. 1990. Taurine concentrations in serum of critically injured patients and age- and sex-matched healthy control subjects. Am J Clin Nutr 52:657-660.

———. 1994. Taurine supplementation at three different dosages and its effects on trauma patients. Am J Clin Nutr 60:203-206.

Page, T. G., Southern, L. L., Ward, T. L., Thompson, D. L. 1993. Effect of chromium picolinate on growth and serum and carcass traits of growing-finishing pigs. J Anim Sci 71:656-662.

Palozza, P., Sgarlata, E., Luberto, C., Piccioni, E., Anti, M., Marra, G., Armelao, F., Franceschelli, P., Bartoli, G. M. 1996. ω-3 fatty acids induce oxidative modification in human erythrocytes depending on dose and duration of dietary supplementation. Am J Clin Nutr 64:297-304.

Paniagua, R., Claure, R., Amato, D., Flores, E., Perez, A., Exaire, E. 1995. Effects of oral administration of zinc and diiodohydroxyquinolein on plasma zinc levels of uremic patients. Nephron 69:147-150.

Pekarek, R. S., Powanda, M. C., Wannemacher, R. W. 1972. The effect of leukocytic endogenous mediator (LEM) on serum copper and ceruloplasmin concentrations in the rat. Proc Soc Exptl Biol Med 141:1029-1031.

Pekarek, R. S., Sandstead, H. H., Jacob, R. A., Barcome, D. F. 1979. Abnormal cellular immune responses during acquired zinc deficiency. Am J Clin Nutr 32:1466-1471.

Pence, B. C. 1991. Dietary selenium and antioxidant status: Toxic effects of 1,2-dimethylhydrazine in rats. J Nutr 121:138-144.

Petersson, B., Waller, S. O., Vinnars, E., Wernerman, J. 1994. Long-term effect of glycyl-glutamine after elective surgery on free amino acids in muscle. J Parent Enter Nutr 18:320-325.

Pion, P. D., Kittleson, M. D. 1990. Taurine's role in clinical practice. J Sm Anim Pract 31:510-518.

Pion, P. D., Kittleson, M. D., Rogers, Q. R., Morris, J. G. 1987. Myocardial failure in cats associated with low plasma taurine: A reversible cardiomyopathy. Science 237:764-768.

Pion, P. D., Kittleson, M. D., Thomas, W. P., Delellis, L. A., Rogers, Q. R. 1992. Response of cats with dilated cardiomyopathy to taurine supplementation. J Am Vet Med Assoc 201:275-284.

Pion, P. D., Lewis, J., Greene, K., Rogers, Q. R., Morris, J. G., Kittleson, M. D. 1991. Effect of meal-feeding and food deprivation on plasma and whole blood taurine concentrations in cats. J Nutr 121:S177-S178.

Podoll, K. L., Bernard, J. B., Ullrey, D. E., DeBar, S. R., Ku, P. K., Magee, W. T. 1992. Dietary selenate versus selenite for cattle, sheep, and horses. J Anim Sci 70:1965-1970.

Polson, R. J., Kenna, J. G., Shears, I. P., Bomford, A., Williams, R. 1988. Measurement of ferritin in serum by an indirect competitive enzyme-linked immunosorbent assay. Clin Chem 34:661-664.

Pomposelli, J. J., Flores, E., Blackburn, G. L., Hirschberg, Y., Zeisel, S. H., Bistrian, B. R. 1991. Diets enriched with ω-3 fatty acids ameliorate lactic acidosis by improving endotoxin-induced tissue hypoperfusion in guinea pigs. Ann Surg 213:166-176.

Pomposelli, J. J., Flores, E., Hirschberg, Y., Teo, T. C., Blackburn, G. L., Zeisel, S. H., Bistrian, B. R. 1990. Short-term TPN containing ω-3 fatty acids ameliorate lactic acidosis induced by endotoxin in guinea pigs. Am J Clin Nutr 52:548-552.

Prabowo, A., Spears, J. W., Goode, L. 1988. Effects of dietary iron on performance and mineral utilization in lambs fed a forage-based diet. J Anim Sci 66:2028-2035.

Prasad, A. S. 1979. Clinical, biochemical, and pharmacological role of zinc. Ann Rev Pharmacol 20:393-426.

Preuss, H. G. 1971. Ammonia production from glutamine and glutamate in isolated dog renal tubules. Am J Physiol 220:54-58.

Prince, T. J., Hays, V. W., Cromwell, G. L. 1984. Interactive effects of dietary calcium, phosphorus, and copper on performance and liver stores of pigs. J Anim Sci 58:356-361.

Prisco, D., Filippini, M., Francalanci, I., Paniccia, R., Gensini, G. F., Abbate, R., Serneri, G. G. N. 1996. Effect of ω-3 polyunsaturated fatty acid intake on phospholipid fatty acid composition in plasma and erythrocytes. Am J Clin Nutr 63:25-32.

Prohaska, J. R. 1991. Changes in Cu, Zn-superoxide dismutase, cytochrome c oxidase, glutathione peroxidase, and glutathione transferase activities in copper-deficient mice and rats. J Nutr 121:355-363.

Prohaska, J. R., Lukasewycz, O. A. 1981. Copper deficiency suppresses the immune response of mice. Science 213:559-561.

Raclot, T., Groscolas, R. 1994. Individual fish oil ω-3 polyunsaturated fatty acid deposition and mobilization rates for adipose tissue of rats in a nutritional steady state. Am J Clin Nutr 60:72-78.

Radack, K., Deck, C., Huster, G. 1991. The effects of low doses of ω-3 fatty acid supplementation on blood pressure in hypertensive subjects. Arch Int Med 151:1173-1180.

Radecki, S. V., Ku, P. K., Bennink, M. R., Yokoyama, M. T., Miller, E. R. 1992. Effect of dietary copper on intestinal mucosa enzyme activity, morphology, and turnover rates in weanling pigs. J Anim Sci 70:1424-1431.

Rassin, D. K., Gaull, G. E., Jarvenpaa, A. L., Raiha, N. C. 1983. Feeding the low birth weight infant: II. Effects of taurine and cholesterol supplementation on amino acid cholesterol. Pediatrics 71:179-186.

Reddy, B. S., Burill, C., Rigotty, J. 1991. Effects of diets high in ω-3 and ω-6 fatty acids on initiation and postinitiation stages of colon carcinogenesis. Cancer Res 51:487-491.

Reece, W. O., Self, H. L., Hotchkiss, D. K. 1984. Injection of iron in newborn beef calves: Erythrocyte variables and weight gains with newborn-dam correlations. Am J Vet Re 45:2119-2122.

Reffet, J. K., Spears, J. W., Brown, T. T. 1988. Effect of dietary selenium and vitamin E on the primary and secondary immune response in lambs challenged with $parainfluenza_3$ virus. J Anim Sci 66:1520-1528.

Reid, R. L., Jung, G. A., Stout, W. L., Ranney, T. S. 1987. Effects of varying zinc concentrations on quality of alfalfa for lambs. J Anim Sci 64:1735-1742.

Remillad, R. L. 1989. Taurine and other dietary considerations for cats. J Am Vet Med Assoc 194:1679 (letter).

Rioux, F. M., Innis, S. M., Dyer, R., MacKinnon, M. 1997. Diet-induced changes in liver and bile but not brain fatty acids can be predicted from differences in plasma phospholipid fatty acids in formula- and milk-fed piglets. J Nutr 127:370-377.

Roeback, J. R., Hla, K. M., Chambless, L. E., Fletcher, R. H. 1991. Effects of chromium supplementation on serum high-density lipoprotein cholesterol levels in men taking beta-blockers. Ann Int Med 115:917-924.

Rojas, L. X., McDowell, L. R., Cousins, R. J., Martin, F. G., Wilkinson, N. S., Johnson, A. B., Velasquez, J. B. 1995. Relative bioavailability of two organic and two inorganic zinc sources fed to sheep. J Anim Sci 73:1202-1207.

Rose, D. P., Connolly, J. M. 1990. Effects of fatty acids and inhibitors of eicosanoid synthesis on the growth of a human breast cancer cell line in culture. Cancer Res 50:7139-7144.

Rose, D. P., Connolly, J. M., Rayburn, J., Coleman, M. 1995. Influence of diets containing eicosapentaenoic or docosahexaenoic acid on growth and metastasis of breast cancer cells in nude mice. J Natl Cancer Inst 87:587-592.

Rose, D. P., Connolly, J. M., Coleman, M. 1996. Effect of omega-3 fatty acids on the progression of metastases after the surgical excision of human breast cancer cell solid tumors growing in nude mice. Clin Cancer Res 2:1751-1756.

Ruhr, L. P., Nicholson, S. S., Confer, A. W., Blakewood, B. W. 1983. Acute intoxication from a hematinic in calves. J Am Vet Med Assoc 182:616-618.

Saad, M. J. A., Morais, S. L., Saad, S. T. O. 1991. Reduced cortisol secretion in patients with iron deficiency. Ann Nutr Metab 35:111-115.

Salvin, S. B., Rabin, B. S. 1984. Resistance and susceptibility to infection in inbred murine strains. IV. Effects of dietary zinc. Cell Immunol 87:546-552.

Sanders, D. E. 1983. Copper deficiency in food animals. Comp Cont Educ Pract Vet 5:S404-S410.

Sanders, D. E., Koestner, A. 1980. Bovine neonatal ataxia associated with hypocupremia in pregnant cows. J Am Vet Med Assoc 176:728-730.

Sanecki, R. K., Corbin, J. E., Forbes, R. M. 1982. Tissue changes in dogs fed a zinc-deficient ration. Am J Vet Res 43:1642-1646.

———. 1985. Extracutaneous histologic changes accompanying zinc deficiency in pups. Am J Vet Res 46:2120-2123.

Sargent, T., Lim, T. H., Jenson, R. L. 1979. Reduced chromium retention in patients with hemochromatosis, a possible basis for hemochromatotic diabetes. Metabolism 28:70-79.

Scharschmidt, L. A., Gibbons, N. B., McGarry, L., Berger, P., Axelrod, M., Janis, R., Ko, Y. H. 1987. Effects of dietary fish oil on renal insufficiency in rats with subtotal nephrectomy. Kidn Intl 32:700-709.

Schecter, Y., Karlish, S. J. D. 1980. Insulin-like stimulation of glucose oxidation in rat adipocytes by vanadyl (IV) ions. Nature 284:556-558.

Schell, T. C., Kornegay, E. T. 1996. Zinc concentration in tissues and performance of weanling pigs fed pharmacological levels of zinc from ZnO, Zn-methionine, Zn-lysine, or $ZnSO_4$. J Anim Sci 74:1584-1593.

Schroder, J., Wardelmann, E., Fandrich, F., Schweizer, E., Schroeder, P. 1995. Glutamine-dipeptide-supplemented parenteral nutrition reverses gut atrophy, disaccharidase enzyme activity, and absorption in rats. J Parent Enter Nutr 19:502-506.

Schroeder, H. A. 1966. Chromium deficiency in rats: a syndrome simulating diabetes mellitus with retarded growth. J Nutr 88:439-445.

Scott, D. W., Miller, W. H., Reinhart, G. A., Mohammed, H. O., Bagladi, M. S. 1997. Effect of an omega-3/omega-6 fatty acid-containing commercial lamb and rice diet on pruritus in atopic dogs: results of a single-blinded study. Can J Vet Res 61:145-153.

Shaw, N. S., Chin, C. J., Pan, W. H. 1995. A vegetarian diet rich in soybean products compromises iron status in young students. J Nutr 125:212-219.

Shearer, T. R., Kolstad, D. L., Suttie, J. W. 1978. Bovine dental fluorosis: Histologic and physical characteristics. An J Vet Res 39:597-602.

Shrock, H., Goldstein, L. 1981. Interorgan relationships for glutamine metabolism in normal and acidotic rats. Am J Physiol 240:E519-E525.

Shupe, J. L. 1980. Clinicopathologic features of fluoride toxicosis in cattle. J Anim Sci 51:746-758.

Shupe, J. L., Olson, A. E. 1971. Clinical aspects of fluorosis in horses. J Am Vet Med Assoc 158:167-174.

Shurson, G. C., Ku, P. K., Waxler, G. L., Yokoyama, M. T., Miller, E. R. 1990. Physiological relationships between microbiological status and dietary copper levels in the pig. J Anim Sci 68:1061-1071.

Singh, R. K., Kooreman, K. M., Babbs, C. F., Fessler, J. F., Salaris, S. C., Pham, J. 1992. Potential use of simple manganese salts as antioxidant drugs in horses. Am J Vet Rers 53:1822-1829.

Smith, J. E., Moore, K., Cipriano, J. E., Morris, P. G. 1984. Serum ferritin as a measure of stored iron in horses. J Nutr 114:677-681.

Smith, J. E., Moore, K., Schoneweis, D. 1981. Coulometric technique for iron determinations. Am J Vet Res 42:1084-1085.

Snyder, S. L., Walker, R. I. 1976. Inhibition of lethality in endotoxin-challenged mice treated with zinc chloride. Infec Immun 13:998-1000.

Sobocinski, P. Z., Canterbury, W. J., Mapes, C. A., Dinterman, R. E. 1978. Involvement of hepatic metallothioneins in hypozincemia associated with bacterial infection. Am J Physiol 234:E399-E406.

Sobocinski, P. Z., Canterbury, W. J., Powanda, M. C. 1977. Differential effect of parenteral zinc on the course of various bacterial infections. Proc Soc Exptl Biol Med 156:334-339.

Soli, N. E. 1980. Chronic copper poisoning in sheep. Nord Vet Med 32:75-89.

Souba, W. W. 1991. Glutamine: a key substrate for the splanchnic bed. Ann Rev Nutr 11:285-308.

———. 1993. Glutamine and cancer. Ann Surg 218:715-728.

Spears, J. W., Harvey, R. W., Brown, T. T. 1991. Effects of zinc methionine and zinc oxide on performance, blood characteristics, and antibody titer response to viral vaccination in stressed feeder calves. J Am Vet Med Assoc 199:1731-1733.

Sprecher H., Luthria D. L., Mohammed B. S., Baykousheva S. P. Reevaluation of the pathways for the biosynthesis of polyunsaturated fatty acids. J Lipid Res 1995;36:2471-2477.

Stabel, J. R., Spears, J. W., Brown, T. T. 1993. Effect of copper deficiency on tissue, blood characteristics, and immune function of calves challenged with infectious bovine rhinotracheitis virus and *Pasteurella hemolytica.* J Anim Sci 71:1247-1255.

Starcher, B. C., Glauber, J. G., Madaras, J. G. 1980. Zinc absorption and its relationship to intestinal metallothioneins. J Nutr 110:1391-1397.

Stehle, P., Zander, J., Mertes, N., Albers,, S., Puchstein, C., Lawin, P., Furst, P. 1989. Effect of parenteral glutamine peptide supplements on muscle glutamine loss and nitrogen balance after major surgery. Lancet 1(8632):231-233.

Stowe, H. D., Herdt, T. H. 1992. Clinical assessment of selenium status of livestock. J Anim Sci 70:3928-3933.

Stowe, H. D., Thomas, J. W., Johnson, T., Marteniuk, J. V., Morrow, D. A., Ullrey, D. E. 1988. Responses of dairy cattle to long-term and short-term supplementation with oral selenium and vitamin E. J Dairy Sci 71:1830-1839.

Sture, G. H., Lloyd, D. H. 1995. Canine atopic disease: therapeutic use of an evening primrose oil and fish oil combination. Vet Rec 137:169-170.

Sturman, J. A., Moretz, R. C., French, J. H., Wisniewski, H. M. 1985. Taurine deficiency in the developing cat: Persistence of the cerebellar external granule layer. J Neuroscience Res 13:405-416.

Su, L. C., Ravanshad, S., Owen, C. A., McCall, J. T., Zollman, P. E., Hardy, R. M. 1982a. A comparison of copper-loading disease in Bedlington terriers and Wilson's disease in humans. Am J Physiol 243:G226-G230.

Su, L. C., Owen, C. A., Zollman, P. E., Hardy, R. M. 1982b. defect of biliary excretion of copper in copper-laden Bedlington terriers. Am J Physiol 243:G231-G236.

Suttie, J. W. 1980. Nutritional aspects of fluoride toxicosis. J Anim Sci 51:759-766.

Suttle, N. F. 1987. Safety and effectiveness of cupric oxide particles for increasing liver copper stores in cattle. Res Vet Sci 42:224-227.

———. 1991. The interactions between copper, molybdenum, and sulphur in ruminant nutrition. Ann Rev Nutr 11:121-140.

Swanson, E. W., Miller, J. K., Mueller, F. J., Patton, C. S., Bacon, J. A., Ramsey, N. 1990. Iodine in milk and meat of dairy cows fed different amounts of potassium iodide or ethylenediamine dihydroiodide. J Dairy Sci 73:398-405.

Swecker, W. S., Eversole, D. E., Thatcher, C. D., Blodgett, D. J., Schurig, G. G., Meldrum, J. B. 1989. Influence of supplemental selenium on humoral immune responses in weaned beef calves. Am J Vet Res 50:1760-1763.

Swinkels, J. W. G. M., Kornegay, E. T., Zhou, W., Lindemann, M. D., Webb, K. E., Vestegen, M. W. A. 1996. Effectiveness of a zinc amino acid chelate and zinc sulfate in restoring serum and soft tissue zinc concentrations when fed to zinc-depleted pigs. J Anim Sci 74:2420-2430.

Tamura, H., Hirose, S., Watanabe, O., Arai, K. I., Murakawa, M., Matsumura O., Isoda K. 1994. Anemia and neutropenia due to copper deficiency in enteral nutrition. J Parent Ent Nutr 18:185-189.

Tanner, D. Q., Stednick, J. D., Leininger, W. C. 1988. Minimal herd sample size for determination of blood copper status of cattle. J Am Vet Med Assoc 192:1074-1076.

Tennant, B., Harrold, D., Reina-Guerra, M., Kaneko, J. J. 1975. Hematology of the neonatal calf. III. Frequency of congenital iron deficiency anemia. Cornell Vet 65:543-556.

Thornburg, L. P., Rottinghaus, G., Dennis, G., Crawford, S. 1996. The relationship between hepatic copper content and morphologic changes in the liver of West Highland White terriers. Vet Pathol 33:656-661.

Tisdale, M. J., Dhesi, J. K. 1990. Inhibition of weight loss by ω-3 fatty acids in an experimental cachexia. Cancer Res 50:5022-5026.

Tocco-Bradley, R., Kluger, M. J. 1984. Zinc concentration and survival in rats infected with *Salmonella typhimurium.* Infec Immun 45:332-338.

Toft, I., Bonna, K. H., Ingebretsen, O. C., Norday, A., Jenssen, T. 1995. Effects of ω-3 polyunsaturated fatty acids on glucose homeostasis and blood pressure in essential hypertension. Ann Intern Med 123:911-918.

Traub-Dargatz, J. L., Hamar, D. W. 1986. Selenium toxicity in horses. Comp Cont Educ Pract Vet 8:771-776.

Trautwein, E. A., Hayes, K. C. 1990. Taurine concentrations in plasma and whole blood in humans: Estimation of error from intra- and inter-individual variation and sampling technique. Am J Clin Nutr 52:758-764.

Tremel, H., Kienle, B., Weilemann, L. S., Stehle, P., Furst, P. 1994. Glutamine dipeptide-supplemented parenteral nutrition maintains intestinal function in the critically ill. Gastroenterology 107:1595-1601.

Twedt, D. C., Sternlieb, I., Gilbertson, S. R. 1979. Clinical, morphologic, and chemical studies of copper toxicosis of Bedlington terriers. J Am Vet Med Assoc 175:269-275.

Unverferth, D. V., Croskery, R. W., Leier, C. V., Altschuld, R., Pipers, F. S., Thomas, J., Magorien, R. D., Hamlin, R. L. 1983. Canine cobalt cardiomyopathy: A model for the study of heart failure. Am J Vet Res 44:989-995.

van Heugten, A., Spears, J. W. 1997. Immune response and growth of stressed weanling pigs fed diets supplemented with organic or inorganic forms of chromium. J Anim Sci 75:409-416.

Van Lente, F., Daher, R. 1992. Plasma selenium concentrations in patients with euthyroid sick syndrome. Clin Chem 38:1885-1888.

Van Vleet, J. F., Kennedy, S. 1989. Selenium-vitamin E deficiency in swine. Comp Cont Educ Prac Vet 11:662-668.

Vaughn, D. M., Reinhart, G. A., Swaim, S. F., Lauten, S. D., Garner, C. A., Boudreaux, M. K., Spano, J. S., Hoffman, C. E., Conner, B. 1994. Evaluation of effects of dietary ω-6 to ω-3 fatty acid ratios on leukotriene B synthesis in dog skin and neutrophils. Vet Dermatol 5:163-173.

Vestweber, J. G., Leipold, H. W., Steffen, D. J. 1994. Difficult dermatologic diagnosis. Parakeratosis in two female Angus calves. J Am Vet Med Assoc 204:1567-1568.

Vinary, P., Allignet, E., Pichette, C., Watford, M., Lemieux, G., Gougoux, A. 1980. Changes in renal metabolite profile and ammoniagenesis during acute and chronic metabolic acidosis in dog and rat. Kidn Intl 17:312-325.

Voyatzoglou, V., Mountokalakis, T., Tsata-Voyatzoglou, V., Koutselinis, A., Skalkeas, G. 1982. Serum zinc levels and urinary zinc excretion in patients with bronchogenic carcinoma. Am J Surg 144:355-358.

Vruwink, K. G., Fletcher, M. P., Keen, C. L., Golub, M. S., Hendrick, A. G., Gershwin, M. E. 1991. Moderate zinc deficiency in rhesus monkeys. An intrinsic defect of neutrophil chemotaxis corrected by zinc repletion. J Immunol 146:244-249.

Wallace, J. M. W., Turley, I., Gilmore, W. S., Strain, J. J. 1995. Dietary fish oil supplementation alters leukocyte function and cytokine production in healthy women. Arterio Thromb Vasc Biol 15:185-189.

Wang, J. H., Redmond, H. P., Watson, W. G., Condron, C., Bouchier-Hayes, D. 1996. The beneficial effect of taurine on the prevention of human endothelial cell death. Shock 6:331-338.

Ward, J. D., Spears, J. W. 1993. Comparison of copper lysine and copper sulfate as copper sources for ruminants using in vitro methods. J Dairy Sci 76:2994-2998.

Ward, J. D., Spears, J. W., Kegley, E. B. 1996. Bioavailability of copper proteinate and copper carbonate relative to copper sulfate in cattle. J Dairy Sci 79:127-132.

Wasa, M., Satani, M., Tanano, H., Nezu, R., Takagi, Y., Okada, A. 1994. Copper deficiency with pancytopenia during total parenteral nutrition. J Parent Ent Nutr 18:190-192.

Watkins, J. B., Jarvenpaa, A. L., Szczepanik-Van Leeuwen, P., Klein, P. D., Rassin, D. K., Gaull, G., Raiha, N. C. 1983. Feeding the low birth weight infant: V. Effects of taurine, cholesterol, and human milk on bile acid kinetics. Gastroenterol 85:793-800.

Wedekind, K. J., Baker, D. H. 1990. Zinc bioavailability in feed-grade sources of zinc. J Anim Sci 68:684-689.

Wedekind, K. J., Lewis, A. J., Giesemann, M. A., Miller, P. S. 1994. Bioavailability of zinc from inorganic and organic sources for pigs fed corn-soybean meal diets. J Anim Sci 72:2681-2689.

Weeks, B. R., Smith, J. E., Nothrop, J. K. 1989. Relationship of serum ferritin and iron concentrations and serum total iron-binding capacity to nonheme iron stores in dogs. Am J Vet Res 50:198-200.

Weinberg, E. D. 1974. Iron and susceptibility to infectious disease. Science 184:952-956.

Weiser, M. G., Kociba, G. J. 1983. Sequential changes in erythrocyte volume distribution and microcytosis associated with iron deficiency anemia in kittens. Vet Pathol 20:1-12.

Weiser, M. G., O'Grady, M. 1983. Erythrocyte volume distribution analysis and hematologic changes in dogs with iron deficiency anemia. Vet Pathol 20:230-241.

Weiss, W. P., Colenbrander, V. F., Cunningham, M. D., Callahan, C. J. 1983. Selenium/vitamin E: Role in disease prevention and weight gain of neonatal calves. J Dairy Sci 66:1101-1107.

Weiss, W. P., Todhunter, D. A., Hogan, J. S., Smith, K. L. 1990. Effect of duration of supplementation of selenium and vitamin E on periparturient dairy cows. J Dairy Cows 73:3187-3194.

Welles, E. G., Boudreaux, M. K., Tyler, J. W. 1993. Platelet, antithrombin, and fibrinolytic activities in taurine-deficient and taurine-replete cats. Am J Vet Res 54:1235-1243.

Wheeler, D. C., Nair, D. R., Persaud, J. W., Jeremy, J. Y., Chappell, M. E., Varghese, Z., Moorhead, J. F. 1991. Effects of dietary fatty acids in an animal model of focal glomerulosclerosis. Kidn Intl 39:930-937.

Wiren, M., Magnusson, K. E., Larsson, J. 1995. Enteral glutamine increases growth and absorptive capacity of intestinal mucosa in the malnourished rat. Scand J Gastroenterol 30:146-152.

Wong-Valle, J., Henry, P. R., Ammerman, C. B., Rao, P. V. 1989. Estimation of the relative bioavailability of manganese sources for sheep. J Anim Sci 67:2409-2414.

Wooliscroft, J., Barbosa, J. 1977. Analysis of chromium induced carbohydrate intolerance in the rat. J Nutr 107:1702-1706.

Wright, C. E., Tallan, H. H., Lin, Y. Y. 1986. Taurine: Biological update. Ann Rev Biochem 55:427-453.

Xin, Z., Waterman, D. F., Hemken, R. W., Harmon, R. J. 1991a. Effects of copper status on neutrophil function, superoxide dismutase, and copper distribution in steers. J Dairy Sci 74:3078-3085.

Xin, Z., Waterman, D. F., Hemken, R. W., Harmon, R. J., Jackson, J. A. 1991b. Effects of copper sources and dietary cation-anion balance on copper availability and acid-base status in dairy calves. J Dairy Sci 74:3167-3173.

Yang, B., Saldeen, T. G. P., Nichols, W. M., Mehta, J. L. 1993. Dietary fish oil supplementation attenuates myocardial dysfunction and injury caused by global ischemia and reperfusion in isolated rat hearts. J Nutr 123:2067-2074.

Yen, J. T., Pond, W. G. 1981. Effect of dietary vitamin C addition on performance, plasma vitamin C and hematinic iron status in weanling pigs. J Anim Sci 53:1292-1296.

SECTION 10

Chemotherapy of Microbial Diseases

39 ANTISEPTICS AND DISINFECTANTS

MARK C. HEIT AND JIM E. RIVIERE

Cleansers
Antiseptics and Disinfectants
  Alcohol
  Halogens
  Chlorhexidine
  Aldehydes
  Hydrogen Peroxide
  Phenols
  Gases
Factors Affecting Efficacy of Antiseptics
  Concentration
  Temperature
  pH
  Contamination
  Organism Type
Microbial788
 Resistance to Disinfectants and Antiseptics
Antiseptic Usage in Veterinary Medicine
  Skin Cleansers
  Treatment of Open Wounds
  Teat Antisepsis
Disinfectant Usage in Veterinary Medicine
  General Principles
  Special Considerations in Specific Applications

Long before the ability to view microorganisms with a microscope and three centuries before Koch and Pasteur, Fracastoro postulated that germs caused infections. In the 1840s, Ignaz Semmelweis, a Hungarian obstetrician, demonstrated the beneficial effects of hand washing between patients as well as the antiseptic effect of chlorine in the form of chlorinated lime. Following Pasteur's identification of infective agents as the cause of disease, Joseph Lister suggested the use of antiseptics in the field of surgery. His treatment of the hands with 1:20 carbolic lotion and his initiation of methods for chemical sterilization of bandages, dressings, and surgical instruments and for antisepsis of wounds began aseptic surgery. Although originally targeted toward the surgeon, general cleanliness and the use of antiseptics and disinfectants have spread to all fields of the medical, dental, and veterinary professions.

Cleansers, antiseptics, and disinfectants are differentiated by their intended use and characteristic properties and not by their chemical content. A cleanser aids in physical removal of foreign material and is not a germicide. An antiseptic is a germicide applied to living tissue, and a disinfectant is a germicide applied to inanimate objects. Because certain antiseptics may be inactivated on inanimate surfaces and because certain disinfectants are hazardous to living tissue, the two should not be used interchangeably. Even products with the identical active chemical moiety may be formulated in such a way to prevent their interchangeable use. Products to be used on inanimate surfaces, objects, or instruments are regulated by the Environmental Protection Agency (EPA), whereas chemicals in antiseptics for use on the human body must be registered with the Food and Drug Administration (FDA).

CLEANSERS. Cleansers (surfactants, detergents) remove dirt and contaminating organisms by solubilization and physical means. Cleaning an area to remove gross contamination prior to disinfection or antisepsis treatment maximizes their efficacy. Cleansers can be classified into three types based on the position of the hydrophobic portion of the molecule: anionic, cationic, and nonionic.

Soaps are anionic surfactants of the general structure $R\text{-}COO^-Na^+$. Dissociation in water to $R\text{-}COO^-$ liberates a molecule with both a hydrophilic and a hydrophobic portion that can emulsify and solubilize hydrophobic dirt, fat, and protoplasmic membranes. Once solubilized, this contamination can be rinsed away with water. The ability to solubilize membranes renders soaps antibacterial against gram-positive and acid-fast bacteria. The anionic nature of soaps, however, causes them to be inactivated in the presence of certain positive ions such as free Ca^+ in hard water and in the presence of cationic detergents. The mixture of soaps and quaternary ammonium compounds (QACs) forms a precipitate that terminates the activity of both compounds. Inclusion of antiseptic compounds in soap preparations has given them a wider antibacterial spectrum.

The QACs are examples of cationic surfactants with germicidal activity. These compounds have been widely used as disinfectants. Cationic surfactants combine readily with proteins, fats, and phosphates and are thus of limited value in the presence of serum, blood, and other tissue debris (Huber 1988). In addition, use with materials such as gauze pads and cotton balls makes them less microbicidal owing to adsorption of the active ingredients. For these reasons, and because several outbreaks of infections have been associated with use of contaminated solutions, the Centers for Disease Control (CDC) no longer recommend cationic surfactants for antisepsis.

Second- and third-generation QACs are less affected by hard water and other anions. These quaternaries are fungicidal, bactericidal, and virucidal against lipophilic viruses but are not sporicidal, tuberculocidal, or active against hydrophilic viruses. Benzalkonium chloride, the first commercially available quaternary compound, has been shown to cause chemical burns when used undiluted (Bilbrey et al. 1989).

ANTISEPTICS AND DISINFECTANTS. An antiseptic is a chemical agent that reduces the microbial population on skin and other living tissues. Because, in most cases, its mechanism of action involves nonspecific disruption of cellular membranes or enzymes, caution must be taken not to harm host tissue. An ideal antiseptic would have a broad spectrum of activity, low toxicity, and high penetrability, would maintain activity in the presence of pus and necrotic tissue, and would cause little skin irritation or interference with the normal healing process.

The use of antiseptics has been suggested in situations that require maximal reduction of bacterial contamination (Larson 1987), such as when defense mechanisms are compromised after surgery, during catheterization or insertion of other invasive implants, and in immunocompromised states due to immune defects, cytotoxic drug therapy, extreme old or young age, or extensive skin damage (burns and wounds).

Disinfection is the elimination of many or all pathogenic organisms, excluding spore forms, from an inanimate object. The treatment of objects that are too large to soak in disinfectant, such as cabinets, exam tables, chairs, lights, and cages, is considered surface disinfection. Immersion disinfection, sometimes wrongly referred to as cold sterilization, is the immersion of smaller objects in disinfectant for sufficient time to kill the majority of contaminating organisms. True chemical sterilization necessitates the use of an EPA-registered agent capable of killing all infective organisms, including fungal and bacterial spores, usually within 10 hours. Chemical sterilization should not replace heat-pressure sterilization.

The ideal characteristics of a disinfectant include a broad spectrum, fast action, activity in the presence of organic material (including blood, sputum, and feces), compatibility with detergents, low toxicity, and residual surface activity. Disinfectants should not corrode instruments or metallic surfaces or disintegrate rubber, plastic, or other materials, and they should be odorless and economical (Molinari et al. 1982).

Microorganisms can be ranked from least to most resistant to disinfectant killing as follows: vegetative bacteria, medium-size lipid-coated viruses, fungi, small nonlipid enveloped viruses, *Mycobacterium tuberculosis,* and bacterial endospores. Using these different resistances, disinfection can be further divided into three levels. Low-level disinfection kills most bacteria, some viruses, and some fungi, but not tubercle bacilli or bacterial spores. Intermediate-level disinfection inactivates *M. tuberculosis,* most viruses and fungi, but not necessarily bacterial spores. High-level disinfection destroys all microorganisms except high numbers of bacterial spores.

A second classification system divides instruments and patient-care items into three categories based on risk of infection involved in their use (Spaulding 1968). In this system, items are classified as (1) critical—those that enter or penetrate skin or mucous membranes (e.g., needles, scalpels); (2) semicritical—those that touch intact mucous membranes (e.g., anesthesia equipment, endoscopes); and (3) noncritical—those that do not touch mucous membranes but may contact intact skin (e.g., cages, tables, food bowls). In general, items classified as critical should be sterilized, semicritical items require high-level disinfection, and noncritical items require low- to intermediate-level disinfection.

The following is a discussion of local anti-infective agents categorized by the active chemical entity. Where appropriate, considerations and recommendations for their use as cleansers, disinfectants, or antiseptics are noted.

Alcohol. Although many alcohols are germicidal, the two most commonly used are ethyl and isopropyl alcohol. These compounds are both lipid solvents and protein denaturants. They kill organisms by solubilizing the lipid cell membrane and by denaturing membrane cellular proteins. Alcohols are most effective when diluted with water to a final concentration of 70% ethyl or 50% isopropyl alcohol by weight. It is thought that at greater concentrations, initial dehydration of cellular proteins makes them resistant to the denaturing effect (Molinari and Runnel 1991). The alcohols have excellent antibacterial activity against most vegetative gram-positive, gram-negative, and tubercle bacillus organisms but do not inactivate bacterial spores. They are active against many fungi and viruses, principally enveloped viruses due to alcohol's lipid-solubilizing action. They are active against cytomegalovirus and herpes simplex and human immunodeficiency viruses.

Both isopropyl and ethyl alcohols are commonly used, effective antiseptics, with only subtle differences in their action. Because their effectiveness is drastically reduced by organic matter such as excreta, mucus, and blood, they are most effective on "clean" skin. Of all agents, they produce the most rapid and largest reduction in bacterial counts (Lowbury et al. 1974), with contact times of 1–3 minutes resulting in elimination of almost 80% of organisms. Rapid evaporation limits contact time; however, residual decreases in bacterial counts are seen to occur after the alcohol has evaporated from the skin. Although alcohols are among the safest antiseptics, toxic reactions have been reported in children. Alcohol is very drying to the skin and can cause local irritation. In efforts to minimize this drying effect, emollients such as glycerine have been added with good results (Larson et al. 1986).

The alcohols are not recommended for high-level disinfection or chemical sterilization due to their inactivity against bacterial spores and reduced efficacy in the presence of protein or other bioburden. Blood proteins are denatured by alcohol and will adhere to instruments being disinfected. Fatal *Clostridium* spp. infections have occurred postoperatively that were the result of contaminated surgical instruments that had been disinfected with alcohol containing bacterial spores (Nye and Mallory 1923). After repeated and prolonged use, alcohols can damage the shellac mounting of lensed instruments, can swell or harden rubber and certain plastic tubing (Rutala 1990), and can be corrosive to metal surfaces. Alcohols are flammable; thus caution must be taken in their storage and when used prior to electrocautery or laser surgery. In deciding between ethyl and isopropyl alcohol, it is important to consider isopropyl's inactivity against hydrophilic viruses, its less corrosive nature, and the abuse potential for ethyl alcohol (grain alcohol).

Halogens. Elemental iodine has activity against gram-positive and gram-negative bacteria, bacterial spores, fungi, and most viruses. It exerts these lethal effects by diffusing into the cell and interfering with metabolic reactions and by disrupting protein and nucleic acid structure and synthesis. Iodine has a characteristic odor and is corrosive to metals. It is insoluble in water and thus is prepared in alcohol (tincture) or with solubilizing surfactants ("tamed" iodines). Tincture of iodine, used as early as 1839, in the French Civil War, is most effectively formulated as a 1–2% iodine solution in 70% ethyl alcohol. In this form, most (~90%) bacteria are killed within 3 minutes of application. The antibacterial activity of this combination is greater than that of the alcohol alone. Tincture of iodine, however, is irritating and allergenic, corrodes metals, and stains skin and clothing. It is also painful when applied to open wounds and is harmful to host tissue; therefore, it can delay healing and thereby increase the chance of infection. For these reasons, this preparation has fallen out of favor as an antiseptic or disinfectant. Strong tinctures of iodine have been used as blistering agents in the equine industry.

Efforts to reduce the undesirable aspects of tinctures while retaining the powerful killing action of iodine have led to the introduction of tamed iodines known as iodophors. In this preparation, iodine is solubilized by surfactants, which allow it to remain in a dissociable form. Application of this product allows for slow continual release of free iodine to exert its germicidal effects. The iodophors have a similar spectrum of activity to aqueous solution; are less irritating, allergenic, corrosive, and staining; and have prolonged activity after application (4–6 hours). Common solubilizing carriers include polyvinylpyrrolidone (called PVP-iodine or povidone-iodine [PI]) as well as other nonionic surfactants, making iodophors excellent cleansing agents as well as antiseptics and disinfectants. Iodophor solutions retain their activity in the presence of organic matter at pH < 4 (Huber 1988). The water-soluble carriers have been postulated to interact with epithelial surfaces to increase tissue permeability, thereby enhancing iodine's killing efficacy.

Free iodine released by the iodophor complex is apparently responsible for its germicidal activity. Proper dilution to 1% iodine is necessary for maximum killing effect and minimal toxicity. More-concentrated solutions are actually less efficacious, presumably due to stronger complexation preventing free iodine release. It takes approximately 2 minutes of contact time for release of free iodine (Lavelle et al. 1975). Literature reports indicate that iodophors are quickly bactericidal, virucidal, and mycobactericidal but may require prolonged contact times to kill certain fungi and bacterial spores. Iodophors formulated as antiseptics are not suitable as hard-surface disinfectants, due to insufficient concentrations of iodine.

Consideration must be taken of iodine's ability to be systemically absorbed through the skin and especially mucous membranes. The extent of absorption is related to the concentration used, frequency of application, and status of renal function (the principal excretory route) (Swaim and Lee 1987). Complications of systemic iodophor absorption include increased serum enzyme levels, renal failure, metabolic acidosis (Pretsch and Meakins 1976), and increased serum free iodide. If renal function is normal, serum iodine concentrations quickly return to normal. Clinical hyperthyroidism and thyroid hyperplasia have been reported after treatment with PI (Scheider et al. 1976; Altemeier 1976). Chap. 53 should be consulted for further details.

Chlorine-containing solutions were first introduced by Dakin in the early 1900s in the chemical form of sodium hypochlorite. They are effective antibacterial, fungicidal, virucidal, and protozoacidal agents. The chemical forms most commonly used today include the hypochlorites (sodium and calcium) and organic chlorides (chloramine-T). In either form, the germicidal activity is due to release of free chlorine and formation of hypochlorous acid (HOCl) from water. The mechanisms of action of these compounds include inhibition of cellular enzymatic reactions, protein denaturation, and inactivation of nucleic acids (Dychdala 1983). Dissociation of HOCl to the less microbicidal hypochlorite ion (OCl^-) increases as pH increases, and thus the solution may be rendered ineffective above pH 8.0 (Weber 1950). Mixing NaOCl with acid liberates toxic chlorine gas, and NaOCl decomposes when exposed to light.

Low concentrations of free chlorine are active against *M. tuberculosis* (50 ppm) and vegetative bacteria (<1 ppm) within seconds. Concentrations of 100 ppm destroy fungi in less than 1 hour, and many viruses are inactivated in 10 minutes at 200 ppm. Household bleach is 5.25% (52,500 ppm); thus dilutions of 1:100–1:250 should result in effective germicidal concentrations, although more-concentrated solutions are often recommended (1:10–1:100).

The use of the hypochlorites as disinfectants is limited by several characteristics. Chlorine solutions are corrosive to metals and destroy many fabrics. Because chlorine solutions are unstable to light, they must be prepared fresh daily. Hypochlorites are inactivated by the presence of blood more so than are the organic chlorides (Bloomfield and Miller 1989). They have a strong odor and are not suitable for enclosed spaces. Despite these shortcomings, chlorine solutions are commonly used as low-level disinfectants to sanitize dairy equipment, animal housing quarters, hospital floors, and other noncritical items. Of 12 disinfectant solutions evaluated for their ability to kill the dermatophyte *Microsporum canis,* those containing hypochlorite were most effective. Also found effective were benzalkonium chloride- and glutaraldehyde-based products; phenolics and anionic detergents were considered inadequate (Rycroft and McLay 1991). The hypochlorites are not recommended for use as antiseptics because they are very irritating to skin and other tissues and they delay healing.

Several compounds from a class called N-halamines (oxazolidinones and imidazolidinones) have been developed that are water-soluble solids and have been shown to be bactericidal, fungicidal, virucidal, and protozoacidal in water disinfection at low total halogen concentrations (1–10 mg/L). They are noncorrosive and tasteless and odorless in water. They are extremely stable in water even in the presence of organic loads. Their potential use in poultry processing to control *Salmonella* organisms has been evaluated (Smith et al. 1990).

Chlorhexidine. Chlorhexidine (Chx) is a synthetic cationic compound (1-1′-hexamethylenebis[5-(*p*-chlorophenyl)biguanide]) with better activity against gram-positive organisms than against gram-negative ones. It was found to be superior to PI against *Staphylococcus aureus* infection in dogs (Amber et al. 1983), but some gram-negative bacteria were found to be resistant (Russel 1986). Chlorhexidine kills bacteria by disrupting the cell membrane and precipitating cell contents. It has also been suggested that membrane bound adenosine triphosphatases, specifically inhibition of the F1 ATPase, may be a primary target for Chx (Gayle et al. 1981). It is active against fungi, fairly active against *M. tuberculosis,* but poorly active against viruses. The antibacterial activity of Chx is not as rapid as that of the alcohols; however, as a 0.1% aqueous solution, significant killing action is evident after only 15 seconds. Additionally, Chx solutions have the longest residual activity, remaining chemically active for 5–6 hours and retaining their activity in the presence of blood and other organic material. Being cationic, it is inactivated by hard water, nonionic surfactants, inorganic anions, and soaps. Dilution with saline causes precipitation, and its activity is pH dependent. It has extremely low toxicity even when used on intact skin of newborns (O'Neill et al. 1982).

Chlorhexidine is available in a detergent base as a 4% solution or as a 2% liquid foam. It is widely used as a presurgical antiseptic, wound flush, and teat dip. Its use as a disinfectant has not been described.

Aldehydes. Two related aldehyde disinfectants are formaldehyde and glutaraldehyde (GLT). Formaldehyde has antimicrobial activity both as a gas (see below) and in liquid form. Formalin, the aqueous form, is 37% formaldehyde by weight. It inactivates microorganisms by alkylating the amino and sulfhydryl groups of proteins and ring nitrogen atoms of purine bases (Favero 1983). Formaldehyde is an effective but slow bactericide, virucide, and fungicide, requiring 6–12 hours' contact time. It is effective against *M. tuberculosis,* bacterial spores, and most animal viruses, including foot-and-mouth disease virus. Its action is not affected by organic matter, and it is relatively noncorrosive to metals, paint, and fabric. Formaldehyde alone is considered a high-level disinfectant and in combination with alcohol can be used as a chemical sterilant for surgical instruments. However, due to irritating fumes and pungent odor at low concentrations (~1 ppm), and because the National Institute for Occupational Safety and Health requires it to be handled as a potential carcinogen, thereby limiting worker exposure time, formaldehyde's use as a disinfectant has been limited to certain veterinary applications (see below).

GLT, a saturated dialdehyde, is similar to formaldehyde but without some of its shortcomings. GLT has better bactericidal, virucidal, and sporicidal activity than formaldehyde. Its biocidal activity is related to its ability to alkylate sulfhydryl, hydroxyl, carboxyl, and amino groups affecting RNA, DNA, and protein synthesis (Scott and Gorman 1983). Acidic GLT solutions are not sporicidal; thus, they must be "activated" by alkalinizing agents to a pH between 7.5 and 8.5. Once activated, these solutions have a limited shelf life (14 days) due to polymerization of the GLT molecules (Rutala 1990). Newer formulations (stabilized alkaline GLT, potentiated acid GLT, GLT-phenate) have increased shelf life (28–30 days) and excellent germicidal activity (Pepper 1980).

GLT has gained wide acceptance in high-level disinfection and chemical sterilization due to several favorable properties, including wide spectrum of activity. Low surface tension allows GLT to penetrate blood and exudate without coagulating proteins. It retains its biocidal activity in the presence of organic matter. It is noncorrosive to metal, rubber, and plastic and does not damage lensed instruments. GLT solutions must be used in well-ventilated areas, since air concentrations of 0.2 ppm are irritating to the eyes and nasal passages (CDC 1987).

Contact times of less than 2 minutes for vegetative bacteria, 10 minutes for fungi, and 3 hours for bacterial spores were necessary using a 2% aqueous alkaline GLT solution (Stonehill et al. 1963). Activity against the tubercle bacillus was found to be somewhat variable; at least 20 minutes at room temperature is needed to reliably kill these organisms with 2% GLT. When used as a high-level disinfectant, a minimum of 1% GLT should be used. GLT-phenate formulations should be used with caution since they were shown to be less effective than other aldehyde solutions in decreasing bacterial counts from some medical instruments (Ayliffe et al. 1986). GLT disinfectants were found to more effectively reduce duck hepatitis B virus infectivity when they contained additives such as alcohol, an ammonium chloride derivative, and a surfactant (Murray et al. 1991).

The caustic nature of both formaldehyde and GLT makes them inappropriate as antiseptics, and in fact, protective gloves should be worn when using the aldehyde disinfectants.

Hydrogen Peroxide. Conflicting reports concerning hydrogen peroxide's efficacy as a germicide make evaluating its utility in disinfection and antisepsis difficult. Although it has been reported to have bactericidal (Schaeffer et al. 1980), virucidal (Mentel and Schmidt 1973), and fungicidal (Turner 1983) activity, others believe it to be more effective against bacterial spores (Reybrouk 1985; Baldry 1983) than against vegetative bacteria. For this reason, one author suggests that hydrogen peroxide antiseptic use be restricted to initial treatment of recently contaminated wounds suspected of containing clostridial spores (Reybrouk 1985). Because 3% hydrogen peroxide has been shown to be damaging to tissues including fibroblasts (Lineweaver et al. 1982), it is not considered suitable for routine wound care. It is, however, considered a stable and effective disinfectant and is used in the disinfection of soft contact lenses.

Phenols. Carbolic acid, a phenol, is the oldest example of an antiseptic compound. However, due to severe local and systemic toxicity, it is no longer appropriate for use as an antiseptic. These agents act as cytoplasmic poisons by penetrating and disrupting microbial cell walls. Most commercially available phenolic products contain two or more compounds that act synergistically, resulting in a wider spectrum of activity, including against *M. tuberculosis*. Sodium o-phenylphenol is effective against staphylococci, pseudomonads, mycobacteria, fungi, and lipophilic viruses and against ascarids, strongyles, and tichurids. Cresols are substituted phenols and are more bactericidal and less toxic and caustic than phenols. Phenolics are not recommended for disinfection of anything other than noncritical items, because residual disinfectant on porous materials can cause tissue irritation even when the items have been thoroughly rinsed, because of strong odors, and because of absorption into feed.

Gases. Gases are used primarily as disinfectants for large spaces and for sterilization of sensitive surgical equipment. Ethylene oxide (C_2H_4O) is a water-soluble flammable gas used for gas sterilization. Mixing ethylene oxide with carbon dioxide or fluorocarbons reduces its flammability. Ethylene oxide kills bacteria, fungi, yeasts, viruses, and spores. Bacterial spores are only 2–10 times more resistant to the killing activity than are vegetative cells. It has been shown that the relative humidity of the microenvironment is critical to microbial susceptibility to ethylene oxide. Activity is decreased in the presence of organic matter due to interaction with proteins and nucleic acids. Care must be used to contain the gas, as it has an irritant effect on the skin and eyes and may cause headaches and nausea.

Formaldehyde gas inactivates viruses, fungi, bacteria, and bacterial spores. Its activity is dependent on relative humidity, and its efficacy is thought to peak at less than 50% relative humidity. Formaldehyde has been used for disinfection of hospital linen and for terminal disinfection in certain food-producing industries (see below).

Popriolactone, methyl bromide, and propylene oxide have also been used as gas disinfectants.

FACTORS AFFECTING EFFICACY OF ANTISEPTICS. Several factors influence the efficacy of antiseptics and disinfectants, including concentration and contact time, temperature, pH, presence of organic or other material, type and concentration of offending organism.

Concentration. The time to effectively kill an organism is inversely dependent upon antimicrobial concentration. For certain compounds (Fig. 39.1, compound A), small decreases in concentration may result in large increases in the time required for killing, whereas other compounds (compound B) are less sensitive to changes in concentration. In this example it would be much more critical to achieve the appropriate concentration of compound A to ensure adequate antisepsis/disinfection. Alcohols and phenolics are very concentration dependent, whereas QACs, aldehydes, and Chx are less sensitive.

Temperature. Increased temperature results in increased antimicrobial activity. This relationship can be described by $Q_{T_2-T_1}$ = (time to kill at T_1) ÷ (time to kill at T_2), where T_2 and T_1 are two different temperatures in centigrade degrees. This equation is commonly referred to as the Q_{10} coefficient and describes the change in activity caused by a 10° C rise in temperature. Table 39.1 lists the Q_{10} coefficients of certain disinfectant compounds.

pH. The pH at the site of action may affect a compound's activity by influencing the compound itself or the microbial cell. Certain molecules (e.g., phenols) and certain acids (e.g., hypochlorous acid [bleach]) are effective only in the un-ionized form; thus, as pH increases they become less efficacious. GLT is more potent at alkaline pH but is more stable at acid pH. Increased pH results in higher numbers of negative charges on cell surfaces with which positively charged molecules, such as QACs and Chx, can interact, thereby increasing their activity. Lastly, in a process similar to absorption through any cell membrane, pH can effect partitioning from the bathing solution into the cell's interior.

Contamination. The most important step in attempting to maximize the efficacy of antisepsis and disinfection is thorough cleansing of the site. Organic matter such as blood, pus, feces, soil, food, and milk are believed to directly reduce the activity of antimicrobial compounds via a chemical reaction that results in a smaller amount of compound available for killing microorganisms or by spatial nonreaction (the inability

TABLE 39.1—Q_{10} coefficients for selected disinfectant/antiseptic compounds

Compound	Q_{10} coefficient
Formaldehyde	1.5
β-Propriolactone	2–3
Ethylene oxide	2.7
Phenol and cresol	3–5
Aliphatic alcohols	30–40

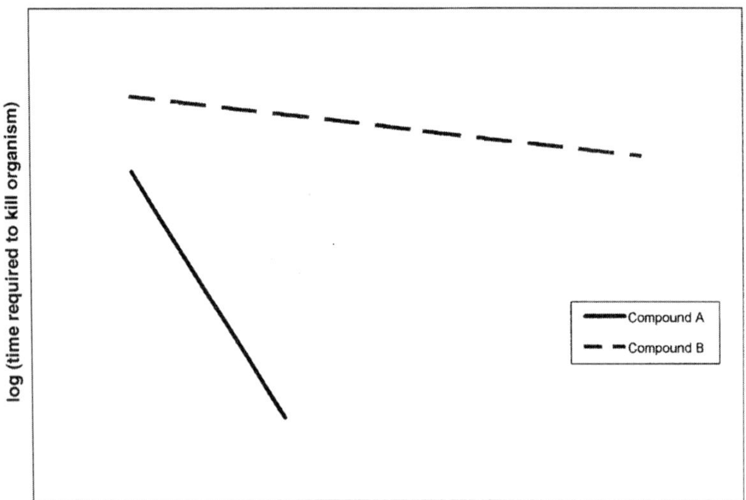

FIG. 39.1—The relationship of the concentration of two theoretical antimicrobial agents to the time required to kill a theoretical organism. The efficacy of compound A is more sensitive to change in concentration than that of compound B.

of the disinfectant molecule to get to the organism). Certain compounds (hypochlorites and iodines) are more susceptible to this type of interference than others. GLT is less affected by organic contamination than other compounds and is therefore useful for instruments whose surface or design makes them impossible to thoroughly clean. Soil contamination can make large-animal facilities difficult to disinfect and may require removal of surface layers of soil and bedding for complete treatment. The presence of inorganic ions (Ca^{+2}, Mg^{+2}, Na^{+}, and Cl^{-}) may be physically incompatible with certain antiseptics/disinfectants, and therefore dilution with either hard water or saline solutions may render these formulations ineffective.

Organism Type. The sensitivity of different classes (bacteria, fungus, virus, etc.) of organisms has been previously discussed. Within each group, however, differences in sensitivities to the various chemical compounds exist that may render a particular disinfection process ineffective against certain microbes while effective against others. Gram-positive bacteria are in general less resistant to disinfectant/antiseptic compounds than are gram-negative organisms due to a less complex and less lipid-rich outer membrane. Staphylococci are less susceptible to alcohols, glycols, and ethylene oxide than are other cocci. Of the gram-negative bacteria, *Pseudomonas aeruginosa, Escherichia coli,* and *Klebsiella* spp. seem to be more resistant to antimicrobial agents, especially QACs and Chx, than other species. Mycobacteria, due to the hydrophobic nature of their cell walls, are highly resistant to many compounds. *Mycobacterium tuberculosis* is resistant to Chx, acids, and alkalis, while QACs are tuberculostatic. The tuberculosis organism is killed by alcohols, formaldehyde (GLT, but slower killing), and ethylene oxide. Bacterial sporicides include the aldehydes, hydrogen peroxide, hypochlorites, iodine, acid alcohol, and ethylene oxide. By inhibiting germination or spore outgrowth, phenols, QACs, biguanides, and alcohols are sporostatic. The efficacy of most germicides against bacterial spores increases with temperature; however, the most effective method against bacterial spores is moist heat (115° C autoclaving). Fungi are sensitive to chlorine, phenols, iodine compounds, ethylene oxide, and the aldehydes, whereas QACs are fungistatic. Fungal spores are resistant to most disinfectants. The sensitivity of viruses to disinfectant compounds relates to the composition of the viral envelope. The lipid-enveloped viruses are readily inactivated by lipophilic agents such as ether, chloroform, phenols, QACs, and even detergents. The nonenveloped viruses are resistant to these agents but are sensitive to chlorine and the aldehydes. Formaldehyde and β-propriolactone are used to inactivate viruses in the production of viral vaccines utilized in veterinary medicine.

MICROBIAL RESISTANCE TO DISINFECTANTS AND ANTISEPTICS. Bacterial resistance to antibiotics is a well-researched phenomenon. Recent evidence suggests a similar emergence of microbial resistance to actions of certain antiseptics and disinfectants, termed "acquired resistance." This type of resistance is the result of acquisition of either a plasmid or a chromosomal mutation and usually involves previous exposure to the chemical agent. A second type, termed "intrinsic resistance," is most frequently due to the biochemical makeup of the organism or cellular components making them inherently resistant to certain molecules. As an example, the cell walls of gram-negative bacteria and mycobacteria may act as absorption barriers to certain agents, thereby protecting deeper sensitive cellular targets. Bacterial spores similarly exhibit intrinsic resistance to many disinfectants. Table 39.2 illustrates examples of, and suspected mechanisms responsible for, resistance to disinfectant agents. The significance of such resistance in clinical practice is uncertain because unlike with systemic antibiotics, very high concentrations of compound are easily and safely achievable.

ANTISEPTIC USAGE IN VETERINARY MEDICINE. The role of antiseptics in veterinary medicine includes their use in skin cleansers, wound scrubs, and teat dips.

TABLE 39.2—Examples of intrinsic and acquired resistance to certain germicidal agents and suspected mechanisms for each (when known)

Agent	Intrinsic resistance	Mechanism	Acquired resistance	Mechanism
Alcohol	Mycobacteria		*E. coli* K12 mutants	Increase in acidic phopholipids
Phenols			*Staphylococcus aureus*	Lipid enhanced
Quaternary ammonium compounds	Most gram-negative organisms, especially *Pseudomonas aeruginosa;* mycobacteria	Outer membrane	Methycillin-resistant *Staphylococcus aureus*	Plasmid mediated
			Serratia marcescens	Increase in cellular lipid content
Chlorhexidine			*Serratia marcescens*	Alteration of inner cytoplasmic membrane
Hexachlorophane	Gram-negative organisms		*Pseudomonas aeruginosa*	Plasmid conferred

Skin Cleansers. Skin cleansers are important in the presurgical antisepsis of both the surgeon and the patient. The recommendations of the Association of Practitioners of Infection Control for presurgical antisepsis of the surgeon include two alternatives. The first involves an initial water-and-soap cleansing followed by use of an alcohol emollient scrub for at least 5 minutes. The second and more traditional method consists of a 5-minute Chx or iodophor hand scrub. This second method has the advantage that the active agents have residual bactericidal activity under surgical gloves. The presence of organic material and dirt can decrease the effectiveness of most antiseptics; thus removal of gross contamination should precede any antiseptic scrub. Additionally, an important reservoir of dirt and bacteria that needs to be specifically addressed is the subungual space (McHinley et al. 1988).

Preoperative preparation of the veterinary patient varies depending on the surgical environment, yet attempts to achieve the optimal antiseptic cleansing can aid in limiting postsurgical infections. Contrary to human surgery, hair removal from the operative site is almost always a necessity with animal patients. Clipping hair is superior to shaving since it causes less damage and less favorable conditions for bacterial colonization of the surgical skin site (Alexander et al. 1983). Removal of gross contamination and dirt should precede use of antiseptics for previously mentioned reasons. Gentle antiseptic scrubbing should begin at the incision site and move outward over the entire surgical area. Proper antiseptic contact times should be considered. A final antiseptic spray is often applied and left to dry on the surgical site. Despite even the most careful presurgical preparation, up to 20% of skin-resident bacteria may be unaffected by skin antiseptic cleansing (Smeak and Olmstead 1984).

Three antiseptic combinations were evaluated for surgical preparation of canine paws (Swaim et al. 1991): 7.5% PI scrub/10% PI solution, 2% Chx acetate scrub/2% Chx diacetate solution, and tincture of green soap/70% isopropyl alcohol combinations were each shown to effectively reduce bacterial colony counts. The first two combinations were also effective in residual killing for 24 hours when applied under a sterile bandage. However, no significant advantage of applying the antiseptics 24 hours prior to surgery was shown. This is in contrast to results in human patients, where antiseptic cleaning the night prior to surgery has resulted in fewer wound infections (Garibaldi et al. 1988). A similar technique involving prophylactic antiseptic cleansing and wrapping of a limb overnight has been stated to reduce contamination of equine orthopedic surgical sites (Stewart 1984). Antibacterial agents found in shampoos were shown to prevent infections caused by *S. intermedius* in a skin infection model in beagles. Shampoo containing 3% benzoyl peroxide was most effective, followed by shampoos containing 0.5% Chx acetate and iodine (1.0% polyalkyleneglycol-iodine) (Kwochka and Kowalski 1991).

Treatment of Open Wounds. The treatment of open wounds is an important clinical entity in veterinary medicine. The important processes involved in wound healing and proper wound care have been reviewed (Swaim and Wihalf 1985; Berk et al. 1992). Issues involved in the decision of how to properly treat a wound include host age and general health status, and the age, cause, size, and extent of contamination of the wound. Treatment options include surgical closure, bandaging (of different types), and irrigation or application of a varied group of topical agents, including saline, antiseptics, antibiotics, and local anesthetics. It is important to recognize that each wound has different characteristics, and thus treatment must be individualized. For all wounds, however, a basic principle to which all caregivers should adhere is "above all, do no harm"; i.e., any agent chosen should not impede the healing process. When treating a wound topically, a general guideline would be not to apply anything that should not be placed in the patient's conjunctival sac (Peacock 1984).

The literature is divided concerning the utility of antiseptics in routine wound care. Some authors contend that this practice reduces the incidence of infections as a complication (Zukin and Simon 1987), while others believe that any benefit is outweighed by the potential for these agents to cause tissue damage (Oberg and Lindsey 1987). It is our opinion that in the initial care of grossly contaminated wounds, antiseptic application may be beneficial. Once the healing process has begun, however, the use of more-benign agents may be indicated. Saline has been shown to be an effective means of eliminating debris and lowering bacterial counts (Stevenson et al. 1976). Hypertonic saline has also been proposed as a wound dressing (Lowthian and Oke 1993). Archer et al. (1990) report that surface colonization of wounds does not impede healing and thus recommend a move away from potentially damaging antiseptics.

Many reports in the literature discuss potential toxic and harmful effects of antiseptics on fragile healing tissues, making their use controversial. A 5% PI solution inhibited local leukocyte migration, fibroblast activity, and wound cellularity (Viljanto 1980). In vitro, neutrophil migration was inhibited at concentrations greater than 0.05% (Tvedten and Till 1985), whereas 1% PI killed fibroblasts and resulted in weaker wound breaking strength (Lineweaver et al. 1985). Detergent scrubs containing PI and other surfactants were found to damage wound tissue and therefore are not recommended for wound care (Rodheaver et al. 1982). A maximum of 1% PI solution has been recommended as the most effective and least tissue-toxic dilution for wound irrigation (Swaim and Lee 1987). Because antibacterial activity lasts 4–6 hours, repeated treatment is necessary for optimal results.

Chlorhexidine's residual activity (possibly by binding to proteins of the stratum corneum) and its activity against many organisms make it a useful wound treatment. In an experimental wound infection model, wounds irrigated with 0.05–0.1% Chx diacetate solution had fewer infections than those treated with 0.1–0.5% PI. Concentrations of Chx gluconate 0.5% or greater were effective against *S. aureus* in vitro; however, concentrations above 0.05% were lethal to equine fibroblasts (Redding and Booth 1991) and in a wound model in pigs. Unfortunately, it also delayed healing to a greater extent than other solutions tested, including PI (Archer et al. 1990).

Chlorine solution, such as sodium hypochlorite, was used as an effective wound flush in World War I. Full-strength Dakin's solution (0.5% NaOCl) kills bacteria and fibroblasts, as well as retarding epithelialization in vivo in rats (Lineweaver et al. 1985). Other studies have shown low concentrations (0.025–0.0025%) to be toxic to neutrophils, fibroblasts, and endothelial cells, prompting one author to recommend abandoning the use of NaOCl as an irrigant (Kozol et al. 1988). In contrast, a concentration of 0.025% NaOCl was shown to be bactericidal while having no in vitro and in vivo tissue toxicity, suggesting a modified Dakin's solution may be a safe and effective fluid dressing (Heggers et al. 1991). Chloramine-T (Chlorazene) was shown to reduce in vitro *P. aeruginosa* growth and the ability of the bacteria to colonize experimentally created wounds in guinea pigs. Additionally, Chlorazene did not delay the healing of these wounds at a concentration of 0.03% (Henderson et al. 1989). Thus, it was concluded that this preparation should have no effect on healing of wounds when used to sanitize hydrotherapy units.

Teat Antisepsis. Postmilking teat antisepsis is one of the most effective procedures for reducing clinical and subclinical mastitis during lactation (Bramley and Dodd 1984). An ideal teat dip kills bacteria left on the skin after milking, prevents colonization of the teat orifice by pathogens, and cleans teat lesions without irritating the skin (Pankey et al. 1984). Many products exist with proven efficacy against intramammary infections (IMI) caused by *Streptococcus agalactiae* and *S. aureus.* Mastitis caused by environmental pathogens such as coliforms and non–*S. agalactiae Streptococcus* spp. is more difficult to combat. Since the environment is the reservoir for these organisms, residual activity of an antibacterial is necessary for infection control. In a natural-exposure trial (Oliver et al. 1990), a 0.35% Chx/glycerine emollient was shown to lower new infections caused by non–*S. agalactiae Streptococcus* spp. This combination was also effective against coagulase-negative *Staphylococcus* spp. and *Corynebacterium bovis.* No irritation or chapping of the quarters resulted.

The in vitro germicidal activity of nine commercial teat dips was tested (Larocque et al. 1992). All products tested were found to be effective against *E. coli, S. aureus,* and *S. agalactiae.* Chx acetate was found to be only bacteriostatic against *Nocardia* organisms; thus, dips containing this compound should not be used if this organism is present on a farm. The automatic application of an iodine-containing teat dip through the milking machine cluster appeared to be as effective as manual teat dipping in preventing IMI under conditions of artificially high levels of bacterial exposure (Grindal and Priest 1989).

Chlorous acid and chlorine dioxide reduced IMI caused by *Streptococcus uberis* and *S. aureus* significantly better when used for premilk and postmilk dipping than when used as a postmilking teat dip alone. There were no treatment differences against gram-negative bacteria, coagulase-negative *Staphylococcus* spp., and *C. bovis* (Oliver et al. 1993). These authors warn against assuming all teat dips to be safe and effective as premilking dips. Correct use of a premilk dip requires careful drying of the udder since studies have shown that cleaning liquid containing bacteria can drain into the teat cups after milk machine attachment (Galton et al. 1986). These bacteria can both increase milk bacterial counts and cause mastitis. In addition, premilk dip liquid runoff may leave chemical residues in milk. In an attempt to avoid these pitfalls, a 0.5% iodophor-containing gel was developed and compared to routine udder preparation and to premilk dipping with a 0.5% iodophor solution. Gel treatment resulted in low bacterial contamination of milk and teat ends, low somatic cell counts, low milk iodine content, and reduced mastitis. In addition, parlor throughput was higher than with standard predip therapy (Ingawa et al. 1992).

DISINFECTANT USAGE IN VETERINARY MEDICINE. Disinfectants are widely used in veterinary medicine as hospital disinfectants on floors, tables, and walls, on surgical equipment and other instruments before storage, and for disinfection of animal housing facilities. For effective germicidal activity, manufacturer recommendations regarding contact time, dilution, and useful life of a disinfectant solution should be followed. The best disinfectant for a particular situation will depend on the surface's shape, structure, chemical reactivity, and use as well as on the type of contaminating organisms anticipated. It is beyond the scope of this chapter to provide guidelines for disinfectant use in all circumstances; however, a short discussion of their use in production medicine with emphasis on distinguishing features is worthwhile.

A newer disinfectant finding widespread application in over-the-counter human products is triclosan (Irgasan DP300). This compound is incorporated into hand cleansers, dermatologic creams, and even toys. The compound is essentially nontoxic, although data are not available on its relative efficacy compared to the existing compounds described above. It is likely that triclosan will be incorporated into veterinary products.

General Principles. In order to best target disinfection procedures, knowledge of the most likely agent responsible for a clinical outbreak is paramount. Using a compound to which the causative agent is resistant is wasted effort and money. Contamination caused by certain etiologic agents is more easily controlled than contamination by others (e.g., disinfection following *Salmonella* outbreak, a bacteria, compared to Aujeszky's disease, which is caused by a virus). It is also important to understand the mode of transmission of a disease outbreak since this will help identify other measures necessary for control. For example, a disease spread via insect vector would require a different approach than one spread via fomites or direct animal-to-animal contact. Knowledge of the causative agent also allows predictions of its survival in the environment. This would again impact the decision regarding how disinfection should proceed. For instance, survival time of most microorganisms is increased with humidity and in the presence of organic soiling.

For certain diseases (e.g., reportable diseases), a disinfection procedure has been outlined that should be followed to prevent the spread of highly contagious diseases (e.g., foot-and-mouth disease, bluetongue, vesicular stomatitis). This procedure includes the following:

1. Set up to prevent further spread of agent: shut down fans, block water runoff; establish perimeter area for showering in/out.
2. Preliminary disinfection: using low-pressure sprayer, cover all areas to damp down and control infective dust, etc., minimize pooling of disinfectant.
3. Equipment: all portable equipment should be disinfected by soaking; equipment used for decontaminating should be disinfected as well.
4. Removal of gross contamination: manure, soiled bedding, unused feed, insulation, top layer of dirt floors should be scraped and removed.
5. Cleaning: hot water with detergent or disinfectant should be used to remove soiling, starting from the top of the room and working downward; manual scrubbing may be necessary.
6. Water system: if applicable, the water system should be drained and disinfected.
7. Disinfection: following drying, the room should be disinfected again with the appropriate compound at the appropriate dilution.
8. Drying: the room should be allowed to fully dry.
9. Flaming: for some agents (e.g., swine vesicular disease) a flame gun may be necessary on stone or metal surfaces; surfaces should be wetted initially so that areas that have been completed are easily identified.
10. Fumigation: may be necessary for certain persistent agents (foot-and-mouth disease); it should be attempted only if the room can be sealed; formaldehyde is commonly used.

Although considered necessary for control of highly infective, easily spread pathogens, the above listed steps are valuable for the control of other organisms as well.

Special Considerations in Specific Applications

FOOD PRODUCTION AREAS. Two categories of food products exist. Low-risk products are stored at room temperature or need further cooking prior to eating; high-risk products require refrigeration, have short shelf lives, or are eaten without further cooking. Cleaning is necessary to maximize disinfection efficiency. The nature of possible pathogens and the appropriate cleaning agent depend upon the chemical nature of the food being prepared (e.g., sugars are water soluble whereas fats are not). Periodic routine cleaning/disinfecting is recommended to prevent the buildup of soil. Heat is the best disinfectant but impractical in certain situations. Surface-active (attach to surface to prolong contact time) amphoteric and QACs have been suggested as appropriate. See Holah 1995 for further information on disinfection of food production areas.

DAIRY PARLOR. The price of milk is dependent upon bacterial contamination in many countries, which illustrates the importance of hygiene in the dairy industry. Milk is sterile when secreted from the udder. Cleanliness and disinfection of the udder, milking equipment, and environment have been suggested to be more important to limiting contamination of raw milk than refrigeration during storage. The implementation of automated milking and three-times-daily milking have created increased conditions for contamination. The discussion of mastitis is beyond the scope of this chapter; however, it is important to note that the two major classifications of pathogens causing mastitis are those that are contagious and are found principally in the udder and those found in the environment. Control of contagious organisms should be focused on the cow, milking parlor, and barn using pre- and postmilk teat dipping and dry cow treatment. Chlorine, Chx, and iodophors have all been used effectively as teat antiseptics. It should be noted that teat disinfection should not be a substitute for adequate cleaning of the udder. Control of environmental pathogens is accomplished with general cleanliness, effective ventilation, fly control, and adequate sanitation of the milking apparatus (the main source of milk contamination). Procedures for disinfection of equipment vary with the type of equipment but in general will include manual cleaning, descaling, and heat/disinfectant treatment. Disinfectants used for this application, alone or in combination with detergents, include sodium hypochlorite, chlorine-releasing compounds, QACs, and iodophors. See Saran 1995 for further information on disinfection of dairy parlors.

STOCKYARDS. Stockyards, defined as places where groups of animals are brought temporarily before returning to their original housing or moving to new premises, present several unique obstacles to disinfection. Animals being transported to these areas are subject to shipping stresses and therefore decreased immunity. In some circumstances, different species are housed in proximity to one another, allowing the opportunity for organisms to spread to naive hosts. In public situations (e.g., fairs, exhibition centers), large numbers of visitors aid in the spread of infectious organisms. The procedures for disinfection of such areas are not unique, although areas must be vacated to allow successful decontamination. See Fotheringham 1995b for further information on disinfection of stockyards.

LIVESTOCK PRODUCTION AREAS. Livestock areas are where breeding, birth, and feeding of various species of food animals for economic profit occur. Most of the animals housed in such areas (newborns, pregnant and lactating females) have reduced resistance to infection, making proper hygiene of the area critical in preventing disease outbreaks. In addition, current practices have resulted in increased stocking densities in attempts to maximize profits. Procedures to accomplish disinfection will vary with the species and raising practices. For example, in beef and calf units and pig farms, as opposed to sheep facilities, there may be no vacant period during which long-term disinfection can be performed. The farrowing house presents particular problems in that it usually contains complex structures that are difficult to clean/disinfect, such as bars, crates, gates, electrical equipment, etc. (Owen 1995). General principles for effective disease control include routine planned disinfection rather than reacting to disease outbreaks, isolation of replacement animals, rotation of housing units to allow at least 10 days of "downtime," and "all-in/all-out" procedures. Whenever possible, access to outdoors tends to decrease microbial load. As has been stated, the disinfectant compound of choice depends upon the most likely pathogens that will be encountered, which, in turn, depends upon species. See Fotheringham 1995a for further information on disinfection of livestock production areas.

EQUINE FACILITIES. Equine facilities necessitate special considerations regarding disinfection due to the construction materials most commonly used. The porous and irregular surface of raw wood and absorptive nature of dirt or sand floors make complete disinfection extremely difficult. Because most equine pathogens are spread in organic material (e.g., rotavirus and *Salmonella* organisms in feces, influenza virus and *S. equi* in nasal secretions), it is imperative to consider disinfectant activity in the presence of such materials. Rotavirus, one of the pathogens responsible for foal diarrhea, is nonenveloped and therefore quite difficult to inactivate. A disinfectant that is effective against rotavirus will most likely be effective against other equine pathogens. Phenols are considered good disinfectants because they are effective against rotavirus and maintain their activity in the presence of organic matter. Although iodophors have similar characteristics, they are not routinely used to disinfect equine facilities. In contrast, QACs do not kill rotavirus nor are they active in the presence of organic material and therefore they should be avoided.

POULTRY PRODUCTION/HATCHERIES. The vast majority of hatchery sanitation is dependent upon proper design, management, and cleanliness rather than disinfection procedures. The control of dust, insects, and rodents and prevention of reexposure from soiled bedding and carcasses also need to be addressed. A major source of contamination of the hatchery is unsanitary eggs; therefore, eggs should be disinfected as soon as possible after collection to prevent microorganisms from penetrating the shell.

The disinfection program should be effective against *Salmonella* spp, *Pseudomonas* spp., *Proteus* spp., *Staphylococcus* spp., *Streptococcus* spp., and *Aspergillus* spp. (Magwood and Marr 1964). Formaldehyde fumigation is extensively used in the poultry industry to reduce microbiological contamination of eggs, hatchery machinery, and housing. For maximal efficacy special attention should be paid to temperature, humidity, time of use, and concentration. Other compounds that have use in the hatchery are chlorine dioxide foam (barns, eggs, and hatchery equipment), phenols (footbaths and floor disinfectants), QACs (floors, walls, and incubator trays), ozone (eggshells, setters, and hatchers; overexposure results in high embryo mortality), and hydrogen peroxide (eggs).

Poultry production facility management is similar to other food-producing operations, and therefore similar disinfection programs apply. In general, it is best to use the all-in/all-out method to allow for routine and complete cleaning and disinfection before introducing new animals. Disinfection of virtually all spaces and surfaces of the poultry house is performed, including heating system and ductwork, water systems, ceiling, walls, and floors, as well as all machinery and workers' clothes. It is fairly common to allow 2 weeks before new animals are brought in. Again, formaldehyde (4% formalin) disinfection is common; however, chlorine- and iodine-based disinfectants can be used. See Samberg and Meroz 1995 for further information on disinfection of poultry production facilities.

AQUACULTURE. Disinfection in aquaculture poses several challenges not found in other veterinary industries. The pathogenic organisms are quite different, and often less is known about them with regard to susceptibility to commonly used chemicals. In addition, the housing infrastructure, including ponds, tanks, and floating installations, as well as the use of boats and tanks for transportation, requires special considerations when cleaning and disinfection procedures are devised. In situ treatment is difficult due to dilution of added chemicals, low temperatures of use, and sensitivity of the fish to certain compounds. See Torgersen and Hastein 1995 for further information on disinfection in aquaculture.

ZOOS. Because of their diverse population, the principles utilized for disinfection of zoos will be a conglomeration of the above-described situations. Virtually all methods and compounds have utility for certain species and housing practices. Additionally, most modern zoos have onsite veterinary hospitals with surgical capabilities, which are reliant upon good hygiene and disinfection procedures.

REFERENCES

Alexander, J. W., Fisher, J., Boyajiani, M., Palmquist, J., and Morris, M. J. 1983. The influence of hair removal methods on wound infections. Arch Surg 118:347–349.

Altemeier, W. A. (ed.). 1976. Manual on Control of Infection in Surgical Patients, p. 212. Philadelphia: J. P. Lippincott.

Amber, E. I., Henderson, R. A., Swaim, S. F., and Gray B. W. 1983. A comparison of antimicrobial efficacy and tissue reaction of four antiseptics on canine wounds. Vet Surg 12:63–68.

Archer, H. G., Barrett, S., Irving, S., Middleton, K. R., and Seal, D. V. 1990. A controlled model of moist wound healing: comparison between semipermeable film, antiseptics and sugar paste. J Exp Path 71:155–170.

Ayliffe, G. A. J., Babb, J. R., and Bradley, C. R. 1986. Disinfection of endoscopes. J Hosp Infect 7:296–299.

Baldry, M. G. C. 1983. The bactericidal, fungicidal, and sporicidal properties of hydrogen peroxide and peracetic acid. J Appl Bacteriol 54:417–423.

Berk, W. A., Welch, R. D., Brooks, B. F. 1992. Controversial issues in clinical management of the simple wound. Annal Emerg Med 21:72–80.

Bilbrey, S. A, Dulisch, J. L, and Stallings, B. 1989. Chemical burns caused by benzalkonium chloride in eight surgical cases. J Am Anim Hosp Assoc 25:31–34.

Bloomfield, S. F., and Miller, E. A. 1989. A comparison of hypochlorite and phenolic disinfectants for disinfection of clean and soiled surfaces and blood spillages. J Hosp Infect 13:231–239.

Bramley, A. J., and Dodd, F. H. 1984. Reviews of the progress of dairy science: mastitis control— progress and prospects. J Dairy Res 51:481–512.

Centers for Disease Control (CDC). 1987. Symptoms of irritation associated with exposure to glutaraldehyde. Colorado MMWR 36:190–191.

Dychdala, G. R. 1983. Chlorine and chlorine compounds. In S. S. Block, ed., Disinfection, Sterilization, and Preservation, 3rd ed., pp. 157–182. Philadelphia: Lea & Febiger.

Favero, M. S. 1983. Chemical disinfection of medical and surgical materials. In S. S. Block, ed., Disinfection, Sterilization, and Preservation, 3rd ed., pp. 469–492. Philadelphia: Lea & Febiger.

Fotheringham, V. J. C. 1995a. Disinfection of livestock production premises. Rev Sci Tech Off Int Epiz 14(1):191–205.

———. 1995b. Disinfection of stockyards. Rev Sci Tech Off Int Epiz 14(2):293–307.

Galton, D. M., Petersson, L. G., and Merril, W. G. 1986. Effects of premilking udder preparation practices on bacterial counts in milk and on teats. J Dairy Sci 69:260–266.

Garibaldi, R. A., Skolnick, D., and Lerer, T. 1988. The impact of preoperative skin disinfection on preventing intraoperative wound contamination. Infect Control Hosp Epidemiol 9:109–113.

Gayle, E. F., Cundliffe, E., Reynolds, P. E., Richmond, M. H., and Waring, M. J. 1981. Molecular Basis of Antibiotic Action. London: John Wiley & Sons.

Grindal, R. J., and Priest, D. J. 1989. Automatic application of teat disinfectant through the milking machine cluster. J Dairy Res 56:579–585.

Heggers, J. P., Sazy, J. A., Stenberg, B. D., Strock, L. L., McCauley, R. L., Herndon, D. N., and Robson, M. C. 1991. Bactericidal and wound healing properties of sodium hypochlorite solutions: the 1991 Lindberg Award. J Burn Care Rehabil 12:420–424.

Henderson, J. D., Leming, J. T., and Melon-Niksa, D. B. 1989. Chloramine-T solutions: effect on wound healing in guinea pigs. Arch Phys Med Rehabil 70:628–631.

Holah, J. T. 1995. Disinfection of food production area. Rev Sci Tech Off Int Epiz 14(2):343–363.

Huber, W. G. 1988. Antiseptics and disinfectants. In N. H. Booth and L. E. McDonald, eds., Veterinary Pharmacology and Therapeutics, 6th ed., pp. 765–784. Ames: Iowa State Univ Press.

Ingawa, K. H., Adkinson, R. W., and Hough, R. H. 1992. Evaluation of a gel teat cleaning and sanitizing compound for premilking hygiene. J Dairy Sci 75:1224–1232.

Kozol, R. A., Gillies, C., and Elgebaly, S. A. 1988. Effects of sodium hypochlorite (Dakin's solution) on cells of the wound module. Arch Surg 123:420–423.

Kwochka, K. W., and Kowalski, J. J. 1991. Prophylactic efficacy of four antibacterial shampoos against *Staphylococcus intermedius* in dogs. Am J Vet Res 52(1):115–118.

Larocque, L., Malik, S. S., Landry, D. A., Presseault, S., Sved, S., and Matula, T. 1992. In vitro germicidal activity of teat dips against *Nocardia asteroides* and other udder pathogens. J Dairy Sci 75:1233–1240.

Larson, E. 1987. Draft guidelines for the use of topical antimicrobial agents. (Abstr.) Am J Infec Control 15:25–30.

Larson, E. L., Eke, P. I., and Laughon, B. E. 1986. Efficacy of alcohol based hand rinses under frequent use conditions. Antimicrob Agents Chemother 30:542–544.

Lavelle, K. J., Doedus, D. J., Kleit, S. A., and Forney, R. B. 1975. Iodine absorption in burn patients treated topically with povidone iodine. Clin Pharmacol Ther 17:355–356.

Lineweaver, W., Howard, R., Soucy, D., McMorris, S., Freeman, J., Crain, C., Robertson, J., and Rumley, T. 1985. Topical antimicrobial toxicity. Arch Surg 120:267–270.

Lineweaver, W., McMorris, S., and Howard, R. 1982. Effects of topical disinfectants and antibiotics on human fibroblasts. Surg Forum 33:37–39.

Lowbury, E. J. L., Lilly, H. A., and Ayliffe, G. A. J. 1974. Preoperative disinfection of surgeon's hands: use of alcoholic solutions and effects of gloves on skin flora. Br Med J 4:369–372.

Lowthian, P., and Oke, S. 1993. Hypertonic saline solution as a disinfectant. Lancet 341:182.

Magwood, S. E., and Marr H. 1964. Studies in hatchery sanitation 2. A simplified method for assessing bacterial populations on surfaces within hatcheries. Poult Sci 43:1558–1566.

McHinley, K. J., Larson, E. L., and Leyden, J. J. 1988. Composition and density of microflora in the subungual space of the hand. J Clin Microbiol 26:950–953.

Mentel, R., and Schmidt, J. 1973. Investigations on rhinovirus inactivation by hydrogen peroxide. Acta Virol 17:351–354.

Molinari, J. A., Campbell, M. D., and York, J. J. 1982. Minimizing potential infections in dental practice. Michigan Dental Assoc 64:411–416.

Molinari, J. A., and Runnel, R. R. 1991. Role of disinfectants in infection control. Dental Clin North Am 35(2):323–337.

Murray, S. M., Freiman, J. S., Vickery, K., Lim, D., Cossart, T. E., and Whiteley, R. K. 1991. Duck hepatitis B virus: a model to assess efficacy of disinfectants against hepadnavirus infectivity. Epidemiol Infect 106:434–443.

Nye, R. N., and Mallory, T. B. 1923. A note on the fallacy of using alcohol for the sterilization of surgical instruments. Boston Med Surg J 189:561–563.

Oberg, M. S., and Lindsey, D. 1987. Do not put hydrogen peroxide or povidone-iodine into wounds. Am J Dis Child 141:27–28.

Oliver, S. P., King, S. H., Lewis, M. J., Torre, P. M., Matthews, K. R., and Dowlen, H. H. 1990. Efficacy of chlorhexidine as a postmilking teat disinfectant for the prevention of bovine mastitis during lactation. J Dairy Sci 73:2230–2235.

Oliver, S. P., Lewis, M. J., Ingle, T. L., Gillespie, B. E., and Matthews, K. R. 1993. Prevention of bovine mastitis by a premilking teat disinfectant containing chlorous acid and chlorine dioxide. J Dairy Sci 76:287–292.

O'Neill, J., Hosmer, M., Challup, R. M., Driscoll, J., Speck, W., and Sprunt, K. 1982. Percutaneous absorption potential of chlorhexidine in neonates. Curr Ther Res 31:485–487.

Owen, J. M. 1995. Disinfection of farrowing pens. Rev Sci Tech Off Int Epiz 14:381–391.

Pankey, J. W., Eberhart, R. J., Cuming, A. L., Dagget, R. D., Farnsworth, R. J., and McDuff, C. K. 1984. Update on postmilking antisepsis. J Dairy Sci 67:1336–1353.

Peacock, E. E., Jr. 1984. Wound Repair, 3rd ed., pp. 141–186. Philadelphia: W. B. Saunders.

Pepper, R. E. 1980. Comparison of the activities and stabilities of alkaline glutaraldehyde sterilizing solutions. Infect Control 1:90–92.

Pretsch, J., and Meakins, J. L. 1976. Complications of povidone-iodine absorption in topically treated burn patients. Lancet 1:280–282.

Redding, W. R., and Booth, L. C. 1991. Effects of chlorhexidine gluconate and chlorous acid–chlorine dioxide on equine fibroblasts and *Staphylococcus aureus*. Vet Surg 20(5):306–310.

Reybrouk, G. 1985. The bactericidal activity of aqueous disinfectants applied on living tissues. Pharm Weekbl (Sci) 7:100–103.

Rodheaver, G, Bellamy, W, Kody, M, Spatafora, G, Fitton, L, Leyden, K, and Edlich, R. 1982. Bacterial activity and toxicity of iodine-containing solutions in wounds. Arch Surg 117:181–186.

Russel, A. D. 1986. Chlorhexidine: antibacterial action and bacterial resistance. Infection 14:212–215.

Rutala, W. A. 1990. APIC guideline for selection and use of disinfectants. Am J Inf Control 18(2):99–117.

Rycroft, A. N., and McLay, C. 1991. Disinfectants in the control of small animal ringworm due to *Microsporum canis*. Vet Rec 129:239–241.

Samberg, Y., and Meroz, M. 1995. Application of disinfectants in poultry hatcheries. Rev Sci Tech Off Int Epiz 14(2):365–380.

Saran, A. 1995. Disinfecton in the dairy parlour. Rev Sci Tech Off Int Epiz 14(1):207–224.

Schaeffer, A. J., Jones, J. M., and Amundsen, S. K. 1980. Bactericidal effect of hydrogen peroxide on urinary tract pathogens. Appl Environ Microbiol 40:337–340.

Scheider, W., Ahuja, S., and Klebe, I. 1976. Clinical and bacteriological studies of the polyvinylpyrrolidone-iodine complex. In World Congress on Antisepsis, pp. 79–81. New York: PH Publishing.

Scott, E. M., and Gorman, S. P. 1983. Sterilization with glutaraldehyde. In S. S. Block, ed., Disinfection, Sterilization, and Preservation, 3rd ed., pp. 65–68. Philadelphia: Lea & Febiger.

Smeak, D. O., and Olmstead, M. L. 1984. Infections in clean wounds: the roles of the surgeon, environment, and the host. Comp Contin Educ Pract Vet 6:629–634.

Smith, M. S., Williams, D. E., and Worley, S. D. 1990. Potential uses of combined halogen disinfectants in poultry processing. Poultry Sci 69:1590–1594.

Spaulding, E. H. 1968. Chemical disinfection of medical and surgical materials. In C. A. Lawrence and S. S. Block, eds., Disinfection, Sterilization, and Preservation, pp. 517–531. Philadelphia: Lea & Febiger.

Stevenson, T. R., Thacker, J. G., and Rodheaver, G. T. 1976. Cleansing the traumatic wound by high pressure irrigation. J Am Col Emer Phys 141:357–362.

Stewart, K. 1984. Equine intensive care: preoperative, intraoperative, and postoperative procedures. Vet Tech 5:177–180.

Stonehill, A. A., Krop, S., and Borick, P. M. 1963. Buffered glutaraldehyde: a new chemical sterilizing solution. Am J Hosp Pharm 20:458–465.

Swaim, S. F., and Lee, A. H. 1987. Topical wound medications: a review. JAVMA 190(12):1588–1592.

Swaim, S. F., Riddell, K. P., Geiger, M. S., Hathcock, T. L., and McHuire, J. A. 1991. Evaluation of surgical scrub and antiseptic solutions for surgical preparation of canine paws. JAVMA 198(11):1941–1945.

Swaim, S. F., and Wihalf, D. 1985. The physics, physiology, and chemistry of bandaging open wounds. Comp Cont Educ Pract Vet 7(2):146–156.

Torgersen, T., and Hastein, T. 1995. Disinfection in aquaculture. Rev Sci Tech Off Int Epiz 14(2):419–434.

Turner, F. J. 1983. Hydrogen peroxide and other oxidant disinfectants. In S. S. Block, ed., Disinfection, Sterilization, and Preservation, 3rd ed., pp. 240–250. Philadelphia: Lea & Febiger.

Tvedten, H. W., and Till, G. O. 1985. Effect of povidon, povidone-iodine and iodide on locomotion (in vitro) of neutrophils from people, rats, dogs and rabbits. Am J Vet Res 46:1797–1800.

Viljanto, J. 1980. Disinfection of surgical wounds without inhibition of normal healing. Arch Surg 115:253–256.

Weber, G. R. 1950. Effect of concentration and reaction (pH) on germicidal activity of chloramine T. Public Health Rep 65:503–512.

Zukin, D. D., and Simon, R. R. 1987. Emergency Wound Care: Principles and Practice, pp. 30–31. Rockville, MD: Aspen Publishers.

40 SULFONAMIDES

JERRY W. SPOO AND JIM E. RIVIERE

Pharmacology of Sulfonamides
General
Mechanism of Action
Clinical Uses and Microbial Susceptibility
Pharmacokinetics of Sulfonamides
Absorption
Distribution
Metabolism
Excretion
Toxicity
Resistance
Commonly Used Sulfonamides
Sulfadimethoxine
Sulfamethazine (Sulfadimidine)
Sulfaquinoxaline
Sulfamerazine
Sulfathiazole
Sulfasalazine (Salicylazosulfapyridine)
Sulfadiazine
Sulfabromomethazine
Sulfaethoxypyridazine
Sulfisoxazole
Sulfachlorpyridazine
Other Sulfonamides
Potentiated Sulfonamides
Mechanism of Action
Absorption, Distribution, Metabolism, Excretion
Clinical Uses and Pharmacokinetics
Residues in Food Animals

The sulfonamides are one of the oldest groups of antimicrobial compounds still in use today. Sulfanilamide, an amide of sulfanilic acid, was the first sulfonamide used clinically. It was derived from the azo dye Prontosil, and all other sulfonamides produced since have structurally resembled it. Sulfonamides have been in clinical use for 50 years, and widespread resistance has developed against some of them. Sulfonamide-diaminopyrimidine combinations have been used to reduce the incidence of sulfonamide resistance, and this combination has all but replaced single or combination sulfonamide treatment regimens. In addition to microbial resistance, recent concern has focused on the possible carcinogenicity of some sulfonamides in laboratory animals, which may eventually preclude their widespread use in food-producing animals. Previous editions of this text should be consulted for a review of this extensive historical database.

PHARMACOLOGY OF SULFONAMIDES

General. All sulfonamides are derivatives of sulfanilamide (structurally similar to para-aminobenzoic acid), which was, in the 1940s, the first sulfonamide discovered to have antimicrobial activity (see Fig. 40.1). Since then, many structural derivatives of sulfanilamide with differing pharmacokinetic and antimicrobial spectrums have been used in veterinary medicine to treat microbial infections of the respiratory, urinary, gastrointestinal, and central nervous systems. Susceptible organisms include many bacteria, coccidia, chlamydia, and protozoal organisms, including *Toxoplasma* spp.

Sulfonamides are white crystalline powders that are weak organic acids, are relatively insoluble in water, and have a wide range of pK_a values, as shown in Table 40.1. They also show great variability in the extent to which they bind to plasma proteins (15–90%) with respect to individual drugs and species. Sulfonamides are more soluble in alkaline than in neutral or acidic pHs; solubility is enhanced when the sulfonamides are formulated as sodium salts or when in solution in more alkaline environments. Some sulfonamide solutions have pHs between 9 and 10, prohibiting extravascular use. Sulfonamides in general are relatively insoluble in water and tend to undergo crystallization in the urine (acid pH) in vivo, especially in animals that are overdosed, dehydrated, acidotic from disease, or given large doses of a sulfonamide by bolus injection. To minimize crystalluria and obtain high blood or urine levels of the sulfonamides, they are often given in combination with each other. Each sulfonamide in a mixture of sulfonamides exhibits its own solubility in solution (law of independent solubility); i.e., sulfonamides do not significantly affect the solubility of each other, which has important clinical considerations in the excretion of parent compound and any metabolites. However, the antimicrobial effect is additive; thus the use of "triple-sulfas" (three sulfonamides formulated in solution together) allows increased efficacy without a significant increased risk of adverse effects (Prescott and Baggot 1993; Bevill 1988).

$H_2N-C_6H_4-SO_2NH_2$

FIG. 40.1—Sulfanilamide

TABLE 40.1—pK$_a$ values for some sulfonamides

Compound	pK$_a$
Sulfanilamide	10.4
Sulfamethazine	7.4
Sulfadiazine	6.4
Sulfadoxine	6.1
Sulfamethoxazole	6.0
Sulfadimethoxine	6.0
Sulfachlorpyridazine	NA
Sulfaquinoxaline	5.5
Sulfamethazine (sulfadimidine)	2.65, 7.4
Sulfabromomethazine	NA
Sulfaethoxypyridazine	NA
Sulfamerazine	NA
Sulfamethazole	5.45
Sulfathiazole	7.1
Sulfisoxazole	4.7
Phthalylsulfathiazole	NA

Sources: Data from Prescott and Baggot 1993 and Riviere et al. 1986.
Note: NA = data not available.

Mechanism of Action. For sulfonamides to be therapeutically effective, organisms must intracellularly synthesize their own folic acid. Sulfonamides are antimetabolites, interfering with the normal production of RNA, protein synthesis, and microbial replication mechanisms. Sulfonamides inhibit intermediary metabolism by interfering with the production of folic acid, while the diaminopyrimidines (discussed later in this chapter) interfere in later steps of this metabolic cascade by arresting the production of tetrahydrofolic acid (THFA). Sulfonamides used in the absence of diaminopyrimidines are bacteriostatic. The existing folic acid supply within the susceptible organisms must be consumed before any metabolic effects can begin, which usually occurs within 4–6 hours after administration.

A simplified version of folic acid metabolism is presented in Fig. 40.2.

Para-aminobenzoic acid (PABA), pteridines, glutamic acid, and the enzyme dihydropterate synthase interact to form dihydropteroic acid, the immediate precursor to dihydrofolic acid. Dihydropteroic acid is enzymatically converted to dihydrofolic acid by dihydrofolate synthase, followed by another enzymatic conversion of dihydrofolic acid to THFA via dihydrofolate reductase (DHFR). THFA continues on in this pathway to permit RNA production and bacterial reproduction. PABA and sulfanilamide bear a strong enough structural resemblance for one to be chemically mistaken for the other in the folic acid production pathway. Sulfanilamide, and all sulfonamides, inhibit the biosynthesis of folic acid by being mistakenly substituted for

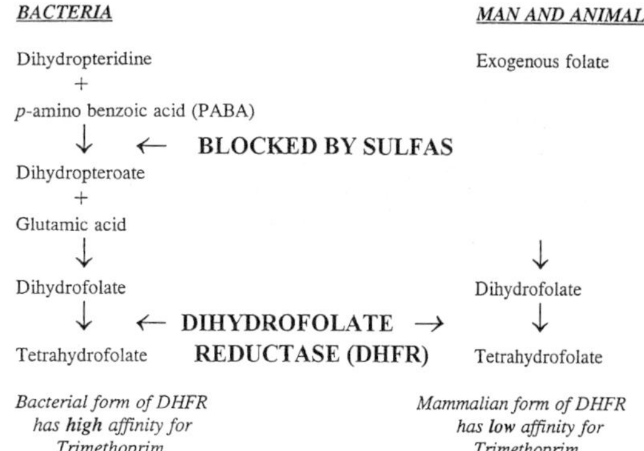

FIG. 40.2—Schematic representation of the mechanism of action of the sulfonamides and trimethoprim. (Adapted from Davis and Jackson 1973.)

PABA. However, there are sufficient structural differences between the sulfonamides and PABA to not allow the conversion to dihydropteroic acid, hence inhibiting bacterial protein synthesis. Folic acid synthesis can be restored by flooding the system with excess PABA. Mammalian cell metabolic pathways are not inhibited, because mammalian cells utilize preformed folic acid obtained from the diet. Sulfonamides have little effect on those microbial organisms that, like mammalian cells, can utilize preformed folic acid (Prescott and Baggot 1993; Bevill 1988).

Clinical Uses and Microbial Susceptibility. The spectrum of activity for the sulfonamides is broad, affecting gram-positive, gram-negative, and many protozoal organisms, and is bacteriostatic rather than bactericidal. As stated earlier, sulfonamides have been used clinically for approximately 50 years, with many organisms once quite susceptible to the sulfonamides now being resistant. Combining sulfonamides with diaminopyrimidines has markedly increased the spectrum of activity and is the most common sulfonamide preparation used in veterinary antimicrobial therapy today. Single or combination sulfonamide therapy is common in food-animal medicine, with sulfonamide-diaminopyrimidine combinations being used more frequently in large animals. Specific microbial susceptibility patterns for each sulfonamide will be discussed in more detail later in this chapter; however, Table 40.2 illustrates the general susceptibility/resistance patterns of most sulfonamides, trimethoprim, and trimethoprim-sulfamethoxazole combinations against the most commonly encountered veterinary pathogens. In vitro susceptibility patterns of many pathogens (Van Duijkeren et al. 1994b) and more specifically *Salmonella* spp. (Van Duijkeren et al. 1994a) that affect the horse have been recently reported.

Sulfonamides are used to treat infections of the CNS, respiratory tract, gastrointestinal tract (among a variety

TABLE 40.2—Comparative activity of sulfonamides, trimethoprim, and trimethoprim-sulfamethoxazole against selected microorganisms

Organism	Sulfonamide[a]	Trimethoprim	Trimethoprim-sulfamethoxazole[b]
A. pyogenes	30	10	0.15
C. pseudotuberculosis	NA	NA	≤0.5
C. renale	>50	NA	NA
E. rhusiopathiae	10	0.15	0.05
L. monocytogenes	10	0.06	0.01
N. asteroides	128	128	8/160
R. equi	>100	50	32/608
S. aureus	30	1.5	0.2
S. agalactia	30	0.5	0.05
S. dysgalactia	>250	3.1	0.05
S. uberis	>100	3	0.5
β-hemolytic streptococci	>100	10	1.5
C. perfringens	16	50	
Actinobacillus spp.	64	NA	≤0.05
A. pleuropneumonia	≥100	2	8
B. bronchiseptica	400	NA	≤0.05
B. abortus	15	3	0.05
B. canis	1.6	NA	NA
C. jejuni	≥256	≥512	≥512
E. coli	≥128	1	≤0.5
H. somnus	≥100	NA	NA
K. pneumoniae	>100	3.1	≤0.5
M. bovis	>60	>75	<0.15
P. multocida	>128	3.1	NA
Proteus spp.	>1000	6.3	≤0.5
P. aeruginosa	>1000	1000	100
Salmonella spp.	128	1000	100
T. equigenitalis	>100	3	0.5
Y. enterocolitica	>128	1	8

Source: Adapted from Prescott and Baggot 1993.
[a]The sulfonamide in most instances was sulfadimethoxine.
[b]Single values refer to trimethoprim concentration; second figure refers to sulfamethoxazole. Trimethoprim:sulfamethoxazole ratio is usually 1:20.
Note: Concentrations are MIC_{90}'s in µg/mL. MIC_{90} = the minimum inhibitory concentration that inhibits 90% of the microbes.

of other soft tissues), and, in particular, the urinary tract. Prescott and Baggot (1993) have grouped veterinary urinary pathogens into three categories according to their susceptibility to sulfonamides:

Good susceptibility: Actinomyces spp., *Bacillus* spp., *Brucella* spp., *E. rhusiopathiae, L. monocytogenes, Streptococcus* spp., *Chlamydia* spp., many coccidia, *Pneumocystis carinii, Cryptosporidium* spp.

Moderate susceptibility: Gram-positive aerobes, such as staphylococci and enterococci, and gram-negative aerobes, such as *Enterobacter* spp., *E. coli, Klebsiella* spp., *Proteus* spp., *Actinobacillus* spp., *Hemophilus* spp., *Pasteurella* spp., *Pseudomonas* spp. Also included in this category are *Actinomyces* spp., *Bacteroides* spp., *Fusobacterium* spp., and perhaps some *Clostridium* spp.

Resistant: Includes *Mycobacterium* spp., *Mycoplasma* spp., *Rickettsia* spp., *P. aeruginosa,* and spirochetes.

These groupings are only correct for sulfonamides used against microbial urinary tract infections, since concentrations obtained in the urine can exceed by several times the MIC_{90} values reported in Table 40.2.

PHARMACOKINETICS OF SULFONAMIDES

Absorption. Sulfonamides in general are rapidly absorbed from the gastrointestinal tract when administered orally. A few exceptions do exist, such as phthalylsulfathiazole, which has poor water solubility and is slowly absorbed from the gastrointestinal tract. Sulfasalazine is not absorbed as a whole molecule to any extent but rather is cleaved into two more-active compounds by native resident colonic bacteria. Phthalylsulfathiazole and other related sulfonamides are of little use for susceptible systemic infections but have found clinical use in treating susceptible microbial infections that are limited to the gastrointestinal tract. Animals given sulfonamides either intramuscularly or subcutaneously require that the solution be buffered prior to administration to prevent perivascular reactions due to the inherent alkalinity of most sulfonamides. Sulfonamides are well absorbed when administered intraperitoneally. Topical administration to the skin and mucous membranes is not recommended, because they cause delayed wound healing, sensitivity reactions, and competition from PABA in some wound exudates. How-

TABLE 40.3—Classification of sulfonamides based on plasma concentration versus time profiles

Short-acting sulfonamides	Intermediate-acting sulfonamides	Long-acting sulfonamides	Enteric sulfonamides
Sulfacetamide	Sulfadimethoxine	Sulfamethylphenazole	Succinylsulfathiazole
Sulfamethazole	Sulfisoxazole	Sulfabromomethazine	Sulfaguanidine
Trisulfapyrimidine (triple sulfas)	Sulfamethoxazole	Sulfabromethazine	Sulfaquinoxaline
	Sulfapyridine	Sulfadimethoxine	Phthalylsulfathiazole (sulfathalidine)
Sulfathiazole	Sulfachlorpyridazine	Sulfamethazine	
	Sulfamethazine	Sulfaethoxypyridazine	Sulfasalazine
Sulfisoxazole	Sulfadiazine		

ever, diaminopyrimidine-sulfonamide combinations have been successful when administered orally or parenterally to treat susceptible microbial skin infections. Silver sulfadiazine and mafenide are the only two sulfonamides that may be used topically. Only sulfonamides with neutral or near-neutral pHs (e.g., sulfacetamide) can be used in ophthalmic preparations.

Sulfonamides are also classified as short-, intermediate-, and long-acting according to plasma concentration-time profile. Sulfonamides are considered short-acting if after one therapeutic dose, blood concentrations remain above 50 μg/mL for less than 12 hours after dosing, intermediate if these plasma levels are obtained between 12 and 24 hours, and long-acting if obtained 24 hours after dosing. A fourth class, the enteric sulfonamides, are not absorbed (or minimally absorbed) from the gastrointestinal tract after oral administration but act locally within the lumen of the gastrointestinal tract. Sulfonamides that are used in veterinary medicine are classified using this method in Table 40.3.

Distribution. Sulfonamides are widely distributed throughout the body and into many soft tissues, including the CNS (cerebrospinal fluid) and joints (synovial fluid), making these compounds one of the few antimicrobials that can obtain therapeutic concentrations of drug in these environments. Binding to plasma proteins, usually to albumin, varies from sulfonamide to sulfonamide and from species to species and ranges from 15 to 90% (USPDI 1998). High protein binding markedly increases the half-life of sulfonamides; however, only the un-ionized and non-protein-bound sulfonamide is pharmacologically active. Since the sulfonamides are weak acids, their pHs generally do not support significant partitioning into milk; however, passive diffusion does occur to some extent. Concentrations are generally low, making them of limited use for the treatment of mastitis in most mammals.

Metabolism. Acetylation (mainly occurring in the liver and lung) is the major pathway by which sulfonamides are metabolized in most species. Ruminants metabolize sulfonamides by acetylation pathways, and apparently acetylated metabolites are the major urinary metabolites in cattle, sheep, and swine. The canine lacks the ability to acetylate aromatic amines, relying on alternative metabolic pathways to convert sulfonamides to less active forms. Acetylated metabolites are less soluble than the parent compounds and increase the risks of renal tubular damage due to precipitation and crystal formation. Glucuronide conjugation and aromatic hydroxylation are two additional metabolic pathways by which sulfonamides are metabolized in animals. Glucuronide metabolites are highly water soluble and are generally excreted quickly without the possibility of precipitation in the urine. Deacetylation, oxidation, deamination, conjugation with sulfate, and cleavage of heterocyclic rings of sulfonamide molecules have also been reported (Bevill 1988). Regardless of the metabolic pathway taken, all metabolites either display reduced therapeutic activity (hydroxy metabolite) or are therapeutically inactive (N_4-acetyl metabolite).

Excretion. Sulfonamides that are capable of obtaining therapeutic blood concentrations (i.e., all sulfonamides except the enteric, or "gut-active," compounds) are excreted by the kidneys, either as the parent compound or as metabolites by way of glomerular filtration (unbound to plasma proteins), active carrier-mediated proximal tubular excretion, or passive absorption of the nonionized drug from the distal tubular fluid. Sulfonamides are also excreted in the tears, feces, bile, milk, and sweat. Low urine pHs favor tubular reabsorption and hence longer half-lives of the sulfonamides, whereas alkalinization of the urine increases urinary excretion by slowing this pH-dependent passive reabsorption in the tubules. Many of the long-acting sulfonamides, with extended half-lives in the body, undergo extensive tubular reabsorption in addition to some enterohepatic recycling. Enteric sulfonamides are primarily eliminated via the feces, with little of the active or metabolized drug being absorbed systemically to be excreted by these renal mechanisms.

Toxicity. Sulfonamide-induced toxicoses may be classified as nonimmunologic or immunologic in etiology. A retrospective evaluation of dermal adverse reactions due to trimethoprim-sulfonamide combinations used in male dogs and cats has been presented by Noli et al. (1995). Of the immunologic sulfonamide-induced toxicoses, most have been documented in the canine. Brief descriptions of possible sulfonamide toxicoses are given below.

CRYSTALLURIA. Crystalluria, hematuria, and renal tubule blockage can occur due to precipitation of the sulfonamide in the glomerular filtrate of the kidney. Crystalluria occurs when the animal becomes dehydrated and the sulfonamide concentration increases beyond its solubility point in water, resulting in high rates of crystal formation. A similar reaction may occur if the more water-insoluble sulfonamides are used therapeutically. Aciduria can also alter the ionization state of sulfonamides and decrease drug solubility, resulting in crystal formation. Crystalluria can be minimized or prevented by keeping the patient well hydrated during therapy, by using the more water-soluble sulfonamides, and by keeping the urine alkalinized using Na_2CO_3 therapy when necessary.

KERATOCONJUNCTIVITIS SICCA (KCS). Several cases of sulfonamide-induced KCS have been reported in dogs treated with sulfasalazine, sulfadiazine, and sulfamethoxazole (Morgan and Bachrach 1982; Slatter and Blogg 1978; Collins et al. 1986). Sulfonamide-induced KCS does not seem to affect any particular breed of dog, and the precise mechanism behind the induction of KCS is not known; however, it is believed to be the result of a hypersensitivity reaction due to a direct lacrimotoxic effect of the nitrogen-containing pyridine ring on the lacrimal acinar cells (Collins et al. 1986; Slatter and Blogg 1978). Berger et al. (1995) observed 33 dogs of various breeds for the occurrence of KCS after trimethoprim-sulfadiazine treatment, as characterized by changes in the Schirmer tear test (STT) values. The average age of the dogs was 5 years (range = 6 months to 13 years); the group included both sexes (20 females, 13 males), ranged in weight from 2 kg to 56 kg, and received 8.6 mg/kg to 104 mg/kg of the trimethoprim-sulfadiazine combinations. It was found that 15.2% of the dogs developed KCS and that the incidence of the disease was closely correlated with the weight of the dog. Dogs weighing less than 12 kg were apparently at greater risk for developing KCS than those weighing more than 12 kg. Of note is the fact that 63.6% of the dogs receiving the trimethoprim-sulfadiazine had decreased STT values compared to pretreatment values but were still within the normal range. The data from this study suggest that dogs being treated with trimethoprim-sulfadiazine who weigh less than 12 kg are at the greatest risk for developing KCS during treatment. For every 10 kg decrease in dog weight, there is a 2.5 times greater risk for developing KCS during trimethoprim-sulfadiazine therapy.

Once sulfonamide-induced KCS is recognized, the prognosis for returning the tear production to normal is dependent on the age of the dog and the duration of therapy, with a better prognosis for young dogs having undergone short durations of sulfonamide drug therapy. Reversal of KCS may or may not occur once sulfonamide therapy has been discontinued.

HEPATIC NECROSIS. Trimethoprim-sulfadiazine and trimethoprim-sulfamethoxazole combination therapy in dogs has resulted in hepatic necrosis (Twedt et al. 1997; Dodds 1997). Hepatic necrosis and reversible cholestatic hepatitis have been reported in humans. The exact mechanism responsible for this pathology is not known but may result from damage directed specifically at the liver or via a hypersensitivity reaction. Hepatotoxicity may be a result of an abnormal metabolic pathway which allows the production or accumulation of hepatotoxic metabolites. Sulfonamides are metabolized in many ways, including acetylation. Slow acetylation can lead to increased sulfonamide dehydroxylamine metabolites, which may result in hepatic injury. Although dogs are known to be slow acetylators, there is no conclusive proof that this is the mechanism by which dogs may succumb to hepatic injury.

HYPOPROTHROMBINEMIA. Hypoprothrombinemia has been reported in dogs (Neer and Savant 1992; Patterson and Grenn 1975), in coyote pups (Brown et al. 1982), and in Leghorn chickens (Daft et al. 1989) given sulfaquinoxaline. Sulfaquinoxaline is unique among the sulfonamides in that it can induce hypoprothrombinemia in animals within 24 hours after dosing by lengthening prothrombin times. It is thought that this adverse effect is unrelated to the individual sulfonamide or to the quinoxaline portion of the sulfaquinoxaline molecule but occurs when the two entities are combined into a single molecule. Sulfaquinoxaline is not an anticoagulant in vitro, nor does it destroy or otherwise inactivate prothrombin. Nevertheless, recent studies have reported that sulfaquinoxaline is a potent inhibitor of vitamin K epoxide reductase, and this inhibition is the most likely reason for the hypothrombinemic reaction seen in the reported cases of sulfaquinoxaline toxicosis. Treatment is by vitamin K_1 administration for 4–7 days, and recovery is usually uneventful.

APLASTIC ANEMIA AND THROMBOCYTOPENIA. Aplastic anemia presumably induced by drug therapy with trimethoprim-sulfadiazine has been reported (Weiss and Adams 1987; Weiss and Klausner 1990; Stockner 1993). Mammals derive their folic acid preformed either in the diet or from bacteria that produce the vitamin in the intestinal tract. The anemia induced by either the sulfadiazine, the trimethoprim, or a combination of the two drugs has been reported to decrease serum folate reductions, presumably by inhibiting the folate production by intestinal bacteria or by blocking its reduction to tetra- and dihydrofolate, resulting in lowered serum folate concentrations in the animal's serum that eventually induce an anemia. Thrombocytopenia has been reported in animals and in humans (Sullivan et al. 1992; Dodds 1993). The thrombocytopenia in animals, as in humans, is probably associated with an immune-mediated component that may resolve after the drug is discontinued.

OTHER IDIOSYNCRATIC REACTIONS. Other idiosyncratic reactions have been reported in dogs and summarized by Cribb (1989). These reactions include polyarthritis and fever (Giger et al. 1985), cutaneous eruptions, and hepatitis (Cribb 1989; Rowland et al. 1992), all believed to be linked to an immunologic component. These idiosyncratic reactions have been observed most frequently in Doberman Pinschers. Some less commonly used sulfonamides have been linked to hypoglycemia in ducks and dogs (Kajinuma et al. 1974).

Sulfonamides are also known to interfere with thyroid hormone synthesis by blocking the conversion of iodide to iodine and may increase thyroid-releasing hormone or thyroid-stimulating hormone. Hall et al. (1993) reported that trimethoprim-sulfamethoxazole combinations may cause iatrogenic hypothyroidism in some dogs with pyoderma. Iatrogenic hypothyroidism has been reported after high-dose (3–5 times label) potentiated sulfonamide administration and is marked by reduced T_4 and thyrotropin stimulation tests with normal T_3 (USPDI 1998).

CARCINOGENESIS. Sulfamethazine (discussed later in this chapter) has been demonstrated to induce thyroid hyperplasia in rats (Astwood et al. 1943; MacKenzie and MacKenzie 1943; Swarm et al. 1973) but has more recently been shown to induce specific types of thyroid cancer in both mice and rats. Fullerton et al. (1987) found that male and female Fischer 344 rats fed diets containing 1200 or 2400 ppm of sulfamethazine had significantly increased thyroid weights than controls and that these increased weights were most likely due to thyroid hyperplasia related to increased thyroid-stimulating hormone levels. Littlefield et al. (1989) fed sulfamethazine to $B6C3F_1$ mice at up to 4800 ppm in the diet for up to 24 months. In that study, sulfamethazine was found to induce follicular cell adenomas of the thyroid gland after 24 months of continuous feeding at the 4800 ppm dose in both males (33% incidence) and females (26% incidence), with focal follicular cell hyperplasia and other organ aberrations being noted at some of the lower doses of sulfamethazine. In a similar study, sulfamethazine was fed to Fischer 344/N rats at doses of 0–2400 ppm, with these rats sacrificed at regular intervals over a 24-month period. The study determined that there was a statistically significant increase in the incidence of thyroid follicular cell adenocarcinomas in rats sacrificed after 24 months of continuous feeding of sulfamethazine, with other non-neoplastic lesions of the thyroid also being reported in other treatment groups.

Resistance. Resistance by many bacterial and protozoal organisms has become widespread due to the extensive use of sulfonamides over many years. Resistance occurs via chromosomal and plasmid-mediated mechanisms. Chromosomal resistance tends to occur slowly and confers resistance via impaired drug penetration into the microbial cell, producing an insensitive dihydropteroate enzyme and an increased production of PABA. Plasmid-mediated resistance, the most commonly encountered form of sulfonamide resistance, occurs quickly and manifests itself via the impaired drug penetration mechanism in addition to producing sulfonamide-resistant dihydropteroate synthase enzymes. If an organism becomes resistant to one sulfonamide, it is generally resistant to all other sulfonamides.

COMMONLY USED SULFONAMIDES

Sulfadimethoxine. The chemical structure of sulfadimethoxine is shown in Fig. 40.3. Sulfadimethoxine is a low-dose, rapidly absorbed, long-acting sulfonamide that has been used for a number of years by itself or in combination with ormetoprim for the treatment of susceptible microbial infections of cattle, swine, horses, and dogs, in addition to many other vertebrate and invertebrate animals.

Sulfadimethoxine pharmacokinetics in cattle has been described by many investigators. Bourne et al. (1981) dosed adult cattle with 107 mg/kg either intravenously (IV) or orally. In the IV study, sulfadimethoxine plasma concentrations peaked at 0.5 hours after administration and slowly declined over time, with the parent compound, acetylsulfadimethoxine, and a "polar" metabolite being found in the urine for at least 48 hours after the IV dose. The volume of distribution (V_d) was determined to be 0.315 L/kg in those cattle. In the oral study, plasma concentrations of sulfadimethoxine started low at 0.5 hours and gradually peaked at 10 hours after dose and then began to drop, with detectable levels of parent compound and all metabolites being found in the urine for at least 84 hours after dosing. Bioavailability of sulfadimethoxine was calculated to be 59.1%. Boxenbaum et al. (1977) administered 55 mg/kg IV sulfadimethoxine (40% solution) or 55 mg/kg orally to cattle, followed by 27.5 mg/kg sulfadimethoxine administered orally at 24, 48, and 72 hours after the initial loading dose. After IV injection, the half-life of sulfadimethoxine was determined to be 12.5 hours, with $V_d = 0.31$ L/kg. This study also confirmed that adequate plasma concentrations (>50 μg/mL) maintained the plasma concentrations achieved from the initial, higher oral dose throughout the oral-dosing study and this method would be useful in treating cattle with susceptible microbial infections when IV administration could not be utilized. By comparison, a study by Wilson et al. (1987) demonstrated that sulfadimethoxine (27.5 mg/kg) in combination with ormetoprim (5.5 mg/kg) administered IV to cattle had a shorter half-life, 7.91 hours, and $V_d = 0.185$ L/kg. When given the same dose orally, bioavailability of sulfadimethoxine was 56.6%.

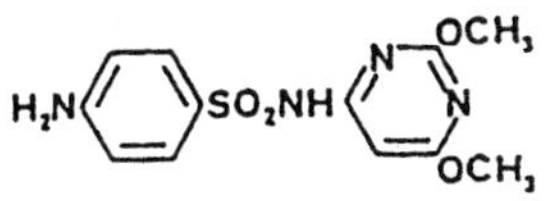

H_2N–C_6H_4–SO_2NH–(pyrimidine with OCH_3, OCH_3)

FIG. 40.3—Sulfadimethoxine

Sulfadimethoxine has been formulated with ormetoprim to enhance the spectrum of antimicrobial activity against some bovine pathogens. This combination has been shown to be highly effective in treating calves with experimentally induced *Pasteurella hemolytica* pneumonia. Wilson et al. (1987) investigated the potential efficacy of a sulfadimethoxine-ormetoprim combination administered orally and IV to treat *Moraxella bovis* infections in cattle. In cattle, sulfadimethoxine-ormetoprim administered IV was effective in maintaining sufficiently high concentrations of both drugs in the tears to exceed the known MICs of 13 *Moraxella bovis* isolates and in maintaining those concentrations for approximately 6 hours. However, when the same concentration of sulfadimethoxine-ormetoprim was administered orally, sulfadimethoxine appeared in low concentrations and ormetoprim in very low or trace concentrations in the tears, indicating this combination of drugs when administered orally is not suitable for treating *Moraxella bovis* infections in cattle.

Studies by Righter et al. (1979) examined the pharmacokinetics of sulfadimethoxine in mature, growing, and suckling pigs. Mature pigs dosed with 20, 50, or 100 mg/kg of sulfadimethoxine IV had V_d values of 0.178, 0.258, and 0.331 L/kg and total body clearance of 4.21, 5.54, and 7.37 mL/hr/kg, respectively. The pharmacokinetic parameters of 55 mg/kg sulfadimethoxine given IV to growing and suckling pigs have also been reported. Suckling pigs (1–2 weeks old) had sulfadimethoxine half-lives of 16.16 hours, V_d = 0.483 L/kg, and total body clearance of 20.9 mL/kg/hr. In contrast, growing pigs (11–12 weeks old) had sulfadimethoxine half-lives of 9.35 hours, V_d = 0.347 L/kg, and total body clearance of 26.1 mL/kg/hr, indicating an age-related effect of sulfadimethoxine pharmacokinetics in young pigs. Weanling pigs consuming water dosed with 0.05 g sulfadimethoxine/100 mL showed mean plasma concentrations of 80 ppm 12 hours after introduction of the medicated water, with plasma concentrations declining to approximately 50 ppm thereafter. Total water consumption was not affected, indicating sulfadimethoxine may be of therapeutic use in swine provided that water consumption is maintained throughout the medication period. Mengelers et al. (1995) dosed 34–40 kg healthy and febrile (inoculated endobronchially with *A. pleuropneumoniae* toxins) pigs with 25 mg/kg sulfadimethoxine and 5 mg/kg trimethoprim IV. Sulfadimethoxine plasma half-lives for both healthy and pneumonic pigs were not significantly different (approximately 13 hr). Trimethoprim half-lives were not significantly different between healthy and pneumonic pigs (approximately 2.7 hr); however, the half-lives were significantly shorter than the half-life of sulfadimethoxine. In addition, the V_d values of healthy and pneumonic pigs receiving sulfadimethoxine were not significantly different (approximately 0.25 L/kg), but trimethoprim did show significant differences between healthy (1.21 L/kg) and pneumonic (1.49 L/kg) pigs. The mean area under the curve (AUC) of trimethoprim was decreased and the total body clearance was increased in the febrile pigs, but with no significant changes in these sulfadimethoxine pharmacokinetic parameters.

The in vitro susceptibility of some porcine pathogens to sulfadimethoxine, other sulfonamides, and other antimicrobial agents has been reported (Mengelers et al. 1990). Sulfadimethoxine has also been implicated as being goitrogenic to swine fetuses in late gestation (Blackwell et al. 1989).

Fewer reports are available on the pharmacokinetics of sulfadimethoxine in horses. Brown et al. (1989) administered sulfadimethoxine-ormetoprim (45.8 mg/kg:9.2 mg/kg) orally, followed by lower oral doses (22.9 mg/kg:4.6 mg/kg) at 24-hour intervals, to healthy adult mares. Sulfadimethoxine showed peak plasma concentrations 8 hours after the initial dose, and plasma concentrations above 50 μg/mL were maintained for the entire dosing schedule. Significant concentrations were also found in the synovial fluid, peritoneal fluid, endometrium, and urine, with a small amount (2.1 μg/mL) appearing in the cerebrospinal fluid approximately 100 hours after the initial dose.

The pharmacokinetic parameters of sulfadimethoxine-ormetoprim were determined in 1- to 3-day-old foals given a sulfadimethoxine-ormetoprim dose (17.5 mg/kg:3.5 mg/kg) orally (Brown et al. 1993). In the foals, sulfadimethoxine concentrations peaked at 8 hours (55 μg/mL) after the oral dose and declined to 37.6 μg/mL 24 hours after the dose.

Sulfadimethoxine usage has also been described in species in which sulfadimethoxine is less commonly used, including turkeys (Epstein and Ashworth 1989), dogs (Yagi et al. 1981; Fish et al. 1965; Dunbar and Foreyt 1985; Imamura et al. 1986; Imamura et al. 1989), primates (Adamson et al. 1970; Bridges et al. 1968), lobsters (James and Barron 1988), channel catfish (Squibb et al. 1988), and rainbow trout (Kleinow and Lech 1988). A promising method for detecting violative levels of sulfadimethoxine residues in channel catfish has also been reported (Walker and Barker 1993).

Sulfamethazine (Sulfadimidine). The chemical structure of sulfamethazine (sulfadimidine) is shown in Fig. 40.4. Sulfamethazine, like many sulfonamides, has been utilized for decades in veterinary medicine; hence, the veterinary literature contains many reports on its usage in a wide variety of animals, including cattle, horses, swine, poultry, small ruminants, and rabbits (among others). Table 40.4 summarizes some of the pharmacokinetic parameters of sulfamethazine in animals.

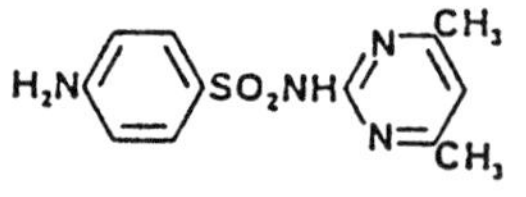

FIG. 40.4—Sulfamethazine (sulfadimidine)

TABLE 40.4—Some pharmacokinetic parameters of sulfamethazine (sulfadimidine) in animals

Species	Dose (mg/kg)	Route	V_d (L/kg)	$t_{1/2}$ (hr)	Clearance (mL/hr/kg)	Reference
Cattle	107	IV	0.346	NR	NR	Bevill et al. 1977a
Cattle (male)	200	IV	0.37	5.82	45	Witcamp et al. 1992
Cattle (female)	200	IV	0.24	3.64	54	Witcamp et al. 1992
Calves (62-70 days old)	10	IV	NR	5.2	NR	Nouws et al. 1988c
Calves (68-76 days old)	100	IV	NR	5.7	NR	Nouws et al. 1988c
Cows (4-5 yr old)	10	IV	NR	4	NR	Nouws et al. 1988c
Cows (3-5 yr old)	100	IV	NR	5.9	NR	Nouws et al. 1988c
Cows (5-6 yr old)	200	IV	NR	5.5	NR	Nouws et al. 1988c
Pigs (9 wk old)	50	IV	0.51	16	21	Sweeney et al. 1993
Pigs (10 wk old)	20	IV	0.604	10	42	Nouws et al. 1989a
Pigs (10 wk old, given in drench)	20	PO	NR	11.9	NR	Nouws et al. 1989a
Pigs (10 wk old, given in medicated feed)	20	PO	NR	16.6	NR	Nouws et al. 1989a
Pigs (male, 18-32 kg)	20	IV	0.55	12.4	25	Nouws et al. 1989a
Gilts (12-13 wk old)	107.5	IA	0.493	15.61	NR	Duffee et al. 1984
Barrows (12-13 wk old)	107.5	IA	0.614	17.7	NR	Duffee et al. 1984
Boars (12-13 wk old)	107.5	IA	0.542	16.63	NR	Duffee et al. 1984
Pigs (normal castrated males and intact females)	50	IV	0.50	15	23	Yuan et al. 1997
Pigs (castrated males and intact females infected with *S. suum*)	50	IV	0.52	20	17	Yuan et al. 1997
Goat	100	IV	0.316	2.77	81	Elsheikh et al. 1991
Goats (adult and fed)	100	IV	0.9	4.75	135.6	Abdullah and Baggot 1988
Goats (adult and fasted)	100	IV	0.897	7.03	69.6	Abdullah and Baggot 1988
Goats (adult male)	20	IV	0.28	8.7	20	Witcamp et al. 1992
Goats (adult female)	20	IV	0.18	2.13	70	Witcamp et al. 1992
Goats (12 wk old)	100	IV	0.43	1.97	134	Nouws et al. 1989b
Goats (18 wk old)	100	IV	0.507	2.56	106	Nouws et al. 1989b
Sheep	100	IV	0.297	4.72	44.6	Elsheikh et al. 1991
Sheep (male)	100	IV	0.4	4.5	90	Srivastava and Rampal 1990
Ewes	100	IV	0.474	9.51	35.07	Youssef et al. 1981
Ewes (dosed in summer months)	100	IV	0.37	3.64	63	Nawaz and Nawaz 1983
Ewes (dosed in winter months)	100	IV	0.49	3.92	85	Nawaz and Nawaz 1983
Sheep (ewes and rams)	100	IV	0.41	10.8	41	Bulgin et al. 1991
Sheep (ewes and rams)	100	PO	NR	4.3	NR	Bulgin et al. 1991
Sheep (ewes and rams)	391	PO	NR	14.3	NR	Bulgin et al. 1991
Sheep (ewes and rams)	100	IV	0.37	3.64	NR	Bulgin et al. 1991
Sheep (ewes and rams)	107.5	IV	0.293	5.87	NR	Bulgin et al. 1991
Sheep (ewes and rams)	107.5	IV	0.327	7.09	NR	Bulgin et al. 1991
Ponies (breed unknown)	160	IV	0.63	11.4	42.1	Wilson et al. 1989
Ponies (Shetland)	20	IV	0.33	5.4	55.2	Nouws et al. 1987
Mare (2 yr old)	20	IV	0.47	5	65	Nouws et al. 1985a
Mare (2 yr old)	200	IV	0.56	6	67	Nouws et al. 1985a
Mare (22 yr old)	20	IV	0.38	9.5	28	Nouws et al. 1985a
Mare (22 yr old)	200	IV	0.36	14.6	27	Nouws et al. 1985a
Stallion (1.5 yr old)	20	IV	0.44	9.5	32	Nouws et al. 1985a
Stallion (1.5 yr old)	200	IV	0.65	11	41	Nouws et al. 1985a
Dogs (normal)	100	IV	0.628	16.2	22.4	Riffat et al. 1982
Dogs (febrile)	100	IV	0.495	16.7	20.2	Riffat et al. 1982
Rabbits (male)	35	IV	0.42	0.4	73.6	Witcamp et al. 1992
Rabbits (female)	35	IV	0.23	0.39	40.8	Witcamp et al. 1992
Carp (10° C)	100	IV	1.15	50.3	16.14	van Ginneken et al. 1991
Carp (20° C)	100	IV	0.9	25.6	24.66	van Ginneken et al. 1991
Rainbow trout (10° C)	100	IV	1.2	20.6	41.1	van Ginneken et al. 1991
Rainbow trout (20° C)	100	IV	0.83	14.7	39.9	van Ginneken et al. 1991
Camel	50	IV	0.73	13.2	40	Younan et al. 1989
Camel	100	IV	0.394	7.36	40.9	Elsheikh et al. 1991
Buffalo (female)	200	IV	1.23	12.36	193.2	Singh et al. 1988

Note: NR = not reported; IV = intravenously; IA = intra-arterially; PO = orally.

Sulfamethazine has been utilized extensively in cattle and swine for a number of years. Sulfamethazine has been formulated for use in the drinking water (Church et al. 1979) and as a feed additive, an extended-release bolus, and an IV preparation. Sulfamethazine has been marketed by itself and in combination with other antimicrobials, such as other sulfonamides, tylosin, chlortetracycline, and procaine penicillin G. The basic pharmacokinetic parameters of sulfamethazine in cattle have been reported by Bevill et al. (1977a) and Nouws et al. (1988), among many others. Of particular interest are the oral forms of sulfamethazine that have been formulated in extended-release (sustained-release) form for cattle. Several reports on the efficacy and clinical uses of the extended-release form of sulfamethazine in cattle are available (Clark et al. 1966; Ellison et al. 1967; Miller et al. 1969; Carlson et al. 1976). This sustained-release formulation has been reported to achieve therapeutic blood levels (i.e., 50 μg/mL) within 6–12 hours after oral administration and to maintain or exceed that level for 2–5 days after dosing. The sustained-release formulation of sulfamethazine has been reported to be highly efficacious in the treatment of shipping fever pneumonia, diphtheria, and pneumonia in cattle (Carlson et al. 1976; Clark et al. 1966). Clearance of sulfamethazine and its metabolites in cattle are age and dose dependent (Nouws et al. 1986a; Lapka et al. 1980; Nouws et al. 1985; Nouws et al. 1983). Several metabolites of sulfamethazine have been identified and described in both adult cattle and calves (Nouws et al. 1988c).

The pharmacokinetics of sulfamethazine and its metabolites are of particular interest in swine. Sulfonamides had been one of the most common causes of food-residue violations reported by the US Food Safety Inspection Service, with swine being the food-animal species with the greatest number of residue violations (Sweeney et al. 1993). Sulfamethazine and its metabolites are most often associated with violative levels in pork products because of sulfamethazine's widespread use as a swine feed additive. Sulfamethazine has been used extensively to treat a host of susceptible microbial infections in swine, including *Salmonella typhisuis* (Fenwick and Olander 1987) and *Bordetella bronchiseptica* (Kobland et al. 1984). Pharmacokinetic parameters have been described by Sweeney et al. (1993) and others (see Table 40.4), including its metabolites (Nouws et al. 1989a; Nouws et al. 1986b). Several studies have used radiolabeled (Mitchell et al. 1986; Mitchell and Paulson 1986) and nonradiolabeled (Biehl et al. 1981; Ashworth et al. 1986) sulfamethazine to determine the elimination patterns of sulfamethazine and its metabolites from the tissues in swine. Other studies have shown that the major metabolites produced from sulfamethazine metabolism in swine are sulfamethazine (parent compound), N_4-acetylsulfamethazine, N_4-glucose conjugate of sulfamethazine, and desaminosulfamethazine (Mitchell et al. 1986). Studies using pigs fed 110 ppm of ^{14}C-sulfamethazine in the feed for 3–7 days, euthanized, and their tissues examined for total radioactivity and metabolite content found the highest concentration of radioactivity in the gut (undigested feed). Blood, kidney, urine, and liver all had high concentrations of radioactivity (i.e., parent compound and metabolite). Adipose tissue contained the least amount of radioactivity of all tissues assayed (Mitchell et al. 1986). Specific metabolites found in these and other tissues of swine given ^{14}C-labeled sulfamethazine in the feed have been reported by Mitchell and Paulson (1986). Other studies have also reported on sulfamethazine residues in swine (Ashworth et al. 1986; Biehl et al. 1981).

Cattle and swine are the two major species in which sulfamethazine is approved for use. There are fewer reports on the clinical use of sulfamethazine in other domestic animals. Pharmacokinetic parameters and/or tissue-depletion kinetics of sulfamethazine and metabolites have been established in ponies (Wilson et al. 1989; Nouws et al. 1987) and horses (Nouws et al. 1985a). Studies have focused on the pharmacokinetic parameters of sulfadimidine in goats (Abdullah and Baggot 1988; Witcamp et al. 1992; Nouws et al. 1989b; Elsheikh et al. 1991; Youssef et al. 1981; van Gogh et al. 1984; Witcamp et al. 1993; Nouws et al. 1988b), sheep (Srivastava and Rampal 1990; Bourne et al. 1977; Bevill et al. 1977c; Bulgin et al. 1991; Nawaz and Nawaz 1983), dogs (Riffat et al. 1982), chickens (Righter et al. 1971; Nouws et al. 1988a; Goren et al. 1987), rabbits (Yuan and Fung 1990), mice (Littlefield et al. 1989), buffalo (Singh et al. 1988), camels (Younan et al. 1989), and carp and rainbow trout (van Ginneken et al. 1991).

A recent report by Lashev et al. (1995) described altered pharmacokinetics in roosters treated with a single 50 mg/kg IV dose of sulfadimidine only or IV sulfadimidine after two weeks of four 3.5 mg/kg subcutaneous (SC) testosterone treatments. Normal and castrated roosters provided no significant differences in $t_{1/2\alpha}$ values, which ranged from 7.62 hours (castrated) to 9.38 hours (intact). Roosters pretreated with testosterone and then dosed with sulfadimidine had a $t_{1/2\alpha}$ value of 23.85 hours, as well as significantly decreased Cl_B and $V_{d(area)}$ values. Chickens metabolize sulfadimidine in relatively equal parts through hydroxylation and acetylation. It was hypothesized in this study that the acetylation pathway of sulfadimidine metabolism was retarded by the testosterone treatments and resulted in the prolonged half-lives.

Sulfaquinoxaline. The chemical structure of sulfaquinoxaline is shown in Fig. 40.5. Sulfaquinoxaline has primarily been utilized in poultry for control of coccidia and some susceptible bacterial diseases. The veterinary literature also contains a few reports of sulfaquinoxaline use in rabbits (Eppel and Thiessen 1984; Joyner et al. 1983) and canines (Brown et al. 1982; Patterson and Grenn 1975).

Sulfaquinoxaline alone or in combination with a diaminopyrimidine has been used extensively to con-

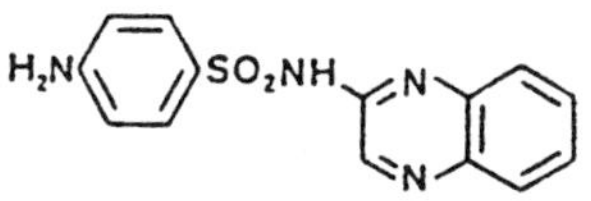

FIG. 40.5—Sulfaquinoxaline

trol coccidiosis in poultry in the United States. Mathis and McDougald (1984) described the therapeutic effectiveness of sulfaquinoxaline and sulfaquinoxaline-pyrimethamine against several species of *Eimeria* coccidia. It was determined from that study that both sulfaquinoxaline and sulfaquinoxaline-pyrimethamine were highly effective against *E. acervulina* but less effective against *E. tenella.* In addition, the potentiated mixture was determined to be more effective against *E. tenella* than sulfaquinoxaline alone, although neither mixture was found to be particularly effective against any cecal coccidia. Amprolium was found to be efficacious against cecal-dwelling forms of coccidia; hence amprolium has been combined with sulfaquinoxaline or sulfaquinoxaline-pyrimethamine to enhance the spectrum of activity. Ineffectiveness of sulfaquinoxaline-pyrimethamine against *E. tenella* has also been documented in another study (Chapman 1989), underlining the importance of correct coccidia species identification before instituting anticoccidial therapy with sulfaquinoxaline or any other sulfonamide.

Banerjee et al. (1974) reported that hens receiving 275 mg/kg PO once had average mean peak blood levels of 16.1 mg/dL of free drug 12 hours after administration, with this level decreasing to 12.7 mg/dL by 24 hours (8–10 mg/dL was considered to be therapeutically effective). In that same study, sulfaquinoxaline was found in high concentrations in the liver, kidney, and cecum, with the lowest concentrations found in the yolk sac and brain. A single oral dose of ^{35}S-labeled sulfaquinoxaline in 1-week-old chicks showed rapid uptake from the gastrointestinal tract and wide distribution throughout the body, including crossing of the blood-brain barrier. At 0.5 hours after dosing, autoradiography showed that all tissues (brain, lung, liver, kidney, fat, and muscle) except the lens of the eye had measurable concentrations of sulfaquinoxaline. Similar findings resulted from IV administration of ^{35}S-labeled sulfaquinoxaline, and it was also found that excretion of sulfaquinoxaline by the bile and secretion by the cecal mucosa, crop, and gizzard probably occur. Interestingly, oral dosing with sulfaquinoxaline of chickens with *E. acervulina* and *E. tenella* increases the absorption of the drug approximately 3.5 times over that found in uninfected birds (Williams et al. 1995). A study by Qiao et al. (1995) found that in 7- to 8-week-old male and female broilers given a single 200 mg/kg oral dose of sulfaquinoxaline, peak concentration times in plasma and liver were similar (4 hr) but were longer in the heart, kidney, and muscle (6 hr). The half-life of sulfaquinoxaline was the shortest in the muscle (4.5 hr), with significantly longer half-lives in the heart (10 hr), plasma (11 hr), liver (13 hr), and kidney (18 hr).

The safety and efficacy of sulfaquinoxaline alone or in combination with trimethoprim (trimethoprim:sulfaquinoxaline = 1:3) have been reported in poultry (White and Williams 1983; Piercy et al. 1984; Sainsbury 1988). A total dose of 30 mg/kg/day PO satisfactorily controlled experimentally induced colisepticemia and pasteurellosis in addition to 5 species of coccidia (White and Williams 1983). A wide margin of safety has been shown for the 1:3 combination of trimethoprim:sulfaquinoxaline in poultry, although decreased appetite and water consumption and lowered egg production, egg weight, and hatchability were noted when these antimicrobials were incorporated in the feed or water in higher than recommended concentrations (Piercy et al. 1984).

Toxicosis from sulfaquinoxaline use in animals has been infrequently reported. Toxicity from sulfaquinoxaline has occurred in Leghorn chickens (Daft et al. 1989), where a mortality of 47% was reported in a commercial flock given a 0.05% concentration of sulfaquinoxaline in the feed. Lesions included mildly enlarged livers; swollen and pale livers; hemorrhages on the epicardium, kidney, oviduct, small intestine, and cecum; pale bone marrow; and gangrenous dermatitis; and some lung involvement was present. Patterson and Grenn (1975) reported a situation where 12 adult Miniature Poodles that received 3.16 g/L of sulfaquinoxaline in the drinking water as treatment for coccidiosis suffered similar lesions as described above in poultry, in addition to depressed body temperature, pale mucous membranes, microscopic hemorrhages of the jejunum and ileum, and prolonged prothrombin times. Treatment with vitamin K was efficacious in all dogs treated. Although the exact mechanism has not been reported, sulfaquinoxaline possesses an ability to produce a marked hypothrombinemia, even in animals receiving balanced diets containing adequate amounts of vitamin K. It is thought that this adverse effect is not related to the individual sulfonamide or quinoxaline portion of the sulfaquinoxaline molecule but occurs only when the two entities are combined. A similar toxicosis has also been reported in coyote pups treated with sulfaquinoxaline (Brown et al. 1982).

Sulfamerazine. The chemical structure of sulfamerazine is shown in Fig. 40.6. Sulfamerazine has primarily been utilized in adult sheep and lambs to treat susceptible microbial infections. Sulfamerazine has been used alone or in combination with other

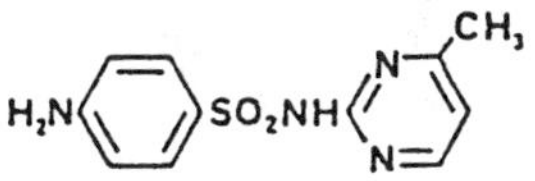

FIG. 40.6—Sulfamerazine

antibiotics (tylosin) and other sulfonamides (sulfamethazine, sulfadiazine).

The pharmacokinetics of sulfamerazine has been described for ewes and lambs. Hayashi et al. (1979) described the pharmacokinetics of sulfamerazine in ewes dosed IV or PO with 107 mg/kg. In the IV studies, the V_d was 0.266 L/kg, and the half-life calculated to be 2.55 hours. The biological half-life was determined to be 6.6 hours. For the oral study, the bioavailability of sulfamerazine administered as a 12.5% oral solution was 81 ± 19%. Urinary concentrations of parent compound and metabolites were also reported for both IV- and PO-dosing studies. Both routes produced appreciable concentrations of sulfamerazine and three metabolites in the urine (described as acetylsulfamerazine, "polar" metabolite, and third metabolite as determined by thin-layer chromatography). IV sulfamerazine produced more parent compound in the urine than did the PO route (31% vs. 21%), and more polar metabolite was produced via the PO route than via the IV route (19% vs. 10%). More parent compound was found in the IV study due to lack of rumen metabolism, while more metabolite than parent compound was found in the PO study due to rumen metabolism. In a similar pharmacokinetic study, Garwacki et al. (1991) administered 60 mg/kg sulfamerazine IV in fasted sheep and in sheep fed ad libitum. That study determined that sheep fed ad libitum had a sulfamerazine $t_{1/2}$ of 5.72 hours and a V_d of 0.40 L/kg, while those sheep that were fasted had a $t_{1/2}$ of 6.91 hours and a V_d of 0.41 L/kg. The authors proposed that since sulfamerazine is an acidic drug ($pK_a = 7$), it preferred the ruminal pH environment in the fasted state, and hence a reservoir of drug was established in the rumen that resulted in the prolonged half-life.

The pharmacokinetics of sulfamerazine has also been reported in neonatal and young lambs (Debacker et al. 1982). Lambs from birth to 16 weeks of age were dosed either IV or PO with 100 mg/kg of sulfamerazine. In the IV study, it was found that the sulfamerazine half-life was longest in the first week of life (9–14 hours) and decreased to 4–7 hours by 9–16 weeks of age. Likewise V_d was highest during the first week of life and steadily decreased with age, while clearance of sulfamerazine was lowest in the first week of life (20–40 mL/kg/hr) and steadily increased with age up to 9–16 weeks of age (50–80 mL/kg/hr). In the oral study, plasma concentrations of sulfamerazine tended to decrease more slowly after dosing in the early weeks of life (<4 weeks of age), with plasma clearance of the drug steadily increasing after 4 weeks of age until 16 weeks, when it approached the adult values.

Sulfathiazole. The chemical structure of sulfathiazole is shown in Fig. 40.7. Sulfathiazole has been used in veterinary medicine since its synthesis (Koritz et al. 1977), but today it is formulated in combination with chlortetracycline HCl and procaine penicillin G. Few recent reports are available on its use and thus earlier editions of this text should be consulted for more details. A few reports have described the pharmacokinetics of sulfathiazole in sheep and swine.

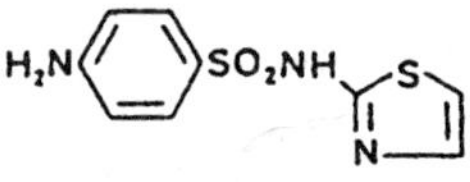

H_2N–[benzene ring]–SO_2NH–[thiazole ring: S, N]

FIG. 40.7—Sulfathiazole

Sulfathiazole pharmacokinetics in sheep has been outlined by Koritz et al. (1977), and sulfathiazole tissue residues in sheep have been described by Bevill et al. (1977b). When 36 or 72 mg/kg of 5% aqueous solution of sulfathiazole sodium IV was given to ewe lambs, it cleared quickly from the plasma, having V_d values of 0.34 and 0.59 L/kg and half-lives of 1.2 and 1.4 hours, respectively. Ewes given 214 mg/kg orally of a 12.5% aqueous solution of sulfathiazole sodium cleared the drug from plasma much more slowly than by the IV route, with the systemic bioavailability being approximately 73%, with a half-life of approximately 18 hours. Both PO and IV routes resulted in parent compound accompanied by acetylsulfathiazole and a third "polar" metabolite in the urine of these sheep. In the study by Bevill et al. (1977b), sheep given IV doses of 36 mg/kg sulfathiazole sodium had a lower mean V_d value than the 72 mg/kg dose (0.389 L/kg), but a comparable half-life to that found by Koritz (1.1 hours). Sulfathiazole residues in sheep 2 hours after a 72 mg/kg IV dose were also determined, with the highest concentrations of drug found in the kidney (308 ppm), followed by the liver (40 ppm), heart (34 ppm), shoulder muscle (23 ppm), leg and loin muscle (22 ppm), body fat (11 ppm), and omental fat (6.7 ppm). Residues quickly dropped to very low (<0.13 ppm) or to nondetectable levels by 24 hours after dosing in all tissues tested.

Pharmacokinetic parameters have also been reported for swine. Pigs given 72 mg/kg of sulfathiazole sodium IV had quick plasma elimination of the drug, with mean V_d of 0.54 L/kg and a biological half-life of 1.39 hours, similar to those for sheep. Given 214 mg/kg orally, sulfathiazole had a V_d of 0.32 L/kg and a systemic bioavailability of 73%, identical to that of sheep.

Sulfasalazine (Salicylazosulfapyridine). The chemical structure of sulfasalazine is shown in Fig. 40.8. Sulfasalazine was originally developed as a possible treatment for rheumatoid arthritis in humans. It was found, however, to be more effective in the treatment of inflammatory bowel disease. Few reports are available in the veterinary literature on the pharmacokinetics and use of sulfasalazine in animals. It has been used with some success in some animals (mainly dogs) to treat various forms of colitis (Aronson and Kirk 1983). Many forms of inflammatory bowel diseases (most commonly ulcerative colitis and Crohn's disease) have been treated with sulfasalazine in humans.

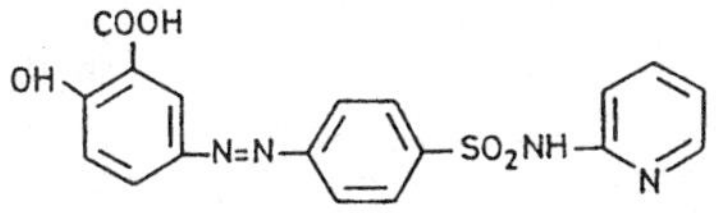

FIG. 40.8—Sulfasalazine

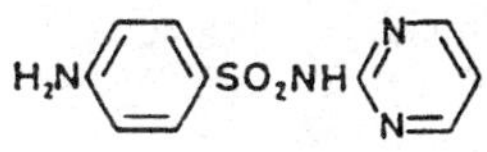

FIG. 40.9—Sulfadiazine

Sulfasalazine consists of two components, 5-aminosalicylic acid and sulfapyridine, which are linked by an azo bond. After oral administration, sulfasalazine is partly absorbed in the small intestine, where it undergoes enterohepatic circulation (unmetabolized by the liver), and it is then excreted in the urine. The majority of the remaining drug (70%) is retained in the lumen of the intestine, where it is presented to bacteria in the colon, which split the drug's azo bond and liberate the two compounds from one another. The sulfapyridine is quickly absorbed into the blood, metabolized, and excreted in the urine. The exact mechanism behind sulfasalazine's effect on inflammatory bowel disease is unclear. However, many believe that its effects are due to the 5-aminosalicylic acid acting locally on the bowel mucosa as a topical anti-inflammatory delivered in much higher concentrations in sulfasalazine formulation than if 5-aminosalicylic acid had been given orally by itself (no conjugation with sulfapyridine). Its anti-inflammatory effects may be due to prostaglandin inhibition (Hoult and Moore 1978), interacting with oxygen free radicals (Del Soldato et al. 1985) or with sulfhydryls (Garg et al. 1991). Several metabolites of sulfasalazine have been identified in rats and humans (Das and Dubin 1976), and its possible effects on male fertility have been described (Giwercman and Skakkebaek 1986). More in-depth information on the pharmacokinetic parameters of sulfasalazine is available for humans than for animals (Shafii et al. 1982; Eastwood 1980; Das and Dubin 1976; Das et al. 1979). Sulfasalazine should be used with caution (if at all) in cats because of the toxicity that the salicylate portion of this drug can induce in this species.

Phthalylsulfathiazole acts topically in the bowel and has similar indications as sulfasalazine. However, its intact molecule is longer acting, with very little (if any) systemic absorption, is excreted in the feces, and is especially effective against coliforms (Aronson and Kirk 1983). Phthalylsulfathiazole is hydrolyzed in the bowel by bacteria into phthalic acid and sulfathiazole, with sulfathiazole being the active component. Succinylsulfathiazole is another sulfonamide used in animals, is poorly absorbed systemically, is hydrolyzed into the succinic (inactive) and sulfathiazole (active) drugs by colonic bacteria, and is used for the treatment of bacterial bowel infections (colitis) (Bevill 1988).

Sulfadiazine. The chemical structure of sulfadiazine is shown in Fig. 40.9. Table 40.5 summarizes some of the pharmacokinetic parameters of sulfadiazine in several species of animals.

Sulfadiazine has enjoyed widespread use in cattle and in small animals (dogs and cats) for several years.

TABLE 40.5—Some pharmacokinetic parameters of sulfadiazine in animals

Species	Dose (mg/kg)	Route	V_d (L/kg)	$t_{1/2}$ (hr)	Clearance (mL/hr/kg)	Reference
Pigs	25/5[a]	PO	NR	3.1–4.31	NR	Soli et al. 1990
Pigs	20	IV	0.54	4.0[b]	140	Nielsen and Gyrd-Hansen 1994
Pigs (fed)	40	PO	NR	11.5[b]	NR	Nielsen and Gyrd-Hansen 1994
Pigs (fasted)	40	PO	NR	8.1[b]	NR	Nielsen and Gyrd-Hansen 1994
Carp (10° C)	100/20[a]	IV	0.53	47.1	7.9	Nouws et al. 1993
Carp (20° C)	100/20[a]	IV	0.60	33	12.2	Nouws et al. 1993
Ewes	100	IV	0.39	37.15	38.75	Youssef et al. 1981
Dogs	100/20[a]	PO	NR	9.84	NR	Sigel et al. 1981
Calves (milk diet, 7 wk)	25/5[a]	SC	NR	3.4	NR	Shoaf et al. 1987
Calves (milk diet, 13 wk)	25/5[a]	SC	SC	3.4	NR	Shoaf et al. 1987
Calves (grain diet, 7 wk)	25/5[a]	SC	NR	4.4	NR	Shoaf et al. 1987
Calves (grain diet, 13 wk)	25/5[a]	SC	NR	3.6	NR	Shoaf et al. 1987
Calves (8-20 days)	20	IV	NR	6.2	NR	Nouws et al. 1988c
Calves (0.5 yr)	100	IV	NR	7	NR	Nouws et al. 1988c
Cattle (5 yr)	10	IV	NR	4.1	NR	Nouws et al. 1988c
Calves (male, 1 day)	25/5[a]	IV	0.72	5.78	5.8	Shoaf et al. 1989
Calves (male, 7 days)	25/5[a]	IV	0.67	4.4	102	Shoaf et al. 1989
Calves (male, 42 days)	25/5[a]	IV	0.59	3.6	112.8	Shoaf et al. 1989
Calves (7 days, with synovitis)	25/5[a]	IV	28.7	24.44	102	Shoaf et al. 1986

Note: NR = not reported; IV = intravenously; PO = orally; SC = subcutaneously.
[a]Sulfadiazine-trimethoprim dose.
[b]Reported as mean residence time (MRT).

It is usually found in the potentiated form with trimethoprim and may be combined with other antimicrobials such as sulfamethazine, sulfamerazine, and tylosin for use in food-producing animals. The trimethoprim-sulfadiazine combination (TMS) in a 1:5 ratio was found to be clinically useful in dogs and cats against a wide variety of pathogens, in particular *Staphylococcus* spp., *Streptococcus* spp., *Corynebacterium* spp., *Clostridium* spp., and several gram-negative organisms, such as *Proteus* spp., *Salmonella* spp., *Pasteurella* spp., and *Klebsiella* spp., among many others (Cannon 1976; McCaig 1970; Craig and White 1976). Toxicologic studies confirmed its safety in both dogs and cats (Craig and White 1976). In the Craig and White study, dogs were dosed with up to 300 mg/kg/day orally (10 times the normal dose) of TMS for as long as 20 days with no abnormal clinical signs or blood or serum chemistry abnormalities reported. Cats were dosed with 30–300 mg/kg/day orally for 10–30 days and were more sensitive to the TMS combination. The cats receiving the 300 mg/kg dose showed signs of lethargy, anorexia, anemia, leukopenia, and altered blood urea nitrogen (BUN). Despite these alterations, both dogs and cats have a wide margin of safety when administered TMS.

TMS combinations have been used to treat urinary tract infections in dogs and cats (Ling et al. 1984). TMS has been shown to be effective in treating urinary tract infections caused by *Staphylococcus intermedius* (Turnwald et al. 1986) as well as the more common pathogens such as *E. coli, Proteus mirabilis, Klebsiella pneumoniae,* and *Streptococcus* spp. (Ling and Ruby 1979; Ling et al. 1984). Beagle dogs treated with 40 mg:200 mg TMS or that dose divided into two were found to have high concentrations of both sulfadiazine and trimethoprim in their urine that greatly exceeded the MIC values for most susceptible pathogens (Sigel et al. 1981).

In addition to being of value in treating urinary tract infections, TMS has also demonstrated usefulness in the treatment of many bacterial skin diseases. Success rates of 90% (skin diseases either cured or improved) in bacterial skin infections, foot infections, interdigital abscesses, anal abscesses, and infections of the eye, ear, and mouth in dogs have been reported. A similar success rate was reported in cats (89%) with bites and other infections. An overall success rate of 85% was reported in dogs and cats treated with a TMS combination for microbial diseases involving the alimentary, respiratory, urogenital, skin, and other systems (Craig 1972). Dogs administered 30 mg/kg of TMS orally at 12- or 24-hour intervals were found to attain therapeutically useful concentrations of both trimethoprim and sulfadiazine in the skin (Pohlenz-Zertuche et al. 1992).

Sulfadiazine has also demonstrated an ability to control plaque and gingivitis in Beagles (Howell et al. 1989) and has attained concentrations in the cerebrospinal fluid (when administered IV) above the reported MIC values for many of the Enterobacteriaceae family (Vergin et al. 1984). TMS has also been reported to be of potential therapeutic use in cases of *Streptococcus zooepidemicus* (McCandlish and Thompson 1979) and *Bordetella bronchiseptica* (Powers et al. 1980) in dogs and in ocular infections (Sigel et al. 1981).

Sulfadiazine pharmacokinetics in dog prostates has also been reported (Robb et al. 1971). In that study, sulfadiazine (a weak acid) was found to penetrate the prostate to approximately 11% that of the mean plasma concentration. The penetration abilities of other sulfonamides (including sulfadiazine) are strongly pK_a dependent, with those sulfonamides with higher pK_a values penetrating at accelerated rates. Trimethoprim (a weak base with a pK_a of 7.3) penetrated the prostatic environment at a concentration 380% higher than that of plasma.

TMS has found similar uses in the treatment of susceptible microbial infections in cattle (Slaughter 1972). No difference in trimethoprim or sulfadiazine concentrations in the synovial fluid of normal neonatal calves administered TMS IV or in those calves with experimentally induced synovitis has been demonstrated (Shoaf et al. 1986). The pharmacokinetics of sulfadiazine and trimethoprim has been studied extensively in calves and in cattle (see Tables 40.5 and 40.6). Age and diet can markedly affect trimethoprim and oral sulfadiazine disposition in calves (Guard et al. 1986; Shoaf et al. 1987). Orally administered sulfadiazine (30 mg/kg) was absorbed very slowly in those calves fed milk diets, with absorption slightly higher in ruminating calves. Calves given sulfadiazine subcutaneously (30 mg/kg) had a rapid absorption of the drug; age and diet had no effect on sulfadiazine or trimethoprim disposition in those calves (Shoaf et al. 1987). In another study by Guard et al. (1986), calves 1 day of age showed higher serum and synovial fluid concentrations of trimethoprim and sulfadiazine than did calves of 1 week or 6 weeks of age. Sulfadiazine is acetylated to a great degree in calves and cows, with lower concentrations of the 4-hydroxysulfadiazine being observed and with no glucuronide or 5-hydroxy derivatives detected in this species (Nouws et al. 1988c). TMS concentrations can also be obtained in the cerebrospinal fluid of neonatal calves (Shoaf et al. 1989). A pharmacokinetic model has been developed for determining the metabolic depletion of sulfadiazine (Woolly and Sigel 1982).

Sulfadiazine's use has also been reported in pigs (Soli et al. 1990; Guise et al. 1986), carp (Nouws et al. 1993), ewes (Youssef et al. 1981), and horses (White and Prior 1982; Divers et al. 1981; Bertone et al. 1988). Trimethoprim (8 mg/kg)-sulfadiazine (40 mg/kg) was administered orally to pigs to determine bioavailability and other pharmacokinetic parameters. Bioavailability of sulfadiazine was 89% and 85% in fasted and fed pigs, respectively, while the trimethoprim resulted in bioavailabilities of 90% and 92%. After IV administration of trimethoprim (4 mg/kg)-sulfadiazine (20 mg/kg), sulfadiazine was detectable in plasma up to 30 hours after administration, while the trimethoprim was

TABLE 40.6—Some pharmacokinetic parameters of trimethoprim in animals

Species	Dose[a] (mg/kg)	Route	V_d (L/kg)	$t_{1/2}$ (hr)	Clearance (mL/hr/kg)	Reference
Cows	8/40	IV	NR	1.18	NR	Davitiyananda and Rasmussen 1974
Pigs	4	IV	1.8	3.3[b]	0.55	Nielsen and Gyrd-Hansen 1994
Pigs (fed)	8	PO	NR	10.6[b]	NR	Nielsen and Gyrd-Hansen 1994
Pigs (fasted)	8	PO	NR	6.5[b]	NR	Nielsen and Gyrd-Hansen 1994
Calves (male, 1 day old)	5/25	IV	1.67	8.4	2.8	Shoaf et al. 1989
Calves (male, 7 days old)	5/25	IV	2.23	2.11	2.0	Shoaf et al. 1989
Calves (male, 42 days old)	5/25	IV	2.36	0.9	28.9	Shoaf et al. 1989
Calves (7 wk old, milk diet)	5/25	SC	NR	3.4	126.0	Shoaf et al. 1987
Calves (13 wk old, milk diet)	5/25	SC	NR	3.4	124.8	Shoaf et al. 1987
Calves (7 wk old, grain diet)	5/25	SC	SC	4.4	105.6	Shoaf et al. 1987
Calves (13 wk old, grain diet)	5/25	SC	NR	3.6	112.2	Shoaf et al. 1987
Calves (7 days old)	5/25	IV	28.72	4.44	102.0	Shoaf et al. 1986
Carp (10° C)	20/100	IV	3.1	40.7	47.0	Nouws et al. 1993
Carp (20° C)	20/100	IV	4.0	20.0	141.0	Nouws et al. 1993
Broilers	4/2[c]	PO	NR	0.63	NR	Dagorn et al. 1991
Quail (*Coturnix coturnix japonica;* male and female)	10	PO	NR	2.98	NR	Lashev and Mihailov 1994
Quail (*Coturnix coturnix japonica;* male and female)	4	IV	2.99	2.38	1.129	Lashev and Mihailov 1994
Pigs	5/25 (Tribrissen 12%)	PO	NR	3.35	NR	Soli et al. 1990
Pigs	5/25 (Trimazin 12%)	PO	NR	4.86	4.86	Soli et al. 1990
Pigs	5/25 (Trimazin Forte 24%)	PO	NR	5.92	NR	Soli et al. 1990

Note: NR = not reported; IV = intravenously; SC = subcutaneously; PO = orally.
[a]First dose is trimethoprim; second dose is sulfadiazine (except for Davitiyananda and Rasmussen 1974 reference, in which the sulfonamide is sulfadoxine).
[b]Reported as mean residence time (MRT).
[c]Dose reported in mg/kg/24 hr.

found in the plasma only during the first 12 hours after dosing. The authors concluded that IV administration of TMS was a practical and efficient route and was not significantly affected by fasting (Nielsen and Gyrd-Hansen 1994).

Sulfabromomethazine. The chemical structure of sulfabromomethazine is shown in Fig. 40.10. Sulfabromomethazine is the brominated derivative of sulfamethazine and is considered a long-acting sulfonamide. Sulfabromomethazine has a lower solubility than sulfamethazine, and single oral doses of the drug have been used to treat calf diphtheria and pneumonia, metritis, foot rot, and septic mastitis in cattle, with a repeated dose 48 hours later sometimes required. Use of sulfabromomethazine during the last 3 months of pregnancy should be avoided (Bevill 1988).

FIG. 40.10—Sulfabromomethazine

Sulfaethoxypyridazine. The chemical structure of sulfaethoxypyridazine is shown in Fig. 40.11. Few recent literature reports exist on the use of sulfaethoxypyridazine in animals. It is rapidly absorbed after oral administration to swine, sheep, and cattle and is extensively bound to plasma proteins. The parent compound and the N_4-acetylated metabolite and another unidentified glucuronide conjugate seem to be the major urinary excretion products (Bevill 1988). Sulfaethoxypyridazine has also been reported to induce cataracts at some doses when fed to dogs and rats over a period of 27 and 118 weeks, respectively (Ribelin et al. 1967).

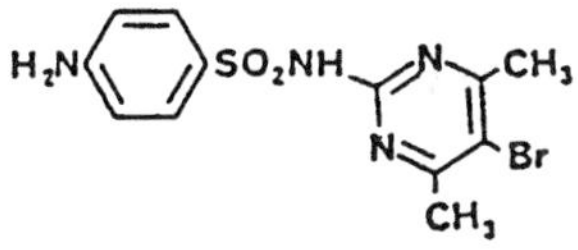

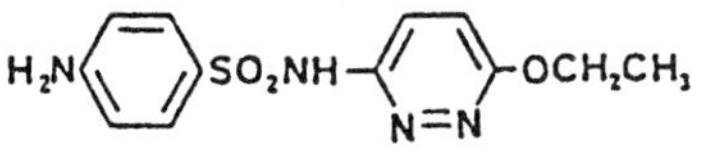

FIG. 40.11—Sulfaethoxypyridazine

Sulfisoxazole. The chemical structure of sulfisoxazole is shown in Fig. 40.12. Sulfisoxazole has limited use today but has found some application in the treatment

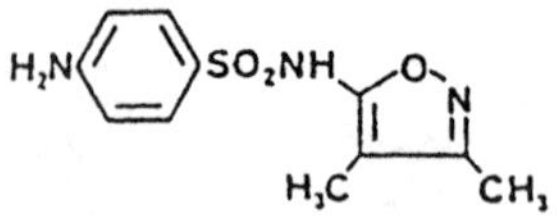

FIG. 40.12—Sulfisoxazole

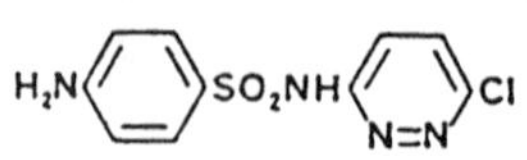

FIG. 40.13—Sulfachlorpyridazine

of urinary tract infections in the dog and cat, especially infections caused by *E. coli, Proteus vulgaris, Pseudomonas aeruginosa,* and some gram-positive cocci (Bevill 1988). The pharmacokinetics of sulfisoxazole has been studied in dogs, swine, and humans (Suber et al. 1981) as well as its delivery across the skin using iontophoresis (Inada et al. 1989).

Sulfachlorpyridazine. The chemical structure of sulfachlorpyridazine is shown in Fig. 40.13. Horses intravenously given 5 mg/kg trimethoprim and 25 mg/kg sulfachlorpyridazine revealed an elimination $t_{1/2}$ of 2.57 hours (trimethoprim) and 3.78 hours (sulfachlorpyridazine) and a $V_{d(steady\ state)}$ of 1.51 L/kg (trimethoprim) and 0.26 L/kg (sulfachlorpyridazine). Bioavailability of the same dose of sulfachlorpyridazine in a powder formulation administered in the feed was about 46%. Interestingly, oral absorption appeared to be delayed, with the first peak appearing 1 hour after dosing and the second appearing 8–10 hours postdosing. Dual absorption peaks were not found after nasogastric administration. This phenomenon may be due to a number of reasons, such as differences in the time span of drug administration, physical barriers from the feed, biphasic gastric emptying, or recirculation/reabsorption of the drugs excreted in the bile. It was the authors' contention that the physical presentation (formulation) of the drug was likely the cause of the two absorption peaks (van Duijkerne et al. 1995).

Sulfachlorpyridazine is rapidly eliminated from the plasma following IV administration. Intramuscular injections in swine result in maximum blood concentrations within 30 minutes after injection, which are maintained for up to 3 hours (Bevill 1988). A single 50 mg/kg IV dose of sulfachlorpyridazine demonstrated significantly different $V_{d(area)}$ in cocks (0.34 L/kg) versus hens (0.36 L/kg), with the sulfonamide being more slowly excreted in hens (Lashev et al. 1995).

The pharmacokinetics of sulfachlorpyridazine after oral and intracardiac administrations has also been described in the channel catfish (*Ictalurus punctatus*), and the drug has been found to have a potential use in aquaculture (Alavi et al. 1993).

Other Sulfonamides. This chapter has discussed the major sulfonamides in use in veterinary medicine today. However, other sulfonamides do exist that are not currently or are no longer used in the US markets. Other sulfonamides that may be of interest include sulfadimethoxypyrimidine (Walker and Williams 1972), sulfasomidine and sulfamethomidine (Bridges et al. 1969), sulfamethoxypyridazine (Garg and Uppal 1997), sulfamethoxydiazine (Weijkamp et al. 1994), and sulfamethylphenazole (Austin and Kelly 1966). Sulfadimethoxine-sulfamethoxazole use in healthy and pneumonic pigs (Mengelers et al. 1995), trimethoprim-sulfamethoxazole in goats (kids) (Koudela and Bokova 1997), and trimethoprim-sulfamethoxazole combinations in Japanese quails (Lashev and Mihailov 1994) have also been reported. Previous editions of this textbook or the individual references listed above may be consulted for more in-depth information on the older and less commonly used sulfonamides not discussed in this chapter.

POTENTIATED SULFONAMIDES. The combination of sulfonamides with other antimicrobial drugs (most commonly trimethoprim) has been repeatedly shown to be therapeutically useful in treating veterinary microbial infections in both small and large animals. These combinations were discussed under the individual drug sections above. Sulfonamide and trimethoprim combinations have been reviewed in some depth by Bushby (1980), Van Miert (1994), and in the 1998 USPDI monograph on this subject. An extensive review of trimethoprim-sulfonamide combinations in the horse is also available (Van Duijkeren et al. 1994b). Combinations of a sulfonamide with trimethoprim (2,4-diamino-5-(3,4,5-trimethoxybenzyl) pyrimidine), aditoprim (2,4-diamino-5-[4-(dimethylamino)-3,5-dimethoxybenzyl] pyrimidine), ormetoprim (2,4-diamino-5-[4,5-dimethoxy-2-methylbenzyl] pyrimidine), or tetroxoprim (2,4-diamino-5-[3,5-dimethoxy-4(2-methoxy ethoxy)benzyl] pyrimidine), among others, are commonly termed "potentiated sulfonamides." The chemical structures of trimethoprim and ormetoprim are shown in Figs. 40.14 and 40.15. Potentiated sulfonamides have the desirable property of reducing, by several-fold, the MIC of both the sulfonamide and the diaminopyrimidine against a wide range of pathogenic organisms. Lowered MICs needed to control infections result in small doses of drugs used in each animal and thereby a reduction in the total dose of drug administered to the animal (Craig 1972).

Mechanism of Action. As seen in Fig. 40.2, the synthesis of dihydrofolic acid from PABA is blocked by competitive inhibition of PABA with a sulfonamide. Trimethoprim and other diaminopyrimidine analogs block the synthesis of tetrahydrofolic acid from dihydrofolic acid by competitive inhibition of dihydrofolate reductase. Trimethoprim and sulfonamides, each used separately, are bacteriostatic. By blocking both steps of

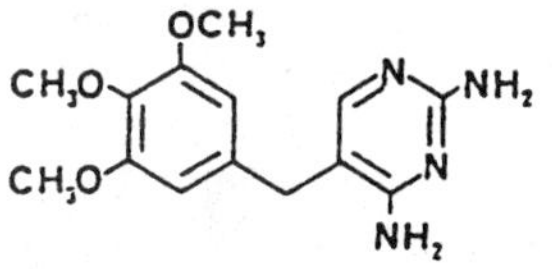

FIG. 40.14—Trimethoprim

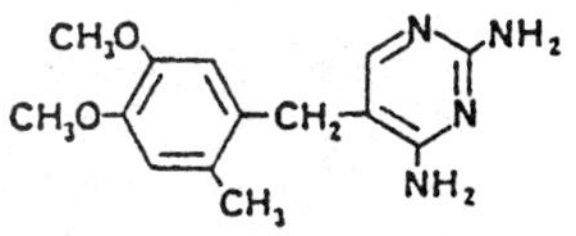

FIG. 40.15—Ormetoprim

folic acid metabolism, the combination becomes bactericidal and increases the spectrum of antimicrobial activity. Both mammals and bacteria use dihydrofolate reductase in folic acid metabolic pathways. However, trimethoprim and the other diaminopyrimidine analogs have a very low affinity for the enzyme in mammals and preferentially inhibit to a great extent the bacterial form of the enzyme at normal therapeutic doses.

Absorption, Distribution, Metabolism, Excretion. Trimethoprim is a lipid-soluble organic base that distributes to most tissues of the body and tends to concentrate in tissues with a greater acidity than plasma (e.g., prostate). Metabolism is by oxidation and conjugation reactions in the liver. Both parent compound and metabolites are excreted in the urine. Aditoprim has pharmacokinetic advantages over trimethoprim in that it has a larger V_d, longer $t_{1/2}$, and overall better tissue penetration.

Clinical Uses and Pharmacokinetics. The diaminopyrimidines are most commonly used in conjunction with sulfonamides to increase the antimicrobial spectrum of activity; rarely are they used alone in veterinary therapy due to the quick development of bacterial resistance. The therapeutic uses of trimethoprim and the other diaminopyrimidine analogs have been discussed with the individual sulfonamides they are used with in previous sections of this chapter and will not be covered in great detail here, except to delineate some of their general pharmacokinetic properties in animals. The pharmacokinetic parameters of trimethoprim and other diaminopyrimidines have been established for some species and are listed in Tables 40.6 and 40.7.

Readers requiring more information on specific properties of these diaminopyrimidines should consult Ascalone et al. 1986, Mengelers et al. 1990, Lohuis et al. 1992, Sutter et al. 1993, Wilson et al. 1987, Brown et al. 1989, Iversen et al. 1984, Vergin et al. 1984, or Aschhoff 1979.

RESIDUES IN FOOD ANIMALS. Tissue residues from sulfonamide use in food-producing animals are a concern of both US government agencies and the end consumers. The US Department of Agriculture (USDA)

TABLE 40.7—Some pharmacokinetic parameters of aditoprim, ormetoprim, tetroxoprim, and metioprim in animals

Species	Dose (mg/kg)	Route	V_d (L/kg)	$t_{1/2}$ (hr)	Clearance (mL/hr/kg)	Reference
		Aditoprim:				
Calves (80 kg, milk fed)	5.0	IV	10.44	13.0	11.03	Sutter et al. 1993
Calves (80 kg, conventionally fed)	5.0	IV	9.72	14.8	8.20	Sutter et al. 1993
Calves (160 kg, milk fed)	5.0	IV	9.64	10.7	12.17	Sutter et al. 1993
Calves (160 kg, conventionally fed)	5.0	IV	6.29	8.8	10.29	Sutter et al. 1993
Calves (210 kg, conventionally fed)	5.0	IV	7.16	7.2	13.75	Sutter et al. 1993
Calves (80 kg, milk fed)	5.0	PO	NR	11.6	NR	Sutter et al. 1993
Calves (80 kg, conventionally fed)	5.0	PO	NR	11.60	NR	Sutter et al. 1993
Calves (160 kg, milk fed)	5.0	PO	NR	10.2	NR	Sutter et al. 1993
Calves (160 kg, conventionally fed)	5.0	PO	NR	NR	NR	Sutter et al. 1993
Calves (210 kg, conventionally fed)	10.0	PO	NR	16.6	NR	Sutter et al. 1993
Dairy cows (3–7 yr old)	5.0	IV	6.28	7.26	820.0	Lohuis et al. 1992
Dairy cows (3–7 yr old, mammary endotoxin)	5.0	IV	12.25	about 7 hr	1000.0	Lohuis et al. 1992
		Ormetoprim:				
Calves (6-8 months old)	5.5/27.5[a]	IV	1.450	1.37	13.71	Wilson et al. 1987
Mare[b]	9.2/45.8[a]	IV	1.66	1.19	671.0	Brown et al. 1989
		Tetroxoprim:				
Dogs	5.0	IV	NR	5.45	NR	Vergin et al. 1984
		Metioprim:				
Dogs	5.0	IV	NR	3.07	NR	Vergin et al. 1984

Note: NR = not reported; IV = intravenously; PO = orally.
[a]First dose is trimethoprim; second dose is sulfadimethoxine.
[b]One mare studied.

has been charged with the task of inspecting meat and poultry destined for interstate sale. Both the Federal Insecticide, Fungicide, and Rodenticide Act of 1947 and the Toxic Substances Act authorize the USDA to test tissues of animals for drug residues and to determine if those tissues are in violation of federal residue guidelines. In 1973, the Food Safety Inspection Service (FSIS) of the USDA established the National Residue Program to be responsible for monitoring drug residues in animal tissues available for human consumption (Bevill 1989). FARAD (Food Animal Residue Avoidance Databank), a computerized databank of scientific and regulatory data, is available to assist the veterinarian, producer, and other individuals in solving drug- and chemical-residue problems in food-producing animals (Riviere et al. 1986) and also provides some excellent detection methods for sulfonamides and metabolites (Sharma et al. 1976; Agarwal 1992).

Sulfonamide residues were a problem in the United States for at least 25 years, having produced more drug-residue violations than any other drug, with the highest incidence occurring in pork, followed by veal and poultry. Residues in animal tissues consumed by humans are considered to be potential health hazards to humans. Toxic or allergic reactions to the sulfonamide class of antimicrobials have been reported in humans receiving therapeutic doses of sulfonamides. However, we are aware of no reports in the open literature about toxicity or other adverse reactions in humans consuming animal products containing trace amounts of sulfonamides or its metabolites. These trace amounts of drug may select for drug resistance to sulfonamides, especially those bacteria in the family Enterobacteriaceae, although the problem of transfer of drug-resistant strains of bacteria from animals to humans still needs further investigation (Bevill 1989). Recent evidence indicating that sulfonamides (in particular, sulfamethazine) may be carcinogenic in humans consuming small amounts over long periods of time (based on in vivo rat and mouse data) has heightened the FSIS's concern for controlling sulfonamide residues in food animals (USDA 1988).

The highest rate of sulfonamide-residue violations has historically occurred in swine. Sulfamethazine and sulfathiazole are the two most commonly used sulfonamides in swine feeds today. However, sulfamethazine is responsible for most of the sulfonamide-residue violations (97%) due to its mass incorporation in swine feeds and its longer half-life when compared to that of sulfathiazole (12.7 vs. 1.2 hr). The primary reasons for the occurrence of violative levels of sulfonamides in pork were failure to observe drug withdrawal time, improper feed mixing, and improper cleaning of feed-mixing equipment, causing a cross-contamination of feed (Bevill 1984, 1989). During the late 1970s, 13% of swine livers were found to be in violation of federal sulfonamide tissue concentrations. At that time the maximum amount of sulfonamide (parent compound) permitted in animal tissues was 0.1 ppm, with a 7-day withdrawal period. Drug manufacturers at this time increased the withdrawal time for sulfonamides used in animal feed from 7 to 15 days, and by 1980, the violation rate in liver tissue had fallen to 4%. In 1987, the rate was reported to be 3.8% (Augsburg 1989), with the rate decreasing significantly by the end of the 1990s.

In veal calves presented for slaughter, similar problems with sulfamethazine residues have been reported. The prevalence rate of sulfamethazine violations in veal calves was 1.9% in 1979 and 2.9% in 1981. Reasons for violations in this species include administering the drug to calves by individuals unaware of the drug withdrawal time constraints, unknowingly selling calves treated with sulfonamides, not following drug label directions, not seeking professional advice regarding drug use, and failing to maintain drug use records (Bevill 1989).

More information about residues in food-producing animals is presented in Chap. 58 of this textbook and also in previous editions. Several references are also available on this subject (Kaneene and Miller 1992; Bevill 1984; Dalvi 1988; Rosenberg 1985).

REFERENCES

Abdullah, A.S., and Baggot, J.D. 1988. The effect of food deprivation on the rate of sulfamethazine elimination in goats. Vet Res Commun 12:441–446.

Adamson, R.H., Bridges, J.W., Kibby, M.R., Walker, S.R., and Williams, R.T. 1970. The fate of sulfphdimethoxine in primates compared with other species. Biochem J 118:41–45.

Agarwal, V.K. 1992. High-performance liquid chromatographic methods for the determination of sulfonamides in tissue, milk, and eggs. J Chromatography 624:411–423.

Alavi, F.K., Rolf, L.L., and Clarke, C.R. 1993. The pharmacokinetics of sulfachlorpyridazine in channel catfish, *Icthlurus punctatus*. J Vet Pharmacol Therap 16:232–236.

Ames, T.R., Casagranda, C.L., Werdin, R.E., and Hanson, L.J. 1987. Effect of sulfadimethoxine-ormetroprim in the treatment of calves with induced Pasteurella pneumonia. AJVR 48(1):17–20.

Aronson, A.L., and Kirk, R.W. 1983. Antimicrobial drugs. In Textbook of Veterinary Internal Medicine: Diseases of the Dog and Cat. SJ Ettinger, Ed. WB Saunders Co., Philadelphia, pp. 338–366.

Ascalone, V., Jordan, J.C., and Ludwig, B.M. 1986. Determination of aditoprim, a new dihydrofolate reductase inhibitor, in the plasma of cows and pigs. J Chromatography 383:111–118.

Aschhoff, H.S. 1979. Tetroxoprim: A new inhibitor of bacterial dihydrofolate reductase. J Antimicrob Chemotherapy 5(Suppl B):19–25.

Ashworth, R.B., Epstein, R.L., Thomas, M.H., and Frobish, L.T. 1986. Sulfamethazine blood/tissue correlation study in swine. AJVR 47(12):2596–2603.

Astwood, E.B., Sullivan J., Bissell, A., and Tyslowitz, R. 1943. Action of certain sulfonamides and thiourea upon the thyroid gland of the rat. Endocrinology 32:210–225.

Augsberg, J.K. 1989. Sulfa residues in pork: An update. J Anim Sci 67:2817–2821.

Austin, F.H., and Kelly, W.R. 1966. Sulphamethylphenazole: A new long-acting sulphonamide. II. Some pharmacodynamic aspects in dogs, pigs and horses. Vet Rec 78(6):192–195.

Azad Kahn, A.K., Guthrie, G., Johnston, H.H., Truelove, S.C., Williamson, D.H. 1983. Tissue and bacterial splitting of sulphasalazine. Clin Sci 64(3):349–354.

Banerjee, N.C., Yadava, K.P., and Jha, H.N. 1974. Distribution of sulphaquinoxaline in tissues of poultry. Ind J Physiol Pharmacol 18(4):361–363.

Berger, S.L., Scagliotti, R.H., Lund, E.M. 1995. A quantitative study of the effects of tribrissen on canine tear production. JAAHA 31:236–241.

Bertone, A.L., Jones, R.L., and McIlwraith, C.W. 1988. Serum and synovial fluid steady-state concentrations of trimethoprim and sulfadiazine in horses with experimentally induced infectious arthritis. AJVR 49(10):1681–1687.

Bevill, R.F. 1984. Factors influencing the occurrence of drug residues in animal tissues after the use of antimicrobial agents in animal feeds. JAVMA 185(10):1124–1126.

———. 1988. Sulfonamides. In N.H. Booth and L.E. McDonald, eds., Veterinary Pharmacology and Therapeutics, 6th ed., pp. 785–795. Ames: Iowa State Univ Press.

———. 1989. Sulfonamide residues in domestic animals. J Vet Pharmacol Therap 12:241–252.

Bevill, R.F., Dittert, L.W., and Bourne, D.W.A. 1977a. Disposition of sulfonamides in food-producing animals IV: Pharmacokinetics of sulfamethazine in cattle following administration of an intravenous dose and three oral dosage forms. J Pharm Sci 66(5):619–623.

Bevill, R.F., Koritz, G.D., Dittert, L.W., and Bourne, W.A. 1977b. Disposition of sulfonamides in food-producing animals. V. Disposition of sulfathiazole in tissue, urine, and plasma of sheep following intravenous administration. J Pharm Sci 66(9):1297–1300.

Bevill, R.F., Sharma, R.M., Meachum, S.H., Wozniak, S.C., Bourne, D.W.A., and Dittert, L.W. 1977c. Disposition of sulfonamides in food-producing animals: Concentrations of sulfamethazine and its metabolites in plasma, urine, and tissues of lambs following intravenous adminstration. AJVR 38:973–977.

Biehl, L.G., Bevill, R.F., Limpoka, and Koritz, G.D. 1981. Sulfamethazine residues in swine. J Vet Pharmacol Therap 4:285–290.

Blackwell, T.E., Werdin, R.E., Eisenmenger, M.C., and FitzSimmons, M.A. 1989. Goitrogenic effects in offspring of swine fed sulfadimethoxine and ormetoprim in late gestation. JAVMA 194(4):519–523.

Bourne, D.W.A., Bevill, R.F., Sharma, R.M., Gural, R.P., and Dittert, L.W. 1977. Disposition of sulfonamides in food-producing animals: pharmacokinetics of sulfamethazine in lambs. AJVR 38:967–972.

Bourne, D.W.A., Bialer, M., Kittert, L.W., Hayashi, M., Rudawsky, G., Koritz, G.D., and Bevill, R.F. 1981. Disposition of sulfadimethoxine in cattle: inclusion of protein binding factors in a pharmacokinetic model. J Pharm Sci 70(9):1068–1074.

Boxenbaum, H.G., Fellig, J., Hanson, L.J., Snyder, W.E., and Kaplan, S.A. 1977. Pharmacokinetics of sulphadimethoxine in cattle. Res Vet Sci 23:24–28.

Bridges, J.W., Kibby, M.R., Walker, S.R., and Williams, R.T. 1968. Species differences in the metabolism of sulfadimethoxine. Biochem J 109:851–856.

Bridges, J.W., Walker, S.R., and Williams, R.T. 1969. Species differences in the metabolism and excretion of sulphasomidine and sulphamethomidine. Biochem J 111:173–179.

Brown, M.J., Wojcik, B., Burgess, E.D., and Smith, G.J. 1982. Adverse reactions to sulfaquinoxaline in coyote pups. JAVMA 181(11):1419–1420.

Brown, M.P., Gronwall, R.R., Cook, L.K., and Houston, A.E. 1993. Serum concentrations of ormetoprim/sulfadimethoxine in 1-3-day-old foals after a single dose of oral paste combination. Eq Vet J 25(1):73–74.

Brown, M.P., Gronwall, R.R., and Houston, A.E. 1989. Pharmacokinetics and body fluid and endometrial concentrations of ormetoprim-sulfadimethoxine in mares. Can J Vet Res 53:12–16.

Bulgin, M.S., Lane, V.M., Archer, T.E., Baggot, and Craigmill, A.L. 1991. Pharmacokinetics, safety and tissue residues of sustained-release sulfamethazine in sheep. J Vet Pharmacol Therap 14:36–45.

Bushby, S.R.M. 1980. Sulfonamide and trimethoprim combinations. JAVMA 176(10):1049–1053.

Cannon, R.W. 1976. Clinical evaluation of tribrissen: New antibacterial agent for dogs and cats. VMSAC 71(8):1090–1095.

Carlson, A., Rupe, B.D., Buss, D., Homman, C., and Leaton, J. 1976. Evaluation of a new prolonged-release sulfamethazine bolus for use in cattle. VMSAC 71(5):693–696.

Chapman, H.D. 1989. Chemotherapy of caecal coccidiosis: efficacy of toltrazuril, sulphaquinoxalin/pyrimethamine and amprolium/ethopabate, given in drinking water, against field isolated *Eimeria tenella.* Res Vet Sci 46:419–420.

Church, T.L., Janzen, E.D., Sisodia, C.S., and Radostits, O.M. 1979. Blood levels of sulfamethazine achieved in beef calves on medicated drinking water. Can Vet J 20:41–44.

Clark, J.G., Mackey, D.R., and Scheel, E.H. 1966. Evaluation of sustained-release sulfamethazine in infectious diseases of cattle. VMSAC 11:1103–1104.

Collins, B.K., Moore, C.P., and Hagee, J.H. 1986. Sulfonamide-associated keratoconjunctivitis sicca and corneal ulceration in a dysuric dog. JAVMA 189(8):924–926.

Cordle, M.K. 1989. Sulfonamide residues in pork: past, present, and future. J Anim Sci 67(10):2810–2816.

Craig, G.R. 1972. The place for potentiated trimethoprim in the therapy of diseases of the skin in dogs and cats. J Small Animal Pract 13:65–70.

Craig, G.R., and White, G. 1976. Studies in dogs and cats dosed wtih trimethoprim and sulphadiazine. Vet Rec 98(5):82–86.

Cribb, A.E. 1989. Idiosyncratic reactions to sulfonamides in dogs. JAVMA 195(11):1612–1614.

Daft, B.M., Bickford, A.A., and Hammarlund, M.A. 1989. Experimental and field sulfaquinoxaline toxicosis in Leghorn chickens. Avian Dis 33:30–34.

Dagorn, M., Moulin, G., Laurentie, M., and Delmas, J.M. 1991. Plasma and lung pharmacokinetics of trimethoprim and sulphadiazine combinations administered to broilers. Acta Veterinaria Scandinavica 87:273–277.

Dalvi, R.F. 1988. Comparative in vitro and in vivo drug metabolism in major and minor food-producing species. Vet Human Toxicol 30(Suppl 1):22–25.

Das, K.M., Chowdhury, J.R., Zapp, B., and Fara, J.W. 1979. Small bowel absorption of sulfasalazine and its hepatic metabolism in human beings, cats, and rats. Gastroenterology 77:280–284.

Das, K.M., and Dubin, R. 1976. Clinical pharmacokinetics of sulphasalazine. Clin Pharmacokinetics 1:406–425.

Davis, R.E., and Jackson, J.M. 1973. Trimethoprim/sulphmethoxazole and folate metabolism. Pathology 5:23–29.

Davitiyananda, D., and Rasmussen F. 1974. Half-lives of sulfadoxine and trimethoprim after a single intravenous infusion in cows. Acta Vet Scand 15:356–365.

Debacker, P., Belpaire, F.M., Bogaert, M.G., and Debackere, M. 1982. Pharmacokinetics of sulfamerazine and antipyrine in neonatal and young lambs. AJVR 43(10):1744–1751.

Del Soldato, P., Campieri, M., Brignola, C., Bazzocchi, G., Gionchetti, P., Lanfranchi, G.A., and Tamba, M. 1985. A possible mechanism of action of sulfasalazine and

5-aminosalicylic acid in inflammatory bowel disease: interaction with oxygen free radicals. Gastroenterology 89(5):1215–1216.

Divers, J., Byars, T.D., Murch, O., and Sigel, C.W. 1981. Experimental induction of *Proteus mirabilis* cystitis in the pony and evaluation of therapy with trimethoprim-sulfadiazine. AJVR 42:1203–1205.

Dodds, W.J. 1993. Hemorrhagic complications attributable to certain drugs. JAVMA 202(5):702–703.

———. 1997. Letter to the Editor. J Vet Internal Med 11:267–268.

Duffee, E., Bevill, R.F., Thurmon, J.C., Luther, H.G., Nelson, D.E., and Hacker, F.E. 1984. Pharmacokinetics of sulfamethazine in male, female, and castrated male swine. J Vet Pharmacol Therap 7:203–211.

Dunbar, R., and Foreyt, W.J. 1985. Prevention of coccidiosis in domestic dogs and captive coyotes (*Canis latrans*) with sulfadimethoxine-ormetoprim combination. AJVR 46(9):1899–1902.

Eastwood, M.A. 1980. Pharmacokinetic patterns of sulfasalazine. Therapeutic Drug Monitoring 2:149–152.

Ellison, T., Scheidy, S.F., Tucker, S., Scott, G.C., and Bucy, C.B. 1967. Blood concentration studies in cattle of a sustained-release form of sulfamethazine. JAVMA 150(6):629–633.

Elsheikh, H.A., Ali, B.H., Homeida, A.M., Hassan, T., and Hapke, H.J. 1991. Pharmacokinetics of antipyrine and sulphadimidine (sulfamethazine) in camels, sheep, and goats. J Vet Pharmacol Therap 14:269–275.

Eppel, J.G., and Thiessen, J.J. 1984. Liquid chromatographic analysis of sulfaquinoxaline and its application to pharmacokinetic studies in rabbits. J Pharm Sci 73(11):1635–1638.

Epstein, R.L., and Ashworth, R.B. 1989. Tissue sulfonamide concentration and correlation in turkeys. AJVR 50(6):926–928.

Fenwick, B.W., and Olander, H.J. 1987. Experimental infection of weanling pigs with *Salmonella typhisuis:* effect of feeding low concentrations of chlortetracycline, penicillin, and sulfamethazine. AJVR 48(11):1568–1573.

Fish, J.G., Morgan, D.W., and Horton, C.R. 1965. Clinical experiences with sulfadimethoxine in small animal practice. VMSAC 60(12):1201–1203.

Fullerton, F.R., Kushmaul, R.J., Suber, R.L., and Littlefield, N.A. 1987. Influence of oral administration of sulfamethazine on thyroid hormone levels in Fischer 344 rats. J Toxicol Environ Health 22:175–185.

Garg, G.P., Cho, C.H., and Ogle, C.W. 1991. The role of the gastric mucosal sulphydryls in the ulcer-protecting effects of sulfasalazine. J Pharm Pharmacol 43:733–734.

Garg, S.K., and Uppal, R.P. 1997. Bioavailability of sulfamethoxypyridazine following intramuscular or subcutaneous administration in goats. Vet Res 28:101–104.

Garwacki, S., Hornik, H., Karlik, W., and Dabrowski, J. 1991. Pharmacokinetics of sulfamerazine in sheep fed ad libitum and fasted. Acta Veterinaria Scandinavica 87:145–146.

Giger, U., Werner, L.L., Millichamp, N.J., and Gorman, N.T. 1985. Sulfadiazine-induced allergy in six Doberman Pinschers. JAVMA 186(5):479–484.

Giwercman, A., and Skakkebaek, N.E. 1986. The effect of salicylazosulphapyridine (sulfasalazine) on male fertility. A review. Inter J Andrology 9:38–52.

Gomez-Bautista, M., and Rojo-Vazauez, F.A. 1986. Chemotherapy and chemoprophylaxis of hepatic coccidiosis with sulphadimethoxine and pyrimethamine. Res Vet Sci 41:28–32.

Goren, E., de Jong, W.A., and Doornenbal, P. 1987. Additional studies on the therapeutic efficacy of sulphadimidine sodium in experimental *Eschericha coli* infection of broilers. Vet Quarterly 9(1):86–87.

Guard, C.L., Schwark, W.S., Friedman, D.S., Blackshear, P., and Haluska, M. 1986. Age-related alterations in trimethoprim-sulfadiazine disposition following oral or parenteral administration in calves. Can J Vet Res 50:342–346.

Guise, H.J., Penny, H.C., and Petherick, D.J. 1986. Streptococcal meningitis in pigs: field trial to study the prophylactic effect of trimethoprim/sulphadiazine medication in feed. Vet Rec 119(16):395–400.

Hall, I.A., Campbell, K.L., Chambers, M.D., and Davis, C.N. 1993. Effect of trimethoprim/sulfamethoxazole on thyroid function in dogs with pyoderma. JAVMA 202:1959–1962.

Hayashi, M., Bourne, D.W.A., Bevill, R.F., and Koritz, G.D. 1979. Disposition of sulfonamides in food-producing animals: pharmacokinetics of sulfamerazine in ewe lambs. AJVR 49(11):1578–1582.

Hoult, J.R.S., and Moore, P.K. 1978. Sulphasalazine is a potent inhibitor of prostaglandin 15-hydroxydehydrogenase: possible basis for therapeutic action in ulcerative colitis. Br J Pharmacol 64:6–8.

Howell, T.H., Reddy, M.S., Weber, H.P., Li, K.L., Alfano, M.C., Vogel, R, Tanner, ACR, and Williams, RC. 1989. Sulfadiazines prevent plaque formation and gingivitis in beagles. J Periodont Res 25:197–200.

Imamura, Y., Nakamura, H., and Otagiri, M. 1986. Effect of phenylbutazone on serum protein binding of sulfadimethoxine in different animal species. J Pharmacobio-Dyn 9:694–696.

———. 1989. Effect of phenylbutazone on serum protein binding and pharmacokinetic behavior of sulfadimethoxine in rabbits, dogs and rats. J Pharmacobio-Dyn 12:208–215.

Inada, H., Endoh, M., Katayama, K., Kakemi, M., and Koizumi, T. 1989. Factors affecting sulfisoxizole transport through excised rat skin during iontophoresis. Chem Pharm Bull 37(7):1870–1873.

Iverson, P., Vergin, H., and Madsen, P.O. 1984. Renal handling and lymph concentration of tetroxoprim and metioprim: An experimental study in dogs. J Urology 132:362–362.

James, M.O., and Barron, M.G. 1988. Disposition of sulfadimethoxine in the lobster (*Homarus americanus.* Vet Human Toxicol 30(Suppl 1): 36–40.

Joyner, L.P., Catchpole, J., and Berrett, S. 1983. *Eimeria stiedai* in rabbits: The demonstration of responses to chemotherapy. Res Vet Sci 34:64–67.

Kajinuma, H., Kuzuya, T., and Ide, T. 1974. Effects of hypoglycemic sulfonamides on glucagon and insulin secretion in ducks and dogs. Diabetes 23(5):412–417.

Kaneene, J.B., and Miller, R. 1992. Description and evaluation of the influence of veterinary presence on the use of antibiotics and sulfonamides in dairy herds. JAVMA 201(1):68–76.

Khan, A.K.A., Guthrie, G., Johnston, H.H., Truelove, S.C., and Williamson, D.H. 1983. Tissue and bacterial splitting of sulphasalazine. Clin Sci 64:349–354.

Kleinow, K.M., and Lech, J.J. 1988. A review of the pharmacokinetics and metabolism of sulfadimethoxine in the rainbow trout. Vet Human Toxicol 30(Suppl 1):26–30.

Kobland, J.D., Gale, G.O., Maddock, H.M., Garces, T.R., and Simkins, K.L. 1984. Comparative efficacy of sulfamethazine and sulfathiazole in feed for control of *Bordetella bronchiseptica* infection in swine. AJVR 45(4):720–723.

Koritz, G.D., Bevill, R.F., Bourne, D.W.A., and Dittert, L.W. 1978. Disposition of sulfonamides in food-producing animals: pharmacokinetics of sulfathiazole in swine. AJVR 39(3):481–484.

Koritz, G.D., Bourne, D.W.A., Dittert, L.W., and Bevill, R.F. 1977. Disposition of sulfonamides in food-producing

animals: pharmacokinetics of sulfathiazole in sheep. AJVR 38:979–982.
Koudela, B., and Bokova, A. 1997. The effect of cotrimoxazole on experimental *Cryptosporidium parvum* infection in kids. Vet Res 28:405–412.
Lapka, R., Urbanova, Z., Raskova, H., Cerny, J., Sykora, Z., Vanecek, J., Ploak, L., and Kubicek, A. 1980. Acetylation of sulphadimidine in calves. Gen Pharmacol 11:147–148.
Lashev, L.D., Bochukov, A.K., and Penchev, G. 1995. Effect of testosterone on the pharmacokinetics of sulphadimidine and sulphachloropyrazine in roosters: a preliminary report. Br Vet J 151:331–336.
Lashev, L.D., and Mihailov, R. 1994. Pharmacokinetics of sulphamethoxazole and trimethoprim administered intravenously and orally to japanese quails. J Vet Pharmacol Therap 17:327–330.
Li, T., Qiao, G.L., Hu, G.Z., Meng, F.D., Qiu, U.S., Zhang, X.Y., Guo, W.X., Yie, H.L., Li, S.F., and Li, S.Y. 1995. Comparative plasma and tissue pharmacokinetics and drug residue profiles of different chemotherapeutants in fowls and rabbits. J Vet Pharmacol Therap 18:260–273.
Ling, G.V., Rohrich, P.J., Ruby, A.L., Johnson, D.L., and Jang, S.S. 1984. Canine urinary tract infections: a comparison of in vitro antimicrobial susceptibility test results and response to oral therapy with ampicillin or with trimethoprim-sulfa. JAVMA 185(3):277–281.
Ling, G.V., and Ruby, A.L. 1979. Trimethoprim in combination with a sulfonamide for oral treatment of canine urinary tract infections. JAVMA 174(9):1003–1005.
Littlefield, N.A., Gaylor, D.W., Blackwell, B.N., and Allen, R.R. 1989. Chronic toxicity/carcinogenicity studies of sulphamethazine in B6C3F$_1$ mice. Fd Chem Toxicol 27(7):455–463.
Littlefield, N.A., Sheldon, W.G., Allen, R., and Gaylor, D.W. 1990. Chronic toxicity/carcinogenicity studies of sulphamethazine in Fischer 344/N rats: Two-generation exposure. Food Chem Toxicol 28(3):157–167.
Lohuis, J.A.C.M., Sutter, H.M., Graser, T., Ludwig, B., van Miert, A.S.J.P.A.M., Rehm, W.F., Rohde, E., Schneider, B., Wanner, and van Werven, T. 1992. Effects of endotoxin-induced mastitis on the pharmacokinetic properties of aditoprim in dairy cows. AJVR 53(12):2311–2314.
MacKenzie, C.G., and MacKenzie, J.B. 1943. Effect of sulfonamides and thiourea on thyroid gland and basal metabolism. Endocrinology 32:185–209.
Mathis, G.F., and McDougald, L.R. 1984. Effectiveness of therapeutic anticoccidial drugs against recently isolated coccidia. Poultry Sci 63:1149–1153.
McCaig, J. 1970. A clinical trial using trimethoprim-sulphadiazine in dogs and cats. Vet Rec 87(9):265–266.
McCandlish, I.A.P., and Thompson, H. 1979. Canine bordetellosis: chemotherapy using a sulphadiazine-trimethoprim combination. Vet Rec 105(3):51–54.
Mengelers, M.J.B., van Klingeren, B., and van Miert, A.S.J.P.A.M. 1990. In vitro susceptibility of some porcine respiratory tract pathogens to aditoprim, trimethoprim, sulfadimethoxine, sulfamethoxazole, and combinations of these agents. AJVR 51(11):1860–1864.
Mengelers, M.J.B., van Gogh, E.R., Kuiper, H.A., Pijpers, A., Verheijden, J.H.M., and Van Miert, A.S.J.P.A.M. 1995. Pharmacokinetics of sulfadimethoxine and sulfamethoxazole in combination with trimethoprim after intravenous administration to healthy and pneumonic pigs. J Vet Pharmacol Therap 18:243–253.
Miller, G.E., Stowe, C.M., Jegers, A., and Bucy, C.B. 1969. Blood concentration studies of a sustained release form of sulfamethazine in cattle. JAVMA 154(7):733–779.
Mitchell, AD, and Paulson, GD. 1986. Depletion kinetics of 14C-sulfamethazine {4-amino-N-(4,6-dimethyl-2-pyr}midinyl)benzene[U-14C]sulfonamide metabolism in swine. Drug Metabol Disposition 14(2):161–165.
Mitchell, A.D., Paulson, G.D., and Zaylskie, R.G. 1986. Steady state kinetics of 14C-sulfamethazine {4-amino-N-(4,6-dimethyl-2-pyr}midinyl)benzene[U-14C]sulfonamide metabolism in swine. Drug Metabol Disposition 14(2):155–160.
Morgan, R.V., and Bachrach, A. 1982. Keratoconjunctivitis sicca associated with sulfonamide therapy in dogs. JAVMA 180(4):432–434.
Nawaz, M., and Nawaz, R. 1983. Pharmacokinetics and urinary excretion of sulphadimidine in sheep during summer and winter. Vet Rec 112(16):379–381.
Neer, T.M., and Savant, R.L. 1992. Hypoprothrombinemia secondary to administration of sulfaquinoxaline to dogs in a kennel setting. JAVMA 200(9):1344–1345.
Nielsen, P., and Gyrd-Hansen, N. 1994. Oral bioavailability of sulphadiazine and trimethoprim in fed and fasted pigs. Res Vet Sci 56:48–52.
Noli, C., Koeman, J.P., and Willemse, T. 1995. A retrospective evaluation of adverse reactions to trimethoprim-sulphonamide combinations in dogs and cats. Vet Quarterly 17:123–128.
Nouws, J.F.M., Firth, E.C., Vree, T.B., and Baakman, M. 1987. Pharmacokinetics and renal clearance of sulfamethazine, sulfamerazine, and sulfadiazine and their N4-acetyl and hydroxy metabolites in horses. AJVR 48(3):392–402.
Nouws, J.F.M., Geertsma, M.F., Grondel, J.L., Aerts, M.M.L., Vree, T.B., and Kan, C.A. 1988a. Plasma disposition and renal clearance of sulphadimidine and its metabolites in laying hens. Res Vet Sci 44:202–207.
Nouws, J.F.M., Meesen, B.P.W., van Gogh, H., Korstanje, C., van Miert, A.S.J.P.A.M., Vree, T.B., and Degen, M. 1988b. The effect of testosterone and rutting on the metabolism and pharmacokinetics of sulphadimidine in goats. J Vet Pharmacol Therap 11:145–154.
Nouws, J.F.M., Mevius, D., Vree, T.B., Baakman, M., and Degen, M. 1988c. Pharmacokinetics, metabolism, and renal clearance of sulfadiazine, sulfamerazine, and sulfamethazine and of their N_4-acetyl and hydroxy metabolites in calves and cows. AJVR 49(7):1059–1065.
Nouws, J.F.M., Mevius, D., Vree, T.B., and Degen, M. 1989a. Pharmacokinetics and renal clearance of sulphadimidine, sulphamerazine, and sulphadiazine and their N4-acetyl and hydroxy metabolites in pigs. Vet Quarterly 11(2):78–86.
Nouws, J.F.M., van Ginneken, J.T., Grondel, J.L., and Degen, M. 1993. Pharmacokinetics of sulphadiazine and trimethoprim in carp (*Cyprinus carpio* L.) acclimated at two different temperatures. J Vet Pharmacol Therap 16:110–113.
Nouws, J.F.M., Vree, T.B., Baakman, M., and Tijhuis, M. 1983. Effect of age on the acetylation and deacetylation reactions of sulphadimidine and N4-acetylsulphadimidine in calves. J Vet Pharmacol Therap 6:13–22.
Nouws, J.F.M., Vree, T.B., Baakman, M., Driessens, F., Breukink, H.J., and Mevius, D. 1986a. Age and dosage dependency in the plasma disposition and the renal clearance of sulfamethazine and its N4-acetyl and hydroxy metabolites in calves and cows. AJVR 47(3):642–649.
Nouws, J.F.M., Vree, T.B., Baakman, M., Driessens, F., Smulders, A., and Holtkamp, J. 1985a. Disposition of sulfadimidine and its N_4-acetyl and hydroxy metabolites in horse plasma. J Vet Pharmacol Therap 8:303–311.
Nouws, J.F.M., Vree, T.B., Baakman, M., Driessens, F., Vellenga, L., and Mevius, D.J. 1986b. Pharmacokinetics, renal clearance, tissue distribution, and residue aspects of sulphadimidine and its N_4-acetyl metabolite in pigs. Vet Quarterly 8(2):123–135.
Nouws, J.F.M., Vree, T.B., Breukink, H.J., Baakman, M., Driessens, F., and Smulders, A. 1985b. Dose dependent disposition of sulphadimidine and of its N_4-acetyl and

hydroxy metabolites in plasma and milk of dairy cows. Vet Quarterly 7(3):177–186.
Nouws, J.F.M., Watson, A.D.J., van Miert, A.S.J.P.A.M., Degen, M., van Gogh, H., and Vree, T.B. 1989b. Pharmacokinetics and metabolism of sulphadimidine in kids at 12 and 18 weeks of age. J Vet Pharmacol Therap 12:19–24.
Patterson, J.M., and Grenn, H.H. 1975. Hemorrhage and death in dogs following the administration of sulfaquinoxaline. Can Vet J 16(9):265–268.
Piercy, D.W.T., Williams, R.B., and White, G. 1984. Evaluation of a mixture of trimethoprim and sulphaquinoxaline for the treatment of poultry: safety and palatability studies. Vet Rec 114(3):60–62.
Pohlenz-Zertuche, H.O., Brown, M.P., Gronwall, R., Kunkle, G.A., and Merritt, K. 1992. Serum and skin concentrations after multiple-dose oral administration of trimethoprim-sulfadiazine in dogs. AJVR 53(7):1273–1276.
Powers, T.E., Powers, J.D., Garg, R.C., Scialli, V.T., and Hajian, G.H. 1980. Trimethoprim and sulfadiazine: Experimental infection of beagles. AJVR 41(7):1117–1122.
Prescott, J.F., and Baggot, J.D., eds. 1993. Sulfonamides, trimethoprim, ormetoprim, and their combinations. In Antimicrobial Therapy in Veterinary Medicine, 2d ed., pp. 229–251. Ames: Iowa State Univ Press.
Ribelin, W.E., Owen, G., Rubin, L.F., Levinskas, G.J., and Agersborg, H.P.K. 1967. Development of cataracts in dogs and rats from prolonged feeding of sulfaethoxypyridazine. Toxicol Appl Pharmacol 10:557–564.
Riffat, S., Nawaz, M., and Rehman, Z.U. 1982. Pharmacokinetics of suphadimidine in normal and febrile dogs. J Vet Pharmacol Therap 5:131–135.
Righter, H.F., Worthington, J.M., and Mercer, H.D. 1971. Tissue-residue depletion of sulfamethazine in calves and chickens. AJVR 32(7):1003–1006.
Righter, H.R., Showalter, D.H., and Teske, R.H. 1979. Pharmacokinetic study of sulfadimethoxine depletion in suckling and growing pigs. AJVR 49(5):713–715.
Riviere, J.E., Craigmill, A.L., and Sundlof, S.F. 1986. Food animal residue avoidance databank (FARAD): an automated pharmacologic databank for drug and chemical residue avoidance. J Food Protection 49(10):826–830.
Robb, C.A., Carroll, P.T., Tippett, L.O., and Langston, J.B. 1971. The diffusion of selected sulfonamides, trimethoprim, and diaveridine into prostatic fluid of dogs. Invest Urology 8(6):679–685.
Rosenberg, M.C. 1985. Update on the sulfonamide residue problem. JAVMA 187(7):704–705.
Rowland, P.H., Center, S.A., and Dougherty, S.A. 1992. Presumptive trimethoprim-sulfadiazine-related hepatotoxicosis in a dog. JAVMA 200(3):348–350.
Sainsbury, D.W.B. 1988. Potentiated sulphaquinoxaline used as "strategic medication" for broiler poultry. Vet Rec 122(16):395.
Scheidy, S.F., and Bucy, C.B. 1967. Evaluation of a prolonged-acting oral dose form of sulfamethazine in cattle. VMSAC 62(12):1161–1164.
Shafii, A., Chowdhury, J.R., and Das, K.M. 1982. Absorption, enterohepatic circulation, and excretion of 5-aminosalicylic acid in rats. Am J Gastroenterology 77(5):297–299.
Sharma, J.P., Perkins, E.G., and Bevill, R.F. 1976. High-pressure liquid chromatographic separation, identification, and determination of sulfa drugs and their metabolites in urine. J Pharm Sci 1606–1608.
Shimoda, M., Kokue, E., Itani, M., Hayama, T., and Vree, T.B. 1989. Nonlinear pharmacokinetics of intravenous sulphadimethoxine and its dosage regimen in pigs. Vet Quarterly 11(4):242–250.
Shoaf, S.E., Schwark, W.S., and Guard, C.L. 1987. The effect of age and diet on sulfadiazine/trimethoprim disposition following oral and subcutaneous administration to calves. J Vet Pharmacol Therap 10:331–345.
———. 1989. Pharmacokinetics of sulfadiazine/trimethoprim in neonatal male calves: effect of age and penetration into cerebrospinal fluid. AJVR 50(3):396–403.
Shoaf, S.E., Schwark, W.S., Guard, C.L., and Schwartsman, R.V. 1986. Pharmacokinetics of trimethoprim/sulfadiazine in neonatal calves: influence of synovitis. J Vet Pharmacol Therap 9:446–454.
Sigel, C.W., Ling, G.V., Bushby, R.M., Woolley, J.L., DeAngelis, D., and Eure, S. 1981. Pharmacokinetics of trimethoprim and sulfadiazine in the dog: urine concentrations after oral administration. AJVR 42(6): 996–1001.
Sigel, C.W., Macklin, A.W., Grace, M.E., and Tracy, C.H. 1981. Trimethoprim and sulfadiazine concentrations in aqueous and vitreous humors of the dog. VMSAC 76(7):991–993.
Singh, M.K., Jayachandran, C., Roy, G.P., and Banerjee, N.C. 1988. Pharmacokinetics and distribution of sulphadimidine in plasma, milk and uterine fluid of female buffaloes. Vet Res Commun 12:41–46.
Slatter, D.H., and Blogg, J.R. 1978. Keratoconjunctivitis sicca in dogs associated with sulphonamide administration. Aust Vet J 54:444–446.
Slaughter, R.E. 1972. Potentiated trimethoprim for the therapy of calf scours. New Zealand Vet J 20:221–223.
Slavik, D., Oehme, F.W., and Schoneweis, D.A. 1980. Plasma levels of sulfadimethoxine in swine given the medication in their water. VMSAC 75(6):1035–1038.
Soli, N.E., Framstad, T., Skjerve, E., Sohlberg, S., and Odegaard, S.A. 1990. A comparison of some of the pharmacokinetic parameters of three commercial sulfphadiazine/trimethoprim combined preparations given orally to pigs. Vet Res Commun 14:403–410.
Squibb, K.S., Michel, C.M.F., Zelikoff, J.T, and O'Conner, J.M. 1988. Sulfadimethoxine pharmacokinetics and metabolism in the channel catfish (*Ictalurus punctatus*). Vet Human Toxicol 30(Suppl 1):31–35.
Srivastava, A.K., and Rampal, S. 1990. Disposition kinetics and dosage regimen of sulphamethazine in sheep (*Ovis aries*. Br Vet J 146:239–242.
Stampa, S. 1986. A field trial comparing the efficacy of sulphamonomethoxine, penicillin, and tarantula poison in the treatment of pododermatitis circumspecta of cattle. J So African Vet Assn 57(2):91–93.
Stockner, P.K. 1993. More on hemorrhagic complications attributable to certain drugs. JAVMA 202:1547.
Suber, R.L., Lee, C., Torosian, G., and Edds, G.T. 1981. Pharmacokinetics of sulfisoxazole compared to humans and two monogastric species. J Pharm Sci 70(9):981–984.
Sullivan, P.S., Arrington, K., West, R., and McDonald, T.P. 1992. Thrombocytopenia associated with administration of trimethoprim/sulfadiazine in a dog. JAVMA 201(11):1741–1744.
Sutter, H.M., Riond, J.L., and Wanner, M. 1993. Comparative pharmacokinetics of aditoprim in milk-fed and conventionally fed calves of different ages. Res Vet Sci 54:86–93.
Swarm, R.L., Robers, G.K.S., Levy, A.C., and Hines, L.R. 1973. Observations on the thyroid gland in rats following the administration of sulfamethoxazole and trimethoprim. Toxicol Appl Pharmacol 24:351–363.
Sweeney, R.W., Bardalaye, P.C., Smith, C.M., Soma, L.R., and Uboh, C.E. 1993. Pharmacokinetic model for predicting sulfamethazine disposition in pigs. AJVR 54(5):750–754.

Turnwald, G.H., Gossett, K.A., Cox, H.U., Kearney, M.T., Roy, A.F., Thomas, D.E., and Troy, G.C. 1986. Comparison of single-dose and conventional trimethoprim-sulfadiazine therapy in experimental *Staphylococcus intermedius* cystitis in the female dog. AJVR 47(12):2621–2623.

Twedt, D.C., Kiehl, K.J., Lappin, M.R., and Getzy, D.M. 1997. Association of hepatic necrosis with trimethoprim sulfonamide administration in 4 dogs. J Vet Internal Med 11:20–23.

Ueda, M., Tsurui, Y., and Koizumi, T. 1972. Studies on metabolism of drugs. XII. Quantitative separation of metabolites in human and rabbit urine after oral administration of sulfamonomethoxine and sulfamethomidine. Chem Pharm Bull 20:2042–2046.

Uno, T., Kushima, T., and Hiraoka, T. 1967. Studies on the metabolism of sulfadimethoxine. II. Determinations of metabolites in human and rabbit urine after oral administration of sulfadimethoxine. Chem Pharm Bull 15:1272–1276.

USDA Food Safety Inspection Service, Residue Evaluation and Planning Division. 1988. Program Report: Sulfamethazine (SMZ) Control Program, part 1: Mar 7–June 13, 1988.

USPDI. 1998. Potentiated Sulfonamides. In USPDI Vols. I and II Update, pp. 1503–1518. Sept. US Pharmacopeial Convention, Rockville, MD.

Van Duijkeren, E., van Klingeren, B., Vulto, A.G., van Oldruitenborgh-Oosterbann, M.M.S., Breukink, H.J., van Miert, A.S.J.P.A.M. 1994a. In vitro susceptibility of equine *Salmonella* strains to trimethoprim and sulfonamide alone or in combination. Am J Vet Res 55:1386–1390.

Van Duijkeren, E., Vulto, A.G., and Van Miert, A.S.J.P.A.M. 1994b. Trimethoprim/sulfonamide combination in the horse: a review. J Vet Pharmacol Therap 17:64–73.

Van Duijkeren, E., Vulto, A.G., van Oldruitenborgh-Oosterbann, M.M.S., Kessels, B.G.F., van Miert, A.S.J.P.A.M., and Breukink, H.J. 1995. Pharmacokinetics of trimethoprim/sulphachlorpyridazine in horses after oral, nasogastric and intravenous administration. J Vet Pharmacol Therap 18:47–53.

van Ginneken, V.J.T., Nouws, J.F.M., Grondel, J.L., Driessens, F., and Degen, M. 1991. Pharmacokinetics of sulphadimidine in carp (*Cyprinus carpio* L.) and rainbow trout (*Salmo gairdneri* Richardson) acclimated at two different temperature levels. Vet Quarterly 13(2):88–96.

van Gogh, R., van Deurzen, E.J.M., van Duin, C.T.M., and van Miert, A.S.J.P.A.M. 1984. Effect of staphylococcal enterotoxin B–induced diarrhoea on the pharmacokinetics of sulphadimidine in the goat. J Vet Pharmacol Therap 7:303–305.

Van Miert, A.S.J.P.A.M. 1994. The sulfonamide-diaminopyrimidine story. J Vet Pharmacol Therap 17:309–316.

Van Miert, A.S.J.P.A.M., Peters, R.H.M., Basudde, C.D.K., Nijmeijer, S.N., Van Duin, C.T.M., Van Gogh, H., and Korstanje, C. 1988. Effect of trenbolone and testosterone on the plasma elimination rates of SMZ, trimethoprim, and antipyrine in female dwarf goats. AJVR 49(12):2060–2064.

Vergin, H., Bishop-Freudling, G.B., Foing, N., Szelenyi, I., Armengaud, H., and van Tho, T. 1984. Diffusion of metioprim, tetroxoprim and sulphadiazine in the cerebrospinal fluid of dogs with healthy meninges and dogs with experimental meningitis. Chemotherapy 30:297–304.

Walker, C.C., and Barker, S.A. 1994. Extraction and enzyme immunoassay of sulfadimethoxine residues in channel catfish (*Ictalurus punctatus*) muscle. JAOAC Internat 77:908–916.

Walker, S.R., and Williams, R.T. 1972. The metabolism of sulphadimethoxypyrimidine. Xenobiotica 2(1):69–75.

Weijkamp, K., Faghihi, S.M., Nijmeijer, S.M., Witkamp, R.F., and van Miert, A.S.J.P.A.M. 1994. Oral bioavailability of sulphamethoxydiazine, sulphathiazole and sulphamoxazole in dwarf goats. Vet Quarterly 16:33–37.

Weiss, D.J., and Adams, L.G. 1987. Aplastic anemia associated with trimethoprim-sulfadiazine and fenbendazole adminstration in a dog. JAVMA 191(9):1119–1120.

Weiss, D.J., and Klausner, J.S. 1990. Drug-associated aplastic anemia in dogs: Eight cases. 1984–1988. JAVMA 196(3):472–475.

White, G., and Prior, S.D. 1982. Comparative effects of oral administration of trimethoprim/sulphadiazine or oxytetracycline on the faecal flora of horses. Vet Rec 111(14):316–318.

White, G., and Williams, R.B. 1983. Evaluation of a mixture of trimethoprim and sulphaquinoxaline for the treatment of bacterial and coccidial diseases of poultry. Vet Rec 113(26–27):608–612.

Williams, R.B., Farebrother, D.A., and Latter, V.S. 1995. Coccidiosis: a radiological study of sulphaquinoxaline distribution in infected and uninfected chickens. J Vet Pharmacol Therap 18:172–179.

Wilson, R.C., Hammond, L.S., Clark, C.H., and Ravis, W.R. 1989. Bioavailability and pharmacokinetics of sulfamethazine in the pony. J Vet Pharmacol Therap 12:99–102.

Wilson, W.D., George, L.W., Baggot, J.D., Adamson, P.J.W., Hietala, S.K., and Mihalyi, J.E. 1987. Ormethoprim-sulfadimethoxine in cattle: pharmacokinetics, bioavailability, distribution to the tears, and in vitro activity against *Moraxella bovis.* AJVR 48(3):407–414.

Witcamp, R.F., van't Klooster, G.A.E., Nijmeijer, S.M., Kolker, H.J., Noordhoek, J., and van Miert, A.S.J.P.A.M. 1993. Hormonal regulation of oxidative drug metabolism in the dwarf goat: the effect of sex hormonal treatment on plasma disposition and metabolite formation of sulphadimidine. J Vet Pharmacol Therap 16:55–62.

Witcamp, R.F., Yun, H.-I., van't Klooster, G.A.E., van Mosel, J.F., van Mosel, M., Ensink, J.M., Noordhoek, J., and van Miert, A.S.J.P.A.M. 1992. Comparative aspects and sex differentiation of plasma sulfamethazine elimination and metabolite formation in rats, rabbits, dwarf goats, and cattle. AJVR 53(10):1830–1835.

Woolly, J.L., and Sigel, C.W. 1982. Development of pharmacokinetic models for sulfonamides in food animals: metabolic depletion profile of sulfadiazine in the calf. AJVR 43(5):768–774.

Yagi, N., Agata, I., Kawamura, T., Tanaka, Y., Sakamoto, M., Itoh, M., Sekikawa, H., and Takada, M. 1981. Fundamental pharmacokinetic behavior of sulfadimethoxine, sulfamethazole and their biotransformed products in dogs. Chem Pharm Bull 29(12):3741–3747.

Younan, W., Nouws, J.F.M., Homeid, A.M., Vree, T.B., and Degen, M. 1989. Pharmacokinetics and metabolism of suphadimidine in the camel. J Vet Pharmacol Therap 12:327–329.

Youssef, S.A.H., el-Gendi, A.Y.I., el-Sayed, M.G.A., Atef, M., and Abdel, S.A. 1981. Some pharmacokinetic and biochemical aspects of sulphadiazine and sulphadimidine in ewes. J Vet Pharmacol Therap 4:173–182.

Yuan, Z.-H., and Fung, K.-F. 1990. Pharmacokinetics of sulfadimidine and its N4-acetyl metabolite in healthy and diseased rabbits infected with *Pasteurella multocida.* J Vet Pharmacol Therap 13:192–197.

Yuan, Z.-H., Miao, X.-Q., and Yin, Y.-H. 1997. Pharmacokinetics of ampicillin and sulfadimidine in pigs infected experimentally with Streptococcus suum. J Vet Pharmacol Therap 20:318–322.

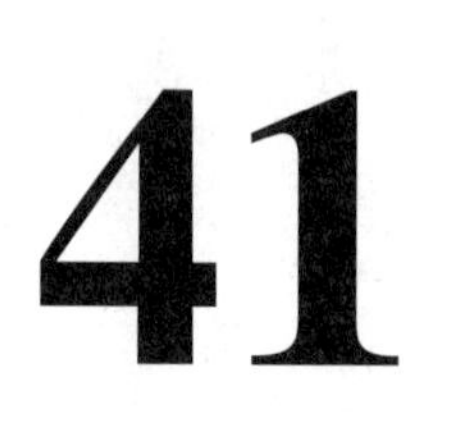

PENICILLINS AND RELATED β-LACTAM ANTIBIOTICS

SHELLY L. VADEN AND JIM E. RIVIERE

Mechanism of Action of β-Lactam Antibiotics
Microbial Resistance to β Lactams
Penicillins
Cephalosporins
Other β-Lactam Antibiotics

In 1928, Alexander Fleming observed that a *Penicillium* mold contaminating a Petri dish culture of staphylococci colonies was surrounded by a clear zone free of growth. Fleming cultured the contaminating mold on a special medium and demonstrated that the culture broth contained a potent antibacterial substance that was effective against a variety of gram-positive organisms and was relatively nontoxic to animals. He named the substance penicillin. In 1940, penicillin was isolated in the form of a brown, impure powder and was the most powerful chemotherapeutic agent known at that time. Since then, more than 40 penicillins have been identified. Some occur naturally; others are biosynthesized.

In 1945, *Cephalosporium acremonium* was isolated from raw sewage. The first cephalosporin, cephalosporin C, was derived from this fungus. All other cephalosporins are semisynthetic antibiotic derivatives of cephalosporin C. The first cephalosporin was available for clinical use in 1964.

Although penicillins and cephalosporins are still the most commonly used β-lactam antibiotics, much progress has been made in the development of new β lactams during recent years. Most notably, these include the β-lactamase inhibitors (e.g., clavulanic acid), the carbapenems (e.g., imipenem), and the monobactams (e.g., aztreonam) (Abraham 1987).

MECHANISM OF ACTION OF β-LACTAM ANTIBIOTICS. Beta-lactam antibiotics exert their bacteriocidal effects by preventing bacterial cell wall synthesis and disrupting bacterial cell wall integrity. Beta lactams bind to a series of enzymes, known as penicillin-binding proteins, which are involved in the final stages of cell wall synthesis. The β-lactam ring is a structural analog to the final peptide bridge (D-alanine-D-alanine) that cross-links the peptidoglycan chains that compose the bacterial cell wall. Penicillin-binding proteins vary between bacterial species. The affinity of various β-lactam antibiotics for the different penicillin-binding proteins may explain differences in spectra of activity of β-lactam antibiotics that are not caused by the presence or absence of β lactamases (AHFS Drug Information 1994b). Gram-negative bacteria can have up to seven different penicillin-binding proteins on their cell membranes, each of which is involved in a different catalytic reaction. The binding of a β-lactam antibiotic to a penicillin-binding protein leads to the formation of defective cell walls that are osmotically unstable. Cell death usually results from lysis, which may be mediated by bacterial autolysins. The β-lactam antibiotics demonstrate a postantibiotic effect against gram-positive cocci but not against gram-negative bacilli (Zhanel et al. 1991).

MICROBIAL RESISTANCE TO β LACTAMS. Three independent factors determine the bacterial susceptibility to β-lactam antibiotics: production of β lactamases, permeability of cell wall, and the sensitivity of the penicillin-binding protein (Frere et al. 1991). The elaboration of β lactamases, enzymes that inactivate the drugs by hydrolyzing the β-lactam ring, is the major mechanism of drug resistance. Different bacteria produce β lactamases that differ in physical, chemical, and functional properties. Some β lactamases are specific for penicillins (penicillinases), some are specific for cephalosporins (cephalosporinases), while still others have affinity for both groups. There are two mechanisms of β-lactamase production: chromosomal and plasmid. Chromosomally derived β lactamases are species and genus specific and can be induced by the presence of any β-lactam compound. Plasmid-derived β lactamases can be transferred between bacteria, increasing the number of bacteria resistant to the antibiotic (Graham et al. 1992).

Gram-positive bacteria generally produce chromosomally derived β lactamases. Those produced by gram-negative bacteria are chromosomally derived or plasmid mediated. The chromosomally derived β lactamases produced by gram-negative bacteria are primarily cephalosporinases while the plasmid-mediated ones are generally broader spectrum (Caprile 1988; Sanders and Sanders 1988). Gram-negative bacteria secrete small amounts of β lactamases into their periplasmic space, allowing for optimal location of the enzyme to degrade the β lactam upon entry into the organism. Newer agents have increasing resistance to β lactamases. For example, the cephamycins (cefoxitin and cefotetan) are apparently stable to chromosomally mediated β lactamases, which may give them their excellent activity against anaerobic gram-negative rods (Williams 1987).

Gram-negative bacteria can produce a cell wall with a modified outer membrane that is no longer permeable to β-lactam antibiotics. While this mechanism can enhance resistance produced by the elaboration of β lactamases, it is usually not sufficient to markedly increase resistance by itself. Finally, some bacteria have an intrinsic resistance to β lactams because of reduced sensitivity of the penicillin-binding proteins and failure of the drugs to inhibit the operative pathways of cell wall formation.

PENICILLINS

General Pharmacology. The international unit (IU) for penicillin has been identified as the amount of activity present in 0.6 mg of the international pure crystalline standard sodium salt of penicillin G; 1 mg contains 1667 Oxford units. The dose of more recent β-lactam antibiotics is expressed in milligrams per unit of body weight rather than in international units.

The essential penicillin molecule contains a fused ring system, the β-lactam thiazolidine (Fig. 41.1). The physical and chemical properties, especially solubilities, of penicillins are related to the structure of the acyl side chain and the cations used to form salts.

Hydrolysis is the main cause of penicillin degradation and can take place in the syringe when penicillin is mixed with another drug. Some penicillins are rapidly hydrolyzed by gastric acid, making them unsuitable for oral administration. Aqueous solutions of the alkaline sodium salts of sulfonamides inactivate penicillin. Penicillin is incompatible with heavy metal ions, oxidizing agents, and strong concentrations of alcohol.

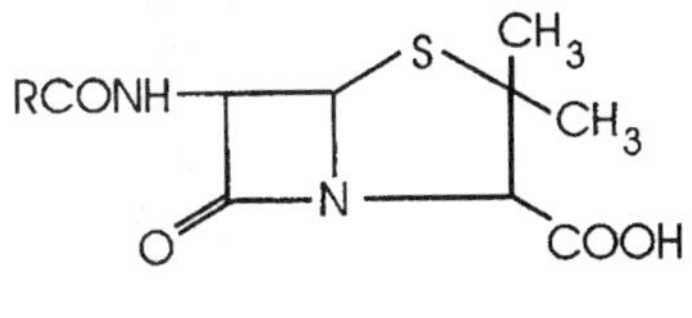

FIG. 41.1—Chemical structure of penicillins.

There are four groups of penicillins (Table 41.1):

1. Natural penicillins (e.g., penicillin G) are produced by mold cultures, then extracted and purified.
2. Aminopenicillins (e.g., amoxicillin) are semisynthetic derivatives that have a free amino group at the α position at R on the penicillin nucleus.
3. Penicillinase-resistant penicillins (e.g., oxacillin, cloxacillin) have a ring structure attached to the carbonyl carbon of the amide side chain. Substituents on the ring protect the lactam ring from β lactamases.
4. Extended-spectrum penicillins (e.g., ticarcillin, carbenicillin) have either a carboxylic acid group or a basic group at the α position at R, which gives these drugs a wider spectrum of activity than the other three groups of penicillins.

Microbial Susceptibility. The natural penicillins are active against many *Streptococci* spp. and non-penicillinase-producing *Staphylococci* spp. They are active against some gram-positive and gram-negative bacilli, including *Corynebacterium, Listeria monocytogenes, Pasteurella multocida,* and *Haemophilus influenzae.* These drugs are active against many gram-positive and gram-negative anaerobic bacteria, including *Fusobacterium, Peptococcus, Peptostreptococcus,* and some strains of *Bacteroides* and *Clostridium.* These drugs are also active against most spirochetes, including *Leptospira* and *Borrelia burgdorferi.* Natural penicillins are inactive against *Pseudomonas,* most Enterobacteriaceae, and penicillinase-producing *Staphylococcus* spp.

Aminopenicillins are generally active against the microbes that are susceptible to natural penicillins. They are also active against some Enterobacteriaceae, including strains of *E. coli, Proteus mirabilis,* and *Salmonella.* Aminopenicillins are inactive against *Pseudomonas, Bacteroides fragilis,* and penicillinase-producing *Staphylococcus* spp.

The penicillinase-resistant penicillins are active against many penicillinase-producing *Staphylococcus* spp. which are resistant to the natural penicillins and the aminopenicillins. They also have some activity against other gram-positive and gram-negative bacteria and spirochetes. However, they are generally less effective than the other penicillins.

Extended-spectrum penicillins have the most activity against gram-negative aerobic and anaerobic bacteria of all of the penicillin groups. The drugs are active

TABLE 41.1—Penicillins

Natural penicillins	Aminopenicillins	Penicillinase-resistant penicillins	Extended-spectrum penicillins
Penicillin G	Amoxicillin	Cloxacillin	Azlocillin
Penicillin V	Ampicillin	Dicloxacillin	Carbenicillin
	Hetacillin	Methicillin	Mezlocillin
		Nafcillin	Piperacillin
		Oxacillin	Ticarcillin

TABLE 41.2—Pharmacokinetic parameters of selected penicillins in domestic species

Drug	Species	V_d* (L/kg)	Clearance (mL/kg/min)	Elimination half-life (hr)	Reference
Penicillin G (sodium or potassium)	Dogs	0.16	3.6	0.50	Huber 1988
	Horses	0.65	8.5	0.88	Huber 1988
	Cattle			0.50	Huber 1988
Procaine penicillin G	Dogs	0.16	3.6	0.50	Huber 1988
	Horses	0.65	3.6	0.88	Huber 1988
	Sheep			1.42	Huber 1988
Benzathine penicillin	Horses	0.65		0.88	Huber 1988
	Sheep	0.23	12.4		Oukessou et al. 1990a
	Camels	0.15	4.9		Oukessou et al. 1990b
Ampicillin	Dogs	0.20	1.9	1.25	Huber 1988
	Horses	0.18		0.62	Sarasola and McKella 1993
	Cattle			1.20	Huber 1988
	Sheep	6.39	50.0	1.58	Nawaz and Kahn 1991
	Goats	7.15	57.0	1.58	Nawaz et al. 1990
Amoxicillin	Dogs	0.20	1.9	1.25	Huber 1988
	Foals	0.27	5.7	0.74	Baggot 1988
	Horses	0.33	5.7	0.66	Wilson et al. 1988
	Sheep	0.22	10.1	0.77	Craigmill et al. 1992
	Goats	0.47	11.4	1.12	Craigmill et al. 1992
Oxacillin	Dogs	0.30	6.9	0.50	Huber 1988
	Horses	0.60	11.6	0.60	Huber 1988
Cloxacillin	Dogs	0.20	4.6	0.50	Huber 1988
Dicloxacillin	Dogs	0.20	3.5	0.67	Huber 1988
Methicillin	Cattle			0.30	Huber 1988
Carbenicillin	Dogs	0.19	1.8	1.25	Huber 1988
	Horses	0.40	4.6	1.00	Huber 1988
Ticarcillin	Dogs	0.34	4.3	0.95	Huber 1988
	Horses			0.90	Huber 1988

*V_d = volume of distribution.

against many strains of Enterobacteriaceae and some strains of *Pseudomonas.* Carbenicillin and ticarcillin are active against some strains of *E. coli, Morganella morganii, Proteus* spp., and *Salmonella.* In addition to these organisms, mezlocillin and piperacillin are active against some strains of *Enterobacter, Citrobacter, Klebsiella,* and *Serratia.* The extended-spectrum penicillins have some activity against gram-positive aerobic and anaerobic bacteria but are generally less effective against these organisms than are the natural penicillins and aminopenicillins. Extended-spectrum penicillins are generally more active against *Bacteroides fragilis* than are other available penicillins.

Pharmacokinetics. Table 41.2 lists the pharmacokinetic parameters of several penicillins in domestic species and Table 41.3 lists recommended dosages. Most penicillins are rapidly absorbed when injected in aqueous suspension by the IM or SC route. Maximum blood concentrations result in 15-30 minutes. IM injection is the most common route of administration. It is necessary to orally administer 5 times the amount of penicillin G necessary for IM injections to produce comparable blood concentrations, because of inactivation by the gastric acid and enteric bacteria.

Some absorption of penicillin occurs during the first few hours after intramammary infusion. Blood concentrations are consistently higher when penicillin is infused in infected quarters than when infused into normal quarters. Serum plays a significant role in transfer of penicillin from treated to untreated quarters. There is systemic absorption of sodium benzylpenicillin and procaine benzylpenicillin administered intrauterine to horses and cattle, respectively.

Sodium or potassium penicillin suspended in an inert oil prolongs absorption of penicillin from the site of infection for approximately 18 hours. Incorporation of the poorly soluble procaine penicillin in oil prolongs absorption for 24 or more hours. Addition of 2% aluminum monosterate to a suspension of penicillin in oil produces a gel with a high degree of water repellency, which markedly slows absorption of procaine penicillin suspended in the medium. Although the use of an oil vehicle helps prolong the duration of therapeutic blood concentrations, undesirable physical properties limit widespread use. Horses may show unfavorable acute and chronic tissue reactions to the parenteral administration of an antibiotic in an oil vehicle.

Procaine penicillin G is a buffered aqueous suspension available for IM injection. Absorption of penicillin from this preparation is prolonged. Absorption of procaine may become problematic in drug-testing programs used in racing horses. A small amount of sodium or potassium penicillin G may be added to establish a

TABLE 41.3—Recommended dosages for penicillins

Drug	Species	Dose	Route	Interval (hr)
Penicillin G (sodium or potassium)	Horses	20,000–60,000 IU/kg	IM, IV	6–8
	Dogs and cats	22,000–55,000 IU/kg	IM, IV, SQ	6–8
Procaine penicillin G	Horses	20,000–100,000 IU/kg	IM	12
	Cattle	10,000–66,000 IU/kg	IM, SQ	12–24
	Swine	40,000 IU/kg	IM	24
	Dogs and cats	20,000 IU/kg	IM, SQ	12–24
Benzathine penicillin	Horses	50,000 IU/kg	IM	48
	Cattle	10,000–66,000 IU/kg	IM, SQ	48
	Dogs and cats	40,000–50,000 IU/kg	IM	120
Penicillin V (potassium)	Horses	66,000–110,000 IU/kg	PO	6–8
	Dogs and cats	5.5–11 mg/kg	PO	6–8
Ampicillin	Horses	10–22 mg/kg	IV, IM	8
	Cattle	11–22 mg/kg	SQ, IM	12
		4–10 mg/kg	PO	12–24
	Dogs and cats	10–20 mg/kg	IV, SQ	6–8
		22–33 mg/kg	PO	8
	Swine	6–8 mg/kg	SQ, IM	8
Amoxicillin	Horses	20–30 mg/kg	IM, PO	6–2
	Cattle	6–11 mg/kg	IM, SC	12–24
	Dogs and cats	10–22 mg/kg	PO	8
		5–11 mg/kg	IM, IV, SQ	8
Amoxicillin + Cavulanate	Dog	12.5–25 mg/kg	PO	8–12
	Cat	62.5 mg/kg	PO	8–12
Cloxacillin	Dogs and cats	20–40 mg/kg	IM, IV, PO	8
Dicloxacillin	Dogs and cats	10–50 mg/kg	PO	8
Oxacillin	Horses	20–50 mg/kg	IM, IV	6–8
	Dogs and cats	20–40 mg/kg	PO	8
		5.5–11 mg/kg	IV, IM	4–8
Carbenicillin	Dogs and cats	55–100 mg/kg	IV, PO	8
Ticarcillin	Dogs and cats	40–110 mg/kg	IV, IM, SC	6

therapeutic concentration immediately following IM injection. Benzathine penicillin G is a repository salt of penicillin. Absorption of this compound may be prolonged for 7 or more days.

Diffusion of penicillin into the tissues and fluids occurs as long as the unbound plasma concentration exceeds that of the tissues and fluids. High concentrations of penicillins are generally reached in kidneys, liver, and lung. Penicillins do not penetrate the CNS to any great extent. Penicillin will diffuse across the placenta, into the fetal circulation. Tissue residues of penicillin in slaughtered animals are considered a public health hazard because of potential hypersensitivity reactions in people.

Penicillin G, penicillin V, nafcillin, ticarcillin, and the aminopenicillins are metabolized to some extent by hydrolysis of the β-lactam ring. The metabolites are microbiologically inactive. Penicillins and their metabolites are excreted in the urine by tubular secretion. Most of the drug is excreted in the urine within 1 hour of IM injection of sodium or potassium penicillin in aqueous solution. Probenecid competitively inhibits renal tubular secretion of penicillins. Penicillin is also eliminated in milk.

Compounds

NATURAL PENICILLINS. Only penicillin G and penicillin V are currently used clinically. The phenoxymethyl group on penicillin V imparts more acid stability, allowing for oral administration, but less antibacterial activity. Penicillin G is commercially available as a benzathine, procaine, potassium, or sodium salt. Penicillin V is available as a potassium salt. The potassium and sodium salts of the drugs are soluble in water while the benzathine and procaine salts are less soluble in water. Penicillin G can be injected IV, IM, or SC. Procaine penicillin G should not be administered IV, because procaine can adversely affect the cardiac conduction system. Oral administration of penicillin V is more applicable to humans and small animals than to food-producing animals. Penicillin is usually not administered orally to herbivores because it suppresses bacterial metabolism in the digestive tract. The exception are those herbivores that are very young or animals that require suppression of bacterial fermentation to prevent bloat.

Penicillin is administered via both intramammary and systemic routes to treat bovine mastitis. Milk contaminated with antibiotics may cause public health problems as well as inhibit the cheese-making process. Penicillin in milk and milk products may sensitize susceptible humans, with subsequent penicillin therapy more likely to produce an allergic reaction. Recommended withdrawal times must be adhered to. The type of vehicle used in intramammary infusion preparation is a factor that also determines time required for elimination of antibiotics via the milk. In general, penicillin in fat-soluble ointments or mineral oil vehicles persists longer in the bovine udder than penicillin administered in an aqueous vehicle. In contrast, aqueous vehicles favor rapid release of antibiotics to attain maximum therapeutic concentrations. This information is provided on the label.

AMINOPENICILLINS. Ampicillin and amoxicillin have been used in the treatment of a variety of diseases in domestic animals. The half-life of all aminopenicillins is approximately 60-90 minutes. Tissue drug concentrations may be higher than serum concentrations. Following oral administration, ampicillin is more quickly absorbed when mixed with water or glucose solutions than when added to milk or milk replacer. Amoxicillin differs from ampicillin by the addition of a parahydroxy group. It has greater resistance to gastric acid and is more completely absorbed than ampicillin. Hetacillin is prepared by a reaction of ampicillin with acetone. When administered as an aqueous solution, it is rapidly converted back to ampicillin and acetone. Thus the spectrum of activity is identical to that of ampicillin.

PENICILLINASE-RESISTANT PENICILLINS. Methicillin sodium is a water-soluble penicillinase-resistant penicillin that produces therapeutic concentrations in the CNS. Methicillin is primarily used as an antistaphylococcal drug. However, methicillin is a powerful inducer of penicillinase, and staphylococci may develop resistance by nonpenicillinase mechanisms. Methicillin is given by the IV or IM route and is usually well tolerated. Occasionally some pain may be observed following IM injection. Oxacillin, cloxacillin, dicloxacillin, and nafacillin resist acid hydrolysis and can be administered orally.

EXTENDED-SPECTRUM PENICILLINS. Carbenicillin and other members of this group have the major advantage that they are effective against *Pseudomonas, Proteus,* and other gram-negative bacteria resistant to other penicillins. Carbenicillin has a broad range of antibacterial activity that has been related to the carboxyl group substituted on the α carbon of the benzyl side chain. Carbenicillin is acid labile and must be administered parenterally. Carbenicillin indanyl, the indanyl ester of carbenicillin, is acid stable and suitable for oral administration. It is rapidly absorbed from the small intestine and peak plasma concentrations are achieved within 1 hour of oral administration. Carbenicillin is primarily eliminated by the renal tubules, with approximately 80% of the dose appearing in the urine within 9 hours. Peak serum carbenicillin concentrations achieved following oral administrations are low, and many infections are not treatable with this drug unless confined to the lower urinary tract. Ticarcillin and mezlocillin are not absorbed orally and must be administered IV or IM.

Toxicity. Penicillins are very safe drugs, with relative few adverse effects reported. Acute allergic reactions are the most common untoward effect in people. Acute anaphylaxis, collapse, hypersalivation, shaking, vomiting, urticaria, fever, eosinophilia, neutropenia, agranulocytosis, thrombocytopenia, leukopenia, anemia, and lymphadenopathy can occur in sensitized animals. Coomb's-positive hemolytic anemia has been reported in horses following penicillin administration (Blue et al. 1987; Step et al. 1991).

The IV administration of hypertonic solutions of sodium benzylpenicillin has resulted in ataxia and convulsions in cats and dogs. Procaine can also cause anaphylaxis and CNS disorders (Neilsen et al. 1988). Guinea pigs, chinchillas, birds, snakes, and turtles are sensitive to procaine penicillin (Jenkins 1987).

Anorexia, vomiting, and diarrhea can occur when penicillins are given orally. Changes in the intestinal flora induced by penicillin administration can also lead to diarrhea.

The extended-spectrum penicillins have been associated with coagulopathies in humans. The incidence of this is unknown in veterinary patients.

CEPHALOSPORINS

General Pharmacology. Cephalosporins contain a 7-aminocephalosporanic acid nucleus which is composed of a β-lactam ring fused with a 6-membered dihydrothiazine ring (Fig. 41.2). Additions of various groups at the R positions form derivatives with differences in antimicrobial activity, stability against β lactamases, protein binding, intestinal absorption, metabolism, and toxicity.

The cephalosporins are usually divided into 3 classes: first, second, and third generation (Table 41.4). Although this division is based largely on the chronological development of the drugs, some generalities can be made about the spectrum of antimicrobial activity of each generation, as given below. Cefoxitin, cefotetan, and loracarbef are cephamycins, and moxalactam is an oxa-β-lactam, but these agents are generally included with the cephalosporins because of their similar pharmacologic behavior.

Unless frozen, most cephalosporins are stable in solution for only short time periods. Some drugs, such as aminoglycosides, are potentially incompatible with cephalosporins when mixed in solution. Specific references should be consulted for compatibility information.

Microbial Susceptibility. There are substantial differences between cephalosporins with regard to microbial susceptibility. The National Committee for Clinical Laboratory Standards (NCCLS) uses cephalothin susceptibility as an indicator for all first-generation cephalosporins. The activity of the first-generation cephalosporins is essentially identical when given parenterally, except that cefazolin has somewhat lesser activity against staphylococci and somewhat greater

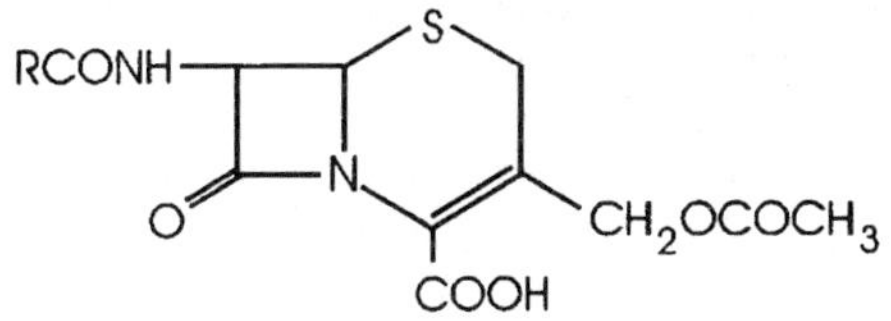

FIG. 41.2—Chemical structure of cephalosporins.

TABLE 41.4—Cephalosporins

First generation	Second generation	Third generation
Cefadroxil	Cefaclor	Cefixime
Cefazolin	Cefamandole	Cefoperazone
Cephalexin	Cefmetazole	Cefotaxime
Cephalothin	Cefonicid	Cefpodoxime
Cephapirin	Ceforanide	Ceftazidime
Cephradine	Cefotetan	Ceftiofur
	Cefoxitin	Ceftizoxime
	Cefprozil	Ceftriaxone
	Cefuroxime	Moxalactam
	Loracarbef	

activity against gram-negative organisms. In general, first-generation cephalosporins are active against *Staphylococci* spp., *Streptococci* spp., *Escherichia coli, Proteus mirabilis,* and *Klebsiella* spp. This makes the spectrum of activity similar to that of the aminopenicillins, with the exception of their excellent activity against *Staphylococci* spp. First-generation cephalosporins do not generally have activity against anaerobic bacteria, *Pseudomonas* spp., *Enterococcus* spp., *Enterobacter* spp., other *Proteus,* and *Serratia.*

Second-generation cephalosporins tend to be active against the same bacteria as first-generation cephalosporins. However, the activity of these drugs, with the exception of cefaclor, against gram-negative bacteria increases. Second-generation cephalosporins may be active against some strains of *Enterobacter, E. coli, Klebsiella, Proteus,* and *Serratia* that are resistant to first-generation cephalosporins. Cefoxitin, cefotetan, cefmetazole, and cefamandole possess some activity against anaerobic bacteria. Of the second-generation cephalosporins, cefuroxime has somewhat greater β-lactamase stability.

Third-generation cephalosporins typically have less activity against staphylococci but greater gram-negative activity than the other cephalosporins. Third-generation cephalosporins may be active against some strains of *Enterobacter, E. coli, Klebsiella, Proteus,* and *Serratia* that are resistant to first- and second-generation cephalosporins. Most third-generation cephalosporins also have some activity against *Pseudomonas* spp. Cefixime, ceftriaxome, and ceftazidime have limited anaerobic activity, whereas cefotaxime possesses good anaerobic activity. Of the third-generation cephalosporins, cefotaxime has slightly better gram-positive activity and ceftizoxime has somewhat better anaerobic activity than the others.

Methicillin-resistant *Staphylococcus* spp. and *Enterococci* spp. are resistant to cephalosporins.

Pharmacokinetics. Table 41.5 lists pharmacokinetic parameters derived after the administration of several cephalosporins to domestic species, and Table 41.6 lists recommended dosages. A two-compartment open model usually characterizes the disposition of cephalosporins following IV administration. Cephalosporins are rapidly absorbed following IM or SC administration. The bioavailability varies with the drug and species. Absorption following oral administration is also variable but less well characterized. For example, cefadroxil administered orally to dogs results in high serum concentrations, whereas cefadroxil is poorly and erratically absorbed following oral administration to horses (Caprile 1988). Variations in protein binding and rate of renal elimination lead to varied pharmacokinetic profiles of the different cephalosporins.

The cephalosporins are widely distributed throughout the body, achieving high concentrations in blood, urine, bile, pleural fluid, pericardial fluid, synovial fluid, cortical bone, and cancellous bone. Although most first- and second-generation cephalosporins fail to cross the blood-brain barrier, cefuroxime, cefotaxime, cefizoxime, ceftriaxome, and ceftazidime reach high concentrations in the cerebrospinal fluid when the meninges are inflamed. Cephalosporins have poor penetration into prostatic tissue and aqueous and vitreous humors.

The chief route of excretion for most cephalosporins is renal filtration. In people, most cephalosporins are eliminated unchanged. The exceptions include cephalothin, cephaprin, and cefotaxime, which are deacetylated. The deacetylated metabolite of cefotaxime has a longer half-life than the parent compound and has considerable antimicrobial activity. Ceftriaxome and cefoperazone are eliminated chiefly by the biliary system in people, resulting in longer half-lives. As much as 17% of administered cefotetan undergoes biliary excretion in the dog.

Compounds

FIRST-GENERATION CEPHALOSPORINS. This group of cephalosporins is composed of the primary cephalosporins used in veterinary practice. Cephradine, cephalexin monohydrate, and cefadroxil are the first-generation cephalosporins available for oral administration, whereas cephalothin sodium, cefazolin sodium, cephapirin sodium, and cephradine are available for parenteral administration. Formulations of cephapirin sodium and cephapirin benzathine are available for intramammary infusion in lactating cows and dry cows, respectively.

SECOND-GENERATION CEPHALOSPORINS. Second-generation cephalosporins available for oral administration include cefuroxime axetil and cefaclor, while

TABLE 41.5—Pharmacokinetic parameters of selected cephalosporins in domestic species

Drug	Species	V_d[a] (L/kg)	Clearance (mL/kg/min)	Elimination half-life (hr)	Reference
Cephapirin	Foals[b]	1.06	18.4	0.70	Brown et al. 1987
	Horses	0.17	10.0		Brown et al. 1986a
	Cows[c]		12.7		Prades et al. 1988
	Dogs	0.32	8.9	0.42	Cabana et al. 1976
Cephalothin	Horses	0.15	13.6	0.25	Ruoff and Sams 1985
Cefadroxil	Horses	0.46	7.0	0.77	Wilson et al. 1985
Cefazolin	Foals	0.45	0.4	1.37	Duffee et al. 1989
	Horses	0.19	5.5	0.67	Sams and Ruoff 1985
	Calves	0.17	5.8	0.62	Soback et al. 1987
	Dogs	0.70	10.4	0.80	
Cephalexin	Calves	0.32	1.9	2.00	Garg et al. 1992
	Cows	0.39	10.5	0.58	Soback et al. 1988
	Sheep	0.17	5.0	1.20	Villa et al. 1991
Cefoxitin	Calves			1.12	Soback 1988
	Horses	0.12	4.3	0.82	Brown 1986b
Cepfaronide	Sheep	0.39	2.7		Guerrini et al. 1985
Ceftriaxone	Dogs			0.85	Matsui et al. 1984
	Sheep	0.30	3.7		Guerrini et al. 1985
	Calves			1.40	Soback and Ziv 1988
Ceftazidime	Dogs			0.82	Matusi et al. 1984
	Sheep	0.36		1.60	Rule et al. 1991
Cefoperazone	Calves			0.89	Carli et al. 1986
	Sheep	0.16	2.7		Guerrini et al. 1985
Moxalactam	Calves			2.40	Soback 1989

[a]V_d = volume of distribution.
[b]Neonatal.
[c]Lactating.

TABLE 41.6—Recommended dosages for cephalosporins

Drug	Species	Dose (mg/kg)	Route	Interval (hr)
Cefadroxil	Dogs/Cats	22	PO	8–12
	Horses	25	PO	4
Cephalexin	Horses	22–33	PO	6
	Dogs/Cats	22	PO	8
Cephapirin	Horses	20–30	IM, IV	8–12
	Dogs/Cats	10–30	IV, IM, SC	6–8
Cephalothin	Horses	11–20	IV, IM	6
	Cattle	55	SC	6
	Dogs/Cats	10–30	IM, IV, SC	6–8
Cefazolin	Horse	15–20	IV, IM	8
	Dogs/Cats	20–35	IM, IV, SC	6–8
Cefoxitin	Dogs/Cats	30	IV	8
	Foals	20	IV	4–6
Cefotetan	Dogs/Cats	30	IV	8
Cefotaxime	Dogs/Cats	25–50	IV, IM, SC	8
	Foals	20–30	IV	6
	Goats	50	IV	12
Ceftiofur	Cattle	1	IM	24

cefamandole nafate, cefonicid sodium, ceforanide, cefuroxime sodium, cefoxitin sodium, and cefotetan disodium are available for parenteral administration. With the exception of cefotetan disodium and cefoxitin sodium, second-generation cephalosporins are less commonly used in veterinary medicine because of their expense.

THIRD-GENERATION CEPHALOSPORINS. This class of drugs was developed for use in specialized situations where antibiotic-resistant, gram-negative infections are common and safety is of prime concern. These drugs are very expensive and, with few exceptions, are infrequently used in veterinary medicine. Cefixime is an orally administered third-generation cephalosporin; the remaining compounds are available for parenteral administration. Ceftiofur sodium is approved for parenteral administration in nonlactating cattle. A product containing cefoperazone in an oil base for intramammary infusion is available in the United Kingdom but is not licensed for use in the United States. The nonirritant properties of cefoperazone plus the persistence of therapeutic concentrations of the drug in treated quarters for 3-4 milkings make this drug very useful for the treatment of bovine mastitis; however, its persistence also prolongs the milk-discard time because of residue concerns (Holmgren et al. 1985).

Toxicity. As a group, cephalosporins have a favorable toxicity profile in comparison with other antibiotics. Local reactions account for the majority of adverse reactions to cephalosporins reported in humans. Pain, sterile abscess formation, and tissue sloughing following IM injection and thrombophlebitis following IV injection have occurred in people. These reactions are usually mild and do not lead to discontinuation of drug administration (Caprile 1988). There is one report of a horse having a serious local reaction and acute laminitis following the IM administration of cefoxitin (Brown et al. 1986b).

Oral administration of cephalosporins can cause vomiting and diarrhea. Administration of cephalosporins with food may decrease these effects.

Hypersensitivity reactions to cephalosporins have been reported in people but appear to be uncommon in the domestic species. Patients who are allergic to penicillins may also be allergic to cephalosporins.

Hypersensitivity reactions can also lead to the development of nephropathies. Although some cephalosporins have a direct toxic effect on the proximal tubule, this only occurs at doses in excess of 100 times those commonly used in clinics. The only cephalosporin that produced direct toxicity at therapeutic doses was cephaloridine, which is no longer in use. Following controlled trials in people, concern was raised about the potential of cephalothin and the aminoglycosides to interact synergistically to produce renal damage. Other controlled trials failed to show synergistic nephrotoxicity. Cephalothin can interfere with a standard laboratory assay for serum creatinine (Jaffe technique), and it is unclear how many of these reports may have been following false creatinine increases and how many were due to true renal insufficiency (Goldberg 1987). Nevertheless, it is prudent to adjust doses or dosage intervals in patients with renal failure (Zhanel 1990).

Cephalosporins in the urine can cause a false-positive reaction for glucosuria (copper-reduction technique) and proteinuria (sulfosalicylic turbidimetric test).

Cefoperazone, cefamandole, and moxalactam inhibit the vitamin K-dependent pathway for the synthesis of clotting factors. This can lead to hypoprothrombinemia and coagulopathy. High-dose and/or prolonged cephalosporin administration has the potential to cause neutropenia, thrombocytopenia, agranulocytosis, positive Coomb's test, hepatopathy, and neuropathy (Caprile 1988).

OTHER β-LACTAM ANTIBIOTICS

β-Lactamase Inhibitors

CLAVULANIC ACID. Clavulanic acid, like penicillins and cephalosporins, contains a β-lactam ring and is able to fit into the catalytic center of the β-lactamase enzyme. With time, clavulanic acid becomes more firmly attached than the β lactam and blocks the β-lactamase binding site. This prevents any degradation of simultaneously administered penicillins. Clavulanic acid has minimal antimicrobial efficacy if administered alone; however, it augments β lactam's effects by protecting it from breakdown by β lactamases (Rolinson 1991).

Amoxicillin is combined with potassium clavulanate in a 4:1 ratio and is available for oral administration. This preparation is not destroyed by gastric or intestinal secretions and is rapidly absorbed. Both drugs distribute well to blood, tissue fluid, and skin (Bywater et al. 1985). A formulation of ticarcillin and potassium clavulanate is also available and has been used in dogs and cats. This formulation can be administered only by the IV route.

SULBACTAM. Sulbactam is a penicillanic acid sulfone and, like clavulanic acid, has little antibacterial activity by itself. It is a chemically stable β-lactamase inhibitor that synergistically increases the activity of β-lactam antibiotics against β-lactamase-producing bacteria. Sodium sulbactam and ampicillin, when used in combination, synergistically rendered ampicillin-resistant strains of *Pasteurella* spp., *Haemophilus pleuropneumoniae,* and *Staphylococcus aureus* sensitive to ampicillin in vitro (Girard et al. 1987). Sodium sulbactam-ampicillin is available for IV administration.

Carbapenems. Carbapenems are structurally different from penicillin in that they have a carbon on the five-membered ring instead of a sulfur. Imipenem, a thienamycin antibiotic, is the only drug of this class that is currently available. Because of renal toxicity and poor urinary concentrations, imipenem was combined with cilastatin, a renal enzyme inhibitor. This combination has a broad spectrum of microbial susceptibility, with activity against gram-negative aerobic and anaerobic bacteria, including *Pseudomonas* spp. The recommended dose for imipenem-cilastatin in dogs and cats is 2 mg/kg given IV every 6-8 hours by slow infusion.

Monobactams. Unlike other β-lactam antibiotics, which are bicyclic, monobactams are monocyclic β-lactam antibiotics. Aztreonam is the prototype of this class of drugs. The pattern of microbial susceptibility to aztreonam can be characterized by potent activity against gram-negative bacteria, including *Pseudomonas aeruginosa,* but little to no activity against gram-positive bacteria and anaerobic bacteria. Aztreonam is stable against hydrolysis by many β lactamases. Equally as important, aztreonam is a poor inducer of β-lactamase production (AHFS Drug Information 1994b; Thompson 1987). Little is known about the pharmacokinetics, clinical usage, and toxicity of aztreonam in domestic species. Aztreonam has been advocated for use in penicillin-allergic patients because it has a low immunogenic profile and is less likely to cross-react with penicillins and cephalosporins (Saxon 1989).

REFERENCES

Abraham, E. P. 1987. Cephalosporins, 1945-1986. Drugs 34:1-14.

AHFS Drug Information. 1994a. Cephalosporins. 95-101.

———. 1994b. Miscellaneous β-lactam antibiotics: aztreonam. 164-172.

———. 1994c. Penicillins. 213-308.

Baggot, J. D. 1988. Bioavailability and disposition kinetics of amoxicillin in neonatal foals. Equine Vet J 20:125-127.

Baggot, J. D., Love, D., Love, R. J., Raus, J., and Rose, R. J. 1990. Oral dosage of penicillin V in adult horses and foals. Equine Vet J 22:290-291.

Blue, J. T., Dinsmore, R. P., and Anderson, K. L. 1987. Immune-mediated hemolytic anemia induced by penicillin in horses. Cornell Vet 77:263-276.

Brown, M. P., Gronwall, R. R., Gossman, T. B., and Houston, A. E. 1987. Pharmacokinetics and serum concentrations of cephapirin in neonatal foals. Am J Vet Res 48:805-806.

Brown, M. P., Gronwall, R. R., and Houston, A. E. 1986a. Pharmacokinetics and body fluid and endometrial concentrations of cephapirin in mares. Am J Vet Res 47:784-788.

———. 1986b. Pharmacokinetics and body fluid and endometrial concentrations of cefoxitin in mares. Am J Vet Res 47:1734-1737.

Bywater, R. J., Palmer, G. H., Buswell, J. F., and Stanton, A. 1985. Clavulanate-potentiated amoxycillin: activity in vitro and bioavailability in the dog. Vet Record 116:33-36.

Cabana, B. C., VanHarken, D. R., and Hottendorf, G. H. 1976. Comparative pharmacokinetics and metabolism of cephapirin in laboratory animals and humans. Antimicrob Agents Chemotherap 10:307-317.

Caprile, K. A. 1988. The cephalosporin antimicrobial agents: a comprehensive review. J Vet Pharmacol Therap 11:1-32.

Carli, S., Montesissa, C., Sonzogni, O., and Madonna, M. 1986. Pharmacokinetics of sodium cefoperazone in calves. Pharmacol Res Commun 18:481-490.

Craigmill, A. L., Pass, M. A., and Wetzlich, S. 1992. Comparative pharmacokinetics of amoxicillin administered intravenously to sheep and goats. J Vet Pharmacol Therap 15:72-77.

Dorrestein, G. M., van Gogh, H., and Rinzema, J. D. 1984. Pharmacokinetic aspects of penicillins, aminoglycosides and chloramphenicol in birds compared to mammals: a review. Vet Quarterly 6(4):216-224.

Duffee, N. E., Christensen, J. M., and Craig, A. M. 1989. The pharmacokinetics of cefadroxil in the foal. J Vet Pharmacol Therap 12:322-326.

Frere, J. M., Joris, B., Granier, B., Matagne, A., Jacob, F., and Bourguignon-Bellefroid, C. 1991. Diversity of the mechanisms of resistance to β-lactam antibiotics. Res Microbiol 142:705-710.

Garg, S. K., Chaudhary, R. K., and Srivastava, A. K. 1992. Disposition kinetics and dosage of cephalexin in cow calves following intramuscular administration. Annales de Recherches Veterinaires 23:399-402.

Girard, A. E., Schelkly, W. U., Murphy, K. T., and Sawyer, P. S. 1987. Activity of β-lactamase inhibitor subactam plus ampicillin against animal isolates of Pasterurella, Haemophilus, and Staphylococcus. Am J Vet Res 48:1678-1683.

Goldberg, D. M. 1987. The cephalosporins. Med Clin North Am 71:1113-1133.

Graham, J. M., Oshiro, B. T., and Blanco, J. D. 1992. Limited-spectrum (first-generation) cephalopsorins. Obstet Gynecol Clin North Am 19:449-459.

Guerrini, V. H., Filippich, L. J., Cao, G. R., English, P. B., and Bourne, D. W. 1985. Pharmacokinetics of cefaronide, ceftriaxone, and cefoperazone in sheep. J Vet Pharmacol Therap 8:120-127.

Holmgren, N., Haggmar, B., and Tolling, S. 1985. A field trial evaluating the use of cefoperazone in the treatment of bovine clinical mastitis. Nord Vet Med 37:228-233.

Huber, W. G. 1988. Penicillins. In L. E. McDonald and N. H. Booth, eds., Veterinary Pharmacology and Therapeutics, 6th ed., pp. 796-812. Ames: Iowa State Univ Press.

Jayachandran, C., Singh, M. K., and Banerjee, N. C. 1990. Pharmacokinetics and distribution of ampicillin in plasma, milk and uterine fluid of female buffaloes. Vet Res Commun 14:47-51.

Jenkins, W. L. 1987. The penicillins. In D. E. Johnston, ed., The Bristol Veterinary Handbook of Antimicrobial Therapy, pp. 243-248.

Lee, F. H., Pfeffer, M., VanHarken, D. R., Smyth, R. D., and Hottendorf, G. H. 1980. Comparative pharmacokinetics of ceforanide (BL-S786R) and cefazolin in laboratory animals and humans. Antimicrob Agents Chemotherap 17:188-192.

Matsui, H., Komiya, M., Ikeda, C., and Tachibana, A. 1984. Comparative pharmacokinetics of YM-13115, ceftriaxone, and ceftazidime in rats, dogs, and rhesus monkeys. Antimicrob Agents Chemotherap 26:204-207.

Nawaz, M., and Kahn, H. 1991. Bioavailability, elimination kinetics, renal clearance and excretion of ampicillin following intravenous and oral administration in sheep and goats. Acta Veterinaria Scandinavica 8:131-132.

Nawaz, M., Tabassum, R., Iqbal, T., and Perveen, Z. 1990. Disposition kinetics, renal clearance and excretion of ampicillin after oral administration in goats. Zentralblatt für Veterinarmedizin 37:247-252.

Neilsen, I. L., Jacobs, K. A., Huntington, P. J., Chapman, C. B., and Lloyd, K. C. 1988. Adverse reaction to procaine penicillin G in horses. Australian Vet J 65:181-185.

Oukessou, M., Benlamlih, S., and Toutain, P. L. 1990a. Benylpenicillin kinetics in the ewe: influence of pregnancy and lactation. Res Vet Sci 49(2):190-193.

Oukessou, M., Hossaini, J., Zine-Filali, R., and Toutain, P. L. 1990b. Comparative benzylpenicillin pharmacokinetics in the dromedary *Camelus dromedarius* and in sheep. J Vet Pharmacol Therap 13:298-303.

Prades, M., Brown, M. P., Gronwall, R., and Miles, N. S. 1988. Pharmacokinetics of sodium cephapirin in lactating dairy cows. Am J Vet Res 49:1888-1890.

Rolinson, G. N. 1991. Evolution of beta-lactamase inhibitors. Surg Gyn Obstet 172:11-16.

Rule, R., Rubio, M., and Perelli, M. C. 1991. Pharmacokinetics of ceftazidime in sheep and its penetration into tissue and peritoneal fluids. Res Vet Sci 51:233-238.

Ruoff, W. W., and Sams, R. A. 1985. Pharmacokinetics and bioavailability of cephalothin in horse mares. Am J Vet Res 46:2085-2090.

Sams, R. A., and Ruoff, W. W. 1985. Pharmacokinetics and bioavailability of cefazolin in horses. Am J Vet Res 46:348-352.

Sanders, W. E., and Sanders, C. C. 1988. Inducible β-lactamases: clinical and epidemiologic implications for use of newer cephalosporins. Rev Infect Dis 10:830-838.

Sarasola, P., and McKella, Q. A. 1993. Pharmacokinetics and applications of ampicillin sodium as an intravenous infusion in the horse. J Vet Pharmacol Therap 16:63-69.

Saxon, A. 1989. Aztreonam in the management of gram-negative infections in penicillin-allergic patients: a review. Pediatr Infect Dis J 8:S124-S127.

Soback, S. 1988. Pharmacokinetics of single doses of cefoxitin given by the intravenous and intramuscular routes to unweaned calves. J Vet Pharmacol Therap 11:155-162.

———. 1989. Pharmacokinetics of single-dose administration of moxolactam in unweaned calves. Am J Vet Res 50:498-501.

Soback, S., Bor, A., and Ziv, G. 1987. Clinical pharmacology of cefazolin in calves. J Vet Med Assoc 34:25-32.

Soback, S., and Ziv, G. 1988. Pharmacokinetics and bioavailability of ceftriaxone administered intravenously and intramuscularly to calves. Am J Vet Res 49:535-538.

Soback, S., Ziv, G., Bor, A., and Shapira, M. 1988. Pharmacokinetics of cephalexin glycinate in lactating cows and ewes. J Vet Med Assoc 35:755-760.

Step, D. L., Blue, F. T., and Dill, S. G. 1991. Penicillin-induced hemolytic anemia and acute hepatic failure following treatment of tetanus in a horse. Cornell Vet 81:13-18.

Thompson, R. L. 1987. Cephalosporin, carbapenem, and monobactam antibiotics. Mayo Clin Proc 62:821-834.

Villa, R., Carli, S., Montesissa, C., and Sonzogni, U. 1991. Influence of probenecid on cephalexin pharmacokinetics in sheep. Acta Veterinaria Scandinavica 8:124-126.

Wilson, W. D., Baggot, J. D., Adamson, P. J., Hirsh, D. C., and Hietala, S. K. 1985. Cefadroxil in the horse: pharmacokinetics and in vitro antibacterial activity. J Vet Pharmacol Therap 8:246-253.

Wilson, W. D., Spensley, M. S., Baggot, J. D., and Hietala, S. K. 1988. Pharmacokinetics and estimated bioavailability of amoxicillin in mares after intravenous, intramuscular, and oral administration. Am J Vet Res 49:1688-1694.

Williams, J. D. 1987. Drugs 34:15-22.

Zhanel, G. G. 1990. Cephalosporin-induced nephrotoxicity: does it exist? DICP 24:262-265.

Zhanel, G. G., Hoban, D. J., and Harding, G. K. 1991. The postantibiotic effect: a review of in vitro and in vivo data. DICP 25:153-163.

42

TETRACYCLINE ANTIBIOTICS

JIM E. RIVIERE AND JERRY W. SPOO

General Pharmacology of Tetracyclines
Mechanism of Action
Absorption
Distribution
Metabolism and Excretion
Clinical Uses
Toxicity and Adverse Side Effects
Commonly Used Tetracyclines
Chlortetracycline
Tetracycline
Oxytetracycline
Doxycycline
Minocycline

GENERAL PHARMACOLOGY OF TETRACYCLINES. The tetracycline antibiotics were isolated from various species of *Streptomyces* in the late 1940s and early 1950s. Since that time, many semisynthetic structural modifications have been made on the tetracycline molecule to yield other tetracyclines with differing pharmacokinetic properties and antimicrobial activities.

The tetracyclines are a group of four-ringed amphoteric compounds that differ by specific chemical substitutions at different points on the rings. As a group, the tetracyclines are acidic, hygroscopic compounds in aqueous solutions and easily form salts with acids and bases, which are how they are commonly marketed. The most common salt form is the hydrochloride formulation; however, as is the case with oxytetracycline, combining the base compound with certain carriers will result in prolonged serum and tissue half-lives. Some of the chemical and physical properties of the tetracyclines used in veterinary medicine today are listed in Table 42.1.

TABLE 42.1—Chemical and physical properties of tetracyclines

Drug	Molecular weight	pK_a
Chlortetracycline	478.88	3.3, 7.4, 9.3
Doxycycline	462.46	NA
Minocycline	457.48	2.8, 5.0, 7.8, 9.3
Oxytetracycline	460.44	NA
Tetracycline	444.43	8.3, 10.2

Note: NA = information not available.

Mechanism of Action. Tetracyclines possess antimicrobial activity by binding to the 30S ribosomal subunit of susceptible organisms. After binding to the ribosome, the tetracyclines interfere with the binding of aminoacyl-tRNA to the messenger RNA molecule/ribosome complex, thereby interfering with bacterial protein synthesis in growing or multiplying organisms (Gale and Folkes 1953; Suzuka et al. 1966). Tetracyclines have much less affinity for mammalian ribosomes, but some amount of inhibition does occur in mammals given tetracyclines. When inhibition of mammalian protein synthesis occurs, it is referred to as the "catabolic effect." Tetracyclines are bacteriostatic and broad spectrum at therapeutic concentrations.

Absorption. Tetracyclines can be administered intravenously (most tetracyclines) or intramuscularly (oxytetracycline), but the oral route is the preferred route in most animals to minimize adverse side effects (see the section Toxicity and Adverse Side Effects below). Generally, the tetracyclines are well absorbed from the gastrointestinal tract. However, absorption can vary between species and between oral formulations. Half-lives range from 7 to 19 hours. Tetracyclines can easily chelate to polyvalent cations, which decreases their absorption several-fold. Thus, tetracycline absorption in general can be decreased with the coadministration of food, dairy products, polyvalent cations (i.e., Ca^{++}, Mg^{++}, Fe^{++}, Al^{3+}), kaolin/pectin preparations, and antacids (Weinberg 1957; Waisbren and Hueckel 1950; Aronson 1980; Harcourt and Hamburger 1957; Neuvonen et al. 1970; Hagermark and Hoglund 1974; Gothoni et al. 1972). Therapeutic doses of tetracyclines given orally should not be administered to ruminants or horses due to the severe disruptions of intestinal microflora that may ensue. However, tetracyclines can be added in subtherapeutic concentrations to feed rations (in particular, chlortetracycline) for various uses (Zinn 1993; Jones et al. 1983; Dawson et al. 1983; Williams et al. 1978; Quarles et al. 1977; Richey et al. 1977; Nivas et al. 1976).

Distribution. Once absorbed, tetracyclines bind to plasma proteins to varying degrees in each species. Tetracyclines are widely distributed throughout most tissues of the body after oral and intravenous administrations and accumulate in the liver and kidneys. Distribution in the body is a function of lipid solubility; therefore, some tetracyclines penetrate some tissues better than others. For example, minocycline and doxycycline penetrate brain, spinal fluid, and prostate better than other tetracyclines, such as oxytetracycline or chlortetracycline. Minocycline is found in high concentrations in the bronchial secretions (Kelly and Kanegis 1967a; MacCulloch et al. 1974), prostate (Fair 1974), brain (Barza et al. 1975), thyroid, saliva, and tears (Hoeprich and Warshauer 1974) and may be of greater use than other tetracyclines in treating susceptible microbial infections in those organs.

Metabolism and Excretion. With the exception of minocycline and doxycycline, the tetracyclines are not metabolized to a significant extent in the body (Aronson 1980). Approximately 60% of the dose is eliminated in the urine via glomerular filtration, with the other 40% eliminated in the feces. The glomerular filtration pathway does not appear to be of importance with doxycycline, as most of the dose is excreted in the large intestine. Enterohepatic circulation does occur with the tetracyclines, with up to 20 times the plasma concentration of tetracyclines being present in the bile (Kunin and Finland 1961; Schach von Wittenau and Twomey 1971). Resistance occurs in bacteria due to R-plasmids.

Clinical Uses. The tetracyclines are broad-spectrum antibiotics and, as a class, inhibit the growth of a wide variety of bacteria, protozoa, and many intracellular organisms such as mycoplasma, chlamydia, and rickettsia. Differences in antimicrobial spectrum of the tetracyclines in vivo result mainly from differences in lipid solubility, which influences the absorption, distribution, metabolism/excretion, and concentration of a specific tetracycline within the cell. Higher concentrations of the tetracycline within the organism or cell (as is the case with the more lipid soluble doxycycline and minocycline) usually result in an increase in antimicrobial activity and better clinical efficacy.

Tetracyclines in general have good or moderate activity against the following organisms: *Bacillus* spp., *Corynebacterium* spp., *Erysipelothrix rhusiopathiae, Listeria monocytogenes,* streptococci, *Actinobacillus* spp., *Bordetella* spp., *Brucella* spp., *Francisella tularensis, Hemophilus* spp., *Pasteurella multocida, Yersinia* spp., *Campylobacter fetus, Borrelia* spp., *Leptospira* spp., *Actinomyces* spp., *Fusobacterium* spp., *Mycoplasma* spp., *Chlamydia* spp., *Rickettsia,* some protozoa, and *Anaplasma* spp. Some staphylococcus and enterococcus species and members of the family Enterobacteriaceae (*Enterobacter* spp., *E. coli, Klebsiella* spp., *Proteus* spp., *Salmonella* spp.) and some anaerobes (such as *Bacteroides* spp. and *Clostridium* spp.) have shown variable susceptibility. Commonly resistant to the tetracyclines are those infections involving *Mycobacterium* spp., *Proteus vulgaris, Pseudomonas aeruginosa, Serratia* spp., and some *Mycoplasma* spp. (Prescott and Baggot 1993). Increased activity against staphylococcus has been reported when doxycycline or minocycline has been used, presumably due to their increased ability to permeate the cell wall of this organism, which results in higher intracellular concentrations of drug.

Toxicity and Adverse Side Effects. Numerous side effects have been reported for the tetracyclines, although in general the tetracyclines are considered a relatively safe class of antimicrobials for use in animals. As stated earlier, glomerular filtration is the main pathway for elimination of most tetracyclines. Animals with renal insufficiency have impaired abilities to eliminate tetracyclines and may be at risk for tetracycline toxicosis.

The most commonly reported side effect of the tetracyclines, in both humans and animals, is gastrointestinal upset that results from irritation of the stomach and the upper small intestine, where the bulk of the tetracyclines is absorbed after oral administration. Hepatotoxicity may result from accumulation of tetracyclines when they are not eliminated quickly enough by the kidneys or by administration of frequent and/or large doses above recommended therapeutic dosages. In mice, tetracycline-induced toxicosis resulted in increased transaminases, alkaline phosphatase, urea, and total and conjugated bilirubin, in addition to decreased cholesterol (Bocker et al. 1982; Hopf et al. 1985). Acceptable alternatives in avoiding toxicosis include lowering the dose and lengthening the time between doses of the tetracycline used or selecting a tetracycline that does not depend on glomerular filtration for elimination (i.e., doxycycline).

Tetracyclines administered by rapid intravenous injection may cause the animal to collapse, possibly due either to high initial blood concentrations or to chelation with calcium in the blood. To avoid this side effect, the tetracycline should be administered slowly over a period of several minutes or administered diluted in normal saline or other fluid free of polyvalent cations. Most tetracyclines are also too irritating and absorption is too erratic and too painful to be administered by routes other than the intravascular or oral routes. The exception is oxytetracycline, which has been formulated to be a sustained-release form of this drug, although its long half-live is related to irritation at the intramuscular injection site. Doxycycline is fatal in horses (Riond et al. 1989a; Riond et al. 1992).

Tooth mottling/discoloration occurs when tetracyclines are administered during pregnancy when tooth development is occurring or when administered during the first postnatal month. The discoloration is related to the chelation of tetracyclines to the calcium deposits in the developing teeth in the dentin (where it is mostly visible) and to a lesser extent in the enamel (Hamp 1967; Hennon 1965; Finerman and Milch 1963; Moffit et al. 1974).

Of particular interest in horses and ruminants is the ability of orally administered (and, in the case of minocycline, parenterally administered) tetracyclines to alter the gastrointestinal tract flora by inducing a widespread suppression of these bacteria, resulting in a wide range of digestive disturbances. This suppression of gut bacteria is a leading reason why tetracyclines should be avoided in the equine.

Phototoxicity has been reported in humans and presumably may occur in animals. The most common lesion reported is dermatitis. Onycholysis has also been reported (Segal 1963; Harber et al. 1961).

Superinfections (new infections that develop during the course of antibiotic therapy that are resistant to that antibiotic) occur with many antibiotics and have been reported for the tetracyclines. The bacteria that colonize these sites are usually tetracycline resistant, and therefore, another antibiotic needs to be selected to combat the tetracycline-induced superinfection.

COMMONLY USED TETRACYCLINES

Chlortetracycline. Chlortetracycline was the first tetracycline discovered and was first introduced for clinical use in 1948 (see Fig. 42.1). Chlortetracycline has historically been used to treat several of the susceptible organisms listed above. Chlortetracycline is not utilized to any significant degree in small-animal medicine for treatment of disease, but it is still in use today in some feed and water additives for food-producing animals. Chlortetracycline is marketed alone or in combination with other antimicrobials (penicillin G, sulfonamides); amprolium, ethopabate, buquinolate, decoquinate, robenidine, and monensin are some of the preparations available. Some of the pharmacokinetic parameters of chlortetracycline in food-producing animals are listed in Table 42.2.

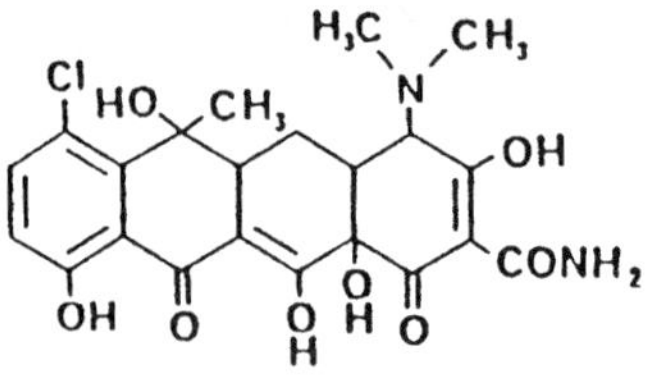

FIG. 42.1—Chemical structure of chlortetracycline.

The absorption, distribution, metabolism, and excretion of chlortetracycline in animals is as described previously for the tetracyclines in general. In a study by Kelly and Kanegis (1967b), ^{14}C-labeled chlortetracycline was administered intravenously (10 mg/kg) to dogs, which were then sacrificed to determine the extent of penetration of the radiolabeled chlortetracycline in the tissues. Four and one-half hours after administration, colon contents, ileal contents, bile (gallbladder), urine and jejunal contents, liver, and kidney all showed high accumulations of the drug. Significant amounts of drug accumulated in most tissues of the body except for the cerebrospinal fluid (CSF), vitreous and aqueous humors, and fat deposits. In cattle, chlortetracycline given intravenously at 2.27 mg/kg showed blood levels of 1.0-4.4 μg/mL for at least 12 hours after injection and low levels present in serum in some animals for 48 hours after administration. Chlortetracycline appeared in milk at 1-3 μg/mL for 4-12 hours following intravenous injection of 2.5 g/cow. At the 2.27 mg/kg dose, milk concentration of chlortetracycline was between 2.5 and 5 μg/mL between 2 and 8 hours postadministration, with levels slowly falling off to 0.25 μg/mL at 48 hours after dose (Schipper 1965).

Chlortetracycline has been fed orally at varying concentrations to food animals such as pigs, calves, cattle, chickens, and turkeys. As a feed additive, 350 mg of chlortetracycline per animal daily resulted in significant increases in daily weight gain (Perry et al. 1971; Brown et al. 1975). Tylosin and chlortetracycline have been compared with respect to their ability to prevent liver abscesses in feedlot cattle (Brown et al. 1975). In that study, chlortetracycline reduced the number of liver abscesses by about 12% compared to controls, but tylosin was better than chlortetracycline at preventing these abscesses. Low levels of chlortetracycline have been fed to cattle at a dose of 1.1 mg/kg for 120 days to eliminate latent infections of anaplasmosis as determined using complement-fixation testing (Richey et al. 1977). In contrast, Royal et al. (1970) reported that chlortetracycline fed at levels of 50 mg or 100 mg daily did not alter the excretion patterns of *Salmonella typhimurium* in calves.

Chlortetracycline has been used in pigs as a feed additive for promotion of growth as well as being used

TABLE 42.2—Some pharmacokinetic parameters of chlortetracycline in some food-animal species

Species	Dose (mg/kg)	Route	V_d (L/kg)	$t_{1/2}$ (hr)	Clearance (mL/min/kg)	Reference
Turkey	0.9	IV	0.2284	0.877	3.77	Dyer 1989
Pigs	11.0	IV	1.3883	NR	0.3071	Kilroy et al. 1990
Calves (milk fed)	11.0	IV	3.34	8.89	260.52 L/hr/kg	Bradley et al. 1982
Calves (conventionally fed)	11.0	IV	1.93	8.25	162.12 L/hr/kg	Bradley et al. 1982

Note: NR = information not reported; IV = intravenous.

orally for the treatment of *Salmonella typhimurium* (Jones et al. 1983; Williams et al. 1978), coccidiosis (Onawunmi and Todd 1976), and many other porcine diseases. Similar infections have been treated with chlortetracycline in poultry (Fagerberg et al. 1978; Nivas et al. 1976; Quarles et al. 1977; Landgraf et al. 1981; Dawson et al. 1983). Chlortetracycline has been reported to decrease the breeding rate of sows, although it did increase conception and farrowing rates. Birth weights, overall litter weights of pigs born alive, and weights of pigs at weaning were also significantly higher than unmedicated controls (Soma and Speer 1975).

Tetracycline. The chemical structure of tetracycline is shown in Fig. 42.2. The drug was first introduced for clinical use in 1952 and is still used today, primarily in small animals and some exotic species, although some use occurs in food-producing animals. Relatively little has been published recently on the pharmacokinetics of tetracycline; however, the absorption, distribution, metabolism, and excretion of tetracycline in animals is as described previously for the tetracyclines in general. Some of the more recent pharmacokinetic information on tetracycline is presented in Table 42.3; older information on tetracycline pharmacokinetics in other species can be obtained from previous editions of this text.

In a study by Kelly and Kanegis (1967b), ^{3}H-labeled tetracycline was administered intravenously (10 mg/kg) to dogs, which were then sacrificed to determine the extent of penetration of the radiolabeled tetracycline in the tissues. Four and one-half hours after administration, colon contents, ileal contents, bile (gallbladder), urine and jejunal contents, liver, and kidney all showed high accumulations of the drug. Significant amounts of drug accumulated in most tissues of the body except for the CSF, vitreous and aqueous humors, and fat deposits. This same study was repeated with ^{14}C-labeled chlortetracycline, and although the penetration of tetracycline and chlortetracycline was similar, the tissue penetration of tetracycline was found to be somewhat less than that of chlortetracycline in the dog. Jun and Lee (1980) studied the distribution of tetracycline in the red blood cells of dogs and humans and determined that tetracycline enters red blood cells quickly, forming a steady-state equilibrium with the extracellular fluid within 10 minutes. Hypoalbuminemia in the dog seemed to accelerate the uptake of tetracycline into the red blood cell. Tetracycline has also been explored for use in parakeets (Schachter et al. 1984). These and other studies have shown that tetracycline is absorbed and distributed well to many tissues.

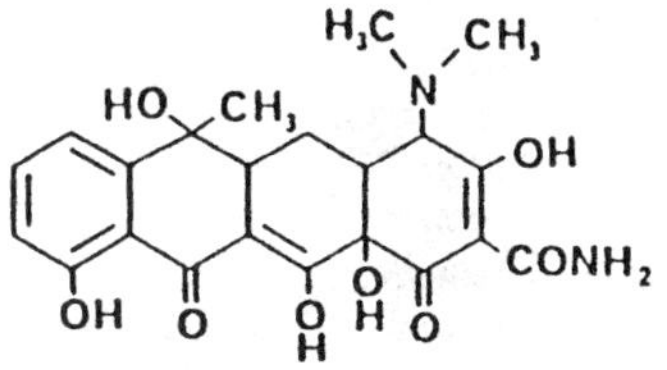

Tetracycline has been used in small animals to treat various diseases such as *Rickettsia rickettsii* (Rocky Mountain spotted fever). A study by Breitschwerdt et al. (1991) determined that tetracycline, chloramphenicol, and enrofloxacin were all equally effective in treating this disease in dogs experimentally infected with the causative organism. Tetracycline was also found to be efficacious in the treatment of canine ehrlichiosis (*E. canis*). Amyx et al. (1971) found that oral administrations of tetracycline at 30 mg/lb (13.6 mg/kg) resulted in the remission of the clinical signs associated with the disease. In addition, tetracycline administered at the dose of 3 mg/lb (1.36 mg/kg) was adequate as a prophylactic agent for the prevention of the disease. In a later study by Davidson et al. (1978), oral treatments of dogs with canine ehrlichiosis in Thailand at a dose of 66 mg/kg for 14 days caused remission of the clinical signs of this disease. However, another report (Price and Dolan 1980) found that tetracycline was rather ineffective at clearing ehrlichiosis in dogs compared to imidocarb dipropionate. Many are now using doxycycline to treat cases of ehrlichiosis in dogs due to better penetration and higher concentrations of drug within the cell. Tetracycline (10 mg/kg every 8 hr) has also been reported to be efficacious in other intracellular infections, such as *Brucella canis* (Lewis et al. 1973), as well as in treating canine urinary tract infections caused by *Pseudomonas aeruginosa* (Ling et al. 1981) in otherwise healthy dogs (Ling et al. 1980). The combination tetracycline-niacinamide has been used to treat autoimmune skin disease in dogs (White et al. 1992). Tetracycline and the other tetracyclines can be

FIG. 42.2—Chemical structure of tetracycline.

TABLE 42.3—Some pharmacokinetic parameters of tetracycline recently reported in some species

Species	Dose (mg/kg)	Route	V_d (L/kg)	$t_{1/2}$ (hr)	Clearance (mL/min/kg)	Reference
Gilts	11	IA	1.06	NR	0.4	Kniffen et al. 1989
Chickens	65	IV	0.174	2.772	1.632	Anadon et al. 1985
Rabbits (male and female)	10	IV	1.047	2	6.1	Percy and Black 1988
Channel catfish (*Ictalurus punctatus*) (27° C)	4	IV	0.513	16.5	0.365	Plakas et al. 1988

Note: NR = information not reported; IV = intravenous; IA = intra-arterial.

useful in treating borreliosis, chlamydiosis (especially in cats and poultry), *Mycoplasma* spp. *Leptospira* spp., and *Listeria* spp.

The toxicology of tetracycline has also been reported. Rats and mice given 0, 12,500, and 25,000 ppm of tetracycline in their feed for 2 years showed no evidence of carcinogenicity (Dietz et al. 1991). The use of tetracycline in conjunction with methoxyflurane anesthesia has been implicated as a causative factor in nephrotoxicosis, causing severe kidney failure and death in people and dogs. However, a study by Fleming and Pedersoli (1980) did not support the previous reports that the simultaneous use of tetracycline and methoxyflurane had deleterious effects on kidney function. Renal tubular nephrotoxicosis has also been reported when outdated tetracycline preparations were administered to humans and to calves. The degradation products of the tetracyclines have been found to be nephrotoxic and are formed in the presence of heat, low pH, and moisture (Cleveland et al. 1965; Teuscher et al. 1982; Lowe and Tapp 1966; Riond and Riviere 1989a).

Adverse reactions to tetracycline have also been reported. Tetracycline has been reported to induce anaphylactic shock in dogs after intravenous injection (Ward et al. 1982) as well as possibly increasing alanine transaminase activity in the cat (Kaufman and Greene 1993). The cardiovascular effects of tetracycline in cattle have also been reported (Gyrd-Hansen et al. 1981). Cattle were administered 5 or 10 mg/kg of tetracycline, with the total amount administered over a 10-, 60-, or 300-second time period. No cows collapsed when either dose of tetracycline was given slowly over a 300-second period, but 1 cow in 7 collapsed when given the 5 mg/kg dose over a 10-second period, and 2 cows in 7 collapsed when given the same dose over a 60-second period. For the 10 mg/kg dose, 2 cows in 7 collapsed when given the dose over a 10-second period, and 4 cows in 7 collapsed when given the dose over a 60-second period. Collapse at either dose and at any injection time was prevented when the cows were premedicated with calcium borogluconate, indicating that tetracycline may decrease the amount of calcium available to the heart for its role in contraction to the point of producing collapse of the animals. Other reports of the toxicity of tetracycline are available (McPherson et al. 1974; Wivagg et al. 1976).

Oxytetracycline. By far the most commonly used tetracycline in veterinary practice today is oxytetracycline. Numerous reports are available in the literature on the uses of oxytetracycline in veterinary medicine. Its chemical structure is shown in Fig. 42.3.

The clinical usefulness of oxytetracycline has been studied in most domestic species of animals in recent years. Previous editions of this textbook should be consulted for historic work on oxytetracycline. Recently, oxytetracycline has been used to treat ehrlichiosis in dogs (Adawa et al. 1992) and in horses (Palmer et al. 1992). A long-acting formulation of oxytetracycline, administered intramuscularly with piroxicam, was found to be effective in treating canine ehrlichiosis, while the piroxicam minimized the pain and swelling associated with oxytetracycline injections. The study by Palmer et al. (1992) also found that low-dose oxytetracycline given once, instead of twice, daily (administered intravenously) was effective in eliminating *Ehrlichia risticii* in horses. Oxytetracycline has also been recently studied in normal and diseased ovine lung tissue (Baxter and McKellar 1990) and in calves with pneumonic pasteurellosis (Burrows et al. 1986). Long-acting oxytetracycline has also found clinical usefulness in the treatment of *Moraxella bovis*/infectious bovine keratoconjunctivitis infections in calves (Smith and George 1985; George and Smith 1985; George et al. 1985; George et al. 1988). The distribution of oxytetracycline in the genital tracts of cows has also been reported (Bretzlaff et al. 1982; Bretzlaff et al. 1983a,b). Absorption of oxytetracycline is known to vary with injection site in calves. A report by Nouws and Vree (1983) found that site-to-site intramuscular injection bioavailability varied widely at 52 hours postinjection, with bioavailability being 79% in the buttock, 86% in the neck, and 98% in the shoulder.

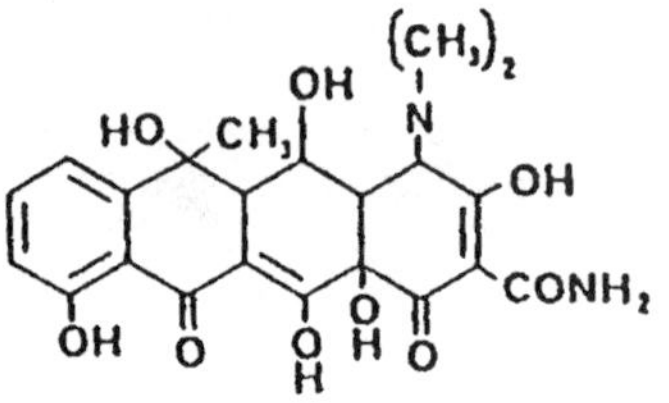

FIG. 42.3—Chemical structure of oxytetracycline.

Oxytetracycline use in the horse has also been reported. Larson and Stowe (1981) reported high serum concentrations obtained in clinically normal horses given 10 mg/kg oxytetracycline intravenously, with serum concentrations peaking at 30 minutes postinjection (16.85 μg/mL) and high concentrations persisting through at least 240 minutes (4.67 μg/mL). In addition to the high serum concentrations, oxytetracycline was demonstrated to penetrate well into pulmonary and renal tissue, as well as into bronchial fluid. In another study of oxytetracycline in horses, Brown et al. (1981) used a dose of 5 mg/kg intravenously and found a peak concentration of oxytetracycline in the serum at 0.5 hours after dose, with a steady decline in serum levels through 36 hours after dose and no detection of oxytetracycline apparent 48 hours after dose. Similar fluid-concentration versus time profiles were also demonstrated for oxytetracycline detected in the synovial fluid, peritoneal fluid, and urine after intravenous injection, suggesting that oxytetracycline crosses those membranes easily and that the concentrations obtained would be adequate for combating such infections as *Corynebacterium equi, Streptococcus zooepidemicus,* and *Actinobacillus* spp., with limited efficacy in treat-

TABLE 42.4—Some pharmacokinetic parameters of oxytetracycline in some species

Species	Dose (mg/kg)	Route	V_d (L/kg)	$t_{1/2}$ (hr)	Clearance (mL/min/kg)	Reference
Horses	10	IV	0.6728	12.953	0.6583	Horspool and McKellar 1990
Ponies	10	IV	1.0482	14.949	1.013	Horspool and McKellar 1990
Donkeys	10	IV	0.7765	6.464	1.523	Horspool and McKellar 1990
Horses (adult)	2.5	IV	1.35	10.5	NR	Pilloud 1973
Pigs	10	IV	1.49	5.99	2.88	Pijpers et al. 1991
Pigs (normal)	50	PO	1.44	5.92		Pijpers et al. 1991
Pigs (pneumonia)	50	PO	1.9	14.1		Pijpers et al. 1991
Pigs	20	IV	5.18	3.68	4.15	Mevius et al. 1986b
Cows (adult)	2.5	IV	1.04	9.12	NR	Pilloud 1973
Dairy cows	5	IV	0.917	2.63	1.24	Nouws et al. 1985a,b
Dairy cows[a]	5.23	IV	1.01	2.58	1.45	Nouws et al. 1985a,b
Veal calves	40	IV	18.144	7.34	2.246	Meijer et al. 1993a
Veal calves	20	IV	18.541		2.167	Meijer et al. 1993a
Calves (3 wk old)	7.54	IV	2.48	13.5		Nouws et al. 1983
Calves (12 wk old)	6.88	IV	1.52	8.8		Nouws et al. 1983
Calves (14 wk old)	17	IV	1.83	10.8		Nouws et al. 1983
Buffalo calves (female)	22	IV	0.32	3.6	1.02	Varma and Paul 1983
Dogs	5	IV	2.096	6.02	4.23	Baggot et al. 1977
Rabbits	10	IV	0.668	1.32	14.6	McElroy et al. 1987
Turkeys	1	IV	3.622	0.7298	3.6579	Dyer 1989
Rainbow trout	5	IV	2.988	81.5	0.423	Black et al. 1991
African catfish	60	IV	1.33	80.3	0.19	Grondel et al. 1989
Red-necked wallaby	40	IV	2.041	11.4	NR	Kirkwood et al. 1988

Note: NR = information not reported; IV = intravenous; PO = per os. All formulations were reported to be or are assumed to be HCl unless otherwise noted.
[a]Oxytetracycline dihydrate formulation tested.

ing some *Staphylococcus aureus, Escherichia coli,* and *Salmonella* spp., and no efficacy in treating common *Pseudomonas aeruginosa* pathogens.

The pharmacokinetic parameters of oxytetracycline for some species are shown in Table 42.4. More information on the pharmacokinetics of oxytetracycline is available for dogs (Baggot et al. 1977; Cooke et al. 1981), calves (Burrows et al. 1987; Banting et al. 1985; Schifferli et al. 1982; Meijer et al. 1993a,c), horses (Larson and Stowe 1981; Brown et al. 1981), chickens (Black 1977), swine (Hall et al. 1989; Pijpers et al. 1990), sheep (Immelman and Dreyer 1986), and other species (Teare et al. 1985; Martinsen et al. 1992).

Oxytetracycline is exceptional among the tetracyclines for having a conventional as well as long-acting formulations, the differences in formulation being in the different vehicles and solvent systems used to suspend the oxytetracycline for injection. Several solvent systems are available around the world that produce a long-acting effect for oxytetracycline, but only one long-acting formulation, oxytetracycline and 2-pyrrolidone, is approved for veterinary use in the United States. These solvent systems induce varying degrees of local irritation at the site of injection in calves, pigs, and sheep and, coupled with the high dose used, are responsible for the "long-acting" pharmacokinetic behavior of all these oxytetracycline formulations (Nouws et al. 1990; Nouws 1984).

Use of a long-acting formulation, particularly in food animals, has the main advantage of obtaining clinically useful sustained serum and tissue concentrations for long periods of time (up to 3-5 days) without frequent dosing. Several studies have described the differing pharmacokinetic patterns of the conventional and long-acting formulations in dogs, sheep, cattle, and pigs. Toutain and Raynaud (1983) examined the pharmacokinetic parameters of oxytetracycline with the 2-pyrrolidone carrier (long-acting formulation) injected intramuscularly in young beef cattle. This intramuscular formulation resulted in rapid development of serum concentrations of 4 μg/mL within 60-90 minutes, followed by persistence of these levels for approximately 12 hours. Serum half-life was calculated to be 21.8 hours, and bioavailability was 51.5%. Extended serum concentrations exceeding 0.5 μg/mL were found to persist for approximately 87 hours, in contrast to approximately 52 hours for the conventional formulation in another study using cattle (Mevius et al. 1986a). Davey et al. (1985) injected cattle with the conventional oxytetracycline HCl or the long-acting formulation, both at a standard 20 mg/kg dose, and found that although the long-acting formulation had lower peak serum concentrations when compared to the conventional formulation, the long-acting formulation had a longer serum $t_{1/2}$ (36.9 hr) than the conventional formulation (11.1 hr). In addition, the time it took for serum concentrations to drop below 0.5 μg/mL was 86.8 hours for the long-acting formulation and 51.5 hours for the conventional formulation. Similar findings have been reported for dairy cows (Nouws et al. 1985b), calves (Nouws and Vree 1983), pigs (Nouws et al. 1990; Xia et al. 1983; Nouws 1984), dogs (Immelman and Dreyer 1981), and sheep (Nouws et al. 1990).

Adverse reactions to oxytetracycline have been reported in dogs (Abdullahi and Adeyanju 1985; Stevenson 1980) and calves (Gross et al. 1981). The report by Abdullahi and Adeyanju describes one case where the dog may have had a hypersensitivity reaction to oxytetracycline after an intramuscular injection and later by intraocular therapy. However, this is the only literature report of this event by these routes. In a case report by Stevenson (1980), two dogs were given two doses of oxytetracycline 24 hours apart at a dose of 130 mg/kg. Both dogs died and both had evidence of acute renal tubular necrosis, indicating that high doses of oxytetracycline can induce a nephrotoxicosis. In calves, Gross et al. (1981) studied the cardiovascular effects of both oxytetracycline and the different vehicles used for injection (propylene glycol, saline, polyvinylpyrrolidine). They determined that the cardiovascular responses observed were due to the vehicles used and not the oxytetracycline. The propylene glycol vehicle studied resulted in increased pulmonary arterial pressures and a decrease in cardiac output and stroke volume. Aortic pressure and heart rates were also depressed in association with vehicle. Using histamine, antihistamine, and propylene glycol in some of the calves, it was determined that the cardiovascular effects observed were due to the endogenous release of histamine after propylene glycol injection and this histamine release was not dependent on the animal being sensitized prior to exposure. No discernible cardiovascular effects were observed after injection with the oxytetracycline-saline combination, while the polyvinylpyrrolidine preparation and vehicle resulted in higher aortic pressure, heart rate, and overall systemic resistance.

Doxycycline. Doxycycline, like all other derivatives of tetracycline, is a structural isomer of the parent molecule and is synthesized from oxytetracycline or methacycline. Doxycycline and minocycline (discussed later in this chapter) differ from tetracycline, oxytetracycline, and chlortetracycline in that they are more lipophilic (5- to 10-fold increase), resulting in higher tissue penetration, larger volumes of distribution, and better overall antimicrobial properties. Doxycycline is unique in that it is excreted in the feces as an inactive conjugate or chelate and, in this form, has little impact on the lower intestinal microbial flora. Doxycycline also has greater plasma protein binding than the other tetracyclines, which produces a prolonged half-life of the drug in humans and animals. The chemical structure of doxycycline is shown in Fig. 42.4.

The pharmacokinetics of doxycycline has been studied in dogs and cats (Wilson et al. 1988; Riond et al. 1990), pigs (Riond and Riviere 1990a,b), calves (Meijer et al. 1993b; Riond et al. 1989b), goats (Jha et al. 1989), rhesus monkeys (Kelly et al. 1992), and birds (Prus et al. 1992; Greth et al. 1993). Some of the pharmacokinetic data for doxycycline for commonly encountered species of animals are listed in Table 42.5.

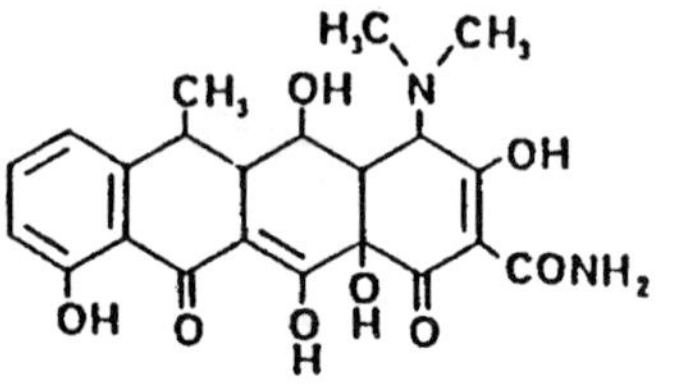

FIG. 42.4—Chemical structure of doxycycline.

Doxycycline pharmacokinetics has been extensively studied in humans and to a lesser degree in animals. An excellent review of doxycycline's use in humans is available (Cunha et al. 1982). Riond et al. (1990) compared the pharmacokinetics of doxycycline in dogs and cats given 5 mg/kg intravenously. In dogs, a peak serum concentration of 11.56 μg/mL was detected in serum 0.17 minutes after injection, steadily falling to 0.33 μg/mL 32 hours after injection and to nondetectable serum levels at 44 hours and beyond. Similar serum pharmacokinetics have been reported in dogs by others (Wilson et al. 1988). In cats, the peak serum concentration was 22.89 μg/mL and fell to 0.89 μg/mL 20 hours after injection, falling to nondetectable levels at 32 hours and beyond. Doxycycline was more extensively bound to serum proteins in cats than in dogs. Protein binding was reported to be 98.35% in cats and 91.40% in dogs, with albumin binding being 76.46% in cats and 53.87% in dogs (Riond et al. 1990). Doxycycline pharmacokinetics has been reported in pigs (Riond and Riviere 1990a). The $t_{1/2}$ for doxycycline in this species was significantly shorter than that in other food-producing animals. Also, no doxycycline biotransformation was detected in those pigs, and no metabolites were detected in calves (Riond et al. 1989b). Bioavailability in calves of doxycycline fed orally with milk replacer was approximately 70%, with an elimination $t_{1/2}$ of 9.5 (±3.0) hours. Plasma concentrations after repeated oral doses of doxycycline in those calves indicated doxycycline may be a potentially valuable drug in food-animal medicine (Meijer et al. 1993b). Doxycycline use in the goat has also been reported (Jha et al. 1989). The pharmacokinetics of doxycycline is easily extrapolated across species using allometric procedures (Riond and Riviere 1990b).

Riond and Riviere (1989b) reported on the binding of doxycycline to plasma albumin in dogs, sheep, cats, cows, pigs, and humans by measuring the association constants (Ka, L/mol). Doxycycline is associated with less gastrointestinal tract irritation and superinfection, and it has been suggested that intravenous doxycycline may be suitable for use in the equine because tetracycline-induced colitis may be avoided or minimized using this route. However, two reports have shown that even subtherapeutic doses of doxycycline in a proprietary vehicle administered via a slow intravenous injection induced collapse and death within 15 minutes in

TABLE 42.5—Some pharamcokinetic parameters of doxycycline in some species

Species	Dose (mg/kg)	Route	V_d (L/kg)	$t_{1/2}$ (hr)	Clearance (mL/min/kg)	Reference
Pigs (9 wk old)	20	IV	0.53	4.04	1.67	Riond and Riviere 1989b
Calves	5	IV	NR	9.5	1.2 (mg/L)	Meijer et al. 1993b
Calves (functional rumen)	20	IV	1.31	14.9	1.07	Riond et al. 1989b
Calves (nonfunctional rumen)	20	IV	1.81	9.9	2.2	Riond et al. 1989b
Cats	5	IV	0.34	4.56	1.09	Riond et al. 1990
Dogs	5	IV	0.93	6.99	1.72	Riond et al. 1990
Dogs	5	IV	1.468	10.36	1.68	Wilson et al. 1988
Goats (lactating)	5	IV	9.78	16.63	6.91	Jha et al. 1989

Note: IV = intravenous; NR = information not reported.

two horses, whereas injection of just the proprietary vehicle produced no ill effects. Similar effects were seen in doxycycline given intravenously at doses above the recommended therapeutic dose in a saline vehicle in horses. Due to these adverse cardiovascular effects in horses induced by doxycycline, it is strongly recommended that doxycycline use in this species be avoided (Riond et al. 1989a; Riond et al. 1992). In dogs and cats, nausea and vomiting have been reported to occur and can be minimized if the doxycycline tablet is administered with food.

Few recent clinical reports are available on the use of doxycycline in animals. Doxycycline has been used to treat a variety of extracellular and intracellular infections in dogs, in particular ehrlichiosis (*Ehrlichia canis*), and other infections in other species, including respiratory tract disease and systemic colibacillosis in poultry (Migaki and Babcock 1977; George et al. 1977), psittacosis in avians, and anaplasmosis in splenectomized calves (Kutter and Simpson 1978). Other susceptible organisms may include *Haemobartonella* spp., *Mycoplasma* spp., *Rickettsia* spp., *Campylobacter* spp., and *Leptospira* spp. Doxycycline and minocycline have increased activity against susceptible intracellular-dwelling microbes because of their high penetration into cells due to increased lipophilicity. Because of the unique way doxycycline is eliminated (fecal), concentrations of doxycycline do not tend to accumulate in the blood of human patients experiencing renal failure. Doxycycline is thus ideal for treating susceptible infections when renal failure or renal insufficiency is a complicating factor in antimicrobial therapy (Shaw and Rubin 1986). Doxycycline accumulation in normal and diseased kidneys in dogs and humans has been studied (Whelton et al. 1975). Recent work by Yu et al. (1992) has indicated that doxycycline administered prophylactically markedly reduced the severity of osteoarthritis in dogs with surgically induced transactions of the anterior cruciate ligament. Inhibition of classical lesions in that model was felt to be due to doxycycline's ability to inhibit (chelate) metalloproteases (collagenase, gelatinase, stromelysin) in the degenerating cartilage of the canine knee.

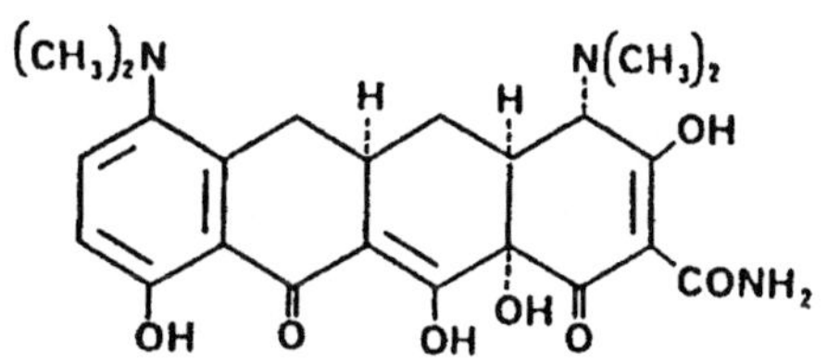

FIG. 42.5—Chemical structure of minocycline.

Minocycline. Like doxycycline, minocycline is a product of chemical manipulations of the tetracycline base molecule that enhance antimicrobial action by improving gastrointestinal tract absorption, prolonging the half-life, and increasing the tissue penetration of the drug. The chemical structure of minocycline is shown in Fig. 42.5. Increased penetration of minocycline into bacterial cells results in more activity against penicillinase-resistant strains of *Staphylococcus aureus* and a variety of other gram-positive and gram-negative organisms (Jonas and Cunha 1982). The increased concentration of the drug within the cell, which results in an overall increase in pharmacologic activity, is the primary advantage of minocycline.

Little recent information on the clinical use of minocycline in animals is available. In humans, minocycline is rapidly and completely absorbed from the gastrointestinal tract, which results in high bioavailability by this route and serves to minimize disturbance of the normal bacterial flora of the gastrointestinal tract. As with other tetracyclines, food, milk, and iron decrease the absorption of minocycline, but not to as great an extent (Leyden 1985). A high degree of protein binding occurs with minocycline in the plasma, with 80% protein binding reported for sheep serum (Wilson and Green 1986).

Some studies have been performed with minocycline in dogs. A toxicologic study performed by Noble et al. (1967) examined the use of minocycline in Beagles administered a daily dose of 5, 10, 20, or 40 mg/kg intravenously for 1 month. Significant weight loss occurred in the dogs treated with the 40 mg/kg dose

TABLE 42.6—Some pharmacokinetic parameters of minocycline HCl in some species

Species	Dose (mg/kg)	Route	V_d (L/kg)	$t_{1/2}$ (hr)	Clearance (mL/min/kg)	Reference
Dogs (2-compartment model)	5	IV	1.952	6.93	3.347	Wilson et al. 1985
Dogs (3-compartment model)	5	IV	2.001	7.24	3.424	Wilson et al. 1985
Sheep (normal)	2.2	IV	1.32	2.58	5.94	Wilson and Green 1986
Sheep (hypoproteinemic)	2.2	IV	1.67	2.91	5.60	Wilson and Green 1986

Note: IV = intravenous.

and in one dog given the 20 mg/kg dose of minocycline. In most dogs receiving any of the doses of minocycline, there was erythema of the skin and mucous membranes, characterized by papules around the eyes, muzzle, ears, and abdomen; the intensity of these lesions was directly proportional to the dose administered. Dogs administered the high dose of minocycline (40 mg/kg) showed increased glutamic-oxalacetic acid and glutamic-pyruvate and a decrease in serum protein-bound iodine values. Decreases in red blood cell packed cell volumes, hemoglobin concentrations, and red cell counts were noted in dogs receiving 10 mg/kg or more of minocycline intravenously. Similar adverse effects was noted by Wilson et al. (1985). Other toxicologic studies with minocycline have been performed in dogs, rats, mice, and monkeys (Benitz et al. 1967).

Minocycline is highly lipid soluble; therefore, it has a great ability to penetrate many tissues of the body and has far better tissue penetration than other tetracyclines. Tissue distribution studies in dogs given a 10 mg/kg intravenous dose of minocycline showed that the drug penetrated most tissues very well, much like the other tetracyclines (Kelly and Kanegis 1967a). High concentrations are found in the bile, brain, CSF, upper respiratory tract secretions, lung, skin, reproductive organs, thyroid gland, milk, and prostate of the human, with similar penetration patterns likely present in animals. Minocycline is unique in that excretion seems to be independent of renal function, indicating that renal excretion of minocycline is a minor route of eliminating the drug from the body, which may be of importance for veterinary patients undergoing minocycline therapy with concurrent renal dysfunction. Minocycline is extensively bound to plasma proteins, which may in part account for its prolonged biological half-life. Minocycline in humans is partly degraded to inactive metabolites, with the parent compound concentrating in the bile, where enterohepatic circulation is likely and may account in part (in addition to its high lipid solubility) for its prolonged half-life in the body compared to other tetracyclines. Other evidence suggests that metabolism may not play a major role in the elimination of minocycline in the rat or dog (Wilson and Green 1986). The major route of elimination for minocycline appears to be through the feces.

The pharmacokinetics of minocycline in some species is summarized in Table 42.6. Pharmacokinetic parameters of other tetracycline analogs (including minocycline) have also been reported in dairy cows and ewes (Ziv and Sulman 1974) and in rabbits (Nicolau et al. 1993).

REFERENCES

Abdullahi, S. U., and Adeyanju, J. B. 1985. Adverse reaction to oxytetracycline in a dog. Vet Hum Toxicol 27(5):390.

Adawa, D. A. Y., Hassan, A. Z., Abdullah, S. U., Ogunkoya, A. B., Adeyanju, J. B., and Okoro, J. E. 1992. Clinical trial of long-acting oxytetracycline and piroxicam in the treatment of canine ehrlichiosis. Vet Quarterly 14(3):118-120.

Amyx, H. L., Huxsoll, D. L., Zeiler, D. C., and Hildebrandt, P. K. 1971. Therapeutic and prophylactic value of tetracycline in dogs infected with the agent of tropical canine pancyctopenia. JAVMA 159(11):1428-1432.

Anadon, A., Martinez-Larranaga, M. R., and Diaz, M. J. 1985. Pharmacokinetics of tetracycline in chickens after intravenous administration. Poultry Sci 64:2273-79.

Aronson, A. L. 1980. Pharmacotherapeutics of the newer tetracyclines. JAVMA 176(10):1061-68.

Baggot, J. D., Powers, T. E., Powers, J. D., Kowalski, J. J., and Kerr, K. M. 1977. Pharmacokinetics and dosage of oxytetracycline in dogs. Res Vet Sci 24:77-81.

Banting, A. de L., Duval, M., and Gregoire, S. 1985. A comparative study of serum kinetics of oxytetracycline in pigs and calves following intramuscular administration. J Vet Pharmacol Therap 8:418-20.

Barza, M., Brown, R. B., Shanks, C., Gamble, C., and Weinstein, L. 1975. Relation between lipophilicity and pharmacological behavior of minocycline, doxycycline, tetracycline, and oxytetracycline in dogs. Antimicrob Agents Chemotherapy 8(6):713-20.

Baxter, P., and McKellar, Q. A. 1990. Distribution of oxytetracycline in normal and diseased ovine lung tissue. J Vet Pharmacol Therap 13:428-31.

Benitz, K.-F.., Roberts, G. K. S., and Yusa, A. 1967. Morphologic effects of minocycline in laboratory animals. Toxicol Appl Pharmacol 11:150-70.

Black, W. D. 1977. A study of the pharmacokinetics of oxytetracycline in the chicken. Poultry Sci 56:1430-34.

Black, W. D., Ferguson, H. W., Byrne, P., and Claxton, M. J. 1991. Pharmacokinetic and tissue distribution study of oxytetracycline in rainbow trout following bolus intravenous administration. J Vet Pharmacol Therap 14:351-58.

Bocker, R., Estler, C. J., Muller, S., Pfandzelter, C., and Spachmuller, B. 1982. Comparative evaluation of the effects of tetracycline, rolitetracycline and doxycycline on some blood parameters related to liver function. Arzneim Forsch 32(1):237-41.

Bradley, B. D., Allen, E. H., Showalter, D. H., and Colaianne, J. J. 1982. Comparative pharmacokinetics of chlortetracycline in milk-fed versus conventionally fed calves. J Vet Pharmacol Therap 5:267-78.

Breitschwerdt, E. B., Davidson, M. G., Aucoin, D. P., Levy, M. G., Szabados, N. S., Hegarty, B. C., Kuehne, A. L., and James, R. L. 1991. Efficacy of chloramphenicol, enrofloxacin, tetracycline for treatment of experimental rocky mountain spotted fever in dogs. Antimicrob Agents Chemotherapy 35(11):2375-81.

Bretzlaff, K. N., Ott, R. S., Koritz, G. D., Bevill, R. F., Gustafsson, B. K., and Davis, L. E. 1983a. Distribution of oxytetracycline in the genital tract tissues of postpartum cows given the drug by intravenous and intrauterine routes. AJVR 44(5):764-69.

———. 1983b. Distribution of oxytetracycline in the healthy and diseased postpartum genital tract of cows. AJVR 44:760-63.

Bretzlaff, K. N., Ott, R. S., Koritz, G. D., Lock, T. F., Bevill, R. F., Shawley, R. V., Gustafsson, B. K., and Davis, L. E. 1982. Distribution of oxytetracycline in the genital tract of cows. AJVR 43:12-16.

Brown, H., Bing, R. F., Grueter, H. P., McAskill, J. W., Cooley, C. O., and Rathmacher, R. P. 1975. Tylosin and chlortetracycline for the prevention of liver abscesses, improved weight gains and feed efficiency in feedlot cattle. J Anim Sci 40(2):207-13.

Brown, M. P., Stover, S. M., Kelly, R. H., Farber, T. B., and Knight, H. D. 1981. Oxytetracycline hydrochloride in the horse: serum, synovial, peritoneal and urine concentrations after single dose intravenous administration. J Vet Pharmacol Therap 4:7-10.

Burrows, G. E., Barto, P. B., and Martin, B. 1987. Comparative pharmacokinetics of gentamicin, neomycin and oxytetracycline in newborn calves. J Vet Pharmacol Therap 10:54-63.

Burrows, G. E., Barto, P. B., and Weeks, B. R. 1986. Chloramphenicol, lincomycin and oxytetracycline disposition in calves with experimental pneumonic pasteurellosis. J Vet Pharmacol Therap 9:213-22.

Cleveland, W. W., Adams, W. C., Mann, J. B. 1965. Acquired fanconi syndrome following degraded tetracycline. J Pediatr 66:333-42.

Cooke, R. G., Knifton, A., Murdoch, D. B., and Yacoub, I. S. 1981. Bioavailability of oxytetracycline dihydrate tables in dogs. J Vet Pharmacol Therap 4:11-13.

Cunha, B. A., Sibley, C. M., and Ristuccia, A. M. 1982. Doxycycline. Therap Drug Monit 4:115-35.

Davey, L. A., Ferber, M. T., and Kaye, B. 1985. Comparison of the serum pharmacokinetics of a long acting and a conventional oxytetracycline injection. Vet Rec 117:426-29.

Davidson, D. E., Jr., Dill, G. S., Jr., Tingpalapong, M., Premabutra, S., Nguen, P. L., Stephenson, E. H., and Ristic, M. 1978. Prophylactic and therapeutic use of tetracycline during an epizootic of ehrlichiosis among military dogs. J Am Vet Med Assoc 172(6):697-700.

Dawson, K. A., Langlois, B. E., Stahly, T. S., and Cromwell, G. L. 1983. Multiple antibiotic resistance in fecal, cecal and colonic coliforms from pigs fed therapeutic and subtherapeutic concentrations of chlortetracycline. J Anim Sci 57(5):1225-34.

Dietz, D. D., Abdo, K. M., Haseman, J. K., Eustis, S. L., and Huff, J. E. 1991. Comparative toxicity and carcinogenicity studies of tetracycline and oxytetracycline in rats and mice. Fund Appl Toxicol 17:335-46.

Dyer, D. C. 1989. Pharmacokinetics of oxytetracycline in the turkey: evaluation of biliary and urinary excretion. AJVR 50(4):522-24.

Fagerberg, D. J., Quarles, C. L., George, B. A., Fenton, J. M., Rollins, L. D., Williams, L. P., and Hancock, C. B. 1978. Effect of low level chlortetracycline feeding on subsequent therapy of *Escherichia coli* infection in chickens. J Anim Sci 46(5):1397-1412.

Fair, W. R. 1974. Diffusion of minocycline into prostatic secretions in dogs. Urology 3:339-44.

Finerman, G. A. M., and Milch, R. A. 1963. In vitro binding of tetracyclines to calcium. Nature 198:486-87.

Fleming, J. T., and Pedersoli, W. M. 1980. Serum inorganic fluoride and renal function in dogs after methoxyflurane anesthesia, tetracycline treatment, and surgical manipulation. AJVR 41:2025-29.

Gale, E. F., and Folkes, J. P. 1953. The assimilation of amino acids by bacteria: actions of antibiotics on nucleic acid and protein synthesis in *Staphylococcus aureus*. Biochem J 53:493-98.

George, B. A., Fagerberg, D. J., Quarles, C. L. 1977. Comparison of therapeutic efficacy of doxycycline, chlortetracycline and lincomycin-spectinomycin on *E. coli* infection of young chickens. Poultry Sci 56:452-58.

George, L., Mihalyi, J., Edmondson, A., Daigneault, J., Kagonyera, G., Willits, N., and Lucas, M. 1988. Topically applied furazolidone or parenterally administered oxytetracycline for the treatment of infectious bovine keratoconjunctivitis. JAVMA 192(10):1415-22.

George, L. W., and Smith, J. A. 1985. Treatment of *Moraxella bovis* infections in calves using a long-term oxytetracycline formulation. J Vet Pharmacol Therap 8:55-61.

George, L. W., Smith, J. A., and Kaswan, R. 1985. Distribution of oxytetracycline into ocular tissues and tears of calves. J Vet Pharmacol Therap 8:47-54.

Gothoni, G., Neuvonen, P. J., Mattila, M. 1972. Iron-tetracycline interaction: effect of time interval between the drugs. Acta Med Scand 191:409-11.

Greth, A., Gerlach, H., Gerbermann, H., Vassart, M., and Richez, P. 1993. Pharmacokinetics of doxycycline after parenteral administration in the Houbara Bustard (*Chlamydotis undulata*). Avian Dis 37:31-36.

Grondel, J. L., Nouws, J. F. M., Schutte, A. R., and Driessens, F. 1989. Comparative pharmacokinetics of oxytetracycline in rainbow trout (*Salmo gairdneri*) and African catfish (*Clarias gariepinus*). J Vet Pharmacol Therap 12:157-62.

Gross, D. R., Dodd, K. T., Williams, J. D., and Adams, H. R. 1981. Adverse cardiovascular effects of oxytetracycline preparations and vehicles in intact awake calves. AJVR 42(8):1371-77.

Gyrd-Hansen, N., Rasmussen, F., and Smith, M. 1981. Cardiovascular effects of intravenous administration of tetracycline in cattle. J Vet Pharmacol Therap 4:15-25.

Hagermark, O., and Hoglund, S. 1974. Iron metabolism in tetracycline-treated acne patients. Acta Derm Venereol 54:45-48.

Hall, W. F., Kniffen, T. S., Bane, D. P., Bevill, R. F., and Koritz, G. D. 1989. Plasma concentrations of oxytetracycline in swine after administration of the drug intramuscularly and orally in feed. JAVMA 194(9):1265-68.

Hamp, S. E. 1967. The tetracyclines and their effect on teeth: a clinical study. Odontologisk Tidskrift 75:33-49.

Harber, L. C., Tromovitch, T. A., and Baer, R. L. 1961. Studies on photosensitivity due to demethylchlortetracycline. J Invest Dermatol 37:189-93.

Harcourt, R. S., and Hamburger, M. 1957. The effect of magnesium sulfate in lowering tetracycline blood levels. J Lab Clin Med 50:464-68.

Hennon, D. K. 1965. Dental aspects of tetracycline therapy: literature review and results of a prevalence survey. J Indiana Dent Assoc 44:484-92.

Hoeprich, P. D., and Warshauer, D. M. 1974. Entry of four tetracyclines into saliva and tears. Antimicrob Agents Chemotherapy 5:330-36.

Hopf, G., Bocker, R., and Estler, C. J. 1985. Comparative effects of tetracycline and doxycycline on liver function of young adult and old mice. Arch Int Pharmacodyn 278:157-68.

Horspool, L. J. I., and McKellar, Q. A. 1990. Disposition of oxytetracycline in horses, ponies and donkeys after intravenous administration. Eq Vet J 22(4):284-85.

Immelman, A., and Dreyer, G. 1981. Oxytetracycline plasma levels in dogs after intramuscular administration of two formulations. J S African Vet Assoc 52(3):191-93.

———. 1986. Oxytetracycline concentration in plasma and semen of rams. J S African Vet Assoc 57(2):103-104.

Jha, V. K., Jayachandran, C., Singh, M. K., and Singh, S. D. 1989. Pharmacokinetic data on doxycycline and its distribution in different biological fluids in female goats. Vet Res Commun 13:11-16.

Jonas, M., and Cunha, B. A. 1982. Minocycline. Therap Drug Monitoring 4(2):137-45.

Jones, F. T., Langlois, B. E., Cromwell, G. L., and Hays, V. W. 1983. Effect of feeding chlortetracycline or virginiamycin on shedding of salmonellae from experimentally-infected swine. J Anim Sci 57(2):279-85.

Jun, H. W., and Lee, B. H. 1980. Distribution of tetracycline in red blood cells. J Pharm Sci 69(4):455-57.

Kaufman, A. C., and Greene, C. E. 1993. Increased alanine transaminase activity associated with tetracycline administration in a cat. JAVMA 202(4):628-30.

Kelly, D. J., Chulay, J. D., Mikesell, P., and Friedlander, A. M. 1992. Serum concentrations of penicillin, doxycycline, and ciprofloxacin during prolonged therapy in rhesus monkeys. J Infect Dis 166:1184-87.

Kelly, R. G., and Kanegis, L. A. 1967a. Metabolism and tissue distribution of radioisotopically labeled minocycline. Toxicol Appl Pharmacol 11:171-83.

———. 1967b. Tissue distribution of tetracycline and chlortetracycline in the dog. Toxicol Appl Pharmacol 11:114-20.

Kilroy, C. R., Hall, W. F., Bane, D. P., Bevill, R. F., and Koritz, G. D. 1990. Chlortetracycline in swine: bioavailability and pharmacokinetics in fasted and fed pigs. J Vet Pharmacol Therap 13:49-58.

Kirkwood, J. K., Gulland, F. M. D., Needham, J. R., and Vogler, M. G. 1988. Pharmacokinetics of oxytetracycline in clinical cases in the red-necked walaby (*Macropus rufogriseus*). Res Vet Sci 44:335-37.

Kniffen, T. S., Bane, D. P., Hall, W. F., Koritz, G. D., and Bevill, R. F. 1989. Bioavailability, pharmacokinetics, and plasma concentration of tetracycline hydrochloride fed to swine. AJVR 50(4):518-21.

Kunin, C. M., and Finland, M. 1961. Clinical pharmacology of the tetracycline antibiotics. Clin Pharmacol Ther 2:51-69.

Kutter, K. L., and Simpson, J. E. 1978. Relative efficacy of two oxytetracycline formulations and doxycycline in the treatment of acute anaplasmosis in splenectomized calves. AJVR 39:347-49.

Landgraf, W. W., Ross, P. F., Cassidy, D. R., and Clubb, S. L. 1981. Concentration of chlortetracycline in the blood of yellow-crowned Amazon parrots fed medicated pelleted feeds. Avian Dis 26(1):14-17.

Larson, V. L., and Stowe, C. M. 1981. Plasma and tissue concentrations of oxytetracycline in the horse after intravenous administration. AJVR 42(12):2165-66.

Lewis, G. E., Crumrine, M. H., Jennings, P. B., and Fariss, B. L. 1973. Therapeutic value of tetracycline and ampicillin in dogs infected with *Brucella canis*. JAVMA 163:239-41.

Leyden, J. J. 1985. Absorption of minocycline hydrochloride and tetracycline hydrochloride. J Am Acad Dermatol 12:308-12.

Ling, G. V., Conzelman, G. M., Franti, C. E., and Ruby, A. L. 1980. Urine concentrations of chloramphenicol, tetracycline, and sulfisoxazole after oral administration to healthy adult dogs. AJVR 41(6):950-52.

Ling, G. V., Creighton, S. R., and Ruby, A. L. 1981. Tetracycline for oral treatment of canine urinary tract infection caused by *Pseudomonas aeruginosa*. JAVMA 179(6):578-79.

Lowe, M. B., and Tapp, E. 1966. Renal damage caused by anhydro-4-epitetracycline. Arch Pathol 81:362-64.

MacCulloch, D., Richardson, R. A., and Allwood, G. K. 1974. The penetration of doxycycline, oxytetracycline and minocycline into sputum. NZ Med J 80:300-302.

Martinsen, B., Oppegaard, H., Wichstrom, R., and Myhr, E. 1992. Temperature-dependent in vitro antimicrobial activity of four 4-quinolones and oxytetracycline against bacteria pathogenic to fish. Antimicrob Agents Chemotherapy 36(8):1738-43.

McElroy, D. E., Ravis, W. R., and Clark, C. H. 1987. Pharmacokinetics of oxytetracycline hydrochloride in rabbits. AJVR 48(8):1261-63.

McPherson, J. C., Ellison, R. G., Davis, H. N., Hawkridge, F. M., Ellison, L. T., and Hall, W. K. 1974. The metabolic acidosis resulting from intravenous tetracycline administration (37829). Proc Soc Exper Biol Med 145:450-55.

Meijer, L. A., Ceyssens, G. F., deJong, W. T., and de Greve, B. I. J. A. C. 1993a. Correlation between tissue and plasma concentrations of oxytetracycline in veal calves. J Toxicol Environ Health 40:35-45.

Meijer, L. A., Ceyssens, K. G. F , de Greve, B. I. J. A. C., and de Bruijn, W. 1993b. Pharmacokinetics and bioavailability of doxycycline hyclate after oral administration in calves. Vet Quarterly 15(1):1-5.

Meijer, L. A., Ceyssens, K. G. F., deJong, W. T., and deGreve, B. I. J. A. C. 1993c. Three phase elimination of oxytetracycline in veal calves: the presence of an extended terminal elimination phase. J Vet Pharmacol Therap 16:214-22.

Mevius, D. J., Nouws, J. F. M., Breukink, H. J., Vree, T. B., Driessens, F., and Verkaik, R. 1986a. Comparative pharmacokinetics, bioavailability and renal clearance of five parenteral oxytetracycline-20% formulations in dairy cows. Vet Quarterly 8(4):285-94.

Mevius, D. J., Vellenga, L., Breukink, H. J., Nouws, J. F. M., Vree, T. B., and Driessens, F. 1986b. Pharmacokinetics and renal clearance of oxytetracycline in piglets following intravenous and oral administration. Vet Quarterly 8(4):274-84.

Migaki, T. T., and Babcock, W. E. 1977. Efficacy of doxycycline against experimental complicated chronic respiratory disease compared with commercially available water medicants in broilers. Poutry Sci 56:1739.

Moffit, J. M., Cooley, R. O., and Olsen, N. H. 1974. Prediction of tetracycline-induced tooth discoloration. J Am Dental Assoc 88:547-52.

Neuvonen, P. J., Gothoni, G., Hackman, R., and Bjorksten, K. 1970. Interference of iron with the absorption of tetracyclines in man. Brit Med J 4:532-34.

Nicolau, D. P., Freeman, C. D., Nightingale, C. H., and Quintiliani, R. 1993. Pharmacokinetics of minocycline and vancomycin in rabbits. Lab An Sci 43(3):222-25.

Nivas, S. C., York, M. D., and Pomeroy, B. S. 1976. Effects of different levels of chlortetracycline in the diet of turkey poults artificially-infected with *Salmonella typhimurium*. Poultry Sci 55:2176-89.

Noble, J. F., Kanegis, L. A., and Hallesy, D. W. 1967. Short-term toxicity and observations on certain aspects of the pharmacology of a unique tetracycline—minocycline. Toxicol Appl Pharmacol 11:128-49.

Nouws, J. F. M. 1984. Irritation, bioavailability, and residue aspects of ten oxytetracycline formulations administered intramuscularly to pigs. Vet Quarterly 6(2):80-84.

Nouws, J. F. M., Breukink, H. J., Binkhorst, G. J., Lohuis, J., van Lith, P., Mevius, D. J., and Vree, T. B. 1985a. Comparative pharmacokinetics and bioavailability of eight parenteral oxytetracycline-10% formulations in dairy cows. Vet Quarterly 7(4):306-14.

Nouws, J. F. M., Smulders, A., and Rappalini, M. 1990. A comparative study on irritation and residue aspects of five oxytetracycline formulations administered intramuscularly to calves, pigs and sheep. Vet Quarterly 12(3):129-38.

Nouws, J. F. M., van Ginneken, C. A. M., and Ziv, G. 1983. Age-dependent pharmacokinetics of oxytetracycline in ruminants. J Vet Pharmacol Therap 6:59-66.

Nouws, J. F. M., and Vree, T. B. 1983. Effect of injection site on the bioavailability of an oxytetracycline formulation in ruminant calves. Vet Quarterly 5(4):165-70.

Nouws, J. F. M., Vree, T. B., Termond, E., Lohuis, J., van Lith, P., Binkhorse, G. J., and Breukink, H. J. 1985b. Pharmacokinetics and renal clearance of oxytetracycline after intravenous and intramuscular administration to dairy cows. Vet Quarterly 7(4):296-305.

Onawunmi, O. A., and Todd, A. C. 1976. Suppression and control of experimentally induced porcine coccidiosis with chlortetracycline combination, buquinolate, and lincomycin hydrochloride. AJVR 37:657-60.

Palmer, J. E., Benson, C. E., and Whitlock, R. H. 1992. Effect of treatment with oxytetracycline during the acute stages of experimentally induced equine ehrlichial colitis in ponies. AJVR 53(12):2300-2304.

Percy, D. H., and Black, W. D. 1988. Pharmacokinetics of tetracycline in the domestic rabbit following intravenous or oral administration. Can J Vet Res 52:5-11.

Perry, T. W., Beeson, W. M., Mohler, M. T., and Harrington, R. B. 1971. Value of chlortetracycline and sulfamethazine for conditioning feeder cattle after transit. J Anim Sci 32(1):137-40.

Pijpers, A., Schoevers, E. J., van Gogh, H., van Leengoed, L. A. M. G., Visser, I. J. R., van Miert, A. S. J. P. A. M., and Verheijden, J. H. M. 1990. The pharmacokinetics of oxytetracycline following intravenous administration in healthy and diseased pigs. J Vet Pharmacol Therap 13:320-26.

———. 1991. The influence of disease on feed and water consumption and on pharmacokinetics of orally administered oxytetracycline in pigs. J Anim Sci 69:2947-54.

Pilloud, M. 1973. Pharmacokinetics, plasma protein binding and dosage of oxytetracycline in cattle and horses. Res Vet Sci 15:224-30.

Plakas, S. M., McPhearson, R. M., and Guarino, A. M. 1988. Disposition and bioavailability of 3H-tetracycline in the channel catfish (*Ictalurus punctatus*). Xenobiotica 18(1):83-93.

Prescott, J. F., and Baggot, J. D. (eds.) 1993. Tetracyclines. In Antimicrobial Therapy in Veterinary Medicine, 2nd ed., pp. 215-228. Ames: Iowa State Univ Press.

Price, J. E., and Dolan, T. T. 1980. A comparison of the efficacy of imidocarb dipropionate and tetracycline hydrochloride in the treatment of canine ehrlichiosis. Vet Rec 107:275-77.

Prus, S. E., Clubb, S. L., Flammer, K. 1992. Doxycycline plasma concentrations in macaws fed a medicated corn diet. Avian Dis 36:480-83.

Quarles, C. L., Fagerberg, D. J., and Greathouse, G. A. 1977. Effect of low level feeding chlortetracycline on subsequent therapy of chicks infected with *Salmonella typhimurium*. Poultry Sci 56:1674-75.

Richey, E. J., Brock, W. E., Kliewer, I. O., and Jones, E. W. 1977. Low levels of chlortetracycline for anaplasmosis. AJVR 38(2):171-72.

Riond, J.-L., and Riviere, J. E. 1988. Pharmacology and toxicology of doxycycline. Vet Human Toxicol 30(5):431-43.

———. 1989a. Effects of tetracyclines on the kidney in cattle and dogs. JAVMA 195(7):995-97.

———. 1989b. Doxycycline binding to plasma albumin of several species. J Vet Pharmacol Therap 12:253-60.

———. 1990a. Pharmacokinetics and metabolic inertness of doxycycline in young pigs. AJVR 51(8):1271-75.

———. 1990b. Allometric analysis of doxycycline pharmacokinetic parameters. J Vet Pharmacol Therap 13:404-07.

Riond, J.-L., Duckett, W. M., Riviere, J. E., Jernigan, A. D., and Spurlock, S. L. 1989a. Concerned about intravenous use of doxycycline in horses. JAVMA 195(7):846-47.

Riond, J.-L., Tyczkowska, K., and Riviere, J. E. 1989b. Pharmacokinetics and metabolic inertness of doxycycline in calves with mature or immature rumen function. AJVR 50(8):1329-33.

Riond, J.-L., Vaden, S. L., and Riviere, J. E. 1990. Comparative pharmacokinetics of doxycycline in cats and dogs. J Vet Pharmacol Therap 13:415-24.

Riond, J.-L., Riviere, J. E., Duckett, W. M., Atkins, C. E., Jernigan, A. D., Rikihisa, Y., and Spurlock, S. L. 1992. Cardiovascular effects and fatalities associated with intravenous administration of doxycycline to horses and ponies. Eq Vet J 24(1):41-45.

Royal, W. A., Robinson, R. A., and Loken, K. I. 1970. The influence of chlortetracycline feeding on *Salmonella typhimurium* excretion in young calves. Vet Rec 86:67-69.

Schach von Wittenau, M., and Delahunt, C. S. 1966. The distribution of tetracycline in tissues of dogs after repeated oral administration. J Pharmacol Exp Therap 152:164-69.

Schach von Wittenau, M., and Twomey, T. M. 1971. The disposition of doxycycline by man and dog. Chemotherapy 16:217-28.

Schachter, J., Bankowski, R. A., Sung, M. L., Miers, L., and Strassburger, M. 1984. Measurement of tetracycline levels in parakeets. Avian Dis 28(1):295-302.

Schifferli, D., Galeazzi, R. L., Nicolet, J., and Wanner, M. 1982. Pharmacokinetics of oxytetracycline and therapeutic implications in veal calves. J Vet Pharmacol Therap 5:247-57.

Schipper, I. A. 1965. Milk and blood levels of chemotherapeutic agents in cattle. JAVMA 147(12):1403-7.

Segal, B. M. 1963. Photosensitivity, nail discoloration, and onycholysis: side effect of tetracycline therapy. Arch Int Med 112:165-67.

Shaw, D. H., and Rubin, S. I. 1986. Pharmacologic activity of doxycycline. JAVMA 189(7):808-10.

Smith, J. A., and George, L. W. 1985. Treatment of acute ocular *Moraxella bovis* infections in calves with a parenterally administered long-acting oxytetracycline formulation. AJVR 46(4):804-7.

Soma, J. A., and Speer, V. C. 1975. Effects of pregnant mare serum and chlortetracycline on the reproductive efficiency of sows. J Anim Sci 41(1):100-105.

Stevenson, S. 1980. Oxytetracycline nephrotoxicosis in two dogs. JAVMA 176(6):530-31.

Suzuka, I., Kaji, H., and Kaji, A. 1966. Binding of specific sRNA to 30S ribosomal subunits: effect of 50S ribosomal subunits. Proc Natl Acad Sci 55:1483-86.

Teare, A., Schwark, W. S., Shin, S. J., and Graham, D. L. 1985. Pharmacokinetics of a long-acting oxytetracycline preparation in ring-necked pheasants, great horned owls, and Amazon parrots. AJVR 46(12):2639-43.

Teuscher, E., Lamothe, P., Tellier, P., and Lavallee, J.-C. 1982. A toxic nephrosis in calves treated with a medication containing tetracycline degradation products. Can Vet J 23:327-31.

Toutain, P. L., and Raynaud, J. P. 1983. Pharmacokinetics of oxytetracycline in young cattle: comparison of conventional vs. long-acting formulations. AJVR 44:1203-9.

Varma, K. J., and Paul, B. S. 1983. Pharmacokinetics and plasma protein binding (in vitro) of oxytetracycline in buffalo (*Bubalus bubalis*). AJVR 44(3):497-99.
Waisbren, B. A., and Hueckel, J. S. 1950. Reduced absorption of Aureomycin caused by aluminum hydroxide gel (Amphojel). Proc Soc Exp Biol Med 73:73-74.
Ward, G. S., Guiry, C. C., and Alexander, L. L. 1982. Tetracycline-induced anaphylactic shock in a dog. JAVMA 180(7):770-71.
Weinberg, E. D. 1957. The mutual effects of antimicrobial compounds and metallic cations. Bacteriol Rev 21:4-68.
Whelton, A., Nightingale, S. D., Carter, G. G., Gordon, L. S., Bryant, H. H., and Walker, W. G. 1975. Pharmacokinetic characteristics of doxycycline accumulation in normal and severely diseased kidneys. J Infect Dis 132(4):467-71.
White, S. D., Rosychuk, A. W., Reinke, S. I., and Paradis, M. 1992. Use of tetracycline and niacinamide for treatment of autoimmune skin disease in 31 dogs. JAVMA 200(10):1497-1500.
Williams, R. D., Rollins, L. D., Pocurull, D. W., Selwyn, M., and Mercer, H. D. 1978. Effect of feeding chlortetracycline on the reservoir of *Salmonella typhimurium* in experimentally infected swine. Antimicrob Agents Chemotherapy 14(5):710-19.
Wilson, R. C., and Green, N. K. 1986. Pharmacokinetics of minocycline hydrochloride in clinically normal and hypoproteinemic sheep. AJVR 47(3):650-52.
Wilson, R. C., Kemp, D. T., Kitzman, J. V., and Goetsch, D. D. 1988. Pharmacokinetics of doxycycline in dogs. Can J Vet Res 52:12-14.
Wilson, R. C., Kitzman, J. V., Kemp, D. T., and Goetsch, D. D. 1985. Compartmental and noncompartmental pharmacokinetic analyses of minocycline hydrochloride in the dog. AJVR 46(6):1316-18.
Wivagg, R. T., Jaffe, J. M., and Colaizzi, J. L. 1976. Influence of pH and route of injection on acute toxicity of tetracycline in mice. J Pharm Sci 65(6):916-18.
Xia, W., Gyrd-Hanson, N., and Nielsen, P. 1983. Comparison of pharmacokinetic parameters for two oxytetracycline preparations in pigs. J Vet Pharmacol Therap 6:113-20.
Yu, L. P., Smith, G. N., Brandt, K. D., Myers, S. L., O'Connor, B. L., and Brandt, D. A. 1992. Reduction of the severity of canine osteoarthritis by prophylactic treatment with oral doxycycline. Arthritis and Rheum 35(10):1150-59.
Zinn, R. A. 1993. Influence of oral antibiotics on digestive function in Holstein steers fed a 71% concentrate diet. J Anim Sci 71(1):213-17.
Ziv, G., and Sulman, F. G. 1974. Analysis of pharmacokinetic properties of nine tetracycline analogues in dairy cows and ewes. AJVR 35:1197-1201.

43 AMINOGLYCOSIDE ANTIBIOTICS

JIM E. RIVIERE AND JERRY W. SPOO

Pharmacology of Aminoglycosides
Pharmacokinetics of Aminoglycosides
Aminoglycoside Toxicity
Gentamicin
Amikacin
Kanamycin
Apramycin
Tobramycin
Neomycin
Dihydrostreptomycin
Paromomycin

Aminoglycoside antibiotics constitute a very important weapon in the veterinarian's armamentarium against gram-negative infections. As a group, they are the drugs of choice for the treatment of serious gram-negative infections in animals. Aminoglycosides are a therapeutically essential class of antibiotics whose usefulness is often restricted by their nephrotoxic and ototoxic potential. This chapter reviews the pharmacokinetics, toxicity, and tissue disposition of aminoglycoside antibiotics in various species.

PHARMACOLOGY OF AMINOGLYCOSIDES

General. Aminoglycosides are a class of antimicrobial compounds produced from strains of *Streptomyces* spp., *Micromonospora* spp., and *Bacillus* spp. Chemically, they are aminocyclitols: hydroxyl and amino or guanidine substituted cyclohexane with amino sugars joined by glycosidic linkages to one or more of the hydroxyl groups. These molecules have excellent water, but poor lipid, solubility, are thermodynamically stable over a wide range of pH values and temperatures (Lancini and Parenti 1982; Leitner and Price 1982; Nagabhusban et al. 1982; Pechere and Dugal 1979), and have molecular weights ranging from 400 to 500 g/mol. The aminoglycosides are basic polycations with pK_a values that range from 7.2 to 8.8 (Ziv and Sulman 1974; Katzung 1984; Prescott and Baggot 1988).

The authors would like to extend their appreciation to Dr. S. A. Brown as the coauthor of a review of the aminoglycosides (Brown and Riviere 1991) that served as the basis for some of this chapter.

The chemical structures of some of the commonly used aminoglycosides are shown in Fig. 43.1. Chemical structure is important in determining antimicrobial activity, resistance patterns, and inherent propensity to cause toxicosis. The various mechanisms of nephrotoxicity (binding to proximal tubule brush-border vesicles and phospholipids, inhibition of mitochondrial function, etc.) may be related to an increased number of free amino groups on the aminoglycoside molecule. In general, the most ionized aminoglycosides (i.e., neomycin, with six groups) are more toxic and show greater binding affinity than the least ionized aminoglycosides of the class (i.e., streptomycin, with three groups) (Bendirdjian et al. 1982; Cronin 1979; Feldman et al. 1981; Humes et al. 1982; Just and Habermann 1977; Kunin 1970; Lipsky and Lietman 1982; Luft and Evan 1980a,b; Weinberg et al. 1980). Other structural characteristics may account for differences in toxicity within groups of drugs with similar total ionization potentials (i.e., netilmicin, tobramycin, and gentamicin, all with five ionizable groups). More specific information on aminoglycoside structure-toxicity relationships is not presently available.

Mechanism of Action. Aminoglycosides exert their antibacterial action by irreversibly binding to one or more receptor proteins on the 30S subunit of the bacterial ribosome and thereby interfering with several mechanisms in the mRNA translation process. These include disrupting an initiation complex between the mRNA and the 30S subunit, blocking further translation and thereby causing premature chain termination, or causing incorporation of an incorrect amino acid in the protein product. It is significant that most antimicrobials that interfere with ribosomal protein synthesis are bacteriostatic, while aminoglycosides are bactericidal. The postulated mechanism for this effect is either this ribosomal misreading or interference with the initiation of DNA replication (Busse et al. 1992; Jawetz 1984). However, the exact mechanism of the bactericidal effect on bacteria presently remains unclear.

The mechanism of bacterial penetration by the aminoglycoside through the cell membrane is biphasic. Drug diffuses through the outer membrane of gram-negative bacteria through aqueous channels formed by the porin proteins. Once in the periplasmic space, an oxygen-requiring transport process transports the drug into the cell, where it interacts with the ribosome. The

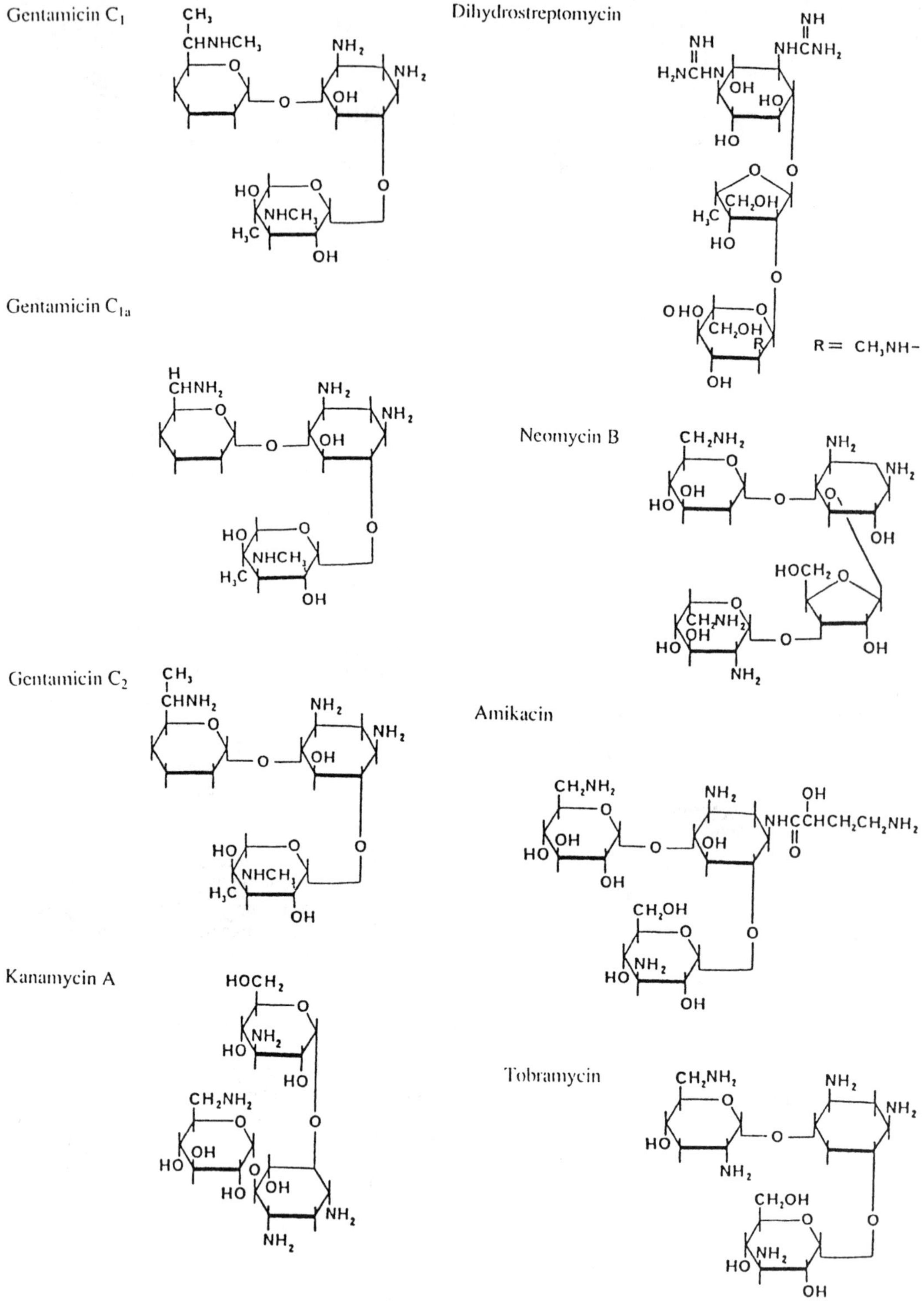

Gentamicin C_1

Dihydrostreptomycin

R= CH_3NH-

Gentamicin C_{1a}

Neomycin B

Gentamicin C_2

Amikacin

Kanamycin A

Tobramycin

FIG. 43.1—Chemical structures of the commonly used aminoglycosides.

oxygen-dependent transport is linked to an electron transport system, which causes the bacterial cytoplasm to be negatively charged with respect to the periplasm and external environment. Anaerobic bacteria are therefore resistant to the antibacterial effects of aminoglycosides. The positively charged aminoglycosides are attracted electrostatically into the bacterial cytoplasm. Some divalent cations (such as calcium and magnesium) are competitive inhibitors of this transport system. This proton-motive force also functions in the lysosomes and mitochondria in which aminoglycosides accumulate and may also be a factor in the intralysosomal accumulation of the aminoglycosides. The same factors that decrease uptake of aminoglycosides into bacteria unfortunately also decrease their uptake into proximal tubular cells, a factor that has been demonstrated to be associated with nephrotoxicity in animals.

A characteristic of aminoglycoside activity is that bacterial killing is concentration dependent, and a postantibiotic effect (PAE) is evident. By definition, the PAE is a persistent suppression of bacterial growth following the removal of an antimicrobial agent. Bactericidal action persists after serum concentrations fall below minimum inhibitory concentrations (MICs). This has ramifications for the design of clinical dosage regimens.

Clinical Uses. Table 43.1 lists some aminoglycosides used clinically (presently or historically). The only ones used to any extent in veterinary medicine are amikacin, gentamicin, kanamycin, neomycin (topically only), and streptomycin. Netilmicin, sisomicin, and dibekacin are newer compounds which may be used clinically in the future.

Aminoglycosides are still considered to be the drug of choice for treating serious aerobic gram-negative infections in veterinary medicine, although newer and less toxic antimicrobials (i.e., the fluoroquinolones) may soon replace the use of aminoglycosides for certain bacterial infections. Not all aminoglycosides are equal in their ability to combat these serious infections. Neomycin is too toxic to be used systemically but is still used to treat some forms of bacterial skin disease. Kanamycin, first introduced in the late 1950s, has a primarily gram-negative spectrum of antimicrobial activity. However, many organisms are now resistant to this aminoglycoside and its use has subsequently declined. Gentamicin, introduced in the 1960s, has a broader spectrum and is less resisted than kanamycin. It covers many more aerobic gram-negative organisms (including some *Pseudomonas* spp.) as well as some gram-positive organisms (in particular, *Staphylococcus* spp.) and certain mycobacteria. Amikacin, a semisynthetic derivative of kanamycin, was introduced clinically in the 1970s, has the broadest spectrum of activity of all the aminoglycoside antibiotics used clinically to date, and is the preferred antibiotic in severe gram-negative infections that are resistant to gentamicin or tobramycin.

TABLE 43.1—Selected common aminoglycosides

Amikacin	Lividomycin	Seldomycin
Butikacin	Neomycin	Sisomicin
Butirosin	Netilmicin	Sorbistin
Dibekacin	Paromomycin (aminosidine)	Streptomycin
Fortimicin	Propikacin	Tobramycin
Gentamicin	Ribostamycin	Apramycin
Kanamycin	Sagamycin (gentamicin C_{2b})	

Table 43.2 lists the current recommended dosage regimens for gentamicin, kanamycin, apramycin, and amikacin. It is important to note that these are *recommended doses* that should be modified proportionately to correct for age, clinical or subclinical disease processes, renal insufficiency, or any of the other factors that may predispose the patient to aminoglycoside toxicosis (see Aminoglycoside Toxicity below). Alterations in the dose can be best determined by monitoring serum creatinine concentrations or optimally by monitoring aminoglycoside serum concentrations at predetermined time points after dosing.

Single Daily Dose Administration. Recent studies in humans, laboratory animals, and veterinary species suggest that single daily dosing (SID) of aminoglycosides may be as efficacious as administering the same dose divided over 24 hours. The concept of single daily dosing of aminoglycosides has been utilized and generally accepted within the human medical community (Bass et al. 1998; Christensen et al. 1997; Freeman et al. 1997; Karachalios et al. 1998; Rodvold et al. 1997). A report from a guinea pig infection model indicates that the recommended total daily dose of gentamicin given SID (6-12 mg/kg/day) has the same antibacterial efficacy as BID or TID therapy (Campbell et al. 1996). The efficacy of single dose administration is rooted in the PAE. Because of the PAE phenomenon, the aminoglycoside can be given less frequently (SID vs. BID or TID) and will continue to inhibit bacterial growth after levels fall below the MIC for the organism. Fortuitously, as will be discussed later relative to nephrotoxicity, aminoglycoside dosage regimens that produce high peak and low trough concentrations also have less propensity to induce renal toxicity than multiple-dose regimens, which produce lower peak but higher trough concentrations. For example, in a classic study rats given gentamicin at a dose of 40 mg/kg/day SID had significantly lower serum creatinine concentrations than rats given the same dose of gentamicin divided BID or TID, indicating that the SID induced less renal damage than the lower, divided dosing scheme (Bennett et al. 1979).

The PAE and efficacy of SID therapy have also been suggested for the horse (Godber et al. 1995). SID therapy resulted in higher tissue concentrations, was more efficacious, produced a prolonged killing of susceptible bacteria, and had a lower risk of nephrotoxicosis. In another supporting study (Magdesian et al. 1998) healthy horses were dosed at 6.6 mg/kg SID gentamicin by both intravenous (IV) and intramuscular (IM)

TABLE 43.2—Recommended dosage regimens based on target maximum concentrations of 10–12 μg/mL for gentamicin and 30–40 μg/mL for kanamycin, apramycin, and amikacin and target minimum concentrations of 1–2 μg/mL for gentamicin and 2.5–5 μg/mL for kanamycin, apramycin, and amikacin

Species	Dosage regimen	Reference
Gentamicin		
Dogs (juvenile)	2–4 mg/kg q6h IV	Riviere and Coppoc 1981a
Cats	3 mg/kg q8h IV	Jernigan et al. 1988a-e
	3 mg/kg q6h IM/SC	Jernigan et al. 1988a-e
Ponies	4 mg/kg q8h IV/IM	Haddad et al. 1985a,b
	5 mg/kg q8h IM	
Horses	4.2 mg/kg q8-12h IV/IM	Pedersoli et al. 1980
Horses (adult)	2 mg/kg q8h IV/IM	Sojka and Brown 1986
Horses (foals)	3 mg/kg q12h IV/IM	Sojka and Brown 1986
Cows	5 mg/kg q8h IV/IM	Haddad et al. 1987
Cows (lactating)	3.5 mg/kg q8h IM	Haddad et al. 1986
Birds of prey	2.5 mg/kg q8h IM	Bird et al. 1983
Catfish	3.5 mg/kg q33h IM	Setzer 1985
	1.6 mg/kg q33h	Setzer 1985
Roosters	2 mg/kg q12h IM	Pedersoli et al. 1990
Kanamycin		
Dogs	10 mg/kg q6-8h IM/IV	Baggot 1978
Apramycin		
Calves	20 mg/kg q12h IM	Ziv et al. 1985
Amikacin		
Cats	10 mg/kg q8h IV/IM/SC	Jernigan et al. 1988a
Dogs	10 mg/kg q8h IM/SC	Baggot et al. 1985
Dogs[a]	10 mg/kg q12h IM/SC	Baggot et al. 1985

Source: Adapted from Brown and Riviere 1991.
[a]Urinary tract infections; based on IV infusion of 0.35 mg/kg/hr and a half-life of 2.5 hr.

routes. Peak plasma gentamicin levels occurred at 0 hours (72 μg/mL) after IV injection and 1.3 hours (22 μg/mL) after IM injection, well above the conventional blood concentration targets of 10-12 μg/mL. Such high blood concentrations would likely maximize the PAE. Packed-cell volume, creatinine, plasma total protein, urine specific gravity, and a number of other urinalysis data indicated no significant changes in these parameters based on predosing data. Based on this preliminary information, the authors suggested that horses could safely receive a SID dose of gentamicin; however, further work clearly needs to be performed in clinically ill horses to conclusively prove this supposition.

PHARMACOKINETICS OF AMINOGLYCOSIDES

General. A comprehensive review of aminoglycoside pharmacokinetics has been reported by Brown and Riviere (1991) and serves as the basis for this review. The pharmacokinetics of the aminoglycosides is similar across species lines, but the variability within each animal population is large, indicating a significant amount of heterogeneity in aminoglycoside disposition in both diseased and normal animals (Sojka and Brown 1986; Frazier et al. 1988). In addition, the inherent variability caused by many different disease states necessitates close monitoring of serum or plasma concentrations to optimize efficacy and minimize toxicosis. A similarly large variability in aminoglycoside pharmacokinetics has also been reported in humans (Kaye et al. 1974; Sawchuk et al. 1977; Zaske et al. 1982; Blaser et al. 1983).

Although there is variability in aminoglycoside pharmacokinetic parameters, the therapeutic range for all of the aminoglycosides is relatively narrow, and the potential for toxicosis is greater than for most other classes of antimicrobials. Serum or plasma concentrations may easily be higher or lower than desired within each dosing interval in normal animals. Altered physiologic or pathologic states such as pregnancy (Lelievre-Pegorier et al. 1985), obesity (Sketris et al. 1981), subnormal body weight (Tointon et al. 1987), renal disease (Frazier and Riviere 1987), dehydration (LeCompte et al. 1981), immaturity (Sojka and Brown 1986), sepsis (Mann et al. 1987), endotoxemia (Wilson et al. 1984; Jernigan et al. 1988c), and intraindividual variability (Mann et al. 1987), among many others, may alter the distribution, clearance, and half-life of aminoglycosides by as much as 1000-fold between individuals in a single study (Zaske et al. 1982). In order to achieve target therapeutic concentrations, dosage adjustment seems to be required in 80-90% of both human and equine patient populations receiving aminoglycosides therapeutically (Bauer and Blouin 1981; Sojka and Brown 1986), with therapeutic drug monitoring highly recommended for any patient receiving multiple doses of parenteral aminoglycosides (Sveska et al. 1985; Sojka and Brown 1986; Frazier et al. 1988). Timing of blood sampling is critical, with consistent sampling times near 1-1.5 hours after dose and immediately prior to the next dose being optimal in most instances (Blaser et al. 1985). This variability expressed in terms of underlying physiological parameters was recently incorporated into a so-called population pharmacokinetic model for gentamicin in horses (Martin et al. 1998) where pharmacokinetic parameters could be expressed with significantly less variability if the individual animal's creatinine and body weight were known. This approach holds much promise for increasing the ability to tailor aminoglycoside dosage regimens to specific clinical scenarios (Martin and Riviere 1998).

Absorption. Aminoglycosides are not appreciably absorbed from the gastrointestinal tract because of their highly polar and cationic nature. However, if there is significant disruption of the intestinal mucosa from necrotizing enteritis (i.e., parvovirus infections) (Gemer et al. 1983; Miranda et al. 1984), some absorption may occur. This lack of absorption in the normal gastrointestinal tract is relevant to achieving therapeutically effective plasma concentrations of drug but may not be accurate if tissue residues are the relevant end point. The aminoglycosides are not inactivated in the intestine and are eliminated in the feces unchanged after oral administration to normal animals. This lack of significant absorption through the gastrointestinal tract requires that all aminoglycosides be given by parenteral routes if therapeutic plasma concentrations are desired. Aminoglycoside absorption is practically complete after IM or subcutaneous (SC) injection. The peak serum concentrations after extravascular injection occur 14-120 minutes after the dose (Blaser et al. 1983; Ristuccia 1984). Absorption is extremely rapid and complete if aminoglycosides are instilled into body cavities which contain serosal surfaces; administration by this route closely mimics IV administration (Jawetz 1984; Sande and Mandell 1985).

Distribution. The distribution of aminoglycoside antibiotics after an IV bolus dose is virtually complete within 1 hour. Because of the polycationic nature of these antibiotics, the penetration of aminoglycosides across membranous barriers by simple diffusion is very limited; therefore, very low concentrations of aminoglycosides are found in cerebrospinal fluid or in respiratory secretions (Riviere and Coppoc 1981b; Strausbaugh and Brinker 1983). Aerosol or intratracheal administration of gentamicin produces negligible serum concentrations in both dogs and sheep, although substantial bronchial and pulmonary concentrations can be achieved (Riviere et al. 1981b; Wilson et al. 1981). Plasma protein binding is generally less than 20% in all species studied (Riond et al. 1986) and has a minimal effect on distribution from the vascular compartment. Binding to erythrocytes has been suggested to be approximately 10%, which is considered insignificant for aminoglycoside disposition (Lee et al. 1981). The molecular weight of aminoglycosides is small enough to allow unhindered passage through the capillary fenestrae and gap junctions of the vasculature (Huber 1982; Ristuccia 1984; Sande and Mandell 1985). Aminoglycoside distribution increases in lean and/or cachectic humans (Tointon et al. 1987) because of decreased plasma protein production leading to extravasation of fluid and resultant edema. A similar phenomenon probably occurs in animals, which may also require a concurrent dose adjustment.

Metabolism and Excretion. Whole animal and human renal clearance (Black et al. 1963; Chiu et al. 1976; Chung et al. 1980; Gyselynck et al. 1971; Schentag and Jusko 1977; Silverman and Mahon 1979), isolated perfused rat kidney (Collier et al. 1979; Mitchell et al. 1977), and micropuncture studies (Pastoriza-Munoz et al. 1979; Senckjian et al. 1981; Sheth et al. 1981) have clearly demonstrated that aminoglycosides are eliminated nonmetabolized from the body in all animal species studied so far, primarily by renal glomerular filtration. The sole route of excretion for all aminoglycosides is the kidney. Some degree of proximal tubular reabsorption does occur and results in an intracellular sequestration or storage in the tubule cells without a significant transepithelial flux from the intraluminal to peritubular space. Net aminoglycoside secretion along more distal nephron segments may also occur. Proximal tubule luminal absorption of aminoglycoside appears quantitatively to be the primary mechanism of intracellular uptake; however, selective peritubular or basolateral reabsorption, evident in isolated tissue slice studies, does occur and may be of toxicologic significance in specific situations. Reabsorption requires metabolic energy and occurs along the midconvoluted and straight portions of the proximal tubule (Barza et al. 1980; Bennett et al. 1982; Hsu et al. 1977; Kaloyanides and Pastoriza-Munoz 1980; Kluwe and Hook 1978a,b; Kuhar et al. 1979; Pastoriza-Munoz et al. 1979; Senckjian et al. 1981; Silverblatt 1982; Silverblatt and Kuehn 1979; Silverman and Mahon 1979; Tulkens and Trouet 1978; Vandewalle et al. 1981; Williams et al. 1981a,b; Zaske 1980). Several laboratories have demonstrated that renal cortical uptake of the aminoglycosides is dose dependent up to a threshold concentration; then, cortical accumulation increases at a progressively slower rate as the dose is increased. Cumulative uptake of aminoglycosides in tissues indicates that the kidney is the major site of drug sequestration, although other organs with larger volumes (e.g., liver) may also contain substantial total drug (Brown et al. 1985).

Aminoglycoside disposition generally follows a three-compartment pharmacokinetic model with a three-phase plasma concentration-time profile curve (α, β, γ) as shown in Fig. 43.2. Using those parameters, the $t_{1/2\alpha}$ represents the distribution half-life, the $t_{1/2\beta}$ reflects the classic elimination phase governed largely by renal elimination, and $t_{1/2\gamma}$ reflects the slow release of drug sequestered in tissues (i.e., renal cortex and liver). Typically, the α phase occurs within the first hour after IV dosing, the β phase occurs between 1 and 24 hours after IV dosing (and probably the most useful in determining dose adjustments in clinical situations),

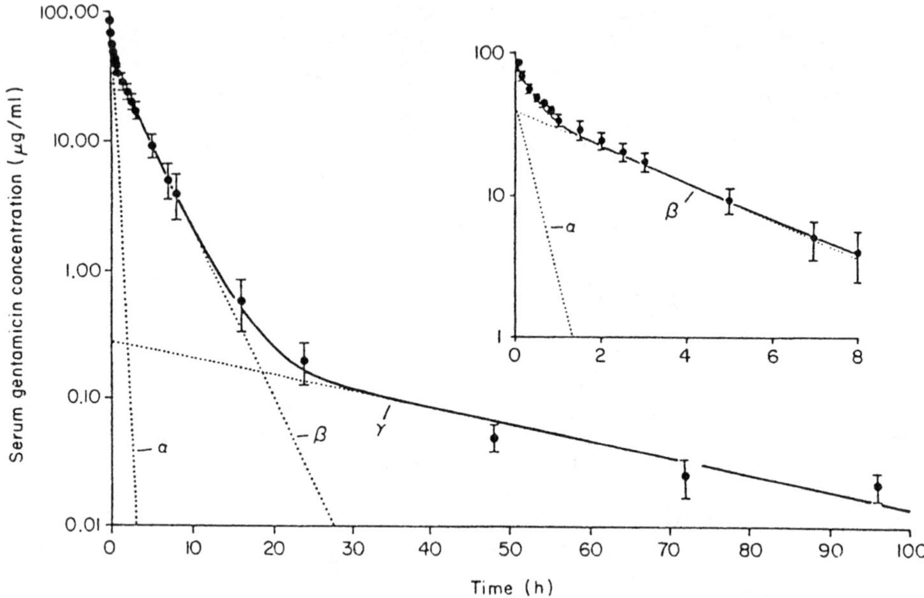

FIG. 43.2—Graphic representation of the three elimination curves associated with aminoglycoside excretion. (From Brown et al. 1991, reproduced by permission.)

and the γ phase occurs 24 hours after dosing and is the most important part of the elimination curve of aminoglycosides when considering drug residues in food-producing animals. The primary determinant of aminoglycoside disposition is reflected in the phase which correlates to renal glomerular filtration. The primary difference in kinetics between species is related to the glomerular filtration rate (GFR), which decreases on a weight basis in larger animals. Larger animals tend to have prolonged half-lives and require smaller doses on a mg/kg basis. In contrast, doses are similar across all species if based on a body surface area or a measure of basal metabolic rate (0.75 mg/kg) (Riviere 1985; Riviere et al. 1997).

The prolonged terminal elimination phase of aminoglycosides has major implication for veterinary therapeutics in food-producing animals. As discussed above, aminoglycosides accumulate in the renal cortex for prolonged periods of time, resulting in violative tissue residues even after short periods of administration. In some cases, aminoglycosides such as gentamicin may be detected for a year after parenteral administration! The veterinary profession had originally recommended a withdrawal time of 18 months for cattle treated with gentamicin but now suggests that the drug not be used in adult food-producing animals. Piglets may be treated up to 3 days of age, but even in this case the withdrawal time is 40 days.

TABLE 43.3—Selected risk factors that predispose to aminoglycoside toxicosis

Age	Peak and trough serum concentrations
Volume contraction (shock)	Hepatic disease
Acidosis	Total dose of drug administered
Sodium or potassium depletion	Duration of treatment
Sepsis	Concurrent administration of loop diuretics
Renal transplantation	Methoxyflurane anesthesia
Prior renal insufficiency	Cephalosporin antibiotics
Prior aminoglycoside exposure	Nephrotoxic drugs
Cumulative dose of aminoglycoside	

AMINOGLYCOSIDE TOXICITY. Aminoglycoside toxicity in domestic and laboratory animals has been reviewed by Riviere (1985). The possible risk factors that may predispose a patient to aminoglycoside toxicity are shown in Table 43.3.

Aminoglycosides can induce ototoxicity and nephrotoxicity because both organs have higher-than-normal concentrations of phospholipid (in particular, phosphatidylinositol) (Sastrasinh et al. 1982a; Sastrasinh et al. 1982b) in their cellular matrixes. Cationic aminoglycosides are chemically attracted to anionic membrane phospholipids, the so-called aminoglycoside receptors. The two tissues into which gentamicin preferentially accumulates (renal cortex and cochlear tissue) have disproportionately high amounts of phosphatidylinositol in their membranes compared with other tissues of the body (Hauser and Eichberg 1973). Basolateral membranes of the renal proximal tubular epithelium also have a higher capacity for binding aminoglycosides than brush-border membranes because of their higher phosphatidylinositol content (Josepovitz et al. 1985). This nearly twofold lower uptake in brush-border membranes is even lower in female rats than in male rats (Williams and Hottendorf 1985, 1986). Ototoxicity studies in a variety of species have shown a progressive accumulation of the aminoglycoside in the perilymph and endolymph of the inner ear that may affect both auditory and vestibular function due to destruction of the sensory hair cells in the cochlea and vestibular labyrinth. The likelihood of inducing ototoxicity is mainly dependent on the duration of treatment, cumulative dose, average daily dose, peak and trough serum concentration, concurrent diuretic use, underlying disease status, and previous exposure to aminoglycoside therapy. Ototoxicity may be irreversible in some cases (Johnson and Hardin 1992). Of pertinence to veterinary medicine, dogs tend to present with auditory toxicity, and cats tend to present with vestibular toxicity, although both usually occur after nephrotoxicity has ensued.

More complete information is available on the toxicosis of the aminoglycosides in the kidney (Ali et al. 1992; Beauchamp et al. 1992; Riviere 1985). Controversy exists as to the precise mechanism by which aminoglycosides initially damage proximal renal tubule cells. All aminoglycosides initiate toxicosis by perturbation of the renal proximal tubular cell membrane structure. The cationic aminoglycosides are chemically attracted to the anionic phospholipids (i.e., phosphoinositides—in particular, phosphatidylinositol), the aminoglycoside receptors, found in high concentrations in the cell membranes of the proximal renal tubular cells. The interaction between the cationic aminoglycosides and the anionic phospholipids appears to be electrostatic and proportional to the cationic charge of the drug. This interaction is saturable and is competitively inhibited by divalent cations (magnesium and calcium), spermine, poly-L-lysine, and other aminoglycosides. After binding, the aminoglycoside is internalized into the cell by pinocytosis (Bennett et al. 1982; Elliott et al. 1982; Feldman et al. 1981; Humes et al. 1982; Lipsky et al. 1980; Lipsky and Lietman 1982; Pastoriza-Munoz et al. 1979; Schacht 1978), where concentrations of the aminoglycoside can reach as high as 50 times the concentrations achieved in serum or plasma. Cytosegresomes are formed and are the primary locus of intracellular aminoglycoside storage. This intralysosomal binding within the proximal tubules results in drug sequestration and is primarily responsible for the prolonged half-life and extended withdrawal times of aminoglycosides, which are pertinent to food-animal tissue residues, and is seen in the renal cortical tissue. The uptake of aminoglycosides into lysosomes is competitive and is dependent in part upon the charge density of the aminoglycoside molecule, which is a function of the number of amino groups. For example, neomycin (valence + 4.37 at pH 7.40) accumulates in the renal cortex more than gentamicin (valence + 3.46 at pH 7.40) due to a higher cationic charge. This highly concentrated packet of drug is slowly transported back into the urine in the form of multilamellar phospholipid structures known as myeloid bodies after proximal tubule cell death.

Because the renal proximal tubules and inner-ear tissues actively take up aminoglycosides, concentrations in the renal cortex and cochlear tissues are far greater than those observed concurrently in the serum and other tissues. In emergency-slaughtered ruminants, renal cortical concentrations of dihydrostreptomycin or neomycin ranged from 4.1 to 237 μg/g of renal cortex (Nouws and Ziv 1978). Studies have also demonstrated a substantially higher renal cortical concentration of other aminoglycosides compared with other tissues in humans (Schentag et al. 1977b; Schentag and Jusko 1977), rats (Luft and Kleit 1974; Fabre et al. 1976; Luft et al. 1978), dogs (Cowan et al. 1980), cats (Jernigan et al. 1988c), sheep (Brown et al. 1985; Brown et al. 1986b; Brown and Garry 1988), lambs (Weisman et al. 982), cattle (Haddad et al. 1987), pigs (Riond and Riviere 1988), and birds (Bush et al. 1981). Endotoxemia increases the renal concentrations of aminoglycosides above normal (Bergeron and Bergeron 1986). Substantial concentrations are also found in the renal medulla, liver, spleen, and lungs in sheep (Brown et al. 1985; Brown et al. 1986b), cattle (Haddad et al. 1987), birds (Bush et al. 1981), and rats (Cowan et al. 1980). Occasionally renal medullary concentrations are substantially higher than the concentrations found in liver, spleen, and lungs (Schentag and Jusko 1977). This may be a result of sloughed renal cortical cells lodging as casts in the loops of Henle or the collecting ducts. A significant correlation exists between urine and renal cortical aminoglycoside concentrations, although the correlation accounts for only 30% of the variability in renal cortical concentrations (Nouws and Ziv 1978). This is an important consideration in food-animal medicine when on-the-farm urine residue screening tests are employed by the veterinarian to assess aminoglycoside tissue-withdrawal times.

Diabetic animals do not accumulate aminoglycosides in their renal cortex to the same extent as normal animals (Teixeira et al. 1982; Vaamonde et al. 1984; Pastoriza-Munoz et al. 1987; Ramsammy et al. 1987). Streptozotocin-induced diabetes mellitus in laboratory rats substantially decreases the renal uptake of aminoglycosides by depressing the uptake and accumulation process of renal proximal tubular cells (Vaamonde et al. 1984; Ramsammy et al. 1987). As an apparent result, single-dose gentamicin disposition in diabetic dogs does not show a γ phase at all, whereas normal dogs do exhibit that terminal elimination phase, with a $t_{1/2\gamma}$ of several days (Brown et al. 1991). This abolition of the γ phase, noted in alloxan-induced diabetic dogs and in dogs with naturally occurring diabetes mellitus, was observed in spite of exogenous insulin therapy to control hyperglycemia. Other endocrine disorders such as familial hypothyroidism also affect the terminal elimination phase (and perhaps renal accumulation) of certain aminoglycosides in certain species (Riond et al. 1986; Riviere and Carver 1984).

As stated previously, the exact mechanism behind aminoglycoside nephrotoxicosis is unknown, with controversy existing over the precise mechanism by which aminoglycosides initially damage the proximal renal tubule cells (Swann et al. 1990; Schumacher et al. 1991; Beauchamp et al. 1992). Abundant evidence suggests that lysosomal dysfunction is a component of this early phase of cellular injury (Carbon et al. 1978; Feldman et al. 1982; Hull et al. 1981; Kaloyanides and Pastoriza-Munoz 1980; Laurent et al. 1982; Lipsky and Lietman 1982; Mazze 1981; Meisner 1981; Morin et al. 1980; Morin et al. 1981; Tulkens and Trouet 1978). This view is consistent with the idea that lysosomes are the primary locus of aminoglycoside sequestration in proximal tubule cells. Lysosomes are also the first organelle to demonstrate morphologic changes (myeloid body or cytosegresome formation) after exposure to the drugs (Riviere et al. 1981a). Studies have demonstrated that lysosomal enzyme activities (i.e., sphingomyelinase, cathepsin B, α-D-galactosidase) are decreased and that the structural latency of lysosomes, reflected by leakage of *N*-acetyl-β-D-glucosaminadase in the cytosol is increased. Inhibition of lysosomal enzymes may cause an intralysosomal accumulation of membrane-associated lipids which would be reflected morphologically as myeloid body formation. However, this process by itself should not be acutely lethal to the cell. Decreased lysosomal function may also result in a decreased ability to degrade endogenous intracellular proteins and exogenous low-molecular weight proteins reabsorbed from the tubular filtrate, events that would perturb nephron function (Cojocel et al. 1983; Cojocel and Hook, 1983). The increase in lysosomal permeability could result in proximal tubule cell dysfunction, although this event is probably a late change in aminoglycoside-induced toxic nephropathy occurring after cell necrosis has been initiated by another factor (Humes et al. 1982). Myeloid body formation is most likely a marker of aminoglycoside exposure rather than toxicosis. The appearance of lysosomal enzymes in the urine of aminoglycoside-induced toxic nephropathy patients is secondary to proximal tubule cell necrosis, apical plasma membrane damage, or lysosome exocytosis.

Mitochondria are a second possible target of aminoglycosides because, both in vitro and in vivo, aminoglycosides decrease mitochondrial respiration, thereby impairing the tubule cell's bioenergetic profile (Appel and Neu 1977; Cuppage et al. 1977; Kaloyanides and Pastoriza-Munoz 1980; Kluwe and Hook 1978a; Sastrasinh et al. 1982b; Simmons et al. 1980; Weinberg et al. 1980; Weinberg and Humes 1980; Weinberg et al. 1990). This could selectively produce tubule dysfunction which would initially be detectable biochemically but not morphologically. The mechanism of this toxicity may be secondary to a direct aminoglycoside interaction with mitochondrial membrane phospholipids, to a competitive interaction with the divalent cations magnesium or calcium, or to an alteration in the intracellular milieu that would indirectly affect mitochondrial function. The magnitude of aminoglycoside effects on mitochondrial respiration is *roughly* correlated to the net positive charge of the specific drug.

The third possible site of initial intracellular aminoglycoside interaction is the proximal tubule cell plasma membrane's phospholipids and enzymes (Feldman et al. 1981; Humes et al. 1982; Knauss et al. 1983; Lullmann and Vollmer 1982; Sastrasinh et al. 1982a; Sastrasinh et al. 1982b; Schacht 1979; Silverman and Mahon 1979; Williams et al. 1981a,b). Binding of aminoglycosides to membrane polyphosphoinositides could perturb the regulation of membrane permeability, thereby promoting cellular dysfunction. Aminoglycosides induce a phospholipidosis that may be secondary to inhibition of cytoplasmic phospholipase activity. This event affecting multiple membrane systems may affect other cellular metabolic processes. Aminoglycosides also inhibit basolateral membrane Na^+,K^+-ATPase activity in vitro and in vivo when used at high doses or incubating concentrations (Appel 1982; Chahwala and Harpur 1982; Cronin et al. 1982). Aminoglycosides have also been found to inhibit adenylate cyclase activity in proximal tubule basolateral membranes and in toad bladder epithelium in vitro (Humes and Weinberg 1980; Ross et al. 1980; Souliere et al. 1978). The enzyme interactions at the basolateral membrane could result in significant cellular dysfunction by altering intracellular electrolyte balance or osmolality.

A final possible site of aminoglycoside interaction with the nephron is at the level of the glomerulus, where gentamicin has been demonstrated to reduce the glomerular ultrafiltration coefficient and to reduce the number and size of glomerular endothelial fenestrae (Avasthi et al. 1981; Huang et al. 1979; Luft and Evan 1980a,b; Luft et al. 1978). These effects may be mediated by a charge interaction between the cationic aminoglycosides and the anionic endothelial cell surfaces or, alternatively, could be a feedback response to a primary tubular injury. The mediator of this mechanism is not known.

The relative contributions of the lysosomal, mitochondrial, and membrane tubular mechanisms and glomerular injury to clinical aminoglycoside-induced toxic nephropathy is not known. The relative importance of each as a primary insult is largely a function of the pattern of intracellular distribution of toxicologically active aminoglycosides. In all probability, cellular dysfunction is a result of a combination of the above processes. Whatever the mechanism, dysfunction of the proximal tubule cell ultimately results in a decrease in nephron function, the sum of which determines whole kidney function.

Aminoglycoside-induced nephropathy has been studied in many species of animals. In general, the syndrome is similar across species lines, with any peculiarities being a result of pharmacokinetic factors or inherent differences in underlying renal morphology or physiology.

Dogs. Aminoglycosides are used in the dog to treat a variety of susceptible bacteria populations. Toxicosis may occur at the recommended therapeutic doses if given to dogs for protracted lengths of time. In veterinary medicine, a dose of 6-9 mg/kg/day is the recommended canine clinical dose (Burrows 1979; Conzelman 1980; Riviere 1982). However, in a clinical study a dose of 6.6 mg/kg/day for 6 days caused an elevation in serum urea nitrogen in only 2 of 16 dogs for which posttreatment renal function was monitored (Ling and Ruby 1979).

In a controlled study, 8 mg/kg/day, divided every 12 hours, produced a statistically significant decrease in urine osmolarity by day 7, an increase in fractional sodium excretion by day 8, an increase in serum urea nitrogen concentration by day 17, and an increase in serum creatinine concentration by day 18. The decrease in urine osmolarity, accompanied by polyuria, was preceded by an increase in the urinary excretion of prostaglandin E_2 and followed by an increase in plasma renin activity. Urinary prostaglandin E_2 activity decreased prior to azotemia, at which time the fractional excretion of sodium greatly increased (McNeil et al. 1983). The increase in urinary prostaglandin excretion was suggested to have induced a state of nephrogenic diabetes insipidus which caused the decreased urine osmolarity. This study documents a bimodal course of aminoglycoside-induced toxic nephropathy in the dog administered low-dose gentamicin therapy: an initial subclinical (subazotemic) phase marked by a urinary concentrating defect followed by a clinical (azotemic) phase. It also serves as the basis for simple noninvasive clinical monitoring for toxicosis since urinary changes preceded the more irreversible systemic changes.

Urine GGT (γ-glutamyl transferase):creatinine and NAG (*N*-acetyl-β-D-glucosaminidase):creatinine ratios may be useful tools in the diagnosis of early gentamicin nephrotoxicosis (Grauer et al. 1995). Young Beagle dogs were fed diets containing low (9.4%), medium (13.7%), and high (27.3%) amounts of dietary protein for 21 days and then administered 10 mg/kg gentamicin IM TID for 8 days. Endogenous creatinine clearance and 24-hour urinary excretions of NAG and GGT were calculated on days 2, 4, 6, and 8 of gentamicin administration. Urinary excretion of GGT increased through day 6 of administration in all three treatment groups. Urinary excretion of NAG increased through day 8 of treatment for all groups, while creatinine clearance tended to decrease in all groups during the study period. Similarly, Rivers et al. (1996) found that in dogs dosed with gentamicin at 3 mg/kg and 30 mg/kg for 10 days, urine GGT:creatinine ratios in the 30 mg/kg dose group were approximately 3 times that of baseline values. The elevated GGT:creatinine ratio indicator preceded clinically significant elevations in serum creatinine, urine specific gravity, and urine protein:creatinine ratios. The authors concluded that urine GGT:creatinine ratios were a much earlier indicator of aminoglycoside-induced renal toxicity and may have potential applications in detecting early gentamicin-induced nephrotoxicity in dogs. Other studies have also examined the effect of dietary protein on nephrotoxicity of aminoglycosides (Behrend et al. 1994).

High-dose studies of 30 mg/kg/day, divided every 8 hours, administered for 10-12 days, produced clinically significant increases in serum creatinine and serum urea nitrogen 9-12 days after the start of drug administration. Increases in urine enzyme excretion of β-glucuronidase and *N*-acetylglucosaminidase were noted as early as 2 days into the regimen. Glucosuria and urine osmolarity declined by day 7. Again, monitoring of urine parameters in a veterinary clinic would detect these changes prior to changes in blood chemistry. Plasma potassium and calcium concentrations were significantly depressed (Adelman et al. 1979; Cronin et al. 1980). Almost complete recovery occurred in dogs taken off gentamicin for 28 days, with only focal, tubulointerstitial nephritis being present on histopathologic examination (Cronin et al. 1980). Dogs dosed at 40 mg/kg/day IM for 15 days became moribund and were euthanized, the necropsy revealing extensive proximal tubular necrosis (Black et al. 1963). In this study, dogs given 8 mg/kg/day for 50 days developed aminoglycoside-induced toxic nephropathy marked by elevated serum urea nitrogen concentrations and histologic evidence of tubular necrosis (Black et al. 1963). In dogs given 5.6 mg/kg/day for 50 days, only cloudy swelling of the renal tubule cells was present histologically. In a recent study dosing gentamicin at 60 or 75 mg/kg/day for 10 days, dogs either died or became anuric (Powell et al. 1983). All of these studies suggest that prolonged low-dose or very high-dose therapy may produce deleterious results.

A number of drugs can have ototoxicity as a side effect (Pickerell et al. 1993). Aminoglycosides, chlorhexidine, polymyxin B, ethacrynic acid, furosemide, salicylates, and cisplatin are all drugs that can result in some degree of ototoxicity under certain conditions. Ototoxicity in dogs, manifested as either vestibulotoxic and/or ototoxic effects, can occur after systemic aminoglycoside therapy, but toxicity after topical use of aminoglycosides is apparently rare. Strain et al. (1995) attempted to detect ototoxicity in dogs treated with topically administered gentamicin using brain stem auditory evoked potential (BAEP). Greyhounds received 7 drops of a 3 mg/mL buffered aqueous solution of gentamicin instilled into one ear twice a day for 3 weeks. Auditory (using BAEP) and vestibular function (eye movements, head tilt, nystagmus, ataxia, etc.) evaluations were performed throughout the study. None of the dogs developed detectable changes in cochlear or vestibular function. Each dog then underwent a unilateral myringotomy, followed by instillation of 7 drops of the 3 mg/mL buffered aqueous solution of gentamicin instilled into one ear twice a day for 3 weeks. Again all dogs failed to develop detectable changes in cochlear or vestibular function.

Cats. Cats administered 50 mg/kg/day of gentamicin for 65 days had markedly elevated serum urea nitrogen concentrations. In 6 cats given 35 mg/kg/day, serum urea nitrogen concentrations were 50 mg/dL or greater after 6-13 days. Tubular necrosis was present on histologic examination (Welles et al. 1973). Cats administered gentamicin at a daily dose of 60 mg/kg/day died after an average of 17 days of dosing from renal tubular necrosis. A total of 4 of 5 cats receiving 40 mg/kg/day died at 18-27 days into the dosing from acute renal failure. A total of 3 of 4 cats given 20 mg/kg/day survived for 70 days. On necropsy, only mild or no tubular damage was present (Waitz et al. 1971). Cats are primarily used as the animal model to study aminoglycoside ototoxicity (primarily vestibular) and have not been utilized to study aminoglycoside-induced toxic nephropathy. Gentamicin and other aminoglycosides not only can induce neuromuscular blockade by itself but also can potentiate a neuromuscular blockade when administered with atracurium in cats (Forsyth et al. 1990). It must be noted that in comparison to other species, cats appear to have a relatively more concentrated urine and retain the ability to produce concentrated urine even when the GFR is significantly reduced (Ross and Finco 1981), making urine monitoring less successful than in dogs.

Nephrotoxicosis associated with the topical use of gentamicin has been reported in cats (Mealey and Boothe 1994). A cat was administered 10 mL of an undiluted gentamicin injectable solution (50 mg/mL) to lavage an open wound twice. The cat eventually progressed to an azotemic state and was euthanized. Histologically, the kidneys showed severe acute proximal tubular necrosis compatible with aminoglycoside toxicosis. Elevated serum levels of gentamicin were noted as late as 96 hours after administration. Although a number of factors may have contributed to the death of this cat, the topical administration of such large quantities of gentamicin was most likely the major determinant. Gentamicin toxicity has also been reported in the North American cougar (Johnson et al. 1993).

Horses. Aminoglycoside toxic nephropathy as well as ototoxicity (Nostrandt et al. 1991) has been studied in horses. Clinically, aminoglycoside-induced toxic nephropathy appears to be restricted to young animals, with toxicity rarely reported in adults (Riviere et al. 1982; Tobin 1979). The effect of neomycin on the kidneys of adult horses has been studied (Fuentes et al. 1997). Horses (4-7 years old) dosed with 10 mg/kg IM BID for 15 days failed to demonstrate liver or renal histopathology by the end of the dosing period. There was no significant change in serum and urinary values of creatinine. There was, however, a significant increase in urinary GGT beginning on or about the third day of treatment, peaking between 12 and 15 days, and decreasing through the end of the study, indicative of damage to the brush border of the proximal tubular cells of the nephron. The use of GGT as a biomarker for nephrotoxicity in horses has been debated. Rossier et al. (1995) studied three groups of horses: normal horses, normal horses treated with 2.2 mg/kg gentamicin IV QID for 10 days, and sick horses (pleuropneumonia) treated with 2.2 mg/kg gentamicin IV QID for 10 days. All groups had urinary GGT, urinary creatinine, and plasma creatinine measured at days 1, 3, and 10 of treatment. Sick horses had significantly higher mean urinary GGT:urinary creatinine ratios than either of the other groups. There was no significant difference between the urinary GGT:urinary creatinine ratios in normal (untreated) horses and normal horses treated with gentamicin. The study further concluded that, at least with horses, the urinary GGT:urinary creatinine ratio could, but does not necessarily, correspond to clinically significant changes in renal function due to aminoglycoside toxicity, mainly due to assay methodology and variability in normal baseline values. High urinary GGT:urinary creatinine ratios may occur early in gentamicin therapy and subsequently decrease over time. This factor reduces the urinary GGT:urinary creatinine ratio's clinical usefulness since it would not provide a useful barometer for determining whether gentamicin therapy should be continued or stopped.

Daily doses of 8.8 mg/kg/day for 5-14 days induced toxic nephropathy marked by elevations in serum creatinine and serum urea nitrogen (Tobin 1979; Riviere 1982). In an experimental study of aminoglycoside-induced toxic nephropathy in young horses, 1 of 3 horses given 8.8 mg/kg/day and 1 of 3 given 17.6 mg/kg/day for 14 days developed elevated serum urea nitrogen and creatinine concentrations and decreased urine osmolarity (Riviere et al. 1983). Three foals given 4.4 mg/kg/day for 14 days did not develop functional evidence of aminoglycoside-induced toxic nephropathy. All foals in this study had dose-related histopathologic evidence of proximal tubular nephrosis including tubular necrosis and regeneration. Ultrastructurally, cytosegresomes were present in gentamicin-treated animals. The clinical and pathologic expression of aminoglycoside-induced toxic nephropathy appeared similar to that in other species. Gentamicin trough serum concentrations increased in the foals exhibiting aminoglycoside-induced toxic nephropathy. These studies suggest that unlike other species, young foals are not resistant to aminoglycoside-induced toxic nephropathy, although a mechanism for this phenomenon is not known. The severity of the aminoglycoside-induced toxic nephropathy seen at the low dose above is expected since the human-equivalent equine dose predicted using allometry (0.75 mg/kg) would be only 2-3 mg/kg/day. Once per day dosing (6.6 mg/kg/day IV for 10 days) did not produce signs of nephrotoxicosis (elevated blood urea nitrogen, serum creatinine, urine GGT, etc.) in adult animals (Godber et al. 1995), suggesting again that a SID regimen may be preferred both for efficacy and for reduced toxicity.

Ruminants. Calves given 5 or 9 mg/kg/day neomycin IM for 12-13 days developed aminoglycoside-induced toxic nephropathy marked by increased serum creatinine and urea nitrogen concentrations, decreased creatinine clearance, decreased urine specific gravity, cylindruria, proteinuria, and enzymuria (γ-glutamyltranspeptidase and alanine aminopeptidase) (Crowell et al. 1981). On histopathologic examination, tubular hyaline droplet change, degeneration, and necrosis were present. This apparent sensitivity is again primarily due to the large body size of cows, for which 5-9 mg/kg/day is an overdosage on a 0.75 mg/kg basis. Finally, neomycin concentrations in the renal cortex ranged from approximately 200 to 400 μg/g. Gentamicin-induced toxic nephropathy was not detected in adult sheep given 9 mg/kg/day for 7 days when serum creatinine and urea nitrogen concentrations were monitored and tissues were examined at necropsy by light microscopy (Brown et al. 1985). Sheep have recently been advocated as a stable animal model for human renal diseases (Eschbach et al. 1980). They may be a useful animal model of gentamicin toxic nephropathy because body weight is essentially identical to that seen in humans and the pharmacokinetic parameters describing gentamicin disposition are also similar. The use of urinary enzyme indices as a function of aminoglycoside nephrotoxicosis has been reported (Garry et al. 1990a,b).

GENTAMICIN. Gentamicin has been the most widely studied aminoglycoside antibiotic to date. Gentamicin is a combination of four components produced by *Micromonospora purpurea,* which all cross-react in common immunoassay procedures and are usually considered a single antimicrobial entity.

The plasma elimination phase (β phase) is correlated well with GFR in dogs and horses (Sojka and Brown, 1986; Frazier et al. 1988). Selected pharmacokinetic data for gentamicin in animals are shown in Tables 43.4 and 43.5.

The parenteral absorption patterns of gentamicin have been studied in several species of animals. Bioavailability (*F*) of gentamicin from IM sites is reported to be 68 ± 13% in cats (Jernigan et al. 1988e), 92 ± 15% in cows (Haddad et al. 1986), 87 ± 14% in horses (Haddad et al. 1985b), 95 ± 20% in dogs (Wilson et al. 1989), 95 ± 18% in roosters (Pedersoli et al. 1990), 21% in turkeys (Pedersoli et al. 1989), ≥95% in hawks and owls (Bird et al. 1983), ≥70% in eagles (Bird et al. 1983), and 60% in catfish (Setzer 1985). Bioavailability from different IM sites is considered identical (Wilson et al. 1989) and bioavailability from SC sites is similar to IM bioavailability (Gilman et al. 1987; Jernigan et al. 1988e; Wilson et al. 1989). The maximum concentration after SC administration is usually lower and occurs later after injection than that observed after an equivalent IM dose (Jernigan et al. 1988a; Wilson et al. 1989), which is most likely due to less blood flow to the SC injection sites than to the IM injection sites, resulting in a slower *rate* of absorption but not altering the *extent* of absorption. Systemic availability from intrauterine (IU) administration is 30% in normal cows, with maximum plasma concentrations of 3.70 mg/L and 17.5 mg/L being observed 30 minutes after IU doses of 2 and 4 mg/kg, respectively (al-Guedawy et al. 1983). Oral availability is near 0% in normal animals with intact intestinal mucosa, although necrotizing enteritis and/or diarrhea have been reported to increase availability in humans (Gemer et al. 1983; Miranda et al. 1984). Concentrations in renal tissue are observed after oral doses of 1 mg/kg/day for 7 days, for 10 days (>0.1 μg/g of renal tissue), and for 30 days (>0.02 μg/g of renal tissue) after the last dose in calves (Takahashi et al. 1985). Serum concentrations after IU dosing were minimal in normal horses; however, in horses treated with progesterone, systemic availability was 8-10 times higher, with greater penetration into endometrial tissue (Pedersoli et al. 1985). Estradiol also increased the systemic availability and endometrial penetration after IU infusion, but not to the same extent as that observed after progesterone. Gentamicin's use in the treatment of coliform mastitis in dairy cattle has also been investigated (Erskine et al. 1992; Jones and Ward 1990). The pharmacokinetics of gentamicin administered IM in budgerigars (*Melopsittacus undulatus*) (Itoh and Okada 1993) and cockatiels (Ramsay and Vulliet 1993) has also been described.

Several studies have shown that after multiple parenteral doses, pharmacokinetic values derived from blood samples taken within 8 hours of drug administration do not change appreciably in cats (Short et al. 1986; Jernigan et al. 1988a), although there is some evidence that shows a systematic circadian rhythm of peak and trough serum gentamicin concentrations, with peak and trough concentrations after the second and third doses of each day consistently higher than those obtained after the first daily dose.

Age appreciably affects gentamicin disposition. Because neonatal and infant animals have a larger proportion of their body weight as extracellular fluid, gentamicin volume of distribution (V_d) is larger in immature animals than in adults. For example, $V_{d(area)}$ of gentamicin in juvenile dogs is 0.35 L/kg (Riviere and Coppoc 1981a), whereas $V_{d(area)}$ in normal dogs is 0.227 L/kg (Brown et al. 1991). Foals less than 3 months of age exhibited a V_d of 0.344 L/kg, whereas adult horses in the same study had V_d of 0.184 L/kg (Sojka and Brown 1986). Another study, in young horses 2-3 months old, demonstrated $V_{d(ss)}$ of 0.306 L/kg (Riviere et al. 1983). Clarke et al. (1992) reported that the $t_{1/2}$, $V_{d(area)}$, and Cl_B (clearance) of gentamicin (3 mg/kg IV, once) did not change appreciably between groups of horses ranging from 0 to 10, 10 to 20, and 20 to 30 years of age and there was no pharmacologic reason to adjust the dose in older animals. However, it was noted in that study that the γ phase of gentamicin elimination was not studied and that the effect of advanced age on this phase of elimination is presently unknown.

Clearance of gentamicin is notably dependent upon renal function and has been shown to be so in (among

TABLE 43.4—Single-dose intravenous serum or plasma pharmacokinetics of gentamicin in various species

Species	Dose (mg/kg)	$V_{d(area)}$ (L/kg)	$V_{d(ss)}$ (L/kg)	Cl_B (mL/min/kg)	$t_{1/2(\beta)}$ (hr)	$t_{1/2(\gamma)}$ (hr)	Reference
Dogs (juvenile)	10	0.354 (0.036)	ND	4.08 (0.62)	1.01 (0.12)	N/A	Riviere and Coppoc 1981a
Dogs	10	0.38 (0.029)	ND	4.20 (0.70)	1.05 (0.13)	N/A	Riviere et al. 1981a; Riviere et al. 1981b
Dogs	10	0.30 (0.06)	ND	3.44 (0.38)	1.01 (0.08)	N/A	Rivierie et al. 1981a; Riviere et al. 1981b
Dogs	10	0.335 (0.094)	ND	2.94 (0.67)	1.36 (0.09)	N/A	Baggot 1977
Dogs	4.4	0.227 (0.076)	0.175 (0.033)	2.27 (0.41)	1.09[a]	N/A	Brown et al. 1991
Dogs	4.4	NR	8.56 (4.48)	1.45 (0.11)	1.04[a]	154.3[a]	Brown et al. 1991
Dogs	4	0.255	ND	3.33	1.06	N/A	Batra et al. 1983
Dogs	3	NR	0.172 (0.025)	2.29 (0.48)	0.91 (0.25)	N/A	Wilson et al. 1989
Cats	4.4	0.190	0.180	1.61	1.36	N/A	Short et al. 1986
Cats	5	ND	0.14 (0.20)	1.38 (0.35)	1.25 (0.30)	86[a]	Jernigan et al. 1988e
Cows	5	0.19 (0.04)	0.16 (0.032)	1.32 (0.17)	1.83 (0.18)	N/A	Haddad et al. 1986
Cattle (1 day old)	4.4	0.393 (0.040)	0.376 (0.041)	1.92 (0.43)	2.49 (0.73)	N/A	Clarke et al. 1985
Cattle (5 days old)	4.4	0.413 (0.050)	0.385 (0.044)	2.44 (0.34)	1.99 (0.33)	N/A	Clarke et al. 1985
Cattle (10 days old)	4.4	0.341 (0.021)	0.323 (0.020)	2.02 (0.27)	1.97 (0.21)	N/A	Clarke et al. 1985
Cattle (15 days old)	4.4	0.334 (0.039)	0.311 (0.029)	2.10 (0.32)	1.85 (0.13)	N/A	Clarke et al. 1985
Cattle (4-5 weeks old)	3	1.95 (1.24)	0.75 (0.20)	4.9 (1.9)	3.96 (1.67)	N/A	Ziv et al. 1982
Cattle (adult)	4.4	0.140 (0.020)	0.140 (0.020)	1.29 (0.26)	1.26 (0.19)	N/A	Clarke et al. 1985
Horses	5	0.254 (0.031)	0.24 (0.03)	2.54 (0.33)	2.54 (0.33)	N/A	Pedersoli et al. 1980
Horses (2-3 months old)	4.5	ND	0.306 (0.094)	1.65 (0.79)	3.23 (0.62)	N/A	Riviere et al. 1983
Horses	2.2	ND	0.15 (0.001)	0.87 (0.05)	3.85 (0.40)	N/A	Bowman et al. 1986
Horses	2.2	ND	1.74 (0.59)	0.68 (0.17)	3.51 (0.59)	142 (31)	Bowman et al. 1986
Horses	3	0.202 (0.028)	0.173 (0.012)	1.41 (0.19)	1.66 (0.06)	N/A	Wilson et al. 1983
Ponies	5	0.20 (0.01)	0.19 (0.01)	1.27 (0.18)	1.82 (0.22)	N/A	Haddad et al. 1985b
Mammoth asses[d]	2.2	0.12 (0.025)	ND	1.22 (0.18)	2.07	ND	Miller et al. 1994
Mammoth asses[e]	2.2	0.088 (0.028)	ND	1.29 (0.07)	0.84	5.12	Miller et al. 1994
Sheep	2.2	0.194 (0.059)	ND	1.56 (0.40)	1.44 (0.085)	N/A	Wilson et al. 1981
Sheep	3	ND	0.408 (0.196)	0.660 (0.256)	1.33[a]	41.9 (18.5)	Brown et al. 1986b
Sheep	10	ND	0.243 (0.026)	1.03 (0.015)	2.4 (0.5)	30.4 (18.9)	Brown et al. 1985
Sheep	10	ND	0.384 (0.195)	0.805 (0.317)	1.72[a]	88.9 (19.8)	Brown et al. 1986b
Sheep	20	ND	0.709 (0.751)	0.882 (0.342)	1.77[a]	167.2 (42.7)	Brown et al. 1986b
Sheep (Desert)	3	0.27	ND	0.07	4.20	ND	Elsheikh et al. 1997
Goat	3	0.22	ND	0.08	1.041	ND	Elsheikh et al. 1997
Pigs	2	0.32 (0.032)	0.24 (0.03)	1.66 (0.12)	1.9 (1.47–4.89)	20.2 (13.9–34.6)	Riond and Riviere 1988
Pigs (newborn)	5	ND	0.80	ND	5.19	ND	Giroux et al. 1995
Pigs (42 days)	5	ND	0.50	ND	3.50	ND	Giroux et al. 1995
Rabbits	20	ND	0.52–0.95[b]	2.90–4.0	0.98–1.15	11.4–15.1	Huang et al. 1979
Rabbits	3.5	ND	0.114 (0.020)	2.82 (0.97)	0.74	ND	Ogden et al. 1995

TABLE 43.4—Single-dose intravenous serum or plasma pharmacokinetics of gentamicin in various species (*continued*)

Species	Dose (mg/kg)	$V_{d(area)}$ (L/kg)	$V_{d(ss)}$ (L/kg)	Cl_B (mL/min/kg)	$t_{1/2(\beta)}$ (hr)	$t_{1/2(\gamma)}$ (hr)	Reference
Hawks[c]	10	0.24 (0.03)	N/A	2.09 (0.16)	1.35 (0.18)	N/A	Bird et al. 1983
Owls[c]	10	0.23 (0.02)	N/A	1.41 (0.10)	1.93 (0.24)	N/A	Bird et al. 1983
Eagles[c]	10	0.21 (0.01)	N/A	1.01 (0.06)	2.46 (0.32)	N/A	Bird et al. 1983
Catfish	1	0.156	NR	0.126	12.2	N/A	Setzer 1985
Catfish	10	0.176	ND	0.215	11.87	N/A	Rolf et al. 1986
Guinea pigs	40	ND	ND	3.4	1.01	1.01	Chung et al. 1982
Buffalo calves	5	0.43	ND	54.61	5.69	ND	Garg et al. 1991a,b
Turkeys	5	0.190	0.172	49.8	2.570	ND	Pedersoli et al. 1989
Roosters	5	0.228 (0.019)	0.209 (0.013)	0.775 (0.132)	3.38 (0.62)	N/A	Pedersoli et al. 1990

Source: Adapted from Brown and Riviere 1991.
Note: Values reported as arithmetic mean followed by SD or SEM in parentheses. N/A = not applicable (inappropriate term for the model used); ND = not determined; NR = not reported.
[a]Harmonic mean; data are IV and IM data pooled together.
[b]Range.
[c]One-compartment model used.
[d]Best described using a two-compartment open model
[e]Best described using a three-compartment open model.

TABLE 43.5—Terminal (γ) elimination half-lives of gentamicin from different species (mean ± SD unless otherwise specified)

Species	Dose (mg/kg)	Route	Interval (hr)	No. of doses	$t_{1/2\gamma}$ (hr)	Reference
Cattle	3.5	IM	8	30	44.9 ± 9.4	Haddad et al. 1987
Sheep	10	IV	NA	1	30.4 ± 18.9	Brown et al. 1985
Sheep	3	IM	8	21	82.1 ± 17.8	Brown et al. 1985
Sheep	3	IV	8	21	129.5[a]	Brown et al. 1986a
Sheep	3	IV	NA	1	42.6[a]	Brown et al. 1986a
Sheep	10	IV	NA	1	107.6[a]	Brown et al. 1986a
Sheep	20	IV	NA	1	164.2[a]	Brown et al. 1986a
Dogs	4.4	IV	NA	1	154.3[a]	Brown et al. 1991
Dogs (diabetic)	4.4	IV	NA	1	NF	Brown et al. 1991
Pigs	6	IV	NA	1	10.6 ± 1.8	Riond et al. 1986
Pigs	2	IV	8	21	13.9 ± 34.6	Riond and Riviere 1988
Rabbits	20	IV	NA	1	11.4 ± 15.1	Huang et al. 1979
Cats	5	IV	NA	1	86.6[a]	Jernigan et al. 1988e
Horses	2.2	IV	NA	1	142 ± 31	Bowman et al. 1986
Dogs	10	IV	NA	1	31 ± 10	Riviere and Carver 1984
Dogs (hypothyroid)	10	IV	NA	1	5.6 ± 4.1	Riviere and Carver 1984
Pigs	6	IV	NA	1	11.0 ± 0.4	Riond et al. 1986

Source: Adapted from Brown and Riviere 1991.
Note: NF = not found in diabetic dogs (only 1 out of 7 dogs had a detectable $t_{1/2\gamma}$ = 46.8 hr); NA = not applicable.
[a]Harmonic mean; range.

others) horses (Sojka and Brown 1986; Sweeney et al. 1992), dogs (Frazier et al. 1988), and pigs (Riond et al. 1986). As predicted by allometric principles, on a mL/min/kg basis, gentamicin clearance decreases as body weight increases. This also strongly suggests that dosages must be reduced in the face of renal dysfunction.

Recovery of gentamicin in the urine has been reported to be 91 ± 28% within the first 24 hours in sheep (Brown et al. 1985; Brown et al. 1986a; Brown et al. 1986b), 96% in the first 5 hours in dogs (Chisholm et al. 1968), 83 ± 8% in the first 8 hours in adult cattle (Haddad et al. 1986), and 90% recovered in the first 24 hours in 4- to 5-week-old calves (Ziv et al. 1982). Urinary recovery data of gentamicin appears to indicate that the β phase of elimination accounts for the majority of gentamicin elimination from the body. The urinary excretion patterns of gentamicin in buffalo calves (*Bubalus bubalis*) has also been reported (Garg and Garg 1989).

Gentamicin disposition is altered in obese patients, with the patient's excess weight (that above lean body weight, LBW) contributing only 0.05 L/kg to the V_d

(Sketris et al. 1981). When converted to LBW, gentamicin V_d is increased from 0.19 L/kg LBW in normal patients to 0.24 L/kg LBW in obese patients. Also, dehydration in rats reduces the V_d from normal (0.19 L/kg and 0.26 L/kg) (LeCompte et al. 1981). Similar results have been reported in dehydrated cattle (Hunter et al. 1991). Gentamicin pharmacokinetics changes appreciably between lean and obese cats (Wright et al. 1991). Obese cats given a 3 mg/kg IV dose of gentamicin had significantly lower $V_{d(ss)}$ and Cl values compared to lean cats. Bioavailability and $t_{1/2}$ values for obese cats were unchanged when compared to the values obtained in lean cats. These changes were attributed to the chemical characteristics of gentamicin, in that the poorly lipid soluble gentamicin fails to distribute adequately into the excess adipose tissue, resulting in reduced V_d values and necessitating a dose adjustment based on the cat's estimated lean body mass and not its overall body mass. In a related study, obese rats were found to sustain more nephrotoxicity due to increased renal uptake and retention of gentamicin in the kidneys than did their lean counterparts (Salazar et al. 1992).

Gentamicin disposition has been extensively studied in animals given IV endotoxin. Endotoxemia decreased plasma gentamicin concentrations in dogs by approximately 20-30% (Pennington et al. 1975) and reduced the area under the plasma concentration-time curve (AUC) after IM dosing in cats from 1620 ± 390 μg/min/mL to 1170 ± 400 μg/min/mL (Jernigan et al. 1988c). Other conditions that have been shown to alter gentamicin disposition include endocrinopathies, pregnancy, and other concurrent drug administrations.

In dogs, familial hypothyroidism effectively abolishes the phase of serum disposition (Riviere and Carver 1984), as does experimentally induced and naturally occurring diabetes mellitus (Brown et al. 1991). In rats, hypoparathyroidism (Holohan et al. 1987) and streptozotocin-induced diabetes mellitus (Ramsammy et al. 1987) reduce the renal accumulation of gentamicin without affecting the number or affinity of the gentamicin binding sites (Holohan et al. 1987). In pigs, hypothyroidism reduced mean (±SEM) gentamicin Cl_B from 2.51 ± 0.17 (normal pigs) to 1.52 ± 0.12 mL/min/kg (Riond et al. 1986), an effect caused by reduction in the GFR. Finally, horses under halothane anesthesia showed longer gentamicin $t_{1/2}$ than when in the awake state (4.03 hours vs. 2.01 hours), as a result of reduced GFR during anesthesia.

Limited work has been done with gentamicin and regional limb perfusion to treat joint infections in horses (Whitehair et al. 1992a, Whitehair et al. 1992b). In another study, where horses were being treated for bacterial infections (pleuropneumonia, peritonitis, pericarditis, abscess, etc.) with gentamicin, it was found that an IV dose of 2.2 mg/kg QID resulted in satisfactory serum levels in most horses, but dose adjustments seem to be necessary to account for individual gentamicin disposition in both normal and diseased horses. Gentamicin clearance was also found to be correlated with the plasma creatinine concentration in both healthy and clinically ill horses (Sweeney et al. 1992), allowing serum creatinine concentrations to be used to individualize gentamicin doses in horses (Martin et al. 1998). The disposition of gentamicin in equine plasma, synovial fluid, and lymph has also been reported (Anderson et al. 1995). Horses had a subcutaneous lymph vessel on the medial aspect of the metatarsus cannulated and were then given a single 2.2 mg/kg IV dose of gentamicin. Plasma and lymph samples were collected together at predetermined times after dosing. The $t_{1/2}$ of gentamicin in the plasma was 2.17 hours (range = 1.92-2.5), and the $t_{1/2}$ in the lymph was 3.03 hours (range = 2.63-3.57). It was concluded that the plasma concentration of gentamicin was a reliable predictor of concentration in lymph fluid and that plasma-based pharmacokinetics could be used with a good degree of confidence to predict the concentrations that would be obtained in the lymph in horses.

Gentamicin is accumulated in renal proximal tubules to concentrations several-fold higher than in serum or any other tissue in every species investigated (Schentag and Jusko 1977; Riviere et al. 1981a; Aronoff et al. 1983; Trnovec et al. 1984; Brown et al. 1985; Brown et al. 1986b; Haddad et al. 1987; Jernigan et al. 1988c). Concentrations in normal calf kidney have accounted for 46% of the dose 4 hours after administration and 6.3% of the dose 48 hours after IV injection (Ziv et al. 1982); in dogs, less than 2% of the dose was present in the renal cortex 1-2 hours after the start of a continuous infusion to maintain blood levels at 11.1 ± 0.5 μg/mL (Chiu et al. 1976).

Renal uptake is inhibited by urinary alkalinization with sodium bicarbonate, theoretically because gentamicin is less ionized and therefore is less able to bind to the acidic phospholipids of the proximal tubular membranes (Chiu et al. 1979). On the other hand, alkalinization with acetazolamide does not reduce gentamicin uptake, presumably because acetazolamide acidifies the proximal tubular lumen (Chiu et al. 1979). High proteinuria due to high-protein diet or diabetes mellitus and proteinuria induced primarily by renal disorders reduce gentamicin uptake into renal proximal tubules (Pattyn et al. 1988), although factors other than proteinuria may also play a role (Ramsammy et al. 1987). In sheep, diet may also play a significant role in gentamicin pharmacokinetics. A study by Oukessou and Toutain (1992) reported that sheep fed a low-protein diet (25 g/day) had significantly lower $V_{d(ss)}$ and Cl values for gentamicin (4 mg/kg IV) than did sheep fed a high-protein (120 g/day), while AUC values were higher in the sheep fed the low-protein diet, indicating higher overall serum concentrations of gentamicin in this treatment group. Coupled with IV insulin clearance data, it was surmised that the protein content of the diet can appreciably modify the distribution of body water and also modulate kidney function, resulting in altered gentamicin kinetics. A similar study in horses found that horses fed a diet of oats (low in calcium and potassium) had a higher incidence of gentamicin-induced nephrotoxicosis than horses fed an all-alfalfa hay diet high in vitamins and minerals (Schumacher et al. 1991). Based on these results, anorectic horses or horses consuming diets low in mineral content are seemingly predisposed to aminoglycoside nephrotoxicosis. A pharmacokinetic model of IM gentamicin has also been described for sheep (Errecalde and Marino 1990).

Gentamicin also reaches therapeutic concentrations in a number of other tissues in addition to the kidney and inner ear. Studies of a variety of wild birds and game birds, including the greater sandhill crane, rosy-bill duck, pigeon, eastern bobwhite quail, argus pheasant, North American wood duck, ruddy shelduck, pintail duck, and emu, as well as laboratory rats show a similar rank order of tissue concentrations of gentamicin, with skeletal muscle concentrations being either very low or nondetectable (Bush et al. 1981; LeCompte et al. 1981). After 5 mg/kg gentamicin every 8 hours in ponies, after 4 and 7 days, the endometrial concentrations were 5.02 ± 3.3 μg/g and 12.7 ± 1.6 μg/g (Haddad et al. 1985a). Milk concentrations after 30 IM doses of 3.5 mg/kg gentamicin were 0.47 ± 0.08 μg/mL 30 minutes after the last dose and 0.19 ± 0.02 μg/mL 14 hours after the last dose (Haddad et al. 1987). In that same study, negligible concentrations were observed in the brain after doses of either 3.5 or 5 mg/kg.

Gentamicin residues can be found in milk after IV, IM, or intramammary (IMM) administration. Pedersoli et al. (1995) administered a single IV or IM dose of gentamicin (5 mg/kg) or a single 500 mg dose of gentamicin to the udder of lactating cows and followed the elimination of the drug via the milk over several days. After a single IMM infusion, the gentamicin levels did not fall below a safe level (≤30 ng/mL) until the seventh milking, 84 hours after treatment. Single IV or IM doses of gentamicin yielding safe milk levels of gentamicin occurred at the third milking, 36 hours after dosing. In another experiment, the cows were given two IV or IM doses of gentamicin (5 mg/kg) or two 500 mg doses of gentamicin to the udders of lactating cows for 5 days. Gentamicin levels did not fall below a safe level (≤30 ng/mL) until the eleventh milking, 132 hours after treatment. Single IV doses again produced safe milk levels of gentamicin at 36 hours after dosing. Because of concerns about residues, gentamicin is not recommended for use in cattle.

Although gentamicin does not partition into and sequester in skeletal muscle (Brown et al. 1986b; Haddad et al. 1987; Riond and Riviere 1988), substantial retention of gentamicin did occur at the site of IM injections (Haddad et al. 1987), reaching concentrations of 16.7 ± 11.3 μg/g at the IM injection site in sheep (Brown et al. 1986b).

Urine concentrations are reported to be as high as 107 ± 33 μg/mL after 2.2 mg/kg every 8 hours in dogs (Ling et al. 1981), and 362 ± 163 μg/mL 3 hours after 3 mg/kg in cats (Jernigan et al. 1988b). Urine concentrations in animals with pyelonephritis (Bergeron et al. 1982) and endotoxemia (Jernigan et al. 1988b) are lower than in control animals given gentamicin, perhaps in part due to retention in the renal medulla (Jernigan et al. 1988b). Changes in urine parameters have been reported in sheep (Garry et al. 1990a,b).

There is some information on the use of gentamicin in sheep and goats. Elsheikh et al. (1997) dosed male Nubian goats and male desert sheep with 3 mg/kg gentamicin IV and found no significant differences in V_d, clearance, and elimination half-lives between the species. Gaddi goats were administered 5 mg/kg gentamicin by IV, IM, and SC routes (Garg et al. 1995). The elimination half-lives were 0.96, 2.37, and 3.56 hours for IV, IM, and SC routes, respectively. The study did show that the half-lives of gentamicin do not appear to be route dependent, as they are in the feline. The pharmacokinetics of gentamicin in normal and febrile goats has also been examined (Ahmad et al. 1994). Healthy and febrile female goats received a single 5 mg/kg IV dose of gentamicin, and its kinetics was examined. Differences in blood serum concentrations between normal and febrile goats were not observed. Apparent volumes of distribution and clearance values did not differ between the groups; however, the median value of gentamicin blood half-life was shorter in normal goats (103.6 min) than in febrile goats (136.0 min). Based on these data, the authors suggested small adjustments in IV doses based on steady-state and peak and trough serum concentrations.

AMIKACIN. Tables 43.6 and 43.7 list some selected pharmacokinetic parameters for amikacin in various species of animals. The parenteral absorption patterns of amikacin have been studied in several species of animals, including red-tailed hawks (*Buteo jamaicensis*) (Bloomfield et al. 1997). Bioavailability of amikacin ranges from 90% after IM and 100% after SC doses in cats (Jernigan et al. 1988d). Mean absorption time is 55 ± 36 minutes after IM doses and 53 ± 19 minutes after SC doses in cats (Jernigan et al. 1988d). The availability of amikacin after IU infusion in horses is minimal; however, availability after intraperitoneal (IP) administration (via instillation in continuous ambulatory peritoneal dialysis) was 53 ± 14% in humans, with therapeutic IP concentrations obtained for 72 hours after an IP dose of 7.5 mg/kg (Smeltzer et al. 1988). The absorption $t_{1/2}$ is 5.7 ± 2.8 hours after IM dosing in snakes and is independent of the ambient temperature (Mader et al. 1985).

In dogs and calves, amikacin concentrations peak at approximately 0.5-0.85 hours (Cabana and Taggart 1973; Ziv 1977), with plasma depletion half-lives slightly longer after IM dosing and particularly after SC dosing than after an IV dose (Baggot et al. 1985; Carli et al. 1990). The urine amikacin concentration in dogs after 15 mg/kg divided into three daily doses was 342 ± 153 μg/mL when obtained as a 6- to 9-hour collection after dosing (Ling et al. 1981). Amikacin use has also been investigated in gopher tortoises (Caligiuri et al. 1990). The V_d of amikacin in tortoises at 20° C (0.221 L/kg) was not appreciably different from that

TABLE 43.6—Single-dose intravenous pharmacokinetics of amikacin in various species

Species	Dose (mg/kg)	$V_{d(area)}$ (L/kg)	$V_{d(ss)}$ (L/kg)	Cl_B (mL/min/kg)	$t_{1/2\beta}$ (hr)	Reference
Cats	5	0.134 (0.008)	NR	110 (15)	NR	Shille et al. 1985
Cats	10	0.14 (0.008)	NR	121 (22)	NR	Shille et al. 1985
Cats	20	0.18 (0.022)	NR	138 (2.6)	NR	Shille et al. 1985
Cats	5	NR	0.17 (0.02)	1.46 (0.26)	79[b] (19)	Jernigan et al. 1988c
Horses	4.4	0.20 (0.05)	NR	89.3 (23.4)	1.44[b]	Orsini et al. 1985
Horses	6.6	0.17 (0.03)	NR	76.6 (11.3)	1.57[b]	Orsini et al. 1985
Horses	11	0.14 (0.02)	NR	84.7 (13.4)	1.14	Orsini et al. 1985
Horses	6	0.214	0.207	0.75	2.8	Horspool et al. 1994
Ponies	6	0.191	0.162	1.37	1.6	Horspool et al. 1994
Donkeys	6	0.156	0.150	0.97	1.9	Horspool et al. 1994
Dogs[a]	5	0.26 (0.23–0.29)	NR	2.82 (2.29–3.22)	1.07 (0.95–1.22)	Baggot et al. 1985
Dogs[a]	10	0.239 (0.18–0.27)	NR	2.66 (2.32–2.89)	0.98 (0.90–1.07)	Baggot et al. 1985
Dogs[a]	20	0.36 (0.32–0.38)	NR	3.57 (3.31–4.73)	1.03 (0.90–1.33)	Baggot et al. 1985
Calves	7.5	350	NR	1.5	150.5	Carli et al. 1990
Sheep	7.5	200	NR	0.7	115.5	Carli et al. 1990
African grey parrots	5	289	233	188	1.06	Gronwall et al. 1989
African grey parrots	10	184	122	142	0.90	Gronwall et al. 1989
African grey parrots	20	444	308	229	1.34	Gronwall et al. 1989
Dogs	25	0.25	NR	34	0.85	Cabana and Taggart 1973
Humans	125	16.26 (1.7)	NR	81 (6)	2.8 (0.26)	Yates et al. 1978

Source: Adapted from Brown and Riviere 1991.
Note: NR = not reported.
[a]Median (range); total dose (mg); mL/min.
[b]Harmonic mean (±SD).

when the body temperature was at 30° C (0.241 L/kg); however, Cl_B in the 30° C tortoises was markedly higher (10.65 mL/min/kg) than in the 20° C animals (5.27 mL/min/kg). Similar differences were also noted for mean residence time and AUC values, indicating that amikacin (like many other drugs in cold-blooded animals) is temperature dependent. The pharmacokinetic profiles for three doses of amikacin have been reported in African grey parrots (Gronwall et al. 1989).

Pharmacokinetic parameters for amikacin in normal, premature, uremic, and hypoxic foals have been reported (Wichtel et al. 1992; Adland-Davenport et al. 1990; Green et al. 1992). In one report, the $t_{1/2}$, V_d, and Cl for amikacin in premature foals (3.5 hr, 0.48 L/kg, and 98.2 mL/hr/kg, respectively) were not very different from the values for full-term nonuremic foals (3.3 hours, 0.40 L/kg, and 85.8 mL/hr/kg, respectively). However, full-term uremic foals less than 4 days old had higher values for two out of three of these parameters (20.1 hr, 0.80 L/kg, and 38.4 mL/hr/kg, respectively) when given 7 mg/kg (IV or IM) either BID or TID. Septic foals (less than 1 week old) with high septic scores appear to have increased amikacin AUC and mean residence times and lower values for clearance when compared to clinically normal foals of similar age. The effects of hypoxia and azotemia on amikacin pharmacokinetics in the neonatal foal have also been reported (Green et al. 1992).

The pharmacokinetics of IV vs. intraosseous (IO) administration of amikacin was studied in 3- and 5-day-old foals (Golenz et al. 1994). Foals were given 7 mg/kg amikacin IV or IO (tibia) and blood samples taken at predetermined times. Radiographic studies confirmed the proper placement of the IO catheter used to administer the amikacin. The pharmacokinetics of amikacin administered IV and IO were almost identical in these foals. Peak concentrations in plasma after IV (34.17 μg/mL) and IO (34.17 μg/mL) administration both occurred during the first sample collected (3 minutes after injection). The mean bioavailability of amikacin after IO administration was 98.1%, indicating nearly complete absorption from the site of administration. No significant differences were noted between the major pharmacokinetic parameters of IV and IO

TABLE 43.7—Nonintravenous disposition values for amikacin in various species (means with standard deviations in parentheses)

Species	Dose (mg/kg)	Route	V_d/F (L/kg)	Cl_B/F (mL/min/kg)	$t_{1/2}$ (hr)	F (%)	Reference
Horses	4.4	IM	NR	NR	NR	100	Orsini et al. 1985
Horses	6.6	IM	NR	NR	NR	100	Orsini et al. 1985
Horses	11	IM	NR	NR	NR	100	Orsini et al. 1985
Cats	5	IM	0.16 (0.004)	132[a] (13)	NR	NR	Shille et al. 1985
Cats	10	IM	0.2 (0.02)	150[a] (10)	NR	NR	Shille et al. 1985
Cats	20	IM	0.19 (0.02)	121[a] (21)	NR	NR	Shille et al. 1985
Cats	5	SC	0.19 (0.01)	138[a] (13)	NR	NR	Shille et al. 1985
Cats	10	SC	0.21 (0.01)	117[a] (6)	NR	NR	Shille et al. 1985
Cats	20	SC	0.19 (0.01)	141[a] (21)	NR	NR	Shille et al. 1985
Cats	5	IM	ND	ND	119	90 (36)	Jernigan et al. 1988d
Cats	5	SC	ND	ND	118	100 (19)	Jernigan et al. 1988d
Sheep	7.5	IM	ND	ND	1.96	87	Carli et al. 1990
Calves	7.5	IM	ND	ND	1.94	99	Carli et al. 1990
African grey parrot	5	IM	ND	ND	1.08	98	Gronwall et al. 1989
African grey parrot	10	IM	ND	ND	1.04	61	Gronwall et al. 1989
African grey parrot	15	IM	ND	ND	0.97	106	Gronwall et al. 1989
Gopher snake (25° C)	5	IM	0.29 (0.04)	2.8 (0.29)	1.2 (0.17)	ND	Mader et al. 1985
Gopher snake (37° C)	5	IM	0.63 (0.31)	5.83 (1.6)	1.25 (0.5)	ND	Mader et al. 1985

Source: Adapted from Brown and Riviere 1991.
ND = not determined; NR = not reported.
[a]mL/min.

amikacin in this study. Five-day-old foals did have statistically significant higher Cl_B values than the 3-day-old foals. The study concluded by stating that the IO infusion methodology in neonatal foals is a safe and effective technique for drug delivery when the IV route cannot be used, particularly in cases of circulatory collapse. Amikacin, like other aminoglycosides, is poorly absorbed from the gastrointestinal tract of the horse. Horspool et al. (1994) administered a single dose of amikacin IV and two PO doses to horses, ponies, and donkeys. Detectable blood levels of amikacin were not found in any of the animals dosed orally with amikacin; likewise, no amikacin was found in the fecal material of animals dosed with amikacin by the IV route. Amikacin had little, if any, effect on the numbers of viable bacteria of the normal gastrointestinal flora of these study animals. Given the mode of action of the aminoglycosides, amikacin appears to have negligible effects in the anaerobic environment of the gastrointestinal tract.

Serum concentrations of amikacin have also been studied in mares in estrus. After induction of estrus, mares were dosed with 1.0 or 2.0 g amikacin by intrauterine (IU) infusion every 24 hours for 3 days, or given an IM injection of either 9.7 or 14.5 mg/kg every 24 hours for 3 days. Amikacin was not detected in the serum of mares given the 1 g IU dose of drug. Low blood levels (0.51-0.71 μg/mL) were detected at 1, 2, and 4 hours after IU infusion after the first and third treatments. As expected, IM injections produced detectable serum levels of amikacin, with peak concentrations attained at 1 hour (9.7 mg/kg) and 2 hours (14.5 mg/kg) after dosing.

KANAMYCIN. Because of the structural similarities between kanamycin and amikacin (amikacin is synthesized from kanamycin), the pharmacokinetics of kanamycin and amikacin are very similar. Lashev et al. (1992) studied species differences in the pharmacokinetics of kanamycin in sheep, goats, rabbits, adult chickens, and pigeons given a 10 mg/mL IV dose of kanamycin. The differences in the V_d in these animals were small, all being between 0.254 and 0.292 L/kg. Eighteen-day-old chicks had the largest V_d (0.671 L/kg). In calves, IM doses of 10, 25, and 50 mg/kg produced peak concentrations at 30 minutes of 31 ± 3.1 μg/mL, 57.3 ± 4.9 μg/mL, and 64 ± 14 μg/mL, respectively. The kanamycin elimination half-lives of 2 hours in all three instances were identical to amikacin (Ziv 1977). Similar half-lives of 1.80 ± 0.17 hours were observed in horses (Baggot et al. 1981) and sheep (Andreini and Pignatelli 1972). IM availability (F) of kanamycin in horses has been reported to be approximately 100% (Baggot et al. 1981). After a dose of 25 mg/kg of either kanamycin or amikacin IV in dogs, V_d was 0.23-0.25 L/kg, and after IM dosing in that same study, absorption $t_{1/2}$ were 0.4-0.75 hours, with apparent elimination $t_{1/2}$ of 0.9-1.2 hours for both amikacin and kanamycin (Cabana and Taggart 1973). The kanamycin $t_{1/2}$ in dogs after a 10 mg/kg IV dose was 0.97 ± 0.31 hours; after IM dosing, the *F* mean was 89 ± 16%, with an absorption $t_{1/2}$ of 0.15 ± 0.003 hours (Baggot 1978). Synovial fluid kanamycin concentrations in horses were equivalent to serum concentrations 4 hours after a 5 mg/kg dose IM, whereas peritoneal kanamycin concentrations were equal to or higher than serum kanamycin concentrations at 3 hours postadministration. The maximum serum concentrations of 12.6 ± 1.89 (mean ± SEM) were observed 1 hour after IM dosing (Brown et al. 1981). Although a γ phase was observed in the bloodstream of horses, the drug apparently did not penetrate into the peritoneal or synovial fluid, because after 12 hours those concentrations did not parallel serum concentrations (Brown et al. 1981). Firth et al. (1993) gave adult ponies a single 10 mg/kg kanamycin dose IM. At 2 and 5 hours after dosing, the metacarpophalangeal, intercarpal, radiocarpal, tibiotarsal, and metatarsophalangeal joints underwent arthrocentesis to determine kanamycin concentrations in the synovial fluid. There was considerable variation between joints sampled at each time point, and the authors reported that the variations were not consistent between animals and that these variations were not statistically significant. At 2 hours after dosing, synovial fluid concentrations fluctuated between joints but averaged 50% that of serum concentration. At 5 hours, synovial fluid concentrations were approximately 145% of plasma concentrations. Urine concentrations of kanamycin in dogs given 5.5 mg/kg twice a day were 473 ± 306 μg/mL urine when obtained as a 6-hour collection after dosing (Ling et al. 1981).

APRAMYCIN. Apramycin, an aminoglycoside derived from *Streptomyces tenebrarius* (Ryden and Moore 1977), is the newest aminoglycoside introduced for veterinary use. Administration of 10 mg/kg apramycin IV to preruminant dairy calves resulted in a $V_{d(ss)}$ of 0.71 ± 0.042 L/kg, a V_c of 0.34 ± 0.065 L/kg, a Cl_B of 3.22 ± 0.44 mL/min/kg, and a $t_{1/2}$ of 4.4 ± 1.2 hours (Ziv et al. 1985). Urine recovery of apramycin accounted for approximately 85% of the dose after 24 hours. Apramycin peak concentrations after IM doses of 10 and 20 mg/kg were 19 and 40 μg/mL, respectively, although peak concentrations occurred somewhat later after the larger dose. There was no plasma accumulation when IM doses of 10 or 20 mg/kg were given daily. Bioavailability of apramycin from IM sites was quite variable, ranging from 50 to 100% (Ziv et al. 1985).

Apramycin pharmacokinetics has also been described in lactating cows, ewes, and goats (Ziv et al. 1995). The IV pharmacokinetics of 20 mg/kg apramycin was very similar in the lactating cow, ewe, and goat, with an elimination $t_{1/2}$ of about 2 hours, a V_d between 1.26 and 1.5 L/kg, and an IM absorption bioavailability between 60% and 70%. All species had higher penetration of apramycin in the milk from inflamed udders than from clinically normal (nonmastitic) udders. The pharmacokinetics of apramycin in Japanese quails has also been described (Lashev and Mihailov 1994).

Pharmacokinetic data for apramycin in selected species are presented in Table 43.8.

TOBRAMYCIN. Tobramycin is produced by *Streptomyces tenebrarius* and is structurally similar to kanamycin. Tobramycin is not extensively used in veterinary medicine, although it is used occasionally in dogs and cats because of its enhanced efficacy against most *Pseudomonas aeruginosa* organisms. In cats, tobramycin possesses a Cl_B of 2.21 ± 0.59 and 1.69 ± 0.36 mL/min/kg after doses of 5 mg/kg and 3 mg/kg IV, respectively, and a $V_{d(ss)}$ of 0.19 ± 0.03 and 0.18 ± 0.03 L/kg, respectively (Jernigan et al. 1988b). In that same study, IV doses of 3 mg/kg and 5 mg/kg resulted in mean residence time (MRT) of 90 ± 16 and 108 ± 21 minutes, respectively. Bioavailability after IM and SC tobramycin administration in cats was reported as

TABLE 43.8—Selected pharmacokinetic parameters of apramycin

Species	$V_{d(ss)}$ (L/kg)	Cl_B (L/kg/hr)	$t_{1/2}$ (hr)	Reference
Sheep	0.167	0.078	90.96	Lashev et al. 1992
Cow (lactating)	1.263	12.164[a]	2.10	Ziv et al. 1995
Ewe (lactating)	1.446	14.142[a]	1.85	Ziv et al. 1995
Goat (lactating)[a]	1.357	11.68[a]	2.14	Ziv et al. 1995
Rabbits	0.284	0.258	48.06	Lashev et al. 1992
Adult chickens	0.182	0.078	100.54	Lashev et al. 1992
18-day-old chicks	0.254	0.218	48.0	Lashev et al. 1992
Japanese quail	0.133[b]	0.186	0.50	Lashev and Mihailov 1994
Pigeons	0.077	0.210	15.24	Lashev et al. 1992

[a]Value in mL/kg/min.
[b]V_d is area, not steady state.

greater than 100%, most likely caused by residual drug left in tissue depots from previous tobramycin administrations (Jernigan et al. 1988*d*). The mean absorption times were 35 and 60 minutes, respectively. Urine tobramycin concentrations following 2.2 mg/kg 3 times a day were 66 ± 39 μg/mL when urine was obtained as a 6-hour collection in dogs (Ling et al. 1981).

Camels (*Camelus dromedarius*) have been dosed with IV and IM tobramycin and their pharmacokinetics described (Hadi et al. 1994). After a single IV dose of tobramycin (1.3 mg/kg), the distribution phase half-life ($t_{1/2\alpha}$) was 10.8 minutes, followed by an elimination phase ($t_{1/2\beta}$) of 189 minutes. The apparent V_d (area method) was 245 mL/kg and $V_{d(ss)}$ was 228 mL/kg. Clearance was measured at 0.9 mL/min/kg. After a 1.0 mg/kg IM dose of tobramycin, bioavailability was almost 91%, with an elimination half-life ($t_{1/2\beta}$) of 201 minutes. The disposition kinetics of IV tobramycin in all camels evaluated was best described by a two-compartment open model, whereas all but one of the camels were best described by a one-compartment open model after IM dosing. In humans, using a three-compartment model, tobramycin $V_{d(ss)}$ and Cl_B decreased and $t_{1/2}$ increased slightly with decreasing renal function (Schentag et al. 1978).

NEOMYCIN. Neomycin is not used systemically in human medicine. Pharmacokinetic information about neomycin's use in human and veterinary medicine is very limited. In calves administered 12 mg/kg IV, $V_{d(B)}$ was 0.39 ± 0.13 L/kg, and $t_{1/2\beta}$ was reported as 167 ± 48 minutes (Black et al. 1983) although half-lives of approximately 1 hour have been observed (Drury 1952). Bioavailability after IM dosing of neomycin was 56 ± 5.4% in calves (Black et al. 1983) and 74 ± 27% in horses (Baggot et al. 1981). The pharmacokinetics of IV, IM, single PO, and repeated PO neomycin in ruminating Holstein calves has been described (Pedersoli et al. 1994). Variable absorption rates were also observed. In horses, a $t_{1/2\beta}$ of 2.1 ±1.0 hours has been reported, in addition to a V_d(area) of 0.232 ± 0.061 L/kg and a Cl_B of 1.3 ± 0.4 mL/min/kg (Baggot et al. 1981). Neomycin did not accumulate in inner-ear tissue as did other aminoglycosides (Desrochers and Schacht 1982) but was more potent than any other clinically used aminoglycoside at displacing gentamicin from renal binding sites (Josepovitz et al. 1982). Concentrations in guinea pig tissues other than the kidney continued to increase during 3 weeks of treatment with a dosing regimen of 100 mg/kg/day administered SC (Desrochers and Schacht 1982). Terminal half-lives have been estimated in cattle to be between 55 and 65 hours after single parenteral doses (Siddique et al. 1965). Neomycin's use today is limited to topical antibacterial therapy (see Chap. 53).

DIHYDROSTREPTOMYCIN. Pharmacokinetic studies are sparse for dihydrostreptomycin, the first aminoglycoside used clinically. After IM doses of 5.5 mg/kg dihydrostreptomycin, maximum concentrations ranged from 5.1 to 17.0 μg/mL, with peak concentrations occurring earlier and more variable from the commercial preparation containing procaine penicillin G, dihydrostreptomycin, dexamethasone, and chlorpheniramine than from the commercial product containing only dihydrostreptomycin and procaine penicillin G (Rollins et al. 1972). Half-lives range from 2.35-4.50 hours in cattle to 1.5-9.3 hours in horses, with a calculated γ-phase half-life of 6.3 hours in horses to a protracted 40 hours in cattle (Hammond 1953; Mercer et al. 1971; Riviere et al. 1990). Streptomycin (*not* dihydrostreptomycin) in horses had a $t_{1/2\beta}$ of 3.4 ± 0.4 hr, a $V_{d(area)}$ of 0.231 ± 0.041 L/kg, and a Cl_B of 0.77 ± 0.14 mL/min/kg (Baggot et al. 1981). Because streptomycin and dihydrostreptomycin are chemically very similar, their dispositions also may be nearly identical. Dihydrostreptomycin has been used successfully in the treatment of cows infected with *Leptospira interrogans* serovar *hardjo* subtype *hardjobovis* (Gerritsen et al. 1994).

PAROMOMYCIN. Paromomycin is a wide-spectrum aminoglycoside antibiotic produced by *Streptomyces rimosus* var. *paromomycinus* and, unlike others in this class, has both gram-positive and gram-negative activity. Paromomycin is poorly absorbed from the gastrointestinal tract, which is clearly an advantage if used to treat certain bacterial or protozoal gastrointestinal infections. The pharmacokinetics of paromomycin in the dog has been described by Belloli et al. (1996); see Table 43.9.

Giardia, Leishmania, Entamoeba histolytica, and *Balantidium coli* have all been demonstrated to be susceptible to paromomycin (Barr et al. 1994; Belloli et al. 1996). Paromomycin has been used to treat cryptosporidiosis in a cat (Barr et al. 1994) and leishmaniasis (*Leishmania infantum*) in the canine (Poli et al. 1997). However, a retrospective case study in cats treated with high-dose oral paromomycin (165 mg/kg) suggested that 4 of 31 individuals developed acute nephrotoxicity, deafness, and/or possible cataract

TABLE 43.9—Pharmacokinetic parameters of paromomycin in the dog

Parameter	IV	IM	SC
$t_{1/2\alpha}$	21.54	15.31	12.43
$t_{1/2\beta}$	91.03	114.22	120.86
V_d (L/kg)	0.51	ND	ND
V_{ss} (L/kg)	0.33	ND	ND
Cl_B (L/min/kg)	0.0037	ND	ND
C_{max} (μg/mL)	ND	32.1	36.3
F	ND	>0.99	>0.99
MRT (min)	98.7	204.8	203.8
K_{el} (min^{-1})	0.0186	0.0061	0.0057

Source: Belloli et al. 1996.
Note: ND = not determined.

formation (Gookin, et al., 1999), implying that enough oral absorption occurred for this large and highly charged aminoglycoside to exert an adverse effect. Therefore, use of this drug at these high doses should be approached with caution until further data are available.

REFERENCES

Adelman, R.D., Spangler, W.L., Beasom, F., Ishizaki, G., and Conzelman, G. 1979. Furosemide enhancement of experimental gentamicin nephrotoxicity, comparison of functional-morphological changes with activities of urinary enzymes. J Infect Dis 140:342-352.

Adland-Davenport, P., Brown, M.P., Robinson, J.D., and Derendorf, H.C. 1990. Pharmacokinetics of amikacin in critically ill neonatal foals treated for presumed or confirmed sepsis. Equine Vet J 22(1):18-22.

Ahmad, A.H., Bahga, H.S., and Sharma, L.D. 1994. Pharmacokinetics of gentamicin following single dose intravenous administration in normal and febrile goats. J Vet Pharmacol Therap 17:369-373.

al-Guedawy, S.S., Neff-Davis, C.A., Davis, L.E., Whitmore, H.L., and Gustafusson, B.K. 1983. Disposition of gentamicin in the genital tract of cows. J Vet Pharmacol and Therap 6:85-92.

Ali, B.H., Abdel Gayoum, A.A., and Bashir, A.A. 1992. Gentamicin nephrotoxicity in rats: some biochemical correlates. Pharmacol and Toxicol 70:419-423.

Anderson, B.H., Firth, E.C., and Whittem, T. 1995. The disposition of gentamicin in equine plasma, synovial fluid and lymph. J Vet Pharmacol Therap 18:124-131.

Andreini, G., and Pignatelli, P. 1972. Kanamycin blood levels and residues in domestic animals. Veterinaria 21:51-72.

Appel, G.B. 1982. Aminoglycoside nephrotoxicity: physiologic studies of the sites of nephron damage. In A. Whelton and H.C. Neu, eds., The Aminoglycosides: Microbiology, Clinical Use and Toxicology, pp. 269-382. New York: Marcel Dekker.

Appel, G.B., and Neu, H.C. 1977. The nephrotoxicity of antimicrobial agents. N Engl J Med 296:722-728.

Aronoff, G.R., Pottratz, S.T., Brier, M.E., et al. 1983. Aminoglycoside accumulation kinetics in rat renal parenchyma. Antimicrob Agents Chemotherapy 23:74-78.

Avasthi, P.S., Evan, A.P., Huser, J.W., and Luft, F.C. 1981. Effect of gentamicin on glomerular ultrastructure. J Lab Clin Med 98:444-454.

Baggot, J.D. 1977. Principles of Drug Disposition in Domestic Animals. Philadelphia: W.B. Saunders.

———. 1978. Pharmacokinetics of kanamycin in dogs. J Vet Pharmacol and Therap 1:163-170.

Baggot, J.D., Ling, G.V., Chatfield, R.C., and Raus, J. 1985. Clinical pharmacokinetics of amikacin in dogs. Am J Vet Res 46:1793-1796.

Baggot, J.D., Love, D.N., Rose, R.J., and Raus, J. 1981. The pharmacokinetics of some aminoglycoside antibiotics in the horse. J Vet Pharmacol and Therap 4:277-284.

Barr, S.C., Jamrosz, G.F., Hornbuckle, W.E., Bowman, D.D., and Fayer, R. 1994. Use of paromomycin for treatment of cryptosporidiosis in a cat. JAVMA 205(12):1742-1743.

Barza, M., Murray, T., and Hamburger, R.J. 1980. Uptake of gentamicin by separated, viable renal tubules from rabbits. J Infect Dis 141:510-517.

Bass, K.D., Larkin, S.E., Paap, C., and Haase, G.M. 1998. Pharmacokinetics of once-daily gentamicin dosing in pediatric patients. J Ped Surg 33(7):1104-1107.

Batra, V.K., Morrison, J.A., and Hoffman, T.R. 1983. Pharmacokinetics of piperacillin and gentamicin following intravenous administration to dogs. J Pharmaceut Sci 72:894-898.

Bauer, L.A., and Blouin, R.A. 1981. Influence of age on tobramycin pharmacokinetics in patients with normal renal function. Antimicrob Agents Chemother 20:587-589.

Beauchamp, D., Gourde, P., Theriault, G., and Bergeron, M.G. 1992. Age-dependent gentamicin experimental nephrotoxicity. J Pharmacol Exp Therap 260(2):444-449.

Behrend, E.N., Grauer, G.F., Greco, D.S., Fettman, M.J., and Allen, T.A. 1994. Effects of dietary protein conditioning on gentamicin pharmacokinetics. J Vet Pharmacol Therap 17:259-264.

Belloli, C., Crescenzo, G., Carli, S., Villa, R., Sonzogni, O., Carelli, G., and Ormas, P. 1996. Pharmacokinetics and dosing regimen of aminosidine in the dog. Vet Res Commun 20:533-541.

Bendirdjian, J.P., Fillastre, J.P., and Foucher, B. 1982. Mitochondria modifications with the aminoglycosides. In A. Whelton and H.C. Neu, eds., The Aminoglycosides: Microbiology, Clinical Use and Toxicology, pp. 325-354. Whelton, A, and Neu, H, eds. New York: Marcel Dekker.

Bennett, W.M., Plamp, C.E., Elliott, W.C., Parker, R.A., and Porter, G.A. 1982. Effect of basic amino acids and aminoglycosides on 3H gentamicin uptake in cortical slices of rat and human kidney. J Lab Clin Med 99:156-162.

Bennett, W.M., Plamp, C.E., Gilbert, D.N., Parker, R.A., and Porter, G.A. 1979. The influence of dosage regimen on experimental gentamicin nephrotoxicity: dissociation of peak serum levels from renal failure. J Infect Dis 140(4):576-580.

Bergeron, M.G., Bastille, A., Lessard, C., and Gagnon, P.M. 1982. Significance of intrarenal concentrations of gentamicin for the outcome of experimental pyelonephritis in rats. J Infect Dis 146:91-96.

Bergeron, M.G., and Bergeron, Y. 1986. Influence of endotoxin on the intrarenal distribution of gentamicin, netilmicin, tobramycin, amikacin, and cephalothin. Antimicrob Agents Chemother 29:7-12.

Bird, J.E., Miller, K.W., Larson, A.A., and Duke, G.E. 1983. Pharmacokinetics of gentamicin in birds of prey. Am J Vet Res 44:1245-1247.

Black, J., Calesnick, B., Williams, D., and Weinstein, M. 1963. Pharmacology of gentamicin, a new broad spectrum antibiotic. Antimicrob Agents Chemother 3:138-147.

Black, W.D., Holt, J.D., and Gentry, R.D. 1983. Pharmacokinetic study of neomycin in calves following intravenous and intramuscular administration. Canad J Comparative Med 47:433-435.

Blantz, R.C. 1980. The glomerulus, passive filter or regulatory organ? Klin Wochenschr 58:957-964.

Blaser, J., Rieder, H., Niederer, P., and Lüthy, R. 1983. Biological variability of multiple dose pharmacokinetics of netilmicin in man. Europ J Clin Pharmacol 24:359-406.

Blaser, J., Simmon, H.P., Gonzenbach, H.R., Sonnabend, W., and Luthy, R. 1985. Aminoglycoside monitoring: timing of peak levels is critical. Therapeutic Drug Monitoring 7:303-307.

Bloomfield, R.B., Brooks, D., and Vulliet, R. 1997. The pharmacokinetics of a single intramuscular dose of amikacin in red-tailed hawks (*Buteo jamaicensis*). J Zoo Wildlife Med 28(1):55-61.

Bowman, K.F., Dix, L.P., Riond, J.-L., and Riviere, J.E. 1986. Prediction of pharmacokinetic profiles of ampicillin sodium, gentamicin sulfate, and combination ampicillin sodium-gentamicin sulfate in serum and synovia of healthy horses. Am J Vet Res 47:1590-1596.

Brown, M.P., Stover, S.M., Kelly, R.H., and Farver, T.B. 1981. Kanamycin sulfate in the horse: serum, synovial fluid, peritoneal fluid, and urine concentrations after single-dose intramuscular administration. Am J Vet Res 42:1823-1825.

Brown, S.A., Coppoc, G.L., and Riviere, J.E. 1986a. Effects of dose and duration of therapy on gentamicin tissue residues in sheep. Am J Vet Res 47:2373-2379.

Brown, S.A., Coppoc, G.L., Riviere, J.E., and Anderson, V.L. 1986b. Dose-dependent pharmacokinetics of gentamicin in sheep. Am J Vet Res 47:789-794.

Brown, S.A., and Garry, F.B. 1988. Comparison of serum and renal gentamicin concentrations and fractional urinary excretion tests as indicators of nephrotoxicity. J Vet Pharmacol Therap 11:330-337.

Brown, S.A., Nelson, R.W., and Scott-Moncrieff, C. 1991. Pharmacokinetics of gentamicin in diabetic dogs. J Vet Pharmacol Therap 14:90-95.

Brown, S.A., and Riviere, J.E. 1991. Comparative pharmacokinetics of aminoglycoside antibiotics. J Vet Pharmacol Therap 14:1-35.

Brown, S.A., Riviere, J.E., Coppoc, G.L., Hinsman, E.J., Carlton, W.W., and Steckel, R.R. 1985. Single intravenous and multiple intramuscular dose pharmacokinetics and tissue residue profile of gentamicin in sheep. Am J Vet Res 47:69-74.

Burrows, G.E. 1979. Gentamicin. JAVMA 175:301-302.

Bush, M., Locke, D., Neal, L.A., and Carpenter, J.W. 1981. Gentamicin tissue concentrations in various avian species following recommended dosage therapy. Am J Vet Res 46:2114-2116.

Busse, H.J., Wostmann, C., and Bakker, E.P. 1992. The bacterial action of streptomycin: Membrane permeabilization caused by the insertion of mistranslated proteins into the cytoplasmic membrane of *Escherichia coli* and subsequent caging of the antibiotic inside the cells due to degradation of these proteins. J Gen Microbiol 138(Pt3):551-561.

Cabana, B.E., and Taggart, J.G. 1973. Comparative pharmacokinetics of BB-K8 and kanamycin in dogs and humans. Antimicrob Agents Chemotherapy 3:478-483.

Caligiuri, R., Kollias, G.V., Jacobson, E., McNab, B., Clark, C.H., and Wilson, R.C. 1990. The effects of ambient temperature on amikacin pharmacokinetics in gopher tortoises. J Vet Pharmacol Therap 13:287-291.

Campbell, B.G., Bartholow, S., and Rosin, E. 1996. Bacterial killing by use of once daily gentamicin dosage in guinea pigs with *Escherichia coli* infection. AJVR 57(11):1627-1630.

Campbell, B.G., and Rosin, E. 1992. Optimal gentamicin dosage regimen in dogs (Abstr). Vet Surgery 21(5):385.

Carbon, C., Contrepois, A., and Lamotte-Barrillon, S. 1978. Comparative distribution of gentamicin, tobramycin, sisomicin, netilmicin, and amikacin in interstitial fluid in rabbits. Antimicrob Agents Chemother 13:368-372.

Carli, S., Montesissa, C., Sonzogni, O., Madonna, M., and Said-Faqi, A. 1990. Comparative pharmacokinetics of amikacin sulphate in calves and sheep. Res Vet Sci 48:231-234.

Chahwala, S.B., and Harpur, E.S. 1982. An investigation of the effects of aminoglycoside antibiotics on Na-K ATPase as a possible mechanism of toxicity. Res Commun Chem Pathol Pharmacol 35:63-78.

Chisholm, G.D., Calnan, J.S., Waterworth, P.M., and Reis, N.D. 1968. Distribution of gentamicin in body fluids. Brit Med J 2:22-24.

Chiu, P.T.S., Brown, A., Miller, G., et al. 1976. Renal extraction gentamicin in anesthetized dogs. Antimicrob Agents Chemother 10:227-282.

Chiu, P.T.S., Miller, G.H., Long, J.F., and Waitz, J.A. 1979. Renal uptake and nephrotoxicity of gentamicin during urinary alkalinization in rats. Clin and Experim Pharmacol and Physiol 6:317-326.

Christensen, S., Ladefoged, K., and Frimodt-Moller, N. 1997. Experience with once daily dosing of gentamicin: considerations regarding dosing and monitoring. Chemotherapy 43:442-450.

Chung, M., Costello, R., and Symchowicz, S. 1980. Comparison of netilmicin and gentamicin pharmacokinetics in humans. Antimicrob Agents Chemother 17:184-187.

Chung, M., Parravicini, L., Assael, B.M., Cavanna, G., Radwanski, E., and Symchowicz, S. 1982. Comparative pharmacokinetics of aminoglycoside antibiotics in guinea pigs. Antimicrob Agents Chemother 10:1017-1021.

Clarke, C.R., Lochner, F.K., and Bellamy, J. 1992. Pharmacokinetics of gentamicin and antipyrine in the horse-effect of advancing age. J Vet Pharmacol Therap 15:309-313.

Clarke, C.R., Short, C.R., Hsu, R.-C., and Baggot, J.D. 1985. Pharmacokinetics of gentamicin in the calf: developmental changes. Am J Vet Res 46:2461-2466.

Cojocel, C., Dociu, N., Malta, K., Sleight, S.D., and Hook, J.B. 1983. Effects of aminoglycosides on glomerular permeability, tubular reabsorption, and intracellular catabolism of the cationic low-molecular weight protein lysozyme. Toxicol Appl Pharmacol 68:96-109.

Cojocel, C., and Hook, J.B. 1983. Aminoglycoside nephrotoxicity. Trends Pharmacol Sci 4:174-179.

Collier, V.U., Lictman, P.S., and Mitch, W.E. 1979. Evidence for luminal uptake of gentamicin in the perfused rat kidney. J Pharmacol Exp Ther 210:247-251.

Conzelman, G.M. 1980. Pharmacotherapeutics of aminoglycoside antibiotics. JAVMA 176:1078-1084.

Cowan, R.H., Jukkola, A.F., and Arant, B.S. 1980. Pathophysiologic evidence of gentamicin nephrotoxicity in neonatal puppies. Pediatric Res 14:1204-1211.

Cronin, R.E. 1979. Aminoglycoside nephrotoxicity, pathogenesis and nephotoxicity. Clin Nephrol 11:251-256.

Cronin, R.E., Bulger, R.E., Southeru, P., and Henrich, W.L. 1980. Natural history of aminoglycoside nephotoxicity in the dog. J Lab Clin Med 95:463-474.

Cronin, R., Nix, K., and Ferguson, E. 1982. Renal cortex ion composition and Na-K ATPase activity in early gentamicin nephrotoxicity. Am J Physiol 242:F477-F483.

Crowell, N.A., Divers, T.J., Byars, T.D., Marshall, A.E., Nusbaum, K.E., and Larsen, L. 1981. Neomycin toxicosis in calves. Am J Vet Res 42:29-34.

Cuppage, F.E., Setter, K., Sullivan, L.P., Reitzes, E.J., and Meinykovych, A.D. 1977. Gentamicin nephrotoxicity 11: Physiological, biochemical and morphological effects of prolonged administration to rats. Virchows Arch B 24:121-138.

Desrochers, C.S., and Schacht, J. 1982. Neomycin concentrations in inner ear tissues and other organs of the guinea pig after chronic drug administration. Acta Otalarygologica 93:233-236.

Drury, A.R. 1952. Evaluation of neomycin sulfate in treatment of bovine mastitis. Vet Med 47:407-411.

Easter, J.L., Hague, B.A., Brumbaugh, G.W., Nguyen, J., Chaffin, M.K., Honnas, C.M., and Kemper, D.L. 1997. Effects of postoperative peritoneal lavage on pharmacokinetics of gentamicin in horses after celiotomy. AJVR 58(10):1166-1170.

Elliott, W.C., Gilbert, D.N., DeFehr, J., Bennett, W.M., and McCarron, D.A. 1982. Protection from experimental gentamicin toxicity by dietary calcium loading. Kidney Int 21:216.

Elsheikh, H.A., Osman, L.A., and Ali, B.H. 1997. Comparative pharmacokinetics of ampicillin trihydrate, gentamicin sulphate and oxytetracycline hydrochloride in Nubian goats and desert sheep. J Vet Pharmacol Therap 20:262-266.

Errecalde, J.O., and Marino, E.L. 1990. A discriminatory study of pharmacokinetic models for intramuscular gentamicin in sheep. Vet Res Commun 14:53-58.

Erskine, J., Wilson, R.C., Riddell, M.G., Tyler, W., and Spears, H.J. 1992. Intramammary administration of gentamicin as treatment for experimentally induced *Escherichia coli* mastitis in cows. Am J Vet Res 53(3):375-381.

Eschbach, J.W., Adamson, J.W., and Dennis, M.B. 1980. Physiologic studies in normal and uremic sheep 1: the experimental model. Kidney Int 18:725-731.

Fabre, J., Rudhardt, M., Blanchard, P., and Regamey, C. 1976. Persistence of sisomicin and gentamicin in renal cortex and medulla compared with other organs and serum of rats. Kidney Int 10:444-449.

Feldman, S., Josepovitz, C., Scott, M., Pastoriza, E., and Kaloyanides, G.J. 1981. Inhibition of gentamicin uptake in rat kidney by polycations. Kidney Int 19:222.

Feldman, S., Wang, M.Y., and Kaloyanides, G.J. 1982. Aminoglycosides induce a phosphaolipidosis in the renal cortex of the rat: an early manifestation of nephrotoxicity. J Pharmacol Exp Ther 220:514-520.

Firth, E.C., Whittem, T., and Nouws, J.F.M. 1993. Kanamycin concentrations in synovial fluid after intramuscular administration in the horse. Aust Vet J 70(9):324-325.

Forsyth, S.F., Ilkiw, J.E., and Hildebrand, S.V. 1990. Effect of gentamicin administration on the neuromuscular blockade induced by atracurium in cats. Am J Vet Res 51(10):1675-1678.

Frazier, D.L., Aucoin, D.P., and Riviere, J.E. 1988. Gentamicin pharmacokinetics and nephrotoxicity in naturally acquired and experimentally induced disease in dogs. JAVMA 192:57-63.

Frazier, D.L., and Riviere, J.E. 1987. Gentamicin dosing strategies for dogs with subclinical renal dysfunction. Antimicrob Agents Chemother 31:1929-1934.

Freeman, C.D., Nicolau, D.P., Belliveau, P.P., and Nightingale, C.H. 1997. Once-daily dosing of aminoglycosides: review and recommendation for clinical practice. J Antimicrob Chemother 39:677-686.

Fuentes, V.O., Gonzalez, H., Sanchez, V., Fuentes, P., and Rosiles, R. 1997. The effect of neomycin on the kidney function of the horse. J Vet Med 44:201-205.

Garg, S.K., and Garg, B.D. 1989. Disposition kinetics and urinary excretion of gentamicin in buffalo bulls (*Bubalus bubalis*). Vet Res Commun 13:331-337.

Garg, S.K., Verma, S.P., and Garg, B.D. 1991a. Disposition kinetics of gentamicin in buffalo calves (*Bubalus bubalis*) following single intravenous administration. J Vet Pharmacol Therap 14:335-340.

———. 1991b. Pharmacokinetics and urinary excretion of gentamicin in *Bubalus bubalis* calves following intramuscular administration. Res Vet Sci 50:102-105.

Garg, S.K., Verma, S.P., and Uppal, R.P. 1995. Pharmacokinetics of gentamicin following single-dose parenteral administration to goats. Br Vet J 151:453-458.

Garry, F., Chew, D.J., Hoffsis, G.F. 1990a. Urinary indices of renal function in sheep with induced aminoglycoside nephrotoxicosis. Am J Vet Res 51(3):420-427.

———. 1990b. Enzymuria as an index of renal damage in sheep with induced aminoglycoside nephrotoxicosis. Am J Vet Res 51(3):428-432.

Gemer, O., Zaltztein, E., and Gorodischer, R. 1983. Absorption of orally administered gentamicin in infants with diarrhea. Pediatric Pharmacol 3:119-123.

Gerber, A.U., Craig, W.A., Brugger, H.-P., Feller, C., Vastola, A.P., and Brandel, J. 1983. Impact of dosing intervals on activity of gentamicin and ticarcillin against *Pseudomonas aeruginosa* in granulocytopenic mice. J Infect Dis 147:910-917.

Gerritsen, M.J., Koopmans, M.J., Dekker, T.C.E.M., De Jong, M.C.M., Moerman, A., and Olyboek, T. 1994. Effective treatment with dihydrostreptomycin of naturally infected cows shedding *Leptospira interrogans* serovar *hardjo* subtype *hardjobovis*. Am J Vet Res 55(3):339-343.

Gilman, J.M., Davis, L.E., Neff-Davis, C.A., Koritz, G.D., and Baker, G.J. 1987. Plasma concentrations of gentamicin after intramuscular or subcutaneous administration to horses. J Vet Pharmacol Therap 10:101-103.

Giroux, D., Sirois, G., and Martineau, G.P. 1995. Gentamicin pharmacokinetics in newborn and 42-day-old male piglets. J Vet Pharmacol Therap 18:407-412.

Godber, L.M., Walker, R.D., Stein, G.E., Hauptman, J.G., and Derksen, F.J. 1995. Pharmacokinetics, nephrotoxicosis, and in vitro antibacterial activity associated with single versus multiple (three times) daily gentamicin treatments in horses. Am J Vet Res 56(5):613-220.

Golenz, M.R., Wilson, W.D., Carlson, G.P., Craychee, T.J., Mihaly, J.E., and Knox, L. 1994. Effect of route of administration and age on the pharmacokinetics of amikacin administered by the intravenous and intraosseous routes to 3- and 5-day-old foals. Eq Vet J 26:367-373.

Gookin, J.L., Riviere, J.E., Gilger, B.C., and Papich, M.G. 1999. Acute renal failure in four cats treated with paromomycin. JAVMA 215:1821-1823.

Grauer, G.F., Greco, D.S., Behrend, E.N., Mani, I., Fettman, M.J., and Allen, T.A. 1995. Estimation of quantitative enzymuria in dogs with gentamicin-induced nephrotoxicosis using urine enzyme/creatinine ratios from spot urine samples. J Vet Int Med 9(5):324-327.

Green, S.L., Conlon, P.D., Mama, K., and Baird, J.D. 1992. Effects of hypoxia and azotaemia on the pharmacokinetics of amikacin in neonatal foals. Equine Vet J 24(6):475-479.

Gronwall, R., Brown, M.P., and Clubb, S. 1989. Pharmacokinetics of amikacin in African grey parrots. Am J Vet Res 50(2):250-252.

Gyselynck, A.M., Forrey, A., and Cutler, R. 1971. Pharmacokinetics of gentamicin distribution and plasma and renal clearance. J Infect Dis 124S:70-76.

Haddad, N.S., Pedersoli, W.M., Ravis, W.R., Fazeli, M.H., and Carson, R.L., Jr. 1985a. Pharmacokinetics of gentamicin at steady-state in ponies: serum, urine, and endometrial concentrations. Am J Vet Res 46:1268-1271.

———. 1985b. Combined pharmacokinetics of gentamicin in pony mares after a single intravenous and intramuscular administration. Am J Vet Res 46:2004-2007.

Haddad, N.S., Ravis, W.R., Pedersoli, W.M., and Carson, R.L., Jr. 1986. Pharmacokinetics of single doses of gentamicin given by intravenous and intramuscular routes to lactating cows. Am J Vet Res 47:808-813.

———. 1987. Pharmacokinetics and residues of gentamicin in lactating cows after multiple intramuscular doses are administered. Am J Vet Res 48:21-27.

Hadi, A.A., Wasfi, I.A., Gadir, F.A., Amir, M.H., Bashir, A.K., and Baggot, J.D. 1994. Pharmacokinetics of tobramycin in the camel. J Vet Pharmacol Therap 17:48-51.

Hammond, P.B. 1953. Dihydrostreptomycin dose-serum level relationships in cattle. JAVMA 122:203-206.

Hauser, G., and Eichberg, J. 1973. Improved conditions for the preservation and extraction of polyphosphoinositides. Biochimica et Biophysiologica Acta 326:201-209.

Holohan, P.D., Elliot, W.C., Grace, E., and Ross, C.R. 1987. Effect of parathyroid hormone on gentamicin plasma membrane binding and tissue accumulation. J Pharmacol Exp Therap 243:893-986.

Horspool, L.J.I., Taylor, D.J., and Mckellar, Q.A. 1994. Plasma disposition of amikacin and interactions with gastrointestinal microflora in Equidae following intravenous and oral administration. J Vet Pharmacol Therap 17:291-298.

Hottendorf, G.H., and Gordon, L.L. 1980. Comparative low-dose nephrotoxicities of gentamicin, tobramycin, and amikacin. Antimicrob Agents Chemother 18:176-181.

Hsu, C.H., Kurtz, T.W., and Weller, J.M. 1977. In vitro uptake of gentamicin by rat renal cortical tissue. Antimicrob Agents Chemother 19:192-194.

Huang, S.M., Huang, Y.C., and Chiou, W.L. 1979. Triexponential disposition pharmacokinetics of gentamicin in rabbits. Res Commun in Chem Pathol and Pharmacol 26:115-127.

Huber, W.G. 1982. Aminoglycosides, macrolides, lincosamides, polymyxins, chloramphenicol, and antibacterial drugs. In N.H. Booth and L.E. McDonald, eds., Veterinary Pharmacology and Therapeutics, 5th ed., pp. 748-756. Ames: Iowa State Univ Press.

Hull, J.H., Hak, L.J., Koch, G.G., Wargin, W.A., Chi, S.L., and Mattocks, AM. 1981. Influence of range of renal function and liver disease on the predictability of creatinine clearance. Clin Pharmacol Ther 29:516-521.

Humes, H.D., and Weinberg, J.M. 1980. Importance of membrane bound calcium on the hydroosmotic water flow response of ADH in toad urinary bladder. Clin Res 28:449.

Humes, H.D., Weinberg, J.M., and Knauss, T.C. 1982. Clinical and pathophysiologic aspects of aminoglycoside nephrotoxicity. Am J Kidney Dis 2:5-29.

Hunter, R.P., Brown, S.A., Rollins, J.K., and Nelligan, D.F. 1991. The effects of experimentally induced bronchopneumonia on the pharmacokinetics and tissue depletion of gentamicin in healthy and pneumonic calves. J Vet Pharmacol and Therap 14:276-292.

Itoh, N., and Okada, H. 1993. Pharmacokinetics and potential use of gentamicin in budgerigars (*Melopsittacus undulatus*). J Vet Med 40:194-199.

Jawetz, E. 1984. Aminoglycosides and polymyxins. In B.G. Katzung, ed., Basic and Clinical Pharmacology, 2nd ed., pp. 538-545. Los Altos, CA: Lange Medical Publications.

Jernigan, A.D., Hatch, R.C., Brown, J., and Crowell, W.A. 1988a. Pharmacokinetic and pathological evaluation of gentamicin in cats given a small intravenous dose repeatedly for five days. Can J Vet Res 52:177-180.

Jernigan, A.D., Hatch, R.C., and Wilson, R.C. 1988b. Pharmacokinetics of tobramycin in cats. Am J Vet Res 49:608-612.

Jernigan, A.D., Hatch, R.C., Wilson, R.C., Brown, J., and Tulelr, S.M. 1988c. Pharmacokinetics of gentamicin in cats given *Escherichia coli* endotoxin. Am J Vet Res 49:603-607.

Jernigan, A.D., Wilson, R.C., and Hatch, R.C. 1988d. Pharmacokinetics of amikacin in cats. Am J Vet Res 49:355-358.

Jernigan, A.D., Wilson, R.C., Hatch, R.C., and Kemp, D.T. 1988e. Pharmacokinetics of gentamicin after intravenous, intramuscular, and subcutaneous administration in cats. Am J Vet Res 49:32-35.

Johnson, J.G., and Hardin, T.C. 1992. Aminoglycosides, imipenem, and aztreonam. Clinics in Podiatric Medicine and Surgery 9(2):443-464.

Johnson, J.H., Wolf, A.M., Johnson, T.L., and Jensen, J. 1993. Gentamicin toxicosis in a North American cougar. JAVMA 203(6):854-856.

Jones, G.F., and Ward, G.E. 1990. Evaluation of systemic administration of gentamicin for treatment of coliform mastitis in cows. JAVMA 197(6):731-735.

Josepovitz, C., Levine, R., Farraggulla, T., Lane, B., and Kaloyanides, G.J. 1985. [3H]netilmicin binding constants and phospholipid composition of renal plasma membranes of normal and diabetic rats. J Pharmacol Exp Therapeutics 233:298-303.

Josepovitz, C., Pastoriza-Munoz, E., Timmerman, D., Scott, M., Feldman, S., and Kaloyanides, G.J. 1982. Inhibition of gentamicin uptake in rat renal cortex in vivo by aminoglycosides and organic polycations. J Pharmacol Exp Therapeutics 223:314-321.

Just, M., and Habermann, E. 1977. The renal handling of polybasic drugs II: in vitro studies with brush border and lysosomal preparations. Naunyn Schmiedebergs Arch Pharmacol 300:67-76.

Kaloyanides, G.J., and Pastoriza-Munoz, E. 1980. Aminoglycoside nephrotoxicity. Kidney Int 18:571-582.

Karachalios, G.N., Houpas, P., Tziviskou, E., Papalimneou, V., Georgiou, A., Karachaliou, I., and Halkiadake, D. 1998. Prospective randomized study of once-daily versus twice-daily amikacin regimens in patients with systemic infections. Internat J Clin Pharmacol Therap 36(10):561-564.

Katzung, B.G. 1984. Introduction. In B.G. Katzung, ed., Basic and Clinical Pharmacology, 2d ed., p. 2. Los Altos, CA: Lange Medical Publications.

Kaye, D., Levison, M.E., and Labovitz, E.D. 1974. The unpredictability of serum concentrations of gentamicin: pharmacokinetics of gentamicin in patients with nomal and abnormal renal function. J Infect Dis 130:150-154.

Kluwe, W.M., and Hook, J.B. 1978a. Analysis of gentamicin uptake by rat renal cortical slices. Toxicol Appl Pharmacol 45:531-539.

———. 1978b. Functional nephrotoxicity of gentamicin in the rat. Toxicol Appl Pharmacol 45:163-175.

Knauss, T.C., Weinberg, J.M., and Humes, U.D. 1983. Alterations in renal cortical phospholipid content induced by gentamicin, time course, specificity, and subcellular localization. Am J Physiol 244F:535-536.

Kuhar, M.J., Mak, L.I., and Lietman, P.S. 1979. Autoradiographic localization of 3H gentamicin in the proximal renal tubules of mice. Antimicrob Agents Chemother 15:131-133.

Kunin, C.M. 1970. Binding of antibiotics to tissue homogenates. J Infect Dis 121:55-64.

Lancini, G., and Parenti, F., eds. 1982. Antibiotics: An Integrated View, pp. 169-196. New York: Marcel Dekker.

Lashev, L.D., and Mihailov, R. 1994. Pharmacokinetics of apramycin in Japanese quails. J Vet Pharmacol Therap 17:394-395.

Lashev, L.D., Pashov, D.A., and Marinkov, T.N. 1992. Interspecies differences in the pharmacokinetics of kanamycin and apramycin. Vet Res Commun 16:293-300.

Laurent, G., Carlier, M.B., Rollman, B., Van Hoof, F., and Tulkens, P. 1982. Mechanisms of aminoglycoside-induced lysosomal phospholipidosis, in vitro and in vivo studies with gentamicin and amikacin. Biochem Pharmacol 31:3861-3870.

LeCompte, J., Dumont, L., DuSouich, P., and LeLorier, J. 1981. Effect of water deprivation and rehydration on gentamicin disposition in the rat. J Pharmacol Exp Therapeutics 218:231-236.

Lee, M.G., Chen, M.-L., Huang, S.-M., and Chiou, W.L. 1981. Pharmacokinetics of drugs in blood I: unusual distribution of gentamicin. Biopharmaceutics and Drug Disposition 2:89-97.

Leitner, F., and Price, K.E. 1982. Aminoglycosides under development. In A. Whelton and H.C. Neu, eds., The Aminoglycosides: Microbiology, Clinical Use and Toxicology, pp. 29-64. New York: Marcel Dekker.

Lelievre-Pegorier, M., Sagly, R., Meulemans, A., and Merlet-Benichou, C. 1985. Kinetics of gentamicin in plasma of nonpregnant, pregnant, and fetal guinea pigs and its distribution in fetal tissues. Antimicrob Agents Chemother 28:565-569.

Ling, G.V., Conzelman, G.M., Franti, C.E., and Ruby, A.L. 1981. Urine concentrations of gentamicin, tobramycin, amikacin, and kanamycin after subcutaneous administration to healthy dogs. Am J Vet Res 42:1792-1974.

Ling, G.V., and Ruby, A.L. 1979. Gentamicin for treatment of resistant urinary tract infections in dogs. JAVMA 175:480-481.

Lipsky, J.J., Cheng, L., Sacktor, B., and Lietman, P.S. 1980. Gentamicin uptake by renal tubule brush border membrane vesicles. J Pharmacol Exp Ther 215:390-393.

Lipsky, J.J., and Lietman, P.S. 1980. Neomycin inhibition of adenosine triphosphatase, evidence for a neomycin-phospholipid interaction. Antimicrob Agents Chemother 18:532-535.

———. 1982. Aminoglycoside inhibition of a renal phosphatidylinositol phospholipase C. J Pharmacol Exp Ther 220:287-292.

Luft, F.C., Bloch, R., Sloan, R.S., Yum, M.N., Costello, R., and Maxwell, D.R. 1978. Comparative nephrotoxicity of aminoglycoside antibiotics in rats. J Infect Dis 138:541-545.

Luft, F.C., and Evan, A.P. 1980a. Comparative effects of tobramycin and gentamicin on glomerular ultrastructure. J Infect Dis 142:910-914.

———. 1980b. Glomerular filtration barrier in aminoglycoside induced nephrotoxic acute renal failure. Renal Physiol 3:265-271.

Luft, F.C., and Kleit, S.A. 1974. Renal parenchymal accumulation of aminoglycoside antibiotics in rats. J Infect Dis 130:656-659.

Luft, F.C., Patel, V., Yum, M.N., Patel, B., and Kleit, S.A. 1975. Experimental aminoglycoside nephrotoxicity. J Lab Clin Med 86:213-220.

Lullmann, H., and Vollmer, B. 1982. An interaction of aminoglycoside antibiotics with Ca binding to lipid monolayers and to biomembranes. Biochem Pharmacol 31:3769-3773.

Mader, D.R., Conzelman, G.M., Jr, and Baggot, J.D. 1985. Effects of ambient temperature on the half-life and dosage regimen of amikacin in the gopher snake. JAVMA 187:1134-1136.

Magdesian, K.G., Hogan, P.M., Cohen, N.D., Brumbaugh, G.W., and Bernard, W.V. 1998. Pharmacokinetics of a high dose of gentamicin administered intravenously or intramuscularly to horses. J Am Vet Med Assoc 213(7):1007-1011.

Mann, H.J., Fuhs, D.W., Awang, R., Ndemo, F.A., and Cerra, F.B. 1987. Altered aminoglycoside pharmacokinetics in critically ill patients with sepsis. Clin Pharmacol 6:148-153.

Martin, T., Papich, M., and Riviere, J.E. 1998. Population pharmacokinetics of gentamicin in horses. Am J Vet Res 59:1589-1598.

Martin, T., and Riviere, J.E. 1998. Population pharmacokinetics in veterinary medicine: potential uses for therapeutic drug monitoring and prediction of tissue residues. J Vet Pharmacol Therap 21:167-189.

Mazze, R.I. 1981. Methoxyflurane nephropathy. In J.B. Hook, ed., Toxicology of the Kidney, pp. 135-149. New York: Raven Press.

McNeil, J.S., Jackson, B., Nelson, L., and Butkas, D.E. 1983. The role of prostaglandins in gentamicin induced nephrotoxicity in the dog. Nephron 33:202-207.

Mealey, K.L., and Boothe, D.M. 1994. Nephrotoxicosis associated with topical administration of gentamicin in a cat. JAVMA 204(12):1919-1921.

Meisner, H. 1981. Effect of gentamicin on the subcellular distribution of renal beta-*N*-acetylglucosaminidase activity. Biochem Pharmacol 30:2949-2952.

Mercer, H.D., Rollins, K.D., Garth, M.A., and Carter, G.C. 1971. A residue study and comparison of penicillin and dihydrostreptomycin concentration in cattle. JAVMA 158:776-779.

Miller, S.M., Matthews, N.S., Mealey, K.L., Taylor, T.S., and Brumbaugh, G.W. 1994. Pharmacokinetics of gentamicin in mammoth asses. J Vet Pharmacol Therap 17:403-406.

Miranda, J.C., Schimmel, M.S., Mimms, G.M., et al. 1984. Gentamicin absorption during prophylactic use for necrotizing enterocolitis. Development Pharmacol and Therapeut 7:303-306.

Mitchell, C.J., Bullock, S., and Ross, B.D. 1977. Renal handling of gentamicin and other antibiotics by the isolated perfused rat kidney, mechanisms of nephrotoxicity. J Antimicrob Chemother 3:593-600.

Morin, J.P., Viotte, G., Vandewalle, A., Van Hoof, F., Tulkens, P., and Fillastre, J.P. 1980. Gentamicin-induced nephrotoxicity, a cell biology approach. Kidney Int 18:583-590.

Morin, J.P., Viotte, G., Van Hoof, F., Tulkens, P., Godin, M., and Fillastre, J.P. 1981. Functional, biochemical and morphological events related to gentamicin therapy in rats. Drugs Exp Clin Res 7:345-348.

Nagabhusban, T.L., Miller, G.H., and Weinstein, M.J. 1982. Structure-activity relationships in aminoglycoside-aminocyclitol antibiotics. In A. Whelton and H.C. Neu, eds., The Aminoglycosides: Microbiology, Clinical Use and Toxicology, pp. 3-27. New York: Marcel Dekker.

Nostrandt, A.C., Pedersoli, W.M., Marshall, A.E., Ravis, W.R., and Robertson, B.T. 1991. Ototoxic potential of gentamicin in ponies. Am J Vet Res 52(3):494-498.

Nouws, J.F.M., and Ziv, G. 1978. Tissue distribution and residues of benzylpenicillin and aminoglycoside antibiotics in emergency-slaughtered ruminants. Tijdschrift voor Diergeneeskunde 102:140-151.

Ogden, L., Wilson, R.C., Clark, C.H., and Colby, E.D. 1995. Pharmacokinetics of gentamicin in rabbits. J Vet Pharmacol Therap 18:156-159.

Orsini, J.A., Park, M.I., and Spencer, P.A. 1996. Tissue and serum concentrations of amikacin after intramuscular and intrauterine administration to mares in estrus. Can Vet J (37):157-160.

Orsini, J.A., Soma, L.R., Rourke, J.E., and Park, M. 1985. Pharmacokinetics of amikacin in the horse following intravenous and intramuscular administration. J Vet Pharmacol Therap 8:194-201.

Oukessou, M., and Toutain, P.L. 1992. Effect of dietary nitrogen intake on gentamicin disposition in sheep. J Vet Pharmacol Therap 15:416-420.

Pastoriza-Munoz, E., Bowman, R.L., and Kaloyanides, G.J. 1979. Renal tubular transport of gentamicin in the rat. Kidney Int 16:440-450.

Pastoriza-Munoz, E., Josepovitz, C., Ramsammy L., and Kaloyanides, G.J. 1987. Renal handling of netilmicin in the rat with streptozotocin-induced diabetes mellitus. J Pharmacol Exp Therap 241:166-173.

Pattyn, V.M., Verpooten, G.A., Guiliano, R.A., Aheng, F., and DeBroe, M.E. 1988. Effect of hyperfiltration, proteinuria and diabetes mellitus on the uptake kinetics of gentamicin in the kidney cortex of rats. J Pharmacol Exp Therap 244:694-698.

Pechere, J.C., and Dugal, R.D. 1979. Clinical pharmacokinetics of aminoglycoside antibiotics. Clin Pharmacokinet 4:170-199.

Pedersoli, W.M., Belmonte, A.A., Purohit, R.C., and Ravis, W.R. 1980. Pharmacokinetics of gentamicin in the horse. Am J Vet Res 41:351-354.

Pedersoli, W.M., Fazeli, M.H., Haddad, N.S., Ravis, W.R., and Carson, R.L., Jr. 1985. Endometrial and serum gentamicin concentrations in pony mares given repeated intrauterine infusions. Am J Vet Res 46:1025-1028.

Pedersoli, W.M., Jackson, J., and Frobish, R.A. 1995. Depletion of gentamicin in the milk of Holstein cows after single and repeated intramammary and parenteral treatments. J Vet Pharmacol Therap 18:457-463.

Pedersoli, W.M., Ravis, W.R., Askins, D.R., et al. 1990. Pharmacokinetics of single-dose intravenous and intramuscular administration of gentamicin in roosters. Am J Vet Res 51:286-289.

Pedersoli, W.M., Ravis, W.R., Askins, D.R., Krista, L.M., Spano, J.S., Whitesides, J.F., and Tolbert, D.S. 1989. Pharmacokinetics of single doses of gentamicin given intravenously and intramuscularly to turkeys. J Vet Pharmacol Therap 12:124-132.

Pedersoli, W.M., Ravis, W.R., Jackson, J., and Shaikh, B. 1994. Disposition and bioavailability of neomycin in Holstein calves. J Vet Pharmacol Therap 17:5-11.

Pennington, J.E., Dale, D.C., Reynolds, H.Y., and MacLowry, J.D. 1975. Gentamicin sulfate pharmacokinetics: lower levels of gentamicin in blood during fever. J Infect Dis 132:270-275.

Pickerell, J.A., Oehme, F.W., and Cash, W.C. 1993. Ototoxicity in dogs and cats. Sem Vet Med Surg (Small Animal) 8(1):42-49.

Poli, A., Sozzi, S., Guidi, G., Bandinelli, and Mancianti, F. 1997. Comparison of aminosidine (paromomycin) and sodium stibogluconate for treatment of canine leishmaniasis. Vet Parasitol 71:263-271.

Powell, S., Thompson, W.L., Luthe, M.A., Stern, R.C., Grossniklaus, D.A., Bloxham, D.D., Groden, D.L., et al. 1983. Once-daily vs. continuous aminoglycoside dosing, efficacy, and toxicity in animal and clinical studies of gentamicin, netilmicin and tobramycin. J Infect Dis 147:918-932.

Prescott, J.F., and Baggot, J.D. 1988. Antimicrobial Therapy in Veterinary Medicine. Boston: Blackwell Scientific Publications.

Ramsammy, L.S., Josepovitz, C., Jones, D., Ling, K.-Y., Lane, B.P., and Kaloyanides, G.J. 1987. Induction of nephrotoxicity by high doses of gentamicin in diabetic rats. Proc Soc Exper and Biol Med 186:306-312.

Ramsay, E.C., and Vulliet, R. 1993. Pharmacokinetic properties of gentamicin and amikacin in the cockatiel. Avian Dis 37:628-634.

Riond, J.-L., Dix, L.P., and Riviere, J.E. 1986. Influence of thyroid function on the pharmacokinetics of gentamicin in pigs. Am J Vet Res 47:2142-2146.

Riond, J.-L., and Riviere, J.E. 1988. Multiple intravenous dose pharmacokinetics and residue depletion profile of gentamicin in pigs. J Vet Pharmacol Therap 11:210-214.

Ristuccia, A.M. 1984. Aminoglycosides. In A.M. Ristuccia and B.A. Cunha, eds., Antimicrobial Therapy, pp. 305-328. New York: Raven Press.

Rivers, B.J., Walter, P.A., O'Brien, T.D., King, V.L., and Polzin, D.J. 1996. Evaluation of urine gamma-glutamyl transpeptidase-to-creatinine ratio as a diagnostic tool in an experimental model of aminoglycoside-induced acute renal failure in the dog. J Am Animal Hosp Assn 32:323-336.

Riviere, J.E. 1982. The Aminoglycosides. In The Bristol Veterinary Handbook of Antimicrobial Therapy, 186-189. Johnston, DE, ed. Syracuse: Veterinary Learning Systems.

———. 1985. Aminoglycoside-induced toxic nephropathy. In S.R. Ash and S.A. Thornhill, eds., CRC Handbook of Animal Models of Renal Failure, pp. 145-182. Boca Raton, FL: CRC Press.

Riviere, J.E., and Carver, M.P. 1984. Effects of familial hypothyroidism and subtotal nephrectomy on gentamicin pharmacokinetics in Beagle dogs. Chemotherapy 30:216-220.

Riviere, J.E., and Coppoc, G.L. 1981a. Pharmacokinetics of gentamicin in the juvenile dog. Am J Vet Res 42:1621-1623.

———. 1981b. Determination of cerebrospinal fluid gentamicin in the Beagle using an indwelling cerebral ventricular cannula. Chemotherapy 27:309-312.

Riviere, J.E., Coppoc, G.L., Hinsman, E.J., Carlton, W.W., and Traver, D.S. 1983. Species-dependent gentamicin pharmacokinetics and nephrotoxicity in the young horse. Fundamental and Applied Toxicology 3:448-457.

Riviere, J.E., Craigmill, A.L., and Sundlof, S.F. 1990. Handbook of Comparative Pharmacokinetics and Tissue Residues of Veterinary Antimicrobial Drugs. Boca Raton, FL: CRC Press.

Riviere, J.E., Hinsman, E.J., Coppoc, G.L., and Carlton, W.W. 1981a. Single dose gentamicin nephrotoxicity in the dog: Early functional and ultrastructural changes. Res Commun Chem Pathol Pharmacol 33:403-418.

Riviere, J.E., Martin, T., Sundlof, S., and Craigmill, A.L. 1997. Interspecies allometric analysis of the comparative pharmacokinetics of 44 drugs across veterinary and laboratory species. J Vet Pharmacol Therap 20:453-463.

Riviere, J.E., Silver, G.R., Coppoc, G.L., and Richardson, R.C. 1981b. Gentamicin aerosol therapy in 18 dogs: failure to induce detectable serum concentrations of the drug. JAVMA 179:166-168.

Riviere, J.E., Traver, D.S., and Coppoc, G.L. 1982. Gentamicin toxic nephropathy in horses with disseminated bacterial infection. JAVMA 180:648-651.

Rodvold, K.A., Danziger, L.H., and Quinn, J.P. 1997. Single daily doses of aminoglycosides. Lancet 350:1412.

Rolf, L.L., Setzer, M.D., and Walker, J.L. 1986. Pharmacokinetics and tissue residues in channel catfish, *Ictalurus pluctatus,* given intracardiac and intramuscular injections of gentamicin sulfate. Veterinary and Human Toxicology 28(Suppl 1):25-30.

Rollins, L.D., Teske, R.H., Condon, R.J., and Carter, G.G. 1972. Serum penicillin and dihydrostreptomycin concentrations in horses after intramuscular administration of selected preparations containing those antibiotics. JAVMA 161:490-493.

Ross, L.A., and Finco, D.R. 1981. Relationship of selected clinical renal function tests to glomerular filtration rate and renal blood flow in cats. Am J Vet Res 42:1704-1710.

Ross, M., Parker, R.A., and Elliot, W.C. 1980. Gentamicin induced resistance to ADH stimulated water flow in the toad bladder explained by drug induced pH changes. Clin Res 28:46-64.

Rossier, Y., Divers, T.J., and Sweeney, R.W.W. 1995. Variations in urinary gamma glutamyl transferase/urinary creatinine ratio in horses with or without pleuropneumonia treated with gentamicin. Equine Vet J 27(3):217-220.

Ryden, R., and Moore, B.J. 1977. The in vitro activity of apramycin, a new aminocyclitol antibiotic. J Antimicrob Chemother 3:609-613.

Salazar, D.E., Schentag, J.J., and Corcoran, G.B. 1992. Obesity as a risk factor in drug-induced organ injury: toxicokinetics of gentamicin in the obese overfed rat. Drug Metabol Disposition 20(3):402-406.

Sande, M.A., and Mandell, G.L. 1985. Antimicrobial agents: the aminoglycosides. In A.G. Gilman, L.S. Goodman, T.W. Rall, and F. Murad, eds., The Pharmacological Basis of Therapeutics, 7th ed., pp. 1157-1169. New York: Macmillan.

Sastrasinh, M., Knauss, T.C., Weinberg, J.M., and Humes, H.D. 1982a. Identification of the aminoglycoside binding site in rat renal brush border membranes. J Pharmacol Exp Therap 222:350-355.

Sastrasinh, M., Weinberg, J.M., and Humes, H.D. 1982b. Effect of gentamicin on calcium uptake by renal mitochondria. Life Sci 26:2309-2315.

Sawchuk, R.J., Zaske, D.E., Cipolle, R.J., Wargin, W.A., and Strate, R.G. 1977. Kinetic model for gentamicin dosing with the use of the individual patient parameters. Clin Pharmacol and Therapeut 21:362-369.

Schacht, J. 1978. Purification of polyphosphoinositides by chromatography on immobilized neomycin. J Lipid Res 19:1063-1067.

———. 1979. Isolation of an aminoglycoside receptor from guinea pig inner ear tissues and kidney. Arch Otorhinolarynol 224:129-134.

Schentag, J.J., and Jusko, W.J. 1977. Renal clearance and tissue accumulation of gentamicin. Clinical Pharmacology and Therapeutics 22:364-370.

Schentag, J.J., Jusko, W.J., Plaut, M.E., Cumbo, T.J., Vance, J.W., and Abrutyn, E. 1977a. Tissue persistence of gentamicin in man. JAVMA 238:327-329.

Schentag, J.J., Jusko, W.J., Vance, J.W., et al. 1977b. Gentamicin disposition and tissue accumulation on multiple dosing. J Pharmacokinetics and Biopharmaceutics 5:559-579.

Schentag, J.J., Lasezkay, G., Cumbo, T.J., Plaut, M.E., and Jusko, W.J. 1978. Accumulation pharmacokinetics of tobramicin. Antimicrob Agents Chemother 13:649-656.

Schumacher, J., Wilson, R.C., Spano, J.S., Hammond, L.S., McGuire, J., Duran, S.H., Kemppainene, R.J., and Hughes, F.E. 1991. Effect of diet on gentamicin-induced nephrotoxicosis in horses. Am J Vet Res 52(8):1274-1278.

Senckjian, H.O., Knight, T.F., and Weinman, E.J. 1981. Micropuncture study of the handling of gentamicin by the rat kidney. Kidney Int 19:416-423.

Setzer, M.D. 1985. Pharmacokinetics of gentamicin in channel fish (*Ictalurus punctatus*). Am J Vet Res 46:2558-2561.

Sheth, A.V., Senckjian, H.O., Babino, H., Knight, T.F., and Weinman, E.J. 1981. Renal handling of gentamicin by the Munich-Wistar rat. Am J Physiol 241F:645-648.

Shille, V.M., Brown, M.P., Gronwall, R., and Hock, H. 1985. Amikacin sulfate in the cat: serum, urine, and uterine tissue concentrations. Theriogenology 23:829-839.

Short, C.R., Hardy, M.L., Clarke, C.R., Taylor, W., and Baggot, J.D. 1986. The nephrotoxic potential of gentamicin in the cat: a pharmacokinetic and histopathologic investigation. J Vet Pharmacol Therap 9:325-329.

Siddique, I.H., Loken, K.I., and Hoyt, H.H. 1965. Concentrations of neomycin, dihydrostreptomycin and polymyxin in milk after intramuscular or intramammary administration. JAVMA 146:594-599.

Silverblatt, F.J. 1982. Autoradiographic studies of intracellular aminoglycoside disposition in the kidney. In A. Whelton and H.C. Neu, eds., The Aminoglycosides: Microbiology, Clinical Use, and Toxicology, pp. 223-233. New York: Marcel Dekker.

Silverblatt, F.J., and Kuehn, C. 1979. Autoradiography of gentamicin uptake by the rat proximal tubule cell. Kidney Int 15:335-345.

Silverman, M., and Mahon, W. 1979. Gentamicin interaction in vivo with luminal and antiluminal nephron surfaces of dog kidney. Abstracts-Am Soc Nephrol 12:89A.

Simmons, C.F., Jr, Bogusky, R.T., and Humes, H.D. 1980. Inhibitory effects of gentamicin on renal mitochondria oxidative phosphorylation. J Pharmacol Exp Ther 214:709-715.

Sketris, I., Lesar, T., Zaske, D.E., and Cipolle, R.J. 1981. Effect of obesity on gentamicin pharmacokinetics. J Clin Pharmacol 21:288-293.

Smeltzer, B.D., Schwartzman, M.S., and Bertino, J.S., Jr. 1988. Amikacin pharmacokinetics during continuous peritoneal dialysis. Antimicrob Agents Chemother 32:236-240.

Sojka, J.E., and Brown, S.A. 1986. Pharmacokinetic adjustment of gentamicin dosing in horses with sepsis. JAVMA 189:784-789.

Souliere, C.R., Goodman, D.B.P., and Appel, G.B. 1978. Gentamicin selectively inhibits antidiuretic hormone induced water flow in the toad urinary bladder. Kidney Int 14:733.

Strain, G.M., Merchant, S.R., Neer, T.M., and Tedford, B.L. 1995. Ototoxicity assessment of a gentamicin sulfate otic preparation in dogs. Am J Vet Res 56(4):532-538.

Strausbaugh, L.J., and Brinker, G.S. 1983. Effect of osmotic blood-brain disruption on gentamicin penetration into the cerebrospinal fluid and brain of normal rats. Antimicrob Agents Chemother 24:147-150.

Sveska, K.J., Roffe, B.D., Solomon, D.K., and Hoffmann, R.P. 1985. Outcome of patients treated by an aminoglycoside pharmacokinetic dosing service. Am J Hospital Pharmacy 42:2472-2478.

Swann, J.D., Ulrich, R., and Acosta, D. 1990. Lack of changes in cytosolic ionized calcium in primary cultures of rat kidney cortical cells exposed to cytotoxic concentrations of gentamicin. Toxicol Appl Pharmacol 106:38-47.

Sweeney, R.W., Divers, T.J., and Rossier, Y. 1992. Disposition of gentamicin administered intravenously to horses with sepsis. JAVMA 200(4):503-506.

Takahashi, Y., Kido, Y., Naoi, M., and Kokue, E.-I. 1985. The serial biopsy technique for estimation of drug residue in calf kidney using gentamicin as a model drug. Jap J Vet Sci 47:179-183.

Teixeira, R.B., Kelley, J., Alpert, H., Pardo, V., and Vaamonde, C.A. 1982. Complete protection from gentamicin-induced acute renal failure in the diabetes mellitus rat. Kidney Int 21:600-612.

Tobin, T. 1979. Pharmacology review: streptomycin, gentamicin and the aminoglycoside antibiotics. J Equine Med Surg 4:206-212.

Tointon, M.M., Job, M.L., Pletier, T.T., Murphy, J.E., and Ward, E.S. 1987. Alterations in aminoglycoside volume of distribution in patients below ideal body weight. Clin Pharmacy 6:160-162.

Trnovec, T., Bezek, S., Kállay, Z., Durisová, M., and Navarová, J. 1984. Non-linear accumulation of gentamicin in guinea-pig kidney. J Animicrob Ther 14:543-548.

Tulkens, P., and Trouet, A. 1978. The uptake and intracellular accumulation of aminoglycoside antibiotics in lysosomes of cultured rat fibroblasts. Biochem Pharmacol 27:415-424.

Vaamonde, C.A., Bier, R.T., Guovea, W., Alpert, H., Kelley, J., and Pardo, V. 1984. Effect of duration of diabetes on the protection observed in the diabetic rat against gentamicin-induced acute renal failure. Mineral and Electrolyte Metab 10:209-216.

Vandewalle, A., Farman, N., Morin, J.P., Fillastre, J.P., Liatt, P.Y., and Bonvalet, J.P. 1981. Gentamicin incorporation along the nephron, autoradiographic study on isolated tubules. Kidney Int 19:529-539.

Waitz, J.A., Moss, E.L., and Weinstein, M.J. 1971. Aspects of the chronic toxicity of gentamicin sulfate in cats. J Infect Dis 124S:125-129.

Weinberg, J.M., Harding, P.G., and Humes, H.D. 1980. Mechanisms of gentamicin induced dysfunction of renal cortical mitochrondria II: effects on mitochondrial monovalent cation transport. Arch Biochem Biophys 205:232-239.

Weinberg, J.M., and Humes, B.D. 1980. Mechanisms of gentamicin induced dysfunction of renal cortical mitochondria I: effects on mitochondrial respiration. Arch Biochem Biophys 205:222-231.

Weinberg, J.M., Simmons, C.F., Jr, and Humes, H.D. 1990. Alterations of mitochondrial respiration induced by aminoglycoside antibiotics. Res Commun Chem Pathol Pharmacol 27:521-531.

Weisman, D., Herrig, J., and McWeeny, O. 1982. Tissue distribution of gentamicin in lambs: effect of postnatal age and acute hapoxemia. Develop Pharmacol and Therapeut 5:194-206.

Welles, J.S., Emmerson, J.L., Gibson, W.R., Nickander, R., Owen, N.V., and Anderson, R.C. 1973. Preclinical toxicology studies with tobramycin. Toxicol Appl Pharmacol 25:398-409.

Whitehair, K.J., Blevins, T.L., Fessler, J.F., Van Sickle, D.C., White, M.R., and Bill, R.P. 1992a. Regional perfusion of the equine carpus for antibiotic delivery. Vet Surg 21(4):279-285.

Whitehair, K.J., Bowersock, T.L., Blevins, W.E., Fessler, J.F., White, M.R., and Van Sickle, D.C. 1992b. Regional limb perfusion for antibiotic treatment of experimentally induced septic arthritis. Vet Surg 21(5):367-373.

Wichtel, M.G., Breuhaus, B.A., and Aucoin, D. 1992. Relation between pharmacokinetics of amikacin sulfate and sepsis score in clinically normal and hospitalized neonatal foals. JAVMA 200(9):1339-1343.

Williams, P.D., Holohan, P.D., and Ross, C.R. 1981a. Gentamicin nephrotoxicity I: acute biochemical correlates in rats. Toxicol Appl Pharmacol 61:234-242.

———. 1981b. Gentamicin nephrotoxicity II: plasma membrane changes. Toxicol Appl Pharmacol 61:243-251.

Williams, P.D., and Hottendorf, G.H. 1985. Inhibition of renal membrane binding and nephrotoxicity of gentamicin by polysaparagine and polyaspartic acid in the rat. Res Communic in Chem Pathol and Pharmacol 47:317-320.

———. 1986. [3H]Gentamicin uptake in brush border and basolateral membrane vesicles from rat kidney cortex. Biochem Pharmacol 35:2253-2256.

Wilson, R.C., Duran, S.H., Horton, C.R., Jr, and Wright, L.C. 1989. Bioavailability of gentamicin in dogs after intramuscular or subcutaneous injections. Am J Vet Res 50:1748-1750.

Wilson, R.C., Goetsch, D.D., and Huber, T.L. 1984. Influence of endotoxin-induced fever on the pharmacokinetics of gentamicin in ewes. Am J Vet Res 45:2495-2497.

Wilson, R.C., Moore, J.N., and Eakle, N. 1983. Gentamicin pharmacokinetics in horses given small doses of *Escherichia coli* endotoxin. Am J Vet Res 44:1746-1749.

Wilson, R.C., Whelan, S.C., Coulter, D.B., Mahaffey, E.A., Mahaffey, M.B., and Huber, T.L. 1981. Kinetics of gentamicin after intravenous, intramuscular, and intratracheal administration in sheep. Am J Vet Res 42:1901-1904.

Wright, L.C., Horton, C.R., Jernigan, A.D., Wilson, R.C., and Clark, C.H. 1991. Pharmacokinetics of gentamicin after intravenous and subcutaneous injection in obese cats. J Vet Pharmacol Therap 14:96-100.

Yates, R.A., Mitchard, M., and Wise, R. 1978. Disposition studies with amikacin after rapid intravenous and intramuscular administration to human volunteers. J Antimicrob Chemother 4:335-341.

Zaske, D.E. 1980. Aminoglycosides. In W.E. Evans, J.J. Schentag, and W.J. Jusko, eds., Applied Pharmacokinetics and Therapeutics, pp. 210-239. San Francisco.

Zaske, D.E., Cipolle, R.J., Rotschafer, J.C., Solem, L.D., Mosier, N.R., and Strate, R.G. 1982. Gentamicin pharmacokinetics in 1,640 patients: method for control of serum concentrations. Antimicrob Agents Chemother 21:407-411.

Ziv, G. 1977. Comparative clinical pharmacology of amikacin and kanamycin in dairy calves. Am J Vet Res 38:337-340.

Ziv, G., Bor, A., Soback, S., Elad, D., and Nouws, J.F.M. 1985. Clinical pharmacology of apramycin in calves. J Vet Pharmacol Therap 8:95-104.

Ziv, G., Kurtz, B., Risenberg, R., and Glickman, A. 1995. Serum and milk concentrations of apramycin in lactating cows, ewes and goats. J Vet Pharmacol Therap 18:346-351.

Ziv, G., Nouws, J.F.M., and Van Ginneken, C.A.M. 1982. The pharmacokinetics and tissue levels of polymyxin B, colistin, and gentamicin in calves. J Vet Pharmacol Therap 5:45-58.

Ziv, G., and Sulman, F.G. 1974. Distribution of aminoglycoside antibiotics in blood and milk. Res in Vet Sci 17:68-71.

44 CHLORAMPHENICOL AND DERIVATIVES, MACROLIDES, LINCOSAMIDES, AND MISCELLANEOUS ANTIMICROBIALS

MARK G. PAPICH AND JIM E. RIVIERE

Chloramphenicol
- Chemical Features
- Drug Formulations
- Mechanism of Action
- Spectrum of Activity
- Bacterial Resistance
- Pharmacokinetics
- Adverse Effects and Precautions
- Drug Interactions
- Clinical Use

Chloramphenicol Derivatives
- Thiamphenicol
- Florfenicol

Macrolide Antibiotics
- Source and Chemistry
- Drug Formulations
- Mechanism of Action
- Spectrum of Activity
- Pharmacokinetics
- Adverse Effects and Precautions
- Drug Interactions
- Clinical Use of Erythromycin
- Tylosin
- Tilmicosin
- Clarithromycin
- Azithromycin

Lincosamides
- Lincomycin
- Clindamycin

Miscellaneous Antibiotics
- Bacitracin
- Novobiocin
- Thiostrepton
- Rifampin
- Nitrofurans
- Virginiamycin
- Carbadox
- Vancomycin
- Methenamine
- Polymyxins

Several of the drugs discussed in this chapter do not fit into other categories or are not important enough for a separate chapter. They are grouped together here because they have certain features in common: they inhibit protein synthesis in bacteria (with macrolides, lincosamides, and chloramphenicol acting at a similar site), are relatively broad spectrum, and have a large volume of distribution (i.e., they achieve effective concentrations in most tissues).

Some of these drugs are not as common or as available as in previous years. Some older drugs have given way to newer derivatives. For example, newer macrolides such as azithromycin have replaced erythromycin for some uses in small-animal medicine, and florfenicol has replaced chloramphenicol for use in cattle. Earlier editions of this text should be consulted for more in-depth discussion of these older agents.

CHLORAMPHENICOL

Chemical Features. Chloramphenicol chemically is D-(−)-threo-1-*p*-nitrolphenyl-2-dichloroacetamido 1,3-propanediol (Fig. 44.1), has a pK_a of 5.5, and was first isolated from the soil organism *Streptomyces venezuelae* in 1947. The chloramphenicol used today is manufactured synthetically. Chloramphenicol is slightly soluble in water and freely soluble in propylene glycol and organic solvents. Chloramphenicol is a broad-spectrum antibiotic, affecting gram-positive and gram-negative organisms, aerobic and anaerobic bacteria, and many intracellular organisms. Chloramphenicol has three functional groups that largely determine its biological activity: the *p*-nitrophenol group, the dichloroacetyl group, and the alcoholic group at the third carbon of the propanediol chain (Yunis 1988). Replacement of the *p*-NO_2 group by a methylsulfonyl (HC_3-SO_2) moiety produces thiamphenicol and a substantial change in biological activity, while modification of the propanediol

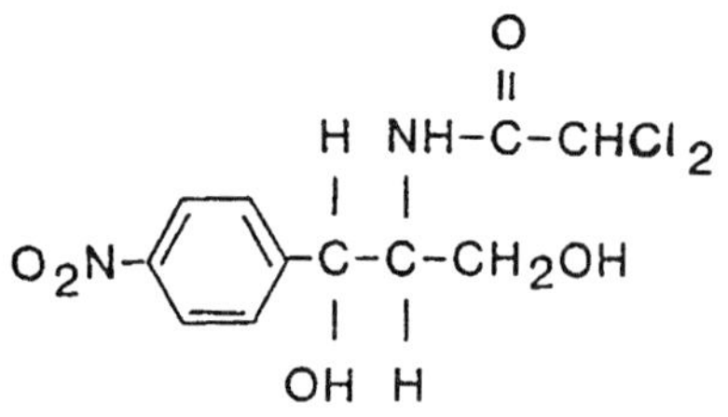

O
II
H NH−C−$CHCl_2$
O_2N−(benzene ring)−C−C−CH_2OH
OH H

FIG. 44.1—The chemical structure of chloramphenicol

group by the addition of a fluorine atom results in the synthesis of florfenicol. Both thiamphenicol and florfenicol will be discussed in more detail later in this chapter. Loss of the dichloroacetyl group altogether results in loss of biological activity (Yunis 1988; Hird and Knifton 1986).

Drug Formulations. Three formulations of chloramphenicol have been administered for systemic therapy in animals. Chloramphenicol base is the unconjugated form of chloramphenicol and is available only in an oral formulation. Chloramphenicol base has a bitter taste, so to increase the palatability, the ester chloramphenicol palmitate was manufactured as an alternative oral formulation. Chloramphenicol palmitate is insoluble in water but soluble in acetone and ether. Before systemic absorption, chloramphenicol palmitate is hydrolyzed in the small intestine by esterases, which release the free base form of chloramphenicol to systemic circulation. Similarly, chloramphenicol succinate is a formulation for parenteral use that requires hydrolysis reactions in the plasma to produce the active drug (Ambrose 1984). The succinate form of the drug is freely soluble in water and can be administered intravenously (IV) or intramuscularly (IM). Topical formulations of chloramphenicol have been used for otic and ophthalmic use. Because of the decreased use of chloramphenicol in human medicine, some of the formulations mentioned above are not as readily available today, if at all.

Mechanism of Action. Chloramphenicol inhibits protein synthesis. Its biologic activity is due to interference with peptidyltransferase activity at the 50S ribosomal subunit, which is near the site of action of macrolide antibiotics and for which there can be competition (Yunis 1988). Because of the interaction with peptidyltransferase, binding with the amino acid substrate cannot occur, and peptide bond formation is inhibited. Chloramphenicol affects mammalian protein synthesis to some degree, especially mitochondrial protein synthesis. Mammalian mitochondrial ribosomes have a strong resemblance to bacterial ribosomes (both are 70S), with the mitochondria of the bone marrow especially susceptible. Prolonged administration to animals has been associated with a dose-related bone marrow suppression, especially in cats (Watson 1980).

Spectrum of Activity. Chloramphenicol has a broad spectrum of activity. It is active against *Staphylococcus intermedius, S. aureus,* streptococci, and some gram-negative bacteria, such as *Pasteurella multocida, P. haemolytica,* and *Haemophilus somnus. Escherichia coli, Proteus vulgaris,* and *Salmonella* spp. may be susceptible, but resistance can occur with many gram-negative bacteria, especially the Enterobacteraceae. Resistance by staphylococci may occur with increased use. Anaerobic bacteria, *Mycoplasma* spp., and many rickettsiae also are susceptible. The National Committee for Clinical Laboratory Standards (NCCLS) approved breakpoint for susceptibility is ≤4 μg/mL for streptococci and ≤8 μg/mL for other organisms (Watts et al. 1999).

Bacterial Resistance. Four mechanisms of resistance to chloramphenicol have been described (Yunis 1988). The most important is plasmid mediated due to the presence of the chloramphenicol acetyltransferase enzyme, which catalyzes a reaction that modifies the hydroxyl groups. Chloramphenicol acetyltransferase was reviewed by Shaw and Leslie (1991). Other mechanisms of resistance include decreased bacterial cell wall permeability, altered binding capabilities at the 50S ribosomal subunit, and inactivation by nitroreductases.

Pharmacokinetics

ABSORPTION AND DISTRIBUTION. The pharmacokinetic parameters of chloramphenicol have been studied in several animal species and are summarized in Table 44.1. Chloramphenicol in animals is well absorbed via both oral and parenteral routes, with a few notable species exceptions. Plasma half-lives vary, ranging from 0.9 hours in ponies to 5.1 hours in the cat (Davis et al. 1972). Watson (1992) reports that fasted cats showed differences in absorption between the chloramphenicol tablets and the chloramphenicol palmitate suspension. The liquid formulation showed a lower systemic drug availability, indicating that hydrolysis of the palmitate form is necessary and that there is a higher risk of drug failure when the palmitate suspension is used to treat sick cats that are also not eating. In ruminants, microflora present in the ruminant forestomach tend to metabolize chloramphenicol faster than it can be absorbed, making chloramphenicol administered orally of little systemic therapeutic use in ruminant animals. This point is rather moot since administration of chloramphenicol to food animals in the United States is currently illegal (discussed in more detail later in the chapter). In most animals, 30–46% of chloramphenicol is bound to plasma proteins, leaving much of the drug in the free and active form. Chloramphenicol is widely distributed to many areas of the body due to its nonionized state and high lipophilicity, enabling it to cross lipid bilayers quite easily. The volume of distribution (V_d) is typically greater than 1.0 L/kg and has been measured at 1–2.5 L/kg (Table 44.1). Chloramphenicol reaches sufficient concentrations in most tissues of the body, including the eye, central nervous system (CNS), heart, lung, prostate, saliva, liver, and spleen, among others (Ambrose 1984; Hird and Knifton 1986). Chloramphenicol concentrations in cerebrospinal fluid (CSF) are approximately 50% of corresponding plasma concentrations. In horses, because of rapid elimination rates, tissue fluid concentrations persisted for only 3 hours after IV administration of chloramphenicol sodium succinate (Brown et al. 1984). Chloramphenicol can also cross

TABLE 44.1—Selected serum pharmacokinetic parameters of chloramphenicol in animals

Species	Dose (mg/kg)	Route	Formulation	Half-life ($t_{1/2\beta}$) (hr)	(l/kg)V_d	Comments	Reference
Dogs	22	IV	Base	4.2	1.77	Dissolved in 50% aqueous solution of N,N,di-methyl-acetamide	Davis et al. 1972
Felines	22	IV	Base	5.1	2.36	Dissolved in 50% aqueous solution of N,N,di-methyl-acetamide	Davis et al. 1972
Sheep	30	IV	Base	1.702	0.691		Dagorn et al. 1990
	30	SC	Base	17.93	NA		Dagorn et al. 1990
	30	IM	Base	2.71	NA		Dagorn et al. 1990
Adult swine	22	IV	Base	1.3	1.05	Dissolved in 50% aqueous solution of N,N,di-methyl-acetamide	Davis et al. 1972
Piglets	25	IV	Base	12.7	0.9411	Normal piglets	Martin and Weise 1988
	25	IV	Base	17.2	0.9549	Colostrum-deprived piglets	Martin and Weise 1988
Goats	25	IV	Succinate	1.22	1.683	Nonfebrile animals	Kume and Garg 1986
	25	IV	Succinate	1.29	1.962	Febrile animals	Kume and Garg 1986
	25	IM	Succinate	1.46	3.019	Nonfebrile animals	Kume and Garg 1986
	25	IM	Succinate	1.45	2.769	Febrile animals	Kume and Garg 1986
Goats	22	IV	Base	2.0	1.33	Dissolved in 50% aqueous solution of N,N,di-methyl-acetamide	Davis et al. 1972
Goats	10	IV	Succinate	1.47	0.312	Normal animals	Abdullah and Baggot 1986
	10	IV	Succinate	3.97	0.287	Starved animals	Abdullah and Baggot 1986
Goats	22	IV	Base	2.0	1.33	Dissolved in 50% aqueous solution of N,N,di-methyl-acetamide	Davis et al. 1972
Goats	10	IV	Succinate	1.47	0.312	Normal animals	Abdullah and Baggot 1986
	10	IV	Succinate	3.97	0.287	Starved animals	Abdullah and Baggot 1986
Cattle	40	IV	Base	2.81	0.351		Sanders et al. 1988
	90	IM	Base	1.345	NA	2 doses 48 hr apart	Sanders et al. 1988
	90	SC	Base	1.153	NA	2 doses 48 hr apart	Sanders et al. 1988
Calves	30	IV	Base	3.98	1.208	Age not reported; average weight = 73 kg	Guillot and Sanders 1991
Calves							
(1 day old)	25	IV	Base in PG vehicle	7.56	1.031		Burrows et al. 1983
(7 days old)	25	IV	Base in PG vehicle	5.96	0.808		Burrows et al. 1983
(14 days old)	25	IV	Base in PG vehicle	4.0	0.903		Burrows et al. 1983
(28 days old)	25	IV	Base in PG vehicle	3.69	0.69		Burrows et al. 1983
(9 months old)	25	IV	Base in PG vehicle	2.47	1.38		Burrows et al. 1983
Horses	22	IV	Base in PG vehicle	0.51–0.78	0.86–1.26		Varma et al. 1987
Ponies	22	IV	Base	0.9	1.02	Dissolved in 50% aqueous solution of N,N,di-methyl-acetamide	Davis et al. 1972

TABLE 44.1—*Continued*

Species	Dose (mg/kg)	Route	Formulation	Half-life ($t_{1/2\beta}$) (hr)	V_d (l/kg)	Comments	Reference
Foals							
(1 day old)	25	IV	Succinate	5.29	1.1		Adamson et al. 1991
(3 days old)	25	IV	Succinate	1.35	0.759		Adamson et al. 1991
(7 days old)	25	IV	Succinate	0.61	0.491		Adamson et al. 1991
(14 days old)	25	IV	Succinate	0.51	0.426		Adamson et al. 1991
(42 days old)	25	IV	Succinate	0.34	0.362		Adamson et al. 1991
(1-9 days old)	50	IV	Succinate	0.95	1.6	After oral suspension administered oral, availability was 83% and half-life of 2.54 hr	Brumbaugh et al. 1983
Rabbits	100	IV	Succinate	1.1575	NA		Mayers et al. 1991
Chickens	20	IV	Succinate	8.32	0.24	Normal animals	Atef et al. 1991a
	20	IV	Succinate	26.21	0.3	*E. coli*-infected animals	Atef et al. 1991a
	20	IM	Succinate	7.84	0.44		Atef et al. 1991a
	20	PO	Succinate	8.26	0.41		Atef et al. 1991a

Note: NA = data not available; PG = propylene glycol.

the placental barrier in pregnant animals and can diffuse into the milk of nursing animals.

METABOLISM AND EXCRETION. Chloramphenicol is metabolized by the liver after absorption into the systemic circulation. Phase II glucuronidation is the principal pathway for the hepatic biotransformation of chloramphenicol, with the principal metabolite being chloramphenicol glucuronide. A few hydrolysis products have also been identified. Cats excrete chloramphenicol more slowly than other animals, perhaps owing to the cat's deficiency in some glucuronidase enzymes. One report notes that 25% of the total dose of chloramphenicol is excreted in the urine in the active form in cats compared to 6% in normal dogs (Hird and Knifton 1986). Most of the absorbed chloramphenicol (approximately 80%) is excreted into the urine as inactive metabolites via tubular secretion.

When chloramphenicol is administered to young animals, there may initially be reduced excretion. Calves showed decreased hepatic glucuronidation of chloramphenicol soon after birth, but this metabolic pathway matured quickly. Calves also showed higher oral availability than older animals because of immaturity of the rumen, with a marked decrease in oral absorption as the calves age (Burrows et al. 1984). Brumbaugh et al. (1983) found that in neonatal horses, elimination and V_d did not differ from adults. Bioavailability in foals was 83%, with an oral half-life of 2.54 hours. A dose of 50 mg/kg orally every 6 hours should be adequate for treating most susceptible bacteria in foals.

Adverse Effects and Precautions. Bone marrow suppression has been the most important adverse effect associated with chloramphenicol administration to people. Bone marrow injury from chloramphenicol takes two forms (Yunis 1988). The first type is the most common and involves a dose-related suppression of the bone marrow precursor erythroid series. This toxicosis is reversible and usually occurs when blood chloramphenicol levels are greater than 25 μg/mL. The evidence suggests that this bone marrow suppression is the result of mitochondrial injury and the suppression of mitochondrial protein synthesis in bone marrow cells. Studies in animal species have described the pathology of bone marrow cell toxicity as a decreased entry into S phase in dividing bone marrow cells, vacuolation of the myeloid and erythroid series precursor cells, and inhibition of erythroid and granulocytic colony forming units (IARC 1976, 1990).

The second type of bone marrow toxicity, aplastic anemia, has been described in people but not in animals. In people, it is rare and independent of dose and treatment duration, and it causes bone marrow aplasia, chiefly characterized by a profound and persistent pancytopenia. This aplastic anemia occurs in approximately 1:10,000 to 1:45,000 humans who receive chloramphenicol. There may be a genetic predisposition to this form of toxicity. It appears that the para-nitro group of the chloramphenicol molecule is responsible for this more serious form of bone marrow toxicity. The para-nitro group undergoes nitroreduction, leading to the production of nitrosochloramphenicol and other toxic intermediates, which trigger the stem cell damage in humans (IARC 1976, 1990; Yunis 1988). Modification of the molecule to eliminate the para-nitro group to produce either thiamfenicol or florfenicol reduces the risk of chloramphenicol-associated aplastic anemia.

Chloramphenicol-induced aplastic anemia in humans is important from a food-animal residue standpoint. If chloramphenicol is used to treat infections in food animals, it is possible that low concentrations of chloramphenicol in milk, meat, and other edible tissues from the animals will be consumed by people and cause aplastic anemia in susceptible individuals. Chloramphenicol residues have been known to persist for prolonged periods in food animals (Korsrud et al. 1987). Even though the amount consumed may be small, the reaction is not concentration dependent. Thus, there is a public health risk for individuals consuming these products. For this and other reasons, the use of chloramphenicol in food-producing animals has been banned in the United States. *Chloramphenicol is prohibited by the Food and Drug Administration (FDA) for use in food-producing animals in the United States.* The hazards of using chloramphenicol in food animals have been reviewed (Settepani 1984; Lacey 1984).

Other adverse effects caused by chloramphenicol in animals are uncommon. However, young animals and cats are the most sensitive to intoxication due to impaired glucuronidation pathways. Cats given 60 and 120 mg/kg/day PO every eight hours for 21 and 14 days (respectively) showed clinical signs of depression, dehydration, reduced fluid intake, weight loss, emesis, and diarrhea. Bone marrow hypoplasia was also documented in addition to pancytopenia (Watson 1980). Other investigators (Penny et al. 1967, 1970) administered to cats 50 mg/kg/day IM, with the cats showing marked depression and inappetence by day 7 of administration and severe bone marrow changes by day 14 and becoming extremely ill by day 21. Dogs showed milder signs of toxicity, mainly gastrointestinal (GI), but doses required to produce these effects were higher than what was administered to cats (225 mg/kg for 2 weeks). In dogs, no changes were noted in peripheral blood cell populations. In both the dog and the cat, signs of toxicity reverse when chloramphenicol therapy is discontinued. Animals with impaired liver function may also have a higher risk of chloramphenicol intoxication.

Drug Interactions. Chloramphenicol is an inhibitor of the cytochrome P-450 drug-metabolizing enzymes. It is not known which specific family of enzymes is inhibited in animals. However, chloramphenicol administration to dogs has been shown to inhibit drug metabolism, and in dogs and cats, it prolongs pentobarbital anesthesia (Adams and Dixit 1970). Sleeping times may be prolonged by 120% in dogs and 260% in cats due to impaired metabolism of pentobarbital. Chloramphenicol also may inhibit the metabolism of digoxin, phenobarbital, propofol, primidone, and perhaps other drugs metabolized by the same enzymes. Erythromycin and chloramphenicol compete for the same site of action on bacteria, and both drugs used together may produce antibacterial antagonism.

Clinical Use. Chloramphenicol has been used for treatment of a wide range of susceptible microbial infections, including those caused by salmonellae, intracellular and extracellular bacteria, rickettsiae, and mycoplasmata; infections of the eyes and CNS; and infections due to anaerobic organisms (IARC 1976, 1990). One of the reasons for its popularity has been the high lipophilicity. Chloramphenicol readily penetrates cells, making it active against intracellular bacteria, and it penetrates tissues that otherwise are difficult to treat, such as the CNS. Chloramphenicol was shown in one study to be equally effective for treatment of Rocky Mountain spotted fever in dogs as enrofloxacin and tetracyclines (Breitschwerdt et al. 1990). Although less popular than it once was, chloramphenicol has been used to treat infections caused by *Staphylococcus* spp., streptococci, *Brucella* spp., *Pasteurella* spp., *E. coli, Proteus* spp., *Salmonella* spp., *Bacillus anthracis, Corynebacterium pyogenes, Erysipelothrix rhusiopathiae,* and *Klebsiella pneumoniae.* It is consistently active against anaerobic bacteria and has been a rational choice for treating these infections.

Chloramphenicol has been popular for treatment of infections of the CNS (encephalitis, meningitis) because it is able to cross the inflamed or uninflamed blood-brain barrier and attain therapeutic concentrations in the CSF and the brain. Despite the popularity for this use, some experts have suggested that since chloramphenicol is merely bacteriostatic against gram-negative pathogens, and there is a lack of phagocytes or immunoglobulins in CSF, chloramphenicol is not well suited to treat serious infections of the CNS (Rahal and Simberkoff 1979).

Chloramphenicol attains high concentrations in the eye when given systemically or after topical application on the cornea and is useful in treating susceptible bacterial conjunctivitis, panophthalmitis, endophthalmitis, and bacterial diseases of the cornea (Conner and Gupta 1973). Topical formulations are not as readily available owing to the risk of aplastic anemia (discussed previously), which can be caused by topical exposure. Florfenicol has been administered systemically for treating eye infections in cattle (see below.)

Chloramphenicol has been used to treat bacterial infections of the respiratory tract because it may have better penetration across the blood-bronchus barrier into respiratory secretions and respiratory lining fluid than more polar or less lipophilic antibiotics. Respiratory infections are among the infections in horses treated with oral chloramphenicol.

Chloramphenicol is one of the few drugs that can be administered orally to horses with safety. It achieves moderate systemic absorption of 21–40% (Gronwall et al. 1986) and has no serious adverse effects on the equine digestive system. However, oral administration resulted in intestinal mucosal damage and diarrhea in calves and reduced glucose absorption (Rollin et al. 1986). For treatment in horses, tablets or capsules are mixed with substances like molasses or corn syrup to facilitate oral administration. Chloramphenicol has been administered to horses for respiratory infections, pleuritis, CNS infections, and joint infections. Despite this widespread use, because of rapid elimination and poor-to-moderate absorption, one author has discouraged its use (Gronwall et al. 1986), but for foals oral doses of 50 mg/kg every 4–12 hours (frequency of administration was dependent on the minimum inhibitory concentration [MIC] of the pathogen) have been recommended (Brumbaugh et al. 1983).

Chloramphenicol has been administered to exotic animals, especially reptiles and amphibians, to treat a variety of infections (Clark et al. 1985). Chloramphenicol administration in 15 species of birds was examined, and the investigators concluded that after IM injections of 50 mg/kg, chloramphenicol would produce adequate concentrations to treat susceptible bacteria for 8–12 hours, except in pigeons, macaws, and conures because effective concentrations could not be achieved in these birds (Clark et al. 1982). However, oral absorption was poor, and this route of administration was discouraged for all birds.

CHLORAMPHENICOL DERIVATIVES. The ban on the use chloramphenicol in food-producing animals in the mid-1980s left a gap in the veterinarian's armamentarium of effective antimicrobial drugs. Because the idiosyncratic aplastic anemia is associated with the presence of the para-nitro group on the chloramphenicol molecule, attempts were made to modify the chloramphenicol structure to simultaneously retain chloramphenicol's broad spectrum of antimicrobial activity and eliminate the induction of aplastic anemia in people. Compounds synthesized in attempts to accomplish this goal are thiamphenicol and florfenicol. Thiamfenicol is not approved in the United States and will be discussed here only briefly. However, florfenicol has been approved for use in cattle and fish (in some countries) and has been effective for treatment of various infections, especially bovine respiratory disease in cattle intended for human consumption.

Thiamphenicol. Thiamphenicol is a semisynthetic structural analog of chloramphenicol (Fig. 44.2). The major structural difference between chloramphenicol and thiamphenicol is that the para-nitrophenol group has been replaced by the methyl sulfonyl moiety. Thiamphenicol inhibits bacterial protein synthesis at the 50S ribosomal subunit at the same location as does chloramphenicol. Thiamphenicol has an antimicrobial spectrum similar to that of chloramphenicol. However, its structural differences result in different pharmacokinetic properties and decreased potency. Thiamphenicol is more water soluble and less lipid soluble and therefore diffuses more slowly through lipid membranes. It is not metabolized to a significant extent in the liver (Ferrari and Bella 1974) and most of the dose is excreted in the urine as the unchanged active compound (Yunis 1988; Lavy et al. 1991a; Gamez et al. 1992). Resistance to thiamphenicol is also similar to that of chloramphenicol, with bacterial acetylation of the thiamphenicol molecule, but at a rate approximately 50% less than that of chloramphenicol.

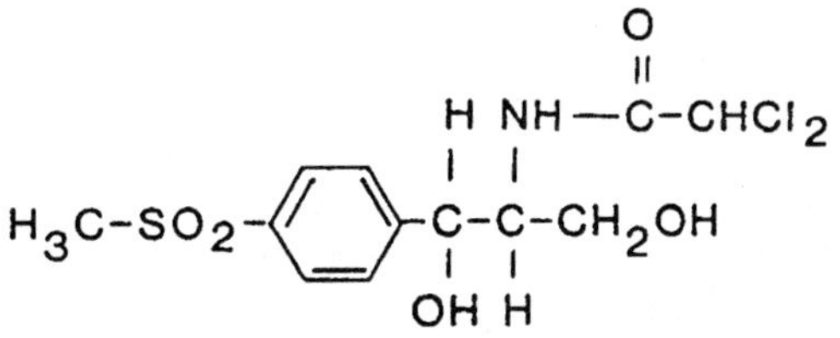

FIG. 44.2—The chemical structure of thiamphenicol.

Few pharmacokinetic studies have been performed on food-producing animals, but thiamphenicol pharmacokinetics has been studied in veal calves (Gamez et al. 1992) and lactating goats (Lavy et al. 1991a). Both studies found thiamphenicol to have a large V_d and to be rapidly eliminated in the urine. In dogs, thiamfenicol had a half-life of 1.7 hours and a V_d of 0.66 L/kg (Castells et al. 1998). In dogs the injection of thiamfenicol was well absorbed, with availability of 97%, but the terminal half-life was longer (5.6 hr), suggesting slow release from the injection site.

Thiamphenicol is considered to be less toxic than chloramphenicol, yet a reversible bone marrow suppression has been reported in humans. However, millions of people have been treated with thiamphenicol in countries in which it is approved, with no reports linking its use to aplastic anemia (Adams et al. 1987). In a thiamphenicol toxicity study in rabbits (Kaltwasser et al. 1974), no changes attributed to thiamphenicol in erythrocyte, reticulocyte, or plasma iron parameters were noted after long-term treatments of up to 90 mg/kg/day. Despite some of the advantages cited here, thiamfenicol is not presently available in North America.

Florfenicol. Florfenicol is structurally related to thiamphenicol; however, florfenicol contains fluorine at the 3′ carbon position (Fig. 44.3). The fluorine molecule substitution at this position also reduces the number of sites available for bacterial acetylation reactions to occur, possibly making the antibiotic more resistant to bacterial inactivation. Florfenicol is as potent or more potent than either chloramphenicol or thiamphenicol against many organisms in vitro. The list of

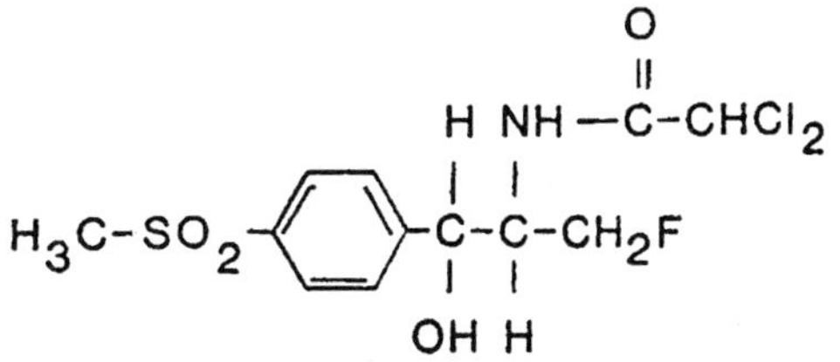

FIG. 44.3—The chemical structure of florfenicol

susceptible bacteria for florfenicol is the same as listed previously for chloramphenicol, except that some bacteria resistant to chloramphenicol due to acetylation may be sensitive to florfenicol. The NCCLS quality control ranges of MIC for florfenicol are 2–8 μg/mL (Marshall et al. 1996). However, *Pasteurella* spp. and *Haemophilus somnus* are several-fold more sensitive in vitro than bacteria of the Enterobacteriaceae, with MIC_{90} for *Pasteurella* and *Haemophilus* in the range of 0.5–1.0 μg/mL. Against these bacteria, florfenicol may actually be bactericidal. No studies have been reported that compare susceptibility or efficacy of florfenicol versus chloramphenicol.

The advantage of florfenicol for administration to food animals is that it lacks the para-nitro group that could contribute to the induction of aplastic anemia associated with chloramphenicol use in humans. Therefore, if residues were to occur in animals treated with florfenicol, no dangerous public health risk would ensue. However, it is possible that florfenicol can still produce a dose-related form of reversible bone marrow suppression with prolonged use or high doses, although such reactions have not been reported from routine use of florfenicol in animals.

PHARMACOKINETICS. The pharmacokinetics of florfenicol are summarized in Table 44.2.

ABSORPTION. Studies in calves (Varma et al. 1986; Adams et al. 1987; Lobell et al. 1994) showed high bioavailability after oral and parenteral administrations, but there was decreased oral absorption when florfenicol was administered with milk. After IM injection in cattle, the absorption is almost complete, with systemic availability of 78%, but absorption is slow, which is demonstrated in cattle by an IV half-life of 2.65 hours but an average of 18 hours after IM injection (Lobell et al. 1994). This suggests that it is more slowly released from an IM injection site, thus prolonging the duration of effective levels. This slow elimination after IM injection in cattle prolongs the effective plasma concentration (above 1 μg/mL for respiratory pathogens) for 23 hours in calves. In horses, florfenicol is absorbed well after oral and IM administration (81% IM and 83% oral) (McKellar and Varma 1996). Oral absorption in Atlantic salmon was 96%.

DISTRIBUTION. Like chloramphenicol, florfenicol has a wide distribution in most tissues of the body (Adams et al. 1987), including high concentrations in the kidney, urine, bile, and small intestine, but less penetration in the CSF, brain, and aqueous humor of the eye than that attained with chloramphenicol. Concentrations in brain and CSF are 1/4 to 1/2, respectively, the corresponding concentrations in plasma. Although in one study the distribution into CSF was only 46% relative to plasma, these levels were high enough to produce concentrations in CSF of cattle to inhibit *Haemophilus somnus* for over 20 hours (DeCraene et al. 1997). Florfenicol was also found to penetrate well into the milk of lactating goats after IV and IM dosing, making it of possible use in the treatment of microbial infections in the udder of lactating animals (Lavy et al. 1991b). The V_d is 0.7–0.9 L/kg in most studies in cattle. Protein binding is low in cattle (13–19%) (Bretzlaff et al. 1987; Lobell et al. 1994) but has not been reported for other species.

ELIMINATION. The elimination half-life is 2–4 hours in cattle (Table 44.2). The half-life of less than 2 hours in horses is shorter than that in cattle.

METABOLISM. Most of the dose administered to cattle is excreted as the parent drug (64%) in the urine. The rest of the drug is excreted as urinary metabolites. Most of the dose was found as unchanged parent compound

TABLE 44.2—Selected pharmacokinetic parameters of florfenicol in animals

Species	Dose mg/kg	Half-life (hr)	Absorption (%)	V_d (L/kg)	C_{MAX} (mcg/mL)	Reference
Cats	22 (all routes)	4 (IV) 7.8 (oral) 5.6 (IM)	> 100 (oral) > 100 (IM)	0.61	57 (IV) 28 (oral) 20 (IM)	Papich 1999
Dogs	20 mg/kg (all routes)	2 (IV) 18 (SC) 9 (IM) 3 (oral)	28 (SC) 16 (IM) > 100 (oral)	1.2	44 (IV) 0.93 (SC) 1.64 (IM) 17 (oral)	Papich 1999
Sea turtles	20 (IM, IV)	2–7.8 hr (IM)	67 (IM)	10-60 L/kg	0.5-0.8 (IM)	Stamper et al 1999
Horses	22 (IV)	1.83	81 (IM) 83 (oral)	0.72	4 (IM) 13 (oral)	McKellar et al 1996
Cattle	50 (IV)	3.2	ND	0.67	157.7	Bretzlaff et al 1987
Feeder calves	20 (IV)	2.65	ND	0.88	73	Lobell et al 1994
Feeder Calves	20 (IM)	18.3	78.5	ND	3.07	Lobell et al 1994
Veal calves	22 (oral)	ND	88	ND	11.3	Varma et al 1986
Veal calves	22 (IV)	2.87	ND	0.78	66	Varma et al 1986
Veal calves	11 (IV)	3.71	ND	0.91	26.35	Adams et al 1987
Veal calves	11 (oral)	3.7	89	ND	5.7	Adams et al 1987

Note: Route of administration used is listed in parentheses. V_d is volume of distribution, C_{MAX} is the maximal concentration after administration with route listed in parentheses. ND = not determined.

in the urine of these animals, possibly indicating its use in the treatment of organisms infecting the genitourinary tract of animals. Florfenicol amine is the metabolite that persists longest in tissues of cattle and is used as the marker residue for withdrawal determination.

STUDIES IN SMALL ANIMALS. In small animals, florfenicol has limited application, but disposition was studied after oral, IM, and subcutaneous (SC) administration (Papich 1999). After IV administration in dogs, the half-life was less than 1 hour for 3 out of 4 dogs and clearance was rapid. After oral administration, inhibitory concentrations were maintained for only 4 hours. In dogs after IM injection, florfenicol mean peak plasma concentrations were 1.64 μg/mL and mean elimination half-life was 9.2 hours. Concentrations were above a MIC of 1.0 μg/mL for only 2 hours. After SC administration, florfenicol was absorbed poorly and inconsistently, with peak concentrations less than 1.0 μg/mL. By contrast, florfenicol solution in cats was absorbed well from both routes, with peak concentrations of 20 μg/mL and 27 μg/mL after IM and oral dose, respectively. Absorption was high from both routes (greater than 100% from IM and oral). IV elimination half-life was 4 hours, and V_d was 0.6 L/kg. The half-life was 5.6 hours and 7.8 hours for IM and oral dose, respectively. In cats, florfenicol produced inhibitory concentrations for 12 hours.

STUDIES IN FISH. Florfenicol has been administered orally for treatment of infections in captive fish and is approved in some countries for this use (Aqua-Flor®). In rainbow trout at a water temperature of 10° C and given an oral dose of 10 mg/kg, florfenicol has a mean residence time of 21 hours and a C_{max} of 3.23 μg/mL and is well distributed to tissues (Pinault 1997). In salmon, florfenicol has a half-life of 12.2 hours at 10.8° C (Martinsen et al. 1993) and is also well distributed (Horsberg et al. 1994), with a V_d of 1.12 L/kg (Martinsen et al. 1993). In salmon the systemic availability of an oral dose is 96.5%.

Clinical Use

FORMULATIONS. There is a 300 mg/mL solution for injection (Nuflor). In some countries, but not the United States, there is a 500 gram per kilogram premix for fish (Aqua-Flor).

CLINICAL EFFICACY. Several studies in cattle have been conducted to support the use of florfenicol for treating bovine respiratory disease. The bacteria involved in this infection usually are *Pasteurella haemolytica, P. multocida,* or *Haemophilus somnus.* Florfenicol has been effective for treating undifferentiated bovine respiratory disease in cattle with doses of 20 mg/kg IM, given every 48 hours and injected in the neck (Hoar et al. 1998; Jim et al. 1999). It is also approved as a single dose for cattle at 40 mg/kg SC in the neck (withdrawal times listed below). Florfenicol has been effective in calves for treating experimentally induced infections and naturally occurring infectious bovine keratoconjunctivitis (Dueger et al. 1999; Angelos et al. 2000). In the naturally occurring case, florfenicol was administered one dose SC at 40 mg/kg or IM two doses 48 hours apart at 20 mg/kg. Concentrations persist in CSF for a long enough period after administration of 20 mg/kg in cattle that concentrations are above MIC for *Haemophilus* for at least 20 hours. When florfenicol was administered by intramammary infusion (750 mg/cow) to cattle (Wilson et al. 1996) with subclinical mastitis, there was poor efficacy, which could, perhaps, be attributed to an interval between treatments that was too long or to a duration of treatment that was too short.

Although some pharmacokinetic studies have been conducted in small animals and exotic animals, there are no reports of efficacy. Pharmacokinetic studies in reptiles and dogs suggest that frequent dosing with high doses would be necessary to maintain plasma concentrations above the MIC for susceptible organisms throughout the dosing interval. In cats, the pharmacokinetic evidence (discussed earlier) indicates that a dose of 22 mg/kg administered every 12 hours orally or parenterally would be adequate to produce sustained plasma concentrations for treatment of susceptible bacteria. There is only one study reporting on florfenicol administration to horses. In that pharmacokinetic study florfenicol had a longer half-life than chloramphenicol, good distribution, and good absorption. However, experimental horses had consistent loose stools and elevated bilirubin (McKellar and Varma 1996). Until adequate studies establish safe doses, florfenicol cannot be recommended for horses.

AQUACULTURE. Florfenicol has been demonstrated to be efficacious against bacteria of fish, especially trout and salmon (Fukui et al. 1987). Florfenicol premix is approved in some countries for treatment of furunculosis in salmon caused by *Aeromonas salmonicida.* Florfenicol has been administered orally for treatment of furunculosis caused by susceptible strains of *Aeromonas salmonicida* in captive fish and is approved in other countries (Aqua-Flor, not available in the United States).

ADVERSE EFFECTS. Effect of florfenicol on bovine pregnancy, reproduction, and lactation have not been determined. Mild diarrhea and elevated bilirubin have been reported from administration to horses (McKellar and Varma 1996). Reversible, dose-related bone marrow suppression is possible but not reported for domestic animals. In cattle, diarrhea and decreased feed consumption have been observed, which are transient. A local tissue reaction from IM or SC injection is possible. When toxic overdoses were administered to calves (200 mg/kg) there was marked anorexia, decrease in body weight, ketosis, and elevated liver enzymes. In dogs administered high doses for prolonged periods there was CNS vacuolation, hematopoietic toxicity, and renal tubule dilation.

REGULATORY INFORMATION. The tolerance for florfenicol is 3.7 ppm for florfenicol amine (the marker residue) in liver and 0.3 ppm in muscle. Withdrawal time for use in salmon is 12 days. After injection to cattle, the withdrawal time for slaughter is 28 days if injected at a dose of 20 mg/kg IM (36 days in Canada). If injected at a dose of 40 mg/kg SC, the withdrawal time for slaughter is 38 days. Do not inject more than 10 mL in one site. Give injections in the neck only (both SC and IM). Do not administer to dairy cows older than 20 months, to calves under 1 month of age, or to calves on an all-milk diet.

MACROLIDE ANTIBIOTICS

Source and Chemistry. The macrolide antibiotics are a group of structurally similar compounds, most of which are derived from various species of *Streptomyces* soil-borne bacteria. Chemically, all the drugs in this group are classified as macrocyclic lactones, with members containing 12–20 atoms of carbon in the lactone ring structure. Attached to this lactone ring are various combinations of deoxy sugars held to the lactone ring by glycosidic linkages. Since erythromycin's discovery in the early 1950s from the soil organism *Streptomyces erythreus,* numerous other macrolides have been isolated or synthesized from the parent molecule erythromycin, including tylosin, roxithromycin, erythromycylamine, tilmicosin, dirithromycin, azithromycin, clarithromycin, spiramycin, and flurithromycin (Kirst and Sides 1989).

Erythromycin, tylosin (see Fig. 44.4), and tilmicosin have found the most clinical applications of the macrolide class in veterinary medicine. New derivatives such as azithromycin are increasing in popularity. Other macrolides such as oleandomycin and carbomycin have been used as feed additives for growth promotion in food animals.

Erythromycin is a large molecule consisting of a 14-atom polyhydroxylactone erythronolide ring and the two sugars clandinose and desosamine. Similarly, tylosin is composed of a 16-atom lactone ring (a tylonolide) to which three sugars, mycinose, mycaminose, and mycarose, are attached (Wilson 1984; Kirst et al. 1982). Other macrolides with 16-member rings include josamycin and spiramycin. Azithromycin is the first drug in the group of azalides, which are semisynthetic derivatives of erythromycin (Lode et al. 1996). Azithromycin has a 15-member ring structure.

Drug Formulations. All macrolides are weak bases, with pK_a's ranging from 6 to 9; erythromycin has a pK_a of 8.7–8.8 and tylosin has a pK_a of 7.1. Erythromycin base is poorly absorbed, and oral formulations are modified to increase absorption and improve oral tolerability. Oral formulations are estolate or ethylsuccinate esters of erythromycin. The esters are absorbed systemically, then hydrolyzed to the erythromycin base by enzymes in the body before they are active. Alternatively, other oral forms of erythromycin are formulated as a salt of stearate or phosphate. After oral administration of the salt, erythromycin dissociates from the salt in the intestine and is absorbed as free drug. There are also oral formulations intended to be added to the feed or drinking water to treat infections for poultry. Examples of these preparations are erythromycin thiocynate premix and erythromycin phosphate powder (Ery-Mycin). In addition, there are formulations of other macrolides to be added to the feed or water of cattle, pigs, or poultry for control of respiratory and other infections. Examples of these formulations are tilmicosin premix (Pulmotil) to be added to feed for pigs, tylosin phosphate premix to be added to feed for cattle, pigs, or poultry, and tylosin tartrate (Tylan soluble) for the drinking water of poultry. Gluceptate (glucoheptonate) and lactobionate forms are intended for IV use. Veterinary forms of erythromycin injectable (e.g., Erythro-100 and Gallimycin-100) are 100 mg/mL formulations intended for IM injection only; they should not be administered SC or IV.

Mechanism of Action. The antibacterial action of macrolides is due to inhibition of protein synthesis by binding to the 50S ribosomal subunit of prokaryote organisms. The binding site on the ribosome is near but not identical to that of chloramphenicol, and antagonism of effect is possible if macrolides are administered with chloramphenicol. Macrolides inhibit translocation of tRNA from the amino acid acceptor site, which disrupts addition of new peptide bonds and thus prevents synthesis of new proteins within the microbial cell. Macrolides can bind to mitochondrial ribosomes but are unable to cross the mitochondrial membrane (in contrast to chloramphenicol) and therefore do not produce bone marrow suppression in mammals. Macrolides in general do not bind to mammalian ribosomes, making them a relatively safe group of drugs for veterinary use.

Although most authors have listed macrolides as bacteriostatic at therapeutic concentrations (Wilson 1984), they can be slowly bactericidal, especially against streptococci. Their bactericidal action is time dependent (Carbon 1998). The antimicrobial action of erythromycin is enhanced by a high pH (Sabath et al. 1968), with the optimum antibacterial effect at a pH of 8. Therefore, in an acidic environment, such as in an abscess, necrotic tissue, or urine, the antibacterial activity is suppressed.

Resistance mechanisms: Resistance to macrolides is usually plasmid mediated, but modification of ribosomes may occur through chromosomal mutation. Resistance can occur from (1) decreased entry into bacteria (most common with the gram-negative organisms), (2) synthesis of bacterial enzymes that hydrolyze the drug, and (3) modification of target (the ribosome in this instance). The ribosomal attenuation involves methylation of the 50S drug receptor site. This resistance may also lead to cross-resistance with other

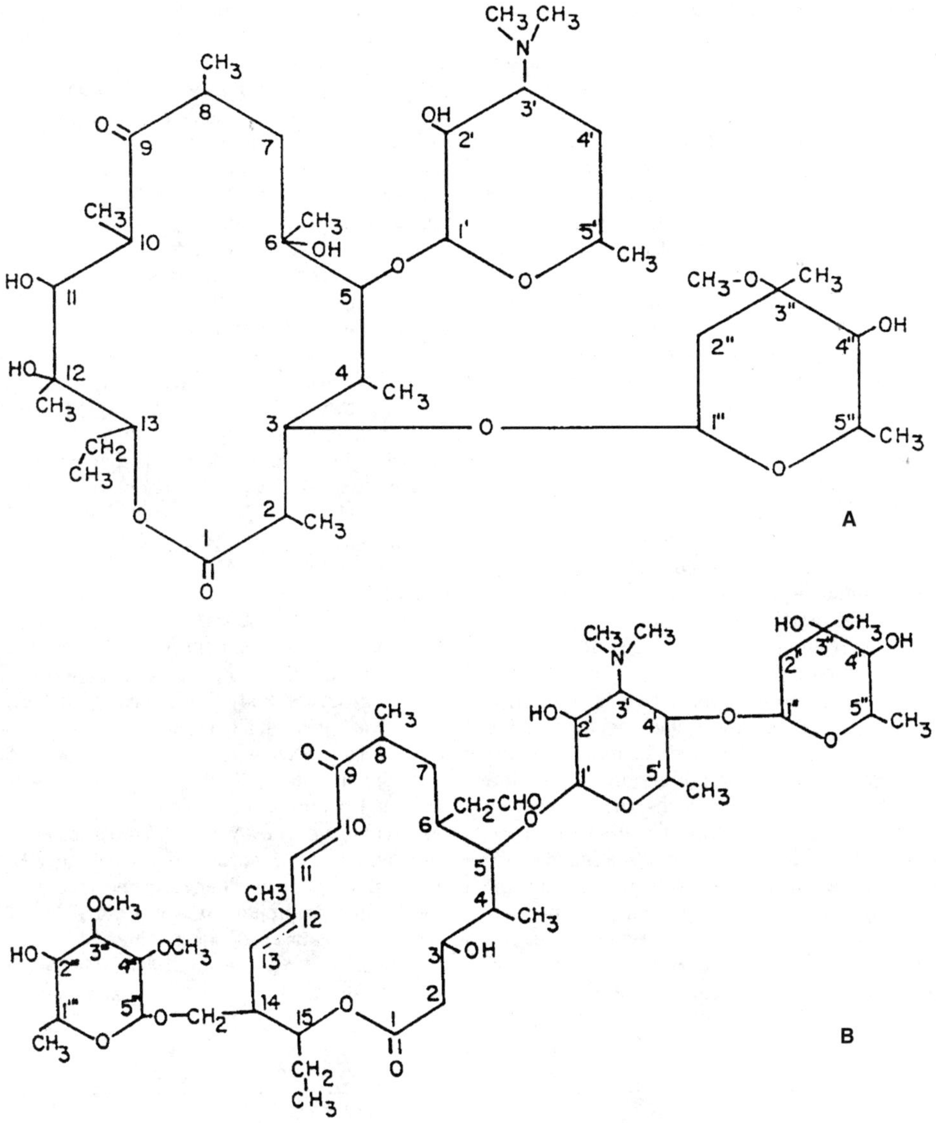

FIG. 44.4—The chemical structures of erythromycin and tylosin.

antibiotics that preferentially bind to these sites, such as other macrolides and lincosamides (Wilson 1984). Resistance to erythromycin in animals in several microorganisms has been discussed in more detail elsewhere (Maguire et al. 1989; Dutta and Devriese 1981, 1982a,b; Leclercq and Courvalin 1991; Devriese and Dutta 1984). In small animals with staphylococcal infections, resistance was more likely if antibiotics had previously been prescribed, especially in cases of recurrent pyoderma (Lloyd et al. 1996; Medleau et al. 1986; Noble and Kent 1992). As summarized by Noli and Boothe (1999), an increasing trend toward resistance to macrolides by staphylocci has been demonstrated when treating pyoderma (increasing from 7 to 22%), whereas in some countries, the incidence of resistance has remained relatively stable at around 22–24%.

Spectrum of Activity. Erythromycin is mainly effective against gram-positive organisms such as streptococci, staphylococci, including staphylococci that may be resistant to β lactams because of β lactamase synthesis or modification of the penicillin-binding protein target. Other organisms that show in vitro susceptibility include *Mycoplasma, Corynebacterium, Erysipelothrix, Bordetella,* and *Bartonella.* Although the spectrum favors the gram-positive group, a few gram-negatives are susceptible, especially *Pasteurella* spp. Activity against anaerobic bacteria is only moderate. Gram-negative anaerobic bacteria often are resistant. Most other gram-negative bacteria, such as those of the Enterobacteriaceae or *Pseudomonas* spp., are resistant. The activity of tilmicosin is similar to that of erythromycin, but most of the in vitro data concern its activity against *Pasteurella* spp. and *Haemophilus somnus,* for which it maintains good activity. Other gram-negative bacteria are resistant to tilmicosin.

The NCCLS guidelines for susceptibility (Watts et al. 1999) list the erythromycin breakpoint for sensitivity as ≤0.25 µg/mL for streptococci and ≤0.5 µg/mL for organisms other than streptococci.

Pharmacokinetics

ABSORPTION AND DISTRIBUTION. Erythromycin pharmacokinetics has been studied in most animals and in humans; some of these parameters are shown in Table 44.3. Oral erythromycin is absorbed well, but inactivation of erythromycin due to gastric acidity is common for the base form of erythromycin, which is the reason that other formulations, such as erythromycin estolate or stearate forms or enteric-coated formulations, are used. They have better bioavailability owing to decreased destruction of erythromycin in the acidic environment of the stomach. The presence of food in the stomach also tends to decrease absorption of erythromycin in most species, including the dog (Wilson 1984; Eriksson et al. 1990). Erythromycin salts (erythromycin-stearate and erythromycin-phosphate) dissociate in the intestine and are absorbed as the active drug. Erythromycin esters (erythromycin-ethylsuccinate and erythromycin-estolate) are absorbed as the esters and hydrolyzed in the body to release active drug. There is no proven difference among these formulations as to which is the most favorable in most animals. However, in horses, it was shown that the salt forms (erythromycin-phosphate or erythromycin-stearate) are preferred for oral administration (Ewing et al. 1994) because they provided the most favorable blood concentrations. Crushed tablets of enteric-coated preparations are substantially degraded in the stomach or are metabolized in the intestine wall and are not recommended for oral administration to animals.

SC or IM injections of erythromycin can be painful and irritating; therefore, the PO route is preferred whenever possible. The only formulations that can be given IV are the glucoptate and lactobionate forms, because these are the only forms soluble in aqueous solution.

Macrolides tend to concentrate in some cells because the basic drug is trapped in cells that are more acidic than plasma. Tissue concentrations for erythromycin, tylosin, and tilmicosin are higher than serum concentrations, especially in the lungs, which is relevant because these drugs are often used to treat respiratory infections. The lung concentrations are so high for tilmicosin that they persist for at least 72 hours after a single dose. In addition to the lungs, erythromycin concentrations are equal to or higher than plasma concentrations in several body fluids such as bile and prostatic, seminal, pleural, and peritoneal fluids, as well as in many tissues, such as the liver, spleen, heart, and kidneys, among others. Erythromycin does not penetrate the blood-brain barrier in high enough concentrations to be therapeutic; however, it can cross the placenta and attain therapeutic concentrations in the fetus. High concentrations are also obtained in the feces of animals due to biliary excretion (Wilson 1984). These high tissue concentrations are reflected in a relatively large V_d of 3–6 L/kg (Riviere et al. 1991). The tylosin V_d is 1–2.5 L/kg for most species of animals. The new

TABLE 44.3—Selected serum pharmacokinetic parameters of erythromycin in animals

Species	Dose (mg/kg)	Route	Formulation	Half-life ($t_{1/2\beta}$) (hr)	V_d (L/kg)	Reference
Cows	12.5	IV	Base	3.16	0.789	Baggot and Gingerich 1976
Calves	15	IV	Base in PG vehicle	2.91	0.835	Burrows et al. 1989
	15	IM	Base in PG vehicle	5.81	NA	Burrows et al. 1989
	15	SC	Base in PG vehicle	26.87	NA	Burrows et al. 1989
Calves	30	IV	Base in PG vehicle	4.09	1.596	Burrows et al. 1989
	30	IM	Base in PG vehicle	11.85	NA	Burrows et al. 1989
	30	SC	Base in PG vehicle	18.3	NA	Burrows et al. 1989
Mice	10	IV	Base	0.65	3.6	Duthu 1985
Rats	25	IV	Base	1.27	9.3	Duthu 1985
Rabbits	10	IV	Base	1.4	6.8	Duthu 1985
Dogs	10	IV	Base	1.72	2.7	Duthu 1985

Note: NA = data not available.

macrolide azithromycin is discussed in more detail later in this section. Its distribution to tissues is higher than other macrolides discussed so far, and its V_d has been measured at over 20 L/kg in animals. Protein binding for macrolides is low, with values of 18–30% for most species.

Tylosin has good absorption from the GI tract, and no enteric coating is required to maintain the stability of the compound in the stomach. It is widely distributed to basically the same tissues as described for erythromycin, metabolized by the liver, and excreted via the bile and feces.

Tilmicosin has slow absorption, 22% bioavailability, a half-life in plasma of 4 hours, and extensive penetration in milk (Ziv et al. 1995). However, because of the high and persistent distribution to tissues, especially lungs, the plasma pharmacokinetics seem to have little correlation to the observed clinical effects (Gourlay et al. 1989).

METABOLISM AND EXCRETION. Metabolism of erythromycin is via hepatic microsomal enzymes, which causes a demethylation of one of the methyl groups on the desosamine sugar moiety of the erythromycin molecule. Little of the antimicrobial action is retained after demethylation by these enzymes. These metabolic enzymes can be induced with phenobarbital; therefore, patients given phenobarbital and erythromycin simultaneously may experience more antimicrobial treatment failures due to increased metabolism. Most (90%) of the drug in the bile is in the metabolized form. Some active erythromycin (2–5%) is found excreted into the urine, with higher levels found in the urine after IV dosing. Renal dysfunction seemingly does not have an appreciable effect on its elimination half-life in the body (Wilson 1984). Although macrolides are not a popular choice for treating urinary tract infections because of their limited spectrum of activity, high urine pH tends to favor antimicrobial activity in the urine environment (Sabath et al. 1968).

Half-lives for erythromycin range from less than 1.0 hour in rodents and rabbits to 3–4 hours in cattle. Tylosin follows a similar pattern, with half-lives of 1–2 hours in most animals.

Adverse Effects and Precautions. Side effects are reported more frequently in humans than in animals. Humans dosed with macrolides (in particular, erythromycin) have experienced nausea and vomiting (oral forms), fever, skin eruptions, cholestatic hepatitis, elevated serum aspartate aminotransferase, epigastric distress, and transient auditory impairment, among many other side effects. Cholestatic hepatitis, most commonly associated with the estolate ester, is the most common of these adverse reactions, with the symptoms starting 10–20 days after beginning therapy and ending a few days after the cessation of therapy. Cholestasis associated with erythromycin use in humans is considered to be a hypersensitivity reaction (Sande and Mandell 1990a). In animals, however, few of these side effects are observed, and hepatitis has not been a reported association. However, regurgitation and/or vomiting has been commonly reported in small animals, especially dogs after oral administration of erythromycin. In one report, erythromycin was the drug that most frequently caused side effects after oral dosing in dogs (Kunkle et al. 1995). Stimulation of GI motility may play a role in small-animal vomiting (discussed below under clinical uses). In horses, erythromycin may induce diarrhea, which stops after therapy is discontinued and is generally not fatal. Although these reactions in the horse may limit its use by some clinicians, erythromycin is still commonly used in horses to treat a variety of infections, especially in the foal.

Drug Interactions. Erythromycin is a well-known hepatic microsomal enzyme inhibitor. Erythromycin is both a substrate and an inhibitor for the cytochrome P-450 enzyme (CYP3A4), which is the enzyme system that is most often involved in drug metabolism. As an inhibitor of the cytochrome P-450 enzyme, it may inhibit metabolism of drugs such as theophylline, cyclosporine, digoxin, and warfarin. Concentrations of these drugs may increase when animals receive erythromycin, resulting in a potentiation of the pharmacologic effect or toxicity.

Clinical Use of Erythromycin. Doses of erythromycin are listed in Table 44.3. Erythromycin is primarily used for treating infections caused by gram-positive organisms. Because of the high distribution into tissues and long persistence in some cells, macrolides are particularly useful for treating some infections caused by bacteria that more-polar or less-lipid-soluble drugs may have difficulty reaching. Erythromycin and other macrolide antibiotics are sometimes used as a penicillin alternative when penicillins have either failed or when there is allergy to penicillins. Infections treated by erythromycin include those caused by *Staphylococcus* spp., *Streptococcus* spp., *Corynebacterium* spp., *Clostridium* spp., *Listeria* spp., *Bacillus* spp., *Erysipelothrix* spp., *Haemophilus* spp., *Brucella* spp., *Fusobacterium* spp., *Pasteurella* spp., *Borrelia* spp., and *Mycoplasma* spp. (Wilson 1984).

In small animals, erythromycin is used to treat pyoderma caused by staphylococci (Noli and Boothe 1999), respiratory infections caused by *Mycoplasma,* and diarrhea caused by *Campylobacter* organisms. When treating *Campylobacter,* erythromycin stopped the shedding but did not eliminate the organism. Respiratory infections are sometimes treated with erythromycin, even when a causative organism has not been identified because erythromycin crosses the blood-bronchus barrier and achieves favorable concentrations in respiratory tract secretions. Erythromycin has also been used as a treatment for undifferentiated bovine respiratory disease and for pig infections caused by *Erysipelothrix* and for pig respiratory infections caused by *Streptococcus* and *Pasteurella.* In poultry, erythromycin is used for treatment of respiratory infections caused by *Mycoplasma.* In foals, erythromycin is used, in combination with rifampin, for treatment of pneumonia caused by *Rhodococcus equi.* However, there is some evidence that erythromycin administered alone may be equally efficacious.

EFFECTS ON GI MOTILITY. Erythromycin is a common cause of vomiting and regurgitation in small animals. In one study erythromycin oral administration produced the most common adverse effects in comparison to other drugs (Kunkle et al. 1995). Although some nausea from the oral preparations is possible, most of this effect is believed to be related to a drug-induced increase in GI motility. This mechanism appears to be related to an increase in activation of motilin receptors, via release of endogenous motilin, or via cholinergic mechanisms in the upper GI tract (Hall and Washabau 1997; Lester et al. 1998). At small doses (1 mg/kg) erythromycin has been considered for use as a motility-stimulating drug in animals. Its clinical benefits for treating GI motility disorders in horses is being explored. Not all macrolide antibiotics exhibit this property.

REGULATORY CONSIDERATIONS. Erythromycin has a 6-day withdrawal time when used according to label in cattle in the United States. Erythromycin added to feed or water for poultry has a withdrawal time of 1–2 days; the specific product label should be consulted for the exact withdrawal time. In the United States erythromycin should not be administered to lactating dairy cattle because macrolides concentrate in the milk for a long time after treatment. However, Canadian labeling lists a milk withholding time of 72 hours after a dose of 2.2–4.4 mg/kg.

Tylosin. Pharmacokinetic data for tylosin are listed in Table 44.4. Tylosin has been used therapeutically to treat "pinkeye" (*Moraxella bovis*) in cattle, respiratory tract infections (Sampson et al. 1974b,c; Ose 1976; Jones 1974; Matsuoka et al. 1980), swine dysentery, pleuropneumonia due to *Haemophilus parahemolyticus,* and a variety of infections such as colitis in dogs (Sampson et al. 1974a) and other infections in cats, chickens (Ose and Tonkinson 1985), quail (Jones et al. 1976), and turkeys (Wilson 1984). Tylosin has been used more extensively as a feed additive to promote growth in food-producing animals, such as swine, cattle, and chickens, among others (Wilson 1984). Residues from tylosin have been discussed in other papers (Knothe 1977a,b; Anderson et al. 1966). After administration to cattle there is a 21- and 14-day withdrawal time for slaughter for cattle and pigs, respectively. Tylosin concentrates in milk for a long time after administration and should not be administered to lactating dairy cattle. Specific product information should be consulted for withholding times when tylosin is administered in feed or water to pigs or poultry because withdrawal times can vary from 0 to 5 days, depending on the use.

Tilmicosin. Tilmicosin is 20-deoxo-20-(3,5-dimethylpiperidin-1-yl)desmycosin, a newer macrolide antibiotic that is closely related to erythromycin. Tilmicosin phosphate (Micotil 300) has been effective for treating bovine respiratory disease and is as effective or more effective than other established treatments, such as ceftiofur, oxytetracycline, or florfenicol (Musser et al. 1996; Hoar et al. 1998; Jim et al. 1999). One study (Ose and Tonkinson 1988) reports that 90% of the *Pasteurella haemolytica* and *Pasteurella multocida* isolates tested were sensitive to tilmicosin at concentrations of ≤6.25 μg/mL, and the drug was also active against *Mycoplasma,* including those from bovine isolates. Other organisms with in vitro susceptibility to tilmicosin include staphylococci and streptococci. Most gram-negative organisms other than *Pasteurella* and *Haemophilus* are resistant.

Tilmicosin (in a 25% propylene glycol carrier) is reported to be effective as a single-dose treatment of neonatal calf pneumonia at dosages of 10, 20, and 30 mg/kg administered subcutaneously. In another study,

TABLE 44.4—Selected serum pharmacokinetic parameters of tylosin in animals

Species	Dose (mg/kg)	Route	Half-life ($t_{1/2\beta}$) (hr)	V_d (L/kg)	Reference
Dogs (Beagle)	10	IV	0.9	1.7	Weisel et al. 1977
Ewes	20	IV	2.05	NA	Ziv and Sulman 1973b
Goats	15	IV	3.04	1.7	Atef et al. 1991b
Cows	12.5	IV	1.62	1.1	Gingerich et al. 1977
Cows	20	IV	2.14	NA	Gingerich et al. 1977
Calves					
(2 days old)	10	IV	2.32	7	Burrows et al. 1983
(1 wk old)	10	IV	1.26	7.2	Burrows et al. 1983
(2 wk old)	10	IV	0.95	11.1	Burrows et al. 1983
(4 wk old)	10	IV	1.53	9	Burrows et al. 1983
(>6 wk old)	10	IV	1.07	11.1	Burrows et al. 1983
Avians (emus)	15	IV	4.7	NA	Locke et al. 1982
Avians (quail, pigeons, cranes)	15	IM	1.2	NA	Locke et al. 1982

Note: NA = data not available.

calves with pneumonia were found to respond better when treated with 10 mg/kg SC tilmicosin than with a 20 mg/kg IM dose of oxytetracycline (Laven and Andrews 1991). In a study by Gourlay et al. (1989) using calves treated with 20 mg/kg SC tilmicosin, the high success rate in treating bovine pneumonia was believed to be due in part to the prolonged presence of therapeutic concentrations of tilmicosin in the lung tissues. Due to high affinity for certain tissues, tilmicosin concentrations remain above the MIC of susceptible organisms for at least 72 hours. Resistance among cattle respiratory pathogens has been recognized (Musser et al. 1996). However, because tilmicosin has such a high concentration in some tissues (e.g., the lung), in vitro measurements of resistance may have little relationship to whether or not the drug produces a cure in cattle with respiratory disease (Musser et al. 1996).

Tilmicosin also has been used as a prophylactic antibiotic for administration to calves entering a feedlot situation. Tilmicosin reduced the incidence of pneumonia in susceptible calves when administered prophylactically as a single 10 mg/kg SC injection (Morck et al. 1993; Schumann et al. 1990). Tilmicosin used as a metaphylactic treatment in newly arrived feedlot calves reduced prevalence of bovine respiratory disease and improved growth of calves (Vogel et al. 1998).

The NCCLS guidelines for tilmicosin susceptibility list a breakpoint of ≤8 μg/mL (Watts et al. 1999). The currently approved dose is 10 mg/kg SC as a single treatment. After treatment with tilmicosin phosphate in cattle, there is a 28-day withdrawal time. Tilmicosin should not be administered to lactating dairy cattle because residues may persist in milk for more than 30 days.

Injections of tilmicosin to horses, goats, swine, or nonhuman primates can be fatal. The heart is the target of toxicity in animals, perhaps mediated via depletion of cardiac intracellular calcium, resulting in a negative inotropic effect (Main et al. 1996). Epinephrine worsens the cardiac toxicity in pigs, but dobutamine has alleviated the cardiac depression in dogs (Main et al. 1996). The effects of toxicity are increased heart rate, arrhythmia, and depressed contractility. Injected doses of 20 and 30 mg/kg to pigs caused death, but oral tilmicosin in pigs produces no toxic effects. In cattle, injected SC doses of 50 mg/kg caused myocardial toxicity; 150 mg/kg was lethal. Doses as low as 10 mg/kg IV have caused cardiac toxicity as well (Ziv et al. 1995).

Tilmicosin phosphate is approved for treatment of swine respiratory disease caused by *Actinobacillus pleuropneumoniae* and *Pasteurella multocida.* This form (Pulmotil) is administered as a feed additive and has been shown to be effective for controlling pneumonia in swine (Moore et al. 1996). When injected in swine, tilmicosin has caused toxic reactions and death due to cardiovascular reactions. Horses should not have access to feeds medicated with swine tilmicosin. There is a 7-day withdrawal time for slaughter when administered to swine.

The only other reports of tilmicosin treatment in animals is for treatment of pasteurellosis in rabbits (McKay et al. 1996). Single doses of 25 mg/kg SC were an effective treatment for pasteurellosis in rabbits. There were no toxic side effects.

Clarithromycin. Clarithromycin (Biaxin®) is a new macrolide that is semisynthetically derived from erythromycin. It is primarily used in people because it is tolerated better than erythromycin, has a broader spectrum, and concentrates in leukocytes. Clarithromycin in combination with ranitidine and bismuth (Tritec®) is currently used to treat *Helicobacter pylori* infections in people. In dogs, clarithromycin does not have pharmacokinetic features that are as favorable as those of azithromycin (the half-life is not as long), and except for pharmacokinetic studies, its use in veterinary medicine has not been reported (Vilmànyi et al. 1996).

Azithromycin. Azithromycin (Zithromax®) is the first drug in the class of azalides. Azalides are derived from erythromycin and their mechanisms of action are similar. (Erythromycin has a 14-member ring structure, and azithromycin has a 15-member ring structure.) Azithromycin has better oral absorption, is better tolerated, has a much longer half-life (especially in tissues), and has a broader spectrum of activity than erythromycin.

Azithromycin is active against gram-positive aerobic bacteria (staphylococci and streptococci) and anaerobes. However, the activity against staphylococci is not as good as erythromycin. It has some activity against gram-negative bacteria such as *Haemophilus* but not against enteric gram-negative bacteria or *Pseudomonas.* It has good activity against many intracellular organisms, including *Chlamydia* and *Toxoplasma.* It is also active against mycobacteria and *Mycoplasma* (Lode et al. 1996)

The primary pharmacokinetic difference between azithromycin and erythromycin is the long half-life and high concentration in tissues. Azithromycin has an extraordinary ability to concentrate in tissues, particularly leukocytes, macrophages, and fibroblasts. The tissue concentration can be as much as 100 times serum concentrations. Concentrations in leukocytes can be at least 200–300 times the concentrations in serum (Panteix et al. 1993). In cats, the serum half-life is 35 hours, tissue half-lives vary from 13 to 72 hours, and the V_d is 23 L/kg (Hunter et al. 1995). In dogs, it also exhibits rapid uptake and persistent concentrations in tissues; the V_d is 12 L/kg, and plasma and tissue half-lives are 29 and 90 hours, respectively (Shepard and Falkner 1990). Oral absorption is high, with bioavailability values of 58% in cats (Hunter et al. 1995) and 97% in dogs (Shepard and Falkner 1990). In people, azithromycin is absorbed much better on an empty stomach (Lode et al. 1996).

Of particular interest is the fact that the intracellular reservoir of azithromycin can apparently produce effective drug concentrations in the interstitial fluids, even after the plasma concentrations have declined below detectable levels (Girard et al. 1990). In fact, plasma pharmacokinetic parameters have little correlation to the in vivo efficacy of azithromycin. Intracellular stores of azithromycin in leukocytes also can serve as a mode of delivery of azithromycin to infected tissues, especially early abscesses, since the leukocytes are attracted to these sites via chemotaxis (Girard et al. 1993). The slow release of azithromycin from leukocytes distinguishes azithromycin from other macrolides and fluoroquinolones, which, despite achieving high concentrations in leukocytes, are released rapidly from cells in a drug-free environment (Panteix et al. 1993).

CLINICAL USE. The therapeutic uses for azithromycin are similar to those of other macrolides such as erythromycin (Lode et al. 1996). The MIC for susceptible organisms is 2 μg/mL. There has been limited use of this drug for treating infections in dogs, cats, and birds, but its popularity is increasing. Results of treatment of intracellular infections caused by *Toxoplasma* spp. and *Mycobacterium* spp. have been conflicting in people and are not yet reported for animals. Because of the long half-life and persistence of drug in tissues, the regimen employed in people is to administer a dose once daily for 3–5 days. Thereafter, effective drug concentrations are expected in tissues for up to 10 days. In dogs, doses of 5–10 mg/kg once daily orally for 1–5 days have been suggested. In cats, doses of 5 mg/kg once daily or every other day or one dose two to three times a week orally have been used.

SAFETY. Azithromycin is generally well tolerated. In people, gastrointestinal disturbances are the most common side effects (nausea, vomiting, diarrhea, abdominal pain). In dogs, high doses may cause vomiting. Erythromycin is well known to decrease the activity of drug-metabolizing enzymes in the liver. This can increase the toxicity of some drugs administered concurrently. Although azithromycin is reported to have less effect on the hepatic enzymes, some caution is needed when combining azithromycin with other drugs.

LINCOSAMIDES. Lincosamides are a group of monoglycoside antibiotics containing an amino-acid-like side chain. There are two antibiotics within this group: lincomycin and clindamycin. Lincomycin and clindamycin are structurally similar. Lincomycin has a hydroxyl moiety at the 7 position of the molecule, and clindamycin contains a chlorine at this position, making clindamycin a more active molecule against bacteria than its parent molecule, lincomycin, and better absorbed orally. The lincosamides, like the macrolides, are used primarily to treat gram-positive infections in cases where there is resistance or intolerance to penicillins. Common infections treated with lincosamides include infections involving *Staphylococcus* spp. and *Streptococcus* spp. (Burrows 1980).

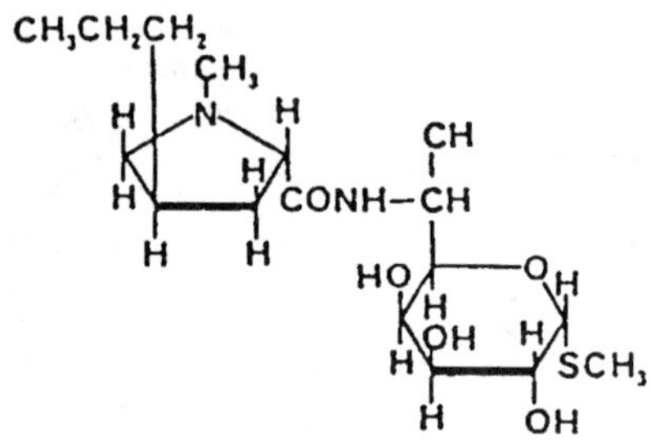

FIG. 44.5—The chemical structure of lincomycin.

Lincomycin

SOURCE AND CHEMISTRY. Lincomycin is the antibiotic produced by *Streptococcus lincolnensis* var. *lincolnensis,* discovered in the 1950s; its name comes from cultures of soil that originated in Lincoln, Nebraska (Fig. 44.5). Lincomycin was first marketed for human clinical use in 1964 and for veterinary use in dogs and cats in 1967. Lincomycin was added to feed premixes for chickens in 1970 and to swine premixes in 1976 for growth promotion. An injectable form was ready for clinical use in swine in 1979 (Ford and Aronson 1985; Kleckner 1984). Lincomycin is a weak base with a pK_a of 7.6 (Riviere et al. 1991).

FORMULATIONS. Lincomycin is available as an oral premix for pigs and chickens (Lincomix), a soluble powder for drinking water (Lincomix), lincomycin hydrochloride oral syrup and tablets for dogs and cats (Lincocin), and lincomycin hydrochloride injection. Ruminants and horses should not be exposed to lincomycin-supplemented feed.

MECHANISM OF ACTION. Lincomycin inhibits protein synthesis in the microbial cell by binding to the 50S ribosomal subunit in much the same way described for macrolides. Other antibiotics, such as erythromycin and clindamycin, function similarly by binding at different sites to the same ribosomal subunit. Concurrent use of these antibiotics typically results in a decrease in the overall efficacy against the microbe due to one bound antibiotic physically overlapping the binding site of another (Burrows 1980).

SPECTRUM OF ACTIVITY. Lincomycin is active against essentially the same bacteria as listed for macrolides.

ABSORPTION AND DISTRIBUTION. Lincomycin is rapidly but incompletely absorbed when administered orally to animals, with one report stating that lincomycin oral absorption in swine given 10 mg/kg is in the range 20–50% (Hornish et al. 1987). Peak serum levels in most animals are reached within 60 minutes after an oral dose and within 2–4 hours after IM injection. Lincomycin is well distributed in the body, with highest tissue concentrations in the liver and kidneys, while very low levels are obtained in the CSF (Burrows 1980; Ford and Aronson 1985; Kleckner 1984). The V_d in animals ranges from 1 to 1.3 L/kg.

METABOLISM AND EXCRETION. The half-life after oral, IM, or IV administration is approximately 2–4 hours. Most of the oral dose, measured as ^{14}C-labeled lincomycin, was recovered in the feces and 14% in the urine after a single oral administration to the dog (Kleckner 1984); thus, biliary secretion of lincomycin appears to be an important route of elimination. After a single IM injection, 38% of the dose was found in the feces and 49% in the urine of the dog. Urine excretion of the radiolabeled drug was complete in 24 hours and fecal excretion was complete within 48 hours for both dosing routes. It is not known whether this radioactivity was associated with an unchanged/unmetabolized lincomycin or with the metabolites of this compound. An unpublished report cited by Hornish et al. (1987) stated the parent drug was the primary form present in the urine of dogs and humans.

Because of the potential for residues in meat, from a food-animal residue viewpoint, the metabolism and excretion of lincomycin have been studied more extensively in swine and chickens (Hornish et al. 1987). When administered to animals, lincomycin concentrations are highest in the liver and kidney, with low, albeit detectable, levels in muscle and skin. Lincomycin can pass unchanged from the body via the bile and feces or urine or can be metabolized to the glucuronide, *N*-demethyl lincomycin, or lincomycin sulfoxide forms by the liver. Swine given oral doses of lincomycin showed that 11–21% was excreted into the urine: 50% unchanged lincomycin, trace amounts of *N*-demethyl lincomycin, no lincomycin sulfoxide or glucuronide forms, and the rest labeled "unidentified substances." The feces contained the remainder of the excreted lincomycin: 17% unchanged lincomycin, possible trace amounts of lincomycin sulfoxide, and 83% uncharacterized metabolites (Hornish et al. 1987). Similarly conducted studies in chickens treated orally for 7 days with lincomycin showed that the excreta contained $\approx$80% lincomycin, $\leq$10% lincomycin sulfoxide, $\leq$5% *N*-demethyl lincomycin.

ADVERSE EFFECTS AND PRECAUTIONS. Dogs and cats have few adverse reactions to lincomycin. Loose stools in the dog and vomiting in the cat have been the major side effects reported (Kleckner 1984). Pigs may occasionally develop diarrhea and/or swelling of the anus within the first 2 days of treatment and will self-correct within a week after withdrawal from the antibiotic.

The most serious adverse effect from lincomycin reported in people is that of pseudomembranous colitis. This is a serious disease in people caused by an overgrowth and production of toxin from *Clostridium difficile,* which may be fatal. In animals with fermenting GI tracts (horses, ruminants, rabbits, hamsters, chinchillas, and guinea pigs) there also is a high risk of GI bacterial overgrowth with *Clostridium* from lincomycin treatment. Severe enteritis, enterocolitis, may lead to diarrhea and death. Other bacteria also have been implicated in this reaction, such as *Salmonella* spp. or *E. coli* (Burrows 1980; Plenderleith 1988). Rehg and Pakes (1982) have implicated *Clostridium difficile* and *Clostridium perfringens* toxins in lincomycin toxicity in rabbits. Lincomycin-induced enterocolitis has been reported for rabbits (Maiers and Mason 1984; Thilsted et al. 1981), horses (Raisbeck et al. 1981; Plenderleith 1988), sheep (Bulgin 1988), and large ruminants (Plenderleith 1988). Lincomycin has been reported to produce ketosis in dairy cows (Rice and McMurray 1983).

CLINICAL USE. Lincomycin is used to treat gram-positive aerobic and anaerobic infections in patients for many of the same indications for which one would use erythromycin or other macrolide. In dogs and cats, lincomycin has been used to treat penicillin-resistant or suspected penicillin-resistant strains of *Staphylococcus* spp. and *Streptococcus* spp. bacteria found in bone, the upper respiratory tract, and the skin. The use for skin infections has been particularly popular (Noli and Boothe 1999). Doses in dogs and cats generally are 22 mg/kg every 12 hours orally. The use of lincomycin to treat bacterial infections in dogs and cats has been largely replaced by clindamycin therapy.

Lincomycin has been utilized to treat bacterial arthritis in swine caused by *Staphylococcus* spp., *Streptococcus* spp., *Erysipelothrix* spp., and *Mycoplasma* spp. and pneumonia caused by *Mycoplasma* spp. Doses in pigs are 11 mg/kg every 24 hours IM. It has also been used as a feed additive (Rainier et al. 1980), drinking-water supplement (Hamdy 1978), and parenteral product (Hamdy and Kratzer 1981) to control or treat swine dysentery.

In broiler chickens, lincomycin has been used as a feed additive to increase the rate of weight gain and improve feed efficiency, in addition to treating necrotic enteritis in this species. The addition of 2 g/ton of lincomycin to the feed of broilers resulted in a significant decrease in the incidence of necrotic enteritis (Maxey and Page 1977). Lincomycin has also been used with success in psittacines (Mandel 1977). Lincomycin use in the eyes of rabbits has also been reported (Kleinberg et al. 1979). Topical corneal administration of 1% lincomycin in water to rabbits showed local therapeutic levels could be maintained from 30–45 minutes to 2 hours postdose in the cornea, aqueous humor, and iris-ciliary body and that deepithelialization of the corneal epithelium served to enhance the ocular topical absorption of this antibiotic.

Sheep, goats, and calves have been treated with parenteral lincomycin-spectinomycin antibiotic combinations for gram-positive and gram-negative respiratory tract infections. The lincomycin-spectinomycin combination (50 mg lincomycin with 100 mg spectinomycin ["Linco-Spectam"] per mL) at a dose of 1 mL/10 kg body weight IM has been used to treat foot rot in sheep caused by *Bacteroides nodosus* with better success than systemic penicillin-streptomycin therapy (Venning et al. 1990).

REGULATORY CONSIDERATIONS. When added to feed for poultry and pigs, the slaughter withdrawal time ranges from 0 to 6 days, depending on the preparation and dose. Consult the package insert for specific recommendations. When injected in pigs, the withdrawal time for slaughter is 2 days.

Clindamycin

SOURCE AND CHEMISTRY. Clindamycin chemically is 7-chlorolincomycin, a derivative of lincomycin and an antibiotic produced by *Streptococcus lincolnensis* var. *lincolnensis.* The replacement of the hydroxyl group at the C7 position of the lincomycin molecule by a chloride results in a more active antibacterial effect when compared to lincomycin. The chemical structure of clindamycin is shown in Fig. 44.6. It is a weak base with a pK_a of 7.6. Both clindamycin hydrochloride (HCl) and clindamycin palmitate are for oral administration. Clindamycin HCl is directly active when administered, whereas the palmitate form must be converted to clindamycin in the small intestine. Clindamycin palmitate is more palatable than clindamycin HCl. Clindamycin phosphate is the parenteral form of clindamycin and must undergo hydrolysis in the plasma for it to become active.

MECHANISM OF ACTION. Clindamycin exerts its antibiotic activity by inhibiting protein synthesis at the 50S ribosomal subunit (Hedstrom 1984) in a manner identical to that described for lincomycin. Plasmid-mediated resistance to clindamycin has been reported in *Bacteroides fragilis* (Tally et al. 1979) and cross-resistance to lincomycin can occur (Harari and Lincoln 1989).

SPECTRUM OF ACTIVITY. Clindamycin is distinguished from the macrolide antibiotics and lincomycin by its high activity against anaerobic bacteria, including gram-negative anaerobes such as *Bacteroides* spp.

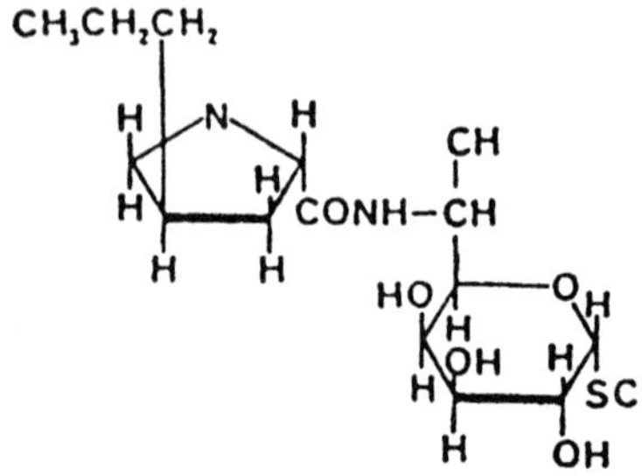

FIG. 44.6—The chemical structure of clindamycin.

In small animals, anaerobic infections are one of the major uses of clindamycin. However, one report (Jang et al. 1997) indicated that only 83% of *Bacteroides* from small animals were sensitive to clindamycin and only 80% of the *Clostridium.* Other than anaerobes, clindamycin is active against the same bacteria previously listed for macrolides and lincomycin. An additional organism for which there is activity is *Toxoplasma.* The clinical use of clindamycin for treating toxoplasmosis in cats is controversial.

PHARMACOKINETICS

ABSORPTION AND DISTRIBUTION. Clindamycin is better absorbed from the GI tract in humans and animals than lincomycin, yielding higher serum concentrations, and is more active than lincomycin due to the chlorine substitution (Nichols and Keys 1984). Brown and coworkers (Brown et al. 1989; Brown et al. 1990) have described the pharmacokinetics of oral clindamycin HCl disposition in the cat. Groups of cats were given oral doses of either 5.5, 11.0, or 22.0 mg/kg once daily of clindamycin (Antirobe), with physical, histologic, and hematologic changes recorded during therapy. Mean residence time was reported to be 276, 274, and 393 minutes, respectively. It was also found that the 5.5 and 11.0 mg/kg oral doses maintained a serum MIC above that necessary for most *Staphylococcus aureus* infections and that the 11.0 and 22.0 mg/kg doses gave serum concentrations above the MIC for many susceptible anaerobes. Clindamycin is distributed well to tissues and attains high intracellular concentrations as exhibited by the high V_d. The apparent V_d in cats was 1.62, 1.76, and 3.06 L/kg for the 5.5, 11, and 22 mg/kg doses, respectively. The highest concentrations of clindamycin were found in the lung, followed by liver, spleen, jejunum, and colon. Although the CSF had very low but detectable levels of clindamycin, the brain had higher than anticipated concentrations. This was most likely due to clindamycin's lipophilic nature, having a greater affinity for the lipid matrix of the brain than for the aqueous CSF. Bone marrow also had appreciable levels of clindamycin accumulation, due to sequestration of clindamycin in the fat, the concentration of clindamycin in the white blood cell precursors, or a combination of both factors.

In the dog (Budsberg et al. 1992; Lavy et al. 1999), clindamycin phosphate was administered IV, IM, and SC at 10 and 11 mg/kg. The elimination half-life was 2–3.2 hours IV but longer (5–7 hr) from IM and SC injection. The V_d was 0.9–1.4 L/kg. The bioavailability of clindamycin in one study after IM injection was 87% (Budsberg et al. 1992), but in another study bioavailability was greater than 100% from an IM dose and over 300% from the SC dose (Lavy et al. 1999). It appears that the prolonged elimination half-life from the SC administration ("flip-flop" effect) resulted in a falsely high estimate of the true availability following IM and SC administration in these studies. In one study, it was reported that clindamycin is too painful for IM administration (Budsberg et al. 1992), but in another study, IM administration of a buffered, more concentrated 20% solution was better tolerated. However, the SC dose was much better tolerated (Lavy et al. 1999) and produced more prolonged concentrations.

Unlike lincomycin, the presence of food does not appear to affect oral absorption of clindamycin. There is good penetration into respiratory secretions, pleural fluid, the prostate, bones, and joints, but with low concentrations appearing in the CSF. The concentrations of clindamycin in phagocytes are 10- to 20-fold (and as high as 40) times the plasma concentrations (Harari and Lincoln 1989). Despite the high intracellular concentrations of clindamycin in phagocytes, intracellular killing is poor (Yancy et al. 1991), perhaps because the drug is sequestered in subcellular sites. Macrophages take up clindamycin by an active transport mechanism and concentrate clindamycin up to 50 times the extracellular concentration (Dhawan and Thadepalli 1982). Because phagocytes are the cells most likely to enter infected tissues, such as abscesses, it is possible for clindamycin to be transported to an abscess and eradicate the bacteria (Yancy et al. 1991). Clindamycin also crosses the placental barrier, but its safety during pregnancy has not been determined.

METABOLISM AND EXCRETION. Clindamycin HCl requires no metabolism to be active once administered orally. Clindamycin phosphate requires hydrolysis to occur in the plasma to be active; similarly, clindamycin palmitate requires the removal of the palmitate moiety in the small intestine to be active.

Clindamycin metabolites are much like those described for lincomycin. In dogs, 36% of the administered dose of clindamycin is excreted unchanged by the bile and urine. The balance of the dose appears to be active or inactive metabolites, 28% excreted by the liver in the glucuronide form (no antimicrobial activity), 28% as clindamycin sulfoxide (25% of the antimicrobial activity of the parent antibiotic), and 9% as *N*-demethyl clindamycin, which has 4–8 times the antimicrobial activity of the parent compound (Dhawan and Thadepalli 1982). The bile is the major excretion route. The colonic contents of humans administered clindamycin were found to suppress microbial activity for as long as 2 weeks after the discontinuation of therapy.

ADVERSE EFFECTS AND PRECAUTIONS. Like lincomycin, the most serious adverse effect in humans is pseudomembranous colitis, from overgrowth of *Clostridium difficile.* This has not been a reported problem in animals. In dogs and cats, vomiting and diarrhea are possible but they are transient and not serious. However, GI problems such as those discussed above for lincomycin in ruminants, horses, rabbits, and rodents are possible, and the same precautions apply that were discussed for lincomycin. Greene et al. (1992) orally administered to cats 25 and 50 mg/kg clindamycin HCl divided in 2 doses and found that diarrhea and vomiting are two clinical signs most often associated with oral therapy. The highest frequency for both of these clinical signs occurred in the 50 mg/kg treatment group and was thought to be related to either a direct irritant effect on the GI tract or some effect on intestinal water absorption. Cats are also reluctant to accept the oral liquid form of clindamycin because of poor palatability.

A study was performed in cats to ascertain the effect of prolonged clindamycin therapy on vitamin K–dependent blood clotting times (Jacobs et al. 1989). The study showed that factor VII levels did not significantly change in cats treated with a total daily dose of 25 mg/kg orally once daily for 6 weeks compared to controls.

CLINICAL USE. Clindamycin possesses an antimicrobial spectrum similar to that of lincomycin, but it is much more extensively used clinically than lincomycin because of higher activity against anaerobes, increased potency, and more complete oral absorption. Clindamycin has been reported to be as much as 20 times more potent than lincomycin in the treatment of *Staphylococcus* and *Streptococcus* infections in humans (Harvey 1985). Clindamycin is active against aerobic species of organisms, including *Staphylococcus, Streptococcus, Actinomyces, Nocardia, Mycoplasma,* and *Toxoplasma.* The anaerobic bacterial spectrum of activity includes *Bacteroides fragilis, Fusobacterium* spp., *Peptostreptococcus* spp., and *Clostridium perfringens* (Harari and Lincoln 1989). Clindamycin has been used to treat wounds, abscesses, osteomyelitis, and periodontal diseases caused by these organisms. Clindamycin is found in high concentrations in the prostate, making it an acceptable choice for treating bacterial prostatitis when caused by gram-positive organisms.

The use of clindamycin for treating toxoplasmosis is controversial. Lappin et al. (1989) performed a retrospective study of cats diagnosed with *Toxoplasma gondii* infections and found that those cats treated with clindamycin resolved all clinical signs of the disease except those lesions involving the eyes. Clindamycin alone or in combination with a corticosteroid helped to resolve the active retinochoroiditis and the anterior uveitis associated with this disease. Even though clindamycin may help clinical signs associated with toxoplasmosis, it may not help to clear organisms from the CNS or the eye. In experimentally infected cats, there was a paradoxical effect in that cats with toxoplasmosis treated with clindamycin had a worsening of clinical signs. As discussed in more detail by Davidson et al. (1996), this paradoxical effect may be due to an inhibition of intracellular killing of organisms by clindamycin.

Clindamycin can be used to treat *Staphylococcus aureus* infections in dogs with experimentally induced posttraumatic osteomyelitis (Braden et al. 1988; Braden et al. 1987). An oral dose 11 mg/kg orally twice daily for 28 days was found to be efficacious in treatment of these infected dogs, resulting in a 94% recovery rate in the clindamycin-treated dogs. Clindamycin also has been shown to be effective for treatment of superficial pyoderma in dogs and is a common choice as an alternative to β-lactam antibiotics (Harvey et al. 1993; Noli and Boothe 1999). In dogs, dosing 11 mg/kg IV every 12 hours should be sufficient for treating most *Staphylococcus* spp. infections, and increasing the frequency of dosing to every 6 or 8 hours should increase serum concentrations sufficiently to combat most susceptible pathogenic anaerobes.

MISCELLANEOUS ANTIBIOTICS

Bacitracin. Bacitracin is a complex labile polypeptide consisting of 5–10 separate chemical components first isolated from a *Bacillus subtillus*–contaminated wound in 1943 (Teske 1984). Bacitracin A ($C_{66}H_{103}N_{17}O_{16}S$) is the major component of this mixture and accounts for most of the antibiotic activities. Bacitracin inhibits peptidoglycan synthesis in bacteria by nonspecifically blocking phosphorylase reactions, some of which occur during cell wall synthesis (Lancini and Parenti 1982). Development of resistance to bacitracin is rare.

Bacitracin is effective against gram-positive organisms when administered topically or parenterally. Bacitracin is not absorbed from the GI tract when given orally. Systemic administration has resulted in a high incidence of nephrotoxicity (albuminuria, cylindruria, azotemia), in addition to pain, induration, and petechiae at the site of injection. In contrast, bacitracin is nonirritating and rarely induces allergic reactions when used topically. Bacitracin (bacitracin, bacitracin methylenedisalicylate, bacitracin manganese, zinc bacitracin) has been used as a feed additive to promote growth in many species of animals, but its most common use today is in topical applications to treat susceptible skin, ear, and eye infections. Bacitracin inhibits many organisms found on skin, such as hemolytic and nonhemolytic *Streptococcus* spp., coagulase-positive *Staphylococcus* spp., and some *Clostridium* spp., and it is often combined with other antibiotics that have a gram-negative spectrum of activity (polymyxin B, neomycin). Zinc bacitracin administered topically may increase the activity of bacitracin due to zinc's astringent properties, which decrease inflammation (Harvey 1985).

Novobiocin. Novobiocin is a dibasic acid (pK_a = 4.3 and 9.1) derived from coumarin and is utilized clinically as a mono- (Na^+) or dibasic (Ca^{++}) salt form. Novobiocin possesses activity against both gram-positive and gram-negative bacteria but is more efficacious against the gram positives, in particular *Staphylococcus aureus.* Other susceptible organisms include *Neisseria* spp., *Haemophilus* spp., *Brucella* spp., and some strains of *Proteus* spp. It may be used as an alternative to penicillins in cases involving penicillin-resistant *Staphylococcus* spp., although other penicillin substitutes (cephalosporins, macrolides, clindamycin) are better clinical choices.

Novobiocin has several toxic effects on bacteria, but its exact mechanism and site of action are unknown. Novobiocin has been shown to cause nonspecific inhibition of cell wall synthesis by inhibiting formation of alternating *N*-acetylmuramic acid pentapeptide and *N*-acetylglucosamine residues; it also inhibits teichuronic acid in some species of bacteria. The concentrations needed to inhibit these cell wall components are greater than the minimal concentration needed to inhibit growth, suggesting these effects on bacteria are secondary effects. DNA and RNA synthesis, protein synthesis (β-galactosidase), respiration, and oxidative phosphorylation are also inhibited in some species of bacteria and in rat liver homogenates (Morris and Russell 1971), with none seemingly being the primary antibiotic effect. Novobiocin is also known to induce an intracellular magnesium deficiency, but there is no direct convincing evidence that this is the mechanism responsible for novobiocin's antimicrobial activity.

Novobiocin is initially highly effective against *Staphylococcus* spp. infections, but resistance to this antibiotic develops quickly (Morris and Russell 1971; Harvey 1985). Synergism occurs when novobiocin is combined with tetracycline. Novobiocin has been combined with tetracycline in a commercial preparation (Delta-Albaplex, Upjohn) to broaden the spectrum of activity and to decrease the resistance to novobiocin. Novobiocin and tetracycline have been reported to be efficacious in cases of canine upper respiratory diseases such as "kennel cough" and tonsillitis (Maxey 1980). Toxic side effects in animals and humans given novobiocin systemically have been reported and include skin rashes, leucopenia, pancytopenia, anemia, agranulocytosis, thrombocytopenia, nausea, vomiting, and diarrhea. Few side effects have been reported for this antibiotic used in its topical form in domestic animals.

Thiostrepton. Thiostrepton is a polypeptide antibiotic produced by *Streptomyces aureus* and has a predominately gram-positive spectrum, although some gram-negative organisms are also affected. Thiostrepton is not absorbed from the GI tract and is used primarily for topical local therapy, usually combined with other antibiotics and/or glucocorticosteroids for dermatologic therapy (Huber 1982).

Rifampin. Rifampin is a complex macrocyclic high-molecular-weight semisynthetic antibiotic derived from rifamycin B, produced by *Nocardia mediterrea.* Rifamycin B is chemically modified to produce rifampin (US and Canadian name), also known as rifampicin in Europe. The chemical structure of rifampin is shown in Fig. 44.7. Rifampin has a high activity against gram-positive bacteria (*Staphylococcus* spp.), *Mycobacterium* spp., *Haemophilus* spp., *Neisseria* spp., and *Chlamydia* spp., and some limited activity against the gram-negative bacteria.

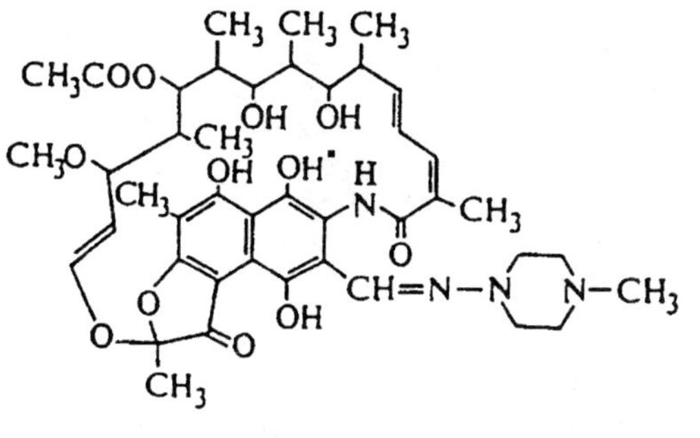

FIG. 44.7—The chemical structure of rifampin.

Rifampin is highly lipid soluble, is stable in acidic environments, and can concentrate in neutrophils and macrophages, which is therapeutically advantageous in diseases involving intracellular organisms (*Brucella, Mycobacterium, Rhodococcus, Chlamydia,* etc.) and chronic granulomatous diseases. Rifampin enters the microbial cell and forms stable complexes with the β subunit of DNA-dependent RNA polymerases of microorganisms. This binding results in inactive enzymes and inhibition of RNA synthesis by preventing chain initiation. This inhibition can also occur in mammalian cells, but much higher concentrations are needed. MICs for gram-positive organisms generally occur at 0.1 μg/mL, while gram negatives have MIC values ranging from 8 to 32 μg/mL. This large disparity in MIC values is attributed to rifampin's ability to more easily permeate the gram-positive organism cell wall than the gram-negative organism cell wall rather than differences in bacterial RNA polymerases.

Rifampin is rapidly absorbed from the GI tract after oral administration in humans, dogs, calves, horses, and foals. Rifampin absorption is highest in an acidic environment; hence the presence of food in the stomach tends to slow its absorption. Sheep also tend to have a prolonged oral absorption due to transit time through the rumen. Rifampin is approximately 80% bound to plasma proteins, with the remainder being widely distributed to all tissues of the body, with particularly high concentrations of the drug found in the lungs, liver, bile, and urine. After oral absorption or parenteral administration, rifampin is primarily metabolized to the bioactive metabolite 25-desacetylrifampin, with some minor glucuronidation products formed in the liver. Both parent and metabolite compounds are excreted in the bile, where enterohepatic circulation occurs for both forms. Both forms are passively filtered through the kidneys, with renal clearance being approximately 12% of total glomerular filtration rate.

Multiple dosing of rifampin often results in decreased, rather than increased, peak serum concentrations. This phenomenon is due to autoinduction of liver enzymes and is known to occur in humans, swine, dogs, calves, and rodents (Frank 1990). Hepatic enzyme induction by rifampin will also alter the disposition of other drugs. Plasma ketoconazole levels decrease and the metabolism of progestin, digitalis, warfarin, glucocorticosteroids, and several other drugs increases when they are concurrently administered with rifampin (Kenny and Strates 1981; Frank 1990).

The pharmacokinetics of rifampin has been studied in humans (Acocella 1983; Kenny and Strates 1981), in the adult horse (Burrows et al. 1985), and in the foal (Castro et al. 1986). Adult horses given 10 mg/kg of rifampin IV, IM, or PO showed a rapid absorption of rifampin by the oral route versus the IM route, but the IM route provided longer detectable plasma concentrations in 50% of the horses than did the oral route. Adult horses given 10 mg/kg IV showed a serum half-life of 6.05 hours and an apparent V_d of 0.7 L/kg. Doses of 10 mg/kg administered IM and PO had half-lives of 7.32 and 5.84 hours, respectively. Oral doses of 25 mg/kg in adult horses had a serum half-life of 4.78 hours. It was determined that the 10 mg/kg PO dose was adequate for susceptible gram-positive infections in the adult horse, whereas the 10 mg/kg IV or the 25 mg/kg PO dose was necessary to treat susceptible gram-negative infections. The rate of excretion in the foal is lower than in the adult horse, mainly due to biliary excretion mechanisms being less developed in the foal. Foals given 10 mg/kg of rifampin orally had a mean serum half-life of 17.5 hours, significantly longer than that found in the adult horse. The authors of that study indicated that 5 mg/kg orally was sufficient in the foal to combat susceptible gram-positive infections and that higher or more-frequent doses were needed to treat susceptible gram-negative infections.

The pharmacokinetics of rifampin has also been studied in sheep (Jernigan et al. 1986), with the recommended dose from that study being 20 mg/kg orally once a day. In sheep administered a 50 mg/kg dose of rifampin IV, the serum half-life was 4.56 hours and the apparent V_d was 0.5 L/kg.

Ciprofloxacin pharmacokinetics in relation to coadministration with rifampin has been described for the rabbit (Barriere et al. 1989). Rifampin is a known inducer of oxidative drug metabolism, causing an increase in smooth endoplasmic reticulum and increased cytochrome P-450 production within the mammalian hepatic cells. Ciprofloxacin undergoes oxidative metabolism in the liver. Rabbits were dosed with 25 mg/kg IV of ciprofloxacin and 2–10 mg/kg of rifampin IM. This study found a substantial decrease in the serum half-life of ciprofloxacin and increases in clearance and V_d of ciprofloxacin after rifampin treatments. Those animals receiving only ciprofloxacin had concentrations in serum that were on average 40% higher than those in animals receiving both rifampin and ciprofloxacin. This study indicates that concurrent administration of rifampin and ciprofloxacin may actually decrease the clinical effectiveness of ciprofloxacin in vivo in the rabbit, with similar effects in other species being possible.

Rifampin has been used to treat a wide variety of microbial infections. Susceptible organisms of interest to veterinarians include *Staphylococcus aureus* and *Staphylococcus epidermidis* (including methicillin-resistant strains), *Streptococcus* spp., *Rhodococcus equi, Corynebacterium pseudotuberculosis,* and most strains of *Bacteroides* spp., *Clostridium* spp., *Neisseria* spp., and *Listeria* spp. Organisms known to be resistant to rifampin are *Pseudomonas aeruginosa, E. coli, Enterobacter* spp., *Klebsiella pneumoniae, Proteus* spp., and *Salmonella* spp. Wilson et al. (1988) obtained samples from clinically ill horses and tested the isolated bacteria for susceptibility to rifampin. It was found that all strains of coagulase-positive *Staphylococcus* spp., *Streptococcus zooepidemicus, Streptococcus equi, Streptococcus equisimilus, Rhodococcus equi,* and *Corynebacterium pseudotuberculosis* were highly susceptible to rifampin at MICs of 0.25 μg/mL. Gram-negative organisms isolated in that study were *Actinobacillus suis, Actinobacillus equuli,* and *Bordetella bronchiseptica,* and MIC values ranged from <0.008 to >16 μg/mL. Other isolates, such as *Pseudomonas aeruginosa, Enterobacter cloacae, Klebsiella pneumoniae, Proteus* spp., and *Salmonella* spp., were found to be resistant, having MICs greater than 4 μg/mL.

Rifampin is used to treat equine diseases of a gram-positive bacterial origin (e.g., *Rhodococcus equi, Streptococcus equi*). However, resistance to rifampin is quickly acquired when administered alone to combat these infections. Resistance is readily accomplished by a single mutation of the amino acid sequence of the β subunit of the DNA-dependent RNA polymerase enzyme. Mutations result in rifampin having less affinity for the RNA polymerase enzyme. Higher concentrations of rifampin are necessary to overcome this resistance in vitro. Resistance can be minimized if other antibiotics are used concurrently with rifampin that will kill the mutant strains of bacteria produced in response to rifampin. Antibiotics that can be so used are erythromycin, most of the β-lactam antibiotics, vancomycin, and gentamicin, depending on the bacterial sensitivity to these drugs (Frank 1990).

Synergism may occur between amphotericin B and rifampin against some fungi, particularly *Saccharomyces cerevisiae, Histoplasma capsulatum,* several species of *Aspergillus,* and *Blastomyces dermatitidis* (Medoff 1983). Increased permeability of rifampin across the fungal cell wall (and hence increased inhibition of RNA polymerases) due to amphotericin B–induced cell wall damage is probably the mechanism responsible for this synergism.

Rifampin is a potent inducer of hepatic microsomal enzymes and is also teratogenic in laboratory animals, so its use in pregnant animals should be restricted. Rifampin has also been reported to turn the urine red. Dogs given the human dose of 10 mg/kg orally developed increases in hepatic enzyme activity, some of which eventually progressed to clinical cases of hepatitis. Hepatitis is the most common reason to discontinue rifampin treatment in dogs. However, lowering the total daily dose of rifampin will decrease the chances of inducing toxic side effects, especially in dogs. Although rare, rifampin can induce thrombocytopenia, hemolytic anemia, anorexia, vomiting, and diarrhea. Preexisting renal disease does not normally require a dose modification of rifampin.

Nitrofurans. Nitrofurans comprise several synthetic compounds derived from 5-nitrofuran and possess antimicrobial activity, the 5-nitro group being required for this activity. Over 3500 nitrofurans have been synthesized to date, with only a handful being useful in animal chemotherapy. Nitrofurans and furazolidone are banned from use in food-producing animals.

Nitrofurans as a group are bacteriostatic and function by blocking oxidative decarboxylation of pyruvate to acetyl coenzyme A, depriving susceptible organisms of vital energy production pathways. Their spectrum of activity encompasses gram-positive and gram-negative bacteria and some protozoans, but they are most effective against the gram-negative bacteria. Nitrofurans can be administered orally or topically. Oral absorption is enhanced when administered with feed; it is widely distributed throughout the body but in low concentrations. Approximately 50% of the total dose of nitrofurans is excreted in the active form. Acidification of the urine promotes tubular reabsorption, which also decreases the overall urine concentration of the drug. An acid environment is required for the nitrofurans to diffuse across the cell membranes. Nitrofurantoin has a broad gram-positive and gram-negative spectrum and also high concentrations in the urine, making it useful as a urinary antiseptic in small animals. Nitrofuran use today is mainly in topical preparations for the eye, ear, mucous membranes, and skin; it finds limited use in treating bacterial GI tract and urinary tract disorders (Ali 1989; Ford and Aronson 1985).

The major disadvantage of nitrofurans to treat systemic infections is that the concentrations needed to reach the MIC also induce systemic toxicity. There are many reports in the veterinary literature on the toxicities induced when the nitrofurans are used systemically (Ali 1983). The toxicology of furazolidone (*N*-5-nitro-2-furfurylidene amino-2-oxazolidinone) has been investigated extensively in laboratory, food, and companion animals as well as in humans and has been reviewed by Ali (1989). The effects of feeding furazolidone to poultry have been reported (Ali 1989; Mustafa et al. 1975; Czarnecki et al. 1974a; Jankus et al. 1972; Czarnecki et al. 1974b).

Furazolidone has also been demonstrated to be carcinogenic when used at a 0.15% w/w concentration in feed for 1 year, inducing mammary tumors in a dose-related manner. Mice fed a 0.03% w/w concentration in feed for life developed bronchial adenocarcinomas in both sexes (Ali 1983). DNA is the principal target of furazolidone in some cells in vivo, causing cuts and mutations in DNA and binding to DNA, hence blocking the replication and transcription processes. Mutagenesis by nitrofurans in general also occurs and has been extensively reviewed by McCalla (1983), who notes several possible metabolic pathways by which nitrofurans can cause mutagenesis in mammalian cells.

Virginiamycin. Virginiamycin is a combination of two chemicals produced by *Streptomyces virginiae,* isolated from soil samples in Belgium in the early 1960s. Virginiamycin is classified as a peptolide antibiotic composed of the predominate M fraction ($C_{28}H_{35}N_3O_7$) and the lesser S fraction ($C_{43}H_{49}NO_{10}$) (Crawford 1984). The optimum ratio of M:S is 4:1 (Gottschall et al. 1988). Administered separately, both M and S fractions have a reversible bacteriostatic action on susceptible bacterial populations; used together, their activity is synergistic, bactericidal, and approximately 100 times that found when used separately. Virginiamycin is not known to be synergistic with other classes of antibiotics. Virginiamycin is primarily active against gram-positive organisms, *Haemophilus* spp., and *Neisseria* spp. and has mild activity against the protozoan *Toxoplasma* spp. It works by inhibiting protein synthesis at the 23S ribosomal subunit, blocking translation but not transcription in susceptible bacteria. Virginiamycin is rapidly absorbed when administered orally, is excreted by the bile with no enterohepatic circulation, and has an affinity for dermal tissues (Crawford 1984). Gottschall et al. (1988) reported that ^{14}C-virginiamycin, specifically the M fraction, was extensively metabolized in the rumen. The S fraction underwent no detectable metabolism in the rumen, and the M fraction metabolites had considerably less antimicrobial activity than the parent compound.

All virginiamycin-like antibiotics fall into one of two groups. Group A consists of polyunsaturated cyclic peptolides that have a molecular weight of approximately 500 and that contain substituted aminodecanoic acid and an oxanzole system. Group B are all cyclic hexadepsipeptides with an approximate molecular weight of 800, and most members contain one molecule of pipecolic acid or its derivative. Both groups have low solubilities in aqueous solvents and are more soluble in organic solvents. All strongly absorb ultraviolet radiation and are therefore degraded in its presence. Virginiamycin-like antibiotics tend to affect gram-positive bacteria more than the gram negatives, with *Mycobacteria* spp. being relatively resistant and *Haemophilus* spp. and *Neisseria* spp. being very sensitive. Differences in bacterial sensitivity to different virginiamycin-like antibiotics are due to each antibiotic's particular ability to permeate that bacteria's cell wall to gain access to the ribosomes (Cocito 1979).

Virginiamycin and virginiamycin-like antibiotics are not commonly used to treat clinical bacterial disease in domestic animals, despite their rather broad spectrum of activity. They have been used to treat swine dysentery (*Treponema hyodysenteriae*) (Olsen and Rodabaugh 1977), but other antibiotics have proven to be more efficacious. Its main use has been as a feed additive for growth promotion in food animals such as swine (Ravindran and Kornegay 1984; Moser et al. 1985), being approved for this use since 1975. Virginiamycin has also been studied in turkeys (Salmon and Stevens 1990), broilers (Miles et al. 1984), and laying hens (Miles et al. 1985) as a growth promotant, all of which experienced either increased weight gain or increased egg production.

Carbadox. Carbadox (methyl 3-(2-quinoxalinylmethylene) carbazate N^1,N^4 dioxide) is a synthetic antibacterial agent primarily active against the gram-positive bacteria, although some gram-negative bacteria are affected as well. Available in 1973, carbadox was marketed as a growth promotant in swine and also for the control of swine dysentery *(Treponema hyodysenteriae)*, bacterial enteritis (in particular, *Salmonella cholerasuis*), and nasal infections of *Bordetella bronchiseptica* in swine (Farrington and Shively 1979; Huber 1982). Carbadox was shown to be better than lincomycin for the treatment of swine dysentery (Anonymous 1980; Rainier et al. 1980). Resistance to carbadox has been reported in *E. coli* via R-plasmids (Ohmae et al. 1981).

The daily feeding of carbadox in feed concentrations of more than 100 ppm for growth promotion in pigs has resulted in toxicities in some weaned pigs, which include growth retardation, dry feces, wasting, dehydration, urine drinking, and a strong interest in salt-containing products (van der Molen et al. 1989a). It is now known that carbadox suppresses aldosterone production, leading to hypoaldosteronism, which then leads to decreased plasma sodium and increased plasma potassium concentrations. These ion alterations are due to stimulation of the renin-angiotensin system with subsequent morphological changes in the zona glomerulosa of the adrenal cortex (van der Molen et al. 1989a; van der Molen et al. 1989b; van der Molen et al. 1989c).

Vancomycin. Of the glycopeptides, vancomycin is the only one used in veterinary medicine. Teicoplanin is used in Europe but is not available in the United States. Vancomycin is not a new antibiotic; it was discovered in the 1950s. In the 1960s and 1970s it was not used much because the penicillins and cephalosporins were active against most gram-positive bacteria. But in the last 10–15 years resistant enterococcal and staphylococcal infections have generated more reliance on vancomycin in human medicine. Vancomycin is a tricyclic glycopeptide having an approximate molecular weight of 1500. It is produced by the soil-borne actinomycete *Streptomyces orientalis.* It is freely soluble in water, odorless, and slightly bitter to the taste. Vancomycin is highly active against gram-positive cocci (in particular, *Staphylococcus* spp. and streptococci), enterococci (*Enterococcus faecium* and *E. faecalis*), as well as *Neisseria* spp. It also is active against gram-positive anaerobic cocci (but not anaerobic gram-negative bacteria) and has been administered to people for diarrhea caused by *Clostridium* spp.

Vancomycin functions as a bactericidal antibiotic by inhibiting the synthesis of the linear peptidoglycan in the bacterial cell wall during replication, resulting in the bacterium's rapid death. Over 80 *n*-alkyl vancomycins have been synthesized by reductive alkylation of vancomycin, with some forms being 5 times more active than vancomycin and with some having longer elimination half-lives (Nagarajan et al. 1989).

ADVERSE EFFECTS. The most common adverse effect is kidney injury. Early formulations of vancomycin were associated with a high incidence of adverse effects. Most of these effects were associated with rapid IV administration, which induced flushing of the skin, pruritus, tachycardia, and other signs attributed to histamine release. Nephrotoxicity and ototoxicity also were reported. Newer formulations are safer, but histamine release still is possible from IV administration. Toxicity studies on vancomycin have been performed in many species of laboratory animals (Wold and Turnipseed 1981). The LD_{50} for the canine was 292 mg/kg, but death did not occur until several days after dosing. Dogs that died typically had blood urea nitrogen (BUN) values between 250 and 300 mg/dL, death presumably being due to acute nephrotoxic renal failure.

CLINICAL USE AND ADMINISTRATION GUIDELINES. Clinical use of vancomycin has been limited in veterinary medicine and most of our clinical recommendations for use are derived from pharmacokinetic studies performed in dogs and recommendations of effective blood concentrations for people. Vancomycin must be administered via IV infusion, although in rare instances intraperitoneal administration has been used. Vancomycin is poorly absorbed orally and this route is not used except to treat intestinal infections. IM administration is painful and irritating.

In dogs the half-life is somewhat shorter and the V_d smaller than in humans (Zaghlol and Brown 1988). In order to keep the plasma concentration within a suggested window of 10–30 μg/mL, the dose rate of 15 mg/kg q6h IV is recommended. (This dose actually produces peaks and troughs of approximately 40 and 5 μg/mL, respectively, but it is the most convenient dose that can be used because of the short half-life in dogs.) This dose should be infused slowly over 30–60 minutes, or a rate of approximately 10 mg/min. The total dose to be administered can be diluted in 0.9% saline or 5% dextrose solution, but not alkalinizing solutions. Vancomycin is available in vials of 500 mg to 5 g (Vancocin, other brands, and generic). If vancomycin is used to treat enterococcal infections, it is strongly recommended to coadminister an aminoglycoside (e.g., amikacin or gentamicin) because when used alone, vancomycin is not bactericidal.

If vancomycin is administered according to the recommended dosing rates, adverse reactions described earlier are rare. A slow infusion is recommended to minimize histamine release. To avoid other toxic reactions, dose recommendations are designed to avoid high plasma concentrations. In people, therapeutic drug monitoring is often performed to ensure that peak concentrations are below 50 μg/mL and the trough concentrations are above 5 μg/mL. If animals have renal disease or unique physiologic changes (e.g., pregnant or a neonatal animal), drug disposition may change, and peak and trough plasma concentrations should be monitored to adjust the dose appropriately.

REGULATORY CONSIDERATIONS. In August 20, 1997, the USFDA prohibited the extralabel use of glycopeptides in food-producing animals for fear of glycopeptide-resistant bacteria being transmitted to humans from treated animals (Bates et al. 1994). Feeding glycopeptides to animals is not legal in the United States.

Methenamine. Methenamine (hexamethylenetetramine) is a urinary antiseptic most commonly used to treat urinary tract infections in small animals. It may be used in conjunction with an antibiotic or occasionally by itself in some cases of bacterial urinary tract infections that have become refractory to conventional antibiotic therapies. Methenamine is activated by a hydrolysis reaction to form formaldehyde and ammonia in acidic urine. It has been proven to be effective against a wide variety of gram-positive and gram-negative organisms but will not affect the growth of *Candida albicans*. It can be either bacteriostatic or bactericidal depending on the pH of the urine (Huber 1982; Harvey 1985).

Methenamine is quickly absorbed when given orally, is excreted via the urine, and is associated with a low systemic toxicity. For this drug to be efficacious, the urine must be at an acidic pH in order to liberate free formaldehyde. Methenamine is often found combined with mandelate (mandelic acid), which assists in lowering the urine pH and also exerts some independent weak antibacterial activity. Concurrent use of other urinary acidifiers, such as ascorbic acid, arginine HCl, methionine, cranberry juice (hippurate), and ammonium chloride, will enhance the antibacterial action of methenamine. Methenamine is most effective when the urine pH is 6 or below. Sulfonamides should not be administered with methenamine due to the formation of insoluble formaldehyde-sulfonamide precipitates. Since methenamine is largely eliminated via the kidney, its use should be restricted or closely monitored in cases of renal insufficiency (Huber 1982; Harvey 1985). Methenamine is less effective for treating infections caused by urea-splitting organisms which increase the urine pH (e.g., *Proteus mirabilis*).

Methenamine mandelate has been used experimentally in the treatment of burn wounds in rats. Topical doses of 5% and 10% were highly efficacious against experimentally induced burns infected with a virulent strain of *Pseudomonas* spp. (Taylor et al. 1970).

Polymyxins. Polymyxins are a group of *N*-monoacetylated decapeptides discovered in 1947 and are produced by *Bacillus polymyxa*. They contain 7 amino acids in a cyclic configuration and have a molecular weight of approximately 1000. Several polymyxins have been isolated and have been named A, B, C, D, E, and M. Of these 6 antibiotics, B and E in their sulfate salt forms are the only ones used clinically. Polymyxin B sulfate is a mixture of polymyxin B_1 ($C_{56}H_{98}N_{16}O_3$) and polymyxin B_2 ($C_{55}H_{96}N_{16}O_{13}$); polymyxin E is more commonly known as colistin (Harvey 1985). Polymyxin B_1 has a pK_a ranging from 8 to 9.

Polymyxins are basic surface-active cationic detergents that interact with the phospholipid within the cell membrane, penetrate that membrane, and then disrupt its structure. This action subsequently induces permeability changes within the cell that result in cell death, giving polymyxins bactericidal properties.

Polymyxins are not absorbed to any extent from the GI tract when administered orally but are rapidly absorbed when given parenterally, with 70–90% plasma protein binding. Polymyxin B is rapidly distributed to the heart, lungs, liver, kidney, and skeletal muscle, with excretion mainly via the urine (Sande and Mandell 1990a). The pharmacokinetics of some of the polymyxins in calves, ewes, rabbits, and dogs is reviewed in greater detail elsewhere (Ziv and Sulman 1973a; Ziv et al. 1982; Craig and Kunin 1973; al-Khayyat and Aronson 1973a,b). Ziv and Sulman (1973a) reported that an IV administration of 5 mg/kg polymyxin B in ewes resulted in a serum half-life of 2.7–4.3 hours and a V_d of 1.29 L/kg.

Polymyxins have a gram-negative antibacterial spectrum, which includes *Aerobacter, Escherichia, Haemophilus, Klebsiella, Pasteurella, Pseudomonas, Salmonella,* and *Shigella. Proteus* spp. and most strains of *Serratia* spp. are not affected by polymyxins, and all gram-positive bacteria are resistant. If bacteria are sensitive to the polymyxins, they rarely acquire resistance. The ability of each antibiotic in this group to kill these bacteria varies (Harvey 1985). The antimicrobial actions of polymyxin B are inhibited by divalent cations, unsaturated fatty acids, debris, purulent exudate, and quaternary ammonium compounds.

Since the polymyxins are not absorbed into the body when given orally, polymyxin B has been used for "bowel sterilization" prior to abdominal surgeries and in irrigation solutions to flush the peritoneal cavities during those procedures. Polymyxins used to be the major drugs for treatment of *Pseudomonas* infections in humans, but since the advent of better penicillins, aminoglycosides, and cephalosporins, their use has declined over time. Nephrotoxicity occurs due to glomerulus and tubular epithelium damage. In addition, respiratory paralysis (usually due to a rapid IV injection, too much peritoneal lavage, or a preexisting renal condition) and CNS dysfunction, including depression, pyrexia, and anorexia, also occur. Polymyxins are mainly used in topical skin, mucous membrane, eye, and ear preparations. No adverse systemic effects have been reported when they are applied to intact or denuded skin surfaces. Polymyxin antibacterial activity is markedly decreased in the presence of pus, in tissues containing acidic phospholipids, and in the presence of anionic detergents or other chemicals that antagonize cationic detergents (Harvey 1985).

In addition to its narrow-spectrum antimicrobial properties, polymyxin B has demonstrated a protective effect against the adverse effects of endotoxin produced by gram-negative bacteria. Mechanistically, the cationic portion of polymyxin B binds to the anionic lipid A portion of this endotoxin. This effectively renders the endotoxin inactive, thereby preventing most of the adverse effects that gram-negative endotoxin has on the mammalian body. The largest use of polymyxin, however, has been in topical ointment preparations.

REFERENCES

Abdullah, A.S., and Baggot, J.D. 1986. Effect of short term starvation on disposition kinetics of chloramphenicol in goats. Res Vet Sci 40:382–385.

Acocella, G. 1983. Pharmacokinetics and metabolism of rifampin in humans. Rev Infect Diseases 5(Suppl 3):S428–S432.

Adams, H.R., and Dixit, B.N. 1970. Prolongation of pentobarbital anesthesia by chloramphenicol in dogs and cats. JAVMA 156:902–905.

Adams, P.E., Varma, K.J., Powers, T.E., and Lamendola, J.F. 1987. Tissue concentrations and pharmacokinetics of florfenicol in male veal calves given repeated doses. Am J Vet Res 48(12):1715–1732.

Adamson, P.J.W., Wilson, W.D., Baggot, J.D., Hietala, S.K., and Mihalyi, J.E. 1991. Influence of age on the disposition kinetics of chloramphenicol in equine neonates. Am J Vet Res 52(3):426–431.

Ali, B.H. 1983. Some pharmcologic and toxicologic properties of furazolidone. Vet Res Commun 6:1–11.

———. 1989. Pharmacology and toxicity of furazolidone in man and animals: some recent research. Gen Pharmac 5:557–563.

Ali, B.H., Hassan, T., Wasfi, I.A., and Mustafa, A. 1984. Toxicity of furazolidone to Nubian goats. Vet Hum Toxicol 26(3):197–200.

al-Khayyat, A.A., and Aronson, A.L. 1973a. Pharmacologic and toxicologic studies with the polymyxins. II. Comparative pharmacologic studies of the sulfate and methanesulfonate salts of polymyxin B and colistin in dogs. Chemotherapy 19:82–97.

———. 1973b. Pharmacologic and toxicologic studies with the polymyxins. III. Considerations regarding clinical use in dogs. Chemotherapy 19:98–107.

Ambrose, P.J. 1984. Clinical pharmacokinetics of chloramphenicol and chloramphenicol succinate. Clin Pharmacokin 9:222–238.

Anderson, R.C., Worth, H.M., Small, R.M., and Harris, P.N. 1966. Toxicologic studies on tylosin: its safety as a food additive. Fd Cosmet Toxicol 4:1–15.

Angelos, J.A., Dueger, E.L., George, L.W. et al. 2000. Efficacy of florfenicol for treatment of naturally occurring infectious bovine keratoconjunctivitis. J Am Vet Med Assoc 216:62–64.

Anonymous. 1980. Carbadox vs. lincomycin in swine dysentery control. Mod Vet Pract 61:152–153.

———. 1990. Chloramphenicol. IARC Monographs 50:169–193.

Atef, M., Atta, A.H., and Amer, A.M. 1991a. Pharmacokinetics of chloramphenicol in normal and *Escherichia coli* infected chickens. Br Poultry Sci 32:589–596.

Atef, M., Youssef, H., Atta, A.H., and el-Maaz, A.A. 1991b. Disposition of tylosin in goats. Br Vet J 147:207–215.

Baggot, J.D., and Gingerich, D.A. 1976. Pharmacokinetic interpretation of erythromycin and tylosin activity in serum after intravenous administration of a single dose to cows. Res Vet Sci 21:318–323.

Baquero, F. 1990. Resistance to quinolones in gram-negative microorganisms: mechanisms and prevention. Eur Urol 17(Suppl 1):3–12.

Barriere, S.L., Kaatz, G.W., and Seo, S.M. 1989. Enhanced elimination of ciprofloxacin after multiple-dose administration of rifampin to rabbits. Antimicrob Agents Chemother 33(4):589–590.

Bates, J., Jordens, J.Z., and Griffiths, D.T. 1994. Farm animals as a putative reservoir for vancomycin-resistant enterococcal infection in man. J Antimicrob Chemother 34:507–516.

Braden, T.D., Johnson, C.A., Gabel, C.L., Lott, G.A., and Caywood, D.D. 1987. Posologic evaluation of clindamycin, using a canine model of posttraumatic osteomyelitis. Am J Vet Res 48(7):1101–1105.

Braden, T.D., Johnson, C.A., Wakenell, P., Tvedten, H.W., and Mostosky, U.V. 1988. Efficacy of clindamycin in the treatment of *Staphylococcus aureus* osteomyelitis in dogs. JAVMA 192(12):1721–1725.

Breitschwerdt, E.B., Davidson, M.G., Aucoin, D.P., Levy, M.G., Szabados, N.S., Hegarty, B.C., Kuehne, A.L., and James, R.L. 1990. Efficacy of chloramphenicol, enrofloxacin, and tetracycline, for treatment of experimental Rocky Mountain spotted fever in dogs. Antimicrob Agents Chemother 35:2375–2381.

Bretzlaff, K.N., Neff-Davis, C.A., Ott, R.S., Koritz, G.D., Gustafsson, B.K., and Davis, L.E. 1987. Florfenicol in non-lactating dairy cows: pharmacokinetics, binding to plasma proteins, and effects on phagocytosis by blood neutrophils. J Vet Pharmacol Therap 10:233–240.

Brown, S.A., Dieringer, T.M, Hunter, R.P., and Zaya, M.J. 1989. Oral clindamycin disposition after single and multiple doses in normal cats. J Vet Pharmacol Therap 12:209–216.

Brown, S.A., Zaya, M.J., Dieringer, T.M, Hunter, R.P., Nappier, J.L., Hoffman, G.A., Hornish, R.E., and Yein, F.S. 1990. Tissue concentrations of clindamycin after multiple oral doses in normal cats. J Vet Pharmacol Therap 13:270–277.

Brown, M.P., Kelly, R.H., Gronwall, R.R., and Stover, S.M. 1984. Chloramphenicol sodium succinate in the horse: serum, synovial, peritoneal, and urine concentrations after single-dose intravenous administration. Am J Vet Res 45:578–580.

Brumbaugh et al. 1983.

Budsberg, S.C., Kemp, D.T., and Wolski, N. 1992. Pharmacokinetics of clindamycin phosphate in dogs after single intravenous and intramuscular administrations. Am J Vet Res 53(12):2333–2336.

Bulgin, M.S. 1988. Losses related to the ingestion of lincomycin-medicated feed in a range sheep flock. JAVMA 192(8):1083–1086.

Burrows, G.E. 1980. Pharmacotherapeutics of macrolides, lincomycins, and spectinomycin. JAVMA 176(10):1072–1077.

Burrows, G.E., Barto, P.B., Martin, B., and Tripp, M.L. 1983. Comparative pharmacokinetics of antibiotics in newborn calves: chloramphenical, lincomycin, and tylosin. Am J Vet Res 44(6):1053–1057.

Burrows, G.E., Griffin, D.D., Pippin, A., and Harris, K. 1989. A comparison of the various routes of administration of erythromycin in cattle. J Vet Pharmacol Therap 12:289–296.

Burrows, G.E., MacAllister, C.G., Beckstrom, D.A., and Nick, J.T. 1985. Rifampin in the horse: comparison of intravenous, intramuscular, and oral administrations. Am J Vet Res 46(2):442–446.

Burrows, G.E., Tyler, R.D., Craigmill, A.L., and Barto, P.B. 1984. Chloramphenicol and the neonatal calf. Am J Vet Res 45(8):1586–1591.

Buss, W.C., Morgan, R., Guttmann, J.G., Barela, T., and Stalter, K. 1978. Rifampin inhibition of protein synthesis in mammalian cells. Science 200(28):432–434.

Carbon, C. 1998. Pharmacodynamics of macrolides, azalides, and streptogramins: effect on extracellular pathogens. Clin Infect Dis 27:28–32.

Castells G, Intorre, L., Franquelo, C., et al. 1998. Pharmacokinetics of thiamfenicol in dogs. Am J Vet Res 59:1473–1475.

Castro, L.A., Brown, M.P., Gronwall, R., Houston, A.E., and Miles, N. 1986. Pharmacokinetics of rifampin given as a single oral dose in foals. Am J Vet Res 47(12):2584–2586.

Christie, P.J., Davidson, J.N., Novick, R.P., and Dunny, G.M. 1983. Effects of tylosin feeding on the antibiotic resistance of selected gram-positive bacteria in pigs. Am J Vet Res 44:126–128.

Clark, C.H., Roger, E.D., and Milton, J.L. 1985. Plasma concentrations of chloramphenicol in snakes. Am J Vet Res 46(12):2654–2657.

Clark, C.H., Thomas, J.E., Milton, J.L., and Goolsby, W.D. 1982. Plasma concentrations of chloramphenicol in birds. Am J Vet Res 43:1249–1253.

Cocito, C. 1979. Antibiotics of the virginiamycin family, inhibitors which contain synergistic components. Microbiologic Rev 43(2):145–198.

Conner, G.H., and Gupta, B.N. 1973. Bone marrow, blood and assay levels following medication of cats with chloramphenicol ophthalmic ointment. VMSAC, Aug:895–899.

Craig, W.A., and Kunin, C.M. 1973. Dynamics of binding and release of the polymyxin antibiotics by tissues. J Pharmacol Exper Therap 184(3):757–765.

Cravedi, J.P., Heuillet, G., Peleran, J.C., and Wal, J.M. 1985. Disposition and metabolism of chloramphenicol in trout. Xenobiotica 15(2):115–121.

Crawford, L.M. 1984. Virginiamycin. In J.H. Steele and G.W. Beran, eds.-in-chief, Handbook Series in Zoonoses, Section D: Antibiotics, Sulfonamides, and Public Health, vol. I, pp. 345–349. Boca Rotan, FL: CRC Press.

Czarnecki, C.M., Jankus, E.R., and Hultgren, B.D. 1974a. Effects of furazolidone on the development of cardiomyopathies in turkey poults. Avian Dis 18(1):125–133.

Czarnecki, C.M., Reneau, J.K., and Jankus, E.F. 1974b. Effect of furazolidone on glycogen deposition in the left ventricle of turkey hearts. Avian Dis 18(4):551–558.

Dagorn, M., Guillot, P., and Sanders, P. 1990. Pharmacokinetics of chloramphenicol in sheep after intravenous, intramuscular and subcutaneous administration. Vet Quart 12(3):166–174.

Davidson, M.G., Lappin, M.R., Rottman, J.R., et al. 1996. Paradoxical effect of clindamycin in experimental, acute toxoplasmosis in cats. Antimicrob Agents Chemother 40:1352–1359.

Davis, L.E., Baggot, J.D., and Powers, T.E. 1972. Pharmacokinetics of chloramphenicol in domesticated animals. Am J Vet Res 33(11):2259–2266.

DeCraene, B.A., Deprez, P., D'Haese, E., et al. 1997. Pharmacokinetics of florfenicol in cerebrospinal fluid and plasma of calves. Antimicrob Agents Chemother 41:1991–1995.

Devriese, L.A., and Dutta, G.N. 1984. Effects of erythromycin-inactivating *Lactobacillus* crop flora on blood levels of erythromycin given orally to chicks. J Vet Pharmacol Therap 7:49–53.

Dhawan, V.K., and Thadepalli, H. 1982. Clindamycin: a review of fifteen years of experience. Rev Infect Dis 4(6):1133–1153.

Dorrestein, G.M., van Gogh, H., and Rinzema, J.D. 1984. Pharmacokinetic aspects of penicillins, aminoglycosides and chloramphenicol in birds compared to mammals: a review. 6(4):216–224.

Dueger, E.L., Angelos, J.A., Cosgrove, S., Johnson, J., and George, L. 1999. Efficacy of florfenicol in the treatment of experimentally induced infectious bovine keratoconjunctivitis. Am J Vet Res 60:960–964.

Duthu, G.S. 1985. Interspecies correlation of the pharmacokinetics of erythromycin, oleandomycin, and tylosin. J Pharm Sci 74(9):943–946.

Dutta, G.N., and Devriese, L.A. 1981. Macrolide-lincosamide-streptogramin resistance patterns in *Clostridium perfringens* from animals. Antimicrob Agents Chemother 19(2):274–278.

———. 1982a. Resistance to macrolide-lincosamide-streptogramin antibiotics in enterococci from the intestine of animals. Res Vet Sci 33:70–72.

———. 1982b. Resistance to macrolide, lincosamide and streptogramin antibiotics and degradation of lincosamide antibiotics in streptococci from bovine mastitis. J Antimicrob Chemother 10:403–408.

Eriksson, A., Rauramaa, V., Happonen, I., and Mero, M. 1990. Feeding reduced the absorption of erythromycin in the dog. Acta Vet Scand 31:497–499.

Ewing, P.J., Burrows, G., Macallister, C., and Clarke, C. 1994. Comparison of oral erythromycin formulations in the horse using pharmacokinetic profiles. J Vet Pharmacol Therap 17:17–23.

Farrington, D.O., and Shively, J.E. 1979. Effect of carbadox on growth, feed utilization, and development of nasal turbinate lesions in swine infected with *Bordetella bronchiseptica.* JAVMA 174(6):597–600.

Ferrari, V., and Bella, D.D. 1974. Comparison of chloramphenicol and thiamphenicol metabolism. Postgrad Med J 50(Suppl 5):17–22.

Finnie, J.W. 1992. Two clinical manifestations of furazolidone toxicity in calves. Aust Vet J 69(1):21.

Fisher, A.A. 1983. Adverse reactions to topical clindamycin, erythromycin and tetracycline. Cutis 32:415–428.

Ford, R.B., and Aronson, A.L. 1985. Antimicrobial drugs and infectious diseases. In Lloyd Davis, ed., Handbook of Small Animal Therapeutics, pp. 45–88. New York: Churchill Livingstone.

Frank, L.A. 1990. Clinical pharmacology of rifampin. JAVMA 197(1):114–117.

Fukui, H., Fujihara, Y., and Kano, T. 1987. In vitro and in vivo antibacterial activities of florfenicol, a new fluorinated analog of thiamfenicol, against fish pathogens. Fish Pathol 22:201–207.

Gamez, A., Perez, Y., Marti, G., Cristofol, C., and Arboix, M. 1992. Pharmacokinetics of thiamphenicol in veal calves. Br Vet J 148:535–539.

George, L., Mihalyi, J., Edmondson, A., Daigneault, J., Kagonyera, G., Willits, N., and Lucas, M. 1988. Topically applied furazolidone or parenterally administered oxytetracycline for the treatment of infectious bovine keratoconjunctivitis. JAVMA 192(10):1415–1422.

Gerken, D.F., and Sams, R.A. 1985. Inhibitory effects of intravenous chloramphenicol sodium succinate on the disposition of phenylbutazone in horses. J Pharmacokin and Biopharmaceutics 13(5):467–476.

Gingerich, D.A., Baggot, J.D., and Kowalski, J.J. 1977. Tylosin antimicrobial activity and pharmacokinetics in cows. Can Vet J 18(4):96–100.

Girard, A.E., Girard, D., and Retsema, J.A. 1990. Correlation of the extravascular pharmacokinetics of azithromycin with in-vivo efficacy in models of localized infection. J Antimicrob Chemother 25(Suppl A):61–71.

Girard, D., Bergeron, J.M., Milisen, W.B., and Retsema, J.A. 1993. Comparison of azithromycin, roxithromycin, and cephalexin penetration kinetics in early and mature abscesses. J Antimicrob Chemother 31(Suppl E):17–28.

Gottschall, D.W., Wang, R., and Kingston, G.I. 1988. Virginiamycin metabolism in cattle rumen fluid. Drug Metab and Dispos 16(6):804–812.

Gourlay, R.N., Thomas, L.H., and Wyld, S.G. 1989. Effect of a new macrolide antibiotic (tilmicosin) on pneumonia experimentally induced in calves by *Mycoplasma bovis* and *Pasteurella haemolytica.* Res Vet Sci 47:84–89.

Greene, C.E., Cook, J.R., and Mahaffey, E.A. 1985. Clindamycin for treatment of *Toxoplasma* polymyositis in a dog. JAVMA 187(6):631–634.

Greene, C.E., Lappin, M.R., and Marks, A. 1992. Effect of clindamycin on clinical, hematological, and biochemical parameters in clinically healthy cats. JAAHA 29:323–326.

Gronwall, R., Brown, M.P., Merritt, A.M., and Stone, H.W. 1986. Body fluid concentrations and pharmacokinetics of chloramphenicol given to mares intravenously or by repeated gavage. Am J Vet Res 47(12):2591–2595.

Guillot, P., and Sanders, P. 1991. Pharmacokinetics of chloramphenicol and oxytetracycline in calves after intravenous and intramuscular administrations. Acta Veterinaria Scandinavica 87:136–138.

Hall, J.A., and Washabau, R.J. 1997. Gastrointestinal prokinetic therapy: motilin-like drugs. Compend Cont Educ Pract 19:281–288.

Hamdy, A.H. 1975. Efficacy of lincomycin and spectinomycin on canine pathogens. Lab An Sci 25(5):570–574.

———. 1978. Therapeutic effects of various concentrations of lincomycin in drinking water on experimentally transmitted swine dysentery. Am J Vet Res 39(7):1175–1180.

Hamdy, A.H., and Kratzer, D.D. 1981. Therapeutic effects of parenteral administration of lincomycin on experimentally transmitted swine dysentery. Am J Vet Res 42(2):178–182.

Harari, J., and Lincoln, J. 1989. Pharmacologic features of clindamycin in dogs and cats. J Am Vet Med Assoc 195(1):124–125.

Harvey, R.G., Noble, W.C., and Ferguson, E.A. 1993. A comparison of lincomycin hydrochloride and clindamycin hydrochloride in the treatment of superficial pyoderma in dogs. Vet Rec 132:351–353.

Harvey, S. 1985. Antimicrobial Drugs. In A. R. Gennaro, ed., Remington's Pharmaceutical Sciences, 17th ed., pp. 1158–1233. Easton, PA: Mack Publishing Co.

Hedstrom, S.A. 1984. Clindamycin as an anti-staphylococcal agent: indications and limitations. Scand J Infect Dis Suppl 43:62–66.

Hird, J.F.R., and Knifton, A. 1986. Chloramphenicol in veterinary practice. Vet Rec 119:248–250.

Hoar, B.R., Jelinski, M.D., Ribble, C.S., et al. 1998. A comparison of the clinical field efficacy and safety of florfenicol and tilmicosin for the treatment of undifferentiated bovine respiratory disease in cattle in western Canada. Can Vet J 39:161–166.

Hornish, R.E., Gosline, R.E., and Nappier, J.M. 1987. Comparative metabolism of lincomycin in the swine, chicken and rat. Drug Metab Rev 18(2–3):177–214.

Horsberg, T.E., Martinsen, B., and Varma, K.J. 1994. The disposition of ^{14}C-florfenicol in Atlantic salmon (*Salmo salar*). Aquaculture 122:97–106.

Huber, W.G. 1982. Aminoglycosides, macrolides, lincomycin, polymyxins, chloramphenicol, and other antibacterial drugs. In N.H. Booth and L.E. McDonald, eds., Veterinary Pharmacology and Therapeutics, 5th ed., pp. 748–771. Ames: Iowa State Univ Press.

Hunter, R.P., Lynch, M.J., Ericson, J.F., et al. 1995. Pharmacokinetics, oral bioavailability and tissue distribution of azithromycin in cats. J Vet Pharmacol Therap 18:38–46.

IARC Monographs on the Evaluation of Carcinogenic Risk of Chemicals to Man. 1976. Chloramphenicol, vol. 10:85–98.

———. 1990. Chloramphenicol, vol. 50:169–193.

Jacobs, G.J., Lappin, M., Marks, A., and Greene, C.E. 1989. Effect of clindamycin on factor-VII activity in healthy cats. Am J Vet Res 50(3):393–395.

Jang, S.S., Breher, J.E., Dabaco, L.A., and Hirsh, D.C. 1997. Organisms isolated from dogs and cats with anaerobic infections and susceptibility to selected antimicrobial agents. J Am Vet Med Assoc 210:1610–1614.

Jankus, E.F., Noren G.R., and Staley, N.A. 1972. Furazolidone-induced cardiac dilatation in turkeys. Avian Dis 16(4):958–961.

Jernigan, A.D., St. Jean, G.D., Rings, D.M., and Sams, R.A. 1986. Pharmacokinetics of rifampin in adult sheep. Am J Vet Res 52(10):1626–1629.

Jim, G.K., Booker, C.W., Guichon, P.T., et al. 1999. A comparison of florfenicol and tilmicosin for the treatment of undifferentiated fever in feedlot calves in western Canada. Can Vet J 40:179–184.

Jones, J.E., Hughes, B.L., and Mulliken, W.E. 1976. Use of tylosin to prevent early mortality in bobwhite quail. Poultry Sci 55:1122–1123.

Jones, P.W. 1974. Treatment of calf pneumonia with tylosin. Vet Rec 94:200.

Kaltwasser, J.P., Werner, E., Simon, B., Bellenberg, U., and Becker, H.J. 1974. The effect of thiamphenicol on normal and activated erythropoiesis in the rabbit. Postgrad Med J 50(Suppl 5):118–122.

Kelly, D.J., Chulay, J.D., Mikesell, P., and Friedlander, A.M. 1992. Serum concentrations of penicillin, doxycycline, and ciprofloxacin during prolonged therapy in rhesus monkeys. J Infect Dis 166:1184–1187.

Kenny, M.T., and Strates, B. 1981. Metabolism and pharmacokinetics of the antibiotic rifampin. Drug Metab Rev 12(1):159–218.

Kirst, H.A., and Sides, G.D. 1989. New directions for macrolide antibiotics: structural modifications and in vitro activity. Antimicrob Agents Chemother 33(9):1413–1418.

Kirst, H.A., Wild, G.M., Baltz, R.H., Hamill, R.L., Ott, J.L., Counter, F.T., and Ose, E.E. 1982. Structure-activity studies among 16-membered macrolide antibiotics related to tylosin. J Antibiotics 35(12):1675–1682.

Kleckner, M.D. 1984. Lincomycin. In J.H. Steele and G.W. Beran, eds.-in-chief, Handbook Series in Zoonoses, Section D: Antibiotics, Sulfonamides, and Public Health, vol. I, pp. 337–345. Boca Rotan, FL: CRC Press.

Kleinberg, J., Dea, F.J., Anderson, J.A., and Leopold, I.H. 1979. Intraocular penetration of topically applied lincomycin hydrochloride in rabbits. Arch Ophthamol 97:933–936.

Knothe, H. 1977a. Medical implications of macrolide resistance and its relationship to the use of tylosin in animal feeds. Infection 5:137–139.

———. 1977b. A review of the medical considerations of the use of tylosin and other macrolide antibiotics as additives in animal feeds. Infection 5:183–187.

Korsrud, G.O., Naylor, J.M., MacNeil, J.D., and Yates, W.D.G. 1987. Persistence of chloramphenicol residues in calf tissues. Can J Vet Res 51:316–318.

Kume, B.B., and Garg, R.C. 1986. Pharmacokinetics and bioavailability of chloramphenicol in normal and febrile goats. J Vet Pharmacol Therap 9:254–263.

Kunkle, G.A., Sundlof, S., and Keisling, K. 1995. Adverse side effects of oral antibacterial therapy in dogs and cats: an epidemiologic study of pet owners' observations. JAAHA 31:46–55.

Lacey, R.W. 1984. Does the use of chloramphenicol in animals jeopardise the treatment of human infections? Vet Rec, Jan 7:6–8.

Lancini, G., and Parenti. 1982. Antibiotics: An Integrated View. New York: Springer-Verlag.

Lappin, M.R., Greene, C.E., Winston, S., Toll, S.L., and Epstein, M.E. 1989. Clinical feline toxoplasmosis: serologic diagnosis and therapeutic management of 15 cases. J Vet Int Med 3:139–143.

Laven, R., and Andrews, A.H. 1991. Long-acting antibiotic formulations in the treatment of calf pneumonia: a comparative study of tilmicosin and oxytetracycline. Vet Rec 129(6):109–111.

Lavy, E., Ziv, G., Lkikman, A., and Ben-Zvi, Z. 1991a. Single-dose pharmacokinetics of thiamphenicol in lactating goats. Acta Veterinaria Scandinavica–Suppl 87:99–102.

Lavy, E., Ziv, G., Shem-Tov, M., Glickman, A., and Dey, A. 1999. Pharmacokinetics of clindamycin HCl administered intravenously, intramuscularly, and subcutaneously to dogs. J Vet Pharmacol Therap 22:261–265.

Lavy, E., Ziv, G., Soback, S., Glickman, A., and Winkler, M. 1991b. Clinical pharmacology of florfenicol in lactating goats. Acta Veterinaria Scandinavica–Suppl 87:133–136.

Leclercq, R., and Courvalin, P. 1991. Intrinsic and unusual resistance to macrolide, lincosamide, and streptogramin antibiotics in bacteria. Antimicrob Agents Chemother 35(7):1273–1276.

Lester, G.D., Merritt, A.M., and Neuwirth, L. 1998. Effect of erythromycin lactobionate on myoelectric activity of ileum, and cecal emptying of radiolabeled markers in clinically normal ponies. Am J Vet Res 59:328–334.

Lloyd, D.H., Lamport, A.I., and Feeney, C. 1996. Sensitivity of antibiotics amongst cutaneous and mucosal isolates of canine pathogenic staphylococci in the UK, 1980–1996. Vet Derm 7:171–175.

Lobell, R.D., Varma, K.J., Johnson, J.C., et al. 1994. Pharmacokinetics of florfenicol following intravenous and intramuscular doses to cattle. J Vet Pharmacol Therap 17:253–258.

Locke, D., Bush, M., and Carpenter, J.W. 1982. Pharmacokinetics and tissue concentrations of tylosin in selected avian species. 43(10):1807–1810.

Lode, H., Borner, K., Koeppe, P., and Schaberg, T. 1996. Azithromycin: review of key chemical, pharmacokinetic, and microbiological features. J Antimicrob Chemother 37(Suppl C):1–8.

Maguire, B.A., Deaves, J.K., and Wild, D.G. 1989. Some properties of 2 erythromycin-dependent strains of *Escherichia coli*. J Gen Micro 135:575–581.

Maiers, J.D., and Mason, S.J. 1984. Lincomycin-associated enterocolitis in rabbits. JAVMA 185(6):670–671.

Main, B.W., Means, J.R., and Rinkema, L.E. 1996. Cardiovascular effects of the macrolide antibiotic tilmicosin, administered alone or in combination with popranolol or dobutamine, in conscious unrestrained dogs. J Vet Pharmacol Therap 19:225–232.

Mandel, M. 1977. Lincomycin in treatment of out-patient psittacines. VMSAC 72:473–474.

Marshall, S.A., Jones, R.N., Wanger, A., et al. 1996. Proposed MIC quality control guidelines for National Committee for Clinical Laboratory Standards susceptibility tests using seven veterinary antimicrobial agents: ceftiofur, enrofloxacin, florfenicol, penicillin G–Novobiocin, pirlimycin, premafloxacin, and spectinomycin. J Clin Microbiol 34:2027–2029.

Martin, K., Wiese, B. 1988. The disposition of chloramphenicol in colostrum-fed and colostrum-deprived newborn pigs. Pharmacol Toxicol 63:16–19.

Martinsen, B., Horsberg, T.E., Varma, K.J., et al. 1993. Single dose pharmacokinetic study of florfenicol in Atlantic salmon (*Salmo salar*) in seawater at 11° C. Aquaculture 112:1–11.

Matsuoka, T., Muenster, O.A., Ose, E.E., and Tonkinson, L. 1980. Orally administered tylosin for the control of pneumonia in neonatal calves. Vet Rec 106:149–151.

Maxey, B.W. 1980. Efficacy of tetracycline/novobiocin combination against canine upper respiratory infections. VMSAC 75:89–92.
Maxey, B.W., and Page, R.K. 1977. Efficacy of lincomycin feed medication for the control of necrotic enteritis in broiler-type chickens. Poultry Sci 56:1909–1913.
Mayers, M., Rush, D., Madu, A., Motyl, M., and Miller, M.H. 1991. Pharmacokinetics of amikacin and chloramphenicol in the aqueous humor of rabbits. Antimicrob Agents Chemother 35(9):1791–1798.
McCalla, D.R. 1983. Mutagenicity of nitrofuran derivative: review. Environmental Mutagenesis 5:745–765.
McKay, S.G., Morck, D.W., Merrill, J.K., et al. 1996. Use of tilmicosin for treatment of pasteurellosis in rabbits. Am J Vet Res 57:1180–1184.
McKellar, Q.A., and Varma, K.J. 1996. Pharmacokinetics and tolerance of florfenicol in Equidae. Equine Vet J 28:209–213.
Medleau L., Long R.E., Brown J., and Miller, W.H. 1986. Frequency and antimicrobial susceptibility of staphylococcus species isolated from canine pyoderma. Am J Vet Res 47:229–231.
Medoff, G. 1983. Antifungal action of rifampin. Rev Infect Dis 5(Suppl 3):S614–S619.
Miles, R.D., Janky, D.M., and Harms, R.H. 1984. Virginiamycin and broiler performance. Poultry Sci 63:1218–1221.
———. 1985. Virginiamycin and laying hen performance. Poultry Sci 64:139–143.
Moore, G.M., Mowrey, D.H., Tonkinson, L.V., et al. 1996. Efficacy dose determination study of tilmicosin phosphate in feed for control of pneumonia caused by *Actinobacillus pleuropneumoniae* in swine. Am J Vet Res 57:220–223.
Morck, D.W., Merrill, J.K., Thorlakson, B.E., Olson, M.E., Tonkinson, L.V., and Costerton, J.W. 1993. Prophylactic efficacy of tilmicosin for bovine respiratory tract disease. JAVMA 202(2):273–277.
Morris, A., and Russell, A.D. 1971. The mode of action of novobiocin. Progress Med Chem 8(1):39–59.
Moser, R.L. Cornelius, S.G. Pettigrew, J.E. Jr., Hanke, H.E., and Hagen, CD. 1985. Response of growing-finishing pigs to decreasing floor space allowance and(or) virginiamycin in diet. J Anim Sci 61(2):337–342.
Musser, J., Mechor, G.D., Grohn, Y.T., et al. 1996. Comparison of tilmicosin with long-acting oxytetracycline for treatment of respiratory tract disease in calves. J Am Vet Med Assoc 208:102–106.
Mustafa, A.I., Ali, B.H., Hassan, T., and Satti, A.M. 1985. Furazolidone concentrations in plasma, milk and some tissues of Nubian goats. J Vet Pharmacol Therap 8:190–193.
Mustafa, A.I., Idris, S.O., Ali, B.H., Mahdi, M., and Elgasim, A.I.A. 1975. Furazolidone poisoning associated with cardiomyopathy in chickens. Avian Dis 19:596.
Nagarajan, R., Schabel, A.A., Occolowitz, J.L., Counter, F.T., Ott, J.T., and Felty-Duckworth, A.M. 1989. Synthesis and antibacterial evaluation of *N*-alkyl vancomycins. J Antibiotics 42(1):63–72.
Nakata, K., Maeda, H., Fujii, A., Arakawa, S., Umezu, K., and Kamidono, S. 1992. In vitro and in vivo activities of sparfloxacin, other quinolones, and tetracyclines against *Chlamydia trachomatis*. Antimicrob Agents Chemother 36(1):188–190.
Neu, H.C. 1992. The crisis in antibiotic resistance. Science 257:1064–1073.
Nichols, D.R., and Keys, T.F. 1984. An historical overview of antibiotics and sulfonamides in society. In J.H. Steele and G.W. Beran, eds.-in-chief, Handbook Series in Zoonoses, Section D: Antibiotics, Sulfonamides, and Public Health, vol. I, pp. 35–43. Boca Rotan, FL: CRC Press.
Noble, W.C., and Kent, L.E. 1992. Antibiotic resistance in *Staphylococcus intermedius* isolated from cases of pyoderma in the dog. Vet Derm 3:71–74.
Noli, C., and Boothe, D.M. 1999. Macrolides and lincosamides. Vet Dermatology 10:217–223.
Ohmae, K., Yonezaw, S., and Terakadok, N. 1981. R plasmid with carbadox resistance from *Escherichia coli* of porcine origin. Antimicrob Agents Chemother 19:86–90.
Olsen, D., and Rodabaugh, D.E. 1977. Evaluation of virginiamycin in feed for treatment and retreatment of swine dysentery. Am J Vet Res 38(10):1485–1490.
Ose, E.E. 1976. Synergistic action of tylosin and oxytetracycline against bovine pasteurella isolates. VM/SAC. 71:92–95.
Ose, E.E., and Tonkinson, L.V. 1985. Comparison of the antimycoplasma activity of two commercially available tylosin premixes. Poultry Sci 64:287–293.
———. 1988. Single-dose treatment of neonatal calf pneumonia with the new macrolide antibiotic tilmicosin. Vet Rec 123(14):367–369.
Panteix, G., Guillaumond, B., Harf, R., et al. 1993. In-vitro concentration of azithromycin in human phagocytic cells. J Antimicrob Chemother 31(Suppl E):1–4.
Papich, M.G. 1999. Florfenicol pharmacokinetics in dogs and cats. Proc 1999 ACVIM Annual Forum.
Penny, R.H.C., Carlisle, C.H., Prescott, C.W., and Davidson, H.A. 1967. Effects of chloramphenicol on the haemopoietic system of the cat. Br Vet J 123(4):145–153.
———. 1970. Further observations on the effect of chloramphenicol on the haemopoietic system of the cat. Br Vet J 126:453–457.
Pinault, L.P., Millot, L.K., Sanders, P.J. 1997. Absolute oral bioavailability and residues of florfenicol in the rainbow trout (*Onchorynchus mykiss*). J Vet Pharmacol Therap 20:297–298.
Plenderleith, R. 1988. Treatment of cattle, sheep and horses with lincomycin: case studies. Vet Rec 122:112–113.
Rahal, J.J., and Simberkoff, M.S. 1979. Bactericidal and bacteriostatic action of chloramphenicol against meningeal pathogens. Antimicrob Agents Chemother 16:13–18.
Rainier, R.H., Harris, D.L., Glock, R.D., Kinyon, J.M., and Brauer, M.A. 1980. Carbadox and lincomycin in the treatment and carrier state of swine dysentery. Am J Vet Res 41(9):1349–1356.
Raisbeck, M.F., Holt, G.R., and Osweiler, G.D. 1981. Lincomycin-associated colitis in horses. JAVMA 179:362–363.
Ravindran, V., and Kornegay, E.T. 1984. Effects of fiber and virginiamycin on nutrient absorption, nutrient retention and rate of passage in growing swine. J Anim Sci 59(2):400–408.
Rehg, J.E., and Pakes, S.P. 1982. Implication of *Clostridium difficile* and *Clostridium perfringens* iota toxins in experimental lincomycin-associated colitis in rabbits. Lab Anim Sci 32(3):253–256.
Renneberg, J., and Walder, M. 1989. Postantibiotic effects of imipenum, norfloxacin, and amikacin in vitro and in vivo. Antimicrob Agents Chemother 33(10):1714–1720.
Rice, D.A., and McMurray, C.H. 1983. Ketosis in dairy cows caused by low levels of lincomycin in concentrate feed. Vet Rec 113:495–496.
Riviere, J.E., Craigmill, A.L., and Sundlof, S.F. 1991. Handbook of Comparative Pharmacokinetics and Residues of Veterinary Antimicrobials. Boca Raton, FL: CRC Press.
Rollin, R.E., Mero, K.N., Kozisek, P.B., Phillips, R.W. 1986. Diarrhea and malabsorption in calves associated with therapeutic doses of antibiotics: absorptive and clinical changes. Am J Vet Res 47:987–991.
Rootman, D.S., Savage, P., Hasany, S.M., Chisholm, L., and Basu, P.K. 1992. Toxicity and pharmacokinetics of intravitreally injected ciprofloxacin in rabbit eyes. Can J Ophthalmol 27(6):277–282.

Sabath, L.D., Gerstein, D.A., Loder, P.B., and Finland, M. 1968. Excretion of erythromycin and its enhanced activity in urine against gram-negative bacilli with alkalinization. J Lab Clin Med 72(6):916–923.
Salmon, R.E., and Stevens, V.I. 1990. Response of large white turkeys to virginiamycin from day-old to slaughter. Poultry Sci 69:1383–1387.
Sampson, G.R., Sauter, R.A., and Gregory, R.P. 1974a. Clinical appraisal of injectable tylosin in swine. Mod Vet Pract 55:261.
———. 1974b. Clinical appraisal of tylosin in dogs. VM/SAC 55:1259–1262.
———. 1974c. Evaluation of injectable tylosin in cattle. Mod Vet Pract 55:10.
Sande, M.A., and Mandell, G.L. 1990a. Antimicrobial agents: tetracyclines, chloramphenicol, erythromycin, and miscellaneous antibacterial agents. In A.G. Goodman, T.W. Rall, A.S. Nies, and P. Taylor, eds., Goodman and Gilman's The Pharmacologic Basis of Therapeutics, 8th ed., pp. 1117–1145. New York: Pergamon Press.
Sanders, P., Guillot, P., and Mourot, D. 1988. Pharmacokinetics of a long-acting chloramphenicol formulation administered by intramuscular and subcutaneous routes in cattle. J Vet Pharmacol Therap 11:183–190.
Schumann, F.J., Janzen, E.D., and McKinnon, J.J. 1990. Prophylactic tilmicosin medication of feedlot calves at arrival. Can Vet J 31:285–288.
Settepani, J.A. 1984. The hazard of using chloramphenicol in food animals. JAVMA 184:930–931.
Shaw, W.V., and Leslie, A.G.W. 1991. Chloramphenicol acetyltransferase. Annu Rev Biophys Chem 20:363–386.
Shepard, R.M., and Falkner, F.C. 1990. Pharmacokinetics of azithromycin in rats and dogs. J Antimicrob Chemother 25(Suppl A):49–60.
Shukla, V.K., Garg, S.K., and Mathur, V.S. 1984. Influence of prednisolone on antipyrine and chloramphenicol disposition in rabbits. Pharmacol 29:117–120.
Smith, M.J. 1966. Efficacy of furazolidone in the treatment of topical bacterial infections in dogs. VM/SAC 61:459–462.
Stern, I.J., Hollifield, R.D., Wilk, S., and Buzard, J.A. 1967. The anti-monoamine oxidase effects of furazolidone. J Pharmacol Exp Therap 156(3):492–499.
Tally, F.P., Snydman, D.R., Gorbach, S.L., and Malamy, M.H. 1979. Plasmid-mediated transferable resistance to clindamycin and erythromycin in *Bacteroides fragilis.* J Infect Dis 139:83–88.
———. 1981. Plasmid-mediated transferable resistance to clindamycin and erythromycin in *Bacteroides fragilis.* Am J Med 139:83–88.
Taylor, J.D., Gibson, J.A., and Yeates, C.E.F. 1991. Furazolidone toxicity in dairy calves. Aust Vet J 68(5):182–183.
Taylor, P.H., Gulupo, P., Naille, R., Heydinger, D.K., and Bowers, J.D. 1970. Experimental use of methanamine mandelate in treatment of burn wounds in rats. J Trauma 10(4):331–333.
Tennent, D.M., and Ray, W.H. 1971. Metabolism of furazolidone in swine. Proc Soc Exper Biology and Med 138(3):808–810.
Teske, R.H. 1984. The polypeptide antibiotics. In J.H. Steele and G.W. Beran, eds.-in-chief, Handbook Series in Zoonoses, Section D: Antibiotics, Sulfonamides, and Public Health, vol. I, pp. 333–335. Boca Raton, FL: CRC Press.
Thilsted, J.P., Newton, W.M, Crandel, R.A., and Bevill, R.F. 1981. Fatal diarrhea in rabbits resulting from the feeding of antibiotic-comtaminated feed. JAVMA 179:360–361.
van der Molen, E.J., Baars, A.J., deGraaf, G.J., and Jager, L.P. 1989a. Comparative study of the effect of carbadox, olaquindox and cyadox on aldosterone, sodium and potassium plasma levels in weaned pigs. Res Vet Sci 47:11–16.
van der Molen, E.J., deGraaf, G.J., and Baars, A.J. 1989b. Persistence of carbadox-induced adrenal lesions in pigs following drug withdrawal and recovery of aldosterone plasma concentrations. J Comp Path 100:295–304.
van der Molen, E.J., van Lieshout, J.H.L.M., Nabuurs, M.J.A., Derkx, F., Michelakis, A. 1989c. Changes in plasma renin activity and renal immunohistochemically demonstrated renin in carbadox treated pigs. Res Vet Sci 46:401–405.
Varma, K.J., Adams, P.E., Powers, T.E., Powers, J.D., and Lamendola, J.F. 1986. Pharmacokinetics of florfenicol in veal calves. J Vet Pharmacol Therap 9:412–425.
Varma, K. J., Powers, T.E., and Powers, J.D. 1987. Single and repeat-dose pharmacokinetic studies of chloramphenicol in horses: values and limitations of pharmacokinetic studies in predicting dosage regimens. Am J Vet Res 48(3):403–406.
Venning, C.M, Curtis, M.A., and Egerton, J.R. 1990. Treatment of virulent footrot with lincomycin and spectinomycin. Aust Vet J 67(6):258–260.
Vernimb, G.D. 1969. A furazolidone aerosol powder in the prevention and treatment of keratoconjunctivitis in cattle and sheep. VM/SAC 64:708–710.
Vilmànyi, E., Küng, K., Riond, J.-L., et al. 1996. Clarithromycin pharmacokinetics after oral administration with or without fasting in crossbred Beagles. J Sm Anim Pract 37:535–539.
Vogel, G.J., Laudert, S.B., Zimmerman, A., et al. 1998. Effects of tilmicosin on acute undifferentiated respiratory tract disease in newly arrived feedlot cattle. J Am Vet Med Assoc 212:1919–1924.
Watson, A.D.J. 1980. Further observations on chloramphenicol toxicosis in cats. Am J Vet Res 41:293–294.
———. 1992. Bioavailability and bioinequivalence of drug formulations in small animals. J Vet Pharmacol Therap 15:151–159.
Watts, J.L., et al. 1999. Performance standards for antimicrobial disk and dilution susceptibility tests for bacteria isolated from animals: approved standard (M31-A). NCCLS 19, no. 11.
Weisel, M.K., Powers, J.D., Powers, T.E., and Baggot, J.D. 1977. A pharmacokinetic analysis of tylosin in the normal dog. Am J Vet Res 38(2):273–275.
Wilson, D.J., Sears, P.M., Gonzalez, R.N., et al. 1996. Efficacy of florfenicol for treatment of clinical and subclinical bovine mastitis. Am J Vet Res 57:526–528.
Wilson, R.C. 1984. The Macrolides. In J.H. Steele, ed.-in-chief, Handbook Series in Zoonoses, Section D: Antibiotics, Sulfonamides, and Public Health, vol. I. Boca Raton, FL: CRC Press.
Wilson, W.D., Spensley, M.S., Baggot, J.D., and Hietala, S.K. 1988. Pharmacokinetics, bioavailablity, and in vitro antibacterial activity of rifampin in the horse. Am J Vet Res 49(12):2041–2046.
Wold, J.S., and Turnipseed, S.A. 1981. Toxicology of vancomycin in laboratory animals. Rev Infect Dis 3:S224–229.
Wolfensohn, S.E. 1991. Clindamycin treatment of mandibular osteomyelitis in a cynomolgus monkey. Vet Rec 129:265–266.
Yancy, R.J., Sanchez, M.S., and Ford, C.W. 1991. Activity of antibiotics against *Staphylococcus aureus* within polymorphonuclear neutrophils. Eur J Clin Microbiol Infect Dis 10:107–113.
Yunis, A.A. 1988. Chloramphenicol: relation of structure to activity and toxicity. Ann Rev Pharmacol Toxicol 28:83–100.

Zaghlol, H.A., and Brown, S.A. 1988. Single- and multiple-dose pharmacokinetics of intravenously administered vancomycin in dogs. Am J Vet Res 49:1637–1640.
Ziv, G., Nouws, J.F.M., and Ginneken, C.A.M. 1982. The pharmacokinetic and tissue levels of polymyxin B, colistin and gentamicin in calves. J Vet Pharmacol Therap 5:45–58.
Ziv, G., Shem-Tov, M., Glickman, A., et al. 1995. Tilmicosin antibacterial activity and pharmacokinetics in cows. J Vet Pharmacol Therap 18:340–345.
Ziv, G., and Sulman, F.G. 1973a. Passage of polymyxins from serum into milk in ewes. Am J Vet Res 34(3):317–322.
———. 1973b. Serum and milk concentrations of spectinomycin and tylosin in cows and ewes. Am J Vet Res 34:329–333.

45

FLUOROQUINOLONE ANTIMICROBIAL DRUGS

MARK G. PAPICH AND JIM E. RIVIERE

Chemical Features
Structure-Activity Relationships
Mechanism of Action
Activity
Susceptibility Testing
Resistance
Clinical Resistance Problems
Human Health Risks
Pharmacokinetics
Oral Absorption
Intramuscular and Subcutaneous Injection
Metabolism
Excretion
Protein Binding
Tissue Distribution
Pharmacodynamics
Flexible Dose Ranges
Clinical Use
Dogs and Cats
Small Mammals
Reptiles
Birds
Fish
Large Animals
Administration to Nursing, Pregnant, or Young Animals
Nursing Animals
Pregnant Animals
Young Animals
Safety
Problems in Young Animals
Effects of Other Diseases or Conditions
Drug Interactions
Formulations Available

The use of the fluoroquinolone antibacterial agents in veterinary medicine has increased tremendously in the last 10 years. The fluoroquinolones are synthetic antibacterial agents introduced in veterinary medicine first as enrofloxacin. Since then, there has been a great deal of research on this class of drugs to better understand their mechanism of action, antimicrobial spectrum, pharmacokinetics in a wide variety of animal species, and clinical use (Brown 1996). In addition, pharmaceutical companies have developed new compounds to increase the number of these drugs available to veterinarians. The advantages of the fluoroquinolones are that they are rapidly bactericidal against a wide variety of clinically important bacterial organisms, are potent, are well-tolerated by animals, and have been administered via a variety of routes (orally via tablets and drinking water, subcutaneously, intramuscularly).

Fluoroquinolones approved for use in veterinary medicine for small animals include enrofloxacin, difloxacin, orbifloxacin, and marbofloxacin. Danofloxacin, enrofloxacin, and sarafloxacin are approved for livestock or poultry. Fluoroquinolones that are labeled for humans and are of potential interest for veterinary medicine include ciprofloxacin, enoxacin, lomefloxacin, and ofloxacin. The newest generation of fluoroquinolones with increased activity against gram-positive cocci and anaerobic bacteria includes grepafloxacin, trovafloxacin, levofloxacin, moxifloxacin, gatifloxacin, and premafloxacin. Grepafloxacin and trovafloxacin already have been discontinued because of toxicities.

CHEMICAL FEATURES. The currently available fluoroquinolones have the same quinolone structure (Fig. 45.1); various chemical substitutions and side groups account for the different physical characteristics of each drug. These differences may account for variations in lipophilicity, volume of distribution (Vd), oral absorption, and elimination rate, but they do not change the antibacterial spectrum appreciably. For example, enrofloxacin has one fluorine substitution, difloxacin has two fluorine substitutions, and orbifloxacin has a three-fluorine substitution, but the presence of more than one fluorine does not increase antibacterial effects (Asuquo and Piddock 1993). When lipid solubility is expressed as the octanyl:water partition coefficient, enrofloxacin and difloxacin have high lipophilicity. Ciprofloxacin has a partition coefficient that is approximately 100-fold less than that of enrofloxacin; the corresponding partition coefficients of orbifloxacin and marbofloxacin are slightly higher than that of ciprofloxacin (Asuquo and Piddock 1993; Takács-Novák et al. 1992). (Some of these octanyl:water partition coefficients were determined in the laboratory of one of the authors and are unpublished.)

No studies are available to show that these chemical differences among the drugs can account for differ-

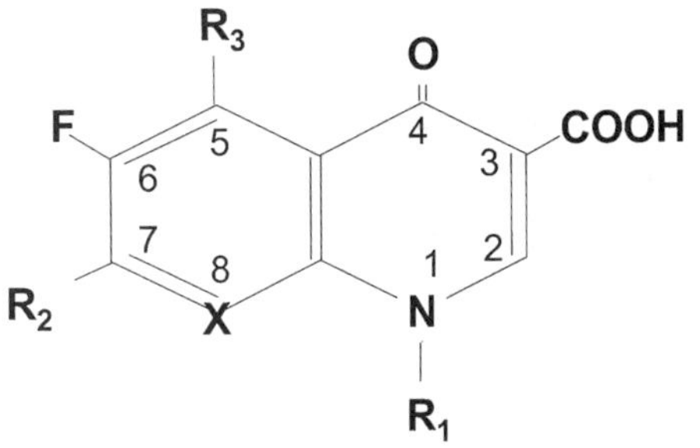

FIG. 45.1—Structure of fluoroquinolone. Features necessary for antibacterial activity are fluorine at position 6, ketone at position 4, and carboxyl at position 3. Addition of cyclopropyl, ethyl, or fluorophenyl at position 1 and of piperazine at position 7 increases the spectrum of antibacterial activity.

ences in clinical response. However, the differences may account for some variation in absorption and distribution. For example, ciprofloxacin oral absorption is approximately one-half that of enrofloxacin in dogs. The less lipid-soluble fluoroquinolones (marbofloxacin, orbifloxacin) have a lower Vd than the ones with higher lipid solubility (enrofloxacin, difloxacin) (Table 45.1). One explanation for this observation is that the more lipid-soluble drugs have higher intracellular concentrations, but higher tissue binding also could explain the differences in Vd.

Quinolones are amphoteric molecules that can be protonated at the carboxyl and the tertiary amine portion of the molecule. The pK_a varies among the drugs slightly, but generally the pK_a for the carboxyl group is 6.0–6.5 (5.5–6.3 in some references) and the pK_a for the nitrogen of the piperazine group is 7.5–8 (Nikaido and Thanassi 1993) (as high as 7.6–9.3 in some references). For two common drugs, enrofloxacin and ciprofloxacin, the pK_a for the carboxyl group is 6.0 and 6.1, respectively, and 8.8 and 7.8 for the amine, respectively. The isoelectric point is midway between the pK_a for each ionizable group. Therefore, at physiologic pH fluoroquinolones exist as zwitterions, in which both of the respective anionic and cationic groups are charged. It is at the isoelectric point that fluoroquinolones are the most lipophilic (Takács-Novák et al. 1992).

Structure-Activity Relationships. Fig. 45.1 shows the basic quinolone structure. The carboxyl group at position 3 and the ketone at position 4 are necessary for the antibacterial activity. The fluorine at position 6 differentiates the quinolones from the fluoroquinolones and accounts for the improved gram-negative and gram-positive activity over the nonfluorinated quinolones, increased potency, and increased entry into bacteria. At position 1, addition of a cyclopropyl (as for enrofloxacin and ciprofloxacin in Fig. 45.2), an ethyl, or a fluorophenyl improve the spectrum of activity against gram-positive and gram-negative bacteria. Addition of a piperazine at position 7, as demonstrated for ciprofloxacin and enrofloxacin (Fig. 45.2), improves the spectrum of activity to include pseudomonads, among other gram-negative bacteria. The change to a carbon from a nitrogen at position 8 decreased some of the adverse central nervous system effects and increased activity against staphylococci.

MECHANISM OF ACTION. Quinolones are bactericidal by inhibiting bacterial DNA replication and transcription. Two-stranded DNA is tightly coiled in the cell and must be separated for transcription and translation. To facilitate coiling, winding, and unwinding, the enzyme DNA gyrase allows the strands to be cut and reconnected. This allows coiling because negative supercoils can be introduced. DNA gyrase, a topoisomerase, consists of A and B subunits. The most common target site for quinolones is the A subunit of DNA gyrase coded by the gene *gyrA*. Mammals are resistant to the killing effects of quinolone antimicrobials because Topoisomerase II in mammalian cells is not inhibited until the drug concentration reaches 100–1000 μg/mL. Bacteria are inhibited by concentrations less than 0.1–10 μg/mL. The National Committee for Clinical Laboratory Standards (NCCLS) breakpoint for ciprofloxacin, the prototypical fluoroquinolone, for susceptible bacteria is ≤1.0 μg/mL. Another target is the Topoisomerase IV enzyme composed of subunits *parC* and *parE*. This site of action is less important for gram-negative bacteria but is a target of fluoroquinolones in some gram-positive bacteria such as streptococci and staphylococci (Ferrero et al. 1995). The action of quinolones on DNA gyrase and Topoisomerase IV has been reviewed in extensive detail by Drlica and Zhao (1997).

ACTIVITY. Fluoroquinolones in general exhibit good activity against most gram-negative bacteria, especially those of the *Enterobacteriaceae*. Representative minimum inhibitory concentration (MIC) values are shown in Table 45.2. *Escherichia coli, Klebsiella* spp., *Proteus* spp., *Salmonella* spp., and *Enterobacter* spp. are usually susceptible. *Pseudomonas aeruginosa* is variably susceptible and, when it is susceptible, usually has a higher MIC than other susceptible organisms. Against *P. aeruginosa,* ciprofloxacin is the most active.

Gram-positive bacteria are variably susceptible. *Staphylococcus aureus* and *Staphylococcus intermedius* usually are susceptible. However, the MIC values for staphylococci typically are higher than for gram-negative bacteria, and staphylococcal resistance to fluoroquinolones has been a problem in human patients. Methicillin-resistant strains of staphylococci (MRSA) may be resistant to fluoroquinolones.

The use of the newest generation of fluoroquinolones has not yet been reported in veterinary medicine, except in experimental studies (Caputo et al. 1997; Watts et al. 1997). These drugs, such as grepafloxacin, trovafloxacin, and premafloxacin, have

TABLE 45.1—Pharmacokinetic comparison of fluoroquinolones

Drug	Dose studied (mg/kg)	Recommended daily dose (mg/kg)	$t_{1/2}$[a] (hr)	Vd (area)[a] (L/kg)	C_{max} (μg/mL)	AUC[a] (μg·hr/mL)	%*F*	Assay[b]	Reference
Dogs									
Enrofloxacin	5.0 IV	5.0	2.7–3	5.0–5.6	—	4.05–4.34	—	HPLC	Intorre et al. 1995
Enrofloxacin	5.0	5.0	2.52	2.5	1.12 (oral)	7.27	72.3	HPLC	Cester et al. 1996
Enrofloxacin	5.8	5.0	4.4 (IV) 2.7 (oral)	4.5	1.44 (oral)	8.2	83.0	HPLC	Monlouis et al. 1997
Enrofloxacin	5.5	2.75–11.0	4.0 (oral)	nd	2.45 (oral)	16.32	nd	Bioassay	Walker et al. 1992
Enrofloxacin	5.0	5.0	2.4	4.5	1.16 (oral)	3.9	100	HPLC	Küng et al. 1993a
Enrofloxacin	5.0	5.0–20.0[c]	4.8	4.2	1.6	8.15	—	HPLC	Stegemann et al. 1996
Ciprofloxacin	5.0	nd	3.17	2.23	0.35	4.18	43.0	HPLC	Cester et al. 1996
Ciprofloxacin	5.8[f]	nd	5.2	nd	0.34	7.2	nd	HPLC	Monlouis et al. 1997
Ciprofloxacin	10.0	10.0–20.0	2.4	3.0	—	12.93	—	HPLC	Abadia et al. 1994
Ciprofloxacin	10.0	10.0–20.0	7.5	—	1.18 (oral)[d]	9.58 (oral)[d]	46[e]	Bioassay	Walker et al. 1990
Difloxacin	5.0	5.0–10.0[c]	9.3	4.63	1.8 (oral)	12.93	96.0	nd	Manufacturer's data
Orbifloxacin	2.5	2.5–7.5[c]	5.6	1.5	2.33 (oral)	14.3	97–100	HPLC	Manufacturer's data
Marbofloxacin	2.0	2.0	12.4–14.0	1.9–2.25	1.38 (oral) 1.52 (SC)	18.6–20.95 99 (SC)	100 (oral)	HPLC	Schneider et al. 1996
Marbofloxacin	2.0	2.0	9.8	1.4	1.35 (oral)	23.31	99.8	HPLC	Cester et al. 1996
Marbofloxacin	5.55 and 2.8 mg/kg	2.75–5.55[c]	9.5 (IV) 11 (oral)	1.27	2.0 at 2.8 mg/kg oral; 4.2 at 5.55 mg/kg oral	59.0	94.0	HPLC	Manufacturer's data
Cats									
Enrofloxacin	4.7	5[c]	6.7	6.3	1.66 (oral)	7.2	100	HPLC	Richez et al. 1997b
Orbifloxacin	2.5	2.5–7.5[c]	5.5	1.4	2.06	10.82	100	HPLC	Manufacturer's data
Horses									
Ciprofloxacin	3.0	Not recommended	4.9 (IV) 10.7 (IM)	0.147	0.77 (IM)	6.97	96.0 (IM)	HPLC	Yun et al. 1994
Ciprofloxacin	5.0	Not recommended	2.6 (IV)	3.88	na	4.83	6.8	Bioassay	Dowling et al. 1995
Enrofloxacin	2.5 and 5.0	5.0 (IV, IM) 5.0–7.5 (oral)	5.9–6.1	0.78 (5 mg/kg)	5.44	58.3	62.5	Bioassay	Giguere et al. 1996
Orbifloxacin	2.5	2.5–5.0 (oral)	5.1	2.4	1.25 (oral)	9.06	68.3 (oral)	HPLC	Manufacturer's data
Enrofloxacin	5.0 (IV, IM)	5.0 (IV or IM)	4.4 (IV) 9.9 (IM)	2.4	1.28 (IM)	13.2	>100% (IM)	HPLC	Pyorala et al. 1994
Enrofloxacin (foals)	5.0	2.5–5.0	16.5	2.31	2.12 (10 mg/kg oral)	48.54	42.0	HPLC	Bermingham et al. 2000
Mice									
Enrofloxacin	10.0	nd	1.48	10.5	nd	2.45	nd	HPLC	Bregante et al. 1999
Rats									
Enrofloxacin	7.5	nd	1.8	4.78	nd	5.65	nc	HPLC	Bregante et al. 1999

Rabbits									
Enrofloxacin	7.5	nd	2.2	4.94	nd	5.52	nd	HPLC	Bregante et al. 1999
Enrofloxacin	7.5 (IV)	nd	1.87	3.97	na	5.38	na	HPLC	Aramayona et al. 1996
Enrofloxacin	5.0 (IV)	5.0	2.18 (IV)	4.4	na	3.89	na	HPLC	Cabanes et al. 1992
Enrofloxacin	5.0 (IM)	5.0	1.8	na	3.04	3.84	92.0	HPLC	Cabanes et al. 1992
Enrofloxacin	5.0 (IV)	5.0	2.5	2.12	na	8.6	na	HPLC	Broome et al. 1991
Enrofloxacin	5.0 (oral)	5.0	2.4	na	0.45	5.4	61.0	HPLC	Broome et al. 1991
Cattle									
Enrofloxacin (1-day-old calves)	2.5	2.5–5 per day or 7.5–12.5 SC once	6.61	1.70	nd	13.94	nd	HPLC	Kaartinen et al. 1997
Enrofloxacin (1-week-old calves)	2.5	2.5–5 per day or 7.5–12.5 SC once	4.87	2.61	nd	6.73	nd	HPLC	Kaartinen et al. 1997
Enrofloxacin (lactating cows)	5.0	nd	1.68 (IV) 5.9 (IM) 5.55 (SC)	1.63	0.73 (IM) 0.98 (SC)	7.42	82.0 (IM) 137.0 (SC)	HPLC	Kaartinen et al. 1995
Enrofloxacin (cows)	2.5	nd	2.82	2.98	nd	5.28	nd	HPLC	Bregante et al. 1999
Enrofloxacin (adult cattle)	5.0	2.5–5 per day or 7.5–12.5 SC once[c]	2.3	1.65	0.73 (SC)	10.08	88.0 (SC)	HPLC	Richez et al. 1997
Enrofloxacin (calves)	5.0	2.5–5 per day or 7.5–12.5 SC once[c]	2.2	1.98	0.87 (SC)	7.99	97.0 (SC)	HPLC	Richez et al. 1997
Ciprofloxacin (calves)	2.8	nd	2.4	2.5	0.27	nd	53.0 (oral)	HPLC	Nouws et al. 1988
Sheep									
Enrofloxacin	2.5	5.0 mg/kg/day SC	3.73	2.18	0.78 (IM)	5.47	85.0 (IM)	HPLC	Mengozzi et al. 1996
Enrofloxacin	2.5	5.0 mg/kg/day SC	3.8	1.3	0.6 (oral)	10.4	60.6 (oral)	Boassay	Pozzin et al. 1997
Enrofloxacin	2.5	nd	2.5	1.53	nd	8.98	nd	HPLC	Bregante et al. 1999
Chickens									
Ciprofloxacin	5.0	5.0–15.0 IM, SC, oral	9.01	2.02	4.67	78.04	70.0	Bioassay	Atta and Sharif 1997
Enrofloxacin	10.0	10.0	5.6 (IV)	5.0	1.88 (oral)	16.17	89.2	HPLC	Knoll et al. 1999
Enrofloxacin	10.0	10.0	10.3 (IV)	4.3	2.44 (oral)	34.51	64.0	HPLC	Anadón et al. 1995
Ciprofloxacin	5.0	5.0	9.0	2.0	4.67	78.04	70.0 (oral)	Bioassay	Atta and Sharif 1997
Camels									
Enrofloxacin	2.5	2.5 IM, SC	3.58	1.4	1.44 (IM)	18.95	85.0 (IM)	Bioassay	Gavrielli et al. 1995
Pigs									
Enrofloxacin	2.5		345	3.34	1.17	5.97	150	HPLC	Zeng and Fung 1997
Enrofloxacin	2.5		7.73	3.5	0.61 (IM)	9.94	95.0 (IM)	HPLC	Richez et al. 1997a
Enrofloxacin	2.5		5.5	3.95	0.75 (IM)	5.03	101 (IM)	Bioassay	Pijpers et al. 1997.
Enrofloxacin	10.0 oral		nd	nd	nd	27.0	73.0–80.0	HPLC	Gyrd-Hansen and Nielsen 1994
Ciprofloxacin	3.06	nd	2.57	3.83	0.17	2.88	37.0	HPLC	Nouws et al. 1988

(continued)

TABLE 45.1—*Continued*

Drug	Dose studied (mg/kg)	Recommended daily dose (mg/kg)	$t_{1/2}$[a] (hr)	Vd (area)[a] (L/kg)	C_{max} (µg/mL)	AUC[a] (µg·hr/mL)	%*F*	Assay[b]	Reference
Dolphins									
Enrofloxacin	5.0	5.0 q24h oral	6.4	nd	1.4	15.4	nd	Bioassay	Linnehan et al. 1999
Fish									
Enrofloxacin trout	5.0 and 10.0	5.0 mg/kg q24h	24.0 and 30.0	3.22 and 2.56	0.945 and 1.28 (15E)	109.2 and 171.3	(oral at 15°) 42 and 49	Bioassay	Bowser et al. 1992
Enrofloxacin (red pacu)	5.0	5.0 mg/kg q48h IM	29.0	nd	1.64 (IM) 0.8 (oral)	46.3 (IM)	57.0 (relative)	HPLC	Lewbart et al. 1997
Enrofloxacin (Atlantic salmon)	10.0	5.0 mg/kg q24h oral	131.0	22.4	0.29 (oral) 0.54 (oral)	84.3 1.3 (IP)	89.0 (IP) 46 (oral)	Bioassay 66 (IM)	Stoffregen et al. 1997

Na = Data not available or not applicable.
Nd = Not determined.
$t_{1/2}$ = Half-life of the terminal portion of the plasma concentration vs. time curve.
Vd = Apparent volume of distribution (area method).
AUC = Area under the curve of the plasma concentration vs. time curve.
C_{max} = Maximum plasma concentration after administration of oral or IM dose.
%*F* = Percentage of oral or IM administered dose absorbed (determined from comparison of IV dose).
[a]Half-life, Vd, and AUC are from an IV dose unless otherwise noted.
[b]Assay type = Assay using HPLC is able to distinguish between enrofloxacin and ciprofloxacin, and values shown in table represent enrofloxacin. Assays performed by bioassay represent the parent drug and active metabolites. Bioassay may include concentrations of ciprofloxacin.
[c]Registered dose with the FDA in the United States. In some European countries doses may vary or may not include the flexible range. In most cases, when treating non-*Pseudomonas* infections, the lowest dose in the range listed is used.
[d]After multiple dosing with ciprofloxacin, the C_{max} was 1.18 mg/mL and the 12 hr AUC was 9.58 mg/hr/mL.
[e]Oral absorption of ciprofloxacin estimated from a comparison of independent oral and IV studies.
[f]These parameters determined after administration of 5.8 mg/kg of enrofloxacin.

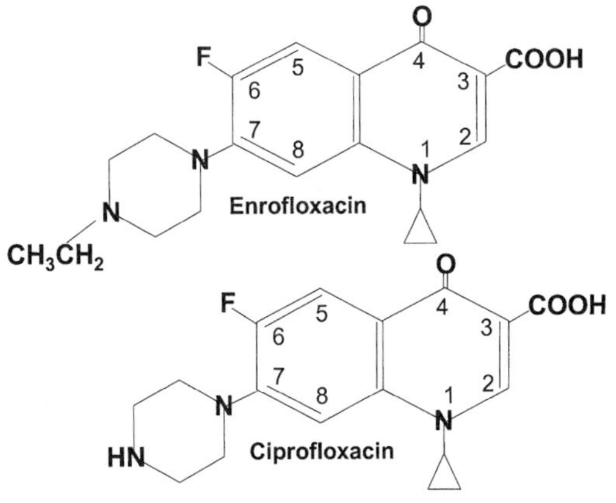

FIG. 45.2—Structure of enrofloxacin and ciprofloxacin.

increased activity against gram-positive cocci and anaerobic bacteria and may have advantages for certain infections (Brighty and Gootz 1997). Premafloxacin, a potential new veterinary drug, has greater activity against gram-positive bacteria than enrofloxacin and also exhibits activity against some methicillin-resistant strains of staphylococci and vancomycin-resistant strains of enterococci. Against gram-negative bacteria, especially *P. aeruginosa,* these drugs are not as active as ciprofloxacin. Despite the increased activity against gram-positive bacteria for this newest generation of fluoroquinolones, their activity against streptococci has been questioned and does not appear to be superior to standard treatment with a β-lactam antibiotic (Legg and Bint 1999).

Factors that may affect activity are cations at the site of infection and low pH. Cations such as Al^{3+}, Mg^{3+}, Fe^{2+}, and Ca^{2+} can bind a carboxyl group to the drug and significantly decrease activity. Low pH at the site of action also can affect the MIC (Ross and Riley 1994), especially for drugs that have a piperazine at position 7 (Fig. 45.1). For example, in urine, the MIC for fluoroquinolones may increase due to the presence of cations in the urine and low pH (Fernandes 1988). This activity in urine may increase the MIC from 4- to 64-fold. Fluoroquinolone activity in an abscess is not diminished despite the observation that in pus there is cellular material that can bind drugs, a low pH, and slow-growing bacteria (Bryant and Mazza 1989). The activity of fluoroquinolones in this milieu may explain its efficacy for treating infections associated with abscessation.

Susceptibility Testing. Susceptibility testing is performed either by the agar-disk-diffusion (ADD) method or broth dilutions (MIC test). The NCCLS has generated standardized breakpoints for some human fluoroquinolones, but they are not yet available for most veterinary quinolones. The breakpoints for the human drug ciprofloxacin are as follows: susceptible, ≤1.0 μg/mL; resistant, ≥4.0 μg/mL; and intermediate, 2.0 μg/mL. For the veterinary fluoroquinolone enrofloxacin, breakpoints are as follows: susceptible, ≤0.5 μg/mL; and resistant, ≥4.0 μg/mL. For enrofloxacin, values of 1.0 and 2.0 μg/mL are categorized as "flexible," which pertains to the Professional Flexible Label. Under the flexible label category, the organism "could be considered as susceptible if appropriate dosing modifications, explained in the package insert, are applied." Breakpoints standardized by the NCCLS are being developed, but are not yet available for the other veterinary fluoroquinolones, but MIC quality-control ranges are available from NCCLS.

RESISTANCE. Resistance develops via the *gyrA* mutation that codes for the A subunit of the DNA gyrase enzyme. A mutation at the serine-83 residue has been one of the most common, but at least 10 additional mutations at the *gyrA* gene have been identified to confer resistance (Ferrero et al. 1995). Mutations in the *parC* gene that codes for Topoisomerase IV enzyme have also been reported. Usually, the *parC* mutation causes a high-level resistance when detected with mutations of *gyrA*. For example, a mutation in *parC* alone has little advantage for *E. coli* (Everett et al. 1996). Among the other mutations identified, a mutation in the gene coded by *grlA* for the enzyme

TABLE 45.2—Comparative microbiological data for common pathogens

	MIC of bacteria (μg/mL)			
Drug	*Pasteurella multocida*	*Escherichia coli*	*Staphylococcus intermedius*	*Pseudomonas aeruginosa*
Ciprofloxacin	0.015	0.03	0.25	0.5
Difloxacin	<0.05	0.11–0.23	0.25–0.91	0.92
Enrofloxacin	0.03	0.03–0.06	0.125	2.0
Marbofloxacin	0.04	0.125–0.25	0.23–0.25	0.94
Orbifloxacin	0.05	0.125–0.39	0.25–0.39	6.25–12.5

Sources: Pirro et al. 1997, 1999; Asuquo and Piddock 1993; Stegemann et al. 1996; Spreng et al. 1995; and manufacturer data.

Note: MIC values listed are MIC_{90} and represent an average from available published literature or manufacturer technical information.

Topoisomerase IV has been found in staphylococci with high-level resistance (Ferrero et al. 1995), a mutation in the outer membrane protein, OmpF, can lead to lack of accumulation of these drugs in bacteria, and other mutations can cause drug efflux (e.g., *mex R, nfx B).*

Resistance can occur through a multistep process (Everett et al. 1996). A single mutation can increase the MIC slightly (perhaps one dilution), and each subsequent mutation produces a progressively higher level resistance in a stepwise fashion. For example, resistant strains of *E. coli* with MIC >8 μg/mL usually have at least 3 mutations for the target genes and may also show enhanced drug efflux. Unlike plasmid-mediated bacterial resistance, in which resistance may disappear after selective antibiotic pressure is removed, chromosomal (mutational) resistance is usually maintained in bacteria after drug administration is discontinued. Plasmid-mediated resistance has been found in *E. coli* and *Klebsiella* organisms, but the clinical significance of plasmid-mediated resistance has not been identified (Martinez-Martinez et al. 1998). Chromosomal mutations, rather than plasmid-mediated resistance, is overwhelmingly the most important mechanism of clinical resistance.

Clinical Resistance Problems. Resistance to fluoroquinolones has become a problem in human medicine that some investigators have attributed to increased prescribing of these drugs. Resistance to fluoroquinolones by *E. coli, Staphylococcus aureus,* and *Streptococcus pneumoniae* has been documented (Chen et al. 1999; Murphy et al. 1997; Sanders et al. 1995; Neu 1992; Peña et al. 1995; Perea et al. 1999; Everett et al. 1996). Clinical resistance in human hospitals among staphylococci appeared relatively quickly after introduction of ciprofloxacin (Neu 1992; Sanders et al. 1995; Hedin and Hambreus 1991). These investigators suggest that increased antibiotic pressure owing to increased prescribing has selected for resistant bacteria. Resistant bacteria also have been identified in companion animals. Resistance in small animals has been documented for *E. coli, P. aeruginosa, Enterobacter, Proteus,* and other gram-negative bacteria. Resistance by staphylococci has also been documented, with a prevalence of 0.9% (Lloyd et al. 1999). In a study of bacteria causing chronic otitis in dogs, 14% of *Staphylococcus intermedius* from the middle ear were resistant to enrofloxacin (Cole et al. 1998).

Pseudomonas organisms have been particularly troublesome because single-step mutations are common for this bacteria, and except for the fluoroquinolones, there are no other oral drugs with which to treat infections caused by *Pseudomonas* organisms. Resistance is primarily caused by a *gyrA* mutation, but an additional mutation in *parC* could cause a high-level resistance (Jalal and Wretlind 1998). Strains with both mutations were significantly more resistant than strains with one mutation. Factors leading to resistant *P. aeruginosa* are an inadequate dosage, low oral absorption, and extended treatment at low doses. From the horizontal and middle ear of dogs with chronic otitis, 87 and 65%, respectively, of the pseudomonads cultured were resistant to enrofloxacin (Cole et al. 1998).

Human Health Risks. Infectious disease experts have warned that frequent usage of fluoroquinolones may lead to increased resistance in animals (World Health Organization 1997). Transfer of fluoroquinolone resistance from animals to people has been suggested to occur for *Campylobacter* species (Endtz et al. 1991) and *Salmonella typhimurium* type DT-104 (Threlfall et al. 1995; Threlfall et al. 1997; Griggs et al. 1994). An increase in the incidence of resistant *Campylobacter jejuni* infecting people was linked to consumption of *Campylobacter*-contaminated chicken. The increased resistance occurred primarily after 1995, which coincides with the time that fluoroquinolones were approved for use in poultry as an additive to drinking water (Smith et al. 1999). Investigators have associated resistance in salmonellae with veterinary use of fluoroquinolones in livestock (Piddock et al. 1998). Resistant strains of *Salmonella typhimurium* may have occurred spontaneously because some of the resistant salmonellae have come from farms in which fluoroquinolones were not administered to animals (Griggs et al. 1994). Nevertheless, some scientists have warned that continued use of fluoroquinolones in livestock is a public health risk because it can potentially lead to resistant mutants of salmonellae being passed on to humans through the food chain. Because of these concerns, there have been limited approvals of fluoroquinolones for food-producing animals, and the extra-label use of fluoroquinolones is prohibited in food-producing animals in the United States.

PHARMACOKINETICS. Pharmacokinetic characteristics such as elimination half-life ($t_{1/2}$), Vd, and oral absorption (*%F*) are listed in Table 45.1. Mammals are relatively consistent in elimination half-life and Vd. Reptiles with lower renal clearance generally demonstrate longer half-lives—as long as 55 and 36 hours for enrofloxacin in alligators and Monitor lizards, respectively (Papich 1999). It has been demonstrated that there are allometric relationships in pharmacokinetic parameters among mammals ranging in size from mice to cattle (Bregante et al. 1999). The allometric relationship was improved considerably when the pharmacokinetic parameters were corrected for the percentage of protein-unbound enrofloxacin in the plasma. In particular, for enrofloxacin the Vd was the most directly proportional to animal body weight, with the animals with largest body weight having the largest Vd.

Among the drugs, there are differences in the pharmacokinetic parameters within species (Table 45.1). Whether or not these differences translate to clinical differences, however, has not been shown, because there are no comparative studies. For example, it does not appear that differences in half-life can account for different clinical results for skin infection treatment in dogs since enrofloxacin, which has the shortest half-life (Table 45.1), and marbofloxacin, which has the longest half-life, have both been reported to be effective when administered once daily (Paradis et al. 1990; Carlotti et al. 1995; Carlotti 1996; Gruet et al. 1997; Koch and Peters 1996; Lloyd 1992; Kwochka 1993; Ihrke 1996, 1998; Cester et al. 1996). Likewise, even though there is a range of values for Vd among the drugs, this has not translated into a superior clinical efficacy. Marbofloxacin and orbifloxacin, which have a Vd in the range of 1–2 L/kg, achieve effective skin concentrations and appear as clinically effective as drugs such as enrofloxacin with a Vd of 2.5–5 L/kg. The data published (Walker et al. 1990, 1992) or available from manufacturer technical information show that all the fluoroquinolones, regardless of their Vd and lipophilicity, achieve concentrations in tissues, except for the central nervous system and eye, that are at least as high as plasma. Differences in Vd, however, account for a range of maximum plasma concentrations (C_{max}) among the drugs (Table 45.1). Drugs with the lowest Vd are diluted less in body fluid and produce higher plasma concentrations than drugs with a higher Vd. The consequence of this difference is reflected in the dose administered. Doses are determined by the following relationship: dose = Vd × C_{max}. Therefore, to achieve the same C_{max}, drugs with high Vd require a higher dose.

Oral Absorption. Oral absorption of fluoroquinolones is high for most animals studied (Table 45.1). Whether fluoroquinolones are administered with or without food has little affect on oral absorption. Fluoroquinolones administered with food may exhibit a slow or a prolonged absorption, but the extent of absorption, determined by either the total AUC (area under the curve of the plasma concentration vs. time curve) or C_{max}, is not affected significantly. Administration with food has prolonged the terminal half-life when enrofloxacin was administered orally to reptiles (Papich 1999), sheep, pigs (Gyrd-Hansen and Nielsen 1994), and chickens (Anadón et al. 1995).

In clinical situations involving animals difficult to dose, fluoroquinolones may be added to a patient's food in order to provide a more convenient dosing form. For example, enrofloxacin tablets were placed in whole fish, which were fed to dolphins to produce good absorption (Linnehan et al. 1999), and enrofloxacin was injected into mice and fed to Monitor lizards to also produce good absorption (Hungerford et al. 1997). Chewable tablets of enrofloxacin (Taste-Tabs) do not affect oral absorption (manufacturer's data).

In dogs, cats and pigs, oral absorption of fluoroquinolones approaches 100% (Table 45.1), but in large animals, extent of absorption has been less. Oral absorption of fluoroquinolones is variable in horses. Ciprofloxacin showed an oral absorption of only 6.8% in ponies (Dowling et al. 1995). But enrofloxacin absorption is 63% (Giguere et al. 1996) in adult horses and 42% in foals (Bermingham et al. 2000). The value reported for adult horses is probably artificially high because the study used a bioassay that overestimates the concentration of enrofloxacin in plasma. Studies in ruminants produce conflicting results on oral absorption. In sheep, oral absorption was reported to be 61% (Pozzin et al. 1997), but absorption in ruminant calves was listed as less than 10% (Vancutsem et al. 1990). Unpublished observations from our laboratory indicated good oral absorption in sheep and bison. In camels (although not a true ruminant), oral absorption is reported to be negligible (Gavrielli et al. 1995).

In birds, oral absorption of enrofloxacin has been reported to be good, with effective levels being achieved by adding the drug to the bird's drinking water. This method of administration has been employed to treat sick pet birds (Flammer 1998) and poultry (Knoll et al. 1999). After continuous medication in the drinking water, steady-state plasma concentrations of enrofloxacin are 0.53 μg/mL (Knoll et al. 1999). In fish enrofloxacin absorption has been estimated to be 40–50% (Lewbart 1998).

Intramuscular and Subcutaneous Injection. Absorption is virtually complete from intramuscular (IM) injection. There have not been many studies that examined subcutaneous (SC) injection, but in the studies that are available, absorption was nearly complete. In some animals there was delayed absorption from IM or SC injections, which produced longer half-lives from these routes compared to IV administration (this is known as "flip-flop" absorption kinetics). In cattle, e.g. (Kaartinen et al. 1995), half-life was 1.68 hours from IV injection of enrofloxacin (5 mg/kg), but 5.9 and 5.55 hours from IM and SC injection, respectively, even though the extent of absorption was high. For danofloxacin, the IV half-life in cattle was 0.9 hours and the IM half-life was 2.26 hours. Delayed absorption from injection is possibly due to a slow release from the injection site caused by tissue binding or tissue injury that disrupts blood flow.

Metabolism. Metabolism of enrofloxacin to ciprofloxacin occurs via deethylation of the ethyl group on the piperazine ring. Other metabolites are produced from further metabolism of ciprofloxacin, but these are minor and do not contribute to the antibacterial effects. There are also minor insignificant metabolites of some of the other drugs. Examination of the extent of metabolism of enrofloxacin to ciprofloxacin in dogs and cats was reported in several studies (Küng et al. 1993a; Monlouis et al. 1997; Cester et al. 1996; Richez et al. 1997b; Kordick et al. 1997; Heinen 1999) in which high-pressure liquid chromatography (HPLC) was used to determine the specific concentrations of enrofloxacin and ciprofloxacin after enrofloxacin administration. An analysis of the data shows that at C_{max} 20 and 10% in dogs and cats, respectively, of the total fluoroquinolone concentration is contributed by ciprofloxacin. (That is, ciprofloxacin accounts for 20 and 10% of enrofloxacin plus ciprofloxacin concentrations.) The proportion of ciprofloxacin in plasma has been measured as high as 25% in cattle (Richez et al. 1994). But in pigs, foals, and some reptiles there were only small traces of ciprofloxacin metabolized from enrofloxacin (Zeng and Fung 1997; Bermingham et al. 2000; Richez et al. 1997a). Studies in fish show that after administration of enrofloxacin, about 2% of the maximal concentration is made up of ciprofloxacin (Lewbart et al. 1997). Difloxacin is metabolized to the active metabolite sarafloxacin by demethylation, but the amount of sarafloxacin from difloxacin in dogs has been small (Heinen 1999).

In chickens, the concentrations of ciprofloxacin in plasma and tissues after administration of enrofloxacin are minimal (Knoll et al. 1999; Anadón et al. 1995). However, one of these studies reported that the ratio of ciprofloxacin:enrofloxacin tissue concentrations was greater than 1.0 after administration of enrofloxacin despite the low plasma concentrations of ciprofloxacin (Anadón et al. 1995). The ciprofloxacin concentration residues were still present in tissues of chickens 12 days after dosing.

If there are active metabolites produced, such as ciprofloxacin from enrofloxacin, this can cause errors in the interpretation of drug assays when a bioassay (microbiological assay) is used because a bioassay does not distinguish parent drug from active metabolite. Pharmacokinetic studies performed using bioassay techniques and compared with HPLC methods have demonstrated that bioassay can overestimate the combined enrofloxacin and ciprofloxacin concentrations in animals by as much as 70% for the AUC and 29% for the C_{max} (Cester et al. 1996). This finding agrees with another study in dogs: a microbiological assay overestimated the total enrofloxacin + ciprofloxacin AUC determined by HPLC by as much as 30–70% (Küng et al. 1993b).

Excretion. The fluoroquinolones are primarily excreted via the kidneys by glomerular filtration and tubular excretion (Bregante et al. 1999). The role of tubular excretion has been demonstrated by showing that probenecid can decrease the clearance for some fluoroquinolones. For most of the drugs a major portion of the parent drug or metabolites can be recovered in the urine, with a smaller amount recovered in the feces. An exception is difloxacin, for which 80% of a dose was recovered in the feces and renal clearance accounted for less than 5% of the total systemic clearance.

Protein Binding. No studies have shown that fluoroquinolones are so highly protein bound that this limits distribution to tissues or causes a protein-binding interaction if displaced by another drug. Table 45.3 shows some of the protein-binding data generated. In most instances protein binding is low, but for animals for which multiple studies are available, as shown in Table 45.3, there is a lack of consistency among studies, which is probably related to differences in technique used to measure protein binding.

TABLE 45.3—Plasma/serum protein binding of fluoroquinolones in animals (% bound)

Animal	Enro-floxacin	Cipro-floxacin	Marbo-floxacin	Orbi-floxacin
Camel	17–24			
Cattle	56, 36–45, 60	31, 70		
Sheep	69			
Horse	22	37		21 (at 1 µg/mL)
Pig	27	23.6, 35		
Dog	15–25, 27, 72	44	9.1	13.24 (at 1 µg/mL)
Rabbit	53, 50, 35, 6.0	33, 28		
Chicken	21	30		
Mouse	42			
Rat	50			

Sources: Villa et al. 1997; Gavrielli et al. 1995; Nouws et al. 1988; Aramayona et al. 1994; and author Papich's unpublished data.

Note: When two or more values are listed, they represent results from independent studies.

Tissue Distribution. Distribution to most tissues is listed for each drug in the manufacturer's package insert or Freedom of Information (FOI) summary. Specific studies for enrofloxacin have been conducted to show that it distributes to bone (Duval and Budsberg 1995), prostate (Dorfman et al. 1995), and skin (DeManuelle et al. 1998). In tissues in which high intracellular distribution does not occur, total tissue concentrations will generally be in equilibrium with drug concentrations in the extracellular fluid (Nix et al. 1991). For example, concentrations of enrofloxacin in canine cortical bone were approximately 30% of the corresponding plasma concentration (determined by bioassay), which approximates the concentration in the extracellular fluid space (Duval and Budsberg 1995).

In tissues in which the fluoroquinolones accumulate intracellularly, high tissue concentrations are reported because measurement of tissue concentrations is typically performed by homogenizing the tissue, which disrupts cells and releases intracellular concentrations. Tissue concentrations measured in this manner represent both intracellular and extracellular concentrations. Some tissues, such as liver and kidney, may have fluoroquinolone concentrations several-fold higher than corresponding plasma concentrations.

Fluoroquinolones attain particularly high intracellular concentrations in macrophages and neutrophils: intracellular concentrations of 4–10 times plasma concentrations can be expected (Pascual et al. 1990; Tulkens 1990; Garaffo et al. 1991; Easmon and Crane 1985). In canine alveolar macrophages, the accumulation of enrofloxacin was 10 times the plasma concentration (Hawkins et al. 1998). The intracellular concentrations occur because fluoroquinolones are sufficiently lipid soluble to cross the cell membrane, or there may be active mechanisms to transport these drugs into cells. Fluoroquinolones also have a slower efflux from these cells. In humans, ciprofloxacin has an intracellular half-life of 6.7 hours in neutrophils versus 3.7 hours in serum (Easmon et al. 1986).

The high intracellular distribution in leukocytes may account for higher drug concentrations of fluoroquinolones in infected tissue compared to healthy tissue. Leukocytes, attracted via chemotaxis, may transport active drug to the site of infection. Dogs with superficial and deep pyoderma had significantly higher enrofloxacin concentrations in affected skin compared to healthy skin from control dogs (DeManuelle et al. 1998). Skin from dogs with deep pyoderma had higher enrofloxacin concentrations than skin from dogs with superficial pyoderma and there was significant correlation between dermal inflammation (dermal inflammatory cell count) and drug concentration.

Concentrations in urine have been several times higher than plasma concentrations. Concentrations of enrofloxacin, marbofloxacin, and orbifloxacin in urine of dogs are listed by the manufacturer to be 43, 40, and 84.5 μg/mL, respectively. One exception to the high urine excretion is difloxacin, of which, according to the manufacturer, less than 5% of the dose is cleared in the urine. Fluoroquinolones are among the few drugs that adequately penetrate the prostate gland in sufficient concentrations to treat infection. Enrofloxacin concentration (determined by bioassay) in the prostatic fluid and prostate tissue exceeded serum concentration at all times after administration (Dorfman et al. 1995). But, there were no differences in tissue concentrations when infected prostate was compared to healthy tissue. Concentrations of other fluoroquinolones in prostate tissue have been reported by the manufacturers to be 3.36, 5.6, and 1.35 μg/gram for difloxacin, marbofloxacin, and orbifloxacin, respectively.

PHARMACODYNAMICS. MIC values for bacteria are listed in Table 45.2. Even though there are differences in potency among the currently available fluoroquinolones, a pattern is apparent: *Pasteurella,* such as the strains found in skin wounds, are the most susceptible; the gram-negative enteric bacilli (e.g., *E. coli* and *Klebsiella*) also have low MIC values. The gram-positive cocci such as the common skin pathogen *Staphylococcus intermedius* have MIC values at a somewhat higher range, and *P. aeruginosa,* if sensitive at all, has MIC values that are among the highest for susceptible bacteria. Although not listed in Table 45.2, streptococci, enterococci, and anaerobic bacteria typically have MIC values high enough that they are usually in the resistant category.

The best pharmacokinetic-pharmacodynamic marker to predict efficacy has been debated for the fluoroquinolones. Most of the evidence suggests that fluoroquinolones are bactericidal and that they act in a concentration-dependent manner rather than a time-dependent manner. The exposure to the bacteria has been measured by using the maximum peak concentration (C_{max}) in relation to the bacteria MIC and expressed as the C_{max}:MIC ratio. Alternatively, the AUC for a 24-hour dose interval in relation to the MIC, expressed as the AUC:MIC ratio, or AUIC, has been used. A C_{max}:MIC ratio that is at least 8–10 (i.e., a peak concentration that is 8–10 times the MIC) or a AUC:MIC ratio of 125–250 has been associated with the optimum antibacterial effect (Lode et al. 1998; Hyatt et al. 1995; Dudley 1991; Nicolau et al. 1995).

These targeted C_{max}:MIC and AUC:MIC ratios were based on in vitro or in vivo studies performed with immunosuppressed laboratory animals or on clinical studies involving people with serious illness (Forrest et al. 1993; Blaser et al. 1987; Sullivan et al. 1993). A study in neutropenic mice showed that the optimum therapeutic effect was attained when the C_{max}:MIC ratio was greater than 10, but at lower drug doses when the C_{max}:MIC ratio was less than 10, the AUC:MIC was better linked to outcome (Drusano et al. 1993). A C_{max}:MIC ratio of at least 8–10 has been associated with a lower incidence of development of resistance (Blaser et al. 1987). When lower ratios were achieved, the mutant strains that occur spontaneously were not suppressed, and resistance was allowed to emerge because these mutant strains have MIC values that are at least 4–8 times that of the parent (wild-type) strain (Drusano et al. 1993). Veterinary studies also have supported a high C_{max}:MIC or AUC:MIC ratio to predict efficacy (Meinen et al. 1995).

Our clinical observations in veterinary patients reveal that we often achieve a cure using standard doses even though we may not achieve these targeted ratios. For example, if one compares the C_{max} or AUC in Table 45.1 to representative MIC values from Table 45.2, an AUC:MIC ratio of 50–60 in some patients appears adequate (Cester et al. 1996). In one model of skin infection in dogs caused by *Staphylococcus intermedius* (MIC 0.5 μg/mL), infections were prevented with C_{max}:MIC ratios of only 3–5.5 μg/mL of marbofloxacin (Gruet et al. 1997). Perhaps a competent immune system or less serious infection accounts for this discrepancy between laboratory studies and clinical observations in veterinary medicine.

FLEXIBLE DOSE RANGES. Despite our uncertainty as to the best pharmacokinetic-pharmacodynamic parameter to use to predict therapeutic efficacy, we usually design dosage regimens to attain a targeted C_{max}:MIC so that we decrease the chance of resistant mutants arising from an infection. Calculated doses listed in Tables 45.1 and 45.4 are based on attaining a C_{max}:MIC ratio of at least 8–10. The basis for the flexible doses listed in Table 45.1 is the wide MIC range among susceptible bacteria, from as low as 0.03 μg/mL, to as high as 1.0 μg/mL. (The flexible dose

TABLE 45.4—Dose recommendations for enrofloxacin in exotic animals

Animal	Dose	Route	Interval	Reference
Alligator	5 mg/kg	IV, oral	Every 96 hr	Helmick et al. 1997
Savanna monitor	5 mg/kg (10 mg/kg for *Pseudomonas* spp.)	IM, oral	Every 96 hr	Hungerford et al. 1997
Burmese python	5 mg/kg (higher doses for *Pseudomonas* spp.)	IM	Every 48 hr	Young et al. 1997
Indian star tortoise	5 mg/kg	IM	Every 24 hr	Raphael et al. 1994
Red-eared slider	5 mg/kg	oral, IM	Every 72 hr (oral), every 48 hr (IM)	James et al. forthcoming
Gopher tortoise	5 mg/kg	IM	Every 24–48 hr	Prezant et al. 1994
Bottlenose dolphin	5 mg/kg	oral	Every 24 hr	Linnehan et al. 1999.
Parrot and cockatoo	7.5–15 mg/kg	oral	Every 12 hr	Flammer 1998
Fish (ornamental)	5 mg/kg	IM, oral, or IP	Every 48 hr	Lewbart 1998

Note: These recommendations are based on an analysis of pharmacokinetic data and limited clinical experience. There have been no well-controlled efficacy studies or safety studies in these animals.

ranges specified by the manufacturers are noted by the superscript "c" in Table 45.1.) The upper dose is limited by safety (such as gastrointestinal effects); the lower dose is determined by efficacy. There is no advantage to frequent dosing (multiple times/day) as long as a sufficiently high C_{max}:MIC or the same AUC:MIC is achieved; therefore, the doses discussed for mammals and listed in Table 45.1 are intended for once-daily administration.

The flexible dose allows relatively low doses of fluoroquinolones to be administered to treat the most susceptible organisms. That is, for susceptible *E. coli* or *Pasteurella* organisms, the lowest approved dose can be administered. To achieve the necessary concentration for some *Staphylococcus* or gram-positive bacteria that have higher MIC values, a higher dose may be needed, e.g., a dose in the middle of the dose range in Table 45.1. When the MIC values are high for organisms such as *P. aeruginosa,* the highest safe dose should be considered (Walker et al. 1992; Meinen et al. 1995).

CLINICAL USE

Dogs and Cats. The administration of fluoroquinolones to dogs and cats constitutes the largest application of these drugs for veterinary medicine. They have been used extensively during the past 10 years for infections of the skin, soft tissue, oral cavity, urinary tract, prostate, external and middle ear, wounds, respiratory tract, and bone (Paradis et al. 1990; Ihrke and DeManuelle 1999; Ihrke 1996; Carlotti et al. 1999; Griffin 1993; Hawkins et al. 1998; Dorfman et al. 1995; Cotard et al. 1995). There has been a decade of experience with enrofloxacin, and veterinarians now have experience with marbofloxacin, orbifloxacin, and difloxacin. The efficacy of the fluoroquinolones has been accepted by virtue of approval by the US Food and Drug Administration (FDA) for the treatment of skin and urinary tract infections (all current drugs) and respiratory infections (enrofloxacin only). In the United States, enrofloxacin and orbifloxacin are approved for dogs and cats; marbofloxacin and difloxacin are registered for dogs only. According to each drug's FOI summary available through the FDA, enrofloxacin, orbifloxacin, marbofloxacin, and difloxacin are efficacious for skin infections and urinary tract infections in dogs at the lowest label dosage.

The efficacy of enrofloxacin and marbofloxacin has been demonstrated specifically for canine pyoderma through published reports (Ihrke and DeManuelle 1999; Ihrke 1996; Paradis et al. 1990; Carlotti et al. 1999). One disease in particular for which enrofloxacin's efficacy has been demonstrated is German Shepherd dog pyoderma when the drug is administered orally once daily at a dose rate of 5–10 mg/kg (Ihrke and DeManuelle 1999; Koch and Peters 1996). The effectiveness of enrofloxacin in the management of this syndrome also may be partially explained by beneficial anti-inflammatory properties (Ihrke and DeManuelle 1999). Quinolones have been shown to diminish tumor necrosis factor production and suppress induced leukotriene generation from neutrophils, lymphocytes, monocytes, and basophils (Bailly et al. 1990; Knöller et al. 1989). German Shepherd dog pyoderma may be associated with a predilection for an exaggerated tissue response to staphylococcal bacteria characterized by an inappropriate release of cytokines and other mediators of inflammation.

In addition to treatment of infections in these common sites, fluoroquinolones also have been used to treat rickettsial infections (Breitschwerdt et al. 1990, 1999) and have been examined for treating *Bartonella* infections in cats (Kordick et al. 1997). Against *Rickettsia rickettsii,* enrofloxacin is equally as effective as doxycycline or chloramphenicol (Breitschwerdt et al. 1990), but the success for eliminating *Bartonella* in cats has been equivocal (Kordick et al. 1997). Enrofloxacin has been used successfully to treat acute ehrlichiosis in dogs caused by *E. canis* and *E. platys* at a dosage of 5 mg/kg once daily for 15 days (Kontos and Athanasiou 1998). However, success in treating chronic ehrlichiosis has not been demonstrated. Fluoroquinolones also have been used to treat infections caused by *Mycoplasma* and *Mycobacteria.* Although the activity against *Mycoplasma* can be variable (Hannan et al. 1997), it has been effective for some opportunistic mycobacterial infections in cats (Studdert and Hughes 1992). Enrofloxacin and danofloxacin were consistently more active against veterinary *Mycoplasma* isolates than flumequine (Hannan et al. 1997).

Small Mammals. Enrofloxacin and other fluoroquinolone antibiotics are used frequently in small mammals such as rabbits, mice, rats, and exotic species for skin and visceral infections (Göbel 1999; Cabanes et al. 1992; Broome and Brooks 1991). One of the reasons fluoroquinolones are popular for treatment in small mammals is the potent activity against gram-negative pathogens affecting these animals and the excellent oral absorption. Another important advantage is the good safety record of the fluoroquinolones in small mammals. Oral tablets of fluoroquinolones have been administered directly or crushed to make a suspension that can be conveniently administered orally to the small mammals mixed with water, fruit, or some other palatable flavoring. Small mammals such as rodents and rabbits are prone to gastrointestinal disturbances and enteritis caused by overgrowth of bacteria, especially *Clostridium* organisms after administration of β-lactam and macrolide antibiotics. Because fluoroquinolones are not active against the anaerobic bacteria that compete with *Clostridium* organisms, bacterial overgrowth of pathogenic opportunistic bacteria has not been a problem as it has with other drugs, such as penicillins or macrolides.

Of the available drugs, enrofloxacin has been the most extensively studied. The doses listed in textbooks and review articles for mice, gerbils, hamsters, rats, and guinea pigs are 2.5–5.0 mg/kg up to 10–20 mg/kg IM, SC, or orally administered twice daily. The pharmacokinetics has been reported (Table 45.1), and there is some experience with the drug's efficacy. In rabbits, e.g., enrofloxacin, after a dose of 5 mg/kg, has been effective for improving clinical signs associated with pasteurellosis. The recommended dose of enrofloxacin for rabbits is 5 mg/kg IM, SC, or oral. Although it does not completely eradicate the bacteria in pasteurellosis in rabbits, it is considered the drug of choice (Göbel 1999; Broome and Brooks 1991).

Reptiles. The use of fluoroquinolones in reptiles has become popular because of their activity, safety, and convenience of administration (Papich 1999; Jacobson 1999; Rosenthal 1999). The only fluoroquinolone studied extensively is enrofloxacin. It is active against gram-negative organisms often implicated in serious infection of reptiles, including *Salmonella* spp., *Aeromonas hydrophilia, Klebsiella* spp., and *P. aeruginosa,* and its pharmacokinetics has been summarized in a review (Papich 1999). It shows remarkable differences among the reptiles, but generally the elimination is longer than in mammals or birds, which allows long dose intervals—as long as every 96 hours in some species. The elimination rate of drugs in reptiles varies with the animal's body temperature, because it affects metabolic rate. When enrofloxacin is administered, there is variable metabolism to the active metabolite ciprofloxacin among the reptiles. Elimination half-life ranged from 55 hours in alligators to 5.1 hours in tortoises (Young et al. 1997; Raphael et al. 1994; Helmick et al. 1997; Hungerford et al. 1997; Prezant et al. 1994; James et al. forthcoming). Monitor lizards, pythons, and turtles had half-lives of 36, 17.6, and 6.4 hours, respectively. Analysis of pharmacokinetic data and appraisal of clinical experience (Jacobson 1999; Papich 1999) suggest a range of doses (Table 45.4), but safety and efficacy studies have not been performed.

Pharmacokinetic studies have shown good absorption of enrofloxacin from IM administration, and this route may prolong the half-life, probably because of delayed absorption from the injection site. Although some authors have suggested that oral administration should be avoided in reptiles because of unreliable absorption, absorption was good after oral administration to alligators, lizards, and turtles (Helmick et al. 1997; Hungerford et al. 1997; James et al. forthcoming). Because of slow gastrointestinal transit time, oral absorption may prolong the half-life.

Birds. The fluoroquinolones are an important group of antibiotics for pet birds and poultry. Administration is via drinking water for bacterial infections in poultry and by injection or orally for pet birds. Fluoroquinolones have the advantage of good activity against bacterial pathogens important to birds, including *E. coli, Klebsiella* spp., *Pseudomonas* spp., *Staphylococcus* spp., and *Chlamydia* spp. Resistance is possible for *E. coli* and *Pseudomonas* spp., however, and activity against gram-positive cocci (e.g., streptococci and enterococci) is low. Although there is in vitro susceptibility of *Chlamydia* to fluoroquinolones, experience suggests that enrofloxacin can decrease clinical signs but not eliminate the infections (Flammer 1998). Therefore, fluoroquinolones are not recommended for mass medication of pet birds, and doxycycline is still the choice for this indication.

For pet birds, the dose is higher than for mammals because the clearance is faster. Pharmacokinetics of enrofloxacin has been studied in some birds (Table 45.1), and from these studies a dose of 15 mg/kg IM or orally every 12 hours has been recommended (Flammer 1998; Flammer et al. 1991). One advantage of enrofloxacin for treating birds is that it has been possible to add it to the drinking water of pet birds so they can be conveniently medicated. Enrofloxacin added to drinking water at a concentration of 0.3–0.5 mg/mL has been used to treat highly susceptible bacteria (Flammer et al. 1990). Enrofloxacin is well absorbed via this route, and as long as the bird is drinking, effective plasma concentrations can be attained. One concern with the IM injection is that it can produce irritation at the site of injection, which is problematic because birds have a limited muscle mass into which one can inject.

Two fluoroquinolones are approved for use in poultry in the United States: enrofloxacin and sarafloxacin. These products are licensed for administration in drinking water for treating infections caused by susceptible organisms such as *E. coli*. Fluoroquinolones are also active against other important pathogens of poultry, such as *Mycoplasma* spp. and *Pasteurella* spp. (Knoll et al. 1999; Jordan et al. 1993). Enrofloxacin oral solution (32.3 mg/mL) has been added to drinking water (25–50 ppm) for 3–7 days. After adding enrofloxacin to drinking water, steady-state plasma concentrations of 0.52 μg/mL were achieved in broiler chickens. Enrofloxacin has been administered to ducks at a dose of 10 mg/kg every 24 hours IM or orally.

Fish. Fluoroquinolones have been considered for treatment of infections in ornamental fish and for use in aquaculture. These drugs are active against important gram-negative bacterial pathogens of fish, and they appear to be well tolerated. Enrofloxacin has been administered orally to Rainbow trout kept in water maintained at 10° and 15° C. Although oral absorption is less than in mammals, it was good enough to produce effective plasma concentrations (Bowser et al. 1992). MIC values for pathogens infecting fish range from 0.0064–0.032 μg/mL for the most sensitive organisms to 0.25–0.45 μg/mL for *Streptococcus* spp. Thus the dose of 5 mg/kg should produce effective plasma concentrations for most susceptible pathogens (Bowser et al. 1992). In Atlantic salmon, enrofloxacin administered at 10 mg/kg intraperitoneally, intramuscularly, intra-arterially, and orally was well absorbed from these routes, with no advantage of one route over another, but it produced a wide range of half-lives and Vd. Oral absorption in salmon was 46%, but the authors concluded that at 5 mg/kg this route would be suitable for therapeutic treatment (Stoffregen et al. 1997). Tissue concentrations were high, with concentrations detected at 120 hours after dosing.

Enrofloxacin has also been studied in red pacu as a model for other ornamental fish (Lewbart et al. 1997). For treatment of bacterial infections in ornamental fish, Lewbart (1998) recommends enrofloxacin at a dose of 5 mg/kg. This can be administered IM, IP, or orally with a recommended interval of every 48 hours, but the IM route produces the most predictable plasma concentrations. The oral dose can be prepared as a mixture of 0.1% in fish food (10 mg per 10 g of food). Enrofloxacin also has been added to water and used as a bath for fish in which the drug is absorbed across the surface area of the gill to produce systemic levels. In this treatment 2.5–5.0 mg enrofloxacin per liter is used as a 5-hour treatment bath repeated every 24 hours (Lewbart et al. 1997). The resulting peak plasma concentration after such a treatment was 0.17 μg/mL. Studies of the stability of enrofloxacin in water at various degrees of salinity and pH showed enrofloxacin to be stable when added to a water bath (unpublished results from the laboratory of one of the authors). However, the effect of the drug on nitrifying bacteria in the water should be considered.

Large Animals. In horses, there is growing interest in the use of fluoroquinolones for treating bacterial infections resistant to other drugs. In cases in which an oral drug is needed, fluoroquinolones are the only drugs that can be administered safely in horses that have the gram-negative spectrum needed. Because fluoroquinolones do not cause much disruption of the intestinal bacterial flora, bacterial overgrowth, enteritis, and diarrhea are not as much of a problem as with other antibiotics in horses.

Enrofloxacin has been studied in horses more than the other quinolones. Orbifloxacin is well absorbed in horses (mean of 68% oral absorption), but clinical use has not been reported. For enrofloxacin, doses of 5 mg/kg orally produces sufficient plasma concentrations for C_{max}:MIC and AUC:MIC ratios high enough for most susceptible bacteria (Langston et al. 1996). Another recommendation, based on measuring plasma concentrations with a bioassay, was a once-daily dose for horses of 5 mg/kg IV or 7.5 mg/kg orally (Giguère et al. 1996). The oral absorption in this study was 62%. Enrofloxacin has achieved high tissue concentrations in horses and has been used for treating joint infections, endometritis, pneumonia, pleuropneumonia, and orthopedic infections caused by organisms resistant to other drugs. Urine concentrations were 170–830 times the plasma concentrations (Giguère et al. 1996). Most bacteria that infect horses are susceptible, but resistance is expected for streptococci and anaerobes. Strains of *P. aeruginosa* may be resistant or only moderately susceptible. *Rhodococcus equi* can be resistant, and success in treating *Rhodococcus* infections in horses with enrofloxacin has not been encouraging.

In cattle and sheep, the pharmacokinetics of enrofloxacin and danofloxacin has been reported (Table 45.1) and doses have been determined. Enrofloxacin is approved for use in cattle in the United States and some European countries. Danofloxacin is approved in some countries outside the United States. Fluoroquinolones can be valuable in ruminants because they are highly active against important pathogens. The MIC_{90} values listed for *Haemophilus somnus, Pasteurella haemolytica,* and *P. multocida* are 0.03, 0.06, and 0.03 μg/mL, respectively, and enrofloxacin is approved for treatment of bovine respiratory disease associated with these pathogens. Extra-label use is not allowed in food-producing animals. The US dose is flexible, with doses ranging from a single SC dose of 7.5–12.5 mg/kg, or treatment for three days at 2.5–5.0 mg/kg, once daily, SC. The withdrawal time is 28 days. It is not approved for lactating cattle or dairy calves, but disposition into milk of lactating cows has been studied. Enrofloxacin is highly excreted in milk. (See the section on administration of fluoroquinolones to nursing animals below.)

Administration to Nursing, Pregnant, or Young Animals

NURSING ANIMALS. Distribution also has been measured for milk in rabbits and cattle. Enrofloxacin is excreted rapidly in the milk after administration. In cattle after administration of enrofloxacin at 5 mg/kg, enrofloxacin concentrations in milk parallel the concentrations in serum, with a C_{max} of 1.3–2.5 μg/mL, but concentrations of the active metabolite ciprofloxacin exceed those of enrofloxacin (Kaartinen et al. 1995; Tyczkowska et al. 1994). Danofloxacin distribution into milk of cows exceeded serum concentrations (Shem-Tov et al. 1998). In rabbits the milk-to-plasma ratios were 3.6 and 2.6 for enrofloxacin and ciprofloxacin, respectively, after administration of 7.5 mg/kg IV (Aramayona et al. 1996). The reason for the high distribution of fluoroquinolones into milk is not known, because these concentrations do not match what is predicted from simple diffusion into milk, even after considering ion trapping. Protein binding is higher in milk, and the milk proteins may act as a reservoir for enrofloxacin and ciprofloxacin (Aramayona et al. 1996). Despite these concentrations of fluoroquinolones in milk, the activity of enrofloxacin in mastitic milk is decreased, possibly owing to lower pH, chelation with cations, or other factors in milk that inhibit fluoroquinolone activity (Kaartinen et al. 1995), and it has not been shown that fluoroquinolones are effective drugs for treating clinical mastitis.

When administering fluoroquinolones to nursing animals, the amount in the milk should be considered because fluoroquinolones may cause arthropathy in some species of young animals (discussed further in the section on safety below). Disposition into milk was studied in two mares after administration, and it was shown that although both ciprofloxacin and enrofloxacin were present in milk at levels that were as high or higher than the mares' plasma concentrations, the total doses administered to the foals via suckling were small, and the plasma concentrations in the foals were negligible (author's observations).

PREGNANT ANIMALS. When administering fluoroquinolones to pregnant animals, there will be some drug transfer across the placenta because these drugs are lipophilic and have low protein binding, and drug transfer is not limited by tissue barriers. Placental transfer has been specifically examined in rabbits, in which it was shown that the more lipophilic drug, enrofloxacin, crossed the placenta to a greater degree (80%) than ciprofloxacin (5% placental transfer), which is less lipophilic (Aramayona et al. 1994). Despite the rather high transfer of enrofloxacin across the placenta, there have been no reports of adverse effects when fluoroquinolones were administered to pregnant animals. Manufacturer studies have not shown any adverse effects on pregnancy or reproduction.

YOUNG ANIMALS. There is a risk that fluoroquinolones may cause damage to the developing cartilage of young animals. This is discussed more thoroughly in the section on safety. There have been few pharmacokinetic comparisons of young animals versus older animals, but the studies available demonstrate that young animals were exposed to more drug than adults because of slower clearance. After administration of enrofloxacin, calves at 1 day of age had smaller Vd, longer half-life, and decreased clearance than at 1 week of age (Kaartinen et al. 1997). There also was a smaller amount of metabolism of enrofloxacin to ciprofloxacin in 1-week-old calves than in older ones. Rabbit pups exhibited lower clearance and longer half-life for enrofloxacin than adult rabbits (Aramayona et al. 1996). This pattern was also seen in horses: foals at 1–2 weeks of age showed little metabolism of enrofloxacin to ciprofloxacin after administration of IV and oral doses. Foals also exhibited slower clearance and longer half-life than adults (Bermingham et al. 2000).

SAFETY. The fluoroquinolones have had a remarkably good safety record. For enrofloxacin, the LD_{50} in laboratory rats is 5000 mg/kg. When high doses were administered to animals during safety testing, one of the most common problems was gastrointestinal disturbances (nausea, vomiting, diarrhea), but these were usually produced at high doses and were not serious. Because these drugs do not alter the anaerobic flora of the gastrointestinal tract, there usually is minimal disruption of the intestinal bacterial population, even when these drugs are administered orally to small rodents. There have been no reports of cutaneous drug reactions resulting from fluoroquinolone usage in the veterinary literature, but some of the FOI summaries from manufacturers report an occasional reddening of the skin of dogs when high doses were administered.

There have been no reports of adverse effects on reproduction or pregnancy from administration of fluoroquinolones. Although the use in pregnant animals has been discouraged because of toxicity to developing cartilage, there have been no clinical reports where this effect has been described in offspring of treated animals.

With very high concentrations, adverse central nervous system (CNS) effects have been observed. The mechanism responsible for the CNS effects is believed to be inhibition of the inhibitory neurotransmitter GABA. Fluoroquinolones injected rapidly IV or administered at high doses can induce CNS excitement. Fluoroquinolones can precipitate convulsions in some animals and should not be administered to animals that are prone to seizures. In cats high doses of fluoroquinolones have caused ocular problems from drug-induced changes in the retina (Corrado et al. 1987). Because of the risk of enrofloxacin causing blindness in cats, doses higher than 5 mg/kg per day are not recommended.

Problems in Young Animals. In young, rapidly growing animals it is well known that fluoroquinolones can produce an arthropathy (Gough et al. 1992). Fluoroquinolones also have caused tendinitis and tendon rupture in people, but this effect has not been reported for animals. The species most susceptible to developmental arthropathy are rats and dogs. Dogs between the ages of 4 and 28 weeks are the most susceptible. Affected dogs may show signs of lameness and joint swelling, but if the drug is discontinued, the lesions may be reversible. Kittens, calves, and pigs are much more resistant to this effect. For example, feeder calves and 23-day-old calves were administered 25 mg/kg for 15 days without evidence of articular cartilage lesions. Young foals also are susceptible to the joint arthropathy from enrofloxacin at 10 mg/kg orally, but adverse effects have not been reported in adult horses.

The risk increases with higher doses and in most instances has been more clinically obvious only when the highest maximum dose was exceeded (e.g., at 25 mg/kg of enrofloxacin); however, even enrofloxacin dosages of 10 mg/kg/day have induced cartilage in young dogs. The use of fluoroquinolones has been discouraged in children, but thousands of children have been treated with these drugs under a compassionate protocol with no reports of joint arthropathy.

Joint arthropathy is best described as a toxicity to the chondrocyte that causes vesicles to form on the articular surface. The mechanism for damage to cartilage apparently is via chelation of magnesium by the drug. Magnesium is necessary for proper development of the cartilage matrix, especially in young, growing animals. Chelation of the magnesium results in a local magnesium deficiency leading to loss of proteoglycan in the articular cartilage. Studies in which magnesium was supplemented to decrease cartilage damage had equivocal results. (Magnesium added to the diet while oral drugs are administered would cause a chelation and significantly decrease oral absorption.)

Effects of Other Diseases or Conditions. There has been limited study of the disposition of fluoroquinolones in animals that have other conditions. In most of these instances, there were no changes in the drug's pharmacokinetics that would necessitate a change in dosage. Since the fluoroquinolones rely on both the kidneys and liver for clearance, insufficiency in one organ may result in compensation by the other clearance route. For example, renal failure may result in more reliance on hepatic clearance. In dogs with renal impairment, clearance of marbofloxacin was only slightly decreased and there was no significant effect on Vd or mean residence time (Lefebvre et al. 1998). In camels that were deprived of water for 14 days and lost 12.5% of their body weight, there was little effect on the distribution, clearance, or half-life of enrofloxacin. Water deprivation resulted in a slower and less complete absorption from a SC injection compared to normal camels or camels injected IM (Gavrielli et al. 1995).

DRUG INTERACTIONS. Combinations with other antibiotics neither antagonize nor enhance the microbiologic effects of fluoroquinolones. The currently used fluoroquinolones will kill bacteria whether or not they are dividing (Lode et al. 1998). Therefore, use of a bacteriostatic agent should not interfere with the action of a fluoroquinolone. Although there is no evidence that other antibiotics produce a synergistic effect when administered with fluoroquinolones, they may produce an additive effect and broaden the spectrum of activity.

Fluoroquinolones are involved in some drug interactions, but few of these are serious. Drugs containing di- and trivalent cations, such as antacids or sucralfate, can inhibit oral absorption (Nix et al. 1989). Fluoroquinolones may inhibit metabolism of some drugs through an interaction with hepatic metabolism. One such example is the inhibition of theophylline metabolism by enrofloxacin (Intorre et al. 1995), in which enrofloxacin significantly increased the C_{max} and decreased systemic clearance of theophylline in dogs. In people, there are reports of an interaction between certain nonsteroidal anti-inflammatory drugs (NSAIDs) and fluoroquinolones (Hori et al. 1989), but this interaction has not been reported in animals.

FORMULATIONS AVAILABLE. Fluoroquinolones licensed for small-animal use are available as oral preparations and may be given to dogs on a once-a-day basis. There are no oral liquid preparations currently available in the United States, but veterinarians have used compounding pharmacists to create oral liquid preparations from tablets dissolved in an aqueous vehicle. The only veterinary fluoroquinolone currently available in an injectable preparation for dogs and cats is enrofloxacin (2.27% solution, 22.7 mg/mL). It is licensed for IM administration, but veterinarians have administered this preparation IV without serious problems. The formulation approved for SC injection in cattle in the United States is 100 mg/mL in an L-arginine base. This preparation may cause tissue irritation if injected in small animals.

Some veterinarians have used topical administration of enrofloxacin for otitis externa caused by pseudomonads (Griffin 1993, 1999; Rosychuk 1994). This is not approved use of this drug, nor has it been clinically evaluated for efficacy, but veterinarians have mixed the 2.27% injectable solution of enrofloxacin with saline, water, or other topical ear solutions in a 1:1 to 4:1 ratio (e.g., 4 parts saline, 1 part enrofloxacin). Stability studies by one of the authors (M.G.P.) with HPLC analysis confirmed these solutions to be stable for 2 weeks at room temperature. When the infection is believed to extend to the middle ear, topical treatment alone is not sufficient, and systemic treatment for pseudomonads should be administered.

REFERENCES

Abadia, A. R., Aramayona, J. J., Munoz, M. J., Pla Delfina, J. M., Saez, M. P., and Bregante, M. A. 1994. Disposition of ciprofloxacin following intravenous administration in dogs. Journal of Veterinary Pharmacology and Therapeutics 17:384–388.

Anadón, A., Martinez-Larranaga, M. R., Diaz, J., Bringas, P., Martinez, M. A., Fernandez-Cruz, M. L., and Fernandez, R. 1995. Pharmacokinetics and residues of enrofloxacin in chickens. American Journal of Veterinary Research 56:501–506.

Aramayona, J. J., Garcia, M. A., Fraile, L., Abadia, A. R., and Bregante, M. A. 1994. Placental transfer of enrofloxacin and ciprofloxacin in rabbits. American Journal of Veterinary Research 55:1313–1318.

Aramayona, J. J., Mora, J., Fraile, L., Garcia, M. A., Abadia, A. R., and Bregante, M. A. 1996. Penetration of enrofloxacin and ciprofloxacin into breast milk, and pharmacokinetics of the drugs in lactating rabbits and neonatal offspring. American Journal of Veterinary Research 57:547–553.

Asuquo, A. E., and Piddock, L. J. V. 1993. Accumulation and killing kinetics of fifteen quinolones for *Escherichia coli, Staphylococcus aureus,* and *Pseudomonas aeruginosa.* Journal of Antimicrobial Chemotherapy 31:865–880.

Atta, A. H., and Sharif, L. 1997. Pharmacokinetics of ciprofloxacin following intravenous and oral administration in broiler chickens. Journal of Veterinary Pharmacology and Therapeutics 20:326–329.

Bailly, S., Fay, M., Roche, Y., and Gougerot-Pocidalo, M. A. 1990. Effect of quinolones on tumor necrosis factor production by human monocytes. International Journal of Immunopharmacology 12:31–36.

Barsanti, J. A. 1995. Diseases of the prostate gland. In C. A. Osborne and D. R. Finco, eds., Canine and Feline Nephrology and Urology, pp. 726–755. Baltimore: Lea & Febiger.

Bermingham, E. C., Papich, M. G., and Vivrette, S. 2000. Pharmacokinetics of enrofloxacin after oral and IV administration to foals. American Journal of Veterinary Research 46(6):

Blaser, J., Stone, B. J., Groner, M. C., and Zinner, S. H. 1987. Comparative study with enoxacin and netilmicin in a pharmacodynamic model to determine importance of ratio of antibiotic peak concentration to MIC for bactericidal activity and emergence of resistance. Antimicrobial Agents and Chemotherapy 31:1054–1060.

Bowser, P. R., Wooster, G. A., St. Leger, J., and Babish, J. G. 1992. Pharmacokinetics of enrofloxacin in fingerling rainbow trout (*Oncorhynchus mykiss).* Journal of Veterinary Pharmacology and Therapeutics 15:62–71.

Bregante, M. A., Saez, P., Aramayona, J. J., Fraile, L., Garcia, M. A., and Solans, C. 1999. Comparative pharmacokinetics of enrofloxacin in mice, rats, rabbits, sheep, and cows. American Journal of Veterinary Research 60:1111–1116.

Breitschwerdt, E. B., Davidson, M. G., Aucoin, D. P., Levy, M. G., Szabados, N. S., Hegarty, B. C., Kuehne, A. L., and James, R. L. 1990. Efficacy of chloramphenicol, enrofloxacin, and tetracycline, for treatment of experimental Rocky Mountain Spotted Fever in dogs. Antimicrobial Agents and Chemotherapy 35:2375–2381.

Breitschwerdt, E. B., Papich, M. G., Hegarty, B. C., Gilger, B., Hancock, S. I., and Davidson, M. G. 1999. Efficacy of doxycycline, azithromycin, or trovafloxacin for treatment of experimental Rocky Mountain Spotted Fever in dogs. Antimicrobial Agents and Chemotherapy. 43:813–821.

Brighty, K. E., and Gootz, T. D. 1997. The chemistry and biological profile of trovafloxacin. Journal of Antimicrobial Chemotherapy 39(Suppl. B):1–14.

Broome, R. L, and Brooks, D. L. 1991. Efficacy of enrofloxacin in the treatment of respiratory pasteurellosis in rabbits. Laboratory Animal Science 41:572–576.

Broome, R. L., Brooks, D. L., Babish, J. G., Copeland, D. D., and Conzelman, G. M. 1991. Pharmacokinetic properties of enrofloxacin in rabbits. American Journal of Veterinary Research 52:1835–1841.

Brown, S. A. 1996. Fluoroquinolones in animal health. Journal of Veterinary Pharmacologic Therapy 19:1–14.

Bryant, E. E., and Mazza, J. A. 1989. Effect of the abscess environment on the antimicrobial activity of ciprofloxacin. American Journal of Medicine 87(Suppl. 5A):23S–27S.

Cabanes, A., Arboix, M., Anton, J. M. A., and Reig, F. 1992. Pharmacokinetics of enrofloxacin after intravenous and intramuscular injection in rabbits. American Journal of Veterinary Research 53:2090–2093.

Caputo, J. F., Brown, S. A., and Papich, M. G. 1997. Pharmacokinetics of premafloxacin following single intravenous, oral solution, or oral capsule dose to healthy Beagle dogs. Journal of Veterinary Pharmacology and Therapeutics 20(Suppl. 1):60–61.

Carlotti, D. N. 1996. New trends in systemic antibiotic therapy of bacterial skin disease in dogs. Compendium on Continuing Education for the Practicing Veterinarian 18(Suppl.):40–47.

Carlotti, D. N., Jasmin, P., Guaguere, E., et al. 1995. Utilisation de la marbofloxacine dans le traitement des pyodermites du chien. Pratique Medicale et Chirurgicale de l'Animal de Compagnie 30:281–293.

Carlotti, D. N., Guaguere, E., Pin, D., et al. 1999. Therapy of difficult cases of canine pyoderma with marbofloxacin: a report of 39 cases. Journal of Small Animal Practice 40:265-270.

Cester, C. C., Schneider, M., and Toutain, P.-L. 1996. Comparative kinetics of two orally administered fluoroquinolones in dog: enrofloxacin versus marbofloxacin. Revue Med Vet 147:703–716.

Chen, D. K., McGeer, A., de Azavedo, J. C., and Low, D. E. 1999. Decreased susceptibility of *Streptococcus pneumoniae* to fluoroquinolones in Canada. New England Journal of Medicine 341:233–239.

Chew, D. J. 1997. An overview of prostatic disease. Compendium of Continuing Education for the Practicing Veterinarian 19:80–85.

Cole, L. K., Kwochka, K. W., Kowalski, J. J., and Hillier, A. 1998. Microbial flora and antimicrobial susceptibility patterns of isolated pathogens from the horizontal ear canal and middle ear in dogs with otitis media. Journal of the American Veterinary Medical Association 212:534–538.

Collins, B. 1994. Antimicrobial drug use in rabbits, rodents, and other small mammals. Proceedings of an International Symposium on Antimicrobial Selection, Orlando: The North American Veterinary Conference, pp. 12–17.

Corrado, M. L., Struble, W. E., Peter, C., et al. 1987. Norfloxacin: review of safety studies. American Journal of Medicine 82(Suppl. 6B):22–26.

Cotard, J. P., Gruet, P., Pechereau, D., Moreau, P., Pages, J. P., Thomas, E. and Deleforge, J. 1995. Comparative study of marbofloxacin and amoxicillin-clavulanic acid in the treatment of urinary tract infections in dogs. Journal of Small Animal Practice 36:349–353.

DeBoer, D. J. 1995. Management of chronic and recurrent pyoderma in the dog. In J. D. Bonagura, ed., Kirk's Current Veterinary Therapy XII, pp. 611–617. Philadelphia: W. B. Saunders.

DeManuelle, T. C., Ihrke, P. J., Brandt, C. M., Kass, P. H., and Vuilliet, P. R. 1998. Determination of skin concentrations of enrofloxacin in dogs with pyoderma. American Journal of Veterinary Research 59:1599–1604.

Dorfman, M., Barsanti, J., and Budsberg, S. C. 1995. Enrofloxacin concentrations in dogs with normal prostate and dogs with chronic bacterial prostatitis. American Journal of Veterinary Research 56:386–390.

Dowling, P. M., Wilson, R. C., Tyler, J. W., and Duran, S. H. 1995. Pharmacokinetics of ciprofloxacin in ponies. Journal of Veterinary Pharmacology and Therapeutics 18:7–12.

Drlica, K., and Zhao, X. 1997. DNA gyrase, Topoisomerase IV, and the 4-quinolones. Microbiology and Molecular Biology Reviews 61:377–392.

Drusano, G. L., Johnson, D. E., Rosen, M., and Stadiford, H. C. 1993. Pharmacodynamics of a fluoroquinolone antimicrobial agent in a neutropenic rat model of *Pseudomonas* sepsis. Antimicrobial Agents and Chemotherapy 37:483–490.

Dudley, M. N. 1991. Pharmacodynamics and pharmacokinetics of antibiotics with special reference to the fluoroquinolones. Ameriacn Journal of Medicine 91(Suppl. 6A):45S–50S.

Duval, J. M., and Budsberg S. C. 1995. Cortical bone concentrations of enrofloxacin in dogs. American Journal of Veterinary Research 56:188–192.

Easmon, C. S. F., and Crane, J. P. 1985. Uptake of ciprofloxacin by macrophages. Journal of Clinical Pathology 38:442–444.

Endtz, H. P., Ruijs, G. J., van Klingeren, B., et al. 1991. Quinolone resistance in campylobacter isolated from man and poultry following the introduction of fluoroquinolones in veterinary medicine. Journal of Antimicrobial Chemotherapy 27:199–208.

Everett, M. J., Jin, Y. F., Ricci, V., and Piddock, L. J. V. 1996. Contributions of individual mechanisms to fluoroquinolone resistance in 36 *Escherichia coli* strains isolated from humans and animals. Antimicrobial Agents and Chemotherapy 40:2380–2386.

Fernandes, P. B. 1988. Mode of action and in vitro and in vivo activities of the fluoroquinolones. Journal of Clinical Pharmacology 28:156–168.

Ferrero, L., Cameron, B., and Crouzet, J. 1995. Analysis of gyrA and grlA mutations in stepwise-selected ciprofloxacin-resistant mutants of *Staphylococcus aureus*. Antimicrobial Agents and Chemotherapy 39:1554–1558.

Flammer, K. 1998. Common bacterial infections and antibiotic use in companion birds. Compendium on Continuing Education for the Practicing Veterinarian 20(Suppl. 3A):34–48.

Flammer, K., Aucoin, D. P., Whitt, D. A., and Prus, S. A. 1990. Plasma concentrations of enrofloxacin in African grey parrots treated with medicated water. Avian Disease 34:1017–1022.

Flammer, K., Aucoin, D. P., and Whitt, D. A. 1991. Intramuscular and oral disposition of enrofloxacin in African grey parrots following single and multiple doses. Journal of Veterinary Pharmacology and Therapeutics 14:359–366.

Forrest, A., Nix, D. E., Ballow, C. H., Goss, T. F., Birmingham, M. C., and Schentag, J. J. 1993. Pharmacodynamics of intravenous ciprofloxacin in seriously ill patients. Antimicrobial Agents and Chemotherapy 37:1073–1081.

Garaffo, R., Jambou, D., Chichmanian, R. M., et al. 1991. In vitro and in vivo ciprofloxacin pharmacokinetics in human neutrophils. Antimicrobial Agents and Chemotherapeutics 35:2215–2218.

Gavrielli, R., Yagil, R., Ziv, G., Creveld, C. V., and Glickman, A. 1995. Effect of water deprivation on the disposition kinetics of enrofloxacin in camels. Journal of Veterinary Pharmacology and Therapeutics 18:333–339.

Giguère, S., Sweeney, R. W., and Belanger, M. 1996. Pharmacokinetics of enrofloxacin in adult horses and concentration of the drug in serum, body fluids, and endometrial tissues after repeated intragastrically administered doses. American Journal of Veterinary Research 57:1025–1030.

Göbel, T. 1999. Bacterial diseases and antimicrobial therapy in small mammals. Compendium on Continuing Education for the Practicing Veterinarian 21(Suppl. 3E):5–20.

Gough, A. W., Kasali, O. B., Sigler, R. E., and Baragi, V. 1992. Quinolone arthropathy: acute toxicity to immature articular cartilage. Toxicological Pathology 20:436–447.

Griffin, C. E. 1993. Otitis externa and otitis media. In C. E. Griffin, K. W. Kwochka, and J. M. MacDonald, eds., Current Veterinary Dermatology: The Science and Art of Therapeutics, pp. 245–262. Philadelphia: W. B. Saunders.

———. 1999. Pseudomonas otitis therapy. In J. D. Bonagura, ed., Current Veterinary Therapy XIII. Philadelphia: W. B. Saunders.

Griggs, D. J., Hall, M. C., Jin, Y. F., and Piddock, J. V. 1994. Quinolone resistance in veterinary isolates of *Salmonella*. Journal of Antimicrobial Chemotherapy 33:1173–1189.

Gruet, P., Richard, P., Thomas, E., and Autefage, A. 1997. Prevention of surgical infections in dogs with a single intravenous injection of marbofloxacin: an experimental model. Veterinary Record 140:199–202.

Gyrd-Hansen, N., and Nielsen, P. 1994. The influence of feed on the oral bioavailability of enrofloxacin, oxytetracycline, penicillin V, and spiramycin in pigs. Proceedings of the 6th EAVPT Congress, pp. 242–243.

Hannan, P. C. T., Windsor, G. D., De Jong, A., Schmeer, N., and Stegemann, M. 1997. Comparative susceptibilities of various animal-pathogenic mycoplasmas to fluoroquinolones. Antimicrobial Agents and Chemotherapy 41:2037–2040.

Hawkins, E. C., Boothe, D. M., Guin, A., et al. 1998. Concentration of enrofloxacin and its active metabolite in alveolar macrophages and pulmonary epithelial lining fluid of dogs. Journal of Veterinary Pharmacology and Therapeutics 21:18–23.

Hedin, G., and Hambreus, A. 1991. Multiply antibiotic-resistant Staphylococcus epidermidis in patients, staff, and environment—a one-week survey in a bone marrow transplant unit. Journal of Hospital Infection 17:95–106.

Heinen, E. 1999. Comparative pharmacokinetics of enrofloxacin and difloxacin as well as their main metabolites in dogs. Compendium for Continuing Education for the Practicing Veterinarian 21(Suppl. 10).

Helmick, K. E., Papich, M. G., Vliet, K. A., et al. 1997. Preliminary kinetics of single dose intravenously administered enrofloxacin and oxytetracycline in the American alligator *(Alligator mississippiensis)*. Proceedings of the American Association of Zoo Veterinarians, pp. 27–28.

Hori, S., Shimada, J., Saito, A., Matsuda, M., and Mitahara, T. 1989. Comparison of the inhibitory effects of new quinolones on gamma aminobutyric acid receptor binding in the presence of anti-inflammatory drugs. Review of Infectious Diseases 11(Suppl. 5):1397–1398.

Hungerford, C., Spelman, L., and Papich, M. G. 1997. Pharmacokinetics of enrofloxacin after oral and intramuscular administration in Savanna monitors *(Varanus exanthematicus)*. Proceedings of the American Association of Zoo Veterinarians, pp. 89–92.

Hyatt, J. M., McKinnon, P. S., Zimmer, G. S., and Schentag, J. J. 1995. The importance of pharmacokinetic/pharmacodynamic surrogate markers to outcome. Clinical Pharmacokinetics 28:143–160.

Ihrke, P. J. 1996. Experiences with enrofloxacin in small animal dermatology. Compendium of Continuing Education for the Practicing Veterinarian 18(2):35–39.

———. 1998. Bacterial infections of the skin. In C. E. Greene, ed., Infectious Diseases of the Dog and Cat, 2nd ed., pp. 541–547. Philadelphia: W. B. Saunders.

Ihrke, P. J., and DeManuelle, T. C. 1999. German Shepherd Dog pyoderma: an overview and antimicrobial management. Compendium of Continuing Education for the Small Animal Practitioner 21(Suppl. 10).

Ihrke, P. J., Papich, M. G., and DeManuelle, T. C. 1999. The use of fluoroquinolones in veterinary dermatology. Veterinary Dermatology 10:193–204.

Intorre, L., Mengozzi, G., Maccheroni, M., Bertini, S., and Soldani, G. 1995. Enrofloxacin-theophylline interaction: influence of enrofloxacin on theophylline steady-state pharmacokinetics in the Beagle dog. Journal of Veterinary Pharmacology and Therapeutics 18:352–356.

Jacobson, E. R. 1999. Antimicrobial therapy in reptiles. Compendium on Continuing Education for the Practicing Veterinarian 21(Suppl. 3E):33–48.

Jalal, S., and Wretlind, B. 1998. Mechanisms of quinolone resistance in clinical strains of *Pseudomonas aeruginosa.* Microbial Drug Resistance 4:257–261.

James, S., Papich, M. G., and Raphael, B. Forthcoming. Pharmacokinetics of enrofloxacin after oral and intramuscular administration in red-eared sliders *(Chrysemys scripts elegans).*

Janbon, F., Jonquet, O., Reynes, J., and Bertrand, A. 1989. Use of pefloxacin in the treatment of rickettsiosis and coxiellosis. Review of Infectious Diseases 11(Suppl.5):990–991.

Jordan, F. T. W., Horrocks, B. K., Jones, S. K., Cooper, A. C., and Giles, C. J. 1993. A comparison of the efficacy of danofloxacin and tylosin in the control of *Mycoplasma gallisepticum* infection in broiler chicks. Journal of Veterinary Pharmacology and Therapeutics 16:79–86.

Kaartinen, L., Salonen, M., Älli, L., and Pyörälä, S. 1995. Pharmacokinetics of enrofloxacin after single intravenous, intramuscular, and subcutaneous injections in cows. Journal of Veterinary Pharmacology and Therapeutics 18:357–362.

Kaartinen, L., Pyörälä, S., Moilanen, M., and Räisänen, S. 1997. Pharmacokinetics of enrofloxacin in newborn and one-week-old calves. Journal of Veterinary Pharmacology and Therapeutics 20:479–482.

Knoll, U., Glunder, G., and Kietzmann, M. 1999. Comparative study of the plasma pharmacokinetics and tissue concentrations of danofloxacin and enrofloxacin in broiler chickens. Journal of Veterinary Pharmacology and Therapeutics 22:239–246.

Knöller, J., Brom, J., Schönfeld, W., and König 1989. Influence of ciprofloxacin on leukotriene generation from various cells in vitro. Journal of Antimicrobial Chemotherapy 25:605–612.

Koch, H.-J., and Peters, S. 1996. Antimicrobial therapy in German Shepherd dog pyoderma (GSP). An open clinical study. Veterinary Dermatology 7:177–181.

Kontos, V. I., and Athanasiou, L. V. 1998. Use of enrofloxacin in the treatment of acute ehrlichiosis. Canine Practice 23:10–14.

Kordick, D., Papich, M. G., and Breitschwerdt, E. B. 1997. Efficacy of enrofloxacin or doxycycline for treatment of *Bartonella henselae* or *Bartonella clarridgeiae* infection in cats. Antimicrobial Agents and Chemotherapy 41:2448–2455.

Küng, K., Riond, J.-L., and Wanner, M. 1993a. Pharmacokinetics of enrofloxacin and its metabolite ciprofloxacin after intravenous and oral administration of enrofloxacin in dogs. Journal of Veterinary Pharmacology and Therapeutics 16:462–468.

Küng, K., Riond, J.-L., Wolfram, S., and Wanner, M. 1993b. Comparison of an HPLC and bioassay method to determine antimicrobial concentrations after intravenous and oral administration of enrofloxacin in four dogs. Research in Veterinary Science 54:247–248.

Kwochka, K. W. 1993. Recurrent pyoderma. In C. E. Griffin, K. W. Kwochka, J. M. MacDonald, eds., Current Veterinary Dermatology, pp. 3–21. St. Louis: Mosby Yearbook.

Langston, V. C., Sedrish, S., and Boothe, D. M. 1996. Disposition of single-dose oral enrofloxacin in the horse. Journal of Veterinary Pharmacology and Therapeutics 19:316–319.

Lefebvre, H. P., Schneider, M., Dupouy, V., Laroute, V., Costes, G., Delesalle, L., and Toutain, P. L. 1998. Effect of experimental renal impairment on disposition of marbofloxacin and its metabolites in the dog. Journal of Veterinary Pharmacology and Therapeutics 21:453–461.

Legg, J. M., and Bint, A. J. 1999. Will pneumococci put quinolones in their place? Journal of Antimicrobial Chemotherapy 44:425–427.

Lewbart, G. A. 1998. Koi medicine and management. Compendium on Continuing Education for the Practicing Veterinarian 20(Suppl. 3A):5–12.

Lewbart, G. A., Vaden, S., Deen, J., et al. 1997. Pharmacokinetics of enrofloxacin in the red pacu *(Colossoma brachypomum)* after intramuscular, oral and bath administration. Journal of Veterinary Pharmacology and Therapeutics 20:124–128.

Ling, G. V. 1995. Lower Urinary Tract Diseases of Dogs and Cats: Diagnosis, Medical Management, Prevention, pp. 116–128. St. Louis: Mosby Yearbook.

Linnehan, R. M., Ulrich, R. W., and Ridgway, S. 1999. Enrofloxacin serum bioactivity in bottlenose dolphins, *Tursiops truncatus,* following oral administration of 5 mg/kg in whole fish. Journal of Veterinary Pharmacology and Therapeutics 22:170–173.

Lloyd, D. H. 1992. Therapy for canine pyoderma. In R. W. Kirk and J. D. Bonagura, eds., Kirk's Current Veterinary Therapy XI, pp. 539–544. Philadelphia: W. B. Saunders.

Lloyd, D. H., Lamport, A. I., Noble, W. C., and Howell, S. A. 1999. Fluoroquinolone resistance in *Staphylococcus intermedius.* Veterinary Dermatology 10:249–251.

Lode, H., Borner, K., and Koeppe, P. 1998. Pharmacodynamics of fluoroquinolones. Clinical Infectious Diseases 27:33–39.

Martinez-Martinez, L., Pascual, A., and Jacoby, G. A. 1998. Quinolone resistance from a transferable plasmid. Lancet 351:797–799.

Meinen, J. B., Rosin, E., and McClure, J. T. 1995. Pharmacokinetics of enrofloxacin in clinically normal dogs and mice and drug pharmacodynamics in neutropenic mice with *Escherichia coli* and staphylococcal infections. American Journal of Veterinary Research 56:1219–1224.

Mengozzi, G., Intorre, L., Bertini S., and Soldani, G. 1996. Pharmacokinetics of enrofloxacin and its metabolite ciprofloxacin after intravenous and intramuscular administration in sheep. American Journal of Veterinary Research 57:1040–1043.

Monlouis, J.-D., DeJong, A., Limet, A., and Richez, P. 1997. Plasma pharmacokinetics and urine concentrations after oral administration of enrofloxacin to dogs. Journal of Veterinary Pharmacology and Therapeutics 20(Suppl. 1):61–63.

Murphy, O. M., Marshall, C., Stewart, D., and Freeman, R. 1997. Ciprofloxacin-resistant Enterobacteriaceae. Lancet 349:1028–1029.

Neu, H. C. 1992. The crisis in antibiotic resistance. Science 257:1064–1073.

Nicolau, D. P., Quintiliani, R., and Nightingale, C. H. 1995. Antibiotic kinetics and dynamics for the clinician. Medical Clinics of North America 79:477–495.

Nikaido, H., and Thanassi, D. G. 1993. Penetration of lipophilic agents with multiple protonation sites into bacterial cells: tetracyclines and fluoroquinolones as examples. Antimicrobial Agents and Chemotherapy 37:1393–1399.

Nix, D. E., Watson, W. A., Lener, M. E., et al. 1989. Effects of aluminum and magnesium antacids and ranitidine on the absorption of ciprofloxacin. Clinical Pharmacology and Therapeutics 46:700–705.

Nix, D. E., Goodwin, S. D., Peloquin, C. A., Rotella, D. L., and Schentag, J. J. 1991. Antibiotic tissue penetration and its relevance: impact of tissue penetration on infection response. Antimicrobial Agents and Chemotherapeutics 35:1953–1959.

Nouws, J. F. M., Mevius, D. J., Vree, T. B., Baars, A. M., and Laurensen, J. 1988. Pharmacokinetics, renal clearance, and metabolism of ciprofloxacin following intravenous and oral administration to calves and pigs. Veterinary Quarterly 10:156–163.

Papich, M. G. 1999. Pharmacokinetics of enrofloxacin in reptiles. Compendium for Continuing Education for the Practicing Veterinarian 21(Suppl. 10).

Paradis, M., Lemay, S., Scott D. W., et al. 1990. Efficacy of enrofloxacin in the treatment of canine bacterial pyoderma. Veterinary Dermatology 1:123–127.

Pascual, A., Garcia, I., and Perea, E. J. 1990. Uptake and intracellular activity of an optically active ofloxacin isomer in human neutrophils and tissue culture cells. Antimicrobial Agents and Chemotherapy 34:277–280.

Peña, C., Albareda, J. M., Pallares, R., Pujol, M., Tubau, F., and Ariza, J. 1995. Relationship between quinolone use and emergence of ciprofloxacin-resistant *Escherichia coli* in bloodstream infections. Antimicrobial Agents and Chemotherapy 39:520–524.

Perea, S., Hidalgo, M., Arcediano, A., et al. 1999. Incidence and clinical impact of fluoroquinolone-resistant *Escherichia coli* in the faecal flora of cancer patients treated with high dose chemotherapy and ciprofloxacin prophylaxis. Journal of Antimicrobial Chemotherapy 44:117–120.

Piddock, L. J. V., Ricci, V., McLaren, I., and Griggs, D. J. 1998. Role of mutation in the *gyrA* and *parC* genes of nalidixic-acid-resistant salmonella serotypes isolated from animals in the United Kingdom. Journal of Antimicrobial Chemotherapy 41:635–641.

Pijpers, A., Heinen, E., DeJong A., and Verheijden, J. H. M. 1997. Enrofloxacin pharmacokinetics after intravenous and intramuscular administration in pigs. Journal of Veterinary Pharmacology and Therapeutics 20(Suppl. 1):42–43.

Pirro, F., Scheer, M., and de Jong, A. 1997. Additive in vitro activity of enrofloxacin and its main metabolite ciprofloxacin. 14th Annual Congress of the ESVD-ECVD, p. 199.

Pirro, F., Edingloh, M., and Schmeer, N. 1999. Bactericidal and inhibitory activity of enrofloxacin and other fluoroquinolones in small animal pathogens. Compendium on Continuing Education for the Practicing Veterinarian 21(Suppl. 10).

Pozzin, O., Harron, D. W. G., Nation, G., Tinson, A. H., Sheen, R., and Dhanasekharan, S. 1997. Pharmacokinetics of enrofloxacin following intravenous/intramuscular/oral administration in Nedji sheep. Journal of Veterinary Pharmacology and Therapeutics 20(Suppl. 1):60.

Prezant, R. M., Isaza, R., and Jacobson, E. R. 1994. Plasma concentrations and disposition kinetics of enrofloxacin in gopher tortoises *(Gopherus polyphemus)*. Journal of Zoo and Wildlife Medicine 25:82–87.

Pyörälä, , S., Panu, S., and Kaartinen, L. 1994. Single dose pharmacokinetics of ciprofloxacin in horses. Proceedings of EAVPT, pp. 45–46.

Raoult, D., and Drancourt, M. 1991. Antimicrobial therapy of rickettsial diseases. Antimicrobial Agents of Chemotherapy 35:2457–2462.

Raphael, B. L., Papich, M. G., and Cook, R. A. 1994. Pharmacokinetics of enrofloxacin after a single intramuscular injection in Indian star tortoises *(Geochelone elegans)*. Journal of Zoo Wildlife Medicine 25:88–94.

Richez, P., Dellac, B., Froyman, R., and DeJong, A. 1994.Pharmacokinetics of enrofloxacin in calves and adult cattle after single and repeated subcutaneous injections. Proceedings of European Association for Veterinary Pharmacology and Toxicology, Proceedings of the 6th International Congress, Deinburgh, UK, 1994, pp. 232-233.

Richez, P., Pedersen Morner, A., DeJong, A., and Monlouis, J. D. 1997a. Plasma pharmacokinetics of parenterally administered danofloxacin and enrofloxacin in pigs. Journal of Veterinary Pharmacology and Therapeutics 20(Suppl. 1):41–42.

Richez, P., Monlouis, J. D., Dellac, B., and Daube, B. 1997b. Validation of a therapeutic regimen for enrofloxacin in cats on the basis of pharmacokinetic data. Journal of Veterinary Pharmacology and Therapeutics 20(Suppl. 1):152–153.

Rosenthal, K. L. 1999. Avian bacterial infections and their treatment. Compendium on Continuing Education for the Practicing Veterinarian 21(Suppl. 3E):21–32.

Ross, D. L., and Riley, C. M. 1994. Dissociation and complexation of the fluoroquinolone antimicrobials—an update. Journal of Pharmaceutical and Biomedical Analysis 12:1325–1331.

Rosychuk, R. A. W. 1994. Management of otitis externa. In R. A. W. Rosychuk and S. R. Merchant, eds., Veterinary Clinics of North America: Small Animal Practice 24(5):921–952.

Sanders, C. C., Sanders, W. E., and Thomson, K. S. 1995. Fluoroquinolone resistance in staphylococci: new challenges. European Journal of Clinical Microbiology and Infectious Disease 14(Suppl. 1):S6–S11.

Schneider, M., Thomas, V., Boisrame, B., and Deleforge, J. 1996. Pharmacokinetics of marbofloxacin in dogs after oral and parenteral administration. Journal of Veterinary Pharmacology and Therapeutics 19:56–61.

Shem-Tov, M., Rav-Hon, O., Ziv, G., Lavi, E., Glickman, A., and Saran, A. 1998. Pharmacokinetics and penetration of danofloxacin from the blood into the milk of cows. Journal of Veterinary Pharmacology and Therapeutics 21:209–213.

Smith, K. E., Besser, J. M., Hedberg, C. W., et al. 1999. Quinolone-resistant Campylobacter jejuni infections in Minnesota, 1992–1998. New England Journal of Medicine 340:1525–1532.

Spreng, M., Deleforge, J., Thomas, V., Boisrame, B., and Drugeon, H. 1995. Antibacterial activity of marbofloxacin: a new fluoroquinolone for veterinary use against canine and feline isolates. Journal of Veterinary Pharmacology and Therapeutics 18:284–289.

Stegemann, M., Heukamp, U., Scheer, M., and Krebber, R. 1996. Kinetics of antibacterial activity after administration of enrofloxacin in dog serum and skin: in vitro susceptibility of field isolates. Compendium on Continuing Education for the Practicing Veterinarian 18(Suppl.):30–34.

Stegemann, M., Wollen, T. S., Ewert, K. M., Terhune, T. N., and Copeland, D. D. 1997. Plasma pharmacokinetics of enrofloxacin administered to cattle at a dose of 7.5 mg/kg. Journal of Veterinary Pharmacology and Therapeutics 20(Suppl. 1):22.

Stoffregen, D. A., Wooster, G. A., Bustos, P. S., Bowser, P. R., and Babish, J. G. 1997. Multiple route and dose pharmacokinetics of enrofloxacin in juvenile Atlantic salmon.

Journal of Veterinary Pharmacology and Therapeutics 20:111–123.

Studdert, V. P., and Hughes, K. L. 1992. Treatment of opportunistic mycobacterial infections with enrofloxacin in cats. Journal of the American Veterinary Medical Association 201:1388–1390.

Sullivan, M. C., Cooper, B. W., Nightingale, C. H., Quintiliani, R., and Lawlor, M. T. 1993. Evaluation of the efficacy of ciprofloxacin against *Streptococcus pneumoniae* by using a mouse protection model. Antimicrobial Agents and Chemotherapy 37:234–239.

Takács-Novák, K., Jozan, M., Hermecz, I., and Szasz, G. 1992. Lipophilicity of antibacterial fluoroquinolones. International Journal of Pharmaceutics 79:89–96.

Threlfall, E. J., Frost, J. A., Ward, L. R., and Rowe, R. 1995. Epidemic in cattle of S typhimurium DT 104 with chromosomally-integrated multiple drug resistance. Veterinary Record 134:577.

Threlfall, E. J., Cheasty, T., Graham, A. and Rowe, B. 1997. High-level resistance to ciprofloxacin in *Escherichia coli*. Lancet 349:403 (Letter).

Tulkens, P. M. 1990. Accumulation and subcellular distribution of antibiotics in macrophages in relation to activity against intracellular bacteria. In R. J. Fass, ed., Ciprofloxacin in Pulmonology, pp. 12–20. Bern: W. Zuckschwerdt Verlag Munchen.

Tyczkowska, K. L., Voyksner, R. D., Anderson, K. L., and Papich, M. G. 1994. Simultaneous determination of enrofloxacin and its primary metabolite ciprofloxacin in bovine milk and plasma by ion-pairing liquid chromatography. Journal of Chromatography B: Biomedical Applications 658:341–348.

Vancutsem, P. M., Babish, J. G., and Schwark, W. S. 1990. The fluoroquinolone antimicrobials: structure, antimicrobial activity, pharmacokinetics, clinical use in domestic animals, and toxicity. Cornell Veterinarian 80:173–186.

Villa, R., Prandini, E., Caloni, F., and Carli, S. 1997. Serum protein binding of some sulfonamides, quinolones, and fluoroquinolones in farm animals and domestic animals. Journal of Veterinary Pharmacology and Therapeutics 20(Suppl. 1):60.34–35.

Walker, R. D., Stein, G. E., Hauptman, J. G., MacDonald, K. H., Budsberg, S. C., and Rosser, E. J. 1990. Serum and tissue cage fluid concentrations of ciprofloxacin after oral administration of the drug to healthy dogs. American Journal of Veterinary Research 51:896–900.

Walker, R. D., Stein, G. E., Hauptman, J. G., and MacDonald, K. H. 1992. Pharmacokinetics evaluation of enrofloxacin administered orally to healthy sdogs. American Journal of Veterinary Research 53:2315–2319.

Watts, J. L., Salmon, S. A., Sanchez, M. S., and Yancey, R. J. 1997. In vitro activity of premafloxacin, a new extended-spectrum fluoroquinolone, against pathogens of veterinary importance. Antimicrobial Agents and Chemotherapy 41:1190–1192.

World Health Organization. 1997. Reduction in use of antimicrobials decreases resistance. WHO Drug Information 11(4):241–243.

Young, L. A., Schumacher, J., Papich, M. G., et al. 1997. Disposition of enrofloxacin and its metabolite ciprofloxacin after intramuscular injection in juvenile Burmese pythons *(Python molurus bivittatus)*. Journal of Zoological and Wildlife Medicine 28:71–79.

Yun, H. I., Park, S. C., Jun, M. H., Hur, W., and Oh, T. K. 1994. Ciprofloxacin in horses: antimicrobial activity, protein binding, and pharmacokinetics. Proceedings of the 6th EAVPT Congress, pp. 28–29.

Zeng, Z., and Fung, K. 1997. Effects of experimentally induced *Escherichia coli* infection on the pharmacokinetics of enrofloxacin in pigs. Journal of Veterinary Pharmacology and Therapeutics 20(Suppl. 1):39–40.

46

ANTIFUNGAL AND ANTIVIRAL DRUGS

MARK G. PAPICH, MARK C. HEIT, AND JIM E. RIVIERE

Antifungal Therapy
- **Characteristics of Fungi**
- **Diseases Caused by Fungi**
- **Antifungal Drugs**
  - **Griseofulvin**
  - **Flucytosine**
  - **Amphotericin B**
  - **Azole Antifungal Drugs**
  - **Terbinafine**
  - **Other Antifungal Agents**
  - **Combination Therapy**

Antiviral Therapy
- **Viral Attachment and Penetration**
- **Transcription**
  - **Idoxuridine and Trifluridine**
  - **Cytarabine and Vidarabine**
  - **Ribavirin**
  - **Acyclovir and Ganciclovir**
  - **Zidovudine**
  - **Foscarnet**
- **Assembly**
  - **Amantadine and Rimantadine**
- **Host Resistance**
  - **Interferon**
- **Other Compounds**

ANTIFUNGAL THERAPY

The need for effective, safe antifungal drugs has become important, especially in small-animal medicine with the recognition of serious systemic fungal diseases and the need for effective drugs to treat skin infections caused by dermatophytes and yeasts. Some animals are at a greater risk of fungal infections because they are immunosuppressed, receiving cancer drugs or radiation therapy, or have received prolonged courses of corticosteroids. Fortunately, there have been good advances in development of antifungal drugs in the last 10 years. Effective oral drugs are more widely used and there are new advances in safe forms of injectable agents.

CHARACTERISTICS OF FUNGI. Fungi are eukaryotic cells and have a true nucleus with several chromosomes. They are considered primitive plants; however, they lack chlorophyll and therefore derive nutrients by means of a saprophytic or parasitic existence. Fungi exist either in a unicellular yeast form (*Candida, Cryptococcus*) or as a multicellular, filamentous mold colony (*Aspergillus, Microsporum, Trichophyton, Mucor, Rhizopus*). Several types of fungi can assume either form depending upon environmental conditions (*Blastomyces, Histoplasma, Coccidioides, Sporothrix*). The fungal cell is surrounded by a cell wall composed primarily of polysaccharide, which provides structural support. Sites of drug action are shown in Fig. 46.1. The cell wall is strongly antigenic, which elicits inappropriate immune reactions in some patients. It is also the site of antigenic specificity, which allows for serologic diagnosis of some fungal infections. The fungal cell membrane is a lipid bilayer whose principal lipid is ergosterol and contains enzymes necessary for normal function. Fungi contain true nuclei that contain several chromosomes.

Fungi may reproduce asexually via budding, sporulation, or hyphal fragmentation. Specialized asexual spores are termed "conidia." Some lower forms of fungi reproduce sexually. Most clinically important fungi in veterinary medicine belong to the Deuteromycetes phylum. Although not yet clearly defined, fungal pathogenesis may involve their ability to adhere to colonizing surfaces, phenotypic switching, production of catalytic enzymes, interaction with endogenous hormone receptors, and iron-scavenging properties. Some have suggested that fungi can suppress the host immune response, which results in worsening of the fungal disease (Vartivarian 1992).

Clinical mycology has lagged behind clinical bacteriology with respect to uniform standardization of susceptibility testing. Some available susceptibility tests are unreliable for predicting in vivo antifungal drug efficacy. This appears to be especially true for azole compounds. Potassium iodide, a systemic antifungal therapy used in large animals, shows no antifungal activity in vitro (Espinel-Ingroff and Shadomy 1989). In vitro antifungal activity can be affected by media, pH, inoculum size, variability of test procedure, and end-point determination (Galgiani 1987; Kobayaashi et al. 1986; Marriot and Richardson 1987) and therefore does not correlate well with in vivo efficacy (Ringel 1990; Troke et al. 1990). Advances in testing are possible with better refinement of clinical laboratory proce-

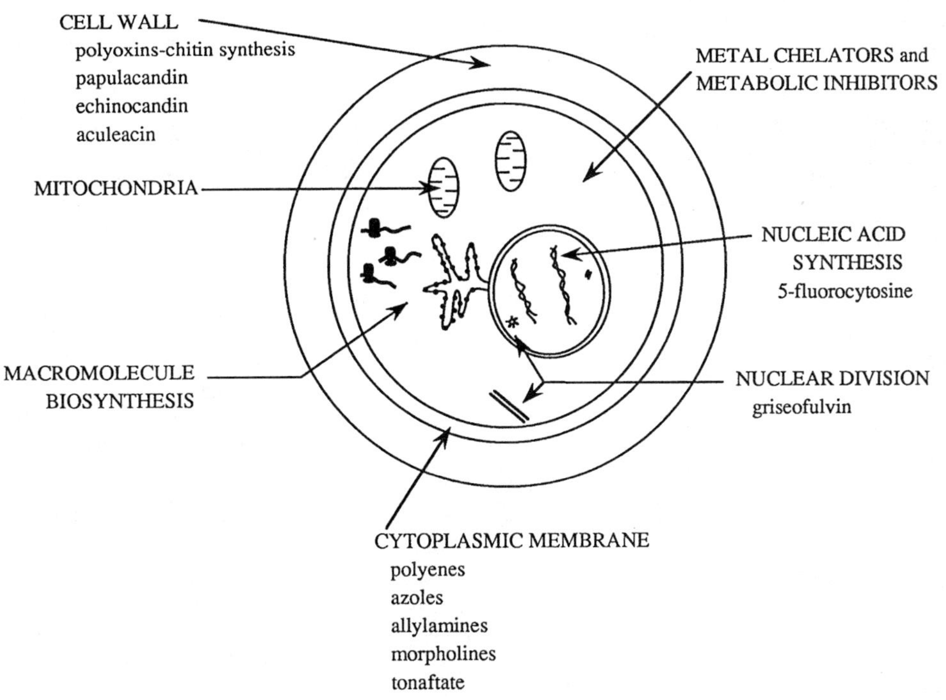

FIG. 46.1—Schematic anatomy of a fungal cell and potential sites where antifungal drugs act.

dures (Galgiani 1990; Graybill 1992). Without readily available susceptibility tests in veterinary medicine, most of the therapeutic choices are empirically based.

The diagnosis of mycotic infection is difficult because clinical signs mimic those of other disease processes, and often clinicians do not initially consider fungal etiologic agents. Definitive diagnosis is difficult owing to the slow and fastidious nature of fungal growth. Additionally, obtaining suitable and sufficient numbers of fungal specimens may be impossible for some of the systemic fungi because the infection may occur in an anatomic location difficult to sample (e.g., central nervous system [CNS] and eye). But advances in immunodiagnosis of systemic mycoses have dramatically improved the ability to diagnose some mycotic diseases (Jackson 1986).

DISEASES CAUSED BY FUNGI. Superficial infections are associated with dermatophytosis and onychomycosis (*Trichophyton, Microsporum*) and thrush (oral candidiasis). Also, yeast infections caused by *Malassezia pachydermatis* (formerly called *Pityrosporum*) are recognized as an important skin infection in dogs.

Subcutaneous or regional lesions are associated with draining sinuses or invasion of bone. These may be introduced traumatically or iatrogenically and can become disseminated. Examples of these infections are mycetomas, chromomycosis, zygomycosis, phycomycosis, sporotrichosis, and rhinosporidiosis.

Systemic fungal infections are often associated with immunocompromised patients, although they may occur in immunocompetent hosts under optimum circumstances. These diseases are serious and often life threatening due to the organ involved and the refractoriness to therapy. These diseases may follow a chronic granulomatous course (e.g., blastomycosis, histoplasmosis, coccidiomycosis, cryptococcosis, aspergillosis) and are often challenging to treat because of the need for potent systemic drugs.

ANTIFUNGAL DRUGS

Griseofulvin. *Griseofulvin,* USP (Fulvicin U/F, Fulvicin P/G, Grifulvin V, Grisactin, Grisactin ultra) (Fig. 46.2), is a fungistatic antibiotic produced by *Penicillium griseofulvin dierckx.* It is colorless, slightly bitter, and virtually insoluble in water. Its selective toxicity is based on an energy-dependent uptake into susceptible fungi that occurs preferentially to uptake into mammalian cells. Once into the cell, griseofulvin disrupts the mitotic spindle by interacting with polymerized microtubules, thus causing mitotic arrest in metaphase. Grossly this may appear as shortened and less branched fungal hyphae, known as the "curling" phenomenon. Griseofulvin may also interfere with cytoplasmic

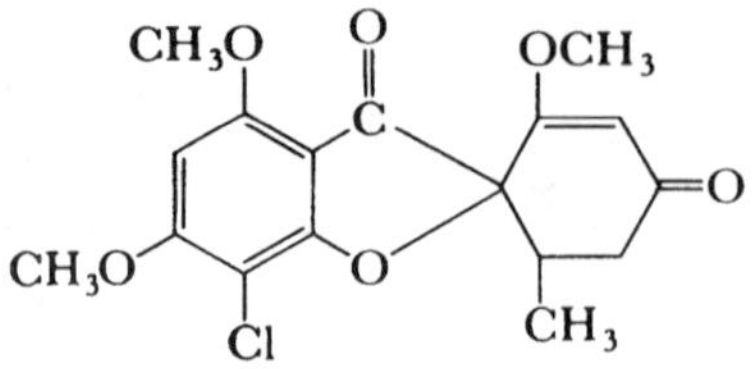

Griseofulvin

FIG. 46.2

tubule formation, thereby inhibiting normal cellular trafficking.

SPECTRUM OF ACTIVITY. Griseofulvin is active against organisms causing dermatophytosis, *Microsporum, Trichophyton,* and *Epidermophyton.* It has no effect on bacteria or on other fungi, yeasts, *Actinomyces,* or *Nocardia.* Fungal resistance to griseofulvin, caused by decreased energy-dependent uptake into the fungal cell, has not been reported to be a clinically important problem in veterinary medicine.

PHARMACOKINETICS. Oral absorption of griseofulvin is variable and dependent on particle size. Microsized preparations are 25–70% absorbed, whereas formulations with smaller particles (ultramicrosized griseofulvin) are virtually 100% absorbed. The ultramicrosized preparations are not used often in veterinary medicine because they are more expensive. If the ultramicrosized form is used, the dose must be decreased to account for differences in absorption. Because of low water solubility, griseofulvin absorption is enhanced when given with a fatty meal. Pharmacokinetic properties were reviewed by Hill et al. (1995). Within hours of oral administration, griseofulvin can be detected in the stratum corneum. It distributes to the keratin of skin, hair, and nails. Only a small fraction of a dose is present in other body fluids or tissues. The plasma half-life in the dog is 47 minutes (Harris and Riegelman 1969); however, the half-life at the site of action, the stratum corneum, is prolonged since drug is bound tightly to keratinocytes and remains in the skin until these cells are shed. Thus, new hair or nail growth is first to become free of disease as fungal-containing keratin is replaced by new cells.

Griseofulvin is metabolized primarily by the liver to demethylgriseofulvin and the glucuronide. It is metabolized approximately 6 times faster in animals than in people, which is the reason animal doses are higher than human doses ($t_{1/2}$ in dogs is less than 1 hour, compared to 20 hours in people) (Shah et al. 1972).

ADVERSE EFFECTS. The most serious adverse effects associated with griseofulvin occur in cats. Problems in cats include leukopenia, anemia, increased hepatic enzyme activity, and neurotoxicosis (Helton et al. 1986). Ataxia has been reported in a kitten receiving griseofulvin (Levy 1991). Griseofulvin caused bone marrow hypoplasia in an 8-year-old cat (Rottman et al. 1991). Prolonged treatment of eight cats with griseofulvin at the high end of the dosage range resulted in no untoward clinical, hematologic, or hepatic side effects, suggesting that griseofulvin toxicity may be idiosyncratic (Kunkle and Meyer 1987). Cats with the feline immunodeficiency virus (FIV) appear to be at increased risk for griseofulvin-associated neutropenia (Shelton et al. 1990); however, toxicity has also been reported in FIV-negative cats (Rottman et al. 1991). The mechanism of this increased risk is unknown but may involve griseofulvin-enhanced binding of immune complexes to granulocytic cells in infected cats (Shelton et al. 1991). Griseofulvin also is extremely teratogenic in cats (Scott et al. 1975; Gruffydd-Jones and Wright 1977) and therefore should not be used in pregnant queens. It has been given to pregnant horses with no apparent ill effect (Hiddleston 1970).

DRUG INTERACTIONS. Griseofulvin is a hepatic enzyme inducer (cytochrome P-450 inducer). This may increase metabolism of coadministered drugs. Despite this precaution, there are few documented cases of these drug interactions in veterinary medicine. Nevertheless, other drugs administered to griseofulvin-treated animals may be metabolized at a faster rate, resulting in diminished therapeutic effect.

CLINICAL USE

SMALL ANIMALS. Griseofulvin is still a popular drug for treating dermatophytosis. The recommended doses have varied, depending on the author. One manufacturer recommends 11–22 mg/kg/day, but recommendations by specialists in dermatology have ranged from 44 mg/kg/day (Sousa and Ihrke 1983) to 110–132 mg/kg/day in divided treatments (Scott 1980). One review suggested a dose of 50 mg/kg once a day of the microsized formulation (Hill et al. 1995), and another review listed 25 mg/kg every 12 hours (deJaham et al. 1999), but the dose can be doubled for refractory cases. A report showed that doses of 50 mg/kg/day for cats was as effective as itraconazole for treatment of dermatophytosis (Moriello and DeBoer 1995).

Griseofulvin is available in 125 and 250 mg capsules; 125, 250, and 500 mg tablets; and an oral 125 mg/mL syrup. Often, at least 4 weeks are needed for successful therapy, and some patients require 3 months (or more) of continuous therapy. As long as 4 months may be necessary to treat onychomycosis.

LARGE ANIMALS. Although use in large animals is not common, griseofulvin has been effective in the prevention and treatment of dermatophytes in cattle (Reuss 1978). It was used in calves at a dose of 0.25 mg/kg given for 7–10 days. A mycelial premix of 10% griseofulvin administered in the diet of 116 infected calves at a dose of 10 mg/kg was found to be as effective, and more practical, than an equal dose of the microsized preparation (Hiddleston 1973). A dose rate of 1 g/100 kg has been recommended for pigs for a duration of 30–40 days (Kielstein and Gottschalk 1970). Griseofulvin at 30 g/day/animal was reported to be effective in curbing a mycotic abortion outbreak due to *Aspergillus fumigatus* and *Cryptococcus neoformans* in buffalo heifers. Considering the concomitant use of intrauterine infusions, these results are difficult to interpret (Shehata 1991).

OTHER SPECIES. Case reports exist of griseofulvin's successful use in the prevention of mycotic dermatitis in ostriches (Onderka and Doornenbal 1992) and in the treatment of *Trichophyton* in small ruminants (Abdel-Halim et al. 1988). In the first report, griseofulvin was added to the drinking water, whereas in the latter it was used as a feed supplement. Griseofulvin was also used as a food supplement at a dose of 7.5 mg/kg to treat an outbreak of ringworm in a flock of 250 housed ewes. The animals were treated for 7 days while all were in their second third of gestation. Lesions resolved within 20 days and were microscopically and culturally negative, and parturition and offspring were normal (McKellar et al. 1987). Griseofulvin was unsuccessful in treating *Trichophyton mentagrophytes* in a commercial rabbitry as a water additive, whereas individual therapy, although potentially effective, was considered impractical and uneconomical (Franklin et al. 1991).

Flucytosine. Flucytosine (*5-Fluorocytosine,* 5-FC, Ancobon) (Fig. 46.3) is a synthetic antifungal agent originally intended as an anticancer agent (Dushchinsky et al. 1957). It was ineffective against tumors, but further screening revealed it possessed antifungal activity in vitro (Berger and Duschinsky 1962). An oral preparation became available in the United States in 1972. To have cytotoxic effects, 5-FC must first be converted to 5-fluorouracil (5-FU). Uptake into the fungal cell is governed by cytosine permeate. Once in the cell, it is converted to the active form by a fungal cytosine deaminase enzyme. Then 5-FU either is incorporated into RNA, disrupting protein synthesis, or is converted to a related compound which inhibits DNA synthesis. The mammalian cell's deficiency in cytosine deaminase is the basis for the selective toxicity of this compound; however, conversion to 5-FU may occur by microbes in the gastrointestinal (GI) tract. 5-FU is not readily absorbed by fungal cells but is toxic to mammalian cells and may lead to anemia, leukopenia, and thrombocytopenia (Bennett 1990).

Flucytosine is active against *Cryptococcus neoformans* and certain species and strains of *Candida.* The majority of *Aspergillus* species are resistant. It has little effect in vitro against *Sporothrix schenckii, Blastomyces dermatitidis, Histoplasma capsulatum, Coccidioides immitis,* and *Rhizopus.* Resistance to flucytosine has developed both in vitro and during therapy, which limits its use as the sole antifungal agent in a therapeutic protocol. This resistance is thought to be due to fungal mutations resulting in either decreased permease or decreased deaminase activity.

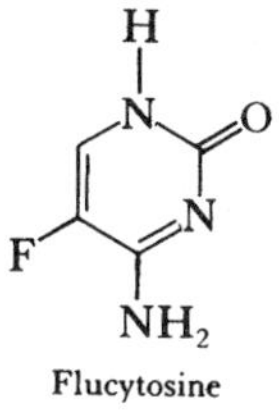

Flucytosine

FIG. 46.3

Flucytosine is used infrequently in veterinary medicine and there is little information available to guide dosing or clinical use. Since few pharmacokinetic data are available, the pharmacokinetics of flucytosine must be inferred from human studies. 5-FC is rapidly and completely absorbed from the (GI) tract. It is minimally bound to plasma proteins such that its volume of distribution approximates total body water. It is present in the cerebrospinal fluid (CSF) at concentrations approximately 65–90% of those in plasma and also appears to penetrate into aqueous humor. The penetration into the CNS has expanded its use to treat CNS fungal infections. Its half-life is between 3 and 6 hours but may be as long as 200 hours in patients in renal failure, as approximately 80% of a dose is excreted unchanged in urine by glomerular filtration.

Due to its previously mentioned limitations, the therapeutic indications for flucytosine are limited to adjunct therapy with amphotericin B in systemic infections caused by *Candida* or *Cryptococcus neoformans.* Synergy between these two medications has been demonstrated, and combination therapy has been successful, particularly in the treatment of cryptococcal meningitis (Utz et al. 1975; Bennet et al. 1979). Flucytosine was shown to be effective in a domestic cat for treating phaeohyphomycosis due to an *Exophiala spinifera* infection that was refractory to both griseofulvin and ketoconazole (Kettlewell et al. 1989). But caution is recommended because combination therapy of flucytosine and ketoconazole was found to be toxic in cats for treatment of this same disease (Pukay and Dion 1984).

Amphotericin B. Amphotericin B (Fungizone) (Fig. 46.4) is a polyene antibiotic first isolated from rotting vegetation in Venezuela in 1956 (Gold et al. 1956). Both amphotericin A and B are natural fermentation products of the actinomycete *Streptomyces nodosus.* Although both forms possess antifungal characteristics, amphotericin B was developed, and current preparations are almost devoid of amphotericin A (less than 2%). As its name implies, it is an amphoteric compound whose molecular structure consists of a large macrolide ring with a hydrophobic conjugated double-bond chain and a hydrophilic hydroxylated carbon

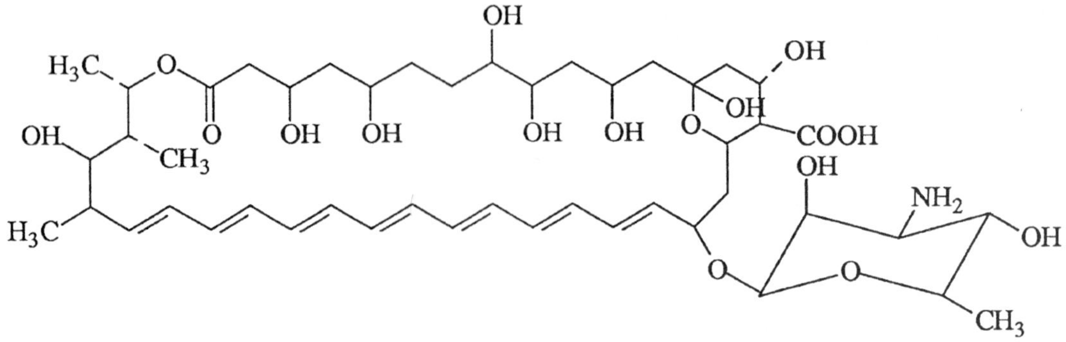

FIG. 46.4—Amphotericin B.

chain and attached sugar (Mechlinsk et al. 1970). It is prepared as a yellowish powder which is insoluble in water and somewhat unstable (Bennett 1990). When reconstituted in a vial, the commercial formulation (Fungizone) is a micellar complex of amphotericin B and a bile salt (sodium dexoxycholate).

MECHANISM OF ACTION. The action of amphotericin B on fungal cells may involve more than one mechanism (Brajtburg et al. 1990). A major action of amphotericin B is to bind ergosterol in the fungal plasma cell membrane, thereby making the membrane more permeable. Increased permeability results, among other actions, in leakage of cell electrolytes, resulting in cell death. At high concentrations, amphotericin B is thought to cause oxidative damage to the fungal cell (Warnock 1991) or disruption of fungal cell enzymes. The selective toxicity of amphotericin B is based on its decreased binding to the major cell membrane sterol of mammalian cells (cholesterol) as compared to that of fungal cells (ergosterol).

SPECTRUM OF ACTIVITY. The growth of strains of most veterinary fungal pathogens is inhibited in vitro at amphotericin B concentrations between 0.05 and 1.0 μg/mL. Sensitive fungi include *H. capsulatum, C. neoformans, C. immitis, B dermatitidis, Candida* spp., and many strains of *Aspergillus*. Amphotericin B has been indicated for treatment of mucormycosis, sporotrichosis, and phycomycosis (Drouhet and Dupont 1987). Most strains of *Pseudallescheria boydii* as well as some agents causing chromoblastomycosis and phaeohyphomycosis have minimum inhibitory concentration (MIC) values greater than 2.0 μg/mL and are therefore considered resistant. Although MIC values are not typically measured for clinically isolated fungi, there is good correlation between the MIC values and clinical response to amphotericin B (O'Day et al. 1987). Clinical fungal resistance to amphotericin B, either primary or acquired, does not appear to occur commonly, although resistant strains occur in vitro. In most cases, these resistant strains contain decreased levels of membrane ergosterol (Pierce et al. 1978); increased catalase levels may allow these fungi to be resistant to oxidative dependent damage (Sokol-Anderson et al. 1988). Treatment failure due to fungal resistance has rarely been reported in humans; however, MIC concentrations were found to be increased in certain patient populations, such as neutropenic patients (Dick et al. 1980), transplant patients (Powderly et al. 1988), and patients undergoing cytotoxic therapy.

CHEMICAL PROPERTIES AND PHARMACOKINETICS. Despite its long history of use, much is still unknown concerning the pharmacokinetics of amphotericin B, especially in the veterinary population. It is poorly absorbed from the GI tract and not administered orally except for local treatment of oral yeast infections. Whether binding in the GI tract, failure to cross the intestinal mucosa, or first-pass hepatic metabolism is responsible for poor systemic absorption is uncertain. Amphotericin B must be given intravenously or intrathecally.

To achieve solubility for injection, current preparations contain sodium deoxycholate, which forms a suspension. This form should not be admixed with electrolytes in solutions or inactivation will occur. Following infusion, amphotericin B separates from the deoxycholate and binds extensively (~95%) to serum proteins, mainly β lipoprotein (Bennett 1977). Much of the drug is thought to leave the vascular space and bind to cholesterol-containing membranes. The highest concentrations are found in liver, spleen, kidney, and lungs, with little accumulation in either muscle or adipose tissue. Concentrations of amphotericin B in fluids from inflamed pleura, peritoneum, and synovium and in aqueous humor are about two-thirds of those in serum. Amphotericin B readily crosses the human placenta. Penetration into normal or inflamed meninges, vitreous humor, and normal amniotic fluid is poor. This differential distribution may explain treatment failures for infections in some tissues. Although amphotericin B binds ergosterol with higher affinity than cholesterol, it was suggested that because there are more binding sites for cholesterol in the body than for ergosterol, this may sequester amphotericin B from its site of action (Bennett 1977).

Amphotericin B is slowly excreted in human urine, with only 3% excreted unchanged (Atkinson and Bennett 1978). Bile may be a major route of elimination (Craven et al. 1979) although metabolic pathways are not known. Drug can be detected for 6–7 weeks in urine after cessation of therapy; however, accumulation does not appear to be a problem in patients with impaired renal function (Feldman et al. 1973).

ADVERSE EFFECTS. The most important clinical toxicosis associated with amphotericin B therapy is that of nephrotoxicity. It is a dose-related, predictable toxic effect that occurs in almost every animal treated with the conventional formulation. Direct tubular damage occurs because amphotericin B binds to cholesterol in the tubular cells, which results in electrolyte leakage from the cells (primarily K^+ loss) and renal tubular acidosis (Bennett 1990). Induced renal vasoconstriction and impaired acid excretion may also contribute to amphotericin B's renal toxicity (Greene 1990). Renal vasoconstriction may be caused by induced increases in the eicosanoid synthesis in renal blood vessels. The tubular damage, along with the renal vasoconstriction, leads to both an acute and a chronic cumulative renal toxicosis. Clinically, the signs of renal toxicosis are seen as increases in creatinine and blood urea nitrogen (BUN). Electrolyte loading, fluid dieresis, and slow infusion of amphotericin B have all been shown to decrease the severity and the rate of development of renal toxicity. Therefore, common protocols for administration of amphotericin B to animals include pretreatment with sodium chloride IV solution and a slow infusion. The renal toxicity of amphotericin B can be ameliorated by pretreatment with sodium-loading fluids (Rubin 1986) and with concurrent mannitol administration (Legendre 1984).

Careful clinical monitoring will help decrease the risk of permanent renal injury. Urine sediment evaluation has been suggested to detect renal toxicity earlier than serum biochemical alterations (Greene 1990); thus, urine should be evaluated for proteinuria, cylinduria, and hematuria, as well as specific gravity. In addition, BUN, creatinine, and electrolyte concentrations should be monitored. Therapy should be temporarily discontinued when active urine sediment is detected or the serum creatinine increases. After stopping therapy, patients may undergo a fluid diuresis to decrease the azotemia. If BUN and creatinine return to near-normal reference values, treatment may be resumed. If azotemia does not improve, one should consider an alternative treatment.

Other adverse effects from amphotericin that are frequently observed in animals include phlebitis, fever, nausea, and vomiting. Measures to prevent the nausea and vomiting have including administration of antiemetic drugs such as chlorpromazine or metoclopramide prior to infusion.

CLINICAL PROTOCOLS. A variety of dosage protocols for amphotericin B have been described in the veterinary literature. One should strive for a total cumulative dose of 4–8 mg/kg given on an every-other-day schedule. Fluid loading with sodium-containing fluids appears to decrease the renal injury. Also, slow infusion of amphotericin B rather than a fast bolus IV appears to decrease the nephrotoxicosis. In the protocol described by Rubin (1986), patients are pretreated with fluid therapy (0.9% sodium chloride solution) and receive the infusion at a slow rate (over 4–6 hr). During infusion, it must be mixed with 5% dextrose solution because if it is added to an electrolyte solution the drug will precipitate. A commonly cited dose for therapy is a test dose of 0.25 mg/kg for the first treatment, then 0.5 mg/kg administered every other day until a total cumulative dose of 4–8 mg/kg has been given. Some references have suggested doses of 1 mg/kg for each dose to increase efficacy. The total cumulative dose is limited by nephrotoxicosis. If the dose administered during a single infusion exceeds 1 mg/kg, acute renal injury is likely (Butler 1964).

Amphotericin B has been used successfully to treat canine histoplasmosis and blastomycosis (Ausherman 1973). A dose of 0.5 mg/kg in 2 L of 5% dextrose given twice weekly for 7 weeks followed by maintenance ketoconazole therapy was ineffective in treating equine coccidioidomycosis (Ziemer et al. 1992).

Other methods of administration have been investigated. Malik and coworkers (1996) have reported on the administration of amphotericin B subcutaneously (SC). In their report, amphotericin was administered to dogs and cats SC at cumulative doses of 8–26 mg/kg. Except for local irritation, injections were well tolerated, and higher doses were administered without producing azotemia as compared to the IV route.

NEW FORMULATIONS. New formulations of amphotericin B have been used in people but have not gained widespread use in veterinary medicine due to their high cost. However, they have distinct advantages over the traditional formulations; the most important is that they are less toxic. These new formulations are lipid-based complexes or cholesteryl complexes of amphotericin B that allow higher doses to be administered with less nephrotoxicosis (Plotnick 2000).

The traditional formulation of amphotericin B is a micellar complex with the bile salt deoxycholate. Amphotericin B lipid complex (ABELCET) is a suspension of amphotericin B complexed with two phospholipids at a concentration of 100 mg/20 mL. This formulation was shown to be safe and effective for treating blastomycosis in dogs at a cumulative dose of 8–12 mg/kg when administered at 1 mg/kg every other day (Krawiec et al. 1996).

Amphotericin B cholesteryl sulfate complex (Amphotec, ABCD) is a colloidal dispersion of amphotericin B. It has been effective in studies in which it was administered at doses higher than those used for the traditional amphotericin B formulation.

The liposomal complex of amphotericin B (AmBisome) is a unilamellar liposomal formulation. This was the first liposomal formulation available. When reconstituted, it produces small vesicles of encapsulated amphotericin B. This formulation has been used safely and effectively in some dogs for blastomycosis (Plotnick 2000). This liposomal complex of amphotericin B was used in another study of 13 dogs for treatment of *Leishmania infantum* at a dose of 3–3.3 mg/kg. Although there was rapid clinical improvement, dogs remained positive for *Leishmania* (Oliva et al. 1995).

The advantage of these lipid-based formulations of amphotericin B is that in comparison to the conventional formulation of amphotericin B (amphotericin B deoxycholate), they can be given at higher doses to produce greater efficacy with less toxicity (Hiemenz and Walsh 1996). Doses of lipid complex formulations of amphotericin B have been 3 mg or more per kilogram (compared to 0.25–0.5 mg/kg of the conventional formulation) (Walsh et al. 1999; Ringden et al. 1991; Graybill et al. 1982; Hostetler et al. 1992). Decreased toxicity is attributed to a selective transfer of the lipid complex amphotericin B, releasing the drug directly to the fungal cell membrane and sparing the mammalian cell membranes. Reduced drug concentrations in the kidneys and diminished release of inflammatory cytokines from amphotericin lipid complex compared to the conventional formulation also may prevent adverse reactions. It is possible that doses used for veterinary patients have been too conservative, and based on experience in people, higher doses may be tolerated.

Azole Antifungal Drugs. The azole antifungal drugs include the imidazoles and triazoles. They are broad-spectrum antifungal agents that also show some activity against gram-positive bacteria (although they are never used therapeutically for treating bacterial infections in animals). In the early 1970s, the first imidazole compound with antifungal activity, clotrimazole, was discovered. Unfortunately, autoinduction of hepatic degrading enzymes caused undetectable plasma concentrations after several days of therapy. In 1977 miconazole, also an azole compound, was introduced and was found to be effective against some fungi refractive to amphotericin B. Rapid clearance and poor oral absorption necessitate frequent IV infusions during hospitalization. In addition, the solubilizing agent in the parenteral form induces histamine-related toxic side effects, making its use hazardous. The current uses of both clotrimazole and miconazole have been primarily restricted to topical treatment of localized superficial infections. The first orally active imidazole antifungal, approved for use in 1979, was ketoconazole. More recently the introduction of two triazoles, fluconazole and itraconazole, has presented the clinician with several safe, effective alternatives to amphotericin B for the treatment of serious fungal infections.

MECHANISM OF ACTION. All azoles exert their antifungal effect on the cell membrane of the fungus by inhibiting synthesis of primary sterol of the fungal cell membrane, ergosterol. Inhibition of the P-450-dependent lanosterol C_{14}-demethylase enzyme results in depletion of ergosterol and accumulation of C_{14}-methyl sterols in the cytoplasmic membrane (Fig. 46.5). Inhibition of the P-450 enzyme occurs via binding of the nitrogen (N_3 of imidazoles and N_4 of azoles) to the heme iron atom of ferric cytochrome P-450. This prevents the formation of the superoxide Fe^{+++} complex ($Fe^{+++}O^-$) needed for hydroxylation of methyl sterols. The result is an inability to demethylate C_{14}-methyl sterols and reduced synthesis of ergosterol. Incorporation into the membrane of sterols that are less planar than ergosterol changes membrane fluidity and interferes with the barrier function of the membrane and with membrane-bound enzymes.

Azole drugs are generally fungistatic at concentrations achieved clinically. Fungicidal action can occur via direct interaction with the cell membrane barrier (miconazole) and accumulation of toxic peroxides resulting from alterations in oxidative metabolism and inhibition of cellular respiration (Polak 1990).

PHARMACODYNAMICS. The potency of each azole drug is related to its affinity for binding the P-450 enzyme. The selective toxicity of each compound is directly dependent upon its specificity for binding fungal P-450 more readily than mammalian P-450. Imidazoles are less specific than triazoles and produce side effects in animals attributed to inhibition of P-450 enzymes such as synthesis of cortisol and reproductive steroid hormones. Azoles may decrease cholesterol, cortisol, androgen, and testosterone biosynthesis and may interfere with several liver enzymes necessary for inactivation of toxic and carcinogenic agents (Polak 1990).

KETOCONAZOLE. Ketoconazole (Nizoral) (Fig. 46.6), one of the imidazoles, became available in 1979, with results of its successful use in veterinary medicine being published shortly thereafter (Legendre et al. 1982; Medleau et al. 1985). Ketoconazole is most effective against yeast and dimorphic fungi such as *Candida, Malassezia (Pityrosporum) pachydermatis, C. immitis, H. capsulatum, B. dermatitidis,* as well as most dermatophytes with MIC values less than 0.5 µg/mL. It is less effective against *C. neoformans, S. schenckii,* and *Aspergillus* spp., with MIC values varying from 6 to >100 µg/mL (Hume and Kerkering 1983).

PHARMACOKINETICS. The advantages over older azole compounds include increased solubility in an acid environment, good tissue distribution, and reasonably long half-life (Daneshmend and Warnock 1988). Ketoconazole is well absorbed from an acid environment and when given with a meal. Ketoconazole is highly protein bound (>98%) and therefore does not penetrate into the cerebrospinal, seminal, or ocular fluid to a significant degree; however, it is found in

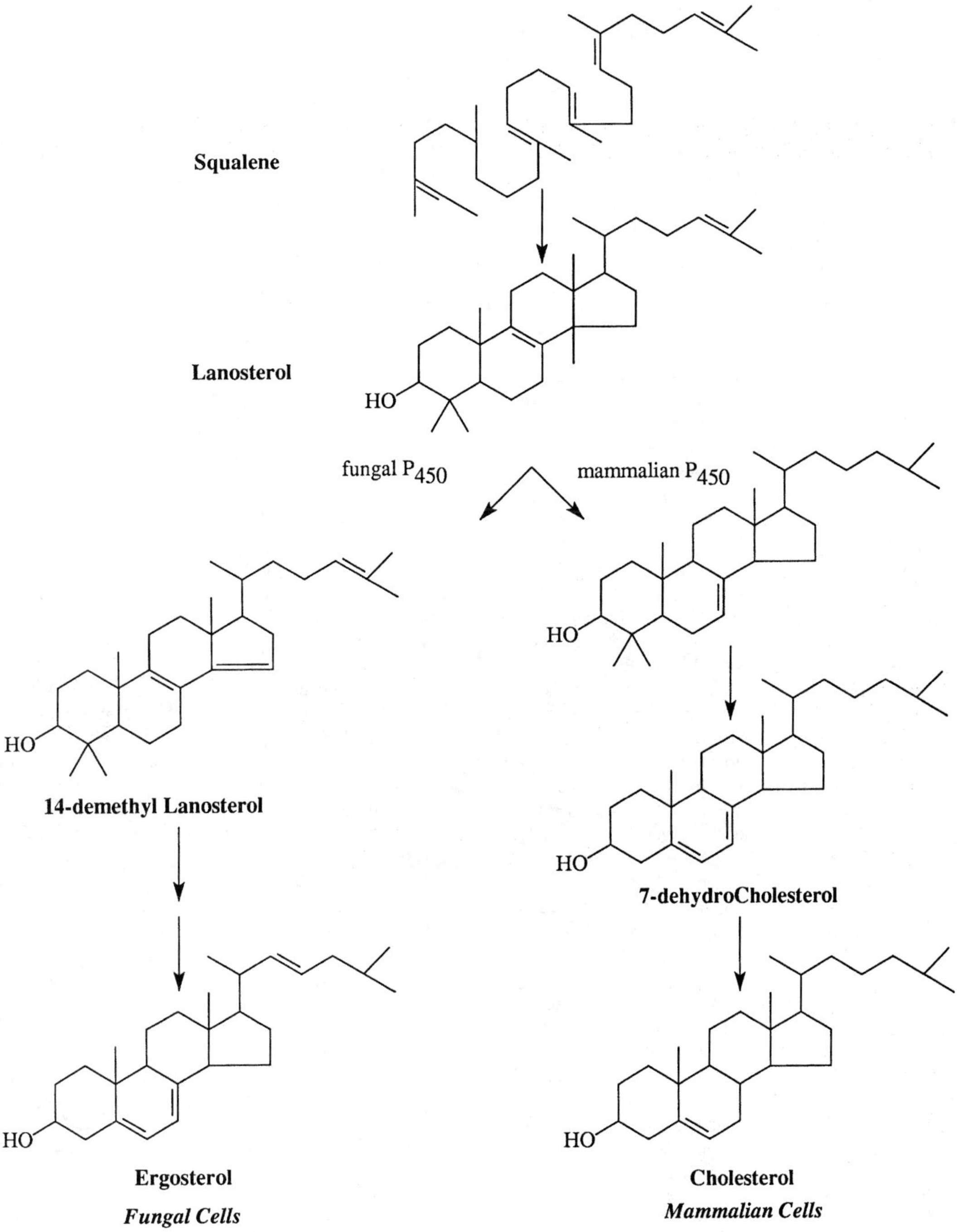

Squalene

Lanosterol

HO

fungal P_{450}

mammalian P_{450}

HO

HO

14-demethyl Lanosterol

HO

7-dehydroCholesterol

HO

HO

Ergosterol

Fungal Cells

Cholesterol

Mammalian Cells

FIG. 46.5—Simplified scheme of fungal and mammalian biosynthesis of the major sterol in the cell membrane. The affinity with which an azole antifungal binds to each P-450 enzyme determines its potency and selective toxicity.

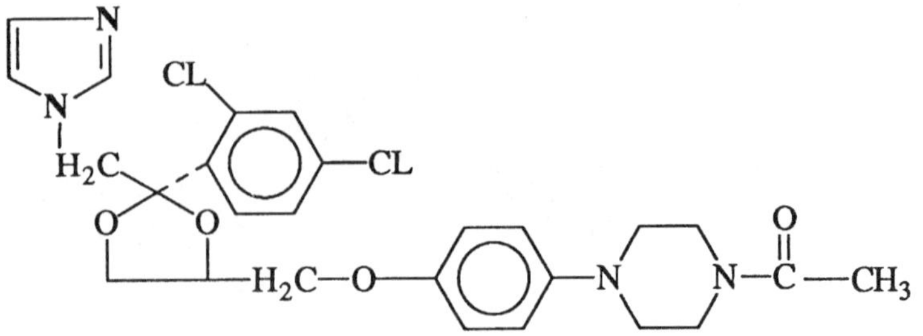

FIG. 46.6—Ketoconazole.

mother's milk. It distributes throughout the skin and subcutaneous tissue, making it effective for treatment of superficial and systemic fungal skin infections. The drug demonstrates nonlinear absorption and elimination kinetics, most probably due to saturation of metabolizing enzymes. It is biotransformed in the liver via O-dealkylation and aromatic hydroxylation and excreted mainly in the bile. Significant drug interactions occur when patients also receive drugs that inhibit or induce these enzymes (e.g., phenytoin, rifampin, barbiturates, and cyclosporine) (Graybill 1990). Elimination half-life is approximately 2 hours in dogs.

Because ketoconazole is only soluble in acid aqueous environments (pH <3), gastric alkalizing agents (e.g., antacids, H_2 blockers, and parietal cell proton pump inhibitors) or diseases resulting in achlorhydria will decrease its dissolution and oral absorption. Because of lack of consistent gastric acidity, ketoconazole is absorbed poorly in horses. When ketoconazole was administered at 30 mg/kg to horses in corn syrup, the drug was not detected in serum (Prades et al. 1989). When it was administered with 0.2 N hydrochloric acid intragastrically, oral absorption increased but was still only 23%. Peak serum concentrations were 3.76 μg/mL in horses.

ADVERSE EFFECTS. Nausea, anorexia, vomiting are the most common adverse effects. They are usually dose related and may be diminished by decreasing the dose, dividing the total dose into smaller doses, and administering each dose with food. Side effects such as anorexia, vomiting, and diarrhea necessitated discontinuation of therapy in three cats (Medleau and Chalmers 1992). With chronic therapy pruritus, alopecia, lightening and drying of the hair coat, and weight loss may occur (Greene 1990). Elevations in hepatic enzymes may occur with therapy. Slight to moderate elevations of inducible enzymes are expected and may not be accompanied by hepatic injury. However, high elevations in hepatic enzymes, accompanied by other parameters (elevations in bilirubin and clinical signs consistent with hepatic disease), may indicate hepatotoxicosis. Therefore, patients should be monitored. Idiosyncratic hepatitis has been reported in animals and people (Janssen and Symoens 1983).

Cats appear to be more sensitive to ketoconazole liver toxicity than are dogs but are less sensitive to the hormonal suppressive side effects (Willard et al. 1986a,b). Ketoconazole has been shown to be teratogenic in the rat and has resulted in mummified fetuses and stillbirths in dogs. It is therefore not recommended for use in pregnant or lactating animals. Ketoconazole is very potent at inhibiting fungal P-450, but it also inhibits mammalian P-450 at relatively low concentrations; therefore, side effects and drug interactions can occur. Dose-related inhibition of testosterone has resulted in gynecomastia, sexual impotence, and azoospermia. Inhibition of corticosteroid biosynthesis has been utilized for the short-term treatment of canine hyperadrenocorticism (Feldman et al. 1990; Bruyette and Feldman 1988).

Cataracts have been reported after long-term ketoconazole therapy in dogs (da Costa et al. 1996). The average duration of therapy in affected dogs was 15 months, and dosages ranged from 6 to 31 mg/kg/day. These dogs were not diabetic. The mechanism of this reaction is not known.

DRUG INTERACTIONS. Ketoconazole may inhibit metabolism of other drugs because it is a potent cytochrome P-450 inhibitor and will inhibit drug-metabolizing enzymes. It also is an inhibitor of the membrane protein p-glycoprotein, which is a membrane efflux pump that is present in many tissues, including the intestine and blood-brain barrier. Ketoconazole also will inhibit metabolism and increase concentrations of cisapride, cyclosporine, and anticonvulsant drugs. In people it was shown that when used in combination with cyclosporine, the cyclosporine concentrations increased. Patients were more responsive to the immunosuppressive action of cyclosporine when it was administered with ketoconazole, and some clinicians have administered ketoconazole with cyclosporine to reduce the cost of cyclosporine therapy. The effect on cyclosporine is caused by both inhibition of p-glycoprotein in the intestine as well as reduction of hepatic cytochrome P-450 metabolism. Because ketoconazole also is a substrate for the cytochrome P-450 enzyme, administration of enzyme inducers will increase clearance. For example, use with rifampin will increase clearance. Do not administer with antacids, H_2 blockers (cimetidine), or omeprazole because they may inhibit absorption.

CLINICAL USE. Owing to ketoconazole's efficacy, safety, cost (generic forms are less expensive than other antifungal drugs), and ease of administration, it is a popular antifungal agent in veterinary medicine (Moriello 1986). Ketoconazole is effective for the treatment of yeasts such as *Malassezia* (*Pityrosporum*) *pachydermatis* and infections caused by *Histoplasma, Coccidioides,* and *Blastomyces.* It is less effective for *Aspergillus* infections. It has been used alone to treat infections caused by *Coccidioides* and *Histoplasma,* but severe infections caused by *Blastomyces* are first treated with amphotericin B.

Ketoconazole is available in 200 mg tablets (Nizoral). For dermatophytosis in cats, 10 mg/kg/day has been used (Medleau and Chalmers 1992). For candidiasis, 10 mg/kg/day for 6–8 weeks is recommended. For canine blastomycosis, histoplasmosis, cryptococcosis, and coccidioidomycosis, the dosage is 10–20 mg/kg every 12 hours. For *Malassezia* dermatitis, dosages of 5–10 mg/kg/day have been recommended (Hill et al. 1995). The duration of treatment is highly variable. Four to six weeks is probably a minimum for most diseases; many patients with blastomycosis are treated for a minimum of 2 months and as long as 6 months. If there is CNS involvement, for mycotic infection such as cryptococcosis, higher doses (40 mg/kg) may be necessary to improve penetration into the CNS. Cats have been successfully treated for cryptococcosis with a dosage of 10–15 mg/kg/day (Pentlarge and Martin 1986; Legendre et al. 1982; Medleau et al. 1985). As complete eradication of the fungal organism is difficult, relapse is common. For this reason, infections should be treated well beyond the time clinical signs have resolved. Ketoconazole was effective in treating nasal cryptococcosis in a dog at a dose of 10 mg/kg/day (Noxon et al. 1986).

Ketoconazole is not absorbed well in horses because an acidic stomach is necessary for absorption (Prades et al. 1986). Unless ketoconazole is administered by oral gavage with an acid solution, absorption in horses is not high enough for effective treatment and it is not recommended. Doses of ketoconazole of 3–6 mg/kg for 26–96 days were ineffective in treating equine coccidiomycosis (Ziemer et al. 1992).

ENILCONAZOLE. Enilconazole (Imaverol) (Fig. 46.7), also called imazalil in some countries, has excellent antifungal activity and a residual effect after application. It has been used in other countries for the topical treatment of dermatophyte infections in dogs and horses. For this treatment, a 10% solution is diluted 50:1 to form an emulsion. It may be sponged on the animal every 3 or 4 days for 4 treatments. It may be applied to the premises as well to prevent recurring infections. In an evaluation of topical therapies for treatment of dermatophyte infections in dogs and cats (White-Weithers and Medleau 1995), enilconazole was more effective than chlorhexidine, povidone iodine, ketoconazole, sodium hypochlorite, and Captan. The safety of enilconazole has been demonstrated in dogs, even at high doses. One study also showed that enilconazole is safe for treatment of dermatophytes in Persian cats (De Jaham 1996).

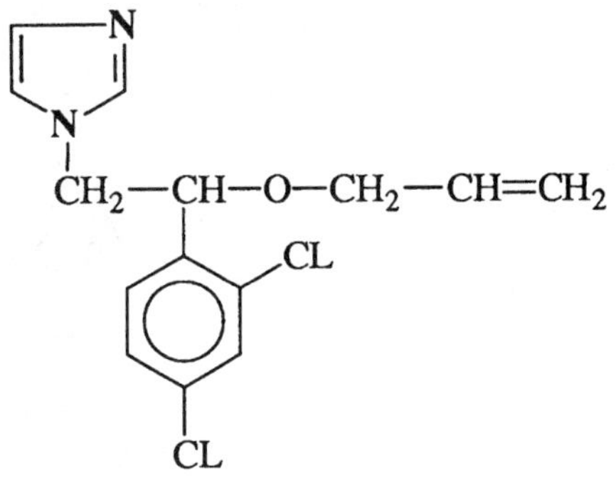

FIG. 46.7—Enilconazole.

CLINICAL USE. Enilconazole is used topically for dermatophytes. Enilconazole also has been used to treat nasal aspergillosis in dogs. It is reported to have a vapor effect and, if instilled into the nasal cavity of dogs, will control fungal growth (Sharp et al. 1991; Sharp and Sullivan 1992). A dose of 10 mg/kg in a volume of 5–10 mL is infused twice a day for 7–14 days. In one study using this protocol (Sharp et al. 1993) 26 of 29 affected dogs became asymptomatic.

Another form of enilconazole (Cinafarm-EC) is 13.8% enilconazole. In the United States enilconazol is available as Clinafarm-EC (imazalil). (It should not be confused with Clinafarm-EG, which are canisters of enilconazole used as a smoke generator in poultry houses.) Clinafarm-EC is available in a 750 mL bottle containing 13.8% (138 mg/mL) enilconazole. The other ingredients listed on the Material Safety Data Sheet are benzyl alcohol and dioctyl sodium sulfosuccinate. It also contains ethoxylated castor oil. The Canadian formulation of Imaverol contains polysorbate 20 and sorbitan monolaurate as its inert ingredients, with 10% enilconazole as the active drug.

The Clinafarm-EC formulation is registered for controlling *Aspergillus* organisms in poultry facilities and equipment by making a 1:100 dilution and spraying or fogging the area to be treated. Topical 0.2% enilconazole (Clinafarm EC) was well tolerated in cats. A 50:1 dilution has been applied topically to dogs and cats at some veterinary hospitals.

ITRACONAZOLE. Itraconazole (Sporanax) (Fig. 46.8) was approved for use in the United States in 1992. Of several triazole compounds screened, itraconazole, first synthesized in 1980, was selected for further clinical

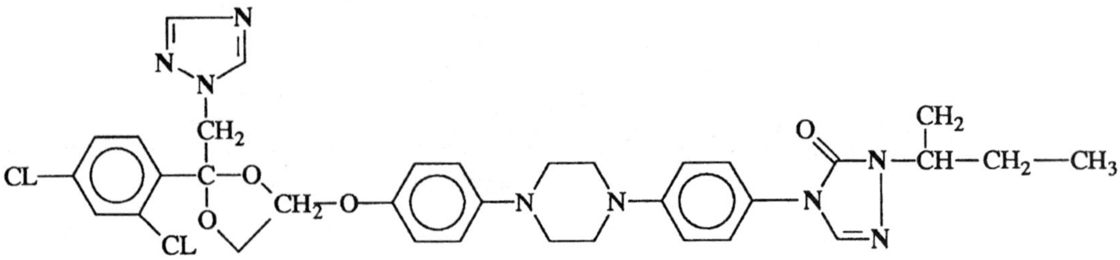

FIG. 46.8—Itraconazole.

development due to several criteria: (1) 5–100 times better in vitro and in vivo potency than ketoconazole, (2) good activity against *Aspergillus* spp., (3) activity against meningeal cryptococcosis in animal models, (4) few adverse side effects, and (5) encouraging pharmacokinetics (Cauwenbergh et al. 1987).

ACTIVITY. Itraconazole has been tested both in vitro and in vivo against a wide variety of fungi (for review see Perfect et al. 1986; VanCutsem et al. 1987; VanCutsem 1990; Cauwenbergh and DeDonker 1987). It was found to be effective against virtually all medically important fungi, including *Microsporum, Trichophyton, Candida, Malassezia* (*Pityrosporum*), *Sporothrix, Pythium, Histoplasma, Aspergillus, Blastomyces, Coccidioides,* and *Cryptococcus.* It is a weak base (pK_a = 3.7), is highly lipophilic (log P = 5.66), and is virtually insoluble in water.

PHARMACOKINETICS. Absorption is increased by an acid environment and when taken with meals (Graybill 1990) and is less variable than ketoconazole absorption. Bioavailability increases from 40% after fasting to 99.8% when given with a meal (VanCauteren et al. 1987). Itraconazole is highly (99.8%) plasma bound (95% to albumin and 5% to red blood cells) (Heykants et al. 1987); however, due to its lipophilicity and even higher affinity for tissue proteins, it is extensively distributed throughout the body. Tissue to plasma concentration ratios range from 1:1 in brain to 8:1 in keratin to 25:1 in fat stores. Highest tissue levels are seen in the liver and adrenal cortex (Heykants et al. 1987). High tissue binding also results in a very large volume of distribution (11–17 L/kg) (Troke et al. 1990; Heykants et al. 1990) and in low plasma concentrations.

Although it does not reach high concentrations in the CSF compared to fluconazole, itraconazole was found to be effective in treating meningeal cryptococcosis in both mouse and guinea pig models (Perfect et al. 1986).

Itraconazole is extensively metabolized, with less than 1% of the active drug and approximately 35% of inactive drug (as more than 10 metabolites) excreted in the urine. The predominant route of elimination for itraconazole is in the bile. Due to the increased metabolic stability of the triazole ring versus the imidazole ring (Richardson et al. 1990), itraconazole has a longer half-life (17–25 hr) than ketoconazole (8 hr) in humans. There is disagreement about the elimination rate since the terminal half-life in the dog has been reported to be 8–12 hours (VanCauteren et al. 1987) and 44–58 hours (Heykants et al. 1987). Differences in study methods and pharmacokinetic analysis may account for this discrepancy. More important than plasma half-life, therapeutically active concentrations are maintained much longer in tissues than in plasma. For example, itraconazole can be detected for 4 days in vaginal epithelium and for 4 weeks in skin and nails after cessation of therapy. Itraconazole, like ketoconazole, exhibits nonlinear pharmacokinetics; steady-state concentrations were found to be three times higher after 14 days of therapy than those predicted by a single dose, and the half-life was seen to increase from 24 to 36 hours (Heykants et al. 1990).

CLINICAL USE. In one study in cats (Moriello and De Boer 1995), itraconazole (10 mg/kg q24h) was compared to griseofulvin (50 mg/kg once daily) for treatment of dermatophytosis. Both drugs were equally effective, but itraconazole achieved cures faster (56 days). There were no adverse effects of itraconazole in the cats. In another study (Mancianti et al. 1998), cats with dermatophyte infections were treated successfully with itraconazole at a dose of 3 mg/kg once daily.

Itraconazole has been compared to ketoconazole in the treatment of experimentally induced feline disseminated cryptococcosis (Medleau et al. 1990). After three months of therapy, the infection had been cleared by both drugs as determined by cryptococcal antigen titers and CSF culture. Three months following therapy all animals remained clinically normal, and titers and CSF cultures remained negative. Although both antifungals brought about resolution of the disease, all cats receiving ketoconazole became anorectic and lost weight, requiring dosage adjustments. This was not seen with itraconazole, and in fact the animals receiving this drug gained weight during the study. Itraconazole has also been used in naturally occurring cryptococcal infections (Medleau 1990). Itraconazole has been successfully used in the treatment of a superficial dermatophyte infection that was refractory to griseofulvin and ketoconazole, and in two subcutaneous dermatophyte infections (pseudomycetoma) in cats (Mundell 1990).

In dogs, the most extensive study has been for treatment of blastomycosis (Legendre et al. 1996). In a study of 112 dogs, 5 mg/kg/day was as effective as 10 mg/kg/day. With a 60-day course of therapy, 54% of dogs were cured.

Itraconazole has been used to treat ocular and systemic blastomycosis in dogs. When given 5 mg/kg itraconazole twice a day for 60 days, 76% of eyes with posterior segment disease other than optic neuritis and 18% and 13% of eyes with anterior uveitis or endophthalmitis, respectively, recovered (Brooks et al. 1992).

Itraconazole has been successfully used in both the prevention and the treatment of aspergillosis in caged birds. A dose of 20 mg/kg daily for at least 30 days was used to successfully treat 5 of 12 presumed cases of *Aspergillus* infections in penguins. This same author suggests its prophylactic use in penguin chicks (Shannon 1992). A different treatment protocol was recommended for aspergillosis in raptors. Birds are treated with 10 mg/kg twice daily in combination with amphotericin B nebulization three times a day for 20 minutes. Treatment for some cases lasted as long as 6 weeks. These authors also recommend the prophylactic use of itraconazole whenever the clinician expects increased risk for the disease (Forbes et al. 1992).

DOSES. Dosages used in dogs have been 2.5–5 mg/kg/day and as high as 5–10 mg/kg/day for the treatment of blastomycosis. The most commonly recommended dose is 5 mg/kg/day (Legendre 1995) and may be as effective as high doses with less toxicity. In cats it has been used to treat dermatophytosis at a dose of 10 mg/kg once daily (Moriello and DeBoer 1995), but 3 mg/kg once daily may be just as effective. Itraconazole is available as 100 mg capsules. The granules in these capsules may be added to food for convenience. It also is available as a 10 mg/mL cherry-flavored oral liquid formulation.

ADVERSE EFFECTS. Itraconazole is probably better tolerated in dogs and cats than ketoconazole. Nevertheless, toxic reactions are still possible. Since most adverse effects are dose related, one is advised to lower the dose in animals in which adverse effects are observed. According to Legendre (1995) about 10% of dogs receiving recommended doses develop hepatic toxicosis. Liver enzyme elevations may occur in 10–15% of dogs. Hepatic toxicosis is also possible in cats. Anorexia may occur as a complication of treatment, especially with high doses and high serum concentrations. It usually develops in the second month of therapy in dogs. In cats there seem to be dose-related GI effects of anorexia and vomiting (Mancianti et al. 1998).

Dogs chronically administered itraconazole (2.5, 10, or 40 mg/kg daily for 3 months) had no significant alterations in mortality rate, behavior, appearance, food consumption, body weight, hematologic values, serum and urine chemistry, or gross pathology (VanCauteren et al. 1987b). Subacute toxicity studies in rats revealed increased adrenal gland weight and the accumulation of proteinaceous material in the mononuclear phagocyte system at doses of 40 and 160 mg/kg. Since the mononuclear phagocyte system is responsible for ridding the body of a fungal infection, the clinical importance of this toxic effect remains to be seen. Although not teratogenic at 10 mg/kg, maternal toxicity, embryo toxicity, and teratogenicity were observed at 40 and 160 mg/kg in rats (VanCauteren et al. 1987b); therefore, its use in pregnant animals is not recommended. Itraconazole has been well tolerated by clinically ill cats, although one case of fatal drug-induced hepatitis has been reported (Medleau 1990).

Itraconazole exhibits the highest affinity and selectivity for the fungal cytochrome P-450 enzyme of all known azoles. It is up to 125 times more selective for fungal P-450 systems than mammalian liver enzymes in certain in vitro preparations (Vanden Bossche 1987). Not only is itraconazole efficacious in vitro, but it also does not inhibit P-450 systems in the testis, adrenal, or liver in vivo (Vanden Bossche et al. 1990). In clinical studies, 100 mg of itraconazole given to humans each day for 30 days had no effect on serum testosterone or cortisol levels (DeCoster et al. 1987). Similarly, there were no changes in testosterone and cortisol concentrations in rats and dogs receiving daily itraconazole for at least 1 month.

The biochemical basis for the specificity of itraconazole toward fungal P-450 is thought to be dependent upon the hydrophobic nonligand portion of the molecule and its affinity for the apoprotein portion of the cytochrome molecule (Vanden Bossche et al. 1990). The resulting lack of significant inhibition of liver microsomal enzymes results in itraconazole's inability to affect other drugs' metabolism. Although the clinical significance is as yet unknown, drugs that can inhibit or stimulate liver degradative enzymes are able to alter the pharmacokinetics of itraconazole. Even though itraconazole is primarily cleared by hepatic metabolism, there appears to be no need for dosage adjustments in patients with liver disease (Heykants et al. 1987). As with ketoconazole, itraconazole's oral absorption is pH dependent; therefore, dosage adjustments may be necessary when gastric pH is increased.

DRUG INTERACTIONS. Like ketoconazole, itraconazole absorption is decreased when the stomach is less acidic. Do not administer with antacids, H_2 blockers, or omeprazole. Oral capsules of itraconazole should be taken with food to increase absorption. The oral solution (10 mg/mL Sporanox solution), on the other hand, is absorbed better on an empty stomach. In a study in cats, itraconazole oral solution appeared to be much better absorbed than a capsule, but cats were fed with each medication.

Some cytochrome P-450 inhibition occurs (CYP3A4) and itraconazole may increase concentrations of cyclosporine, digoxin, and cisapride, when used concurrently. However, enzyme inhibition is much less in comparison to ketoconazole.

FLUCONAZOLE. Like itraconazole, fluconazole (Diflucan) has replaced ketoconazole in small animals and birds for many indications. Fluconazole (Fig. 46.9) is a synthetic bistriazole that was licensed in the United States by the Food and Drug Administration in January 1990 for use in human cryptococcal and candidial infections.

In attempts to overcome some of the deficiencies seen with earlier imidazole compounds, it was found that replacing the imidazole ring with a triazole ring increased in vivo activity despite being four times less potent in vitro than the original imidazole. This suggested that due to the triazole ring's decreased nucleophilicity, it possessed an increased resistance to metabolic attack. Addition of a second triazole group resulted in in vivo potencies 100 times that of ketoconazole and in relatively low lipophilicity. Aqueous solubility dramatically increased (from <1 mg/mL to 8 mg/mL) (Richardson et al. 1990) by replacing the dichlorophenyl substituent in ketoconazole with a difluorophenyl group. The resulting compound has good efficacy in animal models and pharmacokinetics differing from previous azole antifungals.

Fluconazole has been shown to be effective in animal models of *Blastomyces, Candida, Coccidioides, Cryptococcus,* and *Histoplasma* infections and variably effective against *Aspergillus* infection.

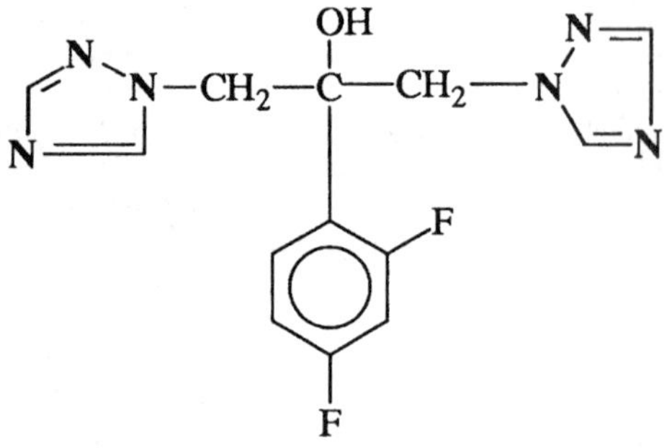

FIG. 46.9—Fluconazole.

PHARMACOKINETICS. Fluconazole has different solubility characteristics than ketoconazole and itraconazole and is absorbed well regardless of the circumstances. Feeding or formulation (liquid vs. tablet) does not affect absorption. Fluconazole absorption is complete in animals. Fluconazole tablets (Diflucan) and oral suspension (10 mg/mL) are absorbed well, and the oral dose is similar to the IV dose.

Fluconazole demonstrates linear absorption kinetics, with bioavailability greater than 90% (Brammer et al. 1990); thus, oral and IV dosages are identical. Maximum fluconazole concentrations are reached 1–4 hours after an oral dose. Unlike other azole antifungals, fluconazole is not highly protein bound. Humphrey et al. (1985) found plasma protein binding to be between 10 and 12% at concentrations of 0.1 and 1 mg/L in mice, rats, dogs, and humans. Fluconazole's low molecular weight, water solubility, and high unbound fraction allow it to be readily distributed throughout the body, including pharmacokinetically privileged spaces. Drug concentrations in saliva, sputum, skin, nails, blister fluid, and vaginal tissue and secretions were found to be similar to plasma concentrations. The advantages of fluconazole lie in its ability to produce higher CSF concentrations than ketoconazole or itraconazole, and therefore, it may be useful for treating mycotic meningitis (Kowalsky and Dixon 1991). Fluconazole CSF/plasma or serum concentration ratios range from 0.5 to 0.9 in humans (Brammer et al. 1990), rabbits (Perfect et al. 1986), and rhesus monkeys (Arndt et al. 1988). Fluconazole has a volume of distribution that approximates total body water, ≈0.7 L/kg (Humphrey et al. 1985).

Due to its polarity, low molecular weight, and metabolic stability, fluconazole is eliminated principally by the kidney. A unique feature of fluconazole is that this drug is the only one of the azoles that is water soluble and excreted in the urine in an active form. Therefore, it may be one of the few drugs useful for treating fungal cystitis. Approximately 80% of the dose is excreted as active drug in the urine. Estimates of renally excreted metabolites range from 4 to 11%, whereas fecal excretion was negligible in the dog but composed 10 and 2% of the dose in mice and humans, respectively. Half-lives were 4–5 hours in mice and rats, ≈14 hours in dogs and cats (Craig et al. 1993), and 22–30 hours in humans. The disparity between renal fluconazole clearance and creatinine clearance suggests that net tubular reabsorption is responsible for the extended half-life. Steady-state levels are achieved in 5–7 days; thus, the manufacturer suggests a two times loading dose during the first 12–24 hours (Dudley 1990). The lack of significant hepatic metabolism allows for linear elimination kinetics; i.e., half-life is independent of dose.

In cats, fluconazole has a long half-life of 25 hours, with good absorption and distribution to the CSF and aqueous humor (Vaden et al. 1997). The volume of distribution was determined to be ~1 L/kg. Based on these results the authors suggest a cat would require 100 mg fluconazole per day, as a single dose or divided, to produce an effective clinical response (Craig et al. 1993).

The pharmacokinetics of fluconazole was investigated in horses recently (author's unpublished data). Briefly, fluconazole administered orally to horses was well absorbed with bioavailability of 100%. The long half-life of 36 hours and good distribution (1 L/kg) indicate the potential utility of this drug in treating fungal infections. Concentrations in the CSF, synovial joint fluid, and aqueous humor of horses in this study were 96, 90, and 73%, respectively, of plasma concentrations. Based on results of this study, a dose of 5 mg/kg once daily orally was calculated.

CLINICAL USE. Extensive experimentation has been done in vitro and in various animal models using various species of fungi (for reviews, see Saag and Dismukes 1988; Troke 1987; Graybill 1987). Based on fluconazole's tissue distribution, certain predictions can be made regarding its clinical applications both in human and in veterinary medicine. High CSF/serum ratios provide a promising alternative to intrathecal use of other antifungals (Foulds et al. 1988). Encouraging results have been seen with fluconazole's use in cryptococcal meningitis either in acute management or in prevention of recurrence in AIDS patients. High penetration into sputum suggests that high enough concentrations exist in pulmonary secretions to be effective against pulmonary mycotic infections. Fluconazole has been used in pulmonary or disseminated coccidioidomycosis with a favorable response in 86% of patients; it had variable success with fungal pneumonia caused by *Aspergillus* spp. (Cantazaro et al. 1990). Penetration into skin and vaginal tissue allow for fluconazole's use in dermatophytosis and vulvovaginal candidiasis. Since the drug is renally excreted, urinary concentrations are approximately 10 times that in serum, suggesting its use for fungal urinary tract infections.

Fluconazole has been used in the treatment of an abdominal eumycetoma caused by *Madurella mycetomatis*. Following surgical excision of the main mass, a 7-month course of fluconazole was initiated. Three weeks into therapy, celiotomy and ultrasonography confirmed no regrowth of the mass, but smaller granulomas were present. Seven months after diagnosis these granulomas had increased in size and number, and the dog was euthanized (Lambrechts et al. 1991).

Fluconazole has also been used to treat canine nasal aspergillosis and penicilliosis. Ten affected dogs were treated with 2.5–5 mg/kg fluconazole orally for 8 weeks. Six dogs became free of disease 2–4 weeks after cessation of therapy and remained free of disease for at least 6 months. Serum alkaline phosphatase and alanine transaminase activity remained within normal ranges throughout the treatment period, and adverse side effects were not noted (Sharp 1991).

Fluconazole was used to control an outbreak of coccidioidomycosis in Japanese Macaque monkeys in the South Texas Primate Observatory. Previous success was seen with liposomal amphotericin B; however, it required anesthesia of the animals. Fluconazole was administered by placing 25 (for juveniles) or 50 mg (for adults) in caramel candies. Of 14 animals treated, 8 improved rapidly while the others had no response. Discontinuation of therapy resulted in relapse of signs in 4 of the surviving monkeys. The authors conclude that fluconazole has a role in the treatment of coccidioidomycosis; however, the dose may exceed the 2–3 mg/kg used in this outbreak, and a protracted duration of therapy may be necessary for fungal eradication (Graybill et al. 1990).

DOSES. For cats with systemic cryptococcosis, clinical studies have shown a benefit from a dose of 100 mg/cat/day in one or two divided doses. Other reported doses are 2.5–5 mg/kg once a day (Hill et al. 1995). Pharmacokinetic studies support a dose of 50 mg/cat per day (Vaden et al. 1997). In dogs the dose is 10–12 mg/kg/day orally. Fluconazole is available in tablets, oral suspension, and IV injection. Oral absorption in horses has been studied; 5 mg/kg q24h in horses produces sufficient concentrations in plasma and tissues.

ADVERSE EFFECTS. Fluconazole has been generally well tolerated, with mild adverse effects being reported in 5–30% of cases. The GI tract was most frequently involved, followed by the CNS and skin. Mild elevations in hepatic enzymes are sometimes seen, and two cases of hepatic necrosis and death occurred in association with fluconazole therapy (Kowalsky and Dixon 1991). There seems to be little evidence of testosterone or other steroid biosynthesis inhibition in vitro (Shaw et al. 1987) or in human or animal patients (VanCauteren et al. 1987). Hematologic abnormalities, including anemia, leukopenia, neutropenia, and thrombocytopenia, have been reported (AHFS Drug Information 1992). In subacute toxicity studies in dogs the highest dose tested (30 mg/kg) caused slight increases in liver weight, hepatic fat, and plasma transaminase activity. Although there is no evidence of mutagenicity or carcinogenicity, its use in pregnant patients is not recommended.

INTERACTIONS WITH OTHER DRUGS OR DISEASES. Unlike ketoconazole or itraconazole, fluconazole's aqueous solubility is acid independent; hence, drugs that raise gastric pH were not found to have any significant effects on fluconazole pharmacokinetics. As can be expected with a renally excreted drug, renal dysfunction affects fluconazole's elimination such that dose adjustments are necessary. When patients with normal renal function were compared with those with severe renal insufficiency, fluconazole's elimination half-life nearly tripled (from 30.1 hr to 84.5 hr) (Dudley 1990). Reduced dosages as well as extended dosing intervals have been recommended in renal insufficiency.

Terbinafine. Terbinafine (Lamisil®) is reported to be a highly fungicidal antifungal agent. It is a synthetic drug of the allylamine class. A closely related drug of the same class is naftifine (Naftin®), which is used as a topical cream for dermatophyte infections in people. Terbinafine inhibits squalene epoxidase to decrease synthesis of ergosterol. Fungal cell death results from disruption of cell membrane (Balfour and Faulds 1992).

ACTIVITY. Terbinafine is active against yeasts and a wide range of dermatophytes. It is fungicidal against

Trichophyton spp., *Microsporum* spp., and *Aspergillus* spp. It is also active against *Blastomyces dermatitidis, Cryptococcus neoformans, Sporothrix schenckii, Histoplasma capsulatum, Candida,* and *Pityrosporum* yeast. In people, it was more effective than griseofulvin for treating dermatophytes, with less relapse (Hoffman et al. 1995). There may be some activity against protozoa (e.g., *Toxoplasma*).

ABSORPTION AND DISTRIBUTION. Terbinafine has high availability in people after oral administration (not reported for dogs and cats). It's lipophilic nature results in high concentration in tissues such as stratum corneum, hair follicles, sebum-rich skin, and nails. In people, after 12 days of therapy, the concentrations in stratum corneum exceed those in plasma by a factor of 75. Concentrations in skin may be detected in people as early as 24 hours after oral administration, but maximum concentrations are reached at 7 days. Fungicidal concentrations in nails may require 3 weeks of treatment.

ADVERSE EFFECTS. In dogs treated with 30 mg/kg, serum ALT concentrations were mildly to moderately elevated in 4 of 10 dogs and Alk Phos was increased in 2 of 10 dogs. Terbinafine does not bind to P-450 enzymes as do other antifungal drugs; therefore, it does not cause drug interactions or inhibition of steroid synthesis in animals. In people, there is a rare incidence of hepatitis and loss of taste. In people there are no effects on pregnancy, as with other antifungal drugs.

CLINICAL USE. Clinical use has been sparse in veterinary medicine. Doses in people are 125 mg twice daily (approx. 1.8 mg/kg q12h). The pediatric dose has been in the range of 4–8 mg/kg once a day, most often administered at the lower dose of 4 mg/kg (Jones 1995). Preliminary results so far suggest that doses in cats are much higher than what is required for people (e.g., 20 mg/kg q24h). It is available as a 1% topical cream (Lamisil) and as 125 and 250 mg tablets.

Other Antifungal Agents

MORPHOLINE DERIVATIVES. Amorolfine is the only morpholine derivative in clinical use. It exhibits antifungal activity against plant and animal fungal pathogens. It is fungicidal against dermatophytes at very low concentrations (MIC = 0.06 μg/mL). Grossly, this agent causes changes in fungal growth similar to the azoles. Its mechanism of action involves inhibition of two steps in the pathway of ergosterol biosynthesis, specifically a reductase and an isomerase enzyme (Polak 1990). Since the reduction reaction is earlier in the pathway, this first inhibition may be more important in achieving its antifungal effect (Baloch and Mercer 1987).

THIOCARBAMATE ANTIFUNGALS. Tonaftate (Tinactin) and tolciclate exhibit strong antifungal activity against dermatophytes (MIC = 0.1–1 μg/kg). However, yeast cells are considered resistant (MIC >100 μg/kg). The mechanism of action of thiocarbamate antifungals is similar to that of allylamine derivatives.

Combination Therapy. In vitro synergism of two antifungal compounds, seen as a fourfold reduction in the MIC when given alone, was first identified between amphotericin B and flucytosine in 1971 (Medoff et al. 1971). One explanation of this synergism involves the membrane-permeabilizing effects of amphotericin B facilitating flucytosine's entrance into the cell cytoplasm (Medoff et al. 1972). This combination of antifungal drugs is more effective than amphotericin B alone in the treatment of cryptococcal meningitis (Bennet et al. 1979; Utz et al. 1975). Advantages of this combination include a reduction in the amphotericin B dose, thereby limiting nephrotoxicity, as well as prevention of mutants to flucytosine (Drouhet and Dupont 1987). This combination has also been suggested for therapy of acute hematogenously disseminated candidiasis (Horn et al. 1985).

Combinations of amphotericin B and azole antifungals have been less successful. Azole-induced depletion of fungal cell membrane ergosterol results in fewer binding sites on which polyene antifungals can exert their effect. Antagonism and synergism between these two classes of antifungal agents have been reported experimentally (Polak et al. 1982; Dupont and Drouhet 1979). Because of the slower onset of action of azole antifungals, many clinicians recommend initial therapy of serious systemic fungal infections with amphotericin B, followed by a weaning to a sole azole therapeutic protocol.

As previously discussed, the combination of flucytosine and ketoconazole proved toxic to cats (Pukay and Dion 1984). Although not investigated, caution should be used with the combination of 5-FC with any azole. The combination of multiple azole antifungal drugs has not been investigated.

ANTIVIRAL THERAPY

The development of specific antiviral drugs is difficult due to the limited number of potential target sites and processes which distinguish virus from host. As an obligate intracellular pathogen, viruses must utilize host cell biochemical machinery to synthesize new viral proteins and genetic material. It is difficult to inhibit viral functions without also inhibiting those of the host; thus, the most severe constraint limiting the use of antiviral drugs is not lack of efficacy but toxicity in the mammalian cell (poor selective toxicity). Combating an intracellular infection also means a compound not only must be able to reach the site of infection but also must be able to get inside the host cell to achieve its desired effect. Over the past two decades identification of specific viral enzymes and proteins has allowed development of antiviral therapeutics and

TABLE 46.1—Suggested antifungal drugs and dosages for treating systemic fungal infections in the dog and cat

Disease	Treatment	Daily dose (mg/kg)		Frequency	Comment
		Dog	Cat		
Blastomycosis[a]	Am B initially	0.5	0.25	3 times/week	For life- threatening disease
	then KTZ	10–15	10	12–24 hr	
	ITZ[b]	5	5	12 hr	For non-life-threatening disease
Histoplasmosis[c]	KTZ	10–15	50	12–24 hr	
	Concurrent Am B	0.25–0.5	0.25–0.5	48 hr	Drugs started together; KTZ given alone after condition improves
	and KTZ	10–15	50	12–24 hr	
Cryptococcosis	Am B	0.25–0.5	0.1–0.5	3 times/week	For CNS infections initially
	5–FC	30	30	6 hr	For CNS infections initially
		50	50	8 hr	
		75	75	12 hr	
	FLZ[d]	10–20	10–20	12–24 hr	For CNS infections initially
	KTZ	5–30	5–20	12–24 hr	For maintenance
	FLZ	5–10	5–10	12 hr	For maintenance
Coccidioidomycosis	KTZ	5–10	50	8–24 hr	Not useful in meningitis
	Am B	0.4–0.5		48–72 hr	If CNS is involved
	FLZ	5–10	5–10	12 hr	
	ITZ	5	5	12 hr	
Aspergillosis[e]	FLZ	5–10	5–10	12 hr	For systemic disease
	Enilconazole	10		12 hr	Topical-direct infusion at infection site
Candidiasis	KTZ	5–11	50–100	12–24 hr	For systemic disease
	ITZ	5–7	5–7	12 hr	For systemic disease
	Nystatin				For local mucocutaneous disease
	Miconazole				Applied topically
	Clotimazole				Applied topically
	Am B cream				Applied topically

Source: Greene 1990, Chaps. 63–72.
Note: Am B = amphotericin B; ITZ = itraconazole; KTZ = ketoconazole; FLZ = fluconazole; 5–FC = fluorocytosine.
[a]Fluconazole not effective, not recommended.
[b]Itraconazole may replace ketoconazole therapy.
[c]Human studies suggest itraconazole and fluconazole to be as effective as ketoconazole-amphotericin B combination therapy.
[d]More rapid cerebrospinal fluid sterilization occurs with amphotericin B-5-fluorocytosine therapy than with fluconazole.
[e]Itraconazole not effective in nasal aspergillosis.

specific treatment of viral diseases in human patients (Crumpacker 1989). In addition, at no other time in history has more emphasis and support been placed on development of antiviral compounds, the result of the epidemic of an invariably fatal infection, HIV.

The treatment of viral disease in the veterinary population is made somewhat problematic due to the infrequency with which definitive diagnosis of a disease attributed to a specific viral agent is made. Viral cultures are not routinely performed and, when done, take a long time, so results are often obtained after the disease has taken its course. Many of the antiviral drugs are toxic and may worsen the condition of an already debilitated infected individual. In chronic viral infections, such as those caused by the feline leukemia or the feline immunodeficiency virus, the ability of the virus to become latent makes eradication of the disease virtually impossible (Huraux et al. 1990). All of the presently available antiviral drugs are virostatic. Thus, an intact immune system is required to maintain the suppression of many viral infections (an additional problem in FeLV and FIV infection). It would appear that the clinicians' best defense against viral disease remains preventing infection (vaccination) rather than attempting to specifically treat an already existing viral infection.

The following discussion of antiviral drugs considers all compounds available, but greater emphasis is placed on those with veterinary significance. An overview of the physiology and biochemistry involved in viral replication is necessary to identify target sites at which antiviral agents are directed. The viral replicative cycle can be divided into eight steps (Fig. 46.10):

1. *Attachment:* The virus particle must attach to the host cell membrane, often to a specific protein receptor.
2. *Penetration:* The virus particle penetrates the host cell membrane.
3. *Uncoating:* The viral protein coat is broken, releasing the viral genetic material into the host cell cytoplasm.
4. *Transcription:* A mRNA strand is made from the viral genetic material.
5. *Translation:* Viral mRNA attaches to host ribosomes, and nucleic acids are translated into viral proteins.
6. *Replication:* Duplicate strands of genetic material are produced from the original viral template.

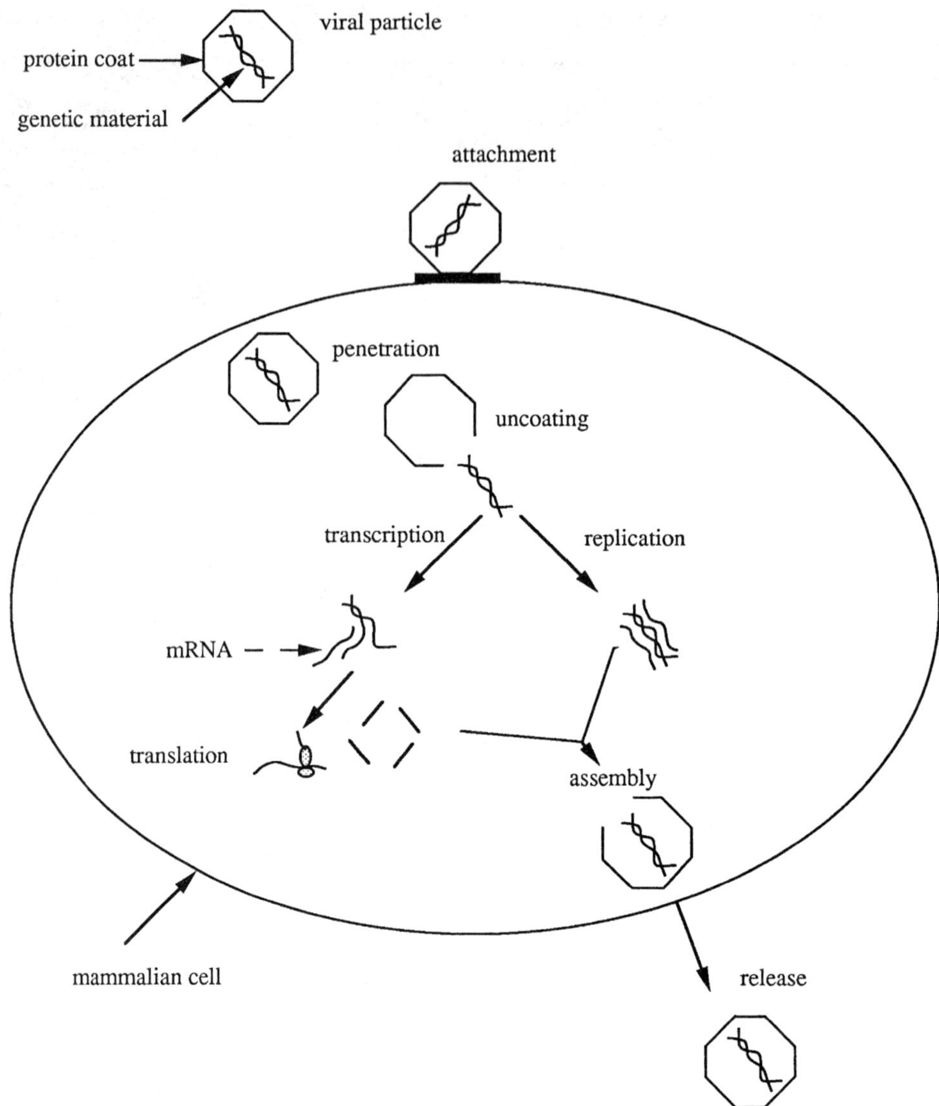

FIG. 46.10—Schematic diagram of the replicative cycle of a viral particle.

7. *Assembly:* Viral proteins/protein coats and newly formed viral genetic material combine to form mature virus particles.

8. *Release:* New virus particles either bud from the host cell membrane or are released as the host cell bursts, allowing infection of other cells.

These steps are common to both RNA and DNA viruses. However, transcription occurs via different mechanisms. In DNA viruses, the DNA template is used to form mRNA via a RNA transcriptase (DNA-dependent RNA polymerase). In positive-strand (+)RNA viruses, the original template can be used as the mRNA. In (–)RNA viruses, replication of a complementary strand must precede translation. In retroviruses, the RNA genetic material is first converted to DNA via reverse transcriptase, which is then transcribed to the mRNA strand. Potential sites for inhibition by exogenous compounds exist at each step in the replication cycle except for translation and protein synthesis. Since viral and host protein synthesis would be similarly inhibited, these compounds would be as toxic to the host as to the virus.

VIRAL ATTACHMENT AND PENETRATION. The attachment and penetration of virus into the host cell often requires the specific interaction of viral coat proteins with "receptor" proteins of the host cell membrane. Strategies for coating specific viral attachment proteins with monoclonal antibody to prevent attachment are limited by the fact that antibody must coat virus prior to infection and hence requires knowledge of exposure or prophylactic use. Analog viral binding proteins can bind host cell receptor proteins, thereby competing with actual viral particle binding. Unfortunately, the host cell proteins often have other physiologic functions which preclude this approach. Host cell protein receptor analogs which attach to the viral coat protein have been conjugated to compounds which enhance opsonization and phagocytosis by macrophages, thereby preventing viral replication.

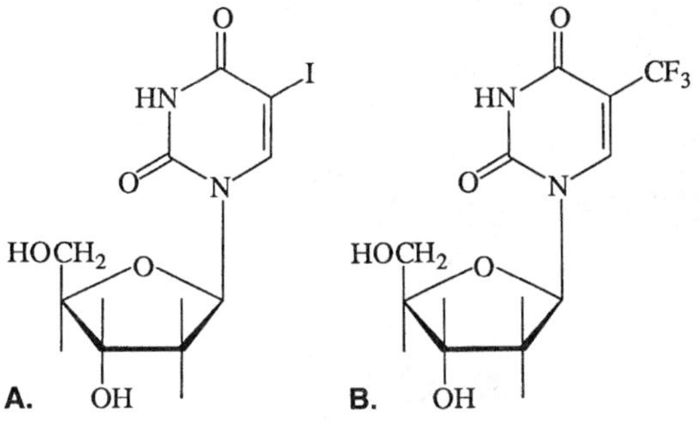

TRANSCRIPTION

Idoxuridine and Trifluridine. *Idoxuridine,* USP (5-iodo-2′-deoxyuridine, Herplex, Stoxil) (Fig. 46.11A), and *Trifluridine,* USP (5-trifluoromethyl-2′-deoxyuridine, Viroptic) (Fig. 46.11B), are thymidine analogs and therefore are only active against DNA viruses, primarily herpesvirus and poxvirus. The compound is phosphorylated inside the host cell and is then incorporated into growing mammalian and viral strands. This DNA is thought to be more susceptible to breakage and results in faulty proteins if transcribed. The fluorinated compound (trifluridine) is thought to have higher affinity for viral DNA than mammalian, as well as being more active. Both compounds are used topically in the treatment of herpetic keratitis. Given the cost of these medications, idoxuridine should be used initially, and if no response is seen within 1 week, trifluridine therapy should be initiated (Martin 1990). Toxic side effects, including leukopenia, hepatotoxicity, and GI signs, have precluded their systemic use.

Cytarabine and Vidarabine. *Cytarabine,* USP (cytosine arabinoside 1-β-D-arabinofuranosylcytosine, Ara-C) (Fig. 46.12A), and *Vidarabine,* USP (adenine arabinoside, 9-β-D-arabinofuranosyladenine, Ara-A) (Fig. 46.12B), are nucleoside analogs of cytosine and adenine, respectively. They have in vitro activity against certain DNA viruses, including herpesviruses, poxviruses, vaccinia, rabies, cytomegalovirus, and probably hepatitis B virus. Cellular enzymes convert these compounds to the triphosphate form, which then act as competitive inhibitors of DNA polymerase. Herpes-induced DNA polymerase seems to be more sensitive to this inhibition than the mammalian cellular counterpart.

Vidarabine is poorly soluble so must be given intravenously in large fluid volumes over 12 hours. Vidarabine and its active metabolite, hypoxanthine arabinoside, are widely distributed in body fluids and tissues, including the brain and cerebrospinal fluid. Cytarabine is biotransformed to an inactive metabolite and is therefore less effective than vidarabine. Major

FIG. 46.11—(A) Idoxuridine; (B) trifluridine.

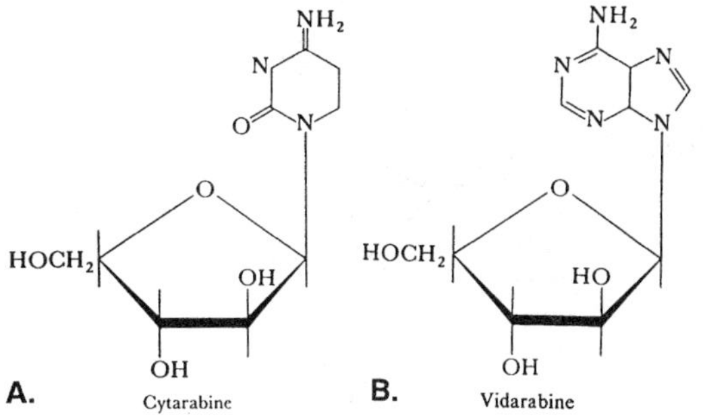

FIG. 46.12

side effects include GI, neurologic, and hematologic toxicity and teratogenicity.

These compounds have been used topically in the treatment of herpes keratitis and systemically in herpes simplex encephalitis. In human medicine, vidarabine's role has been suggested to be as a "backup" drug for resistant infections of herpes simplex virus and varicella-zoster virus (Hirsch and Schooley 1989). Vidarabine demonstrated significant antiviral activity in vitro against the feline infectious peritonitis virus. However, this effect was only seen if the compound was used as a pre- or cotreatment with viral inoculation (Barlough and Scott 1990).

Ribavirin. Ribavirin (Virazole) (Fig. 46.13) is a triazole purine nucleoside analog that inhibits the replication of a wide range of RNA and DNA viruses in vitro. Its strongest antiviral activity is against RNA respiratory viruses (influenza A and B) and herpesviruses but also includes myxoviruses, paramyxoviruses, arenaviruses, bunyaviruses, retroviruses, adenoviruses, and poxviruses. Ribavirin is thought to have multiple sites of action. After being monophosphorylated to ribavirin 5′-monophosphate (RMP) by adenosine kinase, it is able to indirectly inhibit synthesis of guanine nucleotides. Further phosphorylation to RTP allows it

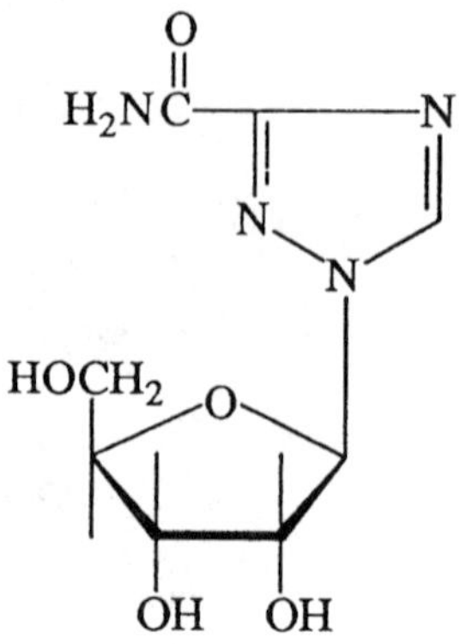

FIG. 46.13—Ribavirin.

to competitively inhibit ATP and GTP binding to RNA polymerase.

Ribavirin can be administered by oral, intravenous, and aerosol routes. When administered by the first two routes, anemia due to extravascular hemolysis, bone marrow suppression, GI toxicity, and central nervous signs may occur. In addition these two routes have been shown to be ineffective in the treatment of influenza A infection (Smith et al. 1980). Aerosolized ribavirin is generally well tolerated (Hall et al. 1983) and is therefore the preferred route for treating susceptible respiratory infections. Ribavirin is used to treat respiratory syncytial virus (RSV) and parainfluenza virus infections in neonate, infants, and young children. Although there is not complete agreement of its indication in RSV (Steele 1988) it has been shown to shorten the duration of virus shedding and improve arterial oxygen saturation in treated infants (Rodriguez et al. 1987). In addition, it may prevent long-term complications of RSV infection such as asthma and other chronic respiratory conditions (Betts 1991).

Oral ribavirin was seen to worsen the condition of cats experimentally infected with calicivirus. Bone marrow suppression, weight loss, increased hepatic enzymes, and icterus were seen (Povey 1978). These side effects were not seen in dogs when given 60 mg/kg for 2 weeks (Canonico 1985). Ribavirin was shown to have in vitro antiviral activity against the FIP virus at concentrations 150 μg/mL (Barlough and Scott 1990).

Acyclovir and Ganciclovir. *Acyclovir,* USP (Zovirax, 9-(2-hydroxyethoxymethyl)guanine) (Fig. 46.14A), and *Ganciclovir,* USP (Cytovene, 9-(1,3-dihydroxy-2-propocymethyl)guanine) (Fig. 46.14B), are synthetic nucleoside analogs of deoxyguanosine, whose antiviral activities are restricted to herpesviruses. Acyclovir is particularly active against herpes simplex 1 and 2 viruses and varicella-zoster virus and is less active against Epstein-Barr and cytomegaloviruses (CMV). Ganciclovir is 25–100 times more active against CMV than acyclovir. Both compounds are more potent in vitro against certain herpesviruses than idoxuridine and vidarabine.

Acyclovir is monophosphorylated by viral thymidine kinase 200 times easier than by the similar mammalian enzyme, which contributes to its good selective toxicity and high therapeutic index. Cellular enzymes then form the di- and triphosphate form, which selectively inhibits the viral DNA polymerase by competing with deoxyguanosine triphosphate. Acyclo-GTP that is incorporated into viral DNA strands causes termination of elongation. Virally infected cells are 40–100 times more efficient in converting acyclo-GMP to acyclo-GTP than are noninfected cells. The mechanism of action for ganciclovir is essentially identical except that initial phosphorylation can be carried out by cellular enzymes, a fact that makes acyclovir-resistant thymidine kinase-deficient strains of virus less resistant to ganciclovir. Intracellular concentrations of ganciclovir are somewhat higher than those achieved with acyclovir.

Pharmacokinetic data are available for human patients. Acyclovir is available as a topical, oral, and intravenous preparation, whereas ganciclovir can only be give IV due to its poor absorption. Oral acyclovir bioavailability is only 15-30% and may decrease with increasing dose (Davey 1990). They are minimally protein bound (9–33% acyclo-; 1–2% ganciclo-) such that volume of distribution approximates total body water. Concentrations in the cerebrospinal fluid and aqueous humor are only one-third to one-half those in plasma. Both compounds are minimally metabolized with >70% excreted unchanged in the urine. Half-lives are approximately 2.5–3.6 hours in patients with normal renal function. Dosage adjustments are necessary in cases of renal impairment.

Acyclovir is indicated in many herpesvirus infections, including chronic and recurrent mucocutaneous

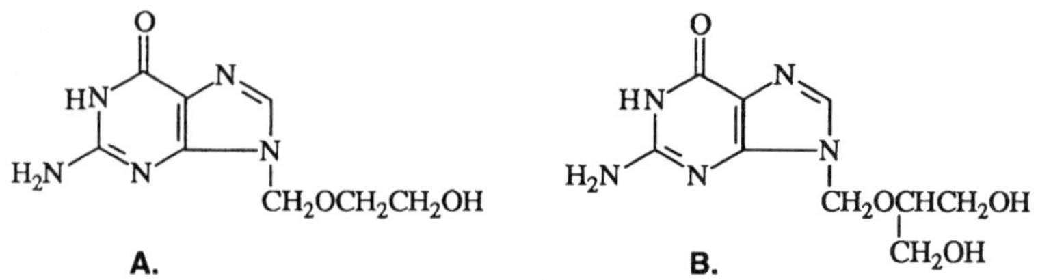

FIG. 46.14—(A) Acyclovir; (B) ganciclovir.

forms, primary and secondary genital herpes, neonatal herpes, and herpes simplex encephalitis (Douglas 1990). It is especially useful in varicella-zoster infections in immunocompromised hosts. Systemic absorption of topically applied acyclovir is limited, although plasma concentrations are measurable (Corey and Holmes 1983). Ganciclovir's toxicity currently limits its use to treatment of life- or sight-threatening cytomegalovirus infections in immunocompromised hosts. Unlike acyclovir, which has few side effects (obstructive nephropathy if given too rapidly, local irritation/phlebitis), bone marrow suppression has been reported in ganciclovir-treated patients, where ~40% develop neutropenia and ~20% thrombocytopenia. Central nervous signs such as headache, behavioral changes, and convulsions have also been described. It is teratogenic and mutagenic and thought to cause infertility, which is permanent in females.

The veterinary use of these antiviral agents is largely unknown although acyclovir has been used to treat experimental herpesvirus encephalitis. Orally administered acyclovir at 80 mg/kg 24 hours after herpesvirus infection in Quaker parakeets was shown to be more effective in preventing death than either low or high dose (40 or 250 mg/kg) intramuscular injections. At the highest dose tested, acyclovir toxicity, as seen by local muscular necrosis, was thought to contribute to bird mortality (Norton et al. 1991). Acyclovir has been shown to decrease mortality in psittacine birds with herpesviral infections if the drug is administered prior to onset of clinical signs (Smith 1987).

Zidovudine. Zidovudine (Azidothymidine, AZT, Retrovir, 3′-azido-3′-deoxythmydine) (Fig. 46.15) is a thymidine analog in which the 3′ hydroxy of the deoxyribose sugar has been replaced with an azido group. It was first synthesized in hopes of having anticancer activity (Horowitz et al. 1964) but was later discovered to have activity against the Friend leukemia virus. Mitsuya et al. (1985) discovered its activity against the HIV virus, thus propelling AZT into national recognition and making it the most important antiviral agent available to treat this epidemic.

AZT is phosphorylated by cellular enzymes to the triphosphate analog. This form inhibits viral reverse transcriptase (RNA-dependent DNA polymerase) as well as causing chain termination due to the unavailability of a 3′-hydroxyl moiety. AZT inhibits the viral enzyme with greater affinity (~100 times) than mammalian DNA polymerases, resulting in selective activity and low mammalian toxicity.

AZT can be given orally or IV in humans. Its oral bioavailability is 60–65%, and peak concentrations are achieved in about 1 hour. Only 25% of the drug is bound to plasma, and concentrations in the cerebrospinal fluid are similar to plasma concentrations. AZT is quickly metabolized to the 5′glucuronide, and metabolite and parent compound are eliminated in urine with a half-life of ~1 hour.

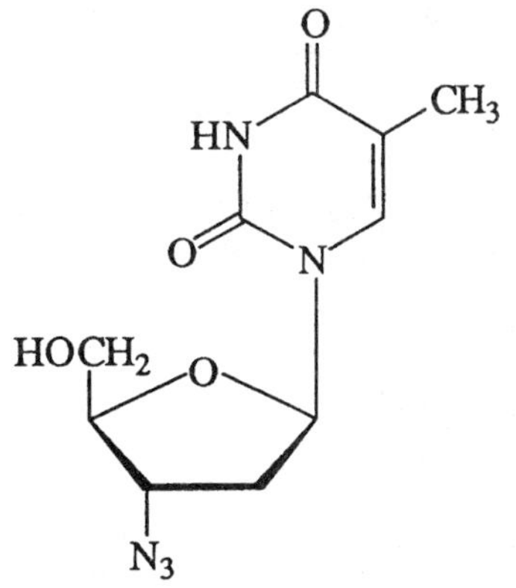

O
HN
CH_3
O
N
$HOCH_2$
O
N_3

FIG. 46.15—Zidovudine.

Major toxicities of AZT include anemia and granulocytopenia, which occur in up to 45% of treated patients (Richman et al. 1987). Drugs that inhibit glucuronyl transferase, such as acetaminophen, aspirin, and indomethacin, increase the risk of hematologic toxicity. It could be surmised that cats, having poor glucuronidation capability, might be sensitive to these effects.

The clinical use of AZT in humans is beyond the scope of this chapter. Its use, however, has been investigated in cats both as a clinical therapy for FIV and experimentally, using FIV as an animal model of HIV infection. Reverse transcriptase from FIV and HIV-1 viruses was shown to be nearly identical in sensitivity to several antiviral agents, including AZT. In addition, similar concentrations of AZT were required to inhibit replication of these viruses (North et al. 1989). Bovine leukemia virus has also been suggested as a possible animal model for investigation of retroviral infection. AZT inhibition of BLV reverse transcriptase was similar to that of FIV-RT (Reimer et al. 1989).

AZT has been shown to reduce clinical signs when given to two FIV-positive cats at a dose of 10 mg/kg/d twice a day subcutaneously for a period of 3 weeks (Egberink et al. 1991). Although not able to eradicate the infection, the authors suggest it is of clinical benefit and should extend the life of FIV-infected cats. AZT has also been advanced as a potential treatment of another retrovirus infection (Cotter 1992). In experimental FeLV infections, when treated with AZT within 1 week after virus challenge, cats are protected from bone marrow infection and viremia. Viremia persisted in cats treated later but before 3 weeks; however, antigen load in the blood was reduced (Tavares et al. 1987). AZT alone, or in combination with interferon or interleukin, was shown to prevent infection in cats challenged with virulent FeLV virus for a period of 6 weeks (Zeidner et al. 1989). Although not well characterized, side effects of AZT in the feline population probably include anemia and hepatotoxicity (Cotter 1992).

O
||
$(NaO)_2PCOONa$

FIG. 46.16—Foscarnet.

Foscarnet. Foscarnet (trisodium phosphonoformate hexahydrate; PFA) (Fig. 46.16) is a pyrophosphate analog which exhibits antiviral activity against a variety of DNA and RNA viruses. It inhibits DNA and RNA polymerases as well as reverse transcriptase. The mechanism of foscarnet differs from those of the preceding antiviral agents in that it inhibits these enzymes by binding at the pyrophosphate binding site rather than at a base binding site. Thus, inhibition is noncompetitive rather than competitive (Oberg 1989). Because phosphorylation by viral kinases is unnecessary for antiviral activity, it has potential for use in thymidine kinase-deficient herpesvirus infections (Teich et al. 1992). Viruses inhibited include avian myeloblastosis, Moloney murine leukemia, Rauscher leukemia, visna, influenza, bovine leukemia, African swine fever, baboon endogenous, simian sarcoma, human herpes, and human immunodeficiency viruses (Swenson et al. 1991).

Although viral replication has been shown to be inhibited at concentrations achievable in plasma, these concentrations often vary widely. In addition, variable interindividual pharmacokinetics in humans make optimal dosage regimes difficult to identify (Lietman 1992). The pharmacokinetics of PFA have been investigated in the cat (Straw et al. 1992). PFA was only 8% bioavailable, was found to have a terminal half-life of ~3 hours, and was not metabolized, resulting in a total clearance of 1.88 mL/min/kg. The related compound thiofoscarnet (thiophosphonoformate, TPFA) had greater bioavailability (22–44%) and a shorter plasma half-life (42 minutes) and was metabolized to the active PFA, suggesting its possible use as a prodrug. The percutaneous absorption of PFA was studied in rabbits and dogs to ensure its safe topical use in herpetic mucocutaneous conditions. Systemic absorption after vaginal application was found to be 14% in the rabbit and 34% in the dog, whereas 12% (rabbit) and 3% (dog) of the dose entered the systemic circulation after topical administration (Hussain and Ritschel 1989).

Foscarnet is more effective than vidarabine in the treatment of acyclovir-resistant herpes simplex virus infections. It is as effective as ganciclovir for treating CMV retinitis in AIDS patients. It has the advantage of having intrinsic anti-HIV activity, and it is better tolerated than ganciclovir when given in combination with AZT (Jacobson et al. 1991; Palestine et al. 1991). Foscarnet therapy may result in renal impairment, and lifelong intermittent therapy may be necessary to prevent recurrent CMV infection, but myelosuppressive toxicity is avoided. For these reasons, it may replace ganciclovir in this application (Minor and Baltz 1991) except in patients with decreased renal function (SOCA 1992). The prophylactic and therapeutic use of PFA has been suggested in the cat (Swenson et al. 1991). It is suggested that long-term PFA administration to FeLV-infected cats may limit spread of infection within and between hosts via extracellular inactivation of newly produced virus particles. The authors also suggest PFA may have a role as a viral disinfectant for blood, blood products, supplies, and equipment.

ASSEMBLY

Amantadine and Rimantadine. *Amantadine hydrochloride,* USP (1-adamantanamine hydrochloride, Symmetrel) (Fig. 46.17A), and *Rimantadine* (Flumadine) (Fig. 46.17B) are water-soluble cyclic amines with antiviral activity against a narrow range of RNA viruses, including myxoviruses, paramyxoviruses, togaviruses, and most strains of influenza A virus. Rimantadine has approximately 3–4 times greater in vitro activity against influenza A than amantadine (Betts 1991). The mechanism of these two related compounds has been debated. They were thought at one time to prevent viral penetration and uncoating (Hoffman et al. 1965), but this has been refuted more recently (Couch and Six 1986). Their antiviral activity is now thought to involve inhibition of late-stage assembly of the virus.

Both compounds are absorbed well from the human GI tract. Serum concentrations of amantadine are greater than those of rimantadine, but the latter achieves greater concentrations in secretions (Hayden et al. 1985). The volume of distribution of amantadine is significantly less than that of rimantadine. Amantadine is excreted unchanged in urine, with an elimination half-life of ~16 hours, whereas rimantadine is 85% metabolized and eliminated with a 24–36 hour half-life. Neither agent has bone marrow, renal, or hepatic side effects, but amantadine may be neurotoxic, causing jitters, difficulty in concentrating, and seizures in certain patient populations. CNS side effects are less

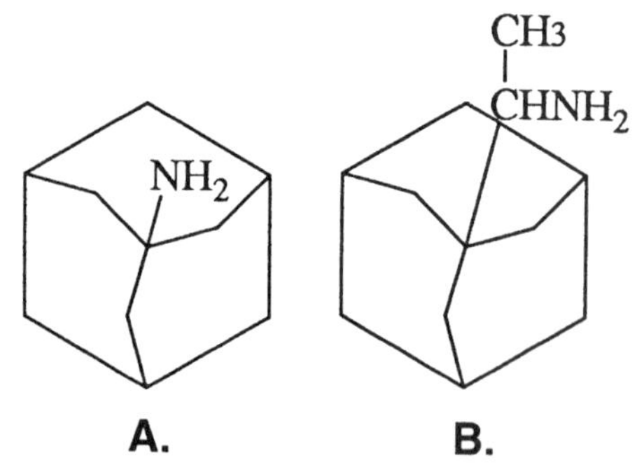

FIG. 46.17—(A) Amantadine; (B) rimantadine.

frequent with rimantadine. The combination of greater in vitro efficacy, greater distribution and terminal half-life, and less toxicity suggests rimantadine has greater clinical potential. Both compounds are equally effective in the prophylactic prevention of respiratory infections caused by influenza A virus, although not as effective as vaccination. They have also been used to treat flu outbreaks, resulting in shorter duration fever and more rapid resolution of symptoms (VanVoris et al. 1981). Experimentally infected chicks that received amantadine via the drinking water were one-half as likely to die as untreated controls (Obrosova-Serova et al. 1976). Amantadine had no inhibitory effect on FIP virus replication in vitro at the highest concentration tested (Barlough and Scott 1990).

HOST RESISTANCE

Interferon. A complete discussion of the biochemistry, physiology, and immunological function of interferon-$\alpha_{2a,2b}$ (Roferon-A, Intron A) is beyond the scope of this chapter. Interferons are glycopolypeptide molecules produced by certain mammalian cells in response to viral infections as well as other stimuli. They are potent cytokines that possess antiviral, immunomodulating, and anticancer properties (Pestka et al. 1987). Three classes of interferons exist: alpha, beta, and gamma, with the last being produced solely by T lymphocytes. Interferons affect RNA and DNA viral replication via multiple mechanisms which act at different stages of the viral replicative cycle. They bind specific cell-surface receptors, inhibiting binding, and may prevent penetration and uncoating. Interferon can inhibit synthesis or methylation of mRNA, translation, and viral assembly and release (Whitaker-Dowling and Younger 1987). Interferons are thought to inhibit viral protein synthesis indirectly by inducing an enzyme that indirectly activates a ribonuclease that degrades mRNA. They may also induce a protein kinase that phosphorylates and inactivates a viral initiation protein (Douglas 1990).

Being peptides, interferons are orally inactive and must be given parenterally. Peak plasma concentrations occur 4–8 hours following subcutaneous or intramuscular injection. Distribution half-life is 40 minutes and the terminal half-life is ~4–5 hours; however, biologic half-life is extended (24 hours). Penetration into the cerebrospinal fluid, brain, and eye is poor (Cantell and Pyhala 1976).

Interferon therapy has shown efficacy in many human clinical situations, including viral infections caused by influenza virus, rhinovirus, herpesvirus, and papilloma virus. Treatment of FeLV with interferon has had mixed results. Although shown to inhibit replication in vitro (Jameson and Essex 1983), this did not carry over to in vivo (Beck 1985). When given at the same time as experimental FeLV virus challenge, interferon-α ameliorated the clinical course and improved survival rates, although it did not affect viremia (Cummins et al. 1989). In contrast to these results, interferon had no protective effect against FeLV challenge unless given in combination with AZT (Zeidner et al. 1989). Bovine interferon-α_1 was able to inhibit replication of the transmissible gastroenteritis virus in vitro but, due to GI instability, was unable to prevent infection in vivo (MacLachlan and Anderson 1986). Human leukocyte interferon-α has been used for prophylactic treatment of bovine herpesvirus type I–associated shipping fever (Baker 1990).

OTHER COMPOUNDS. As previously mentioned, the research and development of antiviral compounds is occurring at an unprecedented pace. Many compounds that, at the time of printing, are only experimental may become available for clinical use.

2′-3′-dideoxyinosine (ddI) and 2′-3′-dideoxycytidine (ddC) are nucleoside analogs under development for the treatment of AIDS. Incorporation of the triphosphate form of these molecules is thought to result in termination of chain elongation and interruption of DNA synthesis. The ability of these compounds to interfere with FeLV infection in vitro and in vivo has been studied (Tavares et al. 1989). The intravenous pharmacokinetics of ddI were found to be nonlinear in the dog (Kaul et al. 1991).

The acyclic purine nucleoside analog 9-2(phosphonomethoxyethyl)adenine (PMEA) has been studied in the treatment of both FeLV and FIV infections in cats. PMEA was found to inhibit replication of FeLV in vitro and prevented the development of persistent antiginemia and the induction of the immunodeficiency disease in cats exposed to the virus (Hoover et al. 1991). PMEA exhibited similar effects against FIV infection. Seropositive cats with symptoms of opportunistic infection showed improvement of clinical signs during PMEA therapy at 5 mg/kg/day (Egberink et al. 1990).

Ribozymes have recently been added to the antiviral armamentarium. Ribozymes are small, single-stranded catalytic RNAs which are capable of destroying specific RNA target sequences. These antisense molecules have the ability to interfere with the virus at an early step in its replicative cycle and have adequate specificity such that host metabolic processes may be spared (Sarver 1991). Aspects of ribozymes currently under investigation include target accessibility, stability, methods for delivery, and intracellular localization (Rossi et al. 1991).

Dextran sulfate is a glucose homopolymer with a molecular weight of 7000–8000 and contains 17–20% sulfur in the form of sulfate. It has been shown to inhibit replication of the HIV virus and other retroviruses in vitro, including the FIV (Tanabe-Tochikura et al. 1992) and the FeLV virus. Dextran sulfate was unable to prevent FeLV infection and development of persistent viremia in challenged cats at a dosage that did not cause toxicity. Toxicity of dextran sulfate at 24 mg/kg/day was seen as GI ulceration, anemia, and death (Mathes et al. 1991).

TABLE 46.2—Antiviral drugs of potential veterinary importance (in most cases doses are experimental, necessitating further clinical study)

Drug	Preparation	Brand (manufacturer)	Route	Dosage	Interval (hr)
Idoxuridine	0.1% ophthalmic solution	Herplex Liquifilm (Allergen); Stoxil (SKF)	Ocular, topical	1 drop	5–6
	0.5% ophthalmic ointment	Stoxil (SKF)	Ocular, topical	Ointment	1–2
Trifluridine	1% ophthalmic solution	Viroptic (Burroughs Wellcome)	Topical	1 drop	2
			IV	1.5, 2.9 mg (humans)	4–8, 4
Vidarabine	3% ophthalmic ointment	Vira-A (Parke-Davis)	Ocular, topical	1 cm ointment	5–6
	200 mg/mL suspension for injection		IV	10–30 mg/kg	24 as a continuous drip for 12–24 hr
Ribavirin	6 g/100 mL vial powder	Virazole (ICN Pharmaceuticals)	Inhalation	Using SPAG-2 nebulizer only	8–18 hr period daily
Acyclovir	5% cutaneous ointment	Zovirax (Burroughs Wellcome)	Topical	Cover lesion adequately	3 hr, 6 times/day
	200 mg capsules or tablets		PO	200 mg (humans)	4 hr, 5 times/day
	200 mg/5 mL suspension				
	500 mg/vial powder		IV	250–500 mg/m^2	8 (infused over at least 1 hr)
	1 g/vial powder			5–10 mg/kg (humans)	8
Ganciclovir	500 mg/vial powder	Cytovene (Syntex)	IV	2–5 (humans)	8–12
Zidovudine	100 mg capsules	Retrovir (Burroughs Wellcome)	PO	100–200 mg (humans)	4
				10–20 mg/kg	
	Syrup 10 mg/mL		PO	200 mg (humans)	4
	10 mg/mL single-use vial		IV	1–2 mg/kg	Infused over 1 hr
Foscarnet			IV	60 mg/kg	8 (CMV initiation therapy)
				90–120 mg/kg	24 (CMV maintenance therapy)
				40 mg/kg	8 (for HSV and VZV infections)
Amantadine	100, 500 mg capsules	Symmetrel (Dupont)	PO	100 mg total (humans)	12–24
	Syrup 10 mg/mL		PO	100 mg total (juveniles)	24
Rimantadine		Flumadine	PO	200–300 mg total (humans)	24
				100–200 mg total (juveniles)	24
Interferon-α_{2a}	3×10^6 IU/vial	Roferon-A (Roche)	SC, IM	3×10^6 IU (humans)	24
Interferon-α_{2b}	3×10^6 IU/vial	Intron A (Schering)	SC, IM	3×10^6 IU (humans)	24

Other potential antiviral agents include glycoprotein-processing inhibitors (Elbein 1991), viral protease inhibitors (Kleina and Grubman 1992), and even neurotransmitter antagonists (Tsiang et al. 1991). The future use of these and other compounds remains to be seen. Table 46.2 lists potentially useful antiviral agents in veterinary medicine. In most cases, doses are experimental and require further clinical trials to verify.

REFERENCES

Abdel-Halim, M., Youssef, H.M., Ramadan, A.A., and Refai, M. Dermatophytosis in Egyptian sheep and goats. 1988. Vet Med J-Giza 36(2)199-206.

AHFS Drug Information. Fluconazole. In McEvoy, G.K. (ed). American Society of Hospital Pharmacists pub. Bethesda, MD. 1992:72-78.

Arndt, C.A., Walsh, T.J., McCullly, C.L., Balis, F.M., Pizzo, P.A., and Poplack, D.G. Fluconazole penetration into cerebrospinal fluid: implications for treating fungal infections of the central nervous system. 1988. J Infect Dis 157(1):8-9.

Atkinson, A.J., and Bennett, J.E. Amphotericin B pharmacokinetics in humans. 1978. Antimicrob Agents Chemother 13:271-276.

Ausherman, R.J. Treatment of blastomycosis and histoplasmosis in the dog. 1973. J Am Vet Med Assoc 163(9):1048-1049.

Baker, J.C. Viral respiratory diseases. In Smith B.P. (Ed.) Large Animal Internal Medicine. St. Louis, MO, C.V. Mosby Co., 1990. p. 576.

Balfour, J.A., and Faulds, D. Terbinafine: a review of its pharmacodynamic and pharmacokinetic properties and therapeutic potential in superficial mycoses. 1992. Drugs 43:258-284.

Baloch, R.I., and Mercer, E.I. Inhibition of sterol ^{8}- ^{7}-isomerase and ^{14}-reductase by fenpropimorph, tridemorph and fenprpidin in cell-free enzyme systems from *Saccharomyces cerevisiae.* 1987. Phytochem 26:663-668.

Barlough, J.E. and Scott, F.W. Effectiveness of three antiviral agents against FIP virus in vitro. 1989. Vet Rec 126:556-558.

Beck, E.R. Clinical and experimental interferon therapy in the cat. 1985. Proc Vet Cancer Soc 21.

Bennett, J.E. Amphotericin B binding to serum β-lipoprotein. 1977. In Iwala K (ed) Recent advances in medical and veterinary mycology. Proc 6th ISHAM University Park Press, Baltimore, USA, pp. 107-109.

———. Antimicrobial agents: antifungal agents. In The Pharmacological Basis of Therapeutics. Gilman, A.G., Rall, T.W., Nies, A.S. and Taylor, P. (Eds) Pergamon Press, New York, 1990; pp. 1165-1181.

Bennet, J.E., Dismukes, W.E., Duma, R.F., Medoff, G., Sande, M.A., Gallis, H., Leonard, J., Fields, B.T., Bradshaw, M., Haywood, H., McGee, Z.A., Cate, T.R., Cobbs, C.G., Warner, J.F., and Alling, D.W. A comparison of amphotericin B alone and combined with flucytosine in the treatment of cryptococcal meningitis. 1979. N Engl J Med 301:126-131.

Berger, J., and Duschinsky, R. Control of fungi with 5-fluorocytosine. 1962. US Pat Appl Ser No 181, p 822.

Betts, R.F. Antiviral agents in respiratory infections. 1991 Sem Resp Infect 6(3):146-157.

Brajtburg, J., Powderly, W.G., Kobayashi, G.S., and Medoff, G. Amphotericin B: current understanding of mechanisms of action. 1990. Antimicrob Agents Chemother 34:183-188.

Brammer, K.W., Farrow, P.R., and Faulkner, J.K. Pharmacokinetics and tissue penetration of fluconazole in humans. 1990. Rev Infect Dis 12(S3):318-326.

Brooks, D.E., Legendre, A.M., Gum, G.G., Laratta, L.J., Abrams, K.L., and Morgan, R.V. The treatment of canine ocular blastomycosis with systemically administered itraconazole. 1992 Prog Vet Comp Ophth 4:263-268.

Bruyette, D.S., and Feldman, E.C. Ketoconazole and its use in the management of canine Cushing's disease. 1988. Compen Contin Educ Prac Vet 10(12):1379-1386.

Butler, W.T., and Hill, G.J. Intravenous administration of amphotericin B in the dog. J Am Vet Med Assoc 1964. 144:399-402.

Cacciapuoti, A., Loebenberg, D., Parmegiani, R., Antonacci, B., Norris, C., Moss, Jr., E.L., Menzel, Jr., F., Tarosh-Tomaine, T., Hare, R.S., and Miller, G.H. Comparison of SCH 39304, fluconazole, and ketoconazole for treatment of systemic infections in mice. 1992. Antimicrob Agents Chemother 36(1):64-67.

Canonico, P.G. Efficacy, toxicity and clinical application of ribavirin against virulent RNA viral infections. 1985 Antiviral Res (suppl 1):75-81.

Cantanzaro, A., Fierer, J., and Fieldman, P.J. Fluconazole in the treatment of persistent coccidioidomycosis. 1990. Chest 97:666-669.

Cantell, K. and Pyhala, L. Pharmacokinetics of human leukocyte interferon. 1976. J Infect Dis 133(Suppl):A6-A12.

Cauwenbergh, G. and DeDoncker, P. The clinical use of itraconazole in superficial and deep mycoses. In Fromtling RA (ed). Recent trends in the discovery, development and evaluation of antifungal agents. JR Prous Publishers, Barcelona 1987;273-284.

Cauwenbergh, G., Doncker, P.D., Stoops, K., DeDier, A.M., Goyvaerts, H. and Schuermans, V. Itraconazole in the treatment of human mycoses:Review of three years of clinical experience. 1987. Rev Infect Dis 9(S1):146-152.

Corey, L., and Holmes, K.K. Genital herpes simplex virus infections: current concepts in diagnosis, therapy, and prevention. 1983. Ann Intern Med 93:914-923.

Cotter, S.M. Feline leukemia virus: pathophysiology, prevention, and treatment. 1992. Cancer Invest 10(2):173-181.

Couch, R.B., and Six, H.R. The antiviral spectrum and mechanism of action of amantadine and rimantadine. In Antiviral Chemotherapy: New Directions for Clinical Applications and Research. (Mills, J., and Corey, L., eds) Elsevier, New York, 1986. pp.50-57.

Craig, A., Malik, R., and Ramzan, I. Pharmacokinetics of fluconazole in the cat. 1993. J Am Col Vet Int Med 7(2):137.

Craven, P.C., Ludden, T.M., Drutz, D.J., Rogers, W., Haegele, K.A., and Skrdlant, H.B. Excretion pathways of amphotericin B. 1979. J Infect Dis 140:329-341.

Crumpacker, C.S., Molecular targets of antiviral therapy. 1989. N Engl J Med 321:163-172.

Cummins, J.M., Tompkins, M.B., Olsen, R.G., Tompkins, W.A., and Lewis, M.G. The oral use of human interferons in cats. 1988 J Biol Response Mod 7:513-523.

Dallman, M.J., Dew, T.L., Tobias, L., and Doss, R. Disseminated aspergillosis in a dog with diskospondylitis and neurologic deficits. 1992. J Am Vet Med Assoc 200(4):511-514.

Daneshmend, T.K., and Warnock, D.W. Clinical Pharmacokinetics of Ketoconzole. 1988. Clin Pharmacokin 14:13-34.

Davey, P.G. New antiviral and antifungal drugs. 1990. Br Med J 300:793-798.

de Costa, P.D., Merideth, R.E., and Sigler, R.L. Cataracts in dogs after long-term ketoconazole therapy. 1996. Vet Comp Ophthalmol 6:176-180.

DeCoster, R., Beerens, D., Haelterman, C., and Doolaege, R. Effects of itraconazole on the pituitary-testicular-adrenal axis: an overview of preclinical and clinical studies In Fromtling RA (ed). Recent trends in the discovery, development and evaluation of antifungal agents. JR Prous Publishers, Barcelona 1987;251-261.

deJaham, C. Toxicity study of enilconazole emulsion in the treatment of dermatophyosis in Persian cats. 1996. St. Hyacinthe, Quebec, Dermatology Meeting Proceedings.

deJaham, C., Paradis, M., and Papich, M.G. Antifungal therapy in small animal dermatology. 2000 (in press). Comp on Cont Educ Pract Vet.

Dick, J.D., Merz, W.G., and Saral, R. Incidence of polyene-resistant yeasts recovered from clinical specimens. 1980. Anitmicrob Agents Chemother 18:158-163.

Douglas Jr. R.G. Antimicrobial agents: antiviral agents In The Pharmacological Basis of Therapeutics. Gilman, A.G., Rall, T.W., Nies, A.S. and Taylor, P. (Eds) Pergamon Press, New York, 1990;1182-1201.

Drouhet, E., and Dupont, B. Evolution of antifungal agents: past, present and future. 1987. Rev Infect Dis 9(Suppl1):4-13.

Drusano, G.L. Role of pharmacokinetics in the outcome of infections. 1988. Antimicrob Agents Chemother 32:289-297.

Dudley, M.N. Clinical pharmacology of fluconazole. 1990. Pharmacotherapy 6(S10):141-145.

Dupont, B., and Drouhet, E. in vitro synergy and antagonism of antifungal agents against yeast-like fungi. 1979. Postgrad Med J 55:683-686.

Duschinsky, R., Pleven, E., Heidelberger. C. The synthesis of 5-fluoropyrimidines. 1957. J Am Chem Soc 79:4559-4560.

Egberink, H., Borst, M., Niphuis, H., Balzarini, J., Neu, H., Schellekens, H., DeClerq, E., Horzinek, M., and Koolen, M. Suppression of feline immunodeficiency virus infection in vitro by 9-2(phosphonomethoxyethy)ladenine. 1990. Proc Natl Acad Sci USA 87(8):3087-3091.

Egberink, H.F., Hartman, D., and Horzinek, M.C. Chemotherapy of feline immunodeficiency virus infection. 1991. J Am Vet Med Assoc 199(10):1485-1487.

Elbein, A.D. Glycosidase inhibitors as antivial and/or antitumor agents. 1991. Sem Cell Bio 2(5):309-317.

Ellis, W.G., Sobel, R.A., and Nielsen, S.L. Leukoencephalopathy in patients treated with amphotericin B methyl ester. 1982. J Infect Dis 146:125-137.

Espinel-Ingroff, A., and Shadomy, S. In vitro and in vivo evaluation of antifungal agents. 1989. Eur J Clin Microbiol Infect Dis 84352-361.

Feldman, E.C., Bruyette, D.S., Nelson, R.W., and Farver, T.B. Plasma cortisol response to ketoconazole administration in dogs with hyperadrenocorticism. 1990. J Am Vet Med Assoc 197(1):71-78.

Feldman, H.A., Hamilton, J.D., and Gutman, R.A. Amphotericin B therapy in an anephric patient. 1973. Antimicrob Agents Chemother 4:402-405.

Foil, C.S. Dermatophytosis In Infectious diseases of the dog and cat. Greene, C.E. (Ed.) 1990. W.B. Sauders Co. Phila, PA.

Forbes, N.A., Simpson, G.N., and Goudswaard, M.F. Diagnosis of avian aspergillosis and treatment with itraconazole. 1992. Vet Rec 130(23):519-520.

Foulds, G., Brennan, D.R., Wajszczuk, C., Catanzaro, A., Garg, D.C., Knopf, W., Rinaldi, M., and Weidler, D.J. Fluconazole penetration into cerebrospinal fluid in humans. 1988 J Clin Pharmacol 28:363-366.

Franklin, C.L., Gibson, S.V., Caffrey, C.J., Wagner, J.E., and Steffen, E.K. Treatment of *Trichophyton mentagrophytes* infection in rabbits. 1991. J Am Vet Med Assoc 198(9):1625-1630.

Galgiani, J. Antifungal susceptibility tests. 1987. Antimicrob Agents Chemother 31:1867-1870.

Galgiani, J.N. Susceptibility of Candida albicans and other yeasts to fluconazole: relation between in vitro and in vivo studies. 1990. Rev Infect Dis 12(S3):272-275.

Gerkins, J.F., Heidemann, H.T., Jackson, E.K., and Branch, R.A. Effect of aminophylline on amphotericin B nephrotoxicity in the dog. 1983. J Pharmacol Exp Ther 224(3):609-613.

Gold, W., Stout, H.A., Pagano, J.F., and Donovick, R. Amphotericins A and B, antifungal antibiotics produced by a streptomycete. I. in vitro studies. 1956. In Welch, H., Marti-Ibanez, F. (eds) Antibiotics Annual 1955-1956. Medical Encyclopedia Inc., New York, pp 579-586.

Graybill, J.R. Fluconazole efficacy in animal models of mycotic diseases. In Fromtling RA (ed). Recent trends in the discovery, development and evaluation of antifungal agents. JR Prous Publishers, Barcelona 1987;113-124.

———. Systemic azole antifungal drugs-into the 1990s. In Ryley JF (ed). Handbook of Experimental Pharmacology: Chemotherapy of Fungal Diseases. Springer-Verlag, Berlin 1990;96:455-482.

———. Future directions of antifungal chemotherapy. 1992. Clin Infect Dis 14(S1):170-179.

Graybill, J.R., Craven, P.C., Taylor, R.L. Williams, D.M., and Magee, W.E. Treatment of murine cryptococcosis with liposome-associated amphotericin B. 1982. J Infect Dis 146:748-752.

Graybill, J.R., Griffith, L., and Sun, S.H. Fluconazole therapy for coccidioidomycosis in Japanes Macaques. 1990. Rev Infect Dis 12(suppl3):286-290.

Greene, C.E. Antifungal chemotherapy. In Infectious diseases of the dog and cat. Greene, C.E. (Ed.) 1990. W.B. Saunders, Philadelphia

Gregoriadis, G. Overview of liposomes. 1991. J Antimicrob Chemother 28(Suppl B):39-48.

Gruffydd-Jones, T.J., and Wright, A.I. Deformed kittens [letter]. 1977. Vet Rec 100:206.

Hall, C.B., McBride, J.T., Walsh, E.E., Bell, D.M., Gala, C., Hildreth, S. TenEyck, L.G., and Hall, W.J. Aerosolized ribavirin treatment of infants with respiratory syncytial viral infection. 1983. N Engl J Med 308:1443-1447.

Harris, P.A., and Riegelman S. Metabolism of griseofulvin in dogs. 1969. J Pharm Sci 58:93-96.

Hauser, W.E. and Remington, J.S. The effect of antibiotics on the humoral and cell-mediated immune responses. 1982 Action of Antibiotics in Patients (Sabath, L.D., Ed) pp 127-147 Huber, Bern.

Hayden, F.G., Minocha, A., Spyker, D.A., and Hoffman, H.E. Comparative single-dose pharmacokinetics of amantadine hydrochloride and rimantadine hydrochoride in young and elderly adults. 1985. Antimicrob Agent Chemother 28:216-221.

Helton K.A., Nesbitt, G.H., and Caciolo, P.L. Griseofulvin toxicity in cats: literature review and report of seven cases. 1986. J Am Anim Hosp Assoc 22:453-458.

Heykants, J., Michiels, M., Meuldermans, W., Monbaliu, J., Lavrijsen, K., VanPeer, A., Levron, J.C., Woestenborghs, R., and Cauwenbergh, G. In Fromtling RA (ed). The pharmacokinetics of itraconazole in animals and man: an overview. Recent trends in the discovery, development and evaluation of antifungal agents. JR Prous Publishers, Barcelona 1987.

Heykants, J., Peer, A.V., Lavrijsen, K., Meuldermans, W., Woestenborghs, R., and Cauwenbergh, G. Pharmacokinetics of oral antifungals and their clinical implications. 1990. Br J Clin Pract Sump Suppl 71:50-56.

Hiddleston, W.A. The use of Griseofulvin Mycelium in equine animals [letter]. 1970. Vet Rec 87:119.

———. The treatment of bovine ringworm. 1973. Vet Rec 92:123.

Hiemenz, J.W., and Walsh, T.J. Lipid formulations of amphotericin B: recent progress and future directions. 1996. Clin Infect Dis 22(suppl 2):S133-S144.

Hill, P.B., Moriello, K.A., and Shaw, S.E. A review of systemic antifungal agents. 1995. Vet Derm 6:59-66.

Hirsh, M.S., and Schooley, R.T. Resistance to antiviral drugs: the end of innocence. 1989. N Engl J Med 320:313-314.

Hoffmann, C.E., Neumayer, E.M., Haff, R.F., and Goldsby, R.A. Mode of action of the antiviral activity of amantadine in tissue culture. 1965. J Bacteriol 90:623-628.

Hofmann, H., Brautigam, M., Weidinger, G., et al. Treatment of toenail onychomycosis: a randomized, double-blind study with terbinafine and griseofulvin. 1995. Arch Dermatol 131:919-922.

Hoover, E.A., Ebner, J.P., Zeidner, N.S. and Mullins, J.I. Early therapy of feline leukemia virus infection (FeLV-FAIDS) with 9-2(phosphonylmethoxyethyl)-adenine (PMEA). 1991. Antiviral Res 16(1):77-92.

Horn, R., Wong, B. Kiehn, T.E., and Armstrong, D. Fungemia in a cancer hospital: changing frequency, earlier onset, and results of therapy. 1985. Rev Infect Dis 7:646-655.

Horowitz, J.P., Chua, J., and Noel, M. Nucleosides 5. The monomesylates of 1-2′-deoxy-β-D-lyxofuranosyl thymine. 1964. J Org Chem 29:2076-2080.

Hostetler, J.S., Clemons, K.V., Hanson, L.G., and Stevens, D.A. Efficacy and safety of amphotericin B colloidal dispersion compared with those of amphotericin B deoxycholate suspension for treatment of disseminated murine cryptococcosis. 1992. Antimicrob Agents Chemother 36(12):2656-2660.

Hume, A.L., and Kerkering, T.M. Ketoconazole 1983. Drug Intell Clin Pharm 17:169-174.

Humphrey, M.J., Jevons, S., and Tarbit, M.H. Pharmacokinetic evaluation of UK-49858, a metabolically stable trazole antifungal drug, in animals and humans. 1985. Antimicrob Agents Chemother 28(5):648-653.

Huraux, J.M., Ingrand, D., and Agut, G. Perpectives in antiviral chemotherpay. 1990. Fund Clin Pharm 4(4):357-372.

Hussain, A.S., and Ritschel, W.A. "Body burden" of phophonoformic acid after topical and vaginal administration to rabbits and beagle dogs. 1989. Meth Find Exp Clin Pharm 11(2):111-114.

Jackson, J.A. Immunodiagnosis of systemic mycoses in animals: A review. 1986. J Am Vet Med Assoc 188(7):702-705.

Jacobson, M.A., Vanderhorst, C., Causey, D.M., et al. In vivo additive antiretroviral effect of combined zidovudine and foscarnet therapy for humane immunodeficiency virus infection (ACTG Protocol 053). 1991. J Infect Dis 163:1219-1222.

Jameson, P., and Essex, M. Inhibition of FeLV replication by human leukocyte interferon. 1983. Antiviral Res 3:115-120.

Janssen, P.A.J., and Symoens, J.E. Hepatic reactions during ketoconazole treatement. 1983. Am J Med 74(S1B):80-85.

Jones, T.C. Overview of the use of terbinafine (Lamisil) in children. 1995 Br J Derm 132:683-689.

Kaul, S., Knupp, D.A., Dandekar, K.A., and Barbhaiya, R.H. Pharmacokinetics of 2′3′dideoxyinosine (BMY-40900), a new anti-human immunodeficiency virus agent, after administration of single intravenous doses to beagle dogs. 1991. Antimicrob Agent Chemother 35(4):610-614.

Kettlewell, P., McGinnis, M.R., and Wilkinson, G.T. Phaeohyphomycosis caused by *Exophiala spinifera* in two cats. 1989. J Med Vet Mycol 27(4):257-264.

Kielstein, P. and Gottschalk, C. *Trichophyton metagrophytes* infection in a breeding-swine herd. 1970. Mh VetMed 25:127-130.

Kleina, L.G., and Grubman, M.J. Antiviral effects of a thiol protease inhibitor on foot-and-mouth disease virus. 1992. J Virol 66(12):7168-7175.

Kobayashi, G.S., Travis, S.F., Medoff, G. Comparison of the in vitro and in vivo activity of the bis-triazole derivative UK 49,858 with that of Amphotericin B against *Histoplasma capsulatum.* 1986. Antimicrob Agents Chemother 29:660-662.

Kowalsky, S.F., and Dixon, D.M. Fluconazole:A new antifungal agent. 1991. Clin Pharmacy 10:9-194.

Krawiec, D.R., McKiernan, B.C., Twardock, A.R., et al. Use of an amphotericin B lipid complex for treatment of blastomycosis in dogs. 1996. J Am Vet Med Assoc 209:2073-2075.

Kunkle, G.A., and Meyer, D.F. Toxicity of high doses of griseofulvin in cats. 1987. J Am Vet Med Assoc 191(3):322-323.

Lambrechts, N., Collett, M.G., and Henton, M. Black grain eumycetoma (*Madurella mycetomatis*) in the abdominal cavity of a dog. 1991. J Med Vet Mycol 29:211-214.

Legendre, A.M. Antimycotic drug therapy. In Bonagura, J.D. (ed.), Current Veterinary Therapy XII. 1995, pp. 327-331. Philadelphia: W.B. Saunders.

Legendre, A.M., Gompf, R., and Bone, D. Treatment of feline cryptococcosis with ketoconazole. 1982. J Am Vet Med Assoc 181:1541-1542.

Legendre, A.M., Rohrbach, B.W., Toal, R.L., et al. Treatment of blastomycosis with itraconazole in 112 dogs. 1996. J Vet Int Med 10:365-371.

Legendre, A.M., Selcer, B.A., Edwards, D.F., and Stevens, R. Treatment of canine blastomycosis with amphotericin B and ketoconazole. 1984. J Am Vet Med Assoc 184(10):1249-1254.

Lenarduzzi, R.F., and Varns, G.M. Adverse reactions of cats treated with griseofulvin, fenthion, and praziquantel. 1986. Mod Vet Prac 67(2):153.

Levitz S.M. Overview of host defenses in fungal infections. 1992. Clin Infect Dis 14(S1):37-42.

Levy, J.K. Ataxia in a kitten treated with griseofulvin. 1991. 198(1):105.

Lietman, P.S. Clinical pharmacology: foscarnet. 1992. Am J Med 92(2A):8S-11S.

MacGregor, R.R., Bennett, J.E. and Ersley, A.J. Erythropoietin concentration in amphotericin B-induced anemia. 1978. Antimicrob Agents Chemother 14:270-273.

MacLachlan, N.J., and Anderson, K.P. Effect of recombinant DNA-derived bovine α-1 interferon on transmissible gastroenteritis virus infection in swine. 1986. Am J Vet Res 47(5):1149-1152.

Malik, R., Craig, A.J., Wigney, D.I., Martin, P., and Love, D.N. Combination chemotherapy of canine and feline cryptococcosis using subcutaneously administered amphotericin B. 1996. Aust Vet J 73:124-128.

Mancianti, F., Pedonese, F., and Zullino, C. Efficacy of oral administration of itraconazole to cats with dermatophytosis caused by *Microsporum canis.* 1998. J Am Vet Med Assoc 213:993-995.

Marriot, M.S., Richardson, K. The discovery and mode of action of fluconazole. In Fromtling RA (ed). Recent trends in the discovery, development and evaluation of antifungal agents. JR Prous Publishers, Barcelona 1987;157-161.

Martin, C.L. Ocular infections. In Infectious diseases of the dog and cat. Greene, C.E. (Ed.) 1990. W.B. Saunders, Philadelphia.

Marx, M.B., Eastin, C.E., Turner, C., Smith, C.D., Roeckell, I., and Furcolow, M.L. The influence of amphotericin B upon *Histoplasma* infection. 1970 Arch Environ Health 21(5):649-655.

Mathes, L.E., Hayes, K.A., Swenson, C.L., Posas, P.J., Weisbrode, S.E., and Koeiba, G.J. Evaluatio of antiviral activity and toxicity of dextran sulfate in feline leukemia virus-infected cats. 1991. Antimicrob Agent Chemother 35(10):2147-2150.

Mayer, V.H. Therapy of dermatomycoses in the horse. 1983. Berl Munch Tierarztl Wochenschr 96(12):458-459.

McKellart, Q., Fishwick, G., and Rycroft, A. Ringworm in housed sheep. 1987. Vet Rec 121(8):168-169.

Mechlinsk, W., Schaffner, C.P., Ganis, P. and Avitabile, G. Structure and absolute configuration of the polyene macrolide amphotericin B. 1970. Tetrahedron Letters 44:3873-3876.

Medleau, L. Recently described feline dermatoses. 1990. Vet Clinic North Am: Sm Anim Prac 20(6):1615-1632.

Medleau, L., and Chalmers, S.A. Ketoconazole for treatment of dermatophytosis in cats. 1992. J Am Vet Med Assoc 200(1):77-78.

Medleau, L., and White-Weithers, N.E. Dermatophytosis in cats. 1991. Compen Contin Educ Pract Vet 13(4):557-562.

Medleau, L., Greene, C.E., and Rakich, P.M. Evaluation of ketoconazole and itraconazole for treatment of disseminated cryptococcosis in cats. 1990. Am J Vet Res 51(9):1454-1458.

Medleau, L., Hall, E.J., Goldschmidt, M.H., Irby, N. Cutaneous cryptococcosis in three cats. 1985 J Am Vet Med Assoc 187:169-170.

Medoff, G., Comfort, M., and Kobayashi, G.S. Synergistic action of amphotericin B and 5-fluorocytosin against yeast-like organisms. 1971. Proc Soc Exp Bio Med 138:571-574.

Medoff, G., Kobayashi, G.S., Kwan, C.N., Schlessinger, D., and Venkov, P. Potentiation of rifampicin and 5-fluorocytosine as antifungal antibiotics by amphotericin B. 1972. Proc Nat Acad Sci USA 69:196-199.

Mieth, H., and Petranyi, G. Preclinical evaluation of terbinafine in vivo. 1989. Clin Exp Dermatol 14:104-107.

Minor, J.R., and Baltz, J.K. Foscarnet sodium. 1991. DICP 25(1):41-47.

Mitsuya, H., Weinhold, K.J., Furman, P.A., St. Clair, M.H., Lehrman, S.N., Gallo, R.C., Bofognesi, D., Barry, D.W., and Broder, S. 3′-Axido-3′-deoxythmidine (BW A509U): an antiviral agent that inhibits the infectivity and cytopathic effect of human T-lymphotrophic virus type III/lymphadenopathy-associated virus in vitro. 1985. Proc Natl Acad Sci USA 82:7096-7100.

Moriello, K.A. Ketoconazole: clinical pharmacology and therapeutic recommendations. 1986. J Am Vet Med Assoc 188(3):303-306.

Moriello, K.A., and DeBoer, D.J. Efficacy of griseofulvin and itraconazole in the treatment of experimentally induced dermatophytosis in cats. 1995. JAVMA 207:439-444.

Mundell, A.C. New therapeutic agents in veterinary dermatology. 1990. Vet Clinic North Am: Sm Anim Prac 20(6):1541-1556.

North, T.W., North, G.L.T., and Pedersen, N.C. Feline immunodeficiency virus, a model for reverse tyreanscriptase-targeted chemotherapy for acquired immune deficiency syndrome. 1989. Antimicrob Agent Chemother 33(6):915-919.

Norton, T.M., Gaskin, J., Kollias, G.V., Homer, B., Clark, C.H., and Wilson, R. Efficacy of acyclovir against herpesvirus infection in Quaker parakeets. 1991. Am J Vet Res 52(12):2007-2009.

Noxon, J.O., Monroe, W.E., and Chinn, D.R. Ketoconazole therapy in canine and feline cryptococcosis. 1986. J Am Anim Hosp Assoc 22:179-183.

Oberg, B. Antiviral effects of phosphonoformate (PFA, Foscarnet sodium). 1989. Pharmacol Ther 2:213-285.

Obrosova-Serova, N.P., Kupryasjina, L.M., Isachenko, V.A., Vorontsova, R.M., and Utkin, V.G. Experience with prevention of chicken influenza with amantadine. 1976. Veterinariia 11:62-63.

O'Day, D.M., Ray W. A., Robinson, R.Dl, Head, W.S. and Savage, A. The influence of yeast growth phase in vivo on the efficacy of topical polyenes. 1987. Curr Eye Res 6:363-368.

Oliva, G., Gradoni, L., Ciaramella, P., et al. Activity of liposomal amphotericin B (AmBisome) in dogs naturally infected with *Leishmania infantum.* 1995. J Antimicrob Chemother 36:1013-1019.

Onderka, D.K. and Doornenbal, E.C. Mycotic dermatitis in ostriches. 1992. Can Vet J 33:547-548.

Palestine, A.G., Polis, M.A., DeSmet, M.D., Baird, B.F., Falloon, J., Kovacs, J.A., Davey, R.T., Zurlo, J.J., Zunich, K.M., Davis, M., et al. A randomized controlled trial of foscarnet in the treatment of cytomegalovirus retinitis in patients with AIDS. 1991. Ann Intern Med 115:665-673.

Pappagianis, D., Zimmer, B.L., Theodoropoulos, G., Plempel, M., and Hector, R.F. Therapeutic effect of the triazole Bay R 3783 in mouse models of coccidioidomycosis, blastomycosis, and histoplasmosis. 1990. Antimicrob Agents Chemother 34(6):1132-1138.

Patterson, T.F., George, D. Miniter, P. and Andriole, V.T. Saperconazole terapy in a rabbit model of invasive aspergillosis. 1992. Antimicrob Agents Chemother 36(12):2681-2685.

Pentlarge, V.W., and Martin, R.A. Treatment of cryptococcosis in three cats, using ketoconazole. 1986. J Am Vet Med Assoc 188(5):536-538.

Perfect, J.R., Savani, D.V., and Durack, D.T. Comparison of itraconazole and fluconazole in treatment of cryptococcal meningitis and candida pyelonephritis in rabbits. 1986. Antimicrob Agents Chemother 29(4):579-583.

Pestka, S., Langer, J.A., Zoon, K.C., and Samuel, S.A. Interferons and their actions. 1987. Ann Rev Biochem 56:727-777.

Pierce A.M., Pierce, H.D., Unrau, A.M. and Oehlschlger, A.C. Lipid composition and polyene antibiotic resistance of *Candida albicans* mutants. 1978. Can J Biochem 56:135-142.

Plotnick, A.N. Lipid-based formulations of amphotericin B. 2000. J Am Vet Med Assoc 216:838-841.

Polak, A. Mode of Action Studies. In Ryley JF (ed). Handbook of Experimental Pharmacology: Chemotherapy of Fungal Diseases. Springer-Verlag, Berlin 1990;96:153-182.

Polak, A., Scholer, H.J., and Wall, M. Combination therapy of experimental candidiasis, cryptococcosis and aspergillosis in mice. 1982 Chemotherapy 28:461-479.

Povey, R.C. Effect of orally administered ribavirin on experimental feline calicivirus infection in cats. 1978. 39:1337-1341.

Powderly, W.G., Kobayashi, G.S., Herzig, G.P. and Medoff, G. Amphotericin B-resistant yeast infection in severely immunocomprimised patients. 1988. Am J Med 84:826-832.

Prades, M., Brown, M.P., Gronwall, R., and Houston, A.E. Body fluid and endometrial concentrations of ketoconazole in mares after intravenous injection or repeated gavage. 1989. Equine Vet J 21:211-214.

Puccini, S., Valdre, A., Papini, R., and Mancianti, F. in vitro susceptibility to antimycotics of *Microsporum canis* isolates from cats. 1992. J Am Vet Med Assoc 201(9):1375-1377.

Pukay, B.P. and Dion, W.M. Feline phaeohyphomycosis: treatment with ketoconazole and 5-fluorocytosine. 1984. Can Vet J 25:130-134.

Reimer, K., Matthes, E., Scholz, D., and Rosenthal, H.A. Effects of suramin, HPA-23 and 3′-azidothymidine triphosphate on the reverse transcriptase of bovine leukaemia virus. 1989 Acta Virologica 33(1):43-49.

Reuss, U. Management of trichophytosis in horses. 1978a. DTW 85:231.

———. Treatment of cattle trichophytosis with griseofulvin. 1978b. Tieraerztl Umschau 33:85-90.

Richardson, K., Cooper, K., Marriott, M.S., Tarbit, M.H., Troke, P.F., and Whittle P.J. Discovery of fluconazole, a novel antifungal agent. 1990. Rev Infect Dis 12(S3):267-271.

Richman, D.D. The toxicity of azidothymidine (AZT) in the treatment of patients with AIDS and AIDS-related complex. 1987. N Engl J Med 317:192-197.

Ringden, O., Meunier, F., Tollemar, J., Ricci, P., Tura, S., Kuse, E., Viviani, M.A., Gorin, N.C., Klastersky, J., Fenaux, P., Prentice, H.G., and Ksionski, G. Efficacy of amphotericin B encapsulated in liposomes (AmBisome) in the treatment of invasive fungal infections in immunocompromised patients. 1991. J Antimicrob Chemother 28(Suppl B):73-82.

Ringel, S.M. New antifungal agents for the systemic mycoses. 1990. Mycopathologia 109:75-87.

Rodriguez. W.J., Kim, H.W., Brandt, C.D., Fink, R.J., Getson, P.R., Arrobio, J., Murphy, T.M., McCarthy, V., and Parott, R.H. Aerosolized ribavirin in the treatment of patients with respiratory syncytial virus disease 1987. Pediatr Infect Dis 6:159-163.

Rossi, J.J., Elkins, D., Taylor, N., Zaia, J., Sullivan, S., and Deshler, J.O. Exploring the use of antisense, enzymatic RNA molecules (ribozymes) as therapeutic agents. 1991. Antisense Res Dev 1(3):285-288.

Rottman, J.B., English, R.V., Breitschwerdt, E.B., and Duncan, D.E. Bone marrow hypoplasia in a cat treated with griseofulvin. 1991. J Am Vet Med Assoc 198(3):429.

Rubin, S.I. Nephrotoxicity of amphotericin B. In Kirk, R.W. (Ed.), Current Veterinary Therapy IX. 1986, pp. 1142-1145. Philadelphia: W.B. Saunders.

Ryder, N., and Dupont, M.C. Inhibition of squalene epoxidase by allylamine antimycotic compounds. A comparative study of the fungal and mammalian enzymes. 1990. Biochem J 230:765-770.

Saag, M.S., and Dismukes, W.E. Azole antifungal agents: emphasis on new triazoles. 1988. Antimicrob Agents Chemother 32(1):1-8.

Sarver, N. Ribozymes: a new fronteir in anti-HIV strategy. 1991. Antisense Res Dev 1(4):373-378.

Schaffner A., Douglas H., and Braude A. Selective protection against conidia by mononuclear and against mycelia by polymorphonuclear phagocytes in resistance to *Aspergillus:* observations on these two lines of defense in vivo and in vitro with human and mouse phagocytes. 1982. J Clin Invest 69:617-631.

Schowengerdt C.G., Suyemoto R. and Main F.B. Granulomatous and fibrous mediastinitis: a review and analysis of 180 cases. 1969. J Thorac Cardiovas Surg 57:365-379.

Scott, D.W. Fungal disorders. Feline dermatology, 1900-1978: a monograph. 1980. J Am Anim Hosp Assoc 16:349-356.

Scott, F.W., deLahunta, A. Schultz, R.D. Bistner, S.I., and Riis, R.C. Teratogenesis in cats associated with griseofulvin therapy. 1975. Teratology 11(1):79-86.

Shah, V.P., Riegelman, S., and Epstein, W.L. Determination of griseofulvin in skin, plasma, and sweat. 1972. J Pharm Sci 61:634-636.

Shannon, D. Treatment with itraconazole of penguins suffering from aspergillosis. 1992. Vet Rec 130(21):479.

Sharp, N.J.H. Treatment of canine nasal aspergillosis/penicilliosis with fluconazole (UK-49,858). 1991. J Small Anim Prac 32:513-516.

Sharp, N.J.H. and Sullivan, M. Treatment of nasal aspergillosis. 1992. In Practice 14(1):26-31.

Sharp, N.J.H., Harvey, C.E., and Sullivan, M. Canine nasal aspergillosis and penicilliosis. 1991. Compen Contin Educ Pract Vet 13:41-49.

Sharp, N.J.H., Sullivan, M., Harvey, C.E., and Webb, T. Treatment of nasal aspergillosis with enilconazole. 1993. J Vet Int Med 7(1):40-43.

Shaw, J.T.B., Tarbit, M.H., and Troke, P.F. Cytochrome P-450 mediated sterol synthesis and metabolism: differences in sensitivity to fluconazole and other azoles. In Fromtling RA (ed). Recent trends in the discovery, development and evaluation of antifungal agents. JR Prous Publishers, Barcelona 1987;125-139.

Shehata, S.H. Treatment and control of mycotic abortion among buffalo-heifers. 1991. Assiut Vet Med J 25(49):236-240.

Shelton, G.H., Grant, C.K., Linenberger, M.L., and Abkowitz J.L. Severe neutropenia associated with griseofulvin therapy in cats with feline immunodeficiency virus infection. 1990. J Vet Int Med 4:317-319.

Shelton, G.H., Linenberger, M.L., and Abkowitz J.L. Hematologic abnormalities in cats seropositive for feline immunodeficiency virus. 1991. J Am Vet Med Assoc 199(10):1353-1357.

Smith, C.B., Charette, R.P., Fox, J.P., Cooney, M.K., and Hall, C.E. Lack of effect of oral ribavirin in naturally occurring influenza A virus (H1N1) infection. 1980 J Infect Dis 141:548-554.

Smith, C.G. Use of acyclovir in an outbreak of Pacheco's parrot disease. 1987. Assoc Avian Vet Today 1:55-57.

Smith, E.K. Dermatohpytosis in pets: avoiding misdiagnosis. 1989. Vet Med 6:554-564.

SOCA. See Studies of Ocular Complications of AIDS Research Group.

Sokol-Anderson M., Sligh, J.E., Elberg, S., Brajtburg, J., Kobayashi, G.S. and Medoff, G. Role of cell defense against oxidative damage in the resistance of *Candida albicans* to the killing effect of amphotericin B. 1988. Am J Med 84:826-832.

Sousa, C.A., and Ihrke, P.J. Superficial fungal infections. In Pratt, P.W. (Ed.), Feline Medicine. 1983, pp. 567-570. Santa Barbara, Calif.: American Vet Pub.

Steele, R.W. Antiviral agents for respiratory infections. 1988. Ped Infect Dis J 7:457-461.

Straw, J.A., Loo, T.L., deVera, C.C., Nelson, P.D., Tompkins, W.A., and Bai, S.A. Pharmacokinetics of potential anti-AIDS agents thiofoscarnet and foscarnet in the cat. 1992. J Acquired Def Syn 5(9):936-942.

Studies of Ocular Complications of AIDS Research Group (SOCA), in collaboration with the AIDS Clinical Trials Group. Mortality in patients with the acquired immunodeficiency syndrome treated with either foscarnet or ganciclovir for cytomegalovirus retinitis. 1992. N Engl J Med 326:213-220.

Swenson, C.L., Polas, P.J., Cheney, C.M. Kociba, G.J., and Mathes, L.E. Prophylactic and therapeutic effects of phosphonoformate against feline leukemia virus in vivo. 1991. Am J Vet Res 52(12):2010-2015.

Tanabe-Tochikura, A., Tochikura, T.S., Blakeslee, J.R., Olsen, R.G., Mathes, L.E. Anti-human immunodeficiency virus (HIV) agents are also potent and selective inhibitiors of feline immunodeficiency virus (FIV) -induced cytopathic effect: development of a new method for screening of anti-FIV substances in vitro. 1992. Antiviral Res 19(2):161-172.

Tavares, L., Roneker, C., Johnston, K., Lehrman, S.N., and deNoronha, F. 3′-azido-3-deoxythymidine in feline leukemia virus-infected cats: a model for therapy and prophylaxis of AIDS. 1987. Cancer Res 47:3190-3194.

Tavares, L., Roneker, C., Postie, L., and deNoronha, F. Testing of mucleoside analogues in cats infected with feline leukemia virus: a model. 1989. Intervirology 30(Suppl1):26-35.

Teich, S.A., Cheung, T.W., and Friedman, A.H. Systemic antiviral drugs used in ophthalmolgy. 1992. Surv Ophth 37(1):19-53.

Thienpont, D., VanCutsem, J., VanCauteren, H., and Marsboom, R. The biological and toxicological properties of imazalil. 1981. Arzneimittel-Forschung 31(2):309-315.

Troke, P.F. Efficacy in animal models of superficial and opportunistic systemic fungal infection. In Fromtling RA (ed). Recent trends in the discovery, development and evaluation of antifungal agents. JR Prous Publishers, Barcelona 1987:103-112.

Troke, P.F., Andrews, R.J., Pye, G.W. Fluconazole and other azoles: translation of in vitro activity to in vivo clinical efficacy. 1990. Rev Infect Dis 12(S3):276-280.

Tsiang, H., Ceccaldi, P-E., Ermine, A., Lockhart, B., and Guillemer, S. Inhibition of rabies virus infection in cultrured rat cortical neurons by an N-methyl-D-aspartate noncompetitive antagonist, MK-801. 1991. Antimicrob Agent Chemother 35(3):572-574.

Utz, J.P., Garriques, I.L., Sande, M.A., Warner, J.F., Mandell, G.L., McGehee, R.F., Duma, R.J., and Shadomy, S. Therapy of cryptococcosis with a combination of flucytosine and amphotericin B. 1975. J Infect Dis 132:368-373.

Vaden, S.L., Heit, M.C., Hawkins, E.C., et al. Fluconazole in cats: pharmacokinetics following intravenous and oral administration and penetration into cerebrospinal fluid, aqueous humour and pulmonary epithelial lining fluid. 1997. J Vet Pharmacol Therap 20(3):181-186.

VanCauteren, H., Heykants, J., DeCoster, R., and Cauwenbergh, G. Itraconazole: pharmacologic studies in animals and humans. 1987a. Rev Infect Dis 9(S1):43-46.

VanCauteren, H., Coussement, W., Vandenberghe, J., Herin, V., Vanparys, P., and Marsboom, R. The toxicological properties of itraconazole. In Fromtling RA (ed). Recent trends in the discovery, development and evaluation of antifungal agents. JR Prous Publishers, Barcelona 1987b;263-271.

VanCutsem, J. Oral and parenteral treatment with itraconazole in various superficial and systemic experimental fungal infections. Comparisons with other antifungals and combination therapy. 1990. Br J Clin Pract Sump Suppl 71:32-40.

VanCutsem, J., VanGerven, F., and Janssen, P.A.J. Activity of orally, topically, and parenterally administered itraconazole in the treatment of superficial and deep mycoses: animal models.1987. Rev Infect Dis 9(S1):15-32.

———. Oral and parenteral therapy with saperconazole (R66905) of invasive Aspergillosis in normal and immunocompromised animals. 1989. Antimicrob Agents Chemother 33(12):2063-2068.

Vanden Bossche, H. Itraconazole:A selective inhibitor of the cytochrome P-450 dependent ergosterol biosynthesis. In Fromtling RA (ed). Recent trends in the discovery, development and evaluation of antifungal agents. JR Prous Publishers, Barcelona 1987;207-221.

Vanden Bossche, H., Marichal, P., Gorrens, J., and Coene, M.C. Biochemical basis for the activity and selectivity of oral antifungal drugs. 1990. Br J Clin Pract Suppl 71:41-46.

vanOosterhoust, I.C.A.M., and Venker-van Haagen, A.J. Aspergillosis: Report on diagnosis and treatment. 1991. Tijdschrift Voor Diergeneeskunde 116(S1):37-38.

VanVoris, L.P., Betts, R.F., Hayden, F.G., Christmas, W.A., and Douglas, R.G. Jr. Successful treatment of naturally occurring influenza A/USSR/77 H1N1. 1981. J Am Med Assoc 245(11):1128-1131.

Vartivarian S.E. Virulence properties and nonimmune pathogenetic mechanisms of fungi. 1992. Clin Infect Dis 14(S1):30-36.

Walsh, T.J., Finberg, R.W., Arndt, C., et al. Liposomal amphotericin B for empirical therapy in patients with persistent fever and neutropenia. 1999. New Engl J Med 340:764-771.

Warnock, D.W. Amphotericin B: an introduction. 1991. J Antimicrob Chemother 28(suppl B):27-38.

Whitaker-Dowling, P., and Younger, J.S. Antiviral effects of interferon in different virus-host cell systems In Mechanisms of Interferon Actions, Vol. 1 (Pfeffer, L.M. ed.) CRC Press, Boca Raton, Fla. 1987 pp. 83-98.

Whitely, R.J., Alford, C.A., and Hirsch, M.S. Vidarabine versus acyclovir therapy in herpes simplex encephalitis. 1986. New Engl J Med 314:144-149.

White-Weithers, N., and Medleau, L. Evaluation of topical therapies for the treatment of dermatophyte-infected hairs from dogs and cats. 1995. J Am Anim Hosp Assoc 31:250-252.

Willard M.D., Nachreiner, R., McDonald R., and Roudebush, P. Ketoconazole-induced changes in selected canine hormone concentrations. 1986a. Am J Vet Res 47:2504-2509.

Willard M.D., Nachreiner, R.F., Howard, V.C., and Fooshee, S.K. Effect of long-term administration of ketoconazole in cats. 1986b. Am J Vet Res 47:2510-2513.

Zeidner, N.S., Mathiason-Dubard, C.K., Rose, L.M., et al. Zidovudine in combination with alpha interferon, interleukin-2, and activated immune lymphocytes as therapy for FeLV-induced immunodeficiency syndrome (FeLV-FAIDS). 1989. Proc XIVth Int Symp Comp Res Leukemia and Related Diseases p. 94.

Ziemer, E.L., Pappagianis, D., Madigan, J.E., Mansmann, R.A., and Hoffman, K.D. Coccidioidomycosis in horses: 15 cases (1975-1984). 1992. J Am Vet Med Assoc 201(6):910-916.

SECTION 11

Chemotherapy of Parasitic Diseases

47 ANTINEMATODAL DRUGS

CRAIG R. REINEMEYER AND CHARLES H. COURTNEY

Benzimidazoles
Probenzimidazoles
  Netobimin
  Febantel
Imidazothiazoles
  Butamisole Hydrochloride
  Levamisole
Tetrahydropyrimidines
  Pyrantel
  Morantel
Organophosphate Compounds
  Dichlorvos
Macrocyclic Lactones (Macrolide Endectocides)
  Avermectins
    Ivermectin
    Abamectin
    Doramectin
    Eprinomectin
    Selamectin
  Milbemycins
    Milbemycin Oxime
    Moxidectin
Heterocyclic Compounds
  Phenothiazine
  Piperazine
  Diethylcarbamazine Citrate
Heartworm adulticides
  Thiacetarsamide Sodium
  Melarsomine
Miscellaneous Nematocidal Compounds
Resistance to Nematocides

Due to their macroscopic nature, nematodes were likely among the first infectious organisms for which therapeutic interventions were attempted. Anthropologists have documented that many primitive and developing cultures recognize internal parasites and employ herbal and other natural remedies to expel them from human and animal patients.

Veterinary medicine relied on such natural remedies for nematode control until the middle of the present century, when synthetic chemistry began to provide more effective and reliable compounds. Some of the earliest antinematodal drugs appeared during the 1930s (phenothiazine) and 1950s (thiabendazole) and remained in common use until recently.

During the past half-century, nematocides have undergone rapid expansion and improvement. This drug class has been transformed from a collection of relatively unsafe compounds with modest efficacy against limited spectra of parasites. Modern antinematodal compounds compose a pharmaceutical armamentarium with a wide therapeutic index, efficacies that approach 100% against literally dozens of species of internal nematode and external arthropod parasites, and excellent activity whether administered orally, parenterally, or topically. In addition, many compounds offer persistent protection from reinfection for several weeks following treatment, and some have no slaughter or milk withdrawal times following treatment.

Modern antinematodal compounds are truly remarkable drugs that set the standard for pharmaceutical development. Realistically, very little improvement of most nematocides is expected or necessary. However, this therapeutic and prophylactic group sorely needs greater chemical diversity. As this chapter will demonstrate, the available nematocidal drugs for most host species belong to only a few chemical classes. Therefore, the number of feasible therapeutic and prophylactic alternatives diminishes rapidly whenever an entire family of dewormers is rendered useless by anthelmintic side-resistance. Anthelmintic resistance has been described as the greatest challenge to parasite control in this millennium.

The compounds described and discussed in the following pages are essential tools for managing nematode parasitism. However, they should be regarded as precious resources to be used sparingly and strategically, because overuse of any tool ultimately renders it dull and ineffectual.

BENZIMIDAZOLES. The introduction of thiabendazole (TBZ) in the early 1960s marked the beginning of the modern era of broad-spectrum anthelmintics that were safe and effective against a wide variety of nematode parasites and could be given in versatile regimens. TBZ was used extensively in a wide range of hosts (sheep, cattle, goats, pigs, horses, birds, and humans). TBZ could be given in a single, therapeutic dose or administered prophylactically at lower doses in the feed for an extended period. In addition to its broad-spectrum activity, TBZ has larvicidal and ovicidal properties.

Based on the success of TBZ, extensive programs were launched to modify it and develop structurally related drugs with improved properties. Of several hundred compounds synthesized, those selected for further development on the basis of overall safety and efficacy included albendazole, cambendazole, fenbendazole, flubendazole, mebendazole, oxfendazole, oxibendazole, parbendazole, and thiophanate. Each of these compounds was produced commercially for anthelmintic use in various countries.

Chemistry. All benzimidazoles (BZDs) have the same central structure (i.e., 1,2-diaminobenzene). The other BZDs differ from TBZ and thiophanate in having a substitution on carbon 5 of the benzene ring (Table 47.1). TBZ, flubendazole, cambendazole, fenbendazole, albendazole, oxfendazole, oxibendazole, and parbendazole are white crystalline powders; mebendazole is an off-white to yellowish amorphous powder; and thiophanate is a pale, yellowish-brown crystalline solid. All are insoluble or only slightly soluble in water. Albendazole, oxfendazole, cambendazole, and parbendazole are soluble in alcohols, but TBZ is only slightly so. Flubendazole and mebendazole are soluble in formic acid, fenbendazole in dimethylsulfoxide, and thiophanate in cyclohexanone.

Pharmacokinetics. Except for TBZ, albendazole, and oxfendazole, only limited amounts of any of the BZDs are absorbed from the gastrointestinal (GI) tract of the host. The limited absorption is probably related to the poor water solubility of these drugs. The little absorption that occurs is generally rapid. Peak plasma levels occur within 2–7 hours after dosing with TBZ, flubendazole, or mebendazole, and within 6–30 hours after dosing with albendazole, fenbendazole, oxfendazole, oxibendazole, parbendazole, or thiophanate, depending on the species. Plasma levels are generally never greater than 1% of the dose administered regardless of the type (paste, suspension, granules, or bolus) of oral formulation. The amount of food in the stomach at the time of treatment influences bioavailability of the drug (e.g., a full stomach is recommended when treating dogs with fenbendazole). Albendazole evidently is absorbed to a much greater degree than the other BZDs because 47% of the administered dose can be recovered in urine over a 9-day period (28% within the first 24 hr). Plasma levels are increased and anthelmintic activity is enhanced when BZDs are retained in the rumen rather than passed directly into the abomasum via closure of the esophageal groove.

Metabolism of the BZDs is variable. Mebendazole is poorly metabolized, and most is excreted unchanged in feces within 24–48 hours. Between 5 and 10% is excreted in urine, and only a small portion is excreted as the decarboxylated derivative of mebendazole. Forty-four to 50% of fenbendazole is excreted unchanged in feces of sheep, cattle, and pigs, and less than 1% in urine. The principal metabolite in ruminants results from hydroxylation of the phenyl ring; some de-ethoxycarbonylation also occurs. Hennessy et al. (1993) reviewed the biliary excretion and enterohepatic recycling of fenbendazole metabolites in sheep. McKellar et al. (1990) reviewed the pharmacokinetics of fenbendazole in Beagle dogs.

TBZ and cambendazole are rapidly metabolized into degradation products, and less than 1% of TBZ and less than 5% of cambendazole are excreted intact. Excretion of these two drugs and their metabolites occurs via both feces and urine within 72 hours and 48 hours of dosing, respectively. Albendazole is metabolized primarily to its sulfoxide and sulfone derivatives, which are excreted mostly through urine. Oxfendazole is

TABLE 47.1—Names and formulas of benzimidazole anthelmintics

Compound	Trade name	Chemical name	Structural formula
Albendazole, INN	Valbazen	Methyl [5-(propylthio)-*H*-benzimidazole-2-yl] carbamate	$CH_3CH_2CH_2$—S— ; H, N, N ; NH—C(=O)—O—CH_3
Fenbendazole, INN	Panacur Safeguard Axilur EnProAl	Methyl 5 (phenylthio)-2-benzimidazolecarbamate	S ; H, N, N ; NH—C(=O)—O—CH_3
Flubendazole, BAN	Flubenol	Methyl [5-(4-fluorobenzoyl)-1*H*-benzimidazole-2-yl] carbamate	F— ; C(=O) ; H, N, N ; NH—C(=O)—O—CH_3
Mebendazole, INN	Telmin Telmintic Vermox (USSR) Multispec Ovitelmin Mebenvet	Methyl 5-benzoyl-2-benzimidazole-carbamate	C(=O) ; H, N, N ; NH—C(=O)—O—CH_3
Oxfendazole, INN	Benzelmin Systamex Synanthic	Methyl 5(6)-phenylsulfinyl-2-benzimidazole-carbamate	S(=O) ; H, N, N ; NH—C(=O)—O—CH_3
Oxibendazole, INN	Anthelcide EQ Loditac	Methyl-5-*n*-propoxy-2-benzimidazolecarbamate	$CH_3CH_2CH_2O$; H, N, N ; NH—C(=O)—O—CH_3
Parbendazole, INN	Verminum Worm Guard Helmatac	Methyl 5-butyl-2-benzimidazole-carbamate	H_9C_4 ; H, N, N ; NH—C(=O)—O—CH_3
Thiophanate, BAN	Nemafax	1,2-bis(3-ethoxycarbonyl-2-thioureido)benzene	$NHCSNHCOOC_2H_5$; $NHCSNHCOOC_2H_5$

Note: → denotes position of carbon 5 in structural formula.
INN = international nonproprietary name; BAN = British approved name.

excreted primarily through urine of monogastric animals and through feces (65%) of ruminants. Less absorption occurs in ruminants than in monogastric animals, but ruminant absorption is increased in animals fed concentrates and hay versus those that ingest forage while grazing. Major metabolites of oxfendazole involve hydroxylation at the 4′-carbon of the thiophenyl group, hydrolysis of the methyl carbamate moiety, and oxidation or reduction of the sulfoxide. The 4′-hydroxy metabolites are excreted as urinary glucuronides and sulfates. Metabolites of flubendazole, a fluoride analog of mebendazole, result from carbamate hydrolysis and reduction of the ketone; metabolites of the former process are found in both feces and urine; those of the latter only in urine. Small amounts of the BZDs are excreted for as long as 10 days after dosing.

Residues of BZDs in most tissues of treated animals approach the lower limit of detection (0.05 mg/kg) within 2 days. However, residual quantities are detectable in the liver by radioisotope techniques at 2 weeks after dosing and occur in the range of 0.3 μg or less/g tissue. Such residues mandate a withdrawal period before slaughter, and most BZDs should not be administered to lactating animals whose milk is to be used for human consumption.

Mode of Action. The BZDs act primarily by binding to nematode tubulin. Specifically, BZDs bind to β-tubulin, which in turn prevents its dimerization with α-tubulin and the polymerization of tubulin oligomers into microtubules. Microtubules are essential structural units of many organelles and are necessary for numerous cellular processes, including mitosis, protein assembly, and energy metabolism.

Mammals also rely on tubulin for cellular metabolism, but BZDs have a higher affinity for nematode tubulin at the normal body temperature range of mammals. This may explain some of their selective action in domestic animals. The β-tubulin isotypes of BZD-resistant nematodes have much lower affinity for BZDs. This change may be attributable to base-pair replacements in the DNA sequence coding β-tubulin isotype.

Anthelmintic Spectrum

HORSES. Thiabendazole and most of the substituted BZDs (fenbendazole, oxfendazole, oxibendazole, albendazole, and parbendazole) have high efficacy (>90%) against adult large strongyles, cyathostomes, mature *Oxyuris equi,* small pinworms (*Probstmayria vivipara*), and *Trichostrongylus axei* of horses. Ascarids (*Parascaris equorum*) and immature *Oxyuris* are more effectively eliminated by the substituted BZDs than by TBZ; but piperazine can be added to TBZ to enhance removal of the latter two nematodes.

In the USA, the only currently marketed BZD with label claims against *Strongyloides westeri* infection is oxibendazole at an elevated dosage (15 mg/kg).

At regular, therapeutic dosages, BZDs have little to no activity against several equine parasites, including *Habronema* spp., *Draschia megastoma,* and *Gasterophilus* spp. Elevated, multiple doses of fenbendazole (10 mg/kg for 5 days) are approved for treatment of migrating *Strongylus vulgaris* and *S. edentatus* larvae and against encysted third- and fourth-stage cyathostome larvae.

Mebendazole and albendazole demonstrate activity against equine lungworms (*Dictyocaulus arnfieldi*) at elevated dosages of 15–20 mg/kg/day and 25 mg/kg twice daily, respectively. Both regimens must be administered for 5 consecutive days.

CATTLE AND SHEEP. The substituted BZDs are markedly effective against adults and larvae of many species of GI nematodes of ruminants and can be used to control lungworms of cattle and sheep. In particular, fenbendazole, albendazole, and oxfendazole are effective for lungworm infections with *Dictyocaulus* spp. Fenbendazole has 99% efficacy against adult and 6- and 13-day-old larval stages of *Dictyocaulus viviparus* in cattle. Low dosages of fenbendazole (1.4 mg/kg/day for 4 days) give better results against *Dictyocaulus filaria* in sheep than a single therapeutic dose, and this regimen is highly effective against inhibited *Ostertagia* larvae. *Muellerius* infection of goats and sheep is cleared with a single dose of fenbendazole at 15 mg/kg.

All of the major GI nematodes of ruminants (*Haemonchus, Ostertagia, Trichostrongylus, Marshallagia, Cooperia, Nematodirus, Bunostomum, Chabertia, Oesophagostomum, Strongyloides*) are eliminated by the substituted BZDs. TBZ is less efficacious than the substituted BZDs for *Ostertagia, Cooperia,* and *Nematodirus.* Adult forms of GI parasites are most susceptible to BZDs, but immature stages are eliminated as well. Fenbendazole, albendazole, oxfendazole, and thiophanate eliminate greater than 90% of the fourth stage and immature fifth stage of all major GI parasites of ruminants.

Albendazole and fenbendazole are especially efficacious against the tissue stages of *Ostertagia.* Treatment with either drug results in approximately 95% reduction of 3-, 7-, and 10-day-old developing larval stages of *Ostertagia.*

Inhibited fourth-stage larvae of *Ostertagia* are more difficult to treat. Among the BZDs, albendazole and oxfendazole (at the label dosage) and fenbendazole (at twice the label dosage) are ~85% effective against this stage. The degree of efficacy, however, may depend on the level of metabolic activity of the larvae. Miller (1993) reported higher efficacy of oxfendazole during induction of inhibition in March (89.4%) and during emergence from the abomasal mucosa in September (94.3%). In contrast, drug efficacy during the depth of arrestment was only 41.5% in May and 68.5% in July. The level of metabolic activity was presumably higher during the months of changing life cycle status, and Miller hypothesized that some of the reported variability in anthelmintic efficacy against hypobiotic *Ostertagia* may be related to the metabolic activity of larvae at the time of treatment. Prichard and Ranjan (1993) have prepared a general review of cattle anthelmintics and their effectiveness against inhibited *Ostertagia.*

In general, the BZDs have limited activity against ruminant whipworms (*Trichuris* spp.) and filarial parasites (*Onchocerca, Setaria*). Notable exceptions include flubendazole, oxibendazole, and oxfendazole, which are useful for whipworms.

SWINE. In swine, TBZ is highly effective against *Hyostrongylus rubidus, Strongyloides ransomi,* and *Oesophagostomum dentatum* but shows poor activity against ascarids (*Ascaris suum*). In contrast, the substituted BZDs are generally effective against all of these parasites of swine.

Efficacy of BZDs against swine whipworms (*Trichuris suis*) is variable at regular therapeutic doses. Parbendazole (20–50 mg/kg) expels 83–97% of *T. suis,* and fenbendazole (15 mg/kg) only 65%. Multiple dosing with fenbendazole (3 mg/kg on each of 6 consecutive days), albendazole (40 ppm in feed for 5–10 days), or mebendazole or flubendazole (each at 30 ppm in feed for 10 days) expels greater than 99% of swine whipworms.

Fenbendazole is highly effective (99–100%) against the kidney worm (*Stephanurus dentatus*) and lungworms (*Metastrongylus* spp.) of swine. The labeled dosage regimen for these parasites is 3 mg/kg/day for 3 days. This regimen is also completely effective for swine ascarids, nodular worms, and whipworms and 81% effective against *S. ransomi.* Similar efficacy against lungworms can be achieved with a single dose of 25 mg/kg fenbendazole. Albendazole is also effective against swine lungworms. Better efficacy is obtained when this drug is administered in the feed (10 ppm) for 5 days rather than by single dosing.

As the previous examples suggest, BZDs generally are more effective when given at lower dosages for several days rather than as larger, single doses. For example, single doses of thiophanate at 50–100 mg/kg are quite effective against adult and larval stages of *Oesophagostomum, Trichuris, Hyostrongylus,* and *Strongyloides* in pigs and against all major GI nematodes of ruminants. When given in feed over several days, however, thiophanate maintains efficacy against these species and is additionally effective against ascarids in pigs (6 mg/kg/day for 14 days) and against inhibited larvae of *Ostertagia ostertagi* in cattle (20 mg/kg/day for 5 days).

It is difficult to assess the comparative values of BZDs against the larval and immature fifth stages of the GI parasites of swine because many reports on efficacy do not include this information. In general, however, efficacy against these stages parallels activity against adult forms. None of the BZDs claims efficacy against spirurid stomach worms or *Macracanthorhynchus hirudinaceus.*

DOGS AND CATS. The activities of mebendazole and fenbendazole have been evaluated extensively in dogs and cats. Mebendazole is approved for use in dogs against adult hookworms, ascarids, and whipworms. Nematodes are satisfactorily expelled by a 3-day course of 22 mg/kg/day. Mebendazole has similar activity against similar parasites of cats but is not approved in this host species.

Fenbendazole also has excellent activity for the same parasites of dogs and cats. It is administered as granular, powder, or suspension formulations at a dosage of 50 mg/kg/day for 3 days for common nematodes. It currently has FDA approval for dogs but not cats. Additionally, administration of fenbendazole at 50 mg/kg daily from the 40th day of pregnancy through the 14th day after whelping provides excellent reduction of hookworm (>99%) and ascarid (>90%) burdens of pups that were infected lactogenically or prenatally, respectively (Burke and Roberson 1983). Albendazole and oxfendazole are apparently effective against somatic ascarid and hookworm larvae when similarly used in infected bitches during the last third of pregnancy (Stoye 1992). Digestion of musculature from dogs, rats, and mice somatically infected with these parasites suggests that fenbendazole kills larval forms of canine ascarids and hookworms. Controlled studies in dogs suggest greater than 94% effectiveness in reducing developing third- and fourth-stage larvae of canine ascarids (*T. canis* and *T. leonina*) following a 30-day regimen at 50 mg/kg/day (Fisher et al. 1993).

The efficacy of albendazole against common GI nematodes of dogs and cats has not been investigated thoroughly. Albendazole's activity for canine ascarids (70%), hookworms (18%), and whipworms (8%) is limited when given as a single dose of 15 mg/kg. A higher, single dose (20 or 25 mg/kg) is 100% effective for *T. canis* but still limited (66–73%) against *Ancylostoma caninum.* Daily dosing (3 days at 15 mg/kg/day) is 100% effective for both *T. canis* and *A. caninum.*

Albendazole apparently is active against some of the less common nematode parasites such as *Filaroides hirthi* and *Capillaria plica.* In dogs with clinical signs (hematuria, dysuria, pollakiuria) associated with *C. plica* infection, a prolonged, high-dose regimen of albendazole (50 mg/kg orally every 12 hr for 12–14 days) is required to achieve efficacy. Anorexia may occur 5–10 days after initiation of treatment. Fenbendazole is reportedly effective against this parasite at its regular therapeutic dosage (50 mg/kg for 3 days) and has no side effects.

Albendazole (25–50 mg/kg every 12 hr for 5 days) is apparently almost totally effective in treating *F. hirthi.* Tracheal infections of *Filaroides osleri* in dogs have been treated by repeated use of oxfendazole (10 mg/kg/day for 28 days) or TBZ (70 mg/kg/day for 2 days, then 140 mg/kg/day for 21 days). Albendazole or fenbendazole may be effective against this parasite with less demanding regimens. Fenbendazole appears to be particularly suited for treatment of the cat lungworm (*Aelurostrongylus abstrusus*) as well as the stomach worm (*Ollulanus tricuspis*). Treatment regimens are 20–50 mg/kg/day for 5 days or 3 days, respectively.

Interested readers are referred to earlier editions of this text for detailed discussions of the activity of BZDs against *Strongyloides stercoralis* infections in dogs (Courtney and Roberson 1995).

A combination of oxibendazole and diethylcarbamazine (Filaribits Plus) is administered daily to dogs for prevention of hookworm and heartworm and for removal of whipworms and ascarids.

BIRDS. Mebendazole and fenbendazole can be used effectively against parasites of the GI and respiratory tracts of birds. Mebendazole in a single dose of 50 mg/kg or fenbendazole at 8 mg/kg/day in feed for 6 consecutive days effectively eliminates ascarid and capillarid infections of birds. Turkeys require fenbendazole at 45 ppm in feed for 6 days to effect 100% removal of ascarids, *Heterakis,* and *Capillaria obsignata.* Single treatments with fenbendazole at 350 mg/kg are fully effective against ascarids. Parbendazole is effective against both ascarids and heterakids at a single dose of 30 mg/kg or as a 0.05% preparation in food for 2 days. Treatment with parbendazole is not recommended during the laying period.

Treatment of zoo birds is generally accomplished with lower daily dosages over a long period to ensure safety and compliance. Mebendazole is used in feed at 60 ppm for 7 days in chickens, turkeys, and guinea fowl and at 120 ppm for 14 days in pheasants, partridges, geese, and ducks. Fenbendazole is used at 60 ppm for 6 days in all these species.

FERAL, ZOO, AND LABORATORY ANIMALS. The BZDs have been used successfully in zoo and game mammals, birds, reptiles, and amphibians. Dosages and safety in these hosts appear to be similar to those of their domesticated counterparts. Fenbendazole, in two formulations, has FDA approval for numerous types of zoo and game animals. Unfortunately, worms resistant to fenbendazole (and presumably to other BZDs) are prevalent in many species of ungulates, especially antelopes. In addition to these FDA-approved uses, fenbendazole has been used widely in primates at 20 mg/kg/day for 5 days. The latter treatment is even effective in removing *Physaloptera* and acanthocephalans (*Prosthenorchis*). Most GI parasites of reptiles and amphibians are eliminated by a single dose of 30–50 mg/kg. However, spirurids, oxyurids, and *Capillaria* require either a higher single dose (50–100 mg/kg) or 2- to 7-day dosing at 30–50 mg/kg/day. Either the granulated, powder, or suspension formulations can be given to reptiles and amphibians in food. A single dose at 10 times the therapeutic dosage or repeated daily treatments for 14 days (10–30 mg/kg/day) have not caused side effects in amphibians and reptiles. Other zoo animals appear to tolerate overdoses of fenbendazole equally well. A distinct advantage of this drug is its palatability; medicated feed is readily consumed by even the most fastidious species.

BZDs have been used in treating parasitic infections of subhuman primates and pet laboratory animals (rabbits, guinea pigs, hamsters, and tortoises). Of particular interest is the use of mebendazole in treating infections of *Strongyloides fuelleborni* and *S. stercoralis*. Infection with the latter nematode is sometimes fatal. Successful treatment has been accomplished only by repeated oral administration of mebendazole at 25 mg/kg twice daily for days 1–7 and 29–35 and 50 mg/kg twice daily on days 15–21, with two 7-day rest periods from days 8–14 and 22–28.

Pinworm (*Syphacia muris*) infections, which are common in laboratory rats and mice, can be controlled by fenbendazole-medicated feed (150 ppm to effect an 8–12 mg/kg/day dose) given for two 7-day periods with an intervening 7-day rest period.

TRICHINELLA SPIRALIS. Several BZDs have activity against *Trichinella spiralis,* at least in laboratory mouse models. Most studies indicate that the greatest chemotherapeutic effect occurs when BZDs are given during the intestinal (first week) or the migratory (subsequent 3 weeks) phase after infection. Treatment of the encysted stage (4 weeks or longer after exposure) is less successful.

Fenbendazole, albendazole, and oxibendazole have relatively good activity against preadult *Trichinella* stages in the intestine of mice but limited efficacy (approximately 50%) against encysted larvae in the regimens tested. A 14-day treatment with mebendazole in the feed (125 ppm) gives 100% reduction of encysted larvae in mouse tissues. Similar tests using flubendazole in feed (32–125 ppm) reduced encysted larvae in swine by 100%.

Based on these encouraging results, successful treatment of human cases of trichinellosis has been accomplished with mebendazole, flubendazole, and albendazole.

LARVICIDAL ACTIVITY. Humans with hookworm-induced cutaneous larva migrans have been treated successfully by oral administration of TBZ or albendazole for 5 days. Topical application to the cutaneous track seems to be as effective as oral administration. Formulations for topical use can be made as a 15% aqueous suspension or as a cream consisting of 0.5 g TBZ in 5 g petrolatum. Either preparation is applied to the affected site daily for 2–3 weeks.

Albendazole is recommended for treatment of human cases of visceral and ocular larva migrans due to animal ascarid larvae. The usual dosage is 5 mg/kg twice daily for 5 days.

OVICIDAL ACTIVITY. Reductions in the viability of parasite eggs in feces following treatment of animals with BZDs suggest that these drugs have ovicidal properties. This effect has been demonstrated against eggs of ruminant trichostrongylids, swine stomach worms (*Hyostrongylus*), chicken ascarids, and canine and human hookworms and whipworms. Production of eggs by female worms is inhibited within 1 hour of BZD administration, and occasional eggs may be distorted in shape. The ovicidal properties of BZDs have led to the development of in vitro egg hatch assays for detection of nematode strains that are resistant to BZD compounds. In these assays, eggs of resistant nematode strains are able to develop and hatch in higher concentrations of soluble BZDs than eggs from strains known to be susceptible.

SAFETY AND TOXICITY. The BZDs are extremely well tolerated by domestic and wild animals in general. They are characteristically free of side effects at therapeutic doses even when administered to young, sick, or debilitated animals.

The minimum lethal dose of fenbendazole in cattle is 750 mg/kg (i.e., 150 times the therapeutic dose). Consecutive daily dosing with fenbendazole is tolerated well by dogs (30 days at 250 mg/kg/day and 90 days at 125 mg/kg/day) and sheep (30 days at 45 mg/kg/day). Multiple dosing of dogs with albendazole (2 or 10 mg/kg daily for 3 months) or oxfendazole (up to 6 mg/kg daily for 3 months) is well tolerated. In ruminants and horses, a single 10-times overdose of oxfendazole did not cause detectable toxic effects, nor did 8 successive administrations of 3 times the recommended dose at 4-day intervals in ruminants. Sheep tolerate a 20-times overdose of oxfendazole, but a 50-times overdose caused inappetance, fever, diarrhea, and 16% mortality. Similarly, thiophanate is tolerated by sheep and cattle in single doses of 25–30 times the regular therapeutic dose or in repeated daily doses of 100 mg/kg for 7 days. Oxibendazole caused no ill effects in horses in a single treatment equal to 60 times the therapeutic dose or in 9 repeated administrations of 5 times the therapeutic dose at approximately 1-week intervals. Similar levels of oxibendazole are also safe for cattle, sheep, and dogs. Mebendazole is tolerated in horses when given as a single dose equal to 40 times the therapeutic dose or as daily, 6-times doses for 15 days. Parbendazole may cause transient diarrhea in horses treated at doses as low as 2.5 mg/kg but is tolerated well in pigs at 10,000 mg/kg. Mebendazole is tolerated in chickens at 2000 mg/kg. In dogs, treatment with this drug at therapeutic doses occasionally results in acute hepatic necrosis with jaundice.

Acute and chronic LD_{50} values have not been established for the BZDs in some domestic animals. A single 200 mg/kg dose of albendazole is lethal for cattle, as parbendazole (600 mg/kg) occasionally is for sheep. The LD_{50} for mebendazole in dogs, cats, and guinea pigs is 640 mg/kg; its LD_{50} in horses is not known, but daily treatment of horses with a standard dose of 5 g mebendazole for 19–74 days had no ill effects. Mebendazole in standard-size particles (10–20 μm) has an LD_{50} of 3.56 g/kg for mice, but in smaller particles (3–5 μm) it is five times more toxic for mice (LD_{50} = 0.62 g/kg). Acute LD_{50} values of oxfendazole are greater than 1600 mg/kg for dogs and greater than 6400 mg/kg for both mice and rats. The LD_{50} value of flubendazole in mice, rats, and guinea pigs exceeds 2560 mg/kg. Attempts to cause fatalities by poisoning small laboratory animals with fenbendazole or oxibendazole have been unsuccessful because rats and mice tolerate the maximum quantities (10,000 mg/kg) that physically can be administered.

Contraindications. Because of the potential for tissue and milk residues, slaughter clearance times are required, and milk of treated animals may not be used for human consumption. A notable exception is fenbendazole in dairy cattle, which requires no milk withdrawal following treatment with 5 mg/kg. A 10-day withdrawal time is recommended for both cattle and sheep following treatment with oxfendazole. Persons administering anthelmintics to food-producing animals should consult the label instructions concerning withdrawal requirements and contraindications.

Another major contraindication for use of some of the substituted BZDs is early pregnancy. Parbendazole and cambendazole exert teratogenic effects when given to pregnant ewes during the second to fourth weeks of gestation. The period of greatest teratogenic potential coincides with the time that normal embryonic limb development begins (i.e., around the 20th day of pregnancy). Principal reported malformations include rotational and flexural deformities of the limbs, overflexion of the carpal joints, and abnormalities of posture and gait. Incidences of malformed lambs born to ewes treated on the 21st and 24th days of gestation were 27 and 47%, respectively. No abnormalities occur if the drugs are administered as early as the 10th or 14th days of pregnancy, but treatment at this time reduces the lambing rate (67% for drug-treated ewes vs. 84% for nontreated controls). There is no restriction on use of cambendazole in ewes following the fourth week of pregnancy.

Although cambendazole is no longer marketed in the USA, its use was reported to cause occasional congenital limb deformities in foals. Interested readers are referred to earlier editions of this text for further details of teratogenic effects of BZD anthelmintics.

There are no known teratogenic effects of mebendazole, fenbendazole, flubendazole, oxibendazole, or thiophanate, and repeated, multiple therapeutic doses of fenbendazole have not caused adverse effects in pregnant ewes, cows, mares, bitches, or laboratory animals.

All BZDs are compatible with other drugs administered simultaneously except that oxfendazole and fenbendazole should not be administered concurrently with bromsalan flukicides. This combination has produced abortions in some cattle and deaths in sheep.

Dosage and Administration. BZDs are almost always administered orally, generally as a paste or suspension for drenching or as a powder or granules for administration in feed or incorporation in a salt- or feed-block carrier. Controlled-release devices (intraruminal bolus) have been developed for sheep and cattle, and oxfendazole can be injected directly into the rumen through the left paralumbar fossa of cattle.

PROBENZIMIDAZOLES. Two probenzimidazole compounds, netobimin and febantel, are converted in the GI tract to albendazole and fenbendazole, respectively, and their subsequent sulfone and sulfoxide metabolites. The parent probenzimidazole compounds have no apparent anthelmintic activity in vivo and are effective only after metabolic conversion. Worms resistant to other BZDs are resistant to the probenzimidazoles as well.

Netobimin. *Netobimin* (Hapadex) is a broad-spectrum probenzimidazole anthelmintic having nematocidal activity in horses and ruminants as well as cestocidal and fasciolicidal activity in ruminants. Netobimin is found only briefly in the GI tract following administration, being replaced by albendazole and albendazole sulfoxide, which are thought to account for its anthelmintic activity. Netobimin is effective against the common GI nematodes (including hypobiotic larvae of *Ostertagia ostertagi*), lungworms, and *Fasciola hepatica.* In horses, it is effective against ascarids as well as large strongyles and cyathostomes.

Febantel. *Febantel* (Rintal) is a broad-spectrum probenzimidazole anthelmintic that has FDA approval for use in horses, dogs, and cats and has broad-spectrum efficacy against nematodes of ruminants, swine, and a variety of species of zoo animals. Febantel is found only briefly in the GI tract following administration, being replaced by fenbendazole and its sulfoxide, oxfendazole, which are thought to account for febantel's anthelmintic activity. Febantel (Rintal Tabs) is approved for use against hookworms (*A. caninum, U. stenocephala*), ascarids (*T. cati, T. leonina*), and whipworms (*T. vulpis*) of dogs, and against ascarids (*T. cati*) and hookworms (*A. tubaeforme*) of cats. The recommended dosage is 10 mg/kg daily for 3 consecutive days. Rintal should be administered at 15 mg/kg and on a full stomach to pups and kittens less than 6 months of age. Febantel is also combined with praziquantel (Vercom Paste) for dogs and cats or with both praziquantel and pyrantel pamoate (Drontal Plus) to expand the antinematodal spectrum to include cestodes as well.

CHEMISTRY. Febantel is a colorless powder that is soluble in acetone, chloroform, tetrahydrofuran, and methylenechloride. It is insoluble in water and alcohols. The chemical name is dimethyl [[2-(2-methoxyacetamido)-4-(phenylthio) phenyl]imidocarbonyl]-dicarbamate. Structurally, it is a guanidine (Fig. 47.1), although it bears structural similarity to the BZDs.

PHARMACOKINETICS. Following oral administration of therapeutic doses of febantel (7.5 mg/kg) to sheep or cattle, the drug is metabolized quickly, and unchanged febantel is present in plasma only at low concentrations. Of 10 identified metabolites, those of interest are chemically identical to fenbendazole and oxfendazole. Maximum plasma concentrations of these compounds occur between 6 and 18 hours in sheep and between 12 and 24 hours in cattle following oral administration. Anthelmintic activity is thought to be due to these two metabolites rather than to their precursor, febantel, and the teratogenic effect of high doses of febantel (45 mg/kg) in pregnant sheep has been ascribed to its oxfendazole metabolite.

ANTHELMINTIC SPECTRUM. Febantel is highly active against a variety of equine parasites, including adult large strongyles (*Strongylus vulgaris, S. edentatus, S. equinus*) and cyathostomes; adult and early fifth-stage ascarids (*Parascaris equorum*); and adult, early fifth-stage, and fourth-stage pinworms (*Oxyuris equi*). At the regular therapeutic dose (6 mg/kg), febantel is not effective against *Trichostrongylus axei* or *Gasterophilus* larvae in the stomach, nor is it effective against larval forms of *S. vulgaris* in the mesenteric arteries. A dose of 10 mg febantel/kg is reported to be effective in killing the eyeworm, *Thelazia lacrymalis*, in horses.

One commercial anthelmintic (Vercom) used for dogs and cats in the USA is a paste formulation containing febantel for nematodes and praziquantel for cestodes. In dogs and cats over 6 months of age, a dose of 10 mg febantel (1 mg praziquantel)/kg is used once daily for 3 consecutive days. Efficacy in pups and kittens less than 6 months of age is improved by using a dose of 15 mg febantel (1.5 mg praziquantel)/kg on a full stomach for 3 consecutive days. These dosages are effective in expelling adult and prepatent infections of *Ancylostoma caninum, A. tubaeforme,* and *Uncinaria stenocephala* (>91%); *Toxocara canis, T. cati,* and *Toxascaris leonina* (98%); *Trichuris vulpis* (100%); and *Taenia* spp., *T. taeniaeformis,* and *Dipylidium caninum* (100%). A more recent product (Drontal Plus) for dogs is administered as a single dose of 35.8 mg febantel, 7 mg pyrantel pamoate, and 7 mg praziquantel/kg. It has similar efficacy for canine ascarids (98%) and tapeworms (100%), greater efficacy for hookworms (>99%), and somewhat lower activity against whipworms (94%). Drontal Plus is 100% effective for both *Echinococcus granulosus* and *E. multilocularis* but is only approved against the former species.

Tests in other hosts suggest satisfactory activity against common GI parasites and lung parasites of sheep, cattle, and swine. Activity against whipworms in these hosts is erratic. The usual dose is 10 mg/kg for ruminants and 20 mg/kg for swine. The drug is also promising in treatment of encysted *Trichinella spiralis.* A dose of 200 mg febantel/kg is 97% effective against the muscle stage in mice.

SAFETY AND TOXICITY. Febantel has a wide margin of safety. The LD_{50} in mice, rats, and dogs is greater than 10,000 mg/kg. In rabbits, the LD_{50} is 1250 mg/kg. There are no known contraindications for use of febantel in horses, cats, or dogs. The combination of febantel and praziquantel, however, causes an increase in frequency of early abortion, and therefore, use of Vercom Paste and Drontal Plus products is contraindicated in pregnant dogs and cats.

In pregnant ewes, febantel is safe at the oral dose of 10 mg/kg. However, when the drug is administered at a higher dose (45 mg/kg) on day 17 of gestation, more than 10% of lambs can be expected to have renal and skeletal abnormalities.

Febantel was formerly marketed in the USA for use in horses. For additional information about potential applications in equids, interested readers are referred to earlier editions of this text (Courtney and Roberson 1995).

Dogs and cats older than 6 months of age require 10 mg febantel/kg for 3 days; pups and kittens, 15 mg/kg for 3 days (Vercom Paste). The single Drontal Plus dose is 35.8 mg/kg for dogs of more than 1 kg body weight or older than 3 weeks.

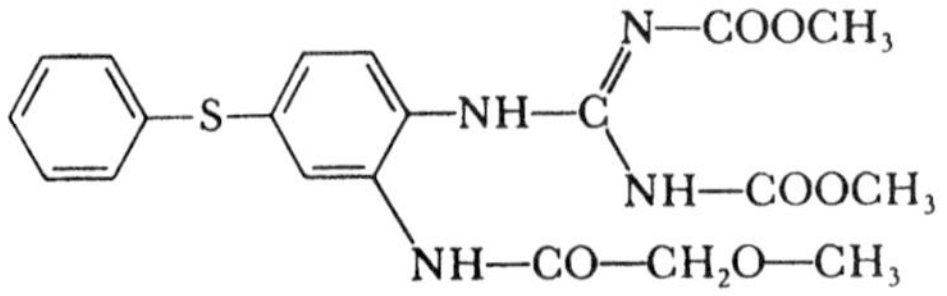

N—COOCH$_3$
S
NH—C
NH—COOCH$_3$
NH—CO—CH$_2$O—CH$_3$

FIG. 47.1—Febantel.

IMIDAZOTHIAZOLES

Butamisole Hydrochloride. *Butamisole Hydrochloride,* INN (Styquin), is an injectable anthelmintic used to treat dogs for whipworm (*Trichuris vulpis*) and hookworm (*Ancylostoma caninum*) infections. It is no longer marketed in the USA. Interested readers are referred to earlier editions of this text (Courtney and Roberson 1995) for additional information about butamisole.

Levamisole. *Levamisole,* INN (Levasole, Tramisol, Totalon), is an antinematodal drug with a broad range of activity in numerous host species (sheep, cattle, swine, horses, chickens, dogs). It is approved and marketed in the USA only for use in cattle, sheep, and swine. Major advantages of levamisole are its efficacy against nematodes of the lungs and GI tract, and optional routes of administration (oral, parenteral, or topical).

CHEMISTRY AND RELATION TO *dl*-TETRAMISOLE. Levamisole is the *l* isomer of *dl*-tetramisole. The latter drug was introduced as an anthelmintic in 1966 and is a racemic mixture of two optical isomers: *s*(−)tetramisole (= *l*-tetramisole = levamisole) rotates plane polarized light to the left; *R*(+)tetramisole (= *d*-tetramisole) rotates light to the right. The mixture of isomers, known as *Tetramisole,* INN, or *dl*-tetramisole (Nemicide, Nilverm, Ripercol), was marketed throughout the world as an anthelmintic for sheep, cattle, and various other hosts.

Following approval of the racemic mixture, pharmaceutical scientists were able to develop a process for separating the *dl*-tetramisole into its two isomers. Upon testing the separated components, it was found that the anthelmintic activity of the mixture was attributable almost solely to the *l* isomer. Thus it was determined that using the *l* isomer alone could reduce the dosage by 50%. Reducing the dosage also increased the safety margin since both components of tetramisole are similarly toxic. The compound currently available in the USA and in many other countries is levamisole rather than the parent tetramisole. Most of the following discussion addresses the *l* isomer.

The chemical name of levamisole is (−)-2,3,5,6-tetrahydro-6-phenylimidazo[2,1-*b*]thiazole. The marketed form is either the hydrochloride (bolus, drench, or paste) or phosphate (injectable) salt. Levamisole hydrochloride, a white crystalline compound, is highly soluble in water. This solubility facilitates the formulation of an injectable solution and a stable drench.

MODE OF ACTION. Levamisole hydrochloride is a direct cholinergic and paralyzes nematodes by sustained muscle contraction. Levamisole acts as a ganglionic stimulant (cholinomimetic). This conclusion is supported by the fact that levamisole-induced contractions of *Ascaris suum* are blocked by the autonomic ganglion-blocking agents mecamylamine and pempidine.

PHARMACOKINETICS. Absorption and excretion of levamisole are rapid following oral administration of the radioactive-labeled drug to rats at a dose of 15 mg/kg. Approximately 40% is excreted in urine within 12 hours. Thereafter, urinary excretion decreases and only another 8% is eliminated over the next 8 days. Elimination in feces over an 8-day period accounts for approximately 41% of the dose, the bulk of which passes in 12–24 hours. A small amount is expelled in respired gases (i.e., 0.2% of the dose during a 48-hour period immediately following dosing).

Tissue residues of the drug are not appreciable. Approximately 0.9% of the initial dose is found in tissues (principally degradative and excretory organs like the liver and kidney) at 12–24 hours after dosing. By 7 days after dosing, levamisole is not detectable in muscle, liver, kidney, fat, blood, or urine of rats or other animals tested. On this basis, a 2- to 11-day slaughter clearance time is mandated, depending on the formulation used. The identified metabolites of levamisole are much less toxic than the parent compound, so the parent drug is sought in analysis of tissue samples.

The pharmacodynamic actions of levamisole (or tetramisole) in the host suggest that the drug exerts both muscarinic and nicotinic effects. Signs of levamisole intoxication (salivation, defecation, and respiratory distress from smooth muscle contraction) are like those of organophosphate poisoning. Indeed, evidence suggests that some of the toxicity of this drug may be concerned with cholinesterase inhibition, leading to manifestations of the muscarinic action of acetylcholine (ACh) (i.e., constriction of pupils and respiratory bronchioles, acceleration of motility of the digestive tract, slowing of the heart rate, and other autonomic actions).

It is suggested that levamisole additionally produces effects consistent with the nicotinic action of ACh (i.e., initial stimulation but subsequent blocking of ganglionic and skeletal neuromuscular transmission). Clinical signs of pronounced nicotinic action of ACh are an initial rise in blood pressure followed by a fall in arterial pressure and simultaneous respiratory paralysis. These nicotinic manifestations are only slightly represented in levamisole toxicosis; the muscarinic manifestations of the drug markedly predominate.

MODULATION OF THE HOST IMMUNE SYSTEM. In addition to its anthelmintic activity, levamisole also apparently enhances immune responsiveness. This characteristic has caused considerable excitement in both veterinary and human medicine. For a discussion of these properties, interested readers are referred to the 7th edition of this text (Courtney and Roberson 1995).

FORMULATIONS AND ADMINISTRATION. Levamisole is administered as a bolus, drench, feed additive, subcutaneous (SC) injectable solution, or topical pour-on. The drug for drenching ruminants is marketed in powder form to which water can be added. Drench solution is quite stable and can be held for as long as 12 days without loss of anthelmintic activity.

Two formulations of levamisole hydrochloride are prepared for administration in feed of ruminants. One incorporates the drug in a pelleted, ready-to-use, dehydrated alfalfa carrier (the pellets should be mixed with one-half the regular daily ration and fed at one time). The second, a medicated premix containing 50% levamisole, is for use by feed mills in manufacturing a deworming supplement (0.8% levamisole) for cattle and sheep. Feed should be withheld overnight. The following morning the medicated supplement can be mixed with one-half the daily ration.

Administration of levamisole in drinking water is used routinely only for swine and poultry. The drug intended for this use is marketed as a powder to be added to water and consumed at the rate of 3.8 L/45.4 kg in a 24-hour period. After mixing, the solution is stable up to 3 months if stored in a tightly capped bottle. For poultry, the medicated drinking water is prepared by calculating the total amount of tetramisole needed to provide a dose of 40 mg/kg. This quantity is used to prepare a 0.01% (approximate) solution that should be consumed by the birds within 12 hours.

Levamisole has wide appeal as an injectable anthelmintic for cattle. The original, aqueous solution of levamisole hydrochloride was administered by intramuscular (IM) or SC injection. The hydrochloride, however, proved to be irritating to tissues, and IM injection resulted in moderate to severe reactions at the injection site. The monobasic phosphoric acid salt of levamisole was found to be less irritating to tissues; thus, levamisole phosphate is now regularly used for SC injections.

The pour-on formulation contains 10% levamisole as base, which is readily absorbed through the skin following application to the midline of the back. Blood levels of levamisole following pour-on application are similar to those obtained after either SC or oral administration. Ease of administration by this method makes treatment more practical than by conventional methods.

Anthelmintic Spectrum

CATTLE AND SHEEP. The efficacy of levamisole in ruminants is essentially equal regardless of whether the bolus, drench, pellet, injectable, or pour-on formulations are used. The pour-on formulation appears to be slightly less effective than other preparations of the drug, which seems to be a common characteristic of other anthelmintics as well. Adult stages of the major ruminant parasites of the abomasum (*Haemonchus, Ostertagia*), small intestine (*Cooperia, Trichostrongylus, Bunostomum*), large intestine (*Oesophagostomum*), and lungs (*Dictyocaulus*) are satisfactorily removed by this broad-spectrum drug. Activity against whipworms is poor or inconsistent. Levamisole is 98% effective for both mature and immature lungworms of ruminants.

Larval and immature stages of the GI parasites of ruminants are effectively removed by levamisole. More than 87% of the lumen-dwelling late fourth-stage and immature adults of *Ostertagia* and *Haemonchus* are removed from treated cattle. Immature adults of *Cooperia* are completely eliminated. Studies using cattle with natural *Ostertagia* infections reported an average 56% reduction in inhibited fourth-stage larvae following treatment with levamisole.

Levamisole also has been successful in treating eyeworms (*Thelazia*) of cattle.

SWINE. The convenient and most widely used method for deworming swine with levamisole is to add the drug to the drinking water or feed. When administered orally, efficacies for levamisole approach 99% for ascarids (*Ascaris suum*), threadworms (*Strongyloides ransomi*), and lungworms (*Metastrongylus* spp.). The nodular worm (*Oesophagostomum dentatum*) is also effectively expelled, but efficacies in separate studies range from 72 to 99%; kidney worms (*Stephanurus dentatus*) are removed from the urinary tract, but larval stages in other parts of the body are not affected. Levamisole is approved in the USA only for the above parasites of swine. Activity of levamisole for swine whipworms is variable, but higher efficacy can be obtained with the injectable formulation (95%) than with oral medication in feed (40%).

Larval stages of certain swine parasites are readily eliminated by levamisole. More than 90% of the third, fourth, and immature adult stages of *Metastrongylus* spp. and the fourth stage and immature adults of *Oesophagostomum* spp. and *Ascaris* spp. are destroyed by the drug. Less than 65% of the third stage of the latter two parasites are eliminated.

POULTRY. Levamisole can be administered to chickens in half the daily consumption of drinking water at either 36 or 48 mg/kg. This dose clears more than 95% of adult forms of *Ascaridia galli, Heterakis gallinarum,* and *Capillaria obsignata* and apparently eliminates a high percentage of the immature adults and larval stages of these parasites as well. At this dosage, the drug is palatable and without toxic signs in birds. Oral administration of levamisole via drinking water is also an effective means of eliminating the fowl eyeworm (*Osyspirura mansoni*). Application of several drops of a 10% solution directly to the eye is nonirritating to the bird, yet completely and rapidly effective in killing the parasites.

Tetramisole is effective against the gapeworm (*Syngamus trachea*). Practically all worms will be expelled from the mouths of turkeys about 16 hours after they have access to medicated water. The water should provide 3.6 mg tetramisole/kg/day and treatment should be continued for 3 days.

DOGS. Although levamisole is not approved for use in dogs, oral treatment with 10 mg tetramisole/kg/day for 2 days removed more than 95% of ascarids (*Toxocara, Toxascaris*) and hookworms (*Ancylostoma, Uncinaria*). Levamisole is not effective against canine whipworms (*Trichuris vulpis*).

Levamisole (Tramisol Sheep Wormer oblet) has been used in dogs as a heartworm microfilaricide at a dosage of 5.5 mg/kg twice daily (12-hr interval) for 6 days (or up to 15 days for persistent microfilaremias). Vomiting and other adverse reactions frequently accompany this regimen. Levamisole's utility as a microfilaricide largely has been displaced by extra-label use of macrocyclic lactones for the same purpose.

ZOO ANIMALS. The anthelmintic activity of tetramisole and levamisole has been tested in a variety of zoo animals. For such applications, critical trials involving necropsy are not possible, so the percentage of efficacy is usually based on parasite egg count reductions. Several major ruminant parasites (*Haemonchus, Bunostomum, Bosicola, Cooperia*) are removed (90–100%) by either oral or SC administration of tetramisole (5 mg/kg).

SAFETY AND TOXICITY. Tetramisole and levamisole have a much narrower safety range than the BZD anthelmintics. Nevertheless, tetramisole itself has a safety margin variously estimated to be two to six times the therapeutic dose of 15 mg/kg; the safety factor of levamisole is about twice that of the parent compound because levamisole is similarly active against parasites at half the dosage.

Tetramisole is lethal to sheep at a dose of 90 mg/kg. Signs suggestive of organophosphate poisoning (salivation, lacrimation, head shaking, muscle tremors, mild excitability) occur in sheep at a dose of 45 mg/kg. An occasional sheep dies even at doses of only 30–50 mg/kg. Repeated daily doses of 20 mg/kg orally or 15 mg/kg subcutaneously in lambs cause no evidence of cumulative effect over a period of 1 month.

Side effects or death are more likely to occur when tetramisole is administered parenterally. The acute oral and SC LD_{50}'s in the mouse are 253 and 100 mg/kg, respectively. Cattle appear to be somewhat more tolerant of parenteral administration of tetramisole than sheep. A twofold overdose of injectable levamisole phosphate may cause about two-thirds of treated cattle to lick their lips and to develop temporary foaming of the muzzle.

The pour-on formulation has been tested on several thousand cattle with only occasional dermal irritation. Lesions include scaling, fissures, and sloughing of necrotic epidermal layers. Healing occurs without scar formation.

Levamisole given to pigs at three times the recommended dosage causes only occasional vomiting. Vomiting as well as coughing may be seen following therapeutic doses if pigs are infected with mature lungworms (*Metastrongylus* spp.). In such cases, reaction is due to expulsion of the worms and should terminate in several hours. The LD_{50} of SC levamisole in pigs is 40 mg/kg. Simultaneous administration of dichlorvos (an organophosphate) does not alter the LD_{50} value, but simultaneous administration of pyrantel tartrate (a nicotine-like drug) enhances toxicity by lowering the levamisole LD_{50} value to 27.5 mg/kg.

Chickens tolerate tetramisole and levamisole very well. The LD_{50} for chickens is quite high (2.75 g tetramisole/kg), and minimum toxic levels of the drug in chickens exceed 640 mg/kg. In geese, however, a dosage of 300 mg/kg is known to be toxic. In chickens, therapeutic doses of levamisole (36–40 mg/kg) cause no undesirable side effects, and egg production, fertility, and hatchability are not affected adversely. Captive birds in general do not seem to tolerate levamisole as well as chickens; 66 mg/kg may be lethal for some birds.

Tetramisole has a narrow margin of safety in horses and is not approved for use in this species. A single dose of 20 mg/kg may cause deaths.

Dogs and cats are much more tolerant of oral than parenteral administration of tetramisole. When given orally to dogs, doses of 20 mg/kg are well tolerated, and even 40 and 80 mg/kg are not fatal, although vomiting occurs. When given subcutaneously, however, tetramisole at 40 mg/kg is fatal to dogs in 10–15 minutes; even at 20 mg/kg, the drug causes severe reactions in dogs, although they persist for only about 20 minutes. On the basis of these findings, the oral route of administration is recommended for dogs and cats.

CONTRAINDICATIONS. Neither tetramisole nor levamisole should be administered within specified time periods before slaughtering swine, cattle, or sheep. Milk from dairy cows apparently is free of residues of levamisole or tetramisole within 48 hours, but the FDA has not established a withdrawal time for lactating dairy cows. Consequently, products containing these drugs should not be administered to lactating cattle producing milk for human consumption.

There are no specific contraindications in administration of levamisole or tetramisole with other drugs. Some commercial preparations have combined two drugs for oral administration; e.g., Nilzan contains tetramisole and oxyclozanide, a fasciolicide.

DOSAGE AND ADMINISTRATION. In cattle, sheep, goats, and pigs, a dosage of 15 mg/kg tetramisole is recommended, but not to exceed a total of 4.5 g for cattle in a single oral or SC dose.

In cattle, sheep, goats, and pigs, a dose of 8 mg/kg levamisole is recommended in a single oral or SC dose and 10 mg/kg as a pour-on for cattle.

TETRAHYDROPYRIMIDINES

Pyrantel. *Pyrantel,* INN, was introduced as a broad-spectrum anthelmintic in 1966, initially for use against GI parasites of sheep. It subsequently has been developed for use in cattle, swine, horses, dogs, and cats. It has FDA approval for all of the above species except cattle.

CHEMISTRY. Pyrantel is an imidazothiazole derivative. Its chemical formula is *E*-1,4,5,6-tetrahydro-1-methyl-2[2-(2-thienyl)vinyl]-pyrimidine. It is prepared

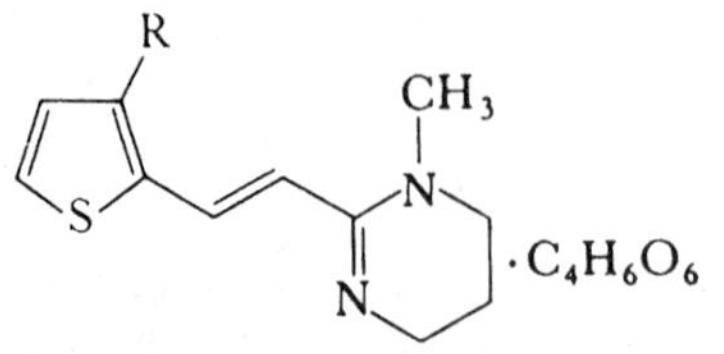

Pyrantel tartrate, R = H
Morantel tartrate, R = CH_3

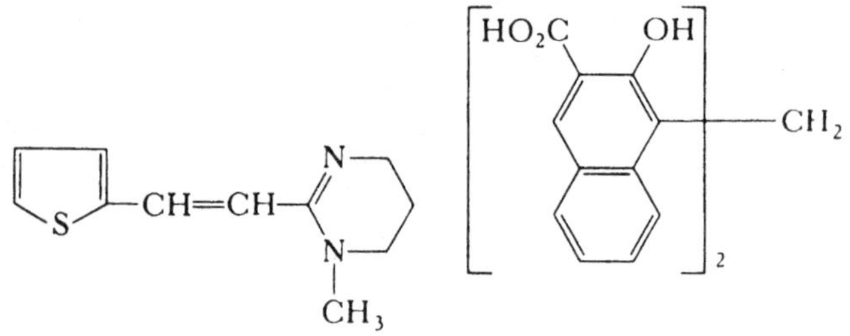

Pyrantel pamoate

FIG. 47.2

for commercial use as the tartrate (Banminth, Strongid, Strongid C) or pamoate salt (*Pyrantel Pamoate,* USP, Strongid Paste, Pyraminth, Nemex-2, Anthelban). The structural formulas of the tartrate and pamoate salts of pyrantel and the methyl-substituted analog morantel are given in Fig. 47.2.

Pyrantel salts are relatively stable in the solid phase; aqueous solutions, however, are subject to photoisomerization upon exposure to light, with resultant loss of potency. It is recommended that drench suspensions be used immediately after preparation.

PHARMACOKINETICS. Following oral administration, pyrantel tartrate is well absorbed in the pig, dog, and rat. There is less absorption of the drug by ruminants. Concentrations of radioactivity from labeled drug are maximal in plasma of the dog and pig at 2–3 hours after dosing but are highly variable in ruminants. The dog achieves the highest plasma levels (4.3 μg/mL). The drug is quickly metabolized in the body, little surviving intact by the time it is excreted.

Urinary excretion of pyrantel accounts for about 40% of the dose in the dog and 34% in the pig, most of which is excreted as metabolites. The dog is the only species excreting more of the drug or its metabolites in urine than in feces. In ruminants, urinary excretion accounts for about 25% of the original dose, much of the remainder passing unchanged in feces. In rats, urinary excretion of the drug is minor; bile is the major route of excretion of metabolites of the absorbed drug.

The pamoate salt of pyrantel is poorly soluble in water, which offers the advantage of reduced absorption from the gut. This allows the drug to reach the lower end of the intestine and to exert activity against parasites in that locale, such as pinworms. Formulations of pyrantel pamoate are beneficial for use against pinworm infections of humans and horses.

Pharmacologic effects of pyrantel tartrate on the host are similar to effects of levamisole, diethylcarbamazine citrate, and morantel tartrate. All of these anthelmintics share biologic properties with ACh and act essentially by mimicking the effects of excessive amounts of this natural neurotransmitter. In physiologic amounts, ACh serves as a neurotransmitter by stimulating all autonomic ganglia, the adrenal medullas, the chemoreceptors of the carotid and aortic bodies, and the neuromuscular junction. With excess amounts of ACh, however, these sites are paralyzed. Pyrantel, morantel, levamisole, and diethylcarbamazine mimic this paralytic action. It is similar to the paralytic effect caused by nicotine; thus the action of these anthelmintics is referred to as nicotine-like. In anesthetized dogs, use of these anthelmintics results in a precipitous pressor response and enhancement of rate and depth of respiration. These effects are antagonized by hexamethonium, and the pressor responses are nullified by the adrenergic blocking agent phentolamine.

MODE OF ACTION. Pyrantel tartrate is a depolarizing neuromuscular blocking agent in nematode parasites and the vertebrate host. The drug probably produces paralysis of worms by causing contracture of the musculature similar to the action of ACh. Pyrantel and morantel are 100 times more potent than ACh, although slower in initiating contraction. The effect of ACh is easily reversible; that of pyrantel or morantel is not.

FORMULATIONS AND ADMINISTRATION. Both the tartrate and pamoate salts of pyrantel are used for treating horses. Pyrantel tartrate is generally administered as a top-dressed pellet. The amount of pellet formulation necessary to yield a single dose of 12.5 mg/kg is mixed in an amount of feed normally consumed at one feeding. Pyrantel tartrate as Strongid C is formulated for continuous, daily administration over prolonged periods of parasite exposure. The medicated alfalfa/molasses pellets are fed once a day with the grain ration to effect a daily dosage of 2.64 mg/kg body weight.

Pyrantel pamoate can be administered in suspension or paste formulations, as well as by mixing with feed. Regardless of the method of administration, a dose of 6.6 mg pyrantel base/kg should be used. The compound contains 34.6% base activity.

A powdered premix formulation containing 10.6% pyrantel tartrate is available for treating parasitic infections of swine via medicated feed. A dosage of 22 mg/kg is used for a single therapeutic treatment. It is recommended that a sufficient quantity (i.e., 0.88 g/40 kg) of the powder formulation be added to a 1 kg meal ration (nonpelleted) after an overnight fast. Large quantities of medicated feed for the single therapeutic treatment can be prepared by adding 800 g of pyrantel tartrate to 900 kg feed. A hog consuming 1 kg medicated feed/40 kg essentially receives a dose of 22 mg/kg. Swine consume the medicated feed without reluctance. Water should be available ad libitum during the fasting and treatment periods.

Pyrantel premix also is used to prepare medicated feed that is used to prevent swine parasites. A 0.016% medicated feed (96 g pyrantel/900 kg feed) can be fed to swine continuously as an aid in prevention of migration and establishment of *Ascaris suum* and *Oesophagostomum* infections.

Formulations of pyrantel pamoate for dogs include a suspension form (Nemex-2) and a tablet form (Purina Tablets), both administered at 5–10 mg/kg. Pyrantel pamoate (5 mg/kg) is also combined with febantel (25 mg/kg) and praziquantel (5 mg/kg) in a tablet form for dogs as Drontal Plus. Each of the above formulations is given to dogs as a single dose. A higher dose of pyrantel pamoate (20 mg/kg) is combined with praziquantel (5 mg/kg) as Drontal for cats.

Administration with food delays passage through the digestive tract, prolongs contact time of the drug with parasites, and thereby increases efficacy. Autoradiography studies (Mackenstedt et al. 1993) with adult and preadult stages of *Toxocara canis* proved that preadult nematodes continuously absorbed the drug through the whole body surface and that duration of exposure to the drug is more important in efficacy than variations in dosage.

A third formulation for dogs is a beef-based chewable form that combines ivermectin (6–12 μg/kg) for control of heartworms and pyrantel pamoate (5–10 mg/kg) for control of hookworms and ascarids. This form (Heartgard-30 Plus) is administered once a month.

Anthelmintic Spectrum

HORSES. In general, activity of pyrantel on GI parasites of the horse and pony is independent of the method of administration or the salt, i.e., tartrate or pamoate. Activity of each of the two salts is characterized by consistently high efficacies for *Parascaris equorum* (mature worms, 86–100%; immature worms, 100%), *Strongylus vulgaris* (92–100%), *Strongylus equinus* (100%), and the pinworm *Probstmayria vivipara* (93–99%). Lower efficacy exists against *Strongylus edentatus* (42–100%), small strongyles (69–99%), and mature (7–100%) and immature (33–100%) *Oxyuris equi.*

Pyrantel is ~95% effective against the ileocecal tapeworm (*Anoplocephala perfoliata*) at double the regular therapeutic dosage (i.e., 13.2 mg/kg). It has little activity against equine stomach worms (*Habronema muscae, Draschia megastoma,* and *Trichostrongylus axei*) or *Strongyloides westeri.* It is also inactive against botfly larvae (*Gasterophilus* spp.).

Administration of pyrantel tartrate (Strongid C) in the feed on a daily basis is very effective in controlling adult and fourth-stage larval infections of the large strongyles, small strongyles, ascarids, and pinworms in equids and effectively reduces pasture contamination. Its efficacy against the early larval stages of *Strongylus vulgaris* and *Parascaris equorum* reduces migratory damage in the mesenteric arteries and liver/lungs, respectively. Foals can begin prophylaxis with this drug at 2 or 3 months of age, when grain intake is sufficient, and can be maintained indefinitely. However, reports of decreased efficacy of daily pyrantel tartrate in young horses suggest that rotation to other drug classes annually is prudent.

As a general caveat, continuous use of a single drug class may select for anthelmintic resistance, and prolonged use of a prophylactic regimen may result in antigenic naivete of host animals. Exposure to infective stages of nematode parasites seems to impart some degree of resistance, even if those infections are subsequently aborted by anthelmintic treatment directed against preadult stages. Foals that have been reared on daily Strongid C appear to be more susceptible to parasite challenge than foals treated bimonthly or never treated previously.

SWINE. Pyrantel tartrate is used in swine principally for its activity against infections of *Ascaris* and *Oesophagostomum.* When offered in the feed at a dosage of 22 mg/kg, it is effective against *A. suum* adults and histotrophic stages, as well as infective ascarid larva that hatch in the gut lumen from ingested eggs. By killing ascarid larvae before they penetrate the gut wall, liver scarring associated with larval migration is reduced. Thus pyrantel tartrate provides prophylactic as well as therapeutic benefits against swine ascarids, especially when fed continuously at low levels (96 g/900 kg feed).

The same dosage is effective against developing *Oesophagostomum* larvae in the walls of the intestine. Development of larval nodular worms negatively impacts the health and productivity of growing swine, and the associated lesions ("pimply gut") render the gut unsuitable for use as sausage casings. A single therapeutic dose of the drug is reported to be 99% effective for the lumen stages of *Oesophagostomum* organisms but ineffective for swine whipworms. The citrate salt of pyrantel has similar efficacy to that of pyrantel tartrate in swine and is marketed in some countries.

SHEEP AND CATTLE. Pyrantel tartrate is effective as a broad-spectrum anthelmintic in ruminants. Specifically, it is effective in sheep, cattle, and goats against *Haemonchus contortus* (including BZD-resistant strains), *Ostertagia ostertagi* and *O. circumcincta, Trichostrongylus axei* and *T. colubriformis, Nematodirus battus* and *N. spathiger, Cooperia* spp., and *Bunostomum* spp. Its activity against *Oesophagostomum* spp. and *Chabertia* spp. is usually but not consistently good.

The activity of pyrantel against immature and larval stages of many ruminant parasites is not known. It has been determined, however, that the therapeutic dose of 25 mg/kg is more than 99% effective against 7-day-old, 81% effective against 14-day-old, and 94% effective against 21-day-old stages of *T. colubriformis* in sheep. It is less effective against these same stages in cattle. The drug is 100% effective for *N. battus,* whether the parasites are 7, 14, or 21 days of age.

For *Ostertagia* infections, pyrantel is highly effective against mature worms and any immature stages that dwell in the lumen. Nevertheless, pyrantel has low activity (42%) against 7-day-old histotrophic stages of *Ostertagia* spp. in sheep and is even less effective against the same stage in cattle.

In addition to its therapeutic use, pyrantel can be used prophylactically in sheep at a dosage of 3 mg/kg/day. Approximately 97% fewer GI worms occurred in medicated sheep than in untreated controls examined after a 50-day period.

DOGS AND CATS. Pyrantel pamoate is effective (95%) against the common hookworms (*Ancylostoma caninum, Uncinaria stenocephala*) and ascarids (*Toxocara canis, Toxascaris leonina*) of dogs at single doses of 5 mg base/kg. Efficacy is inconsistent in pups, so a higher dose (15 mg/kg) is recommended 30 minutes after a light meal. Pups can be treated while suckling (e.g., 2, 4, 6, and 8 weeks of age) to control parasites acquired prenatally or lactogenically.

Pyrantel pamoate has limited efficacy against canine whipworms and no activity against tapeworms or heartworms. By combining pyrantel pamoate with praziquantel and febantel (Drontal Plus), tapeworms as well as whipworms can be eliminated from dogs, in addition to hookworms and ascarids. Drontal Plus is approved for use in dogs as young as 3 weeks of age. Treatment can be repeated at 2-week intervals during exposure to infective stages of parasites from the bitch or environment.

In cats, pyrantel pamoate at 20 mg/kg is effective against the common hookworm (*Ancylostoma tubaeforme*) and ascarid (*T. cati*) and is clinically safe in 4- to 6-week-old kittens at 100 mg/kg for 3 consecutive days. Pyrantel pamoate (20 mg/kg) is combined with praziquantel (5 mg/kg) in tablet form (Drontal) to control hookworm, ascarid, and tapeworm infections in cats.

SAFETY AND TOXICITY. In general, the salts of pyrantel are free of toxic effects in all hosts at doses up to approximately 7 times the therapeutic dose. The oral LD_{50} of pyrantel tartrate is 175 mg/kg in mice and 170 mg/kg in rats. In dogs, the acute oral LD_{50} for pyrantel pamoate is greater than 690 mg/kg (138 times the therapeutic dose). In chronic toxicity studies, dogs showed ill effects when administered pyrantel tartrate at 50 or more mg/kg/day for 3 months but no adverse effects when the dosage was reduced to 20 mg/kg/day for the same period.

Pyrantel is safe for horses and ponies of all ages, including sucklings, weanlings, pregnant mares, and stallions. At 20 times the recommended dose in horses, ponies, and foals, pyrantel pamoate shows no adverse clinical effects or changes in blood cell values or serum chemistry parameters.

Pyrantel tartrate is slightly less tolerated in horses than the pamoate salt. The tartrate salt (100 mg/kg) produced death in one of three horses. Toxic signs preceding death included a marked increase in respiration rate, profuse sweating, and incoordination. No signs of toxicosis occurred following administration of 75 mg/kg. Ataxia is seen in some cattle treated with a high dose of pyrantel tartrate (200 mg/kg). The toxic dose of the drug in pigs is not known.

CONTRAINDICATIONS. Pyrantel is not recommended for use in severely debilitated animals, presumably because its pharmacologic action (cholinergic) may be more pronounced in these hosts.

Withdrawal periods exist for swine and ruminants designated for slaughter. Because of lack of metabolism data in horses, the drug should not be used in horses intended for human consumption.

Despite its cholinergic properties, there is no clinical evidence that simultaneous use of organophosphates increases toxicity. Thus labeling for pyrantel products indicates safety for simultaneous use with insecticides, tranquilizers, muscle relaxants, and central nervous system (CNS) depressants.

DOSAGE. Dosages for Pyrantel tartrate are as follows:

Horses: single therapeutic dose, 12.5 mg/kg; continuous dosing, 2.64 mg/kg/day

Swine: 22 mg/kg; maximum of 2 g/animal

Sheep, cattle, goats: 25 mg/kg

Dosages for Pyrantel pamoate are as follows:

Horses: 6.6 mg base/kg

Dogs: suspension and chewable form, 5 mg base/kg; tablets, 5 mg/kg for dogs over 2.2 kg but 10–15 mg/kg for dogs less than 2.2 kg (with a light meal)

Morantel. *Morantel,* INN (Banminth II), is the methyl ester analog of pyrantel; it is primarily formulated as the tartrate salt for veterinary anthelmintic use. The structural formula of morantel tartrate is presented in Fig. 47.2.

The salts of morantel have greater anthelmintic activity than the parent compound, pyrantel; but their pharmacologic properties are similar. Efficacy of the tartrate salt is quite good against adult and immature stages of *Haemonchus, Ostertagia, Trichostrongylus, Cooperia,* and *Nematodirus* organisms of ruminants. In the USA, morantel tartrate is marketed as a type A medicated premix (Morantel Premix-88) containing 88 g morantel/lb. Sufficient premix is added to a ration to provide from 0.44 to 4.4 g per pound of complete feed, which is fed to deliver 0.44 g/100 lb body weight. Slaughter withdrawal periods are 14 and 30 days for cattle and goats, respectively.

A sustained-release bolus of morantel tartrate (Paratect Flex Diffuser) for both dairy and beef cattle is widely used in Europe and has been approved in the USA. The drug (11.8 g morantel base) is packaged in a cylindrical trilaminate cartridge, which is administered orally by a special delivery device and is retained in the rumen/reticulum. The permeable wall allows continuous release of morantel tartrate (approximately 150 mg/day) into the rumen/reticulum fluid for at least 90 days. Administration of the cartridge is recommended at the beginning of the grazing season so that as overwintered larvae are acquired from pasture, they will be prevented from establishing patent infections in cattle. Existing adult worm burdens in cattle are also eliminated. The ultimate effect is marked reduction in pasture contamination for a prolonged period, e.g., 90 days of drug release and benefits that extend for another 90 days. Numerous field studies in Europe, the UK, Canada, and the USA have demonstrated significantly greater weight gains and less parasite-induced production loss in cattle during their first and second grazing seasons than in nontreated controls. Inhibited *Ostertagia* larvae are not killed by this method of treatment, but lowered pasture contamination helps prevent development of type II ostertagosis.

Pharmacologically, morantel tartrate is a safer drug than pyrantel tartrate. The oral LD_{50} of pyrantel for mice is only 170 mg/kg while that of morantel is 5 g/kg. Chronic toxicity studies indicate that doses up to 4 times the therapeutic dose for sheep for 60 days and 2.5 times that for cattle for 20 days produce no toxic signs. Following a single therapeutic dose (10 mg/kg) via medicated feed (Rumatel), the drug is barely detectable (<0.05 mg/mL) in plasma or milk of lactating cattle and goats. That which is absorbed from the abomasum and proximal small intestine is quickly metabolized, presumably in the liver, and excreted in the urine within 96 hours; the remainder of the dose is excreted in feces.

Negligible or absent levels of morantel tartrate in plasma and milk following single or sustained administration allow use of this drug in lactating dairy animals without a milk withdrawal restriction.

ORGANOPHOSPHATE COMPOUNDS. In general, organophosphate compounds had their origins as pesticides and only subsequently found use as anthelmintics. Six such compounds have been used as anthelmintics in domestic animals: dichlorvos, trichlorfon, haloxon, coumaphos, naphthalophos, and crufomate. The first two were used primarily in horses, and the latter four in ruminants.

Mode of Action. The main effect of organophosphate compounds on nematode parasites is inhibition of acetylcholinesterase (AChE), leading to interference with neuromuscular transmission and subsequent paralysis. Nematodes utilize ACh as a neurotransmitter, and the enzyme acetylcholinesterase (AChE) serves to terminate transmission by destroying ACh. In very dilute amounts, organophosphate drugs are able to bind the AChE of nematodes. In the absence of functional AChE, the neurotransmission initiated by ACh persists, and coordinated feeding activities cease. These assumptions are made because a direct correlation is known to exist between inhibition of AChE of certain parasites by organophosphate drugs and toxicity of the same drug for the parasite. Knowles and Casida (1966) tested a large number of organophosphates in *Ascaris.* Drugs that were poisonous to the parasite also inhibited parasite AChE. Conversely, drugs that did not inhibit AChE were not toxic.

Acetylcholinesterases of host and parasite and of different species of parasites vary in their affinity for, and susceptibility to, organophosphate drugs. For example, AChE of *Haemonchus contortus* forms an irreversible complex with the organophosphate haloxon, which results in toxicity to the worm and eventual expulsion from treated cattle. Conversely, AChE of ascarids is not as susceptible to haloxon as that of *Haemonchus.* Ascarid AChE is bound by haloxon, but it is a reversible complex, and the ascarid enzymatic activity recovers to near pretreatment levels within 32 hours after treatment with haloxon. Nevertheless, this is sufficient time for worms to be expelled effectively by peristalsis. Even shorter periods of incapacitation result when the drug is used against *Nematodirus* and *Oesophagostomum columbianum,* and the efficacy of haloxon for these parasites is generally poor.

The relative safety of various organophosphates is probably correlated to lack of binding susceptibility of host AChE for the drug. The complex formed between sheep erythrocyte AChE and haloxon, for example, is quickly reversible, which may account for the lack of toxicity of therapeutic doses in sheep. Conversely, haloxon is very toxic to geese; indeed, the brain AChE of geese is found to be irreversibly complexed by the drug. These findings illustrate that the AChE enzymes differ among vertebrate hosts and certainly between hosts and their nematode parasites. An attempt has been made to exploit this information in the development of organophosphate anthelmintics in order to produce compounds with maximum anthelmintic efficacy but minimal host toxicity.

General Efficacy. Organophosphate compounds generally remove the principal parasites of horses, pigs, and dogs but are somewhat deficient in their activity against parasites of ruminants. In cattle and sheep, the organophosphates generally have satisfactory efficacy for nematode parasites of the abomasum (especially *Haemonchus*) and small intestine but lack satisfactory efficacy for parasites of the large intestine (*Oesophagostomum, Chabertia*). Where the latter infections are prevalent, it is recommended that cattle or sheep be treated with a nonorganophosphate, broad-spectrum anthelmintic after two consecutive treatments with organophosphate compounds (e.g., haloxon or naphthalophos). It is also advisable to alternate organophosphate anthelmintics with dewormers of other classes to prevent development of organophosphate resistance by target parasites.

Safety and Toxicity. Certain precautions should be followed when using organophosphate anthelmintics. Animals should not be treated simultaneously (or within a few days) with other AChE-inhibiting drugs (e.g., eserine and prostigmine), pesticides, organophosphate or carbamate insecticides, muscle relaxants (e.g., succinylcholine), or certain sedatives (e.g., acepromazine). In cases where concurrent use of an organophosphate anthelmintic and some topical insecticide is indicated, the insecticidal options should be limited to pyrethrins, pyrethroids, certain botanical compounds, or chlorinated hydrocarbons.

The margin of safety of organophosphate anthelmintics is generally less than that of the broad-spectrum anthelmintics (BZDs, macrocyclic lactones, and imidazothiazoles), so strict attention to dosing is necessary. This is important not only for safety of the animal but also because higher than normal doses can result in illegal residues of the drug in animal tissues and milk. Due to the potential for residues, most organophosphate compounds (except coumaphos) are not approved for use in lactating dairy animals, and a withdrawal time of at least 7 days is required before slaughter. Use of organophosphates within 30 days of parturition is not recommended, especially in horses.

Toxic signs of organophosphate poisoning include frequent defecation and urination, plus vomiting (especially in dogs and cats), watering of eyes, and muscular twitching. Subsequently, salivation, diarrhea, and muscular weakness occur. Toxic signs are more likely to develop in sick or stressed animals, such as those recently shipped, dehorned, castrated, or weaned within the preceding 3 weeks. Use of organophosphate anthelmintics is usually contraindicated in such animals. When toxic signs occur, atropine or 2-PAM (pralidoxime) are antidotal.

Specific Organophosphate Anthelmintics. Numerous organophosphate anthelmintics have been marketed for use in domestic animals over the years. These include dichlorvos and trichlorfon for horses, and coumaphos, naphthalophos, haloxon, and crufomate for ruminants. Organophosphate anthelmintics have come into disfavor in recent years for several reasons. Efficacy of organophosphates typically is not broad spectrum, these compounds have a narrower margin of safety than many other drug classes, and their use is associated with more contraindications. Some nematodes of sheep and goats have developed resistance to organophosphates, and therapeutic doses are no longer effective.

The only currently used organophosphate compound to be discussed here is dichlorvos in dogs, cats, and swine. For detailed discussions of specific organophosphate dewormers, interested readers are referred to the 7th edition of this text (Courtney and Roberson 1995).

DICHLORVOS. *Dichlorvos,* INN (Atgard, Task, Task Tabs), is very volatile and degrades rapidly in the proximal alimentary tract. This fate can be delayed by incorporating dichlorvos into polyvinyl chloride resin pellets. This formulation allows dichlorvos to be released slowly from the indigestible pellets as they travel with ingesta and provides for therapeutic concentrations throughout the digestive tract. This slow-release formulation of dichlorvos also provides a safety factor for the host because drug can be detoxified gradually as it is absorbed over a 2- to 3-day period, rather than as a sudden, concentrated dose.

Dichlorvos is principally used as an anthelmintic in dogs, cats, and swine. A chief advantage of dichlorvos over other anthelmintics in dogs and swine is its efficacy against whipworms (*Trichuris* spp.). Dichlorvos was formerly used for equine internal parasites, including ascarids, large and small strongyles, pinworms, and *Gasterophilus* larvae, but its manufacture and distribution in the USA have been discontinued.

CHEMISTRY. Dichlorvos (or dichlorovos) chemically is *O,O*-dimethyl *O*-(2,2-dichlorovinyl) phosphate (DDVP). It is a volatile substance easily destroyed by oxidizing agents and/or moisture (hydrolysis). It must be stored below temperatures of 27° C to ensure proper shelf life. The compound is prepared by reacting trimethylphosphite with chloral. Analogs of DDVP can be prepared by reaction of chloral with other trialkyl phosphites. Vinyl phosphates are generally recognized for their insecticidal properties; DDVP has efficacy against nematodes as well.

FORMULATIONS. The process of incorporating DDVP or other liquids into vinyl resins (usually polyvinyl chloride) is called plasticization. This procedure permits DDVP to be incorporated into a plastic (resin) vehicle, which is then cut into small pellets to prepare a stable, slow-release formulation. When an animal ingests medicated pellets, diffusion of the volatile DDVP from pellets results in a concentration gradient of the active drug. As the indigestible pellets traverse the GI tract, DDVP continues to diffuse into the surrounding fluid medium, which allows the drug to come into contact with helminths located throughout the alimentary tract. Continual depletion of the drug gradually reduces the concentration gradient, so there is a corresponding decrease in the diffusion rate. Pellets containing 20% DDVP formulated for a moderate release rate will release approximately 48% of the incorporated DDVP in a 48-hour period as they traverse the digestive tract of swine. When passed in feces 48–96 hours after ingestion, the pellets still contain approximately 45–50% of the original quantity of DDVP. The drug continues to be released into the fecal mass, and residual dichlorvos may be sufficient to act as an insecticide against filth fly larvae.

The geometry, size, and method of formulation of the pellet, plus the quantity of DDVP incorporated, allow for a range of diffusion rates suitable for different host animals. For example, pellets formulated for dogs (Task) are smaller in size to allow faster release of the drug in the short canine digestive tract, in comparison to larger pellets (Atgard V) that have a moderate release rate in the longer digestive tract of swine.

ANTHELMINTIC SPECTRUM

Dogs and Cats. DDVP causes total expulsion of canine and/or feline hookworms (*Ancylostoma caninum, A. braziliense, A. tubaeforme, Uncinaria stenocephala*) and ascarids (*Toxocara canis, T. cati, Toxascaris leonina*).

Canine whipworms (*Trichuris vulpis*) are removed by granule and capsule formulations (which contain resin pellets) but not by tablets. Greater than 90% efficacy results when canine whipworm numbers are fewer than approximately 100. When the burden exceeds 100 worms, effectiveness of DDVP often is reduced and retreatment may be necessary.

Swine. DDVP was the first broad-spectrum anthelmintic for use in swine. Different formulations of DDVP at the recommended dosage are effective in removing greater than 90% of the fourth-stage larvae, juveniles, and mature adults of *Ascaris suum,* the swine nodular worm (*Oesophagostomum*), the whipworm (*Trichuris suis*), and mature forms of two stomach worms (*Hyostrongylus rubidus, Ascarops strongylina*). DDVP is 71–100% effective against mature *Strongyloides ransomi* but is not effective in treatment for the thorny-headed worm (*Macracanthorhynchus hirudinaceus*). There is little or no activity against larval nematodes migrating or buried in the intestinal mucosa. Hatchability of strongylid eggs passed in swine feces is not affected by the presence of DDVP resin pellets. However, there is a detrimental effect upon a portion of the freshly hatched and free-living *Oesophagostomum* larvae.

Other. For additional information about the spectrum of activity of dichlorvos in other host species, please refer to the 7th edition of this text (Courtney and Roberson 1995).

MACROCYCLIC LACTONES (MACROLIDE ENDECTOCIDES). As the latter name implies, this class of compounds has activity against both internal and external parasites, specifically nematodes and arthropods. They are not panaceas, however, and have no activity against cestodes, trematodes, or protozoa. The macrocyclic lactones are fermentation products, or derivatives thereof, from soil-dwelling fungi of the genus *Streptomyces.* In addition to having broad-spectrum activity, they are effective at very low concentrations.

Chemistry. The macrocyclic lactones comprise two major groups, the avermectins and milbemycins. The avermectins are fermentation products of *Streptomyces avermitilis* and have the 16-membered macrocycle replaced by a spiroketal unit at C-17 to C-28, a hexahydrobenzofuran at C-2 to C-8a, and a bisoleandrosyl oxydisaccharide at C-13. The milbemycins, fermentation products of two species of fungi, are similar to the avermectins but lack the C-13 disaccharide substituent. Both milbemycin D and milbemycin oxime are produced by *Streptomyces hygroscopicus aureolacrimosus.* The nemadectins, a subgroup of milbemycins, are fermentation products of *Streptomyces cyanogriseus noncyanogenus.* Nemadectins differ from the milbemycins proper in that they contain a trisubstituted double bond at C-26 in their side chains. Five avermectins (abamectin, doramectin, eprinomectin, ivermectin, and selamectin) and two milbemycins (milbemycin oxime and moxidectin) are currently marketed.

Mode of action. It was originally believed that the macrolide endectocides increased the release of γ-aminobutyric acid (GABA) from synaptosomes of the nervous system. This, in turn, opened GABA-gated chloride channels. It is now known that the macrocyclic lactones bind selectively and with high affinity to glutamate-gated chloride ion channels in invertebrate nerve and muscle cells. These channels may occur in close anatomic proximity to GABA-gated sites. Macrocyclic lactones may potentiate GABA-gated sites as well at higher dosages. About 50% of the effect of a macrocyclic lactone can be reversed with picrotoxin, a GABA antagonist active at the chloride channel. In nematodes, the synapse between inhibitory interneurons and excitatory motor neurons is the primary site of action, whereas the myoneural junction is the primary site in arthropods. In either case, chloride ion influx lowers cell membrane resistance and causes a slight hyperpolarization of the resting potential of postsynaptic cells. This interferes with transmission of neural stimuli to muscles, resulting in flaccid paralysis of affected parasites, followed by their death or expulsion.

Macrocyclic lactones also interfere with the reproduction of nematode and arthropod parasites, but the mechanisms of this action are poorly understood. Examples of this activity include reduced oviposition by ticks, abnormal egg formation by nematodes of ruminants, and sterility of both male and female filarial nematodes.

Toxicity. Mammalian GABA-mediated neurotransmission occurs only in the CNS. Because macrocyclic lactones do not readily cross the mammalian blood-brain barrier, they have a wide margin of safety in most mammals. Nevertheless, toxicity may accompany overdosage in any species. Dogs of the Collie breed and certain lines of Australian Shepherds appear to be unusually sensitive to certain macrocyclic lactone anthelmintics.

Resistance. Both experimentally induced and naturally occurring avermectin-resistant strains have been reported among certain nematodes of small ruminants and arthropod pests of horticultural and agronomic crops. The degree of side-resistance among the avermectins and milbemycins is not clear, but the modes of activity are considered identical (Conder et al. 1993). Some studies have reported that ivermectin- or abamectin-resistant nematodes were susceptible to moxidectin, a milbemycin. However, Shoop (1994) argues that if dose titration studies had been designed appropriately, side-resistance between ivermectin and moxidectin would have been apparent.

Avermectins

IVERMECTIN. The avermectins are a group of chemically related macrocyclic lactones produced by fermentation of the actinomycete *Streptomyces avermitilis.* Avermectin is a complex of eight such fermentation products, each having nematocidal activity but lacking significant antibacterial or antifungal properties. Ivermectin (Cardomec, Double Impact, Equimectrin, Eqvalan, Heartgard-30, Ivomec, Mectizan, Oramec, Rotectin 1, Topline, Ultramectrin, Zimecterin) is a semisynthetic derivative of avermectin that has a broad spectrum of activity against a wide variety of arthropods and nematodes of domestic animals and humans.

CHEMISTRY. Avermectin is a mixture of four major components (avermectin A_{1a}, A_{2a}, B_{1a}, and B_{2a}) and four minor components recovered in smaller quantities (avermectin A_{1b}, A_{2b}, B_{1b}, and B_{2b}). Of these, the B_{1a} component is recovered in greatest quantity along with its B_{1b} minor homolog. Ivermectin, derived from this mixture of B_1 avermectins by saturation of the double bond between C-22 and C-23, consists of not less than 80% 22,23-dihydroavermectin B_{1a} and not more than 20% 22,23-dihydroavermectin B_{1b} (Fig. 47.3). Ivermectin (as its major component, 22,23-dihydroavermectin B_{1a}) is an off-white powder that is highly lipophilic and hydrophobic. It dissolves in most organic solvents but is poorly soluble in water. It is stable at room temperature in nonacidic solutions but is degraded by ultraviolet light.

PHARMACOKINETICS. Pharmacokinetic studies with ivermectin were summarized by Fink and Porras (1989). The pharmacokinetics of ivermectin is affected by the specific formulation used, the route of administration, and the animal species to which it is administered. The biological half-life ($t_{1/2}$) of ivermectin in plasma following IV administration of 300 μg/kg to cattle is 2.8 days. IV administration to sheep gives a similar biological half-life (2.7 days) but a lower plasma concentration due to a greater volume of distribution in sheep than in cattle (1.9 vs. 4.6 L/kg). Ivermectin is eliminated more rapidly in dogs ($t_{1/2}$ = 1.6–1.8 days).

SC administration of the commercial formulation of ivermectin to cattle at a dosage of 200 μg/kg results in a longer biological half-life ($t_{1/2}$ = 8 days) than IV administration, due to slow absorption from the injection site. A peak plasma concentration (C_p) of 44 ng/mL occurs at 2 days (T_p) after SC injection. Clinically significant anthelmintic efficacy persists for approximately 2 weeks after SC injection, depending upon parasite species. Oral dosing in sheep results in a $t_{1/2}$ of 3–5 days and T_p within 1 day. Oral dosing of dogs (100 μg/kg as a tablet) resulted in a C_p of 40 ng/mL within 2–4 hours. In a comparative bioavailability study, oral dosing of dogs with ivermectin (6 μg/kg) as a chewable tablet, either alone or in combination with pyrantel pamoate, resulted in an essentially identical C_p of about 2.4 ng/mL. Area under the plasma concentration versus time curve (AUC) was about 71 ng-hr/g, although the T_p was significantly longer for the ivermectin–pyrantel pamoate combination than for ivermectin alone (7.6 vs. 5.2 hr) (Clark et al. 1992). Studies in swine show that plasma concentrations peaked faster after oral (oral T_p = 0.5 days) than after SC (SC T_p = 2 days) administration. However, SC injection results in greater bioavailability than oral administration; the AUC for oral administration was only 41% of that for SC administration. Similarly, a pronounced difference in bioavailability was seen in horses between oral administration of a paste and an aqueous micelle formulation. The micelle attained a more rapid peak

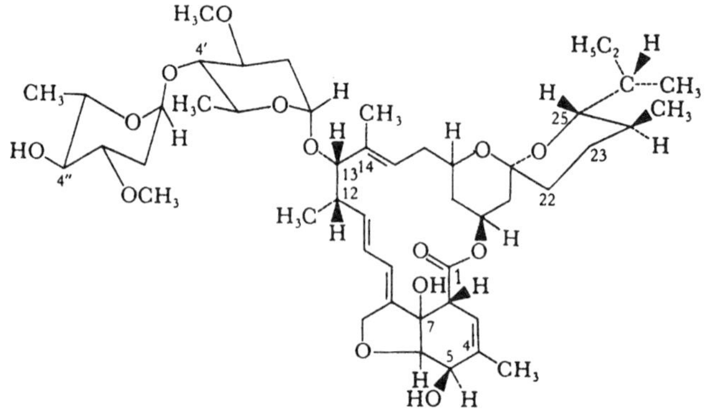

FIG. 47.3—Structure of 22,23-dihydroavermectin B_{1a}, the major component of ivermectin. Ivermectin also contains not more than 20% 22,23-dihydroavermectin B_{1b}, which is identical except that the substituent in the 25 position is *iso* propyl instead of *sec* butyl. Abamectin consists of two components identical to those of ivermectin except the bond between C-22 and C-23 in each abamectin component is not saturated.

concentration (micelle T_p = 4–5 hr; paste T_p = 15 hr) and greater bioavailability than the paste (AUC 20% greater for the micelle).

Following administration, ivermectin residues are lowest in brain and highest in liver, bile, and fat (Chiu and Lu 1989). Depletion half-lives were 4.8 and 7.6 days for liver and fat, respectively, in cattle. Tissue redistribution patterns are similar for sheep, swine, and rats, but depletion half-lives for liver and fat are shorter in sheep and rats than in cattle or swine. Tissue redistribution is not affected by route of administration (SC, intrarumenal, or oral) in cattle. The parent drug is the major liver residue for 3, 5, 7, and 14 days after dosing in rats, sheep, swine, and cattle, respectively. This pattern is identical for fat except that the parent drug is the major metabolite for only 3 days in sheep. In cattle, sheep, and rats, the major liver metabolites are 24-hydroxy-methyl-22,23-dihydroavermectin-B_{1a} and its monosaccharide and B_{1b} equivalents. The major metabolites in swine, 3″-*O*-desmethyl derivatives of 22,23-dihydroavermectin-B_{1a} and -B_{1b}, are identical in liver and fat. Fecal excretion is the main route of elimination, accounting for more than 98% of excreted ivermectin, with the remainder appearing in the urine. In lactating females, up to 5% of the dose may be excreted in milk.

MODE OF ACTION. See the previous general discussion on mode of action of macrocyclic lactones.

FORMULATIONS. Various regulatory agencies have approved ivermectin for use in humans, horses, cattle, sheep, pigs, dogs, cats, reindeer, bison, and camels. Additionally, extensive extra-label use is made of ivermectin in various minor domestic species as well as in captive and free-ranging wildlife.

Ivomec Injection (Double Impact; Ultramectrin) is a sterile solution containing 1% ivermectin (*w/v*) in an organic vehicle containing 60% propylene glycol and 40% glycerol formal for administration by SC injection to cattle, sheep, and swine. A 0.27% (*w/v*) injectable formulation is used in young pigs. Ivomec (or Oramec) oral solution for sheep contains 0.08% ivermectin (*w/v*) in an aqueous micelle used as a drench. An intraruminal bolus (Ivomec SR Bolus for Cattle) contains 1.72 g ivermectin in a wax vehicle that is extruded by an osmotic pump mechanism at a rate of 12 mg/day of ivermectin for 135 days. Eqvalan (Phoenectin) liquid contains 1% ivermectin (*w/v*) in an aqueous micelle for administration to horses either as an oral drench or by nasogastric tube. Eqvalan paste (Zimecterin; Equimectrin; Rotectin 1) contains 1.87% ivermectin (*w/v*) in a vehicle of 79% propylene glycol plus inert binders for oral use in horses. Ivomec Pour-On for Cattle (Topline; Ultramectrin) contains 0.5% ivermectin (*w/v*) in an 80% isopropyl alcohol vehicle for topical administration. Ivermectin Type A Medicated Feed Article contains 0.6% ivermectin (*w/w*) and is mixed to a final maximum ivermectin concentration of 1.8 g/ton in a type C medicated feed for swine. Heartgard-30 tablets and Heartgard-30 Chewables (chewable cubes) for dogs contain either 68, 136, or 272 μg of ivermectin. Heartgard for Cats chewables contain either 55 or 165 μg of ivermectin. Heartgard-30 Plus Chewables (chewable cubes) for dogs contain either 68, 136, or 272 μg of ivermectin and 57, 114, or 227 mg of pyrantel pamoate, respectively.

ANTHELMINTIC SPECTRUM. Extremely small quantities (less than 1 mg/kg) of ivermectin are sufficient for anthelmintic activity by either the oral or the parenteral route of administration. Confirmation tests with ivermectin have indicated a wide range of efficacy against nematodes and many arthropods (Campbell and Benz 1984). The following parasites are eliminated by ivermectin: all major GI and lung nematodes and certain ectoparasites of cattle, sheep, horses, and swine; intestinal nematodes, ear mites, and sarcoptic mange of dogs; infective-stage heartworm and microfilariae of dogs; and certain GI nematodes and ectoparasites of chickens.

Cattle and Sheep. Ivermectin is administered at dosages of 0.2 mg/kg to sheep (orally) and cattle (orally or subcutaneously) or 0.5 mg/kg to cattle (topically). These regimens provide efficacies of 97–100% against adult and fourth-stage larvae of respective species of *Haemonchus, Ostertagia* (including inhibited EL_4 in cattle), *Cooperia, Trichostrongylus* (including *T. axei*), *Strongyloides, Bunostomum, Nematodirus, Trichuris, Oesophagostomum, Dictyocaulus,* and *Chabertia ovina.* Arthropod parasites controlled by this dosage of ivermectin include oestrid larvae (*Hypoderma bovis, H. lineatum, Oestrus ovis*), mites (*Sarcoptes bovis, Psoroptes ovis*), and sucking lice (*Linognathus vituli, Hematopinus eurysternus,* and *L. pedalis*). It is slightly less effective in controlling chewing lice (*Damalinia* spp.) and the sheep ked (*Melophagus ovinus*). Similar high efficacies for nematodes and arthropods have been found when cattle are treated with an intraruminal sustained-release bolus designed to release 12 mg ivermectin daily for 135 days.

Ivermectin has substantial activity against ticks and dung-breeding flies. It does not result in prompt death or detachment of ticks but does interrupt feeding, molting, and egg production, thereby reducing the ticks' reproductive potential. This is especially true of ticks when they are experimentally applied to animals within a 5-day period before a single 0.2 mg/kg SC treatment or during daily low-level (0.01 mg/kg) treatment. Some degree of control of dung-breeding flies is also provided by a single SC treatment at 0.2 mg/kg. For 9 days after treatment of cattle, feces of treated animals failed to support larval development of face flies, *Musca autumnalis*. For a further 5 days, the propagation of the fly is greatly reduced through abnormal pupation and diminished maturation of adults. Development of the horn fly (*Haematobia irritans*) is similarly diminished for 4 weeks after treatment at this dosage.

Horses. In horses, oral administration at 0.2 mg/kg is highly effective (95–100%) against adult and most fourth-stage larvae of cyathostomes, large strongyles (*Strongylus vulgaris, S. equinus, S. edentatus*), ascarids (*Parascaris equorum*), pinworms (*Oxyuris equi*), stomach worms (*Draschia megastoma, Habronema* spp., *Trichostrongylus axei*), threadworms (*Strongyloides westeri*), and lungworm (*Dictyocaulus arnfieldi*). The 0.2 mg/kg dose is also effective against first-, second-, and third-instar larvae of *Gasterophilus* spp. and is effective in resolving skin lesions caused by *Onchocerca* microfilariae and in killing the third-stage larvae of *Draschia* and *Habronema* spp. that cause "summer sores." Resolution of the latter lesions may require a second treatment approximately 1 month after the initial therapeutic application.

It is noteworthy that the therapeutic dosage of ivermectin (0.2 mg/kg) is approximately 99% effective against early and late fourth-stage larvae of *S. vulgaris* migrating in the intima of the mesenteric arterial system. Resolution of lesions occurs in about 28 days.

Swine. Ivermectin administered subcutaneously at 0.3 mg/kg is suitable for broad-spectrum use in swine. This dose provides 94–100% reduction in immature and adult stages of *Ascaris suum, Hyostrongylus rubidus, Strongyloides ransomi, Oesophagostomum* spp., *Metastrongylus* spp., *Stephanurus dentatus,* and the intestinal (but not muscular) stages of *Trichinella spiralis.* Treatment of pregnant sows 4–16 days before farrowing apparently disrupts transcolostral transmission of *S. ransomi* to piglets. Sucking lice (*Hematopinus suis*) and mange mites (*Sarcoptes scabiei* var. *suis*) are controlled by the label dosage of ivermectin.

Dogs and Cats. Three ivermectin products are approved in the USA as preventives for heartworm (*Dirofilaria immitis*) in dogs and cats. Two products (Heartgard-30; Heartgard for Cats) contain only ivermectin; the other (Heartgard-30 Plus) contains both ivermectin and pyrantel pamoate. All are chewable formulations designed to be given once monthly at a dosage of ≥0.006 mg ivermectin/kg (dogs) or ≥0.024 mg ivermectin/kg (cats). This dosage is 100% effective in killing third- and fourth-stage developing larvae of *D. immitis* acquired during the previous 45–55 days. The addition of pyrantel pamoate at >5.0 mg/kg in Heartgard-30 Plus provides monthly treatment for canine hookworms (*Ancylostoma caninum, Uncinaria stenocephala*) and ascarids (*Toxocara canis, Toxascaris leonina*), for which the product is reported to be more than 96% effective. Ivermectin is also effective against heartworm microfilariae (0.05 mg/kg orally) but is not approved for this purpose. Single doses apparently have no effect against adult heartworms.

Experimental studies indicate that higher dosages of ivermectin have a wide spectrum of activity for other canine parasites. Single SC doses of 0.05 mg/kg eliminate both fourth-stage larvae and adults of various parasites (*Ancylostoma caninum, A. braziliense,* and *Uncinaria stenocephala*). Dosages of 0.1 mg/kg or 0.2 mg/kg were required to remove *Trichuris vulpis* and *Toxocara canis,* respectively. SC administration of 0.2 mg/kg is only 69% effective for *Toxascaris leonina;* oral administration at the same dosage improves efficacy to above 95%. Dramatic (approximately 100%) reduction in prenatal and transmammary transmission of *T. canis* and *A. caninum* from nursing bitches to their pups can be achieved by treating the dam 10 days before and 10 days after whelping with 0.5 mg ivermectin/kg SC each time. Single SC doses are reportedly effective in eliminating *Capillaria aerophila* (*Eucoleus aerophilus*) (0.2 mg/kg) and *Oslerus* (*Filaroides*) *osleri* (0.4 mg/kg) in dogs. Oral or SC administration at 0.2 mg/kg twice, 2 weeks apart, is reported to be 95–100% effective against intestinal stages of *Strongyloides stercoralis* in dogs.

Several arthropod parasites of dogs and cats are susceptible to treatment with ivermectin. Two SC doses (0.2 mg/kg) are reported to clear infestations of otodectic, sarcoptic, and notoedric mange as well as *Pneumonyssoides caninum* nasal mites in dogs and cats. The same two-treatment schedule using 0.3 mg/kg each time is effective against infestations of *Cheyletiella* spp. The drug is also suggested to be beneficial in the control of demodectic mange of dogs at higher dosages and prolonged regimens.

Fowl. Ivermectin also has potential use in birds. Studies indicate that single doses of the drug at 0.2–0.3 mg/kg SC or orally are effective against nematodes (*Ascaridia galli* and *Capillaria obsignata* but not *Heterakis gallinarum*) and certain arthropods (the scaly leg mite [*Cnemidocoptes mutans*] and quill and feather mites) in various species of birds.

SAFETY AND TOXICITY. In general, ivermectin has at least a 10-fold safety margin in ruminants, horses, swine, and most dog breeds except Collies and some Australian Shepherds. A 10-fold overdose causes occasional mydriasis in dogs treated orally and, if given orally on 2 consecutive days to horses, results in transient impaired vision. An acute toxic syndrome occurs in horses given IM doses equal to 60 times the therapeutic dose, in dogs given oral or SC doses equal to 200 times the heartworm preventive dose, and in swine given SC doses equal to 40 times the therapeutic dose. The syndrome consists of lethargy, ataxia, recumbency, and possible death. The principal clinical pathologic change in reactive cases is a decrease in serum iron concentrations. This syndrome is not seen in sheep. Sheep tolerate oral doses of the micelle (polysorbate 80) formulation up to 4 mg/kg without adverse reactions, but oral administration of the drug at this dose in propylene glycol may cause ataxia and hemoglobinuria, which persist up to 3 days. This reaction seems to be due to propylene glycol because vehicle-treated sheep develop comparable signs.

Certain Collies are susceptible to ivermectin toxicity at doses of 0.1 mg/kg or higher. Adverse reactions have not been recorded, however, when Collies were given the heartworm preventive dosage (0.006–0.012 mg/kg) or even 10 times the preventive dose monthly for 1 year. For dogs, the efficacy and safety of formulations designed for other species should not be assumed.

Ivermectin is safe for use in breeding and pregnant animals (Campbell and Benz 1984). In general, twofold increase in dosage and multiple dosing have not adversely affected spermatogenesis, conception, longevity of gestation, or fetal development.

Transient pruritus and cutaneous edema may occur in horses following IM or oral treatment. These signs can be attributed to death of microfilariae of *Onchocerca cervicalis* and usually resolve within 3–4 days.

DOSAGE AND ADMINISTRATION. Single-treatment dosages are given below:

Cattle: Pour-on, 0.5 mg/kg; SC or oral, 0.2 mg/kg
Sheep: Oral, 0.2 mg/kg
Horses: Oral, 0.2 mg/kg
Swine: SC, 0.3 mg/kg
Dogs: Oral, 0.006–0.012 mg/kg
Cats: Oral, 0.024–0.048 mg/kg

ABAMECTIN. Abamectin (Avomec) is a naturally occurring fermentation product of *Streptomyces avermitilis*. Abamectin is used in cattle to control adult and larval GI nematodes, lungworms, sucking lice, and ticks, and in horses to control large and small strongyles, ascarids, pinworms, and other nematode internal parasites. Abamectin is also sold as a pesticide under other brand names (Affirm, Agri-Mek, Avid, Vertimec). Abamectin has a broad range of activity against insect and mite pests of horticultural and agronomic crops as well as the imported fire ant.

CHEMISTRY. Abamectin consists of a mixture of not less than 80% avermectin B_{1a} and not more than 20% avermectin B_{1b}. It differs from ivermectin (Fig. 47.3) in that the double bond between C-22 and C-23 is not saturated in abamectin. Abamectin (as its major component, avermectin B_{1a}) is an off-white powder that is highly lipophilic. It dissolves in most organic solvents but is poorly soluble in water. It is stable at room temperature in nonacidic solutions but is degraded by ultraviolet light.

MODE OF ACTION. See the previous general discussion on mode of action of macrocyclic lactones.

FORMULATIONS. Avomec injectable is a sterile solution of 1.0% *w/v* abamectin. It is administered SC to cattle, immediately in front of or behind the shoulder, at a dosage of 200 μg abamectin/kg body weight (1 mL/50 kg).

ANTHELMINTIC SPECTRUM. Abamectin is an endectocide with activity against both nematode and arthropod parasites of cattle (reviewed by Benz and Cox 1989). At the recommended dosage of 200 μg/kg SC in cattle, abamectin is greater than 99% effective against adults and developing fourth-stage larvae of *Ostertagia ostertagi, Haemonchus placei, Cooperia* spp., and *Dictyocaulus viviparus.* Abamectin is similarly effective against hypobiotic larvae of *O. ostertagi* and against adult *Trichostrongylus axei.* Abamectin prevents reinfection with *Ostertagia* spp., *H. placei, Cooperia* spp., and *O. radiatum* for at least 7 days after treatment, and with *D. viviparus* for at least 14 days after treatment. Cattle treated with abamectin remain free of sucking lice (*Linognathus vituli*) for at least 56 days after administration. Abamectin reduces the number of engorged female *Boophilus microplus* ticks from cattle for at least 21 days following treatment, and egg production is reduced in any surviving female ticks.

Abamectin is also effective against larvae of some dung-breeding Diptera. Feces collected from cattle for up to 21 days after SC injection with 200 μg/kg of abamectin would not suport development of the buffalo fly (*Haematobia irritans exigua*).

SAFETY AND TOXICITY. Clinical signs of toxicity include tremors and/or coma in most species, mydriasis in dogs, and emesis in monkeys. Abamectin is slightly more toxic than ivermectin, with an oral LD_{50} in mice of 14–24 mg/kg (vs. 25–40 mg/kg for ivermectin) and a minimum-effect level in dogs of 0.5 mg/kg/day (vs. 1.0 mg/kg/day for ivermectin). Cleft palates are seen at or near maternotoxic doses in developmental toxicology studies with both drugs. The no-effect level for abamectin fed to dogs in 1-year oral toxicity studies was 0.25 mg/kg/day. Two-year carcinogenicity studies at the maximum tolerated dosage in rats and mice demonstrated a lack of carcinogenicity, as did the lack of genotoxic activity in microbial and mammalian genetic toxicity assays.

Cattle tolerate a maximum dose of 1.0 mg/kg abamectin by SC injection. Lethargy and ataxia are early signs of toxicity. At higher doses (2 to >8 mg/kg), cattle show signs of ataxia that progress to paresis, recumbency, decreased lip and tongue tone, drooling, mydriasis, coma, and death. Reproductive safety studies in cows and bulls with 300 μg/kg abamectin showed no negative effects. Adverse reactions, some of which were related to overdosing, have been reported in calves aged 1 week to 4 months; thus the label warns against treating calves under 4 months of age. In Australia, idiosyncratic toxic reactions were reported in one herd of Murray Grey cattle, which may be analogous to idiosyncratic toxicity with ivermectin in Collies.

The avermectins are largely excreted in the feces, and these excreted products have been shown to suppress larvae of some dung-breeding Diptera. Thus, there has been concern about their potential for damage to pasture populations of beneficial dung-destroying insects. Fecal residues resulting from a single SC injection of 200 μg/kg of abamectin apparently have little effect on adult dung beetles (*Onthophagus gazella*). However, dung beetle larvae failed to develop in feces collected for up to 21 days after treatment, although development was unaffected in feces collected 28 days after treatment (reviewed by Roncalli 1989). Similar experiments with a second species of dung beetle (*O. binodis*) again showed no effect on adults although the development and survival of immature beetles were affected in feces collected up to 4 weeks following treatment. Adverse effects on dung beetle populations could result if abamectin were used intensively and simultaneously over a wide geographical area. However, the use of abamectin at infrequent intervals in individual herds should not significantly affect dung beetle populations, because only part of one generation of beetles will be affected and considerable recruitment of beetles will take place from neighboring pastures grazed by untreated herds.

In the environment, abamectin is quickly degraded (half-life of 4–21 hr) by oxidative and photo-oxidative mechanisms when exposed to light in water, on soil particles, or as a thin film on biological surfaces such as leaves. Abamectin is essentially an immobile pesticide that strongly binds to soil particles. When protected from light within the soil, its major component, avermectin B_{1a}, is degraded by aerobic microbial metabolism and has a half-life of 20–47 days, depending on soil type. Abamectin does not bioconcentrate in individual organisms nor does it bioaccumulate in the local food chain, whether terrestrial or aquatic.

DORAMECTIN. Doramectin (Dectomax) is a novel avermectin prepared by mutational biosynthesis. It has a broad range of activity against GI nematodes, lungworms, eyeworms, sucking lice, grubs, ticks, mites, and screwworms in cattle. Doramectin's efficacy against the agents of myiasis is unique among the macrocyclic lactones. In swine, doramectin has excellent efficacy against ascarids, nodular worms, lungworms, sucking lice, and sarcoptic mange mites. Much of the following information is summarized from a review of doramectin edited by Vercruysse (1993).

CHEMISTRY. The structure of doramectin is given in Fig. 47.4. It differs from ivermectin and abamectin in having a cyclohexyl substituent in the C-25 position.

PHARMACOKINETICS. When administered intravenously as an aqueous micelle, plasma concentrations of doramectin were approximately 2-fold higher than those of a similar formulation of dihydroavermectin B_{1a}, the principal component of ivermectin. Also, the plasma half-life with this formulation of doramectin was approximately twice that of the dihydroavermectin B_{1a}. A vehicle formulation consisting of 90:10 (*v*/*v*) sesame oil/ethyl oleate was subsequently found to improve efficacy by reducing the rate of absorption of doramectin following SC administration. This resulted in prolonged plasma concentrations and a higher AUC for doramectin during the first 12 days after injection. SC injection of doramectin in the sesame oil–ethyl oleate vehicle results in clinically significant plasma levels of doramectin for at least 12 days following injection. Efficacy against reinfection persists for at least 12 days for *Cooperia oncophora,* 21 days for *Ostertagia ostertagi,* and for up to 35 days for highly sensitive parasites such as *Dermatobia hominis.*

The identical doramectin injectable formulation is also labeled for IM use in swine.

MODE OF ACTION. See the previous general discussion on mode of action of macrocyclic lactones.

FORMULATIONS. Dectomax is a sterile 1% solution of doramectin in a sesame oil–ethyl oleate (90:10 *v*/*v*) vehicle. It is administered to cattle at a dosage of 200 μg/kg by SC injection and to swine at a dosage

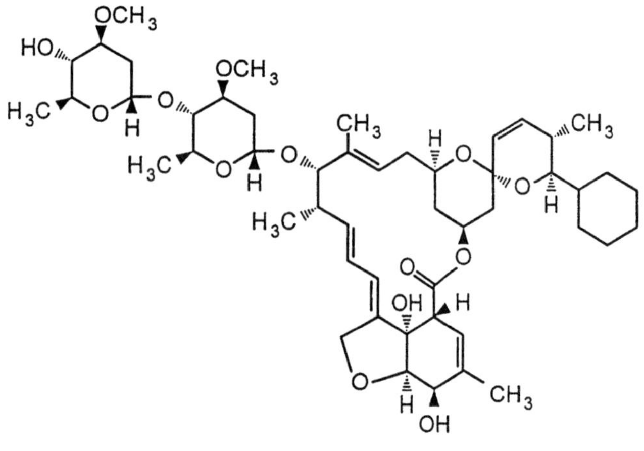

FIG. 47.4—Doramectin.

of 300 μg/kg by IM injection. Dectomax Pour-on is a topical 5% solution in a nonaqueous base and is administered at a dose of 0.5 mg/kg.

ANTHELMINTIC SPECTRUM. In controlled studies in Europe, North America, and South America, doramectin was shown to be greater than 99% effective against mature and immature stages of *Ostertagia ostertagi* (including hypobiotic larvae), *O. lyrata, Haemonchus placei* (including hypobiotic larvae), *H. contortus, H. similis, Trichostrongylus axei* (including hypobiotic larvae), *T. colubriformis, Cooperia oncophora* (including hypobiotic larvae), *C. punctata, C. pectinata, C. spatulata, C. surnabada, Bunostomum phlebotomum, Strongyloides papillosus,* and *Oesophagostomum radiatum* (including hypobiotic larvae). Efficacy was inconsistent against *Trichostrongylus longispicularis;* greater than 93% in one study, but greater than 99% in a second. Doramectin was less effective against *Trichuris* spp. (92.3–94.6%) and *Nematodirus spathiger* (96.5%). *Nematodirus helvetianus* was the dose-limiting species, with efficacy against adult and fourth-stage larvae reported as 73.3% and 75.5%, respectively, in one study but 97.9% in a second trial. Doramectin treatment reduced experimentally administered and naturally acquired burdens of eyeworms (*Thelazia skrjabini* and *T. gulosa*) in calves by 100%.

Like ivermectin and moxidectin, doramectin persists in activity for several weeks following injection. Worm burdens in cattle experimentally challenged with larvae of *Cooperia oncophora* each day for 14 or 21 days following doramectin treatment were reduced by 99.2% and 90.7%, respectively. Reductions for *Ostertagia ostertagi* were 99.9 and 93.7% after daily challenge for 21 and 28 days, respectively, following treatment. Similarly, reductions for *Dictyocaulus viviparus* were 100% and 99.9% after 21 and 28 days, respectively. In natural-grazing experiments, doramectin delayed the appearance of worm eggs in feces of worm-free cattle turned out to graze pastures contaminated with larvae of *O. ostertagi* and *C. oncophora* by 19–22 days compared to untreated control calves.

Doramectin is also efficacious against a variety of arthropod parasites of cattle. Efficacy was 100% against naturally acquired *Psoroptes bovis, Sarcoptes scabiei, Hematopinus eurysternus, Linognathus vituli, Solenopotes capillatus, Hypoderma bovis* (first, second, and third instars), and *Dermatobia hominis.* Furthermore, cattle were protected from new infection with *D. hominis* for at least 35 days following doramectin treatment. As with the other avermectins, the efficacy of doramectin was reduced (82%) against chewing lice (*Damalinia bovis*). Unlike the other avermectins, doramectin is highly effective against the New World screwworm, *Cochliomyia hominivorax.* Doramectin was 100% effective in preventing experimental infections of calves with this parasite for at least 14 days following treatment.

In swine, doramectin has greater than 99% efficacy against *Ascaris suum,* nodular worms (*Oesophagostomum dentatum*), lungworms (*Metastrongylus* spp.), kidney worms (*Stephanurus dentatus*), as well as *Hyostrongylus rubidus* and *Strongyloides ransomi.* Efficacies were 100% against sucking lice (*Hematopinus suis*) and mange mites (*Sarcoptes scabiei* var. *suis*).

EPRINOMECTIN. Eprinomectin (Ivomec Eprinex) is a modified fermentation product of *Streptomyces avermitilis.* It is used in beef and dairy cattle to control most GI nematodes and lungworms and also is highly effective against biting and sucking lice, chorioptic mange mites, cattle grubs, and horn flies.

CHEMISTRY. Eprinomectin is a modified avermectin with an epi-acetylamino substitution at the 4″ position (Fig. 47.5). As marketed, eprinomectin is a racemic mixture of compounds that comprises not less than 90% of the major component (4″-*epi*-acetylamino-4″-deoxy-avermectin B_{1a}) (R = C_2H_5) and not more than 10% of the minor component (4″-*epi*-acetylamino-4″-deoxy-avermectin B_{1b}) (R = CH_3).

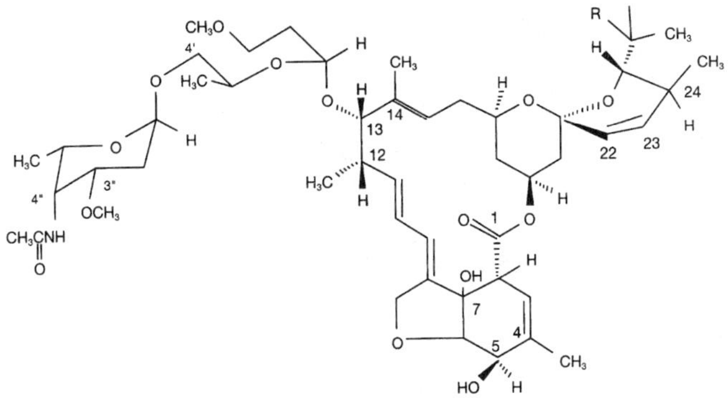

FIG. 47.5—Eprinomectin.

PHARMACOKINETICS AND METABOLISM. Eprinomectin is absorbed soon after topical administration, and achieves peak plasma concentrations of 22.5 ng/mL within 2–5 days after treatment. Plasma concentrations decline to 1 ng/mL within 21 days after administration. The majority of a topical dose is absorbed within 7–10 days.

Eprinomectin is not metabolized extensively, and parent compound makes up 90% of residues in tissues and more than 85% in feces. The major residue is eprinomectin B_{1a}, which is also the major component of the parent compound.

Eprinomectin has an extremely low milk-plasma coefficient, indicating greater partitioning of compound away from milk and into plasma. No meat or milk withdrawal periods are required after treatment with eprinomectin.

MODE OF ACTION. See the previous general discussion on mode of action of macrocyclic lactones.

FORMULATIONS. Eprinomectin has been marketed only as a 5% pour-on formulation (Ivomec Eprinex) for use on beef and dairy cattle. It is administered along the topline, from withers to tail head, as doses of 1 mL/10 kg body weight. The formulation is nonaqueous and very stable in various climatic conditions, including extremely heavy rainfall immediately after application.

ANTIPARASITIC SPECTRUM. Eprinomectin has greater than 99% efficacy against the common nematode genera in the bovine GI tract (including *Nematodirus helvetianus,* arrested early fourth-stage larvae of *Ostertagia ostertagi,* and *Dictyocaulus viviparus*) and greater than 97% efficacy against adult whipworms (*Trichuris* spp.). It exhibits persistent activity against reinfection with lungworms for 21 days after treatment. Eprinomectin has very high efficacy against chewing lice (*Bovicola bovis*), three genera of sucking lice (*Hematopinus, Solenopotes, Linognathus*), the mange mites *Chorioptes* and *Sarcoptes,* and both species of cattle grubs in North America (*Hypoderma bovis, H. lineatum*). Eprinomectin also controls horn flies (*Haematobia irritans*) and has residual activity against these pests for 7 days after administration.

SAFETY AND TOXICITY. The safety of eprinomectin was evaluated by treating 6 calves with a single administration of 10 times the recommended therapeutic dosage (i.e., 5000 μg/kg). The only adverse effect noted was mydriasis in 1 of the 6 calves from 4 to 7 days after the overdose.

Toxicity of eprinomectin was also evaluated by treating calves with up to 5 times the recommended dosage (i.e., 2500 μg/kg) on three occasions at 7-day intervals. No adverse effects were noted.

SELAMECTIN. Selamectin (Revolution) is derived by chemical modification of a precursor avermectin that is produced by fermentation of a new strain of *Streptomyces avermitilis.* Selamectin is used in dogs and cats to prevent heartworm, to kill fleas, and to treat and control a variety of ectoparasitic infections (Bruce et al., 1999). It is also effective against roundworm and hookworm infection in cats.

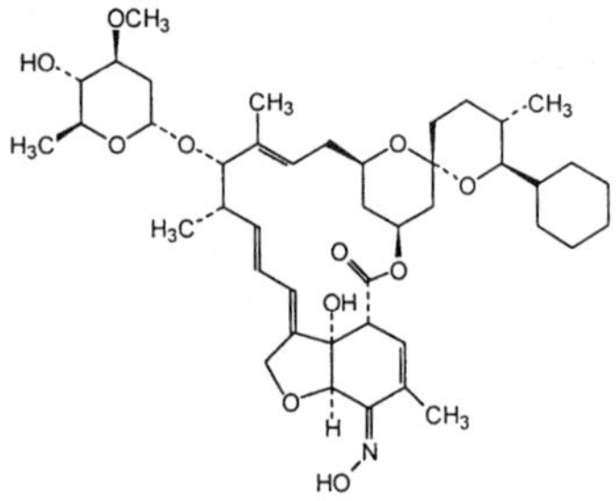

FIG. 47.6—Selamectin.

CHEMISTRY. Selamectin is a modified avermectin (Fig. 47.6) with the chemical name (5Z,25S)-25-cyclohexyl-4′-*O*-de(2,6-dideoxy-3-*O*-methyl-α*bino*-hexopyranosyl)-5-demethoxy-25-de(l-methylpropyl)-22,23-dihydro-5-hydroxyiminoavermectin A_{1a}.

PHARMACOKINETICS AND METABOLISM. Selamectin is absorbed fairly rapidly after administration and achieves peak plasma concentrations approximately 8 hours or 3 days after treatment by the oral or topical routes, respectively. The half-life of a single topical treatment of 24 mg/kg was approximately 11 days in dogs. Selamectin persists at clinically effective levels in dogs and cats for at least 30 days after a single topical treatment.

Following topical administration, selamectin is absorbed into the bloodstream and a portion of the compound is excreted into the intestinal tract. Substantial amounts of circulating selamectin are deposited in the sebaceous glands, which then act as reservoirs to provide persistent activity against various ectoparasitic infections.

MODE OF ACTION. See the general discussion on mode of action of macrocyclic lactones.

FORMULATIONS. Selamectin is marketed as a 6% or 12% topical formulation (Revolution) packaged for dogs and cats of various weight ranges. It is administered in a single spot at the base of the neck, cranial to the shoulder blades. The formulation is nonaqueous, and persistent efficacy is not compromised by bathing or wetting of the animal's haircoat.

ANTIPARASITIC SPECTRUM. Selamectin (6 mg/kg) had 100% efficacy against infective stages of heartworm (*Dirofilaria immitis*) for up to 60 days after exposure. A reduced dosage (3 mg/kg) was protective for up to 45 days. At label dosages (6 to 12 mg/kg) in cats, a single application of selamectin was 84.7% to 99.7% effective against *Ancylostoma tubaeforme* and 100% effective against *Toxocara cati.* Although selamectin demonstrated good efficacy against *Toxocara canis* infections in dogs, it is not currently labeled for that use.

SAFETY AND TOXICITY. The safety of selamectin was evaluated by treating kittens with up to 367.4 mg/kg and puppies with up to 114 mg/kg at 28-day intervals for a total of seven treatments. No adverse reactions were observed. Similarly, selamectin was shown to be safe in breeding cats and dogs, as well as in pregnant and lactating bitches and queens. When administered to dogs with *D. immitis* microfilaremia, selamectin caused no adverse reactions and resulted in a rapid and persistent reduction in microfilaria counts. Selamectin use was also safe in ivermectin-sensitive Collies.

Milbemycins

MILBEMYCIN OXIME. Milbemycin oxime (Interceptor, Sentinel) is a fermentation product of *Streptomyces hygroscopicus aureolacrimosus* and has activity against certain arthropods and nematodes. A second milbemycin, milbemycin D, was marketed in Japan for prophylaxis of canine heartworm (*Dirofilaria immitis*), but it was subsequently replaced by milbemycin oxime because the latter compound has a greater margin of safety in ivermectin-sensitive Collies and in microfilaremic dogs.

CHEMISTRY. As formulated in Interceptor, milbemycin oxime consists of a mixture of not less than 80% A_4 milbemycin oxime and not more than 20% A_3 milbemycin oxime (Fig. 47.7). The drug has low solubility in water.

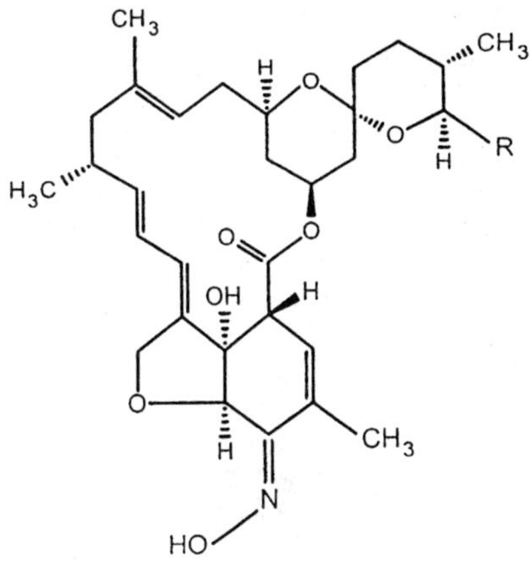

PHARMACOKINETICS AND METABOLISM. Following oral administration, approximately 90–95% of the dose passes through the gut unchanged. The remaining 5–10% is absorbed and subsequently excreted in the bile. Nearly the entire dose is eliminated in feces.

MODE OF ACTION. See the previous general discussion on mode of action of macrocyclic lactones.

FORMULATIONS. Milbemycin oxime is sold as a chewable tablet (Interceptor Palatab) for dogs. Tablets come in four sizes, containing 2.3, 5.75, 11.5, or 23.0 mg of milbemycin oxime. Milbemycin oxime is also marketed as Interceptor Flavor Tabs for Cats in tablet sizes containing 5.75, 11.5, or 23.0 mg of active compound. Milbemycin oxime is administered orally once a month. The recommended dosages are 0.5–0.99 mg/kg for dogs and 2.0 mg/kg for cats.

Recently, milbemycin oxime has been combined with lufenuron in a chewable tablet formulation (Sentinel) that provides simultaneous prevention and control of flea infestations in addition to protection against heartworms and other internal nematodes. Sentinel tablets are available in four sizes, containing the following amounts of milbemycin oxime/lufenuron (all quantities in mg): 2.3/46, 5.75/115, 11.5/230, and 23.0/460.

A_3 Oxime: $R = CH_3$
A_4 Oxime: $R = C_2H_5$

FIG. 47.7—Milbemycin oxime.

ANTHELMINTIC SPECTRUM. Milbemycin oxime is considered an endectocide, having activity against both internal parasites (nematodes) and external parasites (*Demodex canis*). It is effective against nematode parasites at a relatively low dosage (0.5 mg/kg or less). Developing larvae of the dog heartworm are susceptible to milbemycin oxime. It is marketed in Australia, Canada, Italy, Japan, New Zealand, and the USA for prevention of canine dirofilariasis and control of the intestinal nematodes *Toxocara canis, Trichuris vulpis,* and *Ancylostoma* spp. Despite its efficacy against hookworms of the genus *Ancylostoma,* milbemycin oxime does not reliably control hookworms of the genus *Uncinaria.* When administered to cats at 2.0 mg/kg at 30-day intervals, milbemycin prevents feline heartworm and removes *T. cati* and *A. tubaeforme* infections.

The efficacy of the milbemycin/lufenuron combination (Sentinel) against nematodes and fleas, respectively, is equivalent to that of the components used separately. Sentinel is administered to pups older than 4 weeks and heavier than 2 lb body weight at a dosage of 0.5–0.99 mg/kg milbemycin and 10–20 mg/kg lufenuron.

In dogs, a single oral dose of 0.5 mg/kg milbemycin oxime at 30 or 45 days after infection with third-stage larvae of *Dirofilaria immitis* completely prevents development of infection. A single treatment at 60 or 90 days after infection is not completely effective, but two or more monthly treatments beginning at 60 days after infection consistently prevent infection with *D. immitis* (Grieve et al. 1989). Cats treated monthly with an oral dose of 0.5–0.9 mg/kg are completely protected against the establishment of experimental infections with *D. immitis* (Stewart et al. 1992).

Milbemycin oxime is a potent microfilaricide in dogs. A single, oral dose of 0.25 mg/kg or greater results in a precipitous decline (>98%) in microfilaremia within a few days (Blagburn et al. 1992). Because of milbemycin's apparent blockade of embryogenesis, nearly all microfilaremic, *D. immitis*–infected dogs given milbemycin oxime prophylaxis once monthly will become amicrofilaremic within 6–9 months. Most will remain amicrofilaremic for at least 4–6 months after prophylaxis is discontinued (Lok et al. 1992; Bowman et al. 1992).

Milbemycin oxime is moderately effective against *Demodex canis,* and treatment (1.0–4.6 mg/kg/day for at least 60–90 days) of dogs with generalized demodicosis resulted in a temporary improvement for nearly all. This regimen effected a permanent (i.e., nonrelapsing) cure in more than half the cases treated (Miller et al. 1993). The prognosis for a permanent cure may be more favorable for dogs with juvenile-onset demodicosis than for those with adult-onset demodicosis.

Parasitic nematode populations resistant to milbemycin oxime have not been reported. However, this drug has been used only in dogs, a host in which anthelmintic-resistant nematodes are rare.

SAFETY AND TOXICITY. In chronic toxicity studies, dogs tolerated up to 2.5 mg/kg (5 times the monthly dosage) administered on 3 consecutive days each month for 10 months. Bitches were dosed daily with 3 times the normal monthly dose from 2 months prior to mating until 1 week prior to whelping, and male dogs were similarly dosed until mating without effect on the dogs or their offspring. Eight-week-old puppies tolerated up to 6 times the monthly dose each day for 3 consecutive days without ill effect, but transient trembling and ataxia were observed at 30 times the daily dose.

Because milbemycin oxime is a potent and fast-acting microfilaricide, treatment is commonly accompanied by mild reactions characterized by lethargy, salivation, coughing, tachypnea, or emesis (Blagburn et al. 1992). Treatment of dogs with high levels of *D. immitis* microfilaremia occasionally results in shocklike reactions with profound circulatory collapse. Mild and severe adverse reactions reportedly respond to aggressive treatment with corticosteroids and IV fluids.

Milbemycin oxime is not known to interact adversely with any other drug used in small-animal practice.

MOXIDECTIN. Moxidectin (Cydectin, Equest, Moxidec, Quest, Vetdectin) is a chemically modified derivative of the macrocyclic lactone nemadectin, a fermentation product of *Streptomyces cyanogriseus noncyanogenus.* Moxidectin has a broad range of activity against nematode and arthropod parasites of dogs, cattle, sheep, and horses.

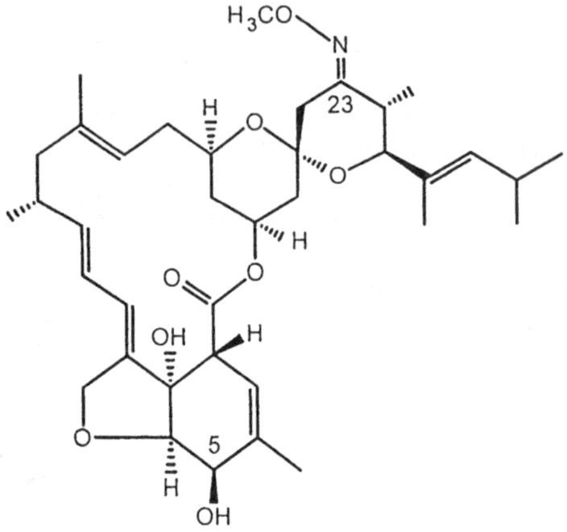

FIG. 47.8—Moxidectin.

CHEMISTRY. Moxidectin is produced by chemical modification of nemadectin, the principal component of the LL-F28249 antibiotic complex produced by *Streptomyces cyanogriseus noncyanogenus.* Unlike ivermectin, abamectin, and milbemycin oxime, moxidectin is essentially a single compound rather than a mixture of two closely related compounds (Fig. 47.8).

PHARMACOKINETICS. Moxidectin is even more lipophilic and hydrophobic than ivermectin, and as a result, therapeutically effective tissue levels persist somewhat longer. Like ivermectin and abamectin, moxidectin is excreted mainly in feces.

MODE OF ACTION. See the previous general discussion on mode of action of macrocyclic lactones.

FORMULATIONS. Moxidectin is marketed for control of internal and external parasites of various ruminants in Australia, New Zealand, South Africa, and Latin America (Cydectin, Vetdectin). Formulations include 0.1% and 0.2% oral drenches for sheep, a 1.0% injection for cattle, and a 0.5% pour-on solution for cattle and deer. The drenches and injection are aqueous formulations containing propylene glycol and solubilizers, whereas the pour-on uses an oil vehicle. The drench and injection are administered at a dosage of 200 μg/kg and the pour-on is administered at a dosage of 500 μg/kg. In Japan, moxidectin is sold as tablets (Moxidec) containing 7.5, 15, and 30 μg of moxidectin for monthly administration as a heartworm prophylactic for dogs at a dosage of 3 μg/kg.

ANTHELMINTIC SPECTRUM. Moxidectin is an endectocide, having activity against both internal parasites (nematodes) and external parasites (arthropods) at a relatively low dosage (0.5 mg/kg or less). All major GI and lung nematodes of domestic ruminants and horses, certain arthropod parasites of ruminants, and developing larvae of the dog heartworm are susceptible.

Ruminants. In cattle, moxidectin (as the injection or pour-on) is highly efficacious (>99%) against *Ostertagia ostertagi* adults and hypobiotic larvae, *O. lyrata* adults, *Haemonchus placei* adults, *Trichostrongylus axei* adults, *T. colubriformis* adults, *Trichuris discolor* adults, *Oesophagostomum radiatum* adults, *Bunostomum phlebotomum* adults and fourth-stage larvae, and *Dictyocaulus viviparus* adults. Moxidectin is slightly less efficacious against *Nematodirus helvetianus* adults (>95%) and *Cooperia* spp., with efficacies of 92–100% against adults and larvae of *Cooperia oncophora, C. punctata, C. pectinata,* and *C. mcmasteri* and against *C. spatulata* adults. Reinfection with nematodes of the genera *Ostertagia, Haemonchus, Trichostrongylus,* and *Oesophagostomum* is prevented for up to 28 days following a single injection or topical application of moxidectin, but such activity persists for no more than 7 days for *Nematodirus* and *Cooperia.* A single SC injection of moxidectin will completely eliminate mites of the genera *Sarcoptes* and *Psoroptes* and will markedly suppress, but not entirely eliminate, *Chorioptes* mites. A single topical application will eliminate mites of the genus *Psoroptes,* but data are not available for the other genera. *Boophilus microplus* tick populations are reduced by more than 95% following a single SC injection of moxidectin, and tick populations are suppressed for up to 32 days. Although both formulations control sucking lice (99–100% efficacious against *Haematopinus eurysternus, Linognathus vituli,* and *Solenopotes capillatus*) and cattle grubs (*Hypoderma lineatum*), the pour-on formulation provides much better control of the chewing louse (*Damalinia bovis*) than the injectable (Chick et al. 1993).

In sheep, orally administered moxidectin is highly efficacious (>99%) against adult and larval nematodes of the genera *Haemonchus, Ostertagia, Trichostrongylus, Cooperia, Oesophagostomum, Chabertia,* and *Dictyocaulus,* as well as adult *Nematodirus.* Additionally, good control is obtained for the sheep itch mite, *Psorergates ovis.*

In New Zealand, moxidectin pour-on is approved for use in ranch-raised deer, in which it is more than 99% effective against nematodes of the genera *Haemonchus, Ostertagia, Trichostrongylus, Oesophagostomum,* and *Dictyocaulus.*

Horses. Moxidectin is reported effective against the common internal parasites of the horse at a dose of 400 μg/kg, although its activity against bots may be erratic. At a dose of 300 μg/kg, an experimental gel formulation of moxidectin was more than 99% effective against adult and larval *Habronema muscae,* adult and larval *Parascaris equorum,* adult and larval *Oxyuris equi,* adult *Strongylus vulgaris* and *S. edentatus,* and adult *Triodontophorus* spp. Moxidectin removed more than 97% of adult and lumen-dwelling fourth-stage larval cyathostomes and was more than 79% effective against late third-stage and developing fourth-stage cyathostome larvae. In North American trials, moxidectin did not exhibit consistent efficacy against early third-stage cyathostome larvae. Efficacy against *Gasterophilus nasalis* is 100%, but efficacy against *G. intestinalis* is variable (57–100%) and apparently less than that of ivermectin (Xiao et al. 1993).

Dogs. Similar to milbemycin oxime, moxidectin is highly effective against *Ancylostoma caninum* but less effective against *Uncinaria stenocephala.* A single oral dose of 25 μg/kg will remove *Ancylostoma,* but a dose of at least 150 μg/kg is necessary for similar efficacy against *Uncinaria.* Whipworms are not controlled by doses up to 300 μg/kg (Supakorndej et al. 1993). Like ivermectin, moxidectin is an effective heartworm prophylactic at a remarkably low dose. Moxidectin is 100% effective against both 1- and 2-month-old larvae of *Dirofilaria immitis* at a dose of 3.0 μg/kg (McTier et al. 1992).

SAFETY AND TOXICITY. No adverse reactions occurred in sheep drenched at 2 or 5 times the recommended dose (0.4 or 1.0 mg/kg). Likewise, no adverse reactions occurred with repeated treatments at twice the normal dose. No deaths occurred when *Bos indicus* and *Bos taurus* cattle were injected SC with up to 10 times the recommended dose (2.0 mg/kg). However, extra care must be taken to use the correct dose in calves under 100 kg body weight because they may be susceptible to overdosing. No adverse reactions, either local or systemic, occurred when cattle were treated with up to 10 times the recommended dose (5.0 mg/kg) or when red deer fawns were treated with up to 5 times the recommended dose (2.5 mg/kg) of a pour-on formulation of moxidectin. The pour-on formulation likewise caused no damage to hides of cattle at the recommended dose (0.5 mg/kg). Known ivermectin-sensitive Collies and microfilaremic, *Dirofilaria immitis*–infected dogs tolerate at least 15 μg/kg moxidectin (5 times the recommended dose for heartworm prophylaxis) (Paul et al. 1992; Hendrix et al. 1992).

Moxidectin is safe in breeding animals. At 3 times the recommended dose (0.6 mg/kg), no adverse effects on reproductive performance of bulls and pregnant cows were observed. Up to 3 times the recommended dose (0.6 mg/kg) had no effect on reproductive performance of cows and heifers when injected during each trimester of pregnancy (Rae et al. 1994).

Residues excreted in feces of animals treated with moxidectin are less toxic to dung beetle larvae than those of animals treated with ivermectin and thus do not impact survival of dung beetles or their development to maturity.

HETEROCYCLIC COMPOUNDS

Phenothiazine. *Phenothiazine,* INN, was perhaps the first anthelmintic to demonstrate a fairly wide range of activity against GI nematodes. Phenothiazine (PTZ) was synthesized as early as 1885 but was not found to possess anthelmintic activity until 1938. In the subsequent years, it was used extensively in sheep, cattle, goats, horses, and chickens. Toxicity limited its use in swine and precluded its use in dogs, cats, and humans. The emergence of PTZ-resistant strains of ruminant and equine nematodes in the 1960s and competition from other broad-spectrum drugs markedly reduced the utility of this compound in subsequent years.

For additional information regarding phenothiazine and its use in domestic animals, readers are referred to the 6th edition of this text (Roberson 1988).

Piperazine. *Piperazine,* USP, was recognized as having anthelmintic properties during the 1950s, and numerous salts of piperazine have been developed since that time. All piperazine derivatives have similar profiles of efficacy: good for ascarid and nodular worm infections of all species of domestic animals, moderate for pinworm infections, and zero to variable for other veterinary helminths. Piperazine compounds have a wide margin of safety in all domestic animals.

CHEMISTRY. Chemically, piperazine is diethylenediamine. It has a simple ring structure that is freely soluble in water and glycerol, less soluble in alcohol, and insoluble in ether. It is a strong base and easily absorbs water and carbon dioxide; therefore, containers of piperazine should be closed tightly and protected from light. Piperazine easily forms the hexahydrate in the presence of moisture, and the resulting colorless crystals are soluble in water and very unstable.

Piperazine can be stabilized through the formation of simple salts (adipate, citrate, hydrochloride, phosphate, sulfate, and tartrate); all are more stable than the piperazine base. Most piperazine salts are white crystalline powders that are readily soluble in water. Exceptions are adipate, which only dissolves to a maximum concentration of 5% in water, and phosphate, which is insoluble.

The antiparasitic activity of various salts of piperazine is attributed to the presence of piperazine base. The amount of base varies among different salts, as reflected by different dosages of each. The hexahydrate of piperazine contains 44% base, and dosages of piperazine salts customarily are expressed in terms of the hydrate equivalent. Thus, 100 mg piperazine hydrate is approximately equivalent to 120 mg piperazine adipate, 125 mg piperazine citrate, and 104 mg piperazine phosphate.

PHARMACOKINETICS. Piperazine and its simple salts are readily absorbed from the proximal GI tract. Some piperazine base is metabolized in tissues, and the remainder (approximately 30–40%) is excreted in urine. Piperazine base is detectable in urine as early as 30 minutes after the drug is administered. The excretion rate is maximal at 1–8 hours, and urinary excretion is practically complete within 24 hours.

MODE OF ACTION. Piperazine blocks transmission by hyperpolarizing nerve membranes at the neuromuscular junction and induces flaccid paralysis. Mature worms are more susceptible to the action of piperazine than younger stages. Immature adults and lumen-dwelling larvae are sufficiently susceptible to be at least partially eliminated. Larval stages in host tissues, however, are relatively insusceptible. Because of subsequent larval development, repeated treatments are generally indicated within 2 weeks for carnivores and within 4 weeks for swine and horses.

TOXICITY. Experience over many years has confirmed the safety of piperazine; it is almost nontoxic under ordinary circumstances. The oral median lethal dose (LD_{50}) of piperazine adipate in mice is 11.4 g/kg, which indicates a wide margin of safety. Very young animals (e.g., 2-week-old pups) can be treated without adverse effects.

Large oral doses of piperazine produce emesis, diarrhea, incoordination, and head pressing in cats and dogs. Adult horses and foals tolerate 5–6 times the therapeutic dose of piperazine without side effects. Forced oral administration of 5 times the therapeutic dose of piperazine to swine results in semifluid feces and impaired appetite but no lasting effects.

The only contraindication to the use of piperazine salts is long-standing renal or liver disease. In extremely heavy ascarid infections, treatment with piperazine may immobilize veritable masses of worms and cause an intestinal impaction. Emergency surgery may be necessary to remove the bolus of dead worms and to evaluate the viability of compromised bowel.

ANTHELMINTIC SPECTRUM

DOGS AND CATS. Several salts of piperazine are used in small domestic animals for removal of ascarids (*Toxocara canis, T. cati,* and *Toxascaris leonina*). Efficacy against these parasites varies from 52 to 100%. Piperazine has no activity against whipworms or tapeworms in carnivores.

Dogs and cats are usually dosed with tablets, but powder and liquid formulations have been available commercially. Treatment of nursing pups with piperazine at 2, 4, 6, and 8 weeks of age is more than 90% effective in removing prenatally acquired *T. canis* infections.

HORSES. Piperazine salts provide excellent activity against equine ascarids and some activity against cyathostomes and pinworms. Piperazine adipate has been used most widely in horses, but other piperazine compounds (citrate, phosphate) are also effective. Nearly 100% of ascarid burdens are eliminated from horses treated with any of the piperazine compounds. Repeated treatment of juvenile horses at 8-week intervals is warranted to prevent reestablishment of patent *Parascaris equorum* populations.

Approximately 80% of mature pinworms (*Oxyuris equi*) are eliminated by piperazine adipate, but there is little activity against immature pinworms. Retreatment within 3–4 weeks is recommended.

Piperazine compounds effectively remove cyathostomes. Piperazine also provides approximately 60% activity against *Strongylus vulgaris* and *Triodontophorus,* but there is no activity against the other *Strongylus* species or against stomach worms (*Habronema*).

Historically, piperazine was added to phenothiazine and thiabendazole to supplement their deficient activity against equine ascarids. In recent years, however, piperazine is most often combined with BZD drugs to increase activity against BZD-resistant cyathostomes that might survive treatment if a BZD were used alone.

SWINE. Piperazine compounds have been used extensively in swine because of their excellent efficacy against ascarids and nodular worms. Approximately 100% of the lumen-dwelling stages of both ascarids and nodular worms can be eliminated by a single treatment with piperazine. Retreatment 1–2 months later may be necessary to remove worms that were migrating through tissues during the initial treatment. Piperazine formulations can be administered to swine via drinking water or feed, either of which should be consumed in an 8- to 12-hour period.

RUMINANTS. Piperazine compounds are seldom used in cattle and sheep because their activity in these hosts is limited to nodular worms (*Oesophagostomum* spp.).

CHICKENS. *Ascaridia galli* is highly susceptible to piperazine, and citrate and adipate salts have been used most commonly to control this parasite in chickens. The cecal worm (*Heterakis gallinarum*) apparently is not susceptible to piperazine.

Piperazine compounds are usually administered to chickens in the feed (citrate or adipate salts) or drinking water (hexahydrate) over a 2-day period.

DOSAGE. Dosages are presented here by the amount of piperazine base. Product information should be consulted for specific information about various salts of piperazine.

Dogs and cats: 45–65 mg/kg

Horses: 110 mg/kg

Swine, cattle, sheep, goats: 110 mg/kg

Poultry: 32 mg/kg (approximately 0.3 g for each adult) given in each of 2 successive feedings or in drinking water for 2 days

Diethylcarbamazine Citrate. *Diethylcarbamazine Citrate,* USP, INN (Caricide, Dirocide, Filaribits, Filaricide), is a piperazine derivative. Diethylcarbamazine (DEC) is a colorless, odorless, crystalline solid that is highly soluble in water, alcohol, and chloroform but insoluble in most organic solvents. It is stable under varied conditions of climate and moisture.

FORMULATIONS AND ADMINISTRATION. DEC is formulated as tablets or chewables that are sold under several trade names as a preventive for heartworm disease in dogs. DEC should be administered daily throughout the mosquito vector season and continued for 2 months following. Young pups can begin a preventive program of daily DEC as soon as they are weaned and eating solid foods consistently.

In addition to heartworm prevention, a combination of DEC and oxibendazole (Filaribits Plus) also prevents the establishment of *Ancylostoma caninum* infections in dogs and removes or controls *Toxocara canis, Toxascaris leonina,* and *Trichuris vulpis.*

DEC apparently is active against *D. immitis* larvae only during 24- to 48-hour periods when they are molting. Thus, DEC kills developing larvae as they molt from the L_3 to the L_4 stage at approximately 2 weeks after infection and again at approximately 8 weeks after infection when the L_4 stage molts to the L_5. Because the latter event represents the last opportunity for DEC to prevent establishment, it is usually recommended that DEC prophylaxis be continued for 2 months after the local mosquito season ends.

DEC also has marked microfilaricidal properties, and dogs that are infected with heartworms must first be cleared of adult stages and microfilariae before DEC prophylaxis is instituted. The microfilaricidal activity often causes severe adverse reactions, especially in dogs with high numbers of circulating microfilariae at the time of treatment. These reactions develop rapidly and are frequently fatal. Consequently, use of DEC in microfilaria-positive dogs is strictly contraindicated.

DEC also can be used as a preventive for heartworms in sea lions and in ferrets. *Dirofilaria immitis* infections are common among captive sea lions, and DEC (7.7 mg/kg/day) in the food prevents infection and has no effect on host fertility. A dose of 2.75–5.5 mg DEC/kg/day is recommended as a preventive regimen for pet ferrets.

DOSAGE. Tablets or chewables used in prophylactic heartworm schedules are administered to dogs daily at 6.6 mg/kg.

PHARMACOKINETICS AND TOXICITY. DEC is absorbed rapidly from the gut. The peak concentration in blood occurs about 3 hours after oral administration and falls to zero within 48 hours. DEC is distributed to all organs and tissues except fat.

Excretion of DEC occurs almost entirely through urine; 70% of the dose is eliminated in this manner within 24 hours of administration. Only 10–25% of the drug is excreted unchanged; the remainder is excreted as one of four known metabolites, all of which contain an intact piperazine ring.

Rapid metabolism and excretion of DEC probably account for its low toxicity. Side effects rarely occur at the low dosage (6.6 mg/kg) used for heartworm prevention.

DEC apparently has no adverse effects on fertility of male dogs. Several studies in the USA to evaluate continued daily use in males have concluded that the drug causes no significant deterioration in quantity, morphology, motility, or viability of spermatozoa.

HEARTWORM ADULTICIDES. Adult stages of *Dirofilaria immitis* cause the major damage associated with heartworm infection in domestic dogs and other carnivores. Removal of adults is the key stage in heartworm therapy, but complete management includes elimination of microfilariae and prevention of new infections. Two compounds are currently approved as *Dirofilaria* adulticides, and both are organic arsenicals.

Thiacetarsamide Sodium. *Thiacetarsamide Sodium,* INN (Caparsolate sodium, Filaramide, Arsenamide), chemically consists of the disodium salt of *S,S*-diester of *p*-carbamoyldithiobenzenearsonous acid with mercaptoacetic acid.

ADMINISTRATION AND DOSAGE. Because thiacetarsamide sodium is hepatotoxic and nephrotoxic, normal kidney and liver function should be ascertained prior to initiating a therapeutic regimen.

Thiacetarsamide is administered intravenously because it is very irritating to tissues. Caution must be exercised to avoid perivascular leakage because extreme local swelling and possible sloughing of affected tissues can result. In the event of leakage or inadvertent perivascular administration, injecting steroids into the area helps to reduce the inflammatory reaction.

The recommended regimen of thiacetarsamide therapy is 2.2 mg/kg twice daily for 2 days. This dosage provides 0.44 mg of elemental arsenic/kg body weight and should not be reduced for large-breed dogs.

Feeding the patient about 1 hour before each treatment is recommended. Interest in eating provides some indication of the dog's general condition, and treatment may be continued if the dog is eating well. Treatment should be discontinued if the dog develops severe anorexia, persistent vomiting, or other indications of hepatic or renal disease.

Arsenic toxicity is manifested as persistent vomiting, icterus, and orange-colored urine. When arsenical treatment must be suspended, a 6-week rest period is recommended before initiating another thiacetarsamide regimen. Severe toxic reactions to thiacetarsamide can be treated with dimercaprol (8.8 mg/kg/day in 4 divided doses).

CLINICAL EFFICACY. Following the four therapeutic injections of thiacetarsamide, adult worms usually die within 5–7 days, but full efficacy may require 2 weeks. Arsenicals have no effect against circulating microfilariae. Dead or dying worms are swept out of the heart and lodge in the branches of the pulmonary arteries, especially those supplying the diaphragmatic lobes. Dead worms are resorbed from the pulmonary vasculature during the subsequent 2–3 months.

In the first 2 months following treatment, the embolic shower of whole or partially phagocytized worms poses a distinct threat to the animal. Absolute rest during the first 2 weeks (the most critical period) is necessary, and only limited exercise should be allowed during the subsequent 6 weeks. Increased body temperature and coughing indicate a pulmonary reaction to embolism.

The proportion of fatalities during or following thiacetarsamide therapy is directly related to the clinical severity of the patients' heartworm disease. Hundreds of asymptomatic dogs are treated without a single loss. Among mildly symptomatic patients, approximately 30% fatality is expected. The poorest risks are dogs in which advanced heartworm disease has resulted in cachexia and ascites; 50% mortality can be expected in this group during or immediately following therapy.

Cats are potential, but not ideal, hosts for *Dirofilaria immitis,* and the prevalence of feline infections is usually about 10% of that in the local dog population. Infections with adult heartworms are far more pathogenic in cats than in dogs. Nevertheless, adulticidal treatment of infected cats with thiacetarsamide cannot be recommended due to the frequency of fatal adverse reactions in treated cats.

Melarsomine. Melarsomine (Immiticide) is a trivalent arsenical of the melanonyl thioarsenite family with activity against adult and 4-month-old heartworms (*Dirofilaria immitis*) in dogs. Its structure is presented in Fig. 47.9.

ADMINISTRATION AND DOSAGE. Melarsomine is marketed as a sterile, lyophilized white powder containing the dihydrochloride salt. It must be reconstituted with 0.9% saline prior to use. Melarsomine is administered to dogs at 2.5 mg/kg (0.1 mL/kg) as two IM doses given 24 hours apart. Deep injections in the lumbar musculature are recommended; injections should be given in alternate sides of the animal on subsequent days. Adult and 4-month-old (L_5) worms appear to be equally sensitive to melarsomine.

A single, two-dose course of treatment kills all male worms and approximately 96% of female heartworms. Treatment completely clears all worms from 60–81% of treated dogs (Keister et al. 1992). When indicated in individual dogs by a lack of seroconversion and per-

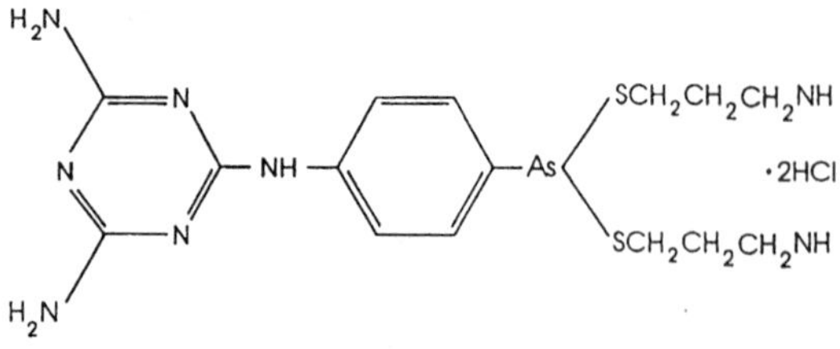

FIG. 47.9—Melarsomine dihydrochloride.

sistent clinical signs, the full, two-dose schedule may be repeated after 90 to 120 days. The described sequence of 2 two-dose regimens 4 months apart is reported to result in complete removal of all adult heartworms in approximately 98% of treated dogs.

Dogs with severe heartworm disease may be given a single dose of 2.5 mg/kg and then rested for at least 1 month, after which time the full, two-dose regimen can be administered. In this sequence, the initial, single treatment is predictably 50% effective, and partial removal of the dog's adult heartworms (88% of males; 17% of females) provides some relief of clinical signs while reducing the complications from pulmonary embolism (Vezzoni et al. 1992).

PHARMACOKINETICS. Following IM injection, melarsomine has a mean absorption half-life of 2.6 minutes and a peak concentration in blood at 8 minutes. Because of its greater bioavailability, melarsomine is adulticidal at approximately half the arsenic equivalent of thiacetarsamide and has approximately twice the therapeutic index. The mean arsenic retention time is about 5 times longer and the body clearance is about 3 times lower for melarsomine than thiacetarsamide (Raynaud 1992). Additionally, melarsomine and its metabolites are free in plasma, unlike thiacetarsamide, which binds to red blood cells. Melarsomine provides higher plasma levels of arsenic for a longer time than thiacetarsamide.

TOXICITY. IM injection of 1–5% solutions of melarsomine results in only minor tissue reactions characterized by mild, localized edema. Overdosage (2 doses of 4.4 mg/kg 3 hours apart) results in distress, restlessness, pawing, salivation, glazed corneas, tachycardia, tachypnea, dyspnea with hilar crackles, abdominal pain and guarded abdomen, hindlimb weakness, recumbency, and difficulty in rising. Signs develop within 30 minutes of overdose administration, and most signs are present by 60 minutes. Severe cases terminate in circulatory collapse, orthopnea, coma, and death. Toxicity can be reversed within 3 hours by IM injection of 3 mg/kg dimercaprol (BAL) administered when the first clinical signs of toxicity appear. However, treatment of clinical toxicity with BAL may reduce the efficacy of melarsomine (Atwell et al. 1989).

Interested readers are referred to the American Heartworm Society, Batavia, Illinois, for authoritative and current recommendations for heartworm diagnosis, management, and prevention.

MISCELLANEOUS NEMATOCIDAL COMPOUNDS. In addition to the major drug classes discussed previously, several chemically distinct anthelmintics have been marketed for a variety of uses in domestic animals. Some of these compounds (disophenol and thenium closylate) have activity that is limited to hookworms in carnivores; neither disophenol nor thenium closylate is still marketed in the USA. Other unique chemicals (*n*-butyl chloride and toluene) also have limited activity but continue to be marketed as over-the-counter products. Hygromycin B is another minor compound that has been displaced by modern drugs with greater efficacy, broader spectra of activity, more flexible regimens, and fewer side effects. For further information about these compounds, readers are referred to an earlier edition of this text (Courtney and Roberson 1995).

RESISTANCE TO NEMATOCIDES. Several species of nematode parasites of domestic animals have developed resistance to certain commonly used anthelmintics (Table 47.2). Resistance may appear whenever antiparasitic drugs are used intensively against parasites that have high biotic potential and for which the host develops little acquired immunity. Horses and small ruminants acquire little immunity to cyathostomes or trichostrongylids, respectively, and the most serious examples of anthelmintic resistance are demonstrated by these nematodes. In contrast, cattle develop good immunity to trichostrongylids, and reports of anthelmintic resistance in nematode parasites of cattle are few.

Nematodes develop resistance to a mode of activity rather than to a specific chemical compound. The entire BZD family is plagued by side-resistance, wherein resistance to one compound essentially imparts resistance to other members of the same chemical family, including those to which the parasites have never been exposed. Side-resistance also occurs between levamisole and morantel in small ruminants.

Other drug classes to which resistance has developed include pyrantel salts and piperazine in equine cyathostomes and imidazothiazoles, organophosphates, and ivermectin in ovine and caprine trichostrongylids.

Resistance generally appears on better-managed farms with a history of intensive anthelmintic use. The development of resistance is directly related to the frequency of deworming. Resistance should be suspected when fecal egg counts remain high or when clinical signs persist following anthelmintic treatment. A veterinarian can make a strong presumptive diagnosis of resistance in a herd by a simple fecal egg count reduction test.

TABLE 47.2—Resistance to antinematodal drugs in veterinary medicine

Host species	Parasites	Parasiticides
Horses	Cyathostomes	Benzimidazoles, phenothiazine, piperazine, pyrantel salts
Small ruminants	Trichostrongylid nematodes	Benzimidazoles, phenothiazine, levamisole/morantel, organophosphates, macrocyclic lactones

If resistance is diagnosed, the herd should be treated with an unrelated compound for which target nematodes are still susceptible. In the USA, small-ruminant producers essentially have three broad categories to choose from (BZDs, macrocyclic lactones, imidazothiazoles), and horse owners have four (piperazine, macrocyclic lactones, pyrantel salts, BZDs).

Once the use of an anthelmintic class has been discontinued, reversion of resistant worm populations to susceptibility is an extremely slow process. Apparently, the genes conferring resistance may be permanent in the absence of selection.

When designing anthelmintic treatment programs, thought should be given to the prevention of resistance. One major strategy recommended by veterinarians is rotation of anthelmintics. Rotation is defined as alternating among anthelmintic classes and not just between different compounds. For example, switching from fenbendazole to oxfendazole is not true rotation because both chemicals are BZDs. Experts differ on recommendations for frequency of rotation. One school promotes rapid rotation, which essentially means that different drug classes are used for each deworming. Still others recommend slow rotation, in which a single drug class is used for an entire calendar year or for an interval that is related to the generation length of the target nematode(s). Some researchers who promote slow rotation have even suggested that an anthelmintic should be used until it is no longer effective. Recent computer models have shown that the eventual onset of anthelmintic resistance can be delayed longest by the concurrent use of two effective anthelmintics each time the host animal is dewormed.

The other major component of selection for anthelmintic resistance is frequency of treatment. Every attempt should be made to use anthelmintics strategically, getting optimal impact from a minimum number of treatments that are timed to disrupt key events in the annual cycle of parasite transmission.

REFERENCES

Atwell, R. B., Sheridan, A. D., Buoro, I. B. J., Kingston, J., and Seton, J. E. 1989. Effective reversal of induced arsenic toxicity using BAL therapy. In G. F. Otto, ed., Proceedings of the Heartworm Symposium `89, pp. 155–158. Washington, DC: American Heartworm Society.

Benz, G. W., and Cox, J. L. 1989. Use of abamectin in cattle. In W. C. Campbell, ed., Ivermectin and Abamectin, pp. 230–233. New York: Springer-Verlag.

Blagburn, B. L., Hendrix, C. M., Lindsay, D. S., Vaughan, J. L., and Hepler, D. I. 1992. Post-adulticide milbemycin oxime microfilaricidal activity in dogs naturally infected with *Dirofilaria immitis.* In M. D. Soll, ed., Proceedings of the Heartworm Symposium `92, pp. 159–164. Batavia, IL: American Heartworm Society.

Bowman, D. D., Johnson, R. C., Ulrich, M. E., Neumann, N., Lok, J. B., Zhang, Y., and Knight, D. H. 1992. Effects of long-term administration of ivermectin and milbemycin oxime on circulating microfilariae and parasite antigenemia in dogs with patent heartworm infections. In M. D. Soll, ed., Proceedings of the Heartworm Symposium `92, pp. 151–158. Batavia, IL: American Heartworm Society.

Bruce, C. I., Bishop, B. F., Evans, N. A., Goudie, A. C., Gration, K. A. F., Gibson, S. P., Pacey, M. S., Petty, D. A., Walshe, N. D. A., and Witty, M. J. 1999. The identification of selamectin: A novel avermectin endectocide for dogs and cats. Proc 44th Ann Mtg Am Assoc Vet Parasitol, p. 55.

Burke, T. M., and Roberson, E. L. 1983. Fenbendazole treatment of pregnant bitches to reduce prenatal and lactogenic infections of *Toxocara canis* and *Ancylostoma caninum* in pups. J Am Vet Med Assoc 183:987–990.

Campbell, W. C., and Benz, G. W. 1984. Ivermectin: a review of efficacy and safety. J Vet Pharmacol Ther 7:1–16.

Chick, B., McDonald, D., Cobb, R., Kieran, P. J., and Wood, I. 1993. The efficacy of injectable and pour-on formulations of moxidectin against lice on cattle. Aust Vet J 70:212–213.

Chiu, S.-H. L., and Lu, A. Y. H. 1989. Metabolism and tissue residues. In W. C. Campbell, ed., Ivermectin and Abamectin, pp. 131–143. New York: Springer-Verlag.

Clark, J. N., Pulliam, J. D., and Daurio, C. P. 1992. Safety and pharmacokinetics of ivermectin in combination with pyrantel in dogs. In M. D. Soll, ed., Proceedings of the Heartworm Symposium `92, pp. 193–196. Batavia, IL: American Heartworm Society.

Conder, G.A., Thompson, D.P., and Johnson, S.S. 1993. Demonstration of co-resistance of *Haemonchus contortus* to ivermectin and moxidectin. Vet Rec 132:651-2.

Courtney, C. H., and Roberson, E. L. 1995. Antinematodal drugs. In H. R. Adams, ed., Veterinary Pharmacology and Therapeutics, 7th ed., pp. 885–932. Ames: Iowa State University Press.

Fink, D. W., and Porras, A. G. 1989. Pharmacokinetics of ivermectin in animals and humans. In W. C. Campbell, ed., Ivermectin and Abamectin, pp. 113–130. New York: Springer-Verlag.

Fisher, M. A., Jacobs, D. E., Hutchinson, M. J., and Abbott, E. M. 1993. Efficacy of fenbendazole and piperazine against developing stages of *Toxocara* and *Toxascaris* in dogs. Vet Rec 132:473–475.

Grieve, R. B., Frank, G. R., Steward, V. A., Parsons, J. C., Abraham, D., MacWilliams, P. S., and Hepler, D. I. 1989. Effect of dosage and dose timing on heartworm (*Dirofilaria immitis*) chemoprophylaxis with milbemycin. In G. F. Otto, ed., Proceedings of the Heartworm Symposium `89, pp. 121–124. Washington, DC: American Heartworm Society.

Hendrix, C. M., Blagburn, B. L., Bowles, J. V., Spano, J. S., and Aguilar, R. 1992. The safety of moxidectin in dogs infected with microfilariae and adults of *Dirofilaria immitis.* In M. D. Soll, ed., Proceedings of the Heartworm Symposium `92, pp. 183–187. Batavia, IL: American Heartworm Society.

Hennessy, D. R., Steel, J. W., and Prichard, R. K. 1993. Biliary secretion and enterohepatic recycling of fenbendazole metabolites in sheep. J Vet Pharmacol Therap 16:132–140.

Keister, D. M., Dzimianski, M. T., McTier, T. L., McCall, J. W., and Brown, J. 1992. Dose selection and confirmation of RM 340, a new filaricide for the treatment of dogs with immature and mature *Dirofilaria immitis.* In M. D. Soll, ed., Proceedings of the Heartworm Symposium `92, pp. 225–229. Batavia, IL: American Heartworm Society.

Knowles, C. O., and Casida, J. E. 1966. Mode of action of organophosphate anthelmintics: cholinesterase inhibition in *Ascaris lumbricoides.* J Agric Food Chem 14:566–572.

Lok, J. B., Knight, D. H., LaPaugh, D. A., and Zhang, Y. 1992. Kinetics of microfilaremia suppression in *Dirofilaria immitis*–infected dogs during and after a prophylactic regimen of milbemycin oxime. In M. D. Soll, ed., Proceedings of the Heartworm Symposium `92, pp. 143–149. Batavia, IL: American Heartworm Society.

Mackenstedt, U., Schmidt, S., Mehlhorn, H., Stoye, M., and Traeder, W. 1993. Effects of pyrantel pamoate on adult and preadult *Toxocara canis* worms: an electron microscope and autoradiography study. Parasitol Res 79:567–578.

McKellar, Q. A., Harrison, P., Galbraith, E. A., and Inglis, H. 1990. Pharmacokinetics of fenbendazole in dogs. J Vet Pharmacol Therap 13:386–392.

McTier, T. L., McCall, J. W., Dzimianski, M. T., Aguilar, R., and Wood, I. 1992. Prevention of experimental heartworm infection in dogs with single oral doses of moxidectin. In M. D. Soll, ed., Proceedings of the Heartworm Symposium `92, pp. 165–168. Batavia, IL: American Heartworm Society.

Miller, J. E. 1993. In E. I. Williams, ed., Proceedings of the Am Assoc Bovine Pract 26:150–153. Alburquerque, NM: Frontier Printers.

Miller, W. H., Scott, D. W., Wellingon, J. R., and Panic, R. 1993. Clinical efficacy of milbemycin oxime in the treatment of generalized demodicosis in adult dogs. J Am Vet Med Assoc 203:1426–1429.

Paul, A. J., Tranquilli, W. J., Todd, K. S., and Aguilar, R. 1992. Evaluation of the safety of moxidectin in collies. In M. D. Soll, ed., Proceedings of the Heartworm Symposium `92, pp. 189–191. Batavia, IL: American Heartworm Society.

Prichard, R. K., and Ranjan, S. 1993. Anthelmintics. Vet Parasitol 46:113–120.

Rae, D. O., Larsen, R. E., and Wang, G. T. 1994. Safety assessment of moxidectin 1% injectable on reproductive performance in beef cows. Am J Vet Res 55:251–253.

Raynaud, J. P. 1992. Thiacetarsamide (adulticide) versus melarsomine (RM 340) developed as a macrofilaricide (adulticide and larvicide) to cure canine heartworm infection in dogs. Ann Rech Vet 23:1–25.

Roberson, E. L. 1988. Antinematodal drugs. In N. H. Booth and L. E. McDonald, eds., Veterinary Pharmacology and Therapeutics, 6th ed., pp. 882–885. Ames: Iowa State University Press.

Roncalli, R. A. 1989. Environmental aspects of use of ivermectin and abamectin in livestock: effects on cattle dung fauna. In W. C. Campbell, ed., Ivermectin and Abamectin, pp. 173–181. New York: Springer-Verlag.

Shoop, W. L. 1994. Ivermectin resistance. Parasitol Today 9:154–159.

Stewart, V. A., Blagburn, B. L., Hendrix, C. M., Hepler, D. I., and Grieve, R. B. 1992. Milbemycin oxime as an effective preventative of heartworm (*Dirofilaria immitis*) infection in cats. In M. D. Soll, ed., Proceedings of the Heartworm Symposium `92, pp. 127–131. Batavia, IL: American Heartworm Society.

Stoye, M. 1992. Biology, pathogenicity, diagnosis, and control of *Ancylostoma caninum*. Dtsch-Tierarztl-Wochenschr 99:315–321.

Supakorndej, P., McTier, T. L., and McCall, J. W. 1993. Evaluation of single oral dosages of moxidectin against hookworms, ascarids, and whipworms in dogs. Proc 38th Ann Mtg Am Assoc Vet Parasitol, p. 35.

Vercruysse, J., ed. 1993. Doramectin—a novel avermectin. Vet Parasitol 49:1–119.

Vezzoni, A., Genchi, C., and Raynaud, J. P. 1992. Adulticide efficacy of RM 340 in dogs with mild and severe natural infections. In M. D. Soll, ed., Proceedings of the Heartworm Symposium `92, pp. 231–240. Batavia, IL: American Heartworm Society.

Xiao, L., Herd, R. P., and Majewski, G. A. 1993. Efficacy of moxidectin equine gel against internal parasite infections in equids with special attention to hypobiotic cyathostomes. Proc 38th Ann Mtg Am Assoc Vet Parasitol, p. 32.

48 ANTICESTODAL AND ANTITREMATODAL DRUGS

CRAIG R. REINEMEYER AND CHARLES H. COURTNEY

ANTICESTODAL DRUGS
Natural Organic Compounds
Inorganic Compounds
Synthetic Organic Compounds
Bunamidine Hydrochloride
Niclosamide
Dichlorophen
Hexachlorophene
Resorantel
Bithionol
Praziquantel
Epsiprantel
Benzimidazoles
Anticestodal Drugs for Horses
ANTITREMATODAL DRUGS
Fasciolosis
Drugs Effective against Adult Flukes
Hexachloroparaxylene
Hexachlorophene
Bithionol Sulfoxide
The Bromsalans
Oxyclozanide
Niclofolan
Nitroxynil
Rafoxanide
Bromophenophos
Clorsulon
Brotianide
Closantel
Benzimidazoles
Drugs with Principal Activity against Immature Flukes
Diamphenethide
Paramphistomosis
Paragonimosis

ANTICESTODAL DRUGS. Anticestodal (antitapeworm) drugs that cause the death of the tapeworm in situ are referred to as taeniacides. Compounds that cause or facilitate tapeworm expulsion are termed taeniafuges. Taeniafuges interfere with the ability of tapeworms to maintain their position in the digestive tract by mucosal attachment of the scolex and by undulation.

Many of the older antitapeworm drugs are natural organic compounds that act as taeniafuges. These drugs paralyze tapeworms at least temporarily, but if tapeworms recover prior to expulsion, they may be able to reattach to the gut. Therefore, the administration of taeniafuges is routinely accompanied by purgation. The disadvantages of purgation plus the demand for greater efficacy have fostered the discovery and development of taeniacidal drugs that are widely used today. Gemmell and Johnstone (1981) have written an excellent review of historical anticestodal compounds used in human and veterinary medicine.

The objective of successful tapeworm treatment is removal of the complete parasite. Because the cestode scolex is capable of regenerating an entire organism, drugs that merely remove the proglottids and soma but leave the scolex intact (i.e., "destrobilization") are unsatisfactory. The usual interval from destrobilization to patency is approximately 3 weeks, so the recommended interval for evaluating tapeworm therapy is ~3 weeks after initial drug treatment.

Virtually all cestodes of veterinary importance have indirect life cycles, so control of intermediate hosts is essential to prevent reinfection following treatment. Examples include controlling the fleas and lice that vector *Dipylidium caninum* in dogs and cats and denying carnivores access to mammalian intermediate hosts to preclude *Taenia* infections. Controlling the oribatid soil mites that vector ruminant and equine tapeworms, however, is currently impractical.

Natural Organic Compounds. The earliest anticestodal drugs used in human and veterinary medicine were of plant origin. Interested readers are referred to the previous edition of this text (Roberson and Courtney 1995) for an expanded discussion of natural compounds such as cucurbitine, male fern extract, kamala, arecoline, and nicotine sulfate.

Inorganic Compounds. The principal inorganic compounds used for their anticestodal properties were tin compounds and lead arsenate. For a discussion of these outmoded compounds, interested readers are referred to the previous edition of this text (Roberson and Courtney 1995).

Synthetic Organic Compounds

BUNAMIDINE HYDROCHLORIDE. *Bunamidine,* INN, was developed in the 1960s and its hydrochloride salt was widely used for treatment of common cestode infections in dogs and cats. Another compound, bunamidine hydroxynapththoate, was effective against *Moniezia* infections in small ruminants.

Although superior to its organic and inorganic natural precursors, bunamidine hydrochloride demonstrated inconsistent efficacy against *Dipylidium caninum* infections, required fasting before treatment (with emesis after treatment a frequent consequence), and occasionally caused fatal adverse reactions in large dogs. Modern cestocidal compounds with greater efficacy and milder side effects have displaced bunamidine, which is no longer marketed in the United States. A thorough discussion of bunamidine can be found in the previous edition of this text (Roberson and Courtney 1995).

NICLOSAMIDE. Niclosamide was widely used for treatment of cestode infections of dogs and cats from the 1960s to the 1980s. It was administered after a 12-hour fast and demonstrated inconsistent efficacy against *Dipylidium* spp. and cestodes other than *Taenia* spp. Like its contemporary, bunamidine, niclosamide has been replaced in small-animal practice by modern cestocides. Interested readers are referred to the previous edition of this text (Roberson and Courtney 1995) for a thorough discussion of the pharmaceutical and therapeutic properties of niclosamide.

DICHLOROPHEN. *Dichlorophen,* INN, has been used as a taeniacide in veterinary medicine for many years. For additional coverage of the chemical properties of dichlorophen, readers are referred to Roberson and Courtney 1995.

Dichlorophen is a taeniacide with efficacy against *Taenia* and *Dipylidium* spp. in the dog and cat, and with limited efficacy against *Moniezia expansa* in sheep. Despite certain disadvantages (frequent vomiting, colic, diarrhea, bulky dose), dichlorophen is still widely used in small-animal practice because it is combined with other antinematodal drugs to formulate several proprietary mixtures. Such mixtures are convenient because they treat both nematodes and cestodes simultaneously. Notable among these mixtures is the combination of dichlorophen with toluene (Vermiplex, Tri-Plex, Difolin) employed for dogs and cats. This combination removes 95% of ascarids, 82% of hookworms, 72% of *Taenia* organisms, and 85% of *Dipylidium* organisms.

HEXACHLOROPHENE. The antitrematodal properties of *hexachlorophene,* USP, will be discussed later in this chapter. In other countries, hexachlorophene enjoys minor use as a cestocide for sheep, cattle, dogs, and poultry. For further discussion of the anticestodal properties of hexachlorophene, readers are referred to Roberson and Courtney 1995.

RESORANTEL. *Resorantel,* INN (Terenol), is an anticestodal compound for ruminants that is now commercially available in parts of Europe. It is a hydroxybenzanilide, chemically named 4′-bromo-γ-resorcylanilide. Resorantel is highly effective (95–100%) against *Moniezia* spp. in both sheep and cattle and against *Thysaniezia giardi* and *Avitellina* spp. in sheep at a dosage of 65 mg/kg. Field trials with large numbers of lambs have demonstrated improved weight gains following removal of tapeworm burdens.

An additional advantage of resorantel is efficacy of approximately 90% against rumen flukes (*Paramphistomum* spp.) in sheep and cattle. Paramphistomosis is discussed later in this chapter.

Little is known about the pharmacodynamics of resorantel. It is excreted rapidly, and serum levels of the drug are undetectable at 48 hours after treatment. Within 3 days of treatment, the total body residue is less than 0.1% of the dose administered. Some minimal blood changes observed in sheep given a 3 times therapeutic dose are rapidly reversible. Side effects of therapeutic doses are limited to slight diarrhea in an occasional animal for 36 hours following treatment. Resorantel is well tolerated, even in ewes treated 2–3 days before lambing.

BITHIONOL. *Bithionol,* INN (Bithin, Lorothidol), is a phenolic compound that is used outside North America for treatment of tapeworm infections of dogs, cats, and poultry, and for tapeworm and rumen fluke infections of sheep, cattle, and goats. For a complete discussion of bithionol's pharmaceutical and therapeutic properties, see Roberson and Courtney 1995.

PRAZIQUANTEL. *Praziquantel,* INN (Droncit), is a novel anthelmintic with excellent activity against a wide spectrum of adult and larval cestodes of animals and humans and against all species of schistosome trematodes that are pathogenic to humans.

CHEMISTRY. Praziquantel is a synthetic isoquinolinepyrazine derivative with the chemical name 4*H*-pyrazino[2,1-a]isoquinolin-4-1,2-(cyclohexylcarbonyl)-1,2,3,6,7,11b-hexahydro-. Its structural formula is shown in Fig. 48.1. Praziquantel is a colorless, almost odorless crystalline compound with a bitter taste. It is soluble in most organic solvents and only sparingly soluble in water.

PHARMACOKINETICS. Praziquantel is quickly and almost completely absorbed from the alimentary tract following oral administration. Significant absorption occurs from the stomach of rats but primarily from the duodenum of mice. Maximum plasma concentrations are obtained after 5 minutes in the mouse, after 15–30 minutes in rats and hamsters, after 30–120 minutes in dogs, and after 2 hours in sheep. The drug is distributed to all organs, crossing the blood-brain barrier of rats (and presumably of other animals) and passing into bile of dogs. The ubiquitous distribution of praziquantel is an asset for activity against larval cestodes that can be located in various organs of the host (musculature, brain, viscera, peritoneal cavity).

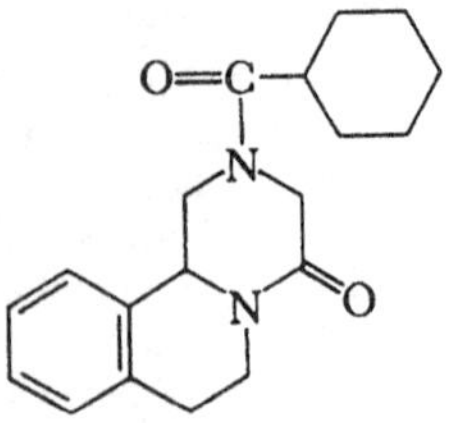

FIG. 48.1—Praziquantel.

Praziquantel is quickly metabolized into inactive forms within the liver. Following an oral dose of 300 mg/kg in rats, the mean drug concentration in portal blood was 21.2 μg/mL, while that in peripheral blood was 6.2 μg/mL. This difference suggests very quick metabolic inactivation of praziquantel by the liver. Plasma concentrations persist longer after intramuscular (IM) or subcutaneous (SC) injection than after oral administration of the same dose. About 80% of ^{14}C-labeled praziquantel administered intravenously to rats, dogs, and rhesus monkeys is eliminated as inactive metabolites, principally in urine, within 24 hours. The half-life of elimination of total radioactivity from the blood of dogs is 3 hours. Only trace amounts of the unchanged dose are excreted in urine and feces (0.3% in mice and dogs, 0.1% in sheep).

MODE OF ACTION. In both in vitro and in vivo studies, praziquantel was absorbed rapidly by cestodes and trematodes. The primary effect is instantaneous: tetanic contraction of parasite musculature and rapid vacuolization of the syncytial tegument. These effects occur within 30 seconds after in vitro contact with the drug at a concentration equivalent to therapeutic serum levels (about 0.3μg/mL) and occur within 15 minutes after in vivo dosing. Rapid contraction apparently is related to increased cell membrane permeability to calcium, with subsequent muscular paralysis.

Vacuolization of the tegument is restricted to the anterior region of the strobila of tapeworms but is scattered over the body surface of trematodes. Vacuoles start at the syncytial layer, increase in size with time, and result in visible blobs above the tegument surface. These burst and create lesions through which neutrophilic and eosinophilic granulocytes enter the parasite tissue and cause lysis within ~4 hours after treatment.

Although the phenomena of muscular contraction and tegument vacuolization appear to be calcium dependent, knowledge of the mode of action of praziquantel on a molecular level is still incomplete. See Andrews and Thomas 1983 for details of the pharmacokinetics of praziquantel.

DOSAGE AND ANTHELMINTIC SPECTRUM. Praziquantel is unique in having extremely high activity against adult stages of all species of tapeworms tested (Thomas and Andrews 1977; Thomas and Gonnert 1978); it also has good activity against larval cestodes (Thomas and Andrews 1977). The method of administration (oral, SC, or IM) affects efficacy slightly, and the SC route is least efficacious. In dogs, 1 mg/kg by any route is 100% effective against adult *Taenia pisiformis;* the same dosage in cats completely clears *Taenia (Hydatigera) taeniaeformis* and *Joyeauxiella pasqualei.* A single treatment of 2 mg/kg clears dogs of *T. hydatigena* and probably *T. ovis* and *T. multiceps,* but 2.5–5 mg/kg is required to completely eliminate *Dipylidium caninum.* A dosage of 5–10 mg/kg is required to obtain 100% removal of *Mesocestoides corti, Echinococcus granulosus,* and *E. multilocularis.* A dosage of 10 mg/kg is required for efficacy against juvenile forms of these parasites. The 5 mg/kg dosage, however, is generally recommended for elimination of the common cestode species of dogs and cats, except *Spirometra mansonoides* and *Diphyllobothrium erinacea,* which require 25 mg/kg on each of 2 consecutive days.

Lung fluke (*Paragonimus*) infections of dogs have been treated successfully with high doses of praziquantel (25 mg/kg) on each of 3 consecutive days. Praziquantel has no efficacy against nematodes but has been combined with febantel in a commercial paste (Vercom), with pyrantel pamoate in a tablet formulation (Drontal), and with both febantel and pyrantel pamoate in a tablet formulation (Drontal Plus) for broad-spectrum use in small animals.

Consistently excellent results against *Echinococcus* make praziquantel ideal for use in eradication programs to reduce the incidence of human hydatid disease. In the United States, Utah has an unusually high incidence of hydatidosis, and much of the investigation with this drug was conducted in that state (Andersen et al. 1978).

Praziquantel is also highly effective against cestodes of ruminants, poultry, and snakes and against certain flukes. All species of *Moniezia, Stilesia,* and *Avitellina* of sheep and/or goats are eliminated by a single dose of 10–15 mg/kg. The pancreatic fluke (*Eurytrema pancreaticum*) of sheep and the intestinal fluke (*Fasciolopsis buski*) of swine have been treated effectively in China with single oral doses of 50–70 and 30 mg/kg, respectively. The common tapeworms of chickens and snakes are expelled by doses of 10 and 3.5–7.0 mg/kg, respectively, without side effects. The skin fluke (*Gyrodactylus aculeatus*) of fish can be removed successfully by placing fish in small tanks for 3 hours in a concentration of 10 mg praziquantel/L water.

Human infections with *Taenia saginata, T. solium,* and *Diphyllobothrium pacificum* are eliminated by oral doses of 10 mg/kg. Removal of *D. latum* and *Schistosoma* spp. requires 25 mg/kg and 40 mg/kg, respectively. The efficacy of 25 mg/kg against *Hymenolepis nana* is incomplete if larval cestodes exceed 5 days of age. De Rezende (1983) and Goldsmith (1988) have reviewed the use of praziquantel against human parasites.

The efficacy of praziquantel against cestode larvae in the intermediate host has been evaluated extensively.

TABLE 48.1—Efficacy of praziquantel against various metacestode stages

Parasite, metacestode	Test host	Regimen		Daily minimum effective dosage	Parasite reduction
		Days	Route	(mg/kg)	(%)
Taenia saginata, cysticercus	Cattle	1	Oral	50	100
		10	Oral	10	100
T. taeniaeformis, strobilocercus	Mice	1	Oral	250	100
				100	0
		5	Oral	50	100
				25	63
		1	SC	250	100
				50	25
		5	SC	25	100
				10	40
T. pisiformis, cysticercus	Rabbit	1	SC	50	Sterilized
		5	SC	25	100
T. hydatigena, cysticercus	Sheep	1	Oral	50	100
		1	SC	50	100*
T. ovis, cysticercus	Sheep	1	SC	50	100
Echinococcus granulosus, hydatid	Sheep	1	SC	50	0
		42	Oral	10	100
	Mice	1	SC	500	**
		5	SC	500	**
Hymenolepis nana, cysticercoid	Mice	1	Oral	25	100

*100% efficacy when fewer than 100 cysts; incomplete when more than 100 cysts.
**Some degeneration of scolices and disruption of germinal epithelium, but no reduction in number or size of cysts.

Table 48.1 lists intermediate stages of tapeworms against which praziquantel has been tested. Of particular interest is its complete efficacy in cattle against the intermediate stage of the human beef tapeworm (*T. saginata*). The endemicity of this zoonotic agent validates the need for a drug that is effective against the metacestode stage (*Cysticercus bovis*).

Although praziquantel is highly effective against adult and juvenile *Echinococcus* organisms in the intestine of carnivores, its activity against the larval stage (hydatid cyst) is disappointing (Table 48.1). The persistent prevalence of human hydatid infections in many parts of the world fuels the search for a cestocidal drug that is totally effective against this stage in humans. Recently, albendazole has given encouraging results and is now undergoing extensive evaluation in the treatment of human hydatid disease.

SAFETY AND TOXICITY. Acute and chronic toxicity studies indicate a wide margin of safety for praziquantel (Muermann et al. 1976). The oral median lethal dose (LD_{50}) in mice and rats is between 2000 and 3000 mg/kg. The LD_{50} is even higher when the drug is given subcutaneously. An acute, oral LD_{50} has not been established in dogs because they vomit when dosages exceed 200 mg/kg. The single therapeutic dose is 3.8–12.5 mg/kg in dogs and 4.2–12.7 mg/kg in cats. Overdoses of up to fivefold are tolerated without adverse effect. Tenfold overdoses may cause transitory vomiting and depression in both dogs and cats. Twentyfold overdoses (200 mg/kg) may be fatal to cats. Dogs given daily dosages of 20, 60, or 180 mg/kg exhibit no changes in hematologic or clinicochemical parameters, except an occasional increase in alkaline phosphatase levels with the highest regimen. Dermal and eye tests in rabbits, guinea pigs, and/or humans indicate that praziquantel does not sensitize the skin or cause irritation.

Studies in pregnant rats and rabbits detected no embryotoxic or teratogenic effects of this drug when given orally at dosages of 30, 100, and 300 mg/kg from the 6th day to the 15th day (rat) or 18th day (rabbit) after copulation. Similar tests in dogs and cats support the use of praziquantel in breeding and pregnant animals without restrictions. Some changes in nuclear structures of treated animals suggest that at some levels praziquantel may have genotoxic effects possibly leading to development of neoplasia (Montero and Ostrosky 1997).

EPSIPRANTEL. *Epsiprantel*, INN (Cestex), is marketed solely as an anticestodal drug. It is chemically related to praziquantel and is a parazino benzazepine with the chemical name 2-(cyclohexylcarbonyl)-4-oxo-l,2,3,4,6,7,8,12b-octahydropyrazino-[2,1-a][2]benzazepine. It is an acid-stable white powder that is sparingly soluble in water. The structural formula of epsiprantel is shown in Fig. 48.2.

PHARMACOKINETICS. Following oral administration, only trace amounts of epsiprantel are absorbed from the gastrointestinal (GI) tract, and most is eliminated in the feces. Mean peak drug plasma levels of 0.13 μg/mL (range, <0.5–0.36 μg/mL) occur in dogs 1 hour after oral dosing with 5.5 mg/kg. After the same dosage, plasma levels are not detected in 83% of cats, and detectable drug concentrations reached only 0.21 μg/mL 30 minutes after dosing. Less than 0.1% of the

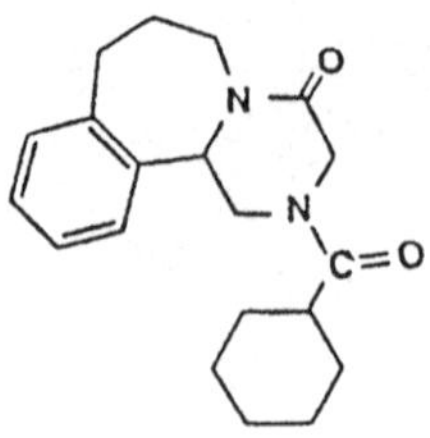

FIG. 48.2—Epsiprantel.

administered dose is recovered in the urine of dogs. There are no metabolites. In contrast, praziquantel is readily absorbed after oral administration, reaches much higher plasma levels, is metabolized to inactive forms by the liver, and is excreted via the bile.

MODE OF ACTION. The mode of action of epsiprantel is apparently similar to that of praziquantel. Although molecular details are unknown, epsiprantel affects tapeworm regulation of calcium and other cations, and the parasite undergoes tetanic contraction. Epsiprantel also damages the tegument of the tapeworm, making it vulnerable to lysis and digestion by the host.

DOSAGE AND ANTHELMINTIC SPECTRUM. Epsiprantel is used specifically for treatment of the common tapeworms of dogs (*Dipylidium caninum, Taenia pisiformis*) and cats (*D. caninum, T. taeniaeformis*). Label dosages of epsiprantel are virtually 100% effective against these cestodes.

The activity of epsiprantel against canine infection by *Echinococcus granulosus* has been evaluated. At a dosage of 5 mg/kg in dogs, the drug is 94% effective against immature (7-day-old) worms and more than 99% effective against 28- and 41-day-old mature stages of *E. granulosus.* Total clearance of mature worms can be achieved with a dosage of 7.5 mg/kg. (Thompson et al. 1991).

The effectiveness of epsiprantel against other GI cestodes or trematodes has not been reported. Due to its low absorption from the GI tract, it is not likely to be effective against extraintestinal helminths such as lung flukes or larval cestodes.

SAFETY AND TOXICITY. Cats tolerate 5 times the therapeutic dose of epsiprantel once daily for 3 days without side effects. Vomiting has been reported in cats administered 40 times the therapeutic dose daily for 4 days.

Beagle puppies (7–10 weeks of age) given 100 mg/kg once (18 times the recommended dosage) exhibited no signs of toxicity. Also, adult dogs treated once with a 36 times overdose were not adversely affected. Daily dosing at 3 times the recommended dosage for 3 consecutive days also is not toxic to pups. Similar studies in Collies and Greyhounds have not produced drug-related side effects. Repeated daily treatment of dogs for 14 days, however, produces occasional emesis at a wide range of dosages from 1.8 to 90 times the single recommended dose.

Benzimidazoles. Benzimidazole anthelmintics are used primarily for their activity against nematodes (Chap. 47). However, some of the substituted benzimidazoles are effective against certain tapeworms and flukes (see below under antitrematodal drugs). Among the notable cestocidal benzimidazoles are mebendazole (Telmintic), fenbendazole (Panacur), oxfendazole (Synanthic), and albendazole (Valbazen).

Mebendazole (22 mg/kg/day for 5 days) and fenbendazole (50 mg/kg/day for 3 days) have good activity against *Taenia* tapeworms of dogs and cats. Mebendazole (two doses of 20 mg/kg q48h; single dose of 160 mg/kg) is also reported to be effective against adult *Echinococcus granulosus* in dogs. Albendazole is effective against *Mesocestoides corti,* an uncommon tapeworm of dogs, at 50 mg/kg q12h for four treatments or 100 mg/kg given once. None of the benzimidazoles is effective against *Dipylidium caninum* in small animals.

In ruminants, albendazole and oxfendazole have satisfactory activity against *Moniezia* tapeworms at the regular therapeutic dosage. Elevated dosages (15 mg/kg) of fenbendazole clear *Moniezia* infections in cattle and sheep. Mebendazole also is effective against *Moniezia* infections at a single dose of 20 mg/kg. Fenbendazole (10 mg/kg) is effective against *Thysanosoma actinioides* of sheep, and oxfendazole is effective against adult (7.5 mg/kg) and immature (10 mg/kg) stages of *Raillietina tetragona* of chickens.

In addition to their effects against adult tapeworms, some of the substituted benzimidazoles are effective against larval forms of tapeworms. For instance, mebendazole kills almost all cysticerci of *Taenia ovis* and *T. hydatigena* in heavily infected sheep. Successful regimens vary but include mebendazole at 50 mg/kg orally for 14 consecutive days, 50 mg/kg/day for 5 consecutive days, or 25 mg/kg for 5 consecutive days (Oguz 1977; Heath and Lawrence 1978). Longer treatment regimens also retard growth of *E. granulosus* cysts in sheep and swine.

Transmission of *T. saginata* tapeworms to humans occurs by ingestion of undercooked beef containing infective cysticerci (*Cysticercus bovis*). Only a few benzimidazoles exhibit activity against the intermediate stages in cattle. Mebendazole was only marginally effective against cysticerci in 10 daily oral doses of 5 mg/kg or in single intraperitoneal (IP) doses of 40 or 100 mg/kg. Better results were obtained with fenbendazole (50 mg/kg) and cambendazole (34 mg/kg), which reduced the number of cysts in beef tissues by 100% after a single oral dose. Flubendazole (10 mg/kg for 10 days) eliminated the larval stage (*Cysticercus cellulosae*) of the human pork tapeworm (*Taenia solium*). A single dose of oxfendazole is effective against *Cysticercus cellulosae* (Gonzalez et al. 1996).

Mebendazole has demonstrated positive results against larval stages of *T. pisiformis* in rabbits, *T. hydatigena* in pigs, and *E. granulosus* and *E. multilocularis* in mice. A brief regimen of treatment (25 mg/kg/day for 5 days) was totally effective for *Taenia* cysticerci in rabbits and pigs. A much longer regimen (60–120 days, 500 ppm mebendazole in food) is necessary for 96% reduction of hydatid cysts of *Echinococcus* in mice. Similar or better results can be obtained against hydatid cysts in mice by giving IP doses of mebendazole (150 mg/kg/day for 3 days) or by oral treatment with fenbendazole (500 ppm in food for 16 weeks). Studies indicate that mebendazole readily crosses the cyst wall by simple diffusion. Protoscolices appear to be more sensitive to the drug than the germinal epithelium of the hydatid cyst. These results have encouraged use of mebendazole (Vermox, USSR) against hydatid disease in humans. Previously, surgical removal of cysts has been only 10% successful.

Mebendazole is also effective against the intermediate stage (tetrathyridium) of *Mesocestoides corti* in mice. Adults and tetrathyridia of *Mesocestoides* can infect dogs, and the latter stage may cause fatal, verminous peritonitis. Five of 6 infected dogs were successfully cleared of larval *Mesocestoides* infections by protracted regimens of fenbendazole at 100 mg/kg twice daily for 14–60 days (Crosbie et al. 1998).

Anticestodal Drugs for Horses. Historically, horses have not been treated routinely for cestode (*Anoplocephala perfoliata*) infections, but public interest in equine tapeworms is definitely increasing. Management of equine tapeworm infections has been hampered by the lack of sensitive diagnostic techniques and by a dearth of biological information about the tapeworm and its oribatid mite vectors. Little is known about the seasonal patterns of transmission, so strategic treatment recommendations to disrupt the annual cycle of reinfection are purely speculative at present.

No products are currently labeled in the United States specifically for treatment of equine cestode infections. Limited tests have shown that pyrantel pamoate (13.2 mg/kg), pyrantel tartrate (2.64 mg/kg daily for 30 days), niclosamide (88 mg/kg), dichlorophen (20 mg/kg), bithionol (7 mg/kg), mebendazole (20 mg/kg), and praziquantel (0.5–1.5 mg/kg) (Lyons et al. 1995; Lyons et al. 1998) are effective and safe cestocides for horses.

ANTITREMATODAL DRUGS. Fasciolosis (infection with *Fasciola hepatica*) is the most common and most economically important trematode disease of domestic animals worldwide. Most of the antitrematodal drugs discussed in this section are compounds used in treatment of fasciolosis. Brief attention also will be given to treatment of infections caused by rumen flukes (*Paramphistomum*) in cattle and sheep and by lung flukes (*Paragonimus*) in dogs and cats.

Fasciolosis. Liver-dwelling trematodes adversely affect the health of sheep and cattle in the United Kingdom, Australia, southern and western United States, and some tropical regions of the world. The United Kingdom has experienced three major outbreaks of acute and chronic fasciolosis in sheep since World War II. In the United States, liver fluke disease is typically more chronic and subclinical in nature.

Both immature and mature flukes damage the host liver. After metacercariae are ingested by grazing sheep or cattle, the immature fluke emerges from its cyst, penetrates the wall of the small intestine, traverses the peritoneal cavity, and penetrates the liver capsule within 4 days of infection. During the next several weeks, immature flukes tunnel through liver tissues, feeding and increasing rapidly in size. The extensive damage and resultant hemorrhaging of the liver often result in clinical signs of acute fasciolosis within 6–8 weeks after infection. This stage is often fatal. During the eighth week of infection, flukes begin to penetrate the main bile ducts, where they attain sexual maturity by ~10–12 weeks after infection. The flukes are most susceptible (or perhaps most accessible) to fasciolicidal drugs at this stage.

Adult flukes, often in pairs, lodge within a bile canal, causing biliary hyperplasia and progressive occlusion. Heavily infected areas may become walled off from the rest of the liver by connective tissue. Such areas become progressively less penetrable by therapeutic agents and consequently more difficult to treat.

The severity of *F. hepatica* infections in sheep may be enhanced by the fluke's potential role in disseminating enteric bacteria (*Clostridium novyi*) in the liver during migration. The resultant infectious, necrotic hepatitis (black disease) can be fatal. A vaccine against *C. novyi,* however, is helpful in controlling the disease.

DRUGS EFFECTIVE AGAINST ADULT FLUKES. Since the introduction of carbon tetrachloride for treatment of helminth infections of animals in the 1920s, numerous other compounds have been investigated for efficacy against *F. hepatica.*

On the basis of chemical structure, the fasciolicidal drugs can be separated into several groups: (1) the halogenated hydrocarbons (carbon tetrachloride, hexachloroethane, tetrachlorodifluoroethane, hexachloroparaxylene) were reviewed in the 6th edition of this text (Roberson 1988), (2) the bisphenolic compounds (hexachlorophene, bithionol sulfoxide, the bromsalans, oxyclozanide, clioxanide), (3) the nitrophenolic compounds (disophenol, niclofolan, nitroxynil), (4) the newer salicylanilides (closantel, brotianide), (5) sulfonamides (clorsulon), and (6) benzimidazoles (albendazole, triclabendazole). A common feature of the first three drug groups is the presence of halogen atoms. It is unknown whether the halogen atom presents a common mechanism for fasciolicidal activity of these drugs, but this is considered unlikely (Fowler 1971).

The flukicides discussed below are marketed in most livestock-producing areas, including Europe, Africa, and Australia. Richards et al. (1990) in Australia compared the efficacies of many antitrematodal drugs against immature and mature stages of *F. hepatica* in cattle. The drugs tested were triclabendazole, albendazole, clorsulon, nitroxynil, oxyclozanide, and rafoxanide. Earlier, Losson (1988) reviewed these drugs as well as closantel and diamphenethide. Among these compounds, however, only albendazole and clorsulon have Food and Drug Administration (FDA) approval for use against fluke infections in the United States.

Fasciolicidal drugs historically have targeted adult-stage flukes. Consequently, immature flukes in the liver parenchyma largely escaped therapeutic activity until the introduction of diamphenethide in 1971. This drug demonstrates greatest efficacy against young flukes, and its effectiveness diminishes as the flukes age.

HEXACHLOROPARAXYLENE. Hexachloroparaxylene is a chlorinated derivative of benzene. For a brief discussion of this compound, readers are referred to the 7th edition of this text (Roberson and Courtney 1995).

HEXACHLOROPHENE. Hexachlorophene is not approved for use in the United States. It has good efficacy against adult flukes but no effect against immature flukes less than 8 weeks of age. Hexachlorophene is discussed in the 7th edition of this text (Roberson and Courtney 1995).

BITHIONOL SULFOXIDE. Bithionol has activity against rumen flukes (*Paramphistomum* spp.) and liver flukes (*Fasciola* and *Fascioloides* spp.) of ruminants and also has some anticestodal properties. Roberson and Courtney (1995) offer further coverage of bithionol.

THE BROMSALANS. The bromsalans are available in some countries for the treatment of mature and immature *Fasciola* infections. These compounds are discussed by Roberson and Courtney (1995).

OXYCLOZANIDE. *Oxyclozanide,* INN (Zanil), was introduced over 30 years ago for use against adult fluke infections and in some countries is formulated together with levamisole to offer broad-spectrum helminth treatment. Oxyclozanide is discussed further by Roberson and Courtney (1995).

NICLOFOLAN. *Niclofolan,* INN (Bilevon, Distolon, Dertil, Menichlopholan), is a nitrosubstituted analog of hexachlorophene. Its chemical formula is 4,4′-dichloro-6,6′-dinitro-*o,o*-biphenol. In addition to the typical adulticidal spectrum, niclofolan has some efficacy against immature *Fasciola* organisms, but only at dosages that are clinically unsafe. Further discussion of niclofolan's properties is included in the 7th edition of this text (Roberson and Courtney 1995).

NITROXYNIL. *Nitroxynil,* INN (Dovenix, Trodax), has the chemical name 4-hydroxy-3-iodo-5-nitrobenzonitrile.

Nitroxynil was developed in the United Kingdom in the late 1960s as an injectable fasciolicide for sheep and cattle. It can be administered orally but is more effective when administered by the SC or IM route. SC or IM administration provides similar efficacy for liver flukes, but the SC route has become the method of choice in practice. It is injected in the side of the neck of cattle and at any convenient site in sheep. The ease of SC administration gives nitroxynil an advantage over fasciolicides that must be administered orally. This compound stains wool or hair yellow; thus, care must be exercised to avoid spilling. Local tolerance at the site of injection is satisfactory, although transitory inflammatory swellings are occasionally observed in cattle.

Nitroxynil is effective against mature *F. hepatica* and *F. gigantica,* but not paramphistomes in sheep and cattle. It also can be used to treat haemonchosis and *Parafilaria bovicola* infections in these hosts. Nitroxynil is more than 99% effective against ivermectin- and benzimidazole-resistant *Haemonchus contortus* of sheep.

Nitroxynil has high activity against mature liver flukes at 10 mg/kg, and its activity against immature flukes reduces mortality from acute fasciolosis in sheep. Efficacy drops off, however, against flukes that are younger than 6 weeks. Nitroxynil is well tolerated at the therapeutic dosage of 10 mg/kg, but higher dosages are not recommended because of potential adverse reactions.

RAFOXANIDE. *Rafoxanide,* INN (Flukanide, Ranide), is a halogenated salicylanilide. Its chemical formula is 3′-chloro-4′-(*p*-chlorophenoxy)-3,5-diiodosalicylanilide. It is an off-white crystalline powder and is commercially formulated for use as a bolus or drenching suspension.

Indications and Effectiveness. Rafoxanide was developed in 1969 and subsequently has been used extensively against fasciolosis and haemonchosis in sheep and cattle in the United Kingdom, Europe, Australia, Brazil, and South Africa. Its principal use is as an adulticide for *F. hepatica* and *F. gigantica,* but it also has respectable efficacy against immature flukes. A single therapeutic dose (7.5 mg/kg) in sheep provides the following efficacies for various ages of *F. hepatica:* nearly 100% for 12-week-old flukes, 86–99% for 6-week-old flukes, and 50–98% for 4-week-old flukes. The same dosages afford similar efficacies against *F. hepatica* in cattle. The reliable efficacy of this drug against 4- and 6-week-old flukes gives rafoxanide an advantage over strictly adulticidal drugs in the treatment of acute fasciolosis. Repeat treatment is advised at 3-week intervals to eliminate maturing flukes that may have escaped earlier treatment.

Rafoxanide is also indicated in the treatment of haemonchosis, bunostomosis, and sheep nasal bots. Greater than 96% efficacy is reported against adult *Haemonchus* and *Bunostomum* in cattle, and against adult and immature forms of these parasites in sheep. Rafoxanide also appears to be highly effective (98%) against all parasitic larval stages of the sheep nasal bot (*Oestrus ovis*).

Pharmacokinetics and Mode of Action. Following oral dosing, rafoxanide is absorbed (presumably from the small intestine) into the bloodstream. Peak plasma levels occur between 24 and 48 hours. The drug is not metabolized to any detectable degree by cattle or sheep. It is extensively bound (>99%) to plasma proteins and has a long (16.6-day) terminal half-life. Perhaps some of the efficacy of rafoxanide against immature flukes is due to its prolonged persistence in the plasma, with subsequent effects on maturing flukes as they reach the bile ducts. Following a single oral dose of 15 mg/kg in cattle, no residue of the compound is detectable in edible tissues at 28 days after treatment.

The mode of action of rafoxanide apparently is as a proton ionophore, transporting cations across cell membranes and ultimately uncoupling oxidative phosphorylation within parasitic mitochondria (Martin 1997).

BROMOPHENOPHOS. *Bromophenophos,* INN (Acedist), is an organophosphoric acid ester. Its chemical formula is 4,4′,6,6′-tetrabromo-2,2′ biphenyldiol mono (dihydrogen phosphate).

Bromophenophos is used to treat *F. hepatica* infections in cattle. Its efficacy for adult flukes is 85–100%, and it has reasonably good activity against immature flukes. Bromophenophos is administered orally to cattle at a dosage of 12 mg/kg.

CLORSULON. *Clorsulon* (Curatrem) is a benzenesulfonamide with the chemical formula 4-amino-6-trichloroethenyl-1,3-benzenedisulfonamide. Its structural formula is shown in Fig. 48.3. Clorsulon is formulated commercially as a drench for sheep and cattle and as a SC injection for cattle (in combination with ivermectin). In the United States, clorsulon and albendazole are the only drugs approved by the FDA for treatment of *F. hepatica* infections. Albendazole is approved for beef and nonlactating dairy cattle; clorsulon is approved for beef and dairy cattle, regardless of lactation status. Neither drug is approved for sheep in the United States.

Indications and Effectiveness. Oral administration of 3.75 mg/kg clorsulon provides 100% efficacy against adult *F. hepatica* (14 or 16 weeks old) in both sheep and cattle. Higher dosages are needed to attain similar levels of efficacy against younger flukes. A single dose of 15 mg/kg clorsulon was 92–99.5% effective against 6- and 8-week-old flukes; 30 mg/kg removed 99.7% of 3-week-old infections and 85.3% of 2-week-old infections. Based on these data, the label dosage of 7 mg/kg is predicted to be approximately 88% effective for immature flukes and 99% effective for mature forms of *F. hepatica* in sheep and cattle. In one endemic area of

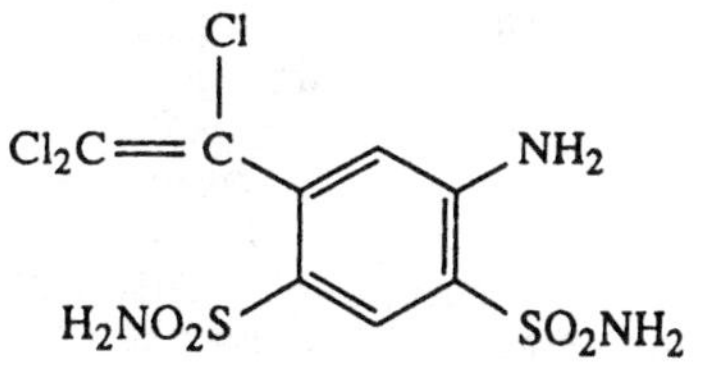

Cl

$Cl_2C{=}C$ — NH_2

H_2NO_2S — SO_2NH_2

FIG. 48.3—Clorsulon.

the United States (Florida) where snail vectors are present on pasture from December to June, it is suggested that treatment with clorsulon in late fall and again in early spring should prevent most transmission of *Fasciola* organisms (Courtney et al. 1985).

The combination of clorsulon with ivermectin in a SC injectable formulation (Ivomec Plus) was designed for simultaneous treatment of *Fasciola* and nematode infections of cattle. The oral formulation of clorsulon (Curatrem) also can be used concurrently with other anthelmintics (e.g., ivermectin, fenbendazole) with no reduction in efficacy of the individual products (Malone et al. 1990).

The efficacy of clorsulon has been tested against infections with several other fluke species in ruminants. It is reasonably effective (>92%) against immature (8-week-old) *Fascioloides magna* in cattle and sheep at an elevated dosage of 21 mg/kg orally. It is not so effective (74%), however, against older (16-week-old) *F. magna* in these atypical hosts. Daily dosing at 7 mg/kg for 5 consecutive days has been 100% effective against adult and 92% effective against immature *Fasciola gigantica* in cattle. Clorsulon has poor efficacy against the rumen fluke, *Paramphistomum.*

Pharmacokinetics and Mode of Action. Schulman et al. (1979) used radiolabeling techniques to determine that clorsulon enters the blood rapidly after treatment and attains maximum concentration approximately 4 hours later, when 75% of the circulating drug is in the plasma and 25% is in erythrocytes. Drug concentration within flukes peaks at 8–12 hours after dosing.

Residue studies indicate a short half-life of clorsulon in tissues and milk. Milk taken from treated animals within 72 hours (six milkings) after treatment should not be used for human consumption, and beef animals should not be slaughtered within 8 days of treatment.

The mode of action of clorsulon has been studied by measuring its effect on glycolytic enzymes of *F. hepatica.* Inhibition of 3-phosphoglycerate kinase and phosphoglyceromutase occurred. This enzymatic inhibition effectively blocks the Embden-Myerhof glycolytic pathway and thereby deprives the fluke of its main source of metabolic energy.

Safety and Toxicity. Acute toxicity of clorsulon has been assessed in mice, rats, sheep, and cattle. The LD_{50} in mice is an IP dose of 761 mg/kg and more than

10,000 mg/kg orally. The latter dose causes no apparent toxicity in rats. Sheep infected with flukes have been dosed repeatedly with 5 mg/kg daily for 28 days or with single doses of 100 mg/kg with no apparent effect. Uninfected sheep tolerated 200 or 400 mg/kg without adverse reactions. A toxic dosage has not been identified in cattle. Oral doses of 7 mg (label) and 21 mg/kg on 3 consecutive days and single oral doses of 7, 70, and 175 mg/kg (i.e., up to 25 times the label dosage) have not affected weight gains, feed consumption, or clinical or histopathologic parameters adversely. In uninfected goats, experimental dosages up to 35 mg/kg every other day for 3 doses did not cause adverse reactions.

Clorsulon is considered safe for use in breeding and pregnant animals. Teratology studies and male fertility studies in laboratory animals have not demonstrated any drug effect. Also, studies in cattle (monthly double doses for 4 months before breeding and monthly during the last two trimesters of pregnancy) have not demonstrated adverse effects on conception or parturition.

Dosage. The recommended dosage of clorsulon for cattle (and sheep where approved) is 7 mg/kg by oral drench. In commercial combination with ivermectin, clorsulon is administered SC to cattle at a rate of 2 mg/kg and ivermectin at 0.2 mg/kg.

BROTIANIDE. *Brotianide,* INN (Dirian), is a salicylanilide derivative that is marketed in parts of Western and Eastern Europe, the former Soviet Union, Madagascar, New Zealand, and Australia to treat fluke infections of *Fasciola hepatica, Fasciola gigantica,* and *Paramphistomum* spp. in sheep and cattle. Roberson and Courtney (1995) discuss brotianide in greater detail in the 7th edition of this text.

CLOSANTEL. *Closantel,* INN (Flukiver), is a salicylanilide, like rafoxanide, oxyclozanide, and brotianide. It is used in the United Kingdom, Australia, and South Africa for its activity against *Fasciola hepatica, Haemonchus contortus,* and certain arthropods of sheep and/or cattle. Its chemical formula is *N*-[5-chloro-4-[(4-chlorophenyl)cyanomethyl]-2-methylphenyl]-2-hydroxy-3,5-diiodobenzamide. Metabolic studies indicate that the drug uncouples oxidative phosphorylation by increasing parasite mitochondrial permeability (i.e., proton ionophore).

Closantel is principally a flukicide for sheep and cattle. At an oral dosage of 10 mg/kg, its efficacy in either host is more than 92.8% against 8-week-old and adult *F. hepatica.* It is less active against younger stages of this parasite, i.e., 70–77% efficacy for 6-week-old flukes migrating in the liver. It is also effective (94.6–97.7%) against 8-week-old *Fascioloides magna* in sheep at oral dosages of 15 mg/kg or IM dosages of 7.5 mg/kg. Closantel is not effective, however, against paramphistome flukes.

In addition to activity for flukes, closantel is active against certain other helminths and arthropods. Notably, it is effective against *Haemonchus contortus* of sheep and has been used successfully against ivermectin-, benzimidazole-, levamisole/morantel-, and rafoxanide-resistant strains of this parasite. Certain strains of *H. contortus,* however, have developed resistance to closantel. The drug can be used against the adult stage of *Ancylostoma caninum,* but is not effective against the somatic larvae of this hookworm. Closantel also has been used in horses to prevent or reduce infections of *Strongylus vulgaris* and *Gasterophilus* spp. A regimen of 8 mg/kg orally every 2 months prevents establishment of bots in the stomach and reduces numbers of larval *S. vulgaris* in the mesenteric arteries by ~86%.

As with other salicylanilides, closantel is extensively bound (>99%) to plasma proteins, mainly albumin, and has a long terminal half-life of 14.5 days. This persistence profile helps prevent *Haemonchus* infections of sheep for up to 60 days after treatment and is thought to enhance efficacy against *F. hepatica* as newly matured flukes enter the bile duct. The drug is excreted primarily (80%) in feces, and less than 0.5% is excreted in the urine. Tissue concentrations are minute, and their decline mirrors decreases in plasma concentration.

Closantel is well tolerated. In sheep, repeated dosing orally or SC at 10 or 40 mg/kg or IM at 20 mg/kg every 4 weeks over a 40-week period did not cause adverse reactions. Extensive reproductive studies in rams, ewes, and bulls indicate that closantel poses no risk to reproductive parameters.

BENZIMIDAZOLES. Among the benzimidazoles, albendazole (Valbazen; *see* Table 47.1) is unique in having therapeutic activity against adult forms of *F. hepatica* (76–100%) and *Fascioloides magna* (63–99%) at single doses of 10 mg/kg in cattle or 7.5 mg/kg in sheep. At these dosages, the activity for immature (3-week-old) *Fasciola* organisms is only 25%, but this can be increased to 75% with an elevated dosage of 50 mg/kg in cattle (Knight and Colglazier 1977). Even greater efficacy has been achieved in sheep (but not cattle) by using albendazole prophylactically in small daily doses of 3 mg/kg/day for 35 days (Rew and Knight 1980; Fetterer et al. 1982). Sheep exposed to infective metacercariae of *Fasciola hepatica* during the first week of this prophylactic regimen have 98% fewer flukes and minimal, if any, hepatic fibrosis or necrosis in comparison to unmedicated controls. More recently an intraruminal slow-release capsule (Proftril-Captec) has been developed that protects sheep against establishment of infection with *F. hepatica* and *Dicrocoelium dentriticum.* Albendazole (15 mg/kg) is also effective against *Dicrocoelium* organisms in sheep and against *F. hepatica* in goats.

Fenbendazole is not as effective as albendazole against *F. hepatica* but apparently has good activity against *Dicrocoelium* organisms in sheep at a single dose of 100 mg/kg. Adult and migrating immature stages of rumen flukes (*Paramphistomum*) of cattle are partially susceptible (~75%) to treatment with fenbendazole (7.5 mg/kg in feed for 6 days). *Fasciola gigantica* infection in sheep is reduced (95%) by a single treatment with fenbendazole at 5 mg/kg. Dogs experimentally infected with the blood fluke *Heterobilharzia americana* have been cleared of infection by using fenbendazole at a daily regimen of 40 mg/kg for 10 consecutive days. In addition, there is one report of successful treatment of pancreatic fluke (*Eurytrema procyonis*) in a cat by using fenbendazole at 30 mg/kg/day for 6 days.

Triclabendazole (Fasinex) has been investigated as a fasciolicide for cattle, sheep, and goats in Europe, the United Kingdom, Australia, South Africa, and the United States. Although the drug is principally active against adult flukes, higher doses are effective for immature forms. Efficacies of 98–100% against *F. hepatica* in sheep can be obtained with doses of 15 mg/kg for 1-day-old flukes, 12.5 mg/kg for 1- to 4-week-old flukes, 10 mg/kg for 6- to 8-week-old flukes, 5 mg/kg for 10-week-old flukes, and 2.5 mg/kg for 12-week-old flukes. In general, doses of 5 mg/kg for goats, 10 mg/kg for sheep, and 12 mg/kg for cattle are recommended for acute, subacute, or chronic fasciolosis. The maximum tolerated dosage in sheep is 200 mg/kg. This criterion has not been reported for cattle or goats.

Triclabendazole also has been successful in the treatment of *F. hepatica* in horses (12 mg/kg), *F. gigantica* in cattle (12 mg/kg), and *Fascioloides magna* in white-tailed deer (10 mg/kg), sheep (20 mg/kg), and wapiti (50–60 mg/kg). It can be used simultaneously with antinematodal drugs such as fenbendazole without adverse effects.

The pharmacokinetics of triclabendazole were investigated by Hennessy et al. (1987) and Kinabo and Bogan (1988). In general, the drug is metabolized rapidly to its sulfoxide and sulfone derivatives after oral or intrarumenal administration. Maximum plasma concentrations are achieved in approximately 12–36 hours. Triclabendazole derivatives are bound to albumin and persist at measurable concentrations in plasma for up to 7 days. Excretion is principally via bile (approximately 50%). The binding of triclabendazole to plasma albumin likely influences the duration of exposure of flukes to the anthelmintic activity of this drug.

Netobimin is a probenzimidazole with primary antinematodal activity at a dosage of 7.5 mg/kg. At elevated dosages (15 and 20 mg/kg), it is effective against adult stages of flukes, including *Dicrocoelium dendriticum* (92–98.9% efficacy) and *F. hepatica* (90.7% efficacy). It is not effective at 15 mg/kg, however, against rumen flukes.

DRUGS WITH PRINCIPAL ACTIVITY AGAINST IMMATURE FLUKES

DIAMPHENETHIDE. *Diamphenethide,* INN (Coriban), possesses exceptionally high activity against the youngest stages of *F. hepatica,* but its activity decreases with aging of the fluke. This is in direct contrast to other currently used fasciolicides, which tend to be less active against younger flukes. The development of diamphenethide offers promise for a potential prophylactic program against liver fluke disease in sheep.

Chemistry. Chemically, diamphenethide is β,β′-*bis*(4-acetamidophenyloxy)ethyl ether. Its structural formula is shown in Fig. 48.4.

Pharmacokinetics. Following oral administration, diamphenethide is absorbed into the blood and distributed throughout the body. At 3 days after dosing, its concentration is greatest in the liver and gallbladder, especially in gallbladder contents. It should be noted that adult flukes reside in intimate association with the biliary system. At 7 days after dosing, concentrations of diamphenethide in these sites are reduced approximately 10-fold, to a range of only 0.1–0.5 ppm, while concentrations in the musculature are approximately 0.02 ppm. In the United Kingdom, animals intended for human consumption are permitted to be slaughtered 7 days after treatment.

Mode of Action. The efficacy of diamphenethide appears to depend upon deacylation of the drug by liver enzymes (deacylases) to an amine metabolite that is active against liver flukes. Diamphenethide is not active against liver flukes in vitro unless incubated in the presence of enzymatically functional liver cells. High concentrations of the amine metabolite are produced in liver parenchyma, where immature flukes are found until at least 7 weeks after infection. It is thought that the metabolite is also rapidly destroyed in the liver. Small amounts of the metabolite may escape into the bloodstream but become diluted. The quantity of active metabolite reaching mature flukes in the bile ducts is small; therefore, efficacy against adult stages is reduced. Anderson and Fairweather (1988) have described drug-induced changes in the integument of flukes and have suggested potential modes of action. Safety of this drug for the host can be explained on the basis of destruction of the toxic metabolite by the liver and dilution in blood so that only small quantities reach other tissues of the body.

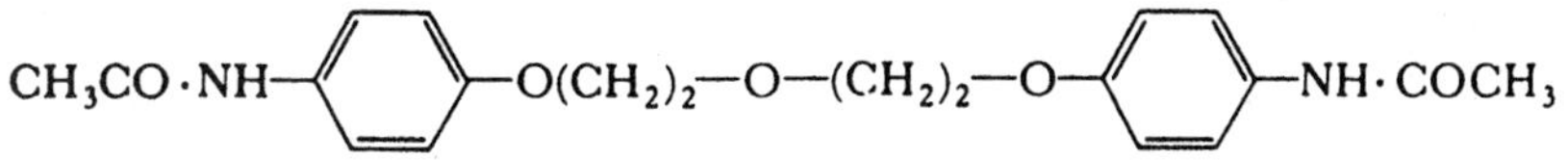

$$CH_3CO \cdot NH-C_6H_4-O(CH_2)_2-O-(CH_2)_2-O-C_6H_4-NH \cdot COCH_3$$

FIG. 48.4—Diamphenethide.

Treatment of Acute Fasciolosis. Diamphenethide is used for treatment of acute fasciolosis resulting from immature forms of *F. hepatica* migrating through the liver parenchyma of sheep. A dosage of 100 mg/kg diamphenethide is almost 100% effective against flukes from 1 to 63 days of age.

The activity of diamphenethide against 10-week-old (i.e., recently mature) flukes diminishes to 78%, and the efficacy for flukes 12 weeks of age or older is 70% or less. Accordingly, a single treatment normally eliminates all the young flukes but leaves at least 30% of the mature population to continue shedding eggs and contaminating pastures.

Prophylaxis. The fundamental prerequisites for successful prevention of fasciolosis include elimination of the existing fluke population in toto; halting contamination of pastures with fluke eggs; and prevention of acute, chronic, or subclinical fasciolosis. To accomplish all these prerequisites, an ideal fasciolicide must be highly efficacious against all parasitic stages of *F. hepatica.* Of the current drugs, only the combination of rafoxanide (with efficacy that spans 4-week-old to adult flukes) and diamphenethide (effective against 1-day-old to 10-week-old flukes) most closely approaches the ideal fasciolicide and therefore offers the best chance for successful chemoprophylaxis.

The value of rafoxanide for prophylaxis of fasciolosis has been demonstrated in Scotland (Armour and Corba 1972; Whitelaw and Fawcett 1981). Drenching of ewes twice (in the spring and early summer) at an interval of 6 weeks kept the test pastures virtually clear of fluke eggs over the vital periods of snail breeding and infection by miracidia. Two further treatments in the fall (6 weeks apart) reduced infection in ewes to negligible proportions in the winter. Armour and Corba (1972) and Rowlands et al. (1985) have proposed that treatments with diamphenethide at 6- to 8-week intervals (twice in the spring and twice in the fall) should provide excellent control of fasciolosis.

Toxicity. The usual oral dosage of 100 mg/kg in sheep apparently is safe. A single oral dose four times the therapeutic dosage (400 mg/kg) produces no toxic signs. At higher dosages, toxic effects include temporary impairment of vision and loss of wool. Pastured sheep are less susceptible to toxic effects than housed sheep. At a dosage of 1600 mg/kg, diamphenethide produces a low incidence of mortality. An acute LD_{50} value for sheep apparently has not been established.

Contraindications. There appear to be no significant contraindications for use of diamphenethide. Pregnant ewes dosed with 200 mg/kg once weekly on 2, 3, or 4 consecutive occasions during the 21-week gestation period exhibited no adverse effects on fertility or teratogenic effects in their offspring. Adverse effects on fertility have not been reported in ewes and rams dosed during the mating period.

Administration and Dosage. Diamphenethide is marketed as a suspension for oral administration to sheep in a single dose of 100 mg/kg. The same dosage is effective and safe for use in goats.

Paramphistomosis. Rumen fluke (*Paramphistomum* spp.) infections are common in cattle and sheep throughout the world. Adult flukes attach to the rumen wall and are of little consequence to the health of the animal. Large numbers of the immature stages, however, can be seriously pathogenic as they migrate within the gut lumen from the duodenum to the rumen. Symptoms are more pronounced in young, previously uninfected sheep or cattle and include severe anorexia, polydipsia, and watery, fetid diarrhea that ultimately results in reduced production or death.

Intestinal paramphistomosis generally responds well to treatment with drugs that are effective against liver fluke and/or cestode infections in ruminants. These include niclosamide, niclofolan, resorantel, and bithionol. Concurrent treatment of infected dairy cows with oxyclozanide and oxfendazole increased milk production by 0.4 liters/day (Spence et al. 1996). Roberson and Courtney (1995) discuss therapy of paramphistomosis at length.

Paragonimosis. Lung fluke (*Paragonimus* spp.) infection is diagnosed occasionally in dogs and cats in the Americas and in the Far East. Four drugs are apparently efficacious against *Paragonimus* organisms: bithionol, praziquantel, albendazole, and fenbendazole. The oral dose of bithionol for dogs and cats is 100 mg/kg every other day for a total of 10–15 treatments. The efficacy of bithionol is rather unpredictable (15–85% reduction in number of flukes), and the drug has undesirable side effects in small animals.

Praziquantel is effective against *Paragonimus* infection in dogs when given at 25 mg/kg on each of 3 consecutive days. The efficacy of praziquantel against *Paragonimus* infection in cats has not been evaluated.

Albendazole, at a dosage of 25 mg/kg twice daily for 14 days, is highly effective against *Paragonimus* infection in both cats and dogs. The twice-daily regimen is crucial; otherwise, single daily doses of 100 mg/kg for 14 days are required to effect a cure (Dubey et al. 1978).

Fenbendazole kills adult flukes in dogs and reduces lung lesions without side effects (Dubey et al. 1979). Effective doses include 50 mg/kg twice daily for 10 days and 25 mg/kg twice daily for 14 days. Shedding of fluke eggs in feces ceased 3 and 8 days after initiation of the respective regimens.

REFERENCES

Andersen, F. L., Conder, G. A., and Marsland, W. P. 1978. Efficacy of injectable and tablet formulations of praziquantel against mature *Echinococcus granulosus.* Am J Vet Res 39:1861–1862.

Anderson, H. R., and Fairweather, I. 1988. *Fasciola hepatica:* Scanning electron microscopic observations of juvenile flukes following treatment in vitro with the deacetylated (amine) metabolite of diamphenethide (DAMD). Int J Parasitol 18:827–837.

Andrews, P., and Thomas, H. 1983. Praziquantel. Med Res Rev 3:147–200.

Armour, I., and Corba, J. 1972. The anthelmintic efficiency of diamphenethide against *Fasciola hepatica* in sheep. Vet Rec 91:211–213.

Courtney, C. H., Shearer, I. K., and Plue, R. E. 1985. Efficacy and safety of clorsulon used concurrently with ivermectin for control of *Fasciola hepatica* in Florida beef cattle. Am J Vet Res 46:1245–1246.

Crosbie, P. R., Boyce, W. M., Platzer, E. G., Nadler, S. A., and Kerner, C. 1998. Diagnostic procedures and treatment of eleven dogs with peritoneal infections caused by *Mesocestoides* spp. J Am Vet Med Assoc 213:1578–1583.

De Rezende, G. L. 1983. Praziquantel: Experiencia clinica mundial. Bol Chil Parasitol 38:52–63.

Dubey, I. P., Hoover, E. A., Stromberg, P. C., et al. 1978. Albendazole therapy for experimentally induced *Paragonimus kellicotti* infection in cats. Am J Vet Res 39:1027–1031.

Dubey, I. P., Miller, T. B., and Sharma, S. P. 1979. Fenbendazole for treatment of *Paragonimus kellicotti* infection in dogs. J Am Vet Med Assoc 174:835–837.

Fetterer, R., Rew, R. S., and Knight, R. 1982. Comparative efficacy of albendazole against *Fasciola hepatica* in sheep and calves: relationship to serum drug metabolite levels. Vet Parasitol 11:309–316.

Fowler, I. S. L. 1971. Toxicity of carbon tetrachloride and other fasciolicidal drugs in sheep and chickens. Br Vet J 127:304–312.

Gemmell, M. A., and Johnstone, P. D. 1981. Cestodes. In H. Schonfeld, ed., Antibiotics and Chemotherapy: Antiparasitic Chemotherapy, vol. 30, pp. 54–114. Basel, Switzerland: S. Karger.

Goldsmith, R. S. 1988. Recent advances in the treatment of helminthic infections: ivermectin, albendazole, and praziquantel. In J. H. Leech, M. A. Sande, and R. K. Root, eds., Parasitic Infections, pp. 327–347. New York: Churchill Livingstone.

Gonzalez, A. E., Garcia, H. H., Gilman, R. H., Gavidia, C. M., Tsang, V. C., Bernal, T., Falcon, N., Romero, M., Lopez-Urbina, M. T. 1996. Effective, single-dose treatment of porcine cysticercosis with oxfendazole. Am J Trop Med Hyg 54:391–394.

Heath, D. D., and Lawrence, S. B. 1978. The effect of mebendazole and praziquantel on the cysts of *Echinococcus granulosus, Taenia hydatigena* and *T. ovis* in sheep. NZ Vet J 26:11–15.

Hennessy, D. R., Lacey, E., and Steel, J. W. 1987. The kinetics of triclabendazole disposition in sheep. J Vet Pharmacol Ther 10:6–72.

Kinabo, L. D., and Bogan, J. A. 1988. Pharmacokinetics and efficacy of triclabendazole in goats with induced fasciolosis. J Vet Pharmacol Ther 11:254–259.

Knight, R. A., and Colglazier, M. L. 1977. Albendazole as a fasciolicide in experimentally infected sheep. Am J Vet Res 37:807–808.

Losson, B. 1988. A review of the different anthelmintics available against *Fasciola hepatica,* with particular reference to nitroxynil, rafoxanide, closantel, diamphenethide, clorsulon, albendazole and triclabendazole. Annal de Med Vet 132:93–106.

Lyons, E. T., Tolliver, S. C., Stamper, S., Drudge, J. H., Granstrom, D. E., and Collins, S. S. 1995. Activity of praziquantel (0.5 mg/kg) against *Anoplocephala perfoliata* (Cestoda) in equids. Vet Parasitol 56:255–257.

Lyons, E. T., Tolliver, S. C., and Ennis, L. E. 1998. Efficacy of praziquantel (0.25 mg/kg) on the cecal tapeworm (*Anoplocephala perfoliata*) in horses. Vet Parasitol 78:287–289.

Malone, J. B., Williams, J. C., Lutz, M., et al. 1990. Efficacy of concomitant early summer treatment with fenbendazole and clorsulon against *Fasciola hepatica* and gastrointestinal nematodes in calves in Louisiana. Am J Vet Res 51:133–136.

Martin, R. J. 1997. Modes of action of anthelmintic drugs. Vet J 154:11–34.

Montero, R., and Ostrosky, P. 1997. Genotoxic activity of praziquantel. Mutat Res 387:123–129.

Muermann, P., Von Eberstein, M., and Frohberg, H. 1976. Notes on the tolerance of Droncit. Vet Med Rev 2:142–153.

Oguz, T. 1977. The therapeutic effects of Embay 8440 (Bayer) and mebendazole (Jansen) in lambs experimentally infected with *Cysticercus tenuicollis.* Summ 1st Mediterr Conf Parasitol, pp. 122–123.

Rew, R. S., and Knight, R. A. 1980. Efficacy of albendazole for prevention of fascioliasis in sheep. J Am Vet Med Assoc 176:1353–1354.

Richards, R. J., Bowen, F. L., Essenwein, F., et al. 1990. The efficacy of triclabendazole and other anthelmintics against *Fasciola hepatica* in controlled studies in cattle. Vet Rec 126:213–216.

Roberson, E. L. 1988. Anticestodal and antitrematodal drugs. In N. H. Booth and L. E. McDonald, eds., Veterinary Pharmacology and Therapeutics, 6th ed., pp. 928–949. Ames: Iowa State Univ Press.

Roberson, E. L., and Courtney, C. H. 1995. Anticestodal and antitrematodal drugs. In H. R. Adams, ed., Veterinary Pharmacology and Therapeutics, 7th ed., pp. 933–954. Ames: Iowa State Univ Press.

Rowlands, D., Clampitt, R. B., and MacPherson, I. S. 1985. The ability of diamphenethide to control immature *Fasciola hepatica* in sheep at a lower than standard dose level. Vet Rec 116:182–184.

Schulman, M. D., Valentino, D., Cifelli, R., et al. 1979. A pharmacokinetic basis for the efficacy of 4-amino-6 trichloroethenyl-1,3-benzenedisul fonamide against *Fasciola hepatica* in the rat. J Parasitol 65:555–561.

Spence, S. A., Fraser, G. C., and Chang, S. 1996. Responses in milk production to control of gastrointestinal nematodes and paramphistome parasites in dairy cattle. Aust Vet J 74:456–459.

Thomas, H., and Andrews, P. 1977. Praziquantel: a new cestocide. Pest Sci 8:556–560.

Thomas, H., and Gonnert, R. 1978. The efficacy of praziquantel against cestodes in cats, dogs, and sheep. Res Vet Sci 24:20–25.

Thompson, R. C., Reynoldson, J. A., and Manger, B. R. 1991. In vitro and in vivo efficacy of epsiprantel against *Echinococcus granulosus.* Res Vet Sci 51:332–334.

Whitelaw, A., and Fawcett, A. R. 1981. Further studies in the control of ovine fascioliasis by strategic dosing. Vet Rec 109:118–119.

49

ANTIPROTOZOAN DRUGS

DAVID S. LINDSAY AND BYRON L. BLAGBURN

PHYLUM SARCOMASTIGOPHORA: The Amoebae and Flagellates
Drugs Effective Against Amoebae and Flagellates
Nitroimidazoles
Metronidazole
Other Nitroimidazoles
Pentavalent Antimonials
Sodium Stibogluconate
Meglumine Antimonate
Arsenicals
Benzimidazoles
Albendazole
Fenbendazole
Febantel
Paromomycin
Nifurtimox
Tetracyclines
PHYLUM APICOMPLEXA: The Coccidia, Haemosporozoans, and Piroplasms
Suborder Eimeriorina: Intestinal and Extraintestinal Coccidia
Timing and Mode of Action of Anticoccidial Agents
Anticoccidial Drug Resistance
New Anticoccidial Drug Targets
Anticoccidials Used for Controlling Coccidiosis in Chickens
Hydroxyquinolones and Naphthoquinones
Clopidol
Robenidine
Amprolium
Nitrobenzamides
Nicarbazin
Halofuginone
Polyether Ionophores
Diclazuril
Toltrazuril
Sulfonamides
Dihydrofolate Reductase/Thymidylate Synthase (DHFR/TS) Inhibitors
Combinations of Sulfonamides and DHFR/TS Inhibitors
Turkey Coccidiosis
Game Bird Coccidiosis
Treatment of Coccidiosis in Mammals
Cattle Coccidiosis
Sheep Coccidiosis
Goat Coccidiosis
Pig Coccidiosis
Dog Coccidiosis
Cat Coccidiosis
Rabbit Coccidiosis
Cryptosporidiosis
Toxoplasmosis and Extraintestinal Coccidia
Feline intestinal toxoplasmosis
Disseminated toxoplasmosis
Canine Neosporosis
Equine Protozoal Myeloencephalitis
Suborder Haemospororina: The Haemosporozoans
Canine Hepatozoonosis
Subclass Piroplasmasina: The Piroplasms
Babesiosis
Diamidine Derivatives
Tetracyclines
Theileriosis
Cytauxzoonosis
PHYLUM CILIOPHORA: The Ciliates
Ciliates of Mammals
Ciliates of Fish
PHYLUM MICROSPORA

Protozoa are ubiquitous unicellular organisms. Most of the more than 65,000 species in this subkingdom are free-living. As parasites, protozoa serve as important disease agents of humans and many domesticated animals. To appreciate their importance, one need only examine the list of animal diseases for which they are responsible. Among them are coccidiosis, giardiasis, cryptosporidiosis, trichomoniasis, babesiosis, toxoplasmosis, trypanosomiasis, leishmaniasis, and amoebiasis. Certain protozoal diseases (e.g., malaria and trypanosomiasis) have rendered millions of acres of arable farmland noninhabitable or have influenced the outcome of wars and the development of civilizations. A significant few are capable of infecting both animals and human beings (e.g., *Toxoplasma gondii, Cryptosporidium parvum, Leishmania* spp., *Trypanosoma cruzi,* African trypanosomes). These zoonotic agents are of particular interest to veterinary and animal scientists for not only do they affect the health of infected animals, but they also place human beings associated with them at risk.

Numerous chemotherapeutic agents are known to possess activity against parasitic protozoa. Antiprotozoal activity is characteristic of many different chemical groups; however, most possess a rather narrow spectrum of activity. This is in contrast to antibacterial agents, which are effective against a wide variety of organisms.

Antiprotozoal agents will be presented on the basis of the taxonomy of organisms. We will first deal with agents effective against the amoebae and flagellates (amoebaflagellates). This will be followed by those effective against the apicomplexans, the ciliates, and the microsporidans. No attempt will be made to include all compounds with antiprotozoal activity. Information presented in the following pages will characterize antiprotozoal modalities effective against the more important protozoal disease agents of domesticated animals.

PHYLUM SARCOMASTIGOPHORA: THE AMOEBAE AND FLAGELLATES

The protozoan phylum Sarcomastigophora contains the amoebae and flagellates. All parasitic members reproduce asexually. The amoebae are in the subphylum Sarcodina and move by means of pseudopodia but may have flagellated stages in their life cycles. Amoebae usually are transmitted by resistant cyst stages that are excreted into the environment. The flagellates are in the subphylum Mastigophora and move by means of flagella. Blood- or tissue-dwelling flagellates are usually transmitted by insect vectors, whereas mucosa-dwelling flagellates may be transmitted by direct contact or may have resistant cyst stages in the environment.

Few amoebae are of veterinary importance, and clinical disease is seldom associated with these organisms.

Mucosal flagellates are the most important flagellate parasites of animals in the United States. *Giardia* infection causes intestinal disease in companion and, rarely, large animals. Clinical signs include nausea and mucoid to mildly bloody diarrhea and may be intermittent. The binucleate, octaflagellated trophozoite attaches to intestinal cells by a special adhesive disk. A tetranucleated cyst stage is excreted in the feces. The role of animals in the transmission of *Giardia* to human beings is not clear. Trichomonads are mucosal parasites of the digestive and urogenital tracts. They are uninucleate and classified based on the numbers of anterior flagella. They do not produce environmentally resistant cyst stages and are transmitted directly. *Tritrichomonas foetus* is found in the reproductive tract of bovines and causes early abortion, pyometra, and sterility. *Cochlosoma anatis* is a trichomonad-like flagellate that is increasingly being associated with enteritis in turkeys (Lindsay et al. 1998). *Histomonas meleagridis* causes necrotic cecitis and hepatitis in turkeys, chickens, and other birds. It exists as a flagellated parasite in the cecum but becomes amoeboid in the liver. This protozoan is unusual in that it does not produce a resistant cyst stage but is transmitted in the egg of a nematode parasite, *Heterakis gallinarum.*

Few blood- or tissue-dwelling flagellates are important parasites in the United States. Clinical trypanosomiasis in the Americas is caused by *Trypanosoma cruzi.* It is transmitted by reduviid. The parasite multiplies as spherical, uninucleate amastigote stages in reticuloendothelial cells, cardiac and smooth muscle cells, and occasionally neural cells. Eventually these stages are released into the circulatory system. They either find and develop in other host cells or change into the elongate trypomastigote stage. The trypomastigote stage of *Try. cruzi,* unlike other trypanosomes, does not divide in the host. *Trypanosoma theileri* occurs in the blood of cattle in the Americas, but it is of little clinical importance.

Leishmaniasis is caused by *Leishmania* spp. and the clinical signs are usually characteristic for a particular species, although many variations occur and speciation is often difficult. These parasites multiply as amastigotes in macrophages in the host's tissues and are transmitted by a wide variety of sandfly species. They do not form trypomastigote stages in the host. Leishmaniasis is primarily a human disease, with canines serving as a reservoir host and also suffering from clinical disease. Leishmaniasis is most common in Central and South America, Africa, Asia, and Mediterranean countries. Canine cases of apparently endogenously acquired visceral leishmaniasis have been reported in the United States.

DRUGS EFFECTIVE AGAINST AMOEBAE AND FLAGELLATES

Nitroimidazoles. Several nitroimidazoles have activity against amoebae and flagellates and include metronidazole, tinidazole, dimetridazole, ronidazole, and ipronidazole (Table 49.1). Many of these important agents were used in the treatment of poultry flagellates, and all except metronidazole have been removed from the market in the United States. Nitroimidazoles are suspected mutagens and carcinogens. Metronidazole is the most commonly used agent in this group and the most studied.

METRONIDAZOLE. Metronidazole (Flagyl) occurs in pure form as cream-colored crystals that are sparingly soluble in water and ethanol but are soluble in dilute acids. Metronidazole is not approved for veterinary use by the Food and Drug Administration (FDA) but is currently used in veterinary medicine for the treatment of giardiasis and bovine genital trichomoniasis. It is absorbed well from the gastrointestinal (GI) tract and reaches high concentrations in the tissues and therefore is active against both luminal and extraluminal protozoa (Finch and Synder 1986). It has a half-life of about 8 hours, and less than 20% binds to plasma proteins. It

TABLE 49.1—Nitroimidazoles

Name	Chemical name (Empirical formula) [Molecular weight]	Chemical structure
Dimetridazole	1,2-dimethyl-5-nitro-1*H*-imidazole ($C_5H_7N_3O_2$) [141.13]	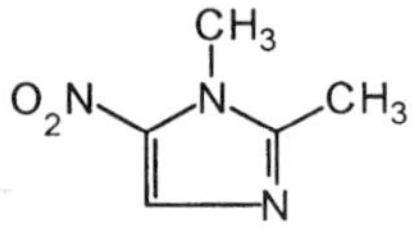 CH_3 O_2N N CH_3 N
Ipronidazole	1-methyl-2-(1-methylethyl)-5-nitro-1*H*-imidazole ($C_7H_{11}N_3O_2$) [169.18]	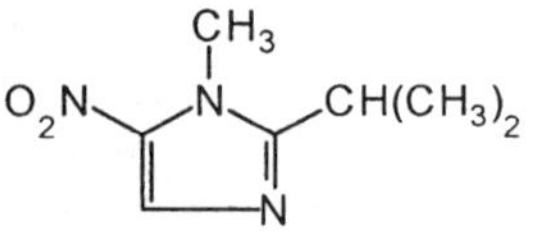 CH_3 O_2N N $CH(CH_3)_2$ N
Metronidazole	1-(2-hydroxyethyl)-2-methyl-5-nitroimidazole ($C_6H_9N_3O_3$) [171.16]	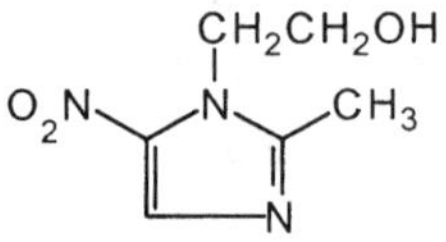 CH_2CH_2OH O_2N N CH_3 N
Ronidazole	1-methyl-2-[(carbamoyloxy)methyl]-5-nitroimidazole ($C_6H_8N_4O_4$) [200.16]	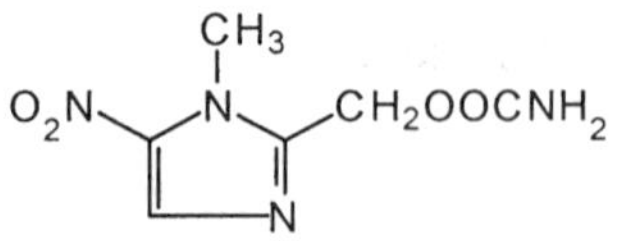 CH_3 O_2N N CH_2OOCNH_2 N
Tinidazole	1-[2-(ethylsufonyl)ethyl]-2-methyl-5-nitro-1*H*-imidazole ($C_8H_{13}N_3O_4S$) [247.26]	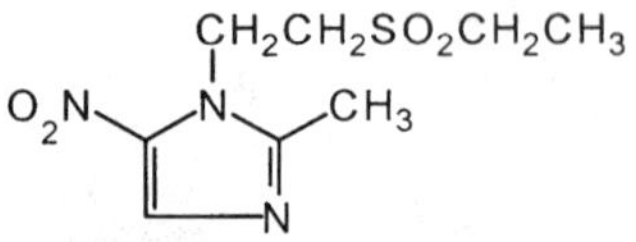 $CH_2CH_2SO_2CH_2CH_3$ O_2N N CH_3 N

is metabolized in the liver by oxidation and glucuronide formation and is excreted primarily by the kidneys, but small amounts may be found in saliva and breast milk (Finch and Synder 1986). The urine may be discolored and appear dark red or reddish brown. Metronidazole is usually well tolerated, but potential adverse reactions include glossitis, stomatitis, nausea, and emesis, and at elevated dosages neurological signs may occur (Longhofer 1988).

It is convenient to think of the mode of action of metronidazole as occurring in four successive steps (Finegold and Mathisen 1990). First is entry into the protozoan cell, second is reductive activation, third is toxic effect of reduced intermediates, and forth is release of inactive end products. The protozoal toxicity is due to short-lived intermediates or free radicals that produce damage by interacting with DNA and possibly other molecules. The cytotoxic intermediates decompose to nontoxic and inactive compounds.

Metronidazole is widely used to treat *Giardia* infections in animals (Table 49.2). Dosages above 100 mg/kg body weight (BW) may result in adverse reactions such as tremors, muscle spasms, weakness, incoordination, and ataxia in dogs.

Bovine genital trichomoniasis is treated with metronidazole and other nitroimidazoles. It has been suggested that the use of penicillin 2 days prior to treatment of bulls will increase the effectiveness of the treatment because the penicillin will reduce the numbers of preputial bacteria and prevent them from metabolizing the nitroimidazoles. Bovine genital trichomoniasis is treated by intravenous (IV) administration of metronidazole at the rate of 75 mg/kg BW daily for 3 days.

TABLE 49.2—Treatment of *Giardia* infections in animals

Agent*	Host	Dose and duration
Albendazole	Dog	25 mg/kg BW twice daily for 2 days
Albendazole	Calf	30 mg/kg BW daily for 3 days
Febantel	Dog	27–35 mg/kg BW daily for 3 days
Fenbendazole	Dog	50 mg/kg BW daily for 3 days
Fenbendazole	Calf	20 mg/kg BW daily for 3 days
Metronidazole	Dog	15–30 mg/kg BW twice daily for 5–7 days
Metronidazole	Cat	10–25 mg/kg BW twice daily for 5–7 days
Metronidazole	Foal	5 mg/kg BW trice daily for 10 days

*None of these agents are approved for the treatment of *Giardia*. None are approved for use in cats. Metronidazole is not approved for use in any of the species listed.

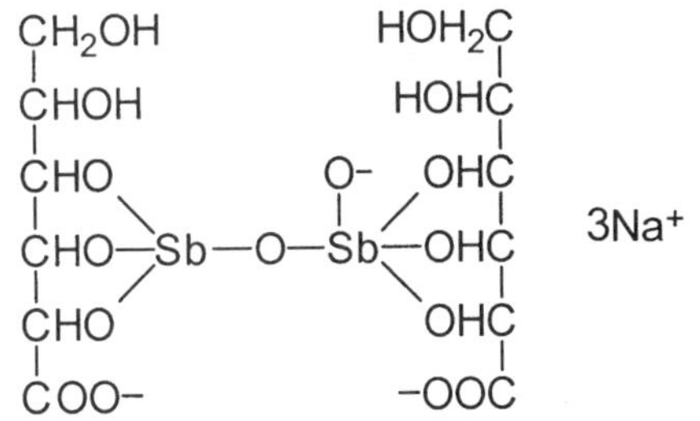

Sodium stibogluconate

FIG. 49.1

OTHER NITROIMIDAZOLES. Dimetridazole (Emtrymix) is no longer available in the United States. It was given orally or intramuscularly (IM) at 60–100 mg/kg BW for 5 days to treat bovine genital trichomoniasis. Ipronidazole (Ipropan) is no longer available in the United States. It was given as a single IM dose of 30 g followed by oral doses of 15 g daily for 2 days.

Pentavalent Antimonials. Sodium stibogluconate (Pentostam) and meglumine antimonate (Glucantime) are pentavalent antimonial compounds that are effective against *Leishmania* spp.

SODIUM STIBOGLUCONATE. Sodium stibogluconate (Fig. 49.1) was made available in the United States from the Centers for Disease Control in 1968 for treatment of leishmaniasis in human beings. It is in aqueous solution at a concentration of 330 mg/mL of agent, which is equivalent to 100 mg/mL pentavalent antimony. Clinical formulations consist of multiple uncharacterized molecular forms, some of which have higher molecular weights than the compound shown in Fig. 49.1. Both sodium stibogluconate and meglumine antimonate are administered on the basis of their antimony content. In human beings, most of a single dose of sodium stibogluconate is excreted by the kidneys in the urine within 24 hours regardless of whether given IV or IM. Antimony compounds are eliminated faster if given IM than SC or IV in dogs, and it is important to maintain serum levels of the compound to treat leishmaniasis. Pentavalent antimonials are relatively well tolerated. Adverse reactions include pain at the injection site, GI symptoms, delayed muscle pain, and joint stiffness.

Pentavalent antimonials have been shown to inhibit topoisomerase (Lucumi et al. 1998) and thereby interfere with parasite replication. They also inhibit enzymes involved in the synthesis of nucleotides and inhibit phosphofructokinase. The in vivo mode of action of the pentavalent antimonials is still unclear.

Canine leishmaniasis is treated with sodium stibogluconate to deliver 30–50 mg/kg BW pentavalent antimony by either IV or SC administration at daily intervals for 3–4 weeks (Slappendel and Teske 1997). Relapses may occur a few months to a year after treatment and should be treated with another round of pentavalent antimony. In general, canine visceral leishmaniasis is more difficult to treat than the human form of the disease. The use of pentavalent antimonials is contraindicated in patients with myocarditis, hepatitis, or nephritis.

MEGLUMINE ANTIMONATE. Meglumine antimonate is not available in the United States. Meglumine antimonate may be less likely to cause toxic side effects than sodium stibogluconate. It is available in a solution that contains 85 mg/mL antimony. Canine leishmaniasis is treated with meglumine antimonate given IV or SC at 100 mg/kg BW for 3–6 weeks (Slappendel and Teske 1997). No advantage is provided by IV administration. Relapses will occur in long-term survivors and require retreatment.

Arsenicals. Carbarsone, nitarsone (Histostat-50), and roxarsone are older compounds that were used at one time for the prevention and treatment of histomoniasis and coccidiosis in turkeys (Table 49.3). Carbarsone is no longer available as a feed additive. Nitarsone is fed at 0.01875% for prevention of histomoniasis in turkeys and chickens. It is not active if birds have been infected for more than 4 days. A 5-day withdrawal is required for nitarsone. Overdosing or lack of adequate water may result in leg weakness and paralysis in birds. Nitarsone is dangerous for ducks, geese, and dogs. Roxarsone is fed at 0.0025–0.005% to promote growth and prevent coccidiosis. A 5-day withdrawal is required for roxarsone. Like nitarsone, overdosing or lack of adequate water may result in leg weakness and paralysis in birds.

Benzimidazoles. The benzimidazoles are a group of agents that are widely used in the treatment of helminth parasites of large and small animals (see Chap. 47). Some have excellent activity against *Giardia* spp. This group lacks or has little antibacterial activity and unlike other antigiardial agents is unlikely to interfere with intestinal microflora during treatment. The benzimidazoles are known to bind to β-tubulin subunits of microtubules and interfere with microtubule polymerization. This causes structural changes in *Giardia* trophozoites consistent with microtubule damage to the adhesive disk and internal microtubule cytoskeleton but not the external flagella.

ALBENDAZOLE. Albendazole (Valbazen), methyl [5-(propylthio)-1*H*-benzimidazole-2-yl]-carbamate (Fig. 49.2), is available in 11.36% liquid and 30% paste formulations. It has been evaluated as successful against *Giardia* in human beings, mice, and dogs. Albendazole is poorly absorbed from the intestinal tract and has low toxicity but is potentially teratogenic. Dogs treated orally with albendazole at 25 mg/kg BW every 12 hours for 2 days cleared *Giardia* cysts from their feces

TABLE 49.3—Arsenicals

Name	Chemical name (Empirical formula) [Molecular weight]	Chemical structure
Carbarsone	[4-[(aminocarbonyl)amino]phenyl]-arsonic acid ($C_7H_9AsN_2O_4$) [260.07]	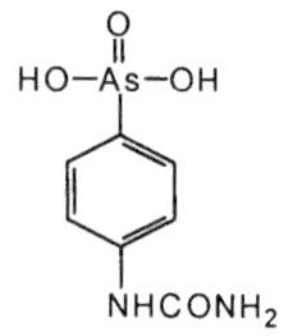
Nitarsone	4-nitrophenylarsonic acid ($C_6H_6AsNO_5$) [247.04]	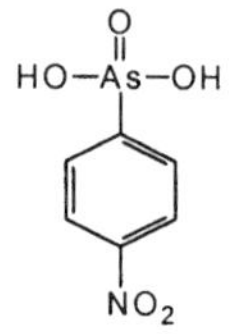
Roxarsone	4-hydroxy-3-nitrophenylarsonic acid ($C_6H_6AsNO_6$) [263.03]	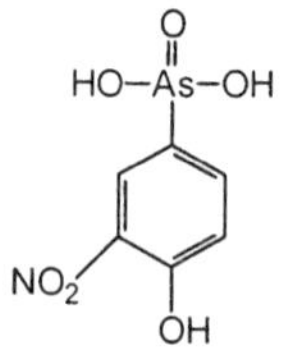

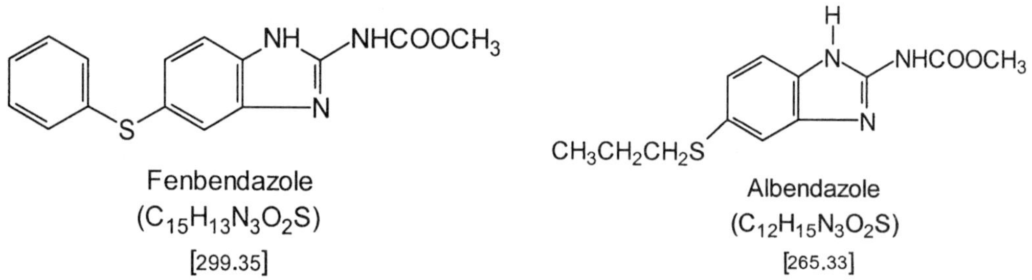

Fenbendazole
($C_{15}H_{13}N_3O_2S$)
[299.35]

Albendazole
($C_{12}H_{15}N_3O_2S$)
[265.33]

FIG. 49.2

(Barr et al. 1993). A single oral 25 mg/kg BW treatment did not clear cysts from the feces of dogs. None of 32 dogs treated for *Giardia* with albendazole developed adverse reactions (Barr et al. 1993). Albendazole given at 30 mg/kg BW orally for 3 days reduced cyst production by >90% in naturally infected calves (Xiao et al. 1996).

FENBENDAZOLE. Fenbendazole (Panacur, Safeguard, Axilur), methyl 5(phenylthio)-2-benzimidazole-carbamate (Fig. 49.2), is effective against *Giardia* organisms in dogs if given at 50 mg/kg BW every 24 hours for 3 days (Zajac et al. 1998). It is also effective against *Giardia* organisms in calves when given orally at 5–20 mg/kg BW every 24 hours for 3 days (O'Handley et al. 1997; Xiao et al. 1996).

FEBANTEL. Febantel (Drontal-Plus), dimethyl [[2-(2-methoxyacetamido)-4-(phenylthio)phenyl]-imidocarbonyl]-dicarbamate, is a benzimidazole available in a combination product for the treatment of intestinal nematodes and cestodes in dogs. This combination has been shown to be effective against canine *Giardia* infections when given orally for 3 days to provide 27–35 mg/kg BW of the febantel component (Barr et al. 1998).

Paromomycin (Aminosidine). Paromomycin sulfate (syn. aminosidine) (Humatin), *O*-2-amino-2-deoxy-α-D-glucopyranosyl-(1→4)-*O*-[*O*-2,6-diamino-2,6-dideoxy-β-L-idopyranosyl-(1→3)-β-D-ribofuranosyl-(1→5)]-2-deoxy-D-streptamine (Fig. 49.3), is an aminoglycoside antibiotic that is produced by *Strepto-*

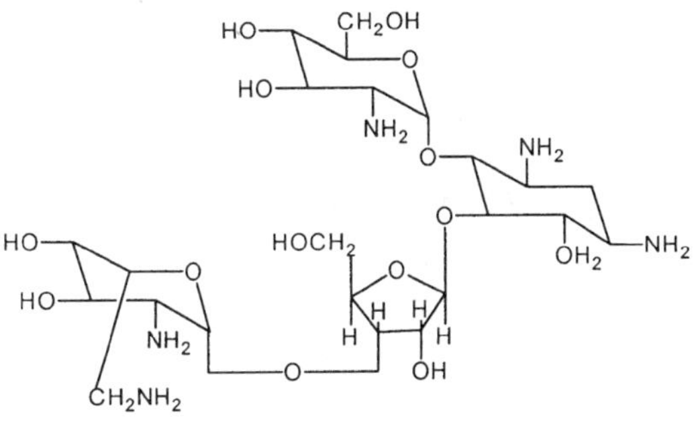

Paromomycin
($C_{23}H_{45}N_5O_{14}$)
[615.65]

FIG. 49.3

myces rimosus. It is used in the treatment of luminal amoebiasis, leishmaniasis, and cryptosporidiosis. It is poorly absorbed following oral administration and has little activity against intestinal bacteria. Side effects include nausea, vomiting, abdominal cramps, and diarrhea. Although little is absorbed from the intestinal tract, it is eliminated via the kidneys, so its use is contraindicated in patients with renal disease. It also has the potential to cause reversible and irreversible vestibular, cochlear, and renal toxicity when given parenterally. Paromomycin levels peak in the serum of dogs at 30 μg/mL about 60 minutes after IM or SC administration of a 15 mg/kg BW dose (Belloli et al. 1996). About 4% is bound to serum proteins.

Paromomycin given IM at 20 mg/kg BW daily for 15 days will greatly improve clinical signs of visceral leishmaniasis in dogs (Vexenat et al. 1998). However, relapses may occur within 50–100 days. Treatment IM with 40 mg/kg daily for 30 days may enhance the cure rate of dogs (Vexenat et al. 1998).

If paromomycin is administered SC with antimony, there is no effect on the kinetics of paromomycin but there is a marked effect on the kinetics of antimony (Belloli et al. 1995). Serum levels of antimony remain higher, and the dose should be adjusted to prevent toxic levels of the metal from appearing in the blood.

Paromomycin interferes with bacterial protein synthesis by binding to 16S rRNA at the amino-acyl-tRNA binding site, which causes a conformational change and subsequent misreading of the mRNA and inhibition of translocation (Fourmy et al. 1998). Its anti-*Leishmania* mode of action is not known, but it has been suggested that it interferes with parasite mitochondrial activity (Maarouf et al. 1997).

NIFURTIMOX. Nifurtimox (Lampit, Bayer 2502), tetrahydro-3-methyl-4-[(5-nitrofurfurylidene)amino]-2*H*-1,4-thiazine 1,1-dioxide, is a nitrofuran derivative (Fig. 49.4) that is the most widely used agent for the treatment of human *Try. cruzi* infections (Van Reken

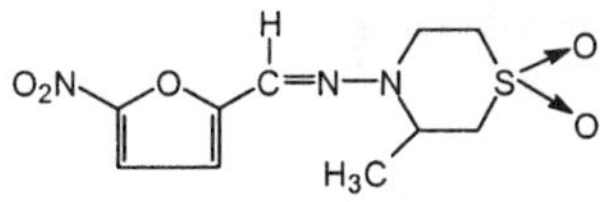

Nifurtimox
($C_{10}H_{13}N_3O_5S$)
[287.29]

FIG. 49.4

and Pearson 1990) and is effective against natural and experimental disease in dogs (Barr 1990). It is marketed as 100 mg tablets and, in the United States, must be obtained from the Centers for Disease Control. It has activity against amastigote and trypomastigote stages.

Its likely mode of action is through the production of activated forms of oxygen. It is reduced to the nitro anion radical in the presence of pyridine nucleotides. The anion then reacts with oxygen to produce superoxide and regeneration of nifurtimox (Finch and Snyder 1986). This cycle continues, and the activated oxygen molecules exert their toxic effects on the parasites. In human beings, nifurtimox is well absorbed after oral administration, but only low concentrations are found in the plasma and little is found in the tissues or urine (Webster 1990). It is excreted in the urine in the form of metabolites. Adverse side effects occur in up to 50% of human beings treated and are associated with GI and central nervous system signs.

Canine *Try. cruzi* infections are treated with 2–7 mg/kg BW nifurtimox orally at 6-hour intervals for 3–5 months (Barr 1990). This is effective in preventing death from acute disease and extending life, but most dogs will still develop chronic cardiac disease, which is usually fatal (Barr 1990).

TETRACYCLINES. Tetracyclines represent a broad group of antiprotozoal agents, some of which have activity against amoebae, mucosal flagellates, piroplasms, and ciliates. See Chap. 42 of this book for the pharmacology of tetracyclines.

PHYLUM APICOMPLEXA: THE COCCIDIA, HAEMOSPOROZOANS, AND PIROPLASMS

All members of this phylum are obligatory parasites. Coccidiosis, cryptosporidiosis, toxoplasmosis, equine protozoal myeloencephalitis (EPM), and piroplasmosis are important diseases of animals caused by apicomplexan parasites.

SUBORDER EIMERIORINA: INTESTINAL AND EXTRAINTESTINAL COCCIDIA. Coccidiosis is generally an enteric disease caused by *Eimeria* or

Isospora spp. Coccidiosis is extremely important in the poultry industry. It is estimated that 350 million dollars worldwide and about 80 million in the United States are spent on anticoccidial agents a year (Long 1993). Economic losses also occur in the cattle, sheep, goat, rabbit, and swine production industries, but the use of anticoccidial agents is less frequent in these industries. Coccidiosis can also occur in humans, other primates, dogs, and cats. Members of the genera *Eimeria* and *Isospora* generally are host specific and complete their entire life cycle in a single animal.

The coccidial life cycle is complex. It begins when sporulated oocysts containing sporozoites are ingested from the environment in contaminated food or water. The sporozoites undergo excystation in the intestine and are liberated from the oocysts. The sporozoites then actively penetrate host cells in the intestinal tract. The sporozoite transforms into a trophozoite, which undergoes multiple karyokinesis and eventually produces numerous merozoites. This sequence of developmental events occurs a predetermined number of times, and each cycle is called a generation. Eventually the merozoites produced by the terminal generation of merozoites transform into sexual stages. Macrogamonts are uninucleate and are the female gamete, while microgamonts become multinucleate and produce flagellated microgametes (sperm). The microgametes fertilize the macrogamonts, and the resulting zygote produces an oocyst. The oocyst is excreted in the feces, usually in the unsporulated condition. Sporulation occurs in the environment.

Members of the genus *Cryptosporidium* can be recognized as serious intestinal and respiratory pathogens of humans and domestic animals. Their life cycles are similar to the *Eimeria* and *Isospora* spp. A notable difference is that the parasite develops in the microvilli of host enterocytes.

Toxoplasma gondii, Neospora caninum, and *Sarcocystis* spp. are related parasites that cause abortion, death, and production losses in ruminants and other animals. These parasites have two hosts in their life cycles. Sexual stages are present in the definitive host, and asexual stages (tachyzoites, merozoites, tissue cysts) are present in the intermediate host. *Sarcocystis*-induced encephalitis is seen in several species of animals and is particularly important in horses, where the causative agent is *S. neurona. Neospora caninum* causes encephalitis and paralysis in dogs and abortions in ruminants. *Hepatozoon americanum* has emerged as the cause of often fatal disease in dogs in the southern United States (Macintire et al. 1997; Vincent-Johnson et al. 1997).

Timing and Mode of Action of Anticoccidial Agents. Anticoccidial drugs can act on extracellular stages (sporozoites, merozoites) to prevent penetration of cells or on the intracellular stages to stop or inhibit development. A few anticoccidials affect the sporulation of oocysts after they are excreted, and a few effect excystation (under experimental conditions). Anticoccidials can act at specific times during the life cycle or exert their effects at several phases. Anticoccidials are classified as coccidiostatic if they arrest the development of the parasite but do not kill the coccidial stages and as coccidiocidal if they kill most of the coccidial stages. The distinction between coccidiostatic versus coccidiocidal is often not clear. Factors such as length of time on medication, dosage, and species of coccidia can cause a compound to appear as coccidiostatic in some instances but coccidiocidal in others.

Anticoccidial Drug Resistance. Development of resistance to anticoccidial drugs is a major problem in the poultry industry. Anticoccidial drug resistance occurs when a coccidial parasite can multiply or survive in the presence of concentrations of an anticoccidial that normally destroy parasites of the same species or prevent their multiplication (Chapman 1997). The speed of development of drug resistance depends on the mode of action of the agent. Resistance to some anticoccidials has appeared in as early as weeks to months, while others require years before resistant strains appear. Cross-resistance to anticoccidials with the same mode of action from the same chemical class is common. The spectrum of activity of an anticoccidial agent must be taken into account when examining resistance.

Development of resistance to an agent does not mean that its use as an anticoccidial is completely abolished. Combination with other agents can improve activity. Also, once a product has been removed from routine use for several years, the drug-resistant coccidia will disappear due to lack of drug pressure.

Rotational and shuttle programs can be used to slow the development of drug resistance. Rotational programs change the agents between grow-out periods, and shuttle programs change anticoccidials during a single grow-out period.

New Anticoccidial Drug Targets. A vestigial, non-photosynthetic plastid has recently been described in apicomplexan parasites (Köhler et al. 1997). It probably was acquired by secondary endosymbiosis of a green alga. The function of the plastid is not known but it is essential for parasite survival. In plants, the plastids are the site for many biochemical pathways, including the biosynthesis of folate, amino acids, ubiquinone, haem, nucleotides, lipid, and starch (Roberts et al. 1998). The shikimate pathway has been found in apicomplexan parasites (Roberts et al. 1998). The enzymes of the shikimate pathway are encoded in the nucleus, made in the cytoplasm, and targeted to the apicoplast (chloroplast). The seven enzymes involved in this pathway are attractive drug targets because vertebrate cells lack the shikimate pathway. Glyphosphate—*N*-(phosphonomethyl)glycine is a well-studied inhibitor of shikimate pathway enzyme 5-enolpyruvyl shikimate 3-phosphate synthase—inhibits development of apicomplexan parasites (Roberts et al. 1998), strengthening the hypothesis that this pathway and this organelle will prove to be good drug targets in the future. The apicoplast may also be important in fatty acid biosynthesis because several proteins involved in fatty acid biosynthesis accumulate in the apicoplast (Waller et al. 1998). Thiolactomycin, a fatty acid biosynthesis inhibitor, inhibits development of malarial parasites, indicating a vital role for the apicoplast and fatty acid biosynthesis. Clindamycin and ciprofloxacin—1-cyclopropyl-6-fluoro-1,4-dihydro-4-oxo-7-(1-piperazinyl)-3-quinolinecarboxylic acid—have also been shown to act on the apicoplast and inhibit development of *Toxo. gondii* (Fichera and Roos 1997). Much research is presently being done on the apicoplast and its potential as a drug target.

The mannitol cycle has been identified in *Eimeria tenella* (Schmatz 1997) and all other *Eimeria* spp. that infect chickens (Liberator et al. 1998). It is an attractive drug target because it is not present in the chicken host. The mannitol pathway is important in the formation of oocysts, and mannitol functions as the endogenous energy source for sporulating oocysts. Nitrophenide—*bis*(3-nitrophenyl)disulphide—inhibits an enzyme needed in the biosynthesis of mannitol and will prevent the formation of oocysts. If nitrophenide is used at lower levels, the oocysts will not sporulate. Additional enzymes involved in the mannitol cycle are probably going to be attractive drug targets.

Anticoccidials used for Controlling Coccidiosis in Chickens. Because the vast majority of anticoccidial agents are intended for use in chickens, we will discuss them first in relation to these birds and then consider additional animal species separately.

HYDROXYQUINOLONES AND NAPHTHOQUINONES. Buquinolate, decoquinate (Deccox), and nequinate are quinolone (4-hydroxyquinolones) anticoccidials (Table 49.4). These compounds are coccidiostatic and allow penetration of sporozoites but not development. These inhibited sporozoites have the ability to resume development after the agents are removed. Little anticoccidial immunity develops in chickens on these medications. Recent evidence indicates that decoquinate can have an anticoccidial effect on first-generation schizonts of *E. tenella,* adversely affect sporulation, and permit the development of immunity if fed at levels that are lower than its coccidiostatic levels (Williams 1997). Buquinolate and nequinate are not presently used in the United States.

Decoquinate is a cream to pale buff, microcrystalline powder with a slight odor. It is practically insoluble in water and is stable for about 4 years if stored under appropriate conditions. Decoquinate is poorly absorbed from the intestinal tract, and what is absorbed is rapidly cleared from the blood and tissues. Decoquinate is fed at 0.003% for prevention of coccidiosis in broilers. It should be fed for at least 28 days when development of coccidiosis is likely. Do not feed to laying chickens. No withdrawal is required.

The quinolone anticoccidials inhibit coccidial respiration by interfering with cytochrome-mediated electron transport in the parasites' mitochondria. The site of action of quinolone anticoccidials is probably within the bc_1 complex, where the electrons are transferred from ubiquinone to cytochrome c.

Atovaquone (Mepron suspension) has broad-spectrum antiprotozoal activity and was developed for use in human beings. It is a yellow crystalline solid that is practically insoluble in water. Atovaquone is supplied as a bright yellow suspension of microfine particles at a concentration of 150 mg atovaquone/mL. It is highly lipophilic and administering it with food increases its absorption twofold. It was originally developed for the treatment of drug-resistant strains of malaria and *Pneumocystis carinii* pneumonia and is discussed here because it was also found to have excellent activity against *Toxo. gondii.* It also has activity against *Eimeria* spp. Atovaquone is also thought to affect the mitochondrial bc_1 complex because a mutant resistant to atovaquone is also resistant to decoquinate (Pfefferkorn et al. 1993).

Parvaquone and buparvaquone are naphthoquinones that are used for the treatment of piroplasmosis and will be discussed below in that section.

CLOPIDOL. Clopidol (Coyden 25), 3,5-dichloro-2,6-dimethyl-4-pyridinol, is the only pyridinol to be used as an anticoccidial (Fig. 49.5). It is practically insoluble in water. It is active against the sporozoite stage, allowing host cell penetration but not parasite development. It also has activity against second-generation schizogony, gametogony, and sporulation. Sporozoites can resume development after the medication is removed. Little anticoccidial immunity develops in chickens receiving this agent.

Long (1993) suggested that the mode of action of clopidol was similar to that of the quinolone anticoccidials because of similar structure and biological activity of the agents. However, cross-resistance between clopidol and quinolone anticoccidials does not occur (Long 1993).

Clopidol is fed at 0.0125–0.0250% for prevention of coccidiosis. A 5-day withdrawal is required if the 0.0250% level is used. This level may be lowered to 0.0125% 5 days before withdrawal and fed. Clopidol is transmitted to the eggs of hens that are fed clopidol-containing diets (Long 1971).

ROBENIDINE. Robenidine (Cycostat, Robenz), 1,3-*bis* [(*p*-chlorobenzylidene)amino]-guanidine hydrochloride (Fig. 49.6), is a synthetic anticoccidial derivative of guanidine. It is active against the first-generation schizont of *E. tenella* by preventing formation of merozoites. Robenidine is fed at 33 ppm for the prevention of coccidiosis. Finish feeds must be fed within 50 days of manufacture. Do not feed with bentonite. Do not feed to layers. A 5-day withdrawal is required. If robenidine is not withdrawn 5 days before slaughter, the flesh of medicated birds will have an unpleasant taste. Robenidine is transmitted to the eggs of hens (Long et al. 1981), and these eggs may have an

TABLE 49.4—Hydroxyquinolones and naphthoquinones

Name	Chemical name (Empirical formula) [Molecular weight]	Chemical structure
Buquinolate	4-hydroxy-6,7-diisobutoxy-3-quinoline-carboxylic acid ethyl ester ($C_{20}H_{27}NO_5$) [361.42]	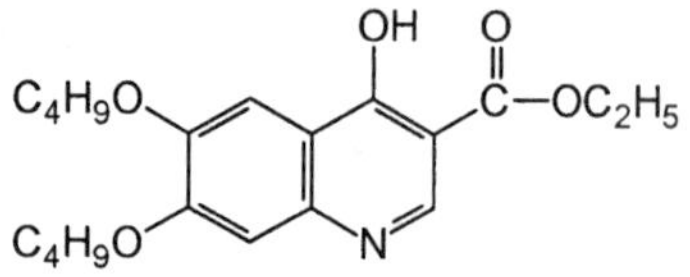
Decoquinate	6-declyoxy-ethoxy-4-hydroxy-3-quinoline-carboxylic acid ethyl ester ($C_{24}H_{35}NO_5$) [417.53]	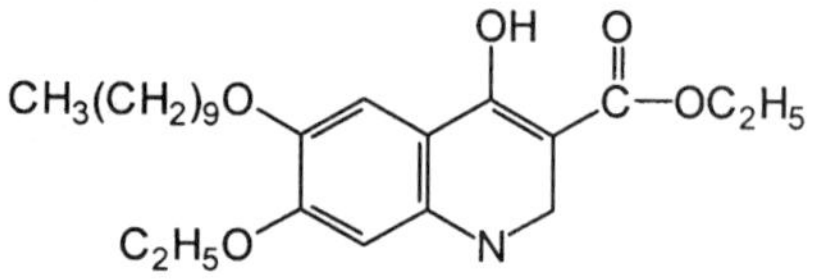
Nequinate	7-(benzyloxy)-6-*n*-butyl-1,4-dihydro-4-oxo-3-quinoline-carboxylic acid methyl ester ($C_{22}H_{23}NO_4$) [365.43]	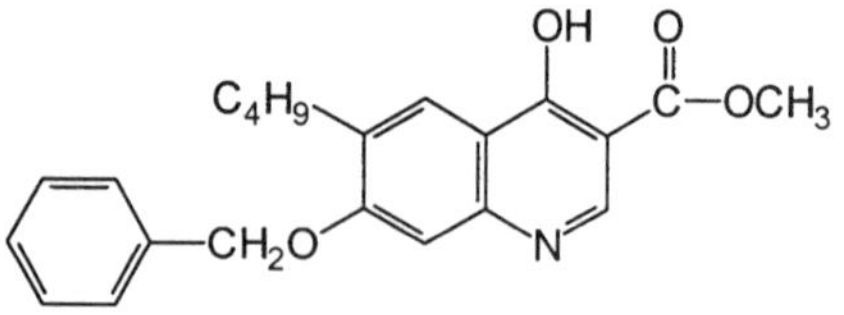
Buparvaquone	2-*trans*(4-*t*-butylcyclohexyl)methyl-3-hydroxy-1,4-naphthoquinone ($C_{21}H_{26}O_3$) [326.44]	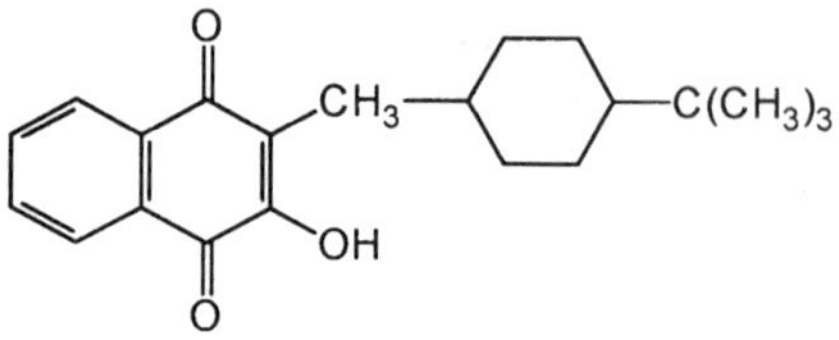
Parvaquone	2-cyclohexyl-3-hydroxy-1,4-naphthoquinone ($C_{16}H_{16}O_3$) [256.30]	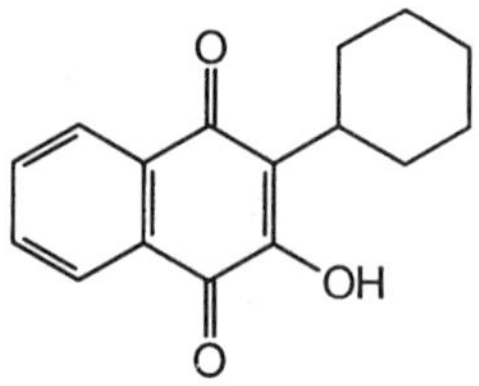
Atovaquone	2-[*trans*-4-(4-chlorophenyl)cyclohexyl]-3-hydroxy-1,4-naphthoquinone ($C_{22}H_{19}ClO_3$) [366.69]	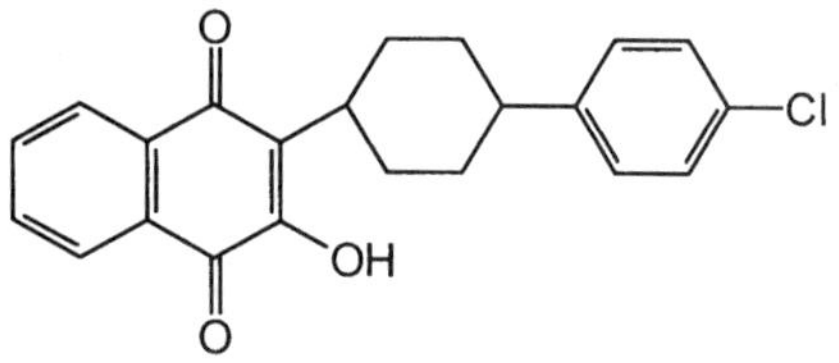

unpleasant taste. The ability of humans to taste robenidine is apparently under genetic control. It does not have any other adverse effects on egg production or quality.

AMPROLIUM. Amprolium (Amprol, Corid), 1-[(4-amino-2-propyl-5-pyrimidyl)-methyl]-2-picolinium chloride, is structurally related to the vitamin thiamine (Fig. 49.7). Amprolium is freely soluble in water. Because amprolium lacks the hydroxyethyl function of thiamine it is not phosphorylated to a pyrophosphate analog (Looker et al. 1986). Amprolium acts on the first-generation schizont to prevent merozoite production and has some activity against sexual stages and the sporulating oocyst. Amprolium-resistant strains of chicken and turkey *Eimeria* spp. are prevalent. Amprolium is often combined with other agents to increase activity. It competitively inhibits the active transport of thiamine. There is a 50-fold greater sensitivity of the parasite system compared with the host system.

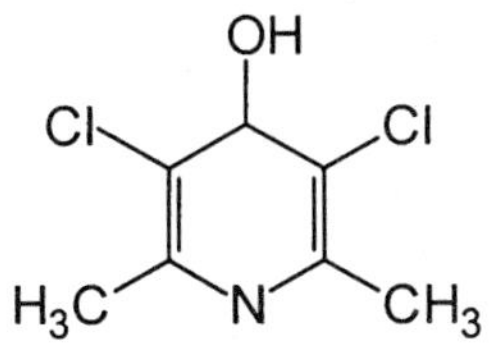

Clopidol
($C_7H_7Cl_2NO$)
[192.06]

FIG. 49.5

Several formulations of amprolium are available. Amprolium is used for the prevention of coccidiosis in chickens and fed at 36.3–113.5 g/ton feed or given in the drinking water at 0.012%. No withdrawal is required.

NITROBENZAMIDES. Aklomide and dinitolamide (syn. zoalene) (Zoamix) are nitrobenzamide anticoccidial agents (Table 49.5). These agents act primarily on the first-generation schizonts, and dinitolmide inhibits sporulation of oocysts (Mathis and McDougald 1981). Dinitolmide is coccidiostatic if given for 6 days but is coccidiocidal if given for longer periods (Long 1993). The nitrobenzamides are often combined with other agents. Nitrobenzamide-resistant strains of coccidia are common. The anticoccidial mode of action of nitrobenzamides is not known.

Alkomide is not currently marketed as a single agent in the United States. It is still used in combination with other agents.

Dinitolmide is fed at 0.0125% to prevent coccidiosis in chickens. Do not feed to layers or birds over 14 weeks of age. No withdrawal is required.

NICARBAZIN. Nicarbazin (Nicarb, Cycarb) is an equimolecular complex of 4,4′-dinitrocarbanilide and 2-hydroxy-4,6dimethylpyrimidine (Fig. 49.8). Dry crystals are strongly electrostatic and present some dry-mixing problems. The agents are absorbed separately from the chicken digestive tract, and both are needed for anticoccidial activity. The precise mode of action of nicarbazin is not known. Nicarbazin is fed at 125 ppm for the prevention of coccidiosis. Do not feed to layers. Do not use for treatment of coccidiosis. A 4-day withdrawal is required. Nicarbazin causes reduced egg production, depressed egg weight, reduced eggshell thickness, and egg-yolk mottling when fed to white leghorn layers at 125 ppm (Jones et al. 1990). It also causes poor hatchability and depigmentation of brown-shelled eggs. Nicarbazin is usually restricted in use to the starting period because of potential growth-suppressing effects and to cooler months of the year because of its potential to enhance the effects of heat distress (McDougald 1993).

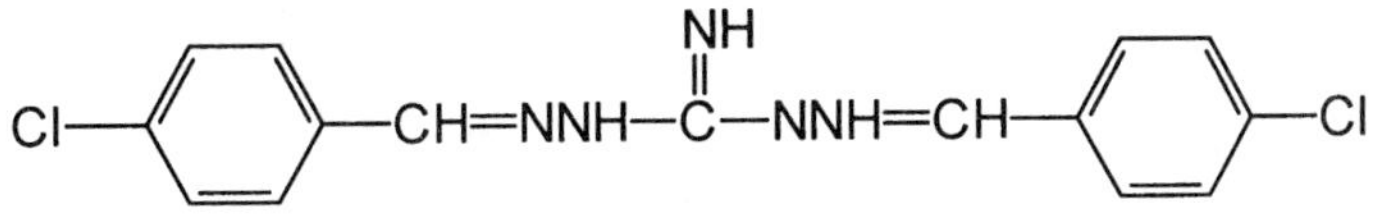

Robenidine
($C_{15}H_{13}Cl_2N_5$)
[334.21]

FIG. 49.6

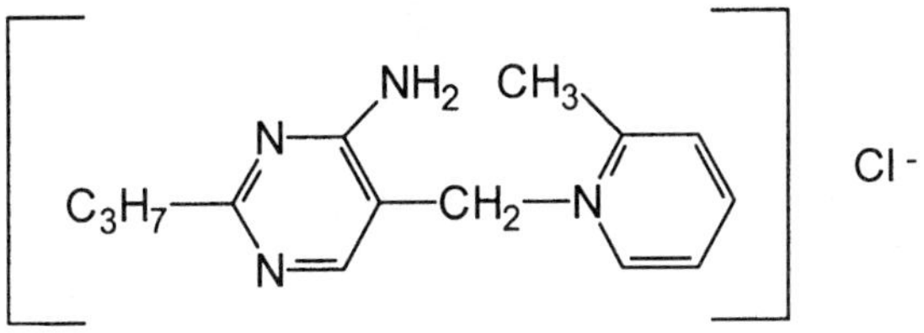

Amprolium
($C_{14}H_{19}ClN_4$)
[278.78]

FIG. 49.7

TABLE 49.5—Nitrobenzamides

Name	Chemical name (Empirical formula) [Molecular weight]	Chemical structure
Aklomide	2-chloro-4-nitrobenzamide ($C_7H_5ClN_2O_3$) [200.60]	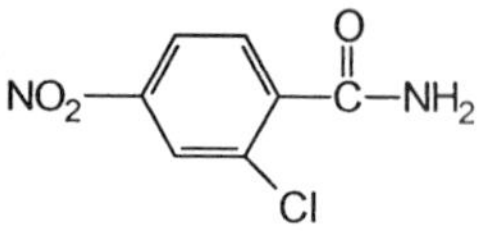
Dinitolmide	2-methyl-3,5-dinitrobenzamide ($C_8H_7N_3O_5$) [225.16]	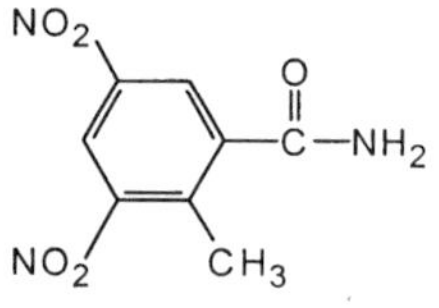

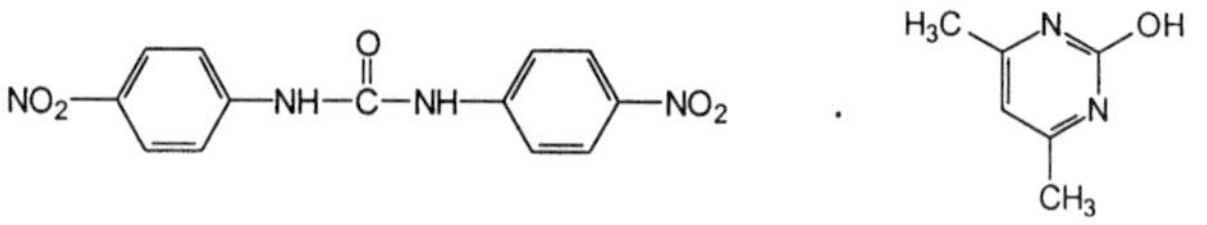

Nicarbazin
($C_{19}H_{18}N_6O_6$)
[426.38]

FIG. 49.8

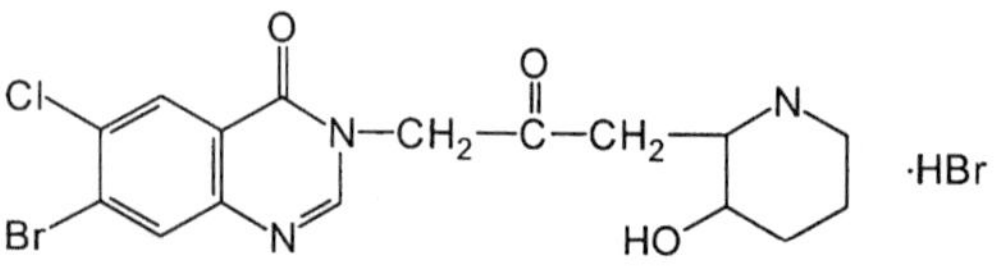

Halofuginone
($C_{16}H_{18}Br_2ClN_3O_3$)
[495.50]

FIG. 49.9

HALOFUGINONE. Halofuginone hydrobromide (Stenerol), (±)-*trans*-7-bromo-6-chloro-3-[3-(3-hydroxy-2-piperidyl)acetonyl]-4(3*H*)-quinazolinone (Fig. 49.9), is an alkaloid originally isolated from the plant *Dichroa febrifuga*. Halofuginone is active against the asexual stages of coccidia. Its anticoccidial mode of action is not known.

Halofuginone is used for the prevention of coccidiosis and fed at 0.03% (3 ppm). Do not feed to layers. A 4-day withdrawal is required. Halofuginone is transmitted to eggs from hens that have been fed halofuginone for 1 week (Long et al. 1981), but no adverse effects on egg production or egg quality are associated with it (Jones et al. 1990). Halofuginone has been associated with skin tears in chickens, and it has been shown to be an inhibitor of collagen type I synthesis in avian and mammalian cells (Granot et al. 1993). Halofuginone is toxic to fish and other aquatic life and must not be fed to waterfowl. Halofuginone is a skin and eye irritant, and appropriate precautions should be taken when handling this agent.

POLYETHER IONOPHORES. The polyether ionophorous antibiotics were first discovered in the early 1950s, and their anticoccidial activities were recognized in the late 1960s (Table 49.6). Because of their broad spectrum of activity and the development of drug resistance to other agents, the ionophores gained widespread usage in the poultry industry soon after their introduction. Polyether ionophores fall into one of five classes: monovalent, monovalent glycosides, divalent, divalent glycosides, or divalent pyrole ethers. The mode of action of ionophores is related to their ability to form lipophilic complexes with alkali metal cations and to transport these cations across biological membranes. Different ionophores may have different affinities for different cations. Ionophores that have anticoccidial activity are thought to act against extracellular

TABLE 49.6—Ionophorous antibiotics

Name	Chemical name (Empirical formula) [Molecular weight]	Chemical structure
Lasalocid	6-[7*R*-[5*S*-Ethyl-5-(5*R*-ethyltetra-hydro-5-hydroxy-6 *S*-methyl-2*H*-pyran-2*R*-yl) tetrahydro-3*S*-methyl-2*S*-furanyl]-4*S*-hydroxy-3*R*,5*S*-dimethyl-6-oxonon-yl]-2-hydroxy-3-methylbenzoic acid ($C_{34}H_{54}O_8$) [590.80]	
Maduramicin	(3*R*,4*S*,5*S*,6*R*,7*S*,22*S*)-23,27-Didemethoxy-2,6,22-tridemethyl-11-*O*-demethyl-22-[(2,6-dideoxy-3,4-di-*O*-methyl-β-L-arabino-hexopyranosyl)oxy]-6-methyl-oxylonomycin A monoammonium salt ($C_{47}H_{83}NO_{17}$) [934.17]	
Monensin	2-[5-Ethyltetrahydro-5-[tetrahydro-3-methyl-5-[tetrahydro-6-hydroxy-6-(hydromethyl)-3,5-dimethyl-2*H* -pyran-2-yl]-2-furyl]-2-furyl]-9-hydroxy-β-methoxy-α, γ, 2,8-tetramethyl-1,6-dioxaspiro [4.5] decane-7-butyric acid ($C_{36}H_{62}O_{11}$) [670.90]	
Narasin	(αβ,2β,3α,5α,6α)-α-ethyl-6-[5-[5-(5α-ethyltetrahydro-5β-hydroxy-6α-methyl-2*H*-pyran-2β-yl)-3″α,4,4″,5,5″α,6″-hexahydro-3′β-hydroxy-3″β,5α,5″β-trimethylspiro] furan-2(3*H*),2′-[2*H*]pyran-6′(3′*H*),2″-[2*H*]pyran]6″α-yl]2α-hydroxy-1α,3β-dimethyl-4-oxoheptyl]-tetrahydro-3,5-dimethyl-2*H*-pyran-2-acetic acid ($C_{43}H_{72}O_{11}$) [765.05]	
Semduramicin	(2*R*,3*S*,4*S*,5*R*,6*S*)-tetrahydro-2,4-dihydroxy-6-[(1*R*)-1-[(2*S*,5*R*,7*S*,8*R*,9*S*)--9-hydroxy-2,8-dimethyl-2-[(2*R*,6*S*)-tetrahydro-5-methyl-5-[(2*R*,3*S*,5*R*)-tetrahydro-5[(2*S*,3*S*,5*R*,6*S*)-tetrahydro-6-hydroxy-3,5,6-trimethyl-2*H*-pyran-2-yl]-3-[[(2*S*,5*S*,6*R*)-tetrahydro-5-methoxy-6-methyl-2*H*-pyran-2-yl]oxy]-2-furyl]-2-furyl]-1,6-dioxaspirol [4.5]dec-7-yl]ethyl]-5-methoxy-3-methyl-2*H*-pyran-2-acetic acid ($C_{44}H_{77}O_{16}$) [748.47]	

sporozoites and merozoites. Extracellular stages develop membrane blebs indicating alterations in membrane integrity and in internal osmolality. Because coccidia have no osmoregulatory organelles, this change in internal osmotic conditions would adversely affect the parasites.

Because of the unique mode of action of ionophores, development of anticoccidial resistance to ionophores was slow to occur in the field and difficult to produce under experimental conditions. In the mid- to late 1980s ionophore-resistant strains of chicken *Eimeria* spp. were documented in the United States, and ionophore resistance is now common. Cross-resistance between ionophores is common, although strain differences in response to specific ionophores have been demonstrated. In general, resistance to a monovalent polyether ionophore confers some cross-resistance to other monovalent polyether ionophores, but susceptibility to monovalent monoglycoside and divalent polyether ionophores may be retained.

Ionophores are potentially toxic for highly susceptible species, such as horses and other equines. Care should always be taken to prevent highly susceptible animals from gaining access to feeds containing these products.

MONENSIN. Monensin (Coban, Rumensin) is a monovalent polyether ionophore that is a fermentation product of *Streptomyces cinnamonensis.* Monensin (Coban) is fed at 99–121 ppm for prevention of coccidiosis in broilers. Do not feed to layers or chickens over 16 weeks of age. No withdrawal is required. Tiamulin (Tiamutin), [(2-(diethylamino)ethyl) ethyl thio] acetic acid 6-ethenyldecahydro-5-hydroxy-4,6,9,10-tetramethyl-1-oxo-3a,9-propano-3a*H*-cyclopentacycloocten-8-yl ester, may interfere with the metabolism of monensin in chickens and cause weight suppression (Meingasser et al. 1979). Monesin is apparently not transmitted to eggs of hens fed monensin for 1 week, nor does it adversely affect egg production or quality. Mature turkeys and guinea fowl should not have access to monensin-containing diets. Monensin will cause deaths in horses that ingest feeds containing it.

LASALOCID. Lasalocid (Avatec, Bovatec) is a divalent polyether ionophore that is a fermentation product of *Streptomyces lasaliensis* and was the second ionophore marketed in the United States. Lasalocid is fed at 0.0075–0.0125% (75–125 ppm) for the prevention of coccidiosis. Lasalocid is well tolerated when fed with tiamulin (Meingasser et al. 1979). Lasalocid is transmitted to eggs of hens that have been fed lasalocid for 1 week. Lasalocid does not appear to accentuate heat distress, but its usage has been associated with wet litter at the higher dosage levels.

SALINOMYCIN. Salinomycin (Bio-Cox) is a monovalent polyether ionophore that is a fermentation product of *Streptomyces albus* and was the third ionophore marketed in the United States. Salinomycin is active against sporozoites and early and late asexual stages of chicken coccidia (Conway et al. 1993). Salinomycin is fed at 66 ppm for prevention of coccidiosis in broilers. Do not feed to layers. It is not for use with pellet binders. No withdrawal is required. Salinomycin does not adversely affect egg production or egg quality. Tiamulin may interfere with the metabolism of salinomycin in chickens and cause weight suppression (Meingasser et al. 1979). Salinomycin will cause deaths in horses and adult turkeys that ingest feeds containing it.

NARASIN. Narasin (Monteban) is a monovalent polyether ionophore that is a fermentation product of *Streptomyces aureofaciens.* It is structurally similar to salinomycin, differing only in the presence of a methyl group in narasin that is not present in salinomycin. Narasin is fed at 70 ppm for the prevention of coccidiosis in broilers. It is for broilers only and should not be fed to other types of chickens. No withdrawal is required. It does not adversely affect egg production or egg quality. Narasin may cause fatalities in horses that ingest it, and it should not be fed to adult turkeys. Tiamulin may interfere with the metabolism of narasin in chickens and cause weight suppression (Meingasser et al. 1979).

A combination of narasin and nicarbazin (Maxiban) is fed at 40 ppm for prevention of coccidiosis in broilers. It is for broilers only and should not be fed to other types of chickens. A 4-day withdrawal period is required. The use of this combination has been associated with increased mortality of broilers in times of heat distress. Feed containing this combination may cause fatalities in horses that ingest it, and it should not be fed to adult turkeys.

MADURAMICIN. Maduramicin (Cygro) is a monovalent monoglycoside polyether ionophore that is a fermentation product of *Actinomadura yumaense.* It is no longer available in the United States. It is used for the prevention of coccidiosis in broilers and fed at 5 ppm. It is for broilers only and should not be fed to other types of chickens. A 5-day withdrawal period is required. Maduramicin does not adversely affect egg production or egg quality (Jones et al. 1990). Maduramicin is well tolerated when fed with tiamulin (Meingasser et al. 1979). If maduramicin is fed at 6 ppm, an adverse effect on growth and feathering may occur.

SEMDURAMICIN. Semduramicin (Aviax) is a monovalent monoglycoside polyether ionophore that is a fermentation product of a mutant of *Actinomadura roseorufa* (Ricketts et al. 1992). The parent produced a diglycoside form of semduramicin that had to be semisynthetically modified. Both forms of the monoglycoside agent have identical activity. It is fed at 25 ppm for prevention of coccidiosis in broiler chickens. No withdrawal time is required. It is well tolerated when coadministered with tiamulin (Ricketts et al. 1992).

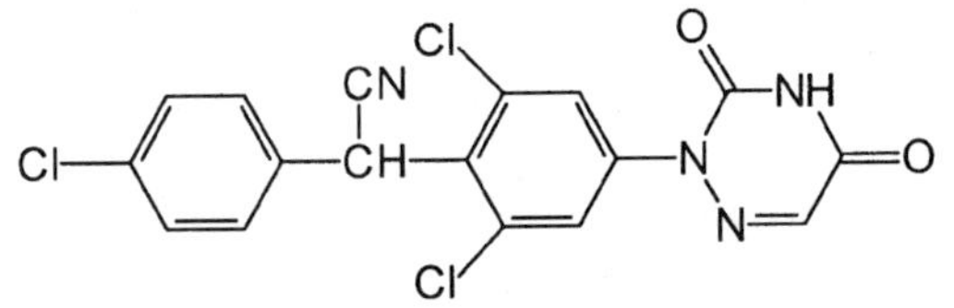

Diclazuril
($C_{17}H_9Cl_3N_4O_2$)
[407.64]

FIG. 49.10

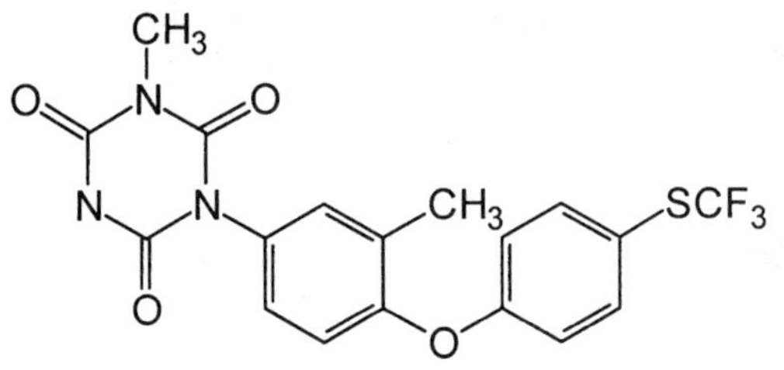

DICLAZURIL. Diclazuril (Clinicox), 2,6-dichloro-α-(4-chlorophenyl)-4-(4,5-dihydro-3,5-dioxo-1,2,4-triazin-2(3*H*)-yl)benzeneacetonitrile (Fig. 49.10), is a benzeneacetonitrile that has potent anticoccidial activity when fed at low levels in the feed. Technical diclazuril is a slightly yellowish to beige powder, and it is almost insoluble in water. It has not yet received approval for use in the United States (as of 1999) but is approved for use in many other countries. It may also be useful in the treatment of toxoplasmosis and EPM.

TOLTRAZURIL. Toltrazuril (Baycox), 1-methyl-3-[3-methyl-4-[4-[(trifluoromethyl)thio]phenyl]-1,3,5-triazine-2,4,6(1*H*,3*H*,5*H*)-trionne, is a triazinon drug (Fig. 49.11) that has broad-spectrum anticoccidial and antiprotozoal activity. It is not commercially available in the United States. It is active against both asexual and sexual stages of coccidia by inhibiting nuclear division of schizonts and microgamonts and the wall-forming bodies of macrogamonts.

It may also be useful in the treatment of neonatal porcine coccidiosis, EPM, and canine hepatozoonosis.

SULFONAMIDES. Sulfonamides were the first effective anticoccidials used. Sulfonamides can be either coccidiostatic or coccidiocidal.

Sulfonamides are produced by chemical synthesis. They are usually white powders, and their sodium salts are usually water soluble. See Chap. 40 of this book for detailed information on the pharmacology of these agents. The structure of sulfonamides is similar to para-aminobenzoate (para-aminobenzoic acid, PABA), which is required by bacteria in the synthesis of folate (folic acid). Sulfonamides interfere in the early phases of folate synthesis. Mammalian and avian cells use preformed folate and are therefore not affected by the sulfonamide treatments. Sulfonamides are often used in combination with dihydrofolate reductase/thymidylate synthase (DHFR/TS) inhibitors because of the observed synergistic effects due to activity at two places in folate biosynthesis. Sulfonamides have most activity against the asexual stages and lesser activity against the sexual stages of coccidia.

Toltrazuril
($C_{18}H_{14}F_3N_3O_4S$)
[425.38]

FIG. 49.11

Sulfonamides used in veterinary medicine for the treatment or prevention of coccidia and coccidia-like parasites include sulfaguanidine, sulfadiazine, sulfadimethoxine, sulfadoxine, sulfamethazine (syn. sulfadimidine), sulfamethoxazole, sulfanitran, and sulfaquinoxaline (Table 49.7). Many are used in combination with other products that have antibacterial or growth-promoting properties. Several are used in combination with DHFR/TS inhibitors because of true synergism.

Because of the development of superior agents and fear of generation of resistant bacterial strains, no sulfonamides were marketed as single feed additives for the prevention or treatment of coccidiosis in chickens in 1998. Sulfonamides still are used in the treatment of coccidiosis in dogs, cats, rabbits, and ruminants.

Dihydrofolate Reductase/Thymidylate Synthase Inhibitors. In protozoa, unlike other eukaryotic cells, the dihydrofolate reductase and thymidylate synthase enzymes do not exist as separate molecular entities, but instead these enzymes are part of a bifunctional DHFR/TS complex that has both DHFR and TS activity (Roos 1993). The best-known and most often used members of this group are trimethoprim, ormetoprim, and pyrimethamine (Table 49.8). All are white to cream, bitter-tasting crystalline powders and are produced by chemical synthesis.

Several formulations of trimethoprim and trimethoprim combinations are available for oral or parenteral administration. Trimethoprim is readily absorbed from the digestive tract after oral administration, and peak serum levels occur 1–4 hours later. The half-life is 3.8 hours in the horse, 3.0 hours in the dog, and 10.6 hours in human beings. Coadministration of sulfonamide does not affect the rate of absorption of trimethoprim. Trimethoprim is widely distributed in tissues. Levels of trimethoprim in cerebral spinal fluid are about 40% of those in the serum (Zinner and Mayer 1990). Trimethoprim is almost completely (60–80%) excreted by the kidneys within 24 hours, and some is also excreted in

TABLE 49.7—Sulfonamides

Name	Chemical name (Empirical formula) [Molecular weight]	Chemical structure
Sulfadiazine	4-amino-*N*-2-pyrimidinylbenzenesulfonamide ($C_{10}H_{10}N_4O_2S$) [250.28]	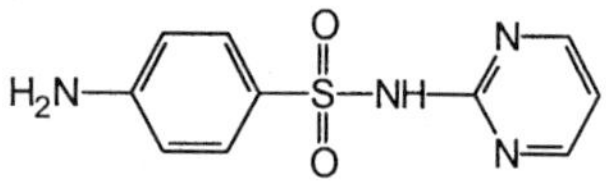
Sulfadimethoxine	4-amino-*N*-(2,6-dimethoxy-4-pyrimidinyl)-benzenesulfonamide ($C_{12}H_{14}N_4O_4S$) [310.33]	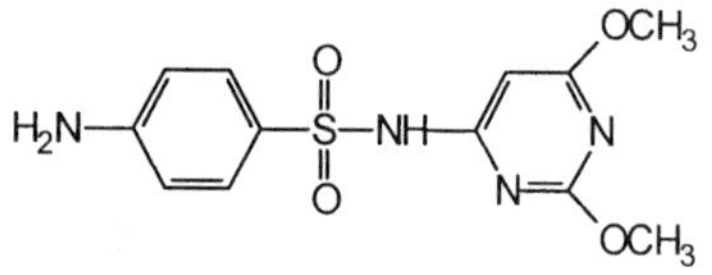
Sulfadoxine	4-amino-*N*-(5,6-dimethoxy-4-pyrimidinyl)-benzenesulfonamide ($C_{12}H_{14}N_4O_4S$) [310.34]	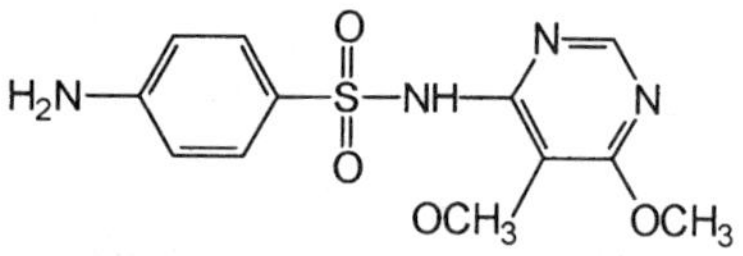
Sulfaguanidine	4-amino-*N*-(aminoiminomethyl)-benzenesulfonamide ($C_7H_{10}N_4O_2S$) [214.24]	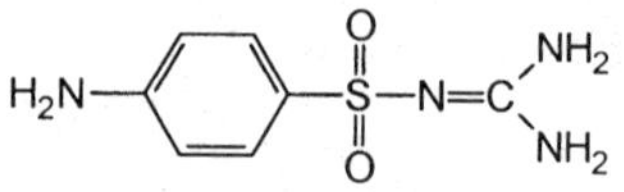
Sulfamethazine	4-amino-*N*-(4,6-dimethyl-2-pyrimidinyl)-benzenesulfonamide ($C_{12}H_{14}N_4O_2S$) [278.32]	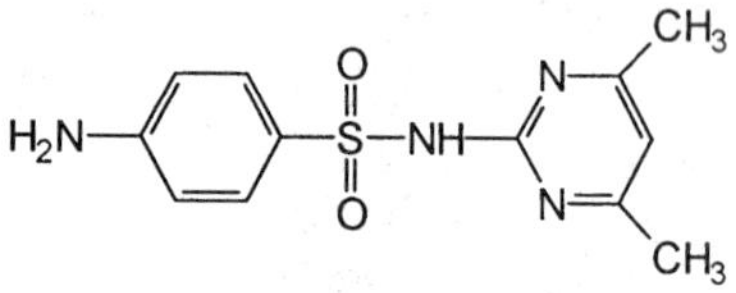
Sulfamethoxazole	4-amino-*N*-(5-methyl-3-isoxazolyl)-benzenesulfonamide ($C_{10}H_{11}N_3O_3S$) [253.31]	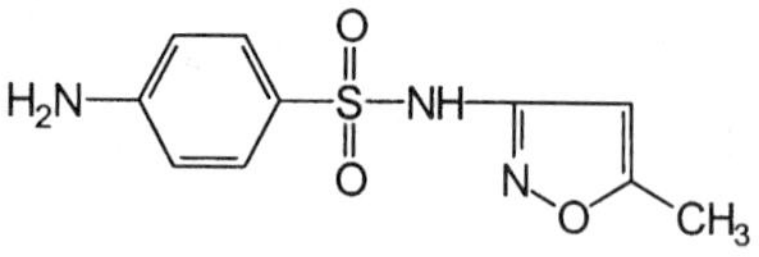
Sulfaquinoxaline	4-amino-*N*-2-quinoxalinyl-benzenesulfonamide ($C_{14}H_{12}N_4O_2S$) [300.33]	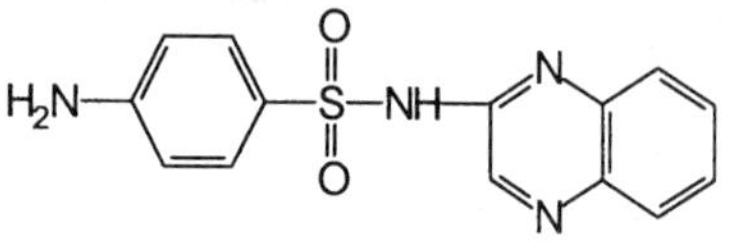
Sulfanitran	4′-[(*p*-nitrophenyl)sulfamoyl]acetanilide ($C_{14}H_{13}N_3O_5S$) [335.34]	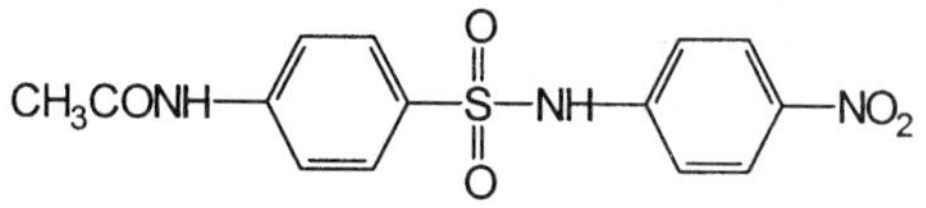

the bile. The remainder is excreted as metabolites by the kidneys. Use of trimethoprim and other DHFR/TS inhibitors is associated with adverse effects on bone marrow. Administration of folinic acid usually will counteract these adverse effects (see toxoplasmosis, EPM below).

Pyrimethamine is available in 25 mg tablets (Daraprim). Pyrimethamine is well absorbed after oral administration and is slowly but extensively metabolized. Less than 3% is excreted in the urine in the first 24 hours, and the half-life is 4–6 days in human beings (Van Reken and Pearson 1990). It accumulates in the kidneys, lungs, liver, and spleen. It is excreted in urine as metabolites, but some pyrimethamine can be found in the milk. Very high doses of pyrimethamine are teratogenic in laboratory animals.

Combinations of Sulfonamides and DHFR/TS Inhibitors. Ormetoprim combined with sulfadimethoxine (Rofenaid 40) is the only combination

TABLE 49.8—Dihydrofolate reductase/thymidylate synthase inhibitors

Name	Chemical name (Empirical formula) [Molecular weight]	Chemical structure
Trimethoprim	2,4-diamino-5-(3,4,5-trimethoxybenzyl)pyrimidine ($C_{14}H_{18}N_4O_3$) [290.32]	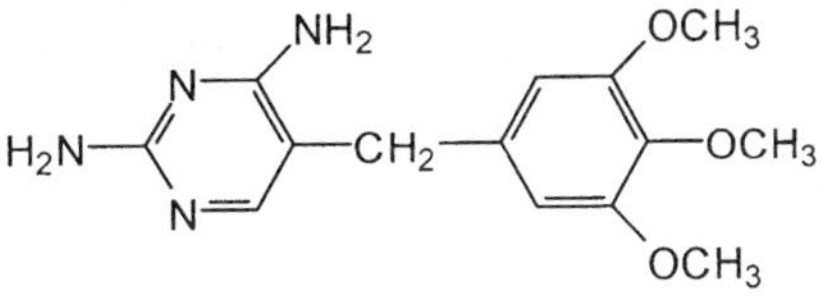
Pyrimethamine	2,4-diamino-5-(*p*-chlorophenyl)-6-ethylpyrimidine ($C_{12}H_{13}ClN_4$) [248.71]	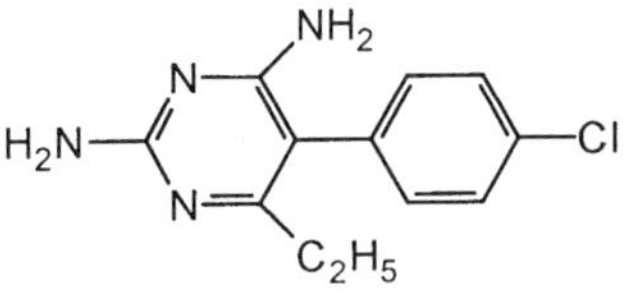
Diaveridine	2,4-diamino-5-veratrylpyrimidine ($C_{13}H_{16}N_4O_2$) [260.29]	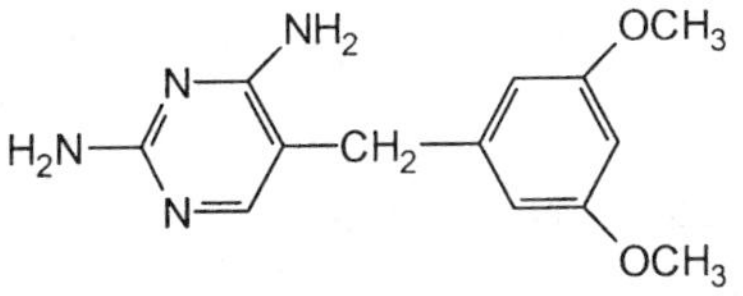
Ormetoprim	2,4-diamino-5-(4,5-dimethoxy-2-methylbenzyl)-pyrimidine ($C_{13}H_{15}N_4O_2$) [259.17]	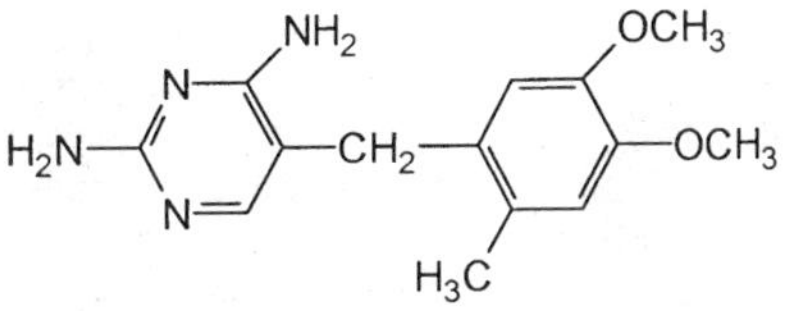

DHFR/TS-sulfonamide presently available in the United States for poultry. It is fed to chickens at 0.0075% ormetoprim and 0.0125% sulfadimethoxine to prevent coccidiosis in broiler chickens. Do not feed to birds producing eggs for food. A 5-day withdrawal is required.

Other combinations are intended for use in human beings, equines, and small animals. Ormetoprim is also available in combination with sulfadimethoxine in the ratio of 1 part ormetoprim plus 5 parts sulfadimethoxine (Primor) in various size tablets. Pyrimethamine is available in tablets that contain 25 mg pyrimethamine and 500 mg sulfadoxine (Fansidar), and in tablets that contain 12.5 mg pyrimethamine and 100 mg dapsone (Maloprim). Trimethoprim is available in several tablet, liquid, and paste formulations in combination with sulfamethoxazole (Cotrimethoxazole, Bactrim, Septra) or sulfadiazine (Di-Trim, Tribrissen) that are usually in the ratio of 1 part trimethoprim to 5 parts sulfamethoxazole or sulfadiazine. These agents are used in treatment of coccidiosis, toxoplasmosis, neosporosis, EPM, and malaria. Adverse reactions to these agents are similar to those of the individual constituents. These combinations should not be used in animals with liver disease, blood dyscrasias, or a history of sulfonamide sensitivity. Precautions normally observed when animals are taking sulfonamides should be observed. Toxicity of these agents is low. The safety of ormetoprim-sulfadimethoxine has not been established in pregnant dogs, but studies indicate that the use of trimethoprim-sulfadiazine is safe in pregnant dogs.

TURKEY COCCIDIOSIS. Ormetoprim combined with sulfadimethoxine (Rofenaid 40) is fed to turkeys at 0.00375% ormetoprim and 0.00625% sulfadimethoxine to prevent coccidiosis. Do not feed to birds producing eggs for food. A 5-day withdrawal is required.

Amprolium is used for the treatment and prevention of coccidiosis in turkeys and fed continuously at 0.0125–0.0.025%. No withdrawal is required. Resistance to amprolium is common.

Clopidol is used for prevention of coccidiosis in turkeys and fed at 0.0125–0.0250%. A 5-day withdrawal is required.

Dinitolamide is used for prevention of coccidiosis in turkeys and fed at 0.0125–0.01875%. Do not feed to birds producing eggs for human consumption. No withdrawal is required.

Halofuginone is approved for the prevention of coccidiosis in growing turkeys. It is fed at 0.03%. A 7-day withdrawal is required. It must not be fed to layers or waterfowl.

Monensin is used for prevention of coccidiosis and is fed at 99 ppm. Do not feed to turkeys over 10 weeks old. No withdrawal is required.

Lasalocid is approved for the prevention of coccidiosis in growing turkeys and is fed at 0.0075–0.0125%. No withdrawal is required.

GAME BIRD COCCIDIOSIS. Monensin is approved for use in bobwhite quail for prevention of coccidiosis and is fed at 73 g/ton from 1 day to 10 weeks old. No withdrawal is required. Salinomycin is approved for prevention of coccidiosis in bobwhite quail and is fed at 55 ppm.

Lasalocid is approved for the prevention of coccidiosis in chukar partridges. It is fed at 0.0125% until the birds are 8 weeks old. No withdrawal is required.

Amprolium is approved for use in the prevention of coccidiosis in pheasants and is fed continuously at 0.0175%. It must not be used in feeds containing bentonite.

Treatment of Coccidiosis in Mammals

CATTLE COCCIDIOSIS. About 17 species of *Eimeria* have been described in cattle throughout the world, and 13 of these occur in the United States. However, only 2 species, *E. bovis* and *E. zuernii,* are commonly associated with outbreaks of clinical disease. Clinical coccidiosis is normally observed in animals under 1 year of age. Moderately infected animals have diarrhea that may or may not have blood; severely infected animals may have watery, bloody diarrhea that may contain portions of sloughed intestinal mucosa. Outbreaks of coccidiosis in feedlots often occur after severe cold, rainy weather, and the ensuing environmental stress placed on the cattle.

Six anticoccidials are approved for use against coccidiosis in cattle in the United States. Sulfamethazine is used to treat coccidiosis by oral administration of two 5 g boluses/45 kg for 1 day, followed by one 5 g bolus/45 kg for up to 4 consecutive days. An 11-day withdrawal is required. Do not feed to calves to be slaughtered under 1 month old or to lactating dairy cattle. Sulfaquinoxaline is used to treat coccidiosis by oral administration of 2.7 mg/kg BW for 3–5 days. A 10-day withdrawal time is required. Do not feed to calves to be slaughtered under 1 month old or use in lactating dairy cattle. Amprolium is given in the feed, drinking water, or orally at 5 mg/kg BW for 21 days to prevent coccidiosis or at 10 mg/kg BW for 21 days to treat coccidiosis. A 1-day withdrawal is required. Lasalocid is used to prevent coccidiosis and is fed at 1 mg/kg BW, with a maximum of 360 mg/animal/day. No withdrawal time is required. Do not use in breeding animals. Monensin is used to prevent coccidiosis and is fed to provide 100–360 mg/animal/day. No withdrawal time is required. Decoquinate is used to prevent coccidiosis and is fed at 0.5–2 mg/kg BW for at least 28 days. Do not feed to lactating dairy cows. No withdrawal time is required.

SHEEP COCCIDIOSIS. There are about 15 species of *Eimeria* that infect sheep. Clinical coccidiosis is seen in lambs about 2–3 weeks after they are weaned or after they are placed in feedlots. Outbreaks often occur after animals are stressed. Watery diarrhea is the main clinical sign; it usually is not bloody.

Only three anticoccidials are approved for use in sheep in the United States. Lasalocid is fed in the ration to sheep at 0.0022–0.0033% (provides 15–70 mg/animal/day) and is used in the prevention of coccidiosis. Do not use with breeding animals. No withdrawal is required. Decoquinate is fed to sheep to provide 0.5 mg/kg BW for at least 28 days to prevent coccidiosis. Do not feed to sheep producing milk for human consumption. No withdrawal is required. Sulfaquinoxaline is given in the drinking water at 0.025% for 2–5 days for treatment of coccidiosis in lambs and at 0.015% for 3–5 days for other animals. A 10-day withdrawal is required.

GOAT COCCIDIOSIS. About 10 species of *Eimeria* are found in goats, with *E. alijevi, E. arloingi, E. christenseni,* and *E. ninakohlyakimovae* being the most pathogenic species. Coccidiosis is often a serious problem in young goats, and in some herds up to 15% of kids may die from coccidiosis or its indirect effects. Diarrhea is the main clinical sign in these animals.

There are two anticoccidials approved for use in goats in the United States. Decoquinate is fed to goats to provide 0.5 mg/kg BW for at least 28 days to prevent coccidiosis. Do not feed to goats producing milk for human consumption. No withdrawal is required. Monensin is fed at 20 g/ton for the prevention of coccidiosis in confinement-reared goats. Do not feed to goats producing milk for human consumption. No withdrawal is required.

PIG COCCIDIOSIS. Coccidiosis in pigs is a disease of nursing pigs that are from 7 to 14 days of age and is caused by *Isospora suis* (Lindsay et al. 1997a). None of the approximately 13 species of *Eimeria* infecting pigs are serious pathogens.

No anticoccidial agents are approved for use in pigs. The feeding of coccidiostats to sows does not appear to aid in prevention of infection in their nursing young because sows do not excrete detectable numbers of *I. suis* oocysts in their feces, and pigs nursing drug-treated sows often develop clinical coccidiosis. Most sows do have *Eimeria* oocysts in their feces, and several anticoccidials will eliminate these oocysts from the sows' feces. Amprolium, decoquinate, and monensin have been used in sow feeds.

Anticoccidial medication of nursing pigs poses several problems because the pigs are not eating or drinking adequate amounts to make food or water a viable treatment source (Lindsay et al. 1997a). Therefore, each pig must be dosed individually. This is often too labor intensive for a large farrowing operation. Controlled studies in nursing pigs experimentally inoculated with *I. suis* have failed to demonstrate benefits of treatment with amprolium, furazolidone, or monensin.

Toltrazuril, although not available in the United States, has been shown to reduce the signs of coccidiosis in naturally infected nursing pigs when a single oral 20–30 mg/kg BW dose is given to 3- to 6-day-old pigs (Driesen et al. 1995). Clinical signs were reduced from 71 to 22% of nursing pigs, and diarrhea and oocyst excretion were also decreased by the single oral treatment.

DOG COCCIDIOSIS. Oocysts of four *Isospora* spp. (*I. canis, I. ohioensis, I. neorivolta,* and *I. burrowsi*) can be found in the feces of dogs (Lindsay et al. 1997a). Additionally, oocysts of *Cryptosporidium, Hammondia,* and *Neospora* spp. and sporocysts of *Sarcocystis* spp. are found in the feces of dogs. These usually are not associated with disease.

Clinical signs of canine coccidiosis caused by *Isospora* spp. are bloody or mucoid diarrhea, abdominal pain, dehydration, anemia, anorexia, weight loss, and emesis, as well as neurologic and respiratory signs. Animals that are nursing, recently weaned, or immunocompromised are most likely to develop clinical signs of disease. Coccidiosis can cause severe problems in some kennels, and the stress of shipping may cause outbreaks of coccidiosis in young dogs.

Several agents have been used for the treatment of intestinal coccidiosis in dogs (Lindsay et al. 1997a), but only sulfadimethoxine is approved by the FDA for this usage. Sulfadimethoxine is used for treatment of coccidiosis at 50 mg/kg BW for 10 days or at 55 mg/kg BW for 1 day, then at 27.5 mg/kg BW until clinical signs disappear. Sulfadimethoxine is combined with ormetoprim (Primor) and used as a treatment for coccidiosis at 11 mg/kg BW ormetoprim plus 55 mg/kg BW sulfadimethoxine for up to 23 days.

Sulfadiazine is combined with trimethoprim (Tribrissen, Di-Trim) and used as a treatment for coccidiosis at 5–10 mg/kg BW trimethoprim combined with 25–50 mg/kg BW of sulfadiazine and given for 6 days to dogs over 4 kg BW; dogs under 4 kg BW are given half this dosage for 6 days.

Amprolium is used in the treatment of coccidiosis at 300–400 mg/kg BW for 55 days or at 110–220 mg/kg BW for 7–12 days. Amprolium is also used in the drinking water (sole source) at 1.5 tbsp/gal for up to 10 days. Amprolium can be combined with sulfadimethoxine and used for the treatment of coccidiosis at 150 mg/kg BW amprolium and 25 mg/kg BW sulfadimethoxine for 14 days.

CAT COCCIDIOSIS. Oocysts of two *Isospora* spp. are found in cats (Lindsay et al. 1997a). Additionally, oocysts of *Toxo. gondii, Hammondia hammondi, Besnoitia* spp., *Cryptosporidium parvum,* and *Sarcocystis* spp. (sporocysts) are found in the feces of cats. Clinical signs are usually not associated with the presence of these oocysts.

Clinical coccidiosis in cats is similar to that seen in dogs. No agents are approved by the FDA for the treatment of coccidiosis in cats. Agents and dosages used for the treatment of canine coccidiosis are also used for the treatment of feline coccidiosis.

RABBIT COCCIDIOSIS. Intestinal and hepatic coccidiosis in rabbits is one of the most economically important diseases of commercially reared rabbits. *Eimeria stiedai* is the cause of hepatic coccidiosis, and important intestinal species include *E. flavescens* and *E. intestinalis.* Traditionally, the sulfonamides have been used extensively in prophylaxis and treatment. However, resistant strains have developed, limiting the effectiveness of these agents in some facilities. Sulfaquinoxaline is used at 0.03% in the drinking water for 10 days for treatment of coccidiosis. A 10-day withdrawal is required. Lasalocid is approved for use in the prevention of hepatic coccidiosis in rabbits and is fed at 0.0125% until the rabbits are 6.5 weeks old. No withdrawal is required.

Cryptosporidiosis. The life cycle of this coccidian is direct. It is unusual in that it develops in the microvillous borders of a variety of epithelial tissues and produces fully sporulated oocysts. *Cryptosporidium parvum* causes intestinal disease in immunocompetent human beings and other mammals (Fayer et al. 1997). Respiratory and biliary tract infections and disease occur in immunocompromised humans and nonhuman primates. *Cryptosporidium baileyi* causes respiratory disease in chickens and other avian species, and *C. meleagridis* causes intestinal and respiratory disease in turkeys (Fayer et al. 1997).

Cryptosporidial infections are remarkably resistant to treatment with most anticoccidials and other antimicrobial agents. Blagburn and Soave (1997) reported that over 100 therapeutic agents have been examined against cryptosporidiosis in humans and animals with little success. The most promising agent identified to date is paromomycin. A naturally infected cat with cryptosporidial diarrhea was successfully treated with oral paromomycin given at 165 mg/kg BW every 12 hours for 5 days (Barr et al. 1994). Treatment of calves with oral paromomycin at 50, 25, or 12.5 mg/kg BW twice daily was effective in preventing oocyst production (50 mg/kg dose) or in delaying the onset of oocyst production and in greatly reducing the numbers of oocysts excreted (12.5–25 mg/kg BW doses) when started 1 day before inoculation and continued for 10 days (Fayer and Ellis 1993). Treatment of 2- to 4-day-old goat kids with oral paromomycin at 50 mg/kg BW twice daily for 10 days was effective in preventing cryptosporidiosis (Mancassola et al. 1995).

The anticryptosporidial activity of paromomycin apparently does not involve trafficking through the host cell cytoplasm but involves movement of the agent through altered apical membranes that surround the developing parasites (Griffiths et al. 1998). Paromomycin does not exert its effects on extracellular stages of *C. parvum* (Griffiths et al. 1998).

Experimental studies demonstrate that *C. baileyi* of chickens is refractory to treatment with approved anticoccidials. Monensin, lasalocid, salinomycin, and halofuginone were fed at recommended anticoccidial levels and had little effect on respiratory or digestive tract diseases when fed 5 days before experimental inoculations and continuously until necropsy 14 days after inoculation (Lindsay et al. 1987).

Toxoplasmosis and Extraintestinal Coccidia

FELINE INTESTINAL TOXOPLASMOSIS. Cats are the only hosts that shed *Toxo. gondii* oocysts in their feces. Clinical disease in cats is associated with fever, dyspnea, polypnea, abdominal pain, icterus, central nervous system signs, and weight loss (Lindsay et al. 1997b). These intestinal infections are usually asymptomatic. Clindamycin, pyrimethamine plus sulfonamides, monensin, and toltrazuril have been used experimentally to treat or prevent oocyst excretion in cats.

DISSEMINATED TOXOPLASMOSIS IN CATS AND DOGS. Clindamycin (Cleocin, Antirobe) is the drug of choice for the treatment of disseminated toxoplasmosis in cats and dogs (Lindsay et al. 1997b). It is a semisynthetic compound produced by alteration of the parent molecule lincomycin, which is produced by *Streptomyces lincolnensis.* It differs from lincomycin in having a chlorine group at C-7 rather than a hydroxyl group (Table 49.9). The dosages used against *Toxo. gondii* are higher than for the treatment of the anaerobic infections for which it is marketed. Oral and parenteral formulations of clindamycin have similar activity. The drug is almost completely absorbed after oral administration in both dogs and cats, and peak serum concentrations occur within 75 minutes (Harari and Lincoln 1989). The half-life is about 5 hours after oral or IV administration. Clindamycin is widely distributed in many tissues and fluids and crosses the placenta. It is metabolized in the liver and excreted in the bile and urine as parent agent and metabolites. Clindamycin is active against tachyzoites of *Toxo. gondii* and is initially coccidiostatic but becomes coccidiocidal after a few days of treatment. Cats are treated with clindamycin at 10–12 mg/kg BW orally every 12 hours for 4 weeks or treated with 12.5–25 mg/kg BW clindamycin IM every 12 hours for 4 weeks. Dogs are treated with 3–13 mg/kg BW orally or IM every 8 hours for 2 weeks or with 10–20 mg/kg BW orally or IM every 12 hours for 2 weeks. Clindamycin is also combined with pyrimethamine and used for the treatment of toxoplasmic encephalitis in human beings; such combinations might have applications in veterinary medicine.

Cats and dogs are treated orally with 0.25–0.5 mg/kg BW pyrimethamine and 30 mg/kg BW sulfonamide (preferably, sulfadiazine) every 12 hours for 2–4 weeks. Bone marrow suppression can occur with the synergistic use of pyrimethamine and sulfonamides and can be corrected by the addition of folinic acid (5 mg/day) or by the addition of yeast (100 mg/kg BW daily) to the animal's diet.

Canine Neosporosis. Dogs have recently been recognized as both intermediate and definitive hosts for *Neospora caninum* (McAllister et al. 1998). In dogs

TABLE 49.9—Lincosamides

Name	Chemical name (Empirical formula) [Molecular weight]	Chemical structure
Clindamycin	(2*S-trans*)-methyl-7-chloro-6,7,8-trideoxy-6-[[(1-methyl-4-propyl-2-pyrrolidinyl)carbonyl]-amino]-1-thio-L-threo-α-D-galacto-octopyranoside ($C_{18}H_{33}ClN_2O_5S$) [424.98]	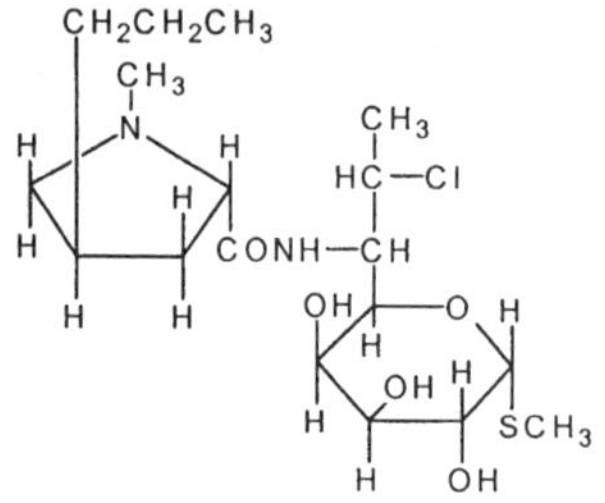 $CH_2CH_2CH_3$; CH_3; N; H; H; H; H; H; H; CH_3; HC—Cl; CONH—CH; OH; O; H; H; OH; H; H; SCH_3; H; OH
Lincomycin	methyl 6,8-dideoxy-6-[[(-1-methyl-4-propyl-2-pyrrolidinyl) carbonyl]amino]-1-thio-D-erythro-α-D-galacto-octopyranoside ($C_{18}H_{34}N_2O_6S$) [406.56]	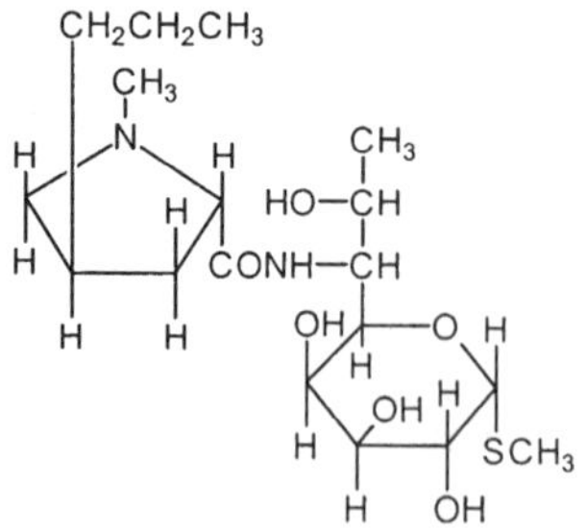 $CH_2CH_2CH_3$; CH_3; N; H; H; H; H; H; H; CH_3; HO—CH; CONH—CH; OH; O; H; H; OH; H; H; SCH_3; H; OH

this disease is most severe in congenitally infected pups, causing posterior paralysis, encephalitis, polymyocitis, and polyradiculoneuritis. *Neospora caninum* also causes abortions in cattle and other animals (Dubey and Lindsay 1996). Neonatal canine neosporosis is treated with 12.5–18.5 mg/kg BW clindamycin orally twice daily for 2–4 weeks (Dubey et al. 1998). Death may be prevented in pups with severe hindlimb involvement, but hindlimb functions usually do not return to normal.

Canine neosporosis will also respond to the above regimens of DHFR/TS inhibitors and sulfonamides used to treat canine toxoplasmosis. The amount of clinical improvement will depend on the degree of paralysis that has occurred.

No drugs will remove the tissue cysts of *N. caninum.* This means that treatment of bitches will not prevent transmission to their pups. Treatment of natural infections with *N. caninum* in animals other than dogs has not been attempted.

Equine Protozoal Myeloencephalitis. Equine protozoal myeloencephalitis is the most important protozoal disease of horses in the United States. It was first recognized in the early 1970s. In 1991, it was grown in cell culture and proven to be a member of the genus *Sarcocystis.* It was named *S. neurona* (Dubey et al. 1991). The opossum is the definitive host (Dubey and Lindsay 1998).

Clinical signs are variable depending on where in the central nervous system the parasite is growing. Head tilt, ataxia, muscle weakness and atrophy, urinary incontinence, and constipation are common findings.

Treatment is most likely to be effective if initiated as soon as EPM is suspected. Brain disease is more likely to resolve clinically than is spinal cord disease, and any muscle atrophy is likely to be permanent. Clinical signs usually begin to improve within 1 week after treatment, and it is estimated that 50–70% of treated horses will improve after chemotherapy.

Current treatment recommendations include trimethoprim-sulfonamide at 15–20 mg/kg BW orally twice daily combined with oral pyrimethamine at 1 mg/kg BW once daily for 30 days after clinical signs have stopped improving. The presence of food may adversely affect the absorption of DHFR/TS inhibitors, and food should be withheld 1–2 hours before and after treatment. As noted, specific anti-EPM treatment should be continued for at least 30 days after clinical improvement has ceased. Twelve weeks is about the average length of treatment time. Relapse is possible if horses are not treated long enough, and reactivation of the infection may occur during periods of unusual stress. These findings indicate that present chemotherapy regimens do not completely remove all parasites from the central nervous system. Cell culture studies have shown that pyrimethamine kills developing *S. neurona* at 1.0 µg/mL and trimethoprim kills it at 5.0 µg/mL (Lindsay and Dubey 1999). These levels of agent probably are not reached in the treated horses. It has been suggested that intermittent (every 2 or 4 weeks) single EPM treatment may help prevent clinical relapse in horses recovering from EPM (MacKay et al. 1992).

If relapse does occur, the entire treatment regimen should be repeated.

Inflammation is responsible for many of the clinical signs observed in acute infections, and the use of anti-inflammatory agents is beneficial. Flunixin meglumine at 1.1 mg/kg BW twice daily parenterally or phenylbutazone orally at 4.4 mg/kg BW twice daily can be helpful. Intravenous dimethylsulfoxide (DMSO) at 1 mg/kg BW once daily in a 10% solution for 3 days is also recommended. Corticosteroid use should be avoided if possible and restricted to 1–3 days of dexamethasone (0.05 mg/kg) in severely affected horses. Vitamin E supplementation (8000–9000 IU/day) may have beneficial anti-inflammatory effects and promote healing of damaged nervous tissue.

A recent study of 12 horses with EPM on a farm with an EPM outbreak indicated that DHFR/TS and DS treatment resulted in transient fever, anorexia, and depression in 2; acute worsening of ataxia in 2; mild anemia in 4; and abortions in 3 (Fenger et al. 1997). Prolonged use of DHFR/TS inhibitors has long been known to result in bone marrow suppression. Therefore, horses should be examined periodically (about every 2 weeks) for anemia and leukopenia. If the neutrophil counts drop below 3000 cells/µL, treatment should be discontinued until the counts recover (MacKay et al. 1992). Supplementation with 40 mg/day of folinic acid is recommended in horses with bone marrow suppression. Pregnant mares should be supplemented routinely with folinic acid while on EPM treatment, and the dose of pyrimethamine should be dropped to 0.5 mg/kg BW to reduce the risks to the fetus.

Diclazuril, toltrazuril, and other agents are currently under investigation for the treatment of EPM.

SUBORDER HAEMOSPORORINA: THE HAEMOSPOROZOANS. The haemosporozoans include *Plasmodium, Leucocytozoon,* and *Haemoproteus* spp. These parasites multiply asexually in various tissues (liver, lung, muscle, etc.) before entering the host's blood cells. Plasmodia undergo asexual and sexual multiplication in the host's erythrocytes, while *Haemoproteus* and *Leucocytozoon* organisms undergo only sexual development in the host's blood cells. *Haemoproteus* organisms develop only in erythrocytes, while *Leucocytozoon* organisms develop in both erythrocytes and leukocytes. Fertilization and sporogony occur in insect hosts. Vectors of these parasites include blackflies, mosquitoes, pigeon flies, and midges. The prevalence and distribution of these parasites depend on the biology and distribution of the insect vectors.

Malaria is caused by *Plasmodium* spp. and it is arguably the most important infectious disease of humans. It is less important in veterinary medicine.

Most of the chemotherapeutic agents used to treat malaria in human beings were first evaluated against malaria in birds. Chloroquine, 7-chloro-4-(4-diethylamino-1-methylbutylamino)quinoline, has been used in the treatment of avian malaria. *Plasmodium relictum* causes clinical malaria in penguins that are kept in zoos or aquaria. It is treated with an oral loading dose of 10 mg/kg BW chloroquine, followed by oral doses of 5 mg/kg BW given 6, 18, and 24 hours later (Clubb 1986).

Leucocytozoon spp. occur only in birds and most are nonpathogenic. *Leucocytozoon smithi* of turkeys, *Leu. simondi* of ducks and geese, and *Leu. caulleryi* of chickens are the most important and pathogenic species. Anemia and enlargement of the liver and spleen are the clinical signs associated with these pathogenic species. *Leucocytozoon simondi* occurs in North America, Europe, and parts of Asia, and *Leu. smithi* occurs in the United States. *Leucocytozoon caulleryi* occurs mainly in southern and eastern Asia. Pyrimethamine (1 ppm) combined with sulfadimethoxine (10 ppm) will prevent but not cure *Leu. caulleryi* infections. Clopidol is approved for the prevention of *Leu. smithi* infections when fed at its anticoccidial levels (0.0125–0.0250%).

Haemoproteus spp. are usually nonpathogenic. Treatment of *Haemoproteus* infections in most birds is not justified because of the minor impact on health.

Canine Hepatozoonosis. *Hepatozoon canis* is a normally nonpathogenic species found in dogs in many regions of the world, including Asia, Africa, southern Europe, the Middle East, Japan, Malaysia, and the Philippines. Diagnosis is made by demonstrating stages in infected leukocytes. Its primary vector is *Rhipicephalus sanquineous,* the brown dog tick. Dogs eat the tick and become infected.

Hepatozoon americum causes canine hepatozoonosis in the Americas (Vincent-Johnson et al. 1997). In the southern United States, *H. americanum* infections are being identified more frequently (Macintire et al. 1997). It is transmitted by *Amblyoma maculatum,* the Gulf Coast tick (Mathew et al. 1998). Clinical signs include fever, stiffness, gait abnormalities, marked lethargy, weight loss, and mucopurulent ocular discharge. A marked leukocytosis is present but no or few gamont stages are present in the blood. Asexual stages are present in muscle tissues, and a pyogranulomatous myositis develops. Periostial bone growth can often be documented on radiographs. Diagnosis is made by demonstrating stages in muscle biopsy or occasionally demonstrating gamonts in blood smears. Relapse is common and most untreated cases are fatal. Toltrazuril given orally at 5 mg/kg BW every 12 hours for 5 days and toltrazuril given orally at 10 mg/kg BW every 12 hours for 10 days caused remission of clinical signs in naturally infected dogs in 2–3 days (Macintire et al. 2000). Unfortunately, most treated dogs relapsed and eventually died from hepatozoonosis. The response of *H. americanum*–infected dogs to treatment with a combination of trimethoprim plus sulfadiazine (orally 15 mg/kg BW every 12 hours) plus clindamycin (orally 10 mg/kg BW every 8 hours) plus pyrimethamine (orally 0.25 mg/kg BW daily) (TCP therapy) for 14 days demonstrated that remission of clinical signs in naturally infected dogs occurred in 2–3 days, but most treated dogs relapsed and eventually died from hepatozoonosis (Macintire et al. 2000). The best results have been seen in dogs that have undergone TCP therapy and then been placed on a daily oral treatment program with 10–20 mg/kg BW decoquinate. The decoquinate treatment must be continued because once it is stopped, relapse and clinical disease occur (Macintire et al. 2000). Dogs have tolerated this treatment and survived for over 18 months.

SUBCLASS PIROPLASMASINA: THE PIROPLASMS. Piroplasms are tick-transmitted protozoans that include the genera *Babesia, Theileria,* and *Cytauxzoon.* Asexual multiplication occurs in the vertebrate host's blood cells (*Babesia*) and host's lymphoid cells and blood cells (*Theileria* and *Cytauxzoon*). Sexual stages and sporulation occur in the tick host. Animals become infected when the tick feeds and injects sporozoites. Tick control programs and vaccination are used in conjunction with chemotherapy to prevent and treat animal infections.

Babesiosis. Clinical signs associated with babesiosis are hemolytic anemia, anorexia, jaundice, fever, central nervous system signs, and hemoglobinuria. Death may result from infection with some of the highly pathogenic species. Babesiosis has the greatest economic impact on cattle and is one of the most important diseases of tropical and subtropical regions, where approximately 600 million cattle are at risk of infection. *Babesia bigemina, Bab. bovis,* and *Bab. divergens* are the causative agents of bovine babesiosis. Bovine babesiosis has been eradicated from the United States.

Equine babesiosis is caused by *Bab. equi* and *Bab. caballi* and is widely distributed throughout the Tropics and, less frequently, the Subtropics. The movements of infected horses are restricted; carrier horses must be cleared of infection before being imported into areas free of the disease.

Canine babesiosis is caused primarily by *Bab. canis* and is transmitted by *Rhipicephalus sanguineous* in the United States. *Babesia gibsoni* has recently been documented in dogs in the United States and is much harder to treat.

Babesia felis and *Bab. herpailuri* cause babesiosis in cats in South Africa.

Babesia infection in wild ruminants is common but its significance is unknown.

Several drugs are used to treat *Babesia* infections and most are potentially toxic for the host. Treatment of species having large piroplasms is generally more successful than treatment of species that have small piroplasms. Treated animals may become carriers. Agent selection and treatment dosage are influenced by the objectives of treatment: relief of clinical signs, elimination of infection, or prevention of infection.

DIAMIDINE DERIVATIVES. Diamidine derivatives are either aromatic (diminazene diaceturate, pentamidine isethionate, phenamidine isethionate) or carbanilide (amicarbalide, imidocarb dipropionate) (Table 49.10). These diamidine derivatives bind to DNA and interfere with parasite replication (Pilch et al. 1995; Patrick et al. 1997).

Most bovine and equine *Babesia* infections can be treated with diminazene diaceturate (Berenil, Ganaseg) at 3–5 mg/kg BW IM, but 6–12 mg/kg BW is required for *Bab. equi* in horses. As little as 0.5 mg/kg BW can be effective against *Bab. bigemina.* Diminazene at 5.0 mg/kg BW will eliminate *Bab. caballi* from horses if given twice during a 24-hour period (Kuttler 1988). A single 3.5 mg/kg BW SC treatment with diminazene is effective against canine babesiosis caused by *Bab. canis,* but 7 mg/kg BW is required for *Bab. gibsoni.* Higher doses may potentially produce central nervous system signs. Diminazene is not effective against *Bab. felis* but is effective against *Bab. herpailuri* in cats.

Pentamidine isethionate (Lomidine, Pentam 300) is useful in programs that are attempting to produce immunity in cattle by abbreviating infections. When given SC during the acute phase at 0.5–2 mg/kg BW, pentamidine usually produces a clinical cure, but as much as 5 mg/kg BW will not completely eradicate the parasite from cattle. Pentamidine is effective against canine babesiosis when given IM at 16.5 mg/kg BW on 2 consecutive days but may cause adverse reactions, including pain at the injection site, hypotension, tachycardia, and vomiting.

Bovine and equine *Babesia* infections are treated IM with 8–13 mg/kg BW phenamidine isethionate (Lomadine). Phenamidine at 8.8 mg/kg BW will eliminate *Bab. caballi* from horses if given twice during a 24-hour period (Kuttler 1988). Phenamidine isethionate given IM at 10 and 5 mg/kg BW, 3 days apart, is effective against canine babesiosis caused by *Bab. gibsoni;* a single dose of 8–13 mg/kg is effective against *Bab. canis.*

Amicarbalide (Diampron) is effective against bovine babesiosis when given IM at 5–10 mg/kg BW. Amicarbalide at 8.8 mg/kg BW will eliminate *Bab. caballi* from horses if given twice during a 24-hour period but will not eliminate *Bab. equi* when used at levels of 22 mg/kg BW, which approaches toxic levels (Kuttler 1988).

Imidocarb (Imizol) is effective against bovine babesiosis when given at 1–3 mg/kg BW IM or SC.

TABLE 49.10—Diamidine derivatives

Name	Chemical name (Empirical formula) [Molecular weight]	Chemical structure
Amicarbalide	3,3′-(Carbonyldiimino)*bis*-benzene-carboximidamide $(C_{15}H_{16}N_6O)$ [296.34]	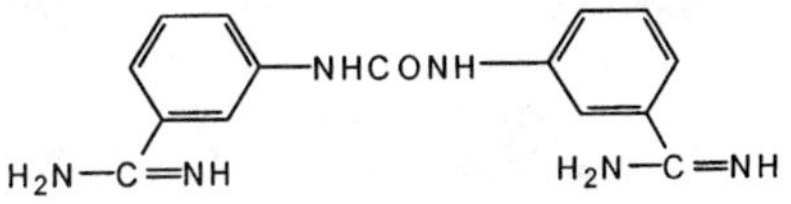 NHCONH; $H_2N-C=NH$; $H_2N-C=NH$
Diminazene	*N*-acetylglycine compounded with 4,4′-(1-triazene-1,3-diyl) *bis*-(benzenecarboximidamide) $(C_{22}H_{29}N_9O_6)$ [515.54]	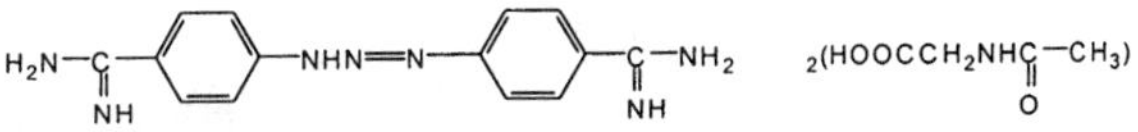 $H_2N-C(=NH)-$; NHN=N; $-C(=NH)-NH_2$; $2(HOOCCH_2NHC(=O)-CH_3)$
Imidocarb	3,3′-di-2-imidazolin-2-yl-carbanilide $(C_{19}H_{20}N_6O)$ [348.41]	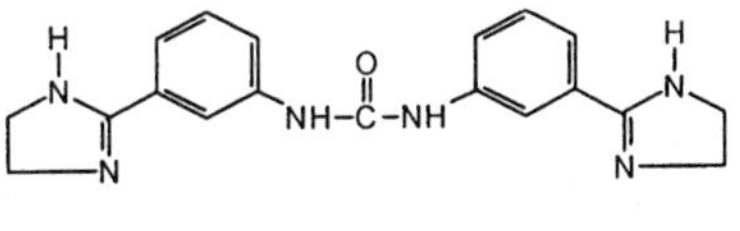 H, N, N; NH-C(=O)-NH; H, N, N
Pentamidine	4,4′-[1,5-pentanediylbis(oxy)]*bis*-benzenecarboximidamide $(C_{19}H_{24}N_4O_2)$ [340.43]	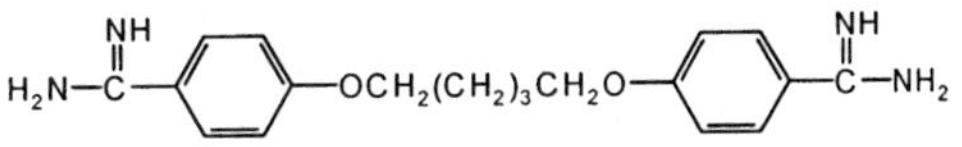 $H_2N-C(=NH)-$; $OCH_2(CH_2)_3CH_2O$; $-C(=NH)-NH_2$
Phenamidine	4,4′-oxybisbenzenecarboximidamide $(C_{14}H_{14}N_4O)$ [254.29]	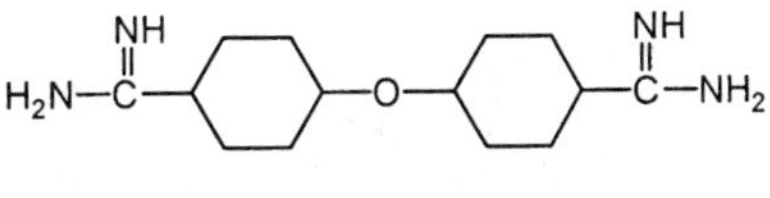 $H_2N-C(=NH)-$; O; $-C(=NH)-NH_2$

Imidocarb given at 1–2 mg/kg BW will eliminate *Bab. caballi* from horses if given twice during a 24-hour period (Kuttler 1988). A single 7.5 mg/kg BW SC imidocarb treatment will completely clear *Bab. canis* infections in dogs (Penzhorn et al. 1995). Feline babesiosis is refractory to treatment with imidocarb.

A single dose of 3.5 mg/kg BW SC diminazene, followed the next day by a single dose of 7.5 mg/kg BW SC imidocarb, will completely clear *Bab. canis* infections in dogs (Penzhorn et al. 1995).

TETRACYCLINES. A long-acting formulation of oxytetracycline (LA/200) is useful in prophylaxis of bovine *Bab. divergens* infection if 20 mg/kg BW is given IM every 4 days for 3 weeks after exposure; 15–10 mg/kg BW given IM every 4 days causes moderation in the clinical signs (Kuttler 1988). Chlortetracycline may be effective against *Bab. equi* infection in horses if 0.5–2.6 mg/kg BW is given IV daily for 6 days early in the infection (Kuttler 1988). Doxycycline is effective at preventing clinical *Bab. canis* infections in dogs if given at 10 mg/kg BW twice daily for 11 days (Vercammen et al. 1996).

Theileriosis. Theileriosis is a severe disease of cattle in Africa and is caused by *Theileria parva.* Several *Theileria* spp. infect wild ruminants in the United States, but none of these causes serious illness.

Parvaquone (Clexon) (Table 49.4) is given IM at 20 mg/kg BW for a single treatment and is curative for *Theileria* infections in cattle. It acts on the macroschizonts and intraerythrocytic piroplasms.

Buparvaquone (Butalex) (Table 49.4) is given IM at 2.5 mg/kg BW for 1–2 treatments and is curative for *Theileria* infections in cattle. It acts on the macroschizonts and intraerythrocytic piroplasms.

Halofuginone is given orally at 1–2 mg/kg BW for a single treatment and is curative for *Theileria* infections in cattle. At 2 mg/kg BW transient diarrhea may occur.

Tetracyclines can also be used to treat *Theileria* infections in cattle but are less effective and must be given in large doses early in the infection and used for longer periods of treatment.

Cytauxzoonosis. *Cytauxzoon felis* infections in cats are treated with parvaquone IM or SC at 10–30 mg/kg BW daily for 2–3 days (Kier 1990). However, only 2 of 18 treated cats survived, indicating that *C. felis* is less sensitive to this agent than are the cattle *Theileria* spp.

Buparvaquone is not effective against *C. felis* in cats when given IM or SC at 10 mg/kg BW daily for 2–3 days (Kier 1990).

PHYLUM CILIOPHORA: THE CILIATES

CILIATES OF MAMMALS. Ciliates move by means of cilia. Ciliates of mammals are generally commensal and cause little harm. They reproduce asexually by transverse binary fission, and most form cyst stages. *Balantidium coli* rarely causes GI disease in human beings, nonhuman primates, pigs, and dogs. Metronidazole and tetracycline are active against *Bal. coli. Balantidium coli* infections in human beings are treated orally with 500 mg tetracycline 4 times a day for 10 days.

CILIATES OF FISH. Ciliates are the most important parasites of farm-raised fish and include the well-known *Ichthyopthirius multifiliis,* the causative agent of "Ich" or "white spot" disease. Other important ciliates include *Ambiphrya* spp., *Chilodonella* spp., *Trichodina* spp., and *Trichophyra* spp. These protozoans infect the gills and skin and cause respiratory problems. The agents used to treat fish protozoans are limited because of the lack of approval. Formalin (Formalin-F, Paracide-F) is approved for use in commercially reared food-fish. Water conditions and chemistry as well as host species are important considerations. Copper sulfate can be toxic in acidic water.

Formalin, dyes (malachite green, methylene blue), and salts are used in the treatment of *Ichthyopthirius* infections, and many of these treatments are designed to kill stages in the environment (tomites) and do not directly kill intradermal or intralamellar stages (trophozoites). The external mucus layer of the fish makes penetration of these agents difficult. Treatment regimes that are effective for *Ichthyopthirius* are also effective for other ciliates and many flagellates ectoparasitic on fish. Formalin is used at 200 mg/L in a bath for 1 hour or at 20 mg/L for 5 days. Malachite green is used at 1.5 mg/L in a bath for 6–24 hours. Methylene blue is used at 1–3 mg/L in a bath for 3 days. Potassium permanganate is used at 4 mg/L in a bath for 30–60 minutes. Sodium chloride is used at 30,000 mg/L in a bath for 1 hour for 7 days.

PHYLUM MICROSPORA

The phylum Microspora is made up of a group of obligatorily intracellular spore-producing parasites that have a direct life cycle. They are important pathogens of insects and cultured fish but are of little importance in veterinary medicine. *Encephalitozoon cuniculi* occasionally causes central nervous system and renal lesions in laboratory rabbits. It can cause central nervous system disease in young dogs. Several new species of this phylum have been recognized as causes of ocular, pulmonary, biliary, intestinal, and muscular disease in human beings that have AIDS. Albendazole given at 400 mg twice daily for 3 weeks has been shown to clear *Enceph. intestinalis* infections in human AIDS patients (Molina et al. 1998).

REFERENCES

Barr, S. C. 1990. American trypanosomiasis, In C. E. Greene, ed., Infectious Diseases of the Dog and Cat, pp. 763–768. Philadelphia: W. B. Saunders.

Barr, S. C., Bowman, D. D., Heller, R. L., and Erb, H. N. 1993. Efficacy of albendazole against giardiasis in dogs. Am J Vet Res 54:926–927.

Barr, S. C., Jamrosz, G. F., Hornbuckle, W. E., Bowman, D. D., and Fayer, R. 1994. Use of paromomycin for treatment of cryptosporidiosis in a cat. J Am Vet Med Assoc 205:1742–1743.

Barr, S. C., Bowman, D. D., Frongillo, M. F., and Joseph, S. L. 1998. Efficacy of a drug combination of praziquantel, pyrantel pamoate, and febantel against giardiasis in dogs. Am J Vet Res 59:1134–1136.

Belloli, S. C., Ceci, L., Carli, S., Montesissa, C., de Natale, G., Marcotrigiano, G., and Ormas, P. 1995. Disposition of antimony and aminosidine in dogs after administration separately and together: implications for therapy of leishmaniasis. Res Vet Sci 58:123–127.

Belloli, S. C., Grescenzo, G., Carli, S., Villa, R., Sonzogni, O., Carelli, G., and Ormas, P. 1996. Pharmacokinetics and dosing regimen of aminosidine in the dog. Vet Res Com 20:533–541.

Blagburn, B. L., and Soave, R. 1997. Prophylaxis and chemotherapy: human and animal. In R. Fayer, ed., Cryptosporidium and Cryptosporidiosis, pp. 111–128. Boca Raton, Fla.

Chapman, H. D. 1997. Biochemical, genetic and applied aspects of drug resistance in *Eimeria* parasites of the fowl. Avian Pathol 26:221–244.

Clubb, S. L. 1986. Therapeutics. In G. J. Harrison and L. R. Harrison, eds., Clinical Avian Medicine and Surgery, pp. 327–355. Philadelphia: W. B. Saunders.

Conway, D. P., Johnson, J. K., Guyonnet, V., Long, P. L., and Smothers, C. D. 1993. Efficacy of semduramicin and salinomycin against different stages of *Eimeria tenella* and *E. acervulina* in the chicken. Vet Parasitol 45:215–229.

Driesen, S. J., Fahy, V. A., and Carland, P. G. 1995. The use of toltrazuril for the prevention of coccidiosis in piglets. Aust Vet J 72:139–141.

Dubey, J. P., and Lindsay, D. S. 1996. A review of *Neospora caninum* and neosporosis. Vet Parasitol 67:1–59.

———. 1998. Isolation of *Sarcocystis neurona* from opossum (*Didelphis virginiana*) faeces in immunodeficient mice and its differentiation from *Sarcocystis falcatula.* Int J Parasitol 29:1823–1828.

Dubey, J. P., Davis, S. W., Speer, C. A., Bowman, D. D., de Lahunta, A., Granstrom, G. E., Topper, M. J., Hamir, A. N., Cummings, J. F., and Suter, M. M. 1991. *Sarcocystis neurona* n. sp. (Protozoa: Apicomplexa): the etiological agent of equine protozoal myeloencephalitis. J Parasitol 77:212–218.

Dubey, J. P., Dorough, K. R., Jenkins, M. C., Liddell, S., Speer, C. A., Kwok, O. C. H., and Shen, S. K. 1998. Canine neosporosis: clinical signs, diagnosis, treatment and isolation of *Neospora caninum* in mice and cell cultures. Int J Parasitol 28:1293–1304.

Fayer, R., and Ellis, W. 1993. Paromomycin is effective as prophylaxis for cryptosporidiosis in dairy calves. J Parasitol 79:771–774.

Fayer, R., Speer, C. A., and Dubey, J. P. 1997. The general biology of *Cryptosporidium.* In R. Fayer, ed., Cryptosporidium and Cryptosporidiosis, pp. 1–29. Boca Raton, Fla.

Fenger, C. K., Granstrom, D. E., Langemeier, J. L., and Stamper, S. 1997. Epizootic of equine protozoal myeloencephalitis on a farm. J Am Vet Med Assoc 210:923–927.

Fichera, M. E., and Roos, D. S. 1997. A plastid organelle as a drug target in apicomplexan parasites. Nature 390:407–409.

Finch, R. G., and Snyder, I. S. 1986. Antiprotozoan drugs. In C. R. Craig and R. E. Stitzel, eds., Modern Pharmacology, 2nd ed., pp. 729–740. Boston: Little, Brown.

Finegold, S. M., and Mathisen, G. E. 1990. Metronidazole. In G. L. Mandell, R. G. Douglas, and J. E. Bennett, eds., Principles and Practice of Infectious Diseases, 3rd ed., pp. 303–308. New York: Churchill Livingstone.

Fourmy, D., Yoshizawa, S., and Puglis, J. D. 1998. Paromomycin binding induces a local conformational change in the A-site of the 16 S rRNA. J Mol Biol 277:333–345.

Granot, I., Halevy, O., Hurwitz, S., and Pines, M. 1993. Halofuginone: an inhibitor of collagen type I synthesis. Biochem Biophys Acta 1156:107–112.

Griffiths, J. K., Balakrishnan, Widmer, G., and Tzipori, S. 1998. Paromomycin and genticin inhibit intracellular *Cryptosporidium parvum* without trafficking through the host cell cytoplasm: implications for drug delivery. Infect Immun 66:3874–3883.

Harari, J., and Lincoln, J. 1989. Pharmacologic features of clindamycin in dogs and cats. J Am Vet Med Assoc 195:124–125.

Jones, J. E., Solis, J., Hughes, B. L., Castaldo, D. J., and Toler, J. E. 1990. Production and egg-quality responses of white leghorn layers to anticoccidial agents. Poult Sci 69:378–387.

Kier, A. B. 1990. Cytauxzoonosis. In C. E. Greene, ed., Infectious Diseases of the Dog and Cat, pp. 792–795. Philadelphia: W. B. Saunders.

Köhler, S., Delwiche, C. F., Denny, P. W., Tilney, L. G., Webster, P., Wilson, R. M. J., Palmer, J. D., and Roos, D. S. 1997. A plastid of probable green algal origin in apicomplexan parasites. Science 275:1485–1489.

Kuttler, K. L. 1988. Chemotherapy of babesiosis. In M. Ristic, ed., Babesiosis of Domestic Animals and Man, pp. 227–243. Boca Raton, Fla.: CRC Press.

Liberator, P., Anderson, J., Feiglin, M., Sardana, M., Griffin, P., Schmatz, D., and Myers, R. W. 1998. Molecular cloning and functional expression of mannitol-1-phosphatase from the apicomplexan parasite *Eimeria tenella.* J Biol Chem 273:4237–4244.

Lindsay, D. S., and Dubey, J. P. 1999. Determination of the activity of pyrimethamine, trimethoprim and sulfonamides and combinations of pyrimethamine and sulfonamides against *Sarcocystis neurona* in cell cultures. Vet Parasitol. 82:205–210.

Lindsay, D. S., Blagburn, B. L., Sundermann, C. A., and Ernest, J. A. 1987. Chemoprophylaxis of cryptosporidiosis in chickens, using halofuginone, salinomycin, lasalocid, or monensin. Am J Vet Res 48:354–355.

Lindsay, D. S., Dubey, J. P., and Blagburn, B. L. 1997a. Biology of *Isospora* spp. from humans, nonhuman primates, and domestic animals. Clin Microbiol Rev 10:19–34.

Lindsay, D. S., Blagburn, B. L., and Dubey, J. P. 1997b. Feline toxoplasmosis and the importance of the *Toxoplasma gondii* oocyst. Comp Cont Ed Pract Vet 19:448–461.

Lindsay, D. S., Larsen, C. T., Zajac, A. M., and Pierson, F. W. 1998. Experimental *Cochlosoma anatis* infections in poultry. Vet Parasitol. 81:21–27.

Long, P. L. 1971. Maternal transfer of anticoccidial drugs in the chicken. J Comp Pathol 81:373–382.

———. 1993. Avian coccidiosis. In J. P. Kreier, ed., Parasitic Protozoa, vol. 4, 2nd ed., pp. 1–88. San Diego: Academic Press.

Long, P. L., Sheridan, K., and McDougald, L. R. 1981. Maternal transfer of some anticoccidial drugs in the chicken. Poult Sci 60:2342–2345.

Longhofer, S. L. 1988. Chemotherapy of rickettsial, protozoal, and chlamydial diseases. Vet Clin N Amer Sm Anim Pract 18:1183–1196.

Looker, D. L., Marr, J. J., and Stotish, R. L. 1986. Modes of action of antiprotozoal agents. In W. L. Campbell and R. S. Rew, eds., Chemotherapy of Parasitic Diseases, pp. 193–207. New York: Plenum Press.

Lucumi, A., Robledo, S., Gama, V., and Saravia, N. G. 1998. Sensitivity of *Leishmania viannia panamensis* to pentavalent antimony is correlated with the formation of cleavable DNA-protein complexes. Antimicrob Agents Chemother 42:1990–1995.

Maarouf, M., de Kouchkovsky, Y., Brown, S., Petit, P. X., and Robert-Gero, M. 1997. In vivo interference of paromomycin with mitochondrial activity of *Leishmania.* Exp Cell Res 232:339–348.

Macintire, D. K., Vincent-Johnson, N., Lindsay, D. S., Kane, C., Blagburn, B. L., and Dillon, A. R. 2000. Treatment of hepatozoonosis in dogs: 54 cases (1989–1998). J Am Vet Med Assoc (in press).

Macintire, D. K., Vincent-Johnson, N., Dillon, A. R., Blagburn, B. L., Lindsay, D. S., Whitley, E. M., Lenz, S. D., Morris, D. C., and Banfield, C. 1997. Canine hepatozoonosis: a retrospective study of 22 naturally occurring cases (1989–1994). J Am Vet Med Assoc 210:916–922.

MacKay, R. L., Davis, S. W., and Dubey, J. P. 1992. Equine protozoal myeloencephalitis. Comp Cont Ed Pract Vet 14:1359–1366.

Mancassola, R., Reperant, J. M., Naciri, M., and Chartier, C. 1995. Chemoprophylaxis of *Cryptosporidium parvum* infection with paromomycin in kids and immunological study. Antimicrob Agents Chemother 39:75–78.

Mathew, J. S., Ewing, S. A., Panciera, R. J., and Woods, J. P. 1998. Experimental transmission of *Hepatozoon americanum* to dogs by the Gulf Coast tick, *Amblyoma americanum* Koch. Vet Parasitol 80:1–14.

Mathis, G. F., and McDougald, L. R. 1981. Experimental development of resistance to amprolium or dinitolmide in *Eimeria acervulina* and its effect on inhibition of sporulation of oocysts. J Parasitol 67:956–957.

McAllister, M. M., Dubey, J. P., Lindsay, J. P., Jolley, W. R., Wills, R. A., and McGuire, A. M. 1998. Dogs are definitive hosts of *Neospora caninum.* Int J Parasitol 28:1473–1478.

McDougald, L. R. 1993. Chemotherapy of coccidiosis. Proc 6th Int Coccid Conf, Guelph, Canada, pp. 45–47.

Meingasser, J. G., Schmook, F. P., Czok, R., and Meith, H. 1979. Enhancement of the anticoccidial activity of polyether antibiotics in chickens by tiamulin. Poult Sci 58:308–313.

Molina, J. M., Chastang, C., Goguel, J., Michiels, J. F., Sarfati, C., Desportes-Livage, I., Horton, J., Derouin, F., and Modai, I. 1998. Albendazole for treatment and prophylaxis of microsporidiosis due to *Encephalitozoon intestinalis* in patients with AIDS: a randomized double-blind control trial. J Infect Dis 177:1373–1377.

O'Handley, R. M., Olsen, M. E., McAllister, T. A., Morck, D. W., Jelinski, M., Royan, G., and Cheng, K. J. 1997. Efficacy of fenbendazole for treatment of giardiasis in calves. Am J Vet Res 58:384–388.

Patrick, D. A., Boykin, D. W., Wilson, D. W., Tanious, F. A., Spychala, J., Bender, B. C., Hall, J. E., Dykstra, C. C., Ohemeng, K. A., and Tidwell, R. R. 1997. Anti-*Pneumocystis carinii* pneumonia activity of dicationic carbazoles. Eur J Med Chem 32:781–783.

Penzhorn, B. L., Lewis, B. D., de Waal, D.T., and Lopez-Rebollar, L. M. 1995. Sterilization of *Babesia canis* infections by imidocarb alone or in combination with diminazene. J S Afr Vet Assoc 66:157–159.

Pfefferkorn, E. R., Borotz, S. E., and Nothnagal, R. F. 1993. Mutants of *Toxoplasma gondii* resistant to atovaquone (566C80) or decoquinate. J Parasitol 79:559–564.

Pilch, D. S., Kirolos, M. A., Liu, X., Plum, G. E., and Breslauer, K. J. 1995. Berenil [1,3-Bis(4′-amidinophenyl)triazene] binding to DNA duplexes and to RNA duplex: evidence for both intercalative and minor grove binding properties. Biochemistry 34:9962–9976.

Ricketts, A. P., Glazer, E. A., Migaki, T. T., and Olson, J.A. 1992. Anticoccidial efficacy of semduramicin in battery studies with laboratory isolates of coccidia. Poult Sci 71:98–103.

Roberts, F., Roberts, C. W., Johnson, J. J., Kyle, D. E., Krell, T., Coggins, J. R., Coombs, G. H., Milhous, W. K., Tzipori, S., Ferguson, D. J. P., Chakrabarti, and McLeod, R. 1998. Evidence for the shikimate pathway in apicomplexan parasites. Nature 393:801–805.

Roos, D. S. 1993. Primary structure of the dihydrofolate reductase-thymidylate synthase gene from *Toxoplasma gondii.* J Biol Chem 268:6269–6280.

Schmatz, D. M. 1997. The mannitol cycle in *Eimeria.* Parasitology 114S:S81–S89.

Slappendel, R. J., and Teske, E. 1997. The effect of intravenous or subcutaneous administration of meglumine antimonate (Glucantime) in dogs with leishmaniasis: a randomized clinical trial. Vet Quart 19:10–13.

Van Reken, D. E., and Pearson, R. D. 1990. Antiparasitic agents. In G. L. Mandell, R. G. Douglas, and J. E. Bennett, eds., Principles and Practice of Infectious Diseases, 3rd ed., pp. 398–427. New York: Churchill Livingstone.

Vercammen, F., De Deken, R., and Maes, L. 1996. Prophylactic treatment of experimental canine (*Babesia canis*) with doxycycline. Vet Parasitol 66:251–255.

Vexenat, J. A., Olliaro, P. L., Castro, J. A. F., Cavalcante, R., Campus, J. H. F., Travares, J. P., and Miles, M. A. 1998. Clinical recovery and limited cure in canine visceral leishmaniasis treated with aminosidine (paromomycin). Am J Trop Med Hyg 58:448–453.

Vincent-Johnson, N. A., Macintire, D. K., Lindsay, D. S., Lenz, S. D., Baneth, B., Shkap, V., and Blagburn, B. L. 1997. A new *Hepatozoon* species from dogs: description of the causative agent of canine hepatozoonosis in North America. J Parasitol 83:1165–1172.

Waller, R. F., Keeling, P. I., Donald, R. G. K., Striepen, B., Handman, E., Lang-Unnasch, N., Cowman, A. F., Besra, G. S., Roos, D. S., and McFadden, G. I. 1998. Nuclear-encoded proteins target to the plastid in *Toxoplasma gondii* and *Plasmodium falciparum.* Proc Natl Acad Sci USA 95:12352–12357.

Webster, L. T. 1990. Drugs used in chemotherapy of protozoal infections: leishmaniasis, trypanosomiasis, and other protozoal infections. In A. G. Gilman, T. W. Rall, A. S. Nies, and P. Taylor, eds., The Pharmacological Basis of Therapeutics, 8th ed., pp. 1008–1017. New York: Pergamon Press.

Williams, R. B. 1997. The mode of action of anticoccidial quinolones (6-decyloxy-4-hydroxyquinoline-3-carboxylates) in chickens. Int J Parasitol 27:101–111.

Xiao, L., Saeed, K., and Herd, R. P. 1996. Efficacy of albendazole and fenbendazole against *Giardia* infection in cattle. Vet Parasitol 61:165–170.

Zajac, A. M., LaBranche, T. P., Donoghue, A. R., and Chu, T. C. 1998. Efficacy of fenbendazole in the treatment of experimental *Giardia* infection in dogs. Am J Vet Res 59:61–63.

Zinner, S. H., and Mayer, K. H. 1990. Sulfonamides and trimethoprim. In G. L. Mandell, R. G. Douglas, and J. E. Bennett, eds., Principles and Practice of Infectious Diseases, 3rd ed., pp. 325–334. New York: Churchill Livingstone.

50 ECTOPARASITICIDES

BYRON L. BLAGBURN AND DAVID S. LINDSAY

Botanicals
- **Pyrethrins and Synthetic Pyrethroids**
- **Rotenone**
- ***d*-Limonene and Linalool**

Chlorinated Hydrocarbons (Organochlorines)
- **Lindane**
- **Methoxychlor**

Organophosphates
- **Chlorpyrifos**
- **Coumaphos**
- **Diazinon**
- **Dichlorvos**
- **Ethion**
- **Famphur**
- **Fenthion**
- **Malathion**
- **Phosmet**
- **Pirimiphos-Methyl**
- **Tetrachlorvinphos**
- **Trichlorfon**

Carbamates
- **Carbaryl**
- **Propoxur**

Formamidines

Miscellaneous Ectoparasiticides
- **Benzyl Benzoate and Lime Sulfur**
- **Insect Growth Regulators and Insect Development Inhibitors**
- **Macrocyclic Lactones**

Synergists and Repellents

Resistance to Ectoparasiticides

Regulation of Ectoparasiticide Approval and Registration in the United States and Canada

Arthropods include a large and diverse group of parasites of domestic animals. Parasitic arthropods of veterinary importance include insects (fleas, lice, flies) and acarines (mites and ticks). Insects not normally considered parasites, such as blister beetles or assassin bugs, also may cause irritation either by inflicting painful bites or by producing toxic substances that irritate the skin or mucosal surfaces of animals exposed to them. Mechanisms of ectoparasite-induced diseases or means by which parasitic arthropods affect animal health include (1) loss of blood, resulting in anemia, (2) physical damage and irritation to skin and hides, (3) allergic reactions to venoms and toxins, (4) decreased resistance to other diseases, (5) reductions in weight gains, milk and egg production, and feed conversion efficiencies in food-producing animals, (6) reduction in reproduction efficiency, and (7) transmission of other disease agents (Loomis 1986).

Impacts of ectoparasitism are also of economic concern to veterinarians, livestock producers, and pet owners. For example, one estimate of annual losses imposed by arthropod pests on livestock, excluding horses, exceeded $3 billion (Drummond et al. 1988). This estimate did not include the costs of control of arthropod pests. Another estimate predicted that losses from arthropod parasites in the beef and dairy cattle production industry, combined with the costs of control, would reach $2 billion (Loomis 1986). In the companion animal arena, control of flea infestations on pet animals and in premises is estimated to cost pet owners in excess of $750 million per year. Given the increases in costs of animal production and veterinary care, today's estimates of ectoparasite impacts and cost to producers and pet owners would certainly exceed those estimates of more than a decade ago.

Chemicals commonly used to control external parasites are known as ectoparasiticides. Chemically, they are a heterogeneous group of agents that act through various mechanisms. Ectoparasiticidal agents are classified on the basis of either their chemistry or their mechanisms of action. The major groups of ectoparasiticides are the plant-derived agents (botanicals), the synthetic pyrethroids, the chlorinated hydrocarbons, the organophosphates, the carbamates, the formamidines, and the miscellaneous compounds comprising the inorganics, the growth regulators and development inhibitors, and macrocyclic lactones (avermectins and milbemycins). Several of the new miscellaneous agents are currently entering the marketplace.

Information presented in this chapter will deal primarily with the chemistry, pharmacology, and toxicology of ectoparasiticides of domestic animals, excluding poultry. It is not the intention of the authors to review the biology of ectoparasites. For those who require a review of common and important arthropod parasites of domestic animals, there are several excellent treatises to which we refer you: Soulsby 1982; Urquhart et al. 1996; Bowman 1999.

BOTANICALS. The botanical ectoparasiticides are derived from the flowers, leaves, stems, or roots of plants. Plant oils or resins have been exploited for many years for their attractant, repellent, or toxic effects on arthropods. Several plant derivatives, such as the pyrethrins, limonene, linalool, and rotenone, have been commercialized as potent ectoparasiticidal or repellent agents. It is conventional practice to group the synthetic pyrethroids with the botanical agents, because their chemistry is based on the constituent esters of natural pyrethrins.

Pyrethrins and Synthetic Pyrethroids. The pyrethrins are a collection of six natural insecticidal esters derived from the flower head of the pyrethrum plant, *Chrysanthemum cinerariaefolium,* or from certain related species. Their excellent knockdown properties and low mammalian toxicity have led to their extensive development and use as ectoparasiticidal agents. Although they remain popular as the active ingredient in numerous commercial formulations, the discovery and synthesis of other classes of agents such as the synthetic pyrethroids, the organophosphates, the carbamates, the phenylpyrazoles, the chloronicotinyls, and avermectins have resulted in the decreased use of pyrethrins.

Synthetic pyrethroids are synthetic analogs of prototype pyrethrin molecules. Pyrethroids retain the knockdown activity of the pyrethrins but are more stable molecules with longer residual activity.

CHEMISTRY. The pyrethrins (pyrethrin I, pyrethrin II, jasmolin I, jasmolin II, cinerin I, and cinerin II) are obtained from extracts and powdered preparations of *C. cinerariaefolium* and closely related plant species (Table 50.1). Purified pyrethrins are viscous, nonpolar liquids, easily decomposed by ultraviolet light, acid, and alkali. Pyrethrins are insoluble in water but are very soluble in kerosene. The acute oral LD_{50} value of pyrethrins in the rat is 200–1500 mg/kg body weight (BW). First-generation pyrethroids (e.g., allethrin) are synthetic esters of chrysanthemic acid. Structural modification of the pyrethroids, including the addition of nitrogen, sulfur, and halogens to the carbon, hydrogen, and oxygen present in the pyrethrin molecule, has led to the development of pyrethroids and pyrethroid analogs (lacking the cyclopropane ring) with excellent stability and potency (Table 50.2). The pyrethrins and pyrethroid insecticides commonly are used with synergists and/or repellents to enhance their activities and effects. Pyrethrins and pyrethroids are used widely in veterinary medicine for control of a broad spectrum of ectoparasitic fleas, lice, ticks, mites, and flies (Tables 50.9–50.13). The chemistry of common pyrethroids and pyrethroid analogs is discussed in more detail below.

MODE OF ACTION. Pyrethrins and pyrethroids exert their effects primarily by modulating gating kinetics of sodium channels in nerves (Hart 1986). This action results in either repetitive discharges or membrane depolarization and subsequent death of the target arthropod. Recent research also indicates that pyrethroid insecticides suppress γ-aminobutyric acid (GABA) and glutamate receptor–channel complexes and voltage-activated Ca^{++} channels (Narahashi 1992)

TABLE 50.1—Botanical compounds

Name	Chemical name (Empirical formula) [Molecular weight]	Chemical structure
Limonene	1-methyl-4-(1-methylethenyl)cyclohexene ($C_{10}H_{16}$) [136.23]	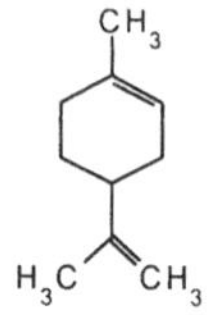 CH_3 … H_3C CH_3
Pyrethrins	Mixture of active constituents: pyrethrins I and II; cinerins I and II; jasmolins I and II	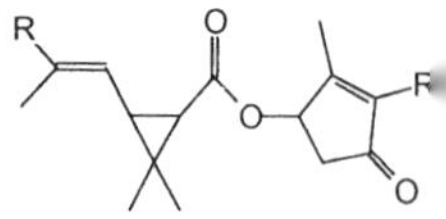 R O O R O
Rotenone	[2*R*-(2α,6aα,12aα)]-1,2,12,12a-tetrahydro-8,9-dimethoxy-2-(1-methylethenyl)-[1]-benzopyrano-[3, 4-b]furo[2,3-h][1]benzopyran-6(6a*H*)-one ($C_{23}H_{22}O_6$) [394.41]	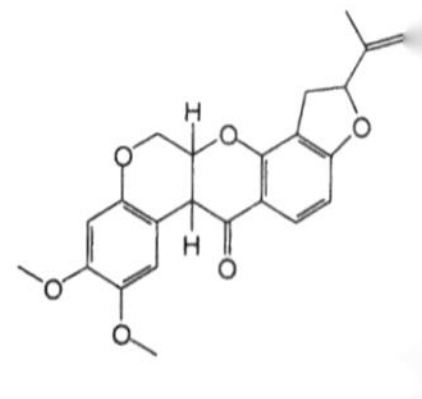 H O O H O O O

TABLE 50.2—Synthetic pyrethroid compounds

Name	Chemical name (Empirical formula) [Molecular weight]	Chemical structure
Allethrin	2,2-dimethyl-3-(2-methyl-1-propenyl)cyclo-propanecarboxylic acid 2-methyl-4-oxo-3-(2-propenyl)-2-cyclopentenl-1-yl ester ($C_{19}H_{26}O_3$) [302.40]	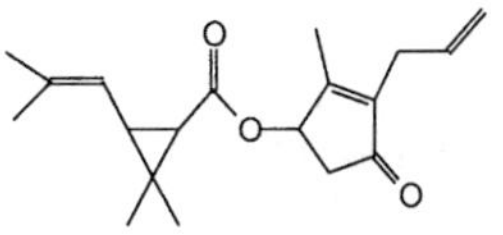
Cyfluthrin	3-(2,2-dichloroethenyl)-2,2-dimethylcyclopropane-carboxylic acid cyanol(4-fluoro-3-phenoxyphenyl)-methyl ester ($C_{22}H_{18}Cl_2FNO_3$) [434.29]	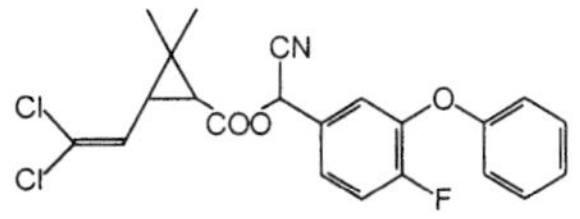
Cyhalothrin	3-(2-chloro-3,3,3-trifluoro-l-propenyl)-2,2-dimethyl-cyclopropanecarboxylic acid cyano(3-phenoxy-phenyl)methyl ester ($C_{23}H_{19}ClF_3NO_3$) [449.86]	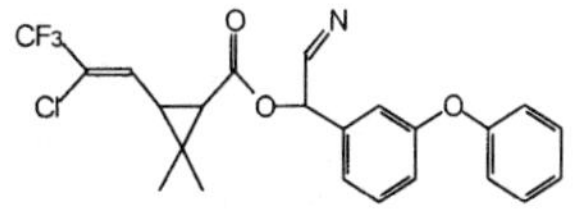
Cypermethrin	3-(2,2-dichloroethenyl)-2,2-dimethylcyclopropane-carboxylic acid cyano(3-phenoxyphenyl)-methyl ester ($C_{22}H_{19}Cl_2NO_3$) [416.30]	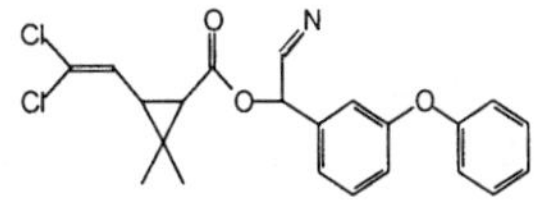
Fenvalerate	4-chloro-α-(l-methylethyl)benzeneacetic acid cyano(3-phenoxyphenyl)methyl ester ($C_{25}H_{22}ClNO_3$) [419.92]	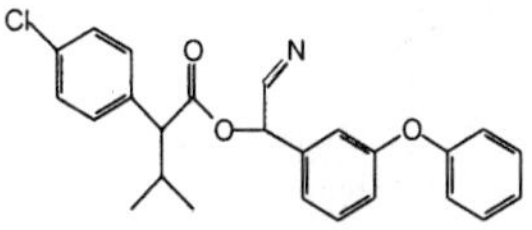
Permethrin	3-(2,2-dichloroethenyl)-2,2-dimethyl-cyclopropane-carboxylic acid (3-phenoxyphenyl)methyl ester ($C_{21}H_{20}Cl_2O_3$) [391.29]	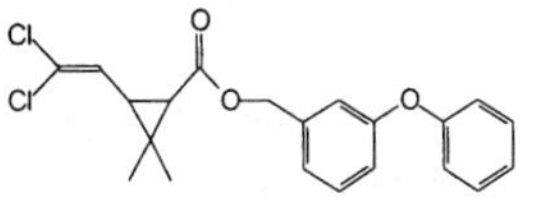
Resmethrin	[5-(phenylmethyl)-3-furanyl]methyl 2,2-dimethyl-3-(2-methyl-l-propenyl)cyclopropanecarboxylate ($C_{22}H_{26}O_3$) [338.40]	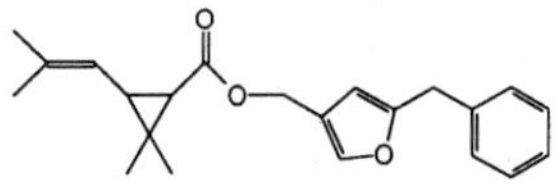

Pyrethroids are classified on the basis of symptoms and neurophysiological effects on target organisms (Gammon et al. 1981). Pyrethroids whose actions result in rapid onset of hyperactivity and repetitive action potentials are type I compounds (e.g., permethrin, resmethrin). Those whose lethal effects are observed at very low doses and with few behavior changes are classified as type II compounds (e.g., fenvalerate, cypermethrin; Hart 1986).

TOXICITY. Pyrethrins and pyrethroids are among the safest of the ectoparasiticides. The selectivity ratio of the pyrethrins and pyrethroids, which compares their toxicity in mammals to their toxicity in insects, generally exceeds 1000 (Table 50.14). In contrast, agents such as the organochlorines, organophosphates, and carbamates have selectivity ratios of 100 or less.

Mechanisms of toxicity of pyrethrins and pyrethroids in mammals are similar to those described for insects. As a result, clinical signs of pyrethrin and pyrethroid toxicity are exemplary of nerve and muscle disorders (Table 50.15; Valentine 1990). Clinical signs in mildly affected dogs and cats include hypersalivation, vomiting, diarrhea, mild tremors, hyperexcitability, or depression. In severely affected animals, signs include hyperthermia, hypothermia, disorientation, and seizures. The period of onset of clinical signs varies from several to many hours, depending on the agent and route of exposure.

ALLETHRIN. Allethrin is one of several first-generation pyrethroids; another is resmethrin. Allethrin, a mixture of several isomers, is a clear, amber-colored, viscous liquid that is insoluble in water but freely soluble in alcohol. The acute oral LD_{50} value for allethrin in the rat is greater than 900 mg/kg BW. The esters of the natural, dextrorotatory (1*R*)-*trans*-chrysanthemic acid are known as bioallethrins. In shampoos for control of fleas and ticks on dogs, *d-trans* allethrin is the active ingredient.

PERMETHRIN. Permethrin, a third-generation pyrethroid, occurs either as a colorless crystalline powder or as a pale yellow, viscous liquid. It is a mixture of *trans* (60%) and *cis* (40%) isomers. The acute oral LD_{50} value of permethrin in the rat is 3800 mg/kg BW. Permethrin is a widely used pyrethroid. It is an active ingredient in collars, sprays, shampoos, dips, and topical concentrates for control of fleas and ticks on dogs and cats; in sprays, dusts, roll-ons, pour-ons, and ear tags for control of flies, lice, ticks, and mites on cattle; in sprays and pour-ons for control of flies, lice, ticks, and keds on sheep and goats; in sprays, paints, dips, and dusts for control of flies, lice, mites, and ticks in swine; and in sprays, wipes, and dusts for control of flies and ticks on horses. The superior stability of permethrin results in residual activity of up to 28 days for some formulations (MacDonald and Miller 1986).

FENVALERATE. Fenvalerate, a type II pyrethroid, occurs as a clear, yellow, viscous liquid, with an acute oral LD_{50} value of 451 mg/kg BW in the rat. Fenvalerate is the active ingredient in ear tags for control of flies on cattle; in sprays and pour-ons for control of lice and keds on sheep and goats; in sprays and pour-ons for control of lice and mites on swine; and in sprays for control of flies, lice, and ticks on horses.

CYPERMETHRIN. Commercial cypermethrin, a viscous semisolid material, is a mixture of eight different isomers. The acute oral LD_{50} value of cypermethrin in the rat is 250–4123 mg/kg BW. Cypermethrin is combined with chorpyrifos as the active ingredients in ear tags for control of flies and ticks on cattle.

ZETAMETHRIN. Zetamethrin is beta-cypermethrin. Zetamethrin is very similar in structure to cypermethrin. However, its oral LD_{50} (106 mg/kg) is less than that of cypermethrin. Beta-cypermethrin is the active ingredient in ear tags for the control of horn flies, face flies, ticks, and lice on cattle.

RESMETHRIN. Resmethrin is a waxy, white to tan, solid material, with a chrysanthemum-like odor. It is insoluble in water but moderately soluble in kerosene. The safety of resmethrin is evident in its very low mammalian toxicity. The acute oral LD_{50} of resmethrin in the rat is in excess of 4000 mg/kg BW. The activity of resmethrin is not enhanced by synergists. It is the only active ingredient in sprays and shampoos for control of fleas and ticks on dogs and cats.

Λ CYHALOTHRIN. Λ Cyhalothrin is a white, odorless, crystalline solid that is virtually insoluble in water. Its acute oral LD_{50} value in the rat is 50.8–75.3 mg/kg BW. Λ Cyhalothrin is the active ingredient in ear tags for control of flies on cattle.

CYFLUTHRIN. Cyfluthrin is a fluorinated pyrethroid that occurs as a yellow-brown oil. Its acute oral LD_{50} value in the rat is 500–800 mg/kg BW. Cyfluthrin is the active ingredient in ear tags for control of flies and ticks on cattle.

Rotenone. Rotenone is an extract of certain plants of the genus *Derris,* principally *Derris elliptica.* It is also known as derris root, tuba-root, and aker-tuba. The extract is a white, odorless, crystalline material that is insoluble in water but is soluble in many organic solvents. The acute oral LD_{50} value for rotenone in the rat is 132–150 mg/kg BW. It exerts its effects by inhibiting the target ectoparasites' respiratory systems, specifically nicotinamide adenine dinucleotide (NADH) oxidation and subsequent generation of adenosine triphosphate (ATP) (Fukami 1976). Rotenone is more toxic to mammals than either the pyrethrins or the pyrethroids but is still considered safe for use in dogs and cats (MacDonald and Miller 1986). It is prohibitively toxic to swine, fish, and snakes and should not be used on these hosts. Rotenone is an active ingredient in ear drops and dips for control of fleas, ticks, lice, and mites on dogs and cats (Table 50.9). It is sometimes formulated with pyrethrins or synergists to potentiate its ectoparasiticidal activity.

***d*-Limonene and Linalool.** Limonene and linalool are natural insecticidal products found in the volatile oil expressed from the peel of oranges and other citrus fruits. A monoterpene, *d*-limonene is a fast-acting agent, immobilizing insects within minutes of exposure. The vapors of *d*-limonene are toxic to target insects; hence, direct contact with the insect is unnecessary for the agent to exert its effect. *d*-Limonene evaporates completely from treated animals, leaving no residual insecticide on their hair coats. It is a safe insecticide, although toxicoses have been reported in cats following its use (Hooser 1990; Table 50.15). The acute oral LD_{50} value in the rat is greater than 5000 mg/kg BW. *d*-Limonene and linalool are active ingredients in sprays, shampoos, and dips for control of fleas on dogs (Table 50.9).

CHLORINATED HYDROCARBONS (ORGANOCHLORINES). The term "chlorinated hydrocarbon insecticide" connotes to many a sole agent with a history of controversy. That agent of course is dichlorodiphenyltrichloroethane, or DDT. Few can forget Rachel Carson's 1962 book *Silent Spring,* which initiated widespread discussion on the environmental problems associated with its use. In reality, widespread resistance to DDT probably contributed as much to its decline as did its persistence in the environment. At the height of its production, 400,000 tons of DDT were used annually in worldwide pest control programs.

The chlorinated hydrocarbons are divided into four chemical groups: the DDT group, the diene-organochlorine group, the hexachlorocyclohexane

TABLE 50.3—Chlorinated hydrocarbon compounds

Name	Chemical name (Empirical formula) [Molecular weight]	Chemical structure
Lindane	1α,2α,3β,4α,5α,6β-hexachlorocyclohexane ($C_6H_6Cl_6$) [290.85]	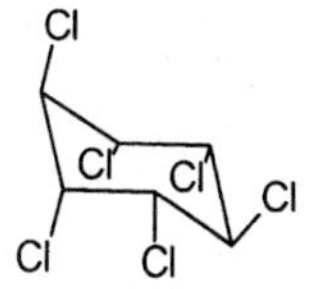
Methoxychlor	1,1′-(2,2,2-trichloroethylidene) *bis*[4-methoxylbenzene] ($C_{16}H_{15}Cl_3O_2$) [345.65]	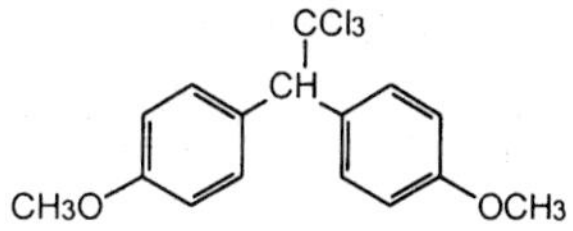

group, and the polychloroterpene group (Brooks 1974). The chlorinated hydrocarbon agents currently in use in veterinary medicine include the hexachlorocyclohexane compound lindane and the DDT analog methoxychlor (Table 50.3). Lindane and methoxychlor do not possess the persistence characteristics of DDT and, as a result, have enjoyed some continued use.

Mechanism of Action. The exact mode of action of methoxychlor and other DDT analogs remains unknown. It is known that the ectoparasite's nervous system is the primary target, and that these agents affect ion channels, most notably sodium ion channels controlled by voltage change (Hart 1986). Research suggests that lindane and cyclodiene agents induce an altered receptor-ionophore complex involving GABA (Ghiasuddin and Matsumura 1982). Studies using cockroach muscle indicate that lindane reduces the GABA-dependent uptake of chloride ions.

Toxicity. Because the chlorinated hydrocarbon agents act on the nervous systems of target organisms, signs of toxicosis in nontarget organisms reflect nervous system dysfunction (Table 50.15). Clinical signs may be immediate in onset or may be delayed for several days. Because the chlorinated hydrocarbons are stored in body fat, signs of toxicosis may be protracted over several days. Procedures for combating chlorinated hydrocarbon toxicosis are outlined in Table 50.15.

Lindane. Lindane (gamma isomer of benzene hexachloride) is the active agent among eight stereoisomers of hexachlorocyclohexane. It is a crystalline powder that is slightly soluble in alcohols, ether, and chloroform. The acute oral LD_{50} value for lindane in the rat is 88–270 mg/kg BW. Because of its lack of persistence in the environment, lindane has remained in use for a longer period of time than other chlorinated hydrocarbon agents. It is the active ingredient in sprays and dips for control of fleas, lice, mites, and ticks on dogs, and in sprays for control of ear ticks and screwworms in cattle, sheep, goats, swine, and horses (Tables 50.9–50.13).

Methoxychlor. Methoxychlor is a dimorphic crystalline powder that is practically insoluble in water but is soluble in most alcohols. The oral LD_{50} value of methoxychlor in the rat is 6000 mg/kg BW. Methoxychlor is an active ingredient in sprays and powders for control of fleas and ticks on dogs, and in sprays and wipes for control of flies on horses (Tables 50.9, 50.13).

ORGANOPHOSPHATES. The organophosphates comprise a large and diverse group of chemicals with insecticidal, acaricidal, and helminthicidal properties (Table 50.4). Some organophosphate compounds also possess herbicidal or fungicidal properties. Organophosphates were at one time the dominant class of insecticides in use, with annual production exceeding 100 million pounds (Chambers 1992). Although they remain an essential component of our pesticidal armamentarium, their use has declined due to the introduction of newer compounds.

Chemistry. Most organophosphate compounds are derivatives of phosphoric acid. The true organophosphates are triesters of phosphoric acid, in which all atoms surrounding the phosphorus atom are oxygen (e.g., dichlorvos, tetrachlorvinphos). The more numerous sulfur-containing organophosphates contain either one sulfur and three oxygen atoms bound to phosphorus (phosphorothioates) or two sulfur and two oxygen atoms bound to the central phosphorus atom (phosphorodithioates). Examples of sulfur-containing organophosphates are chlorpyrifos, coumaphos, diazinon, famphur, fenthion, malathion, and phosmet.

Mechanism of Action. Organophosphates act principally by binding to and inhibiting acetylcholinesterase (AChE), an enzyme widely distributed in nerves, muscles, and fluid and formed elements of blood. Its

Table 50.4—Organophosphate compounds

Name	Chemical name (Empirical formula) [Molecular weight]	Chemical structure
Chlorfenvinphos	phosphoric acid 2-chloro-1-(2,4-dichlorophenyl)-ethenyl diethyl ester ($C_{12}H_{14}Cl_3O_4P$) [359.56]	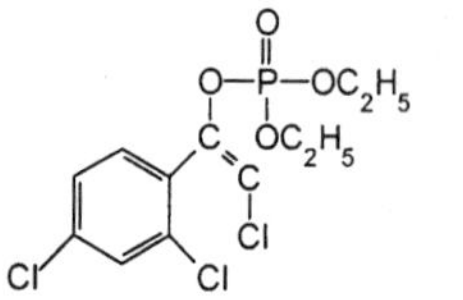
Chlorpyrifos	phosphorothioic acid O,O-diethyl O-(3,5,6-trichloro-2-pyridinyl) ester ($C_9H_{11}Cl_3NO_3PS$) [350.57]	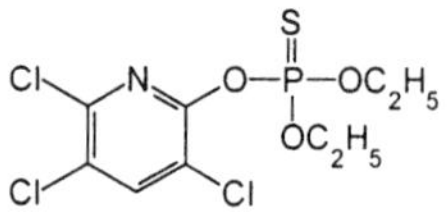
Coumaphos	phosphorothioic acid O-(3-chloro-4-methyl-2-oxo-2*H*-1-benopyran-7-yl) O,O-diethyl ester ($C_{14}H_{16}ClO_5PS$) [362.78]	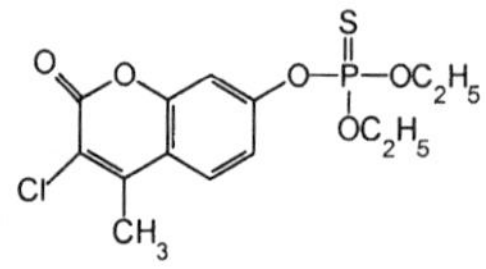
Diazinon	phosphorothioic acid O,O-diethyl O-[6-methyl-2-(1-methylethyl)-4-pyrimidinyl] ester ($C_{12}H_{21}N_2O_3PS$) [304.36]	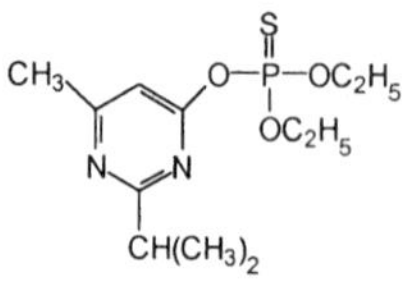
Dichlorvos	phosphoric acid 2,2-dichloroethenyl dimethyl ester ($C_4H_7Cl_2O_4P$) [220.98]	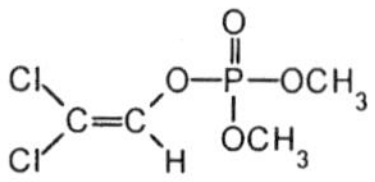
Ethion	O,O,O,O-tetraethyl S,S-methylene bisphosphorodithioate ($C_9H_{22}O_4P_2S_4$) [384.48]	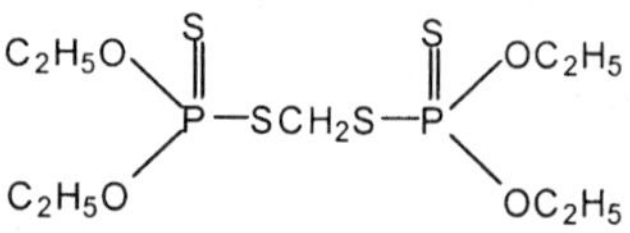
Famphur	phosphorothioic acid O-[4-[(dimethyl-amino)-sulfonyl] phenyl] O,O-dimethyl ester ($C_{10}H_{16}NO_5PS_2$) [325.36]	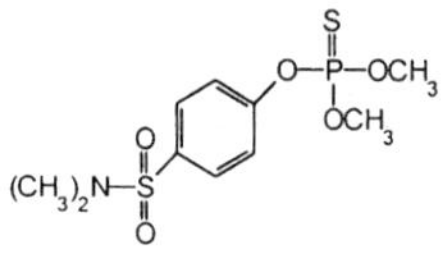
Fenthion	phosphorothioic acid O,O-dimethyl O-[3-methyl-4-(methylthio)phenyl] ester ($C_{10}H_{15}O_3PS_2$) [278.34]	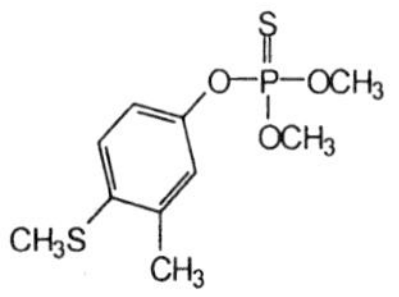
Malathion	[(dimethoxy phosphinothioyl)thio] butanedioic acid diethyl ester ($C_{10}H_{19}O_6PS_2$) [330.36]	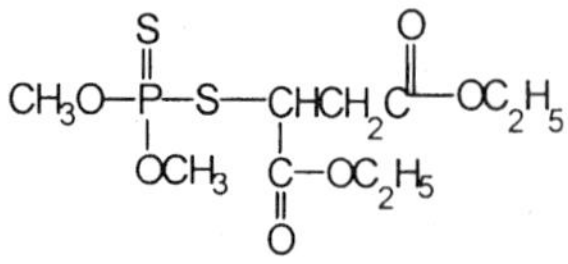

(continued)

TABLE 50.4—(continued)

Name	Chemical name (Empirical formula) [Molecular weight]	Chemical structure
Phosmet	phosphorodithioic acid S-[(1,3-dihydro-1,3-dioxo-2H-isoindol-2-yl)methyl] O,O-dimethyl ester ($C_{11}H_{12}NO_4PS_2$) [317.32]	N–CH$_2$–S–P(=S)–OCH$_3$, OCH$_3$
Primiphos	O-[2-(diethylamino)-6-methyl-4-pyrimidinyl]phosphorothioic acid O,O-dimethyl ester ($C_{11}H_{20}N_3O_3PS$) [277.28]	
Tetrachlorvinphos	phosphoric acid 2-chloro-1-(2,4,5-trichlorophenyl)-ethenyl dimethyl ester ($C_{10}H_9Cl_4O_4P$) [365.95]	$(CH_3O)_2P(=O)–O–C(=ClCH)$–; Cl, Cl, Cl
Trichlorfon	(2,2,2-trichloro-1-hydroxyethyl)-phosphonic acid dimethyl ester ($C_4H_8Cl_3O_4P$) [257.48]	$Cl_3C(OH)CH–P(=O)(OCH_3)–OCH_3$

function is to regulate neurotransmission at synapses by destroying the neurotransmitter acetylcholine (ACh). AChE terminates the activity of ACh by hydrolyzing ACh in the synaptic space. Inhibition is achieved because the organophosphate compound mimics the structure of ACh. The binding of AChE and organophosphates results in transphosphorylation of the enzyme. The activity of organophosphate compounds is determined for the most part by the degree of phosphorylation that occurs. Organophosphates are often characterized as irreversible inhibitors of AChE, although this is not entirely correct. Eventually phosphorylated AChE is hydrolyzed, yielding a recovered or reversed enzyme. Organophosphates are also known to react with cholinergic receptors. However, it is their ability to react with AChE that determines their lethality to target and nontarget organisms.

Pharmacokinetics. Systemic concentrations achieved by organophosphates are determined by their rates of absorption and elimination. The rate of absorption is determined principally by the route (oral or topical) by which the agent is administered. Organophosphates undergo metabolism by oxidative and hydrolytic systems (Carrera and Periquet 1991). A variety of enzymes, including mixed-function oxidases, glutathione transferases, and A- and B-esterases, function in their biometabolism (Chambers 1992).

Toxicity. Organophosphate compounds vary widely in their potential toxicities. Toxicosis results primarily from the inhibition of AChE and may be represented by either muscarinic or nicotinic effects (Table 50.15). Clinical signs of toxicosis resulting from accumulation of ACh at cholinergic receptors in the central nervous system (CNS) are also observed. Infrequently, a non-anti-AChE effect, referred to as organophosphate ester–induced delayed neuropathy (OPIDN), is reported (Fikes 1990; Richardson 1992). Onset of OPIDN is generally delayed 7–21 days following exposure, hence the name. Clinical signs, which are usually more severe in young animals, include weakness, ataxia, and proprioceptive deficits, generally affecting the hindlimbs. The condition has been reproduced experimentally in several species, including dogs, cats, rabbits, and guinea pigs (Johnson 1975).

A wasting syndrome, with death often delayed a week or more after exposure, has also been observed (Chambers 1992). Toxicity is attributed to a by-product of compound synthesis that remains in the formulated product. A specific gross or biochemical lesion has not been described.

Several organophosphate compounds possess teratogenic potential. In most instances the teratogenic effects were seen at rates comparable to the maternally toxic dose (Fikes 1990).

Accepted strategies for treatment of toxicosis resulting from the anti-AChE effects of organophosphate insecticides are detailed in Table 50.15.

Chlorpyrifos. Chlorpyrifos is a colorless crystal readily soluble in several organic solvents. It is sparingly soluble in water. The acute oral LD_{50} value in the rat is 135–163 mg/kg BW. Chlorpyrifos is rapidly metabolized in animals. It is an active ingredient in sprays, shampoos, dips, collars, and streakers for control of fleas, ticks, and mites on dogs and cats, as an ear tag (with diazinon) for control of flies, lice, and ticks, and as liquid for control of ear ticks and screwworms on cattle (Tables 50.9–50.10). Chlorpyrifos is also widely used as a premise insecticide.

Coumaphos. Coumaphos is a crystalline powder soluble in organic solvents but practically insoluble in water. It possesses a low toxicity for mammals. The acute oral LD_{50} value of coumaphos in the rat is 90–110 mg/kg BW. Coumaphos is the active ingredient in wettable powders, liquids, and dusts for control of flies, lice, ticks, mites, or grubs on cattle; in liquids and dusts for control of lice on swine; and in liquids for control of flies, lice, ticks, and screwworms on horses (Tables 50.10, 50.12–50.13). Coumaphos is also used as an anthelmintic.

Diazinon. Diazinon is a reddish-brown liquid miscible in several organic solvents. It is slightly soluble in water. The acute oral LD_{50} value of diazinon in the rat is 600 mg/kg (BW). Diazinon is converted to diazoxon in the treated animal's body. Diazinon is the active ingredient in flea and tick collars for dogs and cats, and in ear tags for control of flies on cattle (Tables 50.9–50.10). It is also widely used as a premise ectoparasiticide.

Dichlorvos. Dichlorvos is a colorless to amber-colored liquid. It is miscible with most organic solvents and to a slight extent with water. The acute oral LD_{50} value for dichlorvos in the rat is 50–108 mg/kg BW. Dichlorvos is a potent organophosphate with a high toxicity potential for mammals and birds. It is the active ingredient in flea and tick collars for dog and cats and in sprays for control of flies, lice, mites, ticks, and grubs on cattle (Tables 50.9–50.10). Dichlorvos also has potent anthelmintic properties.

Ethion. Ethion is a liquid aliphatic organophosphorus insecticide. Its oral LD_{50} in rats in 47 mg/kg. Its dermal toxicity is 155 mg/kg. Ethion is only slightly soluble in water but is soluble in numerous organic solvents. Ethion is the active ingredient in ear tags for control of horn flies, face flies, stable flies, lice, and ticks on cattle (Table 50.10).

Famphur. Famphur is a crystalline powder that is slightly soluble in water but freely soluble in chlorinated hydrocarbons. The acute oral LD_{50} value for famphur in the rat is 35 mg/kg BW. Famphur is the active ingredient in liquids for pour-on treatment of grubs and lice on cattle (Table 50.10).

Fenthion. Technical fenthion is a brownish oil; the formulated product is a colorless liquid. It is readily soluble in most organic solvents but is less soluble in water. The acute oral LD_{50} value for fenthion in the rat is 190–315 mg/kg BW. Fenthion is the active ingredient in ear tags and topical solutions for control of lice, flies, and grubs on cattle (Table 50.10).

Malathion. Malathion is an amber-colored liquid, miscible with organic solvents. It is only moderately soluble in petroleum distillates but is minimally soluble in water. Malathion is among the least toxic of organophosphate compounds, with an acute oral LD_{50} value in the rat of 1500 mg/kg BW. It is rapidly degraded in the animal's body. Malathion is the active ingredient in dips for control of fleas, ticks, and mites on dogs and cats; in sprays for control of flies, lice, and ticks on cattle; in sprays for control of flies, ticks, and lice on horses; in sprays for control of lice, keds, and ticks on sheep and goats; and sprays for control of lice and mites on swine (Tables 50.9–50.13). It is also widely used as a premise insecticide.

Phosmet. Phosmet is an off-white, crystalline powder that is soluble in most organic solvents (not aliphatic hydrocarbons) but sparingly soluble in water. The oral LD_{50} value for the rat is 147–316 mg/kg BW. Phosmet is the active ingredient in dips for control of fleas, ticks, and mites on dogs (Table 50.9).

Pirimiphos-Methyl. Pirimiphos is a member of the group of heterocyclic organophosphate compounds. Pirimiphos-methyl is a straw-colored liquid that is miscible with most organic solvents. The ethyl analog of pirimiphos has an oral LD_{50} in rats of 140 mg/kg. Pirimiphos is the active ingredient in ear tags for control of horn flies and face flies on cattle (Table 50.10).

Tetrachlorvinphos. Tetrachlorvinphos is a white, crystalline powder slightly soluble in water and soluble in most organic solvents. Tetrachlorvinphos possesses a low mammalian toxicity, with an acute oral LD_{50} value of 1000 mg/kg BW in the rat. It is the active ingredient in wettable powders, oral premixes, and dusts for control of flies, lice, and ticks on cattle, and in sprays and dusts for control of lice on swine. Tetrachlorvinphos is also combined with methoprene in collars for control of fleas and ticks on dogs (Tables 50.9–50.10, 50.12).

Trichlorfon. Trichlorfon is a white, crystalline powder that is soluble in chloroform and alcohols. It is only moderately soluble in water. The oral LD_{50} value of trichlorfon is 630 mg/kg in the rat. After treatment, trichlorfon is converted to dichlorvos in the animal's body. It is the active ingredient in sprays and dust bags for control of flies, lice, and ticks on cattle (Table 50.10).

CARBAMATES

Chemistry. Early carbamate insecticides were derivatives of dithiocarbamic acid. Continued development led to the synthesis of the substituted-phenyl monomethylcarbamates, several of which possessed excellent insecticidal potential. A major milestone in insecticide chemistry was achieved when the methylcarbamates were successfully synthesized (Kuhr and Dorough 1976). Thousands of methylcarbamate insecticides have been synthesized, although only about a dozen have been developed successfully as commercial agents (Ivie and Rowe 1986).

Mechanism of Action. Carbamates inhibit the action of the enzyme AChE in a manner somewhat different from that of the organophosphates. Carbamates compete for enzyme-active sites utilizing a process known as carbamylation, a reaction that blocks the action of the enzyme without changing it structurally. When the bond joining the carbamate insecticide and AChE is hydrolyzed, the fully active enzyme is released. Carbamate agents are considered slowly reversible inhibitors of AChE (Fikes 1990). This terminology, as discussed above with the organophosphates, is somewhat misleading in that the carbamate agent undergoes hydrolysis during the reaction. True reversible inhibitors are not destroyed during their reactions with target molecules. Regardless of the mechanism of inhibition of AChE, the effects on target organisms and signs of toxicosis in nontarget mammalian hosts are the same.

Toxicity. The nature and severity of carbamate-induced toxicosis are quite variable. Characteristics and severity depend upon the carbamate agent involved, its route of exposure, its affinity for AChE, and its pharmacokinetics in the host. In general, signs of toxicosis and interventional strategies are similar to those discussed for the organophosphates (Table 50.15).

Carbaryl. Carbaryl occurs as a white, crystalline solid material with an extremely low solubility in water (Table 50.5). However, carbaryl is readily solubilized in nonpolar organic solvents. Its acute oral LD_{50} value in the rat is 850 mg/kg BW. It is widely used in products for control of ectoparasites of companion animals. It is the active ingredient in shampoos, sprays, dusts, and ear drops for control of fleas, ticks, mites, and lice on dogs and cats. Carbaryl-containing products also often contain organophosphates, pyrethrins, synergists, or repellents to enhance their activity and effects (Table 50.9).

Propoxur. Propoxur is a white to tan, crystalline solid material (Table 50.5). It is virtually insoluble in water but is readily soluble in polar organic solvents. The acute oral LD_{50} value of propoxur in the rat is 100 mg/kg BW. Propoxur is the active ingredient in flea and tick collars for use on dogs (Table 50.9).

FORMAMIDINES. The formamidines are a novel group of acaricides that exert their effects in part by inhibiting the enzyme monoamine oxidase. Monoamine oxidase is responsible for metabolism of neurotransmitter amines present in the nervous system of susceptible ticks and mites (Atkinson et al. 1974). Treatment with formamidines leads to detachment of blood-feeding arthropods (Stone and Knowles 1974). Amitraz in the only formamidine ectoparasiticide currently used in veterinary medicine. Amitraz (Table 50.6) is a straw-colored, crystalline material, slightly soluble in water but freely soluble in most organic solvents. The acute oral LD_{50} value for amitraz in the rat is 800 mg/kg BW. Amitraz is the active ingredient in dips and collars for control of mites and ticks on dogs (Table 50.9). Toxicosis in dogs following overexposure to liquids (dips) or after consumption of collars has been reported (Table 50.15). Lethargy and transient sedation are the signs most commonly associated with intoxication. Amitraz is also the active ingredient in sprays for control of lice, ticks, and mites on cattle, and in liquids for the control of lice and mites on swine (Tables 50.10, 50.12).

TABLE 50.5—Carbamate compounds

Name	Chemical name (Empirical formula) [Molecular weight]	Chemical structure
Carbaryl	1-naphthalenol methylcarbamate ($C_{12}H_{11}NO_2$) [201.22]	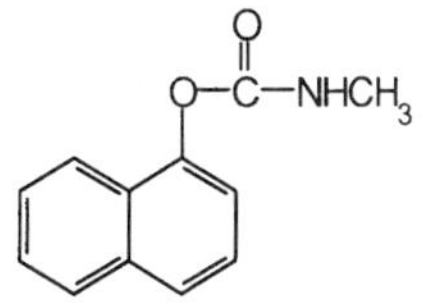 O=C(–NHCH$_3$)–O– on naphthalene ring
Propoxur	2-(1-methylethoxy)phenol methylcarbamate ($C_{11}H_{15}NO_3$) [209.24]	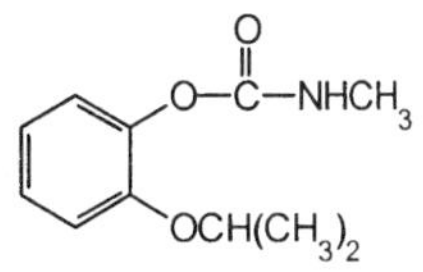 O=C(–NHCH$_3$)–O– and OCH(CH$_3$)$_2$ on benzene ring

TABLE 50.6—Formamidine compound

Name	Chemical name (Empirical formula) [Molecular weight]	Chemical structure
Amitraz	*N*-methyl-*N*′-2,4-xylyl-*N*(*N*-2,4-xylylformimidoyl)-formamidine ($C_{19}H_{23}N_3$) [293.41]	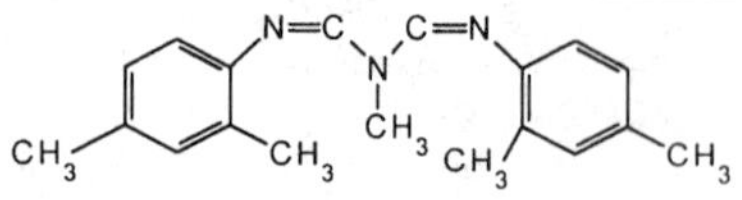

MISCELLANEOUS ECTOPARASITICIDES

Benzyl Benzoate and Lime Sulfur. Early ectoparasiticides consisted of herbals, inorganics, aromatics, petroleum derivatives, and botanical moieties (Ivie and Rowe 1986). All but a few of these agents have been abandoned in favor of more modern synthetic chemicals. However, lime sulfur and benzyl benzoate (benzyl ester of benzoic acid) are still currently used (albeit infrequently) to control canine and feline acariases. Benzyl benzoate lotion is still recommended and used as a spot treatment for demodectic acariasis in dogs (Bowman 1999). Dilute lime sulfur (2–5% in water) remains a reliable scabicide for control of sarcoptiform scabies and cheyletiellosis (MacDonald and Miller 1986; Moriello 1993). The mechanism of action of these agents remains unknown (Hart 1986). Both benzyl benzoate and lime sulfur generally are safe for use on companion animals. However, caution should be exercised when using diluted lime sulfur in dips. Scalding of the skin can result when this agent is administered at inappropriately high concentrations.

Insect Growth Regulators and Insect Development Inhibitors. Ectoparasiticides that exert their effects primarily on the developing stages of insects and other arthropods are becoming increasingly popular as control agents. Such compounds differ from traditional toxicants in several ways. The insect growth regulators (IGRs) and insect development inhibitors (IDIs) have no exploitable adulticidal properties at their commercial use rates. Because they affect preadult stages of insects and acarines, effective control is generally not achieved for several weeks following their use. It is paramount that veterinarians understand the modes of action of these agents if they are to be used knowledgeably and effectively.

IGRs function by mimicking the effects of endogenous insect growth hormone. This hormone, commonly referred to as juvenile hormone, is important in the regulation of insect development and metamorphosis (Williams 1956). Juvenile hormone functions to maintain the larval stage of the insect and thus prevents its subsequent maturation to pupa and adult. Development proceeds only after levels of juvenile hormone in the insect's hemolymph decrease. This decrease is the signal for the organism to continue its development and maturation (Garg and Donahue 1989). IGRs (also known as juvenile hormone analogs or juvenoids), as mimics of juvenile hormone, falsely signal the target organism to remain in its present immature stage. Inability of the insect to molt and develop to subsequent stages results in its death. Examples of IGRs currently in use include methoprene, cyromazine, and piriproxyfen (Table 50.7).

IDIs also target the immature stages of insects but, in contrast to the IGRs, do not mimic the effects of juvenile hormone. Examples of IDIs are the benzoylphenyl urea (BPU) compounds, whose mode of action is interference with development of the insect's exoskeleton by inhibiting chitin synthesis or deposition pathways (Table 50.7; Cohen 1987). Compounds currently in use against animal ectoparasites include diflubenzuron and lufenuron.

METHOPRENE. Methoprene is a terpenoid juvenile hormone mimic with an extremely low toxicity for mammals. An oral dose of up to 34,600 mg/kg BW in the rat did not result in acute toxicosis. The oral LD_{50} in the dog is 5000–10,000 mg/kg BW. Following oral administration, methoprene is metabolized to simple acetates that are incorporated into fatty acids, lactose, and cholesterol (Garg and Donahue 1989). Unmetabolized methoprene is excreted principally in the feces. Methoprene-containing sprays and collars are also available for use on dogs or cats (Table 50.9). It is often combined with adulticidal compounds for premise flea control.

PYRIPROXYFEN. Pyriproxyfen is a white or light yellow solid or a colorless or light yellow liquid. It is stable in most organic solvents. Pyriproxyfen is a juvenoid compound that is structurally unrelated to insect growth hormone. It induces biological effects in target insects that mimic those induced by endogenous insect growth hormone (Palma et al. 1993). It is used to control fleas (*Ctenocephalides felis*) on animals or in their infested environments. Pyriproxyfen possesses potent ovicidal and larvicidal properties at very low concentrations. Pyriproxyfen is not effective against adult fleas at its marketed use rate. Pyriproxyfen is an active ingredient in sprays, liquid concentrates (spot-ons), collars, and stripe-ons for control of fleas in dogs and cats. Pyriproxyfen is combined with permethrin in some formulations. Pyriproxyfen is also the active ingredient in several environmental products.

CYROMAZINE. Cyromazine is a triazine IGR with a mode of action that is likely similar to methoprene and

TABLE 50.7—Miscellaneous compounds

Name	Chemical name (Empirical formula) [Molecular weight]	Chemical structure
Lufenuron (IDI)	*N*-[2,5-dichloro-4-(1,1,2,3,3,3-hexafluoropropoxy)-phenylaminocarbonyl]-2,6-difluorobenzamide ($C_{17}H_8Cl_2F_8N_2O_3$) [511.15]	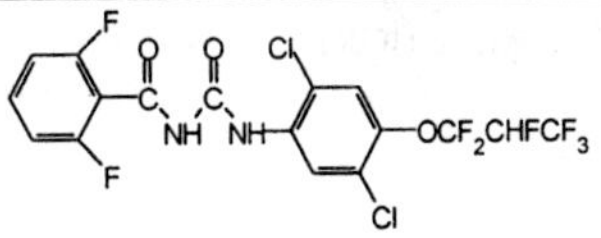
Diflubenzuron (IDI)	*N*-[[(4-chlorophenyl)amino]carbonyl]-2,6-difluoro-benzamide ($C_{14}H_9ClF_2N_2O_2$) [310.68]	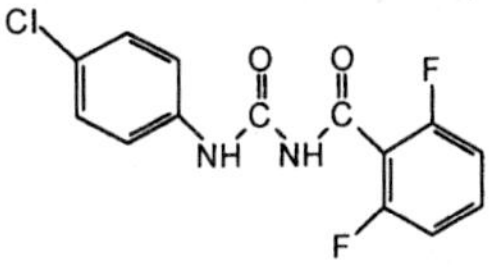
Ivermectin	22,23-dihydroavermectin B_1 ($C_{48}H_{74}O_{14}$) [875.10]	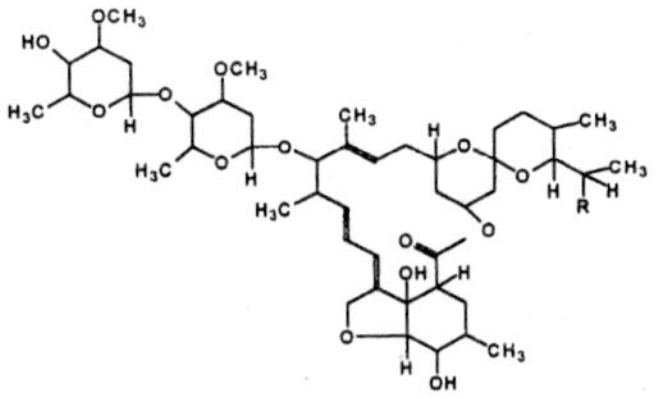 $R=C_2H_5$ B_{1a}; $R=CH_3$ B_{1b}
Milbemycin oxime	5-didehydromilbemycin (oxime derivative) 80% A_4, 20% A_3 ($C_{31}H_{43}NO_7$) A_3 [541.68] ($C_{32}H_{45}NO_7$) A_4 [555.71]	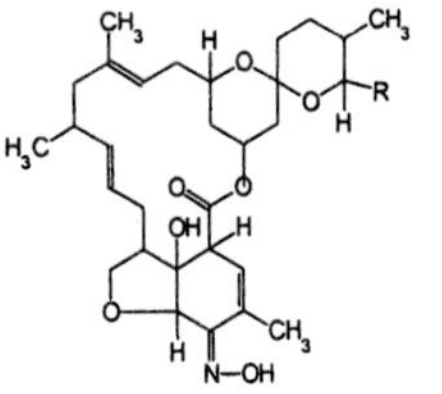 R: CH_3 A_3 oxime; C_2H_5 A_4 oxime
Pyriproxifen (IGR)	2-[1-methyl-2-(4-phenoxyphenoxy)ethox]pyridine ($C_{20}H_{19}NO_3$) [321.37]	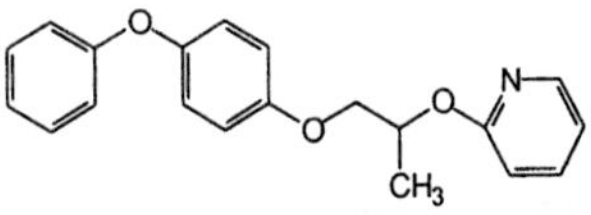
Fipronil	5-amino-1-[2,6-dichloro-4-(trifluoro-methyl)phenyl]-4-[(trifluoromethyl)sulfinyl]-1*H*-pyrazole-3-carbonitrile ($C_{12}H_4Cl_2F_6N_4OS$) [437.15]	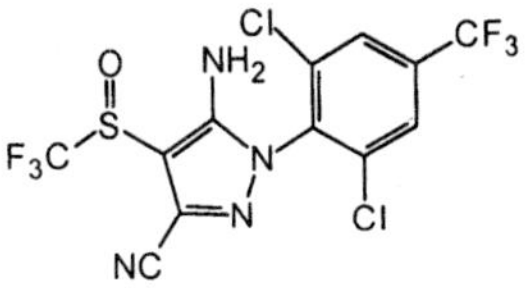
Imidacloprid	1-[(6-chloro-3-pyridinyl)methyl]-4,5-dihydro-*N*-nitro-1*H*-imidazol-2-amine ($C_9H_{10}ClN_5O_2$) [255.66]	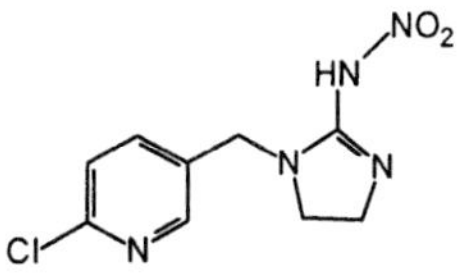

(continued)

TABLE 50.7—(continued)

Name	Chemical name (Empirical formula) [Molecular weight]	Chemical structure
Methoprene (IGR)	11-methoxy-3,7,11-trimethyl-2,4-dodecadienoic acid 1-methylethyl ester ($C_{19}H_{34}O_3$) [310.48]	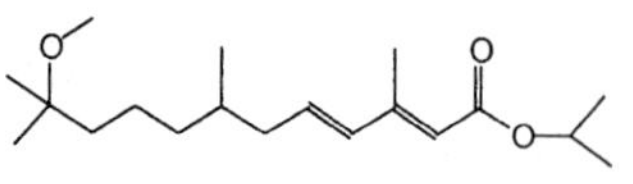
Cyromazine (IGR)	*N*-cyclopropyl-1,3,5-triazine-2,4,6-triamine ($C_6H_{10}N_6$) [166.18]	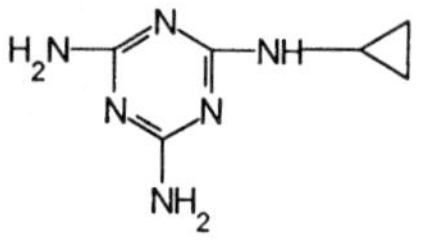
Doramectin	25-cyclohexyl-5-*O*-demethyl-25-de-(1-methylpropyl) avermectin A_{1a} ($C_{50}H_{74}O_{14}$) [899.13]	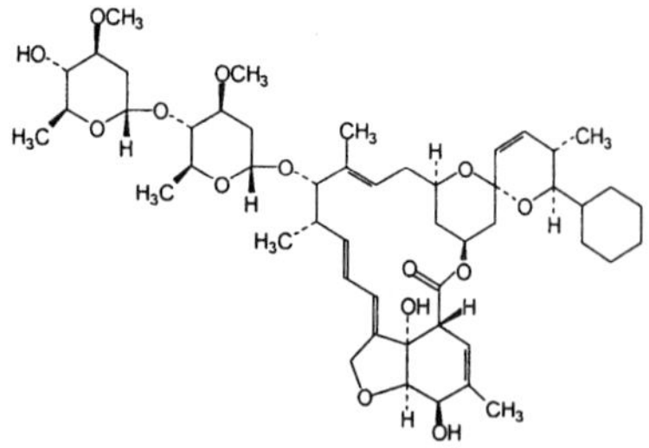
Eprinomectin	(4″R)-4″-epi-(acetylamino)-4″-deoxyavermectin B_1 Component B1a, ($C_{50}H_{75}NO_{14}$) Component B1b, ($C_{49}H_{73}NO_{14}$)	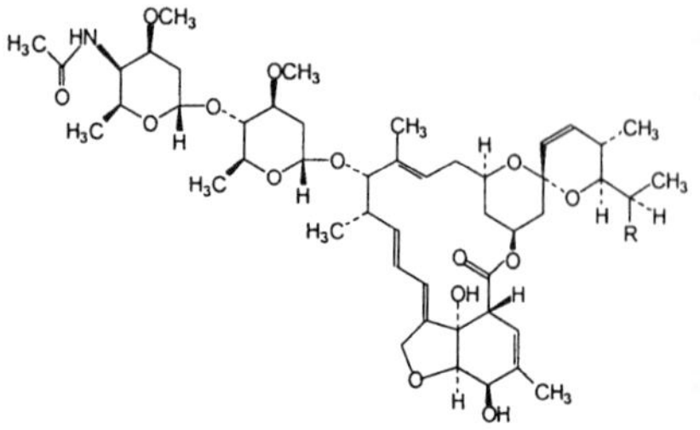 component B_{1a}, R = C_2H_5 component B_{1b}, R = CH_3
Moxidectin	[6*R*,23*E*,25*S*(E)]-5-*O*-demethyl-28-deoxy-25-(1,3-dimethyl-1-butenyl)-6,28-epoxy-23-(methoxyimino) milbemycin B ($C_{37}H_{53}NO_8$) [639.83]	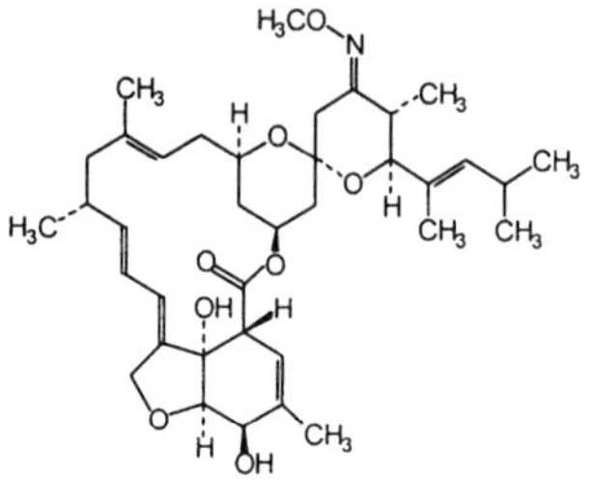
Selamectin	(5Z,25*S*)-25-cyclohexyl-4′-*O*-de(2,6-dideoxy-3-*O*-methyl-*a*-L-*arabino*-hexopyranosyl)-5-demethoxy-25-de(2-methylpropyl)-22,23-dihydro-5-hydroxyiminoavermectin A_{1a} ($C_{43}H_{63}NO_{11}$) [770.00]	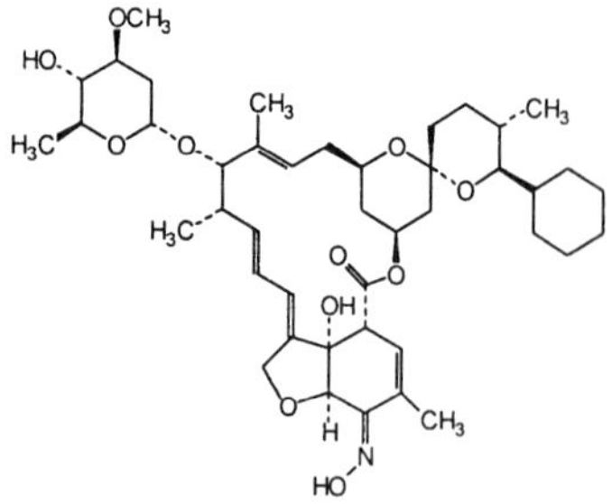
Benzyl benzoate	benzoic acid phenylmethyl ester ($C_{14}H_{12}O_2$) [212.24]	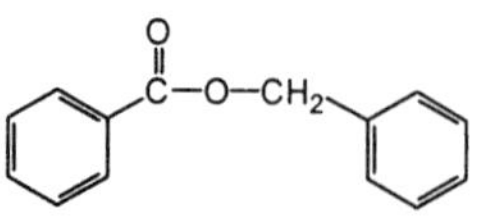

pyriproxyfen. Cyromazine is a white crystalline solid that is soluble in water and methanol but sparingly soluble in most organic solvents. The acute oral LD_{50} value of cyromazine in the rat is 3387 mg/kg BW. Cyromazine is effective against ova and larvae of manure-breeding flies. It is approved and used in the United States for feed-through fly control in poultry.

DIFLUBENZURON AND LUFENURON. Diflubenzuron occurs as odorless crystals that are insoluble in water but moderately soluble in polar organic solvents. Diflubenzuron is safe for use in mammals, as evidenced by its acute oral LD_{50} value of greater than 10,000 mg/kg BW in the rat. The majority (80%) of orally administered drug passes unchanged in the treated animal's feces.

Technical lufenuron occurs as colorless crystals that are insoluble in water but soluble in methanol, acetonitrile, methylene chloride, xylene, and toluene. Lufenuron is a strongly lipophilic compound that accumulates in the adipose tissues of treated animals. The acute oral LD_{50} value for lufenuron in the rat is greater than 2000 mg/kg BW.

Diflubenzuron and lufenuron interfere with development of the target insect's tegument by inhibiting the incorporation of chitin in the exoskeleton. Diflubenzuron is used to control manure-breeding flies in cattle (Table 50.10). Following oral ingestion, active drug passes unchanged in the animal's feces, where it contacts the egg and larval stages of developing flies. Lufenuron is the active ingredient in oral (dog and cat) and injectable formulations (cat only) to control fleas (*Ctenocephalides felis*) when administered at 1-month (dog and cat) or 6-month intervals (cats only) (Table 50.9). Lufenuron is highly lipophilic and, as such, accumulates readily in the target animal's adipose tissues. The release of lufenuron from fat tissues allows maintenance of effective blood levels of drug for weeks after administration (Hink et al. 1991; Zakson et al. 1992; Blagburn et al. 1994; Blagburn et al. 1999). A broad-spectrum combination of lufenuron and milbemycin oxime is also available for use in dogs.

FIPRONIL. Fipronil, a phenylpyrazol compound (Table 50.7), is a relatively new addition to the companion animal ectoparasiticide armamentarium. First developed as a crop protection agent, fipronil is related in mode of action to the avermectins in that it acts as a blocker of GABA-regulated chloride ion channels in nerve cell membranes. Fipronil is a white solid that is only slightly soluble in water (2 mg/L). Fipronil is a safe compound, with an LD_{50} in rats of 100 mg/kg when administered orally. When administered dermally to rats, its LD_{50} is 2000 mg/kg. Fipronil is the active ingredient in spot-ons and sprays for control of fleas and ticks on dogs and cats (Table 50.9). Fipronil's long period of residual activity following topical administration is due to its accumulation in the oils of the skin and hair follicles of treated animals. It is released over a period of time, permitting relatively long intervals between treatments.

IMIDACLOPRID. Imidacloprid, a chloronicotinyl compound, is a member of the nitroguanidine class of insecticides (Table 50.7). It too was first developed as a crop protection insecticide and was later developed for use as a companion animal agent. Imidacloprid inhibits nerve transmission in insects by irreversibly binding to nicotinic acetylcholine receptors on postsynaptic membranes. Imidacloprid is a crystalline solid that is only slightly soluble in water (500 mg/L). Imidacloprid is a safe compound with an oral LD_{50} in rats of approximately 400 mg/kg. Its dermal toxicity exceeds 5000 mg/kg. Imidacloprid is the active ingredient in spot-ons for control of fleas on dogs and cats (Table 50.9). Similar to fipronil, imidacloprid remains in the skin for long periods of time following topical administration.

Macrocyclic Lactones

IVERMECTIN. The avermectins are complex 16-membered lactones, many members of which have potent ectoparasiticidal properties. The best known of the avermectins, ivermectin (Table 50.7), possesses a broad spectrum of activity against many parasitic helminths and arthropods. Details of its chemistry, pharmacology, toxicology, and applications in veterinary medicine are found elsewhere in this textbook (see Chap. 47). We need only comment here that ivermectin is the active ingredient in injectable and oral premix formulations for swine for control of lice and mites; in injectable, pour-on, and sustained-release bolus formulations for cattle for control of grubs, lice, mites, and horn flies; in drench formulations for sheep for control of sheep keds; and in liquid and paste formulations for horses for control of gastric stages of horse botfly larvae (Tables 50.10–50.13).

Results of experimental studies indicate that ivermectin is effective against ear mites (*Otodectes cynotis*) in dogs and cats following subcutaneous injections at dosages of 200, 400, or 666 μg/kg BW (Campbell 1989). Likewise, two subcutaneous injections at 200 μg/kg BW given 14 days apart were completely effective against *Sarcoptes scabiei* in dogs. Ivermectin is also effective against *Demodex canis* in dogs when administered daily at 600 μg/kg BW for up to 210 days (Paradis and Laperriere 1992). A single subcutaneous injection of ivermectin at 1000 μg/kg BW was effective in controlling an outbreak of *Notoedres cati*–induced acariasis in cats (Bigler et al. 1984). Ivermectin also was shown to be effective against *Cheyletiella yasguri* and *Cheyletiella blakei* infestations in dogs and cats (Paradis and Villeneuve 1988; Paradis et al. 1990). The pour-on formulation of ivermectin is reported to aid in the control of one-host ticks on cattle. Efficacies against multihost ticks are too erratic to make definitive efficacy claims (Benz et al. 1989).

MILBEMYCIN OXIME. The milbemycins are 16-membered macrocyclic lactones that are structurally similar to the avermectins. They differ in the absence of the disaccharide substituent at carbon 13 (Table 50.7). The potent ectoparasiticidal properties of the milbemycins were actually discovered before those of the avermectins (Fisher and Mrozik 1989). It was the later discovery of the avermectins' anthelmintic properties that led to their development as parasiticides. The oxime derivative of milbemycin is currently approved and marketed for prevention of heartworm infection and control of major intestinal nematode infections in dogs (see Chap. 47). Little published information is available regarding its efficacies against ectoparasitic arthropods. One therapeutic arena in which milbemycin oxime is receiving considerable attention is in the treatment of recalcitrant generalized demodicosis (Miller and Scott 1991; Kwochka 1993). Data suggest that in cases of amitraz-resistant generalized demodicosis in dogs, daily oral milbemycin oxime therapy can be effective in ameliorating clinical signs and in eradicating mites. Miller and Scott (1991) administered milbemycin oxime daily at 0.5–1.0 mg/kg BW for a minimum of 30 days or until mites could not be demonstrated on repeated skin scrapings. Treatment was then continued for an additional 30 days. In a similar study (Reedy and Garfield 1991), successful treatment was apparently achieved in over 60% of the treatment subjects. On the basis of results obtained thus far, it is likely that 50–60% of animals with amitraz-resistant demodicosis will respond positively to treatment with milbemycin oxime (Kwochka 1993). As stated above, ivermectin is also effective against demodicosis and also should be considered in cases in which amitraz is ineffective.

DORAMECTIN. Doramectin (Table 50.7) is also a member of the avermectin class of compounds. It is more accurately described as a mutational biosynthetic agent, presumably because it is a fermentation product obtained from a mutant strain of *Streptomyces avermitilis*. Nonetheless, much of what was stated for ivermectin will also apply to doramectin. One distinct difference between ivermectin and doramectin is their different elimination times. Doramectin has an elimination half-life that is approximately twice that of ivermectin. Doramectin is the active ingredient in both injectable and pour-on formulations for control of grubs, mites, and biting and sucking lice on cattle (Table 50.10). Doramectin is also the active ingredient in an injectable formulation for use in the control of lice and mites on swine (Table 50.12).

EPRINOMECTIN. Eprinomectin (Table 50.7) is another representative of the avermectin class of molecules. It is a mixture of semisynthetic avermectins and is composed of greater than 90% of component B1a and less than 10% of component B1b. Its mechanism of action is similar to that described for ivermectin. Eprinomectin is a crystalline solid with an oral LD_{50} in mice of 24 mg/kg. Eprinomectin is the active ingredient in a pour-on for control of horn flies, grubs, mites, and biting and sucking lice of cattle. Eprinomectin has a very broad spectrum of activity and is unique among this class of compounds in that it has a zero time withdrawal for meat and milk.

MOXIDECTIN. Moxidectin (Table 50.7) is the methyloxime analog of nemadectin. It is structurally more similar to the milbemycins than to the avermectins, although its spectrum of activity is similar to other endectocides such as ivermectin, eprinomectin, and doramectin. Moxidectin is a product of *Streptomyces noncynogenus*. The marketed product represents a chemically altered version of the natural product. Moxidectin is the active ingredient in a pour-on for use in cattle for control of horn flies, grubs, mites, and biting and sucking lice, and in an oral gel for control of stomach bots in horses (Tables 50.10, 50.13).

SELAMECTIN. Selamectin is a new semisynthetic avermectin compound derived by modification of a precursor molecule produced by fermentation of a new strain of *Streptomyces avermitilis* (Table 50.7). As mentioned for other avermectins, selamectin induces muscular paralysis in target parasites by modulating movement of chloride ions through membrane ion channels. It remains unresolved as to whether modulation of chloride ion channel function is a GABA- or a glutamate-mediated event. Pharmacokinetics data indicate that selamectin enters the vascular compartment following topical administration. The estimated terminal-phase half-life following topical administration was approximately 11 days in dogs and 8 days in cats. Since this was substantially longer than the observed half-life following intravenous administration, it appears as though selamectin is continuously absorbed from the skin and subcutaneous tissues. Selamectin is the active ingredient in a 6% or 12% liquid (spot-on) for control of flea, tick, and mite infestations on dogs and cats (Table 50.9).

SYNERGISTS AND REPELLENTS

Synergists. Synergists (Table 50.8) enhance the activity of ectoparasiticides by inhibiting oxidative and hydrolytic enzymes responsible for their degradation. In so doing, synergists potentiate the activity of the active ingredients and extend their periods of knockdown. Synergists not only improve the performance of active agents but also permit their incorporation into formulations at lower rates than would be required without synergism. In addition, they are generally less toxic than active ingredients, thereby improving the safety of formulated products. Synergists are commonly employed in products containing pyrethrins, synthetic pyrethroids, organophosphates, chlorinated hydrocarbons, and carbamates.

TABLE 50.8—Synergists and repellents

Name	Chemical name (Empirical formula) [Molecular weight]	Chemical structure
MGK 264 (synergist)	*N*-octyl bicycloheptene dicarboximide ($C_{17}H_{25}NO_2$) [275.40]	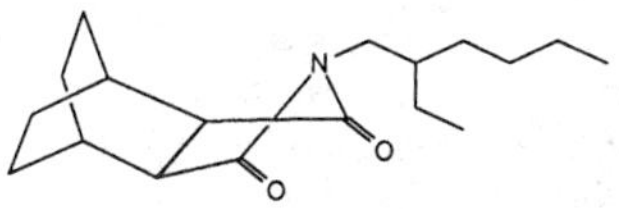
Piperonyl butoxide (synergist)	5-[[2-(2-butoxyethoxy)ethoxy]-methyl]-6-propyl-1,3-benzodioxole ($C_{19}H_{30}O_5$) [338.43]	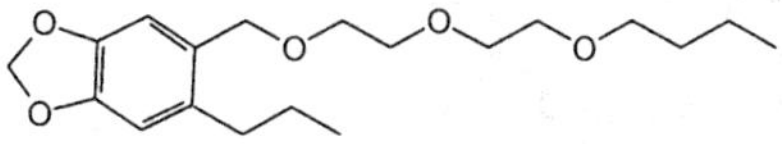
DEET (repellent)	*N,N*-diethyl-*m*-toluamide ($C_{12}H_{17}NO$) [191.26]	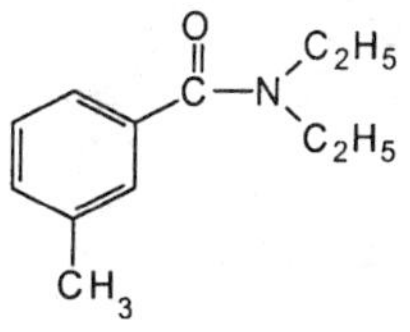
MGK 326 (repellent)	di-*N*-propyl isocinchomeronate ($C_{13}H_{17}NO_4$) [251.30]	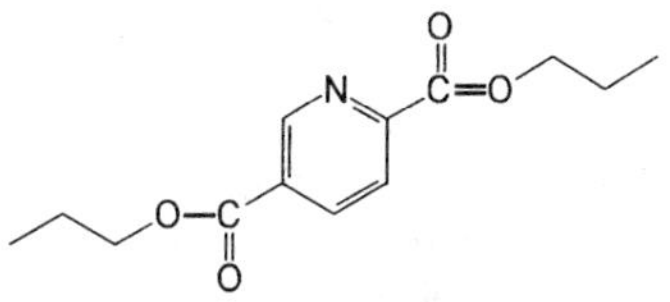
Butoxypolypropylene glycol (repellent)		$CH_3CH_2CH_2CH_2—O—(CH_2CH_2CH_2O)_n—H$

PIPERONYL BUTOXIDE. Piperonyl butoxide, a pale yellow liquid, is freely soluble in organic solvents. Its potential for toxicity to mammals is generally quite low. The acute oral LD_{50} value of piperonyl butoxide in the rat is 7500 mg/kg BW. Caution should be taken when using products containing piperonyl butoxide in cats. Preliminary evidence suggests that at concentrations equal to or exceeding 1.5%, the likelihood of neurologic side effects increases (MacDonald and Miller 1986). The activity of numerous agents, including chlorinated hydrocarbons, organophosphates, carbamates, pyrethrins, synthetic pyrethroids, and rotenone, is synergized by piperonyl butoxide.

N-OCTYL BICYCLOHEPTENE DICARBOXIMIDE (MGK 264). MGK 264 is a colorless liquid, miscible with kerosenes, aliphatic alcohols, and benzol and halogenated hydrocarbons but poorly miscible with water. Its acute oral LD_{50} value in the rat is 4980 mg/kg BW. MGK 264 synergizes the effects of pyrethrins and numerous synthetic pyrethroids. It also enhances the repellency of MGK 326 (see below) when combined with it in ectoparasiticide formulations.

Repellents. Repellents (Table 50.8) are added to formulations of ectoparasiticides to induce ectoparasites to move away from treated animals. They are popular in products used by humans to repel mosquitoes and other flies but are generally too costly for routine use in products to be applied to animals. Although many repellents possess some ectoparasiticidal properties, most are ineffective ectoparasiticides and are not used for that purpose. They are common additives to products intended for use on companion animals and horses. Very few are approved for use on food-animal species. Repellents generally are very stable molecules, capable of extending the apparent life of a product whose active ingredient is easily degraded.

BUTOXYPOLYPROPYLENE GLYCOL (STABILENE). Stabilene is a monohydric alcohol made by polymerizing ethylene oxide to butanol (Table 50.8). It is a relatively colorless liquid and is freely miscible with petroleum distillates. It is particularly effective in repelling flies. It is added to products containing pyrethrins, synthetic pyrethroids, and rotenone for use against ectoparasites of companion animals and horses (Tables 50.9, 50.13).

DI–*N*-Propyl Isocinchomeronate (MGK 326). MGK 326 is a colorless to light yellow liquid, completely miscible with petroleum distillates and other organic solvents but poorly miscible with water. Although water-base formulations of MGK 326 have been prepared, they are generally unstable. MGK 326 is a safe agent, with an acute oral LD_{50} value in the rat of 5200–7200 mg/kg BW. It is widely used in companion-animal ectoparasiticides. MGK 326 is incorporated into many collars, sprays, dusts, shampoos, dips, or topical concentrates, together with synergists and active ectoparasiticides such as pyrethrins and pyrethroids for control of fleas, ticks, mites, and lice on dogs and cats (Table 50.9).

N,N-Diethyl-*m*-Toluamide (DEET). DEET is an odorless liquid, soluble in water, alcohol, ether, and benzene but insoluble in petroleum ether. The acute oral LD_{50} value for DEET in the rat is 1800–2200 mg/kg BW. DEET is employed as a repellent in sprays for control of fleas and ticks on dogs. Apparent toxicoses in dogs and cats treated with DEET/fenvalerate-containing sprays have been reported (Dorman 1990). Clinical signs included vomiting, tremors, excitation, ataxia, and seizures. Therapy consisted of decontamination of the skin and hair coat and concurrent use of drugs to abolish seizure activity.

RESISTANCE TO ECTOPARASITICIDES. The ability of insects and other arthropods to resist the lethal effects of insecticides following continuous exposure has been known for almost a century. Ectoparasiticide resistance is an increasingly prevalent problem facing industry and agriculture. To date, more than 500 species of insects, mites, or ticks are resistant to one or more insecticides (Roush 1993). Resistance is not restricted to a single or even a few chemical classes of insecticides but has been demonstrated for many inorganic and synthetic organic compounds (Brown and Pal 1971). The majority of ectoparasites with demonstrated resistance to pesticides are crop pests. However, approximately 40% of resistant species are either parasites of humans or other animals (Roush 1993).

Mechanisms of resistance to ectoparasiticides have been classified as either behavioral or physiological (Nolan and Schnitzerling 1986). Physiological mechanisms are likely the most important and as such most significantly affect selection and effective use of insecticides. Physiological mechanisms include decreased penetration into the target organism, increased metabolism (detoxification) of insecticides, and decreased sensitivity of the target site (Roush 1993; Nolan and Schnitzerling 1986).

Decreased penetration of insecticides is reportedly a common phenomenon, although resistance by this mechanism normally is less than 5-fold (Roush 1993).

Detoxification of insecticides is mediated by enhanced activity of enzymes such as esterases, monooxygenases, and glutathione-*s*-transferases (Roush 1993; Soderland 1997). Increased enzyme activity, especially esterase activity, is probably due to gene amplification. Increased esterase activity mediates resistance to organophosphate and synthetic pyrethroid insecticides. Glutathione transferases are likely mediators of resistance to some organophosphates and to DDT.

Decreased target site sensitivity is known to occur for several organophosphate compounds and in several target species, including mosquitoes, ticks, and houseflies. In this instance, the target enzyme, AChE, appears less sensitive to the effects of the insecticide (Nolan and Schnitzerling 1986). As yet uncharacterized changes in axonal sodium channels are responsible for decreased sensitivity of certain insects and ticks to DDT and some synthetic pyrethroids. Insensitivity of this nature in the common housefly is attributable to a single gene (Roush 1993). In fact, it is possible, if not likely, that insecticide resistance mechanisms generally involve one gene. In some cases of resistance, a combination of detoxification and insensitivity of the target site is known to occur.

A number of strategies can be applied to prevent or delay development of resistance to ectoparasiticides (summarized here, with modifications, from Roush 1993). These include (1) appropriate selection of insecticides, (2) reduction in the number of treatments, (3) use of pesticide rotations, mosaics, and mixtures, (4) limited interactions with agricultural pesticides, and (5) resistance monitoring. Selection of agents should target chemistry that does not favor a higher level of resistance and/or agents that are less persistent. Reduction of treatments is best achieved by an integrated approach to pest management in which chemicals are allied with other means of controlling pests. A decision to use rotation, mixing, or mosaics of ectoparasiticides depends upon the circumstances. Mixing of agents usually results in redundant killing in which each agent is used at a rate that would kill susceptible organisms if used alone. On the other hand, mixtures often are variable in their persistence following administration, resulting in a shorter period of redundant efficacy. Mosaic use of agents varies the location of use rather than time (rotation) or combination (mixtures). Current strategies suggest that rotation of chemicals across several generations of target ectoparasite may be superior to either mosaic use or rotation over single generations. Increased frequency of exposure of target ectoparasites to agricultural chemicals is likely to speed development of resistance. It is prudent to consider integrating procedures for managing agricultural and animal pests to avoid promoting resistance against currently effective agents. Resistance monitoring can be useful in determining continuing efficacy of agents or the effectiveness of resistance management programs. Resistance monitoring is less useful in detecting resistance in natural populations of ectoparasites because of the magnitude of resistance necessary before established methods can detect it.

At present, sufficient knowledge of resistance mechanisms exists to successfully manage most situations in which resistance has developed or has the potential to develop. A more relevant limitation is our unwillingness to presume inevitable resistance to new agents and

TABLE 50.9—Ectoparasiticides for use on dogs and cats

Compound(s)	Marketed formulation(s)	Target animal(s)	Target parasite(s)
d-trans Allethrin (some formulations contain PBO[a], MGK 264[b] or sumethrin)	Shampoo	Dog, cat	Fleas, ticks
Amitraz	Dip	Dog	Mites
	Collar	Dog	Ticks
Benzyl benzoate	Lotion	Dog	Mites
Carbaryl (some formulations contain methoxychlor, PBO, BPG[c], MGK 326[d], and/or pyrethrins)	Shampoo	Dog, cat	Fleas, ticks, mites (some products claim efficacy against lice; see specific product labels)
	Spray	Dog, cat	
	Dust	Dog and/or cat	
	Ear drops	Dog, cat	
Chlorpyrifos (some formulations contain methoprene PBO, pyrethrins, or MGK 264)	Spray	Dog	Fleas, ticks
	Dip	Dog	Fleas, ticks, mites
	Collar		Fleas, ticks, mites
	Shampoo	Dog or cat	Fleas, ticks, mites
	Streaker (for back and chest streak treatment)	Dog	Fleas
Diazinon	Collar	Dog or cat	Fleas, ticks
Dichlorvos	Collar	Dog or cat	Fleas, ticks
Fipronil	Liquid (spot-on)	Dog, cat	Fleas, ticks
	Spray	Dog, cat	Fleas, ticks
Imidacloprid	Liquid (spot-on)	Dog, cat	Fleas
d-Limonene (some formulations contain linalool)	Spray	Dog, cat	Fleas
	Shampoo	Dog, cat	Fleas
	Dip (also may be added to shampoo)	Dog, cat	Fleas
Linalool (some formulations contain *d*-limonene)	Spray`	Dog, cat	Fleas
Lindane	Dip, spray, bath	Dog	Fleas, ticks, lice, mites
Lufenuron (also combined with milbemycin oxime for dogs)	Tablet	Dog, cat	Fleas
	Six-month injectable	Cat	Fleas
Malathion	Liquid	Dog, cat	Fleas, ticks, lice
Methoprene (some formulations contain permethrin, chlorpyrifos or tetrachlorvinphos	Collar	Dog or cat	Fleas, ticks
	Liquid (spot-on)	Dog	Fleas, ticks
Methoxychlor (some formulations contain carbaryl)	Powder	Dog, cat	Fleas, ticks
	Collar	Dog	Fleas, ticks
Permethrin (some formulations contain PBO, MGK 264, MGK 326[b], pyrethrins, pyriproxyfen or BPG)	Collar, spray, shampoo, dip, cream rinse or topical concentrate (spot-on)	Dog and/or cat (see specific product labels)	Fleas, ticks (see specific product labels)
Phosmet	Dip	Dog	Fleas, ticks, mites
Propoxur	Collar	Dog	Fleas, ticks
Pyrethrins (some formulations contain PBO, MGK 264, MGK 326, BPG, permethrin, carbaryl, or rotenone)	Spray, foam, dust, shampoo, dip, or ear drops	Dog and/or cat (see specific product labels)	Fleas, ticks, or mites (some products claim efficacy against lice; see specific product labels)
Pyriproxyfen (combined with permethrin in certain formulations)	Spray, collar, liquid (spot-on), strip-on	Dog or cat	Fleas (combinations may control additional ectoparasites)
Resmethrin	Shampoo	Dog, cat	Fleas, ticks
Rotenone (some formulations contain pyrethrins)	Ear drops	Dog, cat	Mites
	Dip	Dog	Fleas, ticks, lice
Selamectin	Liquid (spot-on)	Dog	Fleas, ticks, mites
		Cat	Fleas, mites

[a]PBO = piperonyl butoxide (synergist).
[b]MGK 264 = *N*-octyl bicycloheptene dicarboximide (synergist).
[c]BPG = butoxypolypropylene glycol (repellent).
[d]MGK 326 = di-*n*-propyl isocinchomeronate (repellent).

TABLE 50.10—Extoparasiticides for use on cattle

Compound(s)	Marketed formulation(s)	Method of application	Target parasite(s)
Amitraz	Liquid	Spray	Lice, ticks, mites
Chlorpyrifos	Liquid	Spray	Screwworm, ear ticks
Chlorpyrifos, diazinon	Ear tag	One tag in each ear	Horn flies, face flies, stable flies, house flies, lice, ticks
Coumaphos	Wettable powder	Spray or dip	Horn flies, lice, ticks, grubs, screwworms, mites
	Liquid	Spray or dip	Horn flies, lice, mites, ticks, grubs
	Dust	Dust bag or shaker can	Horn flies, face flies, ticks
Cyfluthrin	Ear tag	One tag in each car	Horn flies, face flies, Gulf Coast ticks, ear ticks
Λ Cyhalothrin	Ear tag	One tag in each ear	Horn flies, face flies
	Pour-on	Backline treatment	Horn flies, lice
Cypermethrin, chlorpyrifos	Ear tag	One tag in each ear	Horn flies, face flies, Gulf Coast ticks, ear ticks
Beta-cypermethrin (zetamethrin)	Ear tag	One tag in each ear	Horn flies, face flies, ticks, lice
Diazinon, chlorpyrifos	Ear tag	One tag in each ear	Horn flies, face flies, stable flies, houseflies, lice, ticks
Dichlorvos (some formulations contain pyrethrins)	Liquid	Spray	Stable flies, horn flies, houseflies, mosquitoes, gnats
Diflubenzuron	Bolus	1 bolus per 1,100 lb	Horn flies, face flies, houseflies, stable flies
Doramectin	Injectable solution	Inject subcutaneously	Grubs, mites, biting and sucking lice
	Pour-on	Backline treatment	
Eprinomectin	Pour-on	Backline treatment	Grubs, mites, biting and sucking lice, horn flies
Ethion	Ear tag	One tag in each ear	Horn flies, face flies, stable flies, lice, ticks
Famphur	Pour-on	Backline treatment	Grubs, lice
	Liquid	Spray, spot-on, backrubber	Horn flies, lice, mites, ticks (spectrum depends on formulation)
Fenthion	Pour-on	Backline treatment	Lice, horn flies
	Ear tag	One tag in each ear	Horn flies, face flies
	Low-volume pour-on	Spot treatment on the backline	Grubs, lice
	Pour-on	Backline treatment	Grubs, lice
Fenvalerate	Ear tag	One tag in each ear	Horn flies, face flies, stable flies, houseflies, ticks, lice
Invermectin	Injectable solution	Inject subcutaneously	Grubs, mites, sucking lice
	Pour-on	Backline treatment	Grubs, mites, biting and sucking lice, horn flies
	Sustained-release bolus	Oral	Grubs, sucking lice, mites, ticks
Lindane	Spray	Direct application to infested site	Ear ticks, screwworms
Malathion	Liquid	Spray, backrubber	Horn flies, lice, ticks
Moxidectin	Pour-on	Backline treatment	Grubs, mites, biting and sucking lice, horn flies
Permethrin	Liquid	Spray	Horn flies, face flies, mites, ticks, lice, various other flies
	Liquid	Spray	Horn flies, face flies, stable flies, horseflies, lice, ticks, mites
	Wettable powder	Spray	Horn flies, face flies, stable flies, horse flies, lice, ticks, mites
	Dust	Direct application	Horn flies, face flies, lice
	Ear tag	One or two tags	Horn flies, face flies (generally two tags), Gulf Coast ticks, ear ticks (some tags do not claim horn flies)
	Roll-on paste	Roll on to different body areas	Horn flies, face flies, stable flies, black flies, houseflies, botflies

TABLE 50.10—(continued)

Compound(s)	Marketed formulation(s)	Method of application	Target parasite(s)
Permethrin, chlorpyrifos	Ear tag	One or two tags	Horn flies, face flies (generally two tags), Gulf Coast ticks, ear ticks
Permethrin	Pour-on	Backline treatment	Horn flies, face flies, lice
Pirimiphos	Ear tag	One tag in each ear	Horn flies, face flies
Tetrachlorvinphos	Premix	Mix in feed	Horn flies, face flies, houseflies, stable flies
	Wettable powder	Spray	Horn flies, lice, ticks
	Dust	Dust bag, shaker can	Horn flies, lice, face flies
Trichlorfon	Dust	Dust bag	Horn flies, face flies, ticks
	Wettable powder	Spray	Horn flies, lice, ticks

Note: Some products also may contain synergists and/or repellents.
Refer to label directions for compounds approved for lactating dairy cattle and for compound withdrawal period prior to slaughter.

TABLE 50.11—Ectoparasiticides for use on sheep and goats

Compound(s)	Marketed formulation(s)	Method of application	Target parasite(s)
Fenvalerate	Liquid	Spray, pour-on	Lice, keds
Ivermectin	Drench (sheep only)	Oral drench	Nasal bots
Lindane	Spray	Direct application	Ear ticks, screwworms
Malathion	Emulsifiable concentrate	Spray	Lice, keds, ticks
Permethrin	Liquid	Spray	Lice, ticks (some formulations also claim activity against keds or various flies)
	Pour-on	Pour-on	Lice, keds
	Emulsifiable concentrate	Spray	Lice, ticks, blowflies

Note: Refer to label directions for compounds approved for lactating goats and for compound withdrawal period prior to slaughter.

TABLE 50.12—Ectoparasiticides for use on swine

Compound(s)	Marketed formulation(s)	Method of application	Target parasite(s)
Amitraz	Liquid	Ears and backline treatment	Lice, mites
Coumaphos	Dust	Shaker can	Lice
	Liquid	Spray	Lice
Doramectin	1% injectable solution	Inject subcutaneously	Lice, mites
Fenthion	Pour-on	Pour-on	Lice
Fenvalerate	Liquid	Spray, pour-on	Lice, mites (pour-on only for lice)
Ivermectin	1% injectable solution	Inject subcutaneously	Lice, mites
	0.27% injectable solution	Inject subcutaneously	Lice, mites
	Pre-mix	Mix with feed	Lice, mites
Lindane	Spray	Direct application	Ear ticks, screwworms
Malathion	Liquid	Spray	Lice, mites
Permethrin	Liquid	Spray, paint, dip	Lice, mites (some formulations also claim horn flies, and ticks
	Dust	Direct application	Lice (some formulations also claim horn flies, ticks, and mites)
	Wettable powder	Spray, paint, dip	Horn flies, lice, ticks, mites
Tetrachlorvinphos	Wettable powder	Spray	Lice
	Dust	Direct application	Lice

Note: Refer to label directions for compound withdrawal period prior to slaughter.

TABLE 50.13—Ectoparasiticides for use on horses

Compound(s)	Marketed formulation(s)	Method of application	Target parasite(s)
Coumaphos	Liquid	Spray	Horseflies, ticks, screwworms, lice
	Emusifiable concentrate	Spray	Horseflies, ticks, screwworms, lice
Fenvalerate	Liquid	Spray	Horn flies, face flies, stable flies, houseflies
Ivermectin	Paste	Oral	Botfly larvae
	Liquid	Oral	Botfly larvae
Lindane	Spray	Direct application	Ear ticks, screwworms
Malathion	Liquid	Spray	Horn flies, lice, ticks
Methoxychlor, pyrethrins	Liquid	Spray, wipe	Horn flies, horseflies, stable flies, deerflies
Moxidectin	Gel	Oral	Botfly larvae
Permethrin (some formulations also contain pyrethrins)	Liquid	Spray, wipe	Horn flies, face flies, horseflies, stable flies, deerflies, mosquitoes, biting gnats, ticks
	Dust	Direct application	
Pyrethrins	Liquid	Spray	Horn flies, face flies, houseflies, horseflies, stable flies, deerflies, mosquitoes, biting gnats, ticks

TABLE 50.14—Benefit-risk ratios of selected classes of ectoparasiticides

Class of ectoparasiticide	Mammalian toxicity (mg/kg)	Insect toxicity (mg/kg)	Benefit-risk ratio*
Carbamates	45	2.8	16
Organophosphates	67	2.0	33
Chlorinated hydrocarbons	230	2.6	91
Synthetic pyrethroids	2000	0.45	4500

Source: MacDonald and Miller 1986.
*Safety factor in mammals (usually oral LD_{50} in rat) ÷ toxicity to insect (usually contact LD_{50} in flies).

to adopt the strategies necessary to delay it. Interest in developing long-term strategies to combat resistance does seem to be growing. Insecticide resistance action committees have been established to develop strategies to combat resistance to crop protection chemicals. Similar initiatives are in the planning stages for pesticides marketed for use in food and companion animals.

REGULATION OF ECTOPARASITICIDE APPROVAL AND REGISTRATION IN THE UNITED STATES AND CANADA. Ectoparasiticides are evaluated and subsequently approved by either the US Food and Drug Administration (USFDA) or the US Environmental Protection Agency (USEPA). The agency responsible for reviewing supportive data and subsequent approval or registration of a new product is determined by the product's method of contact with the target parasite. Agents that are administered either orally or topically but exert their effects following systemic distribution are classified as drugs and are evaluated by the USFDA. New agents that are applied topically to target animals and are active by surface contact with target parasites (pesticides) are evaluated by the USEPA.

Although the regulatory processes are somewhat different, similar types of supportive data are required from the regulatory agencies. It begins with the discovery or synthesis of a new agent or a proposed new use for an existing agent. After conducting preliminary safety and efficacy studies, the sponsor applies for either an Investigational New Animal Drug Application (INADA) through the USFDA (pharmaceutical) or an Experimental Use Permit (EUP) through the USEPA (pesticides). Preliminary data are not sufficient for new-product registration or approval. Preliminary efficacy and safety studies are followed by detailed tissue residue studies (food animals) to determine in which tissues the drug accumulates and at what rate it is depleted from these tissues. Reproductive studies confirm the safety of the drug in pregnant animals and its effects on the embryo or fetus. Reproductive studies are not required for all drugs. Studies must be conducted only if the sponsor seeks to use the candidate agent in reproducing animals. Stability studies provide information on the storage properties of the drug or pesticide. The

TABLE 50.15—Clinical signs and treatment of ectoparasiticide toxicosis

Ectoparasiticide group	Clinical signs of toxicosis	Treatment
Carbamates	Abdominal cramping, vomiting, diarrhea, miosis, dyspnea, cyanosis, muscle twitching seizures; rarely tetany followed by weakness and paralysis	Atropine sulfate: 0.2–0.5 mg/kg to effect (mydriasis and reduced salivation) usually 1/4 dose IV and 3/4 SC; may need to repeat at 3–6 hr for 1–2 days depending on response; 2–PAM (pralidoxime) is contraindicated
Chlorinated hydrocarbons	Onset can be minutes to days after exposure, usually several hours; signs include apprehension, exaggerated response to stimuli, vomiting, muscle twitching of face and head that progresses posteriorly to severe fasciculations and tremors; clonic and tonic seizures; elevated body temperature; chlorinated hydrocarbons are stored in fat; therefore, course may be protracted	Emesis (may induce seizures), gastric lavage; no specific antidote; seizures may be controlled with diazepam at 2.5–20 mg IV as needed; barbituate to effect; do *not* use phenothiazines, because they lower seizure threshold; calcium gluconate 10% at 2–10 mL given slowly IV and vitamin B complex IM to protect liver function; critical period, 24–36 hr
d-limonene, linalool, crude citrus oil extracts	(Cats) Hypersalivation, ataxia, and muscle tremors; hypothermia in some animals	Supportive therapy; wash agent from hair coat with nondetergent-, nonalcohol-containing shampoo; external warming for hypothermia
Formamidines	Lethargy, hypotension, hyperglycemia, mydriasis, hypothermia, bradycardia; ataxia, vomiting, and diarrhea have also been reported	Emesis, activated charcoal after oral ingestion (collar); wash agent from hair coat with nondetergent-, nonalcohol-containing shampoo (dip); yohimbine 0.1 mg/kg IV
Organophosphates	*Muscarinic:* salivation, lacrimation, diarrhea, abdominal cramping, miosis, pallor, cyanosis, dyspnea, emesis	Atropine as for carbamates
	Nicotinic: twitching of facial and tongue muscles progressing to generalized twitching followed by paralysis	2-PAM (pralidoxime): 20 mg/kg IV twice per day; give over 5-min duration; if poisoned for less than 24 hr, treatment is necessary for 1–2 days; if longer, therapy may be required for several days
	Central nervous system: depression, tonic/clonic seizures, death is due to hypoxia from respiratory muscle paralysis, bronchoconstriction, excessive pulmonary secretions, pulmonary edema, and bradycardia	Diphenhydramine hydrochloride: animal becomes depressed, decrease 4 mg/kg IV (dogs) or IM (dogs or cats) every 8 hr until asymptomatic; if animal becomes depressed, decrease dose to 1–mg/kg
Pyrethrins, synthetic pyrethroids	Only at very high doses; hypersalivation, vomiting, diarrhea, ataxia, CNS excitation and seizures, hyperthermia, hypothermia	Supportive as for chlorinated hydrocarbons; wash agent from hair coat with nondetergent-, nonalcohol-containing shampoo, monitor and control body temperature
Rotenone	Vomiting, nausea, diarrhea, respiratory stimulation, convulsions, followed by respiratory depression, coma, respiratory failure and death; in humans, causes irritant dermatitis	Emesis, gastric lavage before convulsive state; warmth, quiet; assist respiration; diazepam, calcium gluconate and B complex vitamins as for chlorinated hydrocarbons

Source: Modified from Kwochka 1987.

USEPA also requires a product chemistry package for pesticides that includes specific pesticide composition and characteristics. Also in the case of pesticides, resistance studies may be necessary to determine how easy it will be for the target parasite to develop resistance to the drug. Studies must also be conducted for many drugs and for all pesticides to determine their potential impact on the environment. Efficacy of the candidate drug must be evaluated in detailed laboratory studies and in realistic use situations. This is achieved by conducting numerous laboratory studies and clinical field trials in different geographic regions of the country, although according to the new Food and Drug Administration Modernization Act, field trials are not always required by the USFDA. If required, clinical field trials generally are conducted by either veterinarians or scientists in collaboration with animal owners or producers to obtain detailed information on the performance of the product under realistic use conditions. If new label claims or formulation changes are sought for a drug which is currently approved for use, many of the safety and efficacy studies can be waived if the new formulation is shown by properly conducted studies to be pharmacologically equivalent to the existing formulation.

After all necessary research has been conducted, the sponsor of a new animal drug must arrange all data in a package for presentation to the appropriate regulatory agency. Such a comprehensive data package is referred to as a New Animal Drug Application (NADA) if filed with the USFDA or an Application for Pesticide Registration (APR) if submitted to the USEPA. For pesticides, data also must be reviewed and evaluated by some state agencies before approval is granted in those states. If approval is granted at the federal level, the approval file is maintained by the reviewing agency; it contains all of the information on procedures used to evaluate the efficacy, safety, and environmental impact of the drug as well as the information on manufacture, formulations, drug specification, package labeling, and evidence of compliance with either Good Laboratory, Good Clinical, or Good Manufacturing Practices. Notice of approval of new pharmaceuticals and pesticides is published in the *Federal Register,* a government publication detailing information of a legislative and regulatory nature. A Freedom of Information (FOI) summary describing the safety and efficacy studies conducted to support marketing approval of a drug can be obtained from the USFDA following drug approval. Continued monitoring of approved drugs and pesticides is required to ensure efficacy and safety in the marketplace.

Approval procedures for pharmaceuticals and pesticides in Canada are similar to those required in the United States. The Health Protection Branch of Health and Welfare Canada is responsible for licensing pharmaceuticals. The Plant Industry Directorate oversees licensing of pesticides. In some cases, as in the United States, pesticides may have to undergo provincial review and approval in addition to federal review.

REFERENCES

Atkinson, P. W., Binnington, K. C., and Roulston, W. J. 1974. High monoamine oxidase activity in the tick *Boophilus microplus* and inhibition by chlordimeform and related compounds. J Aust Entomol Soc 13:207–210.

Benz, G. W., Roncalli, R. A., and Gross, S. J. 1989. Use of ivermectin in cattle, sheep, goats, and swine. In W. C. Campbell, ed., Ivermectin and Abamectin, pp. 215–229. New York: Springer-Verlag.

Bigler, B., Waber, S., and Pfister, K. 1984. Successful treatment of *Notoedres cati* infestation with ivermectin. Schweiz Arch Tierheilkd 126:365–367.

Blagburn, B. L., Vaughan, J. L., Lindsay, D. S., and Tebbit, G. L. 1994. Lufenuron: efficacy dosage titration against developmental stages of the cat flea (*Ctenocephalides felis felis*) in cats. Am J Vet Res 55:98–101.

Blagburn, B. L., Vaughan, J. L., Butler, J. M., and Parks, S. C. 1999. Dose titration of an injectable formulation of lufenuron in cats experimentally infested with fleas. Am J Vet Res 60: in press.

Bowman, D. D. 1999. Georgi's Parasitology for Veterinarians. 7th ed. Philadelphia: W. B. Saunders.

Brooks, G. T. 1974. Chlorinated Insecticides. Vol. 1, Technology and Application. Cleveland: CRC Press.

Brown, A. W., and Pal, R. 1971. Insecticide Resistance in Arthropods. WHO Monograph Series no. 38. Geneva: World Health Organization.

Campbell, W. C. 1989. Use of ivermectin in dogs and cats. In W. C. Campbell, ed., Ivermectin and Abamectin, pp. 245–259. New York: Springer-Verlag.

Carrera, G., and Periquet, A. 1991. Metabolism and toxicokinetics of pesticides in animals. In T. S. S. Dikshith, ed., Toxicology of Pesticides in Animals, pp. 67–118. Boca Raton, Fla.: CRC Press.

Chambers, H. W. 1992. Organophosphorus compounds: an overview. In J. E. Chambers and P. E. Levi, eds., Organophosphates: Chemistry, Fate, and Effects, pp. 3–17. New York: Academic Press.

Cohen, E. 1987. Interference with chitin biosynthesis in insects. In J. E. Wright and A. Retnakaran, eds., Chitin and Benzoylphenyl Ureas, Series Entomologica, vol. 38, pp. 43–73. Dordrecht, Netherlands: Dr. W. Junk.

Dorman, D. C. 1990. Diethyltoluamide (DEET) insect repellent toxicosis. In V. R. Beasely, ed., Toxicology of Selected Pesticides and Chemicals. Vet Clin N Am Small Anim Pract 20:387–391.

Drummond, R. O., George, J. E., and Kunz, S. E. 1988. Effects of arthropod pests on livestock production. In R. O. Drummond, J. E. George, and S. E. Kunz, eds., Control of Arthropod Pests of Livestock: A Review of Technology, pp. 1–28. Boca Raton, Fla.: CRC Press.

Fikes, J. D. 1990. Organophosphorus and carbamate insecticides. In V. R. Beasely, ed., Toxicology of Selected Pesticides and Chemicals. Vet Clin N Am Small Anim Pract 20:353–367.

Fisher, M. H., and Mrozik, H. 1989. Chemistry. In W. C. Campbell, ed., Ivermectin and Abamectin, pp. 1–23. New York: Springer-Verlag.

Fukami, J. 1976. Insecticides as inhibitors of respiration. In C. F. Wilkinson, ed., Insect Biochemistry and Physiology, pp. 353–396. New York: Plenum Press.

Gammon, D. W., Brown, M. A., and Casida, J. E. 1981. Two classes of pyrethroid action in the cockroach. Pestic Biochem Physiol 15:181–191.

Garg, R. C., and Donahue, W. A. 1989. Pharmacologic profile of methoprene, an insect growth regulator in cattle, dogs, and cats. J Am Vet Med Assoc 194(3):410–412.

Ghiasuddin, S. M., and Matsumura, F. 1982. Inhibition of GABA induced chloride uptake by γ-BHC and heptachlor epoxide. Comp Biochem Physiol 73:141–144.

Hart, R. J. 1986. Mode of action of agents used against arthropod parasites. In W. C. Campbell and R. S. Rew, eds., Chemotherapy of Parasitic Diseases, pp. 585–601. New York: Plenum Press.

Hink, W. F., Drought, D. C., and Barnett, S. 1991. Effect of an experimental systemic compound, CGA-184699, on life stages of the cat flea (Siphonaptera: Pulicidae). J Med Entomol 28:424–427.

Hooser, S. B. 1990. *d*-Limonene, linalool, and crude citrus oil extracts. In V. R. Beasely, ed., Toxicology of Selected Pesticides and Chemicals. Vet Clin N Am Small Anim Pract 20:383–385.

Ivie, G. W., and Rowe, L. D. 1986. Drugs used against arthropod parasites. In W. C. Campbell and R. S. Rew, eds., Chemotherapy of Parasitic Diseases, pp. 507–529. New York: Plenum Press.

Johnson, M. K. 1975. The delayed neuropathy caused by some organophosphorus esters: mechanism and challenge. CRC Crit Rev Toxicol 3:289–316.

Kuhr, R. J., and Dorough H. W. 1976. Development and use. In R. J. Kuhr and H. W. Dorough, eds., Carbamate Insecticides: Chemistry, Biochemistry, and Toxicology, pp. 1–13. Cleveland: CRC Press.

Kwochka, K. W. 1987. Fleas and flea related diseases. In R. B. Grieve, ed., Veterinary Clinics of North America, Small Animal Practice, Parasitic Infections 17:1235–1262.

———. 1993. Demodicosis. In C. E. Griffin, K. W. Kwochka, and J. M. MacDonald, eds., Current Veterinary Derma-

tology: The Science and Art of Therapy, pp. 72–84. St Louis: Mosby.
Loomis, E. C. 1986. Ectoparasites of cattle. In R. P. Herd, H. C. Gibbs, and K. D. Murrell, eds., Parasites: Epidemiology and Control. Vet Clin N Am Food Anim Pract 2:299–321.
MacDonald, J. M., and Miller, T. A. 1986. Parasiticide therapy in small animal dermatology. In R. W. Kirk, ed., Current Veterinary Therapy IX, Small Animal Practice, pp. 571–596. Philadelphia: W. B. Saunders.
Miller, W. H., and Scott, D. W. 1991. Milbemycin in the treatment of generalized demodicosis in the dog. In Proc Ann Meet Am Assoc Vet Dermatologists, American College of Veterinary Dermatology, p. 41.
Moriello, K. A. 1993. Cheyletiellosis. In C. E. Griffin, K. W. Kwochka, and J. M. MacDonald, eds., Current Veterinary Dermatology: The Science and Art of Therapy, pp. 90–95. St. Louis: Mosby.
Narahashi, T. 1992. Nerve membrane Na^+ channels as targets of insecticides. Trends Pharmacol Sci 13:236–241.
Nolan, J., and Schnitzerling, H. J. 1986. Drug resistance in arthropod parasites. In W. C. Campbell and R. S. Rew, eds., Chemotherapy of Parasitic Diseases, pp. 603–620. New York: Plenum Press.
Palma, K. G., Meola, S. M., and Meola, R. M. 1993. Mode of action of piriproxyfen and methoprene on eggs of *Ctenocephalides felis* (Siphonaptera: Pulicidae). J Med Entomol 30:421–426.
Paradis, M., and Laperriere, E. 1992. Efficacy of daily ivermectin treatment in a dog with amitraz-resistant generalized demodicosis. Vet Dermatol 3:85–88.
Paradis, M., and Villeneuve, A. 1988. Efficacy of ivermectin against *Cheyletiella yasguri* infestation in dogs. Can Vet J 29:633–635.
Paradis, M., Scott, D. M., and Villeneuve, A. 1990. Efficacy of ivermectin against *Cheyletiella blakei* infestation in cats. J Am Anim Hosp Assoc 26:125–128.
Reedy, L. M., and Garfield, R. A. 1991. Results of a clinical study with an oral antiparasitic agent in generalized demodicosis. In Proc Ann Meet Am Assoc Vet Dermatologists, American College of Veterinary Dermatology, p. 43.
Richardson, R. J. 1992. Interactions of organophosphorus compounds with neurotoxic esterase. In J. E. Chambers and P. E. Levi, eds., Organophosphates: Chemistry, Fate, and Effects, pp. 299–323. New York: Academic Press.
Roush, R. T. 1993. Occurrence, genetics and management of insecticide resistance. Parasitol Today 9(5):174–179.
Soderland, D. M. 1997. Molecular mechanisms of insecticide resistance. In W. Ebing, ed., Chemistry of Plant Protection, vol. 13, Molecular Mechanisms of Resistance to Agrichemicals, pp. 21–56. Berlin: Springer.
Soulsby, E. J. L. 1982. Helminths, Arthropods, and Protozoa of Domesticated Animals, 7th ed., pp. 357–540. Philadelphia: Lea & Febiger.
Stone, B. F., and Knowles, C. O. 1974. A laboratory method for evaluation of chemicals causing detachment of the cattle tick *Boophilus microplus.* J Aust Entomol Soc 12:163–172.
Urquhart, G. M., Armour, J., Duncan, J. L., Jennings, F. W., and Dunn, A. M. 1996. Veterinary Parasitology. 2nd ed. Cambridge, Mass.: Blackwell Science.
Valentine, W. M. 1990. Pyrethrin and pyrethoid insecticides. In V. R. Beasely, ed., Toxicology of Selected Pesticides and Chemicals, Vet Clin N Am Small Anim Pract 20:375–382.
Williams, C. M. 1956. The juvenile hormone of insects. Nature 178:212–213.
Zakson, M., Hink, W. F., and MacKichan, J. J. 1992. Fate of the benzoylphenyl urea CGA-184699 in the cat flea *Ctenocephalides felis.* Pestic Sci 35:117–123.

SECTION 12

Specialty Areas of Pharmacology

51 DRUGS AFFECTING GASTROINTESTINAL FUNCTION

DAWN M. BOOTHE

Functions of the Digestive System
Appetite Stimulants
Emetics
- **The Vomition Reflex**
- **Peripherally Acting, or Reflex, Emetics**
- **Centrally Acting Emetics**

Antiemetics
- **Centrally Acting Antiemetics**
- **Peripherally Acting Antiemetics**

Antiulcer Drugs
- **Physiology of Gastric Acid Secretion**
- **Mucosal Defenses**
- **Gastroduodenal Ulceration**
- **Gastric Antisecretory Drugs**
- **Cytoprotective Drugs**

Modulators of Gastric Motility
- **Prokinetics**

Modulation of Intestinal Motility and Secretion
- **Anticholinergic Agents**
- **Opioids**
- **Miscellaneous Antisecretory Drugs**

GI Protectants and Adsorbents
Laxatives and Cathartics
- **Emollient Laxatives**
- **Simple Bulk Laxatives**
- **Osmotic Cathartics**
- **Irritant Cathartics**
- **Neuromuscular Purgatives**
- **Enemas**

Agents Promoting Digestive Functions
Drugs Affecting the Liver
- **Cholagogues and Choleretics**
- **Liver Protectants and Hepatotropic Agents**

FUNCTIONS OF THE DIGESTIVE SYSTEM. Normal digestive function depends upon prehension, mastication, deglutition, and subsequent maceration and decomposition of the ingested food into smaller solubilized forms within the gastrointestinal (GI) tract. These particles are further degraded enzymatically by either the host or symbiotic microorganisms into molecular forms that are conveniently transferred across the GI epithelium into the body. Although the end products are generally similar, the digestive process may vary considerably in different domestic animals, so an appreciation of the comparative aspects of gastroenterology is essential for rational use of drugs that influence the digestive tract.

Major processes involved in digestion include motility of the GI tract, glandular and epithelial secretion, enzymatic action, absorption of end products, and elimination of materials not absorbed from the gut. Mechanical events that occur lead primarily to propulsion of the nutrients from one part of the tract to the next. Absorptive functions depend upon mucosal structure, metabolism, and circulation. Several factors influence digestive processes, including metabolic and electrophysiologic responses that take place in mucosal, glandular, or smooth muscle cells and hemodynamic events that occur in the GI circulation. In addition, GI functions are carefully regulated by intrinsic nerves and the extrinsic autonomic nervous system as well as by circulating and locally acting hormones. Agents used therapeutically because of their actions on the digestive tract modify or influence one or more of the physiologic functions noted above.

APPETITE STIMULANTS. Appetite is controlled primarily but not exclusively by the ventral and lateral nuclei of the hypothalamus (Sugrue 1987). Several major neurotransmitters have been identified in the control of appetite (Sugrue 1987). Stimulatory mediators include norepinephrine (through α_2 receptors) and dopamine (possibly through D_1 receptors), while serotonin (5-HT) is inhibitory. Gamma-aminobutyric acid (GABA) also stimulates appetite, although its effect is controversial and may vary with route of administration (Sugrue 1987). Several neuropeptides have also been implicated in the control of appetite, because of their ability to modulate neurotransmitter release. Opiate and pancreatic polypeptides are associated with increased appetite. Other neuropeptides, such as calcitonin, cholecystokinin, and corticotrophin-releasing factor, inhibit appetite (Sugrue 1987).

Studies on the pharmacologic control of appetite have traditionally focused on decreased food intake in humans, whereas in veterinary medicine it is more often necessary to increase appetite. The role of cachexia associated with weight loss and anorexia in human cancer patients has stimulated a renewed interest in appetite stimulants (Spaulding 1989). Drugs that inhibit gluconeogenesis, such as hydrazine sulfate, or that promote gastric emptying, such as metoclopramide, have been used successfully to stimulate food intake in some patients (Spaulding 1989). Megestrol acetate has caused appetite stimulation in human patients with advanced cancer and is preferred to anabolic steroids, which are associated with more adverse side effects (Spaulding 1989).

The benzodiazepines diazepam (Valium) and oxazepam, a metabolite of diazepam (Serax), have been used successfully to induce appetite in cats, probably through GABA-induced effects and central inhibition of the satiety center in the hypothalamus (Macy and Gasper 1985). Diazepam is administered intravenously or orally, and oxazepam is administered orally. Of the two drugs, diazepam may be more effective, although sedation will be greater. The benzodiazepines do not stimulate appetite in the dog as effectively as they do in the cat.

Cyproheptadine, an antihistamine with antiserotonin properties, has caused weight gain in geriatric human patients and in adults and younger patients afflicted with eating disorders. Its mechanism probably reflects inhibition of serotoninergic receptors which control appetite. Serotonin antagonists also increase food intake in cats (Sugrue 1987), and clinically, cyproheptadine has been used to stimulate the appetite of some anoretic cats. Both glucocorticoids and B vitamins have been used to nonspecifically stimulate the appetites of animals. Drugs used to treat depression and psychosis in human patients are associated with appetite increase and weight gain (Bernstein 1988). They antagonize a variety of receptors, although their clinical potency is related to dopamine antagonism. These drugs, which include tricyclic antidepressants and lithium, have not been studied as appetite stimulants in animals.

EMETICS

The Vomition Reflex. Emesis is a complex, protective reflex that is not well developed in all species (Johnson 1985, 1984; Andrews et al. 1988). Carnivores, primates, swine, certain birds, and reptiles are capable of emesis. Horses and ruminant animals as well as rodents, guinea pigs, and rabbits are unable to vomit effectively.

Emesis is controlled through the emetic center, which is located in the lateral reticular formation of the medulla, where it is protected by the blood-brain barrier (Fig. 51.1) (Johnson 1984; Andrews et al. 1988; Merrifield and Chaffee 1989). Although several afferent pathways may be responsible for initiating emesis, all signals are coordinated by the emetic center. Impulses to the emetic center in the medulla may arise from higher centers, such as the cerebral cortex and limbic system. Psychogenic vomiting and that arising from visual and olfactory stimuli originate in the cerebral cortex, while head injuries and increased intracranial pressure initiate emesis via limbic pathways. Acetylcholine (ACh) is the primary afferent neurotransmitter mediating emesis from these higher centers, although histamine acts as a secondary transmitter via H_1 receptors (Merrifield and Chaffee 1989).

Blood-borne chemical compounds may stimulate the chemoreceptor trigger zone (CTZ), which is located in the area postrema in the lateral walls of the 3rd ventricle (Johnson 1984; Merrifield and Chaffee 1989). This area does not possess a complete blood-brain barrier and thus is more readily accessible than the emetic center to substances such as drugs or toxins present in circulating blood. The neurons of the CTZ are also more responsive to the presence of blood- and cerebrospinal

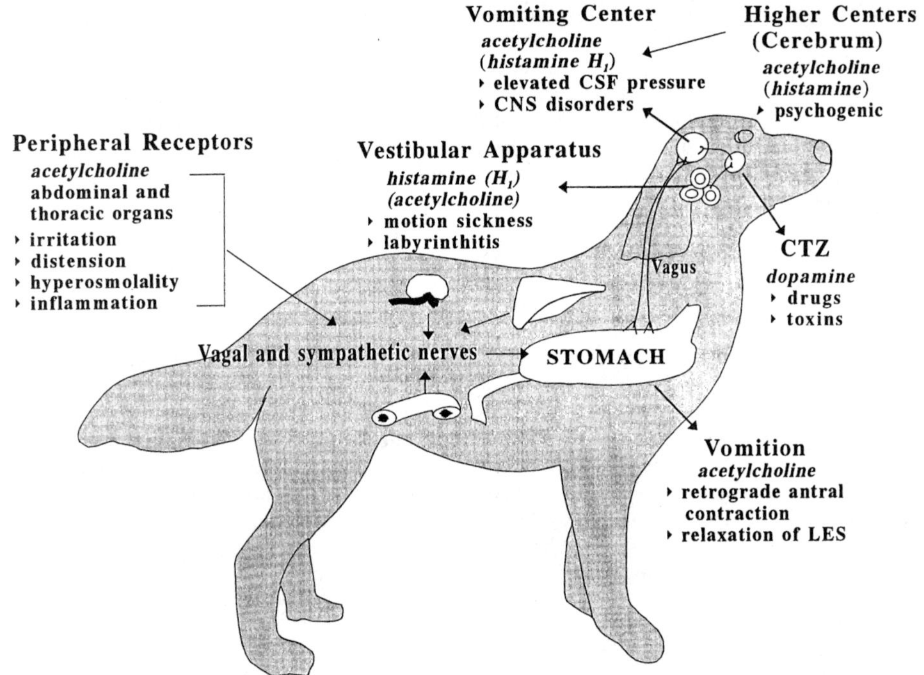

FIG. 51.1—Sites that mediate the emetic reflex. The major neurotransmitter responsible for mediating the reflex at each site is noted in italics; secondary neurotransmitters at each site are in parentheses. Stimuli that mediate emesis at each site are listed below the neurotransmitter.

fluid (CSF)-borne chemical compounds because free nerve endings directly contact the CSF. Free nerve endings reach the CSF either via ependymal pores or in the sheath surrounding fenestrated capillaries. Emesis caused by blood-borne mediators (e.g., uremia, pyometra, liver disease, endotoxemia, and those associated with radiation sickness disease) and drugs (e.g., digitalis glycosides, apomorphine, narcotic analgesics, and estrogens) is mediated by the CTZ. Stimulation of the CTZ is initiated by dopaminergic receptors that respond to agonists such as dopamine and apomorphine (Merrifield and Chaffee 1989). Alpha$_2$ receptors associated with the area postrema also induce emesis in dogs (Hikasa et al. 1992) and cats (Hikasa et al. 1989). Serotonin may also be important in this area (Kohler and Goldspiel 1991). Histamine via H_1 receptors acts as a secondary neurotransmitter at the CTZ. As with dopaminergic receptors, H_1 receptors may also be competitively and noncompetitively inhibited by antagonists.

Impulses originating from the semicircular canals of the vestibular apparatus are transmitted by the 8th cranial nerve to the vestibular nuclei and then via the CTZ and uvula and nodulus of the cerebellum to the emetic center. This pathway, mediated by histaminergic (subtype H_1) receptors, is responsible for eliciting the emesis that accompanies motion sickness and labyrinthitis (Peroutka and Snyder 1982).

Peripheral impulses causing vomition which arise from stimulation of the pharynx and fauces are transmitted by afferent nerves in the 9th cranial nerve to the emetic center. Other peripheral afferent pathways include those arising from stimulation (i.e., irritation or distension) of various visceral organs and tissues. Impulses may be carried by sympathetic or vagal afferents from the heart, stomach, duodenum, small intestine, liver, gallbladder, peritoneum, kidneys, ureter, urinary bladder, and uterus. ACh is the primary neurotransmitter mediating the afferent limb of the emesis reflex from peripheral causes. Muscarinic receptors initiate the impulse which travels to the emetic center via the vagus nerve. Efferent signals which stimulate the emetic reflex travel back to the stomach by the 10th cranial (vagus) nerve. ACh also acts as the primary efferent neurotransmitter in the vagus and in the smooth muscle of the stomach.

Clinically, emesis is pharmacologically induced in order to empty the anterior portion of the digestive tract. Indications include induction of general anesthesia if there is any possibility of food being in the stomach, or ingestion of noncorrosive poisons.

Peripherally Acting, or Reflex, Emetics. Distension of the pharynx, esophagus, stomach, or duodenum (hollow organs) with warm water, hydrogen peroxide, or saline can induce the emetic response. In addition, in the case of toxin ingestion, administration of warm water by stomach tube may help dilute poisons. Although their efficacy and safety vary, a number of substances induce emesis by irritating the epithelium of the GI tract. Emesis can be induced in dogs by oral administration of a solution of warm saturated (strong) sodium chloride or by pharyngeal placement of a small amount of plain table salt or neutral salt crystals, such as Sodium Carbonate, NF. Orally administered hydrogen peroxide (3%) often induces emesis rapidly in cats and dogs, although fatal aspiration of hydrogen peroxide foam is possible. Ipecac syrup is an over-the-counter emetic commonly recommended to induce emesis in human pediatric patients. It contains the alkaloid emetine, which increases lachrymation, salivation, and bronchial secretions. Emesis usually, but not consistently, occurs as a result of both peripheral and central stimulation. However, if repeated use fails to induce emesis, gastric lavage may be indicated to remove potentially toxic doses of the drug. Although ipecac syrup or powder has been used as an emetic for many years in cats, it has been known to induce toxic effects, including death.

Centrally Acting Emetics. Although a number of drugs are capable of stimulating the CTZ centrally, certain opiates, particularly apomorphine, are the most commonly used. Apomorphine Hydrochloride, USP, is a synthetic derivative of morphine with only marginal depressant activity. Its emetic activity predominates over other morphine-like actions and reflects stimulation of dopaminergic receptors in the CTZ. Apomorphine can be administered by almost any route, although oral doses are greater in order to compensate for reduced oral bioavailability. Emesis generally occurs in 2-10 minutes following subcutaneous or conjunctival administration. Although apomorphine stimulates vomiting at the CTZ, it also directly depresses the emetic center, and subsequent doses are less likely to induce emesis even if emesis does not occur following the first dose. Excessive doses of apomorphine can depress the central nervous system (CNS), particularly the respiratory center, and are contraindicated in the presence of existing central depression.

Xylazine (Rompun) is an α_2 agonist used most commonly for its sedative analgesic properties. However, emesis mediated by α_2 stimulation consistently occurs in cats when xylazine is administered at recommended doses (Hikasa et al. 1989). Emesis can also be induced at low doses (0.05 mg/kg) not associated with sedation. Emesis also occurs in dogs, but not as consistently as in cats. The incidence of emesis induced by xylazine is also somewhat lower following IV than IM administration and may be reduced further by fasting prior to use.

ANTIEMETICS. Antiemetics control emesis by either a central or a peripheral action. Both actions depend on and can be correlated to blockade of neurotransmission at receptor sites (Peroutka and Snyder 1982; Costall and Naylor 1992).

Centrally Acting Antiemetics. Antiemetic agents possess either a limited or a broad effect depending on which centers are depressed. Centrally acting antiemetics block impulses at higher centers and at the emetic center and include muscarinic anticholinergics; antidopaminergics which block dopaminergic receptors at the CTZ; and antihistaminergics which block H_1 receptors at the vestibular apparatus and secondarily at the CTZ and the emetic center.

VESTIBULAR APPARATUS. Vomition caused by motion sickness or inner ear disease is mediated by the vestibular apparatus. Motion sickness in dogs and cats can be controlled for several hours (8-12) by administering antihistaminics such as cyclizine hydrochloride, meclizine hydrochloride, or diphenhydramine hydrochloride. Although efficacy depends on a direct effect on neural pathways arising in the vestibular apparatus, it appears to be independent of antihistaminic or sedative potencies. Emesis produced by other stimuli is not controlled by these drugs. Drowsiness and xerostomia are typical side effects encountered with use of this group of drugs.

ANTIMUSCARINICS. Selected antimuscarinic agents are used to control motion sickness in dogs. The belladonna alkaloids, especially hyoscine (scopolamine), and synthetic compounds such as dicyclomine hydrochloride and isopropamide iodide are effective antiemetics. Their duration of action is short (up to 6 hr), and xerostomia, drowsiness, and other side effects should be anticipated. These drugs are not generally used in cats, because of potential adverse reactions.

DRUGS ACTIVE AT THE CTZ

PHENOTHIAZINES. These broad-spectrum antiemetics control emesis induced by most central causes other than labyrinthine stimulation. Phenothiazines block emesis mediated by the CTZ at low doses because of their antidopaminergic and antihistaminergic effects. At higher (perhaps nonpharmacologic) doses, their anticholinergic effects may also act at other central sites, including the emetic center. A variety of phenothiazine derivatives, e.g., chlorpromazine, prochlorperazine, triflupromazine, perphenazine, trifluoperazine, and mepazine, are used in small animals as antiemetics. The primary adverse effects associated with their use as antiemetics are sedation and hypotension due to peripheral α blockade. Selection of a particular phenothiazine may be based on avoidance of adverse reactions. Fluid replacement therapy should be instituted if necessary prior to use of a phenothiazine.

BUTYROPHENONE DERIVATIVES. Haloperidol (Haldol) and droperidol (Inapsine), which are also used as major tranquilizers, are potent antiemetics because of their antidopaminergic activity. Possible side effects are similar to those encountered with the phenothiazine group.

METOCLOPRAMIDE. Metoclopramide effectively blocks emesis mediated by the CTZ. Although its potent antagonism of dopamine was thought to be responsible for the inhibition of the CTZ, more recent evidence indicates that antagonism of 5-HT_3 receptors is more likely (Tyers 1992). Metoclopramide effectively antagonizes apomorphine-induced emesis (Reynolds 1989) and is 20 times as potent as phenothiazines (Burrows 1983). The peripheral effects of metoclopramide on emesis due to prokinesis are discussed with the prokinetic drugs. Metoclopramide is indicated for control of emesis induced by a wide variety of blood-borne and peripheral causes (Urbie et al. 1985; Albibi and McCallum 1983). High doses of metoclopramide, particularly when combined with dexamethasone, have been used to treat emesis associated with cancer chemotherapy in human patients (Shinkai et al. 1989; Gralla et al. 1981; Howard et al. 1985).

TRIMETHOBENZAMIDE HYDROCHLORIDE. Trimethobenzamide hydrochloride (Tigan) is a weak antihistaminic and powerful antidopaminergic antiemetic that suppresses the CTZ without affecting the emetic center. It has been used to control vomiting caused by radiation sickness, drugs, infections, anesthesia, and uremia. Clinically it has not been as effective as other antidopaminergics.

SEROTONIN ANTAGONISTS. Serotonin antagonists reportedly are useful for their antiemetic effects mediated at the CTZ, especially when emesis is induced by chemotherapeutic agents (Gamse 1990). Ondansetron has been useful in dogs, cats, and ferrets to control emesis induced by cisplatin, other chemotherapeutic agents, and radiation treatment (Costall and Naylor 1992). As a 5-HT_3 receptor antagonist, odansetron also may affect vagally mediated peripheral motility of the stomach. However, the impact of this effect on the peripheral control of vomiting has not yet been documented (Itoh et al. 1991). Ondansetron is a potent antiemetic in human cancer patients undergoing chemotherapy (Burrows 1990; Tyers 1992). Cyproheptadine is the only serotonin antagonist which has been cited for use in small animals. In addition to its antiserotonin effects, cyproheptadine is anticholinergic and antihistaminergic. It has been used to control vomiting and diarrhea (the latter associated with spasticity) in humans.

Sedatives such as the barbiturates and the benzodiazepines have also been used to control psychogenic and behavioral vomiting.

Peripherally Acting Antiemetics. Occasionally, some drugs that protect the GI epithelium from further irritation might be used as antiemetics. Drugs that modulate gastric acid secretion might also provide antiemetic effects. These drugs will be discussed as antiulcer drugs. Demulcents, antacids, and protectants such as kaolin, pectin, and bismuth salts are of limited benefit in the control of emesis. Distension or initial irritation of the stomach by these agents may exacerbate emesis. Antacids may be effective in certain cases. Other peripherally acting antiemetics are drugs that affect gastric motility, including anticholinergic drugs and prokinetic drugs such as metoclopramide and domperidone (prokinetic drugs are discussed in a later section).

ANTICHOLINERGICS. Anticholinergic drugs that block muscarinic receptors in the emetic center also inhibit peripheral cholinergic transmission. The anticholinergic drugs that do not cross the blood-brain barrier well and thus act primarily peripherally include glycopyrrolate, propantheline, methscopolamine, and isopropamide. Of these, methscopolamine should not be used in cats. The ability of anticholinergics to suppress emesis is probably related to inhibition of afferent vagal impulses, relief of GI smooth muscle spasms, and the inhibition of gastroenteric secretions. Delayed gastric emptying caused by these drugs may itself cause emesis, and anticholinergics should not be used for longer than 3 days in the vomiting patient.

ANTIULCER DRUGS

Physiology of Gastric Acid Secretion. Gastric acid secretion occurs in four phases. The first three phases, referred to as cephalic, gastric, and intestinal, are stimulated by food and mediated by gastrin. Secretion is persistent during these phases, and gastric pH progressively decreases as nutrients traverse the GI tract. Gastrin secretion is inhibited as gastric pH declines to 3.5 and is completely inhibited at a pH of 1.5, to begin again only when pH is approximately 3.0-3.5. The fourth phase of gastric acid secretion is basal and occurs in the absence of external stimuli. The amount of basal secretion varies among animals. In humans, basal secretion follows a circadian rhythm, reaching a peak at midnight and a nadir at 7 A.M. (Wolfe and Soll 1988).

Gastric acid secretion at the cellular level involves the generation and subsequent secretion of hydrogen ions by the parietal (oxyntic) cells of the gastric mucosa (Fig. 51.2) (Wolfe and Soll 1988). The hydrogen ion pump, located at the apical membrane and associated with the smooth endoplasmic reticulum, is unique in that it is a hydrogen-potassium ATPase exchange system. Three distinct pathways are capable of stimulating gastric acid. Each acts through chemical mediators, which in turn interact with receptors on the parietal cell membrane. The neurocrine pathway delivers transmitters such as ACh that interact with muscarinic receptors located on the parietal cell and other sites; the endocrine pathway delivers hormones such as gastrin that may interact with gastrin receptors; and the paracrine pathway delivers autocoids or tissue factors such as histamine that interact with H_2 receptors on the parietal cell (Fig. 51.2) (Wolfe and Soll 1988).

Potentiation of the effects of gastrin and ACh by histamine has been observed in a number of animals.

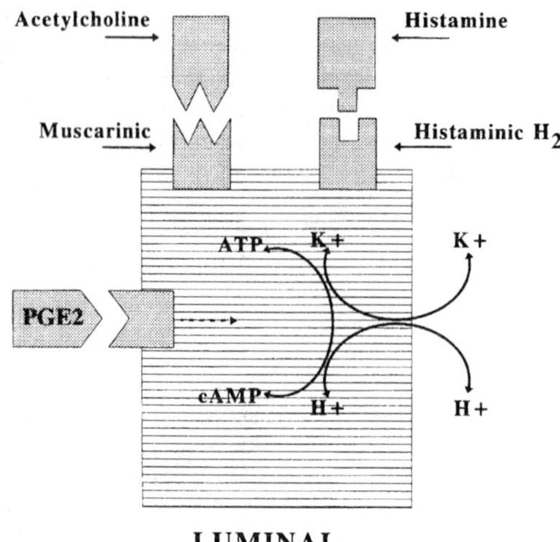

FIG. 51.2—Receptor interactions that mediate gastric acid secretion by the parietal cell include acetylcholine with muscarinic receptors and histamine with H_2 receptors. Gastrin may interact with either receptor. Receptor stimulation activates the K^+,H^+-ATPase pump and exchange of potassium for hydrogen into the lumen. Prostaglandin E_2 modulates gastric acid secretion by inhibiting cAMP.

Intracellular messengers mediating gastric acid secretion vary with the receptor stimulated. Histamine increases cAMP production, which subsequently activates cAMP-dependent protein kinases. Gastrin and muscarinic stimulation by cholinergic drugs increases cytosolic calcium, probably by increased influx through selective receptor-activated calcium channels in the cell membrane. Prostaglandins of the E series (PGEs) modulate these effects, inhibiting gastric acid secretion by blocking cAMP production (Wolfe and Soll 1988).

Mucosal Defenses. Defenses of the GI mucosa which act to prevent or repair GI ulceration include (1) secretion of bicarbonate into the lumen and neutralization of hydrochloric acid in the lumen; (2) secretion of a thick, alkaline mucus which traps and neutralizes inward-moving hydrogen ions; (3) a gastric epithelial barrier comprising active phospholipids, a lipoprotein cell membrane, and tight junctional complexes, all of which prevent hydrogen ion back-diffusion; (4) mucosal blood flow, which, first, provides nutrients and oxygen to mucosal cells and, second, removes hydrogen ions that have penetrated the gastric barrier; (5) rapid replication of mucosal epithelial cells; and (6) production of cytoprotective agents (Fig. 51.3) (Baker 1966; Toutain et al. 1983; Shorrock and Rees 1988). Local secretion of PGE_2 is an important defense mechanism because it modulates hydrochloric acid secretion, increases bicarbonate and mucus production, and enhances mucosal blood flow and epithelialization (Miller 1983; Charlet et al. 1985). Sulfhydryls also produced locally may act as scavengers of oxygen and other tissue-damaging radicals (Szelenyi and Brune 1986).

Gastroduodenal Ulceration. The events leading to gastroduodenal ulceration are complex and reflect interactions between acid-secreting and defense mechanisms of the GI mucosa (Robert and Kauffman 1989; Moreland 1988). Regardless of the cause of GI erosion or ulceration, the basic pathologic mechanism is similar. Gastric acid secretion is a prerequisite for damage to the GI mucosa (Kleiman et al. 1988; Moreland 1988), although damage does not usually occur if luminal pH is greater than 7.0. Pepsin and bile acids can contribute to mucosal damage. Damage is exacerbated when the mucosa loses its ability to sufficiently protect itself through secretion of bicarbonate and mucus and epithelialization. Deceased mucosal blood flow can profoundly affect the injured mucosa's ability to heal itself. Drugs used to control or treat GI erosion and/or ulceration include drugs used to inhibit gastric acid secretion and cytoprotective drugs.

Gastric Antisecretory Drugs. Drugs used to prevent or modulate gastric acid secretion include anticholinergics, H_2 receptor antagonists, proton pump inhibitors, and PGE_2 (Whittle and Garner 1988; Wolfe and Soll 1988; Miller 1983; Muir 1990). Drugs which modify gastric acid (e.g., antacids) are discussed in the section on cytoprotective drugs. All drugs that modify gastric pH can cause complications of achlorhydria when used chronically. Although both gastric acid and pepsin are required for hydrolysis of proteins and other foods, achlorhydria is rarely accompanied by malabsorption unless bacterial overgrowth occurs. Achlorhydria can lead to malabsorption of certain nutrients (e.g., vitamin B_{12} and iron).

ANTICHOLINERGICS. Despite the role of muscarinic receptors in gastric acid secretion, anticholinergics have not proven effective for the control of GI ulceration in animals. In humans, these drugs reduce food-induced gastric acid secretion by 30% and potentiate the inhibitory effect of H_2 receptor antagonists (see below). Side effects, as previously described, further limit their usefulness. Side effects are reduced, however, when selective drugs for muscarinic receptors of the M_1 subtype are used. Pirenzepine, an M_1 antagonist, inhibits food-induced secretion by 50-60%, with fewer antimuscarinic side effects (Wolfe and Soll 1988).

H_2 RECEPTOR ANTAGONISTS. H_2 receptor antagonists are reversible, competitive antagonists that reduce gastric secretion of both hydrochloric acid (HCl) and pepsin (Krishna and Ulrich 1988) induced by a variety of secretogogues (Hirschowitz and Gibson 1987). Cimetidine and ranitidine and, to a lesser degree, famotidine have been used to control gastric acid secretion in animals. Nizatidine is the newest of the H_2 receptor antagonists. Each drug varies in potency, duration of

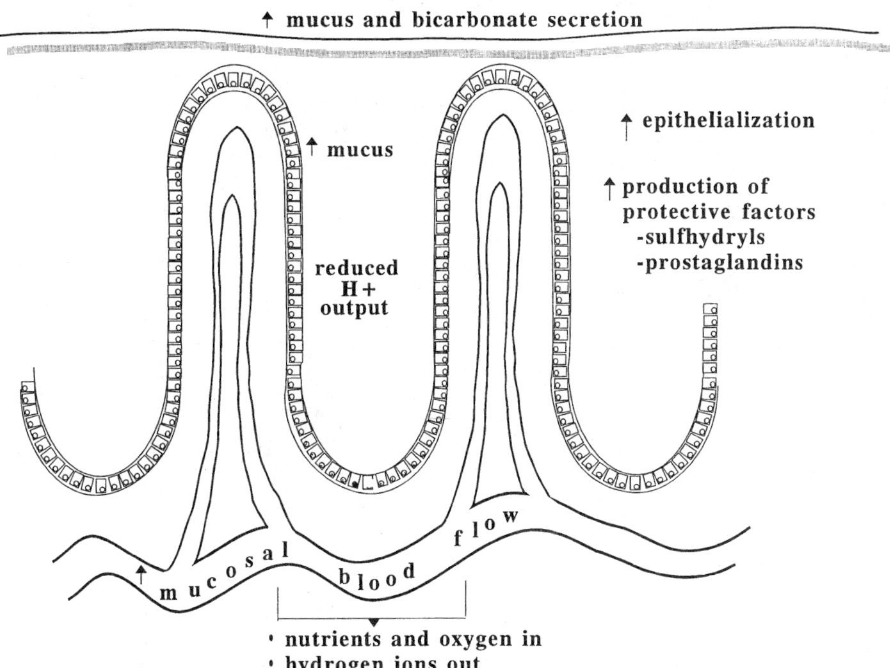

FIG. 51.3—Protective mechanisms against gastroduodenal ulceration provide targets for drug therapy. Bicarbonate secretion neutralizes gastric acid; mucus protects against hydrochloric and bile acids. The rapid turnover of epithelial cells is paramount for rapid healing if damage occurs. Mucosal blood flow not only provides critical oxygen and nutrients necessary for epithelialization but also removes H^+ ions that have penetrated the protective barrier. Other protective factors include mechanisms to control gastric hydrochloric acid secretion and to scavenge mediators capable of cell damage.

action, disposition, and drug interactions (Bemis et al. 1989). Ranitidine is 5-12 times more potent as an inhibitor of gastric acid secretion than cimetidine, while famotidine is 9 times more potent than ranitidine and 32 times more potent than cimetidine. Famotidine has the longest duration of action (Howard et al. 1985). In animal models including dogs, nizatidine is more potent than cimetidine (Price and Brogden 1988).

DISPOSITION. Cimetidine, the oldest of the clinically used H_2 receptor antagonists, is rapidly absorbed from the GI tract, although food will delay the process. The drug undergoes hepatic metabolism and is about 70% bioavailable following oral administration. It is excreted in the urine, primarily in an unchanged form. The plasma half-life is about 1 hour but may be prolonged in the presence of liver or kidney disease.

Ranitidine is less bioavailable (50%) than cimetidine following oral administration. Its elimination half-life is approximately 2.5 hours. Absorption is not impaired by food as it is with cimetidine. Ranitidine is minimally protein bound (15%). Hepatic elimination is responsible for 30% of an IV dose and 73% of an oral dose (Brogden et al. 1982).

Famotidine is only 37% bioavailable after oral administration, due to poor oral absorption. In contrast, nizatidine is rapidly and completely absorbed (Krishna and Ulrich 1988). Both drugs are eliminated unchanged in urine (Krishna and Ulrich 1988). Nizatidine is almost exclusively eliminated by renal excretion, which suggests it might be the preferred H_2 receptor antagonist in patients with hepatic disease. Its efficacy apparently has not been studied clinically in animals, although its safety has been established in healthy dogs (Bemis et al. 1989).

Ranitidine has been studied in dogs and horses. In Beagle dogs receiving 5 mg/kg, ranitidine was characterized by an elimination half-life of 4 hours. Bioavailability after oral administration was 73%, yielding peak concentrations of 2000 ng/mL. Elimination appears to reflect both hepatic metabolism and, for 40% of each dose, renal elimination (Eddershaw et al. 1996). In adult horses, following IV administration of 2.2 mg/kg, ranitidine reached a concentration of 5175 ng/mL and was characterized by a mean residence time of 113 minutes. Following oral administration, mean absorption time was 59 minutes and bioavailability was 27% (Holland et al. 1997).

DRUG INTERACTIONS. Cimetidine can be involved in a number of drug interactions (Ames and Patterson 1984). It impairs oral absorption of a number of drugs either directly or due to alteration of GI pH. It is a potent microsomal enzyme inhibitor and will decrease the metabolism of concurrently administered drugs (Sedman 1984; Gibaldi 1992). Occasionally, this effect may be clinically useful, as in the prevention of acetaminophen intoxication in cases of accidental overdose (Jackson 1982). Cimetidine also reduces hepatic blood flow by about 20% and has been shown to reduce the clearance of flow-limited drugs such as propranolol and lidocaine (Jackson 1981). Unlike cimetidine, ranitidine has limited effects on hepatic blood flow, on the metabolism of other drugs, or on androgenic activity. Drugs can interfere with renal elimination of the H_2-receptor blockers. In Beagle dogs, probenecid decreased renal clearance of ranitidine by close to 50% (Boom et al. 1998). Drug interactions involving famotidine and nizatidine are rare.

ADVERSE REACTIONS. The side effects seen with cimetidine are generally minor even at relatively high doses. Thrombocytopenia has been reported. Although there have been a number of reported side effects for ranitidine in the human, limited experience to date in animals has not indicated any serious toxic manifestations from ranitidine. Famotidine and nizatidine are devoid of many of the side effects of cimetidine. Antiandrogenic effects are most notably absent (Price and Brogden 1988).

A clinically important disadvantage of H_2 receptor antagonists described in humans is relapse of gastroduodenal ulceration after H_2 receptor antagonist therapy is discontinued. Although several explanations for relapse have been offered, rebound hypersecretion of gastric acid appears to be most plausible (Guharoy 1991; Ledger et al. 1992; Fullarton et al. 1991). Suppression of gastric acid by H_2 receptor antagonists results in increased plasma gastrin concentrations as early as 3 hours after a single dose. Subsequent stimulation of gastric mucosal G cells results in gastric acid hypersecretion which becomes evident when the drugs are discontinued. The likelihood of hypersecretion is compounded by increased parietal cell receptor sensitivity, which apparently characterizes patients afflicted with ulcers (Marks et al. 1991). Among the H_2 receptor antagonists studied, cimetidine seems to be the most likely, and famotidine or nazitidine the least likely, to cause rebound gastric acid hypersecretion (Marks et al. 1991; Yamaji et al. 1991; Fullarton et al. 1991).

CLINICAL USE. H_2 receptor antagonists are used principally to treat uremic gastritis, gastric and duodenal ulcers, stress-related erosive gastritis, and hypersecretory conditions such as gastrinoma or systemic mastocytosis. Ranitidine was effective in minimizing ulceration of gastric squamous epithelium experimentally induced by feed deprivation in adult horses (Murray and Eichorn 1996). Although H_2 receptor antagonists can be used to treat drug-induced (e.g., nonsteroidal anti-inflammatory drug; NSAID) ulceration, their efficacy is controversial, and other, more-specific antidotes (i.e., PGE_1) might first be administered (Larsen et al. 1992). Cimetidine and ranitidine also appear to be effective in controlling upper GI bleeding when hemorrhage is not due to erosion of major blood vessels. Histamine (H_2) receptor antagonists have also been used in gastroesophageal reflux disorders, esophagitis, and duodenal gastric reflux. In exocrine pancreatic insufficiency, cimetidine or ranitidine, if given about 30 minutes prior to feeding, will prevent enzymatic and acid hydrolysis of replacement pancreatic enzymes added to food upon their contact with gastric secretions.

PROTON PUMP INHIBITORS

MECHANISM OF ACTION. Omeprazole is the commercially available member of the newest group of gastric antisecretory drugs, the substituted benzimidazoles. These drugs are potent antagonists of the H^+,K^+-ATPase proton pump, the final step in gastric acid secretion stimulated by any secretagogue. Omeprazole is approximately 30 times more potent as an antacid than cimetidine (Lampkin et al. 1990). As a weak base, the drug is unstable in an acid environment and thus is formulated as encapsulated enteric-coated granules (Lampkin et al. 1990). Drug dissolution occurs in the alkaline environment of the small intestine. Because oral bioavailability increases with environmental intestinal pH, plasma drug concentrations tend to increase the first 4-5 days of therapy (Lampkin et al. 1990). Omeprazole selectively partitions from systemic circulation into the acidic environment of parietal cells (pK_a 1) compared to other cells (pK_a 5). In the acidic environment, the drug is protonated and subsequently further transformed to the active inhibitor. Potassium-adenosine triphosphate (H^+, K^+- ATPase), the energy source for the proton pump, is potently and irreversibly inhibited (Lampkin et al. 1990). As a result, the drug not only no longer accumulates but is inactivated when its antacid effects have been achieved. The net effect is a negative feedback (Moreland 1988). Because the drug accumulates in parietal cells, there may be a lag time of 3-5 days before maximum effect is realized (Lampkin et al. 1990; Larsson et al. 1988). In addition, efficacy will be maintained at low plasma drug concentrations and for some time after the drug is discontinued. Because of these characteristics, omeprazole can be administered once a day (Larsson et al. 1988). Secretory volume is not as affected as is acidity (Lampkin et al. 1990). In humans, omeprazole is highly (96%) bound to serum albumin and α_1-acid glycoprotein. Its apparent volume of distribution is 0.31 L/kg (Lampkin et al. 1990). In humans, drug elimination is dependent on hepatic metabolism to inactive metabolites, and elimination half-life is short (52 minutes) (Lampkin et al. 1990). Omeprazole has been studied in dogs and horses (Jenkins and DeNovo 1990). In horses the elimination half-life of omeprazole is 30 minutes. Oral bioavailability is reduced although therapeutic concentrations can be achieved.

ADVERSE REACTIONS. Adverse reactions caused by omeprazole are limited since the drug is selective for the H^+,K^+-ATPase pump. Diarrhea and transient fluctuations in liver enzymes have been reported. Hypergastrinemia has been documented in human patients (Lampkin et al. 1990) following therapy with omeprazole, but rebound hypersecretion of gastric acid has apparently not been studied. Hypertrophy of gastric mucosa has been reported. Compared to cimetidine, omeprazole is less likely to be involved in drug interactions. Partial inhibition of drugs eliminated by selected cytochrome P-450 enzymes has been reported for omeprazole (Andersson 1991).

CLINICAL USE. Omeprazole is the drug of choice for the treatment of the Zollinger-Ellison syndrome. In humans without gastrinomas, extended use of omeprazole is associated with complete antiacidity, which induces hypergastrinemia and gastric hypertrophy. Omeprazole has been used to control gastric acid secretion that has not responded to H_2 receptor antagonists, although its superiority to these and other antacid drugs has not been firmly established. However, generally studies support the superiority of omeprazole compared to cimetidine for treatment of GI ulceration, including amelioration of pain (Lampkin et al. 1990).

PROSTAGLANDINS. In addition to receptor antagonism, gastric acid secretion can also be modulated by prostaglandins of the E series. Their actions appear to be mediated by interaction with a basolateral membrane receptor. Intracellular concentrations of cAMP decrease, which in turn decreases protein kinase activity and hydrogen ion concentration (Wolfe and Soll 1988). Misoprostol is a methyl ester analog of PGE_1. As such it is pharmacologically active following oral administration, with effects lasting longer than those of endogenous prostaglandins (PGs) (Misoprostol monograph 1990). Its action tends to be restricted to the local environment, with systemically absorbed drug rapidly metabolized by the liver (Jones and Bailey 1989). Misoprostol does not appear to alter serum gastrin levels, and rebound acid hypersecretion has not been reported (Jenkins and DeNovo 1990). Basal, nocturnal, and food-induced gastric acid secretion is inhibited by misoprostol. However, the drug may not be as effective as selected H_2 receptor antagonists in decreasing intraluminal pH and appears less effective in controlling pain. Unabsorbed drug which reaches the intestine can have adverse effects in the intestinal tract (Misoprostol monograph 1990). PGEs cause intestinal secretion, smooth muscle contraction, and thus diarrhea, but these side effects may be resolved after several days (Misoprostol monograph 1990).

Cytoprotective Drugs

ANTACIDS. Antacids chemically neutralize HCl present in the gastric lumen so that luminal pH is increased to an acceptable level (Morrissey and Barreras 1974). Inactivation of pepsin and binding of bile salts by some products (e.g., aluminum hydroxide) are also important in the treatment of peptic ulcers. Finally, some products (aluminum hydroxide) also induce the local synthesis of mucosal protectants (e.g., PGs and sulfhydryls) (Vergin and Kori-Lindner 1990; Szelenyi and Brune 1986). Since pepsin activity for peptic digestion is optimal at pH 2-3, effective antacids should raise the pH of gastric fluids to at least 3 or 4 without causing systemic alkalosis. The action of gastric antacids is usually transient and lasts only 1-2 hours. Neutralization of acid in the stomach antrum removes negative-feedback control of gastrin release, which in turn leads to elevated gastrin levels and enhanced HCl secretion, with increased tone of the lower esophageal sphincter. These drugs must be administered frequently or with a meal to avoid this rebound effect. Factors complicating rationale antacid therapy are rate of acid secretion; duration of time the antacid remains in the stomach; the potency of the antacid; and adverse effects (Siepler et al. 1986).

Systemic antacids such as sodium bicarbonate are water soluble, and part of the unneutralized anionic portion is absorbed. However, even though the gastric pH may increase to alkaline levels, the duration of action is short, and rapid liberation of carbon dioxide may lead to gastric distension; acid rebound effects often occur. Part of the systemic alkalosis is caused by the alkaline tide phenomenon.

The major nonsystemic antacids used in veterinary medicine are salts of aluminum, magnesium, and calcium; they are used either alone or in combination with each other or with various protectants, adsorbents, and astringents. One gram of these compounds will generally neutralize 20-35 mEq of acid in vitro. Aluminum hydroxide is a good adsorbent as well as an antacid. In addition, it stimulates local PG production in the intestinal mucosa (Vergin and Kori-Lindner 1990). Other aluminum salts employed as antacids include aluminum magnesium silicate and aluminum phosphate. Aluminum preparations tend to cause constipation and are often mixed with magnesium salts to prevent this side effect. Aluminum hydroxide decreases phosphate absorption by forming insoluble aluminum phosphates in the intestine and is used to control serum phosphorus in patients with renal disease.

Magnesium-containing products can raise gastric pH higher than aluminum-containing antacids (9.0 vs. 4.0) (Morrissey and Barreras 1974). Magnesium hydroxide is the most commonly used form of magnesium, although magnesium oxide, magnesium silicates, and other magnesium salts are also used in various preparations. Magnesium salts tend to be laxative and are often found in combination with aluminum and calcium salts. Their cathartic effects result from soluble but unabsorbed magnesium salts that remain in the intestine and retain water. The neutralizing effect of magnesium hydroxide is prompt and prolonged, with gastric pH reaching high levels (about 7). Up to 20% of the magnesium is absorbed in normal circumstances and in the presence of renal dysfunction; repeated administration can result in hypermagnesia. Combination antacid products containing both aluminum and magnesium are often used to balance the adverse effects of each cation or bowel function (Siepler et al. 1986). Calcium Carbonate, USP, is a rapidly acting, potent antacid with a prolonged duration. However, slowly developing metabolic alkalosis, gastric acid rebound, hypercalcemia, and calciuria with metastatic calcification and urolithiasis, hypophosphatemia, and constipation are potential side effects that may occur following chronic administration of calcium carbonate (Siepler et al. 1986).

Gastric hyperacidity, peptic ulcer, gastritis, reflux esophagitis, and chronic renal failure (uremia) are the more common indications for antacid preparations in veterinary medicine. Pyloric and duodenal peptic ulcers which may be related to gastric hyperacidity have been reported in dogs and foals, and abomasal ulceration is a well-recognized syndrome in cattle. Another major use of antacids in veterinary medicine is in treatment and prevention of ruminal acidosis from grain overload. Antacids are capable of altering oral absorption of other drugs (Steinberg et al. 1982).

PROSTAGLANDIN E_1. PGE_1 (Misoprostol), previously discussed as an antisecretory drug, is also a cytoprotectant (Miller 1983; Misoprostol monograph 1990; Jones and Bailey 1989). In addition to controlling HCl secretion, it increases mucus and bicarbonate secretion and enhances epithelialization of the mucosa and mucosal blood flow (Wilson 1987; Robert 1987). Misoprostol also stabilizes mast cells destroyed by ulcerogens (Jones and Bailey 1989). Although misoprostol may not be as effective as H_2 receptor antagonists in increasing gastric pH, it is often superior for gastroduodenal ulcer healing (Jones and Bailey 1989). Direct indications for PGE_1 include preventive therapy or treatment of GI damage associated with NSAID therapy (Misoprostol monograph 1990; Richter 1990). Misoprostol was effective in preventing gastric hemorrhage induced by aspirin in 4 out of 5 dogs (35 mg/kg body weight, orally q 8 hr for 10 days). Diarrhea occurred in dogs receiving 15 μg of misoprostol/kg body weight but not in dogs receiving 7.5 μg/kg body weight (Bowersox et al. 1996).

SUCRALFATE. Sucralfate is an orally administered disaccharide (sucrose) aluminum hydroxide product which binds to and protects the ulcerated site from acid, bile, and pepsin activity (McCarthy 1991; Tarnawski et al. 1987; Hickey et al. 1991; Hollander and Tarnawski 1990). In the acid environment of the stomach, the sucrose is freed from the aluminum hydroxide and cross-polymerizes and binds to exposed (damaged) anions of GI epithelial cell membranes (Konturek et al. 1991). Binding occurs in the base of ulcer craters and is greater in duodenal ulcers than in gastric ulcers. Sucralfate also binds to and inactivates bile acids and pepsin (Jensen and Jensen 1992). In addition to binding and protection of cells, the polymerized sucrose prevents exudation of protein and electrolytes into the gastric lumen. Although the amount of aluminum hydroxide will not effectively neutralize gastric acidity, it appears to be the stimulus for potentiated formation of local mediators which protect the gastric mucosa, such as PGs (Jensen and Jensen 1992; Hollander and Tarnawski 1990) and possibly sulfhydryl ions. Sucralfate binds epidermal growth factor, thus causing it to accumulate in ulcerated lesions (Hollander and Tarnawski 1990). Sucralfate also increases mucosal blood flow, either by inducing local nitric oxide or PG production (Konturek et al. 1992) or by directly stimulating mucosal angiogenesis (Szabo et al. 1991). PG synthesis is enhanced by sucralfate (Slomiany et al. 1991).

Sucralfate is minimally absorbed following oral administration and is associated with few, if any, side effects. Sucralfate is recognized to be the safest drug available for treatment of gastroduodenal ulcers (Jensen and Jensen 1992). The maximum protective effects of sucralfate depend on an acid environment ($pH < 5$) for activation (Konturek et al. 1991). Sucralfate binds and inhibits cimetidine. Thus, these two drugs probably should be alternated (i.e., administer sucralfate 1-2 hr prior to cimetidine) in patients receiving both drugs. In addition to cimetidine, sucralfate will bind to and prevent the absorption of a number of other orally administered drugs and should not be administered simultaneously with another oral drug. Currently, sucralfate is recommended for treatment of gastroduodenal ulceration, regardless of the cause. Its use prophylactically is also recommended for illnesses associated with ulceration such as renal or liver disease, mastocytosis, and inflammatory bowel diseases for which prolonged use of anti-PG is indicated. Sucralfate also appears beneficial prophylactically in patients receiving NSAID therapy (Konturek et al. 1991). Sucralfate is effective for treatment of acid-induced esophagitis (Katz et al. 1988).

MODULATORS OF GASTRIC MOTILITY. The regulation of electrical and mechanical activity of GI smooth muscle can be subdivided into three levels: the extrinsic system, comprising vagal and sympathetic nerves; the enteric, or intrinsic, system of nerves and ganglia located between the longitudinal and smooth muscles; and the receptors—at least 10—located on the smooth muscle cell. Both neurotransmitters and neuropeptides interact with the receptors with variable effects (Demol et al. 1989).

Cholinergic receptors are excited by ACh. Muscarinic (M_2) receptors regulate phasic bowel movements during fasting. Adrenergic receptors include α_1, β_1, and β_2, located postsynaptically, and α_2, located presynaptically; they regulate ACh release from the myenteric plexus. The net effect is stimulation of peristalsis to stimulate ACh release, whereas α_2 receptor stimulation inhibits ACh release (Demol et al. 1989). Both H_1 and H_2 receptors have been identified in the GI tract. They are located both prejunctionally, where they control ACh release, and postjunctionally. Stimulation of H_1 receptors induces smooth muscle contraction, whereas H_2 receptor stimulation induces relaxation (Demol et al. 1989). Serotoninergic receptor stimulation results in complex neural and myogenic responses in the GI tract. Presynaptically, these receptors inhibit ACh release, activation of cholinergic neurons in the myenteric plexus, and activation of the noncholinergic, nonadrenergic inhibitory neurons responsible for bowel relaxation (Demol et al. 1989). Prostanoids, and specifically PGE receptors, have been identified in the gastric fundus and ileum. PGE receptors are thought to be important in the modulation of GI motility from the esophagus to the colon (Demol et al. 1989). Generally, PGE inhibits mechanical activity of circular smooth muscle, while PGs of the D and F series are stimulatory. At high doses, PGEs stimulate peristaltic activity, although this may represent mechanical response to excess watery fluid in the intestinal lumen (Demol et al. 1989). Several agents promote the functional activity of the stomach by increasing secretions and motility.

Prokinetics. Prokinetics enhance the transit of intraluminal contents (Reynolds 1989). The mechanisms of action of these drugs are varied and are not completely understood. Their effect on intestinal functions generally reflects either promotion of an agonist, such as ACh by muscarinic drugs, or inhibition of an inhibitory transmitter, such as dopamine (Reynolds 1989). Organ- and species-specific differences complicate our comprehension of these drugs (Reynolds 1989). Clinically, the use of these drugs is limited by their tendency to cause systemic effects.

CHOLINERGICS. Bethanechol is a cholinergic agonist. As an ester derivative of choline, it acts almost exclusively at muscarinic (M_2) receptors (Demol et al. 1989). Bethanechol will enhance the amplitude of contractions throughout the GI tract, including the lower esophageal sphincter (Demol et al. 1989; Reynolds 1989). However, its effects on the coordination of small-intestinal contraction may be minimal, and thus it is often not considered to be a prokinetic agent (Reynolds 1989). Adverse effects reflect direct enhanced parasympathomimetic stimulation and include abdominal cramps, diarrhea, salivation, and bradycardia (Reynolds 1989).

METOCLOPRAMIDE. Metoclopramide is a lipid-soluble derivative of para-aminobenzoic acid. It is structurally related to procainamide, a cardiac antiarrhythmic (Reynolds 1989). In addition to its central antidopaminergic (antiemetic) effects, metoclopramide acts peripherally both as an antidopaminergic and as a direct and indirect stimulator of cholinergic receptors (Reynolds 1989; Burrows 1983). Although clinically its effects appear to be limited to the upper intestinal tract (Hunt and Gerring 1986; Wingate et al. 1980; Burrows 1983; Albibi and McCallum 1983; Hunt and Gerring 1986), in vitro studies suggest that the most dramatic effects of metoclopramide are on the colon. The peripheral effects of metoclopramide apparently reflect enhanced release of ACh from intrinsic cholinergic neurons. These effects are completely inhibited by pretreatment with atropine (Reynolds 1989; Albibi and McCallum 1983; Sojka et al. 1988). Peripheral effects may also be mediated by effects on other local neurotransmitters such as dopamine and serotonin (Reynolds 1989). Dopamine has an inhibitor effect on smooth muscle of the stomach, duodenum, and colon and has been implicated as a mediator of receptive relaxation in dogs (Reynolds 1989). Dopamine may exert its inhibitor effect through inhibition of ACh, thus explaining the complex mechanism of metoclopramide (Reynolds 1989). Peripheral antidopaminergic effects of metoclopramide appear to reflect interaction with D_2 receptors (Reynolds 1989). Metoclopramide physiologically antagonizes emesis by increasing the tone in the lower esophageal sphincter, increasing the force and frequency of gastric antral contractions (gastrokinetic effect), relaxing the pyloric sphincter, and promoting peristalsis in the duodenum and jejunum, resulting in accelerated gastric emptying and upper intestinal transit (Burrows 1983).

Metoclopramide is well absorbed orally but undergoes significant first-pass metabolism, with a bioavailability in the 50-70% range. Tissue distribution is rapid, and excretion is both renal and hepatic. The plasma half-life in the dog is only 90 minutes, and metoclopramide has a short duration of action (Burrows 1983). Dose-dependent CNS side effects range from nervousness and restlessness to listlessness, depression, and disorientation (Reynolds 1989; Clark and Becht 1987; Burrows 1983). Extrapyramidal antidopaminergic effects include tremors and motor restlessness. Gynecomastia due to enhanced release of prolactin has been reported in humans (Reynolds 1989). GI disorders may also be observed, with constipation being common with long-term use. As an antiemetic, the main indications of metoclopramide include severe and intractable emesis caused by chemotherapy or other blood-borne toxins, nausea and vomition associated with delayed gastric emptying, gastroesophageal reflux, reflux gastritis, and peptic ulceration. As a prokinetic, metoclopramide is indicated for treatment of a variety of gastric motility disorders, including gastric dilatation, volvulus, postoperative ileus, gastric ulceration, and idiopathic gastroparesis (Albibi and McCallum 1983). Metoclopramide is contraindicated in GI obstruction or perforation, in epilepsy, and in patients receiving neuroleptics. Because of their anticholinergic effects, atropine and the opioid analgesics will antagonize the action of metoclopramide.

Metoclopamide appears to competitively antagonize dopamine-induced renal arterial relaxation. The effect has been documented in renal perfusion models of several species (Brodde 1982). In the anesthetized dog, 1 mg/kg of metoclopramide reduced renal vasodilatory response to dopamine by 42%; 10 mg/kg attenuated essentially all vasodilatory response (Hahn and Wardell 1980). The effect of the clinically recommended dose of metoclopramide on renal vasculature has not been documented. In contrast, in human volunteers, metoclopramide had no effect on basal renal vascular resistance (Manara et al. 1991).

DOMPERIDONE. Domperidone is a dopamine antagonist whose prokinetic properties are similar to metoclopramide (Takahashi et al. 1991). It has no cholinergic activity and is not inhibited by atropine. Domperidone does not cross the blood-brain barrier as readily as metoclopramide. However, like metoclopramide, domperidone can affect central dopamine receptors and thus modulate temperature control, prolactin secretion, and activity at the CTZ (Reynolds 1989). Extrapyramidal side effects are rare. It acts peripherally to coordinate antroduodenal contractions. Its peripheral effects accelerate small-intestinal transit, but colonic activity is apparently unaffected (Clark and Becht 1987).

CISAPRIDE. Cisapride has the broadest spectrum of action of the prokinetic agents (McCallum et al. 1988). It causes dose-dependent increased activity at all sites (stomach, jejunum, ileum, small and large colon) in horses (King and Gerring 1988). Because it does not interact with dopamine receptors, its use is not associated with extrapyramidal side effects (Demol et al. 1989). Its prokinetic actions appear to reflect indirect stimulation of cholinergic nerves. Because secretion is not enhanced, stimulation probably occurs at the level of the myenteric plexus (Reynolds 1989; Edelbroek et al. 1995). Like metoclopramide and domperidone, cisapride also enhances antroduodenal contractility (Reynolds 1989). Prokinetic effects have been documented in the esophagus, stomach, small bowel, and colon (Reynolds 1989). Well absorbed following oral administration, cisapride undergoes first-pass metabolism; oral bioavailability in human beings is 50%. Metabolites are apparently inactive. Volume of distribution is large (2.4 L/kg) in humans and elimination half-life is 10 hours. Elimination may be prolonged in the presence of liver disease (McCallum et al. 1988).

Cisapride kinetics have been described in adult horses. After IV administration of 0.1 mg/kg, peak plasma concentration was 221 ng/mL and elimination half-life was 1.9 hours. Rectal administration also has been studied, although bioavailability was only 1.23% (Cook et al. 1997).

Cisapride appears to coordinate GI motility in horses and cows by acting on 5-hydroxytryptamine receptors (Steiner and Roussel 1995). In horses, cisapride has proven useful for selected disorders of GI motility (Dart and Hodgson 1998; Milne et al. 1996; Steiner and Roussel 1995).

MODULATION OF INTESTINAL MOTILITY AND SECRETION. Diarrhea may be associated with intestinal hypomotility as well as hypermotility. Ordered intestinal motility results from a balance between hormonal, myogenic, and neurogenic factors. It is a complex, physiologic event (Crema and De Ponti 1989). Several forms of coordinated movement occur in the intestine which mix the liquefied contents and propel it in an aboral direction. Rhythmic segmentations are caused by simple nonprogressive contractions of circular muscle. They result in mixing movements and promote absorption of intestinal lumen contents by narrowing the effective diameter of the intestinal lumen, thus impeding flow of fluid intestinal contents. Contraction of longitudinal smooth muscle results in peristaltic movements and aboral movement of intestinal contents. Although peristaltic activity is mainly propulsive, it also ensures mixing and successful absorption. Both longitudinal and circular smooth muscles are involved in peristaltic movements. Activity in the small bowel differs from that in the large bowel. Generally, slow waves occur continuously and propagate aborally. In the colon, slow waves are sometimes absent and propagation may be variable (Crema and De Ponti, 1989). Intestinal motility is integrated at several levels: locally, at autonomic ganglia; and in the CNS, at both spinal and supraspinal levels (Crema and De Ponti 1989). Several types of muscarinic receptors have been identified (M_1, M_2, and M_3) in the GI tract. M_1 receptors present in the myenteric plexus may inhibit motility via GABA-mediated mechanisms. M_2 receptors located pre- and postsynaptically mediate presynaptic inhibition of ACh release. M_3 receptors appear to be located on smooth muscle cells (Crema and De Ponti 1989).

Absorption in the small intestine occurs first by passive sodium absorption across the luminal membrane and second by active secretion of the sodium across the basolateral membrane. Water osmotically follows sodium into the lateral intracellular space. The electrochemical gradient caused by sodium movement facilitates chloride diffusion into the cell (Hughes 1983). A specific brush-border carrier for NaCl cotransport accomplishes absorption. However, nutrients such as glucose and other organic solutes facilitate a solvent drag of water and electrolytes as they enter cells (Hughes 1983).

Secretion in crypt cells of the intestinal epithelium is initiated by intracellular signaling (cAMP) or calcium. Increased chloride conductance into the lumen results in sodium recycling, first through the lateral intercellular space and second into the lumen. Although NaCl cotransport is inhibited, NaCl movement due to solvent drag (i.e., that mediated by nutrients) is not (Hughes 1983).

Increased amounts of fecal water reflect either diminished absorption or a net secretion (accumulation) of fluid into the lumen of the intestine. In all diarrheal states, increased fecal water loss is associated with an overall secretion of electrolytes and water in selected segments of the GI tract. The absorptive capacity of the alimentary canal is overwhelmed distal to the site of secretion. Sodium-absorbing cells are present predominantly on the villi, and chloride-secreting cells are located primarily in the crypts. Increased intestinal cell cyclic 3′5′ adenosine monophosphate, cyclic guanosine 3′5′ monophosphate, and Ca^{++} (through calmodulin) all have similar effects on sodium-absorptive and chloride-secretory cells, producing diminished sodium absorption and increased chloride secretion with a net efflux of water into the lumen. Cholera enterotoxin is the best known intestinal secretagogue (Hughes 1983), but several hormones, including vasoactive intestinal peptide (VIP), gastric inhibitory peptide, cholecystokinin, secretin, glucagon, and PGE_1, are also associated with net fluid accumulation, as are other infectious agents (e.g., *E. coli, Staphylococcus* spp.) (Hughes 1983). Several laxative agents such as bile acids and ricinoleic acid are also thought to act through this mechanism. The exact role of intestinal motility in the alteration of fluid and electrolyte movement is still unclear. The role of mucosal permeability or mucosal damage in the genesis of fluid accumulation within the gut lumen is still obscure.

Substantial evidence exists linking GI secretion with GI motility (Greenwood et al. 1987). Increased motility is usually accompanied by increased fluid and electrolyte secretion (Greenwood et al. 1987).

Rehydration followed by oral replacement therapy has received a lot of attention as the preferred treatment for diarrheas associated with infectious agents (Hughes 1983). Suitable solutions contain K^+, HCO_3^-, Na^+, and glucose in sufficient quantities to replace stool losses (Hughes 1983).

A pyrrazolone derivative, methampyrone (dipyrone), is used for treatment of equine colic and of GI hypermotility or spasm in several species. However, other than for bradykinin-induced spasm, methampyrone has little effect on spontaneous intestinal motility or intestinal spasm produced by a variety of stimulants (Gray and Yano 1975).

Anticholinergic Agents. Parasympatholytic, or antimuscarinic, agents diminish motor and secretory activity of the GI tract. Tone and propulsive movements are decreased, and these agents will often relax spasm of visceral smooth muscle. Such antimuscarinic drugs are known as antispasmodics or spasmolytics. Although cholinolytic agents are commonly used as spasmolytics in antidiarrheal mixtures, severe forms of diarrhea may occur in the presence of drug-induced intestinal paralysis or ileus. The main benefit of anticholinergic agents may be related to their ability to reduce intestinal secretions. This group of drugs should not be used indiscriminately to control diarrhea, especially in the horse.

Antimuscarinic agents used as spasmolytics include the belladonna alkaloids (atropine and hyoscine), their congeners (atropine methonitrate, homatropine methobromide, hyoscine butylbromide, anisotropine methylbromide), and synthetic cholinolytics (aminopentamide, dicyclomine, glycopyrrolate, mepenzolate, oxyphenonium, propantheline, benzetimide, pipenzolate, clidinium, camylofine). Many of the belladonna alkaloid derivatives are substituted tertiary amines and thus may have undesirable CNS and other systemic effects. The synthetic groups are mostly substituted quaternary amines and are devoid of CNS effects. Xerostomia, loss of lens accommodation, urinary retention, constipation, tachycardia, and CNS stimulation are potential side effects that may be encountered when parasympatholytics are administered.

Opioids

ENDOGENOUS OPIATES. Opiates have been used since antiquity to control diarrhea. Opioids appear to influence normal GI physiology (Kromer 1988). Opioids may stimulate GI motility both locally and by central effects in the brain or spinal cord (Demol et al. 1989). Both opioid peptides and opioid receptors have been identified throughout the GI tract. The number and type vary with the species. Endogenous opioids are present in high concentrations in the intestinal wall. Biosynthesis of enkephalins has been demonstrated in the myenteric plexus of some species. In addition, antral G cells are thought to be capable of synthesizing enkephalins or endorphins. Beta endorphin and dynorphin have also been detected. In cats, enkephalin has been detected in both myenteric and submucosal plexuses. In contrast to other species, the predominant location of enkephalin neurons in dogs is the submucosal plexus. Opioid nerve fibers have also been documented in the lower esophagus, pyloric junction, and cardiac and ileocecal regions. Specific degradative enzymes for the opioid peptides have also been identified in similar locations (Kromer 1988).

Location of opioid receptors in the GI tract has been based on the physiologic effects of opioid agonists and antagonists (Kromer 1988; Allescher et al. 1989; Shook et al. 1989). Both in vitro and in vivo preparations have been studied, often with conflicting results. High-affinity, reversible, and saturable binding of opioid receptors has been identified in longitudinal and circular smooth muscles and the myenteric and submucosal plexuses. Binding has also been noted in the muscularis mucosae. Although multiple opioid receptors have been identified, mu- and delta-type opioid binding sites appear to predominate. Morphine stimulates mu receptors of the myenteric plexus, thus inducing migrating motor activity in the duodenum and jejunum. The relative importance of different receptor types in the control of intestinal peristalsis has not been established.

GI MOTILITY. In vitro studies indicate that normal functions attributed to endogenous opioids in the GI tract include modulation of GI motility and gastrin release. In vitro peristalsis results from phasic circular muscle contractions which travel down the intestinal segment, thereby expelling contents distally. It is easily distinguished from in vitro pendular movements or segmentations. Exogenous opioids depress the normal peristaltic reflex and thus appear to control normal peristalsis. This effect has been repetitively demonstrated with the use of the pure antagonist naloxone, which consistently increases peristaltic activity. Naloxone increases the duration of rhythmic peristaltic intervals; terminates the interval if applied at the appropriate time; shortens the interval; and increases the frequency of peristaltic waves. The net effect is enhancement of overall peristalsis. Control of peristalsis is thought to be at the neuronal level. The intestinal opioid mechanism has been documented throughout the intestinal tract by in vitro studies, although its functional role appears to increase from duodenum to ileum. Endogenous opioids may thus be partially responsible for the "gradient of intestine," a term describing the oral-to-aboral phenomenon of decreasing frequency of peristaltic waves and decreasing sensitivity to distension stimuli (Kromer 1988). GI opioids are thought to be subject to feedback control (Kromer 1988).

Although most studies have documented an inhibitory role for endogenous opioids in peristaltic activity, opioids are associated with both excitatory and inhibitory mechanisms, depending on the region, the opioid, and the motility pattern studied. Similarly, the effect of opioids on GI sphincters varies. The net effect may be dose dependent. For example, excitation (contraction) of the choledochoduodenal junction in dogs occurs at doses lower than those causing inhibition. Although species differences have been documented for the sites of action, for the receptor populations, and for the motility caused by opioids, these differences are more often quantitative rather than qualitative (Kromer 1988).

The widely accepted mechanism of opioid actions in the GI tract is inhibition of ACh release. However, modulation of the effects of ACh already released is thought to be important for the effects of opioids on peristalsis. Intracellular mechanisms may involve increased calcium-dependent potassium conductance and hyperpolarization. The spasmogenic effect caused by opioids is antagonized by atropine. Opioids also reduce calcium entry during the action potential and deplete neurons of calcium. Although ACh is generally recognized to be the predominate neurotransmitter modulated by the opioids, modulation of other endogenous mediators such as serotonin is also likely (Kromer 1988).

GI SECRETION. As with motility, the effect of opioids on gastric acid secretion varies with the study, species, and opioid. Opioids enhance gastric acid secretion mediated by histamine in in vitro studies, but the effect on ACh-induced secretion varies in in vivo studies. Dose dependency may account for some of the variability, with excitation or enhancement of basal secretion occurring at lower doses and inhibition at higher doses. A dual effect on stimulated gastric acid secretion appears to be mediated both peripherally and centrally (Kromer 1988).

In contrast to gastric secretion, the effect of opioids on intestinal secretion appears to be consistent among the species (Kromer, 1988). Opioids stimulate the net absorption of water and electrolytes in enterocytes of both small and large intestines in a variety of species. In vitro studies indicate that these peripheral effects are mediated by delta receptors. However, receptor types may vary with the site. These effects, which may reflect facilitated absorption or inhibited secretion, are largely responsible for the antidiarrheal properties of the opioids. Several mediators, acting both centrally and peripherally, may signal the antisecretory effect of the opioids. The ability of opioids to modulate secretion is likely to vary with the chemical mediator. Presynaptic inhibition of ACh release and inhibition of PG-mediated adenylate cyclase activity have been implicated as the site of inhibition. Sodium, but not chloride, appears to be the ion negatively influenced. Bicarbonate-increased sensitization of the GI tract to blood flow has been implicated in the dog, perhaps due to release of histamine. Modulation of the sympathetic nervous system has also been implicated in the central antisecretory effects of the opioids. Antisecretory effects may involve norepinephrine and its effects on vasoinhibitory peptide, PGE, or ACh (Demol et al. 1989). Although the actual mechanism for these effects has not been described, decreased intracellular free calcium has been implicated as a possibility. Studies usually focus on enterocytes, but antisecretory effects may also result from actions at the neuronal plexuses. Opioids increase bicarbonate, rather than water and electrolyte, secretion from the gastric and duodenal mucosa (Kromer 1988).

Diphenoxylate hydrochloride is a meperidine derivative used specifically to control diarrhea. It is often administered in combination with atropine-like compounds. Its action is largely dependent on a direct peripheral effect on the GI wall. Loperamide hydrochloride, a butyramide derivative, is an orally active and effective antidiarrheal agent used in symptomatic control of acute and chronic nonspecific diarrhea. Unlike with diphenoxylate, systemic opiate agonist effects do not appear to occur following oral administration of loperamide, and there are few side effects. Although loperamide has some structural similarities to diphenoxylate, it does not cross the blood-brain barrier, and it differs both qualitatively and quantitatively from diphenoxylate and difenoxin in its pharmacologic actions (Schiller et al. 1984). Intestinal transit time and intestinal luminal capacity increase following treatment with loperamide (Demol et al. 1989).

Miscellaneous Antisecretory Drugs. There are a number of potentially useful drugs that have not been extensively studied but for which there is some evidence of clinical benefit. Glucocorticoids have been found to be beneficial in treating refractory chronic diarrheal disease as well as chronic inflammatory diseases of the intestinal tract. Glucocorticoids stimulate active sodium absorption in the jejunum, ileum, cecum, and colon. Because of many undesirable side effects when used chronically, the glucocorticoids should not be used on a routine basis to treat diarrhea. Adrenergic agents appear to act predominantly by increasing basal fluid absorption and do so at very low concentrations. The mechanisms involved are unclear. Clonidine and other α_2-adrenergic agonists are potentially useful in this regard. Calcium-calmodulin antagonists may act by stimulating active absorption as well as by inhibiting intestinal secretion, but the precise mode of action of these drugs is not clear. Several drugs with this effect have been found to be useful in the control of certain forms of secretory diarrhea. Examples include chlorpromazine and trifluoperazine. NSAIDs such as aspirin, indomethacin, flunixin, and the subsalicylate of bismuth inhibit the cyclooxygenase pathway of arachidonic acid metabolism and thereby suppress the formation of PG mediators. The roles of various PGs in intestinal motility as well as in absorption and secretory processes are complex, and the inhibition of PG synthesis does not consistently influence secretory diarrheal states. However, NSAIDs may prove to be therapeutically beneficial in some acute and chronic diarrheal syndromes. A sulftidine (sulfasalazine) is a product that is metabolized to 5-aminosalicylic acid and sulfadiazine by colonic microbes (Robinson 1989). Either of the two components (i.e., anti-inflammatory or antimicrobial) may be efficacious in the treatment of chronic inflammatory bowel diseases such as ulcerative colitis. As with all aspirin-containing compounds, caution is indicated when a sulfasalazine is used in the cat since salicylic acid released in the colon can be subsequently absorbed.

Cholestyramine resin is a resin that binds bile acids and endotoxin within the lumen of the intestine. It has been used in humans principally for control of hypercholesterolemic syndromes and for treatment of intractable diarrhea.

GI PROTECTANTS AND ADSORBENTS. Compounds that are not absorbed from the GI tract and either line the mucosal surface or adsorb toxic compounds are often incorporated into antidiarrheal mixtures. The protectants seemingly produce a coating of the GI epithelium that prevents irritation or erosion by potentially harmful substances. The adsorbents physically bind chemical compounds, which precludes their absorption, and they are then eliminated in the feces. Use of these two therapeutic classes is obviously directed at potentially harmful agents of either inorganic or organic nature. However, adsorbents will also bind concurrently administered drugs used for therapeutic purposes.

Many protectants and adsorbents possess both properties to varying degrees. Those most frequently used are magnesium trisilicate, hydrated magnesium aluminum trisilicate (activated attapulgite), kaolin (natural hydrated aluminum silicate), aluminum hydroxide and phosphate, bismuth salts, calcium carbonate, pectin (natural polygalacturonic acids), and activated charcoal.

The combination kaolin-pectin product is dissolved in 20 parts water. Described as a demulcent and adsorbent, the drug supposedly binds and removes bacteria and their metabolic products and toxins. These effects are controversial. While stool consistency may improve, studies do not indicate that fluid and electrolyte imbalance is corrected, nor is the course of disease shortened (Wilcke and Turner 1987).

The insoluble bismuth salts have been used for over 400 years (DuPont 1987). Products include bismuth subcarbonate, bismuth subnitrate, and bismuth subsalicylate. Bismuth subsalicylate is a crystalline 1:1 trivalent bismuth and salicylate compound. It is chemically transformed throughout the GI tract to bismuth and salicylate. The drug has been shown to have both antisecretory and antimicrobial effects in several species (DuPont 1987). The subsalicylate fraction has been shown to have anti-PG synthetase effects, which would enhance its action in controlling diarrheal syndromes (Hughes 1983). In people and cats, nearly all the salicylate is systemically available (Papich et al. 1987; DuPont 1987). Caution is recommended in order to prevent salicylate toxicity in cats receiving this drug.

Activated charcoal has primarily adsorbent properties. Because of its broad spectrum of adsorptive activity and its rapidity of action, it is one of the most valuable agents for emergency treatment of certain cases of poisoning. It forms a stable complex with many substances and permits their evacuation from the body. Charcoal preparations vary according to the source of base material, surface area, capacity for drug binding, and affinity and avidity of drug binding (Watson 1987). Source materials are usually lignite, wood, or peat. Activation forms more pores and enlarges the surface area. Activation time is directly correlated to the molecular size of compounds adsorbed. Since most drugs are of an intermediate molecular weight, charcoals with pore sizes between 10 and 20 Å (100 and 200 nm) are most appropriate (Wilcke and Turner 1987). Administration with a cathartic, such as sorbitol, is a common practice and facilitates rapid movement of the charcoal-toxin complex (Watson 1987). Activated charcoal loses its efficacy as the time interval between treatment and toxin ingestion increases. The optimal dose and interval for administration of activated charcoal has not been well established (Watson 1987), although a charcoal-to-toxicant ratio of 10:1 has been recommended (Wilcke and Turner 1987). One source suggests treatment at 6-hour intervals (Watson 1987). Powders are superior to tablets (Wilcke and Turner 1987). Food generally decreases the efficacy of these products. In the common domestic species, 20-120 mg/kg powdered activated charcoal are usually administered as a drench after mixing with water. An activated charcoal suspension may be used for gas lavage in simple-stomached animals.

Cholestyramine is a basic anion exchange resin that binds to acidic side chains such as those occurring in bile acids. In order to increase the number of basic binding sites, cholestyramine is attached to a polystyrene matrix which can act as a nonspecific adsorbent. As bile salts are bound in the GI tract, lipoprotein, cholesterol, and neutral fat absorption are also decreased. Although specifically indicated for pruritus associated with increased bile acids, cholestyramine has also been used to symptomatically treat diarrhea. Nausea, constipation, steatorrhea, and decreased fat-soluble vitamin absorption are reported undesirable effects. The product should be administered in food or water (Wilcke and Turner 1987).

LAXATIVES AND CATHARTICS. Laxatives and cathartics promote defecation by increasing frequency of defection or fecal volume or consistency (Clark and Becht 1987; Dimski 1989; Horn 1987; Burrows 1984). Laxatives (or aperients) promote elimination of a soft-formed stool, whereas cathartics (or purgatives) tend to produce a more fluid evacuation. The difference between these two effects may be just a matter of dose, but in some instances laxatives are only capable of increasing the hydration or softness of the fecal mass without ever inducing catharsis. The enhanced intestinal transit times that occur with use of some of these cathartics are usually due to intrinsic local myenteric reflexes within the visceral smooth muscle or to stimulation of the cholinergic receptors of the extrinsic parasympathetic nervous system. Although a traditional classification of the group will be presented here, it should be noted that many cathartics alter intestinal electrolyte transport to increase fecal water excretion, so the grouping of these compounds should perhaps more logically follow their effects on intestinal electrolyte movement (Thompson 1980).

Emollient Laxatives. The emollient laxatives (lubricant laxatives, mechanical laxatives, fecal softeners) act unchanged. They are not absorbed to any appreciable extent and simply soften and lubricate the fecal mass, which in turn facilitates expulsion. Though not always reliable, particularly in the ruminant, they are used in all species.

Mineral oil (liquid paraffin) is very commonly employed as a lubricant laxative. Mineral oil is bland and generally safe to use, but a few untoward effects may be encountered. Chronic administration may impair absorption of fat-soluble vitamins, other nutrients, and coadministered therapeutic agents. Decreased irritability of the intestinal mucosa becomes evident with protracted use and, paradoxically, chronic constipation may ensue. Lipid pneumonitis, following maladministration into the trachea and bronchial tree, is a serious complication. Following prolonged use, limited absorption of mineral oil, principally into the intestinal lymphatics but also into the intestinal wall and even the liver, does take place. The subsequent tissue reaction leads to development of granulomatous lesions. Anal leakage of mineral oil may be a nuisance in a house pet and will interfere with healing of wounds in the anorectal area. Administration of mineral oil to confirm or treat intestinal obstruction has a shortcoming; the oil may easily bypass a partial obstruction, and its presence in the anal area may lead to a false conclusion. White or yellow soft paraffins are also used as lubricant laxatives (e.g., cats with hair balls).

Several anionic surfactants are employed as fecal softeners. Examples include docusate sodium (previously named dioctyl sodium sulfosuccinate) and dioctyl calcium sulfosuccinate.

Simple Bulk Laxatives. The simple bulk laxatives are hydrophilic in nature and are not digested within the GI tract. They absorb water and swell, and an emollient gel forms. The increased volume or bulk leads to distension, with resultant reflex contraction producing peristaltic activity. The feces remain soft and hydrated. Methylcellulose, carboxymethylcellulose sodium, and plantago seed (psyllium seed) are examples of simple bulk purgatives. Wheat bran, prunes, and other fruits also belong in this group. Besides the bulk action of these laxatives, it should be noted that the celluloses and hemicelluloses present are fermented in the hind gut by bacteria to produce volatile fatty acids and other products that in turn exert an osmotic effect and thus enhance laxative action. Meteorism and a very fluid stool often result from the use of simple bulk laxatives.

Osmotic Cathartics. The osmotic cathartics (saline purgatives) consist of salts or compounds that either are not absorbed at all or are only slowly and incompletely absorbed from the GI tract. They retain or attract water into the intestinal lumen mainly by osmotic forces, although enhanced mucosal secretion of fluid may contribute to their effect. It is imperative that drinking water be made freely available to an animal that has been dosed with an osmotic cathartic; use of this group of purgatives is contraindicated in dehydrated animals. In monogastric animals an effect may generally be anticipated in 3-12 hours, and in ruminants within about 18 hours of dosing.

Magnesium salts are frequently used as saline purgatives. Magnesium ions also bring about release of CCK, which will increase peristaltic activity. Magnesium sulfate (Epsom salts), isotonic in a 6% solution, magnesium hydroxide, magnesium oxide (milk of magnesia), and magnesium citrate are the magnesium salts most commonly employed. The solutions need not be hypertonic to produce an effect. About 20% of the magnesium ions are absorbed when magnesium sulfate is dosed orally, and if purgation does not occur, additional amounts of magnesium may be absorbed with subsequent depression of the excitable tissues in the body. This is even more likely to occur if renal function is impaired. Magnesium sulfate is not often used in horses.

Salts such as sodium sulfate (Glauber's salt), sodium phosphate, potassium sodium tartrate (Rochelle salt), and even large quantities of sodium chloride are effective saline purgatives.

The sugar alcohols mannitol and sorbitol will also induce an osmotic catharsis as will the synthetic disaccharide lactulose, which is not digested in the small intestine because no specific enteric enzyme is present. It passes to the large intestine, where saccharolytic microflora ferment lactulose to produce acetic, lactic, and other organic acids, which in turn lower the pH of the colonic content and exert an osmotic effect. Water is attracted, the fecal mass softens, and colonic peristalsis ensues. Lactulose is used for chronic constipation and treatment of hepatic encephalopathy. Acidification of the content of the large intestine favors greater formation of the nonabsorbable ammonium ion than the readily absorbable ammonia molecule, which requires detoxification in the liver by the urea cycle. Hyperammo-nemia is thus prevented to some degree. Absorption of other toxic amines from the hind gut is also reduced by acidification of the contents. Some meteorism may be evident following administration of lactulose.

Irritant Cathartics. Contact or irritant purgatives were thought to stimulate the mucosal lining of the GI tract and thereby initiate local myenteric reflexes that would enhance intestinal transit. However, it now seems that members of this group also provoke fluid accumulation in the lumen by activating secretory mechanisms. Irritant cathartics are regarded as direct acting or indirect acting depending on whether a metabolic alteration is first required to form an active product.

Several bland vegetable oils act as irritant purgatives. Their action is based on hydrolysis by pancreatic lipase in the small intestine and subsequent formation of sodium and potassium salts of the released fatty acids. These are then irritant soaps, which differ in potency depending on the oil used. Castor oil produces highly irritant ricinoleates; raw linseed oil leads to formation of less irritant linoleates; and olive oil leads to rather mild oliveates. The response to castor oil is prompt, and evacuation of the whole intestinal tract occurs, leading to an almost complete emptying. Moist bulky feeds are needed following purgation with castor oil. It is used mainly in nonruminants and is often employed in calves and foals. The effect occurs in 4-8 hours in small animals and 12-18 hours in large animals.

Another group belonging in this class includes the diphenylmethane cathartics, which appear to have a greater effect on the large intestine. Their precise mechanism of action is unclear. An effect is usually seen within 6-8 hours, and excessive catharsis may occur with overdosage. Phenolphthalein, the well-known indicator, is a potent purgative but only in primates and swine. Bisacodyl also is a diphenylmethane cathartic that inhibits glucose absorption and Na^+,K^+-ATPase activity as well as altering motor activity of the visceral smooth muscle. Only about 5% of any dose of bisacodyl is absorbed. This agent is used both orally and by enema.

Anthraquinone cathartics, also known as the emodin purgatives, exert an indirect secondary purgative action. They are mainly of plant origin, but a synthetic compound, to which all the anthraquinone derivatives are related, is the prototype of the group. This substance is 1,8-dihydroxyanthraquinone, or danthron. The other anthraquinones are precursor glycosides, which may be absorbed from the intestinal tract to some extent, but the portion remaining in the gut is hydrolyzed by bacterial enzymes in the large intestine to release the active aglycones known as emodins. These cathartics are not effective if transit through the small intestine is delayed. Their action is principally on the large intestine, where the myenteric plexuses are stimulated. With prolonged use of these agents, these myenteric plexuses actually degenerate, with a resultant loss in intestinal motility. The effect of danthron may be manifested within 6-14 hours in small animals and within 12-36 hours in large animals. Repeated dosing should be avoided in large animals because of the long latent period. A too hasty second administration may lead to severe superpurgation, especially in the horse. Sufficient anthraquinone can distribute into milk to affect nursing young. Urine color may show changes following administration of members of this group. The naturally occurring anthraquinone glycosides include senna and other sennosides from *Cassia* spp., cascara sagrada from *Rhamnus* spp., and aloins from *Aloe* spp.

Some purgatives are so highly irritant that they may cause severe colic and superpurgation.

Neuromuscular Purgatives. Cholinergic agents with muscarinic actions will initiate hypermotility of the GI tract and promote defecation and urination. Peristaltic activity increases within 10-30 minutes following parenteral administration and within 2-4 hours following oral administration. Neostigmine, physostigmine, bethanecol, and carbachol have been used for this purpose. Neostigmine has fewer side effects than the others. Colic may be precipitated, so care should always be taken when using these agents when a mechanical obstruction is present or viability of the bowel is doubtful. Several other substances will also stimulate visceral smooth muscle to contract, either directly or indirectly. Vasopressin, oxytocin, $PGF_{2\alpha}$, and other PG analogs are capable of promoting evacuation of the rectum. Oxytocin and neostigmine have been shown to stimulate release of VIP from the intestine, so the mechanism of action of this group may be more complex than at first believed.

A number of deleterious effects may occur with excessive or constant use of cathartics. Severe, continuous diarrhea and abdominal colic, leading to dehydration and even shock, may follow overdosage. Other potentially harmful effects include decreased sensitivity of the intestinal mucosa, megacolon, flatulence, loss of electrolytes (especially sodium, potassium, chloride, and bicarbonate), secondary aldosteronism, melanosis coli (anthraquinones), steatorrhea, protein-losing gastroenteropathy, excessive calcium loss with resultant osteomalacia, and exacerbation of inflammatory intestinal disease. Several drugs can also distribute into milk and adversely affect suckling young.

Enemas. Introduction of solutions or suppositories into the rectum to initiate the defecation reflex is a useful and simple method to correct constipation.

Many preparations have successfully served as enemas, including soapy water (soft anionic soap), isotonic or hypertonic sodium chloride solutions, sorbitol, glycerol, surfactants such as sodium lauryl sulfoacetate, mineral oil, and olive oil. Enema preparations that contain phosphate should not be used in cats indiscriminately, since they can precipitate potentially fatal hyperphosphatemia, hypocalcemia, and hypernatremia in cats (Atkins et al. 1985) or debilitated animals.

AGENTS PROMOTING DIGESTIVE FUNCTIONS. Several preparations are used therapeutically to control specific GI diseases by promoting digestive processes. These digestants generally consist of normal digestive enzymes or related substances that are used for replacement therapy in deficiency states.

Pepsin preparations are administered with HCl to treat gastric achylia. Pancreatic extracts that simulate or replace deficient pancreatic exocrine secretions are of therapeutic benefit in cases of chronic pancreatitis and pancreatic hypoplasia where glandular function is diminished or destroyed. Pancreatin (Panteric, Stamyl, Viokase) obtained from hog pancreas is the major ingredient of most commercial pancreatic enzyme preparations. Products should be administered as the powder or crushed non-enteric-coated tablets. Enteric-coated tablets should be avoided since they may not be effectively dissolved in an alkaline pH (Strombeck 1990). Dosage is adjusted to obtain a normal stool. Simultaneous administration of nonsystemic alkalinizing agents to maintain an optimal pH range for enzyme activity has not proved to be successful clinically. However, the administration of cimetidine about half an hour before dosing with pancreatic extract does limit gastric inactivation of the enzymes. Proper dietary control is also essential for the successful management of pancreatic insufficiency.

Bile acids and their salts promote absorption of long-chain fatty acids and fat-soluble vitamins. They also act as choleretics (discussed in the next section). Examples include dehydrocholic acid (Decholin) and chenodiol (previously named chenodeoxycholic acid).

Diastases are amylolytic enzymes obtained from malt and *Aspergillus oryzae* and are used for replacement of pancreatic α-amylase and to control flatulence caused by gas produced from soluble carbohydrates by bacterial flora.

DRUGS AFFECTING THE LIVER

Cholagogues and Choleretics. Substances that cause contraction of the gallbladder are called cholagogues. The resistance of the sphincter of Oddi decreases as bile flows freely into the duodenum. Dietary fat and concentrated magnesium sulfate introduced directly into the duodenum through a tube exert a cholagogue effect through release of CCK-pancreozymin from the upper small intestine. Vagus stimulation will also promote contraction of the gallbladder.

Substances that increase secretion of bile by the hepatocytes are known as choleretics. A drug that stimulates the liver to increase output of bile of low specific gravity is called a hydrocholeretic. Production of bile is enhanced by stimulation of the vagus nerves and by the hormone secretin, which increases the water and bicarbonate content of bile. However, physiologically, bile acid salts are mainly responsible for bile secretion: the so-called bile salt-dependent flow. A number of natural bile salts and several partially synthetic derivatives are used therapeutically as choleretics, including dehydrocholic acid, which is the most potent hydrocholeretic agent. Naturally occurring bile acid conjugates such as glycocholate and taurocholate enhance bile flow to a lesser extent. Bile salts used therapeutically have a dual action in directly promoting fat absorption and stimulating biliary secretion after they have been absorbed. Overdosage with these compounds will tend to cause diarrhea.

Ursodeoxycholic acid (UDCA) is a natural bile acid constituting a very small portion of the bile acid pool. It is a degradation production of chenodeoxycholic acid. Among the bile acids, UDCA has the lowest hydrophobic-hydrophilic balance, the lowest capacity to make micelles, and the least potential for cholestatic or cellular membrane toxicity. Since cholestatic liver disease may be associated with accumulation of toxic bile acids, treatment with UDCA is appealing. Its efficacy in a variety of chronic liver diseases has been established. Its mechanism of action is not well understood but is probably related to bile acid metabolism (Heller et al. 1991). The use of UDCA in dogs suffering from selected cholestatic liver diseases has been documented (Meyer and Thompson 1992). The disposition of UDCA has been studied in healthy cats (Nicholson et al. 1989). Sporadic vomiting and diarrhea were reported, but otherwise the drug appears to be safe. Scientific studies establishing its safety and efficacy in diseased animals are indicated.

Liver Protectants and Hepatotropic Agents. A comprehensive review of treatment and management of hepatic disease is beyond the purview of this chapter. However, a selection of the drugs for treatment of liver failure will be listed and the rationale for their use noted. The major pharmacologic properties of many of these substances are discussed elsewhere in the text. Hepatotropic agents are those having a special affinity for the liver or for exerting a specific effect in the liver.

Lipotropic agents hasten removal of fat or decrease its deposition in the liver.

CHOLINE. Choline is an indispensable metabolite of the body. It forms part of a number of endogenous compounds, particularly phospholipids. Phosphatidylcholine, lysophospholipids, plasmalogens, and sphingomyelins are phospholipids that contain choline. The mode of action of choline as a lipotropic agent is unknown. It may promote conversion of liver fat into choline-containing phospholipids, which are more rapidly transferred from the liver into blood. Choline is also essential for synthesis of phospholipids that are used in intracellular membranes concerned with lipoprotein synthesis. It is thought that the lipotropic agents methionine, betaine, and lecithin are effective because they contain choline or promote choline synthesis. The requirement for choline is well recognized in all conditions predisposing to fatty infiltration of the liver, including diabetes mellitus, malnutrition, and cirrhosis. Greater than normal quantities of choline seem to be needed for prevention of a fatty liver when the liver is already damaged. Choline deficiency is not the only cause of fatty liver in these conditions, nor will choline supplementation alone restore the liver to full functional competence. However, choline is extremely valuable in the multitherapeutic approach to prevention and cure of fatty liver.

METHIONINE. Methionine (L-methionine) readily donates its terminal methyl group for methylation of various compounds. Methionine is the principal methyl donor of the body and supplies its labile methyl group to ethanolamine to form choline. In addition to its methyl group, methionine (and cysteine) contains a sulfhydryl group, which appears to protect the liver against the noxious action of certain poisons. Orally administered methionine can, however, aggravate hepatic coma. Bacterial flora may convert methionine to mercaptan derivatives such as methanethiol and ethanethiol, which are themselves capable of inducing coma.

S-adenosyl-L-methionine (SAMe) is a naturally occurring endogenous methyl donor which in animal studies and clinical human studies improves biochemical parameters of liver function (Osman et al. 1993). Endogenous concentrations are reduced in cirrhotic liver disease patients. Production of sulfated compounds and phosphatidylcholine is subsequently reduced. In animal studies, SAMe improved bile secretion impaired by a variety of toxins and pregnancy. Drug-induced hepatotoxicity and chronic liver disease were also reduced, without occurrence of serious side effects. Although absorbed well following oral administration, SAMe undergoes extensive first-pass metabolism (Osman et al. 1993).

LECITHIN. Lecithin contains choline as part of the molecule, which is liberated upon hydrolysis; it has been used in the dog as a lipotropic agent.

VITAMIN B_{12}. Hydroxocobalamin (previously named vitamin B_{12}) is stored in the liver, mainly in mitochondria, but there is also a microsomal fraction. This microsomal vitamin may be of importance in hepatic protein metabolism. Microsomal cell fractions from the livers of vitamin B_{12}-deficient animals are defective in the incorporation of methionine and alanine into protein. General liver protein synthesis is depressed in hydroxocobalamin deficiency.

Hydroxocobalamin has a lipotropic effect. It is involved in metabolism of labile methyl groups and in formation of choline. Hydroxocobalamin is also necessary for overall utilization of fat. However, when intake is low, the demand for this vitamin in hemopoiesis exceeds that for any other clinically recognizable physiologic function.

Use of lipotropic agents (choline, methionine, cysteine, betaine, lecithin, hydroxocobalamin) to increase mobilization of hepatic lipids is of proven value only in cases in which deficiencies of these substances exist. Deficiencies may be present in hepatic disease as a result of anorexia or insufficient dietary protein. Patients receiving and consuming a nutritious diet with adequate amounts of protein do not require supplementation with lipotropic agents, but their use has not been shown to be detrimental.

SELENIUM AND VITAMIN E. Selenium is now known to be essential for tissue respiration and to protect against dietary hepatic necrosis. It is extremely active and is only required in minute amounts. Vitamin E enhances the action of selenium, but both are required.

Selenium is an essential component of glutathione peroxidase, which catalyzes oxidation of reduced glutathione.

(2) glutathione–SH + H_2O_2 →
(reduced form)
glutathione–S–S glutathione + $2H_2O$
(oxidized form)

This glutathione peroxidase catalyzes removal of hydrogen peroxide and fatty acid hydroperoxides and so exerts a protective effect on all cells, but especially on muscle, liver, and erythrocytes. The essential substances required for removal of peroxides are reduced glutathione and glutathione peroxidase. Vitamin E maintains glutathione in the reduced form by preventing formation of hydroperoxides; it is an antioxidant and so reduces the amount of glutathione peroxidase required. Cysteine (*N*-acetylcysteine) is required for the reduced sulfhydryl radical of glutathione and is generally present in adequate quantities. Selenium and vitamin E enhance each other's action and together protect cells, especially hepatocytes, against harmful buildup of peroxides.

GLUCOSE AND FRUCTOSE. The liver resists many forms of injury when its stores of carbohydrate and protein are adequate; its efficiency is impaired when hepatocytes are laden with fat. Administration of a

TABLE 51.1—Doses of various agents used to treat gastrointestinal disorders

	Dose		Dose
Aluminum hydroxide		Domperidone	
Dogs	100–200 mg	Dogs	0.1–10.5 mg/kg IM 0.5–1 mg/kg PO
Cats	50–100 mg	Isopropamide iodide, USP	0.1–1.2 mg/kg
Cattle	30 g	Lecithin	1–5 g
Apomorphine		Magnesium hydroxide	
Dog	0.04 mg/kg IV 0.07 mg/kg IM 0.25 mg/kg (conjunctival sac)	Dogs	1–20 mL
		Cats	1–5 mL
		Calves and foals	30–60 mL
Calcium carbonate		Magnesium sulfate	
Dogs	0.5–4 g	Cows	500 g
Sheep and swine	8–15 g	Dogs	2–60 g
Cattle	60–360 g	Meclizine hydrochloride	
Horses	30–60 g	Dogs	2–10 mg/kg up to 10 kg or 2–6 mg/kg over 10 kg PO
Carafate®			
Dogs	40 mg/kg PO, TID		
Cats	100–200 mg/cat PO QID–TID	Methionine	
		Dogs	25 mg/kg
Castor oil		Cats	100–400 mg
Calves	60–90 mL	Cattle	20–30 g
Foals	60–90 mL	Horses	12.5 g
Choline		Methylcellulose	
Dogs	40–50 mg/kg	Dogs	0.5–5 g
Cats	100 mg	Cats	1.5–1 g
Cattle	1–8 g	Metoclopramide	
Horses	3–4 g	Dogs and cats	0.1–0.3 mg/kg/TID orally or SC, parenterally 0.02 mg/kg/hr IV
Cimetidine			
Dogs	5–10 mg/kg/6–8 hr PO 10 mg/kg/6 hr, IV, preferably infused slowly over 30–40 minutes	Mineral oil	
		Dogs	2–60 mL
		Cats	2–10 mL
		Cattle and horses	0.5–2 L
Cyclizine hydrochloride		Calves and foals	60–120 mL
Dog	25–100 mg PO	Misoprostol	1–3 μg/kg PO q 12 hr
Danthron		Omeprazole	0.7 mg/kg PO q 24 hr
Dogs	300–400 mg	Naloxone	
Cats	100–250 mg	Dogs	0.04 mg/kg IV
Sheep	2.5–5 g/50 kg	Pancreatin	
Cattle	20–45 g	Dogs	0.5–6 g
Horses	15–40 g	Cats	0.5–2 g
Dehydrocholic acid	100 mg/kg	Pepsin	
Dicyclomine hydrochloride		Dogs	0.2–1 g
Dogs	5–10 mg orally	Cats	100–300 mg
Dioctyl sodium sulfosuccinate		Calves and foals	4 g
Dogs	15–120 mg	Periactin	
Cats	15–30 mg	Cats	1 mg/cat PO
Cattle and horses	5–15 g	Pimozide	
Diphenhydramine hydrochloride		Dogs	0.025–0.1 mg/kg PO
Dogs	2–5 mg/kg PO	Ranitidine	0.5 mg/kg/12 hr
Diphenoxylate hydrochloride		Sulfasalazine	
Cats and dogs	0.5–1 mg/kg every 8–12 hr	Dogs	15–20 mg/kg/8 hr for 3–4 weeks

hypertonic solution of glucose and fructose produces favorable responses in a variety of hepatic abnormalities. A high glycogen content appears to protect liver cells from damage, and inhibition of gluconeogenesis (as occurs with administration of both insulin and glucose) may play an important role. Under the influence of insulin, hepatocytes undergo glycogen storage, hypertrophy, and hyperplasia. Insulin has a major anabolic effect on the liver.

VITAMINS. In the presence of liver disease, the fat-soluble vitamin K should be supplemented, since hepatic stores may be quite rapidly depleted. The water-soluble vitamins of the B-complex group are frequently employed in therapeutic regimens for hepatic insufficiency. Few controlled studies have been carried out in this regard, but the rationale behind their clinical use is based on ensuring an adequate supply of metabolic cofactors.

REFERENCES

Albibi, R., and McCallum, R. W. 1983. Metoclopramide: pharmacology and clinical application. Arch Intern Med 98:86-95.

Allescher, H. D., Ahmad, S., Kostka, P., et al. 1989. Distribution of opioid receptors in canine small intestine: implications for function. Am J Physiol 256:G966-G974.
Ames, T. R., and Patterson, E. B. 1984. Pharmacokinetics of a long-acting oxytetracycline injectable in healthy and diseased calves. Proc 13th World Cong Dis Cattle 2:931-935.
Andersson, T. 1991. Omeprazole drug interaction studies. Clin Pharmacokinet 21:195-212.
Andrews, P. L. R., Rapeport, W. G., and Sanger, G. J. 1988. Neuropharmacology of emesis induced by anti-cancer therapy. TIPS 9:334-341.
Atkins, C. E., Tyler, R., and Greenlee, P. 1985. Clinical, biochemical, acid-base, and electrolyte abnormalities in cats after hypertonic sodium phosphate enema administration. Am J Vet Res 46:980-988.
Baker, K. J. 1966. Binding of sulfobromophthalein sodium and indocyanine green by plasma alpha 1 lipoproteins. Proc Soc Exp Biol and Med 122:957-963.
Bemis, K., Bendele, A., Clemens, J., et al. 1989. General pharmacology of nizatidine in animals. Drug Res 39:240-250.
Bernstein, J. G. 1988. Psychotropic drug induced weight gain: mechanisms and management. Clin Neuropharmacol 11:S194-S206.
Boom, S. P., Meyer, I., Wouterse, A. C., and Russel, F. G. 1998. A physiologically based kidney model for the renal clearance of ranitidine and the interaction with cimetidine and probenecid in the dog. Biopharmaceutics & Drug Disposition 19(3):199-208.
Bowersox, T. S., Lipowitz, A. J., Hardy, R. M., Johnston, G. R., Hayden, D. W., Schwartz, S., and King, V. L. 1996. The use of a synthetic prostaglandin E_1 analog as a gastric protectant against aspirin-induced hemorrhage in the dog. J Am Anim Hosp Assoc 32(5):401-407.
Brodde, O. E. 1982. Vascular dopamine receptors: demonstration and characterization by in vitro studies. Life Sci 31(4):289-306.
Brogden, R. N., Carmine, A. A., Heel, R. C., et al. 1982. Ranitidine: a review of its pharmacology and therapeutic use in peptic ulcer disease and other allied diseases. Drugs 24:267-303.
Burrows, C. F. 1983. Metoclopramide. J Am Vet Med Assoc 183:1341-1343.
———. 1984. Gastrointestinal pharmacology. AAHA's Annual Meeting 51:197-200.
———. 1990. Ondansetron: a new drug to control nausea and emesis in cancer patients. Vet Clin Briefs 8:3.
Charlet, N., Gallo-Torres, H. E., Bounameaux, Y., et al. 1985. Prostaglandins and the protection of the gastroduodenal mucosa in humans: a critical review. J Clin Pharmacol 25:564-582.
Clark, E. S., and Becht, J. L. 1987. Clinical pharmacology of the gastrointestinal tract. Vet Clin North Am Equine Pract 3:101-123.
Cook, G., Papich, M. G., Roberts, M. C., Bowman, K. F. 1997. Pharmacokinetics of cisapride in horses after intravenous and rectal administration. Am J Vet Res 58(12):1427-1430.
Costall, B., and Naylor, R. J. 1992. Neuropharmacology of emesis in relation to clinical response. Br J Cancer Suppl 19:S2-S8.
Crema, A., and De Ponti, F. 1989. Recent advances in the physiology of intestinal motility. Pharmacol Res 21:67-73.
Dart, A. J., and Hodgson, D. R. 1998. Role of prokinetic drugs for treatment of postoperative ileus in the horse. Austr Vet J 76(1):25-31.
Demol, P., Ruoff, H.-J., and Weihrauch, T. R. 1989. Rational pharmacotherapy of gastrointestinal motility disorders. Eur J Pediatr 148:489-495.
Dimski, D. S. 1989. Constipation: pathophysiology, diagnostic approach, and treatment. Sem Vet Med Surg 4:247-254.
DuPont, H. L. 1987. Bismuth subsalicylate in the treatment and prevention of diarrheal disease. DICP: Annals of Pharmacotherapy 21:687-693.
Eddershaw, P. J., Chadwick, A. P., Higton, D. M., Fenwick, S. H., Linacre, P., Jenner, W. N., Bell, J. A., and Manchee, G. R. 1996. Absorption and disposition of ranitidine hydrochloride in rat and dog. Xenobiotica 26(9):947-956.
Edelbroek, M., Schuurkes, J., De Ridder, W., Horowitz, M., Dent, J., and Akkermans, L. 1995. Effect of cisapride on myoelectrical and motor responses of antropyloroduodenal region during intraduodenal lipid and antral tachygastria in conscious dog. Digestive Diseases and Sciences 40(4):901-911.
Fullarton, G. M., MacDonald, A. M. I., and McColl, K. E. L. 1991. Rebound hypersecretion after H2-antagonist withdrawalCa comparative study with nizatidine, ranitidine and famotidine. Aliment Pharmacol Therap 5:391-398.
Gamse, R. 1990. Antiemetic action of 5-HT3 receptor antogonists: review of preclinical and clinical results with ICS 205-930. Cancer Treat Rev 17:301-305.
Gibaldi, M. 1992. Drug interactions, part I. Ann Pharmacother 26:709-713.
Gralla, R. J., Itri, L. M., Pisko, S. E., et al. 1981. Antiemetic efficacy of high-dose metoclopramide: randomized trials with placebo and prochlorperazine in patients with chemotherapy-induced nausea and vomiting. N Engl J Med 305:905-909.
Gray, G. W., and Yano, B. L. 1975. A study of the actions of methampyrone and of a commercial intestinal extract preparation on intestinal motility. Am J Vet Res 36:201-208.
Greenwood, B., and Davison, J. S. 1987. The relationship between gastrointestinal motility and secretion. Am J Physiol 252:G1-G7.
Guharoy, S. R. 1991. Streptokinase versus recombinant tissue-type plasminogen activator. DICP: Annals of Pharmacotherapy 25:1271-1272 (Abstr).
Hahn, R. A., and Wardell, J. R. 1980. Antagonism of the renal vasodilator activity of dopamine by metoclopramide. Naunyn-Schmiedebergs Archives of Pharmacology 314(2):177-182.
Heller, F. R., Martinet, J. P., Henrion, J., et al. 1991. The rationale for using ursodeoxycholic acid in chronic liver disease. Proc Natl Acad Sci USA 88:9543-9547.
Hickey, A. R., Wenger, T. L., Carpenter, V. P., et al. 1991. Digoxin immune fab therapy in the management of digitalis intoxication: safety and efficacy results of an observational surveillance study. J Am Coll Cardiol 17:590-598.
Hikasa, Y., Ogasawara, S., and Takase, K. 1992. Alpha adrenoceptor subtypes involved in the emetic action in dogs. J Pharmacol Exp Ther 261:746-754.
Hikasa, Y., Takase, K., and Ogasawara, S. 1989. Evidence for the involvement of alpha-adrenoceptors in the emetic action of xylazine in cats. Am J Vet Res 50:1348-1350.
Hirschowitz, B. I., and Gibson, R. G. 1987. Effect of cimetidine on stimulated gastric secretion and serum gastrin in the dog. Am J Gastroenterol 70:437-447.
Holland, P. S., Ruoff, W. W., Brumbaugh, G. W., and Brown, S. A. 1997. Plasma pharmacokinetics of ranitidine HCl in adult horses. J Vet Pharmacol Therap 20(2):145-152.
Hollander, D., and Tarnawski, A. 1990. The protective and therapeutic mechanisms of sucralfate. Scand J Gastroenterol 25(Supp 173):1-5.
Horn, D. 1987. The impact of fecal impactions. Cornell Fel Health Cent Info Bull 2:1-8.

Howard, J. M., Chremos, A. N., Collen, M. J., et al. 1985. Famotidine, a new, potent, long-acting histamine H2-receptor antagonist: comparison with cimetidine and ranitidine in the treatment of Zollinger-Ellison syndrome. Gastroenterology 88:1026-1033.

Hughes, S. 1983. Acute secretory diarrhoeas: current concepts in pathogenesis and treatment. Drugs 26:80-90.

Hunt, J. M., and Gerring, E. L. 1986. A preliminary study of the effects of metoclopramide on equine gut activity. J Vet Pharmacol Therap 9:109-112.

Itoh, Z., Mizumoto, A., Iwanaga, Y., Yoshida, N., Torii, K., and Wakabayashi, K. 1991. Involvement of 5-hydroxytryptamine 3 receptors in regulation of interdigestive gastric contractions by motilin in the dog. Gastroenterology 100(4):901-908.

Jackson, J. E. 1981. Reduction of liver blood flow by cimetidine. N Engl J Med 307:99-101.

———. 1982. Cimetidine protects against acetaminophen toxicity. Life Sci 31:31-35.

Jenkins, C. J., and DeNovo, R. C. 1990. OmeprazoleCa new anti-ulcer agent. Proc ACVIM 8:437-439.

Jensen, S. L., and Jensen, P. F. 1992. Role of sucralfate in peptic disease. Dig Dis 10:153-161.

Johnson, S. E. 1984. Clinical pharmacology of antiemetics and antidiarrheals. Proc of the Kal Kan Waltham Symp for the Treatment of Small Animal Diseases 8:7-15.

Jones, J. B., and Bailey, R. T., Jr 1989. Misoprostol: a prostglandin E1 analog with antisecretory and cytoprotective properties. DICP: Annals of Pharmacotherapy 23:276-282.

Katz, P. O., Geisinger, K. R., Hassan, M., et al. 1988. Acid-induced esophagitis in cats is prevented by sucralfate but not synthetic prostaglandin E. Dig Dis Sci 33:217-224.

King, J. N., and Gerring, E. L. 1988. Actions of the novel gastrointestinal prokinetic agent cisapride on equine bowel motility. J Vet Pharmacol Therap 11:314-321.

Kleiman, R. L., Adair, C. G., and Ephgrave, K. S. 1988. Stress ulcers: current understanding of pathogenesis and prophylaxis. DICP: Annals of Pharmacotherapy 22:452-460.

Kohler, D. R., and Goldspiel, B. R. 1991. Ondansetron: a serotonin recepter (5-HT3) antagonist for antineoplastic chemotherapy-induced nausea and vomiting. Ann Pharmacother 25:367-380.

Konturek, S. J., Brzozowski, T., Drozdowicz, D., et al. 1991. Role of acid milieu in the gastroprotective and ulcer-healing activity of sucralfate. Am J Med 91(Suppl 2A):20S-29S.

Konturek, S. J., Brzozowski, T., Majka, J., et al. 1992. Role of nitric oxide and prostaglandins in sucralfate-induced gastroprotection. Eur J Pharmacol 211:277-279.

Krishna, D. R., and Ulrich, K. 1988. Newer H2-receptor antagonists clinical pharmacokinetics and drug interaction potential. Clin Pharmacokinet 15:205-215.

Kromer, W. 1988. Endogenous and exogenous opioids in the control of gastrointestinal motility and secretion. Pharmacol Rev 40:121-162.

Lampkin, T. A., Ouellet, D., Hak, L. J., et al. 1990. Omeprazole: a novel antisecretory agent for the treatment of acid-peptic disorders. DICP: Annals of Pharmacotherapy 24:393-402.

Larsen, K. R., Dajani, E. Z., and Ives, M. M. 1992. Antiulcer drugs and gastric mucosal integrity effects of misoprostol, 16,16-dimethyl PGE2, and cimetidine on hemodynamics and metabolic rate in canine gastric mucosa. Dig Dis Sci 37:1029-1037.

Larsson, H., Mattsson, H., and Carlsson, E. 1988. Gastric acid antisecretory effect of two different dosage forms of omeprazole during prolonged oral treatment in the gastric fistula dog. Scand J Gastroenterol 23:1013-1019.

Ledger, P. W., Gale, R., and Yum, S. I. 1992. In H. Mukhtar, ed., Pharmacology of the Skin, Transdermal Drug Delivery System, pp. 73-85. Boca Raton, Fla.: CRC Press.

Macy, D. W., and Gasper, P. W. 1985. Diazepam-induced eating in anorexic cats. J Am Anim Hos Assoc 21:17-20.

Manara, A. R., Bolsin, S., Monk, C. R., Hartnell, G., and Harris, R. A. 1991. Metoclopramide and renal vascular resistance. Brit J Anaesth 66(1):129-130.

Marks, I. N., Johnston, D. A., and Young, G. O. 1991. Acid secretory changes and early relapse following duodenal ulcer healing with ranitidine or sucralfate. Am J Med 91(Suppl 2A):95S-100S.

McCallum, R. W., Prakash, C., Campoli-Richards, D. M., et al. 1988. Cisapride: a preliminary review of its pharmacodynamics and pharmacokinetic properties, and therapeutic use as a prokinetic agent in gastrointestinal motility disorders. Drugs 36:652-681.

McCarthy, D. M. 1991. Sucralfate. Drug Therapy 325:1017-1023.

Merrifield, K. R., and Chaffee, B. J. 1989. Recent advances in the management of nausea and vomiting caused by antineoplastic agents. Clin Pharm 8:187-199.

Meyer, D. J., and Thompson, M. B. 1992. Bile acidsCbeyond their value as a liver function test. Biochem J 285:929-932.

Miller, T. A. 1983. Protective effects of prostaglandins against gastric mucosal damage: current knowledge and proposed mechanisms. Am J Physiol 245:G601-G623.

Milne, E. M., Doxey, D. L., Woodman, M. P., Cuddeford, D., Pearson, R. A. 1996. An evaluation of the use of cisapride in horses with chronic grass sickness (equine dysautonomia). Brit Vet J 152(5):537-549.

Misoprostol monograph. 1990. Misoprostol: Preclinical and Clinical Review. Glenview, Ill.: Physicians and Scientists Publishing Co.

Moreland, K. J. 1988. Ulcer disease of the upper gastrointestinal tract in small animals: pathophysiology, diagnosis and management. Compendium on Continuing Education 10:1265-1279.

Morrissey, J. F., and Barreras, R. F. 1974. Drug therapy, antacid therapy. N Engl J Med 290:550-554.

Muir, W. W. 1990. Small volume resuscitation using hypertonic saline. Cornell Vet 80:7-12.

Murray, M. J., and Eichorn, E. S. 1996. Effects of intermittent feed deprivation, intermittent feed deprivation with ranitidine administration, and stall confinement with ad libitum access to hay on gastric ulceration in horses. Am J Vet Res 57(11):1599-1603.

Nicholson, B. T., Center, S. A., Rowland, P. J., et al. 1989. Evaluation of the safety of ursodeoxycholic acid in healthy cats. Mech Ageing Dev 48:145-155.

Osman, E., Owen, J. S., and Burroughs, A. K. 1993. Review article: S-adenosyl-L-methionine—new therapeutic agent in liver disease. Aliment Pharmacol Therap 7:21-28.

Papich, M. G., Davis, C. A., and Davis, L. E. 1987. Absorption of salicylate from an antidiarrheal preparation in cats and dogs. J Am Anim Hos Assoc 23:221-228.

Peroutka, S. J., and Snyder, S. H. 1982. Antiemetics: neurotransmitter receptor binding predicts therapeutic actions. Lancet 1982:658-659.

Price, A. H., and Brogden, R. N. 1988. Nizatidine: a preliminary review of its pharmacodynamic and pharmacokinetic properties, and its therapeutic use in peptic ulcer disease. Drugs 36:521-539.

Reynolds, J. C. 1989. Prokinetic agents: a key in the future of gastroenterology. Gastroenterol Clin North Am 18:437-457.

Richter, K. P. 1990. Update on the use of newer gastrointestinal drugs in small animals. Proc ACVIM 8:141-144.

Robert, A. 1987. Effect of drugs on gastric secretion. In L. R. Johnson, ed., Physiology of the Gastroenterology Tract, 2nd ed., pp. 1071-1088. New York: Raven Press.

Robert, A., and Kauffman, G. L., Jr. 1989. Stress ulcers, erosions and gastric mucosal injury. In M. H. Sleisenger and

J. S. Fordtran, eds., Gastrointestinal Diseases: Pathophysiology, Diagnosis, Management, 4th ed., pp. 773-855. Philadelphia: W. B. Saunders.

Robinson, M. G. 1989. New oral salicylates in therapy of chronic idiopathic inflammatory bowel disease. Gastroenterol Clin North Am 18:43-50.

Schiller, L. R., Santa Ana, C. A., Morawski, S. G., et al. 1984. Mechanism of the antidiarrheal effect of loperamide. Gastroenterology 86:1475-1480.

Sedman, A. J. 1984. Cimetidine-drug interactions. Am J Med 76:109-114.

Shinkai, T., Saijo, N., Eguchi, K., et al. 1989. Control of cisplatin-induced delayed emesis with metoclopramide and dexamethasone: a randomized controlled trial. Jpn J Clin Oncol 19:40-44.

Shook, J. E., Lemcke, P. K., Gehrig, C. A., et al. 1989. Antidiarrheal properties of supraspinal Mu and Delta and peripheral Mu, Delta and Kappa opioid receptors: inhibition of diarrhea without constipation. J Pharmacol Exp Ther 249:83-90.

Shorrock, C. J., and Rees, W. D. W. 1988. Overview of gastroduodenal mucosal protection. Am J Med 84(Suppl 2A):25-34.

Siepler, J. K., Mahakian, K., and Trudeau, W. T. 1986. Current concepts in clinical therapeutics: peptic ulcer disease. Clin Pharm 5:128-142.

Slomiany, B. L., Piotrowski, J., Tamura, S., et al. 1991. Enhancement of the protective qualities of gastric mucus by sucralfate: role of phosphoinositides. Am J Med 91(Suppl 2A):30S-36S.

Sojka, J. E., Adams, S. B., Lamar, C. H., et al. 1988. Effect of butorphanol, pentazocine, meperidine, or metoclopramide on intestinal motility in female ponies. Am J Vet Res 49:527-529.

Spaulding, M. 1989. Recent studies of anorexia and appetite stimulation in the cancer patient. Oncology 3(Suppl 8):17-23.

Steinberg, W. M., Lewis, J. H., and Katz, D. M. 1982. Antacid inhibit absorption of cimetidine. N Engl J Med 307:400-404.

Steiner, A., and Roussel, A. J. 1995. Drugs coordinating and restoring gastrointestinal motility and their effect on selected hypodynamic gastrointestinal disorders in horses and cattle. Zentralblatt fur Veterinarmedizin, Reihe A. 42(10):613-631.

Strombeck, D. R., and Guilford, W. G. 1990. Small Animal Gastroenterology, 2nd ed., pp. 297-302. Davis, Calif.: Stonegate Publishing.

Sugrue, M. F. 1987. Neuropharmacology of drugs affecting food intake. Pharmacol Ther 32:145-182.

Szabo, S., Vattay, P., Scarbough, E., et al. 1991. Role of vascular factors, including angiogenesis, in the mechanisms of action of sucralfate. Am J Med 91(Suppl 2A):158S-160S.

Szelenyi, I., and Brune, K. 1986. Possible role of sulfhydryls in mucosal protection induced by aluminum hydroxide. Dig Dis Sci 31:1207-1210.

Takahashi, T., Kurosawa, S., Wiley, J. W., et al. 1991. Mechanism for the gastrokinetic actions of domperidone. Gastroenterology 101:703-710.

Tarnawski, A., Hollander, D., and Gergely, H. 1987. The mechanism of protective, therapeutic and prophylactic actions of sucralfate. Scand J Gastroenterol 22(Suppl 140):7-13.

Thompson, W. G., 1980. Laxatives: clinical pharmacology and rational use. Drugs 19:49-58.

Toutain, P. L., Alvinerie, M., and Ruckebusch, Y. 1983. Pharmacokinetics of dexdamethasone and its effect on adrenal gland function in the dog. Am J Vet Res 44:212-217.

Tyers, M. B. 1992. Pharmacology and preclinical antiemetic properties of ondansetron. Sem Oncol 19(Suppl 10):1-8.

Urbie, M., Ballesteros, A., Strauss, R., et al. 1985. Successful administration of metoclopramide for the treatment of nausea in patients with advanced liver disease. Gastroenterology 88:757-762.

Vergin, H., and Kori-Lindner, C. 1990. Putative mechanisms of cytoprotective effect of certain antacids and sucralfate. Dig Dis Sci 35:1320-1327.

Watson, W. A. 1987. Factors influencing the clinical efficacy of activated charcoal. DICP: Annals of Pharmacotherapy 21:160-166.

Whittle, B. J. R., and Garner, A. 1988. New targets for antiulcer drugs. TIPS 9:187-189.

Wilcke, J. R., and Turner, J. C. 1987. The use of absorbents to treat gastrointestinal problems in small animals. Sem Vet Med Surg 2:266-273.

Wilson, D. E. 1987. Antisecretory and mucosal protective actions of misoprostal. Am J Med 83(Suppl 1A):2-7.

Wingate, D., Pearce, E., Hutton, M., et al. 1980. Effect of metoclopramide on interdigestive myoelectric activity in the conscious dog. Dig Dis Sci 25:15-21.

Wolfe, M. M., and Soll, A. H. 1988. The physiology of gastric acid secretion. N Engl J Med 319:1707-1715.

Yamaji, Y., Abe, T., Omata, T., et al. 1991. Effects of successive doses of nizatidine, cimetidine and ranitidine on serum gastrin level and gastric acid secretion. Drug Res 41:954-957.

52 CHEMOTHERAPY OF NEOPLASTIC DISEASES

KENITA S. ROGERS AND GORDON L. COPPOC

Treatment Perspectives
Cancer Biology
- **Cell Cycle**
- **Tumor Growth Rate**
- **Chemotherapy of the Cancer Cell**
- **Drug Toxicity**
- **Therapist Safety**
- **Drug Dosage**
- **Resistance**
- **Selection of Regimens**
- **Combination Chemotherapy**
- **Multimodal Therapy**

Drugs
- **Alkylating Agents**
- **Antimetabolites**
- **Natural Products**
- **Platinum Coordination Complexes**
- **Hormones and Miscellaneous Agents**

Administration of chemotherapy for treatment of pets with cancer has become an integral skill in many small-animal hospitals. Proper use of these drugs requires a working understanding of their unique pharmacology and range of expected toxicities, as well as current recommendations regarding safe drug handling. Treatment of many cancers remains a challenging task because, despite increased experience with the use of chemotherapeutic agents, therapy is often not curative. Expense of the drugs with appropriate monitoring and the supportive care required in the event of toxicity may discourage some owners from pursuing treatment of their pet with chemotherapy. However, with careful patient selection and monitoring and client discussions designed to be informative and outline realistic goals, chemotherapy can be a rational means of improving the patient's quality and/or quantity of life.

TREATMENT PERSPECTIVES. Cancer is defined as *cured* when all cancer cells that have the capacity for tumor regeneration have been eradicated. While cancer cure is the ideal goal, producing remission and/or palliation is often more readily achievable. A cancer is said to be in *remission* when all clinical evidence of cancer has disappeared but microscopic foci of cancer cells may remain. *Palliative treatment* refers to the treatment of cancer (when cure is unlikely) to reduce pain, improve the sense of well being, or correct some physiological malfunction. The therapeutic regimen selected must be consistent with the goal for the patient (i.e., cure, remission, or palliation).

For most solid tumors, the lower limit of clinical or radiologic detection is about 1 gram of tissue, or approximately 10^9 cells (Tannock and Goldenberg 1998). Recognizing the need to continue aggressive treatment in the face of apparent complete remission ($<10^9$ cells) was one of the factors leading to success in the treatment of many acute childhood leukemias and lymphomas. Unfortunately, for most solid tumors, a drug-resistant subpopulation emerges and eventually leads to relapse. *Adjuvant chemotherapy* is given to patients with no overt evidence of residual cancer after local treatment with surgery or radiation. This strategy derives from past experience with similar patients who have shown a high rate of relapse from local microscopic or distant micrometastatic disease and from the failure of chemotherapy or combined-modality treatment to ultimately cure these patients after recurrence of disease (Kaufman and Chabner 1996). In addition, there is experimental evidence to support the hypothesis that neoplasms are most sensitive to chemotherapy at their earliest stages of growth, probably due to their higher growth fraction and shorter cell cycle times. *Neoadjuvant therapy* refers to adjuvant therapy that is started in patients before treatment of the primary tumor with surgery or radiation. A complete response (CR) is defined as the disappearance of all clinical evidence of tumor (Morrison 1998a). A partial response (PR) is defined as at least a 50% regression of all measurable lesions. Stable disease (SD) is defined as a less than 50% increase in measurable tumor volume with no new tumor lesions, and progressive disease (PD) is defined as a greater than 50% increase in measurable tumor volume or the appearance of new tumor lesions.

Chemotherapy may be broadly defined as the application of drugs to kill or inhibit the growth of viruses or foreign cells, such as bacteria, in the body. Cancer cells can be considered "foreign" in this sense. Cancer chemotherapy was first successfully practiced when nitrogen mustards used as war gases were found to inhibit tumor growth. Unfortunately, they were also extremely toxic for the patient. Effective chemotherapy with more specific agents was not widely used prior to

TABLE 52.1—Examples of factors determining therapeutic goals

Patient
Species
Breed
Age
Sex
Health status
Function/role
Neoplasm
Histologic type
Natural history
Stage (extent)
Grade
Location
Facilities/treatments available
Primary modalities
Secondary support for follow-up care
Proximity
Owner
Ability to care for animal
Relationship with pet
Living circumstances
Commitment
Financial status

the 1960s. Use of chemotherapy in cancer patients grew markedly in the 1970s, providing a means of curing some cancers and lengthening life expectancy with others. In contrast to radiation and surgery, where the limitations are damage to local vital structures and access to metastatic lesions, chemotherapy is principally limited by the presence of a population of resistant cells. The probability that resistant cells will be present within a tumor is correlated to the number of cells present and tumor volume. Thus, it has been found in human medicine that it is difficult to completely cure many solid tumors consisting of more than 1 million cells (approximately 1 mg of tissue) with chemotherapy alone.

The decision to use one or several of the treatment modalities for a patient with cancer rests on factors such as those listed in Table 52.1. Detailed recommendation of specific treatment protocols is beyond the scope of this chapter. Protocols for timing and dosage of drug combinations have been published (Morrison 1998d; Ogilvie and Moore 1995). Veterinary practitioners may also seek the advice of an experienced medical oncologist before instituting therapy with the drugs to be discussed. Cancer chemotherapy should be approached in a judicious manner because the disease process is often intractable and the drugs are frequently toxic. However, carefully planned and monitored therapy can prolong an animal's life while improving quality of life and can be a positive and rewarding experience for both the pet owner and the veterinarian.

CANCER BIOLOGY.

A brief review of certain aspects of cancer biology will aid in understanding the rationale behind treatment protocols and the limitations of chemotherapy. Discovery of qualitative differences between normal and cancerous cells would facilitate development of more selective drugs, i.e., drugs that have relatively lower toxicity for normal tissues. Selectivity is currently based primarily on quantitative differences. That is, both normal and cancer cells have essentially the same ongoing biochemical processes, but the rates and timing may be very different. For most tumors, the success of chemotherapy depends on having drugs that are taken up more avidly by tumor cells, that bind more tightly to some tumor cell constituent, or that affect processes that occur more rapidly in tumor cells, thus enhancing their effect on cancer cells relative to normal cells.

Cell Cycle. The *cell cycle* is the progression of a dividing cell through phases from one mitosis to the next. G1, a presynthetic phase, immediately follows mitosis and is extremely variable in duration, depending on the cell type and the presence or absence of nutrients, growth factors, and metabolic by-products. During this phase, normal cellular events, including protein and ribonucleic acid (RNA) synthesis, occur, in preparation for deoxyribonucleic acid (DNA) synthesis during the S phase. Control of initiation of the S phase, as well as other events in the cell cycle, has been intensively investigated for clues to unique reactions that could be targets of anticancer drugs. The S phase may require between 8 and 20 hours for completion. Constituents required for mitosis are synthesized during the next phase, G2, which may last 3 hours. Mitosis (M phase) typically requires 1 hour for completion to end the cell cycle.

For a variety of reasons, as tumors mature, certain cells may stop traversing the cell cycle. Others may traverse it so slowly that for purposes related to cancer therapy, they are not in the population of actively dividing cells. Operationally, these cells may be grouped and referred to as being in the G0 phase. Such cells are not part of the "growth fraction" of the tumor. However, under proper growth conditions, those that were merely traversing the cycle extremely slowly may be "recruited" back into the pool of actively dividing cells. Cells that have stopped dividing because of differentiation to more mature cell types are less likely to be recruited into the population of dividing cells. One line of anticancer research is investigating means of inducing such terminal differentiation.

Tumor Growth Rate. The apparent growth rate of a tumor does not necessarily reflect the rate at which cells traverse the cell cycle. If it did, and the tumor consisted of only one immortal cell type, tumor growth could be described by a simple geometric progression; i.e., the number of cells would double after an interval equal to the cell cycle time. If this were the case, and if 10^9 cells were required for diagnosis of a tumor, approximately 32 cell cycle times would be required for a single cancer cell to result in a clinically apparent tumor.

In an experimental tumor system it was observed that the time required for the number of cells to double increased from 4 days to over 100 days as the mass grew from approximately 0.3 to 10 g. The growth fraction of the tumor decreased from 80 to 10%, and the time required for cells to complete a cycle increased from 0.8 to 1.6 days. From studies similar to this example and much clinical experience, it has been established that tumor growth rate is complex and that the "fractional" growth rate tends to decrease as the tumor matures. Depending on the growth conditions and tumor type, the time required to complete a cell cycle may range from less than 24 hours to several days. Because of cell death, decreasing growth fraction, and extended cell cycle times as tumors grow larger, cell cycle time rarely equals doubling time over the course of a tumor's life span. Mean clinical doubling times for some human tumors range from 2 to 5 days for Burkitt's lymphoma to 34 days for osteogenic sarcoma to 134 days for adenocarcinoma of the lung (Shackney 1993).

Another level of complexity is introduced when it is appreciated that the stem cell population itself is likely to be quite heterogeneous (Chambers and Hill 1998). Because of heterogeneity, stem cells in the growth fraction may be sensitive or insensitive to a particular drug, and there could be many different categories of cells in a tumor with respect to drug sensitivity. The existence of several populations of cells within a tumor complicates therapy. Most cytotoxic anticancer drugs are effective against rapidly growing tumors with large growth fractions. Thus, small tumors should be most sensitive and large tumors least sensitive to drugs, as has been established clinically. Whether such behavior extends to very small, invisible foci such as metastases is unknown.

The *log cell-kill* hypothesis states that the entire population of cancer cells in a patient must be eradicated to produce a cure. A large number of experimental studies have indicated that drug-induced cell kill is a first-order process; i.e., a constant proportion of the cells present, both normal and cancerous, are killed with each round of therapy. Recall that differences between cancer cells and cells of some normal tissues are often not great. The magnitude of the problem is dramatized by the following example.

It has been estimated that a 20 kg child with acute lymphoblastic leukemia has 10^{10} cancer cells when clinical signs lead to diagnosis, 10^{9} when declared to be in remission (i.e., the leukemia can no longer be clinically detected), and 10^{12} at death. One gram of tumor contains 10^{9} cells. An antitumor agent that killed 99.9% of the cells in a patient with 10^{12} cells would leave 10^{9} cells behind. To kill the remaining cells would require additional courses of therapy, but these would have to be spaced to allow for recovery of tissues such as bone marrow and gut epithelium or the patient would die from drug toxicity. The magnitude of the problem is illustrated by the fact that reduction of the normal cell population by 2–3 log units (i.e., 99–99.9%) may be fatal. Clinically successful chemotherapy requires that there be a significant difference between the proportion of cancerous and normal cells killed and that normal cells rebound more rapidly from the therapeutic insult.

Chemotherapy of the Cancer Cell. Chemotherapeutic agents may be divided into three classes with respect to their dependence on the cell cycle. Some drugs (e.g., alkylating agents) are said to be non-cell-cycle-specific. Although they are toxic to all cells, they are especially toxic to proliferating cells. Other drugs are cell-cycle-specific. Cells must be proliferating for these drugs to be effective. Cell-cycle-specific drugs may also be cell-cycle-phase-specific; such drugs may be active in only one stage of the cell cycle. Vincristine, which binds to a tubulin subunit and thereby interferes with microtubular function, primarily inhibits cells undergoing mitosis. Cytarabine and hydroxyurea are most, although not exclusively, active in the S phase. Dactinomycin and doxorubicin are most active in G1. Bleomycin is active in all phases but especially in the S phase and in mitosis. Knowledge regarding activity in various phases of the cell cycle provides an understanding of why tumors with large growth fractions and rapid generation times usually respond more dramatically to therapy and guides drug selection in development of new protocols. For example, drugs like vincristine may not be very effective against slowly growing tumors with small growth fractions that undergo mitosis infrequently.

Drug Toxicity. Chemotherapy agents are most toxic to cells rapidly traversing the cell cycle, but unfortunately many cancers have smaller growth fractions than certain normal tissues, particularly bone marrow and intestinal epithelium. Although normal tissues recover more rapidly than tumor cells, the chemotherapist must be prepared to provide supportive treatment for transient conditions that develop secondary to drug administration, including cytopenias, sepsis, and gastrointestinal (GI) disturbances.

Although there are important exceptions, the characteristic toxicity to various body tissues produced by antitumor compounds is related to tissue growth rate. Lymphocytes and bone marrow cells are most profoundly affected; the expected consequences are anemia, leukopenia, and thrombocytopenia. Although anemia and thrombocytopenia secondary to chemotherapy administration are rarely life-threatening, neutropenia can be profound and result in an increased risk of sepsis. Indeed, increased susceptibility to infection is the most common bone marrow sequela in patients being treated with chemotherapy. Close monitoring of absolute neutrophil counts is an integral part of managing chemotherapy patients, especially when non-cell-cycle-specific drugs such as alkylating agents are being administered. It is imperative to routinely check blood counts because patients can have dangerously low neutrophil counts and be clinically asymptomatic.

The ideal drug dose does not lower the absolute neutrophil count below 2000–2500/mm^{3}, because the risk of developing sepsis increases dramatically with lower counts. There is evidence that biological response modifiers such as recombinant canine granulocyte colony-stimulating factor (rcG-CSF) and agents that induce it may antagonize the myelosuppression of some anticancer agents (Ogilvie et al. 1992). Because of the longevity of erythrocytes, anemia does not appear as rapidly as myelosuppression and is often mild. Most cytotoxic drugs may produce myelosuppression and some degree of thrombocytopenia, but L-asparaginase, vincristine, prednisone, and bleomycin are minimally toxic in this regard when used as solitary agents.

Mucosal cells of the GI tract have a high growth fraction with a turnover time on the order of 5 days. Many anticancer drugs can produce diarrhea, vomition, anorexia, and mucositis, which may manifest as ulcerative stomatitis and enteritis. These disorders can be more disconcerting to the patient and owner than the less obvious, but potentially more life-threatening, effects on cells derived from the bone marrow. GI signs appear to be less prevalent in animals than humans but should be regarded seriously when they occur. Severe vomiting and diarrhea are cause for temporary cessation of therapy, because they may result in dehydration or presage serious mucositis, which could be life-threatening.

Basal cells of the skin and especially of the hair follicle are also highly susceptible because of high growth fraction in some breeds. Hair loss in breeds with continuously growing hair (e.g., Poodles, Terriers, Schnauzers, and Old English Sheepdogs) may occur, especially in association with doxorubicin therapy. In breeds that shed, the hair coat may thin, but complete alopecia is uncommon. Cats tend to lose their whiskers and outer guard hairs when treated with chemotherapy. Notable hair loss may begin 1 month after therapy. In most cases, hair growth returns to normal once therapy is stopped, often beginning within 1–3 months. Change of coat color in a Standard Poodle has been reported (Simonson and Madewell 1992). Other toxicities related to the skin are not dependent on rate of cell growth and include hyperpigmentation and direct tissue damage with extravasation. Hyperpigmentation has been reported after therapy with doxorubicin, busulfan, cyclophosphamide, methotrexate, and bleomycin.

Drugs such as doxorubicin, actinomycin D, mitoxantrone, cisplatin, vincristine, and vinblastine are notable for the severe phlebitis, cellulitis, and necrosis that follow extravasation (Ogilvie and Moore 1995). It is imperative that an intravenous infusion set placed by a "clean first-stick" technique be used for the injection of these drugs. If a butterfly catheter is used for injection of the small volumes of vincristine, the animal must be restrained properly to avoid inadvertent displacement of the needle. If extravasation occurs, as much of the drug as possible should be removed through the administration needle or catheter. Various compounds have been used for treating accidental extravasation, and the recommended treatment varies with the drug. Sodium bicarbonate, corticosteroids, hyaluronidase, sodium thiosulfate, dimethylsulfoxide (DMSO), and DHM3 have all been shown to be of value clinically or experimentally for specific extravasation injuries.

Liver and kidney cells respond to anticancer drugs in ways frequently unrelated to proliferation. Cisplatin is directly nephrotoxic in dogs, and cats are at a greater risk than dogs for renal damage after receiving doxorubicin. Acute tumor lysis syndrome has been reported in dogs, typically lymphoma patients, and can lead to renal failure (Brooks 1995). This life-threatening metabolic crisis is usually precipitated by cytotoxic chemotherapy that results in massive cell death and release of intracellular substances leading to hyperuricemia, hyperkalemia, hyperphosphatemia, and azotemia.

As a group, the cells of the central nervous system (CNS) are least affected by cytotoxic antitumor drugs because of the blood-brain barrier and their slow growth rate. Nevertheless, some of the drugs cause CNS toxicosis, and it is sometimes difficult to separate a direct drug effect on behavior from the combined effects of the tumor, debris from dying cells, poor nutritional status, and the therapeutic regimen. CNS toxicity may be seen with vincristine, but peripheral neuropathies are more likely (Hamilton et al. 1991a). Serious CNS toxicity is more prevalent in dogs and cats than humans treated with 5-fluorouracil, and L-asparaginase may cause neurotoxicity associated with accumulation of ammonia.

Long-term hazards of certain anticancer therapies are their properties of oncogenesis, mutagenesis, and teratogenesis. Recognition of this potential is important not only for the patient but also for individuals involved in reconstituting and administering these drugs.

Therapist Safety. Anticancer drugs constitute potential hazards to those who handle and administer them, so great caution and good technique should always be observed. Accidental exposure via the skin, respiratory system, or digestive system must be prevented by strict adherence to specific safety protocols. The US Department of Labor's Occupational Safety and Health Administration has issued guidelines for training of personnel in the storage, handling, and disposal of cytotoxic antineoplastic drugs (OSHA Instruction PUB 8-1.1, 1986). A complete discussion of personnel safety is beyond the scope of this chapter, but one can consult the following references for more information: Bonney and Knapp 1993; Morrison 1998c; Fox 1996.

Drug Dosage. Anticancer drugs are frequently dosed on the basis of surface area rather than body weight. A conversion of weight to surface area can be made with the following formula:

$$\text{surface area} = \text{body weight}^{0.67} \times K/10^4$$

where surface area is given in square meters and body weight in grams. For cats and dogs, K is a constant with the value of 10.0 and 10.1, respectively. Conversion tables are widely available, but a few values will give a perspective on the relationship. The following values for the dog list the weight in kilograms followed by the surface area in square meters: 1, 0.1; 10, 0.46; 20, 0.74; 30, 0.96; 40, 1.17; and 50, 1.36. Obviously, failure to convert the patient's weight from pounds to kilograms prior to using the conversion table will result in an approximately doubled dosage being administered to the patient. For many drugs, this calculation error could be fatal.

For several drugs, it has been shown that using body surface area for dose calculation rather than weight may lead to inappropriate drug levels and toxicities, particularly in smaller patients (Arrington et al. 1994; Page et al. 1988). For further discussion of the use of body surface area–based dose calculations, see Price and Frazier 1998 and Frazier and Price 1998.

As one might predict, drug dosage, interval between doses, and duration of therapy are crucial factors in determining the success of cancer therapy. It is important to realize that drugs must be used at the maximum dose possible to achieve optimal therapeutic effects. If the dose of a drug is decreased to the point that it does not produce clinical toxicity, the regimen will likely fail.

Resistance. Despite increasing success in treating cancer, particularly in producing initial responses, too often the long-term result remains failure. Although drug resistance can be viewed from the perspective of the whole tumor, ultimately drug effectiveness will depend on the response of each individual cell to the drug. Resistance to drugs by individual cells can be temporary or permanent and can be present when therapy is begun or arise during its course. Resistance mechanisms can be divided into three broad categories: low concentration of drug in the tumor (pharmacokinetic resistance); small fraction of cells in a susceptible state (kinetic resistance); and biochemical resistance of the tumor cells to the drug even in normally susceptible phases (genetic resistance).

Pharmacokinetic resistance can occur in response to changes in absorption, distribution, biotransformation, and elimination of drugs. Distribution to tumor cells is one of the most important of these. Blood flow to tumors is not as well regulated as it is to normal tissues. In fact, tumors may outgrow their blood supply, leading to extremely slow growth in affected portions of the tumor due to lack of nutrients, including oxygen, and a buildup of metabolic by-products. Under these conditions, drug delivery to many parts of the tumor may be impaired, and further, drug that does reach these sites may find fewer responsive cells because under unfavorable conditions, cells may leave the growth fraction.

As mentioned earlier in this chapter, most cytotoxic drugs are more effective against cells that are rapidly moving through the cell cycle, as would occur in tumors with a large growth fraction. Since the growth fraction is generally inversely proportional to the tumor volume, it is not surprising that cytotoxic drug therapy is less effective on large tumors due, in part, to the decreased growth fraction. This type of resistance has been termed *kinetic resistance* and is considered to be reversible. In this type of resistance, large numbers of cells may become resistant at once.

As important as pharmacokinetic and kinetic resistances may be, they are ultimately less responsible for drug failure than *genetic resistance,* where the trait for the particular resistance is passed to daughter cells and is irreversible. This type of resistance arises from a single mutant cell and may be present before therapy is begun or may appear during therapy. By the time they are diagnosed, most tumors have at least a few cells that are resistant to a particular chemotherapeutic regimen. Regardless of how or when resistant cells appear, as sensitive cells are killed, the resistant cells constitute an increasing proportion of the total number of tumor cells. After they become the predominant cell type, what was originally a "clinically sensitive" tumor becomes a "clinically resistant" tumor.

The *Goldie-Coldman model* assumes that genetic resistance is a permanent all-or-none phenomenon and predicts that once a single cell within a tumor becomes resistant to the current course of therapy, that therapy is ultimately doomed to failure. This assumption has been challenged, however, by the finding that in at least one in vitro tumor model, resistance is associated with shifts in the dose-response curve to the right, i.e., to requiring higher doses of drug (Kuczek and Chan 1992). Nevertheless, the Goldie-Coldman model is valuable because it highlights the importance of early, aggressive therapy to minimize the time available for resistant cells to appear. Biochemical mechanisms of genetic drug resistance in tumor cells are similar to those of bacteria. The following mechanisms have been listed: decreased intracellular accumulation of drug, defective transport, defective drug activation, altered DNA repair, gene amplification, altered target protein, increased drug detoxification, and defective apoptosis (Kaufman and Chabner 1996).

Decreased intracellular accumulation of drug is the ultimate result of a well-known phenomenon called *multidrug resistance* (MDR), which leads to resistance to structurally different drugs, e.g., anthracyclines, epipodophyllotoxins, and vinca alkaloids. Other mechanisms of MDR continue to be investigated, including alteration of DNA topoisomerase activity, alteration of glutathione metabolism, increased lung-resistance protein, increase in DNA-repair associated protein, inhibition of apoptosis, and multiresistance protein-associated MDR (Goldie and Coldman 1998; Kaufman and Chabner 1996; Tannock and Goldenberg 1998). The following discussion will focus on the best-studied example, membrane-bound p-glycoprotein (Gp170) activity.

Decreased accumulation of drug in MDR cells is associated with overexpression of p-glycoprotein (Gp170), which acts as a membrane transporter for a variety of molecular structures from the interior of the cell. This membrane glycoprotein pumps drugs out of cells by a mechanism that requires ATP. Substrates for the transporter tend to be hydrophobic lipid-soluble organic cations. Genes controlling the expression of p-glycoprotein are strongly conserved across species. A variety of normal tissues in mammals have been found to express the protein in an inducible form (kidney, liver, small intestine, colon, uterine secretory epithelium, and adrenal gland), but much higher levels of expression are seen in a variety of tumors, especially those that have regrown after previous treatment by drugs known to be substrates for p-glycoprotein. Probable failure due to MDR has been well predicted by measuring p-glycoprotein expression in some childhood tumors (Chan et al. 1993). See Gatmaitan and Arias 1993 for more information on the normal function of this protein.

It has been shown that for a variety of tumors, there is a high correlation between the presence of p-glycoprotein and drug failure ending in patient death. Attempts to reverse the resistance by inhibiting the transporter have led to clinical trials of drugs known as *chemosensitizers.* Drugs known to work in vitro and being tested in clinical trials in human medicine include verapamil, tamoxifen, quinidine, and analogs of cyclosporin A. While moderate restoration of drug sensitivity has been seen in clinical trials, dramatic responses have not been observed. This is probably due to the multifactorial basis for drug resistance in advanced tumors (Goldie and Coldman 1998). Indeed, in a small number of drug-resistant canine lymphomas, a trial of verapamil and quinine as chemosensitizers produced equivocal results (Klein and Dalton 1992). Consult the following reviews for additional information on this topic: Chan et al. 1993; Georges et al. 1990.

Attempts have also been made to augment anticancer drug action in sensitive cells and to reverse resistance in other cells. An example of one approach is to inhibit efflux of drug from tumor cells. Dipyridamole inhibits membrane nucleoside transport, which occurs in both directions. If one were to administer an anticancer drug transported by this system and follow it an optimal period of time later with dipyridamole, perhaps one could maintain a much higher concentration of the drug within the cell.

Selection of Regimens. Selection of a treatment regimen for an individual patient is empirical and is based largely on the results of clinical trials of drugs in similar cases. Use of in vitro tests for drug efficacy as guides for drug selection have been controversial, and there has been little scientific evidence to show that these tests are helpful in veterinary medicine. These tests are apparently better at predicting drug failure than at identifying drugs that will have clinical efficacy.

The relationship between growth rate, tumor size, and treatment effectiveness implies that tumor size and location(s) are crucial prognostic determinants. Thus, various approaches for "staging" tumors have been developed (Henderson et al. 1995). Drug trials must compare efficacy in tumors of similar susceptibility (i.e., similar stage) for any observed differences to be meaningful.

Combination Chemotherapy. Combination chemotherapy is commonplace in the treatment of cancer because of results of clinical trials using agents singly and in combination. A *combination chemotherapy* treatment regimen entails the use of two or more chemotherapeutic agents at specified dosages and intervals. Combination protocols to be tested in clinical trials are carefully designed using knowledge of pharmacology and toxicology of drugs and their effects on tumors as individual entities.

The rationale of combination therapy is based on the facts that additive effects on tumors are frequently more pronounced than on normal tissues, there is a decreased tendency toward the development of resistance, a combination may be less toxic than an equivalently effective single agent, and heterogeneous stem cell populations usually fail to respond uniformly to a single agent. Some commonsense rules guiding selection of combinations are that each drug should be active on the tumor, drugs should have different mechanisms of action, toxicities should overlap minimally, and each drug should be administered at its optimal dosage and schedule. Drugs should be given at consistent time intervals; the treatment-free interval between cycles should be the shortest time necessary for recovery of the most sensitive normal target tissue, usually bone marrow (Morrison 1998a).

Because combination chemotherapeutic regimens frequently cause complete initial responses followed by relapses, it has been concluded that resistant cells were present at the time therapy was initiated or arose by mutation during the course of therapy. *Multiregimen therapy* is an attempt to overcome this limitation and refers to the rapid alternation of non-cross-resistant therapeutic regimens. Although not completely proven, it appears that multiregimen therapy does not improve the long-term results of therapy if small numbers of genetically resistant cells are present at the beginning of therapy. There is evidence that this approach may improve results against tumors in which mutations lead to resistance during therapy (Shackney 1993).

Multimodal Therapy. Classic modalities of cancer therapy include surgery, radiation, and chemotherapy, although today many new modalities are being used as well. Examples of these include immunotherapy, hyperthermia, and use of biological response modifiers.

Although techniques such as surgery and radiation continue to improve, it is still apparent that many patients die of cancer after the primary tumor has been "successfully" removed. As early as 1957, it was shown that 0% of mice were cured of adenocarcinoma 755 (a model system) after surgery, saline, or chemotherapy alone. When surgery and chemotherapy were combined, the rate of cure was 57% (Shapiro and Fugmann 1957). Multimodal (or adjuvant) therapy is now advocated for many human tumors as a result of the failure of a therapeutic modality to cure cancer when used alone. It appears that full doses of adjuvant therapy should be started at the time of or before primary tumor removal. It is tempting to use low doses because no tumor is visible. Controversy over the advocacy of adjuvant therapy arises because of the potential for producing needless toxicity in patients (if no micrometastases are present) and because of the carcinogenic potential of some drugs. Thus the decision to use multimodal therapy will depend on the tumor type and extent, as well as patient factors discussed earlier. A good clinical example of the use of adjuvant chemotherapy in veterinary medicine is the postoperative use of cisplatin, carboplatin, or doxorubicin following limb amputation or a limb salvage procedure in dogs with appendicular osteosarcoma (Straw et al. 1991; Bergman et al. 1996). Lengthened survival times have been shown repeatedly over surgery alone.

DRUGS. Drug groups and individual drugs are discussed in this section. Typical doses, formulations, and some notable facts about the most frequently used drugs are summarized in Morrison 1998b. Practical information on storage of these expensive drugs for veterinary medicine has been published (Rosenthal 1991).

Alkylating Agents. Alkylating agents were shown to produce a dramatic response in Hodgkin's disease in 1943, making them the first nonhormonal drugs to be used successfully in the treatment of cancer. They are highly reactive molecules in their active state. Alkylating agents undergo strongly electrophilic chemical reactions through formation of carbonium ion intermediates or transition complexes with the target molecules. The intermediates then react with strongly nucleophilic substituents in the cell (e.g., phosphate, amino, sulfhydryl, hydroxyl, carboxyl, imidazole groups) to form covalent bonds. The target molecule is then said to have been alkylated. Alkylation of DNA is the effect primarily responsible for the cytotoxic activity. Such alkylation, of which the 7-nitrogen atom of guanine is an important site, may lead to covalent cross-linking of DNA strands or linking of DNA to a closely associated protein if the drug is a bifunctional alkylating agent. Alkylation of guanine may also shift its electron configuration so that it base-pairs with thymine rather than cytosine, ultimately resulting in the substitution of an adenine-thymine pair in place of a guanine-cytosine pair. Labilization of the imidazole ring may cause the guanine to be lost from the DNA strand, with resultant breaking of the chain. It is not difficult to see how the alkylating agents could be mutagenic and carcinogenic.

Alkylating agents are not regarded as being cell-cycle-specific, because they have more-profound effects on nonproliferating cells than many of the other groups of drugs. However, they are still most effective against cells rapidly traversing the cell cycle, i.e., in tumors with a high growth fraction. For this reason they are much more toxic to bone marrow than to such organs as liver and kidney. Infertility in both males and females may be a problem.

Alkylating agents are frequently referred to as radiomimetic drugs because their action in causing DNA-strand breaks resembles that of radiation. Their action is also conceptually similar to that of cisplatin. Alkylating agents have a relatively wide spectrum of antitumor activity and are very useful in treating tumors of lymphoreticular tissues, with more limited activity against sarcomas and carcinomas.

Tumors commonly, but slowly, develop resistance that may extend across the class of alkylating, or "DNA cross-linking," agents. Several major mechanisms are involved. There may be an increase in the concentration of intracellular nucleophilic substrates (e.g., metallothionein or glutathione) that can compete with DNA for the drugs; thus, the drugs are inactivated by conjugation. There may be increased concentration of aldehyde dehydrogenase in the case of cyclophosphamide. There may be increased activity of DNA repair systems. Reduced intracellular drug accumulation may be a factor due to decreased transport into the cell or increased removal. Resistance to one alkylating agent does not necessarily imply resistance to the others. For example, melphalan is transported into cells by the leucine transport system, whereas mechlorethamine is taken in by the choline transport system. If resistance was due to a change in one of these mechanisms, cross-resistance would be unexpected.

NITROGEN MUSTARDS. Commonly used nitrogen mustards, all of which are bifunctional alkylating agents, include mechlorethamine, cylophosphamide, ifosfamide, melphalan, and chlorambucil. Major differences in the nitrogen mustards are pharmacokinetic. Mechlorethamine is so unstable that it must be given intravenously (IV), freshly prepared. Its serum half-life is on the order of minutes. Conversely, chlorambucil and cyclophosphamide are so stable they can be given orally; cyclophosphamide, a pro-drug, must be activated in the liver.

The mustards are especially toxic to lymphocytes and bone marrow cells. In affected cells, mitosis is stopped and disintegration of formed elements of lymphoid tissue and bone marrow is evident within hours of a therapeutic dose. Immunosuppression and myelosuppression can be profound and a dose-limiting factor in therapy. Although large doses of the mustards can be severely toxic to the GI tract, proportionately this tendency is less severe than with other groups of drugs.

Mechlorethamine Hydrochloride, USP (nitrogen mustard, Mustargen), is a severe vesicant that was the first agent to be used in clinical oncology. In contrast to the other mustards, it has significant GI toxicity, including nausea and vomiting. Myelosuppression is also a major toxicity, as expected from its classification as a nitrogen mustard. Other toxicities include irregularities in reproduction, fetal abnormalities, and CNS effects, e.g., convulsions, paralysis, and cholinomimetic effects. It is rarely used in veterinary medicine.

Cyclophosphamide, USP (Cytoxan), is widely used in veterinary medicine, especially in combination with other drugs, but requires multistep activation in the liver. The first step in the activation of cyclophosphamide is accomplished by a hepatic cytochrome P-450 mixed-function oxidase. One of the metabolites, aldophosphamide, may be converted to phosphoramide mustard and acrolein in target cells. Phosphoramide mustard alkylates and cross-links DNA strands. Increased aldehyde dehydrogenase concentrations have been documented in some tumors resistant to cyclophosphamide.

When used clinically, the dose-limiting side effect of cyclophosphamide is bone marrow suppression, leading to leukopenia and thrombocytopenia. The nadir occurs 7–10 days following oral or IV administration. Sterile necrotizing hemorrhagic cystitis, probably caused by the metabolite acrolein, has been associated with administration of cyclophosphamide in both cats and dogs (Crow et al. 1977) and is a cause for stopping therapy with the drug. To decrease the incidence of this toxicity, which is manifested by bloody urine, dysuria, and frequent secondary bacterial infections, the oral drug should be administered in the morning (if the pet can be let out during the day) so that the animal can be allowed to urinate frequently. Water intake may be encouraged by lightly salting the food and, in some instances, by the concurrent administration of corticosteroids. Sterile hemorrhagic cystitis has developed after a single IV dose of cyclophosphamide (Peterson et al. 1992). In addition, cyclophosphamide has been associated with the development of transitional cell carcinoma of the urinary bladder (Macy et al. 1983).

Ifosfamide is a structural analog of cyclophosphamide that has been proven to have some efficacy against canine lymphoma (Frimberger et al. 1995). It is also similar to cyclophosphamide in that it must be converted to cytotoxic metabolites in the liver. One of these metabolites, phosphoramide mustard, can alkylate and cross-link DNA chains. Currently, ifosfamide is not a first-line drug. Its propensity to cause dysuria, frequent urination, and other signs of bladder irritation is even greater than that of cyclophosphamide. Bladder irrigation with thiol compounds may help, and systemically administered *N*-acetylcysteine may also be of value. It is highly recommended that mesna be concurrently administered (Elias et al. 1990; Frimberger et al. 1995). Mesna (sodium 2-mercaptoethanesulfonate, Mesnex) is an injectable used prophylactically and specifically to reduce the incidence of cystitis. The physically inert mesna disulfide (administered form) is reduced by renal tubules to mesna. Mesna binds to and detoxifies urotoxic metabolites of cyclophosphamide and ifosfamide (Elias et al. 1990) Myelosuppression (neutropenia and milder thrombocytopenia) remains a dose-limiting toxicity.

Melphalan, USP (L-Phenylalanine mustard, Alkeran), has been used primarily for treatment of multiple myeloma. It may produce anorexia, nausea, and vomiting but tends to be well tolerated. Leukopenia, thrombocytopenia, and anemia are the dose-limiting toxicities.

Chlorambucil, USP (Leukeran), is used in cases of chronic lymphocytic leukemia and small cell lymphoma, as well as inflammatory disorders characterized by lymphocyte infiltration in dogs and cats. It is also used as a substitute for cyclophosphamide, particularly when hemorrhagic cystitis has developed. It can be used orally and is the slowest acting of the mustards. Its toxic effects are bone marrow suppression, including leukopenia and delayed thrombocytopenia, but it is typically well tolerated by dogs and cats. High doses may cause cerebellar necrosis and atrophy. Nausea, vomiting, diarrhea, and skin pigmentation are rare.

ALKYLSULFONATES. *Busulfan,* USP (Myleran), is the only significant member of the alkylsulfonates. It is used to treat chronic granulocytic leukemia and polycythemia vera in people. Therapeutic doses produce myelosuppression; in humans, the leukocyte count begins to fall after approximately 10 days of therapy and continues to fall for 2 weeks after discontinuation of the drug. Thrombocytopenia and anemia may also be evident. It may produce so-called busulfan lung, in which pulmonary fibrosis is the end result. Skin hyperpigmentation occasionally occurs.

NITROSOUREAS. The nitrosoureas include carmustine and lomustine. Streptozotocin, another nitrosourea, is rarely used in treatment of animal cancers due to nephrotoxicity but has been used to treat insulinomas in dogs (Meyer 1976, 1977). The nitrosoureas are primarily bifunctional alkylating agents but also act by carbamoylation of lysine residues of proteins. Because they are highly lipid soluble, they have proven useful against tumors of the canine CNS, as well as relapsed canine lymphoma (Dimski and Cook 1990; Fulton and Steinberg 1990; Hamilton et al. 1991b; Moore et al. 1995a). There are reports of its use for unresectable mast cell tumors in dogs.

Limiting toxicities of this group are severe: cumulative myelosuppression and thrombocytopenia. Delayed and cumulative bone marrow suppression is a noteworthy characteristic of the nitrosoureas. In humans the nadir is reached in 4–6 weeks. There is no cross-resistance with other alkylating agents, and the drugs are not cell-cycle-specific. The nitrosoureas have extremely short plasma half-lives; in humans the α and β half-lives are 6 and 68 minutes, respectively. In humans, the drugs are primarily metabolized in the liver.

Carmustine, *N,N-bis*(2-chloroethyl)-*N*-nitrosourea (BiCNU, BCNU), is used in humans with meningeal leukemia and other brain tumors. The treatment interval, dosage, or both are altered if myelosuppression is severe or persistent. The infusion rate must be slow (dose given over 1–2 hr) to prevent local pain. Nausea and vomiting are major problems and occur about 2 hours after drug administration. Hepatotoxicity is manifested by increased serum glutamic pyruvic transaminase (SGPT), alkaline phosphatase, and bilirubin. In addition to the already mentioned bone marrow suppression, there may be renal toxicity. Lomustine

(CeeNU, CCNU) has been evaluated in canine patients with brain masses with some success (Fulton and Steinberg 1990). The most common side effect noted was bone marrow suppression with this orally administered drug.

TRIAZINES. *Dacarbazine,* USP, 5-(3,3-dimethyl-1-triazenyl)-1*H*-imidazole-4-carboxamide (DTIC), is the only triazine compound used in tumor therapy. Because of its structural resemblance to 5-aminoimidazole-4-carboxamide (AIC), which can be converted to inosinic acid, dacarbazine was thought to be an antimetabolite. However, the drug must be activated by a hepatic microsomal cytochrome P-450–dependent *N*-demethylation. An alkylating moiety may then be spontaneously released in the target cells along with AIC. Dacarbazine appears to inhibit RNA and protein synthesis more than DNA synthesis, is not cell-cycle-specific, and seems to kill cells slowly.

Dacarbazine has been used to treat human tumors such as malignant melanoma, sarcomas, and, in a second-line regimen, Hodgkin's lymphoma. Its use in relapsed canine lymphoma has been investigated (Van Vechten et al. 1990). Bone marrow suppression is usually the dose-limiting toxicity and includes leukopenia, thrombocytopenia, and lymphoid depletion. Anemia is uncommon and hepatotoxicity is rare. Although injections are painful, the drug may be given IV over 5 minutes. Extravasation may cause tissue damage. Nausea and vomiting are produced within a few hours of administration in more than 90% of human patients and may last up to 12 hours. Alopecia and an "influenza-like" syndrome consisting of malaise and myalgia have also been reported to occur in humans. Anorexia, debility, and malaise have been observed in the dog.

Antimetabolites. Antimetabolites resemble normal cellular substituents and either compete with them in enzymatic reactions to slow key cellular processes or replace them as substrates, leading to false products that then interfere with important cellular processes. Some antimetabolites are pro-drugs; i.e., they must be biochemically converted to their active form. Clinically useful antimetabolites ultimately inhibit DNA synthesis as their major anticancer mechanism, although their site of action may be several steps removed. In some cases, such as 5-FU, inhibition of RNA processing may also be important. The relative importance of altered DNA versus RNA synthesis and function may be dependent on tumor type. Antimetabolites profoundly inhibit replication of bone marrow cells, and some cause even greater GI toxicity. As their parent category implies, these agents are highly cell-cycle-specific when inhibition of DNA synthesis is the dominant effect. Because cells are far more sensitive to some antimetabolites while in the S phase, those antimetabolites are further categorized as phase-specific.

FOLIC ACID ANALOGS. *Methotrexate,* USP (Amethopterin), is a folic acid analog used against a wide variety of neoplasms, including lymphoreticular neoplasms and human choriocarcinoma (where it produced the first cure of cancer). It is most commonly used in veterinary medicine in protocols treating lymphoma (Bortnowski and Rosenthal 1991; Vonderhaar and Morrison 1998).

After being transported into cells, methotrexate binds strongly to dihydrofolate reductase (DHFR). The resulting inhibition of DHFR depletes cellular tetrahydrofolates (THF), which function as a donor of 1-carbon moieties important in the synthesis of nucleic acids. A possible second mechanism of action is inhibition of thymidylate synthase and other folate-dependent enzymes by accumulation of the derivative polyglutamyl-methotrexate (polyglutamyl-MTX), which has a high affinity for these enzymes. Decreased THF concentration impairs nucleic acid synthesis by decreasing conversion of deoxyuridine monophosphate (dUMP) to thymidine monophosphate (TMP) by thymidylate and by disrupting the de novo synthesis of the purine inosinic acid, a precursor of adenine and guanine nucleotides. Methotrexate is specific to the S phase.

Methotrexate is actively transported into cells by a saturable, carrier-mediated system, so it is active at extremely low concentrations in some cell systems. It does not readily enter cells by passive diffusion and crosses the blood-brain barrier poorly. Because some tumor cells have poor transport systems, it may be difficult to produce therapeutically effective concentrations in them. In fact, impaired transport of methotrexate constitutes one of the mechanisms of acquired resistance. Two others are production of DHFRs that have decreased affinity for the drug and increased concentrations of the reductase through gene amplification.

Some human tumors have been treated with large doses of methotrexate that would be fatal if an antidote were not given within several hours. *Leucovorin rescue* is accomplished by giving *Leucovorin Calcium,* USP (*N*5-formyl THF, folinic acid, citrovorum factor), a fully functional donor of 1-carbon fragments that is more rapidly transported into normal cells than into tumor cells, thus providing selective relief from methotrexate toxicity. High-dose therapy is controversial in human medicine and is rarely, if ever, used in veterinary medicine because of the potential for severe toxicity and the need for intensive monitoring.

Myelosuppression and GI mucositis are the most important side effects of methotrexate. Hepatotoxicity may be noted and it may be advisable to monitor renal function prior to and during therapy because methotrexate produces renal tubular necrosis when given in high doses. In humans, more than 90% of methotrexate is excreted unchanged, primarily by the kidneys. If renal function is impaired, fatal accumulation may occur. Maintenance of an alkaline urine with high volume flow is important to decrease toxicity, especially with high doses. In veterinary medicine, most drug combinations use methotrexate at modest doses.

PYRIMIDINE ANALOGS. *Cytarabine,* USP (β-cytosine arabinoside, arabinosyl cytosine, Ara-C, Cytosar), is a pyrimidine analog that is well established in the treatment of acute leukemia in humans, as the sole agent and in combinations. It has also been used for lymphoreticular and myeloproliferative disorders in dogs and cats, particularly when the CNS is involved. It has been reported to cause remission in a cat with megakaryocytic leukemia (Hamilton et al. 1991c).

Cytarabine enters cells via a membrane transporter. It inhibits DNA synthesis and is, therefore, active in the S phase of the cell cycle. It must be activated to Ara-cytidine triphosphate (Ara-CTP) to inhibit DNA synthesis. The first step in the activation of Ara-C is phosphorylation catalyzed by deoxycytidine kinase to form Ara-cytidine monophosphate (Ara-CMP), the 5′-monophosphate nucleotide. Ara-CMP is then converted to Ara-CTP, which serves as a substrate for DNA synthesis. DNA polymerase is inhibited by Ara-CTP, but the dominant cytotoxic effect stems from incorporation of Ara-CTP into the DNA chain, where it terminates chain growth.

Acquired or de novo resistance may be related to increased intracellular concentration of cytidine deaminase, which converts cytarabine to a less toxic form, Ara-U. Resistant mutants that lack deoxycytidine kinase, the activating enzyme, have been identified. Some resistant mutants have been shown to have high intracellular concentrations of deoxycytidine triphosphate (dCTP), causing decreased activation (phosphorylation) of cytarabine.

Bone marrow suppression is the dose-limiting toxicity. It is manifest by leukopenia, thrombocytopenia, anemia, and megaloblastosis. The leukocyte count may drop within 2 days and continue to fall for up to a week after treatment is stopped. Rapid IV injection is especially likely to induce anorexia, nausea, and vomiting. In contrast to fluorouracil, stomatitis is uncommon. Mild, reversible hepatic dysfunction may occur. The drug should be given by IV infusion for best results but has been administered subcutaneously in animals.

Cytarabine is included in many protocols for treatment of CNS leukemia and lymphoma in dogs and cats. A pharmacokinetic study revealed that cytarabine did cross the blood-brain barrier and that therapeutic doses could produce effective concentrations in the cerebrospinal fluid (CSF) of dogs (Scott-Moncrieff et al. 1991). The plasma elimination half-life in dogs was approximately 64–69 minutes, whereas the half-life of cytarabine in CSF was 165 minutes. The peak concentration of cytarabine in CSF was 29 μM.

Fluorouracil, USP, 5-fluoro-2,4(1*H*,3*H*)-pyrimidinedione (5-FU, Efudex, Adrucil), is a pyrimidine analog used in people for carcinomas of the mammary gland, GI tract (colorectal carcinomas), and ultraviolet light–induced tumors of the skin. Some exploratory work has been done in dogs with GI tract tumors. The topical preparation of 5-flourouracil has been used on cutaneous squamous cell carcinomas in dogs and horses (Madewell and Theilen 1987; Fortier and Harg 1994).

Both DNA synthesis and RNA synthesis and function are altered by 5-FU metabolites. The pro-drug, 5-FU, is metabolized intracellularly to 5′-fluorouridine monophosphate (FUMP) and then to 5′-fluorodeoxyuridine monophosphate (FdUMP). FdUMP, a potent inhibitor of thymidylate synthase, decreases the synthesis of DNA precursors. Fluorouracil is also incorporated into RNA. It is highly cell-cycle-specific, but no clear association with a particular phase has been demonstrated. The relative importance of inhibition of DNA synthesis versus effects on RNA synthesis appears to be tumor dependent.

Fluorouracil is most toxic to bone marrow and oral and GI mucosa. Thus, bone marrow suppression manifested by neutropenia, thrombocytopenia, and anemia can be severe and is the major dose-limiting factor. Anorexia, nausea, and vomiting are frequently seen. Diarrhea and stomatitis are indications for the interruption of therapy. CNS toxicity is regarded as unusual in humans but may be more common in animals (Morrison 1998b). The signs include dementia, excitement, tremors, and ataxia, sometimes followed by opisthotonos, tonic-clonic convulsions, dyspnea, shock, and death. Unexpected neurotoxicity was reported when 5-FU was used in combination with dactinomycin and cyclophosphamide (Hammer et al. 1994a). The drug is contraindicated in cats due to neurotoxicity (Morrison 1998b). Other manifestations of toxicity include skin rash, alopecia, hyperpigmentation, photosensitization, and mild tissue irritation. A cream formulation has been shown to be very toxic if accidentally eaten. A report on 5-FU toxicity in dogs has been published (Dorman et al. 1990).

Fluorouracil is unpredictably absorbed from the GI tract and is usually given by IV injection. The drug is highly metabolized and readily enters the CSF. Fluorouracil is supplied in ampules containing 500 mg of drug for IV injection and as a 5% cream (Efudex). The cream is intended for actinic keratoses and superficial basal or squamous cell carcinoma.

PURINE ANALOGS. *Mercaptopurine,* USP (6-mercaptopurine, 6-MP, Purinethol), is a purine analog used mainly to treat lymphoreticular tumors in humans and has been rarely used to treat leukemias in dogs. Its close relative, *Azathioprine,* USP (Imuran), is used as an immunosuppressive agent.

6-Mercaptopurine must be activated in vivo. It is a substrate for hypoxanthine-guanine phosphoribosyltransferase (HGPRT) and is converted to the corresponding ribonucleotides. The product of the HGPRT reaction with 6-MP, 6-thioinosine-5′-phosphate, inhibits conversion of IMP to AMP and GMP, possibly the cytotoxic effect. Acquired resistance is not shared with other neoplastic agents and may be most often caused by a deficiency of the enzyme HGPRT. Other mechanisms, including decreased uptake by target cells, have been reported. Leukopenia, anemia, and a less severe thrombocytopenia may occur. GI toxicity includes frequent nausea, vomiting, and anorexia.

Stomatitis and diarrhea are rare. Reversible cholestatic jaundice is fairly frequent. Mercaptopurine is variably absorbed after oral administration.

Natural Products

VINCA ALKALOIDS. The vinca alkaloids are large, complex substances derived from the periwinkle plant (*Vinca rosea* L.). Although similar in structure, *Vincristine Sulfate,* USP (Oncovin), and *Vinblastine Sulfate,* USP (Velban, Velsar), differ considerably in antitumor efficacy as well as in the doses that produce toxic effects. These drugs, especially vincristine, are widely used in veterinary medicine in combination with others. Vincristine is the drug of choice for treating transmissible venereal tumor and is commonly used against lymphoreticular neoplasms in a variety of combination protocols. In addition, it may be used in combination with doxorubicin and cyclophosphamide to treat soft-tissue sarcomas. While vincristine has not proven particularly effective, vinblastine has been used with some success to treat unresectable canine mast cell tumors (McCaw et al. 1997; Thamm et al. 1999). Vinca alkaloids are specific to the M phase.

Vinca alkaloids are taken into cells by an energy-dependent carrier-mediated transport system. Both produce a colchicine-like arrest in metaphase. They bind to tubulin, a key protein in microtubules, and cause their dissolution. Microtubules are important for maintaining structural integrity of cells, as conduits for transport of solutes and neurotransmitters, and for secretion of some hormones, such as insulin and thyroid hormones. They are also important for mitotic spindle formation. Inability to segregate chromosomes may be the cytotoxic effect, but the alteration of transport processes may underlie some of the adverse effects. Both colchicine and podophyllotoxin bind to tubulin, but apparently at sites different from the vinca alkaloids. Taxol, an exploratory anticancer drug, also binds to tubulin, but the effect is to increase stability of microtubules rather than to cause their dissolution. It is remarkable that although structurally similar, there is no cross-resistance between vincristine and vinblastine. The vinca alkaloids are, however, susceptible to the MDR phenomenon related to the presence of p-glycoprotein in affected cell membranes (Georges et al. 1990).

Vinblastine may produce a dose-limiting leukopenia, the nadir of which occurs at 5–10 days. Hematologic effects of vincristine are mild, but neutropenia is occasionally seen (Hahn et al. 1996). Thrombocytopenia and anemia are rare with both drugs. Indeed, vincristine induces thrombocytosis and is used to treat severe cases of immune-mediated thrombocytopenia. Both are severe tissue irritants.

Vincristine is much more likely than vinblastine to produce neurotoxicity, although entry of either drug into the brain and CSF is minimal. This difference is paradoxic because vinblastine is more lipid soluble. One hypothetical explanation is that the slower elimination of vincristine relative to vinblastine may lead to prolonged exposure of nerve tissue to high concentrations of vincristine. Mild sensory neuropathy presenting with sensory impairment and paraesthesia is common in humans and is not dose-limiting. Peripheral neuropathy manifested as paresis, voice change, or muscle wasting may be noted in animals (Hamilton et al. 1991a; Morrison 1998b).

In dogs, vinca alkaloids are eliminated by biliary excretion into the feces (Golden and Langston 1988). Both drugs are bound rapidly after injection by platelets, leukocytes, and other tissues rich in tubulin, which probably contributes to their rapid clearance from plasma. Because of the vesicant action of the vinca alkaloids, they should be carefully administered through a butterfly or indwelling catheter.

TAXOL. Taxol (paclitaxel) is the subject of intense interest because it has shown antitumor activity in drug-refractory ovarian and breast carcinomas in people (Horwitz 1992). Its source, the bark of the slowly growing yew, *Taxus brevifolia,* found only in old-growth forests of the Pacific Northwest, made its use problematic. Many trees had to be destroyed to obtain sufficient bark for a limited number of doses. However, supplies of the drug are now more plentiful due to successful efforts to synthetically produce the drug. Veterinary applications have not yet been extensively developed.

The mechanism of taxol promises new approaches to therapy. It is most effective as an inhibitor of cell replication in late G2 and M phases of the cell cycle. Taxol binds specifically and reversibly to tubulin subunits, preferentially to the β subunit. In the presence of microtubule-associated proteins, it can polymerize tubulin into stable microtubules. Ordinarily, microtubules are formed at 37° with expenditure of GTP. Calcium ions and reduced temperature (4°) depolymerize microtubules, but taxol converts the polymer into a stable form that will not depolymerize. Because polymers must continually be formed and broken down to meet changing needs of cells, taxol-induced stability of microtubules is obviously toxic.

Resistance to taxol stems from alterations in α and β subunits of tubulin and from the p-glycoprotein transport system associated with MDR. An interesting observation is that some cells with altered α and β subunits are actually dependent on taxol. This is reminiscent of bacteria that may be sensitive, resistant, or dependent on streptomycin depending on which one of three specific amino acids has been incorporated at a specific location in a ribosomal subunit.

In preclinical normal dog studies, sensitivity to the vehicle used to keep the drug in solution, cremophor EL plus alcohol, was manifested as pruritus, anaphylaxis, hypotension, and edema (Ogilvie et al. 1993a; Ogilvie 1994). Myelosuppression may be the dose-limiting toxicity and occurs on days 3–7. Although slowing the IV infusion rate may also lessen acute side effects, hypersensitivity reactions can be minimized by pretreating the patient with corticosteroids, cimetidine, and diphenhydramine 1 hour before administering paclitaxel (Morrison 1998b). Cats receiving the drug may develop anorexia that can last several days.

EPIPODOPHYLLOTOXINS. Podophyllotoxin is an extract of the mandrake plant that has led to the development of two synthetic derivatives: teniposide (VM-26) and etoposide (VP-16, VP-16-213, VePesid). Etoposide has become an important agent in the treatment of some human tumors. The mechanism of action of these drugs is apparently quite different from that of their parent, which is a spindle poison and produces metaphase arrest. Protein-linked single-strand breaks in DNA have been observed after exposure to etoposide. It inhibits nucleoside transport into cells as well as RNA and DNA synthesis. Etoposide binding to topoisomerase II may be responsible for the cytotoxic effect. Topoisomerase II catalyzes topological alterations in chromosomes that allow replication, transcription, and repair of DNA. Etoposide acts primarily in the G2 phase but may also act in late S or M phases. Increased expression of the p-glycoprotein associated with MDR has been observed in some tumors resistant to this drug. In a study of 13 dogs with lymphoma, only 2 had a response after treatment with etoposide (Hohenhaus and Matus 1990).

In people, the predominant dose-limiting adverse effect is hematologic, particularly neutropenia. The nadir occurs during the second week and recovery occurs during the third week. Nausea and vomiting are usually mild, and hair loss is common. Peripheral neuropathy has been observed and may be additive with that caused by other anticancer drugs. Parenterally administered etoposide should be given by infusion to avoid hypotension. Dogs receiving etoposide become hypotensive and exhibit a cutaneous reaction characterized by moderate to severe pruritus, urticaria, and swelling of the head and extremities attributed to the drug vehicle, polysorbate 80 (Ogilvie et al. 1988; Hohenhaus and Matus 1990).

Etoposide is highly lipophilic but still produces a low concentration in CSF. Approximately half of the dose is eliminated in the urine, of which 30% is inactive as metabolites. The remainder is eliminated by hepatic biotransformation and biliary secretion. Severe hepatic dysfunction is an indication for dose reduction. Half-lives after a single IV dose are 2.8 and 15.1 hours in humans (Slevin 1991). Etoposide may be given orally or IV. Oral bioavailability is approximately 50% but is not linear with dose.

ANTIBIOTICS. Clinically useful antineoplastic antibiotics were obtained by screening the broth of *Streptomyces* organisms for antitumor activity. All of the drugs in this series interact with DNA and/or RNA but may act on other cellular substituents as well. Currently, it is believed that most of the toxicity and antitumor activity is the result of free-radical formation or inhibition of topoisomerase II, which causes DNA fragmentation (Morrison 1998a). In addition, alteration of the DNA helical structure that occurs with DNA intercalation may trigger enhanced topoisomerase II activity and provide a more vulnerable target for anthracycline activity. Dosage does not appear to be as schedule dependent as with the antimetabolites, so the antibiotics may be less cell-cycle-phase-dependent, but their major activity is still evident during the S phase. It is difficult to generalize about the toxicity of this group. All except bleomycin must be given IV because they produce tissue necrosis.

The three *anthracycline* derivatives used in clinical oncology are doxorubicin, daunorubicin, and mitoxantrone. Mitoxantrone differs from the other two in that it is semisynthetic and lacks a sugar moiety.

Doxorubicin Hydrochloride, USP (Adriamycin), is one of the most important chemotherapy agents in veterinary medicine and has antitumor activity against a wide variety of tumors, including solid tumors (Ogilvie et al. 1989a). It is included in many sequential combination drug protocols and is also used as a solitary agent.

The anthracyclines are tetracycline ring structures substituted with the sugar daunosamine. Doxorubicin intercalates between base pairs of DNA. Because of the lack of correlation between intercalation in DNA and cytotoxicity, it has been argued that drugs said to act by "intercalating" actually interfere with the topoisomerase II reaction. As a result, it has been suggested that these drugs should be referred to as "DNA topoisomerase II poisons" (Schneider et al. 1990).

Inhibition of DNA-dependent RNA synthesis as a result of interactions described above is only one of the reputed mechanisms of action of doxorubicin. It is also well established that generation of free radicals by the electron-accepting and electron-donating quinone and hydroquinone moieties of doxorubicin cause membrane damage and DNA strand breaks.

Doxorubicin enters cells by a passive transport process. It is now well established that one cause of resistance to anthracyclines is excess activity of the p-glycoprotein transport system. The p-glycoprotein pumps anthracyclines and other drugs out of cells, leading to decreased intracellular concentration. Other causes of resistance to doxorubicin include changes in the cell membrane, changes in intracellular generation of free radicals, gene amplification, and decreased affinity of topoisomerase II for the drug. Calcium antagonists have been noted to reverse resistance in some model tumors. Other approaches to modulating MDR include encapsulation of drug in liposomes, which may alter its intracellular distribution (Thierry et al. 1993).

Toxicoses caused by doxorubicin have been reviewed and classified as acute, short-term, or chronic (Ogilvie et al. 1989b). Acute toxicosis manifests as head shaking, localized urticaria along the course of the vein used for administration of the drug, and signs associated with histamine release, including generalized blushing of the skin and acute collapse. Short-term reactions include weight loss, anorexia, diarrhea, vomiting, myelosuppression, bone marrow hypoplasia, lymphoid atrophy, and alopecia. Chronic toxicosis is associated with hair loss, testicular atrophy, and dose-dependent cardiac toxicosis leading to arrhythmias and cardiomyopathy. Ogilvie et al. also documented that the probability of doxorubicin-induced toxicity decreased significantly in an inverse relationship to body weight, and that dogs developing signs of toxicosis after their first dose of doxorubicin were 17 times more likely to develop toxicoses after a second dose.

Hematologic changes are the short-term dose-limiting manifestation of toxicity, although cardiac toxicity limits the maximum cumulative dose. Neutropenia, reaching a nadir 7–10 days after treatment and returning to normal by 3 weeks, is common. Less commonly, one may see thrombocytopenia (nadir between 3 and 8 days) and anemia that follow the same pattern. Poikilocytosis occurs in cats receiving doxorubicin (O'Keefe and Schaeffer 1992). Anorexia, nausea, and vomiting are usually mild to moderate. Stomatitis and GI ulceration leading to colitis and diarrhea may occur. The diarrhea may become apparent 3–5 days after treatment, later than with some other anticancer drugs.

Doxorubicin appears to release histamine if administered too rapidly. In dogs this manifests as severe pruritus and swelling, especially about the face, during administration. Rapid administration may result in acute GI upset (anorexia, vomiting, and bloody diarrhea) within 12–24 hours. Histamine-related signs may be decreased by pretreating dogs with diphenhydramine hydrochloride (Benadryl) at 1.0 mg/kg intramuscularly or slowly IV. An increased frequency of acute reactions has been reported with the use of a particular generic formulation of the drug (Phillips et al. 1998).

Anthracyclines cause two types of cardiac toxicity, one immediate and the other cumulative. During IV administration, one may see cardiac arrest preceded by electrocardiographic changes such as T-wave flattening, S-T segment depression, voltage reduction, and arrhythmias. This is usually brief and is not necessarily an indication to stop using doxorubicin. If the changes are minor, some clinicians cautiously continue with slower administration of drug. Others recommend discontinuing therapy with doxorubicin until a later time. Cardiac arrest can usually be avoided by premedication with antihistamines, which may be considered if an animal has previously shown a tendency to arrhythmias.

Cumulative myocardial toxicity is more severe and necessitates permanently stopping doxorubicin therapy. Most cardiac damage from doxorubicin exposure has been attributed to free-radical damage to the myocardium. Toxicity is manifested by arrythmias and congestive heart failure secondary to diffuse cardiomyopathy. The risk of congestive heart failure is thought to increase sharply above 250 mg/m^2 total dose in dogs, although the value used in people is 550–600 mg/m^2. For this reason, one should maintain a record of the total amount of doxorubicin given, stop therapy when the limit is reached, and watch carefully for signs of congestive heart failure. Echocardiographic (ECG) changes consistent with doxorubicin-induced cardiomyopathy occurred in 4 of 6 cats treated with 30 mg/m^2 after cumulative doses of 170–240 mg/m^2 body surface area (O'Keefe et al. 1993). Although clinical heart disease and ECG changes were not observed, subsequent histological examination revealed myocyte vacuolization and myocytolysis in all 6 hearts. Clinical cardiac abnormalities developed in 32 of 175 dogs treated with doxorubicin for a variety of malignancies (Mauldin et al. 1992). Thirty-one dogs had ECG abnormalities and 7 had congestive heart failure. All dogs with congestive heart failure died within 90 days. At necropsy, 13 of 32 affected dogs had noninflammatory myocardial degeneration. Reduction of doxorubicin-induced cardiotoxicity has been reported with dexrazoxane (ICRF-187) (Imondi et al. 1996). ICRF-187 is an analog of ethylenediaminetetraacetic acid (EDTA) and prevents cardiotoxicity by chelating iron and decreasing formation of hydroxyl radicals. There has been no large-scale evaluation of ICRF-187 in cancer-bearing dogs treated with doxorubicin.

Newer antitumor anthracycline derivatives, including epirubicin and idarubicin, with less cardiotoxicity have been studied, but none has replaced doxorubicin (Vonderhaar et al. 1994; Moore et al. 1995b). In an attempt to increase the effectiveness and reduce toxicity, the dose of doxorubicin was changed from every 3 weeks at 30 mg/m^2 to once per week at 10 mg/m^2. The regimen appeared safe but was not effective in the treatment of canine malignant lymphoma (Ogilvie et al. 1991a). Other attempts to increase effectiveness and reduce toxicity have included incorporation of doxorubicin into canine erythrocytes prior to administration. Following IV infusion, the area under the time versus drug concentration plot was increased to 734 μg × hr/L for erythrocyte-encapsulated drug from 136 μg × hr/L for free drug (Tonetti et al. 1991). Erythrocyte-encapsulated drug may be preferentially distributed to organs such as the liver and spleen. The effect of encapsulation on toxicity and efficacy remains to be established. A liposome-encapsulated form of doxorubicin has received considerable clinical attention (Vail et al. 1997; Kisseberth et al. 1995). This formulation appears to be well tolerated at doses comparable to those for free doxorubicin in tumor-bearing dogs. The drug is associated with an unusual dose-limiting toxicity that is cutaneous rather than myelosuppression.

The standard dose for dogs weighing more than 10 kg is 30 mg/m^2 IV every 3 weeks, while dogs weighing less than 10 kg and cats should receive 1 mg/kg IV at 3-week intervals. If smaller animals are dosed based upon body surface area, they tend to be overdosed relative to their body size and often experience greater toxicity (Morrison 1998b). Doxorubicin is a severe tissue irritant (vesicant) and causes mild alopecia and hyperpigmentation in the axillary and inguinal regions. Urine may be colored red while significant quantities of the drug and its metabolites are being eliminated. This is medically harmless and temporary.

Renal disease has been reported after administration of doxorubicin in normal cats and those with malignancies (Cotter et al. 1985; O'Keefe et al. 1993). In 6 cats treated with 30 mg/m^2 at 21-day intervals to a cumulative dose of 300 mg/m^2, histologic evidence of renal disease was identified at necropsy. Mean creatinine clearance values also decreased significantly throughout the study. Doxorubicin is biotransformed to less toxic doxorubicinol in the liver. It would seem that decreased hepatic function would necessitate dosage reduction, but specific guidelines are not available.

Doxorubicin is available in a sterile preparation in vials containing 10 or 50 mg of the drug. Heparin-containing solutions should be avoided during administration because heparin may cause precipitates to form. Doxorubicin should be administered through a well-placed indwelling catheter over 15–20 minutes with direct supervision.

Daunorubicin hydrochloride (daunomycin, Cerubidine) differs from doxorubicin only by having a proton in place of a hydroxyl group. It is similar to doxorubicin in mechanism and toxicity except that it has more pronounced cardiomyopathic effects. It is not effective against solid tumors and seems to have primary utility in treatment of acute lymphocytic and granulocytic leukemias in combination with cytarabine.

Mitoxantrone hydrochloride (Navantrone) is a completely synthetic dihydroxyquinone derivative of anthracene. It does not produce reactive free radicals, so its capacity to trigger topoisomerase II–dependent DNA cleavage is preserved but there is less cardiotoxicity. Another interesting difference is staining of the urine and sclera blue-green during early stages of therapy. The drug has shown activity against a variety of malignancies in dogs and cats (Ogilvie et al. 1991b; Ogilvie et al. 1993b). While it is not as effective as doxorubicin in many cases, it may benefit some patients. Toxicoses associated with its use include GI disturbances and sepsis secondary to neutropenia (Ogilvie et al. 1991c; Ogilvie et al. 1994b). The pharmacokinetics of mitoxantrone in cats has been investigated (Kochevar et al. 1995).

Sterile *Bleomycin Sulfate,* USP (Blenoxane), is actually a mixture of glycopeptides in which bleomycin AV2V and BV2V are dominant in the commercial form. Over 200 congeners have been isolated. This glycopeptide has an amino-terminal tripeptide (S tripeptide) able to bind to DNA and a heavy-metal (copper and iron) binding component located at the opposite end. Bleomycin has produced excellent results in humans in treatment of lymphoma and embryonal testicular tumors and good results in tumors of the head, neck, and skin, including squamous cell carcinoma. It has shown activity against squamous cell carcinoma in dogs and cats. It is highly valued in multidrug regimens because its toxicity does not overlap that of other anticancer drugs.

Bleomycin causes chromosomal abnormalities. The S tripeptide intercalates between guanine-cytosine base pairs of DNA. Superoxide or hydroxyl radicals resulting from the interaction of heavy metal (iron or copper) and bleomycin in direct contact with the base pairs may attack the phosphodiester bonds of the DNA backbone, causing release of free bases and DNA strand scission. This is followed by spontaneous oxidation of ferrous iron to the ferric state (or cuprous to cupric state) and the reduction of molecular oxygen to superoxide or hydroxyl radicals. Bleomycin is cell-cycle-phase-specific. It is most active in G2 but is also active in late G1, early S, and M phases.

Bleomycin is unique in that it causes no clinically significant toxicity to the bone marrow or GI tract. The dose-limiting toxicity of bleomycin in approximately 10% of human patients is pulmonary fibrosis, which may become apparent 4–10 weeks after initiation of therapy. Part of the explanation for this tissue selectivity may be that bleomycin is metabolized by an aminopeptidase B–like enzyme called bleomycin hydrolase, which is present in most tissues except the skin and lung. Thus, signs of toxicity are related to the skin and lung, where drug concentration is highest.

Pulmonary fibrosis may be due to redistribution of procollagen type I mRNAs in fibroblasts or to a direct action of bleomycin on cell types such as macrophages, lymphocytes, or type I and II epithelial cells, causing them to stimulate or inhibit release of secondary products that affect collagen deposition by fibroblasts. If the endothelial lining is damaged or if the drug is given intratracheally and if significant bleomycin reaches the interstitium of the lungs or macrophages, it may be possible to produce pulmonary fibrosis with a single low dose. In dogs, bleomycin initially produces interstitial pneumonia and, after intensive treatment, causes pleural scarring and pulmonary fibrosis. Risk factors include total dose, age, and concomitant use of other drugs. In humans, risk increases as total dose exceeds 400 units. Treatment should be stopped immediately if impairment of pulmonary function is noted. In veterinary patients, the duration of treatment is usually short due to limited remissions, making chronic toxicities less common (Morrison 1998b).

Toxic effects on the skin include desquamation, hyperpigmentation, and pruritic erythema. In humans, hardening and tenderness of the fingertips, ridging of the nails, and occasional bulla formation over pressure points have been noted. Stomatitis, nausea, vomiting, and anorexia may be seen. In humans, the incidence of hypersensitivity reactions is high, ranging from 20% to 50% of patients. Severity of reactions ranges from fever and chills to anaphylaxis. Bleomycin should be used with caution in the presence of renal or pulmonary disease. Bleomycin is distributed widely throughout the body after parenteral administration but does not enter the CSF. Decreased renal function slows elimination and necessitates dosage reduction in humans and, presumably, animals. Bleomycin is not active orally.

Dactinomycin, USP (actinomycin D, Cosmegen), is an antitumor antibiotic that acts by intercalation of DNA that prevents DNA, RNA, and protein synthesis. In humans it has antitumor activity against choriocarcinoma, Wilm's tumor, testicular tumors, nephroblastoma, rhabdomyosarcomas, and a variety of soft-tissue sarcomas. It has also been used against lymphoreticular neoplasms and malignant melanoma. This drug has been evaluated in tumor-bearing dogs, and there have been conflicting reports of its efficacy, particularly in canine lymphoma patients (Hammer et al. 1994b; Moore et al. 1994).

Plicamycin, USP (mithramycin, Mithracin), is a highly toxic antibiotic that has been used for treatment of testicular carcinoma in humans. Its action is similar to that of dactinomycin. It has a hypocalcemic effect that may be the result of a direct action on bone; in fact, it has been used therapeutically to treat hypercalcemia. This drug has received little attention in veterinary medicine.

Mitomycin (mitomycin C, Mutamycin) is a quinone antibiotic that must be reduced to an active form; i.e., it is a pro-drug. It has been used in palliative treatment of certain solid tumors in human medicine but has been used only sparingly in veterinary medicine.

ENZYMES. L-Asparaginase (L-asparagine amidohydrolase, Elspar) is an enzyme that can be derived from the organisms *Escherichia coli* and *Erwinia carotovera.* It has primarily been used to treat canine lymphoma (Rogers 1989). It hydrolyzes asparagine to aspartic acid and ammonia. Many malignant cells have very low concentrations of L-asparagine synthase, the enzyme that synthesizes asparagine. To survive, these cells must scavenge asparagine from the extracellular fluids. The destruction of circulating asparagine causes death of these cells. This was long held to be an example of a qualitative difference between normal and susceptible cells, but it is now known that many normal tissues require preformed asparagine. Lack of asparagine impairs the synthesis of such proteins as insulin, prothrombin, albumin, and parathyroid hormone.

Toxicity is related to transient inhibition of protein synthesis and antigenicity of the enzyme, although some oncologists use the drug for short courses of treatment with little evidence of hypersensitivity. Alteration of the form in which the drug is given, e.g., as a conjugate with polyethylene glycol, decreases the occurrence of hypersensitivity by preventing uptake of the protein into reticuloendothelial cells (Teske et al. 1990; MacEwen et al. 1992); conjugation does not interfere with enzymatic activity. Allergic reactions include chills, urticaria, fever, and, in severe cases, anaphylactic shock. The prevalence of anaphylaxis in dogs receiving the drug for the first time is extremely low (Ogilvie et al. 1994a). Inhibition of protein synthesis can result in decreased AT III, fibrinogen, and other factors, which can lead to clotting and hemorrhagic complications. Biochemical evidence of hepatotoxicity is present in some patients. Hemorrhagic pancreatitis may rarely occur.

L-Asparaginase is supplied as a dry powder derived from *E. coli* and other bacteria such as *Erwinia* spp. L-Asparaginase from the various sources apparently does not cross-react immunologically, so one can continue therapy in a patient who has become allergic to one of the preparations.

Platinum Coordination Complexes. Cisplatin (*cis*-diamminedichloroplatinum II, Platinol, Cis-platinum) was first shown to have antitumor activity in 1969 and is one of the most important drugs in clinical oncology. It is a platinum coordination complex that is unique among anticancer drugs in being an inorganic compound.

Cisplatin has been incorporated into treatment of several solid tumors, including those of the testis, ovary, bladder, head, and neck in humans. In dogs, activity has been demonstrated against transitional cell carcinoma, squamous cell carcinoma, osteosarcoma, and nasal adenocarcinoma (Knapp et al. 1988). Intralesional administration of cisplatin has been utilized successfully in veterinary medicine (Theon et al. 1993; Theon et al. 1994; Kitchell et al. 1994; Kitchell et al. 1995). Cisplatin-impregnated materials used at tumor surgical sites have been extensively evaluated and determined to be safe (Straw et al. 1994; Buss et al. 1999). Additionally, intracavitary chemotherapy with cisplatin has been associated with palliation and control of malignant pleural and/or abdominal effusions in dogs (Moore et al. 1991).

Cisplatin enters cells by passive diffusion. It is activated by sequential aquation of the chloride moieties, which then react with N-7 of guanine residues and other nucleophiles in DNA. Cisplatin resembles the alkylating agents in its mechanism of action. It inhibits DNA synthesis much more than RNA and protein synthesis. It is bifunctional by virtue of the two chloride moieties and can form intrastrand (rapidly) and interstrand (slowly) cross-links in DNA. DNA-protein cross-links may also be formed. Only the *cis* configuration is active. Cytotoxicity is correlated with the number of intrastrand cross-links formed. Cisplatin kills cells at any phase of the cell cycle and is said to be non-phase-specific, although there is evidence that it may be most effective in the G1 phase of the cycle.

Cisplatin is given as a rapid IV infusion. It has a biphasic plasma-decay curve with an initial half-life of 22 minutes (probably distribution) and a terminal half-life of 5 days (probably elimination) in dogs. It is known that intracellular half-life in humans may be as long as 30 days. This presumably represents drug bound to tissue macromolecules. High tissue concentrations have been found in kidney, liver, ovary, testis, and uterus.

Nephrotoxicity is a dose-limiting adverse effect of cisplatin in dogs (Morrison 1998b). Other major toxicities include intractable nausea and vomiting even when antiemetics are used, ototoxicity with hearing loss, anaphylactic-like reactions, and neurotoxicity. Myelosuppression is mild relative to alkylating agents, but thrombocytopenia and granulocytopenia may be observed by days 7–9 and days 17–19 after injection, respectively. GI toxicity manifested as diarrhea and anorexia may also be observed.

Nephrotoxicity is dose related, cumulative, and apparently irreversible in some cases, and primarily affects the proximal tubules. Decreased renal concentrating ability, abnormal numbers of granular casts in the urine sediment, and azotemia suggest toxicity that may warrant suspending treatment (Morrison 1998b). Histopathologic lesions include tubular degeneration, loss of brush border, and necrosis and mineralization of tubular epithelial cells. In dogs, blood urea nitrogen may be elevated by days 7–9 after injection. Diuresis reduces nephrotoxicity and allows the administration of higher doses (Ogilvie et al. 1991d; Ogilvie et al. 1993c). Hypersalination (i.e., induction of forced diuresis with infusion with hypertonic sodium chloride solution) is also useful in reducing nephrotoxicity (Forrester et al. 1993). The antithyroid drug methimazole has been found to provide some protection against nephrotoxicity in dogs receiving cisplatin (Vail et al. 1993). The time of day at which cisplatin is administered has been shown to affect toxicity. Bolus IV infusion of cisplatin (90 mg/m^2) over 5 minutes at 8:00 A.M. appeared to be more nephrotoxic than the same dose given at 4:00 P.M. (Hardie et al. 1991).

Transient nausea and vomiting are severe, almost universal, and may cause cessation of treatment. Cisplatin is extremely toxic to cats, causing a primary pulmonary toxicity resulting in vasculitis in alveolar capillaries, hydrothorax, and pulmonary and mediastinal edema (Knapp et al. 1987). These severe side effects appear to be abrogated in cats when a liposome-encapsulated form of the drug is administered (Thamm and Vail 1998; Fox et al. 1999).

Cisplatin is supplied as a lyophilized powder in vials that contain 10 mg of the drug. Once reconstituted, the solution should be kept at room temperature. Although the search for more convenient and practical administration methods continues, the dose of cisplatin is given by IV push approximately 3–5 hours after initiation of saline loading. After administration of cisplatin, the saline infusion is continued and the animal is watched carefully to ensure that it is well hydrated in the postinfusion period. Cisplatin should not be prepared with or administered through an aluminum needle because aluminum reacts with and inactivates the drug. Ideally, the dog is fasted 12 hours prior to drug administration to decrease nausea and vomiting associated with this drug.

Carboplatin (Paraplatin) is an analog of cisplatin that is effective in treating human ovarian tumors. It has the same mechanism of action as cisplatin, with which cross-resistance has been reported. It has been found to be effective in animal tumors, including postsurgical osteosarcoma. Unlike cisplatin, carboplatin has shown no efficacy in the treatment of canine transitional cell carcinoma. One of the expected advantages over cisplatin is that it can be used more conveniently on an outpatient basis. Its major toxicity is bone marrow suppression. In dogs, leukopenia and thrombocytopenia may be severe at approximately 2 weeks after administration of high doses (Page et al. 1993). Nausea and vomiting, although common, are less severe than with cisplatin. In contrast to cisplatin, carboplatin is not regarded as nephrotoxic, although it did reduce glomerular filtration rate of dogs in one study. Diuresis is not required. Because it is primarily eliminated via the kidney, preexisting renal disease can significantly increase toxicity (Kraegel 1989–1990). Importantly, carboplatin can be safely administered to cats without developing evidence of pulmonary toxicity; the dose-limiting toxicity in this species is also neutropenia (Hahn et al. 1997).

Hormones and Miscellaneous Agents. Estrogens, progestins, androgens, glucocorticoids, and thyroid hormones have been used in the treatment of cancer but are essentially only palliative. Pharmacologic doses are usually required for antitumor effects, so one should expect adverse reactions to be those of hormone excess.

Estrogens such as *Diethylstilbestrol,* USP, and *Estradiol Cypionate,* USP, have been used in the treatment of prostatic hyperplasia and carcinoma and perianal gland neoplasms. Toxic effects include bone marrow suppression, feminization with gynecomastia, and fluid retention. Antiestrogens such as tamoxifen citrate (Nolvadex) may be used in the treatment of estrogen-dependent disseminated mammary gland cancer. Adverse effects of tamoxifen are mild bone marrow suppression (leukopenia, thrombocytopenia, and anemia), skin rash, alopecia, and stump pyometra.

Mitotane, USP (*o,p′*-DDD, Ortho para′DDD, Lysodren), is closely related to the insecticides DDD and DDT. It is the prototype of a drug with selective antitumor activity in that it is used as an antitumor drug only against adrenal carcinoma. It is also highly toxic to normal adrenal cortex. Its dose-limiting toxicities are on the GI tract (nausea and vomiting are common) and the CNS, where it produces depression and vertigo. It may also produce diarrhea, visual disturbances, and dermatitis. In veterinary medicine, many adrenal tumors are handled surgically, so this drug is used most commonly for adrenal hyperplasia. It is supplied as 500 mg tablets.

Adrenocortical hormones, most commonly *Prednisone,* USP, have been used in cancer therapy for two types of action. For nonlymphoid tumors like brain tumors, they are palliative by decreasing inflammation and swelling. For lymphoreticular neoplasms and possibly mast cell tumors, they may be cytotoxic. Resistance develops rapidly in most patients. Ideally, glucocorticoids should be used in large doses for the minimal time required to produce remission, then tapered as rapidly as possible. Long-term use at high doses leads to toxicity (often without benefit to the patient) and iatrogenic hyperadrenocorticism. Toxicity includes gastric ulceration, osteoporosis, and increased susceptibility to infection. Polydipsia, polyuria, polyphagia, and excessive panting are especially common and troublesome when patients are maintained chronically on these drugs. Another use of these drugs, as stated above, is for management of secondary complications of cancer (i.e., to elevate mood, stimulate appetite, and decrease reaction to dying cells). In addition, they are useful in the management of tumor-associated pain, hypercalcemia, hypoglycemia, and increased intracranial pressure.

Hydroxyurea, USP (Hydrea), may act as an antimetabolite by inhibiting ribonucleotide reductase, thus limiting the availability of deoxyribonucleotides needed for DNA synthesis. Hydroxyurea is cell-cycle-phase-specific, acting on the S phase. It has been used for resistant chronic myelogenous leukemia. Hematologic changes constitute the dose-limiting toxicity, but recovery is usually rapid after cessation of treatment. The hematologic toxicity has been used therapeutically in the treatment of polycythemia vera in animals. Leukopenia, thrombocytopenia, and megaloblastosis all occur. Other toxic signs seen in dogs include anorexia, mild nausea, vomiting, stomatitis, and abnormalities of the nails. Alopecia is uncommon.

Piroxicam (Feldene) and other nonsteroidal anti-inflammatory drugs may have antitumor activity against naturally acquired cancer, although this activity is unlikely to be a direct cytotoxicity (Knapp et al. 1992; Knapp et al. 1995). The drug appears to be most active against transitional cell carcinoma (Knapp et al. 1994).

REFERENCES

Arrington, K. A., Legendre, A. M., and Tabeling, G. S. 1994. Comparison of body surface area–based and weight-based dosage protocols for doxorubicin administration in dogs. Am J Vet Res 55:1587–1592.

Bergman, P. J., MacEwen, E. G., Kurzman, I. D., et al. 1996. Amputation and carboplatin for treatment of dogs with osteosarcoma: 48 cases (1991–1993). J Vet Intern Med 10:76–81.

Bonney, P. L., and Knapp, D. W. 1993. Chemotherapy safety: a guide for veterinary practitioners. Feline Health Topics for Veterinarians 8(4):1–2.

Bortnowski, H. B., and Rosenthal, R. C. 1991. Preclinical evaluation of L-asparaginase and methotrexate administered at intermediate doses in dogs. Am J Vet Res 52(10):636–638.

Brooks, D. G. 1995. Acute tumor lysis syndrome in dogs. Compend Cont Educ Pract Vet 17:1103–1106.

Buss, M. S., Henry, C. J., Tyler, J. W., et al. 1999. Systemic and tissue chamber fluid platinum concentrations released from *cis*-diamminedichloroplatinum II–impregnated polymethylmethacrylate in healthy dogs. Am J Vet Res 60:280–283.

Chambers A. F., and Hill R. P. 1998. Tumor progression and metastasis. In I. F. Tannock and R. P. Hill, eds., The Basic Science of Oncology, 3rd ed., pp. 219–239. New York: McGraw-Hill.

Chan, H. S. L., Thorner, P. S., Haddad, G., DeBoer, G., Gallie, G. L., and Ling, V. 1993. Multidrug resistance in cancers of childhood: clinical relevance and circumvention. Adv Pharmacol 24:157–197.

Cotter, S. M., Kanki, P. J., and Simon, M. 1985. Renal disease in five tumor-bearing cats treated with adriamycin. J Am Anim Hosp Assoc 21:405–409.

Crow, S. E., Theilen, G. H., Madewell, B. R., Weller, R. E., and Henness, A. M. 1977. Cyclophosphamide-induced cystitis in the dog and cat. J Am Vet Med Assoc 171(3):259–262.

Dimski, D. S., and Cook, J. R. 1990. Carmustine-induced partial remission of an astrocytoma in a dog. J Am Vet Med Assoc 26:179–182.

Dorman, D. C., Coddington, K. A., and Richardson, R. C. 1990. 5-Fluorouracil toxicosis in the dog. J Vet Intern Med 4(5):254–257.

Elias, A. D., Eder, J. P., Shea, T., Frei, E., III, and Antman, K. H. 1990. High-dose ifosfamide with mesna uroprotection: a phase I study. J Clin Oncol 8(1):170–178.

Forrester, S. D., Fallin, E. A., Saunders, G. K., and Kenny, J. E. 1993. Prevention of cisplatin-induced nephrotoxicosis in dogs, using hypertonic saline solution as the vehicle of administration. Am J Vet Res 54(12):2175–2178.

Fortier, L. A., and Harg, M. A. M. 1994. Topical use of 5-fluorouracil for treatment of squamous cell carcinoma of the external genitalia of horses: 11 cases (1988–1992). J Am Vet Med Assoc 205:1183–1185.

Fox, L. E. 1996. Chemotherapy safety for the practicing veterinarian. Perspectives, May/June:8–15.

Fox, L. E., Toshach, K., and Calderwood-Mays, et al. 1999. Evaluation of liposome-encapsulated *cis-bis*–neodecaoata-*trans-R,R*-1,2-diaminocyclohexane platinum (II) in clinically normal cats. Am J Vet Res 60:257–263.

Frazier, D. L., and Price, G. S. 1998. Use of body surface area to calculate chemotherapeutic drug dose in dogs: II. Limitations imposed by pharmacokinetic factors. J Vet Intern Med 12:272–278.

Frimberger, A. E., Moore, A. S., Cotter, S. M., et al. 1995. Initial clinical evaluation of ifosfamide in dogs. Proc Vet Cancer Soc 15:25–26.

Fulton, L. M., and Steinberg, H. S. 1990. Preliminary study of lomustine in the treatment of intracranial masses in dogs following localization by imaging techniques. Semin Vet Med Surg 5:241–245.

Gatmaitan, Z. C., and Arias, I. M. 1993. Structure and function of p-glycoprotein in normal liver and small intestine. Adv Pharmacol 24:77–97.

Georges, E., Sharom, F. J., and Ling, V. 1990. Multidrug Resistance and chemosensitization: therapeutic implications for cancer chemotherapy. Adv Pharmacol 21:185–220.

Golden, D. L., and Langston, V. C. 1988. Uses of vincristine and vinblastine in dogs and cats. J Am Vet Med Assoc 193:1114–1117.

Goldie, J. H., and Coldman, A. J. 1998. Molecular aspects of drug resistance. In J. H. Goldie and A. J. Coldman, eds., Drug Resistance in Cancer: Mechanisms and Models, pp. 59–89. Cambridge: Cambridge Univ Press.

Hahn, K. A., Fletcher, C. M., and Legendre, A. M. 1996. Marked neutropenia in five tumor-bearing cats one week following single-agent vincristine sulfate chemotherapy. Vet Clin Pathol 25:121–123.

Hahn, K. A., McEntee, M. F., Daniel, G. B., et al. 1997. Hematologic and systemic toxicoses associated with carboplatin administration in cats. Am J Vet Res 58:677–679.

Hamilton, T. A., Cook, J. R., Braund, K. G., et al. 1991a. Vincristine-induced peripheral neuropathy in a dog. J Am Vet Med Assoc 198:635–638.

Hamilton, T. A., Cook, J. R., Scott-Moncrieff, C., et al. 1991b. Carmustine chemotherapy for canine brain tumors. Proc Vet Cancer Soc 11:43–44.

Hamilton, T. A., Morrison, W. B., and DeNicola, D. B. 1991c. Cytosine arabinoside chemotherapy for acute megakaryocytic leukemia in a cat. J Am Vet Med Assoc 199:359–361.

Hammer, A. S., Carothers, M. A., Harris, C. L., et al. 1994a. Unexpected neurotoxicty in dogs receiving a cyclophosphamide, dactinomycin, and 5-fuorouracil chemotherapy protocol. J Vet Intern Med 8:240–243.

Hammer, A. S., Couto, C. G., Ayl, R. D., et al. 1994b. Treatment of tumor-bearing dogs with actinomycin D. J Vet Intern Med 8:236–239.

Hardie, E. M., Page, R. L., Williams, P. L., and Fischer, W. D. 1991. Effect of time of cisplatin administration on its toxicity and pharmacokinetics in dogs. Am J Vet Res 52(11):1821–1825.

Henderson, R. A., Brawner, W. R., Brewer, W. G., et al. 1995. Clinical staging. In K. A. Hahn and R. C. Richardson, eds., Cancer Chemotherapy: A Veterinary Handbook, pp. 23–45. Baltimore: Williams & Wilkins.

Hohenhaus, A. E., and Matus, R. E. 1990. Etoposide (VP-16): retrospective analysis of treatment of 13 dogs with lymphoma. J Vet Intern Med 4:239–241.

Horwitz, S. B. 1992. Mechanism of action of taxol. Trends in Pharmacol 13(4):134–135.

Imondi, A. R., Torre, P. D., Mazue, G., et al. 1996. Dose-response relationship of dexrazone for prevention of doxorubicin-induced cardiotoxicity in mice, rats, and dogs. Cancer Res 56:4200–4204.

Kaufman, D., and Chabner, B. A. 1996. Clinical strategies for cancer treatment: the role of drugs. In B. A. Chabner and D. L. Longo, eds., Cancer Chemotherapy and Biotherapy: Principles and Practice, 2nd ed., pp. 1–16. Philadelphia: Lippincott-Raven.

Kisseberth, W. C., MacEwen, E. G., Helfand, S. C., et al. 1995. Response to liposome-encapsulated doxorubicin (TLC D-99) in a dog with myeloma. J Vet Intern Med 9:425–428.

Kitchell, B. E., Brown, D. M., Luck, E. E., et al. 1994. Intralesional implant for treatment of primary oral malignant melanoma in dogs. J Am Vet Med Assoc 204:229–236.

Kitchell, B. K., Orenber, E. K., Brown, D. M., et al. 1995. Intralesional sustained-release chemotherapy with therapeutic implants for the treatment of canine sun-induced squamous cell carcinoma. Eur J Cancer 31A:2093–2098.

Klein, M. K., and Dalton, W. S. 1992. Verapamil and quinine as modifiers of drug resistance in canine lymphoma. Vet Cancer Soc Newsletter 16(1):7–8.

Knapp, D. W., Richardson, R. C., DeNicola, D. B., Long, G. G., and Blevins, W. E. 1987. Cisplatin toxicity in cats. J Vet Intern Med 1(1):29–35.

Knapp, D. W., Richardson, R. C., Bonney, P. L., and Hahn, K. 1988. Cisplatin therapy in 41 dogs with malignant tumors. J Vet Intern Med 2(1):41–46.

Knapp, D. W., Richardson, R. C., Bottoms, G. D., et al. 1992. Phase I trial of piroxicam in 62 dogs bearing naturally occurring tumors. Cancer Chemother Pharmacol 29:214–218.

Knapp, D. W., Richardson, R. C., Chan, T. C. K., et al. 1994. Piroxicam therapy in 34 dogs with transitional cell carcinoma of the urinary bladder. J Vet Intern Med 8:273–278.

Knapp, D. W., Chan, T. C. K., Kuczek, T., et al. 1995. Evaluation of in vitro cytotoxicity of nonsteroidal anti-inflammatory drugs against canine tumor cells. Am J Vet Res 56:801–805.

Kochevar, D. T., Middendorf, D. L., Mealey, K. L., et al. 1995. Pharmacokinetics and haematological effects of a single intravenous dose of mitoxantrone in cats. J Vet Pharmacol Therap 18:471–475.

Kraegel, S. A. 1989–1990. Carboplatin. Vet Cancer Soc Newsletter 13(4):5.

Kuczek, T., and Chan, T. C. K. 1992. Mechanism-based model for tumor drug resistance. Cancer Chemother Pharmacol 30:355–359.

MacEwen, E. G., Rosenthal, R. C., Fox, L. E., Loar, A. S., and Kurzman, I. D. 1992. Evaluation of L-asparaginase: polyethylene glycol conjugate versus native L-asparaginase combined with chemotherapy: a randomized double-blind study in canine lymphoma. J Vet Intern Med 6(4):230–234.

Macy, D. W., Withrow, S. J., and Hoopes, J. 1983. Transitional cell carcinoma of the bladder associated with cyclophosphamide administration. J Am Anim Hosp Assoc 19:965–969.

Madewell, B. R., and Theilen, G. H. 1987. Tumors and tumor-like conditions of epithelial origin. In G. H. Thielen and B. R. Madewell, eds., Veterinary Cancer Medicine, 2nd ed., pp. 240–266. Philadelphia: Lea & Febiger.

Mauldin, G. E., Fox, P. R., Patnaik, A. K., et al. 1992. Doxorubicin-induced cardiotoxicosis: clinical features in 32 dogs. J Vet Intern Med 6:82–88.

McCaw, D. L., Miller, M. A., Bergman, P. J., et al. 1997. Vincristine therapy for mast cell tumors in dogs. J Vet Intern Med 11:375–378.

Meyer, D. J. 1976. Pancreatic islet cell carcinoma in a dog treated with streptozotocin. Am J Vet Res 37:1221–1223.

———. 1977. Temporary remission of hypoglycemia in a dog with an insulinoma after treatment with streptozotocin. Am J Vet Res 38:1201–1204.

Moore, A. S., Kirk, C., and Cardona, A. 1991. Intracavitary cisplatin chemotherapy experience with six dogs. J Vet Intern Med 5:227–231.

Moore, A. S., Ogilvie, G. K., and Vail, D. M. 1994. Actinomycin D for reinduction of remission in dogs with resistant lymphoma. J Vet Intern Med 8:343–344.

Moore, A. S., London, C. A., Wood, C. A., et al. 1995a. Preliminary report on the use of lomustine (CCNU) for treatment of relapsed lymphoma in dogs. Proc Vet Cancer Soc 15:39–40.

Moore, A. S., Ruslander, D., Cotter, S. M., et al. 1995b. Efficacy of, and toxicoses associated with, oral idarubicin administration in cats with neoplasia. J Am Vet Med Assoc 206:1550–1554.

Morrison, W. B. 1998a. Chemotherapy. In W. B. Morrison, ed., Cancer in Dogs and Cats: Medical and Surgical Management, pp. 351–358. Baltimore: Williams & Wilkins.

———. 1998b. Cancer drug pharmacology and clinical experience. In W. B. Morrison, ed., Cancer in Dogs and Cats: Medical and Surgical Management, pp. 359–378. Baltimore: Williams & Wilkins.

———. 1998c. Providing chemotherapy safely. In W. B. Morrison, ed., Cancer in Dogs and Cats: Medical and Surgical Management, pp. 379–385. Baltimore: Williams & Wilkins.

———, ed. 1998d. Cancer in Dogs and Cats: Medical and Surgical Management. Baltimore: Williams & Wilkins.

Ogilvie, G. K. 1994. New chemotherapeutics: taxol and beyond. Proc ACVIM 12:866–869.

Ogilvie, G. K., and Moore, A. S., eds. 1995. Managing the Veterinary Cancer Patient. Trenton: Veterinary Learning Systems.

Ogilvie, G. K., Cockburn, C. A., Tranquilli, W. J., et al. 1988. Hypotension and cutaneous reactions associated with intravenous administration of etoposide in the dog. Am J Vet Res 49:1367–1370.

Ogilvie, G. K., Reynolds, H. A., Richardson, R. C., Withrow, S. J., Norris, A. M., Henderson, R. A., Klausner, J. S., Fowler, J. D., and McCaw, D. 1989a. Phase II evaluation of doxorubicin for treatment of various canine neoplasms. J Am Vet Med Assoc 195(11):1580–1583.

Ogilvie, G. K., Richardson, R. C., Curtis, C. R., Withrow, S. J., Reynolds, H. A., Norris, A. M., Henderson, R. A., Klausner, J. S., Fowler, J. D., and McCaw, D. 1989b. Acute and short-term toxicoses associated with the administration of doxorubicin to dogs with malignant tumors. J Am Vet Med Assoc 195(11):1584–1587.

Ogilvie, G. K., Vail, D. M., Klein, M. K., et al. 1991a. Weekly administration of low-dose doxorubicin for treatment of malignant lymphoma in dogs. J Am Vet Med Assoc 198:1762–1764.

Ogilvie, G. K., Obradovich, J. E., Elmslie, R.E., et al. 1991b. Efficacy of mitoxantrone against various neoplasms in dogs. J Am Vet Med Assoc 198:1618–1621.

Ogilvie, G. K., Obradovich, J. E., and Elmslie, R. E. 1991c. Toxicoses associated with administration of mitoxantrone to dogs with malignant tumors. J Am Vet Med Assoc 198(9):1613–1617.

Ogilvie, G. K., Straw, R. C., Powers, B. E., et al. 1991d. Prevalence of nephrotoxicosis associated with a short-term saline diuresis protocol for the administration of cisplatin to dogs with malignant tumors: 61 cases (1987–1989). J Am Vet Med Assoc 199:613–616.

Ogilvie, G. K., Obradovich, J. E., Cooper, M. F., Walters, L. M., Salman, M. D., and Boone, T. C. 1992. The use of recombinant canine granulocyte colony-stimulating factor to decrease myelosuppression associated with the administration of mitoxantrone in the dog. J Vet Intern Med 6(1):44–47.

Ogilvie, G. K., Walters, L. M., Powers, B. E., et al. 1993a. Organ toxicity of NBT taxol in the rat and dog: a preclinical study. Proc Vet Cancer Soc 13:90–91.

Ogilvie, G. K., Moore, A. S., Obradovich, J. E., et al. 1993b. Toxicoses and efficacy associated with administration of mitoxantrone to cats with malignant tumors. J Am Vet Med Assoc 202:1839–1844.

Ogilvie, G. K., Straw, R. C., Jameson, V. J., et al. 1993c. Prevalence of nephrotoxicosis associated with a four-hour saline solution diuresis protocol for the administration of cisplatin to dogs with naturally developing neoplasms. J Am Vet Med Assoc 202:1845–1848.

Ogilvie, G. K., Atwater, S. W., Ciekot, P. A., et al. 1994a. Prevalence of anaphylaxis associated with the intramuscular administration of L-asparaginase to 81 dogs with cancer: 1989–1991. J Am Anim Hosp Assoc 30:62–65.

Ogilvie, G. K., Moore, A. S., Chen, C., et al. 1994b. Toxicoses associated with administration of mitoxantrone to dogs with malignant tumors: a dose escalation study. J Am Vet Med Assoc 205:570–573.

Ogilvie, G. K., and Moore, A. S. 1995. Extravasation of chemotherapeutic agents. In G. K. Ogilvie and A. S. Moore., eds., Managing the Veterinary Cancer Patient, pp. 186–188. Trenton: Veterinary Learning Systems.

O'Keefe, D. A., and Schaeffer, D. J. 1992. Hematologic toxicosis associated with doxorubicin administration in cats. J Vet Intern Med 6:276–282.

O'Keefe, D. A., Sisson, D. D., Gelberg, H. B., et al. 1993. Systemic toxicity associated with doxorubicin administration in cats. J Vet Intern Med 7:309–317.

OSHA Instruction PUB 8-1.1. 1986. Subject: Guidelines for Cytotoxic (Antineoplastic) Drugs. Office of Occupational Medicine, Assistant Secretary for Occupational Safety and Health Administration, US Department of Labor, Washington, D.C.

Page, R. L., Macy, D. W., Thrall, D. E., et al. 1988. Unexpected toxicity associated with the use of body surface area for dosing melphalan in the dog. Cancer Res 48:288–290.

Page, R. L., McEntee, M. C., George, S. L., Williams, P. L., Heidner, G. L., Novotney, C. A., Riviere, J. E., Dewhirst, M. W., and Thrall, D. E. 1993. Pharmacokinetic and phase I evaluation of carboplatin in dogs. J Vet Intern Med 7(4):235–240.

Peterson, J. L., Couto, C. G., Hammer, A. S., et al. Acute sterile hemorrhagic cystitis after a single intravenous administration of cyclophosphamide in three dogs. J Am Vet Med Assoc 201:1572–1574.

Phillips, B. S., Kraegel, S. A., Simonson, E., et al. 1998. Acute reactions in dogs treated with doxorubicin: increased frequency with the use of a generic formulation. J Vet Intern Med 12:171–172.

Price, G. S., and Frazier, D. L. 1998. Use of body surface area (BSA)–based dosages to calculate chemotherapeutic drug dose in dogs: I. Potential problems with current BSA formulae. J Vet Intern Med 12:267–271.

Rogers, K. S. 1989. L-Asparaginase for treatment of lymphoid neoplasia in dogs. J Am Vet Med Assoc 194:1626–1630.

Rosenthal, R. C. 1991. Storage of expensive anticancer drugs. J Am Vet Med Assoc 198(1):144–146.

Schneider, E., Hsiang, Y.-H., and Liu, L. F. 1990. DNA topoisomerases as anticancer drug targets. Adv Pharmacol 21:149–183.

Scott-Moncrieff, J. C. R., Chan, T. C. K., Samuels, M. L., Cook, J. R., Coppoc, G. L., DeNicola, D. B., and Richardson, R. C. 1991. Plasma and cerebrospinal fluid pharmacokinetics of cytosine arabinoside in dogs. Cancer Chemother Pharmacol 29:13–18.

Shackney, S. E. 1993. Tumor growth, cell cycle kinetics, and cancer treatment. In P. Calabresi and P. S. Schein, eds., Medical Oncology: Basic Principles and Clinical Management of Cancer, 2nd ed., pp. 43–60. New York: McGraw-Hill.

Shapiro, D. M., and Fugmann, R. A. 1957. A role for chemotherapy as an adjunct to surgery. Cancer Res 17:1098–1101.

Simonson, E., and Madewell, B. R. 1992. Chemotherapy-induced change in coat color in a Standard Poodle dog. Vet Cancer Soc Newsletter 16(2):4.

Slevin, M. L. 1991. The clinical pharmacology of etoposide. Cancer 67(Suppl 1):319–329.

Straw, R. C., Withrow, S. J., Richter, S. L., et al. 1991. Amputation and cisplatin for treatment of canine osteosarcoma. J Vet Intern Med 5:205–210.

Straw, R. C., Withrow, S. J., Douple, E. B., et al. 1994. Effects of *cis*-diamminedichloroplatinum II released from D,L-polylactic acid implanted adjacent to cortical allografts in dogs. J Orthop Res 12:871–877.

Tannock, I. F., and Goldenberg, G. J. 1998. Drug resistance and experimental chemotherapy. In I. F. Tannock and R. P. Hill, eds., The Basic Science of Oncology, 3rd ed., pp. 392–419. New York: McGraw-Hill.

Teske, E., Rutteman, G. R., van Heerde, P., et al. 1990. Polyethylene glycol-L-asparaginase versus native L-asparaginase in canine non-Hodgkin's lymphoma. Eur J Cancer 26(8):891–895.

Thamm, D. H., and Vail, D. M. 1998. Preclinical evaluation of a sterically stabilized liposome-encapsulated cisplatin in clinically normal cats. Am J Vet Res 59:286–289.

Thamm, D. H., Mauldin, E. A., and Vail, D. M. 1999. Prednisone and vinblastine chemotherapy for canine mast cell tumor: 41 cases (1992–1997). J Vet Intern Med 13:491–497.

Theon, A. P., Pascoe, J. R., Carlson, G. P., et al. 1993. Intratumoral chemotherapy with cisplatin in oily emulsion in horses. J Am Vet Med Assoc 202:261–267.

Theon, A. P., Pascoe, J. R., and Meagher, D. M. 1994. Perioperative intratumoral administration of cisplatin for treatment of cutaneous tumors in Equidae. J Am Vet Med Assoc 205:1170–1176.

Thierry, A. R., Vige, D., Coughlin, S. S., Beli, J. A., Dritschilo, A., and Rahman, A. 1993. Modulation of doxorubicin resistance in multidrug-resistant cells by liposomes. FASEB J 7:572–579.

Tonetti, M., Astroff, A. B., Satterfield, W., De Flora, A., Benatti, U., and DeLoach, J. R. 1991. Pharmacokinetic properties of doxorubicin encapsulated in glutaraldehyde-treated canine erythrocytes. Am J Vet Res 52(10):1630–1635.

Vail, D. M., Elfarra, A. A., Cooley, A. J., et al. 1993. Methimazole as a protectant against cisplatin-induced nephrotoxicity using the dog as a model. Cancer Chemother Pharmacol 33:25–30.

Vail, D. M., Kravis, L. D., Cooley, A. J., et al. 1997. Preclinical trial of doxorubicin entrapped in sterically stabilized liposomes in dogs with spontaneously arising malignant tumors. Cancer Chemother Pharmacol 39:410–416.

Van Vechten, M., Helfand, S. C., and Jeglum, K. A. 1990. Treatment of relapsed canine lymphoma with doxorubicin and dacarbazine. J Vet Intern Med 4:187–191.

Vonderhaar, M. A., and Morrison, W. B. 1998. Lymphosarcoma. In W. B. Morrison, ed., Cancer in Dogs and Cats: Medical and Surgical Management, pp. 667–695. Baltimore: Williams & Wilkins.

Vonderhaar, M. A., Morrison, W. B., Glickman, N. W., et al. 1994. Cardiac effects of doxorubicin and epirubicin as single-agent therapy for canine malignant lymphoma. Proc Vet Cancer Soc 14:29–30.

53 DERMATOPHARMACOLOGY: DRUGS ACTING LOCALLY ON THE SKIN

JIM E. RIVIERE AND JERRY W. SPOO

Anatomy and Histology
- **The Epidermis**
- **The Dermis**
- **Species Differences**

Biochemistry
- **Energy Production and Utilization**
- **Drug Biotransformation**
- **Lipid Metabolism**
- **Protein Metabolism**

Principles of Percutaneous Absorption: Skin Permeability

Topical Vehicles
- **Other Factors Affecting Percutaneous Absorption**
- **Penetration Enhancers**
- **Electrically Assisted Transdermal Drug Delivery**

Classification of Dermatologic Vehicles
- **Adsorbents and Protectives**
- **Demulcents**
- **Emollients**
- **Astringents**
- **Rubefacients, Irritants, and Vesicants**
- **Caustics and Escharotics**
- **Keratolytics, Keratoplastics, and Antiseborrheics**

Classes of Medicated Applications
- **Ointments**
- **Poultices**
- **Pastes**
- **Powders**
- **Dressings**
- **Plasters**
- **Suspensions**
- **Lotions**

Antimicrobials
- **Topical Antibiotics**
- **Antifungal Agents**

Glucocorticosteroid Use in Dermatology

Pesticides

A large number of cases seen in the everyday practice of small- and large-animal veterinary medicine involve lesions of the skin or its appendages. This chapter reviews the salient features of the general anatomy, histology, and biochemistry of skin relevant to the treatment of dermatologic disease, acquaints the practitioner with the features of percutaneous drug absorption relevant to the treatment of skin disease, and discusses the categories of pharmacologic preparations available on the veterinary market to treat skin diseases in domestic animals.

Only in the last few decades have scientists begun to understand how the skin functions in normal and diseased states, to understand the skin's barrier function in terms of water loss and drug delivery, and to attempt to improve the delivery of pharmaceutical agents through the skin by temporarily adjusting that barrier to deliver the drug. In order to successfully minimize the skin's ability to block the absorption of drugs in the treatment of dermatologic disease in domestic animals, it is imperative to understand the normal functional anatomy and biochemistry of the skin. In veterinary medicine, transdermal delivery is widely employed, as when pesticides are applied monthly to a single area of skin for the control of fleas and ticks over the entire body. Transdermal fentanyl patches are widely used for postsurgical analgesia. This topical port of drug delivery will see increased use for other therapeutic indications. However, most drugs applied to the skin are not intended to be absorbed systemically but are used to elicit a local therapeutic effect in the treated skin.

The characteristic which separates dermatologic therapy from other components of veterinary pharmacology is this use of topical dosage formulations to target the underlying skin. A full understanding of the biological factors that modulate absorption and of the pharmaceutical composition of dermatologic formulations (e.g., vehicles) is essential to a proper understanding of dermatopharmacology. The drugs incorporated into these formulations are the same as those used to treat diseases of other systems and will not be extensively dealt with in this chapter.

ANATOMY AND HISTOLOGY. The skin is the largest organ of the body, with the integument of the dog accounting for 24% of the overall body weight in the puppy and 12% in the adult dog (Pavletic 1991). The skin has the responsibility of protecting the internal organs of the body from extremes in temperature fluctuations, allergens, pollutants, toxic chemicals, and organisms such as bacteria, fungi, parasites, and viruses found ubiquitously in the environment.

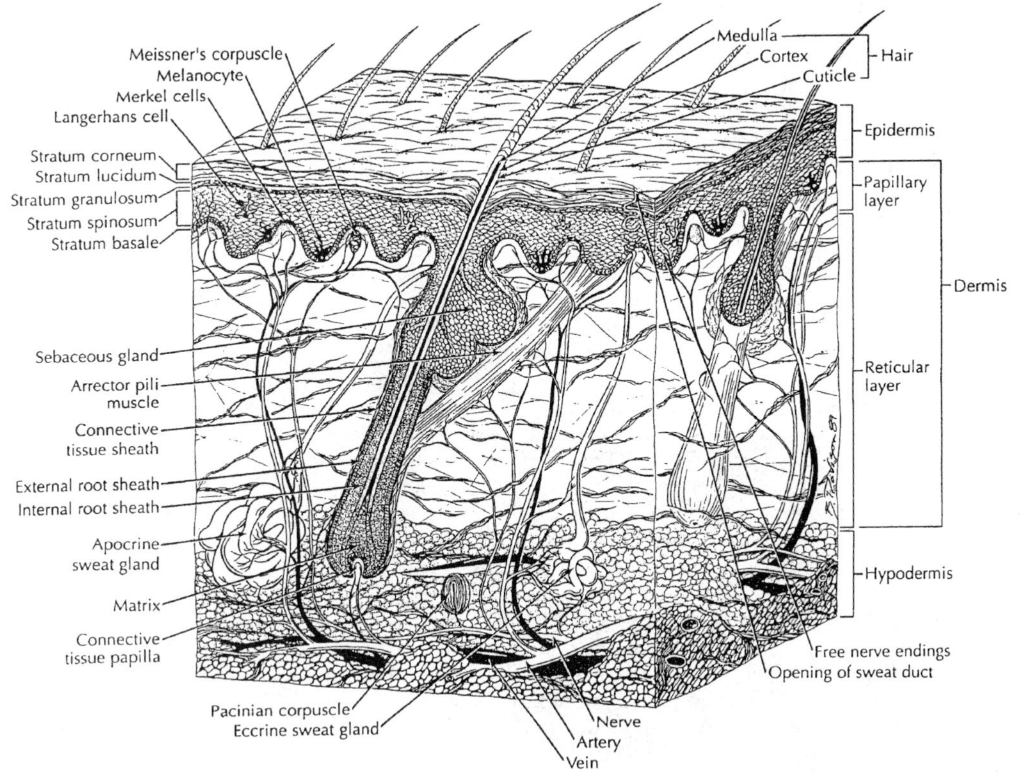

FIG. 53.1—A schematic view of the epidermis and dermis of the skin. (Monteiro-Riviere 1991)

The skin of domestic animals is quite similar in gross and histologic morphology across species lines and is usually thickest over the head, dorsum of the neck, back, and sacrum and on the plantar and palmar surfaces of the feet (Pavletic 1991), thinner on the ventral abdomen, the medial surfaces of the limbs, and the inner pinnae, and thinnest over the scrotum of male animals and the earlobe of the human. Perforating the skin are several types of appendages (depending on the species), such as hair follicles, sebaceous and sweat glands, spines, quills, scales, spurs, horns, claws, nails, and hooves (Montagna 1967). The specific anatomy of skin and hair has been reviewed extensively elsewhere (Monteiro-Riviere et al. 1993b; Blackburn 1965; Lloyd et al. 1979a; Lloyd et al. 1979b; Sar and Calhoun 1966; Kozlowski and Calhoun 1969; Strickland and Calhoun 1963; Talukdar et al. 1972; Pavletic 1991; Montagna 1967; Amakiri 1973).

The Epidermis. On the histological level, the skin can be divided into two distinct units: the epidermis and the dermis. The epidermis consists of stratified squamous keratinized epithelium that undergoes a programmed proliferation and differentiation that will eventually result in the formation of the major barrier to drug penetration: the stratum corneum. Two primary cell types exist in the epidermis: those of keratinocyte origin and those of nonkeratinocyte origin.

Five distinct layers of keratinocytes can be present in the epidermis, as shown in Fig. 53.1. Listed from the deepest layer of the epidermis to the most superficial, they are (1) stratum basale (basal layer), (2) stratum spinosum (prickle layer), (3) stratum granulosum (granular layer), (4) stratum lucidum (clear layer), and (5) stratum corneum (horny layer). Each cell layer has its point of origin at the stratum basale. The stratum basale is a single layer of cuboidal or columnar cells that rest on the basal lamina. These cells are attached to the basal lamina by hemidesmasomes, and to each other and to the cells of the stratum spinosum by desmasomes. The stratum basale cells continuously divide, with some remaining as basal cells and others beginning to move more superficially and mature by changing their intracellular content through the process called keratinization. The next more superficial layer next to the stratum basale, the stratum spinosum, is composed of irregularly shaped polyhedral cells that make up much of the bulk thickness of the epidermis. The next layer composes the stratum granulosum, which consists of several layers of cells that begin to flatten horizontally. Of primary interest are the lamellated granules within these cells, which contain polar phospholipids, such as glycosphingolipids and free steroids, and numerous hydrolytic enzymes, including acid phosphatase, proteases, lipases, and glycosidases. As these intracellular products accumulate, these cells will exocytose their intracellular products and fill in the intercellular spaces, eventually forming the extracellular lipid matrix of the stratum corneum. As these epidermal cells continue their migration, they form the stratum lucidum, a translucent line of cells found only in areas having very thick skin, such as plantar and palmar surfaces (foot pads) and the planum nasale. These cells are translucent because both nuclei and cytoplasmic organelles are missing (Monteiro-Riviere 1991; Monteiro-Riviere et al. 1993b; Idsen 1975; Montagna 1967).

The stratum corneum is the final and most superficial layer of the epidermis and is the most important layer when considering the feasibility of topical drug therapy since it is the primary barrier to percutaneous absorption. In addition to the barrier function for xenobiotics trying to enter the body from the environment, the stratum corneum also provides a barrier to insensible water loss, an evolutionary adaptation that allows terrestrial animals to exist in a nonaquatic environment. In fact, most veterinary dermatologic vehicles are targeted at this action. The stratum corneum consists of several dead layers of cells, organized into vertical columns in a tetrakaidecahedral (14-sided) configuration, the thickness of which varies depending on location (Monteiro-Riviere 1991). This particular cell shape provides a minimal surface-to-volume ratio and also minimizes systemic water loss through the skin (transepidermal water loss). Each cell is ingrained in the lipid matrix produced by the lamellated granules when the cells were still in the stratum granulosum layer. These dead cells are also surrounded by a thick plasma membrane with a submembranous layer of involucrin, also produced earlier in development. With intracellular and intercellular barriers firmly in place, the stratum corneum has the ability to constrain the passage of unwanted chemicals and toxins from the environment. Unfortunately, the stratum corneum does not discriminate between these unwanted substances and the pharmaceuticals the veterinarian may wish to penetrate the skin for topical drug therapy for the treatment of dermatologic disease.

Melanocytes are cells located in the basal layer of the epidermis and contain dark cytoplasmic granules called melanosomes. These cells impart color to the skin, the color and intensity determined by the number, size, distribution, and degree of melanization of the melanosomes. Merkel cells are also located in the basal region of the epidermis and are thought to function as slow-adapting mechanoreceptors for touch. Langerhans cells are located in the stratum spinosum but can also be present in dermal lymph vessels, lymph nodes, and dermis. The Langerhans cells' primary function is to present antigen to lymphocytes; they may also be the initial receptors for cutaneous immune responses.

The Dermis. The dermis is composed of connective tissue consisting of collagen, elastin, and reticular fibers dispersed in an amorphous ground substance and can be divided into two rather poorly demarcated areas. The papillary layer consists of loose connective tissue and connects the epidermis (stratum basale/basal lamina) to the deeper reticular layer of the dermis. The reticular layer consists of dense connective tissue connected to the hypodermis, which is composed mostly of fat.

Dispersed throughout both layers of the dermis is a network of arterial and venous blood vessels needed to nourish the cells of the epidermis and dermis as well as to take part in the last stages of the percutaneous absorption of compounds. Lymph vessels, nerves, apocrine and eccrine sweat glands, sebaceous glands, Pacinian (pressoreceptor), Meissner's (touch receptor), and Ruffini (mechanical receptor) corpuscles, hair follicles, and smooth muscles (arrector pili) are the other major structures found in the dermis. Two types of arteries, musculocutaneous and direct cutaneous, supply the needed nutrients to the epidermis. Direct cutaneous arteries run parallel to the skin, directly supplying the skin with blood, while musculocutaneous arteries supply both the skin and underlying musculature and run perpendicular to the skin. Cutaneous blood supply by each type of artery varies with species and location. Cutaneous blood flow rates may be one of the factors affecting the passive percutaneous absorption of chemicals. Table 53.1 clearly demonstrates this by comparing laser Doppler cutaneous blood flow parameters in nine species of domestic animals (Monteiro-Riviere et al. 1990).

Species Differences. As a general rule, skin structure and function are similar across species lines. However, some minor differences are apparent.

Avian integument possesses the most-profound differences in skin morphology from other domestic species. The four layers of the epidermis are, from the deepest to the most superficial, the stratum basale, the stratum intermedium (stratum spinosum), the stratum transitivum (stratum granulosum), and the stratum corneum (stratum germinativum). Unlike mammals, avians possess no skin glands (Monteiro-Riviere et al. 1993b).

The skin of aquatic mammals has a very thick stratum corneum resembling parakeratosis and there is no stratum granulosum (Montagna 1967).

Pig skin is similar histologically to human skin (Monteiro-Riviere and Stromberg 1985) and has been used experimentally to reliably predict the percutaneous absorption of chemicals in humans. With respect to cutaneous circulation, musculocutaneous arteries are the primary vascular supply to the skin of humans, apes, and swine. Loose-skinned animals (canines and felines) lack musculocutaneous arteries; all vessels involved in cutaneous circulation travel parallel to the skin (Pavletic 1991). Recent studies of piroxicam (a nonsteroidal anti-inflammatory drug) in pigs suggest

TABLE 53.1—Cutaneous blood flow measurements in nine species of domestic animals

Species	Buttocks	Pinnae	Humeroscapular joint	Thoracolumbar joint	Ventral abdomen
Feline	1.82 ± 0.59	6.46 ± 2.30	1.86 ± 0.70	2.39 ± 0.35	6.19 ± 0.94
Bovine	6.03 ± 1.84	6.98 ± 2.19	5.51 ± 2.32	5.49 ± 1.49	10.5 ± 2.13
Canine	2.21 ± 0.67	5.21 ± 1.53	5.52 ± 1.31	1.94 ± 0.27	8.78 ± 1.40
Equine	3.16 ± 1.22	NA	6.76 ± 1.49	2.99 ± 0.86	8.90 ± 1.46
Primate	3.12 ± 0.58	20.9 ± 5.37	8.49 ± 3.28	2.40 ± 0.82	3.58 ± 0.41
Mouse	3.88 ± 0.92	1.41 ± 0.48	10.1 ± 3.51	20.6 ± 4.69	36.9 ± 8.14
Porcine	3.08 ± 0.48	11.7 ± 3.02	6.75 ± 2.09	2.97 ± 0.56	10.7 ± 2.14
Rabbit	3.55 ± 0.93	8.38 ± 1.53	5.38 ± 1.06	5.46 ± 0.94	17.3 ± 6.31
Rat	4.20 ± 1.05	9.13 ± 4.97	6.22 ± 1.47	9.56 ± 2.17	11.4 ± 5.53

Source: Adapted from Monteiro-Riviere et al. 1990.
Note: Values are mL/min/100 g tissue, ± standard error of the mean. NA = data not available.

that the type of cutaneous circulation may affect the local tissue concentrations of topically applied drug (Monteiro-Riviere et al. 1993a).

BIOCHEMISTRY

Energy Production and Utilization. The skin, specifically the epidermis, is mostly an anaerobic organ. The absence of capillaries directly feeding oxygen to the epidermal cells makes the epidermal cells relatively oxygen poor in the normal state when compared to other tissues with a more direct blood supply. Due to this low oxygen tension, the epidermis produces 70–80% of its total energy requirements (adenosine triphosphate) through the anaerobic metabolic pathway (glycolysis), with lactic acid being the end product of glucose utilization. The epidermal cells, the most active of which are those in the single layer of the stratum basale, are the primary cells involved in this energy production, with the lactic acid end product passively diffusing into the dermis and then into the blood vasculature, eventually recycled by the liver back into glucose. Although the glycolytic pathway produces most of the energy requirements of the epidermis, other energy pathways (tricarboxylic acid cycle and pentose phosphate shunt) are also utilized to lesser degrees in some phases of epidermal growth (Freinkel 1983).

Some topically applied drugs may have an effect on energy production pathways within the epidermis. One study (Spoo et al. 1993) showed that in vitro weanling porcine skin flaps had large increases in epidermal cell glucose utilization when the skin was dosed with benzoyl peroxide. In addition to drugs, vehicles (discussed in more detail later) may also have similar effects.

Drug Biotransformation. The stratum corneum is the primary line of defense to prevent percutaneous absorption of drugs. However, any drug passing through the stratum corneum may face a metabolic, rather than a physical, barrier. The skin has a remarkable ability to metabolize xenobiotics. These metabolic reactions consist mainly of oxidation, reduction, hydrolysis, and the phase I and II conjugation reactions. Enzymes present within the extracellular lipid matrix include acid lipase, phospholipase A, sphingomyelinase, glycosidases, acid phosphatases, cathepsins, and carboxypeptidases (Elias 1992). Some of these reactions are major pathways for the metabolism of topical steroids as well as other drugs such as norepinephrine, benzoyl peroxide, and benzo(a)pyrene.

Skin has been shown to metabolize organophosphate parasiticides. When parathion is topically applied to the skin and penetration through the stratum corneum occurs, it undergoes significant metabolism within the epidermis to the bioactive metabolite paraoxon and/or *p*-nitro phenol, both of which will enter the systemic circulation to possibly affect other organ systems (Riviere and Chang 1992). Additional studies have demonstrated the metabolic capabilities of skin when topically exposed to caffeine, testosterone, butylated hydroxytoluene, salicylic acid, norepinephrine, benzo(a)pyrene, and benzoyl peroxide—to name only a few—in many species of laboratory animals, as well as in human skin. Benzoyl peroxide, a popular veterinary drug used as a keratolytic and degreasing agent, is metabolized almost 100% to benzoic acid within the epidermis. In addition, the cytochrome P-450 enzyme system, most commonly associated with the liver, is present and is inducible in skin (depending on the compound that was applied topically) and is the pathway that is responsible for the conversion of parathion into paraoxon in porcine skin (Riviere and Chang 1992; Mukhtar 1992). Glutathione S-transferase, aryl hydrocarbon hydroxylase, and 7-ethoxycoumarin have also been demonstrated to exist in rat and mice epidermal cell homogenates (Raza et al. 1992). These studies all show that the skin has formidable metabolic functions as well as the traditional barrier functions.

Lipid Metabolism. In addition to its metabolic activities, skin also has a marked ability to synthesize lipid, which is used to construct the extracellular epidermal barrier. Epidermal cells manufacture a variety of neutral lipids, ceramides, glycosylceramides, gangliosides, sterol esters, fatty acids, alkanes, and phospholipids, which are largely found in the extracellular barrier of the stratum corneum. Some of these lipids tend to be site-specific, with phospholipids and sterols residing mostly in the basal cell layers and some sterols and neutral lipids occupying the upper regions of the epidermis, mainly the stratum corneum. The effects on percutaneous absorption by the intercellular lipid structure have been discussed in greater detail elsewhere (Wertz 1992; Potts and Francoeur 1992; Hadgraft et al. 1992; Swartzendruber 1992; Elias and Feingold 1992). It is now accepted that this complex intercellular lipid matrix provides the primary barrier to drug penetration. It is important to realize that in some skin disease states, the overall production of lipids by the epidermal cells may be altered due to altered intracellular metabolism, subsequently followed by some alterations in the percutaneous absorption patterns of many drugs. Alterations in the epidermal cell's plasma membrane (primarily composed of lipid), whether due directly to a drug(s), the vehicle a drug was delivered in, or a disease process, may incite inflammatory reactions due to the release of inflammatory mediators (eicosanoids) from the epidermal cells or from the underlying cutaneous vasculature. Eicosanoids are a group of biologically active compounds derived enzymatically from eicosatetraenoic acid (arachidonic acid). Prostaglandins, leukotrienes, thromboxanes, and hydroxyeicosatetraenoic acids can be produced in minute quantities from arachidonic acid and have powerful proinflammatory effects on skin and the surrounding tissues. Eicosanoids are found in nearly every tissue in the mammalian body (Spannhake et al. 1981; Dunn and Hood 1977; Goldyne 1986), with some cells specializing in a certain type of eicosanoid. Skin produces several prostaglandins, including PGE_2, $PGF_{2\alpha}$, and PGI_2, as well as the lipoxygenase product leukotriene B_4.

PGE_2 induces vasodilation by elevating cyclic adenosine monophosphate in vascular smooth muscle cells, while $PGF_{2\alpha}$ causes vasoconstriction of the cutaneous vasculature by elevating cyclic guanosine monophosphate levels in vascular smooth muscle cells. In contrast to PGE_2, increased $PGF_{2\alpha}$ concentrations in skin enhance the leukocytes' response to chemotactic stimuli. $PGF_{2\alpha}$ has many effects on organs other than the skin, most notably in the reproductive tract of both humans and domestic animals. PGI_2 is a potent vasodilator produced mainly by vascular endothelial cells; it also inhibits vascular platelet aggregation. PGI_2 can be released from skin in response to some vehicles—namely, alcohols such as methanol, ethanol, and 2-propanol (Landolfi and Steiner 1984; Karanian et al. 1985). Cutaneous vasodilation has been observed in humans orally consuming alcohol (ethanol), presumably due to release of PGI_2 from vascular endothelial cells in contact with the alcohol-containing blood (Landolfi and Steiner 1984).

Leukotriene B_4 (LTB_4) is an inflammatory mediator produced from arachidonic acid via 5-lipoxygenase enzyme activity (Ford-Hutchinson 1985). Like $PGF_{2\alpha}$, LTB_4 is a potent chemotactic agent (Paulissen et al. 1990; Van de Kerkhof et al. 1991) and may also be a potent vasodilator and cause significant increases in vascular permeability when coadministered with PGE_2 (Ford-Hutchinson 1985). Although LTB_4 is most commonly produced by leukocytes, skin contains some inherent 5-lipoxygenase activity as determined from studies using stimulated human keratinocytes in culture as well as human and murine epidermal homogenates (Ruzicka 1990). These inflammatory mediator–induced changes in cutaneous blood flow may impact the absorption and cutaneous distribution of topically applied drugs.

Protein Metabolism. The primary protein product of the skin is keratin, which is the main intracellular component of the stratum corneum. In tandem with extracellular lipid, keratin forms the major component of the epidermal barrier. Keratin primarily consists of cystine, serine, glutamic acid, arginine, aspartic acid, and glycine amino acid residues. Of significance within the keratin molecule structure is the intrachain cystine disulfide bridging that further strengthens the overall keratin macrostructure. Keratin is the major protein foundation of hair (Monteiro-Riviere 1991; Monteiro-Riviere et al. 1993b).

PRINCIPLES OF PERCUTANEOUS ABSORPTION: SKIN PERMEABILITY. Prior to the 20th century, many scientists believed that skin was an impermeable barrier to all substances, except possibly gases. The science of dermatology has since advanced to reveal that many substances can enter the systemic circulation via the skin. Four pathways by which substances can gain this access to the rest of the body have been postulated and are schematically shown in Fig. 53.2.

The percutaneous absorption of drugs is important from two perspectives. Veterinary clinicians should be concerned about how much of a drug actually penetrates the skin to achieve a pharmacologic effect in treating diseases of the skin. This can be a function of several factors, including vehicle selection, hydration state of the stratum corneum, partition coefficient of the drug from vehicle into the stratum corneum lipids, the integrity of the stratum corneum, and cutaneous blood flow. The other reason to know the extent of percutaneous absorption pertains to public health and food consumption. Many compounds used in food animals are applied to and absorbed through the skin and enter the systemic circulation. Many of these compounds are stored in edible tissues (fat, muscle) for long periods of time, causing concern about residues in these tissues (Baynes et al. 1997; Riviere 1992).

The stratum corneum is accepted to be the major barrier, but not the only barrier, to percutaneous penetration in most species of animals. Passive diffusion is defined here as the movement of matter from one space to another space by random molecular motion. No known active transport processes are used by the stratum corneum to modulate percutaneous absorption. To

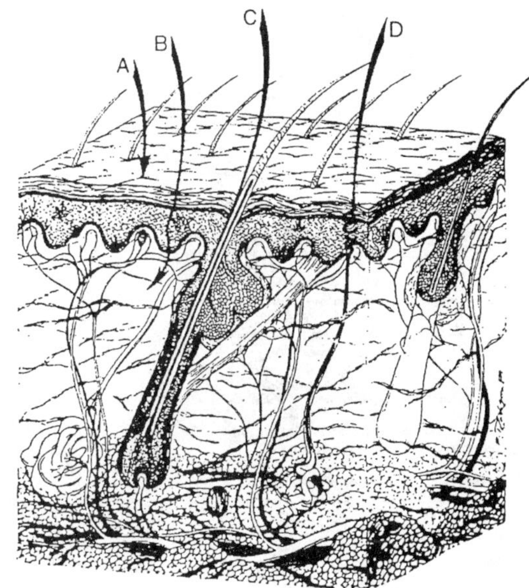

FIG. 53.2—A schematic view of the skin and the four routes of drug penetration. Drugs can penetrate through the stratum corneocytes (A), between the stratum corneocytes (B), transfollicularly via any hair follicle (C), or via an eccrine sweat gland or sebaceous gland (D).

better understand how substances diffuse through the stratum corneum, it is convenient to think of the stratum corneum as a wall in a "brick and mortar" configuration (Elias 1983), with the bricks representing the stratum corneocytes and the mortar representing the lipid matrix around them, as shown in Fig. 53.3. Permeation through the stratum corneum might occur via two routes. The first involves the drug traversing through the stratum corneocytes ("bricks") and extracellular lipid matrix ("mortar"), through the cells of the deeper epidermal cells, and then into the systemic circulation. The second route involves the chemical maneuvering its way through the stratum corneum via the intercellular lipid matrix only. It is generally accepted that the primary route of penetration is via the intercellular pathway. Because of the structure of the stratum corneum and the metabolic capabilities of the lower epidermal cells, the veterinarian must be aware that only a small percentage of the drug that is topically applied is going to actually penetrate the stratum corneum. This small fraction of the total dose will need to be able to affect the disease process occurring in the underlying layers of the epidermis.

The molecular structure of the intercellular lipid matrix throughout the epidermis is in a liquid crystalline configuration, consisting of fatty acids, ceramides, triglycerides, sterols, sterol esters, cholesterol sulfate, and miscellaneous alkanes. As epidermal cells migrate superficially and transform into the cells of the stratum corneum, the lipid content surrounding these cells changes from polar to more neutral in nature. Specifically, phospholipids and triglycerides tend to decrease while fatty acids, cholesterol, cholesterol sulfate, ceramides, and sphingolipids increase as the epidermal cells differentiate (Elias 1992). Enzymes are also present within this matrix of lipid. These lipids organize themselves into a lipid bilayer structure, with the hydrophobic ends of the molecules orienting themselves with other hydrophobic ends, and the hydrophilic ends orienting themselves in a similar fashion. More than one lipid bilayer can be formed within the intercellular matrix, leading to the formation of hydrophilic and hydrophobic channels, as illustrated in Fig. 53.4. One might assume that this complex lipid barrier would result in very low absorption profiles for hydrophilic (water soluble) compounds since these molecules would have difficulty crossing a hydrophobic barrier, but some studies have shown that many hydrophilic compounds penetrate the epidermis in much higher quantities than predicted, implying that there are other mechanisms whereby hydrophilic compounds permeate the stratum corneum. The primary mechanism by which this is accomplished is for hydrophilic molecules to penetrate through fluctuations, or "kinks," in the lipid alkyl chains (Potts and Francoeur 1992; Potts et al. 1992). Further, the permeation of hydrophilic molecules (such as water, methanol, ethanol, etc.) through the lipid matrix is due to their small size and molecular weight, which aid them in traveling through the lipid matrix through passages established by the lipid alkyl chains. This view is supported by the observation that larger hydrophilic molecules have lower percutaneous absorptions than their smaller molecular weight counterparts. Alternatively, penetration may also occur through the aqueous channels formed between the polar head groups of the lipid layers.

Chemicals may also permeate the skin using the skin appendageal route, mostly by way of hair follicles and sweat ducts. The importance of the transappendageal route on percutaneous absorption is controversial, but some studies indicate that the importance of this route tends to be species specific (Pitman and Rostas 1981). Generally, those animals possessing a sparse number of hair follicles per area of skin (humans, pigs) are considered to have little, if any, absorption of topically applied compounds via this route when compared to animals having a high density of hair follicles (cattle, sheep). In these latter animals, the stratum corneum barrier is just as impermeable to drugs as that of their less-haired counterparts, but the drug permeates the skin barrier via the hair follicles, sweat ducts, or other openings in the stratum corneum, increasing the percutaneous absorption of the chemical. It has been demonstrated that transappendageal absorption is high initially, then becomes insignificant, due to the small surface area of follicles and glands in relation to the total surface area of the stratum corneum. Topical delivery of pesticides to domestic livestock has been used for many years for the control of external as well

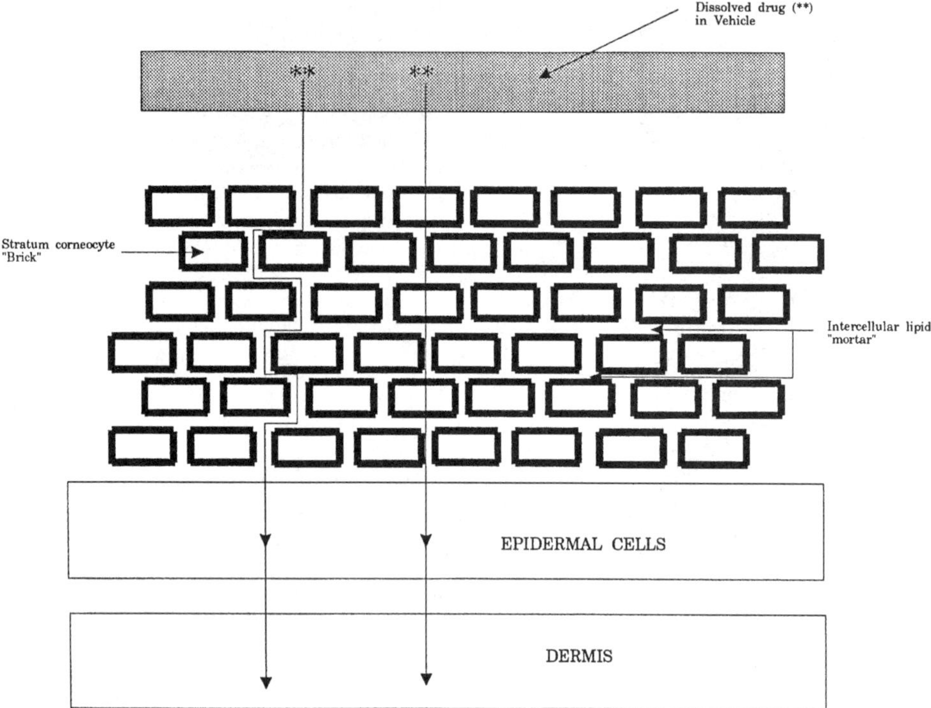

FIG. 53.3—Simplistic "brick and mortar" model of the skin. Drugs can penetrate by traveling around the stratum corneocytes through the lipid matrix, or drugs can pass through each corneocyte via the lipid matrix.

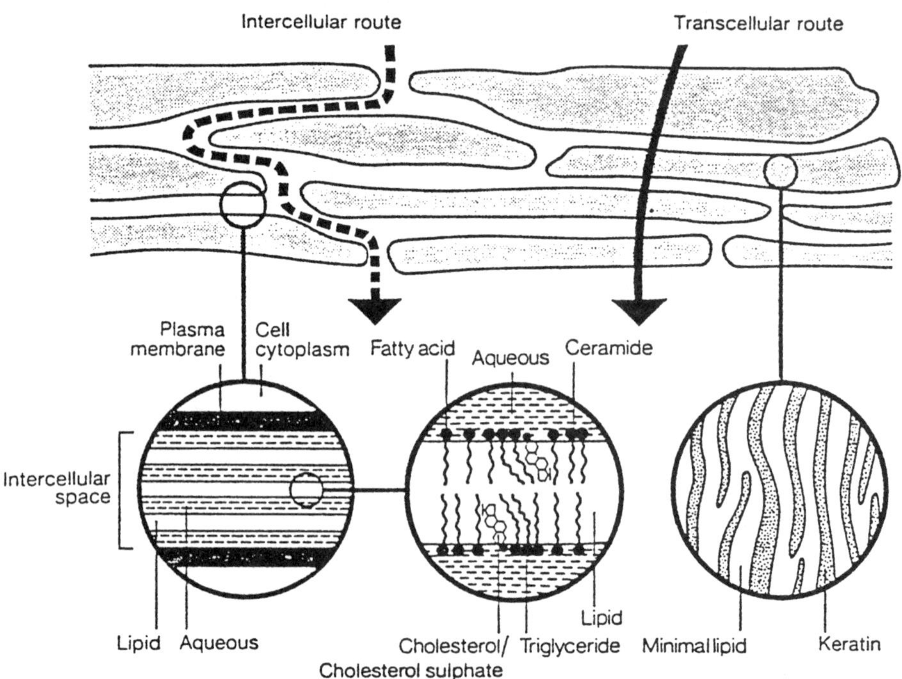

FIG. 53.4—The lipid bilayer model of the stratum corneum.

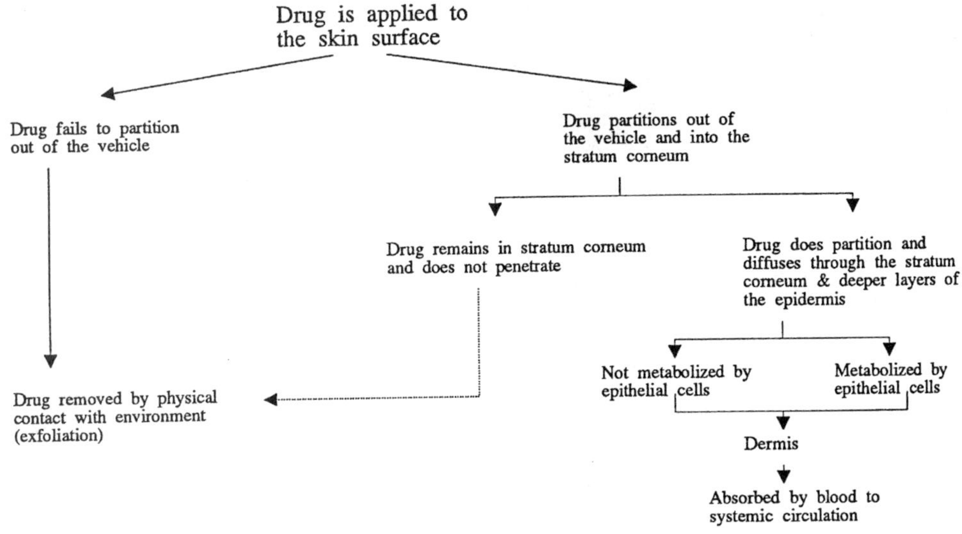

FIG. 53.5—Schematic representation of the fate of topically applied drugs.

as internal parasites of these animals, indicating that enough of the pesticide is absorbed systemically to kill some internal parasites while not harming the host animal (Riviere 1992).

Two events must occur for a drug to be successfully delivered to the epidermis under the stratum corneum: (1) the drug must diffuse out of the vehicle and onto the surface of the stratum corneum and (2) the drug must be able to penetrate the stratum corneum (Idson 1983). Restated, the vehicle in which the topical drug is being delivered should have significantly less affinity for that drug than for the stratum corneum. In actuality, many factors enter into the release of drug from the vehicle and its penetration through the stratum corneum. These factors have been mathematically described for steady-state kinetics in Fick's first law of diffusion (Idson 1983):

$$\frac{dQ}{dt} = \frac{(PC)C_V DA}{h}$$

where dQ/dt is a steady rate of penetration, PC is the drug's partition coefficient between the vehicle and the stratum corneum, C_v is the concentration of the drug dissolved in the vehicle, D is the diffusion coefficient, A is the area of skin to which the drug is applied, and h is the diffusion path length through the stratum corneum. In short, Fick's law states that the driving force causing the transfer of a drug from regions of high concentration to areas of low concentration is proportional to the concentration gradient (Idsen 1975). The diffusion coefficient is primarily correlated to the partition coefficient of the penetrant and can also be predicted from a knowledge of the drug's molecular volume and hydrogen bond activity (Potts and Guy 1995).

Only the nonionized moiety of a weak acid or base is available for diffusion across the stratum corneum. The pH of skin is variable and sensitive to hydration state. The typical pH of skin ranges from 4.2 to 7.3. For drugs with pK_a values within this range, the ionized fraction may vary according to the principles governed by the Henderson-Hasselbach equation, which would alter the amount of drug available for absorption. This is usually controlled for in the dermatologic formulation by use of buffering systems.

TOPICAL VEHICLES. A vehicle is defined as the medium in which a medicinally active agent is topically administered. It is a gross misconception that the vehicle in which topical drugs are dissolved is inert and has little effect on the skin; in fact, the physical and chemical properties of the vehicle will largely determine how successfully the drug will penetrate the skin. This has been clearly demonstrated with the pesticide carbaryl in pigs (Baynes and Riviere 1998). The vehicle may penetrate the stratum corneum to some extent and change the solubility of the intercellular lipid matrix. A simplistic view of the fate of topically applied drugs has been outlined in Fig. 53.5.

The partition coefficient is a unitless measure of the relative affinity of a compound between a highly hydrophobic phase (usually octanol) and a hydrophilic phase (water) and is a physicochemical factor that has a major role in determining the percutaneous absorption of a chemical. As the partition coefficient increases, the compound has a greater affinity for the lipid phase and less affinity for the water phase. As discussed earlier, the intercellular matrix of the skin consists of several different types of lipid, the ratios of which may vary from site to site.

Skin penetration of many chemicals has often been correlated to the partition coefficient of the penetrant. Generally, as the log of the partition coefficient increases, lipid solubility increases and there is an overall increase in the percutaneous absorption of the compound through the skin. This scenario is not always the case, however; some poorly lipid soluble compounds (i.e., low partition coefficients) sometimes penetrate the skin much easier than compounds with higher partition coefficients. Once penetration into the skin occurs, the molecule must eventually leave the lipid phase to be able to reach the systemic circulation. Compounds with high partition coefficients tend to remain within the lipid of the skin and form a reservoir rather than pass through; this is a well-documented phenomenon in skin. It has been shown that a log partition coefficient of 1–2 is desirable for skin penetration of most compounds.

Absorption of the vehicle into the stratum corneum is another factor to consider, since the vehicle may cause some disruptions in the composition and orientation of the intercellular lipid matrix. Partition coefficients for use in predicting the percutaneous absorption of topically applied drugs should ideally measure the index of affinity of a drug between the vehicle the drug is being delivered in and the lipid/vehicle composition of the stratum corneum. Unfortunately, few measurements of this kind are in existence because interaction of the vehicle with the stratum corneum lipids invalidates its determination. The role of partition coefficients in skin has been extensively reviewed elsewhere (Surber et al. 1990a; Sloan et al. 1986; Aungst et al. 1990; Surber et al. 1990b).

The optimal vehicle is one in which the drug is soluble enough to enter into solution but has less affinity for the vehicle than for the stratum corneum lipids, thereby favoring partitioning from the vehicle into the epidermis. Optimal delivery for a polar drug may thus be a relatively hydrophobic vehicle that has sufficient solubility to dissolve the drug. However, if a drug is too soluble in a vehicle relative to the stratum corneum, the drug may persist in the vehicle and only slowly release drug into the skin for as along as the vehicle stays on the skin.

The ability of the vehicle to stay on the skin surface long enough to allow passive absorption of the drug to occur is an important factor in passive drug absorption. The vehicle can be removed by three mechanisms: (1) absorption of the vehicle through the stratum corneum, (2) evaporation from the skin surface into the surrounding air, or (3) physical removal (rubbing, licking, scratching, etc). If the vehicle penetrates the stratum corneum more quickly than the drug, the concentration of the drug in the vehicle left on the surface of the stratum corneum will increase, which would increase the concentration of drug driving absorption but would also have the potential of inducing precipitation of the drug onto the skin's surface. The vehicle may also change the permeability of the lipid matrix (e.g., function as an enhancer). Evaporation of the vehicle will result in a similar scenario.

Vehicles may also affect the hydration state of the stratum corneum, which in turn may affect the rate at which topically applied compounds can penetrate the stratum corneum. Occlusion of the skin significantly increases the penetration of parathion (Chang and Riviere 1993) and other compounds. The vehicle can accomplish this by modulating insensible cutaneous water loss or skin transpiration. "Transpiration" is the term used to describe the passage of water vapor from the body, through the epidermis, and out to the surrounding environment. The act of transpiration is an important factor in determining percutaneous absorption of chemicals. In the normal state, the epidermal cells below the stratum corneum are highly hydrated compared to the stratum corneum. The water in and around these epidermal cells tends to slowly "percolate" upward, following the decreasing concentration gradient of water toward the less hydrated stratum corneum, eventually passing through the stratum corneum and into the environment. This phenomenon can be noninvasively assessed by measuring transepidermal water loss and has been correlated to the stratum corneum permeability of hydrophilic drugs. The stratum corneum normally maintains a 10–20% hydration state. When hydration of the stratum corneum occurs, which may reach 60–80% of the total stratum corneum's mass, this water "opens" the compact substance of the stratum corneum and reduces the density of the intracellular structures, thereby decreasing the cells' resistance to passive diffusion and allowing substances to permeate more readily than in the normal, dehydrated state. Hydration of the stratum corneum can be accomplished by slowing the rate of epidermal water loss to the environment by applying occlusive emollients to the skin (petrolatum, lanolin, etc.), by applying a non-water-permeable membrane (patch), by soaking the skin in water, or by increasing the relative humidity of the air surrounding the skin (Blank et al. 1984). An increase in percent hydration from 10 to 50% in the stratum corneum can result in as much as a 10-fold increase in diffusion constants (Idson 1983). This effect of environmental humidity and occlusion of the absorption of parathion through pig skin was clearly demonstrated (Chang and Riviere 1993).

Even when fully hydrated, the stratum corneum is one of the most water-impermeable biological membranes found in nature (Idsen 1975). Similarly, decreasing the hydration of the stratum corneum can decrease percutaneous absorption of substances. Dehydration of stratum corneum cells below the normal 10–15% usually results in "dry skin" and is a secondary symptom of many dermatologic diseases. Decreased stratum corneum hydration often results in a rugged and rough feeling to the skin, along with cracking, increased desquamation of the stratum corneum, and possible secondary septic or aseptic dermatitis. Dry skin can be treated by (1) treating the underlying condition causing the disease and/or (2) applying agents that will increase the hydration of the stratum corneum by slowing transepidermal water loss. Applying keratolytics (discussed later in this chapter) is also of use. This discussion should point out that selecting a vehicle that increases the amount of water in the stratum corneum will most likely result in more permeation of drug to the underlying affected tissues, an important factor in successful dermatologic therapy. In diseases involving dry skin, returning the stratum corneum to its normal hydration state should also be a goal of dermatologic therapy.

In summary, the vehicle, not just the choice of drug, plays a crucial role in determining the success or failure of dermatologic therapy. No "ideal vehicle" exists; the veterinary clinician must evaluate the patient's skin lesion and should determine what drug is indicated and which vehicle would best augment that therapy. Both factors may markedly influence the success of therapy.

Other Factors Affecting Percutaneous Absorption. Other factors that may enhance or hinder percutaneous absorption are the molecular weight of the chemical, temperature, blood flow, and skin age. Increasing the blood flow through the dermis would suggest a more rapid removal of drugs absorbed from the epidermis (Riviere and Williams 1992). Vasoconstriction of these vessels has been shown to significantly decrease percutaneous absorption of 6-methylprednisolone and testosterone (Malkinson 1958). The temperature of the air surrounding the skin plays a role in blood flow, with warmer environmental temperatures or skin showing one of the cardinal signs of inflammation (heat) increasing the blood flow to the skin and cooler temperatures decreasing cutaneous blood flow. An inverse relationship appears to exist between absorption rate and the molecular weight of the drug (Idsen 1975). Although smaller molecules tend to increase total topical dose absorbed through the skin, there is considerable variability in the amounts percutaneously absorbed among compounds of similar molecular weights (Idsen 1975; Tragear 1966).

Penetration Enhancers. The stratum corneum has been portrayed as a formidable and almost impenetrable barrier to the absorption of lipophilic, hydrophilic, and amphoteric xenobiotics. Many efforts have been made to adjust the barrier of the stratum corneum to increase the percutaneous absorption of topically applied xenobiotics, for the most part with only limited success. The barrier function of the stratum corneum can be structurally modified using a relatively small class of compounds, collectively known as penetration enhancers or penetration accelerants, that increase the percutaneous absorption of many compounds.

Many reports exist in the human and veterinary literature of various agents that have been shown to accelerate penetration of compounds through the skin, but few describe the precise mechanism by which an individual penetration enhancer performs this function. One theory, the lipid-protein-partitioning concept, has been proposed for the mechanism of action of all the known penetration enhancers, including penetration via the intercellular as well as the intracellular routes (Barry 1991). For both routes, this theory acknowledges that polar (hydrophilic) molecules permeate the skin via polar channels (either by aqueous pores or by alkyl group modulation), which are different from the channels used by nonpolar (hydrophobic) molecules. After application to the skin surface, the drug molecules diffuse out of the vehicle and into the stratum corneum and begin to traverse the many aqueous and lipid barriers found in the intercellular matrix (see Fig. 53.4) in order to reach the rest of the body via the systemic circulatory system. Penetration enhancers are hypothesized to modify these lipid and aqueous bilayers of the intercellular lipid matrix and allow topically applied compounds to penetrate the stratum corneum more readily by disrupting the normally very organized structure of the lipid layers.

It is convenient to organize the known penetration enhancers into four common subgroups: azone and its derivatives, urea and its derivatives (1-dodecylurea, 1,3 didodecylurea, 1,3 diphenyl urea, propylene glycol, dimethylisosorbide), the terpenes (carvone, pulegone, piperitone, menthone, cyclohenene oxide, terpinen-4-ol, and others), and the aprotic solvents (dimethylsulfoxide, demethyl formamide, decylmethyl sulfoxide, 2-pyrrolidone, and others). At the present time, the first three groups are used almost exclusively in human pharmaceutical products and research and will not be discussed here. The most extensively used penetration enhancer in veterinary medicine is dimethylsulfoxide (DMSO).

DMSO is a product from the processing of wood pulp and is a dipolar and aprotic solvent. DMSO is also produced by phytoplankton and is present in many foods (Herschler 1982). DMSO has been used to treat a myriad of skin ailments, including otitis externa, interdigital cysts, lick granulomas, superficial burns, skin grafts, and snakebites, and to reduce the engorgement of the mammary glands of the nursing bitch (Knowles 1982). Other less common veterinary uses for DMSO have also been described (Jacob et al. 1965; Jacob 1982; Knowles 1982). In addition to penetration enhancement, DMSO is also bacteriostatic, vasodilatory, fibrinolytic, and anti-inflammatory and produces some degree of topical analgesia. DMSO produces a thermal effect after direct application to the skin, which may function to alleviate pain in the skin and in the underlying muscle and bone. The transient erythema that is induced after topical administration of DMSO is due to the release of histamine (Jacob et al. 1965). These effects are considered transient and reversible and will not generally increase in severity after multiple treatments, indicating no need to discontinue therapy. Potential skin irritation occurs at concentrations of greater than 70% (see the 6th edition of this text for more information on DMSO).

DMSO has the potential to enhance the percutaneous absorption of a number of topically applied compounds.

The exact mechanism of this percutaneous absorption enhancement has not been clearly elucidated. DMSO appears to produce only minor morphological changes in the skin. Penetration enhancement of topically applied chemicals dissolved in DMSO does not appear significant until the DMSO concentrations approach 50–60%, with overall permeability of the compound tending to increase as the concentration of DMSO applied to the skin approaches 100% (Kurihara-Bergstrom et al. 1987). Many mechanisms have been proposed to attempt to explain why DMSO enhances the percutaneous absorption of such a wide variety of compounds. Possible mechanisms include elution of stratum corneum lipids and delamination of the horny layer by stress resulting from crosscurrents of highly water interactive DMSO and water (Kurihara-Bergstrom et al. 1986). Sharata and Burnette (1988) determined that in nude mice skin, DMSO transformed the highly compact cell contents of the basal stratum corneum (keratin) into a looser meshwork of filamentous bundles, resulting in much more porous intracellular structure with an increase in intracellular surface areas, which they believed might increase percutaneous transport. Whatever the mechanism, DMSO has been shown to enhance the percutaneous absorption of many compounds, including water, hydrocortisone, salicylic acid, tubocurarine HCl, multiple glucocorticosteroids and antibiotics, estradiol, hexachlorophene, phenylbutazone, and a host of other topically applied chemicals.

Electrically Assisted Transdermal Drug Delivery. An alternative approach to overcome the stratum corneum permeability barrier is by using electrical (iontophoresis) or ultrasonic (phonophoresis) energy, rather than the concentration gradient of diffusion, to drive drug through the skin (Riviere and Heit 1997). These techniques hold the most promise for delivering large drugs such as peptides and oligonucleotides that now can be administered only by intravascular injection. With these techniques, dose is based on the application surface area and the amount of energy required to actively deliver drug across the skin. In iontophoresis, this amounts to a dose being expressed in mA/cm^2. Formulation factors are also very different, since many of the components used are also delivered by the applied electrical current in direct molar proportion to the active drug. Finally, a recent but related strategy is to employ very short duration high-voltage electrical pulses (electroporation) to reversibly break down the stratum corneum barrier, allowing larger peptides, and even small proteins, to be delivered systemically (Riviere et al. 1995). These approaches, if applied to veterinary medicine, could have implications for the use of controlled transdermal delivery as a viable method of drug delivery.

CLASSIFICATION OF DERMATOLOGIC VEHICLES. As discussed in the introduction to this chapter, the defining difference between dermatologic and other treatment areas of veterinary pharmacology is the topical route of administration coupled with the overriding influence that the dosage vehicle exerts on absorption and activity of the applied drug. The vehicles used as veterinary dermatologics have been historically classified into seven broad categories (Harvey 1985a,b; Block 1985; Rippie 1985; Swinyard 1985; Swinyard and Lowenthal 1985; Nairn 1985).

Adsorbents and Protectives. Adsorbents and protectives are used extensively in many veterinary pharmaceutical preparations. Adsorbents act by binding gases, toxins, and some organisms (such as bacteria) to prevent exposure to the damaged skin surface. Protectives function by providing an occlusive layer of protection from the external environment or by providing mechanical support to the affected area. Protectives and adsorbents can be further divided into two subclasses: dusting powders and mechanical protectives.

Dusting powders are generally inert and innocuous substances. They include starch, calcium carbonate, talc, titanium dioxide, zinc oxide, and boric acid. Many are used in drug formulations alone or as a vehicle for the delivery of other drugs. If the powder particle has a smooth surface, it will act mainly to prevent friction, thus protecting abraded and raw skin surfaces; powder particles with rough or porous surfaces act on the skin by absorbing moisture. Water-absorbing powders tend to coalesce and eventually occlude the skin's surface when wetted and therefore should not be used on wet, moist, or highly exudative skin surfaces. Powders that also contain starch or other carbohydrates that are allowed to cake onto these moist skin surfaces give bacteria and fungi (mainly *Candida* spp.) a source of energy, allowing them to proliferate. This may lead to a secondary bacterial and/or fungal skin infection or exacerbation of an existing microbial skin infection. Powders should not be used within body cavities (thorax, abdomen) or in skin abscesses, especially those powders containing talc. Talc has been shown to promote severe granulomatous reactions when used in these areas but is relatively innocuous when used on intact skin surfaces.

Mechanical protectives provide an occlusive film that protects the underlying skin from irritants present in the external environment (ultraviolet radiation, contact irritants, toxins), provide mechanical support, and are popular vehicles for many drugs. Many members of this subgroup are used to treat cutaneous ulcers and other hard-to-heal cutaneous wounds. Compounds in this group include kaolin, lanolin, anhydrous lanolin, mineral oil, olive oil, peanut oil, petrolatum, zinc stearate, and recently a number of synthetic polymers.

Demulcents. Demulcents are generally high molecular weight compounds that are water soluble and function by alleviating irritation (*demulcere,* "to smooth"). Like the compounds listed in the protectives group, demulcents can coat the surface of damaged skin and protect the stratum corneum and underlying cellular structure of the epidermis by forming a protective barrier against the surrounding environment. They differ from protectives in that they inherently reduce the irritation from these external stimuli. This group comprises a large and diverse number of chemicals, including mucilages, gums, dextrins, starches, polymeric polyhydric glycols, glycerin, gelatin, hydroxypropyl cellulose, hydroxypropyl methylcellulose, hydroxyethyl cellulose, methyl cellulose, and polyvinyl alcohol. The dried gum extracts from the acacia and tragacanth plants can readily dissolve in water to form mucilages (see the 6th edition of this text for more detail). The most commonly used demulcents in veterinary dermatology today are glycerin, propylene glycol, and the polyethylene glycols.

Glycerin is a hygroscopic, trihydric alcohol prepared from propylene and has been used for many years as a suppository, with high concentrations of this vehicle relieving constipation by drawing water from the body and into the colon. Glycerin is a clear, colorless liquid that is miscible with water and alcohol and has been used neat to reduce corneal edema and to facilitate ophthalmoscopic examinations. Used in high concentrations topically on the skin, glycerin may dehydrate and irritate the skin, thereby increasing transepidermal water loss. Lower concentrations of glycerin absorbed into the skin hydrate the stratum corneum because of glycerin's hygroscopic nature. Despite its side effects, glycerin makes an excellent vehicle for topical drug delivery when used at lower concentrations.

Propylene glycol (1,2 propanediol) is a hygroscopic, colorless, odorless water-soluble liquid that is miscible with many compounds (water, alcohols, acetone, many volatile oils) and is also bacteriostatic, fungistatic, and nonocclusive. It was first considered for use in 1932 to be used with a drug to treat human syphilis and has since been used as a nontoxic antifreeze in dairies and beer breweries (Catanzaro and Smith 1991). Propylene glycol is an ideal medium for the topical delivery of many drugs in animals and humans, as well as for many oral and parenteral drug formulations, such as antitussives and shampoos. Propylene glycol spreads evenly onto the skin's surface and has a very low evaporation rate; it is not greasy to the touch, does not stain clothing or hair, and has some effect on slowing transepidermal water loss, thereby hydrating the stratum corneum to some extent. Topical hypersensitization and other toxicities are rare but have been reported (Catanzaro and Smith 1991).

Polyethylene glycols are a group of structurally similar compounds that differ in molecular weight. The larger the number, the higher the molecular weight and the more viscous the formulation becomes. At ambient temperature, polyethylene glycols 200, 300, 400, and 600 are clear viscous liquids; polyethylene glycols 900 to 9000 are semihard waxy solids at room temperature. As a group, the polyethylene glycols do not easily hydrolyze and are nontoxic, bland, highly water soluble, and nonvolatile.

TABLE 53.2—Emollients in use today

Official vegetable oils	Animal fats	Hydrocarbons
Olive oil	Lanolin (wool fat with water added)	Paraffin
Cottonseed oil	Anhydrous wool fat (no water added)	Petrolatum
Corn oil	Lard	White petrolatum (vasoline)
Almond oil	Whale oil	Mineral oil
Peanut oil		White/yellow waxes (beeswax)
Persic oil		Spermaceti
Cocoa butter		

Emollients. Emollients are bland, fatty materials often used to soften or moisten the skin. Emollients are particularly useful when treating skin conditions resulting from water-soluble irritants and airborne bacteria because of their ability to act as a protectant, sequestering the damaged skin away from these noxious stimuli. When used topically, emollients soften skin by decreasing transepidermal water loss, or transpiration, and increasing the hydration of the stratum corneum. A recent addition to this class are silicone-based polymers such as dimethicone. Therefore, this is a useful group of compounds for treating dermatologic conditions involving dry, crusty, or flaky lesions of the epidermis. Emollients are used today as vehicles for many lipid-soluble drugs. Examples of commonly used emollients are listed in Table 53.2.

Astringents. Astringents precipitate protein, toughen the skin, promote healing, and dry the skin when applied topically. When used to coagulate blood, astringents are said to be styptic and elicit a mildly uncomfortable sensation when applied to small open wounds. Most of the chemicals in this group are inorganic salts of aluminum, zinc, potassium, and silver and include aluminum chloride, aluminum sulfate, calamine (a combination of Fe_2O_3 and ZnO_2), potassium permanganate, silver nitrate, zinc chloride, zinc oxide, zirconium chlorhydrate, and tannic acid. There are many germicidal agents that also have astringent activity. Other astringents are of vegetable origin, most of these preparations owing their activity to tannic acid (gallotannic acid). Astringents in the vegetable-derivative group include gallic acid, kino, krameria, and rubus (blackberry). Astringents have limited uses in veterinary medicine today.

Rubefacients, Irritants, and Vesicants. Chemicals in this class are used to induce hyperemia (rubefacients), hyperemia and inflammation (irritants), or cutaneous blisters (vesicants). Heat applied to the skin via a hot-water bottle, heat lamp, moist hot pack, or an electric heating pad are acceptable rubefacients and are extensively used in human medicine. Chemical rubefacients are more commonly used in veterinary medicine, mainly due to the difficulty in applying the heat sources listed above for extended lengths of time. An abbreviated list of chemicals that are known rubefacients, irritants, or vesicants includes anthralin, camphor, coal tar, creosote, ichthamnol, menthol, methyl salicylate, resorcinol, cantharidin, black mustard, iodine, mercuric iodide, capsicum, chloroform, alcohols, turpentine, thymol, and pine tar. With the exception of coal tar, most members of the chemical group are not commonly used in modern veterinary practice because of their potential toxicity. Coal tar is a component found in many veterinary dermatology preparations (especially shampoos) and is a by-product of the distillation of bituminous coal. Photosensitization has been reported to occur. Coal tar should not be used on cats, because of frequent irritant or allergic reactions. Camphor is a rubefacient that has been used in some topical preparations and has some mild analgesic activity. It is of limited use in the treatment of mild pruritus. Similarly, menthol stimulates sensory nerve endings, inducing a feeling of coolness, induces mild analgesia, and is also a mild antipruritic (Harvey 1985a).

Caustics and Escharotics. Caustics (also known as corrosives) are agents that will destroy tissue after one or more applications. Escharotics are corrosive and will also precipitate proteins, leading to the formation of a scab and eventually a permanent scar. As with the rubefacient, irritant, and vesicant group, many of the caustics and escharotics have few uses in veterinary dermatology today. Historically, caustics have been used to induce desquamation of the stratum corneum (keratolytic) and to treat warts, keratoses, and other hyperplastic skin diseases. Escharotics have also been used to seal cutaneous ulcers and wounds. Examples of this group include glacial acetic acid, alum, aluminum chloride, gentian violet, phenol, potassium hydroxide, salicylic acid, and silver nitrate.

Keratolytics, Keratoplastics, and Antiseborrheics. Keratolytics function by loosening keratin, which facilitates the desquamation of the stratum corneum, whereas keratoplastics attempt to "normalize" keratinization by slowing basal cell proliferation through inhibition of DNA synthesis. Other mechanisms may also contribute to this effect. Antiseborrheics attempt to modulate sebum production in the skin. Many of the keratolytics available today are also keratoplastic and/or antiseborrheic; therefore, these functions are discussed together. Most keratolytics and antiseborrheics are also cutaneous irritants, which may, in some cases, preclude their use on diseased skin in some animals (Shanley 1990). Several keratolytics and antiseborrheics used in veterinary dermatology are discussed below.

Salicylic acid (2-hydroxybenzoic acid) is used topically as a keratolytic, keratoplastic, and antiseborrheic agent and has some mild antibacterial and antifungal actions. Salicylic acid (2–10%) causes the dead or dying cells of the stratum corneum to hydrate, swell, and soften, thereby hastening their desquamation, and solubilizes the intercellular lipid layer, releasing the cells of the stratum corneum from each other. Salicylic acid is used extensively in veterinary dermatology to treat many keratoproliferative diseases. Topical use of salicylic acid may cause an irritant dermatitis in animals and has been studied extensively in both humans and many animal models (Weirich 1975; Nook 1987; deMare et al. 1988; Sloan et al. 1986; Roberts and Horlock 1978).

Benzoyl peroxide is a keratolytic and antiseborrheic agent that is also a strong oxidizer, free-radical generator, and antimicrobial and has been used in veterinary and human dermatology for many years. The majority of topically applied benzoyl peroxide is metabolized to benzoic acid by the viable epidermal cells during penetration through the skin (Holzmann et al. 1979; Nacht et al. 1981). Benzoyl peroxide in high concentrations can cause skin irritation and was identified as being a skin tumor promoter in SENCAR mice if used in tandem with 7,12-dimethylbenz(a)-anthracene (Slaga et al. 1981; Epstein 1988; Schweizer et al. 1987). The bactericidal activity associated with benzoyl peroxide comes from its ability to generate free radicals, which disrupt bacterial cell membranes. Due to its bactericidal activities, benzoyl peroxide is indicated in the treatment of pyodermas (Ihrke 1980a,b) as well as in diseases that cause keratosis. Transient stinging or burning sensations after application to the affected site have been reported in humans.

Resorcinol (*m*-dihydroxybenzene) is a keratolytic agent that also has bactericidal and fungicidal properties. Like urea (discussed below), it acts as a protein precipitant and promotes hydration of the keratin, resulting in its keratolytic function. Resorcinol may be used alone or compounded with other mild keratolytic agents, such as sulfur or salicylic acid.

Sulfur is a keratolytic, keratoplastic, and antiseborrheic agent used in a variety of topical agents. Sulfur is also antibacterial and antipruritic and has a mild follicular flushing action. The keratolytic activity of elemental sulfur is thought to be related to an inflammatory process that ultimately causes a sloughing of the stratum corneum. The formation of hydrogen sulfide and pentathionic acid is responsible for some of its keratolytic and antibacterial properties. The keratoplastic effect is most likely similar to that of the coal tars, being cytostatic (Miller 1986).

Retinoids are a class of naturally occurring or synthetically manufactured compounds that have vitamin A–like (retinoic acid) activity. Retinol (vitamin A alcohol) is the most potent analog and is metabolized to two other retinols: retinal and retinoic acid. In the early 20th century, researchers documented the importance of vitamin A in reproduction, vision, and epidermal cell growth promotion, along with its functions in differentiation and maintenance of epithelial cell surface structure, including that of the skin (Kwochka 1989). It was also found that *some* dyskeratotic skin diseases could be correlated to low levels of vitamin A, which eventually led to the therapeutic use of vitamin A to treat these skin diseases. The use of vitamin A was limited, however, as the levels needed to induce a clinical improvement of the lesions often induced signs of hypervitaminosis A. This side-effect dilemma prompted research into vitamin A substitutes, which led to the discovery and testing of over 1500 retinoids. Three retinoids—tretinoin, isotretinoin, and etretinate—are available for clinical use today.

The retinoids, like vitamin A, act as growth and differentiation regulators in the skin when administered orally or topically. Although the exact mechanism by which the retinoids exert these effects is not completely understood, it is theorized that retinoids alter RNA synthesis within the cell, in turn altering protein synthesis and prostaglandin production, and also affecting some enzymes, such as ornithine decarboxylase and collagenase (Power and Ihrke 1990). The overall effect of the retinoids is to "normalize" the epithelium in those diseases responsive to these drugs.

In humans, the retinoids are used to treat severe recalcitrant cystic acne, psoriasis, Darier's disease, pityriasis rubra pilaris, and various other disorders of keratinization. Retinoids also have an ability to control malignant transformations in some tissues that are caused by chemical carcinogens, ionizing radiation, growth factors, and viruses. Naturally occurring retinoids have been shown to protect animals against skin papillomas and carcinomas of the skin and other organs (Griffiths and Vorhees 1994; Kwochka 1989). Numerous side effects have been associated with retinoid use in humans, including cheilitis, xerosis of the skin, pruritus, dryness of mucous membranes, epistaxis, thinning of the hair, palmoplantar desquamation, conjunctivitis, headache, ataxia, fatigue, psychologic changes, and visual disturbances. Teratogenicity is a serious problem in women who take isotretinoin during pregnancy. Symptoms of hypervitaminosis A may also occur, which is characterized by demineralization and thinning of the long bones, cortical hyperostosis, periostitis, and premature closure of the epiphyses (Kwochka 1989).

As of this date, retinoids are not used to a great extent in veterinary medicine (Werner and Power 1994). Reported uses of any of the retinoids in dogs and cats are few, and the recommendations for use and possible toxicities and side effects are based on a very small number of animals. Indications for veterinary use remain rather vague, in part because the skin diseases that retinoids may be efficacious in treating humans do not have exact analogs in domestic animals. There is also a lack of formal studies conducted on large populations of dogs or cats. Reported uses for the retinoids in domestic animals are in disorders of keratinization, which may include primary idiopathic seborrhea in Cocker Spaniels, sebaceous adenitis, canine lamellar ichthyosis, Schnauzer comedo syndrome, and epidermal inclusion cysts, among others (Power and Ihrke 1990; Kwochka 1989). The use of retinoids in cats with neoplastic disorders, specifically squamous cell carcinoma and epidermal dysplasia, has been investigated and found to be of limited value (Evans et al. 1985). Toxicities to the retinoids in animals seem to be few, but it should be made clear that the reported side effects and toxicities are based on a small population of clinically ill animals treated for short periods of time with these compounds, and these observations may prove to be inaccurate if the use of these compounds increases. Out of 29 dogs treated with isotretinoin in one study (Kwochka 1989), 4 dogs developed conjunctivitis that was observed to be reversible after treatments ended. There is no formal information available as to the existence of skeletal anomalies in dogs given retinoids for long periods of time (Power and Ihrke 1990). Birth defects involving the central nervous system, skeleton, thymus, and heart do occur, as seen with high doses of vitamin A during pregnancy. Cats appear to have a higher incidence of side effects associated with retinoid treatment. Cats treated with isotretinoin were observed to develop periocular erythema, periocular crusting, epiphora, and blepharospasm (Kwochka 1989).

Tretinoin (*trans*–retinoic acid), also known as Retin-A, is an oxidation product of vitamin A. Applied topically, tretinoin causes inflammation, thickening of the epidermis, and localized intercellular edema. This edema leads to epidermal cell separation and an increase in exfoliation of the epidermal cells, resulting in an overall keratolytic action of the treated area. Used systemically, tretinoin will induce hypervitaminosis A (Power and Ihrke 1990).

Isotretinoin (Accutane, Roche; 13-*cis*-retinoic acid) and etretinate (Tegison, Roche) are two systemically used retinoids that also have potential veterinary applications. Power and Ihrke (1990) describe several cases where these two retinoids have been used to treat several skin diseases in dogs, with variable success. Isotretinoin is the most effective inhibitor of sebum production known (Kwochka 1989), making it potentially useful in treating primary idiopathic seborrhea and comedo syndromes. Although retinoids are associated with less toxicity than vitamin A, toxicities can occur. Etretinate may be associated with fewer toxic side effects than isotretinoin. Insufficient data are available for dogs or cats to determine its efficacy or toxicity.

Coal tar is another pharmaceutical that has keratolytic as well as keratoplastic and antiseborrheic activity. Its mechanism of action and general uses have been discussed previously. Coal tar products should not be used in the feline due to frequent irritant and allergic reactions.

Urea is a product of protein metabolism that, when used topically, acts as a protein denaturant, promoting the hydration of keratin. Once the treated areas of keratin swell, mild keratolysis ensues. The use of urea alone as a keratolytic agent is not common in veterinary dermatology today.

Selenium sulfide is an externally applied antiseborrheic, keratolytic, and keratoplastic compound that also has some antidandruff activities. Selenium sulfide exerts these actions by its antimitotic activity, slowing cell proliferation and sebum production, and tends to be irritating (especially if used in long-term treatment protocols) and also stains hair. It also causes irritation of the mucous membranes, so care should be taken to avoid contact with these tissues. Percutaneous absorption is minimal if applied to intact skin.

CLASSES OF MEDICATED APPLICATIONS. Pharmaceuticals can also be classified by the type of base they are formulated in. There are eight classes of medicated applications (Harvey 1985a; Block 1985; Rippie 1985; Swinyard 1985; Swinyard and Lowenthal 1985; Nairn 1985).

Ointments. Ointments are semisolid preparations that usually (but not always) contain drugs used to treat dermatologic diseases. There are five classes of ointments commonly used in veterinary medicine.

HYDROCARBON BASES. These emollient ointment bases usually are composed of vegetable oils and animal fats. Common members of this subset include spermaceti, cetyl esters wax ("synthetic spermaceti"), oleic acid, olive oil, paraffin, petrolatum, white petrolatum, white wax, and yellow wax. Hydrocarbon base ointments are emollient and generally hydrophobic and occlusive, causing an increase in the hydration of the stratum corneum and underlying epidermal cell structure by decreasing transepidermal water loss, making them useful in rehydrating or softening the skin. Disadvantages include greasiness and their ability to stain clothing; also, they cannot be washed off in water, making them difficult to completely remove from the skin.

ANHYDROUS ABSORPTION BASES. This type of ointment base contains very little (if any) water after preparation but differs from the hydrocarbon bases in that it will readily accept any water molecules it comes in contact with. Absorbent ointment bases can absorb large quantities of water and still keep their thick consistency. Examples of this subgroup include hydrophilic petrolatum and anhydrous lanolin, both of which are emollient, occlusive, and greasy.

WATER-OIL EMULSION BASES. Emulsions, by definition, are oil and water combinations. Water-in-oil emulsion bases (creams) are water-washable bases that are easily removed from the skin surface and contain more oil than water on a percentage basis. The oil phase usually consists of petrolatum or liquid petrolatum and perhaps an alcohol (cetyl or stearyl alcohol). The aqueous phase may consist of water; however, other aqueous vehicles may be used, such as propylene glycol, polyethylene glycol, or glycerin, to which various preservatives (such as paraben derivatives) are usually added. Water-in-oil bases are emollient (due to the higher percentage of oil than aqueous phase), occlusive, greasy, and may absorb some water, but not to the same degree as the anhydrous absorption bases. Other common components of water-in-oil emulsion bases include glyceryl monosterate and stearic acid.

OIL-WATER EMULSION BASES. Oil-in-water emulsions are manufactured in the same manner as the water-in-oil bases, with the exception that the aqueous phase is in a higher percentage than the oil component. The same ingredients are also used to make the oil-in-water bases. Because of the higher water (or other aqueous phase) content, oil-in-water bases are water-washable, nongreasy, and nonocclusive.

WATER-SOLUBLE BASES. As the name implies, these bases have lost their hydrophobic lipid base components. These demulcent bases are primarily composed of polymers that are completely water soluble and usually anhydrous, do not easily hydrolyze, do not support mold growth, and are nongreasy, nonocclusive, and nonvolatile. If the components of a preparation contain water-soluble bases in a gelled medium, they are referred to as gels. Gels are a combination of propylene glycol, propylene gallate, disodium ethylenediaminetetraacetic acid (EDTA), and carboxypolymethylene that results in a clear, water-miscible, and relatively greaseless formulation. A commonly used drug in a gel formulation is DMSO (Domoso, Diamond). Glucocorticosteroids may also be formulated in this way.

Poultices. A poultice (or cataplasm) is a soft moist mass of materials applied locally to an affected area and was historically composed of roots, herbs, seeds, and even mud in a gruel-like base. The poultice was intended to be a topical wound treatment serving as a counterirritant and absorptive/adsorptive sink. Poultices are rarely used in veterinary medicine today.

Pastes. Pastes are absorptive powders placed in a gelatinous base, usually petrolatum or hydrophilic petrolatum. Pastes have been used to adhere to the skin and thereby act as a "sponge" to absorb exudates and moisture and also as a physical barrier to protect the skin from the external environment. Pastes are easily removed from the skin and can be used on moist lesions of the skin.

Powders. Powders have been discussed earlier in this chapter as a class of vehicle for the delivery of topical drugs to the skin. Powders are commonly used in veterinary medicine to deliver pesticides (carbaryl, permethrins, etc.) for the control of external parasites (mainly fleas) and in large-animal veterinary dermatology to deliver antibiotics, such as nitrofurazone, to wounds.

Dressings. Dressings are external applications of some previously discussed compounds (petrolatum, ointments) on an application device such as plastic wrap or sterile gauze and are placed over wound sites to protect the skin lesion from external environmental trauma. Dressings may also contain antimicrobial agents, such as nitrofurazone.

Plasters. Plasters are similar to dressings; however, they are attached to the skin via some adhesive material. They protect skin lesions from the external environment and provide an occlusive environment. Plasters have limited use in veterinary medicine today.

Suspensions. A suspension is a two-phase system composed of a finely divided solid that is dispersed in a liquid, usually water. Suspensions are not utilized to any great degree in veterinary dermatology today. They are more commonly used in oral drug preparation schemes. The most common type of suspension currently used topically is captan (Orthocide, Chevron Chemical), which is used to treat some types of superficial fungal infections and which also has some limited bacteriostatic properties.

Lotions. Lotions are powders dissolved in a liquid, usually water or an alcohol. Lotions, like powders, tend to be cooling, drying, and somewhat mildly antipruritic. Lotions have limited applications in veterinary medicine but are used extensively in human over-the-counter skin-care products.

ANTIMICROBIALS. Bacterial skin infections are a frequent cause of dermatitis in animals. Antimicrobial therapy is thus a mainstay to treat bacterial skin disease. Like other tissues, healthy skin is associated with normal microbial flora. By and large, this group causes no adverse effects unless the skin is in some way compromised, that is, by trauma, parasitism, or iatrogenic intervention (surgery). There are two approaches to treating bacterial skin disease: systemic administration of antibiotics or application of topical agents to the affected skin site. The drugs used for systemic treatment are the same as those fully discussed in the antimicrobial chapters of this text and will not be discussed further. The requirement for successful systemic treatment includes use of a drug with an appropriate spectrum of activity coupled with a favorable distribution to the skin.

Topical Antibiotics. A select few of the antibiotics used in systemic therapy are also used in topical preparations to treat bacterial skin infections, including sulfonamides, chloramphenicol, polymyxins, and neomycin. Agents that are only used topically include bacitracin, mupromycin, nitrofurazone, povidone iodine, and chlorhexidine (Harvey 1985b; Block 1985; Rippie 1985; Swinyard 1985; Swinyard and Lowenthal 1985; Nairn 1985; Bennett 1995).

When used topically, the percutaneous absorption of the aminoglycosides may be slowed by their large molecular structure, positive charge, and binding to pus. When topically administering any antibiotic combination containing an aminoglycoside, cleaning the affected area of exudate before application will increase efficacy. Nephrotoxicity and ototoxicity are rarely observed when aminoglycosides are applied topically because of the minimal absorption of these large hydrophilic molecules.

Polymyxin B and polymyxin E (colistin) are gram-negative bactericidal antibiotics that labilize the cellular membrane of susceptible bacteria, in particular *Pseudomonas* spp. and *Proteus* spp. Both are used in topical formulations only, since systemic use of these antibiotics is not recommended due to the high incidence of nephrotoxicity and respiratory paralysis. Oral doses may induce "sterile bowel" syndrome. Polymyxins are safe for topical use (no appreciable side effects) and are found in many topical prescription and over-the-counter preparations to control mainly gram-negative bacterial skin infections. Bacitracin is another large polypeptide antibiotic that is used safely in many topical preparations but is toxic if administered systemically. The protective barrier offered by the stratum corneum allows large charged drugs such as polymyxins and bacitracin to be safely used in topical formulations.

Nitrofurans—mainly nitrofurazone (5-nitro-2-furaldehyde semicarbazone) and furazolidone (*N*-(5-nitro-2-furfurylidene)-3-amino-2-oxazolidone)—are a class of broad-spectrum antimicrobials that presumably inhibit the conversion of pyruvate to acetyl coenzyme A by blocking oxidative decarboxylation at this step of energy metabolism. Nitrofurans can be bactericidal or bacteriostatic, depending on the concentration used. Used topically, nitrofurans are not significantly absorbed through the intact skin unless formulated in an oil, ointment, or organic solvent base, making them ideal for treating superficial bacterial infections. Nitrofurazone has been reported to have no effect on wound contraction and reepithelialization when topically applied to open wounds, but other studies show that nitrofurazone slows this process by as much as 30% in pigs, and yet other studies show a more efficient wound-healing process (St. Omer 1978). In spite of this controversy, the nitrofurans, in particular nitrofurazone, remain a popular, safe, and effective class of antibiotic to topically prevent or treat bacterial skin infections in a variety of species.

Iodine is one of the oldest and most widely used topical antimicrobials. Iodine is bactericidal, sporicidal, fungicidal, viricidal, and protozoacidal. Elemental iodine is only slightly soluble in water, resulting in the use of other vehicles to increase its solubility. Tincture of iodine contains 2% iodine and 2.4% sodium iodide diluted in 50% ethanol; Lugol's solution contains 5% iodine and 10% potassium iodide in water. It should be noted that the highest concentration of elemental iodine (the "active" form) that can be obtained in a water base is 0.15%. Addition of sodium iodide or potassium iodide to water containing elemental iodine causes the formation of I^{3-}, which functions as a reservoir for I^2. Iodines are used to treat a variety of skin infections, are highly efficacious, and have a very low toxicity to animal skin. Disadvantages include staining of the skin and clothing that iodine comes in contact with and some pain when iodine comes in contact with raw and abraded skin surfaces (tincture more so than aqueous). In order to circumvent these disadvantages and preserve the high efficacy and safety of iodine, povidone-iodine was formulated.

Povidone-iodine is elemental iodine coupled with a polyvinylpyrrolidone molecule. This particular complex serves as a sustained-release form for elemental iodine while simultaneously preventing staining of the skin and clothing it may come in contact with. A 10% povidone-iodine solution contains approximately 1% "available" or total iodine, with free iodine (dissociated from the povidone complex) being 0.001%. As the povidone-iodine solution is diluted, more free iodine dissociates from the polyvinylpyrrolidone molecules, increasing the free iodine content in the solution. Bactericidal activity tends to increase as the dilution increases. Many povidone-iodine preparations are commercially available for preventing and treating topical microbial infections, wounds, abscesses, and other skin injuries. Povidone-iodine solutions are also used to prepare skin prior to surgical procedures. A potential for systemic absorption exists (*see* Chap. 39).

Chlorhexidine is another commonly utilized topical antimicrobial used in veterinary dermatology. Chlorhexidine is highly bactericidal, is not virucidal, and is relatively unaffected by organic debris (blood, pus, necrotic tissue, etc). Chlorhexidine gluconate has a sustained residual activity; when applied to the surface of the skin, it binds to the protein portion of the stratum corneum and cannot be removed with ethanol treatment. Systemic absorption and toxicity of chlorhexidine are minimal, and it can be used as an effective antimicrobial to treat skin wounds and to flush abscesses, and as a presurgical antiseptic scrub. It is in shampoos for treating bacterial pyodermas.

Thiostrepton is an antibiotic produced by a strain of *Streptomyces aureus.* A polypeptide antibiotic, thiostrepton is not absorbed from the gastrointestinal tract and is used in some topical antibiotic preparations. It has activity against both gram-positive and gram-negative bacteria and is usually found in combination with another antibiotic, an antifungal, and a glucocorticosteroid in an ointment or cream formulation.

Antifungal Agents. Fungal infections in domestic animals are commonly encountered in veterinary dermatology. The systemic treatment of fungal infections is discussed in greater detail in Chap. 46. Cutaneous mycotic infections, like bacterial infections, can be treated by both topical and systemic routes, depending on the location and severity of the lesions. Common antifungal drugs used topically include benzalkonium chloride, zinc, miconazole, copper naphthanate, povidone-iodine, nystatin, tolnaftate, clotrimazole, and thiabendazole. The 7th edition of this text should be consulted for an in-depth discussion of these drugs.

GLUCOCORTICOSTEROID USE IN DERMATOLOGY. Glucocorticosteroids are inflammatory modulators found in many topical skin preparations, either alone or in combination with antibiotics or antifungal preparations. Glucocorticosteroids have definite indications for treating many dermatologic disorders in domestic animals. Glucocorticosteroids are indicated for the treatment of many allergic dermatoses, notably allergies ("fleabite" dermatitis, food allergies), contact dermatitis, autoimmune diseases manifesting themselves with cutaneous lesions (pemphigus, pemphigoid, lupus erythematosus, eosinophilic granuloma complex), and pyotraumatic dermatitis ("hot-spots").

Glucocorticosteroids have functions other than controlling inflammation and inducing immunosuppression. Many skin diseases have neutrophil infiltration in the dermis and/or epidermis. Glucocorticosteroids have a marked ability to stabilize lysosomal membranes within neutrophils, thereby inhibiting the release of enzymes that result in dermatitis. Fibroblast inhibition also occurs, which may retard healing of the skin if high doses are used frequently and for extended periods of time. Many endogenously produced compounds, such as histamine (and its metabolite *N*-methyl histamine) and complement, have their production inhibited in the presence of glucocorticosteroids. In addition, phospholipase A_2, which is responsible for liberating arachidonic acid from epidermal cells and vascular endothelial cells, is also blocked, resulting in decreased production of the many prostaglandins and leukotrienes discussed previously. Prolonged use in humans results in thinning of the viable epidermal layer. Use of these immunosuppressive compounds may also potentiate secondary bacterial infections. Glucocorticosteroids often increase thirst and appetite and have other systemic side effects. It is beyond the scope of this chapter to review all the physiologic and biochemical effects of all the glucocorticosteroids available to the veterinarian (see Chap. 33). However, because glucocorticosteroids have effects on other body systems when being used to treat skin diseases, we offer some general guidelines here for their use in dermatology:

1. *Be sure of the diagnosis.* Glucocorticosteroids are generally used to relieve the symptom of pruritus. This symptom has an underlying cause, and it is important to make the effort to determine it. Not performing the routine measures to determine the underlying cause of pruritus may lead to more serious systemic side effects.
2. *Use the least amount of steroid to achieve the clinical effect.* The dose of steroid cannot be specified for each skin disease. Rather, the dose of steroid must be adjusted for the individual animal, taking into account individual biological variability, the severity of the disease, the overall improvement in the clinical condition of the animal when treated, and the intensity of side effects observed at that dose of steroid. Steroid use above the clinical effect threshold will not improve the animal's overall condition or speed the recovery but may increase the chances of deleterious side effects (i.e., Cushing's disease). This caveat refers not only to the orally administered glucocorticosteroids but also to

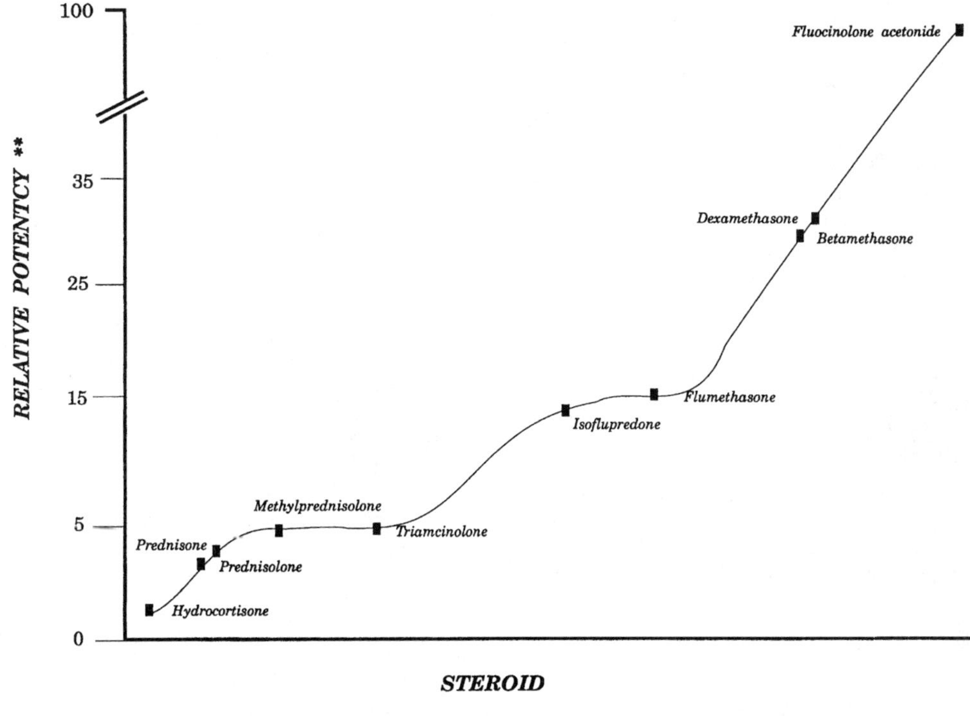

FIG. 53.6—Comparison of the relative potencies of some glucocorticosteroids (compared with hydrocortisone) used in veterinary dermatology.

the topically administered glucocorticosteroids. Glucocorticosteroids applied topically can be absorbed through damaged, as well as normal, skin.

3. *Use the least potent steroid to achieve the clinical effect.* As shown in Fig. 53.6, there is a wide range of potency among the topical glucocorticosteroids, ranging from hydrocortisone (which has the same potency as the endogenously produced cortisol) to the extremely potent fluocinolone acetonide (100 times the potency of hydrocortisone). The more potent glucocorticosteroids should be reserved for the more severe cases of skin disease requiring steroid therapy, while milder cases should be treated with the less potent forms. The least amount as well as the least potent topical steroid should be used to control the symptoms of the disease being treated.

4. *Choose the route of steroid administration according to the type and severity of the lesion being treated.* The route of administration will depend greatly on the skin disease being treated, temperament of the animal, owner compliance, severity of the lesion(s), and whether the lesions are focal or multifocal. Oral or injectable steroid therapies are generally used when lesions are multifocal and/or involve the deeper layers of skin, cover large areas of skin (hot-spots), or involve moderate to severe pruritus, or when immunosuppression is indicated (pemphigus, lupus, eosinophilic granulomas, indolent ulcers, etc.). Topical therapy alone is usually efficacious when a few superficial lesions are present, if mild pruritus is present, and if an anti-inflammatory effect is required.

Antihistamines and nonsteroidal anti-inflammatory drugs have also been used to treat pruritic conditions. Chapters 19–22 of this text should be consulted for further details.

PESTICIDES. Pesticides are widely used in agriculture and home gardening and in the control of many internal and external parasites in both humans and domestic animals. Pesticide use today is important for three reasons: (1) the toxicity that they may induce in the host animal, (2) residues that may accumulate in the food animal and then later be consumed by humans, and (3) environmental effects. All three areas have a formidable literature data base. Chapter 50 of this text should be consulted for a detailed discussion of these agents.

Most pesticides, like many of the drugs and vehicles discussed previously in this chapter, are able to permeate the skin. The skin is the primary route of exposure for pesticides, followed closely by inhalation and ingestion. In fact, the skin is often used as a route for systemic delivery of many veterinary products (Defend, Spot-On, ProSpot), which implies that veterinary medicine is actually far ahead of human medicine in the transdermal drug delivery area. Percutaneous absorption of these compounds, therefore, is an important consideration given the seriousness of side effects that can occur. The topic of pesticide use for veterinary application was recently reviewed (Riviere and Baynes 1998). Finally, in food-producing animals, attention must be paid to the potential of producing residues in their edible products after topical treatment (Baynes et al. 1997).

REFERENCES

Amakiri, S. F. 1973. A comparative study of the thickness of the stratum corneum in Nigerian breeds of cattle. Br Vet J 129:277–281.

Aungst, B. J., Blake, J. A., and Hussain, M. A. 1990. Contributions of drug solubilization, partitioning, barrier disruption, and solvent permeation to the enhancement of skin permeation of various compounds with fatty acids and amines. Pharm Res 7(7):712–718.

Barry, B. W. 1991. Modern methods of promoting drug absorption through the skin. Molecular Aspects Med 12:195–241.

Baynes, R. E., Craigmill, A. L., and Riviere, J. E. 1997. Residue avoidance after topical application of veterinary drugs and parasiticides. J Am Vet Med Assoc 210:1288–1289.

Baynes, R. E., and Riviere, J. E. 1998. Influence of inert ingredients in pesticide formulations on dermal absorption of carbaryl. Am J Vet Res 59:168–175.

Bennett, K., ed. 1995. Compendium of Veterinary Products. 3rd ed. Port Huron, Mich.: North American Compendiums and Adrian J. Bayley.

Blackburn, P. S. 1965. The hair of cattle, horse, dog and cat. In A. J. Rook and G. S. Walton, eds., Comparative Physiology and Pathology of the Skin, pp. 201–210. Oxford: Blackwell.

Blank, I. H., Moloney, J., Emslie, A. G., and Simon, I. 1984. The diffusion of water across the stratum corneum as a function of its water content. J Invest Dermatol 82(2):188–194.

Block, L. H. 1985. Medicated applications. In A. R. Gennara, ed., Remington's Pharmaceutical Sciences, 17th ed., pp. 1567–1584. Easton, PA: Mack Publishing.

Catanzaro, J. M., and Smith, J. G. 1991. Propylene glycol dermatitis. J Am Acad Dermatol 24:90–95.

Chang, S. K., and Riviere, J. E. 1993. Effect of humidity and occlusion on the percutaneous absorption of parathion in vitro. Pharm Res 10(1):152–155.

deMare, S., Calis, N., den Hartog, G., van Erp, P. E. J., and van de Kerkhof, P. C. M. 1988. The relevance of salicylic acid in the treatment of plaque psoriasis with dithranol creams. Skin Pharmacol 1:259–264.

Dunn, M. J., and Hood, V. L. 1977. Prostaglandins and the kidney. Am J Physiol 233(3):F169–F184.

Elias, P. M. 1983. Epidermal lipids, barrier functions and desquamation. J Invest Dermatol 80:44–47.

———. 1992. Role of lipids in barrier function of the skin. In Hasan Mukhtar, ed., Pharmacology of the Skin, pp. 29–40. Boca Raton, FL: CRC Press.

Elias, P. M., and Feingold, K. R. 1992. Lipids and the epidermal water barrier: metabolism, regulation, and pathophysiology. In H. I. Maibach, editor in chief, Seminars in Dermatology 11(2):176–182. Philadelphia: W. B. Saunders.

Epstein, J. H. 1988. Photocarcinogenesis promotion studies with benzoyl peroxide (BPO) and croton oil. J Invest Dermotol 91:114–116.

Evans, A. G., Madewell, B. R., and Stannard, A. A. 1985. A trial of 13-*cis*-retinoic acid for treatment of squamous cell carcinoma and preneoplastic lesions of the head in cats. Am J Vet Res 46(12):2553–2557.

Ford-Hutchinson, A. W. 1985. Leukotrienes: their formation and role as inflammatory mediators. Fed Proc 44(1):25–29.

Freinkel, R. K. 1983. Carbohydrate metabolism of the epidermis. In L. A. Goldsmith, ed., Biochemistry and Physiology of the Skin, pp. 328–337. New York: Oxford Univ Press.

Goldyne, M. E. 1986. Eicosanoids and human skin. Progress in Dermatol 20:1–8.

Griffiths, C. E. M., and Vorhees, J. J. 1994. Human in vivo pharmacology of topical retinoids. Arch Dermatol Res 287:53–60.

Hadgraft, J., Walters, K. A., and Guy, R. H. 1992. Epidermal lipids and topical drug delivery. In H. I. Maibach, editor in chief, Seminars in Dermatology 11(2):139–144. Philadelphia: W. B. Saunders.

Harvey, S. C. 1985a. Topical drugs. In A. R. Gennara, ed., Remington's Pharmaceutical Sciences, 17th ed., pp. 773–791. Easton, PA: Mack Publishing.

Harvey, S. C. 1985b. Antimicrobial drugs. In A. R. Gennara, ed., Remington's Pharmaceutical Sciences, 17th ed., pp. 1158–1233. Easton, PA: Mack Publishing.

Herschler, R. 1982. Proceedings of the symposium on dimethyl sulfoxide. 2. Chemistry and biologic effects. VMSAC 77:367–369.

Holzmann, H., Morsches, B., and Benes, P. 1979. The absorption of benzoyl peroxide from leg ulcers. Drug Res 29(11):1180–1183.

Idsen, I. 1975. Percutaneous absorption. J Pharm Sci 64(6):901–924.

Idson, B. 1983. Vehicle effects in percutaneous absorption. Drug Metabol Rev 14(2):207–222.

Ihrke, P. J. 1980a. Topical therapy—specific topical pharmacologic agents, dermatologic therapy (part II). J Comp Cont Ed 156(2):156–164.

———. 1980b. Topical therapy—uses, principles and vehicles, dermatologic therapy (part I). J Comp Cont Ed 156(1):28–35.

Jacob, S. 1982. Proceedings of the symposium on dimethyl sulfoxide. 1. Mode of action and biologic effects. VMSAC 77:365–366.

Jacob, S. W., Herschler, R. J., and Rosenbaum, E. E. 1965. Dimethyl sulfoxide (DMSO): laboratory and clinical evaluation. JAVMA 147(12):1350–1359.

Karanian, J. W., Stojanov, M., and Salem, N. 1985. Effect of ethanol on prostacyclin and thromboxane A_2 synthesis in rat aortic rings in vitro. Prostaglandins, Leukotrienes, and Medicine 20(2):175–186.

Knowles, R. 1982. Proceedings of the symposium on dimethyl sulfoxide. 3. Clinical applications in veterinary medicine. VMSAC 77:369–373.

Kozlowski, G. P., and Calhoun, M. L. 1969. Microscopic anatomy of the integument of sheep. Am J Vet Res 30(8):1267–1279.

Kunkle, G. A. 1986. Progestagens in dermatology. In R. W. Kirk, ed., Current Veterinary Therapy IX: Small Animal Practice, pp. 601–605. Philadelphia: W. B. Saunders.

Kurihara-Bergstrom, T., Flynn, G. L., and Higuchi, W. I. 1986. Physiochemical study of percutaneous absorption enhancement by dimethyl sulfoxide: kinetic and thermodynamic determinants of dimethyl sulfoxide mediated mass transfer of alkanols. J Pharm Sci 75(5):479–486.

———. 1987. Physicochemical study of percutaneous absorption enhancement by dimethylsulfoxide: dimethyl sulfoxide mediation of vidarabine (ara-A) permeation of hairless mouse skin. J Invest Dermatol 89:274–280.

Kwochka, K. W. 1989. Retinoids in dermatology. In R. W. Kirk, ed., Current Veterinary Therapy X: Small Animal Practice, pp. 553–560. Philadelphia: W. B. Saunders.

Landolfi, R., and Steiner, M. 1984. Ethanol raises prostacyclin in vivo and in vitro. Blood 64(3):679–682.

Lloyd, D. H., Amakiri, S. F., and Jenkinson, D. M. 1979a. Structure of the sheep epidermis. Res Vet Sci 26:180–182.

Lloyd, D. H., Dick, W. D. B., and Jenkinson, D. M. 1979b. Structure of the epidermis in Ayrshire bullocks. Res Vet Sci 26:172–179.

Malkinson, F. D. 1958. The percutaneous absorption of carbon-14 labeled steroids by use of the gas-flow cell. J Invest Dermatol 31.

Miller, W. H. 1986. Antiseborrheic agents in dermatology. In R. W. Kirk, ed., Current Veterinary Therapy IX: Small Animal Practice, pp. 596–601. Philadelphia: W. B. Saunders.

Miller, W. H., Scott, D. W., and Wellington, J. R. 1992. Nonsteroidal management of canine pruritus with amitriptyline. Cornell Vet 82:53–57.

Montagna, W. 1967. Comparative anatomy and physiology of the skin. Arch Dermatol 96:357–363.

Monteiro-Riviere, N. A. 1991. Comparative anatomy, physiology, and biochemistry of mammalian skin. In D. W. Hobson, ed., Dermal and Ocular Toxicology Fundamentals and Methods. Boca Raton, FL: CRC Press.

Monteiro-Riviere, N. A., Bristol, D. G., Manning, T. O., Rogers, R. A., and Riviere, J. E. 1990. Interspecies and interregional analysis of the comparative histologic thickness and laser doppler blood flow measurements at five cutaneous sites in nine species. J Invest Dermatol 95(5):582–586.

Monteiro-Riviere, N. A., Inman, A. O., Riviere, J. E., McNeill, S. C., and Francoeur, M. L. 1993a. Topical penetration of piroxicam is dependent on the distribution of the local cutaneous vasculature. Pharm Res 10:1326–1331.

Monteiro-Riviere, N. A., Stinson, A. W., and Calhoun, H. L. 1993b. Integument. In H. Dieter Dellman, ed., Textbook of Veterinary Histology. Philadelphia: Lea & Febiger.

Monteiro-Riviere, N. A., and Stromberg, M. W. 1985. Ultrastructure of the integument of the domestic pig (*Sus scrofa*) from one through fourteen weeks of age. Anat Histol Embryol 14:97–115.

Mukhtar, H. 1992. Cutaneous cytochrome P-450. In H. Mukhtar, ed., Pharmacology of the Skin, pp. 139–150. Boca Raton, FL: CRC Press.

Nacht, S., Yeung, D., Beasley, H. N., and Anjo, M. D. 1981. Benzoyl peroxide: percutaneous penetration and metabolic disposition. J Am Acad Dermatol 4:31–37.

Nairn, J. G. 1985. Solutions, emulsions, suspensions and extractives. In A. R. Gennara, ed., Remington's Pharmaceutical Sciences, 17th ed., pp. 1492–1517. Easton, PA: Mack Publishing.

Nook, T. H. 1987. In vivo measurement of the keratolytic effect of salicylic acid in three ointment formulations. Br J Dermatol 117:243–245.

Paulissen, M., Peereboom-Stegeman, C. P., and Van de Kerkhof, P. 1990. An ultrastructural study of transcutaneous migration of polymorphonuclear leukocytes following application of leukotriene B_4. Skin Pharmacol 3:236–247.

Pavletic, M. M. 1991. Anatomy and circulation of canine skin. Microsurgery 12:103–112.

Pitman, I. H., and Rostas, S. J. 1981. Topical drug delivery to cattle and sheep. J Pharm Sci 70(11):1181–1193.

Potts, R. O., Bommannan, D. B., and Guy, R. H. 1992. Percutaneous absorption. In H. Mukhtar, ed., Pharmacology of the Skin, pp. 13–28. Boca Raton, FL: CRC Press.

Potts, R. O., and Francoeur, M. L. 1992. Physical methods for studying stratum corneum lipids. In H. I. Maibach, editor in chief, Seminars in Dermatology 11(2):129–138. Philadelphia: W. B. Saunders.

Potts, R. O., and Guy, R. H. 1995. A predictive algorithm for skin permeability: The effects of molecular size and hydrogen bond activity. Pharmaceutical Res 12:1628–1633.

Power, H. T., and Ihrke, P. J. 1990. Synthetic retinoids in veterinary dermatology. Vet Clinics No Am: Small Anim Pract 20(6):1525–1539.

Raza, H., Agarwal, R., and Mukhtar, H. 1992. Cutaneous glutathione-s-transferase. In H. Mukhtar, ed., Pharmacology of the Skin, pp. 131–138. Boca Raton, Fla: CRC Press.

Rippie, E. G. 1985. Powders. In A. R. Gennara, ed., Remington's Pharmaceutical Sciences, 17th ed., pp. 1585–1602. Easton, PA: Mack Publishing.

Riviere, J. E. 1992. Dermal absorption and metabolism of xenobiotics in food-producing animals. In D. H. Hutson et al., eds., Xenobiotics and Food-Producing Animals: Metabolism and Residues, pp. 88–97. American Chemical Society Symposium Series 503. Washington, DC.

Riviere, J. E., and Baynes, R. E. 1998. Dermal absorption and toxicity assessment. In M. S. Roberts and K. Walters, eds., Dermal Absorption and Toxicity Assessment, pp. 625–645. New York: Marcel Dekker.

Riviere, J. E., and Chang, S. K. 1992. Transdermal penetration and metabolism of organophosphate insecticides. In J. E. Chambers and P. E. Levi, eds., Organophosphates: Chemistry, Fate, and Effects, pp. 241–253. New York: Academic Press.

Riviere, J. E., and Heit, M. 1997. Electrically-assisted transdermal drug delivery. Pharmaceutical Res. 14: 691–701.

Riviere, J. E., Monteiro-Riviere, N. A., Rogers, R. A., Bommannan, D., Tamada, J., and Potts, R. O. 1995. Pulsatile transdermal delivery of LHRH using electroporation. J Controlled Release 36:229–233.

Riviere, J. E., and Williams, P. L. 1992. Pharmacokinetic implications of changing blood flow to the skin. J Pharm Sci 81:601–602.

Roberts, M. S., and Horlock, E. 1978. Effect of repeated skin application on percutaneous absorption of salicylic acid. J Pharm Sci 67(12):1685–1687.

Ruzicka, T. 1990. Arachidonic acid metabolism in normal skin. In Thomas Ruzicka, ed., Eicosanoids and the Skin, pp. 23–31. Boca Raton, FL: CRC Press.

Sar, M., and Calhoun, M. L. 1966. Microscopic anatomy of the integument of the common American goat. Am J Vet Res 27:444–456.

Schweizer, J., Loehrke, H., Edler, L., and Goerttler, K. 1987. Benzoyl peroxide promotes the formation of melanotic tumors in the skin of 7,12-dimethylbenz[a]anthracene initiated Syrian golden hamsters. Carcinogenesis 8:479–482.

Shanley, K. J. 1990. The seborrheic disease complex: an approach to underlying causes and therapies. Vet Clin No Am: Small Anim Pract 20(6):1557–1577.

Sharata, H. H., and Burnette, R. R. 1988. Effect of dipolar aprotic permeability enhancers on the basal stratum corneum. J Pharm Sci 77(1):27–32.

Slaga, T. J., Klein-Szanto, A. J. P., Triplett, L. L., and Yotti, L. P. 1981. The tumor-promoting activity of benzoyl peroxide, a widely used free radical–generating compound. Science 213:1023–1025.

Sloan, K. B., Siver, K. G., and Koch, S. A. M. 1986. The effect of vehicle on the diffusion of salicylic acid through hairless mouse skin. J Pharm Sci 75(8):744–749.

Spannhake, E. M., Hyman, A. L., and Kadowitz, P. J. 1981. Bronchoactive metabolites of arachidonic acid and heir role in airway function. Prostaglandins 22(6):1013–1026.

Spoo, J. W., Rogers, R. A., and Monteiro-Riviere, N. A. 1993. Effects of formaldehyde, DMSO, benzoyl peroxide and sodium lauryl sulfate on isolated perfused porcine skin. Vitro Toxicol 5(4):251–260.

St. Omer, V. V. 1978. Efficacy and toxicity of furazolidone in veterinary medicine: a review. VMSAC, Sept.

Strickland, J. H., and Calhoun, M. L. 1963. The integumentary system of the cat. Am J Vet Res 24:1018–1029.

Surber, C., Wilhelm, K. P., Maibach, H. I., Hall, L. L., and Guy, R. H. 1990a. Partitioning of chemicals into human stratum corneum: implications for risk assessment following dermal exposure. Fund Appl Toxicol 15:99–107.

Surber, C., Wilhelm, K. P., Maibach, H. I., Hori, M., and Guy, R. H. 1990b. Optimization of topical therapy: partitioning of drugs into stratum corneum. Pharm Res 7(12):1320–1324.

Swartzendruber, D. C. 1992. Studies of epidermal lipids using electron microscopy. In H. I. Maibach, editor in chief, Seminars in Dermatology 11(2):157–161. Philadelphia: W. B. Saunders.

Swinyard, E. A. 1985. Local anesthetics. In A. R. Gennara, ed., Remington's Pharmaceutical Sciences, 17th ed., pp. 1048–1058. Easton, PA: Mack Publishing.

Swinyard, E. A. and Lowenthal, W. 1985. In A. R. Gennara, ed., Remington's Pharmaceutical Sciences, 17th ed., pp. 1278–1320. Easton, PA: Mack Publishing.

Talukdar, A. H., Calhoun, M. L., and Stinson, A. W. 1972. Microscopic anatomy of the skin of the horse. Am J Vet Res 33(12):2365–2390.

Tragear, R. T. 1966. The permeability of skin to albumin, dextrans, and polyvinyl pyrrolidone. J Invest Dermatol 46:24–27.

Van de Kerkhof, P., Peereboom-Stegeman, J., and Boeijen, J. 1991. An ultrastructural study of the response of normal skin to epicutaneous application of leukotriene B_4. J Dermatol 18:271–276.

Weirich, E. G. 1975. Dermatopharmacology of salicylic acid. I. Range of dermatotherapeutic effects of salicylic acid. Dermatologica 151:268–273.

Werner, A. H., and Power, H. T. 1994. Retinoids in veterinary dermatology. Clinics in Dermatology 12:579–586.

Wertz, P. W. 1992. Epidermal lipids. In H. I. Maibach, editor in chief, Seminars in Dermatology 11(2):106–113. Philadelphia: W. B. Saunders.

54

DRUGS AFFECTING THE RESPIRATORY SYSTEM

DAWN M. BOOTHE

Normal Respiratory Physiology
Airway Caliber Changes
Respiratory Defense Mechanisms
Pathogenesis of Inflammatory Respiratory Diseases
Bronchodilators and Anti-inflammatories
β-Receptor Agonists
Methylxanthine Derivatives
Anticholinergics
Mast Cell Stabilizers
Other Anti-inflammatory Drugs
Antitussives
Centrally Active Antitussives
Peripheral Bronchodilators
Mucokinetics
***N*-Acetyl-L-Cysteine**
Expectorants
Iodide Preparations
Stimulant Expectorants
Decongestants

NORMAL RESPIRATORY PHYSIOLOGY

Airway Caliber Changes. Nervous innervation to the smooth muscle of the respiratory tract is complex. The parasympathetic system provides the primary efferent innervation, with acetylcholine as the primary neurotransmitter (Moses and Spaulding 1985; Slonim and Hamilton 1987). These fibers are responsible for the baseline tone of mild bronchoconstriction which characterizes the normal respiratory tract. The sympathetic system balances these effects by stimulating through β_2 receptors to induce bronchodilation (Scott et al. 1991; Gustin et al. 1989; Chand and Deroth 1979). In contrast, α-adrenergic stimulation can contribute to bronchoconstriction (Moise and Spaulding 1981; Slonim and Hamilton 1987; Gustin et al. 1989). A third, largely understood nervous system, referred to as the nonadrenergic-noncholinergic (NANC) system, or purinergic system, also innervates bronchial smooth muscle (Inque et al. 1989; Moses and Spaulding 1985). This system mediates bronchodilation via vagal stimulation. The afferent fibers of this system are probably irritant receptors, and although the neurotransmitter has not yet been conclusively identified, vasoactive intestinal peptide has been implicated in the cat (Altiere and Diamond 1984; Altiere et al. 1984). Malfunction of this system has been associated with bronchial hyperreactivity, which often characterizes asthma (Inque et al. 1989).

The intracellular mechanisms which transmit signals from the nervous system to smooth muscle depend, in part, upon changes in the intracellular concentration of cyclic adenosine monophosphate (cAMP) and cyclic guanosine monophosphate (cGMP) (Fig. 54.1). The effects of these two secondary messengers are reciprocal: increased intracellular concentrations of one are associated with decreased concentrations of the other. Cyclic AMP is decreased by α-adrenergic stimulation and increased by β_2-receptor stimulation (Scott et al. 1991). In contrast, cGMP is increased by stimulation of muscarinic (cholinergic) and, indirectly, histaminergic receptors (Fig. 54.1). The relative sensitivity of bronchial smooth muscle to histamine- and acetylcholine-induced bronchoconstriction varies with the location and species (Chand and Deroth 1979; Derksen et al. 1985; Downes et al. 1986). Peripheral airways in dogs are more susceptible than those in cats to acetylcholine. Cat airways, in general, are more sensitive to acetylcholine than to histamine (Colebatch et al. 1966). Airways of horses suffering from chronic obstructive pulmonary disease (COPD) are hyperreactive to histamine (Derksen et al. 1985) and acetylcholine (Chand and Deroth 1979). Smooth muscle receptors are also susceptible to stimulation by a variety of chemical mediators (Fig. 54.1) which may also modulate cAMP and cGMP (Townley et al. 1989; Soler et al. 1990; Gray et al. 1989).

Control of bronchial smooth muscle tone is very complex and depends upon input from sensory receptors. At least five types of sensory receptors have been identified in cat lungs, all of which can be classified as either irritant (mechanoreceptor), stretch, or J receptors (Inque et al. 1989). All appear to be innervated by the parasympathetic system. Irritant receptors, located beneath the respiratory epithelium, occur in the upper airways (Slonim and Hamilton 1987) and, in cats, as far peripherally as the alveoli (Moses and Spaulding 1985). Physical, mechanical, or chemical stimulation of these receptors results in tachypnea, bronchoconstriction, and/or cough. Airflow velocity appears to be the most critical factor determining stimulation of irritant receptors in the upper airways (Moses and Spaulding 1985). Airway constriction sufficient to cause air-

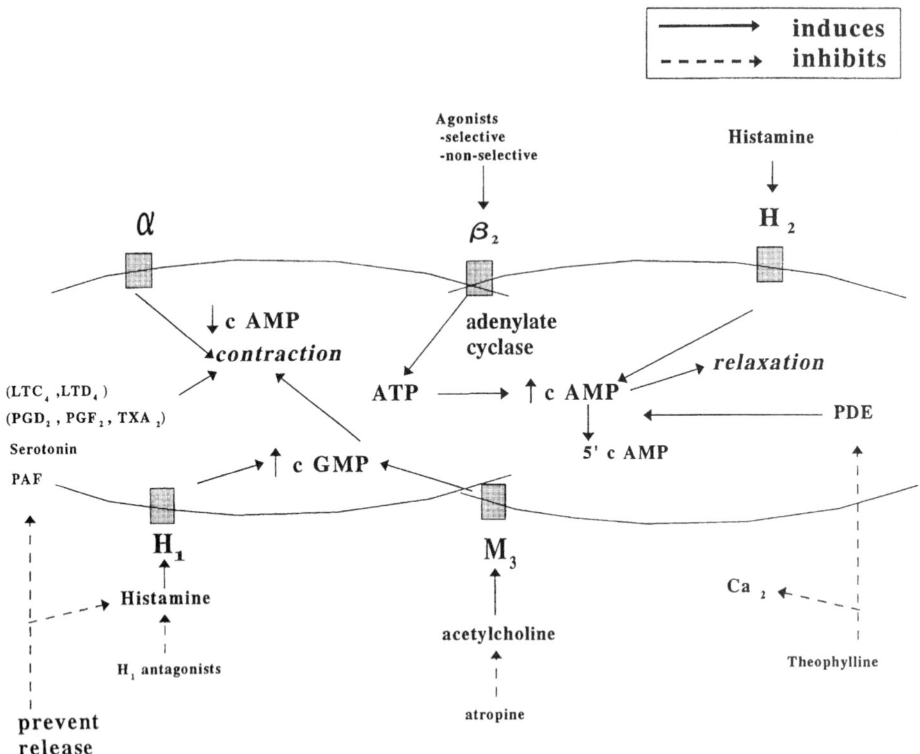

FIG. 54.1—Factors determining bronchial smooth muscle tone. Reciprocal changes in cyclic adenosine monophosphate (cAMP) and cyclic guanosine monophosphate (cGMP) determine muscle tone. Contraction occurs when cAMP levels are decreased by events such as α-adrenergic stimulation or when cGMP levels increase in response to muscarinic-receptor (M_3) stimulation by acetylcholine or H_1-receptor stimulation by histamine. Calcium (Ca^{++}) and several mediators can also induce bronchoconstriction. Increased cAMP levels induced by β_2-adrenergic or histamine-receptor (H_2) stimulation will counteract muscle contraction. Inhibition of phosphodiesterases (PDEs) will also increase cAMP levels. Although the effects of most inflammatory mediators are best counteracted by preventing their release (Fig. 54.3), several drugs can be used to antagonize smooth muscle contraction regardless of the etiology. (LT = leukotriene; PG = prostaglandin; TXA = thromboxane; PAF = platelet-activating factor; PDE = phosphodiesterases.) (Reproduced, with permission, from *Sheba Symposium Proceedings,* 1990, Veterinary Learning Systems.)

flow velocity to exceed a specific threshold results in a vagally mediated cough reflex and bronchoconstriction. Airways can also be occluded by mucus and edema or by chemical mediators released during upper-airway infections (Inque et al. 1989).

Respiratory Defense Mechanisms. In addition to the cough and sneeze reflexes, two other systems provide the major defense of the respiratory tract against invading organisms or foreign materials: the mucociliary apparatus and the respiratory mononuclear phagocyte system (MPS) (Slonim and Hamilton 1987). The mucociliary apparatus is the first major defense and consists of the ciliary lining of the tracheobronchial tree and the fluid blanket surrounding the cilia. Nervous innervation to the cilia has not yet been identified. Although ciliary activity increases with β-adrenergic stimulation, this may simply reflect the sequelae of β-adrenergic stimulation on respiratory secretions (Blair and Woods 1969). Two types of secretions form the fluid blanket of the respiratory tract. The cilia must be surrounded by a low-viscosity, watery medium to maintain their rhythmic beat. A more mucoid layer lies on top of the cilia. The synchronous motion of the cilia causes the cephalad movement of the mucus layer and any trapped materials. Changes in the viscoelastic properties of mucus such that it becomes either too watery or too rigid will result in mucus transport that is less than optimal (Slonim and Hamilton 1987). Mucus released by goblet cells results from direct irritation (Slonim and Hamilton 1987) and is not amenable to pharmacologic manipulation. Surface goblet cells, which are uniquely prominent in feline bronchioles (Gallagher et al. 1975), increase in number with chronic disease. Submucosal glands of the bronchi secrete both a serous and a mucoid fluid. The secretions tend to be more fluid than those of the goblet cells, but the degree varies with the stimulus. The nor-

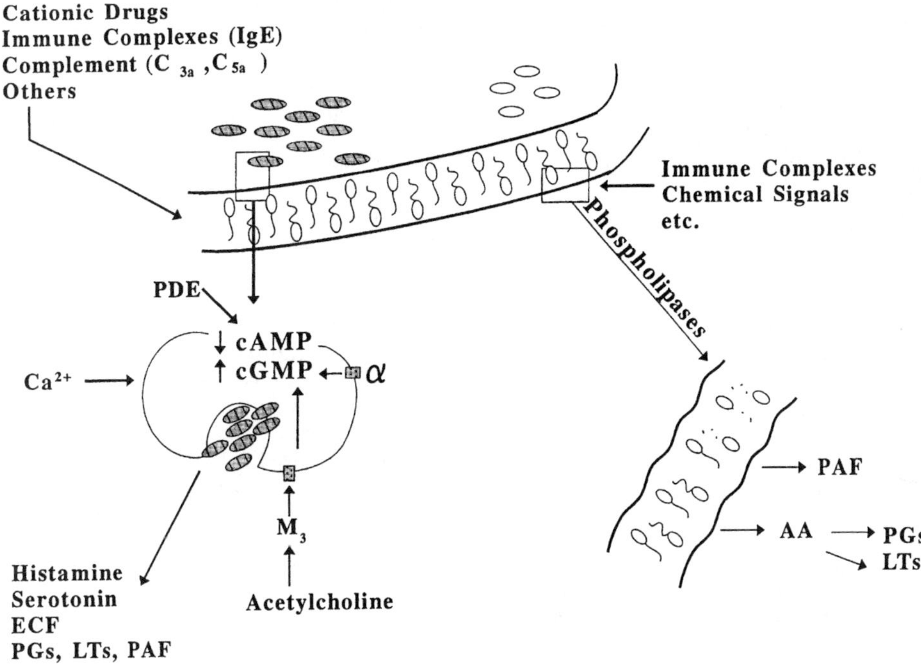

FIG. 54.2—The formation of mediators important in the pathogenesis of respiratory disease. Leukocytes and other cells release arachidonic acid (AA) metabolites and platelet-activating factor (PAF) following activation of phospholipases by a variety of stimuli. Mast cell degranulation induced by both immune and nonimmune stimuli is also accompanied by AA metabolism as well as the release of preformed mediators which are stored in the granules. Intracellular mechanisms that induce mast cell degranulation include increased calcium (Ca^{++}), increased cyclic guanosine monophosphate (cGMP) mediated by muscarinic (M_3) receptors, or decreased cyclic adenosine monophosphate (cAMP) mediated by α-adrenergic receptor stimulation. (PDE = phosphodiesterases; PGs = prostaglandins; LTs = leukotrienes; ECF = eosinophil chemotactic factor.) (Reproduced, with permission, from *Sheba Symposium Proceedings,* 1990, Veterinary Learning Systems.)

mal composition of the combined secretions of the tracheobronchial tree is 95% water, 2% glycoprotein, 1% carbohydrate, and less than 1% lipid (Slonim and Hamilton 1987). Glycoproteins increase the viscosity of the secretions, providing protection and lubrication. Infection and chronic inflammatory diseases can have a profound effect on respiratory secretions. The glycoprotein component tends to be replaced by degradative products of inflammation such as deoxyribonucleic acid. Goblet cell numbers increase, with a subsequent increase in the viscosity of respiration secretion. Parasympathetic, cholinergic stimulation increases mucus secretion, whereas β-adrenergic stimulation causes secretion of both mucus and electrolytes and water (Blair and Woods 1969; Slonim and Hamilton 1987).

The second major component of the pulmonary defense system is the respiratory MPS. In cats, calves, pigs, sheep, and goats, this includes both alveolar macrophages and the pulmonary intravascular macrophages (PIMs) (Winkler 1988). The PIMs are resident cells that are characterized by phagocytic properties and thus cause the release of inflammatory mediators. The clearance of blood-borne bacteria and particulate matter in these species is accomplished by PIMs rather than hepatic Kupffer cells and splenic macrophages as in most other species (Winkler 1988). The pharmacologic significance of the MPS reflects its role in inflammation (Fig. 54.2). A number of preformed (e.g., histamine and serotonin) and in situ (e.g., prostaglandins, leukotrienes, and platelet-activating factor) mediators are released by inflammation cells (Townley et al. 1989; Soler et al. 1990; Gray et al. 1989). Each is capable of inducing a variety of adverse effects which tend to decrease airway caliber size: edema, chemotaxis, increased mucus production, and bronchoconstriction (Table 54.1). The involvement of PIMs in both experimental and natural respiratory diseases of animals suggests that release of chemical mediators from these cells may be important in the pathogenesis of bronchial diseases.

PATHOGENESIS OF INFLAMMATORY RESPIRATORY DISEASES. The interaction of sensory receptors and mediators of bronchial tone is intricately balanced in the normal lung. However, a series of pathological disturbances severely disrupts the balance

TABLE 54.1—Effects of mediators of inflammation

Mediator	BC	BD	VD	VP	CT	MS
Histamine	+		+	+	+	+
Serotonin	+			+		
LTB_4					+	
LTC_4	+			+		+
LTD_4	+			+		+
PGD_2	+		+		+	+
PGE_2	+	+				
PGF_2	+					+
PAF	+			+	+	+

Note: LT = leukotriene, PG = prostaglandin, PAF = platelet-activating factor, BC = bronchoconstriction, BD = bronchodilation, VD = vasodilation, VP = vascular permeability, CT = chemotaxis, MS = mucus secretion.

in bronchial asthma. Asthma is a pathological state of the lungs characterized by marked bronchoconstriction and inflammation (Barnes 1989, 1988; Gold et al. 1977; Norn and Clementson 1988; Wanner and Rao 1980). Mediators released during inflammation are the major contributors to the pathogenesis (Table 54.1) (Barnes 1989; Barnes 1988; Barnes et al. 1988; Bauer 1986; Norn and Clementson 1988; Wanner and Rao 1980). Studies in several species have shown that stimulation of mast cells, macrophages, and other cells lining the airways causes changes in mucosal epithelial permeability. Airways are often characterized by hypersensitivity to selected mediators (e.g., histamine and cholinergic stimulants) (Chand and Deroth 1979; Derksen et al. 1985). As permeability increases, histamine and other inflammatory mediators are better able to reach and stimulate inflammatory cells located in the submucosa. The release of more mediators is associated with stimulation of afferent nerve endings in the mucosa and reflex cholinergic bronchoconstriction. Mediators also increase microvascular permeability, induce chemotaxis, and stimulate mucus secretion. The release of cytotoxic proteins and toxic oxygen radicals further damages the respiratory epithelium, and the bronchial tree becomes hypersensitive. Mediators can also inhibit mucociliary function (Norn and Clementson 1988). Airway obstruction in chronic disease reflects bronchoconstriction, bronchial wall edema, and accumulation of mucus and cells. As the disease progresses, airways eventually become plugged and ultimately collapse. Chronic inflammation leads to fibrosis, which contributes to the collapse, and air trapped within the alveoli can result in emphysema.

The syndrome of chronic bronchial disease is best treated by breaking the inflammatory cycle while immediately relieving bronchoconstriction. Thus, anti-inflammatories and bronchodilators are the cornerstone of therapy in many bronchial diseases. Other categories of drugs that are effective for the management of respiratory diseases, particularly in small animals, include antitussives, respiratory stimulants, and decongestants.

BRONCHODILATORS AND ANTI-INFLAMMATORIES. Because of a shared mechanism of action, most drugs that induce bronchodilation also reduce inflammation. Bronchodilators reverse airway smooth muscle contraction by increasing cAMP, decreasing cGMP, or decreasing calcium ion concentrations (Fig. 54.1). In addition, these drugs also decrease mucosal edema and are anti-inflammatory because they tend to prevent mediator release from inflammatory cells (Fig. 54.3). Rapidly acting bronchodilators include β-receptor agonists, methylxanthines, and cholinergic antagonists.

β-Receptor Agonists. Beta-receptor agonists are the most effective bronchodilators because they act as functional antagonists of airway constriction, regardless of the stimulus (Barnes 1988; Daemen et al. 1988; Papich 1986a; Reed and Kelly 1990). Large numbers of β_2 receptors are located on several cell types in the lung, including smooth muscle and inflammatory cells (Scott et al. 1991). The interaction between a β agonist and receptor causes a conformational change in the receptor and subsequent activation of adenylate cyclase on the inner cell membrane (Fig. 54.1). Adenylate cyclase converts adenosine triphosphate (ATP) to cAMP, which in turn serves as a second messenger for activation of specific protein kinases. The kinases activate the enzymes which cause relaxation of airway smooth muscle. Beta-receptor agonists are most effective in states of bronchoconstriction. In the inflammatory cell, increased cAMP inhibits mediator release (Fig. 54.2). Beta receptors also stimulate secretion of airway mucus, resulting in a less-viscous secretion and enhanced ciliary activity (Barnes 1989, 1988; Reed and Kelly 1990). Drugs that block β_2 receptors, such as propranolol, are contraindicated in animals with bronchial disease.

NONSELECTIVE β-RECEPTOR AGONISTS. The nonselective β-receptor agonists (i.e., capable of both β_1 and β_2 stimulation), such as epinephrine, ephedrine, and isoproterenol, are used for acute and chronic therapy of respiratory diseases. Epinephrine and isoproterenol can be administered parenterally to achieve rapid effects; drugs that can be given orally for chronic therapy include isoproterenol and ephedrine (Moise and Spaulding 1981). Both epinephrine and ephedrine cause α-adrenergic activity, which may cause vasoconstriction and systemic hypertension and contribute to airway constriction (Gustin et al. 1989). Nonselective β agonists may cause adverse cardiac effects due to β_1-receptor stimulation. Aerosolization reduces the adverse effects of nonselective β-adrenergic agonists by increasing β_2 selectivity, since only these β receptors appear to line the airways.

β-SELECTIVE AGONISTS. At appropriate doses, β_2-selective agonists are not generally associated with the undesirable effects of β_1-adrenergic stimulation. However, few of these drugs have been used in animals.

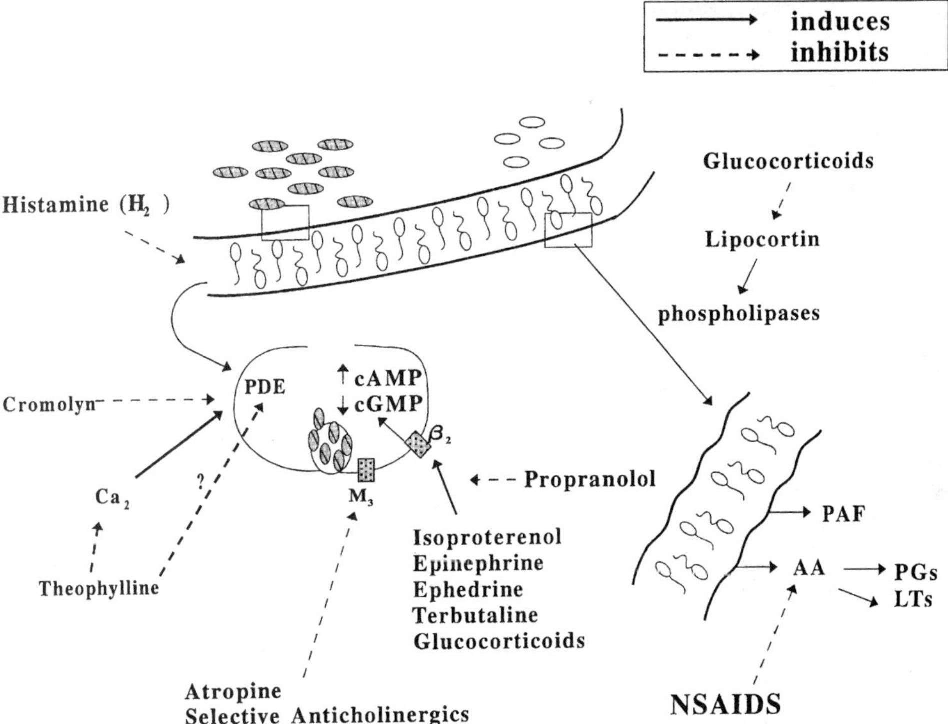

FIG. 54.3—Drugs used to prevent mediator release. Glucocorticoids are among the few drugs that can prevent activation of phospholipases (mediated by lipocortin) and thus release of AA metabolites and PAF. Inhibition of PG synthesis by nonsteroidal anti-inflammatories may prove beneficial. Mast cell degranulation can be prevented by stimulating β_2-adrenergic receptors, inhibiting calcium influx or PDE, or preventing muscarinic-receptor (M_3) stimulation. Drugs that block β_2-adrenergic receptors are contraindicated in most respiratory diseases. (Reproduced, with permission, from *Sheba Symposium Proceedings,* 1990, Veterinary Learning Systems.)

Metaproterenol, a derivative of isoproterenol, and its analog, terbutaline (Bauer 1986; Moise and Spaulding 1981; Papich 1986a), have been used safely in small animals. Rapid first-pass metabolism of both these drugs results in reduced systemic bioavailability following oral administration. Oral doses are thus higher than parenteral doses. Both drugs, but particularly metaproterenol, can cause β_1 side effects at high doses. Albuterol and isoetharine are examples of β_2-selective agonists which have been administered by aerosolization in small animals (Bauer 1986; Papich 1986a). Chronic use of β-adrenergic agonists can result in refractoriness due to down-regulation (i.e., reduced numbers) of β receptors. This problem is largely avoided in people by using proper doses (Reed and Kelly 1990).

Methylxanthine Derivatives

PHARMACOLOGIC EFFECTS. Theophylline has been the cornerstone of long-term bronchodilatory therapy in animals. Its mode of action was originally attributed to inhibition of phosphodiesterase (PDE) and increased concentrations of cAMP (Fig. 54.1) (Hendeles and Weinberger 1983). However, this mechanism is controversial since theophylline does not inhibit PDE at therapeutic concentrations. PDE exists as various isoenzymes located in different sites within the cell, some of which are inaccessible to drugs (Barnes 1989, 1988). Although theophylline may not affect total PDE, it may inhibit a specific isoenzyme, resulting in bronchodilation. Another possible mechanism is antagonism of the inhibitory neurotransmitter adenosine, which induces bronchoconstriction during hypoxia. However, the most likely mechanism by which theophylline induces bronchodilation is through interference of calcium mobilization (Barnes 1989, 1988).

As with β agonists, theophylline is equally effective in large and small airways. Theophylline has other effects in the respiratory system which are important to its clinical efficacy (Barnes 1989, 1988; Hendeles and Weinberger 1983). In addition to its bronchodilatory effects, it inhibits mast cell degranulation and thus mediator release (Mizus et al. 1985) (Fig. 54.2), increases mucociliary clearance, and prevents microvascular leakage (Short 1987). A major advantage of theophylline, compared to other bronchodilators, is increased strength of respiratory muscles and thus a decrease in the work associated with breathing (Hendeles and Weinberger 1983; Murciano et al. 1984; Viires et al. 1984). This may be important to animals with chronic bronchopulmonary disease.

DISPOSITION. Theophylline is one of the few drugs active in the respiratory tract whose disposition has been studied in animals. Because theophylline is not water soluble, it can only be given orally. Salt preparations of theophylline are available for either oral or parenteral administration. Dosing of the various salt preparations must be based on the amount of active theophylline (Table 54.2). Aminophylline, an ethylenediamine salt, is 80% theophylline; oxytriphylline is 65% theophylline; and glycinate and salicylate salts are only 50% theophylline. Regular aminophylline is well absorbed (bioavailability of at least 90%) following oral administration in both dogs and cats (Brumbaugh et al. 1990; Love et al. 1981). In dogs, peak plasma drug concentrations for the theophylline base (approximately 8 μg/mL following a dose of 9.4 mg/kg) occur 1.5 hours following oral administration (McKiernan et al. 1981). In horses, peak plasma theophylline concentrations following intragastric administration of aminophylline occur in 1.5 hours or less. Bioavailability is 100% (Errecalde et al. 1984; McKiernan et al. 1981).

Slow-release preparations have been studied in dogs (Koritz et al. 1986), cats (Koritz et al. 1986), and horses (Errecalde and Landoni 1992). The rate of oral absorption of slow-release products in dogs is apparently faster than in people. The extent of absorption varies with the preparation. Bioavailability of slow-release preparations varies from 30% (anhydrous theophylline 24-hour capsules; Theo-24, Searle and Co., San Juan, Puerto Rico) to 76% (anhydrous theophylline tablets; Theo-Dur, Key Pharmaceuticals, Miami). Oxytriphylline enteric-coated capsules (Choledyl-SA Tablets; Parke-Davis, Morris Plains, New York) and a 12-hour capsular anhydrous theophylline (Slobid Gyrocaps; William H. Rorer, Inc., Fort Washington) are approximately 60% bioavailable. The minimum effective level recommended in people (10 μg/mL) may not be reached by all slow-release products. Plasma drug concentrations during a 12-hour dosing interval vary, being almost 120% for the oxytriphylline product but only 48% for the anhydrous tablet (Koritz et al. 1986). Of the four preparations that have been studied in dogs, the anhydrous theophylline tablet (Theo-Dur) is preferred. Although the mean residence time (MRT) of the slow-release preparations was significantly longer, 1-2 hours, than that of the regular preparation in both dogs and horses, the clinical significance of this difference is questionable (Koritz et al. 1986; Errecalde and Landoni 1992). However, the longer release time may allow twice daily rather than thrice daily dosing. Two sustained-release theophylline products have been evaluated in the cat (Eiser et al. 1981). Once-daily administration has been recommended to achieve the human therapeutic level (Table 54.2). Based on a chronopharmacokinetic study of these sustained-release products, dosing in the evening rather than in the morning appears to be associated with better bioavailability and less peak plasma theophylline concentration fluctuation (Gallagher et al. 1975). A disadvantage of the slow-release products in small animals is the limited dose sizes available. The product cannot be divided for more accurate dosing without altering the kinetics of slow release.

Although it is not distributed to all body tissues, theophylline is characterized by a relatively large volume of distribution in dogs (0.7 L/kg) and cows (0.8 L/kg) and a smaller volume in cats (0.41 L/kg) (Koritz et al. 1986; McKiernan et al. 1981; Langston et al. 1989). Unlike in human beings, distribution of theophylline is not limited by binding to serum proteins in dogs or horses; serum protein binding is less than 12% (Munsiff et al. 1988a; Larsson et al. 1989). Volume of distribution is even larger in horses, ranging from 0.74 to 1 L/kg. The larger volume of distribution in horses has been attributed to binding to tissue or, more plausibly, decreased binding to plasma protein. The elimination half-life is subsequently longer in horses (15-18 hr) since clearance (0.61-0.86 mL/min/kg) is comparable to other species. A greater percentage of total drug present as free and therefore active drug in the plasma has been cited as the reason therapeutic concentrations are apparently lower in horses compared to humans (Errecalde et al. 1984; McKiernan et al. 1981; Larsson et al. 1989). Elimination of theophylline is not dose dependent in dose ranges of 3-15 mg/kg.

Theophylline is metabolized by demethylation in the liver. Theobromine may be an active metabolite in some species. Different rates of metabolism result in variable clearance rates and drug elimination half-lives among animals, and doses consequently vary (Langston et al. 1989; Larsson et al. 1989; Errecalde and Landoni 1992). For example, the elimination rate constant of theophylline is less in cats (0.089/hr) (McKiernan et al. 1983) than in dogs (0.12/hr), thus necessitating a smaller dose in cats (Koritz et al. 1986). Theophylline concentrations can be affected—most commonly increased—by a number of drugs, including fluorinated quinolones (Rybak et al. 1987) and cimetidine (Cremer et al. 1989).

ADVERSE REACTIONS. Theophylline is associated with a wide range of adverse effects, including central nervous excitation (manifested as restlessness, tremors, and seizures), gastrointestinal upset (nausea and vomiting), diuresis, and cardiac stimulation (e.g., tachycardia). Therefore, its intravenous use is limited to patients who have not responded to β-agonist therapy. Compared to the salt preparations, theophylline is more irritating to the gastrointestinal tract than aminophylline (Bauer 1986; Hendeles and Weinberger 1983; Papich 1986a). Rapid infusions or infusions of undiluted aminophylline can cause cardiac arrhythmias, hypotension, nausea, tremors, and acute respiratory failure

TABLE 54.2—Doses of drugs used to treat respiratory diseases

Drug	Route[a]	Dose[b] (mg/kg)	Frequency (hr)
β agonists[c]			
Epinephrine	IM, IV, SC	20 µg/kg of .01% solution	
	SC	0.01 mL/kg of 0.1 solution	0.5[d]
Ephedrine	IM, PO	2–5 mg total (C)	
		5–15 mg (total) (D)	
Isoproterenol	PO	0.44	6–12
	IM, SC, IV	0.1–0.2 mg total	6
	Aerosol	0.5 cc of 1:200 dilution	4 × 3
Metaproterenol	PO	0.5	6
	Aerosol		4 × 3
Albuterol	Aerosol	200 µg[e]	
Terbutaline	PO	1.25 mg total	12
Isoetherine	Aerosol	0.5–1.0 mL of 1:3 saline dilution	8
Anticholinergics			
Atropine	IV, IM, SC	0.02–0.04	Prn
Glycopyrrolate	IV, IM, SC	0.01–0.02	Prn
Methylxanthines		10 (D)	6–8 (D)
Aminophylline	PO	5–6 (C)	12 (C)
	IV infusion[f]	2–5	8–12
			Over 0.5–1 hr
Theophylline base	PO	4 (C)[g]	12 (C)
		5–10 (D)	6–8 (D)
		5 (H)	12 (H)
		20 (C)	12 (C)
Oxytriphylline	PO	10–15[h]	8–12
Glucocorticoids			
Prednisolone	PO	1–2	6–12[i]
Prednisolone sodium succinate	IV, IM[i]	2–4	4–6
Dexamethasone	IV, IM[i]	0.2–2.2	
Triamcinolone	PO	0.25–0.5 mg total	24[i]
Beclomethasone dipropionate	Inhalant	200 µg total[e]	6–8
Megestrol acetate	PO	5 mg total	24 × 4, then weekly × 4
Antitussives			
Codeine	PO	1–2	8
		0.2–2 g (H)	
		15–60 mg (P)	
Hydrocodone	PO	0.22	6–12
Butorphanol tartrate	SC, IM	0.055–0.11	Prn
	PO	0.5–1.0	6–12
	SC	0.55	
Dextromethorphan	PO	1–2	6–8
Morphine	IM, SC	0.1	6–12
Decongestants			
Chlorpheniramine	PO	0.22 mg/kg (D)	8
	PO	2–4 mg total (C)	24
		1/4 to 1/2 slow release (C)	24
Diphenhydramine	PO	2–4	8
Dimenhydrinate	PO	12.5 mg total (C)	8
	PO	8 (D)	
Hydroxyzine	PO	2 (D)	6–8

[a]IV = intravenous, IM = intramuscular, SC = subcutaneous, PO = orally.
[b]C = cat, D = dog, H = horse, P = pig.
[c]Use cautiously in cats with cardiac disease.
[d]Up to a total dose of 0.5 mL.
[e]Human dose.
[f]Emergency treatment.
[g]Based upon 80% theophylline.
[h]Based upon 65% theophylline.
[i]Taper doses to minimum effective dose.

(Bauer 1986; Papich 1986a). Concentrations between 10 and 15 μg/mL have been recommended in horses (Button et al. 1985; Errecalde et al. 1984).

Adverse effects, including central nervous stimulation, sweating, and tremors, occur in horses if serum concentration surpasses 15 μg/mL (Larsson et al. 1989). The application of therapeutic drug monitoring (TDM) to guide therapy will assist in identifying the most appropriate dosing regimen. Although a therapeutic range has not been established in small animals, the range recommended in people (10-20 μg/mL) can be extrapolated until a more definitive range has been established. Dogs are apparently more tolerant of theophylline toxicity than people. In one study, toxicity manifested as tachycardia, central nervous stimulation (restlessness and excitement), and vomition did not occur until plasma theophylline concentrations reached 37-60 μg/mL. Doses of 80-160 mg/kg of a sustained-release preparation were required to induce toxicity (Munsiff et al. 1988b). In cats, concentrations as high as 40 μg/mL do not induce adverse reactions (Love et al. 1981), although salivation and vomiting are common following administration of more than 50 mg/kg and seizures may occur at doses greater than 60 mg/kg (Persson and Ergefalt 1982).

The side effects of theophylline are dose dependent and might be avoided to a large degree by appropriate dosing. TDM should facilitate design of proper dosing regimens to prevent toxicity.

Anticholinergics

PHARMACOLOGIC EFFECTS. Anticholinergic drugs compete with acetylcholine at muscarinic receptor sites (Gross and Skorodin 1984). In the respiratory tract, they reduce the sensitivity of irritant receptors and antagonize vagally mediated bronchoconstriction. In horses, atropine IV appears to minimally affect resting bronchomotor tone but has a major effect on tone in horses suffering from clinical signs of COPD (Broadstone et al. 1988). The site of action of these drugs in the respiratory tract is controversial. In some studies, bronchodilation is reported throughout the airways in asthmatic human patients and cats, but other investigators feel the effects are confined to large airways (Gross and Skorodin 1984). The route by which anticholinergics are administered influences their bronchodilatory effects. Despite their effect on bronchial airways, the anticholinergics have not proven clinically effective in the treatment of bronchial diseases in animals. The lack of clinical efficacy of anticholinergics may reflect nonselective drug-receptor interaction (Barnes 1989, 1988). Thus far, three types of muscarinic receptors have been identified in airways. M_3 receptors release acetylcholine, and M_2 receptors block its release. Nonselective blockade of muscarinic receptors by atropine and ipratropium may actually potentiate acetylcholine release by antagonizing the effects of M_2-receptor stimulation. Drugs specific for M_3 receptors may ultimately lead to successful treatment of bronchial disease with anticholinergics (Barnes 1989, 1988).

ATROPINE. Aerosolized atropine, a prototype anticholinergic drug, affects predominantly the central airways, whereas both central and peripheral airways are affected if the drug is administered intravenously (Barnes 1989, 1988). Because atropine is highly specific for all muscarinic receptors, it causes a number of systemic side effects, including tachycardia, mydriasis, and altered gastrointestinal and urinary tract function (McKiernan et al. 1981). In the respiratory tract, atropine reduces ciliary beat frequency, mucus secretion, and electrolyte and water flux into the trachea. The net effect is decreased mucociliary clearance, which is undesirable in patients with chronic lung disease (McKiernan et al. 1981). Aerosolization of atropine does not reduce the incidence of adverse reactions. Atropine is well absorbed (in humans) following oral administration. In humans, atropine has proven most useful for treatment of chronic bronchitis and emphysema, diseases which are characterized by increased intrinsic vagal tone (Gross and Skorodin 1984). However, its adverse effects on respiratory secretions and ciliary activity negate its benefits to bronchial tone during long-term administration in animals. The primary indication of atropine in small animals is facilitation of bronchodilation in acutely dyspneic animals. It is the treatment of choice for life-threatening respiratory distress induced by anticholinesterases. Combining atropine with either β-adrenergic agonists or glucocorticoids causes better bronchodilation than using either of the latter drugs alone (Gross and Skorodin 1984).

IPRATROPIUM BROMIDE. This synthetic anticholinergic is pharmacodynamically superior to atropine. While the two drugs are equipotent, ipratropium does not cross the blood-brain barrier. It is not well absorbed following aerosolization, which limits the likelihood of adverse effects. Ipratropium has been studied in the dog but not in the cat (Gross and Skorodin 1984). Of the anticholinergics studied in dogs, ipratropium appears to cause the greatest bronchodilation (twice as much as atropine) with the least change in salivation (Gross and Skorodin 1984). Unlike atropine, it does not alter mucociliary transport rates.

GLYCOPYRROLATE. Glycopyrrolate can be used as a bronchodilator in small animals. Although its onset of action is slower than that of atropine (Bauer 1986; Papich 1986a), its half-life is 4-6 hours compared to 1-2 hours for atropine. The potency of the two drugs following systemic therapy has apparently not been compared, although glycopyrrolate is twice as potent when aerosolized. Systemic side effects of glycopyrrolate are minimal.

Mast Cell Stabilizers. Drugs that stabilize mast cells are most effective in syndromes associated with marked mast cell activity. The stabilizing effects of β-adrenergic agonists, methylxanthines, and glucocorticoids on inflammatory cells have been discussed.

CROMOGYLATE. Although the mechanism of action of cromogylate has not been determined with certainty, it appears to inhibit calcium influx into mast cells, thus preventing mast cell degranulation and the release of histamine and other inflammatory mediators (Fig. 54.2) (Barnes 1989, 1988; Murphy and Kelly 1987). At high concentrations, cromogylate inhibits IgE-triggered mediator release from mast cells (Holgate 1989). Some studies suggest that the activation of inflammatory cells other than the mast cells (e.g., macrophages, neutrophils, and eosinophils) is also inhibited by cromogylate (Kay et al. 1987). Cromogylate is most useful as a preventative prior to activation of inflammatory cells. It is not significantly absorbed following oral administration and is characterized by a short half-life (Papich 1986a). Thus, effective therapy is dependent upon frequent aerosolization, which limits its utility in the treatment of small-animal diseases. Currently, cromogylate is the safest drug used to manage asthma in people (Murphy and Kelly 1987). It is associated with only minor side effects and its discovery has revolutionized the management of bronchial asthma in people. Because of its wide therapeutic window and its apparent efficacy in control of many inflammatory cells, its use in the control of small-animal bronchial disease warrants further investigation.

CALCIUM ANTAGONISTS. The use of calcium antagonists for the management of asthma has yet to be identified (Massey and Hendeles 1987). Their potential benefits include prevention of mediator release, smooth muscle contraction, vagus nerve conduction, and infiltration of inflammatory cells (Creese 1983; Massey and Hendeles 1987). Most studies indicate that calcium antagonists have only a modest effect on airway smooth muscle contraction. Their effects as anti-inflammatories may ultimately prove of greater benefit.

Other Anti-inflammatory Drugs

DRUGS THAT TARGET LEUKOTRIENES. Leukotrienes are among the mediators released by inflammatory cells (Townley et al. 1989; Soler et al. 1990; Gray et al. 1989). These 20-carbon-chain derivatives are synthesized exclusively from the membranes of myeloid cells when oxygen reacts with the polyunsaturated fatty acids (arachidonic acid, AA) of the cell membrane. Lipoxygenase enzymes lodged within cells can metabolize AA to leukotrienes (Hochberg 1989; Newcombe 1988). In this family of enzymes, 5-lipoxygenase appears to be the most important (Robinson 1989). The enzyme adds oxygen to AA to form 5-hydroperoxyeicosatetraenoic acid (HPETE) and subsequently the cysteinyl-containing leukotrienes (LT) LTC_4, LTD_4, and LTE_4. These mediators are 100-1000 times more potent than histamine and decrease airway caliber size, cause edema, and induce chemotaxis, mucus production, and bronchoconstriction (Drazen 1997; Robinson 1989; Hochberg 1989). LTs also are largely responsible for the effects of platelet-activating factor, another potent inflammatory mediator in the lungs (Drazen 1997). The importance of these mediators in the pathophysiology of inflammatory lung disease has been well established in human and animal models and in spontaneously occurring asthma in humans (Drazen 1997; Pauwels et al. 1997; Hay 1997; Byrne 1997).

Two classes of drugs that target LTs recently have been introduced in human medicine. Zafurlikast represents drugs that competitively antagonize cysteinyl-containing LT receptors, and zileuton represents drugs that irreversibly inhibit 5-lipoxygenase activity. Both drugs have proven effective for treatment of human asthma based on resolution of clinical signs, indices of respiratory function, and reduction in doses of glucocorticoids or β-adrenergic agonists. Although zileuton has been suggested to offer better therapeutic advantages than zafurlikast, differential efficacy has not been established in human asthmatic patients (Wenzel 1998), and some patients who do not respond to one will respond to the other. Treatment of inflammatory lung diseases in dogs, cats, and horses is likely to be facilitated by a similar choice of options.

Both zafurlikast and zileuton have proven to be safe in human patients. No reports exist regarding the disposition and safety of these drugs in animals, although drug concentrations established in human pharmacokinetic studies might provide a basis for effective target concentrations in dogs and cats. In humans, the disposition of each drug is characterized by good to excellent oral absorption, although bioavailability can be markedly impacted by food. Each is highly protein bound and eliminated by hepatic metabolism, with an approximately 10-hour half-life, which is conducive to twice-daily dosing (Kelloway 1997). The disposition of these drugs is accomplished by mechanisms that are likely to markedly vary between humans and dogs, and although the drugs have been used clinically in dogs and cats with apparent success, scientific studies are warranted.

NONSTEROIDAL ANTI-INFLAMMATORY DRUGS. The role of nonsteroidal anti-inflammatory drugs (NSAIDs) in the treatment of respiratory inflammatory diseases needs to be defined (Parratt and Sturgess 1974; Wasserman 1988). Both LTs and prostaglandins (PGs) are important in the pathophysiology of inflammatory diseases. While NSAIDs effectively block PGs through inhibition of cyclooxygenase, they do not appear to have any effect on lipoxygenase and therefore production of LTs. They have no effect on other chemical mediators of inflammation. Additionally, NSAIDs nonselectively block all PGs, including those that provide some protection during periods of bronchoconstriction (Walker et al. 1982). Some studies have shown that LT production increases in response to NSAID therapy, perhaps by providing more AA for lipoxygenase metabolism. Currently, the use of NSAIDs for the treatment of respiratory diseases in small animals is limited to aspirin therapy as treatment for thromboembolism associated with heartworm disease (Keith 1983; Rawlings et al. 1983). Aspirin is the preferred NSAID because at low doses it irreversibly inhibits thromboxane (TXA_2), an important contributor to pulmonary arterial vasoconstriction which accompanies thromboembolism. Current efforts in NSAID research are oriented toward identifying drugs which successfully inhibit both arms of the AA metabolic cascade or specific PG or LT inhibitors. The use of selective TXA_2 inhibitors in selected feline respiratory diseases is an example (McNamara et al. 1989).

ANTIHISTAMINES. Antihistaminergic drugs have not proven clinically useful in the control of small-animal or human respiratory diseases (Eiser et al. 1981; Moise and Spaulding 1981; Zenoble 1980). Several observations support their lack of efficacy. Although not proven, the number of histamine receptors located in the airways and the proportion of H_1 to H_2 receptors may not be sufficient to induce a response similar to that in disease. Antihistaminergic drugs act to block target receptors from responding to histamine; however, the drugs do nothing to prevent release of histamine or other mediators from any inflammatory cell. This may in fact be the major reason for lack of clinical efficacy of antihistaminergic drugs; mediators other than histamine released during mast cell degranulation and by other inflammatory cells are often much more potent than histamine (Krauer and Krauer 1977). Finally, blockade of histamine receptors is competitive and can be overwhelmed by high concentrations of histamine. The use of H_1 blockers may be detrimental in animals with chronic disease because of their effects on airway secretions (Barnes et al. 1988). The role of H_2 receptors in bronchodilation, mucus secretion, and inflammation suggests that H_2-receptor blockers should also be used with caution (Barnes et al. 1988; Chand 1981).

ANTITUSSIVES. The goal of antitussive therapy is to decrease the frequency and severity of cough without impairing mucociliary defenses. Whenever possible, the underlying cause should be identified and treated. Cough suppressants should be used cautiously and are contraindicated if the cough is productive (Slonim and Hamilton 1987). Irritant, and perhaps chemo- and stretch, receptors initiate the cough reflex (McKiernan 1983; Slonim and Hamilton 1987). Bronchoconstriction is probably the most frequent and important cough stimulus. The cough reflex can be blocked peripherally, either by facilitating removal of the irritant, using mycolytics or expectorants, or by blocking peripheral receptors to induce bronchodilation, or it can be blocked centrally at the cough center in the medulla (Roudebush 1982; Slonim and Hamilton 1987).

Centrally Active Antitussives. Centrally active antitussives are classified as narcotic and nonnarcotic drugs (Roudebush 1982; Irwin et al. 1993).

NARCOTIC ANTITUSSIVES. Narcotic antitussives depress the cough center sensitivity to afferent stimuli. However, they can be associated with strong sedative properties, as well as constipation when administered chronically. Morphine, codeine, and hydrocodone are the narcotics most commonly used to control coughing. As Schedule II drugs, they are subject to the Controlled Substances Act of 1970. They can be used for cough suppression in both dogs and cats.

CODEINE. Codeine is the prototype narcotic antitussive and is one of the most effective drugs available to suppress the cough reflex. Codeine phosphate and codeine sulfate can be used either alone or in combination with either peripheral cough suppressants or decongestants. Over-the-counter preparations are available for human use. Compared to morphine, codeine is equally effective as a cough suppressant but is less suppressing to other central centers and causes less constipation. Side effects of codeine include nausea and constipation.

HYDROCODONE. Hydrocodone is a more potent antitussive than codeine but causes less respiratory depression. It is probably the most commonly used antitussive in dogs. Hydrocodone bitartrate is a hydrolysis product of dihydrothebaine.

NONNARCOTIC ANTITUSSIVES. Nonnarcotic antitussives commonly used in veterinary medicine include the narcotic agonist-antagonist butorphanol and dextromethorphan.

BUTORPHANOL. Butorphanol tartrate is probably more commonly used as an analgesic. Classified as a Schedule IV drug, it is not subject to the Controlled Substances Act. It is approved for use as an antitussive in dogs. As an antitussive, it is 100 times more potent than codeine and 4 times more potent than morphine (Gingerich et al. 1983). In dogs, following subcutaneous (SC) administration, butorphanol concentrations peak at 1 hour. Mean half-life is 1.7 hours, with a duration of activity of 4 hours or more. Butorphanol is characterized by a wide safety margin. The LD_{50} in dogs after intramuscular (IM) administration is 20 mg/kg (Christie et al. 1980). Therapeutic concentrations cause minimal cardiac or respiratory depression. Side effects include sedation, which can be significant and desirable, nausea, some diarrhea, and appetite suppression. Butorphanol tartrate is a potent antitussive when given orally or parenterally in dogs and cats (Hosgood 1990).

DEXTROMETHORPHAN. Dextromethorphan hydrobromide is a semisynthetic derivative of opium which lacks its narcotic properties. Sedation is unusual following its use. Only the *l*-isomer has antitussive activity, which is similar to codeine in potency. Its onset of action is rapid, being fully effective within 30 minutes after oral administration. Dextromethorphan is a nonnarcotic opioid commonly found in over-the-counter cough preparations. It is used in small animals with minimal sedation and its antitussive efficacy is equal to codeine. It can be used safely in cats. Studies in humans have shown that the combination of dextromethorphan with a bronchodilator is superior to dextromethorphan alone (Tukianinen et al. 1986).

NOSCAPINE. Noscapine is a nonaddictive opium alkaloid (benzylisoquinolones) which has antitussive effects similar to codeine (Brain 1983). Its use in small animals appears to be limited.

Peripheral Bronchodilators. Bronchodilators (previously discussed) are powerful peripheral antitussives because they relieve irritant-receptor stimulation induced by mechanical deformation of the bronchial wall during bronchoconstriction. Ephedrine peripherally induces bronchodilation, and as both a bronchodilator and decongestant is a common constituent of over-the-counter cough preparations. Theophylline and isoproterenol are also common ingredients found in some preparations. Other peripheral antitussives include mucokinetic agents and hydrating agents (Roudebush 1982).

MUCOKINETICS. Mucokinetic drugs facilitate the removal of secretions from the respiratory tree. They are indicated in conditions associated with viscous to inspissated pulmonary secretions such as are commonly associated with chronic bronchial diseases. Mucokinesis can be induced by drugs which improve ciliary activity (e.g., β-receptor agonists and methylxanthines) or by drugs that improve the mobility of bronchial secretions by changing viscosity. Viscosity of bronchial secretions can be decreased by hydration (e.g., sterile or bacteriostatic water or saline), increasing pH (e.g., sodium bicarbonate), increasing ionic strength (sodium bicarbonate and saline), or rupturing sulfur (S-S) linkages in the mucus (e.g., acetylcysteine or iodine). Hydrating agents can be administered parenterally (i.e., isotonic crystalloids) or by aerosolization. Home aerosolization can be easily achieved with a humidifier or steamed bathroom or with a commercially available aerosolizer. The efficacy of aerosolization in liquefying airway secretions is controversial (Wanner and Rao 1980), with greatest benefit occurring in upper airways. Bland aerosols such as water and saline can actually be detrimental to mucociliary function (Wanner and Rao 1980). The efficacy of ionic solutions or alkaline solutions, compared to water, on enhanced mucus mobility is controversial (Wanner and Rao 1980).

N-Acetyl-L-Cysteine

PHARMACOLOGIC EFFECTS. Acetylcysteine (*N*-acetyl-L-cysteine) is the most widely used mucolytic drug in humans (Wanner and Rao 1980; Ziment 1988). While it appears to be efficacious following aerosolization, more recently oral administration has become the preferred route (Ziment 1988). In Europe, the drug is available in solid and powder dosing forms. Unfortunately, only the solution, which is unpalatable and malodorous, is approved for use in the United States. Regardless of the route of administration, the mechanism of acetylcysteine reflects destruction of mucoprotein of the disulfide bonds by a free sulfhydryl group. Smaller molecules are less viscid and not able to efficiently bind to inflammatory debris. In addition, *N*-acetylcysteine serves as a precursor to glutathione, a major scavenger of free oxygen radicals associated with inflammation. The drug also appears to induce respiratory tract secretions, probably via a gastropulmonary reflex. At higher oral doses, acetylcysteine will also induce vomition (Ziment 1986). Acetylcysteine is often used in combination with aerosolized antimicrobials because it may improve antibacterial penetration of infected mucus (Ziment 1988). Acetylcysteine improved gas exchange in a study of dogs with experimentally induced methacholine bronchoconstriction (Ueno et al. 1989).

DISPOSITION. In humans, acetylcysteine is rapidly absorbed from the gastrointestinal tract and extensively distributed to the liver, kidneys, and lungs, where it may accumulate. It is rapidly metabolized by the liver to the natural amino acids cysteine and cystine (Ziment 1986, 1988). The indications for oral acetylcysteine therapy in people include toxic inhalants (including tobacco smoke), bronchitis, COPD, cystic fibrosis, asthma, tuberculosis, pneumonia, emphysema, and the adult respiratory distress syndrome. Installation of a 10-20% solution has also been used to clean and treat chronic sinusitis (Ziment 1988). Similar uses are indicated in veterinary patients. Physiotherapy will enhance the efficacy of acetylcysteine.

ADVERSE EFFECTS. Acetylcysteine therapy is associated with few adverse affects. In humans, doses as high as 500 mg/kg are well tolerated (Ziment 1986), although vomition and anorexia can occur. The median LD_{50} in dogs following oral use is 1 g/kg, and parenterally 700 mg/kg. Because it is metabolized to sulfur-containing products, it should be used cautiously in animals suffering from liver disease characterized by hepatic encephalopathy. Aerosolization of *N*-acetylcysteine can cause reflex bronchoconstriction due to irritant-receptor stimulation and should be preceded by administration of bronchodilators.

EXPECTORANTS. Expectorants such as potassium iodide are common ingredients in over-the-counter cough preparations. Expectorants increase the fluidity of respiratory secretions through several possible mechanisms and are often used as adjuvants for the management of cough because they facilitate removal of the inciting cause. Bronchial secretions are increased by vagal reflex following gastric mucosa irritation (iodide salts), and directly through sympathetic stimulation or by volatile oils which are partially eliminated via the respiratory tract. Although the combination of expectorants with antitussives in over-the-counter cough preparations may seem irrational, the antitussive drugs in these combination products do not appear to prevent stimulation of the cough reflex by liquified secretions induced by expectorants. Their mechanism of action is uncertain although they may be ineffective at the doses used in cough preparations (Papich 1986b).

Iodide Preparations. Potassium iodide is a saline expectorant capable of increasing secretions by 150%. Ethylenediamine dihydroiodide, used as a nutritional source of iodine in cattle, may be useful for the treatment of mild respiratory diseases. Iodide preparations should not be used in pregnant or hyperthyroid animals or in milk-producing animals. Demulcents such as syrup are often used as the vehicle for cough medicaments, but they have no apparent expectorant value. They may, however, be useful for treatment of cough caused by pharyngeal irritation.

Stimulant Expectorants. Stimulant expectorants are used more commonly for coughing associated with chronic bronchial diseases. *Guaiacol,* NF, and its glyceryl ether *Guaifenesin,* USP (glyceryl guaiacolate), are wood tar derivatives. Neither the viscosity nor the volume of respiratory secretions appears to change following treatment with guaifenesin, although airway particle clearance increases in bronchitic human patients.

DECONGESTANTS. The indications for decongestants include sinusitis of allergic or viral etiologies and reverse sneezing or other complications of postnasal drip. Information regarding the use of decongestants in animals is largely based on extrapolation from human patients, for whom allergic rhinitis and the common cold are the more common indications. Often decongestants are administered as a single drug combined with expectorants.

The two major categories of drugs used as decongestants are the histamine-receptor (H_1) antagonists (e.g., dimenhydrinate, diphenhydramine, chlorpheniramine, hydroxyzine) and the sympatho-mimetic drugs, i.e., α-adrenergic agonists (e.g., ephedrine [EDE], pseudoephedrine [PDE], and phenylephrine [PNE]) (Hendeles 1993; Johnson and Hricik 1993; Kanfer et al. 1993). These drugs can be given topically in order to avoid systemic effects associated with oral therapy.

Stimulation of α_2 receptors concentrated on precapillary arterioles results in vascular smooth muscle vasoconstriction. Blood flow to the nasal mucosal capillary bed is reduced; excess extracellular fluid associated with congestion and a "runny" nose is thus decreased. Alpha$_1$ receptors are concentrated on the postcapillary venules; when stimulated, the venules act as capacitance vessels which reduce blood volume in the mucosa. Mucosal volume decreases, reducing congestion. Sympathomimetic drugs mimic norepinephrine (NE). Direct-acting agents stimulate one (PNE: α_1) or both types of α receptors, depending on drug chemistry. Indirect-acting agents (PDE) displace NE from nerve terminals and/or block its reuptake, effectively increasing its action on postjunctional α receptors. Some drugs are both direct and indirect in their actions (e.g., PDE, EDE). Prolonged use of agents that act indirectly, such as EDE, may deplete storage granules, and the animal may become refractory to its effects. Alternatively, down-regulation of receptors (tachyphylaxis) may result in refractoriness (Johnson and Hricik 1993; Kanfer et al. 1993).

Topical agents containing sympathomimetic drugs (i.e., nasal sprays) act within minutes, with minimal side effects. In contrast, rebound hyperemia is common, particularly with extended use of the drugs. The mechanism of rebound hyperemia is not clear but may result from secondary β-adrenergic effects as β receptors up-regulate or from desensitization of α receptors. Regardless of the cause, repeated contraction of the vasculature can result in ischemia and mucosal damage, perhaps due to loss of nutrition. Oral treatment with sympathomimetic drugs can be associated with a number of adverse reactions. Systemic vasoconstriction may cause hypertension; cardiac stimulation may result in tachycardia or reflex bradycardia. Stimulation of the central nervous system may also prove problematic, particularly with lipid-soluble agonists such as ephedrine. Stimulation of urinary sphincter α receptors may result in urinary retention. Mydriasis may decrease aqueous humor exit and can prove detrimental in patients with glaucoma. Because of their effects on endocrine and other organs associated with metabolic function, these drugs should be avoided in patients with metabolic disorders, including thyroid disease and diabetes mellitus. There appears to be minimal relationship between plasma drug concentrations and nasal decongestant efficacy with the α agonists, suggesting that topical therapy is as efficacious. In addition, oral administration of some drugs (e.g., PNE) is limited by first-pass metabolism, which prevents therapeutic concentrations of the drug from being reached. Thus, topical therapy may be the preferred route for sympathomimetic drugs. Note, however, that (in the United States) PDE is an "old drug" and, as such, is exempt from FDA regulation, which includes various topical formulations.

Antihistamines are effective for treatment of allergic rhinitis in human patients. In this scenario, they relieve and prevent itching and rhinorrhea but not nasal "stuffiness." Thus, antihistamines are frequently combined with sympathomimetic drugs. The efficacy of these drugs for treatment of symptoms related to the common cold (and, presumably, unknown microbial causes in animals) has not been proven. Sedation is the most common side effect of the first-generation antihistamines (diphenhydramine). Newer antihistamines (e.g., chlorpheniramine) are associated with minimal sedation. In contrast to other causes of rhinitis, topical decongestants may be more of a risk in patients with allergic rhinitis because of the risk of drug reaction (rhinitis medicamentosa). This side effect is avoided with systemic therapy. Since the antihistamines are safer than sympathomimetic drugs following oral administration, this may be the preferred route for antihistamines (Hendeles 1993).

Formulations of topical preparations can influence drug efficacy. Controlled-release polymers can decrease the rate of drug dissolution (and thus its ability to reach cellular targets). Although these differences may not be clinically relevant, it is important to realize that bioequivalency of the topical decongestant products containing older drugs may vary. The major disadvantage of topical agents is their short duration of action.

REFERENCES

Altiere, R. J., and Diamond, L. 1984. Comparison of vasoactive intestinal peptide and isoproterenol relaxant effects in isolated cat airways. J Appl Physiol 56:986-992.

Altiere, R. J., Szarek, J. L., and Diamond, L. 1984. Neuronal control of relaxation in cat airway"s smooth muscle. J Appl Physiol 57:1536-1544.

Barnes, P. J. 1988. The drug therapy of asthma: directions for the 21st century. Agents and Actions 23(Suppl):293-313.

———. 1989. Our changing understanding of asthma. Respir Med 83(Suppl):17-23.

Barnes, P. J., Chung, K. F., and Page, C. P. 1988. Inflammatory mediators and asthma. Pharmacol Rev 40:49-84.

Bauer, T. 1986. In R. W. Kirk, ed., Current Veterinary Therapy IX, Pulmonary hypersensitivity disorders, pp. 369-376. Philadelphia: W. B. Saunders.

Blair, A. M., and Woods, A. 1969. The effects of isoprenaline, atropine, and disodium cromoglycate on ciliary motility and mucous flow in vivo measured in cats. Br J Pharmacol 35:P379-P380.

Brain, J. D. 1983. Factors influencing deposition of inhaled particles. Proc 3rd Annu Comp Respir Soc Symp 3:232.

Broadstone, R. V., Scott, J. S., Derksen, F. J., et al. 1988. Effects of atropine in ponies with recurrent airway obstruction. J Appl Physiol 65:2720-2725.

Brumbaugh, G. W., Davis, L. E., Thurmon, J. C., et al. 1990. Influence of rhodococcuc equi on the respiratory burst of resident alveolar macrophages from adult horses. Am J Vet Res 51:766-771.

Button, C., Errecalde, J. O., and Mulders, M. S. G. 1985. Loading and maintenance dosage regimens for theophylline in horses. J Vet Pharmacol Therap 8:328-330.

Byrne, P. M. 1997. Leukotrienes in the pathogenesis of asthma. Chest 111:27S-34S.

Chand, N. 1981. Reactivity of isolated trachea, bronchus, and lung strip of cats to carbachol, 5-hydroxytryptamine and histamine: evidence for the existence of methylsergide-sensitive receptors. Br J Pharmacol 73:853-857.

Chand, N., and Deroth, L. 1979. Responses to automatic and autacoid agents on horse lung strip. J Vet Pharmacol Therap 2:87-89.

Christie, G. J., Strom, P. W., and Rourke, J. E. 1980. Butorphanol tartrate: a new antitussive agent for use in dogs. Vet Med Small Anim Clin 75:1559-1562.

Colebatch, H. J. H., Olsen, C. R., and Nadel, J. A. 1966. Effect of histamine, serotonin, and acetylcholine on the peripheral airways. J Appl Physiol 21:217-226.

Creese, B. R. 1983. Calcium ions, drug action and airways obstruction. Pharmacol Ther 20:357-375.

Cremer, K. F., Secor, J., and Speeg, K. V. 1989. The effect of route of administration on the cimetidine-theophylline drug interaction. J Clin Pharmacol 29:451-456.

Daemen, M. J. A. P., Smits, J. F. M., Thijssen, H. H. W., et al. 1988. Pharmacokinetic considerations in target-organ directed drug delivery. TIPS 9:138-141.

Derksen, F. J., Robinson, N. E., Armstrong, P. J., et al. 1985. Airway reactivity in ponies with recurrent airway obstruction (heaves). J Appl Physiol 58:598-604.

Downes, H., Austin, D. R., Parks, C. M., et al. 1986. Comparison of drug responses in vivo and in vitro in airways of dogs with and without airway hyperresponsiveness. J Pharmacol Exp Ther 237:214-219.

Drazen, J. M. 1997. Pharmacology of leukotriene receptor antagonists and 5-lipoxygenase inhibitors in the management of asthma. Pharmacotherapy 17:22S-30S.

Eiser, N. M., Mills, J., Snashall, P. D., et al. 1981. The role of histamine receptors in asthma. Clin Sci 60:363-370.

Errecalde, J. O., Baggot, J. D., Mulders, M. S. G., et al. 1984. Pharmacokinetics and bioavailability of theophylline in horses. J Vet Pharmacol Therap 7:255-263.

Errecalde, J. O., and Landoni, M. F. 1992. The pharmacokinetics of a slow-release theophylline preparation in horses after intravenous and oral administration. Vet Res Commun 16:131-138.

Gallagher, J. T., Kent, P. W., Passatore, M., et al. 1975. The composition of tracheal mucus and the nervous control of its secretion in the cat. Proc Royal Soc London 192:49-76.

Gingerich, D. A., Rourke, J. E., and Strom, P. W. 1983. Clinical efficacy of butorphanol injectable and tablets. Vet Med Small Anim Clin 78:179-182.

Gold, W. M., Meyers, G. L., Dain, D. S., et al. 1977. Changes in airway mast cells and histamine caused by antigen aerosol in allergic dogs. J Appl Physiol 43:271-275.

Gray, P. R., Derksen, F. J., Robinson, N. E., et al. 1989. The role of cyclooxygenase products in the acute airway obstruction and airway hyperreactivity of ponies with heaves. Am Rev Respir Dis 140:154-160.

Gross, N. J., and Skorodin, M. S. 1984. Anticholinergic, antimuscarinic bronchodilators. Am Rev Respir Dis 129:856-870.

Gustin, P., Dhem, A. R., Lekeux, P., et al. 1989. Regulation of bronchomotor tone in conscious calves. J Vet Pharmacol Therap 12:58-64.

Hay, D. W. 1997. Pharmacology of leukotriene receptor antagonists. Chest 111:35S-45S.

Heel, R. C., Brogden, R. N., Speight, T. M., et al. 1977. Buprenorphine: a review of its pharmacological properties and therapeutic efficacy. Drugs 17:81-110.

Hendeles, L. 1993. Selecting a decongestant. Pharmacother 13:129S-134S.

Hendeles, L., and Weinberger, M. 1983. Theophylline: a state of the art review. Pharmacotherapy 3:2-44.

Hochberg, M. C. 1989. NSAIDs: mechanisms and pathways of action. Hos Pract 15:185-198.

Holgate, S. T. 1989. Reflections on the mechanisms of action of sodium cromoglycate (Intal) and the role of mast cells in asthma. Respir Med 83(Suppl):25-31.

Hosgood, G. 1990. Pharmacologic features of butorphanol in dogs and cats. J Am Vet Med Assoc 196:135-136.

Inque, H., Masakazu, I., Motohiko, M., et al. 1989. Sensory receptors and reflex pathways of nonadrenergic inhibitory nervous system in feline airways. Am Rev Respir Dis 139:1175-1178.

Irwin, R. S., Curlye, F. J., and Bennett, F. M. 1993. Appropriate use of antitussives and protussives: a practical review. Drugs 46:80-91.

Johnson, D. A., and Hricik, J. G. 1993. The pharmacology of alpha-adrenergic decongestants. Pharmacother 13:110S-115S.

Kanfer, I., Dowse, R., and Vuma, V. 1993. Pharmacokinetics of oral decongestants. Pharmacother 13:116S-128S.

Kay, A. B., Walsh, G. M., Moqbel, R., et al. 1987. Disodium cromoglycate inhibits activation of human inflammatory cells in vitro. J Allergy Clin Immun 80:1-8.

Keith, J. C. 1983. Pulmonary thromboembolism during therapy of dirofilariasis with thiacetarsamide: modification with aspirin or prednisolone. Am J Vet Res 44:1278-1283.

Kelloway, J. S. 1997. Zafirlukast: the first leukotriene-receptor antagonist approved for the treatment of asthma. Ann Pharmacother 31:1012-1021.

Koritz, G. D., McKiernan, B. C., Davis, C. A. N., et al. 1986. Bioavailability of four slow-release theophylline formulations in the beagle dog. J Vet Pharmacol Therap 9:293-302.

Krauer, B., and Krauer, F. 1977. Drug kinetics in pregnancy. Clin Pharmacokinet 2:167-181.

Langston, V. C., Koritz, G. D., Davis, L. E., et al. 1989. Pharmacokinetic properties of theophylline given intravenously and orally to ruminating calves. Am J Vet Res 50:493-497.

Larsson, C. I., Kallings, P., Persson, S., et al. 1989. Pharmacokinetics and cardio-respiratory effects of oral theophylline in exercised horses. J Vet Pharmacol Therap 12:189-199.

Love, D. N., Jones, R. F., and Bailey, M. 1981. Characterization of bacteroides species isolated from soft tissue infections in cats. J Appl Bacteriol 50:567-575.

Massey, K. L., and Hendeles, L. 1987. Calcium antagonists in the management of asthma: breakthrough or ballyhoo? DICP: The Annals of Pharmacotherapy 21:505-508.

McKiernan, B. C. 1983. In R. W. Kirk, ed., Current Veterinary Therapy VIII: Small Animal Practice, Principles of respiratory therapy, pp. 216-221. Philadelphia: W. B. Saunders.

McKiernan, B. C., Davis, C. A. N., Koritz, G. D., et al. 1981. Pharmacokinetic studies of theophylline in dogs. J Vet Pharmacol Therap 4:103-110.

McKiernan, B. C., Koritz, G. D., Davis, L. E., et al. 1983. Pharmacokinetic studies of theophylline in cats. J Vet Pharmacol Therap 6:99-104.

McNamara, D. B., Harrington, J. K., Bellan, J. A., et al. 1989. Inhibition of pulmonary thromboxane A2 synthase activity and airway responses by CGS 13080. Mol Cell Biochem 85:29-41.

Mizus, I., Summer, W., Farrkuhk, I., et al. 1985. Isoproterenol or aminophylline attenuate pulmonary edema after acid lung injury. Am Rev Respir Dis 131:256-259.

Moise, N. S., and Spaulding, G. L. 1981. Feline bronchial asthma: pathogenesis, pathophysiology, diagnostics, and therapeutic considerations. Comp on Cont Educ 3:1091-1103.

Moses, B. L., and Spaulding, G. L. 1985. Chronic bronchial disease of the cat. Vet Clin North Am Small Anim Pract 15:929-949.

Munsiff, I. J., Koritz, G. D., McKiernan, B. C., et al. 1988a. Plasma protein binding of theophylline in dogs. J Vet Pharmacol Therap 11:112-114.

Munsiff, I. J., McKiernan, B. C., Davis, C. A. N., et al. 1988b. Determination of the acute oral toxicity of theophylline in conscious dogs. J Vet Pharmacol Therap 11:381-389.

Murciano, D., Aubier, M., Lecocguic, Y., et al. 1984. Effects of theophylline on diaphragmatic strength and fatigue in patients with chronic obstructive pulmonary disease. N Engl J Med 311:349-353.

Murphy, S., and Kelly, H. W. 1987. Cromolyn sodium: a review of mechanisms and clinical use in asthma. DICP: The Annals of Pharmacotherapy 21:22-35.

Newcombe, D. S. 1988. Leukotrienes: regulation of biosynthesis, metabolism, and bioactivity. J Clin Pharmacol 28:530-549.

Norn, S., and Clementson, P. 1988. Bronchial asthma: pathophysiological mechanisms and corticosteroids. Allergy 43:401-405.

Papich, M. G. 1986a. In R. W. Kirk, ed., Current Veterinary Therapy IX: Small Animal Practice, Bronchodilator therapy, pp. 278-284. Philadephia: W. B. Saunders.

———. 1986b. Current concepts in pulmonary pharmacology. Sem Vet Med Surg 1:289-301.

Parratt, J. R., and Sturgess, R. M. 1974. The effect of indomethacin on the cardiovascular and metabolic responses to *E. coli* endotoxin in the cat. Br J Pharmacol 50:177-183.

Pauwels, R. A., et al. 1997. Cytokine manipulation in animal models of asthma. Am J Respir Crit Care Med 156:S78-S81.

Persson, C. G. A., and Ergefalt, I. 1982. Seizure activity in animals given enprofylline and theophylline, two xanthines with partly different mechanisms of action. Arch Int Pharmacodyn 258:267-282.

Rawlings, C. A., Keith, J. C., Lewis, R. E., et al. 1983. Aspirin and prednisolone modification of radiographic changes caused by adulticide treatment in dogs with heartworm infection. J Am Vet Med Assoc 183:131-132.

Reed, M. T., and Kelly, H. W. 1990. Sympathomimetics for acute severe asthma: should only beta2-selective agonists be used? DICP: The Annals of Pharmacotherapy 24:868-873.

Robinson, D. R. 1989. Eicosanoids, inflammation, and anti-inflammatory drugs. Clin Exp Rheumatol 7:155-161.

Roudebush, P. 1982. Antitussive therapy in small companion animals. J Am Vet Med Assoc 180:1105-1107.

Rybak, M. J., Bowles, S. K., Chandrasekar, P. H., et al. 1987. Increased theophylline concentrations secondary to ciprofloxin. Drug Intell Clin Pharm 21:879-881.

Scott, J. S., Berney, C. E., Derksen, F. J., et al. 1991. β-adrenergic receptor activity in ponies with recurrent obstructive pulmonary disease. Am J Vet Res 52:1416-1422.

Short, C. E. 1987. Telazol: a new injectable anesthetic. Cornell Fel Health Cent Info Bull 2:1-3.

Slonim, N. F., and Hamilton, L. H. 1987. In D. Carson, ed., Respiratory Physiology, 5th ed., Development and functional anatomy of the bronchopulmonary system, pp. 27-47. St. Louis: C. V. Mosby.

Soler, M., Mansour, E., Fernandez, A., et al. 1990. PAF-induced airway responses in sheep: effects of a PAF antagonist and nedocromil sodium. J Allergy Clin Immun 67:661-668.

Townley, R. G., Hopp, R. J., Agrawal, D. K., et al. 1989. Platelet-activating factor and airway reactivity. J Allergy Clin Immun 83:997-1011.

Tukianinen, H., Silvasti, M., Flygare, U., et al. 1986. The treatment of acute transient cough: a placebo-controlled comparison of dextromethorphan and dextromethorphan-beta2-sympathomimetic combination. Eur J Respir Dis 69:95-99.

Ueno, O., Lee, L.-N., and Wagner, P. D. 1989. Effect of *N*-acetylcyteine on gas exchange after methocholine challenge and isoprenaline inhalation in the dog. Eur Respir J 2:238-246.

Viires, N., Aubier, M., Murciano, D., et al. 1984. Effects of aminophylline on diaphragmatic fatigue during acute respiratory failure. Am Rev Respir Dis 129:396-402.

Walker, B. R., Voelkel, N. F., and Reeves, J. T. 1982. Pulmonary pressor response after prostaglandin synthesis inhibition in concious dogs. J Appl Physiol 52:705-709.

Wanner, A., and Rao, A. 1980. Clinical indications for and effects of bland, mucolytic, and antimicrobial aerosols. Am Rev Respir Dis 122:79-87.

Wasserman, M. A. 1988. Modulation of arachidonic acid metabolites as potential therapy of asthma. Agents and Actions 23(Suppl):95-111.

Wenzel, S. E. 1998. New approaches to anti-inflammatory therapy for asthma. Am J Med 104:287-300.

Winkler, G. 1988. Pulmonary intravascular macrophages in domestic animal species: review of structural and functional properties. Am J Anat 181:217-234.

Zenoble, R. D. 1980. Respiratory pharmacology and therapeutics. Comp on Cont Educ 2:139-147.

Ziment, I. 1986. Acetylcysteine: a drug with an interesting past and a fascinating future. Respiration 50(Suppl 1):26-30.

———. 1988. Acetylcysteine: a drug that is much more than a mucokinetic. Biomed Pharmacother 42:513-520.

55 OPHTHALMIC PHARMACOLOGY

CECIL P. MOORE

Delivery of Ophthalmic Drugs
Local Anesthetics
Diagnostic Agents
Ocular Irrigating Solutions
Anti-inflammatory and Antimetabolite Agents
Antimicrobial Agents
Autonomic Ocular Pharmacologic Responses
Topical Hypotensive Agents
Mydriatic/Cycloplegic Agents
Nonautonomic Hypotensive Agents
Tear Substitutes and Stimulants
Miscellaneous Agents

DELIVERY OF OPHTHALMIC DRUGS

Routes of Administration. Therapeutic agents used to treat the eye may be administered locally by topical, subconjunctival, retrobulbar, or intraocular routes or they may be given systemically. The appropriate route of administration for an ophthalmic drug depends upon characteristics of the drug (solubility, available formulations), pathophysiology of the disease process (severity and location of the disease, presence or absence of normal ocular barriers), patient factors (species, animal's behavior), and human factors (ability to administer treatments at recommended frequencies, costs of treatments). A combination of two or more routes of administration may be desirable in some circumstances.

Topical ophthalmic drugs are administered directly to the ocular surface. Drugs intended for topical use are formulated as solutions, suspensions, ointments, or emulsions, or are incorporated within special drug delivery systems (see below). Dilution of the drug and washout by lacrimal secretions account for the fate of most topically administered ophthalmic preparations. Reflex tearing results in loss of topically applied drug either by nasolacrimal drainage or by overflow onto the eyelid margins. Evaporation also occurs but accounts for a relatively small loss of available drug. A portion of absorbed drug will be carried away by the conjunctival circulation.

Since topically applied drugs retained on the eye (unlost portion) encounter the multilayered conjunctival and corneal epithelia, which are formidable barriers to absorption, biphasic aqueous-lipid solubility enhances penetration. Means of enhancing passage of drugs through the cornea include (1) stimulating penetration with electrical current (iontophoresis), (2) disrupting the corneal epithelium, and (3) improving drug formulation and solubility.

Subconjunctival administration involves injecting an aqueous solution or suspension under the bulbar conjunctiva, thereby forming a subconjunctival bleb. In animal patients the subconjunctival space located between the conjunctival epithelium and Tenon's fascia usually accommodates volumes of 0.25-1.0 cc depending on the specific drug and the size of the eye; typical volumes are 0.25-0.50 cc for small domestic species and 0.50-1.0 cc for large animals. A drug is usually administered subconjunctivally when a high initial level (bolus effect) is desired. Subconjunctival injections are often used as an adjunct to other routes of administration. When injected subconjunctivally, drugs gain entry into the eye transcorneally via leakage from the injection site and by transscleral diffusion. Since a substantial portion of a subconjunctival injection is absorbed into peripheral vasculature, the possibility of systemic effects must be recognized.

Whereas aqueous-based preparations injected subconjunctivally are absorbed relatively rapidly (within 6 hr), repositol preparations are absorbed over a period of several days, resulting in a more prolonged therapeutic effect. Preparations for subconjunctival injection should be nonirritating and essentially isotonic. Use of subconjunctival administration for multiple or repeated injections may be limited by the volume of preparation and local irritation occurring at the injection site(s). Injecting drugs under the tarsoconjunctiva is probably less effective in treating ocular disease because of rapid systemic absorption and reduced local effect.

Difficulties encountered with subconjunctival injections usually relate to repositol preparations. Injection of some repositol preparations may result in granuloma formation at the injection site (Hakanson et al. 1991). Another concern is that a clinical condition may change after repositol injection, and treatment may therefore also need to change; however, the repositol material injected for the original problem remains at the site and has a prolonged undesirable effect. For example, when repositol corticosteroid has been injected subconjunctivally for treatment of uveitis and ulcerative keratitis subsequently develops, it is not possible to negate the detrimental effects that the existing corticosteroid has on corneal healing.

Retrobulbar injection involves inserting a needle through the eyelids and orbital fascia and depositing a drug behind the globe into the retrobulbar space. Although retrobulbar injections may be used for local deposition of therapeutic agents, such as antibiotics or corticosteroids for treatment of orbital disease, the most common use for this route is regional anesthesia of the orbit or face. Beyond this application, retrobulbar injections are not commonly used in veterinary medicine. Since therapeutic agents injected in this manner diffuse throughout the retrobulbar space and are absorbed systemically, any benefit derived from retrobulbar injection over systemic therapy is equivocal. Possible complications of retrobulbar injections include damage to orbital structures such as the optic nerve and exacerbation of any preexisting exophthalmos.

Intracameral administration is the placement of an agent into the anterior chamber. General anesthesia is necessary for intracameral injections. Indications for intracameral injection include intraoperative irrigation or postoperative inflation of the anterior chamber, injection of fibrinolytic agents to lyse anterior chamber fibrin, or injection of antimicrobial agents to treat severe intraocular infections (endophthalmitis). Intracamerally injected drugs are either absorbed, metabolized locally by intraocular tissues, diluted and removed by aqueous humor, or acted upon by a combination of these events. When administering intracameral drugs, necessary precautions must be taken to avoid physical or chemical damage to intraocular structures such as the corneal endothelium, iris, or lens.

Intravitreal injection is used in the treatment of infectious endophthalmitis, for chemical ablation of the ciliary epithelium in cases of chronic glaucoma, and for delivery of substances to tamponade the retina in cases of retinal separation. Following heavy sedation or general anesthesia, a needle is inserted 3-4 mm posterior to limbus and directed toward the posterior pole of the globe. Drugs administered by intravitreal injection may diffuse into the anterior chamber, where they are removed with the outflow of aqueous humor. Alternatively, some intravitreally administered agents are directly eliminated by an active transretinal pump (Ben-Nun et al. 1989). As with intracameral injections, physical or chemical damage to intraocular structures is a concern.

Systemic administration of therapeutic agents via oral, subcutaneous, intramuscular, or intravenous methods is often indicated in the management of ophthalmic disease. Intravenous therapy is the preferred method for achieving rapid peak drug levels. Barriers to intraocular penetration of many systemically administered drugs are the blood-aqueous and blood-retinal barriers. Inflammatory processes compromise these barriers and allow or accelerate intraocular deposition of drug. Systemic administration may be indicated for intraocular infection or inflammation, adnexal diseases, or orbital diseases. Most systemic drugs are metabolized by the liver and excreted by the kidneys. When treating eye disease with systemic medications, the clinician must be aware of the potential for adverse systemic side effects.

Drug Delivery Systems. *Lavage systems* are used to facilitate ocular treatments in animals requiring frequent topical treatments or animals that are difficult to treat with topical ophthalmic medications. Used predominantly in equine patients, lavage systems allow infusion of liquid medications into polyethylene or silastic tubing some distance away from the eye. Either subpalpebral or nasolacrimal units may be installed. A subpalpebral system involves inserting tubing through the upper or lower eyelid, and a nasolacrimal system involves tube placement into the nasal orifice of the nasolacrimal duct.

Ocular inserts are devices placed on the cornea or in the conjunctival cul-de-sac to allow constant release of medication onto the ocular surface. Ocular inserts may be dissolvable or nondissolvable. Dissolvable (or erodable) devices include pellets and collagen shields, while nondissolvable (or nonerodable) devices include pellets and hydrophilic contact lenses.

Liposomes are membrane-like vesicles that may be formed with concentric, alternating lipid-aqueous bilayers which can be used to incorporate and release both lipophilic and hydrophilic drugs. The potential of liposomes for delivering drugs to the ocular surface appears promising. However, commercial production for widespread use has not yet occurred.

LOCAL ANESTHETICS. Locally administered anesthetic agents are commonly used for ocular diagnostic and therapeutic procedures, including minor surgery. A combination of local and regional anesthesia (with or without sedation) may provide an alternative for high-risk patients in which general anesthesia is undesirable. Local anesthetic agents reversibly block nerve conduction without damaging nerves, allowing complete recovery of nerve function. These agents are weak bases that form stable water-soluble salts in solution. Bioactivity of local anesthetic agents is pH-dependent and related to their degree of ionization. Most are in the nonionized form at the pH of tears and the interstitial tissue spaces.

Topical Anesthetics. Topical anesthetics are commonly used for a variety of procedures requiring ocular surface analgesia such as tonometry, electroretinography, examination for and removal of foreign bodies, diagnostic or therapeutic scrapings, and nasolacrimal flushing. Two synthetic agents commonly used clinically as topical agents are *proparacaine* and *tetracaine,* which are commercially available as 0.5% solutions. *Oxybuprocaine* has been used for corneal anesthesia in human patients undergoing cataract surgery.

When applied to the cornea, topical anesthetic solutions result in corneal anesthesia within a minute and anesthesia lasts between 10 and 20 minutes. To anesthetize the conjunctiva, 4-5 administrations over 2-3 minutes are usually necessary to achieve adequate analgesia. During the anesthetic period, tear production and blink reflex will be suppressed. Therefore, a lubricant ointment should be applied to the eye at the conclusion of the procedure. Topical anesthetics should not be used continuously for treating ocular pain since these agents are damaging to the corneal epithelium and may delay corneal wound healing. Excessive applications should also be avoided since cardiac and respiratory toxicities, although unlikely, are possible with these lipid-soluble agents.

Injectable Local Anesthetics. Injectable agents may be used for local (eyelid) or regional (orbital) anesthesia in ophthalmic patients and are particularly useful in large herbivores. *Lidocaine* (1-2%), *bupivacaine* (0.25-0.75%), and *mepivacaine* (1-2%) are most commonly used for infiltration anesthesia of the periocular area. The duration of action is the major difference between these agents, with lidocaine having the shortest duration of action (40-60 min), mepivacaine an intermediate duration (2 hr), and bupivacaine the longest duration (4-6 hr). Epinephrine is sometimes added to cause local vasoconstriction, which prolongs absorption and delays the action of the local anesthetic agent. Epinephrine can prolong the duration of action of lidocaine up to 2 hours. Hyaluronidase may also be added to enhance diffusion of local anesthetic. Injectable local and topical agents are frequently used concurrently to achieve the desired degree of local anesthesia.

DIAGNOSTIC AGENTS. *Fluorescein* dye is used extensively in veterinary ophthalmology, with its most frequent and important use being its application to the ocular surface for detecting corneal ulceration. To ensure sterility of topical ophthalmic dyes, individual sterile strips are moistened with sterile eyewash solution or physiologic fluid. This liberates the dye from the sterile strips and allows its instillation onto the eye.

Since the corneal stroma is hydrophilic, water-soluble fluorescein has a marked affinity for exposed stroma. Positive staining is noted as an area of yellow-gold stain retention with room light or when a focal white light is used. A cobalt blue filter or an ultraviolet light source will excite the fluorescein, and any area(s) of positive staining will appear bright green. Topically applied fluorescein will not stain intact epithelial surfaces or Descemet's membrane. Topical fluorescein solution is also useful for determining patency of the nasolacrimal drainage system.

Injectable sodium fluorescein solution may be given intravenously to study intraocular circulation. Anterior segment fluorescein angiography allows evaluation of conjunctival, scleral, and iridal blood vessels. Retinal and choroidal circulation may also be studied following intravenous injection of sodium fluorescein. Breakdown of either the blood-aqueous or the blood-retinal barrier will allow leakage of fluorescein, which can be quantified or photographed:

Rose Bengal is useful in ophthalmic diagnostics because it is retained by abnormal ocular surface cells in the absence of overt ulceration. Although a more sensitive indicator of surface pathology than topical fluorescein, it may cause mild ocular discomfort in some animals. Because devitalized corneal or conjunctival epithelial cells will stain a deep red, subtle surface cell abnormalities such as occur in early cases of keratoconjunctivitis sicca (KCS) are detectable with Rose Bengal. It is also used to detect dendritic epithelial defects in feline corneas resulting from acute herpesvirus keratitis. Like fluorescein, Rose Bengal is best utilized as individual sterile strips moistened with sterile physiologic fluid.

Phenol red has recently been described for tear measurement by placing a small thread impregnated with this dye into the ventral conjunctival fornix for 15 seconds. A normal range of 30-38 mm of wetting per 15 seconds has been determined (Brown et al. 1996).

OCULAR IRRIGATING SOLUTIONS

Ocular Surface Irrigants. Irrigants are used to rinse away ocular surface debris and to reduce numbers of conjunctival bacteria. Only low-pressure lavage should be used for the ocular surface; therefore, an adequate volume of irrigating solution is important. Sterile physiologic saline is a commonly used and acceptable irrigant. Commercially prepared eyewashes are available and also frequently used to flush the ocular surface. These products are polyionic and buffered for ocular use but also have preservatives, which, with repeated use, may cause minor irritation in the eyes of some patients. Sterile distilled water is not recommended as an ocular irrigant because of its hypotonicity.

Adding an antiseptic or antibiotic to the irrigating solution may be useful in further reducing surface bacteria. The efficacy of this practice is dependent on the susceptibility of the resident or contaminating organisms to the specific agent. Also, the choice of agent and the concentration used should be such that the lavage solution has antimicrobial effects without causing tissue damage. A potentially serious error is the addition of an excessively high concentration of the active agent to the irrigating fluids, thereby causing tissue toxicity.

Antiseptic Solutions. Povidone-iodine antiseptic solutions are widely used in veterinary medicine. The advantage of povidone-iodine is its broad spectrum of activity and its wide range of safety to surface tissues. For cutaneous use, a concentration of 1% or less is recommended; a 1:10 dilution of a stock solution results in a 1.0% solution of povidone-iodine. More of the active-free iodine occurs in lower concentrations of povidone-iodine. Roberts et al. studied the effectiveness of various dilute povidone-iodine solutions in eliminating resident bacterial flora from eyes of dogs when used as a presurgical irrigant (Roberts et al. 1986). Disinfection with 1:2, 1:10, and 1:50 povidone-iodine dilutions was effective in eliminating bacteria from canine eyes. The use of a 1:50 povidone-iodine solution was as effective as more concentrated solutions without causing appreciable tissue reactions. Disadvantages of povidone-iodine antiseptics include acidity, possible influence on thyroid function, reduced residual activity, and reduced efficacy in the presence of organic matter. Therefore, povidone-iodine may not be the best choice for heavily contaminated wounds or where devitalized tissue is present.

Chlorhexidine is another effective antiseptic solution. A 1:40 dilution in water of the 2% concentrate is used (final concentration of 0.05%) for cutaneous antisepsis. In a light microscopy study, 2% chlorhexidine was nontoxic to rabbit corneal epithelium or endothelium when applied topically (Gassett and Ishii 1975). Advantages of chlorhexidine are that bacterial resistance has not been documented, it is affected less by organic material than povidone-iodine, and good initial kill of bacteria occurs with excellent residual activity. A disadvantage of chlorhexidine is its potential for irritating the cornea and conjunctiva when higher than recommended strengths contact the ocular surface (MacRae et al. 1984). Chlorhexidine is also unstable in saline solution.

Soaps and detergents are damaging to ocular surface tissues and should *not* be used around the eyes. An exception to this generalization is the possible use of commercial infant hair shampoos as a surgical scrub for the eyelids.

Intraocular Irrigation. Intraocular irrigation is necessary to maintain integrity of the eye during surgery and to flush unwanted material such as lens fragments or blood cells from intraocular compartments. It is essential that intraocular irrigating fluid be isotonic (290-300 mOsm), have a physiologic pH (7.4), and be nonirritating to intraocular tissues, particularly the corneal endothelium. Calcium, bicarbonate, and glutathione are important components of intraocular irrigant solutions for maintaining corneal endothelium health particularly in instances where surgery is prolonged (Glasser et al. 1985; Araie et al. 1990). Polyionic solutions such as lactated Ringer's solution or balanced salt solution are satisfactory solutions for short-term irrigation (Nasisse et al. 1986). Normal physiologic saline (0.9%), when used intraoperatively to irrigate the anterior chamber, has been associated with postoperative corneal edema resulting from loss of corneal endothelium (Edelhauser et al. 1976). Therefore, physiologic saline is not recommended for routine use as an intraocular irrigant.

ANTI-INFLAMMATORY AND ANTIMETABOLITE AGENTS. Steroidal or nonsteroidal anti-inflammatory agents are frequently indicated for treating noninfectious and infectious eye diseases of domestic species. Inflammatory processes of the eye and adnexa may cause progressive deterioration of the eye with loss of vision. Spontaneous immune-mediated diseases affecting the eye may be particularly serious and require short- or long-term anti-inflammatory therapy. In these immune-mediated processes, ocular damage may be controlled or prevented only with appropriate use of topical and/or systemic anti-inflammatory agents.

Corticosteroids

TOPICAL CORTICOSTEROIDS. Topical corticosteroids are used to treat both ocular surface and intraocular inflammatory diseases. The choice of a specific agent depends on penetrability, combination with antibiotic(s), and cost. Because of its lipid solubility, *prednisolone acetate* penetrates the cornea quite effectively and, therefore, is used extensively in therapy of intraocular diseases, particularly for treating anterior uveitis. Prednisolone acetate is commercially available as 0.125% or 1.0% suspensions and is also available as an ointment in combination with antibiotics. The combination of prednisolone acetate and chloramphenicol is often chosen for topical therapy in cases of septic uveitis because of the solubility properties of each drug. Neonatal ophthalmitis resulting from bacterial septicemia and rickettsial disease-associated uveitis are examples of infectious uveitides that respond to this topical combination administered concurrently with appropriate systemic therapy.

Dexamethasone suspension formulated in combination with neomycin and polymyxin also penetrates the cornea well and is effective in treating uveitis of domestic species. However, the antibiotics in this particular combination do not penetrate the eye well. Although *dexamethasone sodium phosphate* is commercially available as an uncombined product, dexamethasone suspension penetrates the cornea more effectively and, therefore, is preferred in therapy of uveitis. Combination solutions of gentamicin and *betamethasone* or neomycin, polymyxin, and *flumethasone* are available commercially. These are effective and less expensive alternatives for treating ocular surface inflammation. However, prednisolone and dexamethasone with or without accompanying antibiotics are generally preferred in the treatment of uveitis. A comparison of different forms of some topical corticosteroids in corneal epithelial penetration and suppression of corneal inflammation is given in Table 55.1.

In the topical treatment of diseases of the external eye, such as blepharitis, conjunctivitis, or keratitis, antibiotic-corticosteroid combinations are commonly administered. A less potent corticosteroid such as *hydrocortisone acetate* may be an effective, economical alternative that may be less likely to cause systemic side effects. Hydrocortisone is also available as an ointment in combination with triple antibiotic or in combination with chloramphenicol and polymyxin B.

TABLE 55.1—Comparison of different topical corticosteroids in suppressing rabbit corneal inflammation

	Corneal epithelium	
Corticosteroid	Intact (% decrease)	Absent (% decrease)
Prednisolone acetate 1%	51	53
Dexamethasone alcohol 0.1%	40	42
Prednisolone sodium phosphate 1%	28	47
Fluoromethalone alcohol 0.1%	31	37
Dexamethasone sodium phosphate 0.1%	19	22
Dexamethasone sodium phosphate ointment 0.05%	13	—

Source: Modified from Leibowitz and Kupferman 1980.

TABLE 55.2—Corticosteroids for topical ophthalmic use

Agent	Dosage form	Concentration
Dexamethasone	Suspension	0.1%
	Sodium phosphate solution	0.1%
	Sodium phosphate ointment	0.05%
Prednisone	Acetate suspension	0.125%, 1.0%
	Sodium phosphate solution	0.125%, 1.0%
Betamethasone	Acetate solution	0.1%
Flumethasone	Solution	0.01%
Hydrocortisone	Acetate ointment	1.0%
Fluorometholone	Suspension	0.1%, 0.25%
	Ointment	0.1%
Medrysone	Suspension	1.0%
Rimexolone	Suspension	1.0%

Medrysone 1.0% is a synthetic corticosteroid marketed for topical ophthalmic anti-inflammatory use in humans. It has less anti-inflammatory potency than 0.1% dexamethasone. Studies in human patients with increased intraocular pressure (IOP) and in those susceptible to a rise in IOP indicate that there is less effect on pressure with medrysone than with either dexamethasone or betamethasone.

Fluorometholone is a progesterone-like corticosteroid developed as an anti-inflammatory agent for human patients who respond adversely to conventional topical corticosteroid therapy by developing an increased IOP. When compared to topical dexamethasone, topical fluorometholone decreases the tendency for increased IOP in human steroid-responders. Although clinical experience indicates that fluorometholone is an effective anti-inflammatory agent when used in animals, there is no evidence that animals treated with topical corticosteroids develop ocular hypertension or glaucoma.

Rimexolone is a recently marketed ophthalmic corticosteroid with the manufacturer's claim of few side effects, including low risk of IOP increase. In clinical trials rimexolone has been similar to fluorometholone in percentage of human patients who demonstrated a significant IOP rise. Produced as a 1% suspension, rimexolone carries a label indication for postoperative inflammation following ocular surgery and for the treatment of anterior uveitis. Topical ophthalmic corticosteroids are summarized in Table 55.2.

The primary contraindication for topical corticosteroid therapy is in the presence of ulcerative keratitis, where topical corticosteroid may delay corneal healing by impairing fibroblastic and keratocytic activity, predispose to infection, and enhance activity of degradative proteases, including collagenases. Topical corticosteroids also are contraindicated for ocular surface viral infections.

SYSTEMIC CORTICOSTEROIDS. Systemic corticosteroids may be used alone or in combination with topical corticosteroids. Common indications for systemic corticosteroids in ophthalmology are for treatment of blepharitis, scleritis/episcleritis, uveitis, chorioretinitis, optic neuritis, and orbital inflammatory diseases. Systemic corticosteroids can be used following traumatic rupture or laceration of the globe when topical corticosteroids are contraindicated because of corneal damage. Systemic corticosteroids may also be used to treat severe uveitis which may be present concurrently with ulcerative keratitis. It is important to remember that both topically and systemically administered corticosteroids may cause adrenal suppression (Roberts et al. 1984; Glaze et al. 1988; Murphy et al. 1990; Moore et al. 1992). Therefore, gradual reduction of systemic corticosteroid therapy is recommended to reduce the likelihood of adrenal complications while preventing recurrence of the ocular condition. For further information on systemic corticosteroids, refer to Chap. 33.

Nonsteroidal Anti-inflammatory Drugs. Nonsteroidal anti-inflammatory drugs (NSAIDs) inhibit prostaglandin-mediated inflammation by inhibiting the cyclooxygenase (COX) enzymes, also referred to as prostaglandin endoperoxide synthases, responsible for converting arachidonic acid to eicosanoids and subsequently prostanoids. Two COX enzymes occur in tissues. COX-1 is most common and promotes release of prostaglandins that regulate normal cell activity, while COX-2 is found in resting cells and is only released in response to noxious stimuli (Vane and Botting 1995). As a result of their action on the inflammatory cascade, NSAIDs have antipyretic and analgesic properties. The primary indication for NSAIDs in ophthalmology is for the treatment of uveitis, although administration of NSAIDs may reduce symptoms of other inflammatory diseases such as blepharitis, conjunctivitis, or keratitis. Since NSAIDs interfere with platelet aggregation, they are contraindicated in cases of hyphema or when systemic bleeding disorders are present.

TOPICAL NONSTEROIDAL DRUGS. Topical NSAIDs, which are both COX-1 and COX-2 inhibitors, are used frequently in therapy of veterinary ophthalmic patients. *Flurbiprofen* 0.03% solution may be administered to prevent intraoperative miosis (Millichamp et al. 1991a), which may be a serious complicating factor during cataract surgery. It may also be used following cataract surgery and in select cases of uveitis where topical corticosteroids are contraindicated. In a fluorophotometric study comparing a number of topical agents, flurbiprofen was found to be as effective as prednisolone acetate in stabilizing the blood-aqueous barrier in a canine model (Ward et al. 1992). Flurbiprofen may delay corneal wound healing (Hersh et al. 1990) and is not recommended in patients with coexisting herpesvirus keratitis. A decrease in aqueous outflow has been noted after topical flurbiprofen administration to cannulated canine eyes (Millichamp et al. 1991b). This effect was more marked in inflamed eyes. Flurbiprofen effectively decreases fluorescein leakage in the anterior chamber of dogs compared to controls and corticosteroids (Dziezyc et al. 1995). Similar to flurbiprofen, *suprofen* 1% solution shows considerable promise as a topical NSAID.

Diclofenac is another topical NSAID advocated for the postoperative treatment of cataract surgery patients. In a study comparing topical 0.01%, 0.05%, or 0.1% diclofenac to 1% prednisolone sodium phosphate, diclofenac was more effective than prednisolone in expediting reestablishment of the blood-aqueous barrier following cataract surgery (Kraff et al. 1990). Although no differences in postoperative inflammation were detected among the three concentrations of diclofenac solution studied, the commercial formulation is available as a 0.1% solution. Ward (1996) has shown that 1% diclofenac was comparable or superior to comparable concentrations of flurbiprofen and suprofen in controlling experimentally induced blood-aqueous barrier disruption in dogs.

Indomethacin prepared as a 1% solution in artificial tears is an effective anti-inflammatory agent when topically applied. Indomethacin has been shown to enhance sliding and spreading of corneal endothelial cells, promoting covering of endothelial wound defects (Joyce and Neufeld 1990). Topically administered indomethacin has been shown to be effective in reducing protein concentrations in normal Beagle eyes following aqueocentesis (Speiss et al. 1991). In experimental dogs, 0.1% indomethacin solution was as effective as topical 1% suspension in preventing the increased permeability of the blood-aqueous barrier and the miotic response induced by aqueous paracentesis (Regnier et al. 1995). Topical ophthalmic indomethacin is not available commercially in the United States, although it is marketed in some countries as a 0.1% preparation.

Ketorolac tromethamine is an NSAID approved for ophthalmic use in human patients as a 0.5% solution. Topical ocular administration has been demonstrated to reduce prostaglandin E_2 levels in aqueous humor.

TABLE 55.3—Nonsteroidal anti-inflammatory drugs for topical ophthalmic use

Diclofenac	
Ophthalmic solution	0.1%
Flurbiprofen	
Ophthalmic Solution*	0.03%
Ketorolac	
Ophthalmic Solution	0.5%
Suprofen	
Ophthalmic Solution*	1%

*Indicated for intraoperative miosis only.

Ketorolac has no inherent effect upon IOP although experimentally it prevents development of increased IOP induced in rabbits after topical application of arachidonic acid. Its primary use in human ophthalmology is in relieving ocular itching caused by seasonal allergic conjunctivitis. For this purpose the recommended dose is 1 drop (0.25 mg) 4 times daily. Long-term efficacy in treating allergic conjunctivitis has not been established. Topical NSAIDs available commercially in the United States are summarized in Table 55.3.

Although topically applied NSAIDs may delay corneal epithelial healing, they do not appear to potentiate enzymatic destruction of the corneal stroma as do topical corticosteroids. The use of topical NSAIDs in treatment of herpetic keratitis is controversial and is not recommended (Nasisse 1991). Krohne et al. (1998a) demonstrated that topical NSAID administration inhibits aqueous flare, hypotony, and miosis in dogs with pilocarpine-induced uveitis. Because topical NSAID administration increases IOP in normal dogs, use of these topical agents is discouraged in treating glaucomatous eyes. The safety, efficacy, and possible systemic side effects of topical NSAIDs in domestic animal species warrant further investigation.

SYSTEMIC NONSTEROIDAL DRUGS. Systemic NSAIDs are routinely used as an adjunct to topical agents for treating ocular inflammation, especially in dogs and horses. *Aspirin, phenylbutazone, flunixin meglumine,* and *carprofen* are the most commonly administered systemic NSAIDs for ophthalmic conditions. Systemic NSAIDs must be used cautiously in patients receiving systemic corticosteroids due to the risk of gastrointestinal complications (Dow et al. 1990). Aspirin dosages for dogs range from 10 mg/kg twice daily to 30 mg/kg three times daily. Equine dosages range from 15 to 35 mg/kg every 12 hours. NSAIDs must be used with extreme caution in cats. Aspirin may be administered to cats at a dose of 10 mg/kg every 48 hours.

Phenylbutazone is an effective NSAID, particularly in horses. For horses with acute uveitis, a loading dose of 4.4 mg/kg twice daily for two doses is usually followed by administering 2.2 mg/kg twice daily for 2-5 days. Thereafter, the dose is further decreased to 2.2

mg/kg once daily and eventually to 1.1 mg/kg once daily. These once-daily doses may be safely administered for several weeks if appetite, gastrointestinal function, and plasma total solids remain normal. Phenylbutazone may be administered to dogs at a dose of 5-10 mg/kg every 8 hours, not to exceed 0.8 g daily.

Flunixin meglumine is FDA approved only for horses. The equine dosage is 1.1 mg/kg given either orally or intravenously. The duration of treatment with flunixin for ocular inflammation in the horse is usually short term, i.e., for 1-5 days, although it has been used safely for longer periods. Flunixin is not approved for use in small companion animals; however, it has been commonly administered as a preoperative treatment immediately prior to cataract surgery in dogs. In a study evaluating the relative stabilizing influences of flunixin and dexamethasone, Krohne and Vestre (1987) found that a combination treatment had a greater inhibitory effect on postoperative aqueous humor protein levels than either drug administered alone. The dose for dogs is 0.5-1.0 mg/kg given as a single intravenous bolus. Dehydration and impaired renal function are contraindications for administering flunixin, and caution is advised when administering flunixin during or immediately following methoxyflurane anesthesia in dogs.

Carprofen, a relatively new NSAID approved for use in dogs, functions as a potent free-radical scavenger and blocks suppressor T-cell inhibition. Besides being useful as a postoperative analagesic, it has been shown to decrease aqueous humor flare, a prostaglandin-mediated inflammatory response. In canine studies, oral carprofen treatment resulted in a 68% inhibition of flare induced by a pilocarpine irrative model and compared favorably with previous studies in which other systemic anti-inflammatory agents were used (Krohne et al. 1998b). The authors indicate that carprofen, at the manufacturer's recommended dose of 2.2 mg/kg twice daily, may be effectively used as a systemically administered ocular anti-inflammatory drug.

Ketoprofen is a relatively new NSAID approved for use in horses. In addition to blocking the cyclooxygenase pathway, ketoprofen may also affect the lipoxygenase pathway. However, data are not available on the effect of ketoprofen on the equine lipoxygenase pathway. The dose of ketoprofen for horses is 1.1 mg/kg administered daily. Horses may be maintained safely on this dose for several days. In a study comparing the adverse effects of phenylbutazone, flunixin meglumine, and ketoprofen in normal adult horses, the toxic potential was greatest for phenylbutazone, less for flunixin meglumine, and least for ketoprofen (MacAllister et al. 1993). Doses administered in that study exceeded the manufacturer's recommended doses.

The effects of two additional NSAIDs, *sulindac* and *tolfenamic acid,* administered orally for control of surgically induced inflammation have been studied in dogs. While tolfenamic acid significantly inhibited experimentally induced blood-aqueous barrier disruption in dogs, sulindac did not (Ward et al. 1992; Roze et al. 1996).

Chemotherapeutic Immunosuppressant Drugs. Locally and systemically administered chemotherapeutic agents have become increasingly useful in veterinary ophthalmology.

Cyclosporine is an immunosuppressive drug which has recently been shown to be an effective topical therapy for dry eye (or KCS) in dogs. Cyclosporine acts primarily through inhibition of T-cell lymphocytes, yet other mechanisms also appear to be involved (see section on lacrimostimulants below). Cyclosporine reduces both inflammation of lacrimal glands (Bounous et al. 1995) and ocular surface inflammation (Read 1995) when administered topically. Besides KCS, chronic superficial keratitis (pannus) and nonspecific pigmentary keratitis are additional corneal inflammatory diseases that have responded well to cyclosporine administered topically 2-3 times daily either along or in combination with topical corticosteroids (Miller 1990; Jackson et al. 1991; Williams et al. 1995). Whitcup et al. (1996) have demonstrated that cyclosporine inhibits the development of mast cell-mediated allergic conjunctivitis in animal (mice) studies. Because intraocular penetration of topically applied cyclosporine is relatively poor, it is not highly effective as the sole treatment of uveitis.

Azathioprine is a systemic immunosuppressive drug used in therapy of various immune-mediated ocular disorders. Azathioprine has been used most commonly in therapy of intractable scleritis or uveitis cases that have been unresponsive to conventional corticosteroid therapy. Canine uveo-dermatologic syndrome (VKH-like syndrome) is an example of a uveitis that may be refractory to corticosteroid therapy alone but may respond to a combination of azathioprine and corticosteroid treatment. An additional indication for the use of azathioprine is for nodular granulomatous episclerokeratitis, which occurs most commonly in Collie dogs. Intermittent blood cell counts, including platelet counts, and liver enzyme determinations are recommended due to potential myelosuppressive and hepatotoxic effects of this drug. The recommended initial dose of azathioprine for the dog is 2 mg/kg/day for 3-5 days, followed by reduction to 1 mg/kg/day for 10 days, and then 0.5 mg/kg/day as a maintenance dose, if necessary. Azathioprine has been used in the cat at a dose of 1.1 mg/kg every other day.

Miscellaneous Anti-inflammatory Agents. Topical antihistamines are not commonly used in veterinary ophthalmology. A combination decongestant (naphazoline) and antihistamine (pheniramine) is frequently used by human patients to relieve symptoms of "red eyes." As a vasoconstrictor, *naphazoline* provides symptomatic treatment for conjunctival hyperemia, whereas *pheniramine* has its primary therapeutic effect by virtue of its antihistamine properties. This combination has occasionally been used in small companion animals at a frequency of 3 times daily when signs of chronic conjunctivitis would not improve with other therapy. A topical, selective histamine antagonist is available for human use and is reported to be effective and well tolerated by children with allergic conjunctivitis (Wultrich and Gerber 1995).

Cromolyn sodium is a mast cell stabilizer that has been used topically and systemically in human patients to prevent signs of allergic conjunctivitis. Because it is most effective when used just prior to exposure to offending allergins rather than after clinical signs are already present, it has not been widely used in veterinary ophthalmology.

Megestrol acetate is a progesterone analog which has been effective in treating feline eosinophilic and proliferative keratopathies. The precise mechanism of its anti-inflammatory action is undetermined. The dosage is 5 mg orally daily for 5 days, then 5 mg every other day for one week, followed by 5 mg weekly as maintenance therapy. Megestrol acetate is not FDA approved for cats, and caution is advised when administering to cats since known side effects include endometritis, pyometra, diabetes mellitus, weight gain, adrenocortical suppression, and behavioral changes.

The combination of *tetracycline* and *niacinamide* has been used to successfully treat sterile granulomatous ocular adnexal diseases in dogs. Tetracycline (500 mg PO q8h) and niacinamide (500 mg PO q8h) are administered until remission of granulomatous swelling is noted. Then, frequency of treatment is tapered to q12h and finally to q24h over several weeks. Eventually all treatments are discontinued. Although the specific mechanism is not understood, the combination of these agents is known to have immunomodulating and anti-inflammatory effects (Rothstein et al. 1997).

ANTIMICROBIAL AGENTS. Antimicrobial drugs are routinely used for treating ophthalmic diseases of domestic animals. Selection of a particular therapeutic agent is based on the known antimicrobial spectrum for a given drug, knowledge of likely offending organisms, and results of specific susceptibility tests. Selection may also be influenced by physiologic barriers and the desired site(s) of action, drug compatibilities, potential toxicity, and specific formulations available (i.e., solution, suspension, ointment).

In cases of ulcerative keratitis where the corneal epithelial barrier is lost, corneal penetration becomes possible for drugs that would not typically move across the epithelium. However, if the primary objective is treatment of deep intraocular or orbital infection, then systemic therapy is indicated. Unique properties of the normal blood-aqueous barrier may limit the intraocular penetration of many antimicrobial agents given systemically. Antimicrobial therapy is frequently warranted in cases of uveitis, whereby intraocular inflammation enhances penetration of systemically administered drugs. Orbital tissues achieve antibiotic levels of systemically administered drugs comparable to those of other soft tissues.

Subconjunctival injection of nonirritating antimicrobials may be used to achieve high local levels of a drug for up to 6 hours for most aqueous-based preparations. Only parenteral antimicrobial preparations should be used for subconjunctival injections. Some injectables, such as oxytetracycline and amphotericin, are extremely irritating and are not recommended for subconjunctival use. Antibiotics which can be safely injected subconjunctivally are given in Table 55.4. Combining antimicrobial therapy may be beneficial in some instances. In therapy of deep corneal disease or uveitis, it is common to combine topical, subconjunctival, and systemic therapy. Alternatively, to enhance antimicrobial activity, more than one drug may be delivered by the same route. If more than one antimicrobial is applied to the eye at one dosing, some minimal amount of time (e.g., 5 min) should be allowed between each instillation to avoid dilution or chemical incompatibility.

Because of the limited availability of antimicrobials approved for topical ophthalmic use in animals, extralabel use of human ophthalmic products or compounding topical preparations from injectable formulations is often necessary to adequately treat animal eye diseases.

Aminoglycosides. Gentamicin, neomycin, tobramycin, kanamycin, and amikacin are aminoglycoside antibiotics commonly used in ophthalmology. Although aminoglycosides penetrate the intact eye poorly, they are extremely useful for treating ocular surface infections that cause or complicate conjunctivitis and ulcerative keratitis. They are particularly effective when used to treat serious gram-negative infections of the eye, specifically those caused by *Pseudomonas aeruginosa.* Aminoglycosides have a broad antibacterial spectrum against a variety of gram-positive and gram-negative bacteria; however, streptococci are notoriously resistant to these drugs. When injected subconjunctivally at recommended doses, the aqueous humor concentrations of aminoglycosides are sufficient to achieve bactericidal levels. Although renal and auditory toxicities are important side effects of systemically administered aminoglycosides, these side effects have not been observed with local ocular administration.

Topical *gentamicin* is recommended as initial therapy when gram-negative bacterial infections are suspected or confirmed. Gentamicin is generally highly effective against *Pseudomonas aeruginosa* and *Staphylococcus* spp. (Moore et al. 1983; Gerding et al. 1988). Gentamicin is commercially available as a 0.3% topical ophthalmic solution and as an ophthalmic ointment. Fortified solutions of gentamicin can be prepared by adding gentamicin injectable to artificial tear solution. For example, 2 mL of gentamicin injectable (50 mg/mL) may be added to 13 mL of artificial tears to make a final concentration of 0.67% gentamicin (6.7 mg/mL); or, alternatively, 5 mL of the same injectable may be added to 12.5 mL of artificial tears to make a

TABLE 55.4—Use of antimicrobial solutions for topical ophthalmic and subconjunctival use

	Topical concentration	Reference	Subconjunctival dose	Reference
Antibacterials				
Gentamicin	10–20 mg/mL	Hyndiuk and Snyder 1987	20–40 mg	Regnier 1991
Tobramycin	10–20 mg/mL	Hyndiuk and Snyder 1987	20–40 mg	Nasisse and Nelms 1992
Amikacin	10 mg/mL	Regnier and Toutain 1991	25 mg	Hyndiuk and Snyder 1987
Kanamycin	10 mg/mL	Moore 1995	10–20 mg	Hyndiuk and Snyder 1987
Cefazolin	50 mg/mL	Hyndiuk and Snyder 1987	100 mg	Hyndiuk and Snyder 1987
Chloramphenicol	5–10 mg/mL	Hyndiuk and Snyder 1987 Regnier and Toutain 1991	100 mg	Hyndiuk and Snyder 1987
Penicillin G	100,000 U/mL	Nasisse and Nelms 1992	500,000 U	Regnier and Toutain 1991
Ampicillin	10 mg/mL	Regnier and Toutain 1991	100 mg	Regnier and Toutain 1991
Methicillin	—	—	100 mg	Regnier and Toutain 1991
Ticarcillin	6.3 mg/mL	Baum 1980	100 mg (comparable to carbenicillin)	Hyndiuk and Snyder 1987
Bacitracin	10,000 U/mL	Nasisse and Nelms 1992	10,000 U	Regnier and Toutain 1991
Antifungals				
Amphotericin B	1.0–2.5 mg/mL (0.10–0.25%)	Forster 1987	0.5–1.0 mg	Forster 1987
Nystatin	50,000 U/mL	Forster 1987	—	—
Miconazole	10 mg/mL (1%)	Forster 1987	5–10 mg	Forster 1987
Ketoconazole	10–20 mg/mL	Forster 1987	—	—
Flucytosine	10 mg/mL (1%)	Forster 1987	—	—
Clotrimazole	1% in peanut oil	Davidson 1991	—	—
Itraconazole	1% in 30% DMSO ointment	Ball 1997	—	—

final concentration of 1.4% gentamicin (14 mg/mL) (Kern 1990). A subconjunctival dose of 10-12.5 mg of gentamicin may be given for small animals or 25 mg for large animals. For subconjunctival use, the 40 mg/mL or 50 mg/mL injectable solutions of gentamicin are preferred over the 100 mg/mL solution, which contains the preservative benzyl alcohol, which may cause local irritation. Gentamicin is incompatible with sulfonamides and chloramphenicol.

Neomycin is an aminoglycoside commonly applied to the eye in combination with bacitracin (or gramicidin) and polymyxin B. This triple antibiotic combination maximizes the spectrum of antibacterial activity against both gram-positive and gram-negative organisms. Triple antibiotic is an excellent first choice for acute external ocular infections or for prophylaxis against surface infection. Neomycin hypersensitivity may occur with chronic therapy and manifests as persistent conjunctival hyperemia in the absence of infection. If neomycin hypersensitivity is suspected, the drug is discontinued and it is replaced with a non-aminoglycoside antibiotic.

Tobramycin has been suggested to be 4 times more effective against *Pseudomonas* organisms than gentamicin (Havener 1983) and, like gentamicin, is effective against penicillinase-producing staphylococci. Tobramycin is available commercially as an ophthalmic ointment or solution and may be used as an alternative to gentamicin, particularly in cases of resistant *Pseudomonas* spp.

Kanamycin is an aminoglycoside that is active against many gram-negative pathogens and is particularly useful when treating coliform or *Klebsiella* spp. infections of the equine eye. Kanamycin has been demonstrated to be highly active against *Moraxella bovis* (minimum inhibitory concentration less than 0.5 μg/mL) (George et al. 1986). *Amikacin* is an acetylated kanamycin and is an alternative aminoglycoside for use against gentamicin- or tobramycin-resistant *Pseudomonas* spp. The acetyl moiety renders amikacin more resistant to bacterial enzyme inactivation. Solutions for topical ophthalmic use may be prepared by adding 3 mL (50 mg/mL) of injectable amikacin or kanamycin to 12 mL of artificial tears for a final concentration of 1.0%. Kanamycin or amikacin injectable (50 mg/mL) can each be given subconjunctivally (Table 55.4). Subconjunctival injections of 100 mg of kanamycin in calves produced local levels exceeding 1 μg/mL for 4 hours, resulting in successful treatment of infectious bovine keratoconjunctivitis (IBK) (George et al. 1986).

Cephalosporins. Cephalosporins are β-lactam bactericidal antibiotics similar in spectrum to penicillins except that this group of agents is generally effective against penicillinase-producing organisms. Local administration of a cephalosporin to the eyes of domestic animals has usually been limited to cases where serious gram-positive infection has been confirmed, e.g., *Streptococcus* spp., or when specifically indicated by bacterial culture and susceptibility results. Most systemically administered cephalosporins are not highly effective in penetrating the normal blood-aqueous barrier. Cross-allergic reactions between the cephalosporins and the penicillins are possible.

Although there is no approved cephalosporin preparation for direct application to the eye, first-generation cephalosporins have been commonly used as topical ophthalmic solutions. A topical cephalosporin preparation can be formulated by reconstituting 1 g of *cefazolin* to 20 mL artificial tears for a final concentration of 50 mg/mL. The subconjunctival dose for cefazolin is 100 mg. Aqueous solutions of second- or third-generation cephalosporins may be similarly formulated for topical or subconjunctival ophthalmic use as dictated by in vitro susceptibility data.

Chloramphenicol and Related Antimicrobials. *Chloramphenicol* is a broad-spectrum bacteriostatic antibiotic effective against a variety of organisms, including most resident ocular bacterial flora, chlamydia, mycoplasma, rickettsia, and spirochetes, but it is usually ineffective against *Pseudomonas* spp. Chloramphenicol works by binding to microbial ribosomes, an action inhibited by macrolide antibiotics, and therefore, it is antagonistic to erythromycin, lincomycin, and clindamycin. Gentamicin and chloramphenicol are also antagonistic.

Chloramphenicol is both aqueous and lipid soluble and penetrates corneal and blood-aqueous barriers extremely effectively and, therefore, is considered the drug of choice for treating intraocular infections. Chloramphenicol is also indicated for treating corneal stromal abscesses sequestered by intact epithelium (Rebhun 1982), eyes affected with septic uveitis, cases of suspected aminoglycoside hypersensitivity, and feline infectious conjunctivitis. Because of its activity against anaerobic bacteria, systemic chloramphenicol is also a good choice for treating orbital infections. Chloramphenicol may be injected subconjunctivally, and the dose of the sodium succinate preparation is 50-100 mg.

Because chloramphenicol has been linked to a rare form of aplastic anemia in humans, it has been banned from use in food-producing animals. Research efforts have focused on modifying the basic structure of the chloramphenicol molecule to eliminate the potentially toxic p-NO_2 group while retaining the compound's broad antimicrobial spectrum. Two products have been derived that are related compounds and have shown promise: *thiamphenicol* and *florfenicol*. Although thiamphenicol is not presently available in North America, florfenicol has recently been marketed for use in food animals as an injectable solution. Florfenicol contains a fluorine at the 3′ carbon position and has been found to be as potent or more potent than chloramphenicol against many organisms in vitro. It is nontoxic and is eliminated rapidly. Although it is well distributed to most tissues, florfenicol does not penetrate the CNS or aqueous humor as well as chloramphenicol. Florfenicol's use in treating ocular infections of ruminants merits investigation.

Fluoroquinolones. Fluoroquinolones are bactericidal agents active against both aerobic gram-positive and gram-negative organisms but generally ineffective against obligate anaerobes. Plasmid-mediated resistance has not been detected with fluoroquinolones. Rarely do they show synergy or antagonism with other antimicrobial agents such as β lactams or aminoglycosides. *Enrofloxacin* and *orbifloxacin* are approved for veterinary use and have proven extremely valuable as systemic agents for treating serious infections in domestic and exotic animals, birds, rodents, reptiles, and fish. *Ciprofloxacin, norfloxacin,* and *ofloxacin* are fluoroquinolone antibiotics approved for topical ophthalmic use in humans. Hyndiuk et al. (1996) report that ciprofloxacin ophthalmic solution (0.3%) is equivalent to fortified tobramycin-cefazolin for topical therapy of bacterial corneal ulcers in human patients and produces less discomfort than the combination treatment. In veterinary ophthalmology, fluoroquinolones are used topically to treat gram-negative corneal infections, particularly aminoglycoside-resistant *pseudo-monas.* Rebhun has indicated successful treatment with ciprofloxacin of three cases of refractory equine keratitis caused by acid-fast organisms (Rebhun 1992). Routine use of topical fluoroquinolones is discouraged, with application of these drugs being dictated by susceptibility results.

Penicillins. Penicillins are used in ophthalmology most often as systemic therapy complementing other locally administered antibiotics. Penicillins may be used locally in the eye as topical solutions or subconjunctival injections. Ocular penetration of penicillins following systemic therapy varies considerably with the specific drug (Havener 1983). In experimental animals treated systemically, good aqueous levels were achieved with ampicillin, whereas amoxicillin exhibited intermediate penetration, and carbenicillin, methicillin, and penicillin G penetrated the normal blood-aqueous barrier poorly. However, as with other antibiotics, ocular penetration is enhanced by loss of corneal epithelium, with uveal inflammation, or by subconjunctival injection.

All penicillins are bactericidal; the early-generation antibiotics have primarily a gram-positive spectrum, whereas newer semisynthetic derivatives are also effective against gram-negative bacteria. Potassium *penicillin G* may be given systemically or injected subconjunctivally as adjunctive therapy for streptococcal keratitis. Locally administered penicillin achieves substantially higher levels in corneal tissues than via systemic administration. Experimental injection of 1 million units of penicillin G subconjunctivally achieves effective intraocular levels for 48 hours (Havener 1983). Although Allen et al. (1995) reported that all 333 *Moraxella bovis* isolates recovered from cattle with infectious keratoconjunctivitis (IBK) were susceptible to 0.3 U of penicillin/mL, subconjunctival treatment with procaine-penicillin G, alone or in combination with dexamethasone, did not significantly affect the outcome of naturally developing IBK.

Penicillin G may be mixed with artificial tears for topical administration; however, its potency is reduced to 74% in 3 days and to 25% after 7 days (Osborn et al. 1976). Therefore, penicillin G in artificial tear solution should be replaced after 3 days at room temperature. *Ampicillin* has broad-spectrum antibacterial activity and may be reconstituted as a 100 mg/mL solution and administered topically after adding 1.75 mL to 15 cc artificial tears (10 mg/mL) or injected subconjunctivally directly (100 mg/mL) as prophylaxis or definitive therapy for streptococcal keratitis or IBK. Ampicillin may be administered parenterally when broad-spectrum systemic therapy is desired. Amoxicillin, which is comparable in spectrum to ampicillin, is often prescribed when prophylaxis or empirical broad-spectrum systemic therapy is desired because of its availability and convenient oral dosage forms. Amoxicillin or amoxicillin-clavulanate combination are excellent first choices for therapy of orbital infections.

Carbenicillin, a semisynthetic penicillin effective against gram-negative infections, including *Pseudomonas, Proteus,* and *Escherichia coli,* is therapeutically synergistic with gentamicin, tobramycin, and amikacin but is no longer commercially available. *Ticarcillin* has a comparable antibacterial spectrum to carbenicillin and is available as a reconstitutable powder in sterile 1 g vials. Although therapeutically synergistic, ticarcillin should not be mixed with aminoglycoside solutions. Therefore, when used simultaneously, these agents should be administered separately.

Methicillin, unlike penicillin, ampicillin, amoxicillin, and ticarcillin, is resistant to destruction by penicillinase and is, therefore, effective against resistant staphylococci. However, methicillin is very unstable and must be used immediately after reconstitution. Like methicillin, *cloxacillin* is also active against staphylococci and other penicillinase-producing bacteria. Benzathine cloxacillin has been documented to be effective against *Moraxella bovis,* the cause of IBK. A single topical administration of an intramammary preparation of benzathine cloxacillin has been used to successfully treat IBK (Daigneault and George 1990). The concentration of cloxacillin in tears should exceed 2 μg/mL for 12 hours to be effective. An apparent affinity of benzathine cloxacillin for cornea and conjunctiva may contribute to its efficacy in treating IBK (Daigneault et al. 1990).

Polypeptide Antibiotics. *Bacitracin* and *polymyxin B* are bactericidal polypeptide antibiotics commonly used in ophthalmology in combination with neomycin. Inclusion of bacitracin in the triple antibiotic combination enhances its spectrum against streptococci, while inclusion of polymyxin B expands efficacy against gram-negative organisms. Like neomycin, bacitracin and polymyxin B do not penetrate the intact cornea. Bacitracin has a range of activity similar to penicillin, but bacterial resistance and allergic reactions against it are much less common than with penicillin. Bacitracin is too toxic for systemic use and, therefore, is used only topically. Bacitracin is water soluble and a 10,000 IU/mL solution may be injected subconjunctivally (up to 1 mL) (Regnier and Toutain 1991).

Polymyxin B is effective against most gram-negative bacteria, including many *Pseudomonas* spp. The presence of polymyxin B makes the triple antibiotic combination preferable to chloramphenicol in therapy of uncomplicated corneal ulcers because of its expanded efficacy against *Pseudomonas* infection. Although *Proteus* spp. are typically resistant to polymyxin B, the neomycin present in the triple antibiotic combination generally is effective against *Proteus.* Polymyxin B has recently been combined with trimethoprim, producing a broad-spectrum preparation for topical ophthalmic use. Polymyxin B should not be injected subconjunctivally since it may cause severe chemosis and conjunctival necrosis.

Like polymyxin B, *colistin* (polymyxin E) is a polypeptide antibiotic which is highly effective in inhibiting gram-negative organisms, including *Pseudomonas aeruginosa,* but has little effect against gram-positive organisms or *Proteus* spp. Colistin is nonirritating when topically applied to the cornea or conjunctiva and, unlike polymyxin B, may be given subconjunctivally without irritation. When administered systemically, both colistin and polymyxin B may produce severe renal and neural toxicity.

Sulfonamides. Sulfonamides are relatively broad-spectrum bacteriostatic antimicrobial agents that demonstrate activity against most gram-positive and a variety of gram-negative organisms, including some *Pseudomonas* spp. *Sulfacetamide* and *sulfisoxazole* are available as human ophthalmic preparations but are not commonly used in veterinary ophthalmology because of more effective and more readily available topical alternatives. In human patients, sulfacetamide is effective therapy for ocular surface infections caused by *Staphylococcus.*

The combination of *trimethoprim-sulfadiazine* is frequently used systemically as an adjunct to topical therapy for ocular infections. Trimethoprim-sulfadiazine is reported to be effective against ocular toxoplasmosis. In the presence of uveitis, the aqueous concentration following systemic administration of trimethoprim-sulfadiazine approximates that in the blood stream. Sulfonamides also show some activity against chlamydia, and therefore, trimethoprim-sulfadiazine may be an effective alternative to systemic tetracycline therapy in young cats with conjunctivitis and respiratory disease. Prolonged systemic therapy with sulfonamides may cause dry eye in the dog due to a direct toxic effect on the lacrimal gland (Morgan and Bachrach 1982; Collins et al. 1986). This effect may be reversible if therapy is discontinued. Sulfonamide activity is inhibited by purulent exudate, topical anesthetic agents, and benzalkonium chloride, which is a common preservative in ophthalmic preparations. Sulfacetamide is antagonistic to the inhibition of *Pseudomonas* by gentamicin. In human patients, topical sulfonamides may cause local allergic or photosensitization reactions, and similar reactions are possible in animals.

Tetracyclines. The tetracycline group of antibiotics are broad-spectrum bacteriostatic agents effective against a variety of organisms including chlamydia, mycoplasma, and rickettsia. However, *Proteus, Pseudomonas,* and many strains of *Staphylococcus* are frequently resistant to tetracyclines. This group includes the topical ophthalmic products *oxytetracycline* (combined with polymyxin B), *chlortetracycline,* and *tetracycline.* Any one of these preparations is a good first choice for treating infectious conjunctivitis in cats. Tetracyclines applied topically to an eye may achieve inhibitory levels in the aqueous humor.

Penetration of the blood-aqueous barrier is primarily related to lipophilicity. Inhibitory levels of tetracycline and oxytetracycline are not achieved in the aqueous humor by systemic administration in the noninflamed eye. However, *doxycycline* and *minocycline* do achieve excellent intraocular levels. Minocycline has been reported to be effective against experimental ocular toxoplasmosis. Doxycycline is recommended for treatment of rickettsial diseases such as ehrlichiosis and Rocky Mountain spotted fever, which are frequently accompanied by signs of uveitis.

Intramuscular injection of long-acting oxytetracycline is effective in treating IBK and ovine keratoconjunctivitis. Subconjunctival injection of oxytetracycline may produce therapeutic levels of drug in the tears of calves; however, because it is extremely irritating, this method of administration cannot be recommended. Oral tetracycline has been used to decrease tear staining in dogs. A recommended dose is 20 mg/kg daily in divided doses for 2-3 days. Tear staining will normally reappear in 2-3 weeks. Tetracyclines are contraindicated in pregnant or young animals since the drug is concentrated in the dentine and enamel of unerupted teeth. Because of antibiotic-induced enteritis, systemic tetracyclines are generally not recommended for horses.

Lincosamides and Macrolides. Although there are structural differences in these two groups, similar spectrums and mechanisms merit including them in one discussion. Drugs in these categories include erythromycin and azithromycin (macrolides) and lincomycin and clindamycin (lincosamides) antibiotics with varied bacterial spectra and ocular penetrations. *Erythromycin,* which is well tolerated as an ophthalmic ointment, has primarily a gram-positive spectrum and, therefore, is particularly useful in treating streptococcal infections. Erythromycin is also effective against chlamydia, mycoplasma, and rickettsial organisms. Erythromycin 0.5% ophthalmic ointment is commercially available and is well tolerated when applied to the animal eye. Clinicians should be aware that staphylococcal resistance to erythromycin frequently occurs.

Azithromycin is a macrolide antibiotic which, when given orally, achieves prolonged high levels in conjunctival tissue. This property raises the possibility that it may be useful for treatment of conjunctivitis caused by chlamydiae and other susceptible organisms (Tabbara et al. 1998).

Lincomycin may be given by subconjunctival injection at 50-150 mg; however, it is not commonly used in ophthalmic therapy. *Clindamycin* is a chlorinated analog of lincomycin that has a better spectrum of activity than lincomycin. Oral clindamycin in divided doses of 25 mg/kg daily has been used effectively in cats to treat ocular toxoplasmosis (Lappin et al. 1989).

Miscellaneous Antibiotics. *Metronidazole* is a nitroimidazole antimicrobial agent initially introduced as an antiprotozoal agent for use in humans. Metronidazole is not approved for veterinary use in the United States but is currently used to treat a number of protozoal and bacterial infections in animals. It is well absorbed from the gastrointestinal tract of animals and is, therefore, active against both luminal and extraluminal protozoa. It is also effective in treating obligate anaerobic infections.

Rifampin is a broad-spectrum antibiotic widely used in human medicine as part of combination therapy for treating mycobacterial diseases. Rifampin has been used in combination with other antibiotics to treat equine infections caused by *Rhodococcus* and *Staphylococcus.* Rebhun has described using oral rifampin at a dose of 4.4 mg/kg twice daily in conjunction with topical aminoglycosides to treat an insidious chronic keratitis of horses believed to be caused by opportunistic acid-fast organisms (Rebhun 1992). Because microbial resistance may develop rapidly to rifampin, it should always be combined with other antimicrobial agents. Rifampin has demonstrated marked synergism with amphotericin B against a variety of fungi (Stern 1978).

Because of changing susceptibilities of ocular microbes, new antibiotics are of great interest to clinicians, particularly those that demonstrate efficacy against typically resistant gram-negative bacteria. *Ceftazidime* is a third-generation semisynthetic cephalosporin which is promising for ophthalmic use because of its activity against *Pseudomonas* and coliforms. Studies indicate that ceftazidime and aminoglycosides may be additive or synergistic against some strains of these organisms. Ceftazidime is slightly less active in vitro against common gram-positive bacteria compared to most other currently available cephalosporins.

Aztreonam is a synthetic mono-bactam antibiotic that is active against many gram-negative aerobic bacteria, including most strains of *Pseudomonas aeruginosa* and enterobacteria. Aztreonam has little or no activity against gram-positive bacteria. Ceftazidime and aztreonam are commercially available as sterile powders for reconstitution and injection in 500 mg, 1 g, and 2 g vials. The principal advantage of these new-generation antibiotics is their decreased vulnerability to hydrolysis by β lactamase and their lack of nephrotoxicity. The potential usefulness of these and other newer generation antibiotics for treating eye infections of animals merits in vitro and clinical investigations.

Imipenem is a β-lactam antibiotic that is highly resistant to all β-lactamase enzymes and can penetrate most gram-negative bacteria. It has been used primarily for serious, resistant infections that would otherwise require multiple drugs, including animoglycosides. Imipenem has the broadest antibacterial action in comparison to other β lactams, even surpassing many third-generation cephalosporins. It is one of the newest and most expensive antibiotics currently available.

Fusidic acid, or fusidin, is a steroidal antibiotic chemically related to cephalosporin P. It is effective against a wide range of gram-positive organisms, especially against staphylococci (both β-lactamase positive and negative) and some gram-negative bacteria. It is marketed as a 1% viscous topical agent in Europe and Great Britain for treatment of bacterial conjunctivitis of dogs. The sustained-release vehicle allows it to be used effectively with once- or twice-daily administration. Although it is not presently licensed for use in cats, it is reportedly well tolerated in cats and is undergoing investigation as a possible treatment for feline conjunctivitis.

Antifungals

POLYENE ANTIBIOTICS. *Natamycin,* a tetraene polyene antibiotic, is the only antifungal agent presently FDA approved for topical ophthalmic use in humans. It is available commercially as a 5% suspension, which is well tolerated by the mammalian eye and may be safely applied topically as frequently as every 1-2 hours for several days in cases of keratomycosis. Natamycin has a broad antifungal spectrum against both filamentous fungi and yeast and is the preferred treatment for *Fusarium* infections of the cornea (Beech and Sweeney 1983). Use of natamycin in veterinary medicine has been limited somewhat by the cost of the product. However, this should not be considered a major deterrent given other expenses incurred in treatment of serious corneal infections of animals, particularly in equids.

Amphotericin B may be used as a topical solution (0.10-0.25%) in cases of keratomycoses when there is known or suspected resistance to other antifungal agents. Only sterile water or 5% dextrose solution should be used as diluents since amphotericin B is incompatible with saline or other electrolyte solutions. Amphotericin B is extremely irritating when injected, and therefore, subconjunctival administration is not recommended. Reconstituted amphotericin B solution should be stored in a dark container and refrigerated to prevent photodegradation.

Nystatin, a polyene antibiotic with high efficacy against yeasts, is widely used in the treatment of localized candidiasis in humans. Nystatin is available in nonocular forms, including tablets, creams, and ointments. Tablets must be dissolved to formulate a solution containing 50,000 U/mL for topical application (Forster 1987). Dermatologic or mucous-membrane creams or ointments may be applied directly to the eye. Although nystatin is relatively nontoxic to ocular surface tissues, its use is somewhat limited because of its limited antifungal spectrum.

IMIDAZOLE AGENTS. *Miconazole* is an imidazole derivative with broad antifungal activity against common fungal infections. Miconazole is often used as the initial treatment for cases of confirmed or suspected fungal keratitis in the horse. A 1% miconazole intravenous solution was historically used directly on the eye 4-6 times daily or even more frequently in severe or rapidly progressive cases of keratomycoses. Miconazole solution *should not* be mixed with artificial tears or other ophthalmic preparations. Unfortunately, 1% miconazole intravenous solution is presently not commercially available. Miconazole 2% creams, available for human and veterinary use, are well tolerated by the equine eye. The author has applied the veterinary dermatologic cream to equine eyes affected with fungal keratitis up to 4 times daily for 3 weeks without adverse effects. Miconazole dermatologic lotions or sprays containing ethyl alcohol *should not* be applied to the eye. Miconazole and amphotericin B are antagonistic and should not be used concurrently.

Fluconazole is a synthetic broad-spectrum imidazole agent with demonstrated fungistatic activity against *Aspergillus flavus* and *A. fumigatus* infections in laboratory animals (Troke et al. 1987). Fluconazole is available as a 0.2% (2 mg/mL) injectable solution, which the author has applied topically to the equine eye and injected subconjunctivally (1 mL) without adverse reaction. As with most antifungal drugs, it should not be mixed with other solutions. *Clotrimazole,* used as a 1% dermatologic cream, has been well tolerated by the equine eye. An anthelmintic paste form of *thiabendazole* has been applied to infected equine eyes and was reportedly effective in treating fungal keratitis (Joyce 1983). *Ketoconazole* and *econazole* are available as 2% and 1% dermatologic creams, respectively; however their tolerance by the equine eye has not been established. *Itraconazole* is commercially available in 100 mg capsules and has been compounded in an ointment with dimethyl sulfoxide and applied topically as effective treatment for equine keratomycosis (Ball et al. 1997) infected with fungi. Oral itraconazole may be useful in treating canine ocular blastomycosis (Brooks et al. 1991). See Table 55.4 for a summary of extralabel formulations of antifungal solutions for local ophthalmic administration.

MISCELLANEOUS ANTIFUNGAL AGENTS. *Flucytosine* (5 fluorocytosine, 5-FC) is an antifungal antimetabolite most commonly used in combination with amphotericin B to treat systemic mycoses in humans. When dictated by in vitro susceptibility testing, flucytosine may be formulated for topical use in the equine eye by dissolving contents of oral capsules in sterile water to form a 1% solution. *Silver sulfadiazine* is a bactericidal dermatologic cream used to treat human burn patients. It also has antifungal properties and has been reported to be safe and effective for treatment of human keratomycosis (Mohan et al. 1988). Silver sulfadiazine has also been used to treat equine keratomycoses; it is well tolerated and appears to be effective. Lower cost and ready availability are the primary reasons for its use as an antifungal agent for treatment of equine eyes. *Iodines,* organic solutions or 7% tincture, are used to treat infectious keratitis in horses. Although more irritating than organic iodine, 7% tincture penetrates the cornea more effectively and serves as a stimulus for fibrovascular infiltrates (Moore et al. 1995). However, iodine tincture must be applied with discretion, as it is capable of causing moderately severe epibulbar hyperemia and chemosis if it inadvertently contacts the conjunctiva.

Antiviral Agents. Antiviral agents applicable to treatment of animal eye disease may be categorized as pyrimidine nucleoside analogs, cytokines, or amino acid (lysine).

Pyrimidine nucleoside analogs include the antiviral drugs *idoxuridine, trifluridine, vidarabine,* and *acyclovir.* These drugs act by substitution reactions within the viral DNA molecule to render the virus ineffective. In veterinary ophthalmology, these antiviral agents are most commonly used for therapy of herpesvirus infections, especially feline herpesvirus 1 (FHV-1) conjunctivitis and keratitis. An in vitro study of FHV-1 sensitivity to a number of antiviral agents indicated the relative potency to be trifluridine > idoxuridine > vidarabine > acyclovir (Nasisse et al. 1989). Although clinical studies to corroborate these in vitro efficacy results are not available, anecdotal accounts indicate trifluridine is the drug of choice for treating feline herpesvirus ocular disease. However, because trifluridine is relatively expensive and available only as a topical solution, idoxuridine is often used as the initial therapy.

Historically, idoxuridine has been commercially available as an ointment or solution. However, it is currently unavailable commercially but may be specially compounded. Vidarabine, available commercially as an ophthalmic ointment, demonstrated some efficacy in Nasisse's in vitro herpesvirus study. Acyclovir, an effective drug for treatment of human patients suffering from herpesvirus infections, appears to have little in vitro efficacy against the FHV-1. *Valacyclovir,* given orally to experimental cats, causes toxicity characterized by bone marrow suppression and renal insufficiency (Nasisse et al. 1997).

When administering topical antiviral agents for ocular herpesvirus infections, solutions are applied every 2-4 hours the first day of therapy and then 4-5 times daily thereafter until clinical improvement is noted. Ointments should be applied a minimum of 4 times daily to be effective.

Interferons (IFNs) are cytokines produced by lymphoid cells and serve as the principal source of macrophage activation. As part of the natural immune system, IFNs offer potential for treating viral diseases. Preparations of recombinant human IFN-α (5-25 U/day) may be administered orally or topically to cats with FHV-1 infections; when given empirically in such cases, this treatment appears to reduce the severity of FHV-1 infections. Recombinant IFN-α has been administered orally in combination with topical antiviral agents in the management of feline herpesvirus ocular disease (Stiles 1995); however, beneficial effects could not be documented.

The amino acid L-lysine, given orally at a dose of 250 mg/day, has been suggested as adjunctive treatment for persistent or severe feline herpesvirus ocular infections (Collins et al. 1995). An in vitro increase in the lysine/arginine ratio reduces herpesvirus replication.

Antiparasiticides. Thelaziasis is a common ocular parasitic condition of large domestic herbivores. Avermectins have been demonstrated to be effective in eliminating organisms from the eye. In experimentally infected cattle, a single dose of ivermectin was 100% effective in eliminating *Thelazia skrjabini* (Kennedy 1992). In a similar study, doramectin was highly effective in treating two *Thelazia* spp., *T. skrjabini* and *T. gulosa* (Kennedy and Phillips 1993). Each drug was administered subcutaneously at a dosage of 200 μg/kg. Ivermectin was also effective against *T. rhodesii* (Soll et al. 1992). Lyons et al. found that oral levamisole was effective against *T. skrjabini* and *T. gulosa;* however, the injectable formulation was not effective against *T. skrjabini* (Lyons et al. 1981).

AUTONOMIC OCULAR PHARMACOLOGIC RESPONSES

Cholinergic Responses. Parasympathomimetic, or cholinergic, agents work either by mimicking endogenous acetylcholine or by binding acetylcholine esterase, which allows endogenous acetylcholine to accumulate and to stimulate cholinoreceptive sites. Therefore, cholinergic agents are divided into direct-acting agents and indirect-acting agents (cholinesterase inhibitors).

Whether direct or indirect acting, the ocular effects of cholinergic stimulation are increased tearing, miosis, and reduction of intraocular pressure (IOP). These effects result from stimulation of lacrimal glands, iris sphincter muscle, and ciliary body muscles, respectively. Additional ocular effects are vasodilation and increased capillary permeability of iris and ciliary vessels with resultant increase in permeability of the blood-aqueous barrier. Myopia (nearsightedness) may be induced or augmented by cholinergic drugs.

Reduction of IOP by parasympathomimetics occurs primarily by decreasing resistance to the outflow of aqueous humor. Constriction of the pupil (miosis), which may be observed after parasympathetic stimulation, is not directly responsible for the observed drop in IOP. Stimulated contraction of ciliary body musculature opens the drainage spaces and thereby reduces resistance to the outflow of aqueous humor.

In veterinary ophthalmology cholinergic agents have been used primarily to lower IOP in animals with glaucoma. Pharmacologic testing of pupillomotor deficits and stimulation of aqueous tear production in cases of deficiency of the preocular tear film (KCS) are other ocular indications for parasympathomimetic agents.

Adrenergic Responses. Ocular effects of adrenergic stimulation are mydriasis, retraction of the third eyelid, and orbital smooth muscle activity resulting in slight exophthalmos. Interestingly, drugs that either stimulate or block the sympathetic innervation to the eye may lower IOP. Although adrenergic mechanisms for modulating IOP are only partially understood, adrenergic drugs have been demonstrated to reduce aqueous humor secretion, increase the outflow facility, or, with some agents, produce both effects. Therefore, these agents are commonly used to treat glaucoma in small companion animals.

An enzyme system within the ciliary epithelium is one site of action of adrenergic agents on IOP. The mechanism involves ciliary epithelial adenylate cyclase, which regulates the formation of the intracellular messenger cyclic adenosine monophosphate (cAMP). Increased cAMP production results in increased aqueous humor production. Activation of β receptors stimulates cAMP production, whereas α_2-adrenergic receptor activation inhibits the synthesis of cAMP. Therefore, either a β blocker or an α_2 agonist will diminish cAMP production, resulting in reduced aqueous flow.

TOPICAL HYPOTENSIVE AGENTS

Cholinergic Drugs

DIRECT-ACTING PARASYMPATHOMIMETICS. *Pilocarpine,* the prototype direct-acting parasympathomimetic agent, is commercially available in topical ophthalmic preparation strengths of 0.5-8.0%. In small-animal patients, 1% or 2% solutions are most commonly prescribed. Vehicles for delivering pilocarpine to the eye include methylcellulose, polyvinyl alcohol, high-viscosity acrylic gels, and extended-delivery ocular inserts. A single dose of topical pilocarpine will reduce IOP 30-40% for 6 hours in normotensive Beagles (Gwin et al. 1977). A greater response is noted in glaucomatous eyes. The observed response is independent of the concentration of the pilocarpine. Pilocarpine will induce miosis within 10-15 minutes and last for 6-8 hours. A single administration of 4% pilocarpine gel reduces IOP in dogs for 24 hours (Carrier and Gum 1989).

Effects of topical 2% pilocarpine have been studied in normotensive feline eyes (Wilkie and Latimer 1991c). A single dose of 2% pilocarpine resulted in reduced IOP in the treated eye and the untreated fellow eye. Effects on IOP were noted 4 hours after instillation, with 15% reduction in the treated eye and 9% in the untreated fellow eye. Pupil size was also reduced in both eyes, with a greater effect in the treated eye. Pupillary effects of pilocarpine in horses are minimal compared to dogs (van der Woerdt et al. 1998). The same equine study reported slightly elevated IOPs in animals treated with topical pilocarpine, suggesting a depressant effect on uveoscleral outflow in the horse.

Topical pilocarpine is synergistic with adrenergic agents, carbonic anhydrase inhibitors, and systemic hyperosmotic agents. Pilocarpine may cause local irritation within a few minutes after topical administration. The reaction is characterized by local conjunctival hyperemia, epiphora, third-eyelid protrusion, and blepharospasm. Curiously, this appears to be more severe during the first 72 hours of treatment. Ocular side effects of direct-acting parasympathomimetics are conjunctival vasodilation, miosis, and ciliary spasm. Systemic side effects include salivation, bronchospasm, cardiac arrhythmia, syncope, vomiting, and diarrhea.

INDIRECT-ACTING PARASYMPATHOMIMETICS (CHOLINESTERASE INHIBITORS). Two potent organophosphate compounds are available for ophthalmic use: *isoflurophate* and *echothiophate.* A single instillation of either of these solutions into the eye may result in reduction of IOP and miosis which last for several days. Isoflurophate is available as either a 0.125% or 0.25% solution. Echothiophate iodide may be reconstituted and used as a 0.03%, 0.06%, 0.125%, or 0.25% solution. Although data from use of these agents in dogs are limited, topical instillation of 1 drop of either of these drugs every 12-48 hours has been recommended for maintenance therapy of primary canine glaucoma. An adaptation phenomenon has been reported in dogs receiving echothiophate whereby a diminished response occurs with chronic use. This adaptation may explain recurrences in apparently well-controlled glaucoma cases.

Demecarium bromide is a carbamate inhibitor that affects the eye for 12-48 hours. Demecarium bromide is available commercially as 0.125% and 0.25% solutions. In human patients a single instillation results in a significant reduction of IOP for up to 3 days. In normotensive and glaucomatous Beagles, a single dose of demecarium bromide induced miosis and a significant decrease in IOP and was comparable in its effects to echothiophate iodide (Gum et al. 1993).

Indirect-acting parasympathomimetics may cause irritation when instilled into the eye. Spasms of ocular smooth muscles may occur, resulting in intense miosis and ciliary spasm. Ophthalmic organophosphates should not be used concurrently with topical or systemic organophosphate parasiticide drugs, because systemic toxicity may result. Systemic side effects of cholinesterase inhibitors include salivation, vomiting, diarrhea, and abdominal cramps. Following long-term use of indirect-acting parasympathomimetic ophthalmic agents in human patients, ocular side effects include cataracts, iris cysts, disrupted blood-aqueous barrier, and retinal separation.

Adrenergic Drugs

ADRENERGIC AGONISTS. *Epinephrine,* an α- and β-adrenergic agonist, both reduces the production of aqueous humor (early effect) and increases the outflow facility (prolonged effect). Reduced aqueous production results from α_2-receptor stimulation and reduced intracellular cAMP (Erickson et al. 1994). The α-receptor effect also causes vasoconstriction of ciliary vessels. The effect on outflow has been associated with an increase in aqueous cAMP, probably a β-mediated effect.

Epinephrine is used clinically as a 1% or 2% solution which may be used concurrently with other hypotensive agents such as pilocarpine, timolol, and carbonic anhydrase inhibitors. Ocular side effects of epinephrine include formation of rust-colored deposits on the cornea, conjunctiva, and eyelids, and mydriasis. Rust discoloration and facial tear staining is due to accumulation of adrenochrome pigment, an oxidative product of epinephrine. Systemic cardiovascular effects reported in human patients after topical administration of epinephrine include arrhythmias, tachycardia, and hypertension.

Dipivefrin hydrochloride is an epinephrine prodrug produced by the addition of two pivalic acid groups to the parent epinephrine molecule. This configuration results in increased lipophilicity of the dipivefrin molecule, allowing it to penetrate the cornea more readily. Once absorbed, dipivefrin is converted by tissue esterases to epinephrine, which produces the observed hypotensive effects. In Beagle dogs, topical 0.5% dipivefrin has hypotensive and mydriatic effects similar to those of 2% epinephrine (Gwin et al. 1978). Topical administration of the 0.5% solution will cause local irritation, mild conjunctivitis, and tearing in some animals.

Dipivefrin is commercially prepared as a 0.1% topical solution. Twice-daily administration of 0.1% dipivefrin in human patients produces hypotensive effects equivalent to those of 4-times-daily topical 2% pilocarpine. Infrequent ocular side effects in humans include slight discomfort (burning or stinging), mild mydriasis, and rare allergic reactions.

Apraclonidine hydrochloride, a clonidine derivative, is an α agonist approved for use in human patients prior to laser iridotomy and laser trabeculoplasty to prevent postoperative rises in IOP (Brown et al. 1988). Apraclonidine reduces IOP by reducing aqueous humor formation (Gharagozloo et al. 1988). Although the mechanism by which it decreases aqueous humor production is presumably through α_2-receptor agonist activity, the precise mechanism is unknown. Vasoconstriction of afferent arterioles supplying the ciliary body may also contribute to its hypotensive effect. Ocular side effects of apraclonidine in human patients are infrequent but include conjunctival blanching, upper eyelid elevation, mydriasis, and allergic responses.

Effects of topical administration of 0.5% apraclonidine have been studied in clinically normal dogs and cats. In cats, apraclonidine reduced IOP, pupil size, and resting heart rate while causing miosis (Miller and Rhaesa 1996). By contrast, this drug resulted in mydriasis in dogs while also lowering IOP and exhibiting less predictable depressant effects on heart rate (Miller et al. 1996). No information is currently available on the efficacy or safety of apraclonidine in treating spontaneous glaucomas of animal patients.

Brimonidine is an α_2-adrenergic receptor agonist that reduces intraocular pressure probably both by reducing aqueous humor production and by increasing uveoscleral outflow. In human patients, the recommended dose is one drop 3 times daily, whereby the ocular hypotensive effects are generally equivalent to those of timolol. Local ocular irritation is the most common side effect and occurs in 3-9% of human patients receiving this drug. Fatigue or drowsiness has also been reported.

ADRENERGIC ANTAGONISTS. Beta-blocking agents effectively lower IOP in human and animal glaucoma patients. There are a number of β-blocking drugs approved for human antiglaucoma therapy, including *timolol, betaxolol, carteolol, metipranolol,* and *levobunolol.* In veterinary medicine timolol is the most widely used ophthalmic β-blocking agent, blocking both β_1 and β_2 receptors. Two concentrations are available, 0.25% and 0.50% solutions. Experimentally in rabbits, cats, and dogs, timolol produces a relatively short duration, dose-dependent lowering of the IOP (Potter 1981; Svec and Strosberg 1986). In multiple-dose studies in glaucomatous Beagles, timolol significantly reduced IOP, with increasing concentrations yielding more profound reduction in IOP (Gum et al. 1991).

Timolol is used to treat both primary and secondary glaucomas. Timolol reduces IOP by inhibiting aqueous humor formation rather than by any effects on aqueous humor outflow. The β-blocking effect diminishes cAMP production and thereby reduces aqueous humor formation. In experiments performed in rabbits, timolol also reduced the blood flow to the ciliary body, which resulted in a decrease in aqueous humor production (Watanabe and Chiou 1983). In humans, the acute effect of timolol on aqueous humor production diminishes when the drug is used chronically. The mechanism of adaptation in the chronically β-blocked eye is unclear. The hypotensive effects of timolol are additive with parasympathomimetic and carbonic anhydrase inhibitors.

Effects of topical administration of a single dose of timolol maleate on IOP and pupil diameter were evaluated in normal cats (Wilkie and Latimer 1991b).

Topical treatment with 0.5% timolol resulted in reduction of IOP in treated and nontreated fellow eyes and reduced pupil diameter in only the treated eye. When this experiment was performed in dogs, similar effects on IOPs were found in that both treated and nontreated eyes had reduced IOP (Wilkie and Latimer 1991a). In both cats and dogs the treated eye had a greater reduction of IOP than the untreated eye. In dogs, both treated and untreated eyes had reduced pupil diameter, with the treated eye being more miotic. In Beagles with glaucoma, Gelatt et al. (1995) demonstrated that 4% and 6% timolol reduced IOP to a greater extent when combined with 2% pilocarpine. In this study, a 10% decrease in mean heart rate was found.

Topical timolol is generally well tolerated in small companion animals but may cause systemic side effects in patients with preexisting cardiovascular, respiratory, or metabolic disease. Bradycardia, arrhythmias, hypotension, and cardiac arrest have been reported in humans. In human patients with preexisting bronchospasms, dyspnea and respiratory failure have occurred. Timolol may also mask signs of hypoglycemia associated with diabetes mellitus and certain clinical signs of hyperthyroidism, such as tachycardia. In patients exhibiting side effects, use of a selective blocking agent, e.g., betaxolol, will minimize cardiopulmonary effects.

MYDRIATIC/CYCLOPLEGIC AGENTS. The two mechanisms by which drugs produce pupillary dilation are (1) paralysis of the iris sphincter muscle and (2) stimulation of the dilator muscle of the iris. Cholinergic antagonists paralyze iris and ciliary muscles by inhibiting the action of acetylcholine. Adrenergic agonists stimulate the dilator muscle by mimicking the action of norepinephrine. Adrenergic drugs have no appreciable affect on the ciliary muscle.

Ophthalmic uses of these drugs include mydriasis for complete lens and fundus examination, treatment of anterior uveitis, preoperative and postoperative management of intraocular surgical cases, and diagnosis of autonomic dysfunction, such as Horner's syndrome. Cholinergic antagonists are contraindicated for most types of glaucoma.

Cholinergic Antagonists. *Atropine,* a naturally occurring alkaloid, is a potent anticholinergic mydriatic/cycloplegic agent. Mydriasis accompanied by cycloplegia is desirable for treatment of anterior segment inflammation. In cases of ulcerative keratitis or anterior uveitis, intraocular pain is attributable to ciliary spasm. In cases of iridocyclitis, in addition to the cycloplegic effects which reduce the signs of ocular pain (e.g., squinting, tearing, and photophobia), mydriasis decreases the sequelae of posterior synechiae. Atropine is available in strengths of 0.25-5.0% as sterile ophthalmic solutions or 0.5 and 1.0% ophthalmic ointments. Concentrations of 0.5-2.0% are commonly used clinically, with 1% being the most widely used. Following instillation of 1% atropine in normal animal eyes, mydriasis is maximal within 1 hour and may last for several days.

Atropine is the mydriatic/cycloplegic agent of choice for treating anterior uveitis. When severe anterior uveitis is present, it may initially be necessary to instill atropine 4-6 times daily to induce mydriasis. Once pupil dilation is achieved, the frequency is reduced to the minimum frequency necessary for maintenance of moderate mydriasis. Because of its relatively long duration of action, atropine is not usually the mydriatic drug chosen for routine ophthalmic examinations.

Topical atropine will increase IOP, and therefore, its use is contraindicated in hypertensive eyes. Atropine must be used with caution in chronically inflamed eyes that may have volatile IOPs because of synechiae or inflammatory infiltrates. For this reason, monitoring IOP is important in eyes being treated long term with atropine. Aqueous tear secretions are reduced with atropine administration, and topical atropine may exacerbate signs of marginal tear deficiency, precipitating acute KCS. Therefore, it is prudent to periodically measure Schirmer tear values during the course of topical atropine therapy. Systemic absorption of topically applied atropine may occur and can cause reduced gastrointestinal motility and tachycardia. Because of the bitter taste of the alkaloid following nasolacrimal drainage of tear fluid, salivation may be noted immediately after administering atropine topically.

Tropicamide is a short-acting cholinergic antagonist that has a greater mydriatic than cycloplegic effect. It is the drug of choice for diagnostic procedures such as slit-lamp biomicroscopy of the lens and funduscopic examination. Within 20 minutes of topical application of tropicamide, mydriasis is achieved. Following dilation with tropicamide, the pupil returns to normal size within 4-6 hours. In normal canine eyes, one or two doses of topical 1% tropicamide do not significantly affect IOP. Salivation following topical administration is uncommon in dogs but is occasionally seen in cats.

Cyclopentolate, another anticholinergic drug, has an onset of action and duration intermediate between tropicamide and atropine. Cyclopentolate has stronger cycloplegic action than does tropicamide. Maximal mydriasis and cycloplegia usually occur within 30-45 minutes following instillation. While complete recovery from mydriasis may take several days, recovery from cycloplegia takes 6-24 hours. Cyclopentolate is available in 0.5 and 1.0% solutions. Following topical administration, slight irritation may occur and manifest as mild chemosis and conjunctival hyperemia.

Adrenergic Agonists. *Phenylephrine* is a potent α-adrenergic stimulant with little β-receptor activity. A 10% ophthalmic solution is most commonly used clinically for its mydriatic effect. In dogs, maximal mydriasis occurs within 2 hours and lasts up to 18 hours. Phenylephrine has a weaker mydriatic effect than cholinergic antagonists. The efficacy of phenylephrine as a mydriatic in horses has been questioned (Hacker et al. 1987). It has been used as an adjunct to atropine therapy in cases of anterior uveitis with severe miosis. In cats, phenylephrine is ineffective by itself as a mydriatic agent.

Phenylephrine is used in the diagnosis of sympathetic denervation syndromes, e.g., Horner's syndrome, whereby an affected eye exhibits a denervation hypersensitivity due to functional destruction of postganglionic sympathetic neurons. In such cases, instillation of low concentrations of phenylephrine, such as 0.1-1.0%, will stimulate pupillary dilation. In cases of conjunctival hyperemia, topical phenylephrine causes blanching of conjunctival vessels and, therefore, may be used to differentiate between conjunctivitis and uveitis. In cases of sympathetic denervation, application of phenylephrine will result in symptomatic improvement by stimulating retraction of the third eyelid. Repeated administration of 10% phenylephrine to an eye may cause conjunctival irritation and corneal epithelial damage.

Topical ophthalmic *epinephrine,* used mainly as an antiglaucoma agent, has limited clinical application as a mydriatic in animals. Similar to phenylephrine, dilute epinephrine (0.10-0.01% solution) will result in mydriasis in cases of Horner's syndrome. A positive response confirms a postganglionic lesion of the sympathetic neuron. Concentrations of epinephrine normally used to treat glaucoma (1-2% solutions) produce moderate mydriasis in dogs given a single dose but have no apparent effects in cats. During intraocular surgery, intracameral solutions of 0.01% epinephrine aid in maintaining mydriasis and controlling minor bleeding. Intracameral epinephrine solution should not be used with halothane anesthesia.

Adrenergic Antagonist (Mydriasis Reversal). *Dapiprazole* is a recently synthesized α-adrenolytic agent which produces miosis by blocking the α receptors of the dilator muscle of the iris. Dapiprazole has been used to reverse the effects of diagnostic mydriatics. A topical solution containing 0.5% dapiprazole has been demonstrated to safely and effectively reverse mydriasis induced by 1% tropicamide and 2.5% phenylephrine in human patients (Allinson et al. 1990). Although dapiprazole caused short-term conjunctival vascular injection in some patients, no effects on IOP, visual acuity, blood pressure, or heart rate were noted (Allinson et al. 1990).

Contraindications and Cautions with Use of Topical Autonomic Agents. *Miotics* are contraindicated when constriction of the pupil is undesirable, such as with acute iritis or anterior lens luxations. In inflamed eyes, cholinergic agents may exacerbate signs of inflammation. Indirect-acting cholinergic drugs should not be used concurrently with topical or systemically administered organophosphates.

Adrenergic agents must be used cautiously in patients with cardiac arrhythmias. Timolol is contraindicated when bradycardia or hypotension is present or in patients with bronchospasm. Timolol should be used cautiously in cases with metabolic disease, such as diabetes mellitus or hyperthyroidism. Epinephrine or propine should not be used in animals with tachycardia or hypertension.

Anticholinergic *mydriatic drugs,* e.g., atropine, should not be used in instances where the IOP is elevated. Topical atropine will exacerbate aqueous tear deficiency and is, therefore, contraindicated in cases of KCS. Systemic absorption of topically administered atropine may potentiate preexisting gastrointestinal hypomotility and result in gut stasis, particularly in horses.

NONAUTONOMIC HYPOTENSIVE AGENTS

Carbonic Anhydrase Inhibition. Carbonic anhydrase, present in both pigmented and nonpigmented layers of the ciliary epithelium, is an enzyme essential to the production of aqueous humor. The reversible carbonic anhydrase reaction produces bicarbonate, which binds to sodium and results in the secretion of both ions into the posterior chamber. Sodium molecules osmotically attract water from the vessels of the ciliary stroma, contributing to aqueous humor formation. Carbonic anhydrase inhibitor (CAI) diuretics suppress bicarbonate formation by ciliary epithelium and, therefore, prevent transport of sodium from ciliary stroma to aqueous humor. The net effect of CAI administration is lowering of the IOP. Systemic acidosis induced by CAIs may also inhibit aqueous humor formation and enhance the pressure-lowering effect of these drugs.

For additive hypotensive effects in managing primary or secondary glaucomas, CAIs are usually administered in combination with other agents. CAIs may be used both for short-term treatment to control acute increases in IOP and for long-term therapy of chronic glaucoma. Reduced response to CAI drugs may occur with prolonged use. In some cases systemic side effects, such as metabolic acidosis, gastrointestinal signs, panting, hypokalemia, and behavioral changes, may limit the use of these agents. Therefore, dosage alterations or changes in combination therapy may be needed in the course of glaucoma treatment.

Selection of a systemic CAI diuretic is based on familiarity with a given product, relative side effects, individual patient tolerance, and cost. *Acetazolamide,* a first-generation CAI, is available in oral and injectable forms. An intravenous dose of 5-10 mg/kg is recommended for emergency treatment of acute glaucoma. Oral dosage forms include 125 mg and 500 mg tablets and 500 mg time-released capsules. A dose of 10-25 mg/kg 2-3 times daily is the usual dose for canine glaucoma. In glaucomatous Beagles the effect of a single dose of acetazolamide lasts 8 hours. In cats the hypotensive effect of a single dose lasts about 5 hours.

Although acetazolamide is the least expensive of the CAI drugs, adverse side effects are common, especially when used long term. *Ethoxyzolamide* has essentially the same mechanisms of action, therapeutic activity, and side effects as acetazolamide. For prolonged treatment of glaucoma in small animals *dichlorphenamide* or *methazolamide* is preferred over acetazolamide or ethoxyzolamide because of reduced side effects. Dichlorphenamide presently is not commercially available. Methazolamide is available only as 50 mg tablets; the oral dose for dogs is 2.0-10.0 mg/kg 2-3 times daily.

Topical CAIs, such as the sulfonamide derivative *dorzolamide,* have been developed to minimize or eliminate systemic complications (Maren et al. 1997). Dorzolamide was evaluated for its ocular hypotensive activity in normotensive and glaucomatous Beagles (King et al. 1992). Single administrations of 2% and 4% solutions significantly lowered IOP in eyes of normotensive and glaucomatous Beagles. In multiple-dose studies using topical 2% dorzolamide, IOP was significantly decreased in normotensive and glaucomatous Beagles, with the maximal effect observed by day 4. Topical administration of dorzolamide also reduces IOP in normotensive rabbits and in rabbits with α-chymotrypsin-induced ocular hypertension (Sugrue et al. 1988). Eyes of cynomolgus monkeys with laser-induced ocular hypertension also responded with reduction of IOP following dorzolamide treatment (Wang et al. 1990). Topical 2% dorzolamide, which significantly lowers IOP and aqueous humor flow rate in normal dogs, can be considered for three times per day use in the medical management of canine glaucoma (Cawrse et al. 1999).

Furosemide, a diuretic that works through a different mechanism of action, is *not* effective in reducing IOP.

Osmotic Agents. Systemic osmotic (or hyperosmotic) agents (1) reduce the rate of plasma ultrafiltration within ciliary blood vessels, thereby inhibiting aqueous humor formation, and (2) produce osmotic gradients that stimulate diffusion of water from the intraocular fluids into the plasma, causing reduction of vitreous volume. In addition shrinkage of the vitreous allows the lens to move posteriorly and the iridocorneal angle to open for better drainage. The result of these combined effects is to reduce the IOP.

Osmotic agents are most often used for rapid reduction of IOP following an episode of acute pressure increase. *Mannitol,* a 6-carbon sugar, is the most rapidly acting of the osmotic agents and is excreted in the urine unmetabolized. Given intravenously at a dose of 1-2 g/kg at a rate of 1 mL/kg/min, mannitol will reduce IOP in 30 minutes in dogs (Lorimer et al. 1989). The maximal hypotensive effect with mannitol occurs in 90 minutes, with a declining effect over a period of 6 hours.

Mannitol administration enhances retinal adhesive force in rabbits possibly by increasing the viscosity of the interphotoreceptor matrix and/or increased retinal pigment epithelium permeability with enhanced outward flow of subretinal fluid (Kita and Marmor 1991). Therefore, mannitol may have clinical applications in the prevention or management of retinal detachments.

Glycerin (or glycerol) is a trihydric alcohol rapidly absorbed from the gastrointestinal tract after oral administration. Glycerin is available in flavored commercial preparations of 50% or as 95% Glycerin, USP. The dose of glycerin is 1-2 g/kg given directly by mouth or in the food. Palatability of Glycerin, USP, may be improved by mixing with milk or syrup. The ocular hypotensive effect of glycerin starts within 1 hour and lasts up to 10 hours in dogs (Lorimer et al. 1989). Because glycerin is metabolized readily into glucose, it may cause hyperglycemia and glycosuria. Glycerin is a less potent osmotic agent than mannitol because it is metabolized, whereas mannitol is excreted unaltered. Vomition may occur following administration, contributing to variable and unpredictable effects.

Isosorbide, a dihydric alcohol, is available as a 50% oral preparation. Although similar to glycerin in dosage and hypotensive effect, isosorbide is not metabolized and does not cause hyperglycemia. A canine dose of 1.5 g/kg has been recommended; however, its efficacy has not been documented in the dog (Dugan et al. 1989).

Following dosing with an osmotic agent, water is usually withheld for 4-6 hours to allow the maximal hyperosmotic effect.

Prostaglandin and Prostaglandin Analogs. *Latanoprost,* a prostaglandin $F_{2\alpha}$ analog, is believed to reduce the intraocular pressure by increasing the outflow of aqueous humor. Studies in humans and animals suggest the main mechanism of action is increased uveoscleral outflow (Toris et al. 1993). As one of the newer ocular hypotensive agents, latanoprost is prescribed for human patients because of its unique pharmacologic effects, its once-daily administration, and its lack of significant cardiovascular effects. Local ocular irritation is the most common immediate side effect. Latanoprost may gradually change iris color when used for several months or years by increasing the number of melanosomes in iris melanocytes, resulting in permanent iridal color changes. Besides altering ocular appearance, the consequence of this change is currently unknown. Prostaglandin $F_{2\alpha}$ injected into the anterior chamber of normal dogs has a potent miotic effect and results in a significant breakdown of the blood-aqueous barrier (Dziezyc et al. 1992).

Ethacrynic Acid. Originally developed as a diuretic, ethacrynic acid is a sulhydryl reactive drug that results in increased outflow facility in mammalian eyes. Topical ethacrynic acid, used as a 1.5% ophthalmic ointment, reduced IOP 22% in normotensive monkeys with a 40% increase in outflow facility (Croft and Kaufman 1995). Side effects include conjunctival hyperemia and eyelid and corneal edema. Ethacrynic acid merits further investigation particularly as a potential treatment for spontaneous canine glaucomas.

Contraindications and Cautions with Systemic Hypotensive Agents. *Systemic carbonic anhydrous inhibitors* are contraindicated in patients with respiratory or metabolic acidosis and must be used with caution in animals with cardiovascular or renal disease.

Osmotic agents are contraindicated in patients with cardiopulmonary disease, preexisting dehydration, or anuric renal failure. The use of mannitol prior to methoxyflurane anesthesia is discouraged (Brock et al. 1985). Mannitol should be used cautiously in patients with head trauma since leakage of mannitol into an area of subdural hemorrhage can exacerbate subdural hematoma. Glycerin may cause nausea and vomiting shortly after administration. Glycerin should be avoided in patients with diabetes mellitus.

TEAR SUBSTITUTES AND STIMULANTS

Lacrimostimulants

CYCLOSPORINE. Topically applied cyclosporine, a specific T-cell immunosuppressant, increases tearing, decreases mucopurulent conjunctivitis, and decreases corneal granulation in spontaneous cases of canine KCS (Kaswan et al. 1989). Topical 2% cyclosporine has been demonstrated to improve 75-82% of idiopathic (presumed immune-mediated) cases of KCS in dogs (Salisbury et al. 1990). When topically applied to the eyes of live rabbits, cyclosporine penetrates lacrimal glandular tissue (Kaswan et al. 1988). After exposure of early helper T cells to lacrimal gland antigens, cyclosporine blocks the T-cell response, preventing interleukin-2, IFN-γ, and other cytokines from being synthesized.

The marked lacrimomimetic effects of cyclosporine cannot be attributed solely to immunosuppression of overzealous immune mechanisms, because normal Beagle dogs treated with topical cyclosporine show an almost immediate increase in tear secretion (Kaswan et al. 1989). Furthermore, cyclosporine applied directly to ex vivo rat lacrimal glands enhances secretions. Cyclosporine has been demonstrated to regulate cell growth and differentiation by affecting cytosolic enzymes, calmodulin and cyclophilin. These enzymes regulate DNA transcription in response to interleukins and other cell surface activators. A natural ligand for cyclophilin, prolactin is found in lacrimal acini and may be an important tear regulator. Therefore, it has been hypothesized that cyclosporine, via cyclophilin, regulates prolactin receptors in lacrimal tissue (Russell et al. 1985; Kaswan et al. 1989).

Although cyclosporine causes tear secretion in dogs with KCS, a recurrence of the disease is noted promptly following cessation of cyclosporine treatment. In cases where one eye has clinical signs of KCS, both eyes are treated since subsequent involvement of the second eye is typical. Canine KCS is treated initially by administering topical 0.2-2% cyclosporine twice daily. Other symptomatic therapies, such as artificial tears, lubricant ointments, and topical antibiotics, are often used concurrently with topical cyclosporine. As improvement in lacrimation and reduction of clinical signs are observed, the concurrent symptomatic therapy is reduced or eliminated. This is usually possible over a period of 3-6 weeks. Reduction in the frequency of cyclosporine to 1 drop daily or 1 drop every other day may be possible in some cases exhibiting an optimal response.

Local irritation from 2% cyclosporine in oil was noted following initial use in the eyes of some dogs. Irritation observed in such cases may have been due to use of an unpurified olive oil vehicle. Purified olive oil and other purified vegetable oils, particularly corn oil, are well tolerated and have been used with very infrequent signs of ocular irritation. Although ocular irritation has occurred with spontaneous breakdown of oil vehicles that form oxidative products, irritation has not been attributed to the cyclosporine molecule.

Systemic toxicity of cyclosporine is dose dependent, with renal toxicity being the most common serious side effect. Renal toxicity has not been seen in dogs, despite extensive toxicity testing. No reports have indicated any ocular toxicity, in humans or experimental animals, related to systemic administration of cyclosporine. Application of 1 drop (50 μL) of 2% cyclosporine (20 mg/mL) to the eyes twice daily provides 200 μL (4 mg) per patient per day. In the event there was complete systemic absorption of ophthalmically administered cyclosporine, this would represent merely 1-2% of the recommended safe dose of systemically administered cyclosporine in a 50-100 kg human patient.

Cyclosporine is presently widely used for the treatment of KCS in dogs. A 0.2% cyclosporine ointment for canine use is commercially available. Compounding of higher concentrations (0.5–2.0%) is commonly done when 0.2% is not effective in increasing tear production.

PILOCARPINE. Secretions of the lacrimal glands may be increased by parasympathetic stimulation with topical or oral cholinergic agents. Pilocarpine has most commonly been used for this purpose. A positive response depends upon having functional lacrimal tissue present. Since the effectiveness of cyclosporine has been documented, pilocarpine is used less frequently than cyclosporine as a primary stimulant therapy for KCS.

Lacrimomimetics. Lacrimomimetics, also referred to as tear substitutes or artificial tears, may be divided into aqueous substitutes, mucinomimetics, and lipid replacements. Table 55.5 provides a list of commercially available tear substitute products.

AQUEOUS SOLUTIONS. *Methylcellulose* is a semisynthetic cellulose derivative in colloid form that is water soluble, viscous, and virtually inert. Methylcellulose is nonirritating to the eye and is compatible with most

TABLE 55.5—Tear substitutes

Product	Viscosity agents/ concentrations	Preservative	Source
Polyvinyl alcohol solutions			
AKWA Tears	PVA 1.40%	BAC, EDTA	Akorn
Artificial Tears	PVA 1.40%	BAC, EDTA	Generic (many)
Dry Eyes	PVA 1.40%	BAC, EDTA	Bausch & Lomb
Liquifilm Forte	PVA 3%	Thimerosal, EDTA	Allergan
Liquifilm Tears	PVA 1.40%	Chlorobutanol	Allergan
Ocu-tears PF	PVA 0.10%	None	Ocumed
Cellulose-based solutions			
Cellufresh	CMC 0.50%	None	Allergan
Celluvisc	CMC 1%	None	Allergan
Comfort Tears	HEC	BAC, EDTA	Barnes-Hinds
Isopto Alkaline	HPMC 1%	BAC, EDTA	Alcon
Isopto Tears Plain	HPMC 0.50%	BAC, EDTA	Alcon
Murocel	MC 1%	Methylparaben Propylparaben	Bausch & Lomb
Refresh plus	CMC 0.50%	None	Allergan
TearGard	HPMC 0.50%	Sorbic acid, EDTA	Med Tech
Tearisol	HPMC 0.50%	BAC, EDTA	Iolab
Polymer combinations			
Adsorbotear	HEC 0.40%, povidone 1.67%, Adsorbobase	Thimerosal, EDTA	Alcon
Aqua Site	PEG-400 0.20%, DEX 0.10%	EDTA	Ciba
Bion Tears	DEX 0.10%, HPMC 0.30%	None	Alcon
Hypotears	PVA 1%, HEC, DEX	BAC, EDTA	Iolab
Hypotears PF	PVA 1%, HEC, DEX 3.30%	EDTA	Iolab
Lacril	HPMC 0.50%, GEL 0.01%, PSB	Chlorobutanol	Allergan
Lubrifair Solution	DEX-70, HPMC	None	Pharmafair
Lubri Tears	HPMC 0.50%, DEX 0.10%	BAC, EDTA	Bausch & Lomb
Murine Eye Lubricant	PVA 1.40%, povidone 0.60%	BAC, EDTA	Ross
Moisture Drops	HPMC 0.50%, DEX 0.10%, povidone 0.10%, glycerin 0.20%	BAC, EDTA	Bausch & Lomb
Nature's Tears	HPMC 0.40%, DEX	BAC, EDTA	Rugby
Refresh	PVA 1.40%, povidone 0.60%	None	Allergan
Tears Naturale	HPMC 0.30%, DEX 0.10%	BAC, EDTA	Alcon
Tears Naturale II	HPMC 0.30%, DEX-70 0.10%	POLYQUAD, EDTA	Alcon
Tears Naturale Free	HPMC 0.30%, DEX 0.10%	None	Alcon
Tears Plus	PVA 1.40%, povidone 0.60%	Chlorobutanol	Allergan
Tears Renewed	HPMC 0.30%, DEX-70 0.10%	BAC, EDTA	Akorn
Vasoclastic products			
Hylashield	Hylan 0.15%	None	I-Med
Hylashield Nite	Hylan 0.40%	None	I-Med
Glycerin products			
Dry Eye Therapy	Glycerin 0.30%	None	Bausch & Lomb
Eye-Lube-A	Glycerin 0.25%	BAC, EDTA	Optoptics
Ointments			
AKWA Tears Ointment	White petrolatum, MO	None	Akorn
Dry Eyes	White petrolatum, MO	None	Bausch & Lomb
Duolube	White petrolatum 80%, MO 20%	None	Bausch & Lomb
Duratears Naturale	White petrolatum, lanolin, MO	None	Alcon
Hypo Tears	White petrolatum 85%, lanolin, MO 15%	None	Iolab
Lacri-Lube	White petrolatum 55%, lanolin, MO 41.50%	Chlorobutanol	Allergan
Lacri-Lube NP	White petrolatum 55%, lanolin, MO 42.50%	None	Allergan
Lacri-Lube S.O.P.	White petrolatum 55%, MO 41.50%, 2% nonionic lanolin derivatives	Chlorobutanol	Allergan
Lipotears	White petrolatum, MO	None	Coopervision
Lubri Tears	White petrolatum, lanolin, MO	Chlorobutanol	Bausch & Lomb
Ocutube	White petrolatum	Methylparaben	Ocumed
Paralube	White petrolatum, lanolin 2%, MO	None	Fourgera
Refresh PM	White petrolatum 56.80%, lanolin, MO 41.50%	None	Allergan

Note: Percentage composition given where information available.

BAC = benzalkonium chloride; CMC = carboxymethyl cellulose; DEX = dextran; EDTA = ethylenediaminetetraacetic acid; GEL = gelatin; HEC = hydroxyethyl cellulose; HPMC = hydroxypropyl methylcellulose; MC = methylcellulose; MO = mineral oil; PEG = polyethylene glycol; POLYQUAD = polyquaternium-1; PSB = polysorbate 80; PVA = polyvinyl alcohol.

drugs. It does not significantly delay healing of corneal epithelial wounds. *Polyvinyl alcohol* is a synthetic hydrophilic resin that is less viscous than methylcellulose but has good corneal adhesive properties. Available as a 1.4% solution, polyvinyl alcohol is the primary ingredient in a number of artificial tear products.

MUCINOMIMETICS. Linear polymers, such as dextran and polyvinylpyrrolidone, have mucomimetic properties. Patented polymers are often combined with buffered solutions of substituted cellulose esters to form preparations for treating deficiencies of aqueous and mucin components of the preocular tear film.

Viscoelastic substances that have mucinomimetic properties include sodium hyaluronate, chondroitin sulfate, and methylcellulose. Sodium hyaluronate is a naturally occurring, high-molecular-weight glycosaminoglycan that has excellent viscoelastic and lubricating properties. Sodium hyaluronate has been diluted with artificial tear to make a 0.04% solution that may be applied topically every 4 hours initially and then reduced to 2-4 times daily in treating eyes of patients with KCS (Schadler 1987). Treated eyes were markedly improved, although Schirmer tear test values were not improved with this treatment. A hyaluron-derivative viscoelastic tear supplement is available commercially in Canada as either a 0.15% or a 0.40% drop. This product has been particularly useful in managing severe cases of KCS in dogs. Chondroitin sulfate is a glycosaminoglycan polymer made up of disaccharide units. Chondroitin sulfate is not as viscous as sodium hyaluronate. Hydroxypropylmethylcellulose in concentrations of 1-2% has been proposed as a less expensive substitute for sodium hyaluronate and chondroitin sulfate.

LIPOPHILIC AGENTS. *Lanolin* and *petrolatum* are commonly used as bases for ophthalmic lubricant ointments. These ingredients mimic the function of naturally occurring meibomian lipids by preventing evaporation and preserving existing tears. Nonmedicated ophthalmic ointments containing lanolin and/or petrolatum are used to lubricate and protect eyes in instances where corneal exposure is a problem, i.e., during anesthesia and surgery or in cases of eyelid paresis or eyelid swelling. Lanolin and petrolatum vehicles provide prolonged corneal and conjunctival contact for other agents, such as corticosteroids and antibiotics.

MISCELLANEOUS AGENTS. A variety of therapeutic agents have recently been developed for ophthalmic use. Because these agents do not fit into established categories of ophthalmic pharmaceutical agents, they are discussed separately here.

Adhesives. *Cyanoacrylate* adhesives have the unique property of rapidly solidifying by anionic polymerization at room temperature without catalysts, solvents, or application of pressure. Corneal uses of tissue adhesive include sealing of perforations, covering epithelial erosions, and inhibiting progression of noninfectious stromal ulceration. Although cyanoacrylates have been shown to possess bactericidal properties, corneal infections may be masked by these adhesives (Cavanaugh and Gottsch 1991). Adverse effects of cyanoacrylates are related to rapid degradation rate and release of irritating breakdown products, such as formaldehyde. Local tissue toxicity may compromise the host's immune barriers, enhancing development of infections.

Aldose Reductase Inhibitors. Aldose reductase inhibitors, such as *sorbinil,* have been shown to prevent and reverse cataracts in galactosemic rats (Tsuju et al. 1990). However, effective use of aldose reductase inhibitors to prevent or reverse spontaneous cataracts in domestic animals has not been reported. Aldose reductase inhibition has been demonstrated to prevent retinal capillary basement membrane thickening in galactosemic rats, and therefore, use of inhibitor agents may prove to be beneficial in prevention of diabetic retinopathy (Das et al. 1990).

Anticoagulants. By activating antithrombin, *heparin* can minimize intraocular fibrin formation and the associated undesirable sequelae of synechiae, i.e., anterior capsular lens opacities and fibrin in the trabecular meshwork of the drainage angle. Heparin is frequently diluted to 2-5 U/mL in irrigating solutions used for intraocular procedures. Heparin has a half-life of 5 hours, and its action can be stopped by protamine sulfate. Aspirin and other nonsteroidal anti-inflammatory agents often used to treat uveitis in animals suppress the aggregation of platelets and reduce the adherence of platelets to the vascular wall, interfering with plug formation. Therefore, for patients receiving nonsteroidal anti-inflammatory therapy preoperatively, it may be prudent to discontinue administration several days prior to planned intraocular surgery (Moll et al. 1989).

Anticollagenases and Antiproteases. Because *N-acetylcysteine* has both anticollagenase and mucinolytic properties, it has been commonly used in veterinary ophthalmology to treat ulcerative keratitis and KCS. Excessive collagenase, produced by epithelial and stromal tissue, inflammatory cells, and ocular surface bacteria, is destructive to stromal collagen and can contribute to progressive ulceration and perforation. Acetylcysteine inhibits collagenase activity by chelating available free calcium cations essential for enzyme activation. Other agents used topically for their protease-inhibiting activity include cysteine, sodium ethylenediaminetetraacetic acid (Na-EDTA), heparin, and serum.

Denatured mucous harbors microorganisms and surface debris and loses it viscoelastic properties, becoming tenacious and inhibiting normal ocular cleansing and lubrication. Since free sulfhydryl groups reduce the viscosity of mucoproteins, increasing concentrations of acetylcysteine decrease the viscosity of mucus.

A dose-related effect of acetylcysteine on conjunctival mucus has been demonstrated (Thermes et al. 1991).

Ophthalmic solutions containing acetylcysteine can be stored at ambient temperatures without a decrease in efficacy (Costa and Slatter 1983). The anticollagenase activity of acetylcysteine is not affected by combining it with pilocarpine, atropine, gentamicin, and artificial tears. However, preparations combining chloramphenicol and acetylcysteine are less stable and show reduced anticollagenase activity (Costa and Slatter 1983). Frequent administration of acetylcysteine solutions can be irritating to the ocular surface, and a 20% concentration has caused superficial necrosis and cellular infiltration in rabbit conjunctiva and corneas (Thermes et al. 1991). A 5% acetylcysteine solution appears to be well tolerated in eyes of domestic species at frequencies not exceeding 4 times daily for several days.

Antifibrinolytics. Recurrent intraocular bleeding with associated hyphema may lead to secondary glaucoma, corneal staining, and lens opacities with subsequent loss of vision. Since uncontrolled IOP may occur after rebleeding, prevention of secondary hemorrhage becomes a primary concern in managing patients with hyphema. The antifibrinolytic agents *tranexamic acid* and *epsilonaminocaproic acid,* which competitively inhibit factors promoting clot lysis, have been used effectively in human patients to reduce the rate of secondary hemorrhage (Gottsch 1990). The human dose of aminocaproic acid is 50 mg/kg every 4-5 hours for 5 days, with the total dose not exceeding 30 g/day. Aminocaproic acid is contraindicated in patients with blood dyscrasias or clotting disorders. Effective use of either tranexamic or aminocaproic acid in recurrent hyphemas in domestic animal species has not been reported.

Antiproliferative Agents. Antiproliferative agents have been used in human ophthalmic surgery to reduce the amount of scarring associated with glaucoma-filtration surgery (Lee 1994). Subconjunctival fibroplasia has been recognized as a major limiting factor in the success of glaucoma filtration surgery. Results from rabbit studies indicate that *5-fluorouracil* (5-FU) or *mitomycin C* (MMC), given as a single subconjunctival dose, will prolong the effectiveness of filtration surgery (Khaw et al. 1993). Filtration bleb survival times were greater for eyes treated with MMC than for those treated with 5-FU. The potential usefulness and applicability of MMC to filtration surgery in dogs were investigated by Glover et al. (1995). Results of this study in clinically normal dogs indicated that MMC suppresses but does not prevent fibrosis around silicone filtering implants. Damji evaluated the response of subconjunctival fibroblasts to a variety of antiproliferative agents (Damji et al. 1990). The agents tested (in order of decreasing potency), using an in vitro wound assay, were cytosine arabinoside, doxorubicin, colchicine, 5-FU, cytochalasin B, cyclosporine, 6-mercaptopurine, and dexamethasone. Colchicine and cytochalasin B were effective in arresting wound closure at doses well below those documented to produce ocular toxicity. Antiprotease agents and methotrexate were not effective in suppressing fibroplasia.

Enzymes. Glycosaminoglycans within the iridocorneal angle appear to play a role in regulation of aqueous humor outflow. Therefore, the IOP-altering effects of testicular *hyaluronidase,* which degrades hyaluronic acid and some chondroitin sulfates, has been tested. Hyaluronidase has been shown to increase aqueous humor outflow when injected into the anterior chamber of the eyes of several animal species. Although hyaluronidase is effective in decreasing resistance to aqueous outflow in normotensive canine eyes, it did not affect aqueous humor outflow rates in eyes of glaucomatous Beagle dogs (Gum et al. 1992), suggesting that the glycosaminoglycan moieties may change or form conjugates in glaucomatous eyes that resist enzymatic degradation.

Fibrinolytics. Breakdown of the blood-aqueous barrier following ocular surgery, trauma, or inflammation can result in intraocular fibrin formation, causing vision-threatening complications. Injection of the fibrinolytic agent *tissue plasminogen activator* (tPA) is advocated for treatment of intraocular fibrin to prevent severe consequences. Tissue plasminogen activator forms a complex with fibrin and activates plasminogen into plasmin, which then lyses fibrin, fibrinogen, and other procoagulant proteins into soluble degradation products. Recombinant tPA is effective in lysing intraocular fibrin with minimal complications. Since the plasma half-life of tPA is very short and very low concentrations of tPA are necessary for intraocular fibrinolysis, there is virtually no risk of systemic plasminogen activation.

In a study using experimental dogs, a mean decrease of greater than 90% of the clot size was detected 2 hours after a single intracameral injection with 0.01 mL of 25 μg/100 μL tPA (Gerding et al. 1992b). In normal dogs, adverse effects were not detected on either corneal endothelium or on intraocular pressure following intracameral injection of 25 μg/100 μL tPA (Gerding et al. 1992a). Intraocular activity of topically administered tPA (5 mg/mL) was evaluated using an enzyme substrate-based microassay (Gerding and Eurell 1993). Single and multiple topical doses of tPA entered the canine eye and were enzymatically active. Repeated administration (3 doses at 10 min intervals) of 50 μL of tPA (5 mg/mL) resulted in a 1.5-fold increase in activity compared to the single-dose administration. Subconjunctival delivery of 0.4 mL of tPA (1 mg/mL and 10 mg/mL) has also been reported experimentally in rabbits (Lim et al. 1993), with the average aqueous tPA concentration being similar to that found after topical tPA delivery. Martin et al. (1993) reported that tPA (25 μg/100 μL) injected into the anterior chamber of animals with aqueous fibrin clots was effective in lysing clots when given within 1-3 days of fibrin formation.

Fibronectin. Fibronectin is a ubiquitous glycoprotein found in plasma, extracellular tissue matrices, and basement membranes. Many different cell types have been shown to produce fibronectin, including epithelium, fibroblasts, macrophages, and vascular endothelium. Fibronectin is a substrate for plasmin and plasminogen activators and functions in mobilization, migration, and cell-to-substratum adhesion for a variety of cells, including corneal epithelium. Although fibronectin has generated considerable interest as a possible therapeutic agent for treatment of corneal epithelial erosions, its efficacy in treating this disorder has been equivocal (Suzuki et al. 1989).

Growth Stimulants. Epidermal growth factor (EGF) acts through specific cell surface receptors to exert a potent mitogenic effect on cells. Addition of EGF to growing cultures of rabbit corneal endothelial cells induces cell division and a dose-dependent shape change (spindle rather than polygonal). EGF also stimulates the cells to be highly motile and unusually elongated (Joyce and Neufeld 1990). The precise role of EGF in the normal healing process has yet to be established. In rabbits with full-thickness corneal wounds, significant wound strength enhancement was demonstrated following topical treatment with EGF once or twice daily for 9 days (Leibowitz et al. 1990). This suggests a potential postoperative use of EGF as a local therapeutic agent.

Immunostimulants. In oncotherapy of animal patients, a number of biological substances have been used as nonspecific immunostimulants (or immunomodulators. The rationale for immunotherapy is based on the property of bacteria-derived lipopolysaccharides and polysaccharides to stimulate host immunity, including an enhanced response to tumor-associated antigens. Activation of T lymphocytes (natural killer cells) and macrophages and an increase in serum interferon levels are the desired outcomes of immunostimulation that characterize the antineoplastic responses. Organisms most widely used as immunostimulants are mycobacterial (bacillus Calmette-Guérin, or BCG) and *Propionibacterium acnes.* Recently, yeast-derived polysaccharides (acemannan) have been beneficial in treating spontaneous canine and feline neoplasms, especially fibrosarcomas (Harris et al. 1991).

Concerning ocular and periocular tumors, immunotherapy has been used most commonly in large domestic species for treating equine sarcoid and squamous cell carcinoma of horses and cattle (Klein 1990). Intralesional administration of a purified BCG cell-wall extract has been reported to be particularly effective in treating periocular sarcoid of Equidae (Lavach et al. 1985). Multiple injections at 2- to 4-week intervals are usually necessary for successful treatment of periocular sarcoid. The volume of BCG cell-wall extract varies considerably, from 1 to 65 mL, depending upon the size of the tumor (Lavach et al. 1985). Considerable swelling is anticipated following each injection, and necrosis and suppuration at the injection site are often noted. Although results of treating ocular squamous cell carcinoma of large domestic species with BCG seem to be less predictable, successful treatment of an ocular carcinoma metastatic from the eye to a regional lymph node has been reported (McCalla et al. 1992).

Inert Gases. Expandable inert fluorocarbon gases are injected into the vitreous cavity to tamponade and stabilize retinal separations. Referred to as pneumatic retinopexy, this technique is used in combination with other retinopexy procedures (Boyd 1986). Gases administered for pneumatic retinopexy include sulfur hexafluoride and perfluoropropane, which may expand from 2.5 to 4 times, respectively, their original volumes within 24 hours after injection. Complications include postoperative increase in IOP.

Photodynamic Substances. Photodynamic therapy is a modality of tumor treatment utilizing an injectable photosensitizing agent which is activated by a specific wavelength of light, usually delivered by laser irradiation. Selective tumor destruction occurs because of greater photosensitizer concentration in tumor tissues and localized irradiation of the tumor site. Once activated, the photosensitizing agent reacts with oxygen to form products that are cytotoxic to tumor cells. In a recent study, aluminum phthalocyanine tetrasulfonate was used as the photosensitizing substance to treat nasal and aural squamous cell carcinomas of cats. The study found treatments to be safe, well tolerated, and reasonably successful (Peaston et al. 1993). The authors indicate that treated animals should be kept out of sunlight for 2 weeks after treatment. Although no ocular squamous cell carcinomas were included in this study, results suggest that this protocol should also be investigated for treatment of periocular squamous cell carcinomas of cats and other domestic species.

Silicone Oil. Retinal separations are sometimes treated with intravitreal injection of silicone oil to tamponade and stabilize the retina. Complications reported with this procedure include corneal damage, IOP elevation, and retinal toxicity (Suzuki et al. 1990).

Viscoelastics. Viscoelastic substances have become an integral component of intraocular surgery, where their use can prevent mechanical damage to tissue, provide a wider space for surgical manipulation, and minimize postoperative adhesions (Liesegang 1990). The chemical and physical characteristics (e.g., viscosity, elasticity, pseudoplasticity, cohesiveness, and coatability) of viscoelastic substances make them useful for a variety of ophthalmic procedures. Since viscoelastic agents vary in composition and physical characteristics, an understanding of their properties allows the surgeon to select the viscoelastic material best suited to a particular surgical procedure. Viscoelastic products may vary considerably in cost; therefore, economic considerations may also influence which product is used.

The first viscoelastic material introduced commercially was sodium hyaluronate, and therefore, it is generally the standard to which other similar products are compared. Sodium hyaluronate is a large polysaccharide molecule that is present in nearly all vertebrate connective tissues. It is also a component of the capsular material surrounding streptococcal organisms. Sodium hyaluronate is extracted from a number of natural sources, including the dermis of rooster combs, umbilical cords, and cultures of streptococcal organisms. Sodium hyaluronate has also been produced using genetic engineering techniques.

Sodium hyaluronate is used widely in cataract surgery and intraocular lens implantation. Because autoclaving causes depolymerization and a change in viscosity, preparation of a sterile and stable compound is technologically demanding. This accounts for its relatively high cost. After intraocular use, a transient postoperative increase in IOP frequently occurs.

Highly purified hydroxypropylmethylcellulose (HPMC), commonly referred to simply as methylcellulose, has long been used as a 2% solution for ocular surface lubrication in gonioscopic solutions and as a base for eyedrops. A newer use has been to lubricate intraocular lenses for implantation following cataract removal. Although methylcellulose products have excellent viscoadherent properties, they have relatively poor viscoelasticity, requiring larger cannulas and higher pressures for injection.

Medical-grade methylcellulose is manufactured from raw wood pulp; production processing to form ophthalmic HPMC includes multiple filtration steps that result in a highly purified synthetic nonprotein substance which is nontoxic. The potential advantages of HPMC over other viscoelastic materials are the availability of raw materials, relative ease in manufacturing, ability to withstand autoclaving, and low cost. However, production procedures necessary to purify the material prior to intraocular use can substantially increase the cost. Also, since it is not a natural animal product, the fate of HPMC in the body is unknown.

Chondroitin sulfate is a polysaccharide, similar to sodium hyaluronate, that is harvested from shark fin cartilage. It differs from sodium hyaluronate by being sulfated. This results in an extra negative charge per repeating unit that may allow it to coat the positively charged tissue or implant surface and thus decrease the electrostatic interaction between the implant and the endothelium. A product with one part 4% chondroitin sulfate and three parts 3% sodium hyaluronate is commercially available. The manufacturer believes this product combines the advantages of each compound, i.e., the higher viscosity and chamber-maintaining properties of sodium hyaluronate with the coating and cell protection properties of chondroitin sulfate.

The effects of intracameral injection of viscoelastic solutions on IOP and corneal endothelium have been evaluated in dogs. Following anterior chamber injection of sodium hyaluronate 1%, combined sodium chondroitin sulfate 4% and sodium hyaluronate 3%, and HPMC 2%, IOP, corneal endothelial integrity, and corneal thickness were evaluated (Gerding et al. 1989; Gerding et al. 1990). These studies revealed that the viscoelastic products evaluated caused relatively minor transient effects on IOP and corneal thickness, suggesting that these substances may be used safely in canine patients undergoing intraocular surgery.

Besides their use in cataract surgery and intraocular implant procedures, other ophthalmic uses of these viscoelastic substances include trauma repair, corneal transplantation, glaucoma filter surgery, and vitreoretinal surgery. Viscoelastic substances are also used in the medical therapy of tear-deficient states. Human placental collagen, synthetic polyacrylamide, and other viscoelastic polymers are being investigated for general medical and ophthalmic uses.

REFERENCES

Allen LJ, George LW, Willith NH: Effect of penicillin or penicillin and dexamethasone in cattle with infectious bovine keratoconjunctivitis. J Am Vet Med Assoc 1995, 206:1200-1203.

Allinson RW, Gerber DS, Bieber S, Hodes BL: Reversal of mydriasis by dapiprazole. Ann Ophthalmol 1990, 22:131-138.

Araie M, Shirasawa E, Ohashi T: Intraocular irrigating solutions and permeability of the blood aqueous barrier. Arch Ophthalmol 1990, 108:882-885.

Ball MA, Rebhun WC, Gaarder JE, Patten V: Evaluation of itraconazole-dimethylsulfoxide ointment for treatment of keratomycosis in 9 horses. J Am Vet Med Assoc 1997, 211:199-203.

Barletta JP, Angella G, Balch KC, et al.: Inhibition of pseudomonal ulceration in rabbit corneas by a synthetic matrix metalloproteinase inhibitor. Invest Ophthalmol Vis Sci 1996, 37:20-28.

Baum JL: Antibiotic use in ophthalmology. In Duane TD (ed.), Clinical Ophthalmology, vol. 4. Hagerstown, MD, Harper & Row, 1980, chap. 26.

Beech J, Sweeney CR: Keratomycoses in 11 horses. Equine Vet J (Suppl 2), 1983, 39-38.

Ben-Nun J, Joyce DA, Cooper RL, Cringle SJ, Constable IJ: Pharmacokinetics of intravitreal injection. Invest Ophthalmol Vis Sci 1989, 30:1055-1061.

Bounous DI, Carmichael KP, Kaswan RL, Hirsh S, Stiles J: Effects of ophthalmic cyclosporine on lacrymal gland pathology and function in dogs with keratoconjunctivitis sicca. Vet Comp Ophthalmol 1995, 5:5-12.

Boyd BF: Pneumatic retinopexy. Highlights Ophthalmol Letter 1986, 14:1-14.

Brock KA, Thurman JC, Benson GJ, et al.: Selected hemodynamic and renal effects of intravenous infusions of hypertonic mannitol in dogs anesthetized with methoxyflurane in oxygen. J Am Anim Hosp Assoc 1985, 21:207-214.

Brooks DE, Legendre AM, Gum GG, Laratta LJ, Abrams KL, Morgan RV: The treatment of canine ocular blastomycosis with systemically administered itraconazole. Progress Vet Compar Ophthalmol 1991, 1(4):263-268.

Brown MH, Galland JC, Davidson HJ, Brightman AH: The phenol red thread tear test in dogs. Vet Compar Ophthalmol 1996, 6:274-277.

Brown RH, Stewart RH, Lynch MG, et al.: ALO 2145 reduces the intraocular pressure elevation after anterior segment laser surgery. Ophthalmology 1988, 95:378-384.

Carrier M, Gum GG: Effects of 4% pilocarpine gel on normotensive and glaucomatous canine eyes. Am J Vet Res 1989, 50(2):239-244.

Cavanaugh TB, Gottsch JD: Infectious keratitis and cyanoacrylate adhesive. Am J Ophthalmol 1991, 111:466-472.

Cawrse MA, Ward DA, Hendrix DVH. 1999. Effects of topically applied 2% dorzolamide on intraocular pressure and aqueous humor flow in normal dogs. Proc Am Coll Vet Ophthalmol 30th Ann Meeting, p. 68.

Collins BK, Moore CP, Hagee JH: Sulfonamide-associated keratoconjunctivitis sicca and corneal ulceration in a dysuric dog. J Am Vet Med Assoc 1986, 189(8):924-926.

Collins BK, Nasisse MP, Moore CP. In vitro efficacy of L-lysine against feline herpesvirus type-A. Proc Am Coll Vet Ophthalmol 1995, 26:141.

Costa ND, Slatter DH: Potency of *n*-acetylcysteine as a collagenase inhibitor in pharmaceutical preparations: effects of temperature and storage. Aust Vet J 1983, 60(6):195-196.

Croft MA, Kaufman PL: Effect of daily topical ethacrynic acid on aqueous humor dynamics in monkeys. Curr Eye Res 1995, 14:777-781.

Daigneault J, George LW: Topically applied benzathine cloxacillin for treatment of experimentally induced infectious bovine keratoconjunctivitis. Am J Vet Res 1990, 51(3):376-380.

Daigneault J, George LW, Baggot JD: Ocular and serum disposition kinetics of cloxacillin and intravenous administration of sodium cloxacillin to calves. Am J Vet Res 1990, 51(3):381-385.

Damji KF, Rootman J, Palcic B: Pharmacological modulation of human subconjunctival fibroblast behavior in vitro. Ophthalmic Surg 1990, 21:31-43.

Das A, Frank RN, Zhang NL, Samadani E: Increases in collagen type IV and laminin in galactose-induced retinal capillary basement membrane thickening-prevention by an aldose reductase inhibitor. Exp Eye Res 1990, 50:269-280.

Davidson MG: Equine ophthalmology. In Gelatt KN (ed.), Veterinary Ophthalmology, 2nd ed. Philadelphia: Lea & Febiger, 1991, pp. 576-610.

Dow SW, Rosychuk RA, McChesney AE, Curtis CR: Effects of flunixin and flunixin plus prednisone on the gastrointestinal tract of dogs. Am J Vet Res 1990, 51(7):1131-1138.

Dugan SJ, Roberts SM, Severin GA: Systemic osmotherapy for ophthalmic disease in dogs and cats. J Am Vet Med Assoc 1989, 194(1):115-118.

Dziezyc J, Millichamp NJ, Keller DB, Smith WB: Effects of prostaglandin $F_{2\alpha}$ and leukotriene D4 on pupil size intraocular pressure, and blood-aqueous barrier in dogs. Am J Vet Res 1992, 53:1302.

Dziezyc J, Millichamp NJ, Smith WB: Effect of flurbiprofen and corticosteroids on the ocular irritative response in dogs. Vet Comp Ophthalmol 1995, 5:42-45.

Edelhauser HF, VanHorn OL, Schultz RO, Hyndiuk RA: Comparative toxicity of intraocular irrigating solutions on the corneal endothelium. Am J Ophthalmol 1976, 81:474-481.

Erickson K, Liang LL, Shum P, Nathanson JA: Adrenergic regulation of aqueous outflow. J Ocul Pharmacol 1994, 10:241-252.

Forster RK: Fungal diseases. In Smolin G and Thoft RA (eds.), The Cornea, 2nd ed. Boston: Little, Brown, & Co., 1987, pp. 228-240.

Gassett AR, Ishii Y: Cytotoxicity of chlorhexidine. Can J Ophthalmol 1975, 10:98.

Gelatt KN, Larocca RD, Gelatt JK, Strubbe T, MacKay EO: Evaluation of multiple doses of 4% and 6% timolol, and timolol combined with 2% pilocarpine in clinically normal Beagles and Beagles with glaucoma. Am J Vet Res 1995, 56:1325-1331.

George LW, Reina-Guerra M, Baggot JD, Mihalyi J: Distribution of kanamycin in ocular tissues of calves. J Vet Pharmac Therap 1986, 9(2):183-191.

Gerding PA, McLaughlin SA, Troop MW: Pathogenic bacteria and fungi associated with external ocular diseases in dogs: 131 cases (1981-1986). J Am Vet Med Assoc 1988, 193(2):242-244.

Gerding PA, McLaughlin SA, Brightman AH, Essex-Sorlie D, Helper LC: Effects of intracameral injection of viscoelastic solutions on intraocular pressure in dogs. Am J Vet Res 1989, 50(5):624-628.

Gerding PA, McLaughlin SA, Brightman AH, Essex-Sorlie D, Laing RA, Hirokawa K: Effects of intracameral injection of viscoelastic solutions on corneal endothelium in dogs. Am J Vet Res 1990, 51(7):1086-1088.

Gerding PA, Essex-Sorlie D, Yack R, Vasaune S: Effects of intracameral injection of tissue plasminogen activator on corneal endothelium and intraocular pressure in dogs. Am J Vet Res 1992a, 53(6):890-893.

Gerding PA, Essex-Sorlie D, Vasaune S, Yack R: Use of tissue plasminogen activator for intraocular fibrinolysis in dogs. Am J Vet Res 1992b, 53(6):894-896.

Gerding PA, Eurell TE: Evaluation of intraocular penetration of topically administered tissue plasminogen activator in dogs. Am J Vet Res 1993, 54(6):836-839.

Gharagozloo NZ, Relf SJ, Brubaker RF: Aqueous flow is reduced by the alpha-adrenergic agonist, apraclonidine hyperchloride (ALO 2145). Ophthalmology 1988, 95:1217-1220.

Glasser DB, Matsuda M, Ellis JG, Edelhauser HF: Effects of intraocular irrigating solutions on the corneal endothelium after in vivo anterior chamber irrigation. Am J Ophthalmol 1985, 99:321-328.

Glaze MB, Crawford MA, Nachreiner RF, Casey HW, Nafe LA, Kearney MT: Ophthalmic corticosteroid therapy: systemic effects in the dog. J Am Vet Med Assoc 1988, 192(1):73-75.

Glover TL, Nasisse MP, Davidson MG: Effects of topically applied mitomycin-C on intraocular pressure, facility of outflow, and fibrosis after glaucoma surgery in clinically normal dogs. Am J Vet Res 1995, 56:936-940.

Gottsch JK: Hyphema: diagnosis and management. Retina 1990, 10:Suppl 1, 65-71.

Gum GG, Larocca RD, Gelatt KN, Mead JP, Gelatt JK: The effect of topical timolol maleate on intraocular pressure in normal Beagles and Beagles with inherited glaucoma. Progress Vet Compar Ophthalmol 1991, 1(3):141-149.

Gum GG, Samuelson DA, Gelatt KN: Effect of hyaluronidase on aqueous outflow resistance in normotensive and glaucomatous eyes of dogs. Am J Vet Res 1992, 53(5):767-770.

Gum GG, Gelatt KN, Gelatt KJ, Jones R: Effect of topically applied demecarium bromide and echothiophate iodide on intraocular pressure and pupil size in Beagles with normotensive eyes and Beagles with inherited glaucoma. Am J Vet Res 1993, 54(2):287-293.

Gwin RM, Gelatt KN, Gum GG, et al.: The effect of topical pilocarpine on intraocular pressure and pupil size in the normotensive and glaucomatous Beagle. Invest Ophthalmol Vis Sci 1977, 16:1143-1148.

Gwin RM, et al.: Effects of topical l-epinephrine and dipivalyl epinephrine on intraocular pressure and pupil size in the normotensive and glaucomatous Beagle. Am J Vet Res 1978, 39:83-86.

Hacker DV, Buyukmihci NC, Franti CE, Bellorn RW: Effect of topical phenylephrine on the equine pupil. Am J Vet Res 1987, 48(2):320-322.

Hakanson N, Shively JN, Merideth RE: Granuloma formation following subconjunctival injections of triamcinolone in two dogs. J Am Anim Hosp Assoc 1991, 27(1):89-92.
Harris C, Pierce K, King G, Yates KM, Hall J, Tizard I: Efficacy of acemannan in treatment of canine and feline spontaneous neoplasms. Mol Biother 1991, 3:207-213.
Havener WH: Antibiotics. In Ocular Pharmacology, 5th ed. St. Louis: CV Mosby Co., 1983, pp. 164-178.
Hersh PS, Rice BA, Baer JC, Wells PA, Lynch SE, McGuigan LJB, Foster CS: Topical nonsteroidal agents and corneal wound healing. Arch Ophthalmol 1990, 108:577-583.
Hyndiuk RA, Snyder RW: Bacterial keratitis. In Smolin G and Thoft RA (eds.), The Cornea, 2nd ed. Boston: Little, Brown & Co., 1987, pp. 193-319.
Hyndiuk RA, Eiferman RA, Caldwell DR, et al.: Comparison of ciprofloxacin ophthalmic solution 0.3% to fortified tobramycin-cefazolin in treating bacterial corneal ulcers. Ophthalmol 1996, 103:1854-1863.
Jackson PA, Kaswan RL, Merideth RE, Barret PM: Chronic superficial keratitis in dogs: a placebo controlled trial of topical cyclosporine treatment. Progress Vet Compar Ophthalmol 1991, 1(4):269-275.
Joyce JR: Thiabendazole therapy of mycotic keratitis in horses. Equine Vet J (Suppl 2), 1983:45-47.
Joyce NC, Neufeld AH: Pharmacology of the corneal endothelium. N Eng J Optometry 1990, 42:6-8.
Kaswan RL, Kaplan HJ, Martin CL: Topically applied cyclosporin for modulation of induced immunogenic uveitis in rabbits. Am J Vet Res 1988, 49(10):1757-1759.
Kaswan RL, Salisbury MA, Ward DA: Spontaneous canine keratoconjunctivitis sicca. A useful model for human keratoconjunctivitis sicca: treatment with cyclosporine eye drops. Arch Ophthalmology 1989, 107(8):1210-1216.
Kennedy MJ: The efficacy of ivermectin against the eyeworm, *Thelazia skrjabini,* in experimentally infected cattle. Vet Parasitol 1992, 45(1/2):127-131.
Kennedy MJ, Phillips FE: Efficacy of doramectin against eyeworms (*Thelazia* spp.) in naturally and experimentally infected cattle. Vet Parasitol 1993, 49(1):61-66.
Kern TJ: Ulcerative keratitis. Vet Clin N Am (Small Anim Prac) 1990, 20:643-666.
Khaw PT, Doyle JW, Sherwood MB, Smith MF, McGorray S: Effects of intraoperative 5-fluorouracil or mitomycin C on glaucoma filtration surgery in rabbits. Ophthalmology 1993, 100:367-372.
King TC, Gum GS, Gelatt KN: Evaluation of topically administered carbonic anhydrase inhibitor (MK-927) in normotensive and glaucomatous beagles. Am J Vet Res 1992, 52(12):2067-2070.
Kita M, Marmor MF: Systemic mannitol increases the retinal adhesive force in vivo. Arch Ophthalmol 1991, 109(10):1449-1450.
Klein WR: Immunotherapy of squamous cell carcinoma of the bovine eye and of equine sarcoid. Tijdschrift voor Diergeneeskunde 1990, 115(24):1149-1155.
Kraff MC, Sanders DR, McGuigan L, Raanan MG: Inhibition of blood-aqueous barrier breakdown with diclofenac. Arch Ophthalmol 1990, 108(3):380-383.
Krohne SDB, Vestre WA: Effects of flunixin meglumine and dexamethasone on aqueous protein values after intraocular surgery in the dog. Am J Vet Res 1987, 48(3):420-422.
Krohne SG: Effect of topically applied 2% pilocarpine and 0.25% demecarium bromide on blood-aqueous barrier permeability in dogs. Am J Vet Res 1994, 55:1729-1733.
Krohne SG, Gionfrido JR, Morrison EA: Inhibition of pilocarpine-induced aqueous humor flare, hypotny, and miosis by topical administration of anti-inflammatory and anesthetic drugs to dogs. Am J Vet Res 1998a, 59:482-488.
Krohne S, Blair MJ, Bingaman D, Gionfrido JR: Carprofen inhibition of flare in the dog measured by laser flare photometry. Vet Ophthalmol 1998b, 1(2-3):81-84.
Lappin MR, Greene CE, Winston S, Toll SL, Epstein ME: Clinical feline toxoplasmosis: serologic diagnosis and therapeutic management of 15 cases. J Vet Inter Med 1989, 3(3):139-143.
Lavach JD, Sullins KE, Roberts SM, Severin GA: BCG treatment of periocular sarcoid. Equine Vet J 1985, 17:445-448.
Lee DA: Antifibrosis agents and glaucoma surgery. Invest Ophthalmol Vis Sci 1994, 35:3789-3791.
Leibowitz HM, Kupferman A: Anti-inflammatory medications. Int Ophthalmol Clin 1980, 20:117.
Leibowitz HM, Morello S, Stern M, Kupferman A: Effect of topically administered epidermal growth factor on corneal wound strength. Arch Ophthalmol 1990, 108(5):734-737.
Liesegang TJ: Viscoelastic substances in ophthalmology. Surv Ophthalmol 1990, 34:268-293.
Lim JI, Maguire AM, John G, Mohler MA, Fiscella RG: Intraocular tissue plasminogen activator concentrations after subconjunctival delivery. Ophthalmology 1993, 100:373-376.
Lorimer DW, Hakanson NE, Pion PD, Merideth RE: The effects of intravenous mannitol or oral glycerol on intraocular pressure in dogs. Cornell Vet 1989, 79(3):249-258.
Lyons ET, Drudge JH, Tolliver SC, Hemken RW, Button FS: Preliminary tests for activity of levamisole against natural infections of eyeworms in dairy calves. Vet Med Small Anim Clin 1981, 1199-1201.
MacAllister CG, Morgan SJ, Borne AT, Pollet RA: Comparison of adverse effects of phenylbutazone, flunixin meglumine, and ketoprofen in horses. J Am Vet Med Assoc 1993, 202:71-77.
MacRae SM, Brown B, Edelhauser HF: The corneal toxicity of presurgical skin antiseptics. Am J Ophthalmol 1984, 97:221-232.
Maren TH, Conroy CW, Wynns GC, Levy NS: Ocular absorption, blood levels, and excretion of dorzolamide, a topically active carbonic anhydrase inhibitor. J Ocul Pharmacol Ther 1997, 12:23-30.
Martin C, Kaswan R, Gratzek A, Champagne E, Salisbury MA, Ward D: Ocular use of tissue plasminogen activator in companion animals. Prog Vet Comp Ophthalmol 1993, 3:29-36.
McCalla TL, Moore CP, Collier LL: Immunotherapy of periocular squamous cell carcinoma with metastasis in a pony. J Am Vet Med Assoc 1992, 200:1678-1681.
Miller PE, Nelson NJ, Rhaesa SL: Effects of topical administration of 0.5% aproclonidine on intraocular pressure, pupil size, and heart rate in clinically normal dogs. Am J Vet Res 1996, 57:79-82.
Miller PE, Rhaesa SL: Effects of topical administration of 0.5% aproclonidine on intraocular pressure, pupil size, and heart rate in clinically normal cats. Am J Vet Res 1996, 57:83-86.
Miller WW: Cyclosporine in ocular diseases: an alternative to glucocorticoid therapy. Vet Med Report 1990, 2(1):86-88.
Millichamp NJ, Dziezyc J, Rohde BH, Chiou GC, Smith WB: Acute effects of anti-inflammatory drugs on neodymium:yttrium aluminum garnet laser-induced uveitis in dogs. Am J Vet Res 1991a, 52(9):1279-1284.
Millichamp NJ, Dziezyc J, Olsen JW: Effects of flurbiprofen on facility of aqueous outflow in the eyes of dogs. Am J Vet Res 1991b, 52(9):1448-1451.
Mohan M, Gupta SK, Kalra VK, Vajpayee RB, Sachdev MS: Topical silver sulphadiazine: a new drug for oc-

ular keratomycosis. Brit J Ophthalmol 1988, 72(3): 192-195.

Moll AC, Van Rij G, Van Der Loos ThLJM: Anticoagulant therapy and cataract surgery. Documenta Ophthalmologica 1989, 72:367-373.

Moore CP, Fales WH, Whittington P, et al.: Bacterial and fungal isolates from Equidae with ulcerative keratitis. J Am Vet Med Assoc 1983, 182:600-603.

Moore CP, Collins BK, Fales WH, Halenda RM: Antimicrobial agents for equine infectious keratitis. J Am Vet Med Assoc 1995, 207:855-862.

Moore GE, Mahaffey EA, Hoenig M: Hematologic and serumbiochemical effects of long-term administration of anti-inflammatory doses of prednisone in dogs. Am J Vet Res 1992, 53(6):1033-1037.

Morgan RV, Bachrach A: Keratoconjunctivitis sicca associated with sulfonamide therapy in dogs. J Am Vet Med Assoc 1982, 180:422.

Murphy CJ, Feldman E, Bellhorn R: Iatrogenic Cushing's syndrome in a dog caused by topical ophthalmic medications. J Am Anim Hosp Assoc 1990, 26(6):640-642.

Nasisse MP, Cook CS, Harling DE: Response of the canine corneal endothelium to intraocular irrigation with saline solution, balanced salt solution, and balanced salt solution with glutathione. Am J Vet Res 1986, 47(10):2261-2265.

Nasisse MP: Anti-inflammatory therapy in herpesvirus keratoconjunctivitis. Prog Vet Comp Ophthalmol 1991, 1:63-65.

Nasisse MP, Guy JS, Davidson MG, et al.: In vitro susceptibility of feline herpesvirus-1 to vidarabine, idoxuridine, trifluridine, acyclovir, or bromovinyldeoxyuridine. Am J Vet Res 1989, 50:158.

Nasisse MP, Nelms S: Equine ulcerative keratitis. Vet Clin North Am (Equine Pract) 1992, 8:537-555.

Nasisse PM, Dorman DC, Jamison KC, Weigler BJ, Hawkins EC, Stevens JB: Effects of valacyclovir in cats infected with feline herpesvirus. Am J Vet Res 1997, 58:114.

Osborn E, Baum JL, Crnst C, et al.: The stability of ten antibiotics in artificial tear solutions. Am J Ophthalmol 1976, 82:775-779.

Peaston AE, Leach MW, Higgins RJ: Photodynamic therapy for nasal and aural squamous cell carcinoma in cats. J Am Vet Med Assoc 1993, 202:1261-1265.

Potter DE: Adrenergic pharmacology of aqueous humor dynamics. Pharmacol Rev 1981, 33:133.

Read RA: Treatment of canine nictitans plasmacytic conjunctivitis with 0.2% cyclosporin ointment. J Small Anim Pract 1995, 36:50-56.

Rebhun WC: Corneal stromal abscesses in the horse. J Am Vet Med Assoc 1982, 181:677-679.

———: Corneal stromal infections in horses. Compend Cont Educ Pract Vet 1992, 14:363-371.

Regnier A, Toutain PL: Ocular pharmacology and therapeutics. In Gelatt KN (ed.), Veterinary Ophthalmology, 2nd ed. Philadelphia: Lea & Febiger, 1991, pp. 162-194.

Regnier AM, Dossin O, Cutzach EE, Gelatt KN: Comparative effects of two formulations of indomethacin eyedrops on the paracentesis-induced inflammatory response in the canine eye. Vet Compar Ophthalmol 1995, 5:242-246.

Roberts SM, Lavach JD, Macy DW, et al.: Effect of ophthalmic prednisolone on the canine adrenal gland and hepatic function. Am J Vet Res 1984, 45:1711-1714.

Roberts SM, Severin GA, Lavach JD: Antibacterial activity of dilute povidone-iodine solutions used for ocular surface disinfection in dogs. Am J Vet Res 1986, 47(6):1207-1210.

Rothstein E, Scott DW, Riis RC: Tetracycline and niacinamide for the treatment of sterile pyogranuloma/granuloma syndrome in a dog. J Am Anim Hosp Assoc 1997, 33:540-543.

Roze M, Thomas E, Davot JL: Tolfenamic acid in the control of ocular inflammation in the dog: pharmacokinetics and clinical results obtained in an experimental model. J Small Anim Pract 1996, 37:371-375.

Russell DH, Kibler R, Martrisian L, Larson DF, Poulos B: Prolactin receptors on human T and B lymphocytes: antagonism of prolactin-hindering by cyclosporine. J Immunol 1985, 134:3027-3031.

Salisbury MA, Kaswan RL, Ward DA, Martin CL, Ramsey JM, Fischer CA: Topical application of cyclosporine in the management of keratoconjunctivitis sicca in dogs. J Am Anim Hosp Assoc 1990, 26(3):269-274.

Schadler HJ: An alternative treatment for keratoconjunctivitis sicca. Vet Med 1987, 71:1145-1148.

Soll MD, Carmichael IH, Scherer HR, Gross SJ: The efficacy of ivermectin against *Thelazia rhodesii* (Desmarest, 1828) in the eyes of cattle. Vet Parasitol 1992, 42(1-2):67-71.

Speiss BM, Mathis GA, Franson KL, Leber A: Kinetics of uptake and effects of topical indomethacin application on protein concentration in the aqueous humor of dogs. Am J Vet Res 1991, 52(7):1159-1163.

Stern GA: In vitro antibiotic synergism against ocular fungal isolates. Am J Ophthalmol 1978, 86:359.

Stiles J: Treatment of cats with ocular disease attributable to herpesvirus infection: 17 cases (1983-1993). J Am Vet Med Assoc 1995, 207:599-603.

Sugrue MF, Gautheron P, Grove J, et al.: MK-927: a topically effective ocular hypotensive carbonic anhydrase (C) inhibitor in rabbits. Invest Ophthalmol Vis Sci 1988, 29(Suppl):81.

Suzuki M, Ando K, Miyata K: Topical fibronectin treatment in 56 cases of corneal epithelial lesion. Folia Ophthalmol Jpn 1989, 40:2699-2703.

Suzuki M, Okada T, Takeuchi S, Yamashita H, Hori S: The effect of silicone oil on the ocular tissues. Acta Soc Ophthalmol Jpn 1990, 94:160-166.

Svec AL, Strosberg AM: Therapeutic and systemic side effects of ocular β-adrenergic antagonists in anesthetized dog. Invest Ophthalmol Vis Sci 1986, 27:401.

Tabbara KF, al-Kharashi SA, al-Mansouri SM, al-Omar OM, Cooper H, el-Asrar AMA, Foulds G: Ocular levels of azithromycin. Arch Ophthalmol 1998, 166:1625-1628.

Thermes F, Molon-Noblot S, Grove J: Effects of acetylcysteine on rabbit conjunctival and corneal surfaces. Invest Ophthalmol Vis Sci 1991, 32:2958-2963.

Toris CB, Camras CB, Yablonski ME: Effects of PhXa41, a new prostaglandin $F_{2\alpha}$ analog, on aqueous humor dynamics in human eyes. Ophthalmol 1993, 100:1297-1304.

Troke PF, Andrews RJ, Marriott MS, Richardson K: Efficacy of fluconazole (UK-49,858) against experimental aspergillosis and cryptococcosis in mice. J Antimicrob Chemother 1987, 19:663-670.

Tsuju T, Matsumoto Y, Mori K, Ikebe H, Terubayashi H, Akagi Y, Tanimoto T: Preventional and therapeutic effects of aldose reductase inhibitor FR 74366 on rat galactose cataract. Acta Soc Ophthalmol Jap 1990, 94:120-127.

van der Woerdt A, Gilger BC, Wilkie D, Strauch SM, Orczeck SM: Normal variation in, and effect of 2% pilocarpine on, intraocular pressure and pupil size in female horses. Am J Vet Res 1998, 59:1459-1462.

Vane JR, Botting RM: Overview: mechanisms of action of anti-inflammatory drugs. In Vane J, Botting J, Botting R, eds. Improved nonsteroidal anti-inflammatory drugs: cox-2 enzyme inhibitors. Dordrecht: Kluwer Academic Publishers, 1995:1-27.

Wang RF, Serle JB, Podos SM, Sugrue MF: The effect of MK-927, a topical carbonic anhydrase inhibitor, on IOP in glaucomatous monkeys. Curr Eye Res 1990, 9:163-168.

Ward DA: Comparative efficacy of topically applied flurbiprofen, diclovenac, tolmetin, and suprofen for the treatment of experimentally induced blood-aqueous barrier disruption in dogs. Am J Vet Res 1996, 5:242-246.

Ward DA, Ferguson DC, Ward SL, Green K, Daswan RL: Comparison of the blood-aqueous barrier stabilizing effects of steroidal and nonsteroidal anti-inflammatory agents in the dog. Progress Vet Comp Ophthalmol 1992, 2(3):117-124.

Watanabe K, Chiou GCY: Action mechanism of timolol to lower the intraocular pressure in rabbits. Ophthalmic Res 1983, 15:160.

Whitcup SM, Chan CC, Luyo DA, Bo P, Li Q: Topical cyclosporine inhibits mast cell-mediated conjunctivitis. Invest Ophthalmol Vis Sci 1996, 37:2686-2693.

Wilkie DA, Latimer CA: Effects of topical administration of timolol maleate on intraocular pressure and pupil size in dogs. Am J Vet Res 1991a, 52(3):432-435.

———: Effects of topical administration of timolol maleate on intraocular pressure and pupil size in cats. Am J Vet Res 1991b, 52(3):436-440.

———: Effects of topical administration of 2.0% pilocarpine on intraocular pressure and pupil size in cats. Am J Vet Res 1991c, 52(3):441-444.

Williams DL, Hoey AJ, Smitherman P: Comparison of topical cyclorsporin and desamethasone for the treatment of chronic superficial keratitis in dogs. Vet Rec 1995, 137:635-639.

Wultrich B, Gerber M: Levocabastine eye drops are effective and well tolerated for the treatment of allergic conjunctivitis in children. Mediators Inflamm 1995, 4:516-520.

SECTION 13

Regulatory Considerations

56 LEGAL CONTROL OF VETERINARY DRUGS

STEPHEN F. SUNDLOF

Legislative Milestones in the Development of Laws Pertaining to the Regulation of Animal Drugs
Drug Compendia

There are indications that the regulation of drugs in America began with the earliest colonies. For example, records of the Massachusetts Bay Colony tell of Nicholas Knopf, who in 1630 was sentenced to pay a fine or be whipped for selling "a water of no worth nor value" as a cure for scurvy. However, federal controls over drugs did not begin until 1848, when the Import Drug Act was passed to stop the adulteration of quinine used to treat American troops who had contracted malaria in Mexico. The Import Drug Act was the first federal statute to guarantee the quality of medicines, and US Customs laboratories were established to administer the law. The mission of the new Customs laboratories was to enforce the purity and potency standards of the *US Pharmacopeia,* which had been compiled in 1820 by trade and professional leaders. Subsequently support dwindled and the program gradually faded away. There was no organizational connection with the agency now known as the Food and Drug Administration.

The first state pure food and drug law was passed by California in 1850. During subsequent years many other states enacted similar legislation, but the need for regulation on an interstate basis was becoming more and more evident.

LEGISLATIVE MILESTONES IN THE DEVELOPMENT OF LAWS PERTAINING TO THE REGULATION OF ANIMAL DRUGS. In 1880, Mr. Peter Collier, chief of the Division of Chemistry, US Department of Agriculture (USDA), began advocating enactment of a national food and drug law. In 1883 Dr. Harvey W. Wiley succeeded Collier as chief chemist and continued and broadened his efforts advocating a national food and drug law. Initially there was little interest in this kind of reform. Advocates were generally regarded as cranks and radicals. Over 100 bills were to be introduced in the US Congress before the first Federal Food and Drugs Act (and the Meat Inspection Act) of 1906 was enacted.

Conditions in the drug industry can scarcely be imagined today. The great advances in bacteriology were just beginning to have an impact on infectious diseases. Milk was still unpasteurized and cows were not tested for tuberculosis. Thousands of so-called patent medicines such as Kickapoo Sagwa Renovator for Stomach, Liver, and Kidney, Dr. Shreve's Anti-Gallstone Remedy, and Hamlin's Wizard Oil—Cures All Pain in Man or Beast flooded the marketplace. "Medicine-men" competed with circuses, minstrel shows, and "Wild West" shows to entertain the public and sell their products. Medicines containing opium, morphine, heroin, and cocaine were sold without restriction and without even any indication of the presence of the drugs in the product. Preparations that were otherwise harmless, other perhaps than being alcohol-based, were labeled for the cure of every disease or symptom of man and beast. Labels did not list ingredients, and warnings against misuse were virtually nonexistent. Of course, such practices were by no means universal, and many firms were producing reliable and wholesome products. However, there was no lack of material for investigation and disclosure by Dr. Wiley's chemists. In order to generate support for his cause, Dr. Wiley took their findings to the public, speaking frequently at women's clubs and civic and business organizations. Crusading reporters (muckrakers), organized women's clubs, and farsighted businessmen became his strong supporters. In 1903, Dr. Wiley captured the attention of the public by establishing his now famous volunteer "poison squad" of young men who agreed to eat only foods treated with measured amounts of chemical preservatives, in order to evaluate the safety of such products. Thanks to the publicity engendered by Dr. Wiley's work, public concern began to build. It reached a climax with the publication of Upton Sinclair's book *The Jungle,* a brutally graphic novel which focused national attention on the unsanitary conditions in US meatpacking plants. As a result the first federal food and drug law, the Food and Drugs Act of 1906, was passed by Congress and signed into law by President Theodore Roosevelt on June 30, 1906.

Basically the law banned from interstate commerce any traffic in adulterated or misbranded food or drugs. The act defined "drug" to include all medicines and preparations recognized in the *US Pharmacopeia* or *National Formulary* for internal or external use and any substance or mixture of substances intended to be used for the cure, mitigation, or prevention of disease in either humans or other animals.

Drugs were to be deemed "adulterated" if they were sold under or by a name recognized in the official compendia (the *US Pharmacopeia* and the *National Formulary*) but failed to meet the standards set forth therein, except that a recognized drug not meeting the official standard would not be deemed adulterated if it met its own standard of strength, quality, and purity as stated on the container. A drug was deemed "misbranded" if the label bore any statement, design, or device regarding the contents which was false or misleading, or if the drug was falsely branded as to the state, territory, or country in which it was manufactured. Drugs would also be misbranded if they were an imitation of, or offered for sale under the name of, another article or if the original contents had been removed in whole or in part and/or other contents added. Drugs would also be misbranded if their labels failed to disclose any quantities of alcohol, narcotics, and other specified substances present in the product.

Although the 1906 law represented a great step forward, there were obvious weaknesses. In 1911, the Supreme Court ruled that the labeling provisions of the act prohibited *only* false statements about the identity of the drug product but not false therapeutic claims. The Congress responded by passing the Shirley Amendment of 1912, which outlawed false *and fraudulent* curative or therapeutic claims. Under the Shirley Amendment, the government was required to prove that a false claim was also fraudulent, that is, that the promoter *intended* to deceive the purchaser. A defendant had only to show that he personally believed in his patent medicine to escape prosecution. This remained a major weakness in the law for 26 years.

The USDA's Bureau of Chemistry enforced the law until 1927, when the bureau was reorganized in order to separate law enforcement functions from agricultural research and development. The Food, Drug, and Insecticide Administration was formed. It was renamed the Food and Drug Administration (FDA) in 1931, and in 1940 the FDA was transferred from the USDA to the Federal Security Agency, in order to eliminate recurring conflicts between consumer interests and producer interests. In 1953, the Federal Security Agency became the Department of Health, Education, and Welfare—now the Department of Health and Human Services (DHHS).

An interesting side note, FDA's budget (appropriations), because of its origins in the USDA, comes through the House and Senate Agricultural Appropriations committees. Amendments to the Federal Food, Drug, and Cosmetic Act, however, come under the jurisdiction of the Senate Committee on Labor and Human Resources and the House Committee on Energy and Commerce.

By the early 1930s it was evident that there were serious shortcomings in the 1906 act. False advertising in print and on the radio was blatant, and manufacturers had found many ways to circumvent the law. Technological advancements were revolutionizing the production and marketing of foods, drugs, and related products, making the 1906 law obsolete.

In 1933, Walter Campbell, then chief of the FDA, seized an opportunity to work with Rexford Tugwell, a member of newly elected president Franklin D. Roosevelt's "brain trust" who had been appointed assistant secretary of agriculture, in developing a complete revision of the Food and Drugs Act. When the resulting "Tugwell bill" was introduced in Congress, it was a legislative disaster. Opposition to this New Deal legislation by industry and advertising interests was total. This was due in part to Rexford Tugwell's reputation in the business community and to some extent in Congress. The Columbia University economics professor, who believed in and advocated a planned economy, was greatly feared in business circles. The Senate sponsor of the bill, Royal S. Copeland, M.D., of New York, aided by FDA officials, consumer-minded congressmen, attorneys, and staffers, began the laborious process that was to become a bitter 5-year battle for new legislation.

As before, public opinion was to play a major role in pushing Congress to act, and again organized club women were very important in generating and molding public support. Public opinion was aroused by a shocking and tragic drug disaster which resulted in over 100 deaths. The drug involved was "Elixir of Sulfanilamide," sulfanilamide dissolved in diethylene glycol. Sulfanilamide had only recently become available, and salesmen reported that there was a demand for a liquid form. Since sulfanilamide is poorly soluble in water, the manufacturer dissolved the drug in diethylene glycol and added coloring and flavoring. The solution was tested for flavor, appearance, and fragrance, but since existing laws did not require manufacturers to demonstrate that their products were safe, no safety or toxicity testing was done. Before the product could be identified and recalled, it had claimed 107 lives in 15 states from Virginia to California.

Shortly after the sulfanilamide disaster, Congress adopted portions of the Copeland bill and it was passed as the Federal Food, Drug, and Cosmetic Act (FFD&C Act) of 1938, also referred to as the Copeland Act.

Under the 1938 act, interstate commerce in a new drug (for humans or animals) was prohibited unless it had been adequately tested to show that it was safe for use under the conditions of use prescribed on its label. Thus, it was illegal to ship a drug across state lines unless it had been shown to be safe. An exemption to this requirement was provided for a drug intended solely for investigational use by qualified scientific experts.

The 1938 act also required labels to bear adequate directions for use and to include warnings against unsafe use, where drugs (or devices) might be injurious to health. It required official drugs to be packaged and labeled as prescribed by the official compendia; required the labels of nonofficial drugs to list active ingredients; and required precautionary labeling of drugs subject to deterioration. Note that the 1938 act still did not require demonstrated proof of effectiveness of drugs.

The new law, and World War II, greatly expanded the FDA's workload. This period was characterized by the development of many new "wonder drugs," especially antibiotics, which were made subject to FDA testing beginning with penicillin in 1945. Fortunately the law required premarket approval of new drugs, but there were no premarket clearance requirements for a host of new chemicals of unknown safety. The law prohibited poisonous substances but provided no requirement that food ingredients be shown to be safe. The law did provide for exemptions and establishment of safe tolerances for unavoidable or necessary poisons such as pesticides, but when the FDA attempted to set a pesticide tolerance, the courts ruled that the lengthy procedure required by law was unworkable. The FDA was able to stop the use of known poisons where they posed a hazard (and did so in many cases) but the vast research effort needed to ensure that all food chemicals were safe was clearly beyond available resources.

During the 1940s there was a substantial increase in the use of commercial pesticides in the growing of agricultural products and in the use of chemicals for flavoring, coloring, preserving, and packaging of processed foods. In 1950, the House of Representatives adopted a resolution creating a Select Committee to Investigate the Use of Chemicals in Foods. Representative James T. Delaney of New York served as its chairman. The committee began extensive hearings, which were to go on for 2 years. As a result of the committee's work and the work of the FDA and others, three very significant amendments to the FFD&C Act were enacted: the Pesticide Amendment (1954), the Food Additives Amendment (1958), and the Color Additives Amendment (1960).

The Food Additives Amendment of 1958 was particularly significant in terms of its impact on the regulation of animal drugs since animal drugs approved for use in food animals were considered to be food additives and thus had to meet not only the drug standards of the act but also the food additive standards. Further, since the 1958 amendment required the premarket clearance of food additives, this meant that for the first time, sponsors of drugs indicated for use in food animals were required to demonstrate, as a condition of approval, the safety to humans of any residues present in food products derived from treated animals. A direct result of this provision has been the development, within veterinary pharmacology and toxicology, of a whole new subdiscipline, that of residue sciences.

This was also significant because it brought animal drugs for use in food animals under the provisions of the "Delaney anticancer clause," which provided that no additive will be deemed to be safe if it is found to induce cancer in humans or animals. The Delaney anticancer clause as it applied to animal drugs was amended in 1962 to include a provision that permits administration of a compound known to induce cancer in humans or animals to food-producing animals when it has been shown that "no residue" will occur in food products. Specifically, this exception, known as the DES Proviso, required that no residue will be found by methods of examination prescribed or approved by the secretary of the DHHS. Initially, the "no residue" provision was met simply by applying the most sensitive analytical methods available. However, it was recognized in doing so that "no residue" did not mean "zero residue" but rather was defined by the sensitivity of the analytical method employed. This was unacceptable. As a result, FDA developed a regulation commonly referred to as the Sensitivity-of-Method procedure, or SOM, now known as the animal drug safety policy, which defined "no residue" in terms of the level of residue that presents an insignificant risk of cancer to the consuming public. The safe level is then described with a finite number in parts per million (ppm) or parts per billion (ppb).

The regulation defines an insignificant risk of cancer as a 1 in 1 million increase in risk over the normal lifetime risk of cancer. Further, the regulation spells out how the level of residue that represents an insignificant risk of cancer is determined. The method to be used in monitoring for residues of the compound then must be sensitive enough to detect the level of residue determined to represent an insignificant risk.

During this period two other amendments to the FFD&C Act were to have a significant impact on veterinary medicine. The first was the Durham-Humphrey Amendment of 1951, which for the first time defined the kinds of drugs for human use that may be dispensed by a pharmacist only upon the prescription of a "practitioner licensed by law to administer such drugs." This was very significant because it created and defined the category of prescription drugs. Under previous law, a drug manufacturer decided whether a given drug would be available by prescription or over the counter. The language of the Durham-Humphrey Amendment specifically restricted the term "prescription" to drugs and medical devices for human use by replacing a section of the 1938 FFD&C Act that contained explicit reference to a "prescription signed by a physician, dentist, or veterinarian." Language in both the Senate and House reports that accompanied the amendment, however, recognized the need for a similar category of "prescription" animal drugs which the FDA had established by regulation. The FDA's authority to restrict a drug to use "by or on the order of a licensed veterinarian" has been upheld by the courts on several occasions, but statutory recognition of the prescription provision pertaining to animal drugs was not codified in the law until the enactment of the Generic Animal Drug Patent Term Restoration Act of 1988.

The Kefauver-Harris Drug Amendments of 1962 were also to have a significant impact on veterinary medicine. The Drug Amendments of 1962, like the 1938 act, were enacted into law following a disaster involving drugs: the "thalidomide disaster." Thalidomide, a sedative that was prescribed to pregnant women, is a potent teratogen causing severe deformities called phocomelia. Although the FDA never approved thalidomide for commercial marketing in the United States, it was distributed to selected doctors for experimental purposes, and it was approved and widely used in Europe.

The 1962 amendments extended, expanded, and strengthened the FDA's regulatory authority with respect to drugs. For the first time manufacturers were required to provide "substantial evidence" of the effectiveness of new drugs, as well as of their safety, as a condition of approval. Labeling now had a material bearing on the matter of new drug approval in that it must not be false or misleading in any particular. With respect to drugs already on the market, the manufacturer was required to report promptly to the FDA any information concerning adverse effects and other clinical experience or data relating in any way to safety and effectiveness.

Relative to effectiveness, the amendments also included a provision which enabled the FDA to require an effectiveness review of every new drug introduced between 1938 and 1962. The program, which began in the late 1960s, was called the Drug Efficacy Study Implementation (DESI) program. As a result of the DESI program, many older products, particularly those with multiple ingredients, were removed from the market. Those products remaining had labeling claims that could be substantiated through adequate studies and thus met the FDA standard for effectiveness.

In 1968, legislation was passed to consolidate provisions of the FFD&C Act with respect to the regulation of animal drugs. Prior to 1968 the act generally did not distinguish between human drugs and animal drugs. Both the House and the Senate reports on the amendment pointed out that, in many cases, the requirements for clearance of new animal drugs were more complicated than the clearance procedures for drugs for humans. This was because animal drugs indicated for use in food animals were required to meet not only the drug standards of the act but also the food additives standards. In fact, ensuring that food products from animals treated with a particular animal drug pose no risk to public health is often the most expensive and time-consuming part of the developmental process for a new animal drug intended for use in food animals.

It is important to note two additional aspects of food and drug legislation. First of all, the Food Additive Amendments of 1958 included language prohibiting the use of an animal drug other than in accord with its approved uses. This reflected congressional concern for human food safety, but it also made extra-label drug use in animals illegal under the act. At the same time Congress was also operating on the principle that animal drugs should be routinely available to farmers to treat their animals, i.e., to protect their property. The act requires that for an animal drug to be legally marketed in the United States, it must bear adequate directions for use by a layperson. Animal drugs that do not or cannot bear such directions for use are considered to be misbranded. The FDA, as noted above, had recognized the need for an exception to this requirement and had, by regulation, provided for the marketing of "prescription" animal drugs which could be used safely by or on the order of a licensed veterinarian, but for which adequate directions for lay use cannot be written.

The congressional bias in favor of the availability of animal drugs direct to farmers was to have a profound effect on the drug development and approval process and ultimately on veterinary pharmacology in the United States. It is reflected in the history of the FDA approvals of drugs for food animals. Even after establishing a category of prescription animal drugs in 1988, most drugs approved for food animals, with the exception of therapeutic antimicrobial agents, are classified as over-the-counter, whereas most drugs approved for companion animals are classified as prescription.

This focus on OTC drugs (and the attendant need to be able to provide labeling that can be reasonably followed by laypersons) has led to the approval of OTC drugs that are labeled for very specific and limited indications and that have directions for use which provide little or no flexibility in how the product can be used. As a result, there are many animal species for which there are no drugs approved, and for others the number of approved drugs is very limited and does not include drugs such as anesthetics, anti-inflammatory agents, or other drugs with low market potential.

Faced with an insufficient armamentarium of drugs approved for all of the various animal species-disease combinations encountered in veterinary practice, veterinarians historically have exercised considerable judgment in utilizing therapeutic agents, often going beyond the limits of approved labeling. Prior to 1994, veterinarians who engaged in extra-label drug use technically were in violation of federal law, unlike their physician counterparts, who were not prohibited by the act from using or prescribing drugs for use in humans as they deemed appropriate. In spite of the fact that the act clearly specifies that an animal drug must be used in strict accordance with the indications and directions for use contained in its labeling, FDA policy was very permissive in this regard.

During the late 1970s and early 1980s the FDA recognized the need for a more structured policy regarding such use, one that would define the conditions under which such use would not ordinarily result in regulatory action while at the same time drawing attention to the responsibilities incurred by the veterinary practitioner electing to use a drug in an extra-label fashion, especially in a food-producing animal. The policy took the form of a Compliance Policy Guide (CPG). CPGs are used to provide guidance regarding regulatory initiatives and enforcement priorities to FDA field and headquarters personnel. CPG 7125.06, titled "Extra-Label Use of New Animal Drugs in Food-Producing Animals," communicated the FDA's recognition that the extra-label use of a drug in food-producing animals may be considered by a veterinarian when the health of animals is immediately threatened and suffering or death would result from failure to treat the affected animal(s). In instances of this nature, regulatory action would not ordinarily be considered provided that several criteria were met (see Chap. 58).

The FDA also recognized that in the case of companion animals (non-food animals) veterinarians had become reliant on a number of drugs approved for use in humans but for which no counterparts were approved for use in animals. Examples of human drugs widely used in companion animals include digitalis derivatives, insulin, and anticancer drugs. CPG 7125.35, "Human Drugs Distributed to Veterinarians for Use in Animals," basically provides that as long as such distribution of a human drug is initiated (ordered) by a licensed veterinarian and is *not* intended for use in food-producing animals, the FDA would *not* ordinarily consider regulatory action. However, it should be noted that the manufacturers are *not* permitted to advertise or otherwise promote the use of human-labeled drugs for use in animals.

Although CPGs generally discourage the use of human drugs in food animals, certain exceptions are recognized. These include certain poison antidotes, insulin for use in the treatment of ketosis, and certain anesthetics and analgesics for use in surgical cases and for relief of pain and suffering.

Despite the efforts of the FDA to establish policies that recognized the needs of animals while protecting the public's health, such policies were based on the agency's authority to exercise discretion in deciding whether or not to enforce certain provisions of the act. The fact that the FDA elected not to take enforcement actions against veterinarians who administered drugs in an extra-label manner in no way conferred legal status to such practices. Concerned by the notion that veterinarians, unlike the members of any other licensed profession, were forced to repeatedly break the law in order to responsibly carry out their professional duties, the American Veterinary Medical Association actively petitioned Congress to amend the act.

In 1994, Congress, in an effort to decriminalize the everyday practice of veterinary medicine, passed the Animal Medicinal Drug Use Clarification Act of 1994. This legislation allows licensed veterinarians to use and prescribe, under specified conditions, animal and human drugs for extra-label purposes. In general the legislation is intended to codify in law and regulations the conditions and restrictions for extra-label use provided in CPG 7125.06 and CPG 7125.35 as outlined above. It also recognized compounding of animal drugs from FDA-approved human or animal drugs as a form of extra-label drug use. Such compounding is permissible by a veterinarian or a pharmacist on the order of a veterinarian provided that (1) there is no approved new animal or new human drug that, when used as labeled and in the available dosage form and concentration, appropriately treats the condition diagnosed; (2) the compounding is performed by a licensed pharmacist or veterinarian within the scope of a professional practice; (3) adequate procedures and processes are followed that ensure the safety and effectiveness of the compounded product; (4) the scale of the compounding operation is commensurate with the established need for compounded products (e.g., similar to that of comparable practices); and (5) all relevant state laws relating to the compounding of drugs for use in animals are followed. Compounding from a human drug for use in food-producing animals is not permitted if an approved animal drug can be used for compounding. Compounding from bulk drugs is not permitted under the act; however, the FDA on occasion has exercised regulatory discretion in allowing compounding from bulk drugs where the need was great and the risk to animals and the public was small. Additional information on compounding of drugs for use in animals is published in CPG 7125.40.

Although the Animal Medicinal Drug Use Clarification Act provided psychologic relief to veterinarians by codifying into law practices previously permitted by the FDA under more tenuous compliance policy guides, it did not address the underlying problem that necessitated extra-label use: the insufficiency of drugs available to treat animals. This sentiment was reflected in the Congressional Record immediately following passage of the bill in the Senate. At that time Senator Coates of Indiana stated that the bill "does nothing to expedite the review process of the FDA and CVM." "Through future legislative initiatives, we now need to address the animal drug availability deficiencies." Shortly after the passage of the Animal Medicinal Drug Use Clarification Act, the Coalition for Animal Health formed with the purpose of increasing the availability of animal drugs through statutory changes to the FFD&C Act. The Coalition, made up of veterinarians, animal producer organizations, the animal feed industry, and the animal drug industry, drafted proposed legislation, which eventually was signed into law on October 9, 1996. The Animal Drug Availability Act (ADAA) introduced major reforms in the way that the FDA evaluates and approves new animal drugs. These reforms are intended to facilitate the approval of new animal drugs and medicated feeds by building greater flexibility into the existing animal drug review processes. Such flexibility does not compromise the FDA's authority to ensure that animal drugs are safe for the animal patient and for the public consuming animal-derived foods.

Most of the reform measures brought about by the ADAA addressed the standard for determining whether a new animal drug is effective for its specified conditions of use. The FFD&C Act provides that the FDA may refuse to approve a new animal drug if it finds that there is a lack of *substantial evidence* that the drug will have the effect it claims under the conditions of use prescribed, recommended, or suggested in the proposed labeling. Prior to ADAA, the FDA had interpreted the phrase *substantial evidence* in fairly rigid terms, requiring a fixed minimum number of field studies (generally 3) conducted at geographically distinct locations. (Field studies are clinical studies conducted under conditions that closely approximate the conditions under which the new animal drug, if approved, is intended to be applied or administered.) With the changes effected by the ADAA, it is now possible that even a single *adequate and well-controlled* study may provide substantial evidence of effectiveness. Furthermore, in certain cases a field investigation may not be necessary to allow the FDA to conclude that the drug is effective.

The ADAA further allowed the FDA to redefine the phrase "adequate and well-controlled" as it applies to field investigations. Because field studies are conducted under field conditions (e.g., on farms or commercial livestock production facilities), it is recognized that the level of control over some study conditions need not or should not be the same as the level of control in laboratory studies. Under the ADAA, the FDA will balance the need to control study conditions with the need to observe the true effect of the drug under closely approximated actual-use conditions in determining whether a field study is adequate and well controlled.

Prior to the ADAA, products containing two or more drugs (combination drugs) were required to meet the same rigorous standard for effectiveness as products containing a single drug, even when the individual drugs in the combination product had been previously proven to be effective. The ADAA streamlined the process for approving a combination new animal drug if each of the drugs used in the combination has been previously approved separately for the uses for which it is intended in the combination. In such cases, additional studies for effectiveness and animal safety are often not required.

The FFD&C Act required that the FDA approve new animal drugs based on the concept of a single optimal dose (i.e., a single dosage that does not exceed the amount reasonably required to accomplish the drug's intended effect). This "optimal dose" concept left little flexibility for veterinarians to exercise professional judgment in the treatment of their patients. Furthermore, for certain drugs such as antimicrobial and antiparasitic agents, the approved "optimal dose" may become ineffective over time. Determining the optimal dose is a time-consuming and costly practice requiring pharmaceutical companies to conduct dose titration studies. The ADAA amended the FFD&C Act to allow the FDA to approve any effective dosage regimen as long as it is safe for the patient and does not result in a residue that exceeds the tolerance (see Chap. 58). Labeling animal drug products with dosage ranges rather than a single fixed dose will allow veterinarians to select a dosing regimen tailored to the specific needs of each patient.

The ADAA defined an entirely new class of drugs, differentiating them from over-the-counter and prescription classifications. Veterinary Feed Directive (VFD) drugs are intended for use in or on animal feed and are limited by approved application to use under the professional supervision of a licensed veterinarian. Previously, all feed additive drugs were available through over-the-counter channels. VFD drugs and animal feeds containing them must be labeled with a cautionary statement, and an animal feed containing a VFD drug can be used only by a licensed veterinarian or upon the lawful VFD issued by a licensed veterinarian. Because veterinary supervision is required, the VFD classification allows the FDA to approve potent new therapeutic drugs for administration to animals via feed.

Another area of drug regulation directly affecting the veterinarian is the Comprehensive Drug Abuse Prevention and Control Act of 1970, commonly called the Controlled Substances Act (CSA). At the turn of the century in the United States, opium, morphine, cocaine, and other such drugs were freely available to the public. In fact, as noted previously, many of the nostrums and patent medicines available at that time contained such drugs even though labels gave no hint of their presence. Although the Food and Drugs Act of 1906 required that the presence of such substances be specified on labels, it was clear that the ready availability of such substances had to be restricted. Thus, in 1914, the Congress enacted the Harrison Narcotic Act, which restricted narcotic drugs such as the opiates, cocaine, and ecgonine and any substances containing such compounds to legitimate medical uses. These drugs could be dispensed by pharmacists only on the basis of a prescription written by a veterinarian, physician, or dentist who was registered with the US Treasury Department. It later became apparent that there were dangers inherent in the distribution and use of many nonnarcotic drugs. Accordingly, in 1965, drug abuse amendments to control traffic in barbiturates, amphetamines, and other abused drugs were added to the FFD&C Act. In 1968, the FDA's Bureau of Drug Abuse Control was transferred to the Department of Justice, where it was consolidated, along with the Treasury Department's Bureau of Narcotics, into the current Drug Enforcement Agency (DEA).

Under the 1970 act, controlled substances include opiates, barbiturates, hallucinogens, methadone, stimulants such as amphetamines, and other addictive or habituating drugs. This act regulates the manufacturing, distribution, and dispensing of controlled substances by providing for a closed system of registered people (manufacturers and distributors, pharmacists, licensed practitioners, and others) authorized to handle such compounds. A veterinarian licensed to practice by a state and wishing to use or prescribe controlled substances must register annually with the DEA. Controlled drugs and drug products are categorized in five schedules, and an applicant requests certification for those schedules or categories of drugs that he or she expects to purchase, store, dispense, and use. The registered person or hospital is given a DEA certificate for display, a registration number, and official forms which must be used in ordering and purchasing controlled substances. The registration number must be used on all prescriptions and order forms. Registrants (and those authorized under a registration) must keep accurate records of orders, receipts, and uses of controlled substances. Current inventory must be reconcilable with amounts received and used or dispensed. All records and activities are subject to inspection by DEA personnel at any time. Both the veterinarian and the pharmacist are legally responsible for the proper prescribing and dispensing of drugs covered by the CSA. Further, controlled substances must be stored in a locked cabinet or preferably in a safe secured to a concrete floor.

The manufacturers and distributors are required to identify a controlled substance on the label of original containers by a symbol corresponding to the schedules specified by DEA for each controlled substance. The symbol is a capital C (for controlled substance), followed by the Roman numeral corresponding to the schedule to which the substance is assigned (i.e., C-I, C-II, C-III, C-IV, or C-V).

Schedule I (C-I) drugs have a high abuse potential and are not currently accepted in the United States for use in any practice situation, although they may be obtained for research or instructional use. Examples are heroin, LSD, mescaline, dihydromorphine, and morphine methylsulfonate.

Schedule II (C-II) drugs have a high abuse potential; their use can produce severe psychic or physical dependence in humans, and they apparently have similar effects in animals. These are the former Class A narcotic drugs plus certain stimulant drugs. Examples are opium, morphine, hydromorphone (Dilaudid), codeine, methadone, meperidine (Demerol), and cocaine; phenmetrazine (Preludin), methylphenidate (Ritalin), and methaqualone (Quaalude) and its salts; and the barbiturates amobarbital (Amytal), pentobarbital (Nembutal), and secobarbital (Seconal) and their salts. The amphetamines are no longer available under Schedule II for veterinary use.

Schedule III (C-III) drugs have less abuse potential than those in Schedules I and II. Abusive use of C-III drugs leads to moderate or low physical dependence but often high psychological dependence in humans. These drugs were formerly known as Class B narcotics (any preparation containing limited amounts of opium, morphine, ethylmorphine, codeine, dihydrocodeine, or hydrocodone) and some nonnarcotic drugs such as glutethimide (Doriden), nalorphine, phencyclidine, ketamine, benzphetamine, paregoric, and barbiturates (except those specified in another schedule).

Schedule IV (C-IV) drugs have a low abuse potential that can lead to limited physical or psychological dependence in humans. Included here are barbital, phenobarbital, methylphenobarbital, chloralhydrate, ethinomate, meprobamate (Miltown, Equanil), chlordiazepoxide (Librium), and diazepam (Valium).

Schedule V (C-V) drugs have a lesser abuse potential and include those preparations formerly known as exempt narcotics, except for paregoric.

Anabolic steroids were added to the list of controlled substances in 1991, under the Anabolic Steroids Control Act (ASCA) (Federal Register [56 FR 5753, February 13, 1991]). Certain veterinary products fall under the ASCA and have been classified as Schedule III (C-III) drugs under the CSA. These products include boldenone, mibolerone, stanozolol, testosterone, and trenbolone and their salts, esters, and isomers. Estrogens and progesterones are not subject to the ASCA or the CSA.

Implants in the final dosage form, if expressly intended for use in cattle or other nonhuman species, in accordance with their approvals under the FFD&C Act, are exempted from the scheduling requirements. However, any person or firm engaged, or proposing to engage, in the production of such implants must comply with the Schedule III requirements of the CSA and must register with the DEA.

DRUG COMPENDIA. It is critically important to the veterinarian, pharmacist, and physician and their patients and clients that the drugs they employ are of uniform potency, purity, and quality. Without such standardization, rational pharmacotherapy would be impossible. Such assurance is a basic objective of the laws and regulations described above and is the purpose of the *US Pharmacopeia* (USP)-*National Formulary* (NF). The USP-NF is the legally recognized drug compendium for the United States. The USP was originally compiled and first published in 1820 and has been regularly and continuously revised by the US Pharmacopeial Convention, which is composed of elected delegates representing human medicine, pharmacy, veterinary medicine, dentistry, and nursing. The *National Formulary* was a separate official compendium published by the American Pharmaceutical Association to serve the need of pharmacists for standardization of certain pure drugs that were not used widely enough to be included in the USP. During the 1975-80 USP revision period these two official compendia were "unified" into a single USP-NF compendium. At that time the scope of the two components was changed in that the USP covered all drug substances and drug products, while the NF was devoted exclusively to pharmaceutic ingredients.

In addition to USP and NF designations, a drug may be given an International Nonproprietary Name (INN).

The USP and NF derive their official status from the FFD&C Act. Standards promulgated by the Committee of Revision of the USP Convention are enforceable by the FDA.

57

DOSAGE FORMS, DRUG PRESCRIPTION ORDERS, AND VETERINARY FEED DIRECTIVES

SCOTT ANTHONY BROWN

Dosage Forms
Nomenclature
Prescription Writing
  Form of the Prescription
  Abbreviations
  Metrology
  Writing the Prescription
  Responsibilities of the Veterinarian
Veterinary Feed Directive
  Requirements
  VFD Form
Incompatibilities

Selection of an appropriate drug for therapy begins with establishment of an accurate diagnosis. Once the veterinarian is satisfied that the disease or dysfunction present in the patient has been determined, a decision is reached on the available options for subsequent therapy based on an understanding of the disease process and the pharmacology of possible choices of drugs (if drug therapy is appropriate). If a drug is chosen, the veterinarian must then decide the route by which to administer the medicament to the animal, what dosage form to use, and what the dose and the dosage interval should be. The client must then be provided with a supply of the medication (dispensed or prescribed) as well as specific instructions on how to administer the drug.

DOSAGE FORMS. Appropriate understanding of dosage forms requires an appreciation for the various routes of administration. The reader is referred to Chap. 3 for a description of the various routes of administration.

Dosage forms are preparations of drugs compounded in such a manner as to provide a convenient means of administering a drug dose to the patient. Such pharmaceutical preparations are designed for inhalation, oral administration, parenteral injection, or external application to the body.

Most commonly used medicinal preparations for oral administration are various solid dosage forms. They have advantages of ease of administration; stability, which provides a long shelf life; and uniformity with respect to drug content. The simplest solid oral dosage form is a simple mixture of powders (drugs) packaged in appropriately sized packets. Generally, these are employed by adding the powder to the drinking water or feed. Compressed tablets are the most commonly employed oral dosage form. These consist of an active drug combined with one or more binders and excipients. The mixture is compressed into appropriately sized tablets by machine. Tablets may be scored on both surfaces to facilitate fractionization for providing smaller doses. Official tablets must meet USP-NF standards for uniformity of weight and content of active ingredients and for rate of disintegration. Tablets of drugs that are irritating to the stomach or destroyed by gastric juice may be coated with phenylsalicylate (salol) or other substance that is insoluble in acid but will dissolve in the alkaline small intestine. These are so-called enteric-coated tablets. Boluses are large compressed tablets that are rectangular or oblong in shape. These are used for horses and cattle to provide the larger amount of drug required in the dose without increasing the cross-sectional size of the dosage form to a dimension that cannot be easily swallowed. Capsules are containers made of a mixture of gelatin and glycerin and are suitable for drugs in powdered form and certain liquid drugs. These have an advantage in that the drug, which may have a very unpalatable taste, does not contact the oral mucosa prior to swallowing. A major disadvantage is that the contained dose cannot be fractionated for smaller animals.

Several liquid preparations are available for oral administration (mixtures, emulsions, syrups, elixirs). Mixtures are aqueous solutions or suspensions intended for oral administration. Because of the possibility of contamination by bacteria or molds, mixtures generally have a preservative added (benzoic acid or chlorobutanol) to inhibit such growth. Aqueous suspensions of solids, also called magmas, generally contain a dispersing agent (tragacanth or methylcellulose) to delay settling. The label on the dispensed bottle should contain the phrase "Shake well before using" to ensure uniformity of dosage. Syrups are solutions of medicinal agents, flavoring, and coloring agents in an 85% sucrose solution. These are generally employed as cough remedies. Elixirs are hydroalcoholic solutions of medicinal substances that have been sweetened and flavored. Because of their high alcohol content, they often have better storage properties than mixtures. Emulsions consist of oily substances dispersed in an aqueous medium with acacia, lecithin, or methylcellulose added to stabilize the dispersion.

Two types of dosage forms are available for parenteral administration: injections and implants. Injections are sterile solutions or suspensions in an aqueous (sometimes an oil) vehicle. Most injections are heat sterilized or, if unstable to heat, are sterilized by filtration or irradiated. Some drugs are unstable in solution and are packaged aseptically in vials. These products are reconstituted with sterile water immediately before use for injection. A somewhat similar situation is that of tablet triturates, which are small, loosely packed tablets to be dissolved in water immediately before injection. Injections must be free of particulate foreign substances and pyrogens and should be nearly isotonic. They may be supplied in ampules, multiple-dose vials, or large-volume capped bottles or IV bags to which an intravenous infusion set may be attached. Syringes and needles for parenteral administration of drugs must be clean and sterile and the needles must be sharp. One may use either glass or disposable plastic syringes. However, it is best to use disposable needles since they are convenient, economical, and always sharp. Injections should not be stored in syringes for any length of time prior to use unless instructed to do so by the manufacturer, as some drugs will adsorb to either the glass (insulin) or plastic (diazepam) walls of the syringe and inadequate doses will be delivered. Disposable syringes and needles should be promptly destroyed and disposed of after use, and syringes and needles should be kept out of sight to keep them out of the hands of people who would use them for self-abuse for administration of addictive drugs. Specific regulations now exist for proper disposal of biohazard material.

Repository forms of drugs are designed to prolong effective drug concentration in the body by providing for sustained release from the dosage form. Sustained-release forms of injections are prepared by modifying the chemical nature of the drug to decrease its solubility, altering its physical form, or modifying its vehicle. Implants are very hard, sterile pellets inserted under the skin where they dissolve very slowly. Oral sustained-release preparations have not been as reliable because of individual differences in GI absorption and transit times. Capsules are available in which drug particles are coated with materials having different dissolution rates. Other methods are layered tablets and incorporation of ion exchange resins with the drug in tablets or capsules.

Several external dosage forms can be applied to the skin surface for various purposes. Liniments or braces are liquid or semisolid preparations to be applied to the skin with inunction (rubbing). These generally contain counterirritants to relieve muscle or tendon pain. Lotions are solutions or suspensions of soothing substances to be applied to the skin without friction (calamine lotion). Ointments are semisolid greasy preparations in which the drug is dissolved or dispersed in a suitable base, the nature of which may vary from an oleaginous substance such as petrolatum to a completely water-soluble base such as polyethylene glycol. Creams incorporate a drug in a water-oil emulsion; water will evaporate following application, leaving the drug and a thin film of oil on the skin. Dusting powders are mixtures of drugs in powder form for application to external surfaces. These may be applied for their adsorbent (cornstarch) or lubricant (talcum) properties. Aerosols are drugs incorporated in a suitable solvent and packaged under pressure with a propellant such as fluorinated hydrocarbon or nitrogen. Topical insecticides and wound dressings are frequently prepared as aerosols.

NOMENCLATURE. Names of drugs are often a source of confusion to the novice, partly because most drugs have at least three different names: a chemical name, a nonproprietary name, and one or more proprietary names. The chemical name provides scientific and technical personnel with a precise and unambiguous description of the substance in accordance with rules of chemical nomenclature established by the International Union of Pure and Applied Chemistry (commonly abbreviated IUPAC). Generally, such names are too complex and cumbersome to meet the everyday needs of the pharmacist, prescriber, and regulatory bodies. Accordingly, official nonproprietary names (incorrectly termed generic names) are designated to identify particular drug entities. Drug names appearing throughout this text and other discussions in pharmacology are principally nonproprietary names. A given drug entity may have a number of proprietary names that are brand names assigned and possibly trademarked by different manufacturers; e.g., POLYOTIC® Oblets, TET-SOL® 10, SOLUTET® Soluble Powder, TETRABAC® 324, ACHROMYCIN® V Capsules, TOPICYCLINE® for Topical Solution, HELIDAC® Therapy, and PANMYCIN® 500 Boluses are all proprietary names used to describe forms of tetracycline. An example of the complete nomenclature for a single entity is as follows: the nonproprietary, or generic, name for a certain sedative drug is diazepam, one proprietary name for a diazepam product is Valium® Tablets, and the chemical name is 7-chloro-1,3-dihydro-1-methyl-5-phenyl-2*H*-1,4-benzodiazepin-2-one. Technically, the proprietary term is an adjective that modifies a dosage form of the drug (e.g., NAXCEL® Sterile Powder, or NAXCEL® brand of Ceftiofur Sodium Sterile Powder).

Some order has been brought to the matter of drug nomenclature by the US Pharmacopeial Convention. A compilation of the United States Adopted Names (USAN) is published annually as the *USAN and the USP Dictionary of Drug Names.* Each entry of the compilation includes the US Adopted Name, the year of publication as a USAN, a pronunciation guide, the molecular formula, the chemical name, the registry number, the pharmacologic and therapeutic activity claim, the proprietary names and manufacturers, and the structural formula. An additional problem for the student is that there may be different nonproprietary names for the same drug in different countries; e.g., an analgesic drug is named meperidine in the United States, pethidine in the United Kingdom (UK), and dolantin in Germany. Similarly, barbiturates have the suffix *-al* in the United States and *-one* in the UK; e.g., pentobarbital is the same compound as pentobarbitone. Sulfamethazine in the United States is sulfadimidine in the UK. These differences are soon learned when practicing in a different country.

PRESCRIPTION WRITING. A prescription is an order to a pharmacist written by a licensed veterinarian, physician, or dentist to prepare the prescribed medicine, affix the directions, and sell the preparation to the client or patient. The prescription is a legally recognized document, and the writer is held responsible for its accuracy. Dispensing, on the other hand, is the preparation and distribution of medicines to those who are to use them. As a licensed practitioner, the veterinarian is entitled by law to dispense, administer, or prescribe medications for animal patients. Veterinarians have tended toward dispensing products rather than prescribing drugs. Knapp (1955) enumerated several good reasons for the veterinarian to become adept at prescription writing and employ the services of a registered pharmacist:

1. The veterinarian can charge just about the same fee as when drugs are dispensed; payment for services and knowledge rather than just payment for the remedy should receive higher priority.
2. Writing a prescription eliminates the cost of the dispensed item so that subtraction from the fee is obviated.
3. Prescribing provides the practicing veterinarian with a supply of pharmaceuticals that might not always be available on the shelves of the clinic.
4. Prescription writing reduces the investment tied up in drug inventory when one dispenses drugs.
5. If a client does not pay the bill, cost of the medicines dispensed are not lost.
6. Prescribing can bring about improved cooperation between the pharmaceutical and veterinary medical professions.
7. The client is frequently more inclined to pay for two smaller fees than one large fee.
8. Prescription writing provides a means for learning, including an appreciation of drugs and their actions, indications, and dosages; individuals adept in prescription writing usually have more detailed information at their command than those who are not.

The veterinarian should weigh the relative advantages between dispensing and prescribing and do what is best for the particular circumstances. In any case, every veterinarian should be able to write a prescription.

Form of the Prescription. The essential parts of a classic prescription consist of the following:

1. The *date* of writing the prescription.
2. The *identity* and *address* of owner and patient.
3. The *superscription,* Rx, is an abbreviation of the Latin word *recipe* meaning "take thou of." A portion of this superscription is the symbol of the Roman god Jupiter and is a relic of the times when all prescriptions were begun with a prayer to Jupiter asking his help in making them effective in the cure of disease.
4. The *inscription* lists the names and amounts of drugs to be incorporated in the prescription. Names of the drugs should be written in English and the total amounts required should be written in the metric system, which is preferred and official in the USP-NF. (In the past, the apothecaries' system of measurement and Latin terminology were preferred for prescription writing.) The modern tendency in therapeutics is to employ as few drugs as possible and strive for specific therapy. The complicated and useless mixtures ("shotgun" prescriptions) of earlier decades have been discarded in favor of single drugs or simple combinations of drugs. Most of the drugs needed by the practitioner are listed in the USP-NF.
5. The *subscription* gives the instructions to the pharmacist. These instructions may be entirely in English or with Latin abbreviations.
6. The *signa* (Sig. or S.) consists of instructions for administration of the medicine, which the pharmacist writes or types on the label.
7. The *signature* of the practitioner must appear on the prescription to make it a legal document.

Abbreviations. Names of drugs to be included in the prescription should not be abbreviated but should be written out in full to avoid possible errors. Chemical formulas must not be used in prescription writing because of the greatly increased probability of error.

Abbreviations of Latin words are commonly used in writing a prescription because they save time and are readily understood by the pharmacist. Commonly used abbreviations that should be memorized are provided in Table 57.1.

Dosage regimens have been expressed in a number of ways that have caused confusion and misunderstanding; e.g., dosage may be recommended as 22 mg/kg t.i.d., 22 mg/kg to be divided for t.i.d. administration, 66 mg/kg to be divided for t.i.d. administration, or 22 mg/kg q8h. As you can see, serious misunderstandings can arise if a drug is employed with a low margin of safety; e.g., if you gave 66 mg/kg three times between 0800 and 2200. It has been recommended (Aronson 1980) that dosage regimens be expressed as mg/kg and the time interval be expressed in hours, e.g., q4h, q8h, q12h. Thus abbreviations of s.i.d., b.i.d., t.i.d. and q.i.d. would be abandoned. This makes good sense, because three doses of a drug could be given within an hour and technically the animal would have received t.i.d. medication.

Metrology. Metrology is the study of weights and measures. The use of different or mixed systems of

TABLE 57.1—Abbreviations commonly used in prescribing

Abbreviation	Latin	Meaning
ad lib.	*ad libitum*	freely as wanted
ā ā	*ana*	of each
ā	*ante*	before
a.c.	*ante cibum*	before meals
aq.	*aqua*	water
b.i.d. (or BID)	*bis in die*	twice a day
cap.	*capula*	capsule
c̄	*cum*	with
div.	*divide*	divide
dos.	*dosis*	a dose
eq. pts.	*equalis partis*	equal parts
ft.	*fiat*	make
gtt.	*gutta*	a drop
haust.	*haustus*	drench
h.	*hora*	hour
M.	*misce*	mix
n.r.	*non repetatur*	not to be repeated
no.	*numero*	number
O.	*octarius*	pint
o.d.	*omne die*	every day
p.c.	*post cibum*	after meals
p.r.n.	*pro re nata*	as occasion requires
Q.R.	*quantum rectum*	correct quantities
q.s.	*quantum sufficiat*	sufficient quantity
q4h	*quaque 4 hora*	every 4 hours
q6h	*quaque 6 hora*	every 6 hours
q.i.d. (or QID)	*quater in die*	four times a day
s.i.d. (or SID)	*semel in die*	once a day
s̄ s̄	*semisse*	half
Sig., S.	*signa*	write on the label
s̄	*sine*	without
s.o.s.	*si opus sit*	if necessary
sol.	*solutio*	solution
stat.	*statim*	immediately
tab.	*tabella*	a tablet
t.i.d. (or TID)	*ter in die*	three times a day

metrology should be avoided, and the metric system is preferred worldwide. Appendix Table A57.1 lists commonly used weights and measures.

In the United States the weight/volume method (W/V) of measuring solids and liquids is employed; i.e., the masses of solids are weighed and the volumes of liquids are measured. The weight/weight method (W/W) is employed in continental Europe; i.e., both liquids and solids are weighed in prescription compounding. The completely gravimetric method is more accurate because it compensates for differences in specific gravity of liquids. However, for most purposes the weight by volume method employed in this country proves satisfactory.

The metric system uses Arabic numerals to indicate the quantities of drug required. The Arabic numeral is followed by the unit of measurement. A single vertical line may be substituted for aligned decimal points on successive lines. The figures to the left of the line are whole numbers, while those to the right are decimal fractions. In the metric system the quantities automatically indicate grams (g) for solids and milliliters (mL) for liquids without specific designation.

The veterinarian must be familiar with basic apothecary units in the United States for conversion to the metric system because a number of older dosage forms are still provided in the apothecaries' system of weights and measures by pharmaceutical companies. Conversion factors can be found in Appendix Table A57.2.

Writing the Prescription. Several examples of prescription writing are given in this section. The prescription is often very simple and requires little writing and calculation. In the one shown in Fig. 57.1, dosage is not important because the lotion would be applied by the owner in quantity sufficient to cover the lesions on the skin. The amount of 480 mL of lotion was chosen for dispensing because this volume exactly fills a 16-oz prescription bottle. The veterinarian should know that prescription bottles are available in the following volumes in fluid ounces: 1, 2, 3, 4, 6, 8, 12, 16, and 32. Bottles are also available calibrated in the metric system (i.e., mL). The veterinarian should prescribe appropriate volumes because the client is often better satisfied when paying for a full bottle.

Some drugs are not soluble in the common solvents and must be administered as solids. Powders may be administered as such when sprinkled on the animal's solid feed. Many powders are distasteful and must be masked by some flavoring agent or administered in a more palatable form. A common way of administering powders is by packing into a hard gelatin capsule. The capsule is tasteless, readily swallowed, and disintegrates rapidly in the stomach. Hard gelatin capsules are available in two series of sizes. The smallest is known as No. 5. In order of increasing size, capsules are numbered as 5, 4, 3, 2, 1, 0, 00, 000. Another numbering scheme is used for the next series of hard gelatin capsules, which increase in size from the last mentioned. In order of increasing size they are 13, 12, 11, and 10. In addition, there are infrequently used sizes 9, 8, and 7. The weight of drug contained in a capsule varies too widely with the ingredient to be of significance, but the No. 10 gelatin capsule is commonly referred to as the 1-oz size, the No. 11 as the 1/2-oz, the No. 12 as the 1/4-oz, and the No. 13 as the 1/8-oz capsule.

Assume that you have examined a toy poodle weighing 11 lb and have decided that the patient will benefit from a drug that will dilate the bronchioles. You elect to write a prescription for aminophylline tablets. You find that the dosage rate is 10 mg/kg to be given every 8 hours. Furthermore, you consult a reference to learn that aminophylline is available in 100- and 200-mg scored tablets. You want to prescribe enough medication for 2 weeks, after which you want to reexamine the patient. Your calculations would be as follows: the dog weighs 11 lb or $11 \div 2.2 = 5$ kg; the dose is 10 mg/kg $\times$ 5 kg = 50 mg; this is to be given every 8 hours for 14 days. The nearest-sized tablet is 100 mg, so each dose would be one-half tablet. The number of 100 mg tablets needed is 21. You would write:

Telephone (999) 123-456 Date:____________

JAMES J. SMITH, D. V. M.

2511 Broad Street Columbus, Ohio

Client's name *Mr. Ross Barnes* Address *Rt. 3. Columbus, Ohio*

Patient *horse (Standardbred)* Age *2 years* Sex *Female*

Rx	g	or ml
Calamine lotion, USP	480	0
M		
Label: Apply daily to skin lesions		

DEA No. XX1234 Refills______ ____________D.V.M.

FIG. 57.1—A sample prescription form.

Aminophylline tabs, Rx, 100 mg
Dispense 21
Sig.: Give one-half tab. q8h
For veterinary use only.

You wish to prescribe a cough syrup with codeine for a dog weighing 35 lb at a dosage rate for the codeine of 2 mg/kg. You advise the owner to treat the animal every 3 hours for 4 doses each day for a total of 6 days. The veterinarian should calculate and state the total amount of ingredients needed. The calculations are as follows:

35 lb ÷ 2.2 = approx. 15 kg
2 mg/kg × 15 kg = 30 mg codeine/dose
4 doses × 6 days = 24 doses
24 × 30 = 720 mg codeine phosphate needed

The next step is to measure the dose. Household measures, such as teaspoonfuls or tablespoonfuls, are commonly used in prescriptions for human use. It is difficult for an owner to administer medication to an animal from a spoon. Consequently, it is useful to show the client how to give liquid medication orally by means of a plastic syringe and include the dispensing of an appropriate size in your prescription. In the example, you decide that 5 mL of syrup would be a convenient single dose. You now calculate the volume of the vehicle needed:

24 doses × 5 mL = 120 mL of vehicle

This is equivalent to 4 fluid oz, which you recall is a common sized bottle for dispensing. You now have sufficient information to write the prescription.

Codeine phosphate, USP	0	720
Syrup of cherry q.s.	120	0

ft. sol. Dispense 5-mL plastic
syringe for oral dosing.
Sig.: 5 mL q3h for 4 doses daily.
For veterinary use only.

When writing a prescription, write in ink (preferably blue or black), write deliberately, avoid rewriting, and use simple ingredients. Do not use chemical formulas or abbreviations for ingredients and do not use prescription blanks with the name of a drugstore on them. Avoid conversation while writing so you do not make errors due to distractions.

Many modern prescriptions stipulate proprietary pharmaceutical preparations. There is no objection to their use if there is no parallel preparation in the USP-NF. Use of a proprietary rather than an official preparation increases the cost of the medicine considerably, because official preparations are more commonly and widely produced in a competitive market. When a proprietary preparation is stipulated in a prescription, the ingredient is identified by the name of the manufacturer and the trademark name of the preparation.

If a veterinarian writes a prescription to be filled by a pharmacist, it cannot be refilled unless authorized by the prescriber, who should indicate on the prescription the number of times it may be refilled. Prescriptions containing drugs regulated by the Controlled Substances Act of 1970 must have appended the registration number obtained by the veterinarian from the Drug Enforcement Administration of the US Department of Justice. The full name and address of both the veterinarian and the owner, as well as the identity of the animal patient, must be on all such prescription forms along with the permit number issued to the practitioner. Prescriptions for controlled substances in Schedule II must be typewritten or written in ink or indelible pencil and signed by the registered practitioner. Prescription orders for Schedule II drugs must be limited to a 34-day supply and cannot be refilled. Prescription orders for Schedule III or IV drugs may be issued orally or in writing by a practitioner and may be refilled when authorized but not more than five times and not later than 6 months after the date of writing the prescription. Thereafter, a new prescription authorization must be issued. Drugs in Schedule V can be prescribed like those of Schedules III and IV, and some may be sold over the counter by a pharmacist under specified conditions.

The label on the container of any controlled substance in Schedules II, III, or IV when dispensed for animal use must contain the following warning: "Caution: Federal law prohibits the transfer of this drug to any person other than the (client and) patient for whom it was prescribed."

Responsibilities of the Veterinarian. Whether the veterinarian administers, dispenses, or prescribes a drug, he or she has the ultimate responsibility for the welfare of the patient and the best interests of the client. Responsibilities include proper dosage, selection, and administration of drugs; providing clients with adequate information for proper usage of a drug; testing for allergy when such is indicated; proper storage and packaging of drugs to be dispensed; maintenance of adequate records concerning drugs used; and maintenance of the security of controlled substances used in the practice.

The veterinarian must be particularly careful to dispense drugs in safe containers with proper labeling. Veterinary drugs are often dispensed to households that have small children. The US Congress passed the Poison Prevention Packaging Act in 1970, which allocated responsibility to the Food and Drug Administration to require special packaging for drugs that may be dangerous to small children. Broadly, this is to be a container that cannot be readily opened by children, but adults should be able to open and close packages easily. These rather stringent requirements arose from recognition by the National Clearinghouse for Poison Control Centers in its 1970 report of an excessive number of hospitalizations of children under 5 years of age from ingestion of amphetamines, barbiturates, meprobamate, and methadone, which are among the more toxic agents ingested. At present, the regulations apply only to drug manufacturers and pharmacists and not to veterinarians; nevertheless, veterinarians should be guided by these regulations for the protection of their clients and to protect themselves against legal actions. One case of a 23-month-old girl dying following ingestion of digitoxin prescribed for her babysitter's pet was described (Anon. 1977). Such tragedies can be prevented by use of childproof containers.

In cases of poisoning of either children or pets by drugs, prompt treatment is facilitated by proper labeling of the dispensed medication. Information to appear on the label is dictated by state and federal laws. The following information should be adequate for labeling in any state (Fillingim 1980): (1) name and address of the place of business from which drug is dispensed; (2) name or initials of authorized person who dispenses the medication; (3) date on which medication is dispensed; (4) prescription serial number, if applicable; (5) last name of prescriber; (6) directions for use; (7) owner's name, animal's name, species, and clinic number; (8) name, strength, and quantity of drug; and (9) any necessary auxiliary labels and warnings.

If instructions for use are lengthy, you can type on the label "Use as directed on the dosage schedule" and provide the detailed instructions on a separate sheet of paper marked "dosage schedule." The label must be attached to the container that directly holds the medication. For example, do not place an unlabeled dropper bottle of ear medication in a box and then place the label on the box, because the two are likely to be separated.

The veterinarian clearly has ethical and legal responsibilities that go along with the privileges of the profession. By careful attention to details of acquisition, storage, dispensing, prescribing, administration, and record keeping, the veterinarian should be able to avoid most grounds for malpractice or other unpleasant legal actions in our modern, litigious society.

VETERINARY FEED DIRECTIVE. Veterinary Feed Directive (VFD) is a new category of medicated feeds created by the Animal Drug Availability Act of 1996 (ADAA). It provides an alternative to prescription status for certain therapeutic drugs for use in feed, while ensuring the participation of the veterinarian, who issues a directive to enable producers to acquire VFD medicated feeds. In 1996, the Center for Veterinary Medicine (CVM) of the Food and Drug Administration (FDA) expressed a need for greater control over the use of certain new therapeutic antimicrobial medicated feeds. The purposely added professional control is to ensure that VFD medicated feeds are fed correctly and are effective for as long as possible. In some ways, the VFD is similar to a prescription; you must get it from a veterinarian after a careful diagnosis is made. However, a VFD allows producers to obtain VFD medicated feeds through normal feed supply channels without involving a pharmacist or having to deal with diverse state pharmacy laws.

The VFD is not a prescription for feed. The VFD is an alternative to prescription classification. A prescription status for feeds would lead to major disruptions of existing marketplace practices for drug sponsors, feed manufacturers, and animal producers. Among other problems, the prescription status would have triggered state pharmacy laws and regulations that were intended to apply only to the dispensing of other dosage forms, not to medicated animal feed. Similarly, it would have triggered statutory limitations on labeling and marketing practices and, therefore, would have placed covered drugs and feeds at a commercial disadvantage compared with over-the-counter (OTC) medicated feeds. The VFD applies only to those specific drugs that are newly approved as VFD medicated feeds. As with other medicated feeds, the extra-label use of VFD drugs is prohibited.

As in the past, all animal drugs must be approved by the FDA. The determination of whether a product will be approved as a VFD drug or as an OTC drug is made by the FDA's CVM. Currently, the CVM states that all new antimicrobials for therapeutic use in feed will be provided as VFD drugs.

Requirements. A veterinarian, in a professional veterinarian-client-patient relationship, examines and diagnoses animal conditions and determines whether a condition warrants administration of a VFD drug. If so, the veterinarian will issue a signed VFD on a preprinted, multipart form. The veterinarian provides the form to the producer, who, in turn, orders the VFD feed from his or her feed supplier. A VFD feed may not be distributed to a producer without a signed VFD form.

Three groups must be involved:

1. The person or firm supplying a VFD to a producer must receive and retain a copy of the signed VFD form issued by a producer's veterinarian.
2. Licensed feed manufacturers and distributors who ship a VFD feed to a downstream distributor or retailer for inventory must receive and retain a copy of written acknowledgment stating that the VFD feed will be further distributed only in accordance with FDA requirements.
3. All distributors and retailers who *do not* hold a Feed Mill license must, within 30 days, notify the FDA of their initial VFD feed shipment.

VFD Form. The form for the Veterinary Feed Directive is generally provided to the veterinarian by the sponsor of the type A medicated feed that is produced by the pharmaceutical company (Fig. 57.2). Information the veterinarian must supply on the VFD form will normally include

1. The producer's name, address, and telephone number.
2. The species, location, number of and description of animals, and the condition being treated.
3. The date of treatment and, if different, the date of issuing the VFD form.
4. The name of the animal drug, the level of the drug in the feed, and the amount of feed to be manufactured.
5. The directions for mixing and feeding (including dilution) and amount or length of time to be fed, withdrawal time, and any cautionary statements.
6. The expiration date and the number of refills, if permitted, by approval.
7. The veterinarian's name, address, license number, state of licensing, and signature.

A producer may not buy VFD products and store them on the farm unless the producer holds a valid feed mill license or is a distributor of VFD feeds and has complied with all requirements for distributors.

The valid veterinarian-client-patient relationship, as defined by the American Veterinary Medical Association, exists when

1. The veterinarian has assumed the responsibility for making medical judgments regarding the health of the animals and the need for medical treatment, and the client (owner or caretaker) has agreed to follow the instructions of the veterinarian.
2. There is sufficient knowledge of the animals by the veterinarian to initiate at least a general or preliminary diagnosis of the medical condition of the animals. This means that the veterinarian has recently seen, or is personally acquainted with, the keeping and care of the animals by virtue of examination of the animals and/or by medically appropriate and timely visits to the premises where the animals are kept.
3. The practicing veterinarian is readily available or has arranged for emergency coverage for follow-up in case of adverse reactions or failure of the regimen of therapy.

INCOMPATIBILITIES. Incompatibility of two or more drugs in a mixture or in a patient can reduce drug safety or efficacy. Three types of incompatibility may be encountered in practice: therapeutic, chemical, or pharmaceutical. Knowledge of these is necessary for the veterinarian to avoid unnecessary problems with therapy and to be able to antagonize certain drug effects. It is impossible to discuss all possible specific incompatibilities, so this discussion is limited to a general description. Tables of commonly encountered incompatibilities have been published elsewhere (Davis 1981).

Therapeutic incompatibilities occur as a result of antagonistic pharmacologic actions in the patient or interference with drug absorption following administration; e.g., a therapeutic incompatibility will arise if you simultaneously administer physostigmine and atropine in the eye. Physostigmine constricts the pupil, whereas atropine dilates it. You might be treating a dog with propranolol for a cardiac dysrhythmia and decide to treat an asthmatic attack with isoproterenol. The propranolol will block the response of bronchioles to the isoproterenol. Drug incompatibilities can occur following oral medication, e.g., antacids or dairy products will impair the absorption of tetracyclines and kaolin will have a similar effect when administered with erythromycin or digoxin.

Chemical incompatibilities will manifest themselves in a number of ways (precipitation, change in color, evolution of gas, gelatinization, inactivation without any visible change). This may be the result of the drugs undergoing a chemical reaction, pH changes in the dosage forms, interactions with preservatives or solvents in the dosage form, and combination of divalent

Veterinary Feed Directive

Client Address	Veterinarian Address
Phone	Phone

Animals to be treated (number and location):

VFD Drug: **HEALWELL**® (anyglycoside)

Mixing Direction: *(See reverse for additional mixing information)*
Mix into type C Medicated Feed to provide: 200 ☐ 300 ☐ 400 ☐ g/ton
(Check only one)

WARNING: Feeds containing anyglycoside must be withdrawn 9 days prior to slaughter.

Feeding Instructions: Feed continuously as the sole ration for 21 days beginning with the onset of symptoms.

Special Instructions: ______________________

Expiration date: ______________________ Refills (if permitted): __________
Month/Day/Year

Total amount of Type C feed to be received under this VFD: __________ tons

Veterinarian's Signature: ______________________ Date: __________

License Number: ______________________ State: __________

This VFD drug will be obtained from: ______________________

See reverse side for important product information.
HEALWELL® is the registered trademark of Know Animal Health.

FIG. 57.2—An example of a Veterinary Feed Directive form.

cations with components of the mixture. Incompatibilities should be a major consideration when the practitioner mixes different drugs in the same syringe (which is an extremely bad practice), formulates solutions for intramammary or intrauterine therapy, and adds drugs to solutions for intravenous infusion. Before doing these things, one should consult a pharmacist or reference on drug incompatibilities. Alkaloids, iodine, arsenic, iron salts, mercury salts, permanganate, salicylates, silver salts, strong acids or alkalis, and tannic acid are frequently incompatible with other agents and should not be mixed. We take advantage of this effect when we lavage the stomach with tannic acid or potassium permanganate solutions in the treatment of alkaloid poisoning or administer copper sulfate solution to an animal that has swallowed phosphorus. Adverse examples are: addition of sodium bicarbonate to calcium-containing solutions will result in the precipitation of calcium carbonate; 5% dextrose solution is acidic (pH 5.0) and will inactivate added potassium penicillin.

Pharmaceutical incompatibilities are usually of a physical nature, e.g., incomplete solutions resulting from low solubility of drug in a given solvent, immiscibility of liquids mixed together, and precipitation. One can readily avoid these problems by thoroughly understanding the actions of drugs used in therapy, using the services of a pharmacist, refraining from mixing different medicaments in the same syringe prior to administration, and being parsimonious in use of drugs.

REFERENCES

Anon. 1977. J Am Vet Med Assoc 171:1028.

———. 1997. VFD Facts. American Feed Industry Association.

Aronson, A. L. 1980. J Am Vet Med Assoc 176:1047.

Davis, L. E. 1981. In W. Guin, ed., Veterinary Values, pp. 60–73. New York: Ag Resources.

Fillingim, D. V. 1980. In C. E. Aronson, ed., Proceedings of the Symposium on Veterinary Pharmacology and Therapeutics, pp. 266–80. Philadelphia: Univ of Pennsylvania.

Knapp, W. A. 1955. Southeast Vet 7:11.

Vogel, L. P. 1997. How the Veterinary Feed Directive Will Impact the Use of Antibiotic Feed Medications. Forum on the Use of Antibiotics in Food Production.

APPENDIX TABLES

TABLE A57.2—Conversion equivalents and factors for obtaining approximate equivalents

	Conversion Equivalents	
	Exact	**Approximate**
1 milligram	1/65 grain	(1/60)
1 gram	15.432 grains	(15)
1 kilogram	2.2 pounds (avoirdupois)	
1 milliliter	16.23 minims	(15)
1 liter	1.06 quarts or 33.8 fluid ounces	
1 grain	65.0 milligrams	(60)
1 dram	3.88 grams	(4)
1 ounce	31.1 grams	(30)
1 avoirdupois pound	454 grams	
1 minim	0.062 milliliter	(0.06)
1 fluid dram	3.7 milliliters	(4)
1 fluid ounce	29.57 milliliters	(30)
1 pint	473 milliliters	(500)
1 quart	946 milliliters	(1000)
1 drop		1 minim
1 teaspoonful		5 milliliters
1 dessertspoonful		8 milliliters
1 tablespoonful		15 milliliters
To convert	**To**	**Multiply by**
gr/lb	mg/lb	64.8
gr/lb	mg/kg	143.0
mg/lb	gr/lb	0.015
mg/lb	mg/kg	2.2
mg/kg	gr/lb	0.007
mg/kg	mg/lb	0.454

Note: Where possible, use suitable units rather than decimal fractions, e.g., 10 mg not 0.010 g. When a decimal fraction is used, the decimal point must be preceded by a zero, e.g., 0.5 not .5.

TABLE A57.1—Weights and measures used in prescribing

	The Metric System	
Weight	1 picogram (pg)	= 10^{-12} gram
	1000 picograms	= 1 nanogram (ng) or 10^{-9} gram
	1000 nanograms	= 1 microgram (µg) or 10^{-6} gram
	1000 micrograms	= 1 milligram (mg) or 10^{-3} gram
	1000 milligrams	= 1 gram (g)
	1000 grams	= 1 kilogram (kg)
Volume	1000 milliliters (mL)	= 1 liter (L)
	The Apothecaries' System	
Weight	20 grains (gr)	= 1 scruple (℈)
	3 scruples	= 1 dram (ʒ) or 60 grains
	8 drams	= 1 ounce (℥) or 480 grains
Volume	60 minims (min.)	= 1 fluid dram (f.ʒ)
	8 fluid drams	= 1 fluid ounce (f. ℥)
	16 fluid ounces	= 1 pint (O.)

58 CHEMICAL RESIDUES IN TISSUES OF FOOD ANIMALS

JIM E. RIVIERE AND STEPHEN F. SUNDLOF

The Concern over Residues in Food
Regulation of Drug Residues in Animals
The Veterinarian and Extra-Label Drug Use
Pharmacokinetics and Residues
Drugs Prohibited from Extra-Label Use
Residue Prevention

Most of this textbook has focused on describing the pharmacodynamics and pharmacokinetics of drugs in animals. In both human medical and companion-animal veterinary practices, the primary concern in drug selection and use is the therapeutic end point, whether or not the drug is efficacious against the disease being treated. Doses are usually administered at label recommendations, and if greater than label doses are administered, only potential toxicity is of concern. While this line of reasoning is also true to a large degree in food-animal production, veterinarians and producers involved in the treatment of disease in food animals bear the additional concern of the persistence of drug residues in the edible tissues after the disease process has been treated. Adulteration of the food supply with antimicrobial agents, pesticides, environmental contaminants, and other chemicals has been a growing source of concern to the general public and special-interest groups in recent years.

The importance of chemical residues in the edible tissues of food-producing animals has been thoroughly reviewed elsewhere (Sundlof 1989; Riviere 1991, 1992a; Van Dresser and Wilcke 1989; Mercer 1990; Kindred and Hubbert 1993; Bevill 1989). The purpose of this chapter is to acquaint the veterinarian with the legal and regulatory issues concerning the control of drug and other chemical residues in the United States, and to review some of the pharmacokinetic parameters used to determine withdrawal times for drugs and other chemicals in food animals. The primary parameter used by veterinarians to prevent violative tissue residues is the length of the withdrawal time, or the time required for a drug to be depleted from the animal before the animal's meat can be marketed for human consumption. In dairy practice, this is the milk discard time. Recently, government regulation and control have necessitated more stringent adherence to withdrawal times, and on-site monitoring for many drugs has been instituted. This may have an economic impact on production costs. Unlike in previous editions of this text, withdrawal times will not be tabulated, because they are subject to constant regulatory revision. Extensive tables of tissue depletion pharmacokinetic data are published elsewhere (Riviere et al. 1991; Craigmill et al. 1994).

THE CONCERN OVER RESIDUES IN FOOD. A great deal of concern has been demonstrated over the last 40 years about the presence of chemical adulterants or residues, mainly antimicrobials and pesticides, in the meat, poultry, and milk supplies of the United States. By definition, a chemical residue is either the parent compound or a metabolite of the parent compound that may accumulate, deposit, or otherwise be stored within the cells, tissues, organs, or edible products (e.g., milk, eggs) of an animal following its use to prevent, control, or treat animal disease or to enhance production. Residues can also result from unintentional administration of drugs or food additives. Finally, accidental exposure to chemicals in the environment can also result in tissue residues.

Concerns over food residues are economic as well as public health related. For example, the contamination of milk with antibiotics, most commonly penicillin, can affect starter cultures used to make fermented milk products such as cheeses, buttermilk, sour cream, etc., which can result in economic losses to those processors. From a public-health viewpoint, both the US government and producer associations have taken active roles in minimizing antibiotic residues in meats and milk. Penicillin, for example, is known to induce allergic reactions in some sensitive people, and therefore, penicillin-tainted milk poses a health risk for these individuals. Similarly, chloramphenicol has been reported to induce blood dyscrasias that may lead to death; hence, its use in food-producing animals has been prohibited by the Food and Drug Administration (FDA). The FDA has also prohibited the use of nitrofurans in food-producing animals because recent data have shown them to be carcinogenic. Not only therapeutic drugs but pesticides create residue problems. Most pesticides are administered topically, allowing some amount of percutaneous absorption and sequestration in edible tissues (see Chap. 53 of this text). Lindane has been detected in the fat deposits of sheep dipped in a 0.0125% lindane emulsion 12 weeks after topical exposure (Collett and Harrison 1963). Other studies have shown lindane residues in sheep, goats (Jackson et al. 1959), and lactating cows (Oehler et al. 1969). In addition to lindane, many common pesticides (organochlorines, organophosphates, botanicals, pyrethrins, etc.) and herbicides used in agriculture today that are applied topically have been shown to produce residues in food-producing animals. Environmental contaminants (e.g., heavy metals, PCB, mycotoxins) are also of major concern today. Tissue residue violations detected by governmental monitoring programs have been summarized by Sundlof (1989). More information on xenobiotics in food-producing animals is available in Riviere 1992a. Both public-health and economic concerns have been the major driving forces in the United States and in other countries behind the search for ways to minimize the threat of residue contamination of the public food supply.

Contamination of the food supply with chemical residues is rarely an intentional act and usually results either from failure to observe the correct meat withdrawal or milk discard time for a drug after it has been used to treat a disease in food animals or from accidental contamination of feed by chemicals or drugs. A study by Van Dresser and Wilcke (1989) provides some interesting insight on drug residue problems in food-producing animals. In that study, streptomycin, penicillin, sulfamethazine, and oxytetracycline were the four most common antibiotics found in tissues, with sulfamethazine being the most commonly found sulfonamide in animal tissues. Long-acting formulations of these drugs (i.e., penicillin and oxytetracycline) had the highest association with violative residues in the animals involved in the study. Injectable drugs were more likely to be associated with residue problems than were feed additives and boluses. Most of these residues were found in veal calves, cows, and market barrows and gilts. The most frequently cited reason for violative residues was failure to observe the correct withdrawal time for the drug. Failure to observe the correct withdrawal time was cited as the most common reason for violative drug residue levels in a study performed by the FDA in the 1970s (Bevill 1984) and continued to be the most common cause of residue violations in the 1990s. Interestingly, in this study the producer was found to be the responsible party in 80% of the cases investigated for violative levels of drug found in edible tissues (when the responsible party could be identified); unapproved drug use (extra-label drugs) is not considered a major cause of drug residues in animals. Ways to prevent drug residues will be discussed later in this chapter.

The FDA and Environmental Protection Agency (EPA) establish tolerances for a drug, pesticide, or other chemical in the relevant tissues of the food-producing animals. The tolerance is the tissue concentration below which a marker residue for the drug or chemical must fall in the target tissue before that animal's edible tissues (meat, milk, or eggs) are considered safe for human consumption (Riviere 1991). The marker residue may be the parent compound or a metabolite and reflects a known relationship to the total residues of the drug or chemical (parent and all metabolites). The target tissue is an edible tissue, frequently liver or kidney, which, when the compound has depleted below the tolerance, assures that all edible tissues are safe for human consumption. Tolerances for different tissues are considered legal end points for which drug withdrawal times are established. Tolerances are established based on extensive toxicologic studies of the potential hazard of consumption to humans. Oral toxicity studies are conducted in animals leading to the determination of an acceptable daily intake (ADI) for the compound in the human diet. These studies consider the compound's carcinogenic potential and its systemic, reproductive, and developmental toxicity and incorporate various safety factors. A safe concentration for human consumption is calculated using an equation that accounts for the amount of a specific food consumed by a person representing a high-consuming population (e.g., 19-year-old males) so that a safe concentration of the drug in this food (e.g., meat, milk, eggs) can be established. Various safety factors and statistical considerations are built into these determinations, and a tolerance for this drug in the specific tissue is established where appropriate and is published. For example, safety factors reflect the duration of exposure and the nature of the toxic effects associated with the chemical. A teratogen requires a larger safety factor than a nonteratogen, and ADIs based on a short-term subchronic study use a larger safety factor than ADIs based on chronic studies. The tolerance is for a specific drug or chemical entity and reflects both the inherent toxicity of the chemical and assumptions about the human consumption of the tissue for which the tolerance is established. Tolerances are determined for the active ingredient (the drug substance or its metabolite) and are not established for the specific formulation of the commercial drug product. A full discussion of this process has recently been reviewed (Baynes et al. 1999) and can be found in toxicology or risk assessment texts. It is important for the veterinarian to realize that the end point for determining withdrawal times, the tolerance, is a combined scientific and legal concept and therefore is ultimately controlled by *regulatory* and not medical practices.

The actual withdrawal time appearing on a drug label is also a function of the experimental design that the manufacturer used in the research studies submitted to the FDA for approval. Thus, although the science governing the withdrawal time is based on the pharmacokinetic principles discussed below, the withdrawal time is actually determined based on experimental data. Generally, a drug is administered to healthy animals, groups of the animals are slaughtered at sequential time intervals, and their edible tissues are analyzed for drug concentrations. The withdrawal time is the time from cessation of treatment to the time it takes for the residues of the drug to deplete below the safe concentration.

A statistical method is used to determine the time at which the marker residue depletes to the tolerance in the target tissue. The method determines the time, rounded to the next whole day, at which the upper bound of the marker residue tissue concentration is below the established tolerance in the target tissue (where the upper bound is statistically determined to represent with 95% confidence the 99th percentile of the population). Withdrawal times for the FDA-approved drugs for use in food animals are only valid for the specified species, dose, route, and frequency of administration. They are also specific to the manufacturer's product and formulation; thus, a drug substance (the active ingredient) may have different withdrawal times when present in the differently formulated drug products. An analogous process occurs in establishing milk discard times and in determining the withdrawal times for drugs administered to egg-laying poultry (although presently, all drugs approved in the United States for use in laying hens have a 0-day withdrawal).

REGULATION OF DRUG RESIDUES IN ANIMALS. Producers, veterinarians, and other persons involved with chemicals and food-animal production should be acquainted with a few terms and the agencies involved in drug residue control in order to better understand the drug residue problem and how withdrawal times are determined.

The use of drugs in veterinary medicine, especially in food-producing animals, is closely regulated in the United States by the FDA under the Department of Health and Human Services. The FDA is charged, through the Federal Food, Drug, and Cosmetic Act of 1938 (amended in 1968), with regulating the use of drugs in humans and in animals as well as requiring that the safety and efficacy of a drug be established before the product can be approved for use in animals, including those products added to animal feeds. The FDA also regulates human biologics, medical devices, drugs, and food safety. The FDA's Center for Veterinary Medicine (FDA-CVM) is responsible for the regulation of drugs, medical devices, and feeds intended for animals. The FDA is charged with the responsibility for establishing withdrawal times of drugs and the tolerances of drugs. The FDA and the EPA share responsibility for establishing tolerances for pesticide residues in animal-derived foods.

Whereas the FDA establishes safety guidelines for drug use in food animals, it is the responsibility of the US Department of Agriculture (USDA) to enforce the standards established by the FDA and the EPA. The USDA, through authorization by the Federal Meat Inspection Act of 1906 and the Poultry Inspection Act of 1967, inspects meat and poultry for sale through interstate commerce. The USDA is also authorized to test the tissues of food-producing animals through provisions in the Federal Insecticide, Fungicide and Rodenticide Act of 1947 in order to determine if violative levels of residues of chemicals and drugs are present. The Food Safety Inspection Service (FSIS), a division of the USDA, monitors these tissues through the National Residue Program (NRP) and identifies problems with drug and chemical residues. The NRP has been in action for over 25 years and has concentrated on individual, as well as population, sampling for monitoring and surveying possible residue problems in slaughter animals. In 1992, the NRP estimated they would collect some 350,000 specimens that year to analyze for antimicrobial and pesticide residues (Kindred and Hubbert 1993). The FSIS is the largest food safety inspection force in the federal government (Norcross and Post 1990).

The FSIS uses several rapid tests for determining contamination of animal products. Among these are the Swab Test on Premises (STOP) for antibiotic and sulfonamide residues, the Overnight Rapid Beef Identification Test (ORBIT) for species identification of meat, the Calf Antibiotic and Sulfa Test (CAST), the Sulfa-on-Site (SOS), and a variety of enzyme-linked immunosorbent assays (ELISAs) (Norcross and Post 1990). Rapid screening tests for residues have been summarized (Sundlof 1989). Milk in bulk tanks and from individual animals is assayed for antibiotic residues using various testing strategies: Charm Tests (Charm Sciences, Inc.), *Bacillus stearmothemophilus* disk assay (Charm Sciences, Inc.), SNAP Beta-lactam (IDEXX Laboratories, Inc.), LakTek tests, and Delvo tests (Gist-Brocades Food Ingredients, Inc.), to name only a few. This area is difficult to adequately summarize because rapid advances in analytical screening methodologies have led to the rapid development of new tests.

Other federal government agencies have defined roles in regulating the sale and use of drugs in animals, including the Drug Enforcement Agency (a division of the Department of Justice), the Animal and Plant Health Inspection Service (a part of the USDA), the EPA (mainly for pesticides), and the Department of Transportation. On a state level, the Department of Public Safety, Department of Health, the Animal Health Commission, Boards of Veterinary Medical Licensing, and Pharmacy Boards all have some regulatory influence over the use of drugs in food-producing, as well as companion, animals.

The Veterinarian and Extra-Label Drug Use. The FDA approves new animal drugs for specific indications in a particular species or subclass of animals (e.g., dairy cattle, weanling pigs). Occasionally, veterinarians may encounter diseases or conditions in animals for which there are no FDA-approved drugs. Under such circumstances, veterinarians often administer drugs that are not approved for use in food animals or they administer approved drugs in nonapproved ways, practices commonly referred to as "extra-label" usage. Extra-label drug use is defined as the use of a drug in a manner that is inconsistent with its FDA-approved labeling, a practice that, until 1994, was technically illegal. Recognizing that the Food, Drug, and Cosmetic

Act (FD&C) placed veterinarians in the untenable position of having to choose between providing for relief of animal suffering or complying with the law, the US Congress passed the Animal Medicinal Drug Use Clarification Act (AMDUCA) in 1994. AMDUCA amended the FD&C Act to allow veterinarians to prescribe and administer drugs in an extra-label manner under specific conditions. Under AMDUCA, veterinarians may resort to the extra-label use of approved animal and human pharmaceuticals provided that the following conditions are met:

1. There is no approved new animal drug that is labeled for the intended use and that contains the same active ingredient in the required dosage form and concentration, except where a veterinarian finds, within the context of a valid veterinarian-client-patient relationship, that the approved new animal drug is clinically ineffective for its intended use.
2. Prior to prescribing or dispensing an approved new animal or human drug for an extra-label use in food animals, the veterinarian must
   - make a careful diagnosis and evaluation of the conditions for which the drug is to be used;
   - establish a substantially extended withdrawal period prior to marketing of milk, meat, eggs, or other edible products that is supported by appropriate scientific information, if applicable;
   - institute procedures to ensure that the identity of the treated animal or animals is carefully maintained; and
   - take appropriate measures to ensure that assigned time frames for withdrawal are met and no illegal drug residues occur in any food-producing animal subjected to extra-label treatment.

The following additional conditions must be met for a permitted extra-label use in food-producing animals of an approved *human* drug or of an animal drug approved only for use in animals not intended for human consumption:

1. Such use must be accomplished in accordance with an appropriate medical rationale.
2. If scientific information on the human food safety aspect of the use of the drug in food-producing animals is not available, the veterinarian must take appropriate measures to ensure that the animal and its food products will not enter the human food supply.
3. Extralabel use of an approved human drug in a food-producing animal is not permitted if an animal drug approved for use in food-producing animals can be used in an extra-label manner for the particular use.

Implicit in these regulations are that the veterinarian makes every effort to first use an approved drug at an approved dosage, that an individual veterinarian-client-patient relationship exists between the producer and the veterinarian, that proper animal identification and documentation are maintained, and that the veterinarian makes every effort to determine an extended withdrawal time for this usage (e.g., consult with a databank such as the Food Animal Residue Avoidance Databank; FARAD), which the producer must adhere to. The regulation prohibits extra-label use for routine production purposes, for routine disease prevention, or as feed additives.

PHARMACOKINETICS AND RESIDUES. Pharmacokinetics is the science of quantitating the change in drug concentration in the body over time as a function of the administered dose. Although this discipline has been covered in earlier chapters and in a recent text (Riviere 1999), it is important to review some principles here since pharmacokinetics is the basis for understanding withdrawal times. As can be appreciated from Fig. 58.1, the overall disposition of a drug in the body is complex (Riviere 1992b).

How a drug or combination of drugs behaves in the body after administration not only is important from a therapeutic point of view but is of paramount importance to the producer and veterinarian in order to prevent residues in the edible tissues after the disease process has been resolved and the animal is slaughtered. For therapeutic usefulness and drug residue determinations, a known amount of drug is administered to a healthy animal. Serum concentration data are collected and mathematical models are created so that the overall disposition of the drug in the body can be evaluated in relation to absorption, distribution, metabolism, and elimination. Parameters for these models are estimated by fitting regression lines to the observed serum concentration versus time profiles, an example of which is shown in Fig. 58.2.

The slopes of the three lines shown in Fig. 58.2, when plotted on a semilogarithmic plot, represent distribution (α), short-term elimination (β), and long-term elimination (γ) from the body. The α and β phases of the serum concentration versus time profile are the only phases that are usually present when serum concentrations are monitored over a short period of time after dosing and are typically used to predict therapeutic drug concentrations. When serum concentrations are monitored for longer periods of time after drug administration using more sensitive assay methods, however, the γ phase of elimination appears for certain compounds. This can be present for several days or several months after the last administered dose, depending on the drug's physicochemical properties, the amount of drug administered, and the species in which it was administered. This γ phase reflects drug disposition in the so-called deep compartments. Alternatively, for prolonged-action depot preparations (e.g., benzathine penicillin), this terminal phase may actually reflect the rate-limiting absorption phase (flip-flop phase). For purposes of determining withdrawal times of drugs that may be used in food-producing animals, we will focus our discussion on the terminal phase of drug elimination to determine the half-life ($t_{1/2}$) of the drug in the body, since this is the measurement that is relevant in determining drug withdrawal times.

In the actual research studies conducted to determine a withdrawal time, it is the half-life of drug in the

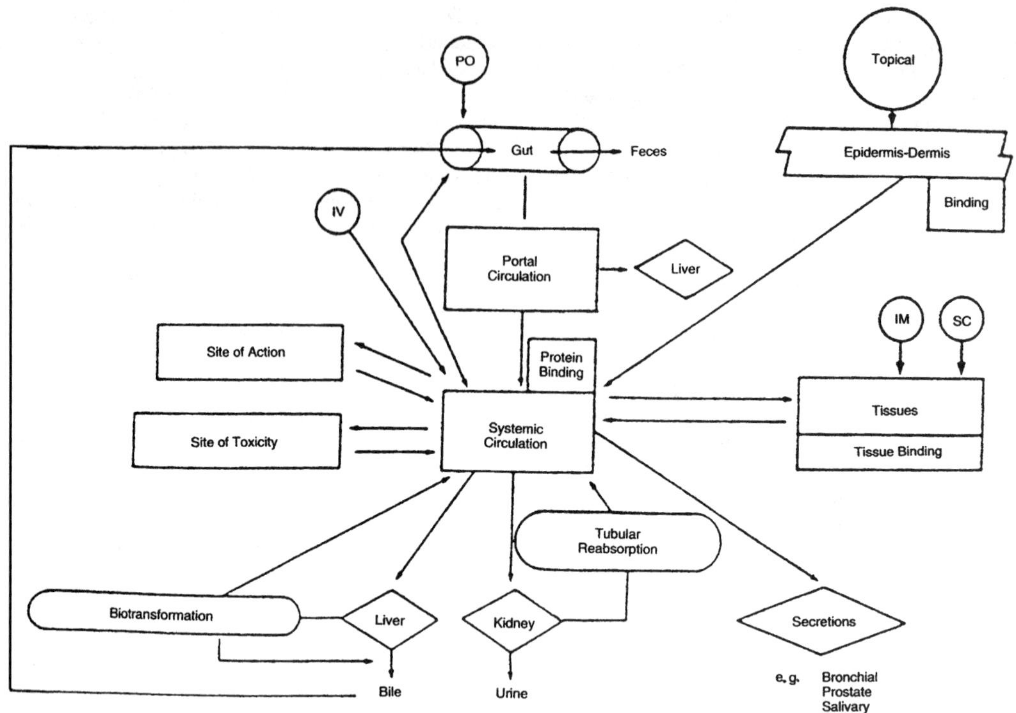

FIG. 58.1—Schematic diagram of how a drug can distribute in the body.

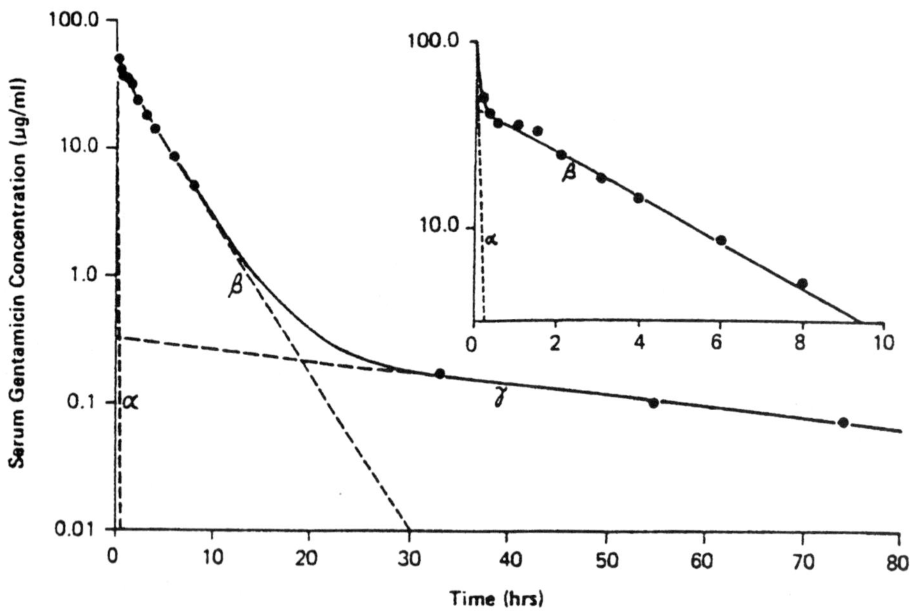

FIG. 58.2—A typical serum concentration-time profile for gentamicin after intravenous administration in a food-producing animal. Note the terminal-phase (γ) half-life of gentamicin, which is useful in predicting tissue withdrawal times. (Reprinted, with permission, from Riviere 1988.)

specific tissue that is of paramount importance. This information is not available to the veterinarian. Additionally, tissue pharmacokinetics is exceedingly complex, and a discussion here of terminal half-lives will be sufficient to illustrate the concepts involved. For more in-depth information on the clinical application of pharmacokinetics and how pharmacokinetic parameters can affect clinical parameters, readers should consult Chaps. 3 and 4 of this textbook.

The half-life of the drug or chemical in the body is the primary biological measurement used to determine withdrawal times of drugs and chemicals in food-producing animals; however, this parameter can be influenced by many biological factors. The $t_{1/2}$ of the γ phase of a drug by definition is the time it takes for 50% of the drug in the animal to be eliminated from the body and is the primary part of the elimination curve shown in Fig. 58.2 used to determine the withdrawal time of a drug. The $t_{1/2}$ is calculated using the equation

$$t_{1/2} = \frac{\ln 2}{\text{slope}} \quad \text{or} \quad t_{1/2} = \frac{0.693}{\text{slope}}$$

If the concentration of a drug in the muscle of a food animal after dosing is 100 parts per million (ppm), then the time it takes for the concentration in the muscle to decrease to 50 ppm would be the biological half-life of the drug in the muscle. Extrapolated out, the amount of drug in the muscle after 10 half-lives would be 0.1 ppm, or, put in other terms, 99.9% of the drug would have been eliminated from the muscle after 10 half-lives. If the dose is doubled and the beginning concentration in the muscle is now 200 ppm, only 1 additional half-life would be required to reach the 0.1 ppm concentration. On the other hand, if the half-life of the drug in the muscle is doubled, perhaps due to a disease state, then the elimination half-life would also double, thereby increasing the risk of violative drug residues in the edible tissues of that animal.

As stated above, the elimination half-life can be influenced by many biological factors. The half-life of a drug or chemical in the body is influenced by how well it distributes in the body and how quickly it is eliminated from the body. The physicochemical properties of a drug can influence its disposition in the body—in particular, how well it distributes into certain tissues or whether or not it penetrates intracellularly or whether it permeates the blood-brain barrier. The volume of distribution (V_d) is the quantitative estimate of the extent of the distribution of the drug in the body and can therefore directly influence the $t_{1/2}$ of the drug. It is a proportionality constant relating the concentration of drug in the serum to the total amount of drug in the body. For an intravenous injection of a drug, the equation for calculating V_d is

$$V_d = \frac{\text{amount of drug in the body}}{\text{serum drug concentration}}$$

It is important to point out that the V_d, typically reported in L/kg, does not actually refer to any specific physiologic space or body area; rather, it gives a good indication of how well a drug in general distributes throughout the body. A drug that has a large V_d typically has good tissue distribution throughout the body (tetracyclines), whereas a drug with a small V_d has less penetration into the body tissues as a whole, perhaps being confined to the extracellular spaces due to one or more of its physicochemical properties (not lipid soluble, fixed charge). While V_d may give an indication of the overall distribution of a drug, some drugs may not be uniformly distributed throughout the body. In this case, a drug may seek specific cells or organs or be bound to tissue macromolecules, resulting in a large V_d measurement and yet a relatively poor overall distribution in a majority of the body's tissues. Some drugs may have prolonged withdrawal times due to a large V_d.

In addition to V_d, the clearance (Cl) of the drug also plays an important part in determining the withdrawal time of the drug. Clearance quantitates the efficiency of the elimination processes and is defined as the rate of drug elimination from the body relative to the concentration of drug in the serum by the equation

$$Cl = \frac{\text{rate of elimination}}{\text{serum drug concentration}}$$

Drugs that have a slow rate of elimination from the body will tend to have protracted half-lives, whereas those that are eliminated quickly will have shorter half-lives.

The $t_{1/2}$ is dependent on two functions: V_d and Cl. By combining terms, an equation can be derived that reflects the influence of V_d and Cl on the $t_{1/2}$ of a drug:

$$t_{1/2} = \ln 2 \times \frac{V_d}{Cl} \quad \text{or} \quad t_{1/2} = 0.693 \times \frac{V_d}{Cl}$$

Several physiologic events can occur to change V_d or Cl and can therefore influence the $t_{1/2}$ of the drug in the body. For example, if renal function is impaired, the drug's clearance may be reduced and the $t_{1/2}$ prolonged by several hours or several days, in turn prolonging the withdrawal time of the drug. If the animal's fluid balance changes, the V_d may change accordingly. Factors such as the age, nutritional status, percentage of body fat, species, presence of other drugs, and extent of protein binding can all have a significant role in determining the V_d and Cl and hence the $t_{1/2}$ of any drug introduced into the body. For more information on the pharmacokinetics, readers are encouraged to consult Chaps. 3 and 4.

The pharmacokinetic behavior and efficacy of the drug or chemical used to treat a disease process are of major concern early on in the successful management of herd health in food animals. For residue control in food-animal species, the primary purpose of knowing the pharmacokinetic behavior of the drug (i.e., the terminal elimination half-life) is to determine the withdrawal time to prevent residue accumulation in those tissues consumed by humans. A knowledge of what physiological processes affect the half-life is thus essential to determine when a withdrawal time might need to be modified due to disease-induced prolongation of the withdrawal time.

Theoretically, if a tissue tolerance and the dose of drug were known, pharmacokinetic techniques could be used to calculate an individual withdrawal time. For an oral drug, this requires knowing the fraction of the dose administered that is absorbed into the body (e.g., bioavailability). This amount, divided by the V_d, is the initial concentration of drug in the body (C^0). If one were to assume that the loss of drug from the body were only dependent upon the terminal withdrawal time, then

$$\text{withdrawal time} = 1.44 \ln (C^0/\text{tolerance})(t_{1/2})$$

Of course, this is an oversimplification. In reality, this equation would work if C^0 were the concentration of drug in the target tissue at the end of drug administration, as this amount is dependent upon the β-phase elimination processes. Complex pharmacokinetic models can be used to calculate this number. Then the above equation would be valid. Officially established withdrawal times must take into account all interanimal variability, and thus statistical processing of these data establishes the withdrawal time for the worst-case scenario (Riviere et al. 1998).

The above equation is useful to gain a perspective on what the withdrawal time is relative to the terminal half-life. Assume that for most antibiotics a "therapeutic" concentration is 10 μg/mL and the tissue tolerance is 0.01 ppm (0.01 μg/mL). One also must assume homogeneous distribution of the drug throughout the body. Thus, withdrawal time equals $1.44[\ln(10/0.01)]t_{1/2}$, or $9.94t_{1/2}$. A withdrawal time for this drug would be equal to 10 half-lives. If the drug has a short half-life (e.g., penicillin), the withdrawal time is short. However, if the drug has a prolonged tissue half-life (e.g., an aminoglycoside), the withdrawal time could exceed a year in the target tissue. Similarly, a drug with a very low tissue tolerance has a longer withdrawal time because $\ln(C^0/\text{tolerance})$ is now greater. If a drug is metabolized, the metabolite may determine the withdrawal time ("marker residue") since its half-life is rate limiting.

This "rule of 10" can be derived by assuming that 10 half-lives are required to eliminate 99.9% of an administered dose. An examination of half-lives and withdrawal times for a number of approved pharmaceutics confirms this relation. Using a divisor of 5 would be even more conservative since the additional time added to the withdrawal time would be longer. This relationship is important to consider when one administers an increased dose of drug. If the dose is doubled, then withdrawal time should just be increased by a single half-life. In the above example, the calculation would be $1.44 [\ln(20/0.01)]t_{1/2}$, or 10.94 half-lives, which confirms this concept. However, if a disease process changed the half-life by either increasing V_d or decreasing clearance (e.g., kidney disease), causing the half-life to double, then withdrawal time should be doubled. This phenomenon supports the observation that seriously ill animals with altered pharmacokinetics deserve increased attention to ensure complete drug withdrawal. It is also important to note that withdrawal time is determined in healthy animals, and thus serious disease conditions may cause residues even when the approved dose and official withdrawal time are used. *It is critical for a veterinarian to have a conceptual understanding of this relationship between withdrawal time and half-life before doses are modified in food-producing animals.* When such a withdrawal time is calculated, the animal should be checked with the appropriate rapid-screening test.

For lactating dairy cows and goats, the identical principles apply to determining the milk discard times. The milk discard or withholding time is the time after drug administration when the milk cannot be used for human consumption. This is determined by administering the drug and collecting and analyzing milk until drug concentrations are below the milk tolerance established for that drug. Like withdrawal times, the discard time is product and species dependent. In this case, it is based on the half-life of the drug in the milk. If one knows the concentration of the drug in the milk at the end of drug administration, the milk half-life, and milk tolerance, the above equation can be used to precisely calculate withdrawal. This has been particularly useful when valuable dairy cows have been accidentally exposed to pesticides (e.g., heptachlor) and pharmacokinetic data were used to determine milk discard times since approved withdrawal times do not exist. In this case, the relevant parameter is the half-life of drug in milk. All of the principles discussed above relative to meat withdrawal apply. The half-life in milk is a function of how the drug is excreted into the milk after systemic administration (or oral or interuterine) or is retained in the udder after intramammary infusion. For example, basic drugs such as erythromycin have longer discard times than acidic drugs such as penicillin because the former tend to distribute more readily into milk due to the pH partitioning phenomenon. Similarly, lipophilic drugs will tend to have longer milk discard times. Discard times are different for these different routes of administration. One must be sure that a drug used as dry cow therapy is not inadvertently administered to a lactating cow, because the residue concerns differ since most dry cow formulations are long-acting preparations.

DRUGS PROHIBITED FROM EXTRA-LABEL USE. Certain drugs are prohibited from extra-label use in food animals under AMDUCA (Table 58.1). The FDA may prohibit the extra-label use of an approved new animal or human drug or class of drugs in food animals if the FDA determines that the extra-label use of the drug or class of drugs presents a risk to the public health, or if an acceptable analytical method has not been established. A prohibition may be a general ban on the extra-label use of the drug or class of drugs or may

TABLE 58.1—Drugs prohibited from extra-label use in food animals

Chloramphenicol
Clenbuterol
Diethylstilbestrol (DES)
Dimetridazole
Ipronidazole
Other nitroimidazoles
Furazolidone
Nitrofurazone
Sulfonamide drugs in lactating cows[a]
Fluoroquinolones[b]
Glycopeptides

[a]Prohibition does not apply to approved uses of sulfadimethoxine, sulfabromomethazine, and sulfaethoxypyridazine.

[b]Prohibition does not apply to approved uses of fluoroquinolones.

be limited to a specific species, indication, dosage form, route of administration, or combination of factors. These are fully discussed elsewhere (Payne et. al., 1999).

RESIDUE PREVENTION. Although public awareness of the drug residue problem in food is high and several governmental agencies spend large amounts of time attempting to control this problem, residues in animal tissues are still an important concern today. The responsibility for residue control and prevention cannot lie solely within a governmental agency; rather, the responsibility must be shared by the government, producers, veterinarians, teachers and academicians, marketing associations, and other interested parties, who must strive for both healthy and efficiently grown animals as well as a residue-free food supply. Several approaches can be taken to achieve this goal.

The first step in residue prevention is to make individuals and organizations aware of the problem through education. Education of laypersons can be accomplished through a variety of mechanisms: available open lay and veterinary medical literature, computer databases, consultations with veterinary medical personnel, or the efforts of national organizations. A number of national producer organizations have firm initiatives in place to prevent harmful residues in food-producing animals, including dairy (Adams 1993), beef (Wilkes 1993), pork (Lautner 1993), and veal (Wilson and Dietrich 1993) organizations. Awareness has also been raised concerning some species of companion animals (Macomber 1993; Kay 1993).

Failure to observe the correct withdrawal time of a drug was the leading cause of tissue residue violations in two studies (Van Dresser and Wilcke 1989; Bevill 1984). Once the importance of residue control in the US food supply is made clear and the importance of observing the correct legal withdrawal times for the drugs used in food-producing animals is understood, the incidence of tissue residue violations will (theoretically) decrease dramatically. Many have reported on other possible ways to reduce or prevent residues from occurring in food animals (Riviere 1991; Marteniuk et al. 1988; Sundlof 1989; Kindred and Hubbert 1993; Mercer 1990). Rapid-screening test technology has advanced significantly in the past few years and has been used to detect low levels of residue contamination in slaughtered animals in a quick manner. As these tests become more sensitive and more widely used, animals with residue contamination can be isolated and removed before reaching the end consumer, further decreasing the residue problem.

Several rapid-screening tests available today are summarized in Sundlof 1989. They are powerful tools for the veterinarian using a drug in an extra-label manner or in a seriously diseased animal. Once the veterinarian establishes a putative withdrawal time using the principles discussed above, the animal should be tested with the appropriate rapid-screening assay to ensure that the prediction is accurate. If a residue is detected, a prolonged withdrawal time should be recommended until a negative screening value is observed. If this practice is followed, the veterinarian will have done everything possible to ensure a residue-free product.

The FARAD is a USDA-supported computerized databank of scientific and regulatory information, established in 1982 and reauthorized by the US Congress in 1998, and can assist the veterinarian, producer, or other individuals in making rational choices in preventing drug and pesticide residues in food animals. It is a collaboration of the University of California at Davis, North Carolina State University, and the University of Florida at Gainesville. FARAD contains information on veterinary drug registration information; current label information; foreign registration and safety data; tolerances for drugs and pesticides for tissues, eggs, and milk; withdrawal information; physicochemical properties; pharmacokinetic and toxicokinetic information; residue test information; bibliographic citations; as well as other information useful in preventing drug residues in food animals. The database is regularly updated to provide users with the most current information available. FARAD is easily accessed by voice telephone (888-USFARAD), fax, and electronic mail at two regional access centers (North Carolina State University, University of California—Davis). By contacting an access center, users can obtain any of the current information listed above. FARAD services are free to clientele. FARAD also publishes periodic updates on extra-label drug withdrawal time estimates and issues as a regular feature in the *Journal of the American Veterinary Medical Association* (FARAD Digests). The program's Website (www.farad.org) should be consulted for orientation to its services and current access information. More information on FARAD is available elsewhere (Riviere et al. 1986; Payne et al. 1999).

Other sources of drug information pertaining to residues in food animals are also available. The FARAD pharmacokinetic data have been published in book form (Riviere et al. 1991; Craigmill et al. 1994; Sundlof et al. 1996). The Joint FAO/WHO Expert

Committee on Food Additives (JECFA) has evaluated several drugs and has published monographs that list toxicity, metabolism, acceptable daily intakes, maximum residue levels permitted for different tissues, and biological fate of drugs in food-producing animals. The *United States Pharmacopoeia* (USP) also publishes monographs (similar to the monographs for human drugs) that go into more detail about expanded (extralabel) pharmaceutical usage and pharmacokinetic variables that can alter withdrawal times in food-producing animals (Sundlof 1993).

The prevention of harmful residues in the edible tissues of our food-producing animals is the responsibility of many producers, veterinarians, professional and layperson associations, and governmental agencies. All of these groups must continue to strive to regulate and utilize the drugs used to prevent or cure animal diseases in a responsible manner in order to prevent the accumulation of harmful amounts of residues in the food supply.

REFERENCES

Adams, J. B. 1993. Assuring a residue-free food supply: milk. JAVMA 202(10):1723–1725.

Baynes, R. A., Martin, T., Craigmill, A. L., and Riviere, J. E. 1999. Strategies for estimating provisional acceptable residues (PAR) for extralabel drug use in livestock. Reg Toxicol Pharmacol 29.

Bevill, R. F. 1984. Factors influencing the occurrence of drug residues in animal tissues after the use of antimicrobial agents in animal feeds. JAVMA 185(10):1124–1126.

———. 1989. Sulfonamide residues in domestic animals. J Vet Pharmacol Therap 12:241–252.

Collett, J. N., and Harrison, D. L. 1963. Lindane residues in sheep following dipping. NZ J Agric Res 6:39–42.

Craigmill, A. L., Sundlof, S. F., and Riviere, J. E. 1994. Handbook of Comparative Pharmacokinetics and Residues of Veterinary Therapeutic Drugs. Boca Raton, FL: CRC Press.

Freese, W. R. 1993. Responsibilities of food animal practitioner regarding extra-label use of drugs. JAVMA 202(10):1733–1734.

Geyer, R. E. 1993. Implications for the FDA/Center for Veterinary Medicine (CVM). JAVMA 202(10):1718–1719.

Guest, G. B., and Solomon S. M. 1993. FDA extra-label use policy: 1992 revisions. JAVMA 202(10):1620–1623.

Jackson, J. B., Ivey, M. C., Roberts, R. H., and Radeleff, R. D. 1959. Residue studies in sheep and goats dipped in 0.025% lindane. J Econ Entomol 52(5):1031–1032.

Jenkins, W. L. 1993. Professional responsibilities. JAVMA 202(10):1742–1743.

Kay, W. J. 1993. Responsibilities under an amended Food, Drug, and Cosmetic Act: companion animal practitioners. JAVMA 202(10):1736–1737.

Kindred, T. P., and Hubbert, W. T. 1993. Residue prevention strategies in the United States. JAVMA 202(1):46–49.

Lautner, B. 1993. Assuring a residue-free food supply: pork. JAVMA 202(10):1727–1729.

Macomber, L. E. 1993. Responsibilities under an amended Food, Drug, and Cosmetic Act: equine practitioners. JAVMA 202(10):1735.

Marteniuk, J. V., Alwynelle, S. A., and Bartlett, P. C. 1988. Compliance with recommended drug withdrawal requirements for dairy cows sent to market in Michigan. JAVMA 193(4):404–407.

Mercer, H. D. 1990. How to avoid the drug residue problem in cattle. Comp Contin Educ Pract Vet—Food Animal 12(1):124–126.

Norcross, M. A., and Post, A. R. 1990. New food safety initiatives in the Food Safety and Inspection Service, US Department of Agriculture. J An Sci 68:863–869.

Oehler, D. D., Eschle, J. L., Miller, J. A., Claborn, H. V., and Ivey, M. C. 1969. Residues in milk resulting from ultra-low volume sprays of malathion, methoxychlor, coumaphos, ronnel, or gardona for control of the horn fly. J Econ Ento 62(6):1481–1483.

Payne, M. A. 1991. Extralabel drug use and withdrawal times in dairy cattle. In The Compendium North American Edition (Food Animal), pp. 1341–1351.

Payne, M. A., Baynes, R. E. Sundlof, S. F., Craigmill, A. L., Webb, A. L., and Riviere, J. E. 1999. Drugs prohibited from extralabel use in food animals. JAVMA 215:28–32.

Payne, M. A., Craigmill, A. L., Riviere, J. E., Webb, A., Baynes, R. A., and Sundlof, S. F. 1999. Food Animal Residue Avoidance Databank. Vet Clinics No Am 15:75–88.

Riviere, J. E. 1991. Pharmacologic principles of residue avoidance for veterinary practitioners. JAVMA 198(5):809–815.

———. 1992a. Dermal absorption and metabolism of xenobiotics in food-producing animals. In D. H. Hutson et al., eds., Xenobiotics and Food-Producing Animals: Metabolism and Residues, pp. 88–97. American Chemical Society Symposium Series 503. Washington, DC.

———. 1992b. Practical aspects of the pharmacology and antimicrobial drug residues in food animals. Agri-Practice 13(6):11–16.

———. 1999. Comparative Pharmacokinetics: Principles, Techniques, and Applications. Ames: Iowa State Univ Press.

Riviere, J. E., Craigmill, A. L., and Sundlof, S. F. 1986. Food Animal Residue Avoidance Databank (FARAD): an automated pharmacologic databank for drug and chemical residue avoidance. J Food Protection 49(10):826–830.

———. 1991. Handbook of Comparative Pharmacokinetics and Residues of Veterinary Antimicrobials. Boca Raton, FL: CRC Press.

Riviere, J. E., Webb, A.L., and Craigmill, A. L. 1998. A primer on estimating withdrawal times after extralabel drug use. JAVMA 213:966–968.

Sundlof, S. F. 1989. Drug and chemical residues in livestock. Vet Clinics No Am: Food Anim Pract 5(2):411–449.

———. 1993. Availability and use of existing scientific information for responsible drug prescribing. JAVMA 202(10):1696–1699.

Sundlof, S. F., Riviere, J. E., and Craigmill, A. L. 1996. Handbook of Comparative Veterinary Pharmacokinetics and Residues of Pesticides and Environmental Contaminants. Boca Raton, FL: CRC Press.

Teske, R. H. 1993. Current FDA policy on use of human-labeled drugs in animals. JAVMA 202(10):1632–1633.

Van Dresser, W. R., and Wilcke, J. R. 1989. Drug residues in food animals. JAVMA 194(12):1700–1710.

Wilkes, D. 1993. Assuring a residue-free food supply: beef. JAVMA 202(10):1725–1727.

Wilson, L. L., and Dietrich, J. R. 1993. Assuring a residue-free food supply: special-fed veal. JAVMA 202(10):1730–1733.

INDEX

Abamectin, 967–68
Abbokinase, 583
Abbreviations, in prescriptions, 1159–60
Abortifacients
ergoline derivatives, 622
estrogens, 613, 618
$PGF_{2\alpha}$, 617–18, 620–21
RU-486, 621–22
Absorbable Gelatin Sponge, USP, 576
Absorption, drug
administration route and, 19–23
bioavailability, 20, 24–25
definition of, 19
gastrointestinal, 21–23
interspecies variations, 15, 23
local anesthetics, 346
percutaneous, 19, 20–21, 1088–94
pharmacokinetics, 23–24, 26–27
pulmonary, 21
rate of, 24
solubility and, 19
Acarbose, 678–79
Acaricides, 1025. *See also* Ectoparasiticides
Acedist, 987
Acepromazine Maleate, INN, 307–12
doxapram antagonism of, 374
ketamine and, 249, 253–55
yohimbine antagonism of, 378
Acetaminophen, 445–46
biotransformation of, 33
toxicity, 61
in cats, 33, 445
Acetazolamide, 539, 1137
Acetylation reactions, 37
Acetyl-β-methylcholine, 122
Acetylcholine, 75, 82. *See also* Autonomic nervous system; Neurohumoral transmission
AChE hydrolysis of, 78
barbiturates and, 219
cardiovascular effects, 120–21
in CNS, 121, 156–57, 384
emesis mediation, 1042
function of, 117
mechanism of action, 117–19
muscarinic and nicotinic effects, 121–22. *See also* Muscarinic receptors; Nicotinic receptors
muscle effects, 121, 122
nicotinic receptors and, 137, 139
storage sites, 139
structure-activity relationship, 119–20
Acetylcholinesterase, 78, 82, 140
Acetylcysteine, 1115, 1141–42
Acetylsalicylic acid. *See* Aspirin
ACh. *See* Acetylcholine
AChE. *See* Acetylcholinesterase
Acid-base metabolism, 514–16
analysis of, 516–19
calcium/phosphorus balance and, 723
disorders of, 519–23
magnesium and, 736
potassium and, 732
Acid Citrate Dextrose, USP, 579
Acidifying solutions, for ketoacidosis, 522
Acidosis
hyperkalemia-associated, 732
metabolic, 519–22
bone mineral deposition and, 723
sodium bicarbonate for, 730
respiratory, 522
bone mineral deposition and, 723
Actase, 582
ACTH. *See* Adrenocorticotropin
ACTH stimulation test, 598, 664
Actinomycin D, 1078
Action potentials
myocardial, 455, 459, 482–88
nerve fibers, 77
nicotinic receptors, 137–39
Activated charcoal, 1055–56
Active transport, 18
blood-brain barrier and, 160
Acute-phase proteins, IL-6 induction of, 431
Acyclovir, USP, 936
ophthalmic uses, 1133
Addiction, cocaine, 351
Addison's disease, 665
ADE. *See* Adverse drug experiences
Adenine arabinoside, 935
Adenosine 3′, 5′-monophosphate. *See* Cyclic AMP
Adenosine diphosphate, 572
Adenosine receptors, 376
S-adenosyl-L-methionine, 1059
Adenylyl cyclase, 87, 156
catecholamines and, 88, 97, 100
Adequan, 446–47
ADH, 537, 606–8
Adhesives, ophthalmic, 1141
Aditoprim, 810–11
Administration routes
approved/nonapproved, 59–60
effect on absorption, 19–23
effect on drug half-life, 42
Adrenaline. *See* Epinephrine
Adrenal medulla, 70, 73–74
ACh effects on, 122
Adrenergic agonists, 1136–37. *See also* Catecholamines
α. *See* Alpha-adrenergic agonists
β, 106, 1108–9
down regulation of, 106
noncatecholamines, 104–6
ophthalmic uses, 1134, 1135–36
receptors, 92–95
structure-activity relationships, 91–92
Adrenergic antagonists, 107–15
α. *See* Alpha-adrenergic antagonists
β. *See* Beta-adrenergic antagonists
ophthalmic uses, 1135–36, 1137
Adrenergic neurohumoral transmission, 78–82
Adrenergic neuron-blocking drugs, 114
Adrenergic receptors, 81–82, 91. *See also* Alpha-adrenergic receptors; Beta-adrenergic receptors
and cAMP, 87
in CNS, 106
subtypes, 81–82, 92–95
Adrenocorticotropin, 596–98, 650
ACTH stimulation test, 598, 664
Adrenolytic drugs, 666–67. *See also* Adrenergic antagonists
Adriamycin, 1075–76
Adrucil, 1073
Adsorbents, topical, 1094
Adverse drug experiences, 60–62
Aerosols, 1158
Aerrane, 198
Affinity, definition of, 9
Age, effect on biotransformation of drugs, 39, 64
Aggressiveness, azaperone for, 334–35. *See also* Behavior modifying drugs
Agonists, definition of, 10
Aklomide, 1001

Albendazole
antinematodal activity, 950–53
antiprotozoan activity, 1014
cestocidal activity, 984–85, 990
for fasciolosis, 988
for giardiasis, 995–96
Albumin, plasma, binding capacity, 28
Albuterol, 1109
Alcaine, 355
Alcohol, as antiseptic, 785
Alcohol dehydrogenase, 35–36
Alcuronium, 141, 146
Aldactone, 549
Aldehyde dehydrogenase, 35–36
Aldehydes, as disinfectants, 786–87
Aldose reductase inhibitors, 1141
Aldosterone, 731
antagonists, 549–50
carbadox suppression of, 889
Alfenta, 286
Alfentanil Hydrochloride, USP, 268, 286
Algesics, kinins, 418
Alkalosis
hypokalemia-associated, 732
metabolic, 522, 729
respiratory, 522
Alkeran, 1071
Alkylating agents
alyklsulfonates, 1071
nitrogen mustards, 1070–71
nitrosureas, 1071–72
triazines, 1072
Alkyl pyrophosphates, 127, 130
Alkylsulfonates, 1071
Allergies
aminophylline for, 410
antihistamines for, 410
drug reactions, 61
ephedrine for, 410
epinephrine for, 98, 101
glucocorticoids for, 153, 661–62
histamine and, 405
isoproterenol for, 410
to local anesthetics, 351
PABA, 351
Allethrin, 1019–20
Allometric scaling, 51–53
Allopurinol, 176
Allyl-trenbolone, 614
Alopecia, 637
Alpha-adrenergic agonists
α_2-selective, 106
adrenoceptors, 106, 313–14
detomidine, 321–23
dexmedetomidine, 324
for diarrhea, 1055
medetomidine, 323
as preanesthetics, 166
romifidine, 323–24
as tranquilizers, 313–25
xylazine, 314–21
as decongestants, 1116–17
Alpha-adrenergic antagonists
α_1-selective, 111–12
side effects, 61
α_2-selective, 112, 377–79
atipamezole, 324–25
tolazoline, 324, 378–79
yohimbine, 324, 377–79
ergot alkaloids, 107–9
nonselective, 111
synthetic, 109–11
as vasodilators, 471–72
Alpha-adrenergic receptors, 81–82, 87, 91, 95–99, 106
blockade, 107
subtypes, 92–93, 94–95
Alpha blockers. *See* Alpha-adrenergic antagonists
Alprenolol, 489
Alternate day therapy, glucocorticoids, 662–63
Althesin, 243–45
clinical uses, 245–46
contraindications, 246–47
Altrenogest, 614–15
Alum, 577
Aluminum hydroxide, 1049
Aluminum hydroxide/phosphate, 1055
Aluminum phthalocyanine tetrasulfonate, 1143
Aluminum salts
as antacids, 1049
as astringents, 1095
Alveolar ventilation, 191
Amantadine Hydrochloride, USP, 938–39
Ambenonium Chloride, USP, 126
Americaine, 355
Amicar, 582
Amicarbalide, 1013
Amidate, 239
Amidone, 284
Amikacin, 855–57
Amiloride, 548
Amino acids
in CNS, 157–58
sulfur-containing, 736–38
Aminoamide local anesthetics, 355–57
Aminocaproic Acid, USP, 582
Aminoester local anesthetics, 353–55
Aminoglycosides, 841–60
ACh inhibition, 141
amikacin, 855–57
apramycin, 858
bioavailability of, 21
in cats, 850
chemistry, 841–42
dihydrostreptomycin, 859
in dogs, 849
gentamycin, 851–55
in horses, 850
kanamycin, 857–58
mechanism of action, 841–43
microbial susceptibility, 843
monitoring, 65–66
neomycin, 859
neuromuscular blocking agent interactions, 148
ophthalmic uses, 1127–28
paromomycin, 859–60
antiprotozoal activity, 996–97
pentobarbital interaction, 218
pharmacokinetics, 844–46
receptors, 846–47
residues, 846
in ruminants, 850–51
single daily dosing, 843–44
tobramycin, 858–59
topical, 1099
toxicity, 61, 846–51
Aminopenicillins, 822
Aminopentamide, 1053
Aminophylline, USP, 376–77
for allergy reactions, 410
cardiac effects, 479
4-Aminopyridine, 150, 333, 377
5-Aminosalicylic acid, 440
Aminosidine, 996–97
Amiodarone, 489–90, 496–97
Amitraz, 1025
Amitriptyline, 390
Amoebae, 993–97
Amorolfine, 932
Amoxicillin, 822
bioavailability of, 21
ophthalmic uses, 1129
potassium clavulanate and, 825
Amphetamine Sulfate, USP, 105–6
biotransformation of, 33
CNS effects, 76, 81, 99
phenothiazines for overdose, 301
Amphotec, 923
Amphotericin B, 921–24
flucytosine and, 932
interspecies scaling profile, 52
ophthalmic uses, 1132
preparations, 923–24
rifampin synergism, 888
Ampicillin, 822
bioavailability of, 21
ophthalmic uses, 1130
sulbactam and, 825
Amprol, 1000
Amprolium, 1000–1001, 1007–10
Amrinone, 471
Analeptic agents, 373–77
Analgesia
mediation of, 159
NSAIDs for, 438
opioids for, 295
Analgesic nephropathy, 439
Analgesics. *See* Alpha-adrenergic agonists, α_2-selective; Anesthetics, dissociative; Nonsteroidal anti-inflammatory drugs; Opioids
Anaphylactic shock, 101–2
Anaphylaxis
due to drug reactions, 62
histamine and, 405
Ancobon, 921
Androgenization, 613
Anectine, 141
Anemias
aplastic
chloramphenicol-induced, 871–72
sulfonamide-induced, 800
blood loss, 560, 563–65
chronic hemorrhage, 561, 564
copper deficiency, 562
folic acid deficiency, 559, 712
hemolytic, 561–62, 565
immune-mediated, 562
zinc toxicoses and, 759

iron deficiency, 558, 561, 562–63, 751–52
vitamin A and, 686
morphological classification of, 559–60, 561
nonregenerative, 560, 562, 565
regenerative, 560
vitamin B_{12} deficiency, 558–59, 714
Anesthesia
epidural. *See* Epidural nerve blocks
induction of, 19–20. *See also* specific drugs
local, 162
principles of, 160
regional, 162
topical, 352
Anesthesia, general, 162–64
depth of, 167–70
drug combinations, 166
effect on fluid balance, 531
maintenance of, 167–68
monitoring equipment, 187
neuromuscular blocking agents and, 148–49
preanesthesia, 165–67
recovery from, 167–68
Anesthetics, dissociative, 247
ketamine, 247–58
phencyclidine, 247
as preanesthetics, 166
tiletamine, 258–61
Anesthetics, inhalation, 184–85
adjuvant drugs, 198
biotransformation of, 35, 193
blood solubility of, 21
characteristics of, 185–87
for euthanasia, 399–400
lipid solubility, 163
minimum alveolar concentration, 193–94
occupational exposure to, 204–5, 399, 401
pharmacodynamics, 194–204
pharmacokinetics, 190–94
phenothiazines and, 301
properties of, 187–89
recovery from, 192–93
reversal of, 163
solubility, 189–90, 191–92
vasodilation by, 531
Anesthetics, injectable, 213–14. *See also* Anesthetics, dissociative; Barbiturates
althesin, 243–47
chloralose, 261
etomidate, 239–40
guaifenesin, 241–43
metomidate, 262
propanidid, 261
propofol, 237–39
urethane, 261
Anesthetics, local, 343–44
absorption of, 346
agents
benzocaine, 355
bupivacaine, 357
chloroprocaine, 355
cocaine, 353–54
etidocaine, 357
lidocaine, 355–56
mepivacaine, 356–57
prilocaine, 356
procaine, 354–55
proparacaine, 355
ropivacaine, 357
tetracaine, 355
biotransformation, 347
clinical pharmacology, 351–52
clinical uses, 352–53
distribution, 346–47
EMLA, 356
mechanism of action, 347–49
ophthalmic, 355, 1121–22
properties of, 244–46
systemic toxicity, 349–50
tissue toxicity, 350
Angiotensin, 413–16
Angiotensin-converting enzyme inhibitors, 473–75, 513
Angiotensin I, 505
Angiotensin II, 505
Anhidrosis, 729
Animal Drug Availability Act, 1154
Animal drugs, legislation concerning, 1152–55
Animal facilities, disinfection of, 792–94
Animal Medicinal Drug Use Clarification Act (1994), 58, 1153–54
Animal safety studies, 60
Anion gap, blood, 517–18
Anipryl, 668
Antacids, 1049–50
Antagonil, 324
Antagonists, drug, 10, 63
Anthelban, 958
Anthelmintics. *See also* Anticestodal drugs; Antinematodal drugs; Antitrematodal drugs
benzimidazoles, 988–89, 995–96
copper oxide wire, 748
Anthracycline derivatives, 1075–77
Anthraquinone glycosides
activation of, 38
as cathartics, 1057
Antiadrenergic drugs. *See* Adrenergic antagonists
Antianemic agents, 563–68. *See also* Anemias
Antiarrhythmic drugs
amiodarone, 489–90, 496–97
aprinidine, 488, 495–96
atropine as, 490
β-blockers as, 489, 492–93
bretylium, 490, 494–95
calcium-channel blockers, 490
classification of, 488–90
digitalis as, 463–64, 490
disopyramide, 488, 495
dosages, 497–98
encainide, 488, 496
epinephrine as, 490
flecainide, 488, 496
lidocaine, 488–89, 492
lorcainide, 488, 496
mexiletine, 488, 495
phenytoin, 488–89, 491–92
procainamide, 488, 491
propanolol, 107, 112–13, 489, 492–93
quinidine, 488, 490–91
tocainide, 488, 495
Antibiotics. *See also* Antifungal drugs; Antiviral agents
absorption of from GI tract, 21–23
aminoglycosides, 841–60
antineoplastic, 1075–78
bacitracin, 886, 1130
barbiturate interactions, 223, 224
β-lactam, 61, 818–25
carbadox, 889
chloramphenicol. *See* Chloramphenicol
concentration-dependent, 49
coumarin potentiation, 581
excretion of, 40
fluoroquinolones, 898–913, 1129
lincosamides, 882–86, 1010, 1131
macrolides, 21, 876–82, 1131
methenamine, 890
in milk, 18, 19, 1166. *See also* Milk
nitrofurans, 888–89, 997, 1099
novobiocin, 886
ophthalmic uses, 1127–32
penicillins, 61, 818–22, 1129–30
polymyxins, 890–91, 1099, 1130
rifampin, 886–88, 1131
side effects of, 61
sulfonamides. *See* Sulfonamides
tetracyclines. *See* Tetracyclines
thiostrepton, 886, 1100
topical, 891, 1099–1110
toxicity of, 224
vancomycin, 889–90
virginiamycin, 889
and vitamin B requirements, 709, 711, 713
Anticarcinogens
omega-3 fatty acids, 764–65
vitamin A, 686–87
vitamin E, 694
Anticestodal drugs
benzimidazoles as, 984–85
bithionol, 981, 990
bunamidine, 980–81
dichlorophen, 981
espirantel, 983–84
hexachlorophene, 981
for horses, 985
inorganic compounds, 980
natural organic compounds, 980
niclosamide, 981, 990
praziquantel, 981–83, 990
resorantel, 981
Anticholinergics, 130–33
as antiemetics, 1045
as antispasmodics, 131, 132, 1053
as antiulcer drugs, 1046
as bronchodilators, 1112
as preanesthetics, 166–67
Anticholinesterase agents. *See* Cholinesterase inhibitors
Anticoagulants
heparin, 579–80
natural, 574–75
ophthalmic, 1141
vitamin K antagonists, 580–82
in vitro, 578–79

Anticoccidial drugs
for coccidiosis, 999–1009
for cryptosporidiosis, 1009–10
mechanism of action, 998
new drug targets, 998–99
resistance, 998
sulfaquinoxaline, 805
Anticollagenases, ophthalmic, 1141–42
Anticonvulsants
as behavior modifying drugs, 395
benzodiazepines, 325, 326, 370–72
bromide, 372–73
diazepam as, 328
mechanism of action, 361
pentobarbital as, 373
pharmacokinetics, 361–63
phenobarbital as, 363–66
phenytoin, 368–70
primidone, 366–68
Antidepressants, 389–94
Antidiarrheal agents, 1052–55. *See also* Antispasmodics
Antidiuretic hormone, 504, 537, 550, 606–8
ACTH and, 596, 650
angiotensin and, 414
purgative effect, 2057
Antiemetics
belladonna alkaloids, 1044
centrally acting, 1044–45
droperidol, 333, 1044
peripherally acting, 1045
phenothiazines, 301
prochlorperazine, 312–13, 1044
Antiepileptics, 373. *See also* Anticonvulsants
Antiestrogens, in cancer therapy, 1079
Antifibrinolytics, ophthalmic, 1142
Antifreeze toxicity, 36
Antifungal drugs, 919–32
amorolfine, 932
amphotericin B, 921–24
combination therapy, 932
enilconazole, 927
fluconazole, 930–31
flucytosine, 921
griseofulvin, 919–21
itraconazole, 927–30
ketoconazole, 924–27
naftifine, 931
ophthalmic, 1132–33
terbinafine, 931–32
thiocarbamate, 932
topical, 920–21, 931–32, 1100
Antihistamines, 404, 407–10
as antiemetics, 1044
as behavior modifying drugs, 395
as decongestants, 116–17
respiratory effects, 1114
Anti-inflammatory agents. *See also* Nonsteroidal anti-inflammatory drugs
bronchodilators, 1108–14
glucocorticoids, 650–53, 661–62
omega-3 fatty acids, 763
ophthalmic, 1126–27
for osteoarthritis, 446–48
sulfasalazine, 806–7
Antimetabolites
folic acid analogs, 1072
purine analogs, 1073–74
pyrimidine analogs, 1073, 1133
Antimicrobials. *See* Antibiotics; Antifungal drugs; Antiviral agents
Antimonials, 995
Antimuscarinic agents, 130–33. *See also* Anticholinergics
as antiemetics, 1044
spasmolytic activity, 1053
Antinematodal drugs
abamectin, 967–68
benzimidazoles, 948–53
butamisole, 954–55
n-butyl chloride, 977
dichlorvos, 962–63
diethylcarbamazine, 975–76
doramectin, 968–69
eprinomectin, 969–70
febantel, 953–54
hygromycin B, 977
ivermectin, 964–67
levamisole, 955–57
melarsomine, 976–77
milbemycin, 971–72
morantel, 960–61
moxidectin, 972–73
netobimin, 953
over-the-counter, 977
phenothiazine, 973–74
piperazine, 974–75
pyrantel, 957–60
rafoxanide, 986–87
resistance to, 977–78
selamectin, 970–71
thiacetarsamide, 967
toluene, 977
Antineoplastic agents
alkylating agents, 1070–72
antibiotics, 1075–78
antimetabolites, 1072–74
cancer cell specificity, 1066
combination therapy, 1069
dosage, 1067–68
enzymes, 1078
epidophyllotoxins, 1075
hormones, 1079–80
platinum coordination complexes, 1078–79
resistance, 1069–9
taxol, 1074–75
therapist safety, 1067
toxicity, 1066–67
treatment regimens, 1069
vinca alkaloids, 1074
Antioxidants
β-carotene, 686–87
and erythrocyte production, 559
taurine, 767
vitamin A, 686–87
vitamin C, 718
vitamin E, 693, 694
Antiplatelet drugs, 584
Antiproliferative agents, ophthalmic uses, 1142
Antiprotozoan drugs
for amoebae, 993–97
anticoccidials, 997–1010
antimonials, 995
arsenicals, 995
for babesiosis, 1012–13
benzimidazoles, 995–96
for ciliates, 1014
for cytauxzoonosis, 1014
for equine protozoal myeloencephalitis, 1011
for flagellates, 993–97
for hepatozoonosis, 1012
for malaria, 1011–12
for neosporosis, 1010–11
nifurtimox, 997
paromomycin, 859–60, 996–97
tetracyclines, 997
for theileriosis, 1014
for toxoplasmosis, 1010
Antipsychotics, 385–89
Antipyretics, NSAIDs, 438
Antirobe, 1010
Antiseborrheics, 1096
Antiseptics, 784–88
clinical use, 789–91
efficacy of, 788–89
resistance to, 789
Antispasmodics
anticholinergics as, 131, 132, 1053
diphenoxylate/atropine, 282–83
meperidine, 282–84
morphine as, 279–80
paregoric, 282
Antithrombin III, 575
heparin binding, 579
Antithyroid drugs, 643–46
Antitrematodal drugs
for fasciolosis
benzimidazoles, 988–89
bithionol sulfoxide, 985, 986
bromophenophos, 987
bromsalans, 986
brotianide, 988
clorsulon, 987–88
closantel, 988
diamphenethide, 989–90
hexachloroparaxylene, 986
hexachlorophene, 986
niclofolan, 986, 990
nitroxynil, 986
oxyclozanide, 986, 990
rafoxanide, 986–87
for paragonimosis, 990
for paramphistomosis, 990
Antitussives
codeine as, 280
morphine as, 275
narcotic, 1114
nonnarcotic, 1114–15
peripheral, 1115
Antiulcer drugs
antacids, 1049–50
anticholinergics, 1046
H_2 receptor antagonists, 1046–48
PGEs, 1049
proton pump inhibitors, 1048–49
sucralfate, 1050
Antiviral agents
assembly inhibitors
amantadine, 938–39
rimantadine, 938–39
dextran sulfate, 939

experimental nucleoside analogs, 939
glycoprotein-processing inhibitors, 940
interferon, 939
neurotransmitter antagonists, 940
ophthalmic, 1133
protease inhibitors, 940
ribozymes, 939
transcription inhibitors
acyclovir, 936–37
cytarabine, 935
foscarnet, 938
ganciclovir, 936–37
idoxuridine, 935
ribavirin, 935–36
trifluridine, 935
vidarabine, 935
zidovudine, 937
Anxiolytics, 393–94
Anxioselectives, 394
Anypril, 666
Apomorphine Hydrochloride, USP, 1044
Apoptosis, glucocorticoid-induced, 652, 653
Apothecaries' system, 1165
Appetite, stimulants, 1042
Apraclonidine hydrochloride, 1135
Apramycin, 858
Apresoline, 473
Aprinidine, 488, 495–96
Aprotinin, 417, 582
Aqua-Flor, 875
Aquaretics, 550
Ara-A, 935
Arabinoside, 1073
Ara-C, 935, 1073
Arachidonic acid, 759–62
conversion to HPETE, 423–24
conversion to prostaglandins, 422–23
steroid inhibition of, 652
Aramine, 106
Arecoline, 123–24, 980
Arginine analogs, 85
Arginine vasopressin, 537, 550
Arrhythmias
atropine for, 490
barbiturate-associated, 229–30
from catecholamines, 97, 102, 197–98, 216
causes, 482
cholinergic drugs and, 121
digitalis and, 465–68
from halothane, 197
mechanisms of, 485–88
neuromuscular blocking agents and, 146
Arsenamide, 976
Arsenicals, 995
for heartworms, 975–76
Arteparon, 446
Arthropathy, fluoroquinolone-induced, 912
L-Asparaginase, 1078
Aspartate, in CNS, 158
Aspirin, 439–40
antiplatelet activity, 583–84
bioavailability, 25
dipyridamole synergism, 584
elimination of, 43
and hyperpyrexia, 61
nonspecific COX-inhibition, 424
for ophthalmic conditions, 1125
for respiratory disease, 1113–14
and thiopental, 223
Astemizole, 408, 410
Asthma, 407, 1108
catecholamines for, 98
cromogylate for, 1113
glucocorticoids in, 654
halothane anesthesia with, 198
Astringents, 1095
Ataranalgesia, 329
Atipamezole hydrochloride, 324–25
Atovaquone, 999
Atracurium, 141
Atravet, 307
Atromid, 608
Atromi-S, 582
Atropine Sulfate, USP, 130, 132, 678
as antidote, 129
for arrhythmias, 490
cardiovascular effects, 131
digitalis and, 462, 467
diphenoxylate and, 282–83
gastrointestinal effects, 131, 132
muscarinic effects, 82
ocular effects, 131–32
ophthalmic uses, 1136
preanesthetic use, 132
respiratory effects, 131, 1112
smooth muscle effects, 131–32
spasmolytic activity, 1053
toxicity of, 132
Attapulgite, activated, 1055
AUC, 23–24, 47
AUMC, 24, 47
Autonomic drugs, 88–89
Autonomic ganglionic blocking drugs, 133–35
Autonomic nervous system
afferent nerve tracts, 75–76
cardiac effects, 454
efferent nerve tracts, 70–75
neurohumoral transmission, 75–89
organization of, 70–73
organ responses, 73–75
receptor sites, 82–83
TCAs and, 390–91
Availability, drug. *See* Bioavailability
Avatec, 1004
Avermectins
antinematodal drugs, 964–71
ectoparasiticides, 1029–30
ophthalmic uses, 1133
AV heart block, isoproterenol for, 101, 490
Aviax, 1004
Avomec, 967
Axilur, 996
Axonal conduction, 76–77
Azamethonium, 134
Azaperone, 333–35
Azapirones, 394
Azathioprine, USP, 1073–74
ophthalmic uses, 1126
Azidothymidine, 937
Azithromycin, 881–82
ophthalmic uses, 1131
Azo compounds, biotransformation of, 35
Azole antifungal drugs, 924–31
AZT, 937
Aztreonam, 825
ophthalmic uses, 1131–32

Babesiosis, 1012–13
Bacitracin, 886
ophthalmic uses, 1130
Bacteria, hemolytic anemia-associated, 561–62
Bacteriostatic drugs, dosage, 49
Bactrim, 1007
Balanced anesthesia, 163
Balanced electrolyte solutions, 527
Banminth, 958
Banminth II, 960
Barbiturates
absorption of, 220
agents
hexobarbital, 237
methohexital, 235–36
pentobarbital, 224–29. *See also Pentobarbital Sodium,* USP
phenobarbital, 214, 363–66, 395, 603, 634
secobarbital, 236–37
thialbarbital, 234
thiamylal, 234–35
thiopental, 229–34, 377
antibiotic interactions, 223, 224
cardiovascular effects, 216–18
chemistry of, 214–15
CNS effects, 215–16
coumarin inhibition, 581
diazepam and, 328
distribution of, 220
duration of action, 221–24
for euthanasia, 400
excretion of, 218–19, 220
fetal effects, 219
hepatic metabolism, 220–21
as meperidine antagonists, 283
pentobarbital-blockade, 219
potentiation of, 223–24
respiratory effects, 216
sodium methiodal interaction, 231
species variation, 221
tolerance to, 221
toxicity, 224
xylazine and, 317
Baroreceptor reflex, 198
Basal metabolic rate (BMR), thyroid hormones and, 636
Baycox, 1005
Bayer, 997, 2502
Baypress, 354
BCG extract, 1143
BCNU, 1071
Behavior disorders, 383–84
Behavior modifying drugs, 384
anticonvulsants as, 395
antidepressants, 389–94
antihistamines as, 395
antipsychotics, 385–89
benzodiazepines as, 326, 328, 330
beta-adrenergic blockers as, 395

Behavior modifying drugs (*continued*)
  opioid agonists/antagonists as, 395
  progestins, 395
  stimulants as, 395
Belladonna alkaloids
  spasmolytic activity, 1044, 1053
  toxicity, 132
Benadryl, 408
Benefit-risk assessment, 60
Benzalkonium chloride, 1100
Benzetimide, 1053
Benzimidazoles
  antinematodal, 948–53
  chemistry, 948
  clinical uses, 950–52
  contraindications, 953
  for fasciolosis, 988–89
  for giardiasis, 995–96
  mechanism of action, 949–50
  pharmacokinetics, 948–49
  safety/toxicity, 952–53
  side resistance, 977–78
Benzocaine, USP, 355
Benzodiazepines, 325–33
  antagonists, 332–33
  as anticonvulsants, 370–72
  as anxiolytics, 393–94
  appetite stimulation, 1042
  chlordiazepoxide, 331–32
  clonazepam, 372
  diazepam, 326–31
  midazolam, 331
  receptors, 325–26
Benzothiadiazines, 547–48, 608
Benzoyl peroxide, 1087, 1096
Benzoylphenyl urea (BPU) compounds, 1026
Benztropine Mesylate, USP, 311
Benzyl benzoate, 1026
Berenil, 1013
Beta-adrenergic agonists, as bronchodilators, 106, 1108–9
Beta-adrenergic antagonists, 112–14
  as antiarrhythmic agents, 489, 492–93
  as behavior modifying drugs, 395
  in congestive heart failure, 473
  hyperkalemia due to, 513
Beta-adrenergic receptors, 81–82, 87, 91–99, 102, 103
  blockade, 107
Beta blockers. *See* Beta-adrenergic antagonists
Beta-carotene, 684
  anticancer/antioxidant activity, 686–87
Beta endorphins, 159
  blocking by naloxone, 288–89
Beta glucuronidase, 38
Beta-lactam antibiotics, 818–25
  β-lactamase inhibitors, 825
  carbapenems, 825
  cephalosporins, 822–25
  cross-reactivity of, 61
  mechanism of action, 818
  microbial resistance, 818–19
  monobactams, 825
  penicillins, 819–22
Beta-lactamases, 818–19
  inhibitors, 825
Betamethasone, 655–58, 662–63
  ophthalmic, 1123
Bethanechol, 119, 122–23
  as purgative, 1057
Biaxin, 881
Bicarbonate
  in acid-base metabolism, 514–19
  intraocular irrigation solutions, 1123
Biguanidine, 582
Bile salts, 1058
Bilevon, 986
Biliary excretion, 40–41
Bioavailability
  definition of, 24–25
  diet and, 49
  of drugs, 20, 24–25
  interspecies variations, 25
  pharmacokinetics, 25
  systemic, 24–25, 47
Bio-Cox, 1004
Bioequivalence, 25–27, 58
Biophase, 13
Biotin, 710–11
Biotransformation
  age and, 39
  by GI microflora, 37–39
  by skin, 1087
  and ionization, 30
  and lipid solubility, 30
  phase I reactions, 30–36
  phase II reactions, 36–37
  rate of, 39
Bipyridine derivatives, 471–72
Birds. *See also* Poultry
  fluoroquinolones in, 909–10
Bisacodyl, 1057
Bismuth salts, 1055
Bisorbin lactate, 583
Bithin, 981
Bithionol, INN, 981, 985, 986, 990
Blacktongue, 706
Blenoxane, 1077
Bleomycin Sulfate, USP, 1077
Bloat, xylazine-induced, 318
Blocks
  epidural, 159, 318, 352, 353, 355
  intravenous, 353
  spinal (subarachnoid), 353
Blood
  anion gap, 517–18
  gases, 516–17
  whole, 577
Blood-brain barrier, 159–60
  and anesthesia induction, 19–20
  drugs and, 17
  osmotherapy and, 541–42
Blood clotting
  calcium and, 724
  clot formation, 571–72, 573
  coagulation factors, 572–73
  fibrinolysis, 574–75, 582
  vitamin K and, 696–97
Blood-CSF barrier
  and anesthesia induction, 19–20
  passage of drugs through, 17
Blood pressure, angiotensin maintenance of, 415
Blood transfusions, 564
  anticoagulants for, 579
Body clearance, 44–45
Body size/weight
  dosing by, 51
  effect on metabolism, 52
Bolus, IV, 19, 20
Bone demineralization, 723, 724
Bone development
  vitamin A and, 686
  vitamin D and, 690
Bone marrow
  chloramphenicol-induced suppression, 871–72
  erythroid, 554–55
  suppressive chemicals, 562
Boric acid, in topical preparations, 1094
Botulinum toxin, 82, 141
Bovatec, 1004
Bovilene, 616
Bovine somatotropin, 604–5
Braces, 1158
Bradykinin, 416, 417
Breokinase, 583
Bretylium tosylate, 114–15, 490, 494–95
Bretylol, 494
Brevane, 235
Brevimytal, 235
Brevital, 235
Brietal, 235
Brimonidine, 1135
Bromide, as anticonvulsant, 372–73
Bromocriptine, 622
Bromophenophos, INN, 987
Bromsalans, 986
Bronchial disease, chronic, 1108
Bronchoconstriction, histamine and, 407
Bronchodilators
  anticholinergics, 1112
  β-adrenergic agonists, 98, 106, 1108–9
  in congestive heart failure, 470
  effect on cAMP/cGMP, 1108
  mast cell stabilizers, 1112–13
  methylxanthine derivatives, 375–77, 1109–12
Brotianide, INN, 985, 988
Bumetanide, 543
Bumex, 543
Bunamidine, INN, 980–81
α-Bungarotoxin, 138
Buparvaquone, 1014
Bupivacaine Hydrochloride, USP, 357
  ophthalmic, 1122
Buprenex, 291
Buprenorphine Hydrochloride, USP, 291
Buquinolate, 999
Burimamide, 404, 408
Buserelin, 616
Buspirone, 394
Busulfan, USP, 1071
Butalex, 1014
Butamisole Hydrochloride, INN, 954–55
Butorphanol Tartrate, USP, 293–94

antitussive activity, 1114
n-Butyl chloride, 977
Butyrocholinesterase, 82
Butyrophenones
as antiemetics, 1044
as antipsychotics, 387
azaperone, 333–35
droperidol, 333
prolactin secretion increase by, 605

C-10, 141
Cabergoline, 622
Caffeine, USP, 375–77
Calamine, 1095
Calciparine, 579
Calcitriol, 722
Ca/P metabolism, 689–90
in hyperparathyroidism, 565
Calcium, 722–26
and ACh release, 139–40
assessment of, 724–25
blood coagulation factor, 573–74, 724
deficiency, 724
dietary, 691, 724, 725
intraocular irrigation solutions, 1123
metabolism of, 722–23, 725
neuromuscular function and, 723–24
NOS and, 84
preparations, 725–26
sources, 722
toxicity, 726
uptake of, 725
vitamin D and, 689
Calcium borogluconate, 725–26
Calcium carbonate, 1055
in topical preparations, 1094
Calcium channel blockers, 475–76
as antiarrhythmic agents, 490, 493–94
clinical uses, 477–78
precautions, 476–77
Calcium channels, 154, 475, 484–85, 487–88
Calcium chelating agents, for digitalis-induced arrhythmias, 466
Calcium entry blockers, 478
Calcium pantothenate, 709
Calcium salts, as antacids, 1049
Calmodulin, 84
cAMP. *See* Cyclic AMP
Camphor, 1096
Camylofine, 1053
Cancer
cell cycle, 1065
chemotherapy drugs, 1070–80. *See also* Antineoplastic agents
multimodal therapy, 1069–70
treatment perspectives, 1064–65
tumor growth rate, 1065–66
Canrenone, 549
Caparsolate sodium, 976
Capoten, 415
Caprocid, 582
Capsules, 1157
Captan, 927
Captopril, 415, 417–18, 473–75
Carbachol, 119, 122–23
as purgative, 1057
Carbadox, 889
Carbamates, 148, 1025
Carbamazepine, 608
Carbamylcholine chloride, 122
Carbamylmethylcholine, 122–23
Carbapenems, 825
Carbarsone, 995
Carbaryl, 1025
Carbenicillin, 822
ophthalmic uses, 1129, 1130
Carbicarb, 521
Carbimazole, 645
Carbocaine, 356
Carbolic acid, 787
Carbon dioxide, 177–78
in acid-base metabolism, 514–19
for euthanasia, 399
hypercapnia, 178–79
hypocapnia, 179
partial pressure, 516–17
Carbonic anhydrase inhibitors, 539–40, 1137–38, 1139
Carbon monoxide, for euthanasia, 398–99
Carbon tetrachloride, 985
Carboplatin, 1079
Carboxymethylcellulose sodium, 1056
Carcinogens, sulfamethazine, 801
Cardiac output
digitalis and, 459–60
influence on anesthesia, 192
Cardiomyopathies, calcium channel blockers for, 477–78
Cardiovascular system
angiotensin and, 414–15
barbiturates and, 216–18
cardiac function, 454
effects of steroids on, 653–54
electrophysiology, 482–88
histamine and, 406
inhalant anesthetics and, 195–97
local anesthetics and, 350
magnesium and, 734
morphine and, 276
omega-3 fatty acids and, 763, 764
potassium and, 731–32
prostaglandins effects on, 425–26
thyroid hormone effects, 637
Carfentanil Citrate, USP, 268, 286
Caricide, 975
Carmustine, 1071
Carnivores, urine pH, 40
Carotenoids, 684–85
Carprofen, 443, 1126
Carrier-mediated transport, 18–19
in renal excretion, 40
Cascara sagrada, 38
Castor oil, 1057
Catalepsy, ketamine-induced, 250
Catecholamine-depleting agents, 114
Catecholamines. *See also* Alpha-adrenergic agonists; Beta-adrenergic agonists
absorption and biotransformation, 100
and blood-brain barrier, 99
cardiovascular effects, 95–98, 101
dobutamine, 103–4
dopamine, 102–3
gastrointestinal effects, 99
and halothane, 197–98
histamine antagonists, 405, 408
inhalant anesthetics and, 196
metabolic effects, 99–100
ocular effects, 99
phenothiazines and, 301
pilomotor effects, 99
respiratory effects, 98, 101–2
smooth muscle effects, 99
synthesis and function of, 79–82
toxicity of, 102
Catechol-*O*-methyltransferase (COMT), 81
Cathartics
cholinergic agents as, 1057
enemas, 1058
irritant, 1057
osmotic, 1056–57
Cathepsin D, 289
Cats
acetaminophen toxicity, 33, 445
aminoglycosides in, 850
arachidonic acid deficiency, 759
coccidiosis, 1009
diabetes in, 676, 678
fluoroquinolones in, 908–9
glucuronyl transferase deficiency, 37
griseofulvin in, 920
hemoglobin of, 562
hyperthyroidism, 641–42
hypothyroidism, 600
taurine deficiency in, 766–68
toxoplasmosis in, 1010
UDPGA deficiency in, 278
urine pH, 736
viruses, 937, 939
Cattle. *See also* Ruminants
aminoglycosides in, 850–51
bovine somatotropin, 604–5
calving, induced, 617–18
coccidiosis, 1008
fluid therapy in, 530
fluoroquinolones in, 910
ketosis in, 676–77
lactation, induced, 620
Caustics, 1096
CCNU, 1072
Cefaclor, 823–25
Cefadroxil, 823–25
Cefamandole, 824–25
Cefazolin, 823–25
ophthalmic uses, 1129
Cefixime, 824–25
Cefonicid sodium, 824–25
Cefoperazone, 824–25
Ceforanide, 824–25
Cefotetan disodium, 824–25
Cefoxitin sodium, 824–25
Ceftazidime, 1131
Ceftiofur sodium, 27, 824–25
Ceftizoxime, interspecies scaling profile, 52
Cefuroxime, 823–25
Cell injury, hypoxic, 176

Central nervous system
α_2 receptors, 106
anatomy/physiology of, 153–55
antagonists, 377–79
4-aminopyridine, 377
tolazoline, 324
yohimbine, 324, 377–79
barbiturates and, 215–16
chloramphenicol and, 872
cytotoxic chemotherapy and, 1067
dopamine in, 383
first messengers, 155–56
GABA in, 383–84
inhalant anesthetics and, 194–95
local anesthetics and, 349–50
neurotransmitters, 155–59
norepinephrine in, 383
phenothiazines and, 388
second messengers, 154–56
sites of action, 159
steroids effects on, 654
stimulants, 373–74
doxapram, 374–75
methylxanthines, 375–77
taurine content, 767
Cephalexin, 823–25
bioavailability of, 21
Cephalosporins
allergies to, 61
chemistry, 822
first-generation, 823
microbial susceptibility, 822–23
ophthalmic uses, 1128–29
pharmacokinetics, 823
second-generation, 823–24
third-generation, 824–25
toxicity, 825
Cephalothin sodium, 823–25
Cephapirin sodium, 823–25
Cephradine, 823–25
Cerebrospinal fluid, blood-CSF barrier, 17, 19–20
Cerubidine, 1077
Ceruloplasmin, 746–47
Cestex, 983
cGMP. *See* Cyclic GMP
Charcoal, activated, 1055–56
Chelating agents, oxalic acid, 725
Chemoreceptor trigger zone, 1042–43, 1044–45
Chemosensitizers, 1069
Chemotherapy, 6, 1064. *See also* Antineoplastic agents
Chenodiol, 1058
Cheque drops, 622
Chloral Hydrate, USP, 240–41
biotransformation of, 36
coumarin inhibition, 581
for euthanasia, 400
Chloralose, 261
Chlorambucil, USP, 563, 1071
Chloramine-T, 791
Chloramphenicol, 868–73
barbiturates and, 223
bioavailability of, 25
biotransformation of, 38
chemistry, 868–69
clinical use, 872–73
drug interactions, 39, 872
formulations, 869
mechanism of action, 869
microbial susceptibility, 869
ophthalmic uses, 1129
pharmacokinetics, 869–71
phenytoin inhibition, 492
primidone contraindication, 367
toxicity, 871–72
Chloramphenicol derivatives, 873–76
florfenicol, 873–76
thiamphenicol, 873
Chlorazene, 791
Chlordiazepoxide Hydrochloride, USP, 331–32
Chlorhexidine, 1100
as antiseptic, 786, 790–91
ophthalmic, 122–23
Chloride, 726–30
assessment of, 729
deficiency, 729
dietary, 728, 729–30
fluid balance and, 727–29
preparations, 730
renal regulation of, 506–7
Chlorinated hydrocarbon insecticides, 1020–21
Chlorine solutions, antiseptic, 786, 791
Chlorisondamine, 134
Chlormadinone acetate, 622
Chloroform, 185
Chloroprocaine Hydrochloride, USP, 355
Chloroquine, for malaria, 1012
Chlorous acid, 791
Chlorpheniramine, 1116
Chlorpromazine Hydrochloride, USP, 110, 302–3
as antiemetic, 1044
for diarrhea, 1055
Chlorpropamide, 582
for diabetes insipidus, 607–8
Chlorpyrifos, 1024
Chlortetracycline, 830–31
ophthalmic uses, 1131
sulfathiazole and, 806
Chlorthiazide, 547
Cholagogues, 1058–59
Cholecalciferol, 688, 691
Choleretics, 1058–59
Cholesterol, 762–63
Cholestyramine Resin, USP, 467, 1055, 1056
Choline, 117, 716–17, 1059
ACh synthesis and, 140
Choline esters
mechanism of action, 117–19
pharmacological effects, 122–23
structure-activity relationship, 119–20
Cholinergic
agonists, as purgatives, 1051, 1057–58
antagonists, ophthalmic uses, 1136, 1137
definition of, 117
nerves, 75
receptors, 82, 388
Cholinesterase inhibitors, 127–30, 141
antagonism of competitive neuromuscular blockers, 141, 143, 148, 150
enzymatic interactions, 125–26
mechanism of action, 124–25
ophthalmic uses, 1134–35
pharmacological effects, 126
reversible, 126–27
Cholinesterase reactivators, 129
Cholinolytics, synthetic, 1053
Cholinomimetic alkaloids, natural, 123–24
Chondroitin sulfate, 1141
ophthalmic uses, 1144
Chromium, 744–45
Chromium trioxide, 577
Chronic obstructive pulmonary disease, 1105
CIDR-Bovine, 616
Cilastatin, 825
Ciliates, 1014
Cimetidine, 404, 408, 565, 1046–48
for acetaminophen toxicity, 446
drug interactions, 62
Ciprofloxacin, 898–913
ophthalmic uses, 1129
rifampin and, 887
Cisapride, 1052
Cisplatin, 1078–79
Citanest, 356
Citrate-phosphate-dextrose-adenine (CPDA-1), 579
Clarithromycin, 881
Clavulanic acid, 825
Cleansers, 784
Clearance
body, 44–45
and drug interactions, 62
Clenbuterol, 106
Cleocin, 1010
Clexon, 1014
Clidinium, 1053
Clinafarm-EC, 927
Clindamycin, 884–86, 1010
ophthalmic uses, 1131
Clinical pharmacology, 6, 15, 57. *See also* Therapeutic principles
Clinicox, 1005
Clioxanide, 985
Clofibrate, 582, 608
ClomCalm, 391
Clomipramine, 390, 391
Clonazepam, USP, 372
Clonidine, for diarrhea, 1055
Clonopin, 372
Clopidol, 999, 1007
Cloprostenol, 616
Clorazepate, 370–72
Clorsulon, 985, 987
Closantel, INN, 985, 988
Clostridium botulinum paralysis, 141, 377
Clotrimazole, 1100
ophthalmic uses, 1132
Clotting factors, 572–74
prekallikrein activation, 417
Cloxacillin, 822
ophthalmic uses, 1130
Clozapine, 300
Coagulopathies, 575
Coal tar, in topical preparations,

1046, 1047
Cobalt, 714–15, 745–46
Cobalt iron oxide pellets, 745
Coban, 1004
Cocaine Hydrochloride, USP, 81, 115, 353–54
  addiction, 351
  as local anesthetic, 343
Coccidiosis, 997–98. *See also* Anticoccidial drugs
Codeine Phosphate, USP, 280
  antitussive activity, 1114
Coerulein, 418
Cogentin, 311
Colchicine, 1142
Colic, equine
  detomidine for, 322
  flunixin for, 443
  morphine for, 279–80
  pentazocine for, 293
  phenothiazines contraindicated, 306, 308
  xylazine in, 317
Colistin, 1099
  ophthalmic uses, 1130
Collagen, microcrystalline, 577
Colloid solutions, 527–29, 563–64
Colostrokinin, 418
Compartmental analysis, 45–46
Compazine, 312
Competitive antagonism, 10
Competitive inhibition, in carrier-mediated transport, 18
Competitive neuromuscular blocking agents, 137–38, 141
  antagonism, 150
  clinical use, 148–50
  drug interactions, 147–48
  effects of, 143–47
  safety, 149–50
Compliance, lack of, 60
Compound 48/80, 404, 405
  serotonin depletion by, 412
Compounding, 59
COMT, 81
Congestive heart failure
  aldosterone antagonists for, 550
  bronchodilators in, 470
  calcium channel blockers for, 477
  digitalis for, 457–64, 467–68
  lasix for, 545
  loop diuretics in, 478–79
  milrinone for, 472
  morphine in, 479
  sodium restriction, 729
  thiazides for, 548
  vasodilators for, 472–78
Conjugating agents, phase II reactions, 36
Contractility, myocardial, 454–55, 458
Controlled internal drug release (CIDR) devices, 616
Controlled substances, 269, 1154–56
Conversion tables, 1165
Copper, 746–49
  deficiency, 562, 747
  toxicity, 748–49, 759
Copper naphthanate, 1100
Copper oxide wire, 748
Copper sulfate, 275, 1014
Coriban, 989
Corid, 1000
Corticosteroids
  ACTH suppression, 598
  for allergy reactions, 410
  ophthalmic uses, 1123–24
  prostaglandin inhibition, 425
Corticotropin-releasing hormone, 594, 596
  CRH stimulation test, 598
Cortisol, 649, 650
  replacement therapy, 661
Cortisone, 655–58, 662–63
Cortrosyn, 664
Cosmegen, 1078
Cotarnine chloride, 5777
Cotrimethoxazole, 1007
Coumaphos, 961, 1024
Coumarin derivatives, 580–82
COX-1 and 2. *See* Cyclooxygenase
Coyden, 25, 999
Creams, 1158
CRH, 596
Crib biting, narcotic antagonists for, 274, 290, 291
Cromogylate, 1113
Cromolyn sodium
  for asthma, 407
  ophthalmic uses, 1127
Cross-reactivity, of drugs, 61
Crufomate, 961
Cryptorchidism, 623
Cryptosporidiosis, 1009–10
Crystalloid solutions, 527
Crystalluria, sulfonamide-induced, 799–800
Cucurbitine, 980
Cupric sulfate, 748
Cuproenzymes, 746–47
Curare, 82, 137
  histamine release by, 146, 405
Curatrem, 987
Cushing's syndrome, 666, 668
  iatrogenic, 658
Cyanoacrylate, 1141
Cyanocobalamin. *See* Vitamin B_{12}
Cycarb, 1001
Cyclic AMP, 86–88, 1105, 1108
  and histamine release, 405
Cyclic GMP, 88, 1105, 1108
Cyclizine, 408, 1044
Cyclooxygenase, 422–25
  NSAIDs inhibition of, 434–37. *See also* individual agents
Cyclopentolate, 1136
Cyclophosphamide, USP, 1070–71
Cycloplegic agents, 1136–37
Cyclopropane, 185
Cyclosporine
  ketoconazole potentiation of, 926
  topical ophthalmic, 1126, 1139
Cycostat, 999
Cydectin, 972
Cyfluthrin, 1020
Cygro, 1004
Λ Cyhalothrin, 1020
Cypermethrin, 1020
Cyprenorphine, 290
Cyproheptadine, 412
  appetite stimulation, 1042
Cyromazine, 1026–29
L-Cysteinamide, 680
Cysteine, 37
Cystorelin, 616
Cytarabine, USP, 935, 1073
Cytauxzoonosis, 1014
Cytochalasin B, 1142
Cytochrome P-450, 33
  and drug absorption, 2
  inhibitors, azoles, 924–31
  interspecies variations in, 35
Cytokines, 428–31
  glucocorticoid inhibition of, 651
  taurine and, 768
Cytosar, 1073
Cytovene, 936
Cytoxan, 1070

Dacarbazine, USP, 1072
Dactinomycin, USP, 1078
Dakin's solution, 791
Danofloxacin, 898–913
Danthron, 1057
Dapiprazole, 1137
Daranide, 539
Darbazine, 312
Darvon, 287
Daunomycin, 1077
Daunorubicin hydrochloride, 1077
Dazamide, 539
DDAVP, 578, 607
DDVP, 962–63
Decamethonium Bromide, USP, 138, 141
  autonomic effects, 146
  drug interactions, 147
  skeletal muscle effects, 144
Deccox, 999
Decholin, 1058
Decongestants, 1116–17
Decoquinate, 999
Dectomax, 968–69
DEET, 1032
Defend, 1102
Deferoxamine mesylate, 567
Dehydration, 507–8, 541
Dehydrocholic acid, 1058
Delaney anticancer clause, 1151
Delmadinone acetate, 622
Delta-Albaplex, 886
Demadex, 543
Demecarium bromide, 1134
Demerol Pethidine, 281
Demulcents, 1094–95
Depolarizing neuromuscular blocking agents, 137–38, 141–43
  antagonism, 150
  clinical use, 148–50
  drug interactions, 147–48
  effects, 143–47
  safety, 149–50
L-Deprenyl, 666
Dermatologic drugs
  absorption of, 19, 20–21, 1088–94
  antifungal, 920–21, 931–32, 1100
  antimicrobial, 1099–1110
  bases for, 1098–99
  glucocorticoids, 1100–1101
  penetration enhancers, 1093–94

Dermatologic drugs (*continued*)
  pesticides, 1101–2
  transdermal delivery, 1094
  vehicles
    properties of, 1041–43
    types of, 1094–98
Dermatophytoses, 920–21, 931–32
Dermatoses
  allergic, 1100
  vitamin A-responsive, 685
Dermis, 1086
DES, 620, 621, 1079
Desflurane, USP, 189, 201–2
Desmethylimipramine, 115
Desmopressin acetate, 578, 607
Desoxycorticosterone pivalate, 665–66
Detergents, 784
Detomidine hydrochloride, 321–23
Dexamethasone, 655–58, 662–63
  lactation induction by, 620
  ophthalmic suspension, 1123
  parturition induction by, 617
Dexmedetomidine, 324
Dextran
  in colloidal solutions, 527
  in hypertonic solutions, 529
  ophthalmic uses, 1141
Dextran-saline solutions, for blood loss anemias, 563
Dextran sulfate, antiviral activity, 939
Dextroamphetamine, 395
Dextromethorphan, antitussive activity, 1114–15
DFP, 124, 125, 127, 130
Diabetes insipidus, 606–8
  nephrogenic, 728
Diabetes mellitus, 672, 674, 676
  aminoglycosides use in, 847–48
  ketoacidosis in, 521–22
  steroid-induced, 652
  vanadium in, 756
Diabinese, 607
Diagnoses, accurate/specific, 57
Diamidine derivatives, 1013–14
Diaminopyrimidine-sulfonamide, 799
Diamond, 1098
Diamox, 539
Diamphenethide, INN, 989–90
Diampron, 1013
Diarrhea. *See* Antidiarrheal agents; Gastrointestinal tract, intestinal motility modulators
Diastases, 1058
Diazepam, USP, 326–31
  as anticonvulsant, 370–72
  appetite stimulation, 1042
  ketamine and, 253, 255
  pentobarbital and, 227
  xylazine-ketamine and, 320
Diazinon, 1024
Diazoxide, 680
Dibenzyline, 110
Dichloroisoproterenol, 112
Dichlorophen, INN, 981
Dichlorphenamide, 539, 1138
Dichlorvos, INN, 962–63, 1024
Diclazuril, 1005, 1011
Diclofenac, 1125
Dicloxacillin, 822
Dicoumarol, USP, 578, 580–82
Dicyclomine, 1044, 1053
Diet, acidifiers/alkalinizers, 735
Diethylcarbamazine Citrate, USP, INN, 975–76
Diethyl ether, 185, 203
N,N,-Diethyl-*m*-toluamide, 1032
Diethylstilbestrol, USP, 620, 621
  in cancer therapy, 1079
Diffusion
  across cell membranes, 17
  and pH, 17–18
  placental, 63
Difloxacin, 898–913
Diflubenzuron, 1026, 1029
Diflucan, 930
Difolin, 981
Digitalis, 456–57
  for arrhythmias, 490
  cardiovascular effects, 457–58
    action potential, 459
    cardiac output, 459–60
    diuresis, 464
    electrophysiologic, 462–64
    myocardial contractility, 458
    oxygen demand, 460–61
    rate/rhythm, 461–62
  chemistry, 457
  contraindications, 468
  digitalization, 468–69
  dosage schedules, 468–71
  extracirculatory effects, 464–65
  indications for, 467–68
  pharmacokinetics, 465
  preparations, 471
  succinylcholine and, 146
  toxicity, 465–67
Digoxin, 470
  dosage, 49, 51
Dihydrofolate reductase-thymidylate synthase inhibitors, 1005–7, 1011
Dihydrostreptomycin, 859
Diisopropyl fluorophosphate (DFP), 124, 125, 127, 130
Dilantin, 368, 491
Dilaudid, 280
Diltiazem, 477, 493–94
Dimethicone, 1095
Dimethylmorphine, 269
Dimethyl sulfoxide, 59, 176, 1093–94, 1098
  anti-inflammatory effects, 447–48
Dimetridazole, 995
Diminazene diaceturate, 1013
Dinitolmide, 1001, 1007
Dinoprost tromethamine, 616, 617, 619
Diphenhydramine hydrochloride, 408, 1116
  as antiemetic, 1044
Diphenoxylate Hydrochloride, USP, 281
  antidiarrheal, 1054
  atropine and, 282–83
Diphenylhydantoin, effects on T_4, 634
Diphenylmethane cathartics, 1057
Diphenytoin, 491
Dipivefrin hydrochloride, 1135
Diprenorphine, 286–290–91
  etorphine antagonist, 286
Diprivan, 237
Dipyridamole, 584, 1069
Dipyrone, 1053
Dirian, 988
Dirocide, 975
Disinfectants, 784–88
  for animal facilities, 792–94
  clinical use, 791–94
  resistance to, 789
Disophenol, 985
Disopyramide, 488, 495
Dispensing, drugs, 1162
Disposition curve, biphasic, 45–46
Distolon, 986
Distribution, drug, 27–30
Di-Trim, 1007
Diuresis
  alkaline, 40
  digitalization and, 464
Diuretics
  aldosterone antagonists, 549–50
  aminophylline, 376–77
  carbonic anhydrase inhibitors, 539–40
  excretion of, 40
  loop, 478–79, 543–47
  osmotic, 540–43
  potassium-sparing, 548–49
  thiazide, 547–48, 608
  tolerance to, 539
  use of, 538–39
Diuril, 547
DMSO. *See* Dimethyl sulfoxide
DNA viruses, antiviral agents for, 935–37, 939
Dobutamine, 103–4
DOCA, 665–66
Docosahexaenoic acid, 759–66
DOCP, 665–66
Docusate sodium, 1056
Dogs
  aminoglycosides in, 849
  arylamine acetyltransferase deficiency, 37
  coccidiosis in, 1009
  diabetes in, 676
  fluoroquinolones in, 908–9
  hepatozoonosis, 1012
  hypothyroidism in, 599–600, 638
  neosporosis in, 1010–11
  renal excretion of drugs, 43–44
  thyroid replacement therapy, 640–41
  toxoplasmosis in, 1010
Dolantin, 281
Dolophine, 284
Domitor, 323
Domoso, 1098
Domperidone, 1052
L-Dopa, 707
Dopamine, 102–3
  antagonists, 1051–52
  appetite stimulation, 1042
  cardiovascular effects, 102–3
  in CNS, 157, 383
  receptors, 299–300, 387–88
  synthesis and function of, 79–82
Dopram, 374
Doramectin
  antinematodal, 968–69

ectoparasiticide, 1030
ophthalmic uses, 1133
Dormosedan, 321
Doryl, 122
Dorzolamide, 539, 540, 1138
Dosage, 6
calculating, 49
drug, 47–52
fixed, 50
forms, 21–23, 1157–58
intervals, 51
regimen, 49, 59–60
Dose
definition of, 6, 47
loading, 20, 49–50
maintenance, 51
optimum, 47
titration studies, 14
Dose-response relationships, 10–14
Dosing
continuous infusion, 49, 50–51
frequency of, 60
intermittent, 49
Double Impact, 965
Dovenix, 986
Doxapram Hydrochloride, USP, 374–75
Doxorubicin Hydrochloride, USP, 1075–77
Doxycycline, 834–35
and thiopental, 223
Dressings, 1098
Droleptan, 333
Droncit, 981
Drontal-Plus, 959, 996
Droperidol, USP, 333, 1044
Drug Enforcement Agency, 269, 1155
Drug fever, 61
Drug interactions, 62–63
additive effects, 63
compounding, 39
half-life and, 42
Drug-protein complex, 27–30
Drugs
action of, 9, 15–16
compendia, 1156
controlled, 1154–56
definition of, 5
dispensing/packaging, 1162
disposition studies, 49
effects, 9
efficacy of, 9, 10–14, 61
excretion of, 39–41
in geriatric patients, 64
incompatibilities, 1163–65
microbial metabolism of, 37–39
nomenclature, 1158–59
in pediatric patients, 63–64
products of, 19
selection of, 57
DTIC, 1072
Duragesic, 285
Duranest, 357
Dynorphins, 270–71, 277, 1053
Dyrenium, 548

Echothiophate, 1134
Econazole, 1132
Ectoparasiticides
avermectins, 1029–30
benzyl benzoate, 1026
botanicals, 1018–20
carbamates, 1025
chlorinated hydrocarbons, 1020–21
formamidines, 1025
formulations, 1033–36
insect development inhibitors, 1026–29
insect growth regulators, 1026–29
lime sulfur, 1026
organophosphates, 1021–24
repellents, 1031–32
resistance to, 1032, 1036
synergists, 1030–31
toxicity, 1037
ED_{50}, 12–13, 14
Edecrin, 543
Edema
formation of, 538–39
lasix for, 545
potassium-sparing diuretics for, 548–49
Edetate Disodium, USP, 579
EDRF, 83–84, 85–86, 94, 180–81
Edrophonium Chloride, USP, 125, 126–27, 150
EDTA, for digitalis-induced arrhythmias, 466
EFA. *See* Fatty acids
Effective dose, median, 12–13, 14
Efficacy
of drugs, 9, 10–14
lack of, 61
Efudex, 1073
Ehrlichiosis, tetracyclines for, 831, 832, 835
Eicosanoids, 420–21. *See also* Prostaglandins
biosynthesis, 421–24
effects of, 425–28
inhibition of, 424–25
leukotrienes, 423–24, 426
metabolism, 763
NSAIDs inhibition of, 434–37
in skin, 1088
thromboxanes, 422–23, 425–26
Eicosapentaenoic acid, 759–66
Electrical potential, cell membranes, 728
Electrocardiogram
effects of digitalis on, 463–64
potassium disturbances and, 513–14
Electrolyte gradients, cardiac, 454–56, 459, 482–88
Electrolytes
angiotensin and, 415
dehydration and, 541
and digitalis-induced arrhythmias, 466
fluid distribution, 503–4. *See also* Fluid balance
Eledoisin, 418
Elimination of drugs
mechanisms of, 30–41
pharmacokinetics, 41–45
and protein binding, 28
Elixirs, 1157
Emetics
centrally acting, 1044
peripherally acting, 1043–44
vomition reflex, 1042–43
EMLA, 356
Emodin purgatives, 1057
Emollients, 1095
Emtrymix, 995
Emulsions, 1098, 1157
Enalapril maleate, 415, 473–75
Encainide, 488, 496
Endectocides. *See* Macrocyclic lactones
Endoperoxides, 420, 422
and platelet aggregation, 572
Endorphins, 159, 270–71, 1053
immunomodulatory effects, 277
Endothelium-derived relaxing factor (EDRF), 83–84, 85–86, 94, 180–81
Endotoxicosis
eicosanoids effects on, 426
flunixine for, 442
omega-3 fatty acids and, 764
tumor necrosis factor-α and, 429
Endplate potential, 140
End points, monitoring, 65
Endrate, 579
Enemas, 1058
Enflurane, USP, 197, 200–201
Enilconazole, 927
Enkephalins, 159, 270–71
immunomodulatory effects, 277
Enoxacin, 898
Enrofloxacin, 898–913
ophthalmic uses, 1129
Enterocolitis
clindamycin-induced, 885
lincomycin-induced, 883
Enterohepatic circulation, of drugs, 41
Environmental contaminants, tissue residues, 1167
Environmental Protection Agency, 1167, 1168
ectoparasiticide regulation, 1036–38
Enzymes
as antineoplastic drugs, 1078
microsomal, 32–36
Epanutin, 368
EPE, 613
Ephedrine, USP, 104–5, 1115
for allergies, 410
bronchodilation by, 1108
Epidermal growth factor, ophthalmic use, 1143
Epidermis, 1085–86
Epidural nerve blocks, 159, 353
in pregnancy, 352, 355
xylazine for, 318
Epilepsy
biochemistry of, 361
phenytoin-phenobarbital for, 369
Epinephrine, USP, 577
in anaphylaxis, 62, 101
for arrhythmias, 490
biotransformation of, 100
bronchodilation by, 1108
cardiovascular effects, 95–98, 101
in CNS, 157

Epinephrine, USP (*continued*)
  with local anesthetics, 20, 100, 351–52
  local hemostasis, 100–101
  ocular effects, 99
  ophthalmic uses, 1122, 1135, 1137
  phenothiazines contraindicated, 303
  preparations, 100
  respiratory effects, 98
  reversal, 107
  smooth muscle effects, 99
  and sodium bicarbonate incompatibility, 62
  structure of, 92
  synthesis and function of, 79–82
  and thiopental, 223
Epipodophyllotoxins, 1075
Epirubicin, 1076
Epithelium, vitamin A and, 685
Epontol, 261
Eprinomectin, 969–70
  ectoparasiticide, 1030
Epsilon-aminocaproic acid, 1142
Equest, 972
Equilibrium concentration ratio, 18
Equimate, 617
Equimectrin, 965
Equine chorionic gonadotropin, 613
Equine pituitary extract, 613
Equine protozoal myeloencephalitis, 1011
Equivalence, therapeutic, 58
Eqvalan, 965
Ergocalciferol, 688, 691
Ergoline derivatives
  as abortifacients, 622
  for pseudopregnancy, 622–23
Ergonovine, 613
Ergosterol, 688–92
Ergot alkaloids, 107–9
Ery-Mycin, 876
Erythrocytes, 553–54, 558–59
  vitamin E deficiency and, 693, 694
Erythromycin, 876–80
  bioavailability of, 21
  ophthalmic uses, 1131
Erythropoiesis, 554–59
Erythropoietin, 555–56
  recombinant, 566
Escharotics, 1096
Eserine, 126
Espirantel, INN, 983–84
Essential fatty acids. *See* Fatty acids
Estradiol benzoate, 618
Estradiol Cypionate, USP
  in cancer therapy, 1079
  post partum, 618
Estradiol valerate, 613, 615, 618
Estrogens
  as abortifacients, 613, 618
  antinidatory effects, 621
  lactation induction by, 620
  postpartum, 618, 621
  pseudopregnancy and, 619
  toxicity, 621
Estrumate, 616
Estrus
  inducing, 614–17, 620
  prevention, 622
  synchronization of, 613, 615
Ethacrynic acid, 543, 1138
Ethanol
  as disinfectant, 785
  for euthanasia, 400
Ether, USP, 203
  neuromuscular blocking agents and, 148, 150
Ethion, 1024
Ethoxyzolamide, 1138
Ethrane, 200
Ethyl alcohol, 400, 785
Ethylenediamine dihydroiodide, 1116
Ethylenediaminetetraacetic acid. *See* EDTA
Ethylene glycol, biotransformation of, 36
Ethylene oxide, 787
Ethylestrol, 582
Etidocaine Hydrochloride, USP, 357
Etomidate, 239–40
Etoposide, 1075
Etorphine Hydrochloride, INN, 286–87
  acepromazine and, 311
  antagonists, 286, 287
  diprenorphine antagonism, 290–91
  xylazine and, 287, 321
Euthanasia, 397
  drugs contraindicated for, 400
Euthanizing agents
  barbiturates, 400
  carbon dioxide, 399
  carbon monoxide, 398–99
  chloral hydrate, 400
  criteria for, 397
  ethanol, 400
  hydrogen cyanide, 399
  inhalation anesthetics, 399–400
  mechanisms of action, 397–98
  MS-222, 401
  nitrogen, 400
  pentobarbital, 226
  T-61, 400
Evipal sodium, 237
Excitation-secretion coupling, 139–40
Excretion of drugs
  biliary, 40–41
  and lipid solubility, 40
  renal, 39–40
Exercise-induced pulmonary hemorrhage, lasix for, 545–46
Exotics
  chloramphenicol in, 873
  chlordiazepoxide in, 332
  chlorpromazine in, 305
  diazepam in, 330–31
  etorphine (M-99) in, 286–87
  fluoroquinolones in, 909–10
  ketamine in, 256–57
  meperidine in, 284
  pentobarbital in, 229
  promazine in, 307
  thiopental in, 234
  tiletamine-zolazepam in, 260
  xylazine in, 321
Expectorants, 1115–16
Extra-label use of drugs (ELUD), 58, 1168–69
  prohibited drugs, 1172–73
  regulation of, 1152–53
Extravasation, of antineoplastic agents, 1067

Fabantol, 261
Facilitated diffusion, 18–19
Factel, 616
Famotidine, 408, 1046–48
Famphur, 1024
Fansidar, 1007
FARAD, 1169, 1173
Fasciolosis, 985–86
Fasinex, 989
Fat, polyunsaturated, effect on vitamin E, 695
Fatty acids
  chemistry, 759
  dietary requirements, 765–66
  eicosanoid metabolism, 763
  omega, 759–66
  sources, 759–61
Fazadinium, 141
FDA. *See* Food and Drug Administration
Febantel, 953–54
  for giardiasis, 996
Federal Food, Drug, and Cosmetic Act (1938), 1151–55, 1168
Feed, drugs in, 1162–63
Feldene, 1080
Feline immunodeficiency virus (FIV), 937, 939
Feline leukemia virus (FeLV), 937, 939
Fenbendazole, 950–53
  as cestocidal, 984
  for fasciolosis, 988–89
  for giardiasis, 996
Fenprostalene, 616
Fentanyl Citrate, USP, 285
  droperidol and, 166
  naloxone antagonism, 290
  xylazine and, 321
Fenthion, 1024
Fenvalerate, 1020
Ferric chloride, 577
Ferric subsulfate, 577
Ferric sulfate, 577
Ferrous carbonate, 751
Ferrous sulfate, 751
Fertagyl, 616
Fertirelin acetate, 616
Fetus, barbiturates and, 219
Fibrin, 573
Fibrin foam, 576
Fibrinogen, 573
Fibrinolysin, 582–83
Fibrinolysis, 574, 582
Fibrinolytic agents, 582–83
  ophthalmic use, 1142
Fibrogen, 576
Fibronectin, ophthalmic use, 1143
Fight or flight response, 74, 75
Filaramide, 976
Filaribits, 951, 975
Filaricide, 975
Filtration, as transfer mechanism, 17
Finasteride, 623
Fipronyl, 1029
First messenger, 299

First pass effect, 25
Fish
antiprotozoan agents, 1014
euthanasia of, 401
florfenicol in, 875
fluoroquinolones in, 910
sulfachloropyridazine in, 810
UDPGA deficiency, 37
Fish oils, 761, 763–66
vitamin A in, 687–88
FIV, 937, 939
Flagellates, 993–97
Flagyl, 993
Flaxedil, 141
Fleas, control of, 1033–34
Flecainide, 488, 496
Flies, control of, 1033–35
Florfenicol, 873–76, 1129
Florinef, 666
Fluconazole, 930–31
interspecies scaling profile, 52
ophthalmic uses, 1132
Flucytosine, 921
amphotericin B and, 932
ophthalmic uses, 1132–33
Fludrocortisone acetate, 666
Fluid balance
body fluid compartments, 502–3
disorders
dehydration, 507–8
hyperchloremia, 511
hyperkalemia, 512–14
hypernatremia, 508–9
hypochloremia, 511
hypokalemia, 512, 514
hyponatremia, 509–11
fluid/electrolyte distribution, 503–4
glucocorticoid regulation of, 652, 653
renal regulation of, 506–7
water turnover, 504–6
Fluid therapy
monitoring, 523–24
parenteral fluids, 527–30
colloids, 527–29
crystalloids, 527
hypertonic solutions, 529–30
rate of, 526–27
replacement/maintenance volumes, 524–26
route of, 526–27
Flukanide, 986
Flukes
liver. *See* Antitrematodal drugs
lung, 990
rumen, 990
Flukicides. *See* Antitrematodal drugs
Flukiver, 988
Flumadine, 938
Flumazenil, 332–33
Flumethasone, 655–58, 662–63
ophthalmic, 1123
parturition induction by, 617
Flunixin meglumine, 442–43, 1126
Fluorescein dye, 1122
Fluorine, 749–50
Fluorocarbon gases, ophthalmic uses, 1143
Fluorometholone, 1124
Fluoroquinolones. *See also* individual agents
chemistry, 898–99
clinical use, 908–11
dose ranges, 907–8
drug interactions, 921–23
efficacy of, 907
mechanism of action, 899
microbial susceptibility, 899, 903
ophthalmic uses, 1129
pharmacokinetics, 899–903, 904–7
placental transfer, 911
resistance, 903–4
safety, 911–12
Fluorosis, dental, 750
Fluorouracil, USP, 1073, 1142
Fluothane, 197804
Fluoxetine, 392–93
Fluprostenol, 617
Flurbiprofen, 1125
Folacin, 711–13
Folic acid, 559, 711–13
Folic acid analogs, 1072
Follicle stimulating hormone, 612, 613, 619
Food, effect on absorption, 23
Food and Drug Administration
Center for Veterinary Medicine (FDA–CVM), 1168
ectoparasiticide regulation, 1036–37
Food and Drugs Act (1906), 1150
Food Animal Residue Avoidance Databank, 1169, 1173
Food animals, drugs prohibited in, 58–59. *See also* Residues, drug
Food poisoning, fatal, 141
Food Safety Inspection Service, 1169
Forane, 198
Formaldehyde, as disinfectant, 786–87
Formalin, 786
for fish protozoans, 1014
Formamidines, 1025
Formulation, of drugs, 58–59
Foscarnet, 938
Free hormone hypothesis, 631–32
Free radicals, 176
Fructose, hepatotropic effects, 1059–60
FSH, 612, 613, 619
FSH-P, 619
5-FU, 1073, 1142
Fulvicin, 919
Fungi, characteristics of, 918–19
Fungizone, 921
Furazolidone, 888
Furosemide, 543–47
effects on thyroid hormones, 633
Fusidic acid, ophthalmic uses, 1132

GABA. *See* Gamma-aminobutyric acid
GABA receptors, 158, 215–16
benzodiazepines and, 325–26
progestins interaction, 395
Gallamine Triethiodide, USP, 138, 141, 149
cardiovascular effects, 146
pharmacokinetics, 147
skeletal muscle effects, 143
Gallic acid, 1095
Gamma-aminobutyric acid, 83
barbiturates and, 215
benzodiazepine potentiation of, 325–26
in CNS, 157–58, 383–84, 911
phenobarbital and, 363
receptors. *See* GABA receptors
Ganaseg, 1013
Ganciclovir, USP, 936–37
Gases
disinfectant, 787
therapeutic, 172–73
Gastrointestinal tract
adsorbents, 1055–56
antimicrobial suppression of microflora, 61
antisecretory drugs, 1046–49
appetite stimulants, 1042
autonomic control of, 73
cytoprotective drugs, 1049–50
digestants, 1058
and drug absorption, 21–23
and drug biotransformation, 37–39
erythromycin and, 880
function, 1041–42
gastric acid secretion, 1045–46
gastric emptying
alterations in, 62
effect on absorption, 22, 23
gastric motility modulators, 1050–51
cholinergics, 1051
cisapride, 1052
domperidone, 1052
metoclopramide, 1051–52
glutamine utilization, 769
intestinal motility modulators, 1052–53
anticholinergic agents, 1053
opiates, 1053–54
laxatives/cathartics, 1056–58
morphine and, 277
mucosal defenses, 1046
muscarinic receptors, 1052–53
Na/Cl effects on, 727
nitric oxide regulation of, 86
NSAID side effects, 438–39
potassium and, 731
protectants, 1055–56
receptors, 1050–51
tetracyclines and, 829–30
ulceration, 1046
Gatifloxacin, 898
Gecolate, 241
Gelfoam, 576
Generic drugs, 58
bioequivalence of, 25–27
Gentamicin, 851–55
and carbenicillin incompatibility, 62
ophthalmic uses, 1127–28
Geriatric patients, drug therapy in, 64
GHRH, 603
Giardiasis, 994
Glaucoma
carbonic anhydrase inhibitors for, 540, 542

Glaucoma (*continued*)
hypotensive agents for, 1134–39
Glipizide, 677–78
Glucagon, 679
Glucantime, 995
Glucocorticoids. *See also* Mineralocorticoids; Steroids
alternate day therapy, 662–63
anti-inflammatory effects, 650–52, 653
clinical use, 660–65
cortisol, 649, 650
for diarrhea, 1054–55
effect on T_3, 633–34
pharmacological effects, 652–54
physiological effects, 652
preparations, 654–58
topical/ophthalmic, 664–65, 1100–1101
toxicity, 658–60
withdrawal, 663–64
Gluconeogenesis, glutamine and, 769
Glucose
hepatotropic effects, 1059–60
metabolism, glucocorticoids and, 652, 654
Glucuronide conjugates, 36–37
Glutamate, in CNS, 158, 384
Glutamic acid, 361
Glutamine, 769–72
Glutaraldehyde, as disinfectant, 786–87
Glutathione, 37
intraocular irrigation solutions, 1123
Glycerin, 1095
ophthalmic uses, 1138
Glycine, in CNS, 158
Glycopeptides, prohibitions against, 890
p-Glycoprotein
and drug resistance, 1068–69
pump, 22–23
Glycoprotein-processing inhibitors, 940
Glycopyrrolate, NF, 132–33
antiemetic activity, 1045
bronchodilation by, 1112
spasmolytic activity, 1053
Glycosaminoglycan, polysulfated, 446–47
Glycosides, cardiac
amrinone, 471
biotransformation of, 38
digitalis, 456–71
milrinone, 471–72
GnRH, 613, 616
clinical uses, 620
Goats, coccidiosis, 1008
Goitrin, 643
Goitrogens, 643
Gonadorelin, 616
Gonadotropin-releasing hormone, 613, 616
clinical uses, 620
G-protein-coupled receptors, 299, 314–15
G proteins, 155–56, 603
Grepafloxacin, 898
Greyhounds, barbiturates in, 222–23, 229, 232, 235
Grifulvin V, 919
Grisactin, 919
Griseofulvin, USP, 919–21
coumarin inhibition, 581
Growth hormone, 604–5
Growth hormone release-inhibiting hormone, 603
Growth hormone-releasing hormone, 603
Guaiacol, NF, 1116
Guaifenesin, USP, 241–43
as expectorant, 1116
Guanethidine, 114
Guanosine 3′, 5′-monophosphate. *See* Cyclic GMP

H_1 blockers, 404, 408–10. *See also* Antihistamines
H_1 receptors, and vomition reflex, 1042
H_2 blockers, 404, 408–10. *See also* Antihistamines
drug interactions, 62
H_2 receptor antagonists
adverse reactions, 1048
clinical use, 1048
control of gastric acid secretion, 1046–47
drug interactions, 1048
Hageman factor, prekallikrein activation, 417
Haldol, 1044
Half-life
and dosage, 49–50
effect of plasma protein binding on, 27–28
elimination, 41–44
and withdrawal times, 1169–72
Haloalkylamines, 109, 110
Halofuginone, 1002, 1007, 1014
Haloperidol, as antiemetic, 1044
Halothane, USP, 197–98
curare-like drugs and, 148
doxapram antagonism of, 374
elimination of, 30
hepatitis due to, 198
malignant hyperthermia, 196, 198, 308
structure of, 187
Haloxon, 961
Hapadex, 953
HCG, 613, 623
Head-drop test, for muscle paralysis, 148
Heartgard, 965, 966
Heartworms
adulticides, 967
prevention, 975–76
Hematinic drugs, 563–68
Hemicholinium, 140
Hemochromatosis, 567
Hemoglobin, 557–58
carbon monoxide affinity for, 398
oxidative damage, 562
replacement therapy, 564
saturation of, 174–75
Hemo-pak, 576
Hemosiderosis, 567
Hemostasis, 571–75
Hemostatics
systemic, 577–78
topical, 575–76
Henderson-Hasselbalch equation, 516–17, 519
Heparin Sodium, USP, 579–80
coumarin potentiation, 581
ophthalmic uses, 1141
Hepatic microsomal enzymes. *See* Microsomal enzyme system
Hepatotropic agents, 1058–59
Herbivores
drug excretion, 43
urine pH, 40
Herpesviruses, 935–36, 938
Herplex, 935
Hetastarch, 527
Heterocyclic compounds, antinematodal drugs, 973–76
Hexachloroethane, 985
Hexachloroparaxylene, 985, 986
Hexachlorophene, USP, 985
anticestodal, 981
for fasciolosis, 986
Hexamethonium, 134
Hexobarbital Sodium, NF, 237
Histamine, 403
biotransformation, 407
clinical uses, 407
in CNS, 157
effects of, 406–7
emesis mediation, 1042
endogenous, 404, 406
H_1-receptor antagonists, decongestants, 1116
H_2-receptor antagonists, in GI hemorrhage, 565
mechanism of action, 407
putative neurotransmitter, 83
receptors, 388, 403–4, 407–8, 409
and vomition reflex, 1042
release of, 404–5
shock, 404
tubocurarine release of, 146, 405
Histostat-50, 995
Homatropine Hydrobromide, USP, 132, 133
Homocysteine, 712–13
Hormones
as antineoplastic drugs, 1079–80
implants, 20
Horses
aminoglycosides in, 850
anhidrosis, 729
anticestodal drugs in, 985
colic. *See* Colic, equine
digestive physiology and drug absorption, 23
estrous cycle control, 614–15, 617
exercise-induced pulmonary hemorrhage, 545–46
fluid therapy in, 530
fluoroquinolones in, 910
hypothyroidism, 600
parturition induction, 618
protozoal myeloencephalitis, 1011
steroid-induced laminitis, 660
succinylcholine in, 146
5-HT. *See* Serotonin
Human chorionic gonadotropin

(HCG), 613
for cryptorchidism, 623
Human Fibrinogen, USP, 576
Human-label drugs, 58–59
and adverse drug experiences, 60
Humidity, 179–80
Hyaluronic acid, 447
Hyaluronidase
with local anesthetics, 351
ophthalmic use, 1142
Hydantoins, 368–70
Hydralazine Hydrochloride, USP, 473
anti-vitamin B_6 activity, 707
Hydrazine sulfate, appetite stimulation, 1042
Hydrea, 1080
Hydrochlorothiazide, 547, 608
Hydrocodone, antitussive activity, 1114
Hydrocortisone, 655–58, 662–63
ophthalmic, 1123
Hydrodiuril, 608
Hydrogen, in acid-base metabolism, 514–19
Hydrogen cyanide, for euthanasia, 399
Hydrogen peroxide
as disinfectant, 787
as emetic, 1044
Hydromorphone Hydrochloride, USP, 280
12-Hydroperoxyarachidonic acid, 423–24
6-Hydroxydopamine, 115
Hydroxypropylmethylcellulose, 1141
Hydroxyquinolones, anticoccidial, 999
5-Hydroxytryptamine, 411–12
in CNS, 157
neurotransmitter, 83
Hydroxyurea, USP, 563, 1080
Hydrozide, 547
Hygromycin B, 977
Hyoscine, 130
as antiemetic, 1044
spasmolytic activity, 1053
Hyperadrenocorticism, 666–68
Hyperbaric oxygen, 177
Hypercapnia, 178–79
Hypercatabolism, glutamine and, 769–70
Hyperchloremia, 511
Hypercholesterolemia, 637
Hyperglycemia, phenothiazine-induced, 301
Hyperhomocysteinemia, 712–13, 716
Hyperkalemia, 512–14, 731
from potassium-sparing diuretics, 548
Hypernatremia, 508–9
Hyperoxia, 176–77
Hyperparathyroidism
calcitriol supplementation, 565
nutritional secondary, 723, 725, 726
Hyperpyrexia, 61
Hypersensitivity reactions, histamine and, 405
Hypertension, salt and, 728–29
Hyperthermia, malignant halothane-induced, 196, 198
Hyperthermia, seizure-related, 361
acepromazine for, 308
Hyperthyroidism, 626
Hypertonic solutions, for fluid therapy, 529–30
Hyperventilation, 179
Hypervitaminosis A, 688
Hypervitaminosis D, 692
Hypnodil, 262
Hypnomidate, 239
Hypoadrenocorticism, 649
Hypocalcemia, 723–24, 726
Hypocapnia, 179
Hypochloremia, 511
Hypochlorites, as disinfectants, 786
Hypoglycemia, acute, 677, 678
Hypoglycemic agents, oral, 677–78
Hypokalemia, 512, 514, 731
Hypomagnesemia, 734–35
Hyponatremia, 509–11
Hypotension
acepromazine and, 308
and catecholamines, 101
tubocurarine-induced, 146
xylazine-induced, 315, 317, 318
Hypotensive agents, topical, 1133–39
Hypothalamic-pituitary-adrenal axis, 650
Hypothalamic-pituitary-thyroid-extrathyroid axis, 628
Hypothalamus
autonomic regulation, 75–76
effects of glucocorticoids on, 654
hormones, 593–96. *See also* individual hormones
Hypothermia
during anesthesia, 219
morphine-induced, 275
phenothiazine-induced, 301
and thiopental anesthesia, 223–24
Hypothrombinemia, sulfonamide-induced, 800
Hypothyroidism, 626
cats, 600
congenital, 636
dogs, 599–600
horses, 600
juvenile-onset, 636
sulfonamide-induced, 801
Hypovolemia, 560, 563–64
Hypoxemia, 175
Hypoxia, 175–76
altitude and, 176
chronic, 563
and erythropoiesis, 555

Ibuprofen, 444
Idarubicin, 1076
Idiosyncratic reactions, 61
Idoxuridine, USP, 935
ophthalmic uses, 1133
Ifosfamide, 1071
Imaverol, 927
Imidacloprid, 1029
Imidazolidinones, 786
Imidazolines, 109, 110
Imidazothiazoles, antinematodal drugs, 954–57
Imidocarb, 1013–14
Imipenem, 825
ophthalmic uses, 1132
Imipenem-cilastatin, 825
Imipramine, 81, 115, 390
Imizol, 1013
Immiticide, 976
Immobility, 161
Immobilization, neuromuscular blocking agents for, 147
Immune system
copper deficiency and, 747
glutamine effects on, 771
taurine and, 767
vitamin A and, 686
vitamin E and, 693
zinc deficiency and, 757–58
Immunoglobulins, vitamin E and, 693
Immunomodulation, by NSAIDs, 437
Immunostimulants, ophthalmic uses, 1143
Immunosuppressives
azathioprine, 1073–74, 1126
cyclosporine, 926, 1126, 1139
glucocorticoids, 662
ophthalmic, 1126
Implants
dosage form, 1158
regulation of, 1155–56
Imuran, 1073–74, 1126
Inapsine, 333, 1044
Incompatibilities, drug, 62, 1163–65
Inderal, 492
Indomethacin, 445, 1125
Induction, of anesthesia, 19–20
Infiltration, local, 352
Inflammation
chemical mediators of, 433–31
in degenerative joint disease, 446
leukotrienes in, 427
pathophysiology of, 433
prostaglandins in, 427
Infusion rate, 20
Injections, dosage form, 1158
Injury, histamine response to, 405
INN, 1156
Innovar-Vet, 166, 333
Insecticides
carbamates, 1025
development inhibitors, 1026–29
growth regulators, 1026–29
organochlorine, 1020–21
organophosphates, 1021–24
repellents, 1031–32
Insects, β-glucoside conjugation, 37
Insulin
adverse effects, 677
biosynthesis, 672–73
clinical use, 676–77
mechanism of action, 674
metabolism, 674
preparations, 674–75
resistance, 678
secretion of, 673–74
Insulinase, 674
Interceptor, 971
Interferons, 939
ophthalmic uses, 1133
Interleukin-1, 430–31
Interleukin-2, 690
Interleukin-6, 431

International Nonproprietary Name (INN), 1156
International Union of Pure and Applied Chemistry (IUPAC), 1158
Interspecies scaling, 51–52
Intra-articular route, local anesthetics, 353
Intracranial pressure, osmotherapy for, 542
Intramammary infusions, and drug absorption, 19
Intramuscular injection, and absorption, 20
Intraocular irrigation, 1123
Intraocular pressure, osmotherapy for, 540, 542
Intrauterine infusions, and drug absorption, 19
Intraval sodium, 229
Intravenous (IV)
block, 353
infusion, continuous, 20, 47, 49, 50–51
injection, 19–20
Intrinsic sympathomimetic activity (ISA), 113–14
Intubation, neuromuscular blocking agents for, 148
Iodine
as antiseptic, 785–86
deficiency, 627
dietary, 750
metabolism, 626–27
radioactive, 645–46
topical solutions, 1099–1100
Iodine solutions, ophthalmic uses, 1133
Iodophors, 790, 792–93
Ion channels, 154–56
calcium, 475, 484–85, 487–88
as receptors, 9
sodium, 475, 723
Ionophores, polyether, as anticoccidials, 1002–4
Iontophoresis, 1094
Ipecac syrup, 1044
Ipodate, 645
Ipratropium bromide, 1112
Ipronidazole, 993
Irgasan DP300, 791
Iron, 750–51
cycle, 557–58
deficiency, 558, 562–63, 751–52
supplementation, 566–68
toxicity, 567, 752
Iron dextran, 752
Iron oxide, 751
Irrigants, ocular, 1122–23
Irritants, skin, 1095–96
Ischemia-reperfusion injury, 176
Isoetharine, 106, 1109
Isoflurane, USP, 198–200
Isoflurophate, 1134
Isoniazid, 707
Isonicotinic acid hydrazide, 707
Isopropamide, 1044
antiemetic activity, 1045
Isopropyl alcohol, 785
Isoproterenol
for allergy reactions, 410
in AV block, 490
bronchodilation by, 102, 1108
cardiovascular effects, 95–98, 101
gastrointestinal effects, 99
preparations, 100
structure of, 92
and thiopental, 223
Isoptin, 493
Isosorbide, 478, 1138
Itraconazole, 927–30
ophthalmic uses, 1132
Ivermectin, 964–67, 1029
Ivomec, 965
Ivomec Eprinex, 969–70
Ivomec Plus, 987

Juvenile hormone analogs, 1026

Kallidin, 417
Kallikrein inhibitors, 417, 418
Kallikrein-kinin system, and blood coagulation, 574
Kallikreins, 416–17
Kamala, 980
Kanamycin, 857–58
ophthalmic uses, 1128
Kaolin, 1094
Kaolin-pectin, 1055
Keratoconjunctivitis sicca, sulfonamide-induced, 800
Keratolytics, 1096
Keratoplastics, 1096
Ketaject, 247
Ketalar, 247
Ketamine Hydrochloride, USP, 247–50
acepromazine and, 249, 253–55
antagonism of, 250, 258, 377
barbiturates incompatibility, 62
cataleptoid anesthesia, 250
clinical uses, 251–58
contraindications, 250–51
detomidine and, 322
diazepam and, 253, 255, 328
guaifenesin and, 243
pentobarbital and, 227
xylazine and, 249, 251–56, 319–21
Ketanserin, 412
Ketaset, 247
Ketoacidosis, 521–22
Ketoconazole, 924–27
for hyperadrenocorticism, 667–68
ophthalmic uses, 1132
Ketoprofen, 444–45, 1126
Ketorolac, 1125
Kidneys
aminoglycoside-induced nephrotoxicity, 846–51
amphotericin B-associated nephrotoxicity, 923
α-receptors in, 96
cytotoxic chemotherapy and, 1067
digitalization and, 464
drug excretion and, 39–40, 43
drug therapy and, 65
failure, mannitol for, 542
fatty acids and, 763–64
glutamine and, 770–71
inhalant anesthetics and, 196
magnesium regulation, 734
Na/Cl effects on, 727
neuromuscular blocking agents and, 148
parathyroid hormone effects, 690
physiology of, 534–37
potassium balance, 511–12, 731
prostaglandins and, 426–27
regulation of fluid balance, 506–7
renal disease
anemias associated with, 565–66
vitamin D and, 691
Kininases, 417
inhibitors, 417–18
Kininogenase, 417
Kininogens, 417
Kinins, 416–18
Kino, 1095
Krameria, 1095

Labor. *See* Parturition, induced
Lacrimomimetics, 1139–40
Lacrimostimulants, 1139
Lactation, inducing, 620
Lactulose, as cathartic, 1057
Laminitis, steroid-induced, 660
Lamisil, 931
Lampit, 997
Lanolin, 1094
Largactil, 302
Lasalocid, 1004, 1008–10
Lasix, 543–47
Latanoprost, 1138
Lavage systems, ocular, 1121
Laxatives
bulk, 1056
emollient, 1056
LD_{50}, 12–13
Lecithin, 716, 1059
Leishmaniasis, 995
Lentin, 122
Lethal dose, median, 12–13
Lethal synthesis, 32
Lethidrone, 294
Leucovorin Calcium, USP, 1072
Leukeran, 1071
Leukotrienes, 423–24, 426
inflammation and, 427, 1088
NSAIDs effects on, 436–37
Levallorphan Tartrate, USP, 291
Levamisole, INN, 955–56
ophthalmic uses, 1133
Levasole, 956
Levodopa, anti-vitamin B_6 activity, 707
Levofloxacin, 898
Levothyroxine sodium, 638–41
LH, 612–13, 615, 619, 620
Librium, 331
Lice, control of, 1033–35
Lidocaine Hydrochloride, USP, 355–56, 488–89, 492
biotransformation of, 36
ophthalmic, 1122
pentobarbital and, 226
thiopental and, 230
Lime sulfur, 1026
Limonene, 1020
Linalool, 1020
Lincocin, 882

Lincomix, 882
Lincomycin, 882–84
  ophthalmic uses, 1131
Lincosamides
  clindamycin, 884–86
  lincomycin, 882–84
  ophthalmic uses, 1131
  for toxoplasmosis, 1010
Lindane, 1021, 1166–67
Liniments, 1158
Linseed oil, 1057
Lipid metabolism, 762–63
Lipoproteins, 762–63
Liposomes, 1121
Lipotropic agents, 1058–59
Lipoxygenase, 423
Liquid preparations, 1157
Live-and-let-live response, 74, 75
Liver
  biliary excretion, 40–41
  cytotoxic chemotherapy and, 1067
  drug clearance by, 25
  drugs affecting, 1058–60
  flukes. *See* Antitrematodal drugs
  glutamine and, 769
  hepatic insufficiency and drug therapy, 64–65
  inhalant anesthetics and, 196
  pseudocholinesterase synthesis, 148
  sulfonamide-induced necrosis, 800
Loading dose, 20, 49–50
Lomefloxacin, 898
Lomidine, 1013
Lomotil, 283
Lomustine, 1071–72
Loperamide, 22, 1054
Lopressor, 493
Lorcainide, 488, 496
Lorfan, 291
Lorothidol, 981
Lotions, 1098, 1158
Lufenuron, 1026, 1029
Luminal, 363
Lutalyse, 616, 617
Luteinizing hormone, 612–13, 615, 619, 620
Lysine-8-vasopressin, 607
L-Lysine, ophthalmic uses, 1133
Lysodren, 667

M-99, 286
Macrocyclic lactones, 963–64
  abamectin, 967–68
  doramectin, 968–69, 1030, 1133
  eprinomectin, 969–70, 1030
  ivermectin, 964–67, 1029
  milbemycins, 971–73, 1030
  moxidectin, 972–73, 1030
  selamectin, 970–71, 1030
Macrolide antibiotics
  azithromycin, 881–82
  chemistry, 876
  clarithromycin, 881
  drug interactions, 879
  erythromycin, 21, 876–80, 1131
  formulations, 876
  mechanism of action, 877–78
  microbial susceptibility/resistance, 876–78
  ophthalmic uses, 1131
  pharmacokinetics, 878–79
  side effects, 879
  tilmicosin, 880–81
  tylosin, 880
Macrolide endectocides. *See* Macrocyclic lactones
Maduramicin, 1004
Mafenide, 799
Magnesium, 733–36
  ACh and, 141
  assessment of, 735
  and cardiac glycosides, 467
  deficiency, 734–35
  dietary requirements, 735
  preparations, 735–36
Magnesium salts
  as antacids, 1049
  as cathartics, 1056
Magnesium sulfate, chloral hydrate and, 240–41
Magnesium trisilicate, 1055
Malachite green, 1014
Malaria, 1012
Malathion, 30, 1024
Male fern extract, 980
Manganese, 752–53
Mannitol, 540–43
  as cathartic, 1057
  ophthalmic uses, 1138
MAO. *See* Monoamine oxidase (MAO)
MAO inhibitors. *See* Monoamine oxidase inhibitors
Marbofloxacin, 898–913
Marcaine, 357
Marezine, 408
Margin of safety, 60
Mast cells
  degranulation, 404–5
  stabilizers, 1112–13
Mastitis, 791
Materia medica, 6
Mebendazole, 950–53
  as cestocidal, 984–85, 990
Mecamylamine, 134
Mechlorethamine Hydrochloride, USP, 1070
Meclizine hydrochloride, 1044
Meclofenamic acid, 444
Medetomidine hydrochloride, 323
MEDIC, 7
Medroxyprogesterone acetate, 622
Medrysone, 1124
Megestrol acetate
  appetite stimulation, 1042
  ophthalmic uses, 1127
  for prostate hypertrophy, 623
Meglumine antimonate, 995
Melarsomine, 976–77
Melatonin, 614
Melengestrol acetate, 615–16
Melphalan, USP, 563, 1071
Membranes, cell
  calcium channels, 154, 475, 484–85, 487–88
  cardiac action potentials, 482–88
  drug passage across, 15–19
  electrical potential, 728
  fatty acids and, 763
  Na^+, K^+-ATPase pump, 456, 503, 511, 512, 513
Menadione, 696–98
Menthol, 1096
Mepazine, as antiemetic, 1044
Mepenzolate, 1053
Meperidine Hydrochloride, USP
  acepromazine and, 311
  biotransformation, 281–82
  clinical use, 283–84
  effects, 282–83
  toxicity, 283
Mephenesin, secobarbital and, 237
Mepivacaine Hydrochloride, USP, 356–57
  ophthalmic, 1122
Mepron suspension, 999
Mercaptopurine, USP, 1073–74
Messengers, first/second, 299
Mestinon, 126
Metabolism, drug. *See* Biotransformation
Metabolites, activity of, 32
Metalloenzymes
  copper-containing, 753
  molybdenum-containing, 753
  zinc as cofactor, 757
Metamide, 404, 408
Metaproterenol, 106, 1109
Metaraminol Bitartrate, USP, 106
Metformin, 582, 678
Methacholine, 119, 122–23
Methadone Hydrochloride, USP, 284–85
Methampyrone, 1053
Methanechol, 1051
Methantheline Bromide, USP, 133
Methazolamide, 539, 1138
Methemoglobinemia, local anesthetic-induced, 350–51, 356
Methenamine, 890
Methenolone, 582
Methicillin, 822
  ophthalmic uses, 1129, 1130
Methimazole, 643–45
Methionine, 1059
Methiothepin maleate, 250
Methohexital Sodium, USP, 235–36
Methoprene, 1026
Methotrexate, USP, 1072
Methoxamine Hydrochloride, USP, 106
Methoxychlor, 1021
Methoxyflurane, USP, 30, 196, 200
Methscopolamine
  absorption of, 22
  antiemetic activity, 1045
Methylatropine Nitrate, USP, 133
Methyl bromide, 787
Methylcellulose, 1056
  ophthalmic uses, 1139–41, 1144
α-Methyldopa, 115
Methylene blue, 1014
Methylmorphine, 280
α-Methyl-para-tyrosin, 115
Methylprednisolone, 655–58, 662–63

Methylprednisolone sodium succinate, and calcium gluconate incompatibility, 62
Methylxanthines
  bronchodilation by, 1109–12
  cardiovascular effects, 88
  use with β_2 agonists, 106
Metoclopramide
  antiemetic effects, 1045
  appetite stimulation, 1042
  cholinergic effects, 1051–52
  prolactin secretion increase, 605
Metocurine Iodide, USP, 141, 143, 147
Metofane, 200
Metomidate, INN, 262
  azaperone and, 335
Metoprolol Tartrate, USP, 113, 489, 493
Metric system, 1165
Metrology, 6, 1159–62
Metronidazole, 993–94
  ophthalmic uses, 1131
Metubine, 141
Mexiletine, 488, 495
Meyer-Overton rule, 163
Mezlocillin, 822
MGA, 615–16
MGK, 264, 326, 1031–32
Mibolerone, 622
Miconazole, 1100
  ophthalmic uses, 1132
Micotil, 60, 880–81
Micronization, 21
Microsomal enzyme system, 32–36
  inducers, 39, 62, 230
    griseofulvin, 920
    phenytoin, 369
  inhibitors, 39, 62
    chloramphenicol, 367
    erythromycin, 879
  phenobarbital acceleration of, 230, 364–65
Microsomes, 33
Midamor, 548
Midazolam Maleate, INN, 331
Mifepristone, 621–22
Milbemycins
  antinematodal, 971–73
  ectoparasiticide, 1030
Milk
  antibiotics in, 18, 19, 1166
  benzimidazoles residues, 953
  cephalosporins residues, 824–25
  chloramphenicol residues, 872
  drug diffusion into, 18, 19
  erythromycin residues, 880
  fluoroquinolones residues, 911
  gentamycin residues, 855
  levamisole residues, 957
  organophosphates residues, 962
  penicillin residues, 821–22
Milking equipment, disinfection of, 792
Milrinone, 471–72
Mineralocorticoids, 665–66
Mineral oil, 1056
  in topical preparations, 1094
Minerals, supplements, 567–68, 684
Minimal Essential Drug Information Checklist (MEDIC), 7
Minimum alveolar concentration (MAC), 193–94
Minocycline, 835–36
  ophthalmic uses, 1131
Misoprostol, 427, 1049, 1050
Mites, control of, 1033–35
Mithracin, 1078
Mithramycin, 1078
Mitomycin, 1078
Mitotane, USP, 667, 1079
Mitoxantrone hydrochloride, 1077
Mixed-function oxidase reaction, 33
Mixtures, 1157
MMI, 643–45
Molybdenum, 753–54
Monensin, 1004, 1008–10
Monoamine oxidase (MAO), 36
Monoamine oxidase inhibitors, 36, 39, 115
  for behavior modification, 393
Monobactams, 825
Monteban, 1004
Morantel, INN, 960–61
Morphine Sulfate, USP
  antidiuretic effects, 276–77
  antitussive effects, 275
  biotransformation of, 277–78
  cardiovascular effects, 276
  chemistry, 272–73
  clinical uses, 278–80
  CNS effects, 273–75
  contraindications, 278
  emetic effects, 275
  endocrine organ modulation, 277
  GI effects, 277
  immunomodulation, 277
  methylxanthine and, 376
  mydriasis, 276
  phenothiazine and, 301
  for pulmonary edema, 479
  respiratory effects, 276
  semisynthetic derivatives, 273
  thermoregulation, 275–76
  thiopental and, 232
  toxicity, 278
Motion sickness, 1044
Moxidec, 972
Moxidectin, 972–73, 1030
Moxifloxacin, 898
6-MP, 1073
Mucinomimetics, 1141
Mucolytic drugs, 1115
Multidrug resistance, 1068–69
Multiple drug resistance protein, 22–23
Muscarine, 82, 123–24
Muscarinic blocking agents, synthetic, 132–33
Muscarinic receptors, 82–83, 118–19, 120
  gastrointestinal tract, 1052–53
Muscle relaxants, clinical uses, 148. *See also* Neuromuscular blocking agents
Muscle, skeletal
  ACh-induced fasciculations, 122
  barbiturates and, 219–20
Muscular dystrophy, nutritional
  selenium-induced, 754
  vitamin E-induced, 694–95
Mustargen, 1070
Mutamycin, 1078
Mycoses, 919, 933. *See also* Antifungal drugs
Mydriasis, 99, 167
  reversal, 1137
Mydriatic agents, 1136–37
Myelosuppressive drugs, for idiopathic polycythemia, 563
Mylepsin, 366
Myleran, 1071
Myocardial depressant factor (MDF), 289
Myocardium
  contractility, 458
  electrophysiology of, 482–88
  oxygen demand, 454, 460–61
  taurine content, 767
Myopathies, hypothyroidism-associated, 637
Mysoline, 366
Mysuran, 126
Mytelase, 126
Myxedema, 637
Myxedema coma, 643

Na^+, K^+-ATPase pump, 456, 503, 511, 512, 513
Nafcillin, 822
Naftifine, 931
Naftin, 931
Nalbuphine Hydrochloride, USP, 291–92
Nalline, 294
Nalmefene, INN, 291
Nalorphine Hydrochloride, USP, 294–95
Naloxone Hydrochloride, USP
  clinical uses, 290
  effects of, 288–90
  etorphine antagonist, 287
  opioid receptors and, 270
  oxymorphone antagonist, 280
Naltrexone, INN, 291
NANC neurons, 75, 77
Napental, 224, 373
Naphazoline, 1126
Naphthalophos, 961
Naphthoquinones, 696
  anticoccidial, 999
Naproxen, 443–44
Narasin, 1004
Narcotics
  opioid receptors and, 278
  regulation of, 1155
Naropin, 357
Nasal sprays, 1116
Natamycin, ophthalmic uses, 1132
National Formulary (NF), 1150
National Residue Program, 1168
Navantrone, 1077
Nemadectins, 963
Nematodes. *See* Antinematodal drugs
Nembutal, 224, 373
Nemex-2, 958, 959
Neoantergan, 408
Neo-Darbazine, 312
Neomycin, 859
  ophthalmic uses, 1128

Neonates, drug biotransformation in, 42, 63–64
Neosporosis, 1010–11
Neostigmine Bromide, USP
  antagonism of neuromuscular blocking agents, 143, 144, 150
  cholinesterase inhibition, 124, 125, 126–27
  as purgative, 1057
Neo-Synephrine, 106
Nephrotoxicity
  aminoglycoside-induced, 846–51
  amphotericin B-associated, 923
Neptazane, 539
Nequinate, 999
Nerve blocks
  differential, 349
  epidural. *See* Epidural nerve blocks
  peripheral, 352–53
Nerve impulses
  blocking, 348–49
  transmission of, 153–55
Nerves
  adrenergic, 75
  afferent, 75–76
  efferent, 70–75
  nonadrenergic-noncholinergic (NANC), 75, 86
Nesacaine, 355
Netobimin, 953–54, 989
Neurohumoral transmission, 75, 76–89
  adrenergic, 78–82
  axonal conduction, 76–77
  cholinergic, 82, 139–41
  neurotransmitter release, 77–78
  receptors, 78
Neuroleptics. *See* Antipsychotics; Tranquilizers
Neuromuscular blocking agents
  antagonism of, 150
  antibiotic-induced paralysis, 150
  autonomic effects, 145–46
  cardiovascular effects, 146–47
  clinical uses, 137, 148–50
  CNS effects, 146
  competitive, 137–38, 141
  contraindicated for euthanasia, 400
  depolarizing, 137–38, 141–43
  drug interactions, 147–48
  excretion of, 40
  histamine release and, 146
  nicotinic receptors and, 137–41
  ocular effects, 147
  pharmacokinetics, 147
  potassium and, 147
  safety, 149–50
  skeletal muscle effects, 143–44
Neuromuscular disorders, magnesium and, 734–35
Neuromuscular junction, impulse transmission, 139–41
Neurons
  histamine effects on, 406
  NANC, 75, 77
Neuropeptides, 158–59
  appetite control, 1042
Neurotoxins, 138, 141
Neurotransmitter antagonists, as antiviral agents, 940
Neurotransmitters. *See also* specific neurotransmitters
  acetylcholine, 75
  behavior-associated, 373–74
  benzodiazepines and, 327
  catabolism of, 78
  CNS, 155–59
  criteria for, 77
  excitatory, 384
  norepinephrine, 75, 77
  putative, 75, 83–88
  receptors, 78
  release of, 77–78
NF, 1150
Niacin, 705–7
Niacinamide, ophthalmic uses, 1127
Nicarb, 1001
Nicarbazin, 1001
Niclofolan, INN, 985, 986, 990
Niclosamide, 981–90, 985
Nicotinamide, 705, 706
Nicotine, 82, 118
  effects of, 133–34
Nicotine sulfate, 980
Nicotinic acid, 705, 706
Nicotinic receptors, 82, 118, 182
  and neuromuscular blocking agents, 137–41
Nifedipine, 477
  xylazine blocking by, 315
Nifurtimox, 997
Nitarsone, 995
*Nitrendipine,*INN, 354
Nitric oxide, 83–84, 180–81
  administration of, 181
  biosynthesis of, 84–85
  in CNS, 158
  as NANC neurotransmitter, 75, 77
  oxidation of, 78
  proposed roles of, 85–86
  sources of, 85
  therapeutic uses, 181
Nitric oxide synthase (NOS), 84–86
  inhibitors, 85
Nitrobenzamides, anticoccidials, 1001
Nitro compounds, biotransformation of, 35
Nitrofurans, 888–89
  antiprotozoal activity, 997
  topical, 1099
Nitrofurazone, topical, 1099
Nitrogen, for euthanasia, 400
Nitrogen mustards, 1070–71
Nitroglycerin, 478
Nitroimidazoles, 993–95
Nitroprusside, 478
Nitroreductase, 35
Nitrosureas, 1071–72
Nitrous oxide, USP, 203–4
Nitroxynil, INN, 985, 986
Nizatidine, 408, 1046–48
Nizoral, 667, 924
Nociception, 160–61, 270
Noncatecholamines, 104–6
Noncompartmental analysis, 46–47
Noncompetitive antagonism, 10
Nonsteroidal anti-inflammatory drugs
  accidental poisoning, 438
  agents, 439–46
  for diarrhea, 1055
  drug interactions, 438
  effects of, 438
  lasix inhibition by, 543
  mechanism of action, 434–37
  nonspecific COX-inhibition, 424–25
  ophthalmic, 1124–26
  pharmacokinetics, 437–38
  for respiratory disease, 1113–14
  side effects, 61, 434
Norepinephrine, 75, 77
  appetite stimulation, 1042
  biotransformation of, 100
  cardiovascular effects, 95–98, 101
  catabolism of, 78
  in CNS, 157, 383
  ocular effects, 99
  preparations, 100
  smooth muscle effects, 99
  structure of, 92
  synthesis and function of, 79–82
  topical vasoconstriction, 577
Norfloxacin, ophthalmic uses, 1129
Norgestomet, 613
Nororipavine, 290
Noscapine, 1115
Notensil, 307
Novobiocin, 886
Novocaine, 354
Noxious stimuli, perception of, 160–61
NSAIDs. *See* Nonsteroidal anti-inflammatory drugs
Nubain, 291
Nucleoside analogs, 935–37, 939
Nuflor, 875
Numorphan, 280
Nutraceuticals, definition of, 6
Nystatin, 1100
  ophthalmic uses, 1132

Occupational exposure, to inhalation anesthetics, 204–5, 399, 401
Octreotide, 604, 680
Ocular inserts, 1121
Off-patent drugs, 58
Ofloxacin, 898
  ophthalmic uses, 1129
Ointments, 1158, 2098
Olive oil, 1057
  in topical preparations, 1094
Omeprazole, 1048–49
Oncovin, 1074
Ophthalmic drugs
  adhesives, 1141
  aldose reductase inhibitors, 1141
  antibiotics, 1127–32
  anticoagulants, 1141
  anticollagenases, 1141–42
  antifibrinolytics, 1142
  antifungal, 1132–33
  anti-inflammatory agents, 1126–27
  antiparasiticides, 1133
  antiproliferative agents, 1142
  antiproteases, 1141–42

Ophthalmic drugs (*continued*)
antiviral agents, 1133
corticosteroids, 1123–24
delivery of, 1120–21
dyes, 1122
epidermal growth factor, 1143
fibrinolytics, 1142
fibronectin, 1143
fluorocarbon gases, 1143
hyaluronidase, 1142
hypotensive agents, 1133–39
immunostimulants, 1143
immunosuppressants, 1126
local anesthetics, 1121–22
NSAIDs as, 1124–26
ocular irrigants, 1122–23
photosensitizing agents, 1143
silicone oil, 1143
tear stimulants, 1139
tear substitutes, 1139–41
viscoelastics, 1143–44
Ophthetic, 355
Opioids
α_2-adrenergic agonists and, 323
agonist-antagonists, 271–72
butorphanol, 293–94
nalbuphine, 291–92
nalorphine, 294–95
pentazocine, 292–93
agonists
alfentanil, 286
as behavior modifying drugs, 395
carfentanil, 286
codeine, 280
definition, 271
etorphine, 286–87
fentanyl, 285
hydromorphone, 280
meperidine, 281–84
methadone, 284–85
morphine, 272–80
oxymorphone, 280–81
partial, 271, 291
propoxyphene, 287–88
remifentanil, 286
sufentanil, 285
antagonists
as behavior modifying drugs, 395
definition, 271
diprenorphine, 286, 290–91
levallorphan, 291
nalmefene, 291
naloxone, 288–90
naltrexone, 291
efficacy of, 271
endogenous, 270–71
GI tract and, 1053–54
peptides, 159
peripheral analgesia, 295
as preanesthetics, 166
receptors, 159, 269–70, 288
antagonists, 291
GI tract, 1053–54
naloxone binding and, 288
narcotic addiction and, 278
spinal analgesia, 295
Opium, USP, 269
Optimum dose, 47
Oral administration, of drugs, 21–23
Oramec, 965
Orbifloxacin, 898–913
ophthalmic uses, 1129
Organochlorine insecticides, 1020–21
Organon, 664
Organophosphates, 127–28
AChE interaction, 126
agents, 1024
antagonists, 129
antidotes, 129
antinematodal, 961–63
chemistry, 1021–23
clinical uses, 129–30
mechanism of action, 1021–23
neuromuscular blocking agents and, 148
pharmacokinetics, 1023
skin metabolism of, 1087
toxicity, 39, 962, 1023–24
Orgotein, 176, 446
Oripavine, 286
Ormetoprim, 810–11, 1005–7
Osmotic agents, for intraocular pressure reduction, 1138
Osteoarthritis, drugs for, 446–48
Osteocalcin, 697
Osteofluorosis, 750
Osteoporosis
due to excess calcium, 723
steroid-induced, 653
Ototoxicity
aminoglycoside-induced, 846–47, 849–51
drug-induced, 849
loop diuretics and, 544–45
Ouabain, 465, 468
Over-the-counter drugs, 1153, 1154–55
Ovulation, inducing, 619–20
Oxacillin, 822
Oxalic acid, calcium chelation by, 725
Oxazepam, appetite stimulation, 1042
Oxazolidinones, 786
Oxfendazole, 950–52
as cestocidal, 984
in paramphistomosis, 990
Oxibendazole, 950–53
Oxidative reactions, in biotransformation, 32–36
Oxidized Cellulose, USP, 576–77
Oxime reactivators, 129
Oxprenolol, 489
Oxybuprocaine, 1121
Oxycel, 576
Oxyclozanide, INN, 985, 986, 990
Oxygen, 173–75
administration of, 177
hyperbaric, 177
hypoxia, 175–76
therapeutic uses, 177
toxicity, 176–77
Oxymorphone Hydrochloride, USP, 280–81
naloxone antagonism, 290
Oxyphenonium, 1053
Oxypolygelatin, 527
Oxytetracycline, 832–34
ophthalmic uses, 1131
Oxytocin, 608, 613–14
parturition induction by, 618
postpartum, 618–19, 621, 623
purgative effect, 1057

PABA, allergies to, 57, 351
Paclitaxel, 1074
Pain, mechanisms of, 160–61
2-PAM, 129
Panacur, 984, 996
Pancreatin, 1058
Pancuronium, 138, 141
autonomic effects, 146
cardiovascular effects, 146
skeletal muscle effects, 143
Panteric, 1058
Pantothenic acid, 708–10
Para-aminobenzoic acid, 57, 351
Paracide-F, 1014
Paragonimosis, 990
Paralysis, 137, 141–44
antibiotic-induced, 148, 150
Paramphistomosis, 990
Paraoxon, 38
Paraplatin, 1079
Parasites. *See* Anticestodal drugs; Antinematodal drugs; Antitrematodal drugs; Ectoparasiticides; Insecticides; Pesticides
Parasites, blood, anemia-causing, 561–62
Parasympathetic nervous system, 71–73
Parasympatholytic drugs, 130–33, 166–67. *See also* Anticholinergics
Parasympathomimetic agents
direct-acting, 117–24
ophthalmic uses, 1134
as purgatives, 1057–58
Paratect Flex Diffuser, 960
Parathion
biotransformation of, 38
lethal synthesis, 32
Parathyroid hormone
Ca/P metabolism, 722–23
vitamin D and, 689
Paregoric, 282
Parenogen, 576
Parlodel, 623
Paromomycin, 859–60
antiprotozoan activity, 996–97
for cryptosporidiosis, 1009
Partition coefficients, 188–90
blood/gas, 189
oil/gas, 189
topical vehicles, 1091–92
Parturient paresis, 725–26
Parturition, induced
cattle, 617–18
horses, 614, 617
oxytocin for, 614, 617
Parvaquone, 1014
Passive transfer, of drugs, 16–17
Pastes, 1098
Pavulon, 141

Peanut oil, in topical
preparations, 1094
Pectin, 1055
Pediatric patients, drug therapy in,
63–64
Pemoline, 395
Pempidine, 134
Penicillinase, 819, 822
Penicillin G, 819–22
ophthalmic uses, 1129–30
sulfathiazole and, 806
Penicillin G procaine, 58, 355, 820–21
label dose, 58
Penicillins
allergies to, 61
aminopenicillins, 822
chemistry, 819
extended-spectrum, 822
GABA antagonism, 215
microbial susceptibility, 819–20
ophthalmic uses, 1129–30
penicillinase-resistant, 822
pharmacokinetics, 820–21
toxicity, 822
Penicillin V, 21, 819–22
Penile erection, and nitric oxide, 86
Penile prolapse, phenothiazines
and, 311
Pentam 300, 1013
Pentamethonium, 134
Pentamidine isethionate, 1013
Pentastarch, 527
Pentazocine lactate, 292–93
Penthrane, 200
Pentobarbital Sodium, USP, 373
administration of, 224–25
aminoglycosides interaction, 218
blockade, 219
chloramphenicol potentiation
of, 872
clinical uses, 225–29
diazepam and, 227
for euthanasia, 226, 401
in exotics, 229
inducing with, 20
ketamine and, 227
lidocaine and, 226
in nonhuman primates, 228
streptomycin interaction, 218
toxicity, 226
xylazine and, 226
yohimbine antagonism of, 378
Pentobarbitone sodium, 224, 373
Pentolinium, 134
Pentostam, 995
Pentothal sodium, 229
Pepsin, 1058
Percorten-V, 666
Percutaneous absorption, 20–21
Permethrin, 1020
Perphenazine, as antiemetic, 1044
Pesticides. *See also* Ectoparasiticides
carbamates, 1025
organophosphates, 127–30
residues, 1166–67
transdermal delivery, 1101–2
Petrolatum, 1094
PFA, 938
PG-600, 614
PGA-H, 422–27
PGEs, 427, 1049, 1050, 1088
$PGF_{2\alpha}$, 613, 616–17
as abortifacient, 620–21
chemistry, 420
functions, 422–27
parturition induction by, 617
postpartum, 618–19
purgative effects, 1057
in skin, 1088
superovulation induction, 619–20
PGI_2, 422–27, 1088
pH
body, regulation of, 514–19
partition hypothesis, 17–18
Pharmaceutical equivalent, 58
Pharmacodynamics, definition of,
5, 9
Pharmacokinetics
analysis of, 45–47
definition of, 5–6, 15
drug clearance, 41–42, 44–45
drug distribution, 29–30
drug induced changes in, 62–63
terms, 52–54
transmembrane diffusion, 17–18
Pharmacology
clinical. *See* Clinical pharmacology
history of, 3–5
role in veterinary medicine, 6–7
scope of, 5–6
Pharmacotherapy, definition of, 5
Pharmacy, definition of, 6
Phencyclidine hydrochloride, 247
Phenergan, 408
Phenformin, 582
Pheniramine, 1126
Phenobarbital Sodium, USP
as anticonvulsant, 363–66
for behavior modification, 395
effect on thyroid function tests, 603
effects on T_4, 634
Phenobarbitone, 363
Phenolphthalein, 1057
Phenol red, 1122
Phenothiazine, INN, antinematodal,
973–74
Phenothiazines
acepromazine, 307–12
actions of, 300–302
anticholinesterase activity, 148
antiemetic activity, 301, 1044
as antipsychotics, 387–89
chlorpromazine, 302–3
diazepam and, 328
prochlorperazine, 312–13
prolactin secretion increase by, 605
promazine, 305–7
teratogenic effects, 304
as tranquilizers, 299–313
trimeprazine, 313
Phenoxybenzamine Hydrochloride,
USP, 110
Phentolamine Hydrochloride, USP,
107, 110, 111
Phenylbutazone, 440–42
antithyroid effect, 633–34
biotransformation of, 33–35
coumarin potentiation, 581
for ophthalmic conditions,
1125–26
potentiating effects, 39
and thiopental, 223
Phenylephrine, 106
ophthalmic, 1136–37
Phenytoin Sodium, USP, 368–70,
488–89, 491–92
for behavior modification, 395
coumarin inhibition, 582
Phoenectin, 965
Phonophoresis, 1094
Phosmet, 1024
Phosphodiesterase inhibitors, 88
Phospholipase
corticosteroid inhibition of, 425
prostaglandin synthesis and, 422
Phosphorus
assessment of, 724–25
deficiency, 724
dietary, 691, 724, 725
excess, 726
metabolism of, 689, 722–23, 725
neuromuscular function and,
723–24
preparations, 726
radiophosphorus, 563
sources, 722
uptake of, 725
Photosensitizing agents,
ophthalmic, 1143
Phthalylsulfathiazole, 798, 807
Phylloquinone, 696
Physalamin, 418
Physostigmine, USP, 124, 125,
126–27
ophthalmic preparations, 127
as purgative, 1057
Picrotoxin, 215
Pigs. *See* Swine
Pilocarpine, 123–24
ophthalmic uses, 1139
Pimozide, 250
Pindolol, 489
Pink tooth, 218
Pioneer drugs, 58
Pipenzolate, 1053
Piperazine, USP, 974–75
Piperonyl butoxide, 1031
Pirbuterol, 106
Pirenzepine, 1046
Pirimiphos, 1024
Piroplasms, 1012–14
Piroxicam, 445, 1080
Pitressin Synthetic, 607
Pituitary gland, effects of
glucocorticoids on, 654
Pituitary hormones, 593–96. *See
also* individual hormones
Placenta, drug diffusion across, 63
Plantago seed, 1056
Plasma, therapeutic drug
concentration ranges, 47–48, 49
Plasma concentration-time curves
analysis of, 45–47
drug
absorption, 23–24, 26–27
distribution, 29–30
elimination, 41–42, 44–45
monitoring, 65–66
Plasma protein binding, 27–29
effect on drug excretion, 40

Plasmin, 574, 582
Plasminogen, 582
  tissue, 574
Plasters, 1098
Platelet-activating factor, 428
  steroid inhibition of, 652
Platelets
  adhesion, 571
  aggregation, 572, 573
    platelet-activating factor, 428
    thromboxane, 426
  effects of NSAIDs on, 438
  taurine content, 766
Platinol, 1078
Platinum coordination complexes, 1078–79
Plicamycin, USP, 1078
PMEA, 939
PMSG, 613
Podophyllotoxin, 1075
Polycythemia, 563
Polyethylene glycol, 1095
  as a vehicle, 61
Polymyxin B, 1099
  ophthalmic uses, 1130
Polymyxin E, 1099
  ophthalmic uses, 1130
Polymyxins, 890–91
Polysulfated glycosaminoglycan (PSGAG), 446–47
Polyvinyl alcohol, in tear substitutes, 1141
Polyvinylpyrrolidone, ophthalmic uses, 1141
Pontocaine, 355
Porphyria, congenital, 562
Posology, definition of, 6
Postantibiotic effect, aminoglycosides, 843–44
Potassium, 511–14, 730–33
  assessment of, 732–33
  deficiency, 732
  depolarizing neuromuscular agents and, 147
  dietary, 511, 732, 733
  preparations, 733
  sources, 730
Potassium chloride, for digitalis-induced arrhythmias, 466
Potassium iodide, expectorant, 1116
Potassium permanganate, 1014, 1095
Potassium-sparing diuretics, 548–49
  and aldosterone antagonists, 549–50
Potency, definition of, 9
Poultices, 1098
Poultry
  coccidiosis in, 999–1008
  fluoroquinolones in, 901–10
  vitamin D deficiency, 691
  vitamin E deficiency, 695
Povidone-iodine, 785, 790–91, 1100
  ophthalmic, 1122–23
Powders, 1094, 1098, 1157, 1158
Poxvirus, 935
Pralidoxime, 129
Praziquantel, INN, 981–83, 985, 990
Prazosin, 111–12, 472–73
Preanesthetics, 165–67
  acepromazine, 309–10
  atropine, 132
  detomidine, 322
  glycopyrrolate, 132–33
Precose, 678
Prednisolone, 655–58, 662–63
  ophthalmic, 1123
  trimeprazine and, 313
Prednisone, USP, 655–58, 662–63
  in cancer therapy, 1079–80
Pregnancy, drug therapy during, 63
Pregnant mare serum gonadotropin (PMSG), 613, 614
Premafloxacin, 898
Prescription writing, 1159–62
Pressor amines, use of in shock, 101
Pressor effects, inhibition of, 110
PRID, 616
Prilocaine Hydrochloride, USP, 356
Primates, nonhuman
  althesin in, 246
  barbiturates in, 228
  ketamine in, 252
  morphine in, 279
  thiopental in, 234
  tiletamine-zolazepam in, 260
Primidone, USP, 366–68
Primor, 1007
Priscoline hydrochloride, 110, 324, 378
Probenzimidazoles, 953–54
Procainamide Hydrochloride, USP, 36, 488, 491
Procaine Hydrochloride, USP, 354–55
Prochlorperazine, 312–13, 1044
Proftril-Captec, 988
Progesterone
  controlled-release, 616
  lactation induction by, 620
  receptor antagonist, 621–22
Progesterone-releasing intravaginal device (PRID), 616
Progestins, 395, 612–13, 615–16
  for estrus prevention, 613, 622
  long-acting, 622
Proglycem, 680
Prolactin, 605, 620, 623
Proligestone, 622
Promace, 307
Promazine Hydrochloride, USP, 305–7
Pronestyl, 491
Pro-opiomelanocortin (POMC), 594, 596
Propanidid, 261
Propantheline Bromide, USP, 22, 133, 1053
  antiemetic activity, 1045
Proparacaine Hydrochloride, USP, 355
  ophthalmic, 1121
Propflo, 237
Propofol, USP, 237–39
Propoxur, 1025
Propoxyphene Hydrochloride, USP, 287–88
Propranolol Hydrochloride, USP
  β-blockade by, 107, 112–13, 489, 492–93
  renin secretion inhibition by, 416
Proprietary drugs, 1158–59
Propriolactone, 787
Propylene glycol, 1095
  cardiovascular effects, 59
Propylene oxide, 787
Propylthiouracil (PTU), 643–45
Proscar, 623
ProSpot, 1102
Prostacyclin, 422, 422–27, 423, 572
Prostacyclin synthase, 424
Prostaglandin inhibitors, hyperkalemia due to, 513
Prostaglandins. *See also* Eicosanoids
  A-H, 420–28
  biosynthesis, 421–25
  chemistry, 420–21
  clinical use, 427–28
  effects of, 425–27
  Es, 420–28, 1049, 1050, 1088
  $F_{2\alpha}$, 420, 422–27, 613, 616–21, 1057, 1088. *See also* $PGF_{2\alpha}$
  I_2, 420–27, 572, 1088
  inflammation and, 427
  inhibitors, 513
  intestinal motility and, 1055
  for intraocular pressure reduction, 1138–39
  NSAIDs inhibition of, 434–37
  and platelet aggregation, 572
  purgative effect, 1057
  receptors, 427
  skin, 1088
Prostate hypertrophy, 623
Prostigmine, 126
Protamine Sulfate, USP, 578
Protease inhibitors
  ophthalmic, 1141–42
  viral, 940
Protectives, topical, 1094
Protein C, 575, 577
Protein S, 575, 577
Proteins, contractile, 459
Prothrombin, 573
Proton pump inhibitors, 1048–49
Protozoa. *See* Antiprotozoan drugs
Pseudocholinesterase, 30, 82
  inhibition of, 39, 141
  species variation, 144
  synthesis of, 148
Pseudopregnancy
  ergoline derivatives for, 622–23
  estradiol-induced, 619
  testosterone for, 623
Psyllium seed, 1056
Pteroylglutamic acid. *See* Folic acid
PTU, 643–45
Pulmonary absorption, 21
Pulmonary intravascular macrophages, 1107
Purgatives. *See* Cathartics
Purina tablets, 959
Purine analogs, 1073–74
Purinethol, 1073
Puritus, 1100
Pyraminth, 958
Pyrantel, INN, 957–60, 985
Pyrethrins, 1018–20
Pyrethroids, 1018–20
Pyridostigmine Bromide, USP, 126, 150
Pyrilamine, 404, 408
Pyrimethamine, 1005–7

for malaria, 1012
Pyrimidine analogs, 1073
ophthalmic uses, 1133
Pyriproxyfen, 1026

Quaternary amines, 133
Quaternary ammonium compounds, 22, 784
Quelcin, 141
Quest, 972
Quinidine, 488, 490–91
effects on thyroid hormones, 633
Quinine, coumarin potentiation, 581

Rabbits, coccidiosis, 1009
Radiomimetic drugs, 1070
Rafoxanide, INN, 986–87
Ranide, 986
Ranitidine, 408, 565, 1046–48
Rapinovet, 237
Rauwolscine, 112
Rebound intracranial hypertension, 541–42
Receptal, 616
Receptor blockade, 107
Receptors
α-adrenergic, 81–82, 87, 91–99, 106, 107
α-adrenergic agonists, 313–14
adenosine, 376
aminoglycoside, 846–47
angiotensin, 415
autonomic nervous system, 82–83
β-adrenergic, 81–82, 87, 91–99, 102, 103, 107
benzodiazepines, 325–26
cholinergic, 82, 388
dopamine, 299–300, 387–88
down-regulation of, 60
GABA. *See* GABA receptors
gastrointestinal tract, 1050–51
glutamate, 158
histamine, 403–4, 407–8, 409
H_1, 388, 1042
muscarinic, 82–83, 118–19, 120, 1052–53
neurotransmitters, 78
nicotinic, 82, 118, 137–41, 182
opioid, 159, 269–70, 288, 291
GI tract, 1053–54
prostaglandins, 427
serotonin, 383, 394, 411–12
specificity of, 10
steroids, 650–52
TSH, 602
types of, 9
Regitine hydrochloride, 110
Regonol, 126
Regulin, 614
Relefact, 600
Remifentanil Citrate, USP, 268, 286
Renin, 413–16
Renin-angiotensin system, 504–5, 727, 730–31
Repellents, 1031–32
Reproductive system
phenothiazines and, 301
prostaglandins and, 425
thyroid hormone effects, 637–38
vitamin A and, 686
vitamin E/selenium effects, 693
Reptiles, fluoroquinolones in, 909–10. *See also* Exotics
Reserpine, 114, 274
diazepam and, 329
lactation induction by, 620
serotonin depletion by, 412
Reserpine-like drugs, 81
Residues, drug. *See also* Milk
acepromazine, 310, 311
aminoglycosides, 846
benzimidazoles, 953
cephalosporins, 824–25
chloramphenicol, 872
chlorpromazine, 305
doxapram, 374
erythromycin, 880
florfenicol, 876
fluoroquinolone prohibition, 904
in food products, 58, 59
gentamycin, 855
glycopeptide prohibition, 890
lincomycin, 883, 884
lindane, 1166–67
nitrofurans, 1166
organophosphates, 962
penicillins, 821
pesticides, 1166–67
prevention, 1173–74
promazine, 305
regulation of, 1151–52, 1168–69
sulfamethazine, 804
sulfonamides, 811–12
xylazine, 317, 319
Resistance, antineoplastic agents, 1069–9
Resistance transfer, fluoroquinolones and, 904
Resmethrin, 1020
Resorantel, INN, 981
Resorcinol, 1096
Respiration
barbiturates and, 216
inhalant anesthetics and, 195
morphine and, 276
nitric oxide and, 86
Respiratory mononuclear phagocyte system, 1106
Respiratory syncytial viruses, 936
Respiratory tract
antitussives, 1114–15
bronchodilators, 1108–14
decongestants, 1115–17
expectorants, 1115–16
inflammatory diseases, 1107–8
mucolytic drugs, 1115
physiology of, 1105–6
Response, to drugs
dose-response relationships, 10–14
interspecies variation, 15
quantifying, 13–14
Retina, taurine content, 767
Retinoids, in topical preparations, 1096–97
Retinol, 684–88
Retinol-A, 1097
Retrovir, 937
Retroviruses, 937–38, 939
Revivon, 290
Revolution, 970
Rezulin, 678
Ribavirin, 935–36
Riboflavin, 704–5
Ribozymes, antiviral activity, 939
Rickets, 690, 723, 724
Rickettsia
chloramphenicol for, 872
fluoroquinolones for, 908
tetracycline for, 831
Rifampin, 886–88
ophthalmic uses, 1131
Rimantadine, 938–39
Rimexolone, 1124
Ringer's solution, 527
Rintal, 953–54
Ritalin (methylphenidate), 395
RNA viruses, antiviral agents for, 937–39
Robenidine, 999–1000
Robenz, 999
Rodenticides
cholecalciferol, vitamin D toxicity and, 691–92
vitamin K antagonists, 577–78
warfarin, 578, 580
Rofenaid, 40, 1006–7
Romifidine, 324
Rompun, 314
as emetic, 1044
Ronidazole, 993
Ropivacaine Hydrochloride, USP, 357
Rose Bengal, 1122
Rotectin 1, 965
Rotenone, 1020
Routes of administration
approved/nonapproved, 59–60
effect on absorption, 19–23
effect on drug half-life, 42
Roxarsone, 995
RU-486, 621
Rubefacients, 1095–96
Rubus, 1095
Rumen
microflora and drug biotransformation, 38
pH of, 23
Rumensin, 1004
Ruminants. *See also* Cattle
aminoglycosides in, 850–51
digestive physiology and drug absorption, 23
estrous synchronization, 613
fluid therapy in, 530

Safeguard, 996
Saffan, 243
Sagatal, 224, 373
Salbutamol, 98, 99, 106
Salicylates
bioavailability, 25
coumarin potentiation, 581
effects on thyroid hormones, 633
elimination, 43
Salicylazosulfapyridine, 806–7
Salicylic acid, 1096
Saline, 730
hypertonic, 529–30
purgatives, 1056–57

Salinomycin, 1004
Salt, 730
  hypertension and, 728–29
SAMe, 1059
Sarafloxacin, 898–913
Saralasin, 415
Saxitoxin, 141
Sciatic nerve-gastrocnemius muscle
    preparation, 143–44
Scopolamine Hydrobromide, USP,
    130–32, 1044
Scurvy, 718
Secobarbital Sodium, USP, 236–37
Seconal sodium, 236
Second messenger, 299
Sedatives. *See also* individual
    agents; Tranquilizers
  as preanesthetics, 165–66
Seizures
  opioid-induced, 274
  pathophysiology of, 360–61
Selamectin, 970–71, 1030
Selective serotonin-reuptake
    inhibitors (SSRIs), 392–93
Selectivity, definition of, 10
Selegiline hydrochloride, 668
Selenium
  deficiency, 754–55
  hepatotropic effects, 1059
  reproductive function and, 693
  toxicity, 755–56
Selenium sulfide, 1097–98
Semduramicin, 1004
Senna, 38
Sensorcaine, 357
Sepsis, glutamine
    supplementation, 771
Septra, 1007
Serotonin, 411–12
  appetite suppression, 1042
  and behavior disorders, 383
  neurotransmitter, 83
  phenothiazines block of, 301
  receptors, 383, 394, 411–12
Serotonin antagonists, 411–12
  as antiemetics, 1045
  appetite stimulation, 1042
Sevoflurane, 202–3
Sheep, coccidiosis in, 1008
Shock
  calcium channel blockers for, 477
  glucocorticoids for, 661
  omega-3 fatty acids for, 764
  use of pressor amines, 101–2
Side effects, 61
Silicone oil, 1143
Silver nitrate, 577, 1095
Silver sulfadiazine, 799
  ophthalmic uses, 1133
Single daily dosing,
    aminoglycosides, 843–44
SIRS, 528–29
Skeletal muscle
  inhalant anesthetics and, 196
  neuromuscular blocking agents
    and, 143–44
  paralysis of, 137, 141–44
Skin
  anatomy, 1084–85
  cleansers, 790
  dermis, 1086
  energy production, 1087
  epidermis, 1085–86
  lipid synthesis, 1087–88
  metabolic capabilities, 1087
  permeability, 1088–94
  protein synthesis, 1088
  species differences, 1086–87
Small intestine, drug absorption
    in, 22
Soaps, 784
Sodium, 726–30. *See also* Fluid
    balance
  assessment of, 729
  deficiency, 729
  dietary, 479, 506, 728, 729–30
  hyponatremia, 509–11
  preparations, 730
  renal regulation of, 506–7
Sodium Bicarbonate, USP
  for acidosis, 521, 730
  as antacid, 1049
  iron toxicosis lavage, 567
  for urinary alkalization, 218–19
Sodium Carbonate, NF, as emetic,
    1044
Sodium channels, calcium blocking
    of, 475, 723
Sodium chloride
  as emetic, 1044
  for fish protozoans, 1014
  hypertension and, 728–29
Sodium Citrate, USP, 579
  for digitalis-induced
    arrhythmias, 466
Sodium hexametaphosphate, 726
Sodium hyaluronate, 1141, 1144
Sodium hypochlorite, 927
Sodium orthovanadate, 756
Sodium oxalate, 579
Sodium pump, 456, 503, 511,
    512, 513
Sodium response, fast, 483–84,
    487–88
Sodium stibogluconate, 995
Sodium Versenate, 579
Solubility
  coefficient, 189
  and drug absorption, 19
Somatostatin, 603, 679–80
Somatotropin, 604–5
Sometribove, 605
Sorbitol, 1055, 1057
Spare receptor, 9
Sparine, 305
Spasmolytics, 132, 1053. *See also*
    Antispasmodics
Specificity, definition of, 10
Sphingomyelin, 716
Spinal analgesia, opioids for, 295
Spironolactone, 549
Sporanax, 927
Spot-On, 1102
SSRIs, 392–93
Stabilene, 1031
Stadol, 293
Stamyl, 1058
Starch, 1094
Starvation, and ketoacidosis, 521–22
Status epilepticus, 360
  benzodiazepines for, 371–72
  drugs contraindicated in, 373
Steady-state concentration, 47,
    49–51
Stereotypy, 274
Steroids. *See also* Glucocorticoids;
    Mineralocorticoids
  angiotensin increase of, 415
  anti-inflammatory effects,
    650–51, 653
  biosynthesis of, 649–50
  implants, 20
  receptors, 650–52
Steroids, anabolic
  coumarin potentiation, 581
  fibrinolytic activity, 582
  regulation of, 1155
  in renal disease associated
    anemias, 565–66
Steroid synthesis inhibitors
  ketoconazole, 667–68
  L-deprenyl, 668
Stimulants
  as behavior modifying drugs, 395
  CNS, 324–25, 373–74
    doxapram, 374–75
    methylxanthines, 375–77
Stoxil, 935
Streptokinase, 582
Streptomycin, pentobarbital
    interaction, 218
Stresnil, 333
Stress, glucocorticoids
    supplementation for, 664
Strongid, 958
Strychnine poisoning, 216
Styptics, 577, 1095
Styquin, 954
Subcutaneous injection, and
    absorption, 20
Sublimaze, 285
Substance P, 159, 418
Succinylcholine Chloride, USP, 138,
    141–43, 149
  autonomic effects, 145–46
  cardiovascular effects, 146–47
  drug interactions, 147–48
  pharmacokinetics, 147
  skeletal muscle effects, 144
Sucostrin, 141
Sucralfate, 565, 1050
Sufentanil Citrate, USP, 268, 285
Suicalm, 333
Sulbactam, 825
Sulfabromomethazine, 809
Sulfacetamide, 1130
Sulfachloropyridazine, 810
Sulfadiazine, 807–9
  as anticoccidial, 1005
  keratoconjunctivitis sicca from, 800
Sulfadimethoxine, 801–2
  acetyl derivatives of, 37
Sulfadimethoxine-ormetoprim, 802
Sulfadimethoxine-sulfamethoxazole,
    810
Sulfadimethoxypyrimidine, 810
Sulfadimidine, 802–4
Sulfadoxine, acetyl derivatives
    of, 37
Sulfaguanidine, as anticoccidial, 1005

Sulfamerazine, 805–6
Sulfamethazine, 802–4
  as anticoccidial, 1005
  carcinogenicity, 801
Sulfamethomidine, 810
Sulfamethoxazole
  as anticoccidial, 1005
  keratoconjunctivitis sicca from, 800
Sulfamethoxydiazine, 810
Sulfamethoxypyridazine, 809, 810
Sulfamethylphenazole, 810
Sulfanilamides
  acetylation of, 37
  carbonic anhydrase inhibition by, 539–40
Sulfanitran, as anticoccidial, 1005
Sulfapyrimidine, acetyl derivatives of, 37
Sulfaquinoxaline, 804–5, 1005
Sulfasalazine, 439–40, 806–7, 1055
  keratoconjunctivitis sicca from, 800
Sulfasomidine, 810
Sulfate conjugation, 37
Sulfathiazole, 806
Sulfisoxazole, 809–10
  ophthalmic uses, 1130–31
Sulfonamides, 796–812
  agents, 801–10
  as anticoccidials, 1005–10
  biotransformation of, 37
  chemistry, 796
  clinical uses, 797–98
  enteric, 21, 38
  mechanism of action, 797
  microbial resistance/susceptibility, 797–98, 801
  ophthalmic uses, 1130–31
  PABA inhibition by, 57
  pharmacokinetics, 798–91, 803
  potentiated, 810–11
  residues, 811–12
  sensitivity to, 547
  systemic, 21
  and thiopental, 223
  topical, 799
  toxicity, 799–801
Sulfonylureas
  fibrinolytic activity, 582
  insulin secretion stimulation, 677–78
Sulfur, 736–38
  deficiency, 737
  dietary requirements, 737
  preparations, 737
  topical uses, 1096
  toxicity, 738
Sulfur-containing amino acids, 736–38
Sulindac, 1126
Super-Ov, 619
Superovulation, 619–20
Superoxide dismutase, 176, 446
Suprane, 201
Suprofen, 1125
Surfactants, 21, 784
  anionic, 1056
Surgicel, 576
Suspensions, 1098
Sustained-release dosage forms, 20, 1158
Suxamethonium, 141
Sweet clover poisoning, 578, 580
Swine
  azaperone for aggressiveness in, 334–35
  coccidiosis in, 1008–9
  estrous synchronization, 615
  farrowing, induced, 618
  iron deficiency anemia in, 562, 564–65
  somatotropin, 604
  sulfate conjugation in, 37
  sulfonamide residues in, 811–12
Symmetrel, 938
Sympathetic nervous sytem, 70
Sympathoadrenal axis, 73
Sympatholytic drugs. *See* Adrenergic antagonists
Sympathomimetic amines. *See* Adrenergic agonists
Synanthic, 984
Synapses, neuromuscular junction, 139–40
Syncro-Mate B, 615
Syncurine, 141
Synergism, 63
Syrups, 1157
Systemic inflammatory response syndrome (SIRS), 528–29

T_3. *See* Triiodothyronine
T_4. *See* Thyroxine
T-61, 400
Tablets, 1157
Tachyarrhythmias, supraventricular, calcium channel blockers for, 477
Tachyphylaxis, 60, 405
Taeniacides. *See* Anticestodal drugs
Taeniafuges. *See* Anticestodal drugs
Talc, 1094
Talwin-V, 292
Tamoxifen citrate, 1079
Tannic acid, 577, 1095
Taurine, 361, 766–68
Taxol, 1074–75
Tear stimulants, 1139
Tear substitutes, 1139–41
Teat dips, 791
Tegretol, for diabetes insipidus, 608
Telazol, 166, 258–61
Teldrin, 408
Telmintic, 984
Temaril, 313
Teniposide, 1075
Tensilon, 126
TEPP, 127, 130
Teprotide, 417–18
Teratogenic effects, phenothiazines, 304
Terbinafine, 931–32
Terbutaline, 98, 106
  bronchodilation by, 1109
Terenol, 981
Terfenadine, 408, 410
Testosterone
  in cows, 613, 614
  for estrus prevention, 622
Tetracaine Hydrochloride, USP, 355, 1121
Tetrachlorodifluoroethane, 985
Tetrachlorvinphos, 1024
Tetracycline, 831–32
  novobiocin and, 886
  ophthalmic uses, 1127, 1131
Tetracyclines, 828–36
  antiprotozoan activity, 997
  for babesiosis, 1014
  bioavailability of, 21
  chemistry, 828
  chlortetracycline, 830–31
  doxycycline, 834–35
  mechanism of action, 828
  microbial susceptibility, 829
  minocycline, 835–36
  ophthalmic uses, 1131
  outdated, 61
  oxytetracycline, 832–34
  pharmacokinetics, 828–29
  side effects, 829–30
  tetracycline, 831–32, 886, 1127, 1131
  toxicity, 829–30
Tetraethylammonium ions, 134
Tetraethylpyrophosphate (TEPP), 127, 130
Tetrahydropyrimidines, 957–61
Tetramisole, 957
Tetrodotoxin, 141
Tetroxoprim, 810–11
Thebaine, 269
Theileriosis, 1014
Theophylline, 376, 1109–12
Therapeutic concentration range, in plasma, 47–48, 49
Therapeutic drug monitoring, 65–66
Therapeutic effect, and bioequivalence, 26
Therapeutic failure, 58
Therapeutic index, 12, 13, 49
Therapeutic principles, 57–66
  adverse drug experiences, 60–62
  contraindications, 60
  decision making, 57–63
  dosage regimen, 59–60
  drug formulation, 58–59
  drug interactions, 62–63
  margin of safety, 60
  monitoring responses, 65–66
  rational drug therapy, 57
  in special patient populations, 63–65
Therapy
  prolonged, 60
  short-term, 60
Thiabendazole, 1100
Thiacetarsamide Sodium, INN, 976
Thialbarbital Sodium, USP, 234
Thiamin, 702–4
  antagonists, 703
  deficiency, 703
Thiamphenicol, 873, 1129
Thiamylal Sodium, USP, 234–35
Thiazide diuretics, 547–48
  for diabetes insipidus, 608
  sulfonamide sensitivity and, 547
Thiazolidinediones, 678
Thiocarbamate, 932
Thionamides, 643–45
Thiopental Sodium, USP, 229–31
  administration, 231–32

Thiopental Sodium, USP (*continued*)
4-AP antagonism of, 377
clinical use, 232–34
lidocaine and, 230
morphine and, 232
xylazine and, 233
Thiopentone sodium, 229
Thiophanate, 952
Thiostrepton, 886, 1100
Thiouracil, 643
Thioureylenes, 643–45
Thorazine, 302
Thrombin, USP, 576
Thrombocytopenia, sulfonamide-induced, 800
Thrombolysin, 582
Thrombomodulin/protein C/protein S anticoagulant system, 575
Thromboplastin, tissue, 573
Thromboplastin, USP, 576
Thromboxane A_2, 572
Thromboxanes, 422–23, 425–26
Thymoxyethyldiethylamine (929F), 408
Thypinone, 600
Thyrocalcitonin, 689, 722
Ca/P metabolism, 689
Thyroglobulin, 627–28
Thyroid, dysfunction, effect on microsomal enzyme system, 39
Thyroid hormone-binding proteins, 631
Thyroid hormones
effect of drugs on, 633–34
free hormone hypothesis, 631–32
mechanism of action, 634–38
metabolism of, 629–32
alterations in, 632–34
monitoring therapy with, 642–43
plasma binding of, 631
preparations, 638–42
replacement therapy, 640–42
secretion, 628
synthesis, 627–28
thyrotropin (T_4), 600–603, 628–29
toxicity, 642
triiodothyronine (T_3), 627–30, 632, 641
TSH, 628–29
Thyroid imaging, 646
Thyroid peroxidase, 643
Thyroid-stimulating hormone, canine TSH assay, 642
Thyrotoxicosis, 642
Thyrotropin, 600–603, 628–29
receptors, 602
TSH stimulation test, 601–2
Thyrotropin-releasing hormone, 598–600
TRH stimulation test, 600
Thyroxine. *See also* Thyroid hormones
low T_4 syndrome, 632
metabolism of, 629–32
secretion/release of, 628–29
synthesis, 627–28
synthetic, 638–41
Thyroxine-binding globulin, 631
Thyroxine-binding prealbumin, 631
Ticarcillin, 822
ophthalmic uses, 1130
potassium clavulanate and, 825
Tick dips, 1033–34
Ticlopidine, 584
Tiletamine Hydrochloride, INN, 258–61
zolazepam and, 166, 258–61
Tilmicosin, 60, 880–81
Timolol, 489, 1135–36, 1137
Tinactin, 932
Tinidazole, 993
Tissue damage, from local anesthetics, 350
Tissue plasminogen activator, 583
Titanium dioxide, 1094
TNF-α, 429–30
Tobramycin, 858–59
ophthalmic uses, 1128
Tocainide, 488, 495
Tocopherols, 692, 693
Tocopheryl acetate, 695
Tocotrienols, 692
Tolazoline Hydrochloride, USP, 110, 324, 378–79
Tolbutamide, 582
Tolerances, drug/chemical, 1167–68
Tolfenamic acid, 1126
Tolnaftate, 932, 1100
Toltrazuril, 1005, 1009, 1011
Toluene, 977
Tooth discoloration, tetracyclines and, 829
Topical drugs. *See* Dermatologic drugs; Vehicles
Torbugesic, 293
Torbutrol, 293
Torsemide, 543
Total body water, 502–4
Totalon, 956
Toxicants, plant, hemolytic anemia-associated, 562
Toxic drug reactions, 61
Toxicology, definition of, 6
Toxoplasmosis, 1010
clindamycin for, 885
Tramadol Hydrochloride, USP, 291
Tramisol, 956
Tranexamic acid, 1142
Tranquilizers
α_2-adrenergic agonists, 313–25
benzodiazepines, 325–33
butyrophenones, 333–35
phenothiazines, 299–313
as preanesthetics, 165–66
Transdermal drug delivery, 1094
Transition elements, vitamin E stability and, 695
Transmission, nerve impulses, 153–55
local blocking of, 348–49
neurohumoral, 75, 76–89, 139–40
neuromuscular junction, 139–41
Trasylol, 417, 582
Treatment, palliative, 1064
Tretinoin, 1097
Trexan, 291
TRH, 598–600
Triamterene, 548
Triazines, 1072
Tribrissen, 1007
Tricaine methane sulphonate (MS-222), 401
Trichlorfon, 961, 1024
Trichomoniasis, 994–95
Triclabendazole, 985
Triclosan, 791
Tricyclic antidepressants, 389–92
Tricyclic antipsychotics, 387
Triethylcholine, 140
Trifluoperazine
as antiemetic, 1044
for diarrhea, 1055
Triflupromazine
as antiemetic, 1044
oxymorphone and, 280–81
Trifluridine, USP, 935
Triiodothyronine. *See also* Thyroid hormones
low T_3 syndrome, 632, 641
metabolism of, 629–30
reverse T_3, 629–30
secretion/release of, 628–29
synthesis, 627–28
synthetic, 641
T_3 suppression test, 641
Trimeprazine Tartrate, USP, 301, 313
Trimethidinium, 134
Trimethobenzamide hydrochloride, as antiemetic, 1045
Trimethoprim, 810–11, 1005–7
and sulfonamides, 43, 810–11
Trimethoprim-sulfadiazine, 808
hepatic necrosis from, 800
keratoconjunctivitis sicca from, 800
ophthalmic uses, 1130–31
Trimethoprim-sulfamethoxazole, 43, 810
effects on T_4, 634
hepatic necrosis from, 800
Tri-Plex, 981
Tritec, 881
Troclabendazole, 989
Trodax, 986
Troglitazone, 678
Tropicamide, 1136
Troponin, 140
Trovafloxacin, 898
Trusopt, 5391920
TSH, 600–603, 628–29
Tubarine, 141
d-Tubocurarine, 138, 141, 149
autonomic effects, 145
cardiovascular effects, 146
histamine release, 146
neuromuscular blocking effect, 143–44
pharmacokinetics, 147
Tubocurarine Chloride, USP, 141
Tumor necrosis factor-α, 429–30
Tylosin, 830, 880
Tyramine, 81

Ultane, 202
Ultram, 291
Ultramectrin, 965
U.S. Department of Agriculture, 1150
food safety, 1168
U.S. Food and Drug Administration-Center for Veterinary Medicine

(US FDA-CVM)
drug safety, 59
extra-label drug use, 58
United States Pharmacopeia (USP), 5, 6, 1150
extra-label drug use, 1174
National Formulary and, 1156
Urea, 1097
Urecholine, 122–23
Urethane, NF, 261
Uridine diphosphate-glucuronic acid (UDPGA), 36, 37, 278
Urine
alkalization of, 17–18, 40, 540
formation of, 535
pH, 40, 43, 736
Urokinase, 583
Urokinin, 418
Ursodeoxycholic acid, 1058

Vagus nerve, 70, 73
Valacyclovir, ophthalmic uses, 1133
Valbazen, 984, 995
Valium, 326
Vanadium, 756
Vancomycin, 889–90
Vapor pressure, saturated, 187
Vasoactive peptides, 418
Vasoconstrictors, with local anesthetics, 351–52
Vasodilation
and fluid balance, 531
skin, 1088
Vasodilators, 478
calcium channel blockers, 475–76
captopril, 473–75
enalapril, 473–75
hydralazine, 473
kinins, 416, 418
prazosin, 472–73
Vasopressin, USP, 607, 1057. *See also* Antidiuretic hormone
Vasopressin-angiotensin feedback loop, 414
Vasotec, 415
Vasoxyl, 106
Vecuronium, 141, 147
Vehicles, topical
properties of, 1041–43
types of, 1094–98
Velban, 1074
Velsar, 1074
Venoms, kinins of, 417, 418
VePesid, 1075
Verapamil, 477, 493–94
Vermiplex, 981
Versed, 331
Vesicants, 1095–96
Vetalar, 247
Vetdectin, 972
Veterinary drugs, legislation concerning, 1152–55
Veterinary Feed Directive, 1154–56, 1162–63
Vidarabine, USP, 935
ophthalmic uses, 1133
Vinblastine Sulfate, USP, 1074
Vinca alkaloids, 1074
Vincristine Sulfate, USP, 1074
Viokase, 1058
Virazole, 935
Virginiamycin, 889
Viroptic, 935
Viruses
attachment/penetration, 934–35
hemolytic anemia-associated, 562
replication of, 933–34
Viscoelastics, ophthalmic uses, 1143–44
Vision, vitamin A and, 685
Vitamin A, 684–88
deficiency, 687
and erythrocyte production, 559
Vitamin B_1, 702–4
Vitamin B_2, 704–5
Vitamin B_3, 705–7
Vitamin B_6, 707–8
deficiency, 558
phenytoin interaction, 370
Vitamin B_{12}, 713–16, 745
cobalt and, 745
deficiency, 558, 714–15
lipotropic effect, 1059
Vitamin B-complex, in liver disease, 1060
Vitamin C, 717–19
antioxidant activity, 718
and erythrocyte production, 559
Vitamin D, 688–92
deficiency, 690–91
phosphorus metabolism and, 689
preparturition, 726
toxicity, 691–92
Vitamin E, 692–96
deficiency, 694–95
and erythrocyte production, 559
hepatotropic effects, 1059
Vitamin K, 696–98
antagonists, 578, 580–82
deficiency, 697
in liver disease, 1060
for rodenticide intoxication, 577–78
Vitamin-mineral supplements, 567–68, 684
Vitamins
fat soluble, 683–98
water-soluble, 702–19
VM-26, 1075
Volume of distribution (Vd), 29–30, 43, 49
Vomiting
behavioral, 1042, 1045
digitalis-induced, 464
Vomition reflex, 1042–43
von Willebrand factor, 571, 578, 638
VP-16, 1075

Warfarin Sodium, USP, 578, 580–82
Water, body, 502–4. *See also* Fluid balance
turnover, 504–6
Water vapor, 179–80
Weights and measures, 1160, 1165
Win-Kinase, 583
Withdrawal times, 1167–68
determining, 1169–72
Wolff-Chaikoff effect, 627
Wounds, antiseptics for, 790–91

Xanthines, as histamine antagonists, 405, 408
Xenobiotics, conjugation of, 37
Xylazine Hydrochloride, INN, 314–21
4-AP antagonism of, 377
doxapram antagonism of, 374
as emetic, 1044
etorphine and, 287
guaifenesin and, 242–43
ketamine and, 249, 251–56
pentobarbital and, 226
propofol and, 239
thiopental and, 233
tolazoline antagonism of, 378–79
yohimbine antagonism of, 378
Xylocaine, 355, 492

Yohimbine hydrochloride, 112, 324, 377–78
xylazine blocking by, 314

Zafurlikast, 1113
Zanil, 986
Zetamethrin, 1020
Zidovudine, 937
Zileuton, 1113
Zimecterin, 965
Zinc
deficiency, 757–58
topical use, 1094, 1095, 1100
toxicity, 758–59
Zinc bacitracin, 886
Zinc chloride, 577, 1095
Zinc oxide, 1094, 1095
Zinc stearate, 1094
Zinc sulfate, 275
Zirconium chlorhydrate, 1095
Zithromax, 881
Zolazepam, tiletamine and, 258–61
Zovirax, 936

ISBN 0-8138-1743-9